SSIONAL

Current Procedural Coding Expert

CPT® codes with Medicare essentials
for enhanced accuracy

2020

THE NEW WEBSITE HAS
LAUNCHED!
VISIT OPTUM360CODING.COM

Notice

The *2020 Current Procedural Coding Expert, Professional Edition,* is designed to be an accurate and authoritative source of information about the CPT® coding system. Every effort has been made to verify the accuracy of the listings, and all information is believed reliable at the time of publication. Absolute accuracy cannot be guaranteed, however. This publication is made available with the understanding that the publisher is not engaged in rendering legal or other services that require a professional license.

American Medical Association Notice

CPT © 2019 American Medical Association. All rights reserved.

Fee schedules, relative value units, conversion factors and/or related components are not assigned by the AMA, are not part of CPT, and the AMA is not recommending their use. The AMA does not directly or indirectly practice medicine or dispense medical services. The AMA assumes no liability for data contained or not contained herein.

CPT is a registered trademark of the American Medical Association.

Our Commitment to Accuracy

Optum360 is committed to producing accurate and reliable materials.

To report corrections, please email accuracy@optum.com. You can also reach customer service by calling 1.800.464.3649, option 1.

Copyright

Acknowledgments

Gregory A. Kemp, MA, *Product Manager*
Karen Schmidt, BSN, *Technical Director*
Stacy Perry, *Manager, Desktop Publishing*
Lisa Singley, *Project Manager*
Karen Krawzik, RHIT, CCS, AHIMA, AHIMA-approved ICD-10-CM/PCS Trainer, *Clinical/Technical Editor*
Elizabeth Leibold, RHIT, *Clinical/Technical Editor*
Anita Schmidt, BS, RHIA, AHIMA-approved ICD-10-CM/PCS Trainer, *Clinical/Technical Editor*
LaJuana Green, RHIA, CCS, *Clinical/Technical Editor*
Tracy Betzler, *Senior Desktop Publishing Specialist*
Hope M. Dunn, *Senior Desktop Publishing Specialist*
Katie Russell, *Desktop Publishing Specialist*
Kate Holden, *Editor*

About the Contributors

Karen Krawzik, RHIT, CCS, AHIMA, AHIMA-approved ICD-10-CM/PCS Trainer

Ms. Krawzik has expertise in ICD-10-CM, ICD-9-CM, CPT/HCPCS, DRG, and data quality and analytics, with more than 30 years' experience coding in multiple settings, including inpatient, observation, ambulatory surgery, ancillary, and emergency room. She has served as a DRG analyst and auditor of commercial and government payer claims, as a contract administrator, and worked on a team providing enterprise-wide conversion of the ICD-9-CM code set to ICD-10. More recently, she has been developing print and electronic content related to ICD-10-CM and ICD-10-PCS coding systems, MS-DRGs, and HCCs. Ms. Krawzik is credentialed by the American Health Information Management Association (AHIMA) as a Registered Health Information Technician (RHIT) and a Certified Coding Specialist (CCS) and is an AHIMA-approved ICD-10-CM/PCS trainer. She is an active member of AHIMA and the Missouri Health Information Management Association.

Elizabeth Leibold, RHIT

Ms. Leibold has more than 25 years of experience in the health care profession. She has served in a variety of roles, ranging from patient registration to billing and collections, and has an extensive background in both physician and hospital outpatient coding and compliance. She has worked for large health care systems and health information management services companies, and has wide-ranging experience in facility and professional component coding, along with CPT expertise in interventional procedures, infusion services, emergency department, observation, and ambulatory surgery coding. Her areas of expertise include chart-to-claim coding audits and providing staff education to both tenured and new coding staff. She is an active member of the American Health Information Management Association (AHIMA).

Anita Schmidt, BS, RHIA, AHIMA-approved ICD-10-CM/PCS Trainer

Ms. Schmidt has expertise in ICD-10-CM/PCS, DRG, and CPT with more than 15 years' experience in coding in multiple settings, including inpatient, observation, and same-day surgery. Her experience includes analysis of medical record documentation, assignment of ICD-10-CM and PCS codes, and DRG validation. She has conducted training for ICD-10-CM/PCS and electronic health record. She has also collaborated with clinical documentation specialists to identify documentation needs and potential areas for physician education. Most recently she has been developing content for resource and educational products related to ICD-10-CM, ICD-10-PCS, DRG, and CPT. Ms. Schmidt is an AHIMA-approved ICD-10-CM/PCS trainer and is an active member of the American Health Information Management Association (AHIMA) and the Minnesota Health Information Management Association.

LaJuana Green, RHIA, CCS

Ms. Green is a Registered Health Information Administrator with over 35 years of experience in multiple areas of information management. She has proven expertise in the analysis of medical record documentation, assignment of ICD-10-CM and PCS codes, DRG validation, and CPT code assignment in ambulatory surgery units and the hospital outpatient setting. Her experience includes serving as a director of a health information management department, clinical technical editing, new technology research and writing, medical record management, utilization review activities, quality assurance, tumor registry, medical library services, and chargemaster maintenance. Ms. Green is an active member of the American Health Information Management Association (AHIMA).

Optum360 Learning

Education suiting your specialty, learning style and schedule

Optum360® Learning is designed to address exactly what you and your learners need. We offer: several delivery methods developed for various adult learning styles; general public education; and tailor-made programs specific to your organization — all created by our coding and clinical documentation education professionals.

Our strategy is simple — education must be concise, relevant and accurate. Choose the delivery method that works best for you:

eLearning

- **Web-based** courses offered at the most convenient times
- **Interactive**, task-focused and developed around practical scenarios
- **Self-paced** courses include "try-it" functionality, knowledge checks and downloadable resources

Instructor-led training

On-site or remote courses built specifically for your organization and learners
- CDI specialists
- Coders
- Providers

You've worked hard for your credentials, and now you need an easy way to maintain your certification.

Webinars

Online courses geared toward a broad market of learners and delivered in a live setting

WF1151156

Let Optum360 help you find the best product at the best price for your needs.

Optum360® can help you drive financial results across your organization with industry-leading resources that cut through the complexity of medical coding challenges.

The Price Match Program* is an example of one of the ways in which we can impact your bottom line — to the positive. We're committed to providing you with the best quality product in the market, along with the best price.

Let us help you find the best coding solution, at the best price.

Contact your Medallion representative directly or call Customer Service at 1-800-464-3649, option 1. Or explore online, optum360coding.com/pricematch.

PriceMatch Program

*Some restrictions and exclusions apply. Visit optum360coding.com/pricematch to learn more about the conditions, guidelines and exclusions.

© 2018 Optum360, LLC. All rights reserved. WF621697 SPRJ5186 4/18

OPTUM360°®

RENEW THIS BOOK

SAVE UP TO 30%
ON 2020 EDITION CODING RESOURCES.*

ITEM #	TITLE INDICATE THE ITEMS YOU WISH TO PURCHASE	QUANTITY	PRICE PER PRODUCT	TOTAL

	Subtotal	
(AK, DE, MT, NH & OR are exempt)	Sales Tax	
1 item $10.95 • 2–4 items $12.95 • 5+ CALL	Shipping & Handling	
	TOTAL AMOUNT ENCLOSED	

MANY WAYS TO RENEW!

Save up to 30% when you renew online.*

PROMO CODE: RENEW20A

Visit **optum360coding.com** and enter the promo code above at checkout to **save 30%**.

Call **1-800-464-3649, option 1,** and mention the promo code above to **save 20%**.

Fax this order form with purchase order to **1-801-982-4033 to save 20%**.

Optum360 no longer accepts credit cards by fax.

Mail this order form with payment and/or purchase order to **Optum360, PO Box 88050, Chicago, IL 60680-9920** to **save 20%**. *Optum360 no longer accepts credit cards by mail.*

Name _____

Address _____

_____

Customer Number _____ Contact Number _____

○ CHECK ENCLOSED (PAYABLE TO OPTUM360)

○ BILL ME ○ P.O.# _____

Telephone _____

Fax _____

Email _____

Optum360 respects your right to privacy. We will not sell or rent your email address or fax number to anyone outside Optum360 and its business partners. If you would like to remove your name from Optum360 promotions, please call 1-800-464-3649, option 1.

Contents

Introduction

Welcome to Optum360's *Current Procedural Coding Expert, Professional Edition*, an exciting Medicare coding and reimbursement tool and definitive procedure coding source that combines the work of the Centers for Medicare and Medicaid Services, American Medical Association, and Optum360 experts with the technical components you need for proper reimbursement and coding accuracy.

This approach to CPT® Medicare coding utilizes innovative and intuitive ways of communicating the information you need to code claims accurately and efficiently. *Includes* and *Excludes* notes, similar to those found in the ICD-10-CM manual, help determine what services are related to the codes you are reporting. Icons help you crosswalk the code you are reporting to laboratory and radiology procedures necessary for proper reimbursement. CMS-mandated icons and relative value units (RVUs) help you determine which codes are most appropriate for the service you are reporting. Add to that additional information identifying age and sex edits, ambulatory surgery center (ASC) and ambulatory payment classification (APC) indicators, and Medicare coverage and payment rule citations, and *Current Procedural Coding Expert, Professional Edition* provides the best in Medicare procedure reporting.

Current Procedural Coding Expert, Professional Edition includes the information needed to submit claims to federal contractors and most commercial payers, and is correct at the time of printing. However, CMS, federal contractors, and commercial payers may change payment rules at any time throughout the year. *Current Procedural Coding Expert, Professional Edition* includes effective codes that will not be published in the AMA's Physicians' Current Procedural Terminology (CPT) book until the following year. Commercial payers will announce changes through monthly news or information posted on their websites. CMS will post changes in policy on its website at http://www.cms.gov/transmittals. National and local coverage determinations (NCDs and LCDs) provide universal and individual contractor guidelines for specific services. The existence of a procedure code does not imply coverage under any given insurance plan.

Current Procedural Coding Expert, Professional Edition is based on the AMA's Physicians' Current Procedural Terminology coding system, which is copyrighted and owned by the physician organization. The CPT codes are the nation's official, Health Information Portability and Accountability Act (HIPAA) compliant code set for procedures and services provided by physicians, ambulatory surgery centers (ASCs), and hospital outpatient services, as well as laboratories, imaging centers, physical therapy clinics, urgent care centers, and others.

Getting Started with *Current Procedural Coding Expert, Professional Edition*

Current Procedural Coding Expert, Professional Edition is an exciting tool combining the most current material at the time of our publication from the AMA's CPT 2020, CMS's online manual system, the Correct Coding initiative, CMS fee schedules, official Medicare guidelines for reimbursement and coverage, the Integrated outpatient coding Editor (I/OCE), and Optum360's own coding expertise.

These coding rules and guidelines are incorporated into more specific section notes and code notes. Section notes are listed under a range of codes and apply to all codes in that range. Code notes are found under individual codes and apply to the single code.

Material is presented in a logical fashion for those billing Medicare, Medicaid, and many private payers. The format, based on customer comments, better addresses what customers tell us they need in a comprehensive Medicare procedure coding guide.

Designed to be easy to use and full of information, this product is an excellent companion to your AMA CPT manual, and other Optum360 and Medicare resources.

For mid-year code updates, official errata changes, correction notices, and any other changes pertinent to the information in *Current Procedural*

Coding Expert, Professional Edition, see our product update page at https://www.optum360coding.com/ProductUpdates/. The password for 2020 is PROCEDURE2020.

Note: The AMA releases code changes quarterly as well as errata or corrections to CPT codes and guidelines and posts them on their web site. Some of these changes may not appear in the AMA's CPT book until the following year. *Current Procedural Coding Expert, Professional Edition* incorporates the most recent errata or release notes found on the AMA's web site at our publication time, including new, revised and deleted codes. *Current Procedural Coding Expert, Professional Edition* identifies these new or revised codes from the AMA website errata or release notes with an icon similar to the AMA's current new ● and revised ▲ icons. For purposes of this publication, new CPT codes and revisions that won't be in the AMA book until the next edition are indicated with a ● and a ▲ icon. For the next year's edition of *Current Procedural Coding Expert, Professional Edition*, these codes will appear with standard black new or revised icons, as appropriate, to correspond with those changes as indicated in the AMA CPT book. CPT codes that were new for 2019 and appeared in the 2019 *Current Procedural Coding Expert, Professional Edition* but did not appear in the CPT code book until 2020 are identified in appendix B as "Web Release New and Revised Codes."

General Conventions

Many of the sources of information in this book can be determined by color.

- All CPT codes and descriptions and the Evaluation and Management guidelines from the American Medical Association are in **black text**.

- Includes, Excludes, and other notes appear in **blue text**. The resources used for this information are a variety of Medicare policy manuals, the *National Correct Coding Initiative Policy Manual* (NCCI), AMA resources and guidelines, and specialty association resources and our Optum360 clinical experts.

Resequencing of CPT Codes

The American Medical Association (AMA) uses a numbering methodology of resequencing, which is the practice of displaying codes outside of their numerical order according to the description relationship. According to the AMA, there are instances in which a new code is needed within an existing grouping of codes but an unused code number is not available. In these situations, the AMA will resequence the codes. In other words, it will assign a code that is not in numeric sequence with the related codes. However, the code and description will appear in the CPT manual with the other related codes.

An example of resequencing from *Current Procedural Coding Expert, Professional Edition* follows:

	21555	**Excision, tumor, soft tissue of neck or anterior thorax, subcutaneous; less than 3 cm**
#	21552	**3 cm or greater**
	21556	**Excision, tumor, soft tissue of neck or anterior thorax, subfascial (eg, intramuscular); less than 5 cm**
#	21554	**5 cm or greater**

In *Current Procedural Coding Expert, Professional Edition* the resequenced codes are listed twice. They appear in their resequenced position as shown above as well as in their original numeric position with a note indicating that the code is out of numerical sequence and where it can be found. (See example below.)

21554	**Resequenced code. See code following 21556.**

This differs from the AMA CPT book, in which the coder is directed to a code range that contains the resequenced code and description, rather than to a specific location.

Resequenced codes will appear in brackets in the headers, section notes, and code ranges. For example:

> 27327-27329 [27337, 27339] Excision Soft Tissue Tumors Femur/Knee. Codes [27337, 27339] are included in section 27327-27329 in their resequenced positions.
>
> Code also toxoid/vaccine (90476-90749 [90620, 90621, 90625, 90630, 90644, 90672, 90673, 90674, 90750, 90756])

> This shows codes 90620, 90621, 90625, 90630, 90644, 90672, 90673, 90674, 90750, and 90756 are resequenced in this range of codes.

Code Ranges for Medicare Billing

Appendix E identifies all resequenced CPT codes. Optum360 will display the resequenced coding as assigned by the AMA in its CPT products so that the user may understand the code description relationships.

Each particular group of CPT codes in *Current Procedural Coding Expert, Professional Edition* is organized in a more intuitive fashion for Medicare billing, being grouped by the Medicare rules and regulations as found in the official CMS online manuals that govern payment of these particular procedures and services, as in this example:

99221-99233 Inpatient Hospital Visits: Initial and Subsequent

CMS: 100-4,11,40.1.3 Independent Attending Physician Services; 100-4,12,100.1.1 Teaching Physicians E/M Services; 100-4,12,30.6.10 Consultation Services; 100-4,12,30.6.15.1 Prolonged Services With Direct Face-to-Face Patient Contact; 100-4,12,30.6.4 Services Furnished Incident to Physician's Service; 100-4,12,30.6.9 Hospital Visit and Critical Care on Same Day

Icons

● **New Codes**
Codes that have been added since the last edition of the AMA CPT book was printed.

▲ **Revised Codes**
Codes that have been revised since the last edition of the AMA CPT book was printed.

● **New Web Release**
Codes that are new for the current year but will not be in the AMA CPT book until 2021.

▲ **Revised Web Release**
Codes that have been revised for the current year, but will not be in the AMA CPT book until 2021.

Resequenced Codes
Codes that are out of numeric order but apply to the appropriate category.

★ **Telemedicine Services**
Codes that may be reported for telemedicine services. Modifier 95 must be appended to code.

○ **Reinstated Code**
Codes that have been reinstated since the last edition of the book was printed.

Pink Color Bar—Not Covered by Medicare
Services and procedures identified by this color bar are never covered benefits under Medicare. Services and procedures that are not covered may be billed directly to the patient at the time of the service.

Gray Color Bar—Unlisted Procedure
Unlisted CPT codes report procedures that have not been assigned a specific code number. An unlisted code delays payment due to the extra time necessary for review.

Green Color Bar—Resequenced Codes
Resequenced codes are codes that are out of numeric sequence—they are indicated with a green color bar. They are listed twice, in their resequenced position as well as in their

original numeric position with a note that the code is out of numerical sequence and where the resequenced code and description can be found.

INCLUDES **Includes notes**
Includes notes identify procedures and services that would be bundled in the procedure code. These are derived from AMA, CMS, NCCI, and Optum360 coding guidelines. This is not meant to be an all-inclusive list.

EXCLUDES **Excludes notes**
Excludes notes may lead the user to other codes. They may identify services that are not bundled and may be separately reported, OR may lead the user to another more appropriate code. These are derived from AMA, CMS, NCCI, and Optum360 coding guidelines. This is not meant to be an all-inclusive list.

Code Also This note identifies an additional code that should be reported with the service and may relate to another CPT code or an appropriate HCPCS code(s) that should be reported along with the CPT code when appropriate.

Code First Found under add-on codes, this note identifies codes for primary procedures that should be reported first, with the add-on code reported as a secondary code.

◣ **Laboratory/Pathology Crosswalk**
This icon denotes CPT codes in the laboratory and pathology section of CPT that may be reported separately with the primary CPT code.

⚕ **Radiology Crosswalk**
This icon denotes codes in the radiology section that may be used with the primary CPT code being reported.

TC **Technical Component Only**
Codes with this icon represent only the technical component (staff and equipment costs) of a procedure or service. Do not use either modifier 26 (professional component) or TC (technical component) with these codes.

26 **Professional Component**
Only codes with this icon represent the physician's work or professional component of a procedure or service. Do not use either modifier 26 (professional component) or TC (technical component) with these codes.

50 **Bilateral Procedure**
This icon identifies codes that can be reported bilaterally when the same surgeon provides the service for the same patient on the same date. Medicare allows payment for both procedures at 150 percent of the usual amount for one procedure. The modifier does not apply to bilateral procedures inclusive to one code.

80 **Assist-at-Surgery Allowed**
Services noted by this icon are allowed an assistant at surgery with a Medicare payment equal to 16 percent of the allowed amount for the global surgery for that procedure. No documentation is required.

80 **Assist-at-Surgery Allowed with Documentation**
Services noted by this icon are allowed an assistant at surgery with a Medicare payment equal to 16 percent of the allowed amount for the global surgery for that procedure. Documentation is required.

+ **Add-on Codes**
This icon identifies procedures reported in addition to the primary procedure. The icon "**+**" denotes add-on codes. An add-on code is neither a stand-alone code nor subject to multiple procedure rules since it describes work in addition to the primary procedure.

According to Medicare guidelines, add-on codes may be identified in the following ways:

- The code is found on Change Request (CR) 7501 or successive CRs as a Type I, Type II, or Type III add-on code.

- The add-on code most often has a global period of "ZZZ" in the Medicare Physician Fee Schedule Database.

- The code is found in the CPT book with the icon "**+**" appended. Add-on code descriptors typically include the phrases "each additional" or "(List separately in addition to primary procedure)."

⑤⓪ **Optum Modifier 50 Exempt**
Codes identified by this icon indicate that the procedure should not be reported with modifier 50 (Bilateral procedures).

⦸ **Modifier 51 Exempt**
Codes identified by this icon indicate that the procedure should not be reported with modifier 51 (Multiple procedures).

⑤① **Optum Modifier 51 Exempt**
Codes identified by this Optum360 icon indicate that the procedure should not be reported with modifier 51 (Multiple procedures). Any code with this icon is backed by official AMA guidelines but was not identified by the AMA with their modifier 51 exempt icon.

▱ **Correct Coding Initiative (CCI)**
Current Procedural Coding Expert, Professional Edition identifies those codes with corresponding CCI edits. The CCI edits define correct coding practices that serve as the basis of the national Medicare policy for paying claims. The code noted is the major service/procedure. The code may represent a column 1 code within the column 1/column 2 correct coding edits table or a code pair that is mutually exclusive of each other.

▣ **CLIA Waived Test**
This symbol is used to distinguish those laboratory tests that can be performed using test systems that are waived from regulatory oversight established by the Clinical Laboratory Improvement Amendments of 1988 (CLIA). The applicable CPT code for a CLIA waived test may be reported by providers who perform the testing but do not hold a CLIA license.

㊿ **Modifier 63 Exempt**
This icon identifies procedures performed on infants that weigh less than 4 kg. Due to the complexity of performing procedures on infants less than 4 kg, modifier 63 may be added to the surgery codes to inform the payers of the special circumstances involved.

A2 – Z3 **ASC Payment Indicators**
This icon identifies ASC status payment indicators. They indicate how the ASC payment rate was derived and/or how the procedure, item, or service is treated under the revised ASC payment system. For more information about these indicators and how they affect billing, consult Optum360's *Outpatient Billing Editor*.

A2   Surgical procedure on ASC list in 2007; payment based on OPPS relative payment weight.

B5   Alternative code may be available; no payment made.

D5   Deleted/discontinued code; no payment made.

F4   Corneal tissue acquisition; hepatitis B vaccine; paid at reasonable cost.

G2   Non-office-based surgical procedure added in CY 2008 or later; payment based on OPPS relative payment weight.

H2   Brachytherapy source paid separately when provided integral to a surgical procedure on ASC list; payment based on OPPS rate.

J7   OPPS pass-through device paid separately when provided integral to a surgical procedure on ASC list; payment contractor-priced.

J8   Device-intensive procedure; paid at adjusted rate.

K2   Drugs and biologicals paid separately when provided integral to a surgical procedure on ASC list; payment based on OPPS rate.

K7   Unclassified drugs and biologicals; payment contractor-priced.

L1   Influenza vaccine; pneumococcal vaccine. Packaged item/service; no separate payment made.

L6   New technology intraocular lens (NTIOL); special payment.

N1   Packaged service/item; no separate payment made.

P2   Office-based surgical procedure added to ASC list in CY 2008 or later with MPFS nonfacility practice expense (PE) RVUs; payment based on OPPS relative payment weight.

P3   Office-based surgical procedure added to ASC list in CY 2008 or later with MPFS nonfacility PE RVUs; payment based on MPFS nonfacility PE RVUs.

R2   Office-based surgical procedure added to ASC list in CY 2008 or later without MPFS nonfacility PE RVUs; payment based on OPPS relative payment weight.

Z2   Radiology or diagnostic service paid separately when provided integral to a surgical procedure on ASC list; payment based on OPPS relative payment weight.

Z3   Radiology or diagnostic service paid separately when provided integral to a surgical procedure on ASC list; payment based on MPFS nonfacility PE RVUs.

A **Age Edit**
This icon denotes codes intended for use with a specific age group, such as neonate, newborn, pediatric, and adult. This edit is based on age specifications in the CPT code descriptors or the product/service represented by the code *MAY* have age restrictions. Carefully review the code description to ensure the code you report most appropriately reflects the patient's age.

M **Maternity**
This icon identifies procedures that by definition should be used only for maternity patients generally between 12 and 55 years of age based on CMS I/OCE designations.

♀ **Female Only**
This icon identifies procedures designated by CMS for females only based on CMS I/OCE designations.

♂ **Male Only**
This icon identifies procedures designated by CMS for males only based on CMS I/OCE designations.

🚑 **Facility RVU**
This icon precedes the facility RVU from CMS's 2018 physician fee schedule (PFS). It can be found under the code description.

New codes include no RVU information.

🔎 **Nonfacility RVU**
This icon precedes the nonfacility RVU from CMS's 2018 PFS. It can be found under the code description.

New codes include no RVU information.

FUD: Global days are sometimes referred to as "follow-up days" or FUDs. The global period is the time following surgery during which routine care by the physician is considered postoperative and included in the surgical fee. Office visits or other routine care related to the original surgery cannot be separately reported if provided during the global period. The statuses are:

000   No follow-up care included in this procedure

010   Normal postoperative care is included in this procedure for ten days

090   Normal postoperative care is included in the procedure for 90 days

MMM Maternity codes; usual global period does not apply

XXX   The global concept does not apply to the code

YYY   The carrier is to determine whether the global concept applies and establishes postoperative period, if appropriate, at time of pricing

ZZZ   The code is related to another service and is always included in the global period of the other service

CMS: This notation indicates that there is a specific CMS guideline pertaining to this code in the CMS Online Manual System which includes the internet-only manual (IOM) *National Coverage Determinations Manual* (NCD). These CMS sources present the rules for submitting these services to the federal government or its contractors and are included in appendix G of this book.

AMA: This indicates discussion of the code in the American Medical Association's *CPT Assistant* newsletter. Use the citation to find the correct issue. This includes citations for the current year and the preceding six years. In the event no citations can be found during this time period, the most recent citations that can be found are used.

✗   **Drug Not Approved by FDA**
           The AMA CPT Editorial Panel is publishing new vaccine product codes prior to Food and Drug Administration approval. This symbol indicates which of these codes are pending FDA approval at press time.

A–Y   **OPPS Status Indicators (OPSI)**
           Status indicators identify how individual CPT codes are paid or not paid under the latest available hospital outpatient prospective payment system (OPPS). The same status indicator is assigned to all the codes within an ambulatory payment classification (APC). Consult your payer or other resource to learn which CPT codes fall within various APCs.

A   Services furnished to a hospital outpatient that are paid under a fee schedule or payment system other than OPPS. For example:

- Ambulance services
- Separately payable clinical diagnostic laboratory services
- Separately payable non-implantable prosthetics and orthotics
- Physical, occupational, and speech therapy
- Diagnostic mammography
- Screening mammography

B   Codes that are not recognized by OPPS when submitted on an outpatient hospital Part B bill type (12x and 13x)

C   Inpatient procedures

D   Discontinued codes

E1   Items, codes, and services:

- Not covered by any Medicare outpatient benefit category
- Statutorily excluded by Medicare
- Not reasonable and necessary

E2   Items, codes, and services for which pricing information and claims data are not available

F   Corneal tissue acquisition; certain CRNA services and hepatitis B vaccines

G   Pass-through drugs and biologicals

H   Pass-through device categories

J1   Hospital Part B services paid through a comprehensive APC

J2   Hospital Part B services that may be paid through a comprehensive APC

K   Nonpass-through drugs and nonimplantable biologicals, including therapeutic radiopharmaceuticals

L   Influenza vaccine; pneumococcal pneumonia vaccine

M   Items and services not billable to the MAC

N   Items and services packaged into APC rates

P   Partial hospitalization

Q1   STV-packaged codes

Q2   T-packaged codes

Q3   Codes that may be paid through a composite APC

Q4   Conditionally packaged laboratory tests

R   Blood and blood products

S   Procedure or service, not discounted when multiple

T   Procedure or service, multiple procedure reduction applies

U   Brachytherapy sources

V   Clinic or emergency department visit

Y   Nonimplantable durable medical equipment

Appendixes

Appendix A: Modifiers—This appendix identifies modifiers. A modifier is a two-position alpha or numeric code that is appended to a CPT or HCPCS code to clarify the services being billed. Modifiers provide a means by which a service can be altered without changing the procedure code. They add more information, such as anatomical site, to the code. In addition, they help eliminate the appearance of duplicate billing and unbundling. Modifiers are used to increase the accuracy in reimbursement and coding consistency, ease editing, and capture payment data.

Appendix B: New, Revised, and Deleted Codes—This is a list of new, revised, and deleted CPT codes for the current year. This appendix also includes a list of web release new and revised codes, which indicate official code changes in *Current Procedural Coding Expert, Professional Edition* that will not be in the CPT code book until the following year.

Appendix C: Evaluation and Management Extended Guidelines—This appendix presents an overview of evaluation and management (E/M) services that augment the official AMA CPT E/M services. It includes tables that distinguish documentation components of each E/M code and the federal documentation guidelines (1995 and 1997) currently in use by the Centers for Medicare and Medicaid Services (CMS).

Appendix D: Crosswalk of Deleted Codes—This appendix is a cross-reference from a deleted CPT code to an active code when one is available. The deleted code cross-reference will also appear under the deleted code description in the tabular section of the book.

Appendix E: Resequenced Codes—This appendix contains a list of codes that are not in numeric order in the book. AMA resequenced some of the code numbers to relocate codes in the same category but not in numeric sequence.

Appendix F: Add-on, Optum Modifier 50 Exempt, Modifier 51 Exempt, Optum Modifier 51 Exempt, Modifier 63 Exempt, and Modifier 95 Telemedicine Services—This list includes add-on codes that cannot be reported alone, codes that are exempt from modifiers 50 and 51, codes that should not be reported with modifier 63, and codes identified by the ★ icon to which modifier 95 may be appended when the service is provided as a synchronous telemedicine service.

Appendix G: Medicare Internet-only Manual (IOMs)—This appendix contains a verbatim printout of the Medicare Internet Only Manual references that pertain to specific codes. The reference, when available, is listed after the header in the CPT section. For example:

93784-93790 Ambulatory Blood Pressure Monitoring
CMS: 100-3,20.19 Ambulatory Blood Pressure Monitoring (20.19); 100-4,32,10.1 Ambulatory Blood Pressure Monitoring Billing Requirements

Since appendix G contains these references from the *Medicare National Coverage Determinations (NCD) Manual*, Pub 100-3, chapter 20, section 20.19, and the *Medicare Claims Processing Manual*, Pub 100-4, chapter 32, section 10.1, there is no need to search the Medicare website for the applicable reference.

Appendix H: Quality Payment Program (QPP)—Previously, this appendix contained lists of the numerators and denominators applicable to the Medicare PQRS. However, with the implementation of the Quality Payment Program (QPP) mandated by passage of the Medicare Access and Chip Reauthorization Act (MACRA) of 2015, the PQRS system will be obsolete. This appendix now contains information pertinent to that legislation as well as a comprehensive overview of the QPP.

Appendix I: Medically Unlikely Edits—This appendix contains the published medically unlikely edits (MUEs). These edits establish maximum daily allowable units of service. The edits will be applied to the services provided to the same patient, for the same CPT code, on the same date of service when billed by the same provider. Included are the physician and facility edits.

Appendix J: Inpatient-Only Procedures—This appendix identifies services with the status indicator "C." Medicare will not pay an OPPS hospital or ASC when these procedures are performed on a Medicare patient as an outpatient. Physicians should refer to this list when scheduling Medicare patients for surgical procedures. CMS updates this list quarterly.

Appendix K: Place of Service and Type of Service—This appendix contains lists of place-of-service codes that should be used on professional claims and type-of-service codes used by the Medicare Common Working File.

Appendix L: Multianalyte Assays with Algorithmic Analyses—This appendix lists the administrative codes for multianalyte assays with algorithmic analyses. The AMA updates this list three times a year.

Appendix M: Glossary—This appendix contains general terms and definitions as well as those that would apply to or be helpful for billing and reimbursement.

Appendix N: Listing of Sensory, Motor, and Mixed Nerves—This appendix lists a summary of each sensory, motor, and mixed nerve with its appropriate nerve conduction study code.

Note: All data current as of November 11, 2019.

Anatomical Illustrations

Body Planes and Movements

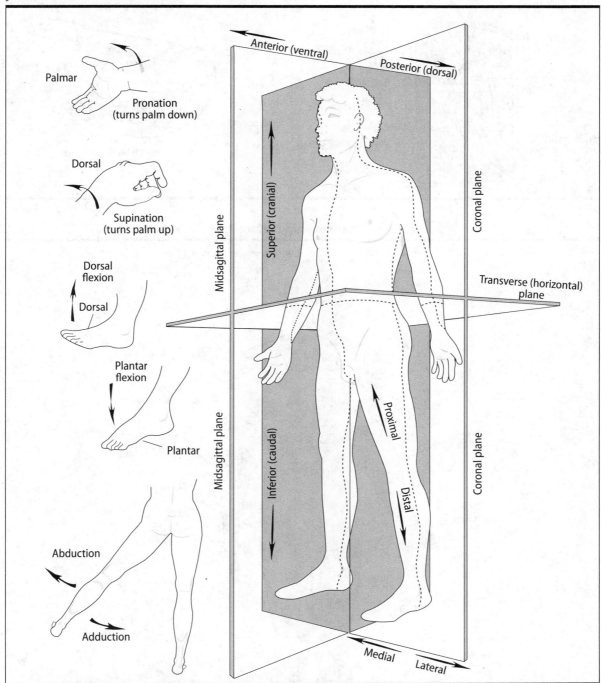

Integumentary System

Skin and Subcutaneous Tissue

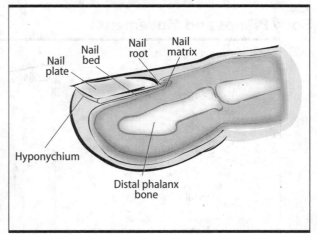

- Hair
- Sebaceous gland
- Hair follicle
- Arrector pili muscle
- Epidermis
- Thick-skin epidermis
- Dermis
- Hair shaft
- Pacinian corpuscle
- Hypodermis (subcutaneous layer)
- Hair matrix
- Sweat (eccrine gland)
- Bulb
- Sensory nerve
- Blood vessels

Nail Anatomy

- Nail plate
- Nail bed
- Nail root
- Nail matrix
- Hyponychium
- Distal phalanx bone

Assessment of Burn Surface Area

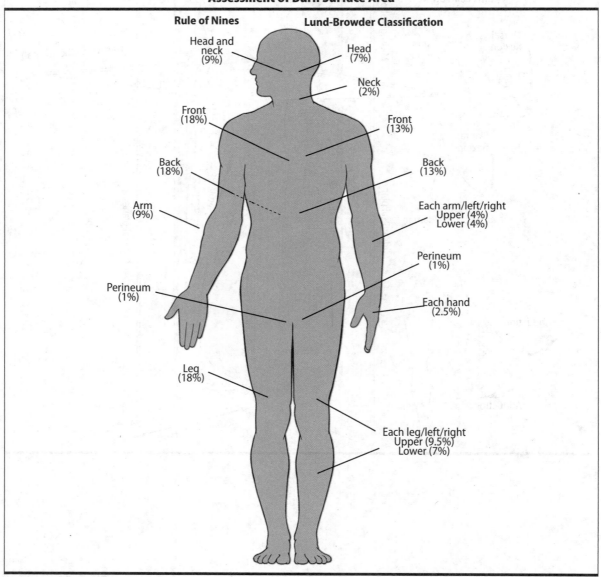

Rule of Nines

- Head and neck (9%)
- Front (18%)
- Back (18%)
- Arm (9%)
- Perineum (1%)
- Leg (18%)

Lund-Browder Classification

- Head (7%)
- Neck (2%)
- Front (13%)
- Back (13%)
- Each arm/left/right Upper (4%) Lower (4%)
- Perineum (1%)
- Each hand (2.5%)
- Each leg/left/right Upper (9.5%) Lower (7%)

Musculoskeletal System

Bones and Joints

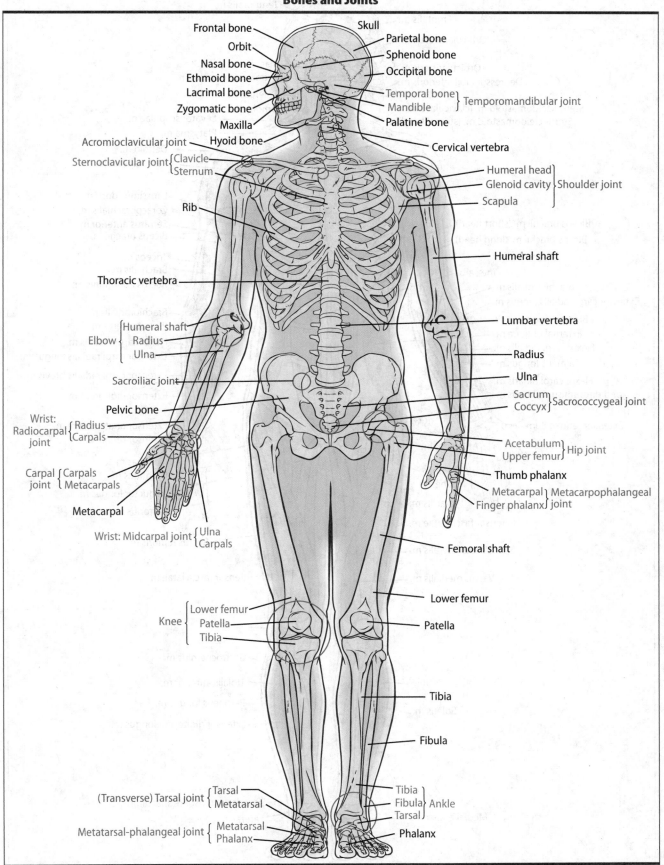

Anatomical Illustrations—Musculoskeletal System

Muscles

- Temporalis m.
- Frontalis m.
- Orbicularis oculi m.
- Orbicularis oris m.
- Masseter m.
- Depressor labii inferioris m.
- Zygomaticus major m.
- Mentalis m.
- Splenius m.
- Sternocleidomastoid m. (clavicular head)
- Omohyoid m.
- Sternocleidomastoid m. (sternal head)
- Levator scapulae m.
- Platysma m.
- Deltoid m.
- Pectoralis major m.
- Latissimus dorsi m.
- Coracobrachialis m.
- Biceps brachii m. (short head)
- Serratus anterior m.
- Biceps brachii m. (long head)
- Biceps brachii m.
- Triceps m.
- Linea alba
- Brachialis m.
- Brachioradialis m.
- Rectus abdominis m.
- Extensor carpi radialis longus m.
- Bicipital aponeurosis
- Brachioradialis m.
- External oblique m.
- Pronator teres m.
- Flexor carpi radialis m.
- Flexor carpi radialis m.
- Palmaris longus m.
- Extensor carpi radialis longus m.
- Flexor carpi ulnaris m.
- Extensor carpi radialis brevis m.
- Flexor digitorum superficialis m.
- Extensor digitorum m.
- Extensor digiti minimi m.
- Extensor retinaculum
- Anterior superior iliac spine
- Extensor retinaculum
- Iliopsoas m.
- Pectineus m.
- Pubic tubercle
- Adductor longus m.
- Gracilis m.
- Sartorius m.
- Tensor fascia latae m.
- Rectus femoris m.
- Vastus lateralis m.
- Vastus medialis m.
- Tensor fascia latae m.
- Patella
- Gastrocnemius m.
- Tibia
- Tibialis anterior m.
- Soleus m.
- Peroneus longus m.
- Extensor digitorum longus m.
- Superior extensor retinaculum
- Medial malleolus
- Lateral malleolus

Head and Facial Bones

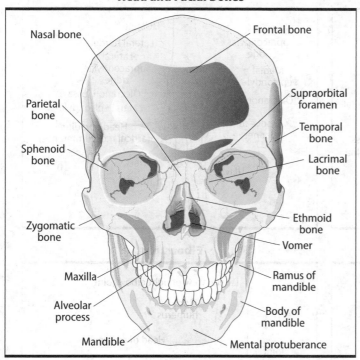

Nasal bone
Frontal bone
Parietal bone
Supraorbital foramen
Sphenoid bone
Temporal bone
Lacrimal bone
Zygomatic bone
Ethmoid bone
Vomer
Maxilla
Ramus of mandible
Alveolar process
Body of mandible
Mandible
Mental protuberance

Nose

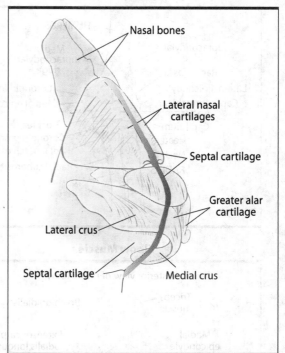

Nasal bones
Lateral nasal cartilages
Septal cartilage
Greater alar cartilage
Lateral crus
Septal cartilage
Medial crus

Shoulder (Anterior View)

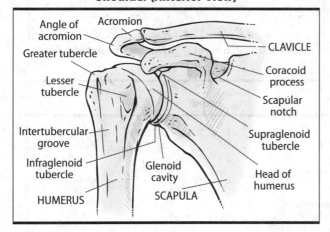

Angle of acromion
Acromion
Greater tubercle
CLAVICLE
Lesser tubercle
Coracoid process
Scapular notch
Intertubercular groove
Supraglenoid tubercle
Infraglenoid tubercle
Glenoid cavity
Head of humerus
HUMERUS
SCAPULA

Shoulder (Posterior View)

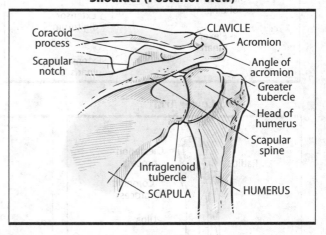

Coracoid process
CLAVICLE
Scapular notch
Acromion
Angle of acromion
Greater tubercle
Head of humerus
Scapular spine
Infraglenoid tubercle
SCAPULA
HUMERUS

Shoulder Muscles

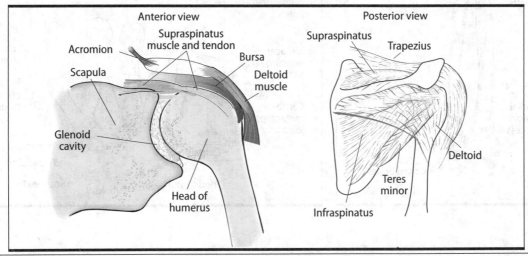

Anterior view
Supraspinatus muscle and tendon
Acromion
Bursa
Scapula
Deltoid muscle
Glenoid cavity
Head of humerus

Posterior view
Supraspinatus
Trapezius
Deltoid
Teres minor
Infraspinatus

Anatomical Illustrations—Musculoskeletal System

Elbow (Anterior View)

Elbow (Posterior View)

Elbow Muscles

Elbow Joint

Lower Arm

Hand

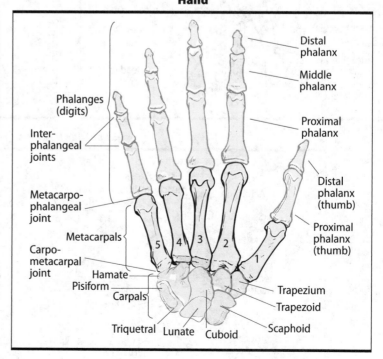

© 2019 Optum360, LLC

Hip (Anterior View)

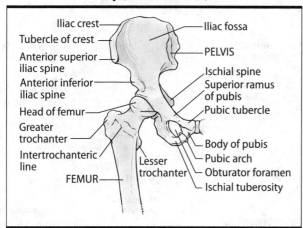

Iliac crest
Tubercle of crest
Anterior superior iliac spine
Anterior inferior iliac spine
Head of femur
Greater trochanter
Intertrochanteric line
FEMUR
Lesser trochanter
Iliac fossa
PELVIS
Ischial spine
Superior ramus of pubis
Pubic tubercle
Body of pubis
Pubic arch
Obturator foramen
Ischial tuberosity

Hip (Posterior View)

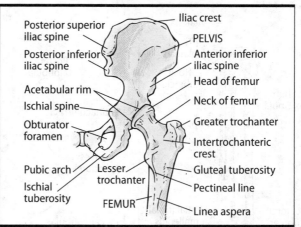

Posterior superior iliac spine
Posterior inferior iliac spine
Acetabular rim
Ischial spine
Obturator foramen
Pubic arch
Ischial tuberosity
Lesser trochanter
FEMUR
Iliac crest
PELVIS
Anterior inferior iliac spine
Head of femur
Neck of femur
Greater trochanter
Intertrochanteric crest
Gluteal tuberosity
Pectineal line
Linea aspera

Knee (Anterior View)

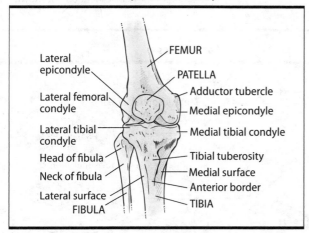

Lateral epicondyle
Lateral femoral condyle
Lateral tibial condyle
Head of fibula
Neck of fibula
Lateral surface
FIBULA
FEMUR
PATELLA
Adductor tubercle
Medial epicondyle
Medial tibial condyle
Tibial tuberosity
Medial surface
Anterior border
TIBIA

Knee (Posterior View)

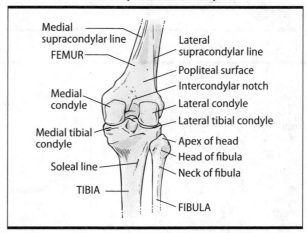

Medial supracondylar line
FEMUR
Medial condyle
Medial tibial condyle
Soleal line
TIBIA
Lateral supracondylar line
Popliteal surface
Intercondylar notch
Lateral condyle
Lateral tibial condyle
Apex of head
Head of fibula
Neck of fibula
FIBULA

Knee Joint (Anterior View)

Patella
Lateral meniscus cartilage
Medial meniscus cartilage

Knee Joint (Lateral View)

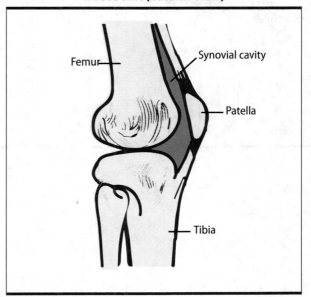

Femur
Synovial cavity
Patella
Tibia

Lower Leg

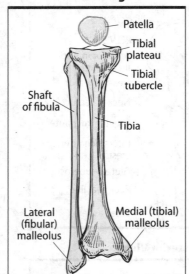

Patella
Tibial plateau
Tibial tubercle
Shaft of fibula
Tibia
Lateral (fibular) malleolus
Medial (tibial) malleolus

Ankle Ligament (Lateral View)

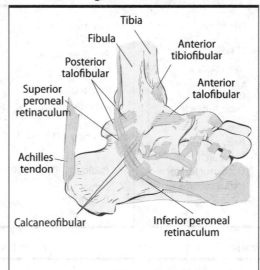

Tibia
Fibula
Posterior talofibular
Anterior tibiofibular
Superior peroneal retinaculum
Anterior talofibular
Achilles tendon
Calcaneofibular
Inferior peroneal retinaculum

Ankle Ligament (Posterior View)

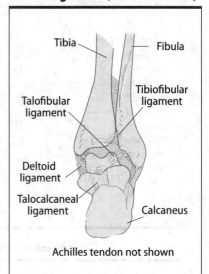

Tibia
Fibula
Talofibular ligament
Tibiofibular ligament
Deltoid ligament
Talocalcaneal ligament
Calcaneus

Achilles tendon not shown

Foot Tendons

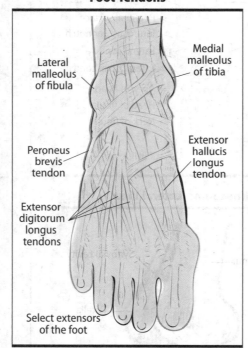

Lateral malleolus of fibula
Medial malleolus of tibia
Peroneus brevis tendon
Extensor hallucis longus tendon
Extensor digitorum longus tendons
Select extensors of the foot

Foot Bones

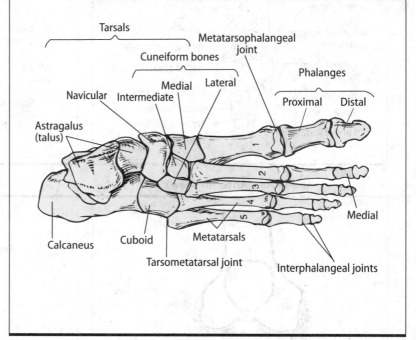

Tarsals
Metatarsophalangeal joint
Cuneiform bones
Medial
Lateral
Phalanges
Navicular
Intermediate
Proximal
Distal
Astragalus (talus)
Calcaneus
Cuboid
Metatarsals
Medial
Tarsometatarsal joint
Interphalangeal joints

Respiratory System

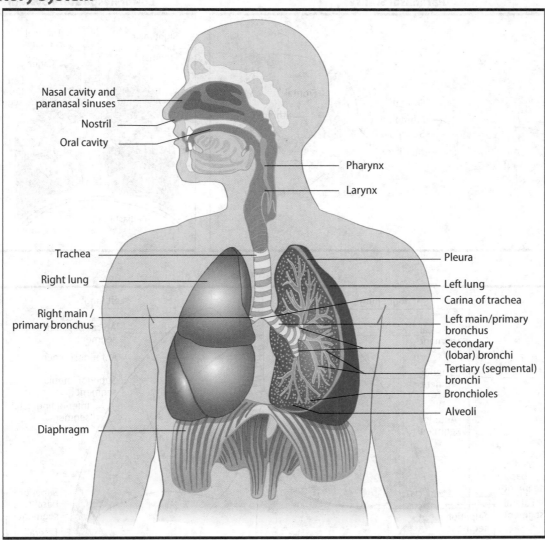

- Nasal cavity and paranasal sinuses
- Nostril
- Oral cavity
- Pharynx
- Larynx
- Trachea
- Right lung
- Right main / primary bronchus
- Diaphragm
- Pleura
- Left lung
- Carina of trachea
- Left main/primary bronchus
- Secondary (lobar) bronchi
- Tertiary (segmental) bronchi
- Bronchioles
- Alveoli

Upper Respiratory System

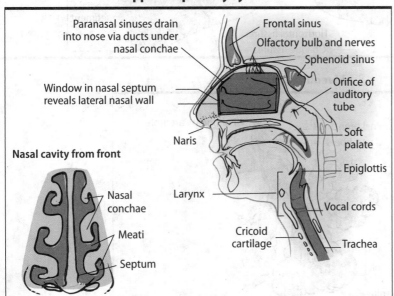

- Paranasal sinuses drain into nose via ducts under nasal conchae
- Window in nasal septum reveals lateral nasal wall
- Naris
- Frontal sinus
- Olfactory bulb and nerves
- Sphenoid sinus
- Orifice of auditory tube
- Soft palate
- Epiglottis
- Larynx
- Vocal cords
- Cricoid cartilage
- Trachea

Nasal cavity from front

- Nasal conchae
- Meati
- Septum

Nasal Turbinates

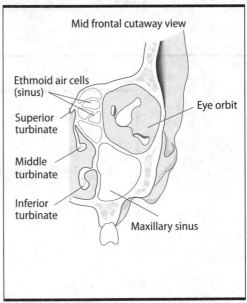

Mid frontal cutaway view

- Ethmoid air cells (sinus)
- Superior turbinate
- Middle turbinate
- Inferior turbinate
- Eye orbit
- Maxillary sinus

Paranasal Sinuses

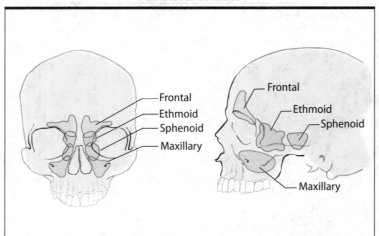

Frontal
Ethmoid
Sphenoid
Maxillary

Frontal
Ethmoid
Sphenoid
Maxillary

Lower Respiratory System

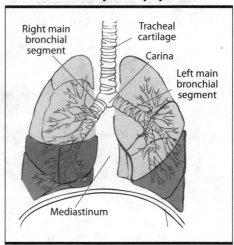

Right main bronchial segment
Tracheal cartilage
Carina
Left main bronchial segment
Mediastinum

Lung Segments

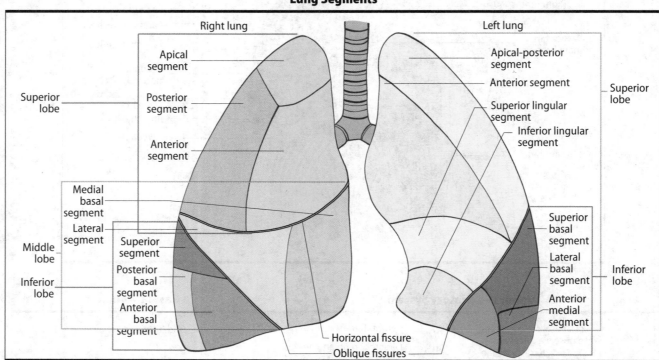

Right lung
Left lung

Apical segment
Superior lobe
Posterior segment
Anterior segment

Medial basal segment
Lateral segment
Middle lobe
Superior segment
Inferior lobe
Posterior basal segment
Anterior basal segment

Horizontal fissure
Oblique fissures

Apical-posterior segment
Anterior segment
Superior lingular segment
Inferior lingular segment
Superior lobe

Superior basal segment
Lateral basal segment
Inferior lobe
Anterior medial segment

Alveoli

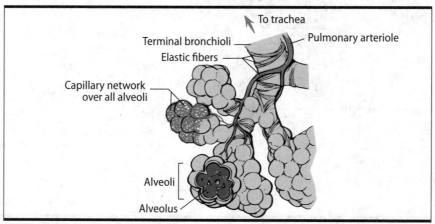

To trachea
Terminal bronchioli
Pulmonary arteriole
Elastic fibers
Capillary network over all alveoli
Alveoli
Alveolus

Arterial System

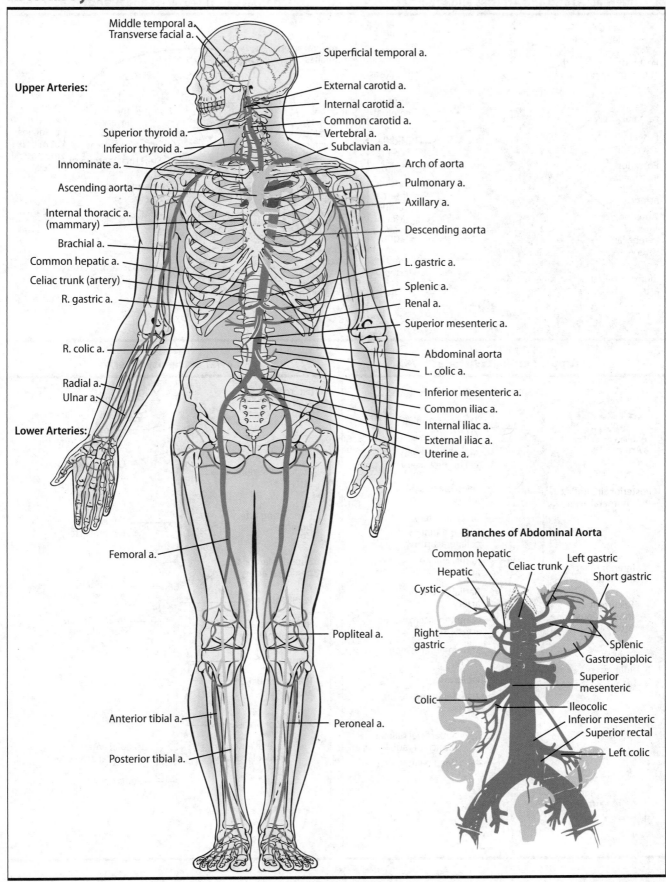

Upper Arteries:

Middle temporal a.
Transverse facial a.
Superficial temporal a.
External carotid a.
Internal carotid a.
Common carotid a.
Superior thyroid a.
Vertebral a.
Inferior thyroid a.
Subclavian a.
Innominate a.
Arch of aorta
Ascending aorta
Pulmonary a.
Internal thoracic a. (mammary)
Axillary a.
Brachial a.
Descending aorta
Common hepatic a.
L. gastric a.
Celiac trunk (artery)
Splenic a.
R. gastric a.
Renal a.
Superior mesenteric a.
R. colic a.
Abdominal aorta
L. colic a.
Radial a.
Inferior mesenteric a.
Ulnar a.
Common iliac a.

Lower Arteries:

Internal iliac a.
External iliac a.
Uterine a.

Femoral a.
Popliteal a.
Anterior tibial a.
Peroneal a.
Posterior tibial a.

Branches of Abdominal Aorta

Common hepatic
Left gastric
Hepatic
Celiac trunk
Cystic
Short gastric
Right gastric
Splenic
Gastroepiploic
Superior mesenteric
Colic
Ileocolic
Inferior mesenteric
Superior rectal
Left colic

Anatomical Illustrations—Arterial System

Internal Carotid and Arteries and Branches

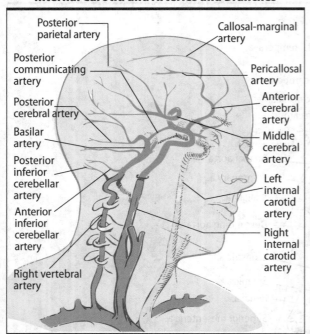

Posterior parietal artery
Callosal-marginal artery
Posterior communicating artery
Pericallosal artery
Posterior cerebral artery
Anterior cerebral artery
Basilar artery
Middle cerebral artery
Posterior inferior cerebellar artery
Left internal carotid artery
Anterior inferior cerebellar artery
Right internal carotid artery
Right vertebral artery

External Carotid Arteries and Branches

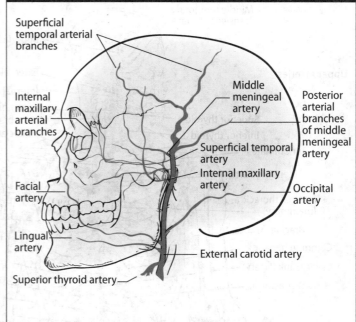

Superficial temporal arterial branches
Middle meningeal artery
Internal maxillary arterial branches
Posterior arterial branches of middle meningeal artery
Superficial temporal artery
Internal maxillary artery
Facial artery
Occipital artery
Lingual artery
External carotid artery
Superior thyroid artery

Upper Extremity Arteries

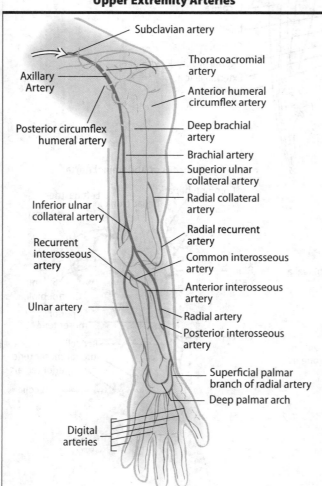

Subclavian artery
Thoracoacromial artery
Axillary Artery
Anterior humeral circumflex artery
Posterior circumflex humeral artery
Deep brachial artery
Brachial artery
Superior ulnar collateral artery
Inferior ulnar collateral artery
Radial collateral artery
Recurrent interosseous artery
Radial recurrent artery
Common interosseous artery
Ulnar artery
Anterior interosseous artery
Radial artery
Posterior interosseous artery
Superficial palmar branch of radial artery
Deep palmar arch
Digital arteries

Lower Extremity Arteries

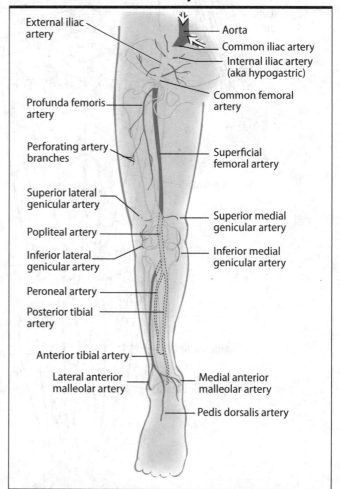

External iliac artery
Aorta
Common iliac artery
Internal iliac artery (aka hypogastric)
Profunda femoris artery
Common femoral artery
Perforating artery branches
Superficial femoral artery
Superior lateral genicular artery
Superior medial genicular artery
Popliteal artery
Inferior lateral genicular artery
Inferior medial genicular artery
Peroneal artery
Posterior tibial artery
Anterior tibial artery
Lateral anterior malleolar artery
Medial anterior malleolar artery
Pedis dorsalis artery

Venous System

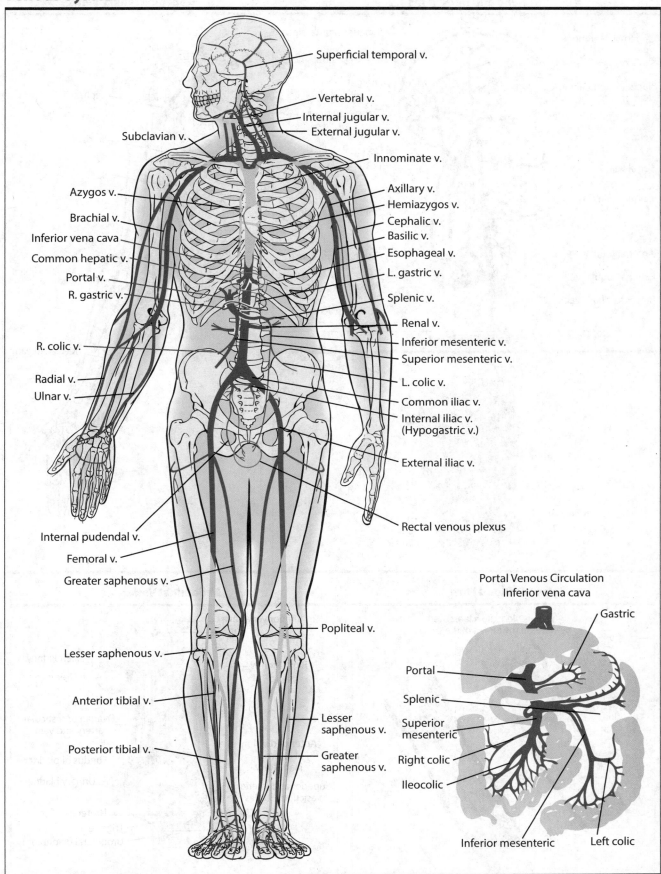

Superficial temporal v.
Vertebral v.
Internal jugular v.
External jugular v.
Subclavian v.
Innominate v.
Azygos v.
Axillary v.
Hemiazygos v.
Brachial v.
Cephalic v.
Inferior vena cava
Basilic v.
Common hepatic v.
Esophageal v.
Portal v.
L. gastric v.
R. gastric v.
Splenic v.
Renal v.
R. colic v.
Inferior mesenteric v.
Superior mesenteric v.
Radial v.
L. colic v.
Ulnar v.
Common iliac v.
Internal iliac v.
(Hypogastric v.)
External iliac v.
Rectal venous plexus
Internal pudendal v.
Femoral v.
Greater saphenous v.
Popliteal v.
Lesser saphenous v.
Anterior tibial v.
Lesser saphenous v.
Posterior tibial v.
Greater saphenous v.

Portal Venous Circulation
Inferior vena cava
Gastric
Portal
Splenic
Superior mesenteric
Right colic
Ileocolic
Inferior mesenteric
Left colic

Anatomical Illustrations—Venous System

Head and Neck Veins

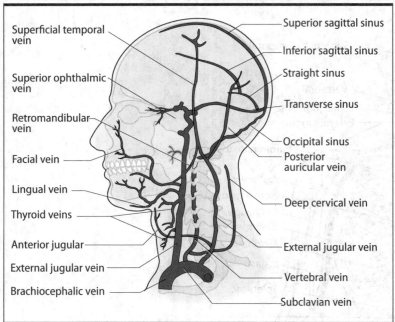

Superficial temporal vein
Superior ophthalmic vein
Retromandibular vein
Facial vein
Lingual vein
Thyroid veins
Anterior jugular
External jugular vein
Brachiocephalic vein

Superior sagittal sinus
Inferior sagittal sinus
Straight sinus
Transverse sinus
Occipital sinus
Posterior auricular vein
Deep cervical vein
External jugular vein
Vertebral vein
Subclavian vein

Venae Comitantes

Artery

Venae comitantes

Upper Extremity Veins

Axillary
Cephalic
Brachial
Basilic
Median cubital
Median forearm

Venous Blood Flow

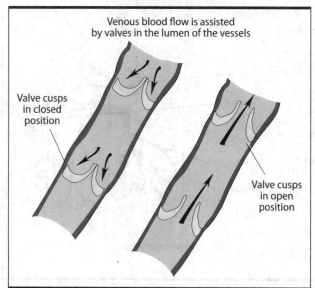

Venous blood flow is assisted by valves in the lumen of the vessels

Valve cusps in closed position

Valve cusps in open position

Abdominal Veins

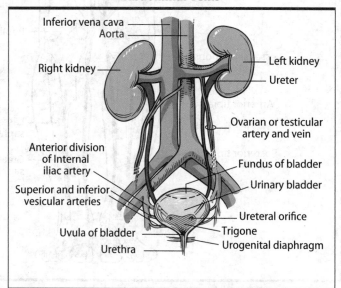

Inferior vena cava
Aorta
Right kidney
Left kidney
Ureter
Ovarian or testicular artery and vein
Anterior division of Internal iliac artery
Fundus of bladder
Urinary bladder
Superior and inferior vesicular arteries
Ureteral orifice
Trigone
Uvula of bladder
Urogenital diaphragm
Urethra

Cardiovascular System

Coronary Veins

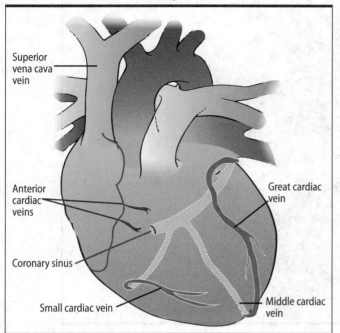

Superior vena cava vein

Anterior cardiac veins

Coronary sinus

Small cardiac vein

Great cardiac vein

Middle cardiac vein

Anatomy of the Heart

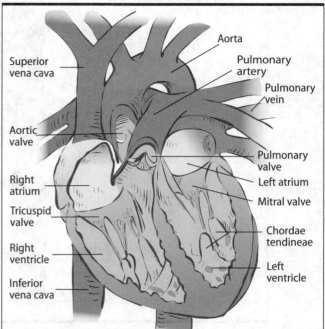

Superior vena cava

Aortic valve

Right atrium

Tricuspid valve

Right ventricle

Inferior vena cava

Aorta

Pulmonary artery

Pulmonary vein

Pulmonary valve

Left atrium

Mitral valve

Chordae tendineae

Left ventricle

Heart Cross Section

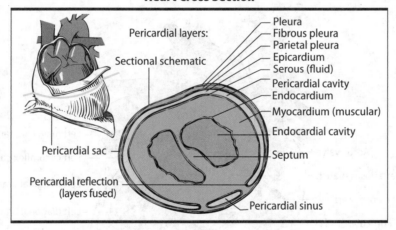

Pericardial layers:

Sectional schematic

Pericardial sac

Pericardial reflection (layers fused)

Pleura
Fibrous pleura
Parietal pleura
Epicardium
Serous (fluid)
Pericardial cavity
Endocardium
Myocardium (muscular)
Endocardial cavity
Septum

Pericardial sinus

Heart Valves

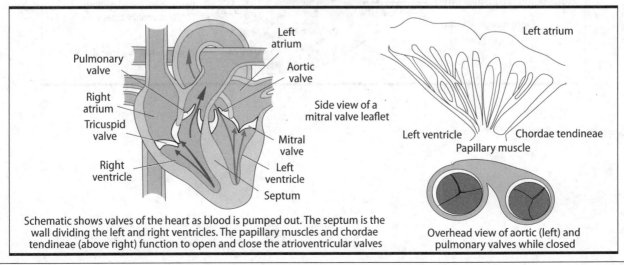

Pulmonary valve

Right atrium

Tricuspid valve

Right ventricle

Left atrium

Aortic valve

Mitral valve

Left ventricle

Septum

Side view of a mitral valve leaflet

Left atrium

Left ventricle

Papillary muscle

Chordae tendineae

Overhead view of aortic (left) and pulmonary valves while closed

Schematic shows valves of the heart as blood is pumped out. The septum is the wall dividing the left and right ventricles. The papillary muscles and chordae tendineae (above right) function to open and close the atrioventricular valves

Anatomical Illustrations—Cardiovascular System

Anatomical Illustrations—Cardiovascular System

Heart Conduction System

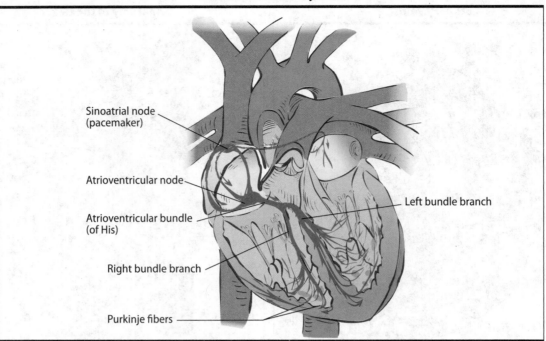

Sinoatrial node (pacemaker)

Atrioventricular node

Atrioventricular bundle (of His)

Right bundle branch

Purkinje fibers

Left bundle branch

Coronary Arteries

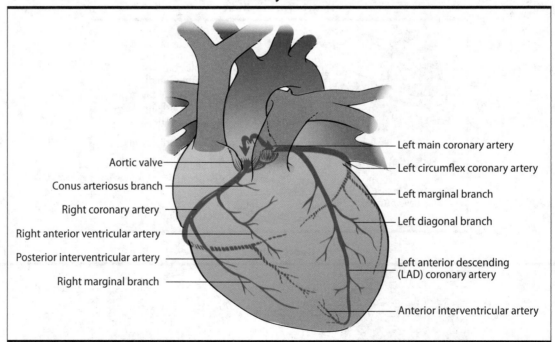

Aortic valve

Conus arteriosus branch

Right coronary artery

Right anterior ventricular artery

Posterior interventricular artery

Right marginal branch

Left main coronary artery

Left circumflex coronary artery

Left marginal branch

Left diagonal branch

Left anterior descending (LAD) coronary artery

Anterior interventricular artery

Lymphatic System

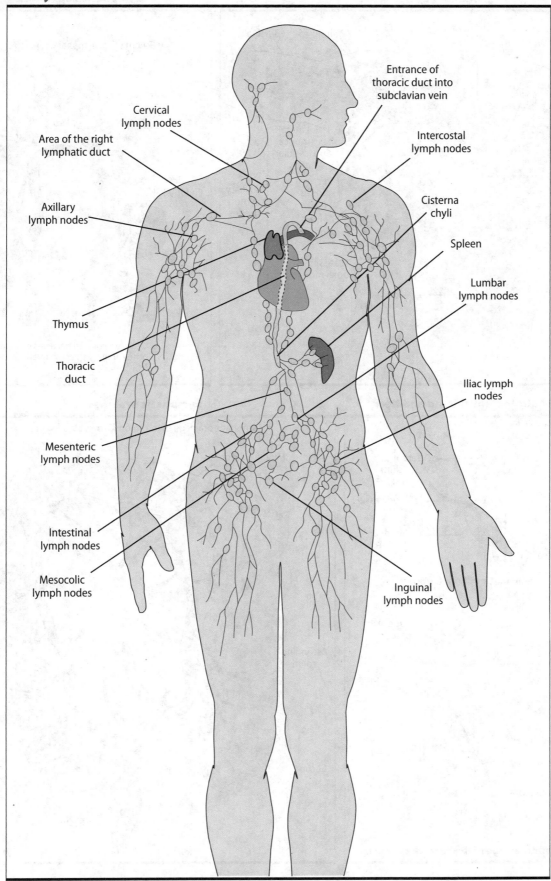

Cervical lymph nodes

Area of the right lymphatic duct

Axillary lymph nodes

Thymus

Thoracic duct

Mesenteric lymph nodes

Intestinal lymph nodes

Mesocolic lymph nodes

Entrance of thoracic duct into subclavian vein

Intercostal lymph nodes

Cisterna chyli

Spleen

Lumbar lymph nodes

Iliac lymph nodes

Inguinal lymph nodes

Axillary Lymph Nodes

Lymphatic Capillaries

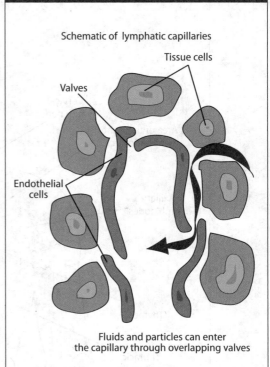

Schematic of lymphatic capillaries

Fluids and particles can enter the capillary through overlapping valves

Lymphatic System of Head and Neck

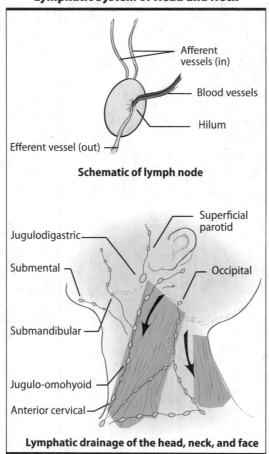

Schematic of lymph node

Lymphatic drainage of the head, neck, and face

Lymphatic Drainage

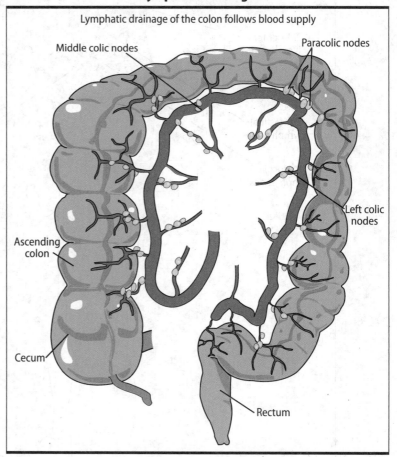

Lymphatic drainage of the colon follows blood supply

Spleen Internal Structures

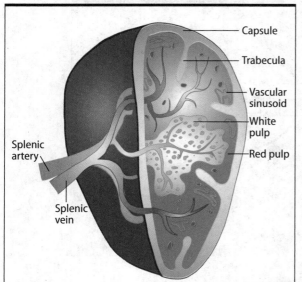

- Capsule
- Trabecula
- Vascular sinusoid
- White pulp
- Red pulp
- Splenic artery
- Splenic vein

Spleen External Structures

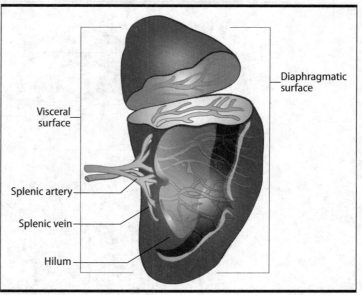

- Diaphragmatic surface
- Visceral surface
- Splenic artery
- Splenic vein
- Hilum

Anatomical Illustrations—Lymphatic System

Digestive System

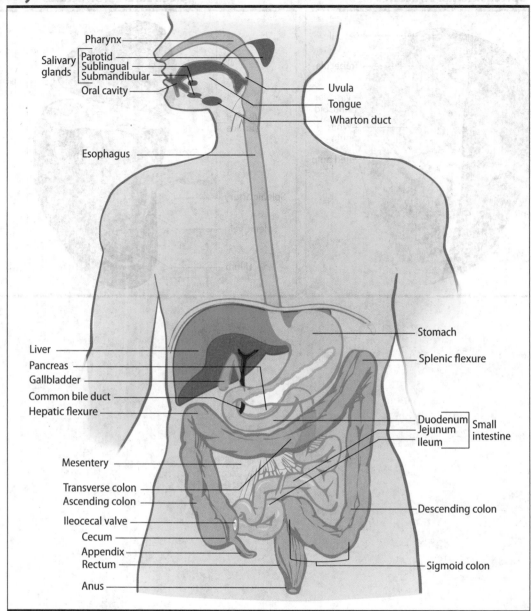

Pharynx

Salivary glands
- Parotid
- Sublingual
- Submandibular

Oral cavity

Uvula

Tongue

Wharton duct

Esophagus

Liver

Pancreas

Gallbladder

Common bile duct

Hepatic flexure

Stomach

Splenic flexure

Duodenum
Jejunum
Ileum

Small intestine

Mesentery

Transverse colon

Ascending colon

Ileocecal valve

Cecum

Appendix

Rectum

Anus

Descending colon

Sigmoid colon

Gallbladder

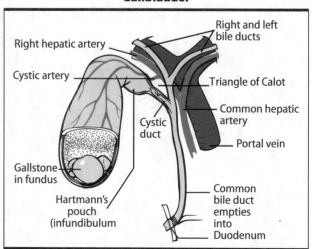

Right hepatic artery

Cystic artery

Right and left bile ducts

Triangle of Calot

Common hepatic artery

Cystic duct

Portal vein

Gallstone in fundus

Hartmann's pouch (infundibulum

Common bile duct empties into Duodenum

Stomach

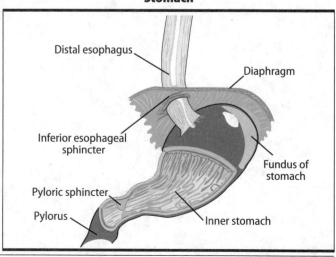

Distal esophagus

Diaphragm

Inferior esophageal sphincter

Pyloric sphincter

Pylorus

Fundus of stomach

Inner stomach

Mouth (Upper)

Mouth (Lower)

Pancreas

Liver

Anus

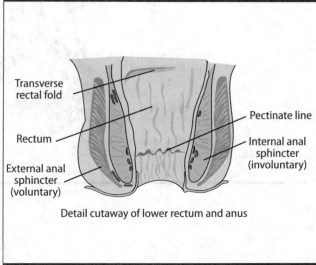

Detail cutaway of lower rectum and anus

Genitourinary System

Urinary System

Nephron

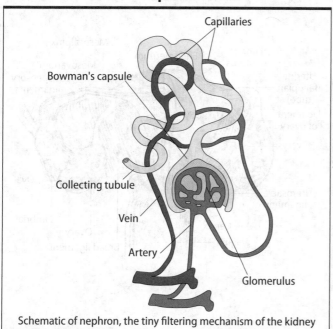

Schematic of nephron, the tiny filtering mechanism of the kidney

Male Genitourinary

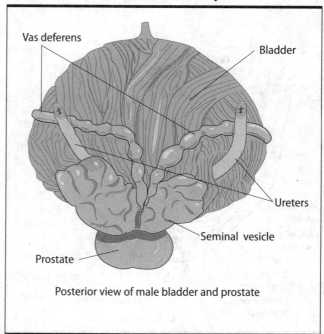

Posterior view of male bladder and prostate

Testis and Associate Structures

Male Genitourinary System

Female Genitourinary

Female Reproductive System

Female Bladder

Female Breast

Endocrine System

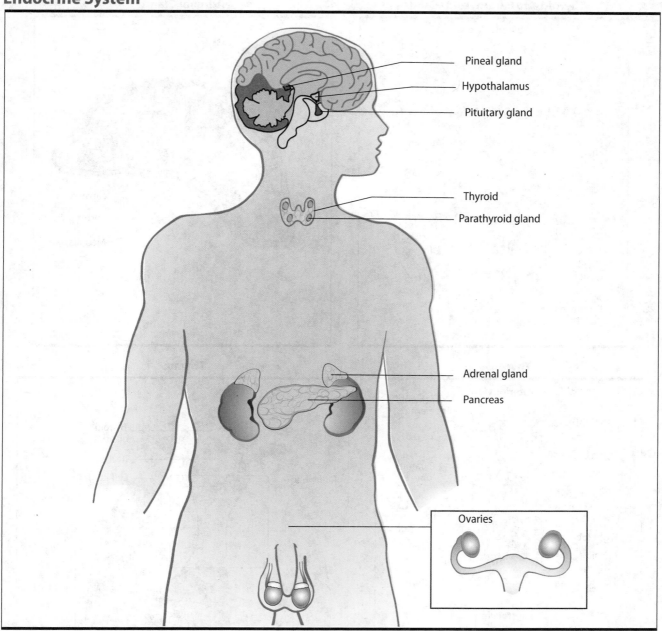

Pineal gland
Hypothalamus
Pituitary gland
Thyroid
Parathyroid gland
Adrenal gland
Pancreas
Ovaries

Structure of an Ovary

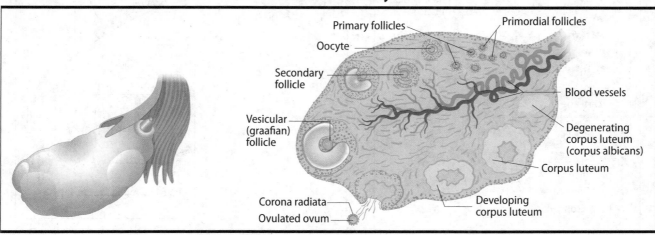

Primary follicles
Primordial follicles
Oocyte
Secondary follicle
Blood vessels
Vesicular (graafian) follicle
Degenerating corpus luteum (corpus albicans)
Corpus luteum
Corona radiata
Developing corpus luteum
Ovulated ovum

Thyroid and Parathyroid Glands

Posterior view

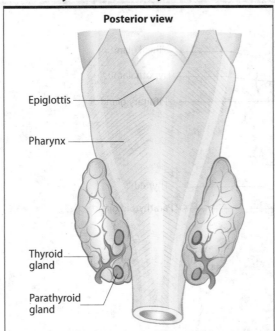

- Epiglottis
- Pharynx
- Thyroid gland
- Parathyroid gland

Adrenal Gland

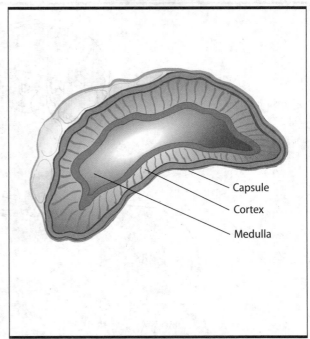

- Capsule
- Cortex
- Medulla

Thyroid

Anterior view

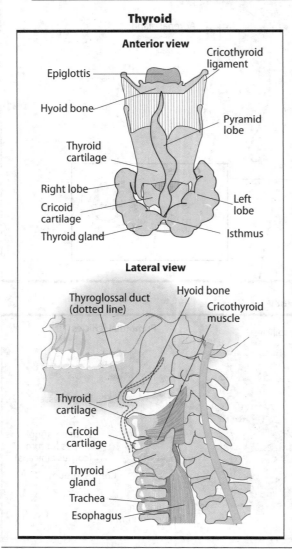

- Epiglottis
- Hyoid bone
- Cricothyroid ligament
- Thyroid cartilage
- Pyramid lobe
- Right lobe
- Cricoid cartilage
- Thyroid gland
- Left lobe
- Isthmus

Lateral view

- Thyroglossal duct (dotted line)
- Hyoid bone
- Cricothyroid muscle
- Thyroid cartilage
- Cricoid cartilage
- Thyroid gland
- Trachea
- Esophagus

Thymus

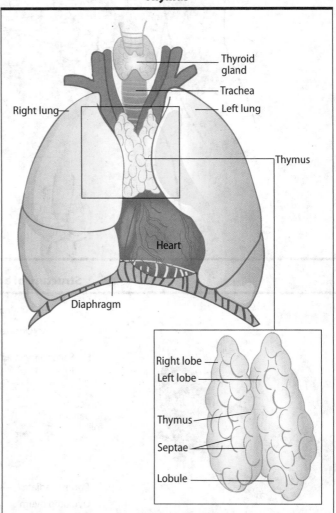

- Thyroid gland
- Trachea
- Left lung
- Right lung
- Thymus
- Heart
- Diaphragm
- Right lobe
- Left lobe
- Thymus
- Septae
- Lobule

Nervous System

Great auricular — Cervical plexus
Lesser occipital
Greater occipital — Cervical nerve
Suboccipital
3rd occipital
Ansa cervicalis
Cervical plexus — Transverse cervical
L. phrenic
Supraclavicular
Dorsal scapular
First intercostal
Subclavian
Brachial plexus — Long thoracic
Axillary
Musculocutaneous
Median
Ulnar
Radial
Thoracic splanchnic
Intercostal nerves
Subcostal
Lumbar splanchnic
Genitofemoral
Iliohypogastric
Ilioinguinal — Lumbar plexus
Obturator
Lateral femoral cutaneous
Sacral — Accessory obturator
Superior gluteal
Inferior gluteal
Sacral splanchnic — Sacral plexus and sacral sympathetic nerves
Pelvic splanchnic
Pudendal
Posterior femoral cutaneous
Posterior scrotal/labial
Femoral
Sciatic
Saphenous
Tibial
Common peroneal
Superficial peroneal
Deep peroneal

Anatomical Illustrations—Nervous System

Brain

Cranial Nerves

© 2019 Optum360, LLC

Spinal Cord and Spinal Nerves

Nerve Cell

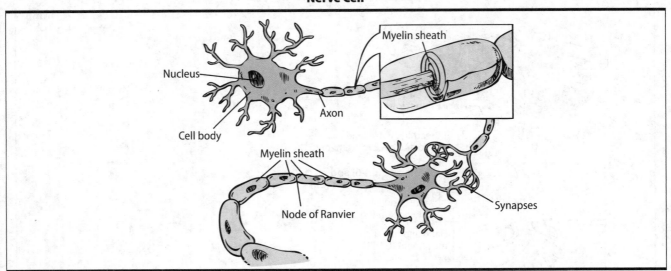

Eye

Eye Structure

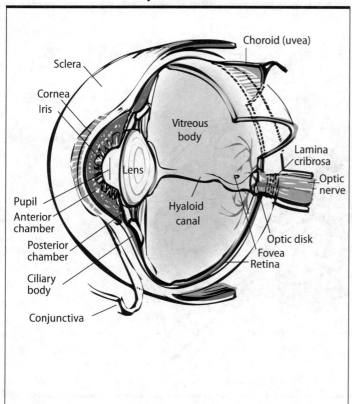

Posterior Pole of Globe/Flow of Aqueous Humor

Eye Musculature

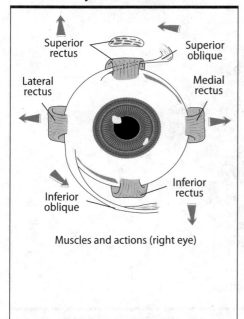

Muscles and actions (right eye)

Eyelid Structures

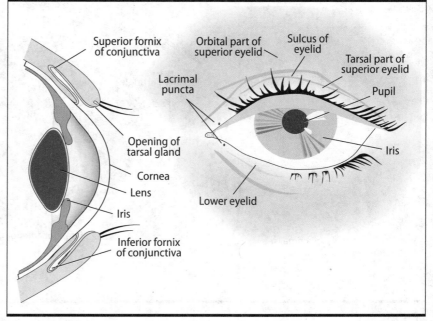

Ear and Lacrimal System

Ear Anatomy

Lacrimal System

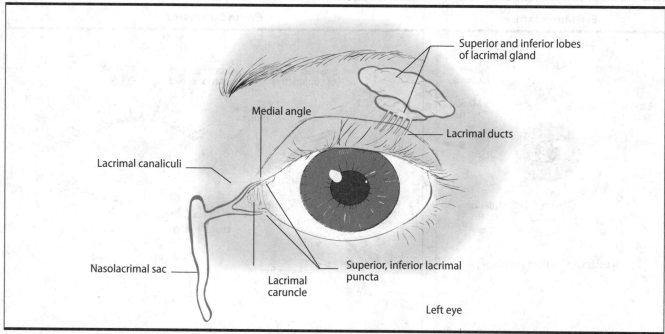

© 2019 Optum360, LLC

Abscess — continued
Arm, Upper
  Incision and Drainage, 23930-23935
Auditory Canal, External, 69020
Bartholin's Gland
  Incision and Drainage, 56420
Bladder
  Incision and Drainage, 51080
Brain
  Drainage by
    Burr Hole, 61150, 61151
    Craniotomy/Craniectomy, 61320, 61321
  Excision, 61514, 61522
  Incision and Drainage, 61320-61321
Breast
  Incision and Drainage, 19020
Carpals
  Incision, Deep, 25035
Clavicle
  Sequestrectomy, 23170
Drainage
  Contrast Injection, 49424
  with X-ray, 75989, 76080
Ear, External
  Complicated, 69005
  Simple, 69000
Elbow
  Incision and Drainage, 23930-23935
  Sequestrectomy, 24136-24138
Epididymis
  Incision and Drainage, 54700
Excision
  Olecranon Process, 24138
  Radius, 24136
  Ulna, 24138
Eyelid
  Incision and Drainage, 67700
Facial Bone(s)
  Excision, 21026
Femur
  Bursa, 27301
  Deep Abscess, 27301
  Hematoma, 27301
  with Opening Bone Cortex, 27303
Finger, 26010-26011
  Incision and Drainage, 26010, 26011, 26034
Foot
  Incision, 28005
Gums
  Incision and Drainage, 41800
Hand
  Incision and Drainage, 26034
Hematoma
  Incision and Drainage, 27603
Hip
  Incision and Drainage, 26990-26992
Humeral Head, 23174
Humerus
  Excision, 24134
  Incision and Drainage, 23935
Kidney
  Incision and Drainage
    Open, 50020
Leg, Lower
  Incision and Drainage, 27603
    Bone Abscess, 27607
Liver
  Incision and Drainage, 47010
    Open, 47010
  Injection, 47015
  Marsupialization, 47300
Lung
  Open Drainage, 32200
Lymph Node, 38300, 38305
  Incision and Drainage, 38300-38305
Lymphocele
  Drainage, 49062
  Sclerotherapy, 49185
Mandible
  Excision, 21025
Mouth
  Dentoalveolar, 41800
  Floor of Mouth
    Extraoral, 41015-41018

Abscess — continued
Mouth — continued
  Floor of Mouth — continued
    Intraoral, 41000-41009
  Incision and Drainage, 40800, 40801, 41005-41009, 41015-41018
  Vestibule, 40800-40801
Nasal
  Incision and Drainage, 30000, 30020
Nasal Septum
  Incision and Drainage, 30020
Neck
  Incision and Drainage, 21501, 21502
Nose
  Incision and Drainage, 30000, 30020
Olecranon Process
  Incision and Drainage, 23930-23935
  Sequestrectomy, 24138
Ovarian
  Incision and Drainage, 58820-58822
    Abdominal Approach, 58822
    Vaginal Approach, 58820
Ovary
  Incision and Drainage
    Abdominal Approach, 58822
    Vaginal Approach, 58820
Palate
  Incision and Drainage, 42000
Paraurethral Gland
  Incision and Drainage, 53060
Parotid Gland
  Drainage, 42300, 42305
Pelvis
  Incision and Drainage, 26990-26992
  Transrectal, 45000
Perineum
  Incision and Drainage, 56405
Perirenal or Renal
  Drainage, 50020
Peritoneum
  Incision and Drainage
    Open, 49020
Pharynx, 42700-42725
Posterior Spine, 22010, 22015
Prostate
  Incision and Drainage, 55720-55725
    Prostatotomy, 55720, 55725
    Transurethral, 52700
Radius
  Bone Abscess, 25035
  Incision and Drainage, 25028
  Incision, Deep, 25035
  Sequestrectomy, 24136
Rectum
  Incision and Drainage, 45005, 45020, 46040, 46060
Retroperitoneal, 49060
  Drainage
    Open, 49060
Salivary Gland
  Drainage, 42300-42320
Scapula
  Sequestrectomy, 23172
Scrotum
  Incision and Drainage, 54700, 55100
Shoulder
  Bone Cortex, 23035
  Incision and Drainage, 23030
Skene's Gland
  Incision and Drainage, 53060
Skin
  Incision and Drainage, 10060-10061
    Complicated, 10061
    Multiple, 10061
    Simple, 10060
    Single, 10060
  Puncture Aspiration, 10160
Soft Tissue
  Catheter Drainage, 10030
Spine
  Incision and Drainage, 22010-22015
Subdiaphragmatic
  Incision and Drainage
    Open, 49040
Sublingual Gland
  Drainage, 42310, 42320

Abscess — continued
Submaxillary Gland
  Drainage, 42310, 42320
Subphrenic, 49040
Testis
  Incision and Drainage, 54700
Thigh
  Incision and Drainage, 27301
    Bone Abscess, 27303
Thoracostomy, 32551
Thorax
  Bone Cortex, 21510
  Incision and Drainage, 21501, 21502
Throat
  Incision and Drainage, 42700-42725
Tongue
  Incision and Drainage, 41000-41006
Tonsil
  Incision and Drainage, 42700
Ulna
  Incision, Deep, 25035
Urethra
  Incision and Drainage, 53040
Uvula
  Incision and Drainage, 42000
Vagina
  Incision and Drainage, 57010
Visceral, 49405
Vulva
  Incision and Drainage, 56405
Wrist
  Excision, 25145
  Incision and Drainage, 25028, 25035
X-ray, 76080
Absolute Neutrophil Count (ANC), 85048
Absorptiometry
  Dual Energy, 77080
    Bone
      Appendicular Skeleton, 77081
      Axial Skeleton, 77078, 77080
      Vertebral, 77080, [77086]
    Ordered and Documented (PQRS), 3095F-3096F
  Dual Photon
    Bone, 78351
  Single Photon
    Bone, 78350
Absorption Spectrophotometry, 82190
  Atomic, 82190
ACADM, 81400-81401
ACADS, 81404-81405
ACADVL, 81406
ACB, 82045
ACBE (Air Contrast Barium Enema), 74280
Accelerometer Data Recording, 3-Axis, 0381T-0386T
Access
  Small Bowel via Biliary Tree, Percutaneous, 47541
Accessory Nerve
  Incision, 63191
  Section, 63191
Accessory, Toes, 28344
ACD, 63075, 63076
ACE (Angiotensin Converting Enzyme)
  See Angiotensin
Acellular Immunization, 90700
Acetabuloplasty, 27120, 27122, [29915]
Acetabulum
  Fracture
    Closed Treatment, 27220, 27222
    Open Treatment, 27226-27228
    with Manipulation, 27222
    without Manipulation, 27220
  Reconstruction, 27120
    with Resection, Femoral Head, 27122
  Tumor
    Excision, 27076
Acetaminophen, [80329, 80330, 80331]
Acetic Anhydrides, 84600
Acetone
  Blood or Urine, 82009, 82010
Acetone Body, 82009, 82010
Acetylcholinesterase
  Blood or Urine, 82013
AcG, 85220

Achilles Tendon
  Incision, 27605, 27606
  Lengthening, 27612
  Repair, 27650-27654
Achillotomy, 27605-27606
ACI, 27412, 29870
Acid
  Adenylic, 82030
  Amino
    Blood or Urine, 82127-82139
  Aminolevulinic
    Urine or Blood, 82135
  Ascorbic
    Blood, 82180
  Bile, 82239
    Blood, 82240
  Deoxyribonucleic
    Antibody, 86225-86226
  Diethylamide, Lysergic, 80299
  Fast Bacilli (AFB)
    Culture, 87116
  Fast Stain, 88312
  Fatty
    Blood, 82725
    Very Long Chain, 82726
  Folic, 82746
    RBC, 82747
  Gastric, 82930
  Glycocholic, 82240
  Lactic, 83605
  N-Acetylneuraminic, 84275
  Perfusion Test
    Esophagus, 91013, 91030
  Phenylethylbarbituric
    Assay, 80184
  Phosphatase, 84060-84066
  Probes, Nucleic
    See Nucleic Acid Probe
  Reflux Test, 91034-91038
  Salic, 84275
  Uric
    Blood, 84550
    Other Source, 84560
    Urine, 84560
Acidity/Alkalinity
  Blood Gasses, 82800-82805
  Body Fluid, Not Otherwise Specified, 83986
  Exhaled Breath Condensate, 83987
ACL Repair
  Arthroscopy aided, 29888
  Open, 27407, 27409
Acne Surgery
  Incision and Drainage
    Abscess, 10060, 10061
      Puncture Aspiration, 10160
    Bulla
      Puncture Aspiration, 10160
    Comedones, 10040
    Cyst, 10040
      Puncture Aspiration, 10160
    Milia, Multiple, 10040
    Pustules, 10040
Acne Treatment
  Abrasion, 15786, 15787
  Chemical Peel, 15788-15793
  Cryotherapy, 17340
  Dermabrasion, 15780-15783
  Exfoliation
    Chemical, 17360
Acoustic
  Evoked Brain Stem Potential, 92585, 92586
  Heart Sounds
    with Computer Analysis, 93799
  Immittance Testing, 92570
  Neuroma
    Brain Tumor Excision, 61510, 61518, 61520, 61521, 61526, 61530, 61545
    Brainstem
      Biopsy, 61575, 61576
      Decompression, 61575, 61576
      Evoked Potentials, 92585
      Lesion Excision, 61575, 61576
    Skull Base Surgery
      Anterior Cranial Fossa
        Bicoronal Approach, 61586

Acoustic — *continued*
  Neuroma — *continued*
    Skull Base Surgery — *continued*
      Anterior Cranial Fossa — *continued*
        Craniofacial Approach, 61580-61583
        Extradural, 61600, 61601
        LeFort I Osteotomy Approach, 61586
        Orbitocranial Approach, 61584, 61585
        Transzygomatic Approach, 61586
      Carotid Aneurysm, 61613
      Craniotomy, 62121
      Dura
        Repair of Cerebrospinal Fluid Leak, 61618, 61619
      Middle Cranial Fossa
        Extradural, 61605-61607
        Infratemporal Approach, 61590, 61591
        Intradural, 61606-61608
        Orbitocranial Zygomatic Approach, 61592
      Posterior Cranial Fossa
        Extradural, 61615
        Intradural, 61616
        Transcondylar Approach, 61596, 61597
        Transpetrosal Approach, 61598
        Transtemporal Approach, 61595
    Recording
      Heart Sounds, 93799
ACP, 84060-84066
Acromioclavicular Joint
  Arthrocentesis, 20605-20606
  Arthrotomy, 23044
    with Biopsy, 23101
  Dislocation, 23540-23552
    Open Treatment, 23550, 23552
  X-ray, 73050
Acromion
  Excision
    Shoulder, 23130
Acromionectomy
  Partial, 23130
Acromioplasty, 23415, 23420
  Partial, 23130
ACTA2, 81405, 81410
ACTC1, 81405
ACTH (Adrenocorticotropic Hormone), 80400-80406, 80412, 80418, 82024
ACTH Releasing Factor, 80412
ActHIB, 90648
Actigraphy, 95803
Actinomyces
  Antibody, 86602
Actinomycosis, 86000
Actinomycotic Infection
  See Actinomycosis
Actinotherapy, 96900
Activated Factor X, 85260
Activated Partial Thromboplastin Time, 85730, 85732
Activation, Lymphocyte, 86353
Activities of Daily Living (ADL), 97535, 99509
  See Physical Medicine/Therapy/ Occupational Therapy
    Training, 97535, 97537
Activity, Glomerular Procoagulant
  See Thromboplastin
ACTN4, 81406
Acupuncture
  One or More Needles
    with Electrical Stimulation, 97813-97814
    without Electrical Stimulation, 97810-97811
Acute Poliomyelitis
  See Polio
Acylcarnitines, 82016, 82017
Adacel, 90715

Adalimumab
  Assay, 80145
Adamantinoma, Pituitary
  See Craniopharyngioma
ADAMTS-13, 85397
Adaptive Behavior
  Assessments, 0362T, [97151], [97152]
  Treatment, 0373T, [97153], [97154], [97155], [97156], [97157], [97158]
Addam Operation, 26040-26045
Adductor Tenotomy of Hip
  See Tenotomy, Hip, Adductor
Adelson
  Crosby Immersion Method, 85999
Adenoidectomy
  Primary
    Age 12 or Over, 42831
    Younger Than Age 12, 42830
  Secondary
    Age 12 or Over, 42836
    Younger Than Age 12, 42835
  with Tonsillectomy, 42820, 42821
Adenoids
  Excision, 42830-42836
    with Tonsillectomy, 42820, 42821
  Unlisted Services and Procedures, 42999
Adenoma
  Pancreas
    Excision, 48120
  Parathyroid
    Injection for Localization, 78808
  Thyroid Gland
    Excision, 60200
Adenosine 3', 5' Monophosphate, 82030
Adenosine Diphosphate
  Blood, 82030
Adenosine Monophosphate (AMP)
  Blood, 82030
Adenovirus
  Antibody, 86603
  Antigen Detection
    Enzyme Immunoassay, 87301-87451
    Immunofluorescence, 87260
Adenovirus Vaccine, 90476-90477
ADH (Antidiuretic Hormone), 84588
ADHD Emotional/Behavioral Assessment, 96127
Adhesion, Adhesions
  Epidural, 62263, 62264
  Eye
    Corneovitreal, 65880
    Incision
      Anterior Segment, 65860-65870
      Posterior Segment, 65875
    Intermarginal
      Construction, 67880
        Transposition of Tarsal Plate, 67882
  Intestinal
    Enterolysis, 44005
      Laparoscopic, 44180
  Intracranial
    Lysis, 62161
  Intranasal Synechia, 30560
  Intrauterine
    Lysis, 58559
  Labial
    Lysis, 56441
  Lungs
    Pneumolysis, 32124, 32940
  Pelvic
    Lysis, 58660, 58662, 58740
  Penile
    Lysis
      Post-circumcision, 54162
  Preputial
    Lysis, 54450
  Urethral
    Lysis, 53500
Adipectomy, 15830-15839, 15876-15879
Adjustment
  External Fixation, 20693, 20696
  Transperineal Periurethral Balloon, 0551T
ADL
  Activities of Daily Living, 97535, 97537
Administration
  Health Risk Assessment, 96160-96161

Administration — *continued*
  Immunization
    with Counseling, 90460-90461
    without Counseling, 90471-90474
  Injection
    Intramuscular Antibiotic, 96372
    Therapeutic, Diagnostic, Prophylactic
      Intra-arterial, 96373
      Intramuscular, 96372
      Intravenous, 96374-96376
      Subcutaneous, 96372
  Occlusive Substance During Bronchoscopy, 31634
  Pharmacologic Agent w/Monitoring
    Endovascular Intracranial
      for Other Than Thrombolysis, 61650-61651
      with Monitoring, 93463
Administrative Codes for Multianalyte Assays with Algorithmic Analyses, 0002M-0004M, 0006M-0009M, 0011M-0013M
ADP (Adenosine Diphosphate), 82030
ADRB2, 81401
Adrenal Cortex Hormone, 83491
Adrenal Gland
  Biopsy, 60540, 60545
  Excision
    Laparoscopy, 60650
    Retroperitoneal, 60545
  Exploration, 60540, 60545
  Nuclear Medicine
    Imaging, 78075
Adrenal Medulla
  See Medulla
Adrenalectomy, 60540
  Anesthesia, 00866
  Laparoscopic, 60650
  with Excision Retroperitoneal Tumor, 60545
Adrenalin
  Blood, 82383, 82384
  Fractionated, 82384
  Urine, 82382, 82384
Adrenaline or Noradrenaline
  Testing, 82382-82384
Adrenocorticotropic Hormone (ACTH), 80400-80406, 80412, 80418, 82024
  Blood or Urine, 82024
  Stimulation Panel, 80400-80406
Adrenogenital Syndrome, 56805, 57335
Adson Test, 95870
Adult T Cell Leukemia Lymphoma Virus I, 86687, 86689
Advance Care Planning, 99497-99498
Advance Directives, 99497-99498
Advanced Life Support
  Emergency Department Services, 99281-99288
  Physician Direction, 99288
Advancement
  Genioglossus, 21199
  Tendon
    Foot, 28238
    Genioglossus, 21199
Advancement Flap
  Skin, Adjacent Tissue Transfer, 14000-14350
AEP, 92585, 92586
Aerosol Inhalation
  Inhalation Treatment, 94640, 94664
  Pentamidine, 94642
AF4/FMR2, 81171-81172
AFB (Acid Fast Bacilli), 87116
AFBG, 35539, 35540, 35646
AFF2, 81171-81172
Afferent Nerve
  See Sensory Nerve
AFG3L2, 81406
AFGE, 66020
AFI, 76815
Afluria, 90655-90658
AFP, 82105, 82106
After Hours Medical Services, 99050-99060
Afterloading Brachytherapy, 77767-77768, 77770-77772
Agents, Anticoagulant
  See Clotting Inhibitors
Agglutinin
  Cold, 86156, 86157

Agglutinin — *continued*
  Febrile, 86000
Aggregation
  Platelet, 85576
AGL, 81407
AGTR1, 81400
AGTT, 82951, 82952
AHG (Antihemophilic Globulin), 85240
AHI1, 81407
Ahmed Glaucoma Valve
  Insertion, 66180
  Removal, 67120
  Revision, 66185
AICD (Pacing Cardioverter-Defibrillator), 0571T-0580T, 33223, 93282, 93289, 93292, 93295
  Heart
    Defibrillator, 33240-33249 [33230, 33231, 33262, 33263, 33264], 93282, 93292, 93295
    Pacemaker, 33212-33214 [33221], 33233-33237 [33227, 33228, 33229]
Aid, Hearing
  Bone Conduction, 69710-69711
  Check, 92590-92595
AIDS
  Antibodies, 86687-86689, 86701-86703
  Virus, 86701, 86703
A-II (Angiotensin II), 82163
Air Contrast Barium Enema (ACBE), 74280
AIRE, 81406
Airway
  Integrity Testing Car Seat/Bed Neonate, 94780-94781
  Resistance by oscillometry, 94728
ALA (Aminolevulinic Acid), 82135
Alanine 2 Oxoglutarate Aminotransferase
  See Transaminase, Glutamic Pyruvic
Alanine Amino (ALT), 84460
Alanine Transaminase
  See Transaminase, Glutamic Pyruvic
Albumin
  Cobalt Binding (ACB), 82045
  Ischemia Modified, 82045
  Other Source, [82042]
  Serum Plasma, 82040
  Urine, 82043-82044
  Whole Blood, 82040
Alcohol, [80320]
  Abuse Screening and Intervention, 99408-99409
  Biomarkers, [80321, 80322]
  Breath, 82075
  Ethylene Glycol, 82693
Alcohol Dehydrogenase
  See Antidiuretic Hormone
Alcohol, Isopropyl
  See Isopropyl Alcohol
Alcohol, Methyl
  See Methanol
ALDH7A1, 81406
Aldolase
  Blood, 82085
Aldosterone
  Blood, 82088
  Suppression Evaluation, 80408
  Urine, 82088
Alexander's Operation, 58400-58410
ALIF (Anterior Lumbar Interbody Fusion), 22558-22585
Alimentary Canal
  See Gastrointestinal Tract
ALK (Automated Lamellar Keratoplasty), 65710
Alkaline Phosphatase, 84075-84080
  Leukocyte, 85540
  WBC, 85540
Alkaloids, [80323]
  See Also Specific Drug
Allergen Bronchial Provocation Tests, 95070-95071
Allergen Challenge, Endobronchial, 95070-95071
Allergen Immunotherapy
  Allergen
    Allergenic Extracts
      Extract Supply with Injection, 95120-95134
      Injection, 95115, 95117

Analysis — *continued*
  Gene — *continued*

ANG, 81403
Angelman Syndrome, 81331, 81402, 81406
ANK2, 81413
ANKRD1, 81405
ANO5, 81406
ANOS1, 81406
Aortic Dysfunction or Dilation, 81410-81411
Aortic Valve Disease, 81407
APC, 81201-81203, 81435
Apert Syndrome, 81404
APOB, 81401, 81407
APOE, 81401
APP, 81406
APTX, 81405
AQP1, 81403
AQP2, 81404
AR, 81204, *[81173, 81174]*
Arrhythmogenic Right Ventricular Dysplasia/Cardiomyopathy, 81406, 81408
ARSA, 81405
ART4, 81403
ARX, 81403-81404
Arylsulfatase A Deficiency, 81405
Ashkenazi Jewish Associated Disorders, 81412, 81443
ASPA, 81200, 81412
Aspartoacylase (ASPA), 81200, 81412
ASPM, 81407
ASS1, 81406
ASXL1, 81175
  Targeted Sequence Analysis (exon 12), 81176
Ataxia, Spinocerebellar, 81178-81183, 81184-81186
ATL1, 81406
ATM, 81408
ATN1, 81177
ATP1A2, 81406
ATP7B, 81406
Atrophy
  Dentatorubral-pallidoloysian, 81177
  Spinal Muscular, 81329
  Spinal/bulbar, 81204
ATXN1, 81178
ATXN10, 81183
ATXN2, 81179
ATXN3, 81180
ATXN7, 81181
ATXN8OS, 81182
Autism Spectrum Disorders, 81404-81405
Autoimmune Disorders
  Polyendocrinopathy Syndrome, 81406
  Rheumatoid Arthritis, 81490
Autosomal Disorders
  Dominant Dopa-Responsive Dystonia, 81405
  Dominant Hyper-IgE Syndrome, 81405
  Dominant Progressive External Ophthalmoplegia, 81406
  Recessive Nonsyndromic Hearing Impairment, 81405
AVPR2, 81404
Bardet-Biedel Syndrome, 81404, 81406
Barth Syndrome, 81406
Bartter Syndrome, 81404, 81406-81407
BBS1, 81406
BBS10, 81404
BBS2, 81406
BCAM, 81403
BCKDHA, 81400, 81405
BCKDHB, 81205, 81406
BCR/ABL1 (t(9;22)), 81206-81208
BCS1L, 81405
Beckwith-Wiedemann Syndrome, 81401
Berardinelli-Seip Congenital Lipodystrophy, 81406
Bernard-Soulier Syndrome Type B, 81404

Analysis — *continued*
  Gene — *continued*

BEST1, 81406
Beta Hemoglobinopathies, 81443
Biotinidase Deficiency, 81404
Blau Syndrome, 81401
BLM, 81209, 81412
Bloom Syndrome, RecQ Helicase-Like (BLM), 81209, 81412, 81443
BMPR1A, 81435
BMPR2, 81405-81406
BRAF (B-Raf proto-oncogene, serine/threonine kinase), 81210, 81406
Brain Small-Vessel Disease, 81408
Branched-Chain Keto Acid Dehydrogenase E1, Beta Polypeptide (BCKDHB), 81205, 81406
Branchio-Oto-Renal (BOR) Spectrum Disorders, 81405-81406
BRCA1, 81212 *[81162, 81163, 81164, 81165, 81166]*, 81215, 81432-81433
BRCA1, BRCA2, 81212, *[81162, 81163, 81164]*
BRCA2, 81167, 81216-81217, 81432-81433
Breast Cancer, 81402, 81406, *[81307]*, *[81308], [81309]*
Breast Cancer 1 and 2, 81212, *[81162, 81163, 81164]*
Breast Cancer Related Genomic Sequence, Hereditary, 81432-81433
Brugada Syndrome, 81404, 81406, 81413-81414
Bruton's Tyrosinekinase, 81233
BSCL2, 81406, *[81448]*
BTD, 81404
BTK, 81233, 81406
C10orf2, 81404
C481F/C481R/CR481S, 81233
CACNA1A, *[81184, 81185, 81186]*
CACNB2, 81406
CALR, 81219
Canavan Disease, 81200, 81412, 81443
CAPN3, 81406
Cardiofaciocutaneous Syndrome, 81406
Cardiomyopathy
  Arrhythmogenic Right Ventricular, 81406, 81439
  Dilated Hypertrophic, 81403, 81405-81406, 81439
  Familial Hypertrophic, 81405-81407
  Hereditary, 81439
  Hypertrophic, 81439
Carnitine Palmitoyltransferase II Deficiency, 81404, 81406
Carnitine-acylcarnitine Translocase Deficiency, 81404-81405
CASQ2, 81405, 81413
CASR, 81405
Catecholaminergic Polymorphic Ventricular Tachycardia, 81405, 81408, 81413-81414
CAV3, 81404, 81413
CBFB/MYH11, 81401
CBS, 81401, 81406
CCAAT/enhancer binding protein [C/EBP], alpha, 81218
CcEe Antigens, 81403
CCHC-type Zinc Finger Nucleic Acid Binding Protein, 81187
CCND1/IGH (BCL1/IgH, t(11;14)), 81401
CCR5, 81400
CD109, *[81112]*
CD40LG, 81404
CDH1, 81406, 81432, 81435
CDH23, 81408, 81430
CDKL5, 81405-81406
CDKN2A, 81404
CDKNDA, 81445, 81455
C/EBP, 81218
CEBPA (CCAAT/enhancer binding protein [C/EBP]), 81218
CEL, 81403
CEP290, 81408

Analysis — *continued*
  Gene — *continued*

Cerebral Autosomal Dominant Arteriopathy, 81406
CFH/ARMS2, 81401
CFTR, 81220-81224, 81412
Charcot-Marie-Tooth, 81324-81326, 81403-81406, *[81448]*
CHARGE Syndrome, 81407
CHD7, 81407
Chimerism Analysis, 81267-81268
Christianson Syndrome, 81406
CHRNA4, 81405
CHRNB2, 81405
Chromosome 1p-/19q, 18q, 81402
Citrullinemia Type I, 81406
CLCN1, 81406
CLCNKB, 81406
Clear Cell Sarcoma, 81401
CLRN1, 81400, 81404, 81430
CNBP, 81187
CNGA1, 81434
CNTNAP2, 81406
Coagulation Factor
  F11 (Factor XI), 81401
  F12 (Factor XII), 81403
  F13B (Factor XIII, B polypeptide), 81400
  F2 (Factor 2), 81240, 81400
  F5 (Factor V), 81241, 81400
  F7 (Factor VII), 81400
  F8 (Factor VIII), 81403, 81406-81407
  F9 (Factor IX), 81405
Cohen Syndrome, 81407-81408
COL1A1, 81408
COL1A1/PDGFB, 81402
COL1A2, 81408
COL3A1, 81410-81411
COL4A1, 81408
COL4A3, 81408
COL4A4, 81407
COL4A5, 81407-81408
COL6A1, 81407
COL6A2, 81406-81407
COL6A3, 81407
Collagen Related Disorders, 81406-81408
Colorectal Cancer, 81210, 81237, 81292-81301 *[81288]*, 81311, 81317-81319, 81401-81402, 81404, *[81309]*
Combined Pituitary Hormone Deficiency, 81404-81405
Comparative Analysis Using Short Tandem Repeat (STR) Markers, 81265-81266
Cone-Rod Dystrophy 2, 81404
Congenital Adrenal Hyperplasia, 81402, 81405
Congenital Disorder Glycosylation 1b, 81405
Congenital Finnish Nephrosis, 81407
Congenital Hypoventilation Syndrome, 81403-81404
Congenital/Infantile Fibrosarcoma, 81401
Corneal Dystrophy, 81333
Coronary Artery Disease, 81493
Costello Syndrome, 81403-81404
Cowden Syndrome, 81321-81323
COX10, 81405
COX15, 81405
COX6B1, 81404
CPOX, 81405
CPT1A, 81406
CPT2, 81404
Craniosynostosis, 81400, 81403-81404
CRB1, 81406, 81434
CREBBP, 81406-81407
Cri-du-chat Syndrome, 81422
Crohn's Disease, 81401
Crouzon Syndrome, 81404
CRX, 81404
CSTB, 81188-81190
CTNNB1, 81403
CTRC, 81405

Analysis — *continued*
  Gene — *continued*

Cutaneous Malignant Melanoma, CDKN2A Related, 81404
CYP11B1, 81405
CYP17A1, 81405
CYP1B1, 81404
CYP21A2, 81402, 81405
CYP2C19, 81225
CYP2C9, 81227
CYP2D6, 81226
CYP3A4, *[81230]*
CYP3A5, *[81231]*
Cystathionine Beta-synthase Deficiency, 81401
Cystatin B, 81188-81190
Cystic Fibrosis, 81412, 81443
  Transmembrane Conductance Regulator (CFTR), 81220-81224
Cytochrome P450, Family 2, Subfamily C, Polypeptide 19 (CYP2C19), 81225
Cytochrome P450, Family 2, Subfamily C, Polypeptide 9 (CYP2C9), 81227
Cytochrome P450, Family 2, Subfamily D, Polypeptide 6 (CYP2D6), 81226
Cytogenomic Microarray Analysis, 81228-81229, 81405, 81407, *[81277]*
DARC, 81403
DAZ/SRY, 81403
DBT, 81405-81406
DCX, 81405
Deafness, Nonsyndromic Sensorineural, 81401
DEK/NUP214 (t(6;9)), 81401
Denys-Drash Syndrome, 81405
Dermatofibrosarcoma Protuberans, 81402
DES, 81405
Desmoid Tumors, 81403
Desmoplastic Small Round Cell Tumor, 81401
DFNB59, 81405
DGUOK, 81405
DHCR7, 81405
DHT, 82642
Diabetes Mellitus, 81401, 81404
Diamond-Blackfan Anemia, 81405
Diffuse Large B-cell Lymphoma, 81237
DiGeorge Syndrome, 81422
Dihydrotestosterone, 82642
DLAT, 81406
DLD, 81406
DM1 Protein Kinase, 81234
DMD (dystrophin), 81408, *[81161]*
DMPK, 81234, *[81239]*
DNMT3A, 81403
DPYD, 81232
Drug Metabolism, 81350
DSC2, 81406
DSG2, 81406, 81439
DSP, 81406
Duplication/Deletion Panel
  Alpha Thalassemia/Hb Bart/HbH Disease, 81257
  Aortic Dysfunction/Dilation, 81411
  APC (Adenomatous Polyposis Coli), 81203
  BRCA1/BRCA2 (Breast Cancer), 81433
  CFTR (Cystic Fibrosis Transmembrane Conductance Regulator), 81222
  FAP (Familial Adenomatosis Polyposis), 81203
  FLT3 (Fms-related tyrosine kinase 3), 81245
  Hearing Loss, 81431
  Hereditary Breast Cancer, 81433
  Hereditary Colon Cancer, 81294, 81297, 81300, 81319, 81436

Index

Analysis — Analysis

[Resequenced]
© 2019 Optum360, LLC

Angioplasty — Antigen

[Resequenced]

Index

Arthroplasty — Atomic Absorption Spectroscopy

Biopsy — continued
Colon–Sigmoid
  Endoscopic, 45305, 45331
Conjunctiva, 68100
Cornea, 65410
Duodenum, 44010
Ear
  External, 69100
  Inner, 69949
  Middle, 69799
Elbow, 24065, 24066, 24101, 29830
  Synovium, 24100
Embryo Blastomere, 89290, 89291
Endometrium, 58100, 58110, 58558
Epididymis, 54800, 54865
Esophagus
  Endoscopic, 43193, 43198, 43202, 43238-43239, 43242
  Forceps, 3150F
  Open, 43499
Eye
  Iris, Prolapsed, 66999
Eye Muscle, 67346
Eyelid, [67810]
Fallopian Tube, 49321
Foot
  Interphalangeal Joint, 28054
  Intertarsal Joint, 28050
  Metatarsophalangeal Joint, 28052
  Tarsometatarsal Joint, 28050
Forearm, Soft Tissue, 25065, 25066
Gallbladder
  Endoscopic, 43261
  Open, 47999
Gastrointestinal, Upper
  Endoscopic, 43239
Glenohumeral Joint, 23105
Gum, 41899
Hand
  Interphalangeal Joint, 26110
  Metacarpophalangeal Joint, 26105, 29900
  Synovium, 26100
Heart, 93505
Hip, 27040, 27041
  Joint, 27052
  Synovium, 29860
Ileum
  Endoscopic, 44382
Interphalangeal Joint
  Finger, 26110
  Finger Synovium, 26110
  Toe, 28054
Intertarsal Joint
  Synovial, 28050
  Toe, 28050
Intervertebral Disc, 62267
Intestines, Small, 44010, 44020, 44100
  Endoscopic, 44361, 44377, 44382, 44386
Intracranial Lesion, 61140, 61750
Kidney, 50200-50205
  Endoluminal, Renal Pelvis, 50606
  Endoscopic, 50555-50557, 50574-50576, 52354
Knee, 27323, 27324
  Synovium, 27330, 29870
Knee Joint
  Synovium, 27330, 29870
Lacrimal Gland, 68510
Lacrimal Sac, 68525
Larynx
  Endoscopy, 31510, 31535, 31536, 31576
Leg
  Lower, 27613, 27614
  Upper, 27323, 27324
Lip, 40490
Liver, 47000, 47001, 47100, 47700
Lung
  Needle, 32405
  Thoracoscopy, 32604-32608
  Thoracotomy, 32096-32097
Lymph Nodes, 38500-38530, 38570
  Injection Procedure
    Identification of Sentinel Node, 38792
    Radioactive Tracer, 38792

Biopsy — continued
Lymph Nodes — continued
  Laparoscopic, 38570-38572
  Mediastinum, 39000-39010, 39401-39402
  Needle, 38505
  Open, 38500, 38510-38530
    Superficial, 38500
  Para-aortic, 57109, 57112, 57531, 58210, 58548
  Prostate, 55812, 55842, 55862
Mediastinum, 39401-39402
  Needle, 39401
Metacarpophalangeal Joint, 26105, 29900
Metatarsophalangeal Joint, 28052
Mouth, 40808, 41108
Muscle, 20200-20206
Nail, 11755
Nasopharynx, 42804, 42806
Neck, 21550
Needle
  Abdomen
    Mass, 49180
Nerve, 64795
Nose
  Endoscopic, 31237
  Intranasal, 30100
Nucleus Pulposus, 62267
Omentum, 49321
Oocyte Polar Body, 89290, 89291
Orbit
  Exploration, 67400, 67450
  Fine Needle Aspiration, 67415
Oropharynx, 42800
Ovary, 49321, 58900
Palate, 42100
Pancreas, 48100-48102
Parathyroid Gland, 60699
Paravertebral Tissue, 62267
Pelvis, 27040, 27041
Penis, 54100
  Cutaneous, 54100
  Deep Structures, 54105
Percutaneous Needle
  Spinal Cord, 62269
Pericardium, 32604
Perineum, 56605, 56606
Periprostatic Tissue, 54699, 55899
Perirenal Tissue, 53899
Peritoneum
  Endoscopic, 49321
Periurethral Tissue, 53899
Perivesical Tissue, 53899
Pharynx, 42800-42806
Pineal Gland, 60699
Pituitary Gland, 60699
Pleura, 32098, 32400, 32609
  Needle, 32400
  Thoracoscopy, 32609
  Thoracotomy, 32098
Prostate, 55700, 55705, 55706
  Lymph Nodes, 55812, 55842, 55862
  mRNA Gene Expression Profiling, 0011M
  with Fluorescence Spectroscopy, 0443T
Rectum, 45100, 45305, 45331
Renal Pelvis, 50606
Retroperitoneal Area, 49010, 49180
Sacroiliac Joint, 27050
Salivary Gland, 42400, 42405
Seminal Vesicles, 54699, 55899
Shoulder
  Deep, 23066
  Glenohumeral Joint, 23105
  Joint, 23100-23101
  Soft Tissue, 23065
  Sternoclavicular Joint, 23106
  Synovium, 29805
Sinus
  Sphenoid, 31050, 31051
Skin Lesion, 11102-11107
Skull Base, 61575-61576
Spinal Cord, 63275-63290
  Needle, 62269
  Percutaneous, 62269
  Transoral, 61575-61576
Spleen, 38999

Biopsy — continued
Stomach, 43605
Tarsometatarsal Joint
  Synovial, 28050
Temporomandibular Joint, 29800
Testis, 54500, 54505
Thigh, 27323-27324
Thorax, 21550
Throat, 42800, 42804-42806
Thymus, 38999, 60699
Thyroid, 60100
Thyroid Gland, 60699
Tongue, 41100, 41105
Tonsils (and Adenoids), 42999
Transcatheter, 37200
Tunica Vaginalis, 54699, 55899
Ureter, 52354
  Endoluminal, 50606
  Endoscopic, 50955-50957, 50974-50976
  Open, 53899
Urethra, 52204, 52250, 52354, 53200
Uterus
  Endometrial, 58100-58110
  Endoscopic, 58558
Uvula, 42100
Vagina, 57100, 57105, 57421
  Endocervical, 57454
Vein, 37200
  Radiological Supervision and Interpretation, 75970
Vertebral Body, 20250-20251
Vulva, 56605, 56606, 56821
with Arthrotomy
  Acromioclavicular Joint, 23101
  Glenohumeral Joint, 23100, 23105
  Sternoclavicular Joint, 23101, 23106
with Cystourethroscopy, 52354
Wrist, 25065-25066, 25100-25101, 29840
Biopsy, Skin
  See Skin, Biopsy
Biostatistics
  See Biometry
Biosterol
  See Vitamin, A
BIOTHRAX, 90581
Biotinidase, 82261
BiPAP, 94660
Birthing Room
  Attendance at Delivery, 99464
  Newborn Care, 99460, 99463-99465
  Resuscitation, 99465
Bischof Procedure
  Laminectomy, Surgical, 63170, 63172
Bismuth, 83015
Bizzozero's Corpuscle/Cell
  See Blood, Platelet
BKA, 27598, 27880-27882
Bladder
  Abscess
    Incision and Drainage, 51080
  Anastomosis
    Ureter to Bladder, 50780, 50782
    with Intestine, 51960
  Anesthesia, 00864, 00870, 00912
  Aspiration, 51100-51102
  Biopsy, 52204
    by Cystourethroscopy, 52204
  Catheterization, 51045, 51102, 51701-51703
  Change Tube, 51705, 51710
  Chemodenervation, 52287
  Creation/Stoma, 51980
  Cuff, 50234-50236, 50650
  Cyst
    Urachal
      Excision, 51500
  Cystometrogram (CMG), 51725-51729
  Cystostomy Tube, 51705-51710
  Cystourethroscopy, 52000
    Biopsy, 52204, 52224, 52250, 52354
    Catheterization, 52005, 52010
    Destruction, 52214, 52224, 52400
    Dilation, 52260, 52265
      Urethra, 52281
    Diverticulum, 52305
    Evacuation
      Clot, 52001

Bladder — continued
Cystourethroscopy — continued
  Excision
    Tumor, 52234-52240, 52355
  Exploration, 52351
  Fulguration, 52214-52224, 52234-52235, 52240, 52250, 52400
  Injection, 52283
  Insertion of Stent, 52332, 52334
  Lithotripsy, 52353
  Radiotracer, 52250
  Removal
    Calculus, 52310, 52315, 52352
    Foreign Body, 52310, 52315
  Sphincter Surgery, 52277
  Tumor
    Excision, 52355
  Ureter Surgery, 52290, 52300
  Urethral Syndrome, 52285
  with Urethrotomy, 52270-52276
Destruction
  Endoscopic, 52214-52240, 52354
Dilation
  Ureter, 52260, 52265
Diverticulum
  Excision, 51525
  Incision, 52305
  Resection, 52305
Endoscopy
  See Cystourethroscopy
Excision
  Partial, 51550-51565
  Total, 51570, 51580, 51590-51597
    with Nodes, 51575, 51585, 51595
  Transurethral of Neck, 52640
  Tumor, 52234-52240
Fulguration, 52214, 52250, 52400
  Tumor(s), 52224, 52234-52235, 52240
Incision
  Catheter or Stent, 51045
  with
    Cryosurgery, 51030
    Destruction, 51020, 51030
    Fulguration, 51020
    Insertion Radioactive, 51020
    Radiotracer, 51020
Incision and Drainage, 51040
Injection
  Radiologic, 51600-51610
Insertion
  Stent, 51045, 52282, 52334
Instillation
  Anticarcinogenics, 51720
  Drugs, 51720
  Interstitial Cystitis, 52260-52265
  with Cystourethroscopy, 52005, 52010
Irrigation, 51700, 52005, 52010
  Clot, 52001
Laparoscopy, 51999
Lesion
  Destruction, 51030
Neck
  Endoscopy
    Injection of Implant Material, 51715
  Excision, 51520
  Remodeling for Incontinence, 53860
Nuclear Medicine
  Residual Study, 78730
Radiotracer, 51020, 52250
Reconstruction
  Radiofrequency Micro-Remodeling, 53860
  with Intestines, 51960
  with Urethra, 51800, 51820
Removal
  Calculus, 51050, 51065, 52310, 52315, 52352
  Foreign Body, 52310, 52315
  Litholapaxy, 52317-52318
  Lithotripsy, 51065, 52353
  Urethral Stent, 52310, 52315
Repair
  Diverticulum, 52305
  Exstrophy, 51940

Blood Vessel(s) — *continued*
Great
  Suture, 33320-33322
Harvest
  Endoscopic, 33508
  Lower Extremity Vein, 35572
  Upper Extremity Artery, 35600
  Upper Extremity Vein, 35500
Kidney
  Repair, 50100
Repair
  Abdomen, 35221, 35251, 35281
    See Aneurysm Repair; Fistula, Re-
      pair
    with Composite Graft, 35681-
      35683
    with Other Graft, 35281
    with Vein Graft, 35251
  Aneurysm, 61705-61710
  Aorta, 33320-33322
  Arteriovenous Malformation, 61680-
    61692, 61705-61710, 63250-
    63252
  Chest, 35211, 35216
    with Composite Graft, 35681-
      35683
    with Other Graft, 35271, 35276
    with Vein Graft, 35241, 35246
  Direct, 35201-35226
  Finger, 35207
  Graft Defect, 35870
  Great Vessels, 33320-33322
  Hand, 35207
  Intraabdominal, 35221, 35251, 35281
  Intrathoracic, 35211, 35216, 35241,
    35246, 35271, 35276
  Kidney, 50100
  Lower Extremity, 35226, 35256, 35286
    with Composite Graft, 35681-
      35683
    with Other Graft, 35281
    with Vein Graft, 35256
  Neck, 35201
    with Composite Graft, 35681-
      35683
    with Other Graft, 35261
    with Vein Graft, 35231
  Upper Extremity, 35206, 35236, 35266
    with Composite Graft, 35681-
      35683
    with Other Graft, 35266
    with Vein Graft, 35236
Shunt Creation
  Direct, 36821
  Thomas Shunt, 36835
  with Bypass Graft, 35686
  with Graft, 36825, 36830
  with Transposition, 36818-36820
Shunt Revision
  with Graft, 36832
Suture Repair, Great Vessels, 33320-33322
Bloom Syndrome
  Chromosome Analysis, 88245
  Gene Analysis, 81209
  Genomic Sequencing Analysis, 81412, 81443
Blot Test, Ink
  See Inkblot Test
Blotting, Western
  See Western Blot
Blount Osteotomy, 27455, 27475-27485
Blow–Out Fracture
  Orbital Floor, 21385-21395
Blue, Dome Cyst
  See Breast, Cyst
BMAC (Breath Methylated Alkane Contour), 0085T
BMPR1A, 81435
BMPR2, 81405-81406
BMT, 38240, 38241, 38242
Boarding Home Care, 99324-99337
Bodies, Acetone
  See Acetone Body
Bodies, Barr
  See Barr Bodies
Bodies, Carotid
  See Carotid Body

Bodies, Ciliary
  See Ciliary Body
Bodies, Heinz
  See Heinz Bodies
Bodies, Inclusion
  See Inclusion Bodies
Bodies, Ketone
  See Ketone Bodies
Body Cast
  Halo, 29000
  Removal, 29700, 29710
  Repair, 29720
  Risser Jacket, 29010, 29015
  Upper Body and One Leg, 29044
  Upper Body Only, 29035
  Upper Body with Head, 29040
  Upper Body with Legs, 29046
Body Fluid
  Crystal Identification, 89060
Body of Vertebra
  See Vertebral Body
Body Section
  X–ray, 76100
    Motion, 76101, 76102
Body System, Neurologic
  See Nervous System
BOH, 93600
Bohler Procedure, 28405
Bohler Splinting, 29515
Boil
  See Furuncle
Boil, Vulva
  See Abscess, Vulva
Bone
  See Specific Bone
Ablation
  Tumor, 20982-20983
Biopsy, 20220-20245, 20250-20251
  with Vertebroplasty, 22510-22512
Conduction Hearing Device
  Implantation, 69710
    Replacement, 69710
  Removal
    Repair, 69711
CT Scan
  Density Study, 77078
Cyst
  Drainage, 20615
  Injection, 20615
Debridement, 11044 *[11047]*
Density Study
  Appendicular Skeleton, 77081
  Axial Skeleton, 77078, 77080
  Pulse-echo Ultrasound, 0508T
  Ultrasound, 76977
  Vertebral Fracture Assessment, *[77085,*
    77086]
Dual Energy X–ray
  Absorptiometry, 77080-77081, *[77085]*
Excision
  Epiphyseal Bar, 20150
  Facial Bones, 21026
  Mandible, 21025
Fixation
  Caliper, 20660
  Cranial Tong, 20660
  External, 20690
  Halo, 20661-20663, 21100
  Interdental, 21110
  Multiplane, 20692
  Pin
    Wire, 20650
  Skeletal
    Humeral Epicondyle
      Percutaneous, 24566
  Stereotactic Frame, 20660
  Uniplane, 20690
Fracture
  Hyoid
    See Hyoid Bone
  Osteoporosis Screening, 5015F
Graft
  Allograft
    Morselized, 20930
    Structural, 20931
    Any Donor Area, 20900-20902

Bone — *continued*
Graft — *continued*
  Augmentation
    Mandibular Body, 21127
  Autograft, 20936
    Morselized, 20937
    Structural, 20932, 20938
  Calcaneal Fracture, 28420
  Clavicle, 23485
  Craniofacial Separation, 21436
  Cranium, 61316, 61559, 62146-62148
  Femur, 27170, 27177, 27470
  Fracture
    Orbit, 21408
  Harvesting, 20900, 20902
  Knee Drilling, 29885
  Malar Area, 21210, 21366
  Mandible, 21127, 21194, 21215
  Mandibular Ramus, 21194
  Maxilla, 21210
  Metacarpal, Nonunion, 26546
  Metatarsal Nonunion, 28322
  Microvascular Anastomosis
    Fibula, 20955
    Iliac Crest, 20956
    Metatarsal Bone, 20957
    Other, 20962
    Rib, 20962
  Midface, 21145-21147, 21150-21151,
    21154-21155, 21159-21160,
    21182-21184, 21188
  Nasal Area, 21210
  Nasomaxillary Complex Fracture, 21348
  Open Treatment
    Craniofacial Separation, 21436
  Orbit
    Blowout Fracture, 21395
    Cleft Palate, 42210
    Fracture, 21408
    Hypertelorism, 21260
    Reconstruction, 21182-21184,
      21256
    Repositioning, 21267
  Osteocutaneous Flap, 20969-20973
  Patella, 27599
  Reconstruction
    Mandibular Ramis, 21194
    Midface, 21145-21160
  Skull, 61316
    Excision, 62148
  Spine Surgery
    Allograft
      Morselized, 20930
      Structural, 20931
    Autograft
      Local, 20936
      Morselized, 20937
      Structural, 20938
      with Arthrodesis, Presacral Inter-
        body Technique, 22586,
        22899
  Toe to Hand Transfer, 26551
  Ulna, 25830
  Vascular Pedicle, 25430
  Vertebra, 0222T
    Cervical, 0219T, 63051
    Lumbar, 0221T
    Thoracic, 0220T
  Wrist, 25805, 25810, 25825
Healing
  Electrical Stimulation
    Invasive, 20975
    Noninvasive, 20974
  Ultrasound Stimulation, 20979
Insertion
  Needle, 36680
  Osseointegrated Implant
    for External Speech Proces-
      sor/Cochlear Stimulator,
      69714-69718
Marrow
  Aspiration, 20939, 38220, 38222
  Biopsy, 38221-38222
  CAR-T Therapy, 0537T-0540T
    Administration, 0540T
    Harvesting, 0537T

Bone — *continued*
Marrow — *continued*
  CAR-T Therapy — *continued*
    Preparation, 0538T-0539T
  Cell Preparation, 38207-38215
  Cell Therapy, 0263T-0265T
  Cytogenic Testing, 3155F
  Harvesting, 38230, 38232
    Allogeneic, 38230
    Autologous, 38232
    Intramuscular Therapy, 0263T,
      0265T
  Magnetic Resonance Imaging (MRI),
    77084
  Nuclear Medicine
    Imaging, 78102-78104
  Smear, 85097
  Surgical Pathology, 88305
  T–Cell
    Transplantation, 38240, 38241,
      38242
  Trocar Biopsy, 38221
Nuclear Medicine
  Density Study, 78350, 78351
  Imaging, 78300-78315
  SPECT, 78803
  Unlisted Services and Procedures, 78399
Osseous Survey, 77074-77075
Osteoporosis
  Pharmacologic Therapy, 4005F
Plate
  Mandible, 21244
Protein, 83937
Pulse-echo Ultrasound, 0508T
Removal
  Fixation Device, 20670, 20680
Replacement
  Osseointegrated Implant
    for External Speech Proces-
      sor/Cochlear Stimulator,
      69717-69718
Spur, 28119
Wedge Reversal
  Osteotomy, 21122
X–ray
  Age Study, 77072
  Dual Energy Absorptiometry (DEXA),
    77080-77081
  Joint Stress, 77071
  Length Study, 77073
  Osseous Survey, 77074-77077
Bone 4–Carboxyglutamic Protein
  See Osteocalcin
Bone, Carpal
  See Carpal Bone
Bone, Cheek
  See Cheekbone
Bone, Facial
  See Facial Bone
Bone, Hyoid
  See Hyoid Bone
Bone Infection
  See Osteomyelitis
Bone Material, Quality Testing, 0547T
Bone, Metatarsal
  See Metatarsal
Bone, Nasal
  See Nasal Bone
Bone, Navicular
  See Navicular
Bone, Scan
  See Bone, Nuclear Medicine; Nuclear Medicine
Bone, Semilunar
  See Lunate
Bone, Sesamoid
  See Sesamoid Bone
Bone, Tarsal
  See Ankle Bone
Bone, Temporal
  See Temporal, Bone
BOOSTRIX, 90715
Bordetella
  Antibody, 86615
  Antigen Detection
    Direct Fluorescent Antibody, 87265
Borrelia (relapsing fever), 86619

Cannulization
See Catheterization
Arteriovenous (AV), 36810, 36815, 36901-36903
Chemotherapy, 36823
Declotting, 36593, 36860, 36861
Dialysis Circuit, 36901-36903
ECMO
Insertion, 33951-33956
Isolated with Chemotherapy Perfusion, 36823
Removal, [33965, 33966, 33969, 33984, 33985, 33986]
Repositioning, 33957-33959 [33962, 33963, 33964]
External
Declotting, 36860-36861
Vas Deferens, 55200
Vein to Vein, 36800
Canthocystostomy
See Conjunctivorhinostomy
Canthopexy
Lateral, 21282
Medial, 21280
Canthoplasty, 67950
Canthorrhaphy, 67880, 67882
Canthotomy, 67715
Canthus
Reconstruction, 67950
Cap, Cervical, 57170
CAPD, 90945, 90947
CAPN3, 81406
Capsule
See Capsulodesis
Ankle, 27612, 27630
Biopsy of Intestine, 44100
Elbow
Arthrotomy, 24006
Excision, 24006
Endoscopy, 0355T, 91110-91111
Eye, 66830
Finger, 26160, 26520, 26525
Foot, 28090, 28260-28264
Heyman, 58346
Hip, 27036
Injection, 27515
Interphalangeal Joint
Foot, 28272
Hand, 26525
Knee, 27435
Leg, 27630
Metacarpophalangeal Joint
Excision, 26160
Incision, 26520
Metatarsophalangeal Joint Release
with Implant, 28291
without Implant, 28289
Shoulder, Incision, 23020
Tenon's, 67515
Toe, 28270, 28272
Wrist
Excision, 25320
Capsulectomy
Breast, Periprosthetic, 19371
Elbow, 24149
Finger, 26160, 26525
Foot, 28090
Hand, 26160, 26520
Hip, 27036
Knee, 27347
Capsulodesis
Blatt, 25320
Metacarpophalangeal Joint, 26516-26518
Capsulorrhaphy
Ankle, 27630
Anterior, 23450-23462
Bankart Procedure, 23455
Bristow Procedure, 23460
Glenohumeral Joint, 23465-23466
Magnuson Type Procedure, 23450
Multi–Directional Instability, 23466
Posterior, 23465
Putti-Platt Procedure, 23450
Shoulder, Arthroscopic, 29806
Thermal, 29999
Wrist, 25320

Capsulotomy
Breast
Periprosthetic, 19370
Eye, 66830
Foot, 28260-28262, 28264
Hip with Release, Flexor Muscles, 27036
Interphalangeal Joint, 28272
Knee, 27435
Leg, 27630
Metacarpophalangeal Joint, 26520
Metatarsophalangeal Joint, 28270
Shoulder, 23020
Toe, 28270, 28272
Wrist, 25085, 25320
Captopril, 80416, 80417
Car Seat Testing, 94780-94781
Car Seat/Bed Neonatal Testing, 94780-94781
Carbamazepine
Assay, 80156-80157
Carbazepin
See Carbamazepine
Carbinol
See Methanol
Carbohydrate Deficient Transferin, 82373
Carbon Dioxide
Blood or Urine, 82374, 82803
Carboxycathepsin
See Angiotensin Converting Enzyme (ACE)
Carboxyhemoglobin, 82375-82376, 88740
Carbuncle
Incision and Drainage, 10060, 10061
Carcinoembryonal Antigen
See Antigen, Carcinoembryonic
Carcinoembryonic Antigen, 82378
Cardiac Arrhythmia, Tachycardia
See Tachycardia
Cardiac Atria
See Atria
Cardiac Catheterization
Angiography
Bypass Graft(s), 93455, 93457, 93459, 93461
Congenital Heart, 93563-93564
Coronary, 93454-93461, 93563, 93571
Left Atrium, 93565
Left Ventricle, 93565
Pulmonary, 93568
Right Atrium, 93566
Right Ventricle, 93566
Combined Left and Right Heart, 93531-93533
Congenital Anomalies, 93530-93533
with Ventriculography, 93453, 93460-93461
Flow Directed, 93503
Flow Measurement, 93571-93572
for Biopsy, 93505
for Congenital Anomalies
Right and Retrograde Left, 93531
Transseptal and Retrograde Left, 93532, 93533
for Dilution Studies, 93561, 93562
for Measurement of O2 Cardiac Output, 93451
for Opacification
Bypass Grafts, 93564
For Supravalvular Aortography, 93567
Imaging, 93452-93461, 93563-93568
Injection, 93452-93461, 93563-93568
Insertion Swan-Ganz, 93503
Left Heart, 93452, 93458-93459
By Transseptal Puncture, 93462
for Transapical Puncture, 93462
with Ventriculography, 93452, 93458-93459, 93565
Right Heart, 93451, 93456-93457
for Congenital Anomalies, 93530
Cardiac Contractility Modulation System, 0408T-0418T
Cardiac Electroversion
See Cardioversion
Cardiac Event Recorder (wearable), 93224-93272
Cardiac Magnetic Resonance Imaging (CMRI)
Morphology and Function, 75557, 75559, 75561, 75563
Stress Imaging, 75559, 75563
Velocity Flow Mapping, 75565
with Contrast, 75561-75563

Cardiac Magnetic Resonance Imaging (CMRI) — *continued*
without Contrast, 75557-75559
Cardiac Massage
Thoracotomy, 32160
Cardiac Output Measurement
by Indicator Dilution, 93561, 93562
Cardiac Pacemaker
See Heart, Pacemaker
Cardiac Rehabilitation, 93797, 93798
Cardiac Rhythm Monitor System
Analysis, 93285, 93291-93292, 93297-93298
Implantation, 93285
Removal, 33286
Cardiac Septal Defect
See Septal Defect
Cardiac Stimulator, Wireless *See* **Wireless Cardiac Stimulator**
Cardiac Transplantation
See Heart, Transplantation
Cardiectomy
Donor, 33930, 33940
Cardio Defibrillator (Implantable)
Transvenous Device
Insertion
Electrode, 33216-33217
Pulse Generator, 33240, [33230, 33231]
System, 33249
Interrogation Device Evaluation, 93289
Periprocedural, 93287
Remote, 93295-93296
Programming Device Evaluation, 93282-93284
Relocation
Skin Pocket, 33223
Removal
Electrode, 33243-33244
Pulse Generator, 33241, [33262, 33263, 33264]
Repair Electrode, 33218, 33220
Reposition Electrode, 33215, 33226
Wearable, 93745
Data Analysis, 93292
Cardioassist, 92970, 92971
Cardio-Fascio-Cutaneous Syndrome, 81442
Cardiolipin Antibody, 86147
Cardiology
Diagnostic
Atrial Electrogram
Esophageal Recording, 93615, 93616
Bioimpedance Analysis, 93701
Cardiac Rhythm Monitor System
Data Analysis, 93291, 93297-93298
Evaluation and Programming, 93285
Echocardiography
Doppler, 93303-93321, 93662
Intracardiac, 93662
Myocardial Contrast Perfusion, 0439T
Strain Imaging, [93356]
Transesophageal, 93318
Transthoracic, 93303-93317, 93350
Electrocardiogram
64 Leads or Greater, 93799
Evaluation, 93000, 93010, 93660
Microvolt T–wave, Alternans, 93025
Patient-Activated, 93268-93272
Recording, 93000-93005, 93224-93229
Rhythm, 93040-93042
Tracing, 93005
Transmission, 93268, 93271
Electrophysiologic
Follow–Up Study, 93624
with Myocardial Contrast Perfusion, 0439T
Endoluminal Imaging, [92978, 92979]
Ergonovine Provocation Test, 93024
Evaluation
Heart Device, 93640
Heart
Stimulation and Pacing, 93623

Cardiology — *continued*
Diagnostic — *continued*
Implantable Defibrillator
Data Analysis, 93289, 93295-93296
Evaluation of Programming, 93282-93284, 93287, 93289, 93292, 93295-93296, 93640-93642
Implantable Monitor
Data Analysis, 93290, 93297-93298
Intracardiac Pacing and Mapping, 93631
3–D Mapping, 93613, 93654
Follow–up Study, 93624
Stimulation and Pacing, 93623
Intracardiac Pacing and Recording
Arrhythmia Induction, 93618, 93620-93622, 93624, 93640-93642, 93653-93656
Bundle of His, 93600, 93619-93620, 93653-93654, 93656
Comprehensive, 93619-93622
Intra–Atrial, 93602, 93610, 93616, 93656
Left Ventricle, 93654
Right Ventricle, 93603, 93653, 93656
Tachycardia Sites, 93609
Ventricular, 93612
M Mode and Real Time, 93307-93321
Pacemaker Testing, 93642
Antitachycardia System, 93724
Data Analysis, 93288, 93293-93294
Dual Chamber, 93280, 93288, 93293-93294
Evaluation of Device Programming, 93279-93281, 93286, 93288, 93290, 93293-93294, 93296
Leads, 93641
Single Chamber, 93279, 93288, 93294
Perfusion Imaging, 78451-78454, 78491-78492
Strain Imaging, [93356]
Stress Tests
Cardiovascular, 93015-93018
Drug Induced, 93024
MUGA (Multiple Gated Acquisition), 78483
Temperature Gradient Studies, 93740
Tilt Table Evaluation, 93660
Vectorcardiogram
Evaluation, 93799
Tracing, 93799
Venous Pressure Determination, 93784, 93786, 93788, 93790
Therapeutic
Ablation, 93650, 93653-93656
Cardioassist, 92970, 92971
Cardiopulmonary Resuscitation, 92950
Cardioversion, 92960, 92961
Endoluminal Imaging, [92978, 92979]
Implantable Defibrillator
Data Analysis, 93289, 93295-93296
Evaluation of Device Programming, 93282-93284, 93287, 93289, 93292, 93295-93296
Initial Set-up and Programming, 93745
Pacing
Transcutaneous, Temporary, 92953
Rehabilitation, 93668, 93797-93798
Thrombolysis
Coronary Vessel, [92975, 92977]
Thrombolysis, Coronary, [92977]
Valvuloplasty
Open, 33390-33391
Percutaneous, 92986, 92990
Cardiomyotomy
See Esophagomyotomy
Cardioplasty, 43320
Cardioplegia, 33999
Cardiopulmonary Bypass
Aortic Valve Replacement, Transcatheter, 33367-33369

[Resequenced]   CPT © 2019 American Medical Association. All Rights Reserved.   © 2019 Optum360, LLC

Cardiopulmonary Bypass — *continued*
Lung Transplant with
Double, 32854
Single, 32852
with Prosthetic Valve Repair, 33496
Cardiopulmonary Exercise Testing, 94621
Cardiopulmonary Resuscitation, 92950
Cardiotomy, 33310, 33315
Cardiovascular Physiologic Monitor System
Analysis, 93290, 93297-93298
Cardiovascular Stress Test
See Exercise Stress Tests
Cardioversion, 92960, 92961
Care, Custodial
See Nursing Facility Services
Care, Intensive
See Intensive Care
Care Management, Psychiatric, 99492-99494, *[99484]*
Care, Neonatal Intensive
See Intensive Care, Neonatal
Care Plan Oversight Services
Extracorporeal Liver Assist System, 0405T
Home Health Agency Care, 99374, 99375
Hospice, 99377, 99378
Nursing Facility, 99379, 99380
Care Planning, Cognitive Impairment, 99483
Care, Self
See Self Care
Care-giver Focused Assessment, 96161
Carneous Mole
See Abortion
Carnitine Total and Free, 82379
Carotene, 82380
Carotid Artery
Aneurysm Repair
Vascular Malformation or Carotid Cavernous Fistula, 61710
Baroreflex Activation Device
Implantation/Replantation, 0266T-0268T
Interrogation Evaluation, 0272T-0273T
Revision/Removal, 0269T-0271T
Excision, 60605
Ligation, 37600-37606
Stenosis Imaging, 3100F
Stent, Transcatheter Placement, 0075T-0076T
Carotid Body
Lesion
Carotid Artery, 60605
Excision, 60600
Carotid Pulse Tracing
with ECG Lead, 93799
Carotid Sinus Baroreflex Activation Device
Implantation, 0266T-0268T
Interrogation Device Evaluation, 0272T, 0273T
Removal, 0269T-0271T
Replacement, 0266T-0268T
Carpal Bone
Arthroplasty
with Implant, 25441-25446
Cyst
Excision, 25130-25136
Dislocation
Closed Treatment, 25690
Open Treatment, 25695
Excision, 25210, 25215
Partial, 25145
Fracture, 25622-25628
Closed Treatment, 25622, 25630, 25635
Open Treatment, 25628, 25645
with Manipulation, 25624, 25635
without Manipulation, 25630
Incision and Drainage, 26034
Insertion
Vascular Pedicle, 25430
Ligament Release, 29848
Navicular (Scaphoid)
Fracture, 25622-25624, 25628, 25630-25635, 25645
Nonunion, 25440
Osteoplasty, 25394
Prosthetic Replacement, 25443-25446
Repair, 25431-25440
Nonunion, 25431, 25440
with Fixation, 25628
with Styloidectomy, 25440

Carpal Bone — *continued*
Sequestrectomy, 25145
Tumor
Excision, 25130-25136
Carpal Tunnel
Injection
Therapeutic, 20526
Carpal Tunnel Syndrome
Decompression, 64721
Arthroscopy, 29848
Injection, 20526
Median Nerve Neuroplasty, 64721
Carpals
Incision and Drainage, 25035
Carpectomy, 25210, 25215
Carpometacarpal Joint
Arthrodesis
Fingers, 26843-26844
Hand, 26843-26844
Thumb, 26841-26844
Wrist, 25800-25810
Arthrotomy, 26070, 26100
Biopsy
Synovium, 26100
Dislocation
Closed Treatment, 26670
with Manipulation, 26675, 26676
Open Treatment, 26685, 26686
Drainage, 26070
Exploration, 26070
Fusion
Hand, 26843, 26844
Thumb, 26841, 26842
Magnetic Resonance Imaging, 73221-73225
Removal
Foreign Body, 26070
Repair, 25447
Synovectomy, 26130
Carpue's Operation, 30400
CAR-T Therapy, 0537T-0540T
Administration, 0540T
Harvesting, 0537T
Preparation, 0538T-0539T
Cartilage, Arytenoid
See Arytenoid
Cartilage, Ear
See Ear Cartilage
Cartilage Graft
Costochondral, 20910
Ear to Face, 21235
Harvesting, 20910, 20912
Mandibular Condyle Reconstruction, 21247
Nasal Septum, 20912
Rib to Face, 21230
Zygomatic Arch Reconstruction, 21255
Cartilaginous Exostosis
See Exostosis
Case Management Services
Anticoagulation Management, 93792-93793
Online, 98970-98972, 99446-99449
Referral, 99451-99452
Team Conferences, 99366-99368
Telephone Calls
Consult Physician, 99446-99449
Nonphysician, 98966-98968
Physician, 99441-99443
CASQ2, 81405
CASR, 81405
Cast
See Brace; Splint
Body
Halo, 29000
Risser Jacket, 29010, 29015
Upper Body and Head, 29040
Upper Body and Legs, 29046
Upper Body and One Leg, 29044
Upper Body Only, 29035
Clubfoot, 29450, 29750
Cylinder, 29365
Figure-of-Eight, 29049
Finger, 29086
Gauntlet, 29085, 29750
Hand, 29085
Hip, 29305, 29325
Leg
Rigid Total Contact, 29445

Cast — *continued*
Long Arm, 29065
Long Leg, 29345, 29355, 29365, 29450
Long Leg Brace, 29358
Minerva, 29040
Patellar Tendon Bearing (PTB), 29435
Removal, 29700-29710
Repair, 29720
Short Arm, 29075
Short Leg, 29405-29435, 29450
Shoulder, 29049-29058
Spica, 29055, 29305, 29325, 29720
Unlisted Services and Procedures, 29799
Velpeau, 29058
Walking, 29355, 29425
Revision, 29440
Wedging, 29740, 29750
Windowing, 29730
Wrist, 29085
Casting
Unlisted Services and Procedures, 29799
Castration
See Orchiectomy
Castration, Female
See Oophorectomy
CAT Scan
See CT Scan
Cataract
Dilated Fundus Evaluation Prior to Surgery, 2020F
Discission, 66820-66821
Excision, 66830
Incision, 66820-66821
Laser, 66821
Stab Incision, 66820
Presurgical Measurements, 3073F
Removal
Extraction
Extracapsular, 66982, 66984
Intracapsular, 66983
Catecholamines, 80424, 82382-82384
Blood, 82383
Fractionated, 82384
Pheochromocytoma Panel, 80424
Urine, 82382
Cathepsin-D, 82387
Catheter
See Cannulization; Venipuncture
Aspiration
Nasotracheal, 31720
Tracheobronchial, 31725
Biopsy, Transcatheter, 37200
Bladder, 51701-51703
Irrigation, 51700
Blood Specimen Collection, 36592, 37799
Breast
for Interstitial Radioelement Application, 19296-19298
Bronchus for Intracavitary Radioelement Application, 31643
Central Venous
Repair, 36575
Replacement, 36580, 36581, 36584
Repositioning, 36597
Cystourethroscopy, 52320-52353 *[52356]*
Declotting, 36593, 36861
Drainage
Biliary, 47533-47537
Peritoneal, 49406-49407
Pleural, 32556-32557
Retroperitoneal, 49406-49407
Spinal, 62272
Ventricular, 62162, 62164
Electrode Array, 63650
Embolectomy, 34001, 34051, 34101-34111, 34151, 34201, 34203
Embolization, 61624, 61626
Peritoneal, 49423
Endovenous Ablation, 0524T
Enteral Alimentation, 44015
Exchange
Drainage, 49423
Nephrostomy, *[50435]*
Peritoneal, 49423
Flow Directed, 93503
Home Visit Catheter Care, 99507

Catheter — *continued*
Infusion
Brachial Plexus, 64416
Femoral Nerve, 64448
Lumbar Plexus, 64449
Saline, 58340
Sciatic Nerve, 64446
Vertebral, 62324-62327
Installation
Fibrinolysis, 32561-32562
Pleurodesis, 32560
Intracatheter
Irrigation, 99507
Obstruction Clearance, 36596
Intraperitoneal
Tunneled
Laparoscopic, 49324
Open, 49421
Percutaneous, 49418-49419
Pericatheter
Obstruction Clearance, 36595
Placement
Brain
Stereotactic, 64999
Breast
for Interstitial Radioelement Placement, 19296-19298, 20555
Bronchus
for Intracavitary Radioelement Placement, 31643
Head and/or Neck, 41019
Muscle and/or Soft Tissue, 20555
Nephrostomy, Percutaneous, *[50432]*
Nephroureteral, *[50433, 50434]*
Radiation Source, 61770
Stent, 33621, 61635
Wireless Physiologic Sensor, 34701-34708
Removal
Central Venous, 36589
Foreign Body, 37197
Nephroureteral, Accessible, 50387
Obstruction, 36595-36596
Peritoneum, 49422
Pleural catheter, 32552
Spinal Cord, 62355
Repair
Central Venous, 36575
Intraperitoneal, 49325
Replacement
Central Venous, 36580-36581, 36584
Nephroureteral, Accessible, 50387
Shunt System, 62230
Subarachnoid, 62194
Subdural, 62194
Ventricular, 62225
Repositioning, 36597
Thrombectomy, 34001, 34051, 34101-34111, 34151, 34201, 34203, 34401, 34421, 34451, 61645
Transcatheter Therapy, 36640, 36660, 62320-62327, *[37211, 37212, 37213, 37214]*
Ureteral
Manometric Studies, 50396, 50686
Ureterography, 50684
Ureteropyelography, 50684
Catheterization
Abdomen, 49324, 49418-49419, 49421
Abdominal Artery, 36245-36248
Aorta, 36160-36215
Arterial
Aorta, 36200, 36221
Translumbar, 36160
Arteriovenous Shunt
Dialysis Circuit, 36901-36903
Cutdown, 36625
Intracatheter/Needle, 36100-36140
Percutaneous, 36620
Selective Placement, 36215-36218, 36222-36252
Superselective Placement, 36253-36254
Arteriovenous Shunt
Dialysis Circuit, 36901-36903
Bile Duct
Change, 47535-47536
Percutaneous, 47533-47534

Circumcision — *continued*
  Repair, 54163
  Surgical Excision
    28 days or less, 54160
    Older than 28 days, 54161
    with Clamp or Other Device, 54150
Cisternal Puncture, 61050, 61055
Cisternography, 70015
  Nuclear, 78630
Citrate
  Blood or Urine, 82507
CK, 82550-82554
  Total, 82550
Cl, 82435-82438
Clagett Procedure
  Chest Wall, Repair, Closure, 32810
Clavicle
  Arthrocentesis, 20605
  Arthrotomy
    Acromioclavicular Joint, 23044, 23101
    Sternoclavicular Joint, 23044, 23101, 23106
  Claviculectomy
    Arthroscopic, 29824
    Partial, 23120
    Total, 23125
  Craterization, 23180
  Cyst
    Excision, 23140
      with Allograft, 23146
      with Autograft, 23145
  Diaphysectomy, 23180
  Dislocation
    Acromioclavicular Joint
      Closed Treatment, 23540, 23545
      Open Treatment, 23550, 23552
    Sternoclavicular Joint
      Closed Treatment, 23520, 23525
      Open Treatment, 23530, 23532
      without Manipulation, 23540
  Excision, 23170
    Partial, 23120, 23180
    Total, 23125
  Fracture
    Closed Treatment
      with Manipulation, 23505
      without Manipulation, 23500
    Open Treatment, 23515
  Osteotomy, 23480
    with Bone Graft, 23485
  Pinning, Wiring, Etc., 23490
  Prophylactic Treatment, 23490
  Repair Osteotomy, 23480, 23485
  Saucerization, 23180
  Sequestrectomy, 23170
  Tumor
    Excision, 23140, 23146, 23200
      with Allograft, 23146
      with Autograft, 23145
    Radical Resection, 23200
  X-ray, 73000
Clavicula
  See Clavicle
Claviculectomy
  Arthroscopic, 29824
  Partial, 23120
  Total, 23125
Claw Finger Repair, 26499
Clayton Procedure, 28114
CLCN1, 81406
CLCNKB, 81406
Cleft, Branchial
  See Branchial Cleft
Cleft Cyst, Branchial
  See Branchial Cleft, Cyst
Cleft Foot
  Reconstruction, 28360
Cleft Hand
  Repair, 26580
Cleft Lip
  Repair, 40700-40761
  Rhinoplasty, 30460, 30462
Cleft Palate
  Repair, 42200-42225
  Rhinoplasty, 30460, 30462

Clinical Act of Insertion
  See Insertion
Clitoroplasty
  for Intersex State, 56805
Closed [Transurethral] Biopsy of Bladder
  See Biopsy, Bladder , Cystourethroscopy
Clostridial Tetanus
  See Tetanus
Clostridium Botulinum Toxin
  See Chemodenervation
Clostridium Difficile Toxin
  Amplified Probe Technique, 87493
  Antigen Detection
    Enzyme Immunoassay, 87324
  by Immunoassay
    with Direct Optical Observation, 87803
  Tissue Culture, 87230
Clostridium Tetani ab
  See Antibody, Tetanus
Closure
  Anal Fistula, 46288
  Appendiceal Fistula, 44799
  Atrial Appendage
    with Implant, 33340
  Atrial Septal Defect, 33641, 33647
  Atrioventricular Valve, 33600
  Cardiac Valve, 33600, 33602
  Cystostomy, 51880
  Diaphragm
    Fistula, 39599
  Enterostomy, 44620-44626
    Laparoscopic, 44227
  Esophagostomy, 43420-43425
  Fistula
    Anal, 46288, 46706
    Anorectal, 46707
    Bronchi, 32815
    Carotid-Cavernous, 61710
    Chest Wall, 32906
    Enterovesical, 44660-44661
    Ileoanal Pouch, 46710-46712
    Kidney, 50520-50526
    Lacrimal, 68770
    Nose, 30580-30600
    Oval Window, 69666
    Rectovaginal, 57305-57308
    Tracheoesophageal, 43305, 43312, 43314
    Ureter, 50920-50930
    Urethra, 53400-53405
    Urethrovaginal, 57310-57311
    Vesicouterine, 51920-51925
    Vesicovaginal, 51900, 57320, 57330
  Gastrostomy, 43870
  Lacrimal Fistula, 68770
  Lacrimal Punctum
    Plug, 68761
    Thermocauterization, Ligation, or Laser Surgery, 68760
  Meningocele, 63700-63702
  Patent Ductus Arteriosus, 93582
  Rectovaginal Fistula, 57300-57308
  Semilunar Valve, 33602
  Septal Defect, 33615
    Ventricular, 33675-33677, 33681-33688, 93581
  Skin
    Abdomen
      Complex, 13100-13102
      Intermediate, 12031-12037
      Layered, 12031-12037
      Simple, 12001-12007
      Superficial, 12001-12007
    Arm, Arms
      Complex, 13120-13122
      Intermediate, 12031-12037
      Layered, 12031-12037
      Simple, 12001-12007
      Superficial, 12001-12007
    Axilla, Axillae
      Complex, 13131-13133
      Intermediate, 12031-12037
      Layered, 12031-12037
      Simple, 12001-12007
      Superficial, 12001-12007

Closure — *continued*
  Skin — *continued*
    Back
      Complex, 13100-13102
      Intermediate, 12031-12037
      Layered, 12031-12037
      Simple, 12001-12007
      Superficial, 12001-12007
    Breast
      Complex, 13100-13102
      Intermediate, 12031-12037
      Layered, 12031-12037
      Simple, 12001-12007
      Superficial, 12001-12007
    Buttock
      Complex, 13100-13102
      Intermediate, 12031-12037
      Layered, 12031-12037
      Simple, 12001-12007
      Superficial, 12001-12007
    Cheek, Cheeks
      Complex, 13131-13133
      Intermediate, 12051-12057
      Layered, 12051-12057
      Simple, 12011-12018
      Superficial, 12011-12018
    Chest
      Complex, 13100-13102
      Intermediate, 12031-12037
      Layered, 12031-12037
      Simple, 12001-12007
      Superficial, 12001-12007
    Chin
      Complex, 13131-13133
      Intermediate, 12051-12057
      Layered, 12051-12057
      Simple, 12011-12018
      Superficial, 12011-12018
    Ear, Ears
      Complex, 13151-13153
      Intermediate, 12051-12057
      Layered, 12051-12057
      2.5 cm or less, 12051
      Simple, 12011-12018
      Superficial, 12011-12018
    External
      Genitalia
        Intermediate, 12041-12047
        Layered, 12041-12047
        Simple, 12001-12007
        Superficial, 12001-12007
    Extremity, Extremities
      Intermediate, 12031-12037
      Layered, 12031-12037
      Simple, 12001-12007
      Superficial, 12001-12007
    Eyelid, Eyelids
      Complex, 13151-13153
      Intermediate, 12051-12057
      Layered, 12051-12057
      Simple, 12011-12018
      Superficial, 12011-12018
    Face
      Complex, 13131-13133
      Intermediate, 12051-12057
      Layered, 12051-12057
      Simple, 12011-12018
      Superficial, 12011-12018
    Feet
      Complex, 13131-13133
      Intermediate, 12041-12047
      Layered, 12041-12047
      Simple, 12001-12007
      Superficial, 12001-12007
    Finger, Fingers
      Complex, 13131-13133
      Intermediate, 12041-12047
      Layered, 12041-12047
      Simple, 12001-12007
      Superficial, 12001-12007
    Foot
      Complex, 13131-13133
      Intermediate, 12041-12047
      Layered, 12041-12047
      Simple, 12001-12007
      Superficial, 12001-12007

Closure — *continued*
  Skin — *continued*
    Forearm, Forearms
      Complex, 13120-13122
      Intermediate, 12031-12037
      Layered, 12031-12037
      Simple, 12001-12007
      Superficial, 12001-12007
    Forehead
      Complex, 13131-13133
      Intermediate, 12051-12057
      Layered, 12051-12057
      Simple, 12011-12018
      Superficial, 12011-12018
    Genitalia
      Complex, 13131-13133
      External
        Intermediate, 12041-12047
        Layered, 12041-12047
        Simple, 12001-12007
        Superficial, 12001-12007
    Hand, Hands
      Complex, 13131-13133
      Intermediate, 12041-12047
      Layered, 12041-12047
      Simple, 12001-12007
      Superficial, 12001-12007
    Leg, Legs
      Complex, 13120-13122
      Intermediate, 12031-12037
      Layered, 12031-12037
      Simple, 12001-12007
      Superficial, 12001-12007
    Lip, Lips
      Complex, 13151-13153
      Intermediate, 12051-12057
      Layered, 12051-12057
      Simple, 12011-12018
      Superficial, 12011-12018
    Lower
      Arm, Arms
        Complex, 13120-13122
        Intermediate, 12031-12037
        Layered, 12031-12037
        Simple, 12001-12007
        Superficial, 12001-12007
      Extremity, Extremities
        Intermediate, 12031-12037
        Layered, 12031-12037
        Simple, 12001-12007
        Superficial, 12001-12007
      Leg, Legs
        Complex, 13120-13122
        Intermediate, 12031-12037
        Layered, 12031-12037
        Simple, 12001-12007
        Superficial, 12001-12007
    Mouth
      Complex, 13131-13133
    Mucous Membrane, Mucous Membranes
      Intermediate, 12051-12057
      Layered, 12051-12057
      Simple, 12011-12018
      Superficial, 12011-12018
    Neck
      Complex, 13131-13133
      Intermediate, 12041-12047
      Layered, 12041-12047
      Simple, 12001-12007
      Superficial, 12001-12007
    Nose
      Complex, 13151-13153
      Intermediate, 12051-12057
      Layered, 12051-12057
      Simple, 12011-12018
      Superficial, 12011-12018
    Palm, Palms
      Complex, 13131-13133
      Intermediate, 12041-12047
      Layered, 12041-12047
      Simple, 12001-12007
      Superficial, 12001-12007
    Scalp
      Complex, 13120-13122
      Intermediate, 12031-12037
      Layered, 12031-12037

[Resequenced]

Index

Consultation — Count, Erythrocyte

Count, Leukocyte
See White Blood Cell, Count
Count, Reticulocyte
See Reticulocyte, Count
Counters, Cell
See Cell Count
Countershock, Electric
See Cardioversion
Coventry Tibial Wedge Osteotomy
See Osteotomy, Tibia
Cowper's Gland
Excision, 53250
COX10, 81405
COX15, 81405
COX6B1, 81404
Coxa
See Hip
Coxiella Brunetii
Antibody, 86638
Coxsackie
Antibody, 86658
CPAP (Continuous Positive Airway Pressure), 94660
CPB, 32852, 32854, 33496, 33503-33505, 33510-33523, 33533-33536
C–Peptide, 80432, 84681
CPK
Isoenzymes, 82252, 82552
Isoforms, 82554
MB Fraction Only, 82553
Total, 82550
CPOX, 81405
CPR (Cardiopulmonary Resuscitation), 92950
CPT1A, 81406
CPT2, 81404
CR, 82565-82575
Cranial Bone
Frontal Bone Flap, 61556-61557
Halo
for Thin Skull Osteology, 20664
Parietal Bone Flap, 61556
Reconstruction
Extracranial, 21181-21184
Temporal Bone
Hearing Device, 69710-69711
Implantation Cochlear Device, 69930
Osseointegrated Implant, 69714-69715
Removal Tumor, 69970
Resection, 69535
Unlisted Procedure, 69979
Tumor
Excision, 61563-61564
Cranial Halo, 20661
Cranial Nerve
Avulsion, 64732-64760, 64771
Decompression, 61458, 61460, 64716
Implantation
Electrode, 64553, 64568-64569
Incision, 64732-64746, 64760
Injection
Anesthetic or Steroid, 64400-64408
Neurolytic, 64600-64610
Insertion
Electrode, 64553, 64568-64569
Neuroplasty, 64716
Release, 64716
Repair
Suture, with or without Graft, 64864, 64865
Section, 61460
Transection, 64732-64760, 64771
Transposition, 64716
Cranial Nerve II
See Optic Nerve
Cranial Nerve V
See Trigeminal Nerve
Cranial Nerve VII
See Facial Nerve
Cranial Nerve X
See Vagus Nerve
Cranial Nerve XI
See Accessory Nerve
Cranial Nerve XII
See Hypoglossal Nerve

Cranial Tongs
Application
Removal, 20660
Removal, 20665
Craniectomy
See Craniotomy
Anesthesia, 00211
Compression
Sensory Root Gasserian Ganglion, 61450
Craniosynostosis, 61558, 61559
Multiple Sutures, 61552, 61558-61559
Single Suture, 61550
Decompression, 61322-61323, 61340-61343
Cranial Nerves, 61458
Sensory Root Gasserian Ganglion, 61450
Drainage of Abscess, 61320-61321
Electrode Placement
Cortical, 61860, 61870
Subcortical, 61863-61864, 61867-61868
Excision
for Osteomyelitis, 61501
of Lesion or Tumor, 61500
Exploratory, 61304-61305, 61458
Section, 61450, 61460
Stenosis Release, 61550-61552
Surgical, 61312-61315, 61320-61323, 61450-61460, 61500-61522
with Craniotomy, 61530
Wound Treatment, 61571
Craniofacial and Maxillofacial
Unlisted Services and Procedures, 21299
Craniofacial Procedures
Unlisted Services and Procedures, 21299
Craniofacial Separation
Bone Graft, 21436
Closed Treatment, 21431
External Fixation, 21435
Open Treatment, 21432-21436
Wire Fixation, 21431-21432
Craniomegalic Skull
Reduction, 62115-62117
Craniopharyngioma
Excision, 61545
Cranioplasty, 62120
Bone Graft Retrieval, 62148
Encephalocele Repair, 62120
for Defect, 62140, 62141, 62145
with Autograft, 62146, 62147
with Bone Graft, 61316, 62146, 62147
Craniostenosis
See Craniosynostosis
Craniosynostosis
Bifrontal Craniotomy, 61557
Extensive Craniectomy, 61558, 61559
Frontal, 61556
Multiple Sutures, 61552
Parietal, 61556
Single Suture, 61550
Craniotomy
Abscess Drainage
Infratentorial, 61321
Supratentorial, 61320
Anesthesia, 00211
Barrel–Stave Procedure, 61559
Bifrontal Bone Flap, 61557
Cloverleaf Skull, 61558
Craniosynostosis, 61556-61557
Decompression, 61322-61323
Orbit Only, 61330
Other, Supratentorial, 61340
Posterior Fossa, 61345
Encephalocele, 62121
Excision Brain Tumor
Benign of Cranial Bone, 61563
with Optic Nerve Decompression, 61564
Cerebellopontine Angle Tumor, 61520
Cyst, Supratentorial, 61516
Infratentorial or posterior fossa, 61518
Meningioma, 61519
Midline at Skull Base, 61521
Supratentorial, 61510
Excision Epileptogenic Focus
with Electrocorticography, 61536
without Electrocorticography, 61534
Exploratory, 61304, 61305

Craniotomy — continued
Exploratory — continued
Orbit with Lesion Removal, 61333
Foreign Body, 61570
Frontal Bone Flap, 61556
Hematoma, 61312-61315
Implant of Neurostimulator, 61850-61870
Implantation Electrodes, 61531, 61533
Stereotactic, 61760
Lobectomy
with Electrocorticography, 61538
Meningioma, 61519
Multiple Osteotomies and Bone Autografts, 61359
Neurostimulators, 61850-61870
Osteomyelitis, 61501
Parietal Bone Flap, 61556
Penetrating Wound, 61571
Pituitary Tumor, 61546
Recontouring, 61559
Removal of Electrode Array, 61535
Suboccipital
for Cranial Nerves, 61458
Subtemporal, 61450
with Cervical Laminectomy, 61343
Surgery, 61312-61323, 61546, 61570-61571, 61582-61583, 61590, 61592, 61760, 62120
Transoral Approach, 61575
requiring Splitting Tongue and/or Mandible, 61576
with Bone Flap, 61510-61516, 61526, 61530, 61533-61545, 61566-61567
for Bone Lesion, 61500
Cranium
See Skull
Craterization
Calcaneus, 28120
Clavicle, 23180
Femur, 27070, 27071, 27360
Fibula, 27360, 27641
Hip, 27070, 27071
Humerus, 23184, 24140
Ileum, 27070, 27071
Metacarpal, 26230
Metatarsal, 28122
Olecranon Process, 24147
Phalanges
Finger, 26235, 26236
Toe, 28124
Pubis, 27070, 27071
Radius, 24145, 25151
Scapula, 23182
Talus, 28120
Tarsal, 28122
Tibia, 27360, 27640
Ulna, 24147, 25150
CRB1, 81406, 81434
C–Reactive Protein, 86140, 86141
Creatine, 82553-82554
Blood or Urine, 82540
Creatine Kinase (Total), 82550
Creatine Phosphokinase
Blood, 82552
Total, 82550
Creatinine
Blood, 82565
Clearance, 82575
Other Source, 82570
Urine, 82570, 82575
Creation
Arteriovenous
Fistula, 35686, 36825, 36830
Catheter Exit Site, 49436
Cavopulmonary Anastomosis, 33622
Colonic Reservoir, 45119
Complete Heart Block, 93650
Cutaneoperitoneal Fistula, 49999
Defect, 40720
Ileal Reservoir, 44158, 44211, 45113
Iliac Artery Conduit, 34833
Lesion
Gasserian Ganglion, 61790
Globus Pallidus, 61720
Other Subcortical Structure, 61735
Spinal Cord, 63600

Creation — continued
Lesion — continued
Thalamus, 61720
Trigeminal Tract, 61791
Mucofistula, 44144
Pericardial Window, 32659, 33025
Recipient Site, 15002-15003, 15004-15005
Shunt
Cerebrospinal Fluid, 62200
Subarachnoid
Lumbar–Peritoneal, 63740
Subarachnoid–Subdural, 62190
Ventriculo, 62220
Sigmoid Bladder, 50810
Speech Prosthesis, 31611
Stoma
Bladder, 51980
Kidney, 50436-50437
Renal Pelvis, 50436-50437
Tympanic Membrane, 69433, 69436
Ureter, 50860
Ventral Hernia, 39503
CREBBP, 81406-81407
CRF, 80412
CRH (Corticotropic Releasing Hormone), 80412
Cricoid Cartilage Split, 31587
Cricothyroid Membrane
Incision, 31605
Cristobalite
See Silica
CRIT, 85013
Critical Care Services
Cardiopulmonary Resuscitation, 92950
Evaluation and Management, 99291-99292, 99468-99476
Interfacility Transport, 99466-99467 [99485] [99486]
Ipecac Administration for Poison, 99175
Neonatal
Initial, 99468
Intensive, 99477
Low Birth Weight Infant, 99478-99479
Subsequent, 99469
Pediatric
Initial, 99471, 99475
Interfacility Transport, 99466-99467 [99485, 99486]
Supervision, [99485, 99486]
Subsequent, 99472, 99476
CRM197, 90734
Cross Finger Flap, 15574
Crossmatch, 86825-86826, 86920-86923
Crossmatching, Tissue
See Tissue Typing
CRP, 86140
Cruciate Ligament
Arthroscopic Repair, 29888-29889
Repair, 27407, 27409
Knee with Collateral Ligament, 27409
CRX, 81404
Cryoablation
See Cryosurgery
Cryofibrinogen, 82585
Cryofixation
Cells, 38207-38209, 88240-88241
Embryo, 89258
for Transplantation, 32850, 33930, 33940, 44132, 47133, 47140, 48550, 50300-50320, 50547
Freezing and Storage, 38207, 88240
Oocyte, 89240
Ovarian Tissue, 89240
Sperm, 89259
Testes, 89335
Thawing
Embryo, 89352
Oocytes, 89353
Reproductive Tissue, 89354
Sperm, 89356
Cryoglobulin, 82595
Cryopreservation
Bone Marrow, 38207-38209
Cells, 38207-38208, 88240, 88241
Embryo, 89258, 89352

[Resequenced]

Cystotomy — *continued*
with Fulguration, 51020
with Insertion
Radioactive Material, 51020
Urethral Catheter, 51045
with Removal Calculus, 51050, 51065
Cystourethrogram, Retrograde, 51610
Cystourethropexy, 51840-51841
Cystourethroplasty, 51800, 51820
Radiofrequency Micro-Remodeling, 53860
Cystourethroscopy, 52000, 52320-52355, 52601, 52647, 52648, 53500
Biopsy, 52204, 52224, 52250, 52354
Brush, 52007
Calibration and/or Dilation Urethral Stricture or Stenosis, 52281, 52630, 52647-52649
Catheterization
Ejaculatory Duct, 52010
Ureteral, 52005
Chemodenervation of Bladder, 52287
Destruction
Lesion, 52400
Dilation
Bladder, 52260, 52265
Intra–Renal Stricture, 52343, 52346
Ureter, 52341, 52342, 52344, 52345
Urethra, 52281, 52285
Evacuation
Clot, 52001
Examination, 52000
Female Urethral Syndrome, 52285
Incision
Bladder Neck, 52285
Congenital Obstructive Mucosal Folds, 52400
Diverticulum, 52305
Ejaculatory Duct, 52402
Urethral Valves, 52400
Injection
for Cystography, 52281
Implant Material, 52327
Insertion
Indwelling Urethral Stent, 52282, 52332
Radioactive Substance, 52250
Ureteral Guide Wire, 52334
Urethral Stent, 52282
Instillation, 52005, 52010
Irrigation, 52005, 52010
Lithotripsy, 52353
with Ureteral Stent, [52356]
Lysis
Urethra, 53500
Urethrovaginal Septal Fibrosis, 52285
Manipulation of Ureteral Calculus, 52330, 52352
Meatotomy
Ureteral, 52290
Urethral, 52281, 52285, 52630, 52647-52649
Removal
Calculus, 52310, 52315, 52320, 52325, 52352
Foreign Body, 52310, 52315
Urethral Stent, 52310, 52315
Resection
Congenital Obstructive Mucosal Folds, 52400
Diverticulum, 52305
Ejaculatory Duct, 52402
External Sphincter, 52277
Prostate, 52601, 52630
Tumor, 52234-52235, 52240, 52355
Ureterocele(s), 52300-52301
Urethral Valves, 52400
Treatment
Lesion(s), 52224
Ureteral Stricture, 52341
Urethral Syndrome, 52285
Vasectomy
Transurethral, 52402, 52630, 52647-52649
Vasotomy
Transurethral, 52402
with Direct Vision Internal Urethrotomy, 52276
with Duct Radiography, 52010

Cystourethroscopy — *continued*
with Ejaculatory Duct Catheterization, 52010
with Fulguration, 52214, 52354
Congenital Obstructive Mucosal Folds, 52400
Lesion, 52224
Polyps, 52285
Tumor, 52234-52240
Ureterocele(s), 52300-52301
Urethral Valves, 52400
with Internal Urethrotomy, 52630, 52647-52649
Female, 52270, 52285
Male, 52275
with Mechanical Dilation, 0499T
with Prostate
Insertion Transprostatic Implant, 52441-52442
Laser Coagulation, 52647
Laser Enucleation, 52649
Laser Vaporization, 52648
with Steroid Injection, 52283
with Ureteropyelography, 52005
with Ureteroscopy, 52351
with Urethral Catheterization, 52005
with Urethral Meatotomy, 52290, 52300, 52305
with Urethral Therapeutic Drug Delivery, 0499T
Cytochrome Gene Analysis, 81225-81227
Cytochrome, Reductase, Lactic
See Lactic Dehydrogenase
Cytogenetic Study
Bone Marrow
Breakage Syndromes
See Chromosome Analysis
Diagnostic, 3155F
Neoplastic Disorder, 88237
Interpretation and Report, 88291
Molecular DNA Probe, 88271-88275, 88291, 88365
Non-neoplastic Disorders
Amniotic Fluid, 88235
Chorionic Villus Cells, 88235
Lymphocyte, 88230
Skin or Tissue Biopsy, 88233
Unlisted Services and Procedures, 88299
Cytogenomic Constitutional Microarray Analysis, 81228-81229, 81406
Cytogenomic Microarray Analysis, 81406
Chromosome 22q13, 81405
Neoplasia, [81277]
X chromosome, 81405
Cytomegalovirus
Antibody, 86644, 86645
Antigen Detection
Direct Fluorescence, 87271
Enzyme Immunoassay, 87332
Nucleic Acid, 87495-87497
Cytometries, Flow
See Flow Cytometry
Cytopathology
Cervical or Vaginal
Requiring Interpretation by Physician, 88141
Thin Layer Prep, 88142-88143, 88174-88175
Concentration Technique, 88108
Evaluation, 88172-88173, [88177]
Hormone Evaluation, 88155
Immediate Cytohistologic Study, 88172 [88177]
Fine Needle Aspirate, 88172-88173 [88177]
Fluids, Washings, Brushings, 88104-88108
Forensic, 88125
Other Source, 88160-88162
Pap, 88164-88167
Selective Cellular Enhancement Technique, 88112
Smears
Brushings, 88104
Cervical or Vaginal, 88141-88155, 88164-88167, 88174-88175
Manual Screen, 88150-88153, 88164-88167
Other Source, 88160-88162
Techniques
Concentration, 88108

Cytopathology — *continued*
Techniques — *continued*
In Situ Hybridization, 88120-88121, 88367-88368
Unlisted Services and Procedures, 88199
Urinary Tract
In Situ Hybridization Technique, 88120-88121
Cytoscopy
See Bladder, Endoscopy
Cytosol Aminopeptidase, 83670
Cytotoxic Screen
Lymphocyte, 86805, 86806
Percent Reactive Antibody (PRA), 86807, 86808
Serum Antibodies, 86807, 86808
Cytotoxicity Assay
Chemotherapeutic Drug, 0564T

D

D and C (Dilation and Curettage), 59840
D and E (Dilation and Evacuation), 59841-59851
D Galactose
See Galactose
D Glucose
See Glucose
D Vitamin
See Vitamin, D
D2, Vitamin
See Calciferol
Dacryoadenectomy
Partial, 68505
Total, 68500
Dacryocystectomy, 68520
Dacryocystogram
See Dacryocystography
Dacryocystography, 68850, 70170
with Nuclear Imaging, 78660
Dacryocystorhinostomy, 68720
Total
with Nasal
Sinus Endoscopy, 31239
Dacryocystostomy, 68420
Daily Living Activities
See Activities of Daily Living
D&C Yellow No. 7
See Fluorescein
Damus–Kaye–Stansel Procedure, 33606
Dana Operation, 63185, 63190
Rhizotomy, 63185, 63190
Dandy Operation, 62200
DAPTACEL, 90700
DARC, 81403
Dark Adaptation Examination, 92284
Dark Field Examination, 87164, 87166
Darrach Procedure, 25240
See Excision, Ulna, Partial
David Procedure, 33864
Day Test, 82270
DAZ/SRY, 81403
DBT, 81405-81406
DCP, 83951
DCR, 31239, 68720
DCX, 81405
DDST, 96112-96116
Death, Brain
See Brain Death
Debridement
Bone, 11044 [11047]
with Open Fracture and/or Dislocation, 11012
Brain, 62010
Burns, 16020-16030
Anesthesia, 01951-01953
Cartilage
Hip, 29862
Knee, 29877, 29880-29881, 29885
Elbow, 29837-29838
with Removal Prosthesis, 24160, 24164
Forearm, 25023, 25025
Infected Inflatable Urethral/Bladder Neck Sphincter, 53448
Infected Tissue, with Removal Penile Implant, 54411, 54417
Knee, 27441, 27443, 27497, 27499
Leg, 27892-27894
Liver, 47361

Debridement — *continued*
Mastoid Cavity
Complex, 69222
Simple, 69220
Metatarsophalangeal Joint, 28289, 28291, 29901-29902
Muscle, 11043-11044 [11046], 11044-11047 [11046]
Infected, 11004-11006, 11008
with Open Fracture and/or Dislocation, 11011-11012
Nails, 11720, 11721
Necrotizing Soft Tissue, 11004-11008
Nonviable Tissue, 25023, 25025, 27497, 27499, 27892-27894
Nose
Endoscopic, 31237
Pancreatic Tissue, 48105
Pathology Analysis, 88304-88305
Shoulder, 29822-29823
with Removal Prosthesis, 23334-23335
Skin
Eczematous, 11000, 11001
Excision, 15920-15999
Infected, 11000-11006
Subcutaneous Tissue, 11042-11047 [11045, 11046]
Infected, 11004-11006, 11008
Necrotized, 49568
with Open Fracture and/or Dislocation, 11010-11012
Sternum, 21627
Subcutaneous, 11042-11047 [11045, 11046]
Thigh, 27497, 27499
Wound
Non–Selective, 97602
Selective, 97597-97598
Wrist
Joint, 29846
Nonviable Tissue, 25023, 25025
Debulking Procedure
Ovary
Pelvis, 58952-58954
Decapsulation
of Kidney, 53899
DECAVAC, 90714
Declotting
Vascular Access Device, 36593
Decompression
Arm, Lower, 24495, 25020-25025
Auditory Canal, Internal, 61591, 69960
Brainstem, 61575, 61576
Buttocks, 27057
Carotid Artery, 61590-61591
Carpal Tunnel, 64721
Cauda Equina, 63011, 63017, 63047, 63048, 63056, 63057, 63087-63091
Colon, 45378
Cranial Nerves, 61458
Esophagogastric Varices, 37181
Facial Nerve, 61590
Intratemporal
Lateral to Geniculate Ganglion, 69720, 69740
Medial to Geniculate Ganglion, 69725, 69745
Total, 69955
Transtemporal, 61595
Fasciotomy
Leg, 27892-27894
Pelvic/Buttock, 27027
with Debridement, 27057
Thigh/Knee, 27496-27499
Finger, 26035
Gasserian Ganglion
Sensory Root, 61450
Gill Type procedure, 63012
Hand, 26035, 26037
Intestines
Small, 44021
Jejunostomy
Laparoscopic, 44186-44187
Leg
Fasciotomy, 27600-27602
Nerve, 64702-64727

Dilation — *continued*
- Nose
  - Balloon, 31295-31297
- Pancreatic Duct
  - Endoscopy, *[43277]*
- Rectum
  - Endoscopy, 45303
  - Sphincter, 45910
- Salivary Duct, 42650, 42660
- Sinus Ostium, 31295-31298
- Trachea
  - Endoscopic, 31630, 31631, 31636-31638
- Transluminal
  - Aqueous Outflow Canal, 66174-66175
  - Ureter, 50436-50437, 50706, 52341-52342, 52344-52346
  - Endoscopic, 50553, 50572, 50575, 50953, 50972
  - Urethra, 52260, 52265
    - Female Urethral Syndrome, 52285
    - General, 53665
    - Suppository and/or Instillation, 53660-53661
    - with Prostate Resection, 52601, 52630, 52647-52649
    - with Prostatectomy, 55801, 55821
  - Urethral
    - Stenosis, 52281
    - Stricture, 52281, 53600-53621
  - Vagina, 57400
- **Dilation and Curettage**
  - *See* Curettage; Dilation
  - Cervical Stump, 57558
  - Cervix, 57520, 57522, 57558, 57800
  - Corpus Uteri, 58120
  - Hysteroscopy, 58558
  - Induced Abortion, 59840
    - with Amniotic Injections, 59851
    - with Vaginal Suppositories, 59856
  - Postpartum, 59160
- **Dilation and Evacuation**, 59841
  - with Amniotic Injections, 59851
  - with Vaginal Suppository, 59856
- **Dimethadione**, *[80339, 80340, 80341]*
- **Dioxide, Carbon**
  - *See* Carbon Dioxide
- **Dioxide Silicon**
  - *See* Silica
- **Dipeptidyl Peptidase A**
  - *See* Angiotensin Converting Enzyme (ACE)
- **Diphenylhydantoin**
  - *See* Phenytoin
- **Diphosphate, Adenosine**
  - *See* Adenosine Diphosphate
- **Diphtheria**
  - Antibody, 86648
  - Immunization, 90696-90698, 90700-90702, 90714-90715, 90723
- **Dipropylacetic Acid**
  - Assay, 80164
  - *See Also* Valproic Acid
- **Direct Pedicle Flap**
  - Formation, 15570-15576
  - Transfer, 15570-15576, 15650
- **Disability Evaluation Services**
  - Basic Life and/or Disability Evaluation, 99450
  - Work–Related or Medical Disability Evaluation, 99455, 99456
- **Disarticulation**
  - Ankle, 27889
  - Elbow, 20999
  - Hip, 27295
  - Knee, 27598
  - Mandible, 61590
  - Shoulder, 23920, 23921
  - Wrist, 25920, 25924
    - Revision, 25922
- **Disarticulation of Shoulder**
  - *See* Shoulder, Disarticulation
- **Disc Chemolyses, Intervertebral**
  - *See* Chemonucleolysis
- **Disc, Intervertebral**
  - *See* Intervertebral Disc
- **Discectomies**
  - *See* Discectomy

Discectomies, Percutaneous
- *See* Discectomy, Percutaneous
Discectomy
- Additional Segment, 22226
- Anterior with Decompression
  - Cervical Interspace, 63075
    - Each Additional, 63076
  - Thoracic Interspace, 63077
    - Each Additional, 63078
- Arthrodesis
  - Additional Interspace, 22534, 22585, 22634
  - Cervical, 22551-22552, 22554, 22585, 22856, 22899, 63075-63076
  - Lumbar, 0163T-0164T, 22533, 22558, 22585, 22630, 22633-22634, 22857, 22899, 62380
  - Sacral, 22586
  - Thoracic, 22532, 22534, 22556, 22585, 63077-63078
- Vertebra
  - Cervical, 22554
- Cervical, 22220
- Endoscopic Lumbar, 62380
- Lumbar, 22224, 22630, 62380
- Percutaneous, 0274T-0275T
- Sacral, 22586
- Thoracic, 22222
  - Additional Segment, 22226
- with Endplate Preparation, 22856
- with Osteophytectomy, 22856
Discharge, Body Substance
- *See* Drainage
Discharge Instructions
- Heart Failure, 4014F
Discharge Services
- *See* Hospital Services
- Hospital, 99238, 99239
- Newborn, 99463
- Nursing Facility, 99315, 99316
- Observation Care, 99217, 99234-99236
Discission
- Cataract
  - Laser Surgery, 66821
  - Stab Incision, 66820
- Hyaloid Membrane, 65810
- Vitreous Strands, 67030
Discography
- Cervical Disc, 72285
- Injection, 62290, 62291
- Lumbar Disc, 62287, 72295
- Thoracic, 72285
Discolysis
- *See* Chemonucleolysis
Disease
- Durand–Nicolas–Favre
  - *See* Lymphogranuloma Venereum
- Erb–Goldflam
  - *See* Myasthenia Gravis
- Heine–Medin
  - *See* Polio
- Hydatid
  - *See* Echinococcosis
- Lyme
  - *See* Lyme Disease
- Ormond
  - *See* Retroperitoneal Fibrosis
- Peyronie
  - *See* Peyronie Disease
- Posada–Wernicke
  - *See* Coccidioidomycosis
Disease/Organ Panel
- *See* Organ/Disease Panel
Diskectomy
- *See* Discectomy
Dislocated Elbow
- *See* Dislocation, Elbow
Dislocated Hip
- *See* Dislocation, Hip Joint
Dislocated Jaw
- *See* Dislocation, Temporomandibular Joint
Dislocated Joint
- *See* Dislocation
Dislocated Shoulder
- *See* Dislocation, Shoulder

Dislocation
- Acromioclavicular Joint
  - Closed Treatment, 23540, 23545
  - Open Treatment, 23550, 23552
- Ankle Joint
  - Closed Treatment, 27840, 27842
  - Open Treatment, 27846, 27848
- Carpal
  - Closed Treatment, 25690
  - Open Treatment, 25695
- Carpometacarpal Joint
  - Closed Treatment, 26641, 26645, 26670
    - with Anesthesia, 26675
  - Open Treatment, 26665, 26685, 26686
  - Percutaneous Fixation, 26676
  - Thumb, 26641
    - Bennett Fracture, 26650, 26665
- Clavicle
  - Closed Treatment, 23540, 23545
  - Open Treatment, 23550, 23552
  - with Manipulation, 23545
  - without Manipulation, 23540
- Elbow
  - Closed Treatment, 24600, 24605
    - Monteggia, 24620, 24635
  - Open Treatment, 24586-24587, 24615
  - with Manipulation, 24620, 24640
- Finger(s)/Hand
  - Interphalangeal, 26770-26785
  - Metacarpal Except Thumb, 26670-26686
- Hand
  - Carpal
    - Closed, 25690
    - Open, 25695
  - Carpometacarpal
    - Closed, 26670, 26675
    - Open, 26685-26686
    - Percutaneous, 26676
    - Thumb, 26641, 26650, 26665
  - Interphalangeal joint
    - Closed, 26770, 26775
    - Open, 26785
    - Percutaneous, 26776
  - Lunate
    - Closed, 25690
    - Open, 26715
    - Percutaneous, 26705
  - Metacarpophalangeal
    - Closed, 26700-26705
    - Open, 26715
    - Percutaneous, 26705
  - Radiocarpal
    - Closed, 25660
    - Open, 25670
  - Thumb
    - *See* Dislocation, thumb
  - Wrist
    - *See* Dislocation, Wrist
- Hip Joint
  - Closed Treatment, 27250, 27252, 27265, 27266
  - Congenital, 27256-27259
  - Open Treatment, 27253, 27254, 27258, 27259
  - without Trauma, 27265, 27266
- Interphalangeal Joint
  - Finger(s)/Hand
    - Closed Treatment, 26770, 26775
    - Open Treatment, 26785
    - Percutaneous Fixation, 26776
  - Toe(s)/Foot, 28660-28675
    - Closed Treatment, 28660, 28665
    - Open Treatment, 28675
    - Percutaneous Fixation, 28666
- Knee
  - Closed Treatment, 27550, 27552
  - Open Treatment, 27556-27558, 27566, 27730
  - Patella, 27560-27562
  - Recurrent, 27420-27424
- Lunate
  - Closed Treatment, 25690
  - Open Treatment, 25695
  - with Manipulation, 25690, 26670-26676, 26700-26706

Dislocation — *continued*
- Metacarpophalangeal Joint
  - Closed Treatment, 26700-26706
  - Open Treatment, 26715
- Metatarsophalangeal Joint
  - Closed Treatment, 28630, 28635
  - Open Treatment, 28645
  - Percutaneous Fixation, 28636
- Patella
  - Closed Treatment, 27560, 27562
  - Open Treatment, 27566
  - Recurrent, 27420-27424
- Pelvic Ring
  - Closed Treatment, 27197-27198
  - Open Treatment, 27217, 27218
  - Percutaneous Fixation, 27216
- Percutaneous Fixation
  - Metacarpophalangeal, 26705
- Peroneal Tendons, 27675, 27676
- Radiocarpal Joint
  - Closed Treatment, 25660
  - Open Treatment, 25670
- Radioulnar Joint
  - Closed Treatment, 25675
    - with Radial Fracture, 25520
  - Galeazzi, 25520, 25525-25526
  - Open Treatment, 25676
    - with Radial Fracture, 25525, 25526
- Radius
  - Closed Treatment, 24640
  - with Fracture, 24620, 24635
    - Closed Treatment, 24620
    - Open Treatment, 24635
- Shoulder
  - Closed Treatment
    - with Manipulation, 23650, 23655
    - with Fracture of Greater Humeral Tuberosity, 23665
    - Open Treatment, 23670
    - with Surgical or Anatomical Neck Fracture, 23675
    - Open Treatment, 23680
  - Open Treatment, 23660
  - Recurrent, 23450-23466
- Sternoclavicular Joint
  - Closed Treatment
    - with Manipulation, 23525
    - without Manipulation, 23520
  - Open Treatment, 23530, 23532
- Talotarsal Joint
  - Closed Treatment, 28570, 28575
  - Open Treatment, 28546
  - Percutaneous Fixation, 28576
- Tarsal
  - Closed Treatment, 28540, 28545
  - Open Treatment, 28555
  - Percutaneous Fixation, 28545, 28546
- Tarsometatarsal Joint
  - Closed Treatment, 28600, 28605
  - Open Treatment, 28615
  - Percutaneous Fixation, 28606
- Temporomandibular Joint
  - Closed Treatment, 21480, 21485
  - Open Treatment, 21490
- Thumb
  - Closed Treatment, 26641, 26645
  - Open Treatment, 26665
  - Percutaneous Fixation, 26650
  - with Fracture, 26645
    - Open Treatment, 26665
    - Percutaneous Fixation, 26650, 26665
  - with Manipulation, 26641-26650
- Tibiofibular Joint
  - Closed Treatment, 27830, 27831
  - Open Treatment, 27832
- Toe
  - Closed Treatment, 26770, 26775, 28630-28635
  - Open Treatment, 28645
  - Percutaneous Fixation, 26776, 28636
- Trans-scaphoperilunar, 25680
  - Closed Treatment, 25680
  - Open Treatment, 25685

Left margin: **Index** **Dilation — Dislocation**

   [Resequenced]

Ear Canal
  See Auditory Canal
Ear Cartilage
  Graft
    to Face, 21230
    to Nose or Ear, 21230, 21235
Ear Lobes
  Pierce, 69090
Ear, Nose, and Throat
  Acoustic, 92568
  Audiometric Group Testing, 92559
  Audiometry
    Conditioning Play, 92582
    Evoked Response, 92585-92586
    Groups, 92559
    Picture, 92583
    Pure Tone, 92552-92553, 0208T-0209T
    Select Picture, 92583
    Speech, 92555-92557, 0210T-0212T
    Tympanotomy and Reflex, 92550
    Visual Reinforcement, 92579
  Bekesy Screening, 92560-92561
  Binocular Microscopy, 92504
  Brainstem Evoked Response, 92585, 92586
  Central Auditory Function Evaluation, 92620-92621
  Comprehensive Audiometry Threshold Evaluation, 92557
  Diagnostic Analysis
    Auditory Brainstem Implant, 92640
    Cochlear Implant, 92601-92604
  Ear Protector Evaluation, 92596
  Electrocochleography, 92584
  Evaluation
    Auditory Rehabilitation Status, 92626-92627, 92630, 92633
    Communication Device
      Non-speech Generating, 92605, [92618]
      Speech Generating, 92607-92608
    Language Comprehensive and Expression, 92523
    Laryngeal Sensory Testing, 92614-92617
    Speech Fluency, 92521
    Speech Sound Production, 92522
    Swallowing, 92610-92613, 92616
    Voice and Resonance Analysis, 92524
  Examination Under Anesthesia, 92502
  Facial Nerve Function Study, 92516
  Filtered Speech, 92571
  Hearing Aid Evaluation, 92590-92595
  Hearing, Language, and Speech Evaluation, 92521-92524
  Immittance Testing, 92570
  Impedance Testing, 92567
  Laryngeal Function Study, 92520
  Lombard Test, 92700
  Loudness Balance, 92562
  Nasal Function Study, 92512
  Nasopharyngoscopy, 92511
  Reflex, 92568
  Screening Test, 92551
  Treatment
    Hearing, Language, Speech Disorder, 92507-92508
    Oral Function for Feeding, 92526
    Swallowing Dysfunction, 92526
Ear Protector Attenuation, 92596
  See Hearing Aid Services
Ear Wax
  See Cerumen
Ebstein Anomaly Repair, 33468
EBV, 86663-86665
ECCE, 66840-66852, 66940
Eccrine Glands
  Chemodenervation
    Axillae, 64650
    Feet, 64999
    Hands, 64999
    Other Areas, 64653
ECG, 0295T-0298T, 93000-93024, 93040-93278
  External, 93224-93272, 0295T-0298T
  Signal-Averaged, 93278
Echinococcosis, 86171, 86280
ECHO, 76825, 93303-93312, 93314, 93315, 93317-93321, 93350, [93356]

Echocardiography
  Cardiac, 93320-93350
    Intracardiac, 93662
    Strain Imaging, [93356]
    Transesophageal, 93318
    Transthoracic, 93303-93317
      with Myocardial Contrast Perfusion, 0439T
      with Stress Test, 93350-93352
  Doppler, 93303-93321, 93350, 93662
  Fetal Heart, 76825-76828
    Doppler
      Complete, 76827
      Follow–up or Repeat Study, 76828
    for Assessment of Myocardial Ischemia/Viability, 0439T
    for Congenital Anomalies
      Transesophageal, 93315-93317
      Transthoracic, 93303, 93304
  Intracardiac, 93662
  M Mode and Real Time, 93306
  Myocardial Contrast Perfusion, 0439T
  Strain Imaging, [93356]
  Stress Test, 93350-93351
    with Contrast, 93352
    with Myocardial Contrast Perfusion, 0439T
  Transesophageal, 93312-93318
    for Congenital Anomalies, 93315-93317
    for Guidance Intracardiac or Great Vessel Intervention, 93355
    for Monitoring Purposes, 93318
  Transthoracic, 93303-93308, 93350-93352
    for Congenital Anomalies, 93303, 93304
    with Myocardial Contrast Perfusion, 0439T
    with Stress Test, 93350-93352
Echoencephalography, 76506
Echography
  Abdomen, 76700-76705
  Arm
    Complete, 76881
    Limited, 76882
  Cardiac, 0439T, 93303-93317, 93320-93321, 93350-93352, 93662
    Guidance for Biopsy, 76932
  Chest, 76604
  Extracranial Arteries, 93880, 93882
  Eyes, 76510-76529
  Follow–Up, 76970
  Head, 76536
  Heart, 0439T, 93303-93317, 93320-93321, 93350-93352, 93662
    Guidance for Biopsy, 76932
  Hip
    Infant, 76885, 76886
  Intracranial Arteries, 93886-93893
  Intraoperative, 76998
  Kidney
    Transplant, 76776
  Leg
    Complete, 76881
    Limited, 76882
  Neck, 76536
  Pelvis, 76856, 76857
  Pregnant Uterus, 76801-76828
  Prostate, 76872-76873
  Retroperitoneal, 76770, 76775
  Scrotum, 76870
  Spine, 76800
  Transrectal, 76872, 76873
  Transvaginal, 76817, 76830
  Unlisted Ultrasound, 76999
  Vagina, 76817, 76830
Echotomography
  See Echography
ECLS (Extracorporeal Life Support Services)
  Cannulization
    Insertion, 33951-33956
    Removal, [33965, 33966, 33969, 33984, 33985, 33986]
    Repositioning, 33957-33959 [33962, 33963, 33964]
  Creation Graft Conduit, [33987]
  Daily Management, 33948-33949
  Initiation, 33946-33947

ECLS (Extracorporeal Life Support Services) — *continued*
    Left Heart Vent Insertion, [33988]
    Left Heart Vent Removal, [33989]
ECMO (Extracorporeal Membrane Oxygenation)
  Cannulization
    Insertion, 33951-33956
    Isolated with Chemotherapy Perfusion, 36823
    Removal, [33965, 33966, 33969, 33984, 33985, 33986]
    Repositioning, 33957-33959 [33962, 33963, 33964]
  Creation Graft Conduit, [33987]
  Daily Management, 33948-33949
  Initiation, 33946-33947
    Left Heart Vent Insertion, [33988]
    Left Heart Vent Removal, [33989]
ECS
  See Emission Computerized Tomography
ECSF (Erythrocyte Colony Stimulating Factor)
  See Erythropoietin
ECT (Emission Computerized Tomography), 78803
ECT (Electroconvulsive Therapy), 90870
Ectasia
  See Dilation
Ectopic Pregnancy
  See Obstetrical Care
  Abdominal, 59130
  Cervix, 59140
  Interstitial
    Partial Resection Uterus, 59136
    Total Hysterectomy, 59135
  Laparoscopy, 59150
    with Salpingectomy and/or Oophorectomy, 59151
  Ovarian
    with Salpingectomy and/or Oophorectomy, 59120
    without Salpingectomy and/or Oophorectomy, 59121
  Tubal
    with Salpingectomy and/or Oophorectomy, 59120
    without Salpingectomy and/or Oophorectomy, 59121
  Uterine
    with Hysterectomy, 59135
    with Partial Uterine Resection, 59136
Ectropion
  Repair
    Blepharoplasty
      Excision Tarsal Wedge, 67916
      Extensive, 67917
    Suture, 67914
    Thermocauterization, 67915
ED, 99281-99288
Education, 99078
  Patient
    Heart Failure, 4003F
    Pediatric Gastroenteritis to Caregiver, 4058F
    Self-management by Nonphysician, 98960-98962
  Services (Group), 99078
  Supplies, 99071
EEG, 95812-95824, 95830, 95955-95958
  See also Electroencephalography
  Long Term Set Up, [95700, 95705, 95706, 95707, 95708, 95709, 95710, 95711, 95712, 95713, 95714, 95715, 95716, 95717, 95718, 95719, 95720, 95721, 95722, 95723, 95724, 95725, 95726]
  Pharmacological/Physical Activation, 95954
EFHC1, 81406
EGD, 43235-43255 [43233], 43257, 43259, [43233], [43266], [43270]
EGFR, 81235
Egg
  See Ova
Eggers Procedure, 27100
EGR2, 81404
Ehrlichia, 86666
EIF2B2, 81406
EIF2B3, 81405-81406
EIF2B4, 81406

EIF2B5, 81406
EKG, 93000-93010
  64-Lead or Greater, 93799
  External, 0295T-0298T, 93224-93272
  Rhythm Strips, 93040-93042
  Routine, 93000-93010
  Signal Averaged, 93278
Elastase, 82656
Elastography
  Magnetic Resonance, 76391
  Ultrasound, Parenchyma, 76981-76983
Elbow
  See Humerus; Radius; Ulna
  Abscess
    Incision and Drainage, 23930, 23935
  Anesthesia, 00400, 01710-01782
  Arthrectomy, 24155
  Arthrocentesis, 20605-20606
  Arthrodesis, 24800, 24802
  Arthrography, 73085
    Contrast Injection, 24220
  Arthroplasty, 24360
    Removal Prosthesis, 24160, 24164
    Revision, 24370-24371
    Total Replacement, 24363
    with Implant, 24361-24362
  Arthroscopy
    Diagnostic, 29830
    Surgical, 29834-29838
  Arthrotomy, 24000
    Capsular Release, 24006
    Drainage, 24000
    Foreign Body Removal, 24000
    with Joint Exploration, 24000, 24101
    with Synovectomy, 24102
    with Synovial Biopsy, 24100, 29830
  Biopsy, 24065-24066, 24101
  Bone Cortex Incision, 23935
  Bursa
    Incision and Drainage, 23931
  Capsule
    Excision, 24006
    Radical Resection, 24149
  Contracture Release, 24149
  Dislocation
    Closed Treatment, 24600, 24605, 24640
    Nursemaid Elbow, 24640
    Open Treatment, 24615
    Partial, 24640
    Subluxate, 24640
  Epicondylitis
    Debridement, 24358-24359
    Percutaneous, 24357
  Excision, 24155
    Bursa, 24105
    Synovium, 24102, 29835-29836
    Tumor
      Soft Tissue, 24077-24079
        Subcutaneous, 24075, [24071]
        Subfascial, 24076, [24073]
  Exploration, 24000-24101 [24071, 24073]
  Fracture
    Monteggia, 24620, 24635
    Open Treatment, 24586, 24587
  Hematoma
    Incision and Drainage, 23930
  Incision and Drainage
    Abscess, Deep, 23930
    Bursa, 23931
    Hematoma, 23930
  Injection
    Arthrography (Radiologic), 24220
  Magnetic Resonance Imaging (MRI), 73221
  Manipulation, 24300
  Prosthesis
    Removal, 24160-24164
  Radical Resection
    Bone Tumor, 24150, 24152
    Capsule, Soft Tissue and Bone with Contracture Release, 24149
    Soft Tissue Tumor, 24077-24079
  Removal
    Foreign Body, 24000, 24101, 24200, 24201, 29834
    Implant, 24160-24164
    Loose Body, 24101, 29834

Elbow — continued

Removal — continued
  Prosthesis, 24160
Repair
  Advancement, 24330-24331
  Epicondylitis, 24357-24359
  Fasciotomy, 24357-24359
  Flexorplasty, 24330
  Graft, 24320
  Hemiepiphyseal Arrest, 24470
  Ligament, 24343-24346
  Muscle, 24341
  Muscle Transfer, 24301, 24320
  Tendon, 24340-24342
    Lengthening, 24305
    Release
      Debridement, 24358-24359
      Percutaneous, 24357
      Repair, 24359
    Repair, 24341, 24359
    Tenodesis, 24340
    Tenotomy, 24310, 24357-24359
  Tennis Elbow, 24357-24359
Seddon-Brookes Procedure, 24320
Steindler Advancement, 24330
Strapping, 29260
Tenotomy, 24357-24359
Tumor
  Excision, 24075-24076 [24071]
  Radical Resection, 24077-24079
Ulnar Neuroplasty, 64718
Unlisted Services and Procedures, 24999
X–ray, 73070, 73080
  with Contrast, 73085

Elbow, Golfer, 24357-24359
Elbow, Tennis, 24357-24359
Electric Countershock
  See Cardioversion
Electric Modulation Pain Reprocessing
  Transcutaneous, 0278T
Electrical Stimulation
  Acupuncture, 97813-97814
  Bone Healing
    Invasive, 20975
    Noninvasive, 20974
  Brain Surface, 95961, 95962
  Cardiac, 93623
    Induction of Arrhythmia, 93618
  Guidance
    Chemodenervation, 95873
  Physical Therapy
    Attended, Manual, 97032
    Unattended, 97014
  Spine, 63650, 63655, 63661-63664, 63685, 63688
Electrocardiogram, 93000-93010
  64-Lead or Greater, 93799
  See Electrocardiography
  External, 0295T-0298T, 93224-93272
  Rhythm Strips, 93040-93042
    Interpretation and Report Only, 93042
    Tracing Only Without Interpretation and Report, 93041
    with Interpretation and Report, 93040
  Routine 12-Lead, 93000-93010
  Signal-Averaged, 93278
Electrocardiography
  12-Lead ECG, 3120F, 93000
  24–hour Monitoring, 93224-93272
  48 Hours up to 21 Days, 0295T-0298T
  64 Leads or Greater, 93799
  Evaluation, 93000, 93010
  Event Monitors, 93268-93272
  External Recording
    24 Hour Attended Monitoring, 0497T-0498T
    in-office Connection, 0497T
    Review and Interpretation, 0498T
    48-Hours Duration, 93224-93229
    Auto Activated, 93268, 93270-93272
    Interpretation, 0295T, 0298T, 93272
    Mobile
      Greater than 24 Hours, 93228-93229
      Patient Activated, 93268, 93270-93272

Electrocardiography — continued

External Recording — continued
  Transmission and Evaluation, 93268, 93270-93271
  Up to 30 Days Download, 93268, 93270-93272
Holter Monitors, 93224-93227
Microvolt T-Wave Alternans, 93025
Mobile Telemetry, 93228-93229
Monitoring
  with Attended Surveillance
    Cardiovascular Telemetry with Physician Review and Report, 93228
    Technical Support, 93229
  Recording, 93224-93272
  Rhythm, 93040
    1-3 Leads, 93040
    Evaluation, 93042
    Interpretation and Report Only, 93042
    Microvolt T-Wave Alternans, 93025
    Recording, 0295T-0296T
    Scanning Analysis with Report, 0295T, 0297T
    Tracing and Evaluation, 93040
    Tracing Only without Interpretation and Report, 93005, 93041
  Routine; at Least 12 Leads, 93000-93010
    Interpretation and Report Only, 93010
    Tracing Only, without Interpretation and Report, 93005
    with Interpretation and Report, 93000
  Signal Averaged, 93278
  Symptom-Related Memory Loop, 93268, 93270-93272
  Tracing, 93005
Electrocautery, 17000-17286
  See Destruction
  Inferior Turbinates, 30801-30802
  Prostate Resection, 52601
  Ureteral Stricture, 52341-52346
Electrochemistry
  See Electrolysis
Electroconvulsive Therapy, 90870
Electrocorticogram, 95836
  Intraoperative, 61536, 61538, 95829
Electrode
  Array
    Intracranial, 61850-61868, 61885-61886, 64568-64570
    Peripheral Nerve, 64555, 64575
    Retinal, 0100T
    Spinal, 63650-63655
  Depth Electrode Implantation, 61760
Electrodesiccation, 17000-17286
  Lesion
    Penis, 54055
Electroejaculation, 55870
Electroencephalography (EEG)
  Brain Death, 95824
  Coma, 95822
  Digital Analysis, 95957
  Electrode Placement, 95830
  Intraoperative, 95955
  Monitoring, 95812, 95813
    Long Term Set Up, [95706, 95707], [95709, 95710], [95712, 95713], [95715, 95716]
    with Drug Activation, 95954
    with Physical Activation, 95954
    with WADA Activation, 95958
  Sleep, 95819, 95822, [95706, 95707], [95712, 95713], [95715, 95716], [95719, 95720, 95721, 95722, 95723, 95724, 95725, 95726]
  Standard, 95816, 95819
Electrogastrography, 91132, 91133
Electrogram, Atrial
  Esophageal Recording, 93615, 93616
Electro–Hydraulic Procedure, 52325
Electrolysis, 17380
Electromyographs
  See Electromyography, Needle
Electromyography
  Anus
    Biofeedback, 90912-90913

Electromyography — continued

Extremity, 95860-95872 [95885, 95886]
Fine Wire, 96004
  Dynamic, 96004
Guidance
  Chemodenervation, 95874
Hemidiaphragm, 95866
Larynx, 95865
Needle
  Extremities, 95861-95872 [95885, 95886, 95887]
  Extremity, 95860
  Face and Neck Muscles, 95867, 95868
  Guidance
    Chemodenervation, 64617, 95874
  Hemidiaphragm, 95866
  Larynx, 95865
  Muscle Supplied by Cranial Nerve, 95867-95868
  Non-extremity, [95887]
  Ocular, 92265
  Other than Thoracic Paraspinal, 95870
  Single Fiber Electrode, 95872
  Thoracic Paraspinal Muscles, 95869
  Nonextremity, [95887]
Rectum
  Biofeedback, 90912-90913
Sphincter Muscles
  Anus, 51784-51785
  Needle, 51785
  Urethra, 51784, 51785
  Needle, 51785
Surface
  Dynamic, 96002-96004
Electron Microscopy, 88348
Electronic Analysis
  Cardiac Rhythm Monitor System, 93285, 93290-93291, 93297-93298
    Data Analysis, 93291, 93297-93298
    Evaluation of Programming, 93285, 93291, 93297-93298
  Cardioverter–Defibrillator
    Evaluation
      in Person, 0575T-0576T, 93289, 93640, 93642
      Remote, 0578T-0579T, 93295-93296
      with Reprogramming, 93282-93284, 93287, 93642, 93644
      without Reprogramming, 93289, 93292, 93295, 93640-93641
  Data Analysis, 93289
  Defibrillator, 93282, 93289, 93292, 93295
  Drug Infusion Pump, 62367-62370, 95990-95991
  Neurostimulator Pulse Generator, 0589T-0590T, 95970-95982 [95983, 95984]
  Pulse Generator, 0589T-0590T, 95970-95982 [95983, 95984]
    Field Stimulation, 64999
    Gastric Neurostimulator, 95980-95982
Electro–oculography, 92270
Electrophoresis
  Hemoglobin, 83020
  High Resolution, 83701
  Immuno–, 86320-86327
  Immunofixation, 86334-86335
  Protein, 84165-84166
  Unlisted Services and Procedures, 82664
Electrophysiology Procedure, 93600-93660
Electroretinography, 0509T, 92273-92274
Electrostimulation, Analgesic Cutaneous
  See Application, Neurostimulation
Electrosurgery
  Anal, 46924
  Penile, 54065
  Rectal Tumor, 45190
  Skin Lesion, 17000-17111, 17260-17286
  Skin Tags, 11200-11201
  Trichiasis
    Correction, 67825
  Vaginal, 57061, 57065
  Vulva, 56501, 56515
Electroversion, Cardiac
  See Cardioversion

Elevation, Scapula, Congenital

See Sprengel's Deformity
Elliot Operation, 66130
  Excision, Lesion, Sclera, 66130
Eloesser Procedure, 32035, 32036
Eloesser Thoracoplasty, 32905
Embolectomy
  Aortoiliac Artery, 34151, 34201
  Axillary Artery, 34101
  Brachial Artery, 34101
  Carotid Artery, 34001
  Celiac Artery, 34151
  Femoral, 34201
  Iliac, 34151, 34201
  Innominate Artery, 34001-34101
  Mesentery Artery, 34151
  Peroneal Artery, 34203
  Popliteal Artery, 34201, 34203
  Pulmonary Artery, 33910-33916
  Radial Artery, 34111
  Renal Artery, 34151
  Subclavian Artery, 34001-34101
  Tibial Artery, 34203
  Ulnar Artery, 34111
Embolization
  Arterial (not hemorrhage or tumor), 37242
  Hemorrhage
    Arterial, 37244
    Venous, 37244
  Infarction, 37243
  Leiomyomata, 37243
  Lymphatic Extravasation, 37244
  Organ Ischemia, 37243
  Tumors, 37243
  Ureter, 50705
  Venous Malformations, 37241
Embryo
  Biopsy, 89290, 89291
  Carcinoembryonic Antigen, 82378
  Cryopreservation, 89258
  Cryopreserved
    Preparation/Thawing, 89352
  Culture, 89250
    Extended Culture, 89272
    with Co–Culture Oocyte, 89251
  Hatching
    Assisted Microtechnique, 89253
  Preparation for Transfer, 89255
  Storage, 89342
Embryo Implantation
  See Implantation
Embryo Transfer
  In Vitro Fertilization, 58970, 58974, 58976
    Intrafallopian Transfer, 58976
    Intrauterine Transfer, 58974
    Preparation for Transfer, 89255
Embryo/Fetus Monitoring
  See Monitoring, Fetal
Embryonated Eggs
  Inoculation, 87250
EMD, 81404-81405
Emergency Department Services, 99281-99288
  See Critical Care; Emergency Department
  Anesthesia, 99140
    in Office, 99058
  Physician Direction of Advanced Life Support, 99288
Emesis Induction, 99175
EMG (Electromyography, Needle), 51784, 51785, 92265, 95860-95872 [95885, 95886, 95887]
EMI Scan
  See CT Scan
Emission Computerized Tomography, 78803
Emission Computerized Tomography, Single–Photon
  See also SPECT
EML4/ALK, 81401
Emmet Operation, 57720
Empyema
  Closure
    Chest Wall, 32810
  Empyemectomy, 32540
  Enucleation, 32540
  Thoracostomy, 32035, 32036, 32551
Empyemectomy, 32540
EMS, 99288

Encephalitis
Antibody, 86651-86654
Encephalitis Virus Vaccine, 90738
Encephalocele
Repair, 62120
Craniotomy, 62121
Encephalography, A–Mode, 76506
Encephalon
See Brain
End Stage Renal Disease Services, 90951-90962, 90967-90970
Home, 90963-90966
Endarterectomy
Coronary Artery, 33572
Anomaly, 33500-33507
Pulmonary, 33916
Endemic Flea–Borne Typhus
See Murine Typhus
End–Expiratory Pressure, Positive
See Pressure Breathing, Positive
Endobronchial Challenge Tests
See Bronchial Challenge Test
Endocavitary Fulguration
See Electrocautery
Endocrine, Pancreas
See Islet Cell
Endocrine System
Unlisted Services and Procedures, 60699, 78099
Endocrinology (Type 2 Diabetes) Biochemical Assays, 81506
Endograft
Aorta, 34701-34706
Iliac Artery, 34707-34711
Infrarenal Artery, 34701-34706
Endolaser Photocoagulation
Focal, 67039
Panretinal, 67040
Endoluminal Imaging, [92978, 92979]
Endolymphatic Sac
Exploration
with Shunt, 69806
without Shunt, 69805
Endometrial Ablation, 0404T, 58353, 58356, 58563
Curettage, 58356
Exploration via Hysteroscopy, 58563
Endometrioma
Abdomen
Destruction, 49203-49205
Excision, 49203-49205
Mesenteric
Destruction, 49203-49205
Excision, 49203-49205
Peritoneal
Destruction, 49203-49205
Excision, 49203-49205
Retroperitoneal
Destruction, 49203-49205
Excision, 49203-49205
Endometriosis, Adhesive
See Adhesions, Intrauterine
Endometrium
Ablation, 0404T, 58353, 58356, 58563
Biopsy, 58100, 58110, 58558
Curettage, 58356
Endomyocardial
Biopsy, 93505
Endonuclease, DNA
See DNAse
Endopyelotomy, 50575
Endorectal Pull–Through
Proctectomy, Total, 45110, 45112, 45120, 45121
Endoscopic Retrograde Cannulation of Pancreatic Duct (ERCP)
See Cholangiopancreatography
Endoscopic Retrograde Cholangiopancreatography
Ablation Lesion/Polyp/Tumor, [43278]
Balloon Dilation, [43277]
Destruction of Calculi, 43265
Diagnostic, 43260
Measure Pressure Sphincter of Oddi, 43263
Placement
Stent, [43274]

Endoscopic Retrograde Cholangiopancreatography — *continued*
Placement — *continued*
Stent — *continued*
with Removal and Replacement, [43276]
Removal
Calculi or Debris, 43264
Foreign Body, [43275]
Stent, [43275]
with Stent Exchange, [43276]
Removal Calculi or Debris, 43264
with Optical Endomicroscopy, 0397T
Endoscopies, Pleural
See Thoracoscopy
Endoscopy
See Arthroscopy; Thoracoscopy
Adrenal Gland
Biopsy, 60650
Excision, 60650
Anal
Ablation
Polyp, 46615
Tumor, 46615
Biopsy, 46606, 46607
Collection of Specimen, 46600-46601
Diagnostic, 46600-46601
Dilation, 46604
Exploration, 46600
Hemorrhage, 46614
High Resolution, 46601, 46607
Removal
Foreign Body, 46608
Polyp, 46610, 46612
Tumor, 46610, 46612
Atria, 33265-33266
Bile Duct
Biopsy, 47553
Cannulation, 43273
Catheterization, 74328, 74330
Destruction
Calculi (Stone), 43265
Tumor, [43278]
Diagnostic, 47552
Dilation, 47555, 47556, [43277]
Exchange
Stent, [43276]
Exploration, 47552
Intraoperative, 47550
Percutaneous, 47552-47556
Removal
Calculi (Stone), 43264, 47554
Foreign Body, [43275]
Stent, [43275]
Specimen Collection, 43260
Sphincter Pressure, 43263
Sphincterotomy, 43262, [43274]
Stent Placement, [43274]
Bladder
Biopsy, 52204, 52250, 52354
Catheterization, 52005, 52010
Destruction, 52354
Lesion, 52400
Polyps, 52285
with Fulguration, 52214
Diagnostic, 52000
Dilation, 52260, 52265
Evacuation
Clot, 52001
Excision
Tumor, 52355
Exploration, 52351
Insertion
Radioactive Substance, 52250
Stent, 52282, 53855
Instillation, 52010
Irrigation, 52010
Lesion, 52224, 52234-52235, 52240, 52400
Litholapaxy, 52317-52318
Lithotripsy, 52353
Neck, 51715
Removal
Calculus, 52310, 52315, 52352
Urethral Stent, 52310, 52315

Endoscopy — *continued*
Bladder Neck
Injection of Implant Material, 51715
Brain
Catheterization, 62160
Dissection
Adhesions, 62161
Cyst, 62162
Drainage, 62162
Excision
Brain Tumor, 62164
Cyst, 62162
Pituitary Tumor, 62165
Removal Foreign Body, 62163
Shunt Creation, 62201
Bronchi
Aspiration, 31645-31646
Biopsy, 31625, 31632, 31633
Computer-assisted Image Guidance, 31627
Destruction
Lesion, 31641, 96570-96571
Tumor, 31641, 96570-96571
Dilation, 31630-31631, 31636-31638
Excision Tumor, 31640
Exploration, 31622
Lavage, 31624
Lesion, 31641
Destruction, 31641, 96570-96571
Needle Biopsy, 31629, 31633
Occlusion, 31634
Placement
Fiducial Marker, 31626
Radioelement Catheter, 31643
Stent, 31631, 31636-31637
Removal
Foreign Body, 31635
Revision
Stent, 31638
Specimen Collection, 31623-31624
Stenosis, 31641
Tracheobronchoscopy, 31615
Tumor
Destruction, 31641, 96570-96571
Ultrasound
Destruction, 31641
Excision, 31640
Cannulization
Papilla, 43273
Capsule, 91111
Cervix
Biopsy, 57421, 57454, 57455, 57460
Curettage, 57454, 57456
Exploration, 57452
Loop Electrode Biopsy, 57460
Loop Electrode Conization, 57461
Chest Cavity
Diagnostic, 32601-32604
Exploration, 32601-32606
Surgical, 32650-32674
with Biopsy, 32607-32609
Colon
Ablation, [44401], [45388]
Band Ligation, [45398]
Biopsy, 44389, 44407, 45380, 45392
Collection of Specimen, 44388, 45378
Decompression, 44408, 45393
Destruction
Lesion, [44401], [45388]
Tumor, [44401], [45388]
Dilation, 44405, 45386
Exploration, 44388, 45378
Hemorrhage, 44391, 45382
Injection, Submucosal, 44404, 45381
Placement
Stent, 44402, 45389
Removal
Foreign Body, 44390, 45379
Polyp, 44392, 44394, 45384-45385
Tumor, 44392, 44394, 45384-45385
Ultrasound, 44406-44407, 45391-45392
via Colotomy, [45399]
via Stoma (Colostomy), 44388-44408 [44401]
Virtual, 74261-74263

Endoscopy — *continued*
Colon–Sigmoid
Ablation
Polyp, [45346]
Tumor, [45346]
Biopsy, 45331
Dilation, 45340
Exploration, 45330
Specimen Collection, 45331
Hemorrhage, 45334
Injection, 45335
Needle Biopsy, 45342
Placement
Stent, 45327, 45347
Removal
Foreign Body, 45332
Polyp, 45333, 45338
Tumor, 45333, 45338
Specimen Collection, 45330
Ultrasound, 45341, 45342
Volvulus, 45321, 45337
Duodenum Ultrasound, 43253
Endomicroscopy
Esophageal, 43206
Gastrointestinal, 43252
Esophagus
Biopsy, 43193, 43198, 43202
Dilation, 43195-43196, 43220, 43220 [43212, 43213, 43214], 43226, 43229, 43248-43249 [43233], [43233]
Exploration, 43191, 43197, 43200
Hemorrhage, 43227
Injection, 43192, 43201, 43204
Varices, 43243
Insertion Stent, [43212]
Mucosal Resection, [43211]
Needle Biopsy, 43232
Removal
Foreign Body, 43194, 43215
Polyp, 43216-43217, 43229
Tumor, 43216-43217, 43229
Specimen Collection, 43197, 43200
Ultrasound, 43231-43232, 43237-43238, 43242, 43253
Vein Ligation, 43205
with Optical Endomicroscopy, 43206
Eye, 66990
Foot
Plantar Fasciotomy, 29893
Gastrointestinal
Ablation
Lesion, [43270]
Photodynamic Therapy, 96570-96571
Polyp, [43270]
Tumor, [43270]
Capsule, 91110-91111
Upper
Biopsy, 43239
Catheterization, 43241
Destruction of Lesion, [43270]
Dilation, 43245, 43248, 43249, [43233]
Drainage of Pseudocyst, 43240
Exploration, 43235, 43252
Foreign Body, 43247
Gastric Bypass, 43644-43645
Gastroenterostomy, 43644-43645
Hemorrhage, 43255
Inject Varices, 43243
Injection, 43236, 43253
Mucosal Resection, 43254
Needle Biopsy, 43232, 43238, 43242
Performance Measures, 3130F-3132F, 3140F-3141F
Referral, 3132F
Removal, 43247, 43250, 43251
Roux–En–Y, 43644
Stent Placement, [43266]
Thermal Radiation, 43257
Tube Placement, 43246
Ultrasound, 43237-43242, 43253, 43259, 76975
Vein Ligation, 43244

 [Resequenced]

Evaluation and Management — *continued*
  Health Behavior — *continued*
    Group Intervention, 0403T, [96164, 96165]
    Individual Intervention, 96158-96159
    Re–assessment, 96156
  Home Services, 99341-99350
  Hospital, 99221-99233
  Hospital Discharge, 99238, 99239
  Hospital Services
    Initial, 99221-99233, 99460-99463, 99477
    Intensive Care
      Low Birth Weight, 99478-99480
      Neonate, 99477
    Observation Care, 99217-99220
    Subsequent, 99231, 99462-99463
  Insurance Examination, 99455-99456
  Internet Communication
    Consult Physician, 99446-99449, [99451]
    Nonphysician, 98970-98972
    Physician, [99421, 99422, 99423]
    Referral, [99452]
  Low Birth Weight Infant, 99468-99469, 99478-99480
  Medical
    Team Conference, 99366-99368
  Neonatal
    Critical Care, 99468-99469
    Intensive Observation, 99477-99480
  Newborn Care, 99460-99465
  Nursing Facility, 99304-99318
    Annual Assessment, 99318
    Discharge, 99315-99316
    Initial Care, 99304-99306
    Subsequent Care, 99307-99310
  Observation Care, 99217-99220
  Occupation Therapy Evaluation, [97165, 97166, 97167]
    Re–evaluation, 97168
  Office and Other Outpatient, 99201-99215
  Online Assessment
    Consult Physician, 99446-99449, [99451]
    Nonphysician, 98970-98972
    Physician, [99421, 99422, 99423]
    Referral, [99452]
  Online Evaluation
    Consult Physician, 99446-99449, [99451]
    Nonphysician, 98970-98972
    Physician, [99421, 99422, 99423]
    Referral, [99452]
  Pediatric
    Critical Care, 99471-99472
    Interfacility Transport, 99466-99467
  Physical Therapy Evaluation, [97161, 97162, 97163]
    Re–evaluation, 97164
  Physician Standby Services, 99360
  Preventive Services, 4000F-4001F, 99381-99429
  Prolonged Services, 99356, 99357
  Psychiatric/Records or Reports, 90885
  Smoking and Tobacco Cessation Counseling, 99406-99407
  Team Conference, 99366-99368
  Telephone Assessment
    Consult Physician, 99446-99449, [99451]
    Nonphysician, 98966-98968
    Physician, 99441-99443
    Referral, [99452]
  Unlisted Service and Procedures, 99499
  Work–Related and/or Medical Disability Evaluation, 99455
Evaluation Studies, Drug, Preclinical
  See Drug Screen
EVAR (Endovascular Aortic Repair), 34701-34713
Everolimus
  Assay, 80169
Evisceration
  Ocular Contents
    with Implant, 65093
    without Implant, 65091
  Repair
    Abdominal Wall, 49900
  Suture
    Abdominal Wall, 49900

Evisceration, Pelvic
  See Exenteration, Pelvis
Evocative/Suppression Test, 80400-80439
  Stimulation Panel, 80410
Evoked Potential
  See Audiologic Function Tests
  Auditory Brainstem, 92585, 92586
  Central Motor
    Transcranial Motor Stimulation, 95928-95929
  Somatosensory Testing, 95925-95927 [95938]
  Visual, CNS, 95930
Ewart Procedure
  Palate, Reconstruction, Lengthening, 42226, 42227
EWSR1/ATF1 (t(12;22)), 81401
EWSR1/ERG (t(21;22)), 81401
EWSR1/FLI1 (t(11;22)), 81401
EWSR1/WT1 (t(11;22)), 81401
Ex Vivo Organ Perfusion System
  Cadaver Donor Lung(s)
    Surgical Preparation and Cannulation, 0494T
Examination
  Anorectal, 45990
  Involved Joint, 2004F
Excavatum, Pectus
  See Pectus Excavatum
Exchange
  Blood, 36450-36455
  Blood Components, 36511-36516
  Drainage Catheter
    under Radiologic Guidance, 49423
  External Fixation, 20697
  Intraocular Lens, 66986
Excision
  See Also Debridement; Destruction
  Abscess
    Brain, 61514, 61522
    Olecranon Process, 24138
    Radius, 24136
    Ulna, 24138
  Acromion, 23130
    Shoulder, 23130
  Adenoids
    Primary
      12 or over, 42831
      Younger Than Age 12, 42830
    Secondary
      12 or over, 42836
      Younger Than Age 12, 42835
    with Tonsils, 42820, 42821
  Adenoma
    Thyroid Gland, 60200
  Adrenal Gland, 60540
    Laparoscopic, 60650
    with Excision Retroperitoneal Tumor, 60545
  Alveolus, 41830
  Anal
    Crypt, 46999
    Fissure, 46200
    Tag, 46230 [46220]
  Aorta
    Coarctation, 33840-33851
  Appendix, 44950-44960
  Arteriovenous Malformation
    Spinal, 63250-63252
  Arytenoid Cartilage, 31400
    Endoscopic, 31560, 31561
  Atrial Septum, 33735-33737
  Bartholin's gland, 56740
  Bladder
    Diverticulum, 51525
    Neck, 51520
    Partial, 51550-51565
    Total, 51570, 51580, 51590-51597
      with Nodes, 51575, 51585, 51595
    Transurethral, 52640
    Tumor, 51530
  Bladder Neck Contracture, Postoperative, 52640
  Bone
    Abscess
      Facial, 21026
      Mandible, 21025

Excision — *continued*
  Bone — *continued*
    Facial, 21026
    Femur, 20150
    Fibula, 20150
    Mandible, 21025
    Radius, 20150
    Tibia, 20150
    Ulna, 20150
  Brain
    Amygdala, 61566
    Epileptogenic Focus, 61536
    Hemisphere, 61543
    Hippocampus, 61566
    Other Lobe, 61323, 61539-61540
    Temporal Lobe, 61537, 61538
  Brain Lobe
    See Lobectomy, Brain
  Breast
    Biopsy, 19100-19101
    Chest Wall Tumor, 21601-21603
    Cyst, 19120-19126
    Lactiferous Duct Fistula, 19112
    Lesion, 19120-19126
      by Needle Localization, 19125, 19126
    Mastectomy, 19300-19307
    Nipple Exploration, 19110
  Bulbourethral Gland, 53250
  Bullae
    Lung, 32141
      Endoscopic, 32655
  Burns, 15002-15003, 15004-15005
  Bursa
    Elbow, 24105
    Excision, 27060
    Femur, 27062
    Ischial, 27060
    Knee, 27340
    Wrist, 25115, 25116
  Bypass Graft, 35901-35907
  Calcaneus, 28118-28120
  Calculi (Stone)
    Parotid Gland, 42330, 42340
    Salivary Gland, 42330-42340
    Sublingual Gland, 42330, 42335
    Submandibular Gland, 42330, 42335
  Carotid Artery, 60605
  Carpal, 25145, 25210, 25215
  Cartilage
    Knee Joint, 27332, 27333
    Shoulder Joint, 23101
    Temporomandibular Joint, 21060
    Wrist, 25107
  Caruncle, Urethra, 53265
  Cataract
    Secondary, 66830
  Cervix
    Electrode, 57460
    Radical, 57531
    Stump
      Abdominal Approach, 57540, 57545
      Vaginal Approach, 57550-57556
    Total, 57530
  Chalazion
    Multiple
      Different Lids, 67805
      Same Lid, 67801
    Single, 67800
    with Anesthesia, 67808
  Chest Wall Tumor, 21601-21603
  Choroid Plexus, 61544
  Clavicle
    Partial, 23120, 23180
    Sequestrectomy, 23170
    Total, 23125
    Tumor
      Radical Resection, 23200
  Coccyx, 27080
  Colon
    Excision
      Partial, 44140-44147, 44160
        with Anastomosis, 44140
      Total, 44150-44156

Excision — *continued*
  Colon — *continued*
    Laparoscopic
      with Anastomosis, 44204, 44207-44208
      with Colostomy, 44206, 44208
      with Ileocolostomy, 44205
  Condyle
    Temporomandibular Joint, 21050
  Condylectomy, 21050
  Constricting Ring
    Finger, 26596
  Cornea
    Epithelium, 65435
      with Chelating Agent, 65436
    Scraping, 65430
  Coronoidectomy, 21070
  Cowper's gland, 53250
  Cranial Bone
    Tumor, 61563, 61564
  Cyst
    See Ganglion Cyst
    Bile Duct, 47715
    Bladder, 51500
    Brain, 61516, 61524, 62162
    Branchial, 42810, 42815
    Breast, 19120
    Calcaneus, 28100-28103
    Carpal, 25130-25136
    Cheekbone, 21030
    Clavicle, 23140
      with Allograft, 23146
      with Autograft, 23145
    Facial Bone, 21030
    Femur, 27065-27067, 27355-27358
    Fibula, 27635-27638
    Finger, 26034, 26160
    Foot, 28090
    Hand, 26160
    Hip, 27065-27067
    Humerus, 23150, 24110
      with Allograft, 23156, 24116
      with Autograft, 23155, 24115
    Ileum, 27065-27067
    Intra-abdominal, 49203-49205
    Kidney, 50280, 50290
    Knee, 27345, 27347
    Lung, 32140
    Mandible, 21040, 21046-21047
    Maxilla, 21030, 21048-21049
    Mediastinum, 32662
    Metacarpal, 26200, 26205
    Metatarsal, 28104-28107
    Mullerian Duct, 55680
    Nose, 30124-30125
    Olecranon (Process), 24120
      with Allograft, 24126
      with Autograft, 24125
    Ovarian, 58925
      See Cystectomy, Ovarian
    Pericardial, 33050
      Endoscopic, 32661
    Phalanges
      Finger, 26210, 26215
      Toe, 28108
    Pilonidal, 11770-11772
    Pubis, 27066, 27067
    Radius, 24120, 25120-25126
      with Allograft, 24126
      with Autograft, 24125
    Salivary Gland, 42408
    Scapula, 23140
      with Allograft, 23146
      with Autograft, 23145
    Seminal Vesicle, 55680
    Sublingual Gland, 42408
    Talus, 28100-28103
    Tarsal, 28104-28107
    Thyroglossal Duct, 60280, 60281
    Thyroid Gland, 60200
    Tibia, 27635-27638
    Toe, 28092
    Ulna, 24120, 25120
      with Allograft, 24126
      with Autograft, 24125

Excision — *continued*
    Cyst — *continued*
        Urachal
            Bladder, 51500
        Vaginal, 57135
    Destruction of the Vestibule of the Mouth
        See Mouth, Vestibule of, Excision, Destruction
    Diverticulum, Meckel's
        See Meckel's Diverticulum, Excision
    Ear, External
        Partial, 69110
        Total, 69120
    Elbow Joint, 24155
    Electrode, 57522
    Embolectomy/Thrombectomy
        Aortoiliac Artery, 34151, 34201
        Axillary Artery, 34101
        Brachial Artery, 34101
        Carotid Artery, 34001
        Celiac Artery, 34151
        Femoral Artery, 34201
        Heart, 33310-33315
        Iliac Artery, 34151, 34201
        Innominate Artery, 34001-34101
        Mesentery Artery, 34151
        Peroneal Artery, 34203
        Popliteal Artery, 34203
        Radial Artery, 34111
        Renal Artery, 34151
        Subclavian Artery, 34001-34101
        Tibial Artery, 34203
        Ulnar Artery, 34111
    Embolism
        Pulmonary Artery, 33910-33916
    Empyema
        Lung, 32540
        Pleural, 32540
    Endometriomas
        Intra-abdominal, 49203-49205
    Epididymis
        Bilateral, 54861
        Unilateral, 54860
    Epiglottis, 31420
    Epikeratoplasty, 65767
    Epiphyseal Bar, 20150
    Esophagus
        Diverticulum, 43130, 43135
        Partial, 43116-43124
        Total, 43107-43113, 43124
    Excess Skin
        Abdomen, 15830
    Eye
        See Enucleation, Eye
    Fallopian Tubes
        Salpingectomy, 58700
        Salpingo–Oophorectomy, 58720
    Fascia
        See Fasciectomy
    Femur, 27360
        Partial, 27070, 27071
    Fibula, 27360, 27455, 27457, 27641
    Fistula
        Anal, 46270-46285
    Foot
        Fasciectomy, 28060
        Radical, 28062
    Gallbladder
        Open, 47600-47620
        via Laparoscopy
            Cholecystectomy, 47562
                with Cholangiography, 47563
                with Exploration Common Duct, 47564
    Ganglion Cyst
        Knee, 27347
        Wrist, 25111, 25112
    Gingiva, 41820
    Gums, 41820
        Alveolus, 41830
        Operculum, 41821
    Heart
        Donor, 33940
    Lung
        Donor, 33930
    Hemangioma, 11400-11446

Excision — *continued*
    Hemorrhoids, 46221, 46250
        Clot, *[46320]*
        Complex, 46260-46262
        Simple, 46255
        with Fissurectomy, 46257, 46258
    Hip
        Partial, 27070, 27071
    Hippocampus, 61566
    Humeral Head
        Resection, 23195
        Sequestrectomy, 23174
    Humerus, 23184, 23220, 24134, 24140, 24150
    Hydrocele
        Spermatic Cord, 55500
        Tunica Vaginalis, 55040, 55041
            Bilateral, 55041
            Unilateral, 55040
    Hygroma, Cystic
        Axillary
            Cervical, 38550, 38555
    Hymenotomy, 56700
        See Hymen, Excision
    Ileum
        Ileoanal Reservoir, 45136
        Partial, 27070, 27071
    Inner Ear
        See Ear, Inner, Excision
    Interphalangeal Joint
        Toe, 28160
    Intervertebral Disc
        Decompression, 62380, 63075-63078
        Hemilaminectomy, 63040, 63043, 63044
        Herniated, 62380, 63020-63044, 63055-63066
    Intestine
        Laparoscopic
            with Anastomosis, 44202, 44203
    Intestines
        Donor, 44132, 44133
    Intestines, Small, 44120-44128
        Transplantation, 44137
    Iris
        Iridectomy
            Optical, 66635
            Peripheral, 66625
            Sector, 66630
            with Corneoscleral or Corneal Section, 66600
            with Cyclectomy, 66605
    Kidney
        Donor, 50300, 50320, 50547
        Partial, 50240
        Recipient, 50340
        Transplantation, 50370
        with Ureters, 50220-50236
    Kneecap, 27350
    Labyrinth
        Transcanal, 69905
        with Mastoidectomy, 69910
    Lacrimal Gland
        Partial, 68505
        Total, 68500
    Lacrimal Sac, 68520
    Laparoscopy
        Adrenalectomy, 60650
    Larynx
        Endoscopic, 31545-31546
        Partial, 31367-31382
        Total, 31360-31365
        with Pharynx, 31390, 31395
    Leg, 27630
    Leg, Lower, 27630
    Lesion
        Anal, 45108, 46922
        Ankle, 27630
            Arthroscopic, 29891
        Arm, 25110
        Arthroscopic
            Ankle, 29891
            Talus, 29891
            Tibia, 29891
        Auditory Canal, External
            Exostosis, 69140
            Radical with Neck Dissection, 69155

Excision — *continued*
    Lesion — *continued*
        Auditory Canal, External — *continued*
            Radical without Neck Dissection, 69150
            Soft Tissue, 69145
        Bladder, 52224
        Brain, 61534, 61536-61540
        Brainstem, 61575, 61576
        Carotid Body, 60600, 60605
        Colon, 44110, 44111
        Conjunctiva, 68110-68130
            over One Centimeter, 68115
            with Adjacent Sclera, 68130
        Cornea, 65400
            without Graft, 65420
        Ear, Middle, 69540
        Epididymis
            Local, 54830
            Spermatocele, 54840
        Esophagus, 43100, 43101
        Eye, 65900
        Eyelid
            Multiple, Different Lids, 67805
            Multiple, Same Lid, 67801
            Single, 67800
            under Anesthesia, 67808
            without Closure, 67840
        Femur, 27062
        Finger, 26160
        Foot, 28080, 28090
        Gums, 41822-41828
        Hand, 26160
        Intestines, 44110
            Small, 43250, 44111
        Intraspinal, 63265-63273
        Knee, 27347
        Larynx
            Endoscopic, 31545-31546
        Meniscus, 27347
        Mesentery, 44820
        Mouth, 40810-40816, 41116
        Nerve, 64774-64792
        Neuroma, 64778
        Orbit, 61333
            Lateral Approach, 67420
            Removal, 67412
        Palate, 42104-42120
        Pancreas, 48120
        Penis, 54060
            Plaque, 54110-54112
        Pharynx, 42808
        Rectum, 45108
        Sclera, 66130
        Skin
            Benign, 11400-11471
            Malignant, 11600-11646
        Skull, 61500, 61615-61616
        Spermatic Cord, 55520
        Spinal Cord, 63300-63308
        Stomach, 43611
        Talus
            Arthroscopic, 29891
        Tendon Sheath
            Arm, 25110
            Foot, 28090
            Hand/Finger, 26160
            Leg/Ankle, 27630
            Wrist, 25110
        Testis, 54512
        Tibia
            Arthroscopic, 29891
        Toe, 28092
        Tongue, 41110-41114
        Urethra, 52224, 53265
        Uterus
            Leiomyomata, 58140, 58545-58546, 58561
        Uvula, 42104-42107
        Wrist Tendon, 25110
    Lip, 40500-40530
        Frenum, 40819
    Liver
        Allotransplantation, 47135
        Biopsy, wedge, 47100

Excision — *continued*
    Liver — *continued*
        Donor, 47133-47142
        Extensive, 47122
        Lobectomy, total
            Left, 47125
            Right, 47130
        Resection
            Partial, 47120, 47125, 47140-47142
            Total, 47133
        Trisegmentectomy, 47122
    Lung, 32440-32445, 32488
        Bronchus Resection, 32486
        Bullae
            Endoscopic, 32655
        Completion, 32488
        Emphysematous, 32491
        Heart
            Donor, 33930
        Lobe, 32480, 32482
        Pneumonectomy, 32440-32445
        Segment, 32484
        Total, 32440-32445
        Tumor
            with Reconstruction, 32504
            with Resection, 32503
        Wedge Resection, 32505-32507
            Endoscopic, 32666-32668
    Lymph Nodes, 38500, 38510-38530
        Abdominal, 38747
        Axillary, 38740
        Complete, 38745
        Cervical, 38720, 38724
        Cloquet's node, 38760
        Deep
            Axillary, 38525
            Cervical, 38510, 38520
            Mammary, 38530
        Inguinofemoral, 38760, 38765
        Limited, for Staging
            Para–Aortic, 38562
            Pelvic, 38562
            Retroperitoneal, 38564
        Mediastinal, 38746
        Pelvic, 38770
        Peritracheal, 38746
        Radical
            Axillary, 38740, 38745
            Cervical, 38720, 38724
            Suprahyoid, 38700
        Retroperitoneal Transabdominal, 38780
        Superficial
            Needle, 38505
            Open, 38500
        Suprahyoid, 38700
        Thoracic, 38746
    Mandibular, Exostosis, 21031
    Mastoid
        Complete, 69502
        Radical, 69511
            Modified, 69505
            Petrous Apicectomy, 69530
        Simple, 69501
    Maxilla
        Exostosis, 21032
    Maxillary Torus Palatinus, 21032
    Meningioma
        Brain, 61512, 61519
    Meniscectomy
        Temporomandibular Joint, 21060
    Metacarpal, 26230
    Metatarsal, 28110-28114, 28122, 28140
        Condyle, 28288
    Mucosa
        Gums, 41828
        Mouth, 40818
    Mucous Membrane
        Sphenoid Sinus, 31288, *[31257], [31259]*
    Nail Fold, 11765
    Nails, 11750
        Finger, 26236
        Toe, 28124, 28160
    Nasopharynx, 61586, 61600
    Nerve
        Foot, 28055
        Hamstring, 27325

Eye — *continued*
  Photocoagulation — *continued*
    Lesion
      Choroid, 67220
      Cornea, 65450
      Retina, 67210, 67227-67228
      Retinal Detachment, 67105, 67107-67108, 67113, 67145
      Retinopathy, 67228-67229
      Vitrectomy, 67039-67040, 67043
    Photodynamic Therapy Choroidal Lesions, 67221, 67225
  Placement
    Pharmacologic Agent, 68399
    Prosthesis, 21077, 65770, 66982-66985
      Loan, 92358
  Pupillometry, Quantitative, 92499
  Radial Keratotomy, 65771
  Reconstruction
    Amniotic Membrane, 65780
    Conjunctiva, 65782
  Removal
    Blood Clot, 65930
    Bone, 65112
    Foreign Body
      Conjunctival Embedded, 65210
      Conjunctival Superficial, 65205
      Corneal with Slit Lamp, 65222
      Corneal without Slit Lamp, 65220
      Intraocular, 65235-65265
    Implant, 65175
      Anterior Segment, 65920
      Muscles not Attached, 65103
      Posterior Segment, 67120, 67121
  Repair
    Conjunctiva
      by Mobilization and Rearrangement with Hospitalization, 65273
      by Mobilization and Rearrangement without Hospitalization, 65272
      Direct Closure, 65270
    Cornea
      Nonperforating, 65275
      Perforating, 65280, 65285
    Muscles, 65290
    Sclera
      Anterior Segment, 66250
      with Graft, 66225
      with Tissue Glue, 65286
    Trabecular Meshwork, 65855
    Wound
      by Mobilization and Rearrangement, 65272, 65273
      Direct Closure, 65270
  Shunt, Aqueous
    into Subconjunctival Space, 0449T-0450T
    into Supraciliary Space, 0474T
    to Extraocular Reservoir, 66179-66180
  Stem Cell Transplantation, 65781
  Tear Film Imaging, 0330T
  Tear Osmolarity, 83861
  Transluminal Dilation
    Aqueous Outflow Canal, 66174-66175
  Ultrasound, 76510-76514
    Biometry, 76516, 76519
    Foreign Body, 76529
  Unlisted Services and Procedures
    Anterior Segment, 66999
    Posterior Segment, 67299
  X-ray, 70030
Eye Socket
  See Orbit; Orbital Contents; Orbital Floor; Periorbital Region
Eyebrow
  Repair
    Ptosis, 67900
Eyeglasses
  See Spectacle Services
Eyelashes
  Repair Trichiasis
    Epilation
      by Forceps Only, 67820
      by Other than Forceps, 67825
    Incision of Lid Margin, 67830

Eyelashes — *continued*
  Repair Trichiasis — *continued*
    Incision of Lid Margin — *continued*
      with Free Mucous Membrane Graft, 67835
Eyelid
  Abscess
    Incision and Drainage, 67700
  Biopsy, [67810]
  Blepharoplasty, 15820-15823
  Chalazion
    Excision
      Multiple, 67801, 67805
      Single, 67800
      with Anesthesia, 67808
  Closure by Suture, 67875
  Drug-eluting Ocular Insert Placement, 0444T-0445T
  Evacuation
    Meibomian Glands, 0207T, [0563T]
  Incision
    Canthus, 67715
  Injection
    Subconjunctival, 68200
    Sutures, 67710
  Lesion
    Destruction, 67850
    Excision
      Multiple, 67801, 67805
      Single, 67800
      with Anesthesia, 67808
      without Closure, 67840
  Meibomian Glands Evacuation, 0207T, [0563T]
  Placement, Drug-eluting Ocular Insert, 0444T-0445T
  Ptosis, 67901-67908
  Reconstruction
    Canthus, 67950
    Total Eyelid
      Conjunctivo-Tarso-Muller's Muscle-Levator Resection, 67908
      Lower, 67973
        Second Stage, 67975
      Upper, 67974
        Second Stage, 67975
      Full Thickness, 67973-67975
    Transfer of Tarsoconjunctival Flap from Opposing Eyelid, 67971
  Removal
    Foreign Body, 67938
  Repair, 21280, 21282
    Blepharoptosis
      Conjunctivo-Tarso-Muller's Muscle-Levator Resection, 67908
      Frontalis Muscle Technique, 67901-67904
      Reduction Overcorrection of Ptosis, 67909
      Superior Rectus Technique with Fascial Sling, 67906
    Ectropion
      Excision Tarsal Wedge, 67916
      Extensive, 67917
      Suture, 67914
      Thermocauterization, 67915
    Entropion
      Excision Tarsal Wedge, 67923
      Extensive, 67924
      Frontalis Muscle Technique, 67901-67904
      Suture, 67921
      Thermocauterization, 67922
    Excisional, 67961
      over One-Fourth of Lid Margin, 67966
    Lagophthalmos, 67912
    Lashes
      Epilation, by Forceps Only, 67820
      Epilation by Other than Forceps, 67825
      Lid Margin, 67830, 67835
    Wound
      Full Thickness, 67935
      Partial Thickness, 67930

Eyelid — *continued*
  Skin Graft
    Delay of Flap, 15630
    Full Thickness, 15260, 15261, 67961
    Pedicle Flap, 15576
    Split, 15120, 15121, 67961
    Suture, 67880
      with Transposition of Tarsal Plate, 67882
    Tissue Transfer, Adjacent, 14060, 14061, 67961
  Unlisted Services and Procedures, 67999
EYS, 81434
EZH2, 81236-81237

F

F11, 81401
F12, 81403
F13B, 81400
F2, 81240, 81400
F5, 81241, 81400
F7, 81400
F8, 81403, 81406-81407
F9, [81238]
Face
  CT Scan, 70486-70488
  Lesion
    Destruction, 17000-17108, 17280-17286
    Magnetic Resonance Imaging (MRI), 70540-70543
  Skin Graft
    Split, 15120, 15121
  Tumor Resection, 21011-21016
Face Lift, 15824-15828
Facial
  Bone
    Abscess
      Excision, 21026
    Anesthesia, 00190, 00192
    Reconstruction
      Secondary, 21275
    Repair, 21208, 21209
    Tumor
      Excision, 21029, 21030, 21034
      Resection
        Radical, 21015
    X-ray
      Complete, Minimum Three Views, 70150
      Less than Three Views, 70140
      Nasal Bones, 70160
  Nerve
    Anastomosis
      to Hypoglossal Nerve, 64868
      to Spinal Accessory Nerve, 64866
    Avulsion, 64742
    Decompression, 61590, 61596
      Intratemporal
        Lateral to Geniculate Ganglion, 69720, 69740
        Medial to Geniculate Ganglion, 69725, 69745
      Total, 69955
    Function Study, 92516
    Incision, 64742
    Injection
      Anesthetic or Steroid, 64999
    Mobilization, 61590
    Paralysis
      Graft, 15840-15845
      Repair, 15840-15845
    Paralysis Repair, 15840-15845
    Repair
      Lateral to Geniculate Ganglion, 69740
      Medial to Geniculate Ganglion, 69745
      Suture with or without Graft, 64864, 64865
    Suture
      Lateral to Geniculate Ganglion, 69740
      Medial to Geniculate Ganglion, 69745
    Transection, 64742
  Prosthesis, 21088
Facial Asymmetries
  See Hemifacial Microsomia

Facial Rhytidectomy
  See Face Lift
Factor
  ACTH Releasing, 80412
  Antinuclear, 86038-86039
  Blood Coagulation
    I, 85384, 85385
    II, 85210
    III, 85730, 85732
    IV, 82310
    IX, 85250
    V, 85220
    VII, 85230
    VIII, 85244, 85247
    X, 85260
    XI, 85270
    XIII, 85290, 85291
  Fitzgerald, 85293
  Fletcher, 85292
  Hyperglycemic-Glycogenolytic, 82943
  Inhibitor Test, 85335
  Intrinsic, 83528, 86340
  Rheumatoid, 86430-86431
  Sulfation, 84305
FAH, 81406
Fallopian Tube
  Anastomosis, 58750
  Catheterization, 58345, 74742
  Destruction
    Endoscopy, 58670
  Ectopic Pregnancy, 59121
    with Salpingectomy and/or Oophorectomy, 59120
  Excision, 58700, 58720
  Ligation, 58600-58611
  Lysis
    Adhesions, 58740
  Occlusion, 0567T, 58565, 58615
    Endoscopy, 58671
    Sonosalpingography Confirmation, 0568T
  Placement
    Implant for Occlusion, 0567T, 58565, 58615
  Repair, 58752
    Anastomosis, 58750
    Creation of Stoma, 58770
  Tumor
    Resection, 58950, 58952-58956
  Unlisted Procedure, Female Genital System, 58999
  X-ray, 74742
Fallopian Tube Pregnancy
  See Ectopic Pregnancy, Tubal
Fallot, Tetralogy of
  See Tetralogy of Fallot
Familial Dysautonomia Genomic Sequence Analysis, 81412
Familial Hyperinsulinism, 81400
Family Psychotherapy
  See Psychotherapy, Family
Fan Type Procedure, 40525
FANCC, 81242, 81412
Fanconi Anemia, 88248
  Chromosome Analysis, 88248
  Complementation Group C Gene Analysis, 81242
  Genomic Sequence Analysis, 81412, 81443
Farr Test, 82784, 82785
Fasanella-Servat Procedure, 67908
Fascia Graft, 15840
  Free Microvascular Anastomosis, 15758
  Harvesting, 20920, 20922
  Open Treatment, Sternoclavicular Dislocation, 23532
Fascia Lata Graft
  Harvesting, 20920, 20922
Fascial Defect
  Repair, 50728
Fascial Graft
  Free
    Microvascular Anastomosis, 15758
    Open Treatment
      Sternoclavicular Dislocation, 23532
Fasciectomy
  Foot, 28060

Fracture Treatment — *continued*
Phalanges — *continued*
Great Toe — *continued*
Percutaneous Fixation — *continued*
without Manipulation, 28496
Open Treatment, 26735, 26746
Distal, 26765
Shaft
Closed Treatment, 26725
Open Treatment, 26735
Percutaneous Fixation, 26727
Toe
Closed Treatment, 28515
Open Treatment, 28525
with Manipulation, 28515
without Manipulation, 28510
Radius
Closed Treatment, 24650, 24655, 25500, 25505, 25515, 25560, 25565, 25600, 25605
Colles, 25600, 25605
Distal, 25600-25609
Open Treatment, 25607, 25608-25609
Smith, 25600-25605, 25606, 25607, 25609
Head/Neck
Closed Treatment, 24650, 24655
Open Treatment, 24665, 24666
Open Treatment, 25515, 25607, 25608-25609
Percutaneous Fixation, 25606
Shaft, 25500, 25525, 25526
Closed Treatment, 25500, 25505, 25520
Open Treatment, 25515, 25525, 25526, 25574
with Manipulation, 25565, 25605
with Ulna, 25560, 25565
Open Treatment, 25575
without Manipulation, 25560, 25600
Rib
Closed Treatment
See E&M codes
Open Treatment, 21811-21813
Scaphoid
Closed Treatment, 25622
Open Treatment, 25628
with Dislocation
Closed Treatment, 25680
Open Treatment, 25685
with Manipulation, 25624
Scapula
Closed Treatment
with Manipulation, 23575
without Manipulation, 23570
Open Treatment, 23585
Sesamoid
Closed Treatment, 28530
Foot, 28530, 28531
Open Treatment, 28531
Shoulder
Closed Treatment
with Greater Tuberosity Fracture, 23620, 23655
with Surgical or Anatomical Neck Fracture, 23600, 23675
Open Treatment, 23630, 23680
Skin Debridement, 11010-11012
Skull, 62000-62010
Sternum
Closed Treatment, 21820
Open Treatment, 21825
Talus
Closed Treatment, 28430, 28435
Open Treatment, 28445
with Manipulation, 28435, 28436
without Manipulation, 28430
Tarsal
Open Treatment, 28465
Percutaneous Fixation, 28456
with Manipulation, 28455, 28456
without Manipulation, 28450

Fracture Treatment — *continued*
Thigh
Femur
Closed Treatment
with manipulation, 27502, 27503, 27510, 27517
without manipulation, 27500, 27501, 27508, 27516, 27520
Open Treatment, 27506, 27507, 27511, 27513, 27514, 27519, 27524
Percutaneous fixation, 27509
Thumb
Closed Treatment, 26645, 26650
Percutaneous Fixation, 26650
with Dislocation, 26645, 26650
Open Treatment, 26665
Tibia
Arthroscopic Treatment, 29855, 29856
Closed Treatment, 27530, 27532, 27538, 27750, 27752, 27760, 27762, 27808, 27810, 27824, 27825
with Traction, 27532, 27825
Distal, 27824-27828
Intercondylar Spines, 27538, 27540
Malformation, 27810
Malleolus, 27760-27766, 27808-27814
Open Treatment, 27535, 27536, 27540, 27758, 27759, 27766, 27814, 27826-27828
Percutaneous Fixation, 27756
Bimalleolar
Closed Treatment, 27808
with Manipulation, 27810
Open Treatment, 27814
Lateral
Closed Treatment, 27786
with Manipulation, 27788
Open Treatment, 27792
Medial
Closed Treatment, 27760
with Manipulation, 27762
Open Treatment, 27766
Trimalleolar
Closed Treatment, 27816
with Manipulation, 27818
Open Treatment, 27822
with Fixation, 27823
Plateau, 27530-27535, 29855, 29856
Bicondylar, 29856
Unicondylar, 29855
Shaft, 27750-27759
with Manipulation, 27752, 27762, 27825
without Manipulation, 27530, 27750, 27760, 27824
with Manipulation, 27752, 27762, 27810
without Manipulation, 27530, 27750, 27760, 27808, 27825
Tibia and Fibula
Malleolar, 27808-27814
Trachea
Endoscopy Repair, 31630
Turbinate
Therapeutic, 30930
Ulna
See Elbow; Humerus; Radius
Closed Treatment, 25560, 25565
Monteggia type, 24620
of Shaft, 25530, 25535
and Radial, 25560
with Manipulation, 25565
with Manipulation, 25535
Proximal end, 24670
with Manipulation, 24675
Ulnar Styloid, 25650
Olecranon
Closed Treatment, 24670, 24675
with Manipulation, 24675
Open Treatment, 24685

Fracture Treatment — *continued*
Ulna — *continued*
Open Treatment, 25574, 25575
Proximal End, 24685
Radial AND Ulnar Shaft, 25574, 25575
Shaft, 25545
Shaft
Closed Treatment, 25530, 25535
Open Treatment, 25545, 25574
Styloid Process
Closed Treatment, 25650
Open Treatment, 25652
Percutaneous Fixation, 25651
with Dislocation, 24620, 24635
Closed Treatment, 24620
Monteggia, 24620, 24635
Open Treatment, 24635
with Manipulation, 25535, 25565
with Radius, 25560, 25565
Open Treatment, 25574-25575
without Manipulation, 25530
Vertebra
Additional Segment
Open Treatment, 22328
Cervical
Open Treatment, 22326
Closed Treatment
with Manipulation, Casting and/or Bracing, 22315
without Manipulation, 22310
Lumbar
Open Treatment, 22325
Posterior
Open Treatment, 22325-22327
Thoracic
Open Treatment, 22327
Vertebral Process
Closed Treatment
See Evaluation and Management Codes
Wrist
with Dislocation, 25680, 25685
Closed Treatment, 25680
Open Treatment, 25685
Zygomatic Arch
Open Treatment, 21356, 21360-21366
with Manipulation, 21355
Fragile–X
Chromosome Analysis, 88248
Mental Retardation 1 Gene Analysis, 81243-81244
Fragility
Red Blood Cell
Mechanical, 85547
Osmotic, 85555, 85557
Frames, Stereotactic
See Stereotactic Frame
Francisella, 86000
Antibody, 86668
Frataxin, 81284-81286
FRAXE, 81171-81172
Frazier-Spiller Procedure, 61450
Fredet–Ramstedt Procedure, 43520
Free E3
See Estriol
Free Skin Graft
See Skin, Grafts, Free
Free T4
See Thyroxine, Free
Frei Disease
See Lymphogranuloma Venereum
Frenectomy, 40819, 41115
Frenoplasty, 41520
Frenotomy, 40806, 41010
Frenulectomy, 40819
Frenuloplasty, 41520
Frenum
See Lip
Lip
Incision, 40806
Frenumectomy, 40819
Frickman Operation, 45550
Friederich Ataxia, 81284-81286
Frontal Craniotomy, 61556

Frontal Sinus
See Sinus, Frontal
Frontal Sinusotomy
See Exploration, Sinus, Frontal
Frost Suture
Eyelid
Closure by Suture, 67875
Frozen Blood Preparation, 86930-86932
Fructose, 84375
Semen, 82757
Fructose Intolerance Breath Test, 91065
Fruit Sugar
See Fructose
FSF, 85290, 85291
FSH, 83001
with Additional Tests, 80418, 80426
FSHMD1A, 81404
FSP, 85362-85380
FT–4, 84439
FTG, 15200-15261
FTI, 84439
FTSG, 15200-15261
FTSJ1, 81405-81406
Fulguration
See Destruction
Bladder, 51020
Cystourethroscopy with, 52214
Lesion, 52224
Tumor, 52234-52240
Ureter, 50957, 50976
Ureterocele
Ectopic, 52301
Orthotopic, 52300
Fulguration, Endocavitary
See Electrocautery
Full Thickness Graft, 15200-15261
Function, Study, Nasal
See Nasal Function Study
Function Test, Lung
See Pulmonology, Diagnostic
Function Test, Vestibular
See Vestibular Function Tests
Functional Ability
See Activities of Daily Living
Functional MRI, 70554-70555
Fundoplasty
Esophagogastric
Laparoscopic, 43279-43280, 43283
Laparotomy, 43327
Thoracotomy, 43328
with Gastroplasty, 43842-43843
Esophagomyotomy
Laparoscopic, 43279
with Fundic Patch, 43325
with Paraesophageal Hernia
Laparoscopic, 43281-43282
with Fundoplication
Laparotomy, 43332-43333
Thoracoabdominal Incisional, 43336-43337
Thoracotomy, 43334-43335
Fundoplication
See Fundoplasty, Esophagogastric
Fungal Wet Prep, 87220
Fungus
Antibody, 86671
Culture
Blood, 87103
Hair, 87101
Identification, 87106
Nail, 87101
Other, 87102
Skin, 87101
Tissue Exam, 87220
Funnel Chest
See Pectus Excavatum
Furuncle
Incision and Drainage, 10060, 10061
Furuncle, Vulva
See Abscess, Vulva
FUS/DDIT3, 81401, 81406
Fusion
See Arthrodesis
Pleural Cavity, 32560
Thumb
in Opposition, 26820

Fusion, Epiphyseal–Diaphyseal
See Epiphyseal Arrest
Fusion, Joint
See Arthrodesis
Fusion, Joint, Ankle
See Ankle, Arthrodesis
Fusion, Joint, Interphalangeal, Finger
See Arthrodesis, Finger Joint, Interphalangeal
FXN, [81284, 81285, 81286], [81289]

G

G6PC, 81250
G6PD, 81247-81249
  Common Variants, 81247
  Full Gene Sequence, 81249
  Known Familial Variants, 81248
GAA, 81406
Gabapentin
  Assay, 80171
GABRG2, 81405
Gago Procedure
  Repair, Tricuspid Valve, 33463-33465
Gait Training, 97116
Galactogram, 77053, 77054
  Injection, 19030
Galactokinase
  Blood, 82759
Galactose
  Blood, 82760
  Urine, 82760
Galactose–1–Phosphate
  Uridyl Transferase, 82775-82776
Galactosemia, 81443
GALC, 81401, 81406
Galeazzi Dislocation
  Fracture
    Closed Treatment, 25520
    Open Treatment, 25525, 25526
Galectin-3, 82777
Gallbladder
  See Bile Duct
  Anastomosis
    with Intestines, 47720-47741
  Cholecystectomy, 47600
    Laparoscopic, 47562
      with Cholangiogram, 47564
    Open, 47600
      with Cholangiogram, 47605
      with Choledochoenterostomy, 47612
      with Exploration Common Duct, 47610
      with Transduodenal Sphincterotomy or Sphincteroplasty, 47620
  Cholecystostomy
    for Drainage, 47480
    for Exploration, 47480
    for Removal of Stone, 47480
    Percutaneous, 47490
  Excision, 47562-47564, 47600-47620
  Exploration, 47480
  Incision, 47490
  Incision and Drainage, 47480
  Nuclear Medicine
    Imaging, 78226-78227
  Removal Calculi, 47480
  Repair
    with Gastroenterostomy, 47741
    with Intestines, 47720-47740
  Unlisted Services and Procedures, 47999
  X-ray with Contrast, 74290
GALT, 81401, 81406
Galvanocautery
  See Electrocautery
Galvanoionization
  See Iontophoresis
Gamete Intrafallopian Transfer (GIFT), 58976
Gamete Transfer
  In Vitro Fertilization, 58976
Gamma Camera Imaging
  See Nuclear Medicine
Gamma Glutamyl Transferase, 82977
Gamma Seminoprotein
  See Antigen, Prostate Specific

Gammacorten
  See Dexamethasone
Gammaglobulin
  Blood, 82784-82787
Gamulin Rh
  See Immune Globulins, Rho (D)
Ganglia, Trigeminal
  See Gasserian Ganglion
Ganglion
  See Gasserian Ganglion
  Cyst
    Aspiration/Injection, 20612
    Drainage, 20612
    Wrist
      Excision, 25111, 25112
  Injection
    Anesthetic, 64505, 64510
Ganglion Cervicothoracicum
  See Stellate Ganglion
Ganglion, Gasser's
  See Gasserian Ganglion
Ganglion Pterygopalatinum
  See Sphenopalatine Ganglion
GARDASIL, 90649
Gardner Operation, 63700, 63702
Gardnerella Vaginalis Detection, 87510-87512
GARS, 81406
Gasser Ganglion
  See Gasserian Ganglion
Gasserian Ganglion
  Sensory Root
    Decompression, 61450
    Section, 61450
  Stereotactic, 61790
Gastrectomy
  Longitudinal, 43775
  Partial, 43631
    Distal with Vagotomy, 43635
    with Gastroduodenostomy, 43631
      with Roux–en–Y Reconstruction, 43633
    with Gastrojejunostomy, 43632
      with Intestinal Pouch, 43634
  Sleeve, 43775
  Total, 43621, 43622
    with Esophagoenterostomy, 43620
    with Intestinal Pouch, 43622
Gastric, 82930
  Acid, 82930
  Analysis Test, 43755-43757
  Electrodes
    Neurostimulator
      Implantation
        Laparoscopic, 43647
        Open, 43881
      Removal
        Laparoscopic, 43648
        Open, 43882
      Replacement
        Laparoscopic, 43647
        Open, 43881
      Revision
        Laparoscopic, 43648
        Open, 43882
  Intubation, 43753-43755
    Diagnostic, 43754-43757
    Therapeutic, 43753
  Lavage
    Therapeutic, 43753
  Restrictive Procedure
    Laparoscopy, 43770-43774
    Open, 43886-43888
  Tests
    Manometry, 91020
Gastric Ulcer Disease
  See Stomach, Ulcer
Gastrin, 82938, 82941
Gastrocnemius Recession
  Leg, Lower, 27687
Gastroduodenostomy, 43810
  Revision of Anastomosis with Reconstruction, 43850
    with Vagotomy, 43855
  with Gastrectomy, 43631, 43632
Gastroenterology, Diagnostic
  Breath Hydrogen Test, 91065

Gastroenterology, Diagnostic — continued
  Colon Motility Study, 91117
  Duodenal Intubation and Aspiration, 43756-43757
  Esophagus Tests
    Acid Perfusion, 91030
    Acid Reflux Test, 91034-91038
    Balloon Distension Provocation Study, 91040
    Intubation with Specimen Collection, 43754-43755
    Manometry, 91020
    Motility Study, 91010-91013
  Gastric Tests
    Manometry, 91020
  Gastroesophageal Reflux Test
    See Acid Reflux, 91034-91038
  Manometry, 91020
  Rectum
    Manometry, 91122
    Sensation, Tone, and Compliance Test, 91120
  Stomach
    Intubation with Specimen Collection, 43754-43755
    Manometry, 91020
    Stimulation of Secretion, 43755
  Unlisted Services and Procedures, 91299
Gastroenterostomy
  for Obesity, 43644-43645, 43842-43848
Gastroesophageal Reflux Test, 91034-91038
Gastrointestinal Endoscopies
  See Endoscopy, Gastrointestinal
Gastrointestinal Exam
  Nuclear Medicine
    Blood Loss Study, 78278
    Protein Loss Study, 78282
    Shunt Testing, 78291
    Unlisted Services and Procedures, 78299
Gastrointestinal Prophylaxis for NSAID Use Prescribed, 4017F
Gastrointestinal Tract
  Imaging Intraluminal
    Colon, 0355T
    Distal Ileum, 0355T
    Esophagus, 91111
    Esophagus Through Ileum, 91110
  Reconstruction, 43360, 43361
  Transit and Pressure Measurements, 91112
  Upper
    Dilation, 43249
    X–ray, 74240, 74248
      Guide Dilator, 74360
      Guide Intubation, 49440, 74340
      with Contrast, 74246, 74248
Gastrointestinal, Upper
  Biopsy
    Endoscopy, 43239
  Dilation
    Endoscopy, 43245
    Esophagus, 43248
  Endoscopy
    Catheterization, 43241
    Destruction
      Lesion, [43270]
    Dilation, 43245
    Drainage
      Pseudocyst, 43240
    Exploration, 43235
    Hemorrhage, 43255
    Inject Varices, 43243
    Needle Biopsy, 43238, 43242
    Removal
      Foreign Body, 43247
      Lesion, 43250-43251
      Polyp, 43250-43251
      Tumor, 43250-43251
    Resection, Mucosa, 43254
    Stent Placement, [43266]
    Thermal Radiation, 43257
    Tube Placement, 43246
    Ultrasound, 43237, 43238, 43242, 43253, 76975
  Exploration
    Endoscopy, 43235

Gastrointestinal, Upper — continued
  Hemorrhage
    Endoscopic Control, 43255
  Injection
    Submucosal, 43236
    Varices, 43243
  Lesion
    Destruction, [43270]
  Ligation of Vein, 43244
  Needle Biopsy
    Endoscopy, 43238, 43242
  Removal
    Foreign body, 43247
    Lesion, 43250-43251
    Polyp, 43250-43251
    Tumor, 43250-43251
  Stent Placement, [43266]
  Tube Placement
    Endoscopy, 43237, 43238, 43246
  Ultrasound
    Endoscopy, 43237, 43238, 43242, 43259, 76975
Gastrojejunostomy, 43860, 43865
  Contrast Injection, 49465
  Conversion from Gastrostomy Tube, 49446
  Removal
    Obstructive Material, 49460
  Replacement
    Tube, 49452
  Revision, 43860
    with Vagotomy, 43865
  with Duodenal Exclusion, 48547
  with Partial Gastrectomy, 43632
  with Vagotomy, 43825
  without Vagotomy, 43820
Gastroplasty
  Collis, 43283, 43338
  Esophageal Lengthening Procedure, 43283, 43338
  Laparoscopic, 43283, 43644-43645
  Restrictive for Morbid Obesity, 43842-43843, 43845-43848
    Other than Vertical Banded, 43843
  Wedge, 43283, 43338
Gastrorrhaphy, 43840
Gastroschisis, 49605
Gastrostomy
  Closure, 43870
  Laparoscopic
    Permanent, 43832
    Temporary, 43653
  Temporary, 43830
    Laparoscopic, 43653
    Neonatal, 43831
  Tube
    Change of, 43762-43763
    Conversion to Gastro-jejunostomy Tube, 49446
    Directed Placement
      Endoscopic, 43246
      Percutaneous, 49440
    Insertion
      Endoscopic, 43246
      Percutaneous, 49440
    Percutaneous, 49440
    Removal
      Obstructive Material, 49460
    Replacement, 49450
    Repositioning, 43761
  with Pancreatic Drain, 48001
  with Pyloroplasty, 43640
  with Vagotomy, 43640
Gastrotomy, 43500, 43501, 43510
Gaucher Disease Genomic Sequence Analysis, 81412, 81443
GBA, 81251, 81412
GCDH, 81406
GCH1, 81405
GCK, 81406
GDAP1, 81405
GDH, 82965
GE
  Reflux, 78262
Gel Diffusion, 86331
Gene Analysis
  See Analysis, Gene

Genioplasty, 21120-21123
  Augmentation, 21120, 21123
  Osteotomy, 21121-21123
Genitalia
  Female
    Anesthesia, 00940-00952
  Male
    Anesthesia, 00920-00938
  Skin Graft
    Delay of Flap, 15620
    Full Thickness, 15240, 15241
    Pedicle Flap, 15574
    Split, 15120, 15121
  Tissue Transfer, Adjacent, 14040, 14041
Genitourinary Sphincter, Artificial
  See Prosthesis, Urethral Sphincter
Genotype Analysis
  See Analysis, Gene
Gentamicin, 80170
  Assay, 80170
Gentiobiase, 82963
Genus: Human Cytomegalovirus Group
  See Cytomegalovirus
GERD
  See Gastroesophageal Reflux Test
German Measles
  See Rubella
Gestational Trophoblastic Tumor
  See Hydatidiform Mole
GFAP, 81405
GGT, 82977
GH, 83003
GH1, 81404
GHb, 83036
GHR, 81405
GHRHR, 81405
GI Tract
  See Gastrointestinal Tract
  X–rays, 74240, 74248, 74250-74251, 74340,
    74360
Giardia
  Antigen Detection
    Enzyme Immunoassay, 87329
    Immunofluorescence, 87269
Giardia Lamblia
  Antibody, 86674
Gibbons Stent, 52332
GIF, 84307
GIFT, 58976
Gill Operation, 63012
Gillies Approach
  Fracture
    Zygomatic Arch, 21356
Gingiva
  See Gums
Gingiva, Abscess
  See Abscess
  Fracture
    See Abscess, Gums; Gums
    Zygomatic Arch
      See Abscess, Gums; Gums,
        Abscess
Gingivectomy, 41820
Gingivoplasty, 41872
Girdlestone Laminectomy
  See Laminectomy
Girdlestone Procedure
  Acetabulum, Reconstruction, 27120, 27122
GJB1, 81403, *[81448]*
GJB2, 81252-81253, 81430
GJB6, 81254
GLA, 81405
Gla Protein (Bone)
  See Osteocalcin
Glabellar Frown Lines
  Rhytidectomy, 15826
Gland
  See Specific Gland
Gland, Adrenal
  See Adrenal Gland
Gland, Bartholin's
  See Bartholin's Gland
Gland, Bulbourethral
  See Bulbourethral Gland
Gland, Lacrimal
  See Lacrimal Gland

Gland, Mammary
  See Breast
Gland, Parathyroid
  See Parathyroid Gland
Gland, Parotid
  See Parotid Gland
Gland, Pituitary
  See Pituitary Gland
Gland, Salivary
  See Salivary Glands
Gland, Sublingual
  See Sublingual Gland
Gland, Sweat
  See Sweat Glands
Gland, Thymus
  See Thymus Gland
Gland, Thyroid
  See Thyroid Gland
Glasses
  See Spectacle Services
Glaucoma
  Cryotherapy, 66720
  Cyclophotocoagulation, 66710, 66711
  Diathermy, 66700
  Fistulization of Sclera, 66150
Glaucoma Drainage Implant
  See Aqueous Shunt
Glenn Procedure, 33622, 33766-33767
Glenohumeral Joint
  Arthrotomy, 23040
    with Biopsy, 23100
    with Synovectomy, 23105
  Exploration, 23107
  Removal
    Foreign or Loose Body, 23107
Glenoid Fossa
  Reconstruction, 21255
Glioblastoma Multiforme, 81345, *[81287]*
GLN, 82127-82131
Globulin
  Antihuman, 86880-86886
  Immune, 90281-90399
  Sex Hormone Binding, 84270
Globulin, Corticosteroid–Binding, 84449
Globulin, Rh Immune, 90384-90386
Globulin, Thyroxine–Binding, 84442
Glomerular Procoagulant Activity
  See Thromboplastin
Glomus Caroticum
  See Carotid Body
Glossectomies, 41120-41155
Glossectomy, 41120-41155
Glossorrhaphy
  See Suture, Tongue
Glucagon, 82943
  Tolerance Panel, 80422, 80424
  Tolerance Test, 82946
Glucose, 80422, 80424, 80430-80435, 95251 *[95249]*
  Blood Test, 82947-82950, 82962
  Body Fluid, 82945
  Hormone Panel, 80430
  Interstitial Fluid
    Continuous Monitoring, 95250-95251
      [95249]
  Interstitial Sensor (implantable), 0446T-0448T
  Tolerance Test, 82951, 82952
Glucose Phosphate Isomerase, 84087
Glucose Phosphate Isomerase Measurement, 84087
Glucose-6-Phosphatase, Catalytic Subunit Gene Analysis, 81250
Glucose–6–Phosphate
  Dehydrogenase, 82955, 82960
Glucosidase, 82963
  Beta Acid Gene Analysis, 81251
Glucuronide Androstanediol, 82154
GLUD1, 81406
Glue
  Cornea Wound, 65286
  Sclera Wound, 65286
Glukagon
  See Glucagon
Glutamate Dehydrogenase, 82965
Glutamate Pyruvate Transaminase, 84460
Glutamic Alanine Transaminase, 84460
Glutamic Aspartic Transaminase, 84450

Glutamic Dehydrogenase, 82965
Glutamine, 82127-82131
Glutamyltransferase, Gamma, 82977
Glutathione, 82978
  Glutathione Reductase, 82979
Glycanhydrolase, N–Acetylmuramide
  See Lysozyme
Glycated Hemoglobins
  See Glycohemoglobin
Glycated Protein, 82985
Glycerol, Phosphatidyl
  See Phosphatidylglycerol
Glycerol Phosphoglycerides
  See Phosphatidylglycerol
Glycerophosphatase
  See Alkaline Phosphatase
Glycinate, Theophylline Sodium
  See Theophylline
Glycocholic Acid
  See Cholylglycine
Glycohemoglobin, 83036-83037
Glycol, Ethylene
  See Ethylene Glycol
Glycols, Ethylene
  See Ethylene Glycol
Glycosaminoglycan
  See Mucopolysaccharides
GNAQ, 81403
GNE, 81400, 81406
Goeckerman Treatment
  Photochemotherapy, 96910-96913
Gold
  Assay, *[80375]*
Goldwaite Procedure
  Reconstruction, Patella, for Instability, 27422
Golfer's Elbow, 24357-24359
Gol–Vernet Operation, 50120
Gonadectomy, Female
  See Oophorectomy
Gonadectomy, Male
  See Excision, Testis
Gonadotropin
  Chorionic, 84702, 84703
  FSH, 83001
  ICSH, 83002
  LH, 83002
Gonadotropin Panel, 80426
Goniophotography, 92285
Gonioscopy, 92020
Goniotomy, 65820
Gonococcus
  See Neisseria Gonorrhoeae
Goodenough Harris Drawing Test, 96112-96116
GOTT
  See Transaminase, Glutamic Oxaloacetic
GP1BA, *[81106]*
GP1BB, 81404
GPUT, 82775-82776
Graefe's Operation, 66830
Graft
  Anal, 46753
  Aorta, 33845, 33852, 33858-33859, 33863-
    33864, 33866, 33871-33877
  Artery
    Coronary, 33503-33505
  Bone
    See Bone Marrow, Transplantation
    Anastomosis, 20969-20973
    Harvesting, 20900, 20902
    Microvascular Anastomosis, 20955-
      20962
    Osteocutaneous Flap with Microvascular
      Anastomosis, 20969-20973
    Vascular Pedicle, 25430
    Vertebra, 0222T
      Cervical, 0219T
      Lumbar, 0221T
      Thoracic, 0220T
  Bone and Skin, 20969-20973
  Cartilage
    Costochondral, 20910
    Ear to Face, 21235
    Harvesting, 20910, 20912
      See Cartilage Graft
    Rib to Face, 21230

Graft — *continued*
  Cartilage — *continued*
    Rib to Face — *continued*
      Three or More Segments
        Two Locations, 35682, 35683
    Composite, 35681-35683
  Conjunctiva, 65782
    Harvesting, 68371
  Cornea
    with Lesion Excision, 65426
  Corneal Transplant
    Allograft Preparation, 0290T, 65757
    Endothelial, 65756
    in Aphakia, 65750
    in Pseudophakia, 65755
    Lamellar, 65710
    Penetrating, 65730
  Dura
    Spinal Cord, 63710
  Eye
    Amniotic Membrane, 65780
    Conjunctiva, 65782
      Harvesting, 68371
    Stem Cell, 65781
  Facial Nerve Paralysis, 15840-15845
  Fascia Graft
    Cheek, 15840
  Fascia Lata
    Harvesting, 20920, 20922
  Gum Mucosa, 41870
  Heart
    See Heart, Transplantation
  Heart Lung
    See Transplantation, Heart–Lung
  Hepatorenal, 35535
  Kidney
    See Kidney, Transplantation
  Liver
    See Liver, Transplantation
  Lung
    See Lung, Transplantation
  Muscle
    Cheek, 15841-15845
  Nail Bed Reconstruction, 11762
  Nerve, 64885-64907
  Oral Mucosa, 40818
  Organ
    See Transplantation
  Osteochondral
    Knee, 27415-27416
    Talus, 28446
  Pancreas
    See Pancreas, Transplantation
  Peroneal-Tibial, 35570
  Skin
    Autograft, 15150-15152, 15155-15157
    Biological, 15271-15278
    Blood Flow Check, Graft, 15860
      See Skin Graft and Flap
    Check Vascular Flow Injection, 15860
    Composite, 15760, 15770
    Delayed Flap, 15600-15630
    Free Flap, 15757
    Full Thickness, Free
      Axillae, 15240, 15241
      Cheeks, Chin, 15240, 15241
      Ears, Eyelids, 15260, 15261
      Extremities (Excluding Hands/Feet),
        15240, 15241
      Feet, Hands, 15240, 15241
      Forehead, 15240, 15241
      Genitalia, 15240, 15241
      Lips, Nose, 15260, 15261
      Mouth, Neck, 15240, 15241
      Scalp, 15220, 15221
      Trunk, 15200, 15201
    Harvesting
      for Tissue Culture, 15040
    Pedicle
      Direct, 15570, 15576
      Transfer, 15650
    Pinch Graft, 15050
    Preparation Recipient Site, 15002, 15004-
      15005
    Split Graft, 15100, 15101, 15120, 15121
    Substitute, 15271-15278

Index

Graft — Hct

Heart — *continued*
- Repair — *continued*
  - Ventricular Tunnel, 33722
  - Wound, 33300, 33305
  - Replacement
    - Artificial Heart, Intracorporeal, 33928
    - Electrode, 33210, 33211, 33217
    - Mitral Valve, 33430
    - Total Replacement Heart System, Intracorporeal, 33928
    - Tricuspid Valve, 33465
    - Ventricular Assist Device, 0459T, 33981-33983
  - Repositioning
    - Aortic Counterpulsation, 0459T, 0460T-0461T
    - Electrode, 33215, 33217, 33226
    - Tricuspid Valve, 33468
  - Resuscitation, 92950
  - Septal Defect
    - Repair, 33782-33783, 33813-33814
    - Ventricular
      - Closure, 33675-33688
      - Open, 33675-33688
      - Percutaneous, 93581
  - Stimulation and Pacing, 93623
  - Thrombectomy, 33310-33315
    - Ventricular Assist Device, 33976
      - Intracorporeal, 33979
  - Transplantation, 33935, 33945
    - Allograft Preparation, 33933, 33944
    - Anesthesia, 00580
  - Tricuspid Valve
    - *See* Tricuspid Valve
  - Tumor
    - Excision, 33120, 33130
  - Ultrasound
    - Myocardial Strain Imaging, [93356]
    - Radiologic Guidance, 76932
  - Unlisted Services and Procedures, 33999
  - Ventriculography
    - *See* Ventriculography
  - Ventriculomyectomy, 33416
  - Ventriculomyotomy, 33416
  - Wound
    - Repair, 33300, 33305

Heart Biopsy
- Ultrasound, Radiologic Guidance, 76932

Heart Vessels
- Angiography, 93454-93461, 93563-93566
- Angioplasty, [92920, 92921], [92928, 92929], [92937, 92938], [92941], [92943, 92944]
- Injection, 93452-93461, 93563-93568
- Insertion
  - Graft, 33330-33335
- Thrombolysis, [92975, 92977]
- Valvuloplasty
  - *See* Valvuloplasty
  - Percutaneous, 92986-92990

Heartsbreath Test, 0085T

Heat Unstable Haemoglobin
- *See* Hemoglobin, Thermolabile

Heavy Lipoproteins
- *See* Lipoprotein

Heavy Metal, 83015, 83018

Heel
- *See* Calcaneus
- Collection of Blood, 36415, 36416
- X-ray, 73650

Heel Bone
- *See* Calcaneus

Heel Fracture
- *See* Calcaneus, Fracture

Heel Spur
- Excision, 28119

Heine Operation
- *See* Cyclodialysis

Heine–Medin Disease
- *See* Polio

Heinz Bodies, 85441, 85445

Helicobacter Pylori
- Antibody, 86677
- Antigen Detection
  - Enzyme Immunoassay, 87338, 87339
- Breath Test, 78267, 78268, 83013
- Stool, 87338

Helicobacter Pylori — *continued*
- Urease Activity, 83009, 83013, 83014

Heller Procedure, 32665, 43279, 43330-43331

Helminth
- Antibody, 86682

Hemagglutination Inhibition Test, 86280

Hemangioma, 17106-17108

Hemapheresis, 36511-36516

Hematochezia, 82270, 82274

Hematologic Test
- *See* Blood Tests

Hematology
- Unlisted Services and Procedures, 85999

Hematoma
- Ankle, 27603
- Arm, Lower, 25028
- Arm, Upper
  - Incision and Drainage, 23930
- Brain
  - Drainage, 61154, 61156
  - Evacuation, 61312-61315
  - Incision and Drainage, 61312-61315
- Drain, 61108
- Ear, External
  - Complicated, 69005
  - Simple, 69000
- Elbow
  - Incision and Drainage, 23930
- Epididymis
  - Incision and Drainage, 54700
- Gums
  - Incision and Drainage, 41800
- Hip, 26990
- Incision and Drainage
  - Neck, 21501, 21502
  - Skin, 10140
  - Thorax, 21501, 21502
- Knee, 27301
- Leg, Lower, 27603
- Leg, Upper, 27301
- Mouth, 41005-41009, 41015-41018
  - Incision and Drainage, 40800, 40801
- Nasal Septum
  - Incision and Drainage, 30020
- Nose
  - Incision and Drainage, 30000, 30020
- Pelvis, 26990
- Puncture Aspiration, 10160
- Scrotum
  - Incision and Drainage, 54700
- Shoulder
  - Drainage, 23030
- Skin
  - Incision and Drainage, 10140
  - Puncture Aspiration, 10160
- Subdural, 61108
- Subungual
  - Evacuation, 11740
- Testis
  - Incision and Drainage, 54700
- Tongue, 41000-41006, 41015
- Vagina
  - Incision and Drainage, 57022, 57023
- Wrist, 25028

Hematopoietic Stem Cell Transplantation
- *See* Stem Cell, Transplantation

Hematopoietin
- *See* Erythropoietin

Hematuria
- *See* Blood, Urine

Hemic System
- Unlisted Procedure, 38999

Hemiephyseal Arrest
- Elbow, 24470

Hemifacial Microsomia
- Reconstruction Mandibular Condyle, 21247

Hemilaminectomy, 63020-63044

Hemilaryngectomy, 31370-31382

Hemipelvectomies
- *See* Amputation, Interpelviabdominal

Hemiphalangectomy
- Toe, 28160

Hemispherectomy
- Partial, 61543

Hemochromatosis Gene Analysis, 81256

Hemocytoblast
- *See* Stem Cell

Hemodialysis, 90935, 90937, 99512
- Blood Flow Study, 90940
- Duplex Scan of Access, 93990
  - Prior to Access Creation, 93985-93986

Hemofiltration, 90945, 90947
- Hemodialysis, 90935, 90937
- Peritoneal Dialysis, 90945, 90947

Hemoglobin
- A1C, 83036
- Analysis
  - O2 Affinity, 82820
- Antibody
  - Fecal, 82274
- Carboxyhemoglobin, 82375-82376
- Chromatography, 83021
- Electrophoresis, 83020
- Fetal, 83030, 83033, 85460, 85461
- Fractionation and Quantitation, 83020
- Glycosylated (A1c), 83036-83037
- Methemoglobin, 83045, 83050
- Non–Automated, 83026
- Plasma, 83051
- Sulfhemoglobin, 83060
- Thermolabile, 83065, 83068
- Transcutaneous
  - Carboxyhemoglobin, 88740
  - Methemoglobin, 88741
- Urine, 83069

Hemoglobin F
- Fetal
  - Chemical, 83030
  - Qualitative, 83033

Hemoglobin, Glycosylated, 83036-83037

Hemoglobin (Hgb) quantitative
- Transcutaneous, 88738-88741

Hemogram
- Added Indices, 85025-85027
- Automated, 85025-85027
- Manual, 85014, 85018, 85032

Hemolysins, 85475
- with Agglutinins, 86940, 86941

Hemolytic Complement
- *See* Complement, Hemolytic

Hemolytic Complement, Total
- *See* Complement, Hemolytic, Total

Hemoperfusion, 90997

Hemophil
- *See* Clotting Factor

Hemophilus Influenza
- Antibody, 86684
- B Vaccine, 90647-90648, 90748

Hemorrhage
- Abdomen, 49002
- Anal
  - Endoscopic Control, 46614
- Bladder
  - Postoperative, 52214
- Chest Cavity
  - Endoscopic Control, 32654
- Colon
  - Endoscopic Control, 44391, 45382
- Colon–Sigmoid
  - Endoscopic Control, 45334
- Esophagus
  - Endoscopic Control, 43227
- Gastrointestinal, Upper
  - Endoscopic Control, 43255
- Intestines, Small
  - Endoscopic Control, 44366, 44378
- Liver
  - Control, 47350
- Lung, 32110
- Nasal
  - Cauterization, 30901-30906
  - Endoscopic Control, 31238
- Nasopharynx, 42970-42972
- Nose
  - Cauterization, 30901-30906
- Oropharynx, 42960-42962
- Rectum
  - Endoscopic Control, 45317
- Throat, 42960-42962
- Uterus
  - Postpartum, 59160

Hemorrhage — *continued*
- Vagina, 57180

Hemorrhoidectomy
- External, 46250, [46320]
- Internal and External, 46255-46262
- Ligation, 46221 [46945, 46946]
- Whitehead, 46260

Hemorrhoidopexy, [46947]

Hemorrhoids
- Destruction, 46930
- Excision, 46250-46262, [46320]
- Incision, 46083
- Injection
  - Sclerosing Solution, 46500
- Ligation, 45350, 46221 [46945, 46946], [45398]
- Stapling, [46947]

Hemosiderin, 83070

Hemothorax
- Thoracostomy, 32551

Heparin, 85520
- Clotting Inhibitors, 85300-85305
- Neutralization, 85525
- Protamine Tolerance Test, 85530

Heparin Cofactor I
- *See* Antithrombin III

Hepatectomy
- Extensive, 47122
- Left Lobe, 47125
- Partial
  - Donor, 47140-47142
  - Lobe, 47120
- Right Lobe, 47130
- Total
  - Donor, 47133

Hepatic Abscess
- *See* Abscess, Liver

Hepatic Arteries
- *See* Artery, Hepatic

Hepatic Artery Aneurysm
- *See* Artery, Hepatic, Aneurysm

Hepatic Duct
- Anastomosis
  - with Intestines, 47765, 47802
- Exploration, 47400
- Incision and Drainage, 47400
- Nuclear Medicine
  - Imaging, 78226-78227
- Removal
  - Calculi (Stone), 47400
- Repair
  - with Intestines, 47765, 47802
- Unlisted Services and Procedures, 47999

Hepatic Haemorrhage
- *See* Hemorrhage, Liver

Hepatic Portal Vein
- *See* Vein, Hepatic Portal

Hepatic Portoenterostomies
- *See* Hepaticoenterostomy

Hepatic Transplantation
- *See* Liver, Transplantation

Hepaticodochotomy
- *See* Hepaticostomy

Hepaticoenterostomy, 47802

Hepaticostomy, 47400

Hepaticotomy, 47400

Hepatitis A and Hepatitis B, 90636

Hepatitis A Vaccine
- Adolescent
  - Pediatric
    - Three Dose Schedule, 90634
    - Two Dose Schedule, 90633
- Adult Dosage, 90632

Hepatitis Antibody
- A, 86708, 86709
- B core, 86704, 86705
- B Surface, 86706
- Be, 86707
- C, 86803, 86804
- Delta Agent, 86692
- IgG, 86704, 86708
- IgM, 86704, 86705, 86709

Hepatitis Antigen
- B, 87516-87517
- B Surface, 87340, 87341
- Be, 87350
- C, 87520-87522

Hepatitis Antigen — continued
Delta Agent, 87380
G, 87525-87527
Hepatitis B and Hib, 90748
Hepatitis B Immunization, 90739-90748
Hepatitis B Vaccine
Dosage
Adolescent, 90743-90744
Adult, 90739, 90746
Dialysis Patient, 90747
Immunosuppressed, 90740, 90747
Pediatric, 90744
Adolescent, 90743-90744
with Hemophilus Influenza Vaccine, 90748
Hepatitis B Virus E Antibody
See Antibody, Hepatitis
Hepatitis B Virus Surface ab
See Antibody, Hepatitis B, Surface
Hepatitis C Virus Biochemical Assay, 81596
Hepatobiliary System Imaging, 78226
with Pharmacologic Intervention, 78227
Hepatorrhaphy
See Liver, Repair
Hepatotomy
Abscess, 47010
Cyst, 47010
Hereditary Disorders
Breast Cancer, 81432-81433
Colon Cancer, 81435-81436
Neuroendocrine Tumor, 81437-81438
Peripheral Neuropathy, [81448]
Retinal Disorders, 81434
Hernia
Repair
Abdominal, 49560, 49565, 49590
Incisional, 49560
Recurrent, 49565
Diaphragmatic, 39503-39541
Chronic, 39541
Neonatal, 39503
Epigastric, 49570
Incarcerated, 49572
Femoral, 49550
Incarcerated, 49553
Recurrent, 49555
Recurrent Incarcerated, 49557
Reducible, 49550
Incisional, 49561, 49566
Incarcerated, 49561
Inguinal, 49491, 49495-49500, 49505
Incarcerated, 49492, 49496, 49501, 49507, 49521
Infant, Incarcerated
Strangulated, 49496, 49501
Infant, Reducible, 49495, 49500
Laparoscopic, 49650, 49651
Pediatric, Reducible, 49500, 49505
Recurrent, Incarcerated
Strangulated, 49521
Recurrent, Reducible, 49520
Sliding, 49525
Strangulated, 49492
Lumbar, 49540
Lung, 32800
Mayo, 49585
Orchiopexy, 54640
Recurrent Incisional
Incarcerated, 49566
Umbilicus, 49580, 49585
Incarcerated, 49582, 49587
with Spermatic Cord, 55540
Spigelian, 49590
Hernia, Cerebral
See Encephalocele
Hernia, Rectovaginal
See Rectocele
Hernia, Umbilical
See Omphalocele
Heroin Test, [80305, 80306, 80307]
Herpes Simplex Virus
Antibody, 86696
Antigen Detection
Immunofluorescence, 87273, 87274
Nucleic Acid, 87528-87530

Herpes Simplex Virus — continued
Identification
Smear and Stain, 87207
Herpes Smear, 87207
Herpes Virus-6 Detection, 87531-87533
Herpesvirus 4 (Gamma), Human
See Epstein-Barr Virus
Herpetic Vesicle
Destruction, 54050, 54065
Heteroantibodies
See Antibody, Heterophile
Heterologous Transplant
See Xenograft
Heterologous Transplantations
See Heterograft
Heterophile Antibody, 86308-86310
Heterotropia
See Strabismus
Hex B
See b-Hexosaminidase
HEXA, 81255, 81406, 81412
Hexadecadrol
See Dexamethasone
Hexosaminidase A (Alpha Polypeptide) Gene Analysis, 81255
Hexosephosphate Isomerase
See Phosphohexose Isomerase
Heyman Procedure, 27179, 28264
HFE, 81256
Hg Factor
See Glucagon
Hgb, 83036, 83051, 83065, 83068, 85018
HGH (Human Growth Hormone), 80418, 80428, 80430, 83003, 86277
HHV-4
See Epstein-Barr Virus
HIAA (Hydroxyindolacetic Acid, Urine), 83497
Hib Vaccine
Four Dose Schedule
Hib-MenCY, 90644
PRP-T Four Dose Schedule, 90648
Hib, 90647-90648
PRP-OMP
Three Dose Schedule, 90647
Hibb Operation, 22841
Hiberix, 90648
Hickman Catheterization
See Cannulization; Catheterization, Venous, Central Line; Venipuncture
Hicks-Pitney Test
Thromboplastin, Partial Time, 85730, 85732
Hidradenitis
See Sweat Gland
Excision, 11450-11471
Suppurative
Incision and Drainage, 10060, 10061
High Altitude Simulation Test, 94452-94453
High Density Lipoprotein, 83718
High Molecular Weight Kininogen
See Fitzgerald Factor
Highly Selective Vagotomy
See Vagotomy, Highly Selective
Highmore Antrum
See Sinus, Maxillary
Hill Procedure, 43842-43843
Hinton Positive
See RPR
Hip
See Femur; Pelvis
Abscess
Incision and Drainage, 26990
Arthrocentesis, 20610-20611
Arthrodesis, 27284, 27286
Arthrography, 73525
Arthroplasty, 27130, 27132
Arthroscopy, 29860-29863 [29914, 29915, 29916]
Arthrotomy, 27030, 27033
Biopsy, 27040, 27041
Bone
Drainage, 26992
Bursa
Incision and Drainage, 26991
Capsulectomy
with Release, Flexor Muscles, 27036
Cast, 29305, 29325

Hip — continued
Craterization, 27070, 27071
Cyst
Excision, 27065-27067
Denervation, 27035
Echography
Infant, 76885, 76886
Endoprosthesis
See Prosthesis, Hip
Excision, 27070
Excess Skin, 15834
Exploration, 27033
Fasciotomy, 27025
Fusion, 27284, 27286
Hematoma
Incision and Drainage, 26990
Injection
Radiologic, 27093, 27095, 27096
Manipulation, 27275
Reconstruction
Total Replacement, 27130
Removal
Cast, 29710
Foreign Body, 27033, 27086, 27087
Arthroscopic, 29861
Loose Body
Arthroscopic, 29861
Prosthesis, 27090, 27091
Repair
Muscle Transfer, 27100-27105, 27111
Osteotomy, 27146-27156
Tendon, 27097
Saucerization, 27070
Stem Prostheses
See Arthroplasty, Hip
Strapping, 29520
Tenotomy
Abductor Tendon, 27006
Adductor Tendon, 27000-27003
Iliopsoas Tendon, 27005
Total Replacement, 27130, 27132
Tumor
Excision, 27047-27049 [27043, 27045, 27059], 27065-27067, 27075-27078
Ultrasound
Infant, 76885, 76886
X-ray, 73501-73503, 73521-73523
with Contrast, 73525
Hip Joint
Arthroplasty, 27132
Revision, 27134-27138
Arthrotomy, 27502
Biopsy, 27502
Capsulotomy
with Release, Flexor Muscles, 27036
Dislocation, 27250, 27252
Congenital, 27256-27259
Open Treatment, 27253, 27254
without Trauma, 27265, 27266
Manipulation, 27275
Reconstruction
Revision, 27134-27138
Synovium
Excision, 27054
Arthroscopic, 29863
Total Replacement, 27132
Hip Stem Prosthesis
See Arthroplasty, Hip
Hippocampus
Excision, 61566
Histamine, 83088
Histamine Release Test, 86343
Histochemistry, 88319
Histocompatibility Testing
See Tissue Typing
Histoplasma
Antibody, 86698
Antigen, 87385
Histoplasma Capsulatum
Antigen Detection
Enzyme Immunoassay, 87385
Histoplasmin Test
See Histoplasmosis, Skin Test
Histoplasmoses
See Histoplasmosis

Histoplasmosis
Skin Test, 86510
History and Physical
See Evaluation and Management, Office and/or Other Outpatient Services
Pelvic Exam under Anesthesia, 57410
Preventive
Established Patient, 99391-99397
New Patient, 99381-99387
HIV, 86689, 86701-86703, 87389-87391, 87534-87539
Antibody
Confirmation Test, 86689
Antigen HIV-1 with HIV-1 and HIV-2 Antibodies, 87389
HIV Antibody, 86701-86703
HIV Detection
Antibody, 86701-86703
Antigen, 87390, 87391, 87534-87539
Confirmation Test, 86689
HIV-1
Antigen Detection
Enzyme Immunoassay, 87390
HIV-2
Antigen Detection
Enzyme Immunoassay, 87391
HK3 Kallikrein
See Antigen, Prostate Specific
HLA
Antibody Detection, 86828-86835
Crossmatch, 86825-86826
Typing, 86812-86813, 86816-86817, 86821
Molecular Pathology Techniques, 81370-81383
HLCS, 81406
HMBS, 81406
HMRK
See Fitzgerald Factor
HNF1A, 81405
HNF1B, 81404-81405
HNF4A, 81406
Hoffman Apparatus, 20690
Hofmeister Operation, 43632
Holten Test, 82575
Holter Monitor, 93224-93227
Home Services
Activities of Daily Living, 99509
Catheter Care, 99507
Enema Administration, 99511
Established Patient, 99347-99350
Hemodialysis, 99512
Home Infusion Procedures, 99601, 99602
Individual or Family Counseling, 99510
Intramuscular Injections, 99506
Mechanical Ventilation, 99504
New Patient, 99341-99345
Newborn Care, 99502
Postnatal Assessment, 99501
Prenatal Monitoring, 99500
Respiratory Therapy, 99503
Sleep Studies, 95805-95811 [95800, 95801]
Stoma Care, 99505
Unlisted Services and Procedures, 99600
Homocystine, 83090
Urine, 82615
Homogenization, Tissue, 87176
Homologous Grafts
See Graft, Skin
Homologous Transplantation
See Homograft, Skin
Homovanillic Acid
Urine, 83150
Horii Procedure (Carpal Bone), 25430
Hormone Adrenocorticotrophic
See Adrenocorticotropic Hormone (ACTH)
Hormone Assay
ACTH, 82024
Aldosterone
Blood or Urine, 82088
Androstenedione
Blood or Urine, 82157
Androsterone
Blood or Urine, 82160
Angiotensin II, 82163
Corticosterone, 82528
Cortisol
Total, 82533

Hormone Assay — *continued*
Dehydroepiandrosterone, 82626-82627
Dihydrotestosterone, [80327, 80328]
Epiandrosterone, [80327, 80328]
Estradiol, 82670
Estriol, 82677
Estrogen, 82671, 82672
Estrone, 82679
Follicle Stimulating Hormone, 83001
Growth Hormone, 83003
Suppression Panel, 80430
Hydroxyprogesterone, 83498
Luteinizing Hormone, 83002
Somatotropin, 80430, 83003
Testosterone, 84403
Vasopressin, 84588
Hormone, Corticotropin–Releasing
See Corticotropic Releasing Hormone (CRH)
Hormone, Growth
See Growth Hormone
Hormone, Human Growth
See Growth Hormone, Human
Hormone, Interstitial Cell–Stimulation
See Luteinizing Hormone (LH)
Hormone, Parathyroid
See Parathormone
Hormone Pellet Implantation, 11980
Hormone, Pituitary Lactogenic
See Prolactin
Hormone, Placental Lactogen
See Lactogen, Human Placental
Hormone, Somatotropin Release–Inhibiting
See Somatostatin
Hormone, Thyroid–Stimulating
See Thyroid Stimulating Hormone (TSH)
Hormone–Binding Globulin, Sex
See Globulin, Sex Hormone Binding
Hormones, Adrenal Cortex
See Corticosteroids
Hormones, Antidiuretic
See Antidiuretic Hormone
Hospital Discharge Services
See Discharge Services, Hospital
Hospital Services
Inpatient Services
Discharge Services, 99238, 99239
Initial Care New or Established Patient, 99221-99223
Initial Hospital Care, 99221-99223
Neonate, 99477
Newborn, 99460-99465, 99466-99480
Prolonged Services, 99356, 99357
Subsequent Hospital Care, 99231-99233
Normal Newborn, 99460-99463
Observation
Discharge Services, 99234-99236
Initial Care, 99218-99220
New or Established Patient, 99218-99220
Intensive Neonatal, 99477
Same Day Admission
Discharge Services, 99234-99236
Subsequent Newborn Care, 99462
Hot Pack Treatment, 97010
See Physical Medicine and Rehabilitation
House Calls, 99341-99350
Howard Test
Cystourethroscopy, Catheterization, Ureter, 52005
HP, 83010, 83012
HPA-15a/b (S682Y), [81112]
HPA-1a/b (L33P), [81105]
HPA-2a/b (T145M), [81106]
HPA-3a/b (I843S), [81107]
HPA-4a/b (R143Q), [81108]
HPA-5a/b (K505E), [81109]
HPA-6a/b (R489Q), [81110]
HPA-9a/b (V837M), [81111]
HPL, 83632
HRAS, 81403-81404
HSD11B2, 81404
HSD3B2, 81404
HSG, 58340, 74740
HSPB1, 81404

HTLV I
Antibody
Confirmatory Test, 86689
Detection, 86687
HTLV III
See HIV
HTLV–II
Antibody, 86688
HTLV–IV
See HIV–2
HTRA1, 81405
HTT, 81271, [81274]
Hubbard Tank Therapy, 97036
See Physical Medicine/ Therapy/Occupational Therapy
with Exercises, 97036, 97113
Hue Test, 92283
Huggin Operation, 54520
Huhner Test, 89300-89320
Human
Epididymis Protein 4 (HE4), 86305
Growth Hormone, 80418, 80428, 80430
Leukocyte Antigen, 86812-86826
Papillomavirus Detection, [87623, 87624, 87625]
Papillomavirus Vaccine, 90649-90651
Human Chorionic Gonadotropin
See Chorionic Gonadotropin
Human Chorionic Somatomammotropin
See Lactogen, HumanPlacental
Human Cytomegalovirus Group
See Cytomegalovirus
Human Herpes Virus 4
See Epstein–Barr Virus
Human Immunodeficiency Virus
See HIV
Human Immunodeficiency Virus 1
See HIV–1
Human Immunodeficiency Virus 2
See HIV–2
Human Placental Lactogen, 83632
Human Platelet Antigen, [81105, 81106, 81107, 81108, 81109, 81110, 81111, 81112]
1 Genotyping (HPA-1), [81105]
15 Genotyping (HPA-15), [81112]
2 Genotyping (HPA-2), [81106]
3 Genotyping (HPA-3), [81107]
4 Genotyping (HPA-4), [81108]
5 Genotyping (HPA-5), [81109]
6 Genotyping (HPA-6), [81110]
9 Genotyping (HPA-9), [81111]
Human T Cell Leukemia Virus I
See HTLV I
Human T Cell Leukemia Virus I Antibodies
See Antibody, HTLV–I
Human T Cell Leukemia Virus II
See HTLV II
Human T Cell Leukemia Virus II Antibodies
See Antibody, HTLV–II
Humeral Epicondylitides, Lateral
See Tennis Elbow
Humeral Fracture
See Fracture, Humerus
Humerus
See Arm, Upper; Shoulder
Abscess
Incision and Drainage, 23935
Craterization, 23184, 24140
Cyst
Excision, 23150, 24110
with Allograft, 23156, 24116
with Autograft, 23155, 24115
Diaphysectomy, 23184, 24140
Excision, 23174, 23184, 23195, 23220, 24077-24079, 24110-24116, 24134, 24140, 24150
Fracture
Closed Treatment, 24500, 24505
with Manipulation, 23605
without Manipulation, 23600
Condyle
Closed Treatment, 24576, 24577
Open Treatment, 24579
Percutaneous Fixation, 24582
Epicondyle
Closed Treatment, 24560, 24565

Humerus — *continued*
Fracture — *continued*
Epicondyle — *continued*
Open Treatment, 24575
Percutaneous Fixation, 24566
Greater Tuberosity Fracture
Closed Treatment with Manipulation, 23625
Closed Treatment without Manipulation, 23620
Open Treatment, 23630
Open Treatment, 23615, 23616
Shaft
Closed Treatment, 24500, 24505, 24516
Open Treatment, 24515
Supracondylar
Closed Treatment, 24530, 24535
Open Treatment, 24545, 24546
Percutaneous Fixation, 24538
Transcondylar
Closed Treatment, 24530, 24535
Open Treatment, 24545, 24546
Percutaneous Fixation, 24538
with Dislocation, 23665, 23670
Osteomyelitis, 24134
Pinning, Wiring, 23491, 24498
Prophylactic Treatment, 23491, 24498
Radical Resection, 23220, 24077-24079
Repair, 24430
Nonunion, Malunion, 24430, 24435
Osteoplasty, 24420
Osteotomy, 24400, 24410
with Graft, 24435
Resection Head, 23195
Saucerization, 23184, 24140
Sequestrectomy, 23174, 24134
Tumor
Excision, 23150-23156, 23220, 24075-24079 [24071, 24073], 24110-24116
X-ray, 73060
Hummelshein Operation, 67340
Strabismus Repair
Adjustable Sutures, 67335
Extraocular Muscles, 67340
One Horizontal Muscle, 67311
One Vertical Muscle, 67314
Posterior Fixation Suture Technique, 67335
Previous Surgery not Involving Extraocular Muscles, 67331
Release Extensive Scar Tissue, 67343
Superior Oblique Muscle, 67318
Transposition, 67320
Two Horizontal Muscles, 67312
Two or More Vertical Muscles, 67316
Humor Shunt, Aqueous
See Aqueous Shunt
Huntington Disease, 81271, [81274]
HVA (Homovanillic Acid), 83150
Hybridization Probes, DNA
See Nucleic Acid Probe
Hydatid Disease
See Echinococcosis
Hydatid Mole
See Hydatidiform Mole
Hydatidiform Mole
Evacuation and Curettage, 59870
Excision, 59100
Hydration, 96360-96361
Hydrocarbons, Chlorinated
See Chlorinated Hydrocarbons
Hydrocele
Aspiration, 55000
Excision
Bilateral, Tunica Vaginalis, 55041
Unilateral
Spermatic Cord, 55500
Tunica Vaginalis, 55040
Repair, 55060
Hydrocele, Tunica Vaginalis
See Tunica Vaginalis, Hydrocele
Hydrocelectomy, 49495-49501
Hydrochloric Acid, Gastric
See Acid, Gastric

Hydrochloride, Vancomycin
See Vancomycin
Hydrocodone
See Dihydrocodeinone
Hydrogen Ion Concentration
See pH
Hydrolase, Acetylcholine
See Acetylcholinesterase
Hydrolase, Triacylglycerol
See Lipase
Hydrolases, Phosphoric Monoester
See Phosphatase
Hydrotherapy (Hubbard Tank), 97036
See Physical Medicine/Therapy/ Occupational Therapy
with Exercises, 97036, 97113
Hydrotubation, 58350
Hydroxyacetanilide
See Acetaminophen
Hydroxycorticosteroid, 83491
Hydroxyindolacetic Acid, 83497
Urine, 83497
Hydroxypregnenolone, 80406, 84143
Hydroxyprogesterone, 80402, 80406, 83498
Hydroxyproline, 83500, 83505
Hydroxytyramine
See Dopamine
Hygroma, Cystic
Axillary or Cervical Excision, 38550, 38555
Hymen
Excision, 56700
Incision, 56442
Hymenal Ring
Revision, 56700
Hymenectomy, 56700
Hymenotomy, 56442
Hyoid Bone
Fracture
Open Treatment, 31584
Hyperbaric Oxygen Pressurization, 99183
Hypercholesterolemia, 81401, 81405-81407
Hypercycloidal X–ray, 76101, 76102
Hyperdactylies
See Supernumerary Digit
Hyperglycemic Glycogenolytic Factor
See Glucagon
HyperRAB, 90375
HyperTED, 90389
Hypertelorism of Orbit
See Orbital Hypertelorism
Hyperthermia Therapy
See Thermotherapy
Hyperthermia Treatment, 77600-77620
Hypnotherapy, 90880
Hypodermis
See Subcutaneous Tissue
Hypogastric Plexus
Destruction, 64681
Injection
Anesthetic, 64517
Neurolytic, 64681
Hypoglossal Nerve
Anastomosis
to Facial Nerve, 64868
Hypoglossal–Facial Anastomosis
See Anastomosis, Nerve, Facial to Hypoglossal
Hypopharynges
See Hypopharynx
Hypopharynx
Diverticulectomy, 43130, 43180
Hypophysectomy, 61546, 61548, 62165
Hypophysis
See Pituitary Gland
Hypopyrexia
See Hypothermia
Hypospadias
Repair, 54300, 54352
Complications, 54340-54348
First Stage, 54304
Meatal Advancement, 54322
Perineal, 54336
Proximal Penile or Penoscrotal, 54332
One Stage
Meatal Advancement, 54322
Perineal, 54336

[Resequenced] CPT © 2019 American Medical Association. All Rights Reserved. © 2019 Optum360, LLC

Implant — *continued*
Electrode — *continued*
  Gastric Implantation — *continued*
    Open — *continued*
      Neurostimulator, 43881
  Nerve, 64553-64581
  Spinal Cord, 63650, 63655
External Speech Processor/Cochlear Stimulator, 69714-69718
Eye
  Anterior Segment, 65920
    Aqueous Drainage Device, without Reservoir, 66183
    Aqueous Shunt
      into Subconjunctival Space, 0449T-0450T
      into Supraciliary Space, 0474T
      Revision, 66184-66185
      to Extraocular Reservoir, 66179-66180
    Corneal Ring Segments, 65785
    Placement or Replacement of Pegs, 65125
  Posterior Segment
    Extraocular, 67120
    Intraocular, 67121
  Replacement of Pegs, 65125
  Reservoir, 66180
  Vitreous
    Drug Delivery System, 67027
Fallopian Tube, 58565
Fascial Reinforcement
  Abdominal Wall, 0437T
Glaucoma Drainage, 66180
Hearing Aid
  Bone Conduction, 69710
Hip Prosthesis
  See Arthroplasty, Hip
Hormone Pellet, 11980
Iliac Arteriovenous Anastomosis, 0553T
Intraocular Lens
  See Insertion, Intraocular Lens
Intraocular Retinal Electrode Array, 0100T
Intrastromal Corneal Ring Segments, 65785
Joint
  See Arthroplasty
Mesh
  Closure of Necrotizing Soft Tissue Infection, 49568
  Hernia Repair, 49568, 49652-49657
  Vaginal Repair, 57267
Nerve
  into Bone, 64787
  into Muscle, 64787
Neurostimulation System
  Posterior Tibial Nerve, 0587T
Neurostimulator
  Cranial, 61885-61886, 64568
  Gastric, 43647, 43881, 64590
  Spine, 64999
Orbital, 67550
Ovum, 58976
Penile Prosthesis, 54400-54405
Pulsatile Heart Assist System, 33999
Pulse Generator
  Brain, 61885, 61886
  Spinal Cord, 63685
Receiver
  Brain, 61885, 61886
  Nerve, 64590
  Spinal Cord, 63685
Reinforcement Soft Tissue, 15777
Removal, 20670, 20680
  Anesthesia, External Fixation, 20694
  Elbow, 24164
  Radius, 24164
  Sinus Tarsi, 0510T-0511T
  Wire, Pin, Rod, 20670
  Wire, Pin, Rod/Deep, 20680
Reservoir Vascular Access Device
  Declotting, 36593
Retinal Electrode Array, 0100T
Subtalar Joint, Extra-osseous, 0335T
Total Replacement Heart System, Intracorporeal, 33927
Tubouterine, 58752

Implant — *continued*
Ventricular Assist Device, 33976
  Intracorporeal, 0451T-0454T, 33979
Impression, Maxillofacial, 21076-21089
  Auricular Prosthesis, 21086
  Definitive Obturator Prosthesis, 21080
  Facial Prosthesis, 21088
  Interim Obturator, 21079
  Mandibular Resection Prosthesis, 21081
  Nasal Prosthesis, 21087
  Oral Surgical Splint, 21085
  Orbital Prosthesis, 21077
  Palatal Augmentation Prosthesis, 21082
  Palatal Lift Prosthesis, 21083
  Speech Aid Prosthesis, 21084
  Surgical Obturator, 21076
IMRT (Intensity Modulated Radiation Therapy)
  Plan, 77301
  Treatment
    Complex, [77386]
    Plan, 77301
    Simple, [77385]
IMT Testing, 0126T
In Situ Hybridization
  See Nucleic Acid Probe, Cytogenic Studies, Morphometric Analysis
In Vitro Fertilization
  Biopsy Oocyte, 89290, 89291
  Culture Oocyte, 89250, 89251
    Extended, 89272
  Embryo Hatching, 89253
  Fertilize Oocyte, 89250
    Microtechnique, 89280, 89281
  Identify Oocyte, 89254
  Insemination of Oocyte, 89268
  Prepare Embryo, 89255, 89352
  Retrieve Oocyte, 58970
  Transfer Embryo, 58974, 58976
  Transfer Gamete, 58976
In Vivo NMR Spectroscopy
  See Magnetic Resonance Spectroscopy
Incision
  See Incision and Drainage
  Abdomen, 49000
    Exploration, 58960
  Accessory Nerve, 63191
  Anal
    Fistula, 46270, 46280
    Septum, 46070
    Sphincter, 46080
  Ankle, 27607
    Tendon, 27605, 27606
  Anus
    See Anus, Incision
  Aortic Valve, 33390-33391
    for Stenosis, 33415
  Artery
    Nose, 30915, 30920
  Atrial Septum, 33735-33737
  Bile Duct
    Sphincter, 43262, 47460
  Bladder
    Catheterization, 51045
    with Destruction, 51020, 51030
    with Radiotracer, 51020
  Bladder Diverticulum, 52305
  Brachial Artery
    Exposure, 34834
  Brain
    Amygdalohippocampectomy, 61566
    Subpial, 61567
  Breast
    Capsules, 19370
  Bronchus, 31899
  Burn Scab, 16035, 16036
  Cataract
    Secondary
      Laser Surgery, 66821
      Stab Incision Technique, 66820
  Colon
    Exploration, 44025
    Stoma
      Creation, 44320, 44322
      Revision, 44340-44346
  Cornea
    for Astigmatism, 65772

Incision — *continued*
Cornea — *continued*
  for Keratoplasty, 0290T
Corpus Callosum, 61541
Cricothyroid Membrane, 31605
Dentate Ligament, 63180, 63182
Duodenum, 44010
Ear, Inner
  Labyrinthectomy, 61596, 69801, 69905
    with Mastoidectomy, 69910
Elbow, 24000
Esophagus, 43020, 43045
  Esophageal Web, 43499
  Muscle, 43030
Exploration
  Heart, 33310-33315
  Kidney, 50010
Eye
  Adhesions, 65880
    Anterior Segment, 65860, 65865
    Anterior Synechiae, 65870
    Corneovitreal, 65880
    Posterior, 65875
  Anterior Chamber, 65820
  Trabecular, 65850
Eyelid
  Canthus, 67715
  Sutures, 67710
Femoral Artery
  Exposure, 34812, 34813
Fibula, 27607
Finger
  Decompression, 26035
  Tendon, 26060, 26455, 26460
  Tendon Sheath, 26055, 26060, 26455, 26460
Foot
  Bone Cortex, 28005
  Capsule, 28260-28264
  Fascia, 28008
  for Infection, 28002, 28003
  Tendon, 28230, 28234
for Implantation of Neurostimulator, 64568
Gallbladder, 47490
Hand Decompression, 26035, 26037
  Tendon, 26450, 26460
Heart
  Exploration, 33310, 33315
  Incision, Not Specified, 33999
Hemorrhoid
  External, 46083
Hepatic Ducts
  See Hepaticostomy
Hip
  Denervation, 27035
  Exploration, 27033
  Fasciotomy, 27025
  Joint Capsule for Flexor Release, 27036
  Tendon
    Abductor, 27006
    Adductor, 27000-27003
    Iliopsoas, 27005
Hymen
  See Hymen, Incision
Hymenotomy, 56442
Hyoid, Muscle, 21685
Iliac Artery
  Exposure, 34820, 34833
Intercarpal Joint
  Dislocation, 25670
Interphalangeal Joint
  Capsule, 26525
Intestines (Except Rectum)
  See Enterotomy
Intestines, Small, 44010
  Biopsy, 44020
  Creation
    Pouch, 44316
    Stoma, 44300-44314
  Decompression, 44021
  Exploration, 44020
  Incision, 44020
  Removal
    Foreign Body, 44020
  Revision
    Stoma, 44312

Incision — *continued*
Intracranial Vessels, 37799
Iris, 66500, 66505
Kidney, 50010, 50045
  Calculus Removal, 50130
    Complicated, 50135
  Exploration, 50010
  Nephrotomy, with Exploration, 50045
  Pyelotomy, with Exploration, 50120
Knee
  Capsule, 27435
  Exploration, 27310
  Fasciotomy, 27305
  Removal of Foreign Body, 27310
Lacrimal Punctum, 68440
Lacrimal Sac
  See Dacryocystotomy
Larynx, 31300
Leg, Lower
  Fasciotomy, 27600-27602
Leg, Upper
  Fasciotomy, 27025, 27305
  Tenotomy, 27306, 27307, 27390-27392
Lip
  Frenum, 40806
Liver
  See Hepatotomy
Lymphatic Channels, 38308
Mastoid
  See Mastoidotomy
Metacarpophalangeal Joint
  Capsule, 26520
Mitral Valve, 33420, 33422
Muscle
  See Myotomy
Nerve, 64568, 64575-64580, 64585, 64595, 64702-64772
  Foot, 28035
  Root, 63185, 63190
  Sacral, 64581
  Vagus, 43640, 43641
Nose
  See Rhinotomy
Orbit
  See Orbitotomy
Palm
  Fasciotomy, 26040, 26045
Pancreas
  Sphincter, 43262
Penis
  Prepuce, 54000, 54001
  Newborn, 54000
Pericardium, 33030, 33031
  with Clot Removal, 33020
  with Foreign Body Removal, 33020
  with Tube Insertion, 33017-33019
Pharynx
  Stoma, 42955
Pleural Cavity
  Empyema, 32035, 32036
  Pneumothorax, 32551
Prostate
  Exposure
    Bilateral Pelvic Lymphadenectomy, 55865
    Insertion Radioactive Substance, 55860
    Lymph Node Biopsy, 55862
  Transurethral, 52450
Pterygomaxillary Fossa, 31040
Pulmonary Valve, 33470-33474
Pyloric Sphincter, 43520
Retina
  Encircling Material, 67115
Sclera
  Fistulization
    Sclerectomy with Punch or Scissors with Iridectomy, 66160
    Thermocauterization with Iridectomy, 66155
    Trabeculectomy ab Externo in Absence Previous Surgery, 66170
    with Iridectomy, 66160
  Trephination with Iridectomy, 66150
Seminal Vesicle, 55600-55605

Infection — *continued*
Diagnosis
Group A Strep Test, 3210F
Drainage
Postoperative Wound, 10180
Filarioidea, 86280
Immunoassay, 86317, 86318
Rapid Test, 86403, 86406
Treatment
Antibiotics Prescribed, 4045F
Infection, Bone
See Osteomyelitis
Infection, Wound
See Wound, Infection
Infectious Agent Detection
Antigen Detection
Direct Fluorescence
Bordetella, 87265
Chlamydia Trachomatis, 87270
Cryptosporidium, 87272
Cytomegalovirus, 87271
Enterovirus, 87267
Giardia, 87269
Influenza A, 87276
Legionella Pneumophila, 87278
Pertussis, 87265
Respiratory Syncytial Virus, 87280
Treponema Pallidum, 87285
Varicella Zoster, 87290
Direct Probe
Vancomycin Resistance, 87500
Enzyme Immunoassay
Adenovirus, 87301
Aspergillus, 87305
Chlamydia Trachomatis, 87320
Clostridium Difficile Toxin A, 87324
Cryptococcus Neoformans, 87327
Cryptosporidium, 87328
Cytomegalovirus, 87332
Entamoeba Histolytica Dispar
Group, 87336
Entamoeba Histolytica Group,
87337
Escherichia coli 0157, 87335
Giardia, 87329
Helicobacter Pylori, 87338, 87339
Hepatitis B Surface Antigen (HB-
sAg), 87340
Hepatitis B Surface Antigen (HB-
sAg) Neutralization, 87341
Hepatitis Be Antigen (HBeAg),
87350
Hepatitis, Delta Agent, 87380
Histoplasma Capsulatum, 87385
HIV–1, 87390
HIV–2, 87391
Influenza A, 87400
Influenza B, 87400
Multiple Step Method, 87301-
87449, 87451
See specific agent
Not Otherwise Specified, 87449-
87451
Respiratory Syncytial Virus, 87420
Rotavirus, 87425
Shiga–like Toxin, 87427
Single Step Method, 87450
Streptococcus, Group A, 87430
Immunoassay
Adenovirus, 87809
Immunofluorescence, 87260, 87273-
87275, 87279, 87281-87283,
87299-87300
Adenovirus, 87260
Herpes Simplex, 87273, 87274
Influenza B, 87275
Not otherwise Specified, 87299
Parainfluenza Virus, 87279
Pneumocystis Carinii, 87281
Polyvalent, 87300
Rubeola, 87283
Nucleic Acid
Vancomycin Resistance, 87500
Concentration, 87015

Infectious Agent Detection — *continued*
Detection
by Immunoassay
Chlamydia Trachomatis, 87810
Clostridium difficile, 87803
HIV Antigen(s) with HIV-1 and HIV-
2 Antibodies, [87806]
Influenza, 87804
Neisseria Gonorrhoeae, 87850
Not Otherwise Specified, 87899
Respiratory Syncytial Virus, 87807
Streptococcus, Group A, 87880
Streptococcus, Group B, 87802
Trichomonas Vaginalis, 87808
with Direct Optical Observation,
87802-87899
by Nucleic Acid
Bartonella Henselae, 87471-87472
Bartonella Quintana, 87471-87472
Borrelia Burgdorferi, 87475-87476
Candida Species, 87480-87482
Central Nervous System Pathogen,
87483
Chlamydia Pneumoniae, 87485-
87487
Chlamydia Trachomatis, 87490-
87492
Cytomegalovirus, 87495-87497
Gardnerella Vaginalis, 87510-87512
Hepatitis B Virus, 87516-87517
Hepatitis C, 87520-87522
Hepatitis G, 87525-87527
Herpes Simplex Virus, 87528-87530
Herpes Virus–6, 87531-87533
HIV–1, 87534-87536
HIV–2, 87537-87539
HPV, 0500T
Influenza, 87501-87503
Intracellulare, 87560-87562
Legionella Pneumophila, 87540-
87542
Multiple Organisms, 87800, 87801
Mycobacteria Avium-Intracellu-
larae, 87560-87562
Mycobacteria Species, 87550-
87552
Mycobacteria Tuberculosis, 87555-
87557
Mycoplasma Genitalium, 87563
Mycoplasma Pneumoniae, 87580-
87582
Neisseria Gonorrhoeae, 87590-
87592
Not Otherwise Specified, 87797-
87799
Papillomavirus, Human, [87623,
87624, 87625]
Respiratory Syncytial Virus, 87634
Staphylococcus
Aureus, 87640-87641
Streptococcus
Group A, 87650-87652
Group B, 87653
Trichomonas Vaginalis, 87660
Zika Virus, 87662
Enzymatic Activity, 87905
Genotype Analysis
by Nucleic Acid
Hepatitis C Virus, 87902
HIV–1 Protease/Reverse Transcrip-
tase, 87901
Phenotype Analysis
by Nucleic Acid
HIV–1 Drug Resistance, 87903,
87904
HIV–1 Drug Resistance, 87900
Phenotype Prediction
by Genetic Database, 87900
Vancomycin Resistance, 87500
Infectious Mononucleosis Virus
See Epstein–Barr Virus
Inflammatory Process
Localization
Nuclear Medicine, 78800-78803 [78804,
78830, 78831, 78832], [78835]

Inflation
Eustachian Tube
Myringotomy, 69420
Anesthesia, 69424
Influenza A
Antigen Detection
Direct Fluorescent, 87276
Enzyme Immunoassay, 87400
Influenza B
Antigen Detection
Enzyme Immunoassay, 87400
Immunofluorescence, 87275
Influenza B Vaccine, 90647-90648, 90748
Influenza Vaccine, 90653-90668 [90630, 90672,
90673, 90674, 90756], 90682-90689, [90694]
In Combination Vaccines, 90697-90698, 90748
Influenza Virus
Antibody, 86710
Vaccine, 90657-90660
by Immunoassay
with Direct Optical Observation, 87804
Infraorbital Nerve
Avulsion, 64734
Incision, 64734
Transection, 64734
Infrared Light Treatment, 97026
See Physical Medicine/Therapy/ Occupational
Therapy
Infratentorial Craniotomy, 61520, 61521
Infusion
Amnion, Transabdominal, 59072
Cerebral
Intravenous for Thrombolysis, 37195
Chemotherapy, 96413-96417, 96423, 96425
Continuous, by Catheter Paraverte-
bral/Paraspinous Block
Thoracic, [64463]
Hydration, 96360-96361
Intra-Arterial
Chemotherapy or Complex Biological
Agent, 96422-96425
Diagnostic, Prophylactic, Diagnostic,
96373
Unlisted, Intra-arterial, 96379
Intracranial Administration
Pharmacological Agent Other Than
Thrombolysis, 61650-61651
Intracranial for Thrombolysis, 61645
Intraosseous, 36680
IV
Chemotherapy, Complex Biological
Agent, 96413-96417
Diagnostic, Prophylactic, Therapeutic,
96365-96368
Hydration, 96360-96361
Unlisted Intravenous Infusion, 96379
Pump
Electronic Analysis, 62367-62370, 95990-
95991
Insertion
Intraarterial, 36260
Intraarterial
Removal, 36262
Revision, 36261
Intravenous
Insertion, 36563
Removal, 36590
Revision, 36576, 36578
Maintenance, 95990-95991, 96521-
96522
Chemotherapy, Pump Services,
96521-96522
Refill, 62369-62370, 95990-95991
Spinal Cord, 62361-62362, 62367-62370,
95990-95991
Ventricular Catheter, 61215
Radioelement, 77750
Subcutaneous, 96369-96371
Therapy, 62350, 62351, 62360-62362
See Injection, Chemotherapy
Arterial Catheterization, 36640
Chemotherapy, 96401-96542, 96549
Home Infusion Procedures, 99601-99602
Intravenous, 96360-96361, 96365-96368
Pain, 62360-62362, 62367-62368

Infusion — *continued*
Transcatheter Therapy, 75894-75898, [37211,
37212, 37213, 37214]
Inguinal Hernia Repair
See Hernia, Repair, Inguinal
INH
See Drug Assay
Inhalation
Pentamidine, 94642
Inhalation Provocation Tests
See Bronchial Challenge Test
Inhalation Treatment, 94640-94645, 94664, 99503
See Pulmonology, Therapeutic
Inhibin A, 86336
Inhibition, Fertilization
See Contraception
Inhibition Test, Hemagglutination, 86280
Inhibitor
Alpha 1-Protease, 82103-82104
Alpha 2-Plasmin, 85410
of Kappa Light Polypeptide Gene Enhancer in
B-Cells, Kinase Complex-Associated
Protein Gene Analysis, 81260
Inhibitory Concentration, Minimum
See Minimum Inhibitory Concentration
Initial Inpatient Consultations
See Consultation, Initial Inpatient
Injection
Abdomen
Air, 49400
Contrast Material, 49400
Allergen, 95115-95134
Anesthetic
Morton's Neuroma, 64455
Paravertebral Facet, 64490-64495
Paravertebral/Paraspinal Block, [64461,
64462, 64463]
Plantar Common Digit, 64455
Sympathetic Nerves, 64505-64530
Transforaminal, 64479-64484
Angiography
Heart Vessels, 93454-93464, 93563-
93568
Pulmonary, 75746
Ankle, 27648
Antigen (Allergen), 95115-95125, 95145-95170
Aponeurosis, 20550
Application, on-body injector, 96377
Autologous Protein Solution, 0481T
Autologous WBC, 0481T
Bladder
Radiologic, 51600-51610
Bone Marrow, into, 38999
Brain Canal, 61070
Breast
Radiologic, 19030
Brisement, 20550-20551
Bursa, 20600-20611
Cardiac Catheterization, 93452-93461, 93563-
93568
Carpal Tunnel
Therapeutic, 20526
Chemotherapy, 96401-96549
Cistern
Medication or Other, 61055
Contrast
Central Venous Access Device, 36598
Gastrostomy, Duodenostomy, Jejunosto-
my, Gastro-jejunostomy, or Ce-
costomy Tube, Percutaneous,
49465
via Peritoneal Catheter, 49424
Corpora Cavernosa, 54235
Cyst
Bone, 20615
Kidney, 50390
Pelvis, 50390
Thyroid, 60300
Dupuytren's Contracture, 20527
Elbow
Arthrography, Radiologic, 24220
Enzyme
Palmar Fascial Cord, 20527
Epidural, 0228T-0231T, 62281-62282, 62320-
62327, 64479-64484

Laparotomy — *continued*
Exploration, 47015, 49000, 49002, 58960
for Staging, 49220
Hemorrhage Control, 49002
Hiatal Hernia, 43332-43333
Second Look, 58960
Staging, 58960
Surgical, 44050
with Biopsy, 49000
Laparotomy, Exploratory, 47015, 49000-49002
Large Bowel
See Anus; Cecum; Rectum
Laroyenne Operation
Vagina, Abscess, Incision and Drainage, 57010
Laryngeal Function Study, 92520
Laryngeal Sensory Testing, 92614-92617
Laryngectomy, 31360-31382
Partial, 31367-31382
Subtotal, 31367, 31368
Total, 31360, 31365
Laryngocele
Removal, 31300
Laryngofissure, 31300
Laryngopharyngectomy
Excision, Larynx, with Pharynx, 31390, 31395
Laryngoplasty
Burns, 31599
Cricoid Split, 31587
Cricotracheal Resection, 31592
Laryngeal Stenosis, *[31551, 31552, 31553, 31554]*
Laryngeal Web, 31580
Medialization, 31591
Open Reduction of Fracture, 31584
Laryngoscopy
Diagnostic, 31505
Direct, 31515-31571
Exploration, 31505, 31520-31526, 31575
Indirect, 31505-31513
Newborn, 31520
Operative, 31530-31561
Telescopic, 31575-31579
with Stroboscopy, 31579
Laryngotomy
Partial, 31370-31382
Removal
Tumor, 31300
Total, 31360-31368
Larynx
Aspiration
Endoscopy, 31515
Biopsy
Endoscopy, 31510, 31535, 31536, 31576
Dilation
Endoscopic, 31528, 31529
Electromyography
Needle, 95865
Endoscopy
Ablation, *[31572]*
Augmentation, *[31574]*
Destruction, *[31572]*
Direct, 31515-31571
Excision, 31545-31546
Exploration, 31505, 31520-31526, 31575
Indirect, 31505-31513
Injection, Therapeutic, *[31573]*
Operative, 31530-31561
Telescopic, 31575-31579
with Stroboscopy, 31579
Excision
Lesion, Endoscopic, 31512, 31545-31546, 31578
Partial, 31367-31382
Total, 31360, 31365
with Pharynx, 31390, 31395
Exploration
Endoscopic, 31505, 31520-31526, 31575
Fracture
Open Treatment, 31584
Insertion
Obturator, 31527
Pharynx
with Pharynx, 31390
Reconstruction
Burns, 31599
Cricoid Split, 31587

Larynx — *continued*
Reconstruction — *continued*
Other, 31599
Stenosis, *[31551, 31552, 31553, 31554]*
Web, 31580
with Pharynx, 31395
Removal
Foreign Body
Endoscopic, 31511, 31530, 31531, 31577
Lesion
Endoscopic, 31512, 31545-31546, 31578
Repair
Reinnervation Neuromuscular Pedicle, 31590
Stroboscopy, 31579
Tumor
Excision, 31300
Endoscopic, 31540, 31541
Unlisted Services and Procedures, 31599
Vocal Cord
Injection, 31513, 31570, 31571
X-ray, 70370
LASEK, 65760
Laser Surgery
Anal, 46917
Cautery
Burn Fenestration, 0479T-0480T
Esophagus, 43227
Eye
Anterior Segment Adhesions, 65860
Corneovitreal Adhesions, 66821
Iridectomy, 66761
Iridotomy, 66761
Lacrimal Punctum, 68760
Posterior Lens, 66821
Retinal Detachment, 67145
Secondary Cataract, 66821
Vitreous Strands/Adhesions, 67031
Lacrimal Punctum, 68760
Lens
Posterior, 66821
Lesion
Mouth, 40820
Nose, 30117, 30118
Penis, 54057
Skin, 17000-17111, 17260-17286
Prostate, 52647-52649
Scar Fenestration, 0479T-0480T
Spine
Diskectomy, 62287
Tumor
Urethra and Bladder, 52234-52240
Urethra and Bladder, 52214
Laser Treatment, 17000-17286, 96920-96922
See Destruction
Lash Procedure
Tracheoplasty, 31750-31760
LASIK, 65760
Lateral Epicondylitis
See Tennis Elbow
Latex Fixation, 86403, 86406
LATS, 80438, 80439
Latzko Procedure
Colpocleisis, 57120
LAV
See HIV
LAV Antibodies, 86689, 86701-86703
LAV-2, 86702-86703
Lavage
Colon, 44701
Gastric, 43753
Lung
Bronchial, 31624
Total, 32997
Peritoneal, 49084
LCM
Antibody, 86727
LCT, 81400
LD (Lactic Dehydrogenase), 83615
LDB3, 81406
LDH, 83615, 83625
LDL, 83721, 83722
LDLR, 81405-81406
Lead, 83655

Leadbetter Procedure, 53431
Lecithin C
See Tissue Typing
Lecithin-Sphingomyelin Ratio, 83661
Lee and White Test, 85345
LEEP Procedure, 57460
LeFort I Procedure
Midface Reconstruction, 21141-21147, 21155, 21160
Palatal or Maxillary Fracture, 21421-21423
LeFort II Procedure
Midface Reconstruction, 21150, 21151
Nasomaxillary Complex Fracture, 21345-21348
LeFort III Procedure
Craniofacial Separation, 21431-21436
Midface Reconstruction, 21154-21159
LeFort Procedure
Vagina, 57120
Left Atrioventricular Valve
See Mitral Valve
Left Heart Cardiac Catheterization
See Cardiac Catheterization, Left Heart
Leg
Cast
Rigid Total Contact, 29445
Excision
Excess Skin, 15833
Lipectomy, Suction Assisted, 15879
Lower
See Ankle; Fibula; Knee; Tibia
Abscess
Incision and Drainage, 27603
Amputation, 27598, 27880-27882
Revision, 27884, 27886
Angiography, 73706
Artery
Ligation, 37618
Biopsy, 27613, 27614
Bursa
Incision and Drainage, 27604
Bypass Graft, 35903
Cast, 29405-29435, 29450
CT Scan, 73700-73706
Decompression, 27600-27602
Exploration
Blood Vessel, 35860
Fasciotomy, 27600-27602, 27892-27894
Hematoma
Incision and Drainage, 27603
Lesion
Excision, 27630
Magnetic Resonance Imaging, 73718-73720
Repair
Blood Vessel, 35226
with Other Graft, 35286
with Vein Graft, 35256
Fascia, 27656
Tendon, 27658-27692
Skin Graft
Delay of Flap, 15610
Full Thickness, 15220, 15221
Pedicle Flap, 15572
Split, 15100, 15101
Splint, 29515
Strapping, 29580
Tendon, 27658-27665
Tissue Transfer, Adjacent, 14020, 14021
Tumor, 27615-27619 *[27632, 27634]*, 27635-27638, 27645-27647
Ultrasound, 76881-76882
Unlisted Services and Procedures, 27899
Unna Boot, 29580
X-ray, 73592
Upper
See Femur
Abscess, 27301
Amputation, 27590-27592
at Hip, 27290, 27295
Revision, 27594, 27596
Angiography, 73706, 75635
Artery
Ligation, 37618
Biopsy, 27323, 27324
Bursa, 27301
Bypass Graft, 35903

Leg — *continued*
Upper — *continued*
Cast, 29345-29365, 29450
Cast Brace, 29358
CT Scan, 73700-73706, 75635
Exploration
Blood Vessel, 35860
Fasciotomy, 27305, 27496-27499, 27892-27894
Halo Application, 20663
Hematoma, 27301
Magnetic Resonance Imaging, 73718-73720
Neurectomy, 27325, 27326
Pressure Ulcer, 15950-15958
Removal
Cast, 29705
Foreign Body, 27372
Repair
Blood Vessel
with Other Graft, 35286
with Vein Graft, 35256
Muscle, 27385, 27386, 27400, 27430
Tendon, 27393-27400
Splint, 29505
Strapping, 29580
Suture
Muscle, 27385, 27386
Tendon, 27658-27665
Tenotomy, 27306, 27307, 27390-27392
Tumor
Excision, 27327-27328 *[27337, 27339]*, 27364-27365 *[27329]*
Ultrasound, 76881-76882
Unlisted Services and Procedures, 27599
Unna Boot, 29580
X-ray, 73592
Wound Exploration
Penetrating, 20103
Leg Length Measurement X-Ray
See Scanogram
Legionella
Antibody, 86713
Antigen, 87278, 87540-87542
Legionella Pneumophila
Antigen Detection
Direct Fluorescence, 87278
Leiomyomata
Embolization, 37243
Removal, 58140, 58545-58546, 58561
Leishmania
Antibody, 86717
Lengthening
Esophageal, 43338
Radius and Ulna, 25391, 25393
Tendons
Lower Extremities, 27393-27395, 27685-27686
Upper Extremities, 24305, 25280, 26476, 26478
Tibia and Fibula, 27715
Lens
Extracapsular, 66940
Intracapsular, 66920
Dislocated, 66930
Intraocular
Exchange, 66986
Reposition, 66825
Prosthesis
Insertion, 66983
Manual or Mechanical Technique, 66982, 66984
not associated with Concurrent Cataract Removal, 66985
Removal
Lens Material
Aspiration Technique, 66840
Extracapsular, 66940
Intracapsular, 66920, 66930
Pars Plana Approach, 66852
Phacofragmentation Technique, 66850
Lens Material
Aspiration Technique, 66840

Lindholm Operation
See Tenoplasty
Lingual Bone
See Hyoid Bone
Lingual Frenectomy
See Excision, Tongue, Frenum
Lingual Nerve
Avulsion, 64740
Incision, 64740
Transection, 64740
Lingual Tonsil
See Tonsils, Lingual
Linton Procedure, 37760
Lip
Biopsy, 40490
Excision, 40500-40530
Frenum, 40819
Incision
Frenum, 40806
Reconstruction, 40525, 40527
Repair, 40650-40654
Cleft Lip, 40700-40761
Fistula, 42260
Unlisted Services and Procedures, 40799
Lip, Cleft
See Cleft Lip
Lipase, 83690
Lipectomies, Aspiration
See Liposuction
Lipectomy
Excision, 15830-15839
Suction Assisted, 15876-15879
Lipids
Feces, 82705, 82710
Lipo–Lutin
See Progesterone
Lipolysis, Aspiration
See Liposuction
Lipophosphodiesterase I
See Tissue Typing
Lipoprotein
(a), 83695
Blood, 83695, 83700-83721
LDL, 83700-83701, 83721, 83722
Phospholipase A2, 0423T, 83698
Lipoprotein, Alpha
See Lipoprotein
Lipoprotein, Pre–Beta
See Lipoprotein, Blood
Liposuction, 15876-15879
Lips
Skin Graft
Delay of Flap, 15630
Full Thickness, 15260, 15261
Pedicle Flap, 15576
Tissue Transfer, Adjacent, 14060, 14061
Lisfranc Operation
Amputation, Foot, 28800, 28805
Listeria Monocytogenes
Antibody, 86723
LITAF, 81404
Lithium
Assay, 80178
Litholapaxy, 52317, 52318
Lithotripsy
See Extracorporeal Shock Wave Therapy
Bile Duct Calculi (Stone)
Endoscopic, 43265
Bladder, 52353
Kidney, 50590, 52353
Pancreatic Duct Calculi (Stone)
Endoscopic, 43265
Skin Wound, 0512T-0513T
Ureter, 52353
Urethra, 52353
with Cystourethroscopy, 52353
Lithotrity
See Litholapaxy
Liver
See Hepatic Duct
Ablation
Tumor, 47380-47383
Laparoscopic, 47370-47371
Abscess
Aspiration, 47015

Liver — continued
Abscess — continued
Incision and Drainage
Open, 47010
Injection, 47015
Aspiration, 47015
Biopsy, 47100
Anesthesia, 00702
Cholangiography Injection
Existing Access, 47531
New Access, 47532
Cyst
Aspiration, 47015
Incision and Drainage
Open, 47010
Excision
Extensive, 47122
Partial, 47120, 47125, 47130, 47140-47142
Total, 47133
Injection, 47015
Cholangiography
Existing Access, 47531
New Access, 47532
Lobectomy, 47125, 47130
Partial, 47120
Needle Biopsy, 47000, 47001
Nuclear Medicine
Imaging, 78201-78216
Vascular Flow, 78803
Repair
Abscess, 47300
Cyst, 47300
Wound, 47350-47362
Suture
Wound, 47350-47362
Transplantation, 47135
Allograft preparation, 47143-47147
Anesthesia, 00796, 01990
Trisegmentectomy, 47122
Ultrasound Scan (LUSS), 76705
Unlisted Services and Procedures, 47379, 47399
Living Activities, Daily, 97535, 97537
LKP, 65710
L–Leucylnaphthylamidase, 83670
LMNA, 81406
Lobectomy
Brain, 61323, 61537-61540
Contralateral Subtotal
Thyroid Gland, 60212, 60225
Liver, 47120-47130
Lung, 32480-32482
Sleeve, 32486
Parotid Gland, 42410, 42415
Segmental, 32663
Sleeve, 32486
Temporal Lobe, 61537, 61538
Thyroid Gland
Partial, 60210, 60212
Total, 60220, 60225
Total, 32663
Local Excision Mastectomies
See Breast, Excision, Lesion
Local Excision of Lesion or Tissue of Femur
See Excision, Lesion, Femur
Localization
Nodule Radiographic, Breast, 19281-19288
with Biopsy, 19081-19086
Patient Motion, [77387]
Log Hydrogen Ion Concentration
See pH
Lombard Test, 92700
Long Acting Thyroid Stimulator
See Thyrotropin Releasing Hormone (TRH)
Long Chain (C20–C22) Omega–3 Fatty Acids in RBC Membranes, 0111T
Long QT Syndrome Gene Analyses, 81413-81414
Long Term Care Facility Visits
Annual Assessment, 99318
Care Plan Oversight Services, 99379-99380
Discharge Services, 99315-99316
Initial, 99304-99306
Subsequent, 99307-99310
Longmire Operation, 47765

Loopogram
See Urography, Antegrade
Looposcopy, 53899
Loose Body
Removal
Ankle, 27620
Carpometacarpal, 26070
Elbow, 24101
Interphalangeal Joint, 28020
Toe, 28024
Knee Joint, 27331
Metatarsophalangeal Joint, 28022
Tarsometatarsal Joint, 28020
Toe, 28022
Wrist, 25101
Lord Procedure
Anal Sphincter, Dilation, 45905
Lorenz's Operation, 27258
Louis Bar Syndrome, 88248
Low Birth Weight Intensive Care Services, 99478-99480
Low Density Lipoprotein
See Lipoprotein, LDL
Low Frequency Ultrasound, 97610
Low Level Laser Therapy, 0552T
Low Vision Aids
Fitting, 92354, 92355
Lower Extremities
See Extremity, Lower
Lower GI Series
See Barium Enema
Lowsley's Operation, 54380
LP, 62270
LRH (Luteinizing Releasing Hormone), 83727
LRP5, 81406
LRRK2, 81401, 81408
L/S, 83661
L/S Ratio
Amniotic Fluid, 83661
LSD (Lysergic Acid Diethylamide), 80299, [80305, 80306, 80307]
LTH
See Prolactin
Lucentis Injection, 67028
Lumbar
See Spine
Lumbar Plexus
Decompression, 64714
Injection, Anesthetic or Steroid, 64449
Neuroplasty, 64714
Release, 64714
Repair
Suture, 64862
Lumbar Puncture
See Spinal Tap
Lumbar Spine Fracture
See Fracture, Vertebra, Lumbar
Lumbar Sympathectomy
See Sympathectomy, Lumbar
Lumbar Vertebra
See Vertebra, Lumbar
Lumen Dilation, 74360
Lumpectomy, 19301-19302
Lunate
Arthroplasty
with Implant, 25444
Dislocation
Closed Treatment, 25690
Open Treatment, 25695
Lung
Ablation, 32998, [32994]
Abscess
Incision and Drainage, 32200
Angiography
Injection, 93568
Biopsy, 32096-32097, 32100
Bullae
Excision, 32141
Endoscopic, 32655
Cyst
Incision and Drainage, 32200
Removal, 32140
Decortication
Endoscopic, 32651, 32652
Partial, 32225
Total, 32220

Lung — continued
Decortication — continued
with Parietal Pleurectomy, 32320
Empyema
Excision, 32540
Excision
Bronchus Resection, 32486
Completion, 32488
Donor, 33930
Heart Lung, 33930
Lung, 32850
Emphysematous, 32491
Empyema, 32540
Lobe, 32480, 32482
Segment, 32484
Total, 32440-32445
Tumor, 32503-32504
Wedge Resection, 32505-32507
Endoscopic, 32666-32668
Foreign Body
Removal, 32151
Hemorrhage, 32110
Injection
Radiologic, 93568
Lavage
Bronchial, 31624
Total, 32997
Lysis
Adhesions, 32124
Needle Biopsy, 32405
Nuclear Medicine
Imaging, Perfusion, 78580-78598
Imaging, Ventilation, 78579, 78582, 78598
Unlisted Services and Procedures, 78599
Pneumolysis, 32940
Pneumothorax, 32960
Removal
Bilobectomy, 32482
Bronchoplasty, 32501
Completion Pneumonectomy, 32488
Extrapleural, 32445
Single Lobe, 32480
Single Segment, 32484
Sleeve Lobectomy, 32486
Sleeve Pneumonectomy, 32442
Total Pneumonectomy, 32440-32445
Two Lobes, 32482
Volume Reduction, 32491
Wedge Resection, 32505-32507
Repair
Hernia, 32800
Segmentectomy, 32484
Tear
Repair, 32110
Thoracotomy, 32110-32160
Biopsy, 32096-32098
Cardiac Massage, 32160
for Post–Operative Complications, 32120
Removal
Bullae, 32141
Cyst, 32140
Intrapleural Foreign Body, 32150
Intrapulmonary Foreign Body, 32151
Repair, 32110
with Excision–Plication of Bullae, 32141
with Open Intrapleural Pneumonolysis, 32124
Transplantation, 32851-32854, 33935
Allograft Preparation, 32855-32856, 33933
Donor Pneumonectomy
Heart–Lung, 33930
Lung, 32850
Tumor
Removal, 32503-32504
Unlisted Services and Procedures, 32999
Volume Reduction
Emphysematous, 32491
Lung Function Tests
See Pulmonology, Diagnostic
Lupus Anticoagulant Assay, 85705
Lupus Band Test
Immunofluorescence, 88346, [88350]
Luschke Procedure, 45120

LUSCS, 59514-59515, 59618, 59620, 59622
LUSS (Liver Ultrasound Scan), 76705
Luteinizing Hormone (LH), 80418, 80426, 83002
Luteinizing Release Factor, 83727
Luteotropic Hormone, 80418, 84146
Luteotropin, 80418, 84146
Luteotropin Placental, 83632
Lutrepulse Injection, 11980
LVRS, 32491
- **Lyme Disease**, 86617, 86618
Lyme Disease ab, 86617
Lymph Duct
 Injection, 38790
Lymph Node(s)
 Abscess
  Incision and Drainage, 38300, 38305
 Biopsy, 38500, 38510-38530, 38570
  Needle, 38505
 Dissection, 38542
 Excision, 38500, 38510-38530
  Abdominal, 38747
  Inguinofemoral, 38760, 38765
  Laparoscopic, 38571-38573
  Limited, for Staging
   Para–Aortic, 38562
   Pelvic, 38562
   Retroperitoneal, 38564
  Pelvic, 38770
  Radical
   Axillary, 38740, 38745
   Cervical, 38720, 38724
   Suprahyoid, 38720, 38724
  Retroperitoneal Transabdominal, 38780
  Thoracic, 38746
 Exploration, 38542
 Hygroma, Cystic
  Axillary
   Cervical
    Excision, 38550, 38555
 Nuclear Medicine
  Imaging, 78195
 Removal
  Abdominal, 38747
  Inguinofemoral, 38760, 38765
  Pelvic, 38747, 38770
  Retroperitoneal Transabdominal, 38780
  Thoracic, 38746
Lymph Vessels
 Imaging
  Lymphangiography
   Abdomen, 75805-75807
   Arm, 75801-75803
   Leg, 75801-75803
   Pelvis, 75805-75807
  Nuclear Medicine, 78195
 Incision, 38308
Lymphadenectomy
 Abdominal, 38747
 Bilateral Inguinofemoral, 54130, 56632, 56637
 Bilateral Pelvic, 51575, 51585, 51595, 54135,
   55845, 55865
  Total, 38571-38573, 57531, 58210
 Diaphragmatic Assessment, 58960
 Gastric, 38747
 Inguinofemoral, 38760, 38765
 Inguinofemoral, Iliac and Pelvic, 56640
 Injection
  Sentinel Node, 38792
 Limited, for Staging
  Para–Aortic, 38562
  Pelvic, 38562
  Retroperitoneal, 38564
 Limited Para–Aortic, Resection of Ovarian Ma-
   lignancy, 58951
 Limited Pelvic, 55842, 55862, 58954
 Malignancy, 58951, 58954
 Mediastinal, 21632, 32674
 Para-Aortic, 58958
 Pelvic, 58958
 Peripancreatic, 38747
 Portal, 38747
 Radical
  Axillary, 38740, 38745
  Cervical, 38720, 38724
  Groin Area, 38760, 38765
  Pelvic, 54135, 55845, 58548

Lymphadenectomy — continued
 Radical — continued
  Suprahyoid, 38700
 Retroperitoneal Transabdominal, 38780
 Thoracic, 38746
 Unilateral Inguinofemoral, 56631, 56634
Lymphadenitis
 Incision and Drainage, 38300, 38305
Lymphadenopathy Associated Antibodies
 See Antibody, HIV
Lymphadenopathy Associated Virus
 See HIV
Lymphangiogram, Abdominal
 See Lymphangiography, Abdomen
Lymphangiography
 Abdomen, 75805, 75807
 Arm, 75801, 75803
 Injection, 38790
 Leg, 75801, 75803
 Pelvis, 75805, 75807
Lymphangioma, Cystic
 See Hygroma
Lymphangiotomy, 38308
Lymphatic Channels
 Incision, 38308
Lymphatic Cyst
 Drainage
  Laparoscopic, 49323
  Open, 49062
Lymphatic System
 Anesthesia, 00320
 Unlisted Procedure, 38999
Lymphoblast Transformation
 See Blastogenesis
Lymphoblastic Leukemia, 81305
Lymphocele
 Drainage
  Laparoscopic, 49323
  Extraperitoneal
   Open Drainage, 49062
Lymphocyte
 Culture, 86821
 Toxicity Assay, 86805, 86806
 Transformation, 86353
Lymphocyte, Thymus–Dependent
 See T–Cells
Lymphocytes, CD4
 See CD4
Lymphocytes, CD8
 See CD8
Lymphocytic Choriomeningitis
 Antibody, 86727
Lymphocytotoxicity, 86805, 86806
Lymphoma Virus, Burkitt
 See Epstein–Barr Virus
Lynch Procedure, 31075
Lysergic Acid Diethylamide, 80299, [80305, 80306,
   80307]
Lysergide, 80299, [80305, 80306, 80307]
Lysis
 Adhesions
  Bladder
   Intraluminal, 53899
  Corneovitreal, 65880
  Epidural, 62263, 62264
  Fallopian Tube, 58740
  Foreskin, 54450
  Intestinal, 44005
  Labial, 56441
  Lung, 32124
  Nose, 30560
  Ovary, 58740
  Oviduct, 58740
  Penile
   Post–circumcision, 54162
  Spermatic Cord, 54699, 55899
  Tongue, 41599
  Ureter, 50715-50725
   Intraluminal, 53899
  Urethra, 53500
  Uterus, 58559
 Euglobulin, 85360
 Eye
  Goniosynechiae, 65865
  Synechiae
   Anterior, 65870

Lysis — continued
 Eye — continued
  Synechiae — continued
   Posterior, 65875
 Labial
  Adhesions, 56441
 Nose
  Intranasal Synechia, 30560
 Transurethral
  Adhesions, 53899
Lysozyme, 85549

M

MacEwen Operation
 Hernia Repair, Inguinal, 49495-49500, 49505
  Incarcerated, 49496, 49501, 49507,
   49521
  Laparoscopic, 49650, 49651
  Recurrent, 49520
  Sliding, 49525
Machado Test
 Complement, Fixation Test, 86171
MacLean–De Wesselow Test
 Clearance, Urea Nitrogen, 84540, 84545
Macrodactylia
 Repair, 26590
Macroscopic Examination and Tissue Preparation,
   88387
 Intraoperative, 88388
Macular Pigment Optical Density, 0506T
Maculopathy, 67208-67218
Madlener Operation, 58600
Magnesium, 83735
Magnet Operation
 Eye, Removal of Foreign Body
  Conjunctival Embedded, 65210
  Conjunctival Superficial, 65205
  Corneal with Slit Lamp, 65222
  Corneal without Slit Lamp, 65220
  Intraocular, 65235-65265
Magnetic Resonance Angiography (MRA)
 Abdomen, 74185
 Arm, 73225
 Chest, 71555
 Fetal, 74712-74713
 Head, 70544-70546
 Leg, 73725
 Neck, 70547-70549
 Pelvis, 72198
 Spine, 72159
Magnetic Resonance Spectroscopy, 76390
Magnetic Stimulation
 Transcranial, 90867-90869
Magnetocardiography (MCG)
 Interpretation and Report, 0542T
 Single Study, 0541T
Magnetoencephalography (MEG), 95965-95967
Magnuson Procedure, 23450
MAGPI Operation, 54322
Magpi Procedure, 54322
Major Vestibular Gland
 See Bartholin's Gland
Malar Area
 Augmentation, 21270
 Bone Graft, 21210
 Fracture
  Open Treatment, 21360-21366
   with Bone Grafting, 21366
   with Manipulation, 21355
 Reconstruction, 21270
Malar Bone
 See Cheekbone
Malaria Antibody, 86750
Malaria Smear, 87207
Malate Dehydrogenase, 83775
Maldescent, Testis
 See Testis, Undescended
Male Circumcision
 See Circumcision
Malformation, Arteriovenous
 See Arteriovenous Malformation
Malic Dehydrogenase
 See Malate Dehydrogenase
Malignant Hyperthermia Susceptibility
 Caffeine Halothane Contracture Test (CHCT),
   89049

Malleolus
 See Ankle; Fibula; Leg, Lower; Tibia; Tibiofibular
   Joint
 Metatarsophalangeal Joint, 27889
Mallet Finger Repair, 26432
Mallory–Weiss Procedure, 43502
Maltose
 Tolerance Test, 82951, 82952
Malunion Repair
 Femur
  with Graft, 27472
  without Graft, 27470
 Metatarsal, 28322
 Tarsal Joint, 28320
Mammalian Oviduct
 See Fallopian Tube
Mammaplasties
 See Breast, Reconstruction
Mammaplasty, 19318-19325
Mammary Abscess, 19020
Mammary Arteries
 See Artery, Mammary
Mammary Duct
 X–ray with Contrast, 77053, 77054
Mammary Ductogram
 Injection, 19030
 Radiologic Supervision and Interpretation,
   77053-77054
Mammary Node
 Dissection
  Anesthesia, 00406
Mammary Stimulating Hormone, 80418, 84146
Mammilliplasty, 19350
Mammogram
 Diagnostic, 77065-77066
 Guidance for Placement Localization Device,
   19281-19282
 Magnetic Resonance Imaging (MRI) with
  Computer-aided Detection, 77048-
   77049
 Screening, 77067
 with Computer-Aided Detection, 77065-77067
Mammography
 Assessment, 3340F-3350F
 Diagnostic, 77065-77066
 Guidance for Placement Localization Device,
   19281-19282
 Magnetic Resonance Imaging (MRI) with
  Computer-Aided Detection, 77048-
   77049
 Screening, 77067
 with Computer-Aided Detection, 77065-77067
Mammoplasty
 Anesthesia, 00402
 Augmentation, 19324, 19325
 Reduction, 19318
Mammotomy
 See Mastotomy
Mammotropic Hormone, Pituitary, 80418, 84146
Mammotropic Hormone, Placental, 83632
Mammotropin, 80418, 84146
Manchester Colporrhaphy, 58400
Mandated Services
 Hospital, on call, 99026, 99027
Mandible
 See Facial Bones; Maxilla; Temporomandibular
   Joint (TMJ)
 Abscess
  Excision, 21025
 Bone Graft, 21215
 Cyst
  Excision, 21040, 21046, 21047
 Dysostosis Repair, 21150-21151
 Fracture
  Closed Treatment
   with Interdental Fixation, 21453
   with Manipulation, 21451
   without Manipulation, 21450
  Open Treatment, 21454-21470
   External Fixation, 21454
   with Interdental Fixation, 21462
   without Interdental Fixation, 21461
  Percutaneous Treatment, 21452
 Osteotomy, 21198, 21199

Mandible — *continued*
Reconstruction
with Implant, 21244-21246, 21248, 21249
Removal
Foreign Body, 41806
Torus Mandibularis
Excision, 21031
Tumor
Excision, 21040-21047
X–ray, 70100, 70110
Mandibular Body
Augmentation
with Bone Graft, 21127
with Prosthesis, 21125
Mandibular Condyle
Fracture
Open Treatment, 21465, 21470
Reconstruction, 21247
Mandibular Condylectomy
See Condylectomy
Mandibular Fracture
See Fracture, Mandible
Mandibular Rami
Reconstruction
with Bone Graft, 21194
with Internal Rigid Fixation, 21196
without Bone Graft, 21193
without Internal Rigid Fixation, 21195
Mandibular Resection Prosthesis, 21081
Mandibular Staple Bone Plate
Reconstruction
Mandible, 21244
Manganese, 83785
Manipulation
Chest Wall, 94667-94669
Chiropractic, 98940-98943
Dislocation and/or Fracture
Acetabulum, 27222
Acromioclavicular, 23545
Ankle, 27810, 27818, 27860
Carpometacarpal, 26670-26676
Clavicle, 23505
Elbow, 24300, 24640
Epicondyle, 24565
Femoral, 27232, 27502, 27510, 27517
Peritrochanteric, 27240
Fibula, 27781, 27788
Finger, 26725, 26727, 26742, 26755
Greater Tuberosity
Humeral, 23625
Hand, 26670-26676
Heel, 28405, 28406
Hip, 27257
Hip Socket, 27222
Humeral, 23605, 24505, 24535, 24577
Epicondyle, 24565
Intercarpal, 25660
Interphalangeal Joint, 26340, 26770-26776
Lunate, 25690
Malar Area, 21355
Mandibular, 21451
Metacarpal, 26605, 26607
Metacarpophalangeal, 26700-26706, 26742
Metacarpophalangeal Joint, 26340
Metatarsal Fracture, 28475, 28476
Nasal Bone, 21315, 21320
Orbit, 21401
Phalangeal Shaft, 26727
Distal, Finger or Thumb, 26755
Phalanges, Finger/Thumb, 26725
Phalanges
Finger, 26742, 26755, 26770-26776
Finger/Thumb, 26727
Great Toe, 28495, 28496
Toes, 28515
Radial, 24655, 25565
Radial Shaft, 25505
Radiocarpal, 25660
Radioulnar, 25675
Scapula, 23575
Shoulder, 23650, 23655
with Greater Tuberosity, 23665

Manipulation — *continued*
Dislocation and/or Fracture — *continued*
Shoulder — *continued*
with Surgical or Anatomical Neck, 23675
Sternoclavicular, 23525
with Surgical or Anatomical Neck, 23675
Talus, 28435, 28436
Tarsal, 28455, 28456
Thumb, 26641-26650
Tibial, 27532, 27752
Trans–Scaphoperilunar, 25680
Ulnar, 24675, 25535, 25565
Vertebral, 22315
Wrist, 25259, 25624, 25635, 25660, 25675, 25680, 25690
Foreskin, 54450
Globe, 92018, 92019
Hip, 27275
Interphalangeal Joint, Proximal, 26742
Knee, 27570
Osteopathic, 98925-98929
Palmar Fascial Cord, 26341
Physical Therapy, 97140
Shoulder
.Application of Fixation Apparatus, 23700
Spine
Anesthesia, 22505
Stoma, 44799
Temporomandibular Joint (TMJ), 21073
Tibial, Distal, 27762
Manometric Studies
Kidney
Pressure, 50396
Rectum
Anus, 91122
Ureter
Pressure, 50686
Ureterostomy, 50686
Manometry
Anorectal, 90912-90913
Esophageal, 43499
Esophagogastric, 91020
Perineal, 90912-90913
Mantoux Test
Skin Test, 86580
Manual Therapy, 97140
MAP2K1, 81406
MAP2K2, 81406
Mapping
Brain, 96020
for Seizure Activity, 95961-95962
Sentinel Lymph Node, 38900
MAPT, 81406
Maquet Procedure, 27418
Marcellation Operation
Hysterectomy, Vaginal, 58260-58270, 58550
Marrow, Bone
Aspiration, 20939, 38220, 38222
Biopsy, 38221-38222
CAR-T Therapy, 0537T-0540T
Harvesting, 0537T, 38230
Magnetic Resonance Imaging (MRI), 77084
Nuclear Medicine Imaging, 78102-78104
Smear, 85097
T-Cell Transplantation, 38240-38242
Marshall–Marchetti–Krantz Procedure, 51840, 51841, 58152, 58267, 58293
Marsupialization
Bartholin's Gland Cyst, 56440
Cyst
Acne, 10040
Bartholin's Gland, 56440
Laryngeal, 31599
Splenic, 38999
Sublingual Salivary, 42409
Lesion
Kidney, 53899
Liver
Cyst or Abscess, 47300
Pancreatic Cyst, 48500
Skin, 10040
Urethral Diverticulum, 53240

Mass
Kidney
Ablation, 50542
Cryosurgery, 50250
Mass Spectrometry and Tandem Mass Spectrometry
Analyte(s), 83789
Massage
Cardiac, 32160
Therapy, 97124
See Physical Medicine/Therapy/Occupational Therapy
Masseter Muscle/Bone
Reduction, 21295, 21296
Mastectomy
Gynecomastia, 19300
Modified Radical, 19307
Partial, 19301-19302
Radical, 19305-19306
Simple, Complete, 19303
Subcutaneous, 19300, 19318
Mastectomy, Halsted
See Mastectomy, Radical
Masters' 2–Step Stress Test, 93799
Mastoid
Excision
Complete, 69502
Radical, 69511
Modified, 69505
Petrous Apicectomy, 69530
Simple, 69501
Total, 69502
Obliteration, 69670
Repair
by Excision, 69601-69603
Fistula, 69700
with Apicectomy, 69605
with Tympanoplasty, 69604
Mastoid Cavity
Debridement, 69220, 69222
Mastoidectomy
Cochlear Device Implantation, 69930
Complete, 69502
Revision, 69601-69605
Osseointegrated Implant
for External Speech Processor/Cochlear Stimulator, 69715, 69718
Ossicular Chain Reconstruction, 69605
Radical, 69511
Modified, 69505
Revision, 69602, 69603
Revision, 69601
Simple, 69501
with Apicectomy, 69605
with Labyrinthectomy, 69910
with Petrous Apicectomy, 69530
with Skull Base Surgery, 61591, 61597
Decompression, 61595
Facial Nerve, 61595
with Tympanoplasty, 69604, 69641-69646
Ossicular Chain Reconstruction, 69642, 69644, 69646
Mastoidotomy, 69635-69637
with Tympanoplasty, 69635
Ossicular Chain Reconstruction, 69636
and Synthetic Prosthesis, 69637
Mastoids
Polytomography, 76101, 76102
X–ray, 70120, 70130
Mastopexy, 19316
Mastotomy, 19020
Maternity Care and Delivery, 0500F-0502F, 0503F, 59400-59898
See also Abortion, Cesarean Delivery, Ectopic Pregnancy, Vaginal Delivery
Maxilla
See Facial Bones; Mandible
Bone Graft, 21210
CT Scan, 70486-70488
Cyst, Excision, 21048, 21049
Excision, 21030, 21032-21034
Fracture
Closed Treatment, 21345, 21421
Open Treatment, 21346-21348, 21422, 21423
with Fixation, 21345-21347

Maxilla — *continued*
Osteotomy, 21206
Reconstruction
with Implant, 21245, 21246, 21248, 21249
Tumor
Excision, 21048-21049
Maxillary Sinus
Antrostomy, 31256-31267
Dilation, 31295
Excision, 31225-31230
Exploration, 31020-31032
Incision, 31020-31032, 31256-31267
Irrigation, 31000
Skull Base, 61581
Maxillary Torus Palatinus
Tumor Excision, 21032
Maxillectomy, 31225, 31230
Maxillofacial Fixation
Application
Halo Type Appliance, 21100
Maxillofacial Impressions
Auricular Prosthesis, 21086
Definitive Obturator Prosthesis, 21080
Facial Prosthesis, 21088
Interim Obturator Prosthesis, 21079
Mandibular Resection Prosthesis, 21081
Nasal Prosthesis, 21087
Oral Surgical Splint, 21085
Orbital Prosthesis, 21077
Palatal Augmentation Prosthesis, 21082
Palatal Lift Prosthesis, 21083
Speech Aid Prosthesis, 21084
Surgical Obturator Prosthesis, 21076
Maxillofacial Procedures
Unlisted Services and Procedures, 21299
Maxillofacial Prosthetics, 21076-21088
Unlisted Services and Procedures, 21089
Maydl Operation, 45563, 50810
Mayo Hernia Repair, 49580-49587
Mayo Operation
Varicose Vein Removal, 37700-37735, 37780, 37785
Maze Procedure, 33254-33259, 33265-33266
MBC, 87181-87190
MC4R, 81403
McBurney Operation
Hernia Repair, Inguinal, 49495-49500, 49505
Incarcerated, 49496, 49501, 49507, 49521
Recurrent, 49520
Sliding, 49525
McCall Culdoplasty, 57283
McCannel Procedure, 66682
McCauley Procedure, 28240
MCCC1, 81406
MCCC2, 81406
McDonald Operation, 57700
MCG, 0541T-0542T
McKeown Esophagectomy, 43112
McKissock Surgery, 19318
McIndoe Procedure, 57291
MCOLN1, 81290, 81412
McVay Operation
Hernia Repair, Inguinal, 49495-49500, 49505
Incarcerated, 49496, 49501, 49507, 49521
Laparoscopic, 49650, 49651
Recurrent, 49520
Sliding, 49525
MEA (Microwave Endometrial Ablation), 58563
Measles, German
Antibody, 86756
Vaccine, 90707, 90710
Measles Immunization, 90707, 90710
Measles, Mumps, Rubella Vaccine, 90707
Measles Uncomplicated
Antibody, 86765
Antigen Detection, 87283
Measles Vaccine, 90707, 90710
Measurement
Macular Pigment Optical Density, 0506T
Meibomian Gland Near-infrared, 0507T
Ocular Blood Flow, 0198T
Spirometric Forced Expiratory Flow, 94011-94012

Meat Fibers
  Feces, 89160
Meatoplasty, 69310
Meatotomy, 53020-53025
  Contact Laser Vaporization with/without
    Transurethral Resection of Prostate,
    52648
    with Cystourethroscopy, 52281
  Infant, 53025
  Non–Contact Laser Coagulation Prostate,
    52647
  Prostate
    Laser Coagulation, 52647
    Laser Vaporization, 52648
    Transurethral Electrosurgical Resection
      Prostate, 52601
  Ureter, 52290
  Urethral
    Cystourethroscopy, 52290-52305
Meckel's Diverticulum
  Excision, 44800
  Unlisted Services and Procedures, 44899
MECP2, 81302-81304
MED12, 81401
Median Nerve
  Decompression, 64721
  Neuroplasty, 64721
  Release, 64721
  Repair
    Suture
      Motor, 64835
  Transposition, 64721
Median Nerve Compression
  Decompression, 64721
    Endoscopy, 29848
    Injection, 20526
Mediastinoscopy
  with Biopsy, 39401-39402
  with Esophagogastric Fundoplasty, [43210]
Mediastinotomy
  Cervical Approach, 39000
  Transthoracic Approach, 39010
Mediastinum
  See Chest; Thorax
  Cyst
    Excision, 32662, 39200
  Endoscopy
    Biopsy, 39401-39402
    Esophagogastric Fundoplasty, [43210]
    Exploration, 39401
  Exploration, 39000, 39010
  Incision and Drainage, 39000, 39010
  Lymphadenectomy, 32674
  Needle Biopsy, 32405
  Removal
    Foreign Body, 39000, 39010
  Tumor
    Excision, 32662, 39220
  Unlisted Procedures, 39499
Medical Disability Evaluation Services, 99455,
  99456
Medical Genetics
  Counseling, 96040
Medical Nutrition Therapy, 97802-97804
Medical Team Conference, 99366-99368
Medical Testimony, 99075
Medication Therapy Management
  By a Pharmacist
    Initial Encounter, 99605-99606
    Subsequent Encounter, 99607
  Each Additional 15 Minutes, 99607
Medicine, Preventive
  See Preventive Medicine
Medicine, Pulmonary
  See Pulmonology
MEFV, 81402, 81404
MEG (Magnetoencephalography), 95965-95967
MEG3/DLK1, 81401
Meibomian Cyst
  Excision, 67805
    Multiple
      Different Lids, 67805
      Same Lid, 67801
    Single, 67800
    Under Anesthesia, 67808
Meiobomian Gland Near-infrared Imaging, 0507T

Membrane, Mucous
  See Mucosa
Membrane, Tympanic
  See Ear, Drum
MEN1, 81404-81405
Menactra, 90734
MenACWY-CRM, 90734
MenACWY-D, 90734
MenACWY-TT, 90619
MenB-4C, [90620]
MenB-FHbp, [90621]
Meninges
  Tumor
    Excision, 61512, 61519
Meningioma
  Excision, 61512, 61519
  Tumor
    Excision, 61512, 61519
Meningitis, Lymphocytic Benign
  Antibody, 86727
Meningocele Repair, 63700, 63702
Meningococcal Vaccine
  Conjugate, Serogroups A, C, W, Y
    A, C, Y, W-135 Combined, 90733-90734
    CRM197, 90734
    MenACWY-CRM, 90734
    MenACWY-D, diphtheria toxoid carrier,
      90734
    MenACWY-TT, tetanus toxoid carrier,
      90619
  Conjugate, Serogroups C & Y and Hemophilus
    Influenza B, 90644
  Group B, [90620, 90621]
  Recombinant, [90620, 90621]
Meningococcus, 86741
Meningomyelocele
  Repair, 63704-63706
Meniscal Temporal Lobectomy, 61566
Meniscectomy
  Knee Joint, 27332, 27333
  Temporomandibular Joint, 21060
Meniscus
  Knee
    Excision, 27332, 27333
    Repair, 27403
    Transplantation, 29868
Menomune, 90733
Mental Nerve
  Avulsion, 64736
  Incision, 64736
  Transection, 64736
Menveo, 90734
Meprobamate, [80369, 80370]
Mercury, 83015, 83825
Merskey Test
  Fibrin Degradation Products, 85362-85379
Mesenteric Arteries
  See Artery, Mesenteric
Mesentery
  Lesion
    Excision, 44820
  Repair, 44850
  Suture, 44850
  Unlisted Services and Procedures, 44899
Mesh
  Implantation
    Hernia, 49568
  Insertion
    Pelvic Floor, 57267
  Removal
    Abdominal Infected, 11008
Mesh Implantation
  Closure of Necrotizing Soft Tissue Infection,
    49568
  Incisional or Ventral Hernia, 49568
  Vagina, 57267
Metabisulfite Test
  Red Blood Cell, Sickling, 85660
Metabolic Panel
  Calcium Ionized, 80047
  Calcium Total, 80048
  Comprehensive, 80053
Metabolite
  Cocaine, [80353]
  Thromboxane, 84431

Metacarpal
  Amputation, 26910
  Craterization, 26230
  Cyst
    Excision, 26200, 26205
  Diaphysectomy, 26230
  Excision, 26230
    Radical for Tumor, 26250
  Fracture
    Closed Treatment, 26605
      with Fixation, 26607
    Open Treatment, 26615
    Percutaneous Fixation, 26608
    with Manipulation, 26605, 26607
    without Manipulation, 26600
  Ostectomy
    Radical
      for Tumor, 26250
  Repair
    Lengthening, 26568
    Nonunion, 26546
    Osteotomy, 26565
  Saucerization, 26230
  Tumor
    Excision, 26200, 26205
Metacarpophalangeal Joint
  Arthrodesis, 26850, 26852
  Arthroplasty, 26530, 26531
  Arthroscopy
    Diagnostic, 29900
    Surgical, 29901, 29902
  Arthrotomy, 26075
  Biopsy
    Synovium, 26105
  Capsule
    Excision, 26520
    Incision, 26520
  Capsulodesis, 26516-26518
  Dislocation
    Closed Treatment, 26700
    Open Treatment, 26715
    Percutaneous Fixation, 26705, 26706
    with Manipulation, 26340
  Exploration, 26075
  Fracture
    Closed Treatment, 26740
    Open Treatment, 26746
    with Manipulation, 26742
  Fusion, 26516-26518, 26850, 26852
  Removal of Foreign Body, 26075
  Repair
    Collateral Ligament, 26540-26542
  Synovectomy, 26135
Metadrenaline, 83835
Metals, Heavy, 83015, 83018
Metanephrine, 83835
Metatarsal
  See Foot
  Amputation, 28810
  Condyle
    Excision, 28288
  Craterization, 28122
  Cyst
    Excision, 28104-28107
  Diaphysectomy, 28122
  Excision, 28110-28114, 28122, 28140
  Fracture
    Closed Treatment
      with Manipulation, 28475, 28476
      without Manipulation, 28470
    Open Treatment, 28485
    Percutaneous Fixation, 28476
  Free Osteocutaneous Flap with Microvascular
    Anastomosis, 20972
  Repair, 28322
    Lengthening, 28306, 28307
    Osteotomy, 28306-28309
  Saucerization, 28122
  Tumor
    Excision, 28104-28107, 28173
Metatarsectomy, 28140
Metatarsophalangeal Joint
  Arthrotomy, 28022, 28052
  Cheilectomy, 28289, 28291
  Dislocation, 28630, 28635, 28645
    Open Treatment, 28645

Metatarsophalangeal Joint — continued
  Dislocation — continued
    Percutaneous Fixation, 28636
  Exploration, 28022
  Great Toe
    Arthrodesis, 28750
    Fusion, 28750
  Release, 28289, 28291
  Removal
    of Foreign Body, 28022
    of Loose Body, 28022
  Repair
    Hallux Rigidus, 28289, 28291
  Synovial
    Biopsy, 28052
    Excision, 28072
  Toe, 28270
Methadone, [80358]
Methamphetamine, [80359]
Methbipyranone, 80436
Methemalbumin, 83857
Methemoglobin, 83045, 83050, 88741
Methenamine Silver Stain, 88312
Methopyrapone, 80436
Methoxyhydroxymandelic Acid, 84585
Methsuximide, [80339, 80340, 80341]
Methyl Alcohol, [80320]
Methyl CpG Binding Protein 2 Gene Analysis,
  81302-81304
Methylamphetamine, [80359]
Methylfluorprednisolone, 80420
Methylmorphine
  See Codeine
Metroplasty, 58540
Metyrapone, 80436
MFN2, 81406, [81448]
Mg, 83735
MGMT, [81287]
MIC (Minimum Inhibitory Concentration), 87186
MICA, 81403
Microalbumin
  Urine, 82043, 82044
Microbiology, 87003-87999 [87623, 87624, 87625,
  87806, 87906, 87910, 87912]
Microdissection, 88380-88381
Microfluorometries, Flow, 88182-88189
  Diagnostic/Pretreatment, 3170F
Microglobulin, Beta 2
  Blood, 82232
  Urine, 82232
Micrographic Surgery
  Mohs Technique, 17311-17315
Micro–Ophthalmia
  Orbit Reconstruction, 21256
Micropigmentation
  Correction, 11920-11922
Micro-Remodeling Female Bladder, 53860
Microsatellite Instability Analysis, 81301
Microscope, Surgical
  See Operating Microscope
Microscopic Evaluation
  Hair, 96902
Microscopies, Electron
  See Electron Microscopy
Microscopy
  Ear Exam, 92504
  Reflectance Confocal (RCM), 96931-96936
Microsomal Antibody, 86376
Microsomia, Hemifacial
  See Hemifacial Microsomia
Microsurgery
  Operating Microscope, 69990
Microvascular Anastomosis
  Bone Graft
    Fibula, 20955
    Other, 20962
  Facial Flap, Free, 15758
  Muscle Flap, Free, 15756
  Osteocutaneous Flap with, 20969-20973
  Skin Flap, Free, 15757
Microvite A, 84590
Microvolt T-Wave Alternans, 93025
Microwave Therapy, 97024
  See Physical Medicine/Therapy/Occupational
    Therapy

Mucosa — *continued*
  Periodontal Grafting, 41870
  Urethra, Mucosal Advancement, 53450
  Vaginal Biopsy, 57100, 57105
Mucosa, Buccal
  See Mouth, Mucosa
Mucosectomy
  Rectal, 44799, 45113
Mucous Cyst
  Hand or finger, 26160
Mucous Membrane
  See Mouth, Mucosa
  Cutaneous
    Biopsy, 11102-11107
    Excision
      Benign Lesion, 11440-11446
      Malignant, 11640-11646
    Layer Closure, Wounds, 12051-12057
    Simple Repair, Wounds, 12011-12018
  Excision
    Sphenoid Sinus, 31288, *[31257]*, *[31259]*
  Lid Margin
    Correction of Trichiasis, 67835
    Nasal Test, 95065
    Ophthalmic Test, 95060
  Rectum
    Proctoplasty for Prolapse, 45505
Mucus Cyst
  See Mucous Cyst
MUGA (Multiple Gated Acquisition), 78453, 78454, 78472-78473, 78483
Muller Procedure
  Attended, 95806
  Unattended, 95807
Multianalyte Assays with Algorithmic Analyses, 0002M-0004M, 0006M-0013M, 81490-81599 *[81522]*
Multifetal Pregnancy Reduction, 59866
Multiple Sleep Latency Testing (MSLT), 95805
Multiple Valve Procedures
  See Valvuloplasty
Mumford Operation, 29824
Mumford Procedure, 23120, 29824
Mumps
  Antibody, 86735
  Immunization, 90707, 90710
  Vaccine
    MMR, 90707
    MMRV, 90710
Muramidase, 85549
Murine Typhus, 86000
Muscle(s)
  See Specific Muscle
  Abdomen
    See Abdominal Wall
  Biofeedback Training, 90912-90913
  Biopsy, 20200-20206
  Chemodenervation
    Extremity, 64642-64645
    Larynx, 64617
    Neck, 64616
    Trunk, 64646-64647
  Debridement
    Infected, 11004-11006
  Heart
    See Myocardium
  Neck
    See Neck Muscle
  Removal
    Foreign Body, 20520, 20525
  Repair
    Extraocular, 65290
    Forearm, 25260-25274
    Wrist, 25260-25274
  Revision
    Arm, Upper, 24330, 24331
    Elbow, 24301
  Transfer
    Arm, Upper, 24301, 24320
    Elbow, 24301
    Femur, 27110
    Hip, 27100-27105, 27111
    Shoulder, 23395, 23397, 24301, 24320

Muscle Compartment Syndrome
  Detection, 20950
Muscle Denervation
  See Chemodenervation
Muscle Division
  Scalenus Anticus, 21700, 21705
  Sternocleidomastoid, 21720, 21725
Muscle Flaps, 15731-15738
  Free, 15756
Muscle Grafts, 15841-15845
Muscle, Oculomotor
  See Eye Muscles
Muscle Testing
  Dynamometry, Eye, 92260
  Extraocular Multiple Muscles, 92265
  Manual, *[97161, 97162, 97163, 97164, 97165, 97166, 97167, 97168, 97169, 97170, 97171, 97172]*
Musculoplasty
  See Muscle, Repair
Musculoskeletal System
  Computer Assisted Surgical Navigational Procedure, 0054T-0055T, 20985
  Unlisted Services and Procedures, 20999, 21499, 24999, 25999, 26989, 27299, 27599, 27899
  Unlisted Services and Procedures, Head, 21499
Musculotendinous (Rotator) Cuff
  Repair, 23410, 23412
Mustard Procedure, 33774-33777
  See Repair, Great Arteries, Revision
MUT, 81406
MutL Homolog 1, Colon Cancer, Nonpolyposis Type 2 Gene Analysis, 81292-81294
MutS Homolog 2, Colon Cancer, Nonpolyposis Type 1 Gene Analysis, 81295-81297
MutS Homolog 6 (E. Coli) Gene Analysis, 81298-81300
MUTYH, 81401, 81406, 81435
MVD (Microvascular Decompression), 61450
MVR, 33430
Myasthenia Gravis
  Cholinesterase Inhibitor Challenge Test, 95857
Myasthenic, Gravis
  See Myasthenia Gravis
MYBPC3, 81407, 81439
Mycobacteria
  Culture, 87116
    Identification, 87118
  Detection, 87550-87562
  Sensitivity Studies, 87190
Mycophenolate
  Assay, 80180
Mycoplasma
  Antibody, 86738
  Culture, 87109
  Detection, 87580-87582
Mycota
  See Fungus
MYD88, 81305
Myectomy, Anorectal
  See Myomectomy, Anorectal
Myelencephalon
  See Medulla
Myelin Basic Protein
  Cerebrospinal Fluid, 83873
Myelodysplastic Syndrome, 81236
Myelography
  Brain, 70010
  Spine
    Cervical, 62302, 72240
    Lumbosacral, 62304, 72265
    Thoracic, 62303, 72255
    Two or More Regions, 62305, 72270
Myeloid Differentiation Primary Response 88, 81305
Myelomeningocele
  Repair, 63704, 63706
  Stereotaxis
    Creation Lesion, 63600
Myeloperoxidase, 83876
Myeloproliferative Neoplasms, 81237
Myelotomy, 63170
MYH11, 81408, 81410-81411
MYH6, 81407
MYH7, 81407, 81439

MYL2, 81405
MYL3, 81405
MYO15A, 81430
MYO7A, 81430
Myocardial
  Imaging, 0331T-0332T, 0541T-0542T, 78466, 78468, 78469, *[93356]*
  Perfusion Imaging, 0439T, 78451-78454, 78491-78492 *[78430, 78431, 78432, 78433]*
    See also Specific Site; Nuclear Medicine
  Positron Emission Tomography (PET), 78459, 78491-78492 *[78430]*, *[78430]*
  Repair
    Postinfarction, 33542
Myocardium, 33140-33141
Myocutaneous Flaps, 15733-15738, 15756
Myofascial Pain Dysfunction Syndrome
  See Temporomandibular Joint (TMJ)
Myofascial Release, 97140
Myofibroma
  Embolization, 37243
  Removal, 58140, 58545-58546, 58561
Myoglobin, 83874
Myomectomy
  Anorectal, 45108
  Uterus, 58140-58146, 58545, 58546
Myoplasty
  Extraocular, 65290, 67346
MYOT, 81405
Myotomy
  Esophagus, 43030
  Hyoid, 21685
  Sigmoid Colon
    Intestine, 44799
    Rectum, 45999
Myotonic Dystrophy, 81187, 81234
Myringoplasty, 69620
Myringostomy, 69420-69421
Myringotomy, 69420, 69421
Myxoid Cyst
  Aspiration/Injection, 20612
  Drainage, 20612
  Wrist
    Excision, 25111-25112

N

N. Meningitidis, 86741
Na, 84295
Nabi-HIB, 90371
Naffziger Operation, 61330
Nagel Test, 92283
Nail Bed
  Reconstruction, 11762
  Repair, 11760
Nail Fold
  Excision
    Wedge, 11765
Nail Plate Separation
  See Onychia
Nails
  Avulsion, 11730, 11732
  Biopsy, 11755
  Debridement, 11720, 11721
  Drainage, 10060-10061
  Evacuation
    Hematoma, Subungual, 11740
  Excision, 11750
    Finger, 26236
    Toe, 28124, 28160
  KOH Examination, 87220
  Removal, 11730, 11732, 11750, 26236, 28124, 28160
  Trimming, 11719
Narcoanalysis, 90865
Narcosynthesis
  Diagnostic and Therapeutic, 90865
Nasal
  Abscess, 30000-30020
  Bleeding, 30901-30906, 31238
  Bone
    Fracture
      Closed Treatment, 21310-21320
      Open Treatment, 21325-21335
      with Manipulation, 21315, 21320
      without Manipulation, 21310

Nasal — *continued*
  Bone — *continued*
    X–ray, 70160
  Deformity Repair, 40700-40761
  Function Study, 92512
  Polyp
    Excision
      Extensive, 30115
      Simple, 30110
  Prosthesis
    Impression, 21087
  Septum
    Abscess
      Incision and Drainage, 30020
    Fracture
      Closed Treatment, 21337
      Open Treatment, 21336
    Hematoma
      Incision and Drainage, 30020
    Repair, 30630
    Submucous Resection, 30520
  Sinuses
    See Sinus; Sinuses
  Smear
    Eosinophils, 89190
  Turbinate
    Fracture
      Therapeutic, 30930
Nasoethmoid Complex
  Fracture
    Open Treatment, 21338, 21339
    Percutaneous Treatment, 21340
  Reconstruction, 21182-21184
Nasogastric Tube
  Placement, 43752
Nasolacrimal Duct
  Exploration, 68810
    with Anesthesia, 68811
  Insertion
    Stent, 68815
  Probing, 68816
  X–ray
    with Contrast, 70170
Nasomaxillary
  Fracture
    Closed Treatment, 21345
    Open Treatment, 21346-21348
    with Bone Grafting, 21348
Nasopharynges
  See Nasopharynx
Nasopharyngoscopy, 92511
Nasopharynx
  See Pharynx
  Biopsy, 42804, 42806
  Hemorrhage, 42970-42972
  Unlisted Services and Procedures, 42999
Natriuretic Peptide, 83880
Natural Killer Cells (NK)
  Total Count, 86357
Natural Ostium
  Sinus
    Maxillary, 31000
    Sphenoid, 31002
Navicular
  Arthroplasty
    with Implant, 25443
  Fracture
    Closed Treatment, 25622
    Open Treatment, 25628
    with Manipulation, 25624
  Repair, 25440
Navigation
  Computer Assisted, 20985, 61781-61783
NDP, 81403-81404
NDUFA1, 81404
NDUFAF2, 81404
NDUFS1, 81406
NDUFS4, 81404
NDUFS7, 81405
NDUFS8, 81405
NDUFV1, 81405
Near-infrared
  Dual Imaging of Meibomian Glands, 0507T
  Spectroscopy Studies
    Lower Extremity Wound, 0493T
NEB, 81400, 81408

NPWT (Negative Pressure Wound Therapy), 97605-97608

NRAS, 81311

NROB1, 81404

NSD1, 81405-81406

NST, 59025

NSVD, 59400-59410, 59610-59614

NTD (Nitroblue Tetrazolium Dye Test), 86384

Nuclear Antigen
Antibody, 86235

Nuclear Imaging
See Nuclear Medicine

Nuclear Magnetic Resonance Imaging
See Magnetic Resonance Imaging (MRI)

Nuclear Magnetic Resonance Spectroscopy
See Magnetic Resonance Spectroscopy

Nuclear Matrix Protein 22 (NMP22), 86386

Nuclear Medicine, 78012-79999 [78429, 78430, 78431, 78432, 78433, 78434, 78804, 78830, 78831, 78832, 78835]
Abscess Localization, 78300, 78305-78306, 78315
Adrenal Gland Imaging, 78075
Bladder, 78730
Blood
Flow Imaging, 78445
Iron
Plasma Volume, 78110, 78111
Platelet Survival, 78191
Red Cell Survival, 78130, 78135
Red Cells, 78120, 78121, 78130-78140
Whole Blood Volume, 78122
Bone
Density Study, 78350, 78351
Imaging, 78300-78315, 78803
SPECT, 78803
Bone Marrow, 78102-78104
Brain
Blood Flow, 78610
Cerebrospinal Fluid, 78630-78650
Imaging, 78600-78609
Vascular Flow, 78610
Diagnostic, 78012-79999 [78429, 78430, 78431, 78432, 78433, 78434, 78804, 78830, 78831, 78832, 78835]
Endocrine Glands, 78012-78099
Esophagus
Imaging (Motility), 78258
Reflux Study, 78262
Gallbladder
Imaging, 78226-78227
Gastrointestinal, 78201-78299
Blood Loss Study, 78278
Gastric Emptying, 78264-78266
Protein Loss Study, 78282
Reflux Study, 78262
Shunt Testing, 78291
Genitourinary System, 78700-78799
Heart, 78414-78499 [78429, 78430, 78431, 78432, 78433, 78434]
Blood Flow, 78414
Blood Pool Imaging, 78472, 78473, 78481, 78483, 78494, 78496
Myocardial Imaging, 78459, 78466-78469, [78429], [78434]
Myocardial Perfusion, 0439T, 78451-78454, 78491-78492 [78430, 78431, 78432, 78433]
Shunt Detection, 78428
Hepatobiliary System, 78226-78227
Inflammatory Process, 78803
Intestines, 78290
Kidney
Blood Flow, 78701-78709
Function Study, 78725
Imaging, 78700-78709
SPECT, 78803
Lacrimal Gland
Tear Flow, 78660
Liver
Imaging, 78201-78227
Vascular Flow, 78216
Lung, 78579-78599
Imaging Perfusion, 78580-78598

Nuclear Medicine — continued
Lung — continued
Imaging Ventilation, 78579, 78582, 78598
Lymphatics, 78102-78199
Musculoskeletal System, 78300-78399
Nervous System, 78600-78699
Parathyroid Glands, 78070-78072
Pulmonary, 78579-78582, 78597-78599
Salivary Gland
Function Study, 78232
Imaging, 78230, 78231
Spleen, 78185, 78215, 78216
Stomach
See Nuclear Medicine, Gastrointestinal
Testes
Imaging, 78761
Therapeutic, 79005-79999
Heart, 79440
Interstitial, 79300
Intra-arterial, 79445
Intra-articular, 79440
Intracavitary, 79200
Intravenous, 79101
Intravenous Infusion, 79101, 79403
Oral Administration, 79005
Radioactive Colloid Therapy, 79200, 79300
Thyroid, 79200, 79300
Thyroid
Imaging, 78012-78014
for Metastases, 78015-78018
Metastases Uptake, 78020
Tumor Imaging
Positron Emission Tomography, 78811-78816
with Computed Tomography, 78814-78816
Tumor Localization, 78800-78803 [78804, 78830, 78831, 78832], [78835]
Urea Breath Test, 78267, 78268
Ureter, 78740
Vein, 78456-78458

Nucleases, DNA
Antibody, 86215

Nucleic Acid Probe
Amplified Probe Detection
Infectious Agent
Bartonella Henselae, 87471
Bartonella Quintana, 87471
Borrelia Burgdorferi, 87476
Candida Species, 87481
Central Nervous System Pathogen, 87483
Chlamydia Pneumoniae, 87486
Chlamydia Trachomatis, 87491
Enterovirus, 87498, 87500
Gardnerella Vaginalis, 87511
Hepatitis B Virus, 87516
Hepatitis C, 87521
Hepatitis G, 87526
Herpes Simplex Virus, 87529
HIV-1, 87535
HIV-2, 87538
Legionella Pneumophila, 87541
Multiple Organisms, 87801
Mycobacteria Avium-Intracellulare, 87561
Mycobacteria Species, 87551
Mycobacteria Tuberculosis, 87556
Mycoplasma Genitalium, 87563
Mycoplasma Pneumoniae, 87581
Neisseria Gonorrhoeae, 87591
Not Otherwise Specified, 87798, 87801
Papillomavirus, Human, [87623, 87624, 87625]
Respiratory Syncytial Virus, 87634
Staphylococcus Aureus, 87640-87641
Streptococcus, Group A, 87651
Streptococcus, Group B, 87653
Zika Virus, 87662
Direct Probe Detection
Infectious Agent
Bartonella Henselae, 87471

Nucleic Acid Probe — continued
Direct Probe Detection — continued
Infectious Agent — continued
Bartonella Quintana, 87471
Borrelia Burgdorferi, 87475
Candida Species, 87480
Chlamydia Pneumoniae, 87485
Chlamydia Trachomatis, 87490
Cytomegalovirus, 87495
Gardnerella Vaginalis, 87510
Gastrointestinal Pathogens, 87505-87507
Hepatitis C, 87520
Hepatitis G, 87525
Herpes Simplex Virus, 87528
Herpes Virus-6, 87531
HIV-1, 87534
HIV-2, 87537
Legionella Pneumophila, 87540
Multiple Organisms, 87800
Mycobacteria Avium-Intracellulare, 87560
Mycobacteria Species, 87550
Mycobacteria Tuberculosis, 87555
Mycoplasma Pneumoniae, 87580
Neisseria Gonorrhoeae, 87590
Not Otherwise Specified, 87797
Papillomavirus, Human, [87623, 87624, 87625]
Streptococcus, Group A, 87650
Trichomonas Vaginalis, 87660
Genotype Analysis
Infectious Agent
Hepatitis C Virus, 87902
HIV-1, 87901
In Situ Hybridization, 88365-88369 [88364, 88373, 88374, 88377]
Nucleic Acid Microbial Identification, 87797-87799
Phenotype Analysis
Infectious Agent
HIV-1 Drug Resistance, 87903, 87904
Quantification
Infectious Agent
Bartonella Henselae, 87472
Bartonella Quintana, 87472
Candida Species, 87482
Chlamydia Pneumoniae, 87487
Chlamydia Trachomatis, 87492
Cytomegalovirus, 87497
Gardnerella Vaginalis, 87512
Hepatitis B Virus, 87517
Hepatitis C, 87522
Hepatitis G, 87527
Herpes Simplex Virus, 87530
Herpes Virus-6, 87533
HIV-1, 87536
HIV-2, 87539
Legionella Pneumophila, 87542
Mycobacteria Avium-Intracellulare, 87562
Mycobacteria Species, 87552
Mycobacteria Tuberculosis, 87557
Mycoplasma Pneumoniae, 87582
Neisseria Gonorrhoeae, 87592
Not Otherwise Specified, 87799
Papillomavirus, Human, [87623], [87624, 87625]
Streptococcus, Group A, 87652

Nucleic Medicine
Vein
Thrombosis Imaging, 78456-78458

Nucleolysis, Intervertebral Disc
See Chemonucleolysis

Nucleophosmin Gene Analysis, 81310

Nucleotidase, 83915

Nudix Hydrolase, [81306]

NUDT15, [81306]

Nursemaid Elbow, 24640

Nursing Facility Services
Annual Assessment, 99318
Care Plan Oversight Services, 99379, 99380
Discharge Services, 1110F-1111F, 99315-99316
Initial, 99304-99306
Subsequent Nursing Facility Care, 99307-99310

Nursing Facility Services — continued
Subsequent Nursing Facility Care — continued
New or Established Patient, 99307-99310
See also Domiciliary Services

Nuss Procedure
with Thoracoscopy, 21743
without Thoracoscopy, 21742

Nutrition Therapy
Group, 97804
Home Infusion, 99601, 99602
Initial Assessment, 97802
Reassessment, 97803

Nystagmus Tests
See Vestibular Function Tests
Optokinetic, 92534, 92544
Positional, 92532, 92542
Spontaneous, 92531, 92541

O

O2 Saturation, 82805-82810, 94760-94762

O-6-Methylguanine-DNA Methyltransferase, [81287]

OAE Test, 92587-92588

Ober-Yount Procedure, 27025

Obliteration
Mastoid, 69670
Vaginal
Total, 57110-57112
Vault, 57120

Obliteration, Total Excision of Vagina, 57110-57112

Obliteration, Vaginal Vault, 57120

Observation
Discharge, 99217
Initial, 99218-99220
Same Date Admit/Discharge, 99234-99236
Subsequent, [99224, 99225, 99226]

Obstetric Tamponade
Uterus, 59899
Vagina, 59899

Obstetrical Care
See Also Abortion; Cesarean Delivery; Ectopic Pregnancy
Abortion
Induced
by Amniocentesis Injection, 59850-59852
by Dilation and Curettage, 59840
by Dilation and Evaluation, 59841
Missed
First Trimester, 59820
Second Trimester, 59821
Spontaneous, 59812
Therapeutic, 59840-59852
Antepartum Care, 59425-59426
Cesarean Section
for Failed VBAC
Only, 59620
Routine (Global), 59618
with Postpartum Care, 59622
Only, 59514
Routine (Global), 59510
with Hysterectomy, 59525
with Postpartum Care, 59515
Curettage
Hydatidiform Mole, 59870
Evacuation
Hydatidiform Mole, 59870
External Cephalic Version, 59412
Miscarriage
Surgical Completion, 59812-59821
Placenta Delivery, 59414
Postpartum Care
Cesarean Delivery, 59510
Following Vaginal Delivery After Prior Cesarean Section, 59610, 59614, 59618, 59622
Postpartum care only, 59430
Vaginal, 59400, 59410
Septic Abortion, 59830
Total (Global), 59400, 59510, 59610, 59618
Unlisted Services and Procedures, 59898-59899
Vaginal Delivery
After C/S-VBAC (Global), 59610
Delivery Only, 59612

Obstetrical Care — *continued*
Vaginal Delivery — *continued*
After C/S–VBAC — *continued*
with Postpartum Care, 59614
Only, 59409
Routine (Global), 59400
with Postpartum Care, 59410
Obstruction
Extracranial, 61623
Fallopian Tube, 58565, 58615
Head/Neck, 61623
Intracranial, 61623
Penis (Vein), 37790
Umbilical Cord, 59072
Obstruction Clearance
Venous Access Device, 36595-36596
Obstruction Colon, 44025-44050
Obstructive Material Removal
Gastrostomy, Duodenostomy, Jejunostomy, Gastro-jejunostomy, or Cecostomy Tube, 49460
Obturator Nerve
Avulsion, 64763-64766
Incision, 64763-64766
Transection, 64763-64766
Obturator Prosthesis
Impression/Custom Preparation
Definitive, 21080
Interim, 21079
Surgical, 21076
Insertion
Larynx, 31527
Occipital Nerve, Greater
Avulsion, 64744
Incision, 64744
Injection
Anesthetic or Steroid, 64405
Transection, 64744
Occlusion
Extracranial/Intracranial, 61623
Fallopian Tubes
Oviduct, 0567T, 58565, 58615
Penis
Vein, 37790
Umbilical Cord, 59072
Ureteral, 50705
Occlusive Disease of Artery, 35001, 35005-35021, 35045-35081, 35091, 35102, 35111, 35121, 35131, 35141, 35151
See Also Repair, Artery; Revision
Occult Blood, 82270-82272
by Hemoglobin Immunoassay, 82274
Occupational Therapy
Evaluation, *[97165, 97166, 97167, 97168]*
OCT (Oxytocin Challenge), 59020
OCT (Optical Coherence Tomography), 0351T-0352T, 0353T-0354T, 0470T-0471T, 0485T-0486T
Endoluminal Imaging Coronary Graft or Vessel, *[92978, 92979]*
Ocular Implant
See Also Orbital Implant
Insertion
in Scleral Shell, 65130
Muscles Attached, 65140
Muscles Not Attached, 65135
Modification, 65125
Reinsertion, 65150
with Foreign Material, 65155
Removal, 65175
Ocular Insert, Drug-eluting, 0444T-0445T
Ocular Muscle, 67311-67399
Ocular Orbit
See Orbit
Ocular Photoscreening, 99174, *[99177]*
Ocular Prosthesis, 21077, 65770, 66982-66985, 92358
Oculomotor Muscle, 67311-67399
Oculopharyngeal Muscular Dystrophy, 81312
Oddi Sphincter
Pressure Measurement, 43263
ODM, 92260
Odontoid Dislocation
Open Treatment
Reduction, 22318
with Grafting, 22319

Odontoid Fracture
Open Treatment
Reduction, 22318
with Grafting, 22319
Odontoid Process
Excisions, 22548
Oesophageal Neoplasm
Endoscopic Removal
Ablation, 43229
Bipolar Cautery, 43216
Hot Biopsy Forceps, 43216
Snare, 43217
Excision, Open, 43100-43101
Oesophageal Varices
Injection Sclerosis, 43204, 43243
Ligation, 43205, 43244, 43400
Oesophagus
See Esophagus
Oestradiol, 82670
Response, 80415
Office and/or Other Outpatient Visits
Consultation, 99241-99245
Established Patient, 99211-99215
New Patient, 99201-99205
Normal Newborn, 99461
Office Visit
Established Patient, 99211-99215
New Patient, 99201-99205
Prolonged Service, 99354-99355
Outpatient Visit
Established Patient, 99211-99215
New Patient, 99201-99205
Prolonged Service, 99354-99355
Office Medical Services
After Hours, 99050
Emergency Care, 99058
Extended Hours, 99051
Office or Other Outpatient Consultations, 99241-99245, 99354-99355
Olecranon
See Also Elbow; Humerus; Radius; Ulna
Bone Cyst
Excision, 24120-24126
Bursa
Arthrocentesis, 20605-20606
Excision, 24105
Tumor, Benign, 25120-25126
Cyst, 24120
Excision, 24125, 24126
Olecranon Process
Craterization, 24147
Diaphysectomy, 24147
Excision
Cyst/Tumor, 24120-24126
Partial, 24147
Fracture
Closed Treatment, 24670-24675
Open Treatment, 24685
Osteomyelitis, 24138, 24147
Saucerization, 24147
Sequestrectomy, 24138
Oligoclonal Immunoglobulin
Cerebrospinal Fluid, 83916
Omentectomy, 49255, 58950-58958
Laparotomy, 58960
Oophorectomy, 58943
Resection Ovarian Malignancy, 58950-58952
Resection Peritoneal Malignancy, 58950-58958
Resection Tubal Malignancy, 58950-58958
Omentum
Excision, 49255, 58950-58958
Flap, 49904-49905
Free
with Microvascular Anastomosis, 49906
Unlisted Services and Procedures, 49999
Omphalectomy, 49250
Omphalocele
Repair, 49600-49611
Omphalomesenteric Duct
Excision, 44800
Omphalomesenteric Duct, Persistent
Excision, 44800
OMT, 98925-98929
Oncology (Ovarian) Biochemical Assays, 81500, 81503-81504

Oncology Cytotoxicity Assay
Chemotherapeutic Drug, 0564T
Oncology mRNA Gene Expression
Breast, 81520-81521
Prostate, 0011M, 81541, 81551
Urothelial, 0012M-0013M
Oncoprotein
Des-Gamma-Carboxy Prothrombin (DCP), 83951
HER–2/neu, 83950
One Stage Prothrombin Time, 85610-85611
Online Internet Assessment/Management
Nonphysician, 98970-98972
Physician, *[99421, 99422, 99423]*
Online Medical Evaluation
Nonphysician, 98970-98972
Physician, *[99421, 99422, 99423]*
ONSD, 67570
Onychectomy, 11750
Onychia
Drainage, 10060-10061
Onychoplasty, 11760, 26236, 28124, 28160
Oocyte
Assisted Fertilization, Microtechnique, 89280-89281
Biopsy, 89290-89291
Cryopreservation, 88240
Culture
Extended, 89272
Less than 4 days, 89250
with Co–Culture, 89251
Identification, Follicular Fluid, 89254
Insemination, 89268
Retrieval
for In Vitro Fertilization, 58970
Storage, 89346
Thawing, 89356
Oophorectomy, 58262-58263, 58291-58292, 58552, 58554, 58661, 58940-58943
Ectopic Pregnancy
Laparoscopic Treatment, 59151
Surgical Treatment, 59120
Oophorectomy, Partial, 58920, 58940-58943
Oophorocystectomy, 58925
Laparoscopic, 58662
OPA1, 81406-81407
Open Biopsy, Adrenal Gland, 60540-60545
Opening (Incision and Drainage)
Acne
Comedones, 10040
Cysts, 10040
Milia, Multiple, 10040
Pustules, 10040
Operating Microscope, 69990
Operation/Procedure
Blalock–Hanlon, 33735
Blalock–Taussig Subclavian–Pulmonary Anastomosis, 33750
Collis, 43283, 43338
Damus-Kaye-Stansel, 33606
Dana, 63185
Dor, 33548
Dunn, 28715
Duvries, 27675-27676
Estes, 58825
Flip-flap, 54324
Foley Pyeloplasty, 50400-50405
Fontan, 33615-33617
Fowler-Stephens, 54650
Fox, 67923
Fredet-Ramstedt, 43520
Gardner, 63700-63702
Green, 23400
Harelip, 40700, 40761
Heine, 66740
Heller, 32665, 43330-43331
Jaboulay Gastroduodenostomy, 43810, 43850-43855
Johannsen, 53400
Krause, 61450
Kuhnt–Szymanowski, 67917
Leadbetter Urethroplasty, 53431
Maquet, 27418
Mumford, 23120, 29824
Nissen, 43280
Norwood, 33611-33612, 33619

Operation/Procedure — *continued*
Peet, 64802-64818
Ramstedt, 43520
Richardson Hysterectomy
See Hysterectomy, Abdominal, Total
Richardson Urethromeatoplasty, 53460
Schanz, 27448
Schlatter Total Gastrectomy, 43620-43622
Smithwick, 64802-64818
Stamm, 43830
Laparoscopic, 43653
SVR, SAVER, 33548
Tenago, 53431
Toupet, 43280
Winiwarter Cholecystoenterostomy, 47720-47740
Winter, 54435
Operculectomy, 41821
Operculum
See Gums
Ophthalmic Biometry, 76516-76519, 92136
Ophthalmic Mucous Membrane Test, 95060
Ophthalmology
Unlisted Services and Procedures, 92499
See Also Ophthalmology, Diagnostic
Ophthalmology, Diagnostic
Color Vision Exam, 92283
Computerized Scanning, 92132-92134
Computerized Screening, 99172, 99174, *[99177]*
Dark Adaptation, 92284
Electromyography, Needle, 92265
Electro–oculography, 92270
Electroretinography, 0509T, 92273-92274
Endoscopy, 66990
Eye Exam
Established Patient, 92012-92014
New Patient, 92002-92004
with Anesthesia, 92018-92019
Gonioscopy, 92020
Ocular Photography
External, 92285
Internal, 92286-92287
Ophthalmoscopy
with Angiography, 92235
with Angioscopy, 92230
with Dynamometry, 92260
with Fluorescein Angiography, 92235
and Indocyanine–Green, 92242
with Fluorescein Angioscopy, 92230
with Fundus Photography, 92250
with Indocyanine–Green Angiography, 92240
and Fluorescein, 92242
with Retinal Drawing and Scleral Depression, 92201-92202
Photoscreening, 99174, *[99177]*
Refractive Determination, 92015
Retinal Polarization Scan, 0469T
Rotation Tests, 92499
Sensorimotor Exam, 92060
Tonometry
Serial, 92100
Ultrasound, 76510-76529
Visual Acuity Screen, 99172-99173
Visual Field Exam, 92081-92083
Visual Function Screen, 99172, 99174, *[99177]*
Ophthalmoscopy
See Also Ophthalmology, Diagnostic
Opiates, *[80361, 80362, 80363, 80364]*
Opinion, Second
See Confirmatory Consultations
Optic Nerve
Decompression, 67570
with Nasal/Sinus Endoscopy, 31294
Head Evaluation, 2027F
Optical Coherence Tomography
Axillary Lymph Node, Each Specimen, Excised Tissue, 0351T-0352T
Breast Tissue, Each Specimen, Excised Tissue, 0351T-0352T
Coronary Vessel or Graft, *[92978, 92979]*
Endoluminal, *[92978, 92979]*
Middle Ear, 0485T-0486T
Skin Imaging, Microstructural and Morphological, 0470T-0471T

Index

ORIF — Osteomyelitis

Index

Osteomyelitis — Palate

[Resequenced]   CPT © 2019 American Medical Association. All Rights Reserved.   © 2019 Optum360, LLC

Phosphotransferase, ADP Phosphocreatine, 82550-82552
Photo Patch
　Allergy Test, 95052
　　See Also Allergy Tests
Photochemotherapies, Extracorporeal, 36522
Photochemotherapy, 96910-96913
　See Also Dermatology
　Endoscopic Light, 96570-96571
Photocoagulation
　Endolaser Panretinal
　　Vitrectomy, 67040
　Focal Endolaser
　　Vitrectomy, 67040
　Iridoplasty, 66762
　Lesion
　　Choroid, 67220
　　Cornea, 65450
　　Retina, 67210, 67228, 67229
　Retinal Detachment
　　Prophylaxis, 67145
　　Repair, 67105, 67107, 67108, 67113
　Retinopathy, 67228-67229
Photodynamic Therapy
　Choroidal Lesions Eye, 67221, 67225
　External, 96567, 96573-96574
Photography
　Ocular
　　Anterior Segment, 92286, 92287
　　External, 92285
　　Fundus, 92250
　Skin, Diagnostic, 96904
Photopheresis
　Extracorporeal, 36522
Photophoresis
　See Actinotherapy; Photochemotherapy
Photoradiation Therapies
　See Actinotherapy
Photoscreen
　Ocular, 99174
Photosensitivity Testing, 95056
　See Also Allergy Tests
Phototherapies
　See Actinotherapy
Phototherapy, Ultraviolet, 96900
PHOX2B, 81403-81404
Phrenic Nerve
　Avulsion, 64746
　Incision, 64746
　Injection
　　Anesthetic or Steroid, 64999
　Transection, 64746
Physical Examination
　Office and/or Other Outpatient Services, 99201-99205
Physical Medicine/Therapy/Occupational Therapy
　See Also Neurology, Diagnostic
　Activities of Daily Living, 97535, 99509
　Aquatic Therapy
　　with Exercises, 97113
　Athletic Training
　　Evaluation, *[97169, 97170, 97171]*
　　Re–evaluation, *[97172]*
　Cognitive Skills Development, 97129-97130
　Community/Work Reintegration, 97537
　Evaluation, *[97161, 97162, 97163, 97164, 97165, 97166, 97167, 97168, 97169, 97170, 97171, 97172]*
　Hydrotherapy
　　Hubbard Tank, 97036
　　Pool with Exercises, 97036, 97113
　Joint Mobilization, 97140
　Kinetic Therapy, 97530
　Manipulation, 97140
　Manual Therapy, 97140
　Modalities
　　Contrast Baths, 97034
　　Diathermy Treatment, 97024
　　Electric Stimulation
　　　Attended, Manual, 97032
　　　Unattended, 97014
　　Hot or Cold Pack, 97010
　　Hydrotherapy (Hubbard Tank), 97036
　　Infrared Light Treatment, 97026
　　Iontophoresis, 97033
　　Microwave Therapy, 97024

Physical Medicine/Therapy/Occupational Therapy — *continued*
　Modalities — *continued*
　　Paraffin Bath, 97018
　　Traction, 97012
　　Ultrasound, 97035
　　Ultraviolet Light, 97028
　　Unlisted Services and Procedures, 97039
　　Vasopneumatic Device, 97016
　　Whirlpool Therapy, 97022
　Orthotics Training, 97760, 97763
　Osteopathic Manipulation, 98925-98929
　Procedures
　　Aquatic Therapy, 97113
　　Direct, 97032
　　Gait Training, 97116
　　Group Therapeutic, 97150
　　Massage Therapy, 97124
　　Neuromuscular Reeducation, 97112
　　Physical Performance Test, 97750
　　Supervised, 97010-97028
　　Therapeutic Exercises, 4018F, 97110
　　Traction Therapy, 97140
　　Work Hardening, 97545, 97546
　Prosthetic Training, 97761
　Sensory Integration, 97533
　Therapeutic Activities, 97530
　Unlisted Services and Procedures, 97139, 97799
　Wheelchair Management, 97542
　Work Reintegration, 97537
Physical Therapy
　See Physical Medicine/Therapy/Occupational Therapy
Physician Services
　Care Plan Oversight Services, 99339-99340, 99374-99380
　　Domiciliary Facility, 99339-99340
　　Extracorporeal Liver Assist System, 0405T
　　Home Health Agency Care, 99374
　　Home/Rest Home Care, 99339-99340
　　Hospice, 99377, 99378
　　Nursing Facility, 99379, 99380
　Case Management Services, 99366-99368
　Direction, Advanced Life Support, 99288
　Online, *[99421, 99422, 99423]*
　Prolonged
　　with Direct Patient Contact, 99354-99357
　　　Outpatient Office, 99354, 99355
　　with Direct Patient Services
　　　Inpatient, 99356, 99357
　　without Direct Patient Contact, 99358, 99359
　Standby, 99360
　Supervision, Care Plan Oversight Services, 0405T, 99339-99340, 99374-99380
　Team Conference, 99367
　Telephone, 99441-99443
Physiologic Recording of Tremor, 95999
PICC Line Insertion, 36568-36569, 36572-36573, 36584
Pierce Ears, 69090
Piercing of Ear Lobe, 69090
PIK3CA, *[81309]*
Piles
　See Hemorrhoids
Pilon Fracture Treatment, 27824
Pilonidal Cyst
　Excision, 11770-11772
　Incision and Drainage, 10080, 10081
Pin
　See Also Wire
　Insertion
　　Removal
　　　Skeletal Traction, 20650
　　Prophylactic Treatment
　　　Femur, 27187
　　　Humerus, 24498
　　　Shoulder, 23490, 23491
Pinch Graft, 15050
Pineal Gland
　Excision
　　Partial, 60699
　　Total, 60699
　Incision, 60699
PINK1, 81405

Pinna
　See Ear, External
Pinworms
　Examination, 87172
Pirogoff Procedure, 27888
Pituitary Epidermoid Tumor
　See Craniopharyngioma
Pituitary Fossa
　Exploration, 60699
Pituitary Gland
　Excision, 61546, 61548
　Incision, 60699
　Tumor
　　Excision, 61546, 61548, 62165
Pituitary Growth Hormone
　See Growth Hormone
Pituitary Lactogenic Hormone
　See Prolactin
Pituitectomy
　See Excision, Pituitary Gland
PKD1, 81407
PKD2, 81406
PKHD1, 81408
PKLR, 81405
PKP, 65730-65755
PKP2, 81406, 81439
PKU, 84030
PL, 80418, 84146
PLA Codes
　see Proprietary Laboratory Analyses (PLA)
Placement
　Adjustable Gastric Restrictive Device, 43770
　Amniotic Membrane
　　Ocular Surface, 65778-65779
　Aqueous Drainage Device, 0191T *[0253T, 0376T]*, 0449T-0450T, 0474T, 66179-66185
　Arteriovenous Implant, Percutaneous Transcatheter, 0553T
　Breast Localization Device
　　with Guidance
　　　Mammographic, 19281-19282
　　　MRI, 19287-19288
　　　Stereotactic, 19283-19284
　　　Ultrasound, 19285-19286
　Bronchial Stent, 31636-31637
　Catheter
　　Aneurysm Sac Pressure Sensor, 34701-34708
　　Bile Duct, 47533-47540
　　Brain for Chemotherapy, 64999
　　Bronchus
　　　for Intracavitary Radioelement Application, 31643
　　　See Catheterization
　　for Interstitial Radioelement Application
　　　Breast, 19296-19298
　　　Genitalia, 55920
　　　Head/Neck, 41019
　　　Muscle, 20555
　　　Pelvic Organs, 55920
　　　Prostate, 55875
　　　Soft Tissue, 20555
　　Pleural, 32550
　　Renal Artery, 36251-36254
　Catheter, Cardiac, 93503
　　See Also Catheterization, Cardiac
　Cecostomy Tube, 44300, 49442
　Colonic Stent, 45327, 45347, 45389
　Dosimeter
　　Prostate, 55876
　Drainage
　　Pancreas, 48001
　Drug-eluting ocular Insert, 0444T-0445T
　Duodenostomy Tube, 49441
　Endovascular Prosthesis
　　Aorta, 33883-33886, 34701-34706
　　Fenestrated Endograft, 34841-34848
　　Iliac Artery, 34707-34711
　Enterostomy Tube, 44300
　Fiducial Markers
　　Duodenum/Jejunum, 43253
　　Esophagus, 43253
　　Intra-abdominal, 49411
　　Intra-pelvic, 49411
　　Intrathoracic, 32553

Placement — *continued*
　Fiducial Markers — *continued*
　　Prostate, 55876
　　Retroperitoneum, 49411
　　Stomach, 43253
　Gastrostomy Tube, 43246, 49440
　Guidance Catheter
　　Abscess, 75989
　　Specimen, 75989
　Interstitial Device
　　Bone, 0347T
　　Intra-abdominal, 49327, 49411-49412
　　Intra-pelvic, 49411
　　Intra-thoracic, 32553
　　Prostate, 55876
　　Retroperitoneum, 49411
　Intrafacet Implant(s), 0219T-0222T
　Intravascular Stent
　　Cervical Carotid Artery, 37215-37216
　　Innominate Artery, 37217-37218
　　Intracranial, 61635
　　Intrathoracic Common Carotid Artery, 37217-37218
　IVC Filter, 37191
　Jejunostomy Tube
　　Endoscopic, 44372
　　Percutaneous, 49441
　Localization Device, Breast, 19281-19288
　Nasogastric Tube, 43752
　Needle
　　Bone, 36680
　　for Interstitial Radioelement Application
　　　Genitalia, 55920
　　　Head, 41019
　　　Muscle, 20555
　　　Neck, 41019
　　　Pelvic Organs, 55920
　　　Prostate, 55875
　　　Soft Tissue, 20555
　　Head and/or Neck, 41019
　　Muscle or Soft Tissue
　　　for Radioelement Application, 20555
　　Pelvic Organs and/or Genitalia, 55920
　　Prostate, 55875-55876
　Needle Wire
　　Breast, 19281-19288
　Orogastric Tube, 43752
　Pharmacological Agent
　　Intravitreal Drug Delivery System, 67027
　Pressure Sensor, 34701-34708
　Prosthesis, Thoracic Aorta, 75958-75959
　Radiation Delivery Device
　　Intracoronary Artery, *[92974]*
　　Intraocular, 67299
　　Pleural Cavity, 32553
　　Therapy Applicator for IORT, 19294
　Sensor, Wireless
　　Endovascular Repair, 34701-34708
　Seton
　　Anal, 46020
　Stereotactic Frame, 20660
　　Head Frame, 61800
　Subconjunctival Retinal Prosthesis Receiver, 0100T
　Tracheal Stent, 31631
　Transcatheter
　　Extracranial, 0075T-0076T
　　Physiologic Sensor, 34701-34708
　Ureteral Stent, 50693-50695, 50947
Placenta
　Delivery, 59414
Placental
　Alpha Microglobulin-1, 84112
　Lactogen, 83632
Placental Villi
　See Chorionic Villus
Plafond Fracture Treatment
　Tibial, 27824
Plagiocephaly, 21175
Planing
　Nose
　　Skin, 30120
Plantar Digital Nerve
　Decompression, 64726

Index

Psychiatric Diagnosis — Quadriceps Repair

Psychiatric Diagnosis — *continued*
  Evaluation, 90791-90792
  Evaluation of Records, Reports, and Tests, 90885
  Major Depressive Disorder (MDD), 3088F-3093F
    Diagnostic and Statistical Manual (DSM) Criteria Documented, 1040F
  Narcosynthesis, 90865
  Psychological Testing, 96116-96121
    Cognitive Performance, 96112-96121, 96125
  Suicide Risk Assessment, 3085F
  Unlisted Services and Procedures, 90899
Psychiatric Treatment
  Adaptive Behavior Treatment
    Exposure Adaptive Behavior Treatment, 0373T
    Family, 97156
    Group, 97154, 97158
    Individual Patient, 97153, 97155
    Multiple Family Group, 97157
  Biofeedback Training, 90875-90876
  Consultation with Family, 90887
  Electroconvulsive Therapy, 4066F, 90870
    Referral Documented, 4067F
  Environmental Intervention, 90882
  Family, 90846-90849, 99510
  Hypnotherapy, 90880
  Individual Psychotherapy
    with Evaluation and Management Service, 90833, 90836, 90838
    without Evaluation and Management Service, 90832, 90834, 90837
  Narcosynthesis
    Analysis, 90865
  Pharmacotherapy
    Antidepressant, 4064F
    Antipsychotic, 4065F
    Management, 90863
  Psychoanalysis, 90845
  Psychotherapy
    Family, 90846-90849
    Group, 90853
    Individual
      with Evaluation and Management Service, 90833, 90836, 90838
      without Evaluation and Management Service, 90832, 90834, 90837
    Interactive Complexity, 90785
  Report Preparation, 90889
  Suicide Risk Assessment, 3085F
  Unlisted Services/Procedures, 90899
Psychoanalysis, 90845
Psychodrama, 90899
Psychophysiologic Feedback, 90875-90876
Psychotherapy
  Adaptive Behavior
    Assessment, 0362T, [97151], [97152]
    Treatment, 0373T, [97153], [97154], [97155], [97156], [97157], [97158]
  Family, 90846-90849, 97156, 99510
  Follow up Behavioral Assessment
    Exposure, 0362T, 0373T, [97153, 97154, 97155, 97156, 97157, 97158]
    Observational, [97151, 97152]
  Group, 90853, 97154, 97158
  Home Visit by Nonphysician for Counseling, 99510
  Individual, 97153, 97155
    for Crisis, 90839-90840
    with Evaluation and Management Service, 90833, 90836, 90838
    without Evaluation and Management Service, 90832, 90834, 90837
  Interactive Complexity, 90785
  Multiple Family Group, 97157
  Pharmacologic Management, 90863
  Referral Documented, 4062F
  Services Provided, 4060F
PT, 85610-85611
PTA (Factor XI), 85270
PTA, 36902-36903, 36905-36906, 37220-37235, 92997-92998, [37246, 37247, 37248, 37249]

PTB, 29435
PTC, 85250
PTC Factor, 85250
PTCA
  Artery, Aortic, [37246, 37247]
PTE (Prolonged Tissue Expansion), 11960, 19357
PTEN, 81321-81323, 81432, 81435, [81448]
Pteroylglutamic Acid, 82746, 82747
Pterygium
  Excision, 65420
    with Graft, 65426
Pterygomaxillary Fossa
  Incision, 31040
Pterygopalatine Ganglion
  Injection
    Anesthetic, 64505
PTH, 83970
PTK, 65400
Ptosis
  See Blepharoptosis; Procidentia
PTPN11, 81406
PTT, 85730, 85732
Ptyalectasis, 42650-42660
Pubic Symphysis, 27282
Pubiotomy, 59899
Pubis
  Craterization, 27070, 27071
  Cyst
    Excision, 27065-27067
  Excision, 27070
  Saucerization, 27070, 27071
  Tumor
    Excision, 27065-27067
PUBS (Percutaneous Umbilical Blood Sampling), 59012
Pudendal Nerve
  Destruction, 64630
  Injection
    Anesthetic or Steroid, 64430
    Neurolytic, 64630
Puestow Procedure, 48548
Pulled Elbow, 24640
Pulmonary, 78579-78582, 78597-78598
Pulmonary Artery, 33690
  Angioplasty, 92997, 92998
  Banding, 33690
  Catheterization, 36013-36015
  Embolism, 33910-33916
    Excision, 33910-33916
  Percutaneous Transluminal Angioplasty, 92997, 92998
  Pressure Sensor
    Insertion, 33289
    Remote Monitoring, 93264
    Reimplantation, 33788
  Repair, 33690, 33917-33920
    Reimplantation, 33788
  Shunt
    from Aorta, 33755, 33762, 33924
    from Vena Cava, 33766, 33767
    Subclavian, 33750
  Transection, 33922
Pulmonary Decortication, 32220, 32225, 32320, 32651-32652
Pulmonary Hemorrhage, 32110
Pulmonary Valve
  Incision, 33470-33474
  Repair, 33470-33474
  Replacement, 33475
Pulmonary Vein
  Repair
    Complete, 33730
    Partial, 33724
    Stenosis, 33726
  Stenosis
    Repair, 33726
Pulmonology
  Diagnostic
    Airway Integrity, 94780-94781
    Airway Resistance, 94728
    Apnea Monitoring, Pediatric, 94774-94777
    Bronchodilation, 94664
    Bronchospasm Evaluation, 94060, 94070
    Carbon Dioxide Response Curve, 94400

Pulmonology — *continued*
  Diagnostic — *continued*
    Diffusing Capacity, 94729
    Expired Gas Analysis
      Carbon Dioxide, 94770
      CO2, 94770
      NO, 95012
      O2 and CO2, 94681
      O2 Uptake, Direct, 94680
      O2 Uptake, Indirect, 94690
      Oxygen and Carbon Dioxide, 94681
      Oxygen Uptake, 94680
      Oxygen Uptake, Indirect, 94690
      Quantitative, 94250
    Flow–Volume Loop, 94375
    Hemoglobin Oxygen Affinity, 82820
    High Altitude Simulation Test (HAST), 94452-94453
    Hypoxia Response Curve, 94450
    Inhalation Treatment, 94640, 94642, 94644-94645, 94664, 99503
    Lung Volume, 94726-94727
    Maximum Breathing Capacity, 94200
    Maximum Voluntary Ventilation, 94200
    Membrane Compliance, 94750
    Oximetry
      Ear or Pulse, 94760-94762
    Resistance to Airflow, 94728
    Spirometry, 94010-94070
      Patient Initiated, 94014-94016
      with Bronchospasm Evaluation, 94070
    Sputum Mobilization with Inhalants, 94664
    Stress Test, 94618-94621
    Unlisted Services and Procedures, 94799
    Vital Capacity, 94150
  Therapeutic
    Expired Gas Analysis, 94250
    Inhalation Treatment, 94640, 94642, 94644-94645, 94664, 99503
    Intrapulmonary Surfactant Administration, 94610
    Manipulation of Chest Wall, 94667-94669
    Pressure Ventilation
      Negative CNPB, 94662
      Positive CPAP, 94660
    Ventilation Assist, 94002-94005, 99504
  Unlisted Noninvasive Vascular Diagnostic Study, 93998
  Unlisted Services and Procedures, 94799
Pulse Generator
  Electronic Analysis, 95970-95972, 95976-95977, 95980-95982, [95983, 95984]
  Heart
    Insertion/Replacement, 33212, 33213
Pulse Rate Increased
  Heart
    Recording, 93609
Pulse-echo Ultrasound, 0508T
Pump
  See Chemotherapy, Pump Services; Infusion Pump
Pump, Infusion
  See Infusion Pump
Pump Services
  Oxygenator/Heat Exchange, 99190-99192
Pump Stomach for Poison, 43753
Punch Graft, 15775, 15776
Puncture
  Artery, 36600
  Chest
    with Imaging Guidance, 32555, 32557
    without Imaging Guidance, 32554, 32556
  Cisternal, 61050-61055
  Lumbar, 62270-62272
  Pericardium, 33016-33019
  Pleural Cavity
    Drainage, 32556-32557
  Skull
    Drain Fluid, 61000-61020
      Cistern, 61050
    Inject Cistern, 61055
    Inject Ventricle, 61026

Puncture — *continued*
  Skull — *continued*
    Shunt
      Drainage of Fluid, 61070
      Injection, 61070
  Spinal Cord
    Diagnostic, 62270
    Drainage of Fluid, 62272
    Lumbar, 62270
  Spleen, 38999
  Tracheal
    Aspiration and/or Injection, 31612
Puncture Aspiration
  Abscess
    Skin, 10160
  Bulla, 10160
  Cyst
    Breast, 19000, 19001
    Skin, 10160
  Hematoma, 10160
Puncturing
  See Puncture
Pupillometry, Quantitative, 92499
Pure–Tone Audiometry, 0208T-0209T, 92552, 92553
Pustules
  Removal, 10040
Putti–Platt Procedure, 23450
PUVA, 96912, 96913
PV, 90713
PVA (Percutaneous Vertebral Augmentation), 22513-22515
PVB (Paraspinous Vertebral Block), Thoracic, [64461, 64462, 64463]
Pyelogram
  See Urography, Intravenous; Urography, Retrograde
Pyelography, 74400, 74425
Pyelolithotomy, 50130
  Anatrophic, 50075
  Coagulum, 50130
Pyeloplasty, 50400, 50405, 50544
  Repair
    Horseshoe Kidney, 50540
    Secondary, 50405
Pyeloscopy
  with Cystourethroscopy, 52351
    Biopsy, 52354
    Destruction, 52354
    Lithotripsy, 52353
    Removal
      Calculus, 52352
    Tumor Excision, 52355
Pyelostolithotomy
  Percutaneous, 50080, 50081
Pyelostomy, 50125, 50400, 50405
  Closure, 53899
Pyelotomy
  Complicated, 50135
  Endoscopic, 50570
  Exploration, 50120
  with Drainage, 50125
  with Removal Calculus, 50130
Pyeloureteroplasty, 50400, 50405, 50544
PYGM, 81401, 81406
Pyloric Sphincter
  Incision, 43520
  Reconstruction, 43800
Pyloromyotomy, 43520
Pyloroplasty, 43800
  with Vagotomy, 43640
Pyothorax
  Incision and Drainage, 21501, 21502
Pyridoxal Phosphate, 84207
Pyrophosphate, Adenosine, 82030
Pyrophosphorylase, UDP Galactose, 82775-82776
Pyruvate, 84210, 84220

Q

Q Fever, 86000, 86638
Q Fever ab, 86638
QSART, 95923
QST (Quantitative Sensory Testing), 0106T-0110T
Quadrantectomy, 19301-19302
Quadriceps Repair, 27430

Radiocarpal Joint
  Arthrotomy, 25040
  Dislocation
    Closed Treatment, 25660
Radiocinematographies
  Esophagus, 74230
  Pharynx, 70371, 74230
  Speech Evaluation, 70371
  Swallowing Evaluation, 74230
  Unlisted Services and Procedures, 76120-76125
Radioelement
  Application, 77761-77772
    Surface, 77789
    with Ultrasound, 76965
  Handling, 77790
  Infusion, 77750
  Placement *See* Radioelement Substance
Radioelement Substance
  Catheter Placement
    Breast, 19296-19298
    Bronchus, 31643
    Head and/or Neck, 41019
    Muscle and/or Soft Tissue, 20555
    Pelvic Organs or Genitalia, 55920
    Prostate, 55875
  Catheterization, 55875
  Needle Placement
    Head and/or Neck, 41019
    Muscle and/or Soft Tissue, 20555
    Pelvic Organs and Genitalia, 55920
    Prostate, 55875
Radiofrequency Spectroscopy
  Parital Mastectomy, 0546T
Radiography
  See Radiology, Diagnostic; X–Ray
Radioimmunosorbent Test
  Gammaglobulin, Blood, 82784-82785
Radioisotope Brachytherapy
  See Brachytherapy
Radioisotope Scan
  See Nuclear Medicine
Radiological Marker
  Preoperative Placement
    Excision of Breast Lesion, 19125, 19126
Radiology
  See Also Nuclear Medicine, Radiation Therapy,
    X–Ray, Ultrasound
  Diagnostic
    Unlisted Services and Procedures, 76499
    Examination, 70030
      Stress Views, 77071
    Joint Survey, 77077
  Therapeutic
    Field Set–Up, 77280-77290
    Planning, 77261-77263, 77299
    Port Film, 77417
Radionuclide Therapy
  Heart, 79440
  Interstitial, 79300
  Intra–arterial, 79445
  Intra–articular, 79440
  Intracavitary, 79200
  Intravascular, 79101
  Intravenous, 79101, 79403
  Intravenous Infusion, 79101, 79403
  Oral, 79005
  Remote Afterloading, 77767-77768, 77770-
    77772
  Unlisted Services and Procedures, 79999
**Radionuclide Tomography, Single–Photon
    Emission–Computed**
  See Specific Site; Nuclear Medicine
Radiopharmaceutical Localization of Tumor,
    78800-78803 [78804, 78830, 78831, 78832],
    [78835]
Radiopharmaceutical Therapy
  Heart, 79440
  Interstitial, 79300
    Colloid Administration, 79300
  Intra-arterial Particulate, 79445
  Intra–articular, 79440
  Intracavitary, 79200
  Intravascular, 79101
  Intravenous, 78808, 79101, 79403
  Oral, 79005
  Unlisted Services and Procedures, 79999

Radiostereometric Analysis
  Lower Extremity, 0350T
  Placement Interstitial Device, 0347T
  Spine, 0348T
  Upper Extremity, 0349T
Radiosurgery
  Cranial Lesion, 61796-61799
  Spinal Lesion, 63620-63621
Radiotherapeutic
  See Radiation Therapy
Radiotherapies
  See Irradiation
Radiotherapy
  Afterloading, 77767-77768, 77770-77772
    Catheter Insertion, 19296-19298
    Planning, 77316-77318
Radiotherapy, Surface, 77789
Radioulnar Joint
  Arthrodesis
    with Ulnar Resection, 25830
  Dislocation
    Closed Treatment, 25525, 25675
    Open Treatment, 25676
    Percutaneous Fixation, 25671
Radius
  See Also Arm, Lower; Elbow; Ulna
  Arthroplasty, 24365
    with Implant, 24366, 25441
  Craterization, 24145, 25151
  Cyst
    Excision, 24125, 24126, 25120-25126
  Diaphysectomy, 24145, 25151
  Dislocation
    Partial, 24640
    Subluxate, 24640
    with Fracture
      Closed Treatment, 24620
      Open Treatment, 24635
  Excision, 24130, 24136, 24145, 24152
    Epiphyseal Bar, 20150
    Partial, 25145
    Styloid Process, 25230
  Fracture, 25605
    Closed Treatment, 25500, 25505, 25520,
      25600, 25605
      with Manipulation, 25605
      without Manipulation, 25600
    Colles, 25600, 25605
    Distal, 25600-25609
      Closed Treatment, 25600-25605
      Open Treatment, 25607-25609
    Head/Neck
      Closed Treatment, 24650, 24655
      Open Treatment, 24665, 24666
    Open Treatment, 25515, 25525, 25526,
      25574
    Percutaneous Fixation, 25606
    Shaft, 25500-25526
      Open Treatment, 25515, 25574-
        25575
    with Ulna, 25560, 25565
      Open Treatment, 25575
  Implant
    Removal, 24164
  Incision and Drainage, 25035
  Osteomyelitis, 24136, 24145
  Osteoplasty, 25390-25393
  Prophylactic Treatment, 25490, 25492
  Repair
    Epiphyseal Arrest, 25450, 25455
    Epiphyseal Separation
      Closed, 25600
      Closed with Manipulation, 25605
      Open Treatment, 25607, 25608-
        25609
      Percutaneous Fixation, 25606
    Malunion or Nonunion, 25400, 25415
    Osteotomy, 25350, 25355, 25370, 25375
      and Ulna, 25365
    with Graft, 25405, 25420-25426
  Saucerization, 24145, 25151
  Sequestrectomy, 24136, 25145
  Subluxation, 24640
  Tumor
    Cyst, 24120

Radius — continued
  Tumor — continued
    Excision, 24125, 24126, 25120-25126,
      25170
RAF1, 81404, 81406
RAI1, 81405
Ramstedt Operation
  Pyloromyotomy, 43520
Ramus Anterior, Nervus Thoracicus
  Destruction, 64620
  Injection
    Anesthetic or Steroid, 64420-64421
    Neurolytic, 64620
Range of Motion Test
  Extremities, 95851
  Eye, 92018, 92019
  Hand, 95852
  Rectum
    Biofeedback, 90912-90913
  Trunk, 97530
Ranula
  Treatment of, 42408
Rapid Heart Rate
  Heart
    Recording, 93609
Rapid Plasma Reagin Test, 86592, 86593
Rapid Test for Infection, 86308, 86403, 86406
  Monospot Test, 86308
Rapoport Test, 52005
Raskind Procedure, 33735-33737
Rastelli Procedure, 33786
Rat Typhus, 86000
Rathke Pouch Tumor
  Excision, 61545
Rays, Roentgen
  See X–Ray
Raz Procedure, 51845
RBC, 78120, 78121, 78130-78140, 85007, 85014,
    85041, 85547, 85555, 85557, 85651-85660,
    86850-86870, 86970-86978
RBC ab, 86850-86870
RBL (Rubber Band Ligation)
  Hemorrhoids, 46221
  Skin Tags, 11200-11201
RCM, 96931-96936
RDH12,, 81434
Reaction
  Lip
    without Reconstruction, 40530
Realignment
  Femur, with Osteotomy, 27454
  Knee, Extensor, 27422
  Muscle, 20999
    Hand, 26989
  Tendon, Extensor, 26437
Reattachment
  Muscle, 20999
  Thigh, 27599
Receptor
  CD4, 86360
  Estrogen, 84233
  Progesterone, 84234
  Progestin, 84234
Receptor Assay
  Endocrine, 84235
  Estrogen, 84233
  Non–Hormone, 84238
  Progesterone, 84234
Recession
  Gastrocnemius
    Leg, Lower, 27687
  Tendon
    Hand, 26989
RECOMBIVAX HB, 90740, 90743-90744, 90746
Reconstruction
  See Also Revision
  Abdominal Wall
    Omental Flap, 49905
  Acetabulum, 27120, 27122
  Anal
    Congenital Absence, 46730-46740
    Fistula, 46742
    Graft, 46753
    Sphincter, 46750, 46751, 46760-46761
  Ankle, 27700-27703
  Apical–Aortic Conduit, 33404

Reconstruction — continued
  Atrial, 33254-33259
    Endoscopic, 33265-33266
    Open, 33254-33259
  Auditory Canal, External, 69310, 69320
  Bile Duct
    Anastomosis, 47800
  Bladder
    from Colon, 50810
    from Intestines, 50820, 51960
    with Urethra, 51800, 51820
  Breast
    Augmentation, 19324, 19325
    Mammoplasty, 19318-19325
      Biesenberger, 19318
    Nipple, 19350, 19355
    Revision, 19380
    Transverse Rectus Abdominis Myocuta-
      neous Flap, 19367-19369
    with Free Flap, 19364
    with Latissimus Dorsi Flap, 19361
    with Other Techniques, 19366
    with Tissue Expander, 19357
  Bronchi
    Graft Repair, 31770
    Stenosis, 31775
    with Lobectomy, 32501
    with Segmentectomy, 32501
  Canthus, 67950
  Cardiac Anomaly, 33622
  Carpal, 25443
  Carpal Bone, 25394, 25430
  Cheekbone, 21270
  Chest Wall
    Omental Flap, 49905
    Trauma, 32820
  Cleft Palate, 42200-42225
  Conduit
    Apical–Aortic, 33404
  Conjunctiva, 68320-68335
    with Flap
      Bridge or Partial, 68360
      Total, 68362
  Cranial Bone
    Extracranial, 21181-21184
  Ear, Middle
    Tympanoplasty with Antrotomy or Mas-
      toidectomy
      with Ossicular Chain Reconstruc-
        tion, 69636, 69637
    Tympanoplasty with Mastoidectomy,
      69641
      Radical or Complete, 69644, 69645
      with Intact or Reconstructed Wall,
        69643, 69644
      with Ossicular Chain Reconstruc-
        tion, 69642
    Tympanoplasty without Mastoidectomy,
      69631
      with Ossicular Chain Reconstruc-
        tion, 69632, 69633
  Elbow, 24360
    Total Replacement, 24363
    with Implant, 24361, 24362
  Esophagus, 43300, 43310, 43313
    Creation
      Stoma, 43351-43352
    Esophagostomy, 43351-43352
    Fistula, 43305, 43312, 43314
    Gastrointestinal, 43360-43361
  Eye
    Graft
      Conjunctiva, 65782
      Stem Cell, 65781
    Transplantation
      Amniotic Membrane, 65780
  Eyelid
    Canthus, 67950
    Second Stage, 67975
    Total, 67973-67975
    Total Eyelid
      Lower, One Stage, 67973
      Upper, One Stage, 67974
    Transfer Tarsoconjunctival Flap from
      Opposing Eyelid, 67971

Index — Repair — Repair

[Resequenced]

Repair — *continued*
  Hernia — *continued*
    Reducible — *continued*
      Initial — *continued*
        Umbilical, 49580, 49585
        Ventral, 49560
      Recurrent
        Femoral, 49555
        Incisional, 49565
        Inguinal, 49520
        Ventral, 49560
      Sliding, 49525
      Spigelian, 49590
      Umbilical, 49580, 49585
        Incarcerated, 49582, 49587
        Reducible, 49580, 49585
      Ventral
        Initial
          Incarcerated, 49561
          Reducible, 49565
      with Mesh, 49568
      with Spermatic Cord, 54640
  Hip
    Muscle Transfer, 27100-27105, 27111
    Osteotomy, 27146-27156
    Tendon, 27097
  Humerus, 24420, 24430
    Osteotomy, 24400, 24410
    with Graft, 24435
  Hypoplasia
    Aortic Arch, 33619
  Hypospadias, 54308, 54312, 54316, 54318, 54322, 54326, 54328, 54332, 54336, 54340, 54344, 54348, 54352
  Ileoanal Pouch, 46710-46712
  Ileostomy, 44310, 45136
    Continent (Kock Pouch), 44316
  Iliac Artery, 34707-34711 [34717, 34718], 35102-35103, 37220-37223
  Interphalangeal Joint
    Volar Plate, 26548
  Intestine
    Large
      Ulcer, 44605
      Wound, 44605
  Intestines
    Enterocele
      Abdominal Approach, 57270
      Vaginal Approach, 57268
    Large
      Closure Enterostomy, 44620-44626
      Diverticula, 44605
    Obstruction, 44615
  Intestines, Small
    Closure Enterostomy, 44620-44626
    Diverticula, 44602, 44603
    Fistula, 44640-44661
    Hernia, 44050
    Malrotation, 44055
    Obstruction, 44025, 44050
    Ulcer, 44602, 44603
    Wound, 44602, 44603
  Introitus, Vagina, 56800
  Iris, Ciliary Body, 66680
  Jejunum
    Free Transfer with Microvascular Anastomosis, 43496
  Kidney
    Fistula, 50520-50526
    Horseshoe, 50540
    Renal Pelvis, 50400, 50405
    Wound, 50500
  Knee
    Cartilage, 27403
    Instability, 27420
    Ligament, 27405-27409
      Collateral, 27405
      Collateral and Cruciate, 27409
      Cruciate, 27407, 27409
    Meniscus, 27403
    Tendons, 27380, 27381
  Laceration, Skin
    Abdomen
      Complex, 13100-13102
      Intermediate, 12031-12037
      Layered, 12031-12037

Repair — *continued*
  Laceration, Skin — *continued*
    Abdomen — *continued*
      Simple, 12001-12007
      Superficial, 12001-12007
    Arm, Arms
      Complex, 13120-13122
      Intermediate, 12031-12037
      Layered, 12031-12037
      Simple, 12001-12007
      Superficial, 12001-12007
    Axilla, Axillae
      Complex, 13131-13133
      Intermediate, 12031-12037
      Layered, 12031-12037
      Simple, 12001-12007
      Superficial, 12001-12007
    Back
      Complex, 13100-13102
      Intermediate, 12031-12037
      Layered, 12031-12037
      Simple, 12001-12007
      Superficial, 12001-12007
    Breast
      Complex, 13100-13102
      Intermediate, 12031-12037
      Layered, 12031-12037
      Simple, 12001-12007
      Superficial, 12001-12007
    Buttock
      Complex, 13100-13102
      Intermediate, 12031-12037
      Layered, 12031-12037
      Simple, 12001-12007
      Superficial, 12001-12007
    Cheek, Cheeks
      Complex, 13131-13133
      Intermediate, 12051-12057
      Layered, 12051-12057
      Simple, 12011-12018
      Superficial, 12011-12018
    Chest
      Complex, 13100-13102
      Intermediate, 12031-12037
      Layered, 12031-12037
      Simple, 12001-12007
      Superficial, 12001-12007
    Chin
      Complex, 13131-13133
      Intermediate, 12051-12057
      Layered, 12051-12057
      Simple, 12011-12018
      Superficial, 12011-12018
    Ear, Ears
      Complex, 13151-13153
      Intermediate, 12051-12057
      Layered, 12051-12057
        2.5 cm or less, 12051
      Simple, 12011-12018
      Superficial, 12011-12018
    External
      Genitalia
        Complex/Intermediate, 12041-12047
        Layered, 12041-12047
        Simple, 12001-12007
        Superficial, 12041-12047
    Extremity, Extremities
      Complex, 13120-13122
      Complex/Intermediate, 12031-12037
      Intermediate, 12051-12057
      Layered, 12031-12037
      Simple, 12001-12007
      Superficial, 12001-12007
    Face
      Complex/Intermediate, 12051-12057
      Layered, 12051-12057
      Simple, 12011-12018
      Superficial, 12011-12018
    Feet
      Complex, 13131-13133
      Intermediate, 12041-12047
      Layered, 12041-12047
      Simple, 12001-12007

Repair — *continued*
  Laceration, Skin — *continued*
    Feet — *continued*
      Superficial, 12001-12007
    Finger, Fingers
      Complex, 13131-13133
      Intermediate, 12041-12047
      Layered, 12041-12047
      Simple, 12001-12007
      Superficial, 12001-12007
    Foot
      Complex, 13131-13133
      Intermediate, 12041-12047
      Layered, 12041-12047
      Simple, 12001-12007
      Superficial, 12001-12007
    Forearm, Forearms
      Complex, 13120-13122
      Intermediate, 12031-12037
      Layered, 12031-12037
      Simple, 12001-12007
      Superficial, 12001-12007
    Forehead
      Complex, 13131-13133
      Intermediate, 12051-12057
      Layered, 12051-12057
      Simple, 12011-12018
      Superficial, 12011-12018
    Genitalia
      Complex, 13131-13133
      External
        Complex/Intermediate, 12041-12047
        Layered, 12041-12047
        Simple, 12001-12007
        Superficial, 12001-12007
    Hand, Hands
      Complex, 13131-13133
      Intermediate, 12041-12047
      Layered, 12041-12047
      Simple, 12001-12007
      Superficial, 12001-12007
    Leg, Legs
      Complex, 13120-13122
      Intermediate, 12031-12037
      Layered, 12031-12037
      Simple, 12001-12007
      Superficial, 12001-12007
    Lip, Lips
      Complex, 13151-13153
      Intermediate, 12051-12057
      Layered, 12051-12057
      Simple, 12011-12018
      Superficial, 12011-12018
    Lower
      Arm, Arms
        Complex, 13120-13122
        Intermediate, 12031-12037
        Layered, 12031-12037
        Simple, 12001-12007
        Superficial, 12001-12007
      Extremity, Extremities
        Complex, 13120-13122
        Intermediate, 12031-12037
        Layered, 12031-12037
        Simple, 12001-12007
        Superficial, 12001-12007
      Leg, Legs
        Complex, 13120-13122
        Intermediate, 12031-12037
        Layered, 12031-12037
        Simple, 12001-12007
        Superficial, 12001-12007
    Mouth
      Complex, 13131-13133
    Mucous Membrane
      Complex/Intermediate, 12051-12057
      Layered, 12051-12057
      Simple, 12011-12018
      Superficial, 12011-12018
    Neck
      Complex, 13131-13133
      Intermediate, 12041-12047
      Layered, 12041-12047
      Simple, 12001-12007

Repair — *continued*
  Laceration, Skin — *continued*
    Neck — *continued*
      Superficial, 12001-12007
    Nose
      Complex, 13151-13153
      Complex/Intermediate, 12051-12057
      Layered, 12051-12057
      Simple, 12011-12018
      Superficial, 12011-12018
    Palm, Palms
      Complex, 13131-13133
      Intermediate, 12041-12047
      Layered, 12041-12047
      Layered Simple, 12001-12007
      Superficial, 12001-12007
    Scalp
      Complex, 13120-13122
      Intermediate, 12031-12037
      Layered, 12031-12037
      Simple, 12001-12007
      Superficial, 12001-12007
    Toe, Toes
      Complex, 13131-13133
      Intermediate, 12041-12047
      Layered, 12041-12047
      Simple, 12001-12007
      Superficial, 12001-12007
    Trunk
      Complex, 13100-13102
      Intermediate, 12031-12037
      Layered, 12031-12037
      Simple, 12001-12007
      Superficial, 12001-12007
    Upper
      Arm, Arms
        Complex, 13120-13122
        Intermediate, 12031-12037
        Layered, 12031-12037
        Simple, 12001-12007
        Superficial, 12001-12007
      Extremity
        Complex, 13120-13122
        Intermediate, 12031-12037
        Layered, 12031-12037
        Simple, 12001-12007
        Superficial, 12001-12007
      Leg, Legs
        Complex, 13120-13122
        Intermediate, 12031-12037
        Layered, 12031-12037
        Simple, 12001-12007
        Superficial, 12001-12007
  Larynx
    Fracture, 31584
    Reinnervation
      Neuromuscular Pedicle, 31590
  Leak
    Cerebrospinal Fluid, 31290-31291
  Leg
    Lower
      Fascia, 27656
      Tendon, 27658-27692
    Upper
      Muscles, 27385, 27386, 27400, 27430
      Tendon, 27393-27400
  Ligament
    Ankle, 27695-27696, 27698
    Anterior Cruciate, 29888
    Collateral
      Elbow, 24343, 24345
      Metacarpophalangeal or Interphalangeal Joint, 26540
    Knee, 27405, 27407, 27409
    Posterior Cruciate Ligament, 29889
  Lip, 40650-40654
    Cleft Lip, 40700-40761
    Fistula, 42260
  Liver
    Abscess, 47300
    Cyst, 47300
    Wound, 47350-47361
  Lung
    Hernia, 32800

Repair — *continued*
Ureter — *continued*
  Suture, 50900
  Urinary Undiversion, 50830
Ureterocele, 51535
Urethra
  Artificial Sphincter, 53449
  Diverticulum, 53240, 53400, 53405
  Fistula, 45820, 45825, 53400, 53405, 53520
  Prostatic or Membranous Urethra, 53415, 53420, 53425
  Stoma, 53520
  Stricture, 53400, 53405
  Urethrocele, 57230
  with Replantation Penis, 54438
  Wound, 53502-53515
Urethral Sphincter, 57220
Urinary Incontinence, 53431, 53440, 53445
Uterus
  Anomaly, 58540
  Fistula, 51920, 51925
  Rupture, 58520, 59350
  Suspension, 58400, 58410
   Presacral Sympathectomy, 58410
Vagina
  Anterior, 57240, 57289
   with Insertion of Mesh, 57267
   with Insertion of Prosthesis, 57267
  Cystocele, 57240, 57260
  Enterocele, 57265
  Episiotomy, 59300
  Fistula, 46715, 46716, 51900
   Rectovaginal, 57300-57307
   Transvesical and Vaginal Approach, 57330
   Urethrovaginal, 57310, 57311
   Vaginoenteric, 58999
   Vesicovaginal, 57320, 57330
  Hysterectomy, 58267, 58293
  Incontinence, 57288
  Pereyra Procedure, 57289
  Postpartum, 59300
  Prolapse, 57282, 57284
  Rectocele, 57250, 57260
  Suspension, 57280-57284
   Laparoscopic, 57425
  Wound, 57200, 57210
Vaginal Wall Prolapse
  Anterior, 57240, 57267, 57289
  Anteroposterior, 57260-57267
  Nonobstetrical, 57200
  Posterior, 57250, 57267
Vas Deferens
  Suture, 55400
Vein
  Angioplasty, *[37248, 37249]*
  Femoral, 34501
  Graft, 34520
  Pulmonary, 33730
  Transposition, 34510
Ventricle, 33545, 33611-33612, 33782-33783
Vulva
  Postpartum, 59300
Wound
  Cardiac, 33300, 33305
  Complex, 13100-13160
  Extraocular Muscle, 65290
  Intermediate, 12031-12057
  Operative Wound Anterior Segment, 66250
  Simple, 12001-12021
Wound Dehiscence
  Abdominal Wall, 49900
  Skin and Subcutaneous Tissue
   Complex, 13160
   Simple, 12020, 12021
  Wrist, 25260, 25263, 25270, 25447
  Bones, 25440
  Carpal Bone, 25431
  Cartilage, 25107
  Muscles, 25260-25274
  Removal
   Implant, 25449
  Secondary, 25265, 25272, 25274
  Tendon, 25280-25316

Repair — *continued*
Wrist — *continued*
  Tendon — *continued*
   Sheath, 25275
  Total Replacement, 25446
Repeat Surgeries
Carotid
  Thromboendarterectomy, 35390
Coronary Artery Bypass
  Valve Procedure, 33530
Distal Vessel Bypass, 35700
Replacement
Adjustable Gastric Restrictive Device, 43773
Aortic Valve, 33405-33413
  Transcatheter, 33361-33369
  with Translocation Pulmonary Valve, 33440
Arthroplasty
  Hip, 27125-27138
  Knee, 0396T, 27447
  Spine, 22856-22857, 22861-22862
Artificial Heart
  Intracorporeal, 33928-33929
Cardio-Defibrillator, 33249, *[33262, 33263, 33264]*
Carotid Sinus Baroreflex Activation Device, 0266T-0268T
Cecostomy Tube, 49450
Cerebrospinal Fluid Shunt, 62160, 62194, 62225, 62230
Chest Wall Respiratory Sensor Electrode or Electrode Array, 0467T
Colonic Tube, 49450
Contact Lens, 92326
  See Also Contact Lens Services
Duodenostomy Tube, 49451
Elbow
  Total, 24363
Electrode
  Heart, 33210, 33211, 33216, 33217
  Stomach, 43647
External Fixation, 20697
Eye
  Drug Delivery System, 67121
Gastro-jejunostomy Tube, 49452
Gastrostomy Tube, 43762-43763, 49450
Hearing Aid
  Bone Conduction, 69710
Heart
  Defibrillator
   Leads, 33249
Hip, 27130, 27132
  Revision, 27134-27138
Implant
  Bone
   for External Speech Processor/Cochlear Stimulator, 69717, 69718
Intervertebral Disc
  Cervical Interspace, 22856, 22899
  Lumbar Interspace, 0163T, 22862
Jejunostomy Tube, 49451
Knee
  Intraoperative Balance Sensor, 0396T
  Total, 27447
Mitral Valve, 33430
Nerve, 64726
Neurostimulator
  Electrode, 63663-63664, 64569
  Pulse Generator/Receiver
   Intracranial, 61885
   Peripheral Nerve, 64590
   Spinal, 63685
Ossicles
  with Prosthesis, 69633, 69637
Ossicular Replacement, 69633, 69637
Pacemaker, 33206-33208, *[33227, 33228, 33229]*
  Catheter, 33210
  Electrode, 33210, 33211, 33216, 33217
  Pulse Generator, 33212-33214 *[33221]*, 33224-33233 *[33227, 33228, 33229]*
Pacing Cardioverter–Defibrillator
  Leads, 33243, 33244
  Pulse Generator Only, 33241

Replacement — *continued*
Penile
  Prosthesis, 54410, 54411, 54416, 54417
Prosthesis
  Skull, 62143
  Urethral Sphincter, 53448
Pulmonary Valve, 33475
Pulse Generator
  Brain, 61885
  Peripheral Nerve, 64590
  Spinal Cord, 63685
  Vagus Nerve Blocking Therapy, 0316T
Receiver
  Brain, 61885
  Peripheral Nerve, 64590
  Spinal Cord, 63685
Skin, 15002-15278
Skull Plate, 62143
Spinal Cord
  Reservoir, 62360
Stent
  Ureteral, 50382, 50385
Strut, 20697
Subcutaneous Port for Gastric Restrictive Procedure, 43888
Tissue Expanders
  Skin, 11970
Total Replacement Heart System
  Intracorporeal, 33928-33929
Total Replacement Hip, 27130-27132
Tricuspid Valve, 33465
Ureter
  Electronic Stimulator, 53899
  with Intestines, 50840
Uterus
  Inverted, 59899
Venous Access Device, 36582, 36583, 36585
  Catheter, 36578
Venous Catheter
  Central, 36580, 36581, 36584
Ventricular Assist Device, 0451T-0454T, 0459T, 33981-33983
Wireless Cardiac Stimulator, 0518T-0520T
Replantation, Reimplantation
Adrenal Tissue, 60699
Arm, Upper, 20802
Digit, 20816, 20822
Foot, 20838
Forearm, 20805
Hand, 20808
Penis, 54438
Scalp, 17999
Thumb, 20824, 20827
Report Preparation
Extended, Medical, 99080
Psychiatric, 90889
Reposition
Toe to Hand, 26551-26556
Repositioning
Canalith, 95992
Central Venous Catheter, Previously Placed, 36597
Defibrillator, *[33273]*
Electrode
  Heart, 0574T, 33215, 33226
Gastrostomy Tube, 43761
Intraocular Lens, 66825
Intravascular Vena Cava Filter, 37192
Tricuspid Valve, 33468
Ventricular Assist Device, 0460T-0461T
Reproductive Tissue
Preparation
  Thawing, 89354
  Storage, 89344
Reprogramming
Infusion Pump, 62369-62370
Peripheral Subcutaneous Field Stimulation
  Pulse Generator, 64999
Shunt
  Brain, 62252
Reptilase
Test, 85635
Time, 85670-85675
Resection
Abdomen, 51597
Aortic Valve Stenosis, 33415

Resection — *continued*
Bladder Diverticulum, 52305
Bladder Neck
  Transurethral, 52500
Brain Lobe, 61323, 61537-61540
Bullae, 32141
Chest Wall, 21601-21603, 32900
Cyst
  Mediastinal, 39200
Diaphragm, 39560-39561
Emphysematous Lung, 32672
Endaural, 69905-69910
Humeral Head, 23195
Intestines, Small
  Laparoscopic, 44202-44203
Lung, 32491, 32503-32504, 32672
Mouth
  with Tongue Excision, 41153
Myocardium
  Aneurysm, 33542
  Septal Defect, 33545
Nasal Septum, Submucous, 30520
Nose
  Septum, 30520
Ovary, Wedge, 58920
Palate, 42120
Pancoast Tumor, 32503-32504
Phalangeal Head
  Toe, 28153
Prostate, Transurethral, 52601, 52630
Radical
  Abdomen, 22904-22905, 51597
  Acetabulum, 27049 *[27059]*, 27076
  Ankle, 27615-27616, 27645-27647
  Arm, Lower, 24152, 25077-25078, 25170
  Arm, Upper, 23220, 24077-24079, 24150
  Back, 21935-21936
  Calcaneus, 27615-27616, 27647
  Elbow, 24077-24079, 24152
   Capsule Soft Tissue, 24149
  Face, 21015-21016
  Femur, 27364-27365 *[27329]*
  Fibula, 27615-27616, 27646
  Finger, 26117-26118, 26260-26262
  Flank, 21935-21936
  Foot, 28046-28047, 28171-28173
  Forearm, 25077-25078, 25170
  Hand, 26117-26118, 26250
  Hip, 27049 *[27059]*, 27075-27078
  Humerus, 23220, 24077-24079
  Innominate, 27049 *[27059]*, 27077
  Ischial, 27049 *[27059]*, 27078
  Knee, 27364-27365 *[27329]*
  Lymph Node(s)
   Abdomen, 38747
   Axillary, 38740, 38745
   Cervical, 38720, 38724
   Groin Area, 38760, 38765
   Pelvic, 38770
   Retroperitoneal, 38780
   Suprahyoid, 38700
   Thoracic, 38746
  Metacarpal, 26117-26118, 26250
  Metatarsal, 28046-28047, 28173
  Mouth
   with Tongue Excision, 41150, 41155
  Neck, 21557-21558
  Ovarian Tumor
   Bilateral Salpingo–Oophorectomy–Omentectomy, 58950-58954
   Omentectomy, 58950-58956
   with Radical Dissection for Debulking, 58952-58954
   with Total Abdominal Hysterectomy, 58951, 58953-58956
  Pelvis, 27049 *[27059]*, 27075-27078
  Peritoneal Tumor
   Bilateral Salpingo–Oophorectomy–Omentectomy, 58952-58954
   with Radical Dissection for Debulking, 58952-58954

Index   **Sclerotherapy**

Index

Risk Score Cancer, mRNA — Sclerotherapy

Risk Score Cancer, mRNA
  Prostate, 0011M
  Urothelial, 0012M-0013M
Risser Jacket, 29010-29015
  Removal, 29710
RK, 65771
Robotic Assistance
  Prostatectomy, 55866
Rocky Mountain Spotted Fever, 86000
Roentgen Rays
  See X–Ray
Roentgenographic
  See X–Ray
Roentgenography
  See Radiology, Diagnostic
ROM, 95851-95852, 97110, 97530
Ropes Test, 83872
Rorschach Test, 96112-96116
Ross Information Processing Assessment, 96125
Ross Procedure, 33413
Ross-Konno Procedure, 33440
Rotarix, 90681
RotaTeq, 90680
Rotation Flap, 14000-14350
Rotator Cuff
  Repair, 23410-23420
Rotavirus
  Antibody, 86759
  Antigen Detection
    Enzyme Immunoassay, 87425
Rotavirus Vaccine, 90680-90681
Round Window
  Repair Fistula, 69667
Round Window Fistula, 69667
Roux–en–Y Procedures
  Biliary Tract, 47740-47741, 47780-47785
  Pancreas, 48540
  Stomach, 43621, 43633, 43644, 43846
    Laparoscopic, 43644
RP1, 81404, 81434
RP2, 81434
RPE65, 81406, 81434
RPGR, 81434
RPP (Radical Perineal Prostatectomy), 55810-55815
RPR, 86592-86593
RPS19, 81405
RRM2B, 81405
RRP (Radical Retropubic Prostatectomy), 55840-55845
RSV
  Antibody, 86756
  Antigen Detection
    Direct Fluorescent Antibody, 87280
    Enzyme Immunoassay, 87420
    Recombinant, 90378
RT3, 84482
Rubber Band Ligation
  Hemorrhoids, 46221
  Skin Tags, 11200-11201
Rubella
  Antibody, 86762
  Vaccine, 90707-90710
Rubella HI Test
  Hemagglutination Inhibition Test, 86280
Rubella Immunization
  MMR, 90707
  MMRV, 90710
Rubeola
  Antibody, 86765
  Antigen Detection
    Immunofluorescence, 87283
Ruiz–Mora Procedure, 28286
RUNX1/RUNX1T1, 81401, *[81334]*
Russell Viper Venom Time, 85612-85613
RYR1, 81406, 81408
RYR2, 81408

S

Sac, Endolymphatic
  Exploration, 69805-69806
Saccomanno Technique, 88108
Sacral Nerve
  Implantation
    Electrode, 64561, 64581

Sacral Nerve — *continued*
  Insertion
    Electrode, 64561, 64581
Sacroiliac Joint
  Arthrodesis, 27280
  Arthrotomy, 27050
  Biopsy, 27050
  Dislocation
    Open Treatment, 27218
  Fusion, 27280
  Injection for Arthrography, 27096
  Stabilization for Arthrodesis, 27279
  X–ray, 72200-72202, 73525
Sacroplasty, 0200T-0201T
Sacrum
  Augmentation, 0200T-0201T
  Pressure Ulcer, 15931-15937
  Tumor
    Excision, 49215
  X–ray, 72220
SAECG, 93278
SAH, 61566
Salabrasion, 15780-15787
Salicylate
  Assay, *[80329, 80330, 80331]*
Saline–Solution Abortion, 59850-59851
Salivary Duct
  Catheterization, 42660
  Dilation, 42650-42660
  Ligation, 42665
  Repair, 42500-42505
    Fistula, 42600
Salivary Gland Virus
  Antibody, 86644-86645
  Antigen Detection
    Direct Fluorescence, 87271
    Enzyme Immunoassay, 87332
    Nucleic Acid, 87495-87497
Salivary Glands
  Abscess
    Incision and Drainage, 42310-42320
  Biopsy, 42405
  Calculi (Stone)
    Excision, 42330-42340
  Cyst
    Drainage, 42409
    Excision, 42408
  Injection
    X–ray, 42550
  Needle Biopsy, 42400
  Nuclear Medicine
    Function Study, 78232
    Imaging, 78230-78231
  Parotid
    Abscess, 42300-42305
  Unlisted Services and Procedures, 42699
  X–ray, 70380-70390
    with Contrast, 70390
Salmonella
  Antibody, 86768
Salpingectomy, 58262-58263, 58291-58292, 58552, 58554, 58661, 58700
  Ectopic Pregnancy
    Laparoscopic Treatment, 59151
    Surgical Treatment, 59120
  Oophorectomy, 58943
Salpingography, 0568T
Salpingohysterostomy, 58752
Salpingolysis, 58740
Salpingoneostomy, 58673, 58770
Salpingo–Oophorectomy, 58720
  Resection Ovarian Malignancy, 58950-58956
  Resection Peritoneal Malignancy, 58950-58956
  Resection Tubal Malignancy, 58950-58956
Salpingostomy, 58673, 58770
  Laparoscopic, 58673
SALT, 84460
Salter Osteotomy of the Pelvis, 27146
Sampling
  See Biopsy; Brush Biopsy; Needle Biopsy
Sang–Park Procedure
  Septectomy, Atrial, 33735-33737
    Balloon (Rashkind Type), 92992
    Blade Method (Park), 92993
Sao Paulo Typhus, 86000
SAST, 84450

Saucerization
  Calcaneus, 28120
  Clavicle, 23180
  Femur, 27070, 27360
  Fibula, 27360, 27641
  Hip, 27070
  Humerus, 23184, 24140
  Ileum, 27070
  Metacarpal, 26230
  Metatarsal, 28122
  Olecranon Process, 24147
  Phalanges
    Finger, 26235-26236
    Toe, 28124
  Pubis, 27070
  Radius, 24145, 25151
  Scapula, 23182
  Talus, 28120
  Tarsal, 28122
  Tibia, 27360, 27640
  Ulna, 24147, 25150
Saundby Test, 82270, 82272
Sauve–Kapandji Procedure
  Arthrodesis, Distal Radioulnar Joint, 25830
SAVER (Surgical Anterior Ventricular Endocardial Restoration), 33548
SBFT, 74246, 74248
SBRT (Stereotactic Body Radiation Therapy), 77373
Scabies, 87220
Scalenotomy, 21700-21705
Scalenus Anticus
  Division, 21700-21705
Scaling
  Chemical for Acne, 17360
Scalp
  Skin Graft
    Delay of Flap, 15610
    Full Thickness, 15220-15221
    Pedicle Flap, 15572
    Split, 15100-15101
    Tissue Transfer, Adjacent, 14020-14021
  Tumor Excision, 21011-21016
Scalp Blood Sampling, 59030
Scan
  See Also Specific Site; Nuclear Medicine
  Abdomen
    Computed Tomography, 74150-74175, 75635
  Computerized
    Ophthalmic, 92132-92134
  CT
    See CT Scan
  MRI
    See Magnetic Resonance Imaging
  PET
    See Specific Site; Nuclear Medicine
  Radionuclide, Brain, 78803
  Retinal Polarization, 0469T
Scanning Radioisotope
  See Nuclear Medicine
Scanogram, 77073
Scaphoid
  Fracture
    Closed Treatment, 25622
    Open Treatment, 25628
    with Manipulation, 25624
Scapula
  Craterization, 23182
  Cyst
    Excision, 23140
      with Allograft, 23146
      with Autograft, 23145
  Diaphysectomy, 23182
  Excision, 23172, 23190
    Partial, 23182
  Fracture
    Closed Treatment
      with Manipulation, 23575
      without Manipulation, 23570
    Open Treatment, 23585
  Ostectomy, 23190
  Repair
    Fixation, 23400
    Scapulopexy, 23400
  Saucerization, 23182

Scapula — *continued*
  Sequestrectomy, 23172
  Tumor
    Excision, 23140, 23210
      with Allograft, 23146
      with Autograft, 23145
    Radical Resection, 23210
  X–ray, 73010
Scapulopexy, 23400
Scarification
  Pleural, 32215
Scarification of Pleura
  Agent for Pleurodesis, 32560
  Endoscopic, 32650
SCBE (Single Contrast Barium Enema), 74270
Schanz Operation, 27448
Schauta Operation, 58285
Schede Procedure, 32905-32906
Scheie Procedure, 66155
Schlatter Operation, 43620
Schlemm's Canal Dilation, 66174-66175
Schlichter Test, 87197
Schocket Procedure, 66180
Schuchardt Procedure
  Osteotomy
    Maxilla, 21206
Schwannoma, Acoustic
  See Brain, Tumor, Excision
Sciatic Nerve
  Decompression, 64712
  Injection
    Anesthetic or Steroid, 64445-64446
  Lesion
    Excision, 64786
  Neuroma
    Excision, 64786
  Neuroplasty, 64712
  Release, 64712
  Repair
    Suture, 64858
Scintigraphy
  See Emission Computerized Tomography
  See Nuclear Medicine
Scissoring
  Skin Tags, 11200-11201
Sclera
  Excision, 66130
    Sclerectomy with Punch or Scissors, 66160
  Fistulization
    Sclerectomy with Punch or Scissors with Iridectomy, 66160
    Thermocauterization with Iridectomy, 66155
    Trabeculectomy ab Externo in Absence of Previous Surgery, 66170
    Trephination with Iridectomy, 66150
  Incision (Fistulization)
    Sclerectomy with Punch or Scissors with Iridectomy, 66160
    Thermocauterization with Iridectomy, 66155
    Trabeculectomy ab Externo in Absence of Previous Surgery, 66170
    Trephination with Iridectomy, 66150
  Lesion
    Excision, 66130
  Repair
    Reinforcement
      with Graft, 67255
      without Graft, 67250
    Staphyloma
      with Graft, 66225
      with Glue, 65286
    Wound (Operative), 66250
      Tissue Glue, 65286
Scleral Buckling Operation
  Retina, Repair, Detachment, 67107-67108, 67113
Scleral Ectasia
  Repair with Graft, 66225
Sclerectomy, 66160
Sclerotherapy
  Percutaneous (Cyst, Lymphocele, Seroma), 49185
  Venous, 36468-36471

© 2019 Optum360, LLC   CPT © 2019 American Medical Association. All Rights Reserved.   *[Resequenced]*   **Index — 117**

Sclerotomy, 66150-66170
SCN1A, 81407
SCN1B, 81404
SCN4A, 81407
SCN5A, 81407
SCNN1A, 81406
SCNN1B, 81406
SCNN1G, 81406
SCO1, 81405
SCO2, 81404
Scoliosis Evaluation, Radiologic, 72081-72084
Scrambler Therapy, 0278T
Screening
  Abdominal Aortic Aneurysm (AAA), 76706
  Developmental, 96110, 96112-96113
  Drug
    Alcohol and/or Substance Abuse, 99408-99409
  Evoked Otoacoustic Emissions, [92558]
  Mammography, 77067
Scribner Cannulization, 36810
Scrotal Varices
  Excision, 55530-55540
Scrotoplasty, 55175-55180
Scrotum
  Abscess
    Incision and Drainage, 54700, 55100
  Excision, 55150
  Exploration, 55110
  Hematoma
    Incision and Drainage, 54700
  Removal
    Foreign Body, 55120
  Repair, 55175-55180
  Ultrasound, 76870
  Unlisted Services and Procedures, 55899
Scrub Typhus, 86000
SDHA, 81406
SDHB, 81405, 81437-81438
SDHC, 81404-81405, 81437-81438
SDHD, 81404, 81437-81438
Second Look Surgery
  Carotid Thromboendarterectomy, 35390
  Coronary Artery Bypass, 33530
  Distal Vessel Bypass, 35700
  Valve Procedure, 33530
Secretory Type II Phospholipase A2 (sPLA2-IIA), 0423T
Section
  See Also Decompression
  Cesarean
    See Cesarean Delivery
  Cranial Nerve, 61460
    Spinal Access, 63191
  Dentate Ligament, 63180-63182
  Gasserian Ganglion
    Sensory Root, 61450
  Nerve Root, 63185-63190
  Spinal Accessory Nerve, 63191
  Spinal Cord Tract, 63194-63199
  Vestibular Nerve
    Transcranial Approach, 69950
    Translabyrinthine Approach, 69915
Sedation
  Moderate, 99155-99157
    with Independent Observation, 99151-99153
Seddon–Brookes Procedure, 24320
Sedimentation Rate
  Blood Cell
    Automated, 85652
    Manual, 85651
Segmentectomy
  Breast, 19301-19302
  Lung, 32484, 32669
Selective Cellular Enhancement Technique, 88112
Selenium, 84255
Self Care
  See Also Physical Medicine/ Therapy/Occupational Therapy
  Training, 97535, 98960-98962, 99509
Sella Turcica
  CT Scan, 70480-70482
  X–ray, 70240

Semen
  Cryopreservation
    Storage (per year), 89343
    Thawing, Each Aliquot, 89353
Semen Analysis, 89300-89322
  Sperm Analysis, 89329-89331
    Antibodies, 89325
    with Sperm Isolation, 89260-89261
Semenogelase, 84152-84154
Semilunar
  Bone
    See Lunate
Seminal Vesicle
  Cyst
    Excision, 55680
  Excision, 55650
  Incision, 55600, 55605
  Mullerian Duct
    Excision, 55680
  Unlisted Services and Procedures, 55899
Seminal Vesicles
  Vesiculography, 74440
  X–ray with Contrast, 74440
Seminin, 84152-84154
Semiquantitative, 81005
Semont Maneuver, 95992
Sengstaaken Tamponade
  Esophagus, 43460
Senning Procedure
  Repair, Great Arteries, 33774-33777
Senning Type, 33774-33777
Sensitivity Study
  Antibiotic
    Agar, 87181
    Disc, 87184
    Enzyme Detection, 87185
    Macrobroth, 87188
    MIC, 87186
    Microtiter, 87186
    MLC, 87187
    Mycobacteria, 87190
  Antiviral Drugs
    HIV–1
      Tissue Culture, 87904
Sensor, Chest Wall Respiratory Electrode or Electrode Array
  Insertion, 0466T
  Removal, 0468T
  Replacement, 0467T
  Revision, 0467T
Sensor, Interstitial Glucose, 0446T-0448T
Sensor, Transcatheter Placement, 34701-34708
Sensorimotor Exam, 92060
Sensory Nerve
  Common
    Repair/Suture, 64834
Sensory Testing
  Quantitative (QST), Per Extremity
    Cooling Stimuli, 0108T
    Heat–Pain Stimuli, 0109T
    Touch Pressure Stimuli, 0106T
    Using Other Stimuli, 0110T
    Vibration Stimuli, 0107T
Sentinel Node
  Injection Procedure, 38792
SEP (Somatosensory Evoked Potentials), 95925-95927 [95938]
Separation
  Craniofacial
    Closed Treatment, 21431
    Open Treatment, 21432-21436
SEPT9, 81327
Septal Defect
  Repair, 33813-33814
  Ventricular
    Closure
      Open, 33675-33688
      Percutaneous, 93581
Septectomy
  Atrial, 33735-33737
    Balloon Type, 92992
    Blade Method, 92993
  Closed, 33735
  Submucous Nasal, 30520
Septic Abortion, 59830
Septin9, 81327

Septoplasty, 30520
Septostomy
  Atrial, 33735-33737
    Balloon Type, 92992
    Blade Method, 92993
Septum, Nasal
  See Nasal Septum
Sequestrectomy
  Calcaneus, 28120
  Carpal, 25145
  Clavicle, 23170
  Forearm, 25145
  Humeral Head, 23174
  Humerus, 24134
  Olecranon Process, 24138
  Radius, 24136, 25145
  Scapula, 23172
  Skull, 61501
  Talus, 28120
  Ulna, 24138, 25145
  with Alveolectomy, 41830
  Wrist, 25145
Serialography
  Aorta, 75625
Serodiagnosis, Syphilis, 86592-86593
Serologic Test for Syphilis, 86592-86593
Seroma
  Incision and Drainage
    Skin, 10140
  Sclerotherapy, Percutaneous, 49185
Serotonin, 84260
Serpin Peptidase Inhibitor, Clade A, Alpha-1 Antiproteinase, Antitrypsin, Member 1 Gene Analysis, 81332
SERPINA1, 81332
SERPINE1, 81400
Serum
  Albumin, 82040
  Antibody Identification
    Pretreatment, 86975-86978
  CPK, 82550
  Serum Immune Globulin, 90281-90284
Serum Globulin Immunization, 90281-90284
Sesamoid Bone
  Excision, 28315
  Finger
    Excision, 26185
  Foot
    Fracture, 28530-28531
  Thumb
    Excision, 26185
Sesamoidectomy
  Toe, 28315
SETX, 81406
Sever Procedure, 23020
Severing of Blepharorrhaphy, 67710
Sex Change Operation
  Female to Male, 55980
  Male to Female, 55970
Sex Chromatin, 88130
Sex Chromatin Identification, 88130-88140
Sex Hormone Binding Globulin, 84270
Sex–Linked Ichthyoses, 86592-86593
SG, 84315, 93503
SGCA, 81405
SGCB, 81405
SGCD, 81405
SGCE, 81405-81406
SGCG, 81404-81405
SGOT, 84450
SGPT, 84460
SH2D1A, 81403-81404
SH3TC2, 81406
Shaving
  Skin Lesion, 11300-11313
SHBG, 84270
Shelf Procedure
  Osteotomy, Hip, 27146-27151
    Femoral with Open Reduction, 27156
Shiga–Like Toxin
  Antigen Detection
    Enzyme Immunoassay, 87427
Shigella
  Antibody, 86771
Shirodkar Operation, 57700
SHOC2, 81400, 81405

Shock Wave Lithotripsy, 50590
Shock Wave (Extracorporeal) Therapy, 0101T-0102T, 0512T-0513T, 20999, 28890, 28899, 43265, 50590, 52353
Shock Wave, Ultrasonic
  See Ultrasound
Shop Typhus of Malaya, 86000
Shoulder
  See Also Clavicle; Scapula
  Abscess
    Drainage, 23030
  Amputation, 23900-23921
  Arthrocentesis, 20610-20611
  Arthrodesis, 23800
    with Autogenous Graft, 23802
  Arthrography
    Injection
      Radiologic, 23350
  Arthroplasty
    with Implant, 23470-23472
  Arthroscopy
    Diagnostic, 29805
    Surgical, 29806-29828
  Arthrotomy
    with Removal Loose or Foreign Body, 23107
  Biopsy
    Deep, 23066
    Soft Tissue, 23065
  Blade
    See Scapula
  Bone
    Excision
      Acromion, 23130
      Clavicle, 23120-23125
      Clavicle Tumor, 23140-23146
    Incision, 23035
    Tumor
      Excision, 23140-23146
  Bursa
    Drainage, 23031
  Capsular Contracture Release, 23020
  Cast
    Figure Eight, 29049
    Removal, 29710
    Spica, 29055
    Velpeau, 29058
  Disarticulation, 23920-23921
  Dislocation
    Closed Treatment
      with Manipulation, 23650, 23655
    Open Treatment, 23660
    with Greater Tuberosity Fracture
      Closed Treatment, 23665
      Open Treatment, 23670
    with Surgical or Anatomical Neck Fracture
      Closed Treatment with Manipulation, 23675
      Open Treatment, 23680
  Excision
    Acromion, 23130
    Torn Cartilage, 23101
  Exploration, 23107
  Hematoma
    Drainage, 23030
  Incision and Drainage, 23040-23044
    Superficial, 10060-10061
  Joint
    X–ray, 73050
  Manipulation
    Application of Fixation Apparatus, 23700
  Prophylactic Treatment, 23490-23491
  Prosthesis
    Removal, 23334-23335
  Radical Resection, 23077
  Removal
    Calcareous Deposits, 23000
    Cast, 29710
    Foreign Body, 23040-23044
      Deep, 23333
      Subcutaneous, 23330
    Foreign or Loose Body, 23107
    Prosthesis, 23334-23335
  Repair
    Capsule, 23450-23466

Index

Spinal Accessory Nerve — Stem Cell

  [Resequenced]   CPT © 2019 American Medical Association. All Rights Reserved.   © 2019 Optum360, LLC

Suture — *continued*

Pancreas, 48545
Pharynx
  Wound, 42900
Rectum
  Fistula, 45800-45825
  Prolapse, 45540, 45541
Removal
  Anesthesia, 15850, 15851
Spleen, 38115
Stomach
  Fistula, 43880
  Laceration, 43501, 43502
  Stoma, 43870
  Ulcer, 43501, 43840
  Wound, 43840
Tendon
  Foot, 28200-28210
  Knee, 27380, 27381
Testis
  Injury, 54670
  Suspension, 54620, 54640
Thoracic Duct
  Abdominal Approach, 38382
  Cervical Approach, 38380
  Thoracic Approach, 38381
Throat
  Wound, 42900
Tongue
  to Lip, 41510
Trachea
  Fistula, 31825
    with Plastic Repair, 31825
    without Plastic Repair, 31820
  Stoma, 31825
    with Plastic Repair, 31825
    without Plastic Repair, 31820
  Wound
    Cervical, 31800
    Intrathoracic, 31805
  Ulcer, 44604-44605
Ureter, 50900, 50940
  Deligation, 50940
  Fistula, 50920-50930
Urethra
  Fistula, 45820-45825, 53520
  Stoma, 53520
  to Bladder, 51840-51841
  Wound, 53502-53515
Uterus
  Fistula, 51920-51925
  Rupture, 58520, 59350
  Suspension, 58400-58410
Vagina
  Cystocele, 57240, 57260
  Enterocele, 57265
  Fistula
    Rectovaginal, 57300-57307
    Transvesical and Vaginal Approach, 57330
    Urethrovaginal, 57310-57311
    Vesicovaginal, 51900, 57320-57330
  Rectocele, 57250-57260
  Suspension, 57280-57283
  Wound, 57200-57210
Vas Deferens, 55400
Vein
  Femoral, 37650
  Iliac, 37660
  Vena Cava, 37619
Wound, 44604-44605
Skin
  Complex, 13100-13160
  Intermediate, 12031-12057
  Simple, 12020-12021
SUZI (Sub-Zonal Insemination), 89280
SVR (Surgical Ventricular Restoration), 33548
Swallowing
  Cine, 74230
  Evaluation, 92610-92613, 92616-92617
  Therapy, 92526
  Video, 74230
Swan-Ganz Catheter Insertion, 93503
Swanson Procedure
  Repair, Metatarsal, 28322
  Osteotomy, 28306-28309

Sweat Collection
  Iontophoresis, 89230
Sweat Glands
  Excision
    Axillary, 11450, 11451
    Inguinal, 11462, 11463
    Perianal, 11470, 11471
    Perineal, 11470, 11471
    Umbilical, 11470, 11471
Sweat Test
  Chloride, Blood, 82435
Swenson Procedure, 45120
Syme Procedure, 27888
Sympathectomy
  Artery
    Digital, 64820
    Radial, 64821
    Superficial Palmar Arch, 64823
    Ulnar, 64822
  Cervical, 64802
  Cervicothoracic, 64804
  Digital Artery with Magnification, 64820
  Lumbar, 64818
  Presacral, 58410
  Renal, 0338T-0339T
  Thoracic, 32664
  Thoracolumbar, 64809
  with Rib Excision, 21616
Sympathetic Nerve
  Excision, 64802-64818
  Injection
    Anesthetic, 64520-64530
Sympathins, 80424, 82382-82384
Symphysiotomy
  Horseshoe Kidney, 50540
Symphysis, Pubic, 27282
Synagis, 90378
Syncytial Virus, Respiratory
  Antibody, 86756
  Antigen Detection
    Direct Fluorescence, 87280
    Direct Optical Observation, 87807
    Enzyme Immunoassay, 87420
Syndactylism, Toes, 28280
Syndactyly
  Repair, 26560-26562
Syndesmotomy
  Coracoacromial
    Arthroscopic, 29826
    Open, 23130, 23415
  Lateral Retinacular
    Endoscopic, 29873
    Open, 27425
  Transverse Carpal, 29848
Syndrome
  Adrenogenital, 56805, 57335
  Ataxia–Telangiectasia
    Chromosome Analysis, 88248
  Bloom
    Chromosome Analysis, 88245
    Genomic Sequence Analysis, 81412
  Carpal Tunnel
    Decompression, 64721
  Costen's
    See Temporomandibular Joint (TMJ)
  Crigler-Najjar, 81404
  Erb–Goldflam, 95857
  Gilbert, 81350
  Ovarian Vein
    Ureterolysis, 50722
  Synechiae, Intrauterine
    Lysis, 58559
  Treacher Collins
    Midface Reconstruction, 21150-21151
  Urethral
    Cystourethroscopy, 52285
Syngesterone, 84144
Synostosis (Cranial)
  Bifrontal Craniotomy, 61557
  Extensive Craniectomy, 61558-61559
  Frontal Craniotomy, 61556
  Parietal Craniotomy, 61556
Synovectomy
  Arthrotomy with
    Glenohumeral Joint, 23105
    Sternoclavicular Joint, 23106

Synovectomy — *continued*

Elbow, 24102
Excision
  Carpometacarpal Joint, 26130
  Finger Joint, 26135-26140
  Hip Joint, 27054
  Interphalangeal Joint, 26140
  Knee Joint, 27334-27335
  Metacarpophalangeal Joint, 26135
  Palm, 26145
  Wrist, 25105, 25115-25119
  Radical, 25115-25116
Synovial
  Bursa
    See Also Bursa
    Joint Aspiration, 20600-20611
  Cyst
    See Also Ganglion
    Aspiration, 20612
  Membrane
    See Synovium
  Popliteal Space, 27345
Synovium
  Biopsy
    Carpometacarpal Joint, 26100
    Interphalangeal Joint, 26110
    Knee Joint, 27330
    Metacarpophalangeal Joint
      with Synovial Biopsy, 26105
  Excision
    Carpometacarpal Joint, 26130
    Finger Joint, 26135-26140
    Hip Joint, 27054
    Interphalangeal Joint, 26140
    Knee Joint, 27334-27335
Syphilis Nontreponemal Antibody, 86592-86593
Syphilis Test, 86592, 86593
Syrinx
  Spinal Cord
    Aspiration, 62268
System
  Auditory, 69000-69979
  Cardiac Contractility Modulation, 0408T-0418T
  Cardiovascular, 33016-37799 *[33221, 33227, 33228, 33229, 33230, 33231, 33262, 33263, 33264, 33270, 33271, 33272, 33273, 33274, 33275, 33440, 33962, 33963, 33964, 33965, 33966, 33969, 33984, 33985, 33986, 33987, 33988, 33989, 34717, 34718, 34812, 34820, 34833, 34834, 36465, 36466, 36482, 36483, 36572, 36573, 37246, 37247, 37248, 37249]*
  Digestive, 40490-49999 *[43211, 43212, 43213, 43214, 43233, 43266, 43270, 43274, 43275, 43276, 43277, 43278, 44381, 44401, 45346, 45388, 45390, 45398, 45399, 46220, 46320, 46945, 46946, 46947]*
  Endocrine, 60000-60699
  Eye/Ocular Adnexa, 65091-68899 *[67810]*
  Genital
    Female, 56405-58999
    Male, 54000-55899
  Hemic/Lymphatic, 38100-38999
  Integumentary, 10040-19499 *[11045, 11046]*
  Mediastinum/Diaphragm, 39000-39599
  Musculoskeletal, 20100-29999 *[21552, 21554, 22858, 22859, 23071, 23073, 24071, 24073, 25071, 25073, 26111, 26113, 27043, 27045, 27059, 27329, 27337, 27339, 27632, 27634, 28039, 28041, 28295, 29914, 29915, 29916]*
  Nervous, 61000-64999 *[64633, 64634, 64635, 64636]*
  Neurostimulator
    Central Sleep Apnea, 0424T-0436T
  Respiratory, 30000-32999 *[31651]*
  Tympanostomy
    Automated Tube Delivery, 0583T
  Urinary, 50010-53899 *[51797, 52356]*

T

T Cell
  Antigen Receptor
    Beta Gene Rearrangement Analysis, 81340-81341
    Gamma Gene Rearrangement Analysis, 81342
  Leukemia Lymphoma Virus I, 86687, 86689
  Leukemia Lymphoma Virus II, 86688
T(9;22) Translocation Analysis, 81206-81208
T(15;17) Translocation Analysis, 81315-81316
T–3, 84480
T3 Free, 84481
T–4
  T Cells, 86360-86361
  Thyroxine, 84436-84439
T4 Molecule, 86360
T4 Total, 84436
T–7 Index
  Thyroxine, Total, 84436
  Triiodothyronine, 84480-84482
T–8, 86360
Taarnhoj Procedure
  Decompression, Gasserian Ganglion, Sensory Root, 61450
Tachycardia
  Heart
    Recording, 93609
TACO1, 81404
Tacrolimus
  Assay, 80197
Tactile Breast Imaging, 0422T
Tag
  Anus, 46230 *[46220]*
  Skin Removal, 11200-11201
TAH, 51925, 58150, 58152, 58200-58240, 58951, 59525
TAHBSO, 58150, 58152, 58200-58240, 58951
Tail Bone
  Excision, 27080
  Fracture, 27200, 27202
Takeuchi Procedure, 33505
Talectomy, 28130
Talotarsal Joint
  Dislocation, 28570, 28575, 28585
  Percutaneous Fixation, 28576
Talus
  Arthrodesis
    Pantalar, 28705
    Subtalar, 28725
    Triple, 28715
  Arthroscopy
    Surgical, 29891, 29892
  Craterization, 28120
  Cyst
    Excision, 28100-28103
  Diaphysectomy, 28120
  Excision, 28120, 28130
  Fracture
    Open Treatment, 28445
    Percutaneous Fixation, 28436
    with Manipulation, 28435, 28436
    without Manipulation, 28430
  Osteochondral Graft, 28446
  Repair
    Osteochondritis Dissecans, 29892
    Osteotomy, 28302
  Saucerization, 28120
  Tumor
    Excision, 27647, 28100-28103
Tap
  Cisternal, 61050-61055
  Lumbar Diagnostic, 62270
TARDBP, 81405
Tarsal
  Fracture
    Percutaneous Fixation, 28456
Tarsal Bone
  See Ankle Bone
Tarsal Joint
  See Also Foot
  Arthrodesis, 28730, 28735, 28740
    with Advancement, 28737
    with Lengthening, 28737
  Craterization, 28122

Testis — *continued*
Repair — *continued*
Suspension, 54620, 54640
Torsion, 54600
Suture
Injury, 54670
Suspension, 54620, 54640
Transplantation
to Thigh, 54680
Tumor
Excision, 54530, 54535
Undescended
Exploration, 54550, 54560
Unlisted Services and Procedures, 54699, 55899
Testosterone, 84402
Bioavailable, Direct, 84410
Response, 80414
Stimulation, 80414, 80415
Total, 84403
Testosterone Estradiol Binding Globulin, 84270
Tetanus, 86280
Antibody, 86774
Immunoglobulin, 90389
Tetanus Immunization, 90698-90702, 90714-90715, 90723
Tetralogy of Fallot, 33692-33697, 33924
TGFBR1, 81405, 81410-81411
TGFBR2, 81405, 81410-81411
TGRBI, 81333
TH, 81406
THA, 27130-27134
Thal–Nissen Procedure, 43325
THAP1, 81404
Thawing
Cryopreserved
Embryo, 89352
Oocytes, 89356
Reproductive Tissue, 89354
Sperm, 89353
Previously Frozen Cells, 38208, 38209
Thawing and Expansion
of Frozen Cell, 88241
THBR, 84479
Theleplasty, 19350
Theophylline
Assay, 80198
TheraCys, 90586
Therapeutic
Abortion, 59850-59852
Apheresis, 36511-36516
Drug Assay
See Drug Assay
Mobilization
See Mobilization
Photopheresis
See Photopheresis
Radiology
See Radiation Therapy
Therapeutic Activities
Music
Per 15 Minutes, 97530
Therapies
Actinotherapy, 96900
Cold
See Cryotherapy
Exercise, 97110-97113
Family, 99510
Psychotherapy, 90846-90849
Interventions
Cognitive Function, 97129-97130
Language, 92507-92508
Milieu, 90882
Occupational
Evaluation, *[97165, 97166, 97167, 97168]*
Photodynamic, 67221, 96567-96571
See Photochemotherapy
Physical
See Physical Medicine/ Therapy/Occupational Therapy
Rhinophototherapy, 30999
Speech, 92507-92508
Tocolytic, 59412
Ultraviolet Light, 96900
Therapy
ACE Inhibitor Therapy, 4010F

Therapy — *continued*
Bone Marrow Cell, 0263T-0264T
Cognitive Function, 97129-97130
Desensitization, 95180
Evaluation
Athletic Training, *[97169, 97170, 97171, 97172]*
Occupational, *[97165, 97166, 97167, 97168]*
Physical, *[97161, 97162, 97163, 97164]*
Hemodialysis
See Hemodialysis
Hot Pack, 97010
Low Level Laser, 0552T
Pharmacologic, for Cessation of Tobacco Use, 4001F
Radiation
Blood Products, 86945
Speech, 92507-92508
Statin Therapy, Prescribed, 4013F
Vagus Nerve, 0312T-0317T
Warfarin, 4012F
Thermocauterization
Ectropion
Repair, 67922
Lesion
Cornea, 65450
Thermocoagulation, 17000-17286
Thermotherapy
Prostate, 53850-53852
High-energy Water Vapor, 0582T
Microwave, 53850
Radiofrequency, 53852
Thiamine, 84425
Thiersch Operation
Pinch Graft, 15050
Thiersch Procedure, 46753
Thigh
Excision
Excess Skin, 15832
Tumor, 27327-27328 *[27337, 27339]*, 27355-27358, 27364-27365 *[27329]*
Fasciotomy, 27025
ThinPrep, 88142
Thiocyanate, 84430
Thompson Procedure, 27430
Thompson Test
Smear and Stain, Routine, 87205
Urinalysis, Glass Test, 81020
Thoracectomy, 32905-32906
Thoracic
Anterior Ramus
Anesthetic or Steroid Injection, 64400-64421
Destruction, 64620
Neurolytic Injection, 64620
Arteries
Catheterization, 36215-36218
Cavity
Bypass Graft Excision, 35905
Endoscopy
Exploration, 32601-32606
Surgical, 32650-32674
Duct
Cannulation, 38794
Ligation, 38380
Abdominal Approach, 38382
Thoracic Approach, 38381
Suture, 38380
Abdominal Approach, 38382
Cervical Approach, 38380
Thoracic Approach, 38381
Empyema
Incision and Drainage, 21501-21502
Surgery
Video–Assisted
See Thoracoscopy
Vertebra
See Also Vertebra, Thoracic
Corpectomy, 63085-63101, 63103
Intraspinal Lesion, 63300-63308
Decompression, 62380, 63055, 63057, 63064-63066
Discectomy, 63077-63078
Excision for Lesion, 22101, 22112

Thoracic — *continued*
Vertebra — *continued*
Injection Procedure
Diagnostic/Therapeutic, 62320-62327
for Discography, 62291
for Neurolysis, 62280-62282
Paravertebral, 64490-64495, *[64461, 64462, 64463]*
Laminectomy, 63003, 63016, 63046, 63048
Wall
See Chest Wall
Thoracoplasty, 32905
with Closure Bronchopleural Fistula, 32906
Thoracoscopy
Biopsy, 32604, 32607-32609
Diagnostic, 32601, 32604, 32606
Surgical, 32650-32674
Control Traumatic Hemorrhage, 32654
Creation Pericardial Window, 32659
Esophagomyotomy, 32665
Excision
Mediastinal Cyst, Tumor and/or Mass, 32662
Pericardial Cyst, Tumor and/or Mass, 32661
Lymphadenectomy, 32674
Parietal Pleurectomy, 32656
Partial Pulmonary Decortication, 32651
Pleurodesis, 32650
Removal
Clot, 32658
Foreign Body, 32653, 32658
Lung, 32671
Single Lobe, 32663
Single Lung Segment, 32669
Two Lobes, 32670
Resection
Thymus, 32673
Resection-Plication
Bullae, 32655
Emphysematous Lung, 32672
Sternum Reconstruction, 21743
Thoracic Sympathectomy, 32664
Total Pulmonary Decortication, 32652
Wedge Resection, 32666-32668
Thoracostomy
Empyema, 32035, 32036
Tube, 32551
Thoracotomy
Biopsy, 32096-32098
Cardiac Massage, 32160
Cyst Removal, 32140
Esophagogastric Fundoplasty, 43328
Exploration, 32100
for Postoperative Complications, 32120
Hemorrhage, 32110
Hiatal Hernia Repair, 43334-43335
Neonatal, 39503
Lung Repair, 32110
Open Intrapleural Pneumolysis, 32124
Removal
Bullae, 32141
Cyst, 32140
Defibrillator, 33243
Electrodes, 33238
Foreign Body
Intrapleural, 32150
Intrapulmonary, 32151
Pacemaker, 33236, 33237
Resection-Plication of Bullae, 32141
Transmyocardial Laser Revascularization, 33140, 33141
Wedge Resection, 32505-32507
Thorax
See Also Chest; Chest Cavity; Mediastinum
Angiography, 71275
Biopsy, 21550
CT Scan, 71250-71275
Incision
Empyema, 32035, 32036
Pneumothorax, 32551
Incision and Drainage
Abscess, 21501, 21502
Deep, 21510

Thorax — *continued*
Incision and Drainage — *continued*
Hematoma, 21501, 21502
Strapping, 29200
Tumor, 21555-21558 *[21552, 21554]*
Unlisted Services and Procedures, 21899
THRB, 81405
Three Glass Test
Urinalysis, Glass Test, 81020
Three–Day Measles
Antibody, 86762
Vaccine, 90707-90710
Throat
See Also Pharynx
Abscess
Incision and Drainage, 42700-42725
Biopsy, 42800-42806
Hemorrhage, 42960-42962
Reconstruction, 42950
Removal
Foreign Body, 42809
Repair
Pharyngoesophageal, 42953
Wound, 42900
Suture
Wound, 42900
Unlisted Services and Procedures, 42999
Thrombectomy
Aortoiliac Artery, 34151, 34201
Arterial, Mechanical, 37184-37185
Arteriovenous Fistula
Graft, 36904-36906
Axillary Artery, 34101
Axillary Vein, 34490
Brachial Artery, 34101
Bypass Graft, 35875, 35876
Noncoronary/Nonintracranial, 37184-37186
Carotid Artery, 34001
Celiac Artery, 34151
Dialysis Circuit, 36904-36906
Dialysis Graft
without Revision, 36831
Femoral, 34201
Femoropopliteal Vein, 34421, 34451
Iliac Artery, 34151, 34201
Iliac Vein, 34401-34451
Innominate Artery, 34001-34101
Intracranial, Percutaneous, 61645
Mesenteric Artery, 34151
Percutaneous
Coronary Artery, *[92973]*
Noncoronary, Nonintracranial, 37184-37186
Vein, 37187-37188
Peroneal Artery, 34203
Popliteal Artery, 34203
Radial Artery, 34111
Renal Artery, 34151
Subclavian Artery, 34001-34101
Subclavian Vein, 34471, 34490
Tibial Artery, 34203
Ulnar Artery, 34111
Vena Cava, 34401-34451
Vena Caval, 50230
Venous, Mechanical, 37187-37188
Thrombin Inhibitor I, 85300-85301
Thrombin Time, 85670, 85675
Thrombocyte (Platelet)
Aggregation, 85576
Automated Count, 85049
Count, 85008
Manual Count, 85032
Thrombocyte ab, 86022-86023
Thromboendarterectomy
See Also Thrombectomy
Aorta, Abdominal, 35331
Aortoiliofemoral Artery, 35363
Axillary Artery, 35321
Brachial Artery, 35321
Carotid Artery, 35301, 35390
Celiac Artery, 35341
Femoral Artery, 35302, 35371-35372
Iliac Artery, 35351, 35361, 35363
Iliofemoral Artery, 35355, 35363
Innominate Artery, 35311

Toe — *continued*
  Reconstruction
    Angle Deformity, 28313
    Extra Digit, 26587
    Extra Toes, 28344
    Hammer Toe, 28285, 28286
    Macrodactyly, 28340, 28341
    Syndactyly, 28345
    Webbed Toe, 28345
  Repair, 26590
    Bunion, 28289-28299 [28295]
    Extra Digit, 26587
    Macrodactylia, 26590
    Muscle, 28240
    Tendon, 28232, 28234, 28240
    Webbed, 28280, 28345
    Webbed Toe, 28345
  Reposition, 20973, 26551-26554
  Reposition to Hand, 26551-26554, 26556
  Strapping, 29550
  Tenotomy, 28010, 28011, 28232, 28234
  Tumor, 28043-28047 [28039, 28041], 28108, 28175
  Unlisted Services and Procedures, 28899
  X–Ray, 73660
Tolerance Test(s)
  Glucagon, 82946
  Glucose, 82951, 82952
  Heparin–Protamine, 85530
  Insulin, 80434, 80435
  Maltose, 82951, 82952
Tomodensitometries
  See CT Scan
Tomographic Scintigraphy, Computed, 78803
Tomographic SPECT
  Myocardial Imaging, 78469
Tomographies, Computed X–Ray
  See CT Scan
Tomography
  Coherence
    Optical
      Axillary Node, Each Specimen, Excised Tissue, 0351T-0352T
      Breast, Each Specimen, Excised Tissue, 0351T-0352T
      Coronary Vessel or Graft, [92978, 92979]
      Middle Ear, 0485T-0486T
      Skin, 0470T-0471T
      Surgical Cavity, Breast, 0353T-0354T
  Computed
    Abdomen, 74150-74175, 75635
    Biomechanical Analysis, 0558T
    Bone Strength and Fracture Risk, 0554T-0557T
    Head, 70450-70470, 70496
    Heart, 75571-75574
Tomosynthesis, Breast
  Bilateral, 77062
  Screening, 77063
  Unilateral, 77061
Tompkins Metroplasty
  Uterus Reconstruction, 58540
Tongue
  Ablation, 41530
  Abscess
    Incision and Drainage, 41000-41006, 41015
  Biopsy, 41100, 41105
  Cyst
    Incision and Drainage, 41000-41006, 41015, 60000
  Excision
    Base
      Radiofrequency, 41530
    Complete, 41140-41155
    Frenum, 41115
    Partial, 41120-41135
    with Mouth Resection, 41150, 41153
    with Radical Neck, 41135, 41145, 41153, 41155
  Hematoma
    Incision and Drainage, 41000-41006, 41015

Tongue — *continued*
  Incision
    Frenum, 41010
  Lesion
    Excision, 41110-41114
  Reconstruction
    Frenum, 41520
    Reduction for Sleep Apnea, 41530
  Repair
    Laceration, 41250-41252
    Suture, 41510
  Suspension, 41512
  Unlisted Services and Procedures, 41599
Tonometry, Serial, 92100
Tonsil, Pharyngeal
  Excision, 42830-42836
    with Tonsillectomy, 42820-42821
  Unlisted Services/Procedures, 42999
Tonsillectomy, 42820-42826
  Primary
    Age 12 or Over, 42826
    Younger Than Age 12, 42825
  Secondary
    Age 12 or Over, 42826
    Younger Than Age 12, 42825
  with Adenoidectomy
    Age 12 or Over, 42821
    Younger Than Age 12, 42820
Tonsils
  Abscess
    Incision and Drainage, 42700
  Excision, 42825, 42826
  Excision with Adenoids, 42820, 42821
    Lingual, 42870
    Radical, 42842-42845
    Tag, 42860
  Lingual
    Destruction, 42870
  Removal
    Foreign Body, 42999
  Unlisted Services and Procedures, 42999
Topiramate
  Assay, 80201
Topography
  Corneal, 92025
TOR1A, 81400, 81404
Torek Procedure
  Orchiopexy, 54650
Torkildsen Procedure, 62180
TORP (Total Ossicular Replacement Prosthesis), 69633, 69637
Torsion Swing Test, 92546
Torula, 86641, 87327
Torus Mandibularis
  Tumor Excision, 21031
Total
  Abdominal Hysterectomy, 58150
    with Colpo-Urethrocystopexy, 58152
    with Omentectomy, 58956
    with Partial Vaginectomy, 58200
  Bilirubin Level, 82247, 88720
  Catecholamines, 82382
  Cystectomy, 51570-51597
  Dacryoadenectomy, 68500
  Elbow Replacement, 24363
  Esophagectomy, 43107-43113, 43124, 43286-43288
  Gastrectomy, 43620-43622
  Hemolytic Complement, 86162
  Hip Arthroplasty, 27130-27132
  Knee Arthroplasty, 0396T, 27447
  Mastectomies
    See Mastectomy
  Ostectomy of Patella, 27424
  Splenectomy, 38100, 38102
Toupet Procedure, 43280
Touroff Operation/Ligation, Artery, Neck, 37615
Toxicology, [80305, 80306, 80307]
Toxin Assay, 87230
  Tissue Culture, 87230
Toxin, Botulinum
  Chemodenervation
    Eccrine Glands, 64650-64653
    Extraocular Muscle, 67345
    Extremity Muscle, 64642-64645
    for Blepharospasm, 64612

Toxin, Botulinum — *continued*
  Chemodenervation — *continued*
    for Hemifacial Spasm, 64612
    Internal Anal Sphincter, 46505
    Neck Muscle, 64616
    Trunk Muscle, 64646-64647
Toxoplasma
  Antibody, 86777, 86778
TP53, 81404-81405, 81432
T–Phyl, 80198
TPM1, 81405
TPMT, 81335
TR3SVR, 33548
Trabeculectomy, 66170
Trabeculectomy Ab Externo
  in Absence of Previous Surgery, 66170
  with Scarring Previous Surgery, 66172
Trabeculoplasty
  by Laser Surgery, 65855
Trabeculotomy Ab Externo
  Eye, 65850
Trachea
  Aspiration, 31720
    Catheter, 31720, 31725
  Dilation, 31630-31631, 31636-31638
  Endoscopy
    via Tracheostomy, 31615
  Excision
    Stenosis, 31780, 31781
  Fistula
    Repair, 31825
      with Plastic Repair, 31825
      without Plastic Repair, 31820
  Fracture
    Endoscopy, 31630
  Incision
    Emergency, 31603, 31605
    Planned, 31600, 31601
    with Flaps, 31610
  Introduction
    Needle Wire, 31730
  Puncture
    Aspiration and
      or Injection, 31612
  Reconstruction
    Carina, 31766
    Cervical, 31750
    Fistula, 31755
    Graft Repair, 31770
    Intrathoracic, 31760
  Repair
    Cervical, 31750
    Fistula, 31755
    Intrathoracic, 31760
    Stoma, 31613, 31614
  Revision/Stoma/Scars, 31830
  Scar
    Revision, 31830
  Stenosis
    Excision, 31780, 31781
    Repair, 31780, 31781
  Stoma
    Repair, 31825
      with Plastic Repair, 31825
      without Plastic Repair, 31820
    Revision
      Scars, 31830
  Tumor
    Excision
      Cervical, 31785
      Thoracic, 31786
  Unlisted Services and Procedures, 31899
    Bronchi, 31899
  Wound
    Suture
      Cervical, 31800
      Intrathoracic, 31805
Tracheal
  Stent
    Placement, 31631
  Tube, 31500
Trachelectomy, 57530
  Radical, 57531
Trachelorrhaphy, 57720
Tracheobronchoscopy
  via Tracheostomy, 31615

Tracheoesophageal Fistula
  Repair, 43305, 43312, 43314
  Speech Prosthesis, 31611
Tracheoplasty
  Cervical, 31750
  Intrathoracic, 31760
  Tracheopharyngeal Fistulization, 31755
Tracheoscopy, 31515-31529
Tracheostoma
  Revision, 31613, 31614
Tracheostomy
  Emergency, 31603, 31605
  Planned, 31600, 31601
  Revision
    Scar, 31830
  Surgical Closure
    with Plastic Repair, 31825
    without Plastic Repair, 31820
  Tracheobronchoscopy through, 31615
  with Flaps, 31610
Tracheotomy
  Tube Change, 31502
Tracking Tests (Ocular), 92545
Tract, Urinary
  X-Ray with Contrast, 74400-74425
Traction Therapy
  Manual, 97140
  Mechanical, 97012
  Skeletal, 20999
Training
  Activities of Daily Living, 97535, 99509
  Athletic, Evaluation, [97169, 97170, 97171, 97172]
  Biofeedback, 90901, 90912-90913
  Cognitive Skills, 97129-97130
  Community
    Work Reintegration, 97537
  Home Management, 97535, 99509
  Management
    Propulsion, 97542
  Orthoptic
    Pleoptic, 92065
  Orthotics, 97760
  Prosthetics, 97761
  Seeing Impaired, 97799
    Braille, or Moon, 97799
    Lead Dog, Use of, 97799
  Self Care, 97535, 99509
  Sensory Integration, 97533
  Walking (Physical Therapy), 97116
  Wheelchair Management
    Propulsion, 97542
TRAM Flap
  Breast Reconstruction, 19367-19369
Transabdominal Endoscopy
  Intestine, Large, [45399]
Transaminase
  Glutamic Oxaloacetic, 84450
  Glutamic Pyruvic, 84460
Transapical Mitral Valve Repair, 0543T
Transbronchial Needle Aspiration (TBNA), 31629, 31633
Transcatheter
  Biopsy, 37200
  Closure
    Left Atrial Appendage, 33340
    Percutaneous, Heart, 93580-93582
  Denervation
    Renal Sympathetic, 0338T-0339T
  Embolization
    Cranial, 61624, 61626
    Vascular, 37241-37244
  Implantation or Replacement
    Mitral Valve
      Percutaneous, 0483T
      Transthoracic, 0484T
  Occlusion
    Cranial, 61624, 61626
    Vascular, 37241-37244
  Placement
    Intravascular Stent(s), 0075T-0076T, 37215-37217, 37236-37239
    Wireless Physiologic Sensor, 34701-34708
  Reconstruction
    Mitral Valve Annulus, 0544T

Transcatheter — continued
Reconstruction — continued
Tricuspid Valve Annulus, 0545T
Removal, Foreign Body, 37197
Therapy
Embolization, 75894
Infusion, 75898, [37211, 37212, 37213, 37214]
Perfusion
Cranial, 61624, 61626
Septal Reduction, 93583
Transcortin, 84449
Transcranial
Doppler Study (TCP), 93886-93893
Stimulation, Motor, 95928-95929
Transcutaneous
Electric Nerve Stimulation, 97014, 97032
Electrical Modulation Pain Reprocessing, 0278T
Transdermal Electrostimulation, 97014, 97032
Transection
Blood Vessel
Kidney, 50100
Brain
Subpial, 61597
Nerve, 64732-64772
Vagus, 43640, 43641
Pulmonary Artery, 33922
Transesophageal
Echocardiography, 93312-93318
Guidance for Intracardiac or Great Vessel Intervention, 93355
Transfer
Adjacent Tissue, 14000-14350
Blastocyst, 58974-58976
Cryopreserved, 89352
Finger Position, 26555
Gamete Intrafallopian, 58976
Jejunum
Free, 43496
with Microvascular Anastomosis Preparation/Embryo, 89255
Toe Joint, 26556
Toe to Hand, 26551-26554, 26556
Tubal Embryo Stage, 58974
Transferase
Aspartate Amino, 84450
Glutamic Oxaloacetic, 84450
Transferrin, 84466
Transformation
Lymphocyte, 86353
Transforming Growth Factor Beta-induced, 81333
Transfusion
Blood, 36430
Exchange, 36450, 36455
Newborn, Partial, 36456
Fetal, 36460
Push
Infant, 36440
Unlisted Services and Procedures, 86999
White Blood Cells, 86950
Transfusion, Blood, Autologous, 86890-86891
Transillumination
Skull
Newborn, 95999
Transitional Care Management, 99495-99496
Translocation
Aortic Root, 33782-33783
Transluminal
Angioplasty
Arterial, 36902-36903, 36905-36906
Coronary, [92920, 92921, 92924, 92925, 92928, 92929, 92933, 92934, 92937, 92938, 92941, 92943, 92944]
Atherectomies, 0234T-0238T, 37227, 37229, 37231, 37233, 37235, [92924, 92925], [92933, 92934], [92937, 92938], [92941], [92943, 92944], [92973]
Transmyocardial Laser Revascularization, 33140, 33141
Transosteal Bone Plate
Reconstruction
Mandible, 21244
Transpeptidase, Gamma–Glutamyl, 82977
Transperineal Periurethral Balloon Device, 0548T-0551T

Transperineal Placement
Biodegradable Material
Periprostatic, 55874
Transplant
See Also Graft
Bone
See Also Bone Graft
Allograft, Spine, 20930-20931
Autograft, Spine, 20936-20938
Hair, 15775-15776
See Hair, Transplant
Islet Cell, 0584T-0586T
Transplantation
See Also Graft
Amniotic Membrane, 65780
Backbench Preparation Prior to Transplantation
Intestine, 44715-44721
Kidney, 50323-50329
Liver, 47143-47147
Pancreas, 48551-48552
Bone Marrow, 38240, 38241
Harvesting, 38230
Cartilage
Knee
Allograft, 20932, 27415, 29867
Autograft, 27412, 29866
Osteoarticular, 20932
Chondrocytes
Knee, 27412
Conjunctiva, 65782
Cornea
Autograft/Homograft
Lamellar, 65710
Penetrating, 65730-65755
for Aphakia, 65750
Eye
Amniotic Membrane, 65780
Conjunctiva, 65782
Stem Cell, 65781
Hair
Punch Graft, 15775, 15776
Strip, 15220, 15221
Heart, 33945
Allograft Preparation, 33933, 33944
Heart–Lung, 33935
Intestines
Allograft Preparation, 44715-44721
Allotransplantation, 44135, 44136
Donor Enterectomy, 44132, 44133
Removal of Allograft, 44137
Islet Cell, 0584T-0586T
Liver, 47135
Allograft Preparation, 47143-47147
Lung
Allograft Preparation, 32855-32856, 33933
Donor Pneumonectomy, 32850
Double with Cardiopulmonary Bypass, 32854
Double, without Cardiopulmonary Bypass, 32853
Single, with Cardiopulmonary Bypass, 32852
Single, without Cardiopulmonary Bypass, 32851
Meniscus
Knee, 29868
Muscle, 15731-15738, 15756
Osteoarticular, 20932
Ovary, 58999
Pancreas, 48550, 48554-48556
Allograft Preparation, 48551-48552
Pancreatic Islet Cell, 0584T-0586T
with Pancreatectomy, 48160
Parathyroid, 60512
Renal
Allograft Preparation, 50323-50329
Allotransplantation, 50360
with Recipient Nephrectomy, 50365
Autotransplantation, 50380
Donor Nephrectomy, 50300, 50320, 50547
Recipient Nephrectomy, 50340

Transplantation — continued
Renal — continued
Removal Transplanted Renal Allograft, 50370
Spleen, 38999
Stem Cells, 38240, 38241, 38242
Cell Concentration, 38215
Cryopreservation, 38207, 88240
Donor Search, 38204
Harvesting, 38205-38206
Plasma Depletion, 38214
Platelet Depletion, 38213
Red Blood Cell Depletion, 38212
T–cell Depletion, 38210
Thawing, 38208, 88241
Tumor Cell Depletion, 38211
Washing, 38209
Testis
to Thigh, 54680
Tissue, Harvesting, 15771-15774, [15769]
Transpleural Thoracoscopy
See Thoracoscopy
Transposition
Arteries
Carotid, 33889, 35691, 35694, 35695
Subclavian, 33889, 35693-35695
Vertebral, 35691, 35693
Cranial Nerve, 64716
Eye Muscles, 67320
Great Arteries
Repair, 33770-33781
Nerve, 64718-64721
Nipple, 19499
Ovary, 58825
Peripheral Nerve
Major, 64856
Vein Valve, 34510
Trans–Scaphoperilunar
Fracture
Dislocation, 25680, 25685
Closed Treatment, 25680
Open Treatment, 25685
Transthoracic Echocardiography, 0439T, 93303-93350, [93356]
Transthyretin, 84134
Transureteroureterostomy, 50770
Transurethral
See Also Specific Procedure
Fulguration
Postoperative Bleeding, 52214
Prostate
Ablation
Waterjet, 0421T
Incision, 52450
Resection, 52601, 52630-52640
Thermotherapy, 53850-53852
High-energy Water Vapor, 0582T
Microwave, 53850
Radiofrequency, 53852
Radiofrequency Micro-Remodeling
Female Bladder, 53860
Transvaginal
Biomechanical Mapping, 0487T
Transversus Abdominis Plane (TAP) Block
Bilateral, 64488-64489
Unilateral, 64486-64487
Trapezium
Arthroplasty
with Implant, 25445
Travel, Unusual, 99082
TRB@, 81340-81341
TRD@, 81402
Treacher–Collins Syndrome
Midface Reconstruction, 21150, 21151
Treatment, Tocolytic, 59412
Trendelenburg Operation, 37785
Trephine Procedure
Sinusotomy
Frontal, 31070
Treponema Pallidum
Antibody, 86780
Antigen Detection
Direct Fluorescent Antibody, 87285
TRF (Thyrotropin Releasing Factor), 80439
TRG@, 81342
TRH, 80438, 80439

Triacylglycerol, 84478
Triacylglycerol Hydrolase, 83690
Triangular Cartilage
Repair with Fracture
Radial shaft, 25526
Triangular Fibrocartilage
Excision, 29846
Tributyrinase, 83690
Trichiasis
Repair, 67825
Epilation, by Forceps, 67820
Epilation, by Other than Forceps, 67825
Incision of Lid Margin, 67830
with Free Mucous Membrane Graft, 67835
Trichina, 86784, 96902
Trichinella
Antibody, 86784
Trichogram, 96902
Trichomonas Vaginalis
Antigen Detection
Nucleic Acid, 87660-87661
Trichrome Stain, 88313
Tricuspid Valve
Excision, 33460
Repair, 0569T-0570T, 33463-33465
Replace, 33465
Repositioning, 33468
Tridymite, 84285
Trigeminal Ganglia, 61450, 61790
Trigeminal Nerve
Destruction, 64600-64610
Injection
Anesthetic or Steroid, 64400
Neurolytic, 64600, 64605
Trigeminal Tract
Stereotactic
Create Lesion, 61791
Trigger Finger Repair, 26055
Trigger Point
Injection
One or Two Muscle Groups, 20552
Two or More Muscle Groups, 20553
Triglyceridase, 83690
Triglyceride Lipase, 83690
Triglycerides, 84478
Trigonocephaly, 21175
Tri-incisional esophagectomy, 43112
Triiodothyronine
Free, 84481
Resin Uptake, 84479
Reverse, 84482
Total, 84480
True, 84480
Triolean Hydrolase, 83690
Trioxopurine, 84550, 84560
Tripcellim
Duodenum, 84485
Feces, 84488-84490
Tripedia, 90700
Trisegmentectomy, 47122
Trocar Biopsy
Bone Marrow, 38221
Trochanter
Pressure Ulcer, 15950-15958
Trochanteric Femur Fracture, 27246-27248
Trophoblastic Tumor GTT, 59100, 59870
Troponin
Qualitative, 84512
Quantitative, 84484
TRPC6, 81406
Trumenba, [90621]
Truncal Vagotomies, 43640
Truncus Arteriosus
Repair, 33786
Truncus Brachiocephalicus
Angioplasty, [37246, 37247]
Atherectomy, 0237T
Catheterization, 36215-36218
Trunk
Lipectomy, Suction Assisted, 15877
Skin Graft
Delay of Flap, 15600
Full Thickness, 15200
Muscle, Myocutaneous, or Fasciocutaneous Flaps, 15734

[Resequenced]

Trunk — *continued*
  Skin Graft — *continued*
    Split, 15100, 15101
    Tissue Transfer, Adjacent, 14000
TRUSP (Transrectal Ultrasound of Prostate), 76873
Trypanosomiases, 86171, 86280
Trypanosomiasis, 86171, 86280
Trypsin
  Duodenum, 84485
  Feces, 84488-84490
Trypsin Inhibitor, Alpha 1–Antitrypsin, 82103-82104
Trypure
  Duodenum, 84485
  Feces, 84488-84490
TSA, 86316
Tsalicylate Intoxication, *[80329, 80330, 80331]*
TSC1, 81405-81406
TSC2, 81406-81407
TSH, 80418, 80438, 84443
TSI, 84445
Tsutsugamushi Disease, 86000
TT, 85670-85675
TT–3, 84480
TT–4, 84436
TTN, 81439
TTPA, 81404
TTR, 81404
Tuba, Auditoria (Auditiva)
  Eustachian Tube Procedures, 69420-69421, 69799
Tubal Embryo Stage Transfer, 58976
Tubal Ligation, 58600
  Laparoscopic, 58670
  Postpartum, 58605
  with Cesarean Section, 58611
Tubal Occlusion
  See Fallopian Tube
  with Cesarean Delivery
    See Fallopian Tube, Occlusion; Occlusion
    Create Lesion
      See Fallopian Tube, Occlusion; Occlusion, Fallopian Tube
Tubal Pregnancy, 59121
  with Salpingectomy and/or Oophorectomy, 59120
Tube Change
  Colonic, 49450
  Duodenostomy, 49451
  Gastro-Jejunostomy, 49452
  Gastrostomy, 43762-43763, 49446
  Jejunostomy, 49451
  Tracheotomy, 31502
  Tube, Fallopian
    See Fallopian Tube
Tube Placement
  Cecostomy, 44300, 49442
  Chest, 32551
  Colonic, 49442
  Duodenostomy, 49441
  Enterostomy, 44300
  Gastrostomy Tube, 43246, 49440
  Jejunostomy, 49441
  Nasogastric Tube, 43752
  Orogastric Tube, 43752
Tube Replacement
  See Tube Change
Tubectomy, 58700, 58720
Tubed Pedicle Flap
  Formation, 15570-15576
  Walking Tube, 15650
Tubercle Bacilli
  Culture, 87116
Tubercleplasty, Anterior Tibial, 27418
Tuberculin Test, 86580
Tuberculosis
  Antigen Response Test, 86480
  Cell Mediated Immunity Antigen, 86480-86481
  Culture, 87116
  Skin Test, 86580
Tuberculosis Vaccine (BCG), 90585, 90586
Tubes
  Chest, 32551
  Endotracheal, 31500
  Gastrostomy, 43246, 49440

Tubes — *continued*
  Gastrostomy — *continued*
    See Also Gastrostomy Tube
Tudor "Rabbit Ear"
  Urethra, Repair
    Diverticulum, 53240, 53400, 53405
    Fistula, 45820, 45825, 53400, 53405, 53520
    Sphincter, 57220
    Stricture, 53400, 53405
    Urethrocele, 57230
    Wound, 53502-53515
Tuffier Vaginal Hysterectomy
  See Hysterectomy, Vaginal
TULIP, 52647-52648
Tumor
  Abdomen
    Destruction
      Excision, 49203-49205
  Abdominal Wall, 22900-22905
  Acetabulum
    Excision, 27076
  Ankle, 27615-27619 *[27632]*
  Arm, Lower, 24152, 25075-25078 *[25071, 25073]*
  Arm, Upper, 23220, 24075-24079 *[24071, 24073]*, 24110-24126, 24150
  Back, 21930-21936
  Bile Duct
    Ablation, *[43278]*
    Extrahepatic, 47711
    Intrahepatic, 47712
  Bladder, 52234-52240
    Excision, 51530, 52355
  Brain, 61510
    Excision, 61518, 61520, 61521, 61526, 61530, 61545, 62164
  Breast
    Cryoablation, 0581T
    Excision, 19120-19126
  Bronchi
    Excision, 31640
  Calcaneus, 28100-28103
    Excision, 27647
  Carpal, 25130-25136
  Chest Wall
    Excision, 21601-21603
  Clavicle
    Excision, 23140, 23200
      with Allograft, 23146
      with Autograft, 23145
  Coccyx, 49215
  Colon
    Destruction, *[44401], [45388]*
    Removal, 44392, 44394, 45384-45385
  Cranial Bone
    Reconstruction, 21181, 21182
  Destruction
    Abdomen, 49203-49205
    Chemosurgery, 17311-17315
    Urethra, 53220
  Ear, Middle
    Extended, 69554
    Transcanal, 69550
    Transmastoid, 69552
  Elbow, 24075-24079 *[24071, 24073]*, 24120-24126, 24152
  Esophagus
    Ablation, 43229
  Excision
    Femur, 27355-27358
    Face, 21011-21016
    Facial Bones, 21029, 21030, 21034
    Fallopian Tube
      Resection, 58950, 58952-58956
    Femoral, 27355-27358
    Excision, 27365
    Femur, 27065-27067
    Excision, 27365
    Fibula, 27635-27638
    Excision, 27646
    Finger
      Excision, 26115-26117 *[26111, 26113]*
      Foot, 28043, 28045, 28046
    Flank, 21930-21936

Tumor — *continued*
  Forearm
    Radical Resection, 25077
  Gums
    Excision, 41825-41827
  Hand, 26115-26117 *[26111, 26113]*
  Heart
    Excision, 33120, 33130
  Hip, 27047-27049 *[27043, 27045]*, 27065-27067
    Excision, 27075, 27076
  Humerus, 23155-23156, 23220, 24115-24116, 24150
  Ileum, 27065-27067
  Immunoassay for Antigen, 86294, 86316
    CA 125, 86304
    CA 15–3, 86300
    CA 19–9, 86301
  Innominate
    Excision, 27077
  Intestines, Small
    Destruction, 44369
    Removal, 44364-44365
  Ischial Tuberosity, 27078
  Kidney
    Excision, 52355
  Knee
    Excision, 27327-27328 *[27337, 27339]*, 27355-27358, 27364-27365 *[27329]*
  Lacrimal Gland
    Excision
      Frontal Approach, 68540
      with Osteotomy, 68550
  Larynx, 31540, 31541
    Excision, 31300
      Endoscopic, 31540, 31541, 31578
    Incision, 31300
  Leg, Lower, 27615-27619 *[27632]*
  Leg, Upper
    Excision, 27327-27328 *[27337, 27339]*, 27355-27358, 27364-27365 *[27329]*
  Liver
    Ablation, 47380-47383
  Localization
    with Nuclear Medicine, 78800-78803 *[78804, 78830, 78831, 78832]*, *[78835]*
  Mandible, 21040-21045
  Maxillary Torus Palatinus, 21032
  Mediastinal
    Excision, 39220
  Mediastinum, 32662
  Meningioma
    Excision, 61519
  Metacarpal, 26200, 26205, 26250
  Metatarsal, 28104-28107
    Excision, 28173
  Neck, 21555-21558 *[21552, 21554]*
  Olecranon Process, 24075-24077 *[24071, 24073]*, 24120-24126
  Ovary
    Resection, 58950, 58952-58954
  Pancreatic Duct
    Ablation, *[43278]*
  Parotid Gland
    Excision, 42410-42426
  Pelvis, 27047-27049 *[27043, 27045]*
  Pericardial
    Endoscopic, 32661
    Excision, 33050
  Peritoneum
    Resection, 58950-58956
  Phalanges
    Finger, 26210, 26215, 26260-26262
    Toe, 28108
      Excision, 28175
  Pituitary Gland
    Excision, 61546, 61548
  Prostate
    Thermotherapy Ablation, 0582T
  Pubis, 27065-27067
  Radiation Therapy, *[77295]*
  Radius, 25120-25126, 25170
    Excision, 24120
      with Allograft, 24126

Tumor — *continued*
  Radius — *continued*
    with Autograft, 24125
  Rectum, 0184T, 45160, 45171-45172, 45190
  Resection
    Face, 21015
    Scalp, 21015
    with Cystourethroscopy, 52355
  Retroperitoneal
    Destruction
      Excision, 49203-49205
  Sacrum, 49215
  Scalp, 21011-21016
  Scapula, 23140
    Excision, 23140, 23210
      with Allograft, 23146
      with Autograft, 23145
  Shoulder, 23075-23078 *[23071, 23073]*
  Skull
    Excision, 61500
  Soft Tissue
    Elbow
      Excision, 24075
    Finger
      Excision, 26115
    Forearm
      Radical Resection, 25077
    Hand
      Excision, 26115
  Spinal Cord
    Excision, 63275-63290
  Stomach
    Excision, 43610, 43611
  Talus, 28100-28103
    Excision, 27647
  Tarsal, 28104-28107
    Excision, 28171
  Temporal Bone
    Removal, 69970
  Testis
    Excision, 54530, 54535
  Thorax, 21555-21558 *[21552, 21554]*
  Thyroid
    Excision, 60200
  Tibia, 27365, 27635-27638
    Excision, 27645
  Torus Mandibularis, 21031
  Trachea
    Excision
      Cervical, 31785
      Thoracic, 31786
  Ulna, 25120-25126, 25170
    Excision, 24120
      with Allograft
        Excision, 24126
      with Autograft
        Excision, 24125
  Ureter
    Excision, 52355
  Urethra, 52234-52240, 53220
    Excision, 52355
  Uterus
    Excision, 58140, 58145
  Vagina
    Excision, 57135
  Vertebra
    Additional Segment
      Excision, 22103, 22116
    Cervical
      Excision, 22100
    Lumbar, 22102
    Thoracic
      Excision, 22101
  Wrist, 25075-25078 *[25071, 25073]*
TUMT (Transurethral Microwave Thermotherapy), 53850
TUNA, 53852
Tunica Vaginalis
  Hydrocele
    Aspiration, 55000
    Excision, 55040, 55041
    Repair, 55060
Turbinate
  Excision, 30130, 30140
  Fracture
    Therapeutic, 30930

[Resequenced] CPT © 2019 American Medical Association. All Rights Reserved. © 2019 Optum360, LLC

© 2019 Optum360, LLC

CPT © 2019 American Medical Association. All Rights Reserved.

[Resequenced]

Index — 135

Index

Uterus — Vagus Nerve

Vagus Nerve — *continued*
  Transection — *continued*
    Truncal, 43651
Valentine's Test
  Urinalysis, Glass Test, 81020
Valproic Acid, 80164
Valproic Acid Measurement, 80164
Valsalva Sinus
  Repair, 33702-33720
Valva Atrioventricularis Sinistra (Valva Mitralis)
  Incision, 33420, 33422
  Repair, 33420-33427
    Transcatheter, 33418-33419
  Replacement, 33430
Valve
  Aortic
    Repair, Left Ventricle, 33414
    Replacement, 33405-33413
  Bicuspid
    Incision, 33420, 33422
    Repair, 33420-33427
      Transcatheter, 33418-33419
    Replacement, 33430
  Mitral
    Incision, 33420, 33422
    Repair, 33420-33427
      Transcatheter, 33418-33419
    Replacement, 33430
  Pulmonary
    Incision, 33470-33474
    Repair, 33470-33474
    Replacement, 33475
  Tricuspid
    Excision, 33460
    Repair, 0569T-0570T, 33463-33465
    Replace, 33465
    Reposition, 33468
Valve Stenosis, Aortic
  Repair, 33415
    Supravalvular, 33417
Valvectomy
  Tricuspid Valve, 33460
Valvotomy
  Mitral Valve, 33420, 33422
  Pulmonary Valve, 33470-33474
  Reoperation, 33530
Valvuloplasty
  Aortic Valve, 33390-33391
  Femoral Vein, 34501
  Mitral Valve, 33425-33427
  Percutaneous Balloon
    Aortic Valve, 92986
    Mitral Valve, 92987
    Pulmonary Valve, 92990
  Prosthetic Valve, 33496
  Reoperation, 33530
  Tricuspid Valve, 0569T-0570T, 33460-33465
Van Den Bergh Test, 82247, 82248
Vancomycin
  Assay, 80202
  Resistance, 87500
Vanillylmandelic Acid
  Urine, 84585
VAQTA, 90632-90633
VAR, 90716
Varicella (Chicken Pox)
  Immunization, 90710, 90716
Varicella–Zoster
  Antibody, 86787
  Antigen Detection
    Direct Fluorescent Antibody, 87290
Varices, Esophageal
  Injection Sclerosis, 43204
  Ligation, 43205, 43400
Varicocele
  Spermatic Cord
    Excision, 55530-55540
Varicose Vein
  Ablation, 36473-36479
  Removal, 37718, 37722, 37735, 37765-37785
  Secondary Varicosity, 37785
  with Tissue Excision, 37735, 37760
VARIVAX, 90716
Vas Deferens
  Anastomosis
    to Epididymis, 54900, 54901

Vas Deferens — *continued*
  Excision, 55250
  Incision, 55200
    for X–Ray, 55300
  Ligation, 55250
  Repair
    Suture, 55400
  Unlisted Services and Procedures, 55899
  Vasography, 74440
  X–Ray with Contrast, 74440
Vascular Flow Check, Graft, 15860
Vascular Injection
  Unlisted Services and Procedures, 36299
Vascular Lesion
  Cranial
    Excision, 61600-61608, 61615, 61616
  Cutaneous
    Destruction, 17106-17108
Vascular Malformation
  Cerebral
    Repair, 61710
  Finger
    Excision, 26115
  Hand
    Excision, 26115
Vascular Procedure(s)
  Angioscopy
    Noncoronary Vessels, 35400
  Brachytherapy
    Intracoronary Artery, [92974]
  Endoluminal Imaging
    Coronary Vessels, [92978, 92979]
  Endoscopy
    Surgical, 37500
  Harvest
    Lower Extremity Vein, 35572
  Thrombolysis
    Coronary Vessels, [92975, 92977]
    Cranial Vessels, 37195
    Intracranial Vessels, 61645
Vascular Rehabilitation, 93668
Vascular Studies
  See Also Doppler Scan, Duplex, Plethysmography
  Angioscopy
    Aorta, 93978, 93979
    Noncoronary Vessels, 35400
  Artery Studies
    Extracranial, 93880-93882
    Extremities, 93922-93924
    Intracranial, 93886, 93888
    Lower Extremity, 93922-93926
    Middle Cerebral Artery, Fetal, 76821
    Umbilical Artery, Fetal, 76820
    Upper Extremity, 93930, 93931
  Blood Pressure Monitoring, 24 Hour, 93784-93790
  Hemodialysis Access, 93990
    Prior to Access Creation, 93985-93986
  Kidney
    Multiple Study with Pharmacological Intervention, 78709
    Single Study with Pharmacological Intervention, 78708
  Penile Vessels, 93980, 93981
  Temperature Gradient, 93740
  Unlisted Services and Procedures, 93799
  Venous Studies
    Extremities, 93970-93971
    Venous Pressure, 93770
    Visceral Studies, 93975-93979
Vascular Surgery
  Arm, Upper
    Anesthesia, 01770-01782
  Elbow
    Anesthesia, 01770-01782
  Endoscopy, 37500
  Unlisted Services and Procedures, 37799
Vasectomy, 55250
  Laser Coagulation of Prostate, 52647
  Laser Vaporization of Prostate, 52648
  Reversal, 55400
  Transurethral
    Cystourethroscopic, 52402
    Transurethral Electrosurgical Resection of Prostate, 52601

Vasectomy — *continued*
  Transurethral Resection of Prostate, 52648
Vasoactive Drugs
  Injection
    Penis, 54231
Vasoactive Intestinal Peptide, 84586
Vasogram, 74440
Vasography, 74440
Vasointestinal Peptide, 84586
Vasopneumatic Device Therapy, 97016
  See Also Physical Medicine/Therapy/ Occupational Therapy
Vasopressin, 84588
Vasotomy, 55200, 55300
  Transurethral
    Cystourethroscopic, 52402
Vasovasorrhaphy, 55400
Vasovasostomy, 55400
VATS
  See Thoracoscopy
VBAC, 59610-59614
VBG (Vertical Banding Gastroplasty), 43842
VCU (Voiding Cystourethrogram), 51600
VCUG (Voiding Cystourethrogram), 51600
VDRL, 86592-86593
Vectorcardiogram
  Evaluation, 93799
  Tracing, 93799
Vein
  Ablation
    Endovenous, 36473-36479
  Adrenal
    Venography, 75840, 75842
  Anastomosis
    Caval to Mesenteric, 37160
    Intrahepatic Portosystemic, 37182-37183
    Portocaval, 37140
    Reniportal, 37145
    Saphenopopliteal, 34530
    Splenorenal, 37180, 37181
    Vein, 34530, 37180, 37181
      to Vein, 37140-37160, 37182-37183
  Angioplasty
    Transluminal, 36902, 36905, 36907, [37248, 37249]
  Arm
    Harvest of Vein for Bypass Graft, 35500
    Venography, 75820, 75822
  Axillary
    Thrombectomy, 34490
  Biopsy
    Transcatheter, 75970
  Cannulization
    to Artery, 36810, 36815
    to Vein, 36800
  Catheterization
    Central Insertion, 36555-36558, 36560-36561, 36563, 36565-36566, 36578, 36580-36583
    Organ Blood, 36500
    Peripheral Insertion, 36568-36569, 36570-36571, 36584-36585, [36572, 36573]
    Removal, 36589
    Repair, 36575
    Replacement, 36578-36581, 36584
    Umbilical, 36510
  Endoscopic Harvest
    for Bypass Graft, 33508
  External Cannula Declotting, 36860, 36861
  Extremity
    Non–Invasive Studies, 93970-93971
  Femoral
    Repair, 34501
  Femoropopliteal
    Thrombectomy, 34421, 34451
  Guidance
    Fluoroscopic, 77001
    Ultrasound, 76937
  Hepatic Portal
    Splenoportography, 75810
    Venography, 75885, 75887
  Iliac
    Thrombectomy, 34401, 34421, 34451

Vein — *continued*
  Injection
    Sclerosing Agent, 36468-36471, [36465, 36466]
  Insertion
    IVC Filter, 37191
  Interrupt
    Femoral Vein, 37650
    Iliac, 37660
    Vena Cava, 37619
  Jugular
    Venography, 75860
  Leg
    Harvest for Vascular Reconstruction, 35572
    Venography, 75820, 75822
  Ligation
    Clusters, 37785
    Esophagus, 43205
    Jugular, 37565
    Perforation, 37760
    Saphenous, 37700-37735, 37780
    Secondary, 37785
  Liver
    Venography, 75860, 75889, 75891
  Neck
    Venography, 75860
  Nuclear Medicine
    Thrombosis Imaging, 78456-78458
  Orbit
    Venography, 75880
  Portal
    Catheterization, 36481
  Pulmonary
    Repair, 33730
  Removal
    Clusters, 37785
    Saphenous, 37700-37735, 37780
    Varicose, 37765, 37766
  Renal
    Venography, 75831, 75833
  Repair
    Angioplasty, [37248, 37249]
    Graft, 34520
  Sampling
    Venography, 75893
  Sinus
    Venography, 75870
  Skull
    Venography, 75870, 75872
  Spermatic
    Excision, 55530-55540
    Ligation, 55500
  Splenic
    Splenoportography, 75810
  Stripping
    Saphenous, 37700-37735, 37780
  Subclavian
    Thrombectomy, 34471, 34490
  Thrombectomy
    Other than Hemodialysis Graft or Fistula, 35875, 35876
  Unlisted Services and Procedures, 37799
  Valve Transposition, 34510
  Varicose
    Ablation, 36473-36479
    Removal, 37700-37735, 37765-37785
    Secondary Varicosity, 37785
    with Tissue Excision, 37735, 37760
  Vena Cava
    Thrombectomy, 34401-34451
    Venography, 75825, 75827
Velpeau Cast, 29058
Vena Cava
  Catheterization, 36010
  Interruption, 37619
  Reconstruction, 34502
  Resection with Reconstruction, 37799
Vena Caval
  Thrombectomy, 50230
Venereal Disease Research Laboratory (VDRL), 86592-86593
Venesection
  Therapeutic, 99195
Venipuncture
  See Also Cannulation; Catheterization

 [Resequenced]

Wrist — *continued*
Arthroplasty — *continued*
with Implant, 25441, 25442, 25444, 25445
Arthroscopy
Diagnostic, 29840
Surgical, 29843-29848
Arthrotomy, 25040, 25100-25105
for Repair, 25107
Biopsy, 25065, 25066, 25100, 25101
Bursa
Excision, 25115, 25116
Incision and Drainage, 25031
Capsule
Incision, 25085
Cast, 29085
Cyst, 25130-25136
Decompression, 25020, 25023
Disarticulation, 25920
Reamputation, 25924
Revision, 25922
Dislocation
Closed Treatment, 25660
Intercarpal, 25660
Open Treatment, 25670
Open Treatment, 25660, 25670, 25676
Percutaneous Fixation, 25671
Radiocarpal, 25660
Open Treatment, 25670
Radioulnar
Closed Treatment, 25675
Percutaneous Fixation, 25671
with Fracture
Closed Treatment, 25680
Open Treatment, 25685
with Manipulation, 25259, 25660, 25675
Excision
Carpal, 25210, 25215
Cartilage, 25107
Tendon Sheath, 25115, 25116
Tumor, 25075-25078 [25071, 25073]
Exploration, 25040, 25101
Fasciotomy, 25020-25025
Fracture, 25645
Closed Treatment, 25622, 25630
Open Treatment, 25628
with Dislocation, 25680, 25685
with Manipulation, 25259, 25624, 25635
Ganglion Cyst
Excision, 25111, 25112
Hematoma, 25028
Incision, 25040, 25100-25105
Tendon Sheath, 25000, 25001
Injection
Carpal Tunnel
Therapeutic, 20526
X-ray, 25246
Joint
See Radiocarpal Joint
Lesion
Excision, 25110
Tendon Sheath, 25000
Magnetic Resonance Imaging, 73221
Reconstruction
Capsulectomy, 25320
Capsulorrhaphy, 25320
Carpal Bone, 25394, 25430
Realign, 25335
Removal
Foreign Body, 25040, 25101, 25248
Implant, 25449
Loose Body, 25101
Prosthesis, 25250, 25251
Repair, 25447
Bone, 25440
Carpal Bone, 25431
Muscle, 25260, 25270
Secondary, 25263, 25265, 25272, 25274
Tendon, 25260, 25270, 25280-25316
Secondary, 25263, 25265, 25272, 25274
Tendon Sheath, 25275
Strapping, 29260
Synovium
Excision, 25105, 25115-25119

Wrist — *continued*
Tendon
Excision, 25109
Tendon Sheath
Excision, 25115, 25116
Tenodesis, 25300, 25301
Tenotomy, 25290
Unlisted Services and Procedures, 25999
X-ray, 73100, 73110
with Contrast, 73115
WT1, 81405

X

X Chromosome Inactivation, [81204]
X, Coagulation Factor, 85260
X, Cranial Nerve
See Vagus Nerve
Xa, Coagulation Factor, 85260
Xenoantibodies, 86308-86310
XI, Coagulation Factor, 85270
XI, Cranial Nerve
See Accessory Nerve
XII, Coagulation Factor, 85280
XII, Cranial Nerve
Hypoglossal Nerve
Anastomosis to Facial Nerve, 64868
XIII, Coagulation Factor, 85290-85291
X-Linked Ichthyoses, 86592-86593
X-ray
Abdomen, 74018-74022
Abscess, 76080
Acromioclavicular Joint, 73050
Ankle, 73600, 73610
Arm, Lower, 73090
Arm, Upper, 73092
Auditory Meatus, 70134
Barium Swallow Test, 3142F, 3200F
Bile Duct
Guide Dilation, 74360
Body Section, 76100
Motion, 76101, 76102
Bone
Age Study, 77072
Dual Energy Absorptiometry, 77080-77081, [77086]
Length Study, 77073
Osseous Survey, 77074-77076
Complete, 77075
Infant, 77076
Limited, 77074
Ultrasound, 76977
Breast, 77065-77067
with Computer-aided Detection, 77065-77067
Calcaneus, 73650
Chest, 71045-71048
Complete (four views)
with Fluoroscopy, 71048, 76000
Partial (two views)
Partial (two views), 71046, 76000
Stereo, 71045
with Computer-Aided Detection, 0174T-0175T
with Fluoroscopy, 71046, 76000
Clavicle, 73000
Coccyx, 72220
Consultation, 76140
Duodenum, 74251
Elbow, 73070, 73080
Esophagus, 74210, 74220
Eye, 70030
Facial Bones, 70140, 70150
Fallopian Tube, 74742
Femur, 73551-73552
Fibula, 73590
Fingers, 73140
Fistula, 76080
Foot, 73620, 73630
Gastrointestinal Tract, 74240, 74248
Guide Dilation, 74360
Guide Intubation, 49440, 74340
Upper, 3142F, 3200F
Hand, 73120, 73130
Head, 70350
Heel, 73650
Hip, 73501-73503, 73521-73523

X-ray — *continued*
Humerus, 73060
Intestines, Small, 74246, 74248, 74250-74251
Guide Intubation, 74355
Jaws, 70355
Joint
Stress Views, 77071
Knee, 73560-73564, 73580
Bilateral, 73565
Larynx, 70370
Leg, 73592
Lumen Dilator, 74360
Mandible, 70100, 70110
Mastoids, 70120, 70130
Nasal Bones, 70160
Neck, 70360
Nose to Rectum
Foreign Body
Child, 76010
Orbit, 70190, 70200
Pelvis, 72170, 72190
Manometry, 74710
Peritoneum, 74190
Pharynx, 70370, 74210
Ribs, 71100-71111
Sacroiliac Joint, 72200, 72202
Sacrum, 72220
Salivary Gland, 70380
Scapula, 73010
Sella Turcica, 70240
Shoulder, 73020, 73030, 73050
Sinus Tract, 76080
Sinuses, 70210, 70220
Skull, 70250, 70260
Specimen
Surgical, 76098
Spine, 72020
Cervical, 72040-72052
Lumbosacral, 72100-72120
Thoracic, 72070-72074
Thoracolumbar, 72080, 72084
Thoracolumbar Junction, 72080
Sternum, 71120, 71130
Teeth, 70300-70320
Tibia, 73590
Toe, 73660
Total Body
Foreign Body, 76010
Unlisted Services and Procedures, 76120, 76125
Upper Gastrointestinal Series (Upper GI Series), 3142F, 3200F
with Contrast
Ankle, 73615
Aorta, 34701-34711 [34717, 34718], 75600-75630
Artery
Abdominal, 75726
Adrenal, 75731, 75733
Arm, 75710, 75716
Arteriovenous Shunt, 36901
Brachial, 75710
Leg, 75710, 75716
Mammary, 75756
Pelvic, 75736
Pulmonary, 75741-75746
Spine, 75705
Transcatheter Therapy, 75894-75898
Angiogram, 75898
Embolization, 75894
with Additional Vessels, 75774
Bile Duct, 74301
Guide Catheter, 74328, 74330
Bladder, 74430, 74450, 74455
Brain, 70010, 70015
Central Venous Access Device, 36598
Colon
Barium Enema, 74270, 74280
Corpora Cavernosa, 74445
Elbow, 73085
Epididymis, 74440
Gallbladder, 74290
Gastrointestinal Tract, 74246-74248
Hip, 73525
Iliac, 34701-34711 [34717, 34718]

X-ray — *continued*
with Contrast — *continued*
Iliofemoral Artery, 75630
Intervertebral Disc
Cervical, 72285
Lumbar, 72295
Thoracic, 72285
Joint
Stress Views, 77071
Kidney
Cyst, 74470
Knee, 73560-73564, 73580
Lacrimal Duct, 70170
Lymph Vessel, 75805, 75807
Abdomen, 75805, 75807
Arm, 75801, 75803
Leg, 75801, 75803
Mammary Duct, 77053-77054
Nasolacrimal Duct, 70170
Oviduct, 74740
Pancreas, 74300, 74301
Pancreatic Duct
Guide Catheter, 74329, 74330
Perineum, 74775
Peritoneum, 74190
Salivary Gland, 70390
Seminal Vesicles, 74440
Shoulder, 73040
Spine
Cervical, 72240
Lumbosacral, 72265
Thoracic, 72255
Total, 72270
Temporomandibular Joint (TMJ), 70328-70332
Ureter
Guide Dilation, 74485
Urethra, 74450, 74455
Urinary Tract, 74400-74425
Uterus, 74740
Vas Deferens, 74440
Vein
Adrenal, 75840, 75842
Arm, 75820, 75822
Hepatic Portal, 75810, 75885, 75887
Jugular, 75860
Leg, 75820, 75822
Liver, 75889, 75891
Neck, 75860
Orbit, 75880
Renal, 75831, 75833
Sampling, 75893
Sinus, 75870
Skull, 75870, 75872
Splenic, 75810
Vena Cava, 75825, 75827
Wrist, 73115
Wrist, 73100, 73110
X-Ray Tomography, Computed
See CT Scan
Xylose Absorption Test
Blood, 84620
Urine, 84620

Y

Yacoub Procedure, 33864
YAG, 66821
Yeast
Culture, 87106
Yellow Fever Vaccine, 90717
Yersinia
Antibody, 86793
YF-VAX, 90717
Y-Plasty, 51800

Z

ZEB2, 81404-81405
Ziegler Procedure
Discission Secondary Membranous Cataract, 66820
ZIFT, 58976
Zinc, 84630
Zinc Manganese Leucine Aminopeptidase, 83670
ZNF41, 81404

Zonisamide
  Assay, 80203
ZOSTAVAX, 90736
Zoster
  Shingles, 90736, [90750]

Z–Plasty, 26121-26125, 41520
Zygoma
  Fracture Treatment, 21355-21366
  Reconstruction, 21270

Zygomatic Arch
  Fracture
    Open Treatment, 21356-21366
    with Manipulation, 21355
  Reconstruction, 21255

[Resequenced]

00100-00126 Anesthesia for Cleft Lip, Ear, ECT, Eyelid, and Salivary Gland Procedures

CMS: 100-04,12,140.1 Qualified Nonphysician Anesthetists; 100-04,12,140.3 Payment for Qualified Nonphysician Anesthetists; 100-04,12,140.3.3 Billing Modifiers; 100-04,12,140.3.4 General Billing Instructions; 100-04,12,140.4.1 Anesthesiologist/Qualified Nonphysican Anesthetist; 100-04,12,140.4.2 Anesthetist and Anesthesiologist in a Single Procedure; 100-04,12,140.4.3 Payment for Medical /Surgical Services by CRNAs; 100-04,12,140.4.4 Conversion Factors for Anesthesia Services; 100-04,12,140.5 Payment for Anesthesia Services Furnished by a Teaching CRNA; 100-04,4,250.3.2 Anesthesia in a Hospital Outpatient Setting

00100 Anesthesia for procedures on salivary glands, including biopsy

🚑 0.00 ⚕ 0.00 **FUD** XXX N ▢

AMA: 2018,Jan,8; 2017,Dec,8; 2017,Jan,8; 2016,Jan,13; 2015,Jan,16; 2014,Aug,5; 2014,Jan,11

00102 Anesthesia for procedures involving plastic repair of cleft lip

🚑 0.00 ⚕ 0.00 **FUD** XXX N ▢

AMA: 2018,Jan,8; 2017,Dec,8; 2017,Jan,8; 2016,Jan,13; 2015,Jan,16; 2014,Aug,5; 2014,Jan,11

00103 Anesthesia for reconstructive procedures of eyelid (eg, blepharoplasty, ptosis surgery)

🚑 0.00 ⚕ 0.00 **FUD** XXX N ▢

AMA: 2018,Jan,8; 2017,Dec,8; 2017,Jan,8; 2016,Jan,13; 2015,Jan,16; 2014,Aug,5; 2014,Jan,11

00104 Anesthesia for electroconvulsive therapy

🚑 0.00 ⚕ 0.00 **FUD** XXX N ▢

AMA: 2018,Jan,8; 2017,Dec,8; 2017,Jan,8; 2016,Jan,13; 2015,Jan,16; 2014,Aug,5; 2014,Jan,11

00120 Anesthesia for procedures on external, middle, and inner ear including biopsy; not otherwise specified

🚑 0.00 ⚕ 0.00 **FUD** XXX N ▢

AMA: 2018,Jan,8; 2017,Dec,8; 2017,Jan,8; 2016,Jan,13; 2015,Jan,16; 2014,Aug,5; 2014,Jan,11

00124 otoscopy

🚑 0.00 ⚕ 0.00 **FUD** XXX N ▢

AMA: 2018,Jan,8; 2017,Dec,8; 2017,Jan,8; 2016,Jan,13; 2015,Jan,16; 2014,Aug,5; 2014,Jan,11

00126 tympanotomy

🚑 0.00 ⚕ 0.00 **FUD** XXX N ▢

AMA: 2018,Jan,8; 2017,Dec,8; 2017,Jan,8; 2016,Jan,13; 2015,Jan,16; 2014,Aug,5; 2014,Jan,11

00140-00148 Anesthesia for Eye Procedures

CMS: 100-04,12,140.1 Qualified Nonphysician Anesthetists; 100-04,12,140.3 Payment for Qualified Nonphysician Anesthetists; 100-04,12,140.3.3 Billing Modifiers; 100-04,12,140.3.4 General Billing Instructions; 100-04,12,140.4.1 Anesthesiologist/Qualified Nonphysican Anesthetist; 100-04,12,140.4.2 Anesthetist and Anesthesiologist in a Single Procedure; 100-04,12,140.4.3 Payment for Medical /Surgical Services by CRNAs; 100-04,12,140.4.4 Conversion Factors for Anesthesia Services; 100-04,12,140.5 Payment for Anesthesia Services Furnished by a Teaching CRNA; 100-04,4,250.3.2 Anesthesia in a Hospital Outpatient Setting

00140 Anesthesia for procedures on eye; not otherwise specified

🚑 0.00 ⚕ 0.00 **FUD** XXX N ▢

AMA: 2018,Jan,8; 2017,Dec,8; 2017,Jan,8; 2016,Jan,13; 2015,Jan,16; 2014,Aug,5; 2014,Jan,11

00142 lens surgery

🚑 0.00 ⚕ 0.00 **FUD** XXX N ▢

AMA: 2018,Jan,8; 2017,Dec,8; 2017,Jan,8; 2016,Jan,13; 2015,Jan,16; 2014,Aug,5; 2014,Jan,11

00144 corneal transplant

🚑 0.00 ⚕ 0.00 **FUD** XXX N ▢

AMA: 2018,Jan,8; 2017,Dec,8; 2017,Jan,8; 2016,Jan,13; 2015,Jan,16; 2014,Aug,5; 2014,Jan,11

00145 vitreoretinal surgery

🚑 0.00 ⚕ 0.00 **FUD** XXX N ▢

AMA: 2018,Jan,8; 2017,Dec,8; 2017,Jan,8; 2016,Jan,13; 2015,Jan,16; 2014,Aug,5; 2014,Jan,11

00147 iridectomy

🚑 0.00 ⚕ 0.00 **FUD** XXX N ▢

AMA: 2018,Jan,8; 2017,Dec,8; 2017,Jan,8; 2016,Jan,13; 2015,Jan,16; 2014,Aug,5; 2014,Jan,11

00148 ophthalmoscopy

0.00 ⚕ 0.00 **FUD** XXX N ▢

AMA: 2018,Jan,8; 2017,Dec,8; 2017,Jan,8; 2016,Jan,13; 2015,Jan,16; 2014,Aug,5; 2014,Jan,11

00160-00326 Anesthesia for Face and Head Procedures

CMS: 100-04,12,140.1 Qualified Nonphysician Anesthetists; 100-04,12,140.3 Payment for Qualified Nonphysician Anesthetists; 100-04,12,140.3.3 Billing Modifiers; 100-04,12,140.3.4 General Billing Instructions; 100-04,12,140.4.1 Anesthesiologist/Qualified Nonphysican Anesthetist; 100-04,12,140.4.2 Anesthetist and Anesthesiologist in a Single Procedure; 100-04,12,140.4.4 Conversion Factors for Anesthesia Services; 100-04,12,140.5 Payment for Anesthesia Services Furnished by a Teaching CRNA; 100-04,4,250.3.2 Anesthesia in a Hospital Outpatient Setting

00160 Anesthesia for procedures on nose and accessory sinuses; not otherwise specified

🚑 0.00 ⚕ 0.00 **FUD** XXX N ▢

AMA: 2018,Jan,8; 2017,Dec,8; 2017,Jan,8; 2016,Jan,13; 2015,Jan,16; 2014,Aug,5; 2014,Jan,11

00162 radical surgery

🚑 0.00 ⚕ 0.00 **FUD** XXX N ▢

AMA: 2018,Jan,8; 2017,Dec,8; 2017,Jan,8; 2016,Jan,13; 2015,Jan,16; 2014,Aug,5; 2014,Jan,11

00164 biopsy, soft tissue

🚑 0.00 ⚕ 0.00 **FUD** XXX N ▢

AMA: 2018,Jan,8; 2017,Dec,8; 2017,Jan,8; 2016,Jan,13; 2015,Jan,16; 2014,Aug,5; 2014,Jan,11

00170 Anesthesia for intraoral procedures, including biopsy; not otherwise specified

🚑 0.00 ⚕ 0.00 **FUD** XXX N ▢

AMA: 2018,Jan,8; 2017,Dec,8; 2017,Jan,8; 2016,Jan,13; 2015,Jan,16; 2014,Aug,5; 2014,Jan,11

00172 repair of cleft palate

🚑 0.00 ⚕ 0.00 **FUD** XXX N ▢

AMA: 2018,Jan,8; 2017,Dec,8; 2017,Jan,8; 2016,Jan,13; 2015,Jan,16; 2014,Aug,5; 2014,Jan,11

00174 excision of retropharyngeal tumor

🚑 0.00 ⚕ 0.00 **FUD** XXX N ▢

AMA: 2018,Jan,8; 2017,Dec,8; 2017,Jan,8; 2016,Jan,13; 2015,Jan,16; 2014,Aug,5; 2014,Jan,11

00176 radical surgery

🚑 0.00 ⚕ 0.00 **FUD** XXX C ▢

AMA: 2018,Jan,8; 2017,Dec,8; 2017,Jan,8; 2016,Jan,13; 2015,Jan,16; 2014,Aug,5; 2014,Jan,11

00190 Anesthesia for procedures on facial bones or skull; not otherwise specified

🚑 0.00 ⚕ 0.00 **FUD** XXX N ▢

AMA: 2018,Jan,8; 2017,Dec,8; 2017,Jan,8; 2016,Jan,13; 2015,Jan,16; 2014,Aug,5; 2014,Jan,11

00192 radical surgery (including prognathism)

🚑 0.00 ⚕ 0.00 **FUD** XXX C ▢

AMA: 2018,Jan,8; 2017,Dec,8; 2017,Jan,8; 2016,Jan,13; 2015,Jan,16; 2014,Aug,5; 2014,Jan,11

00210 Anesthesia for intracranial procedures; not otherwise specified

🚑 0.00 ⚕ 0.00 **FUD** XXX N ▢

AMA: 2018,Jan,8; 2017,Dec,8; 2017,Jan,8; 2016,Jan,13; 2015,Jan,16; 2014,Aug,5; 2014,Jan,11

00211 craniotomy or craniectomy for evacuation of hematoma

🚑 0.00 ⚕ 0.00 **FUD** XXX C ▢

AMA: 2018,Jan,8; 2017,Dec,8; 2017,Jan,8; 2016,Jan,13; 2015,Jan,16; 2014,Aug,5; 2014,Jan,11

00212 subdural taps

🚑 0.00 ⚕ 0.00 **FUD** XXX N ▢

AMA: 2018,Jan,8; 2017,Dec,8; 2017,Jan,8; 2016,Jan,13; 2015,Jan,16; 2014,Aug,5; 2014,Jan,11

00214 burr holes, including ventriculography

🚑 0.00 ⚕ 0.00 **FUD** XXX C ▢

AMA: 2018,Jan,8; 2017,Dec,8; 2017,Jan,8; 2016,Jan,13; 2015,Jan,16; 2014,Aug,5; 2014,Jan,11

● New Code ▲ Revised Code ○ Reinstated ● New Web Release ▲ Revised Web Release + Add-on Unlisted Not Covered # Resequenced
㊿ Optum Mod 50 Exempt ⚕ AMA Mod 51 Exempt �51 Optum Mod 51 Exempt �63 Mod 63 Exempt ⁄ Non-FDA Drug ★ Telemedicine Ⓜ Maternity 🅐 Age Edit

CPT © 2019 American Medical Association. All Rights Reserved.

00215 cranioplasty or elevation of depressed skull fracture, extradural (simple or compound)

🚗 0.00   ⚖ 0.00   **FUD** XXX   C 🖥

AMA: 2018,Jan,8; 2017,Dec,8; 2017,Jan,8; 2016,Jan,13; 2015,Jan,16; 2014,Aug,5; 2014,Jan,11

00216 vascular procedures

🚗 0.00   ⚖ 0.00   **FUD** XXX   N 🖥

AMA: 2018,Jan,8; 2017,Dec,8; 2017,Jan,8; 2016,Jan,13; 2015,Jan,16; 2014,Aug,5; 2014,Jan,11

00218 procedures in sitting position

🚗 0.00   ⚖ 0.00   **FUD** XXX   N 🖥

AMA: 2018,Jan,8; 2017,Dec,8; 2017,Jan,8; 2016,Jan,13; 2015,Jan,16; 2014,Aug,5; 2014,Jan,11

00220 cerebrospinal fluid shunting procedures

🚗 0.00   ⚖ 0.00   **FUD** XXX   N 🖥

AMA: 2018,Jan,8; 2017,Dec,8; 2017,Jan,8; 2016,Jan,13; 2015,Jan,16; 2014,Aug,5; 2014,Jan,11

00222 electrocoagulation of intracranial nerve

🚗 0.00   ⚖ 0.00   **FUD** XXX   N 🖥

AMA: 2018,Jan,8; 2017,Dec,8; 2017,Jan,8; 2016,Jan,13; 2015,Jan,16; 2014,Aug,5; 2014,Jan,11

00300 Anesthesia for all procedures on the integumentary system, muscles and nerves of head, neck, and posterior trunk, not otherwise specified

🚗 0.00   ⚖ 0.00   **FUD** XXX   N 🖥

AMA: 2018,Jan,8; 2017,Dec,8; 2017,Jan,8; 2016,Jan,13; 2015,Jan,16; 2014,Aug,5; 2014,Jan,11

00320 Anesthesia for all procedures on esophagus, thyroid, larynx, trachea and lymphatic system of neck; not otherwise specified, age 1 year or older

🚗 0.00   ⚖ 0.00   **FUD** XXX   N 🖥

AMA: 2018,Jan,8; 2017,Dec,8; 2017,Jan,8; 2016,Jan,13; 2015,Jan,16; 2014,Aug,5; 2014,Jan,11

00322 needle biopsy of thyroid

EXCLUDES   *Cervical spine and spinal cord procedures (00600, 00604, 00670)*

🚗 0.00   ⚖ 0.00   **FUD** XXX   N 🖥

AMA: 2018,Jan,8; 2017,Dec,8; 2017,Jan,8; 2016,Jan,13; 2015,Jan,16; 2014,Aug,5; 2014,Jan,11

00326 Anesthesia for all procedures on the larynx and trachea in children younger than 1 year of age   A

INCLUDES   Anesthesia for patient of extreme age, younger than 1 year and older than 70 (99100)

🚗 0.00   ⚖ 0.00   **FUD** XXX   N 🖥

AMA: 2018,Jan,8; 2017,Dec,8; 2017,Jan,8; 2016,Jan,13; 2015,Jan,16; 2014,Aug,5; 2014,Jan,11

00350-00352 Anesthesia for Neck Vessel Procedures

CMS: 100-04,12,140.1 Qualified Nonphysician Anesthetists; 100-04,12,140.3 Payment for Qualified Nonphysician Anesthetists; 100-04,12,140.3.3 Billing Modifiers; 100-04,12,140.3.4 General Billing Instructions; 100-04,12,140.4.1 Anesthesiologist/Qualified Nonphysican Anesthetist; 100-04,12,140.4.2 Anesthetist and Anesthesiologist in a Single Procedure; 100-04,12,140.4.3 Payment for Medical /Surgical Services by CRNAs; 100-04,12,140.4.4 Conversion Factors for Anesthesia Services; 100-04,12,140.5 Payment for Anesthesia Services Furnished by a Teaching CRNA; 100-04,4,250.3.2 Anesthesia in a Hospital Outpatient Setting

EXCLUDES   *Arteriography (01916)*

00350 Anesthesia for procedures on major vessels of neck; not otherwise specified

🚗 0.00   ⚖ 0.00   **FUD** XXX   N 🖥

AMA: 2018,Jan,8; 2017,Dec,8; 2017,Jan,8; 2016,Jan,13; 2015,Jan,16; 2014,Aug,5; 2014,Jan,11

00352 simple ligation

🚗 0.00   ⚖ 0.00   **FUD** XXX   N 🖥

AMA: 2018,Jan,8; 2017,Dec,8; 2017,Jan,8; 2016,Jan,13; 2015,Jan,16; 2014,Aug,5; 2014,Jan,11

00400-00529 Anesthesia for Chest/Pectoral Girdle Procedures

CMS: 100-04,12,140.1 Qualified Nonphysician Anesthetists; 100-04,12,140.3 Payment for Qualified Nonphysician Anesthetists; 100-04,12,140.3.3 Billing Modifiers; 100-04,12,140.3.4 General Billing Instructions; 100-04,12,140.4.1 Anesthesiologist/Qualified Nonphysican Anesthetist; 100-04,12,140.4.2 Anesthetist and Anesthesiologist in a Single Procedure; 100-04,12,140.4.3 Payment for Medical /Surgical Services by CRNAs; 100-04,12,140.4.4 Conversion Factors for Anesthesia Services; 100-04,12,140.5 Payment for Anesthesia Services Furnished by a Teaching CRNA; 100-04,4,250.3.2 Anesthesia in a Hospital Outpatient Setting

00400 Anesthesia for procedures on the integumentary system on the extremities, anterior trunk and perineum; not otherwise specified

🚗 0.00   ⚖ 0.00   **FUD** XXX   N 🖥

AMA: 2018,Jan,8; 2017,Dec,8; 2017,Jan,8; 2016,Jan,13; 2015,Jan,16; 2014,Aug,5; 2014,Jan,11

00402 reconstructive procedures on breast (eg, reduction or augmentation mammoplasty, muscle flaps)

🚗 0.00   ⚖ 0.00   **FUD** XXX   N 🖥

AMA: 2018,Jan,8; 2017,Dec,8; 2017,Jan,8; 2016,Jan,13; 2015,Jan,16; 2014,Aug,5; 2014,Jan,11

00404 radical or modified radical procedures on breast

🚗 0.00   ⚖ 0.00   **FUD** XXX   N 🖥

AMA: 2018,Jan,8; 2017,Dec,8; 2017,Jan,8; 2016,Jan,13; 2015,Jan,16; 2014,Aug,5; 2014,Jan,11

00406 radical or modified radical procedures on breast with internal mammary node dissection

🚗 0.00   ⚖ 0.00   **FUD** XXX   N 🖥

AMA: 2018,Jan,8; 2017,Dec,8; 2017,Jan,8; 2016,Jan,13; 2015,Jan,16; 2014,Aug,5; 2014,Jan,11

00410 electrical conversion of arrhythmias

🚗 0.00   ⚖ 0.00   **FUD** XXX   N 🖥

AMA: 2018,Jan,8; 2017,Dec,8; 2017,Jan,8; 2016,Jan,13; 2015,Jan,16; 2014,Aug,5; 2014,Jan,11

00450 Anesthesia for procedures on clavicle and scapula; not otherwise specified

🚗 0.00   ⚖ 0.00   **FUD** XXX   N 🖥

AMA: 2018,Jan,8; 2017,Dec,8; 2017,Jan,8; 2016,Jan,13; 2015,Jan,16; 2014,Aug,5; 2014,Jan,11

00454 biopsy of clavicle

🚗 0.00   ⚖ 0.00   **FUD** XXX   N 🖥

AMA: 2018,Jan,8; 2017,Dec,8; 2017,Jan,8; 2016,Jan,13; 2015,Jan,16; 2014,Aug,5; 2014,Jan,11

00470 Anesthesia for partial rib resection; not otherwise specified

🚗 0.00   ⚖ 0.00   **FUD** XXX   N 🖥

AMA: 2018,Jan,8; 2017,Dec,8; 2017,Jan,8; 2016,Jan,13; 2015,Jan,16; 2014,Aug,5; 2014,Jan,11

00472 thoracoplasty (any type)

🚗 0.00   ⚖ 0.00   **FUD** XXX   N 🖥

AMA: 2018,Jan,8; 2017,Dec,8; 2017,Jan,8; 2016,Jan,13; 2015,Jan,16; 2014,Aug,5; 2014,Jan,11

00474 radical procedures (eg, pectus excavatum)

🚗 0.00   ⚖ 0.00   **FUD** XXX   C 🖥

AMA: 2018,Jan,8; 2017,Dec,8; 2017,Jan,8; 2016,Jan,13; 2015,Jan,16; 2014,Aug,5; 2014,Jan,11

00500 Anesthesia for all procedures on esophagus

🚗 0.00   ⚖ 0.00   **FUD** XXX   N 🖥

AMA: 2018,Jan,8; 2017,Dec,8; 2017,Jan,8; 2016,Jan,13; 2015,Jan,16; 2014,Aug,5; 2014,Jan,11

00520 Anesthesia for closed chest procedures; (including bronchoscopy) not otherwise specified

🚗 0.00   ⚖ 0.00   **FUD** XXX   N 🖥

AMA: 2018,Jan,8; 2017,Dec,8; 2017,Jan,8; 2016,Jan,13; 2015,Jan,16; 2014,Aug,5; 2014,Jan,11

00522 needle biopsy of pleura

🚗 0.00   ⚖ 0.00   **FUD** XXX   N 🖥

AMA: 2018,Jan,8; 2017,Dec,8; 2017,Jan,8; 2016,Jan,13; 2015,Jan,16; 2014,Aug,5; 2014,Jan,11

26/TC PC/TC Only   A2-Z3 ASC Payment   50 Bilateral   ♂ Male Only   ♀ Female Only   🚗 Facility RVU   ⚖ Non-Facility RVU   🖥 CCI   ☒ CLIA

FUD Follow-up Days   **CMS:** IOM   **AMA:** CPT Asst   A-Y OPPSI   80/80 Surg Assist Allowed / w/Doc   Lab Crosswalk   Radiology Crosswalk

00524	**pneumocentesis**

0.00   0.00   **FUD** XXX   C

AMA: 2018,Jan,8; 2017,Dec,8; 2017,Jan,8; 2016,Jan,13; 2015,Jan,16; 2014,Aug,5; 2014,Jan,11

00528	**mediastinoscopy and diagnostic thoracoscopy not utilizing 1 lung ventilation**

EXCLUDES   *Tracheobronchial reconstruction (00539)*

0.00   0.00   **FUD** XXX   N

AMA: 2018,Jan,8; 2017,Dec,8; 2017,Jan,8; 2016,Jan,13; 2015,Jan,16; 2014,Aug,5; 2014,Jan,11

00529	**mediastinoscopy and diagnostic thoracoscopy utilizing 1 lung ventilation**

0.00   0.00   **FUD** XXX   N

AMA: 2018,Jan,8; 2017,Dec,8; 2017,Jan,8; 2016,Jan,13; 2015,Jan,16; 2014,Aug,5; 2014,Jan,11

00530 Anesthesia for Cardiac Pacemaker Procedure

CMS: 100-03,10.6 Anesthesia in Cardiac Pacemaker Surgery; 100-04,12,140.1 Qualified Nonphysician Anesthetists; 100-04,12,140.3 Payment for Qualified Nonphysician Anesthetists; 100-04,12,140.3.3 Billing Modifiers; 100-04,12,140.3.4 General Billing Instructions; 100-04,12,140.4.1 Anesthesiologist/Qualified Nonphysican Anesthetist; 100-04,12,140.4.2 Anesthetist and Anesthesiologist in a Single Procedure; 100-04,12,140.4.3 Payment for Medical /Surgical Services by CRNAs; 100-04,12,140.4.4 Conversion Factors for Anesthesia Services; 100-04,12,140.5 Payment for Anesthesia Services Furnished by a Teaching CRNA; 100-04,4,250.3.2 Anesthesia in a Hospital Outpatient Setting

00530	**Anesthesia for permanent transvenous pacemaker insertion**

0.00   0.00   **FUD** XXX   N

AMA: 2018,Jan,8; 2017,Dec,8; 2017,Jan,8; 2016,Jan,13; 2015,Jan,16; 2014,Aug,5; 2014,Jan,11

00532-00550 Anesthesia for Heart and Lung Procedures

CMS: 100-04,12,140.1 Qualified Nonphysician Anesthetists; 100-04,12,140.3 Payment for Qualified Nonphysician Anesthetists; 100-04,12,140.3.3 Billing Modifiers; 100-04,12,140.3.4 General Billing Instructions; 100-04,12,140.4.1 Anesthesiologist/Qualified Nonphysican Anesthetist; 100-04,12,140.4.2 Anesthetist and Anesthesiologist in a Single Procedure; 100-04,12,140.4.3 Payment for Medical /Surgical Services by CRNAs; 100-04,12,140.4.4 Conversion Factors for Anesthesia Services; 100-04,12,140.5 Payment for Anesthesia Services Furnished by a Teaching CRNA; 100-04,4,250.3.2 Anesthesia in a Hospital Outpatient Setting

00532	**Anesthesia for access to central venous circulation**

0.00   0.00   **FUD** XXX   N

AMA: 2018,Jan,8; 2017,Dec,8; 2017,Jan,8; 2016,Jan,13; 2015,Jan,16; 2014,Aug,5; 2014,Jan,11

00534	**Anesthesia for transvenous insertion or replacement of pacing cardioverter-defibrillator**

EXCLUDES   *Transthoracic approach (00560)*

0.00   0.00   **FUD** XXX   N

AMA: 2018,Jan,8; 2017,Dec,8; 2017,Jan,8; 2016,Jan,13; 2015,Jan,16; 2014,Aug,5; 2014,Jan,11

00537	**Anesthesia for cardiac electrophysiologic procedures including radiofrequency ablation**

0.00   0.00   **FUD** XXX   N

AMA: 2018,Jan,8; 2017,Dec,8; 2017,Jan,8; 2016,Jan,13; 2015,Jan,16; 2014,Aug,5; 2014,Jan,11

00539	**Anesthesia for tracheobronchial reconstruction**

0.00   0.00   **FUD** XXX   N

AMA: 2018,Jan,8; 2017,Dec,8; 2017,Jan,8; 2016,Jan,13; 2015,Jan,16; 2014,Aug,5; 2014,Jan,11

00540	**Anesthesia for thoracotomy procedures involving lungs, pleura, diaphragm, and mediastinum (including surgical thoracoscopy); not otherwise specified**

EXCLUDES   *Thoracic spine and spinal cord procedures via anterior transthoracic approach (00625-00626)*

0.00   0.00   **FUD** XXX   C

AMA: 2018,Jan,8; 2017,Dec,8; 2017,Jan,8; 2016,Jan,13; 2015,Jan,16; 2014,Aug,5; 2014,Jan,11

00541	**utilizing 1 lung ventilation**

EXCLUDES   *Thoracic spine and spinal cord procedures via anterior transthoracic approach (00625-00626)*

0.00   0.00   **FUD** XXX   N

AMA: 2018,Jan,8; 2017,Dec,8; 2017,Jan,8; 2016,Jan,13; 2015,Jan,16; 2014,Aug,5; 2014,Jan,11

00542	**decortication**

0.00   0.00   **FUD** XXX   C

AMA: 2018,Jan,8; 2017,Dec,8; 2017,Jan,8; 2016,Jan,13; 2015,Jan,16; 2014,Aug,5; 2014,Jan,11

00546	**pulmonary resection with thoracoplasty**

0.00   0.00   **FUD** XXX   C

AMA: 2018,Jan,8; 2017,Dec,8; 2017,Jan,8; 2016,Jan,13; 2015,Jan,16; 2014,Aug,5; 2014,Jan,11

00548	**intrathoracic procedures on the trachea and bronchi**

0.00   0.00   **FUD** XXX   N

AMA: 2018,Jan,8; 2017,Dec,8; 2017,Jan,8; 2016,Jan,13; 2015,Jan,16; 2014,Aug,5; 2014,Jan,11

00550	**Anesthesia for sternal debridement**

0.00   0.00   **FUD** XXX   N

AMA: 2018,Jan,8; 2017,Dec,8; 2017,Jan,8; 2016,Jan,13; 2015,Jan,16; 2014,Aug,5; 2014,Jan,11

00560-00580 Anesthesia for Open Heart Procedures

CMS: 100-04,12,140.1 Qualified Nonphysician Anesthetists; 100-04,12,140.3 Payment for Qualified Nonphysician Anesthetists; 100-04,12,140.3.3 Billing Modifiers; 100-04,12,140.3.4 General Billing Instructions; 100-04,12,140.4.1 Anesthesiologist/Qualified Nonphysican Anesthetist; 100-04,12,140.4.2 Anesthetist and Anesthesiologist in a Single Procedure; 100-04,12,140.4.3 Payment for Medical /Surgical Services by CRNAs; 100-04,12,140.4.4 Conversion Factors for Anesthesia Services; 100-04,12,140.5 Payment for Anesthesia Services Furnished by a Teaching CRNA; 100-04,4,250.3.2 Anesthesia in a Hospital Outpatient Setting

00560	**Anesthesia for procedures on heart, pericardial sac, and great vessels of chest; without pump oxygenator**

0.00   0.00   **FUD** XXX   C

AMA: 2018,Jan,8; 2017,Dec,8; 2017,Jan,8; 2016,Jan,13; 2015,Jan,16; 2014,Aug,5; 2014,Jan,11

00561	**with pump oxygenator, younger than 1 year of age** A

INCLUDES   Anesthesia complicated by utilization of controlled hypotension (99135)
Anesthesia complicated by utilization of total body hypothermia (99116)
Anesthesia for patient of extreme age, younger than 1 year and older than 70 (99100)

0.00   0.00   **FUD** XXX   C

AMA: 2018,Jan,8; 2017,Dec,8; 2017,Jan,8; 2016,Jan,13; 2015,Jan,16; 2014,Aug,5; 2014,Jan,11

00562	**with pump oxygenator, age 1 year or older, for all noncoronary bypass procedures (eg, valve procedures) or for re-operation for coronary bypass more than 1 month after original operation** A

0.00   0.00   **FUD** XXX   C

AMA: 2018,Jan,8; 2017,Dec,8; 2017,Jan,8; 2016,Jan,13; 2015,Jan,16; 2014,Aug,5; 2014,Jan,11

00563	**with pump oxygenator with hypothermic circulatory arrest**

0.00   0.00   **FUD** XXX   N

AMA: 2018,Jan,8; 2017,Dec,8; 2017,Jan,8; 2016,Jan,13; 2015,Jan,16; 2014,Aug,5; 2014,Jan,11

00566	**Anesthesia for direct coronary artery bypass grafting; without pump oxygenator**

0.00   0.00   **FUD** XXX   N

AMA: 2018,Jan,8; 2017,Dec,8; 2017,Jan,8; 2016,Jan,13; 2015,Jan,16; 2014,Aug,5; 2014,Jan,11

00567	**with pump oxygenator**

0.00   0.00   **FUD** XXX   C

AMA: 2018,Jan,8; 2017,Dec,8; 2017,Jan,8; 2016,Jan,13; 2015,Jan,16; 2014,Aug,5; 2014,Jan,11

00580	**Anesthesia for heart transplant or heart/lung transplant**

0.00   0.00   **FUD** XXX   C

AMA: 2018,Jan,8; 2017,Dec,8; 2017,Jan,8; 2016,Jan,13; 2015,Jan,16; 2014,Aug,5; 2014,Jan,11

00600-00670 Anesthesia for Spinal Procedures

CMS: 100-04,12,140.1 Qualified Nonphysician Anesthetists; 100-04,12,140.3 Payment for Qualified Nonphysician Anesthetists; 100-04,12,140.3.3 Billing Modifiers; 100-04,12,140.3.4 General Billing Instructions; 100-04,12,140.4.1 Anesthesiologist/Qualified Nonphysican Anesthetist; 100-04,12,140.4.2 Anesthetist and Anesthesiologist in a Single Procedure; 100-04,12,140.4.3 Payment for Medical /Surgical Services by CRNAs; 100-04,12,140.4.4 Conversion Factors for Anesthesia Services; 100-04,12,140.5 Payment for Anesthesia Services Furnished by a Teaching CRNA; 100-04,4,250.3.2 Anesthesia in a Hospital Outpatient Setting

00600 Anesthesia for procedures on cervical spine and cord; not otherwise specified

  EXCLUDES *Percutaneous image-guided spine and spinal cord anesthesia services (01935-01936)*
  0.00   0.00   **FUD** XXX   N
  AMA: 2018,Jan,8; 2017,Dec,8; 2017,Jan,8; 2016,Jan,13; 2015,Jan,16; 2014,Aug,5; 2014,Jan,11

00604 procedures with patient in the sitting position
  0.00   0.00   **FUD** XXX   C
  AMA: 2018,Jan,8; 2017,Dec,8; 2017,Jan,8; 2016,Jan,13; 2015,Jan,16; 2014,Aug,5; 2014,Jan,11

00620 Anesthesia for procedures on thoracic spine and cord, not otherwise specified
  0.00   0.00   **FUD** XXX   N
  AMA: 2018,Jan,8; 2017,Dec,8; 2017,Jan,8; 2016,Jan,13; 2015,Jan,16; 2014,Aug,5; 2014,Jan,11

00625 Anesthesia for procedures on the thoracic spine and cord, via an anterior transthoracic approach; not utilizing 1 lung ventilation
  EXCLUDES *Anesthesia services for thoracotomy procedures other than spine (00540-00541)*
  0.00   0.00   **FUD** XXX   N
  AMA: 2018,Jan,8; 2017,Dec,8; 2017,Jan,8; 2016,Jan,13; 2015,Jan,16; 2014,Aug,5; 2014,Jan,11

00626 utilizing 1 lung ventilation
  EXCLUDES *Anesthesia services for thoracotomy procedures other than spine (00540-00541)*
  0.00   0.00   **FUD** XXX   N
  AMA: 2018,Jan,8; 2017,Dec,8; 2017,Jan,8; 2016,Jan,13; 2015,Jan,16; 2014,Aug,5; 2014,Jan,11

00630 Anesthesia for procedures in lumbar region; not otherwise specified
  0.00   0.00   **FUD** XXX   N
  AMA: 2018,Jan,8; 2017,Dec,8; 2017,Jan,8; 2016,Jan,13; 2015,Jan,16; 2014,Aug,5; 2014,Jan,11

00632 lumbar sympathectomy
  0.00   0.00   **FUD** XXX   C
  AMA: 2018,Jan,8; 2017,Dec,8; 2017,Jan,8; 2016,Jan,13; 2015,Jan,16; 2014,Aug,5; 2014,Jan,11

00635 diagnostic or therapeutic lumbar puncture
  0.00   0.00   **FUD** XXX   N
  AMA: 2018,Jan,8; 2017,Dec,8; 2017,Jan,8; 2016,Jan,13; 2015,Jan,16; 2014,Aug,5; 2014,Jan,11

00640 Anesthesia for manipulation of the spine or for closed procedures on the cervical, thoracic or lumbar spine
  0.00   0.00   **FUD** XXX   N
  AMA: 2018,Jan,8; 2017,Dec,8; 2017,Jan,8; 2016,Jan,13; 2015,Jan,16; 2014,Aug,5; 2014,Jan,11

00670 Anesthesia for extensive spine and spinal cord procedures (eg, spinal instrumentation or vascular procedures)
  0.00   0.00   **FUD** XXX   C
  AMA: 2018,Jan,8; 2017,Dec,8; 2017,Jan,8; 2016,Jan,13; 2015,Jan,16; 2014,Aug,5; 2014,Jan,11

00700-00882 Anesthesia for Abdominal Procedures

CMS: 100-04,12,140.1 Qualified Nonphysician Anesthetists; 100-04,12,140.3 Payment for Qualified Nonphysician Anesthetists; 100-04,12,140.3.3 Billing Modifiers; 100-04,12,140.3.4 General Billing Instructions; 100-04,12,140.4.1 Anesthesiologist/Qualified Nonphysican Anesthetist; 100-04,12,140.4.2 Anesthetist and Anesthesiologist in a Single Procedure; 100-04,12,140.4.3 Payment for Medical /Surgical Services by CRNAs; 100-04,12,140.4.4 Conversion Factors for Anesthesia Services; 100-04,12,140.5 Payment for Anesthesia Services Furnished by a Teaching CRNA; 100-04,4,250.3.2 Anesthesia in a Hospital Outpatient Setting

00700 Anesthesia for procedures on upper anterior abdominal wall; not otherwise specified
  0.00   0.00   **FUD** XXX   N
  AMA: 2018,Jan,8; 2017,Dec,8; 2017,Jan,8; 2016,Jan,13; 2015,Jan,16; 2014,Aug,5; 2014,Jan,11

00702 percutaneous liver biopsy
  0.00   0.00   **FUD** XXX   N
  AMA: 2018,Jan,8; 2017,Dec,8; 2017,Jan,8; 2016,Jan,13; 2015,Jan,16; 2014,Aug,5; 2014,Jan,11

00730 Anesthesia for procedures on upper posterior abdominal wall
  0.00   0.00   **FUD** XXX   N
  AMA: 2018,Jan,8; 2017,Dec,8; 2017,Jan,8; 2016,Jan,13; 2015,Jan,16; 2014,Aug,5; 2014,Jan,11

00731 Anesthesia for upper gastrointestinal endoscopic procedures, endoscope introduced proximal to duodenum; not otherwise specified
  EXCLUDES *Combination of upper and lower endoscopic gastrointestinal procedures (00813)*
  0.00   0.00   **FUD** XXX   N
  AMA: 2018,Jan,8; 2017,Dec,8

00732 endoscopic retrograde cholangiopancreatography (ERCP)
  EXCLUDES *Combination of upper and lower endoscopic gastrointestinal procedures (00813)*
  0.00   0.00   **FUD** XXX   N
  AMA: 2018,Jan,8; 2017,Dec,8

00750 Anesthesia for hernia repairs in upper abdomen; not otherwise specified
  0.00   0.00   **FUD** XXX   N
  AMA: 2018,Jan,8; 2017,Dec,8; 2017,Jan,8; 2016,Jan,13; 2015,Jan,16; 2014,Aug,5; 2014,Jan,11

00752 lumbar and ventral (incisional) hernias and/or wound dehiscence
  0.00   0.00   **FUD** XXX   N
  AMA: 2018,Jan,8; 2017,Dec,8; 2017,Jan,8; 2016,Jan,13; 2015,Jan,16; 2014,Aug,5; 2014,Jan,11

00754 omphalocele
  0.00   0.00   **FUD** XXX   N
  AMA: 2018,Jan,8; 2017,Dec,8; 2017,Jan,8; 2016,Jan,13; 2015,Jan,16; 2014,Aug,5; 2014,Jan,11

00756 transabdominal repair of diaphragmatic hernia
  0.00   0.00   **FUD** XXX   N
  AMA: 2018,Jan,8; 2017,Dec,8; 2017,Jan,8; 2016,Jan,13; 2015,Jan,16; 2014,Aug,5; 2014,Jan,11

00770 Anesthesia for all procedures on major abdominal blood vessels
  0.00   0.00   **FUD** XXX   N
  AMA: 2018,Jan,8; 2017,Dec,8; 2017,Jan,8; 2016,Jan,13; 2015,Jan,16; 2014,Aug,5; 2014,Jan,11

00790 Anesthesia for intraperitoneal procedures in upper abdomen including laparoscopy; not otherwise specified
  0.00   0.00   **FUD** XXX   N
  AMA: 2018,Jan,8; 2017,Dec,8; 2017,Jan,8; 2016,Jan,13; 2015,Jan,16; 2014,Aug,5; 2014,Jan,11

00792 partial hepatectomy or management of liver hemorrhage (excluding liver biopsy)
  0.00   0.00   **FUD** XXX   C
  AMA: 2018,Jan,8; 2017,Dec,8; 2017,Jan,8; 2016,Jan,13; 2015,Jan,16; 2014,Aug,5; 2014,Jan,11

00794 pancreatectomy, partial or total (eg, Whipple procedure)
🚫 0.00 ⬡ 0.00 **FUD** XXX [C][▫]
AMA: 2018,Jan,8; 2017,Dec,8; 2017,Jan,8; 2016,Jan,13; 2015,Jan,16; 2014,Aug,5; 2014,Jan,11

00796 liver transplant (recipient)
EXCLUDES *Physiological support during liver harvest (01990)*
🚫 0.00 ⬡ 0.00 **FUD** XXX [C][▫]
AMA: 2018,Jan,8; 2017,Dec,8; 2017,Jan,8; 2016,Jan,13; 2015,Jan,16; 2014,Aug,5; 2014,Jan,11

00797 gastric restrictive procedure for morbid obesity
🚫 0.00 ⬡ 0.00 **FUD** XXX [N][▫]
AMA: 2018,Jan,8; 2017,Dec,8; 2017,Jan,8; 2016,Jan,13; 2015,Jan,16; 2014,Aug,5; 2014,Jan,11

00800 Anesthesia for procedures on lower anterior abdominal wall; not otherwise specified
🚫 0.00 ⬡ 0.00 **FUD** XXX [N][▫]
AMA: 2018,Jan,8; 2017,Dec,8; 2017,Jan,8; 2016,Jan,13; 2015,Jan,16; 2014,Aug,5; 2014,Jan,11

00802 panniculectomy
🚫 0.00 ⬡ 0.00 **FUD** XXX [C][▫]
AMA: 2018,Jan,8; 2017,Dec,8; 2017,Jan,8; 2016,Jan,13; 2015,Jan,16; 2014,Aug,5; 2014,Jan,11

00811 Anesthesia for lower intestinal endoscopic procedures, endoscope introduced distal to duodenum; not otherwise specified
🚫 0.00 ⬡ 0.00 **FUD** XXX [N][▫]
AMA: 2018,Jan,8; 2017,Dec,8

00812 screening colonoscopy
INCLUDES Anesthesia services for all screening colonoscopy irrespective of findings
🚫 0.00 ⬡ 0.00 **FUD** XXX [N][▫]
AMA: 2018,Jan,8; 2017,Dec,8

00813 Anesthesia for combined upper and lower gastrointestinal endoscopic procedures, endoscope introduced both proximal to and distal to the duodenum
🚫 0.00 ⬡ 0.00 **FUD** XXX [N][▫]
AMA: 2018,Jan,8; 2017,Dec,8

00820 Anesthesia for procedures on lower posterior abdominal wall
🚫 0.00 ⬡ 0.00 **FUD** XXX [N][▫]
AMA: 2018,Jan,8; 2017,Dec,8; 2017,Jan,8; 2016,Jan,13; 2015,Jan,16; 2014,Aug,5; 2014,Jan,11

00830 Anesthesia for hernia repairs in lower abdomen; not otherwise specified
EXCLUDES *Anesthesia for hernia repairs on infants one year old or less (00834, 00836)*
🚫 0.00 ⬡ 0.00 **FUD** XXX [N][▫]
AMA: 2018,Jan,8; 2017,Dec,8; 2017,Jan,8; 2016,Jan,13; 2015,Jan,16; 2014,Aug,5; 2014,Jan,11

00832 ventral and incisional hernias
EXCLUDES *Anesthesia for hernia repairs on infants one year old or less (00834, 00836)*
🚫 0.00 ⬡ 0.00 **FUD** XXX [N][▫]
AMA: 2018,Jan,8; 2017,Dec,8; 2017,Jan,8; 2016,Jan,13; 2015,Jan,16; 2014,Aug,5; 2014,Jan,11

00834 Anesthesia for hernia repairs in the lower abdomen not otherwise specified, younger than 1 year of age [A]
INCLUDES Anesthesia for patient of extreme age, younger than 1 year and older than 70 (99100)
🚫 0.00 ⬡ 0.00 **FUD** XXX [N][▫]
AMA: 2018,Jan,8; 2017,Dec,8; 2017,Jan,8; 2016,Jan,13; 2015,Jan,16; 2014,Aug,5; 2014,Jan,11

00836 Anesthesia for hernia repairs in the lower abdomen not otherwise specified, infants younger than 37 weeks gestational age at birth and younger than 50 weeks gestational age at time of surgery [A]
INCLUDES Anesthesia for patient of extreme age, younger than 1 year and older than 70 (99100)
🚫 0.00 ⬡ 0.00 **FUD** XXX [N][▫]
AMA: 2018,Jan,8; 2017,Dec,8; 2017,Jan,8; 2016,Jan,13; 2015,Jan,16; 2014,Aug,5; 2014,Jan,11

00840 Anesthesia for intraperitoneal procedures in lower abdomen including laparoscopy; not otherwise specified
🚫 0.00 ⬡ 0.00 **FUD** XXX [N][▫]
AMA: 2018,Jan,8; 2017,Dec,8; 2017,Jan,8; 2016,Jan,13; 2015,Jan,16; 2014,Aug,5; 2014,Jan,11

00842 amniocentesis [M][♀]
🚫 0.00 ⬡ 0.00 **FUD** XXX [N][▫]
AMA: 2018,Jan,8; 2017,Dec,8; 2017,Jan,8; 2016,Jan,13; 2015,Jan,16; 2014,Aug,5; 2014,Jan,11

00844 abdominoperineal resection
🚫 0.00 ⬡ 0.00 **FUD** XXX [C][▫]
AMA: 2018,Jan,8; 2017,Dec,8; 2017,Jan,8; 2016,Jan,13; 2015,Jan,16; 2014,Aug,5; 2014,Jan,11

00846 radical hysterectomy [♀]
🚫 0.00 ⬡ 0.00 **FUD** XXX [C][▫]
AMA: 2018,Jan,8; 2017,Dec,8; 2017,Jan,8; 2016,Jan,13; 2015,Jan,16; 2014,Aug,5; 2014,Jan,11

00848 pelvic exenteration
🚫 0.00 ⬡ 0.00 **FUD** XXX [C][▫]
AMA: 2018,Jan,8; 2017,Dec,8; 2017,Jan,8; 2016,Jan,13; 2015,Jan,16; 2014,Aug,5; 2014,Jan,11

00851 tubal ligation/transection [♀]
🚫 0.00 ⬡ 0.00 **FUD** XXX [N][▫]
AMA: 2018,Jan,8; 2017,Dec,8; 2017,Jan,8; 2016,Jan,13; 2015,Jan,16; 2014,Oct,14; 2014,Aug,5; 2014,Jan,11

00860 Anesthesia for extraperitoneal procedures in lower abdomen, including urinary tract; not otherwise specified
🚫 0.00 ⬡ 0.00 **FUD** XXX [N][▫]
AMA: 2018,Jan,8; 2017,Dec,8; 2017,Jan,8; 2016,Jan,13; 2015,Jan,16; 2014,Aug,5; 2014,Jan,11

00862 renal procedures, including upper one-third of ureter, or donor nephrectomy
🚫 0.00 ⬡ 0.00 **FUD** XXX [N][▫]
AMA: 2018,Jan,8; 2017,Dec,8; 2017,Jan,8; 2016,Jan,13; 2015,Jan,16; 2014,Aug,5; 2014,Jan,11

00864 total cystectomy
🚫 0.00 ⬡ 0.00 **FUD** XXX [C][▫]
AMA: 2018,Jan,8; 2017,Dec,8; 2017,Jan,8; 2016,Jan,13; 2015,Jan,16; 2014,Aug,5; 2014,Jan,11

00865 radical prostatectomy (suprapubic, retropubic) [♂]
🚫 0.00 ⬡ 0.00 **FUD** XXX [C][▫]
AMA: 2018,Jan,8; 2017,Dec,8; 2017,Jan,8; 2016,Jan,13; 2015,Jan,16; 2014,Aug,5; 2014,Jan,11

00866 adrenalectomy
🚫 0.00 ⬡ 0.00 **FUD** XXX [C][▫]
AMA: 2018,Jan,8; 2017,Dec,8; 2017,Jan,8; 2016,Jan,13; 2015,Jan,16; 2014,Aug,5; 2014,Jan,11

00868 renal transplant (recipient)
EXCLUDES *Anesthesia for donor nephrectomy (00862)*
Physiological support during kidney harvest (01990)
🚫 0.00 ⬡ 0.00 **FUD** XXX [C][▫]
AMA: 2018,Jan,8; 2017,Dec,8; 2017,Jan,8; 2016,Jan,13; 2015,Jan,16; 2014,Aug,5; 2014,Jan,11

00870 cystolithotomy
🚫 0.00 ⬡ 0.00 **FUD** XXX [N][▫]
AMA: 2018,Jan,8; 2017,Dec,8; 2017,Jan,8; 2016,Jan,13; 2015,Jan,16; 2014,Aug,5; 2014,Jan,11

Anesthesia

00872 Anesthesia for lithotripsy, extracorporeal shock wave; with water bath
⚙ 0.00 ⚗ 0.00 **FUD** XXX N ▣
AMA: 2018,Jan,8; 2017,Dec,8; 2017,Jan,8; 2016,Jan,13; 2015,Jan,16; 2014,Aug,5; 2014,Jan,11

00873 without water bath
⚙ 0.00 ⚗ 0.00 **FUD** XXX N ▣
AMA: 2018,Jan,8; 2017,Dec,8; 2017,Jan,8; 2016,Jan,13; 2015,Jan,16; 2014,Aug,5; 2014,Jan,11

00880 Anesthesia for procedures on major lower abdominal vessels; not otherwise specified
⚙ 0.00 ⚗ 0.00 **FUD** XXX N ▣
AMA: 2018,Jan,8; 2017,Dec,8; 2017,Jan,8; 2016,Jan,13; 2015,Jan,16; 2014,Aug,5; 2014,Jan,11

00882 inferior vena cava ligation
⚙ 0.00 ⚗ 0.00 **FUD** XXX C ▣
AMA: 2018,Jan,8; 2017,Dec,8; 2017,Jan,8; 2016,Jan,13; 2015,Jan,16; 2014,Aug,5; 2014,Jan,11

00902-00952 Anesthesia for Genitourinary Procedures

CMS: 100-04,12,140.1 Qualified Nonphysician Anesthetists; 100-04,12,140.3 Payment for Qualified Nonphysician Anesthetists; 100-04,12,140.3.3 Billing Modifiers; 100-04,12,140.3.4 General Billing Instructions; 100-04,12,140.4.1 Anesthesiologist/Qualified Nonphysican Anesthetist; 100-04,12,140.4.2 Anesthetist and Anesthesiologist in a Single Procedure; 100-04,12,140.4.3 Payment for Medical /Surgical Services by CRNAs; 100-04,12,140.4.4 Conversion Factors for Anesthesia Services; 100-04,12,140.5 Payment for Anesthesia Services Furnished by a Teaching CRNA; 100-04,4,250.3.2 Anesthesia in a Hospital Outpatient Setting

EXCLUDES *Procedures on perineal skin, muscles, and nerves (00300, 00400)*

00902 Anesthesia for; anorectal procedure
⚙ 0.00 ⚗ 0.00 **FUD** XXX N ▣
AMA: 2018,Jan,8; 2017,Dec,8; 2017,Jan,8; 2016,Jan,13; 2015,Jan,16; 2014,Aug,5; 2014,Jan,11

00904 radical perineal procedure
⚙ 0.00 ⚗ 0.00 **FUD** XXX C ▣
AMA: 2018,Jan,8; 2017,Dec,8; 2017,Jan,8; 2016,Jan,13; 2015,Jan,16; 2014,Aug,5; 2014,Jan,11

00906 vulvectomy ♀
⚙ 0.00 ⚗ 0.00 **FUD** XXX N ▣
AMA: 2018,Jan,8; 2017,Dec,8; 2017,Jan,8; 2016,Jan,13; 2015,Jan,16; 2014,Aug,5; 2014,Jan,11

00908 perineal prostatectomy ♂
⚙ 0.00 ⚗ 0.00 **FUD** XXX C ▣
AMA: 2018,Jan,8; 2017,Dec,8; 2017,Jan,8; 2016,Jan,13; 2015,Jan,16; 2014,Aug,5; 2014,Jan,11

00910 Anesthesia for transurethral procedures (including urethrocystoscopy); not otherwise specified
⚙ 0.00 ⚗ 0.00 **FUD** XXX N ▣
AMA: 2018,Jan,8; 2017,Dec,8; 2017,Jan,8; 2016,Jan,13; 2015,Jan,16; 2014,Aug,5; 2014,Jan,11

00912 transurethral resection of bladder tumor(s)
⚙ 0.00 ⚗ 0.00 **FUD** XXX N ▣
AMA: 2018,Jan,8; 2017,Dec,8; 2017,Jan,8; 2016,Jan,13; 2015,Jan,16; 2014,Aug,5; 2014,Jan,11

00914 transurethral resection of prostate ♂
⚙ 0.00 ⚗ 0.00 **FUD** XXX N ▣
AMA: 2018,Jan,8; 2017,Dec,8; 2017,Jan,8; 2016,Jan,13; 2015,Jan,16; 2014,Aug,5; 2014,Jan,11

00916 post-transurethral resection bleeding
⚙ 0.00 ⚗ 0.00 **FUD** XXX N ▣
AMA: 2018,Jan,8; 2017,Dec,8; 2017,Jan,8; 2016,Jan,13; 2015,Jan,16; 2014,Aug,5; 2014,Jan,11

00918 with fragmentation, manipulation and/or removal of ureteral calculus
⚙ 0.00 ⚗ 0.00 **FUD** XXX N ▣
AMA: 2018,Jan,8; 2017,Dec,8; 2017,Jan,8; 2016,Jan,13; 2015,Jan,16; 2014,Aug,5; 2014,Jan,11

00920 Anesthesia for procedures on male genitalia (including open urethral procedures); not otherwise specified ♂
⚙ 0.00 ⚗ 0.00 **FUD** XXX N ▣
AMA: 2018,Jan,8; 2017,Dec,8; 2017,Jan,8; 2016,Jan,13; 2015,Jan,16; 2014,Aug,5; 2014,Jan,11

00921 vasectomy, unilateral or bilateral ♂
⚙ 0.00 ⚗ 0.00 **FUD** XXX N ▣
AMA: 2018,Jan,8; 2017,Dec,8; 2017,Jan,8; 2016,Jan,13; 2015,Jan,16; 2014,Aug,5; 2014,Jan,11

00922 seminal vesicles ♂
⚙ 0.00 ⚗ 0.00 **FUD** XXX N ▣
AMA: 2018,Jan,8; 2017,Dec,8; 2017,Jan,8; 2016,Jan,13; 2015,Jan,16; 2014,Aug,5; 2014,Jan,11

00924 undescended testis, unilateral or bilateral ♂
⚙ 0.00 ⚗ 0.00 **FUD** XXX N ▣
AMA: 2018,Jan,8; 2017,Dec,8; 2017,Jan,8; 2016,Jan,13; 2015,Jan,16; 2014,Aug,5; 2014,Jan,11

00926 radical orchiectomy, inguinal ♂
⚙ 0.00 ⚗ 0.00 **FUD** XXX N ▣
AMA: 2018,Jan,8; 2017,Dec,8; 2017,Jan,8; 2016,Jan,13; 2015,Jan,16; 2014,Aug,5; 2014,Jan,11

00928 radical orchiectomy, abdominal ♂
⚙ 0.00 ⚗ 0.00 **FUD** XXX N ▣
AMA: 2018,Jan,8; 2017,Dec,8; 2017,Jan,8; 2016,Jan,13; 2015,Jan,16; 2014,Aug,5; 2014,Jan,11

00930 orchiopexy, unilateral or bilateral ♂
⚙ 0.00 ⚗ 0.00 **FUD** XXX N ▣
AMA: 2018,Jan,8; 2017,Dec,8; 2017,Jan,8; 2016,Jan,13; 2015,Jan,16; 2014,Aug,5; 2014,Jan,11

00932 complete amputation of penis ♂
⚙ 0.00 ⚗ 0.00 **FUD** XXX C ▣
AMA: 2018,Jan,8; 2017,Dec,8; 2017,Jan,8; 2016,Jan,13; 2015,Jan,16; 2014,Aug,5; 2014,Jan,11

00934 radical amputation of penis with bilateral inguinal lymphadenectomy ♂
⚙ 0.00 ⚗ 0.00 **FUD** XXX C ▣
AMA: 2018,Jan,8; 2017,Dec,8; 2017,Jan,8; 2016,Jan,13; 2015,Jan,16; 2014,Aug,5; 2014,Jan,11

00936 radical amputation of penis with bilateral inguinal and iliac lymphadenectomy ♂
⚙ 0.00 ⚗ 0.00 **FUD** XXX C ▣
AMA: 2018,Jan,8; 2017,Dec,8; 2017,Jan,8; 2016,Jan,13; 2015,Jan,16; 2014,Aug,5; 2014,Jan,11

00938 insertion of penile prosthesis (perineal approach) ♂
⚙ 0.00 ⚗ 0.00 **FUD** XXX N ▣
AMA: 2018,Jan,8; 2017,Dec,8; 2017,Jan,8; 2016,Jan,13; 2015,Jan,16; 2014,Aug,5; 2014,Jan,11

00940 Anesthesia for vaginal procedures (including biopsy of labia, vagina, cervix or endometrium); not otherwise specified ♀
⚙ 0.00 ⚗ 0.00 **FUD** XXX N ▣
AMA: 2018,Jan,8; 2017,Dec,8; 2017,Jan,8; 2016,Jan,13; 2015,Jan,16; 2014,Aug,5; 2014,Jan,11

00942 colpotomy, vaginectomy, colporrhaphy, and open urethral procedures ♀
⚙ 0.00 ⚗ 0.00 **FUD** XXX N ▣
AMA: 2018,Jan,8; 2017,Dec,8; 2017,Jan,8; 2016,Jan,13; 2015,Jan,16; 2014,Aug,5; 2014,Jan,11

00944 vaginal hysterectomy ♀
⚙ 0.00 ⚗ 0.00 **FUD** XXX C ▣
AMA: 2018,Jan,8; 2017,Dec,8; 2017,Jan,8; 2016,Jan,13; 2015,Jan,16; 2014,Aug,5; 2014,Jan,11

00948 cervical cerclage ♀
⚙ 0.00 ⚗ 0.00 **FUD** XXX N ▣
AMA: 2018,Jan,8; 2017,Dec,8; 2017,Jan,8; 2016,Jan,13; 2015,Jan,16; 2014,Aug,5; 2014,Jan,11

00950	**culdoscopy** ♀

🛏 0.00   ⚕ 0.00   **FUD** XXX   N 🖥

AMA: 2018,Jan,8; 2017,Dec,8; 2017,Jan,8; 2016,Jan,13;
2015,Jan,16; 2014,Aug,5; 2014,Jan,11

00952	**hysteroscopy and/or hysterosalpingography** ♀

🛏 0.00   ⚕ 0.00   **FUD** XXX   N 🖥

AMA: 2018,Jan,8; 2017,Dec,8; 2017,Jan,8; 2016,Jan,13;
2015,Jan,16; 2014,Aug,5; 2014,Jan,11

01112-01522 Anesthesia for Lower Extremity Procedures

CMS: 100-04,12,140.1 Qualified Nonphysician Anesthetists; 100-04,12,140.3 Payment for Qualified Nonphysician Anesthetists; 100-04,12,140.3.3 Billing Modifiers; 100-04,12,140.3.4 General Billing Instructions; 100-04,12,140.4.1 Anesthesiologist/Qualified Nonphysician Anesthetist; 100-04,12,140.4.2 Anesthetist and Anesthesiologist in a Single Procedure; 100-04,12,140.4.3 Payment for Medical /Surgical Services by CRNAs; 100-04,12,140.4.4 Conversion Factors for Anesthesia Services; 100-04,12,140.5 Payment for Anesthesia Services Furnished by a Teaching CRNA; 100-04,4,250.3.2 Anesthesia in a Hospital Outpatient Setting

01112 **Anesthesia for bone marrow aspiration and/or biopsy, anterior or posterior iliac crest**

🛏 0.00   ⚕ 0.00   **FUD** XXX   N 🖥

AMA: 2018,Jan,8; 2017,Dec,8; 2017,Jan,8; 2016,Jan,13;
2015,Jan,16; 2014,Aug,5; 2014,Jan,11

01120 **Anesthesia for procedures on bony pelvis**

🛏 0.00   ⚕ 0.00   **FUD** XXX   N 🖥

AMA: 2018,Jan,8; 2017,Dec,8; 2017,Jan,8; 2016,Jan,13;
2015,Jan,16; 2014,Aug,5; 2014,Jan,11

01130 **Anesthesia for body cast application or revision**

🛏 0.00   ⚕ 0.00   **FUD** XXX   N 🖥

AMA: 2018,Jan,8; 2017,Dec,8; 2017,Jan,8; 2016,Jan,13;
2015,Jan,16; 2014,Aug,5; 2014,Jan,11

01140 **Anesthesia for interpelviabdominal (hindquarter) amputation**

🛏 0.00   ⚕ 0.00   **FUD** XXX   C 🖥

AMA: 2018,Jan,8; 2017,Dec,8; 2017,Jan,8; 2016,Jan,13;
2015,Jan,16; 2014,Aug,5; 2014,Jan,11

01150 **Anesthesia for radical procedures for tumor of pelvis, except hindquarter amputation**

🛏 0.00   ⚕ 0.00   **FUD** XXX   C 🖥

AMA: 2018,Jan,8; 2017,Dec,8; 2017,Jan,8; 2016,Jan,13;
2015,Jan,16; 2014,Aug,5; 2014,Jan,11

01160 **Anesthesia for closed procedures involving symphysis pubis or sacroiliac joint**

🛏 0.00   ⚕ 0.00   **FUD** XXX   N 🖥

AMA: 2018,Jan,8; 2017,Dec,8; 2017,Jan,8; 2016,Jan,13;
2015,Jan,16; 2014,Aug,5; 2014,Jan,11

01170 **Anesthesia for open procedures involving symphysis pubis or sacroiliac joint**

🛏 0.00   ⚕ 0.00   **FUD** XXX   N 🖥

AMA: 2018,Jan,8; 2017,Dec,8; 2017,Jan,8; 2016,Jan,13;
2015,Jan,16; 2014,Aug,5; 2014,Jan,11

01173 **Anesthesia for open repair of fracture disruption of pelvis or column fracture involving acetabulum**

🛏 0.00   ⚕ 0.00   **FUD** XXX   N 🖥

AMA: 2018,Jan,8; 2017,Dec,8; 2017,Jan,8; 2016,Jan,13;
2015,Jan,16; 2014,Aug,5; 2014,Jan,11

01200 **Anesthesia for all closed procedures involving hip joint**

🛏 0.00   ⚕ 0.00   **FUD** XXX   N 🖥

AMA: 2018,Jan,8; 2017,Dec,8; 2017,Jan,8; 2016,Jan,13;
2015,Jan,16; 2014,Aug,5; 2014,Jan,11

01202 **Anesthesia for arthroscopic procedures of hip joint**

🛏 0.00   ⚕ 0.00   **FUD** XXX   N 🖥

AMA: 2018,Jan,8; 2017,Dec,8; 2017,Jan,8; 2016,Jan,13;
2015,Jan,16; 2014,Aug,5; 2014,Jan,11

01210 **Anesthesia for open procedures involving hip joint; not otherwise specified**

🛏 0.00   ⚕ 0.00   **FUD** XXX   N 🖥

AMA: 2018,Jan,8; 2017,Dec,8; 2017,Jan,8; 2016,Jan,13;
2015,Jan,16; 2014,Aug,5; 2014,Jan,11

01212 **hip disarticulation**

🛏 0.00   ⚕ 0.00   **FUD** XXX   C 🖥

AMA: 2018,Jan,8; 2017,Dec,8; 2017,Jan,8; 2016,Jan,13;
2015,Jan,16; 2014,Aug,5; 2014,Jan,11

01214 **total hip arthroplasty**

🛏 0.00   ⚕ 0.00   **FUD** XXX   C 🖥

AMA: 2018,Jan,8; 2017,Dec,8; 2017,Jan,8; 2016,Jan,13;
2015,Jan,16; 2014,Aug,5; 2014,Jan,11

01215 **revision of total hip arthroplasty**

🛏 0.00   ⚕ 0.00   **FUD** XXX   N 🖥

AMA: 2018,Jan,8; 2017,Dec,8; 2017,Jan,8; 2016,Jan,13;
2015,Jan,16; 2014,Aug,5; 2014,Jan,11

01220 **Anesthesia for all closed procedures involving upper two-thirds of femur**

🛏 0.00   ⚕ 0.00   **FUD** XXX   N 🖥

AMA: 2018,Jan,8; 2017,Dec,8; 2017,Jan,8; 2016,Jan,13;
2015,Jan,16; 2014,Aug,5; 2014,Jan,11

01230 **Anesthesia for open procedures involving upper two-thirds of femur; not otherwise specified**

🛏 0.00   ⚕ 0.00   **FUD** XXX   N 🖥

AMA: 2018,Jan,8; 2017,Dec,8; 2017,Jan,8; 2016,Jan,13;
2015,Jan,16; 2014,Aug,5; 2014,Jan,11

01232 **amputation**

🛏 0.00   ⚕ 0.00   **FUD** XXX   C 🖥

AMA: 2018,Jan,8; 2017,Dec,8; 2017,Jan,8; 2016,Jan,13;
2015,Jan,16; 2014,Aug,5; 2014,Jan,11

01234 **radical resection**

🛏 0.00   ⚕ 0.00   **FUD** XXX   C 🖥

AMA: 2018,Jan,8; 2017,Dec,8; 2017,Jan,8; 2016,Jan,13;
2015,Jan,16; 2014,Aug,5; 2014,Jan,11

01250 **Anesthesia for all procedures on nerves, muscles, tendons, fascia, and bursae of upper leg**

🛏 0.00   ⚕ 0.00   **FUD** XXX   N 🖥

AMA: 2018,Jan,8; 2017,Dec,8; 2017,Jan,8; 2016,Jan,13;
2015,Jan,16; 2014,Aug,5; 2014,Jan,11

01260 **Anesthesia for all procedures involving veins of upper leg, including exploration**

🛏 0.00   ⚕ 0.00   **FUD** XXX   N 🖥

AMA: 2018,Jan,8; 2017,Dec,8; 2017,Jan,8; 2016,Jan,13;
2015,Jan,16; 2014,Aug,5; 2014,Jan,11

01270 **Anesthesia for procedures involving arteries of upper leg, including bypass graft; not otherwise specified**

🛏 0.00   ⚕ 0.00   **FUD** XXX   N 🖥

AMA: 2018,Jan,8; 2017,Dec,8; 2017,Jan,8; 2016,Jan,13;
2015,Jan,16; 2014,Aug,5; 2014,Jan,11

01272 **femoral artery ligation**

🛏 0.00   ⚕ 0.00   **FUD** XXX   C 🖥

AMA: 2018,Jan,8; 2017,Dec,8; 2017,Jan,8; 2016,Jan,13;
2015,Jan,16; 2014,Aug,5; 2014,Jan,11

01274 **femoral artery embolectomy**

🛏 0.00   ⚕ 0.00   **FUD** XXX   C 🖥

AMA: 2018,Jan,8; 2017,Dec,8; 2017,Jan,8; 2016,Jan,13;
2015,Jan,16; 2014,Aug,5; 2014,Jan,11

01320 **Anesthesia for all procedures on nerves, muscles, tendons, fascia, and bursae of knee and/or popliteal area**

🛏 0.00   ⚕ 0.00   **FUD** XXX   N 🖥

AMA: 2018,Jan,8; 2017,Dec,8; 2017,Jan,8; 2016,Jan,13;
2015,Jan,16; 2014,Aug,5; 2014,Jan,11

01340 **Anesthesia for all closed procedures on lower one-third of femur**

🛏 0.00   ⚕ 0.00   **FUD** XXX   N 🖥

AMA: 2018,Jan,8; 2017,Dec,8; 2017,Jan,8; 2016,Jan,13;
2015,Jan,16; 2014,Aug,5; 2014,Jan,11

01360 **Anesthesia for all open procedures on lower one-third of femur**

🛏 0.00   ⚕ 0.00   **FUD** XXX   N 🖥

AMA: 2018,Jan,8; 2017,Dec,8; 2017,Jan,8; 2016,Jan,13;
2015,Jan,16; 2014,Aug,5; 2014,Jan,11

● New Code   ▲ Revised Code   ○ Reinstated   ● New Web Release   ▲ Revised Web Release   + Add-on   Unlisted   Not Covered   # Resequenced
㊿ Optum Mod 50 Exempt   ⊘ AMA Mod 51 Exempt   �51 Optum Mod 51 Exempt   ㊿ Mod 63 Exempt   🗡 Non-FDA Drug   ★ Telemedicine   Ⓜ Maternity   Ⓐ Age Edit

01380 **Anesthesia for all closed procedures on knee joint**
🔧 0.00   ✂ 0.00   **FUD** XXX   N ▣

AMA: 2018,Jan,8; 2017,Dec,8; 2017,Jan,8; 2016,Jan,13; 2015,Jan,16; 2014,Aug,5; 2014,Jan,11

01382 **Anesthesia for diagnostic arthroscopic procedures of knee joint**
🔧 0.00   ✂ 0.00   **FUD** XXX   N ▣

AMA: 2018,Jan,8; 2017,Dec,8; 2017,Jan,8; 2016,Jan,13; 2015,Jan,16; 2014,Aug,5; 2014,Jan,11

01390 **Anesthesia for all closed procedures on upper ends of tibia, fibula, and/or patella**
🔧 0.00   ✂ 0.00   **FUD** XXX   N ▣

AMA: 2018,Jan,8; 2017,Dec,8; 2017,Jan,8; 2016,Jan,13; 2015,Jan,16; 2014,Aug,5; 2014,Jan,11

01392 **Anesthesia for all open procedures on upper ends of tibia, fibula, and/or patella**
🔧 0.00   ✂ 0.00   **FUD** XXX   N ▣

AMA: 2018,Jan,8; 2017,Dec,8; 2017,Jan,8; 2016,Jan,13; 2015,Jan,16; 2014,Aug,5; 2014,Jan,11

01400 **Anesthesia for open or surgical arthroscopic procedures on knee joint; not otherwise specified**
🔧 0.00   ✂ 0.00   **FUD** XXX   N ▣

AMA: 2018,Jan,8; 2017,Dec,8; 2017,Jan,8; 2016,Jan,13; 2015,Jan,16; 2014,Aug,5; 2014,Jan,11

01402 **total knee arthroplasty**
🔧 0.00   ✂ 0.00   **FUD** XXX   C ▣

AMA: 2018,Jan,8; 2017,Dec,8; 2017,Jan,8; 2016,Jan,13; 2015,Jan,16; 2014,Aug,5; 2014,Jan,11

01404 **disarticulation at knee**
🔧 0.00   ✂ 0.00   **FUD** XXX   C ▣

AMA: 2018,Jan,8; 2017,Dec,8; 2017,Jan,8; 2016,Jan,13; 2015,Jan,16; 2014,Aug,5; 2014,Jan,11

01420 **Anesthesia for all cast applications, removal, or repair involving knee joint**
🔧 0.00   ✂ 0.00   **FUD** XXX   N ▣

AMA: 2018,Jan,8; 2017,Dec,8; 2017,Jan,8; 2016,Jan,13; 2015,Jan,16; 2014,Aug,5; 2014,Jan,11

01430 **Anesthesia for procedures on veins of knee and popliteal area; not otherwise specified**
🔧 0.00   ✂ 0.00   **FUD** XXX   N ▣

AMA: 2018,Jan,8; 2017,Dec,8; 2017,Jan,8; 2016,Jan,13; 2015,Jan,16; 2014,Aug,5; 2014,Jan,11

01432 **arteriovenous fistula**
🔧 0.00   ✂ 0.00   **FUD** XXX   N ▣

AMA: 2018,Jan,8; 2017,Dec,8; 2017,Jan,8; 2016,Jan,13; 2015,Jan,16; 2014,Aug,5; 2014,Jan,11

01440 **Anesthesia for procedures on arteries of knee and popliteal area; not otherwise specified**
🔧 0.00   ✂ 0.00   **FUD** XXX   N ▣

AMA: 2018,Jan,8; 2017,Dec,8; 2017,Jan,8; 2016,Jan,13; 2015,Jan,16; 2014,Aug,5; 2014,Jan,11

01442 **popliteal thromboendarterectomy, with or without patch graft**
🔧 0.00   ✂ 0.00   **FUD** XXX   C ▣

AMA: 2018,Jan,8; 2017,Dec,8; 2017,Jan,8; 2016,Jan,13; 2015,Jan,16; 2014,Aug,5; 2014,Jan,11

01444 **popliteal excision and graft or repair for occlusion or aneurysm**
🔧 0.00   ✂ 0.00   **FUD** XXX   C ▣

AMA: 2018,Jan,8; 2017,Dec,8; 2017,Jan,8; 2016,Jan,13; 2015,Jan,16; 2014,Aug,5; 2014,Jan,11

01462 **Anesthesia for all closed procedures on lower leg, ankle, and foot**
🔧 0.00   ✂ 0.00   **FUD** XXX   N ▣

AMA: 2018,Jan,8; 2017,Dec,8; 2017,Jan,8; 2016,Jan,13; 2015,Jan,16; 2014,Aug,5; 2014,Jan,11

01464 **Anesthesia for arthroscopic procedures of ankle and/or foot**
🔧 0.00   ✂ 0.00   **FUD** XXX   N ▣

AMA: 2018,Jan,8; 2017,Dec,8; 2017,Jan,8; 2016,Jan,13; 2015,Jan,16; 2014,Aug,5; 2014,Jan,11

01470 **Anesthesia for procedures on nerves, muscles, tendons, and fascia of lower leg, ankle, and foot; not otherwise specified**
🔧 0.00   ✂ 0.00   **FUD** XXX   N ▣

AMA: 2018,Jan,8; 2017,Dec,8; 2017,Jan,8; 2016,Jan,13; 2015,Jan,16; 2014,Aug,5; 2014,Jan,11

01472 **repair of ruptured Achilles tendon, with or without graft**
🔧 0.00   ✂ 0.00   **FUD** XXX   N ▣

AMA: 2018,Jan,8; 2017,Dec,8; 2017,Jan,8; 2016,Jan,13; 2015,Jan,16; 2014,Aug,5; 2014,Jan,11

01474 **gastrocnemius recession (eg, Strayer procedure)**
🔧 0.00   ✂ 0.00   **FUD** XXX   N ▣

AMA: 2018,Jan,8; 2017,Dec,8; 2017,Jan,8; 2016,Jan,13; 2015,Jan,16; 2014,Aug,5; 2014,Jan,11

01480 **Anesthesia for open procedures on bones of lower leg, ankle, and foot; not otherwise specified**
🔧 0.00   ✂ 0.00   **FUD** XXX   N ▣

AMA: 2018,Jan,8; 2017,Dec,8; 2017,Jan,8; 2016,Jan,13; 2015,Jan,16; 2014,Aug,5; 2014,Jan,11

01482 **radical resection (including below knee amputation)**
🔧 0.00   ✂ 0.00   **FUD** XXX   N ▣

AMA: 2018,Jan,8; 2017,Dec,8; 2017,Jan,8; 2016,Jan,13; 2015,Jan,16; 2014,Aug,5; 2014,Jan,11

01484 **osteotomy or osteoplasty of tibia and/or fibula**
🔧 0.00   ✂ 0.00   **FUD** XXX   N ▣

AMA: 2018,Jan,8; 2017,Dec,8; 2017,Jan,8; 2016,Jan,13; 2015,Jan,16; 2014,Aug,5; 2014,Jan,11

01486 **total ankle replacement**
🔧 0.00   ✂ 0.00   **FUD** XXX   C ▣

AMA: 2018,Jan,8; 2017,Dec,8; 2017,Jan,8; 2016,Jan,13; 2015,Jan,16; 2014,Aug,5; 2014,Jan,11

01490 **Anesthesia for lower leg cast application, removal, or repair**
🔧 0.00   ✂ 0.00   **FUD** XXX   N ▣

AMA: 2018,Jan,8; 2017,Dec,8; 2017,Jan,8; 2016,Jan,13; 2015,Jan,16; 2014,Aug,5; 2014,Jan,11

01500 **Anesthesia for procedures on arteries of lower leg, including bypass graft; not otherwise specified**
🔧 0.00   ✂ 0.00   **FUD** XXX   N ▣

AMA: 2018,Jan,8; 2017,Dec,8; 2017,Jan,8; 2016,Jan,13; 2015,Jan,16; 2014,Aug,5; 2014,Jan,11

01502 **embolectomy, direct or with catheter**
🔧 0.00   ✂ 0.00   **FUD** XXX   C ▣

AMA: 2018,Jan,8; 2017,Dec,8; 2017,Jan,8; 2016,Jan,13; 2015,Jan,16; 2014,Aug,5; 2014,Jan,11

01520 **Anesthesia for procedures on veins of lower leg; not otherwise specified**
🔧 0.00   ✂ 0.00   **FUD** XXX   N ▣

AMA: 2018,Jan,8; 2017,Dec,8; 2017,Jan,8; 2016,Jan,13; 2015,Jan,16; 2014,Aug,5; 2014,Jan,11

01522 **venous thrombectomy, direct or with catheter**
🔧 0.00   ✂ 0.00   **FUD** XXX   N ▣

AMA: 2018,Jan,8; 2017,Dec,8; 2017,Jan,8; 2016,Jan,13; 2015,Jan,16; 2014,Aug,5; 2014,Jan,11

26/TC PC/TC Only   A2-Z3 ASC Payment   50 Bilateral   ♂ Male Only   ♀ Female Only   🔧 Facility RVU   ✂ Non-Facility RVU   ▣ CCI   ✖ CLIA
FUD Follow-up Days   **CMS:** IOM   **AMA:** CPT Asst   A-Y OPPSI   80/80 Surg Assist Allowed / w/Doc   ▣ Lab Crosswalk   ▣ Radiology Crosswalk

8

01610-01680 Anesthesia for Shoulder Procedures

CMS: 100-04,12,140.1 Qualified Nonphysician Anesthetists; 100-04,12,140.3 Payment for Qualified Nonphysician Anesthetists; 100-04,12,140.3.3 Billing Modifiers; 100-04,12,140.3.4 General Billing Instructions; 100-04,12,140.4.1 Anesthesiologist/Qualified Nonphysican Anesthetist; 100-04,12,140.4.2 Anesthetist and Anesthesiologist in a Single Procedure; 100-04,12,140.4.3 Payment for Medical /Surgical Services by CRNAs; 100-04,12,140.4.4 Conversion Factors for Anesthesia Services; 100-04,12,140.5 Payment for Anesthesia Services Furnished by a Teaching CRNA; 100-04,4,250.3.2 Anesthesia in a Hospital Outpatient Setting

INCLUDES
Acromioclavicular joint
Humeral head and neck
Shoulder joint
Sternoclavicular joint

01610 **Anesthesia for all procedures on nerves, muscles, tendons, fascia, and bursae of shoulder and axilla**
0.00   0.00   **FUD** XXX   N
AMA: 2018,Jan,8; 2017,Dec,8; 2017,Jan,8; 2016,Jan,13; 2015,Jan,16; 2014,Aug,5; 2014,Jan,11

01620 **Anesthesia for all closed procedures on humeral head and neck, sternoclavicular joint, acromioclavicular joint, and shoulder joint**
0.00   0.00   **FUD** XXX   N
AMA: 2018,Jan,8; 2017,Dec,8; 2017,Jan,8; 2016,Jan,13; 2015,Jan,16; 2014,Aug,5; 2014,Jan,11

01622 **Anesthesia for diagnostic arthroscopic procedures of shoulder joint**
0.00   0.00   **FUD** XXX   N
AMA: 2018,Jan,8; 2017,Dec,8; 2017,Jan,8; 2016,Jan,13; 2015,Jan,16; 2014,Aug,5; 2014,Jan,11

01630 **Anesthesia for open or surgical arthroscopic procedures on humeral head and neck, sternoclavicular joint, acromioclavicular joint, and shoulder joint; not otherwise specified**
0.00   0.00   **FUD** XXX   N
AMA: 2018,Jan,8; 2017,Dec,8; 2017,Jan,8; 2016,Jan,13; 2015,Jan,16; 2014,Aug,5; 2014,Jan,11

01634 **shoulder disarticulation**
0.00   0.00   **FUD** XXX   C
AMA: 2018,Jan,8; 2017,Dec,8; 2017,Jan,8; 2016,Jan,13; 2015,Jan,16; 2014,Aug,5; 2014,Jan,11

01636 **interthoracoscapular (forequarter) amputation**
0.00   0.00   **FUD** XXX   C
AMA: 2018,Jan,8; 2017,Dec,8; 2017,Jan,8; 2016,Jan,13; 2015,Jan,16; 2014,Aug,5; 2014,Jan,11

01638 **total shoulder replacement**
0.00   0.00   **FUD** XXX   C
AMA: 2018,Jan,8; 2017,Dec,8; 2017,Jan,8; 2016,Jan,13; 2015,Jan,16; 2014,Aug,5; 2014,Jan,11

01650 **Anesthesia for procedures on arteries of shoulder and axilla; not otherwise specified**
0.00   0.00   **FUD** XXX   N
AMA: 2018,Jan,8; 2017,Dec,8; 2017,Jan,8; 2016,Jan,13; 2015,Jan,16; 2014,Aug,5; 2014,Jan,11

01652 **axillary-brachial aneurysm**
0.00   0.00   **FUD** XXX   C
AMA: 2018,Jan,8; 2017,Dec,8; 2017,Jan,8; 2016,Jan,13; 2015,Jan,16; 2014,Aug,5; 2014,Jan,11

01654 **bypass graft**
0.00   0.00   **FUD** XXX   C
AMA: 2018,Jan,8; 2017,Dec,8; 2017,Jan,8; 2016,Jan,13; 2015,Jan,16; 2014,Aug,5; 2014,Jan,11

01656 **axillary-femoral bypass graft**
0.00   0.00   **FUD** XXX   C
AMA: 2018,Jan,8; 2017,Dec,8; 2017,Jan,8; 2016,Jan,13; 2015,Jan,16; 2014,Aug,5; 2014,Jan,11

01670 **Anesthesia for all procedures on veins of shoulder and axilla**
0.00   0.00   **FUD** XXX   N
AMA: 2018,Jan,8; 2017,Dec,8; 2017,Jan,8; 2016,Jan,13; 2015,Jan,16; 2014,Aug,5; 2014,Jan,11

01680 **Anesthesia for shoulder cast application, removal or repair, not otherwise specified**
0.00   0.00   **FUD** XXX   N
AMA: 2018,Jan,8; 2017,Dec,8; 2017,Jan,8; 2016,Jan,13; 2015,Jan,16; 2014,Aug,5; 2014,Jan,11

01710-01860 Anesthesia for Upper Extremity Procedures

CMS: 100-04,12,140.1 Qualified Nonphysician Anesthetists; 100-04,12,140.3 Payment for Qualified Nonphysician Anesthetists; 100-04,12,140.3.3 Billing Modifiers; 100-04,12,140.3.4 General Billing Instructions; 100-04,12,140.4.1 Anesthesiologist/Qualified Nonphysican Anesthetist; 100-04,12,140.4.2 Anesthetist and Anesthesiologist in a Single Procedure; 100-04,12,140.4.3 Payment for Medical /Surgical Services by CRNAs; 100-04,12,140.4.4 Conversion Factors for Anesthesia Services; 100-04,12,140.5 Payment for Anesthesia Services Furnished by a Teaching CRNA; 100-04,4,250.3.2 Anesthesia in a Hospital Outpatient Setting

01710 **Anesthesia for procedures on nerves, muscles, tendons, fascia, and bursae of upper arm and elbow; not otherwise specified**
0.00   0.00   **FUD** XXX   N
AMA: 2018,Jan,8; 2017,Dec,8; 2017,Jan,8; 2016,Jan,13; 2015,Jan,16; 2014,Aug,5; 2014,Jan,11

01712 **tenotomy, elbow to shoulder, open**
0.00   0.00   **FUD** XXX   N
AMA: 2018,Jan,8; 2017,Dec,8; 2017,Jan,8; 2016,Jan,13; 2015,Jan,16; 2014,Aug,5; 2014,Jan,11

01714 **tenoplasty, elbow to shoulder**
0.00   0.00   **FUD** XXX   N
AMA: 2018,Jan,8; 2017,Dec,8; 2017,Jan,8; 2016,Jan,13; 2015,Jan,16; 2014,Aug,5; 2014,Jan,11

01716 **tenodesis, rupture of long tendon of biceps**
0.00   0.00   **FUD** XXX   N
AMA: 2018,Jan,8; 2017,Dec,8; 2017,Jan,8; 2016,Jan,13; 2015,Jan,16; 2014,Aug,5; 2014,Jan,11

01730 **Anesthesia for all closed procedures on humerus and elbow**
0.00   0.00   **FUD** XXX   N
AMA: 2018,Jan,8; 2017,Dec,8; 2017,Jan,8; 2016,Jan,13; 2015,Jan,16; 2014,Aug,5; 2014,Jan,11

01732 **Anesthesia for diagnostic arthroscopic procedures of elbow joint**
0.00   0.00   **FUD** XXX   N
AMA: 2018,Jan,8; 2017,Dec,8; 2017,Jan,8; 2016,Jan,13; 2015,Jan,16; 2014,Aug,5; 2014,Jan,11

01740 **Anesthesia for open or surgical arthroscopic procedures of the elbow; not otherwise specified**
0.00   0.00   **FUD** XXX   N
AMA: 2018,Jan,8; 2017,Dec,8; 2017,Jan,8; 2016,Jan,13; 2015,Jan,16; 2014,Aug,5; 2014,Jan,11

01742 **osteotomy of humerus**
0.00   0.00   **FUD** XXX   N
AMA: 2018,Jan,8; 2017,Dec,8; 2017,Jan,8; 2016,Jan,13; 2015,Jan,16; 2014,Aug,5; 2014,Jan,11

01744 **repair of nonunion or malunion of humerus**
0.00   0.00   **FUD** XXX   N
AMA: 2018,Jan,8; 2017,Dec,8; 2017,Jan,8; 2016,Jan,13; 2015,Jan,16; 2014,Aug,5; 2014,Jan,11

01756 **radical procedures**
0.00   0.00   **FUD** XXX   C
AMA: 2018,Jan,8; 2017,Dec,8; 2017,Jan,8; 2016,Jan,13; 2015,Jan,16; 2014,Aug,5; 2014,Jan,11

01758 **excision of cyst or tumor of humerus**
0.00   0.00   **FUD** XXX   N
AMA: 2018,Jan,8; 2017,Dec,8; 2017,Jan,8; 2016,Jan,13; 2015,Jan,16; 2014,Aug,5; 2014,Jan,11

01760 **total elbow replacement**
0.00   0.00   **FUD** XXX   N
AMA: 2018,Jan,8; 2017,Dec,8; 2017,Jan,8; 2016,Jan,13; 2015,Jan,16; 2014,Aug,5; 2014,Jan,11

● New Code   ▲ Revised Code   ○ Reinstated   ● New Web Release   ▲ Revised Web Release   + Add-on   Unlisted   Not Covered   # Resequenced
50 Optum Mod 50 Exempt   ⊘ AMA Mod 51 Exempt   51 Optum Mod 51 Exempt   63 Mod 63 Exempt   ✗ Non-FDA Drug   ★ Telemedicine   M Maternity   A Age Edit

CPT © 2019 American Medical Association. All Rights Reserved.

01770	**Anesthesia for procedures on arteries of upper arm and elbow; not otherwise specified**

0.00 0.00 **FUD** XXX N ▢

AMA: 2018,Jan,8; 2017,Dec,8; 2017,Jan,8; 2016,Jan,13; 2015,Jan,16; 2014,Aug,5; 2014,Jan,11

01772   **embolectomy**

0.00 0.00 **FUD** XXX N ▢

AMA: 2018,Jan,8; 2017,Dec,8; 2017,Jan,8; 2016,Jan,13; 2015,Jan,16; 2014,Aug,5; 2014,Jan,11

01780   **Anesthesia for procedures on veins of upper arm and elbow; not otherwise specified**

0.00 0.00 **FUD** XXX N ▢

AMA: 2018,Jan,8; 2017,Dec,8; 2017,Jan,8; 2016,Jan,13; 2015,Jan,16; 2014,Aug,5; 2014,Jan,11

01782   **phleborrhaphy**

0.00 0.00 **FUD** XXX N ▢

AMA: 2018,Jan,8; 2017,Dec,8; 2017,Jan,8; 2016,Jan,13; 2015,Jan,16; 2014,Aug,5; 2014,Jan,11

01810   **Anesthesia for all procedures on nerves, muscles, tendons, fascia, and bursae of forearm, wrist, and hand**

0.00 0.00 **FUD** XXX N ▢

AMA: 2018,Jan,8; 2017,Dec,8; 2017,Jan,8; 2016,Jan,13; 2015,Jan,16; 2014,Aug,5; 2014,Jan,11

01820   **Anesthesia for all closed procedures on radius, ulna, wrist, or hand bones**

0.00 0.00 **FUD** XXX N ▢

AMA: 2018,Jan,8; 2017,Dec,8; 2017,Jan,8; 2016,Jan,13; 2015,Jan,16; 2014,Aug,5; 2014,Jan,11

01829   **Anesthesia for diagnostic arthroscopic procedures on the wrist**

0.00 0.00 **FUD** XXX N ▢

AMA: 2018,Jan,8; 2017,Dec,8; 2017,Jan,8; 2016,Jan,13; 2015,Jan,16; 2014,Aug,5; 2014,Jan,11

01830   **Anesthesia for open or surgical arthroscopic/endoscopic procedures on distal radius, distal ulna, wrist, or hand joints; not otherwise specified**

0.00 0.00 **FUD** XXX N ▢

AMA: 2018,Jan,8; 2017,Dec,8; 2017,Jan,8; 2016,Jan,13; 2015,Jan,16; 2014,Aug,5; 2014,Jan,11

01832   **total wrist replacement**

0.00 0.00 **FUD** XXX N ▢

AMA: 2018,Jan,8; 2017,Dec,8; 2017,Jan,8; 2016,Jan,13; 2015,Jan,16; 2014,Aug,5; 2014,Jan,11

01840   **Anesthesia for procedures on arteries of forearm, wrist, and hand; not otherwise specified**

0.00 0.00 **FUD** XXX N ▢

AMA: 2018,Jan,8; 2017,Dec,8; 2017,Jan,8; 2016,Jan,13; 2015,Jan,16; 2014,Aug,5; 2014,Jan,11

01842   **embolectomy**

0.00 0.00 **FUD** XXX N ▢

AMA: 2018,Jan,8; 2017,Dec,8; 2017,Jan,8; 2016,Jan,13; 2015,Jan,16; 2014,Aug,5; 2014,Jan,11

01844   **Anesthesia for vascular shunt, or shunt revision, any type (eg, dialysis)**

0.00 0.00 **FUD** XXX N ▢

AMA: 2018,Jan,8; 2017,Dec,8; 2017,Jan,8; 2016,Jan,13; 2015,Jan,16; 2014,Aug,5; 2014,Jan,11

01850   **Anesthesia for procedures on veins of forearm, wrist, and hand; not otherwise specified**

0.00 0.00 **FUD** XXX N ▢

AMA: 2018,Jan,8; 2017,Dec,8; 2017,Jan,8; 2016,Jan,13; 2015,Jan,16; 2014,Aug,5; 2014,Jan,11

01852   **phleborrhaphy**

0.00 0.00 **FUD** XXX N ▢

AMA: 2018,Jan,8; 2017,Dec,8; 2017,Jan,8; 2016,Jan,13; 2015,Jan,16; 2014,Aug,5; 2014,Jan,11

01860   **Anesthesia for forearm, wrist, or hand cast application, removal, or repair**

0.00 0.00 **FUD** XXX N ▢

AMA: 2018,Jan,8; 2017,Dec,8; 2017,Jan,8; 2016,Jan,13; 2015,Jan,16; 2014,Aug,5; 2014,Jan,11

01916-01936 Anesthesia for Interventional Radiology Procedures

CMS: 100-04,12,140.1 Qualified Nonphysician Anesthetists; 100-04,12,140.3 Payment for Qualified Nonphysician Anesthetists; 100-04,12,140.3.3 Billing Modifiers; 100-04,12,140.3.4 General Billing Instructions; 100-04,12,140.4.1 Anesthesiologist/Qualified Nonphysican Anesthetist; 100-04,12,140.4.2 Anesthetist and Anesthesiologist in a Single Procedure; 100-04,12,140.4.3 Payment for Medical /Surgical Services by CRNAs; 100-04,12,140.4.4 Conversion Factors for Anesthesia Services; 100-04,12,140.5 Payment for Anesthesia Services Furnished by a Teaching CRNA; 100-04,4,250.3.2 Anesthesia in a Hospital Outpatient Setting

01916   **Anesthesia for diagnostic arteriography/venography**

EXCLUDES *Anesthesia for therapeutic interventional radiological procedures involving the arterial system (01924-01926)*

Anesthesia for therapeutic interventional radiological procedures involving the venous/lymphatic system (01930-01933)

0.00 0.00 **FUD** XXX N ▢

AMA: 2018,Jan,8; 2017,Dec,8; 2017,Jan,8; 2016,Jan,13; 2015,Jan,16; 2014,Aug,5; 2014,Jan,11

01920   **Anesthesia for cardiac catheterization including coronary angiography and ventriculography (not to include Swan-Ganz catheter)**

0.00 0.00 **FUD** XXX N ▢

AMA: 2018,Jan,8; 2017,Dec,8; 2017,Jan,8; 2016,Jan,13; 2015,Jan,16; 2014,Aug,5; 2014,Jan,11

01922   **Anesthesia for non-invasive imaging or radiation therapy**

0.00 0.00 **FUD** XXX N ▢

AMA: 2018,Jan,8; 2017,Dec,8; 2017,Jan,8; 2016,Jan,13; 2015,Jan,16; 2014,Aug,5; 2014,Jan,11

01924   **Anesthesia for therapeutic interventional radiological procedures involving the arterial system; not otherwise specified**

0.00 0.00 **FUD** XXX N ▢

AMA: 2018,Jan,8; 2017,Dec,8; 2017,Jan,8; 2016,Jan,13; 2015,Jan,16; 2014,Aug,5; 2014,Jan,11

01925   **carotid or coronary**

0.00 0.00 **FUD** XXX N ▢

AMA: 2018,Jan,8; 2017,Dec,8; 2017,Jan,8; 2016,Jan,13; 2015,Jan,16; 2014,Aug,5; 2014,Jan,11

01926   **intracranial, intracardiac, or aortic**

0.00 0.00 **FUD** XXX N ▢

AMA: 2018,Jan,8; 2017,Dec,8; 2017,Jan,8; 2016,Jan,13; 2015,Jan,16; 2014,Aug,5; 2014,Jan,11

01930   **Anesthesia for therapeutic interventional radiological procedures involving the venous/lymphatic system (not to include access to the central circulation); not otherwise specified**

0.00 0.00 **FUD** XXX N ▢

AMA: 2018,Jan,8; 2017,Dec,8; 2017,Jan,8; 2016,Jan,13; 2015,Jan,16; 2014,Aug,5; 2014,Jan,11

01931   **intrahepatic or portal circulation (eg, transvenous intrahepatic portosystemic shunt[s] [TIPS])**

0.00 0.00 **FUD** XXX N ▢

AMA: 2018,Jan,8; 2017,Dec,8; 2017,Jan,8; 2016,Jan,13; 2015,Jan,16; 2014,Aug,5; 2014,Jan,11

01932   **intrathoracic or jugular**

0.00 0.00 **FUD** XXX N ▢

AMA: 2018,Jan,8; 2017,Dec,8; 2017,Jan,8; 2016,Jan,13; 2015,Jan,16; 2014,Aug,5; 2014,Jan,11

01933   **intracranial**

0.00 0.00 **FUD** XXX N ▢

AMA: 2018,Jan,8; 2017,Dec,8; 2017,Jan,8; 2016,Jan,13; 2015,Jan,16; 2014,Aug,5; 2014,Jan,11

01935 **Anesthesia for percutaneous image guided procedures on the spine and spinal cord; diagnostic**
🔢 0.00   ⚕ 0.00   **FUD** XXX   N ▣
AMA: 2018,Jan,8; 2017,Dec,8; 2017,Jan,8; 2016,Jan,13; 2015,Jan,16; 2014,Aug,5; 2014,Jan,11

01936 **therapeutic**
🔢 0.00   ⚕ 0.00   **FUD** XXX   N ▣
AMA: 2018,Jan,8; 2017,Dec,8; 2017,Jan,8; 2016,Jan,13; 2015,Jan,16; 2014,Aug,5; 2014,Jan,11

01951-01953 Anesthesia for Burn Procedures

CMS: 100-04,12,140.1 Qualified Nonphysician Anesthetists; 100-04,12,140.3 Payment for Qualified Nonphysician Anesthetists; 100-04,12,140.3.3 Billing Modifiers; 100-04,12,140.3.4 General Billing Instructions; 100-04,12,140.4.1 Anesthesiologist/Qualified Nonphysican Anesthetist; 100-04,12,140.4.2 Anesthetist and Anesthesiologist in a Single Procedure; 100-04,12,140.4.3 Payment for Medical /Surgical Services by CRNAs; 100-04,12,140.4.4 Conversion Factors for Anesthesia Services; 100-04,12,140.5 Payment for Anesthesia Services Furnished by a Teaching CRNA; 100-04,4,250.3.2 Anesthesia in a Hospital Outpatient Setting

01951 **Anesthesia for second- and third-degree burn excision or debridement with or without skin grafting, any site, for total body surface area (TBSA) treated during anesthesia and surgery; less than 4% total body surface area**
🔢 0.00   ⚕ 0.00   **FUD** XXX   N ▣
AMA: 2018,Jan,8; 2017,Dec,8; 2017,Jan,8; 2016,Jan,13; 2015,Jan,16; 2014,Aug,5; 2014,Jan,11

01952 **between 4% and 9% of total body surface area**
🔢 0.00   ⚕ 0.00   **FUD** XXX   N ▣
AMA: 2018,Jan,8; 2017,Dec,8; 2017,Jan,8; 2016,Jan,13; 2015,Jan,16; 2014,Aug,5; 2014,Jan,11

+ 01953 **each additional 9% total body surface area or part thereof (List separately in addition to code for primary procedure)**
Code first (01952)
🔢 0.00   ⚕ 0.00   **FUD** XXX   N ▣
AMA: 2018,Jan,8; 2017,Dec,8; 2017,Jan,8; 2016,Jan,13; 2015,Jan,16; 2014,Aug,5; 2014,Jan,11

01958-01969 Anesthesia for Obstetric Procedures

CMS: 100-04,12,140.1 Qualified Nonphysician Anesthetists; 100-04,12,140.3 Payment for Qualified Nonphysician Anesthetists; 100-04,12,140.3.3 Billing Modifiers; 100-04,12,140.3.4 General Billing Instructions; 100-04,12,140.4.1 Anesthesiologist/Qualified Nonphysican Anesthetist; 100-04,12,140.4.2 Anesthetist and Anesthesiologist in a Single Procedure; 100-04,12,140.4.3 Payment for Medical /Surgical Services by CRNAs; 100-04,12,140.4.4 Conversion Factors for Anesthesia Services; 100-04,12,140.5 Payment for Anesthesia Services Furnished by a Teaching CRNA; 100-04,4,250.3.2 Anesthesia in a Hospital Outpatient Setting

01958 **Anesthesia for external cephalic version procedure**   M
🔢 0.00   ⚕ 0.00   **FUD** XXX   N ▣
AMA: 2018,Jan,8; 2017,Dec,8; 2017,Jan,8; 2016,Jan,13; 2015,Jan,16; 2014,Aug,5; 2014,Jan,11

01960 **Anesthesia for vaginal delivery only**   M ♀
🔢 0.00   ⚕ 0.00   **FUD** XXX   N ▣
AMA: 2018,Jan,8; 2017,Dec,8; 2017,Jan,8; 2016,Jan,13; 2015,Jan,16; 2014,Aug,5; 2014,Jan,11

01961 **Anesthesia for cesarean delivery only**   M ♀
🔢 0.00   ⚕ 0.00   **FUD** XXX   N ▣
AMA: 2018,Jan,8; 2017,Dec,8; 2017,Jan,8; 2016,Jan,13; 2015,Jan,16; 2014,Aug,5; 2014,Jan,11

01962 **Anesthesia for urgent hysterectomy following delivery**   M ♀
🔢 0.00   ⚕ 0.00   **FUD** XXX   N ▣
AMA: 2018,Jan,8; 2017,Dec,8; 2017,Jan,8; 2016,Jan,13; 2015,Jan,16; 2014,Aug,5; 2014,Jan,11

01963 **Anesthesia for cesarean hysterectomy without any labor analgesia/anesthesia care**   M ♀
🔢 0.00   ⚕ 0.00   **FUD** XXX   N ▣
AMA: 2018,Jan,8; 2017,Dec,8; 2017,Jan,8; 2016,Jan,13; 2015,Jan,16; 2014,Aug,5; 2014,Jan,11

01965 **Anesthesia for incomplete or missed abortion procedures**   M ♀
🔢 0.00   ⚕ 0.00   **FUD** XXX   N ▣
AMA: 2018,Jan,8; 2017,Dec,8; 2017,Jan,8; 2016,Jan,13; 2015,Jan,16; 2014,Aug,5; 2014,Jan,11

01966 **Anesthesia for induced abortion procedures**   M ♀
🔢 0.00   ⚕ 0.00   **FUD** XXX   N ▣
AMA: 2018,Jan,8; 2017,Dec,8; 2017,Jan,8; 2016,Jan,13; 2015,Jan,16; 2014,Aug,5; 2014,Jan,11

01967 **Neuraxial labor analgesia/anesthesia for planned vaginal delivery (this includes any repeat subarachnoid needle placement and drug injection and/or any necessary replacement of an epidural catheter during labor)**   M ♀
🔢 0.00   ⚕ 0.00   **FUD** XXX   N ▣
AMA: 2018,Jan,8; 2017,Dec,8; 2017,Jan,8; 2016,Jan,13; 2015,Jan,16; 2014,Oct,14; 2014,Aug,5; 2014,Jan,11

+ 01968 **Anesthesia for cesarean delivery following neuraxial labor analgesia/anesthesia (List separately in addition to code for primary procedure performed)** .   M ♀
Code first (01967)
🔢 0.00   ⚕ 0.00   **FUD** XXX   N ▣
AMA: 2018,Jan,8; 2017,Dec,8; 2017,Jan,8; 2016,Jan,13; 2015,Jan,16; 2014,Oct,14; 2014,Aug,5; 2014,Jan,11

+ 01969 **Anesthesia for cesarean hysterectomy following neuraxial labor analgesia/anesthesia (List separately in addition to code for primary procedure performed)**   M ♀
Code first (01967)
🔢 0.00   ⚕ 0.00   **FUD** XXX   N ▣
AMA: 2018,Jan,8; 2017,Dec,8; 2017,Jan,8; 2016,Jan,13; 2015,Jan,16; 2014,Aug,5; 2014,Jan,11

01990-01999 Anesthesia Miscellaneous

CMS: 100-04,12,140.1 Qualified Nonphysician Anesthetists; 100-04,12,140.3 Payment for Qualified Nonphysician Anesthetists; 100-04,12,140.3.3 Billing Modifiers; 100-04,12,140.3.4 General Billing Instructions; 100-04,12,140.4.1 Anesthesiologist/Qualified Nonphysican Anesthetist; 100-04,12,140.4.2 Anesthetist and Anesthesiologist in a Single Procedure; 100-04,12,140.4.3 Payment for Medical /Surgical Services by CRNAs; 100-04,12,140.4.4 Conversion Factors for Anesthesia Services; 100-04,12,140.5 Payment for Anesthesia Services Furnished by a Teaching CRNA; 100-04,4,250.3.2 Anesthesia in a Hospital Outpatient Setting

01990 **Physiological support for harvesting of organ(s) from brain-dead patient**
🔢 0.00   ⚕ 0.00   **FUD** XXX   C ▣
AMA: 2018,Jan,8; 2017,Dec,8; 2017,Jan,8; 2016,Jan,13; 2015,Jan,16; 2014,Aug,5; 2014,Jan,11

01991 **Anesthesia for diagnostic or therapeutic nerve blocks and injections (when block or injection is performed by a different physician or other qualified health care professional); other than the prone position**
EXCLUDES *Bier block for pain management (64999)*
Moderate Sedation (99151-99153, 99155-99157)
Pain management via intra-arterial or IV therapy (96373-96374)
Regional or local anesthesia of arms or legs for surgical procedure
🔢 0.00   ⚕ 0.00   **FUD** XXX   N ▣
AMA: 2018,Jan,8; 2017,Dec,8; 2017,Jan,8; 2016,Jan,13; 2015,Jan,16; 2014,Aug,5; 2014,Jan,11

01992 **prone position**
EXCLUDES *Bier block for pain management (64999)*
Moderate sedation (99151-99153, 99155-99157)
Pain management via intra-arterial or IV therapy (96373-96374)
Regional or local anesthesia of arms or legs for surgical procedure
🔢 0.00   ⚕ 0.00   **FUD** XXX   N ▣
AMA: 2018,Jan,8; 2017,Dec,8; 2017,Jan,8; 2016,Jan,13; 2015,Jan,16; 2014,Aug,5; 2014,Jan,11

01996 **Daily hospital management of epidural or subarachnoid continuous drug administration**

> INCLUDES   Continuous epidural or subarachnoid drug services performed after insertion of an epidural or subarachnoid catheter

🚑 0.00   ⚕ 0.00   **FUD** XXX   N 🔲

AMA: 2018,Jan,8; 2017,Dec,8; 2017,Sep,6; 2017,Jan,8; 2016,Jan,13; 2015,May,10; 2015,Jan,16; 2014,Aug,5; 2014,Jan,11

01999 **Unlisted anesthesia procedure(s)**

🚑 0.00   ⚕ 0.00   **FUD** XXX   N 🔲

AMA: 2018,Jan,8; 2017,Dec,8; 2017,Jan,8; 2016,Jan,13; 2015,May,10; 2015,Jan,16; 2014,Aug,5; 2014,Aug,14; 2014,Jan,11

10004-10012 [10004, 10005, 10006, 10007, 10008, 10009, 10010, 10011, 10012] Fine Needle Aspiration

EXCLUDES Percutaneous localization clip placement during breast biopsy (19081-19086)
Percutaneous needle biopsy of:
Abdominal or retroperitoneal mass (49180)
Bone (20220, 20225)
Bone marrow (38220-38222)
Epididymis (54800)
Kidney (50200)
Liver (47000)
Lung or mediastinum (32405)
Lymph node (38505)
Muscle (20206)
Nucleus pulposus, paravertebral tissue, intervertebral disc (62267)
Pancreas (48102)
Pleura (32400)
Prostate (55700, 55706)
Salivary gland (42400)
Spinal cord (62269)
Testis (54500)
Thyroid (60100)
Soft tissue percutaneous fluid drainage by catheter using image guidance (10030)
Thyroid cyst (60300)

Code also multiple biopsies on same date of service:
FNA biopsies using same imaging guidance: report imaging add-on code for second and successive procedures
FNA biopsies separate lesions, different imaging guidance: append modifier 59 to codes for additional imaging modality used
FNA and core needle biopsy same lesion, same imaging guidance, procedure includes imaging guidance for core needle procedure
FNA and core needle biopsies separate lesions, same or different imaging guidance, append modifier 59 to code for core needle biopsy and imaging guidance

10004	Resequenced code. See code following 10021.
10005	Resequenced code. See code following 10021.
10006	Resequenced code. See code following 10021.
10007	Resequenced code. See code following 10021.
10008	Resequenced code. See code following 10021.
10009	Resequenced code. See code following 10021.
10010	Resequenced code. See code following 10021.
10011	Resequenced code. See code following 10021.
10012	Resequenced code. See code following 10021.

10021 **Fine needle aspiration biopsy, without imaging guidance; first lesion**
(88172-88173)
1.61 2.78 **FUD** XXX T P3 80
AMA: 2019,May,10; 2019,Apr,4; 2019,Feb,8; 2018,Jan,8; 2017,Jan,8; 2016,Jan,13; 2015,Jan,16; 2014,Jan,11

+ # **10004** **each additional lesion (List separately in addition to code for primary procedure)**
EXCLUDES Fine needle biopsy using other imaging methods for same lesion ([10005, 10006, 10007, 10008, 10009, 10010, 10011, 10012])
(88172-88173, [88177])
Code first (10021)
1.25 1.49 **FUD** ZZZ N1 80
AMA: 2019,Apr,4; 2019,Feb,8

10005 **Fine needle aspiration biopsy, including ultrasound guidance; first lesion**
INCLUDES Imaging guidance (76942)
(88172-88173, [88177])
2.10 3.59 **FUD** XXX P3 80
AMA: 2019,May,10; 2019,Feb,8; 2019,Apr,4

+ # **10006** **each additional lesion (List separately in addition to code for primary procedure)**
INCLUDES Imaging guidance (76942)
(88172-88173, [88177])
Code first ([10005])
1.43 1.71 **FUD** ZZZ N1 80
AMA: 2019,Apr,4; 2019,Feb,8

10007 **Fine needle aspiration biopsy, including fluoroscopic guidance; first lesion**
INCLUDES Imaging guidance (77002)
(88172-88173, [88177])
2.70 8.09 **FUD** XXX P3 80
AMA: 2019,Apr,4; 2019,Feb,8

+ # **10008** **each additional lesion (List separately in addition to code for primary procedure)**
INCLUDES Imaging guidance (77002)
(88172-88173, [88177])
Code first ([10007])
1.76 4.56 **FUD** ZZZ N1 80
AMA: 2019,Apr,4; 2019,Feb,8

10009 **Fine needle aspiration biopsy, including CT guidance; first lesion**
INCLUDES Imaging guidance (77012)
(88172-88173, [88177])
3.27 13.2 **FUD** XXX P2 80
AMA: 2019,Apr,4; 2019,Feb,8

+ # **10010** **each additional lesion (List separately in addition to code for primary procedure)**
INCLUDES Imaging guidance (77012)
(88172-88173, [88177])
Code first ([10009])
2.39 7.98 **FUD** ZZZ N1 80
AMA: 2019,Apr,4; 2019,Feb,8

10011 **Fine needle aspiration biopsy, including MR guidance; first lesion**
INCLUDES Imaging guidance (77021)
(88172-88173, [88177])
0.00 0.00 **FUD** XXX R2 80
AMA: 2019,Apr,4; 2019,Feb,8

+ # **10012** **each additional lesion (List separately in addition to code for primary procedure)**
INCLUDES Imaging guidance (77021)
(88172-88173, [88177])
Code first ([10011])
0.00 0.00 **FUD** ZZZ N1 80
AMA: 2019,Apr,4; 2019,Feb,8

10030-10180 Treatment of Lesions: Skin and Subcutaneous Tissues

EXCLUDES Excision benign lesion (11400-11471)

10030 **Image-guided fluid collection drainage by catheter (eg, abscess, hematoma, seroma, lymphocele, cyst), soft tissue (eg, extremity, abdominal wall, neck), percutaneous**
INCLUDES Radiologic guidance (75989, 76942, 77002-77003, 77012, 77021)
EXCLUDES Percutaneous drainage with imaging guidance of:
Peritoneal or retroperitoneal collections (49406)
Visceral collections (49405)
Transvaginal or transrectal drainage with imaging guidance of:
Peritoneal or retroperitoneal collections (49407)
Code also every instance of fluid collection drained using a separate catheter (10030)
3.97 16.2 **FUD** 000 T G2 80
AMA: 2019,Apr,4; 2018,Jan,8; 2017,Aug,9; 2017,Jan,8; 2016,Jan,13; 2015,Jan,16; 2014,May,3; 2014,May,9

Integumentary System

10035 — 11004

10035 Placement of soft tissue localization device(s) (eg, clip, metallic pellet, wire/needle, radioactive seeds), percutaneous, including imaging guidance; first lesion

INCLUDES Radiologic guidance (76942, 77002-77003, 77012, 77021)

EXCLUDES Sites with a more specific code descriptor, such as the breast

Use of code more than one time per site, regardless of the number of markers used

Code also each additional target on the same or opposite side (10036)

⚕ 2.48   ✂ 13.6   **FUD** 000   T N1 80 50 🖵

AMA: 2018,Jan,8; 2017,Jan,8; 2016,Jun,3

+ 10036 each additional lesion (List separately in addition to code for primary procedure)

INCLUDES Radiologic guidance (76942, 77002, 77012, 77021)

EXCLUDES Sites with a more specific code descriptor, such as the breast

Use of code more than one time per site, regardless of the number of markers used

Code first (10035)

⚕ 1.25   ✂ 11.7   **FUD** ZZZ   N N1 80 🖵

AMA: 2018,Jan,8; 2017,Jan,8; 2016,Jun,3

10040 Acne surgery (eg, marsupialization, opening or removal of multiple milia, comedones, cysts, pustules)

⚕ 1.66   ✂ 3.09   **FUD** 010   01 N1 🖵

AMA: 2018,Jan,8; 2017,Jan,8; 2016,Jan,13; 2015,Jan,16; 2014,Jan,11

10060 Incision and drainage of abscess (eg, carbuncle, suppurative hidradenitis, cutaneous or subcutaneous abscess, cyst, furuncle, or paronychia); simple or single

⚕ 2.81   ✂ 3.37   **FUD** 010   T P3 🖵

AMA: 2018,Jan,8; 2017,Jan,8; 2016,Jan,13; 2015,Jan,16; 2014,Jan,11

10061 complicated or multiple

⚕ 5.16   ✂ 5.87   **FUD** 010   T P3 🖵

AMA: 2018,Jan,8; 2017,Jan,8; 2016,Jan,13; 2015,Jan,16; 2014,Jan,11

10080 Incision and drainage of pilonidal cyst; simple

⚕ 2.93   ✂ 5.23   **FUD** 010   T P3 🖵

AMA: 2018,Jan,8; 2017,Jan,8; 2016,Jan,13; 2015,Jan,16; 2014,Jan,11

10081 complicated

EXCLUDES Excision of pilonidal cyst (11770-11772)

⚕ 4.87   ✂ 7.84   **FUD** 010   T P3 🖵

AMA: 2018,Jan,8; 2017,Jan,8; 2016,Jan,13; 2015,Jan,16; 2014,Jan,11

10120 Incision and removal of foreign body, subcutaneous tissues; simple

⚕ 2.96   ✂ 4.32   **FUD** 010   T P3 🖵

AMA: 2018,Jan,8; 2017,Jan,8; 2016,Jan,13; 2015,Jan,16; 2014,Jan,11

10121 complicated

EXCLUDES Debridement associated with a fracture or dislocation (11010-11012)

Exploration penetrating wound (20100-20103)

⚕ 5.32   ✂ 7.77   **FUD** 010   J A2 🖵

AMA: 2018,Jan,8; 2017,Jan,8; 2016,Jan,13; 2015,Jan,16; 2014,Jan,11

10140 Incision and drainage of hematoma, seroma or fluid collection

🩻 (76942, 77002, 77012, 77021)

⚕ 3.40   ✂ 4.77   **FUD** 010   J P3

AMA: 2018,Jan,8; 2017,Jan,8; 2016,Jan,13; 2015,Jan,16; 2014,Nov,5; 2014,Jan,11

Hematoma may be decompressed with a hemostat

Drain may be placed to allow further drainage

10160 Puncture aspiration of abscess, hematoma, bulla, or cyst

🩻 (76942, 77002, 77012, 77021)

⚕ 2.72   ✂ 3.70   **FUD** 010   T P3 🖵

AMA: 2018,Jan,8; 2017,Aug,9; 2017,Jan,8; 2016,Jan,13; 2015,Jan,16; 2014,Jan,11

10180 Incision and drainage, complex, postoperative wound infection

EXCLUDES Wound dehiscence (12020-12021, 13160)

⚕ 5.10   ✂ 7.12   **FUD** 010   J A2 🖵

AMA: 2018,Jan,8; 2017,Jan,8; 2016,Jan,13; 2015,Jan,16; 2014,Nov,5; 2014,Jan,11

11000-11012 Removal of Foreign Substances and Infected/Devitalized Tissue

EXCLUDES Debridement of:
Burns (16000-16030)
Deeper tissue (11042-11047 [11045, 11046])
Nails (11720-11721)
Skin only (97597-97598)
Wounds (11042-11047 [11045, 11046])
Dermabrasions (15780-15783)
Pressure ulcer excision (15920-15999)

11000 Debridement of extensive eczematous or infected skin; up to 10% of body surface

EXCLUDES Necrotizing soft tissue infection of:
Abdominal wall (11005-11006)
External genitalia and perineum (11004, 11006)

⚕ 0.82   ✂ 1.57   **FUD** 000   T P3 🖵

AMA: 2018,Feb,10; 2018,Jan,8; 2017,Jan,8; 2016,Jan,13; 2015,Jan,16; 2014,Jan,11

+ 11001 each additional 10% of the body surface, or part thereof (List separately in addition to code for primary procedure)

EXCLUDES Necrotizing soft tissue infection of:
Abdominal wall (11005-11006)
External genitalia and perineum (11004, 11006)

Code first (11000)

⚕ 0.41   ✂ 0.62   **FUD** ZZZ   N N1 🖵

AMA: 2018,Feb,10; 2018,Jan,8; 2017,Jan,8; 2016,Jan,13; 2015,Jan,16; 2014,Jan,11

11004 Debridement of skin, subcutaneous tissue, muscle and fascia for necrotizing soft tissue infection; external genitalia and perineum

EXCLUDES Skin grafts or flaps (14000-14350, 15040-15770)

⚕ 16.6   ✂ 16.6   **FUD** 000   C 🖵

AMA: 2018,Feb,10; 2018,Jan,8; 2017,Jan,8; 2016,Jan,13; 2015,Jan,16; 2014,Jan,11

11005   **abdominal wall, with or without fascial closure**

> EXCLUDES *Skin grafts or flaps (14000-14350, 15040-15770)*
>
> 🖫 22.6   ⚕ 22.6 **FUD** 000   C 80 ▯
>
> **AMA:** 2018,Feb,10; 2018,Jan,8; 2017,Jan,8; 2016,Jan,13; 2015,Jan,16; 2014,Jan,11

11006   **external genitalia, perineum and abdominal wall, with or without fascial closure**

> EXCLUDES *Orchiectomy (54520)*
>
> *Skin grafts or flaps (14000-14350, 15040-15770)*
>
> *Testicular transplant (54680)*
>
> 🖫 20.4   ⚕ 20.4 **FUD** 000   C ▯
>
> **AMA:** 2018,Jan,8; 2017,Jan,8; 2016,Jan,13; 2015,Jan,16; 2014,Jan,11

+ **11008**   **Removal of prosthetic material or mesh, abdominal wall for infection (eg, for chronic or recurrent mesh infection or necrotizing soft tissue infection) (List separately in addition to code for primary procedure)**

> EXCLUDES *Debridement (11000-11001, 11010-11044 [11045, 11046])*
>
> *Insertion of mesh (49568)*
>
> *Skin grafts or flaps (14000-14350, 15040-15770)*
>
> Code first (10180, 11004-11006)
>
> 🖫 7.96   ⚕ 7.96 **FUD** ZZZ   C 80 ▯
>
> **AMA:** 2019,Jan,14; 2018,Jan,8; 2017,Jan,8; 2016,Jan,13; 2015,Jan,16; 2014,Jan,11

11010   **Debridement including removal of foreign material at the site of an open fracture and/or an open dislocation (eg, excisional debridement); skin and subcutaneous tissues**

> 🖫 8.01   ⚕ 13.8 **FUD** 010   T A2 ▯
>
> **AMA:** 2018,Jan,8; 2017,Jan,8; 2016,Jan,13; 2015,Jan,16; 2014,Jan,11

11011   **skin, subcutaneous tissue, muscle fascia, and muscle**

> 🖫 8.68   ⚕ 15.2 **FUD** 000   T A2 ▯
>
> **AMA:** 2018,Jan,8; 2017,Jan,8; 2016,Jan,13; 2015,Jan,16; 2014,Jan,11

11012   **skin, subcutaneous tissue, muscle fascia, muscle, and bone**

> 🖫 12.1   ⚕ 19.7 **FUD** 000   J A2 ▯
>
> **AMA:** 2018,Jan,8; 2017,Jan,8; 2016,Jan,13; 2015,Jan,16; 2014,Jan,11

11042-11047 [11045, 11046] Removal of Infected/Devitalized Tissue

> INCLUDES Debridement reported by the size and depth
>
> Debridement reported for multiple wounds by adding the total surface area of wounds of the same depth
>
> Injuries, wounds, chronic ulcers, infections
>
> EXCLUDES *Debridement of:*
>
> *Burn (16020-16030)*
>
> *Eczematous or infected skin (11000-11001)*
>
> *Nails (11720-11721)*
>
> *Necrotizing soft tissue infection of external genitalia, perineum, or abdominal wall (11004-11006)*
>
> *Non-elective debridement/active care management of same wound (97597-97602)*
>
> *Dermabrasions (15780-15783)*
>
> *Excision of pressure ulcers (15920-15999)*
>
> Code also each additional single wound of different depths
>
> Code also modifier 59 for additional wound debridement
>
> Code also multiple wound groups of different depths

11042   **Debridement, subcutaneous tissue (includes epidermis and dermis, if performed); first 20 sq cm or less**

> 🖫 1.76   ⚕ 3.46 **FUD** 000   T A2 ▯
>
> **AMA:** 2018,Jan,8; 2017,Jan,8; 2016,Oct,3; 2016,Aug,9; 2016,Feb,13; 2016,Jan,13; 2015,Jan,16; 2014,Nov,5; 2014,Jan,11

+ # **11045**   **each additional 20 sq cm, or part thereof (List separately in addition to code for primary procedure)**

> Code first (11042)
>
> 🖫 0.76   ⚕ 1.18 **FUD** ZZZ   N N1 80 ▯
>
> **AMA:** 2018,Jan,8; 2017,Jan,8; 2016,Oct,3; 2016,Aug,9; 2016,Jan,13; 2015,Jan,16; 2014,Nov,5; 2014,Jan,11

11043   **Debridement, muscle and/or fascia (includes epidermis, dermis, and subcutaneous tissue, if performed); first 20 sq cm or less**

> 🖫 4.45   ⚕ 6.57 **FUD** 000   T A2 ▯
>
> **AMA:** 2018,Jan,8; 2017,Jan,8; 2016,Oct,3; 2016,Aug,9; 2016,Jan,13; 2015,Jan,16; 2014,Nov,5; 2014,Jan,11

+ # **11046**   **each additional 20 sq cm, or part thereof (List separately in addition to code for primary procedure)**

> Code first (11043)
>
> 🖫 1.61   ⚕ 2.09 **FUD** ZZZ   N N1 80 ▯
>
> **AMA:** 2018,Jan,8; 2017,Jan,8; 2016,Oct,3; 2016,Aug,9; 2016,Jan,13; 2015,Jan,16; 2014,Nov,5; 2014,Jan,11

11044   **Debridement, bone (includes epidermis, dermis, subcutaneous tissue, muscle and/or fascia, if performed); first 20 sq cm or less**

> 🖫 6.58   ⚕ 8.93 **FUD** 000   J A2 ▯
>
> **AMA:** 2018,Jan,8; 2017,Jan,8; 2016,Oct,3; 2016,Aug,9; 2016,Jan,13; 2015,Jan,16; 2014,Nov,5; 2014,Jan,11

11045   **Resequenced code. See code following 11042.**

11046   **Resequenced code. See code following 11043.**

+ **11047**   **each additional 20 sq cm, or part thereof (List separately in addition to code for primary procedure)**

> Code first (11044)
>
> 🖫 2.85   ⚕ 3.53 **FUD** ZZZ   N N1 80 ▯
>
> **AMA:** 2018,Jan,8; 2017,Jan,8; 2016,Oct,3; 2016,Aug,9; 2016,Jan,13; 2015,Jan,16; 2014,Nov,5; 2014,Jan,11

11055-11057 Excision Benign Hypertrophic Skin Lesions

> **CMS:** 100-04,32,80.8 CSF Edits: Routine Foot Care
>
> EXCLUDES *Destruction (17000-17004)*

11055   **Paring or cutting of benign hyperkeratotic lesion (eg, corn or callus); single lesion**

> 🖫 0.46   ⚕ 1.59 **FUD** 000   01 N1 ▯
>
> **AMA:** 2018,Jan,8; 2017,Jan,8; 2016,Jan,13; 2015,Jan,16; 2014,Jan,11

11056   **2 to 4 lesions**

> 🖫 0.65   ⚕ 1.90 **FUD** 000   01 N1 ▯
>
> **AMA:** 2018,Jan,8; 2017,Jan,8; 2016,Jan,13; 2015,Jan,16; 2014,Jan,11

11057   **more than 4 lesions**

> 🖫 0.85   ⚕ 2.11 **FUD** 000   T P3 ▯
>
> **AMA:** 2018,Jan,8; 2017,Jan,8; 2016,Jan,13; 2015,Jan,16; 2014,Jan,11

11102-11107 Surgical Biopsy Skin and Mucous Membranes

> INCLUDES Attaining tissue for pathologic exam
>
> EXCLUDES *Biopsies performed during related procedures*
>
> *Biopsy of:*
>
> *Anterior 2/3 of tongue (41100)*
>
> *Conjunctiva (68100)*
>
> *Ear (69100)*
>
> *Eyelid ([67810])*
>
> *Floor of mouth (41108)*
>
> *Penis (54100)*
>
> *Perineum/vulva (56605-56606)*

11102   **Tangential biopsy of skin (eg, shave, scoop, saucerize, curette); single lesion**

> 🖫 1.14   ⚕ 2.80 **FUD** 000   P3 ▯
>
> **AMA:** 2019,Jan,9

+ **11103**   **each separate/additional lesion (List separately in addition to code for primary procedure)**

> Code first different biopsy techniques used for additional separate lesions, when performed (11102, 11104, 11106)
>
> 🖫 0.66   ⚕ 1.51 **FUD** ZZZ   N1 ▯
>
> **AMA:** 2019,Jan,9

11104   **Punch biopsy of skin (including simple closure, when performed); single lesion**

> 🖫 1.43   ⚕ 3.52 **FUD** 000   P2 ▯
>
> **AMA:** 2019,Jan,9

● New Code   ▲ Revised Code   ○ Reinstated   ● New Web Release   ▲ Revised Web Release   + Add-on   Unlisted   Not Covered   # Resequenced

50 Optum Mod 50 Exempt   ⊘ AMA Mod 51 Exempt   51 Optum Mod 51 Exempt   63 Mod 63 Exempt   ⩘ Non-FDA Drug   ★ Telemedicine   M Maternity   A Age Edit

© 2019 Optum360, LLC   CPT © 2019 American Medical Association. All Rights Reserved.   15

+   11105   each separate/additional lesion (List separately in addition to code for primary procedure)
Code first different biopsy techniques used for additional separate lesions, when performed (11104, 11106)
🔧 0.78   ✂ 1.73   **FUD** ZZZ   N1 ▢
AMA: 2019,Jan,9

11106   Incisional biopsy of skin (eg, wedge) (including simple closure, when performed); single lesion
🔧 1.74   ✂ 4.26   **FUD** 000   P3 ▢
AMA: 2019,Jan,9

+   11107   each separate/additional lesion (List separately in addition to code for primary procedure)
Code first (11106)
🔧 0.93   ✂ 2.04   **FUD** ZZZ   N1 ▢
AMA: 2019,Jan,9

11200-11201 Skin Tag Removal - All Techniques

INCLUDES Chemical destruction
Electrocauterization
Electrosurgical destruction
Ligature strangulation
Removal with or without local anesthesia
Sharp excision or scissoring
EXCLUDES *Extensive or complicated secondary wound closure (13160)*

11200   Removal of skin tags, multiple fibrocutaneous tags, any area; up to and including 15 lesions
🔧 2.10   ✂ 2.51   **FUD** 010   01 N1 ▢
AMA: 2018,Jan,8; 2017,Jan,8; 2016,Jan,13; 2015,Jan,16; 2014,Jan,11

+   11201   each additional 10 lesions, or part thereof (List separately in addition to code for primary procedure)
Code first (11200)
🔧 0.48   ✂ 0.54   **FUD** ZZZ   N N1 ▢
AMA: 2018,Jan,8; 2017,Jan,8; 2016,Jan,13; 2015,Jan,16; 2014,Jan,11

11300-11313 Skin Lesion Removal: Shaving

INCLUDES Local anesthesia
Partial thickness excision by horizontal slicing
Wound cauterization

11300   Shaving of epidermal or dermal lesion, single lesion, trunk, arms or legs; lesion diameter 0.5 cm or less
🔧 1.01   ✂ 2.77   **FUD** 000   01 N1 80 ▢
AMA: 2019,Jan,9; 2018,Feb,10; 2018,Jan,8; 2017,Dec,14; 2017,Jan,8; 2016,Jan,13; 2015,Jan,16; 2014,Jan,11

Shave excision of an elevated lesion; technique also used to biopsy

Elliptical excision is often used when tissue removal is larger than 4 mm or when deep pathology is suspected

A punch biopsy cuts a core of tissue as the tool is twisted downward

11301   lesion diameter 0.6 to 1.0 cm
🔧 1.53   ✂ 3.40   **FUD** 000   01 N1 80 ▢
AMA: 2019,Jan,9; 2018,Feb,10; 2018,Jan,8; 2017,Dec,14; 2017,Jan,8; 2016,Jan,13; 2015,Jan,16; 2014,Jan,11

11302   lesion diameter 1.1 to 2.0 cm
🔧 1.80   ✂ 3.98   **FUD** 000   01 N1 80 ▢
AMA: 2019,Jan,9; 2018,Feb,10; 2018,Jan,8; 2017,Dec,14; 2017,Jan,8; 2016,Jan,13; 2015,Jan,16; 2014,Jan,11

11303   lesion diameter over 2.0 cm
🔧 2.13   ✂ 4.39   **FUD** 000   01 N1 80 ▢
AMA: 2019,Jan,9; 2018,Feb,10; 2018,Jan,8; 2017,Dec,14; 2017,Jan,8; 2016,Jan,13; 2015,Jan,16; 2014,Jan,11

11305   Shaving of epidermal or dermal lesion, single lesion, scalp, neck, hands, feet, genitalia; lesion diameter 0.5 cm or less
🔧 1.12   ✂ 2.90   **FUD** 000   01 N1 80 ▢
AMA: 2019,Jan,9; 2018,Feb,10; 2018,Jan,8; 2017,Dec,14; 2017,Jan,8; 2016,Jan,13; 2015,Jan,16; 2014,Jan,11

11306   lesion diameter 0.6 to 1.0 cm
🔧 1.49   ✂ 3.45   **FUD** 000   01 N1 80 ▢
AMA: 2019,Jan,9; 2018,Feb,10; 2018,Jan,8; 2017,Dec,14; 2017,Jan,8; 2016,Jan,13; 2015,Jan,16; 2014,Jan,11

11307   lesion diameter 1.1 to 2.0 cm
🔧 1.92   ✂ 4.09   **FUD** 000   T P2 80 ▢
AMA: 2019,Jan,9; 2018,Feb,10; 2018,Jan,8; 2017,Dec,14; 2017,Jan,8; 2016,Jan,13; 2015,Jan,16; 2014,Jan,11

11308   lesion diameter over 2.0 cm
🔧 2.14   ✂ 4.34   **FUD** 000   01 N1 80 ▢
AMA: 2019,Jan,9; 2018,Feb,10; 2018,Jan,8; 2017,Dec,14; 2017,Jan,8; 2016,Jan,13; 2015,Jan,16; 2014,Jan,11

11310   Shaving of epidermal or dermal lesion, single lesion, face, ears, eyelids, nose, lips, mucous membrane; lesion diameter 0.5 cm or less
🔧 1.36   ✂ 3.23   **FUD** 000   T P3 80 ▢
AMA: 2019,Jan,9; 2018,Feb,10; 2018,Jan,8; 2017,Dec,14; 2017,Jan,8; 2016,Jan,13; 2015,Jan,16; 2014,Jan,11

11311   lesion diameter 0.6 to 1.0 cm
🔧 1.88   ✂ 3.86   **FUD** 000   T P2 80 ▢
AMA: 2019,Jan,9; 2018,Feb,10; 2018,Jan,8; 2017,Dec,14; 2017,Jan,8; 2016,Jan,13; 2015,Jan,16; 2014,Jan,11

11312   lesion diameter 1.1 to 2.0 cm
🔧 2.23   ✂ 4.52   **FUD** 000   T P3 80 ▢
AMA: 2019,Jan,9; 2018,Feb,10; 2018,Jan,8; 2017,Dec,14; 2017,Jan,8; 2016,Jan,13; 2015,Jan,16; 2014,Jan,11

11313   lesion diameter over 2.0 cm
🔧 2.89   ✂ 5.30   **FUD** 000   T P3 80 ▢
AMA: 2019,Jan,9; 2018,Feb,10; 2018,Jan,8; 2017,Dec,14; 2017,Jan,8; 2016,Jan,13; 2015,Jan,16; 2014,Jan,11

11400-11446 Skin Lesion Removal: Benign

INCLUDES Biopsy on same lesion
Cicatricial lesion excision
Full thickness removal including margins
Lesion measurement before excision at largest diameter plus margin
Local anesthesia
Simple, nonlayered closure
EXCLUDES *Adjacent tissue transfer: report only adjacent tissue transfer (14000-14302)*
Biopsy of eyelid ([67810])
Destruction:
  Benign lesions, any method (17110-17111)
  Cutaneous vascular proliferative lesions (17106-17108)
  Destruction of eyelid lesion (67850)
  Malignant lesions (17260-17286)
  Premalignant lesions (17000, 17003-17004)
Escharotomy (16035-16036)
Excision and reconstruction of eyelid (67961-67975)
Excision of chalazion (67800-67808)
Eyelid procedures involving more than skin (67800 and subsequent codes)
Laser fenestration for scars (0479T-0480T)
Shave removal (11300-11313)
Code also complex closure (13100-13153)
Code also each separate lesion
Code also intermediate closure (12031-12057)
Code also modifier 22 if excision is complicated or unusual
Code also reconstruction (15002-15261, 15570-15770)

11400   Excision, benign lesion including margins, except skin tag (unless listed elsewhere), trunk, arms or legs; excised diameter 0.5 cm or less
🔧 2.33   ✂ 3.53   **FUD** 010   T P3 ▢
AMA: 2018,Sep,7; 2018,Feb,10; 2018,Jan,8; 2017,Jan,8; 2016,Apr,3; 2016,Jan,13; 2015,Jan,16; 2014,Mar,4; 2014,Mar,12; 2014,Jan,11

11401   **excised diameter 0.6 to 1.0 cm**
2.99   4.30   **FUD** 010   T P3
AMA: 2018,Sep,7; 2018,Feb,10; 2018,Jan,8; 2017,Jan,8;
2016,Apr,3; 2016,Jan,13; 2015,Jan,16; 2014,Mar,4; 2014,Mar,12;
2014,Jan,11

11402   **excised diameter 1.1 to 2.0 cm**
3.29   4.78   **FUD** 010   T P3
AMA: 2018,Sep,7; 2018,Feb,10; 2018,Jan,8; 2017,Jan,8;
2016,Apr,3; 2016,Jan,13; 2015,Jan,16; 2014,Mar,12; 2014,Mar,4;
2014,Jan,11

11403   **excised diameter 2.1 to 3.0 cm**
4.25   5.53   **FUD** 010   T P3
AMA: 2018,Sep,7; 2018,Feb,10; 2018,Jan,8; 2017,Jan,8;
2016,Apr,3; 2016,Jan,13; 2015,Jan,16; 2014,Mar,12; 2014,Mar,4;
2014,Jan,11

11404   **excised diameter 3.1 to 4.0 cm**
4.67   6.27   **FUD** 010   J A2
AMA: 2018,Sep,7; 2018,Feb,10; 2018,Jan,8; 2017,Jan,8;
2016,Apr,3; 2016,Jan,13; 2015,Jan,16; 2014,Mar,12; 2014,Mar,4;
2014,Jan,11

11406   **excised diameter over 4.0 cm**
7.11   9.02   **FUD** 010   J A2
AMA: 2018,Sep,7; 2018,Feb,10; 2018,Jan,8; 2017,Jan,8;
2016,Apr,3; 2016,Jan,13; 2015,Jan,16; 2014,Mar,4; 2014,Mar,12;
2014,Jan,11

11420   **Excision, benign lesion including margins, except skin tag
(unless listed elsewhere), scalp, neck, hands, feet, genitalia;
excised diameter 0.5 cm or less**
2.33   3.53   **FUD** 010   J P3
AMA: 2018,Sep,7; 2018,Feb,10; 2018,Jan,8; 2017,Jan,8;
2016,Apr,3; 2016,Jan,13; 2015,Jan,16; 2014,Mar,4; 2014,Mar,12;
2014,Jan,11

11421   **excised diameter 0.6 to 1.0 cm**
3.15   4.49   **FUD** 010   T P3
AMA: 2018,Sep,7; 2018,Feb,10; 2018,Jan,8; 2017,Jan,8;
2016,Apr,3; 2016,Jan,13; 2015,Jan,16; 2014,Mar,12; 2014,Mar,4;
2014,Jan,11

11422   **excised diameter 1.1 to 2.0 cm**
3.90   5.06   **FUD** 010   J P3
AMA: 2018,Sep,7; 2018,Feb,10; 2018,Jan,8; 2017,Jan,8;
2016,Apr,3; 2016,Jan,13; 2015,Jan,16; 2014,Mar,12; 2014,Mar,4;
2014,Jan,11

11423   **excised diameter 2.1 to 3.0 cm**
4.48   5.77   **FUD** 010   J P3
AMA: 2018,Sep,7; 2018,Feb,10; 2018,Jan,8; 2017,Jan,8;
2016,Apr,3; 2016,Jan,13; 2015,Jan,16; 2014,Mar,12; 2014,Mar,4;
2014,Jan,11

11424   **excised diameter 3.1 to 4.0 cm**
5.16   6.69   **FUD** 010   J A2
AMA: 2018,Sep,7; 2018,Feb,10; 2018,Jan,8; 2017,Jan,8;
2016,Apr,3; 2016,Jan,13; 2015,Jan,16; 2014,Mar,12; 2014,Mar,4;
2014,Jan,11

11426   **excised diameter over 4.0 cm**
7.93   9.59   **FUD** 010   J A2
AMA: 2018,Sep,7; 2018,Feb,10; 2018,Jan,8; 2017,Jan,8;
2016,Apr,3; 2016,Jan,13; 2015,Jan,16; 2014,Mar,12; 2014,Mar,4;
2014,Jan,11

11440   **Excision, other benign lesion including margins, except skin
tag (unless listed elsewhere), face, ears, eyelids, nose, lips,
mucous membrane; excised diameter 0.5 cm or less**
2.96   3.91   **FUD** 010   T P3
AMA: 2019,Jan,14; 2018,Sep,7; 2018,Feb,10; 2018,Jan,8;
2017,Jan,8; 2016,Apr,3; 2016,Jan,13; 2015,Jan,16; 2014,Mar,12;
2014,Mar,4; 2014,Jan,11

The physician removes
a benign lesion from
the external ear, nose,
or mucous membranes

11441   **excised diameter 0.6 to 1.0 cm**
3.76   4.83   **FUD** 010   T P3
AMA: 2019,Jan,14; 2018,Sep,7; 2018,Feb,10; 2018,Jan,8;
2017,Jan,8; 2016,Apr,3; 2016,Jan,13; 2015,Jan,16; 2014,Mar,12;
2014,Mar,4; 2014,Jan,11

11442   **excised diameter 1.1 to 2.0 cm**
4.16   5.39   **FUD** 010   T P3
AMA: 2019,Jan,14; 2018,Sep,7; 2018,Feb,10; 2018,Jan,8;
2017,Jan,8; 2016,Apr,3; 2016,Jan,13; 2015,Jan,16; 2014,Mar,12;
2014,Mar,4; 2014,Jan,11

11443   **excised diameter 2.1 to 3.0 cm**
5.11   6.42   **FUD** 010   J P3
AMA: 2019,Jan,14; 2018,Sep,7; 2018,Feb,10; 2018,Jan,8;
2017,Jan,8; 2016,Apr,3; 2016,Jan,13; 2015,Jan,16; 2014,Mar,12;
2014,Mar,4; 2014,Jan,11

11444   **excised diameter 3.1 to 4.0 cm**
6.51   8.05   **FUD** 010   J A2
AMA: 2019,Jan,14; 2018,Sep,7; 2018,Feb,10; 2018,Jan,8;
2017,Jan,8; 2016,Apr,3; 2016,Jan,13; 2015,Jan,16; 2014,Mar,12;
2014,Mar,4; 2014,Jan,11

11446   **excised diameter over 4.0 cm**
9.33   11.1   **FUD** 010   J A2
AMA: 2019,Jan,14; 2018,Sep,7; 2018,Feb,10; 2018,Jan,8;
2017,Jan,8; 2016,Apr,3; 2016,Jan,13; 2015,Jan,16; 2014,Mar,12;
2014,Mar,4; 2014,Jan,11

Integumentary System

11450 — 11642

11450-11471 Treatment of Hidradenitis: Excision and Repair

Code also closure by skin graft or flap (14000-14350, 15040-15770)

11450 Excision of skin and subcutaneous tissue for hidradenitis, axillary; with simple or intermediate repair

🚗 7.33   ✂ 11.2   **FUD** 090   J A2 50 ▢

AMA: 2018,Sep,7; 2018,Feb,10; 2018,Jan,8; 2017,Jan,8; 2016,Aug,9; 2016,Jan,13; 2015,Jan,16; 2014,Jan,11

Hidradenitis is a disease process stemming from clogged specialized sweat glands, principally located in the axilla and groin areas

Hair shaft

Hidradenitis of the axilla

Hair matrix

Sweat (eccrine gland)

11451 with complex repair

🚗 9.37   ✂ 14.1   **FUD** 090   J A2 80 50 ▢

AMA: 2018,Sep,7; 2018,Feb,10; 2018,Jan,8; 2017,Jan,8; 2016,Aug,9; 2016,Jan,13; 2015,Jan,16; 2014,Jan,11

11462 Excision of skin and subcutaneous tissue for hidradenitis, inguinal; with simple or intermediate repair

🚗 6.98   ✂ 10.9   **FUD** 090   J A2 80 50 ▢

AMA: 2018,Sep,7; 2018,Feb,10; 2018,Jan,8; 2017,Jan,8; 2016,Aug,9; 2016,Jan,13; 2015,Jan,16; 2014,Jan,11

11463 with complex repair

🚗 9.42   ✂ 14.3   **FUD** 090   J A2 80 50 ▢

AMA: 2018,Sep,7; 2018,Feb,10; 2018,Jan,8; 2017,Jan,8; 2016,Aug,9; 2016,Jan,13; 2015,Jan,16; 2014,Jan,11

11470 Excision of skin and subcutaneous tissue for hidradenitis, perianal, perineal, or umbilical; with simple or intermediate repair

🚗 8.08   ✂ 12.0   **FUD** 090   J A2 ▢

AMA: 2018,Sep,7; 2018,Feb,10; 2018,Jan,8; 2017,Jan,8; 2016,Aug,9; 2016,Jan,13; 2015,Jan,16; 2014,Jan,11

11471 with complex repair

🚗 9.99   ✂ 14.7   **FUD** 090   J A2 80 ▢

AMA: 2018,Sep,7; 2018,Feb,10; 2018,Jan,8; 2017,Jan,8; 2016,Aug,9; 2016,Jan,13; 2015,Jan,16; 2014,Jan,11

11600-11646 Skin Lesion Removal: Malignant

INCLUDES Biopsy on same lesion
Excision of additional margin at same operative session
Full thickness removal including margins
Lesion measurement before excision at largest diameter plus margin
Local anesthesia
Simple, nonlayered closure

EXCLUDES Adjacent tissue transfer. Report only adjacent tissue transfer (14000-14302)
Destruction (17260-17286)
Excision of additional margin at subsequent operative session (11600-11646)
Code also complex closure (13100-13153)
Code also each separate lesion
Code also intermediate closure (12031-12057)
Code also modifier 58 if re-excision is performed during postoperative period
Code also reconstruction (15002-15261, 15570-15770)

11600 Excision, malignant lesion including margins, trunk, arms, or legs; excised diameter 0.5 cm or less

🚗 3.45   ✂ 5.53   **FUD** 010   T P3 ▢

AMA: 2018,Sep,7; 2018,Jan,8; 2017,Jan,8; 2016,Jan,13; 2015,Jan,16; 2014,Mar,4; 2014,Mar,12; 2014,Jan,11

11601 excised diameter 0.6 to 1.0 cm

🚗 4.29   ✂ 6.52   **FUD** 010   T P3 ▢

AMA: 2018,Sep,7; 2018,Jan,8; 2017,Jan,8; 2016,Jan,13; 2015,Jan,16; 2014,Mar,4; 2014,Mar,12; 2014,Jan,11

11602 excised diameter 1.1 to 2.0 cm

🚗 4.70   ✂ 7.06   **FUD** 010   T P3 ▢

AMA: 2018,Sep,7; 2018,Jan,8; 2017,Jan,8; 2016,Jan,13; 2015,Jan,16; 2014,Mar,4; 2014,Mar,12; 2014,Jan,11

11603 excised diameter 2.1 to 3.0 cm

🚗 5.63   ✂ 8.07   **FUD** 010   T P3 ▢

AMA: 2018,Sep,7; 2018,Jan,8; 2017,Jan,8; 2016,Jan,13; 2015,Jan,16; 2014,Mar,4; 2014,Mar,12; 2014,Jan,11

11604 excised diameter 3.1 to 4.0 cm

🚗 6.19   ✂ 8.95   **FUD** 010   T A2 ▢

AMA: 2018,Sep,7; 2018,Jan,8; 2017,Jan,8; 2016,Jan,13; 2015,Jan,16; 2014,Mar,4; 2014,Mar,12; 2014,Jan,11

11606 excised diameter over 4.0 cm

🚗 9.24   ✂ 12.8   **FUD** 010   J A2 ▢

AMA: 2018,Sep,7; 2018,Jan,8; 2017,Jan,8; 2016,Jan,13; 2015,Jan,16; 2014,Mar,4; 2014,Mar,12; 2014,Jan,11

11620 Excision, malignant lesion including margins, scalp, neck, hands, feet, genitalia; excised diameter 0.5 cm or less

🚗 3.49   ✂ 5.57   **FUD** 010   J P3 ▢

AMA: 2018,Sep,7; 2018,Jan,8; 2017,Jan,8; 2016,Jan,13; 2015,Jan,16; 2014,Mar,4; 2014,Mar,12; 2014,Jan,11

11621 excised diameter 0.6 to 1.0 cm

🚗 4.32   ✂ 6.55   **FUD** 010   T P3 ▢

AMA: 2018,Sep,7; 2018,Jan,8; 2017,Jan,8; 2016,Jan,13; 2015,Jan,16; 2014,Mar,4; 2014,Mar,12; 2014,Jan,11

11622 excised diameter 1.1 to 2.0 cm

🚗 4.93   ✂ 7.30   **FUD** 010   T P3 ▢

AMA: 2018,Sep,7; 2018,Jan,8; 2017,Jan,8; 2016,Jan,13; 2015,Jan,16; 2014,Mar,4; 2014,Mar,12; 2014,Jan,11

11623 excised diameter 2.1 to 3.0 cm

🚗 6.10   ✂ 8.55   **FUD** 010   J P3 ▢

AMA: 2018,Sep,7; 2018,Jan,8; 2017,Jan,8; 2016,Jan,13; 2015,Jan,16; 2014,Mar,4; 2014,Mar,12; 2014,Jan,11

11624 excised diameter 3.1 to 4.0 cm

🚗 6.92   ✂ 9.67   **FUD** 010   J A2 ▢

AMA: 2018,Sep,7; 2018,Jan,8; 2017,Jan,8; 2016,Jan,13; 2015,Jan,16; 2014,Mar,4; 2014,Mar,12; 2014,Jan,11

11626 excised diameter over 4.0 cm

🚗 8.48   ✂ 11.6   **FUD** 010   J A2 ▢

AMA: 2018,Sep,7; 2018,Jan,8; 2017,Jan,8; 2016,Jan,13; 2015,Jan,16; 2014,Mar,4; 2014,Mar,12; 2014,Jan,11

11640 Excision, malignant lesion including margins, face, ears, eyelids, nose, lips; excised diameter 0.5 cm or less

EXCLUDES Eyelid excision involving more than skin (67800-67808, 67840-67850, 67961-67966)

🚗 3.61   ✂ 5.74   **FUD** 010   T P3 ▢

AMA: 2018,Sep,7; 2018,Jan,8; 2017,Jan,8; 2016,Jan,13; 2015,Jan,16; 2014,Mar,4; 2014,Mar,12; 2014,Jan,11

11641 excised diameter 0.6 to 1.0 cm

EXCLUDES Eyelid excision involving more than skin (67800-67808, 67840-67850, 67961-67966)

🚗 4.50   ✂ 6.78   **FUD** 010   T P3 ▢

AMA: 2018,Sep,7; 2018,Jan,8; 2017,Jan,8; 2016,Jan,13; 2015,Jan,16; 2014,Mar,4; 2014,Mar,12; 2014,Jan,11

11642 excised diameter 1.1 to 2.0 cm

EXCLUDES Eyelid excision involving more than skin (67800-67808, 67840-67850, 67961-67966)

🚗 5.30   ✂ 7.73   **FUD** 010   T P3 ▢

AMA: 2018,Sep,7; 2018,Jan,8; 2017,Jan,8; 2016,Jan,13; 2015,Jan,16; 2014,Mar,4; 2014,Mar,12; 2014,Jan,11

26/TC PC/TC Only   A2-Z3 ASC Payment   50 Bilateral   ♂ Male Only   ♀ Female Only   🚗 Facility RVU   ✂ Non-Facility RVU   ▢ CCI   ✖ CLIA
FUD Follow-up Days   **CMS:** IOM   **AMA:** CPT Asst   A-Y OPPSI   80/80 Surg Assist Allowed / w/Doc   ▨ Lab Crosswalk   ▨ Radiology Crosswalk

18   CPT © 2019 American Medical Association. All Rights Reserved.   © 2019 Optum360, LLC

11643   **excised diameter 2.1 to 3.0 cm**
EXCLUDES   *Eyelid excision involving more than skin (67800-67808, 67840-67850, 67961-67966)*
⚙ 6.62   ⚗ 9.09   **FUD** 010   J P3 ▣
AMA: 2018,Sep,7; 2018,Jan,8; 2017,Jan,8; 2016,Jan,13; 2015,Jan,16; 2014,Mar,4; 2014,Mar,12; 2014,Jan,11

11644   **excised diameter 3.1 to 4.0 cm**
EXCLUDES   *Eyelid excision involving more than skin (67800-67808, 67840-67850, 67961-67966)*
⚙ 8.21   ⚗ 11.2   **FUD** 010   J A2 ▣
AMA: 2018,Sep,7; 2018,Jan,8; 2017,Jan,8; 2016,Jan,13; 2015,Jan,16; 2014,Mar,4; 2014,Mar,12; 2014,Jan,11

11646   **excised diameter over 4.0 cm**
EXCLUDES   *Eyelid excision involving more than skin (67800-67808, 67840-67850, 67961-67966)*
⚙ 11.3   ⚗ 14.6   **FUD** 010   J A2 ▣
AMA: 2018,Sep,7; 2018,Jan,8; 2017,Jan,8; 2016,Jan,13; 2015,Jan,16; 2014,Mar,4; 2014,Mar,12; 2014,Jan,11

11719-11765 Nails and Supporting Structures

CMS: 100-02,15,290 Foot Care
EXCLUDES   *Drainage of paronychia or onychia (10060-10061)*

11719   **Trimming of nondystrophic nails, any number**
⚙ 0.22   ⚗ 0.41   **FUD** 000   Q1 N1 ▣
AMA: 2018,Jan,8; 2017,Jan,8; 2016,Jan,13; 2015,Jan,16; 2014,Jan,11

11720   **Debridement of nail(s) by any method(s); 1 to 5**
⚙ 0.42   ⚗ 0.94   **FUD** 000   Q1 N1 ▣
AMA: 2018,Jan,8; 2017,Jan,8; 2016,Jan,13; 2015,Jan,16; 2014,Jan,11

11721   **6 or more**
⚙ 0.71   ⚗ 1.29   **FUD** 000   Q1 N1 ▣
AMA: 2018,Jan,8; 2017,Jan,8; 2016,Jan,13; 2015,Jan,16; 2014,Jan,11

11730   **Avulsion of nail plate, partial or complete, simple; single**
⚙ 1.58   ⚗ 3.09   **FUD** 000   Q1 N1 ▣
AMA: 2018,Jan,8; 2017,Jan,8; 2016,Jan,13; 2015,Jan,16; 2014,Jan,11

+ 11732   **each additional nail plate (List separately in addition to code for primary procedure)**
Code first (11730)
⚙ 0.51   ⚗ 0.93   **FUD** ZZZ   N N1 ▣
AMA: 2018,Jan,8; 2017,Jan,8; 2016,Jan,13; 2015,Jan,16; 2014,Jan,11

11740   **Evacuation of subungual hematoma**
⚙ 0.92   ⚗ 1.46   **FUD** 000   Q1 N1 ▣
AMA: 2018,Jan,8; 2017,Jan,8; 2016,Jan,13; 2015,Jan,16; 2014,Jan,11

11750   **Excision of nail and nail matrix, partial or complete (eg, ingrown or deformed nail), for permanent removal;**
EXCLUDES   *Skin graft (15050)*
⚙ 2.92   ⚗ 4.41   **FUD** 010   T P3
AMA: 2018,Jan,8; 2017,Jan,8; 2016,Jan,13; 2015,Jan,16; 2014,Jan,11

11755   **Biopsy of nail unit (eg, plate, bed, matrix, hyponychium, proximal and lateral nail folds) (separate procedure)**
⚙ 1.79   ⚗ 3.47   **FUD** 000   T P3 80 ▣
AMA: 2019,Jan,9; 2018,Jan,8; 2017,Jan,8; 2016,Jan,13; 2015,Jan,16; 2014,Jan,11

11760   **Repair of nail bed**
⚙ 3.27   ⚗ 5.46   **FUD** 010   T G2 ▣
AMA: 2018,Jan,8; 2017,Jan,8; 2016,Jan,13; 2015,Jan,16; 2014,Jan,11

11762   **Reconstruction of nail bed with graft**
⚙ 5.33   ⚗ 8.15   **FUD** 010   T P3 ▣
AMA: 2018,Jan,8; 2017,Jan,8; 2016,Jan,13; 2015,Jan,16; 2014,Jan,11

11765   **Wedge excision of skin of nail fold (eg, for ingrown toenail)**
INCLUDES   Cotting's operation
⚙ 2.67   ⚗ 4.80   **FUD** 010   Q1 N1 ▣
AMA: 2018,Jan,8; 2017,Jan,8; 2016,Jan,13; 2015,Jan,16; 2014,Jan,11

11770-11772 Treatment Pilonidal Cyst: Excision

EXCLUDES   *Incision of pilonidal cyst (10080-10081)*

11770   **Excision of pilonidal cyst or sinus; simple**
⚙ 5.31   ⚗ 8.10   **FUD** 010   J A2 ▣

11771   **extensive**
⚙ 12.6   ⚗ 16.7   **FUD** 090   J A2 ▣

11772   **complicated**
⚙ 16.6   ⚗ 20.1   **FUD** 090   J A2 ▣
AMA: 2018,Jan,8; 2017,Jan,8; 2016,Jan,13; 2015,Sep,12

11900-11901 Treatment of Lesions: Injection

EXCLUDES   *Injection of local anesthesia performed preoperatively*
Injection of veins (36470-36471)
Intralesional chemotherapy (96405-96406)

11900   **Injection, intralesional; up to and including 7 lesions**
⚙ 0.90   ⚗ 1.54   **FUD** 000   Q1 N1 ▣
AMA: 2018,Jan,8; 2017,Jan,8; 2016,Jan,13; 2015,Jan,16; 2014,Jan,11

11901   **more than 7 lesions**
⚙ 1.39   ⚗ 1.95   **FUD** 000   Q1 N1 ▣
AMA: 2018,Jan,8; 2017,Jan,8; 2016,Jan,13; 2015,Jan,16; 2014,Jan,11

11920-11971 Tattoos, Tissue Expanders, and Dermal Fillers

CMS: 100-02,16,10 Exclusions from Coverage; 100-02,16,120 Cosmetic Procedures; 100-02,16,180 Services Related to Noncovered Procedures

11920   **Tattooing, intradermal introduction of insoluble opaque pigments to correct color defects of skin, including micropigmentation; 6.0 sq cm or less**
⚙ 3.24   ⚗ 5.10   **FUD** 000   T P3 80 ▣
AMA: 2018,Jan,8; 2017,Jan,8; 2016,Aug,9

11921   **6.1 to 20.0 sq cm**
⚙ 3.80   ⚗ 5.84   **FUD** 000   T P3 80 ▣
AMA: 2018,Jan,8; 2017,Jan,8; 2016,Aug,9

+ 11922   **each additional 20.0 sq cm, or part thereof (List separately in addition to code for primary procedure)**
⚙ 0.85   ⚗ 1.73   **FUD** ZZZ   N N1 80 ▣
Code first (11921)

11950   **Subcutaneous injection of filling material (eg, collagen); 1 cc or less**
⚙ 1.35   ⚗ 1.95   **FUD** 000   T P3 ▣
AMA: 2019,Aug,10; 2018,Jan,8; 2017,Jan,8; 2016,Jan,13; 2015,Jan,16; 2014,Jan,11

11951   **1.1 to 5.0 cc**
⚙ 1.98   ⚗ 2.80   **FUD** 000   T P3 80 ▣
AMA: 2019,Aug,10; 2018,Jan,8; 2017,Jan,8; 2016,Jan,13; 2015,Jan,16; 2014,Jan,11

11952   **5.1 to 10.0 cc**
⚙ 2.80   ⚗ 3.78   **FUD** 000   T P3 80 ▣
AMA: 2019,Aug,10; 2018,Jan,8; 2017,Jan,8; 2016,Jan,13; 2015,Jan,16; 2014,Jan,11

11954   **over 10.0 cc**
⚙ 3.21   ⚗ 4.41   **FUD** 000   T P3 80 ▣
AMA: 2019,Aug,10; 2018,Jan,8; 2017,Jan,8; 2016,Jan,13; 2015,Jan,16; 2014,Jan,11

11960   **Insertion of tissue expander(s) for other than breast, including subsequent expansion**
EXCLUDES   *Breast reconstruction with tissue expander(s) (19357)*
⚙ 27.7   ⚗ 27.7   **FUD** 090   T A2 ▣
AMA: 1991,Win,1

Integumentary System

11970 — 12014

11970 Replacement of tissue expander with permanent prothesis
🏥 17.4 ⚕ 17.4 **FUD** 090 [J] [A2] [50] [▭]
AMA: 2018,Jan,8; 2017,Jan,8; 2016,Jan,13; 2015,Jan,16; 2014,Jan,11

11971 Removal of tissue expander(s) without insertion of prosthesis
🏥 9.16 ⚕ 13.5 **FUD** 090 [02] [A2] [80] [50] [▭]
AMA: 2018,Jan,8; 2017,Jan,8; 2016,Jan,13; 2015,Jan,16; 2014,Jan,11

11976-11983 Drug Implantation

11976 Removal, implantable contraceptive capsules ♀
🏥 2.68 ⚕ 4.13 **FUD** 000 [02] [P3] [80] [▭]
AMA: 1992,Win,1; 1991,Win,1

11980 Subcutaneous hormone pellet implantation (implantation of estradiol and/or testosterone pellets beneath the skin)
🏥 1.61 ⚕ 2.69 **FUD** 000 [01] [N1] [▭]
AMA: 2018,Jan,8; 2017,Jan,8; 2016,Jan,13; 2015,Jan,16; 2014,Jan,11

11981 Insertion, non-biodegradable drug delivery implant
EXCLUDES Insertion of deep drug-delivery device:
Intra-articular (20704)
Intramedullary (20702)
Subfascial (20700)
🏥 2.40 ⚕ 4.05 **FUD** XXX [01] [N1] [80] [▭]
AMA: 2018,Jan,8; 2017,Jan,8; 2016,Jan,13; 2015,Jan,16; 2014,Jan,11

11982 Removal, non-biodegradable drug delivery implant
🏥 2.87 ⚕ 4.49 **FUD** XXX [01] [N1] [80] [▭]
EXCLUDES Removal of deep drug-delivery device:
Intra-articular (20705)
Intramedullary (20703)
Subfascial (20701)

11983 Removal with reinsertion, non-biodegradable drug delivery implant
🏥 5.12 ⚕ 6.56 **FUD** XXX [01] [N1] [80] [▭]

12001-12021 Suturing of Superficial Wounds

INCLUDES Administration of local anesthesia
Cauterization without closure
Simple:
  Exploration nerves, blood vessels, tendons
  Vessel ligation, in wound
Simple repair that involves:
  Routine debridement and decontamination
  Simple one layer closure
  Superficial tissues
  Sutures, staples, tissue adhesives
  Total length of several repairs in same code category

EXCLUDES Adhesive strips only, see appropriate E&M service
Complex repair nerves, blood vessels, tendons (see appropriate anatomical section)
Debridement:
  Performed separately, no closure (11042-11047 [11045, 11046])
  That requires:
    Comprehensive cleaning
    Removal of significant tissue
    Removal soft tissue and/or bone, no fracture/dislocation (11042-11047 [11045, 11046])
    Removal soft tissue and/or bone with open fracture/dislocation (11010-11012)
Deep tissue repair (12031-13153)
Major exploration (20100-20103)
Repair of nerves, blood vessels, tendons (See appropriate anatomical section. These repairs include simple and intermediate closure. Report complex closure with modifier 59.)
Secondary closure/dehiscence (13160)
Code also modifier 59 added to the less complicated procedure code if reporting more than one classification of wound repair

12001 Simple repair of superficial wounds of scalp, neck, axillae, external genitalia, trunk and/or extremities (including hands and feet); 2.5 cm or less
🏥 1.27 ⚕ 2.53 **FUD** 000 [01] [N1] [▭]
AMA: 2018,Sep,7; 2018,Jan,8; 2017,Dec,14; 2017,Jan,8; 2016,Jan,13; 2015,Jan,16; 2014,Jan,11

12002 2.6 cm to 7.5 cm
🏥 1.67 ⚕ 3.08 **FUD** 000 [01] [N1] [▭]
AMA: 2018,Sep,7; 2018,Jan,8; 2017,Jan,8; 2016,Jan,13; 2015,Jan,16; 2014,Oct,14; 2014,Jan,11

12004 7.6 cm to 12.5 cm
🏥 2.09 ⚕ 3.61 **FUD** 000 [01] [N1] [▭]
AMA: 2018,Sep,7; 2018,Jan,8; 2017,Jan,8; 2016,Jan,13; 2015,Jan,16; 2014,Jan,11

12005 12.6 cm to 20.0 cm
🏥 2.71 ⚕ 4.69 **FUD** 000 [01] [A2] [▭]
AMA: 2018,Sep,7; 2018,Jan,8; 2017,Jan,8; 2016,Jan,13; 2015,Jan,16; 2014,Jan,11

12006 20.1 cm to 30.0 cm
🏥 3.33 ⚕ 5.54 **FUD** 000 [02] [A2] [▭]
AMA: 2018,Sep,7; 2018,Jan,8; 2017,Jan,8; 2016,Jan,13; 2015,Jan,16; 2014,Jan,11

12007 over 30.0 cm
🏥 4.15 ⚕ 6.37 **FUD** 000 [T] [A2] [▭]
AMA: 2018,Sep,7; 2018,Jan,8; 2017,Jan,8; 2016,Jan,13; 2015,Jan,16; 2014,Jan,11

12011 Simple repair of superficial wounds of face, ears, eyelids, nose, lips and/or mucous membranes; 2.5 cm or less
🏥 1.57 ⚕ 3.09 **FUD** 000 [01] [N1] [▭]
AMA: 2018,Sep,7; 2018,Jan,8; 2017,Jan,8; 2016,Nov,7; 2016,Jan,13; 2015,Jan,16; 2014,Jan,11

12013 2.6 cm to 5.0 cm
🏥 1.66 ⚕ 3.23 **FUD** 000 [01] [N1] [▭]
AMA: 2018,Sep,7; 2018,Jan,8; 2017,Jan,8; 2016,Jan,13; 2015,Jan,16; 2014,Jan,11

12014 5.1 cm to 7.5 cm
🏥 2.14 ⚕ 3.88 **FUD** 000 [01] [N1] [▭]
AMA: 2018,Sep,7; 2018,Jan,8; 2017,Jan,8; 2016,Jan,13; 2015,Jan,16; 2014,Jan,11

12015	**7.6 cm to 12.5 cm**				
	🚑 2.69	✂ 4.69	**FUD** 000		01 G2 ▱

AMA: 2018,Sep,7; 2018,Jan,8; 2017,Jan,8; 2016,Jan,13; 2015,Jan,16; 2014,Jan,11

12016	**12.6 cm to 20.0 cm**				
	🚑 3.67	✂ 5.92	**FUD** 000		01 A2 ▱

AMA: 2018,Sep,7; 2018,Jan,8; 2017,Jan,8; 2016,Jan,13; 2015,Jan,16; 2014,Jan,11

12017	**20.1 cm to 30.0 cm**				
	🚑 4.38	✂ 4.38	**FUD** 000		01 A2 80 ▱

AMA: 2018,Sep,7; 2018,Jan,8; 2017,Jan,8; 2016,Jan,13; 2015,Jan,16; 2014,Jan,11

12018	**over 30.0 cm**				
	🚑 4.96	✂ 4.96	**FUD** 000		01 A2 80 ▱

AMA: 2018,Sep,7; 2018,Jan,8; 2017,Jan,8; 2016,Jan,13; 2015,Jan,16; 2014,Jan,11

12020	**Treatment of superficial wound dehiscence; simple closure**

> EXCLUDES *Secondary closure major/complex wound or dehiscence (13160)*

	🚑 5.41	✂ 8.17	**FUD** 010		T A2 ▱

AMA: 2018,Jan,8; 2017,Jan,8; 2016,Jan,13; 2015,Jan,16; 2014,Jan,11

12021	**with packing**

> EXCLUDES *Secondary closure major/complex wound or dehiscence (13160)*

	🚑 3.98	✂ 4.76	**FUD** 010		T A2 ▱

AMA: 2018,Jan,8; 2017,Jan,8; 2016,Jan,13; 2015,Jan,16; 2014,Jan,11

12031-12057 Suturing of Intermediate Wounds

INCLUDES Administration of local anesthesia
Repair that involves:
    Closure of contaminated single layer wound
    Layered closure (e.g., subcutaneous tissue, superficial fascia)
    Limited undermining
    Removal foreign material (e.g. gravel, glass)
    Routine debridement and decontamination
Simple:
    Exploration nerves, blood vessels, tendons in wound
    Vessel ligation, in wound
Total length of several repairs in same code category

EXCLUDES *Debridement:*
    Performed separately, no closure (11042-11047 [11045, 11046])
    That requires:
        Removal soft tissue and/or bone, no fracture/dislocation (11042-11047 [11045, 11046])
        Removal soft tissue/bone due to open fracture/dislocation (11010-11012)
    Major exploration (20100-20103)
    Repair of nerves, blood vessels, tendons (See appropriate anatomical section. These repairs include simple and intermediate closure. Report complex closure with modifier 59.)
    Secondary closure major/complex wound or dehiscence (13160)
    Wound repair involving more than layered closure
Code also modifier 59 added to the less complicated procedure code if reporting more than one classification of wound repair

12031	**Repair, intermediate, wounds of scalp, axillae, trunk and/or extremities (excluding hands and feet); 2.5 cm or less**

	🚑 4.40	✂ 6.98	**FUD** 010		T P2 ▱

AMA: 2018,Sep,7; 2018,Jan,8; 2017,Jan,8; 2016,Jan,13; 2015,Jan,16; 2014,Jan,11

12032	**2.6 cm to 7.5 cm**				
	🚑 5.58	✂ 8.65	**FUD** 010		T P2 ▱

AMA: 2018,Sep,7; 2018,Jan,8; 2017,Jan,8; 2016,Jan,13; 2015,Jan,16; 2014,Jan,11

12034	**7.6 cm to 12.5 cm**				
	🚑 5.96	✂ 9.07	**FUD** 010		T A2 ▱

AMA: 2018,Sep,7; 2018,Jan,8; 2017,Jan,8; 2016,Jan,13; 2015,Jan,16; 2014,Jan,11

12035	**12.6 cm to 20.0 cm**				
	🚑 6.91	✂ 10.9	**FUD** 010		T A2 ▱

AMA: 2018,Sep,7; 2018,Jan,8; 2017,Jan,8; 2016,Jan,13; 2015,Jan,16; 2014,Jan,11

12036	**20.1 cm to 30.0 cm**				
	🚑 8.05	✂ 12.1	**FUD** 010		T A2 ▱

AMA: 2018,Sep,7; 2018,Jan,8; 2017,Jan,8; 2016,Jan,13; 2015,Jan,16; 2014,Jan,11

12037	**over 30.0 cm**				
	🚑 9.41	✂ 13.7	**FUD** 010		T A2 80 ▱

AMA: 2018,Sep,7; 2018,Jan,8; 2017,Jan,8; 2016,Jan,13; 2015,Jan,16; 2014,Jan,11

12041	**Repair, intermediate, wounds of neck, hands, feet and/or external genitalia; 2.5 cm or less**

	🚑 4.29	✂ 6.97	**FUD** 010		02 P2 ▱

AMA: 2018,Sep,7; 2018,Jan,8; 2017,Jan,8; 2016,Jan,13; 2015,Jan,16; 2014,Jan,11

12042	**2.6 cm to 7.5 cm**				
	🚑 5.75	✂ 8.41	**FUD** 010		T P2 ▱

AMA: 2018,Sep,7; 2018,Jan,8; 2017,Jan,8; 2016,Jan,13; 2015,Jan,16; 2014,Jan,11

12044	**7.6 cm to 12.5 cm**				
	🚑 6.17	✂ 10.4	**FUD** 010		T A2 ▱

AMA: 2018,Sep,7; 2018,Jan,8; 2017,Jan,8; 2016,Jan,13; 2015,Jan,16; 2014,Jan,11

12045	**12.6 cm to 20.0 cm**				
	🚑 7.71	✂ 11.4	**FUD** 010		T A2 ▱

AMA: 2018,Sep,7; 2018,Jan,8; 2017,Jan,8; 2016,Jan,13; 2015,Jan,16; 2014,Jan,11

12046	**20.1 cm to 30.0 cm**				
	🚑 9.01	✂ 13.8	**FUD** 010		T A2 80 ▱

AMA: 2018,Sep,7; 2018,Jan,8; 2017,Jan,8; 2016,Jan,13; 2015,Jan,16; 2014,Jan,11

12047	**over 30.0 cm**				
	🚑 10.0	✂ 15.2	**FUD** 010		T A2 80 ▱

AMA: 2018,Sep,7; 2018,Jan,8; 2017,Jan,8; 2016,Jan,13; 2015,Jan,16; 2014,Jan,11

12051	**Repair, intermediate, wounds of face, ears, eyelids, nose, lips and/or mucous membranes; 2.5 cm or less**

	🚑 4.92	✂ 7.55	**FUD** 010		T P2 ▱

AMA: 2018,Sep,7; 2018,Jan,8; 2017,Jan,8; 2016,Jan,13; 2015,Jan,16; 2014,Jan,11

12052	**2.6 cm to 5.0 cm**				
	🚑 5.85	✂ 8.55	**FUD** 010		T P2 ▱

AMA: 2018,Sep,7; 2018,Jan,8; 2017,Jan,8; 2016,Jan,13; 2015,Jan,16; 2014,Jan,11

12053	**5.1 cm to 7.5 cm**				
	🚑 6.26	✂ 10.0	**FUD** 010		T P2 ▱

AMA: 2018,Sep,7; 2018,Jan,8; 2017,Jan,8; 2016,Jan,13; 2015,Jan,16; 2014,Jan,11

12054	**7.6 cm to 12.5 cm**				
	🚑 6.37	✂ 10.4	**FUD** 010		02 A2 ▱

AMA: 2018,Sep,7; 2018,Jan,8; 2017,Jan,8; 2016,Jan,13; 2015,Jan,16; 2014,Jan,11

12055	**12.6 cm to 20.0 cm**				
	🚑 8.67	✂ 13.5	**FUD** 010		T A2 ▱

AMA: 2018,Sep,7; 2018,Jan,8; 2017,Jan,8; 2016,Jan,13; 2015,Jan,16; 2014,Jan,11

12056	**20.1 cm to 30.0 cm**				
	🚑 11.0	✂ 16.0	**FUD** 010		02 A2 80 ▱

AMA: 2018,Sep,7; 2018,Jan,8; 2017,Jan,8; 2016,Jan,13; 2015,Jan,16; 2014,Jan,11

12057	**over 30.0 cm**				
	🚑 12.2	✂ 16.9	**FUD** 010		T A2 80 ▱

AMA: 2018,Sep,7; 2018,Jan,8; 2017,Jan,8; 2016,Jan,13; 2015,Jan,16; 2014,Jan,11

Integumentary System

13100 — 13160

13100-13160 Suturing of Complicated Wounds

INCLUDES Creation of a limited defect for repair
Debridement complicated wounds/avulsions
Repair with layered closure that involves at least one of the following:
Debridement of wound edges
Exposure of underlying structures, such as bone, cartilage, tendon, or named neovascular structure
Extensive undermining
Free margin involvement of helical or nostril rim or vermillion border
Retention suture placement
Simple:
Exploration nerves, vessels, tendons in wound
Vessel ligation in wound
Total length of several repairs in same code category

EXCLUDES Excision (of or for):
Benign lesions (11400-11446)
Extensive debridement of open fracture/dislocation (11010-11012)
Extensive debridement of penetrating or blunt trauma not associated with open fracture/dislocation (11042-11047 [11045, 11046])
Malignant lesions (11600-11646)
Surgical preparation of a wound bed (15002-15005)
Extensive exploration (20100-20103)
Repair of nerves, blood vessel, tendons (See appropriate anatomical section. These repairs include simple and intermediate closure. Report complex closure with modifier 59.)
Code also modifier 59 added to the less complicated procedure code if reporting more than one classification of wound repair

13100 **Repair, complex, trunk; 1.1 cm to 2.5 cm**

EXCLUDES Complex repair 1.0 cm or less (12001, 12031)
🚑 5.90 ✂ 9.66 **FUD** 010 T A2 ▣

AMA: 2018,Sep,7; 2018,Jan,8; 2017,Apr,9; 2017,Jan,8; 2016,Jan,13; 2015,Jan,16; 2014,Jan,11

13101 **2.6 cm to 7.5 cm**

🚑 7.27 ✂ 11.3 **FUD** 010 T A2 ▣

AMA: 2018,Sep,7; 2018,Jan,8; 2017,Apr,9; 2017,Jan,8; 2016,Jan,13; 2015,Jan,16; 2014,Jan,11

+ 13102 **each additional 5 cm or less (List separately in addition to code for primary procedure)**

Code first (13101)
🚑 2.14 ✂ 3.46 **FUD** ZZZ N N1 ▣

AMA: 2018,Sep,7; 2018,Jan,8; 2017,Apr,9; 2017,Jan,8; 2016,Jan,13; 2015,Jan,16; 2014,Jan,11

13120 **Repair, complex, scalp, arms, and/or legs; 1.1 cm to 2.5 cm**

EXCLUDES Complex repair 1.0 cm or less (12001, 12031)
🚑 6.78 ✂ 10.0 **FUD** 010 T A2 ▣

AMA: 2018,Sep,7; 2018,Jan,8; 2017,Jan,8; 2016,Jan,13; 2015,Jan,16; 2014,Jan,11

13121 **2.6 cm to 7.5 cm**

🚑 7.67 ✂ 12.2 **FUD** 010 T A2 ▣

AMA: 2018,Sep,7; 2018,Jan,8; 2017,Jan,8; 2016,Jan,13; 2015,Jan,16; 2014,Jan,11

+ 13122 **each additional 5 cm or less (List separately in addition to code for primary procedure)**

Code first (13121)
🚑 2.47 ✂ 3.78 **FUD** ZZZ N N1 ▣

AMA: 2018,Sep,7; 2018,Jan,8; 2017,Jan,8; 2016,Jan,13; 2015,Jan,16; 2014,Jan,11

13131 **Repair, complex, forehead, cheeks, chin, mouth, neck, axillae, genitalia, hands and/or feet; 1.1 cm to 2.5 cm**

EXCLUDES Complex repair 1.0 cm or less (12001, 12011, 12031, 12041, 12051)
🚑 7.17 ✂ 11.0 **FUD** 010 T A2 ▣

AMA: 2018,Sep,7; 2018,Jan,8; 2017,Apr,9; 2017,Jan,8; 2016,Jan,13; 2015,Jan,16; 2014,Jan,11

13132 **2.6 cm to 7.5 cm**

🚑 9.03 ✂ 13.6 **FUD** 010 T A2 ▣

AMA: 2018,Sep,7; 2018,Jan,8; 2017,Apr,9; 2017,Jan,8; 2016,Jan,13; 2015,Jan,16; 2014,Oct,14; 2014,Jan,11

+ 13133 **each additional 5 cm or less (List separately in addition to code for primary procedure)**

Code first (13132)
🚑 3.77 ✂ 5.06 **FUD** ZZZ N N1 ▣

AMA: 2018,Sep,7; 2018,Jan,8; 2017,Apr,9; 2017,Jan,8; 2016,Jan,13; 2015,Jan,16; 2014,Jan,11

13151 **Repair, complex, eyelids, nose, ears and/or lips; 1.1 cm to 2.5 cm**

EXCLUDES Complex repair 1.0 cm or less (12011, 12051)
🚑 8.25 ✂ 12.1 **FUD** 010 T A2 ▣

AMA: 2018,Sep,7; 2018,Jan,8; 2017,Jan,8; 2016,Jan,13; 2015,Jan,16; 2014,May,3; 2014,Mar,12; 2014,Jan,11

13152 **2.6 cm to 7.5 cm**

🚑 9.99 ✂ 14.4 **FUD** 010 T A2 ▣

AMA: 2018,Sep,7; 2018,Jan,8; 2017,Jan,8; 2016,Jan,13; 2015,Jan,16; 2014,Oct,14; 2014,May,3; 2014,Mar,12; 2014,Jan,11

+ 13153 **each additional 5 cm or less (List separately in addition to code for primary procedure)**

Code first (13152)
🚑 4.07 ✂ 5.50 **FUD** ZZZ N N1 ▣

AMA: 2018,Sep,7; 2018,Jan,8; 2017,Jan,8; 2016,Jan,13; 2015,Jan,16; 2014,May,3; 2014,Mar,12; 2014,Jan,11

13160 **Secondary closure of surgical wound or dehiscence, extensive or complicated**

EXCLUDES Packing or simple secondary wound closure (12020-12021)
🚑 22.9 ✂ 22.9 **FUD** 090 T A2 ▣

AMA: 2018,Jan,8; 2017,Jan,8; 2016,Jan,13; 2015,Jan,16; 2014,Jan,11

26/TC PC/TC Only   A2-Z3 ASC Payment   50 Bilateral   ♂ Male Only   ♀ Female Only   🚑 Facility RVU   ✂ Non-Facility RVU   ▣ CCI   ❌ CLIA
FUD Follow-up Days   **CMS:** IOM   **AMA:** CPT Asst   A-Y OPPSI   80/80 Surg Assist Allowed / w/Doc   Lab Crosswalk   Radiology Crosswalk

22   CPT © 2019 American Medical Association. All Rights Reserved.   © 2019 Optum360, LLC

14000-14350 Reposition Contiguous Tissue

INCLUDES Excision (with or without lesion) with repair by adjacent tissue transfer or tissue rearrangement

Size of defect includes primary (due to excision) and secondary (due to flap design)

Z-plasty, W-plasty, VY-plasty, rotation flap, advancement flap, double pedicle flap, random island flap

EXCLUDES Closure of wounds by undermining surrounding tissue without additional incisions (13100-13160)

Full thickness closure of:
Eyelid (67930-67935, 67961-67975)
Lip (40650-40654)

Code also skin graft necessary to repair secondary defect (15040-15731)

14000 Adjacent tissue transfer or rearrangement, trunk; defect 10 sq cm or less

INCLUDES Burrow's operation

EXCLUDES Excision of lesion with repair by adjacent tissue transfer or tissue rearrangement (11400-11446, 11600-11646)

🚑 14.3 ⚕ 17.8 **FUD** 090 T A2 ▢

AMA: 2018,Jan,8; 2017,Oct,9; 2017,Jan,8; 2016,Jan,13; 2015,Sep,12; 2015,Feb,10; 2015,Jan,16; 2014,Apr,10; 2014,Jan,11

Example of common Z-plasty. Lesion is removed with oval-shaped incision

Two additional incisions (a. and b.) intersect the area

Skin of each incision is reflected back

The flaps are then transposed and the repair is closed

An adjacent flap, or other rearrangement flap, is performed to repair a defect

14001 defect 10.1 sq cm to 30.0 sq cm

EXCLUDES Excision of lesion with repair by adjacent tissue transfer or tissue rearrangement (11400-11446, 11600-11646)

🚑 18.7 ⚕ 22.8 **FUD** 090 T A2 ▢

AMA: 2018,Jan,8; 2017,Oct,9; 2017,Jan,8; 2016,Jan,13; 2015,Feb,10; 2015,Jan,16; 2014,Apr,10; 2014,Jan,11

14020 Adjacent tissue transfer or rearrangement, scalp, arms and/or legs; defect 10 sq cm or less

EXCLUDES Excision of lesion with repair by adjacent tissue transfer or tissue rearrangement (11400-11446, 11600-11646)

🚑 16.2 ⚕ 19.8 **FUD** 090 T A2 ▢

AMA: 2018,Jan,8; 2017,Jan,8; 2016,Jan,13; 2015,Jan,16; 2014,Jan,11

14021 defect 10.1 sq cm to 30.0 sq cm

EXCLUDES Excision of lesion with repair by adjacent tissue transfer or tissue rearrangement (11400-11446, 11600-11646)

🚑 20.5 ⚕ 24.7 **FUD** 090 T A2 ▢

AMA: 2018,Jan,8; 2017,Jan,8; 2016,Jan,13; 2015,Jan,16; 2014,Jan,11

14040 Adjacent tissue transfer or rearrangement, forehead, cheeks, chin, mouth, neck, axillae, genitalia, hands and/or feet; defect 10 sq cm or less

INCLUDES Krimer's palatoplasty

EXCLUDES Excision of lesion with repair by adjacent tissue transfer or tissue rearrangement (11400-11446, 11600-11646)

🚑 18.1 ⚕ 21.7 **FUD** 090 T A2 ▢

AMA: 2018,Jan,8; 2017,Nov,6; 2017,Jan,8; 2016,Jan,13; 2015,Jan,16; 2014,Jan,11

14041 defect 10.1 sq cm to 30.0 sq cm

EXCLUDES Excision of lesion with repair by adjacent tissue transfer or tissue rearrangement (11400-11446, 11600-11646)

🚑 22.3 ⚕ 26.7 **FUD** 090 T A2 ▢

AMA: 2018,Jan,8; 2017,Nov,6; 2017,Jan,8; 2016,Jan,13; 2015,Jan,16; 2014,Jan,11

14060 Adjacent tissue transfer or rearrangement, eyelids, nose, ears and/or lips; defect 10 sq cm or less

INCLUDES Denonvillier's operation

EXCLUDES Excision of lesion with repair by adjacent tissue transfer or tissue rearrangement (11400-11446, 11600-11646)

Eyelid, full thickness (67961-67966)

🚑 19.3 ⚕ 22.1 **FUD** 090 T A2 ▢

AMA: 2018,Jan,8; 2017,Nov,6; 2017,Jan,8; 2016,Jan,13; 2015,Jan,16; 2014,Jan,11

14061 defect 10.1 sq cm to 30.0 sq cm

EXCLUDES Excision of lesion with repair by adjacent tissue transfer or tissue rearrangement (11400-11446, 11600-11646)

Eyelid, full thickness (67961 and subsequent codes)

🚑 23.8 ⚕ 28.7 **FUD** 090 T A2 ▢

AMA: 2018,Jan,8; 2017,Nov,6; 2017,Jan,8; 2016,Jan,13; 2015,Jan,16; 2014,Jan,11

14301 Adjacent tissue transfer or rearrangement, any area; defect 30.1 sq cm to 60.0 sq cm

EXCLUDES Excision of lesion with repair by adjacent tissue transfer or tissue rearrangement (11400-11446, 11600-11646)

🚑 25.2 ⚕ 30.7 **FUD** 090 T G2 80 ▢

AMA: 2018,Jan,8; 2017,Nov,6; 2017,Apr,9; 2017,Jan,8; 2016,Jan,13; 2015,Jan,16; 2014,Jan,11

+ 14302 each additional 30.0 sq cm, or part thereof (List separately in addition to code for primary procedure)

EXCLUDES Excision of lesion with repair by adjacent tissue transfer or tissue rearrangement (11400-11446, 11600-11646)

Code first (14301)

🚑 6.34 ⚕ 6.34 **FUD** ZZZ N N1 80 ▢

AMA: 2018,Jan,8; 2017,Nov,6; 2017,Jan,8; 2016,Jan,13; 2015,Jan,16; 2014,Jan,11

14350 Filleted finger or toe flap, including preparation of recipient site

🚑 19.6 ⚕ 19.6 **FUD** 090 T A2 80 ▢

AMA: 2018,Jan,8; 2017,Jan,8; 2016,Jan,13; 2015,Jan,16; 2014,Jan,11

15002-15005 Development of Base for Tissue Grafting

INCLUDES Add together the surface area of multiple wounds in the same anatomical locations as indicated in the code descriptor groups, such as face and scalp. Do not add together multiple wounds at different anatomical site groups such as trunk and face

Ankle or wrist if code description describes leg or arm

Cleaning and preparing a viable wound surface for grafting or negative pressure wound therapy used to heal the wound primarily

Code selection based on the defect size and location

Percentage applies to children younger than age 10

Removal of nonviable tissue in nonchronic wounds for primary healing

Square centimeters applies to children and adults age 10 or older

EXCLUDES *Chronic wound management on wounds left to heal by secondary intention (11042-11047 [11045, 11046], 97597-97598)*

Necrotizing soft tissue infections for specific anatomical locations (11004-11008)

15002 **Surgical preparation or creation of recipient site by excision of open wounds, burn eschar, or scar (including subcutaneous tissues), or incisional release of scar contracture, trunk, arms, legs; first 100 sq cm or 1% of body area of infants and children**

EXCLUDES *Linear scar revision (13100-13153)*

6.47   9.94   **FUD** 000   T A2 80

AMA: 2018,Jan,8; 2017,Jan,8; 2016,Jan,13; 2015,Jan,16; 2014,Mar,12; 2014,Jan,11

+ 15003 **each additional 100 sq cm, or part thereof, or each additional 1% of body area of infants and children (List separately in addition to code for primary procedure)**

Code first (15002)

1.32   2.11   **FUD** ZZZ   N N1 80

AMA: 2018,Jan,8; 2017,Jan,8; 2016,Jan,13; 2015,Jan,16; 2014,Mar,12; 2014,Jan,11

15004 **Surgical preparation or creation of recipient site by excision of open wounds, burn eschar, or scar (including subcutaneous tissues), or incisional release of scar contracture, face, scalp, eyelids, mouth, neck, ears, orbits, genitalia, hands, feet and/or multiple digits; first 100 sq cm or 1% of body area of infants and children**

7.68   11.3   **FUD** 000   T A2 80

AMA: 2018,Jan,8; 2017,Jan,8; 2016,Jan,13; 2015,Jan,16; 2014,Mar,12; 2014,Jan,11

+ 15005 **each additional 100 sq cm, or part thereof, or each additional 1% of body area of infants and children (List separately in addition to code for primary procedure)**

Code first (15004)

2.64   3.52   **FUD** ZZZ   N N1 80

AMA: 2018,Jan,8; 2017,Jan,8; 2016,Jan,13; 2015,Jan,16; 2014,Mar,12; 2014,Jan,11

15040 Obtain Autograft

INCLUDES Ankle or wrist if code description describes leg or arm

Percentage applies to children younger than age 10

Square centimeters applies to children and adults age 10 or older

15040 **Harvest of skin for tissue cultured skin autograft, 100 sq cm or less**

3.62   7.29   **FUD** 000   T A2

AMA: 2018,Jan,8; 2017,Jan,8; 2016,Jan,13; 2015,Jan,16; 2014,Jan,11

15050 Pinch Graft

INCLUDES Autologous skin graft harvest and application

Current graft removal

Fixation and anchoring skin graft

Simple cleaning

EXCLUDES *Removal of devitalized tissue from wound(s), non-selective debridement, without anesthesia (97602)*

Code also graft or flap necessary to repair donor site

15050 **Pinch graft, single or multiple, to cover small ulcer, tip of digit, or other minimal open area (except on face), up to defect size 2 cm diameter**

12.7   16.1   **FUD** 090   T A2

AMA: 2018,Jan,8; 2017,Jan,8; 2016,Jun,8; 2016,Jan,13; 2015,Jan,16; 2014,Jan,11

15100-15261 Skin Grafts and Replacements

INCLUDES Add together the surface area of multiple wounds in the same anatomical locations as indicated in the code description groups, such as face and scalp. Do not add together multiple wounds at different anatomical site groups such as trunk and face.

Ankle or wrist if code description describes leg or arm

Autologous skin graft harvest and application

Code selection based on recipient site location and size and type of graft

Current graft removal

Fixation and anchoring skin graft

Percentage applies to children younger than age 10

Simple cleaning

Simple tissue debridement

Square centimeters applies to children and adults age 10 or older

EXCLUDES *Debridement without immediate primary closure, when wound is grossly contaminated and extensive cleaning is needed, or when necrotic or contaminated tissue is removed (11042-11047 [11045, 11046], 97597-97598)*

Removal of devitalized tissue from wound(s), non-selective debridement, without anesthesia (97602)

Code also graft or flap necessary to repair donor site

Code also primary procedure requiring skin graft for definitive closure

15100 **Split-thickness autograft, trunk, arms, legs; first 100 sq cm or less, or 1% of body area of infants and children (except 15050)**

20.5   24.5   **FUD** 090   T A2

AMA: 2018,Jan,8; 2017,Jan,8; 2016,Jun,8; 2016,Jan,13; 2015,Jan,16; 2014,Jan,11

+ 15101 **each additional 100 sq cm, or each additional 1% of body area of infants and children, or part thereof (List separately in addition to code for primary procedure)**

Code first (15100)

3.22   5.31   **FUD** ZZZ   N N1

AMA: 2018,Jan,8; 2017,Jan,8; 2016,Jun,8; 2016,Jan,13; 2015,Jan,16; 2014,Jan,11

15110 **Epidermal autograft, trunk, arms, legs; first 100 sq cm or less, or 1% of body area of infants and children**

19.8   22.8   **FUD** 090   T A2

AMA: 2018,Jan,8; 2017,Jan,8; 2016,Jan,13; 2015,Jan,16; 2014,Jan,11

+ 15111 **each additional 100 sq cm, or each additional 1% of body area of infants and children, or part thereof (List separately in addition to code for primary procedure)**

Code first (15110)

3.00   3.32   **FUD** ZZZ   N N1

AMA: 2018,Jan,8; 2017,Jan,8; 2016,Jan,13; 2015,Jan,16; 2014,Jan,11

15115 **Epidermal autograft, face, scalp, eyelids, mouth, neck, ears, orbits, genitalia, hands, feet, and/or multiple digits; first 100 sq cm or less, or 1% of body area of infants and children**

19.6   22.6   **FUD** 090   T A2

AMA: 2018,Jan,8; 2017,Jan,8; 2016,Jan,13; 2015,Jan,16; 2014,Jan,11

+ 15116 **each additional 100 sq cm, or each additional 1% of body area of infants and children, or part thereof (List separately in addition to code for primary procedure)**

Code first (15115)

4.38   4.80   **FUD** ZZZ   N N1

AMA: 2018,Jan,8; 2017,Jan,8; 2016,Jan,13; 2015,Jan,16; 2014,Jan,11

15120 **Split-thickness autograft, face, scalp, eyelids, mouth, neck, ears, orbits, genitalia, hands, feet, and/or multiple digits; first 100 sq cm or less, or 1% of body area of infants and children (except 15050)**

EXCLUDES *Other eyelid repair (67961-67975)*

20.0   24.2   **FUD** 090   T A2

AMA: 2018,Jan,8; 2017,Jan,8; 2016,Jun,8; 2016,Jan,13; 2015,Jan,16; 2014,Jan,11

+ **15121** each additional 100 sq cm, or each additional 1% of body area of infants and children, or part thereof (List separately in addition to code for primary procedure)

EXCLUDES *Other eyelid repair (67961-67975)*
Code first (15120)
⚕ 3.86   ⚖ 5.95   **FUD** ZZZ   N N1 ▭
AMA: 2018,Jan,8; 2017,Jan,8; 2016,Jun,8; 2016,Jan,13; 2015,Jan,16; 2014,Jan,11

15130 **Dermal autograft, trunk, arms, legs; first 100 sq cm or less, or 1% of body area of infants and children**
⚕ 15.9   ⚖ 19.0   **FUD** 090   T A2 ▭
AMA: 2018,Jan,8; 2017,Jan,8; 2016,Jan,13; 2015,Jan,16; 2014,Jan,11

+ **15131** each additional 100 sq cm, or each additional 1% of body area of infants and children, or part thereof (List separately in addition to code for primary procedure)
Code first (15130)
⚕ 2.63   ⚖ 2.85   **FUD** ZZZ   N N1 ▭
AMA: 2018,Jan,8; 2017,Jan,8; 2016,Jan,13; 2015,Jan,16; 2014,Jan,11

15135 **Dermal autograft, face, scalp, eyelids, mouth, neck, ears, orbits, genitalia, hands, feet, and/or multiple digits; first 100 sq cm or less, or 1% of body area of infants and children**
⚕ 21.4   ⚖ 24.5   **FUD** 090   T A2 ▭
AMA: 2018,Jan,8; 2017,Jan,8; 2016,Jan,13; 2015,Jan,16; 2014,Jan,11

+ **15136** each additional 100 sq cm, or each additional 1% of body area of infants and children, or part thereof (List separately in addition to code for primary procedure)
Code first (15135)
⚕ 2.63   ⚖ 2.82   **FUD** ZZZ   N N1 ▭
AMA: 2018,Jan,8; 2017,Jan,8; 2016,Jan,13; 2015,Jan,16; 2014,Jan,11

15150 **Tissue cultured skin autograft, trunk, arms, legs; first 25 sq cm or less**
⚕ 18.3   ⚖ 20.0   **FUD** 090   T A2 ▭
AMA: 2018,Jan,8; 2017,Jan,8; 2016,Jan,13; 2015,Jan,16; 2014,Jan,11

+ **15151** additional 1 sq cm to 75 sq cm (List separately in addition to code for primary procedure)
EXCLUDES *Grafts over 75 sq cm (15152)*
Use of code more than one time per session
Code first (15150)
⚕ 3.19   ⚖ 3.45   **FUD** ZZZ   N N1 ▭
AMA: 2018,Jan,8; 2017,Jan,8; 2016,Jan,13; 2015,Jan,16; 2014,Jan,11

+ **15152** each additional 100 sq cm, or each additional 1% of body area of infants and children, or part thereof (List separately in addition to code for primary procedure)
Code first (15151)
⚕ 3.98   ⚖ 4.25   **FUD** ZZZ   N N1 ▭
AMA: 2018,Jan,8; 2017,Jan,8; 2016,Jan,13; 2015,Jan,16; 2014,Jan,11

15155 **Tissue cultured skin autograft, face, scalp, eyelids, mouth, neck, ears, orbits, genitalia, hands, feet, and/or multiple digits; first 25 sq cm or less**
⚕ 21.0   ⚖ 22.8   **FUD** 090   T A2 ▭
AMA: 2018,Jan,8; 2017,Jan,8; 2016,Jan,13; 2015,Jan,16; 2014,Jan,11

+ **15156** additional 1 sq cm to 75 sq cm (List separately in addition to code for primary procedure)
EXCLUDES *Grafts over 75 sq cm (15157)*
Use of code more than one time per session
Code first (15155)
⚕ 4.38   ⚖ 4.65   **FUD** ZZZ   N N1 ▭
AMA: 2018,Jan,8; 2017,Jan,8; 2016,Jan,13; 2015,Jan,16; 2014,Jan,11

+ **15157** each additional 100 sq cm, or each additional 1% of body area of infants and children, or part thereof (List separately in addition to code for primary procedure)
Code first (15156)
⚕ 4.78   ⚖ 5.17   **FUD** ZZZ   N N1 ▭
AMA: 2018,Jan,8; 2017,Jan,8; 2016,Jan,13; 2015,Jan,16; 2014,Jan,11

15200 **Full thickness graft, free, including direct closure of donor site, trunk; 20 sq cm or less**
⚕ 19.3   ⚖ 23.8   **FUD** 090   T A2 ▭
AMA: 2018,Jan,8; 2017,Jan,8; 2016,Jun,8; 2016,Jan,13; 2015,Jan,16; 2014,Jan,11

+ **15201** each additional 20 sq cm, or part thereof (List separately in addition to code for primary procedure)
Code first (15200)
⚕ 2.26   ⚖ 4.14   **FUD** ZZZ   N N1 ▭
AMA: 2018,Jan,8; 2017,Jan,8; 2016,Jun,8; 2016,Jan,13; 2015,Jan,16; 2014,Jan,11

15220 **Full thickness graft, free, including direct closure of donor site, scalp, arms, and/or legs; 20 sq cm or less**
⚕ 17.6   ⚖ 22.0   **FUD** 090   T A2 ▭
AMA: 2018,Jan,8; 2017,Jan,8; 2016,Jun,8; 2016,Jan,13; 2015,Jan,16; 2014,Jan,11

+ **15221** each additional 20 sq cm, or part thereof (List separately in addition to code for primary procedure)
Code first (15220)
⚕ 2.05   ⚖ 3.87   **FUD** ZZZ   N N1 ▭
AMA: 2018,Jan,8; 2017,Jan,8; 2016,Jun,8; 2016,Jan,13; 2015,Jan,16; 2014,Jan,11

15240 **Full thickness graft, free, including direct closure of donor site, forehead, cheeks, chin, mouth, neck, axillae, genitalia, hands, and/or feet; 20 sq cm or less**
EXCLUDES *Fingertip graft (15050)*
Syndactyly repair fingers (26560-26562)
⚕ 23.0   ⚖ 26.6   **FUD** 090   T A2 ▭
AMA: 2018,Jan,8; 2017,Jan,8; 2016,Jun,8; 2016,Jan,13; 2015,Jan,16; 2014,Jan,11

+ **15241** each additional 20 sq cm, or part thereof (List separately in addition to code for primary procedure)
Code first (15240)
⚕ 3.18   ⚖ 5.22   **FUD** ZZZ   N N1 ▭
AMA: 2018,Jan,8; 2017,Jan,8; 2016,Jun,8; 2016,Jan,13; 2015,Jan,16; 2014,Jan,11

15260 **Full thickness graft, free, including direct closure of donor site, nose, ears, eyelids, and/or lips; 20 sq cm or less**
EXCLUDES *Other eyelid repair (67961-67975)*
⚕ 24.6   ⚖ 28.8   **FUD** 090   T A2 ▭
AMA: 2018,Jan,8; 2017,Jan,8; 2016,Jun,8; 2016,Jan,13; 2015,Jan,16; 2014,Jan,11

+ **15261** each additional 20 sq cm, or part thereof (List separately in addition to code for primary procedure)
EXCLUDES *Other eyelid repair (67961-67975)*
Code first (15260)
⚕ 4.01   ⚖ 6.05   **FUD** ZZZ   N N1 ▭
AMA: 2018,Jan,8; 2017,Jan,8; 2016,Jun,8; 2016,Jan,13; 2015,Jan,16; 2014,Jan,11

● New Code   ▲ Revised Code   ○ Reinstated   ● New Web Release   ▲ Revised Web Release   + Add-on   Unlisted   Not Covered   # Resequenced
⑤⓪ Optum Mod 50 Exempt   ⊘ AMA Mod 51 Exempt   ⑤① Optum Mod 51 Exempt   ⑥③ Mod 63 Exempt   ✗ Non-FDA Drug   ★ Telemedicine   M Maternity   A Age Edit

CPT © 2019 American Medical Association. All Rights Reserved.

15271-15278 Skin Substitute Graft Application

INCLUDES Add together the surface area of multiple wounds in the same anatomical locations as indicated in the code description groups, such as face and scalp. Do not add together multiple wounds at different anatomical site groups such as trunk and face.
Ankle or wrist if code description describes leg or arm
Code selection based on defect site location and size
Fixation and anchoring skin graft
Graft types include:
  Biological material used for tissue engineering (e.g.,scaffold) for growing skin
  Nonautologous human skin such as:
    Acellular
    Allograft
    Cellular
    Dermal
    Epidermal
    Homograft
    Nonhuman grafts
Percentage applies to children younger than age 10
Removing current graft
Simple cleaning
Simple tissue debridement
Square centimeters applies to children and adults age 10 or older

EXCLUDES *Application of nongraft dressing*
Injected skin substitutes
Removal of devitalized tissue from wound(s), non-selective debridement, without anesthesia (97602)
Skin application procedures, low cost (C5271-C5278)
Code also biologic implant for soft tissue reinforcement (15777)
Code also primary procedure requiring skin graft for definitive closure
Code also supply of high cost skin substitute product (C9363, Q4101, Q4103-Q4110, Q4116, Q4121-Q4123, Q4126-Q4128, Q4132-Q4133, Q4137-Q4138, Q4140-Q4141, Q4143, Q4146-Q4148, Q4150-Q4161, Q4163-Q4164, Q4169, Q4173, Q4175, Q4178)

15271 **Application of skin substitute graft to trunk, arms, legs, total wound surface area up to 100 sq cm; first 25 sq cm or less wound surface area**

EXCLUDES *Total wound area greater than or equal to 100 sq cm (15273-15274)*

🔌 2.42   ⚖ 4.14   **FUD** 000   T G2 ▢

AMA: 2018,Jan,8; 2017,Oct,9; 2017,Jan,8; 2016,Jan,13; 2015,Jan,16; 2014,Jun,14; 2014,Jan,11

+ 15272 **each additional 25 sq cm wound surface area, or part thereof (List separately in addition to code for primary procedure)**

EXCLUDES *Total wound area greater than or equal to 100 sq cm (15273-15274)*
Code first (15271)

🔌 0.50   ⚖ 0.76   **FUD** ZZZ   N N1 ▢

AMA: 2018,Jan,8; 2017,Jan,8; 2016,Jan,13; 2015,Jan,16; 2014,Jun,14; 2014,Jan,11

15273 **Application of skin substitute graft to trunk, arms, legs, total wound surface area greater than or equal to 100 sq cm; first 100 sq cm wound surface area, or 1% of body area of infants and children**

EXCLUDES *Total wound surface area up to 100 cm (15271-15272)*

🔌 5.84   ⚖ 8.73   **FUD** 000   T G2 ▢

AMA: 2018,Jan,8; 2017,Jan,8; 2016,Jan,13; 2015,Jan,16; 2014,Jun,14; 2014,Jan,11

+ 15274 **each additional 100 sq cm wound surface area, or part thereof, or each additional 1% of body area of infants and children, or part thereof (List separately in addition to code for primary procedure)**

EXCLUDES *Total wound surface area up to 100 cm (15273)*
Code first (15273)

🔌 1.33   ⚖ 2.15   **FUD** ZZZ   N N1 ▢

AMA: 2018,Jan,8; 2017,Jan,8; 2016,Jan,13; 2015,Jan,16; 2014,Jun,14; 2014,Jan,11

15275 **Application of skin substitute graft to face, scalp, eyelids, mouth, neck, ears, orbits, genitalia, hands, feet, and/or multiple digits, total wound surface area up to 100 sq cm; first 25 sq cm or less wound surface area**

EXCLUDES *Total wound area greater than or equal to 100 sq cm (15277-15278)*

🔌 2.74   ⚖ 4.37   **FUD** 000   T G2 ▢

AMA: 2018,Jan,8; 2017,Jan,8; 2016,Jan,13; 2015,Jan,16; 2014,Jun,14; 2014,Jan,11

+ 15276 **each additional 25 sq cm wound surface area, or part thereof (List separately in addition to code for primary procedure)**

EXCLUDES *Total wound area greater than or equal to 100 sq cm (15277-15278)*
Code first (15275)

🔌 0.73   ⚖ 0.98   **FUD** ZZZ   N N1 ▢

AMA: 2018,Jan,8; 2017,Jan,8; 2016,Jan,13; 2015,Jan,16; 2014,Jun,14; 2014,Jan,11

15277 **Application of skin substitute graft to face, scalp, eyelids, mouth, neck, ears, orbits, genitalia, hands, feet, and/or multiple digits, total wound surface area greater than or equal to 100 sq cm; first 100 sq cm wound surface area, or 1% of body area of infants and children**

EXCLUDES *Total surface area up to 100 sq cm (15275-15276)*

🔌 6.60   ⚖ 9.55   **FUD** 000   T G2 ▢

AMA: 2018,Jan,8; 2017,Jan,8; 2016,Jan,13; 2015,Jan,16; 2014,Jun,14; 2014,Jan,11

+ 15278 **each additional 100 sq cm wound surface area, or part thereof, or each additional 1% of body area of infants and children, or part thereof (List separately in addition to code for primary procedure)**

EXCLUDES *Total surface area up to 100 sq cm (15275-15276)*
Code first (15277)

🔌 1.66   ⚖ 2.54   **FUD** ZZZ   N N1 ▢

AMA: 2018,Jan,8; 2017,Jan,8; 2016,Jan,13; 2015,Jan,16; 2014,Jun,14; 2014,Jan,11

26/TC PC/TC Only   A2-Z3 ASC Payment   50 Bilateral   ♂ Male Only   ♀ Female Only   🔌 Facility RVU   ⚖ Non-Facility RVU   ▢ CCI   ✖ CLIA
FUD Follow-up Days   **CMS:** IOM   **AMA:** CPT Asst   A-Y OPPSI   80/80 Surg Assist Allowed / w/Doc   Lab Crosswalk   Radiology Crosswalk

26

15570-15731 Wound Reconstruction: Skin Flaps

INCLUDES Ankle or wrist if code description describes leg or arm
Code based on recipient site when the flap is attached in the transfer or to a final site and is based on donor site when a tube is created for transfer later or when the flap is delayed prior to transfer
Fixation and anchoring skin graft
Simple tissue debridement
Tube formation for later transfer

EXCLUDES Contiguous tissue transfer flaps (14040-14041, 14060-14061, 14301-14302)
Debridement without immediate primary closure (11042-11047 [11045, 11046], 97597-97598)
Excision of:
Benign lesion (11400-11471)
Burn eschar or scar (15002-15005)
Malignant lesion (11600-11646)
Microvascular repair (15756-15758)
Primary procedure--see appropriate anatomical site
Code also application of extensive immobilization apparatus
Code also repair of donor site with skin grafts or flaps

15570 **Formation of direct or tubed pedicle, with or without transfer; trunk**

INCLUDES Flaps without a vascular pedicle
🚑 21.0   ⚘ 26.0   **FUD** 090   [T] [A2] [□]

AMA: 2018,Jan,8; 2017,Jan,8; 2016,Jan,13; 2015,Jan,16; 2014,Jan,11

Pedicle flap

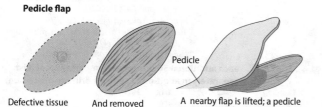

Defective tissue is identified   And removed   A nearby flap is lifted; a pedicle remains attached to provide an intact blood supply

Pedicle

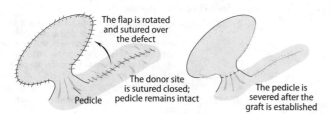

The flap is rotated and sutured over the defect

The donor site is sutured closed; pedicle remains intact

Pedicle

The pedicle is severed after the graft is established

15572 **scalp, arms, or legs**

INCLUDES Flaps without a vascular pedicle
🚑 21.3   ⚘ 25.3   **FUD** 090   [T] [A2] [□]

AMA: 2018,Jan,8; 2017,Jan,8; 2016,Jan,13; 2015,Jan,16; 2014,Jan,11

15574 **forehead, cheeks, chin, mouth, neck, axillae, genitalia, hands or feet**

INCLUDES Flaps without a vascular pedicle
🚑 21.7   ⚘ 25.8   **FUD** 090   [T] [A2] [□]

AMA: 2018,Jan,8; 2017,Jan,8; 2016,Jan,13; 2015,Jan,16; 2014,Jan,11

15576 **eyelids, nose, ears, lips, or intraoral**

INCLUDES Flaps without a vascular pedicle
🚑 19.1   ⚘ 22.9   **FUD** 090   [T] [A2] [□]

AMA: 2018,Jan,8; 2017,Jan,8; 2016,Jan,13; 2015,Jan,16; 2014,Jan,11

15600 **Delay of flap or sectioning of flap (division and inset); at trunk**

🚑 5.91   ⚘ 9.30   **FUD** 090   [T] [A2] [80] [□]

AMA: 2019,Jun,14; 2018,Jan,8; 2017,Jan,8; 2016,Jan,13; 2015,Jan,16; 2014,Jan,11

15610 **at scalp, arms, or legs**

🚑 6.86   ⚘ 10.1   **FUD** 090   [T] [A2] [80] [□]

AMA: 2018,Jan,8; 2017,Jan,8; 2016,Jan,13; 2015,Jan,16; 2014,Jan,11

15620 **at forehead, cheeks, chin, neck, axillae, genitalia, hands, or feet**

🚑 9.27   ⚘ 12.5   **FUD** 090   [T] [A2] [□]

AMA: 2018,Jan,8; 2017,Jan,8; 2016,Jan,13; 2015,Jan,16; 2014,Jan,11

15630 **at eyelids, nose, ears, or lips**

🚑 9.87   ⚘ 13.0   **FUD** 090   [T] [A2] [□]

AMA: 2018,Jan,8; 2017,Jan,8; 2016,Jan,13; 2015,Jan,16; 2014,Jan,11

15650 **Transfer, intermediate, of any pedicle flap (eg, abdomen to wrist, Walking tube), any location**

EXCLUDES Defatting, revision, or rearranging of transferred pedicle flap or skin graft (13100-14302)
Eyelids, ears, lips, and nose - refer to anatomical area
🚑 11.0   ⚘ 14.5   **FUD** 090   [T] [A2] [80] [□]

AMA: 2018,Jan,8; 2017,Jan,8; 2016,Jan,13; 2015,Jan,16; 2014,Jan,11

15730 **Midface flap (ie, zygomaticofacial flap) with preservation of vascular pedicle(s)**

🚑 26.4   ⚘ 43.6   **FUD** 090   [T] [62] [□]

AMA: 2018,Apr,10; 2018,Jan,8; 2017,Nov,6

15731 **Forehead flap with preservation of vascular pedicle (eg, axial pattern flap, paramedian forehead flap)**

EXCLUDES Muscle, myocutaneous, or fasciocutaneous flap of the head or neck (15733)
🚑 28.7   ⚘ 32.0   **FUD** 090   [T] [A2] [80] [□]

AMA: 2018,Jan,8; 2017,Nov,6; 2017,Jan,8; 2016,Jan,13; 2015,Jan,16; 2014,Jan,11

15733-15738 Wound Reconstruction: Muscle Flaps

INCLUDES Code based on donor site
EXCLUDES Contiguous tissue transfer flaps (14040-14041, 14060-14061, 14301-14302)
Microvascular repair (15756-15758)
Code also application of extensive immobilization apparatus
Code also repair of donor site with skin grafts or flaps

15733 **Muscle, myocutaneous, or fasciocutaneous flap; head and neck with named vascular pedicle (ie, buccinators, genioglossus, temporalis, masseter, sternocleidomastoid, levator scapulae)**

INCLUDES Repair of extracranial defect by anterior pericranial flap on vascular pedicle (15731)
🚑 30.1   ⚘ 30.1   **FUD** 090   [T] [A2] [□]

AMA: 2018,Apr,10; 2018,Jan,8; 2017,Nov,6

15734 **trunk**

🚑 43.4   ⚘ 43.4   **FUD** 090   [T] [A2] [80] [□]

AMA: 2018,Aug,10; 2018,Jan,8; 2017,Nov,6; 2017,Jan,8; 2016,Jan,13; 2015,Jan,16; 2014,Apr,10; 2014,Jan,11

15736 **upper extremity**

🚑 35.3   ⚘ 35.3   **FUD** 090   [T] [A2] [□]

AMA: 2018,Jan,8; 2017,Nov,6; 2017,Jan,8; 2016,Jan,13; 2015,Jan,16; 2014,Jan,11

15738 **lower extremity**

🚑 37.6   ⚘ 37.6   **FUD** 090   [T] [A2] [80] [□]

AMA: 2018,Jan,8; 2017,Nov,6; 2017,Jan,8; 2016,Jan,13; 2015,Jan,16; 2014,Jan,11

15740-15758 Wound Reconstruction: Other

INCLUDES Fixation and anchoring skin graft
Routine dressing
Simple tissue debridement

EXCLUDES Adjacent tissue transfer (14000-14302)
Excision of:
    Benign lesion (11400-11471)
    Burn eschar or scar (15002-15005)
    Malignant lesion (11600-11646)
Flaps without addition of a vascular pedicle (15570-15576)
Primary procedure--see appropriate anatomical section
Skin graft for repair of donor site (15050-15278)
Code also repair of donor site with skin grafts or flaps (14000-14350, 15050-15278)

15740 Flap; island pedicle requiring identification and dissection of an anatomically named axial vessel

EXCLUDES V-Y subcutaneous flaps, random island flaps, and other flaps from adjacent areas (14000-14302)

🛠 24.2   ✄ 28.8   **FUD** 090   T A2 ▢

AMA: 2018,Jan,8; 2017,Dec,14; 2017,Jan,8; 2016,Jan,13; 2015,Jan,16; 2014,Jan,11

15750 neurovascular pedicle

EXCLUDES V-Y subcutaneous flaps, random island flaps, and other flaps from adjacent areas (14000-14302)

🛠 26.3   ✄ 26.3   **FUD** 090   T A2 80 ▢

AMA: 2018,Jan,8; 2017,Dec,14

15756 Free muscle or myocutaneous flap with microvascular anastomosis

INCLUDES Operating microscope (69990)

🛠 66.2   ✄ 66.2   **FUD** 090   C 80 ▢

AMA: 2018,Jan,8; 2017,Jan,8; 2016,Feb,12; 2016,Jan,13; 2015,Jan,16; 2014,Jan,11

15757 Free skin flap with microvascular anastomosis

INCLUDES Operating microscope (69990)

🛠 65.5   ✄ 65.5   **FUD** 090   C 80 ▢

AMA: 2018,Jan,8; 2017,Jan,8; 2016,Apr,8; 2016,Feb,12; 2016,Jan,13; 2015,Jan,16; 2014,Jan,11

15758 Free fascial flap with microvascular anastomosis

INCLUDES Operating microscope (69990)

🛠 66.0   ✄ 66.0   **FUD** 090   C 80 ▢

AMA: 2018,Jan,8; 2017,Jan,8; 2016,Feb,12; 2016,Jan,13; 2015,Jan,16; 2014,Jan,11

15760-15774 [15769] Other Grafts

EXCLUDES Adjacent tissue transfer (14000-14302)
Excision of:
    Benign lesion (11400-11471)
    Burn eschar or scar (15002-15005)
    Malignant lesion (11600-11646)
Flaps without addition of vascular pedicle (15570-15576)
Microvascular repair (15756-15758)
Primary procedure (see appropriate anatomical site)
Repair of donor site with skin grafts or flaps (14000-14350, 15050-15278)

15760 Graft; composite (eg, full thickness of external ear or nasal ala), including primary closure, donor area

INCLUDES Fixation and anchoring skin graft
Routine dressing
Simple tissue debridement

🛠 20.2   ✄ 24.2   **FUD** 090   T A2 ▢

AMA: 2018,Jan,8; 2017,Jan,8; 2016,Jan,13; 2015,Jan,16; 2014,Jan,11

15769 Resequenced code. See code following 15770.

15770 derma-fat-fascia

INCLUDES Fixation and anchoring skin graft
Routine dressing
Simple tissue debridement

🛠 19.0   ✄ 19.0   **FUD** 090   T A2 80 ▢

AMA: 2018,Jan,8; 2017,Jan,8; 2016,Jan,13; 2015,Jan,16; 2014,Jan,11

● # 15769 Grafting of autologous soft tissue, other, harvested by direct excision (eg, fat, dermis, fascia)

🛠 0.00   ✄ 0.00   **FUD** 000

INCLUDES Excisional graft harvest and recipient site placement

EXCLUDES Autologous grafts of specific tissue types, such as skin, bone, nerve, tendon, fascia lata, or vessels
Autologous white blood cell concentrate injection (0481T)
Harvesting of adipose tissue for adipose-derived regenerative cell therapy (0489T-0490T)
Platelet-rich plasma injection (0232T)
Suction assisted lipectomy (15876-15879)

● 15771 Grafting of autologous fat harvested by liposuction technique to trunk, breasts, scalp, arms, and/or legs; 50 cc or less injectate

INCLUDES Add together the volume of injectate harvested from each anatomical area indicated in the code description, such as face and neck, to report the total volume. Do not add together injectate harvested from different anatomical site groups, such as trunk and face
Code based on recipient site

EXCLUDES Autologous white blood cell concentrate injection (0481T)
Liposuction not for grafting purposes (15876-15879)
Obtaining tissue for adipose-derived regenerative cell therapy (0489T-0490T)
Platelet-rich plasma injection (0232T)
Subcutaneous injection of filling material, at same anatomical site (11950-11954)
Use of code more than one time per session

● + 15772 each additional 50 cc injectate, or part thereof (List separately in addition to code for primary procedure)

🛠 0.00   ✄ 0.00   **FUD** 000

Code first (15771)

● 15773 Grafting of autologous fat harvested by liposuction technique to face, eyelids, mouth, neck, ears, orbits, genitalia, hands, and/or feet; 25 cc or less injectate

INCLUDES Add together the volume of injectate harvested from each anatomical area indicated in the code description, such as face and neck, to report the total volume. Do not add together injectate harvested from different anatomical site groups, such as trunk and face
Code based on recipient site

EXCLUDES Autologous white blood cell concentrate injection (0481T)
Liposuction not for grafting purposes (15876-15879)
Obtaining tissue for adipose-derived regenerative cell therapy (0489T-0490T)
Platelet-rich plasma injection (0232T)
Subcutaneous injection of filling material, at same anatomical site (11950-11954)
Use of code more than one time per session

● + 15774 each additional 25 cc injectate, or part thereof (List separately in addition to code for primary procedure)

🛠 0.00   ✄ 0.00   **FUD** 000

Code first (15773)

15775-15839 Plastic, Reconstructive, and Aesthetic Surgery

CMS: 100-02,16,10 Exclusions from Coverage; 100-02,16,120 Cosmetic Procedures; 100-02,16,180 Services Related to Noncovered Procedures

15775   Punch graft for hair transplant; 1 to 15 punch grafts

EXCLUDES Strip transplant (15220)

🔲 6.42   ✂ 8.74   **FUD** 000   T A2 80 ▢

AMA: 2018,Jan,8; 2017,Jan,8; 2016,Jan,13; 2015,Jan,16; 2014,Jan,11

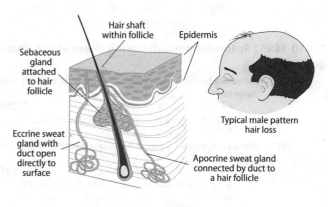

Hair shaft within follicle
Epidermis
Sebaceous gland attached to hair follicle
Eccrine sweat gland with duct open directly to surface
Apocrine sweat gland connected by duct to a hair follicle
Typical male pattern hair loss

15776   more than 15 punch grafts

EXCLUDES Strip transplant (15220)

🔲 9.12   ✂ 12.5   **FUD** 000   T A2 80 ▢

AMA: 2018,Jan,8; 2017,Jan,8; 2016,Jan,13; 2015,Jan,16; 2014,Jan,11

+ **15777   Implantation of biologic implant (eg, acellular dermal matrix) for soft tissue reinforcement (ie, breast, trunk) (List separately in addition to code for primary procedure)**

EXCLUDES Application of skin substitute (high cost) to an external wound (15271-15278)
Application of skin substitute (low cost) to an external wound (C5271-C5278)
Mesh implantation for:
Open repair of ventral or incisional hernia (49560-49566) and (49568)
Repair of devitalized soft tissue infection (11004-11006) and (49568)
Repair of pelvic floor (57267)
Repair anorectal fistula with plug (46707)
Reporting with modifier 50. Report once for each side when performed bilaterally
Soft tissue reinforcement with biologic implants other than in the breast or trunk (17999)
Code also supply of biologic implant
Code also synthetic or non-biological implant to reinforce abdominal wall (0437T)
Code first primary procedure

🔲 6.25   ✂ 6.25   **FUD** ZZZ   50 N N1 ▢

AMA: 2019,Jan,14; 2018,Jan,8; 2017,Jan,8; 2016,Jan,13; 2015,Jan,16; 2014,Jan,11

15780   Dermabrasion; total face (eg, for acne scarring, fine wrinkling, rhytids, general keratosis)

🔲 20.1   ✂ 26.1   **FUD** 090   J P3 80 ▢

AMA: 2018,Jan,8; 2017,Jan,8; 2016,Jan,13; 2015,Jan,16; 2014,Jan,11

15781   segmental, face

🔲 12.3   ✂ 15.7   **FUD** 090   T P2 ▢

AMA: 1997,Nov,1

15782   regional, other than face

🔲 11.9   ✂ 16.3   **FUD** 090   J P3 80 ▢

AMA: 1997,Nov,1

15783   superficial, any site (eg, tattoo removal)

🔲 10.6   ✂ 13.6   **FUD** 090   T P2 80 ▢

AMA: 2018,Jan,8; 2017,Jan,8; 2016,Jan,13; 2015,Jan,16; 2014,Jan,11

15786   Abrasion; single lesion (eg, keratosis, scar)

🔲 3.91   ✂ 6.98   **FUD** 010   Q1 N1 ▢

AMA: 1997,Nov,1

+ **15787   each additional 4 lesions or less (List separately in addition to code for primary procedure)**

Code first (15786)

🔲 0.50   ✂ 1.27   **FUD** ZZZ   N N1 ▢

AMA: 1997,Nov,1

15788   Chemical peel, facial; epidermal

🔲 6.81   ✂ 12.7   **FUD** 090   Q1 N1 ▢

AMA: 1997,Nov,1; 1993,Win,1

15789   dermal

🔲 11.8   ✂ 15.7   **FUD** 090   T P2 ▢

AMA: 1997,Nov,1; 1993,Win,1

15792   Chemical peel, nonfacial; epidermal

🔲 7.02   ✂ 11.8   **FUD** 090   Q1 N1 80 ▢

AMA: 1997,Nov,1; 1993,Win,1

15793   dermal

🔲 10.3   ✂ 14.0   **FUD** 090   Q1 N1 80 ▢

AMA: 1997,Nov,1; 1993,Win,1

15819   Cervicoplasty

🔲 22.7   ✂ 22.7   **FUD** 090   T G2 80 ▢

AMA: 1997,Nov,1

15820   Blepharoplasty, lower eyelid;

🔲 14.5   ✂ 16.2   **FUD** 090   T A2 80 50 ▢

AMA: 2018,Jan,8; 2017,Jan,8; 2016,Jan,13; 2015,Jan,16; 2014,Jan,11

15821   with extensive herniated fat pad

🔲 15.5   ✂ 17.3   **FUD** 090   T A2 80 50 ▢

AMA: 2018,Jan,8; 2017,Jan,8; 2016,Jan,13; 2015,Jan,16; 2014,Jan,11

15822   Blepharoplasty, upper eyelid;

🔲 11.1   ✂ 12.7   **FUD** 090   T A2 50 ▢

AMA: 2018,Jan,8; 2017,Jan,8; 2016,Jan,13; 2015,Jan,16; 2014,Jan,11

15823   with excessive skin weighting down lid

🔲 15.5   ✂ 17.3   **FUD** 090   T A2 50 ▢

AMA: 2018,Jan,8; 2017,Jan,8; 2016,Jan,13; 2015,Jan,16; 2014,Jan,11

15824   Rhytidectomy; forehead

EXCLUDES Repair of brow ptosis (67900)

🔲 0.00   ✂ 0.00   **FUD** 000   T A2 80 50 ▢

AMA: 2018,Jan,8; 2017,Apr,9

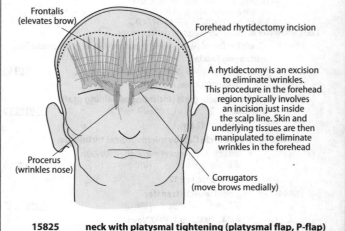

Frontalis (elevates brow)
Forehead rhytidectomy incision
A rhytidectomy is an excision to eliminate wrinkles. This procedure in the forehead region typically involves an incision just inside the scalp line. Skin and underlying tissues are then manipulated to eliminate wrinkles in the forehead
Procerus (wrinkles nose)
Corrugators (move brows medially)

15825   neck with platysmal tightening (platysmal flap, P-flap)

🔲 0.00   ✂ 0.00   **FUD** 000   T A2 80 50 ▢

AMA: 2018,Jan,8; 2017,Apr,9

15826   glabellar frown lines

🔲 0.00   ✂ 0.00   **FUD** 000   T A2 80 50 ▢

AMA: 1997,Nov,1

15828 cheek, chin, and neck
📔 0.00　✂ 0.00　**FUD** 000　　　T A2 80 50 ▭
AMA: 1997,Nov,1

15829 superficial musculoaponeurotic system (SMAS) flap
📔 0.00　✂ 0.00　**FUD** 000　　　T A2 80 50 ▭
AMA: 1997,Nov,1

15830 Excision, excessive skin and subcutaneous tissue (includes lipectomy); abdomen, infraumbilical panniculectomy
📔 33.7　✂ 33.7　**FUD** 090　　　J A2 80 ▭
EXCLUDES　Adjacent tissue transfer, trunk (14000-14001, 14302)
　　　　　Complex wound repair, trunk (13100-13102)
　　　　　Intermediate wound repair, trunk (12031-12032, 12034-12037)
　　　　　Other abdominoplasty (17999)
　　　　Code also (15847)

15832 thigh
📔 26.4　✂ 26.4　**FUD** 090　　　J A2 80 50 ▭
AMA: 1997,Nov,1

15833 leg
📔 25.0　✂ 25.0　**FUD** 090　　　J A2 80 50 ▭
AMA: 1997,Nov,1

15834 hip
📔 25.5　✂ 25.5　**FUD** 090　　　J A2 80 50 ▭
AMA: 1997,Nov,1

15835 buttock
📔 26.8　✂ 26.8　**FUD** 090　　　J A2 80 ▭
AMA: 1997,Nov,1

15836 arm
📔 22.6　✂ 22.6　**FUD** 090　　　J A2 80 50 ▭
AMA: 1997,Nov,1

15837 forearm or hand
📔 20.6　✂ 24.7　**FUD** 090　　　J G2 80 ▭
AMA: 1997,Nov,1

15838 submental fat pad
📔 18.3　✂ 18.3　**FUD** 090　　　J G2 80 ▭
AMA: 1998,Feb,1; 1997,Nov,1

15839 other area
📔 21.1　✂ 25.2　**FUD** 090　　　J A2 80 ▭
AMA: 1997,Nov,1

15840-15845 Reanimation of the Paralyzed Face
INCLUDES　Routine dressing and supplies
EXCLUDES　Intravenous fluorescein evaluation of blood flow in graft or flap (15860)
　　　Nerve:
　　　　Decompression (69720, 69725, 69955)
　　　　Pedicle transfer (64905, 64907)
　　　　Suture (64831-64876, 69740, 69745)
Code also repair of donor site with skin grafts or flaps

15840 Graft for facial nerve paralysis; free fascia graft (including obtaining fascia)
📔 28.8　✂ 28.8　**FUD** 090　　　T A2 ▭
AMA: 1997,Nov,1

15841 free muscle graft (including obtaining graft)
📔 51.2　✂ 51.2　**FUD** 090　　　T A2 80 ▭
AMA: 1997,Nov,1

15842 free muscle flap by microsurgical technique
INCLUDES　Operating microscope (69990)
📔 78.0　✂ 78.0　**FUD** 090　　　T G2 80 ▭
AMA: 2016,Feb,12

15845 regional muscle transfer
📔 28.8　✂ 28.8　**FUD** 090　　　T A2 80 ▭
AMA: 1998,Feb,1; 1997,Nov,1

15847 Removal of Excess Abdominal Tissue Add-on
CMS: 100-02,16,10 Exclusions from Coverage; 100-02,16,120 Cosmetic Procedures; 100-02,16,180 Services Related to Noncovered Procedures

+　**15847** Excision, excessive skin and subcutaneous tissue (includes lipectomy), abdomen (eg, abdominoplasty) (includes umbilical transposition and fascial plication) (List separately in addition to code for primary procedure)
📔 0.00　✂ 0.00　**FUD** YYY　　　N N1 80 ▭
EXCLUDES　Abdominal wall hernia repair (49491-49587)
　　　　　Other abdominoplasty (17999)
　　　Code first (15830)

15850-15852 Suture Removal/Dressing Change: Anesthesia Required
15850 Removal of sutures under anesthesia (other than local), same surgeon
📔 1.19　✂ 2.56　**FUD** XXX　　　T G2 ▭
AMA: 2018,Jan,8; 2017,Jan,8; 2016,Jan,13; 2015,Jan,16; 2014,Jan,11

15851 Removal of sutures under anesthesia (other than local), other surgeon
📔 1.31　✂ 2.85　**FUD** 000　　　T P3 ▭
AMA: 2018,Jan,8; 2017,Jan,8; 2016,Jan,13; 2015,Jan,16; 2014,Jan,11

15852 Dressing change (for other than burns) under anesthesia (other than local)
EXCLUDES　Dressing change for burns (16020-16030)
📔 1.33　✂ 1.33　**FUD** 000　　　Q1 N1 ▭
AMA: 1997,Nov,1

15860 Injection for Vascular Flow Determination
15860 Intravenous injection of agent (eg, fluorescein) to test vascular flow in flap or graft
📔 3.10　✂ 3.10　**FUD** 000　　　Q1 N1 80 ▭
AMA: 2002,May,7; 1997,Nov,1

15876-15879 Liposuction
CMS: 100-02,16,10 Exclusions from Coverage; 100-02,16,120 Cosmetic Procedures; 100-02,16,180 Services Related to Noncovered Procedures
EXCLUDES　Liposuction for autologous fat grafting (15771-15774)
　　　　Obtaining tissue for adipose-derived regenerative cell therapy (0489T-0490T)

15876 Suction assisted lipectomy; head and neck
📔 0.00　✂ 0.00　**FUD** 000　　　T A2 80 ▭
AMA: 2019,Aug,10; 2018,Sep,12

Cannula typically inserted through incision in front of ear

15877 trunk
📔 0.00　✂ 0.00　**FUD** 000　　　T A2 80 ▭
AMA: 2019,Aug,10; 2018,Sep,12; 2018,Jan,8; 2017,Jan,8; 2016,Jan,13; 2015,Jan,16; 2014,Jan,11

15878 upper extremity
📔 0.00　✂ 0.00　**FUD** 000　　　T A2 80 50 ▭
AMA: 2019,Aug,10; 2018,Sep,12

15879   **lower extremity**

🔧 0.00   ⚕ 0.00   **FUD** 000   [T] [A2] [80] [50] 🔲

AMA: 2019,Aug,10; 2018,Sep,12

15920-15999 Treatment of Decubitus Ulcers

Code also free skin graft to repair ulcer or donor site

15920   **Excision, coccygeal pressure ulcer, with coccygectomy; with primary suture**

🔧 17.8   ⚕ 17.8   **FUD** 090   [J] [A2] [80] 🔲

AMA: 2011,May,3-5; 1997,Nov,1

15922   **with flap closure**

🔧 22.5   ⚕ 22.5   **FUD** 090   [T] [A2] [80] 🔲

AMA: 2011,May,3-5; 1997,Nov,1

15931   **Excision, sacral pressure ulcer, with primary suture;**

🔧 19.9   ⚕ 19.9   **FUD** 090   [J] [A2] 🔲

AMA: 2011,May,3-5; 1997,Nov,1

15933   **with ostectomy**

🔧 24.5   ⚕ 24.5   **FUD** 090   [J] [A2] [80] 🔲

AMA: 2011,May,3-5; 1997,Nov,1

15934   **Excision, sacral pressure ulcer, with skin flap closure;**

🔧 27.1   ⚕ 27.1   **FUD** 090   [T] [A2] 🔲

AMA: 2011,May,3-5; 1997,Nov,1

15935   **with ostectomy**

🔧 31.6   ⚕ 31.6   **FUD** 090   [T] [A2] [80] 🔲

AMA: 2011,May,3-5; 1997,Nov,1

15936   **Excision, sacral pressure ulcer, in preparation for muscle or myocutaneous flap or skin graft closure;**

Code also any defect repair with:
Muscle or myocutaneous flap (15734, 15738)
Split skin graft (15100-15101)

🔧 25.7   ⚕ 25.7   **FUD** 090   [T] [A2] 🔲

AMA: 2011,May,3-5; 1998,Nov,1

15937   **with ostectomy**

Code also any defect repair with:
Muscle or myocutaneous flap (15734, 15738)
Split skin graft (15100-15101)

🔧 29.8   ⚕ 29.8   **FUD** 090   [T] [A2] 🔲

AMA: 2011,May,3-5; 1998,Nov,1

15940   **Excision, ischial pressure ulcer, with primary suture;**

🔧 20.1   ⚕ 20.1   **FUD** 090   [J] [A2] 🔲

AMA: 2011,May,3-5; 1997,Nov,1

15941   **with ostectomy (ischiectomy)**

🔧 26.0   ⚕ 26.0   **FUD** 090   [J] [A2] [80] 🔲

AMA: 2011,May,3-5; 1997,Nov,1

15944   **Excision, ischial pressure ulcer, with skin flap closure;**

🔧 25.8   ⚕ 25.8   **FUD** 090   [T] [A2] [80] 🔲

AMA: 2011,May,3-5; 1997,Nov,1

15945   **with ostectomy**

🔧 28.4   ⚕ 28.4   **FUD** 090   [T] [A2] [80] 🔲

AMA: 2011,May,3-5; 1997,Nov,1

15946   **Excision, ischial pressure ulcer, with ostectomy, in preparation for muscle or myocutaneous flap or skin graft closure**

Code also any defect repair with:
Muscle or myocutaneous flap (15734, 15738)
Split skin graft (15100-15101)

🔧 46.8   ⚕ 46.8   **FUD** 090   [T] [A2] 🔲

AMA: 2018,Jan,8; 2017,Jan,8; 2016,Jan,13; 2015,Jan,16; 2014,Jan,11

15950   **Excision, trochanteric pressure ulcer, with primary suture;**

🔧 17.3   ⚕ 17.3   **FUD** 090   [J] [A2] 🔲

AMA: 2011,May,3-5; 1997,Nov,1

15951   **with ostectomy**

🔧 25.3   ⚕ 25.3   **FUD** 090   [J] [A2] [80] 🔲

AMA: 2011,May,3-5; 1997,Nov,1

15952   **Excision, trochanteric pressure ulcer, with skin flap closure;**

🔧 26.0   ⚕ 26.0   **FUD** 090   [T] [A2] [80] 🔲

AMA: 2011,May,3-5; 1997,Nov,1

15953   **with ostectomy**

🔧 28.6   ⚕ 28.6   **FUD** 090   [T] [A2] 🔲

AMA: 2011,May,3-5; 1997,Nov,1

15956   **Excision, trochanteric pressure ulcer, in preparation for muscle or myocutaneous flap or skin graft closure;**

Code also any defect repair with:
Muscle or myocutaneous flap (15734, 15738)
Split skin graft (15100-15101)

🔧 33.3   ⚕ 33.3   **FUD** 090   [T] [A2] 🔲

AMA: 2011,May,3-5; 1998,Nov,1

15958   **with ostectomy**

Code also any defect repair with:
Muscle or myocutaneous flap (15734-15738)
Split skin graft (15100-15101)

🔧 34.0   ⚕ 34.0   **FUD** 090   [T] [A2] 🔲

AMA: 2011,May,3-5; 1998,Nov,1

15999   **Unlisted procedure, excision pressure ulcer**

🔧 0.00   ⚕ 0.00   **FUD** YYY   [T] [80] 🔲

AMA: 2011,May,3-5; 1997,Nov,1

16000-16036 Burn Care

INCLUDES   Local care of burn surface only

EXCLUDES   *Application of skin grafts including all services described in the following codes (15100-15777)*
E&M services
Flaps (15570-15650)
Laser fenestration for scars (0479T-0480T)

16000   **Initial treatment, first degree burn, when no more than local treatment is required**

🔧 1.32   ⚕ 2.00   **FUD** 000   [Q1] [N1] 🔲

AMA: 2018,Jan,8; 2017,Jan,8; 2016,Jan,13; 2015,Jan,16; 2014,Jan,11

16020   **Dressings and/or debridement of partial-thickness burns, initial or subsequent; small (less than 5% total body surface area)**

INCLUDES   Wound coverage other than skin graft

🔧 1.55   ⚕ 2.32   **FUD** 000   [Q1] [N1] 🔲

AMA: 2018,Jan,8; 2017,Jan,8; 2016,Jan,13; 2015,Jan,16; 2014,Jan,11

16025   **medium (eg, whole face or whole extremity, or 5% to 10% total body surface area)**

INCLUDES   Wound coverage other than skin graft

🔧 3.16   ⚕ 4.26   **FUD** 000   [T] [A2] 🔲

AMA: 2018,Jan,8; 2017,Jan,8; 2016,Jan,13; 2015,Jan,16; 2014,Jan,11

16030   **large (eg, more than 1 extremity, or greater than 10% total body surface area)**

INCLUDES   Wound coverage other than skin graft

🔧 3.82   ⚕ 5.40   **FUD** 000   [T] [A2] 🔲

AMA: 2018,Jan,8; 2017,Jan,8; 2016,Jan,13; 2015,Jan,16; 2014,Jan,11

16035   **Escharotomy; initial incision**

EXCLUDES   *Debridement or scraping of burn (16020-16030)*

🔧 5.65   ⚕ 5.65   **FUD** 000   [T] [G2] 🔲

AMA: 2018,Jan,8; 2017,Jan,8; 2016,Jan,13; 2015,Jan,16; 2014,Jan,11

+ **16036**   **each additional incision (List separately in addition to code for primary procedure)**

EXCLUDES   *Debridement or scraping of burn (16020-16030)*

Code first (16035)

🔧 2.36   ⚕ 2.36   **FUD** ZZZ   [C] 🔲

AMA: 2018,Jan,8; 2017,Jan,8; 2016,Jan,13; 2015,Jan,16; 2014,Jan,11

● New Code   ▲ Revised Code   ○ Reinstated   ● New Web Release   ▲ Revised Web Release   + Add-on   Unlisted   Not Covered   # Resequenced
🔟 Optum Mod 50 Exempt   ⊘ AMA Mod 51 Exempt   5️⃣1️⃣ Optum Mod 51 Exempt   6️⃣3️⃣ Mod 63 Exempt   ✗ Non-FDA Drug   ★ Telemedicine   Ⓜ Maternity   🅐 Age Edit

CPT © 2019 American Medical Association. All Rights Reserved.

17000-17004 Destruction Any Method: Premalignant Lesion

CMS: 100-03,140.5 Laser Procedures

EXCLUDES   *Cryotherapy acne (17340)*
    Destruction of:
      Benign lesions other than cutaneous vascular proliferative lesions
        (17110-17111)
      Cutaneous vascular proliferative lesions (17106-17108)
      Malignant lesions (17260-17286)
      Plantar warts (17110-17111)
    Destruction of lesion of:
      Anus (46900-46917, 46924)
      Conjunctiva (68135)
      Eyelid (67850)
      Penis (54050-54057, 54065)
      Vagina (57061, 57065)
      Vestibule of mouth (40820)
      Vulva (56501, 56515)
    Destruction or excision of skin tags (11200-11201)
    Escharotomy (16035-16036)
    Excision benign lesion (11400-11446)
    Laser fenestration for scars (0479T-0480T)
    Localized chemotherapy treatment see appropriate office visit service code
    Paring or excision of benign hyperkeratotic lesion (11055-11057)
    Shaving skin lesions (11300-11313)
    Treatment of inflammatory skin disease via laser (96920-96922)

17000   **Destruction (eg, laser surgery, electrosurgery, cryosurgery, chemosurgery, surgical curettement), premalignant lesions (eg, actinic keratoses); first lesion**
     🚗 1.53   ⚕ 1.85   **FUD** 010   01 N1 ▭
     AMA: 2018,Jan,8; 2017,Dec,14; 2017,Jan,8; 2016,Apr,3; 2016,Jan,13; 2015,Jan,16; 2014,Jan,11

+ 17003   **second through 14 lesions, each (List separately in addition to code for first lesion)**
     Code first (17000)
     🚗 0.07   ⚕ 0.16   **FUD** ZZZ   N N1 ▭
     AMA: 2018,Jan,8; 2017,Dec,14; 2017,Jan,8; 2016,Apr,3; 2016,Jan,13; 2015,Jan,16; 2014,Jan,11

17004   **Destruction (eg, laser surgery, electrosurgery, cryosurgery, chemosurgery, surgical curettement), premalignant lesions (eg, actinic keratoses), 15 or more lesions**
     EXCLUDES   *Use of code for destruction of less than 15 lesions*
         (17000-17003)
     🚗 2.85   ⚕ 4.31   **FUD** 010   🚫 T P3 ▭
     AMA: 2018,Jan,8; 2017,Dec,14; 2017,Jan,8; 2016,Apr,3; 2016,Jan,13; 2015,Jan,16; 2014,Jan,11

17106-17250 Destruction Any Method: Vascular Proliferative Lesion

CMS: 100-02,16,10 Exclusions from Coverage; 100-02,16,120 Cosmetic Procedures

EXCLUDES   *Destruction of lesion of:*
      Anus (46900-46917, 46924)
      Conjunctiva (68135)
      Eyelid (67850)
      Penis (54050-54057, 54065)
      Vagina (57061, 57065)
      Vestibule of mouth (40820)
      Vulva (56501, 56515)
    Treatment of inflammatory skin disease via laser (96920-96922)

17106   **Destruction of cutaneous vascular proliferative lesions (eg, laser technique); less than 10 sq cm**
     🚗 7.93   ⚕ 9.78   **FUD** 090   T P2 ▭
     AMA: 2019,Sep,10; 2018,Jan,8; 2017,Dec,14; 2017,Jan,8; 2016,Apr,3; 2016,Jan,13; 2015,Jan,16; 2014,Jan,11

17107   **10.0 to 50.0 sq cm**
     🚗 10.1   ⚕ 12.6   **FUD** 090   T P2 ▭
     AMA: 2018,Jan,8; 2017,Dec,14; 2017,Jan,8; 2016,Apr,3; 2016,Jan,13; 2015,Jan,16; 2014,Jan,11

17108   **over 50.0 sq cm**
     🚗 15.2   ⚕ 18.3   **FUD** 090   T P3 80 ▭
     AMA: 2018,Jan,8; 2017,Dec,14; 2017,Jan,8; 2016,Apr,3; 2016,Jan,13; 2015,Jan,16; 2014,Jan,11

17110   **Destruction (eg, laser surgery, electrosurgery, cryosurgery, chemosurgery, surgical curettement), of benign lesions other than skin tags or cutaneous vascular proliferative lesions; up to 14 lesions**
     🚗 1.96   ⚕ 3.13   **FUD** 010   01 N1 ▭
     AMA: 2018,Jan,8; 2017,Dec,14; 2017,Jan,8; 2016,Apr,3; 2016,Jan,13; 2015,Jan,16; 2014,Jan,11

17111   **15 or more lesions**
     EXCLUDES   *Destruction of neurofibromas, 50-100 lesions*
         (0419T-0420T)
     🚗 2.41   ⚕ 3.71   **FUD** 010   01 N1 ▭
     AMA: 2018,Jan,8; 2017,Dec,14; 2017,Jan,8; 2016,Apr,3; 2016,Jan,13; 2015,Jan,16; 2014,Jan,11

17250   **Chemical cauterization of granulation tissue (ie, proud flesh)**
     EXCLUDES   *Excision/removal codes for the same lesion*
       Chemical cauterization when applied for hemostasis of
         wound
       Wound care management (97597-97598, 97602)
     🚗 1.05   ⚕ 2.31   **FUD** 000   01 N1 ▭
     AMA: 2018,Jan,8; 2017,Dec,14; 2017,Jan,8; 2016,Jan,13; 2015,Jan,16; 2014,Jan,11

17260-17286 Destruction, Any Method: Malignant Lesion

CMS: 100-03,140.5 Laser Procedures

EXCLUDES   *Destruction of lesion of:*
      Anus (46900-46917, 46924)
      Conjunctiva (68135)
      Eyelid (67850)
      Penis (54050-54057, 54065)
      Vestibule of mouth (40820)
      Vulva (56501-56515)
    Localized chemotherapy treatment see appropriate office visit service code
    Shaving skin lesion (11300-11313)
    Treatment of inflammatory skin disease via laser (96920-96922)

17260   **Destruction, malignant lesion (eg, laser surgery, electrosurgery, cryosurgery, chemosurgery, surgical curettement), trunk, arms or legs; lesion diameter 0.5 cm or less**
     🚗 2.03   ⚕ 2.71   **FUD** 010   01 N1 ▭
     AMA: 2018,Jan,8; 2017,Dec,14; 2017,Jan,8; 2016,Jan,13; 2015,Jan,16; 2014,Jan,11

17261   **lesion diameter 0.6 to 1.0 cm**
     🚗 2.58   ⚕ 4.11   **FUD** 010   01 N1 ▭
     AMA: 2018,Jan,8; 2017,Dec,14; 2017,Jan,8; 2016,Jan,13; 2015,Jan,16; 2014,Jan,11

17262   **lesion diameter 1.1 to 2.0 cm**
     🚗 3.30   ⚕ 5.01   **FUD** 010   01 N1 ▭
     AMA: 2018,Jan,8; 2017,Dec,14; 2017,Jan,8; 2016,Jan,13; 2015,Jan,16; 2014,Jan,11

17263   **lesion diameter 2.1 to 3.0 cm**
     🚗 3.66   ⚕ 5.47   **FUD** 010   01 N1 ▭
     AMA: 2018,Jan,8; 2017,Dec,14; 2017,Jan,8; 2016,Jan,13; 2015,Jan,16; 2014,Jan,11

17264   **lesion diameter 3.1 to 4.0 cm**
     🚗 3.90   ⚕ 5.85   **FUD** 010   T P3 ▭
     AMA: 2018,Jan,8; 2017,Dec,14; 2017,Jan,8; 2016,Jan,13; 2015,Jan,16; 2014,Jan,11

17266   **lesion diameter over 4.0 cm**
     🚗 4.60   ⚕ 6.66   **FUD** 010   T P3 ▭
     AMA: 2018,Jan,8; 2017,Dec,14; 2017,Jan,8; 2016,Jan,13; 2015,Jan,16; 2014,Jan,11

17270   **Destruction, malignant lesion (eg, laser surgery, electrosurgery, cryosurgery, chemosurgery, surgical curettement), scalp, neck, hands, feet, genitalia; lesion diameter 0.5 cm or less**
     🚗 2.84   ⚕ 4.24   **FUD** 010   T P2 ▭
     AMA: 2018,Jan,8; 2017,Dec,14; 2017,Jan,8; 2016,Jan,13; 2015,Jan,16; 2014,Jan,11

17271 lesion diameter 0.6 to 1.0 cm
🚑 3.14 ✂ 4.67 **FUD** 010 [T] [P2] 🖳
AMA: 2018,Jan,8; 2017,Dec,14; 2017,Jan,8; 2016,Jan,13; 2015,Jan,16; 2014,Jan,11

17272 lesion diameter 1.1 to 2.0 cm
🚑 3.63 ✂ 5.33 **FUD** 010 [01] [N1] 🖳
AMA: 2018,Jan,8; 2017,Dec,14; 2017,Jan,8; 2016,Jan,13; 2015,Jan,16; 2014,Jan,11

17273 lesion diameter 2.1 to 3.0 cm
🚑 4.11 ✂ 5.94 **FUD** 010 [T] [P3] 🖳
AMA: 2018,Jan,8; 2017,Dec,14; 2017,Jan,8; 2016,Jan,13; 2015,Jan,16; 2014,Jan,11

17274 lesion diameter 3.1 to 4.0 cm
🚑 5.04 ✂ 7.01 **FUD** 010 [T] [P3] 🖳
AMA: 2018,Jan,8; 2017,Dec,14; 2017,Jan,8; 2016,Jan,13; 2015,Jan,16; 2014,Jan,11

17276 lesion diameter over 4.0 cm
🚑 6.02 ✂ 8.11 **FUD** 010 [T] [P3] 🖳
AMA: 2018,Jan,8; 2017,Dec,14; 2017,Jan,8; 2016,Jan,13; 2015,Jan,16; 2014,Jan,11

17280 Destruction, malignant lesion (eg, laser surgery, electrosurgery, cryosurgery, chemosurgery, surgical curettement), face, ears, eyelids, nose, lips, mucous membrane; lesion diameter 0.5 cm or less
🚑 2.58 ✂ 3.97 **FUD** 010 [01] [N1] 🖳
AMA: 2018,Jan,8; 2017,Dec,14; 2017,Jan,8; 2016,Jan,13; 2015,Jan,16; 2014,Jan,11

17281 lesion diameter 0.6 to 1.0 cm
🚑 3.54 ✂ 5.09 **FUD** 010 [T] [P3] 🖳
AMA: 2018,Jan,8; 2017,Dec,14; 2017,Jan,8; 2016,Jan,13; 2015,Jan,16; 2014,Jan,11

17282 lesion diameter 1.1 to 2.0 cm
🚑 4.10 ✂ 5.84 **FUD** 010 [T] [P3] 🖳
AMA: 2018,Jan,8; 2017,Dec,14; 2017,Jan,8; 2016,Jan,13; 2015,Jan,16; 2014,Jan,11

17283 lesion diameter 2.1 to 3.0 cm
🚑 5.13 ✂ 6.99 **FUD** 010 [T] [P3] 🖳
AMA: 2018,Jan,8; 2017,Dec,14; 2017,Jan,8; 2016,Jan,13; 2015,Jan,16; 2014,Jan,11

17284 lesion diameter 3.1 to 4.0 cm
🚑 5.97 ✂ 7.97 **FUD** 010 [T] [P3] 🖳
AMA: 2018,Jan,8; 2017,Dec,14; 2017,Jan,8; 2016,Jan,13; 2015,Jan,16; 2014,Jan,11

17286 lesion diameter over 4.0 cm
🚑 8.03 ✂ 10.2 **FUD** 010 [T] [P3] 🖳
AMA: 2018,Jan,8; 2017,Dec,14; 2017,Jan,8; 2016,Jan,13; 2015,Jan,16; 2014,Jan,11

17311-17315 Mohs Surgery

INCLUDES The following surgical/pathology services performed by the same physician or other qualified health care provider:
Evaluation of skin margins by surgeon
Pathology exam on Mohs surgery specimen (by Mohs surgeon) (88302-88309)
Routine frozen section stain (88314)
Tumor removal, mapping, preparation, and examination of lesion

EXCLUDES *Frozen section if no prior diagnosis determination has been performed (88331)*
Code also any special histochemical stain on a frozen section, nonroutine (with modifier 59) (88311-88314, 88342)
Code also biopsy (with modifier 59) if no prior diagnosis determination has been performed, if biopsy is indeterminate, or performed more than 90 days preoperatively (11102, 11104, 11106)
Code also complex repair (13100-13160)
Code also flaps or grafts (14000-14350, 15050-15770)
Code also intermediate repair (12031-12057)
Code also simple repair (12001-12021)

17311 Mohs micrographic technique, including removal of all gross tumor, surgical excision of tissue specimens, mapping, color coding of specimens, microscopic examination of specimens by the surgeon, and histopathologic preparation including routine stain(s) (eg, hematoxylin and eosin, toluidine blue), head, neck, hands, feet, genitalia, or any location with surgery directly involving muscle, cartilage, bone, tendon, major nerves, or vessels; first stage, up to 5 tissue blocks
🚑 10.8 ✂ 18.9 **FUD** 000 [T] [P2] 🖳
AMA: 2018,Jan,8; 2017,Jan,8; 2016,Jan,13; 2015,Jan,16; 2014,Oct,14; 2014,Feb,10

+ **17312** each additional stage after the first stage, up to 5 tissue blocks (List separately in addition to code for primary procedure)
Code first (17311)
🚑 5.76 ✂ 11.2 **FUD** ZZZ [N] [N1] 🖳
AMA: 2018,Jan,8; 2017,Jan,8; 2016,Jan,13; 2015,Jan,16; 2014,Oct,14; 2014,Feb,10

17313 Mohs micrographic technique, including removal of all gross tumor, surgical excision of tissue specimens, mapping, color coding of specimens, microscopic examination of specimens by the surgeon, and histopathologic preparation including routine stain(s) (eg, hematoxylin and eosin, toluidine blue), of the trunk, arms, or legs; first stage, up to 5 tissue blocks
🚑 9.70 ✂ 17.7 **FUD** 000 [T] [P2] 🖳
AMA: 2018,Jan,8; 2017,Jan,8; 2016,Jan,13; 2015,Jan,16; 2014,Oct,14; 2014,Feb,10

+ **17314** each additional stage after the first stage, up to 5 tissue blocks (List separately in addition to code for primary procedure)
Code first (17313)
🚑 5.34 ✂ 10.7 **FUD** ZZZ [N] [N1] 🖳
AMA: 2018,Jan,8; 2017,Jan,8; 2016,Jan,13; 2015,Jan,16; 2014,Oct,14; 2014,Feb,10

+ **17315** Mohs micrographic technique, including removal of all gross tumor, surgical excision of tissue specimens, mapping, color coding of specimens, microscopic examination of specimens by the surgeon, and histopathologic preparation including routine stain(s) (eg, hematoxylin and eosin, toluidine blue), each additional block after the first 5 tissue blocks, any stage (List separately in addition to code for primary procedure)
Code first (17311-17314)
🚑 1.52 ✂ 2.26 **FUD** ZZZ [N] [N1] 🖳
AMA: 2018,Jan,8; 2017,Jan,8; 2016,Jan,13; 2015,Jan,16; 2014,Oct,14; 2014,Feb,10; 2014,Jan,11

17340-17999 Treatment for Active Acne and Permanent Hair Removal

CMS: 100-02,16,10 Exclusions from Coverage; 100-02,16,120 Cosmetic Procedures

17340 Cryotherapy (CO2 slush, liquid N2) for acne
🚑 1.40 ✂ 1.49 **FUD** 010 [01] [N1] 🖳
AMA: 2018,Jan,8; 2017,Jan,8; 2016,Jan,13; 2015,Jan,16; 2014,Jan,11

Integumentary System

17360   Chemical exfoliation for acne (eg, acne paste, acid)
🔲 2.77   🔲 3.61   **FUD** 010   `01` `N1` 🔲
AMA: 2018,Jan,8; 2017,Jan,8; 2016,Jan,13; 2015,Jan,16; 2014,Jan,11

17380   Electrolysis epilation, each 30 minutes
EXCLUDES   *Actinotherapy (96900)*
🔲 0.00   🔲 0.00   **FUD** 000   `T` `R2` `80` 🔲
AMA: 2018,Jan,8; 2017,Jan,8; 2016,Jan,13; 2015,Jan,16; 2014,Jan,11

17999   Unlisted procedure, skin, mucous membrane and subcutaneous tissue
🔲 0.00   🔲 0.00   **FUD** YYY   `01` `80` 🔲
AMA: 2019,Sep,10; 2019,Mar,10; 2019,Jan,14; 2018,Jan,8; 2017,Dec,13; 2017,Jan,8; 2016,May,13; 2016,Jan,13; 2015,Jan,16; 2014,Jan,11

19000-19030 Treatment of Breast Abscess and Cyst with Injection, Aspiration, Incision

19000   Puncture aspiration of cyst of breast;
📷 (76942, 77021)
🔲 1.26   🔲 3.12   **FUD** 000   `T` `P3` 🔲
AMA: 2018,Jan,8; 2017,Jan,8; 2016,Jan,13; 2015,Jan,16; 2014,Jan,11

+ 19001   each additional cyst (List separately in addition to code for primary procedure)
Code first (19000)
📷 (76942, 77021)
🔲 0.62   🔲 0.77   **FUD** ZZZ   `N` `N1` 🔲
AMA: 2018,Jan,8; 2017,Jan,8; 2016,Jan,13; 2015,Jan,16; 2014,Jan,11

19020   Mastotomy with exploration or drainage of abscess, deep
🔲 8.84   🔲 13.5   **FUD** 090   `J` `A2` `50` 🔲
AMA: 2018,Jan,8; 2017,Jan,8; 2016,Jan,13; 2014,Dec,16; 2014,Dec,16; 2014,Jan,11

19030   Injection procedure only for mammary ductogram or galactogram
📷 (77053-77054)
🔲 2.23   🔲 4.74   **FUD** 000   `N` `N1` `50` 🔲
AMA: 2018,Jan,8; 2017,Jan,8; 2016,Jan,13; 2015,Jan,16; 2014,Jan,11

19081-19086 Breast Biopsy with Imaging Guidance

CMS: 100-03,220.13 Percutaneous Image-guided Breast Biopsy; 100-04,12,40.7 Bilateral Procedures; 100-04,13,80.1 Physician Presence; 100-04,13,80.2 S&I Multiple Procedure Reduction

INCLUDES   Breast biopsy with placement of localization devices
Fluoroscopic guidance for needle placement (77002)
Magnetic resonance guidance for needle placement (77021)
Radiological examination, surgical specimen (76098)
Ultrasonic guidance for needle placement (76942)

EXCLUDES   *Biopsy of breast without imaging guidance (19100-19101)*
Lesion removal without concentration on surgical margins (19110-19126)
Open biopsy after placement of localization device (19101)
Partial mastectomy (19301-19302)
Placement of localization devices only (19281-19288)
Total mastectomy (19303-19307)
Code also additional biopsies performed with different imaging modalities

19081   Biopsy, breast, with placement of breast localization device(s) (eg, clip, metallic pellet), when performed, and imaging of the biopsy specimen, when performed, percutaneous; first lesion, including stereotactic guidance
🔲 4.85   🔲 18.4   **FUD** 000   `J` `G2` `80` `50` 🔲
AMA: 2019,Apr,4; 2018,Jan,8; 2017,Jan,8; 2016,Jun,3; 2016,Jan,13; 2015,May,8; 2015,Mar,5; 2015,Jan,16; 2014,Jun,14; 2014,May,3

+ 19082   each additional lesion, including stereotactic guidance (List separately in addition to code for primary procedure)
Code first (19081)
🔲 2.44   🔲 15.0   **FUD** ZZZ   `N` `N1` `80` 🔲
AMA: 2019,Apr,4; 2018,Jan,8; 2017,Jan,8; 2016,Jun,3; 2016,Jan,13; 2015,May,8; 2015,Mar,5; 2015,Jan,16; 2014,Jun,14; 2014,May,3

19083   Biopsy, breast, with placement of breast localization device(s) (eg, clip, metallic pellet), when performed, and imaging of the biopsy specimen, when performed, percutaneous; first lesion, including ultrasound guidance
🔲 4.57   🔲 18.0   **FUD** 000   `J` `G2` `80` `50` 🔲
AMA: 2019,Apr,4; 2018,Jan,8; 2017,Jan,8; 2016,Jun,3; 2016,Jan,13; 2015,May,8; 2015,Mar,5; 2015,Jan,16; 2014,Jun,14; 2014,May,3

+ 19084   each additional lesion, including ultrasound guidance (List separately in addition to code for primary procedure)
Code first (19083)
🔲 2.28   🔲 14.4   **FUD** ZZZ   `N` `N1` `80` 🔲
AMA: 2019,Apr,4; 2018,Jan,8; 2017,Jan,8; 2016,Jun,3; 2016,Jan,13; 2015,May,8; 2015,Mar,5; 2015,Jan,16; 2014,Jun,14; 2014,May,3

19085   Biopsy, breast, with placement of breast localization device(s) (eg, clip, metallic pellet), when performed, and imaging of the biopsy specimen, when performed, percutaneous; first lesion, including magnetic resonance guidance
🔲 5.30   🔲 27.3   **FUD** 000   `J` `G2` `80` `50` 🔲
AMA: 2019,Apr,4; 2018,Jan,8; 2017,Jan,8; 2016,Jun,3; 2016,Jan,13; 2015,May,8; 2015,Mar,5; 2015,Jan,16; 2014,Jun,14; 2014,May,3

+ 19086   each additional lesion, including magnetic resonance guidance (List separately in addition to code for primary procedure)
Code first (19085)
🔲 2.65   🔲 21.9   **FUD** ZZZ   `N` `N1` `80` 🔲
AMA: 2019,Apr,4; 2018,Jan,8; 2017,Jan,8; 2016,Jun,3; 2016,Jan,13; 2015,May,8; 2015,Mar,5; 2015,Jan,16; 2014,Jun,14; 2014,May,3

19100-19101 Breast Biopsy Without Imaging Guidance

EXCLUDES   *Biopsy of breast with imaging guidance (19081-19086)*
Lesion removal without concentration on surgical margins (19110-19126)
Partial mastectomy (19301-19302)
Total mastectomy (19303-19307)

19100   Biopsy of breast; percutaneous, needle core, not using imaging guidance (separate procedure)
EXCLUDES   *Fine needle aspiration:*
    With imaging guidance ([10005, 10006, 10007, 10008, 10009, 10010, 10011, 10012])
    Without imaging guidance (10021, [10004])
🔲 2.03   🔲 4.32   **FUD** 000   `J` `A2` `50` 🔲
AMA: 2018,Jan,8; 2017,Jan,8; 2016,Jan,13; 2015,Jan,16; 2014,May,3; 2014,Jan,11

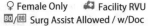

Labels: Clavicle, Deltoid, Tail of Spence area, Brachialis, Parasternal nodes, Lateral nodes, Subscapular nodes, Pectoral nodes, Central nodes, Axillary lymph nodes, Lactiferous ducts and gland lobules, Latissimus dorsi muscle, Areola, Nipple

19101   open, incisional
Code also placement of localization device with imaging guidance (19281-19288)
⚕ 6.39 ⚕ 9.64 **FUD** 010 `J` `A2` `50` 🔲
AMA: 2018,Jan,8; 2017,Jan,8; 2016,Jan,13; 2015,Jan,16; 2014,May,3; 2014,Jan,11

19105 Treatment of Fibroadenoma: Cryoablation
CMS: 100-04,13,80.1 Physician Presence; 100-04,13,80.2 S&I Multiple Procedure Reduction
INCLUDES Adjacent lesions treated with one cryoprobe
Ultrasound guidance (76940, 76942)
EXCLUDES Cryoablation of malignant breast tumors (0581T)

19105   Ablation, cryosurgical, of fibroadenoma, including ultrasound guidance, each fibroadenoma
⚕ 6.13 ⚕ 80.5 **FUD** 000 `J` `J8` `50` 🔲
AMA: 2007,Mar,7-8

19110-19126 Excisional Procedures: Breast
INCLUDES Open removal of breast mass without concentration on surgical margins
Code also placement of localization device with imaging guidance (19281-19288)

19110   Nipple exploration, with or without excision of a solitary lactiferous duct or a papilloma lactiferous duct
⚕ 9.94 ⚕ 13.9 **FUD** 090 `J` `A2` `50` 🔲
AMA: 2018,Jan,8; 2017,Jan,8; 2016,Jan,13; 2015,Jan,16; 2014,Jan,11

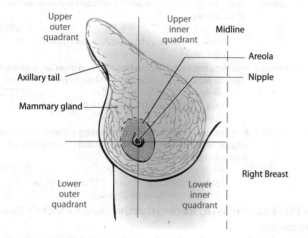

19112   Excision of lactiferous duct fistula
⚕ 9.04 ⚕ 13.1 **FUD** 090 `J` `A2` `80` `50` 🔲
AMA: 2018,Jan,8; 2017,Jan,8; 2016,Jan,13; 2015,Jan,16; 2014,Jan,11

19120   Excision of cyst, fibroadenoma, or other benign or malignant tumor, aberrant breast tissue, duct lesion, nipple or areolar lesion (except 19300), open, male or female, 1 or more lesions
⚕ 11.9 ⚕ 14.3 **FUD** 090 `J` `A2` `50` 🔲
AMA: 2018,Jan,8; 2017,Jan,8; 2016,Jan,13; 2015,Mar,5; 2015,Jan,16; 2014,Mar,13; 2014,Jan,11

19125   Excision of breast lesion identified by preoperative placement of radiological marker, open; single lesion
INCLUDES Intraoperative clip placement
⚕ 13.2 ⚕ 15.8 **FUD** 090 `J` `A2` `50` 🔲
AMA: 2018,Jan,8; 2017,Jan,8; 2016,Jan,13; 2015,Mar,5; 2015,Jan,16; 2014,Jan,11

+ 19126   each additional lesion separately identified by a preoperative radiological marker (List separately in addition to code for primary procedure)
INCLUDES Intraoperative clip placement
Code first (19125)
⚕ 4.68 ⚕ 4.68 **FUD** ZZZ `N` `N1` 🔲
AMA: 2018,Jan,8; 2017,Jan,8; 2016,Jan,13; 2015,Jan,16; 2014,Jan,11

19260-19272 Excisional Procedures: Chest Wall
~~19260   Excision of chest wall tumor including ribs~~
To report, see (21601)
~~19271   Excision of chest wall tumor involving ribs, with plastic reconstruction; without mediastinal lymphadenectomy~~
To report, see (21602)
~~19272   with mediastinal lymphadenectomy~~
To report, see (21603)

19281-19288 Placement of Localization Markers
INCLUDES Placement of localization devices only
EXCLUDES Biopsy of breast without imaging guidance (19100-19101)
Fluoroscopic guidance for needle placement (77002)
Localization device placement with biopsy of breast (19081-19086)
Magnetic resonance guidance for needle placement (77021)
Ultrasonic guidance for needle placement (76942)
Code also open excision of breast lesion when performed after localization device placement (19110-19126)
Code also open incisional breast biopsy when performed after localization device placement (19101)
Code also radiography of surgical specimen (76098)

19281   Placement of breast localization device(s) (eg, clip, metallic pellet, wire/needle, radioactive seeds), percutaneous; first lesion, including mammographic guidance
⚕ 2.91 ⚕ 6.90 **FUD** 000 `Q1` `N1` `80` `50` 🔲
AMA: 2018,Jan,8; 2017,Jan,8; 2016,Jun,3; 2016,Jan,13; 2015,May,8; 2015,Jan,16; 2014,Jun,14; 2014,May,3

+ 19282   each additional lesion, including mammographic guidance (List separately in addition to code for primary procedure)
Code first (19281)
⚕ 1.46 ⚕ 4.82 **FUD** ZZZ `N` `N1` `80` 🔲
AMA: 2018,Jan,8; 2017,Jan,8; 2016,Jun,3; 2016,Jan,13; 2015,May,8; 2015,Jan,16; 2014,Jun,14; 2014,May,3

19283   Placement of breast localization device(s) (eg, clip, metallic pellet, wire/needle, radioactive seeds), percutaneous; first lesion, including stereotactic guidance
⚕ 2.93 ⚕ 7.73 **FUD** 000 `Q1` `N1` `80` `50` 🔲
AMA: 2018,Jan,8; 2017,Jan,8; 2016,Jun,3; 2016,May,13; 2016,Jan,13; 2015,May,8; 2015,Jan,16; 2014,May,3

+ 19284   each additional lesion, including stereotactic guidance (List separately in addition to code for primary procedure)
Code first (19283)
⚕ 1.50 ⚕ 5.87 **FUD** ZZZ `N` `N1` `80` 🔲
AMA: 2018,Jan,8; 2017,Jan,8; 2016,Jun,3; 2016,May,13; 2016,Jan,13; 2015,May,8; 2015,Jan,16; 2014,May,3

19285   Placement of breast localization device(s) (eg, clip, metallic pellet, wire/needle, radioactive seeds), percutaneous; first lesion, including ultrasound guidance
⚕ 2.50 ⚕ 13.7 **FUD** 000 `Q1` `N1` `80` `50` 🔲
AMA: 2018,Jan,8; 2017,Jan,8; 2016,Jun,3; 2016,May,13; 2016,Jan,13; 2015,May,8; 2015,Jan,16; 2014,May,3

+ 19286   each additional lesion, including ultrasound guidance (List separately in addition to code for primary procedure)
Code first (19285)
⚕ 1.25 ⚕ 11.9 **FUD** ZZZ `N` `N1` `80` 🔲
AMA: 2018,Jan,8; 2017,Jan,8; 2016,Jun,3; 2016,May,13; 2016,Jan,13; 2015,May,8; 2015,Jan,16; 2014,May,3

19287   Placement of breast localization device(s) (eg clip, metallic pellet, wire/needle, radioactive seeds), percutaneous; first lesion, including magnetic resonance guidance
⚕ 3.72 ⚕ 23.3 **FUD** 000 `Q1` `N1` `80` `50` 🔲
AMA: 2018,Jan,8; 2017,Jan,8; 2016,Jun,3; 2016,May,13; 2016,Jan,13; 2015,Jan,16; 2014,May,3

Integumentary System

+ 19288   each additional lesion, including magnetic resonance guidance (List separately in addition to code for primary procedure)
Code first (19287)
📷 1.87   ⚗ 18.6   **FUD** ZZZ   N N1 80 ▣
AMA: 2018,Jan,8; 2017,Jan,8; 2016,Jun,3; 2016,May,13; 2016,Jan,13; 2015,Jan,16; 2014,May,3

19294-19298 Radioelement Application

+ 19294   Preparation of tumor cavity, with placement of a radiation therapy applicator for intraoperative radiation therapy (IORT) concurrent with partial mastectomy (List separately in addition to code for primary procedure)
📷 4.71   ⚗ 4.71   **FUD** ZZZ   N N1 80 ▣
Code first (19301-19302)

19296   Placement of radiotherapy afterloading expandable catheter (single or multichannel) into the breast for interstitial radioelement application following partial mastectomy, includes imaging guidance; on date separate from partial mastectomy
📷 6.09   ⚗ 113.   **FUD** 000   J J8 80 50 ▣
AMA: 2018,Jan,8; 2017,Jan,8; 2016,Jan,13; 2015,Jan,16; 2014,Jan,11

+ 19297   concurrent with partial mastectomy (List separately in addition to code for primary procedure)
Code first (19301-19302)
📷 2.75   ⚗ 2.75   **FUD** ZZZ   N N1 80 ▣
AMA: 2019,Apr,10; 2018,Jan,8; 2017,Jan,8; 2016,Jan,13; 2015,Jan,16; 2014,Jan,11

19298   Placement of radiotherapy after loading brachytherapy catheters (multiple tube and button type) into the breast for interstitial radioelement application following (at the time of or subsequent to) partial mastectomy, includes imaging guidance
📷 9.17   ⚗ 28.2   **FUD** 000   J G2 80 50 ▣
AMA: 2018,Jan,8; 2017,Jan,8; 2016,Jan,13; 2015,Jan,16; 2014,Jan,11

19300-19307 Mastectomies: Partial, Simple, Radical

CMS: 100-04,12,40.7 Bilateral Procedures
INCLUDES   Intraoperative clip placement
EXCLUDES   Insertion of prosthesis (19340, 19342)

19300   Mastectomy for gynecomastia   ♂
EXCLUDES   Removal of breast tissue for:
Other than gynecomastia (19318)
Treatment or prevention of breast cancer (19301-19307)
📷 11.9   ⚗ 15.3   **FUD** 090   J A2 50 ▣
AMA: 2018,Jan,8; 2017,Jan,8; 2016,Jan,13; 2015,Jan,16; 2014,Mar,13; 2014,Jan,11

19301   Mastectomy, partial (eg, lumpectomy, tylectomy, quadrantectomy, segmentectomy);
EXCLUDES   Insertion of radiotherapy afterloading balloon during separate encounter (19296)
Code also intraoperative radiofrequency spectroscopy margin assessment and report (0546T)
Code also insertion of radiotherapy afterloading balloon catheter, when performed at same time (19297)
Code also insertion of radiotherapy afterloading brachytherapy catheter, when performed at same time (19298)
Code also tumor cavity preparation with intraoperative radiation therapy applicator, when performed (19294)
📷 18.8   ⚗ 18.8   **FUD** 090   J A2 80 50 ▣
AMA: 2018,Jan,8; 2017,Oct,9; 2017,Jan,8; 2016,Jan,13; 2015,Mar,5; 2015,Jan,16; 2014,Jan,11

19302   with axillary lymphadenectomy
EXCLUDES   Insertion of radiotherapy afterloading balloon during separate encounter (19296)
Code also intraoperative radiofrequency spectroscopy margin assessment and report (0546T)
Code also insertion of radiotherapy afterloading balloon catheter, when performed at same time (19297)
Code also insertion of radiotherapy afterloading brachytherapy catheter, when performed at same time (19298)
Code also tumor cavity preparation with intraoperative radiation therapy applicator, when performed (19294)
📷 25.9   ⚗ 25.9   **FUD** 090   J A2 80 50 ▣
AMA: 2019,Feb,8; 2018,Jan,8; 2017,Jan,8; 2016,Jan,13; 2015,Mar,5; 2015,Jan,16; 2014,Jan,11

19303   Mastectomy, simple, complete
EXCLUDES   Excision of pectoral muscles and axillary or internal mammary lymph nodes
Removal of breast tissue for:
Gynecomastia (19300)
Other than gynecomastia (19318)
📷 27.6   ⚗ 27.6   **FUD** 090   J A2 80 50 ▣
AMA: 2018,Jan,8; 2017,Jan,8; 2016,Jan,13; 2015,Mar,5; 2015,Jan,16; 2014,Jan,11

~~19304~~   ~~Mastectomy, subcutaneous~~

19305   Mastectomy, radical, including pectoral muscles, axillary lymph nodes
📷 32.7   ⚗ 32.7   **FUD** 090   C 80 50 ▣
AMA: 2018,Jan,8; 2017,Jan,8; 2016,Jan,13; 2015,Jan,16; 2014,Jan,11

19306   Mastectomy, radical, including pectoral muscles, axillary and internal mammary lymph nodes (Urban type operation)
📷 34.7   ⚗ 34.7   **FUD** 090   C 80 50 ▣
AMA: 2018,Jan,8; 2017,Jan,8; 2016,Jan,13; 2015,Jan,16; 2014,Jan,11

19307   Mastectomy, modified radical, including axillary lymph nodes, with or without pectoralis minor muscle, but excluding pectoralis major muscle
📷 34.6   ⚗ 34.6   **FUD** 090   J 80 50 ▣
AMA: 2019,Feb,8; 2018,Jan,8; 2017,Jan,8; 2016,Jan,13; 2015,Mar,5; 2015,Jan,16; 2014,Jan,11

19316-19499 Plastic, Reconstructive, and Aesthetic Breast Procedures

CMS: 100-03,140.2 Breast Reconstruction Following Mastectomy; 100-04,12,40.7 Bilateral Procedures
Code also biologic implant for tissue reinforcement (15777)

19316   Mastopexy
📷 22.1   ⚗ 22.1   **FUD** 090   J A2 80 50 ▣
AMA: 2018,Jan,8; 2017,Jan,8; 2016,Jan,13; 2015,Jan,16; 2014,Jan,11

19318   Reduction mammaplasty
INCLUDES   Aries-Pitanguy mammaplasty
Biesenberger mammaplasty
📷 31.5   ⚗ 31.5   **FUD** 090   J A2 80 50 ▣
AMA: 2018,Jan,8; 2017,Jan,8; 2016,Jan,13; 2015,Jan,16; 2014,Apr,10; 2014,Jan,11

19324   Mammaplasty, augmentation; without prosthetic implant
📷 15.2   ⚗ 15.2   **FUD** 090   J A2 80 50 ▣
AMA: 2018,Jan,8; 2017,Jan,8; 2016,Jan,13; 2015,Jan,16; 2014,Jan,11

19325   with prosthetic implant
EXCLUDES   Flap or graft (15100-15650)
📷 18.4   ⚗ 18.4   **FUD** 090   J G2 80 50 ▣
AMA: 2018,Jan,8; 2017,Jan,8; 2016,Jan,13; 2015,Jan,16; 2014,Jan,11

19328   Removal of intact mammary implant
📷 14.2   ⚗ 14.2   **FUD** 090   02 A2 50 ▣
AMA: 2018,Jan,8; 2017,Jan,8; 2016,Jan,13; 2015,Jan,16; 2014,Jan,11

2B/TC PC/TC Only   A2-Z3 ASC Payment   50 Bilateral   ♂ Male Only   ♀ Female Only   📷 Facility RVU   ⚗ Non-Facility RVU   ▣ CCI   ✖ CLIA
FUD Follow-up Days   **CMS:** IOM   **AMA:** CPT Asst   A-Y OPPSI   80/80 Surg Assist Allowed / w/Doc   Lab Crosswalk   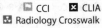 Radiology Crosswalk

                                       © 2019 Optum360, LLC

19330 **Removal of mammary implant material**
📷 18.1 ⚱ 18.1 **FUD** 090 [02] [A2] [50] [▣]
AMA: 2018,Jan,8; 2017,Jan,8; 2016,Jan,13; 2015,Jan,16; 2014,Jan,11

19340 **Immediate insertion of breast prosthesis following mastopexy, mastectomy or in reconstruction**
EXCLUDES Supply of prosthetic implant (99070, L8030, L8039, L8600)
📷 28.6 ⚱ 28.6 **FUD** 090 [J] [A2] [50] [▣]
AMA: 2018,Jan,8; 2017,Jan,8; 2016,Jan,13; 2015,Dec,18; 2015,Jan,16; 2014,Jan,11

19342 **Delayed insertion of breast prosthesis following mastopexy, mastectomy or in reconstruction**
EXCLUDES Preparation of moulage for custom breast implant (19396)
📷 26.5 ⚱ 26.5 **FUD** 090 [J] [A2] [80] [50] [▣]
AMA: 2018,Jan,8; 2017,Jan,8; 2016,Jan,13; 2015,Nov,10; 2015,Jan,16; 2014,Jan,11

19350 **Nipple/areola reconstruction**
📷 19.3 ⚱ 23.6 **FUD** 090 [J] [A2] [50] [▣]
AMA: 2018,Jan,8; 2017,Jan,8; 2016,Aug,9; 2016,Jan,13; 2015,Jan,16; 2014,Jan,11

19355 **Correction of inverted nipples**
📷 17.7 ⚱ 21.5 **FUD** 090 [J] [A2] [80] [50] [▣]
AMA: 2018,Jan,8; 2017,Jan,8; 2016,Jan,13; 2015,Jan,16; 2014,Jan,11

19357 **Breast reconstruction, immediate or delayed, with tissue expander, including subsequent expansion**
📷 43.1 ⚱ 43.1 **FUD** 090 [J] [J8] [80] [50] [▣]
AMA: 2018,Jan,8; 2017,Jan,8; 2016,Jan,13; 2015,Feb,10; 2015,Jan,16; 2014,Jan,11

19361 **Breast reconstruction with latissimus dorsi flap, without prosthetic implant**
EXCLUDES Implant of prosthesis (19340)
📷 45.2 ⚱ 45.2 **FUD** 090 [C] [80] [50] [▣]
AMA: 2018,Jan,8; 2017,Jan,8; 2016,Jan,13; 2015,Feb,10; 2015,Jan,16; 2014,Jan,11

19364 **Breast reconstruction with free flap**
INCLUDES Closure of donor site
Harvesting of skin graft
Inset shaping of flap into breast
Microvascular repair
Operating microscope (69990)
📷 79.2 ⚱ 79.2 **FUD** 090 [C] [80] [50] [▣]
AMA: 2018,Jan,8; 2017,Jan,8; 2016,Feb,12; 2016,Jan,13; 2015,Feb,10; 2015,Jan,16; 2014,Apr,10; 2014,Jan,11

19366 **Breast reconstruction with other technique**
INCLUDES Operating microscope (69990)
Code also implant of prosthesis if appropriate (19340, 19342)
📷 40.3 ⚱ 40.3 **FUD** 090 [J] [A2] [80] [50] [▣]
AMA: 2018,Jan,8; 2017,Jan,8; 2016,Jan,13; 2015,Feb,10; 2015,Jan,16; 2014,Apr,10; 2014,Jan,11

19367 **Breast reconstruction with transverse rectus abdominis myocutaneous flap (TRAM), single pedicle, including closure of donor site;**
📷 51.3 ⚱ 51.3 **FUD** 090 [C] [80] [50] [▣]
AMA: 2018,Jan,8; 2017,Jan,8; 2016,Jan,13; 2015,Feb,10; 2015,Jan,16; 2014,Jan,11

19368 **with microvascular anastomosis (supercharging)**
INCLUDES Operating microscope (69990)
📷 63.2 ⚱ 63.2 **FUD** 090 [C] [80] [50] [▣]
AMA: 2018,Jan,8; 2017,Jan,8; 2016,Feb,12; 2016,Jan,13; 2015,Feb,10; 2015,Jan,16; 2014,Jan,11

19369 **Breast reconstruction with transverse rectus abdominis myocutaneous flap (TRAM), double pedicle, including closure of donor site**
📷 58.6 ⚱ 58.6 **FUD** 090 [C] [80] [50] [▣]
AMA: 2018,Jan,8; 2017,Jan,8; 2016,Jan,13; 2015,Feb,10; 2015,Jan,16; 2014,Jan,11

19370 **Open periprosthetic capsulotomy, breast**
📷 19.7 ⚱ 19.7 **FUD** 090 [J] [A2] [50] [▣]
AMA: 2018,Jan,8; 2017,Jan,8; 2016,Jan,13; 2015,Dec,18; 2015,Jan,16; 2014,Jan,11

19371 **Periprosthetic capsulectomy, breast**
📷 22.5 ⚱ 22.5 **FUD** 090 [J] [A2] [50] [▣]
AMA: 2018,Jan,8; 2017,Jan,8; 2016,Jan,13; 2015,Jan,16; 2014,Jan,11

19380 **Revision of reconstructed breast**
📷 22.2 ⚱ 22.2 **FUD** 090 [J] [A2] [50] [▣]
AMA: 2018,Jan,8; 2017,Dec,13; 2017,Jan,8; 2016,Jan,13; 2015,Dec,18; 2015,Jan,16; 2014,Jan,11

19396 **Preparation of moulage for custom breast implant**
📷 4.17 ⚱ 8.23 **FUD** 000 [J] [62] [80] [50] [▣]
AMA: 2018,Jan,8; 2017,Jan,8; 2016,Jan,13; 2015,Jan,16; 2014,Jan,11

19499 **Unlisted procedure, breast**
📷 0.00 ⚱ 0.00 **FUD** YYY [J] [80] [50] [▣]
AMA: 2019,Aug,10; 2019,Apr,10; 2018,Jan,8; 2017,Jan,8; 2016,Dec,16; 2016,Jan,13; 2015,Mar,5; 2015,Jan,16; 2014,Dec,16; 2014,Dec,16; 2014,Jan,11

20100-20103 Exploratory Surgery of Traumatic Wound

INCLUDES Debridement
Expanded dissection of wound for exploration
Extraction of foreign material
Open examination
Tying or coagulation of small vessels

EXCLUDES Cutaneous/subcutaneous incision and drainage procedures (10060-10061)
Laparotomy (49000-49010)
Repair of major vessels of:
  Abdomen (35221, 35251, 35281)
  Chest (35211, 35216, 35241, 35246, 35271, 35276)
  Extremity (35206-35207, 35226, 35236, 35256, 35266, 35286)
  Neck (35201, 35231, 35261)
Thoracotomy (32100-32160)

20100 Exploration of penetrating wound (separate procedure); neck
🔧 17.5   ⚕ 17.5   **FUD** 010   T 80 50 ▢
AMA: 2018,Jan,8; 2017,Jan,8; 2016,Jan,13; 2015,Jan,16; 2014,Jan,11

20101 chest
🔧 6.05   ⚕ 12.9   **FUD** 010   T ▢
AMA: 2018,Jan,8; 2017,Jan,8; 2016,Jan,13; 2015,Jan,16; 2014,Jan,11

20102 abdomen/flank/back
🔧 7.39   ⚕ 14.0   **FUD** 010   T ▢
AMA: 2018,Jan,8; 2017,Jan,8; 2016,Jan,13; 2015,Jan,16; 2014,Jan,11

20103 extremity
🔧 9.99   ⚕ 16.6   **FUD** 010   T 62 80 ▢
AMA: 2018,Jan,8; 2017,Jan,8; 2016,Jan,13; 2015,Jan,16; 2014,Jan,11

20150 Epiphyseal Bar Resection

20150 Excision of epiphyseal bar, with or without autogenous soft tissue graft obtained through same fascial incision
🔧 29.0   ⚕ 29.0   **FUD** 090   J 62 80 50 ▢
AMA: 1996,Nov,1

20200-20206 Muscle Biopsy

EXCLUDES Removal of muscle tumor (see appropriate anatomic section)

20200 Biopsy, muscle; superficial
🔧 2.73   ⚕ 5.95   **FUD** 000   J A2 ▢

20205 deep
🔧 4.48   ⚕ 8.35   **FUD** 000   J A2 ▢

20206 Biopsy, muscle, percutaneous needle
EXCLUDES Fine needle aspiration (10021, [10004, 10005, 10006, 10007, 10008, 10009, 10010, 10011, 10012])
🔬 (76942, 77002, 77012, 77021)
🔬 (88172-88173)
🔧 1.68   ⚕ 6.71   **FUD** 000   J A2 ▢
AMA: 2019,Apr,4

20220-20225 Percutaneous Bone Biopsy

EXCLUDES Bone marrow aspiration(s) or biopsy(ies) (38220-38222)

20220 Biopsy, bone, trocar, or needle; superficial (eg, ilium, sternum, spinous process, ribs)
🔬 (77002, 77012, 77021)
🔧 2.06   ⚕ 4.79   **FUD** 000   J A2 ▢
AMA: 2018,Jan,8; 2017,Jan,8; 2016,Jan,13; 2015,Jan,16; 2014,Jan,11

20225 deep (eg, vertebral body, femur)
EXCLUDES Percutaneous vertebroplasty (22510-22515)
Percutaneous sacral augmentation (sacroplasty) (0200T-0201T)
🔬 (77002, 77012, 77021)
🔧 3.07   ⚕ 14.7   **FUD** 000   J A2 ▢
AMA: 2018,Jan,8; 2017,Jan,8; 2016,Jan,13; 2015,Jan,8; 2015,Jan,16; 2014,Jan,11

20240-20251 Open Bone Biopsy

EXCLUDES Sequestrectomy or incision and drainage of bone abscess of:
  Calcaneus (28120)
  Carpal bone (25145)
  Clavicle (23170)
  Humeral head (23174)
  Humerus (24134)
  Olecranon process (24138)
  Radius (24136, 25145)
  Scapula (23172)
  Skull (61501)
  Talus (28120)
  Ulna (24138, 24145)

20240 Biopsy, bone, open; superficial (eg, sternum, spinous process, rib, patella, olecranon process, calcaneus, tarsal, metatarsal, carpal, metacarpal, phalanx)
🔧 4.31   ⚕ 4.31   **FUD** 000   J A2 ▢
AMA: 2018,Jan,8; 2017,Jan,8; 2016,Jan,13; 2015,Jan,16; 2014,Jan,11

20245 deep (eg, humeral shaft, ischium, femoral shaft)
🔧 10.1   ⚕ 10.1   **FUD** 000   J A2 ▢
AMA: 2018,Jan,8; 2017,Jan,8; 2016,Jan,13; 2015,Jan,16; 2014,Jan,11

20250 Biopsy, vertebral body, open; thoracic
🔧 11.5   ⚕ 11.5   **FUD** 000   J A2 ▢
AMA: 2018,Jan,8; 2017,Jan,8; 2016,Jan,13; 2015,Jan,16; 2014,Jan,11

20251 lumbar or cervical
🔧 12.4   ⚕ 12.4   **FUD** 010   J A2 80 ▢
AMA: 2018,Jan,8; 2017,Jan,8; 2016,Jan,13; 2015,Jan,16; 2014,Jan,11

20500-20501 Injection Fistula/Sinus Tract

EXCLUDES Arthrography injection of:
  Ankle (27648)
  Elbow (24220)
  Hip (27093, 27095)
  Sacroiliac joint (27096)
  Shoulder (23350)
  Temporomandibular joint (TMJ) (21116)
  Wrist (25246)
  Autologous adipose-derived regenerative cells injection (0490T)

20500 Injection of sinus tract; therapeutic (separate procedure)
🔧 2.45   ⚕ 3.09   **FUD** 010   T P3 ▢
🔬 (76080)

20501 diagnostic (sinogram)
🔧 1.09   ⚕ 3.62   **FUD** 000   N N1 ▢
EXCLUDES Contrast injection or injections for radiological evaluation of existing gastrostomy, duodenostomy, jejunostomy, gastro-jejunostomy, or cecostomy (or other colonic) tube from percutaneous approach (49465)
🔬 (76080)

20520-20525 Foreign Body Removal

20520 Removal of foreign body in muscle or tendon sheath; simple
🔧 4.20   ⚕ 5.87   **FUD** 010   J P3 ▢

20525 deep or complicated
🔧 7.11   ⚕ 13.6   **FUD** 010   J A2 ▢

20526-20561 [20560, 20561] Therapeutic Injections: Tendons, Trigger Points

EXCLUDES Autologous adipose-derived regenerative cells injection (0489T-0490T)
Platelet rich plasma (PRP) injections (0232T)

20526 Injection, therapeutic (eg, local anesthetic, corticosteroid), carpal tunnel
🔧 1.66   ⚕ 2.20   **FUD** 000   T P3 50 ▢
AMA: 2018,Jan,8; 2017,Jan,8; 2016,Jan,13; 2015,Jan,16; 2014,Jan,11

Musculoskeletal System

20527 — 20660

20527 Injection, enzyme (eg, collagenase), palmar fascial cord (ie, Dupuytren's contracture)

> *EXCLUDES* Post injection palmar fascial cord manipulation (26341)
>
> 🖫 1.90 ⚕ 2.39 **FUD** 000 Ⓣ P3 50 ▢
>
> **AMA:** 2018,Jan,8; 2017,Jan,8; 2016,Jan,13; 2015,Jan,16; 2014,Jan,11

20550 Injection(s); single tendon sheath, or ligament, aponeurosis (eg, plantar "fascia")

> *EXCLUDES* Autologous WBC injection (0481T)
> Platelet rich plasma injection (0232T)
> Morton's neuroma (64455, 64632)
>
> ✖ (76942, 77002, 77021)
>
> 🖫 1.13 ⚕ 1.51 **FUD** 000 Ⓣ P3 50 ▢
>
> **AMA:** 2018,Jan,8; 2017,Jan,8; 2016,Jan,13; 2015,Jan,16; 2014,Oct,9; 2014,Jan,11

20551 single tendon origin/insertion

> *EXCLUDES* Autologous WBC injection (0481T)
> Platelet rich plasma injection (0232T)
>
> ✖ (76942, 77002, 77021)
>
> 🖫 1.15 ⚕ 1.53 **FUD** 000 Ⓣ P3 ▢
>
> **AMA:** 2018,Jan,8; 2017,Dec,13; 2017,Jan,8; 2016,Jan,13; 2015,Jan,16; 2014,Oct,9; 2014,Jan,11

20552 Injection(s); single or multiple trigger point(s), 1 or 2 muscle(s)

> *EXCLUDES* Autologous WBC injection (0481T)
> Needle insertion(s) without injection(s) for the same muscle(s) ([20560, 20561])
> Platelet rich plasma injection (0232T)
>
> ✖ (76942, 77002, 77021)
>
> 🖫 1.09 ⚕ 1.57 **FUD** 000 Ⓣ P3 ▢
>
> **AMA:** 2018,Jan,8; 2017,Dec,13; 2017,Jun,10; 2017,Jan,8; 2016,Jan,13; 2015,Jan,16; 2014,Oct,9; 2014,Jan,11

20553 single or multiple trigger point(s), 3 or more muscles

> *EXCLUDES* Needle insertion(s) without injection(s) for the same muscle(s) ([20560, 20561])
>
> ✖ (76942, 77002, 77021)
>
> 🖫 1.24 ⚕ 1.81 **FUD** 000 Ⓣ P3 ▢
>
> **AMA:** 2018,Dec,8; 2018,Dec,8; 2018,Jan,8; 2017,Jun,10; 2017,Jan,8; 2016,Jan,13; 2015,Jan,16; 2014,Oct,9; 2014,Jan,11

● # **20560** Needle insertion(s) without injection(s); 1 or 2 muscle(s)

> 🖫 0.00 ⚕ 0.00 **FUD** 000
>
> *INCLUDES* Dry needling and trigger-point acupuncture

● # **20561** 3 or more muscles

> 🖫 0.00 ⚕ 0.00 **FUD** 000
>
> *INCLUDES* Dry needling and trigger-point acupuncture

20555-20561 Placement of Catheters/Needles for Brachytherapy

Code also interstitial radioelement application (77770-77772, 77778)

20555 Placement of needles or catheters into muscle and/or soft tissue for subsequent interstitial radioelement application (at the time of or subsequent to the procedure)

> *EXCLUDES* Interstitial radioelement:
> Devices placed into the breast (19296-19298)
> Placement of needle, catheters, or devices into muscle or soft tissue of the head and neck (41019)
> Placement of needles or catheters into pelvic organs or genitalia (55920)
> Placement of needles or catheters into prostate (55875)
>
> ✖ (76942, 77002, 77012, 77021)
>
> 🖫 9.49 ⚕ 9.49 **FUD** 000 Ⓙ R2 80 ▢
>
> **AMA:** 2018,Jan,8; 2017,Jan,8; 2016,Jan,13; 2015,Jan,16; 2014,Jan,11

20560 Resequenced code. See code following 20553.

20561 Resequenced code. See code before 20555.

20600-20611 Aspiration and/or Injection of Joint

CMS: 100-03,150.7 Prolotherapy, Joint Sclerotherapy, and Ligamentous Injections with Sclerosing Agents

> *EXCLUDES* Autologous adipose-derived regenerative cells injection (0489T-0490T)
> Ultrasonic guidance for needle placement (76942)

20600 Arthrocentesis, aspiration and/or injection, small joint or bursa (eg, fingers, toes); without ultrasound guidance

> ✖ (77002, 77012, 77021)
>
> 🖫 1.03 ⚕ 1.38 **FUD** 000 Ⓣ P3 50 ▢
>
> **AMA:** 2018,Sep,12; 2018,Jan,8; 2017,Aug,9; 2017,Jan,8; 2016,Jan,13; 2015,Nov,10; 2015,Feb,6; 2015,Jan,16; 2014,Jan,11

20604 with ultrasound guidance, with permanent recording and reporting

> *EXCLUDES* Autologous adipose-derived regenerative cells injection (0489T-0490T)
>
> ✖ (77002, 77012, 77021)
>
> 🖫 1.34 ⚕ 2.10 **FUD** 000 Ⓣ P3 50 ▢
>
> **AMA:** 2018,Sep,12; 2018,Jan,8; 2017,Jan,8; 2016,Jan,13; 2015,Jul,10; 2015,Feb,6

20605 Arthrocentesis, aspiration and/or injection, intermediate joint or bursa (eg, temporomandibular, acromioclavicular, wrist, elbow or ankle, olecranon bursa); without ultrasound guidance

> ✖ (77002, 77012, 77021)
>
> 🖫 1.07 ⚕ 1.44 **FUD** 000 Ⓣ P3 50 ▢
>
> **AMA:** 2018,Jan,8; 2017,Aug,9; 2017,Jan,8; 2016,Jan,13; 2015,Nov,10; 2015,Feb,6; 2015,Jan,16; 2014,Jan,11

20606 with ultrasound guidance, with permanent recording and reporting

> ✖ (77002, 77012, 77021)
>
> 🖫 1.53 ⚕ 2.32 **FUD** 000 Ⓣ P3 50 ▢
>
> **AMA:** 2018,Jan,8; 2017,Jan,8; 2016,Jan,13; 2015,Jul,10; 2015,Feb,6

20610 Arthrocentesis, aspiration and/or injection, major joint or bursa (eg, shoulder, hip, knee, subacromial bursa); without ultrasound guidance

> *EXCLUDES* Injection of contrast for knee arthrography (27369)
>
> ✖ (77002, 77012, 77021)
>
> 🖫 1.32 ⚕ 1.71 **FUD** 000 Ⓣ P3 50 ▢
>
> **AMA:** 2019,Aug,7; 2018,Jan,8; 2017,Apr,9; 2017,Jan,8; 2016,Jan,13; 2015,Nov,10; 2015,Aug,6; 2015,Feb,6; 2015,Jan,16; 2014,Dec,18; 2014,Jan,11

20611 with ultrasound guidance, with permanent recording and reporting

> *EXCLUDES* Injection of contrast for knee arthrography (27369)
>
> ✖ (77002, 77012, 77021)
>
> 🖫 1.75 ⚕ 2.61 **FUD** 000 Ⓣ P3 50 ▢
>
> **AMA:** 2019,Aug,7; 2018,Jan,8; 2017,Jan,8; 2016,Jan,13; 2015,Nov,10; 2015,Aug,6; 2015,Jul,10; 2015,Feb,6

20612-20615 Aspiration and/or Injection of Cyst

> *EXCLUDES* Autologous adipose-derived regenerative cells injection (0489T-0490T)

20612 Aspiration and/or injection of ganglion cyst(s) any location

> 🖫 1.20 ⚕ 1.71 **FUD** 000 Ⓣ P3 ▢
>
> Code also modifier 59 for multiple major joint aspirations or injections

20615 Aspiration and injection for treatment of bone cyst

> 🖫 4.63 ⚕ 6.95 **FUD** 010 Ⓣ P3 ▢

20650-20697 Procedures Related to Bony Fixation

20650 Insertion of wire or pin with application of skeletal traction, including removal (separate procedure)

> 🖫 4.58 ⚕ 6.07 **FUD** 010 Ⓙ A2 ▢

20660 Application of cranial tongs, caliper, or stereotactic frame, including removal (separate procedure)

> 🖫 7.07 ⚕ 7.07 **FUD** 000 02 ▢
>
> **AMA:** 2018,Jan,8; 2017,Jan,8; 2016,Jan,13; 2015,Jan,16; 2014,Jan,11

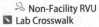

20661 Application of halo, including removal; cranial
🚑 14.5 ⚕ 14.5 **FUD** 090 [C] 🖵
AMA: 2018,Jan,8; 2017,Jan,8; 2016,Jan,13; 2015,Jan,16; 2014,Jan,11

20662 pelvic
🚑 14.7 ⚕ 14.7 **FUD** 090 [J][R2][80] 🖵

20663 femoral
🚑 13.5 ⚕ 13.5 **FUD** 090 [J][R2][80][50] 🖵

20664 Application of halo, including removal, cranial, 6 or more pins placed, for thin skull osteology (eg, pediatric patients, hydrocephalus, osteogenesis imperfecta)
🚑 25.3 ⚕ 25.3 **FUD** 090 [C] 🖵
AMA: 2018,Jan,8; 2017,Jan,8; 2016,Jan,13; 2015,Jan,16; 2014,Jan,11

20665 Removal of tongs or halo applied by another individual
🚑 2.65 ⚕ 3.13 **FUD** 010 [Q1][G2][80] 🖵
AMA: 2018,Jan,8; 2017,Jan,8; 2016,Jan,13; 2015,Jan,16; 2014,Jan,11

20670 Removal of implant; superficial (eg, buried wire, pin or rod) (separate procedure)
🚑 4.19 ⚕ 10.6 **FUD** 010 [Q2][A2] 🖵
AMA: 2018,Jan,3; 2018,Jan,8; 2017,Jan,8; 2016,Jan,13; 2015,Jan,16; 2014,Jan,11

20680 deep (eg, buried wire, pin, screw, metal band, nail, rod or plate)
EXCLUDES Removal and reinsertion sinus tarsi implant ([0511T])
Removal sinus tarsi implant ([0510T])
🚑 12.1 ⚕ 17.6 **FUD** 090 [Q2][A2][80] 🖵
AMA: 2018,Jan,3; 2018,Jan,8; 2017,Jan,8; 2016,Nov,9; 2016,Jan,13; 2015,Nov,10; 2015,Jan,16; 2014,Mar,4; 2014,Jan,11

20690 Application of a uniplane (pins or wires in 1 plane), unilateral, external fixation system
🚑 17.2 ⚕ 17.2 **FUD** 090 [J][J8] 🖵
AMA: 2018,Jan,3; 2018,Jan,8; 2017,Jan,8; 2016,Jan,13; 2015,Jan,16; 2014,Jan,11

20692 Application of a multiplane (pins or wires in more than 1 plane), unilateral, external fixation system (eg, Ilizarov, Monticelli type)
🚑 32.2 ⚕ 32.2 **FUD** 090 [J][J8][80] 🖵
AMA: 2019,May,10; 2018,Jan,8; 2018,Jan,3; 2017,Jan,8; 2016,Jan,13; 2015,Jan,16; 2014,Jan,11

20693 Adjustment or revision of external fixation system requiring anesthesia (eg, new pin[s] or wire[s] and/or new ring[s] or bar[s])
🚑 12.7 ⚕ 12.7 **FUD** 090 [J][A2] 🖵
AMA: 2018,Jan,3; 2018,Jan,8; 2017,Jan,8; 2016,Jan,13; 2015,Jan,16; 2014,Jan,11

20694 Removal, under anesthesia, of external fixation system
🚑 9.73 ⚕ 12.2 **FUD** 090 [Q2][A2] 🖵
AMA: 2018,Jan,3; 2018,Jan,8; 2017,Jan,8; 2016,Jan,13; 2015,Jan,16; 2014,Jan,11

20696 Application of multiplane (pins or wires in more than 1 plane), unilateral, external fixation with stereotactic computer-assisted adjustment (eg, spatial frame), including imaging; initial and subsequent alignment(s), assessment(s), and computation(s) of adjustment schedule(s)
EXCLUDES Application of multiplane external fixation system (20692)
Removal and replacement of each strut (20697)
🚑 34.4 ⚕ 34.4 **FUD** 090 [J][J8][80] 🖵
AMA: 2018,Jan,3; 2018,Jan,8; 2017,Jan,8; 2016,Jan,13; 2015,Jan,16; 2014,Jan,11

20697 exchange (ie, removal and replacement) of strut, each
EXCLUDES Application of multiplane external fixation system (20692)
Exchange of strut for multiplane external fixation system (20697)
🚑 58.9 ⚕ 58.9 **FUD** 000 [⊘][J][P2][80][TC] 🖵
AMA: 2018,Jan,3; 2018,Jan,8; 2017,Jan,8; 2016,Jan,13; 2015,Jan,16; 2014,Jan,11

20700-20705 Drug Delivery Device

● + **20700** Manual preparation and insertion of drug-delivery device(s), deep (eg, subfascial) (List separately in addition to code for primary procedure)
🚑 0.00 ⚕ 0.00 **FUD** 000
INCLUDES Combining therapeutic agents, including antibiotics, with carrier substance during operative episode
Forming resulting mixture into drug delivery devices (beads, nails, spacers)
Insertion therapeutic device/agent once per anatomic location
EXCLUDES Insertion drug delivery implant, non-biodegradable (11981)
Insertion prefabricated drug device
Code first (11010-11012, 11043, [11046], 11044, 11047, 20240-20251, 21010, 21025-21026, 21501-21510, 21627-21630, 22010-22015, 23030-23044, 23170-23184, 23334-23335, 23930-24000, 24134-24140, 24147, 24160, 25031-25040, 25145-25151, 26070, 26230-26236, 26990-26992, 27030, 27070-27071, 27090, 27301-27303, 27310, 27360, 27603-27604, 27610, 27640-27641, 28001-28003, 28020, 28120-28122)

● + **20701** Removal of drug-delivery device(s), deep (eg, subfascial) (List separately in addition to code for primary procedure)
🚑 0.00 ⚕ 0.00 **FUD** 000
INCLUDES Removal therapeutic device/agent once per anatomic location from subfascial tissues
EXCLUDES Removal drug delivery device, performed alone (20680)
Removal drug delivery implant, non-biodegradable (11982)
Code first (11010-11012, 11043, [11046], 11044, 11047, 20240-20251, 21010, 21025-21026, 21501-21510, 21627-21630, 22010-22015, 23030-23044, 23170-23184, 23334-23335, 23930-24000, 24134-24140, 24147, 24160, 25031-25040, 25145-25151, 26070, 26230-26236, 26990-26992, 27030, 27070-27071, 27090, 27301-27303, 27310, 27360, 27603-27604, 27610, 27640-27641, 28001-28003, 28020, 28120-28122)

● + **20702** Manual preparation and insertion of drug-delivery device(s), intramedullary (List separately in addition to code for primary procedure)
🚑 0.00 ⚕ 0.00 **FUD** 000
INCLUDES Combining therapeutic agents, including antibiotics, with carrier substance during operative episode
Forming resulting mixture into drug delivery devices (beads, nails, spacers)
Insertion therapeutic device/agent once per anatomic location into intramedullary spaces
EXCLUDES Insertion drug delivery implant, non-biodegradable (11981)
Insertion prefabricated drug device
Code first (20680-20692, 20694, 20802-20805, 20838, 21510, 23035, 23170, 23180, 23184, 23515, 23615, 23935, 24134, 24138-24140, 24147, 24430, 24516, 25035, 25145-25151, 25400, 25515, 25525-25526, 25545, 25574-25575, 27245, 27259, 27360, 27470, 27506, 27640, 27720)

● + **20703** **Removal of drug-delivery device(s), intramedullary (List separately in addition to code for primary procedure)**
0.00   0.00   **FUD** 000

> INCLUDES Removal therapeutic device/agent once per anatomic location from intramedullary spaces
>
> EXCLUDES Removal drug delivery device, performed alone (20680)
> Removal drug delivery implant, non-biodegradable (11982)
>
> Code first (20690-20692, 20694, 20802-20805, 20838, 21510, 23035, 23170, 23180, 23184, 23515, 23615, 23935, 24134, 24138-24140, 24147, 24430, 24516, 25035, 25145-25151, 25400, 25515, 25525-25526, 25545, 25574-25575, 27245, 27259, 27360, 27470, 27506, 27640, 27720)

● + **20704** **Manual preparation and insertion of drug-delivery device(s), intra-articular (List separately in addition to code for primary procedure)**
0.00   0.00   **FUD** 000

> INCLUDES Combining therapeutic agents, including antibiotics, with carrier substance during operative episode
> Forming resulting mixture into drug delivery devices (beads, nails, spacers)
> Insertion therapeutic device/agent once per anatomic location into intra-articular spaces
>
> EXCLUDES Insertion drug delivery implant, non-biodegradable (11981)
> Insertion prefabricated drug device
> Removal hip prosthesis (27091)
> Removal knee prosthesis (27488)
>
> Code first (22864-22865, 23040-23044, 23334, 24000, 24160, 25040, 25250-25251, 26070-26080, 26990, 27030, 27090, 27301, 27310, 27603, 27610, 28020)

● + **20705** **Removal of drug-delivery device(s), intra-articular (List separately in addition to code for primary procedure)**
0.00   0.00   **FUD** 000

> INCLUDES Removal therapeutic device/agent once per anatomic location from intra-articular space(s)
>
> EXCLUDES Open treatment femoral neck fracture/internal fixation or prosthetic replacement (27236)
> Partial knee replacement (27446)
> Partial or total hip replacement (27125-27130)
> Patella arthroplasty with prosthesis (27438)
> Removal drug delivery device, performed alone (20680)
> Removal drug delivery implant, non-biodegradable (11982)
> Removal hip prosthesis (27091)
> Removal knee prosthesis (27488)
> Removal shoulder prosthesis (23335)
> Revision hip arthroplasty (27134-27138)
> Revision knee arthroplasty (27486-27487)
>
> Code first (22864-22865, 23040-23044, 23334, 24000, 24160, 25040, 25250-25251, 26070-26080, 26990, 27030, 27090, 27301, 27310, 27603, 27610, 28020)

20802-20838 Reimplantation Procedures

> EXCLUDES Repair of incomplete amputation (see individual repair codes for bone(s), ligament(s), tendon(s), nerve(s), or blood vessel(s) and append modifier 52)

20802 **Replantation, arm (includes surgical neck of humerus through elbow joint), complete amputation**
79.6   79.6   **FUD** 090   C 80 50 ▣
AMA: 1997,Apr,4

20805 **Replantation, forearm (includes radius and ulna to radial carpal joint), complete amputation**
94.8   94.8   **FUD** 090   C 80 50 ▣
AMA: 1997,Apr,4

20808 **Replantation, hand (includes hand through metacarpophalangeal joints), complete amputation**
114.   114.   **FUD** 090   C 80 50 ▣
AMA: 1997,Apr,4

20816 **Replantation, digit, excluding thumb (includes metacarpophalangeal joint to insertion of flexor sublimis tendon), complete amputation**
59.6   59.6   **FUD** 090   C 80 ▣
AMA: 2018,Jan,8; 2017,Jan,8; 2016,Jan,13; 2015,Jan,16; 2014,Jan,11

20822 **Replantation, digit, excluding thumb (includes distal tip to sublimis tendon insertion), complete amputation**
51.2   51.2   **FUD** 090   J G2 80 ▣
AMA: 1997,Apr,4

20824 **Replantation, thumb (includes carpometacarpal joint to MP joint), complete amputation**
59.7   59.7   **FUD** 090   C 80 50 ▣
AMA: 1997,Apr,4

20827 **Replantation, thumb (includes distal tip to MP joint), complete amputation**
52.6   52.6   **FUD** 090   C 80 50 ▣
AMA: 1997,Apr,4

20838 **Replantation, foot, complete amputation**
80.6   80.6   **FUD** 090   C 80 50 ▣
AMA: 1997,Apr,4

20900-20926 Bone and Tissue Autografts

> EXCLUDES Acquisition of autogenous bone, bone marrow, cartilage, tendon, fascia lata or other grafts through distinct incision unless included in the code description
> Autologous fat graft obtained by liposuction (15771-15774)
> Bone graft procedures on the spine (20930-20938)
> Other autologous soft tissue grafts (fat, dermis, fascia) harvested by direct excision ([15769])

20900 **Bone graft, any donor area; minor or small (eg, dowel or button)**
5.37   11.7   **FUD** 000   J A2 80 ▣
AMA: 2018,Jul,14; 2018,Jan,8; 2017,Jan,8; 2016,Jan,13; 2015,Jan,16; 2014,Jan,11

20902 **major or large**
8.20   8.20   **FUD** 000   J A2 80 ▣
AMA: 2018,Jul,14; 2018,Jan,8; 2017,Jan,8; 2016,Jan,13; 2015,Jan,16; 2014,Jan,11

20910 **Cartilage graft; costochondral**
> EXCLUDES Graft with ear cartilage (21235)

13.4   13.4   **FUD** 090   T A2 80 ▣
AMA: 2018,Jul,14; 2018,Jan,8; 2017,Jan,8; 2016,Jan,13; 2015,Jan,16; 2014,Jan,11

20912 **nasal septum**
> EXCLUDES Graft with ear cartilage (21235)

13.6   13.6   **FUD** 090   T A2 80 ▣
AMA: 2018,Jul,14

20920 **Fascia lata graft; by stripper**
11.5   11.5   **FUD** 090   T A2 ▣
AMA: 2018,Jul,14; 2018,Jan,8; 2017,Jan,8; 2016,Jan,13; 2015,Jan,16; 2014,Jan,11

20922 **by incision and area exposure, complex or sheet**
14.0   17.0   **FUD** 090   T A2 80 ▣
AMA: 2018,Jul,14; 2018,Jan,8; 2017,Jan,8; 2016,Jan,13; 2015,Jan,16; 2014,Jan,11

20924 **Tendon graft, from a distance (eg, palmaris, toe extensor, plantaris)**
14.5   14.5   **FUD** 090   J A2 80 ▣
AMA: 2018,Jul,14

20926 ~~Tissue grafts, other (eg, paratenon, fat, dermis)~~

20930-20939 Bone Allograft and Autograft of Spine

EXCLUDES Acquisition of autogenous bone, bone marrow, cartilage, tendon, fascia lata, or other grafts through distinct incision unless included in the code description
Autologous fat graft obtained by liposuction (15771-15774)
Other autologous soft tissue grafts (fat, dermis, fascia) harvested by direct excision ([15769])

+ **20930** **Allograft, morselized, or placement of osteopromotive material, for spine surgery only (List separately in addition to code for primary procedure)**
Code first (22319, 22532-22533, 22548-22558, 22590-22612, 22630, 22633-22634, 22800-22812)
🚗 0.00 ⚕ 0.00 **FUD** XXX N N1 ▣
AMA: 2019,May,7; 2018,Jul,14; 2018,Jan,8; 2017,Mar,7; 2017,Jan,8; 2016,Jan,13; 2015,Jan,16; 2014,Jan,11

+ **20931** **Allograft, structural, for spine surgery only (List separately in addition to code for primary procedure)**
Code first (22319, 22532-22533, 22548-22558, 22590-22612, 22630, 22633-22634, 22800-22812)
🚗 3.26 ⚕ 3.26 **FUD** ZZZ N N1 ▣
AMA: 2019,May,7; 2018,Jul,14; 2018,Jan,8; 2017,Mar,7; 2017,Jan,8; 2016,Jan,13; 2015,Jan,16; 2014,Jan,11

+ **20932** **Allograft, includes templating, cutting, placement and internal fixation, when performed; osteoarticular, including articular surface and contiguous bone (List separately in addition to code for primary procedure)**
EXCLUDES Allograft, intercalary (20933-20934)
Injection of contrast for ankle arthrography (27648)
Osteotomy, femur (27448)
Radical resection tumor:
  Clavicle (23200)
  Fibula (27646)
  Ischial tuberosity/greater trochanter femur (27078)
  Radial head or neck (24152)
  Talus or calcaneus (27647)
  Removal hip prosthesis (27090-27091)
Code also insertion of joint prosthesis
Code first (23210, 23220, 24150, 25170, 27075-27077, 27365, 27645, 27704)
🚗 20.5 ⚕ 20.5 **FUD** ZZZ N1 80 ▣
AMA: 2019,May,7

+ **20933** **hemicortical intercalary, partial (ie, hemicylindrical) (List separately in addition to code for primary procedure)**
EXCLUDES Allograft, intercalary, complete (20934)
Allograft, osteoarticular (20932)
Arthroplasty procedures, hip (27130, 27132, 27134, 27138)
Bone graft (20955-20957, 20962)
Excision of cyst with allograft (23146, 23156, 24116, 24126, 25126, 25136, 27356, 27638, 28103, 28107)
Injection of contrast for ankle arthrography (27648)
Open treatment femoral fractures (27236, 27244)
Osteotomy, femur (27448)
Radical resection tumor:
  Clavicle (23200)
  Fibula (27646)
  Ischial tuberosity/greater trochanter femur (27078)
  Radial head or neck (24152)
  Talus or calcaneus (27647)
  Removal hip prosthesis (27090-27091)
Code also insertion of joint prosthesis
Code first (23210, 23220, 24150, 25170, 27075-27077, 27365, 27645, 27704)
🚗 18.8 ⚕ 18.8 **FUD** ZZZ N1 80 ▣
AMA: 2019,May,7

+ **20934** **intercalary, complete (ie, cylindrical) (List separately in addition to code for primary procedure)**
Allograft, intercalary, partial (20933)
Allograft, osteoarticular (20932)
Excision of cyst with allograft (23146, 23156)
Injection of contrast for ankle arthrography (27648)
Osteotomy, femur (27448)
Radical resection tumor:
  Clavicle (23200)
  Fibula (27646)
  Ischial tuberosity/greater trochanter femur (27078)
  Radial head or neck (24152)
  Talus or calcaneus (27647)
  Removal hip prosthesis (27090-27091)
Code also insertion of joint prosthesis
Code first (23210, 23220, 24150, 25170, 27075-27077, 27365, 27645, 27704)
🚗 20.5 ⚕ 20.5 **FUD** ZZZ N1 80 ▣
AMA: 2019,May,7

+ **20936** **Autograft for spine surgery only (includes harvesting the graft); local (eg, ribs, spinous process, or laminar fragments) obtained from same incision (List separately in addition to code for primary procedure)**
Code first (22319, 22532-22533, 22548-22558, 22590-22612, 22630, 22633-22634, 22800-22812)
🚗 0.00 ⚕ 0.00 **FUD** XXX N N1 ▣
AMA: 2018,Jul,14; 2018,Jan,8; 2017,Mar,7; 2017,Jan,8; 2016,Jan,13; 2015,Jan,16; 2014,Jan,11

+ **20937** **morselized (through separate skin or fascial incision) (List separately in addition to code for primary procedure)**
Code first (22319, 22532-22533, 22548-22558, 22590-22612, 22630, 22633-22634, 22800-22812)
🚗 4.88 ⚕ 4.88 **FUD** ZZZ N N1 80 ▣
AMA: 2018,Jul,14; 2018,Jan,8; 2017,Mar,7; 2017,Jan,8; 2016,Jan,13; 2015,Jan,16; 2014,Jan,11

+ **20938** **structural, bicortical or tricortical (through separate skin or fascial incision) (List separately in addition to code for primary procedure)**
EXCLUDES Bone marrow for bone grafting in spinal surgery (20939)
Code first (22319, 22532-22533, 22548-22558, 22590-22612, 22630, 22633-22634, 22800-22812)
🚗 5.40 ⚕ 5.40 **FUD** ZZZ N N1 80 ▣
AMA: 2018,Jul,14; 2018,Jan,8; 2017,Mar,7; 2017,Jan,8; 2016,Jan,13; 2015,Jan,16; 2014,Jan,11

+ **20939** **Bone marrow aspiration for bone grafting, spine surgery only, through separate skin or fascial incision (List separately in addition to code for primary procedure)**
EXCLUDES Bone marrow aspiration for other than bone grafting in spinal surgery (20999)
Diagnostic bone marrow aspiration (38220, 38222)
Platelet rich plasma injection (0232T)
Reporting with modifier 50. Report once for each side when performed bilaterally
Code first (22319, 22532-22534, 22548, 22551-22552, 22554, 22556, 22558, 22590, 22595, 22600, 22610, 22612, 22630, 22633-22634, 22800, 22802, 22804, 22808, 22810, 22812)
🚗 1.92 ⚕ 1.92 **FUD** ZZZ 50 N N1 80 ▣
AMA: 2018,May,3

20950 Measurement of Intracompartmental Pressure

20950 **Monitoring of interstitial fluid pressure (includes insertion of device, eg, wick catheter technique, needle manometer technique) in detection of muscle compartment syndrome**
🚗 2.60 ⚕ 7.41 **FUD** 000 T 62 80 ▣
AMA: 2018,Jan,8; 2017,Jan,8; 2016,Jan,13; 2015,Jan,16; 2014,Jan,11

20955-20973 Bone and Osteocutaneous Grafts

INCLUDES Operating microscope (69990)

20955 **Bone graft with microvascular anastomosis; fibula**
🚗 71.6 ⚕ 71.6 **FUD** 090 C 80 ▣
AMA: 2019,May,7; 2018,Jan,8; 2017,Jan,8; 2016,Feb,12; 2016,Jan,13; 2015,Jan,16; 2014,Jan,11

20956 **iliac crest**
🔧 76.6 ✂ 76.6 **FUD** 090 ☐ C 80 ☐
AMA: 2019,May,7; 2018,Jan,8; 2017,Jan,8; 2016,Feb,12; 2016,Jan,13; 2015,Jan,16; 2014,Jan,11

20957 **metatarsal**
🔧 79.7 ✂ 79.7 **FUD** 090 ☐ C 80 ☐
AMA: 2019,May,7; 2018,Jan,8; 2017,Jan,8; 2016,Feb,12; 2016,Jan,13; 2015,Jan,16; 2014,Jan,11

20962 **other than fibula, iliac crest, or metatarsal**
🔧 77.0 ✂ 77.0 **FUD** 090 ☐ C 80 ☐
AMA: 2019,May,7; 2016,Feb,12

20969 **Free osteocutaneous flap with microvascular anastomosis; other than iliac crest, metatarsal, or great toe**
🔧 79.1 ✂ 79.1 **FUD** 090 ☐ C 80 ☐
AMA: 2018,Jan,8; 2017,Jan,8; 2016,Feb,12; 2016,Jan,13; 2015,Jan,16; 2014,Jan,11

20970 **iliac crest**
🔧 82.8 ✂ 82.8 **FUD** 090 ☐ C 80 ☐
AMA: 2018,Jan,8; 2017,Jan,8; 2016,Feb,12; 2016,Jan,13; 2015,Jan,16; 2014,Jan,11

20972 **metatarsal**
🔧 82.6 ✂ 82.6 **FUD** 090 ☐ J G2 80 ☐
AMA: 2018,Jan,8; 2017,Jan,8; 2016,Feb,12; 2016,Jan,13; 2015,Jan,16; 2014,Jan,11

20973 **great toe with web space**
🔧 87.3 ✂ 87.3 **FUD** 090 ☐ J R2 80 50 ☐
AMA: 2018,Jan,8; 2017,Jan,8; 2016,Feb,12; 2016,Jan,13; 2015,Jan,16; 2014,Jan,11

20974-20979 Osteogenic Stimulation

CMS: 100-03,150.2 Osteogenic Stimulation

20974 **Electrical stimulation to aid bone healing; noninvasive (nonoperative)**
🔧 1.46 ✂ 2.24 **FUD** 000 ⊘ A ☐
AMA: 2018,Jan,8; 2017,Jan,8; 2016,Jan,13; 2015,Jan,16; 2014,Jan,11

20975 **invasive (operative)**
🔧 5.18 ✂ 5.18 **FUD** 000 ⊘ N N1 80 ☐
AMA: 2002,Apr,13; 2000,Nov,8

20979 **Low intensity ultrasound stimulation to aid bone healing, noninvasive (nonoperative)**
🔧 0.93 ✂ 1.49 **FUD** 000 01 N1 ☐
AMA: 2018,Jan,8; 2017,Jan,8; 2016,Jan,13; 2015,Jan,16; 2014,Jan,11

20982-20999 General Musculoskeletal Procedures

20982 **Ablation therapy for reduction or eradication of 1 or more bone tumors (eg, metastasis) including adjacent soft tissue when involved by tumor extension, percutaneous, including imaging guidance when performed; radiofrequency**
🔧 10.5 ✂ 110. **FUD** 000 ☐ J G2 50 ☐
AMA: 2018,Jan,8; 2017,Jan,8; 2016,Jan,13; 2015,Sep,12; 2015,Jul,8

20983 **cryoablation**
🔧 10.1 ✂ 163. **FUD** 000 ☐ J G2 50 ☐
AMA: 2018,Jan,8; 2017,Jan,8; 2016,Jan,13; 2015,Jul,8

+ 20985 **Computer-assisted surgical navigational procedure for musculoskeletal procedures, image-less (List separately in addition to code for primary procedure)**
EXCLUDES *Image guidance derived from intraoperative and preoperative obtained images (0054T-0055T)*
Stereotactic computer-assisted navigational procedure; cranial or intradural (61781-61783)
Code first primary procedure
🔧 4.24 ✂ 4.24 **FUD** ZZZ N N1 80 ☐
AMA: 2018,Jan,8; 2017,Jan,8; 2016,Jan,13; 2015,Jan,16; 2014,Jan,11

20999 **Unlisted procedure, musculoskeletal system, general**
🔧 0.00 ✂ 0.00 **FUD** YYY ☐ T 80 ☐
AMA: 2018,May,3; 2018,Jan,8; 2017,Jan,8; 2016,Jan,13; 2015,Jul,8; 2015,Jan,16; 2014,Oct,9; 2014,Jan,11

21010 Temporomandibular Joint Arthrotomy

21010 **Arthrotomy, temporomandibular joint**
EXCLUDES *Cutaneous/subcutaneous abscess and hematoma drainage (10060-10061)*
Excision of foreign body from dentoalveolar site (41805-41806)
🔧 22.0 ✂ 22.0 **FUD** 090 ☐ J A2 80 50 ☐
AMA: 2002,Apr,13

21011-21016 Excision Soft Tissue Tumors Face and Scalp

INCLUDES Any necessary elevation of tissue planes or dissection
Measurement of tumor and necessary margin at greatest diameter prior to excision
Simple and intermediate repairs
Types of excision:
Fascial or subfascial soft tissue tumors: simple and marginal resection of tumors found either in or below the deep fascia, not including bone or excision of a substantial amount of normal tissue; primarily benign and intramuscular tumors
Radical resection soft tissue tumor: wide resection of tumor involving substantial margins of normal tissue and may include tissue removal from one or more layers; most often malignant or aggressive benign
Subcutaneous: simple and marginal resection of tumors in the subcutaneous tissue above the deep fascia; most often benign

EXCLUDES *Complex repair*
Excision of benign cutaneous lesions (eg, sebaceous cyst) (11420-11426)
Radical resection of cutaneous tumors (eg, melanoma) (11620-11646)
Significant exploration of vessels or neuroplasty

21011 **Excision, tumor, soft tissue of face or scalp, subcutaneous; less than 2 cm**
🔧 7.39 ✂ 10.1 **FUD** 090 ☐ J P3 80 ☐
AMA: 2018,Sep,7; 2018,Jan,8; 2017,Jan,8; 2016,Jan,13; 2015,Jan,16; 2014,Jan,11

21012 **2 cm or greater**
🔧 9.75 ✂ 9.75 **FUD** 090 ☐ J R2 80 ☐
AMA: 2018,Sep,7; 2018,Jan,8; 2017,Jan,8; 2016,Jan,13; 2015,Jan,16; 2014,Jan,11

21013 **Excision, tumor, soft tissue of face and scalp, subfascial (eg, subgaleal, intramuscular); less than 2 cm**
🔧 11.5 ✂ 15.0 **FUD** 090 ☐ J P3 80 ☐
AMA: 2018,Sep,7; 2018,Jan,8; 2017,Jan,8; 2016,Jan,13; 2015,Jan,16; 2014,Jan,11

21014 **2 cm or greater**
🔧 15.0 ✂ 15.0 **FUD** 090 ☐ J R2 80 ☐
AMA: 2018,Sep,7; 2018,Jan,8; 2017,Jan,8; 2016,Jan,13; 2015,Jan,16; 2014,Jan,11

21015 **Radical resection of tumor (eg, sarcoma), soft tissue of face or scalp; less than 2 cm**
EXCLUDES *Removal of cranial tumor for osteomyelitis (61501)*
🔧 20.3 ✂ 20.3 **FUD** 090 ☐ J G2 ☐
AMA: 2018,Sep,7; 2018,Jan,8; 2017,Jan,8; 2016,Jan,13; 2015,Jan,16; 2014,Jan,11

21016 **2 cm or greater**
🔧 29.1 ✂ 29.1 **FUD** 090 ☐ J G2 80 ☐
AMA: 2018,Sep,7; 2018,Jan,8; 2017,Jan,8; 2016,Jan,13; 2015,Jan,16; 2014,Jan,11

  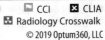
26/TC PC/TC Only   **A2-Z3** ASC Payment   **50** Bilateral   ♂ Male Only   ♀ Female Only   🔧 Facility RVU   ✂ Non-Facility RVU   ☐ CCI   ☒ CLIA
FUD Follow-up Days   **CMS:** IOM   **AMA:** CPT Asst   **A-Y** OPPSI   **80/80** Surg Assist Allowed / w/Doc   Lab Crosswalk   Radiology Crosswalk

44   CPT © 2019 American Medical Association. All Rights Reserved.   © 2019 Optum360, LLC

21025-21070 Procedures of Cranial and Facial Bones

INCLUDES Any necessary elevation of tissue planes or dissection
Measurement of tumor and necessary margins prior to excision
Radical resection of bone tumor involves resection of the tumor (may include entire bone) and wide margins of normal tissue primarily for malignant or aggressive benign tumors
Simple and intermediate repairs

EXCLUDES *Complex repair*
Excision of soft tissue tumors, face and scalp (21011-21016)
Radical resection of cutaneous tumors (e.g., melanoma) (11620-11646)
Significant exploration of vessels, neuroplasty, reconstruction, or complex bone repair

21025   **Excision of bone (eg, for osteomyelitis or bone abscess); mandible**
🚑 21.0   ⚕ 24.8   **FUD** 090   J A2 ▱
AMA: 2018,Sep,7; 2018,Jan,8; 2017,Jan,8; 2016,Jan,13; 2015,Jan,16; 2014,Jan,11

21026   **facial bone(s)**
🚑 13.8   ⚕ 17.0   **FUD** 090   J A2 ▱
AMA: 2018,Sep,7

21029   **Removal by contouring of benign tumor of facial bone (eg, fibrous dysplasia)**
🚑 18.2   ⚕ 22.0   **FUD** 090   J A2 80 ▱
AMA: 2018,Sep,7

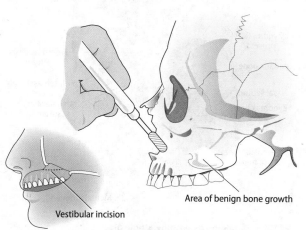

Vestibular incision

Area of benign bone growth

Burrs, files, and osteotomes used to remove bone

21030   **Excision of benign tumor or cyst of maxilla or zygoma by enucleation and curettage**
🚑 11.7   ⚕ 14.6   **FUD** 090   J P3 50 ▱
AMA: 2018,Sep,7; 2018,Jan,8; 2017,Jan,8; 2016,Jan,13; 2015,Jan,16; 2014,Jan,11

21031   **Excision of torus mandibularis**
🚑 8.34   ⚕ 11.3   **FUD** 090   J P3 50 ▱
AMA: 2018,Sep,7

21032   **Excision of maxillary torus palatinus**
🚑 8.21   ⚕ 11.3   **FUD** 090   J P3 ▱
AMA: 2018,Sep,7

21034   **Excision of malignant tumor of maxilla or zygoma**
🚑 33.0   ⚕ 37.5   **FUD** 090   J A2 80 ▱
AMA: 2018,Sep,7; 2018,Jan,8; 2017,Jan,8; 2016,Jan,13; 2015,Jan,16; 2014,Jan,11

21040   **Excision of benign tumor or cyst of mandible, by enucleation and/or curettage**
INCLUDES Removal of benign tumor or cyst without osteotomy
EXCLUDES *Removal of benign tumor or cyst with osteotomy (21046-21047)*
🚑 11.7   ⚕ 14.7   **FUD** 090   J A2 ▱
AMA: 2018,Sep,7; 2018,Jan,8; 2017,Jan,8; 2016,Jan,13; 2015,Jan,16; 2014,Jan,11

21044   **Excision of malignant tumor of mandible;**
🚑 25.0   ⚕ 25.0   **FUD** 090   J A2 80 ▱
AMA: 2018,Sep,7

21045   **radical resection**
Code also bone graft procedure (21215)
🚑 35.1   ⚕ 35.1   **FUD** 090   C 80 ▱
AMA: 2018,Sep,7

21046   **Excision of benign tumor or cyst of mandible; requiring intra-oral osteotomy (eg, locally aggressive or destructive lesion[s])**
🚑 31.5   ⚕ 31.5   **FUD** 090   J A2 80 ▱
AMA: 2018,Sep,7; 2018,Jan,8; 2017,Jan,8; 2016,Jan,13; 2015,Jan,16; 2014,Jan,11

21047   **requiring extra-oral osteotomy and partial mandibulectomy (eg, locally aggressive or destructive lesion[s])**
🚑 37.6   ⚕ 37.6   **FUD** 090   J A2 80 ▱
AMA: 2018,Sep,7; 2018,Jan,8; 2017,Jan,8; 2016,Jan,13; 2015,Jan,16; 2014,Jan,11

21048   **Excision of benign tumor or cyst of maxilla; requiring intra-oral osteotomy (eg, locally aggressive or destructive lesion[s])**
🚑 32.0   ⚕ 32.0   **FUD** 090   J R2 80 ▱
AMA: 2018,Sep,7; 2018,Jan,8; 2017,Jan,8; 2016,Jan,13; 2015,Jan,16; 2014,Jan,11

21049   **requiring extra-oral osteotomy and partial maxillectomy (eg, locally aggressive or destructive lesion[s])**
🚑 34.7   ⚕ 34.7   **FUD** 090   J 80 ▱
AMA: 2018,Sep,7; 2018,Jan,8; 2017,Jan,8; 2016,Jan,13; 2015,Jan,16; 2014,Jan,11

21050   **Condylectomy, temporomandibular joint (separate procedure)**
🚑 25.9   ⚕ 25.9   **FUD** 090   J A2 80 50 ▱
AMA: 2018,Sep,7

21060   **Meniscectomy, partial or complete, temporomandibular joint (separate procedure)**
🚑 23.5   ⚕ 23.5   **FUD** 090   J A2 80 50 ▱
AMA: 2018,Sep,7

21070   **Coronoidectomy (separate procedure)**
🚑 18.3   ⚕ 18.3   **FUD** 090   J A2 80 50 ▱
AMA: 2018,Sep,7

21073 Temporomandibular Joint Manipulation with Anesthesia

21073   **Manipulation of temporomandibular joint(s) (TMJ), therapeutic, requiring an anesthesia service (ie, general or monitored anesthesia care)**
EXCLUDES *Closed treatment of TMJ dislocation (21480, 21485)*
Manipulation of TMJ without general or MAC anesthesia (97140, 98925-98929, 98943)
🚑 7.30   ⚕ 11.0   **FUD** 090   T P3 80 50 ▱
AMA: 2018,Sep,7; 2018,Jan,8; 2018,Jan,3; 2017,Jan,8; 2016,Jan,13; 2015,Jan,16; 2014,Jan,11

21076-21089 Medical Impressions for Fabrication Maxillofacial Prosthesis

INCLUDES Design, preparation, and professional services rendered by a physician or other qualified health care professional
EXCLUDES *Application or removal of caliper or tongs (20660, 20665)*
Professional services rendered for outside laboratory designed and prepared prosthesis

21076   **Impression and custom preparation; surgical obturator prosthesis**
🚑 23.1   ⚕ 27.6   **FUD** 010   T P3 80 ▱
AMA: 2018,Sep,7; 2018,Jan,8; 2017,Jan,8; 2016,Jan,13; 2015,Jan,16; 2014,Jan,11

21077   **orbital prosthesis**
🏥 57.9 ⚕ 68.8 **FUD** 090   J P3 80 50 ▣
AMA: 2018,Sep,7; 2018,Jan,8; 2017,Jan,8; 2016,Jan,13; 2015,Jan,16; 2014,Jan,11

21079   **interim obturator prosthesis**
🏥 38.8 ⚕ 46.6 **FUD** 090   J P3 ▣
AMA: 2018,Sep,7; 2018,Jan,8; 2017,Jan,8; 2016,Jan,13; 2015,Jan,16; 2014,Jan,11

21080   **definitive obturator prosthesis**
🏥 43.3 ⚕ 52.7 **FUD** 090   J P3 ▣
AMA: 2018,Sep,7; 2018,Jan,8; 2017,Jan,8; 2016,Jan,13; 2015,Jan,16; 2014,Jan,11

21081   **mandibular resection prosthesis**
🏥 39.8 ⚕ 48.5 **FUD** 090   J P3 80 ▣
AMA: 2018,Sep,7; 2018,Jan,8; 2017,Jan,8; 2016,Jan,13; 2015,Jan,16; 2014,Jan,11

21082   **palatal augmentation prosthesis**
🏥 36.8 ⚕ 45.3 **FUD** 090   J P3 80 ▣
AMA: 2018,Sep,7; 2018,Jan,8; 2017,Jan,8; 2016,Jan,13; 2015,Jan,16; 2014,Jan,11

21083   **palatal lift prosthesis**
🏥 34.3 ⚕ 43.2 **FUD** 090   J P3 80 ▣
AMA: 2018,Sep,7; 2018,Jan,8; 2017,Jan,8; 2016,Jan,13; 2015,Jan,16; 2014,Jan,11

21084   **speech aid prosthesis**
🏥 39.6 ⚕ 49.5 **FUD** 090   J P3 80 ▣
AMA: 2018,Sep,7; 2018,Jan,8; 2017,Jan,8; 2016,Jan,13; 2015,Jan,16; 2014,Jan,11

21085   **oral surgical splint**
🏥 15.7 ⚕ 21.0 **FUD** 010   T P2 80 ▣
AMA: 2018,Sep,7; 2018,Jan,8; 2017,Sep,14; 2017,Jan,8; 2016,Jan,13; 2015,Jan,16; 2014,Jan,11

21086   **auricular prosthesis**
🏥 42.7 ⚕ 51.1 **FUD** 090   J P3 80 50 ▣
AMA: 2018,Sep,7; 2018,Jan,8; 2017,Jan,8; 2016,Jan,13; 2015,Jan,16; 2014,Jan,11

21087   **nasal prosthesis**
🏥 42.7 ⚕ 51.1 **FUD** 090   J P3 80 ▣
AMA: 2018,Sep,7; 2018,Jan,8; 2017,Jan,8; 2016,Jan,13; 2015,Jan,16; 2014,Jan,11

21088   **facial prosthesis**
🏥 0.00 ⚕ 0.00 **FUD** 090   J R2 80 ▣
AMA: 2018,Sep,7; 2018,Jan,8; 2017,Jan,8; 2016,Jan,13; 2015,Jan,16; 2014,Jan,11

21089   **Unlisted maxillofacial prosthetic procedure**
🏥 0.00 ⚕ 0.00 **FUD** YYY   T ▣
AMA: 2018,Sep,7; 2018,Jan,8; 2017,Jan,8; 2016,Jan,13; 2015,Jan,16; 2014,Jan,11

21100-21110 Application Fixation Device

21100   **Application of halo type appliance for maxillofacial fixation, includes removal (separate procedure)**
🏥 11.3 ⚕ 19.8 **FUD** 090   J A2 80 ▣
AMA: 2018,Sep,7

21110   **Application of interdental fixation device for conditions other than fracture or dislocation, includes removal**
EXCLUDES *Interdental fixation device removal by different provider (20670-20680)*
🏥 19.5 ⚕ 23.3 **FUD** 090   Q2 P2 ▣
AMA: 2018,Sep,7; 2018,Jan,8; 2017,Jan,8; 2016,Jan,13; 2015,Jan,16; 2014,Jan,11

21116 Injection for TMJ Arthrogram

CMS: 100-02,15,150.1 Treatment of Temporomandibular Joint (TMJ) Syndrome; 100-04,13,80.1 Physician Presence; 100-04,13,80.2 S&I Multiple Procedure Reduction

21116   **Injection procedure for temporomandibular joint arthrography**
🔀 (70332)
🏥 1.38 ⚕ 5.08 **FUD** 000   N N1 50 ▣
AMA: 2018,Sep,7; 2018,Jan,8; 2017,Jan,8; 2016,May,13; 2016,Jan,13; 2015,Aug,6

21120-21299 Repair/Reconstruction Craniofacial Bones

EXCLUDES *Cranioplasty (21179-21180, 62120, 62140-62147)*

21120   **Genioplasty; augmentation (autograft, allograft, prosthetic material)**
🏥 15.2 ⚕ 19.3 **FUD** 090   J G2 ▣
AMA: 2018,Sep,7

Nasal bone · Frontal bone · Frontonasal suture · Supraorbital margin · Parietal bone · Zygomatic process · Zygomatic bone · Frontomaxillary suture · Nasal septum · Internasal suture · Zygomaxillary suture · Nasomaxillary suture · Maxilla · Ramus · Alveolar process of maxilla · Body of mandible · Mental foramen

21121   **sliding osteotomy, single piece**
🏥 17.8 ⚕ 20.9 **FUD** 090   J A2 80 ▣
AMA: 2018,Sep,7

21122   **sliding osteotomies, 2 or more osteotomies (eg, wedge excision or bone wedge reversal for asymmetrical chin)**
🏥 22.3 ⚕ 22.3 **FUD** 090   J A2 80 ▣
AMA: 2018,Sep,7

21123   **sliding, augmentation with interpositional bone grafts (includes obtaining autografts)**
🏥 26.1 ⚕ 26.1 **FUD** 090   J A2 80 ▣
AMA: 2018,Sep,7

21125   **Augmentation, mandibular body or angle; prosthetic material**
🏥 21.4 ⚕ 82.8 **FUD** 090   J A2 80 ▣
AMA: 2018,Sep,7

21127   **with bone graft, onlay or interpositional (includes obtaining autograft)**
🏥 24.6 ⚕ 112. **FUD** 090   J A2 80 ▣
AMA: 2018,Sep,7

21137   **Reduction forehead; contouring only**
🏥 21.6 ⚕ 21.6 **FUD** 090   J G2 80 ▣
AMA: 2018,Sep,7

21138   **contouring and application of prosthetic material or bone graft (includes obtaining autograft)**
🏥 26.4 ⚕ 26.4 **FUD** 090   J G2 80 ▣
AMA: 2018,Sep,7

Musculoskeletal System

21139 contouring and setback of anterior frontal sinus wall
32.1 ⚖ 32.1 **FUD** 090 J 62 80 ▢
AMA: 2018,Sep,7

21141 Reconstruction midface, LeFort I; single piece, segment movement in any direction (eg, for Long Face Syndrome), without bone graft
39.4 ⚖ 39.4 **FUD** 090 C 80 ▢
AMA: 2018,Sep,7

21142 2 pieces, segment movement in any direction, without bone graft
40.5 ⚖ 40.5 **FUD** 090 C 80 ▢
AMA: 2018,Sep,7

21143 3 or more pieces, segment movement in any direction, without bone graft
42.3 ⚖ 42.3 **FUD** 090 C 80 ▢
AMA: 2018,Sep,7

21145 single piece, segment movement in any direction, requiring bone grafts (includes obtaining autografts)
46.2 ⚖ 46.2 **FUD** 090 C 80 ▢
AMA: 2018,Sep,7

21146 2 pieces, segment movement in any direction, requiring bone grafts (includes obtaining autografts) (eg, ungrafted unilateral alveolar cleft)
48.2 ⚖ 48.2 **FUD** 090 C 80 ▢
AMA: 2018,Sep,7

21147 3 or more pieces, segment movement in any direction, requiring bone grafts (includes obtaining autografts) (eg, ungrafted bilateral alveolar cleft or multiple osteotomies)
50.8 ⚖ 50.8 **FUD** 090 C 80 ▢
AMA: 2018,Sep,7

21150 Reconstruction midface, LeFort II; anterior intrusion (eg, Treacher-Collins Syndrome)
47.6 ⚖ 47.6 **FUD** 090 J 62 80 ▢
AMA: 2018,Sep,7

21151 any direction, requiring bone grafts (includes obtaining autografts)
52.4 ⚖ 52.4 **FUD** 090 C 80 ▢
AMA: 2018,Sep,7

21154 Reconstruction midface, LeFort III (extracranial), any type, requiring bone grafts (includes obtaining autografts); without LeFort I
56.4 ⚖ 56.4 **FUD** 090 C 80 ▢
AMA: 2018,Sep,7

21155 with LeFort I
62.6 ⚖ 62.6 **FUD** 090 C 80 ▢
AMA: 2018,Sep,7

Bicoronal scalp flap
Lower eyelid
Circum-vestibular

Typical transcutaneous and transoral incisions

LeFort III with LeFort I down-fracture

21159 Reconstruction midface, LeFort III (extra and intracranial) with forehead advancement (eg, mono bloc), requiring bone grafts (includes obtaining autografts); without LeFort I
75.0 ⚖ 75.0 **FUD** 090 C 80 ▢
AMA: 2018,Sep,7

21160 with LeFort I
81.4 ⚖ 81.4 **FUD** 090 C 80 ▢
AMA: 2018,Sep,7

21172 Reconstruction superior-lateral orbital rim and lower forehead, advancement or alteration, with or without grafts (includes obtaining autografts)
EXCLUDES Frontal or parietal craniotomy for craniosynostosis (61556)
60.8 ⚖ 60.8 **FUD** 090 J 80 ▢
AMA: 2018,Sep,7

21175 Reconstruction, bifrontal, superior-lateral orbital rims and lower forehead, advancement or alteration (eg, plagiocephaly, trigonocephaly, brachycephaly), with or without grafts (includes obtaining autografts)
EXCLUDES Bifrontal craniotomy for craniosynostosis (61557)
63.8 ⚖ 63.8 **FUD** 090 J 80 ▢
AMA: 2018,Sep,7

21179 Reconstruction, entire or majority of forehead and/or supraorbital rims; with grafts (allograft or prosthetic material)
EXCLUDES Extensive craniotomy for numerous suture craniosynostosis (61558-61559)
43.8 ⚖ 43.8 **FUD** 090 C 80 ▢
AMA: 2018,Sep,7

21180 with autograft (includes obtaining grafts)
EXCLUDES Extensive craniotomy for numerous suture craniosynostosis (61558-61559)
49.0 ⚖ 49.0 **FUD** 090 C 80 ▢
AMA: 2018,Sep,7

21181 Reconstruction by contouring of benign tumor of cranial bones (eg, fibrous dysplasia), extracranial
21.2 ⚖ 21.2 **FUD** 090 J A2 80 ▢
AMA: 2018,Sep,7

Musculoskeletal System

21182 — 21248

21182 Reconstruction of orbital walls, rims, forehead, nasoethmoid complex following intra- and extracranial excision of benign tumor of cranial bone (eg, fibrous dysplasia), with multiple autografts (includes obtaining grafts); total area of bone grafting less than 40 sq cm
EXCLUDES Removal of benign tumor of the skull (61563-61564)
61.2 ⚕ 61.2 **FUD** 090 C 80 ▢
AMA: 2018,Sep,7

21183 total area of bone grafting greater than 40 sq cm but less than 80 sq cm
EXCLUDES Removal of benign tumor of the skull (61563-61564)
66.7 ⚕ 66.7 **FUD** 090 C 80 ▢
AMA: 2018,Sep,7

21184 total area of bone grafting greater than 80 sq cm
EXCLUDES Removal of benign tumor of the skull (61563-61564)
71.8 ⚕ 71.8 **FUD** 090 C 80 ▢
AMA: 2018,Sep,7

21188 Reconstruction midface, osteotomies (other than LeFort type) and bone grafts (includes obtaining autografts)
48.0 ⚕ 48.0 **FUD** 090 C 80 ▢
AMA: 2018,Sep,7

21193 Reconstruction of mandibular rami, horizontal, vertical, C, or L osteotomy; without bone graft
36.8 ⚕ 36.8 **FUD** 090 J 80 ▢
AMA: 2018,Sep,7; 2018,Jan,8; 2017,Jan,8; 2016,Jan,13; 2015,Jan,16; 2014,Jan,11

21194 with bone graft (includes obtaining graft)
42.3 ⚕ 42.3 **FUD** 090 C 80 ▢
AMA: 2018,Sep,7; 2018,Jan,8; 2017,Jan,8; 2016,Jan,13; 2015,Jan,16; 2014,Jan,11

21195 Reconstruction of mandibular rami and/or body, sagittal split; without internal rigid fixation
41.0 ⚕ 41.0 **FUD** 090 J 80 ▢
AMA: 2018,Sep,7; 2018,Jan,8; 2017,Jan,8; 2016,Jan,13; 2015,Jan,16; 2014,Jan,11

21196 with internal rigid fixation
42.1 ⚕ 42.1 **FUD** 090 C 80 ▢
AMA: 2018,Sep,7; 2018,Jan,8; 2017,Jan,8; 2016,Jan,13; 2015,Jan,16; 2014,Jan,11

21198 Osteotomy, mandible, segmental;
EXCLUDES Total maxillary osteotomy (21141-21160)
33.0 ⚕ 33.0 **FUD** 090 J 62 80 ▢
AMA: 2018,Sep,7; 2018,Jan,8; 2017,Jan,8; 2016,Jan,13; 2015,Jan,16; 2014,Jan,11

21199 with genioglossus advancement
EXCLUDES Total maxillary osteotomy (21141-21160)
30.9 ⚕ 30.9 **FUD** 090 J 62 80 ▢
AMA: 2018,Sep,7; 2018,Jan,8; 2017,Jan,8; 2016,Jan,13; 2015,Jan,16; 2014,Jan,11

21206 Osteotomy, maxilla, segmental (eg, Wassmund or Schuchard)
34.1 ⚕ 34.1 **FUD** 090 J A2 80 ▢
AMA: 2018,Sep,7

21208 Osteoplasty, facial bones; augmentation (autograft, allograft, or prosthetic implant)
23.2 ⚕ 49.9 **FUD** 090 J A2 80 ▢
AMA: 2018,Sep,7

21209 reduction
19.3 ⚕ 25.7 **FUD** 090 J A2 80 ▢
AMA: 2018,Sep,7

21210 Graft, bone; nasal, maxillary or malar areas (includes obtaining graft)
EXCLUDES Cleft palate procedures (42200-42225)
23.9 ⚕ 60.2 **FUD** 090 J A2 ▢
AMA: 2018,Sep,7

21215 mandible (includes obtaining graft)
24.9 ⚕ 114. **FUD** 090 J A2 ▢
AMA: 2018,Sep,7

21230 Graft; rib cartilage, autogenous, to face, chin, nose or ear (includes obtaining graft)
EXCLUDES Augmentation of facial bones (21208)
21.3 ⚕ 21.3 **FUD** 090 J A2 80 ▢
AMA: 2018,Sep,7

21235 ear cartilage, autogenous, to nose or ear (includes obtaining graft)
EXCLUDES Augmentation of facial bones (21208)
16.2 ⚕ 20.7 **FUD** 090 J A2 ▢
AMA: 2018,Sep,7; 2018,Jan,8; 2017,Jan,8; 2016,Jan,13; 2015,Jan,16

21240 Arthroplasty, temporomandibular joint, with or without autograft (includes obtaining graft)
32.1 ⚕ 32.1 **FUD** 090 J A2 80 50 ▢
AMA: 2018,Sep,7

Cutaway view of temporomandibular joint (TMJ)

TMJ syndrome is often related to stress and tooth-grinding; in other cases, arthritis, injury, poorly aligned teeth, or ill-fitting dentures may be the cause

Upper joint space
Lower joint space
Articular disc (meniscus)
Cutaway detail
Condyle
Mandible

Symptoms include facial pain and chewing problems; TMJ syndrome occurs more frequently in women

21242 Arthroplasty, temporomandibular joint, with allograft
30.0 ⚕ 30.0 **FUD** 090 J A2 80 50 ▢
AMA: 2018,Sep,7

21243 Arthroplasty, temporomandibular joint, with prosthetic joint replacement
48.9 ⚕ 48.9 **FUD** 090 J J8 80 50 ▢
AMA: 2018,Sep,7

21244 Reconstruction of mandible, extraoral, with transosteal bone plate (eg, mandibular staple bone plate)
30.0 ⚕ 30.0 **FUD** 090 J J8 80 ▢
AMA: 2018,Sep,7

21245 Reconstruction of mandible or maxilla, subperiosteal implant; partial
27.5 ⚕ 34.9 **FUD** 090 J A2 80 ▢
AMA: 2018,Sep,7

21246 complete
25.4 ⚕ 25.4 **FUD** 090 J A2 80 ▢
AMA: 2018,Sep,7

21247 Reconstruction of mandibular condyle with bone and cartilage autografts (includes obtaining grafts) (eg, for hemifacial microsomia)
47.3 ⚕ 47.3 **FUD** 090 C 80 50 ▢
AMA: 2018,Sep,7

21248 Reconstruction of mandible or maxilla, endosteal implant (eg, blade, cylinder); partial
EXCLUDES Midface reconstruction (21141-21160)
25.3 ⚕ 31.1 **FUD** 090 J A2 ▢
AMA: 2018,Sep,7

26/TC PC/TC Only   A2-Z3 ASC Payment   50 Bilateral   ♂ Male Only   ♀ Female Only   ⚕ Facility RVU   ⚕ Non-Facility RVU   ▢ CCI   ✖ CLIA
FUD Follow-up Days   **CMS:** IOM   **AMA:** CPT Asst   A-Y OPPSI   80/80 Surg Assist Allowed / w/Doc   ▢ Lab Crosswalk   ▢ Radiology Crosswalk

21249 complete

> EXCLUDES Midface reconstruction (21141-21160)

🖐 36.7 🔧 44.9 **FUD** 090   J A2 80 ▭

AMA: 2018,Sep,7

21255 Reconstruction of zygomatic arch and glenoid fossa with bone and cartilage (includes obtaining autografts)

🖐 40.6 🔧 40.6 **FUD** 090   C 80 50

AMA: 2018,Sep,7

21256 Reconstruction of orbit with osteotomies (extracranial) and with bone grafts (includes obtaining autografts) (eg, micro-ophthalmia)

🖐 35.7 🔧 35.7 **FUD** 090   J 80 50 ▭

AMA: 2018,Sep,7

21260 Periorbital osteotomies for orbital hypertelorism, with bone grafts; extracranial approach

🖐 40.1 🔧 40.1 **FUD** 090   J 62 80 ▭

AMA: 2018,Sep,7

21261 combined intra- and extracranial approach

🖐 71.1 🔧 71.1 **FUD** 090   J 80 ▭

AMA: 2018,Sep,7

21263 with forehead advancement

🖐 65.8 🔧 65.8 **FUD** 090   J 80 ▭

AMA: 2018,Sep,7

A frontal craniotomy is performed, the brain retracted, and the orbit approached from inside the skull; frontal bone is advanced and secured

Grafts

Grafts are placed and the bony orbits realigned

Osteotomies are cut 360 degrees around the orbit; portions of nasal and ethmoid bones are removed

21267 Orbital repositioning, periorbital osteotomies, unilateral, with bone grafts; extracranial approach

🖐 47.0 🔧 47.0 **FUD** 090   J A2 80 50 ▭

AMA: 2018,Sep,7

21268 combined intra- and extracranial approach

🖐 58.9 🔧 58.9 **FUD** 090   C 80 50 ▭

AMA: 2018,Sep,7

21270 Malar augmentation, prosthetic material

> EXCLUDES Augmentation procedure with bone graft (21210)

🖐 21.6 🔧 29.0 **FUD** 090   J A2 80 50 ▭

AMA: 2018,Sep,7

21275 Secondary revision of orbitocraniofacial reconstruction

🖐 24.1 🔧 24.1 **FUD** 090   J 62 80 ▭

AMA: 2018,Sep,7

21280 Medial canthopexy (separate procedure)

> EXCLUDES Reconstruction of canthus (67950)

🖐 16.4 🔧 16.4 **FUD** 090   J A2 80 50 ▭

AMA: 2018,Sep,7

21282 Lateral canthopexy

🖐 11.0 🔧 11.0 **FUD** 090   J A2 50 ▭

AMA: 2018,Sep,7

21295 Reduction of masseter muscle and bone (eg, for treatment of benign masseteric hypertrophy); extraoral approach

🖐 5.37 🔧 5.37 **FUD** 090   T A2 80 50 ▭

AMA: 2018,Sep,7

21296 intraoral approach

🖐 11.7 🔧 11.7 **FUD** 090   J A2 80 50 ▭

AMA: 2018,Sep,7

21299 Unlisted craniofacial and maxillofacial procedure

🖐 0.00 🔧 0.00 **FUD** YYY   T 80 ▭

AMA: 2018,Sep,7

21310-21499 Care of Fractures/Dislocations of the Cranial and Facial Bones

> EXCLUDES Closed treatment of skull fracture, report with appropriate E&M service
> Open treatment of skull fracture (62000-62010)

21310 Closed treatment of nasal bone fracture without manipulation

🖐 0.78 🔧 3.76 **FUD** 000   T A2 ▭

AMA: 2019,Sep,3; 2018,Sep,7; 2018,Jan,3

21315 Closed treatment of nasal bone fracture; without stabilization

🖐 4.32 🔧 7.84 **FUD** 010   T A2 ▭

AMA: 2019,Sep,3; 2018,Sep,7; 2018,Jan,3

21320 with stabilization

🖐 3.83 🔧 7.23 **FUD** 010   J A2 ▭

AMA: 2019,Sep,3; 2018,Sep,7

21325 Open treatment of nasal fracture; uncomplicated

🖐 13.3 🔧 13.3 **FUD** 090   J A2 80 ▭

AMA: 2018,Sep,7

21330 complicated, with internal and/or external skeletal fixation

🖐 16.1 🔧 16.1 **FUD** 090   J A2 80 ▭

AMA: 2018,Sep,7

21335 with concomitant open treatment of fractured septum

🖐 20.5 🔧 20.5 **FUD** 090   J A2 ▭

AMA: 2018,Sep,7

21336 Open treatment of nasal septal fracture, with or without stabilization

🖐 18.3 🔧 18.3 **FUD** 090   J A2 ▭

AMA: 2018,Sep,7

21337 Closed treatment of nasal septal fracture, with or without stabilization

🖐 8.42 🔧 11.6 **FUD** 090   J A2 80 ▭

AMA: 2019,Sep,3; 2018,Sep,7

21338 Open treatment of nasoethmoid fracture; without external fixation

🖐 18.8 🔧 18.8 **FUD** 090   J J8 80 ▭

AMA: 2018,Sep,7

21339 with external fixation

🖐 21.3 🔧 21.3 **FUD** 090   J A2 80 ▭

AMA: 2018,Sep,7

21340 Percutaneous treatment of nasoethmoid complex fracture, with splint, wire or headcap fixation, including repair of canthal ligaments and/or the nasolacrimal apparatus

🖐 21.3 🔧 21.3 **FUD** 090   J A2 80 ▭

AMA: 2018,Sep,7

21343 Open treatment of depressed frontal sinus fracture

🖐 30.8 🔧 30.8 **FUD** 090   C 80 ▭

AMA: 2018,Sep,7

21344 Open treatment of complicated (eg, comminuted or involving posterior wall) frontal sinus fracture, via coronal or multiple approaches

🖐 39.7 🔧 39.7 **FUD** 090   C 80 ▭

AMA: 2018,Sep,7

21345 **Closed treatment of nasomaxillary complex fracture (LeFort II type), with interdental wire fixation or fixation of denture or splint**
🚑 17.9   ⚕ 22.2   **FUD** 090   T A2 80 ▭
AMA: 2018,Sep,7

21346 **Open treatment of nasomaxillary complex fracture (LeFort II type); with wiring and/or local fixation**
🚑 26.6   ⚕ 26.6   **FUD** 090   J ▭
AMA: 2018,Sep,7

21347 **requiring multiple open approaches**
🚑 29.0   ⚕ 29.0   **FUD** 090   C 80 ▭
AMA: 2018,Sep,7

21348 **with bone grafting (includes obtaining graft)**
🚑 31.0   ⚕ 31.0   **FUD** 090   C 80 ▭
AMA: 2018,Sep,7

21355 **Percutaneous treatment of fracture of malar area, including zygomatic arch and malar tripod, with manipulation**
🚑 9.17   ⚕ 12.1   **FUD** 010   J A2 80 50 ▭
AMA: 2018,Sep,7

21356 **Open treatment of depressed zygomatic arch fracture (eg, Gillies approach)**
🚑 10.8   ⚕ 14.3   **FUD** 010   J A2 80 50 ▭
AMA: 2018,Sep,7

21360 **Open treatment of depressed malar fracture, including zygomatic arch and malar tripod**
🚑 14.6   ⚕ 14.6   **FUD** 090   J G2 80 50 ▭
AMA: 2018,Sep,7

21365 **Open treatment of complicated (eg, comminuted or involving cranial nerve foramina) fracture(s) of malar area, including zygomatic arch and malar tripod; with internal fixation and multiple surgical approaches**
🚑 31.9   ⚕ 31.9   **FUD** 090   J 80 50 ▭
AMA: 2018,Sep,7

21366 **with bone grafting (includes obtaining graft)**
🚑 36.7   ⚕ 36.7   **FUD** 090   C 80 50 ▭
AMA: 2018,Sep,7

21385 **Open treatment of orbital floor blowout fracture; transantral approach (Caldwell-Luc type operation)**
🚑 21.6   ⚕ 21.6   **FUD** 090   J 80 50 ▭
AMA: 2018,Sep,7

21386 **periorbital approach**
🚑 19.9   ⚕ 19.9   **FUD** 090   J 80 50 ▭
AMA: 2018,Sep,7

21387 **combined approach**
🚑 22.6   ⚕ 22.6   **FUD** 090   J 80 50 ▭
AMA: 2018,Sep,7

21390 **periorbital approach, with alloplastic or other implant**
🚑 22.9   ⚕ 22.9   **FUD** 090   J G2 80 50 ▭
AMA: 2018,Sep,7

21395 **periorbital approach with bone graft (includes obtaining graft)**
🚑 29.0   ⚕ 29.0   **FUD** 090   J 80 50 ▭
AMA: 2018,Sep,7

21400 **Closed treatment of fracture of orbit, except blowout; without manipulation**
🚑 4.59   ⚕ 5.73   **FUD** 090   T A2 80 50 ▭
AMA: 2018,Sep,7

21401 **with manipulation**
🚑 9.23   ⚕ 14.7   **FUD** 090   T A2 80 50 ▭
AMA: 2018,Sep,7

21406 **Open treatment of fracture of orbit, except blowout; without implant**
🚑 16.5   ⚕ 16.5   **FUD** 090   J G2 80 50 ▭
AMA: 2018,Sep,7

21407 **with implant**
🚑 18.5   ⚕ 18.5   **FUD** 090   J G2 80 50 ▭
AMA: 2018,Sep,7

21408 **with bone grafting (includes obtaining graft)**
🚑 25.9   ⚕ 25.9   **FUD** 090   J 80 50 ▭
AMA: 2018,Sep,7

21421 **Closed treatment of palatal or maxillary fracture (LeFort I type), with interdental wire fixation or fixation of denture or splint**
🚑 17.2   ⚕ 20.3   **FUD** 090   J A2 80 ▭
AMA: 2018,Sep,7

21422 **Open treatment of palatal or maxillary fracture (LeFort I type);**
🚑 18.9   ⚕ 18.9   **FUD** 090   C 80 ▭
AMA: 2018,Sep,7

21423 **complicated (comminuted or involving cranial nerve foramina), multiple approaches**
🚑 22.2   ⚕ 22.2   **FUD** 090   C 80 ▭
AMA: 2018,Sep,7

21431 **Closed treatment of craniofacial separation (LeFort III type) using interdental wire fixation of denture or splint**
🚑 20.6   ⚕ 20.6   **FUD** 090   C 80 ▭
AMA: 2018,Sep,7

21432 **Open treatment of craniofacial separation (LeFort III type); with wiring and/or internal fixation**
🚑 20.6   ⚕ 20.6   **FUD** 090   C 80 ▭
AMA: 2018,Sep,7

21433 **complicated (eg, comminuted or involving cranial nerve foramina), multiple surgical approaches**
🚑 50.1   ⚕ 50.1   **FUD** 090   C 80 ▭
AMA: 2018,Sep,7

21435 **complicated, utilizing internal and/or external fixation techniques (eg, head cap, halo device, and/or intermaxillary fixation)**
EXCLUDES *Removal of internal or external fixation (20670)*
🚑 40.4   ⚕ 40.4   **FUD** 090   C 80 ▭
AMA: 2018,Sep,7

21436 **complicated, multiple surgical approaches, internal fixation, with bone grafting (includes obtaining graft)**
🚑 58.8   ⚕ 58.8   **FUD** 090   C 80 ▭
AMA: 2018,Sep,7

21440 **Closed treatment of mandibular or maxillary alveolar ridge fracture (separate procedure)**
🚑 14.0   ⚕ 17.3   **FUD** 090   J P3 80 ▭
AMA: 2018,Sep,7

21445 **Open treatment of mandibular or maxillary alveolar ridge fracture (separate procedure)**
🚑 18.0   ⚕ 22.2   **FUD** 090   J A2 80 ▭
AMA: 2018,Sep,7

21450 **Closed treatment of mandibular fracture; without manipulation**
🚑 13.4   ⚕ 16.4   **FUD** 090   T A2 80 ▭
AMA: 2018,Sep,7

21451 **with manipulation**
🚑 18.2   ⚕ 21.7   **FUD** 090   T A2 80 ▭
AMA: 2018,Sep,7

21452 Percutaneous treatment of mandibular fracture, with external fixation

    🚑 11.4   ⚕ 19.1   **FUD** 090   J A2 80 ▣

    AMA: 2018,Sep,7

Comminuted fractures

Metal or acrylic bar

Rods and pins placed in drilled holes

21453 Closed treatment of mandibular fracture with interdental fixation

    🚑 23.6   ⚕ 27.6   **FUD** 090   J A2 80 ▣

    AMA: 2018,Sep,7; 2018,Jan,8; 2017,Jan,8; 2016,Jan,13; 2015,Jan,16; 2014,Jan,11

21454 Open treatment of mandibular fracture with external fixation

    🚑 15.6   ⚕ 15.6   **FUD** 090   J J8 80 ▣

    AMA: 2018,Sep,7

21461 Open treatment of mandibular fracture; without interdental fixation

    🚑 28.1   ⚕ 59.4   **FUD** 090   J J8 ▣

    AMA: 2018,Sep,7

21462 with interdental fixation

    🚑 31.2   ⚕ 63.3   **FUD** 090   J J8 80 ▣

    AMA: 2018,Sep,7

21465 Open treatment of mandibular condylar fracture

    🚑 25.9   ⚕ 25.9   **FUD** 090   J A2 80 50 ▣

    AMA: 2018,Sep,7

21470 Open treatment of complicated mandibular fracture by multiple surgical approaches including internal fixation, interdental fixation, and/or wiring of dentures or splints

    🚑 34.5   ⚕ 34.5   **FUD** 090   J 80 ▣

    AMA: 2018,Sep,7; 2018,Jan,8; 2017,Jan,8; 2016,Jan,13; 2015,Jan,16; 2014,Jan,11

21480 Closed treatment of temporomandibular dislocation; initial or subsequent

    🚑 0.91   ⚕ 3.07   **FUD** 000   T A2 50 ▣

    AMA: 2018,Sep,7

21485 complicated (eg, recurrent requiring intermaxillary fixation or splinting), initial or subsequent

    🚑 19.5   ⚕ 23.8   **FUD** 090   T A2 80 50 ▣

    AMA: 2018,Sep,7

21490 Open treatment of temporomandibular dislocation

    EXCLUDES   Interdental wiring (21497)

    🚑 25.5   ⚕ 25.5   **FUD** 090   J A2 80 50 ▣

    AMA: 2018,Sep,7

21497 Interdental wiring, for condition other than fracture

    🚑 16.5   ⚕ 19.6   **FUD** 090   T A2 80 ▣

    AMA: 2018,Sep,7; 2018,Jan,8; 2017,Jan,8; 2016,Jan,13; 2015,Jan,16; 2014,Jan,11

21499 Unlisted musculoskeletal procedure, head

    EXCLUDES   Unlisted procedures of craniofacial or maxillofacial areas (21299)

    🚑 0.00   ⚕ 0.00   **FUD** YYY   T 80 ▣

    AMA: 2018,Sep,7

21501-21510 Surgical Incision for Drainage: Chest and Soft Tissues of Neck

EXCLUDES   Biopsy of the flank or back (21920-21925)
Simple incision and drainage of abscess or hematoma (10060, 10140)
Tumor removal of flank or back (21930-21936)

21501 Incision and drainage, deep abscess or hematoma, soft tissues of neck or thorax;

    EXCLUDES   Deep incision and drainage of posterior spine (22010-22015)

    🚑 9.29   ⚕ 13.1   **FUD** 090   J A2 ▣

    AMA: 2018,Sep,7; 2018,Jan,8; 2017,Jan,8; 2016,Jan,13; 2015,Jan,16; 2014,Dec,16; 2014,Dec,16

21502 with partial rib ostectomy

    🚑 14.5   ⚕ 14.5   **FUD** 090   J A2 80 ▣

    AMA: 2018,Sep,7

21510 Incision, deep, with opening of bone cortex (eg, for osteomyelitis or bone abscess), thorax

    🚑 12.7   ⚕ 12.7   **FUD** 090   C 80 ▣

    AMA: 2018,Sep,7

21550 Soft Tissue Biopsy of Chest or Neck

EXCLUDES   Biopsy of bone (20220-20251)
Soft tissue needle biopsy (20206)

21550 Biopsy, soft tissue of neck or thorax

    🚑 4.51   ⚕ 7.46   **FUD** 010   J G2 ▣

    AMA: 2018,Sep,7

21552-21558 [21552, 21554] Excision Soft Tissue Tumors Chest and Neck

INCLUDES   Any necessary elevation of tissue planes or dissection
Measurement of tumor and necessary margin at greatest diameter prior to excision
Resection without removal of significant normal tissue
Simple and intermediate repairs
Types of excision:
    Fascial or subfascial soft tissue tumors: simple and marginal resection of tumors found either in or below the deep fascia, not involving bone or excision of a substantial amount of normal tissue; primarily benign and intramuscular tumors
    Radical resection soft tissue tumor: wide resection of tumor, involving substantial margins of normal tissue and may involve tissue removal from one or more layers; most often malignant or aggressive benign
    Subcutaneous: simple and marginal resection of tumors in the subcutaneous tissue above the deep fascia; most often benign

EXCLUDES   Complex repair
Excision of benign cutaneous lesions (eg, sebaceous cyst) (11400-11426)
Radical resection of cutaneous tumors (eg, melanoma) (11600-11626)
Significant exploration of the vessels or neuroplasty

21552 Resequenced code. See code following 21555.

21554 Resequenced code. See code following 21556.

21555 Excision, tumor, soft tissue of neck or anterior thorax, subcutaneous; less than 3 cm

    🚑 8.78   ⚕ 12.0   **FUD** 090   J G2 ▣

    AMA: 2018,Sep,7; 2018,Jan,8; 2017,Jan,8; 2016,Jan,13; 2015,Jan,16; 2014,Jan,11

\# **21552** 3 cm or greater

    🚑 12.8   ⚕ 12.8   **FUD** 090   J G2 80 ▣

    AMA: 2018,Sep,7

21556 Excision, tumor, soft tissue of neck or anterior thorax, subfascial (eg, intramuscular); less than 5 cm

    🚑 15.1   ⚕ 15.1   **FUD** 090   J G2 ▣

    AMA: 2018,Sep,7

\# **21554** 5 cm or greater

    🚑 21.0   ⚕ 21.0   **FUD** 090   J G2 80 ▣

    AMA: 2018,Sep,7

21557 Radical resection of tumor (eg, sarcoma), soft tissue of neck or anterior thorax; less than 5 cm

    🚑 27.4   ⚕ 27.4   **FUD** 090   J G2 80 ▣

    AMA: 2018,Sep,7; 2018,Jan,8; 2017,Jan,8; 2016,Jan,13; 2015,Jan,16; 2014,Jan,11

21558   **5 cm or greater**
🚑 38.7   ⚬ 38.7   **FUD** 090   J G2 80 ▢
AMA: 2018,Sep,7

21600-21632 Bony Resection Chest and Neck

21600   **Excision of rib, partial**
    EXCLUDES   *Extensive debridement (11044, 11047)*
                Radical resection, chest wall/rib cage for tumor (21601)
🚑 15.8   ⚬ 15.8   **FUD** 090   J A2 80 ▢
AMA: 2018,Sep,7; 2018,Jan,8; 2017,Jan,8; 2016,Jan,13;
2015,Jan,16; 2014,Jan,11

● **21601**   **Excision of chest wall tumor including rib(s)**
    EXCLUDES   *Exploratory thoracotomy (32100)*
                Resection of apical lung tumor (32503-32504)
                Thoracentesis (32554-32555)
                Tube thoracostomy (32551)

● **21602**   **Excision of chest wall tumor involving rib(s), with plastic reconstruction; without mediastinal lymphadenectomy**
    EXCLUDES   *Exploratory thoracotomy (32100)*
                Resection of apical lung tumor (32503-32504)
                Thoracentesis (32554-32555)
                Tube thoracostomy (32551)

● **21603**   **with mediastinal lymphadenectomy**
    EXCLUDES   *Exploratory thoracotomy (32100)*
                Resection of apical lung tumor (32503-32504)
                Thoracentesis (32554-32555)
                Tube thoracostomy (32551)

21610   **Costotransversectomy (separate procedure)**
🚑 35.1   ⚬ 35.1   **FUD** 090   J A2 80 ▢
AMA: 2018,Sep,7

21615   **Excision first and/or cervical rib;**
🚑 17.5   ⚬ 17.5   **FUD** 090   C 80 50 ▢
AMA: 2018,Sep,7; 2018,Jan,8; 2017,Jan,8; 2016,Jan,13;
2015,Jan,16; 2014,Mar,13

21616   **with sympathectomy**
🚑 20.5   ⚬ 20.5   **FUD** 090   C 80 50 ▢
AMA: 2018,Sep,7

21620   **Ostectomy of sternum, partial**
🚑 14.5   ⚬ 14.5   **FUD** 090   C 80 ▢
AMA: 2018,Sep,7

21627   **Sternal debridement**
    EXCLUDES   *Debridement with sternotomy closure (21750)*
🚑 15.4   ⚬ 15.4   **FUD** 090   C 80 ▢
AMA: 2018,Sep,7; 2018,Jan,8; 2017,Jan,8; 2016,Jan,13;
2015,Jan,16; 2014,Jan,11

21630   **Radical resection of sternum;**
🚑 35.4   ⚬ 35.4   **FUD** 090   C 80 ▢
AMA: 2018,Sep,7

21632   **with mediastinal lymphadenectomy**
🚑 34.8   ⚬ 34.8   **FUD** 090   C 80 ▢
AMA: 2018,Sep,7

21685-21750 Repair/Reconstruction Chest and Soft Tissues Neck

EXCLUDES   *Biopsy of chest or neck (21550)*
            Repair of simple wounds (12001-12007)
            Tumor removal of chest or neck (21552-21558 [21552, 21554])

21685   **Hyoid myotomy and suspension**
🚑 28.2   ⚬ 28.2   **FUD** 090   J G2 80 ▢
AMA: 2018,Sep,7; 2018,Jan,8; 2017,Jan,8; 2016,Jan,13;
2015,Jan,16; 2014,Jan,11

21700   **Division of scalenus anticus; without resection of cervical rib**
🚑 10.3   ⚬ 10.3   **FUD** 090   J A2 80 50 ▢
AMA: 2018,Sep,7

21705   **with resection of cervical rib**
🚑 15.4   ⚬ 15.4   **FUD** 090   C 80 50 ▢
AMA: 2018,Sep,7; 2018,Jan,8; 2017,Jan,8; 2016,Jan,13;
2015,Jan,16; 2014,Mar,13

21720   **Division of sternocleidomastoid for torticollis, open operation; without cast application**
    EXCLUDES   *Transection of spinal accessory and cervical nerves (63191, 64722)*
🚑 15.2   ⚬ 15.2   **FUD** 090   J A2 80 ▢
AMA: 2018,Sep,7

21725   **with cast application**
    EXCLUDES   *Transection of spinal accessory and cervical nerves (63191, 64722)*
🚑 15.5   ⚬ 15.5   **FUD** 090   T A2 80 ▢
AMA: 2018,Sep,7

21740   **Reconstructive repair of pectus excavatum or carinatum; open**
🚑 29.8   ⚬ 29.8   **FUD** 090   C 80 ▢
AMA: 2018,Sep,7

21742   **minimally invasive approach (Nuss procedure), without thoracoscopy**
🚑 0.00   ⚬ 0.00   **FUD** 090   J 80 ▢
AMA: 2018,Sep,7

21743   **minimally invasive approach (Nuss procedure), with thoracoscopy**
🚑 0.00   ⚬ 0.00   **FUD** 090   J 80 ▢
AMA: 2018,Sep,7

21750   **Closure of median sternotomy separation with or without debridement (separate procedure)**
🚑 19.7   ⚬ 19.7   **FUD** 090   C 80 ▢
AMA: 2018,Sep,7; 2018,Jan,8; 2017,Jan,8; 2016,Jan,13;
2015,Jan,16; 2014,Jan,11

21811-21825 Fracture Care: Ribs and Sternum

EXCLUDES   *E&M services for treatment of closed uncomplicated rib fractures*

21811   **Open treatment of rib fracture(s) with internal fixation, includes thoracoscopic visualization when performed, unilateral; 1-3 ribs**
🚑 17.1   ⚬ 17.1   **FUD** 000   J 80 50 ▢
AMA: 2018,Sep,7; 2018,Jan,8; 2017,Jan,8; 2016,Jan,13;
2015,Aug,3

21812   **4-6 ribs**
🚑 21.0   ⚬ 21.0   **FUD** 000   J 80 50 ▢
AMA: 2018,Sep,7; 2018,Jan,8; 2017,Jan,8; 2016,Jan,13;
2015,Aug,3

21813   **7 or more ribs**
🚑 28.6   ⚬ 28.6   **FUD** 000   J 80 50 ▢
AMA: 2018,Sep,7; 2018,Jan,8; 2017,Jan,8; 2016,Jan,13;
2015,Aug,3

21820   **Closed treatment of sternum fracture**
🚑 4.10   ⚬ 4.08   **FUD** 090   T A2 ▢
AMA: 2018,Sep,7

21825   **Open treatment of sternum fracture with or without skeletal fixation**
    EXCLUDES   *Treatment of sternoclavicular dislocation (23520-23532)*
🚑 15.5   ⚬ 15.5   **FUD** 090   C 80 ▢
AMA: 2018,Sep,7

21899 Unlisted Procedures of Chest or Neck

CMS: 100-04,4,180.3 Unlisted Service or Procedure

21899   **Unlisted procedure, neck or thorax**
🚑 0.00   ⚬ 0.00   **FUD** YYY   T 80 ▢
AMA: 2018,Sep,7; 2018,Jan,8; 2017,Jan,8; 2016,Jan,13;
2015,Aug,3

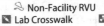

21920-21925 Biopsy Soft Tissue of Back and Flank

EXCLUDES   *Soft tissue needle biopsy (20206)*

21920   **Biopsy, soft tissue of back or flank; superficial**
4.55   7.30   **FUD** 010   `J` `P3`
AMA: 2018,Sep,7

21925   **deep**
10.3   13.1   **FUD** 090   `J` `A2`
AMA: 2018,Sep,7

21930-21936 Excision Soft Tissue Tumors Back or Flank

INCLUDES   Any necessary elevation of tissue planes or dissection
Measurement of tumor and necessary margin at greatest diameter prior to excision
Simple and intermediate repairs
Types of excision:
    Fascial or subfascial soft tissue tumors: simple and marginal resection of tumors found either in or below the deep fascia, not involving bone or excision of a substantial amount of normal tissue; most often benign and intramuscular tumors
    Radical resection soft tissue tumor: wide resection of tumor, involving substantial margins of normal tissue and may include tissue removal from one or more layers; most often malignant or aggressive benign
    Subcutaneous: simple and marginal resection of tumors in the subcutaneous tissue above the deep fascia; most often benign

EXCLUDES   *Complex repair*
Excision of benign cutaneous lesions (eg, sebaceous cyst) (11400-11406)
Radical resection of cutaneous tumors (eg, melanoma) (11600-11606)
Significant exploration of the vessels or neuroplasty

21930   **Excision, tumor, soft tissue of back or flank, subcutaneous; less than 3 cm**
10.4   13.8   **FUD** 090   `J` `G2`
AMA: 2018,Sep,7; 2018,Jan,8; 2017,Jan,8; 2016,Jan,13; 2015,Jan,16; 2014,Jan,11

21931   **3 cm or greater**
13.5   13.5   **FUD** 090   `J` `G2` `80`
AMA: 2018,Sep,7

21932   **Excision, tumor, soft tissue of back or flank, subfascial (eg, intramuscular); less than 5 cm**
19.0   19.0   **FUD** 090   `J` `G2` `80`
AMA: 2018,Sep,7

21933   **5 cm or greater**
21.2   21.2   **FUD** 090   `J` `G2` `80`
AMA: 2018,Sep,7

21935   **Radical resection of tumor (eg, sarcoma), soft tissue of back or flank; less than 5 cm**
29.6   29.6   **FUD** 090   `J` `G2`
AMA: 2018,Sep,7

21936   **5 cm or greater**
40.9   40.9   **FUD** 090   `J` `G2` `80`
AMA: 2018,Sep,7

22010-22015 Incision for Drainage of Deep Spinal Abscess

EXCLUDES   *Incision and drainage of hematoma (10060, 10140)*
Injection:
    Chemonucleolysis (62292)
    Discography (62290-62291)
    Facet joint (64490-64495, [64633, 64634, 64635, 64636])
    Myelography (62284)
Needle/trocar biopsy (20220-20225)

22010   **Incision and drainage, open, of deep abscess (subfascial), posterior spine; cervical, thoracic, or cervicothoracic**
27.7   27.7   **FUD** 090   `C` `80`
AMA: 2018,Sep,7

22015   **lumbar, sacral, or lumbosacral**
EXCLUDES   *Incision and drainage, complex, postoperative wound infection (10180)*
Incision and drainage, open, of deep abscess (subfascial), posterior spine; cervical, thoracic, or cervicothoracic (22010)
Removal of posterior nonsegmental instrumentation (eg, Harrington rod) (22850)
Removal of posterior segmental instrumentation (22852)
27.4   27.4   **FUD** 090   `C`
AMA: 2018,Sep,7

22100-22103 Partial Resection Vertebral Component

EXCLUDES   *Back or flank biopsy (21920-21925)*
Bone biopsy (20220-20251)
Injection:
    Chemonucleolysis (62292)
    Discography (62290-62291)
    Facet joint (64490-64495, [64633, 64634, 64635, 64636])
    Myelography (62284)
Removal of tumor flank or back (21930)
Soft tissue needle biopsy (20206)
Spinal reconstruction with vertebral body prosthesis:
    Cervical (20931, 20938, 22554, 63081)
    Thoracic (20931, 20938, 22556, 63085, 63087)

22100   **Partial excision of posterior vertebral component (eg, spinous process, lamina or facet) for intrinsic bony lesion, single vertebral segment; cervical**
24.8   24.8   **FUD** 090   `J` `80`
AMA: 2018,Sep,7; 2018,Jan,8; 2017,Mar,7; 2017,Jan,8; 2016,Jan,13; 2015,Jan,16

22101   **thoracic**
24.8   24.8   **FUD** 090   `J` `80`
AMA: 2018,Sep,7; 2018,Jan,8; 2017,Mar,7; 2017,Jan,8; 2016,Jan,13; 2015,Jan,16

22102   **lumbar**
Code also posterior spinous process distraction device insertion, if applicable (22867-22870)
23.4   23.4   **FUD** 090   `J` `G2` `80`
AMA: 2018,Sep,7; 2018,Jan,8; 2017,Mar,7; 2017,Jan,8; 2016,Jan,13; 2015,Jan,16

+   **22103**   **each additional segment (List separately in addition to code for primary procedure)**
Code first (22100-22102)
4.10   4.10   **FUD** ZZZ   `N` `N1` `80`
AMA: 2018,Sep,7

22110-22116 Partial Resection Vertebral Component without Decompression

EXCLUDES   *Back or flank biopsy (21920-21925)*
Bone biopsy (20220-20251)
Bone grafting procedures (20930-20938)
Harvest bone graft (20931, 20938)
Injection:
    Chemonucleolysis (62292)
    Discography (62290-62291)
    Facet joint (64490-64495, [64633, 64634, 64635, 64636])
    Myelography (62284)
Osteotomy (22210-22226)
Removal of tumor flank or back (21930)
Restoration after vertebral body resection (22585, 63082, 63086, 63088, 63091)
Spinal restoration with graft:
    Cervical (20931, 20938, 22554, 63081)
    Lumbar (20931, 20938, 22558, 63087, 63090)
    Thoracic (20931, 20938, 22556, 63085, 63087)
Spinal restoration with prosthesis:
    Cervical (20931, 20938, 22554, 22853-22854 [22859], 63081)
    Lumbar (20931, 20938, 22558, 22853-22854 [22859], 63087, 63090)
    Thoracic (20931, 20938, 22556, 22853-22854 [22859], 63085, 63087)
Vertebral corpectomy (63081-63091)

22110   **Partial excision of vertebral body, for intrinsic bony lesion, without decompression of spinal cord or nerve root(s), single vertebral segment; cervical**
30.2   30.2   **FUD** 090   `C` `80`
AMA: 2018,Sep,7; 2018,Jan,8; 2017,Mar,7; 2017,Jan,8; 2016,Jan,13; 2015,Jan,16

22112 **thoracic**
🛏 32.7   ⚕ 32.7   **FUD** 090   C 80 ▭
AMA: 2018,Sep,7; 2018,Jan,8; 2017,Mar,7; 2017,Jan,8;
2016,Jan,13; 2015,Jan,16

22114 **lumbar**
🛏 32.7   ⚕ 32.7   **FUD** 090   C 80 ▭
AMA: 2018,Sep,7; 2018,Jan,8; 2017,Mar,7; 2017,Jan,8;
2016,Jan,13; 2015,Jan,16

+ **22116** **each additional vertebral segment (List separately in addition to code for primary procedure)**
Code first (22110-22114)
🛏 4.12   ⚕ 4.12   **FUD** ZZZ   C 80 ▭
AMA: 2018,Sep,7

22206-22216 Spinal Osteotomy: Posterior/Posterolateral Approach

EXCLUDES *Decompression of the spinal cord and/or nerve roots (63001-63308)*
Injection:
Chemonucleolysis (62292)
Discography (62290-62292)
Facet joint (64490-64495, [64633, 64634, 64635, 64636])
Myelography (62284)
Repair of vertebral fracture by the anterior approach, see appropriate arthrodesis, bone graft, instrumentation codes, and (63081-63091)
Code also arthrodesis (22590-22632)
Code also bone grafting procedures (20930-20938)
Code also spinal instrumentation (22840-22855 [22859])

22206 **Osteotomy of spine, posterior or posterolateral approach, 3 columns, 1 vertebral segment (eg, pedicle/vertebral body subtraction); thoracic**
EXCLUDES *Osteotomy of spine, posterior or posterolateral approach, lumbar (22207)*
Procedures performed at same level (22210-22226, 22830, 63001-63048, 63055-63066, 63075-63091, 63101-63103)
🛏 71.3   ⚕ 71.3   **FUD** 090   C 80 ▭
AMA: 2018,Sep,7; 2018,Jan,8; 2017,Mar,7; 2017,Jan,8;
2016,Jan,13; 2015,Jan,16; 2014,Jan,11

22207 **lumbar**
EXCLUDES *Osteotomy of spine, posterior or posterolateral approach, thoracic (22206)*
Procedures performed at the same level (22210-22226, 22830, 63001-63048, 63055-63066, 63075-63091, 63101-63103)
🛏 69.8   ⚕ 69.8   **FUD** 090   C 80 ▭
AMA: 2018,Sep,7; 2018,Jan,8; 2017,Mar,7; 2017,Jan,8;
2016,Jan,13; 2015,Jan,16; 2014,Jan,11

+ **22208** **each additional vertebral segment (List separately in addition to code for primary procedure)**
EXCLUDES *Procedures performed at the same level (22210-22226, 22830, 63001-63048, 63055-63066, 63075-63091, 63101-63103)*
Code first (22206, 22207)
🛏 17.2   ⚕ 17.2   **FUD** ZZZ   C 80 ▭
AMA: 2018,Sep,7; 2018,Jan,8; 2017,Jan,8; 2016,Jan,13;
2015,Jan,16; 2014,Jan,11

22210 **Osteotomy of spine, posterior or posterolateral approach, 1 vertebral segment; cervical**
🛏 52.0   ⚕ 52.0   **FUD** 090   C 80 ▭
AMA: 2018,Sep,7; 2018,Jan,8; 2017,Mar,7; 2017,Jan,8;
2016,Jan,13; 2015,Jan,16

Patient is stabilized by halo and traction to correct cervical problem

Several sections may be removed

C-6
C-7
T-1

Physician removes spinous processes, lamina

22212 **thoracic**
🛏 43.2   ⚕ 43.2   **FUD** 090   C 80 ▭
AMA: 2018,Sep,7; 2018,Jan,8; 2017,Mar,7; 2017,Jan,8;
2016,Jan,13; 2015,Jan,16; 2014,Jan,11

22214 **lumbar**
🛏 43.4   ⚕ 43.4   **FUD** 090   C 80 ▭
AMA: 2018,Sep,7; 2018,Jan,8; 2017,Mar,7; 2017,Jan,8;
2016,Jan,13; 2015,Jan,16; 2014,Dec,16; 2014,Dec,16; 2014,Jan,11

+ **22216** **each additional vertebral segment (List separately in addition to primary procedure)**
Code first (22210-22214)
🛏 10.6   ⚕ 10.6   **FUD** ZZZ   C 80 ▭
AMA: 2018,Sep,7; 2018,Jan,8; 2017,Jan,8; 2016,Jan,13;
2015,Jan,16; 2014,Jan,11

22220-22226 Spinal Osteotomy: Anterior Approach

EXCLUDES *Corpectomy (63081-63091)*
Decompression of the spinal cord and/or nerve roots (63001-63308)
Injection:
Chemonucleolysis (62292)
Discography (62290-62291)
Facet joint (64490-64495, [64633], [64634], [64635], [64636])
Myelography (62284)
Needle/trocar biopsy (20220-20225)
Repair of vertebral fracture by the anterior approach, see appropriate arthrodesis, bone graft, instrumentation codes, and (63081-63091)
Code also arthrodesis (22590-22632)
Code also bone grafting procedures (20930-20938)
Code also spinal instrumentation (22840-22855 [22859])

22220 **Osteotomy of spine, including discectomy, anterior approach, single vertebral segment; cervical**
🛏 47.0   ⚕ 47.0   **FUD** 090   C 80 ▭
AMA: 2018,Sep,7; 2018,Jan,8; 2017,Mar,7; 2017,Jan,8;
2016,Jan,13; 2015,Jan,16

22222 **thoracic**
🛏 51.1   ⚕ 51.1   **FUD** 090   C 80 ▭
AMA: 2018,Sep,7; 2018,Jan,8; 2017,Mar,7; 2017,Jan,8;
2016,Jan,13; 2015,Jan,16; 2014,Jan,11

22224 **lumbar**
🛏 45.9   ⚕ 45.9   **FUD** 090   C 80 ▭
AMA: 2018,Sep,7; 2018,Jan,8; 2017,Mar,7; 2017,Jan,8;
2016,Jan,13; 2015,Jan,16

+ **22226** **each additional vertebral segment (List separately in addition to code for primary procedure)**
Code first (22220-22224)
🛏 10.5   ⚕ 10.5   **FUD** ZZZ   C 80 ▭
AMA: 2018,Sep,7

22310-22315 Closed Treatment Vertebral Fractures

EXCLUDES Injection:
    Chemonucleolysis (62292)
    Discography (62290-62291)
    Facet joint (64490-64495, [64633], [64634], [64635], [64636])
    Myelography (62284)
    Percutaneous vertebroplasty at same level (22510-22515)
Code also arthrodesis (22590-22632)
Code also bone grafting procedures (20930-20938)
Code also spinal instrumentation (22840-22855 [22859])

22310 **Closed treatment of vertebral body fracture(s), without manipulation, requiring and including casting or bracing**
    🔧 8.17   ⚕ 8.82   **FUD** 090   T A2 ▱
    AMA: 2018,Sep,7; 2018,Jan,8; 2017,Mar,7; 2017,Jan,8; 2016,Jan,13; 2015,Jan,16; 2015,Jan,8; 2014,Jul,8; 2014,Jan,11

22315 **Closed treatment of vertebral fracture(s) and/or dislocation(s) requiring casting or bracing, with and including casting and/or bracing by manipulation or traction**
    EXCLUDES Spinal manipulation (97140)
    🔧 22.2   ⚕ 25.3   **FUD** 090   J A2 ▱
    AMA: 2018,Sep,7; 2018,Jan,8; 2017,Mar,7; 2017,Jan,8; 2016,Jan,13; 2015,Jan,8; 2015,Jan,16; 2014,Jan,11

22318-22319 Open Treatment Odontoid Fracture: Anterior Approach

EXCLUDES Injection:
    Chemonucleolysis (62292)
    Discography (62290-62291)
    Facet joint (64490-64495, [64633, 64634, 64635, 64636])
    Myelography (62284)
    Needle/trocar biopsy (20220-20225)
Code also arthrodesis (22590-22632)
Code also bone grafting procedures (20930-20938)
Code also spinal instrumentation (22840-22855 [22859])

22318 **Open treatment and/or reduction of odontoid fracture(s) and or dislocation(s) (including os odontoideum), anterior approach, including placement of internal fixation; without grafting**
    🔧 47.6   ⚕ 47.6   **FUD** 090   C 80 ▱
    AMA: 2018,Sep,7; 2018,Jan,8; 2017,Mar,7; 2017,Jan,8; 2016,Jan,13; 2015,Jan,16; 2014,Jan,11

22319 **with grafting**
    🔧 53.6   ⚕ 53.6   **FUD** 090   C 80 ▱
    AMA: 2018,Sep,7; 2018,May,3; 2018,Jan,8; 2017,Mar,7; 2017,Jan,8; 2016,Jan,13; 2015,Jan,16; 2014,Jan,11

22325-22328 Open Treatment Vertebral Fractures: Posterior Approach

EXCLUDES Corpectomy (63081-63091)
    Injection:
        Chemonucleolysis (62292)
        Discography (62290-62291)
        Facet joint (64490-64495, [64633], [64634], [64635], [64636])
        Myelography (62284)
    Needle/trocar biopsy (20220-20225)
    Spine decompression (63001-63091)
    Vertebral fracture care by arthrodesis (22548-22632)
    Vertebral fracture care frontal approach (63081-63091)
Code also arthrodesis (22548-22632)
Code also bone grafting procedures (20930-20938)
Code also spinal instrumentation (22840-22855 [22859])

22325 **Open treatment and/or reduction of vertebral fracture(s) and/or dislocation(s), posterior approach, 1 fractured vertebra or dislocated segment; lumbar**
    EXCLUDES Percutaneous vertebral augmentation performed at same level (22514-22515)
           Percutaneous vertebroplasty performed at same level (22511-22512)
    🔧 41.9   ⚕ 41.9   **FUD** 090   C 80 ▱
    AMA: 2018,Sep,7; 2018,Jan,8; 2017,Aug,9; 2017,Mar,7; 2017,Jan,8; 2016,Jan,13; 2015,Jan,16; 2015,Jan,8; 2014,Jan,11

22326 **cervical**
    EXCLUDES Percutaneous vertebroplasty performed at same level (22510, 22512)
    🔧 43.4   ⚕ 43.4   **FUD** 090   C 80 ▱
    AMA: 2018,Sep,7; 2018,Jan,8; 2017,Mar,7; 2017,Jan,8; 2016,Jan,13; 2015,Jan,16; 2014,Jan,11

22327 **thoracic**
    EXCLUDES Percutaneous vertebral augmentation performed at same level (22515)
           Percutaneous vertebroplasty performed at same level (22510, 22512-22513)
    🔧 43.8   ⚕ 43.8   **FUD** 090   C 80 ▱
    AMA: 2018,Sep,7; 2018,Jan,8; 2017,Mar,7; 2017,Jan,8; 2016,Jan,13; 2015,Jan,8; 2015,Jan,16; 2014,Jan,11

+ 22328 **each additional fractured vertebra or dislocated segment (List separately in addition to code for primary procedure)**
    Code first (22325-22327)
    🔧 8.25   ⚕ 8.25   **FUD** ZZZ   C 80 ▱
    AMA: 2018,Sep,7

22505 Spinal Manipulation with Anesthesia

EXCLUDES Manipulation not requiring anesthesia (97140)

22505 **Manipulation of spine requiring anesthesia, any region**
    🔧 3.79   ⚕ 3.79   **FUD** 010   J A2 ▱
    AMA: 2018,Sep,7; 2018,Jan,8; 2017,Jan,8; 2016,Jan,13; 2015,Jan,16; 2014,Jan,11

22510-22515 Percutaneous Vertebroplasty/Kyphoplasty

INCLUDES Bone biopsy when applicable (20225)
    Radiological guidance
EXCLUDES Closed treatment vertebral fractures (22310, 22315)
    Open treatment/reduction vertebral fractures (22325, 22327)
    Sacroplasty/augmentation (0200T-0201T)

22510 **Percutaneous vertebroplasty (bone biopsy included when performed), 1 vertebral body, unilateral or bilateral injection, inclusive of all imaging guidance; cervicothoracic**
    🔧 12.5   ⚕ 49.8   **FUD** 010   J G2 ▱
    AMA: 2018,Sep,7; 2018,Jan,8; 2017,Jan,8; 2016,Jan,13; 2015,Jan,8

22511 **lumbosacral**
    🔧 11.7   ⚕ 49.3   **FUD** 010   J G2 ▱
    AMA: 2018,Sep,7; 2018,Jan,8; 2017,Jan,8; 2016,Jan,13; 2015,Apr,8; 2015,Jan,8

+ 22512 **each additional cervicothoracic or lumbosacral vertebral body (List separately in addition to code for primary procedure)**
    Code first (22510-22511)
    🔧 5.99   ⚕ 25.6   **FUD** ZZZ   N N1 ▱
    AMA: 2018,Sep,7; 2018,Jan,8; 2017,Jan,8; 2016,Jan,13; 2015,Jan,8

22513 **Percutaneous vertebral augmentation, including cavity creation (fracture reduction and bone biopsy included when performed) using mechanical device (eg, kyphoplasty), 1 vertebral body, unilateral or bilateral cannulation, inclusive of all imaging guidance; thoracic**
    🔧 14.9   ⚕ 195.   **FUD** 010   J G2 ▱
    AMA: 2018,Sep,7; 2018,Jan,8; 2017,Jan,8; 2016,Jan,13; 2015,Jan,8

22514 **lumbar**
    🔧 13.9   ⚕ 194.   **FUD** 010   J G2 ▱
    AMA: 2018,Sep,7; 2018,Jan,8; 2017,Jan,8; 2016,Jan,13; 2015,Jan,8

+ 22515 **each additional thoracic or lumbar vertebral body (List separately in addition to code for primary procedure)**
    Code first (22513-22514)
    🔧 6.46   ⚕ 113.   **FUD** ZZZ   N N1 ▱
    AMA: 2018,Sep,7; 2018,Jan,8; 2017,Jan,8; 2016,Jan,13; 2015,Jan,8

22526-22527 Percutaneous Annuloplasty

CMS: 100-04,32,220.1 Thermal Intradiscal Procedures (TIPS)

INCLUDES Fluoroscopic guidance (77002, 77003)
EXCLUDES Needle/trocar biopsy (20220-20225)
Injection:
Chemonucleolysis (62292)
Discography (62290-62291)
Facet joint (64490-64495, [64633], [64634], [64635], [64636])
Myelography (62284)
Procedure performed by other methods (22899)

22526 Percutaneous intradiscal electrothermal annuloplasty, unilateral or bilateral including fluoroscopic guidance; single level

🚑 9.76 ⚕ 65.0 **FUD** 010 [E] 🔲

AMA: 2018,Sep,7; 2018,Jan,8; 2017,Jan,8; 2016,Jan,13; 2015,Jan,8; 2015,Jan,16; 2014,Jan,11

+ 22527 1 or more additional levels (List separately in addition to code for primary procedure)

Code first (22526)

🚑 4.61 ⚕ 54.6 **FUD** ZZZ [E] 🔲

AMA: 2018,Sep,7; 2018,Jan,8; 2017,Jan,8; 2016,Jan,13; 2015,Jan,8; 2015,Jan,16; 2014,Jan,11

22532-22534 Spinal Fusion: Lateral Extracavitary Approach

EXCLUDES Corpectomy (63101-63103)
Exploration of spinal fusion (22830)
Fracture care (22310-22328)
Injection:
Chemonucleolysis (62292)
Discography (62290-62291)
Facet joint (64490-64495, [64633], [64634], [64635], [64636])
Myelography (62284)
Laminectomy (63001-63017)
Needle/trocar biopsy (20220-20225)
Osteotomy (22206-22226)
Code also bone grafting procedures (20930-20938)
Code also spinal instrumentation (22840-22855 [22859])

22532 Arthrodesis, lateral extracavitary technique, including minimal discectomy to prepare interspace (other than for decompression); thoracic

🚑 52.4 ⚕ 52.4 **FUD** 090 [C] 80 🔲

AMA: 2018,Sep,7; 2018,May,3; 2018,Jan,8; 2017,Mar,7; 2017,Feb,9; 2017,Jan,8; 2016,Jan,13; 2015,Jan,16; 2014,Jan,11

22533 lumbar

🚑 48.1 ⚕ 48.1 **FUD** 090 [C] 80 🔲

AMA: 2018,Sep,7; 2018,May,3; 2018,Jan,8; 2017,Mar,7; 2017,Feb,9; 2017,Jan,8; 2016,Jan,13; 2015,Jan,16; 2014,Jan,11

+ 22534 thoracic or lumbar, each additional vertebral segment (List separately in addition to code for primary procedure)

Code first (22532-22533)

🚑 10.5 ⚕ 10.5 **FUD** ZZZ [C] 80 🔲

AMA: 2018,Sep,7; 2018,May,3; 2017,Feb,9

22548-22634 Spinal Fusion: Anterior and Posterior Approach

EXCLUDES Corpectomy (63081-63091)
Exploration of spinal fusion (22830)
Fracture care (22310-22328)
Facet joint arthrodesis (0219T-0222T)
Injection:
Chemonucleolysis (62292)
Discography (62290-62291)
Facet joint (64490-64495, [64633], [64634], [64635], [64636])
Myelography (62284)
Laminectomy (63001-63017)
Needle/trocar biopsy (20220-20225)
Osteotomy (22206-22226)
Code also bone grafting procedures (20930-20938)
Code also spinal instrumentation (22840-22855 [22859])

22548 Arthrodesis, anterior transoral or extraoral technique, clivus-C1-C2 (atlas-axis), with or without excision of odontoid process

EXCLUDES Laminectomy or laminotomy with disc removal (63020-63042)

🚑 57.5 ⚕ 57.5 **FUD** 090 [C] 80 🔲

AMA: 2018,Sep,7; 2018,May,3; 2018,Jan,8; 2017,Mar,7; 2017,Jan,8; 2016,Jan,13; 2015,Jan,16; 2014,Jan,11

22551 Arthrodesis, anterior interbody, including disc space preparation, discectomy, osteophytectomy and decompression of spinal cord and/or nerve roots; cervical below C2

INCLUDES Operating microscope (69990)

🚑 49.6 ⚕ 49.6 **FUD** 090 [J] J8 80 🔲

AMA: 2018,Sep,7; 2018,Aug,10; 2018,May,3; 2018,Jan,8; 2017,Mar,7; 2017,Jan,8; 2016,May,13; 2016,Feb,12; 2016,Jan,13; 2015,Jan,13; 2015,Jan,16; 2014,Jan,11

Typical approach

Herniated disk

Anterior approach

+ 22552 cervical below C2, each additional interspace (List separately in addition to code for separate procedure)

INCLUDES Operating microscope (69990)
Code first (22551)

🚑 11.6 ⚕ 11.6 **FUD** ZZZ [N] N1 80 🔲

AMA: 2018,Sep,7; 2018,Aug,10; 2018,May,3; 2018,Jan,8; 2017,Mar,7; 2017,Jan,8; 2016,Feb,12; 2016,Jan,13; 2015,Jan,16; 2014,Jan,11

22554 Arthrodesis, anterior interbody technique, including minimal discectomy to prepare interspace (other than for decompression); cervical below C2

EXCLUDES Anterior discectomy and interbody fusion during the same operative session (regardless if performed by multiple surgeons) (22551)

Discectomy, anterior, with decompression of spinal cord and/or nerve root(s), cervical (even by separate individual) (63075-63076)

⚕ 36.4   ⚖ 36.4   **FUD** 090   [J] [J8] [80] 🔲

AMA: 2018,Sep,7; 2018,May,3; 2018,Jan,8; 2017,Mar,7; 2017,Jan,8; 2016,Jan,13; 2015,Apr,7; 2015,Jan,16; 2014,Jan,11

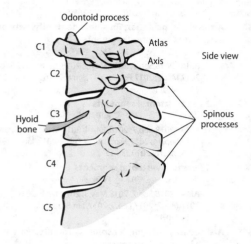

22556 thoracic

⚕ 48.5   ⚖ 48.5   **FUD** 090   [C] [80] 🔲

AMA: 2018,Sep,7; 2018,May,3; 2018,Jan,8; 2017,Mar,7; 2017,Jan,8; 2016,Jan,13; 2015,Jan,16; 2014,Jan,11

22558 lumbar

EXCLUDES Arthrodesis using pre-sacral interbody technique (22586)

⚕ 44.4   ⚖ 44.4   **FUD** 090   [C] [80] 🔲

AMA: 2018,Sep,7; 2018,May,3; 2018,Jan,8; 2017,Mar,7; 2017,Feb,9; 2017,Jan,8; 2016,Jan,13; 2015,Mar,9; 2015,Jan,16; 2014,Jan,11

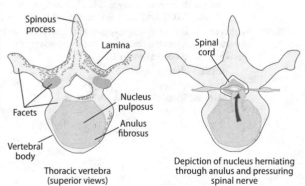

Thoracic vertebra (superior views)

Depiction of nucleus herniating through anulus and pressuring spinal nerve

+ 22585 each additional interspace (List separately in addition to code for primary procedure)

EXCLUDES Anterior discectomy and interbody fusion during the same operative session (regardless if performed by multiple surgeons) (22552)

Discectomy, anterior, with decompression of spinal cord and/or nerve root(s), cervical (even by separate individual) (63075)

Code first (22554-22558)

⚕ 9.55   ⚖ 9.55   **FUD** ZZZ   [N] [N1] [80] 🔲

AMA: 2018,Sep,7; 2018,Jan,8; 2017,Jan,8; 2016,Jan,13; 2015,Jan,16; 2014,Jan,11

22586 Arthrodesis, pre-sacral interbody technique, including disc space preparation, discectomy, with posterior instrumentation, with image guidance, includes bone graft when performed, L5-S1 interspace

INCLUDES Radiologic guidance (77002-77003, 77011-77012)

EXCLUDES Allograft and autograft of spinal bone (20930-20938)

Epidurography, radiological supervision and interpretation (72275)

Pelvic fixation, other than sacrum (22848)

Posterior non-segmental instrumentation (22840)

⚕ 59.6   ⚖ 59.6   **FUD** 090   [C] [80] 🔲

AMA: 2018,Sep,7

22590 Arthrodesis, posterior technique, craniocervical (occiput-C2)

EXCLUDES Posterior intrafacet implant insertion (0219T-0222T)

⚕ 45.9   ⚖ 45.9   **FUD** 090   [C] [80] 🔲

AMA: 2018,Sep,7; 2018,May,3; 2018,Jan,8; 2017,Mar,7; 2017,Jan,8; 2016,Jan,13; 2015,Jan,16; 2014,Jan,11

Skull and cervical vertebrae; posterior view

The physician fuses skull to C2 (axis) to stabilize cervical vertebrae; anchor holes are drilled in the occiput of the skull

22595 Arthrodesis, posterior technique, atlas-axis (C1-C2)

EXCLUDES Posterior intrafacet implant insertion (0219T-0222T)

⚕ 43.8   ⚖ 43.8   **FUD** 090   [C] [80] 🔲

AMA: 2018,Sep,7; 2018,May,3; 2018,Jan,8; 2017,Mar,7; 2017,Jan,8; 2016,Jan,13; 2015,Jan,16; 2014,Jan,11

22600 Arthrodesis, posterior or posterolateral technique, single level; cervical below C2 segment

EXCLUDES Posterior intrafacet implant insertion (0219T-0222T)

⚕ 37.4   ⚖ 37.4   **FUD** 090   [C] [80] 🔲

AMA: 2018,Sep,7; 2018,May,3; 2018,Jan,8; 2017,Mar,7; 2017,Jan,8; 2016,Jan,13; 2015,Jan,16; 2014,Jan,11

22610 thoracic (with lateral transverse technique, when performed)

EXCLUDES Posterior intrafacet implant insertion (0219T-0222T)

⚕ 36.7   ⚖ 36.7   **FUD** 090   [C] [80] 🔲

AMA: 2018,Sep,7; 2018,May,3; 2018,Jan,8; 2017,Mar,7; 2017,Jan,8; 2016,Jan,13; 2015,Jan,16; 2014,Jan,11

22612 lumbar (with lateral transverse technique, when performed)

EXCLUDES Arthrodesis performed at same interspace and segment (22630)

Combined technique at the same interspace and segment (22633)

Posterior intrafacet implant insertion (0219T-0222T)

⚕ 46.0   ⚖ 46.0   **FUD** 090   [J] [62] [80] 🔲

AMA: 2018,Sep,7; 2018,May,3; 2018,Jan,8; 2017,Mar,7; 2017,Feb,9; 2017,Jan,8; 2016,Jan,13; 2015,Jan,16; 2014,Jan,11

● New Code ▲ Revised Code ○ Reinstated ● New Web Release ▲ Revised Web Release + Add-on Unlisted Not Covered # Resequenced

⑤⓪ Optum Mod 50 Exempt ⊘ AMA Mod 51 Exempt ⑤① Optum Mod 51 Exempt ⑥③ Mod 63 Exempt ⚡ Non-FDA Drug ★ Telemedicine [M] Maternity [A] Age Edit

© 2019 Optum360, LLC   CPT © 2019 American Medical Association. All Rights Reserved.   57

+   22614   **each additional vertebral segment (List separately in addition to code for primary procedure)**

INCLUDES   Additional level fusion arthrodesis posterior or posterolateral interbody

EXCLUDES   *Additional level interbody arthrodesis combined posterolateral or posterior with posterior interbody arthrodesis (22634)*

Additional level posterior interbody arthrodesis (22632)

Posterior intrafacet implant insertion (0219T-0222T)

Code first (22600, 22610, 22612, 22630, 22633)

🚑 11.4   ⚕ 11.4   **FUD** ZZZ   N NI 80 ▭

AMA: 2018,Sep,7; 2018,Jan,8; 2017,Feb,9; 2017,Jan,8; 2016,Jan,13; 2015,Jan,16; 2014,Jan,11

22630   **Arthrodesis, posterior interbody technique, including laminectomy and/or discectomy to prepare interspace (other than for decompression), single interspace; lumbar**

EXCLUDES   *Arthrodesis performed at same interspace and segment (22612)*

Combined technique (22612 and 22630) for same interspace and segment (22633)

🚑 45.8   ⚕ 45.8   **FUD** 090   C 80 ▭

AMA: 2018,Sep,7; 2018,May,3; 2018,Jan,8; 2017,Mar,7; 2017,Feb,9; 2017,Jan,8; 2016,Jan,13; 2015,Jan,16; 2014,Jan,11

+   22632   **each additional interspace (List separately in addition to code for primary procedure)**

INCLUDES   Includes posterior interbody fusion arthrodesis, additional level

EXCLUDES   *Additional level combined technique (22634)*

Additional level posterior or posterolateral fusion (22614)

Code first (22612, 22630, 22633)

🚑 9.40   ⚕ 9.40   **FUD** ZZZ   C 80 ▭

AMA: 2018,Sep,7; 2018,Jan,8; 2017,Feb,9; 2017,Jan,8; 2016,Jan,13; 2015,Jan,16; 2014,Jan,11

22633   **Arthrodesis, combined posterior or posterolateral technique with posterior interbody technique including laminectomy and/or discectomy sufficient to prepare interspace (other than for decompression), single interspace and segment; lumbar**

EXCLUDES   *Arthrodesis performed at same interspace and segment (22612, 22630)*

🚑 53.8   ⚕ 53.8   **FUD** 090   C 80 ▭

AMA: 2018,Sep,7; 2018,Jul,14; 2018,May,9; 2018,May,3; 2018,Jan,8; 2017,Mar,7; 2017,Feb,9; 2017,Jan,8; 2016,Oct,11; 2016,Jan,13; 2015,Jan,16; 2014,Jan,11

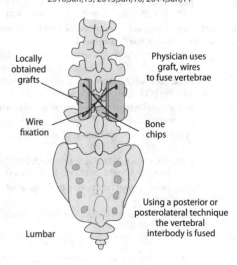

Locally obtained grafts

Physician uses graft, wires to fuse vertebrae

Wire fixation

Bone chips

Lumbar

Using a posterior or posterolateral technique the vertebral interbody is fused

+   22634   **each additional interspace and segment (List separately in addition to code for primary procedure)**

Code first (22633)

🚑 14.4   ⚕ 14.4   **FUD** ZZZ   C 80 ▭

AMA: 2018,Sep,7; 2018,Jul,14; 2018,May,3; 2018,Jan,8; 2017,Mar,7; 2017,Feb,9; 2017,Jan,8; 2016,Jan,13; 2015,Jan,16; 2014,Jan,11

22800-22819 Procedures to Correct Anomalous Spinal Vertebrae

CMS: 100-03,150.2 Osteogenic Stimulation

EXCLUDES   *Facet injection (64490-64495, [64633, 64634, 64635, 64636])*

Code also bone grafting procedures (20930-20938)

Code also spinal instrumentation (22840-22855 [22859])

22800   **Arthrodesis, posterior, for spinal deformity, with or without cast; up to 6 vertebral segments**

🚑 39.3   ⚕ 39.3   **FUD** 090   C 80 ▭

AMA: 2018,Sep,7; 2018,May,3; 2018,Jan,8; 2017,Sep,14; 2017,Mar,7; 2017,Feb,9; 2017,Jan,8; 2016,Jan,13; 2015,Jan,16; 2014,Jan,11

22802   **7 to 12 vertebral segments**

🚑 61.1   ⚕ 61.1   **FUD** 090   C 80 ▭

AMA: 2018,Sep,7; 2018,Jul,14; 2018,May,3; 2018,Jan,8; 2017,Sep,14; 2017,Mar,7; 2017,Feb,9; 2017,Jan,8; 2016,Jan,13; 2015,Jan,16; 2014,Jan,11

22804   **13 or more vertebral segments**

🚑 70.6   ⚕ 70.6   **FUD** 090   C 80 ▭

AMA: 2018,Sep,7; 2018,May,3; 2018,Jan,8; 2017,Sep,14; 2017,Mar,7; 2017,Feb,9; 2017,Jan,8; 2016,Jan,13; 2015,Jan,16; 2014,Jan,11

22808   **Arthrodesis, anterior, for spinal deformity, with or without cast; 2 to 3 vertebral segments**

INCLUDES   Smith-Robinson arthrodesis

🚑 53.7   ⚕ 53.7   **FUD** 090   C 80 ▭

AMA: 2018,Sep,7; 2018,May,3; 2018,Jan,8; 2017,Sep,14; 2017,Mar,7; 2017,Jan,8; 2016,Jan,13; 2015,Jan,16; 2014,Jan,11

22810   **4 to 7 vertebral segments**

🚑 60.2   ⚕ 60.2   **FUD** 090   C 80 ▭

AMA: 2018,Sep,7; 2018,May,3; 2018,Jan,8; 2017,Sep,14; 2017,Mar,7; 2017,Jan,8; 2016,Jan,13; 2015,Jan,16; 2014,Jan,11

22812   **8 or more vertebral segments**

🚑 64.0   ⚕ 64.0   **FUD** 090   C 80 ▭

AMA: 2018,Sep,7; 2018,May,3; 2018,Jan,8; 2017,Sep,14; 2017,Mar,7; 2017,Jan,8; 2016,Jan,13; 2015,Jan,16; 2014,Jan,11

22818   **Kyphectomy, circumferential exposure of spine and resection of vertebral segment(s) (including body and posterior elements); single or 2 segments**

EXCLUDES   *Arthrodesis (22800-22804)*

🚑 62.8   ⚕ 62.8   **FUD** 090   C 80 ▭

AMA: 2018,Sep,7; 2018,Jan,8; 2017,Sep,14

22819   3 or more segments
EXCLUDES Arthrodesis (22800-22804)

🔲 72.2 👤 72.2 **FUD** 090   C 80 ▢

AMA: 2018,Sep,7; 2018,Jan,8; 2017,Sep,14

Excessively kyphotic thoracic spine may be caused by Scheuermann's disease or juvenile kyphosis

Excessive convexity in the thoracic region is known as kyphosis

Excessive concavity in the lumbar region is known as lordosis

Scoliosis is the lateral curvature of the spine; most commonly diagnosed during adolescence; occurrence is higher among females

22830 Surgical Exploration Previous Spinal Fusion

CMS: 100-03,150.2 Osteogenic Stimulation

EXCLUDES Arthrodesis (22532-22819)
Bone grafting procedures (20930-20938)
Facet injection (64490-64495, [64633, 64634, 64635, 64636])
Instrumentation removal (22850, 22852, 22855)
Spinal decompression (63001-63103)
Code also spinal instrumentation (22840-22855 [22859])

22830   Exploration of spinal fusion
🔲 23.6 👤 23.6 **FUD** 090   C 80 ▢

AMA: 2018,Sep,7; 2018,Jan,8; 2017,Jan,8; 2016,Jan,13; 2015,Jan,16; 2014,Jan,11

22840-22848 Posterior, Anterior, Pelvic Spinal Instrumentation

INCLUDES Removal or revision of previously placed spinal instrumentation during same session as insertion of new instrumentation at levels including all or part of previously instrumented segments (22849, 22850, 22852, 22855)

EXCLUDES Arthrodesis (22532-22534, 22548-22812)
Bone grafting procedures (20930-20938)
Exploration of spinal fusion (22830)
Fracture treatment (22325-22328)
Use of more than one instrumentation code per incision

+ **22840** Posterior non-segmental instrumentation (eg, Harrington rod technique, pedicle fixation across 1 interspace, atlantoaxial transarticular screw fixation, sublaminar wiring at C1, facet screw fixation) (List separately in addition to code for primary procedure)
Code first (22100-22102, 22110-22114, 22206-22207, 22210-22214, 22220-22224, 22310-22327, 22532-22533, 22548-22558, 22590-22612, 22630, 22633-22634, 22800-22812, 63001-63030, 63040-63042, 63045-63047, 63050-63056, 63064, 63075, 63077, 63081, 63085, 63087, 63090, 63101-63102, 63170-63290, 63300-63307)
🔲 22.2 👤 22.2 **FUD** ZZZ   N N1 80 ▢

AMA: 2018,Sep,7; 2018,Jan,8; 2017,Jun,10; 2017,Feb,9; 2017,Jan,8; 2016,Jan,13; 2015,Jan,16; 2014,Oct,14; 2014,Jan,11

+ **22841** Internal spinal fixation by wiring of spinous processes (List separately in addition to code for primary procedure)
Code first (22100-22102, 22110-22114, 22206-22207, 22210-22214, 22220-22224, 22310-22327, 22532-22533, 22548-22558, 22590-22612, 22630, 22633-22634, 22800-22812, 63001-63030, 63040-63042, 63045-63047, 63050-63056, 63064, 63075, 63077, 63081, 63085, 63087, 63090, 63101-63102, 63170-63290, 63300-63307)
🔲 0.00 👤 0.00 **FUD** XXX   C ▢

AMA: 2018,Sep,7; 2018,Jan,8; 2017,Feb,9; 2017,Jan,8; 2016,Jan,13; 2015,Jan,16; 2014,Jan,11

+ **22842** Posterior segmental instrumentation (eg, pedicle fixation, dual rods with multiple hooks and sublaminar wires); 3 to 6 vertebral segments (List separately in addition to code for primary procedure)
Code first (22100-22102, 22110-22114, 22206-22207, 22210-22214, 22220-22224, 22310-22327, 22532-22533, 22548-22558, 22590-22612, 22630, 22633-22634, 22800-22812, 63001-63030, 63040-63042, 63045-63047, 63050-63056, 63064, 63075, 63077, 63081, 63085, 63087, 63090, 63101-63102, 63170-63290, 63300-63307)
🔲 22.3 👤 22.3 **FUD** ZZZ   N N1 80 ▢

AMA: 2018,Sep,7; 2018,Jan,8; 2017,Feb,9; 2017,Jan,8; 2016,Jan,13; 2015,Jan,16; 2014,Jan,11

Example of rod hook; may be attached at top and bottom only, or also at segments

Rod

Segment

+ **22843** 7 to 12 vertebral segments (List separately in addition to code for primary procedure)
Code first (22100-22102, 22110-22114, 22206-22207, 22210-22214, 22220-22224, 22310-22327, 22532-22533, 22548-22558, 22590-22612, 22630, 22633-22634, 22800-22812, 63001-63030, 63040-63042, 63045-63047, 63050-63056, 63064, 63075, 63077, 63081, 63085, 63087, 63090, 63101-63102, 63170-63290, 63300-63307)
🔲 23.8 👤 23.8 **FUD** ZZZ   C 80 ▢

AMA: 2018,Sep,7; 2018,Jul,14; 2018,Jan,8; 2017,Jan,8; 2016,Jan,13; 2015,Jan,16; 2014,Jan,11

+ **22844** 13 or more vertebral segments (List separately in addition to code for primary procedure)
Code first (22100-22102, 22110-22114, 22206-22207, 22210-22214, 22220-22224, 22310-22327, 22532-22533, 22548-22558, 22590-22612, 22630, 22633-22634, 22800-22812, 63001-63030, 63040-63042, 63045-63047, 63050-63056, 63064, 63075, 63077, 63081, 63085, 63087, 63090, 63101-63102, 63170-63290, 63300-63307)
🔲 28.8 👤 28.8 **FUD** ZZZ   C 80 ▢

AMA: 2018,Sep,7; 2018,Jan,8; 2017,Jan,8; 2016,Jan,13; 2015,Jan,16; 2014,Jan,11

+ **22845** Anterior instrumentation; 2 to 3 vertebral segments (List separately in addition to code for primary procedure)
INCLUDES Dwyer instrumentation technique
Code first (22100-22102, 22110-22114, 22206-22207, 22210-22214, 22220-22224, 22310-22327, 22532-22533, 22548-22558, 22590-22612, 22630, 22633-22634, 22800-22812, 63001-63030, 63040-63042, 63045-63047, 63050-63056, 63064, 63075, 63077, 63081, 63085, 63087, 63090, 63101-63102, 63170-63290, 63300-63307)
🔲 21.3 👤 21.3 **FUD** ZZZ   N N1 80 ▢

AMA: 2018,Sep,7; 2018,Jan,8; 2017,Mar,7; 2017,Jan,8; 2016,May,13; 2016,Jan,13; 2015,Apr,7; 2015,Mar,9; 2015,Jan,16; 2015,Jan,13; 2014,Nov,14; 2014,Jan,11

+ 22846   4 to 7 vertebral segments (List separately in addition to code for primary procedure)

> INCLUDES   Dwyer instrumentation technique
>
> Code first (22100-22102, 22110-22114, 22206-22207, 22210-22214, 22220-22224, 22310-22327, 22532-22533, 22548-22558, 22590-22612, 22630, 22633-22634, 22800-22812, 63001-63030, 63040-63042, 63045-63047, 63050-63056, 63064, 63075, 63077, 63081, 63085, 63087, 63090, 63101-63102, 63170-63290, 63300-63307)
>
> 🏥 22.1   ⚕ 22.1   **FUD** ZZZ   C 80 ▢

AMA: 2018,Sep,7; 2018,Jan,8; 2017,Jan,8; 2016,May,13; 2016,Jan,13; 2015,Jan,16; 2014,Jan,11

+ 22847   8 or more vertebral segments (List separately in addition to code for primary procedure)

> INCLUDES   Dwyer instrumentation technique
>
> Code first (22100-22102, 22110-22114, 22206-22207, 22210-22214, 22220-22224, 22310-22327, 22532-22533, 22548-22558, 22590-22612, 22630, 22633-22634, 22800-22812, 63001-63030, 63040-63042, 63045-63047, 63050-63056, 63064, 63075, 63077, 63081, 63085, 63087, 63090, 63101-63102, 63170-63290, 63300-63307)
>
> 🏥 23.5   ⚕ 23.5   **FUD** ZZZ   C 80 ▢

AMA: 2018,Sep,7; 2018,Jan,8; 2017,Jan,8; 2016,May,13; 2016,Jan,13; 2015,Jan,16; 2014,Jan,11

+ 22848   Pelvic fixation (attachment of caudal end of instrumentation to pelvic bony structures) other than sacrum (List separately in addition to code for primary procedure)

> Code first (22100-22102, 22110-22114, 22206-22207, 22210-22214, 22220-22224, 22310-22327, 22532-22533, 22548-22558, 22590-22612, 22630, 22633-22634, 22800-22812, 63001-63030, 63040-63042, 63045-63047, 63050-63056, 63064, 63075, 63077, 63081, 63085, 63087, 63090, 63101-63102, 63170-63290, 63300-63307)
>
> 🏥 10.5   ⚕ 10.5   **FUD** ZZZ   C 80 ▢

AMA: 2018,Sep,7; 2018,Jan,8; 2017,Jan,8; 2016,Jan,13; 2015,Jan,16; 2014,Jan,11

22849-22855 [22859] Miscellaneous Spinal Instrumentation

> EXCLUDES   Arthrodesis (22532-22534, 22548-22812)
> Bone grafting procedures (20930-20938)
> Exploration of spinal fusion (22830)
> Facet injection (64490-64495, [64633], [64634], [64635], [64636])
> Fracture treatment (22325-22328)

22849   Reinsertion of spinal fixation device

> INCLUDES   Removal of instrumentation at the same level (22850, 22852, 22855)
>
> 🏥 37.7   ⚕ 37.7   **FUD** 090   C 80 ▢

AMA: 2018,Sep,7; 2018,Jan,8; 2017,Jun,10; 2017,Jan,8; 2016,May,13; 2016,Jan,13; 2015,Jan,16; 2014,Jan,11

22850   Removal of posterior nonsegmental instrumentation (eg, Harrington rod)

> 🏥 21.0   ⚕ 21.0   **FUD** 090   C 80 ▢

AMA: 2018,Sep,7; 2018,Jan,8; 2017,Jun,10; 2017,Jan,8; 2016,May,13; 2016,Jan,13; 2015,Jan,16; 2014,Jan,11

22852   Removal of posterior segmental instrumentation

> 🏥 20.2   ⚕ 20.2   **FUD** 090   C 80 ▢

AMA: 2018,Sep,7; 2018,Jan,8; 2017,Jun,10; 2017,Jan,8; 2016,Jan,13; 2015,Jan,16; 2014,Jan,11

+ 22853   Insertion of interbody biomechanical device(s) (eg, synthetic cage, mesh) with integral anterior instrumentation for device anchoring (eg, screws, flanges), when performed, to intervertebral disc space in conjunction with interbody arthrodesis, each interspace (List separately in addition to code for primary procedure)

> Code also intervertebral bone device/graft application (20930-20931, 20936-20938)
> Code also subsequent disc spaces undergoing device insertion when disc spaces are not connected (22853-22854, [22859])
> Code first (22100-22102, 22110-22114, 22206-22207, 22210-22214, 22220-22224, 22310-22327, 22532-22533, 22548-22558, 22590-22612, 22630, 22633-22634, 22800-22812, 63001-63030, 63040, 63042, 63045-63047, 63050-63056, 63064, 63075, 63077, 63081, 63085, 63087, 63090, 63101-63102, 63170-63290, 63300-63307)
>
> 🏥 7.55   ⚕ 7.55   **FUD** ZZZ   N N1 80 ▢

AMA: 2018,Sep,7; 2018,Jul,14; 2018,Jan,8; 2017,Aug,9; 2017,Mar,7

+ 22854   Insertion of intervertebral biomechanical device(s) (eg, synthetic cage, mesh) with integral anterior instrumentation for device anchoring (eg, screws, flanges), when performed, to vertebral corpectomy(ies) (vertebral body resection, partial or complete) defect, in conjunction with interbody arthrodesis, each contiguous defect (List separately in addition to code for primary procedure)

> Code also intervertebral bone device/graft application (20930-20931, 20936-20938)
> Code also subsequent disc spaces undergoing device insertion when disc spaces are not connected (22853-22854, [22859])
> Code first (22100-22102, 22110-22114, 22206-22207, 22210-22214, 22220-22224, 22310-22327, 22532-22533, 22548-22558, 22590-22612, 22630, 22633-22634, 22800-22812, 63001-63030, 63040, 63042, 63045-63047, 63050-63056, 63064, 63075, 63077, 63081, 63085, 63087, 63090, 63101-63102, 63170-63290, 63300-63307)
>
> 🏥 9.78   ⚕ 9.78   **FUD** ZZZ   N N1 80 ▢

AMA: 2018,Sep,7; 2018,Jan,8; 2017,Mar,7

+ # 22859   Insertion of intervertebral biomechanical device(s) (eg, synthetic cage, mesh, methylmethacrylate) to intervertebral disc space or vertebral body defect without interbody arthrodesis, each contiguous defect (List separately in addition to code for primary procedure)

> Code also intervertebral bone device/graft application (20930-20931, 20936-20938)
> Code also subsequent disc spaces undergoing device insertion when disc spaces are not connected (22853-22854, 22854)
> Code first (22100-22102, 22110-22114, 22206-22207, 22210-22214, 22220-22224, 22310-22327, 22532-22533, 22548-22558, 22590-22612, 22630, 22633-22634, 22800-22812, 63001-63030, 63040-63042, 63045-63047, 63050-63056, 63064, 63075, 63077, 63081, 63085, 63087, 63090, 63101-63102, 63170-63290, 63300-63307)
>
> 🏥 9.78   ⚕ 9.78   **FUD** ZZZ   N N1 80 ▢

AMA: 2018,Sep,7; 2018,Jan,8; 2017,Mar,7

22855   Removal of anterior instrumentation

> 🏥 32.1   ⚕ 32.1   **FUD** 090   C 80 ▢

AMA: 2018,Sep,7; 2018,Jan,8; 2017,Jun,10; 2017,Jan,8; 2016,Jan,13; 2015,Jan,16; 2014,Jan,11

22856-22865 [22858] Artificial Disc Replacement

EXCLUDES Fluoroscopy
Spinal decompression (63001-63048)

22856 Total disc arthroplasty (artificial disc), anterior approach, including discectomy with end plate preparation (includes osteophytectomy for nerve root or spinal cord decompression and microdissection); single interspace, cervical

INCLUDES Operating microscope (69990)

EXCLUDES Application of intervertebral biomechanical device(s) at the same level (22853-22854, [22859])
Arthrodesis at the same level (22554)
Discectomy at the same level (63075)
Insertion of instrumentation at the same level (22845)
Code also arthroplasty more than one interspace, when performed ([22858])

🚑 47.6 ⚕ 47.6 **FUD** 090 J J8 80 ▢

AMA: 2018,Sep,7; 2018,Jan,8; 2017,Jan,8; 2016,Feb,12; 2016,Jan,13; 2015,Apr,7

+ # 22858 second level, cervical (List separately in addition to code for primary procedure)

Code first (22856)

🚑 14.9 ⚕ 14.9 **FUD** ZZZ N N1 80 ▢

AMA: 2018,Sep,7; 2018,Jan,8; 2017,Jan,8; 2016,Feb,12; 2016,Jan,13; 2015,Apr,7

22857 Total disc arthroplasty (artificial disc), anterior approach, including discectomy to prepare interspace (other than for decompression), single interspace, lumbar

INCLUDES Operating microscope (69990)

EXCLUDES Application of intervertebral biomechanical device(s) at the same level (22853-22854, [22859])
Arthrodesis at the same level (22558)
Insertion of instrumentation at the same level (22845)
Retroperitoneal exploration (49010)
Code also arthroplasty more than one interspace, when performed (0163T)

🚑 51.4 ⚕ 51.4 **FUD** 090 C 80 ▢

AMA: 2018,Sep,7; 2016,Feb,12

22858 Resequenced code. See code following 22856.

22859 Resequenced code. See code following 22854.

22861 Revision including replacement of total disc arthroplasty (artificial disc), anterior approach, single interspace; cervical

INCLUDES Operating microscope (69990)

EXCLUDES Procedures performed at the same level (22845, 22853-22854, [22859], 22864, 63075)
Revision of additional cervical arthroplasty (0098T)

🚑 68.4 ⚕ 68.4 **FUD** 090 C 80 ▢

AMA: 2018,Sep,7; 2016,Feb,12

22862 lumbar

EXCLUDES Arthroplasty revision more than one interspace (0165T)
Procedures performed at the same level (22558, 22845, 22853-22854, [22859], 22865, 49010)

🚑 54.9 ⚕ 54.9 **FUD** 090 C 80 ▢

AMA: 2018,Sep,7; 2018,Jan,8; 2017,Jan,8; 2016,Jan,13; 2015,Jan,16; 2014,Jan,11

22864 Removal of total disc arthroplasty (artificial disc), anterior approach, single interspace; cervical

INCLUDES Operating microscope (69990)

EXCLUDES Cervical total disc arthroplasty with additional interspace removal (0095T)
Revision of total disc arthroplasty (22861)

🚑 60.9 ⚕ 60.9 **FUD** 090 C 80 ▢

AMA: 2018,Sep,7

22865 lumbar

EXCLUDES Arthroplasty more than one level (0164T)
Exploration, retroperitoneal area with or without biopsy(s) (49010)

🚑 57.2 ⚕ 57.2 **FUD** 090 C 80 ▢

AMA: 2018,Sep,7; 2018,Jan,8; 2017,Jan,8; 2016,Jan,13; 2015,Jan,16; 2014,Jan,11

22867-22899 Spinal Distraction/Stabilization Device

22867 Insertion of interlaminar/interspinous process stabilization/distraction device, without fusion, including image guidance when performed, with open decompression, lumbar; single level

EXCLUDES Interlaminar/interspinous stabilization/distraction device insertion (22869, 22870)
Procedures at the same level (22532-22534, 22558, 22612, 22614, 22630, 22632-22634, 22800, 22802, 22804, 22840-22842, 22869-22870, 63005, 63012, 63017, 63030, 63035, 63042, 63044, 63047-63048, 77003)

🚑 28.2 ⚕ 28.2 **FUD** 090 J J8 80 ▢

AMA: 2018,Sep,7; 2018,Jan,8; 2017,Feb,9

+ 22868 second level (List separately in addition to code for primary procedure)

EXCLUDES Interlaminar/interspinous stabilization/distraction device insertion (22869-22870)
Procedures at the same level (22532-22534, 22558, 22612, 22614, 22630, 22632-22634, 22800, 22802, 22804, 22840-22842, 22869-22870, 63005, 63012, 63017, 63030, 63035, 63042, 63044, 63047-63048, 77003)

Code first (22867)

🚑 7.06 ⚕ 7.06 **FUD** ZZZ N N1 80 ▢

AMA: 2018,Sep,7; 2018,Jan,8; 2017,Feb,9

22869 Insertion of interlaminar/interspinous process stabilization/distraction device, without open decompression or fusion, including image guidance when performed, lumbar; single level

🚑 13.2 ⚕ 13.2 **FUD** 090 J J8 80 ▢

AMA: 2018,Sep,7; 2018,Jan,8; 2017,Feb,9

+ 22870 second level (List separately in addition to code for primary procedure)

EXCLUDES Procedures at the same level (22532-22534, 22558, 22612, 22614, 22630, 22632-22634, 22800, 22802, 22804, 22840-22842, 63005, 63012, 63017, 63030, 63035, 63042, 63044, 63047-63048, 77003)

Code first (22869)

🚑 3.96 ⚕ 3.96 **FUD** ZZZ N N1 80 ▢

AMA: 2018,Sep,7; 2018,Jan,8; 2017,Feb,9

22899 Unlisted procedure, spine

🚑 0.00 ⚕ 0.00 **FUD** YYY T 80 ▢

AMA: 2018,Sep,7; 2018,May,10; 2018,Jan,8; 2017,Feb,9; 2017,Jan,8; 2016,Jan,13; 2015,Jan,8; 2015,Jan,16; 2014,Oct,14; 2014,Jan,11

22900-22999 Musculoskeletal Procedures of Abdomen

INCLUDES
Any necessary elevation of tissue planes or dissection
Measurement of tumor and necessary margin at greatest diameter prior to excision
Simple and intermediate repairs
Types of excision:
  Fascial or subfascial soft tissue tumors: simple and marginal resection of tumors found either in or below the deep fascia, not involving bone or excision of a substantial amount of normal tissue; primarily benign and intramuscular tumors
  Radical resection soft tissue tumor: wide resection of tumor involving substantial margins of normal tissue and may include tissue removal from one or more layers; most often malignant or aggressive benign
  Subcutaneous: simple and marginal resection of tumors in the subcutaneous tissue above the deep fascia; most often benign

EXCLUDES
Complex repair
Excision of benign cutaneous lesions (eg, sebaceous cyst) (11400-11406)
Radical resection of cutaneous tumors (eg, melanoma) (11600-11606)
Significant exploration of the vessels or neuroplasty

22900 Excision, tumor, soft tissue of abdominal wall, subfascial (eg, intramuscular); less than 5 cm
🔲 16.2   ⚕ 16.2   **FUD** 090   J G2 80 🔲
AMA: 2018,Sep,7

22901 5 cm or greater
🔲 19.2   ⚕ 19.2   **FUD** 090   J G2 80 🔲
AMA: 2018,Sep,7

22902 Excision, tumor, soft tissue of abdominal wall, subcutaneous; less than 3 cm
🔲 9.53   ⚕ 12.8   **FUD** 090   J G2 80 🔲
AMA: 2018,Sep,7

22903 3 cm or greater
🔲 12.6   ⚕ 12.6   **FUD** 090   J G2 80 🔲
AMA: 2018,Sep,7

22904 Radical resection of tumor (eg, sarcoma), soft tissue of abdominal wall; less than 5 cm
🔲 30.4   ⚕ 30.4   **FUD** 090   J G2 80 🔲
AMA: 2018,Sep,7

22905 5 cm or greater
🔲 38.5   ⚕ 38.5   **FUD** 090   J G2 80 🔲
AMA: 2018,Sep,7

22999 Unlisted procedure, abdomen, musculoskeletal system
🔲 0.00   ⚕ 0.00   **FUD** YYY   T 80 🔲
AMA: 2018,Sep,7

23000-23044 Surgical Incision Shoulder: Drainage, Foreign Body Removal, Contracture Release

23000 Removal of subdeltoid calcareous deposits, open
EXCLUDES Arthroscopic removal calcium deposits of bursa (29999)
🔲 10.3   ⚕ 16.0   **FUD** 090   J A2 80 50 🔲
AMA: 2018,Sep,7

23020 Capsular contracture release (eg, Sever type procedure)
EXCLUDES Simple incision and drainage (10040-10160)
🔲 19.8   ⚕ 19.8   **FUD** 090   J A2 80 50 🔲
AMA: 2018,Sep,7

23030 Incision and drainage, shoulder area; deep abscess or hematoma
🔲 7.20   ⚕ 12.4   **FUD** 010   J A2 🔲
AMA: 2018,Sep,7

23031 infected bursa
🔲 5.99   ⚕ 11.4   **FUD** 010   J A2 50 🔲
AMA: 2018,Sep,7

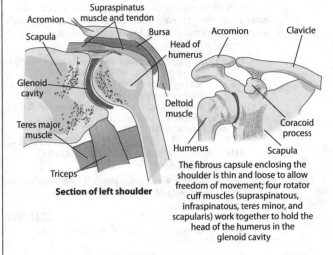

Section of left shoulder

Labels: Supraspinatus muscle and tendon; Acromion; Scapula; Bursa; Head of humerus; Glenoid cavity; Deltoid muscle; Teres major muscle; Humerus; Triceps; Acromion; Clavicle; Coracoid process; Scapula

The fibrous capsule enclosing the shoulder is thin and loose to allow freedom of movement; four rotator cuff muscles (supraspinatous, infraspinatous, teres minor, and scapularis) work together to hold the head of the humerus in the glenoid cavity

23035 Incision, bone cortex (eg, osteomyelitis or bone abscess), shoulder area
🔲 19.4   ⚕ 19.4   **FUD** 090   J A2 80 50 🔲
AMA: 2018,Sep,7

23040 Arthrotomy, glenohumeral joint, including exploration, drainage, or removal of foreign body
🔲 20.6   ⚕ 20.6   **FUD** 090   J A2 80 50 🔲
AMA: 2018,Sep,7

23044 Arthrotomy, acromioclavicular, sternoclavicular joint, including exploration, drainage, or removal of foreign body
🔲 16.3   ⚕ 16.3   **FUD** 090   J A2 50 🔲
AMA: 2018,Sep,7

23065-23066 Shoulder Biopsy

EXCLUDES Soft tissue needle biopsy (20206)

23065 Biopsy, soft tissue of shoulder area; superficial
🔲 4.81   ⚕ 6.34   **FUD** 010   J P3 50 🔲
AMA: 2018,Sep,7

23066 deep
🔲 10.4   ⚕ 16.1   **FUD** 090   J A2 50 🔲
AMA: 2018,Sep,7

23071-23078 [23071, 23073] Excision Soft Tissue Tumors of Shoulder

INCLUDES
Any necessary elevation of tissue planes or dissection
Measurement of tumor and necessary margin at greatest diameter prior to excision
Simple and intermediate repairs
Types of excision:
  Fascial or subfascial soft tissue tumors: simple and marginal resection of tumors found either in or below the deep fascia, not involving bone or excision of a substantial amount of normal tissue; primarily benign and intramuscular tumors
  Radical resection soft tissue tumor: wide resection of tumor, involving substantial margins of normal tissue and may involve tissue removal from one or more layers; most often malignant or aggressive benign
  Subcutaneous: simple and marginal resection of tumors in the subcutaneous tissue above the deep fascia; most often benign

EXCLUDES
Complex repair
Excision of benign cutaneous lesions (eg, sebaceous cyst) (11400-11406)
Radical resection of cutaneous tumors (eg, melanoma) (11600-11606)
Significant exploration of the vessels or neuroplasty

23071 Resequenced code. See code following 23075.

23073 Resequenced code. See code following 23076.

23075 Excision, tumor, soft tissue of shoulder area, subcutaneous; less than 3 cm
9.41 13.9 **FUD** 090   J G2 50
AMA: 2018,Sep,7; 2018,Jan,8; 2017,Jan,8; 2016,Jan,13; 2015,Jan,16; 2014,Jan,11

\# **23071** 3 cm or greater
12.0 12.0 **FUD** 090   J G2 80 50
AMA: 2018,Sep,7

23076 Excision, tumor, soft tissue of shoulder area, subfascial (eg, intramuscular); less than 5 cm
15.6 15.6 **FUD** 090   J G2 50
AMA: 2018,Sep,7; 2018,Jan,8; 2017,Jan,8; 2016,Jan,13; 2015,Jan,16; 2014,Jan,11

\# **23073** 5 cm or greater
20.0 20.0 **FUD** 090   J G2 50
AMA: 2018,Sep,7

23077 Radical resection of tumor (eg, sarcoma), soft tissue of shoulder area; less than 5 cm
32.8 32.8 **FUD** 090   J G2 80 50
AMA: 2018,Sep,7

23078 5 cm or greater
41.4 41.4 **FUD** 090   J G2 80 50
AMA: 2018,Sep,7

23100-23195 Bone and Joint Procedures of Shoulder

INCLUDES Acromioclavicular joint
Clavicle
Head and neck of humerus
Scapula
Shoulder joint
Sternoclavicular joint

23100 Arthrotomy, glenohumeral joint, including biopsy
14.4 14.4 **FUD** 090   J A2 80 50
AMA: 2018,Sep,7

23101 Arthrotomy, acromioclavicular joint or sternoclavicular joint, including biopsy and/or excision of torn cartilage
13.1 13.1 **FUD** 090   J A2 50
AMA: 2018,Sep,7

23105 Arthrotomy; glenohumeral joint, with synovectomy, with or without biopsy
18.3 18.3 **FUD** 090   J A2 80 50
AMA: 2018,Sep,7

23106 sternoclavicular joint, with synovectomy, with or without biopsy
14.3 14.3 **FUD** 090   J A2 50
AMA: 2018,Sep,7

23107 Arthrotomy, glenohumeral joint, with joint exploration, with or without removal of loose or foreign body
19.0 19.0 **FUD** 090   J A2 80 50
AMA: 2018,Sep,7

23120 Claviculectomy; partial
INCLUDES Mumford operation
EXCLUDES Arthroscopic claviculectomy (29824)
16.8 16.8 **FUD** 090   J A2 80 50
AMA: 2018,Sep,7; 2018,Jan,8; 2017,Jan,8; 2016,Jan,13; 2015,Jan,16; 2014,Jan,11

23125 total
20.4 20.4 **FUD** 090   J A2 80 50
AMA: 2018,Sep,7

23130 Acromioplasty or acromionectomy, partial, with or without coracoacromial ligament release
17.6 17.6 **FUD** 090   J A2 50
AMA: 2018,Sep,7; 2018,Jan,8; 2017,Jan,8; 2016,Jan,13; 2015,Mar,7; 2015,Feb,10; 2015,Jan,16; 2014,Jan,11

23140 Excision or curettage of bone cyst or benign tumor of clavicle or scapula;
15.9 15.9 **FUD** 090   J A2 50
AMA: 2018,Sep,7

23145 with autograft (includes obtaining graft)
20.0 20.0 **FUD** 090   J A2 80 50
AMA: 2018,Sep,7

23146 with allograft
17.9 17.9 **FUD** 090   J A2 80 50
AMA: 2019,May,7; 2018,Sep,7

23150 Excision or curettage of bone cyst or benign tumor of proximal humerus;
18.9 18.9 **FUD** 090   J A2 80 50
AMA: 2018,Sep,7

23155 with autograft (includes obtaining graft)
22.9 22.9 **FUD** 090   J A2 80 50
AMA: 2018,Sep,7

23156 with allograft
19.4 19.4 **FUD** 090   J A2 80 50
AMA: 2019,May,7; 2018,Sep,7

23170 Sequestrectomy (eg, for osteomyelitis or bone abscess), clavicle
16.1 16.1 **FUD** 090   J A2 50
AMA: 2018,Sep,7

23172 Sequestrectomy (eg, for osteomyelitis or bone abscess), scapula
16.3 16.3 **FUD** 090   J A2 80 50
AMA: 2018,Sep,7

23174 Sequestrectomy (eg, for osteomyelitis or bone abscess), humeral head to surgical neck
21.9 21.9 **FUD** 090   J A2 80 50
AMA: 2018,Sep,7

23180 Partial excision (craterization, saucerization, or diaphysectomy) bone (eg, osteomyelitis), clavicle
18.9 18.9 **FUD** 090   J A2 50
AMA: 2018,Sep,7

23182 Partial excision (craterization, saucerization, or diaphysectomy) bone (eg, osteomyelitis), scapula
18.9 18.9 **FUD** 090   J A2 80 50
AMA: 2018,Sep,7

23184 Partial excision (craterization, saucerization, or diaphysectomy) bone (eg, osteomyelitis), proximal humerus
21.1 21.1 **FUD** 090   J A2 80 50
AMA: 2018,Sep,7

23190 Ostectomy of scapula, partial (eg, superior medial angle)
16.5 16.5 **FUD** 090   J A2 80 50
AMA: 2018,Sep,7

23195 Resection, humeral head
EXCLUDES Arthroplasty with replacement with implant (23470)
21.4 21.4 **FUD** 090   J A2 80 50
AMA: 2018,Sep,7

23200-23220 Radical Resection of Bone Tumors of Shoulder

INCLUDES Any necessary elevation of tissue planes or dissection
Excision of adjacent soft tissue during bone tumor resection (23071-23078 [23071, 23073])
Measurement of tumor and necessary margin at greatest diameter prior to excision
Radical resection of cutaneous tumors (e.g., melanoma)
Resection of the tumor (may include entire bone) and wide margins of normal tissues primarily for malignant or aggressive benign tumors
Simple and intermediate repairs
EXCLUDES Complex repair
Significant exploration of vessels, neuroplasty, reconstruction, or complex bone repair

23200 Radical resection of tumor; clavicle
43.7 43.7 **FUD** 090   C 80 50
AMA: 2019,May,7; 2018,Sep,7

23210 scapula
51.4 51.4 **FUD** 090   C 80 50
AMA: 2019,May,7; 2018,Sep,7

● New Code   ▲ Revised Code   ○ Reinstated   ● New Web Release   ▲ Revised Web Release   + Add-on   Unlisted   Not Covered   # Resequenced
50 Optum Mod 50 Exempt   AMA Mod 51 Exempt   51 Optum Mod 51 Exempt   63 Mod 63 Exempt   Non-FDA Drug   ★ Telemedicine   M Maternity   A Age Edit

Musculoskeletal System

23220 — 23472

23220   **Radical resection of tumor, proximal humerus**
     56.3   56.3   **FUD** 090   C 80 50
     AMA: 2019,May,7; 2018,Sep,7

23330-23335 Removal Implant/Foreign Body from Shoulder

EXCLUDES   Bursal arthrocentesis or needling (20610)
               K-wire or pin insertion (20650)
               K-wire or pin removal (20670, 20680)

23330   **Removal of foreign body, shoulder; subcutaneous**
     4.79   8.03   **FUD** 010   T A2 80 50
     AMA: 2018,Sep,7; 2018,Jan,8; 2017,Jan,8; 2016,Jan,13; 2015,Jan,16; 2014,Mar,4; 2014,Jan,11

23333   **deep (subfascial or intramuscular)**
     13.2   13.2   **FUD** 090   J G2 80 50
     AMA: 2018,Sep,7; 2018,Jan,8; 2017,Jan,8; 2016,Jan,13; 2015,Jan,16; 2014,Mar,4

23334   **Removal of prosthesis, includes debridement and synovectomy when performed; humeral or glenoid component**
         EXCLUDES   Foreign body removal (23330, 23333)
                  Prosthesis removal and replacement in same shoulder (eg, glenoid and/or humeral components) (23473-23474)
     30.8   30.8   **FUD** 090   J G2 50
     AMA: 2018,Sep,7; 2018,Jan,8; 2017,Jan,8; 2016,Jan,13; 2015,Jan,16; 2014,Mar,4

23335   **humeral and glenoid components (eg, total shoulder)**
         EXCLUDES   Foreign body removal (23330, 23333)
                  Prosthesis removal and replacement in same shoulder (eg, glenoid and/or humeral components) (23473-23474)
     36.8   36.8   **FUD** 090   C 50
     AMA: 2018,Sep,7; 2018,Jan,8; 2017,Jan,8; 2016,Jan,13; 2015,Jan,16; 2014,Mar,4

23350 Injection for Shoulder Arthrogram

23350   **Injection procedure for shoulder arthrography or enhanced CT/MRI shoulder arthrography**
         EXCLUDES   Shoulder biopsy (29805-29826)
         (73040, 73201-73202, 73222-73223, 77002)
     1.47   3.97   **FUD** 000   N N1 50
     AMA: 2018,Sep,7; 2018,Jan,8; 2017,Jan,8; 2016,May,13; 2016,Jan,13; 2015,Aug,6; 2015,Jan,16; 2014,Jan,11

23395-23491 Repair/Reconstruction of Shoulder

23395   **Muscle transfer, any type, shoulder or upper arm; single**
     36.9   36.9   **FUD** 090   J A2 80
     AMA: 2018,Sep,7

23397   **multiple**
     32.6   32.6   **FUD** 090   J A2 80
     AMA: 2018,Sep,7

23400   **Scapulopexy (eg, Sprengels deformity or for paralysis)**
     28.0   28.0   **FUD** 090   J A2 80 50
     AMA: 2018,Sep,7

23405   **Tenotomy, shoulder area; single tendon**
     17.7   17.7   **FUD** 090   J A2 80
     AMA: 2018,Sep,7

23406   **multiple tendons through same incision**
     22.2   22.2   **FUD** 090   J A2 80
     AMA: 2018,Sep,7

23410   **Repair of ruptured musculotendinous cuff (eg, rotator cuff) open; acute**
         EXCLUDES   Arthroscopic repair (29827)
     23.6   23.6   **FUD** 090   J A2 80 50
     AMA: 2018,Sep,7; 2018,Jan,8; 2017,Jan,8; 2016,Jan,13; 2015,Jan,16; 2014,Jan,11

23412   **chronic**
         EXCLUDES   Arthroscopic repair (29827)
     24.5   24.5   **FUD** 090   J A2 80 50
     AMA: 2018,Sep,7; 2018,Jan,8; 2017,Jan,8; 2016,Jan,13; 2015,Jun,10; 2015,Feb,10; 2015,Jan,16; 2014,Jan,11

23415   **Coracoacromial ligament release, with or without acromioplasty**
         EXCLUDES   Arthroscopic repair (29826)
     20.1   20.1   **FUD** 090   J A2 50
     AMA: 2018,Sep,7; 2018,Jan,8; 2017,Jan,8; 2016,Jan,13; 2015,Mar,7

23420   **Reconstruction of complete shoulder (rotator) cuff avulsion, chronic (includes acromioplasty)**
     27.9   27.9   **FUD** 090   J A2 80 50
     AMA: 2018,Sep,7; 2018,Jan,8; 2017,Jan,8; 2016,Jan,13; 2015,Jan,16; 2014,Jan,11

23430   **Tenodesis of long tendon of biceps**
         EXCLUDES   Arthroscopic biceps tenodesis (29828)
     21.4   21.4   **FUD** 090   J A2 80 50
     AMA: 2018,Sep,7

23440   **Resection or transplantation of long tendon of biceps**
     21.7   21.7   **FUD** 090   J A2 80 50
     AMA: 2018,Sep,7

23450   **Capsulorrhaphy, anterior; Putti-Platt procedure or Magnuson type operation**
         EXCLUDES   Arthroscopic thermal capsulorrhaphy (29999)
     27.4   27.4   **FUD** 090   J A2 80 50
     AMA: 2018,Sep,7

23455   **with labral repair (eg, Bankart procedure)**
         EXCLUDES   Arthroscopic repair (29806)
     28.7   28.7   **FUD** 090   J A2 80 50
     AMA: 2018,Sep,7

23460   **Capsulorrhaphy, anterior, any type; with bone block**
         INCLUDES   Bristow procedure
     31.5   31.5   **FUD** 090   J A2 80 50
     AMA: 2018,Sep,7

23462   **with coracoid process transfer**
         EXCLUDES   Open thermal capsulorrhaphy (23929)
     30.3   30.3   **FUD** 090   J A2 80 50
     AMA: 2018,Sep,7

23465   **Capsulorrhaphy, glenohumeral joint, posterior, with or without bone block**
         EXCLUDES   Sternoclavicular and acromioclavicular joint repair (23530, 23550)
     32.3   32.3   **FUD** 090   J G2 80 50
     AMA: 2018,Sep,7

23466   **Capsulorrhaphy, glenohumeral joint, any type multi-directional instability**
     32.1   32.1   **FUD** 090   J A2 80 50
     AMA: 2018,Sep,7

23470   **Arthroplasty, glenohumeral joint; hemiarthroplasty**
     34.5   34.5   **FUD** 090   J 80 50
     AMA: 2018,Sep,7; 2018,Jan,8; 2017,Jan,8; 2016,Jan,13; 2015,Jan,16; 2014,Mar,4

23472   **total shoulder (glenoid and proximal humeral replacement (eg, total shoulder))**
         EXCLUDES   Proximal humerus osteotomy (24400)
                  Removal of total shoulder components (23334-23335)
     41.9   41.9   **FUD** 090   C 80 50
     AMA: 2018,Sep,7; 2018,Jan,8; 2017,Jan,8; 2016,Jan,13; 2015,Jan,16; 2014,Mar,4; 2014,Jan,11

23473 **Revision of total shoulder arthroplasty, including allograft when performed; humeral or glenoid component**
EXCLUDES *Removal of prosthesis only (glenoid and/or humeral component) (23334-23335)*
46.7 46.7 **FUD** 090 J 80 50
AMA: 2018,Sep,7; 2018,Jan,8; 2017,Jan,8; 2016,Jan,13; 2015,Jan,16; 2014,Mar,4; 2014,Jan,11

23474 **humeral and glenoid component**
EXCLUDES *Removal of prosthesis only (glenoid and/or humeral component) (23334-23335)*
50.5 50.5 **FUD** 090 C 80 50
AMA: 2018,Sep,7; 2018,Jan,8; 2017,Jan,8; 2016,Jan,13; 2015,Jan,16; 2014,Mar,4; 2014,Jan,11

23480 **Osteotomy, clavicle, with or without internal fixation;**
23.7 23.7 **FUD** 090 J A2 50
AMA: 2018,Sep,7

23485 **with bone graft for nonunion or malunion (includes obtaining graft and/or necessary fixation)**
27.5 27.5 **FUD** 090 J J8 80 50
AMA: 2018,Sep,7

23490 **Prophylactic treatment (nailing, pinning, plating or wiring) with or without methylmethacrylate; clavicle**
24.6 24.6 **FUD** 090 J A2 80 50
AMA: 2018,Sep,7

23491 **proximal humerus**
29.3 29.3 **FUD** 090 J A2 80 50
AMA: 2018,Sep,7

23500-23680 Treatment of Shoulder Fracture/Dislocation

23500 **Closed treatment of clavicular fracture; without manipulation**
6.37 6.24 **FUD** 090 T A2 50
AMA: 2018,Sep,7

23505 **with manipulation**
9.51 10.1 **FUD** 090 J A2 50
AMA: 2018,Sep,7

23515 **Open treatment of clavicular fracture, includes internal fixation, when performed**
20.7 20.7 **FUD** 090 J J8 80 50
AMA: 2018,Sep,7; 2018,Jan,8; 2017,Jan,8; 2016,Jan,13; 2015,Jan,16; 2014,Jan,11

23520 **Closed treatment of sternoclavicular dislocation; without manipulation**
6.73 6.72 **FUD** 090 J A2 80 50
AMA: 2018,Sep,7

23525 **with manipulation**
10.2 11.1 **FUD** 090 T A2 80 50
AMA: 2018,Sep,7

23530 **Open treatment of sternoclavicular dislocation, acute or chronic;**
16.5 16.5 **FUD** 090 J A2 80 50
AMA: 2018,Sep,7

23532 **with fascial graft (includes obtaining graft)**
18.0 18.0 **FUD** 090 J A2 80 50
AMA: 2018,Sep,7

23540 **Closed treatment of acromioclavicular dislocation; without manipulation**
6.56 6.54 **FUD** 090 T A2 50
AMA: 2018,Sep,7

23545 **with manipulation**
8.93 9.91 **FUD** 090 T A2 80 50
AMA: 2018,Sep,7

23550 **Open treatment of acromioclavicular dislocation, acute or chronic;**
16.3 16.3 **FUD** 090 J A2 80 50
AMA: 2018,Sep,7

23552 **with fascial graft (includes obtaining graft)**
18.8 18.8 **FUD** 090 J J8 80 50
AMA: 2018,Sep,7

23570 **Closed treatment of scapular fracture; without manipulation**
6.83 6.62 **FUD** 090 T A2 50
AMA: 2018,Sep,7

23575 **with manipulation, with or without skeletal traction (with or without shoulder joint involvement)**
10.8 11.5 **FUD** 090 J A2 80 50
AMA: 2018,Sep,7

23585 **Open treatment of scapular fracture (body, glenoid or acromion) includes internal fixation, when performed**
28.2 28.2 **FUD** 090 J A2 80 50
AMA: 2018,Sep,7; 2018,Jan,8; 2017,Jan,8; 2016,Jan,13; 2015,Jan,16; 2014,Jan,11

23600 **Closed treatment of proximal humeral (surgical or anatomical neck) fracture; without manipulation**
8.82 9.37 **FUD** 090 T P2 50
AMA: 2018,Sep,7

23605 **with manipulation, with or without skeletal traction**
12.1 13.3 **FUD** 090 J A2 50
AMA: 2018,Sep,7

23615 **Open treatment of proximal humeral (surgical or anatomical neck) fracture, includes internal fixation, when performed, includes repair of tuberosity(s), when performed;**
25.4 25.4 **FUD** 090 J J8 80 50
AMA: 2018,Sep,7; 2018,Jan,8; 2017,Jan,8; 2016,Jan,13; 2015,Jan,16; 2014,Jan,11

23616 **with proximal humeral prosthetic replacement**
35.7 35.7 **FUD** 090 J J8 80 50
AMA: 2018,Sep,7

23620 **Closed treatment of greater humeral tuberosity fracture; without manipulation**
7.32 7.65 **FUD** 090 T P2 50
AMA: 2018,Sep,7

23625 **with manipulation**
10.0 10.9 **FUD** 090 J A2 50
AMA: 2018,Sep,7

23630 **Open treatment of greater humeral tuberosity fracture, includes internal fixation, when performed**
22.4 22.4 **FUD** 090 J A2 80 50
AMA: 2018,Sep,7

23650 **Closed treatment of shoulder dislocation, with manipulation; without anesthesia**
8.29 9.10 **FUD** 090 T A2 50
AMA: 2018,Sep,7

23655 **requiring anesthesia**
11.5 11.5 **FUD** 090 J A2 50
AMA: 2018,Sep,7

23660 **Open treatment of acute shoulder dislocation**
EXCLUDES *Chronic dislocation repair (23450-23466)*
16.7 16.7 **FUD** 090 J A2 80 50
AMA: 2018,Sep,7; 2018,Jan,8; 2017,Jan,8; 2016,Jan,13; 2015,Jan,16; 2014,Jan,11

23665 **Closed treatment of shoulder dislocation, with fracture of greater humeral tuberosity, with manipulation**
11.3 12.2 **FUD** 090 J A2 50
AMA: 2019,Feb,10; 2018,Sep,7

23670 **Open treatment of shoulder dislocation, with fracture of greater humeral tuberosity, includes internal fixation, when performed**
25.2 25.2 **FUD** 090 J A2 80 50
AMA: 2018,Sep,7

23675 Closed treatment of shoulder dislocation, with surgical or anatomical neck fracture, with manipulation
🔷 14.3   ⚖ 15.7   **FUD** 090   J A2 50 ▣
AMA: 2018,Sep,7

23680 Open treatment of shoulder dislocation, with surgical or anatomical neck fracture, includes internal fixation, when performed
🔷 26.7   ⚖ 26.7   **FUD** 090   J J8 80 50 ▣
AMA: 2018,Sep,7

23700-23929 Other/Unlisted Shoulder Procedures

23700 Manipulation under anesthesia, shoulder joint, including application of fixation apparatus (dislocation excluded)
🔷 5.64   ⚖ 5.64   **FUD** 010   J A2 50 ▣
AMA: 2018,Sep,7; 2018,Jan,8; 2017,Jan,8; 2016,Jan,13; 2015,Jun,10; 2015,Jan,16; 2014,Jan,11

23800 Arthrodesis, glenohumeral joint;
🔷 29.6   ⚖ 29.6   **FUD** 090   J G2 80 50 ▣
AMA: 2018,Sep,7

23802 with autogenous graft (includes obtaining graft)
🔷 37.0   ⚖ 37.0   **FUD** 090   J G2 80 50 ▣
AMA: 2018,Sep,7

23900 Interthoracoscapular amputation (forequarter)
🔷 40.1   ⚖ 40.1   **FUD** 090   C 80
AMA: 2018,Sep,7

23920 Disarticulation of shoulder;
🔷 32.5   ⚖ 32.5   **FUD** 090   C 80 50 ▣
AMA: 2018,Sep,7

23921 secondary closure or scar revision
🔷 13.4   ⚖ 13.4   **FUD** 090   T A2 50 ▣
AMA: 2018,Sep,7

23929 Unlisted procedure, shoulder
🔷 0.00   ⚖ 0.00   **FUD** YYY   T 80 ▣
AMA: 2018,Sep,7

23930-24006 Surgical Incision Elbow/Upper Arm
EXCLUDES   Simple incision and drainage procedures (10040-10160)

23930 Incision and drainage, upper arm or elbow area; deep abscess or hematoma
🔷 6.13   ⚖ 10.1   **FUD** 010   J A2 50 ▣
AMA: 2018,Sep,7

23931 bursa
🔷 4.48   ⚖ 8.19   **FUD** 010   J A2 50 ▣
AMA: 2018,Sep,7

23935 Incision, deep, with opening of bone cortex (eg, for osteomyelitis or bone abscess), humerus or elbow
🔷 14.6   ⚖ 14.6   **FUD** 090   J A2 80 50 ▣
AMA: 2018,Sep,7

24000 Arthrotomy, elbow, including exploration, drainage, or removal of foreign body
🔷 13.7   ⚖ 13.7   **FUD** 090   J A2 80 50 ▣
AMA: 2018,Sep,7

24006 Arthrotomy of the elbow, with capsular excision for capsular release (separate procedure)
🔷 20.5   ⚖ 20.5   **FUD** 090   J A2 80 50 ▣
AMA: 2018,Sep,7

24065-24066 Biopsy of Elbow/Upper Arm
EXCLUDES   Soft tissue needle biopsy (20206)

24065 Biopsy, soft tissue of upper arm or elbow area; superficial
🔷 4.78   ⚖ 7.40   **FUD** 010   J P3 50 ▣
AMA: 2018,Sep,7

24066 deep (subfascial or intramuscular)
🔷 12.0   ⚖ 18.0   **FUD** 090   J A2 50 ▣
AMA: 2018,Sep,7

24071-24079 [24071, 24073] Excision Soft Tissue Tumors Elbow/Upper Arm

INCLUDES   Any necessary elevation of tissue planes or dissection
Measurement of tumor and necessary margin at greatest diameter prior to excision
Types of excision:
   Fascial or subfascial soft tissue tumors: simple and marginal resection of tumors found either in or below the deep fascia, not involving bone or excision of a substantial amount of normal tissue; primarily benign and intramuscular tumors
   Radical resection of soft tissue tumor: wide resection of tumor involving substantial margins of normal tissue and may involve tissue removal from one or more layers; most often malignant or aggressive benign
   Subcutaneous: simple and marginal resection of tumors found in the subcutaneous tissue above the deep fascia; most often benign

EXCLUDES   Complex repair
Excision of benign cutaneous lesion (eg, sebaceous cyst) (11400-11406)
Radical resection of cutaneous tumors (eg, melanoma) (11600-11606)
Significant exploration of vessels or neuroplasty

24071 Resequenced code. See code following 24075.

24073 Resequenced code. See code following 24076.

24075 Excision, tumor, soft tissue of upper arm or elbow area, subcutaneous; less than 3 cm
🔷 9.48   ⚖ 14.4   **FUD** 090   J G2 50 ▣
AMA: 2018,Sep,7

24071 3 cm or greater
🔷 11.7   ⚖ 11.7   **FUD** 090   J G2 80 50 ▣
AMA: 2018,Sep,7

24076 Excision, tumor, soft tissue of upper arm or elbow area, subfascial (eg, intramuscular); less than 5 cm
🔷 15.6   ⚖ 15.6   **FUD** 090   J G2 50 ▣
AMA: 2018,Sep,7

24073 5 cm or greater
🔷 19.9   ⚖ 19.9   **FUD** 090   J G2 80 50 ▣
AMA: 2018,Sep,7

24077 Radical resection of tumor (eg, sarcoma), soft tissue of upper arm or elbow area; less than 5 cm
🔷 29.9   ⚖ 29.9   **FUD** 090   J G2 50 ▣
AMA: 2018,Sep,7

24079 5 cm or greater
🔷 38.2   ⚖ 38.2   **FUD** 090   J G2 80 50 ▣
AMA: 2018,Sep,7

24100-24149 Bone/Joint Procedures Upper Arm/Elbow

24100 Arthrotomy, elbow; with synovial biopsy only
🔷 12.0   ⚖ 12.0   **FUD** 090   J A2 80 50 ▣
AMA: 2018,Sep,7

24101 with joint exploration, with or without biopsy, with or without removal of loose or foreign body
🔷 14.3   ⚖ 14.3   **FUD** 090   J A2 80 50 ▣
AMA: 2018,Sep,7

24102 with synovectomy
🔷 17.7   ⚖ 17.7   **FUD** 090   J A2 80 50 ▣
AMA: 2018,Sep,7

24105 Excision, olecranon bursa
🔷 10.1   ⚖ 10.1   **FUD** 090   J A2 50 ▣
AMA: 2018,Sep,7

24110 Excision or curettage of bone cyst or benign tumor, humerus;
🔷 16.8   ⚖ 16.8   **FUD** 090   J A2 50 ▣
AMA: 2018,Sep,7

24115 with autograft (includes obtaining graft)
🔷 21.2   ⚖ 21.2   **FUD** 090   J J8 80 50 ▣
AMA: 2018,Sep,7

24116 with allograft
🔷 24.8   ⚖ 24.8   **FUD** 090   J A2 80 50 ▣
AMA: 2019,May,7; 2018,Sep,7

| 26/TC PC/TC Only | A2-Z3 ASC Payment | 50 Bilateral | ♂ Male Only | ♀ Female Only | 🔷 Facility RVU | ⚖ Non-Facility RVU | ▣ CCI | ☒ CLIA |
| FUD Follow-up Days | CMS: IOM | AMA: CPT Asst | A-Y OPPSI | 80/80 Surg Assist Allowed / w/Doc | ◪ Lab Crosswalk | ▣ Radiology Crosswalk | | |

66

24120 Excision or curettage of bone cyst or benign tumor of head or neck of radius or olecranon process;
📇 15.2 ⚕ 15.2 **FUD** 090   J A2 80 50 ▱
AMA: 2018,Sep,7

24125 with autograft (includes obtaining graft)
📇 17.8 ⚕ 17.8 **FUD** 090   J A2 80 50 ▱
AMA: 2018,Sep,7

24126 with allograft
📇 18.7 ⚕ 18.7 **FUD** 090   J J8 80 50 ▱
AMA: 2019,May,7; 2018,Sep,7

24130 Excision, radial head
EXCLUDES Radial head arthroplasty with implant (24366)
📇 14.6 ⚕ 14.6 **FUD** 090   J A2 50 ▱
AMA: 2018,Sep,7

24134 Sequestrectomy (eg, for osteomyelitis or bone abscess), shaft or distal humerus
📇 21.5 ⚕ 21.5 **FUD** 090   J A2 80 50 ▱
AMA: 2018,Sep,7

24136 Sequestrectomy (eg, for osteomyelitis or bone abscess), radial head or neck
📇 18.1 ⚕ 18.1 **FUD** 090   J A2 50 ▱
AMA: 2018,Sep,7

24138 Sequestrectomy (eg, for osteomyelitis or bone abscess), olecranon process
📇 19.5 ⚕ 19.5 **FUD** 090   J A2 80 50 ▱
AMA: 2018,Sep,7

24140 Partial excision (craterization, saucerization, or diaphysectomy) bone (eg, osteomyelitis), humerus
📇 20.2 ⚕ 20.2 **FUD** 090   J A2 80 50 ▱
AMA: 2018,Sep,7

24145 Partial excision (craterization, saucerization, or diaphysectomy) bone (eg, osteomyelitis), radial head or neck
📇 17.0 ⚕ 17.0 **FUD** 090   J A2 50 ▱
AMA: 2018,Sep,7

24147 Partial excision (craterization, saucerization, or diaphysectomy) bone (eg, osteomyelitis), olecranon process
📇 17.9 ⚕ 17.9 **FUD** 090   J A2 50 ▱
AMA: 2018,Sep,7

24149 Radical resection of capsule, soft tissue, and heterotopic bone, elbow, with contracture release (separate procedure)
EXCLUDES Capsular and soft tissue release (24006)
📇 33.8 ⚕ 33.8 **FUD** 090   J 62 80 50 ▱
AMA: 2018,Sep,7

24150-24152 Radical Resection Bone Tumor Upper Arm
INCLUDES Any necessary elevation of tissue planes or dissection
Excision of adjacent soft tissue during bone tumor resection (24071-24079 [24071, 24073])
Measurement of tumor and necessary margin at greatest diameter prior to excision
Resection of the tumor (may include entire bone) and wide margins of normal tissue primarily for malignant or aggressive benign tumors
Simple and intermediate repairs
EXCLUDES Complex repair
Significant exploration of vessels, neuroplasty, reconstruction, or complex bone repair

24150 Radical resection of tumor, shaft or distal humerus
📇 44.9 ⚕ 44.9 **FUD** 090   J 80 50 ▱
AMA: 2019,May,7; 2018,Sep,7

24152 Radical resection of tumor, radial head or neck
📇 39.0 ⚕ 39.0 **FUD** 090   J 62 80 50 ▱
AMA: 2019,May,7; 2018,Sep,7

24155 Elbow Arthrectomy
24155 Resection of elbow joint (arthrectomy)
📇 24.6 ⚕ 24.6 **FUD** 090   J A2 80 50 ▱
AMA: 2018,Sep,7

24160-24201 Removal Implant/Foreign Body from Elbow/Upper Arm
EXCLUDES Bursal or joint arthrocentesis or needling (20605)
K-wire or pin insertion (20650)
K-wire or pin removal (20670, 20680)

24160 Removal of prosthesis, includes debridement and synovectomy when performed; humeral and ulnar components
INCLUDES Prosthesis removal and replacement in same elbow (eg, humeral and/or ulnar component(s)) (24370-24371)
EXCLUDES Foreign body removal (24200-24201)
Hardware removal other than prosthesis (20680)
📇 36.4 ⚕ 36.4 **FUD** 090   02 A2 50 ▱
AMA: 2018,Sep,7; 2018,Jan,8; 2017,Jan,8; 2016,Jan,13; 2015,Jan,16; 2014,Mar,4; 2014,Jan,11

24164 radial head
EXCLUDES Foreign body removal (24200-24201)
Hardware removal other than prosthesis (20680)
📇 20.8 ⚕ 20.8 **FUD** 090   02 A2 50 ▱
AMA: 2018,Sep,7; 2018,Jan,8; 2017,Jan,8; 2016,Jan,13; 2015,Jan,16; 2014,Mar,4

24200 Removal of foreign body, upper arm or elbow area; subcutaneous
📇 3.99 ⚕ 6.02 **FUD** 010   J P3 80 50 ▱
AMA: 2018,Sep,7; 2018,Jan,8; 2017,Jan,8; 2016,Jan,13; 2015,Jan,16; 2014,Mar,4

24201 deep (subfascial or intramuscular)
📇 10.4 ⚕ 15.8 **FUD** 090   J A2 50 ▱
AMA: 2018,Sep,7; 2018,Jan,8; 2017,Jan,8; 2016,Jan,13; 2015,Jan,16; 2014,Mar,4

24220 Injection for Elbow Arthrogram
24220 Injection procedure for elbow arthrography
EXCLUDES Injection tennis elbow (20550)
📷 (73085)
📇 1.95 ⚕ 4.71 **FUD** 000   N N1 80 50 ▱
AMA: 2018,Sep,7; 2018,Jan,8; 2017,Jan,8; 2016,May,13; 2016,Jan,13; 2015,Aug,6

24300-24498 Repair/Reconstruction of Elbow/Upper Arm
24300 Manipulation, elbow, under anesthesia
EXCLUDES External fixation (20690, 20692)
📇 12.0 ⚕ 12.0 **FUD** 090   J 62 50 ▱
AMA: 2018,Sep,7

24301 Muscle or tendon transfer, any type, upper arm or elbow, single (excluding 24320-24331)
📇 21.6 ⚕ 21.6 **FUD** 090   J A2 80 ▱
AMA: 2018,Sep,7

24305 Tendon lengthening, upper arm or elbow, each tendon
📇 16.5 ⚕ 16.5 **FUD** 090   J A2 80 ▱
AMA: 2018,Sep,7

24310 Tenotomy, open, elbow to shoulder, each tendon
📇 13.4 ⚕ 13.4 **FUD** 090   J A2 80 ▱
AMA: 2018,Sep,7

24320 Tenoplasty, with muscle transfer, with or without free graft, elbow to shoulder, single (Seddon-Brookes type procedure)
📇 22.5 ⚕ 22.5 **FUD** 090   J A2 80 ▱
AMA: 2018,Sep,7

24330 Flexor-plasty, elbow (eg, Steindler type advancement);
📇 20.7 ⚕ 20.7 **FUD** 090   J A2 80 ▱
AMA: 2018,Sep,7

24331 with extensor advancement
📇 22.6 ⚕ 22.6 **FUD** 090   J A2 80 ▱
AMA: 2018,Sep,7

24332 Tenolysis, triceps
🔧 17.6 ⬥ 17.6 **FUD** 090
⬜ J ⬜ 62 ⬜ 50 ⬜
AMA: 2018,Sep,7

24340 Tenodesis of biceps tendon at elbow (separate procedure)
🔧 17.6 ⬥ 17.6 **FUD** 090
⬜ J ⬜ A2 ⬜ 80 ⬜ 50 ⬜
AMA: 2018,Sep,7

24341 Repair, tendon or muscle, upper arm or elbow, each tendon or muscle, primary or secondary (excludes rotator cuff)
🔧 21.4 ⬥ 21.4 **FUD** 090
⬜ J ⬜ A2 ⬜ 80 ⬜ 50 ⬜
AMA: 2018,Sep,7

24342 Reinsertion of ruptured biceps or triceps tendon, distal, with or without tendon graft
🔧 22.3 ⬥ 22.3 **FUD** 090
⬜ J ⬜ A2 ⬜ 80 ⬜ 50 ⬜
AMA: 2018,Sep,7; 2018,Jan,8; 2017,Apr,9

24343 Repair lateral collateral ligament, elbow, with local tissue
🔧 20.4 ⬥ 20.4 **FUD** 090
⬜ J ⬜ 62 ⬜ 80 ⬜ 50 ⬜
AMA: 2018,Sep,7

24344 Reconstruction lateral collateral ligament, elbow, with tendon graft (includes harvesting of graft)
🔧 31.4 ⬥ 31.4 **FUD** 090
⬜ J ⬜ J8 ⬜ 80 ⬜ 50 ⬜
AMA: 2018,Sep,7

24345 Repair medial collateral ligament, elbow, with local tissue
🔧 20.2 ⬥ 20.2 **FUD** 090
⬜ J ⬜ A2 ⬜ 80 ⬜ 50 ⬜
AMA: 2018,Sep,7

24346 Reconstruction medial collateral ligament, elbow, with tendon graft (includes harvesting of graft)
🔧 31.7 ⬥ 31.7 **FUD** 090
⬜ J ⬜ 62 ⬜ 80 ⬜ 50 ⬜
AMA: 2018,Sep,7

24357 Tenotomy, elbow, lateral or medial (eg, epicondylitis, tennis elbow, golfer's elbow); percutaneous
EXCLUDES Arthroscopy, elbow, surgical; debridement (29837-29838)
🔧 11.9 ⬥ 11.9 **FUD** 090
⬜ J ⬜ 62 ⬜ 80 ⬜ 50 ⬜
AMA: 2018,Sep,7; 2018,Jan,8; 2017,Jan,8; 2016,Jan,13; 2015,Jan,16; 2014,Jan,11

24358 debridement, soft tissue and/or bone, open
EXCLUDES Arthroscopy, elbow, surgical; debridement (29837-29838)
🔧 15.0 ⬥ 15.0 **FUD** 090
⬜ J ⬜ 62 ⬜ 80 ⬜ 50 ⬜
AMA: 2018,Sep,7; 2018,Jan,8; 2017,Jan,8; 2016,Jan,13; 2015,Jan,16; 2014,Jan,11

24359 debridement, soft tissue and/or bone, open with tendon repair or reattachment
EXCLUDES Arthroscopy, elbow, surgical; debridement (29837-29838)
🔧 19.0 ⬥ 19.0 **FUD** 090
⬜ J ⬜ 62 ⬜ 80 ⬜ 50 ⬜
AMA: 2018,Sep,7; 2018,Jan,8; 2017,Jan,8; 2016,Jan,13; 2015,Jan,16; 2014,Jan,11

24360 Arthroplasty, elbow; with membrane (eg, fascial)
🔧 26.0 ⬥ 26.0 **FUD** 090
⬜ J ⬜ A2 ⬜ 80 ⬜ 50 ⬜
AMA: 2018,Sep,7

24361 with distal humeral prosthetic replacement
🔧 29.0 ⬥ 29.0 **FUD** 090
⬜ J ⬜ J8 ⬜ 80 ⬜ 50 ⬜
AMA: 2018,Sep,7

24362 with implant and fascia lata ligament reconstruction
🔧 30.6 ⬥ 30.6 **FUD** 090
⬜ J ⬜ J8 ⬜ 80 ⬜ 50 ⬜
AMA: 2018,Sep,7

24363 with distal humerus and proximal ulnar prosthetic replacement (eg, total elbow)
EXCLUDES Total elbow implant revision (24370-24371)
🔧 41.9 ⬥ 41.9 **FUD** 090
⬜ J ⬜ J8 ⬜ 80 ⬜ 50 ⬜
AMA: 2018,Sep,7; 2018,Jan,8; 2017,Jan,8; 2016,Jan,13; 2015,Jan,16; 2014,Jan,11

24365 Arthroplasty, radial head;
🔧 18.4 ⬥ 18.4 **FUD** 090
⬜ J ⬜ 62 ⬜ 80 ⬜ 50 ⬜
AMA: 2018,Sep,7

24366 with implant
🔧 19.6 ⬥ 19.6 **FUD** 090
⬜ J ⬜ J8 ⬜ 80 ⬜ 50 ⬜
AMA: 2018,Sep,7

24370 Revision of total elbow arthroplasty, including allograft when performed; humeral or ulnar component
EXCLUDES Prosthesis removal without replacement (eg, humeral and/or ulnar component/s) (24160)
🔧 44.7 ⬥ 44.7 **FUD** 090
⬜ J ⬜ J8 ⬜ 80 ⬜ 50 ⬜
AMA: 2018,Sep,7; 2018,Jan,8; 2017,Jan,8; 2016,Jan,13; 2015,Jan,16; 2014,Mar,4

24371 humeral and ulnar component
EXCLUDES Prosthesis removal without replacement (eg, humeral and/or ulnar component/s) (24160)
🔧 51.3 ⬥ 51.3 **FUD** 090
⬜ J ⬜ J8 ⬜ 80 ⬜ 50 ⬜
AMA: 2018,Sep,7; 2018,Jan,8; 2017,Jan,8; 2016,Jan,13; 2015,Jan,16; 2014,Mar,4

24400 Osteotomy, humerus, with or without internal fixation
🔧 23.7 ⬥ 23.7 **FUD** 090
⬜ J ⬜ A2 ⬜ 80 ⬜ 50 ⬜
AMA: 2018,Sep,7; 2018,Jan,8; 2017,Jan,8; 2016,Jan,13; 2015,Jan,16; 2014,Mar,4

24410 Multiple osteotomies with realignment on intramedullary rod, humeral shaft (Sofield type procedure)
🔧 30.5 ⬥ 30.5 **FUD** 090
⬜ J ⬜ 62 ⬜ 80 ⬜ 50 ⬜
AMA: 2018,Sep,7

24420 Osteoplasty, humerus (eg, shortening or lengthening) (excluding 64876)
🔧 28.5 ⬥ 28.5 **FUD** 090
⬜ J ⬜ A2 ⬜ 80 ⬜ 50 ⬜
AMA: 2018,Sep,7

24430 Repair of nonunion or malunion, humerus; without graft (eg, compression technique)
🔧 30.4 ⬥ 30.4 **FUD** 090
⬜ J ⬜ J8 ⬜ 80 ⬜ 50 ⬜
AMA: 2018,Sep,7

24435 with iliac or other autograft (includes obtaining graft)
🔧 31.0 ⬥ 31.0 **FUD** 090
⬜ J ⬜ J8 ⬜ 80 ⬜ 50 ⬜
AMA: 2018,Sep,7

24470 Hemiepiphyseal arrest (eg, cubitus varus or valgus, distal humerus)
🔧 19.3 ⬥ 19.3 **FUD** 090
⬜ J ⬜ A2 ⬜ 80 ⬜ 50 ⬜
AMA: 2018,Sep,7

24495 Decompression fasciotomy, forearm, with brachial artery exploration
🔧 21.3 ⬥ 21.3 **FUD** 090
⬜ J ⬜ A2 ⬜ 80 ⬜ 50 ⬜
AMA: 2018,Sep,7

24498 Prophylactic treatment (nailing, pinning, plating or wiring), with or without methylmethacrylate, humeral shaft
🔧 24.9 ⬥ 24.9 **FUD** 090
⬜ J ⬜ J8 ⬜ 80 ⬜ 50 ⬜
AMA: 2018,Sep,7

24500-24685 Treatment of Fracture/Dislocation of Elbow/Upper Arm

INCLUDES Treatment for either closed or open fractures or dislocations

24500 Closed treatment of humeral shaft fracture; without manipulation
🔧 9.35 ⬥ 10.2 **FUD** 090
⬜ T ⬜ A2 ⬜ 50 ⬜
AMA: 2018,Sep,7

24505 with manipulation, with or without skeletal traction
🔧 12.8 ⬥ 14.2 **FUD** 090
⬜ J ⬜ A2 ⬜ 50 ⬜
AMA: 2018,Sep,7

24515 Open treatment of humeral shaft fracture with plate/screws, with or without cerclage
🔧 25.2 ⬥ 25.2 **FUD** 090
⬜ J ⬜ J8 ⬜ 80 ⬜ 50 ⬜
AMA: 2018,Sep,7

26/TC PC/TC Only   A2-Z3 ASC Payment   50 Bilateral   ♂ Male Only   ♀ Female Only   🔧 Facility RVU   ⬥ Non-Facility RVU   ⬜ CCI   ⬛ CLIA
FUD Follow-up Days   **CMS:** IOM   **AMA:** CPT Asst   A-Y OPPSI   80/80 Surg Assist Allowed / w/Doc   ⬛ Lab Crosswalk   ⬛ Radiology Crosswalk

68   CPT © 2019 American Medical Association. All Rights Reserved.   © 2019 Optum360, LLC

24516 Treatment of humeral shaft fracture, with insertion of intramedullary implant, with or without cerclage and/or locking screws
🔲 24.7   24.7   **FUD** 090   J J8 80 50
AMA: 2018,Sep,7; 2018,Jan,8; 2018,Jan,3; 2017,Jan,8; 2016,Jan,13; 2015,Jan,16; 2014,Jan,11

24530 Closed treatment of supracondylar or transcondylar humeral fracture, with or without intercondylar extension; without manipulation
🔲 9.89   10.8   **FUD** 090   T A2 50
AMA: 2018,Sep,7

24535 with manipulation, with or without skin or skeletal traction
🔲 16.3   17.6   **FUD** 090   J A2 50
AMA: 2018,Sep,7

24538 Percutaneous skeletal fixation of supracondylar or transcondylar humeral fracture, with or without intercondylar extension
🔲 21.5   21.5   **FUD** 090   J A2 50
AMA: 2018,Sep,7; 2018,Jan,8; 2017,Jan,8; 2016,Jan,13; 2015,Jan,16; 2014,Jan,11

24545 Open treatment of humeral supracondylar or transcondylar fracture, includes internal fixation, when performed; without intercondylar extension
🔲 26.7   26.7   **FUD** 090   J J8 80 50
AMA: 2018,Sep,7

24546 with intercondylar extension
🔲 29.9   29.9   **FUD** 090   J J8 80 50
AMA: 2018,Sep,7

24560 Closed treatment of humeral epicondylar fracture, medial or lateral; without manipulation
🔲 8.28   9.29   **FUD** 090   T A2 50
AMA: 2018,Sep,7

24565 with manipulation
🔲 14.1   15.3   **FUD** 090   J A2 50
AMA: 2018,Sep,7

24566 Percutaneous skeletal fixation of humeral epicondylar fracture, medial or lateral, with manipulation
🔲 20.6   20.6   **FUD** 090   J A2 50
AMA: 2018,Sep,7

24575 Open treatment of humeral epicondylar fracture, medial or lateral, includes internal fixation, when performed
🔲 21.0   21.0   **FUD** 090   J A2 80 50
AMA: 2018,Sep,7

24576 Closed treatment of humeral condylar fracture, medial or lateral; without manipulation
🔲 8.75   9.80   **FUD** 090   T A2 50
AMA: 2018,Sep,7

24577 with manipulation
🔲 14.4   15.8   **FUD** 090   J A2 50
AMA: 2018,Sep,7

24579 Open treatment of humeral condylar fracture, medial or lateral, includes internal fixation, when performed
    EXCLUDES *Closed treatment without manipulation (24530, 24560, 24576, 24650, 24670)*
    Repair with manipulation (24535, 24565, 24577, 24675)
🔲 24.0   24.0   **FUD** 090   J J8 80 50
AMA: 2018,Sep,7

24582 Percutaneous skeletal fixation of humeral condylar fracture, medial or lateral, with manipulation
🔲 23.3   23.3   **FUD** 090   J A2 50
AMA: 2018,Sep,7

24586 Open treatment of periarticular fracture and/or dislocation of the elbow (fracture distal humerus and proximal ulna and/or proximal radius);
🔲 31.2   31.2   **FUD** 090   J G2 80 50
AMA: 2018,Sep,7

24587 with implant arthroplasty
    EXCLUDES *Distal humerus arthroplasty with implant (24361)*
🔲 31.4   31.4   **FUD** 090   J J8 80 50
AMA: 2018,Sep,7

24600 Treatment of closed elbow dislocation; without anesthesia
🔲 9.60   10.5   **FUD** 090   T A2 50
AMA: 2018,Sep,7

24605 requiring anesthesia
🔲 13.5   13.5   **FUD** 090   J A2 50
AMA: 2018,Sep,7

24615 Open treatment of acute or chronic elbow dislocation
🔲 20.5   20.5   **FUD** 090   J A2 80 50
AMA: 2018,Sep,7

24620 Closed treatment of Monteggia type of fracture dislocation at elbow (fracture proximal end of ulna with dislocation of radial head), with manipulation
🔲 15.8   15.8   **FUD** 090   J A2 80 50
AMA: 2018,Sep,7

24635 Open treatment of Monteggia type of fracture dislocation at elbow (fracture proximal end of ulna with dislocation of radial head), includes internal fixation, when performed
🔲 19.3   19.3   **FUD** 090   J J8 80 50
AMA: 2018,Sep,7

24640 Closed treatment of radial head subluxation in child, nursemaid elbow, with manipulation
🔲 2.23   2.86   **FUD** 010   T P3 80 50
AMA: 2018,Sep,7

24650 Closed treatment of radial head or neck fracture; without manipulation
🔲 6.89   7.45   **FUD** 090   T P2 50
AMA: 2018,Sep,7

24655 with manipulation
🔲 11.4   12.6   **FUD** 090   J A2 50
AMA: 2018,Sep,7

24665 Open treatment of radial head or neck fracture, includes internal fixation or radial head excision, when performed;
🔲 18.7   18.7   **FUD** 090   J A2 80 50
AMA: 2018,Sep,7

24666 with radial head prosthetic replacement
🔲 21.0   21.0   **FUD** 090   J J8 80 50
AMA: 2018,Sep,7

24670 Closed treatment of ulnar fracture, proximal end (eg, olecranon or coronoid process[es]); without manipulation
🔲 7.53   8.28   **FUD** 090   T A2 50
AMA: 2018,Sep,7

24675 with manipulation
🔲 11.9   13.1   **FUD** 090   J A2 50
AMA: 2018,Sep,7

24685 Open treatment of ulnar fracture, proximal end (eg, olecranon or coronoid process[es]), includes internal fixation, when performed
    EXCLUDES *Arthrotomy, elbow (24100-24102)*
🔲 18.8   18.8   **FUD** 090   J J8 80 50
AMA: 2018,Sep,7; 2018,Jan,3

24800-24999 Other/Unlisted Elbow/Upper Arm Procedures

24800 Arthrodesis, elbow joint; local
🔲 23.9   23.9   **FUD** 090   J A2 80 50
AMA: 2018,Sep,7

24802 with autogenous graft (includes obtaining graft)
🔲 28.9   28.9   **FUD** 090   J G2 80 50
AMA: 2018,Sep,7

24900 Amputation, arm through humerus; with primary closure
🔲 21.2   21.2   **FUD** 090   C 80 50
AMA: 2018,Sep,7

● New Code   ▲ Revised Code   ○ Reinstated   ● New Web Release   ▲ Revised Web Release   + Add-on   Unlisted   Not Covered   # Resequenced
50 Optum Mod 50 Exempt   ⊘ AMA Mod 51 Exempt   51 Optum Mod 51 Exempt   63 Mod 63 Exempt   ✗ Non-FDA Drug   ★ Telemedicine   M Maternity   A Age Edit

    69

Musculoskeletal System

24920 — 25100

24920   open, circular (guillotine)
🚗 21.1   ⅋ 21.1   **FUD** 090   C 80 50 ▭
AMA: 2018,Sep,7

24925   secondary closure or scar revision
🚗 16.3   ⅋ 16.3   **FUD** 090   J A2 80 50 ▭
AMA: 2018,Sep,7

24930   re-amputation
🚗 22.3   ⅋ 22.3   **FUD** 090   C 80 50 ▭
AMA: 2018,Sep,7

24931   with implant
🚗 26.9   ⅋ 26.9   **FUD** 090   C 80 50 ▭
AMA: 2018,Sep,7

24935   Stump elongation, upper extremity
🚗 33.6   ⅋ 33.6   **FUD** 090   J 80 50 ▭
AMA: 2018,Sep,7

24940   Cineplasty, upper extremity, complete procedure
🚗 0.00   ⅋ 0.00   **FUD** 090   C 80 50 ▭
AMA: 2018,Sep,7

24999   Unlisted procedure, humerus or elbow
🚗 0.00   ⅋ 0.00   **FUD** YYY   T 80 50 ▭
AMA: 2018,Sep,7

25000-25001 Incision Tendon Sheath of Wrist

25000   Incision, extensor tendon sheath, wrist (eg, deQuervains disease)
EXCLUDES   Carpal tunnel release (64721)
🚗 9.70   ⅋ 9.70   **FUD** 090   J A2 50 ▭
AMA: 2018,Sep,7

25001   Incision, flexor tendon sheath, wrist (eg, flexor carpi radialis)
🚗 9.88   ⅋ 9.88   **FUD** 090   J G2 50 ▭
AMA: 2018,Sep,7

25020-25025 Decompression Fasciotomy Forearm/Wrist

25020   Decompression fasciotomy, forearm and/or wrist, flexor OR extensor compartment; without debridement of nonviable muscle and/or nerve
EXCLUDES   Brachial artery exploration (24495)
       Superficial incision and drainage (10060-10160)
🚗 16.4   ⅋ 16.4   **FUD** 090   J A2 50 ▭
AMA: 2018,Sep,7

25023   with debridement of nonviable muscle and/or nerve
EXCLUDES   Debridement (11000-11044 [11045, 11046])
       Decompression fasciotomy with exploration brachial artery exploration (24495)
       Superficial incision and drainage (10060-10160)
🚗 31.8   ⅋ 31.8   **FUD** 090   J A2 80 50 ▭
AMA: 2018,Sep,7

25024   Decompression fasciotomy, forearm and/or wrist, flexor AND extensor compartment; without debridement of nonviable muscle and/or nerve
🚗 22.4   ⅋ 22.4   **FUD** 090   J A2 50 ▭
AMA: 2018,Sep,7

25025   with debridement of nonviable muscle and/or nerve
🚗 34.8   ⅋ 34.8   **FUD** 090   J A2 80 50 ▭
AMA: 2018,Sep,7

25028-25040 Incision for Drainage/Foreign Body Removal

25028   Incision and drainage, forearm and/or wrist; deep abscess or hematoma
🚗 15.1   ⅋ 15.1   **FUD** 090   J A2 50 ▭
AMA: 2018,Sep,7

25031   bursa
🚗 10.0   ⅋ 10.0   **FUD** 090   J A2 80 50 ▭
AMA: 2018,Sep,7

25035   Incision, deep, bone cortex, forearm and/or wrist (eg, osteomyelitis or bone abscess)
🚗 16.8   ⅋ 16.8   **FUD** 090   J A2 80 50 ▭
AMA: 2018,Sep,7

25040   Arthrotomy, radiocarpal or midcarpal joint, with exploration, drainage, or removal of foreign body
🚗 16.1   ⅋ 16.1   **FUD** 090   J A2 80 50 ▭
AMA: 2018,Sep,7

25065-25066 Biopsy Forearm/Wrist

EXCLUDES   Soft tissue needle biopsy (20206)

25065   Biopsy, soft tissue of forearm and/or wrist; superficial
🚗 4.64   ⅋ 7.32   **FUD** 010   J P3 50 ▭
AMA: 2018,Sep,7

25066   deep (subfascial or intramuscular)
🚗 10.3   ⅋ 10.3   **FUD** 090   J A2 50 ▭
AMA: 2018,Sep,7

25071-25078 [25071, 25073] Excision Soft Tissue Tumors Forearm/Wrist

INCLUDES   Any necessary elevation of tissue planes or dissection
Measurement of tumor and necessary margin at greatest diameter prior to excision
Simple and intermediate repairs
Types of excision:
     Fascial or subfascial soft tissue tumors: simple and marginal resection of tumors found either in or below the deep fascia, not involving bone or excision of a substantial amount of normal tissue; primarily benign and intramuscular tumors
     Radical resection soft tissue tumor: wide resection of tumor involving substantial margins of normal tissue and may include tissue removal from one or more layers; most often malignant or aggressive benign
     Subcutaneous: simple and marginal resection of tumors in the subcutaneous tissue above the deep fascia; most often benign
EXCLUDES   Complex repair
Excision of benign cutaneous lesions (eg, sebaceous cyst) (11400-11406)
Radical resection of cutaneous tumors (eg, melanoma) (11600-11606)
Significant exploration of vessels or neuroplasty

25071   Resequenced code. See code following 25075.

25073   Resequenced code. See code following 25076.

25075   Excision, tumor, soft tissue of forearm and/or wrist area, subcutaneous; less than 3 cm
🚗 9.09   ⅋ 14.0   **FUD** 090   J G2 50 ▭
AMA: 2018,Sep,7

\# **25071**   3 cm or greater
🚗 12.2   ⅋ 12.2   **FUD** 090   J G2 80 50 ▭
AMA: 2018,Sep,7

25076   Excision, tumor, soft tissue of forearm and/or wrist area, subfascial (eg, intramuscular); less than 3 cm
🚗 14.8   ⅋ 14.8   **FUD** 090   J G2 50 ▭
AMA: 2018,Sep,7

\# **25073**   3 cm or greater
🚗 15.3   ⅋ 15.3   **FUD** 090   J G2 80 50 ▭
AMA: 2018,Sep,7

25077   Radical resection of tumor (eg, sarcoma), soft tissue of forearm and/or wrist area; less than 3 cm
🚗 25.4   ⅋ 25.4   **FUD** 090   J G2 50 ▭
AMA: 2018,Sep,7

25078   3 cm or greater
🚗 33.6   ⅋ 33.6   **FUD** 090   J G2 80 50 ▭
AMA: 2018,Sep,7

25085-25240 Procedures of Bones/Joints Lower Arm/Wrist

25085   Capsulotomy, wrist (eg, contracture)
🚗 12.9   ⅋ 12.9   **FUD** 090   J A2 80 50 ▭
AMA: 2018,Sep,7

25100   Arthrotomy, wrist joint; with biopsy
🚗 9.96   ⅋ 9.96   **FUD** 090   J A2 80 50 ▭
AMA: 2018,Sep,7

26/TC PC/TC Only   A2-Z3 ASC Payment   50 Bilateral   ♂ Male Only   ♀ Female Only   🚗 Facility RVU   ⅋ Non-Facility RVU   ▭ CCI   ☒ CLIA
FUD Follow-up Days   **CMS:** IOM   **AMA:** CPT Asst   A-Y OPPSI   80/80 Surg Assist Allowed / w/Doc   ◼ Lab Crosswalk   ☒ Radiology Crosswalk

70   CPT © 2019 American Medical Association. All Rights Reserved.   © 2019 Optum360, LLC

25101 with joint exploration, with or without biopsy, with or without removal of loose or foreign body
🚗 11.6　⚕ 11.6　**FUD** 090　　J A2 80 50 ▢
AMA: 2018,Sep,7

25105 with synovectomy
🚗 13.8　⚕ 13.8　**FUD** 090　　J A2 80 50 ▢
AMA: 2018,Sep,7

25107 Arthrotomy, distal radioulnar joint including repair of triangular cartilage, complex
🚗 17.7　⚕ 17.7　**FUD** 090　　J A2 80 50 ▢
AMA: 2018,Sep,7

25109 Excision of tendon, forearm and/or wrist, flexor or extensor, each
🚗 15.4　⚕ 15.4　**FUD** 090　　J 62 50 ▢
AMA: 2018,Sep,7

25110 Excision, lesion of tendon sheath, forearm and/or wrist
🚗 9.82　⚕ 9.82　**FUD** 090　　J A2 50 ▢
AMA: 2018,Sep,7

25111 Excision of ganglion, wrist (dorsal or volar); primary
EXCLUDES *Excision of ganglion hand or finger (26160)*
🚗 9.21　⚕ 9.21　**FUD** 090　　J A2 50 ▢
AMA: 2018,Sep,7

Synovial sheaths (blue) of the dorsum of right wrist, containing extensor tendons

Ganglion

Anatomical "snuffbox"

Anatomical "snuffbox"

Ganglions are round cystic swellings usually appearing on the dorsum of the wrist or hand; these swellings often communicate with the synovial sheath

Typical location of ganglion

25112 recurrent
EXCLUDES *Excision of ganglion hand or finger (26160)*
🚗 11.1　⚕ 11.1　**FUD** 090　　J A2 50 ▢
AMA: 2018,Sep,7

25115 Radical excision of bursa, synovia of wrist, or forearm tendon sheaths (eg, tenosynovitis, fungus, Tbc, or other granulomas, rheumatoid arthritis); flexors
EXCLUDES *Finger synovectomy (26145)*
🚗 21.8　⚕ 21.8　**FUD** 090　　J A2 50 ▢
AMA: 2018,Sep,7; 2018,Jan,8; 2017,Jan,8; 2016,Jan,13; 2015,Jan,16

25116 extensors, with or without transposition of dorsal retinaculum
EXCLUDES *Finger synovectomy (26145)*
🚗 17.2　⚕ 17.2　**FUD** 090　　J A2 80 50 ▢
AMA: 2018,Sep,7

25118 Synovectomy, extensor tendon sheath, wrist, single compartment;
EXCLUDES *Finger synovectomy (26145)*
🚗 10.9　⚕ 10.9　**FUD** 090　　J A2 50 ▢
AMA: 2018,Sep,7; 2018,Jan,8; 2017,Jan,8; 2016,Jan,13; 2015,Jun,10; 2015,Jan,16; 2014,Jan,11

25119 with resection of distal ulna
EXCLUDES *Finger synovectomy (26145)*
🚗 14.2　⚕ 14.2　**FUD** 090　　J A2 80 50 ▢
AMA: 2018,Sep,7

25120 Excision or curettage of bone cyst or benign tumor of radius or ulna (excluding head or neck of radius and olecranon process);
EXCLUDES *Removal of bone cyst or tumor of radial head, neck, or olecranon process (24120-24126)*
🚗 14.3　⚕ 14.3　**FUD** 090　　J A2 80 50 ▢
AMA: 2018,Sep,7

25125 with autograft (includes obtaining graft)
🚗 17.0　⚕ 17.0　**FUD** 090　　J A2 80 50 ▢
AMA: 2018,Sep,7

25126 with allograft
🚗 17.2　⚕ 17.2　**FUD** 090　　J J8 80 50 ▢
AMA: 2019,May,7; 2018,Sep,7

25130 Excision or curettage of bone cyst or benign tumor of carpal bones;
🚗 12.8　⚕ 12.8　**FUD** 090　　J A2 80 50 ▢
AMA: 2018,Sep,7

25135 with autograft (includes obtaining graft)
🚗 16.0　⚕ 16.0　**FUD** 090　　J A2 80 50 ▢
AMA: 2018,Sep,7

25136 with allograft
🚗 14.0　⚕ 14.0　**FUD** 090　　J A2 80 50 ▢
AMA: 2019,May,7; 2018,Sep,7

25145 Sequestrectomy (eg, for osteomyelitis or bone abscess), forearm and/or wrist
🚗 14.9　⚕ 14.9　**FUD** 090　　J A2 80 50 ▢
AMA: 2018,Sep,7

25150 Partial excision (craterization, saucerization, or diaphysectomy) of bone (eg, for osteomyelitis); ulna
🚗 16.2　⚕ 16.2　**FUD** 090　　J A2 50 ▢
AMA: 2018,Sep,7

25151 radius
EXCLUDES *Partial removal of radial head, neck, or olecranon process (24145, 24147)*
🚗 16.7　⚕ 16.7　**FUD** 090　　J A2 80 50 ▢
AMA: 2018,Sep,7

25170 Radical resection of tumor, radius or ulna
INCLUDES Any necessary elevation of tissue planes or dissection
Excision of adjacent soft tissue during bone tumor resection (25071-25078 [25071, 25073])
Measurement of tumor and necessary margin at greatest diameter prior to excision
Resection of the tumor (may include entire bone) and wide margins of normal tissue primarily for malignant or aggressive benign tumors
Resection without removal of significant normal tissue
Simple and intermediate repairs
EXCLUDES *Complex repair*
Excision of adjacent soft tissue during bone tumor resection (25076-25078 [25073])
Radical resection of cutaneous tumors (e.g., melanoma) (11600-11646)
Significant exploration of vessels, neuroplasty, reconstruction, or complex bone repair
🚗 42.7　⚕ 42.7　**FUD** 090　　J 80 50 ▢
AMA: 2019,May,7; 2018,Sep,7

25210 Carpectomy; 1 bone
EXCLUDES *Carpectomy with insertion of implant (25441-25445)*
🚗 14.0　⚕ 14.0　**FUD** 090　　J A2 80 ▢
AMA: 2018,Sep,7

25215 all bones of proximal row
🚗 17.7　⚕ 17.7　**FUD** 090　　J A2 80 50 ▢
AMA: 2019,Feb,10; 2018,Sep,7

25230 Radial styloidectomy (separate procedure)
🔲 12.4   ⚖ 12.4   **FUD** 090   J A2 50 ▢
AMA: 2018,Sep,7

25240 Excision distal ulna partial or complete (eg, Darrach type or matched resection)
> EXCLUDES   Acquisition of fascia for interposition (20920, 20922)
>   Implant replacement (25442)
🔲 12.3   ⚖ 12.3   **FUD** 090   J A2 80 50 ▢
AMA: 2018,Sep,7

25246 Injection for Wrist Arthrogram

25246 Injection procedure for wrist arthrography
> EXCLUDES   Excision of superficial foreign body (20520)
> 🔳 (73115)
🔲 2.16   ⚖ 4.88   **FUD** 000   N N1 50 ▢
AMA: 2018,Sep,7; 2018,Jan,8; 2017,Jan,8; 2016,Jan,13; 2015,Aug,6

25248-25251 Removal Foreign Body of Wrist

> EXCLUDES   Excision of superficial foreign body (20520)
>   K-wire, pin, or rod insertion (20650)
>   K-wire, pin, or rod removal (20670, 20680)

25248 Exploration with removal of deep foreign body, forearm or wrist
🔲 11.8   ⚖ 11.8   **FUD** 090   J A2 50 ▢
AMA: 2018,Sep,7

25250 Removal of wrist prosthesis; (separate procedure)
🔲 15.2   ⚖ 15.2   **FUD** 090   02 A2 80 50 ▢
AMA: 2018,Sep,7

25251 complicated, including total wrist
🔲 20.7   ⚖ 20.7   **FUD** 090   02 A2 80 50 ▢
AMA: 2018,Sep,7

25259 Manipulation of Wrist with Anesthesia

25259 Manipulation, wrist, under anesthesia
> EXCLUDES   Application external fixation (20690, 20692)
🔲 12.0   ⚖ 12.0   **FUD** 090   J G2 50 ▢
AMA: 2018,Sep,7; 2018,Jan,8; 2017,Jan,8; 2016,Jan,13; 2015,Jan,16; 2014,Jan,11

25260-25492 Repair/Reconstruction of Forearm/Wrist

25260 Repair, tendon or muscle, flexor, forearm and/or wrist; primary, single, each tendon or muscle
🔲 18.1   ⚖ 18.1   **FUD** 090   J A2
AMA: 2018,Sep,7

25263 secondary, single, each tendon or muscle
🔲 18.1   ⚖ 18.1   **FUD** 090   J A2 80 ▢
AMA: 2018,Sep,7

25265 secondary, with free graft (includes obtaining graft), each tendon or muscle
🔲 21.4   ⚖ 21.4   **FUD** 090   J A2 80 ▢
AMA: 2018,Sep,7

25270 Repair, tendon or muscle, extensor, forearm and/or wrist; primary, single, each tendon or muscle
🔲 14.0   ⚖ 14.0   **FUD** 090   J A2 80 ▢
AMA: 2018,Sep,7

25272 secondary, single, each tendon or muscle
🔲 15.9   ⚖ 15.9   **FUD** 090   J A2 80 ▢
AMA: 2018,Sep,7

25274 secondary, with free graft (includes obtaining graft), each tendon or muscle
🔲 19.1   ⚖ 19.1   **FUD** 090   J A2 80 ▢
AMA: 2018,Sep,7

25275 Repair, tendon sheath, extensor, forearm and/or wrist, with free graft (includes obtaining graft) (eg, for extensor carpi ulnaris subluxation)
🔲 19.2   ⚖ 19.2   **FUD** 090   J A2 80 50 ▢
AMA: 2018,Sep,7

25280 Lengthening or shortening of flexor or extensor tendon, forearm and/or wrist, single, each tendon
🔲 16.1   ⚖ 16.1   **FUD** 090   J A2 80 ▢
AMA: 2018,Sep,7

25290 Tenotomy, open, flexor or extensor tendon, forearm and/or wrist, single, each tendon
🔲 12.5   ⚖ 12.5   **FUD** 090   J A2
AMA: 2018,Sep,7

25295 Tenolysis, flexor or extensor tendon, forearm and/or wrist, single, each tendon
🔲 15.1   ⚖ 15.1   **FUD** 090   J A2
AMA: 2018,Sep,7; 2018,Jan,8; 2017,Jan,8; 2016,Jan,13; 2015,Jan,16; 2014,Jan,11

25300 Tenodesis at wrist; flexors of fingers
🔲 19.5   ⚖ 19.5   **FUD** 090   J A2 80 50 ▢
AMA: 2018,Sep,7

25301 extensors of fingers
🔲 18.4   ⚖ 18.4   **FUD** 090   J A2 80 50 ▢
AMA: 2018,Sep,7

25310 Tendon transplantation or transfer, flexor or extensor, forearm and/or wrist, single; each tendon
🔲 17.7   ⚖ 17.7   **FUD** 090   J A2 80 ▢
AMA: 2018,Sep,7; 2018,Jan,8; 2017,Jan,8; 2016,Jan,13; 2015,Jan,16; 2014,Jan,11

25312 with tendon graft(s) (includes obtaining graft), each tendon
🔲 20.6   ⚖ 20.6   **FUD** 090   J A2 80 ▢
AMA: 2018,Sep,7

25315 Flexor origin slide (eg, for cerebral palsy, Volkmann contracture), forearm and/or wrist;
🔲 22.2   ⚖ 22.2   **FUD** 090   J A2 80 50 ▢
AMA: 2018,Sep,7

25316 with tendon(s) transfer
🔲 26.4   ⚖ 26.4   **FUD** 090   J A2 80 50 ▢
AMA: 2018,Sep,7

25320 Capsulorrhaphy or reconstruction, wrist, open (eg, capsulodesis, ligament repair, tendon transfer or graft) (includes synovectomy, capsulotomy and open reduction) for carpal instability
🔲 28.3   ⚖ 28.3   **FUD** 090   J A2 80 50 ▢
AMA: 2018,Sep,7

25332 Arthroplasty, wrist, with or without interposition, with or without external or internal fixation
> EXCLUDES   Acquiring fascia for interposition (20920, 20922)
>   Arthroplasty with prosthesis (25441-25446)
🔲 24.2   ⚖ 24.2   **FUD** 090   J A2 80 50 ▢
AMA: 2019,Feb,10; 2018,Sep,7; 2018,Jan,8; 2017,Jan,8; 2016,Jan,13; 2015,Jan,16; 2014,Jan,11

25335 Centralization of wrist on ulna (eg, radial club hand)
🔲 27.2   ⚖ 27.2   **FUD** 090   J A2 80 50 ▢
AMA: 2018,Sep,7; 2018,May,10

25337 Reconstruction for stabilization of unstable distal ulna or distal radioulnar joint, secondary by soft tissue stabilization (eg, tendon transfer, tendon graft or weave, or tenodesis) with or without open reduction of distal radioulnar joint
> EXCLUDES   Acquiring fascia lata graft (20920, 20922)
🔲 25.6   ⚖ 25.6   **FUD** 090   J A2 50 ▢
AMA: 2018,Sep,7

25350 Osteotomy, radius; distal third
🔲 19.3   ⚖ 19.3   **FUD** 090   J A2 80 50 ▢
AMA: 2018,Sep,7

25355 middle or proximal third
🔲 22.0   ⚖ 22.0   **FUD** 090   J A2 80 50 ▢
AMA: 2018,Sep,7

26/TC PC/TC Only   A2-Z3 ASC Payment   50 Bilateral   ♂ Male Only   ♀ Female Only   🔲 Facility RVU   ⚖ Non-Facility RVU   ▢ CCI   ✖ CLIA
FUD Follow-up Days   CMS: IOM   AMA: CPT Asst   A-Y OPPSI   80/80 Surg Assist Allowed / w/Doc   🔳 Lab Crosswalk   🔳 Radiology Crosswalk

72   CPT © 2019 American Medical Association. All Rights Reserved.   © 2019 Optum360, LLC

25360 Osteotomy; ulna
18.8   18.8   **FUD** 090   J A2 80 50
AMA: 2018,Sep,7

25365 radius AND ulna
26.4   26.4   **FUD** 090   J A2 80 50
AMA: 2018,Sep,7

25370 Multiple osteotomies, with realignment on intramedullary rod (Sofield type procedure); radius OR ulna
29.0   29.0   **FUD** 090   J A2 80 50
AMA: 2018,Sep,7

25375 radius AND ulna
27.5   27.5   **FUD** 090   J A2 80 50
AMA: 2018,Sep,7

25390 Osteoplasty, radius OR ulna; shortening
22.1   22.1   **FUD** 090   J J8 80 50
AMA: 2018,Sep,7

25391 lengthening with autograft
28.7   28.7   **FUD** 090   J J8 80 50
AMA: 2018,Sep,7

25392 Osteoplasty, radius AND ulna; shortening (excluding 64876)
29.2   29.2   **FUD** 090   J A2 80 50
AMA: 2018,Sep,7

25393 lengthening with autograft
32.6   32.6   **FUD** 090   J A2 80 50
AMA: 2018,Sep,7

25394 Osteoplasty, carpal bone, shortening
22.6   22.6   **FUD** 090   J 62 80 50
AMA: 2018,Sep,7

25400 Repair of nonunion or malunion, radius OR ulna; without graft (eg, compression technique)
23.1   23.1   **FUD** 090   J J8 80 50
AMA: 2018,Sep,7

25405 with autograft (includes obtaining graft)
29.9   29.9   **FUD** 090   J J8 80 50
AMA: 2018,Sep,7

25415 Repair of nonunion or malunion, radius AND ulna; without graft (eg, compression technique)
27.9   27.9   **FUD** 090   J J8 80 50
AMA: 2018,Sep,7

25420 with autograft (includes obtaining graft)
33.7   33.7   **FUD** 090   J J8 80 50
AMA: 2018,Sep,7

25425 Repair of defect with autograft; radius OR ulna
27.8   27.8   **FUD** 090   J A2 80 50
AMA: 2018,Sep,7

25426 radius AND ulna
32.4   32.4   **FUD** 090   J 62 80 50
AMA: 2018,Sep,7

25430 Insertion of vascular pedicle into carpal bone (eg, Hori procedure)
21.0   21.0   **FUD** 090   J 62 50
AMA: 2018,Sep,7

25431 Repair of nonunion of carpal bone (excluding carpal scaphoid (navicular)) (includes obtaining graft and necessary fixation), each bone
22.7   22.7   **FUD** 090   J 62 80 50
AMA: 2018,Sep,7

25440 Repair of nonunion, scaphoid carpal (navicular) bone, with or without radial styloidectomy (includes obtaining graft and necessary fixation)
22.1   22.1   **FUD** 090   J A2 80 50
AMA: 2018,Sep,7

25441 Arthroplasty with prosthetic replacement; distal radius
27.0   27.0   **FUD** 090   J J8 80 50
AMA: 2018,Sep,7; 2018,Jan,8; 2017,Aug,9; 2017,Jan,8; 2016,Jan,13; 2015,Jan,16; 2014,Jan,11

25442 distal ulna
23.2   23.2   **FUD** 090   J J8 80 50
AMA: 2018,Sep,7; 2018,Jan,8; 2017,Aug,9; 2017,Jan,8; 2016,Jan,13; 2015,Jan,16; 2014,Jan,11

25443 scaphoid carpal (navicular)
22.5   22.5   **FUD** 090   J A2 80 50
AMA: 2018,Sep,7; 2018,Jan,8; 2017,Jan,8; 2016,Jan,13; 2015,Jan,16; 2014,Jan,11

25444 lunate
23.8   23.8   **FUD** 090   J J8 80 50
AMA: 2018,Sep,7; 2018,Jan,8; 2017,Jan,8; 2016,Jan,13; 2015,Jan,16; 2014,Jan,11

25445 trapezium
20.7   20.7   **FUD** 090   J J8 50
AMA: 2018,Sep,7; 2018,Jan,8; 2017,Jan,8; 2016,Jan,13; 2015,Jan,16; 2014,Jan,11

25446 distal radius and partial or entire carpus (total wrist)
33.8   33.8   **FUD** 090   J J8 80 50
AMA: 2018,Sep,7; 2018,Jan,8; 2017,Jan,8; 2016,Jan,13; 2015,Jan,16; 2014,Jan,11

25447 Arthroplasty, interposition, intercarpal or carpometacarpal joints
EXCLUDES   Wrist arthroplasty (25332)
23.8   23.8   **FUD** 090   J A2 80 50
AMA: 2018,Sep,7; 2018,Jan,8; 2017,Jan,8; 2016,Jan,13; 2015,Jan,16; 2014,Jan,11

25449 Revision of arthroplasty, including removal of implant, wrist joint
29.7   29.7   **FUD** 090   J A2 80 50
AMA: 2018,Sep,7

25450 Epiphyseal arrest by epiphysiodesis or stapling; distal radius OR ulna
17.7   17.7   **FUD** 090   J A2 50
AMA: 2018,Sep,7

25455 distal radius AND ulna
20.9   20.9   **FUD** 090   J A2 50
AMA: 2018,Sep,7

25490 Prophylactic treatment (nailing, pinning, plating or wiring) with or without methylmethacrylate; radius
20.7   20.7   **FUD** 090   J A2 80 50
AMA: 2018,Sep,7

25491 ulna
21.3   21.3   **FUD** 090   J A2 80 50
AMA: 2018,Sep,7

25492 radius AND ulna
26.1   26.1   **FUD** 090   J A2 80 50
AMA: 2018,Sep,7

25500-25695 Treatment of Fracture/Dislocation of Forearm/Wrist

Code also external fixation (20690)

25500 Closed treatment of radial shaft fracture; without manipulation
7.16   7.87   **FUD** 090   T P2 50
AMA: 2018,Sep,7

25505 with manipulation
13.0   14.2   **FUD** 090   J A2 50
AMA: 2018,Sep,7

25515 Open treatment of radial shaft fracture, includes internal fixation, when performed
19.2   19.2   **FUD** 090   J J8 80 50
AMA: 2018,Sep,7

25520 Closed treatment of radial shaft fracture and closed treatment of dislocation of distal radioulnar joint (Galeazzi fracture/dislocation)
　15.5　16.4　**FUD** 090　J A2 50
　AMA: 2018,Sep,7

25525 Open treatment of radial shaft fracture, includes internal fixation, when performed, and closed treatment of distal radioulnar joint dislocation (Galeazzi fracture/ dislocation), includes percutaneous skeletal fixation, when performed
　22.6　22.6　**FUD** 090　J J8 80 50
　AMA: 2018,Sep,7

25526 Open treatment of radial shaft fracture, includes internal fixation, when performed, and open treatment of distal radioulnar joint dislocation (Galeazzi fracture/ dislocation), includes internal fixation, when performed, includes repair of triangular fibrocartilage complex
　27.5　27.5　**FUD** 090　J A2 80 50
　AMA: 2018,Sep,7

25530 Closed treatment of ulnar shaft fracture; without manipulation
　6.80　7.46　**FUD** 090　T P2 50
　AMA: 2018,Sep,7

25535 with manipulation
　12.9　14.0　**FUD** 090　T A2 50
　AMA: 2018,Sep,7

25545 Open treatment of ulnar shaft fracture, includes internal fixation, when performed
　17.9　17.9　**FUD** 090　J A2 80 50
　AMA: 2018,Sep,7; 2018,Jan,8; 2017,Jan,8; 2016,Jan,13; 2015,Jan,16; 2014,Jan,11

25560 Closed treatment of radial and ulnar shaft fractures; without manipulation
　7.22　8.03　**FUD** 090　T P2 50
　AMA: 2018,Sep,7

25565 with manipulation
　13.2　14.7　**FUD** 090　J A2 50
　AMA: 2018,Sep,7

25574 Open treatment of radial AND ulnar shaft fractures, with internal fixation, when performed; of radius OR ulna
　19.3　19.3　**FUD** 090　J J8 80 50
　AMA: 2018,Sep,7; 2018,Jan,8; 2017,Jan,8; 2016,Jan,13; 2015,Jan,16; 2014,Jan,11

25575 of radius AND ulna
　25.9　25.9　**FUD** 090　J J8 80 50
　AMA: 2018,Sep,7

25600 Closed treatment of distal radial fracture (eg, Colles or Smith type) or epiphyseal separation, includes closed treatment of fracture of ulnar styloid, when performed; without manipulation
　INCLUDES Closed treatment of ulnar styloid fracture (25650)
　8.93　9.40　**FUD** 090　T P2 50
　AMA: 2018,Sep,7; 2018,Jan,8; 2017,Jan,8; 2016,Jan,13; 2015,Jan,16; 2014,Jan,11

25605 with manipulation
　INCLUDES Closed treatment of ulnar styloid fracture (25650)
　14.5　15.4　**FUD** 090　J A2 50
　AMA: 2018,Sep,7; 2018,Jan,8; 2017,Jan,8; 2016,Jan,13; 2015,Jan,16; 2014,Jan,11

25606 Percutaneous skeletal fixation of distal radial fracture or epiphyseal separation
　EXCLUDES Closed treatment of ulnar styloid fracture (25650)
　Open repair of ulnar styloid fracture (25652)
　Percutaneous repair of ulnar styloid fracture (25651)
　19.0　19.0　**FUD** 090　J A2 50
　AMA: 2018,Sep,7

25607 Open treatment of distal radial extra-articular fracture or epiphyseal separation, with internal fixation
　EXCLUDES Closed treatment of ulnar styloid fracture (25650)
　Open repair of ulnar styloid fracture (25652)
　Percutaneous repair of ulnar styloid fracture (25651)
　21.1　21.1　**FUD** 090　J J8 80 50
　AMA: 2018,Sep,7; 2018,Jan,8; 2017,Jan,8; 2016,Jan,13; 2015,Jan,16; 2014,Jan,11

25608 Open treatment of distal radial intra-articular fracture or epiphyseal separation; with internal fixation of 2 fragments
　EXCLUDES Closed treatment of ulnar styloid fracture (25650)
　Open repair of ulnar styloid fracture (25652)
　Open treatment of distal radial intra-articular fracture or epiphyseal separation; with internal fixation of 3 or more fragments (25609)
　Percutaneous repair of ulnar styloid fracture (25651)
　23.7　23.7　**FUD** 090　J J8 80 50
　AMA: 2018,Sep,7; 2018,Jan,8; 2017,Jan,8; 2016,Jan,13; 2015,Jan,16; 2014,Jan,11

25609 with internal fixation of 3 or more fragments
　EXCLUDES Closed treatment of ulnar styloid fracture (25650)
　Open repair of ulnar styloid fracture (25652)
　Percutaneous repair of ulnar styloid fracture (25651)
　30.1　30.1　**FUD** 090　J J8 80 50
　AMA: 2018,Sep,7; 2018,Jan,8; 2017,Jan,8; 2016,Jan,13; 2015,Jan,16; 2014,Jan,11

25622 Closed treatment of carpal scaphoid (navicular) fracture; without manipulation
　7.98　8.70　**FUD** 090　T P2 50
　AMA: 2018,Sep,7

25624 with manipulation
　12.5　13.8　**FUD** 090　J A2 80 50
　AMA: 2018,Sep,7

25628 Open treatment of carpal scaphoid (navicular) fracture, includes internal fixation, when performed
　20.7　20.7　**FUD** 090　J A2 80 50
　AMA: 2018,Sep,7

25630 Closed treatment of carpal bone fracture (excluding carpal scaphoid [navicular]); without manipulation, each bone
　8.04　8.69　**FUD** 090　T P2 50
　AMA: 2018,Sep,7

25635 with manipulation, each bone
　11.9　13.1　**FUD** 090　J A2 80 50
　AMA: 2018,Sep,7

25645 Open treatment of carpal bone fracture (other than carpal scaphoid [navicular]), each bone
　16.4　16.4　**FUD** 090　J A2 80 50
　AMA: 2018,Sep,7

25650 Closed treatment of ulnar styloid fracture
　EXCLUDES Closed treatment of distal radial fracture (25600, 25605)
　Open treatment of distal radial extra-articular fracture or epiphyseal separation, with internal fixation (25607-25609)
　8.57　9.20　**FUD** 090　T P2 50
　AMA: 2018,Sep,7; 2018,Jan,8; 2017,Jan,8; 2016,Jan,13; 2015,Jan,16; 2014,Jan,11

25651 Percutaneous skeletal fixation of ulnar styloid fracture
　13.9　13.9　**FUD** 090　J G2 80 50
　AMA: 2018,Sep,7

25652 Open treatment of ulnar styloid fracture
　17.9　17.9　**FUD** 090　J G2 50
　AMA: 2018,Sep,7; 2018,Jan,8; 2017,Jan,8; 2016,Jan,13; 2015,Jan,16; 2014,Jan,11

25660 Closed treatment of radiocarpal or intercarpal dislocation, 1 or more bones, with manipulation
　11.8　11.8　**FUD** 090　T A2 80 50
　AMA: 2018,Sep,7

25670 Open treatment of radiocarpal or intercarpal dislocation, 1 or more bones
🔲 17.4 ⬡ 17.4 **FUD** 090 [J] [A2] [80] [50] ▣
AMA: 2018,Sep,7

25671 Percutaneous skeletal fixation of distal radioulnar dislocation
🔲 15.1 ⬡ 15.1 **FUD** 090 [J] [A2] [50] ▣
AMA: 2018,Sep,7

25675 Closed treatment of distal radioulnar dislocation with manipulation
🔲 11.3 ⬡ 12.5 **FUD** 090 [T] [A2] [80] [50] ▣
AMA: 2018,Sep,7

25676 Open treatment of distal radioulnar dislocation, acute or chronic
🔲 18.0 ⬡ 18.0 **FUD** 090 [J] [A2] [80] [50] ▣
AMA: 2018,Sep,7

25680 Closed treatment of trans-scaphoperilunar type of fracture dislocation, with manipulation
🔲 15.0 ⬡ 15.0 **FUD** 090 [T] [A2] [80] [50] ▣
AMA: 2018,Sep,7

25685 Open treatment of trans-scaphoperilunar type of fracture dislocation
🔲 21.2 ⬡ 21.2 **FUD** 090 [J] [A2] [80] [50] ▣
AMA: 2018,Sep,7

25690 Closed treatment of lunate dislocation, with manipulation
🔲 13.9 ⬡ 13.9 **FUD** 090 [J] [A2] [80] [50] ▣
AMA: 2018,Sep,7

25695 Open treatment of lunate dislocation
🔲 18.2 ⬡ 18.2 **FUD** 090 [J] [A2] [80] [50] ▣
AMA: 2018,Sep,7

25800-25830 Wrist Fusion

25800 Arthrodesis, wrist; complete, without bone graft (includes radiocarpal and/or intercarpal and/or carpometacarpal joints)
🔲 21.0 ⬡ 21.0 **FUD** 090 [J] [G2] [80] [50] ▣
AMA: 2018,Sep,7

25805 with sliding graft
🔲 24.4 ⬡ 24.4 **FUD** 090 [J] [J8] [80] [50] ▣
AMA: 2018,Sep,7

25810 with iliac or other autograft (includes obtaining graft)
🔲 24.9 ⬡ 24.9 **FUD** 090 [J] [J8] [80] [50] ▣
AMA: 2018,Sep,7

25820 Arthrodesis, wrist; limited, without bone graft (eg, intercarpal or radiocarpal)
🔲 17.8 ⬡ 17.8 **FUD** 090 [J] [J8] [80] [50] ▣
AMA: 2018,Sep,7

25825 with autograft (includes obtaining graft)
🔲 21.9 ⬡ 21.9 **FUD** 090 [J] [J8] [80] [50] ▣
AMA: 2018,Sep,7; 2018,Jan,8; 2017,Jan,8; 2016,Jan,13; 2015,Jan,16; 2014,Jan,11

25830 Arthrodesis, distal radioulnar joint with segmental resection of ulna, with or without bone graft (eg, Sauve-Kapandji procedure)
🔲 27.0 ⬡ 27.0 **FUD** 090 [J] [J8] [80] [50] ▣
AMA: 2018,Sep,7

25900-25999 Amputation Through Forearm/Wrist

25900 Amputation, forearm, through radius and ulna;
🔲 20.4 ⬡ 20.4 **FUD** 090 [C] [80] [50] ▣
AMA: 2018,Sep,7

25905 open, circular (guillotine)
🔲 20.2 ⬡ 20.2 **FUD** 090 [C] [80] [50] ▣
AMA: 2018,Sep,7

25907 secondary closure or scar revision
🔲 17.6 ⬡ 17.6 **FUD** 090 [J] [A2] [80] [50] ▣
AMA: 2018,Sep,7

25909 re-amputation
🔲 19.7 ⬡ 19.7 **FUD** 090 [J] [80] [50] ▣
AMA: 2018,Sep,7

25915 Krukenberg procedure
🔲 33.8 ⬡ 33.8 **FUD** 090 [C] [80] [50] ▣
AMA: 2018,Sep,7

25920 Disarticulation through wrist;
🔲 20.2 ⬡ 20.2 **FUD** 090 [C] [80] [50] ▣
AMA: 2018,Sep,7

25922 secondary closure or scar revision
🔲 17.7 ⬡ 17.7 **FUD** 090 [J] [A2] [80] [50] ▣
AMA: 2018,Sep,7

25924 re-amputation
🔲 19.7 ⬡ 19.7 **FUD** 090 [C] [80] [50] ▣
AMA: 2018,Sep,7

25927 Transmetacarpal amputation;
🔲 23.2 ⬡ 23.2 **FUD** 090 [C] [80] [50] ▣
AMA: 2018,Sep,7

25929 secondary closure or scar revision
🔲 17.1 ⬡ 17.1 **FUD** 090 [T] [A2] [80] [50] ▣
AMA: 2018,Sep,7

25931 re-amputation
🔲 21.3 ⬡ 21.3 **FUD** 090 [J] [G2] [50] ▣
AMA: 2018,Sep,7

25999 Unlisted procedure, forearm or wrist
🔲 0.00 ⬡ 0.00 **FUD** YYY [T] [80] [50] ▣
AMA: 2019,Feb,10; 2018,Sep,7

26010-26037 Incision Hand/Fingers

26010 Drainage of finger abscess; simple
🔲 3.90 ⬡ 7.74 **FUD** 010 [T] [P2] ▣
AMA: 2018,Sep,7

The six synovial sheaths (blue) of the dorsum of the wrist branch into nine extensor tendons

Fibrous sheaths

Synovium

Extensor pollicis longus

Extensor digitorum (five tendons)

Flexor tendons

Tendons typically join in a common synovial sheath

Anatomical "snuffbox"

Extensor retinaculum

Head of ulna

26011 complicated (eg, felon)
🔲 5.28 ⬡ 11.4 **FUD** 010 [J] [A2] ▣
AMA: 2018,Sep,7

26020 Drainage of tendon sheath, digit and/or palm, each
🔲 12.4 ⬡ 12.4 **FUD** 090 [J] [A2] ▣
AMA: 2018,Sep,7

26025 Drainage of palmar bursa; single, bursa
🔲 12.1 ⬡ 12.1 **FUD** 090 [J] [A2] [80] [50] ▣
AMA: 2018,Sep,7

26030 multiple bursa
🔲 14.0 ⬡ 14.0 **FUD** 090 [J] [A2] [80] [50] ▣
AMA: 2018,Sep,7

26034 Incision, bone cortex, hand or finger (eg, osteomyelitis or bone abscess)
🔲 15.6 ⬡ 15.6 **FUD** 090 [J] [A2] ▣
AMA: 2018,Sep,7

● New Code ▲ Revised Code ○ Reinstated ● New Web Release ▲ Revised Web Release + Add-on Unlisted Not Covered # Resequenced
⑤⓪ Optum Mod 50 Exempt Ⓝ AMA Mod 51 Exempt ⑤① Optum Mod 51 Exempt ⑥③ Mod 63 Exempt ⩗ Non-FDA Drug ★ Telemedicine Ⓜ Maternity Ⓐ Age Edit

Musculoskeletal System

26035 — 26123

26035 Decompression fingers and/or hand, injection injury (eg, grease gun)
   🖾 24.7   24.7   **FUD** 090   J G2 80 ▣
    AMA: 2018,Sep,7

26037 Decompressive fasciotomy, hand (excludes 26035)
    EXCLUDES   *Injection injury (26035)*
   🖾 16.2   16.2   **FUD** 090   J G2 80 50 ▣
    AMA: 2018,Sep,7

26040-26045 Incision Palmar Fascia

EXCLUDES   *Enzyme injection fasciotomy (20527, 26341)*
              Fasciectomy (26121, 26123, 26125)

26040 **Fasciotomy, palmar (eg, Dupuytren's contracture); percutaneous**
   🖾 8.96   8.96   **FUD** 090   J A2 50 ▣
    AMA: 2018,Sep,7; 2018,Jan,8; 2017,Jan,8; 2016,Jan,13; 2015,Jan,16; 2014,Jan,11

26045 **open, partial**
   🖾 13.4   13.4   **FUD** 090   J A2 50 ▣
    AMA: 2018,Sep,7; 2018,Jan,8; 2017,Jan,8; 2016,Jan,13; 2015,Jan,16; 2014,Jan,11

26055-26080 Incision Tendon/Joint of Fingers/Hand

26055 **Tendon sheath incision (eg, for trigger finger)**
   🖾 8.91   16.1   **FUD** 090   J A2 ▣
    AMA: 2018,Sep,7

26060 **Tenotomy, percutaneous, single, each digit**
    EXCLUDES   *Arthrocentesis (20610)*
   🖾 7.36   7.36   **FUD** 090   J A2 80 ▣
    AMA: 2018,Sep,7

26070 **Arthrotomy, with exploration, drainage, or removal of loose or foreign body; carpometacarpal joint**
   🖾 9.19   9.19   **FUD** 090   J A2 50 ▣
    AMA: 2018,Sep,7

26075 **metacarpophalangeal joint, each**
   🖾 9.59   9.59   **FUD** 090   J A2 50 ▣
    AMA: 2018,Sep,7; 2018,Jan,8; 2017,Jan,8; 2016,Jan,13; 2015,Jan,16; 2014,Jan,11

26080 **interphalangeal joint, each**
   🖾 11.2   11.2   **FUD** 090   J A2 ▣
    AMA: 2018,Sep,7; 2018,Jan,8; 2017,Jan,8; 2016,Jan,13; 2015,Jan,16; 2014,Jan,11

26100-26110 Arthrotomy with Biopsy of Joint Hand/Fingers

26100 **Arthrotomy with biopsy; carpometacarpal joint, each**
   🖾 9.64   9.64   **FUD** 090   J A2 80 50 ▣
    AMA: 2018,Sep,7

26105 **metacarpophalangeal joint, each**
   🖾 9.71   9.71   **FUD** 090   J A2 80 50 ▣
    AMA: 2018,Sep,7

26110 **interphalangeal joint, each**
   🖾 9.25   9.25   **FUD** 090   J A2 ▣
    AMA: 2018,Sep,7

26111-26118 [26111, 26113] Excision Soft Tissue Tumors Fingers and Hand

INCLUDES   Any necessary elevation of tissue planes or dissection
       Measurement of tumor and necessary margin at greatest diameter prior to excision
       Simple and intermediate repairs
       Types of excision:
           Fascial or subfascial soft tissue tumors: simple and marginal resection of tumors found either in or below the deep fascia, not involving bone or excision of a substantial amount of normal tissue; primarily benign and intramuscular tumors
           Tumors of fingers and toes involving joint capsules, tendons and tendon sheaths
           Radical resection soft tissue tumor: wide resection of tumor, involving substantial margins of normal tissue and may include tissue removal from one or more layers; most often malignant or aggressive benign
           Tumors of fingers and toes adjacent to joints, tendons and tendon sheaths
           Subcutaneous: simple and marginal resection of tumors found in the subcutaneous tissue above the deep fascia; most often benign

EXCLUDES   *Complex repair*
       Excision of benign cutaneous lesions (eg, sebaceous cyst) (11420-11426)
       Radical resection of cutaneous tumors (eg, melanoma) (11620-11626)
       Significant exploration of the vessels or neuroplasty

26111   **Resequenced code. See code following 26115.**

26113   **Resequenced code. See code following 26116.**

26115 **Excision, tumor or vascular malformation, soft tissue of hand or finger, subcutaneous; less than 1.5 cm**
   🖾 9.54   14.8   **FUD** 090   J G2 ▣
    AMA: 2018,Sep,7

\# **26111** **1.5 cm or greater**
   🖾 11.9   11.9   **FUD** 090   J G2 80 ▣
    AMA: 2018,Sep,7

26116 **Excision, tumor, soft tissue, or vascular malformation, of hand or finger, subfascial (eg, intramuscular); less than 1.5 cm**
   🖾 15.1   15.1   **FUD** 090   J G2 ▣
    AMA: 2018,Sep,7; 2018,Jan,8; 2017,Jan,8; 2016,Jan,13; 2015,Jan,16; 2014,Jan,11

\# **26113** **1.5 cm or greater**
   🖾 15.7   15.7   **FUD** 090   J G2 80 ▣
    AMA: 2018,Sep,7

26117 **Radical resection of tumor (eg, sarcoma), soft tissue of hand or finger; less than 3 cm**
   🖾 21.3   21.3   **FUD** 090   J G2 ▣
    AMA: 2018,Sep,7

26118 **3 cm or greater**
   🖾 30.2   30.2   **FUD** 090   J G2 80 ▣
    AMA: 2018,Sep,7

26121-26236 Procedures of Bones, Fascia, Joints and Tendons Hands and Fingers

26121 **Fasciectomy, palm only, with or without Z-plasty, other local tissue rearrangement, or skin grafting (includes obtaining graft)**
    EXCLUDES   *Enzyme injection fasciotomy (20527, 26341)*
              Fasciotomy (26040, 26045)
   🖾 17.1   17.1   **FUD** 090   J A2 50 ▣
    AMA: 2018,Sep,7; 2018,Jan,8; 2017,Jan,8; 2016,Jan,13; 2015,Jan,16; 2014,Jan,11

26123 **Fasciectomy, partial palmar with release of single digit including proximal interphalangeal joint, with or without Z-plasty, other local tissue rearrangement, or skin grafting (includes obtaining graft);**
    EXCLUDES   *Enzyme injection fasciotomy (20527, 26341)*
              Fasciotomy (26040, 26045)
   🖾 24.0   24.0   **FUD** 090   J A2 50 ▣
    AMA: 2018,Sep,7; 2018,Jan,8; 2017,Jan,8; 2016,Jan,13; 2015,Jan,16; 2014,Jan,11

26/**TC** PC/TC Only   **A2-Z3** ASC Payment   **50** Bilateral   ♂ Male Only   ♀ Female Only   🖾 Facility RVU   Non-Facility RVU   ▣ CCI   ☒ CLIA
FUD Follow-up Days   **CMS:** IOM   **AMA:** CPT Asst   **A**-**Y** OPPSI   **80**/**80** Surg Assist Allowed / w/Doc   ◼ Lab Crosswalk   ◼ Radiology Crosswalk

76   CPT © 2019 American Medical Association. All Rights Reserved.   © 2019 Optum360, LLC

+ **26125** **each additional digit (List separately in addition to code for primary procedure)**
> EXCLUDES Enzyme injection fasciotomy (20527, 26341)
> Fasciotomy (26040, 26045)
> Code first (26123)
> 🚑 7.89 ⚕ 7.89 **FUD** ZZZ   N N1
> **AMA:** 2018,Sep,7; 2018,Jan,8; 2017,Jan,8; 2016,Jan,13; 2015,Jan,16; 2014,Jan,11

26130 **Synovectomy, carpometacarpal joint**
> 🚑 13.1 ⚕ 13.1 **FUD** 090   J A2 50
> **AMA:** 2018,Sep,7

26135 **Synovectomy, metacarpophalangeal joint including intrinsic release and extensor hood reconstruction, each digit**
> 🚑 15.8 ⚕ 15.8 **FUD** 090   J A2 80
> **AMA:** 2018,Sep,7

26140 **Synovectomy, proximal interphalangeal joint, including extensor reconstruction, each interphalangeal joint**
> 🚑 14.5 ⚕ 14.5 **FUD** 090   J A2
> **AMA:** 2018,Sep,7

26145 **Synovectomy, tendon sheath, radical (tenosynovectomy), flexor tendon, palm and/or finger, each tendon**
> EXCLUDES Wrist synovectomy (25115-25116)
> 🚑 14.7 ⚕ 14.7 **FUD** 090   J A2
> **AMA:** 2018,Sep,7

26160 **Excision of lesion of tendon sheath or joint capsule (eg, cyst, mucous cyst, or ganglion), hand or finger**
> EXCLUDES Trigger finger (26055)
> Wrist ganglion removal (25111-25112)
> 🚑 9.59 ⚕ 16.6 **FUD** 090   J A2
> **AMA:** 2019,Jul,10; 2018,Sep,7

26170 **Excision of tendon, palm, flexor or extensor, single, each tendon**
> EXCLUDES Excision extensor tendon, with implantation of synthetic rod for delayed tendon graft, hand or finger, each rod (26415)
> Excision flexor tendon, with implantation of synthetic rod for delayed tendon graft, hand or finger, each rod (26390)
> 🚑 11.6 ⚕ 11.6 **FUD** 090   J A2 80
> **AMA:** 2018,Sep,7; 2018,Jan,8; 2017,Jan,8; 2016,Jan,13; 2015,Jan,16

26180 **Excision of tendon, finger, flexor or extensor, each tendon**
> EXCLUDES Excision extensor tendon, with implantation of synthetic rod for delayed tendon graft, hand or finger, each rod (26390)
> Excision flexor tendon, with implantation of synthetic rod for delayed tendon graft, hand or finger, each rod (26390)
> 🚑 12.7 ⚕ 12.7 **FUD** 090   J A2 80
> **AMA:** 2018,Sep,7

26185 **Sesamoidectomy, thumb or finger (separate procedure)**
> 🚑 15.8 ⚕ 15.8 **FUD** 090   J A2 80 50
> **AMA:** 2018,Sep,7

26200 **Excision or curettage of bone cyst or benign tumor of metacarpal;**
> 🚑 12.9 ⚕ 12.9 **FUD** 090   J A2 80
> **AMA:** 2018,Sep,7

26205 **with autograft (includes obtaining graft)**
> 🚑 17.3 ⚕ 17.3 **FUD** 090   J A2
> **AMA:** 2018,Sep,7

26210 **Excision or curettage of bone cyst or benign tumor of proximal, middle, or distal phalanx of finger;**
> 🚑 12.7 ⚕ 12.7 **FUD** 090   J A2
> **AMA:** 2018,Sep,7

26215 **with autograft (includes obtaining graft)**
> 🚑 16.2 ⚕ 16.2 **FUD** 090   J A2
> **AMA:** 2018,Sep,7

26230 **Partial excision (craterization, saucerization, or diaphysectomy) bone (eg, osteomyelitis); metacarpal**
> 🚑 14.3 ⚕ 14.3 **FUD** 090   J A2 80
> **AMA:** 2018,Sep,7

26235 **proximal or middle phalanx of finger**
> 🚑 14.1 ⚕ 14.1 **FUD** 090   J A2 80
> **AMA:** 2019,Jul,10; 2018,Sep,7

26236 **distal phalanx of finger**
> 🚑 12.6 ⚕ 12.6 **FUD** 090   J A2
> **AMA:** 2019,Jul,10; 2018,Sep,7

26250-26262 Radical Resection Bone Tumor of Hand/Finger
> INCLUDES Any necessary elevation of tissue planes or dissection
> Excision of adjacent soft tissue during bone tumor resection (26111-26118 [26111, 26113])
> Measurement of tumor and necessary margin at greatest diameter prior to excision
> Resection of the tumor (may include entire bone) and wide margins of normal tissue primarily for malignant or aggressive benign tumors
> Simple and intermediate repairs
> EXCLUDES Complex repair
> Significant exploration of vessels, neuroplasty, reconstruction, or complex bone repair

26250 **Radical resection of tumor, metacarpal**
> 🚑 30.8 ⚕ 30.8 **FUD** 090   J A2 80
> **AMA:** 2018,Sep,7

26260 **Radical resection of tumor, proximal or middle phalanx of finger**
> 🚑 23.1 ⚕ 23.1 **FUD** 090   J A2 80
> **AMA:** 2018,Sep,7

26262 **Radical resection of tumor, distal phalanx of finger**
> 🚑 18.2 ⚕ 18.2 **FUD** 090   J A2 80
> **AMA:** 2018,Sep,7

26320 Implant Removal Hand/Finger
26320 **Removal of implant from finger or hand**
> EXCLUDES Excision of foreign body (20520, 20525)
> 🚑 9.98 ⚕ 9.98 **FUD** 090   02 A2
> **AMA:** 2018,Sep,7

26340-26548 Repair/Reconstruction of Fingers and Hand
26340 **Manipulation, finger joint, under anesthesia, each joint**
> EXCLUDES Application external fixation (20690, 20692)
> 🚑 9.67 ⚕ 9.67 **FUD** 090   J 62 50
> **AMA:** 2018,Sep,7; 2018,Jan,8; 2017,Jan,8; 2016,Jan,13; 2015,Jan,16; 2014,Jan,11

26341 **Manipulation, palmar fascial cord (ie, Dupuytren's cord), post enzyme injection (eg, collagenase), single cord**
> EXCLUDES Enzyme injection fasciotomy (20527)
> Code also custom orthotic fabrication and/or fitting
> 🚑 2.17 ⚕ 2.90 **FUD** 010   T P3 50
> **AMA:** 2018,Sep,7; 2018,Jan,8; 2017,Jan,8; 2016,Jan,13; 2015,Jan,16; 2014,Jan,11

26350 **Repair or advancement, flexor tendon, not in zone 2 digital flexor tendon sheath (eg, no man's land); primary or secondary without free graft, each tendon**
> 🚑 20.0 ⚕ 20.0 **FUD** 090   J A2
> **AMA:** 2018,Sep,7

26352 **secondary with free graft (includes obtaining graft), each tendon**
> 🚑 23.0 ⚕ 23.0 **FUD** 090   J A2 80
> **AMA:** 2018,Sep,7

26356 **Repair or advancement, flexor tendon, in zone 2 digital flexor tendon sheath (eg, no man's land); primary, without free graft, each tendon**
> 🚑 22.8 ⚕ 22.8 **FUD** 090   J A2
> **AMA:** 2018,Sep,7; 2018,Jan,8; 2017,Dec,14; 2017,Jan,8; 2016,Jan,13; 2015,Jan,16; 2014,Sep,13; 2014,Jan,11

26357 secondary, without free graft, each tendon
25.5 · 25.5 · **FUD** 090 · J A2 80 ▭
AMA: 2018,Sep,7

26358 secondary, with free graft (includes obtaining graft), each tendon
28.3 · 28.3 · **FUD** 090 · J A2 80 ▭
AMA: 2018,Sep,7

26370 Repair or advancement of profundus tendon, with intact superficialis tendon; primary, each tendon
21.2 · 21.2 · **FUD** 090 · J A2 80 ▭
AMA: 2018,Sep,7; 2018,Jan,8; 2017,Jan,8; 2016,Jan,13; 2015,Jan,16; 2014,Jan,11

26372 secondary with free graft (includes obtaining graft), each tendon
25.0 · 25.0 · **FUD** 090 · J A2 80 ▭
AMA: 2018,Sep,7

26373 secondary without free graft, each tendon
23.9 · 23.9 · **FUD** 090 · J A2 80 ▭
AMA: 2018,Sep,7

26390 Excision flexor tendon, with implantation of synthetic rod for delayed tendon graft, hand or finger, each rod
23.6 · 23.6 · **FUD** 090 · J A2 80 ▭
AMA: 2018,Sep,7

26392 Removal of synthetic rod and insertion of flexor tendon graft, hand or finger (includes obtaining graft), each rod
27.5 · 27.5 · **FUD** 090 · J A2 80 ▭
AMA: 2018,Sep,7

26410 Repair, extensor tendon, hand, primary or secondary; without free graft, each tendon
15.8 · 15.8 · **FUD** 090 · J A2 ▭
AMA: 2018,Sep,7

26412 with free graft (includes obtaining graft), each tendon
19.1 · 19.1 · **FUD** 090 · J A2 80 ▭
AMA: 2018,Sep,7

26415 Excision of extensor tendon, with implantation of synthetic rod for delayed tendon graft, hand or finger, each rod
23.0 · 23.0 · **FUD** 090 · J A2 80 ▭
AMA: 2018,Sep,7

26416 Removal of synthetic rod and insertion of extensor tendon graft (includes obtaining graft), hand or finger, each rod
25.0 · 25.0 · **FUD** 090 · J A2 ▭
AMA: 2018,Sep,7; 2018,Jan,8; 2017,Jan,8; 2016,Jan,13; 2015,Jan,16; 2014,Jan,11

26418 Repair, extensor tendon, finger, primary or secondary; without free graft, each tendon
16.2 · 16.2 · **FUD** 090 · J A2 ▭
AMA: 2018,Sep,7; 2018,Jan,8; 2017,Jan,8; 2016,Jan,13; 2015,Jan,16; 2014,Jan,11

26420 with free graft (includes obtaining graft) each tendon
19.9 · 19.9 · **FUD** 090 · J A2 80 ▭
AMA: 2018,Sep,7

26426 Repair of extensor tendon, central slip, secondary (eg, boutonniere deformity); using local tissue(s), including lateral band(s), each finger
14.4 · 14.4 · **FUD** 090 · J A2 ▭
AMA: 2018,Sep,7

26428 with free graft (includes obtaining graft), each finger
21.3 · 21.3 · **FUD** 090 · J A2 80 ▭
AMA: 2018,Sep,7

26432 Closed treatment of distal extensor tendon insertion, with or without percutaneous pinning (eg, mallet finger)
13.9 · 13.9 · **FUD** 090 · J A2 ▭
AMA: 2018,Sep,7

26433 Repair of extensor tendon, distal insertion, primary or secondary; without graft (eg, mallet finger)
EXCLUDES Trigger finger (26055)
14.8 · 14.8 · **FUD** 090 · J A2 ▭
AMA: 2018,Sep,7

26434 with free graft (includes obtaining graft)
EXCLUDES Trigger finger (26055)
18.2 · 18.2 · **FUD** 090 · J A2 80 ▭
AMA: 2018,Sep,7

26437 Realignment of extensor tendon, hand, each tendon
17.5 · 17.5 · **FUD** 090 · J A2 ▭
AMA: 2018,Sep,7

26440 Tenolysis, flexor tendon; palm OR finger, each tendon
17.4 · 17.4 · **FUD** 090 · J A2 ▭
AMA: 2018,Sep,7; 2018,Jan,8; 2017,Jan,8; 2016,Jan,13; 2015,Jun,10; 2015,Jan,16; 2014,Jan,11

26442 palm AND finger, each tendon
27.1 · 27.1 · **FUD** 090 · J A2 ▭
AMA: 2018,Sep,7

26445 Tenolysis, extensor tendon, hand OR finger, each tendon
16.1 · 16.1 · **FUD** 090 · J A2 ▭
AMA: 2018,Sep,7; 2018,Jan,8; 2017,Jan,8; 2016,Jan,13; 2015,Jan,16; 2014,Jan,11

26449 Tenolysis, complex, extensor tendon, finger, including forearm, each tendon
19.9 · 19.9 · **FUD** 090 · J A2 80 ▭
AMA: 2018,Sep,7

26450 Tenotomy, flexor, palm, open, each tendon
11.4 · 11.4 · **FUD** 090 · J A2 80 ▭
AMA: 2018,Sep,7

26455 Tenotomy, flexor, finger, open, each tendon
11.3 · 11.3 · **FUD** 090 · J A2 80 ▭
AMA: 2018,Sep,7

26460 Tenotomy, extensor, hand or finger, open, each tendon
11.1 · 11.1 · **FUD** 090 · J A2 ▭
AMA: 2018,Sep,7

26471 Tenodesis; of proximal interphalangeal joint, each joint
17.3 · 17.3 · **FUD** 090 · J A2 ▭
AMA: 2018,Sep,7

26474 of distal joint, each joint
16.9 · 16.9 · **FUD** 090 · J A2 80 ▭
AMA: 2018,Sep,7

26476 Lengthening of tendon, extensor, hand or finger, each tendon
16.7 · 16.7 · **FUD** 090 · J A2 ▭
AMA: 2018,Sep,7

26477 Shortening of tendon, extensor, hand or finger, each tendon
16.3 · 16.3 · **FUD** 090 · J A2 ▭
AMA: 2018,Sep,7

26478 Lengthening of tendon, flexor, hand or finger, each tendon
17.4 · 17.4 · **FUD** 090 · J A2 80 ▭
AMA: 2018,Sep,7; 2018,Jan,8; 2017,Jan,8; 2016,Jan,13; 2015,Jan,16; 2014,Jan,11

26479 Shortening of tendon, flexor, hand or finger, each tendon
17.6 · 17.6 · **FUD** 090 · J A2 80 ▭
AMA: 2018,Sep,7

26480 Transfer or transplant of tendon, carpometacarpal area or dorsum of hand; without free graft, each tendon
21.1 · 21.1 · **FUD** 090 · J A2 80 ▭
AMA: 2018,Sep,7; 2018,Jan,8; 2017,Jan,8; 2016,Jan,13; 2015,Jan,16; 2014,Jan,11

26483 with free tendon graft (includes obtaining graft), each tendon
23.7 23.7 **FUD** 090 J A2 80
AMA: 2018,Sep,7

26485 Transfer or transplant of tendon, palmar; without free tendon graft, each tendon
22.7 22.7 **FUD** 090 J A2 80
AMA: 2018,Sep,7

26489 with free tendon graft (includes obtaining graft), each tendon
26.4 26.4 **FUD** 090 J A2 80
AMA: 2018,Sep,7

26490 Opponensplasty; superficialis tendon transfer type, each tendon
EXCLUDES *Thumb fusion (26820)*
22.5 22.5 **FUD** 090 J A2 80
AMA: 2018,Sep,7

26492 tendon transfer with graft (includes obtaining graft), each tendon
EXCLUDES *Thumb fusion (26820)*
25.0 25.0 **FUD** 090 J A2 80
AMA: 2018,Sep,7

26494 hypothenar muscle transfer
EXCLUDES *Thumb fusion (26820)*
22.6 22.6 **FUD** 090 J A2 80
AMA: 2018,Sep,7

26496 other methods
EXCLUDES *Thumb fusion (26820)*
24.2 24.2 **FUD** 090 J A2 80
AMA: 2018,Sep,7

26497 Transfer of tendon to restore intrinsic function; ring and small finger
24.5 24.5 **FUD** 090 J A2 80
AMA: 2018,Sep,7

26498 all 4 fingers
32.5 32.5 **FUD** 090 J A2 80
AMA: 2018,Sep,7

26499 Correction claw finger, other methods
23.5 23.5 **FUD** 090 J A2 80
AMA: 2018,Sep,7

26500 Reconstruction of tendon pulley, each tendon; with local tissues (separate procedure)
17.4 17.4 **FUD** 090 J A2 80
AMA: 2018,Sep,7

26502 with tendon or fascial graft (includes obtaining graft) (separate procedure)
20.0 20.0 **FUD** 090 J A2 80
AMA: 2018,Sep,7

26508 Release of thenar muscle(s) (eg, thumb contracture)
17.7 17.7 **FUD** 090 J A2 80 50
AMA: 2018,Sep,7

26510 Cross intrinsic transfer, each tendon
16.7 16.7 **FUD** 090 J A2 80
AMA: 2018,Sep,7

26516 Capsulodesis, metacarpophalangeal joint; single digit
19.7 19.7 **FUD** 090 J A2 80 50
AMA: 2018,Sep,7

26517 2 digits
23.3 23.3 **FUD** 090 J A2 80 50
AMA: 2018,Sep,7

26518 3 or 4 digits
23.6 23.6 **FUD** 090 J A2 80 50
AMA: 2018,Sep,7

26520 Capsulectomy or capsulotomy; metacarpophalangeal joint, each joint
EXCLUDES *Carpometacarpal joint arthroplasty (25447)*
18.2 18.2 **FUD** 090 J A2
AMA: 2018,Sep,7

26525 interphalangeal joint, each joint
EXCLUDES *Carpometacarpal joint arthroplasty (25447)*
18.3 18.3 **FUD** 090 J A2
AMA: 2018,Sep,7; 2018,Jan,8; 2017,Jan,8; 2016,Jan,13; 2015,Jun,10; 2015,Jan,16; 2014,Jan,11

26530 Arthroplasty, metacarpophalangeal joint; each joint
EXCLUDES *Carpometacarpal joint arthroplasty (25447)*
15.4 15.4 **FUD** 090 J A2 80
AMA: 2018,Sep,7

26531 with prosthetic implant, each joint
EXCLUDES *Carpometacarpal joint arthroplasty (25447)*
17.9 17.9 **FUD** 090 J J8 80
AMA: 2018,Sep,7; 2018,Jan,8; 2017,Jan,8; 2016,Jan,13; 2015,Jan,16; 2014,Jan,11

26535 Arthroplasty, interphalangeal joint; each joint
EXCLUDES *Carpometacarpal joint arthroplasty (25447)*
12.3 12.3 **FUD** 090 J A2
AMA: 2018,Sep,7

26536 with prosthetic implant, each joint
EXCLUDES *Carpometacarpal joint arthroplasty (25447)*
20.0 20.0 **FUD** 090 J J8 80
AMA: 2018,Sep,7

26540 Repair of collateral ligament, metacarpophalangeal or interphalangeal joint
18.5 18.5 **FUD** 090 J A2 80
AMA: 2018,Sep,7

26541 Reconstruction, collateral ligament, metacarpophalangeal joint, single; with tendon or fascial graft (includes obtaining graft)
22.5 22.5 **FUD** 090 J A2 80
AMA: 2018,Sep,7; 2018,Jan,8; 2017,Jan,8; 2016,Jan,13; 2015,Jan,16; 2014,Jan,11

26542 with local tissue (eg, adductor advancement)
19.1 19.1 **FUD** 090 J A2 80
AMA: 2018,Sep,7; 2018,Jan,8; 2017,Jan,8; 2016,Jan,13; 2015,Jan,16; 2014,Jan,11

26545 Reconstruction, collateral ligament, interphalangeal joint, single, including graft, each joint
19.9 19.9 **FUD** 090 J A2 80
AMA: 2018,Sep,7

26546 Repair non-union, metacarpal or phalanx (includes obtaining bone graft with or without external or internal fixation)
28.1 28.1 **FUD** 090 J A2 80 50
AMA: 2018,Sep,7

26548 Repair and reconstruction, finger, volar plate, interphalangeal joint
21.4 21.4 **FUD** 090 J A2 80
AMA: 2018,Sep,7

26550-26556 Reconstruction Procedures with Finger and Toe Transplants

26550 Pollicization of a digit
46.8 46.8 **FUD** 090 J A2 80 50
AMA: 2018,Sep,7

26551 Transfer, toe-to-hand with microvascular anastomosis; great toe wrap-around with bone graft
INCLUDES Operating microscope (69990)
EXCLUDES *Big toe with web space (20973)*
94.6 94.6 **FUD** 090 C 80 50
AMA: 2018,Sep,7; 2018,Jan,8; 2017,Jan,8; 2016,Feb,12; 2016,Jan,13; 2015,Jan,16; 2014,Jan,11

● New Code ▲ Revised Code ○ Reinstated ● New Web Release ▲ Revised Web Release + Add-on Unlisted Not Covered # Resequenced
50 Optum Mod 50 Exempt ⚬ AMA Mod 51 Exempt 51 Optum Mod 51 Exempt 63 Mod 63 Exempt ✗ Non-FDA Drug ★ Telemedicine M Maternity A Age Edit

26553 other than great toe, single
INCLUDES Operating microscope (69990)
📷 93.9 ✂ 93.9 **FUD** 090   C 80 50 ▭
AMA: 2018,Sep,7; 2018,Jan,8; 2017,Jan,8; 2016,Feb,12; 2016,Jan,13; 2015,Jan,16; 2014,Jan,11

26554 other than great toe, double
INCLUDES Operating microscope (69990)
📷 109. ✂ 109. **FUD** 090   C 80 50 ▭
AMA: 2018,Sep,7; 2018,Jan,8; 2017,Jan,8; 2016,Feb,12; 2016,Jan,13; 2015,Jan,16; 2014,Jan,11

26555 Transfer, finger to another position without microvascular anastomosis
📷 38.9 ✂ 38.9 **FUD** 090   J A2 80 ▭
AMA: 2018,Sep,7

26556 Transfer, free toe joint, with microvascular anastomosis
INCLUDES Operating microscope (69990)
EXCLUDES Big toe to hand transfer (20973)
📷 97.6 ✂ 97.6 **FUD** 090   C 80 ▭
AMA: 2018,Sep,7; 2018,Jan,8; 2017,Jan,8; 2016,Feb,12; 2016,Jan,13; 2015,Jan,16; 2014,Jan,11

26560-26596 Repair of Other Deformities of the Fingers/Hand

26560 Repair of syndactyly (web finger) each web space; with skin flaps
📷 16.5 ✂ 16.5 **FUD** 090   J A2 80 ▭
AMA: 2018,Sep,7

26561 with skin flaps and grafts
📷 26.8 ✂ 26.8 **FUD** 090   J A2 80 ▭
AMA: 2018,Sep,7

26562 complex (eg, involving bone, nails)
📷 38.1 ✂ 38.1 **FUD** 090   J A2 80 ▭
AMA: 2018,Sep,7

26565 Osteotomy; metacarpal, each
📷 19.0 ✂ 19.0 **FUD** 090   J A2 80 ▭
AMA: 2018,Sep,7

26567 phalanx of finger, each
📷 19.2 ✂ 19.2 **FUD** 090   J A2 80 ▭
AMA: 2018,Sep,7; 2018,Jan,8; 2017,Jan,8; 2016,Jan,13; 2015,Jan,16; 2014,Jan,11

26568 Osteoplasty, lengthening, metacarpal or phalanx
📷 25.4 ✂ 25.4 **FUD** 090   J A2 80 ▭
AMA: 2018,Sep,7

26580 Repair cleft hand
INCLUDES Barsky's procedure
📷 43.0 ✂ 43.0 **FUD** 090   J A2 80 50 ▭
AMA: 2018,Sep,7

26587 Reconstruction of polydactylous digit, soft tissue and bone
EXCLUDES Soft tissue removal only (11200)
📷 30.0 ✂ 30.0 **FUD** 090   J A2 80 ▭
AMA: 2018,Sep,7; 2018,Jan,8; 2017,Jan,8; 2016,Jan,13; 2015,Jan,16; 2014,Jan,11

26590 Repair macrodactylia, each digit
📷 40.0 ✂ 40.0 **FUD** 090   J A2 80 ▭
AMA: 2018,Sep,7; 2018,Jan,8; 2017,Jan,8; 2016,Jan,13; 2015,Jan,16; 2014,Jan,11

26591 Repair, intrinsic muscles of hand, each muscle
📷 12.3 ✂ 12.3 **FUD** 090   J A2 80 ▭
AMA: 2018,Sep,7; 2018,Jan,8; 2017,Jan,8; 2016,Jan,13; 2015,Jan,16; 2014,Jan,11

26593 Release, intrinsic muscles of hand, each muscle
📷 16.9 ✂ 16.9 **FUD** 090   J A2 ▭
AMA: 2018,Sep,7

26596 Excision of constricting ring of finger, with multiple Z-plasties
EXCLUDES Graft repair or scar contracture release (11042, 14040-14041, 15120, 15240)
📷 21.6 ✂ 21.6 **FUD** 090   J A2 80 ▭
AMA: 2018,Sep,7

26600-26785 Treatment of Fracture/Dislocation of Fingers and Hand
INCLUDES Closed, percutaneous, and open treatment of fractures or dislocations

26600 Closed treatment of metacarpal fracture, single; without manipulation, each bone
📷 7.94 ✂ 8.39 **FUD** 090   T P2 ▭
AMA: 2018,Sep,7

26605 with manipulation, each bone
📷 8.38 ✂ 9.24 **FUD** 090   T A2 ▭
AMA: 2018,Sep,7

26607 Closed treatment of metacarpal fracture, with manipulation, with external fixation, each bone
📷 13.4 ✂ 13.4 **FUD** 090   J A2 80 ▭
AMA: 2018,Sep,7

26608 Percutaneous skeletal fixation of metacarpal fracture, each bone
📷 13.7 ✂ 13.7 **FUD** 090   J A2 80 ▭
AMA: 2018,Sep,7

26615 Open treatment of metacarpal fracture, single, includes internal fixation, when performed, each bone
📷 16.5 ✂ 16.5 **FUD** 090   J A2 ▭
AMA: 2018,Sep,7

26641 Closed treatment of carpometacarpal dislocation, thumb, with manipulation
📷 9.72 ✂ 10.7 **FUD** 090   T P2 80 50 ▭
AMA: 2018,Sep,7

26645 Closed treatment of carpometacarpal fracture dislocation, thumb (Bennett fracture), with manipulation
📷 11.2 ✂ 12.3 **FUD** 090   J A2 80 50 ▭
AMA: 2018,Sep,7

26650 Percutaneous skeletal fixation of carpometacarpal fracture dislocation, thumb (Bennett fracture), with manipulation
📷 13.7 ✂ 13.7 **FUD** 090   J A2 50 ▭
AMA: 2018,Sep,7

26665 Open treatment of carpometacarpal fracture dislocation, thumb (Bennett fracture), includes internal fixation, when performed
📷 17.9 ✂ 17.9 **FUD** 090   J A2 50 ▭
AMA: 2018,Sep,7

26670 Closed treatment of carpometacarpal dislocation, other than thumb, with manipulation, each joint; without anesthesia
📷 8.86 ✂ 9.86 **FUD** 090   T P2 80 ▭
AMA: 2018,Sep,7

26675 requiring anesthesia
📷 12.0 ✂ 13.1 **FUD** 090   J A2 80 ▭
AMA: 2018,Sep,7

26676 Percutaneous skeletal fixation of carpometacarpal dislocation, other than thumb, with manipulation, each joint
📷 14.4 ✂ 14.4 **FUD** 090   J A2 ▭
AMA: 2018,Sep,7

26685 Open treatment of carpometacarpal dislocation, other than thumb; includes internal fixation, when performed, each joint
📷 16.4 ✂ 16.4 **FUD** 090   J A2 ▭
AMA: 2018,Sep,7

26686 complex, multiple, or delayed reduction
📷 17.9 ✂ 17.9 **FUD** 090   J A2 80 ▭
AMA: 2018,Sep,7

 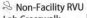

26700 Closed treatment of metacarpophalangeal dislocation, single, with manipulation; without anesthesia
🛠 8.73 ✂ 9.38 **FUD** 090 　 T P2 ▢
AMA: 2018,Sep,7

26705 requiring anesthesia
🛠 10.9 ✂ 11.9 **FUD** 090 　 J A2 80 ▢
AMA: 2018,Sep,7

26706 Percutaneous skeletal fixation of metacarpophalangeal dislocation, single, with manipulation
🛠 12.6 ✂ 12.6 **FUD** 090 　 J A2 ▢
AMA: 2018,Sep,7

26715 Open treatment of metacarpophalangeal dislocation, single, includes internal fixation, when performed
🛠 16.4 ✂ 16.4 **FUD** 090 　 J A2 80 ▢
AMA: 2018,Sep,7

26720 Closed treatment of phalangeal shaft fracture, proximal or middle phalanx, finger or thumb; without manipulation, each
🛠 5.26 ✂ 5.62 **FUD** 090 　 T P2 ▢
AMA: 2018,Sep,7

26725 with manipulation, with or without skin or skeletal traction, each
🛠 8.66 ✂ 9.66 **FUD** 090 　 T P2 ▢
AMA: 2018,Sep,7

26727 Percutaneous skeletal fixation of unstable phalangeal shaft fracture, proximal or middle phalanx, finger or thumb, with manipulation, each
🛠 13.5 ✂ 13.5 **FUD** 090 　 J A2 ▢
AMA: 2018,Sep,7

26735 Open treatment of phalangeal shaft fracture, proximal or middle phalanx, finger or thumb, includes internal fixation, when performed, each
🛠 17.1 ✂ 17.1 **FUD** 090 　 J A2 ▢
AMA: 2018,Sep,7

26740 Closed treatment of articular fracture, involving metacarpophalangeal or interphalangeal joint; without manipulation, each
🛠 6.19 ✂ 6.56 **FUD** 090 　 T P2 ▢
AMA: 2018,Sep,7

26742 with manipulation, each
🛠 9.57 ✂ 10.6 **FUD** 090 　 J A2 ▢
AMA: 2018,Sep,7

26746 Open treatment of articular fracture, involving metacarpophalangeal or interphalangeal joint, includes internal fixation, when performed, each
🛠 21.3 ✂ 21.3 **FUD** 090 　 J A2 ▢
AMA: 2018,Sep,7

26750 Closed treatment of distal phalangeal fracture, finger or thumb; without manipulation, each
🛠 5.28 ✂ 5.25 **FUD** 090 　 T P3 ▢
AMA: 2018,Sep,7

26755 with manipulation, each
🛠 7.77 ✂ 8.99 **FUD** 090 　 T G2 ▢
AMA: 2018,Sep,7

26756 Percutaneous skeletal fixation of distal phalangeal fracture, finger or thumb, each
🛠 11.9 ✂ 11.9 **FUD** 090 　 J A2 80 ▢
AMA: 2018,Sep,7

26765 Open treatment of distal phalangeal fracture, finger or thumb, includes internal fixation, when performed, each
🛠 14.3 ✂ 14.3 **FUD** 090 　 J A2 ▢
AMA: 2018,Sep,7

26770 Closed treatment of interphalangeal joint dislocation, single, with manipulation; without anesthesia
🛠 7.29 ✂ 7.94 **FUD** 090 　 T G2 ▢
AMA: 2018,Sep,7

26775 requiring anesthesia
🛠 9.91 ✂ 10.9 **FUD** 090 　 T P2 ▢
AMA: 2018,Sep,7

26776 Percutaneous skeletal fixation of interphalangeal joint dislocation, single, with manipulation
🛠 12.7 ✂ 12.7 **FUD** 090 　 J A2 ▢
AMA: 2018,Sep,7

26785 Open treatment of interphalangeal joint dislocation, includes internal fixation, when performed, single
🛠 15.7 ✂ 15.7 **FUD** 090 　 J A2 ▢
AMA: 2018,Sep,7

26820-26863 Fusion of Joint(s) of Fingers or Hand

26820 Fusion in opposition, thumb, with autogenous graft (includes obtaining graft)
🛠 22.2 ✂ 22.2 **FUD** 090 　 J J8 80 50 ▢
AMA: 2018,Sep,7

26841 Arthrodesis, carpometacarpal joint, thumb, with or without internal fixation;
🛠 20.4 ✂ 20.4 **FUD** 090 　 J A2 80 50 ▢
AMA: 2018,Sep,7

26842 with autograft (includes obtaining graft)
🛠 22.0 ✂ 22.0 **FUD** 090 　 J A2 80 50 ▢
AMA: 2018,Sep,7

26843 Arthrodesis, carpometacarpal joint, digit, other than thumb, each;
🛠 20.8 ✂ 20.8 **FUD** 090 　 J A2 80 ▢
AMA: 2018,Sep,7; 2018,Jan,8; 2017,Jan,8; 2016,Jan,13; 2015,Jan,16; 2014,Jan,11

26844 with autograft (includes obtaining graft)
🛠 23.1 ✂ 23.1 **FUD** 090 　 J J8 80 ▢
AMA: 2018,Sep,7

26850 Arthrodesis, metacarpophalangeal joint, with or without internal fixation;
🛠 19.4 ✂ 19.4 **FUD** 090 　 J A2 80 ▢
AMA: 2018,Sep,7

26852 with autograft (includes obtaining graft)
🛠 22.4 ✂ 22.4 **FUD** 090 　 J A2 80 ▢
AMA: 2018,Sep,7

26860 Arthrodesis, interphalangeal joint, with or without internal fixation;
🛠 15.9 ✂ 15.9 **FUD** 090 　 J A2 ▢
AMA: 2018,Sep,7; 2018,Jan,8; 2017,Jan,8; 2016,Jan,13; 2015,Jan,16; 2014,Jan,11

+ **26861** each additional interphalangeal joint (List separately in addition to code for primary procedure)
Code first (26860)
🛠 2.98 ✂ 2.98 **FUD** ZZZ 　 N N1 ▢
AMA: 2018,Sep,7; 2018,Jan,8; 2017,Jan,8; 2016,Jan,13; 2015,Jan,16; 2014,Jan,11

26862 with autograft (includes obtaining graft)
🛠 20.4 ✂ 20.4 **FUD** 090 　 J A2 80 ▢
AMA: 2018,Sep,7

+ **26863** with autograft (includes obtaining graft), each additional joint (List separately in addition to code for primary procedure)
Code first (26862)
🛠 6.64 ✂ 6.64 **FUD** ZZZ 　 N N1 80 ▢
AMA: 2018,Sep,7

26910-26989 Amputations and Unlisted Procedures Finger/Hand

26910 Amputation, metacarpal, with finger or thumb (ray amputation), single, with or without interosseous transfer
EXCLUDES Repositioning (26550, 26555)
Transmetacarpal amputation of hand (25927)
🛠 20.4 ✂ 20.4 **FUD** 090 　 J A2 ▢
AMA: 2018,Sep,7

Musculoskeletal System

26951 — 27049

26951 Amputation, finger or thumb, primary or secondary, any joint or phalanx, single, including neurectomies; with direct closure
EXCLUDES *Repair necessitating flaps or grafts (15050-15758)*
Transmetacarpal amputation of hand (25927)
🔧 18.4 🔨 18.4 **FUD** 090 J A2
AMA: 2018,Sep,7

26952 with local advancement flaps (V-Y, hood)
EXCLUDES *Repair necessitating flaps or grafts (15050-15758)*
Transmetacarpal amputation of hand (25927)
🔧 18.1 🔨 18.1 **FUD** 090 J A2
AMA: 2018,Sep,7

26989 Unlisted procedure, hands or fingers
🔧 0.00 🔨 0.00 **FUD** YYY T
AMA: 2018,Sep,7

26990-26992 Incision for Drainage of Pelvis or Hip
EXCLUDES *Simple incision and drainage procedures (10040-10160)*

26990 Incision and drainage, pelvis or hip joint area; deep abscess or hematoma
🔧 18.3 🔨 18.3 **FUD** 090 J A2
AMA: 2018,Sep,7

26991 infected bursa
🔧 15.0 🔨 20.2 **FUD** 090 J A2 80
AMA: 2018,Sep,7

26992 Incision, bone cortex, pelvis and/or hip joint (eg, osteomyelitis or bone abscess)
🔧 27.9 🔨 27.9 **FUD** 090 C 80
AMA: 2018,Sep,7; 2018,Jan,8; 2017,Jan,8; 2016,Jan,13; 2015,Jan,16; 2014,Jan,11

27000-27006 Tenotomy Procedures of Hip

27000 Tenotomy, adductor of hip, percutaneous (separate procedure)
🔧 11.6 🔨 11.6 **FUD** 090 J A2 50
AMA: 2018,Sep,7

27001 Tenotomy, adductor of hip, open
🔧 15.4 🔨 15.4 **FUD** 090 J A2 80 50
AMA: 2018,Sep,7

27003 Tenotomy, adductor, subcutaneous, open, with obturator neurectomy
🔧 17.0 🔨 17.0 **FUD** 090 J A2 80 50
AMA: 2018,Sep,7

27005 Tenotomy, hip flexor(s), open (separate procedure)
🔧 20.8 🔨 20.8 **FUD** 090 C 80 50
AMA: 2018,Sep,7

27006 Tenotomy, abductors and/or extensor(s) of hip, open (separate procedure)
🔧 20.7 🔨 20.7 **FUD** 090 J 80 50
AMA: 2018,Sep,7

27025-27036 Surgical Incision of Hip

27025 Fasciotomy, hip or thigh, any type
🔧 26.3 🔨 26.3 **FUD** 090 C 80 50
AMA: 2018,Sep,7

27027 Decompression fasciotomy(ies), pelvic (buttock) compartment(s) (eg, gluteus medius-minimus, gluteus maximus, iliopsoas, and/or tensor fascia lata muscle), unilateral
🔧 25.4 🔨 25.4 **FUD** 090 J 80 50
AMA: 2018,Sep,7

27030 Arthrotomy, hip, with drainage (eg, infection)
🔧 27.0 🔨 27.0 **FUD** 090 C 80 50
AMA: 2018,Sep,7

27033 Arthrotomy, hip, including exploration or removal of loose or foreign body
🔧 28.0 🔨 28.0 **FUD** 090 J A2 80 50
AMA: 2018,Sep,7; 2018,Jan,8; 2017,Jan,8; 2016,Jan,13; 2015,Jan,16; 2014,Jan,11

27035 Denervation, hip joint, intrapelvic or extrapelvic intra-articular branches of sciatic, femoral, or obturator nerves
EXCLUDES *Transection of obturator nerve (64763, 64766)*
🔧 32.8 🔨 32.8 **FUD** 090 J A2 80 50
AMA: 2018,Sep,7; 2018,Jan,8; 2017,Jan,8; 2016,Jan,13; 2015,Jan,16; 2014,Mar,13

27036 Capsulectomy or capsulotomy, hip, with or without excision of heterotopic bone, with release of hip flexor muscles (ie, gluteus medius, gluteus minimus, tensor fascia latae, rectus femoris, sartorius, iliopsoas)
🔧 29.1 🔨 29.1 **FUD** 090 C 80 50
AMA: 2018,Sep,7

27040-27041 Biopsy of Hip/Pelvis
EXCLUDES *Soft tissue needle biopsy (20206)*

27040 Biopsy, soft tissue of pelvis and hip area; superficial
🔧 5.70 🔨 9.83 **FUD** 010 J A2 50
AMA: 2018,Sep,7

27041 deep, subfascial or intramuscular
🔧 20.1 🔨 20.1 **FUD** 090 J A2 50
AMA: 2018,Sep,7

27043-27059 [27043, 27045, 27059] Excision Soft Tissue Tumors Hip/ Pelvis
INCLUDES Any necessary elevation of tissue planes or dissection
Measurement of tumor and necessary margin at greatest diameter prior to excision
Simple and intermediate repairs
Types of excision:
  Fascial or subfascial soft tissue tumors: simple and marginal resection of tumors found either in or below the deep fascia, not involving bone or excision of a substantial amount of normal tissue; primarily benign and intramuscular tumors
  Radical resection of soft tissue tumor: wide resection of tumor involving substantial margins of normal tissue and may involve tissue removal from one or more layers; mostly malignant or aggressive benign.
  Subcutaneous: simple and marginal resection of tumors found in the subcutaneous tissue above the deep fascia; most often benign
EXCLUDES *Complex repair*
Excision of benign cutaneous lesions (eg, sebaceous cyst) (11400-11406)
Radical resection of cutaneous tumors (eg, melanoma) (11600-11606)
Significant exploration of vessels, neuroplasty, reconstruction, or complex bone repair

27043 Resequenced code. See code following 27047.

27045 Resequenced code. See code following 27048.

27047 Excision, tumor, soft tissue of pelvis and hip area, subcutaneous; less than 3 cm
🔧 10.4 🔨 13.6 **FUD** 090 J 62 50
AMA: 2018,Sep,7

\# **27043** 3 cm or greater
🔧 13.5 🔨 13.5 **FUD** 090 J 62 50
AMA: 2018,Sep,7

27048 Excision, tumor, soft tissue of pelvis and hip area, subfascial (eg, intramuscular); less than 5 cm
🔧 17.6 🔨 17.6 **FUD** 090 J 62 80 50
AMA: 2018,Sep,7

\# **27045** 5 cm or greater
🔧 21.3 🔨 21.3 **FUD** 090 J 62 80 50
AMA: 2018,Sep,7

27049 Radical resection of tumor (eg, sarcoma), soft tissue of pelvis and hip area; less than 5 cm
🔧 38.6 🔨 38.6 **FUD** 090 J 62 80 50
AMA: 2018,Sep,7

27050-27071 Procedures of Bones and Joints of Hip and Pelvis

#	27059	5 cm or greater				
		🚑 52.6	⚕ 52.6	**FUD** 090		J 62 80 50
		AMA: 2018,Sep,7				

27050 Arthrotomy, with biopsy; sacroiliac joint
🚑 11.5　⚕ 11.5　**FUD** 090　　J A2 80 50 📄
AMA: 2018,Sep,7

27052 hip joint
🚑 16.6　⚕ 16.6　**FUD** 090　　J A2 80 50 📄
AMA: 2018,Sep,7

27054 Arthrotomy with synovectomy, hip joint
🚑 19.7　⚕ 19.7　**FUD** 090　　C 80 50 📄
AMA: 2018,Sep,7

27057 Decompression fasciotomy(ies), pelvic (buttock) compartment(s) (eg, gluteus medius-minimus, gluteus maximus, iliopsoas, and/or tensor fascia lata muscle) with debridement of nonviable muscle, unilateral
🚑 29.2　⚕ 29.2　**FUD** 090　　J 80 50 📄
AMA: 2018,Sep,7

27059 *Resequenced code. See code following 27049.*

27060 Excision; ischial bursa
🚑 13.3　⚕ 13.3　**FUD** 090　　J A2 50 📄
AMA: 2018,Sep,7

27062 trochanteric bursa or calcification
EXCLUDES *Arthrocentesis (20610)*
🚑 13.1　⚕ 13.1　**FUD** 090　　J A2 50 📄
AMA: 2018,Sep,7

27065 Excision of bone cyst or benign tumor, wing of ilium, symphysis pubis, or greater trochanter of femur; superficial, includes autograft, when performed
🚑 14.9　⚕ 14.9　**FUD** 090　　J A2 80 50 📄
AMA: 2018,Sep,7

27066 deep (subfascial), includes autograft, when performed
🚑 23.1　⚕ 23.1　**FUD** 090　　J A2 80 50 📄
AMA: 2018,Sep,7

27067 with autograft requiring separate incision
🚑 29.8　⚕ 29.8　**FUD** 090　　J A2 80 50 📄
AMA: 2018,Sep,7

27070 Partial excision, wing of ilium, symphysis pubis, or greater trochanter of femur, (craterization, saucerization) (eg, osteomyelitis or bone abscess); superficial
🚑 24.6　⚕ 24.6　**FUD** 090　　C 80 50 📄
AMA: 2018,Sep,7

27071 deep (subfascial or intramuscular)
🚑 26.6　⚕ 26.6　**FUD** 090　　C 80 50 📄
AMA: 2018,Sep,7

27075-27078 Radical Resection Bone Tumor of Hip/Pelvis

INCLUDES Any necessary elevation of tissue planes or dissection
Excision of adjacent soft tissue during bone tumor resection (27043-27049 [27043, 27045, 27059])
Measurement of tumor and necessary margin at greatest diameter prior to excision
Resection of the tumor (may include entire bone) and wide margins of normal tissue primarily for malignant or aggressive benign tumors
Simple and intermediate repairs
EXCLUDES Complex repair
Significant exploration of vessels, neuroplasty, reconstruction, or complex bone repair

27075 Radical resection of tumor; wing of ilium, 1 pubic or ischial ramus or symphysis pubis
🚑 60.7　⚕ 60.7　**FUD** 090　　C 80 📄
AMA: 2019,May,7; 2018,Sep,7

27076 ilium, including acetabulum, both pubic rami, or ischium and acetabulum
🚑 73.5　⚕ 73.5　**FUD** 090　　C 80 📄
AMA: 2019,May,7; 2018,Sep,7

27077 innominate bone, total
🚑 82.0　⚕ 82.0　**FUD** 090　　C 80 📄
AMA: 2019,May,7; 2018,Sep,7

27078 ischial tuberosity and greater trochanter of femur
🚑 59.8　⚕ 59.8　**FUD** 090　　C 80 50 📄
AMA: 2019,May,7; 2018,Sep,7

27080 Excision of Coccyx

EXCLUDES *Surgical excision of decubitus ulcers (15920, 15922, 15931-15958)*

27080 Coccygectomy, primary
🚑 14.7　⚕ 14.7　**FUD** 090　　J A2 80 📄
AMA: 2018,Sep,7

27086-27091 Removal Foreign Body or Hip Prosthesis

27086 Removal of foreign body, pelvis or hip; subcutaneous tissue
🚑 4.83　⚕ 8.63　**FUD** 010　　J A2 80 50 📄
AMA: 2018,Sep,7; 2018,Jan,8; 2017,Jan,8; 2016,Jan,13; 2015,Jan,16; 2014,Jan,11

27087 deep (subfascial or intramuscular)
🚑 17.6　⚕ 17.6　**FUD** 090　　J A2 80 50 📄
AMA: 2018,Sep,7

A foreign body is removed from the pelvis or hip

27090 Removal of hip prosthesis; (separate procedure)
🚑 23.9　⚕ 23.9　**FUD** 090　　C 80 50 📄
AMA: 2019,May,7; 2018,Sep,7

27091 complicated, including total hip prosthesis, methylmethacrylate with or without insertion of spacer
🚑 46.0　⚕ 46.0　**FUD** 090　　C 80 50 📄
AMA: 2019,May,7; 2018,Sep,7; 2018,Jan,8; 2017,Jan,8; 2016,Jan,13; 2015,Jan,16; 2014,Jan,11

27093-27096 Injection for Arthrogram Hip/Sacroiliac Joint

27093 Injection procedure for hip arthrography; without anesthesia
🔳 (73525)
🚑 2.01　⚕ 5.72　**FUD** 000　　N N1 50 📄
AMA: 2018,Sep,7; 2018,Jan,8; 2017,Jan,8; 2016,Jan,13; 2015,Aug,6; 2015,Jan,16; 2014,Jan,11

27095 with anesthesia
🔳 (73525)
🚑 2.41　⚕ 7.62　**FUD** 000　　N N1 50 📄
AMA: 2018,Sep,7; 2018,Jan,8; 2017,Jan,8; 2016,Jan,13; 2016,Jan,11; 2015,Aug,6; 2015,Jan,16; 2014,Jan,11

27096 Injection procedure for sacroiliac joint, anesthetic/steroid, with image guidance (fluoroscopy or CT) including arthrography when performed

> INCLUDES Confirmation of intra-articular needle placement with CT or fluoroscopy
> Fluoroscopic guidance (77002-77003)
> EXCLUDES *Procedure performed without fluoroscopy or CT guidance (20552)*
> 📟 2.38 ⚕ 4.56 **FUD** 000 B 50 ▢

AMA: 2018,Sep,7; 2018,Jan,8; 2017,Jan,8; 2016,Jan,13; 2015,Aug,6; 2015,Jan,16; 2014,Jan,11

27097-27187 Revision/Reconstruction Hip and Pelvis

> INCLUDES Closed, open and percutaneous treatment of fractures and dislocations

27097 Release or recession, hamstring, proximal
> 📟 19.6 ⚕ 19.6 **FUD** 090 J A2 80 50 ▢
> AMA: 2018,Sep,7

27098 Transfer, adductor to ischium
> 📟 20.0 ⚕ 20.0 **FUD** 090 J A2 80 50 ▢
> AMA: 2018,Sep,7

27100 Transfer external oblique muscle to greater trochanter including fascial or tendon extension (graft)
> INCLUDES Eggers procedure
> 📟 23.6 ⚕ 23.6 **FUD** 090 J A2 80 50 ▢
> AMA: 2018,Sep,7

27105 Transfer paraspinal muscle to hip (includes fascial or tendon extension graft)
> 📟 25.0 ⚕ 25.0 **FUD** 090 J A2 80 50 ▢
> AMA: 2018,Sep,7

27110 Transfer iliopsoas; to greater trochanter of femur
> 📟 28.0 ⚕ 28.0 **FUD** 090 J A2 80 50 ▢
> AMA: 2018,Sep,7

27111 to femoral neck
> 📟 25.9 ⚕ 25.9 **FUD** 090 J A2 80 50 ▢
> AMA: 2018,Sep,7

27120 Acetabuloplasty; (eg, Whitman, Colonna, Haygroves, or cup type)
> 📟 37.5 ⚕ 37.5 **FUD** 090 C 80 50 ▢
> AMA: 2018,Sep,7

27122 resection, femoral head (eg, Girdlestone procedure)
> 📟 31.7 ⚕ 31.7 **FUD** 090 C 80 50 ▢
> AMA: 2018,Sep,7

27125 Hemiarthroplasty, hip, partial (eg, femoral stem prosthesis, bipolar arthroplasty)
> EXCLUDES *Hip replacement following hip fracture (27236)*
> 📟 32.7 ⚕ 32.7 **FUD** 090 C 80 50 ▢
> AMA: 2018,Sep,7; 2018,Jan,8; 2017,Jan,8; 2016,Jan,13; 2015,Jan,16; 2014,Jan,11

Acetabulum remains intact

Prosthesis

27130 Arthroplasty, acetabular and proximal femoral prosthetic replacement (total hip arthroplasty), with or without autograft or allograft
> 📟 39.0 ⚕ 39.0 **FUD** 090 C 80 50 ▢
> AMA: 2019,May,7; 2018,Sep,7; 2018,Jan,8; 2017,Jan,8; 2016,Jan,13; 2015,Jan,16; 2014,Jan,11

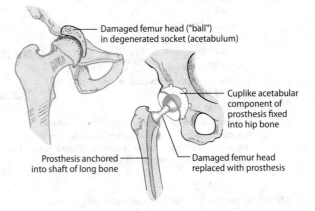

Damaged femur head ("ball") in degenerated socket (acetabulum)

Cuplike acetabular component of prosthesis fixed into hip bone

Prosthesis anchored into shaft of long bone

Damaged femur head replaced with prosthesis

27132 Conversion of previous hip surgery to total hip arthroplasty, with or without autograft or allograft
> 📟 48.3 ⚕ 48.3 **FUD** 090 C 80 50 ▢
> AMA: 2019,May,7; 2018,Sep,7; 2018,Jan,8; 2017,Sep,14; 2017,Jan,8; 2016,Jan,13; 2015,Jan,16; 2014,Jan,11

27134 Revision of total hip arthroplasty; both components, with or without autograft or allograft
> 📟 55.2 ⚕ 55.2 **FUD** 090 C 80 50 ▢
> AMA: 2019,May,7; 2018,Sep,7; 2018,Jan,8; 2017,Jan,8; 2016,Jan,13; 2015,Jan,16; 2014,Jan,11

27137 acetabular component only, with or without autograft or allograft
> 📟 42.4 ⚕ 42.4 **FUD** 090 C 80 50 ▢
> AMA: 2018,Sep,7; 2018,Jan,8; 2017,Jan,8; 2016,Jan,13; 2015,Jan,16; 2014,Jan,11

27138 femoral component only, with or without allograft
> 📟 44.1 ⚕ 44.1 **FUD** 090 C 80 50 ▢
> AMA: 2019,May,7; 2018,Sep,7; 2018,Jan,8; 2017,Jan,8; 2016,Jan,13; 2015,Jan,16; 2014,Jan,11

27140 Osteotomy and transfer of greater trochanter of femur (separate procedure)
> 📟 25.6 ⚕ 25.6 **FUD** 090 C 80 50 ▢
> AMA: 2018,Sep,7

27146 Osteotomy, iliac, acetabular or innominate bone;
> INCLUDES Salter osteotomy
> 📟 36.8 ⚕ 36.8 **FUD** 090 C 80 50 ▢
> AMA: 2018,Sep,7; 2018,Jan,8; 2017,Jan,8; 2016,Jan,13; 2015,Jan,16; 2014,Jan,11

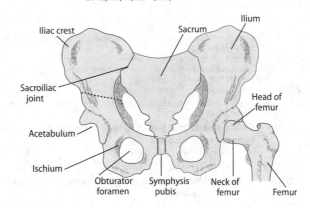

Iliac crest

Sacrum

Ilium

Sacroiliac joint

Acetabulum

Ischium

Head of femur

Obturator foramen

Symphysis pubis

Neck of femur

Femur

27147 **with open reduction of hip**
INCLUDES Pemberton osteotomy
⚙ 42.4 ⚲ 42.4 **FUD** 090
AMA: 2018,Sep,7 ☐C☐80☐50☐

Ilium

Greater trochanter

Acetabulum

Example of innominate osteotomy

Head of femur

Kirschner wires are drilled through the ilium and into lower fragment

Femoral head is reduced into the acetabulum

27151 **with femoral osteotomy**
⚙ 45.9 ⚲ 45.9 **FUD** 090
AMA: 2018,Sep,7 ☐C☐80☐50☐

27156 **with femoral osteotomy and with open reduction of hip**
INCLUDES Chiari osteotomy
⚙ 49.5 ⚲ 49.5 **FUD** 090
AMA: 2018,Sep,7 ☐C☐80☐50☐

27158 **Osteotomy, pelvis, bilateral (eg, congenital malformation)**
⚙ 40.5 ⚲ 40.5 **FUD** 090
AMA: 2018,Sep,7 ☐C☐80☐

27161 **Osteotomy, femoral neck (separate procedure)**
⚙ 35.0 ⚲ 35.0 **FUD** 090
AMA: 2018,Sep,7 ☐C☐80☐50☐

27165 **Osteotomy, intertrochanteric or subtrochanteric including internal or external fixation and/or cast**
⚙ 39.4 ⚲ 39.4 **FUD** 090
AMA: 2018,Sep,7; 2018,Jan,8; 2017,Jan,8; 2016,Jan,13; 2015,Jan,16; 2014,Jan,11 ☐C☐80☐50☐

27170 **Bone graft, femoral head, neck, intertrochanteric or subtrochanteric area (includes obtaining bone graft)**
⚙ 33.8 ⚲ 33.8 **FUD** 090
AMA: 2018,Sep,7; 2018,Jan,8; 2017,Jan,8; 2016,Jan,13; 2015,Jan,16; 2014,Jan,11 ☐C☐80☐50☐

27175 **Treatment of slipped femoral epiphysis; by traction, without reduction**
⚙ 19.2 ⚲ 19.2 **FUD** 090
AMA: 2018,Sep,7 ☐C☐80☐50☐

27176 **by single or multiple pinning, in situ**
⚙ 26.5 ⚲ 26.5 **FUD** 090
AMA: 2018,Sep,7 ☐C☐80☐50☐

27177 **Open treatment of slipped femoral epiphysis; single or multiple pinning or bone graft (includes obtaining graft)**
⚙ 32.2 ⚲ 32.2 **FUD** 090
AMA: 2018,Sep,7 ☐C☐80☐50☐

27178 **closed manipulation with single or multiple pinning**
⚙ 26.5 ⚲ 26.5 **FUD** 090
AMA: 2018,Sep,7 ☐C☐80☐50☐

27179 **osteoplasty of femoral neck (Heyman type procedure)**
⚙ 28.2 ⚲ 28.2 **FUD** 090
AMA: 2018,Sep,7 ☐J☐80☐50☐

27181 **osteotomy and internal fixation**
⚙ 32.4 ⚲ 32.4 **FUD** 090
AMA: 2018,Sep,7 ☐C☐80☐50☐

27185 **Epiphyseal arrest by epiphysiodesis or stapling, greater trochanter of femur**
⚙ 20.7 ⚲ 20.7 **FUD** 090
AMA: 2018,Sep,7 ☐C☐50☐

27187 **Prophylactic treatment (nailing, pinning, plating or wiring) with or without methylmethacrylate, femoral neck and proximal femur**
⚙ 28.6 ⚲ 28.6 **FUD** 090
AMA: 2018,Sep,7; 2018,Jan,8; 2017,Jan,8; 2016,Jan,13; 2015,Jan,16; 2014,Jan,11 ☐C☐80☐50☐

27197-27269 Treatment of Fracture/Dislocation Hip/Pelvis

27197 **Closed treatment of posterior pelvic ring fracture(s), dislocation(s), diastasis or subluxation of the ilium, sacroiliac joint, and/or sacrum, with or without anterior pelvic ring fracture(s) and/or dislocation(s) of the pubic symphysis and/or superior/inferior rami, unilateral or bilateral; without manipulation**
⚙ 3.57 ⚲ 3.57 **FUD** 000
AMA: 2018,Sep,7; 2018,Jan,8; 2017,Jun,9 ☐T☐62☐

27198 **with manipulation, requiring more than local anesthesia (ie, general anesthesia, moderate sedation, spinal/epidural)**
EXCLUDES Closed treatment anterior pelvic ring, pubic symphysis, inferior rami fracture/dislocation--see appropriate E&M codes
⚙ 8.67 ⚲ 8.67 **FUD** 000
AMA: 2018,Sep,7; 2018,Jan,3; 2018,Jan,8; 2017,Jun,9 ☐T☐62☐80☐

27200 **Closed treatment of coccygeal fracture**
⚙ 5.39 ⚲ 5.26 **FUD** 090
AMA: 2018,Sep,7 ☐T☐P3☐

27202 **Open treatment of coccygeal fracture**
⚙ 15.3 ⚲ 15.3 **FUD** 090
AMA: 2018,Sep,7 ☐J☐A2☐80☐

27215 **Open treatment of iliac spine(s), tuberosity avulsion, or iliac wing fracture(s), unilateral, for pelvic bone fracture patterns that do not disrupt the pelvic ring, includes internal fixation, when performed**
⚙ 18.0 ⚲ 18.0 **FUD** 090
AMA: 2018,Sep,7 ☐E☐

27216 **Percutaneous skeletal fixation of posterior pelvic bone fracture and/or dislocation, for fracture patterns that disrupt the pelvic ring, unilateral (includes ipsilateral ilium, sacroiliac joint and/or sacrum)**
EXCLUDES Sacroiliac joint arthrodesis without fracture and/or dislocation, percutaneous or minimally invasive (27279)
⚙ 26.7 ⚲ 26.7 **FUD** 090
AMA: 2018,Sep,7; 2018,Jan,8; 2017,Jan,8; 2016,Jan,13; 2015,Jan,16; 2014,Mar,4 ☐E☐

27217 **Open treatment of anterior pelvic bone fracture and/or dislocation for fracture patterns that disrupt the pelvic ring, unilateral, includes internal fixation, when performed (includes pubic symphysis and/or ipsilateral superior/inferior rami)**
⚙ 25.0 ⚲ 25.0 **FUD** 090
AMA: 2018,Sep,7 ☐E☐

27218 Open treatment of posterior pelvic bone fracture and/or dislocation, for fracture patterns that disrupt the pelvic ring, unilateral, includes internal fixation, when performed (includes ipsilateral ilium, sacroiliac joint and/or sacrum)

EXCLUDES *Sacroiliac joint arthrodesis without fracture and/or dislocation, percutaneous or minimally invasive (27279)*

🔧 34.6   ⚕ 34.6   **FUD** 090   E 🖵

AMA: 2018,Sep,7; 2018,Jan,8; 2017,Jan,8; 2016,Jan,13; 2015,Jan,16; 2014,Mar,4

27220 Closed treatment of acetabulum (hip socket) fracture(s); without manipulation

🔧 15.1   ⚕ 15.3   **FUD** 090   T 62 50 🖵

AMA: 2018,Sep,7

27222 with manipulation, with or without skeletal traction

🔧 28.0   ⚕ 28.0   **FUD** 090   C 50 🖵

AMA: 2018,Sep,7

27226 Open treatment of posterior or anterior acetabular wall fracture, with internal fixation

🔧 30.4   ⚕ 30.4   **FUD** 090   C 80 50 🖵

AMA: 2018,Sep,7

27227 Open treatment of acetabular fracture(s) involving anterior or posterior (one) column, or a fracture running transversely across the acetabulum, with internal fixation

🔧 47.9   ⚕ 47.9   **FUD** 090   C 80 50 🖵

AMA: 2018,Sep,7

27228 Open treatment of acetabular fracture(s) involving anterior and posterior (two) columns, includes T-fracture and both column fracture with complete articular detachment, or single column or transverse fracture with associated acetabular wall fracture, with internal fixation

🔧 54.3   ⚕ 54.3   **FUD** 090   C 80 50 🖵

AMA: 2018,Sep,7

27230 Closed treatment of femoral fracture, proximal end, neck; without manipulation

🔧 13.5   ⚕ 13.7   **FUD** 090   T A2 50 🖵

AMA: 2018,Sep,7

27232 with manipulation, with or without skeletal traction

🔧 21.4   ⚕ 21.4   **FUD** 090   C 50 🖵

AMA: 2018,Sep,7

27235 Percutaneous skeletal fixation of femoral fracture, proximal end, neck

🔧 26.2   ⚕ 26.2   **FUD** 090   J 50 🖵

AMA: 2018,Sep,7; 2018,Jan,8; 2017,Jan,8; 2016,Jan,13; 2015,Jan,16; 2014,Jan,11

27236 Open treatment of femoral fracture, proximal end, neck, internal fixation or prosthetic replacement

🔧 34.4   ⚕ 34.4   **FUD** 090   C 80 50 🖵

AMA: 2019,May,7; 2018,Sep,7; 2018,Jan,8; 2017,Jan,8; 2016,Nov,9; 2016,Jan,13; 2015,Jan,16; 2014,Jan,11

27238 Closed treatment of intertrochanteric, peritrochanteric, or subtrochanteric femoral fracture; without manipulation

🔧 13.2   ⚕ 13.2   **FUD** 090   J A2 50 🖵

AMA: 2018,Sep,7; 2018,Jan,8; 2017,Jan,8; 2016,Jan,13; 2015,Jan,16; 2014,Jan,11

27240 with manipulation, with or without skin or skeletal traction

🔧 27.6   ⚕ 27.6   **FUD** 090   C 50 🖵

AMA: 2018,Sep,7; 2018,Jan,8; 2017,Jan,8; 2016,Jan,13; 2015,Jan,16; 2014,Jan,11

27244 Treatment of intertrochanteric, peritrochanteric, or subtrochanteric femoral fracture; with plate/screw type implant, with or without cerclage

🔧 35.5   ⚕ 35.5   **FUD** 090   C 80 50 🖵

AMA: 2019,May,7; 2018,Sep,7; 2018,Jan,8; 2017,Jan,8; 2016,Jan,13; 2015,Jan,16; 2014,Jan,11

27245 with intramedullary implant, with or without interlocking screws and/or cerclage

🔧 35.4   ⚕ 35.4   **FUD** 090   C 80 50 🖵

AMA: 2018,Sep,7; 2018,Jan,8; 2017,Jan,8; 2016,Jan,13; 2015,Jan,16; 2014,Jan,11

27246 Closed treatment of greater trochanteric fracture, without manipulation

🔧 11.0   ⚕ 11.1   **FUD** 090   T A2 50 🖵

AMA: 2018,Sep,7

27248 Open treatment of greater trochanteric fracture, includes internal fixation, when performed

🔧 21.4   ⚕ 21.4   **FUD** 090   C 80 50 🖵

AMA: 2018,Sep,7

27250 Closed treatment of hip dislocation, traumatic; without anesthesia

🔧 5.17   ⚕ 5.17   **FUD** 000   T A2 50 🖵

AMA: 2018,Sep,7

27252 requiring anesthesia

🔧 21.8   ⚕ 21.8   **FUD** 090   J A2 50 🖵

AMA: 2018,Sep,7

27253 Open treatment of hip dislocation, traumatic, without internal fixation

🔧 27.1   ⚕ 27.1   **FUD** 090   C 80 50 🖵

AMA: 2018,Sep,7

27254 Open treatment of hip dislocation, traumatic, with acetabular wall and femoral head fracture, with or without internal or external fixation

EXCLUDES *Acetabular fracture treatment (27226-27227)*

🔧 36.4   ⚕ 36.4   **FUD** 090   C 80 50 🖵

AMA: 2018,Sep,7

27256 Treatment of spontaneous hip dislocation (developmental, including congenital or pathological), by abduction, splint or traction; without anesthesia, without manipulation

🔧 6.78   ⚕ 8.73   **FUD** 010   T 62 80 50 🖵

AMA: 2018,Sep,7

27257 with manipulation, requiring anesthesia

🔧 10.4   ⚕ 10.4   **FUD** 010   J A2 80 50 🖵

AMA: 2018,Sep,7

27258 Open treatment of spontaneous hip dislocation (developmental, including congenital or pathological), replacement of femoral head in acetabulum (including tenotomy, etc);

INCLUDES Lorenz's operation

🔧 32.1   ⚕ 32.1   **FUD** 090   C 80 50 🖵

AMA: 2018,Sep,7

27259 with femoral shaft shortening

🔧 44.8   ⚕ 44.8   **FUD** 090   C 80 50 🖵

AMA: 2018,Sep,7

27265 Closed treatment of post hip arthroplasty dislocation; without anesthesia

🔧 11.5   ⚕ 11.5   **FUD** 090   T A2 50 🖵

AMA: 2018,Sep,7

27266 requiring regional or general anesthesia

🔧 16.7   ⚕ 16.7   **FUD** 090   J A2 50 🖵

AMA: 2018,Sep,7

27267 Closed treatment of femoral fracture, proximal end, head; without manipulation

🔧 12.4   ⚕ 12.4   **FUD** 090   J 62 80 50 🖵

AMA: 2018,Sep,7; 2018,Jan,8; 2017,Jan,8; 2016,Jan,13; 2015,Jan,16; 2014,Jan,11

27268 with manipulation

🔧 15.5   ⚕ 15.5   **FUD** 090   C 80 50 🖵

AMA: 2018,Sep,7; 2018,Jan,8; 2017,Jan,8; 2016,Jan,13; 2015,Jan,16; 2014,Jan,11

26/TC PC/TC Only   A2-Z3 ASC Payment   50 Bilateral   ♂ Male Only   ♀ Female Only   🔧 Facility RVU   ⚕ Non-Facility RVU   🖵 CCI   ⊠ CLIA
FUD Follow-up Days   CMS: IOM   AMA: CPT Asst   A-Y OPPSI   80/80 Surg Assist Allowed / w/Doc   Lab Crosswalk   Radiology Crosswalk

86   CPT © 2019 American Medical Association. All Rights Reserved.   © 2019 Optum360, LLC

27269 Open treatment of femoral fracture, proximal end, head, includes internal fixation, when performed

EXCLUDES Arthrotomy, hip (27033)

Open treatment of hip dislocation, traumatic, without internal fixation (27253)

⏱ 35.8 ⚕ 35.8 **FUD** 090 C 80 50 ▣

AMA: 2018,Sep,7; 2018,Jan,8; 2017,Jan,8; 2016,Jan,13; 2015,Jan,16; 2014,Jan,11

27275 Hip Manipulation with Anesthesia

27275 Manipulation, hip joint, requiring general anesthesia

⏱ 5.27 ⚕ 5.27 **FUD** 010 J A2 ▣

AMA: 2018,Sep,7; 2018,Jan,8; 2017,Jan,8; 2016,May,13; 2016,Jan,11; 2016,Jan,13; 2015,Jan,16; 2014,Jan,11

27279-27286 Arthrodesis of Hip and Pelvis

27279 Arthrodesis, sacroiliac joint, percutaneous or minimally invasive (indirect visualization), with image guidance, includes obtaining bone graft when performed, and placement of transfixing device

⏱ 19.9 ⚕ 19.9 **FUD** 090 J J8 80 50 ▣

AMA: 2018,Sep,7

27280 Arthrodesis, open, sacroiliac joint, including obtaining bone graft, including instrumentation, when performed

EXCLUDES Sacroiliac joint arthrodesis without fracture and/or dislocation, percutaneous or minimally invasive (27279)

⏱ 39.2 ⚕ 39.2 **FUD** 090 C 80 50 ▣

AMA: 2018,Sep,7; 2018,Jan,8; 2017,Jan,8; 2016,Jan,13; 2015,Jan,16; 2014,Mar,4; 2014,Jan,11

27282 Arthrodesis, symphysis pubis (including obtaining graft)

⏱ 24.7 ⚕ 24.7 **FUD** 090 C 80 ▣

AMA: 2018,Sep,7

27284 Arthrodesis, hip joint (including obtaining graft);

⏱ 46.7 ⚕ 46.7 **FUD** 090 C 80 50 ▣

AMA: 2018,Sep,7

27286 with subtrochanteric osteotomy

⏱ 47.7 ⚕ 47.7 **FUD** 090 C 80 50 ▣

AMA: 2018,Sep,7; 2018,Jan,8; 2017,Jan,8; 2016,Jan,13; 2015,Jan,16; 2014,Jan,11

27290-27299 Amputations and Unlisted Procedures of Hip and Pelvis

27290 Interpelviabdominal amputation (hindquarter amputation)

INCLUDES Pean's amputation

⏱ 47.0 ⚕ 47.0 **FUD** 090 C 80 ▣

AMA: 2018,Sep,7; 2018,Jan,8; 2017,Jan,8; 2016,Jan,13; 2015,Jan,16; 2014,Jan,11

27295 Disarticulation of hip

⏱ 36.3 ⚕ 36.3 **FUD** 090 C 80 50 ▣

AMA: 2018,Sep,7; 2018,Jan,8; 2017,Jan,8; 2016,Jan,13; 2015,Jan,16; 2014,Jan,11

27299 Unlisted procedure, pelvis or hip joint

⏱ 0.00 ⚕ 0.00 **FUD** YYY T 80 50 ▣

AMA: 2018,Sep,7; 2018,Jan,8; 2017,Jan,8; 2016,Jun,8; 2016,Jan,13; 2015,Jan,16; 2014,Mar,13; 2014,Jan,11

27301-27310 Incisional Procedures Femur or Knee

EXCLUDES Superficial incision and drainage (10040-10160)

27301 Incision and drainage, deep abscess, bursa, or hematoma, thigh or knee region

⏱ 14.5 ⚕ 19.3 **FUD** 090 J A2 50 ▣

AMA: 2018,Sep,7; 2018,Jan,8; 2017,Jan,8; 2016,Jan,13; 2015,Jan,16; 2014,Jan,11

27303 Incision, deep, with opening of bone cortex, femur or knee (eg, osteomyelitis or bone abscess)

⏱ 18.4 ⚕ 18.4 **FUD** 090 C 80 50 ▣

AMA: 2018,Sep,7

27305 Fasciotomy, iliotibial (tenotomy), open

EXCLUDES Ober-Yount (gluteal-iliotibial) fasciotomy (27025)

⏱ 13.8 ⚕ 13.8 **FUD** 090 J A2 80 50 ▣

AMA: 2018,Sep,7

27306 Tenotomy, percutaneous, adductor or hamstring; single tendon (separate procedure)

⏱ 9.89 ⚕ 9.89 **FUD** 090 J A2 80 50 ▣

AMA: 2018,Sep,7; 2018,Jan,8; 2017,Aug,9

27307 multiple tendons

⏱ 13.8 ⚕ 13.8 **FUD** 090 J A2 80 50 ▣

AMA: 2018,Sep,7; 2018,Jan,8; 2017,Aug,9

27310 Arthrotomy, knee, with exploration, drainage, or removal of foreign body (eg, infection)

⏱ 21.0 ⚕ 21.0 **FUD** 090 J A2 80 50 ▣

AMA: 2018,Sep,7; 2018,Jan,8; 2017,Jan,8; 2016,Jan,13; 2015,Jan,16; 2014,Jan,11

27323-27324 Biopsy Femur or Knee

EXCLUDES Soft tissue needle biopsy (20206)

27323 Biopsy, soft tissue of thigh or knee area; superficial

⏱ 5.15 ⚕ 7.91 **FUD** 010 J A2 50 ▣

AMA: 2018,Sep,7; 2018,Jan,8; 2017,Jan,8; 2016,Jan,13; 2015,Jan,16; 2014,Jan,11

27324 deep (subfascial or intramuscular)

⏱ 11.5 ⚕ 11.5 **FUD** 090 J A2 50 ▣

AMA: 2018,Sep,7; 2018,Jan,8; 2017,Jan,8; 2016,Jan,13; 2015,Jan,16; 2014,Jan,11

27325-27326 Neurectomy

27325 Neurectomy, hamstring muscle

⏱ 16.1 ⚕ 16.1 **FUD** 090 J A2 80 50 ▣

AMA: 2018,Sep,7

27326 Neurectomy, popliteal (gastrocnemius)

⏱ 14.8 ⚕ 14.8 **FUD** 090 J A2 80 50 ▣

AMA: 2018,Sep,7

27327-27329 [27337, 27339] Excision Soft Tissue Tumors Femur/ Knee

INCLUDES Any necessary elevation of tissue planes or dissection

Measurement of tumor and necessary margin at greatest diameter prior to excision

Simple and intermediate repairs

Types of excision:

Fascial or subfascial soft tissue tumors: simple and marginal resection of tumors found either in or below the deep fascia, not including bone or excision of a substantial amount of normal tissue; primarily benign and intramuscular tumors

Radical resection of soft tissue tumor: wide resection of tumor involving substantial margins of normal tissue and may involve tissue removal from one or more layers; most often malignant or aggressive benign

Subcutaneous: simple and marginal resection of tumors in the subcutaneous tissue above the deep fascia; most often benign

EXCLUDES Complex repair

Excision of benign cutaneous lesions (eg, sebaceous cyst) (11400-11406)

Radical resection of cutaneous tumors (eg, melanoma) (11600-11606)

Significant exploration of vessels or neuroplasty

27327 Excision, tumor, soft tissue of thigh or knee area, subcutaneous; less than 3 cm

⏱ 9.00 ⚕ 13.5 **FUD** 090 J 62 50 ▣

AMA: 2018,Sep,7

\# **27337** 3 cm or greater

⏱ 12.0 ⚕ 12.0 **FUD** 090 J 62 80 50 ▣

AMA: 2018,Sep,7

27328 Excision, tumor, soft tissue of thigh or knee area, subfascial (eg, intramuscular); less than 5 cm

⏱ 17.9 ⚕ 17.9 **FUD** 090 J 62 50 ▣

AMA: 2018,Sep,7; 2018,Jan,8; 2017,Jan,8; 2016,Nov,9

27329 Resequenced code. See code following 27360.

● New Code ▲ Revised Code ○ Reinstated ● New Web Release ▲ Revised Web Release + Add-on Unlisted Not Covered # Resequenced
50 Optum Mod 50 Exempt Ⓢ AMA Mod 51 Exempt 51 Optum Mod 51 Exempt 63 Mod 63 Exempt ✗ Non-FDA Drug ★ Telemedicine M Maternity A Age Edit

CPT © 2019 American Medical Association. All Rights Reserved.

 # 27339   **5 cm or greater**
    21.7   21.7   **FUD** 090   J G2 80 50
    AMA: 2018,Sep,7

27330-27360 Resection Procedures Thigh/Knee

27330   **Arthrotomy, knee; with synovial biopsy only**
    11.9   11.9   **FUD** 090   J A2 50
    AMA: 2018,Sep,7; 2018,Jan,8; 2017,Jan,8; 2016,Jan,13; 2015,Jan,16; 2014,Jan,11

27331   **including joint exploration, biopsy, or removal of loose or foreign bodies**
    13.6   13.6   **FUD** 090   J A2 80 50
    AMA: 2018,Sep,7; 2018,Jan,8; 2017,Jan,8; 2016,Jan,13; 2015,Jan,16; 2014,Jan,11

27332   **Arthrotomy, with excision of semilunar cartilage (meniscectomy) knee; medial OR lateral**
    18.5   18.5   **FUD** 090   J A2 80 50
    AMA: 2018,Sep,7

Lateral meniscus / Posterior cruciate ligament / Medial meniscus / Anterior horns / Patellar ligament / Anterior cruciate ligament / Posterior horns

Overhead view of right knee

Bucket handle tear

Radial tear

Meniscus

27333   **medial AND lateral**
    16.8   16.8   **FUD** 090   J A2 80 50
    AMA: 2018,Sep,7; 2018,Jan,8; 2017,Jan,8; 2016,Jan,13; 2015,Jan,16; 2014,Jan,11

27334   **Arthrotomy, with synovectomy, knee; anterior OR posterior**
    19.7   19.7   **FUD** 090   J A2 80 50
    AMA: 2018,Sep,7

27335   **anterior AND posterior including popliteal area**
    21.9   21.9   **FUD** 090   J A2 80 50
    AMA: 2018,Sep,7

27337   Resequenced code. See code following 27327.

27339   Resequenced code. See code before 27330.

27340   **Excision, prepatellar bursa**
    10.6   10.6   **FUD** 090   J A2 50
    AMA: 2018,Sep,7

27345   **Excision of synovial cyst of popliteal space (eg, Baker's cyst)**
    13.8   13.8   **FUD** 090   J A2 80 50
    AMA: 2018,Sep,7

27347   **Excision of lesion of meniscus or capsule (eg, cyst, ganglion), knee**
    15.1   15.1   **FUD** 090   J A2 80 50
    AMA: 2018,Sep,7

27350   **Patellectomy or hemipatellectomy**
    18.7   18.7   **FUD** 090   J A2 80 50
    AMA: 2018,Sep,7

27355   **Excision or curettage of bone cyst or benign tumor of femur;**
    17.4   17.4   **FUD** 090   J A2 80 50
    AMA: 2018,Sep,7

27356   **with allograft**
    21.3   21.3   **FUD** 090   J G2 80 50
    AMA: 2019,May,7; 2018,Sep,7

27357   **with autograft (includes obtaining graft)**
    23.4   23.4   **FUD** 090   J A2 80 50
    AMA: 2018,Sep,7; 2018,Jan,8; 2017,Jan,8; 2016,Jan,13; 2015,Jan,16; 2014,Jan,11

+ 27358   **with internal fixation (List in addition to code for primary procedure)**
    Code first (27355-27357)
    8.07   8.07   **FUD** ZZZ   N N1 80
    AMA: 2018,Sep,7

27360   **Partial excision (craterization, saucerization, or diaphysectomy) bone, femur, proximal tibia and/or fibula (eg, osteomyelitis or bone abscess)**
    24.7   24.7   **FUD** 090   J A2 80 50
    AMA: 2018,Sep,7

27329-27365 [27329] Radical Resection Tumor Knee/Thigh

INCLUDES Any necessary elevation of tissue planes or dissection
Excision of adjacent soft tissue during bone tumor resection
Measurement of tumor and necessary margin at greatest diameter prior to excision
Radical resection of bone tumor: resection of the tumor (may include entire bone) and wide margins of normal tissue primarily for malignant or aggressive benign tumors
Radical resection of soft tissue tumor: wide resection of tumor involving substantial margins of normal tissue that may include tissue removal from one or more layers; most often malignant or aggressive benign
Simple and intermediate repairs
EXCLUDES Complex repair
Radical resection of cutaneous tumors (eg, melanoma) (11600-11606)
Significant exploration of vessels, neuroplasty, reconstruction, or complex bone repair

 # 27329   **Radical resection of tumor (eg, sarcoma), soft tissue of thigh or knee area; less than 5 cm**
    29.9   29.9   **FUD** 090   J G2 80 50
    AMA: 2018,Sep,7

27364   **5 cm or greater**
    45.2   45.2   **FUD** 090   J G2 80 50
    AMA: 2018,Sep,7

27365   **Radical resection of tumor, femur or knee**
    EXCLUDES Soft tissue tumor excision thigh or knee area (27329, 27364)
    59.6   59.6   **FUD** 090   C 80 50
    AMA: 2019,May,7; 2018,Sep,7

27369 Injection for Arthrogram of Knee

EXCLUDES Arthrocentesis, aspiration and/or injection, knee (20610-20611)
Arthroscopy, knee (29871)

27369   **Injection procedure for contrast knee arthrography or contrast enhanced CT/MRI knee arthrography**
    Code also fluoroscopic guidance, when performed for CT arthrography (73701-73702, 77002)
    (73580, 73701-73702, 73722-73723)
    1.17   4.06   **FUD** 000   N1 50
    AMA: 2019,Aug,7

27372 Foreign Body Removal Femur or Knee

EXCLUDES Arthroscopic procedures (29870-29887)
Removal knee prosthesis (27488)

27372   **Removal of foreign body, deep, thigh region or knee area**
    11.4   17.0   **FUD** 090   J A2 80 50
    AMA: 2018,Sep,7

27380-27499 Repair/Reconstruction of Femur or Knee

27380 Suture of infrapatellar tendon; primary
🚑 17.1 🔗 17.1 **FUD** 090 ⬛J A2 80 50 📁
AMA: 2018,Sep,7

27381 secondary reconstruction, including fascial or tendon graft
🚑 23.0 🔗 23.0 **FUD** 090 ⬛J A2 80 50 📁
AMA: 2018,Sep,7

27385 Suture of quadriceps or hamstring muscle rupture; primary
🚑 16.6 🔗 16.6 **FUD** 090 ⬛J A2 80 50 📁
AMA: 2018,Sep,7; 2018,Jan,8; 2017,Aug,9

27386 secondary reconstruction, including fascial or tendon graft
🚑 23.9 🔗 23.9 **FUD** 090 ⬛J A2 80 50 📁
AMA: 2018,Sep,7

27390 Tenotomy, open, hamstring, knee to hip; single tendon
🚑 12.9 🔗 12.9 **FUD** 090 ⬛J A2 80 50 📁
AMA: 2018,Sep,7

27391 multiple tendons, 1 leg
🚑 16.4 🔗 16.4 **FUD** 090 ⬛J A2 80 📁
AMA: 2018,Sep,7

27392 multiple tendons, bilateral
🚑 20.5 🔗 20.5 **FUD** 090 ⬛J A2 80 📁
AMA: 2018,Sep,7

27393 Lengthening of hamstring tendon; single tendon
🚑 14.6 🔗 14.6 **FUD** 090 ⬛J A2 80 50 📁
AMA: 2018,Sep,7

27394 multiple tendons, 1 leg
🚑 18.5 🔗 18.5 **FUD** 090 ⬛J A2 80 📁
AMA: 2018,Sep,7

27395 multiple tendons, bilateral
🚑 25.3 🔗 25.3 **FUD** 090 ⬛J A2 80 📁
AMA: 2018,Sep,7

27396 Transplant or transfer (with muscle redirection or rerouting), thigh (eg, extensor to flexor); single tendon
🚑 17.7 🔗 17.7 **FUD** 090 ⬛J J8 80 50 📁
AMA: 2018,Sep,7

27397 multiple tendons
🚑 26.4 🔗 26.4 **FUD** 090 ⬛J G2 80 50 📁
AMA: 2018,Sep,7

27400 Transfer, tendon or muscle, hamstrings to femur (eg, Egger's type procedure)
🚑 20.0 🔗 20.0 **FUD** 090 ⬛J A2 80 50 📁
AMA: 2018,Sep,7

27403 Arthrotomy with meniscus repair, knee
EXCLUDES *Arthroscopic treatment (29882)*
🚑 18.4 🔗 18.4 **FUD** 090 ⬛J J8 80 50 📁
AMA: 2019,May,10; 2018,Sep,7

27405 Repair, primary, torn ligament and/or capsule, knee; collateral
🚑 19.4 🔗 19.4 **FUD** 090 ⬛J A2 80 50 📁
AMA: 2018,Sep,7; 2018,Jan,8; 2017,Jan,8; 2016,Jan,13; 2015,Jan,16; 2014,Jan,11

27407 cruciate
EXCLUDES *Reconstruction (27427)*
🚑 22.9 🔗 22.9 **FUD** 090 ⬛J A2 80 50 📁
AMA: 2018,Sep,7

27409 collateral and cruciate ligaments
EXCLUDES *Reconstruction (27427-27429)*
🚑 27.9 🔗 27.9 **FUD** 090 ⬛J A2 80 50 📁
AMA: 2018,Sep,7

27412 Autologous chondrocyte implantation, knee
EXCLUDES *Arthrotomy, knee (27331)*
Autologous fat graft obtained by liposuction (15771-15774)
Manipulation of knee joint under general anesthesia (27570)
Obtaining chondrocytes (29870)
Other autologous soft tissue grafts (fat, dermis, fascia) harvested by direct excision ([15769])
🚑 47.8 🔗 47.8 **FUD** 090 ⬛J 80 50 📁
AMA: 2018,Sep,7

27415 Osteochondral allograft, knee, open
EXCLUDES *Arthroscopic procedure (29867)*
Osteochondral autograft knee (27416)
🚑 38.9 🔗 38.9 **FUD** 090 ⬛J J8 80 50 📁
AMA: 2019,Apr,10; 2018,Sep,7; 2018,Jan,8; 2017,Jan,8; 2016,Jan,13; 2015,Jan,16; 2014,Jan,11

27416 Osteochondral autograft(s), knee, open (eg, mosaicplasty) (includes harvesting of autograft[s])
EXCLUDES *Procedures in the same compartment (29874, 29877, 29879, 29885-29887)*
Procedures performed at the same surgical session (27415, 29870-29871, 29875, 29884)
Surgical arthroscopy of the knee with osteochondral autograft(s) (29866)
🚑 28.3 🔗 28.3 **FUD** 090 ⬛J J8 80 50 📁
AMA: 2018,Sep,7; 2018,Jan,8; 2017,Jan,8; 2016,Jan,13; 2015,Jan,16; 2014,Jan,11

27418 Anterior tibial tubercleplasty (eg, Maquet type procedure)
🚑 23.8 🔗 23.8 **FUD** 090 ⬛J A2 80 50 📁
AMA: 2018,Sep,7; 2018,Jan,8; 2017,Jan,8; 2016,Jan,13; 2015,Jan,16; 2014,Jan,11

27420 Reconstruction of dislocating patella; (eg, Hauser type procedure)
🚑 21.3 🔗 21.3 **FUD** 090 ⬛J A2 80 50 📁
AMA: 2018,Sep,7; 2018,Jan,8; 2017,Jan,8; 2016,Jan,13; 2015,Jan,16; 2014,Jan,11

Patella

Patella

Patellar ligament

Tuberosity is osteotomized

Attachment is shifted and fixed

Patellar tendon insertion point is resected and shifted

27422 with extensor realignment and/or muscle advancement or release (eg, Campbell, Goldwaite type procedure)
🚑 21.3 🔗 21.3 **FUD** 090 ⬛J A2 80 50 📁
AMA: 2018,Sep,7; 2018,Jan,8; 2017,Jan,8; 2016,Jan,13; 2015,Jan,16; 2014,Jan,11

27424 with patellectomy
🚑 21.5 🔗 21.5 **FUD** 090 ⬛J A2 80 50 📁
AMA: 2018,Sep,7

27425 Lateral retinacular release, open

EXCLUDES *Arthroscopic release (29873)*
🔧 12.9 ⚕ 12.9 **FUD** 090   J A2 50 ▭
AMA: 2018,Sep,7; 2018,Jan,8; 2017,Jan,8; 2016,Jan,13; 2015,Nov,7; 2015,Jan,16; 2014,Jan,11

Lateral retinaculum
Patella
Medial retinaculum
Lateral and medial condyles
Normal alignment

Iliotibial tract
Patella
Medial patellar retinaculum
Lateral patellar retinaculum is incised, decreasing lateral pull on patella

Poor alignment

27427 Ligamentous reconstruction (augmentation), knee; extra-articular

EXCLUDES *Primary repair of ligament(s) (27405, 27407, 27409)*
🔧 20.4 ⚕ 20.4 **FUD** 090   J A2 80 50 ▭
AMA: 2018,Sep,7; 2018,Jan,8; 2017,Jan,8; 2016,Jan,13; 2015,Jan,16; 2014,Jan,11

27428 intra-articular (open)

EXCLUDES *Primary repair of ligament(s) (27405, 27407, 27409)*
🔧 32.2 ⚕ 32.2 **FUD** 090   J A2 80 50 ▭
AMA: 2018,Sep,7; 2018,Jan,8; 2017,Jan,8; 2016,Jan,13; 2015,Jan,16; 2014,Jan,11

27429 intra-articular (open) and extra-articular

EXCLUDES *Primary repair of ligament(s) (27405, 27407, 27409)*
🔧 36.2 ⚕ 36.2 **FUD** 090   J J8 80 50 ▭
AMA: 2018,Sep,7; 2018,Jan,8; 2017,Jan,8; 2016,Jan,13; 2015,Jan,16; 2014,Jan,11

27430 Quadricepsplasty (eg, Bennett or Thompson type)

🔧 21.2 ⚕ 21.2 **FUD** 090   J A2 80 50 ▭
AMA: 2018,Sep,7

27435 Capsulotomy, posterior capsular release, knee

🔧 23.2 ⚕ 23.2 **FUD** 090   J A2 80 50 ▭
AMA: 2018,Sep,7

27437 Arthroplasty, patella; without prosthesis

🔧 19.0 ⚕ 19.0 **FUD** 090   J A2 50 ▭
AMA: 2018,Sep,7

27438 with prosthesis

🔧 24.1 ⚕ 24.1 **FUD** 090   J J8 80 50 ▭
AMA: 2018,Sep,7

27440 Arthroplasty, knee, tibial plateau;

🔧 23.0 ⚕ 23.0 **FUD** 090   J J8 80 50 ▭
AMA: 2018,Sep,7

27441 with debridement and partial synovectomy

🔧 23.8 ⚕ 23.8 **FUD** 090   J G2 80 50 ▭
AMA: 2018,Sep,7

27442 Arthroplasty, femoral condyles or tibial plateau(s), knee;

🔧 25.0 ⚕ 25.0 **FUD** 090   J J8 80 50 ▭
AMA: 2018,Sep,7; 2018,Jan,8; 2017,Jan,8; 2016,Jun,8

27443 with debridement and partial synovectomy

🔧 23.4 ⚕ 23.4 **FUD** 090   J A2 80 50 ▭
AMA: 2018,Sep,7

27445 Arthroplasty, knee, hinge prosthesis (eg, Walldius type)

EXCLUDES *Removal knee prosthesis (27488)*
Revision knee arthroplasty (27487)
🔧 36.1 ⚕ 36.1 **FUD** 090   C 80 50 ▭
AMA: 2018,Sep,7

27446 Arthroplasty, knee, condyle and plateau; medial OR lateral compartment

EXCLUDES *Removal knee prosthesis (27488)*
Revision knee arthroplasty (27487)
🔧 33.4 ⚕ 33.4 **FUD** 090   J J8 80 50 ▭
AMA: 2018,Sep,7; 2018,Jan,8; 2017,Dec,13

27447 medial AND lateral compartments with or without patella resurfacing (total knee arthroplasty)

EXCLUDES *Removal knee prosthesis (27488)*
Revision knee arthroplasty (27487)
🔧 39.0 ⚕ 39.0 **FUD** 090   J 80 50 ▭
AMA: 2018,Sep,7; 2018,Jan,8; 2017,Jan,8; 2016,Jan,13; 2015,Jan,16; 2014,Jan,11

27448 Osteotomy, femur, shaft or supracondylar; without fixation

🔧 22.3 ⚕ 22.3 **FUD** 090   C 80 50 ▭
AMA: 2019,May,7; 2018,Sep,7

27450 with fixation

🔧 29.3 ⚕ 29.3 **FUD** 090   C 80 50 ▭
AMA: 2018,Sep,7

27454 Osteotomy, multiple, with realignment on intramedullary rod, femoral shaft (eg, Sofield type procedure)

🔧 37.5 ⚕ 37.5 **FUD** 090   C 80 50 ▭
AMA: 2018,Sep,7

27455 Osteotomy, proximal tibia, including fibular excision or osteotomy (includes correction of genu varus [bowleg] or genu valgus [knock-knee]); before epiphyseal closure

🔧 27.3 ⚕ 27.3 **FUD** 090   C 80 50 ▭
AMA: 2018,Sep,7

27457 after epiphyseal closure

🔧 27.8 ⚕ 27.8 **FUD** 090   C 80 50 ▭
AMA: 2018,Sep,7

27465 Osteoplasty, femur; shortening (excluding 64876)

🔧 36.2 ⚕ 36.2 **FUD** 090   C 80 50 ▭
AMA: 2018,Sep,7

27466 lengthening

🔧 34.0 ⚕ 34.0 **FUD** 090   C 80 50 ▭
AMA: 2018,Sep,7

27468 combined, lengthening and shortening with femoral segment transfer

🔧 38.8 ⚕ 38.8 **FUD** 090   C 80 50 ▭
AMA: 2018,Sep,7

27470 Repair, nonunion or malunion, femur, distal to head and neck; without graft (eg, compression technique)

🔧 33.9 ⚕ 33.9 **FUD** 090   C 80 50 ▭
AMA: 2018,Sep,7

27472 with iliac or other autogenous bone graft (includes obtaining graft)

🔧 36.4 ⚕ 36.4 **FUD** 090   C 80 50 ▭
AMA: 2018,Sep,7

27475 Arrest, epiphyseal, any method (eg, epiphysiodesis); distal femur

🔧 19.0 ⚕ 19.0 **FUD** 090   J G2 50 ▭
AMA: 2018,Sep,7

27477 tibia and fibula, proximal

🔧 21.1 ⚕ 21.1 **FUD** 090   J 50 ▭
AMA: 2018,Sep,7

27479 combined distal femur, proximal tibia and fibula

🔧 26.5 ⚕ 26.5 **FUD** 090   J G2 80 50 ▭
AMA: 2018,Sep,7

27485 Arrest, hemiepiphyseal, distal femur or proximal tibia or fibula (eg, genu varus or valgus)
📖 19.3   ⚕ 19.3   **FUD** 090   J 50 ▢
AMA: 2018,Sep,7

27486 Revision of total knee arthroplasty, with or without allograft; 1 component
📖 40.5   ⚕ 40.5   **FUD** 090   C 80 50 ▢
AMA: 2018,Sep,7; 2018,Apr,10; 2018,Jan,8; 2017,Jan,8; 2016,Jan,13; 2015,Jul,10; 2015,Jan,16; 2014,Jan,11

27487 femoral and entire tibial component
📖 50.7   ⚕ 50.7   **FUD** 090   C 80 50 ▢
AMA: 2018,Sep,7; 2018,Jan,8; 2017,Jan,8; 2016,Jan,13; 2015,Jan,16

27488 Removal of prosthesis, including total knee prosthesis, methylmethacrylate with or without insertion of spacer, knee
📖 34.6   ⚕ 34.6   **FUD** 090   C 80 50 ▢
AMA: 2018,Sep,7; 2018,Jan,8; 2017,Jan,8; 2016,Jan,13; 2015,Jan,16

27495 Prophylactic treatment (nailing, pinning, plating, or wiring) with or without methylmethacrylate, femur
📖 32.5   ⚕ 32.5   **FUD** 090   C 80 50 ▢
AMA: 2018,Sep,7

27496 Decompression fasciotomy, thigh and/or knee, 1 compartment (flexor or extensor or adductor);
📖 15.6   ⚕ 15.6   **FUD** 090   J A2 50 ▢
AMA: 2018,Sep,7

27497 with debridement of nonviable muscle and/or nerve
📖 16.7   ⚕ 16.7   **FUD** 090   J A2 80 50 ▢
AMA: 2018,Sep,7

27498 Decompression fasciotomy, thigh and/or knee, multiple compartments;
📖 18.8   ⚕ 18.8   **FUD** 090   J A2 80 50 ▢
AMA: 2018,Sep,7

27499 with debridement of nonviable muscle and/or nerve
📖 20.1   ⚕ 20.1   **FUD** 090   J A2 80 50 ▢
AMA: 2018,Sep,7

27500-27566 Treatment of Fracture/Dislocation of Femur/Knee

INCLUDES   Closed, percutaneous, and open treatment of fractures and dislocations

27500 Closed treatment of femoral shaft fracture, without manipulation
📖 13.7   ⚕ 14.9   **FUD** 090   T A2 50 ▢
AMA: 2018,Sep,7

27501 Closed treatment of supracondylar or transcondylar femoral fracture with or without intercondylar extension, without manipulation
📖 14.3   ⚕ 14.5   **FUD** 090   T A2 80 50 ▢
AMA: 2018,Sep,7

27502 Closed treatment of femoral shaft fracture, with manipulation, with or without skin or skeletal traction
📖 21.8   ⚕ 21.8   **FUD** 090   J A2 50 ▢
AMA: 2018,Sep,7; 2018,Jan,8; 2017,Jan,8; 2016,Jan,13; 2015,Jan,16; 2014,Jan,11

27503 Closed treatment of supracondylar or transcondylar femoral fracture with or without intercondylar extension, with manipulation, with or without skin or skeletal traction
📖 23.0   ⚕ 23.0   **FUD** 090   J A2 80 50 ▢
AMA: 2018,Sep,7

27506 Open treatment of femoral shaft fracture, with or without external fixation, with insertion of intramedullary implant, with or without cerclage and/or locking screws
📖 38.6   ⚕ 38.6   **FUD** 090   C 80 50 ▢
AMA: 2018,Sep,7; 2018,Jan,8; 2017,Jan,8; 2016,Jan,13; 2015,Jan,16; 2014,Jan,11

27507 Open treatment of femoral shaft fracture with plate/screws, with or without cerclage
📖 28.0   ⚕ 28.0   **FUD** 090   C 80 50 ▢
AMA: 2018,Sep,7

27508 Closed treatment of femoral fracture, distal end, medial or lateral condyle, without manipulation
📖 14.1   ⚕ 15.0   **FUD** 090   T A2 50 ▢
AMA: 2018,Sep,7

27509 Percutaneous skeletal fixation of femoral fracture, distal end, medial or lateral condyle, or supracondylar or transcondylar, with or without intercondylar extension, or distal femoral epiphyseal separation
📖 18.6   ⚕ 18.6   **FUD** 090   J J8 80 50 ▢
AMA: 2018,Dec,10; 2018,Dec,10; 2018,Sep,7

Pins are placed percutaneously

27510 Closed treatment of femoral fracture, distal end, medial or lateral condyle, with manipulation
📖 19.6   ⚕ 19.6   **FUD** 090   J A2 50 ▢
AMA: 2018,Sep,7

27511 Open treatment of femoral supracondylar or transcondylar fracture without intercondylar extension, includes internal fixation, when performed
📖 28.7   ⚕ 28.7   **FUD** 090   C 80 50 ▢
AMA: 2018,Sep,7

27513 Open treatment of femoral supracondylar or transcondylar fracture with intercondylar extension, includes internal fixation, when performed
📖 35.8   ⚕ 35.8   **FUD** 090   C 80 50 ▢
AMA: 2018,Sep,7

27514 Open treatment of femoral fracture, distal end, medial or lateral condyle, includes internal fixation, when performed
📖 27.9   ⚕ 27.9   **FUD** 090   C 80 50 ▢
AMA: 2018,Sep,7

27516 Closed treatment of distal femoral epiphyseal separation; without manipulation
📖 13.7   ⚕ 14.6   **FUD** 090   T A2 50 ▢
AMA: 2018,Sep,7

27517 with manipulation, with or without skin or skeletal traction
📖 19.7   ⚕ 19.7   **FUD** 090   J A2 80 50 ▢
AMA: 2018,Sep,7

27519 Open treatment of distal femoral epiphyseal separation, includes internal fixation, when performed
📖 25.8   ⚕ 25.8   **FUD** 090   C 80 50 ▢
AMA: 2018,Sep,7

27520 Closed treatment of patellar fracture, without manipulation
📖 8.46   ⚕ 9.21   **FUD** 090   T A2 50 ▢
AMA: 2018,Sep,7

● New Code   ▲ Revised Code   ○ Reinstated   ● New Web Release   ▲ Revised Web Release   + Add-on   Unlisted   Not Covered   # Resequenced
50 Optum Mod 50 Exempt   ⊘ AMA Mod 51 Exempt   51 Optum Mod 51 Exempt   63 Mod 63 Exempt   ✗ Non-FDA Drug   ★ Telemedicine   M Maternity   A Age Edit

27524 Open treatment of patellar fracture, with internal fixation and/or partial or complete patellectomy and soft tissue repair
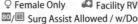 21.6   21.6   **FUD** 090   J 62 80 50
AMA: 2018,Sep,7

27530 Closed treatment of tibial fracture, proximal (plateau); without manipulation
EXCLUDES   *Arthroscopic repair (29855-29856)*
8.05   8.63   **FUD** 090   T A2 50
AMA: 2018,Sep,7

27532 with or without manipulation, with skeletal traction
EXCLUDES   *Arthroscopic repair (29855-29856)*
16.5   17.7   **FUD** 090   J A2 50
AMA: 2018,Sep,7

27535 Open treatment of tibial fracture, proximal (plateau); unicondylar, includes internal fixation, when performed
EXCLUDES   *Arthroscopic repair (29855-29856)*
25.9   25.9   **FUD** 090   C 80 50
AMA: 2018,Sep,7

27536 bicondylar, with or without internal fixation
EXCLUDES   *Arthroscopic repair (29855-29856)*
34.2   34.2   **FUD** 090   C 80 50
AMA: 2018,Sep,7

27538 Closed treatment of intercondylar spine(s) and/or tuberosity fracture(s) of knee, with or without manipulation
EXCLUDES   *Arthroscopic repair (29850-29851)*
12.7   13.6   **FUD** 090   T A2 80 50
AMA: 2018,Sep,7

27540 Open treatment of intercondylar spine(s) and/or tuberosity fracture(s) of the knee, includes internal fixation, when performed
23.4   23.4   **FUD** 090   C 80 50
AMA: 2018,Sep,7

27550 Closed treatment of knee dislocation; without anesthesia
13.8   14.9   **FUD** 090   T A2 80 50
AMA: 2018,Sep,7

27552 requiring anesthesia
18.0   18.0   **FUD** 090   J A2 80 50
AMA: 2018,Sep,7

27556 Open treatment of knee dislocation, includes internal fixation, when performed; without primary ligamentous repair or augmentation/reconstruction
25.3   25.3   **FUD** 090   C 80 50
AMA: 2018,Sep,7

27557 with primary ligamentous repair
30.3   30.3   **FUD** 090   C 80 50
AMA: 2018,Sep,7

27558 with primary ligamentous repair, with augmentation/reconstruction
34.5   34.5   **FUD** 090   C 80 50
AMA: 2018,Sep,7

27560 Closed treatment of patellar dislocation; without anesthesia
EXCLUDES   *Recurrent dislocation (27420-27424)*
9.66   10.5   **FUD** 090   T A2 50
AMA: 2018,Sep,7

27562 requiring anesthesia
EXCLUDES   *Recurrent dislocation (27420-27424)*
13.9   13.9   **FUD** 090   T A2 80 50
AMA: 2018,Sep,7

27566 Open treatment of patellar dislocation, with or without partial or total patellectomy
EXCLUDES   *Recurrent dislocation (27420-27424)*
25.8   25.8   **FUD** 090   J A2 80 50
AMA: 2018,Sep,7

27570 Knee Manipulation with Anesthesia

27570 Manipulation of knee joint under general anesthesia (includes application of traction or other fixation devices)
4.34   4.34   **FUD** 010   J A2 50
AMA: 2018,Sep,7; 2018,Jan,8; 2017,Jan,8; 2016,Jan,13; 2015,Jan,16; 2014,Jan,11

27580 Knee Arthrodesis

27580 Arthrodesis, knee, any technique
INCLUDES   Albert's operation
41.5   41.5   **FUD** 090   C 80 50
AMA: 2018,Sep,7

27590-27599 Amputations and Unlisted Procedures at Femur or Knee

27590 Amputation, thigh, through femur, any level;
22.9   22.9   **FUD** 090   C 80 50
AMA: 2018,Sep,7; 2018,Jan,8; 2017,Dec,13

27591 immediate fitting technique including first cast
27.9   27.9   **FUD** 090   C 80 50
AMA: 2018,Sep,7

27592 open, circular (guillotine)
19.6   19.6   **FUD** 090   C 80 50
AMA: 2018,Sep,7

27594 secondary closure or scar revision
14.6   14.6   **FUD** 090   J A2 50
AMA: 2018,Sep,7

27596 re-amputation
20.7   20.7   **FUD** 090   C 50
AMA: 2018,Sep,7

27598 Disarticulation at knee
INCLUDES   Batch-Spittler-McFaddin operation
    Callander knee disarticulation
    Gritti amputation
20.5   20.5   **FUD** 090   C 80 50
AMA: 2018,Sep,7

27599 Unlisted procedure, femur or knee
0.00   0.00   **FUD** YYY   T 80 50
AMA: 2019,Apr,10; 2018,Dec,10; 2018,Dec,10; 2018,Sep,7; 2018,Apr,10; 2018,Jan,8; 2017,Aug,9; 2017,Mar,10; 2017,Jan,8; 2016,Nov,9; 2016,Jun,8; 2016,Jan,13; 2015,Jan,13; 2015,Jan,16; 2014,Jan,11; 2014,Jan,9

27600-27602 Decompression Fasciotomy of Leg

EXCLUDES   *Fasciotomy with debridement (27892-27894)*
    Simple incision and drainage (10140-10160)

27600 Decompression fasciotomy, leg; anterior and/or lateral compartments only
11.6   11.6   **FUD** 090   J A2 50
AMA: 2018,Sep,7

27601 posterior compartment(s) only
12.8   12.8   **FUD** 090   J A2 50
AMA: 2018,Sep,7

27602 anterior and/or lateral, and posterior compartment(s)
13.9   13.9   **FUD** 090   J A2 80 50
AMA: 2018,Sep,7

27603-27612 Incisional Procedures Lower Leg and Ankle

27603 Incision and drainage, leg or ankle; deep abscess or hematoma
11.1   15.2   **FUD** 090   J A2 50
AMA: 2018,Sep,7

27604 infected bursa
9.61   13.6   **FUD** 090   J A2 80 50
AMA: 2018,Sep,7

27605 Tenotomy, percutaneous, Achilles tendon (separate procedure); local anesthesia
🚗 5.36 ⚒ 9.88 **FUD** 010 J A2 80 50 ▢
AMA: 2018,Sep,14; 2018,Sep,7

27606 general anesthesia
🚗 8.01 ⚒ 8.01 **FUD** 010 J A2 50 ▢
AMA: 2018,Sep,7; 2018,Sep,14

27607 Incision (eg, osteomyelitis or bone abscess), leg or ankle
🚗 17.5 ⚒ 17.5 **FUD** 090 J A2 50 ▢
AMA: 2018,Sep,7

27610 Arthrotomy, ankle, including exploration, drainage, or removal of foreign body
🚗 18.7 ⚒ 18.7 **FUD** 090 J A2 50 ▢
AMA: 2018,Sep,7

27612 Arthrotomy, posterior capsular release, ankle, with or without Achilles tendon lengthening
EXCLUDES *Lengthening or shortening tendon (27685)*
🚗 16.3 ⚒ 16.3 **FUD** 090 J A2 80 50 ▢
AMA: 2018,Sep,7

27613-27614 Biopsy Lower Leg and Ankle
EXCLUDES *Needle biopsy (20206)*

27613 Biopsy, soft tissue of leg or ankle area; superficial
🚗 4.62 ⚒ 7.19 **FUD** 010 J P3 50 ▢
AMA: 2018,Sep,7

27614 deep (subfascial or intramuscular)
🚗 11.6 ⚒ 16.5 **FUD** 090 J A2 50 ▢
AMA: 2018,Sep,7

27615-27634 [27632, 27634] Excision Soft Tissue Tumors Lower Leg/Ankle
INCLUDES Any necessary elevation of tissue planes or dissection
Measurement of tumor and necessary margin at greatest diameter prior to excision
Resection without removal of significant normal tissue
Simple and intermediate repairs
Types of excision:
　　Fascial or subfascial soft tissue tumors: simple and marginal resection of most often benign and intramuscular tumors found either in or below the deep fascia, not involving bone
　　Resection of the tumor (may include entire bone) and wide margins of normal tissue primarily for malignant or aggressive benign tumors
　　Subcutaneous: simple and marginal resection of most often benign tumors found in the subcutaneous tissue above the deep fascia
EXCLUDES *Complex repair*
Excision of benign cutaneous lesions (eg, sebaceous cyst) (11400-11406)
Radical resection of cutaneous tumors (eg, melanoma) (11600-11606)
Significant exploration of vessels or neuroplasty

27615 Radical resection of tumor (eg, sarcoma), soft tissue of leg or ankle area; less than 5 cm
🚗 29.5 ⚒ 29.5 **FUD** 090 J G2 80 50 ▢
AMA: 2018,Sep,7

27616 5 cm or greater
🚗 36.6 ⚒ 36.6 **FUD** 090 J G2 80 50 ▢
AMA: 2018,Sep,7

27618 Excision, tumor, soft tissue of leg or ankle area, subcutaneous; less than 3 cm
🚗 8.83 ⚒ 13.2 **FUD** 090 J G2 50 ▢
AMA: 2018,Sep,7; 2018,Jan,8; 2017,Jan,8; 2016,Jan,13; 2015,Jan,16; 2014,Jan,11

\# **27632** 3 cm or greater
🚗 11.9 ⚒ 11.9 **FUD** 090 J G2 80 50 ▢
AMA: 2018,Sep,7

27619 Excision, tumor, soft tissue of leg or ankle area, subfascial (eg, intramuscular); less than 5 cm
🚗 13.3 ⚒ 13.3 **FUD** 090 J G2 50 ▢
AMA: 2018,Sep,7

\# **27634** 5 cm or greater
🚗 19.5 ⚒ 19.5 **FUD** 090 J G2 80 50 ▢
AMA: 2018,Sep,7

27620-27641 Bone and Joint Procedures Ankle/Leg

27620 Arthrotomy, ankle, with joint exploration, with or without biopsy, with or without removal of loose or foreign body
🚗 13.0 ⚒ 13.0 **FUD** 090 J A2 80 50 ▢
AMA: 2018,Sep,7

27625 Arthrotomy, with synovectomy, ankle;
🚗 16.4 ⚒ 16.4 **FUD** 090 J A2 80 50 ▢
AMA: 2018,Sep,7

27626 including tenosynovectomy
🚗 17.5 ⚒ 17.5 **FUD** 090 J A2 80 50 ▢
AMA: 2018,Sep,7

27630 Excision of lesion of tendon sheath or capsule (eg, cyst or ganglion), leg and/or ankle
🚗 10.4 ⚒ 15.9 **FUD** 090 J A2 50 ▢
AMA: 2018,Sep,7

27632 Resequenced code. See code following 27618.

27634 Resequenced code. See code following 27619.

27635 Excision or curettage of bone cyst or benign tumor, tibia or fibula;
🚗 16.7 ⚒ 16.7 **FUD** 090 J A2 50 ▢
AMA: 2018,Sep,7; 2018,Jan,8; 2017,Jan,8; 2016,Jan,13; 2015,Jan,16; 2014,Jan,11

27637 with autograft (includes obtaining graft)
🚗 21.4 ⚒ 21.4 **FUD** 090 J A2 80 50 ▢
AMA: 2018,Sep,7

27638 with allograft
🚗 22.0 ⚒ 22.0 **FUD** 090 J A2 80 50 ▢
AMA: 2019,May,7; 2018,Sep,7

27640 Partial excision (craterization, saucerization, or diaphysectomy), bone (eg, osteomyelitis); tibia
EXCLUDES *Excision of exostosis (27635)*
🚗 23.9 ⚒ 23.9 **FUD** 090 J A2 50 ▢
AMA: 2018,Sep,7; 2018,Jan,8; 2017,Jan,8; 2016,Jan,13; 2015,Jan,16; 2014,Jan,11

27641 fibula
EXCLUDES *Excision of exostosis (27635)*
🚗 19.0 ⚒ 19.0 **FUD** 090 J A2 50 ▢
AMA: 2018,Sep,7

27645-27647 Radical Resection Bone Tumor Ankle/Leg
INCLUDES Any necessary elevation of tissue planes or dissection
Excision of adjacent soft tissue during bone tumor resection (27615-27619 [27632, 27634])
Measurement of tumor and necessary margin at greatest diameter prior to excision
Resection of the tumor (may include entire bone) and wide margins of normal tissue primarily for malignant or aggressive benign tumors
Simple and intermediate repairs
EXCLUDES *Complex repair*
Significant exploration of vessels, neuroplasty, reconstruction, or complex bone repair

27645 Radical resection of tumor; tibia
🚗 51.4 ⚒ 51.4 **FUD** 090 C 80 50 ▢
AMA: 2019,May,7; 2018,Sep,7

27646 fibula
🚗 44.6 ⚒ 44.6 **FUD** 090 C 80 50 ▢
AMA: 2019,May,7; 2018,Sep,7

27647 talus or calcaneus
🚗 29.3 ⚒ 29.3 **FUD** 090 J A2 80 50 ▢
AMA: 2019,May,7; 2018,Sep,7

● New Code　▲ Revised Code　○ Reinstated　● New Web Release　▲ Revised Web Release　＋ Add-on　Unlisted　Not Covered　\# Resequenced
50 Optum Mod 50 Exempt　Ⓝ AMA Mod 51 Exempt　51 Optum Mod 51 Exempt　63 Mod 63 Exempt　⚹ Non-FDA Drug　★ Telemedicine　M Maternity　A Age Edit

27648 Injection for Ankle Arthrogram

EXCLUDES Arthroscopy (29894-29898)

27648 Injection procedure for ankle arthrography
☒ (73615)
🖥 1.52   ⚖ 5.22   **FUD** 000   N N1 80 50 ▭
AMA: 2019,May,7; 2018,Sep,7; 2018,Jan,8; 2017,Jan,8; 2016,Jan,13; 2015,Aug,6

27650-27745 Repair/Reconstruction Lower Leg/Ankle

27650 Repair, primary, open or percutaneous, ruptured Achilles tendon;
🖥 18.9   ⚖ 18.9   **FUD** 090   J A2 80 50 ▭
AMA: 2018,Sep,7; 2018,Jan,8; 2017,Jan,8; 2016,Jan,13; 2015,Jan,16; 2014,Jul,5

27652 with graft (includes obtaining graft)
🖥 19.3   ⚖ 19.3   **FUD** 090   J A2 50 ▭
AMA: 2018,Sep,7; 2018,Jan,8; 2017,Jan,8; 2016,Jan,13; 2015,Jan,16; 2014,Jul,5

27654 Repair, secondary, Achilles tendon, with or without graft
🖥 20.4   ⚖ 20.4   **FUD** 090   J A2 80 50 ▭
AMA: 2018,Sep,7; 2018,Jan,8; 2017,Jan,8; 2016,Dec,16; 2016,Jan,13; 2015,Jan,16; 2014,Jul,5

27656 Repair, fascial defect of leg
🖥 11.4   ⚖ 18.2   **FUD** 090   J A2 80 50 ▭
AMA: 2018,Sep,7

27658 Repair, flexor tendon, leg; primary, without graft, each tendon
🖥 10.6   ⚖ 10.6   **FUD** 090   J A2 80 ▭
AMA: 2018,Sep,7

27659 secondary, with or without graft, each tendon
🖥 13.5   ⚖ 13.5   **FUD** 090   J A2 80 ▭
AMA: 2018,Sep,7; 2018,Jan,8; 2017,Jan,8; 2016,Jan,13; 2015,Jan,13

27664 Repair, extensor tendon, leg; primary, without graft, each tendon
🖥 10.4   ⚖ 10.4   **FUD** 090   J A2 80 ▭
AMA: 2018,Sep,7; 2018,Jan,8; 2017,Jan,8; 2016,Jan,13; 2015,Jan,13

27665 secondary, with or without graft, each tendon
🖥 11.9   ⚖ 11.9   **FUD** 090   J A2 80 ▭
AMA: 2018,Sep,7

27675 Repair, dislocating peroneal tendons; without fibular osteotomy
🖥 14.1   ⚖ 14.1   **FUD** 090   J A2 80 50 ▭
AMA: 2018,Sep,7

27676 with fibular osteotomy
🖥 17.2   ⚖ 17.2   **FUD** 090   J A2 80 50 ▭
AMA: 2018,Sep,7

27680 Tenolysis, flexor or extensor tendon, leg and/or ankle; single, each tendon
🖥 12.2   ⚖ 12.2   **FUD** 090   J A2 ▭
AMA: 2018,Sep,7; 2018,Jan,8; 2017,Jan,8; 2016,Jan,13; 2015,Jan,16; 2014,Jan,11

27681 multiple tendons (through separate incision[s])
🖥 15.7   ⚖ 15.7   **FUD** 090   J A2 50 ▭
AMA: 2018,Sep,7

27685 Lengthening or shortening of tendon, leg or ankle; single tendon (separate procedure)
🖥 13.3   ⚖ 19.0   **FUD** 090   J A2 80 50 ▭
AMA: 2018,Sep,7; 2018,Sep,14; 2018,Jan,8; 2017,Jan,8; 2016,Jan,13; 2015,Jan,16; 2014,Jan,11

27686 multiple tendons (through same incision), each
🖥 15.7   ⚖ 15.7   **FUD** 090   J A2 50 ▭
AMA: 2018,Sep,7; 2018,Jan,8; 2017,Jan,8; 2016,Jan,13; 2015,Jan,16; 2014,Jan,11

27687 Gastrocnemius recession (eg, Strayer procedure)
🖥 13.0   ⚖ 13.0   **FUD** 090   J A2 80 50 ▭
AMA: 2018,Sep,7

27690 Transfer or transplant of single tendon (with muscle redirection or rerouting); superficial (eg, anterior tibial extensors into midfoot)
INCLUDES Toe extensors considered a single tendon with transplant into midfoot
🖥 18.3   ⚖ 18.3   **FUD** 090   J A2 80 50 ▭
AMA: 2018,Sep,7

27691 deep (eg, anterior tibial or posterior tibial through interosseous space, flexor digitorum longus, flexor hallucis longus, or peroneal tendon to midfoot or hindfoot)
INCLUDES Barr procedure
Toe extensors considered a single tendon with transplant into midfoot
🖥 21.4   ⚖ 21.4   **FUD** 090   J A2 80 50 ▭
AMA: 2018,Sep,7

+ **27692** each additional tendon (List separately in addition to code for primary procedure)
INCLUDES Toe extensors considered a single tendon with transplant into midfoot
Code first (27690-27691)
🖥 3.02   ⚖ 3.02   **FUD** ZZZ   N N1 80 ▭
AMA: 2018,Sep,7

27695 Repair, primary, disrupted ligament, ankle; collateral
🖥 13.6   ⚖ 13.6   **FUD** 090   J A2 50 ▭
AMA: 2018,Nov,11; 2018,Sep,7; 2018,Jan,8; 2017,Jan,8; 2016,Jan,13; 2015,Jan,16; 2014,Mar,13; 2014,Jan,11

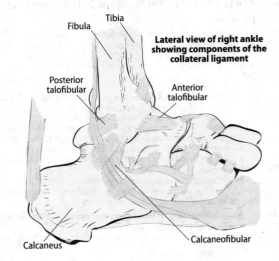

Fibula   Tibia

Posterior talofibular   Anterior talofibular

Lateral view of right ankle showing components of the collateral ligament

Calcaneus   Calcaneofibular

27696 both collateral ligaments
🖥 15.9   ⚖ 15.9   **FUD** 090   J J8 50 ▭
AMA: 2018,Nov,11; 2018,Sep,7; 2018,Jan,8; 2017,Jan,8; 2016,Jan,13; 2015,Jan,16; 2014,Mar,13

27698 Repair, secondary, disrupted ligament, ankle, collateral (eg, Watson-Jones procedure)
🖥 18.3   ⚖ 18.3   **FUD** 090   J A2 80 50 ▭
AMA: 2018,Sep,7; 2018,Jan,8; 2017,Jan,8; 2016,Jan,13; 2015,Jan,16; 2014,Mar,13

27700 Arthroplasty, ankle;
🖥 17.5   ⚖ 17.5   **FUD** 090   J A2 80 50 ▭
AMA: 2018,Sep,7

27702 with implant (total ankle)
🖥 27.7   ⚖ 27.7   **FUD** 090   C 80 50 ▭
AMA: 2018,Sep,7

27703 revision, total ankle
🖥 31.9   ⚖ 31.9   **FUD** 090   C 80 50 ▭
AMA: 2018,Sep,7

27704 **Removal of ankle implant**
🚑 16.5 ⚕ 16.5 **FUD** 090
02 A2 50 ▣
AMA: 2019,May,7; 2018,Sep,7

27705 **Osteotomy; tibia**
EXCLUDES *Genu varus or genu valgus repair (27455-27457)*
🚑 21.8 ⚕ 21.8 **FUD** 090
J J8 80 50 ▣
AMA: 2018,Sep,7

27707 **fibula**
EXCLUDES *Genu varus or genu valgus repair (27455-27457)*
🚑 11.5 ⚕ 11.5 **FUD** 090
J A2 50 ▣
AMA: 2018,Sep,7

27709 **tibia and fibula**
EXCLUDES *Genu varus or genu valgus repair (27455-27457)*
🚑 33.6 ⚕ 33.6 **FUD** 090
J J8 80 50 ▣
AMA: 2018,Sep,7

27712 **multiple, with realignment on intramedullary rod (eg, Sofield type procedure)**
EXCLUDES *Genu varus or genu valgus repair (27455-27457)*
🚑 31.9 ⚕ 31.9 **FUD** 090
C 80 50 ▣
AMA: 2018,Sep,7

27715 **Osteoplasty, tibia and fibula, lengthening or shortening**
INCLUDES Anderson tibial lengthening
🚑 30.9 ⚕ 30.9 **FUD** 090
C 80 50 ▣
AMA: 2018,Sep,7

27720 **Repair of nonunion or malunion, tibia; without graft, (eg, compression technique)**
🚑 25.1 ⚕ 25.1 **FUD** 090
J J8 80 50 ▣
AMA: 2018,Sep,7

27722 **with sliding graft**
🚑 25.7 ⚕ 25.7 **FUD** 090
J 80 50 ▣
AMA: 2018,Sep,7

27724 **with iliac or other autograft (includes obtaining graft)**
🚑 36.4 ⚕ 36.4 **FUD** 090
C 80 50 ▣
AMA: 2018,Sep,7; 2018,Jan,8; 2017,Jan,8; 2016,Jan,13; 2015,Jan,16; 2014,Jan,11

27725 **by synostosis, with fibula, any method**
🚑 35.1 ⚕ 35.1 **FUD** 090
C 80 50 ▣
AMA: 2018,Sep,7

27726 **Repair of fibula nonunion and/or malunion with internal fixation**
INCLUDES Osteotomy; fibula (27707)
🚑 27.7 ⚕ 27.7 **FUD** 090
J J8 50 ▣
AMA: 2018,Sep,7; 2018,Jan,8; 2017,Jan,8; 2016,Jan,13; 2015,Jan,16; 2014,Jan,11

27727 **Repair of congenital pseudarthrosis, tibia**
🚑 29.9 ⚕ 29.9 **FUD** 090
C 80 50 ▣
AMA: 2018,Sep,7

27730 **Arrest, epiphyseal (epiphysiodesis), open; distal tibia**
🚑 16.9 ⚕ 16.9 **FUD** 090
J A2 50 ▣
AMA: 2018,Sep,7

27732 **distal fibula**
🚑 12.9 ⚕ 12.9 **FUD** 090
J A2 50 ▣
AMA: 2018,Sep,7

27734 **distal tibia and fibula**
🚑 18.9 ⚕ 18.9 **FUD** 090
J A2 50 ▣
AMA: 2018,Sep,7

27740 **Arrest, epiphyseal (epiphysiodesis), any method, combined, proximal and distal tibia and fibula;**
EXCLUDES *Epiphyseal arrest of proximal tibia and fibula (27477)*
🚑 20.4 ⚕ 20.4 **FUD** 090
J 62 80 50 ▣
AMA: 2018,Sep,7

27742 **and distal femur**
EXCLUDES *Epiphyseal arrest of proximal tibia and fibula (27477)*
🚑 22.4 ⚕ 22.4 **FUD** 090
J A2 80 50 ▣
AMA: 2018,Sep,7

27745 **Prophylactic treatment (nailing, pinning, plating or wiring) with or without methylmethacrylate, tibia**
🚑 21.7 ⚕ 21.7 **FUD** 090
J J8 80 50 ▣
AMA: 2018,Sep,7

27750-27848 Treatment of Fracture/Dislocation Lower Leg/Ankle

INCLUDES Treatment of open or closed fracture or dislocation

27750 **Closed treatment of tibial shaft fracture (with or without fibular fracture); without manipulation**
🚑 9.11 ⚕ 9.87 **FUD** 090
T A2 50 ▣
AMA: 2018,Sep,7; 2018,Jan,8; 2017,Jan,8; 2016,Jan,13; 2015,Jan,16; 2014,Jan,11

27752 **with manipulation, with or without skeletal traction**
🚑 14.1 ⚕ 15.3 **FUD** 090
J A2 50 ▣
AMA: 2018,Sep,7; 2018,Jan,8; 2018,Jan,3; 2017,Jan,8; 2016,Jan,13; 2015,Jan,16; 2014,Jan,11

27756 **Percutaneous skeletal fixation of tibial shaft fracture (with or without fibular fracture) (eg, pins or screws)**
🚑 16.6 ⚕ 16.6 **FUD** 090
J J8 80 50 ▣
AMA: 2018,Sep,7; 2018,Jan,8; 2017,Jan,8; 2016,Jan,13; 2015,Jan,16; 2014,Jan,11

27758 **Open treatment of tibial shaft fracture (with or without fibular fracture), with plate/screws, with or without cerclage**
🚑 25.7 ⚕ 25.7 **FUD** 090
J J8 80 50 ▣
AMA: 2018,Sep,7; 2018,Jan,8; 2017,Jan,8; 2016,Jan,13; 2015,Jan,16; 2014,Jan,11

27759 **Treatment of tibial shaft fracture (with or without fibular fracture) by intramedullary implant, with or without interlocking screws and/or cerclage**
🚑 28.8 ⚕ 28.8 **FUD** 090
J J8 80 50 ▣
AMA: 2018,Sep,7; 2018,Jan,8; 2017,Jan,8; 2016,Jan,13; 2015,Jan,16; 2014,Jan,11

27760 **Closed treatment of medial malleolus fracture; without manipulation**
🚑 8.72 ⚕ 9.50 **FUD** 090
T A2 50 ▣
AMA: 2018,Sep,7

27762 **with manipulation, with or without skin or skeletal traction**
🚑 12.3 ⚕ 13.6 **FUD** 090
J A2 50 ▣
AMA: 2018,Sep,7

27766 **Open treatment of medial malleolus fracture, includes internal fixation, when performed**
🚑 17.4 ⚕ 17.4 **FUD** 090
J A2 50 ▣
AMA: 2018,Sep,7

27767 **Closed treatment of posterior malleolus fracture; without manipulation**
EXCLUDES *Treatment of bimalleolar ankle fracture (27808-27814)*
Treatment of trimalleolar ankle fracture (27816-27823)
🚑 8.08 ⚕ 8.08 **FUD** 090
T P2 50 ▣
AMA: 2018,Sep,7

27768 **with manipulation**
EXCLUDES *Treatment of bimalleolar ankle fracture (27808-27814)*
Treatment of trimalleolar ankle fracture (27816-27823)
🚑 12.7 ⚕ 12.7 **FUD** 090
J 62 50 ▣
AMA: 2018,Sep,7

27769 **Open treatment of posterior malleolus fracture, includes internal fixation, when performed**
EXCLUDES *Treatment of bimalleolar ankle fracture (27808-27814)*
Treatment of trimalleolar ankle fracture (27816-27823)
🚑 21.0 ⚕ 21.0 **FUD** 090
J 62 50 ▣
AMA: 2018,Sep,7

27780 **Closed treatment of proximal fibula or shaft fracture; without manipulation**
🚑 7.98 ⚕ 8.71 **FUD** 090
T A2 50 ▣
AMA: 2018,Sep,7; 2018,Jan,8; 2017,Jan,8; 2016,Jan,13; 2015,Jan,16; 2014,Jan,11

27781   with manipulation
   11.3   12.3   **FUD** 090   [J] [A2] [50] [▢]
AMA: 2018,Sep,7

27784   Open treatment of proximal fibula or shaft fracture, includes internal fixation, when performed
   20.6   20.6   **FUD** 090   [J] [A2] [50] [▢]
AMA: 2018,Sep,7; 2018,Jan,8; 2017,Jan,8; 2016,Jan,13; 2015,Jan,16; 2014,Jan,11

27786   Closed treatment of distal fibular fracture (lateral malleolus); without manipulation
   8.17   8.97   **FUD** 090   [T] [A2] [50] [▢]
AMA: 2018,Sep,7

27788   with manipulation
   11.0   12.1   **FUD** 090   [T] [A2] [50] [▢]
AMA: 2018,Sep,7

27792   Open treatment of distal fibular fracture (lateral malleolus), includes internal fixation, when performed
   EXCLUDES   *Repair of tibia and fibula shaft fracture (27750-27759)*
   18.6   18.6   **FUD** 090   [J] [J8] [50] [▢]
AMA: 2018,Sep,7; 2018,Jan,8; 2017,Jan,8; 2016,Jan,13; 2015,Jan,16; 2014,Jan,11

27808   Closed treatment of bimalleolar ankle fracture (eg, lateral and medial malleoli, or lateral and posterior malleoli or medial and posterior malleoli); without manipulation
   8.62   9.53   **FUD** 090   [T] [A2] [50] [▢]
AMA: 2018,Sep,7

27810   with manipulation
   12.1   13.3   **FUD** 090   [J] [A2] [50] [▢]
AMA: 2018,Sep,7

27814   Open treatment of bimalleolar ankle fracture (eg, lateral and medial malleoli, or lateral and posterior malleoli, or medial and posterior malleoli), includes internal fixation, when performed
   22.1   22.1   **FUD** 090   [J] [J8] [80] [50] [▢]
AMA: 2018,Sep,7; 2018,Jan,8; 2017,Jan,8; 2016,Feb,13

27816   Closed treatment of trimalleolar ankle fracture; without manipulation
   8.28   9.27   **FUD** 090   [T] [A2] [50] [▢]
AMA: 2018,Sep,7

27818   with manipulation
   12.4   13.9   **FUD** 090   [J] [A2] [50] [▢]
AMA: 2018,Sep,7

27822   Open treatment of trimalleolar ankle fracture, includes internal fixation, when performed, medial and/or lateral malleolus; without fixation of posterior lip
   24.7   24.7   **FUD** 090   [J] [J8] [80] [50] [▢]
AMA: 2018,Sep,7

27823   with fixation of posterior lip
   28.0   28.0   **FUD** 090   [J] [J8] [80] [50] [▢]
AMA: 2018,Sep,7

27824   Closed treatment of fracture of weight bearing articular portion of distal tibia (eg, pilon or tibial plafond), with or without anesthesia; without manipulation
   8.71   9.02   **FUD** 090   [T] [A2] [50] [▢]
AMA: 2018,Sep,7

27825   with skeletal traction and/or requiring manipulation
   14.2   15.7   **FUD** 090   [J] [A2] [80] [50] [▢]
AMA: 2018,Sep,7

27826   Open treatment of fracture of weight bearing articular surface/portion of distal tibia (eg, pilon or tibial plafond), with internal fixation, when performed; of fibula only
   24.2   24.2   **FUD** 090   [J] [A2] [80] [50] [▢]
AMA: 2018,Sep,7

27827   of tibia only
   31.7   31.7   **FUD** 090   [J] [J8] [80] [50] [▢]
AMA: 2018,Sep,7

27828   of both tibia and fibula
   37.8   37.8   **FUD** 090   [J] [J8] [80] [50] [▢]
AMA: 2018,Sep,7; 2018,Jan,8; 2017,Jan,8; 2016,Jan,13; 2015,Jan,16; 2014,Apr,10

27829   Open treatment of distal tibiofibular joint (syndesmosis) disruption, includes internal fixation, when performed
   20.0   20.0   **FUD** 090   [J] [A2] [80] [50] [▢]
AMA: 2018,Sep,7; 2018,Jan,8; 2017,Jan,8; 2016,Feb,13; 2016,Jan,13; 2015,Jan,16; 2014,Jan,11

27830   Closed treatment of proximal tibiofibular joint dislocation; without anesthesia
   10.2   11.0   **FUD** 090   [T] [A2] [80] [50] [▢]
AMA: 2018,Sep,7

27831   requiring anesthesia
   11.5   11.5   **FUD** 090   [J] [A2] [80] [50] [▢]
AMA: 2018,Sep,7

27832   Open treatment of proximal tibiofibular joint dislocation, includes internal fixation, when performed, or with excision of proximal fibula
   21.8   21.8   **FUD** 090   [J] [A2] [80] [50] [▢]
AMA: 2018,Sep,7

27840   Closed treatment of ankle dislocation; without anesthesia
   10.7   10.7   **FUD** 090   [T] [A2] [50] [▢]
AMA: 2018,Sep,7

27842   requiring anesthesia, with or without percutaneous skeletal fixation
   14.0   14.0   **FUD** 090   [J] [A2] [50] [▢]
AMA: 2018,Sep,7

27846   Open treatment of ankle dislocation, with or without percutaneous skeletal fixation; without repair or internal fixation
   EXCLUDES   *Arthroscopy (29894-29898)*
   20.7   20.7   **FUD** 090   [J] [A2] [80] [50] [▢]
AMA: 2018,Sep,7

27848   with repair or internal or external fixation
   EXCLUDES   *Arthroscopy (29894-29898)*
   23.0   23.0   **FUD** 090   [J] [A2] [80] [50] [▢]
AMA: 2018,Sep,7

27860 Ankle Manipulation with Anesthesia

27860   Manipulation of ankle under general anesthesia (includes application of traction or other fixation apparatus)
   4.92   4.92   **FUD** 010   [J] [A2] [80] [50] [▢]
AMA: 2018,Sep,7

27870-27871 Arthrodesis Lower Leg/Ankle

27870   Arthrodesis, ankle, open
   EXCLUDES   *Arthroscopic arthrodesis of ankle (29899)*
   29.5   29.5   **FUD** 090   [J] [J8] [80] [50] [▢]
AMA: 2018,Sep,7

27871   Arthrodesis, tibiofibular joint, proximal or distal
   19.8   19.8   **FUD** 090   [J] [J8] [80] [50] [▢]
AMA: 2018,Sep,7

27880-27889 Amputations of Lower Leg/Ankle

27880   Amputation, leg, through tibia and fibula;
   INCLUDES   Burgess amputation
   26.3   26.3   **FUD** 090   [C] [80] [50] [▢]
AMA: 2018,Sep,7

27881   with immediate fitting technique including application of first cast
   24.9   24.9   **FUD** 090   [C] [80] [50] [▢]
AMA: 2018,Sep,7

27882   open, circular (guillotine)
   17.2   17.2   **FUD** 090   [C] [80] [50] [▢]
AMA: 2018,Sep,7

| 2G/TC PC/TC Only | A2-Z3 ASC Payment | 50 Bilateral | ♂ Male Only | ♀ Female Only | Facility RVU | Non-Facility RVU | CCI | CLIA |
| FUD Follow-up Days | CMS: IOM | AMA: CPT Asst | A-Y OPPSI | 80/80 Surg Assist Allowed / w/Doc | Lab Crosswalk | Radiology Crosswalk |

96   CPT © 2019 American Medical Association. All Rights Reserved.   © 2019 Optum360, LLC

27884   secondary closure or scar revision
      16.4   16.4   **FUD** 090   J A2 50
      AMA: 2018,Sep,7

27886   re-amputation
      18.8   18.8   **FUD** 090   C 50
      AMA: 2018,Sep,7

27888   Amputation, ankle, through malleoli of tibia and fibula (eg, Syme, Pirogoff type procedures), with plastic closure and resection of nerves
      19.0   19.0   **FUD** 090   C 80 50
      AMA: 2018,Sep,7

27889   Ankle disarticulation
      18.6   18.6   **FUD** 090   J A2 50
      AMA: 2018,Sep,7

27892-27899 Decompression Fasciotomy Lower Leg

EXCLUDES   *Decompression fasciotomy without debridement (27600-27602)*

27892   Decompression fasciotomy, leg; anterior and/or lateral compartments only, with debridement of nonviable muscle and/or nerve
      15.8   15.8   **FUD** 090   J A2 80 50
      AMA: 2018,Sep,7

27893   posterior compartment(s) only, with debridement of nonviable muscle and/or nerve
      17.5   17.5   **FUD** 090   J A2 80 50
      AMA: 2018,Sep,7

27894   anterior and/or lateral, and posterior compartment(s), with debridement of nonviable muscle and/or nerve
      24.3   24.3   **FUD** 090   J A2 80 50
      AMA: 2018,Sep,7

27899   Unlisted procedure, leg or ankle
      0.00   0.00   **FUD** YYY   T 80 50
      AMA: 2018,Sep,7; 2018,Jan,8; 2017,Jan,8; 2016,Dec,16; 2016,Jan,13; 2015,Jan,16; 2014,Jan,11

28001-28008 Surgical Incision Foot/Toe

EXCLUDES   *Simple incision and drainage (10060-10160)*

28001   Incision and drainage, bursa, foot
      4.90   8.03   **FUD** 010   J P3
      AMA: 2018,Sep,7

28002   Incision and drainage below fascia, with or without tendon sheath involvement, foot; single bursal space
      9.20   12.7   **FUD** 010   J A2
      AMA: 2018,Sep,7

28003   multiple areas
      16.0   20.1   **FUD** 090   J A2
      AMA: 2018,Sep,7

28005   Incision, bone cortex (eg, osteomyelitis or bone abscess), foot
      16.6   16.6   **FUD** 090   J A2
      AMA: 2018,Sep,7

28008   Fasciotomy, foot and/or toe
        EXCLUDES   *Plantar fascia division (28250)*
                 Plantar fasciectomy (28060, 28062)
      8.46   12.5   **FUD** 090   J A2 50
      AMA: 2018,Sep,7

28010-28011 Tenotomy/Toe

EXCLUDES   *Open tenotomy (28230-28234)*
            Simple incision and drainage (10140-10160)

28010   Tenotomy, percutaneous, toe; single tendon
      5.99   6.69   **FUD** 090   J P3
      AMA: 2018,Sep,7

28011   multiple tendons
      8.14   9.14   **FUD** 090   J A2
      AMA: 2018,Sep,7

28020-28024 Arthrotomy Foot/Toe

EXCLUDES   *Simple incision and drainage (10140-10160)*

28020   Arthrotomy, including exploration, drainage, or removal of loose or foreign body; intertarsal or tarsometatarsal joint
      10.4   15.5   **FUD** 090   J A2
      AMA: 2018,Sep,7

28022   metatarsophalangeal joint
      9.32   14.0   **FUD** 090   J A2
      AMA: 2018,Sep,7

28024   interphalangeal joint
      8.67   13.1   **FUD** 090   J A2
      AMA: 2018,Sep,7

28035 Tarsal Tunnel Release

EXCLUDES   *Other nerve decompression (64722)*
            Other neuroplasty (64704)

28035   Release, tarsal tunnel (posterior tibial nerve decompression)
      10.2   15.2   **FUD** 090   J A2 50
      AMA: 2018,Sep,7

28039-28047 [28039, 28041] Excision Soft Tissue Tumors Foot/Toe

INCLUDES   Any necessary elevation of tissue planes or dissection
          Measurement of tumor and necessary margin at greatest diameter prior to excision
          Simple and intermediate repairs
          Types of excision:
               Fascial or subfascial soft tissue tumors: simple and marginal resection of tumors found either in or below the deep fascia, not involving bone or excision of a substantial amount of normal tissue; primarily benign and intramuscular tumors
               Tumors of fingers and toes involving joint capsules, tendons and tendon sheaths
               Radical resection soft tissue tumor: wide resection of tumor, involving substantial margins of normal tissue and may involve tissue removal from one or more layers; most often malignant or aggressive benign
               Tumors of fingers and toes adjacent to joints, tendons and tendon sheaths
               Subcutaneous: simple and marginal resection of tumors in the subcutaneous tissue above the deep fascia; most often benign

EXCLUDES   *Complex repair*
          Excision of benign cutaneous lesions (eg, sebaceous cyst) (11420-11426)
          Radical resection of cutaneous tumors (eg, melanoma) (11620-11626)
          Significant exploration of vessels, neuroplasty, or reconstruction

28039   Resequenced code. See code following 28043.

28041   Resequenced code. See code following 28045.

28043   Excision, tumor, soft tissue of foot or toe, subcutaneous; less than 1.5 cm
      7.56   11.4   **FUD** 090   J 62 50
      AMA: 2018,Sep,7

\#   **28039**   1.5 cm or greater
      9.94   14.3   **FUD** 090   J 62 80 50
      AMA: 2018,Sep,7

28045   Excision, tumor, soft tissue of foot or toe, subfascial (eg, intramuscular); less than 1.5 cm
      10.0   14.2   **FUD** 090   J 62 80 50
      AMA: 2018,Sep,7

\#   **28041**   1.5 cm or greater
      13.0   13.0   **FUD** 090   J 62 80 50
      AMA: 2018,Sep,7

28046   Radical resection of tumor (eg, sarcoma), soft tissue of foot or toe; less than 3 cm
      20.8   20.8   **FUD** 090   J 62 50
      AMA: 2018,Sep,7

28047   3 cm or greater
      30.1   30.1   **FUD** 090   J 62 80 50
      AMA: 2018,Sep,7

28050-28160 Resection Procedures Foot/Toes

28050 **Arthrotomy with biopsy; intertarsal or tarsometatarsal joint**
🚑 8.05 ⚕ 12.2 **FUD** 090   J A2 50 ▭
AMA: 2002,Apr,13; 1998,Nov,1

28052 **metatarsophalangeal joint**
🚑 8.15 ⚕ 12.8 **FUD** 090   J A2 50 ▭
AMA: 2002,Apr,13

28054 **interphalangeal joint**
🚑 6.77 ⚕ 10.8 **FUD** 090   J A2 80 50 ▭
AMA: 2002,Apr,13

28055 **Neurectomy, intrinsic musculature of foot**
🚑 11.0 ⚕ 11.0 **FUD** 090   J A2 80 50 ▭
AMA: 2002,Apr,13

28060 **Fasciectomy, plantar fascia; partial (separate procedure)**
EXCLUDES Plantar fasciotomy (28008, 28250)
🚑 10.3 ⚕ 15.0 **FUD** 090   J A2 50 ▭
AMA: 2018,Jan,8; 2017,Jan,8; 2016,Jan,13; 2015,Jan,16; 2014,Jan,11

28062 **radical (separate procedure)**
EXCLUDES Plantar fasciotomy (28008, 28250)
🚑 11.7 ⚕ 16.8 **FUD** 090   J A2 50 ▭
AMA: 2002,Apr,13

28070 **Synovectomy; intertarsal or tarsometatarsal joint, each**
🚑 10.2 ⚕ 15.4 **FUD** 090   J A2 ▭
AMA: 2002,Apr,13

28072 **metatarsophalangeal joint, each**
🚑 9.26 ⚕ 14.1 **FUD** 090   J A2 ▭
AMA: 2002,Apr,13

28080 **Excision, interdigital (Morton) neuroma, single, each**
🚑 10.5 ⚕ 15.1 **FUD** 090   J A2 80 ▭
AMA: 2018,Jan,8; 2017,Jan,8; 2016,Jan,13; 2015,Jan,16; 2014,Jan,11

28086 **Synovectomy, tendon sheath, foot; flexor**
🚑 10.3 ⚕ 15.7 **FUD** 090   J A2 80 50 ▭
AMA: 2002,Apr,13

28088 **extensor**
🚑 8.22 ⚕ 13.0 **FUD** 090   J A2 80 50 ▭
AMA: 2002,Apr,13

28090 **Excision of lesion, tendon, tendon sheath, or capsule (including synovectomy) (eg, cyst or ganglion); foot**
🚑 8.86 ⚕ 13.5 **FUD** 090   J A2 50 ▭
AMA: 2002,Apr,13; 1998,Nov,1

28092 **toe(s), each**
🚑 7.79 ⚕ 12.3 **FUD** 090   J A2 ▭
AMA: 2002,Apr,13; 1998,Nov,1

28100 **Excision or curettage of bone cyst or benign tumor, talus or calcaneus;**
🚑 11.9 ⚕ 17.6 **FUD** 090   J A2 80 50 ▭
AMA: 2002,Apr,13

28102 **with iliac or other autograft (includes obtaining graft)**
🚑 17.5 ⚕ 17.5 **FUD** 090   J J8 80 50 ▭
AMA: 2002,Apr,13

28103 **with allograft**
🚑 11.2 ⚕ 11.2 **FUD** 090   J A2 80 50 ▭
AMA: 2019,May,7

28104 **Excision or curettage of bone cyst or benign tumor, tarsal or metatarsal, except talus or calcaneus;**
🚑 10.2 ⚕ 15.4 **FUD** 090   J A2 80 ▭
AMA: 2002,May,7; 2002,Apr,13

28106 **with iliac or other autograft (includes obtaining graft)**
🚑 12.3 ⚕ 12.3 **FUD** 090   J A2 80 ▭
AMA: 2002,May,7; 2002,Apr,13

28107 **with allograft**
🚑 10.0 ⚕ 14.8 **FUD** 090   J A2 80 ▭
AMA: 2019,May,7

28108 **Excision or curettage of bone cyst or benign tumor, phalanges of foot**
EXCLUDES Partial excision bone, toe (28124)
🚑 8.30 ⚕ 12.7 **FUD** 090   J A2 ▭
AMA: 2002,Apr,13

28110 **Ostectomy, partial excision, fifth metatarsal head (bunionette) (separate procedure)**
🚑 8.37 ⚕ 13.4 **FUD** 090   J A2 50 ▭
AMA: 2018,Jan,8; 2017,Jan,8; 2016,Jan,13; 2015,Jan,16; 2014,Jan,11

28111 **Ostectomy, complete excision; first metatarsal head**
🚑 9.32 ⚕ 14.1 **FUD** 090   J A2 50 ▭
AMA: 2002,Apr,13

28112 **other metatarsal head (second, third or fourth)**
🚑 8.99 ⚕ 14.1 **FUD** 090   J A2 50 ▭
AMA: 2002,Apr,13

28113 **fifth metatarsal head**
🚑 12.2 ⚕ 17.0 **FUD** 090   J A2 80 50 ▭
AMA: 2002,Apr,13

28114 **all metatarsal heads, with partial proximal phalangectomy, excluding first metatarsal (eg, Clayton type procedure)**
🚑 23.9 ⚕ 30.7 **FUD** 090   J A2 80 50 ▭
AMA: 2002,Apr,13; 1998,Nov,1

28116 **Ostectomy, excision of tarsal coalition**
🚑 16.6 ⚕ 22.0 **FUD** 090   J A2 50 ▭
AMA: 2002,Apr,13

28118 **Ostectomy, calcaneus;**
🚑 11.9 ⚕ 17.2 **FUD** 090   J A2 80 50 ▭
AMA: 2018,Jan,8; 2017,Jan,8; 2016,Jan,13; 2015,Jan,13; 2015,Jan,16; 2014,Jan,11

28119 **for spur, with or without plantar fascial release**
🚑 10.3 ⚕ 15.1 **FUD** 090   J A2 50 ▭
AMA: 2018,Jan,8; 2017,Jan,8; 2016,Jan,13; 2015,Jan,16; 2014,Jan,11

28120 **Partial excision (craterization, saucerization, sequestrectomy, or diaphysectomy) bone (eg, osteomyelitis or bossing); talus or calcaneus**
INCLUDES Barker operation
🚑 14.3 ⚕ 19.5 **FUD** 090   J A2 50 ▭
AMA: 2018,Jan,8; 2017,Jan,8; 2016,Jan,13; 2015,Jan,16; 2014,Jan,11

28122 **tarsal or metatarsal bone, except talus or calcaneus**
EXCLUDES Hallux rigidus cheilectomy (28289)
Partial removal of talus or calcaneus (28120)
🚑 12.6 ⚕ 17.2 **FUD** 090   J A2 80 50 ▭
AMA: 2002,Apr,13; 1998,Nov,1

28124 **phalanx of toe**
🚑 9.54 ⚕ 13.8 **FUD** 090   J P3 50 ▭
AMA: 2002,Apr,13

28126 **Resection, partial or complete, phalangeal base, each toe**
🚑 7.14 ⚕ 11.4 **FUD** 090   J A2 ▭
AMA: 2018,Jan,8; 2017,Jan,8; 2016,Jan,13; 2015,Mar,9

28130 **Talectomy (astragalectomy)**
INCLUDES Whitman astragalectomy
EXCLUDES Calcanectomy (28118)
🚑 18.3 ⚕ 18.3 **FUD** 090   J A2 80 50 ▭
AMA: 2002,Apr,13

28140 **Metatarsectomy**
🚑 12.5 ⚕ 17.1 **FUD** 090   J A2 ▭
AMA: 2002,Apr,13

28150 **Phalangectomy, toe, each toe**
🚑 8.04 ⚕ 12.2 **FUD** 090   J A2 ▭
AMA: 2002,Apr,13; 1998,Nov,1

28153 Resection, condyle(s), distal end of phalanx, each toe
🚑 7.63 ⚕ 11.9 **FUD** 090 [J] [A2] [▢]
AMA: 2018,Jan,8; 2017,Jan,8; 2016,Jan,13; 2015,Jan,16; 2014,Jan,11

28160 Hemiphalangectomy or interphalangeal joint excision, toe, proximal end of phalanx, each
🚑 7.70 ⚕ 12.0 **FUD** 090 [J] [A2] [▢]
AMA: 2002,Apr,13; 1998,Nov,1

28171-28175 Radical Resection Bone Tumor Foot/Toes

INCLUDES Any necessary elevation of tissue planes or dissection
Excision of adjacent soft tissue during bone tumor resection (28039-28047 [28039, 28041])
Measurement of tumor and necessary margin at greatest diameter prior to excision
Resection of the tumor (may include entire bone) and wide margins of normal tissue primarily for malignant or aggressive benign tumors
Simple and intermediate repairs
EXCLUDES Complex repair
Radical tumor resection calcaneus or talus (27647)
Significant exploration of vessels, neuroplasty, reconstruction, or complex bone repair

28171 Radical resection of tumor; tarsal (except talus or calcaneus)
🚑 32.2 ⚕ 32.2 **FUD** 090 [J] [A2] [80] [▢]
AMA: 2002,Apr,13; 1994,Win,1

28173 metatarsal
🚑 21.3 ⚕ 21.3 **FUD** 090 [J] [A2] [▢]
AMA: 2002,Apr,13; 1994,Win,1

28175 phalanx of toe
🚑 13.7 ⚕ 13.7 **FUD** 090 [J] [A2] [▢]
AMA: 2002,Apr,13

28190-28193 Foreign Body Removal: Foot

28190 Removal of foreign body, foot; subcutaneous
🚑 3.85 ⚕ 7.35 **FUD** 010 [T] [P3] [50] [▢]
AMA: 2018,Jan,8; 2017,Jan,8; 2016,Jan,13; 2015,Jan,16; 2014,Jan,11

28192 deep
🚑 8.99 ⚕ 13.5 **FUD** 090 [J] [A2] [50] [▢]
AMA: 2018,Jan,8; 2017,Jan,8; 2016,Jan,13; 2015,Jan,16; 2014,Jan,11

28193 complicated
🚑 10.6 ⚕ 15.3 **FUD** 090 [J] [A2] [50] [▢]
AMA: 2002,Apr,13

28200-28360 [28295] Repair/Reconstruction of Foot/Toe

INCLUDES Closed, open, and percutaneous treatment of fractures and dislocations

28200 Repair, tendon, flexor, foot; primary or secondary, without free graft, each tendon
🚑 9.32 ⚕ 14.2 **FUD** 090 [J] [A2] [▢]
AMA: 2018,Jan,8; 2017,Jan,8; 2016,Feb,15; 2016,Jan,13; 2015,Jan,16; 2014,Jul,5; 2014,Jan,11

28202 secondary with free graft, each tendon (includes obtaining graft)
🚑 12.4 ⚕ 17.5 **FUD** 090 [J] [A2] [80] [▢]
AMA: 2002,Apr,13

28208 Repair, tendon, extensor, foot; primary or secondary, each tendon
🚑 9.09 ⚕ 13.9 **FUD** 090 [J] [A2] [▢]
AMA: 2002,Apr,13; 1998,Nov,1

28210 secondary with free graft, each tendon (includes obtaining graft)
🚑 12.0 ⚕ 17.0 **FUD** 090 [J] [A2] [80] [▢]
AMA: 2002,Apr,13

28220 Tenolysis, flexor, foot; single tendon
🚑 8.73 ⚕ 13.0 **FUD** 090 [J] [P3] [50] [▢]
AMA: 2002,Apr,13; 1998,Nov,1

28222 multiple tendons
🚑 10.2 ⚕ 14.9 **FUD** 090 [J] [A2] [50] [▢]
AMA: 2002,Apr,13; 1998,Nov,1

28225 Tenolysis, extensor, foot; single tendon
🚑 7.65 ⚕ 12.1 **FUD** 090 [J] [A2] [50] [▢]
AMA: 2002,Apr,13; 1998,Nov,1

28226 multiple tendons
🚑 11.3 ⚕ 17.6 **FUD** 090 [J] [A2] [50] [▢]
AMA: 2002,Apr,13; 1998,Nov,1

28230 Tenotomy, open, tendon flexor; foot, single or multiple tendon(s) (separate procedure)
🚑 8.17 ⚕ 12.5 **FUD** 090 [J] [P3] [50] [▢]
AMA: 2002,Apr,13; 1998,Nov,1

28232 toe, single tendon (separate procedure)
🚑 6.98 ⚕ 11.1 **FUD** 090 [J] [P3] [▢]
AMA: 2018,Jan,8; 2017,Jan,8; 2016,Jan,13; 2015,Mar,9

28234 Tenotomy, open, extensor, foot or toe, each tendon
EXCLUDES Tendon transfer (27690-27691)
🚑 7.59 ⚕ 11.8 **FUD** 090 [J] [A2] [▢]
AMA: 2018,Jan,8; 2017,Jan,8; 2016,Jan,13; 2015,Jan,16; 2014,Jan,11

28238 Reconstruction (advancement), posterior tibial tendon with excision of accessory tarsal navicular bone (eg, Kidner type procedure)
EXCLUDES Extensor hallucis longus transfer with big toe fusion (28760)
Jones procedure (28760)
Subcutaneous tenotomy (28010-28011)
Transfer or transplant of tendon with muscle redirection or rerouting (27690-27692)
🚑 14.0 ⚕ 19.3 **FUD** 090 [J] [A2] [80] [50] [▢]
AMA: 2002,Apr,13; 2002,May,7

28240 Tenotomy, lengthening, or release, abductor hallucis muscle
🚑 8.59 ⚕ 13.2 **FUD** 090 [J] [A2] [50] [▢]
AMA: 2002,Apr,13

28250 Division of plantar fascia and muscle (eg, Steindler stripping) (separate procedure)
🚑 11.5 ⚕ 16.6 **FUD** 090 [J] [A2] [80] [50] [▢]
AMA: 2002,Apr,13; 1998,Nov,1

28260 Capsulotomy, midfoot; medial release only (separate procedure)
🚑 14.6 ⚕ 19.8 **FUD** 090 [J] [A2] [80] [50] [▢]
AMA: 2002,Apr,13

28261 with tendon lengthening
🚑 23.4 ⚕ 29.7 **FUD** 090 [J] [A2] [80] [50] [▢]
AMA: 2002,Apr,13

28262 extensive, including posterior talotibial capsulotomy and tendon(s) lengthening (eg, resistant clubfoot deformity)
🚑 32.5 ⚕ 40.4 **FUD** 090 [J] [J8] [80] [50] [▢]
AMA: 2002,Apr,13; 1998,Nov,1

28264 Capsulotomy, midtarsal (eg, Heyman type procedure)
🚑 22.1 ⚕ 29.1 **FUD** 090 [J] [A2] [80] [50] [▢]
AMA: 2002,Apr,13; 1998,Nov,1

Musculoskeletal System

28270 — 28309

28270 **Capsulotomy; metatarsophalangeal joint, with or without tenorrhaphy, each joint (separate procedure)**
🏥 9.64   ⚕ 14.2   **FUD** 090   J A2 50 ▣
AMA: 2018,Jan,8; 2017,Jan,8; 2016,Jan,13; 2015,Jan,16; 2014,Sep,13; 2014,Jan,11

Tarsals
Metatarsophalangeal joint
Cuneiform bones
Phalanges
Medial   Lateral
Navicular   Intermediate
Proximal   Distal
Astragalus (talus)
Calcaneus
Medial
Cuboid   Metatarsals
Tarsometatarsal joint   Interphalangeal joints

Tenorrhaphy

28272 **interphalangeal joint, each joint (separate procedure)**
🏥 7.27   ⚕ 11.3   **FUD** 090   J P3 50 ▣
AMA: 2018,Jan,8; 2017,Jan,8; 2016,Jan,13; 2015,Jan,16; 2014,Jan,11

28280 **Syndactylization, toes (eg, webbing or Kelikian type procedure)**
🏥 10.0   ⚕ 14.8   **FUD** 090   J A2 80 50 ▣
AMA: 2002,Apr,13; 1998,Nov,1

28285 **Correction, hammertoe (eg, interphalangeal fusion, partial or total phalangectomy)**
🏥 10.9   ⚕ 15.5   **FUD** 090   J A2 50 ▣
AMA: 2018,Jan,8; 2017,Jan,8; 2016,Jun,8; 2016,Jan,13; 2015,Mar,9; 2015,Jan,16; 2014,Jan,11

28286 **Correction, cock-up fifth toe, with plastic skin closure (eg, Ruiz-Mora type procedure)**
🏥 8.57   ⚕ 12.9   **FUD** 090   J A2 50 ▣
AMA: 2002,Apr,13; 1998,Nov,1

28288 **Ostectomy, partial, exostectomy or condylectomy, metatarsal head, each metatarsal head**
🏥 12.4   ⚕ 17.6   **FUD** 090   J A2 ▣
AMA: 2002,Apr,13; 1998,Nov,1

28289 **Hallux rigidus correction with cheilectomy, debridement and capsular release of the first metatarsophalangeal joint; without implant**
🏥 13.2   ⚕ 21.0   **FUD** 090   J A2 80 50 ▣
AMA: 2018,Jan,8; 2017,Jan,8; 2016,Dec,3; 2016,Jan,13; 2015,Sep,12; 2015,Jan,16; 2014,Jan,11

28291 **with implant**
🏥 13.8   ⚕ 21.0   **FUD** 090   J J8 80 50 ▣
AMA: 2018,Jan,8; 2017,Nov,10; 2017,Jan,8; 2016,Dec,3

28292 **Correction, hallux valgus (bunionectomy), with sesamoidectomy, when performed; with resection of proximal phalanx base, when performed, any method**
🏥 13.9   ⚕ 21.3   **FUD** 090   J A2 80 50 ▣
AMA: 2018,Jan,8; 2017,Jan,8; 2016,Dec,3; 2016,Jan,13; 2015,Jan,16; 2014,Jan,11

28295 **Resequenced code. See code following 28296.**

28296 **with distal metatarsal osteotomy, any method**
🏥 14.8   ⚕ 26.3   **FUD** 090   J A2 80 50 ▣
AMA: 2018,Sep,14; 2018,Jan,8; 2017,Jan,8; 2016,Dec,3; 2016,Jan,13; 2015,Jan,16; 2014,Jan,11

28295 **with proximal metatarsal osteotomy, any method**
🏥 15.6   ⚕ 27.6   **FUD** 090   J 62 80 50 ▣
AMA: 2018,Jan,8; 2017,Jan,8; 2016,Dec,3

28297 **with first metatarsal and medial cuneiform joint arthrodesis, any method**
🏥 17.3   ⚕ 30.2   **FUD** 090   J J8 80 50 ▣
AMA: 2018,Jan,8; 2017,Jan,8; 2016,Dec,3; 2016,Jan,13; 2015,Jan,16; 2014,Jan,11

28298 **with proximal phalanx osteotomy, any method**
INCLUDES Akin procedure
🏥 14.3   ⚕ 24.5   **FUD** 090   J A2 80 50 ▣
AMA: 2018,Jan,8; 2017,Jan,8; 2016,Dec,3; 2016,Jan,13; 2015,Jan,16; 2014,Jan,11

28299 **with double osteotomy, any method**
🏥 16.8   ⚕ 29.1   **FUD** 090   J A2 80 50 ▣
AMA: 2018,Jan,8; 2017,Jan,8; 2016,Dec,3; 2016,Apr,8; 2016,Jan,13; 2015,Jan,16; 2014,Jan,11

Hallux valgus bunion
Medial eminence of metatarsal bone
A portion of the metatarsal head is resected
Kirshner wires stabilize the osteotomies
A wedge of the proximal phalanx is resected

28300 **Osteotomy; calcaneus (eg, Dwyer or Chambers type procedure), with or without internal fixation**
🏥 18.7   ⚕ 18.7   **FUD** 090   J J8 80 50 ▣
AMA: 2002,Apr,13; 1998,Nov,1

28302 **talus**
🏥 20.6   ⚕ 20.6   **FUD** 090   J A2 80 50 ▣
AMA: 2002,Apr,13

28304 **Osteotomy, tarsal bones, other than calcaneus or talus;**
🏥 17.3   ⚕ 23.6   **FUD** 090   J A2 80 50 ▣
AMA: 2002,Apr,13; 1998,Nov,1

28305 **with autograft (includes obtaining graft) (eg, Fowler type)**
🏥 19.0   ⚕ 19.0   **FUD** 090   J 62 80 50 ▣
AMA: 2002,Apr,13; 1998,Nov,1

28306 **Osteotomy, with or without lengthening, shortening or angular correction, metatarsal; first metatarsal**
🏥 11.6   ⚕ 17.6   **FUD** 090   J A2 80 50 ▣
AMA: 2018,Jan,8; 2017,Jan,8; 2016,Jan,13; 2015,Jan,16; 2014,Jan,11

28307 **first metatarsal with autograft (other than first toe)**
🏥 12.3   ⚕ 18.5   **FUD** 090   J A2 80 50 ▣
AMA: 2002,Apr,13; 1998,Nov,1

28308 **other than first metatarsal, each**
🏥 10.9   ⚕ 16.4   **FUD** 090   J A2 80 50 ▣
AMA: 2002,Apr,13; 1998,Nov,1

28309 **multiple (eg, Swanson type cavus foot procedure)**
🏥 25.5   ⚕ 25.5   **FUD** 090   J A2 80 50 ▣
AMA: 2018,Jan,8; 2017,Jan,8; 2016,Jan,13; 2015,Jan,16; 2014,Jan,11

28310 Osteotomy, shortening, angular or rotational correction; proximal phalanx, first toe (separate procedure)
   🖬 10.2   ⚕ 15.7   **FUD** 090   J A2 50 ▢
   AMA: 2018,Jan,8; 2017,Jan,8; 2016,Jan,13; 2015,Jan,16

28312 other phalanges, any toe
   🖬 9.11   ⚕ 14.5   **FUD** 090   J A2 ▢
   AMA: 2002,Apr,13

28313 Reconstruction, angular deformity of toe, soft tissue procedures only (eg, overlapping second toe, fifth toe, curly toes)
   🖬 10.1   ⚕ 15.0   **FUD** 090   J A2 ▢
   AMA: 2002,Apr,13; 1998,Nov,1

28315 Sesamoidectomy, first toe (separate procedure)
   🖬 9.37   ⚕ 13.9   **FUD** 090   J A2 50 ▢
   AMA: 2002,Apr,13

28320 Repair, nonunion or malunion; tarsal bones
   🖬 17.5   ⚕ 17.5   **FUD** 090   J J8 80 50 ▢
   AMA: 2002,Apr,13; 1998,Nov,1

28322 metatarsal, with or without bone graft (includes obtaining graft)
   🖬 16.5   ⚕ 22.6   **FUD** 090   J J8 80 ▢
   AMA: 2002,Apr,13

28340 Reconstruction, toe, macrodactyly; soft tissue resection
   🖬 11.8   ⚕ 16.6   **FUD** 090   J A2 ▢
   AMA: 2002,Apr,13

28341 requiring bone resection
   🖬 14.1   ⚕ 19.3   **FUD** 090   J A2 ▢
   AMA: 2002,Apr,13

28344 Reconstruction, toe(s); polydactyly
   🖬 8.07   ⚕ 12.3   **FUD** 090   J A2 50 ▢
   AMA: 2002,Apr,13

28345 syndactyly, with or without skin graft(s), each web
   🖬 10.5   ⚕ 15.0   **FUD** 090   J A2 80 ▢
   AMA: 2002,Apr,13

28360 Reconstruction, cleft foot
   🖬 31.4   ⚕ 31.4   **FUD** 090   J 80 50 ▢
   AMA: 2002,Apr,13

28400-28675 Treatment of Fracture/Dislocation of Foot/Toe

28400 Closed treatment of calcaneal fracture; without manipulation
   🖬 6.52   ⚕ 7.09   **FUD** 090   T A2 50 ▢
   AMA: 2002,Apr,13

28405 with manipulation
   INCLUDES Bohler reduction
   🖬 10.1   ⚕ 11.2   **FUD** 090   T A2 80 50 ▢
   AMA: 2002,Apr,13

28406 Percutaneous skeletal fixation of calcaneal fracture, with manipulation
   🖬 15.1   ⚕ 15.1   **FUD** 090   J A2 80 50 ▢
   AMA: 2002,Apr,13

28415 Open treatment of calcaneal fracture, includes internal fixation, when performed;
   🖬 32.1   ⚕ 32.1   **FUD** 090   J J8 80 50 ▢
   AMA: 2002,Apr,13

28420 with primary iliac or other autogenous bone graft (includes obtaining graft)
   🖬 36.8   ⚕ 36.8   **FUD** 090   J J8 80 50 ▢
   AMA: 2002,Apr,13

28430 Closed treatment of talus fracture; without manipulation
   🖬 6.01   ⚕ 6.81   **FUD** 090   T P2 50 ▢
   AMA: 2002,Apr,13

28435 with manipulation
   🖬 9.29   ⚕ 10.4   **FUD** 090   J A2 80 50 ▢
   AMA: 2002,Apr,13

28436 Percutaneous skeletal fixation of talus fracture, with manipulation
   🖬 12.9   ⚕ 12.9   **FUD** 090   J G2 50 ▢
   AMA: 2002,Apr,13

28445 Open treatment of talus fracture, includes internal fixation, when performed
   🖬 30.2   ⚕ 30.2   **FUD** 090   J A2 80 50 ▢
   AMA: 2002,Apr,13

28446 Open osteochondral autograft, talus (includes obtaining graft[s])
   INCLUDES   Osteotomy; fibula (27707)
             Osteotomy; tibia (27705)
   EXCLUDES   *Arthroscopically aided osteochondral talus graft (29892)*
             Open osteochondral allograft or repairs with industrial grafts (28899)
   🖬 35.3   ⚕ 35.3   **FUD** 090   J G2 80 50 ▢
   AMA: 2018,Jan,8; 2017,Jan,8; 2016,Jan,13; 2015,Jan,16; 2014,Jan,11

28450 Treatment of tarsal bone fracture (except talus and calcaneus); without manipulation, each
   🖬 5.47   ⚕ 6.09   **FUD** 090   T P2 ▢
   AMA: 2018,Jan,8; 2017,Jan,8; 2016,Jan,13; 2015,Jan,16; 2014,Jan,11

28455 with manipulation, each
   🖬 7.41   ⚕ 8.28   **FUD** 090   J P3 80 ▢
   AMA: 2002,Apr,13

28456 Percutaneous skeletal fixation of tarsal bone fracture (except talus and calcaneus), with manipulation, each
   🖬 9.25   ⚕ 9.25   **FUD** 090   J A2 ▢
   AMA: 2002,Apr,13

28465 Open treatment of tarsal bone fracture (except talus and calcaneus), includes internal fixation, when performed, each
   🖬 18.1   ⚕ 18.1   **FUD** 090   J J8 ▢
   AMA: 2019,Aug,10

28470 Closed treatment of metatarsal fracture; without manipulation, each
   🖬 5.83   ⚕ 6.26   **FUD** 090   T P2 ▢
   AMA: 2002,Apr,13

28475 with manipulation, each
   🖬 6.50   ⚕ 7.35   **FUD** 090   T P2 ▢
   AMA: 2002,Apr,13

28476 Percutaneous skeletal fixation of metatarsal fracture, with manipulation, each
   🖬 10.1   ⚕ 10.1   **FUD** 090   J A2 80 ▢
   AMA: 2002,Apr,13

28485 Open treatment of metatarsal fracture, includes internal fixation, when performed, each
   🖬 15.6   ⚕ 15.6   **FUD** 090   J J8 ▢
   AMA: 2019,Aug,10

28490 Closed treatment of fracture great toe, phalanx or phalanges; without manipulation
   🖬 3.57   ⚕ 4.12   **FUD** 090   T P3 50 ▢
   AMA: 2002,Apr,13

28495 with manipulation
   🖬 4.28   ⚕ 5.13   **FUD** 090   T P2 50 ▢
   AMA: 2002,Apr,13

28496 Percutaneous skeletal fixation of fracture great toe, phalanx or phalanges, with manipulation
   🖬 7.03   ⚕ 13.2   **FUD** 090   J A2 50 ▢
   AMA: 2002,Apr,13

28505 Open treatment of fracture, great toe, phalanx or phalanges, includes internal fixation, when performed
   🖬 14.3   ⚕ 19.1   **FUD** 090   J A2 50 ▢
   AMA: 2002,Apr,13

28510 Closed treatment of fracture, phalanx or phalanges, other than great toe; without manipulation, each

🔧 3.43 🔨 3.51 **FUD** 090 T P3 ▨

AMA: 2002,Apr,13

28515 with manipulation, each

🔧 4.08 🔨 4.67 **FUD** 090 T P3 ▨

AMA: 2002,Apr,13

28525 Open treatment of fracture, phalanx or phalanges, other than great toe, includes internal fixation, when performed, each

🔧 11.5 🔨 16.4 **FUD** 090 J A2 80 ▨

AMA: 2002,Apr,13

28530 Closed treatment of sesamoid fracture

🔧 2.95 🔨 3.34 **FUD** 090 T P3 80 50 ▨

AMA: 2002,Apr,13

28531 Open treatment of sesamoid fracture, with or without internal fixation

🔧 5.23 🔨 9.85 **FUD** 090 J A2 50 ▨

AMA: 2002,Apr,13

28540 Closed treatment of tarsal bone dislocation, other than talotarsal; without anesthesia

🔧 5.00 🔨 5.56 **FUD** 090 T P2 80 50 ▨

AMA: 2002,Apr,13

28545 requiring anesthesia

🔧 7.58 🔨 8.60 **FUD** 090 J G2 80 50 ▨

AMA: 2002,Apr,13

28546 Percutaneous skeletal fixation of tarsal bone dislocation, other than talotarsal, with manipulation

🔧 9.82 🔨 16.7 **FUD** 090 J A2 80 50 ▨

AMA: 2002,Apr,13

28555 Open treatment of tarsal bone dislocation, includes internal fixation, when performed

🔧 18.9 🔨 24.9 **FUD** 090 J J8 80 50 ▨

AMA: 2002,Apr,13

28570 Closed treatment of talotarsal joint dislocation; without anesthesia

🔧 5.51 🔨 6.54 **FUD** 090 T P2 80 50 ▨

AMA: 2002,Apr,13

28575 requiring anesthesia

🔧 9.54 🔨 10.5 **FUD** 090 J A2 80 50 ▨

AMA: 2002,Apr,13

28576 Percutaneous skeletal fixation of talotarsal joint dislocation, with manipulation

🔧 11.2 🔨 11.2 **FUD** 090 J A2 80 50 ▨

AMA: 2002,Apr,13

28585 Open treatment of talotarsal joint dislocation, includes internal fixation, when performed

🔧 19.6 🔨 25.0 **FUD** 090 J J8 80 50 ▨

AMA: 2018,Jan,8; 2017,Jan,8; 2016,Jan,13; 2015,Jan,16; 2014,Jan,11

28600 Closed treatment of tarsometatarsal joint dislocation; without anesthesia

🔧 5.35 🔨 6.26 **FUD** 090 T P2 80 ▨

AMA: 2002,Apr,13

28605 requiring anesthesia

🔧 8.51 🔨 9.52 **FUD** 090 T A2 80 ▨

AMA: 2002,Apr,13

28606 Percutaneous skeletal fixation of tarsometatarsal joint dislocation, with manipulation

🔧 11.2 🔨 11.2 **FUD** 090 J A2 ▨

AMA: 2002,Apr,13

28615 Open treatment of tarsometatarsal joint dislocation, includes internal fixation, when performed

🔧 23.2 🔨 23.2 **FUD** 090 J J8 80

AMA: 2002,Apr,13

28630 Closed treatment of metatarsophalangeal joint dislocation; without anesthesia

🔧 3.15 🔨 4.49 **FUD** 010 T P3 80 ▨

AMA: 2002,Apr,13

28635 requiring anesthesia

🔧 3.82 🔨 5.08 **FUD** 010 J A2 80 ▨

AMA: 2002,Apr,13

28636 Percutaneous skeletal fixation of metatarsophalangeal joint dislocation, with manipulation

🔧 5.91 🔨 9.25 **FUD** 010 J A2 ▨

AMA: 2002,Apr,13

28645 Open treatment of metatarsophalangeal joint dislocation, includes internal fixation, when performed

🔧 13.9 🔨 18.9 **FUD** 090 J A2 ▨

AMA: 2018,Jan,8; 2017,Jan,8; 2016,Jan,13; 2015,Jan,16; 2014,Sep,13

28660 Closed treatment of interphalangeal joint dislocation; without anesthesia

🔧 2.56 🔨 3.38 **FUD** 010 T P3 ▨

AMA: 2002,Apr,13

28665 requiring anesthesia

🔧 3.76 🔨 4.45 **FUD** 010 T A2 80 ▨

AMA: 2002,Apr,13

28666 Percutaneous skeletal fixation of interphalangeal joint dislocation, with manipulation

🔧 4.53 🔨 4.53 **FUD** 010 J A2 ▨

AMA: 2002,Apr,13

28675 Open treatment of interphalangeal joint dislocation, includes internal fixation, when performed

🔧 11.5 🔨 16.4 **FUD** 090 J A2 ▨

AMA: 2002,Apr,13

28705-28760 Arthrodesis of Foot/Toe

28705 Arthrodesis; pantalar

🔧 35.5 🔨 35.5 **FUD** 090 J J8 80 50 ▨

AMA: 2002,Apr,13

28715 triple

🔧 27.1 🔨 27.1 **FUD** 090 J J8 80 50 ▨

AMA: 2002,Apr,13; 1998,Nov,1

28725 subtalar

INCLUDES Dunn arthrodesis
Grice arthrosis

🔧 22.4 🔨 22.4 **FUD** 090 J J8 80 50 ▨

AMA: 2018,Jan,8; 2017,Jan,8; 2016,Jan,13; 2015,Jan,16; 2014,Jan,11

28730 Arthrodesis, midtarsal or tarsometatarsal, multiple or transverse;

INCLUDES Lambrinudi arthrodesis

🔧 21.1 🔨 21.1 **FUD** 090 J J8 80 50 ▨

AMA: 2002,Apr,13

28735 with osteotomy (eg, flatfoot correction)

🔧 22.4 🔨 22.4 **FUD** 090 J J8 80 50 ▨

AMA: 2019,May,10

28737 Arthrodesis, with tendon lengthening and advancement, midtarsal, tarsal navicular-cuneiform (eg, Miller type procedure)

🔧 20.0 🔨 20.0 **FUD** 090 J J8 80 50 ▨

AMA: 2002,Apr,13; 2002,May,7

28740 Arthrodesis, midtarsal or tarsometatarsal, single joint

🔧 17.9 🔨 24.3 **FUD** 090 J J8 80 50 ▨

AMA: 2018,Jan,8; 2017,Jan,8; 2016,Jan,13; 2015,Jan,16; 2014,Jan,11

28750 Arthrodesis, great toe; metatarsophalangeal joint

🔧 16.8 🔨 23.1 **FUD** 090 J J8 80 50 ▨

AMA: 2018,Jan,8; 2017,Jan,8; 2016,Dec,3; 2016,Jan,13; 2015,Jan,16; 2014,Jan,11

26/TC PC/TC Only   A2-Z3 ASC Payment   50 Bilateral   ♂ Male Only   ♀ Female Only   🔧 Facility RVU   🔨 Non-Facility RVU   ▨ CCI   ⊗ CLIA
FUD Follow-up Days   **CMS:** IOM   **AMA:** CPT Asst   A-Y OPPSI   80/80 Surg Assist Allowed / w/Doc   Lab Crosswalk   Radiology Crosswalk

© 2019 Optum360, LLC

28755 interphalangeal joint
⚕ 9.56 ⚚ 14.7 **FUD** 090 〔J〕〔A2〕〔50〕▢
AMA: 2002,Apr,13

28760 Arthrodesis, with extensor hallucis longus transfer to first metatarsal neck, great toe, interphalangeal joint (eg, Jones type procedure)
EXCLUDES *Hammer toe repair or interphalangeal fusion (28285)*
⚕ 16.7 ⚚ 22.8 **FUD** 090 〔J〕〔A2〕〔80〕〔50〕▢
AMA: 2002,Apr,13; 1998,Nov,1

28800-28825 Amputation Foot/Toe

28800 Amputation, foot; midtarsal (eg, Chopart type procedure)
⚕ 15.3 ⚚ 15.3 **FUD** 090 〔C〕〔80〕〔50〕▢
AMA: 2002,Apr,13; 1998,Nov,1

28805 transmetatarsal
⚕ 20.9 ⚚ 20.9 **FUD** 090 〔J〕〔80〕〔50〕▢
AMA: 2002,Apr,13; 1997,May,4

28810 Amputation, metatarsal, with toe, single
⚕ 12.3 ⚚ 12.3 **FUD** 090 〔J〕〔A2〕〔80〕▢
AMA: 2002,Apr,13

28820 Amputation, toe; metatarsophalangeal joint
⚕ 11.3 ⚚ 16.1 **FUD** 090 〔J〕〔A2〕▢
AMA: 2002,Apr,13; 1997,May,4

28825 interphalangeal joint
⚕ 10.6 ⚚ 15.4 **FUD** 090 〔J〕〔A2〕▢
AMA: 2002,Apr,13

28890-28899 Other/Unlisted Procedures Foot/Toe

28890 Extracorporeal shock wave, high energy, performed by a physician or other qualified health care professional, requiring anesthesia other than local, including ultrasound guidance, involving the plantar fascia
EXCLUDES *Extracorporeal shock wave therapy of integumentary system not otherwise specified, when performed on the same treatment area ([0512T, 0513T])*
Extracorporeal shock wave therapy of musculoskeletal system not otherwise specified (0101T-0102T)
⚕ 6.40 ⚚ 9.32 **FUD** 090 〔T〕〔P3〕〔50〕▢
AMA: 2018,Dec,5; 2018,Dec,5; 2018,Jan,8; 2017,Jan,8; 2016,Jan,13; 2015,Jan,16; 2014,Jan,11

28899 Unlisted procedure, foot or toes
⚕ 0.00 ⚚ 0.00 **FUD** YYY 〔T〕〔80〕▢
AMA: 2018,Oct,11; 2018,Jan,8; 2017,Nov,10; 2017,Sep,14; 2017,Jan,8; 2016,Dec,3; 2016,Jun,8; 2016,Jan,13; 2015,Nov,10; 2015,Jan,16; 2014,Jan,11

29000-29086 Casting: Arm/Shoulder/Torso

INCLUDES Application of cast or strapping when provided as:
An initial service to stabilize the fracture or injury without restorative treatment
A replacement procedure
Removal of cast
EXCLUDES *Cast or splint material*
E&M services provided as part of the initial service when restorative treatment is not provided
Orthotic supervision and training (97760-97763)

29000 Application of halo type body cast (see 20661-20663 for insertion)
⚕ 5.70 ⚚ 9.90 **FUD** 000 〔T〕〔G2〕〔80〕▢
AMA: 2018,Jan,8; 2018,Jan,3; 2017,Jan,8; 2016,Jan,13; 2015,Jan,16; 2014,Jan,11

29010 Application of Risser jacket, localizer, body; only
⚕ 4.61 ⚚ 7.73 **FUD** 000 〔T〕〔P2〕〔80〕▢
AMA: 2018,Jan,8; 2018,Jan,3; 2017,Jan,8; 2016,Jan,13; 2015,Jan,16; 2014,Jan,11

29015 including head
⚕ 5.21 ⚚ 8.32 **FUD** 000 〔T〕〔P2〕〔80〕▢
AMA: 2018,Jan,8; 2018,Jan,3; 2017,Jan,8; 2016,Jan,13; 2015,Jan,16; 2014,Jan,11

29035 Application of body cast, shoulder to hips;
⚕ 4.14 ⚚ 7.24 **FUD** 000 〔T〕〔P2〕〔80〕▢
AMA: 2018,Jan,8; 2018,Jan,3; 2017,Jan,8; 2016,Jan,13; 2015,Jan,16; 2014,Jan,11

29040 including head, Minerva type
⚕ 4.98 ⚚ 8.29 **FUD** 000 〔T〕〔G2〕〔80〕▢
AMA: 2018,Jan,8; 2018,Jan,3; 2017,Jan,8; 2016,Jan,13; 2015,Jan,16; 2014,Jan,11

29044 including 1 thigh
⚕ 4.81 ⚚ 8.12 **FUD** 000 〔T〕〔P2〕〔80〕▢
AMA: 2018,Jan,8; 2018,Jan,3; 2017,Jan,8; 2016,Jan,13; 2015,Jan,16; 2014,Jan,11

29046 including both thighs
⚕ 5.40 ⚚ 8.91 **FUD** 000 〔T〕〔G2〕〔80〕▢
AMA: 2018,Jan,8; 2018,Jan,3; 2017,Jan,8; 2016,Jan,13; 2015,Jan,16; 2014,Jan,11

29049 Application, cast; figure-of-eight
⚕ 2.00 ⚚ 2.82 **FUD** 000 〔T〕〔P3〕〔80〕▢
AMA: 2018,Jan,3; 2018,Jan,8; 2017,Jan,8; 2016,Jan,13; 2015,Jan,16; 2014,Jan,11

29055 shoulder spica
⚕ 3.98 ⚚ 6.31 **FUD** 000 〔T〕〔P2〕〔80〕▢
AMA: 2018,Jan,8; 2018,Jan,3; 2017,Jan,8; 2016,Jan,13; 2015,Jan,16; 2014,Jan,11

29058 plaster Velpeau
⚕ 2.72 ⚚ 3.54 **FUD** 000 〔T〕〔P3〕〔80〕▢
AMA: 2018,Jan,8; 2018,Jan,3; 2017,Jan,8; 2016,Jan,13; 2015,Jan,16; 2014,Jan,11

29065 shoulder to hand (long arm)
⚕ 1.94 ⚚ 2.72 **FUD** 000 〔T〕〔P3〕〔50〕▢
AMA: 2018,Jan,8; 2018,Jan,3; 2017,Jan,8; 2016,Jan,13; 2015,Jan,16; 2014,Jan,11

29075 elbow to finger (short arm)
⚕ 1.77 ⚚ 2.46 **FUD** 000 〔T〕〔P3〕〔50〕▢
AMA: 2018,Jan,8; 2018,Jan,3; 2017,Jan,8; 2016,Jan,13; 2015,Jan,16; 2014,Jan,11

29085 hand and lower forearm (gauntlet)
⚕ 1.92 ⚚ 2.70 **FUD** 000 〔T〕〔P3〕〔50〕▢
AMA: 2018,Jan,3; 2018,Jan,8; 2017,Jan,8; 2016,Jan,13; 2015,Jan,16; 2014,Jan,11

29086 finger (eg, contracture)
⚕ 1.45 ⚚ 2.24 **FUD** 000 〔T〕〔P3〕〔50〕▢
AMA: 2018,Jan,8; 2018,Jan,3; 2017,Jan,8; 2016,Jan,13; 2015,Jan,16; 2014,Jan,11

29105-29280 Splinting and Strapping: Torso/Upper Extremities

INCLUDES Application of splint or strapping when provided as:
An initial service to stabilize the fracture or dislocation
A replacement procedure
EXCLUDES *E&M services provided as part of the initial service when restorative treatment is not provided*
Orthotic supervision and training (97760-97763)
Splinting and strapping material

29105 Application of long arm splint (shoulder to hand)
⚕ 1.38 ⚚ 2.33 **FUD** 000 〔T〕〔P3〕〔50〕▢
AMA: 2018,Jan,3; 2018,Jan,8; 2017,Jan,8; 2016,Jan,13; 2015,Jan,16; 2014,Jan,11

29125 Application of short arm splint (forearm to hand); static
⚕ 1.13 ⚚ 1.83 **FUD** 000 〔Q1〕〔N1〕〔50〕▢
AMA: 2018,Jan,8; 2018,Jan,3; 2017,Jan,8; 2016,Jan,13; 2015,Jan,16; 2014,Jan,11

29126 dynamic
⚕ 1.39 ⚚ 2.18 **FUD** 000 〔Q1〕〔N1〕〔50〕▢
AMA: 2018,Jan,8; 2018,Jan,3; 2017,Jan,8; 2016,Jan,13; 2015,Jan,16; 2014,Jan,11

29130   **Application of finger splint; static**
🚗 0.83   ✂ 1.17   **FUD** 000   01 N1 50 ▱
AMA: 2018,Jan,8; 2018,Jan,3; 2017,Jan,8; 2016,Jan,13; 2015,Jan,16; 2014,Jan,11

29131   **dynamic**
🚗 0.96   ✂ 1.46   **FUD** 000   01 N1 50 ▱
AMA: 2018,Jan,8; 2018,Jan,3; 2017,Jan,8; 2016,Jan,13; 2015,Jan,16; 2014,Jan,11

29200   **Strapping; thorax**
EXCLUDES   *Strapping of low back (29799)*
🚗 0.54   ✂ 0.91   **FUD** 000   T P3 ▱
AMA: 2018,Jan,8; 2018,Jan,3; 2017,Jan,8; 2016,Jan,13; 2015,Jan,16; 2014,Jan,11

29240   **shoulder (eg, Velpeau)**
🚗 0.54   ✂ 0.87   **FUD** 000   01 N1 50 ▱
AMA: 2018,Jan,3; 2018,Jan,8; 2017,Jan,8; 2016,Jan,13; 2015,Jan,16; 2014,Jan,11

29260   **elbow or wrist**
🚗 0.56   ✂ 0.85   **FUD** 000   01 N1 50 ▱
AMA: 2018,Jan,8; 2018,Jan,3; 2017,Jan,8; 2016,Jan,13; 2015,Jan,16; 2014,Jan,11

29280   **hand or finger**
🚗 0.58   ✂ 0.87   **FUD** 000   01 N1 50 ▱
AMA: 2018,Jan,8; 2018,Jan,3; 2017,Jan,8; 2016,Jan,13; 2015,Jan,16; 2014,Jan,11

29305-29450 Casting: Legs

INCLUDES   Application of cast when provided as:
     An initial service to stabilize the fracture or injury without restorative treatment
     A replacement procedure
     Removal of cast
EXCLUDES   *Cast or splint materials*
     E&M services provided as part of the initial service when restorative treatment is not provided
     Orthotic supervision and training (97760-97763)

29305   **Application of hip spica cast; 1 leg**
EXCLUDES   *Hip spica cast thighs only (29046)*
🚗 4.57   ✂ 7.02   **FUD** 000   T P2 80 ▱
AMA: 2018,Jan,8; 2018,Jan,3; 2017,Jan,8; 2016,Jan,13; 2015,Jan,16; 2014,Jan,11

29325   **1 and one-half spica or both legs**
EXCLUDES   *Hip spica cast thighs only (29046)*
🚗 5.11   ✂ 7.75   **FUD** 000   T P2 80 ▱
AMA: 2018,Jan,8; 2018,Jan,3; 2017,Jan,8; 2016,Jan,13; 2015,Jan,16; 2014,Jan,11

29345   **Application of long leg cast (thigh to toes);**
🚗 2.87   ✂ 3.85   **FUD** 000   T P3 50 ▱
AMA: 2018,Jan,3; 2018,Jan,8; 2017,Jan,8; 2016,Jan,13; 2015,Jan,16; 2014,Jan,11

29355   **walker or ambulatory type**
🚗 3.06   ✂ 4.03   **FUD** 000   T P3 50 ▱
AMA: 2018,Jan,3; 2018,Jan,8; 2017,Jan,8; 2016,Jan,13; 2015,Jan,16; 2014,Jan,11

29358   **Application of long leg cast brace**
🚗 2.99   ✂ 4.57   **FUD** 000   T P3 50 ▱
AMA: 2018,Jan,3; 2018,Jan,8; 2017,Jan,8; 2016,Jan,13; 2015,Jan,16; 2014,Jan,11

29365   **Application of cylinder cast (thigh to ankle)**
🚗 2.51   ✂ 3.49   **FUD** 000   T P3 50 ▱
AMA: 2018,Jan,3; 2018,Jan,8; 2017,Jan,8; 2016,Jan,13; 2015,Jan,16; 2014,Jan,11

29405   **Application of short leg cast (below knee to toes);**
🚗 1.70   ✂ 2.30   **FUD** 000   T P3 50 ▱
AMA: 2018,Jan,3; 2018,Jan,8; 2017,Jan,8; 2016,Jan,13; 2015,Jan,16; 2014,Jan,11

29425   **walking or ambulatory type**
🚗 1.60   ✂ 2.20   **FUD** 000   T P3 50 ▱
AMA: 2018,Jan,3; 2018,Jan,8; 2017,Jan,8; 2016,Jan,13; 2015,Jan,16; 2014,Jan,11

29435   **Application of patellar tendon bearing (PTB) cast**
🚗 2.38   ✂ 3.35   **FUD** 000   T P3 50 ▱
AMA: 2018,Jan,3; 2018,Jan,8; 2017,Jan,8; 2016,Jan,13; 2015,Jan,16; 2014,Jan,11

29440   **Adding walker to previously applied cast**
🚗 0.82   ✂ 1.24   **FUD** 000   T P3 50 ▱
AMA: 2018,Jan,8; 2018,Jan,3; 2017,Jan,8; 2016,Jan,13; 2015,Jan,16; 2014,Jan,11

29445   **Application of rigid total contact leg cast**
🚗 2.94   ✂ 3.73   **FUD** 000   T P3 50 ▱
AMA: 2018,Jan,3; 2018,Jan,8; 2017,Jan,8; 2016,Jan,13; 2015,Jan,16; 2014,Jan,11

29450   **Application of clubfoot cast with molding or manipulation, long or short leg**
🚗 3.26   ✂ 4.15   **FUD** 000   T P3 50 ▱
AMA: 2018,Jan,8; 2018,Jan,3; 2017,Jan,8; 2016,Jan,13; 2015,Jan,16; 2014,Jan,11

29505-29584 Splinting and Strapping Ankle/Foot/Leg/Toes

INCLUDES   Application of splinting and strapping when provided as:
     An initial service to stabilize the fracture or injury without restorative treatment
     A replacement procedure
EXCLUDES   *E&M services provided as part of the initial service when restorative treatment is not provided*
     Orthotic supervision and training (97760-97763)

29505   **Application of long leg splint (thigh to ankle or toes)**
🚗 1.45   ✂ 2.43   **FUD** 000   T P3 50 ▱
AMA: 2018,Jan,3; 2018,Jan,8; 2017,Jan,8; 2016,Jan,13; 2015,Jan,16; 2014,Jan,11

29515   **Application of short leg splint (calf to foot)**
🚗 1.42   ✂ 2.03   **FUD** 000   T P3 50 ▱
AMA: 2018,Jan,8; 2018,Jan,3; 2017,Jan,8; 2016,Jan,13; 2015,Jan,16; 2014,Jan,11

29520   **Strapping; hip**
EXCLUDES   *For treatment of the same extremity:*
     Endovenous ablation therapy of incompetent vein (36473-36479, [36482], [36483])
     Sclerosal injection for incompetent vein(s) ([36465], [36466], 36468-36471)
🚗 0.55   ✂ 0.97   **FUD** 000   01 N1 80 50 ▱
AMA: 2018,Jan,8; 2018,Jan,3; 2017,Jan,8; 2016,Jan,13; 2015,Jan,16; 2014,Jan,11

29530   **knee**
EXCLUDES   *For treatment of the same extremity:*
     Endovenous ablation therapy of incompetent vein (36473-36479, [36482], [36483])
     Sclerosal injection for incompetent vein(s) ([36465], [36466], 36468-36471)
🚗 0.54   ✂ 0.86   **FUD** 000   01 N1 50 ▱
AMA: 2018,Jan,3; 2018,Jan,8; 2017,Jan,8; 2016,Jan,13; 2015,Jan,16; 2014,Jan,11

29540   **ankle and/or foot**
EXCLUDES   *For treatment of the same extremity:*
     Endovenous ablation therapy of incompetent vein (36473-36479, [36482, 36483])
     Multi-layer compression system (29581)
     Sclerosal injection for incompetent vein(s) ([36465], [36466], 36468-36471)
     Unna boot (29580)
🚗 0.52   ✂ 0.82   **FUD** 000   T P3 50 ▱
AMA: 2018,Jan,3; 2018,Jan,8; 2017,Jan,8; 2016,Aug,3; 2016,Jan,13; 2015,Jan,16; 2014,Mar,4; 2014,Jan,11

26/TC PC/TC Only   A2-Z3 ASC Payment   50 Bilateral   ♂ Male Only   ♀ Female Only   🚗 Facility RVU   ✂ Non-Facility RVU   ▱ CCI   ✖ CLIA
FUD Follow-up Days   CMS: IOM   AMA: CPT Asst   A-Y OPPSI   80/80 Surg Assist Allowed / w/Doc   ▱ Lab Crosswalk   ▱ Radiology Crosswalk

104   CPT © 2019 American Medical Association. All Rights Reserved.   © 2019 Optum360, LLC

29550 **toes**

EXCLUDES For treatment of the same extremity:
Endovenous ablation therapy of incompetent vein
(36476-36479, [36482, 36483])
Sclerosal injection for incompetent vein(s) ([36465],
[36466], 36468-36471)

0.33 0.55 **FUD** 000   01 N1 50

AMA: 2018,Jan,8; 2018,Jan,3; 2017,Jan,8; 2016,Jan,13;
2015,Jan,16; 2014,Jan,11

29580 **Unna boot**

EXCLUDES Application of multi-layer compression system (29581)
For treatment of the same extremity:
Endovenous ablation therapy of incompetent vein
(36473-36479, [36482, 36483])
Sclerosal injection for incompetent vein(s) ([36465],
[36466], 36468-36471)
Strapping of ankle or foot (29540)

0.79 1.78 **FUD** 000   T P3 50

AMA: 2018,Jan,3; 2018,Jan,8; 2017,Jan,8; 2016,Aug,3;
2016,Jan,13; 2015,Jan,16; 2014,Mar,4; 2014,Jan,11

29581 **Application of multi-layer compression system; leg (below knee), including ankle and foot**

EXCLUDES For treatment of the same extremity:
Endovenous ablation therapy of incompetent vein
(36473-36479, [36482, 36483])
Sclerosal injection for incompetent vein(s) ([36465],
[36466], 36468-36471)
Strapping (29540, 29580)

0.80 2.47 **FUD** 000   T P3 80 50

AMA: 2018,Mar,3; 2018,Jan,8; 2018,Jan,3; 2017,Jan,8;
2016,Nov,3; 2016,Aug,3; 2016,Jan,13; 2015,Mar,9; 2015,Jan,16;
2014,Oct,6; 2014,Mar,4; 2014,Jan,11

29584 **upper arm, forearm, hand, and fingers**

EXCLUDES For treatment of the same extremity:
Endovenous ablation therapy of incompetent vein
(36473-36479, [36482], [36483])
Sclerosal injection for incompetent vein(s) ([36465],
[36466], 36468-36471)

0.47 2.29 **FUD** 000   T P2 80 50

AMA: 2018,Jan,3; 2018,Jan,8; 2017,Jan,8; 2016,Aug,3;
2016,Jan,13; 2015,Mar,9

29700-29799 Casting Services Other Than Application

INCLUDES Casts applied by treating individual
Removal of casts applied by treating individual

29700 **Removal or bivalving; gauntlet, boot or body cast**

0.96 1.82 **FUD** 000   T P3

AMA: 2018,Jan,3; 2018,Jan,8; 2017,Jan,8; 2016,Jan,13;
2015,Jan,16; 2014,Jan,11

29705 **full arm or full leg cast**

1.33 1.85 **FUD** 000   T P3 50

AMA: 2018,Jan,3; 2018,Jan,8; 2017,Jan,8; 2016,Jan,13;
2015,Jan,16; 2014,Jan,11

29710 **shoulder or hip spica, Minerva, or Risser jacket, etc.**

2.41 3.51 **FUD** 000   T P3 80 50

AMA: 2018,Jan,3; 2018,Jan,8; 2017,Jan,8; 2016,Jan,13;
2015,Jan,16; 2014,Jan,11

29720 **Repair of spica, body cast or jacket**

1.28 2.41 **FUD** 000   T P3

AMA: 2018,Jan,3; 2018,Jan,8; 2017,Jan,8; 2016,Jan,13;
2015,Jan,16; 2014,Jan,11

29730 **Windowing of cast**

1.27 1.79 **FUD** 000   T P3

AMA: 2018,Jan,3; 2018,Jan,8; 2017,Jan,8; 2016,Jan,13;
2015,Jan,16; 2014,Jan,11

29740 **Wedging of cast (except clubfoot casts)**

2.03 2.83 **FUD** 000   T P3

AMA: 2018,Jan,3; 2018,Jan,8; 2017,Jan,8; 2016,Jan,13;
2015,Jan,16; 2014,Jan,11

29750 **Wedging of clubfoot cast**

2.26 3.07 **FUD** 000   T P3 80 50

AMA: 2018,Jan,3; 2018,Jan,8; 2017,Jan,8; 2016,Jan,13;
2015,Jan,16; 2014,Jan,11

29799 **Unlisted procedure, casting or strapping**

0.00 0.00 **FUD** YYY   T 80

AMA: 2018,Jan,8; 2017,Jan,8; 2016,Aug,3;
2016,Jan,13; 2015,Jan,16; 2014,Jan,11

29800-29999 [29914, 29915, 29916] Arthroscopic Procedures

INCLUDES Diagnostic arthroscopy with surgical arthroscopy
Code also modifier 51 if arthroscopy is performed with arthrotomy

29800 **Arthroscopy, temporomandibular joint, diagnostic, with or without synovial biopsy (separate procedure)**

15.2 15.2 **FUD** 090   J A2 80 50

AMA: 2018,Jan,8; 2017,Jan,8; 2016,Jan,13; 2015,Jan,16

29804 **Arthroscopy, temporomandibular joint, surgical**

EXCLUDES Open surgery (21010)

18.4 18.4 **FUD** 090   J A2 80 50

AMA: 2018,Jan,8; 2017,Jan,8; 2016,Jan,13; 2015,Jan,16

29805 **Arthroscopy, shoulder, diagnostic, with or without synovial biopsy (separate procedure)**

EXCLUDES Open surgery (23065-23066, 23100-23101)

13.5 13.5 **FUD** 090   J A2 50

AMA: 2018,Jan,8; 2017,Jan,8; 2016,Jan,13; 2015,Jun,10;
2015,Jan,16

29806 **Arthroscopy, shoulder, surgical; capsulorrhaphy**

EXCLUDES Open surgery (23450-23466)
Thermal capsulorrhaphy (29999)

30.5 30.5 **FUD** 090   J A2 50

AMA: 2018,Jun,11; 2018,Jan,8; 2017,Jan,8; 2016,Jan,13;
2015,Jul,10; 2015,Mar,7; 2015,Jan,16

29807 **repair of SLAP lesion**

29.8 29.8 **FUD** 090   J A2 50

AMA: 2018,Jan,8; 2017,Jan,8; 2016,Jan,13; 2015,Mar,7;
2015,Jan,16

29819 **with removal of loose body or foreign body**

EXCLUDES Open surgery (23040-23044, 23107)

16.8 16.8 **FUD** 090   J A2 50

AMA: 2018,Jun,11; 2018,Jan,8; 2017,Jan,8; 2016,Jan,13;
2015,Mar,7; 2015,Jan,16

29820 **synovectomy, partial**

EXCLUDES Open surgery (23105)

15.3 15.3 **FUD** 090   J A2 80 50

AMA: 2018,Jan,8; 2017,Jan,8; 2016,Jan,13; 2015,Mar,7;
2015,Jan,16

29821 **synovectomy, complete**

EXCLUDES Open surgery (23105)

16.8 16.8 **FUD** 090   J A2 80 50

AMA: 2018,Jan,8; 2017,Jan,8; 2016,Jan,13; 2015,Mar,7;
2015,Jan,16

29822 **debridement, limited**

EXCLUDES Open surgery (see specific shoulder section)

16.3 16.3 **FUD** 090   J A2 80 50

AMA: 2018,Jan,7; 2018,Jan,8; 2017,Jan,8; 2016,Jan,13;
2015,Mar,7; 2015,Jan,16; 2014,Jan,11

29823 **debridement, extensive**

EXCLUDES Open surgery (see specific shoulder section)

17.7 17.7 **FUD** 090   J A2 80 50

AMA: 2018,Jan,7; 2018,Jan,8; 2017,Jan,8; 2016,Dec,16;
2016,Jan,13; 2015,Mar,7; 2015,Jan,16; 2014,Jan,11

29824 **distal claviculectomy including distal articular surface (Mumford procedure)**   *Bone shave*

INCLUDES Mumford procedure
EXCLUDES Open surgery (23120)

19.1 19.1 **FUD** 090   J A2 80 50

AMA: 2018,Jan,8; 2017,Jan,8; 2016,Jan,13; 2015,Mar,7;
2015,Jan,16

● New Code ▲ Revised Code ○ Reinstated ● New Web Release ▲ Revised Web Release + Add-on Unlisted Not Covered # Resequenced
50 Optum Mod 50 Exempt Ⓢ AMA Mod 51 Exempt 51 Optum Mod 51 Exempt 63 Mod 63 Exempt ✗ Non-FDA Drug ★ Telemedicine M Maternity A Age Edit

29825 with lysis and resection of adhesions, with or without manipulation

EXCLUDES Open surgery (see specific shoulder section)

🗲 16.6 ⚕ 16.6 **FUD** 090 [J] [A2] [80] [50] ▭

AMA: 2018,Jan,8; 2017,Jan,8; 2016,Jan,13; 2015,Mar,7; 2015,Jan,16

+ 29826 decompression of subacromial space with partial acromioplasty, with coracoacromial ligament (ie, arch) release, when performed (List separately in addition to code for primary procedure)

EXCLUDES Open surgery (23130, 23415)

Code first (29806-29825, 29827-29828)

🗲 5.07 ⚕ 5.07 **FUD** ZZZ [N] [N1] [80] [50] ▭

AMA: 2018,Jan,8; 2017,Jan,8; 2016,Jan,13; 2015,Mar,7; 2015,Jan,16; 2014,Jan,11

29827 with rotator cuff repair

EXCLUDES Distal clavicle excision (29824)

Open surgery or mini open repair (23412)

Subacromial decompression (29826)

🗲 30.3 ⚕ 30.3 **FUD** 090 [J] [A2] [80] [50] ▭

AMA: 2018,Jan,8; 2017,Jan,8; 2016,Jul,8; 2016,Jan,13; 2015,Mar,7; 2015,Jan,16; 2014,Jan,11

29828 biceps tenodesis

EXCLUDES Arthroscopy, shoulder, diagnostic, with or without synovial biopsy (29805)

Arthroscopy, shoulder, surgical; debridement, limited (29822)

Arthroscopy, shoulder, surgical; synovectomy, partial (29820)

Tenodesis of long tendon of biceps (23430)

🗲 26.1 ⚕ 26.1 **FUD** 090 [J] [62] [80] [50] ▭

AMA: 2018,Jan,8; 2017,Jan,8; 2016,Jul,8; 2016,Jan,13; 2015,Mar,7; 2015,Jan,16; 2014,Jan,11

29830 Arthroscopy, elbow, diagnostic, with or without synovial biopsy (separate procedure)

🗲 13.0 ⚕ 13.0 **FUD** 090 [J] [A2] [50] ▭

AMA: 2018,Jan,8; 2017,Jan,8; 2016,Jan,13; 2015,Jan,16

29834 Arthroscopy, elbow, surgical; with removal of loose body or foreign body

🗲 13.9 ⚕ 13.9 **FUD** 090 [J] [A2] [80] [50] ▭

AMA: 2018,Jan,8; 2017,Jan,8; 2016,Jan,13; 2015,Jan,16

29835 synovectomy, partial

🗲 14.6 ⚕ 14.6 **FUD** 090 [J] [A2] [80] [50] ▭

AMA: 2018,Jan,8; 2017,Jan,8; 2016,Jan,13; 2015,Jan,16

29836 synovectomy, complete

🗲 16.4 ⚕ 16.4 **FUD** 090 [J] [A2] [80] [50] ▭

AMA: 2018,Jan,8; 2017,Jan,8; 2016,Jan,13; 2015,Jan,16

29837 debridement, limited

🗲 15.0 ⚕ 15.0 **FUD** 090 [J] [A2] [80] [50] ▭

AMA: 2018,Jan,8; 2017,Jan,8; 2016,Jan,13; 2015,Jan,16

29838 debridement, extensive

🗲 16.9 ⚕ 16.9 **FUD** 090 [J] [A2] [80] [50] ▭

AMA: 2018,Jan,8; 2017,Jan,8; 2016,Jan,13; 2015,Jan,16

29840 Arthroscopy, wrist, diagnostic, with or without synovial biopsy (separate procedure)

🗲 12.9 ⚕ 12.9 **FUD** 090 [J] [A2] [80] [50] ▭

AMA: 2018,Jan,8; 2017,Jan,8; 2016,Jan,13; 2015,Jan,16

29843 Arthroscopy, wrist, surgical; for infection, lavage and drainage

🗲 13.9 ⚕ 13.9 **FUD** 090 [J] [A2] [80] [50] ▭

AMA: 2018,Jan,8; 2017,Jan,8; 2016,Jan,13; 2015,Jan,16

29844 synovectomy, partial

🗲 14.2 ⚕ 14.2 **FUD** 090 [J] [A2] [80] [50] ▭

AMA: 2018,Jan,8; 2017,Jan,8; 2016,Jan,13; 2015,Jan,16

29845 synovectomy, complete

🗲 16.6 ⚕ 16.6 **FUD** 090 [J] [A2] [80] [50] ▭

AMA: 2018,Jan,8; 2017,Jan,8; 2016,Jan,13; 2015,Jan,16; 2014,Jan,11

29846 excision and/or repair of triangular fibrocartilage and/or joint debridement

🗲 14.9 ⚕ 14.9 **FUD** 090 [J] [A2] [80] [50] ▭

AMA: 2018,Jan,8; 2017,Jan,8; 2016,Jan,13; 2015,Jan,16; 2014,Jan,11

29847 internal fixation for fracture or instability

🗲 15.6 ⚕ 15.6 **FUD** 090 [J] [A2] [80] [50] ▭

AMA: 2018,Jan,8; 2017,Jan,8; 2016,Jan,13; 2015,Jan,16

29848 Endoscopy, wrist, surgical, with release of transverse carpal ligament

EXCLUDES Open surgery (64721)

🗲 14.7 ⚕ 14.7 **FUD** 090 [J] [A2] [50] ▭

AMA: 2018,Apr,10; 2018,Jan,8; 2017,Jan,8; 2017,Jan,6; 2016,Jan,13; 2015,Jul,10; 2015,Jan,16; 2014,Jan,11

29850 Arthroscopically aided treatment of intercondylar spine(s) and/or tuberosity fracture(s) of the knee, with or without manipulation; without internal or external fixation (includes arthroscopy)

🗲 17.9 ⚕ 17.9 **FUD** 090 [J] [A2] [80] [50] ▭

AMA: 2018,Jan,8; 2017,Jan,8; 2016,Jan,13; 2015,Jan,16

29851 with internal or external fixation (includes arthroscopy)

EXCLUDES Bone graft (20900, 20902)

🗲 26.9 ⚕ 26.9 **FUD** 090 [J] [A2] [80] [50] ▭

AMA: 2018,Jan,8; 2017,Jan,8; 2016,Jan,13; 2015,Jan,16

29855 Arthroscopically aided treatment of tibial fracture, proximal (plateau); unicondylar, includes internal fixation, when performed (includes arthroscopy)

EXCLUDES Bone graft (20900, 20902)

🗲 22.5 ⚕ 22.5 **FUD** 090 [J] [J8] [80] [50] ▭

AMA: 2018,Sep,14; 2018,Jan,8; 2017,Jan,8; 2016,Jan,13; 2015,Jan,16

29856 bicondylar, includes internal fixation, when performed (includes arthroscopy)

EXCLUDES Bone graft (20900, 20902)

🗲 28.7 ⚕ 28.7 **FUD** 090 [J] [J8] [80] [50] ▭

AMA: 2018,Jan,8; 2017,Jan,8; 2016,Jan,13; 2015,Jan,16

29860 Arthroscopy, hip, diagnostic with or without synovial biopsy (separate procedure)

🗲 19.2 ⚕ 19.2 **FUD** 090 [J] [A2] [80] [50] ▭

AMA: 2018,Jan,8; 2017,Jan,8; 2016,Jan,13; 2015,Jan,16; 2014,Jan,11

29861 Arthroscopy, hip, surgical; with removal of loose body or foreign body

🗲 20.6 ⚕ 20.6 **FUD** 090 [J] [A2] [80] [50] ▭

AMA: 2018,Jan,8; 2017,Jan,8; 2016,Jan,13; 2015,Jan,16; 2014,Jan,11

29862 with debridement/shaving of articular cartilage (chondroplasty), abrasion arthroplasty, and/or resection of labrum

🗲 23.1 ⚕ 23.1 **FUD** 090 [J] [A2] [80] [50] ▭

AMA: 2018,Jan,8; 2017,Jan,8; 2016,Jan,13; 2015,Jan,16; 2014,Jan,11

29863 with synovectomy

🗲 23.2 ⚕ 23.2 **FUD** 090 [J] [A2] [80] [50] ▭

AMA: 2018,Jan,8; 2017,Jan,8; 2016,Jan,13; 2015,Jan,16; 2014,Jan,11

 # 29914 with femoroplasty (ie, treatment of cam lesion)

🗲 28.3 ⚕ 28.3 **FUD** 090 [J] [62] [80] [50] ▭

AMA: 2018,Jan,8; 2017,Jan,8; 2016,Jan,13; 2015,Jan,16; 2014,Jan,11

 # 29915 with acetabuloplasty (ie, treatment of pincer lesion)

🗲 29.1 ⚕ 29.1 **FUD** 090 [J] [62] [80] [50] ▭

AMA: 2018,Jan,8; 2017,Jan,8; 2016,Jan,13; 2015,Jan,16; 2014,Jan,11

29916   with labral repair

🚑 29.1   ⚕ 29.1   **FUD** 090   J 62 80 50 ▱

AMA: 2018,Jan,8; 2017,Jan,8; 2016,Jan,13; 2015,Jan,16; 2014,Jan,11

29866   Arthroscopy, knee, surgical; osteochondral autograft(s) (eg, mosaicplasty) (includes harvesting of the autograft[s])

EXCLUDES   *Open osteochondral autograft of the knee (27416)*
Procedures performed at the same surgical session (29870-29871, 29875, 29884)
Procedures performed in the same compartment (29874, 29877, 29879, 29885-29887)

🚑 30.3   ⚕ 30.3   **FUD** 090   J 62 80 50 ▱

AMA: 2018,Jan,8; 2017,Jan,8; 2016,Jan,13; 2015,Jan,16

Cylindrical plugs of healthy bone are harvested, usually from a non-weight bearing area of the femur

The technique employs arthroscopy

Recipient holes are drilled and the grafts tamped into position

29867   osteochondral allograft (eg, mosaicplasty)

EXCLUDES   *Procedures performed at the same surgical session (27415, 27570, 29870-29871, 29875, 29884)*
Procedures performed in the same compartment (29874, 29877, 29879, 29885-29887)

🚑 36.9   ⚕ 36.9   **FUD** 090   J 80 50 ▱

AMA: 2018,Jan,8; 2017,Jan,8; 2016,Jan,13; 2015,Jan,16; 2014,Jan,11

29868   meniscal transplantation (includes arthrotomy for meniscal insertion), medial or lateral

EXCLUDES   *Procedures performed at same surgical session (29870-29871, 29875, 29880, 29883-29884)*
Procedures performed in same compartment (29874, 29877, 29881-29882)

🚑 48.4   ⚕ 48.4   **FUD** 090   J 80 50 ▱

AMA: 2018,Jan,8; 2017,Jan,8; 2016,Jan,13; 2015,Jan,16

29870   Arthroscopy, knee, diagnostic, with or without synovial biopsy (separate procedure)

EXCLUDES   *Open procedure (27412)*

🚑 11.7   ⚕ 16.4   **FUD** 090   J A2 50 ▱

AMA: 2018,Jan,8; 2017,Jan,8; 2016,Jan,13; 2015,Jan,16; 2014,Jan,11

29871   Arthroscopy, knee, surgical; for infection, lavage and drainage

EXCLUDES   *Injection of contrast for knee arthrography (27369)*
Osteochondral graft (27412, 27415, 29866-29867)

🚑 14.8   ⚕ 14.8   **FUD** 090   J A2 50 ▱

AMA: 2019,Aug,7; 2018,Jan,8; 2017,Jan,8; 2016,Jan,13; 2015,Aug,6; 2015,Jan,16; 2014,Jan,11

29873   with lateral release

EXCLUDES   *Open procedure (27425)*

🚑 15.1   ⚕ 15.1   **FUD** 090   J A2 50 ▱

AMA: 2018,Jan,8; 2017,Jan,8; 2016,Jan,13; 2015,Nov,7; 2015,Jan,16; 2014,Jan,11

29874   for removal of loose body or foreign body (eg, osteochondritis dissecans fragmentation, chondral fragmentation)

🚑 15.4   ⚕ 15.4   **FUD** 090   J A2 80 50 ▱

AMA: 2018,Jan,8; 2017,Jan,8; 2016,Jan,13; 2015,Jan,16; 2014,Jan,11

29875   synovectomy, limited (eg, plica or shelf resection) (separate procedure)

🚑 14.2   ⚕ 14.2   **FUD** 090   J A2 80 50 ▱

AMA: 2018,Jan,8; 2017,Jan,8; 2016,Jan,13; 2016,Jan,11; 2015,Jan,16; 2014,May,10; 2014,Jan,11

29876   synovectomy, major, 2 or more compartments (eg, medial or lateral)

🚑 18.9   ⚕ 18.9   **FUD** 090   J A2 80 50 ▱

AMA: 2018,Jan,8; 2017,Jan,8; 2016,Jan,13; 2015,Jan,16; 2014,Jan,11

29877   debridement/shaving of articular cartilage (chondroplasty)

EXCLUDES   *Arthroscopy, knee, surgical; with meniscectomy (29880-29881)*

🚑 17.8   ⚕ 17.8   **FUD** 090   J A2 80 50 ▱

AMA: 2018,Jan,8; 2017,Jan,8; 2016,Jan,13; 2015,Jan,16; 2014,Jan,11

29879   abrasion arthroplasty (includes chondroplasty where necessary) or multiple drilling or microfracture

🚑 19.0   ⚕ 19.0   **FUD** 090   J A2 80 50 ▱

AMA: 2018,Jan,8; 2017,Jan,8; 2016,Jan,13; 2015,Jan,16; 2014,Jan,11

29880   with meniscectomy (medial AND lateral, including any meniscal shaving) including debridement/shaving of articular cartilage (chondroplasty), same or separate compartment(s), when performed

🚑 16.1   ⚕ 16.1   **FUD** 090   J A2 80 50 ▱

AMA: 2018,Jan,8; 2017,Jan,8; 2016,Jan,13; 2015,Jan,16; 2014,Jan,11

29881   with meniscectomy (medial OR lateral, including any meniscal shaving) including debridement/shaving of articular cartilage (chondroplasty), same or separate compartment(s), when performed

🚑 15.5   ⚕ 15.5   **FUD** 090   J A2 80 50 ▱

AMA: 2018,Jan,8; 2017,Jan,8; 2016,Jan,13; 2016,Jan,11; 2015,Jan,16; 2014,May,10; 2014,Jan,11

29882   with meniscus repair (medial OR lateral)

EXCLUDES   *Meniscus transplant (29868)*

🚑 20.1   ⚕ 20.1   **FUD** 090   J A2 50 ▱

AMA: 2019,May,10; 2018,Jan,8; 2017,Jan,8; 2016,Jan,13; 2015,Jan,16; 2014,Jan,11

29883   with meniscus repair (medial AND lateral)

EXCLUDES   *Meniscus transplant (29868)*

🚑 24.3   ⚕ 24.3   **FUD** 090   J A2 80 50 ▱

AMA: 2018,Jan,8; 2017,Jan,8; 2016,Jan,13; 2015,Jan,16; 2014,Jan,11

29884   with lysis of adhesions, with or without manipulation (separate procedure)

🚑 17.6   ⚕ 17.6   **FUD** 090   J A2 80 50 ▱

AMA: 2018,Jan,8; 2017,Jan,8; 2016,Jan,13; 2015,Jan,16; 2014,Jan,11

29885   drilling for osteochondritis dissecans with bone grafting, with or without internal fixation (including debridement of base of lesion)

🚑 21.7   ⚕ 21.7   **FUD** 090   J A2 80 50 ▱

AMA: 2018,Jan,8; 2017,Jan,8; 2016,Jan,13; 2015,Jan,16; 2014,Jan,11

● New Code   ▲ Revised Code   ○ Reinstated   ● New Web Release   ▲ Revised Web Release   + Add-on   Unlisted   Not Covered   # Resequenced
50 Optum Mod 50 Exempt   Ⓢ AMA Mod 51 Exempt   51 Optum Mod 51 Exempt   63 Mod 63 Exempt   ✗ Non-FDA Drug   ★ Telemedicine   M Maternity   A Age Edit

29886 drilling for intact osteochondritis dissecans lesion
🦴 18.3 ⚕ 18.3 **FUD** 090 [J] [A2] [50] [▢]
AMA: 2018,Jan,8; 2017,Jan,8; 2016,Jan,13; 2015,Jan,16;
2014,Jan,11

29887 drilling for intact osteochondritis dissecans lesion with
internal fixation
🦴 21.6 ⚕ 21.6 **FUD** 090 [J] [A2] [80] [50] [▢]
AMA: 2018,Jan,8; 2017,Jan,8; 2016,Jan,13; 2015,Jan,16;
2014,Jan,11

29888 Arthroscopically aided anterior cruciate ligament
repair/augmentation or reconstruction
EXCLUDES Ligamentous reconstruction (augmentation), knee
(27427-27429)
🦴 28.3 ⚕ 28.3 **FUD** 090 [J] [J8] [80] [50] [▢]
AMA: 2018,Jan,8; 2017,Jan,8; 2016,Nov,9; 2016,Jan,13;
2015,Jan,16; 2014,Jan,11

29889 Arthroscopically aided posterior cruciate ligament
repair/augmentation or reconstruction
EXCLUDES Ligamentous reconstruction (augmentation), knee
(27427-27429)
🦴 35.3 ⚕ 35.3 **FUD** 090 [J] [A2] [80] [50] [▢]
AMA: 2018,Jan,8; 2017,Jan,8; 2016,Jan,13; 2015,Jan,16;
2014,Jan,11

29891 Arthroscopy, ankle, surgical, excision of osteochondral defect
of talus and/or tibia, including drilling of the defect
🦴 19.3 ⚕ 19.3 **FUD** 090 [J] [A2] [80] [50] [▢]
AMA: 2018,Jan,8; 2017,Jan,8; 2016,Jan,13; 2015,Jan,16

29892 Arthroscopically aided repair of large osteochondritis
dissecans lesion, talar dome fracture, or tibial plafond
fracture, with or without internal fixation (includes
arthroscopy)
🦴 18.8 ⚕ 18.8 **FUD** 090 [J] [A2] [80] [50] [▢]
AMA: 2018,Jan,8; 2017,Jan,8; 2016,Jan,13; 2015,Jan,16;
2014,Jan,11

29893 Endoscopic plantar fasciotomy
🦴 12.3 ⚕ 17.8 **FUD** 090 [J] [A2] [50] [▢]
AMA: 2018,Jan,8; 2017,Jan,8; 2016,Jan,13; 2015,Jan,16

29894 Arthroscopy, ankle (tibiotalar and fibulotalar joints), surgical;
with removal of loose body or foreign body
🦴 14.2 ⚕ 14.2 **FUD** 090 [J] [A2] [80] [50] [▢]
AMA: 2018,Jan,8; 2017,Jan,8; 2016,Jan,13; 2015,Jan,16

29895 synovectomy, partial
🦴 13.4 ⚕ 13.4 **FUD** 090 [J] [A2] [80] [50] [▢]
AMA: 2018,Jan,8; 2017,Jan,8; 2016,Jan,13; 2015,Jan,16;
2014,Jan,11

29897 debridement, limited
🦴 14.4 ⚕ 14.4 **FUD** 090 [J] [A2] [80] [50] [▢]
AMA: 2018,Jan,8; 2017,Jan,8; 2016,Jan,13; 2015,Jan,16

29898 debridement, extensive
🦴 16.1 ⚕ 16.1 **FUD** 090 [J] [A2] [80] [50] [▢]
AMA: 2018,Jan,8; 2017,Jan,8; 2016,Jan,13; 2015,Jan,16

29899 with ankle arthrodesis
EXCLUDES Open procedure (27870)
🦴 29.8 ⚕ 29.8 **FUD** 090 [J] [J8] [80] [50] [▢]
AMA: 2018,Jan,8; 2017,Jan,8; 2016,Jan,13; 2015,Jan,16

29900 Arthroscopy, metacarpophalangeal joint, diagnostic, includes
synovial biopsy
EXCLUDES Arthroscopy, metacarpophalangeal joint, surgical
(29901-29902)
🦴 14.3 ⚕ 14.3 **FUD** 090 [J] [A2] [80] [50] [▢]
AMA: 2018,Jan,8; 2017,Jan,8; 2016,Jan,13; 2015,Jan,16

29901 Arthroscopy, metacarpophalangeal joint, surgical; with
debridement
🦴 15.4 ⚕ 15.4 **FUD** 090 [J] [A2] [80] [50] [▢]
AMA: 2018,Jan,8; 2017,Jan,8; 2016,Jan,13; 2015,Jan,16

29902 with reduction of displaced ulnar collateral ligament (eg,
Stenar lesion)
🦴 16.3 ⚕ 16.3 **FUD** 090 [J] [A2] [80] [50] [▢]
AMA: 2018,Jan,8; 2017,Jan,8; 2016,Jan,13; 2015,Jan,16

29904 Arthroscopy, subtalar joint, surgical; with removal of loose
body or foreign body
🦴 18.4 ⚕ 18.4 **FUD** 090 [J] [G2] [80] [50] [▢]
AMA: 2018,Jan,8; 2017,Jan,8; 2016,Jan,13; 2015,Jan,16

29905 with synovectomy
🦴 14.9 ⚕ 14.9 **FUD** 090 [J] [G2] [80] [50] [▢]
AMA: 2018,Jan,8; 2017,Jan,8; 2016,Jan,13; 2015,Jan,16

29906 with debridement
🦴 19.5 ⚕ 19.5 **FUD** 090 [J] [G2] [80] [50] [▢]
AMA: 2018,Jan,8; 2017,Jan,8; 2016,Jan,13; 2015,Jan,16

29907 with subtalar arthrodesis
🦴 25.3 ⚕ 25.3 **FUD** 090 [J] [J8] [80] [50] [▢]
AMA: 2018,Jan,8; 2017,Jan,8; 2016,Jan,13; 2015,Jan,16

29914 Resequenced code. See code following 29863.

29915 Resequenced code. See code following 29863.

29916 Resequenced code. See code before 29866.

29999 Unlisted procedure, arthroscopy
🦴 0.00 ⚕ 0.00 **FUD** YYY [T] [80] [50] [▢]
AMA: 2018,Jan,8; 2017,Apr,9; 2017,Jan,8; 2016,Dec,16;
2016,Jan,13; 2015,Dec,16; 2015,Jan,16; 2014,Jan,11

| [26]/[TC] PC/TC Only | [A2]-[Z3] ASC Payment | [50] Bilateral | ♂ Male Only | ♀ Female Only | 🦴 Facility RVU | ⚕ Non-Facility RVU | [▢] CCI | [✗] CLIA |
| **FUD** Follow-up Days | **CMS:** IOM | **AMA:** CPT Asst | [A]-[Y] OPPSI | [80]/[80] Surg Assist Allowed / w/Doc | | [▢] Lab Crosswalk | [▢] Radiology Crosswalk | |

108   CPT © 2019 American Medical Association. All Rights Reserved.   © 2019 Optum360, LLC

30000-30115 I&D, Biopsy, Excision Procedures of the Nose

30000 **Drainage abscess or hematoma, nasal, internal approach**
EXCLUDES *Incision and drainage (10060, 10140)*
🔲 3.37 ⚕ 6.83 **FUD** 010 T P2 80 ▢
AMA: 2005,May,13-14; 1994,Spr,24

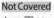

Side view of the pharynx

Nasopharynx region

Oropharynx region

Hypopharynx region

Epiglottis

Larynx

Esophagus

The nasopharynx is the membranous passage above the level of the soft palate; the oropharynx is the region between the soft palate and the upper edge of the epiglottis; the hypopharynx is the region of the epiglottis to the juncture of the larynx and esophagus; the three regions are collectively known as the pharynx

30020 **Drainage abscess or hematoma, nasal septum**
🔲 3.37 ⚕ 6.90 **FUD** 010 T P3 ▢
EXCLUDES *Lateral rhinotomy incision (30118, 30320)*

30100 **Biopsy, intranasal**
EXCLUDES *Superficial biopsy of nose (11102-11107)*
🔲 1.93 ⚕ 4.00 **FUD** 000 T P3 ▢
AMA: 2019,Jan,9

Intranasal biopsy

Suspect tissue is excised for study; some adjacent normal tissue is excised for comparison

Only a wedge of tissue is removed for larger lesions

30110 **Excision, nasal polyp(s), simple**
🔲 3.69 ⚕ 6.65 **FUD** 010 T P3 50 ▢

30115 **Excision, nasal polyp(s), extensive**
🔲 12.4 ⚕ 12.4 **FUD** 090 J A2 50 ▢

30117-30118 Destruction Procedures Nose
CMS: 100-03,140.5 Laser Procedures

30117 **Excision or destruction (eg, laser), intranasal lesion; internal approach**
🔲 9.56 ⚕ 25.6 **FUD** 090 J A2 ▢
AMA: 2019,Jul,10

30118 **external approach (lateral rhinotomy)**
🔲 22.1 ⚕ 22.1 **FUD** 090 J A2 ▢

30120-30140 Excision Procedures Nose, Turbinate

30120 **Excision or surgical planing of skin of nose for rhinophyma**
🔲 12.3 ⚕ 14.6 **FUD** 090 J A2 ▢
AMA: 2018,Jan,8; 2017,Jan,8; 2016,Jan,13; 2015,Jan,16; 2014,Jan,11

30124 **Excision dermoid cyst, nose; simple, skin, subcutaneous**
🔲 8.19 ⚕ 8.19 **FUD** 090 T P2 ▢

30125 **complex, under bone or cartilage**
🔲 17.5 ⚕ 17.5 **FUD** 090 J A2 80 ▢

30130 **Excision inferior turbinate, partial or complete, any method**
EXCLUDES *Ablation, soft tissue of inferior turbinates, unilateral or bilateral, any method (30801-30802)*
Excision middle/superior turbinate(s) (30999)
Fracture nasal inferior turbinate(s), therapeutic (30930)
🔲 11.0 ⚕ 11.0 **FUD** 090 J A2 50 ▢
AMA: 2018,Jan,8; 2017,Jan,8; 2016,Jan,13; 2015,Jan,16; 2014,Jan,11

30140 **Submucous resection inferior turbinate, partial or complete, any method**
EXCLUDES *Ablation, soft tissue of inferior turbinates, unilateral or bilateral, any method (30801-30802)*
Endoscopic resection of concha bullosa of middle turbinate (31240)
Fracture nasal inferior turbinate(s), therapeutic (30930)
Submucous resection:
Nasal septum (30520)
Superior or middle turbinate (30999)
🔲 5.12 ⚕ 7.92 **FUD** 000 J A2 50 ▢
AMA: 2018,Jan,8; 2017,Jan,8; 2016,Jan,13; 2015,Jan,16; 2014,Jan,11

30150-30160 Surgical Removal: Nose
EXCLUDES *Reconstruction and/or closure (primary or delayed primary intention) (13151-13160, 14060-14302, 15120-15121, 15260-15261, 15760, 20900-20912)*

30150 **Rhinectomy; partial**
🔲 22.0 ⚕ 22.0 **FUD** 090 J A2 ▢

30160 **total**
🔲 22.2 ⚕ 22.2 **FUD** 090 J A2 80 ▢

30200-30320 Turbinate Injection, Removal Foreign Substance in the Nose

30200 **Injection into turbinate(s), therapeutic**
🔲 1.66 ⚕ 3.18 **FUD** 000 T P3 ▢
AMA: 2018,Jan,8; 2017,Jan,8; 2016,Jan,13; 2015,Jan,16; 2014,Jan,11

30210 **Displacement therapy (Proetz type)**
🔲 2.82 ⚕ 4.25 **FUD** 010 T P3 ▢
AMA: 2018,Jan,8; 2017,Jan,8; 2016,Jan,13; 2015,Jan,16; 2014,Jan,11

30220 **Insertion, nasal septal prosthesis (button)**
🔲 3.55 ⚕ 8.60 **FUD** 010 T A2 ▢

30300 **Removal foreign body, intranasal; office type procedure**
🔲 3.14 ⚕ 5.26 **FUD** 010 01 N1 ▢
AMA: 2018,Jan,8; 2017,Jan,8; 2016,Jan,13; 2015,Jan,16; 2014,Jan,11

30310 **requiring general anesthesia**
🔲 5.77 ⚕ 5.77 **FUD** 010 J A2 80 ▢

30320 **by lateral rhinotomy**
🔲 13.0 ⚕ 13.0 **FUD** 090 T A2 80 ▢

30400-30630 Reconstruction or Repair of Nose

EXCLUDES Harvesting of bone/tissue/fat grafts ([15769], 15773-15774, 20900-20924, 21210)
Liposuction for autologous fat grafting (15773-15774)

30400 Rhinoplasty, primary; lateral and alar cartilages and/or elevation of nasal tip
🚗 30.9   ✂ 30.9   **FUD** 090   J A2 80 ▣

INCLUDES Carpue's operation
EXCLUDES Reconstruction of columella (13151-13153)

30410 complete, external parts including bony pyramid, lateral and alar cartilages, and/or elevation of nasal tip
🚗 35.8   ✂ 35.8   **FUD** 090   J A2 80 ▣

30420 including major septal repair
🚗 39.4   ✂ 39.4   **FUD** 090   J A2
AMA: 2018,Jan,8; 2017,Nov,11; 2017,Jan,8; 2016,Jul,8

30430 Rhinoplasty, secondary; minor revision (small amount of nasal tip work)
🚗 27.2   ✂ 27.2   **FUD** 090   J A2 80 ▣

30435 intermediate revision (bony work with osteotomies)
🚗 33.7   ✂ 33.7   **FUD** 090   J A2 80 ▣

30450 major revision (nasal tip work and osteotomies)
🚗 44.9   ✂ 44.9   **FUD** 090   J A2 80 ▣

30460 Rhinoplasty for nasal deformity secondary to congenital cleft lip and/or palate, including columellar lengthening; tip only
🚗 23.5   ✂ 23.5   **FUD** 090   J A2 80 ▣
AMA: 2018,Jan,8; 2017,Jan,8; 2016,Jan,13; 2015,Jan,16; 2014,Dec,18

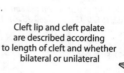

Cleft lip and cleft palate are described according to length of cleft and whether bilateral or unilateral

Complete unilateral cleft lip

Hard palate
Nasal cavity
Nasal septum
Soft palate

Isolated unilateral complete cleft of palate

Bilateral complete cleft of lip and palate

30462 tip, septum, osteotomies
🚗 45.1   ✂ 45.1   **FUD** 090   J A2 80 ▣
AMA: 2018,Jan,8; 2017,Jan,8; 2016,Jan,13; 2015,Jan,16; 2014,Dec,18

30465 Repair of nasal vestibular stenosis (eg, spreader grafting, lateral nasal wall reconstruction)
🚗 28.1   ✂ 28.1   **FUD** 090   J A2 80 ▣

INCLUDES Bilateral procedure
Code also modifier 52 for unilateral procedure

30520 Septoplasty or submucous resection, with or without cartilage scoring, contouring or replacement with graft
EXCLUDES Turbinate resection (30140)
🚗 18.0   ✂ 18.0   **FUD** 090   J A2 ▣
AMA: 2019,Jul,10; 2018,Jan,8; 2017,Jan,8; 2016,Jan,13; 2015,Jul,10; 2015,Jan,16; 2014,Jan,11

30540 Repair choanal atresia; intranasal
🚗 19.8   ✂ 19.8   **FUD** 090   63 J A2 80 ▣

30545 transpalatine
🚗 27.1   ✂ 27.1   **FUD** 090   63 J A2 80 ▣

30560 Lysis intranasal synechia
🚗 3.95   ✂ 7.96   **FUD** 010   T A2 ▣

30580 Repair fistula; oromaxillary (combine with 31030 if antrotomy is included)
🚗 14.2   ✂ 18.3   **FUD** 090   J A2 ▣

30600 oronasal
🚗 12.5   ✂ 16.2   **FUD** 090   J A2 80 ▣

30620 Septal or other intranasal dermatoplasty (does not include obtaining graft)
🚗 18.2   ✂ 18.2   **FUD** 090   J A2 ▣

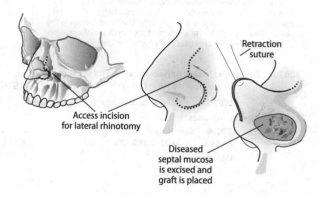

Retraction suture

Access incision for lateral rhinotomy

Diseased septal mucosa is excised and graft is placed

30630 Repair nasal septal perforations
🚗 18.0   ✂ 18.0   **FUD** 090   J A2 80 ▣
AMA: 2018,Jan,8; 2017,Jan,8; 2016,Jan,13; 2015,Jan,16; 2014,Jan,11

30801-30802 Turbinate Destruction

EXCLUDES Ablation middle/superior turbinates (30999)
Cautery to stop nasal bleeding (30901-30906)
Excision inferior turbinate, partial or complete, any method (30130)
Submucous resection inferior turbinate, partial or complete, any method (30140)

30801 Ablation, soft tissue of inferior turbinates, unilateral or bilateral, any method (eg, electrocautery, radiofrequency ablation, or tissue volume reduction); superficial
EXCLUDES Submucosal ablation inferior turbinates (30802)
🚗 3.98   ✂ 6.32   **FUD** 010   T A2 ▣
AMA: 2019,Jul,10

30802 intramural (ie, submucosal)
EXCLUDES Superficial ablation inferior turbinates (30801)
🚗 5.48   ✂ 8.03   **FUD** 010   T A2 ▣
AMA: 2019,Jul,10; 2018,Jan,8; 2017,Jan,8; 2016,Jan,13; 2015,Jan,16; 2014,Jan,11

30901-30920 Control Nose Bleed

30901 Control nasal hemorrhage, anterior, simple (limited cautery and/or packing) any method
🚗 1.62   ✂ 3.91   **FUD** 000   Q1 N1 50 ▣
AMA: 1990,Win,4

26/TC PC/TC Only   A2-Z3 ASC Payment   50 Bilateral   ♂ Male Only   ♀ Female Only   🚗 Facility RVU   ✂ Non-Facility RVU   ▣ CCI   ✖ CLIA
FUD Follow-up Days   CMS: IOM   AMA: CPT Asst   A-Y OPPSI   80/80 Surg Assist Allowed / w/Doc   ▣ Lab Crosswalk   ▣ Radiology Crosswalk

30903 Control nasal hemorrhage, anterior, complex (extensive cautery and/or packing) any method
🔲 2.25 ⚕ 6.16 **FUD** 000 T A2 50 ▫
AMA: 1990,Win,4

30905 Control nasal hemorrhage, posterior, with posterior nasal packs and/or cautery, any method; initial
🔲 3.01 ⚕ 9.36 **FUD** 000 T A2 ▫
AMA: 2018,Jan,8; 2017,Jan,8; 2016,Jan,13; 2015,Jan,16; 2014,Jan,11

30906 subsequent
🔲 3.90 ⚕ 9.79 **FUD** 000 T A2 ▫
AMA: 2002,May,7

30915 Ligation arteries; ethmoidal
🔲 16.5 ⚕ 16.5 **FUD** 090 T A2 ▫
EXCLUDES External carotid artery (37600)

30920 internal maxillary artery, transantral
🔲 24.0 ⚕ 24.0 **FUD** 090 T A2 ▫
EXCLUDES External carotid artery (37600)

30930-30999 Other and Unlisted Procedures of Nose

30930 Fracture nasal inferior turbinate(s), therapeutic
EXCLUDES Excision inferior turbinate, partial or complete, any method (30130)
Fracture of superior or middle turbinate(s) (30999)
Submucous resection inferior turbinate, partial or complete, any method (30140)
🔲 3.43 ⚕ 3.43 **FUD** 010 J A2 50 ▫
AMA: 2018,Jan,8; 2017,Nov,11; 2017,Jan,8; 2016,Jul,8; 2016,Jan,13; 2015,Jan,16; 2014,Jan,11

30999 Unlisted procedure, nose
🔲 0.00 ⚕ 0.00 **FUD** YYY T 80 ▫
AMA: 2018,Jan,8; 2017,Jan,8; 2016,Jan,13; 2015,Jan,16

31000-31230 Opening Sinuses

31000 Lavage by cannulation; maxillary sinus (antrum puncture or natural ostium)
🔲 3.02 ⚕ 5.17 **FUD** 010 T P2 50 ▫
AMA: 2018,Jan,8; 2017,Jan,8; 2016,Jan,13; 2015,Jan,16; 2014,Apr,10

Frontal sinus
Crista galli
Ethmoidal cells
Orbital cavity
Superior, middle, and inferior conchae
Maxillary sinus
Caldwell-Luc approach

Frontal sinus
Posterior ethmoidal cells
Sphenoid sinus
Nostril
Conchae (nasal cavity)
Hard palate

Schematic showing lateral wall of the nasal cavity (above) and coronal section showing nasal and paranasal sinuses (left)

31002 sphenoid sinus
🔲 5.39 ⚕ 5.39 **FUD** 010 T R2 80 50 ▫

31020 Sinusotomy, maxillary (antrotomy); intranasal
🔲 10.4 ⚕ 13.6 **FUD** 090 J A2 50 ▫

31030 radical (Caldwell-Luc) without removal of antrochoanal polyps
🔲 15.0 ⚕ 19.1 **FUD** 090 J A2 50 ▫

31032 radical (Caldwell-Luc) with removal of antrochoanal polyps
🔲 16.5 ⚕ 16.5 **FUD** 090 J A2 50 ▫

31040 Pterygomaxillary fossa surgery, any approach
🔲 22.0 ⚕ 22.0 **FUD** 090 J R2 50 ▫
EXCLUDES Transantral ligation internal maxillary artery (30920)

31050 Sinusotomy, sphenoid, with or without biopsy;
🔲 13.9 ⚕ 13.9 **FUD** 090 J A2 50 ▫

31051 with mucosal stripping or removal of polyp(s)
🔲 18.6 ⚕ 18.6 **FUD** 090 J A2 50 ▫

31070 Sinusotomy frontal; external, simple (trephine operation)
🔲 12.6 ⚕ 12.6 **FUD** 090 J A2 50 ▫
INCLUDES Killian operation
EXCLUDES Intranasal frontal sinusotomy (31276)

31075 transorbital, unilateral (for mucocele or osteoma, Lynch type)
🔲 22.4 ⚕ 22.4 **FUD** 090 J A2 80 50 ▫

31080 obliterative without osteoplastic flap, brow incision (includes ablation)
🔲 29.6 ⚕ 29.6 **FUD** 090 J A2 80 50 ▫
INCLUDES Ridell sinusotomy

31081 obliterative, without osteoplastic flap, coronal incision (includes ablation)
🔲 31.9 ⚕ 31.9 **FUD** 090 J A2 80 50 ▫

31084 obliterative, with osteoplastic flap, brow incision
🔲 33.1 ⚕ 33.1 **FUD** 090 J A2 80 50 ▫

31085 obliterative, with osteoplastic flap, coronal incision
🔲 34.1 ⚕ 34.1 **FUD** 090 J A2 80 50 ▫

31086 nonobliterative, with osteoplastic flap, brow incision
🔲 32.1 ⚕ 32.1 **FUD** 090 J A2 80 50 ▫

31087 nonobliterative, with osteoplastic flap, coronal incision
🔲 30.9 ⚕ 30.9 **FUD** 090 J A2 80 50 ▫

31090 Sinusotomy, unilateral, 3 or more paranasal sinuses (frontal, maxillary, ethmoid, sphenoid)
🔲 29.6 ⚕ 29.6 **FUD** 090 J A2 50 ▫
AMA: 1998,Nov,1; 1997,Nov,1

31200 Ethmoidectomy; intranasal, anterior
🔲 16.7 ⚕ 16.7 **FUD** 090 J A2 50 ▫
AMA: 2018,Jan,8; 2017,Jan,8; 2016,Feb,10

31201 intranasal, total
🔲 21.4 ⚕ 21.4 **FUD** 090 J A2 50 ▫
AMA: 2018,Jan,8; 2017,Jan,8; 2016,Feb,10

31205 extranasal, total
🔲 26.1 ⚕ 26.1 **FUD** 090 J A2 80 50 ▫
AMA: 2018,Jan,8; 2017,Jan,8; 2016,Feb,10

31225 Maxillectomy; without orbital exenteration
🔲 52.8 ⚕ 52.8 **FUD** 090 C 80 50 ▫

31230 with orbital exenteration (en bloc)
🔲 58.3 ⚕ 58.3 **FUD** 090 C 80 50 ▫
EXCLUDES Orbital exenteration without maxillectomy (65110-65114)
Skin grafts (15120-15121)

31231-31235 Nasal Endoscopy, Diagnostic

INCLUDES Complete sinus exam (e.g., nasal cavity, turbinates, sphenoethmoidal recess)
Code also stereotactic navigation, if performed (61782)

31231 Nasal endoscopy, diagnostic, unilateral or bilateral (separate procedure)
🔲 1.86 ⚕ 5.69 **FUD** 000 T P2 ▫
AMA: 2018,Apr,3; 2018,Jan,8; 2017,Jul,7; 2017,Jan,8; 2017,Jan,6; 2016,Dec,13; 2016,Feb,10; 2016,Jan,13; 2015,Jan,16; 2014,Jan,11

▲ **31233** Nasal/sinus endoscopy, diagnostic; with maxillary sinusoscopy (via inferior meatus or canine fossa puncture)
EXCLUDES Nasal/sinus endoscopy, surgical; with dilation of maxillary sinus ostium (31295)
When performed on the same side:
Dilation of maxillary sinus ostium (31295)
Maxillary antrostomy (31256, 31267)
🔲 3.87 ⚕ 7.41 **FUD** 000 T A2 80 50 ▫
AMA: 2018,Apr,3; 2018,Jan,8; 2017,Jan,8; 2016,Jan,13; 2015,Jan,16; 2014,Jan,11

Respiratory System (sidebar)

31235 — 31257 (sidebar)

▲ **31235**   **with sphenoid sinusoscopy (via puncture of sphenoidal face or cannulation of ostium)**

> EXCLUDES   *Insertion of drug-eluting implant performed with biopsy, debridement, or polypectomy (31237)*
> *Insertion of drug-eluting implant without other nasal/sinus endoscopic procedure (31299)*
> *When performed on the same side:*
> *Sinus dilation (31297-31298)*
> *Sphenoidotomy (31287-31288)*
> *Total ethmoidectomy with sphenoidotomy ([31257, 31259])*

🔲 4.58   ⚘ 8.47   **FUD** 000   ☒ J ☒ A2 ☒ 80 ☒ 50 ☒

AMA: 2018,Apr,3; 2018,Jan,8; 2017,Jan,8; 2016,Jan,13; 2015,Jan,16; 2014,Jan,11

31237-31253 Nasal Endoscopy, Surgical

> INCLUDES   Diagnostic nasal/sinus endoscopy
> Unilateral procedure
> EXCLUDES   *Frontal sinus exploration (31276)*
> *Maxillary antrostomy (31256)*
> *Osteomeatal complex (OMC) resection and/or partial (anterior) ethmoidectomy (31254)*
> *Removal of maxillary sinus tissue (31267)*
> *Total (anterior and posterior) ethmoidectomy (31255)*
> Code also stereotactic navigation, if performed (61782)

31237   **Nasal/sinus endoscopy, surgical; with biopsy, polypectomy or debridement (separate procedure)**

> EXCLUDES   *When performed on the same side:*
> *Frontal sinus exploration (31276)*
> *Maxillary antrostomy (31256, 31267)*
> *Nasal hemorrhage control (31238)*
> *Optic nerve decompression (31294)*
> *Orbital wall decompression, medial and/or inferior (31292-31293)*
> *Other total ethmoidectomy procedures ([31253], 31255, [31257], [31259])*
> *Partial ethmoidectomy (31254)*
> *Repair of CSF leak (31290-31291)*
> *Sphenoidotomy (31287-31288)*

🔲 4.58   ⚘ 7.26   **FUD** 000   ☒ J ☒ A2 ☒ 50 ☒

AMA: 2019,Jul,7; 2019,Apr,10; 2018,Apr,3; 2018,Jan,8; 2017,Jan,8; 2016,Feb,10; 2016,Jan,13; 2015,Jan,16; 2015,Jan,13; 2014,Jan,11

31238   **with control of nasal hemorrhage**

> EXCLUDES   *When performed on the same side:*
> *Biopsy, polypectomy, or debridement (31237)*
> *Sphenopalatine artery ligation (31241)*

🔲 4.80   ⚘ 7.17   **FUD** 000   ☒ J ☒ A2 ☒ 80 ☒ 50 ☒

AMA: 2018,Apr,3; 2018,Jan,8; 2017,Jan,8; 2016,Jan,13; 2015,Jan,16; 2014,Jan,11

31239   **with dacryocystorhinostomy**

🔲 17.5   ⚘ 17.5   **FUD** 010   ☒ J ☒ A2 ☒ 80 ☒ 50 ☒

AMA: 2018,Apr,3; 2018,Jan,8; 2017,Jan,8; 2016,Jan,13; 2015,Jan,16; 2014,Jan,11

31240   **with concha bullosa resection**

🔲 4.56   ⚘ 4.56   **FUD** 000   ☒ J ☒ A2 ☒ 80 ☒ 50 ☒

AMA: 2018,Apr,3; 2018,Jan,8; 2017,Jan,8; 2016,Feb,10; 2016,Jan,13; 2015,Jan,16; 2014,Jan,11

31241   **with ligation of sphenopalatine artery**

> EXCLUDES   *Nasal/sinus endoscopy, surgical; with control of nasal hemorrhage, on the same side (31238)*

🔲 12.8   ⚘ 12.8   **FUD** 000   ☒ C ☒ 80 ☒ 50 ☒

AMA: 2018,Apr,3

31253   **Resequenced code. See code following 31255.**

31254-31259 [31253, 31257, 31259] Nasal Endoscopy with Ethmoid Removal

> INCLUDES   Diagnostic nasal/sinus endoscopy
> Sinusotomy, when applicable
> Code also stereotactic navigation, if performed (61782)

31254   **Nasal/sinus endoscopy, surgical with ethmoidectomy; partial (anterior)**

> EXCLUDES   *When performed on the same side:*
> *Biopsy, polypectomy, or debridement (31237)*
> *Optic nerve decompression (31294)*
> *Orbital wall decompression, medial and/or inferior (31292-31293)*
> *Other total ethmoidectomy procedures (31253, 31255, [31257], [31259])*
> *Repair of CSF leak (31290-31291)*

🔲 7.01   ⚘ 11.7   **FUD** 000   ☒ J ☒ A2 ☒ 50 ☒

AMA: 2019,Apr,10; 2018,Apr,3; 2018,Jan,8; 2017,Jan,8; 2016,Feb,10; 2016,Jan,13; 2015,Jan,16; 2014,Jan,11

31255   **with ethmoidectomy, total (anterior and posterior)**

> EXCLUDES   *When performed on the same side:*
> *Biopsy, polypectomy, or debridement (31237)*
> *Frontal sinus exploration (31276)*
> *Optic nerve decompression (31294)*
> *Orbital wall decompression, medial and/or inferior (31292-31293)*
> *Other total ethmoidectomy procedures (31253, [31257], [31259])*
> *Partial ethmoidectomy (31254)*
> *Repair of CSF leak (31290-31291)*
> *Sphenoidotomy (31287-31288)*

🔲 9.33   ⚘ 9.33   **FUD** 000   ☒ J ☒ A2 ☒ 50 ☒

AMA: 2019,Apr,10; 2018,Apr,3; 2018,Apr,10; 2018,Jan,8; 2017,Jan,8; 2016,Feb,10; 2016,Jan,13; 2015,Jan,16; 2014,Jan,11

\# **31253**   **total (anterior and posterior), including frontal sinus exploration, with removal of tissue from frontal sinus, when performed**

> EXCLUDES   *When performed on the same side:*
> *Biopsy, debridement, or polypectomy (31237)*
> *Dilation of sinus (31296, 31298)*
> *Frontal sinus exploration (31276)*
> *Optic nerve decompression (31294)*
> *Orbital wall decompression, medial and/or inferior (31292-31293)*
> *Partial ethmoidectomy (31254)*
> *Repair of CSF leak (31290-31291)*
> *Sinus dilation (31296, 31298)*
> *Total ethmoidectomy (31255)*

🔲 14.4   ⚘ 14.4   **FUD** 000   ☒ J ☒ 62 ☒ 50 ☒

AMA: 2019,Apr,10; 2018,Apr,10; 2018,Apr,3

\# **31257**   **total (anterior and posterior), including sphenoidotomy**

> EXCLUDES   *When performed on the same side:*
> *Biopsy, debridement, or polypectomy (31237)*
> *Diagnostic sphenoid sinusoscopy (31235)*
> *Optic nerve decompression (31294)*
> *Orbital wall decompression, medial and/or inferior (31292-31293)*
> *Other total ethmoidectomy procedures (31255, [31259])*
> *Partial ethmoidectomy (31254)*
> *Repair of CSF leak (31290-31291)*
> *Sinus dilation (31297-31298)*
> *Sphenoidotomy (31287-31288)*

🔲 12.8   ⚘ 12.8   **FUD** 000   ☒ J ☒ 62 ☒ 50 ☒

AMA: 2019,Apr,10; 2018,Apr,10; 2018,Apr,3

\# **31259** total (anterior and posterior), including sphenoidotomy, with removal of tissue from the sphenoid sinus

EXCLUDES *When performed on the same side:*
Biopsy, debridement, or polypectomy (31237)
Diagnostic sphenoid sinusoscopy (31235)
Optic nerve decompression (31294)
Orbital wall decompression, medial and/or inferior (31292-31293)
Other total ethmoidectomy procedures (31255, [31257])
Partial ethmoidectomy (31254)
Repair of CSF leak (31290-31291)
Sinus dilation (31297-31298)
Sphenoidotomy (31287-31288)

🚗 13.6 ⚕ 13.6 **FUD** 000 [J] [62] [50] [▢]

AMA: 2019,Apr,10; 2018,Apr,3

31256-31267 Nasal Endoscopy with Maxillary Procedures

INCLUDES Diagnostic nasal/sinus endoscopy
Nasal/sinus endoscopy, surgical; with dilation of maxillary sinus ostium (31295)
Sinusotomy, when applicable
Code also stereotactic navigation, if performed (61782)

31256 Nasal/sinus endoscopy, surgical, with maxillary antrostomy;

EXCLUDES *When performed on the same side:*
Biopsy, polypectomy, or debridement (31237)
Dilation of maxillary sinus ostium (31295)
Maxillary antrostomy with removal of tissue (31267)
Maxillary sinusoscopy (31233)

🚗 5.19 ⚕ 5.19 **FUD** 000 [J] [A2] [50] [▢]

AMA: 2019,Apr,10; 2018,Apr,3; 2018,Apr,10; 2018,Jan,8; 2017,Jan,8; 2016,Jan,13; 2015,Jan,16; 2014,Jan,11

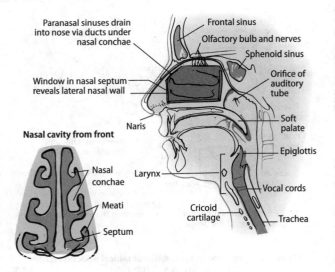

Paranasal sinuses drain into nose via ducts under nasal conchae
Frontal sinus
Olfactory bulb and nerves
Sphenoid sinus
Window in nasal septum reveals lateral nasal wall
Orifice of auditory tube
Naris
Soft palate
Nasal cavity from front
Epiglottis
Larynx
Nasal conchae
Vocal cords
Meati
Cricoid cartilage
Trachea
Septum

Frontal
Frontal
Ethmoid
Sphenoid
Ethmoid
Maxillary
Sphenoid
Maxillary

31257 **Resequenced code. See code following 31255.**

31259 **Resequenced code. See code following 31255.**

31267 with removal of tissue from maxillary sinus

EXCLUDES *When performed on the same side:*
Biopsy, polypectomy, or debridement (31237)
Dilation of maxillary sinus ostium (31295)
Maxillary antrostomy without tissue removal (31256)
Maxillary sinusoscopy (31233)

🚗 7.65 ⚕ 7.65 **FUD** 000 [J] [A2] [50] [▢]

AMA: 2019,Apr,10; 2018,Apr,3; 2018,Jan,8; 2017,Jan,8; 2016,Jan,13; 2015,Jan,16; 2014,Jan,11

31276 Nasal Endoscopy with Frontal Sinus Examination

INCLUDES Diagnostic nasal/sinus endoscopy
Sinusotomy, when applicable
Unilateral procedure
EXCLUDES *When performed on the same side:*
Biopsy, polypectomy, or debridement (31237)
Dilation of frontal or frontal and sphenoid sinus (31296, 31298)
Other total ethmoidectomy procedures (31253, 31255)
Code also stereotactic navigation, if performed (61782)

31276 Nasal/sinus endoscopy, surgical, with frontal sinus exploration, including removal of tissue from frontal sinus, when performed

🚗 10.9 ⚕ 10.9 **FUD** 000 [J] [A2] [50] [▢]

AMA: 2019,Apr,10; 2018,Apr,3; 2018,Apr,10; 2018,Jan,8; 2017,Jan,8; 2016,Jan,13; 2015,Jan,16; 2014,Jan,11

31287-31288 Nasal Endoscopy with Sphenoid Procedures

EXCLUDES *Other total ethmoidectomy procedures (31253, 31255, [31257], [31259])*
Sinus dilation (31297-31298)
Code also stereotactic navigation, if performed (61782)

31287 Nasal/sinus endoscopy, surgical, with sphenoidotomy;

EXCLUDES *When performed on the same side:*
Biopsy, polypectomy, or debridement (31237)
Diagnostic sphenoid sinusoscopy (31235)
Optic nerve decompression (31294)
Other total ethmoidectomy procedures (31255, [31257], [31259])
Repair of CSF leak (31291)
Sphenoidotomy with removal of tissue (31288)

🚗 5.80 ⚕ 5.80 **FUD** 000 [J] [A2] [80] [50] [▢]

AMA: 2019,Apr,10; 2018,Apr,3; 2018,Jan,8; 2017,Jan,8; 2016,Jan,13; 2015,Jan,16; 2014,Jan,11

31288 with removal of tissue from the sphenoid sinus

EXCLUDES *When performed on the same side:*
Biopsy, polypectomy, or debridement (31237)
Diagnostic sphenoid sinusoscopy (31235)
Optic nerve decompression (31294)
Other total ethmoidectomy procedures (31255, [31257], [31259])
Repair of CSF leak (31291)
Sphenoidotomy without removal of tissue (31287)

🚗 6.75 ⚕ 6.75 **FUD** 000 [J] [A2] [80] [50] [▢]

AMA: 2019,Apr,10; 2018,Apr,3; 2018,Jan,8; 2017,Jan,8; 2016,Feb,10; 2016,Jan,13; 2015,Jan,16; 2014,Jan,11

31290-31294 Nasal Endoscopy with Repair and Decompression

INCLUDES Diagnostic nasal/sinus endoscopy
Sinusotomy, when applicable
Code also stereotactic navigation, if performed (61782)

31290 Nasal/sinus endoscopy, surgical, with repair of cerebrospinal fluid leak; ethmoid region

EXCLUDES *When performed on the same side:*
Biopsy, polypectomy, or debridement (31237)
Other total ethmoidectomy procedures ([31253], 31255, [31257], [31259])
Partial ethmoidectomy (31254)

🚗 32.8 ⚕ 32.8 **FUD** 010 [C] [80] [50] [▢]

AMA: 2018,Apr,3; 2018,Jan,8; 2017,Jan,8; 2016,Feb,10; 2016,Jan,13; 2015,Jan,16; 2014,Jan,11

Respiratory System (side tab)

31291 — 31370 (side tab)

31291   **sphenoid region**

EXCLUDES *When performed on the same side:*
Biopsy, polypectomy, or debridement (31237)
Other total ethmoidectomy procedures ([31253],
31255, [31257], [31259])
Partial ethmoidectomy (31254)
Sphenoidotomy (31287-31288)

🔲 34.9 ≈ 34.9 **FUD** 010   C 80 50 ▢

AMA: 2018,Apr,3; 2018,Jan,8; 2017,Jan,8; 2016,Jan,13;
2015,Jan,16; 2014,Jan,11

▲ **31292** **Nasal/sinus endoscopy, surgical, with orbital decompression; medial or inferior wall**

EXCLUDES *When performed on the same side:*
Biopsy, polypectomy, or debridement (31237)
Dilation of frontal sinus only (31296)
Orbital wall decompression, medial and inferior
(31293)
Other total ethmoidectomy procedures ([31253],
31255, [31257], [31259])
Partial ethmoidectomy (31254)

🔲 28.3 ≈ 28.3 **FUD** 010   J 80 50 ▢

AMA: 2018,Apr,3; 2018,Jan,8; 2017,Jan,8; 2016,Jan,13;
2015,Jan,16; 2014,Jan,11

▲ **31293** **medial and inferior wall**

EXCLUDES *When performed on the same side:*
Biopsy, polypectomy, or debridement (31237)
Orbital wall decompression, medial or inferior (31292)
Other total ethmoidectomy procedures ([31253],
31255, [31257], [31259])
Partial ethmoidectomy (31254)

🔲 30.8 ≈ 30.8 **FUD** 010   J 80 50 ▢

AMA: 2018,Apr,3; 2018,Jan,8; 2017,Jan,8; 2016,Jan,13;
2015,Jan,16; 2014,Jan,11

▲ **31294** **Nasal/sinus endoscopy, surgical, with optic nerve decompression**

EXCLUDES *When performed on the same side:*
Biopsy, polypectomy, or debridement (31237)
Other total ethmoidectomy procedures ([31253],
31255, [31257], [31259])
Partial ethmoidectomy (31254)
Sphenoidotomy (31287-31288)

🔲 35.2 ≈ 35.2 **FUD** 010   J 80 50 ▢

AMA: 2018,Apr,3; 2018,Jan,8; 2017,Jan,8; 2016,Jan,13;
2015,Jan,16; 2014,Jan,11

31295-31298 Nasal Endoscopy with Sinus Ostia Dilation

INCLUDES Any method of tissue displacement
Fluoroscopy, when performed
Code also stereotactic navigation, if performed (61782)

▲ **31295** **Nasal/sinus endoscopy, surgical, with dilation (eg, balloon dilation); maxillary sinus ostium, transnasal or via canine fossa**

EXCLUDES *When performed on the same side:*
Maxillary antrostomy (31256-31267)
Maxillary sinusoscopy (31233)

🔲 4.55 ≈ 55.6 **FUD** 000   J P2 80 50 ▢

AMA: 2018,Apr,3; 2018,Jan,8; 2017,Jan,8; 2016,Jan,13;
2015,Jan,16; 2014,Jan,11

▲ **31296** **frontal sinus ostium**

EXCLUDES *When performed on the same side:*
Frontal sinus exploration (31276)
Sinus dilation (31297-31298)
Total ethmoidectomy (31253)

🔲 5.17 ≈ 56.3 **FUD** 000   J P2 80 50 ▢

AMA: 2018,Apr,3; 2018,Jan,8; 2017,Jan,8; 2016,Jan,13;
2015,Jan,16; 2014,Jan,11

▲ **31297** **sphenoid sinus ostium**

EXCLUDES *When performed on the same side:*
Diagnostic sphenoid sinusoscopy (31235)
Sinus dilation (31296, 31298)
Sphenoidotomy (31287-31288)
Total ethmoidectomy procedures ([31257], [31259])

🔲 4.14 ≈ 55.2 **FUD** 000   J P2 80 50 ▢

AMA: 2018,Apr,3; 2018,Jan,8; 2017,Jan,8; 2016,Jan,13;
2015,Jan,16; 2014,Jan,11

▲ **31298** **frontal and sphenoid sinus ostia**

EXCLUDES *When performed on the same side:*
Diagnostic sphenoid sinusoscopy (31235)
Dilation of frontal sinus only (31296)
Dilation of sphenoid sinus only (31297)
Frontal sinus exploration (31276)
Other total ethmoidectomy procedures (31253,
[31257], [31259])
Sphenoidotomy (31287-31288)

🔲 7.37 ≈ 106. **FUD** 000   J 62 80 50 ▢

AMA: 2018,Apr,3

31299 Unlisted Procedures of Accessory Sinuses

CMS: 100-04,4,180.3 Unlisted Service or Procedure

EXCLUDES *Hypophysectomy (61546, 61548)*

31299 **Unlisted procedure, accessory sinuses**

🔲 0.00 ≈ 0.00 **FUD** YYY   T 80 ▢

AMA: 2019,Jul,7; 2019,Apr,10; 2018,Jan,8; 2017,Nov,11;
2017,Jan,8; 2016,Feb,10; 2016,Jan,13; 2015,Jul,10; 2015,Jan,16;
2014,Jan,11

31300-31502 Procedures of the Larynx

31300 **Laryngotomy (thyrotomy, laryngofissure), with removal of tumor or laryngocele, cordectomy**

🔲 36.6 ≈ 36.6 **FUD** 090   J A2 80 ▢

Epiglottis — Hyoid bone — Thyroid cartilage — Cricothyroid ligament — Vocal cord — Cricoid cartilage — Trachea

Vocal cords — Arytenoid cartilage

Overhead schematic showing vocal cords

The larynx is the air passage of the neck area, serving as the voice mechanism as well as the valve to prevent food and other particles from entering the respiratory tract

Frontal view of the major structures of the larynx

31360 **Laryngectomy; total, without radical neck dissection**

🔲 59.8 ≈ 59.8 **FUD** 090   C 80 ▢

AMA: 2018,Jan,8; 2017,Jan,8; 2016,Jan,13; 2015,Jan,16;
2014,Jan,11

31365 **total, with radical neck dissection**

🔲 73.8 ≈ 73.8 **FUD** 090   C 80 ▢

AMA: 2018,Jan,8; 2017,Jan,8; 2016,Jan,13; 2015,Jan,16;
2014,Jan,11

31367 **subtotal supraglottic, without radical neck dissection**

🔲 63.2 ≈ 63.2 **FUD** 090   C 80 ▢

AMA: 2018,Jan,8; 2017,Jan,8; 2016,Jan,13; 2015,Jan,16;
2014,Jan,11

31368 **subtotal supraglottic, with radical neck dissection**

🔲 70.2 ≈ 70.2 **FUD** 090   C 80 ▢

31370 **Partial laryngectomy (hemilaryngectomy); horizontal**

🔲 59.4 ≈ 59.4 **FUD** 090   C 80 ▢

 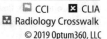

31375	laterovertical
	56.4 56.4 **FUD** 090 `C` `80`

31380	anterovertical
	55.6 55.6 **FUD** 090 `C` `80`

31382	antero-latero-vertical
	61.0 61.0 **FUD** 090 `C` `80`

31390	Pharyngolaryngectomy, with radical neck dissection; without reconstruction
	81.9 81.9 **FUD** 090 `C` `80`

31395	with reconstruction
	86.4 86.4 **FUD** 090 `C` `80`

31400	Arytenoidectomy or arytenoidopexy, external approach
	28.1 28.1 **FUD** 090 `J` `A2` `80`
	EXCLUDES Endoscopic arytenoidectomy (31560)

31420	Epiglottidectomy
	23.5 23.5 **FUD** 090 `J` `A2` `80`

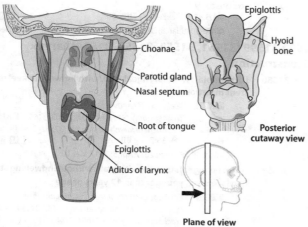

Epiglottis
Hyoid bone
Choanae
Parotid gland
Nasal septum
Root of tongue
Epiglottis
Aditus of larynx
Posterior cutaway view
Plane of view

31500 Intubation, endotracheal, emergency procedure
EXCLUDES Chest x-ray performed to confirm position of endotracheal tube
4.07   4.07   **FUD** 000   ⊘ `T` `G2`
AMA: 2018,Jan,8; 2017,Jan,8; 2016,Oct,8; 2016,May,3; 2016,Jan,13; 2015,Jan,16; 2014,Jan,11

31502 Tracheotomy tube change prior to establishment of fistula tract
1.01   1.01   **FUD** 000   `T` `G2`
AMA: 1990,Win,4

31505-31541 Endoscopy of the Larynx

31505 Laryngoscopy, indirect; diagnostic (separate procedure)
1.39   2.40   **FUD** 000   `T` `P3`
AMA: 2018,Jan,8; 2017,Jan,8; 2016,Jan,13; 2015,Jan,16; 2014,Jan,11

31510 with biopsy
3.46   6.01   **FUD** 000   `J` `A2` `80`
AMA: 2018,Jan,8; 2017,Jan,8; 2016,Jan,13; 2015,Jan,16; 2014,Jan,11

31511 with removal of foreign body
3.78   6.01   **FUD** 000   `T` `A2`
AMA: 2018,Jan,8; 2017,Jan,8; 2016,Jan,13; 2015,Jan,16; 2014,Jan,11

31512 with removal of lesion
3.70   5.92   **FUD** 000   `J` `A2` `80`
AMA: 2018,Jan,8; 2017,Jan,8; 2016,Jan,13; 2015,Jan,16; 2014,Jan,11

31513 with vocal cord injection
3.76   3.76   **FUD** 000   `T` `A2` `80`
AMA: 2018,Jan,8; 2017,Jan,8; 2016,Jan,13; 2015,Jan,16; 2014,Jan,11

31515 Laryngoscopy direct, with or without tracheoscopy; for aspiration
3.12   5.79   **FUD** 000   `T` `A2`
AMA: 1998,Nov,1; 1997,Nov,1

31520 diagnostic, newborn
4.48   4.48   **FUD** 000   `A`
`63` `T` `G2` `80`
AMA: 1998,Nov,1; 1997,Nov,1

31525 diagnostic, except newborn
4.56   7.12   **FUD** 000   `J` `A2`
AMA: 2018,Jan,8; 2017,Jan,8; 2016,Jan,13; 2015,Jan,16; 2014,Jan,11

31526 diagnostic, with operating microscope or telescope
INCLUDES Operating microscope (69990)
4.49   4.49   **FUD** 000   `J` `A2`
AMA: 2018,Jan,8; 2017,Jun,10; 2016,Feb,12

31527 with insertion of obturator
5.58   5.58   **FUD** 000   `J` `A2` `80`
AMA: 1998,Nov,1; 1997,Nov,1

31528 with dilation, initial
4.13   4.13   **FUD** 000   `J` `A2` `80`
AMA: 2002,May,7; 1998,Nov,1

31529 with dilation, subsequent
4.62   4.62   **FUD** 000   `J` `A2` `80`
AMA: 2002,May,7; 1998,Nov,1

31530 Laryngoscopy, direct, operative, with foreign body removal;
5.71   5.71   **FUD** 000   `J` `A2`
AMA: 1998,Nov,1; 1997,Nov,1

31531 with operating microscope or telescope
INCLUDES Operating microscope (69990)
6.08   6.08   **FUD** 000   `J` `A2` `80`
AMA: 2018,Jan,8; 2017,Jun,10; 2016,Feb,12

31535 Laryngoscopy, direct, operative, with biopsy;
5.42   5.42   **FUD** 000   `J` `A2`
AMA: 1998,Nov,1; 1997,Nov,1

31536 with operating microscope or telescope
INCLUDES Operating microscope (69990)
6.04   6.04   **FUD** 000   `J` `A2`
AMA: 2018,Jan,8; 2017,Jun,10; 2016,Feb,12

31540 Laryngoscopy, direct, operative, with excision of tumor and/or stripping of vocal cords or epiglottis;
6.91   6.91   **FUD** 000   `J` `A2`
AMA: 1998,Nov,1; 1997,Nov,1

31541 with operating microscope or telescope
INCLUDES Operating microscope (69990)
7.55   7.55   **FUD** 000   `J` `A2`
AMA: 2019,Sep,10; 2019,Jul,10; 2018,Jan,8; 2017,Jun,10; 2016,Feb,12

31545-31554 Endoscopy of Larynx with Reconstruction

INCLUDES Operating microscope (69990)
EXCLUDES Laryngoscopy, direct, operative, with excision of tumor and/or stripping of vocal cords or epiglottis (31540-31541)
Vocal cord reconstruction with allograft (31599)

31545 Laryngoscopy, direct, operative, with operating microscope or telescope, with submucosal removal of non-neoplastic lesion(s) of vocal cord; reconstruction with local tissue flap(s)
10.3   10.3   **FUD** 000   `J` `A2` `50`
AMA: 2016,Feb,12

Respiratory System

31546   reconstruction with graft(s) (includes obtaining autograft)
> EXCLUDES   Autologous fat graft obtained by liposuction (15771-15774)
> Autologous soft tissue grafts obtained by direct excision ([15769])

🔧 15.7   🔨 15.7   **FUD** 000   J A2 50 ▢

AMA: 2018,Jan,8; 2017,Jan,8; 2016,Feb,12; 2016,Jan,13; 2015,Jan,16; 2014,Jan,11

31551   Resequenced code. See code following 31580.

31552   Resequenced code. See code following 31580.

31553   Resequenced code. See code following 31580.

31554   Resequenced code. See code following 31580.

31560-31571 Endoscopy of Larynx with Arytenoid Removal, Vocal Cord Injection

31560   Laryngoscopy, direct, operative, with arytenoidectomy;
🔧 8.97   🔨 8.97   **FUD** 000   J A2 80 ▢
AMA: 1998,Nov,1; 1997,Nov,1

31561   with operating microscope or telescope
> INCLUDES   Operating microscope (69990)

🔧 9.82   🔨 9.82   **FUD** 000   J A2 80 ▢
AMA: 2018,Jan,8; 2017,Jun,10; 2016,Feb,12

31570   Laryngoscopy, direct, with injection into vocal cord(s), therapeutic;
🔧 6.56   🔨 9.63   **FUD** 000   J A2 ▢
AMA: 2018,Jan,8; 2017,Jan,8; 2017,Jan,6; 2016,Jan,13; 2015,Jan,16; 2014,Jan,6

31571   with operating microscope or telescope
> INCLUDES   Operating microscope (69990)

🔧 7.14   🔨 7.14   **FUD** 000   J A2 ▢
AMA: 2018,Jan,8; 2017,Jun,10; 2017,Jan,8; 2017,Jan,6; 2016,Feb,12; 2016,Jan,13; 2015,Jan,16; 2014,Jan,11; 2014,Jan,6

31572-31579 [31572, 31573, 31574] Endoscopy of Larynx, Flexible Fiberoptic

> EXCLUDES   Evaluation by flexible fiberoptic endoscope:
> Sensory assessment (92614-92615)
> Swallowing (92612-92613)
> Swallowing and sensory assessment (92616-92617)
> Flexible fiberoptic endoscopic examination/testing by cine or video recording (92612-92617)

31572   Resequenced code. See code following 31578.

31573   Resequenced code. See code following 31578.

31574   Resequenced code. See code following 31578.

31575   Laryngoscopy, flexible; diagnostic
> EXCLUDES   Diagnostic nasal endoscopy not through additional endoscope (31231)
> Procedures during same session (31572-31574, 31576-31578, 43197-43198, 92511, 92612, 92614, 92616)

🔧 1.91   🔨 3.31   **FUD** 000   T P3 ▢
AMA: 2018,Jan,8; 2017,Jul,7; 2017,Apr,8; 2017,Jan,8; 2016,Dec,13

31576   with biopsy(ies)
> EXCLUDES   Destruction or excision of lesion (31572, 31578)

🔧 3.39   🔨 7.54   **FUD** 000   J A2 ▢
AMA: 2018,Jan,8; 2017,Jul,7; 2017,Apr,8; 2017,Jan,8; 2016,Dec,13

31577   with removal of foreign body(s)
🔧 3.84   🔨 7.89   **FUD** 000   T A2 80 ▢
AMA: 2018,Jan,8; 2017,Jul,7; 2017,Apr,8; 2017,Jan,8; 2016,Dec,13

31578   with removal of lesion(s), non-laser
🔧 4.27   🔨 8.59   **FUD** 000   J A2 80 ▢
AMA: 2018,Jan,8; 2017,Jul,7; 2017,Apr,8; 2017,Jan,8; 2016,Dec,13

 #   31572   with ablation or destruction of lesion(s) with laser, unilateral
> EXCLUDES   Biopsy or excision of lesion (31576, 31578)
> Swallowing evaluation or sensory testing (92612-92617)

🔧 5.18   🔨 14.4   **FUD** 000   J G2 80 50 ▢
AMA: 2019,Sep,10; 2018,Jan,8; 2017,Jul,7; 2017,Apr,8; 2017,Jan,8; 2016,Dec,13

 #   31573   with therapeutic injection(s) (eg, chemodenervation agent or corticosteroid, injected percutaneous, transoral, or via endoscope channel), unilateral
🔧 4.24   🔨 7.47   **FUD** 000   J P3 80 50 ▢
AMA: 2018,May,7; 2018,Jan,8; 2017,Jul,7; 2017,Apr,8; 2017,Jan,8; 2016,Dec,13

 #   31574   with injection(s) for augmentation (eg, percutaneous, transoral), unilateral
🔧 4.24   🔨 28.8   **FUD** 000   J G2 80 50 ▢
AMA: 2018,May,7; 2018,Jan,8; 2017,Jul,7; 2017,Apr,8; 2017,Jan,8; 2016,Dec,13

31579   Laryngoscopy, flexible or rigid telescopic, with stroboscopy
🔧 3.42   🔨 5.23   **FUD** 000   T P3 ▢
AMA: 2018,Jan,8; 2017,Jul,7; 2017,Apr,8; 2017,Jan,8; 2016,Dec,13

31580-31599 [31551, 31552, 31553, 31554] Larynx Reconstruction

31580   Laryngoplasty; for laryngeal web, with indwelling keel or stent insertion
> EXCLUDES   Keel or stent removal (31599)
> Tracheostomy (31600-31601, 31603, 31605, 31610)
> Treatment of laryngeal stenosis (31551-31554)

🔧 35.7   🔨 35.7   **FUD** 090   J A2 80 ▢
AMA: 2018,Jan,8; 2017,Apr,5; 2017,Mar,10

 #   31551   for laryngeal stenosis, with graft, without indwelling stent placement, younger than 12 years of age   A
> EXCLUDES   Cartilage graft obtained through same incision
> Procedure during same session (31552-31554, 31580)
> Tracheostomy (31600-31601, 31603, 31605, 31610)

🔧 41.2   🔨 41.2   **FUD** 090   J G2 80 ▢
AMA: 2018,Jan,8; 2017,Jul,7; 2017,Apr,5; 2017,Mar,10

 #   31552   for laryngeal stenosis, with graft, without indwelling stent placement, age 12 years or older   A
> EXCLUDES   Cartilage graft obtained through same incision
> Procedure during same session (31551, 31553-31554, 31580)
> Tracheostomy (31600-31601, 31603, 31605, 31610)

🔧 41.4   🔨 41.4   **FUD** 090   J G2 80 ▢
AMA: 2018,Jan,8; 2017,Jul,7; 2017,Apr,5; 2017,Mar,10

 #   31553   for laryngeal stenosis, with graft, with indwelling stent placement, younger than 12 years of age   A
> EXCLUDES   Cartilage graft obtained through same incision
> Procedure during same session (31551-31552, 31554, 31580)
> Stent removal (31599)
> Tracheostomy (31600-31601, 31603, 31605, 31610)

🔧 45.2   🔨 45.2   **FUD** 090   J G2 80 ▢
AMA: 2018,Jan,8; 2017,Jul,7; 2017,Apr,5; 2017,Mar,10

 #   31554   for laryngeal stenosis, with graft, with indwelling stent placement, age 12 years or older   A
> EXCLUDES   Cartilage graft obtained through same incision
> Procedure during same session (31551-31553, 31580)
> Stent removal (31599)
> Tracheostomy (31600-31601, 31603, 31605, 31610)

🔧 47.3   🔨 47.3   **FUD** 090   J G2 80 ▢
AMA: 2018,Jan,8; 2017,Jul,7; 2017,Apr,5; 2017,Mar,10

26/TC PC/TC Only   A2-Z3 ASC Payment   50 Bilateral   ♂ Male Only   ♀ Female Only   🔧 Facility RVU   🔨 Non-Facility RVU   ▢ CCI   ✖ CLIA
FUD Follow-up Days   **CMS:** IOM   **AMA:** CPT Asst   A-Y OPPSI   80/80 Surg Assist Allowed / w/Doc   🔲 Lab Crosswalk   ➕ Radiology Crosswalk

116   CPT © 2019 American Medical Association. All Rights Reserved.   © 2019 Optum360, LLC

31584   **with open reduction and fixation of (eg, plating) fracture, includes tracheostomy, if performed**
EXCLUDES   *Cartilage graft obtained through same incision*
🚑 39.6   ⚕ 39.6   **FUD** 090   J 80 ▢
AMA: 2018,Jan,8; 2017,Apr,5; 2017,Mar,10

31587   **Laryngoplasty, cricoid split, without graft placement**
EXCLUDES   *Tracheostomy (31600-31601, 31603, 31605, 31610)*
🚑 33.2   ⚕ 33.2   **FUD** 090   J 80 ▢
AMA: 2018,Jan,8; 2017,Apr,5; 2017,Mar,10

31590   **Laryngeal reinnervation by neuromuscular pedicle**
🚑 25.0   ⚕ 25.0   **FUD** 090   J A2 80 ▢
AMA: 2018,Jan,8; 2017,Mar,10

31591   **Laryngoplasty, medialization, unilateral**
🚑 30.0   ⚕ 30.0   **FUD** 090   J G2 80 ▢
AMA: 2018,Jan,8; 2017,Jul,7; 2017,Apr,5; 2017,Mar,10

31592   **Cricotracheal resection**
EXCLUDES   *Advancement or rotational flaps performed not requiring additional incision*
Cartilage graft obtained through same incision
Tracheal stenosis excision/anastomosis (31780-31781)
Tracheostomy (31600-31601, 31603, 31605, 31610)
🚑 49.2   ⚕ 49.2   **FUD** 090   J G2 80 ▢
AMA: 2018,Jan,8; 2017,Jul,7; 2017,Apr,5; 2017,Mar,10; 2017,Feb,14

31599   **Unlisted procedure, larynx**
🚑 0.00   ⚕ 0.00   **FUD** YYY   T 80 ▢
AMA: 2018,Jan,8; 2017,Apr,5; 2017,Mar,10; 2017,Jan,8; 2017,Jan,6; 2016,Dec,13; 2016,Jan,13; 2015,Jan,16; 2014,Jan,11

31600-31610 Stoma Creation: Trachea

EXCLUDES   *Aspiration of trachea, direct vision (31515)*
Endotracheal intubation (31500)

31600   **Tracheostomy, planned (separate procedure);**
🚑 8.91   ⚕ 8.91   **FUD** 090   J ▢
AMA: 2019,Sep,10; 2017,Apr,5

31601   **younger than 2 years**
🚑 12.9   ⚕ 12.9   **FUD** 000   A
J 80 ▢
AMA: 2017,Apr,5

31603   **Tracheostomy, emergency procedure; transtracheal**
🚑 9.31   ⚕ 9.31   **FUD** 000   T A2 ▢
AMA: 2017,Apr,5

31605   **cricothyroid membrane**
🚑 9.61   ⚕ 9.61   **FUD** 000   T G2 ▢
AMA: 2017,Apr,5

31610   **Tracheostomy, fenestration procedure with skin flaps**
🚑 27.2   ⚕ 27.2   **FUD** 090   J ▢
AMA: 2017,Apr,5

31611-31614 Procedures of the Trachea

31611   **Construction of tracheoesophageal fistula and subsequent insertion of an alaryngeal speech prosthesis (eg, voice button, Blom-Singer prosthesis)**
🚑 15.2   ⚕ 15.2   **FUD** 090   J A2 80 ▢

31612   **Tracheal puncture, percutaneous with transtracheal aspiration and/or injection**
EXCLUDES   *Tracheal aspiration under direct vision (31515)*
🚑 1.39   ⚕ 2.39   **FUD** 000   J A2 80 ▢
AMA: 1994,Win,1

31613   **Tracheostoma revision; simple, without flap rotation**
🚑 12.6   ⚕ 12.6   **FUD** 090   J A2 ▢

31614   **complex, with flap rotation**
🚑 21.0   ⚕ 21.0   **FUD** 090   J A2 ▢

31615 Endoscopy Through Tracheostomy

INCLUDES   Diagnostic bronchoscopy
EXCLUDES   *Endobronchial ultrasound [EBUS] guided biopsies of mediastinal or hilar lymph nodes (31652-31653)*
Tracheoscopy (31515-31578)
Code also endobronchial ultrasound [EBUS] during diagnostic/therapeutic peripheral lesion intervention (31654)

31615   **Tracheobronchoscopy through established tracheostomy incision**
🚑 3.29   ⚕ 4.83   **FUD** 000   T A2 ▢
AMA: 2018,Jan,8; 2017,Jan,8; 2016,Jan,13; 2015,Jan,16; 2014,Jan,11

31622-31654 [31651] Endoscopy of Lung

INCLUDES   Diagnostic bronchoscopy with surgical bronchoscopy procedures
Fluoroscopic imaging guidance, when performed

31622   **Bronchoscopy, rigid or flexible, including fluoroscopic guidance, when performed; diagnostic, with cell washing, when performed (separate procedure)**
🚑 3.78   ⚕ 6.84   **FUD** 000   J A2 ▢
AMA: 2018,Jan,8; 2017,Jan,8; 2016,Apr,5; 2016,Jan,13; 2015,Jan,16; 2014,Jan,11

31623   **with brushing or protected brushings**
🚑 3.81   ⚕ 7.51   **FUD** 000   J A2 ▢
AMA: 2018,Jan,8; 2017,Jan,8; 2016,Apr,5; 2016,Jan,13; 2015,Jan,16; 2014,Jan,11

31624   **with bronchial alveolar lavage**
🚑 3.86   ⚕ 7.10   **FUD** 000   J A2 ▢
AMA: 2018,Jan,8; 2017,Jun,10; 2017,Jan,8; 2016,Apr,5; 2016,Jan,13; 2015,Jan,16; 2014,Jan,11

31625   **with bronchial or endobronchial biopsy(s), single or multiple sites**
🚑 4.49   ⚕ 9.59   **FUD** 000   J A2 ▢
AMA: 2018,Jan,8; 2017,Jan,8; 2016,Apr,5; 2016,Jan,13; 2015,Jan,16; 2014,Jan,11

31626   **with placement of fiducial markers, single or multiple**
Code also device
🚑 5.72   ⚕ 23.9   **FUD** 000   J G2 80 ▢
AMA: 2018,Jan,8; 2017,Jun,10; 2017,Jan,8; 2016,Apr,5; 2016,Jan,13; 2016,Jun,6; 2015,Jan,16; 2014,Jan,11

+ 31627   **with computer-assisted, image-guided navigation (List separately in addition to code for primary procedure[s])**
INCLUDES   3D reconstruction (76376-76377)
Code first (31615, 31622-31626, 31628-31631, 31635-31636, 31638-31643)
🚑 2.80   ⚕ 37.8   **FUD** ZZZ   N N1 80 ▢
AMA: 2018,Jan,8; 2017,Jan,8; 2016,Jan,13; 2015,Jan,16; 2014,Jan,11

31628   **with transbronchial lung biopsy(s), single lobe**
INCLUDES   All biopsies taken from lobe
EXCLUDES   *Transbronchial biopsies by needle aspiration (31629, 31633)*
Code also transbronchial biopsies of additional lobe(s) (31632)
🚑 5.06   ⚕ 10.1   **FUD** 000   J A2 ▢
AMA: 2018,Jan,8; 2017,Jun,10; 2017,Jan,8; 2016,Apr,5; 2016,Jan,13; 2015,Jan,16; 2014,Jan,11

31629   **with transbronchial needle aspiration biopsy(s), trachea, main stem and/or lobar bronchus(i)**
INCLUDES   All biopsies from same lobe or upper airway
EXCLUDES   *Transbronchial biopsies of lung (31628, 31632)*
Code also transbronchial needle biopsies of additional lobe(s) (31633)
🚑 5.38   ⚕ 12.5   **FUD** 000   J A2 ▢
AMA: 2018,Jan,8; 2017,Jan,8; 2016,Apr,5; 2016,Jan,13; 2015,Jan,16; 2014,Jan,11

31630   **with tracheal/bronchial dilation or closed reduction of fracture**
🚑 5.71   ⚕ 5.71   **FUD** 000   J A2 ▢
AMA: 2018,Jan,8; 2017,Jan,8; 2016,Jan,13; 2015,Jan,16; 2014,Jan,11

31631 with placement of tracheal stent(s) (includes tracheal/bronchial dilation as required)

EXCLUDES *Bronchial stent placement (31636-31637)*
Revision bronchial or tracheal stent (31638)

📷 6.58   ✎ 6.58   **FUD** 000   J A2 ▢

AMA: 2018,Jan,8; 2017,Jan,8; 2016,Jan,13; 2015,Jan,16; 2014,Jan,11

+ 31632 with transbronchial lung biopsy(s), each additional lobe (List separately in addition to code for primary procedure)

INCLUDES All biopsies of additional lobe of lung
Code first (31628)

📷 1.41   ✎ 1.81   **FUD** ZZZ   N N1 ▢

AMA: 2018,Jan,8; 2017,Jan,8; 2016,Jan,13; 2015,Jan,16; 2014,Jan,11

+ 31633 with transbronchial needle aspiration biopsy(s), each additional lobe (List separately in addition to code for primary procedure)

INCLUDES All needle biopsies from another lobe or from trachea
Code first (31629)

📷 1.83   ✎ 2.27   **FUD** ZZZ   N N1 ▢

AMA: 2018,Jan,8; 2017,Jan,8; 2016,Jan,13; 2015,Jan,16; 2014,Jan,11

31634 with balloon occlusion, with assessment of air leak, with administration of occlusive substance (eg, fibrin glue), if performed

EXCLUDES *Bronchoscopy, rigid or flexible, including fluoroscopic guidance, when performed; with balloon occlusion, when performed, assessment of air leak, airway sizing, and insertion of bronchial valve(s), initial lobe (31647, [31651])*

📷 5.53   ✎ 49.4   **FUD** 000   J G2 80 ▢

AMA: 2018,Jan,8; 2017,Jan,8; 2016,Jan,13; 2015,Jan,16; 2014,Jan,11

31635 with removal of foreign body

EXCLUDES *Removal implanted bronchial valves (31648-31649)*

📷 5.06   ✎ 8.03   **FUD** 000   J A2 ▢

AMA: 2018,Jan,8; 2017,Jan,8; 2016,Jan,13; 2015,Jan,16; 2014,Jan,11

31636 with placement of bronchial stent(s) (includes tracheal/bronchial dilation as required), initial bronchus

📷 6.35   ✎ 6.35   **FUD** 000   J J8 ▢

AMA: 2018,Jan,8; 2017,Jan,8; 2016,Jan,13; 2015,Jan,16; 2014,Jan,11

+ 31637 each additional major bronchus stented (List separately in addition to code for primary procedure)

Code first (31636)

📷 2.22   ✎ 2.22   **FUD** ZZZ   N N1 ▢

AMA: 2018,Jan,8; 2017,Jan,8; 2016,Jan,13; 2015,Jan,16; 2014,Jan,11

31638 with revision of tracheal or bronchial stent inserted at previous session (includes tracheal/bronchial dilation as required)

📷 7.21   ✎ 7.21   **FUD** 000   J A2 ▢

AMA: 2018,Jan,8; 2017,Jan,8; 2016,Jan,13; 2015,Jan,16; 2014,Jan,11

31640 with excision of tumor

📷 7.22   ✎ 7.22   **FUD** 000   J A2 ▢

AMA: 2018,Jan,8; 2017,Jan,8; 2016,Apr,5; 2016,Jan,13; 2015,Jan,16; 2014,Jan,11

31641 with destruction of tumor or relief of stenosis by any method other than excision (eg, laser therapy, cryotherapy)

Code also any photodynamic therapy via bronchoscopy (96570-96571)

📷 7.39   ✎ 7.39   **FUD** 000   J A2 ▢

AMA: 2018,Jan,8; 2017,Jan,8; 2016,Jan,13; 2015,Jan,16; 2014,Jan,11

31643 with placement of catheter(s) for intracavitary radioelement application

Code also if appropriate (77761-77763, 77770-77772)

📷 5.09   ✎ 5.09   **FUD** 000   J A2 ▢

AMA: 2018,Jan,8; 2017,Jan,8; 2016,Apr,5; 2016,Jan,13; 2015,Jan,16; 2014,Jan,11

31645 with therapeutic aspiration of tracheobronchial tree, initial (eg, drainage of lung abscess)

EXCLUDES *Bedside aspiration of trachea, bronchi (31725)*

📷 4.21   ✎ 7.42   **FUD** 000   J A2 ▢

AMA: 2018,Jan,8; 2017,Jan,8; 2016,Apr,5; 2016,Jan,13; 2015,Jan,16; 2014,Jan,11

31646 with therapeutic aspiration of tracheobronchial tree, subsequent

EXCLUDES *Bedside aspiration of trachea, bronchi (31725)*

📷 4.09   ✎ 4.09   **FUD** 000   T A2 ▢

AMA: 2018,Sep,3; 2018,Jan,8; 2017,Jan,8; 2016,Apr,5; 2016,Jan,13; 2015,Jan,16; 2014,Jan,11

31647 with balloon occlusion, when performed, assessment of air leak, airway sizing, and insertion of bronchial valve(s), initial lobe

📷 6.10   ✎ 6.10   **FUD** 000   J G2 ▢

AMA: 2018,Sep,3; 2018,Jan,8; 2017,Jan,8; 2016,Jan,13; 2015,Jan,16; 2014,Jan,11

+ # 31651 with balloon occlusion, when performed, assessment of air leak, airway sizing, and insertion of bronchial valve(s), each additional lobe (List separately in addition to code for primary procedure[s])

Code first (31647)

📷 2.13   ✎ 2.13   **FUD** ZZZ   N N1 ▢

AMA: 2018,Sep,3; 2018,Jan,8; 2017,Jan,8; 2016,Jan,13; 2015,Jan,16; 2014,Jan,11

31648 with removal of bronchial valve(s), initial lobe

EXCLUDES *Removal with reinsertion bronchial valve during same session (31647 and 31648) and ([31651])*

📷 5.80   ✎ 5.80   **FUD** 000   J G2 ▢

AMA: 2018,Sep,3; 2018,Jan,8; 2017,Jan,8; 2016,Jan,13; 2015,Jan,16; 2014,Jan,11

+ 31649 with removal of bronchial valve(s), each additional lobe (List separately in addition to code for primary procedure)

Code first (31648)

📷 1.94   ✎ 1.94   **FUD** ZZZ   02 G2 ▢

AMA: 2018,Sep,3; 2018,Jan,8; 2017,Jan,8; 2016,Jan,13; 2015,Jan,16; 2014,Jan,11

31651 Resequenced code. See code following 31647.

31652 with endobronchial ultrasound (EBUS) guided transtracheal and/or transbronchial sampling (eg, aspiration[s]/biopsy[ies]), one or two mediastinal and/or hilar lymph node stations or structures

EXCLUDES *Procedures performed more than one time per session*

📷 6.39   ✎ 27.4   **FUD** 000   J G2 ▢

AMA: 2018,Jan,8; 2017,Jan,8; 2016,Apr,5

31653 with endobronchial ultrasound (EBUS) guided transtracheal and/or transbronchial sampling (eg, aspiration[s]/biopsy[ies]), 3 or more mediastinal and/or hilar lymph node stations or structures

EXCLUDES *Procedures performed more than one time per session*

📷 7.08   ✎ 28.7   **FUD** 000   J G2 ▢

AMA: 2018,Jan,8; 2017,Jan,8; 2016,Apr,5

+ 31654 with transendoscopic endobronchial ultrasound (EBUS) during bronchoscopic diagnostic or therapeutic intervention(s) for peripheral lesion(s) (List separately in addition to code for primary procedure[s])

EXCLUDES Endobronchial ultrasound [EBUS] for mediastinal/hilar lymph node station/adjacent structure access (31652-31653)

Procedures performed more than one time per session

Code first (31622-31626, 31628-31629, 31640, 31643-31646)

1.94 ⚕ 3.53 **FUD** ZZZ N N1 🔲

AMA: 2018,Jan,8; 2017,Jan,8; 2016,Apr,5

31660-31661 Bronchial Thermoplasty

INCLUDES Fluoroscopic imaging guidance, when performed

31660 Bronchoscopy, rigid or flexible, including fluoroscopic guidance, when performed; with bronchial thermoplasty, 1 lobe

5.62 ⚕ 5.62 **FUD** 000 J 🔲

AMA: 2018,Jan,8; 2017,Jan,8; 2016,Jan,13; 2015,Jan,16; 2014,Jan,11

31661 with bronchial thermoplasty, 2 or more lobes

5.93 ⚕ 5.93 **FUD** 000 J 🔲

AMA: 2018,Jan,8; 2017,Jan,8; 2016,Jan,13; 2015,Jan,16; 2014,Jan,11

31717-31899 Respiratory Procedures

EXCLUDES Endotracheal intubation (31500)
Tracheal aspiration under direct vision (31515)

31717 Catheterization with bronchial brush biopsy

3.18 ⚕ 7.98 **FUD** 000 T A2 🔲

AMA: 2018,Jan,8; 2017,Jan,8; 2016,Jan,13; 2015,Jan,16; 2014,Jan,11

31720 Catheter aspiration (separate procedure); nasotracheal

1.43 ⚕ 1.43 **FUD** 000 01 N1 🔲

AMA: 1994,Win,1

31725 tracheobronchial with fiberscope, bedside

2.29 ⚕ 2.29 **FUD** 000 C 🔲

31730 Transtracheal (percutaneous) introduction of needle wire dilator/stent or indwelling tube for oxygen therapy

4.32 ⚕ 34.2 **FUD** 000 J A2 🔲

AMA: 1992,Win,1

31750 Tracheoplasty; cervical

39.5 ⚕ 39.5 **FUD** 090 J A2 80 🔲

31755 tracheopharyngeal fistulization, each stage

49.9 ⚕ 49.9 **FUD** 090 J A2 80 🔲

31760 intrathoracic

39.6 ⚕ 39.6 **FUD** 090 C 80 🔲

31766 Carinal reconstruction

51.4 ⚕ 51.4 **FUD** 090 C 80 🔲

31770 Bronchoplasty; graft repair

38.5 ⚕ 38.5 **FUD** 090 C 80 🔲

EXCLUDES Bronchoplasty done with lobectomy (32501)

31775 excision stenosis and anastomosis

40.4 ⚕ 40.4 **FUD** 090 C 80 🔲

EXCLUDES Bronchoplasty done with lobectomy (32501)

31780 Excision tracheal stenosis and anastomosis; cervical

34.3 ⚕ 34.3 **FUD** 090 C 80 🔲

AMA: 2018,Jan,8; 2017,Apr,5; 2017,Feb,14

31781 cervicothoracic

40.1 ⚕ 40.1 **FUD** 090 C 80 🔲

AMA: 2018,Jan,8; 2017,Apr,5; 2017,Feb,14

31785 Excision of tracheal tumor or carcinoma; cervical

30.9 ⚕ 30.9 **FUD** 090 J 80 🔲

AMA: 2003,Jan,1

31786 thoracic

41.7 ⚕ 41.7 **FUD** 090 C 80 🔲

31800 Suture of tracheal wound or injury; cervical

20.6 ⚕ 20.6 **FUD** 090 C 80 🔲

AMA: 1994,Win,1

31805 intrathoracic

23.5 ⚕ 23.5 **FUD** 090 C 80 🔲

31820 Surgical closure tracheostomy or fistula; without plastic repair

9.35 ⚕ 12.3 **FUD** 090 J A2 80 🔲

EXCLUDES Tracheoesophageal fistula repair (43305, 43312)

31825 with plastic repair

13.7 ⚕ 17.1 **FUD** 090 J A2 80 🔲

EXCLUDES Tracheoesophageal fistula repair (43305, 43312)

31830 Revision of tracheostomy scar

9.87 ⚕ 12.7 **FUD** 090 J A2 80 🔲

Any of a wide variety of scar revision techniques may be employed. A Z-plasty may be used to lengthen or realign the scar line. Revision also serves to neutralize contractures that occur along the scar line

Thyroid cartilage

Cricoid cartilage

1st ring

2nd ring

3rd ring

Tracheostomies typically enter at the second, third, or fourth ring

Example of a common Z-plasty where flaps are rotated to break scar line

A tracheostomy closure scar is revised, usually to make the scar less noticeable

31899 Unlisted procedure, trachea, bronchi

0.00 ⚕ 0.00 **FUD** YYY T 80 🔲

AMA: 2018,Jan,8; 2017,Jan,8; 2016,Jan,13; 2015,Jan,16; 2014,May,10; 2014,Jan,11

32035-32036 Procedures for Empyema

EXCLUDES Wound exploration without thoracotomy for penetrating wound of chest (20101)

32035 Thoracostomy; with rib resection for empyema

20.9 ⚕ 20.9 **FUD** 090 C 80 50 🔲

32036 with open flap drainage for empyema

22.3 ⚕ 22.3 **FUD** 090 C 80 50 🔲

32096-32098 Open Biopsy of Chest and Pleura

INCLUDES Varying amounts of lung tissue excised for analysis
Wedge technique with tissue obtained without precise consideration of margins

EXCLUDES Percutaneous needle biopsy of pleura, lung, and mediastinum (32400, 32405)
Thoracoscopy with biopsy (32607-32609)
Thoracoscopy with diagnostic wedge resection resulting in anatomic lung resection (32668)
Thoracotomy with diagnostic wedge resection resulting in anatomic lung resection (32507)

32096 Thoracotomy, with diagnostic biopsy(ies) of lung infiltrate(s) (eg, wedge, incisional), unilateral

EXCLUDES Procedure performed more than one time per lung
Removal of lung (32440-32445, 32488)

Code also appropriate add-on code for the more extensive procedure at the same location if diagnostic wedge resection results in the need for further surgery (32507, 32668)

23.2 ⚕ 23.2 **FUD** 090 C 80 🔲

AMA: 2018,Jan,8; 2017,Jan,8; 2016,Jan,13; 2015,Jan,16; 2014,Jan,11

Respiratory System

32097—32405

32097   **Thoracotomy, with diagnostic biopsy(ies) of lung nodule(s) or mass(es) (eg, wedge, incisional), unilateral**

> EXCLUDES   *Procedure performed more than one time per lung*
> *Removal of lung (32440-32445, 32488)*
>
> Code also appropriate add-on code for the more extensive procedure in the same location if diagnostic wedge resection results in the need for further surgery (32507, 32668)

🔧 23.1   ⚕ 23.1   **FUD** 090   C 80 ▣

AMA: 2018,Jan,8; 2017,Jan,8; 2016,Jan,13; 2015,Jan,16; 2014,Jan,11

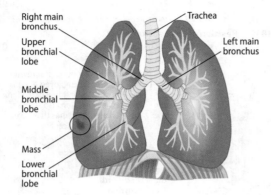

Right main bronchus — Trachea
Upper bronchial lobe — Left main bronchus
Middle bronchial lobe
Mass
Lower bronchial lobe

32098   **Thoracotomy, with biopsy(ies) of pleura**

🔧 21.9   ⚕ 21.9   **FUD** 090   C 80 ▣

AMA: 2018,Jan,8; 2017,Jan,8; 2016,Jan,13; 2015,Jan,16; 2014,Jan,11

32100-32160 Open Procedures: Chest

INCLUDES   Exploration of penetrating wound of chest
EXCLUDES   Lung resection (32480-32504)
            Wound exploration without thoracotomy for penetrating wound of chest (20101)

32100   **Thoracotomy; with exploration**

> EXCLUDES   *Excision of chest wall tumor, when performed (21601-21603)*
> *Extracorporeal membrane oxygenation (ECMO)/extracorporeal life support (ECLS) (33955-33957, [33963, 33964])*
> *Resection of apical lung tumor (32503-32504)*

🔧 23.3   ⚕ 23.3   **FUD** 090   C 80 ▣

AMA: 2018,Jan,8; 2017,Jan,8; 2016,Jan,13; 2015,Jul,3; 2015,Jan,16; 2014,Jan,11

32110   **with control of traumatic hemorrhage and/or repair of lung tear**

🔧 42.4   ⚕ 42.4   **FUD** 090   C 80 ▣

AMA: 2018,Jan,8; 2017,Jan,8; 2016,Jan,13; 2015,Jan,16; 2014,Jan,11

32120   **for postoperative complications**

🔧 25.1   ⚕ 25.1   **FUD** 090   C 80 ▣

32124   **with open intrapleural pneumonolysis**

🔧 26.7   ⚕ 26.7   **FUD** 090   C 80 ▣

AMA: 2018,Jan,8; 2017,Jan,8; 2016,Jan,13; 2015,Jan,16; 2014,Jan,11

32140   **with cyst(s) removal, includes pleural procedure when performed**

🔧 28.6   ⚕ 28.6   **FUD** 090   C 80 ▣

AMA: 2018,Jan,8; 2017,Jan,8; 2016,Jan,13; 2015,Jan,16; 2014,Jan,11

32141   **with resection-plication of bullae, includes any pleural procedure when performed**

> EXCLUDES   *Lung volume reduction (32491)*

🔧 44.0   ⚕ 44.0   **FUD** 090   C 80 ▣

AMA: 2018,Jan,8; 2017,Jan,8; 2016,Jan,13; 2015,Jan,16; 2014,Jan,11

32150   **with removal of intrapleural foreign body or fibrin deposit**

🔧 28.9   ⚕ 28.9   **FUD** 090   C 80 ▣

AMA: 2018,Jan,8; 2017,Jan,8; 2016,Jan,13; 2015,Jan,16; 2014,Jan,11

32151   **with removal of intrapulmonary foreign body**

🔧 29.0   ⚕ 29.0   **FUD** 090   C 80 ▣

32160   **with cardiac massage**

🔧 22.9   ⚕ 22.9   **FUD** 090   C 80 ▣

32200-32320 Open Procedures: Lung

32200   **Pneumonostomy, with open drainage of abscess or cyst**

> EXCLUDES   *Image-guided, percutaneous drainage (eg, abscess, cyst) of lungs/mediastinum via catheter (49405)*
>
> 🔀 (75989)

🔧 32.8   ⚕ 32.8   **FUD** 090   C 80 ▣

AMA: 2013,Nov,9; 1997,Nov,1

32215   **Pleural scarification for repeat pneumothorax**

🔧 22.9   ⚕ 22.9   **FUD** 090   C 80 50 ▣

32220   **Decortication, pulmonary (separate procedure); total**

🔧 45.7   ⚕ 45.7   **FUD** 090   C 80 50 ▣

32225   **partial**

🔧 28.6   ⚕ 28.6   **FUD** 090   C 80 50 ▣

32310   **Pleurectomy, parietal (separate procedure)**

🔧 26.3   ⚕ 26.3   **FUD** 090   C 80 ▣

AMA: 1994,Win,1

32320   **Decortication and parietal pleurectomy**

🔧 46.1   ⚕ 46.1   **FUD** 090   C 80 ▣

AMA: 1994,Fall,1

32400-32405 Lung Biopsy

EXCLUDES   Fine needle aspiration (10004-10012, 10021)
            Open lung biopsy (32096-32097)
            Open mediastinal biopsy (39000-39010)
            Thoracoscopic (VATS) biopsy of lung, pericardium, pleural or mediastinal space (32604-32609)

32400   **Biopsy, pleura, percutaneous needle**

> 🔀 (76942, 77002, 77012, 77021)

🔧 2.50   ⚕ 4.41   **FUD** 000   J A2 ▣

AMA: 2019,Apr,4; 2018,Jan,8; 2017,Jan,8; 2016,Jan,13; 2015,Jan,16; 2014,Jan,11

32405   **Biopsy, lung or mediastinum, percutaneous needle**

> 🔀 (76942, 77002, 77012, 77021)

🔧 2.61   ⚕ 11.1   **FUD** 000   J A2 ▣

AMA: 2019,Apr,4; 2018,Jan,8; 2017,Jan,8; 2016,Jan,13; 2015,Jan,16; 2014,Jan,11

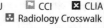

32440-32501 Lung Resection

32440 Removal of lung, pneumonectomy;

Code also excision of chest wall tumor, when performed (21601-21603)

🚑 45.1 ⚕ 45.1 **FUD** 090 C 80 ▣

AMA: 2018,Jan,8; 2017,Jan,8; 2016,Jan,13; 2015,Jan,16; 2014,Jan,11

Removal of entire lung

32442 with resection of segment of trachea followed by broncho-tracheal anastomosis (sleeve pneumonectomy)

Code also excision of chest wall tumor, when performed (21601-21603)

🚑 88.9 ⚕ 88.9 **FUD** 090 C 80 ▣

AMA: 2018,Jan,8; 2017,Jun,10; 2017,Jan,8; 2016,Jan,13; 2015,Jan,16; 2014,Jan,11

32445 extrapleural

Code also empyemectomy with extrapleural pneumonectomy (32540)

Code also excision of chest wall tumor, when performed (21601-21603)

🚑 102. ⚕ 102. **FUD** 090 C 80 ▣

AMA: 2018,Jan,8; 2017,Jan,8; 2016,Jan,13; 2015,Jan,16; 2014,Jan,11

32480 Removal of lung, other than pneumonectomy; single lobe (lobectomy)

EXCLUDES Lung removal with bronchoplasty (32501)

Code also decortication (32320)

Code also excision of chest wall tumor, when performed (21601-21603)

🚑 42.6 ⚕ 42.6 **FUD** 090 C 80 ▣

AMA: 2018,Jan,8; 2017,Jan,8; 2016,Jan,13; 2015,Jan,16; 2014,Jan,11

32482 2 lobes (bilobectomy)

EXCLUDES Lung removal with bronchoplasty (32501)

Code also decortication (32320)

Code also excision of chest wall tumor, when performed (21601-21603)

🚑 45.6 ⚕ 45.6 **FUD** 090 C 80 ▣

AMA: 2018,Jan,8; 2017,Jan,8; 2016,Jan,13; 2015,Jan,16; 2014,Jan,11

32484 single segment (segmentectomy)

EXCLUDES Lung removal with bronchoplasty (32501)

Code also decortication (32320)

Code also excision of chest wall tumor, when performed (21601-21603)

🚑 41.3 ⚕ 41.3 **FUD** 090 C 80 ▣

AMA: 2018,Jan,8; 2017,Jan,8; 2016,Jan,13; 2015,Jan,16; 2014,Jan,11

32486 with circumferential resection of segment of bronchus followed by broncho-bronchial anastomosis (sleeve lobectomy)

Code also decortication (32320)

Code also excision of chest wall tumor, when performed (21601-21603)

🚑 68.1 ⚕ 68.1 **FUD** 090 C 80 ▣

AMA: 2018,Jan,8; 2017,Jun,10; 2017,Jan,8; 2016,Jan,13; 2015,Jan,16; 2014,Jan,11

32488 with all remaining lung following previous removal of a portion of lung (completion pneumonectomy)

Code also decortication (32320)

Code also excision of chest wall tumor, when performed (21601-21603)

🚑 69.3 ⚕ 69.3 **FUD** 090 C 80 ▣

AMA: 2018,Jan,8; 2017,Jan,8; 2016,Jan,13; 2015,Jan,16; 2014,Jan,11

32491 with resection-plication of emphysematous lung(s) (bullous or non-bullous) for lung volume reduction, sternal split or transthoracic approach, includes any pleural procedure, when performed

🚑 42.6 ⚕ 42.6 **FUD** 090 C 80 50 ▣

AMA: 2018,Jan,8; 2017,Jan,8; 2016,Jan,13; 2015,Jan,16; 2014,Jan,11

+ **32501** Resection and repair of portion of bronchus (bronchoplasty) when performed at time of lobectomy or segmentectomy (List separately in addition to code for primary procedure)

INCLUDES Plastic closure of bronchus, not closure of a resected end of bronchus

Code first (32480-32484)

🚑 7.07 ⚕ 7.07 **FUD** ZZZ C 80 ▣

AMA: 1995,Win,1

32503-32504 Excision of Lung Neoplasm

EXCLUDES Excision of chest wall tumor (21601-21603)

Thoracentesis, needle or catheter, aspiration of the pleural space (32554-32555)

Thoracotomy; with exploration (32100)

Tube thoracostomy (32551)

32503 Resection of apical lung tumor (eg, Pancoast tumor), including chest wall resection, rib(s) resection(s), neurovascular dissection, when performed; without chest wall reconstruction(s)

🚑 52.0 ⚕ 52.0 **FUD** 090 C 80 ▣

AMA: 2012,Oct,9-11; 2012,Sep,3-8

32504 with chest wall reconstruction

🚑 59.3 ⚕ 59.3 **FUD** 090 C 80 ▣

AMA: 2012,Oct,9-11; 2012,Sep,3-8

32505-32507 Thoracotomy with Wedge Resection

INCLUDES Wedge technique with tissue obtained with precise consideration of margins and complete resection

Code also resection of chest wall tumor with lung resection, when performed (21601-21603)

32505 Thoracotomy; with therapeutic wedge resection (eg, mass, nodule), initial

EXCLUDES Removal of lung (32440, 32442, 32445, 32488)

Code also a more extensive procedure of the lung when performed on the contralateral lung or different lobe with modifier 59 regardless of intraoperative pathology consultation

🚑 26.8 ⚕ 26.8 **FUD** 090 C 80 ▣

AMA: 2018,Jan,8; 2017,Jan,8; 2016,Jan,13; 2015,Jan,16; 2014,Jan,11

● New Code ▲ Revised Code ○ Reinstated ● New Web Release ▲ Revised Web Release + Add-on Unlisted Not Covered # Resequenced

50 Optum Mod 50 Exempt ⊘ AMA Mod 51 Exempt 51 Optum Mod 51 Exempt 63 Mod 63 Exempt ⁄ Non-FDA Drug ★ Telemedicine M Maternity A Age Edit

© 2019 Optum360, LLC CPT © 2019 American Medical Association. All Rights Reserved. 121

+ 32506 **with therapeutic wedge resection (eg, mass or nodule), each additional resection, ipsilateral (List separately in addition to code for primary procedure)**

Code also a more extensive procedure of the lung when performed on the contralateral lung or different lobe with modifier 59

Code first (32505)

⊞ 4.53 ⚖ 4.53 **FUD** ZZZ C 80 ▣

AMA: 2018,Jan,8; 2017,Jan,8; 2016,Jan,13; 2015,Jan,16; 2014,Jan,11

+ 32507 **with diagnostic wedge resection followed by anatomic lung resection (List separately in addition to code for primary procedure)**

INCLUDES Classification as a diagnostic wedge resection if intraoperative pathology consultation dictates more extensive resection in the same anatomical area

EXCLUDES Diagnostic wedge resection by thoracoscopy (32668)
Therapeutic wedge resection (32505-32506, 32666-32667)

Code first (32440, 32442, 32445, 32480-32488, 32503-32504)

⊞ 4.52 ⚖ 4.52 **FUD** ZZZ C 80 ▣

AMA: 2018,Jan,8; 2017,Jan,8; 2016,Jan,13; 2015,Jan,16; 2014,Jan,11

32540 Removal of Empyema

32540 **Extrapleural enucleation of empyema (empyemectomy)**

EXCLUDES Lung removal code when empyemectomy is performed with lobectomy (see appropriate lung removal code)

Code also appropriate removal of lung code when done with lobectomy (32480-32488)

⊞ 49.6 ⚖ 49.6 **FUD** 090 C 80 ▣

AMA: 1994,Fall,1

32550-32552 Chest Tube/Catheter

32550 **Insertion of indwelling tunneled pleural catheter with cuff**

EXCLUDES Procedures performed on same side of chest with (32554-32557)

⊞ (75989)

⊞ 5.98 ⚖ 21.2 **FUD** 000 J 62 ▣

AMA: 2018,Jan,8; 2017,Jan,8; 2016,Jan,13; 2015,Jan,16; 2014,May,3; 2014,Mar,13; 2014,Jan,11

32551 **Tube thoracostomy, includes connection to drainage system (eg, water seal), when performed, open (separate procedure)**

EXCLUDES Procedures performed on same side of chest with (33020, 33025)

⊞ 4.53 ⚖ 4.53 **FUD** 000 T 50 ▣

AMA: 2018,Jul,7; 2018,Jan,8; 2017,Jun,10; 2017,Jan,8; 2016,Jan,13; 2015,Jan,16; 2014,May,3; 2014,Jan,11

32552 **Removal of indwelling tunneled pleural catheter with cuff**

⊞ 4.55 ⚖ 5.26 **FUD** 010 02 62 80 ▣

AMA: 2018,Jan,8; 2017,Jan,8; 2016,Jan,13; 2015,Jan,16; 2014,Jan,11

32553 Intrathoracic Placement Radiation Therapy Devices

EXCLUDES Percutaneous placement of interstitial device(s) for radiation therapy guidance: intra-abdominal, intrapelvic, and/or retroperitoneal (49411)

Code also device

32553 **Placement of interstitial device(s) for radiation therapy guidance (eg, fiducial markers, dosimeter), percutaneous, intra-thoracic, single or multiple**

⊞ (76942, 77002, 77012, 77021)

⊞ 5.18 ⚖ 14.8 **FUD** 000 S 62 80 ▣

AMA: 2018,Jan,8; 2017,Jan,8; 2016,Jun,3; 2016,Jan,13; 2015,Jun,6; 2015,Jan,16; 2014,Jan,11

32554-32557 Pleural Aspiration and Drainage

EXCLUDES Chest x-ray performed to confirm position of chest tube, complications, adequacy of procedure
Open tube thoracostomy (32551)
Placement of indwelling tunneled pleural drainage catheter (cuffed) (32550)
Radiologic guidance (75989, 76942, 77002, 77012, 77021)

32554 **Thoracentesis, needle or catheter, aspiration of the pleural space; without imaging guidance**

⊞ 2.58 ⚖ 6.01 **FUD** 000 T 62 50 ▣

AMA: 2018,Jan,8; 2017,Jan,8; 2016,Jan,13; 2015,Jan,16; 2014,Jan,11

32555 **with imaging guidance**

⊞ 3.22 ⚖ 8.51 **FUD** 000 T 62 50 ▣

AMA: 2018,Jan,8; 2017,Jan,8; 2016,Jan,13; 2015,Jan,16; 2014,Jan,11

32556 **Pleural drainage, percutaneous, with insertion of indwelling catheter; without imaging guidance**

⊞ 3.55 ⚖ 17.4 **FUD** 000 J 62 50 ▣

AMA: 2018,Jan,8; 2017,Jan,8; 2016,Jan,13; 2015,Jan,16; 2014,Jan,11

32557 **with imaging guidance**

⊞ 4.39 ⚖ 16.0 **FUD** 000 T 62 50 ▣

AMA: 2018,Jan,8; 2017,Jan,8; 2016,Jan,13; 2015,Jan,16; 2014,May,3; 2014,Jan,11

32560-32562 Instillation Drug/Chemical by Chest Tube

EXCLUDES Insertion of chest tube (32551)

32560 **Instillation, via chest tube/catheter, agent for pleurodesis (eg, talc for recurrent or persistent pneumothorax)**

⊞ 2.25 ⚖ 7.17 **FUD** 000 T ▣

AMA: 2018,Jan,8; 2017,Jan,8; 2016,Jan,13; 2015,Jan,16; 2014,Jan,11

32561 **Instillation(s), via chest tube/catheter, agent for fibrinolysis (eg, fibrinolytic agent for break up of multiloculated effusion); initial day**

EXCLUDES Use of code more than one time on the date of initial treatment

⊞ 1.97 ⚖ 2.66 **FUD** 000 T 80 ▣

AMA: 2018,Jan,8; 2017,Jan,8; 2016,Jan,13; 2015,Jan,16; 2014,Jan,11

32562 **subsequent day**

EXCLUDES Use of code more than one time on each day of subsequent treatment

⊞ 1.76 ⚖ 2.38 **FUD** 000 T 80 ▣

AMA: 2018,Jan,8; 2017,Jan,8; 2016,Jan,13; 2015,Jan,16; 2014,Jan,11

32601-32674 Thoracic Surgery: Video-Assisted (VATS)

INCLUDES Diagnostic thoracoscopy in surgical thoracoscopy

32601 **Thoracoscopy, diagnostic (separate procedure); lungs, pericardial sac, mediastinal or pleural space, without biopsy**

⊞ 8.90 ⚖ 8.90 **FUD** 000 J 80 ▣

AMA: 2018,Jan,8; 2017,Jan,8; 2016,Jan,13; 2015,Jan,16; 2014,Jan,11

32604 **pericardial sac, with biopsy**

EXCLUDES Open biopsy of pericardium (39010)

⊞ 13.9 ⚖ 13.9 **FUD** 000 J 80 ▣

AMA: 2018,Jan,8; 2017,Jan,8; 2016,Jan,13; 2015,Jan,16; 2014,Jan,11

32606 **mediastinal space, with biopsy**

⊞ 13.3 ⚖ 13.3 **FUD** 000 J 80 ▣

AMA: 2018,Jan,8; 2017,Jan,8; 2016,Jan,13; 2015,Jan,16; 2014,Jan,11

32607 **Thoracoscopy; with diagnostic biopsy(ies) of lung infiltrate(s) (eg, wedge, incisional), unilateral**

> EXCLUDES Removal of lung (32440-32445, 32488)
> Thoracoscopy, surgical; with removal of lung (32671)
> Use of code more than one time per lung

8.89   8.89   **FUD** 000   J 80

AMA: 2018,Jan,8; 2017,Jan,8; 2016,Jan,13; 2015,Jan,16; 2014,Jan,11

32608 **with diagnostic biopsy(ies) of lung nodule(s) or mass(es) (eg, wedge, incisional), unilateral**

> EXCLUDES Removal of lung (32440-32445, 32488)
> Thoracoscopy, surgical; with removal of lung (32671)
> Use of code more than one time per lung

10.9   10.9   **FUD** 000   J 80

AMA: 2018,Jan,8; 2017,Jan,8; 2016,Jan,13; 2015,Jan,16; 2014,Jan,11

32609 **with biopsy(ies) of pleura**

7.45   7.45   **FUD** 000   J 80

AMA: 2018,Jan,8; 2017,Jan,8; 2016,Jan,13; 2015,Jan,16; 2014,Jan,11

32650 **Thoracoscopy, surgical; with pleurodesis (eg, mechanical or chemical)**

19.1   19.1   **FUD** 090   C 80 50

AMA: 2018,Jan,8; 2017,Jan,8; 2016,Jan,13; 2015,Jan,16; 2014,Jan,11

32651 **with partial pulmonary decortication**

31.6   31.6   **FUD** 090   C 80 50

AMA: 2018,Jan,8; 2017,Jan,8; 2016,Jan,13; 2015,Jan,16; 2014,Jan,11

32652 **with total pulmonary decortication, including intrapleural pneumonolysis**

47.9   47.9   **FUD** 090   C 80 50

AMA: 2018,Jan,8; 2017,Jan,8; 2016,Jan,13; 2015,Jan,16; 2014,Jan,11

32653 **with removal of intrapleural foreign body or fibrin deposit**

30.6   30.6   **FUD** 090   C 80

AMA: 2018,Jan,8; 2017,Jan,8; 2016,Jan,13; 2015,Jan,16; 2014,Jan,11

32654 **with control of traumatic hemorrhage**

33.2   33.2   **FUD** 090   C 80 50

AMA: 2018,Jan,8; 2017,Jan,8; 2016,Jan,13; 2015,Jan,16; 2014,Jan,11

32655 **with resection-plication of bullae, includes any pleural procedure when performed**

> EXCLUDES Thoracoscopic lung volume reduction surgery (32672)

27.5   27.5   **FUD** 090   C 80 50

AMA: 2018,Jan,8; 2017,Jan,8; 2016,Jan,13; 2015,Jan,16; 2014,Jan,11

32656 **with parietal pleurectomy**

23.0   23.0   **FUD** 090   C 80 50

AMA: 2018,Jan,8; 2017,Jan,8; 2016,Jan,13; 2015,Jan,16; 2014,Jan,11

32658 **with removal of clot or foreign body from pericardial sac**

20.6   20.6   **FUD** 090   C 80

AMA: 2018,Jan,8; 2017,Jan,8; 2016,Jan,13; 2015,Jan,16; 2014,Jan,11

32659 **with creation of pericardial window or partial resection of pericardial sac for drainage**

21.1   21.1   **FUD** 090   C 80

AMA: 2018,Jan,8; 2017,Jan,8; 2016,Jan,13; 2015,Jan,16; 2014,Jan,11

32661 **with excision of pericardial cyst, tumor, or mass**

23.0   23.0   **FUD** 090   C 80

AMA: 2018,Jan,8; 2017,Jan,8; 2016,Jan,13; 2015,Jan,16; 2014,Jan,11

32662 **with excision of mediastinal cyst, tumor, or mass**

25.7   25.7   **FUD** 090   C 80

AMA: 2018,Jan,8; 2017,Jan,8; 2016,Jan,13; 2015,Jan,16; 2014,Jan,11

32663 **with lobectomy (single lobe)**

> EXCLUDES Thoracoscopic segmentectomy (32669)

40.4   40.4   **FUD** 090   C 80

AMA: 2018,Jan,8; 2017,Jan,8; 2016,Jan,13; 2015,Jan,16; 2014,Jan,11

32664 **with thoracic sympathectomy**

24.5   24.5   **FUD** 090   C 80 50

AMA: 2018,Jan,8; 2017,Jan,8; 2016,Jan,13; 2015,Dec,16; 2015,Jan,16; 2014,Jan,11

32665 **with esophagomyotomy (Heller type)**

> EXCLUDES Exploratory thoracoscopy with and without biopsy (32601-32609)

35.6   35.6   **FUD** 090   C 80

AMA: 2018,Jan,8; 2017,Jan,8; 2016,Jan,13; 2015,Jan,16; 2014,Jan,11

32666 **with therapeutic wedge resection (eg, mass, nodule), initial unilateral**

> EXCLUDES Removal of lung (32440-32445, 32488)
> Thoracoscopy, surgical; with removal of lung (32671)

Code also a more extensive procedure of the lung when performed on the contralateral lung or different lobe with modifier 59 regardless of pathology consultation

25.1   25.1   **FUD** 090   C 80 50

AMA: 2018,Jan,8; 2017,Jan,8; 2016,Jan,13; 2015,Jan,16; 2014,Jan,11

+ **32667** **with therapeutic wedge resection (eg, mass or nodule), each additional resection, ipsilateral (List separately in addition to code for primary procedure)**

> EXCLUDES Removal of lung (32440-32445, 32488)
> Thoracoscopy, surgical; with removal of lung (32671)

Code also a more extensive procedure of the lung when performed on the contralateral lung or different lobe with modifier 59 regardless of intraoperative pathology consultation

Code first (32666)

4.54   4.54   **FUD** ZZZ   C 80

AMA: 2018,Jan,8; 2017,Jan,8; 2016,Jan,13; 2015,Jan,16; 2014,Jan,11

+ **32668** **with diagnostic wedge resection followed by anatomic lung resection (List separately in addition to code for primary procedure)**

> INCLUDES Classification as a diagnostic wedge resection if intraoperative pathology consultation dictates more extensive resection in the same anatomical area

Code first (32440-32488, 32503-32504, 32663, 32669-32671)

4.54   4.54   **FUD** ZZZ   C 80

AMA: 2018,Jan,8; 2017,Jan,8; 2016,Jan,13; 2015,Jan,16; 2014,Jan,11

32669 **with removal of a single lung segment (segmentectomy)**

38.7   38.7   **FUD** 090   C 80

AMA: 2018,Jan,8; 2017,Jan,8; 2016,Jan,13; 2015,Jan,16; 2014,Jan,11

32670 **with removal of two lobes (bilobectomy)**

46.2   46.2   **FUD** 090   C 80

AMA: 2018,Jan,8; 2017,Jan,8; 2016,Jan,13; 2015,Jan,16; 2014,Jan,11

32671 **with removal of lung (pneumonectomy)**

51.5   51.5   **FUD** 090   C 80

AMA: 2018,Jan,8; 2017,Jan,8; 2016,Jan,13; 2015,Jan,16; 2014,Jan,11

Respiratory System

32672 — 32905

32672 with resection-plication for emphysematous lung (bullous or non-bullous) for lung volume reduction (LVRS), unilateral includes any pleural procedure, when performed

🔧 44.0 ⚖ 44.0 **FUD** 090 [C] [80] [▢]

AMA: 2018,Jan,8; 2017,Jan,8; 2016,Jan,13; 2015,Jan,16; 2014,Jan,11

32673 with resection of thymus, unilateral or bilateral

EXCLUDES Exploratory thoracoscopy with and without biopsy (32601-32609)
Open excision mediastinal cyst (39200)
Open excision mediastinal tumor (39220)
Open thymectomy (60520-60522)

🔧 35.0 ⚖ 35.0 **FUD** 090 [C] [80] [▢]

AMA: 2018,Jan,8; 2017,Jan,8; 2016,Jan,13; 2015,Jan,16; 2014,Jan,11

+ 32674 with mediastinal and regional lymphadenectomy (List separately in addition to code for primary procedure)

INCLUDES Mediastinal lymph nodes:
Left side:
Aortopulmonary window
Inferior pulmonary ligament
Paraesophageal
Subcarinal
Right side:
Inferior pulmonary ligament
Paraesophageal
Paratracheal
Subcarinal

EXCLUDES Mediastinal and regional lymphadenectomy by thoracotomy (38746)
Code first (21601, 31760, 31766, 31786, 32096-32200, 32220-32320, 32440-32491, 32503-32505, 32601-32663, 32666, 32669-32673, 32815, 33025, 33030, 33050-33130, 39200-39220, 39560-39561, 43101, 43112, 43117-43118, 43122-43123, 43287-43288, 43351, 60270, 60505)

🔧 6.24 ⚖ 6.24 **FUD** ZZZ [C] [80] [▢]

AMA: 2018,Jan,8; 2017,Jan,8; 2016,Jan,13; 2015,Jan,16; 2014,May,3; 2014,Jan,11

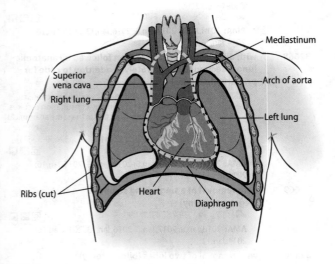

Mediastinum

Superior vena cava

Arch of aorta

Right lung

Left lung

Ribs (cut)

Heart

Diaphragm

32701 Target Delineation for Stereotactic Radiation Therapy

INCLUDES Collaboration between the radiation oncologist and surgeon
Correlation of tumor and contiguous body structures
Determination of borders and volume of tumor
Identification of fiducial markers
Verification of target when fiducial markers are not used

EXCLUDES Fiducial marker insertion (31626, 32553)
Procedure performed by same physician as radiation treatment management (77427-77499)
Radiation oncology services (77295, 77331, 77370, 77373, 77435)
Therapeutic radiology (77261-77799 [77295, 77385, 77386, 77387, 77424, 77425])

32701 Thoracic target(s) delineation for stereotactic body radiation therapy (SRS/SBRT), (photon or particle beam), entire course of treatment

🔧 6.21 ⚖ 6.21 **FUD** XXX [B] [80] [26] [▢]

AMA: 2018,Jan,8; 2017,Jan,8; 2016,Jan,13; 2015,Jun,6

32800-32820 Chest Repair and Reconstruction Procedures

32800 Repair lung hernia through chest wall

🔧 27.0 ⚖ 27.0 **FUD** 090 [C] [80] [▢]

32810 Closure of chest wall following open flap drainage for empyema (Clagett type procedure)

🔧 26.0 ⚖ 26.0 **FUD** 090 [C] [80] [▢]

32815 Open closure of major bronchial fistula

🔧 81.0 ⚖ 81.0 **FUD** 090 [C] [80] [▢]

32820 Major reconstruction, chest wall (posttraumatic)

🔧 38.4 ⚖ 38.4 **FUD** 090 [C] [80] [▢]

32850-32856 Lung Transplant Procedures

INCLUDES Harvesting donor lung(s), cold preservation, preparation of donor lung(s), transplantation into recipient

EXCLUDES Assessment of marginal cadaver donor lungs (0494T-0496T)
Repairs or resection of donor lung(s) (32491, 32505-32507, 35216, 35276)

32850 Donor pneumonectomy(s) (including cold preservation), from cadaver donor

🔧 0.00 ⚖ 0.00 **FUD** XXX [C] [▢]

AMA: 1993,Win,1

32851 Lung transplant, single; without cardiopulmonary bypass

🔧 95.3 ⚖ 95.3 **FUD** 090 [C] [80] [▢]

AMA: 1993,Win,1

32852 with cardiopulmonary bypass

🔧 103. ⚖ 103. **FUD** 090 [C] [80] [▢]

AMA: 2017,Dec,3

32853 Lung transplant, double (bilateral sequential or en bloc); without cardiopulmonary bypass

🔧 133. ⚖ 133. **FUD** 090 [C] [80] [▢]

AMA: 1993,Win,1

32854 with cardiopulmonary bypass

🔧 141. ⚖ 141. **FUD** 090 [C] [80] [▢]

AMA: 2017,Dec,3

32855 Backbench standard preparation of cadaver donor lung allograft prior to transplantation, including dissection of allograft from surrounding soft tissues to prepare pulmonary venous/atrial cuff, pulmonary artery, and bronchus; unilateral

🔧 0.00 ⚖ 0.00 **FUD** XXX [C] [80] [▢]

32856 bilateral

🔧 0.00 ⚖ 0.00 **FUD** XXX [C] [80] [▢]

32900-32997 Chest and Respiratory Procedures

32900 Resection of ribs, extrapleural, all stages

🔧 40.8 ⚖ 40.8 **FUD** 090 [C] [80] [▢]

32905 Thoracoplasty, Schede type or extrapleural (all stages);

🔧 38.6 ⚖ 38.6 **FUD** 090 [C] [80] [▢]

CPT © 2019 American Medical Association. All Rights Reserved.
© 2019 Optum360, LLC

32906	**with closure of bronchopleural fistula**

  🚑 47.7   ⚕ 47.7   **FUD** 090   C 80 ▣

  EXCLUDES   *Open closure of bronchial fistula (32815)*
              Resection first rib for thoracic compression
              (21615-21616)

32940	**Pneumonolysis, extraperiosteal, including filling or packing procedures**

  🚑 35.7   ⚕ 35.7   **FUD** 090   C 80 ▣

32960	**Pneumothorax, therapeutic, intrapleural injection of air**

  🚑 2.63   ⚕ 3.61   **FUD** 000   T 62 ▣

32994	**Resequenced code. See code following 32998.**

32997	**Total lung lavage (unilateral)**

  EXCLUDES   *Broncho-alveolar lavage by bronchoscopy (31624)*

  🚑 9.84   ⚕ 9.84   **FUD** 000   C 50 ▣

  AMA: 2018,Jan,8; 2017,Jan,8; 2016,Jan,13; 2015,Jan,16;
  2014,Jan,11

32998-32999 [32994] Destruction of Lung Neoplasm

32998	**Ablation therapy for reduction or eradication of 1 or more pulmonary tumor(s) including pleura or chest wall when involved by tumor extension, percutaneous, including imaging guidance when performed, unilateral; radiofrequency**

  🚑 12.8   ⚕ 100.   **FUD** 000   J 62 80 50 ▣

  AMA: 2018,Jan,8; 2017,Nov,8

#	*32994*	**cryoablation**

  🚑 13.2   ⚕ 159.   **FUD** 000   J 62 80 50 ▣

  AMA: 2018,Jan,8; 2017,Nov,8

32999	**Unlisted procedure, lungs and pleura**

  🚑 0.00   ⚕ 0.00   **FUD** YYY   T ▣

  AMA: 2018,Jan,8; 2017,Jan,8; 2016,Jan,13; 2015,Dec,16;
  2015,Jun,6; 2015,Jan,16; 2014,Jan,11

33010-33050 Procedures of the Pericardial Sac

EXCLUDES Surgical thoracoscopy (video-assisted thoracic surgery [VATS]) procedures of pericardium (32601, 32604, 32658-32659, 32661)

33010   ~~Pericardiocentesis; initial~~

To report, see (33016-33019)

33011   ~~subsequent~~

To report, see (33016-33019)

33015   ~~Tube pericardiostomy~~

To report, see (33017-33019)

● **33016**   **Pericardiocentesis, including imaging guidance, when performed**

INCLUDES   Imaging guidance for needle placement:
Computed tomography (77012)
Fluoroscopy (77002)
Magnetic resonance (77021)
Ultrasound (76942)

EXCLUDES   Echocardiography for pericardiocentesis guidance (93303-93325)

● **33017**   **Pericardial drainage with insertion of indwelling catheter, percutaneous, including fluoroscopy and/or ultrasound guidance, when performed; 6 years and older without congenital cardiac anomaly**

INCLUDES   Catheters that remain in the patient at the conclusion of the procedure
Imaging guidance for needle placement:
Fluoroscopy (77002)
Magnetic resonance (77021)
Ultrasound (76942)

EXCLUDES   Echocardiography for pericardiocentesis guidance (93303-93325)
Pericardial drainage for patients:
Any age with congenital cardiac anomaly (33018)
Younger than 6 years of age (33018)
Radiologically guided catheter placement for percutaneous drainage (75989)

● **33018**   **birth through 5 years of age or any age with congenital cardiac anomaly**

INCLUDES   Catheters that remain in the patient at the conclusion of the procedure
Imaging guidance for needle placement:
Fluoroscopy (77002)
Magnetic resonance (77021)
Ultrasound (76942)
Patient of age birth to 5 years without congenital cardiac anomaly
Patient of any age with congenital cardiac anomaly, such as heterotaxy, dextrocardia, mesocardia, or single ventricle anomaly, or 90 days following repair of congenital cardiac anomaly

EXCLUDES   CT guided pericardial drainage (33019)
Echocardiography for pericardiocentesis guidance (93303-93325)
Radiologically guided catheter placement for percutaneous drainage (75989)

● **33019**   **Pericardial drainage with insertion of indwelling catheter, percutaneous, including CT guidance**

INCLUDES   Catheters that remain in the patient at the conclusion of the procedure
Imaging guidance for needle placement:
Computed tomography (77012)
Fluoroscopy (77002)
Magnetic resonance (77021)
Ultrasound (76942)

EXCLUDES   Radiologically guided catheter placement for percutaneous drainage (75989)

33020   **Pericardiotomy for removal of clot or foreign body (primary procedure)**

EXCLUDES   Tube thoracostomy if chest tube or pleural drain placed on same side (32551)

🚑 25.3   ⚕ 25.3   **FUD** 090   C 80 ▣

AMA: 1997,Nov,1

33025   **Creation of pericardial window or partial resection for drainage**

INCLUDES   Tube thoracostomy if chest tube or pleural drain placed on same side (32551)

EXCLUDES   Surgical thoracoscopy (video-assisted thoracic surgery [VATS]) creation of pericardial window (32659)

🚑 23.0   ⚕ 23.0   **FUD** 090   C 80 ▣

AMA: 1997,Nov,1

33030   **Pericardiectomy, subtotal or complete; without cardiopulmonary bypass**

INCLUDES   Delorme pericardiectomy

🚑 57.8   ⚕ 57.8   **FUD** 090   C 80 ▣

AMA: 1997,Nov,1; 1994,Win,1

33031   **with cardiopulmonary bypass**

🚑 71.5   ⚕ 71.5   **FUD** 090   C 80 ▣

AMA: 2017,Dec,3

33050   **Resection of pericardial cyst or tumor**

EXCLUDES   Open biopsy of pericardium (39010)
Surgical thoracoscopy (video-assisted thoracic surgery [VATS]) resection of cyst, mass, or tumor of pericardium (32661)

🚑 29.1   ⚕ 29.1   **FUD** 090   C 80 ▣

AMA: 1997,Nov,1

33120-33130 Neoplasms of Heart

Code also removal of thrombus through a separate heart incision, when performed (33310-33315); append modifier 59 to (33315)

33120   **Excision of intracardiac tumor, resection with cardiopulmonary bypass**

🚑 60.6   ⚕ 60.6   **FUD** 090   C 80 ▣

AMA: 2018,Jan,8; 2017,Dec,3; 2017,Jan,8; 2016,Jan,13; 2015,Jan,16; 2014,Jan,11

33130   **Resection of external cardiac tumor**

🚑 39.8   ⚕ 39.8   **FUD** 090   C 80 ▣

AMA: 2018,Jan,8; 2017,Jan,8; 2016,Jan,13; 2015,Jan,16; 2014,Jan,11

33140-33141 Transmyocardial Revascularization

33140   **Transmyocardial laser revascularization, by thoracotomy; (separate procedure)**

🚑 45.5   ⚕ 45.5   **FUD** 090   C 80 ▣

AMA: 2018,Jan,8; 2017,Jan,8; 2016,Jan,13; 2015,Jan,16; 2014,Jan,11

+ **33141**   **performed at the time of other open cardiac procedure(s) (List separately in addition to code for primary procedure)**

Code first (33390-33391, 33404-33496, 33510-33536, 33542)

🚑 3.80   ⚕ 3.80   **FUD** ZZZ   C 80 ▣

AMA: 2018,Jan,8; 2017,Jan,8; 2016,Jan,13; 2015,Jan,16; 2014,Jan,11

33202-33203 Placement Epicardial Leads

INCLUDES Imaging guidance:
Fluoroscopy (76000)
Ultrasound (76942, 76998, 93318)
Temporary pacemaker (33210-33211)
Code also insertion of pulse generator when performed by same physician/same surgical session (33212-33213, [33221], 33230-33231, 33240)

33202 **Insertion of epicardial electrode(s); open incision (eg, thoracotomy, median sternotomy, subxiphoid approach)**

🔲 22.3 ⚕ 22.3 **FUD** 090 C 🖵

AMA: 2019,Mar,6; 2018,Jan,8; 2017,Jan,8; 2016,Aug,5; 2016,May,5; 2016,Jan,13; 2015,May,3; 2015,Jan,16; 2014,Nov,5; 2014,Jan,11

Pacemaker in subcutaneous pocket

Epicardial (on the heart) electrodes

Typical access incisions

Pacemaker

Medial sternotomy

Thoracotomy

Subxiphoid approach

33203 **endoscopic approach (eg, thoracoscopy, pericardioscopy)**

🔲 23.4 ⚕ 23.4 **FUD** 090 C 🖵

AMA: 2019,Mar,6; 2018,Jan,8; 2017,Jan,8; 2016,Aug,5; 2016,May,5; 2016,Jan,13; 2015,May,3; 2015,Jan,16; 2014,Nov,5; 2014,Jan,11

33206-33214 [33221] Pacemakers

INCLUDES Device evaluation (93279-93298 [93260, 93261])
Dual lead: device that paces and senses in two heart chambers
Imaging guidance:
Fluoroscopy (76000)
Ultrasound (76942, 76998, 93318)
Multiple lead: device that paces and senses in three or more heart chambers
Radiological supervision and interpretation for pacemaker procedure
Single lead: device that paces and senses in one heart chamber
Skin pocket revision, when performed
If revision includes incision/drainage of a wound infection or hematoma code also (10140, 10180, 11042-11047 [11045, 11046])
Temporary pacemaker (33210-33211)

EXCLUDES *Electrode repositioning:*
Left ventricle (33226)
Pacemaker (33215)
Insertion of lead for left ventricular (biventricular) pacing (33224-33225)
Leadless pacemaker systems ([33274, 33275])

33206 **Insertion of new or replacement of permanent pacemaker with transvenous electrode(s); atrial**

INCLUDES Pulse generator insertion/single transvenous electrode placement

EXCLUDES *Insertion of transvenous electrode only (33216-33217)*
Removal with immediate replacement of pacemaker pulse generator only, single lead system ([33227])

Code also removal of old pacemaker pulse generator and electrode, when replacement of entire system is performed:
Electrode (33234)
Pulse generator (33233)

🔲 13.1 ⚕ 13.1 **FUD** 090 J J8 🖵

AMA: 2019,Mar,6; 2018,Jan,8; 2017,Jan,8; 2016,Aug,5; 2016,May,5; 2016,Jan,13; 2015,May,3; 2015,Jan,16; 2014,Nov,5; 2014,Jan,11

33207 **ventricular**

INCLUDES Pulse generator insertion/single transvenous electrode placement

EXCLUDES *Insertion of transvenous electrode only (33216-33217)*
Removal with immediate replacement of pacemaker pulse generator only, single lead system ([33227])

Code also removal of old pacemaker pulse generator and electrode, when replacement of entire system is performed:
Electrode (33234)
Pulse generator (33233)

🔲 13.9 ⚕ 13.9 **FUD** 090 J J8 🖵

AMA: 2019,Mar,6; 2018,Jan,8; 2017,Jan,8; 2016,Aug,5; 2016,May,5; 2016,Jan,13; 2015,May,3; 2015,Jan,16; 2014,Nov,5; 2014,Jan,11

33208 **atrial and ventricular**

INCLUDES Pulse generator insertion/dual transvenous electrode placement

EXCLUDES *Insertion of transvenous electrode(s) only (33216-33217)*
Removal with immediate replacement of pacemaker pulse generator only, dual or multiple lead system ([33228, 33229])

Code also removal of old pacemaker pulse generator and electrodes, when replacement of entire system is performed:
Electrodes (33235)
Pulse generator (33233)

🔲 15.1 ⚕ 15.1 **FUD** 090 J J8 🖵

AMA: 2019,Mar,6; 2018,Jan,8; 2017,Jan,8; 2016,Aug,5; 2016,May,5; 2016,Jan,13; 2015,May,3; 2015,Jan,16; 2014,Nov,5; 2014,Jan,11

33210 **Insertion or replacement of temporary transvenous single chamber cardiac electrode or pacemaker catheter (separate procedure)**

🔲 4.76 ⚕ 4.76 **FUD** 000 J G2 🖵

AMA: 2019,Mar,6; 2018,Jan,8; 2017,Jan,8; 2016,Aug,5; 2016,May,5; 2016,Jan,13; 2015,May,3; 2015,Jan,16; 2014,Nov,5; 2014,Jan,11

33211 Insertion or replacement of temporary transvenous dual chamber pacing electrodes (separate procedure)

⚙ 4.95   ⚖ 4.95   **FUD** 000   [J] [J8] 🖥

AMA: 2019,Mar,6; 2018,Jan,8; 2017,Jan,8; 2016,Aug,5; 2016,May,5; 2016,Jan,13; 2015,May,3; 2015,Jan,16; 2014,Nov,5; 2014,Jan,11

33212 Insertion of pacemaker pulse generator only; with existing single lead

EXCLUDES Insertion for replacement of single lead pacemaker pulse generator ([33227])
Insertion of transvenous electrode(s) (33216-33217)
Removal of permanent pacemaker pulse generator only (33233)

Code also placement of epicardial leads by same physician/same surgical session (33202-33203)

⚙ 9.31   ⚖ 9.31   **FUD** 090   [J] [J8] 🖥

AMA: 2019,Mar,6; 2018,Jan,8; 2017,Jan,8; 2016,Aug,5; 2016,May,5; 2016,Jan,13; 2015,May,3; 2015,Jan,16; 2014,Nov,5; 2014,Jan,11

33213 with existing dual leads

EXCLUDES Insertion for replacement of dual lead pacemaker pulse generator ([33228])
Insertion of transvenous electrode(s) (33216-33217)
Removal of permanent pacemaker pulse generator only (33233)

Code also placement of epicardial leads by same physician/same surgical session (33202-33203)

⚙ 9.74   ⚖ 9.74   **FUD** 090   [J] [J8] 🖥

AMA: 2019,Mar,6; 2018,Jan,8; 2017,Jan,8; 2016,Aug,5; 2016,May,5; 2016,Jan,13; 2015,May,3; 2015,Jan,16; 2014,Nov,5; 2014,Jan,11

\# **33221** with existing multiple leads

EXCLUDES Insertion for replacement of multiple lead pacemaker pulse generator ([33229])
Insertion of transvenous electrode(s) (33216-33217)
Removal of permanent pacemaker pulse generator only (33233)

Code also placement of epicardial leads by same physician/same surgical session (33202-33203)

⚙ 10.4   ⚖ 10.4   **FUD** 090   [J] [J8] 🖥

AMA: 2019,Mar,6; 2018,Jan,8; 2017,Jan,8; 2016,Aug,5; 2016,May,5; 2016,Jan,13; 2015,May,3; 2015,Jan,16; 2014,Nov,5; 2014,Jan,11

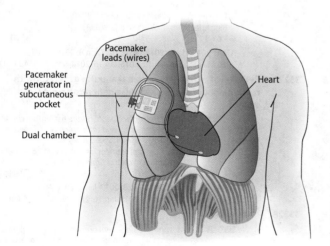

Pacemaker leads (wires)
Pacemaker generator in subcutaneous pocket
Heart
Dual chamber

33214 Upgrade of implanted pacemaker system, conversion of single chamber system to dual chamber system (includes removal of previously placed pulse generator, testing of existing lead, insertion of new lead, insertion of new pulse generator)

EXCLUDES Insertion of transvenous electrode(s) (33216-33217)
Removal and replacement of pacemaker pulse generator (33227-33229)

⚙ 13.9   ⚖ 13.9   **FUD** 090   [J] [J8] [80] 🖥

AMA: 2019,Mar,6; 2018,Jan,8; 2017,Jan,8; 2016,Aug,5; 2016,May,5; 2016,Jan,13; 2015,May,3; 2015,Jan,16; 2014,Nov,5; 2014,Jan,11

33215-33249 [33227, 33228, 33229, 33230, 33231, 33262, 33263, 33264] Pacemakers/Implantable Defibrillator/Electrode Insertion/Replacement/Revision/Repair

INCLUDES Device evaluation (93279-93298 [93260, 93261])
Dual lead: device that paces and senses in two heart chambers
Imaging guidance:
  Fluoroscopy (76000)
  Ultrasound (76942, 76998, 93318)
Multiple lead: device that paces and senses in three or more heart chambers
Radiological supervision and interpretation for pacemaker or pacing cardioverter-defibrillator procedure
Single lead: device that paces and senses in one heart chamber
Skin pocket revision, when performed
  If revision includes incision/drainage of a wound infection or hematoma code also (10140, 10180, 11042-11047 [11045, 11046])
Temporary pacemaker (33210-33211)

EXCLUDES Electrode repositioning:
  Left ventricle (33226)
  Pacemaker or implantable defibrillator (33215)
Insertion of lead for left ventricular (biventricular) pacing (33224-33225)
Removal of leadless pacemaker system ([33275])
Removal of subcutaneous implantable defibrillator electrode ([33272])
Testing of defibrillator threshold (DFT) during follow-up evaluation (93642-93644)
Testing of defibrillator threshold (DFT) during insertion/replacement (93640-93641)

33215 Repositioning of previously implanted transvenous pacemaker or implantable defibrillator (right atrial or right ventricular) electrode

⚙ 9.02   ⚖ 9.02   **FUD** 090   [T] [62] 🖥

AMA: 2019,Mar,6; 2018,Jan,8; 2017,Jan,8; 2016,Aug,5; 2016,May,5; 2016,Jan,13; 2015,May,3; 2015,Jan,16; 2014,Nov,5; 2014,Jan,11

33216 Insertion of a single transvenous electrode, permanent pacemaker or implantable defibrillator

EXCLUDES Insertion or replacement of a lead for a cardiac venous system (33224-33225)
Insertion or replacement of permanent implantable defibrillator generator or system (33249)
Removal and replacement of permanent pacemaker or implantable defibrillator (33206-33208, 33212-33213, [33221], 33227-33229, 33230-33231, 33240, [33262, 33263, 33264])

⚙ 10.7   ⚖ 10.7   **FUD** 090   [J] [J8] 🖥

AMA: 2019,Mar,6; 2018,Jan,8; 2017,Jan,8; 2016,Aug,5; 2016,May,5; 2016,Jan,13; 2015,May,3; 2015,Jan,16; 2014,Nov,5; 2014,Jan,11

33217 Insertion of 2 transvenous electrodes, permanent pacemaker or implantable defibrillator

EXCLUDES Insertion or replacement of a lead for a cardiac venous system (33224-33225)
Insertion or replacement of permanent implantable defibrillator generator or system (33249)
Removal and replacement of permanent pacemaker or implantable defibrillator (33206-33208, 33212-33213, [33221], 33227-33229, 33230-33231, 33240, [33262, 33263, 33264])

⚙ 10.6   ⚖ 10.6   **FUD** 090   [J] [J8] 🖥

AMA: 2019,Mar,6; 2018,Jan,8; 2017,Jan,8; 2016,Aug,5; 2016,May,5; 2016,Jan,13; 2015,May,3; 2015,Jan,16; 2014,Nov,5; 2014,Jan,11

33218 **Repair of single transvenous electrode, permanent pacemaker or implantable defibrillator**

Code also removal of old generator with insertion of new generator replacement, when performed:
Implantable defibrillator ([33262, 33263, 33264])
Pacemaker ([33227, 33228, 33229])

🔓 11.2   ⚕ 11.2   **FUD** 090   [T] [G2] [▭]

AMA: 2019,Mar,6; 2018,Jan,8; 2017,Jan,8; 2016,Aug,5; 2016,May,5; 2016,Jan,13; 2015,May,3; 2015,Jan,16; 2014,Nov,5; 2014,Jan,11

33220 **Repair of 2 transvenous electrodes for permanent pacemaker or implantable defibrillator**

Code also modifier 52 Reduced services, when one electrode of a two-chamber system is repaired
Code also removal of old generator with insertion of new generator replacement, when performed:
Implantable defibrillator ([33263, 33264])
Pacemaker ([33228, 33229])

🔓 11.3   ⚕ 11.3   **FUD** 090   [T] [G2] [▭]

AMA: 2019,Mar,6; 2018,Jan,8; 2017,Jan,8; 2016,Aug,5; 2016,May,5; 2016,Jan,13; 2015,May,3; 2015,Jan,16; 2014,Nov,5; 2014,Jan,11

33221   **Resequenced code. See code following 33213.**

33222 **Relocation of skin pocket for pacemaker**

> INCLUDES Formation of the new pocket
> Procedures related to the existing pocket:
> Accessing the pocket
> Incision/drainage of any abscess or hematoma (10140, 10180)
> Pocket closure (13100-13102)

> EXCLUDES *Debridement, subcutaneous tissue (11042-11047 [11045, 11046])*

Code also removal and replacement of an existing generator

🔓 9.81   ⚕ 9.81   **FUD** 090   [T] [A2] [▭]

AMA: 2019,Mar,6; 2018,Jan,8; 2017,Jan,8; 2016,Aug,5; 2016,May,5; 2016,Jan,13; 2015,May,3; 2015,Jan,16; 2014,Nov,5; 2014,Jan,11

33223 **Relocation of skin pocket for implantable defibrillator**

> INCLUDES Formation of the new pocket
> Procedures related to the existing pocket:
> Accessing the pocket
> Incision/drainage of any abscess or hematoma (10140, 10180)
> Pocket closure (13100-13102)

> EXCLUDES *Debridement, subcutaneous tissue (11042-11047 [11045, 11046])*

Code also removal and replacement of an existing generator

🔓 11.8   ⚕ 11.8   **FUD** 090   [T] [A2] [80] [▭]

AMA: 2019,Mar,6; 2018,Jan,8; 2017,Jan,8; 2016,Aug,5; 2016,Jan,13; 2015,Jan,16; 2014,Nov,5; 2014,Jan,11

33224 **Insertion of pacing electrode, cardiac venous system, for left ventricular pacing, with attachment to previously placed pacemaker or implantable defibrillator pulse generator (including revision of pocket, removal, insertion, and/or replacement of existing generator)**

Code also placement of epicardial electrode when appropriate (33202-33203)

🔓 15.0   ⚕ 15.0   **FUD** 000   [J] [J8] [▭]

AMA: 2019,Mar,6; 2018,Jan,8; 2017,Jan,8; 2016,Aug,5; 2016,May,5; 2016,Jan,13; 2015,May,3; 2015,Jan,16; 2014,Nov,5; 2014,Jan,11

+ **33225** **Insertion of pacing electrode, cardiac venous system, for left ventricular pacing, at time of insertion of implantable defibrillator or pacemaker pulse generator (eg, for upgrade to dual chamber system) (List separately in addition to code for primary procedure)**

Code first (33206-33208, 33212-33213, [33221], 33214, 33216-33217, 33223, 33228-33229, 33230-33231, 33233, 33234-33235, 33240, [33263, 33264], 33249)
Code first (33223) for relocation of pocket for implantable defibrillator
Code first (33222) for relocation of pocket for pacemaker pulse generator

🔓 13.6   ⚕ 13.6   **FUD** ZZZ   [N] [N1] [▭]

AMA: 2019,Mar,6; 2018,Jan,8; 2017,Jan,8; 2016,Aug,5; 2016,May,5; 2016,Jan,13; 2015,May,3; 2015,Jan,16; 2014,Nov,5; 2014,Jan,11

33226 **Repositioning of previously implanted cardiac venous system (left ventricular) electrode (including removal, insertion and/or replacement of existing generator)**

🔓 14.4   ⚕ 14.4   **FUD** 000   [T] [G2] [▭]

AMA: 2019,Mar,6; 2018,Jan,8; 2017,Jan,8; 2016,Aug,5; 2016,May,5; 2016,Jan,13; 2015,May,3; 2015,Jan,16; 2014,Nov,5; 2014,Jan,11

33227   **Resequenced code. See code following 33233.**

33228   **Resequenced code. See code following 33233.**

33229   **Resequenced code. See code before 33234.**

33230   **Resequenced code. See code following 33240.**

33231   **Resequenced code. See code before 33241.**

33233 **Removal of permanent pacemaker pulse generator only**

> EXCLUDES *Removal with immediate replacement of pacemaker pulse generator, without replacement of electrode(s):*
> *Dual lead system ([33228])*
> *Multiple lead system ([33229])*
> *Single lead system ([33227])*

Code also insertion of replacement pacemaker pulse generator with transvenous electrode(s) (total system), when performed:
Pacemaker and dual leads (33208)
Pacemaker and single atrial lead (33206)
Pacemaker and single ventricular lead (33207)
Code also removal of electrode(s), when removal of total system without replacement is performed:
Dual leads (atrial and ventricular) (33235)
Single lead (atrial or ventricular) (33234)

🔓 6.68   ⚕ 6.68   **FUD** 090   [Q2] [G2] [▭]

AMA: 2019,Mar,6; 2018,Jan,8; 2017,Jan,8; 2016,Aug,5; 2016,May,5; 2016,Jan,13; 2015,Jan,16; 2014,Nov,5; 2014,Jan,11

\# **33227** **Removal of permanent pacemaker pulse generator with replacement of pacemaker pulse generator; single lead system**

> EXCLUDES *Removal and replacement of entire system, pacemaker pulse generator and transvenous electrode, use (33206-33207, 33233, 33234)*
> *Removal and replacement for conversion from single chamber to dual chamber system (33214)*

🔓 9.82   ⚕ 9.82   **FUD** 090   [J] [J8] [▭]

AMA: 2019,Mar,6; 2018,Jan,8; 2017,Jan,8; 2016,Aug,5; 2016,May,5; 2016,Jan,13; 2015,Jan,16; 2014,Nov,5; 2014,Jan,11

\# **33228** **dual lead system**

> EXCLUDES *Removal and replacement of entire system, pacemaker pulse generator and transvenous electrode(s), use (33208, 33233, 33235)*

🔓 10.2   ⚕ 10.2   **FUD** 090   [J] [J8] [▭]

AMA: 2019,Mar,6; 2018,Jan,8; 2017,Jan,8; 2016,Aug,5; 2016,May,5; 2016,Jan,13; 2015,Jan,16; 2014,Nov,5; 2014,Jan,11

26/TC PC/TC Only   A2-Z3 ASC Payment   50 Bilateral   ♂ Male Only   ♀ Female Only   🔓 Facility RVU   ⚕ Non-Facility RVU   ▭ CCI   ✖ CLIA
FUD Follow-up Days   CMS: IOM   AMA: CPT Asst   A-Y OPPSI   80/80 Surg Assist Allowed / w/Doc   Lab Crosswalk   Radiology Crosswalk

130   CPT © 2019 American Medical Association. All Rights Reserved.   © 2019 Optum360, LLC

multiple lead system
33229

EXCLUDES *Removal and replacement of entire system, pacemaker pulse generator and transvenous electrode(s), use (33208, 33233, 33235)*

📷 10.8   ⚕ 10.8   **FUD** 090   J J8 🖵

AMA: 2019,Mar,6; 2018,Jan,8; 2017,Jan,8; 2016,Aug,5; 2016,May,5; 2016,Jan,13; 2015,Jan,16; 2014,Nov,5; 2014,Jan,11

33234 **Removal of transvenous pacemaker electrode(s); single lead system, atrial or ventricular**

EXCLUDES *Thoracotomy to remove electrode (33238)*

Code also pacing electrode insertion in cardiac venous system for pacing of left ventricle during insertion of pulse generator (pacemaker or implantable defibrillator) when performed (33225)

Code also removal of old pacemaker pulse generator and insertion of replacement pacemaker pulse generator with transvenous electrode (total system), when performed:
Insertion of pacemaker and atrial lead (33206) OR
Insertion of pacemaker and ventricular lead (33207) AND
Removal of generator (33233)

📷 14.1   ⚕ 14.1   **FUD** 090   Q2 G2 🖵

AMA: 2019,Mar,6; 2018,Jan,8; 2017,Jan,8; 2016,Aug,5; 2016,May,5; 2016,Jan,13; 2015,Jan,16; 2014,Nov,5; 2014,Jan,11

33235 **dual lead system**

EXCLUDES *Thoracotomy to remove electrodes (33238)*

Code also pacing electrode insertion in cardiac venous system for pacing of left ventricle during insertion of pulse generator (pacemaker or implantable defibrillator) when performed (33225)

Code also removal of old pacemaker pulse generator and insertion of replacement pacemaker pulse generator with transvenous electrodes (total system), when performed:
Insertion of generator and dual leads (33208) AND
Removal of generator (33233)

📷 18.5   ⚕ 18.5   **FUD** 090   Q2 G2 🖵

AMA: 2019,Mar,6; 2018,Jan,8; 2017,Jan,8; 2016,Aug,5; 2016,May,5; 2016,Jan,13; 2015,Jan,16; 2014,Nov,5; 2014,Jan,11

33236 **Removal of permanent epicardial pacemaker and electrodes by thoracotomy; single lead system, atrial or ventricular**

EXCLUDES *Removal of implantable defibrillator electrode(s) by thoracotomy (33243)*

Removal of transvenous electrodes by thoracotomy (33238)

Removal of transvenous pacemaker electrodes, single or dual lead system; without thoracotomy (33234, 33235)

📷 22.6   ⚕ 22.6   **FUD** 090   C 80 🖵

AMA: 2019,Mar,6; 2018,Jan,8; 2017,Jan,8; 2016,Aug,5; 2016,May,5; 2016,Jan,13; 2015,Jan,16; 2014,Nov,5; 2014,Jan,11

33237 **dual lead system**

EXCLUDES *Removal of implantable defibrillator electrode(s) by thoracotomy (33243)*

Removal of transvenous electrodes by thoracotomy (33238)

Removal of transvenous pacemaker electrodes, single or dual lead system; without thoracotomy (33234, 33235)

📷 24.3   ⚕ 24.3   **FUD** 090   C 80 🖵

AMA: 2019,Mar,6; 2018,Jan,8; 2017,Jan,8; 2016,Aug,5; 2016,May,5; 2016,Jan,13; 2015,Jan,16; 2014,Nov,5; 2014,Jan,11

33238 **Removal of permanent transvenous electrode(s) by thoracotomy**

EXCLUDES *Removal of implantable defibrillator electrode(s) by thoracotomy (33243)*

Removal of transvenous pacemaker electrodes, single or dual lead system; without thoracotomy (33234, 33235)

📷 27.0   ⚕ 27.0   **FUD** 090   C 80 🖵

AMA: 2018,Jan,8; 2017,Jan,8; 2016,Aug,5; 2016,May,5; 2016,Jan,13; 2015,Jan,16; 2014,Nov,5; 2014,Jan,11

33240 **Insertion of implantable defibrillator pulse generator only; with existing single lead**

EXCLUDES *Insertion of electrode(s) (33216-33217, [33271])*

Removal and replacement of implantable defibrillator pulse generator only ([33262, 33263, 33264])

Code also placement of epicardial leads by same physician/same surgical session as generator insertion (33202-33203)

📷 10.6   ⚕ 10.6   **FUD** 090   J J8 🖵

AMA: 2018,Jan,8; 2017,Jan,8; 2016,Aug,5; 2016,Jan,13; 2015,Jan,16; 2014,Nov,5; 2014,Jan,11

33230 **with existing dual leads**

EXCLUDES *Insertion of a single transvenous electrode, permanent pacemaker or implantable defibrillator (33216-33217)*

Removal and replacement of implantable defibrillator pulse generator only ([33262, 33263, 33264])

Code also placement of epicardial leads by same physician/same surgical session as generator insertion (33202-33203)

📷 11.0   ⚕ 11.0   **FUD** 090   J J8 🖵

AMA: 2019,Mar,6; 2018,Jan,8; 2017,Jan,8; 2016,Aug,5; 2016,Jan,13; 2015,Jan,16; 2014,Nov,5; 2014,Jan,11

33231 **with existing multiple leads**

EXCLUDES *Insertion of a single transvenous electrode, permanent pacemaker or implantable defibrillator (33216-33217)*

Removal and replacement of implantable defibrillator pulse generator only ([33262, 33263, 33264])

Code also placement of epicardial leads by same physician/same surgical session as generator placement (33202-33203)

📷 11.6   ⚕ 11.6   **FUD** 090   J J8 🖵

AMA: 2019,Mar,6; 2018,Jan,8; 2017,Jan,8; 2016,Aug,5; 2016,Jan,13; 2015,Jan,16; 2014,Nov,5; 2014,Jan,11

33241 **Removal of implantable defibrillator pulse generator only**

EXCLUDES *Removal with immediate replacement of implantable defibrillator pulse generator only ([33262, 33263, 33264])*

Removal of substernal implantable defibrillator pulse generator only (0580T)

Code also removal of electrode(s) and insertion of replacement defibrillator with electrode(s) (total system), when performed:
Removal of electrode(s) (33243-33244) AND
Insertion of defibrillator system, single or dual (33249) OR
Removal of subcutaneous electrode ([33272]) AND
Insertion of subcutaneous defibrillator system ([33270])

Code also removal of electrode(s), when total system is removed without replacement:
Subcutaneous electrode ([33272])
Transvenous electrode(s) (33243)

📷 6.24   ⚕ 6.24   **FUD** 090   Q2 G2 🖵

AMA: 2018,Jan,8; 2017,Jan,8; 2016,Aug,5; 2016,Jan,13; 2015,Jan,16; 2014,Nov,5; 2014,Jan,11

33262 **Removal of implantable defibrillator pulse generator with replacement of implantable defibrillator pulse generator; single lead system**

EXCLUDES *Insertion of electrode(s) (33216-33217, [33271])*

Removal and replacement of implantable defibrillator pulse generator and electrode(s) (total system) (33241, 33243-33244, 33249)

Removal and replacement of subcutaneous defibrillator pulse generator and electrode(s) (total system) (33241, [33270], [33272])

Removal of implantable defibrillator pulse generator only (33241)

Repair of implantable defibrillator pulse generator and/or leads (33218, 33220)

Code also electrode(s) removal by thoracotomy (33243)
Code also subcutaneous electrode removal ([33272])
Code also transvenous removal of electrode(s) (33244)

📷 10.8   ⚕ 10.8   **FUD** 090   J J8 🖵

AMA: 2018,Jan,8; 2017,Jan,8; 2016,Aug,5; 2016,Jan,13; 2015,Jan,16; 2014,Nov,5; 2014,Jan,11

● New Code   ▲ Revised Code   ○ Reinstated   ● New Web Release   ▲ Revised Web Release   + Add-on   Unlisted   Not Covered   # Resequenced
50 Optum Mod 50 Exempt   ⊘ AMA Mod 51 Exempt   51 Optum Mod 51 Exempt   63 Mod 63 Exempt   ✗ Non-FDA Drug   ★ Telemedicine   M Maternity   A Age Edit

 # 33263   dual lead system

EXCLUDES *Insertion of a single transvenous electrode, permanent pacemaker or implantable defibrillator (33216-33217)*
Removal and replacement of implantable defibrillator pulse generator and electrode(s) (total system) (33241, 33243-33244, 33249)
Removal and replacement of subcutaneous defibrillator pulse generator and electrode (total system) (33241, [33270], [33272])
Removal of implantable defibrillator pulse generator only (33241)
Repair of implantable defibrillator pulse generator and/or leads (33218, 33220)

Code also removal of electrodes by thoracotomy (33243)
Code also transvenous removal of electrodes (33244)

11.2   11.2   **FUD** 090   J J8

AMA: 2018,Jan,8; 2017,Jan,8; 2016,Aug,5; 2016,Jan,13; 2015,Jan,16; 2014,Nov,5; 2014,Jan,11

 # 33264   multiple lead system

EXCLUDES *Insertion of a single transvenous electrode, permanent pacemaker or implantable defibrillator (33216-33217)*
Removal and replacement of implantable defibrillator pulse generator and electrode(s) (total system) (33241, 33243-33244, 33249)
Removal and replacement of subcutaneous defibrillator pulse generator and electrode(s) (total system) (33241, [33270], [33272])
Removal of implantable defibrillator pulse generator only (33241)
Repair of implantable defibrillator pulse generator and/or leads (33218, 33220)

Code also removal of electrodes by thoracotomy (33243)
Code also transvenous removal of electrodes (33244)

11.7   11.7   **FUD** 090   J J8

AMA: 2018,Jan,8; 2017,Jan,8; 2016,Aug,5; 2016,Jan,13; 2015,Jan,16; 2014,Nov,5; 2014,Jan,11

33243   Removal of single or dual chamber implantable defibrillator electrode(s); by thoracotomy

EXCLUDES *Transvenous removal of defibrillator electrode(s) (33244)*

Code also removal of implantable defibrillator pulse generator and insertion of replacement defibrillator with electrodes (total system), when entire system is being replaced:
Insertion of defibrillator system, single or dual (33249)
Removal of generator (33241)
Code also removal of implantable defibrillator pulse generator, when entire system is removed without replacement (33241)
Code also replacement of implantable defibrillator pulse generator, when performed:
Dual lead system ([33263])
Multiple lead system ([33264])
Single lead system ([33262])

39.6   39.6   **FUD** 090   C 80

AMA: 2018,Jan,8; 2017,Jan,8; 2016,Aug,5; 2016,Jan,13; 2015,Jan,16; 2014,Nov,5; 2014,Jan,11

33244   by transvenous extraction

EXCLUDES *Thoracotomy to remove electrodes (33238, 33243)*

Code also removal of implantable defibrillator pulse generator and insertion of replacement defibrillator with electrodes (total system), when entire system is being replaced:
Insertion of defibrillator system, single or dual (33249)
Removal of generator (33241)
Code also removal of implantable defibrillator pulse generator, when entire system is removed without replacement (33241)
Code also replacement of implantable defibrillator pulse generator, when performed:
Dual lead system ([33263])
Multiple lead system ([33264])
Single lead system ([33262])

25.0   25.0   **FUD** 090   02

AMA: 2018,Jan,8; 2017,Jan,8; 2016,Aug,5; 2016,Jan,13; 2015,Jan,16; 2014,Nov,5; 2014,Jan,11

33249   Insertion or replacement of permanent implantable defibrillator system, with transvenous lead(s), single or dual chamber

EXCLUDES *Insertion of a single transvenous electrode, permanent pacemaker or implantable defibrillator (33216-33217)*

Code also removal of implantable defibrillator pulse generator and removal of electrode(s), when entire system is being replaced:
Removal of electrode(s) (33243-33244)
Removal of generator (33241)
Code also removal of defibrillator generator when upgrading from single to dual-chamber system (33241)

26.6   26.6   **FUD** 090   J J8

AMA: 2018,Jan,8; 2017,Jan,8; 2016,Aug,5; 2016,Jan,13; 2015,Jan,16; 2014,Nov,5; 2014,Jan,11

33270-33275 [33270, 33271, 33272, 33273, 33274, 33275] Subcutaneous Implantable Defibrillator

INCLUDES Programming and interrogation of:
Leadless pacemaker (93279, 93286, 93288, 93294, 93296)
Subcutaneous implantable defibrillator ([93260, 93261])

 # 33270   Insertion or replacement of permanent subcutaneous implantable defibrillator system, with subcutaneous electrode, including defibrillation threshold evaluation, induction of arrhythmia, evaluation of sensing for arrhythmia termination, and programming or reprogramming of sensing or therapeutic parameters, when performed

INCLUDES Electrophysiologic evaluation at time of initial insertion (93644)

EXCLUDES *Insertion of subcutaneous implantable defibrillator electrode only ([33271])*
Insertion/replacement of permanent implantable defibrillator system with substernal electrode (0571T)

Code also electrophysiologic evaluation following replacement of subcutaneous implantable defibrillator, when performed (93644)
Code also removal of subcutaneous implantable defibrillator and removal of subcutaneous electrode, when the entire system is being replaced:
Defibrillator (33241)
Electrode ([33272])

16.4   16.4   **FUD** 090   J J8

AMA: 2018,Jan,8; 2017,Jan,8; 2016,Aug,5; 2016,Jan,13; 2015,Jan,16; 2014,Nov,5

 # 33271   Insertion of subcutaneous implantable defibrillator electrode

EXCLUDES *Insertion of implantable defibrillator pulse generator only, other than subcutaneous:*
Initial insertion (33240)
Removal/replacement ([33262])
Insertion of subcutaneous implantable defibrillator and electrode (total system) ([33270])
Insertion of substernal defibrillator electrode (0572T)

13.2   13.2   **FUD** 090   J J8

AMA: 2018,Jan,8; 2017,Jan,8; 2016,Aug,5; 2016,Jan,13; 2015,Jan,16; 2014,Nov,5

 # 33272   Removal of subcutaneous implantable defibrillator electrode

EXCLUDES *Removal of substernal defibrillator electrode (0573T)*

Code also removal of subcutaneous implantable defibrillator and insertion of replacement implantable subcutaneous defibrillator with electrode (total system), when entire system is being replaced:
Insertion of total system ([33270])
Removal of defibrillator (33241)
Code also removal of implantable defibrillator, when performed:
Removal with replacement ([33262])
Removal without replacement (33241)

10.0   10.0   **FUD** 090   02

AMA: 2018,Jan,8; 2017,Jan,8; 2016,Aug,5; 2016,Jan,13; 2015,Jan,16; 2014,Nov,5

33273
Repositioning of previously implanted subcutaneous implantable defibrillator electrode

EXCLUDES Repositioning of substernal defibrillator electrode (0574T)

🚗 11.6 ⚕ 11.6 **FUD** 090 T G2 📄

AMA: 2018,Jan,8; 2017,Jan,8; 2016,Aug,5; 2016,Jan,13; 2015,Jan,16; 2014,Nov,5

33274
Transcatheter insertion or replacement of permanent leadless pacemaker, right ventricular, including imaging guidance (eg, fluoroscopy, venous ultrasound, ventriculography, femoral venography) and device evaluation (eg, interrogation or programming), when performed

INCLUDES Cardiac catheterization for insertion leadless pacemaker (93451, 93453, 93456-93457, 93460-93461, 93530-93533)
Femoral venography (75820)
Imaging guidance (76000, 76937, 77002)
Right ventriculography (93566)

EXCLUDES Removal permanent leadless pacemaker ([33275])
Services for pacemakers with leads (33202-33203, 33206-33208, 33212-33214 [33221], 33215-33218, 33220, 33233-33237 [33227, 33228, 33229])

🚗 14.2 ⚕ 14.2 **FUD** 090 J8 📄

AMA: 2019,Mar,6

▲ # 33275
Transcatheter removal of permanent leadless pacemaker, right ventricular, including imaging guidance (eg, fluoroscopy, venous ultrasound, ventriculography, femoral venography), when performed

INCLUDES Cardiac catheterization for insertion leadless pacemaker (93451, 93453, 93456-93457, 93460-93461, 93530-93533)
Femoral venography (75820)
Imaging guidance (76000, 76937, 77002)
Right ventriculography (93566)

EXCLUDES Insertion/replacement leadless pacemaker ([33274])
Services for pacemakers with leads (33202-33203, 33206-33208, 33212-33214 [33221], 33215-33218, 33220, 33233-33237 [33227, 33228, 33229])

🚗 15.1 ⚕ 15.1 **FUD** 090 G2 📄

AMA: 2019,Mar,6

33250-33251 Surgical Ablation Arrhythmogenic Foci, Supraventricular

INCLUDES Procedures using cryotherapy, laser, microwave, radiofrequency, and ultrasound

33250
Operative ablation of supraventricular arrhythmogenic focus or pathway (eg, Wolff-Parkinson-White, atrioventricular node re-entry), tract(s) and/or focus (foci); without cardiopulmonary bypass

EXCLUDES Pacing and mapping during surgery by other provider (93631)

🚗 42.4 ⚕ 42.4 **FUD** 090 C 80 📄

AMA: 2018,Jan,8; 2017,Jan,8; 2016,Jan,13; 2015,Jan,16; 2014,Jan,11

33251
with cardiopulmonary bypass

🚗 47.2 ⚕ 47.2 **FUD** 090 C 80 📄

AMA: 2018,Jan,8; 2017,Dec,3; 2017,Jan,8; 2016,Jan,13; 2015,Jan,16; 2014,Jan,11

33254-33256 Surgical Ablation Arrhythmogenic Foci, Atrial (e.g., Maze)

INCLUDES Excision or isolation of the left atrial appendage
Procedures using cryotherapy, laser, microwave, radiofrequency, and ultrasound

EXCLUDES Any procedure involving median sternotomy or cardiopulmonary bypass
Aortic valve procedures (33390-33391, 33404-33415)
Aortoplasty (33417)
Ascending aorta graft (33858-33859, 33863-33864)
Coronary artery bypass (33510-33516, 33517-33523, 33533-33536)
Excision of intracardiac tumor, resection (33120)
Mitral valve procedures (33418-33430)
Outflow tract augmentation (33478)
Prosthetic valve repair (33496)
Pulmonary artery embolectomy (33910-33920)
Pulmonary valve procedures (33470-33477)
Repair aberrant coronary artery anatomy (33500-33507)
Repair aberrant heart anatomy (33600-33853)
Resection of external cardiac tumor (33130)
Temporary pacemaker (33210-33211)
Thoracotomy; with exploration (32100)
Tricuspid valve procedures (33460-33468)
Tube thoracostomy, includes connection to drainage system (32551)
Ventricular reconstruction (33542-33548)
Ventriculomyotomy (33416)

33254
Operative tissue ablation and reconstruction of atria, limited (eg, modified maze procedure)

🚗 39.4 ⚕ 39.4 **FUD** 090 C 80 📄

AMA: 2018,Jan,8; 2017,Jan,8; 2016,Jan,13; 2015,Jan,16; 2014,Jan,11

33255
Operative tissue ablation and reconstruction of atria, extensive (eg, maze procedure); without cardiopulmonary bypass

🚗 47.3 ⚕ 47.3 **FUD** 090 C 80 📄

AMA: 2018,Jan,8; 2017,Jan,8; 2016,Jan,13; 2015,Jan,16; 2014,Jan,11

33256
with cardiopulmonary bypass

🚗 56.1 ⚕ 56.1 **FUD** 090 C 80 📄

AMA: 2018,Jan,8; 2017,Dec,3; 2017,Jan,8; 2016,Jan,13; 2015,Jan,16; 2014,Jan,11

33257-33259 Surgical Ablation Arrhythmogenic Foci, Atrial, with Other Heart Procedure(s)

EXCLUDES Operative tissue ablation and reconstruction of atria (without other cardiac procedure), limited or extensive:
Endoscopic (33265-33266)
Open (33254-33256)
Temporary pacemaker (33210-33211)
Tube thoracostomy, includes connection to drainage system (32551)

+ ### 33257
Operative tissue ablation and reconstruction of atria, performed at the time of other cardiac procedure(s), limited (eg, modified maze procedure) (List separately in addition to code for primary procedure)

🚗 16.8 ⚕ 16.8 **FUD** ZZZ C 80 📄

Code first (33120-33130, 33250-33251, 33261, 33300-33335, 33365, 33390-33391, 33404-33417 [33440], 33420-33430, 33460-33476, 33478, 33496, 33500-33507, 33510-33516, 33533-33548, 33600-33619, 33641-33697, 33702-33732, 33735-33767, 33770, 33877, 33910-33922, 33925-33926, 33975-33983)

+ ### 33258
Operative tissue ablation and reconstruction of atria, performed at the time of other cardiac procedure(s), extensive (eg, maze procedure), without cardiopulmonary bypass (List separately in addition to code for primary procedure)

🚗 18.8 ⚕ 18.8 **FUD** ZZZ C 80 📄

Code first, if performed without cardiopulmonary bypass (33130, 33250, 33300, 33310, 33320-33321, 33330, 33365, 33420, 33470-33471, 33501-33503, 33510-33516, 33533-33536, 33690, 33735, 33737, 33750-33766, 33800-33813, 33820-33824, 33840-33852, 33875, 33877, 33915, 33925, 33981, 33982)

+ 33259 Operative tissue ablation and reconstruction of atria, performed at the time of other cardiac procedure(s), extensive (eg, maze procedure), with cardiopulmonary bypass (List separately in addition to code for primary procedure)

Code first, if performed with cardiopulmonary bypass (33120, 33251, 33261, 33305, 33315, 33322, 33335, 33390-33391, 33404-33410, 33411-33417, 33422-33430, 33460-33468, 33474-33478, 33496, 33500, 33504-33507, 33510-33516, 33533-33548, 33600-33688, 33692-33726, 33730, 33732, 33736, 33767, 33770, 33783, 33786-33788, 33814, 33853, 33858-33877, 33910, 33916-33922, 33926, 33975-33980, 33983)

📋 24.4   ⚕ 24.4   **FUD** ZZZ   C 80 ▢

AMA: 2017,Dec,3

33261-33264 Surgical Ablation Arrhythmogenic Foci, Ventricular

33261 Operative ablation of ventricular arrhythmogenic focus with cardiopulmonary bypass

📋 47.0   ⚕ 47.0   **FUD** 090   C 80 ▢

AMA: 2018,Jan,8; 2017,Dec,3; 2017,Jan,8; 2016,Jan,13; 2015,Jan,16; 2014,Jan,11

Impulse centers that are causing arrhythmia are treated with ablation

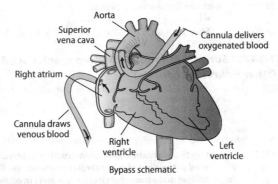

Bypass schematic

33262	Resequenced code. See code following 33241.
33263	Resequenced code. See code following 33241.
33264	Resequenced code. See code before 33243.

33265-33275 Surgical Ablation Arrhythmogenic Foci, Endoscopic

EXCLUDES *Insertion or replacement of temporary transvenous single chamber cardiac electrode or pacemaker catheter (separate procedure) (33210-33211) Tube thoracostomy, includes connection to drainage system (32551)*

33265 Endoscopy, surgical; operative tissue ablation and reconstruction of atria, limited (eg, modified maze procedure), without cardiopulmonary bypass

📋 39.3   ⚕ 39.3   **FUD** 090   C 80 ▢

AMA: 2018,Jan,8; 2017,Jan,8; 2016,Jan,13; 2015,Jan,16; 2014,Jan,11

33266 operative tissue ablation and reconstruction of atria, extensive (eg, maze procedure), without cardiopulmonary bypass

📋 53.4   ⚕ 53.4   **FUD** 090   C 80 ▢

AMA: 2018,Jan,8; 2017,Jan,8; 2016,Jan,13; 2015,Jan,16; 2014,Jan,11

33270	Resequenced code. See code following 33249.
33271	Resequenced code. See code following 33249.
33272	Resequenced code. See code following 33249.
33273	Resequenced code. See code following 33249.
33274	Resequenced code. See code following 33249.
33275	Resequenced code. See code following 33249.

33285-33289 Cardiac Rhythm Monitor System

33285 Insertion, subcutaneous cardiac rhythm monitor, including programming

INCLUDES Implantation of device into subcutaneous prepectoral pocket
Initial programming

EXCLUDES *Successive analysis and/or reprogramming (93285, 93291, 93298)*

📋 2.59   ⚕ 146.   **FUD** 000   J8 ▢

AMA: 2019,Apr,3

33286 Removal, subcutaneous cardiac rhythm monitor

📋 2.54   ⚕ 3.80   **FUD** 000   G2 ▢

AMA: 2019,Apr,3

33289 Transcatheter implantation of wireless pulmonary artery pressure sensor for long-term hemodynamic monitoring, including deployment and calibration of the sensor, right heart catheterization, selective pulmonary catheterization, radiological supervision and interpretation, and pulmonary artery angiography, when performed

INCLUDES Device implantation into subcutaneous pocket
Fluoroscopy (76000)
Pulmonary artery angiography/injection (75741, 75743, 75746, 93568)
Pulmonary artery catheterization (36013-36015)
Radiologic supervision and interpretation
Remote monitoring (93264)
Right heart catheterization (93451, 93453, 93456-93457, 93460-93461, 93530-93533)
Sensor deployment and calibration

📋 9.51   ⚕ 9.51   **FUD** 000   80 ▢

AMA: 2019,Jun,3

33300-33315 Procedures for Injury of the Heart

INCLUDES Procedures with and without cardiopulmonary bypass
EXCLUDES *Cardiac assist services (33946-33949, 33967-33983, 33990-33993)*

33300 Repair of cardiac wound; without bypass

📋 71.0   ⚕ 71.0   **FUD** 090   C 80 ▢

AMA: 1997,Nov,1

33305 with cardiopulmonary bypass

📋 119.   ⚕ 119.   **FUD** 090   C 80 ▢

AMA: 2017,Dec,3

33310 Cardiotomy, exploratory (includes removal of foreign body, atrial or ventricular thrombus); without bypass

EXCLUDES *Other cardiac procedures unless separate incision into heart is necessary in order to remove thrombus*

📋 34.0   ⚕ 34.0   **FUD** 090   C 80 ▢

AMA: 1997,Nov,1

33315 with cardiopulmonary bypass

EXCLUDES *Other cardiac procedures unless separate incision into heart is necessary in order to remove thrombus*

Code also excision of thrombus with cardiopulmonary bypass and append modifier 59 if separate incision is required with (33120, 33130, 33420-33430, 33460-33468, 33496, 33542, 33545, 33641-33647, 33670, 33681, 33975-33980)

📋 55.3   ⚕ 55.3   **FUD** 090   C 80 ▢

AMA: 2018,Jan,8; 2017,Dec,3; 2017,Jan,8; 2016,Jan,13; 2015,Jan,16; 2014,Jan,11

26/TC PC/TC Only   A2-Z3 ASC Payment   50 Bilateral   ♂ Male Only   ♀ Female Only   📋 Facility RVU   ⚕ Non-Facility RVU   ▢ CCI   ☒ CLIA
FUD Follow-up Days   CMS: IOM   AMA: CPT Asst   A-Y OPPSI   80/80 Surg Assist Allowed / w/Doc   ▨ Lab Crosswalk   ▨ Radiology Crosswalk

134

33320-33335 Procedures for Injury of the Aorta/Great Vessels

33320   **Suture repair of aorta or great vessels; without shunt or cardiopulmonary bypass**
30.5   30.5   **FUD** 090   C 80
AMA: 2018,Jun,11; 2018,Jan,8; 2017,Jan,8; 2016,Jan,13; 2015,Jan,16; 2014,Jan,11

33321   **with shunt bypass**
34.6   34.6   **FUD** 090   C 80
AMA: 2018,Jun,11

33322   **with cardiopulmonary bypass**
40.0   40.0   **FUD** 090   C 80
AMA: 2018,Jun,11; 2018,Jan,8; 2017,Dec,3; 2017,Jan,8; 2016,Jan,13; 2015,Jan,16; 2014,Jan,11

33330   **Insertion of graft, aorta or great vessels; without shunt, or cardiopulmonary bypass**
41.5   41.5   **FUD** 090   C 80
AMA: 2018,Jun,11

33335   **with cardiopulmonary bypass**
54.6   54.6   **FUD** 090   C 80
AMA: 2018,Jun,11; 2017,Dec,3

33340 Closure Left Atrial Appendage

EXCLUDES   *Cardiac catheterization except for reasons other than closure left atrial appendage (93451-93453, 93456, 93458-93461, 93462, 93530-93533)*

33340   **Percutaneous transcatheter closure of the left atrial appendage with endocardial implant, including fluoroscopy, transseptal puncture, catheter placement(s), left atrial angiography, left atrial appendage angiography, when performed, and radiological supervision and interpretation**
23.0   23.0   **FUD** 000   C 80
AMA: 2018,Jan,8; 2017,Jul,3

33361-33369 Transcatheter Aortic Valve Replacement

CMS: 100-03,20.32 Transcatheter Aortic Valve Replacement (TAVR); 100-04,32,290.1.1 Coding Requirements for TAVR Services; 100-04,32,290.2 Claims Processing for TAVR/ Professional Claims; 100-04,32,290.3 Claims Processing TAVR Inpatient; 100-04,32,290.4 Payment of TAVR for MA Plan Participants

INCLUDES   Access and implantation of the aortic valve (33361-33366)
Access sheath placement
Advancement of valve delivery system
Arteriotomy closure
Balloon aortic valvuloplasty
Cardiac or open arterial approach
Deployment of valve
Percutaneous access
Temporary pacemaker
Valve repositioning when necessary
Radiology procedures:
    Angiography during and after procedure
    Assessment of access site for closure
    Documentation of completion of the intervention
    Guidance for valve placement
    Supervision and interpretation

EXCLUDES   *Cardiac catheterization procedures included in the TAVR/TAVI service (93452-93453, 93458-93461, 93567)*
Percutaneous coronary interventional procedures
Transvascular ventricular support (33967, 33970, 33973, 33975-33976, 33990-33993, 33999)

Code also cardiac catheterization services for purposes other than TAVR/TAVI
Code also diagnostic coronary angiography at a different session from the interventional procedure
Code also diagnostic coronary angiography at the same time as TAVR/TAVI when:
    A previous study is available, but documentation states the patient's condition has changed since the previous study, visualization of the anatomy/pathology is inadequate, or a change occurs during the procedure warranting additional evaluation of an area outside the current target area
    No previous catheter-based coronary angiography study is available, and a full diagnostic study is performed, with the decision to perform the intervention based on that study
Code also modifier 59 when diagnostic coronary angiography procedures are performed as separate and distinct procedural services on the same day or session as TAVR/TAVI
Code also modifier 62 as all TAVI/TAVR procedures require the work of two physicians

33361   **Transcatheter aortic valve replacement (TAVR/TAVI) with prosthetic valve; percutaneous femoral artery approach**
Code also cardiopulmonary bypass when performed (33367-33369)
39.4   39.4   **FUD** 000   C 80
AMA: 2018,Jan,8; 2017,Jan,8; 2016,Jan,13; 2015,Mar,9; 2015,Jan,16; 2014,Jul,8; 2014,Jan,5; 2014,Jan,11

33362   **open femoral artery approach**
Code also cardiopulmonary bypass when performed (33367-33369)
43.1   43.1   **FUD** 000   C 80
AMA: 2018,Jan,8; 2017,Dec,3; 2017,Jan,8; 2016,Jan,13; 2015,Mar,9; 2015,Jan,16; 2014,Jul,8; 2014,Jan,5; 2014,Jan,11

33363   **open axillary artery approach**
Code also cardiopulmonary bypass when performed (33367-33369)
44.6   44.6   **FUD** 000   C 80
AMA: 2018,Jan,8; 2017,Dec,3; 2017,Jan,8; 2016,Jan,13; 2015,Mar,9; 2015,Jan,16; 2014,Jul,8; 2014,Jan,5; 2014,Jan,11

33364   **open iliac artery approach**
Code also cardiopulmonary bypass when performed (33367-33369)
46.1   46.1   **FUD** 000   C 80
AMA: 2018,Jan,8; 2017,Dec,3; 2017,Jan,8; 2016,Jan,13; 2015,Mar,9; 2015,Jan,16; 2014,Jul,8; 2014,Jan,5; 2014,Jan,11

33365   **transaortic approach (eg, median sternotomy, mediastinotomy)**
Code also cardiopulmonary bypass when performed (33367-33369)
51.8   51.8   **FUD** 000   C 80
AMA: 2018,Jan,8; 2017,Jan,8; 2016,Jan,13; 2015,Mar,9; 2015,Jan,16; 2014,Jul,8; 2014,Jan,5; 2014,Jan,11

33366 transapical exposure (eg, left thoracotomy)

Code also cardiopulmonary bypass when performed (33367-33369)

⚕ 56.0 ⚖ 56.0 **FUD** 000 [C] [80] [▦]

AMA: 2018,Jan,8; 2017,Jan,8; 2016,Jan,13; 2015,Mar,9; 2015,Jan,16; 2014,Jul,8; 2014,Jan,5

+ **33367** cardiopulmonary bypass support with percutaneous peripheral arterial and venous cannulation (eg, femoral vessels) (List separately in addition to code for primary procedure)

EXCLUDES Cardiopulmonary bypass support with open or central arterial and venous cannulation (33368-33369)

Code first (33361-33366, 33418, 33477, 0483T-0484T, 0544T, 0545T, 0569T-0570T)

⚕ 18.2 ⚖ 18.2 **FUD** ZZZ [C] [80] [▦]

AMA: 2018,Jan,8; 2017,Jan,8; 2016,Mar,5; 2016,Jan,13; 2015,Sep,3; 2015,Jan,16

+ **33368** cardiopulmonary bypass support with open peripheral arterial and venous cannulation (eg, femoral, iliac, axillary vessels) (List separately in addition to code for primary procedure)

EXCLUDES Cardiopulmonary bypass support with percutaneous or central arterial and venous cannulation (33367, 33369)

Code first (33361-33366, 33418, 33477, 0483T-0484T, 0544T, 0545T, 0569T-0570T)

⚕ 21.7 ⚖ 21.7 **FUD** ZZZ [C] [80] [▦]

AMA: 2018,Jan,8; 2017,Jan,8; 2016,Mar,5; 2016,Jan,13; 2015,Sep,3; 2015,Jan,16

+ **33369** cardiopulmonary bypass support with central arterial and venous cannulation (eg, aorta, right atrium, pulmonary artery) (List separately in addition to code for primary procedure)

EXCLUDES Cardiopulmonary bypass support with percutaneous or open arterial and venous cannulation (33367-33368)

Code first (33361-33366, 33418, 33477, 0483T-0484T, 0544T, 0545T, 0569T-0570T)

⚕ 28.6 ⚖ 28.6 **FUD** ZZZ [C] [80] [▦]

AMA: 2018,Jan,8; 2017,Jan,8; 2016,Mar,5; 2016,Jan,13; 2015,Sep,3; 2015,Jan,16

33390-33415 [33440] Aortic Valve Procedures

33390 Valvuloplasty, aortic valve, open, with cardiopulmonary bypass; simple (ie, valvotomy, debridement, debulking, and/or simple commissural resuspension)

⚕ 54.9 ⚖ 54.9 **FUD** 090 [C] [80] [▦]

AMA: 2018,Jan,8; 2017,Dec,3

33391 complex (eg, leaflet extension, leaflet resection, leaflet reconstruction, or annuloplasty)

INCLUDES Simple aortic valvuloplasty (33390)

⚕ 66.1 ⚖ 66.1 **FUD** 090 [C] [80] [▦]

AMA: 2018,Jan,8; 2017,Dec,3

33404 Construction of apical-aortic conduit

⚕ 51.0 ⚖ 51.0 **FUD** 090 [C] [80] [▦]

AMA: 2018,Jan,8; 2017,Dec,3; 2017,Jan,8; 2016,Jan,13; 2015,Jan,16; 2014,Jan,11

33405 Replacement, aortic valve, open, with cardiopulmonary bypass; with prosthetic valve other than homograft or stentless valve

⚕ 65.6 ⚖ 65.6 **FUD** 090 [C] [80] [▦]

AMA: 2019,Apr,6; 2018,Jan,8; 2017,Dec,3; 2017,Jan,8; 2016,Jan,13; 2015,Jan,16; 2014,Jan,11

33406 with allograft valve (freehand)

⚕ 83.2 ⚖ 83.2 **FUD** 090 [C] [80] [▦]

AMA: 2019,Apr,6; 2018,Jan,8; 2017,Dec,3; 2017,Jan,8; 2016,Jan,13; 2015,Jan,16; 2014,Jan,11

33410 with stentless tissue valve

⚕ 73.6 ⚖ 73.6 **FUD** 090 [C] [80] [▦]

AMA: 2019,Apr,6; 2018,Jan,8; 2017,Dec,3; 2017,Jan,8; 2016,Jan,13; 2015,Jan,16; 2014,Jan,11

33440 Replacement, aortic valve; by translocation of autologous pulmonary valve and transventricular aortic annulus enlargement of the left ventricular outflow tract with valved conduit replacement of pulmonary valve (Ross-Konno procedure)

INCLUDES Open replacement aortic valve with aortic annulus enlargement (33411-33412)
Open replacement aortic valve with translocation pulmonary valve (33413)

EXCLUDES Aortoplasty for supravalvular stenosis (33417)
Open replacement aortic valve (33405-33406, 33410)
Repair complex cardiac anomaly (except pulmonary atresia) (33608)
Repair left ventricular outlet obstruction (33414)
Repair pulmonary atresia (33920)
Replacement pulmonary valve (33475)
Resection/incision subvalvular tissue for aortic stenosis (33416)

⚕ 98.1 ⚖ 98.1 **FUD** 090 [80] [▦]

AMA: 2019,Apr,6

33411 Replacement, aortic valve; with aortic annulus enlargement, noncoronary sinus

⚕ 97.3 ⚖ 97.3 **FUD** 090 [C] [80] [▦]

AMA: 2019,Apr,6; 2018,Jan,8; 2017,Dec,3; 2017,Jan,8; 2016,Jan,13; 2015,Jan,16; 2014,Jan,11

Overhead schematic of major heart valves

33412 with transventricular aortic annulus enlargement (Konno procedure)

EXCLUDES Replacement aortic valve by translocation pulmonary valve, aortic annulus enlargement, valved conduit pulmonary valve replacement ([33440])
Replacement aortic valve with translocation pulmonary valve (33413)

⚕ 92.1 ⚖ 92.1 **FUD** 090 [C] [80] [▦]

AMA: 2019,Apr,6; 2018,Jan,8; 2017,Dec,3; 2017,Jan,8; 2016,Jan,13; 2015,Jan,16; 2014,Jan,11

33413 by translocation of autologous pulmonary valve with allograft replacement of pulmonary valve (Ross procedure)

EXCLUDES Replacement aortic valve by translocation pulmonary valve, aortic annulus enlargement, valved conduit pulmonary valve replacement ([33440])
Replacement aortic valve with transventricular aortic annulus enlargement (33412)

⚕ 94.3 ⚖ 94.3 **FUD** 090 [C] [80] [▦]

AMA: 2019,Apr,6; 2018,Jan,8; 2017,Dec,3; 2017,Jan,8; 2016,Jan,13; 2015,Jan,16; 2014,Jan,11

33414 Repair of left ventricular outflow tract obstruction by patch enlargement of the outflow tract

⚕ 62.0 ⚖ 62.0 **FUD** 090 [C] [80] [▦]

AMA: 2019,Apr,6; 2018,Jan,8; 2017,Dec,3; 2017,Jan,8; 2016,Jan,13; 2015,Jan,16; 2014,Jan,11

33415 Resection or incision of subvalvular tissue for discrete subvalvular aortic stenosis
58.7   58.7   **FUD** 090   C 80
AMA: 2018,Jan,8; 2017,Dec,3; 2017,Jan,8; 2016,Jan,13; 2015,Jan,16; 2014,Jan,11

33416 Ventriculectomy

CMS: 100-03,20.26 Partial Ventriculectomy

EXCLUDES *Percutaneous transcatheter septal reduction therapy (93583)*

33416 Ventriculomyotomy (-myectomy) for idiopathic hypertrophic subaortic stenosis (eg, asymmetric septal hypertrophy)
58.6   58.6   **FUD** 090   C 80
AMA: 2019,Apr,6; 2018,Jan,8; 2017,Dec,3; 2017,Jan,8; 2016,Jan,13; 2015,Jan,16; 2014,Jan,11

33417 Repair of Supravalvular Stenosis by Aortoplasty

33417 Aortoplasty (gusset) for supravalvular stenosis
48.1   48.1   **FUD** 090   C 80
AMA: 2019,Apr,6; 2018,Jan,8; 2017,Dec,3; 2017,Jan,8; 2016,Jan,13; 2015,Jan,16; 2014,Jan,11

33418-33419 Transcatheter Mitral Valve Procedures

INCLUDES
Access sheath placement
Advancement of valve delivery system
Deployment of valve
Radiology procedures:
  Angiography during and after procedure
  Documentation of completion of the intervention
  Guidance for valve placement
  Supervision and interpretation
Valve repositioning when necessary

EXCLUDES *Cardiac catheterization services for purposes other than TMVR*
Diagnostic angiography at different session from interventional procedure
Percutaneous approach through the coronary sinus for TMVR (0345T)
Percutaneous coronary interventional procedures
Transcatheter mitral valve annulus reconstruction (0544T)
Transcatheter TMVI by percutaneous or transthoracic approach (0483T-0484T)

Code also cardiopulmonary bypass:
  Central (33369)
  Open peripheral (33368)
  Percutaneous peripheral (33367)
Code also diagnostic coronary angiography and cardiac catheterization procedures when:
  No previous study available and full diagnostic study performed
  Previous study inadequate or patient's clinical indication for the study changed prior to or during the procedure
  Use modifier 59 with cardiac catheterization procedures when on same day or same session as TMVR
Code also transvascular ventricular support:
  Balloon pump (33967, 33970, 33973)
  Ventricular assist device (33990-33993)

33418 Transcatheter mitral valve repair, percutaneous approach, including transseptal puncture when performed; initial prosthesis
    Code also left heart catheterization when performed by transapical puncture (93462)
52.3   52.3   **FUD** 090   C 80
AMA: 2018,Jan,8; 2017,Jan,8; 2016,Jan,13; 2015,Sep,3

+ **33419** additional prosthesis(es) during same session (List separately in addition to code for primary procedure)
    EXCLUDES *Procedures performed more than one time per session*
    Code first (33418)
12.3   12.3   **FUD** ZZZ   N N1 80
AMA: 2018,Jan,8; 2017,Jan,8; 2016,Jan,13; 2015,Sep,3

33420-33440 Mitral Valve Procedures

Code also removal of thrombus through a separate heart incision, when performed (33310-33315); append modifier 59 to (33315)

33420 Valvotomy, mitral valve; closed heart
42.3   42.3   **FUD** 090   C
AMA: 2018,Jan,8; 2017,Jan,8; 2016,Jan,13; 2015,Sep,3; 2015,Jan,16; 2014,Jan,11

33422 open heart, with cardiopulmonary bypass
48.5   48.5   **FUD** 090   C 80
AMA: 2018,Jan,8; 2017,Dec,3; 2017,Jan,8; 2016,Jan,13; 2015,Sep,3; 2015,Jan,16; 2014,Jan,11

33425 Valvuloplasty, mitral valve, with cardiopulmonary bypass;
79.0   79.0   **FUD** 090   C 80
AMA: 2018,Jan,8; 2017,Dec,3; 2017,Jan,8; 2016,Jan,13; 2015,Sep,3; 2015,Jan,16; 2014,Jan,11

33426 with prosthetic ring
68.9   68.9   **FUD** 090   C 80
AMA: 2018,Jan,8; 2017,Dec,3; 2017,Jan,8; 2016,Jan,13; 2015,Sep,3; 2015,Jan,16; 2014,Jan,11

33427 radical reconstruction, with or without ring
70.8   70.8   **FUD** 090   C 80
AMA: 2018,Jan,8; 2017,Dec,3; 2017,Jan,8; 2016,Jan,13; 2015,Sep,3; 2015,Jan,16; 2014,Jan,11

33430 Replacement, mitral valve, with cardiopulmonary bypass
81.0   81.0   **FUD** 090   C 80
AMA: 2018,Jan,8; 2017,Dec,3; 2017,Jan,8; 2016,Jan,13; 2015,Sep,3; 2015,Jan,16; 2014,Jan,11

33440 Resequenced code. See code following 33410.

33460-33468 Tricuspid Valve Procedures

EXCLUDES *Transcatheter tricuspid valve annulus reconstruction (0545T)*
Transcatheter tricuspid valve repair (0569T-0570T)
Code also removal of thrombus through a separate heart incision, when performed (33310-33315); append modifier 59 to (33315)

33460 Valvectomy, tricuspid valve, with cardiopulmonary bypass
70.2   70.2   **FUD** 090   C 80
AMA: 2018,Jan,8; 2017,Dec,3; 2017,Jan,8; 2016,Jan,13; 2015,Jan,16; 2014,Jan,11

33463 Valvuloplasty, tricuspid valve; without ring insertion
89.5   89.5   **FUD** 090   C 80
AMA: 2018,Jan,8; 2017,Dec,3; 2017,Jan,8; 2016,Jan,13; 2015,Jan,16; 2014,Jan,11

33464 with ring insertion
70.7   70.7   **FUD** 090   C 80
AMA: 2018,Jan,8; 2017,Dec,3; 2017,Jan,8; 2016,Jan,13; 2015,Jan,16; 2014,Jan,11

33465 Replacement, tricuspid valve, with cardiopulmonary bypass
79.9   79.9   **FUD** 090   C 80
AMA: 2018,Jan,8; 2017,Dec,3; 2017,Jan,8; 2016,Jan,13; 2015,Jan,16; 2014,Jan,11

33468 Tricuspid valve repositioning and plication for Ebstein anomaly
71.2   71.2   **FUD** 090   C 80
AMA: 2018,Jan,8; 2017,Dec,3; 2017,Jan,8; 2016,Jan,13; 2015,Jan,16; 2014,Jan,11

33470-33474 Pulmonary Valvotomy

INCLUDES Brock's operation
Code also the concurrent ligation/takedown of a systemic-to-pulmonary artery shunt (33924)

33470 Valvotomy, pulmonary valve, closed heart; transventricular
35.9   35.9   **FUD** 090   63 C 80
AMA: 2018,Jan,8; 2017,Jan,8; 2016,Jan,13; 2015,Jan,16; 2014,Jan,11

33471 via pulmonary artery
EXCLUDES *Percutaneous valvuloplasty of pulmonary valve (92990)*
38.3   38.3   **FUD** 090   C 80
AMA: 2018,Jan,8; 2017,Jan,8; 2016,Jan,13; 2015,Jan,16; 2014,Jan,11

33474 Valvotomy, pulmonary valve, open heart, with cardiopulmonary bypass
63.2   63.2   **FUD** 090   C 80
AMA: 2017,Dec,3

33475-33476 Other Procedures Pulmonary Valve

Code also the concurrent ligation/takedown of a systemic-to-pulmonary artery shunt (33924)

33475 **Replacement, pulmonary valve**

🔧 67.6   ⚕ 67.6   **FUD** 090   C 80 ▭

AMA: 2019,Apr,6; 2018,Jan,8; 2017,Dec,3; 2017,Jan,8; 2016,Jan,13; 2015,Jan,16; 2014,Jan,11

33476 **Right ventricular resection for infundibular stenosis, with or without commissurotomy**

INCLUDES   Brock's operation

🔧 44.1   ⚕ 44.1   **FUD** 090   C 80 ▭

AMA: 2018,Jan,8; 2017,Dec,3; 2017,Jan,8; 2016,Jan,13; 2015,Jan,16; 2014,Jan,11

33477 Transcatheter Pulmonary Valve Implantation

INCLUDES   Cardiac catheterization, contrast injection, angiography, fluoroscopic guidance and the supervision and interpretation for device placement
Percutaneous balloon angioplasty within the treatment area
Pre-, intra-, and post-operative hemodynamic measurements
Valvuloplasty or stent insertion in pulmonary valve conduit (37236-37237, 92997-92998)

EXCLUDES   *Balloon pump insertion (33967, 33970, 33973)*
Cardiopulmonary bypass performed in the same session (33367-33369)
Extracorporeal membrane oxygenation (ECMO) (33946-33959 [33962, 33963, 33964, 33965, 33966, 33969, 33984, 33985, 33986, 33987, 33988, 33989])
Fluoroscopy (76000)
Injection procedure during cardiac catheterization (93563, 93566-93568)
Percutaneous cardiac intervention procedures, when performed
Procedures performed more than one time per session
Right heart catheterization (93451, 93453-93461, 93530-93533)
Ventricular assist device (VAD) (33990-33993)

Code also the concurrent ligation/takedown of a systemic-to-pulmonary artery shunt (33924)

33477 **Transcatheter pulmonary valve implantation, percutaneous approach, including pre-stenting of the valve delivery site, when performed**

🔧 39.7   ⚕ 39.7   **FUD** 000   C 80 ▭

AMA: 2018,Jan,8; 2017,Jan,8; 2016,Aug,9; 2016,Mar,5

33478 Outflow Tract Augmentation

Code also for cavopulmonary anastomosis to a second superior vena cava (33768)
Code also the concurrent ligation/takedown of a systemic-to-pulmonary artery shunt (33924)

33478 **Outflow tract augmentation (gusset), with or without commissurotomy or infundibular resection**

🔧 45.6   ⚕ 45.6   **FUD** 090   C 80 ▭

AMA: 2018,Jan,8; 2017,Dec,3; 2017,Jan,8; 2016,Jan,13; 2015,Jan,16; 2014,Jan,11

33496 Prosthetic Valve Repair

Code also removal of thrombus through a separate heart incision, when performed (33310-33315); append modifier 59 to (33315)
Code also reoperation if performed (33530)

33496 **Repair of non-structural prosthetic valve dysfunction with cardiopulmonary bypass (separate procedure)**

🔧 48.5   ⚕ 48.5   **FUD** 090   C 80 ▭

AMA: 2018,Jan,8; 2017,Dec,3; 2017,Jan,8; 2016,Jan,13; 2015,Jan,16; 2014,Jan,11

33500-33507 Repair Aberrant Coronary Artery Anatomy

INCLUDES   Angioplasty and/or endarterectomy

33500 **Repair of coronary arteriovenous or arteriocardiac chamber fistula; with cardiopulmonary bypass**

🔧 45.5   ⚕ 45.5   **FUD** 090   C 80 ▭

AMA: 2017,Dec,3

33501 **without cardiopulmonary bypass**

🔧 32.5   ⚕ 32.5   **FUD** 090   C 80 ▭

AMA: 2007,Mar,1-3; 1997,Nov,1

33502 **Repair of anomalous coronary artery from pulmonary artery origin; by ligation**

🔧 37.0   ⚕ 37.0   **FUD** 090   63 C 80 ▭

AMA: 2017,Dec,3

33503 **by graft, without cardiopulmonary bypass**

🔧 38.4   ⚕ 38.4   **FUD** 090   63 C 80 ▭

AMA: 2007,Mar,1-3; 1997,Nov,1

33504 **by graft, with cardiopulmonary bypass**

🔧 42.5   ⚕ 42.5   **FUD** 090   C 80 ▭

AMA: 2017,Dec,3

33505 **with construction of intrapulmonary artery tunnel (Takeuchi procedure)**

🔧 60.0   ⚕ 60.0   **FUD** 090   63 C 80 ▭

AMA: 2017,Dec,3

33506 **by translocation from pulmonary artery to aorta**

🔧 59.7   ⚕ 59.7   **FUD** 090   63 C 80 ▭

AMA: 2017,Dec,3

33507 **Repair of anomalous (eg, intramural) aortic origin of coronary artery by unroofing or translocation**

🔧 50.0   ⚕ 50.0   **FUD** 090   C 80 ▭

AMA: 2018,Jan,8; 2017,Dec,3; 2017,Jan,8; 2016,Jan,13; 2015,Jan,16; 2014,Jan,11

33508 Endoscopic Harvesting of Venous Graft

INCLUDES   Diagnostic endoscopy
EXCLUDES   *Harvesting of vein of upper extremity (35500)*
Code first (33510-33523)

+ **33508** **Endoscopy, surgical, including video-assisted harvest of vein(s) for coronary artery bypass procedure (List separately in addition to code for primary procedure)**

🔧 0.47   ⚕ 0.47   **FUD** ZZZ   N N1 80 ▭

AMA: 1997,Nov,1

33510-33516 Coronary Artery Bypass: Venous Grafts

INCLUDES   Obtaining saphenous vein grafts
Venous bypass grafting only
EXCLUDES   *Arterial bypass (33533-33536)*
Combined arterial-venous bypass (33517-33523, 33533-33536)
Obtaining vein graft:
Femoropopliteal vein (35572)
Upper extremity vein (35500)
Percutaneous ventricular assist devices (33990-33993)
Code also modifier 80 when assistant at surgery obtains grafts

33510 **Coronary artery bypass, vein only; single coronary venous graft**

🔧 55.9   ⚕ 55.9   **FUD** 090   C 80 ▭

AMA: 2018,Jan,8; 2017,Dec,3; 2017,Jan,8; 2016,Jan,13; 2015,Jan,16; 2014,Aug,14; 2014,Jan,11

33511 **2 coronary venous grafts**

🔧 61.4   ⚕ 61.4   **FUD** 090   C 80 ▭

AMA: 2018,Jan,8; 2017,Dec,3; 2017,Jan,8; 2016,Jan,13; 2015,Jan,16; 2014,Aug,14; 2014,Jan,11

33512 **3 coronary venous grafts**

🔧 69.9   ⚕ 69.9   **FUD** 090   C 80 ▭

AMA: 2018,Jan,8; 2017,Dec,3; 2017,Jan,8; 2016,Jan,13; 2015,Jan,16; 2014,Aug,14; 2014,Jan,11

33513 **4 coronary venous grafts**

🔧 72.0   ⚕ 72.0   **FUD** 090   C 80 ▭

AMA: 2018,Jan,8; 2017,Dec,3; 2017,Jan,8; 2016,Jan,13; 2015,Jan,16; 2014,Aug,14; 2014,Jan,11

33514 **5 coronary venous grafts**

🔧 75.7   ⚕ 75.7   **FUD** 090   C 80 ▭

AMA: 2018,Jan,8; 2017,Dec,3; 2017,Jan,8; 2016,Jan,13; 2015,Jan,16; 2014,Aug,14; 2014,Jan,11

33516 **6 or more coronary venous grafts**

🔧 78.9   ⚕ 78.9   **FUD** 090   C 80 ▭

AMA: 2018,Jan,8; 2017,Dec,3; 2017,Jan,8; 2016,Jan,13; 2015,Jan,16; 2014,Aug,14; 2014,Jan,11

33517-33523 Coronary Artery Bypass: Venous AND Arterial Grafts

INCLUDES   Obtaining saphenous vein grafts
EXCLUDES   Obtaining arterial graft:
    Upper extremity (35600)
  Obtaining vein graft:
    Femoropopliteal vein graft (35572)
    Upper extremity (35500)
  Percutaneous ventricular assist devices (33990-33993)
Code also modifier 80 when assistant at surgery obtains grafts
Code first (33533-33536)

+ 33517   Coronary artery bypass, using venous graft(s) and arterial graft(s); single vein graft (List separately in addition to code for primary procedure)
   🚗 5.41   ⚕ 5.41   **FUD** ZZZ   C 80 ▢
   AMA: 2018,Jan,8; 2017,Jan,8; 2016,Jan,13; 2015,Jan,16; 2014,Jan,11

+ 33518   2 venous grafts (List separately in addition to code for primary procedure)
   🚗 11.9   ⚕ 11.9   **FUD** ZZZ   C 80 ▢
   AMA: 2018,Jan,8; 2017,Jan,8; 2016,Jan,13; 2015,Jan,16; 2014,Jan,11

+ 33519   3 venous grafts (List separately in addition to code for primary procedure)
   🚗 15.7   ⚕ 15.7   **FUD** ZZZ   C 80 ▢
   AMA: 2018,Jan,8; 2017,Jan,8; 2016,Jan,13; 2015,Jan,16; 2014,Jan,11

+ 33521   4 venous grafts (List separately in addition to code for primary procedure)
   🚗 18.9   ⚕ 18.9   **FUD** ZZZ   C 80 ▢
   AMA: 2018,Jan,8; 2017,Jan,8; 2016,Jan,13; 2015,Jan,16; 2014,Jan,11

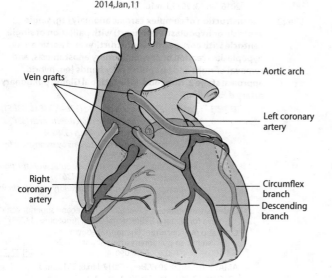

Vein grafts — Aortic arch
Left coronary artery
Right coronary artery — Circumflex branch / Descending branch

+ 33522   5 venous grafts (List separately in addition to code for primary procedure)
   🚗 21.2   ⚕ 21.2   **FUD** ZZZ   C 80 ▢
   AMA: 2018,Jan,8; 2017,Jan,8; 2016,Jan,13; 2015,Jan,16; 2014,Jan,11

+ 33523   6 or more venous grafts (List separately in addition to code for primary procedure)
   🚗 24.0   ⚕ 24.0   **FUD** ZZZ   C 80 ▢
   AMA: 2018,Jan,8; 2017,Jan,8; 2016,Jan,13; 2015,Jan,16; 2014,Jan,11

33530 Reoperative Coronary Artery Bypass Graft or Valve Procedure

EXCLUDES   *Percutaneous ventricular assist devices (33990-33993)*
Code first (33390-33391, 33404-33496, 33510-33536, 33863)

+ 33530   Reoperation, coronary artery bypass procedure or valve procedure, more than 1 month after original operation (List separately in addition to code for primary procedure)
   🚗 15.2   ⚕ 15.2   **FUD** ZZZ   C 80 ▢
   AMA: 2018,Jan,8; 2017,Jan,8; 2016,Jan,13; 2015,Jan,16; 2014,Jan,11

33533-33536 Coronary Artery Bypass: Arterial Grafts

INCLUDES   Obtaining arterial graft (eg, epigastric, internal mammary, gastroepiploic and others)
EXCLUDES   *Obtaining arterial graft:*
    Upper extremity (35600)
  Obtaining venous graft:
    Femoropopliteal vein (35572)
    Upper extremity (35500)
  Percutaneous ventricular assist devices (33990-33993)
  Venous bypass (33510-33516)
Code also for combined arterial venous grafts (33517-33523)
Code also modifier 80 when assistant at surgery obtains grafts

33533   Coronary artery bypass, using arterial graft(s); single arterial graft
   🚗 54.0   ⚕ 54.0   **FUD** 090   C 80 ▢
   AMA: 2018,Jan,8; 2017,Dec,3; 2017,Jan,8; 2016,Jan,13; 2015,Jan,16; 2014,Nov,14; 2014,Jan,11

33534   2 coronary arterial grafts
   🚗 63.6   ⚕ 63.6   **FUD** 090   C 80 ▢
   AMA: 2018,Jan,8; 2017,Dec,3; 2017,Jan,8; 2016,Jan,13; 2015,Jan,16; 2014,Jan,11

33535   3 coronary arterial grafts
   🚗 70.9   ⚕ 70.9   **FUD** 090   C 80 ▢
   AMA: 2018,Jan,8; 2017,Dec,3; 2017,Jan,8; 2016,Jan,13; 2015,Jan,16; 2014,Jan,11

33536   4 or more coronary arterial grafts
   🚗 76.1   ⚕ 76.1   **FUD** 090   C 80 ▢
   AMA: 2018,Jan,8; 2017,Dec,3; 2017,Jan,8; 2016,Jan,13; 2015,Jan,16; 2014,Nov,14; 2014,Jan,11

33542-33548 Ventricular Reconstruction

33542   Myocardial resection (eg, ventricular aneurysmectomy)
   Code also removal of thrombus through a separate heart incision, when performed (33310-33315); append modifier 59 to (33315)
   🚗 76.2   ⚕ 76.2   **FUD** 090   C 80 ▢
   AMA: 2018,Jan,8; 2017,Dec,3; 2017,Jan,8; 2016,Jan,13; 2015,Jan,16; 2014,Jan,11

33545   Repair of postinfarction ventricular septal defect, with or without myocardial resection
   Code also removal of thrombus through a separate heart incision, when performed (33310-33315); append modifier 59 to (33315)
   🚗 89.7   ⚕ 89.7   **FUD** 090   C 80 ▢
   AMA: 2018,Jan,8; 2017,Dec,3; 2017,Jan,8; 2016,Jan,13; 2015,Jan,16; 2014,Jan,11

33548   Surgical ventricular restoration procedure, includes prosthetic patch, when performed (eg, ventricular remodeling, SVR, SAVER, Dor procedures)
   EXCLUDES   *Batista procedure or pachopexy (33999)*
    Cardiotomy, exploratory (33310, 33315)
    Temporary pacemaker (33210-33211)
    Tube thoracostomy (32551)
   🚗 85.7   ⚕ 85.7   **FUD** 090   C 80 ▢
   AMA: 2018,Jan,8; 2017,Dec,3; 2017,Jan,8; 2016,Jan,13; 2015,Jan,16; 2014,Jan,11

Cardiovascular, Hemic, and Lymphatic

33517 — 33548

33572 Endarterectomy with CABG (LAD, RCA, Cx)

Code first (33510-33516, 33533-33536)

+ 33572 Coronary endarterectomy, open, any method, of left anterior descending, circumflex, or right coronary artery performed in conjunction with coronary artery bypass graft procedure, each vessel (List separately in addition to primary procedure)

🚗 6.67   ⚕ 6.67   **FUD** ZZZ   C 80 ▣

AMA: 1997,Nov,1; 1994,Win,1

33600-33622 Repair Aberrant Heart Anatomy

33600 Closure of atrioventricular valve (mitral or tricuspid) by suture or patch

🚗 49.8   ⚕ 49.8   **FUD** 090   C 80 ▣

AMA: 2018,Jan,8; 2017,Dec,3; 2017,Jan,8; 2016,Jan,13; 2015,Jan,16; 2014,Jan,11

33602 Closure of semilunar valve (aortic or pulmonary) by suture or patch

Code also the concurrent ligation/takedown of a systemic-to-pulmonary artery shunt (33924)

🚗 48.4   ⚕ 48.4   **FUD** 090   C 80 ▣

AMA: 2017,Dec,3

33606 Anastomosis of pulmonary artery to aorta (Damus-Kaye-Stansel procedure)

Code also the concurrent ligation/takedown of a systemic-to-pulmonary artery shunt (33924)

🚗 51.6   ⚕ 51.6   **FUD** 090   C 80 ▣

AMA: 2017,Dec,3

33608 Repair of complex cardiac anomaly other than pulmonary atresia with ventricular septal defect by construction or replacement of conduit from right or left ventricle to pulmonary artery

EXCLUDES   *Unifocalization of arborization anomalies of pulmonary artery (33925, 33926)*

Code also the concurrent ligation/takedown of a systemic-to-pulmonary artery shunt (33924)

🚗 52.2   ⚕ 52.2   **FUD** 090   C 80 ▣

AMA: 2019,Apr,6; 2017,Dec,3

33610 Repair of complex cardiac anomalies (eg, single ventricle with subaortic obstruction) by surgical enlargement of ventricular septal defect

Code also the concurrent ligation/takedown of a systemic-to-pulmonary artery shunt (33924)

🚗 51.5   ⚕ 51.5   **FUD** 090   63 C 80 ▣

AMA: 2017,Dec,3

33611 Repair of double outlet right ventricle with intraventricular tunnel repair;

Code also the concurrent ligation/takedown of a systemic-to-pulmonary artery shunt (33924)

🚗 56.7   ⚕ 56.7   **FUD** 090   63 C 80 ▣

AMA: 2017,Dec,3

33612 with repair of right ventricular outflow tract obstruction

Code also the concurrent ligation/takedown of a systemic-to-pulmonary artery shunt (33924)

🚗 58.2   ⚕ 58.2   **FUD** 090   C 80 ▣

AMA: 2017,Dec,3

33615 Repair of complex cardiac anomalies (eg, tricuspid atresia) by closure of atrial septal defect and anastomosis of atria or vena cava to pulmonary artery (simple Fontan procedure)

Code also the concurrent ligation/takedown of a systemic-to-pulmonary artery shunt (33924)

🚗 58.0   ⚕ 58.0   **FUD** 090   C 80 ▣

AMA: 2017,Dec,3

33617 Repair of complex cardiac anomalies (eg, single ventricle) by modified Fontan procedure

Code also cavopulmonary anastomosis to a second superior vena cava (33768)

Code also the concurrent ligation/takedown of a systemic-to-pulmonary artery shunt (33924)

🚗 61.2   ⚕ 61.2   **FUD** 090   C 80 ▣

AMA: 2017,Dec,3

33619 Repair of single ventricle with aortic outflow obstruction and aortic arch hypoplasia (hypoplastic left heart syndrome) (eg, Norwood procedure)

🚗 79.3   ⚕ 79.3   **FUD** 090   63 C 80 ▣

AMA: 2018,Jan,8; 2017,Dec,3; 2017,Jan,8; 2016,Jul,3; 2016,Jan,13; 2015,Jan,16; 2014,Jan,11

33620 Application of right and left pulmonary artery bands (eg, hybrid approach stage 1)

EXCLUDES   *Banding of main pulmonary artery related to septal defect (33690)*

Code also transthoracic insertion of catheter for stent placement with removal of catheter and closure when performed during same session (33621)

🚗 47.9   ⚕ 47.9   **FUD** 090   C 80 ▣

AMA: 2018,Jan,8; 2017,Dec,3; 2017,Jan,8; 2016,Jul,3; 2016,Jan,13; 2015,Jan,16; 2014,Jan,11

33621 Transthoracic insertion of catheter for stent placement with catheter removal and closure (eg, hybrid approach stage 1)

Code also application of right and left pulmonary artery bands when performed during same session (33620)

Code also stent placement (37236)

🚗 27.0   ⚕ 27.0   **FUD** 090   C 80 ▣

AMA: 2018,Jan,8; 2017,Dec,3; 2017,Jan,8; 2016,Jul,3; 2016,Jan,13; 2015,Jan,16; 2014,Jan,11

33622 Reconstruction of complex cardiac anomaly (eg, single ventricle or hypoplastic left heart) with palliation of single ventricle with aortic outflow obstruction and aortic arch hypoplasia, creation of cavopulmonary anastomosis, and removal of right and left pulmonary bands (eg, hybrid approach stage 2, Norwood, bidirectional Glenn, pulmonary artery debanding)

EXCLUDES   *Excision of coarctation of aorta (33840, 33845, 33851)*
     Repair of hypoplastic or interrupted aortic arch (33853)
     Repair of patent ductus arteriosus (33822)
     Repair of pulmonary artery stenosis by reconstruction with patch or graft (33917)
     Repair of single ventricle with aortic outflow obstruction and aortic arch hypoplasia (33619)
     Shunt; superior vena cava to pulmonary artery for flow to both lungs (33767)

Code also anastomosis, cavopulmonary, second superior vena cava for bilateral bidirectional Glenn procedure (33768)

Code also the concurrent ligation/takedown of a systemic-to-pulmonary artery shunt (33924)

🚗 100.   ⚕ 100.   **FUD** 090   C 80 ▣

AMA: 2018,Jan,8; 2017,Dec,3; 2017,Jan,8; 2016,Jul,3; 2016,Jan,13; 2015,Jan,16; 2014,Jan,11

33641-33645 Closure of Defect: Atrium

Code also removal of thrombus through a separate heart incision, when performed (33310-33315); append modifier 59 to (33315)

33641 Repair atrial septal defect, secundum, with cardiopulmonary bypass, with or without patch

🚗 47.3   ⚕ 47.3   **FUD** 090   C 80 ▣

AMA: 2018,Jan,8; 2017,Dec,3; 2017,Jan,8; 2016,Jan,13; 2015,Jan,16; 2014,Jan,11

33645 Direct or patch closure, sinus venosus, with or without anomalous pulmonary venous drainage

EXCLUDES   *Repair of isolated partial anomalous pulmonary venous return (33724)*
     Repair of pulmonary venous stenosis (33726)

🚗 50.2   ⚕ 50.2   **FUD** 090   C 80 ▣

AMA: 2017,Dec,3

26/TC PC/TC Only   A2-Z3 ASC Payment   50 Bilateral   ♂ Male Only   ♀ Female Only   🚗 Facility RVU   ⚕ Non-Facility RVU   □ CCI   ✕ CLIA

FUD Follow-up Days   **CMS:** IOM   **AMA:** CPT Asst   A-Y OPPSI   80/80 Surg Assist Allowed / w/Doc   Lab Crosswalk   Radiology Crosswalk

140   CPT © 2019 American Medical Association. All Rights Reserved.   © 2019 Optum360, LLC

33647 Closure of Septal Defect: Atrium AND Ventricle

EXCLUDES *Tricuspid atresia repair procedures (33615)*
Code also removal of thrombus through a separate heart incision, when performed (33310-33315); append modifier 59 to (33315)

33647 **Repair of atrial septal defect and ventricular septal defect, with direct or patch closure**
🔧 52.8 ⚕ 52.8 **FUD** 090   ⑥③ Ⓒ 80 ▣
AMA: 2017,Dec,3

33660-33670 Closure of Defect: Atrioventricular Canal

33660 **Repair of incomplete or partial atrioventricular canal (ostium primum atrial septal defect), with or without atrioventricular valve repair**
🔧 51.0 ⚕ 51.0 **FUD** 090   Ⓒ 80 ▣
AMA: 2017,Dec,3

33665 **Repair of intermediate or transitional atrioventricular canal, with or without atrioventricular valve repair**
🔧 55.6 ⚕ 55.6 **FUD** 090   Ⓒ 80 ▣
AMA: 2017,Dec,3

33670 **Repair of complete atrioventricular canal, with or without prosthetic valve**
Code also removal of thrombus through a separate heart incision, when performed (33310-33315); append modifier 59 to (33315)
🔧 57.4 ⚕ 57.4 **FUD** 090   ⑥③ Ⓒ 80 ▣
AMA: 2017,Dec,3

33675-33677 Closure of Multiple Septal Defects: Ventricle

EXCLUDES *Closure of single ventricular septal defect (33681, 33684, 33688)*
Insertion or replacement of temporary transvenous single chamber cardiac electrode or pacemaker catheter (33210)
Percutaneous closure (93581)
Thoracentesis (32554-32555)
Thoracotomy (32100)
Tube thoracostomy (32551)

33675 **Closure of multiple ventricular septal defects;**
🔧 57.3 ⚕ 57.3 **FUD** 090   Ⓒ 80 ▣
AMA: 2018,Jan,8; 2017,Dec,3; 2017,Jan,8; 2016,Jan,13; 2015,Jan,16; 2014,Jan,11

33676 **with pulmonary valvotomy or infundibular resection (acyanotic)**
🔧 58.8 ⚕ 58.8 **FUD** 090   Ⓒ 80 ▣
AMA: 2018,Jan,8; 2017,Dec,3; 2017,Jan,8; 2016,Jan,13; 2015,Jan,16; 2014,Jan,11

33677 **with removal of pulmonary artery band, with or without gusset**
🔧 61.1 ⚕ 61.1 **FUD** 090   Ⓒ 80 ▣
AMA: 2018,Jan,8; 2017,Dec,3; 2017,Jan,8; 2016,Jan,13; 2015,Jan,16; 2014,Jan,11

33681-33688 Closure of Septal Defect: Ventricle

EXCLUDES *Repair of pulmonary vein that requires creating an atrial septal defect (33724)*

33681 **Closure of single ventricular septal defect, with or without patch;**
Code also removal of thrombus through a separate heart incision, when performed (33310-33315); append modifier 59 to (33315)
🔧 53.0 ⚕ 53.0 **FUD** 090   Ⓒ 80 ▣
AMA: 2018,Jan,8; 2017,Dec,3; 2017,Jan,8; 2016,Jan,13; 2015,Jan,16; 2014,Jan,11

33684 **with pulmonary valvotomy or infundibular resection (acyanotic)**
Code also concurrent ligation/takedown of a systemic-to-pulmonary artery shunt if performed (33924)
🔧 54.8 ⚕ 54.8 **FUD** 090   Ⓒ 80 ▣
AMA: 2017,Dec,3

33688 **with removal of pulmonary artery band, with or without gusset**
Code also the concurrent ligation/takedown of a systemic-to-pulmonary artery shunt if performed (33924)
🔧 54.8 ⚕ 54.8 **FUD** 090   Ⓒ 80 ▣
AMA: 2017,Dec,3

33690 Reduce Pulmonary Overcirculation in Septal Defects

EXCLUDES *Left and right pulmonary artery banding in a single ventricle (33620)*

33690 **Banding of pulmonary artery**
🔧 34.7 ⚕ 34.7 **FUD** 090   ⑥③ Ⓒ 80 ▣
AMA: 2018,Jan,8; 2017,Jan,8; 2016,Jan,13; 2015,Jan,16; 2014,Jan,11

33692-33697 Repair of Defects of Tetralogy of Fallot

Code also the concurrent ligation/takedown of a systemic-to-pulmonary artery shunt (33924)

33692 **Complete repair tetralogy of Fallot without pulmonary atresia;**
🔧 56.9 ⚕ 56.9 **FUD** 090   Ⓒ 80 ▣
AMA: 2017,Dec,3

33694 **with transannular patch**
🔧 56.7 ⚕ 56.7 **FUD** 090   ⑥③ Ⓒ 80 ▣
AMA: 2017,Dec,3

33697 **Complete repair tetralogy of Fallot with pulmonary atresia including construction of conduit from right ventricle to pulmonary artery and closure of ventricular septal defect**
🔧 59.7 ⚕ 59.7 **FUD** 090   Ⓒ 80 ▣
AMA: 2018,Jan,8; 2017,Dec,3; 2017,Jan,8; 2016,Jan,13; 2015,Jan,16; 2014,Jan,11

33702-33722 Repair Anomalies Sinus of Valsalva

33702 **Repair sinus of Valsalva fistula, with cardiopulmonary bypass;**
🔧 44.8 ⚕ 44.8 **FUD** 090   Ⓒ 80 ▣
AMA: 2018,Jan,8; 2017,Dec,3; 2017,Jan,8; 2016,Jan,13; 2015,Jan,16; 2014,Jan,11

33710 **with repair of ventricular septal defect**
🔧 59.6 ⚕ 59.6 **FUD** 090   Ⓒ 80 ▣
AMA: 2017,Dec,3

33720 **Repair sinus of Valsalva aneurysm, with cardiopulmonary bypass**
🔧 44.9 ⚕ 44.9 **FUD** 090   Ⓒ 80 ▣
AMA: 2017,Dec,3

33722 **Closure of aortico-left ventricular tunnel**
🔧 47.2 ⚕ 47.2 **FUD** 090   Ⓒ 80 ▣
AMA: 2018,Jan,8; 2017,Dec,3; 2017,Jan,8; 2016,Jan,13; 2015,Jan,16; 2014,Jan,11

33724-33732 Repair Aberrant Pulmonary Venous Connection

33724 **Repair of isolated partial anomalous pulmonary venous return (eg, Scimitar Syndrome)**
EXCLUDES *Temporary pacemaker (33210-33211)*
Tube thoracostomy (32551)
🔧 44.2 ⚕ 44.2 **FUD** 090   Ⓒ 80 ▣
AMA: 2018,Jan,8; 2017,Dec,3; 2017,Jan,8; 2016,Jan,13; 2015,Jan,16; 2014,Jan,11

33726 **Repair of pulmonary venous stenosis**
EXCLUDES *Temporary pacemaker (33210-33211)*
Tube thoracostomy (32551)
🔧 59.1 ⚕ 59.1 **FUD** 090   Ⓒ 80 ▣
AMA: 2018,Jan,8; 2017,Dec,3; 2017,Jan,8; 2016,Jan,13; 2015,Jan,16; 2014,Jan,11

33730 **Complete repair of anomalous pulmonary venous return (supracardiac, intracardiac, or infracardiac types)**
EXCLUDES *Partial anomalous pulmonary venous return (33724)*
Repair of pulmonary venous stenosis (33726)
🔧 58.2 ⚕ 58.2 **FUD** 090   ⑥③ Ⓒ 80 ▣
AMA: 2018,Jan,8; 2017,Dec,3; 2017,Jan,8; 2016,Jan,13; 2015,Jan,16; 2014,Jan,11

33732 **Repair of cor triatriatum or supravalvular mitral ring by resection of left atrial membrane**
🔧 47.8 ⚕ 47.8 **FUD** 090   ⑥③ Ⓒ 80 ▣
AMA: 2018,Jan,8; 2017,Dec,3; 2017,Jan,8; 2016,Jan,13; 2015,Jan,16; 2014,Jan,11

● New Code   ▲ Revised Code   ○ Reinstated   ● New Web Release   ▲ Revised Web Release   + Add-on   Unlisted   Not Covered   # Resequenced
㊿ Optum Mod 50 Exempt   ⊘ AMA Mod 51 Exempt   ⑤① Optum Mod 51 Exempt   ⑥③ Mod 63 Exempt   ⁄ Non-FDA Drug   ★ Telemedicine   Ⓜ Maternity   Ⓐ Age Edit

33735-33737 Creation of Atrial Septal Defect

Code also the concurrent ligation/takedown of a systemic-to-pulmonary artery shunt (33924)

33735 **Atrial septectomy or septostomy; closed heart (Blalock-Hanlon type operation)**
Facility RVU 37.5   Non-Facility RVU 37.5   **FUD** 090   63 C 80
AMA: 2018,Jan,8; 2017,Jan,8; 2016,Jan,13; 2015,Jan,16; 2014,Jan,11

33736 **open heart with cardiopulmonary bypass**
Facility RVU 39.6   Non-Facility RVU 39.6   **FUD** 090   63 C 80
AMA: 2017,Dec,3

33737 **open heart, with inflow occlusion**
EXCLUDES   Atrial septectomy/septostomy:
Blade method (92993)
Transvenous balloon method (92992)
Facility RVU 37.6   Non-Facility RVU 37.6   C 80
AMA: 2007,Mar,1-3; 1997,Nov,1

33750-33767 Systemic Vessel to Pulmonary Artery Shunts

Code also the concurrent ligation/takedown of a systemic-to-pulmonary artery shunt (33924)

33750 **Shunt; subclavian to pulmonary artery (Blalock-Taussig type operation)**
Facility RVU 36.6   Non-Facility RVU 36.6   **FUD** 090   63 C 80
AMA: 2017,Dec,3

33755 **ascending aorta to pulmonary artery (Waterston type operation)**
Facility RVU 38.1   Non-Facility RVU 38.1   **FUD** 090   63 C 80
AMA: 2017,Dec,3

33762 **descending aorta to pulmonary artery (Potts-Smith type operation)**
Facility RVU 37.2   Non-Facility RVU 37.2   **FUD** 090   63 C 80
AMA: 2017,Dec,3

33764 **central, with prosthetic graft**
Facility RVU 38.1   Non-Facility RVU 38.1   **FUD** 090   C 80
AMA: 2017,Dec,3

33766 **superior vena cava to pulmonary artery for flow to 1 lung (classical Glenn procedure)**
Facility RVU 38.6   Non-Facility RVU 38.6   **FUD** 090   C 80
AMA: 2017,Dec,3

33767 **superior vena cava to pulmonary artery for flow to both lungs (bidirectional Glenn procedure)**
Facility RVU 41.3   Non-Facility RVU 41.3   **FUD** 090   C 80
AMA: 2018,Jan,8; 2017,Dec,3; 2017,Jan,8; 2016,Jul,3

33768 Cavopulmonary Anastomosis to Decrease Volume Load

EXCLUDES   Temporary pacemaker (33210-33211)
Tube thoracostomy (32551)
Code first (33478, 33617, 33622, 33767)

+ **33768** **Anastomosis, cavopulmonary, second superior vena cava (List separately in addition to primary procedure)**
Facility RVU 12.1   Non-Facility RVU 12.1   **FUD** ZZZ   C 80
AMA: 2018,Jan,8; 2017,Jan,8; 2016,Jul,3; 2016,Jan,13; 2015,Jan,16; 2014,Jan,11

33770-33783 Repair Aberrant Anatomy: Transposition Great Vessels

Code also the concurrent ligation/takedown of a systemic-to-pulmonary artery shunt (33924)

33770 **Repair of transposition of the great arteries with ventricular septal defect and subpulmonary stenosis; without surgical enlargement of ventricular septal defect**
Facility RVU 61.5   Non-Facility RVU 61.5   **FUD** 090   C 80
AMA: 2018,Jan,8; 2017,Dec,3; 2017,Jan,8; 2016,Jan,13; 2015,Jan,16; 2014,Jan,11

33771 **with surgical enlargement of ventricular septal defect**
Facility RVU 63.3   Non-Facility RVU 63.3   **FUD** 090   C 80
AMA: 2017,Dec,3

33774 **Repair of transposition of the great arteries, atrial baffle procedure (eg, Mustard or Senning type) with cardiopulmonary bypass;**
Facility RVU 52.2   Non-Facility RVU 52.2   **FUD** 090   C 80
AMA: 2017,Dec,3

33775 **with removal of pulmonary band**
Facility RVU 53.8   Non-Facility RVU 53.8   **FUD** 090   C 80
AMA: 2017,Dec,3

33776 **with closure of ventricular septal defect**
Facility RVU 56.9   Non-Facility RVU 56.9   **FUD** 090   C 80
AMA: 2017,Dec,3

33777 **with repair of subpulmonic obstruction**
Facility RVU 54.9   Non-Facility RVU 54.9   **FUD** 090   C 80
AMA: 2017,Dec,3

33778 **Repair of transposition of the great arteries, aortic pulmonary artery reconstruction (eg, Jatene type);**
Facility RVU 68.3   Non-Facility RVU 68.3   **FUD** 090   63 C 80
AMA: 2017,Dec,3

33779 **with removal of pulmonary band**
Facility RVU 67.6   Non-Facility RVU 67.6   **FUD** 090   C 80
AMA: 2017,Dec,3

33780 **with closure of ventricular septal defect**
Facility RVU 68.9   Non-Facility RVU 68.9   **FUD** 090   C 80
AMA: 2017,Dec,3

33781 **with repair of subpulmonic obstruction**
Facility RVU 67.3   Non-Facility RVU 67.3   **FUD** 090   C 80
AMA: 2018,Jan,8; 2017,Dec,3; 2017,Jan,8; 2016,Jan,13; 2015,Jan,16; 2014,Jan,11

33782 **Aortic root translocation with ventricular septal defect and pulmonary stenosis repair (ie, Nikaidoh procedure); without coronary ostium reimplantation**
EXCLUDES   Closure of single ventricular septal defect (33681)
Repair of complex cardiac anomaly other than pulmonary atresia (33608)
Repair of pulmonary atresia with ventricular septal defect (33920)
Repair of transposition of the great arteries (33770-33771, 33778, 33780)
Replacement, aortic valve (33412-33413)
Facility RVU 94.0   Non-Facility RVU 94.0   **FUD** 090   C 80
AMA: 2017,Dec,3

33783 **with reimplantation of 1 or both coronary ostia**
Facility RVU 101.   Non-Facility RVU 101.   **FUD** 090   C 80
AMA: 2017,Dec,3

33786-33788 Repair Aberrant Anatomy: Truncus Arteriosus

33786 **Total repair, truncus arteriosus (Rastelli type operation)**
Code also the concurrent ligation/takedown of a systemic-to-pulmonary artery shunt (33924)
Facility RVU 66.2   Non-Facility RVU 66.2   **FUD** 090   63 C 80
AMA: 2018,Jan,8; 2017,Dec,3; 2017,Jan,8; 2016,Jan,13; 2015,Jan,16; 2014,Jan,11

33788 **Reimplantation of an anomalous pulmonary artery**
EXCLUDES   Pulmonary artery banding (33690)
Facility RVU 44.5   Non-Facility RVU 44.5   **FUD** 090   C 80
AMA: 2018,Jan,8; 2017,Dec,3; 2017,Jan,8; 2016,Jan,13; 2015,Jan,16; 2014,Jan,11

33800-33853 Repair Aberrant Anatomy: Aorta

33800 **Aortic suspension (aortopexy) for tracheal decompression (eg, for tracheomalacia) (separate procedure)**
Facility RVU 28.6   Non-Facility RVU 28.6   **FUD** 090   C 80
AMA: 2018,Jan,8; 2017,Jan,8; 2016,Jan,13; 2015,Jan,16; 2014,Jan,11

33802 **Division of aberrant vessel (vascular ring);**
Facility RVU 31.4   Non-Facility RVU 31.4   **FUD** 090   C 80
AMA: 2017,Dec,3

26/TC PC/TC Only   A2-Z3 ASC Payment   50 Bilateral   ♂ Male Only   ♀ Female Only   Facility RVU   Non-Facility RVU   CCI   CLIA
FUD Follow-up Days   CMS: IOM   AMA: CPT Asst   A-Y OPPSI   80/80 Surg Assist Allowed / w/Doc   Lab Crosswalk   Radiology Crosswalk

142   CPT © 2019 American Medical Association. All Rights Reserved.   © 2019 Optum360, LLC

33803 with reanastomosis

🔲 33.4　🔲 33.4　**FUD** 090　　　C 80 🔲

AMA: 2017,Dec,3

33813 Obliteration of aortopulmonary septal defect; without cardiopulmonary bypass

🔲 35.9　🔲 35.9　**FUD** 090　　　C 80 🔲

AMA: 2007,Mar,1-3; 1997,Nov,1

33814 with cardiopulmonary bypass

🔲 44.1　🔲 44.1　**FUD** 090　　　C 80 🔲

AMA: 2017,Dec,3

33820 Repair of patent ductus arteriosus; by ligation

EXCLUDES *Percutaneous transcatheter closure patent ductus arteriosus (93582)*

🔲 27.7　🔲 27.7　**FUD** 090　　　C 80 🔲

AMA: 2018,Jan,8; 2017,Dec,3; 2017,Jan,8; 2016,Jan,13; 2015,Jan,16; 2014,Jan,11

33822 by division, younger than 18 years　　　　　A

EXCLUDES *Percutaneous transcatheter closure patent ductus arteriosus (93582)*

🔲 29.6　🔲 29.6　**FUD** 090　　　C 80 🔲

AMA: 2018,Jan,8; 2017,Dec,3; 2017,Jan,8; 2016,Jul,3; 2016,Jan,13; 2015,Jan,16; 2014,Jan,11

33824 by division, 18 years and older

EXCLUDES *Percutaneous closure patent ductus arteriosus (93582)*

🔲 34.2　🔲 34.2　**FUD** 090　　　C 80 🔲

AMA: 2017,Dec,3

33840 Excision of coarctation of aorta, with or without associated patent ductus arteriosus; with direct anastomosis

🔲 35.9　🔲 35.9　**FUD** 090　　　C 80 🔲

AMA: 2018,Jan,8; 2017,Dec,3; 2017,Jan,8; 2016,Jul,3

33845 with graft

🔲 37.9　🔲 37.9　**FUD** 090　　　C 80 🔲

AMA: 2018,Jan,8; 2017,Dec,3; 2017,Jan,8; 2016,Jul,3

33851 repair using either left subclavian artery or prosthetic material as gusset for enlargement

🔲 36.9　🔲 36.9　**FUD** 090　　　C 80 🔲

AMA: 2018,Jan,8; 2017,Dec,3; 2017,Jan,8; 2016,Jul,3

33852 Repair of hypoplastic or interrupted aortic arch using autogenous or prosthetic material; without cardiopulmonary bypass

EXCLUDES *Hypoplastic left heart syndrome repair by excision of coarctation of aorta (33619)*

🔲 40.5　🔲 40.5　**FUD** 090　　　C 80 🔲

AMA: 2007,Mar,1-3; 1997,Nov,1

33853 with cardiopulmonary bypass

EXCLUDES *Hypoplastic left heart syndrome repair by excision of coarctation of aorta (33619)*

🔲 53.2　🔲 53.2　**FUD** 090　　　C 80 🔲

AMA: 2018,Jan,8; 2017,Dec,3; 2017,Jan,8; 2016,Jul,3; 2016,Jan,13; 2015,Jan,16; 2014,Jan,11

33858-33877 Aortic Graft Procedures

● **33858** Ascending aorta graft, with cardiopulmonary bypass, includes valve suspension, when performed; for aortic dissection

INCLUDES Treatment for aortic dissection

EXCLUDES *Ascending aorta graft:*
For treatment of other aortic disease(s), such as aneurysm (33859)
With remodeling of aortic root (33864)
With replacement of aortic root (33863)

● **33859** for aortic disease other than dissection (eg, aneurysm)

INCLUDES Treatment of aortic disease(s) other than dissection, such as aneurysm

EXCLUDES *Ascending aorta graft:*
For treatment of aortic dissection (33858)
With remodeling of aortic root (33864)
With replacement of aortic root (33863)

33860 ~~Ascending aorta graft, with cardiopulmonary bypass, includes valve suspension, when performed~~

To report, see (33858-33859)

33863 Ascending aorta graft, with cardiopulmonary bypass, with aortic root replacement using valved conduit and coronary reconstruction (eg, Bentall)

EXCLUDES *Ascending aorta graft:*
With remodeling of aortic root (33864)
Without aortic root replacement or remodeling (33858-33859)
Replacement, aortic valve, with cardiopulmonary bypass (33405-33406, 33410-33413)

🔲 91.3　🔲 91.3　**FUD** 090　　　C 80 🔲

AMA: 2018,Jan,8; 2017,Dec,3; 2017,Jan,8; 2016,Jan,13; 2015,Jan,16; 2014,Jan,11

33864 Ascending aorta graft, with cardiopulmonary bypass with valve suspension, with coronary reconstruction and valve-sparing aortic root remodeling (eg, David Procedure, Yacoub Procedure)

EXCLUDES *Ascending aorta graft:*
With replacement of aortic root (33863)
Without aortic root replacement or remodeling (33858-33859)

🔲 93.6　🔲 93.6　**FUD** 090　　　C 80 🔲

AMA: 2018,Jan,8; 2017,Dec,3; 2017,Jan,8; 2016,Jan,13; 2015,Jan,16; 2014,Jan,11

+ **33866** Aortic hemiarch graft including isolation and control of the arch vessels, beveled open distal aortic anastomosis extending under one or more of the arch vessels, and total circulatory arrest or isolated cerebral perfusion (List separately in addition to code for primary procedure)

🔲 29.8　🔲 29.8　**FUD** ZZZ　　　M 80 🔲

INCLUDES Procedure includes:
Extension of ascending aortic graft under arch by creation of beveled anastomosis to distal ascending aorta and aortic arch without crossclamp (open anastomosis)
Incision into the transverse arch that extends under one or more arch vessels (e.g., left common carotid, left subclavian, innominate artery)
Total circulatory arrest or isolated cerebral perfusion (antegrade or retrograde)

EXCLUDES *Complete transverse arch graft (33871)*

Code first (33858-33859, 33863-33864)

33870 ~~Transverse arch graft, with cardiopulmonary bypass~~

To report, see (33871)

● **33871** Transverse aortic arch graft, with cardiopulmonary bypass, with profound hypothermia, total circulatory arrest and isolated cerebral perfusion with reimplantation of arch vessel(s) (eg, island pedicle or individual arch vessel reimplantation)

EXCLUDES *Ascending aortic graft (33858-33859, 33863-33864)*
Hemiarch aortic graft performed in addition to ascending aorta graft (33866)

● New Code　▲ Revised Code　○ Reinstated　● New Web Release　▲ Revised Web Release　+ Add-on　Unlisted　Not Covered　# Resequenced

㊿ Optum Mod 50 Exempt　⊘ AMA Mod 51 Exempt　�51 Optum Mod 51 Exempt　63 Mod 63 Exempt　✒ Non-FDA Drug　★ Telemedicine　M Maternity　A Age Edit

© 2019 Optum360, LLC　　　CPT © 2019 American Medical Association. All Rights Reserved.　　　143

Cardiovascular, Hemic, and Lymphatic

33875 — 33915

33875   **Descending thoracic aorta graft, with or without bypass**
🔧 79.7   🔩 79.7   **FUD** 090   C 80 🖵
AMA: 2017,Dec,3

33877   **Repair of thoracoabdominal aortic aneurysm with graft, with or without cardiopulmonary bypass**
🔧 105.   🔩 105.   **FUD** 090   C 80 🖵
AMA: 2017,Dec,3

33880-33891 Endovascular Repair Aortic Aneurysm: Thoracic

INCLUDES   Balloon angioplasty
Deployment of stent
Introduction, manipulation, placement, and deployment of the device
EXCLUDES   *Additional interventional procedures provided during the endovascular repair*
Carotid-carotid bypass (33891)
Guidewire and catheter insertion (36140, 36200-36218)
Open exposure of artery/subsequent closure ([34812], 34714-34716 [34820, 34833, 34834])
Subclavian to carotid artery transposition (33889)
Substantial artery replacement (35226, 35286)

33880   **Endovascular repair of descending thoracic aorta (eg, aneurysm, pseudoaneurysm, dissection, penetrating ulcer, intramural hematoma, or traumatic disruption); involving coverage of left subclavian artery origin, initial endoprosthesis plus descending thoracic aortic extension(s), if required, to level of celiac artery origin**
    INCLUDES   Placement of distal extensions in distal thoracic aorta
    EXCLUDES   *Proximal extensions*
    🔀 (75956)
    🔧 52.0   🔩 52.0   **FUD** 090   C 80 🖵
    AMA: 2018,Jan,8; 2017,Dec,3; 2017,Jan,8; 2016,Jan,13; 2015,Jan,16; 2014,Jan,11

33881   **not involving coverage of left subclavian artery origin, initial endoprosthesis plus descending thoracic aortic extension(s), if required, to level of celiac artery origin**
    INCLUDES   Placement of distal extensions in distal thoracic aorta
    EXCLUDES   *Procedure where the placement of extension includes coverage of left subclavian artery origin (33880)*
    Proximal extensions
    🔀 (75957)
    🔧 44.6   🔩 44.6   **FUD** 090   C 80 🖵
    AMA: 2018,Jan,8; 2017,Dec,3; 2017,Jan,8; 2016,Jan,13; 2015,Jan,16; 2014,Jan,11

33883   **Placement of proximal extension prosthesis for endovascular repair of descending thoracic aorta (eg, aneurysm, pseudoaneurysm, dissection, penetrating ulcer, intramural hematoma, or traumatic disruption); initial extension**
    EXCLUDES   *Procedure where the placement of extension includes coverage of left subclavian artery origin (33880)*
    🔀 (75958)
    🔧 32.3   🔩 32.3   **FUD** 090   C 80 🖵
    AMA: 2018,Jan,8; 2017,Dec,3; 2017,Jan,8; 2016,Jan,13; 2015,Jan,16; 2014,Jan,11

+ 33884   **each additional proximal extension (List separately in addition to code for primary procedure)**
    Code first (33883)
    🔀 (75958)
    🔧 11.4   🔩 11.4   **FUD** ZZZ   C 80 🖵
    AMA: 2018,Jan,8; 2017,Dec,3; 2017,Jan,8; 2016,Jan,13; 2015,Jan,16; 2014,Jan,11

33886   **Placement of distal extension prosthesis(s) delayed after endovascular repair of descending thoracic aorta**
    INCLUDES   All modules deployed
    EXCLUDES   *Endovascular repair of descending thoracic aorta (33880, 33881)*
    🔀 (75959)
    🔧 27.7   🔩 27.7   **FUD** 090   C 80 🖵
    AMA: 2018,Jan,8; 2017,Dec,3; 2017,Jan,8; 2016,Jan,13; 2015,Jan,16; 2014,Jan,11

Repair of endoleak in descending thoracic aorta

33889   **Open subclavian to carotid artery transposition performed in conjunction with endovascular repair of descending thoracic aorta, by neck incision, unilateral**
    EXCLUDES   *Transposition and/or reimplantation; subclavian to carotid artery (35694)*
    🔧 22.8   🔩 22.8   **FUD** 000   C 80 50 🖵
    AMA: 2018,Jan,8; 2017,Jan,8; 2016,Jan,13; 2015,Jan,16; 2014,Jan,11

33891   **Bypass graft, with other than vein, transcervical retropharyngeal carotid-carotid, performed in conjunction with endovascular repair of descending thoracic aorta, by neck incision**
    EXCLUDES   *Bypass graft (35509, 35601)*
    🔧 27.9   🔩 27.9   **FUD** 000   C 80 50 🖵
    AMA: 2018,Jan,8; 2017,Jan,8; 2016,Jan,13; 2015,Jan,16; 2014,Jan,11

33910-33926 Surgical Procedures of Pulmonary Artery

33910   **Pulmonary artery embolectomy; with cardiopulmonary bypass**
    🔧 76.2   🔩 76.2   **FUD** 090   C 80 🖵
    AMA: 2018,Jan,8; 2017,Dec,3; 2017,Jan,8; 2016,Jan,13; 2015,Jan,16; 2014,Jan,11

33915   **without cardiopulmonary bypass**
    🔧 40.1   🔩 40.1   **FUD** 090   C 80 🖵
    AMA: 2018,Jan,8; 2017,Jan,8; 2016,Jan,13; 2015,Jan,16; 2014,Jan,11

26/TC PC/TC Only   A2-Z3 ASC Payment   50 Bilateral   ♂ Male Only   ♀ Female Only   🔧 Facility RVU   🔩 Non-Facility RVU   CCI   CLIA
FUD Follow-up Days   **CMS:** IOM   **AMA:** CPT Asst   A-Y OPPSI   80/80 Surg Assist Allowed / w/Doc   Lab Crosswalk   Radiology Crosswalk

144   CPT © 2019 American Medical Association. All Rights Reserved.   © 2019 Optum360, LLC

33916 Pulmonary endarterectomy, with or without embolectomy, with cardiopulmonary bypass

123. 123. **FUD** 090 C 80 ▢

AMA: 2018,Jan,8; 2017,Dec,3; 2017,Jan,8; 2016,Jan,13; 2015,Jan,16; 2014,Jan,11

33917 Repair of pulmonary artery stenosis by reconstruction with patch or graft

Code also the concurrent ligation/takedown of a systemic-to-pulmonary artery shunt (33924)

42.2 42.2 **FUD** 090 C 80 ▢

AMA: 2018,Jan,8; 2017,Dec,3; 2017,Jan,8; 2016,Jul,3; 2016,Jan,13; 2015,Jan,16; 2014,Jan,11

33920 Repair of pulmonary atresia with ventricular septal defect, by construction or replacement of conduit from right or left ventricle to pulmonary artery

EXCLUDES *Repair of complicated cardiac anomalies by creating/replacing conduit from ventricle to pulmonary artery (33608)*

Code also the concurrent ligation/takedown of a systemic-to-pulmonary artery shunt (33924)

52.6 52.6 **FUD** 090 C 80 ▢

AMA: 2019,Apr,6; 2018,Jan,8; 2017,Dec,3; 2017,Jan,8; 2016,Jan,13; 2015,Jan,16; 2014,Jan,11

33922 Transection of pulmonary artery with cardiopulmonary bypass

Code also the concurrent ligation/takedown of a systemic-to-pulmonary artery shunt (33924)

40.2 40.2 **FUD** 090 63 C 80 ▢

AMA: 2017,Dec,3

+ **33924** Ligation and takedown of a systemic-to-pulmonary artery shunt, performed in conjunction with a congenital heart procedure (List separately in addition to code for primary procedure)

Code first (33470-33478, 33600-33617, 33622, 33684-33688, 33692-33697, 33735-33767, 33770-33783, 33786, 33917, 33920-33922, 33925-33926, 33935, 33945)

8.31 8.31 **FUD** ZZZ C 80 ▢

AMA: 1997,Nov,1; 1995,Win,1

33925 Repair of pulmonary artery arborization anomalies by unifocalization; without cardiopulmonary bypass

49.9 49.9 **FUD** 090 C 80 ▢

Code also the concurrent ligation/takedown of a systemic-to-pulmonary artery shunt (33924)

33926 with cardiopulmonary bypass

Code also the concurrent ligation/takedown of a systemic-to-pulmonary artery shunt (33924)

70.3 70.3 **FUD** 090 C 80 ▢

AMA: 2017,Dec,3

33927-33945 Heart and Heart-Lung Transplants

INCLUDES Backbench work to prepare the donor heart and/or lungs for transplantation (33933, 33944)
Harvesting of donor organs with cold preservation (33930, 33940)
Transplantation of heart and/or lungs into recipient (33935, 33945)

33927 Implantation of a total replacement heart system (artificial heart) with recipient cardiectomy

EXCLUDES *Implantation ventricular assist device:*
Extracorporeal (33975-33976)
Intracorporeal (33979)
Percutaneous (33990-33991)

74.2 74.2 **FUD** XXX C 80 ▢

AMA: 2018,Jun,3

33928 Removal and replacement of total replacement heart system (artificial heart)

EXCLUDES *Replacement or revision elements of artificial heart (33999)*

0.00 0.00 **FUD** XXX C 80 ▢

AMA: 2018,Jun,3

+ **33929** Removal of a total replacement heart system (artificial heart) for heart transplantation (List separately in addition to code for primary procedure)

Code first (33945)

0.00 0.00 **FUD** ZZZ C 80 ▢

AMA: 2018,Jun,3

33930 Donor cardiectomy-pneumonectomy (including cold preservation)

0.00 0.00 **FUD** XXX C ▢

AMA: 1997,Nov,1

33933 Backbench standard preparation of cadaver donor heart/lung allograft prior to transplantation, including dissection of allograft from surrounding soft tissues to prepare aorta, superior vena cava, inferior vena cava, and trachea for implantation

0.00 0.00 **FUD** XXX C 80 ▢

AMA: 1997,Nov,1

33935 Heart-lung transplant with recipient cardiectomy-pneumonectomy

Code also the concurrent ligation/takedown of a systemic-to-pulmonary artery shunt (33924)

143. 143. **FUD** 090 C 80 ▢

AMA: 2017,Dec,3

33940 Donor cardiectomy (including cold preservation)

0.00 0.00 **FUD** XXX C ▢

AMA: 2018,Jan,8; 2017,Jan,8; 2016,Jan,13; 2015,Jan,16; 2014,Jan,11

33944 Backbench standard preparation of cadaver donor heart allograft prior to transplantation, including dissection of allograft from surrounding soft tissues to prepare aorta, superior vena cava, inferior vena cava, pulmonary artery, and left atrium for implantation

EXCLUDES *Procedures performed on donor heart (33300, 33310, 33320, 33390, 33463-33464, 33510, 33641, 35216, 35276, 35685)*

0.00 0.00 **FUD** XXX C 80 ▢

AMA: 1997,Nov,1

33945 Heart transplant, with or without recipient cardiectomy

Code also the concurrent ligation/takedown of a systemic-to-pulmonary artery shunt (33924)

141. 141. **FUD** 090 C 80 ▢

AMA: 2018,Jun,3; 2017,Dec,3

33946-33989 [33962, 33963, 33964, 33965, 33966, 33969, 33984, 33985, 33986, 33987, 33988, 33989] Extracorporeal Circulatory and Respiratory Support

INCLUDES Cannula repositioning and cannula insertion performed during same procedure
Multiple physician and nonphysician team collaboration
Veno-arterial ECMO/ECLS for heart and lung support
Veno-venous ECMO/ECLS for lung support

Code also extensive arterial repair/replacement (35266, 35286, 35371, 35665)
Code also overall daily management services needed to manage a patient; report the appropriate observation, hospital inpatient, or critical care E/M codes

33946 Extracorporeal membrane oxygenation (ECMO)/extracorporeal life support (ECLS) provided by physician; initiation, veno-venous

EXCLUDES *Daily ECMO/ECLS veno-venous management on day of initial service (33948)*
Repositioning of ECMO/ECLS cannula on day of initial service (33957-33959 [33962, 33963, 33964])

Code also cannula insertion (33951-33956)

8.99 8.99 **FUD** XXX 63 C ▢

AMA: 2018,Jan,8; 2017,Jan,8; 2016,Mar,5; 2016,Jan,13; 2015,Jul,3

33947 **initiation, veno-arterial**

> EXCLUDES   *Daily ECMO/ECLS veno-arterial management on day of initial service (33949)*
>
> *Repositioning of ECMO/ECLS cannula on day of initial service (33957-33959 [33962, 33963, 33964])*
>
> Code also cannula insertion (33951-33956)
>
> 🚑 9.97   ⚕ 9.97   **FUD** XXX   63 C 🖵
>
> **AMA:** 2018,Jan,8; 2017,Jan,8; 2016,Mar,5; 2016,Jan,13; 2015,Jul,3

33948 **daily management, each day, veno-venous**

> EXCLUDES   *ECMO/ECLS initiation, veno-venous (33946)*
>
> 🚑 6.91   ⚕ 6.91   **FUD** XXX   63 C 🖵
>
> **AMA:** 2018,Jan,8; 2017,Jan,8; 2016,Mar,5; 2016,Jan,13; 2015,Jul,3

33949 **daily management, each day, veno-arterial**

> EXCLUDES   *ECMO/ECLS initiation, veno-arterial (33947)*
>
> 🚑 6.72   ⚕ 6.72   **FUD** XXX   63 C 🖵
>
> **AMA:** 2018,Jan,8; 2017,Jan,8; 2016,Mar,5; 2016,Jan,13; 2015,Jul,3

33951 **insertion of peripheral (arterial and/or venous) cannula(e), percutaneous, birth through 5 years of age (includes fluoroscopic guidance, when performed)** A

> INCLUDES   Cannula replacement in same vessel
>
> Cannula repositioning during same episode of care
>
> Code also cannula removal if new cannula inserted in different vessel with ([33965, 33966, 33969, 33984, 33985, 33986])
>
> Code also ECMO/ECLS initiation or daily management (33946-33947, 33948-33949)
>
> 🚑 12.3   ⚕ 12.3   **FUD** 000   C 80 🖵
>
> **AMA:** 2018,Jan,8; 2017,Jan,8; 2016,Mar,5; 2016,Jan,13; 2015,Jul,3

33952 **insertion of peripheral (arterial and/or venous) cannula(e), percutaneous, 6 years and older (includes fluoroscopic guidance, when performed)** A

> INCLUDES   Cannula replacement in same vessel
>
> Cannula repositioning during same episode of care
>
> Code also cannula removal if new cannula inserted in different vessel with ([33965, 33966, 33969, 33984, 33985, 33986])
>
> Code also ECMO/ECLS initiation or daily management (33946-33947, 33948-33949)
>
> 🚑 12.4   ⚕ 12.4   **FUD** 000   C 80 🖵
>
> **AMA:** 2018,Jan,8; 2017,Jan,8; 2016,Mar,5; 2016,Jan,13; 2015,Jul,3

33953 **insertion of peripheral (arterial and/or venous) cannula(e), open, birth through 5 years of age** A

> INCLUDES   Cannula replacement in same vessel
>
> Cannula repositioning during same episode of care
>
> EXCLUDES   *Open artery exposure for delivery/deployment of endovascular prosthesis ([34812], 34714-34716 [34820, 34833, 34834], [34820])*
>
> Code also cannula removal if new cannula inserted in different vessel with ([33965, 33966, 33969, 33984, 33985, 33986])
>
> Code also ECMO/ECLS initiation or daily management (33496-33947, 33948-33949)
>
> 🚑 13.8   ⚕ 13.8   **FUD** 000   C 80 🖵
>
> **AMA:** 2018,Jan,8; 2017,Dec,3; 2017,Jan,8; 2016,Mar,5; 2016,Jan,13; 2015,Jul,3

33954 **insertion of peripheral (arterial and/or venous) cannula(e), open, 6 years and older** A

> INCLUDES   Cannula replacement in same vessel
>
> Cannula repositioning during same episode of care
>
> EXCLUDES   *Open artery exposure for delivery/deployment of endovascular prosthesis ([34812], 34714-34716 [34820, 34833, 34834])*
>
> Code also cannula removal if new cannula inserted in different vessel with ([33965, 33966, 33969, 33984, 33985, 33986])
>
> Code also ECMO/ECLS initiation or daily management (33946-33947, 33948-33949)
>
> 🚑 13.8   ⚕ 13.8   **FUD** 000   C 80 🖵
>
> **AMA:** 2018,Jan,8; 2017,Dec,3; 2017,Jan,8; 2016,Mar,5; 2016,Jan,13; 2015,Jul,3

33955 **insertion of central cannula(e) by sternotomy or thoracotomy, birth through 5 years of age** A

> INCLUDES   Cannula replacement in same vessel
>
> Cannula repositioning during same episode of care
>
> EXCLUDES   *Mediastinotomy (39010)*
>
> *Thoracotomy (32100)*
>
> Code also cannula removal if new cannula inserted in different vessel with ([33965, 33966, 33969, 33984, 33985, 33986])
>
> Code also ECMO/ECLS initiation or daily management (33946-33947, 33948-33949)
>
> 🚑 24.2   ⚕ 24.2   **FUD** 000   C 80 🖵
>
> **AMA:** 2018,Jan,8; 2017,Jan,8; 2016,Mar,5; 2016,Jan,13; 2015,Jul,3

33956 **insertion of central cannula(e) by sternotomy or thoracotomy, 6 years and older**

> INCLUDES   Cannula replacement in same vessel
>
> Cannula repositioning during same episode of care
>
> EXCLUDES   *Mediastinotomy (39010)*
>
> *Thoracotomy (32100)*
>
> Code also cannula removal if new cannula inserted in different vessel with ([33965, 33966, 33969, 33984, 33985, 33986])
>
> Code also ECMO/ECLS initiation or daily management (33946-33947, 33948-33949)
>
> 🚑 24.2   ⚕ 24.2   **FUD** 000   C 80 🖵
>
> **AMA:** 2018,Jan,8; 2017,Jan,8; 2016,Mar,5; 2016,Jan,13; 2015,Jul,3

33957 **reposition peripheral (arterial and/or venous) cannula(e), percutaneous, birth through 5 years of age (includes fluoroscopic guidance, when performed)** A

> INCLUDES   Fluoroscopic guidance
>
> EXCLUDES   *ECMO/ECLS initiation, veno-arterial (33947)*
>
> *ECMO/ECLS initiation, veno-venous (33946)*
>
> *ECMO/ECLS insertion of cannula (33951-33956)*
>
> *Percutaneous access and closure femoral artery for endograft delivery (34713)*
>
> 🚑 5.38   ⚕ 5.38   **FUD** 000   C 80 🖵
>
> **AMA:** 2018,Jan,8; 2017,Jan,8; 2016,Mar,5; 2016,Jan,13; 2015,Jul,3

33958 **reposition peripheral (arterial and/or venous) cannula(e), percutaneous, 6 years and older (includes fluoroscopic guidance, when performed)** A

> INCLUDES   Fluoroscopic guidance
>
> EXCLUDES   *ECMO/ECLS initiation, veno-arterial (33947)*
>
> *ECMO/ECLS initiation, veno-venous (33946)*
>
> *ECMO/ECLS insertion of cannula (33951-33956)*
>
> *Percutaneous access and closure femoral artery for endograft delivery (34713)*
>
> 🚑 5.38   ⚕ 5.38   **FUD** 000   C 80 🖵
>
> **AMA:** 2018,Jan,8; 2017,Jan,8; 2016,Mar,5; 2016,Jan,13; 2015,Jul,3

33959 **reposition peripheral (arterial and/or venous) cannula(e), open, birth through 5 years of age (includes fluoroscopic guidance, when performed)** A

> INCLUDES   Fluoroscopic guidance
>
> EXCLUDES   *ECMO/ECLS initiation, veno-arterial (33947)*
>
> *ECMO/ECLS initiation, veno-venous (33946)*
>
> *ECMO/ECLS insertion of cannula (33951-33956)*
>
> *Open artery exposure for delivery/deployment of endovascular prosthesis ([34812], 34714-34716 [34820, 34833, 34834])*
>
> 🚑 6.84   ⚕ 6.84   **FUD** 000   C 80 🖵
>
> **AMA:** 2018,Jan,8; 2017,Dec,3; 2017,Jan,8; 2016,Mar,5; 2016,Jan,13; 2015,Jul,3

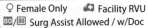

\# 33962 **reposition peripheral (arterial and/or venous) cannula(e), open, 6 years and older (includes fluoroscopic guidance, when performed)** A
- INCLUDES Fluoroscopic guidance
- EXCLUDES *ECMO/ECLS initiation, veno-arterial (33947)*
  ECMO/ECLS initiation, veno-venous (33946)
  ECMO/ECLS insertion of cannula (33951-33956)
  Open artery exposure for delivery/deployment of endovascular prosthesis ([34812], 34714-34716 [34820, 34833, 34834])
- 🚑 6.84 ⚕ 6.84 **FUD** 000 C 80 ▭
- **AMA:** 2018,Jan,8; 2017,Dec,3; 2017,Jan,8; 2016,Mar,5; 2016,Jan,13; 2015,Jul,3

\# 33963 **reposition of central cannula(e) by sternotomy or thoracotomy, birth through 5 years of age (includes fluoroscopic guidance, when performed)** A
- INCLUDES Fluoroscopic guidance
- EXCLUDES *ECMO/ECLS initiation, veno-arterial (33947)*
  ECMO/ECLS initiation, veno-venous (33946)
  ECMO/ECLS insertion of cannula (33951-33956)
  Open artery exposure for delivery/deployment of endovascular prosthesis ([34812], 34714-34716 [34820, 34833, 34834])
- 🚑 13.6 ⚕ 13.6 **FUD** 000 C 80 ▭
- **AMA:** 2018,Jan,8; 2017,Jan,8; 2016,Mar,5; 2016,Jan,13; 2015,Jul,3

\# 33964 **reposition central cannula(e) by sternotomy or thoracotomy, 6 years and older (includes fluoroscopic guidance, when performed)** A
- INCLUDES Fluoroscopic guidance
- EXCLUDES *ECMO/ECLS initiation, veno-arterial (33947)*
  ECMO/ECLS initiation, veno-venous (33946)
  ECMO/ECLS insertion of cannula (33951-33956)
  Mediastinotomy (39010)
  Thoracotomy (32100)
- 🚑 14.4 ⚕ 14.4 **FUD** 000 C 80 ▭
- **AMA:** 2018,Jan,8; 2017,Jan,8; 2016,Mar,5; 2016,Jan,13; 2015,Jul,3

\# 33965 **removal of peripheral (arterial and/or venous) cannula(e), percutaneous, birth through 5 years of age** A
- Code also extensive arterial repair/replacement, when performed (35266, 35286, 35371, 35665)
- Code also new cannula insertion into different vessel (33951-33956)
- 🚑 5.38 ⚕ 5.38 **FUD** 000 C 80 ▭
- **AMA:** 2018,Jan,8; 2017,Jan,8; 2016,Mar,5; 2016,Jan,13; 2015,Jul,3

\# 33966 **removal of peripheral (arterial and/or venous) cannula(e), percutaneous, 6 years and older** A
- Code also extensive arterial repair/replacement, when performed (35266, 35286, 35371, 35665)
- Code also new cannula insertion into different vessel (33951, 33956)
- 🚑 6.91 ⚕ 6.91 **FUD** 000 C 80 ▭
- **AMA:** 2018,Jan,8; 2017,Jan,8; 2016,Mar,5; 2016,Jan,13; 2015,Jul,3

\# 33969 **removal of peripheral (arterial and/or venous) cannula(e), open, birth through 5 years of age** A
- EXCLUDES *Open artery exposure for delivery/deployment of endovascular prosthesis ([34812], 34714-34716 [34820, 34833, 34834])*
  Repair blood vessel (35201, 35206, 35211, 35216, 35226)
- Code also extensive arterial repair/replacement, when performed (35266, 35286, 35371, 35665)
- Code also new cannula insertion into different vessel (33951-33956)
- 🚑 7.98 ⚕ 7.98 **FUD** 000 C 80 ▭
- **AMA:** 2018,Jan,8; 2017,Dec,3; 2017,Jan,8; 2016,Mar,5; 2016,Jan,13; 2015,Jul,3

\# 33984 **removal of peripheral (arterial and/or venous) cannula(e), open, 6 years and older** A
- EXCLUDES *Open artery exposure for delivery/deployment of endovascular prosthesis ([34812], 34714-34716 [34820, 34833, 34834])*
  Repair blood vessel (35201, 35206, 35211, 35216, 35226)
- 🚑 8.25 ⚕ 8.25 **FUD** 000 C 80 ▭
- **AMA:** 2018,Jan,8; 2017,Dec,3; 2017,Jan,8; 2016,Mar,5; 2016,Jan,13; 2015,Jul,3

\# 33985 **removal of central cannula(e) by sternotomy or thoracotomy, birth through 5 years of age** A
- EXCLUDES *Repair blood vessel (35201, 35206, 35211, 35216, 35226)*
- Code also extensive arterial repair/replacement, when performed (35266, 35286, 35371, 35665)
- Code also new cannula insertion into different vessel (33951-33956)
- 🚑 15.0 ⚕ 15.0 **FUD** 000 C 80 ▭
- **AMA:** 2018,Jan,8; 2017,Jan,8; 2016,Mar,5; 2016,Jan,13; 2015,Jul,3

\# 33986 **removal of central cannula(e) by sternotomy or thoracotomy, 6 years and older** A
- EXCLUDES *Repair blood vessel (35201, 35206, 35211, 35216, 35226)*
- Code also extensive arterial repair/replacement, when performed (35266, 35286, 35371, 35665)
- Code also new cannula insertion into different vessel (33951-33956)
- 🚑 15.1 ⚕ 15.1 **FUD** 000 C 80 ▭
- **AMA:** 2018,Jan,8; 2017,Jan,8; 2016,Mar,5; 2016,Jan,13; 2015,Jul,3

+ \# 33987 **Arterial exposure with creation of graft conduit (eg, chimney graft) to facilitate arterial perfusion for ECMO/ECLS (List separately in addition to code for primary procedure)**
- EXCLUDES *Open artery exposure for delivery/deployment of endovascular prosthesis ([34812], 34714-34716 [34820, 34833, 34834])*
- Code first (33953-33956)
- 🚑 6.09 ⚕ 6.09 **FUD** ZZZ C 80 ▭
- **AMA:** 2018,Jan,8; 2017,Dec,3; 2017,Jan,8; 2016,Mar,5; 2016,Jan,13; 2015,Jul,3

\# 33988 **Insertion of left heart vent by thoracic incision (eg, sternotomy, thoracotomy) for ECMO/ECLS**
- 🚑 22.7 ⚕ 22.7 **FUD** 000 C 80 ▭
- **AMA:** 2018,Jan,8; 2017,Jan,8; 2016,Mar,5; 2016,Jan,13; 2015,Jul,3

\# 33989 **Removal of left heart vent by thoracic incision (eg, sternotomy, thoracotomy) for ECMO/ECLS**
- 🚑 14.4 ⚕ 14.4 **FUD** 000 C 80 ▭
- **AMA:** 2018,Jan,8; 2017,Jan,8; 2016,Mar,5; 2016,Jan,13; 2015,Jul,3

33962-33999 Mechanical Circulatory Support

33962 **Resequenced code. See code following 33959.**

33963 **Resequenced code. See code following 33959.**

33964 **Resequenced code. See code following 33959.**

33965 **Resequenced code. See code following 33959.**

33966 **Resequenced code. See code following 33959.**

33967 **Insertion of intra-aortic balloon assist device, percutaneous**
- 🚑 7.56 ⚕ 7.56 **FUD** 000 C 80
- **AMA:** 2018,Jan,8; 2017,Jan,8; 2016,Mar,5; 2016,Jan,13; 2015,Sep,3; 2015,Jul,3; 2015,Jan,16; 2014,Jan,11 ▭

33968 **Removal of intra-aortic balloon assist device, percutaneous**
- EXCLUDES *Removal of implantable aortic counterpulsation ventricular assist system (0455T-0458T)*
- 🚑 0.98 ⚕ 0.98 **FUD** 000 C
- **AMA:** 2018,Jan,8; 2017,Jan,8; 2016,Mar,5; 2016,Jan,13; 2015,Jul,3; 2015,Jan,16; 2014,Jan,11 ▭

33969 **Resequenced code. See code following 33959.**

33970   **Insertion of intra-aortic balloon assist device through the femoral artery, open approach**

> EXCLUDES   *Insertion/replacement implantable aortic counterpulsation ventricular assist system (0451T-0454T)*
>
> *Percutaneous insertion of intra-aortic balloon assist device (33967)*

📇 10.2   ⚗ 10.2   **FUD** 000   C 80 ▣

AMA: 2018,Jan,8; 2017,Jan,8; 2016,Mar,5; 2016,Jan,13; 2015,Sep,3; 2015,Jul,3; 2015,Jan,16; 2014,Jan,11

33971   **Removal of intra-aortic balloon assist device including repair of femoral artery, with or without graft**

> EXCLUDES   *Removal of implantable aortic counterpulsation ventricular assist system (0455T-0458T)*

📇 20.5   ⚗ 20.5   **FUD** 090   C ▣

AMA: 2018,Jan,8; 2017,Jan,8; 2016,Mar,5; 2016,Jan,13; 2015,Jul,3; 2015,Jan,16; 2014,Jan,11

33973   **Insertion of intra-aortic balloon assist device through the ascending aorta**

> EXCLUDES   *Insertion/replacement of implantable aortic counterpulsation ventricular assist system (0451T-0454T)*

📇 15.0   ⚗ 15.0   **FUD** 000   C 80 ▣

AMA: 2018,Jan,8; 2017,Jan,8; 2016,Mar,5; 2016,Jan,13; 2015,Sep,3; 2015,Jul,3; 2015,Jan,16; 2014,Jan,11

33974   **Removal of intra-aortic balloon assist device from the ascending aorta, including repair of the ascending aorta, with or without graft**

> EXCLUDES   *Removal of implantable aortic counterpulsation ventricular assist system (0455T-0458T)*

📇 25.8   ⚗ 25.8   **FUD** 090   C ▣

AMA: 2018,Jan,8; 2017,Jan,8; 2016,Mar,5; 2016,Jan,13; 2015,Jul,3; 2015,Jan,16; 2014,Jan,11

33975   **Insertion of ventricular assist device; extracorporeal, single ventricle**

> INCLUDES   Insertion of the new pump with de-airing, connection, and initiation
>
> Removal of the old pump with replacement of the entire ventricular assist device system, including pump(s) and cannulas
>
> Transthoracic approach
>
> EXCLUDES   *Percutaneous approach (33990-33991)*

Code also removal of thrombus through a separate heart incision, when performed (33310-33315); append modifier 59 to (33315)

📇 37.9   ⚗ 37.9   **FUD** XXX   C 80 ▣

AMA: 2018,Jun,3; 2018,Jan,8; 2017,Dec,3; 2017,Jan,8; 2016,Mar,5; 2016,Jan,13; 2015,Jul,3; 2015,Jan,16; 2014,Jan,11

33976   **extracorporeal, biventricular**

> INCLUDES   Insertion of the new pump with de-airing, connection, and initiation
>
> Removal with replacement of the entire ventricular assist device system, including purnp(s) and cannulas
>
> Transthoracic approach
>
> EXCLUDES   *Percutaneous approach (33990-33991)*

Code also removal of thrombus through a separate heart incision, when performed (33310-33315); append modifier 59 to (33315)

📇 46.4   ⚗ 46.4   **FUD** XXX   C 80 ▣

AMA: 2018,Jun,3; 2018,Jan,8; 2017,Dec,3; 2017,Jan,8; 2016,Mar,5; 2016,Jan,13; 2015,Jul,3; 2015,Jan,16; 2014,Jan,11

33977   **Removal of ventricular assist device; extracorporeal, single ventricle**

> INCLUDES   Removal of the entire device and the cannulas
>
> EXCLUDES   *Removal of ventricular assist device when performed at the same time of insertion of a new device*

Code also removal of thrombus through a separate heart incision, when performed (33310-33315); append modifier 59 to (33315)

📇 32.6   ⚗ 32.6   **FUD** XXX   C 80 ▣

AMA: 2018,Jan,8; 2017,Dec,3; 2017,Jan,8; 2016,Mar,5; 2016,Jan,13; 2015,Jul,3; 2015,Jan,16; 2014,Jan,11

33978   **extracorporeal, biventricular**

> INCLUDES   Removal of the entire device and the cannulas
>
> EXCLUDES   *Removal of ventricular assist device when performed at the same time of insertion of a new device*

Code also removal of thrombus through a separate heart incision, when performed (33310-33315); append modifier 59 to (33315)

📇 38.8   ⚗ 38.8   **FUD** XXX   C 80 ▣

AMA: 2018,Jan,8; 2017,Dec,3; 2017,Jan,8; 2016,Mar,5; 2016,Jan,13; 2015,Jul,3; 2015,Jan,16; 2014,Jan,11

33979   **Insertion of ventricular assist device, implantable intracorporeal, single ventricle**

> INCLUDES   New pump insertion with connection, de-airing, and initiation
>
> Removal with replacement of the entire ventricular assist device system, including pump(s) and cannulas
>
> Transthoracic approach
>
> EXCLUDES   *Insertion/replacement of implantable aortic counterpulsation ventricular assist system (0451T-0454T)*
>
> *Percutaneous approach (33990-33991)*

Code also removal of thrombus through a separate heart incision, when performed (33310-33315); append modifier 59 to (33315)

📇 56.6   ⚗ 56.6   **FUD** XXX   C 80 ▣

AMA: 2018,Jun,3; 2018,Jan,8; 2017,Dec,3; 2017,Jan,8; 2016,Mar,5; 2016,Jan,13; 2015,Jul,3; 2015,Jan,16; 2014,Jan,11

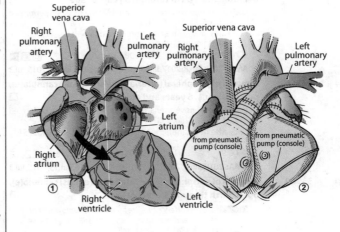

33980   **Removal of ventricular assist device, implantable intracorporeal, single ventricle**

> INCLUDES   Removal of the entire device and the cannulas
>
> EXCLUDES   *Removal of implantable aortic counterpulsation ventricular assist system (0455T-0458T)*
>
> *Removal of ventricular assist device when performed at the same time of insertion of a new device*

Code also removal of thrombus through a separate heart incision, when performed (33310-33315); append modifier 59 to (33315)

📇 51.8   ⚗ 51.8   **FUD** XXX   C 80 ▣

AMA: 2018,Jan,8; 2017,Dec,3; 2017,Jan,8; 2016,Mar,5; 2016,Jan,13; 2015,Jul,3; 2015,Jan,16; 2014,Jan,11

33981 **Replacement of extracorporeal ventricular assist device, single or biventricular, pump(s), single or each pump**

INCLUDES   Insertion of the new pump with de-airing, connection, and initiation
Removal of the old pump
🚑 24.3   ⚕ 24.3   **FUD** XXX   C 80 ▣
AMA: 2018,Jan,8; 2017,Jan,8; 2016,Mar,5; 2016,Jan,13; 2015,Jul,3; 2015,Jan,16; 2014,Jan,11

33982 **Replacement of ventricular assist device pump(s); implantable intracorporeal, single ventricle, without cardiopulmonary bypass**

INCLUDES   New pump insertion with connection, de-airing, and initiation
Removal of the old pump
🚑 57.1   ⚕ 57.1   **FUD** XXX   C 80 ▣
AMA: 2018,Jan,8; 2017,Jan,8; 2016,Mar,5; 2016,Jan,13; 2015,Jul,3; 2015,Jan,16; 2014,Jan,11

33983 **implantable intracorporeal, single ventricle, with cardiopulmonary bypass**

INCLUDES   Removal of the old pump
EXCLUDES   Insertion/replacement of implantable aortic counterpulsation ventricular assist system (0451T-0454T)
Percutaneous transseptal approach (33999)
🚑 67.1   ⚕ 67.1   **FUD** XXX   C 80 ▣
AMA: 2018,Jan,8; 2017,Dec,3; 2017,Jan,8; 2016,Mar,5; 2016,Jan,13; 2015,Jul,3; 2015,Jan,16; 2014,Jan,11

33984   Resequenced code. See code following 33959.

33985   Resequenced code. See code following 33959.

33986   Resequenced code. See code following 33959.

33987   Resequenced code. See code following 33959.

33988   Resequenced code. See code following 33959.

33989   Resequenced code. See code following 33959.

33990 **Insertion of ventricular assist device, percutaneous including radiological supervision and interpretation; arterial access only**

INCLUDES   Initial insertion and replacement of percutaneous ventricular assist device
EXCLUDES   Extensive artery repair/replacement (35226, 35286)
Insertion/replacement of implantable aortic counterpulsation ventricular assist system (0451T-0454T)
Open arterial approach to aid insertion of percutaneous ventricular assist device, when used ([34812], 34714-34716 [34820, 34833, 34834], [34820])
Removal of percutaneous ventricular assist device at time of replacement of the entire system (33992)
Transthoracic approach (33975-33976)
🚑 12.4   ⚕ 12.4   **FUD** XXX   C 80 ▣
AMA: 2018,Jun,3; 2018,Jan,8; 2017,Dec,3; 2017,Jan,8; 2016,Mar,5; 2016,Jan,13; 2015,Sep,3; 2015,Jan,16; 2014,Oct,14; 2014,Jan,11

33991 **both arterial and venous access, with transseptal puncture**

INCLUDES   Initial insertion as well as replacement of percutaneous ventricular assist device
EXCLUDES   Extensive artery repair/replacement (35226, 35286)
Insertion/replacement of implantable aortic counterpulsation ventricular assist system (0451T-0454T)
Open arterial approach to aid with insertion of percutaneous ventricular assist device, when performed ([34812], 34714-34716 [34820, 34833, 34834])
Removal of percutaneous ventricular assist device at time of replacement of the entire system (33992)
Transthoracic approach (33975-33976)
🚑 18.1   ⚕ 18.1   **FUD** XXX   C 80 ▣
AMA: 2018,Jun,3; 2018,Jan,8; 2017,Dec,3; 2017,Jan,8; 2016,Mar,5; 2016,Jan,13; 2015,Sep,3; 2015,Jan,16; 2014,Jan,11

33992 **Removal of percutaneous ventricular assist device at separate and distinct session from insertion**

INCLUDES   Removal of device and cannulas
EXCLUDES   Removal of implantable aortic counterpulsation ventricular assist system (0455T-0458T)
Code also modifier 59 when percutaneous ventricular assist device is removed on the same day as the insertion, but at a different session
🚑 5.80   ⚕ 5.80   **FUD** XXX   C 80 ▣
AMA: 2018,Jan,8; 2017,Jan,8; 2016,Mar,5; 2016,Jan,13; 2015,Sep,3; 2015,Jan,16; 2014,Jan,11

33993 **Repositioning of percutaneous ventricular assist device with imaging guidance at separate and distinct session from insertion**

EXCLUDES   Repositioning of a percutaneous ventricular assist device without image guidance
Repositioning of device/electrode (0460T-0461T)
Repositioning of the percutaneous ventricular assist device at the same session as the insertion (33990-33991)
Skin pocket relocation with replacement implantable aortic counterpulsation ventricular assist device and electrodes (0459T)
Code also modifier 59 when percutaneous ventricular assist device is repositioned using imaging guidance on the same day as the insertion, but at a different session
🚑 5.09   ⚕ 5.09   **FUD** XXX   C 80 ▣
AMA: 2018,Jan,8; 2017,Jan,8; 2016,Mar,5; 2016,Jan,13; 2015,Sep,3; 2015,Jan,16; 2014,Jan,11

33999 **Unlisted procedure, cardiac surgery**
🚑 0.00   ⚕ 0.00   **FUD** YYY   T 80 ▣
AMA: 2019,Apr,10; 2019,Jan,14; 2018,Jun,3; 2018,Jan,8; 2017,Jan,8; 2016,May,5; 2016,Jan,13; 2015,Jan,16; 2014,Dec,16; 2014,Dec,16; 2014,Jan,11

34001-34530 Surgical Revascularization: Veins and Arteries

INCLUDES   Repair of blood vessel
Surgeon's component of operative arteriogram

34001 **Embolectomy or thrombectomy, with or without catheter; carotid, subclavian or innominate artery, by neck incision**
🚑 27.8   ⚕ 27.8   **FUD** 090   C 80 50 ▣
AMA: 1997,Nov,1

Major arteries of the arm: Subclavian artery, Axillary artery, Brachial, Superior ulnar collateral, Radial artery, Posterior ulnar recurrent, Ulnar artery, Common interosseous

Major arteries of the leg: Aorto-femoral artery, Femoral and deep femoral branches, Popliteal artery, Peroneal artery, Anterior tibial artery, Posterior tibial artery

Arteries (red) are usually accompanied by at least one vein (blue)

34051 **innominate, subclavian artery, by thoracic incision**
🚑 28.8   ⚕ 28.8   **FUD** 090   C 80 50 ▣
AMA: 1997,Nov,1

34101 **axillary, brachial, innominate, subclavian artery, by arm incision**
🚑 17.3   ⚕ 17.3   **FUD** 090   T 80 50 ▣
AMA: 1997,Nov,1

34111 **radial or ulnar artery, by arm incision**
🚑 17.3   ⚕ 17.3   **FUD** 090   T 80 50 ▣
AMA: 1997,Nov,1

34151 **renal, celiac, mesentery, aortoiliac artery, by abdominal incision**
  40.4   40.4   **FUD** 090   C 80 50 ▭
  AMA: 1997,Nov,1

34201 **femoropopliteal, aortoiliac artery, by leg incision**
  29.7   29.7   **FUD** 090   T 80 50 ▭
  AMA: 2018,Jan,8; 2017,Jan,8; 2016,Jan,13; 2015,Jan,16; 2014,Jan,11

34203 **popliteal-tibio-peroneal artery, by leg incision**
  27.5   27.5   **FUD** 090   T 80 50 ▭
  AMA: 1997,Nov,1

34401 **Thrombectomy, direct or with catheter; vena cava, iliac vein, by abdominal incision**
  42.4   42.4   **FUD** 090   C 80 50 ▭
  AMA: 1997,Nov,1

34421 **vena cava, iliac, femoropopliteal vein, by leg incision**
  21.3   21.3   **FUD** 090   T 80 50 ▭
  AMA: 2018,Jan,8; 2017,Jan,8; 2016,Jan,13; 2015,Jan,16; 2014,Jan,11

34451 **vena cava, iliac, femoropopliteal vein, by abdominal and leg incision**
  41.4   41.4   **FUD** 090   C 80 50 ▭
  AMA: 1997,Nov,1

34471 **subclavian vein, by neck incision**
  31.1   31.1   **FUD** 090   T 50 ▭
  AMA: 1997,Nov,1

34490 **axillary and subclavian vein, by arm incision**
  18.5   18.5   **FUD** 090   T 62 50 ▭
  AMA: 1997,Nov,1

34501 **Valvuloplasty, femoral vein**
  25.7   25.7   **FUD** 090   T 80 50 ▭
  AMA: 1997,Nov,1

34502 **Reconstruction of vena cava, any method**
  44.6   44.6   **FUD** 090   C 80 ▭
  AMA: 1997,Nov,1

34510 **Venous valve transposition, any vein donor**
  29.4   29.4   **FUD** 090   T 80 50 ▭
  AMA: 1997,Nov,1

34520 **Cross-over vein graft to venous system**
  28.5   28.5   **FUD** 090   T 80 50 ▭
  AMA: 1997,Nov,1

34530 **Saphenopopliteal vein anastomosis**
  27.0   27.0   **FUD** 090   T 80 50 ▭
  AMA: 1997,Nov,1

34701-34713 [34717, 34718] Abdominal Aorta and Iliac Artery Repairs

INCLUDES Closure of artery after delivery of endograft using a sheath size less than 12 French
Treatment with a covered stent for conditions such as:
  Aneurysm
  Aortic dissection
  Arteriovenous malformation
  Pseudoaneurysm
  Trauma
Treatment zones (vessel(s) in which the endograft is deployed):
  Iliac artery(ies) (34707-34708, [34717], [34718])
  Infrarenal aorta (34701-34702)
  Infrarenal aorta and both common iliac arteries (34705-34706)
  Infrarenal aorta and ipsilateral common iliac artery (34703-34704)

EXCLUDES *Treatment of atherosclerotic occlusive disease with covered stent:*
  Aorta (37236-37237)
  Iliac artery(ies) (37221, 37223)
Code also open arterial exposure, when appropriate ([34812], 34714 [34820, 34833, 34834], 34715-34716)
Code also percutaneous closure of artery when endograft is delivered through a sheath 12 French or larger (34713)
Code also selective catheterization of arteries outside target treatment zone

34701 **Endovascular repair of infrarenal aorta by deployment of an aorto-aortic tube endograft including pre-procedure sizing and device selection, all nonselective catheterization(s), all associated radiological supervision and interpretation, all endograft extension(s) placed in the aorta from the level of the renal arteries to the aortic bifurcation, and all angioplasty/stenting performed from the level of the renal arteries to the aortic bifurcation; for other than rupture (eg, for aneurysm, pseudoaneurysm, dissection, penetrating ulcer)**
  INCLUDES Nonselective catheterization
  Code also intravascular ultrasound when performed (37252-37253)
  35.8   35.8   **FUD** 090   C 80 ▭
  AMA: 2018,Jan,8; 2017,Dec,3

34702 **for rupture including temporary aortic and/or iliac balloon occlusion, when performed (eg, for aneurysm, pseudoaneurysm, dissection, penetrating ulcer, traumatic disruption)**
  INCLUDES Nonselective catheterization
  Code also decompressive laparotomy for treatment abdominal compartment syndrome (49000)
  Code also intravascular ultrasound when performed (37252-37253)
  53.5   53.5   **FUD** 090   C 80 ▭
  AMA: 2018,Jan,8; 2017,Dec,3

34703 **Endovascular repair of infrarenal aorta and/or iliac artery(ies) by deployment of an aorto-uni-iliac endograft including pre-procedure sizing and device selection, all nonselective catheterization(s), all associated radiological supervision and interpretation, all endograft extension(s) placed in the aorta from the level of the renal arteries to the iliac bifurcation, and all angioplasty/stenting performed from the level of the renal arteries to the iliac bifurcation; for other than rupture (eg, for aneurysm, pseudoaneurysm, dissection, penetrating ulcer)**
  INCLUDES Endograft extensions ending in the common iliac arteries
   Nonselective catheterization
  Code also intravascular ultrasound when performed (37252-37253)
  40.3   40.3   **FUD** 090   C 80 ▭
  AMA: 2018,Jan,8; 2017,Dec,3

| 26/TC PC/TC Only | A2-Z3 ASC Payment | 50 Bilateral | ♂ Male Only | ♀ Female Only | Facility RVU | Non-Facility RVU | ▭ CCI | ✖ CLIA |
| FUD Follow-up Days | CMS: IOM | AMA: CPT Asst | A-Y OPPSI | 80/80 Surg Assist Allowed / w/Doc | | Lab Crosswalk | Radiology Crosswalk | |

150   CPT © 2019 American Medical Association. All Rights Reserved.   © 2019 Optum360, LLC

34704   for rupture including temporary aortic and/or iliac balloon occlusion, when performed (eg, for aneurysm, pseudoaneurysm, dissection, penetrating ulcer, traumatic disruption)

INCLUDES   Endograft extensions ending in the common iliac arteries
Nonselective catheterization
Code also decompressive laparotomy for treatment abdominal compartment syndrome (49000)
Code also intravascular ultrasound when performed (37252-37253)

🔲 67.2   ✂ 67.2   **FUD** 090   C 80 ▢

AMA: 2018,Jan,8; 2017,Dec,3

34705   Endovascular repair of infrarenal aorta and/or iliac artery(ies) by deployment of an aorto-bi-iliac endograft including pre-procedure sizing and device selection, all nonselective catheterization(s), all associated radiological supervision and interpretation, all endograft extension(s) placed in the aorta from the level of the renal arteries to the iliac bifurcation, and all angioplasty/stenting performed from the level of the renal arteries to the iliac bifurcation; for other than rupture (eg, for aneurysm, pseudoaneurysm, dissection, penetrating ulcer)

INCLUDES   Endograft extensions ending in the common iliac arteries
Nonselective catheterization
Code also intravascular ultrasound when performed (37252-37253)

🔲 44.3   ✂ 44.3   **FUD** 090   C 80 ▢

AMA: 2018,Jan,8; 2017,Dec,3

34706   for rupture including temporary aortic and/or iliac balloon occlusion, when performed (eg, for aneurysm, pseudoaneurysm, dissection, penetrating ulcer, traumatic disruption)

INCLUDES   Endograft extensions ending in the common iliac arteries
Nonselective catheterization
Code also decompressive laparotomy for treatment abdominal compartment syndrome (49000)
Code also intravascular ultrasound when performed (37252-37253)

🔲 66.8   ✂ 66.8   **FUD** 090   C 80 ▢

AMA: 2018,Jan,8; 2017,Dec,3

34707   Endovascular repair of iliac artery by deployment of an ilio-iliac tube endograft including pre-procedure sizing and device selection, all nonselective catheterization(s), all associated radiological supervision and interpretation, and all endograft extension(s) proximally to the aortic bifurcation and distally to the iliac bifurcation, and treatment zone angioplasty/stenting, when performed, unilateral; for other than rupture (eg, for aneurysm, pseudoaneurysm, dissection, arteriovenous malformation)

INCLUDES   Endograft extensions ending in the common iliac arteries
Nonselective catheterization
EXCLUDES   Deployment of iliac branched endograft:
At the time of aorto-iliac graft placement ([34717])
Delayed/separate from aorto-iliac endograft deployment ([34718])
Code also intravascular ultrasound when performed (37252-37253)

🔲 33.4   ✂ 33.4   **FUD** 090   C 80 50 ▢

AMA: 2018,Jan,8; 2017,Dec,3

34708   for rupture including temporary aortic and/or iliac balloon occlusion, when performed (eg, for aneurysm, pseudoaneurysm, dissection, arteriovenous malformation, traumatic disruption)

INCLUDES   Endograft extensions ending in the common iliac arteries
Nonselective catheterization
EXCLUDES   Deployment of iliac branched endograft:
At the time of aorto-iliac graft placement ([34717])
Delayed/separate from aorto-iliac endograft deployment ([34718])
Code also decompressive laparotomy for treatment abdominal compartment syndrome (49000)
Code also intravascular ultrasound when performed (37252-37253)

🔲 53.6   ✂ 53.6   **FUD** 090   C 80 50 ▢

AMA: 2018,Jan,8; 2017,Dec,3

● + # **34717**   **Endovascular repair of iliac artery at the time of aorto-iliac artery endograft placement by deployment of an iliac branched endograft including pre-procedure sizing and device selection, all ipsilateral selective iliac artery catheterization(s), all associated radiological supervision and interpretation, and all endograft extension(s) proximally to the aortic bifurcation and distally in the internal iliac, external iliac, and common femoral artery(ies), and treatment zone angioplasty/stenting, when performed, for rupture or other than rupture (eg, for aneurysm, pseudoaneurysm, dissection, arteriovenous malformation, penetrating ulcer, traumatic disruption), unilateral (List separately in addition to code for primary procedure)**

🔲 0.00   ✂ 0.00   **FUD** 000   50

INCLUDES   Endograft extensions into internal and external iliac, and/or common femoral arteries
EXCLUDES   Delayed deployment of branched iliac endograft, separate from aorto-iliac endograft placement ([34718])
Placement of prosthesis extensions on same side (34709, 34710-34711)
Reporting with modifier 50. Report once for each side when performed bilaterally
Code first (34703-34706)

+   **34709**   **Placement of extension prosthesis(es) distal to the common iliac artery(ies) or proximal to the renal artery(ies) for endovascular repair of infrarenal abdominal aortic or iliac aneurysm, false aneurysm, dissection, penetrating ulcer, including pre-procedure sizing and device selection, all nonselective catheterization(s), all associated radiological supervision and interpretation, and treatment zone angioplasty/stenting, when performed, per vessel treated (List separately in addition to code for primary procedure)**

EXCLUDES   Placement of covered stent (37236-37237)
Placement of iliac branched endograft ([34717], [34718])
Use of code more than one time for each vessel treated
Code first (34701-34708)

🔲 9.38   ✂ 9.38   **FUD** ZZZ   C 80 ▢

AMA: 2018,Jan,8; 2017,Dec,3

● # **34718** **Endovascular repair of iliac artery, not associated with placement of an aorto-iliac artery endograft at the same session, by deployment of an iliac branched endograft, including pre-procedure sizing and device selection, all ipsilateral selective iliac artery catheterization(s), all associated radiological supervision and interpretation, and all endograft extension(s) proximally to the aortic bifurcation and distally in the internal iliac, external iliac, and common femoral artery(ies), and treatment zone angioplasty/stenting, when performed, for other than rupture (eg, for aneurysm, pseudoaneurysm, dissection, arteriovenous malformation, penetrating ulcer), unilateral**

📷 0.00   ⚕ 0.00   **FUD** 000

INCLUDES Endograft extensions into internal and external iliac, and/or common femoral arteries

EXCLUDES *Branched iliac endograft deployed at same session as aorto-iliac endograft placement (34703-34706, [34717])*
Placement of isolated iliac branched endograft, for rupture (37799)
Placement of prosthesis extensions on same side (34709, 34710-34711)

34710 **Delayed placement of distal or proximal extension prosthesis for endovascular repair of infrarenal abdominal aortic or iliac aneurysm, false aneurysm, dissection, endoleak, or endograft migration, including pre-procedure sizing and device selection, all nonselective catheterization(s), all associated radiological supervision and interpretation, and treatment zone angioplasty/stenting, when performed; initial vessel treated**

EXCLUDES *Fenestrated endograft repair (34841-34848)*
Initial endovascular repair by endograft (34701-34709)
Use of code more than one time per procedure
Code also decompressive laparotomy for treatment abdominal compartment syndrome (49000)

📷 23.2   ⚕ 23.2   **FUD** 090   C 80 ▭

AMA: 2018,Jan,8; 2017,Dec,3

+ **34711**   **each additional vessel treated (List separately in addition to code for primary procedure)**

EXCLUDES *Fenestrated endograft repair (34841-34848)*
Initial endovascular repair by endograft (34701-34709)
Use of code more than one time per procedure
Code first (34710)

📷 8.66   ⚕ 8.66   **FUD** ZZZ   C 80 ▭

AMA: 2018,Jan,8; 2017,Dec,3

34712 **Transcatheter delivery of enhanced fixation device(s) to the endograft (eg, anchor, screw, tack) and all associated radiological supervision and interpretation**

EXCLUDES *Use of code more than one time per procedure*

📷 19.8   ⚕ 19.8   **FUD** 090   C 80 ▭

AMA: 2018,Jan,8; 2017,Dec,3

+ **34713** **Percutaneous access and closure of femoral artery for delivery of endograft through a large sheath (12 French or larger), including ultrasound guidance, when performed, unilateral (List separately in addition to code for primary procedure)**

INCLUDES Ultrasound imaging guidance
Unilateral procedure through large sheath of 12 French or larger

EXCLUDES *Reporting with modifier 50. Report once for each side when performed bilaterally*
Code first (33880-33881, 33883-33884, 33886, 34701-34708, [34718], 34710, 34712, 34841-34848)

📷 3.73   ⚕ 3.73   **FUD** ZZZ   50 N N1 80 ▭

AMA: 2018,Jan,8; 2017,Dec,3

34812-34834 [34812, 34820, 34833, 34834] Open Exposure for Endovascular Prosthesis Delivery

INCLUDES Balloon angioplasty/stent deployment within the target treatment zone
Introduction, manipulation, placement, and deployment of the device
Open exposure of femoral or iliac artery/subsequent closure
Thromboendarterectomy at site of aneurysm

EXCLUDES *Additional interventional procedures outside of target treatment zone*
Guidewire and catheter insertion (36140, 36200, 36245-36248)
Substantial artery repair/replacement (35226, 35286)

+ # **34812** **Open femoral artery exposure for delivery of endovascular prosthesis, by groin incision, unilateral (List separately in addition to code for primary procedure)**

INCLUDES Unilateral procedure

EXCLUDES *ECMO/ECLS insertion, removal or repositioning (33953-33954, 33959, [33962], [33969], [33984], [33987])*
Extensive repair of femoral artery (35226, 35286, 35371)
Reporting with modifier 50. Report once for each side when performed bilaterally
Code first (33880-33881, 33883-33884, 33886, 33990-33991, 34701-34708, [34718], 34710, 34712, 34841-34848)

📷 6.00   ⚕ 6.00   **FUD** ZZZ   50 C 80 ▭

AMA: 2018,Jan,8; 2017,Dec,3; 2017,Jan,8; 2016,Jan,13; 2015,Jul,3; 2015,Jan,16; 2014,Jan,11

+ **34714** **Open femoral artery exposure with creation of conduit for delivery of endovascular prosthesis or for establishment of cardiopulmonary bypass, by groin incision, unilateral (List separately in addition to code for primary procedure)**

INCLUDES Unilateral procedure

EXCLUDES *Delivery of endovascular prosthesis via open femoral artery ([34812])*
ECMO/ECLS insertion, removal or repositioning on same side (33953-33954, 33959, [33962], [33969], [33984])
Reporting with modifier 50. Report once for each side when performed bilaterally
Transcatheter aortic valve replacement via open axillary artery (33362)

Code first (32852, 32854, 33031, 33120, 33251, 33256, 33259, 33261, 33305, 33315, 33322, 33335, 33390-33391, 33404-33406, 33410, [33440], 33411-33417, 33422, 33425-33427, 33430, 33460, 33463-33465, 33468, 33474-33476, 33478, 33496, 33500, 33502, 33504-33507, 33510-33516, 33533-33536, 33542, 33545, 33548, 33600-33688, 33692, 33694, 33697, 33702, 33710, 33720, 33722, 33724, 33726, 33730, 33732, 33736, 33750, 33755, 33762, 33764, 33766-33767, 33770-33783, 33786, 33788, 33802-33803, 33814, 33820, 33822, 33824, 33840, 33845, 33851, 33853, 33858-33859, 33863-33864, 33871, 33875, 33877, 33880-33881, 33883-33884, 33886, 33910, 33916-33917, 33920, 33922, 33926, 33935, 33945, 33975-33990, 33983, 33990-33991, 34701-34708, [34718], 34710, 34712, 34841-34848)

📷 7.84   ⚕ 7.84   **FUD** ZZZ   50 N N1 80 ▭

AMA: 2018,Jan,8; 2017,Dec,3

+ # **34820** **Open iliac artery exposure for delivery of endovascular prosthesis or iliac occlusion during endovascular therapy, by abdominal or retroperitoneal incision, unilateral (List separately in addition to code for primary procedure)**

INCLUDES Unilateral procedure

EXCLUDES *ECMO/ECLS insertion, removal or repositioning (33953-33954, 33959, [33962], [33969], [33984])*
Reporting with modifier 50. Report once for each side when performed bilaterally
Code first (33880-33881, 33883-33884, 33886, 33990-33991, 34701-34708, [34718], 34710, 34712, 34841-34848)

📷 10.0   ⚕ 10.0   **FUD** ZZZ   50 C 80 ▭

AMA: 2018,Jan,8; 2017,Dec,3; 2017,Jan,8; 2016,Jan,13; 2015,Jul,3; 2015,Jan,16; 2014,Jan,11

+ # **34833** **Open iliac artery exposure with creation of conduit for delivery of endovascular prosthesis or for establishment of cardiopulmonary bypass, by abdominal or retroperitoneal incision, unilateral (List separately in addition to code for primary procedure)**

INCLUDES   Unilateral procedure

EXCLUDES   *Delivery of endovascular prosthesis via open iliac artery ([34820])*

ECMO/ECLS insertion, removal or repositioning on same side (33953-33954, 33959, [33962], [33969], [33984])

Reporting with modifier 50. Report once for each side when performed bilaterally

Transcatheter aortic valve replacement via open iliac artery (33364)

Code first (32852, 32854, 33031, 33256, 33259, 33261, 33305, 33315, 33322, 33335, 33390-33391, 33404-33406, 33410, [33440], 33411-33417, 33422, 33425-33427, 33430, 33460, 33463-33465, 33468, 33474-33476, 33478, 33496, 33500, 33502, 33504-33514, 33516, 33533-33536, 33542, 33545, 33548, 33600-33688, 33692, 33694, 33697, 33702, 33710, 33720, 33722, 33724, 33726, 33730, 33732, 33736, 33750, 33755, 33762, 33764, 33766-33767, 33770-33783, 33786, 33788, 33802-33803, 33814, 33820, 33822, 33824, 33840, 33845, 33851, 33853, 33858-33859, 33863-33864, 33871, 33875, 33877, 33880-33881, 33883-33884, 33886, 33910, 33916-33917, 33920, 33922, 33926, 33935, 33945, 33975-33980, 33983, 33990-33991, 34701-34708, [34718], 34710, 34712, 34841-34848)

🔲 11.7   ⚖ 11.7   **FUD** ZZZ   ⑤⓪ Ⓒ ⑧⓪ ▱

AMA: 2018,Jan,8; 2017,Dec,3; 2017,Jan,8; 2016,Jan,13; 2015,Jul,3; 2015,Jan,16; 2014,Jan,11

+ # **34834** **Open brachial artery exposure for delivery of endovascular prosthesis, unilateral (List separately in addition to code for primary procedure)**

INCLUDES   Unilateral procedure

EXCLUDES   *ECMO/ECLS insertion, removal or repositioning (33953-33954, 33959, [33962], [33969], [33984])*

Reporting with modifier 50. Report once for each side when performed bilaterally

Code first (33880-33881, 33883-33884, 33886, 33990-33991, 34701-34708, [34718], 34710, 34712, 34841-34848)

🔲 3.75   ⚖ 3.75   **FUD** ZZZ   ⑤⓪ Ⓒ ⑧⓪ ▱

AMA: 2018,Jan,8; 2017,Dec,3; 2017,Jan,8; 2016,Jan,13; 2015,Jul,3; 2015,Jan,16; 2014,Jan,11

+ **34715** **Open axillary/subclavian artery exposure for delivery of endovascular prosthesis by infraclavicular or supraclavicular incision, unilateral (List separately in addition to code for primary procedure)**

INCLUDES   Unilateral procedure

EXCLUDES   *ECMO/ECLS insertion, removal or repositioning on same side (33953-33954, 33959, [33962], [33969], [33984])*

Implantation or replacement of aortic counterpulsation ventricular assist system (0451T-0452T, 0455T-0456T)

Reporting with modifier 50. Report once for each side when performed bilaterally

Transcatheter aortic valve replacement via open axillary artery (33363)

Code first (33880-33881, 33883-33884, 33886, 33990-33991, 34701-34708, [34718], 34710, 34712, 34841-34848)

🔲 8.79   ⚖ 8.79   **FUD** ZZZ   ⑤⓪ Ⓝ N1 ⑧⓪ ▱

AMA: 2018,Jan,8; 2017,Dec,3

+ **34716** **Open axillary/subclavian artery exposure with creation of conduit for delivery of endovascular prosthesis or for establishment of cardiopulmonary bypass, by infraclavicular or supraclavicular incision, unilateral (List separately in addition to code for primary procedure)**

INCLUDES   Unilateral procedure

EXCLUDES   *ECMO/ECLS insertion, removal or repositioning on same side (33953-33954, 33959, [33962], [33969], [33984])*

Implantation or replacement of aortic counterpulsation ventricular assist system (0451T-0452T, 0455T-0456T)

Reporting with modifier 50. Report once for each side when performed bilaterally

Code first (32852, 32854, 33031, 33120, 33251, 33256, 33259, 33261, 33305, 33315, 33322, 33335, 33390-33391, 33404-33406, 33410, [33440], 33411-33417, 33422, 33425-33427, 33430, 33460, 33463-33465, 33468, 33474-33476, 33478, 33496, 33500, 33502, 33504-33514, 33516, 33533-33536, 33542, 33545, 33548, 33600-33688, 33692, 33694, 33697, 33702-33722, 33724, 33726, 33730, 33732, 33736, 33750, 33755, 33762, 33764, 33766-33767, 33770-33783, 33786, 33788, 33802-33803, 33814, 33820, 33822, 33824, 33840, 33845, 33851, 33853, 33858-33859, 33863-33864, 33871, 33875, 33877, 33880-33881, 33883-33884, 33886, 33910, 33916-33917, 33920, 33922, 33926, 33935, 33945, 33975-33980, 33983, 33990-33991, 34701-34708, [34718], 34710, 34712, 34841-34848)

🔲 10.8   ⚖ 10.8   **FUD** ZZZ   ⑤⓪ Ⓝ N1 ⑧⓪ ▱

AMA: 2018,Jan,8; 2017,Dec,3

34717   **Resequenced code. See code following 34708.**

34718   **Resequenced code. See code following 34709.**

+ **34808** **Endovascular placement of iliac artery occlusion device (List separately in addition to code for primary procedure)**

Code first (34701-34704, 34707-34708, 34709, 34710, 34813, 34841-34844)

🔲 6.11   ⚖ 6.11   **FUD** ZZZ   Ⓒ ⑧⓪ ▱

AMA: 2018,Jan,8; 2017,Jan,8; 2016,Jan,13; 2015,Jan,16; 2014,Jan,11

34812   **Resequenced code. See code following 34713.**

+ **34813** **Placement of femoral-femoral prosthetic graft during endovascular aortic aneurysm repair (List separately in addition to code for primary procedure)**

EXCLUDES   *Grafting of femoral artery (35521, 35533, 35539, 35540, 35556, 35558, 35566, 35621, 35646, 35654-35661, 35666, 35700)*

Code first ([34812])

🔲 6.85   ⚖ 6.85   **FUD** ZZZ   Ⓒ ⑧⓪ ▱

AMA: 2018,Jan,8; 2017,Jan,8; 2016,Jan,13; 2015,Jan,16; 2014,Jan,11

34820   **Resequenced code. See code following 34714.**

34830   **Open repair of infrarenal aortic aneurysm or dissection, plus repair of associated arterial trauma, following unsuccessful endovascular repair; tube prosthesis**

🔲 50.9   ⚖ 50.9   **FUD** 090   Ⓒ ⑧⓪ ▱

AMA: 2018,Jan,8; 2017,Jan,8; 2016,Jan,13; 2015,Jan,16; 2014,Jan,11

Abdominal aorta   Renal arteries   The vessel is opened and repaired

Infrarenal aneurysm

Iliac arteries

Prosthesis extends into the femoral arteries

Tube prosthesis   **Aorto-bi-iliac prosthesis**   **Aorto-bifemoral prosthesis**

A tube prosthesis is placed and any associated arterial trauma is repaired

---

34831 **aorto-bi-iliac prosthesis**
 55.9   55.9   **FUD** 090   C 80
AMA: 2018,Jan,8; 2017,Jan,8; 2016,Jan,13; 2015,Jan,16; 2014,Jan,11

34832 **aorto-bifemoral prosthesis**
 54.7   54.7   **FUD** 090   C 80
AMA: 2018,Jan,8; 2017,Jan,8; 2016,Jan,13; 2015,Jan,16; 2014,Jan,11

34833 Resequenced code. See code following 34714.

34834 Resequenced code. See code following 34714.

34839-34848 Repair Visceral Aorta with Fenestrated Endovascular Grafts

INCLUDES   Angiography
Balloon angioplasty before and after deployment of graft
Fluoroscopic guidance
Guidewire and catheter insertion of vessels in the target treatment zone
Radiologic supervision and interpretation
Visceral aorta (34841-34844)
Visceral aorta and associated infrarenal abdominal aorta (34845-34848)

EXCLUDES   *Catheterization of:*
    Arterial families outside treatment zone
    Hypogastric arteries
Distal extension prosthesis terminating in the common femoral, external iliac, or internal iliac artery (34709-34711 [34718])
Insertion of bare metal or covered intravascular stents in visceral branches in the target treatment zone (37236-37237)
Interventional procedures outside treatment zone
Open exposure of access vessels (34713-34716 [34812, 34820, 34833, 34834])
Placement of distal extension prosthesis into internal/external iliac or common femoral artery (34709, [34718], 34710-34711)
Repair of abdominal aortic aneurysm without a fenestrated graft (34701-34708)
Substantial artery repair (35226, 35286)
Code also associated endovascular repair of descending thoracic aorta (33880-33886, 75956-75959)

34839 **Physician planning of a patient-specific fenestrated visceral aortic endograft requiring a minimum of 90 minutes of physician time**
 0.00   0.00   **FUD** YYY   B 80
EXCLUDES   *3D rendering with interpretation and reporting of imaging (76376-76377)*
Endovascular repair procedure on day of or day after planning (34701-34706, 34841-34848)
Planning on day of or day before endovascular repair procedure
Total planning time of less than 90 minutes

34841 **Endovascular repair of visceral aorta (eg, aneurysm, pseudoaneurysm, dissection, penetrating ulcer, intramural hematoma, or traumatic disruption) by deployment of a fenestrated visceral aortic endograft and all associated radiological supervision and interpretation, including target zone angioplasty, when performed; including one visceral artery endoprosthesis (superior mesenteric, celiac or renal artery)**
EXCLUDES   *Endovascular repair of aorta (34701-34706, 34845-34848)*
Physician planning of a patient-specific fenestrated visceral aortic endograft (34839)
 0.00   0.00   **FUD** YYY   C 80
AMA: 2018,Jan,8; 2017,Dec,3; 2017,Jul,3; 2017,Jan,8; 2016,Jan,13; 2015,Jan,16; 2014,Jan,11

34842 **including two visceral artery endoprostheses (superior mesenteric, celiac and/or renal artery[s])**
INCLUDES   Repairs extending from the visceral aorta to one or more of the four visceral artery origins to the level of the infrarenal aorta
EXCLUDES   *Endovascular repair of aorta (34701-34706, 34845-34848)*
Physician planning of a patient-specific fenestrated visceral aortic endograft (34839)
 0.00   0.00   **FUD** YYY   C 80
AMA: 2018,Jan,8; 2017,Dec,3; 2017,Jul,3; 2017,Jan,8; 2016,Jan,13; 2015,Jan,16; 2014,Jan,11

34843 **including three visceral artery endoprostheses (superior mesenteric, celiac and/or renal artery[s])**
INCLUDES   Repairs extending from the visceral aorta to one or more of the four visceral artery origins to the level of the infrarenal aorta
EXCLUDES   *Endovascular repair of aorta (34701-34706, 34845-34848)*
Physician planning of a patient-specific fenestrated visceral aortic endograft (34839)
 0.00   0.00   **FUD** YYY   C 80
AMA: 2018,Jan,8; 2017,Dec,3; 2017,Jul,3; 2017,Jan,8; 2016,Jan,13; 2015,Jan,16; 2014,Jan,11

34844 **including four or more visceral artery endoprostheses (superior mesenteric, celiac and/or renal artery[s])**
INCLUDES   Repairs extending from the visceral aorta to one or more of the four visceral artery origins to the level of the infrarenal aorta
EXCLUDES   *Endovascular repair of aorta (34701-34706, 34845-34848)*
Physician planning of a patient-specific fenestrated visceral aortic endograft (34839)
 0.00   0.00   **FUD** YYY   C 80
AMA: 2018,Jan,8; 2017,Dec,3; 2017,Jul,3; 2017,Jan,8; 2016,Jan,13; 2015,Jan,16; 2014,Jan,11

34845 **Endovascular repair of visceral aorta and infrarenal abdominal aorta (eg, aneurysm, pseudoaneurysm, dissection, penetrating ulcer, intramural hematoma, or traumatic disruption) with a fenestrated visceral aortic endograft and concomitant unibody or modular infrarenal aortic endograft and all associated radiological supervision and interpretation, including target zone angioplasty, when performed; including one visceral artery endoprosthesis (superior mesenteric, celiac or renal artery)**
INCLUDES   Placement of device and extensions into the common iliac arteries
Repairs extending from the visceral aorta into the common iliac arteries
EXCLUDES   *Direct repair aneurysm (35081, 35102)*
Endovascular repair of aorta (34701-34706, 34841-34844)
Physician planning of a patient-specific fenestrated visceral aortic endograft (34839)
Code also iliac artery revascularization when performed outside zone of target treatment (37220-37223)
 0.00   0.00   **FUD** YYY   C 80
AMA: 2018,Jan,8; 2017,Dec,3; 2017,Jul,3; 2017,Jan,8; 2016,Jan,13; 2015,Jan,16; 2014,Jan,11

34846 **including two visceral artery endoprostheses (superior mesenteric, celiac and/or renal artery[s])**
INCLUDES   Placement of device and extensions into the common iliac arteries
Repairs extending from the visceral aorta into the common iliac arteries
EXCLUDES   *Direct repair aneurysm (35081, 35102)*
Endovascular repair of aorta (34701-34706, 34841-34844)
Physician planning of a patient-specific fenestrated visceral aortic endograft (34839)
Code also iliac artery revascularization when performed outside zone of target treatment (37220-37223)
 0.00   0.00   **FUD** YYY   C 80
AMA: 2018,Jan,8; 2017,Dec,3; 2017,Jul,3; 2017,Jan,8; 2016,Jan,13; 2015,Jan,16; 2014,Jan,11

34847   **including three visceral artery endoprostheses (superior mesenteric, celiac and/or renal artery[s])**

INCLUDES   Placement of device and extensions into the common iliac arteries

Repairs extending from the visceral aorta into the common iliac arteries

EXCLUDES   *Direct repair aneurysm (35081, 35102)*

Endovascular repair of aorta (34701-34706, 34841-34844)

Physician planning of a patient-specific fenestrated visceral aortic endograft (34839)

Code also iliac artery revascularization when performed outside zone of target treatment (37220-37223)

🖐 0.00   🖐 0.00   **FUD** YYY   C 80 ▭

AMA: 2018,Jan,8; 2017,Dec,3; 2017,Jul,3; 2017,Jan,8; 2016,Jan,13; 2015,Jan,16; 2014,Jan,11

34848   **including four or more visceral artery endoprostheses (superior mesenteric, celiac and/or renal artery[s])**

INCLUDES   Placement of device and extensions into the common iliac arteries

Repairs extending from the visceral aorta into the common iliac arteries

EXCLUDES   *Direct repair aneurysm (35081, 35102)*

Endovascular repair of aorta (34701-34706, 34841-34844)

Physician planning of a patient-specific fenestrated visceral aortic endograft (34839)

Code also iliac artery revascularization when performed outside zone of target treatment (37220-37223)

🖐 0.00   🖐 0.00   **FUD** YYY   C 80 ▭

AMA: 2018,Jan,8; 2017,Dec,3; 2017,Aug,9; 2017,Jul,3; 2017,Jan,8; 2016,Jul,6; 2016,Jan,13; 2015,Jan,16; 2014,Jan,11

35001-35152 Repair Aneurysm, False Aneurysm, Related Arterial Disease

INCLUDES   Endarterectomy procedures

EXCLUDES   *Endovascular repairs of:*

Abdominal aortic aneurysm (34701-34716 [34717, 34718, 34812, 34820, 34833, 34834])

Thoracic aortic aneurysm (33858-33859, 33863-33875)

Intracranial aneurysms (61697-61710)

Repairs related to occlusive disease only (35201-35286)

35001   **Direct repair of aneurysm, pseudoaneurysm, or excision (partial or total) and graft insertion, with or without patch graft; for aneurysm and associated occlusive disease, carotid, subclavian artery, by neck incision**

🖐 32.2   🖐 32.2   **FUD** 090   C 80 50 ▭

AMA: 2002,May,7; 2000,Dec,1

35002   **for ruptured aneurysm, carotid, subclavian artery, by neck incision**

🖐 32.7   🖐 32.7   **FUD** 090   C 80 50 ▭

AMA: 2002,May,7; 1997,Nov,1

35005   **for aneurysm, pseudoaneurysm, and associated occlusive disease, vertebral artery**

🖐 28.6   🖐 28.6   **FUD** 090   C 80 50 ▭

AMA: 2002,May,7; 1997,Nov,1

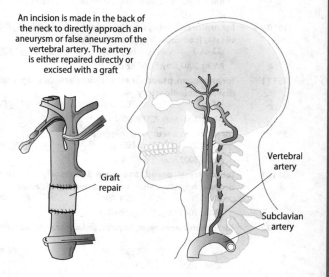

An incision is made in the back of the neck to directly approach an aneurysm or false aneurysm of the vertebral artery. The artery is either repaired directly or excised with a graft

Graft repair

Vertebral artery

Subclavian artery

35011   **for aneurysm and associated occlusive disease, axillary-brachial artery, by arm incision**

🖐 29.0   🖐 29.0   **FUD** 090   T 80 50 ▭

AMA: 2002,May,7; 1997,Nov,1

35013   **for ruptured aneurysm, axillary-brachial artery, by arm incision**

🖐 36.3   🖐 36.3   **FUD** 090   C 80 50 ▭

AMA: 2002,May,7; 1997,Nov,1

35021   **for aneurysm, pseudoaneurysm, and associated occlusive disease, innominate, subclavian artery, by thoracic incision**

🖐 36.6   🖐 36.6   **FUD** 090   C 80 50 ▭

AMA: 2002,May,7; 1997,Nov,1

35022   **for ruptured aneurysm, innominate, subclavian artery, by thoracic incision**

🖐 40.6   🖐 40.6   **FUD** 090   C 80 50 ▭

AMA: 2002,May,7; 1997,Nov,1

35045   **for aneurysm, pseudoaneurysm, and associated occlusive disease, radial or ulnar artery**

🖐 28.4   🖐 28.4   **FUD** 090   T 80 50 ▭

AMA: 2002,May,7; 1997,Nov,1

35081   **for aneurysm, pseudoaneurysm, and associated occlusive disease, abdominal aorta**

🖐 50.2   🖐 50.2   **FUD** 090   C 80 ▭

AMA: 2018,Jan,8; 2017,Jan,8; 2016,Jan,13; 2015,Jan,16; 2014,Jan,11

35082   **for ruptured aneurysm, abdominal aorta**

🖐 63.3   🖐 63.3   **FUD** 090   C 80 ▭

AMA: 2002,May,7; 1997,Nov,1

35091   **for aneurysm, pseudoaneurysm, and associated occlusive disease, abdominal aorta involving visceral vessels (mesenteric, celiac, renal)**

🖐 51.8   🖐 51.8   **FUD** 090   C 80 50 ▭

AMA: 2018,Jan,8; 2017,Jan,8; 2016,Jan,13; 2015,Jan,16; 2014,Jan,11

35092   **for ruptured aneurysm, abdominal aorta involving visceral vessels (mesenteric, celiac, renal)**

🖐 75.5   🖐 75.5   **FUD** 090   C 80 50 ▭

AMA: 2002,May,7; 1997,Nov,1

35102 for aneurysm, pseudoaneurysm, and associated occlusive disease, abdominal aorta involving iliac vessels (common, hypogastric, external)
🔧 54.5 ⚕ 54.5 **FUD** 090 [C] [80] [50] ▭
AMA: 2018,Jan,8; 2017,Jan,8; 2016,Jan,13; 2015,Jan,16; 2014,Jan,11

35103 for ruptured aneurysm, abdominal aorta involving iliac vessels (common, hypogastric, external)
🔧 64.9 ⚕ 64.9 **FUD** 090 [C] [80] [50] ▭
AMA: 2002,May,7; 1997,Nov,1

35111 for aneurysm, pseudoaneurysm, and associated occlusive disease, splenic artery
🔧 38.3 ⚕ 38.3 **FUD** 090 [C] [80] [50] ▭
AMA: 2002,May,7; 1997,Nov,1

35112 for ruptured aneurysm, splenic artery
🔧 47.2 ⚕ 47.2 **FUD** 090 [C] [80] [50] ▭
AMA: 2002,May,7; 1997,Nov,1

35121 for aneurysm, pseudoaneurysm, and associated occlusive disease, hepatic, celiac, renal, or mesenteric artery
🔧 48.3 ⚕ 48.3 **FUD** 090 [C] [80] [50] ▭
AMA: 2002,May,7; 1997,Nov,1

35122 for ruptured aneurysm, hepatic, celiac, renal, or mesenteric artery
🔧 54.6 ⚕ 54.6 **FUD** 090 [C] [80] [50] ▭
AMA: 2002,May,7; 1997,Nov,1

35131 for aneurysm, pseudoaneurysm, and associated occlusive disease, iliac artery (common, hypogastric, external)
🔧 40.2 ⚕ 40.2 **FUD** 090 [C] [80] [50] ▭
AMA: 2018,Jan,8; 2017,Jan,8; 2016,Jan,13; 2015,Jan,16; 2014,Jan,11

35132 for ruptured aneurysm, iliac artery (common, hypogastric, external)
🔧 47.2 ⚕ 47.2 **FUD** 090 [C] [80] [50] ▭
AMA: 2002,May,7; 1997,Nov,1

35141 for aneurysm, pseudoaneurysm, and associated occlusive disease, common femoral artery (profunda femoris, superficial femoral)
🔧 31.9 ⚕ 31.9 **FUD** 090 [C] [80] [50] ▭
AMA: 2002,May,7; 1997,Nov,1

35142 for ruptured aneurysm, common femoral artery (profunda femoris, superficial femoral)
🔧 38.5 ⚕ 38.5 **FUD** 090 [C] [80] [50] ▭
AMA: 2002,May,7; 1997,Nov,1

35151 for aneurysm, pseudoaneurysm, and associated occlusive disease, popliteal artery
🔧 35.8 ⚕ 35.8 **FUD** 090 [C] [80] [50] ▭
AMA: 2002,May,7; 1997,Nov,1

35152 for ruptured aneurysm, popliteal artery
🔧 40.3 ⚕ 40.3 **FUD** 090 [C] [80] [50] ▭
AMA: 2002,May,7; 1997,Nov,1

35180-35190 Surgical Repair Arteriovenous Fistula

35180 Repair, congenital arteriovenous fistula; head and neck
🔧 25.4 ⚕ 25.4 **FUD** 090 [T] [80] ▭
AMA: 2018,Jan,8; 2017,Jan,8; 2016,Jan,13; 2015,Jan,16; 2014,Jan,11

35182 thorax and abdomen
🔧 51.9 ⚕ 51.9 **FUD** 090 [C] [80] ▭
AMA: 2018,Jan,8; 2017,Jan,8; 2016,Jan,13; 2015,Jan,16; 2014,Jan,11

35184 extremities
🔧 27.8 ⚕ 27.8 **FUD** 090 [T] [80] ▭
AMA: 2018,Jan,8; 2017,Jan,8; 2016,Jan,13; 2015,Jan,16; 2014,Jan,11

35188 Repair, acquired or traumatic arteriovenous fistula; head and neck
🔧 37.7 ⚕ 37.7 **FUD** 090 [T] [A2] [80] ▭
AMA: 2018,Jan,8; 2017,Jan,8; 2016,Jan,13; 2015,Jan,16; 2014,Jan,11

35189 thorax and abdomen
🔧 43.5 ⚕ 43.5 **FUD** 090 [C] [80] ▭
AMA: 2018,Jan,8; 2017,Jan,8; 2016,Jan,13; 2015,Jan,16; 2014,Jan,11

35190 extremities
🔧 22.0 ⚕ 22.0 **FUD** 090 [T] [80] ▭
AMA: 2018,Jan,8; 2017,Jan,8; 2016,Jan,13; 2015,Jan,16; 2014,Jan,11

35201-35286 Surgical Repair Artery or Vein

EXCLUDES   *Arteriovenous fistula repair (35180-35190)*
Primary open vascular procedures

35201 Repair blood vessel, direct; neck
EXCLUDES   *Removal ECMO/ECLS of cannula ([33969, 33984, 33985, 33986])*
🔧 27.2 ⚕ 27.2 **FUD** 090 [T] [80] [50] ▭
AMA: 2018,Jan,8; 2017,Jan,8; 2016,Jan,13; 2015,Jul,3; 2015,Jan,16; 2014,Mar,8

35206 upper extremity
EXCLUDES   *Removal ECMO/ECLS of cannula ([33969, 33984, 33985, 33986])*
🔧 22.6 ⚕ 22.6 **FUD** 090 [T] [80] [50] ▭
AMA: 2018,Jan,8; 2017,Jan,8; 2016,Jan,13; 2015,Jul,3; 2015,Jan,16; 2014,Apr,10; 2014,Jan,11

35207 hand, finger
🔧 21.7 ⚕ 21.7 **FUD** 090 [T] [A2] [50] ▭
AMA: 2012,Apr,3-9; 2003,Feb,1

35211 intrathoracic, with bypass
EXCLUDES   *Removal ECMO/ECLS of cannula ([33969, 33984, 33985, 33986])*
🔧 40.0 ⚕ 40.0 **FUD** 090 [C] [80] [50] ▭
AMA: 2015,Jul,3

35216 intrathoracic, without bypass
EXCLUDES   *Removal ECMO/ECLS of cannula ([33969, 33984, 33985, 33986])*
🔧 59.7 ⚕ 59.7 **FUD** 090 [C] [80] [50] ▭
AMA: 2018,Jan,8; 2017,Jan,8; 2016,Jan,13; 2015,Jan,16; 2014,Jan,11

35221 intra-abdominal
🔧 42.4 ⚕ 42.4 **FUD** 090 [C] [80] [50] ▭
AMA: 2012,Apr,3-9; 2003,Feb,1

35226 lower extremity
EXCLUDES   *Removal ECMO/ECLS of cannula ([33969, 33984, 33985, 33986])*
🔧 24.1 ⚕ 24.1 **FUD** 090 [T] [80] [50] ▭
AMA: 2019,Jul,10; 2018,Jan,8; 2017,Aug,10; 2017,Jul,3; 2017,Jan,8; 2016,Jul,6; 2016,Jan,13; 2015,Jul,3; 2015,Jan,16; 2014,Jan,11

35231 Repair blood vessel with vein graft; neck
🔧 35.7 ⚕ 35.7 **FUD** 090 [T] [80] [50] ▭
AMA: 2012,Apr,3-9; 2003,Feb,1

35236 upper extremity
🔧 29.0 ⚕ 29.0 **FUD** 090 [T] [80] [50] ▭
AMA: 2018,Jan,8; 2017,Jan,8; 2016,Jan,13; 2015,Jan,16; 2014,Jan,11

35241 intrathoracic, with bypass
🔧 41.8 ⚕ 41.8 **FUD** 090 [C] [80] [50] ▭
AMA: 2012,Apr,3-9; 2003,Feb,1

35246 intrathoracic, without bypass
🔧 45.6 ⚕ 45.6 **FUD** 090 [C] [80] [50] ▭
AMA: 2012,Apr,3-9; 2003,Feb,1

35251 intra-abdominal
🔧 50.4 ⚕ 50.4 **FUD** 090 [C] [80] [50] ▭
AMA: 2012,Apr,3-9; 2003,Feb,1

35256	**lower extremity**	
	🖭 29.6 🔏 29.6 **FUD** 090	T 80 50 📭
	AMA: 2012,Apr,3-9; 2003,Feb,1	
35261	**Repair blood vessel with graft other than vein; neck**	
	🖭 28.2 🔏 28.2 **FUD** 090	T 80 50 📭
	AMA: 2012,Apr,3-9; 2003,Feb,1	
35266	**upper extremity**	
	🖭 25.1 🔏 25.1 **FUD** 090	T 80 50 📭
	AMA: 2018,Jan,8; 2017,Jan,8; 2016,Jan,13; 2015,Jan,16; 2014,Jan,11	
35271	**intrathoracic, with bypass**	
	🖭 40.0 🔏 40.0 **FUD** 090	C 80 50 📭
	AMA: 2012,Apr,3-9; 2003,Feb,1	
35276	**intrathoracic, without bypass**	
	🖭 42.4 🔏 42.4 **FUD** 090	C 80 50 📭
	AMA: 2012,Apr,3-9; 2003,Feb,1	
35281	**intra-abdominal**	
	🖭 46.8 🔏 46.8 **FUD** 090	C 80 50 📭
	AMA: 2012,Apr,3-9; 2003,Feb,1	
35286	**lower extremity**	
	🖭 26.9 🔏 26.9 **FUD** 090	T 80 50 📭
	AMA: 2019,Jul,10; 2018,Jan,8; 2017,Aug,10; 2017,Jul,3; 2017,Jan,8; 2016,Jul,6; 2016,Jan,13; 2015,Jan,16; 2014,Jan,11	

35301-35372 Surgical Thromboendarterectomy Peripheral and Visceral Arteries

INCLUDES   Obtaining saphenous or arm vein for graft
     Thrombectomy/embolectomy

EXCLUDES   *Coronary artery bypass procedures (33510-33536, 33572)*
     Thromboendarterectomy for vascular occlusion on a different vessel during the same session

35301	**Thromboendarterectomy, including patch graft, if performed; carotid, vertebral, subclavian, by neck incision**	
	🖭 32.7 🔏 32.7 **FUD** 090	C 80 50 📭
	AMA: 2018,Jan,8; 2017,Jan,8; 2016,Jan,13; 2015,Jan,16; 2014,Jan,11	

Plaque

Tool to remove clot and/or plaque

Thrombus (blood clot)

Vertebral

External carotid

Carotid artery

Internal carotid

Subclavian artery

Aorta

35302	**superficial femoral artery**	
	EXCLUDES *Revascularization, endovascular, open or percutaneous, femoral, popliteal artery(s) (37225, 37227)*	
	🖭 32.5 🔏 32.5 **FUD** 090	C 80 50 📭
	AMA: 2018,Jan,8; 2017,Jan,8; 2016,Jan,13; 2015,Jan,16; 2014,Jan,11	
35303	**popliteal artery**	
	EXCLUDES *Revascularization, endovascular, open or percutaneous, femoral, popliteal artery(s) (37225, 37227)*	
	🖭 35.9 🔏 35.9 **FUD** 090	C 80 50 📭
	AMA: 2018,Jan,8; 2017,Jan,8; 2016,Jan,13; 2015,Jan,16; 2014,Jan,11	
35304	**tibioperoneal trunk artery**	
	EXCLUDES *Revascularization, endovascular, open or percutaneous, tibial/peroneal artery (37229, 37231, 37233, 37235)*	
	🖭 37.0 🔏 37.0 **FUD** 090	C 80 50 📭
	AMA: 2018,Jan,8; 2017,Jan,8; 2016,Jan,13; 2015,Jan,16; 2014,Jan,11	
35305	**tibial or peroneal artery, initial vessel**	
	EXCLUDES *Revascularization, endovascular, open or percutaneous, tibial/peroneal artery (37229, 37231, 37233, 37235)*	
	🖭 35.6 🔏 35.6 **FUD** 090	C 80 50 📭
	AMA: 2018,Jan,8; 2017,Jan,8; 2016,Jan,13; 2015,Jan,16; 2014,Jan,11	
+ **35306**	**each additional tibial or peroneal artery (List separately in addition to code for primary procedure)**	
	EXCLUDES *Revascularization, endovascular, open or percutaneous, tibial/peroneal artery (37229, 37231, 37233, 37235)*	
	Code first (35305)	
	🖭 12.9 🔏 12.9 **FUD** ZZZ	C 80 📭
	AMA: 2018,Jan,8; 2017,Jan,8; 2016,Jan,13; 2015,Jan,16; 2014,Jan,11	
35311	**subclavian, innominate, by thoracic incision**	
	🖭 45.4 🔏 45.4 **FUD** 090	C 80 50 📭
	AMA: 1997,Nov,1	
35321	**axillary-brachial**	
	🖭 25.8 🔏 25.8 **FUD** 090	T 80 50 📭
	AMA: 1997,Nov,1	
35331	**abdominal aorta**	
	🖭 42.3 🔏 42.3 **FUD** 090	C 80 50 📭
	AMA: 1997,Nov,1	
35341	**mesenteric, celiac, or renal**	
	🖭 39.9 🔏 39.9 **FUD** 090	C 80 50 📭
	AMA: 1997,Nov,1	
35351	**iliac**	
	🖭 37.0 🔏 37.0 **FUD** 090	C 80 50 📭
	AMA: 1997,Nov,1	
35355	**iliofemoral**	
	🖭 29.8 🔏 29.8 **FUD** 090	C 80 50 📭
	AMA: 1997,Nov,1	
35361	**combined aortoiliac**	
	🖭 43.9 🔏 43.9 **FUD** 090	C 80 50 📭
	AMA: 1997,Nov,1	
35363	**combined aortoiliofemoral**	
	🖭 46.8 🔏 46.8 **FUD** 090	C 80 50 📭
	AMA: 1997,Nov,1	
35371	**common femoral**	
	🖭 23.7 🔏 23.7 **FUD** 090	C 80 50 📭
	AMA: 2018,Jan,8; 2017,Aug,10; 2017,Jul,3; 2017,Jan,8; 2016,Jan,13; 2015,Jan,16; 2014,Jan,11	
35372	**deep (profunda) femoral**	
	🖭 28.3 🔏 28.3 **FUD** 090	C 80 50 📭
	AMA: 2018,Jan,8; 2017,Jan,8; 2016,Jan,13; 2015,Jan,16; 2014,Jan,11	

35390 Surgical Thromboendarterectomy: Carotid Reoperation

Code first (35301)

+ **35390**	**Reoperation, carotid, thromboendarterectomy, more than 1 month after original operation (List separately in addition to code for primary procedure)**	
	🖭 4.61 🔏 4.61 **FUD** ZZZ	C 80 📭
	AMA: 1997,Nov,1; 1993,Win,1	

Cardiovascular, Hemic, and Lymphatic

35400 — 35538

35400 Endoscopic Visualization of Vessels

Code first the therapeutic intervention

+ 35400 **Angioscopy (noncoronary vessels or grafts) during therapeutic intervention (List separately in addition to code for primary procedure)**

🔳 4.32   ✂ 4.32   **FUD** ZZZ   C 80 ▣

AMA: 1997,Dec,1; 1997,Nov,1

35500 Obtain Arm Vein for Graft

EXCLUDES   *Endoscopic harvest (33508)*
Harvesting of multiple vein segments (35682, 35683)
Code first (33510-33536, 35556, 35566, 35570-35571, 35583-35587)

+ 35500 **Harvest of upper extremity vein, 1 segment, for lower extremity or coronary artery bypass procedure (List separately in addition to code for primary procedure)**

🔳 9.29   ✂ 9.29   **FUD** ZZZ   N 80 ▣

AMA: 2018,Jan,8; 2017,Jan,8; 2016,Jan,13; 2015,Jan,16; 2014,Jan,11

35501-35571 Arterial Bypass Using Vein Grafts

INCLUDES   Obtaining saphenous vein grafts
EXCLUDES   *Obtaining multiple vein segments (35682, 35683)*
Obtaining vein grafts, upper extremity or femoropopliteal (35500, 35572)
Treatment of different sites with different bypass procedures during the same operative session

35501 **Bypass graft, with vein; common carotid-ipsilateral internal carotid**

🔳 43.3   ✂ 43.3   **FUD** 090   C 80 50 ▣

AMA: 2018,Jan,8; 2017,Jan,8; 2016,Jan,13; 2015,Jan,16; 2014,Jan,11

35506 **carotid-subclavian or subclavian-carotid**

🔳 36.7   ✂ 36.7   **FUD** 090   C 80 50 ▣

AMA: 2018,Jan,8; 2017,Jan,8; 2016,Jan,13; 2015,Jan,16; 2014,Jan,11

35508 **carotid-vertebral**

INCLUDES   Endoscopic procedure

🔳 38.3   ✂ 38.3   **FUD** 090   C 80 50 ▣

AMA: 1999,Mar,6; 1999,Apr,11

35509 **carotid-contralateral carotid**

🔳 40.8   ✂ 40.8   **FUD** 090   C 80 50 ▣

AMA: 2018,Jan,8; 2017,Jan,8; 2016,Jan,13; 2015,Jan,16; 2014,Jan,11

35510 **carotid-brachial**

🔳 35.5   ✂ 35.5   **FUD** 090   C 80 50 ▣

AMA: 2018,Jan,8; 2017,Jan,8; 2016,Jan,13; 2015,Jan,16; 2014,Jan,11

35511 **subclavian-subclavian**

🔳 32.3   ✂ 32.3   **FUD** 090   C 80 50 ▣

AMA: 2018,Jan,8; 2017,Jan,8; 2016,Jan,13; 2015,Jan,16; 2014,Jan,11

35512 **subclavian-brachial**

🔳 34.8   ✂ 34.8   **FUD** 090   C 80 50 ▣

AMA: 2018,Jan,8; 2017,Jan,8; 2016,Jan,13; 2015,Jan,16; 2014,Jan,11

35515 **subclavian-vertebral**

🔳 38.3   ✂ 38.3   **FUD** 090   C 80 50 ▣

AMA: 1999,Mar,6; 1999,Apr,11

35516 **subclavian-axillary**

🔳 35.2   ✂ 35.2   **FUD** 090   C 80 50 ▣

AMA: 1999,Mar,6; 1999,Apr,11

35518 **axillary-axillary**

🔳 32.9   ✂ 32.9   **FUD** 090   C 80 50 ▣

AMA: 2018,Jan,8; 2017,Jan,8; 2016,Jan,13; 2015,Jan,16; 2014,Jan,11

35521 **axillary-femoral**

EXCLUDES   *Synthetic graft (35621)*

🔳 35.4   ✂ 35.4   **FUD** 090   C 80 50 ▣

AMA: 2018,Jan,8; 2017,Jan,8; 2016,Jan,13; 2015,Jan,16; 2014,Jan,11

35522 **axillary-brachial**

🔳 34.9   ✂ 34.9   **FUD** 090   C 80 50 ▣

AMA: 2018,Jan,8; 2017,Jan,8; 2016,Jan,13; 2015,Jan,16; 2014,Jan,11

35523 **brachial-ulnar or -radial**

🔳 37.1   ✂ 37.1   **FUD** 090   C 80 50 ▣

EXCLUDES   *Bypass graft using synthetic conduit (37799)*
Bypass graft, with vein; brachial-brachial (35525)
Distal revascularization and interval ligation (DRIL), upper extremity hemodialysis access (steal syndrome) (36838)
Harvest of upper extremity vein, 1 segment, for lower extremity or coronary artery bypass procedure (35500)
Repair blood vessel, direct; upper extremity (35206)

35525 **brachial-brachial**

🔳 33.0   ✂ 33.0   **FUD** 090   C 80 50 ▣

AMA: 2018,Jan,8; 2017,Jan,8; 2016,Jan,13; 2015,Jan,16; 2014,Jan,11

35526 **aortosubclavian, aortoinnominate, or aortocarotid**

EXCLUDES   *Synthetic graft (35626)*

🔳 50.5   ✂ 50.5   **FUD** 090   C 80 50 ▣

AMA: 1999,Mar,6; 1999,Apr,11

35531 **aortoceliac or aortomesenteric**

🔳 56.3   ✂ 56.3   **FUD** 090   C 80 50 ▣

AMA: 1999,Mar,6; 1999,Apr,11

35533 **axillary-femoral-femoral**

EXCLUDES   *Synthetic graft (35654)*

🔳 43.4   ✂ 43.4   **FUD** 090   C 80 50 ▣

AMA: 2012,Apr,3-9; 1999,Mar,6

35535 **hepatorenal**

🔳 54.9   ✂ 54.9   **FUD** 090   C 80 50 ▣

EXCLUDES   *Bypass graft (35536, 35560, 35631, 35636)*
Harvest of upper extremity vein, 1 segment, for lower extremity or coronary artery bypass procedure (35500)
Repair blood vessel (35221, 35251, 35281)

35536 **splenorenal**

🔳 48.8   ✂ 48.8   **FUD** 090   C 80 50 ▣

AMA: 2018,Jan,8; 2017,Jan,8; 2016,Jan,13; 2015,Jan,16; 2014,Jan,11

35537 **aortoiliac**

EXCLUDES   *Bypass graft, with vein; aortobi-iliac (35538)*
Synthetic graft (35637)

🔳 60.2   ✂ 60.2   **FUD** 090   C 80 ▣

AMA: 2018,Jan,8; 2017,Jan,8; 2016,Jan,13; 2015,Jan,16; 2014,Jan,11

35538 **aortobi-iliac**

EXCLUDES   *Bypass graft, with vein; aortoiliac (35537)*
Synthetic graft (35638)

🔳 67.5   ✂ 67.5   **FUD** 090   C 80 ▣

AMA: 2018,Jan,8; 2017,Jan,8; 2016,Jan,13; 2015,Jan,16; 2014,Jan,11

Blockage in lower aorta

Aorta

Common iliac

Femoral

Femoral arteries (bilateral graft shown)

26/TC PC/TC Only   A2-Z3 ASC Payment   50 Bilateral   ♂ Male Only   ♀ Female Only   🔳 Facility RVU   ✂ Non-Facility RVU   ▣ CCI   ✖ CLIA
FUD Follow-up Days   CMS: IOM   AMA: CPT Asst   A-Y OPPSI   80/80 Surg Assist Allowed / w/Doc   Lab Crosswalk   Radiology Crosswalk

158   CPT © 2019 American Medical Association. All Rights Reserved.   © 2019 Optum360, LLC

35539   aortofemoral

> EXCLUDES   *Bypass graft, with vein; aortobifemoral (35540)*
> *Synthetic graft (35647)*

🚑 63.3   ⚕ 63.3   **FUD** 090   C 80 50 ▢

AMA: 2018,Jan,8; 2017,Jan,8; 2016,Jan,13; 2015,Jan,16; 2014,Jan,11

35540   aortobifemoral

> EXCLUDES   *Bypass graft, with vein; aortofemoral (35539)*
> *Synthetic graft (35646)*

🚑 70.6   ⚕ 70.6   **FUD** 090   C 50 ▢

AMA: 2018,Jan,8; 2017,Jan,8; 2016,Jan,13; 2015,Jan,16; 2014,Jan,11

35556   femoral-popliteal

🚑 40.5   ⚕ 40.5   **FUD** 090   C 80 50 ▢

AMA: 2018,Jan,8; 2017,Jan,8; 2016,Jan,13; 2015,Jan,16; 2014,Jan,11

35558   femoral-femoral

🚑 35.6   ⚕ 35.6   **FUD** 090   C 80 50 ▢

AMA: 2012,Apr,3-9; 1999,Mar,6

35560   aortorenal

🚑 49.2   ⚕ 49.2   **FUD** 090   C 80 50 ▢

AMA: 2018,Jan,8; 2017,Jan,8; 2016,Jan,13; 2015,Jan,16; 2014,Jan,11

35563   ilioiliac

🚑 38.2   ⚕ 38.2   **FUD** 090   C 80 50 ▢

AMA: 1999,Mar,6; 1999,Apr,11

35565   iliofemoral

🚑 38.1   ⚕ 38.1   **FUD** 090   C 80 50 ▢

AMA: 2012,Apr,3-9; 2004,Oct,6

35566   femoral-anterior tibial, posterior tibial, peroneal artery or other distal vessels

🚑 48.3   ⚕ 48.3   **FUD** 090   C 80 50 ▢

AMA: 2018,Jan,8; 2017,Jan,8; 2016,Jan,13; 2015,Jan,16; 2014,Jan,11

35570   tibial-tibial, peroneal-tibial, or tibial/peroneal trunk-tibial

> EXCLUDES   *Repair of blood vessel with graft (35256, 35286)*

🚑 43.7   ⚕ 43.7   **FUD** 090   C 80 50 ▢

AMA: 2018,Jan,8; 2017,Jan,8; 2016,Jan,13; 2015,Jan,16; 2014,Jan,11

35571   popliteal-tibial, -peroneal artery or other distal vessels

🚑 38.3   ⚕ 38.3   **FUD** 090   C 80 50 ▢

AMA: 2018,Jan,8; 2017,Jan,8; 2016,Jan,13; 2015,Jan,16; 2014,Jan,11

35572 Obtain Femoropopliteal Vein for Graft

> EXCLUDES   *Reporting with modifier 50. Report once for each side when performed bilaterally*

Code first (33510-33523, 33533-33536, 34502, 34520, 35001-35002, 35011-35022, 35102-35103, 35121-35152, 35231-35256, 35501-35587, 35879-35907)

\+   **35572**   Harvest of femoropopliteal vein, 1 segment, for vascular reconstruction procedure (eg, aortic, vena caval, coronary, peripheral artery) (List separately in addition to code for primary procedure)

🚑 10.0   ⚕ 10.0   **FUD** ZZZ   50 N N1 80 ▢

AMA: 2018,Jan,8; 2017,Jan,8; 2016,Jan,13; 2015,Jan,16; 2014,Jan,11

35583-35587 Lower Extremity Revascularization: In-situ Vein Bypass

> INCLUDES   Obtaining saphenous vein grafts
> EXCLUDES   *Obtaining multiple vein segments (35682, 35683)*
> *Obtaining vein graft, upper extremity or femoropopliteal (35500, 35572)*

35583   In-situ vein bypass; femoral-popliteal

Code also aortobifemoral bypass graft other than vein for aortobifemoral bypass using synthetic conduit and femoral-popliteal bypass with vein conduit in situ (35646)

Code also concurrent aortofemoral bypass for aortofemoral bypass graft with synthetic conduit and femoral-popliteal bypass with vein conduit in-situ (35647)

Code also concurrent aortofemoral bypass (vein) for an aortofemoral bypass using a vein conduit or a femoral-popliteal bypass with vein conduit in-situ (35539)

🚑 41.8   ⚕ 41.8   **FUD** 090   C 80 50 ▢

AMA: 2018,Jan,8; 2017,Jan,8; 2016,Jan,13; 2015,Jan,16; 2014,Jan,11

35585   femoral-anterior tibial, posterior tibial, or peroneal artery

🚑 48.4   ⚕ 48.4   **FUD** 090   C 80 50 ▢

AMA: 2018,Jan,8; 2017,Jan,8; 2016,Jan,13; 2015,Jan,16; 2014,Jan,11

35587   popliteal-tibial, peroneal

🚑 39.5   ⚕ 39.5   **FUD** 090   C 80 50 ▢

AMA: 2018,Jan,8; 2017,Jan,8; 2016,Jan,13; 2015,Jan,16; 2014,Jan,11

35600 Obtain Arm Artery for Coronary Bypass

> EXCLUDES   *Transposition and/or reimplantation of arteries (35691-35695)*

Code first (33533-33536)

\+   **35600**   Harvest of upper extremity artery, 1 segment, for coronary artery bypass procedure (List separately in addition to code for primary procedure)

🚑 7.43   ⚕ 7.43   **FUD** ZZZ   C 80 ▢

AMA: 2018,Jan,8; 2017,Jan,8; 2016,Jan,13; 2015,Jan,16; 2014,Jan,11

Median

Ulnar

Radial

An upper extremity artery or segment is harvested for a coronary artery bypass procedure

35601-35671 Arterial Bypass: Grafts Other Than Veins

EXCLUDES *Transposition and/or reimplantation of arteries (35691-35695)*

35601 **Bypass graft, with other than vein; common carotid-ipsilateral internal carotid**

EXCLUDES *Open transcervical common carotid-common carotid bypass with endovascular repair of descending thoracic aorta (33891)*

📋 40.4   ⚕ 40.4   **FUD** 090   C 80 50 ▱

AMA: 2018,Jan,8; 2017,Jan,8; 2016,Jan,13; 2015,Jan,16; 2014,Jan,11

35606 **carotid-subclavian**

EXCLUDES *Open subclavian to carotid artery transposition performed with endovascular thoracic aneurysm repair via neck incision (33889)*

📋 34.0   ⚕ 34.0   **FUD** 090   C 80 50 ▱

AMA: 1997,Nov,1

35612 **subclavian-subclavian**

📋 30.1   ⚕ 30.1   **FUD** 090   C 80 50 ▱

AMA: 1997,Nov,1

35616 **subclavian-axillary**

📋 31.8   ⚕ 31.8   **FUD** 090   C 80 50 ▱

AMA: 1997,Nov,1

35621 **axillary-femoral**

📋 31.7   ⚕ 31.7   **FUD** 090   C 80 50 ▱

AMA: 2018,Jan,8; 2017,Jan,8; 2016,Jan,13; 2015,Jan,16; 2014,Jan,11

35623 **axillary-popliteal or -tibial**

📋 37.9   ⚕ 37.9   **FUD** 090   C 80 50 ▱

AMA: 2012,Apr,3-9; 1997,Nov,1

35626 **aortosubclavian, aortoinnominate, or aortocarotid**

📋 46.0   ⚕ 46.0   **FUD** 090   C 80 50 ▱

AMA: 1997,Nov,1

35631 **aortoceliac, aortomesenteric, aortorenal**

📋 53.7   ⚕ 53.7   **FUD** 090   C 80 50 ▱

AMA: 1997,Nov,1

Vena cava and renal veins / Celiac trunk / Abdominal aorta / Superior mesenteric / Renal / Abdominal aorta as it exits diaphragm / Synthetic graft / Blockage

35632 **ilio-celiac**

📋 52.2   ⚕ 52.2   **FUD** 090   C 80 50 ▱

EXCLUDES *Bypass graft (35531, 35631)*
        Repair of blood vessel (35221, 35251, 35281)

35633 **ilio-mesenteric**

📋 57.8   ⚕ 57.8   **FUD** 090   C 80 50 ▱

EXCLUDES *Bypass graft (35531, 35631)*
        Repair of blood vessel (35221, 35251, 35281)

35634 **iliorenal**

📋 51.0   ⚕ 51.0   **FUD** 090   C 80 50 ▱

EXCLUDES *Bypass graft (35536, 35560, 35631)*
        Repair of blood vessel (35221, 35251, 35281)

35636 **splenorenal (splenic to renal arterial anastomosis)**

📋 46.0   ⚕ 46.0   **FUD** 090   C 80 50 ▱

AMA: 1997,Nov,1; 1994,Win,1

35637 **aortoiliac**

EXCLUDES *Bypass graft (35638, 35646)*

📋 47.9   ⚕ 47.9   **FUD** 090   C 80 ▱

AMA: 2018,Jan,8; 2017,Jan,8; 2016,Jan,13; 2015,Jan,16; 2014,Jan,11

35638 **aortobi-iliac**

EXCLUDES *Bypass graft (35637, 35646)*
        Open placement of aorto-bi-iliac prosthesis after a failed endovascular repair (34831)

📋 50.9   ⚕ 50.9   **FUD** 090   C 80 ▱

AMA: 2018,Jan,8; 2017,Jan,8; 2016,Jan,13; 2015,Jan,16; 2014,Jan,11

35642 **carotid-vertebral**

📋 28.4   ⚕ 28.4   **FUD** 090   C 80 50 ▱

AMA: 1997,Nov,1

35645 **subclavian-vertebral**

📋 27.3   ⚕ 27.3   **FUD** 090   C 80 50 ▱

AMA: 1997,Nov,1

35646 **aortobifemoral**

EXCLUDES *Bypass graft using vein graft (35540)*
        Open placement of aortobifemoral prosthesis after a failed endovascular repair (34832)

📋 49.7   ⚕ 49.7   **FUD** 090   C 80 ▱

AMA: 2018,Jan,8; 2017,Jan,8; 2016,Jan,13; 2015,Jan,16; 2014,Jan,11

35647 **aortofemoral**

EXCLUDES *Bypass graft using vein graft (35539)*

📋 45.0   ⚕ 45.0   **FUD** 090   C 80 50 ▱

AMA: 2018,Jan,8; 2017,Jan,8; 2016,Jan,13; 2015,Jan,16; 2014,Jan,11

35650 **axillary-axillary**

📋 31.3   ⚕ 31.3   **FUD** 090   C 80 50 ▱

AMA: 1997,Nov,1

35654 **axillary-femoral-femoral**

📋 39.6   ⚕ 39.6   **FUD** 090   C 80 ▱

AMA: 2018,Jan,8; 2017,Jan,8; 2016,Jan,13; 2015,Jan,16; 2014,Jan,11

35656 **femoral-popliteal**

📋 31.3   ⚕ 31.3   **FUD** 090   C 80 50 ▱

AMA: 2018,Jan,8; 2017,Jan,8; 2016,Jan,13; 2015,Jan,16; 2014,Jan,11

35661 **femoral-femoral**

📋 31.4   ⚕ 31.4   **FUD** 090   C 80 50 ▱

AMA: 2018,Jan,8; 2017,Jan,8; 2016,Jan,13; 2015,Jan,16; 2014,Jan,11

35663 **ilioiliac**

📋 35.1   ⚕ 35.1   **FUD** 090   C 80 50 ▱

AMA: 1997,Nov,1

35665 **iliofemoral**

📋 34.0   ⚕ 34.0   **FUD** 090   C 80 50 ▱

AMA: 2018,Jan,8; 2017,Jan,8; 2016,Jan,13; 2015,Jan,16; 2014,Jan,11

35666 **femoral-anterior tibial, posterior tibial, or peroneal artery**

📋 36.6   ⚕ 36.6   **FUD** 090   C 80 50 ▱

AMA: 2018,Jan,8; 2017,Jan,8; 2016,Jan,13; 2015,Jan,16; 2014,Jan,11

35671 **popliteal-tibial or -peroneal artery**

📋 32.2   ⚕ 32.2   **FUD** 090   C 80 50 ▱

AMA: 2012,Apr,3-9; 1997,Nov,1

2G/TC PC/TC Only   A2-Z3 ASC Payment   50 Bilateral   ♂ Male Only   ♀ Female Only   📋 Facility RVU   ⚕ Non-Facility RVU   ▱ CCI   ✖ CLIA
FUD Follow-up Days   CMS: IOM   AMA: CPT Asst   A-Y OPPSI   80/80 Surg Assist Allowed / w/Doc   ▤ Lab Crosswalk   ▥ Radiology Crosswalk

160   CPT © 2019 American Medical Association. All Rights Reserved.   © 2019 Optum360, LLC

35681-35683 Arterial Bypass Using Combination Synthetic and Donor Graft

INCLUDES   Acquiring multiple segments of vein from sites other than the extremity for which the arterial bypass is performed
Anastomosis of vein segments to create bypass graft conduits

+   35681   Bypass graft; composite, prosthetic and vein (List separately in addition to code for primary procedure)

EXCLUDES   Bypass graft (35682, 35683)
Code first primary procedure
🔲 2.34   ⚕ 2.34   **FUD** ZZZ   C 80 ▣

AMA: 2018,Jan,8; 2017,Jan,8; 2016,Jan,13; 2015,Jan,16; 2014,Jan,11

+   35682   autogenous composite, 2 segments of veins from 2 locations (List separately in addition to code for primary procedure)

EXCLUDES   Bypass graft (35681, 35683)
Code first (35556, 35566, 35570-35571, 35583-35587)
🔲 10.2   ⚕ 10.2   **FUD** ZZZ   C 80 ▣

AMA: 2018,Jan,8; 2017,Jan,8; 2016,Jan,13; 2015,Jan,16; 2014,Jan,11

+   35683   autogenous composite, 3 or more segments of vein from 2 or more locations (List separately in addition to code for primary procedure)

EXCLUDES   Bypass graft (35681-35682)
Code first (35556, 35566, 35570-35571, 35583-35587)
🔲 11.8   ⚕ 11.8   **FUD** ZZZ   C 80 ▣

AMA: 2018,Jan,8; 2017,Jan,8; 2016,Jan,13; 2015,Jan,16; 2014,Jan,11

35685-35686 Supplemental Procedures

INCLUDES   Additional procedures that may be needed with a bypass graft to increase the patency of the graft
EXCLUDES   Composite grafts (35681-35683)

+   35685   Placement of vein patch or cuff at distal anastomosis of bypass graft, synthetic conduit (List separately in addition to code for primary procedure)

INCLUDES   Connection of a segment of vein (cuff or patch) between the distal portion of the synthetic graft and the native artery
Code first (35656, 35666, 35671)
🔲 5.76   ⚕ 5.76   **FUD** ZZZ   N 80 ▣

AMA: 2018,Jan,8; 2017,Jan,8; 2016,Jan,13; 2015,Jan,16; 2014,Jan,11

+   35686   Creation of distal arteriovenous fistula during lower extremity bypass surgery (non-hemodialysis) (List separately in addition to code for primary procedure)

INCLUDES   Creation of a fistula between the peroneal or tibial artery and vein at or past the site of the distal anastomosis
Code first (35556, 35566, 35570-35571, 35583-35587, 35623, 35656, 35666, 35671)
🔲 4.66   ⚕ 4.66   **FUD** ZZZ   N 80 ▣

AMA: 2018,Jan,8; 2017,Jan,8; 2016,Jan,13; 2015,Jan,16; 2014,Jan,11

35691-35697 Arterial Translocation

CMS: 100-03,160.8 Electroencephalographic Monitoring During Cerebral Vasculature Surgery

35691   Transposition and/or reimplantation; vertebral to carotid artery
🔲 27.2   ⚕ 27.2   **FUD** 090   C 80 50 ▣
AMA: 1997,Nov,1; 1993,Win,1

35693   vertebral to subclavian artery
🔲 24.0   ⚕ 24.0   **FUD** 090   C 80 50 ▣
AMA: 1997,Nov,1; 1994,Sum,29

35694   subclavian to carotid artery
EXCLUDES   Subclavian to carotid artery transposition procedure (open) with concurrent repair of descending thoracic aorta (endovascular) (33889)
🔲 28.5   ⚕ 28.5   **FUD** 090   C 80 50 ▣
AMA: 1997,Nov,1; 1993,Win,1

35695   carotid to subclavian artery
🔲 29.5   ⚕ 29.5   **FUD** 090   C 80 50 ▣
AMA: 1997,Nov,1; 1993,Win,1

+   35697   Reimplantation, visceral artery to infrarenal aortic prosthesis, each artery (List separately in addition to code for primary procedure)
EXCLUDES   Repair of thoracoabdominal aortic aneurysm with graft (33877)
Code first primary procedure
🔲 4.30   ⚕ 4.30   **FUD** ZZZ   C 80 ▣
AMA: 1997,Nov,1

35700 Reoperative Bypass Lower Extremities

Code first (35556, 35566, 35570-35571, 35583, 35585, 35587, 35656, 35666, 35671)

+   35700   Reoperation, femoral-popliteal or femoral (popliteal)-anterior tibial, posterior tibial, peroneal artery, or other distal vessels, more than 1 month after original operation (List separately in addition to code for primary procedure)
🔲 4.42   ⚕ 4.42   **FUD** ZZZ   C 80 ▣
AMA: 2018,Jan,8; 2017,Jan,8; 2016,Jan,13; 2015,Jan,16; 2014,Jan,11

35701-35761 Arterial Exploration without Repair

EXCLUDES   Exploration to identify recipient artery for microvascular anastomosis of free graft/flap of:
Bone (20955-20962)
Jejunum (43496)
Muscle, skin or fascia (15756-15758)
Omentum (49906)
Osteocutaneous (20969-20973)
Exploration without surgical repair of:
Abdominal artery (49000)
Chest artery (32100)
Other arteries not of the neck, upper or lower extremities, chest, abdomen or retroperitoneum (37799)
Retroperitoneal artery (49010)
Code also nonvascular surgical procedures performed in addition to exploration when the exploration is through a separate incision

▲   35701   Exploration not followed by surgical repair, artery; neck (eg, carotid, subclavian)
EXCLUDES   Exploration for postoperative hemorrhage, thrombosis or infection (35800)
Repair of blood vessel on same side of neck (35201, 35231, 35261)
🔲 16.4   ⚕ 16.4   **FUD** 090   C 80 50 ▣
AMA: 1997,Nov,1

●   35702   upper extremity (eg, axillary, brachial, radial, ulnar)
EXCLUDES   Exploration for postoperative hemorrhage, thrombosis or infection in same extremity (35860)
Repair of blood vessel in same extremity (35206-35207, 35236, 35266)

●   35703   lower extremity (eg, common femoral, deep femoral, superficial femoral, popliteal, tibial, peroneal)
EXCLUDES   Exploration for postoperative hemorrhage, thrombosis or infection in same extremity (35860)
Repair of blood vessel in same extremity (35256, 35286)

~~35721~~   ~~femoral artery~~

~~35741~~   ~~popliteal artery~~

~~35761~~   ~~other vessels~~

35800-35860 Arterial Exploration for Postoperative Complication

INCLUDES   Return to the operating room for postoperative hemorrhage

35800   Exploration for postoperative hemorrhage, thrombosis or infection; neck
🔲 20.8   ⚕ 20.8   **FUD** 090   C 80 ▣
AMA: 1997,Nov,1

35820   chest
🔲 58.3   ⚕ 58.3   **FUD** 090   C 80 ▣
AMA: 1997,Nov,1

● New Code   ▲ Revised Code   ○ Reinstated   ● New Web Release   ▲ Revised Web Release   + Add-on   Unlisted   Not Covered   # Resequenced
50 Optum Mod 50 Exempt   ⊘ AMA Mod 51 Exempt   51 Optum Mod 51 Exempt   63 Mod 63 Exempt   ✂ Non-FDA Drug   ★ Telemedicine   M Maternity   A Age Edit

35840 **abdomen**
🖥 34.6 ⚕ 34.6 **FUD** 090
AMA: 1997,May,4; 1997,Nov,1
C 80

35860 **extremity**
🖥 24.2 ⚕ 24.2 **FUD** 090
AMA: 2018,Jan,8; 2017,Jan,8; 2016,Jan,13; 2015,Jan,16; 2014,Apr,10
T 80

35870 Repair Secondary Aortoenteric Fistula

35870 **Repair of graft-enteric fistula**
🖥 35.9 ⚕ 35.9 **FUD** 090
AMA: 1997,Nov,1
C 80

35875-35876 Removal of Thrombus from Graft

EXCLUDES Thrombectomy dialysis fistula or graft (36831, 36833)
Thrombectomy with blood vessel repair, lower extremity, vein graft (35256)
Thrombectomy with blood vessel repair, lower extremity, with/without patch angioplasty (35226)

35875 **Thrombectomy of arterial or venous graft (other than hemodialysis graft or fistula);**
🖥 17.2 ⚕ 17.2 **FUD** 090
AMA: 2018,Jan,8; 2017,Jan,8; 2016,Jan,13; 2015,Jan,16; 2014,Jan,11
T A2

35876 **with revision of arterial or venous graft**
🖥 27.4 ⚕ 27.4 **FUD** 090
AMA: 1999,Mar,6; 1999,Nov,1
T A2 80

35879-35884 Revision Lower Extremity Bypass Graft

EXCLUDES Removal of infected graft (35901-35907)
Revascularization following removal of infected graft(s)
Thrombectomy dialysis fistula or graft (36831, 36833)
Thrombectomy with blood vessel repair, lower extremity, vein graft (35256)
Thrombectomy with blood vessel repair, lower extremity, with/without patch angioplasty (35226)
Thrombectomy with graft revision (35876)

35879 **Revision, lower extremity arterial bypass, without thrombectomy, open; with vein patch angioplasty**
🖥 26.8 ⚕ 26.8 **FUD** 090
AMA: 2018,Jan,8; 2017,Jan,8; 2016,Jan,13; 2015,Jan,16; 2014,Jan,11
T 80 50

35881 **with segmental vein interposition**
EXCLUDES Revision of femoral anastomosis of synthetic arterial bypass graft (35883-35884)
🖥 29.4 ⚕ 29.4 **FUD** 090
AMA: 2018,Jan,8; 2017,Jan,8; 2016,Jan,13; 2015,Jan,16; 2014,Jan,11
T 80 50

35883 **Revision, femoral anastomosis of synthetic arterial bypass graft in groin, open; with nonautogenous patch graft (eg, Dacron, ePTFE, bovine pericardium)**
EXCLUDES Reoperation, femoral-popliteal or femoral (popliteal)-anterior tibial, posterior tibial, peroneal artery, or other distal vessels (35700)
Revision, femoral anastomosis of synthetic arterial bypass graft in groin, open; with autogenous vein patch graft (35884)
Thrombectomy of arterial or venous graft (35875)
🖥 34.8 ⚕ 34.8 **FUD** 090
AMA: 2018,Jan,8; 2017,Jan,8; 2016,Jan,13; 2015,Jan,16; 2014,Jan,11
T 80 50

35884 **with autogenous vein patch graft**
EXCLUDES Reoperation, femoral-popliteal or femoral (popliteal)-anterior tibial, posterior tibial, peroneal artery, or other distal vessels (35700)
Revision, femoral anastomosis of synthetic arterial bypass graft in groin, open; with autogenous vein patch graft (35883)
Thrombectomy of arterial or venous graft (35875-35876)
🖥 35.8 ⚕ 35.8 **FUD** 090
AMA: 2018,Jan,8; 2017,Jan,8; 2016,Jan,13; 2015,Jan,16; 2014,Jan,11
T 80 50

35901-35907 Removal of Infected Graft

35901 **Excision of infected graft; neck**
🖥 13.5 ⚕ 13.5 **FUD** 090
AMA: 1997,Nov,1; 1993,Win,1
C 80

The physician removes an infected graft from the neck and repairs the blood vessel. If a new graft is placed, report the appropriate revascularization code

35903 **extremity**
🖥 16.3 ⚕ 16.3 **FUD** 090
AMA: 2018,Aug,10
T 80

35905 **thorax**
🖥 48.5 ⚕ 48.5 **FUD** 090
AMA: 1997,Nov,1; 1993,Win,1
C 80

35907 **abdomen**
🖥 55.2 ⚕ 55.2 **FUD** 090
AMA: 1997,Nov,1; 1993,Win,1
C 80

36000 Intravenous Access Established

INCLUDES Venous access for phlebotomy, prophylactic intravenous access, infusion therapy, chemotherapy, hydration, transfusion, drug administration, etc. which is included in the work value of the primary procedure

36000 **Introduction of needle or intracatheter, vein**
🖥 0.27 ⚕ 0.77 **FUD** XXX
AMA: 2019,Aug,8; 2018,Mar,3; 2018,Jan,8; 2017,Jan,8; 2016,Nov,3; 2016,Jan,13; 2015,Jan,16; 2014,Oct,6; 2014,Sep,13; 2014,May,4; 2014,Jan,11
N N1

36002 Injection Treatment of Pseudoaneurysm

INCLUDES Insertion of needle or catheter, local anesthesia, injection of contrast, power injections, and all pre- and postinjection care provided
EXCLUDES Arteriotomy site sealant
Compression repair pseudoaneurysm, ultrasound guided (76936)
Medications, contrast material, catheters

36002 **Injection procedures (eg, thrombin) for percutaneous treatment of extremity pseudoaneurysm**
🔀 (76942, 77002, 77012, 77021)
🖥 3.04 ⚕ 4.49 **FUD** 000
AMA: 2018,Mar,3; 2018,Jan,8; 2017,Jan,8; 2016,Nov,3; 2016,Jan,13; 2015,Jan,16; 2014,Oct,6; 2014,Jan,11
T 62 50

36005-36015 Insertion Needle or Intracatheter: Venous

INCLUDES Insertion of needle/catheter, local anesthesia, injection of contrast, power injections, all pre- and postinjection care
EXCLUDES Medications, contrast materials, catheters
Code also catheterization of second order vessels (or higher) supplied by the same first order branch, same vascular family (36012)
Code also each vascular family (e.g., bilateral procedures are separate vascular families)

36005 **Injection procedure for extremity venography (including introduction of needle or intracatheter)**
🔀 (75820, 75822)
🖥 1.40 ⚕ 8.76 **FUD** 000
AMA: 2018,Mar,3; 2018,Jan,8; 2017,Jan,8; 2016,Nov,3; 2016,Jul,6; 2016,Jan,13; 2015,Jan,16; 2014,Oct,6
N N1 80 50

26/TC PC/TC Only	A2-Z3 ASC Payment	50 Bilateral	♂ Male Only	♀ Female Only	🖥 Facility RVU	⚕ Non-Facility RVU	CCI	🔲 CLIA
FUD Follow-up Days	CMS: IOM	AMA: CPT Asst	A-Y OPPSI	80/80 Surg Assist Allowed / w/Doc	Lab Crosswalk	Radiology Crosswalk		

162
CPT © 2019 American Medical Association. All Rights Reserved.
© 2019 Optum360, LLC

36010 **Introduction of catheter, superior or inferior vena cava**

🔲 3.19   🔲 14.2   **FUD** XXX   🔲 🔲 50 🔲

AMA: 2018,Jan,8; 2017,Feb,14; 2017,Jan,8; 2016,Jul,6; 2016,Jan,13; 2015,Jan,16; 2014,Jan,11

36011 **Selective catheter placement, venous system; first order branch (eg, renal vein, jugular vein)**

🔲 4.54   🔲 24.0   **FUD** XXX   🔲 🔲 50 🔲

AMA: 2018,Jan,8; 2017,Jan,8; 2016,Jul,6; 2016,Jan,13; 2015,Jan,16; 2014,Jan,11

36012 **second order, or more selective, branch (eg, left adrenal vein, petrosal sinus)**

🔲 5.03   🔲 24.5   **FUD** XXX   🔲 🔲 50 🔲

AMA: 2018,Oct,3; 2018,Jan,8; 2017,Jan,8; 2016,Jul,6; 2016,Jan,13; 2015,Jan,16; 2014,Jan,11

36013 **Introduction of catheter, right heart or main pulmonary artery**

🔲 3.52   🔲 21.8   **FUD** XXX   🔲 🔲 🔲

AMA: 2019,Jun,3; 2018,Jan,8; 2017,Jan,8; 2016,Jul,6; 2016,Jan,13; 2015,Jan,16; 2014,Jan,11

36014 **Selective catheter placement, left or right pulmonary artery**

🔲 4.38   🔲 23.0   **FUD** XXX   🔲 🔲 50 🔲

AMA: 2019,Jun,3; 2018,Jan,8; 2017,Jan,8; 2016,Jul,6; 2016,Jan,13; 2015,Jan,16; 2014,Jan,11

36015 **Selective catheter placement, segmental or subsegmental pulmonary artery**

EXCLUDES   *Placement of Swan Ganz/other flow directed catheter for monitoring (93503)*
Selective blood sampling, specific organs (36500)

🔲 4.98   🔲 24.9   **FUD** XXX   🔲 🔲 50 🔲

AMA: 2019,Jun,3; 2018,Jan,8; 2017,Jan,8; 2016,Jul,6; 2016,Jan,13; 2015,Jan,16; 2014,Jan,11

36100-36218 Insertion Needle or Intracatheter: Arterial

INCLUDES   Introduction of the catheter and catheterization of all lesser order vessels used for the approach
Local anesthesia, placement of catheter/needle, injection of contrast, power injections, all pre- and postinjection care

EXCLUDES   *Angiography (36222-36228, 75600-75774)*
Angioplasty ([37246, 37247])
Chemotherapy injections (96401-96549)
Injection procedures for cardiac catheterizations (93455, 93457, 93459, 93461, 93530-93533, 93564)
Internal mammary artery angiography without left heart catheterization (36216, 36217)
Medications, contrast, catheters
Transcatheter interventions (37200, 37211, 37213-37214, 37241-37244, 61624, 61626)

Code also additional first order or higher catheterization for vascular families if the vascular family is supplied by a first order vessel that is different from one already coded
Code also catheterization of second and third order vessels supplied by the same first order branch, same vascular family (36218, 36248)

36100 **Introduction of needle or intracatheter, carotid or vertebral artery**

🔲 4.54   🔲 14.8   **FUD** XXX   🔲 🔲 50 🔲

AMA: 2000,Oct,4; 1998,Apr,1

36140 **Introduction of needle or intracatheter, upper or lower extremity artery**

EXCLUDES   *Arteriovenous cannula insertion (36810-36821)*

🔲 2.62   🔲 12.7   **FUD** XXX   🔲 🔲 🔲

AMA: 2018,Jan,8; 2017,Jan,8; 2016,Jan,13; 2015,Jan,16; 2014,Jan,11

36160 **Introduction of needle or intracatheter, aortic, translumbar**

🔲 3.59   🔲 14.6   **FUD** XXX   🔲 🔲 🔲

AMA: 2018,Jan,8; 2017,Jan,8; 2016,Jan,13; 2015,Jan,16; 2014,Jan,11

36200 **Introduction of catheter, aorta**

EXCLUDES   *Nonselective angiography of the extracranial carotid and/or cerebral vessels and cervicocerebral arch (36221)*

🔲 4.05   🔲 16.2   **FUD** 000   🔲 🔲 50 🔲

AMA: 2018,Jan,8; 2017,Mar,3; 2017,Jan,8; 2016,Jul,6; 2016,Jan,13; 2015,Jan,16; 2014,Jan,11

36215 **Selective catheter placement, arterial system; each first order thoracic or brachiocephalic branch, within a vascular family**

INCLUDES   Introduction of catheter into the aorta (36200)

EXCLUDES   *Placement of catheter for coronary angiography (93454-93461)*

🔲 6.16   🔲 29.4   **FUD** 000   🔲 🔲 🔲

AMA: 2018,Jan,8; 2017,Mar,3; 2017,Jan,8; 2016,Jul,6; 2016,Jan,13; 2015,Jan,16; 2014,Jan,11

36216 **initial second order thoracic or brachiocephalic branch, within a vascular family**

🔲 7.93   🔲 31.6   **FUD** 000   🔲 🔲 🔲

AMA: 2018,Jan,8; 2017,Jan,8; 2016,Jul,6; 2016,Jan,13; 2015,Jan,16; 2014,Jan,11

36217 **initial third order or more selective thoracic or brachiocephalic branch, within a vascular family**

🔲 9.51   🔲 53.1   **FUD** 000   🔲 🔲 🔲

AMA: 2018,Jan,8; 2017,Jan,8; 2016,Jul,6; 2016,Jan,13; 2015,Jan,16; 2014,Jan,11

+ **36218** **additional second order, third order, and beyond, thoracic or brachiocephalic branch, within a vascular family (List in addition to code for initial second or third order vessel as appropriate)**

Code also transcatheter therapy procedures (37200, 37211, 37213-37214, 37236-37239, 37241-37244, 61624, 61626)
Code first (36216-36217, 36225-36226)

🔲 1.51   🔲 6.89   **FUD** ZZZ   🔲 🔲 🔲

AMA: 2018,Oct,3; 2018,Jan,8; 2017,Jan,8; 2016,Jul,6; 2016,Jan,13; 2015,Jan,16; 2014,Jan,11

36221-36228 Diagnostic Studies: Aortic Arch/Carotid/Vertebral Arteries

INCLUDES   Accessing the vessel
Arterial contrast injection that includes arterial, capillary, and venous phase imaging, when performed
Arteriotomy closure (pressure or closure device)
Catheter placement
Radiologic supervision and interpretation
Reporting of selective catheter placement based on intensity of services in the following hierarchy:
36226>36225
36224>36223>36222

EXCLUDES   *3D rendering when performed (76376-76377)*
Interventional procedures
Transcatheter intravascular stent placement of common carotid or innominate artery on the same side (37217)
Ultrasound guidance (76937)

Code also diagnostic angiography of upper extremities/other vascular beds during the same session, if performed (75774)

36221 **Non-selective catheter placement, thoracic aorta, with angiography of the extracranial carotid, vertebral, and/or intracranial vessels, unilateral or bilateral, and all associated radiological supervision and interpretation, includes angiography of the cervicocerebral arch, when performed**

EXCLUDES   *Selective catheter placement, common carotid or innominate artery (36222-36226)*
Transcatheter intravascular stent placement of common carotid or innominate artery on the same side (37217)

🔲 5.80   🔲 29.3   **FUD** 000   🔲 🔲 🔲

AMA: 2018,Jan,8; 2017,Jan,8; 2016,Mar,3; 2016,Jan,13; 2015,Nov,3; 2015,May,7; 2015,Jan,16; 2014,Mar,8; 2014,Jan,11

36222 Selective catheter placement, common carotid or innominate artery, unilateral, any approach, with angiography of the ipsilateral extracranial carotid circulation and all associated radiological supervision and interpretation, includes angiography of the cervicocerebral arch, when performed

INCLUDES Unilateral catheterization of artery

EXCLUDES *Transcatheter placement of intravascular stent(s) (37215-37218)*

Code also modifier 59 when different territories on both sides of the body are being studied

🖾 8.22 ⚕ 34.7 **FUD** 000 02 N1 50 ▣

AMA: 2018,Jan,8; 2017,Jan,8; 2016,Mar,3; 2016,Jan,13; 2015,Nov,3; 2015,Nov,10; 2015,May,7; 2015,Jan,16; 2014,Mar,8; 2014,Jan,11

36223 Selective catheter placement, common carotid or innominate artery, unilateral, any approach, with angiography of the ipsilateral intracranial carotid circulation and all associated radiological supervision and interpretation, includes angiography of the extracranial carotid and cervicocerebral arch, when performed

INCLUDES Unilateral catheterization of artery

EXCLUDES *Transcatheter placement of intravascular stent(s) (37215-37218)*

Code also modifier 59 when different territories on both sides of the body are being studied

🖾 9.18 ⚕ 43.9 **FUD** 000 02 N1 50 ▣

AMA: 2018,Jan,8; 2017,Jan,8; 2016,Mar,3; 2016,Jan,13; 2015,Nov,3; 2015,Jan,16; 2014,Mar,8; 2014,Jan,11

36224 Selective catheter placement, internal carotid artery, unilateral, with angiography of the ipsilateral intracranial carotid circulation and all associated radiological supervision and interpretation, includes angiography of the extracranial carotid and cervicocerebral arch, when performed

INCLUDES Unilateral catheterization of artery

EXCLUDES *Transcatheter placement of intravascular stent(s) (37215-37218)*

Code also modifier 59 when different territories on both sides of the body are being studied

🖾 10.4 ⚕ 56.8 **FUD** 000 02 N1 50 ▣

AMA: 2018,Jan,8; 2017,Jan,8; 2016,Mar,3; 2016,Jan,13; 2015,Nov,3; 2015,Jan,16; 2014,Mar,8; 2014,Jan,11

36225 Selective catheter placement, subclavian or innominate artery, unilateral, with angiography of the ipsilateral vertebral circulation and all associated radiological supervision and interpretation, includes angiography of the cervicocerebral arch, when performed

EXCLUDES *Transcatheter placement of intravascular stent(s) (37217)*

🖾 9.16 ⚕ 42.3 **FUD** 000 02 N1 50 ▣

AMA: 2018,Jan,8; 2017,Jan,8; 2016,Mar,3; 2016,Jan,13; 2015,Nov,3; 2015,Jan,16; 2014,Mar,8; 2014,Jan,11

36226 Selective catheter placement, vertebral artery, unilateral, with angiography of the ipsilateral vertebral circulation and all associated radiological supervision and interpretation, includes angiography of the cervicocerebral arch, when performed

EXCLUDES *Transcatheter placement of intravascular stent(s) (37217)*

🖾 10.3 ⚕ 53.7 **FUD** 000 02 N1 50 ▣

AMA: 2018,Jan,8; 2017,Jan,8; 2016,Mar,3; 2016,Jan,13; 2015,Nov,3; 2015,Jan,16; 2014,Mar,8

+ **36227** Selective catheter placement, external carotid artery, unilateral, with angiography of the ipsilateral external carotid circulation and all associated radiological supervision and interpretation (List separately in addition to code for primary procedure)

INCLUDES Unilateral catheter placement/diagnostic imaging of ipsilateral external carotid circulation

EXCLUDES *Reporting with modifier 50. Report once for each side when performed bilaterally*
Transcatheter placement of intravascular stent(s) (37217)

Code first (36222-36224)

🖾 3.41 ⚕ 7.23 **FUD** ZZZ 60 N N1 ▣

AMA: 2018,Jan,8; 2017,Jan,8; 2016,Jan,13; 2015,Nov,10; 2015,Jan,16; 2014,Mar,8; 2014,Jan,11

+ **36228** Selective catheter placement, each intracranial branch of the internal carotid or vertebral arteries, unilateral, with angiography of the selected vessel circulation and all associated radiological supervision and interpretation (eg, middle cerebral artery, posterior inferior cerebellar artery) (List separately in addition to code for primary procedure)

INCLUDES Unilateral catheter placement/imaging of initial and each additional intracranial branch of internal carotid or vertebral arteries

EXCLUDES *Procedure performed more than 2 times per side*
Reporting with modifier 50. Report once for each side when performed bilaterally

Code first (36223-36226)

🖾 7.03 ⚕ 37.6 **FUD** ZZZ 60 N N1 ▣

AMA: 2018,Jan,8; 2017,Jan,8; 2016,Jan,13; 2015,Nov,3; 2015,Jan,16; 2014,Jan,11

36245-36254 Catheter Placement: Arteries of the Lower Body

INCLUDES Introduction of the catheter and catheterization of all lesser order vessels used for the approach
Local anesthesia, placement of catheter/needle, injection of contrast, power injections

EXCLUDES *Angiography (36222-36228, 75600-75774)*
Chemotherapy injections (96401-96549)
Injection procedures for cardiac catheterizations (93455, 93457, 93459, 93461, 93530-93533, 93564)
Internal mammary artery angiography without left heart catheterization (36216-36217)
Medications, contrast, catheters
Transcatheter procedures (37200, 37211, 37213-37214, 37236-37239, 37241-37244, 61624, 61626)

Code also additional first order or higher catheterization for vascular families if the vascular family is supplied by a first order vessel that is different from one already coded
Code also catheterization of second and third order vessels supplied by the same first order branch, same vascular family (36218, 36248)

🖾 (75600-75774)

36245 Selective catheter placement, arterial system; each first order abdominal, pelvic, or lower extremity artery branch, within a vascular family

🖾 6.89 ⚕ 37.4 **FUD** XXX N N1 50 ▣

AMA: 2018,Jan,8; 2017,Jan,8; 2016,Jul,6; 2016,Jan,13; 2015,Jan,16; 2014,Jan,11

36246 initial second order abdominal, pelvic, or lower extremity artery branch, within a vascular family

🖾 7.39 ⚕ 23.8 **FUD** 000 N N1 50 ▣

AMA: 2018,Jan,8; 2017,Jan,8; 2016,Jul,6; 2016,Jan,13; 2015,Jan,16; 2014,Jan,11

36247 initial third order or more selective abdominal, pelvic, or lower extremity artery branch, within a vascular family

🖾 8.78 ⚕ 42.6 **FUD** 000 N N1 50 ▣

AMA: 2018,Jan,8; 2017,Jan,8; 2016,Jul,6; 2016,Jan,13; 2015,Jan,16; 2014,Jan,11

26/TC PC/TC Only   A2-Z3 ASC Payment   50 Bilateral   ♂ Male Only   ♀ Female Only   🖾 Facility RVU   ⚕ Non-Facility RVU   ▣ CCI   ⊠ CLIA
FUD Follow-up Days   **CMS:** IOM   **AMA:** CPT Asst   A-Y OPPSI   80/80 Surg Assist Allowed / w/Doc   ▣ Lab Crosswalk   ⊞ Radiology Crosswalk

+ 36248 additional second order, third order, and beyond, abdominal, pelvic, or lower extremity artery branch, within a vascular family (List in addition to code for initial second or third order vessel as appropriate)

Code first (36246, 36247)

⏱ 1.42 ⚕ 4.11 **FUD** ZZZ N N1 ▭

AMA: 2018,Oct,3; 2018,Jan,8; 2017,Jan,8; 2016,Jul,6; 2016,Jan,13; 2015,Jan,16; 2014,Jan,11

36251 Selective catheter placement (first-order), main renal artery and any accessory renal artery(s) for renal angiography, including arterial puncture and catheter placement(s), fluoroscopy, contrast injection(s), image postprocessing, permanent recording of images, and radiological supervision and interpretation, including pressure gradient measurements when performed, and flush aortogram when performed; unilateral

INCLUDES Closure device placement at vascular access site

EXCLUDES *Transcatheter renal sympathetic denervation, percutaneous approach (0338T-0339T)*

⏱ 7.55 ⚕ 39.2 **FUD** 000 Q2 N1 ▭

AMA: 2018,Jan,8; 2017,Jan,8; 2016,Jan,13; 2015,Jan,16; 2014,Jan,11

36252 bilateral

INCLUDES Closure device placement at vascular access site

EXCLUDES *Transcatheter renal sympathetic denervation, percutaneous approach (0338T-0339T)*

⏱ 10.4 ⚕ 42.4 **FUD** 000 Q2 N1 ▭

AMA: 2018,Jan,8; 2017,Jan,8; 2016,Jan,13; 2015,Jan,16; 2014,Jan,11

36253 Superselective catheter placement (one or more second order or higher renal artery branches) renal artery and any accessory renal artery(s) for renal angiography, including arterial puncture, catheterization, fluoroscopy, contrast injection(s), image postprocessing, permanent recording of images, and radiological supervision and interpretation, including pressure gradient measurements when performed, and flush aortogram when performed; unilateral

INCLUDES Closure device placement at vascular access site

EXCLUDES *Procedure performed on same kidney with (36251)*
Transcatheter renal sympathetic denervation, percutaneous approach (0338T-0339T)

⏱ 10.3 ⚕ 62.6 **FUD** 000 Q2 N1 ▭

AMA: 2018,Jan,8; 2017,Jan,8; 2016,Jan,13; 2015,Jan,16; 2014,Jan,11

36254 bilateral

INCLUDES Closure device placement at vascular access site

EXCLUDES *Selective catheter placement (first-order), main renal artery and any accessory renal artery(s) for renal angiography (36252)*
Transcatheter renal sympathetic denervation, percutaneous approach (0338T-0339T)

⏱ 12.1 ⚕ 60.8 **FUD** 000 Q2 N1 ▭

AMA: 2018,Jan,8; 2017,Jan,8; 2016,Jan,13; 2015,Jan,16; 2014,Jan,11

36260-36299 Implanted Infusion Pumps: Intra-arterial

36260 Insertion of implantable intra-arterial infusion pump (eg, for chemotherapy of liver)

⏱ 18.8 ⚕ 18.8 **FUD** 090 T J8 ▭

AMA: 2018,Jan,8; 2017,Jan,8; 2016,Jan,13; 2015,Jan,16; 2014,Jan,11

36261 Revision of implanted intra-arterial infusion pump

⏱ 11.6 ⚕ 11.6 **FUD** 090 T J8 80 ▭

AMA: 2000,Oct,4; 1997,Nov,1

36262 Removal of implanted intra-arterial infusion pump

⏱ 8.90 ⚕ 8.90 **FUD** 090 Q2 G2 ▭

AMA: 2000,Oct,4; 1997,Nov,1

36299 Unlisted procedure, vascular injection

⏱ 0.00 ⚕ 0.00 **FUD** YYY N 80 ▭

AMA: 2000,Oct,4; 1997,Nov,1

36400-36425 Specimen Collection: Phlebotomy

EXCLUDES *Collection of specimen from:*
A completely implantable device (36591)
An established catheter (36592)

36400 Venipuncture, younger than age 3 years, necessitating the skill of a physician or other qualified health care professional, not to be used for routine venipuncture; femoral or jugular vein A

⏱ 0.53 ⚕ 0.75 **FUD** XXX N N1 ▭

AMA: 2018,Jan,8; 2017,Jan,8; 2016,Jan,13; 2015,Jan,16; 2014,May,4; 2014,Jan,11

36405 scalp vein A

⏱ 0.44 ⚕ 0.66 **FUD** XXX N N1 ▭

AMA: 2018,Jan,8; 2017,Jan,8; 2016,Jan,13; 2015,Jan,16; 2014,May,4; 2014,Jan,11

36406 other vein A

⏱ 0.25 ⚕ 0.47 **FUD** XXX N N1 ▭

AMA: 2018,Jan,8; 2017,Jan,8; 2016,Jan,13; 2015,Jan,16; 2014,May,4; 2014,Jan,11

36410 Venipuncture, age 3 years or older, necessitating the skill of a physician or other qualified health care professional (separate procedure), for diagnostic or therapeutic purposes (not to be used for routine venipuncture) A

⏱ 0.27 ⚕ 0.49 **FUD** XXX N N1 ▭

AMA: 2019,Aug,8; 2018,Mar,3; 2018,Jan,8; 2017,Jan,8; 2016,Nov,3; 2016,Jan,13; 2015,Jan,16; 2014,Oct,6; 2014,Jan,11

36415 Collection of venous blood by venipuncture

⏱ 0.00 ⚕ 0.00 **FUD** XXX 63 Q ▭

AMA: 2019,Aug,8; 2018,Jan,8; 2017,Jan,8; 2016,Jan,13; 2015,Jan,16; 2014,May,4; 2014,Jan,11

36416 Collection of capillary blood specimen (eg, finger, heel, ear stick)

⏱ 0.00 ⚕ 0.00 **FUD** XXX N N1 ▭

AMA: 2008,Apr,-9; 2003,Feb,7

36420 Venipuncture, cutdown; younger than age 1 year A

⏱ 1.35 ⚕ 1.35 **FUD** XXX 63 Q1 N1 80 ▭

AMA: 2018,Jan,8; 2017,Jan,8; 2016,Jan,13; 2015,Jan,16; 2014,Jan,11

36425 age 1 or over A

EXCLUDES *Endovenous ablation therapy of incompetent vein, extremity (36475-36476, 36478-36479)*

⏱ 1.16 ⚕ 1.16 **FUD** XXX Q1 N1 ▭

AMA: 2018,Mar,3; 2018,Jan,8; 2017,Jan,8; 2016,Nov,3; 2016,Jan,13; 2015,Jan,16; 2014,Oct,6

36430-36460 Transfusions

CMS: 100-01,3,20.5 Blood Deductibles; 100-03,110.16 Transfusion in Kidney Transplants; 100-03,110.7 Blood Transfusions; 100-03,110.8 Blood Platelet Transfusions

36430 Transfusion, blood or blood components

EXCLUDES *Infant partial exchange transfusion (36456)*

⏱ 0.99 ⚕ 0.99 **FUD** XXX S P3 ▭

AMA: 2019,Jun,5; 2018,Jan,8; 2017,Jul,3; 2017,Jan,8; 2016,Jan,13; 2015,Jan,16; 2014,Jan,11

36440 Push transfusion, blood, 2 years or younger A

EXCLUDES *Infant partial exchange transfusion (36456)*

⏱ 1.46 ⚕ 1.46 **FUD** XXX S R2 80 ▭

AMA: 2018,Jan,8; 2017,Jul,3; 2017,Jan,8; 2016,Jan,13; 2015,Jan,16; 2014,Jan,11

36450 Exchange transfusion, blood; newborn A

EXCLUDES *Infant partial exchange transfusion (36456)*

⏱ 4.94 ⚕ 4.94 **FUD** XXX 63 S R2 80 ▭

AMA: 2018,Jan,8; 2017,Jul,3

36455 other than newborn A

⏱ 3.68 ⚕ 3.68 **FUD** XXX S G2 ▭

AMA: 2003,Apr,7; 1997,Nov,1

36456   Partial exchange transfusion, blood, plasma or crystalloid necessitating the skill of a physician or other qualified health care professional, newborn   A

EXCLUDES   *Transfusions of other types (36430-36450)*

3.03   3.03   **FUD** XXX   63 S 80

AMA: 2018,Jan,8; 2017,Jul,3

36460   Transfusion, intrauterine, fetal   A ♀

(76941)

9.84   9.84   **FUD** XXX   63 S 80

AMA: 2003,Apr,7; 1997,Nov,1

36465-36466 [36465, 36466] Destruction Spider Veins

INCLUDES   All supplies, equipment, compression stockings or bandages when performed in the physician office

EXCLUDES   *Multi-layer compression system applied to leg (29581, 29584)*
Strapping of leg: ankle, foot, hip, knee, toes of same extremity (29520, 29530, 29540, 29550)
Unna boot (29580)
Use of code more than one time for each extremity treated
Vascular embolization and occlusion (37241-37244)
Vascular embolization vein in same operative field (37241)

36465   Resequenced code. See code following 36471.

36466   Resequenced code. See code following 36471.

36468   Injection(s) of sclerosant for spider veins (telangiectasia), limb or trunk

(76942)

0.00   0.00   **FUD** 000   Q1 N1 80

AMA: 2018,Mar,3; 2018,Jan,8; 2017,Jan,8; 2016,Nov,3; 2016,Jan,13; 2015,Apr,10; 2015,Jan,16; 2014,Oct,6; 2014,Aug,14

36470   Injection of sclerosant; single incompetent vein (other than telangiectasia)

EXCLUDES   *Injection of foam sclerosant with ultrasound guidance for compression maneuvers (36465-36466)*

(76942)

1.11   3.02   **FUD** 000   T P3 50

AMA: 2018,Dec,10; 2018,Dec,10; 2018,Mar,3; 2018,Jan,8; 2017,Jan,8; 2016,Nov,3; 2016,Jan,13; 2015,Nov,10; 2015,Apr,10; 2015,Jan,16; 2014,Oct,6; 2014,Aug,14

36471   multiple incompetent veins (other than telangiectasia), same leg

EXCLUDES   *Injection of foam sclerosant with ultrasound guidance for compression maneuvers (36465-36466)*

(76942)

2.21   5.47   **FUD** 000   T P3 50

AMA: 2018,Dec,10; 2018,Dec,10; 2018,Mar,3; 2018,Jan,8; 2017,Jan,8; 2016,Nov,3; 2016,Jan,13; 2015,Nov,10; 2015,Aug,8; 2015,Apr,10; 2015,Jan,16; 2014,Oct,6; 2014,Aug,14

\#   **36465**   Injection of non-compounded foam sclerosant with ultrasound compression maneuvers to guide dispersion of the injectate, inclusive of all imaging guidance and monitoring; single incompetent extremity truncal vein (eg, great saphenous vein, accessory saphenous vein)

EXCLUDES   *Ablation of vein using chemical adhesive ([36482, 36483])*
Injection of foam sclerosant without ultrasound guidance for compression maneuvers (36470-36471)

3.45   43.6   **FUD** 000   T G2 50

AMA: 2019,Feb,9; 2018,Dec,10; 2018,Dec,10; 2018,Mar,3

\#   **36466**   multiple incompetent truncal veins (eg, great saphenous vein, accessory saphenous vein), same leg

EXCLUDES   *Ablation of vein using chemical adhesive ([36482, 36483])*
Injection of foam sclerosant without ultrasound guidance for compression maneuvers (36470-36471)

4.39   45.8   **FUD** 000   T G2 50

AMA: 2019,Feb,9; 2018,Dec,10; 2018,Dec,10; 2018,Mar,3

36473-36483 [36482, 36483] Vein Ablation

INCLUDES   Multi-layer compression system applied to leg (29581, 29584)
Patient monitoring
Radiological guidance (76000, 76937, 76942, 76998, 77002)
Venous access/injections (36000-36005, 36410, 36425)

EXCLUDES   *Duplex scans (93970-93971)*
Strapping of leg: ankle, foot, hip, knee, toes of same extremity (29520, 29530, 29540, 29550)
Transcatheter embolization (75894)
Unna boot (29580)
Vascular embolization vein in same operative field (37241)

36473   Endovenous ablation therapy of incompetent vein, extremity, inclusive of all imaging guidance and monitoring, percutaneous, mechanochemical; first vein treated

INCLUDES   Local anesthesia

EXCLUDES   *Laser ablation incompetent vein (36478-36479)*
Radiofrequency ablation incompetent vein (36475-36476)

5.15   41.4   **FUD** 000   T P2 50

AMA: 2019,Feb,9; 2018,Mar,3; 2018,Jan,8; 2017,Jan,8; 2016,Nov,3

+   **36474**   subsequent vein(s) treated in a single extremity, each through separate access sites (List separately in addition to code for primary procedure)

INCLUDES   Local anesthesia

EXCLUDES   *Laser ablation incompetent vein (36478-36479)*
Radiofrequency ablation incompetent vein (36475-36476)
Use of code more than one time per extremity
Code first (36473)

2.57   7.87   **FUD** ZZZ   N N1 50

AMA: 2019,Feb,9; 2018,Mar,3; 2018,Jan,8; 2017,Jan,8; 2016,Nov,3

36475   Endovenous ablation therapy of incompetent vein, extremity, inclusive of all imaging guidance and monitoring, percutaneous, radiofrequency; first vein treated

INCLUDES   Tumescent anesthesia

EXCLUDES   *Ablation of vein using chemical adhesive ([36482, 36483])*
Endovenous ablation therapy of incompetent vein (36478-36479)

8.11   40.6   **FUD** 000   T A2 50

AMA: 2018,Mar,3; 2018,Jan,8; 2017,Jan,8; 2016,Nov,3; 2016,Aug,3; 2016,Jan,13; 2015,Apr,10; 2015,Jan,16; 2014,Oct,6; 2014,Aug,14; 2014,Mar,4; 2014,Jan,11

+   **36476**   subsequent vein(s) treated in a single extremity, each through separate access sites (List separately in addition to code for primary procedure)

INCLUDES   Tumescent anesthesia

EXCLUDES   *Ablation of vein using chemical adhesive ([36482, 36483])*
Endovenous ablation therapy of incompetent vein (36478-36479)
Use of code more than one time per extremity
Vascular embolization or occlusion (37242-37244)
Code first (36475)

3.93   8.55   **FUD** ZZZ   N N1 50

AMA: 2018,Mar,3; 2018,Jan,8; 2017,Jan,8; 2016,Nov,3; 2016,Aug,3; 2016,Jan,13; 2015,Apr,10; 2015,Jan,16; 2014,Oct,6; 2014,Aug,14; 2014,Mar,4; 2014,Jan,11

36478   Endovenous ablation therapy of incompetent vein, extremity, inclusive of all imaging guidance and monitoring, percutaneous, laser; first vein treated

INCLUDES   Tumescent anesthesia

EXCLUDES   *Ablation of vein using chemical adhesive ([36482, 36483])*
Endovenous ablation therapy of incompetent vein (36475-36476)

8.06   32.1   **FUD** 000   T A2 50

AMA: 2018,Mar,3; 2018,Jan,8; 2017,Jan,8; 2016,Nov,3; 2016,Aug,3; 2016,Jan,13; 2015,Apr,10; 2015,Jan,16; 2014,Oct,6; 2014,Aug,14; 2014,Mar,4; 2014,Jan,11

 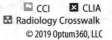

+ 36479 subsequent vein(s) treated in a single extremity, each through separate access sites (List separately in addition to code for primary procedure)

> **INCLUDES** Tumescent anesthesia
> **EXCLUDES** Ablation of vein using chemical adhesive ([36482, 36483])
> Endovenous ablation therapy of incompetent vein (36475-36476)
> Vascular embolization or occlusion (37241)
> Code first (36478)
> ⚡ 3.95 ⚖ 9.03 **FUD** ZZZ N N1 50 ▢

> **AMA:** 2018,Mar,3; 2018,Jan,8; 2017,Jan,8; 2016,Nov,3; 2016,Aug,3; 2016,Jan,13; 2015,Apr,10; 2015,Jan,16; 2014,Oct,6; 2014,Aug,14; 2014,Mar,4; 2014,Jan,11

 # 36482 Endovenous ablation therapy of incompetent vein, extremity, by transcatheter delivery of a chemical adhesive (eg, cyanoacrylate) remote from the access site, inclusive of all imaging guidance and monitoring, percutaneous; first vein treated

> **INCLUDES** Local anesthesia
> **EXCLUDES** Laser ablation incompetent vein (36478-36479)
> Radiofrequency ablation incompetent vein (36475-36476)
> ⚡ 5.12 ⚖ 57.9 **FUD** 000 T G2 50 ▢

> **AMA:** 2019,Feb,9; 2018,Mar,3

+ # 36483 subsequent vein(s) treated in a single extremity, each through separate access sites (List separately in addition to code for primary procedure)

> **INCLUDES** Local anesthesia
> **EXCLUDES** Laser ablation incompetent vein (36478-36479)
> Radiofrequency ablation incompetent vein (36475-36476)
> Use of code more than one time per extremity
> Code first ([36482])
> ⚡ 2.57 ⚖ 4.26 **FUD** ZZZ N N1 50 ▢

> **AMA:** 2019,Feb,9; 2018,Mar,3

36481-36510 Other Venous Catheterization Procedures

> **EXCLUDES** Collection of a specimen from:
> A completely implantable device (36591)
> An established catheter (36592)

36481 Percutaneous portal vein catheterization by any method
> ⊡ (75885, 75887)
> ⚡ 9.67 ⚖ 55.4 **FUD** 000 N N1 ▢

> **AMA:** 2018,Jan,8; 2017,Jan,8; 2016,Jan,13; 2015,Jan,16; 2014,Jan,11

36482 Resequenced code. See code following 36479.

36483 Resequenced code. See code following 36479.

36500 Venous catheterization for selective organ blood sampling
> **EXCLUDES** Inferior or superior vena cava catheterization (36010)
> ⊡ (75893)
> ⚡ 5.30 ⚖ 5.30 **FUD** 000 N N1 ▢

> **AMA:** 2014,Jan,11

36510 Catheterization of umbilical vein for diagnosis or therapy, newborn A
> **EXCLUDES** Collection of a specimen from:
> Capillary blood (36416)
> Venipuncture (36415)
> ⚡ 1.54 ⚖ 2.34 **FUD** 000 63 N N1 80 ▢

> **AMA:** 2018,Jan,8; 2017,Jan,8; 2016,May,3; 2016,Jan,13; 2015,Jan,16; 2014,Jan,11

36511-36516 Apheresis

CMS: 100-03,110.14 Apheresis (Therapeutic Pheresis); 100-04,4,231.9 Billing for Pheresis and Apheresis Services

> **EXCLUDES** Collection of a specimen for therapeutic treatment from:
> A completely implantable device (36591)
> An established catheter (36592)

36511 Therapeutic apheresis; for white blood cells
> ⚡ 3.10 ⚖ 3.10 **FUD** 000 S G2 ▢

> **AMA:** 2018,Jan,8; 2017,Jan,8; 2016,Jan,13; 2015,Jan,16; 2014,Jan,11

36512 for red blood cells
> ⚡ 3.11 ⚖ 3.11 **FUD** 000 S G2 ▢

> **AMA:** 2018,Jan,8; 2017,Jan,8; 2016,Jan,13; 2015,Jan,16; 2014,Jan,11

36513 for platelets
> **EXCLUDES** Collection of platelets from donors
> ⚡ 3.16 ⚖ 3.16 **FUD** 000 S R2 ▢

> **AMA:** 2018,Jan,8; 2017,Jan,8; 2016,Jan,13; 2015,Jan,16; 2014,Jan,11

36514 for plasma pheresis
> ⚡ 2.76 ⚖ 20.5 **FUD** 000 S G2 ▢

> **AMA:** 2018,May,10; 2018,Jan,8; 2017,Jan,8; 2016,Jan,13; 2015,Jan,16; 2014,Jan,11

36516 with extracorporeal immunoadsorption, selective adsorption or selective filtration and plasma reinfusion
> Code also modifier 26 for professional evaluation
> ⚡ 2.46 ⚖ 56.2 **FUD** 000 S P3 ▢

> **AMA:** 2018,Jan,8; 2017,Jan,8; 2016,Jan,13; 2015,Jan,16; 2014,Jan,11

36522 Extracorporeal Photopheresis

CMS: 100-03,110.4 Extracorporeal Photopheresis; 100-04,32,190 Billing for Extracorporeal Photopheresis; 100-04,32,190.2 Extracorporeal Photopheresis; 100-04,32,190.3 Medicare Denial Codes; 100-04,4,231.9 Billing for Pheresis and Apheresis Services

36522 Photopheresis, extracorporeal
> ⚡ 2.79 ⚖ 61.2 **FUD** 000 S G2 ▢

> **AMA:** 2018,May,10; 2018,Jan,8; 2017,Jan,8; 2016,Jan,13; 2015,Jan,16; 2014,Jan,11

Cardiovascular, Hemic, and Lymphatic *(side tab)*

36555 — 36569 *(side tab)*

36555-36573 [36572, 36573] Placement of Implantable Venous Access Device

INCLUDES Devices accessed by an exposed catheter, or a subcutaneous port or pump
Devices inserted via cutdown or percutaneous access:
　Centrally (eg, femoral, jugular, subclavian veins, or inferior vena cava)
　Peripherally (e.g., basilic, cephalic, saphenous vein)
Devices terminating in the brachiocephalic (innominate), iliac, or subclavian veins, vena cava, or right atrium

EXCLUDES *Insertion midline catheter (36400, 36406, 36410)*
Maintenance/refilling of implantable pump/reservoir (96522)
Code also removal of central venous access device (if code available) when a new device is placed through a separate venous access

36555 **Insertion of non-tunneled centrally inserted central venous catheter; younger than 5 years of age** A

　EXCLUDES *Peripheral insertion (36568)*
　▣ (76937, 77001)
　▣ 2.46　▣ 5.33　**FUD** 000　　　　T A2 ▢
　AMA: 2019,May,3; 2018,Jan,8; 2017,Jan,8; 2016,Jan,13; 2015,Jan,16; 2014,Jan,11

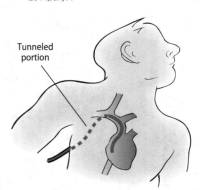

Direct CVC

A non-tunneled centrally inserted CVC is inserted

36556 **age 5 years or older** A

　EXCLUDES *Peripheral insertion (36569)*
　▣ (76937, 77001)
　▣ 2.45　▣ 5.99　**FUD** 000　　　　T A2 ▢
　AMA: 2019,May,3; 2018,Nov,11; 2018,Jan,8; 2017,Jan,8; 2016,Jan,13; 2015,Jan,16; 2014,Jan,11

36557 **Insertion of tunneled centrally inserted central venous catheter, without subcutaneous port or pump; younger than 5 years of age** A

　▣ (76937, 77001)
　▣ 9.21　▣ 29.0　**FUD** 010　　　T A2 80 50 ▢
　AMA: 2018,Jan,8; 2017,Jan,8; 2016,Jan,13; 2015,Jan,16; 2014,Jan,11

Tunneled portion

A tunneled centrally inserted CVC is inserted

36558 **age 5 years or older** A

　EXCLUDES *Peripheral insertion (36571)*
　▣ (76937, 77001)
　▣ 7.54　▣ 21.7　**FUD** 010　　　T A2 80 50 ▢
　AMA: 2018,Jan,8; 2017,Jan,8; 2016,Jan,13; 2015,Jan,16; 2015,Jan,13; 2014,Jan,11

36560 **Insertion of tunneled centrally inserted central venous access device, with subcutaneous port; younger than 5 years of age** A

　EXCLUDES *Peripheral insertion (36570)*
　▣ (76937, 77001)
　▣ 11.0　▣ 37.1　**FUD** 010　　T 62 80 50 ▢
　AMA: 2018,Jan,8; 2017,Jan,8; 2016,Jan,13; 2015,Jan,16; 2014,Jan,11

36561 **age 5 years or older** A

　EXCLUDES *Peripheral insertion (36571)*
　▣ (76937, 77001)
　▣ 9.74　▣ 30.6　**FUD** 010　　　T A2 80 50 ▢
　AMA: 2018,Jan,8; 2017,Jan,8; 2016,Jan,13; 2015,Jan,16; 2014,Jan,11

36563 **Insertion of tunneled centrally inserted central venous access device with subcutaneous pump**

　▣ (76937, 77001)
　▣ 10.6　▣ 34.4　**FUD** 010　　　T A2 80 ▢
　AMA: 2018,Jan,8; 2017,Jan,8; 2016,Jan,13; 2015,Jan,16; 2014,Jan,11

36565 **Insertion of tunneled centrally inserted central venous access device, requiring 2 catheters via 2 separate venous access sites; without subcutaneous port or pump (eg, Tesio type catheter)**

　▣ (76937, 77001)
　▣ 9.63　▣ 24.8　**FUD** 010　　　T A2 80 50 ▢
　AMA: 2018,Jan,8; 2017,Jan,8; 2016,Jan,13; 2015,Jan,16; 2014,Jan,11

36566 **with subcutaneous port(s)**

　▣ (76937, 77001)
　▣ 10.4　▣ 135.　**FUD** 010　　　T A2 80 50 ▢
　AMA: 2018,Jan,8; 2017,Jan,8; 2016,Jan,13; 2015,Jan,16; 2014,Jan,11

36568 **Insertion of peripherally inserted central venous catheter (PICC), without subcutaneous port or pump, without imaging guidance; younger than 5 years of age** A

　EXCLUDES *Centrally inserted placement (36555)*
　Imaging guidance (76937, 77001)
　Peripherally inserted ([36572])
　PICC line removal with codes for removal of tunneled central venous catheters; report appropriate E&M code
　▣ 2.65　▣ 2.65　**FUD** 000　　　T A2
　AMA: 2019,May,3; 2018,Jan,8; 2017,Jan,8; 2016,Jan,13; 2015,Jan,16; 2014,Jan,11

36569 **age 5 years or older** A

　EXCLUDES *Centrally inserted placement (36556)*
　Imaging guidance (76937, 77001)
　Peripherally inserted ([36573])
　PICC line removal with codes for removal of tunneled central venous catheters; report appropriate E&M code
　▣ 2.72　▣ 2.72　**FUD** 000　　　T A2
　AMA: 2019,May,3; 2018,Jan,8; 2017,Jan,8; 2016,Jan,13; 2015,Jan,16; 2014,Sep,13; 2014,Jan,11

Cardiovascular, Hemic, and Lymphatic

36572 — 36589

 # 36572 **Insertion of peripherally inserted central venous catheter (PICC), without subcutaneous port or pump, including all imaging guidance, image documentation, and all associated radiological supervision and interpretation required to perform the insertion; younger than 5 years of age** A

INCLUDES Verification of site of catheter tip (71045-71048)

EXCLUDES *Centrally inserted placement (36555)*
Imaging guidance (76937, 77001)
Peripherally inserted without imaging guidance (36568)

2.65 ⚕ 11.9 **FUD** 000 G2 ▢

AMA: 2019,May,3; 2019,Mar,10

 # 36573 **age 5 years or older** A

INCLUDES Verification of site of catheter tip (71045-71048)

EXCLUDES *Centrally inserted placement (36556)*
Imaging guidance (76937, 77001)
Peripherally inserted without imaging guidance (36569)

2.45 ⚕ 11.2 **FUD** 000 G2 ▢

AMA: 2019,May,3; 2019,Mar,10

36570 **Insertion of peripherally inserted central venous access device, with subcutaneous port; younger than 5 years of age** A

EXCLUDES *Centrally inserted placement (36560)*

9.56 ⚕ 40.8 **FUD** 010 T A2 80 50 ▢

AMA: 2018,Jan,8; 2017,Jan,8; 2016,Jan,13; 2015,Jan,16; 2014,Jan,11

36571 **age 5 years or older** A

EXCLUDES *Centrally inserted placement (36561)*

9.00 ⚕ 35.8 **FUD** 010 T A2 80 50 ▢

AMA: 2018,Jan,8; 2017,Jan,8; 2016,Jan,13; 2015,Jan,16; 2014,Jan,11

36572 Resequenced code. See code following 36569.

36573 Resequenced code. See code following 36569.

36575-36590 Repair, Removal, and Replacement Implantable Venous Access Device

EXCLUDES *Mechanical removal obstructive material, pericatheter/intraluminal (36595, 36596)*

Code also a frequency of two for procedures involving both catheters from a multicatheter device

36575 **Repair of tunneled or non-tunneled central venous access catheter, without subcutaneous port or pump, central or peripheral insertion site**

INCLUDES Repair of the device without replacing any parts

1.01 ⚕ 4.59 **FUD** 000 T A2 80 ▢

AMA: 2018,Jan,8; 2017,Jan,8; 2016,Jan,13; 2015,Jan,16; 2014,Jan,11

36576 **Repair of central venous access device, with subcutaneous port or pump, central or peripheral insertion site**

INCLUDES Repair of the device without replacing any parts

5.33 ⚕ 9.31 **FUD** 010 T A2 80 ▢

AMA: 2018,Jan,8; 2017,Jan,8; 2016,Jan,13; 2015,Jan,16; 2014,Jan,11

36578 **Replacement, catheter only, of central venous access device, with subcutaneous port or pump, central or peripheral insertion site**

INCLUDES Partial replacement (catheter only)

EXCLUDES *Total replacement of the entire device using the same venous access sites (36582-36583)*

5.86 ⚕ 13.0 **FUD** 010 T A2 80 ▢

AMA: 2018,Jan,8; 2017,Jan,8; 2016,Jan,13; 2015,Jan,16; 2014,Jan,11

36580 **Replacement, complete, of a non-tunneled centrally inserted central venous catheter, without subcutaneous port or pump, through same venous access**

INCLUDES Complete replacement (replace all components/same access site)

1.92 ⚕ 6.13 **FUD** 000 T J8 ▢

AMA: 2018,Jan,8; 2017,Jan,8; 2016,Jan,13; 2015,Jan,16; 2014,Jan,11

36581 **Replacement, complete, of a tunneled centrally inserted central venous catheter, without subcutaneous port or pump, through same venous access**

INCLUDES Complete replacement (replace all components/same access site)

EXCLUDES *Removal of old device and insertion of new device using a separate venous access site*

5.31 ⚕ 21.4 **FUD** 010 T J8 80 ▢

AMA: 2018,Jan,8; 2017,Jan,8; 2016,Jan,13; 2015,Jan,16; 2014,Jan,11

36582 **Replacement, complete, of a tunneled centrally inserted central venous access device, with subcutaneous port, through same venous access**

INCLUDES Complete replacement (replace all components/same access site)

EXCLUDES *Removal of old device and insertion of new device using a separate venous access site*

8.38 ⚕ 28.3 **FUD** 010 T A2 80 ▢

AMA: 2018,Jan,8; 2017,Jan,8; 2016,Jan,13; 2015,Jan,16; 2014,Jan,11

36583 **Replacement, complete, of a tunneled centrally inserted central venous access device, with subcutaneous pump, through same venous access**

INCLUDES Complete replacement (replace all components/same access site)

EXCLUDES *Removal of old device and insertion of new device using a separate venous access site*

9.45 ⚕ 35.9 **FUD** 010 T A2 80 ▢

AMA: 2018,Jan,8; 2017,Jan,8; 2016,Jan,13; 2015,Jan,16; 2014,Jan,11

36584 **Replacement, complete, of a peripherally inserted central venous catheter (PICC), without subcutaneous port or pump, through same venous access, including all imaging guidance, image documentation, and all associated radiological supervision and interpretation required to perform the replacement**

INCLUDES Complete replacement (replace all components/same access site)
Imaging guidance (76937, 77001)
Verification of site of catheter tip (71045-71048)

EXCLUDES *Replacement of PICC line without imaging guidance (37799)*

1.73 ⚕ 9.78 **FUD** 000 T A2 ▢

AMA: 2019,May,3; 2019,Mar,10; 2018,Jan,8; 2017,Jan,8; 2016,Jan,13; 2015,Jan,16; 2014,Jan,11

36585 **Replacement, complete, of a peripherally inserted central venous access device, with subcutaneous port, through same venous access**

INCLUDES Complete replacement (replace all components/same access site)

7.80 ⚕ 30.5 **FUD** 010 T A2 80 ▢

AMA: 2018,Jan,8; 2017,Jan,8; 2016,Jan,13; 2015,Jan,16; 2014,Jan,11

36589 **Removal of tunneled central venous catheter, without subcutaneous port or pump**

INCLUDES Complete removal/all components

EXCLUDES *Non-tunneled central venous catheter removal; report appropriate E&M code*

3.96 ⚕ 4.71 **FUD** 010 Q2 A2 80 ▢

AMA: 2018,Jan,8; 2017,Jan,8; 2016,Jan,13; 2015,Nov,10; 2015,Jan,16; 2014,Jan,11

36590 Removal of tunneled central venous access device, with subcutaneous port or pump, central or peripheral insertion

> INCLUDES Complete removal/all components
> EXCLUDES Non-tunneled central venous catheter removal; report appropriate E&M code

🔧 5.49 ⚖ 6.34 **FUD** 010   Q2 A2 80 ▣

AMA: 2018,Jan,8; 2017,Jan,8; 2016,Jan,13; 2015,Jan,16; 2014,Jan,11

36591-36592 Obtain Blood Specimen from Implanted Device or Catheter

> EXCLUDES Use of code with any other service except laboratory services

36591 Collection of blood specimen from a completely implantable venous access device

> EXCLUDES Collection of:
> Capillary blood specimen (36416)
> Venous blood specimen by venipuncture (36415)

🔧 0.69 ⚖ 0.69 **FUD** XXX   Q1 N1 80 TC ▣

AMA: 2019,Aug,8; 2018,Jan,8; 2017,Jan,8; 2016,Jan,13; 2015,Jan,16; 2014,May,4; 2014,Jan,11

36592 Collection of blood specimen using established central or peripheral catheter, venous, not otherwise specified

> EXCLUDES Collection of blood from an established arterial catheter (37799)

🔧 0.77 ⚖ 0.77 **FUD** XXX   Q1 N1 80 TC ▣

AMA: 2018,Jan,8; 2017,Jan,8; 2016,Jan,13; 2015,Jan,16; 2014,Jan,11

36593-36596 Restore Patency of Occluded Catheter or Device

> EXCLUDES Venous catheterization (36010-36012)

36593 Declotting by thrombolytic agent of implanted vascular access device or catheter

🔧 0.89 ⚖ 0.89 **FUD** XXX   T P3 80 TC ▣

AMA: 2018,Jan,8; 2017,Jan,8; 2016,Jan,13; 2015,Jan,16; 2014,Jan,11

36595 Mechanical removal of pericatheter obstructive material (eg, fibrin sheath) from central venous device via separate venous access

> EXCLUDES Declotting by thrombolytic agent (36593)
> 🔄 (75901)

🔧 5.30 ⚖ 17.3 **FUD** 000   T J8 ▣

AMA: 2018,Jan,8; 2017,Jan,8; 2016,Jan,13; 2015,Jan,16; 2014,Jan,11

36596 Mechanical removal of intraluminal (intracatheter) obstructive material from central venous device through device lumen

> EXCLUDES Declotting by thrombolytic agent (36593)
> 🔄 (75902)

🔧 1.28 ⚖ 3.57 **FUD** 000   T G2 ▣

AMA: 2018,Jan,8; 2017,Jan,8; 2016,Jan,13; 2015,Jan,16; 2014,Jan,11

36597-36598 Repositioning or Assessment of In Situ Venous Access Device

36597 Repositioning of previously placed central venous catheter under fluoroscopic guidance

> 🔄 (76000)

🔧 1.77 ⚖ 3.69 **FUD** 000   T G2 ▣

AMA: 2018,Jan,8; 2017,Jan,8; 2016,Jan,13; 2015,Jan,16; 2014,Sep,5; 2014,Jan,11

36598 Contrast injection(s) for radiologic evaluation of existing central venous access device, including fluoroscopy, image documentation and report

> EXCLUDES Complete venography studies (75820, 75825, 75827)
> Fluoroscopy (76000)
> Mechanical removal of pericatheter obstructive material (36595-36596)

🔧 1.06 ⚖ 3.30 **FUD** 000   T P3 80 50 ▣

AMA: 2014,Jan,11

36600-36660 Insertion Needle or Catheter: Artery

36600 Arterial puncture, withdrawal of blood for diagnosis

> EXCLUDES Critical care services

🔧 0.45 ⚖ 0.87 **FUD** XXX   Q1 N1 ▣

AMA: 2019,Aug,8; 2018,Jan,8; 2017,Jan,8; 2016,Jan,13; 2015,Jan,16; 2014,May,4; 2014,Jan,11

36620 Arterial catheterization or cannulation for sampling, monitoring or transfusion (separate procedure); percutaneous

🔧 1.28 ⚖ 1.28 **FUD** 000   🚫 N N1 ▣

AMA: 2018,Jan,8; 2017,Jan,8; 2016,Jan,13; 2015,Jan,16; 2014,Jan,11

36625 cutdown

🔧 3.05 ⚖ 3.05 **FUD** 000   N N1 ▣

AMA: 2018,Jan,8; 2017,Jan,8; 2016,Jan,13; 2015,Jan,16; 2014,Jan,11

36640 Arterial catheterization for prolonged infusion therapy (chemotherapy), cutdown

> EXCLUDES Intra-arterial chemotherapy (96420-96425)
> Transcatheter embolization (75894)

🔧 3.30 ⚖ 3.30 **FUD** 000   T A2 ▣

AMA: 2018,Jan,8; 2017,Jan,8; 2016,Jan,13; 2015,Jan,16; 2014,Jan,11

36660 Catheterization, umbilical artery, newborn, for diagnosis or therapy   A

🔧 1.98 ⚖ 1.98 **FUD** 000   63 C 80 ▣

AMA: 2018,Jan,8; 2017,Jan,8; 2016,Jan,13; 2015,Jan,16; 2014,Jan,11

36680 Percutaneous Placement of Catheter/Needle into Bone Marrow Cavity

36680 Placement of needle for intraosseous infusion

🔧 1.69 ⚖ 1.69 **FUD** 000   Q1 N1 80 ▣

AMA: 2018,Jan,8; 2017,Jan,8; 2016,Jan,13; 2015,Jan,16; 2014,Jan,11

36800-36821 Vascular Access for Hemodialysis

36800 Insertion of cannula for hemodialysis, other purpose (separate procedure); vein to vein

🔧 3.53 ⚖ 3.53 **FUD** 000   T G2 ▣

AMA: 2018,Jan,8; 2017,Jan,8; 2016,Jan,13; 2015,Jan,16; 2014,Jan,11

36810 arteriovenous, external (Scribner type)

🔧 6.05 ⚖ 6.05 **FUD** 000   T A2 ▣

AMA: 2018,Jan,8; 2017,Jan,8; 2016,Jan,13; 2015,Jan,16; 2014,Jan,11

36815 arteriovenous, external revision, or closure

🔧 3.91 ⚖ 3.91 **FUD** 000   T A2 ▣

AMA: 2018,Jan,8; 2017,Jan,8; 2016,Jan,13; 2015,Jan,16; 2014,Jan,11   *vein to artery visa versa*

36818 Arteriovenous anastomosis, open; by upper arm cephalic vein transposition

> INCLUDES Two incisions in the upper arm; a medial incision over the brachial artery and a lateral incision for exposure of a portion of the cephalic vein
> EXCLUDES When performed unilaterally with:
> Arteriovenous anastomosis, open (36819-36820)
> Creation of arteriovenous fistula by other than direct arteriovenous anastomosis (36830)
> Code also modifier 50 or 59, as appropriate, for a bilateral procedure

🔧 20.1 ⚖ 20.1 **FUD** 090   T A2 80 ▣

AMA: 2018,Jan,8; 2017,Mar,3; 2017,Jan,8; 2016,Mar,10; 2016,Jan,13; 2015,Jan,16; 2014,Jan,11

CPT © 2019 American Medical Association. All Rights Reserved.   © 2019 Optum360, LLC

36819   **by upper arm basilic vein transposition**

> EXCLUDES   *When performed unilaterally with:*
> *Arteriovenous anastomosis, open (36818, 36820-36821)*
> *Creation of arteriovenous fistula by other than direct arteriovenous anastomosis (36830)*
> *Code also modifier 50 or 59, as appropriate, for bilateral procedure*

  ⚕ 21.1   ⚑ 21.1   **FUD** 090   [T] [A2] [80] [▣]

  AMA: 2018,Jan,8; 2017,Mar,3; 2017,Jan,8; 2016,Jan,13; 2015,Jan,16; 2014,Jan,11

36820   **by forearm vein transposition**

  ⚕ 21.2   ⚑ 21.2   **FUD** 090   [T] [A2] [80] [50] [▣]

  AMA: 2018,Jan,8; 2017,Mar,3; 2017,Jan,8; 2016,Jan,13; 2015,Jan,16; 2014,Jan,11

36821   **direct, any site (eg, Cimino type) (separate procedure)**

  ⚕ 19.2   ⚑ 19.2   **FUD** 090   [T] [A2] [80] [▣]

  AMA: 2018,Jan,8; 2017,Mar,3; 2017,Jan,8; 2016,Jan,13; 2015,Aug,8; 2015,Jan,16; 2014,Jan,11

36823 Vascular Access for Extracorporeal Circulation

> INCLUDES   Chemotherapy perfusion
> EXCLUDES   *Chemotherapy administration (96409-96425)*
> *Maintenance for extracorporeal circulation (33946-33949)*

36823   **Insertion of arterial and venous cannula(s) for isolated extracorporeal circulation including regional chemotherapy perfusion to an extremity, with or without hyperthermia, with removal of cannula(s) and repair of arteriotomy and venotomy sites**

  ⚕ 40.5   ⚑ 40.5   **FUD** 090   [C] [▣]

  AMA: 2018,Jan,8; 2017,Mar,3; 2014,Jan,11

36825-36835 Permanent Vascular Access Procedures

36825   **Creation of arteriovenous fistula by other than direct arteriovenous anastomosis (separate procedure); autogenous graft**

> EXCLUDES   *Direct arteriovenous (AV) anastomosis (36821)*

  ⚕ 23.0   ⚑ 23.0   **FUD** 090   [T] [A2] [80] [▣]

  AMA: 2018,Jan,8; 2017,Mar,3; 2017,Jan,8; 2016,Jan,13; 2015,Jan,16; 2014,Jan,11

Artery and vein connected by a vein graft in an end-to-side manner, creating an arteriovenous fistula

Radial artery

Radial artery

Graft

Basilic vein

Basilic vein

Artery and vein connected by a synthetic graft

36830   **nonautogenous graft (eg, biological collagen, thermoplastic graft)**

> EXCLUDES   *Direct arteriovenous (AV) anastomosis (36821)*

  ⚕ 19.3   ⚑ 19.3   **FUD** 090   [T] [A2] [80] [▣]

  AMA: 2018,Jan,8; 2017,Mar,3; 2017,Jan,8; 2016,Jan,13; 2015,Jan,16; 2015,Jan,13; 2014,Jan,11

36831   **Thrombectomy, open, arteriovenous fistula without revision, autogenous or nonautogenous dialysis graft (separate procedure)**

  ⚕ 17.8   ⚑ 17.8   **FUD** 090   [T] [A2] [80] [▣]

  AMA: 2018,Jan,8; 2017,Mar,3; 2017,Jan,8; 2016,Jan,13; 2015,Jan,16; 2014,Jan,11

36832   **Revision, open, arteriovenous fistula; without thrombectomy, autogenous or nonautogenous dialysis graft (separate procedure)**

> INCLUDES   Revision of an arteriovenous access fistula or graft

  ⚕ 21.9   ⚑ 21.9   **FUD** 090   [T] [A2] [80] [▣]

  AMA: 2018,Jan,8; 2017,Mar,3; 2017,Jan,8; 2016,Jan,13; 2015,Jan,16; 2014,Jan,11

36833   **with thrombectomy, autogenous or nonautogenous dialysis graft (separate procedure)**

> EXCLUDES   *Hemodialysis circuit procedures (36901-36906)*

  ⚕ 23.5   ⚑ 23.5   **FUD** 090   [T] [A2] [80] [▣]

  AMA: 2018,Jan,8; 2017,Mar,3; 2017,Jan,8; 2016,Jan,13; 2015,Jan,16; 2014,Jan,11

36835   **Insertion of Thomas shunt (separate procedure)**

  ⚕ 13.8   ⚑ 13.8   **FUD** 090   [T] [A2] [▣]

  AMA: 2014,Jan,11

36838 DRIL Procedure for Ischemic Steal Syndrome

> EXCLUDES   *Bypass graft, with vein (35512, 35522-35523)*
> *Ligation (37607, 37618)*
> *Revision, open, arteriovenous fistula (36832)*

36838   **Distal revascularization and interval ligation (DRIL), upper extremity hemodialysis access (steal syndrome)**

  ⚕ 33.1   ⚑ 33.1   **FUD** 090   [T] [80] [50] [▣]

  AMA: 2014,Jan,11

36860-36861 Restore Patency of Occluded Cannula or Arteriovenous Fistula

36860   **External cannula declotting (separate procedure); without balloon catheter**

  ⊞ (76000)

  ⚕ 3.20   ⚑ 7.17   **FUD** 000   [T] [A2] [▣]

  AMA: 2018,Jan,8; 2017,Jan,8; 2016,Jan,13; 2015,Jan,16; 2014,Jan,11

36861   **with balloon catheter**

  ⊞ (76000)

  ⚕ 4.02   ⚑ 4.02   **FUD** 000   [T] [A2] [▣]

  AMA: 2018,Jan,8; 2017,Jan,8; 2016,Jan,13; 2015,Jan,16; 2014,Jan,11

36901-36909 Hemodialysis Circuit Procedures

> EXCLUDES   *Arteriography to assess inflow to hemodialysis circuit when performed (76937)*

36901   **Introduction of needle(s) and/or catheter(s), dialysis circuit, with diagnostic angiography of the dialysis circuit, including all direct puncture(s) and catheter placement(s), injection(s) of contrast, all necessary imaging from the arterial anastomosis and adjacent artery through entire venous outflow including the inferior or superior vena cava, fluoroscopic guidance, radiological supervision and interpretation and image documentation and report;**

> INCLUDES   Access
> Catheter advancement (e.g., imaging of accessory veins, assess all sections of circuit)
> Contrast injection
> EXCLUDES   *Balloon angioplasty of peripheral segment (36902)*
> *Open revision with thrombectomy of arteriovenous fistula (36833)*
> *Percutaneous transluminal procedures of peripheral segment (36904-36906)*
> *Stent placement in peripheral segment (36903)*
> *Use of code more than one time per procedure*

  ⚕ 4.90   ⚑ 16.9   **FUD** 000   [T] [P3] [▣]

  AMA: 2018,Jan,8; 2017,Mar,3

36902 with transluminal balloon angioplasty, peripheral dialysis segment, including all imaging and radiological supervision and interpretation necessary to perform the angioplasty

EXCLUDES *Open revision with thrombectomy of arteriovenous fistula (36833)*
Percutaneous transluminal procedures of peripheral segment (36904-36906)
Stent placement in peripheral segment (36903)
Use of code more than one time per procedure

⚕ 6.98   ⚗ 36.0   **FUD** 000   J 62 ▣

AMA: 2018,Jan,8; 2017,Jul,3; 2017,Mar,3

36903 with transcatheter placement of intravascular stent(s), peripheral dialysis segment, including all imaging and radiological supervision and interpretation necessary to perform the stenting, and all angioplasty within the peripheral dialysis segment

INCLUDES Balloon angioplasty of peripheral segment (36902)
EXCLUDES *Central hemodialysis circuit procedures (36907-36908)*
Open revision with thrombectomy of arteriovenous fistula (36833)
Percutaneous transluminal procedures of peripheral segment (36904-36906)
Use of code more than one time per procedure

⚕ 9.23   ⚗ 152.   **FUD** 000   J J8 ▣

AMA: 2018,Jan,8; 2017,Jul,3; 2017,Mar,3

36904 Percutaneous transluminal mechanical thrombectomy and/or infusion for thrombolysis, dialysis circuit, any method, including all imaging and radiological supervision and interpretation, diagnostic angiography, fluoroscopic guidance, catheter placement(s), and intraprocedural pharmacological thrombolytic injection(s);

EXCLUDES *Open thrombectomy of arteriovenous fistula with/without revision (36831, 36833)*
Use of code more than one time per procedure

⚕ 10.7   ⚗ 53.1   **FUD** 000   J 62 ▣

AMA: 2018,Jan,8; 2017,Jul,3; 2017,Mar,3

36905 with transluminal balloon angioplasty, peripheral dialysis segment, including all imaging and radiological supervision and interpretation necessary to perform the angioplasty

INCLUDES Percutaneous mechanical thrombectomy (36904)
EXCLUDES *Use of code more than one time per procedure*

⚕ 12.9   ⚗ 66.8   **FUD** 000   J 62 ▣

AMA: 2018,Jan,8; 2017,Jul,3; 2017,Mar,3

36906 with transcatheter placement of intravascular stent(s), peripheral dialysis segment, including all imaging and radiological supervision and interpretation necessary to perform the stenting, and all angioplasty within the peripheral dialysis circuit

INCLUDES Percutaneous transluminal balloon angioplasty (36905)
Percutaneous transluminal thrombectomy (36904)
EXCLUDES *Hemodialysis circuit procedures provided by catheter or needle access (36901-36903)*
Use of code more than one time per procedure
Code also balloon angioplasty of central veins, when performed (36907)
Code also stent placement in central veins, when performed (36908)

⚕ 14.9   ⚗ 193.   **FUD** 000   J J8 ▣

AMA: 2018,Jan,8; 2017,Jul,3; 2017,Mar,3

+ **36907** Transluminal balloon angioplasty, central dialysis segment, performed through dialysis circuit, including all imaging and radiological supervision and interpretation required to perform the angioplasty (List separately in addition to code for primary procedure)

INCLUDES All central hemodialysis segment angiography
EXCLUDES *Angiography with stent placement (36908)*
Code first (36818-36833, 36901-36906)

⚕ 4.26   ⚗ 20.4   **FUD** ZZZ   N N1 ▣

AMA: 2018,Jan,8; 2017,Jul,3; 2017,Mar,3

+ **36908** Transcatheter placement of intravascular stent(s), central dialysis segment, performed through dialysis circuit, including all imaging and radiological supervision and interpretation required to perform the stenting, and all angioplasty in the central dialysis segment (List separately in addition to code for primary procedure)

INCLUDES All central hemodialysis segment stent(s) placed
Balloon angioplasty central dialysis segment (36907)
Code first when performed (36818-36833, 36901-36906)

⚕ 6.03   ⚗ 68.0   **FUD** ZZZ   N N1 ▣

AMA: 2018,Jan,8; 2017,Jul,3; 2017,Mar,3

+ **36909** Dialysis circuit permanent vascular embolization or occlusion (including main circuit or any accessory veins), endovascular, including all imaging and radiological supervision and interpretation necessary to complete the intervention (List separately in addition to code for primary procedure)

INCLUDES All embolization/occlusion procedures performed in the hemodialysis circuit
EXCLUDES *Banding/ligation of arteriovenous fistula (37607)*
Use of code more than one time per day
Code first (36901-36906)

⚕ 5.84   ⚗ 54.9   **FUD** ZZZ   N N1 ▣

AMA: 2018,Jan,8; 2017,Mar,3

37140-37181 Open Decompression of Portal Circulation

EXCLUDES *Peritoneal-venous shunt (49425)*

37140 Venous anastomosis, open; portocaval

⚕ 67.4   ⚗ 67.4   **FUD** 090   C ▣

AMA: 2014,Jan,11

37145 renoportal

⚕ 62.5   ⚗ 62.5   **FUD** 090   C 80 ▣

AMA: 2014,Jan,11

37160 caval-mesenteric

⚕ 64.2   ⚗ 64.2   **FUD** 090   C 80 ▣

AMA: 2014,Jan,11

37180 splenorenal, proximal

⚕ 61.7   ⚗ 61.7   **FUD** 090   C 80 ▣

AMA: 2014,Jan,11

37181 splenorenal, distal (selective decompression of esophagogastric varices, any technique)

EXCLUDES *Percutaneous procedure (37182)*

⚕ 67.4   ⚗ 67.4   **FUD** 090   C 80 ▣

AMA: 2014,Jan,11

37182-37183 Transvenous Decompression of Portal Circulation

INCLUDES Percutaneous transhepatic portography (75885, 75887)

37182 Insertion of transvenous intrahepatic portosystemic shunt(s) (TIPS) (includes venous access, hepatic and portal vein catheterization, portography with hemodynamic evaluation, intrahepatic tract formation/dilatation, stent placement and all associated imaging guidance and documentation)

EXCLUDES *Open procedure (37140)*

⚕ 23.7   ⚗ 23.7   **FUD** 000   C 80 ▣

AMA: 2018,Jan,8; 2017,Jan,8; 2016,Jan,13; 2015,Jan,16; 2014,Jan,11

26/TC PC/TC Only   A2-Z3 ASC Payment   50 Bilateral   ♂ Male Only   ♀ Female Only   ⚕ Facility RVU   ⚗ Non-Facility RVU   ▣ CCI   ☒ CLIA
FUD Follow-up Days   CMS: IOM   AMA: CPT Asst   A-Y OPPSI   80/80 Surg Assist Allowed / w/Doc   ▣ Lab Crosswalk   ▣ Radiology Crosswalk

172   CPT © 2019 American Medical Association. All Rights Reserved.   © 2019 Optum360, LLC

37183 Revision of transvenous intrahepatic portosystemic shunt(s) (TIPS) (includes venous access, hepatic and portal vein catheterization, portography with hemodynamic evaluation, intrahepatic tract recanulization/dilatation, stent placement and all associated imaging guidance and documentation)

EXCLUDES *Arteriovenous (AV) aneurysm repair (36832)*
10.8 170. **FUD** 000 [J] [80] [▣]
AMA: 2018,Jan,8; 2017,Jan,8; 2016,Jan,13; 2015,Jan,16; 2014,Jan,11

37184-37188 Removal of Thrombus from Vessel: Percutaneous

INCLUDES Fluoroscopic guidance (76000)
Injection(s) of thrombolytics during the procedure
Postprocedure evaluation
Pretreatment planning
EXCLUDES *Continuous infusion of thrombolytics prior to and after the procedure (37211-37214)*
Diagnostic studies
Intracranial arterial mechanical thrombectomy or infusion (61645)
Mechanical thrombectomy, coronary (92973)
Other interventions performed percutaneously (e.g., balloon angioplasty)
Placement of catheters
Radiological supervision/interpretation

37184 Primary percutaneous transluminal mechanical thrombectomy, noncoronary, non-intracranial, arterial or arterial bypass graft, including fluoroscopic guidance and intraprocedural pharmacological thrombolytic injection(s); initial vessel

EXCLUDES *Intracranial arterial mechanical thrombectomy (61645)*
Mechanical thrombectomy for embolus/thrombus complicating another percutaneous interventional procedure (37186)
Mechanical thrombectomy of another vascular family/separate access site, append modifier 59 to the primary service
Therapeutic, prophylactic, or diagnostic injection (96374)
12.9 60.2 **FUD** 000 [J] [J8] [50] [▣]
AMA: 2019,Sep,5; 2018,Jan,8; 2017,Jan,8; 2016,Jul,6; 2016,Mar,3; 2016,Jan,13; 2015,Nov,3; 2015,Apr,10; 2015,Jan,16; 2014,Jan,11

+ **37185** second and all subsequent vessel(s) within the same vascular family (List separately in addition to code for primary mechanical thrombectomy procedure)

INCLUDES *Treatment of second and all succeeding vessel(s) in same vascular family*
EXCLUDES *Intravenous drug injections administered subsequent to an initial service*
Mechanical thrombectomy for treating of embolus/thrombus complicating another percutaneous interventional procedure (37186)
Therapeutic, prophylactic, or diagnostic injection (96375)
Code first (37184)
4.85 18.5 **FUD** ZZZ [N] [N1] [▣]
AMA: 2019,Sep,5; 2018,Jan,8; 2017,Jan,8; 2016,Jul,6; 2016,Jan,13; 2015,Nov,3; 2015,Apr,10; 2015,Jan,16; 2014,Jan,11

+ **37186** Secondary percutaneous transluminal thrombectomy (eg, nonprimary mechanical, snare basket, suction technique), noncoronary, non-intracranial, arterial or arterial bypass graft, including fluoroscopic guidance and intraprocedural pharmacological thrombolytic injections, provided in conjunction with another percutaneous intervention other than primary mechanical thrombectomy (List separately in addition to code for primary procedure)

INCLUDES *Removal of small emboli/thrombi prior to or after another percutaneous procedure*
EXCLUDES *Primary percutaneous transluminal mechanical thrombectomy, noncoronary, non-intracranial (37184-37185)*
Therapeutic, prophylactic, or diagnostic injection (96375)
Code first primary procedure
7.10 37.4 **FUD** ZZZ [N] [N1] [▣]
AMA: 2019,Sep,5; 2018,Jan,8; 2017,Jan,8; 2016,Jul,6; 2016,Jan,13; 2015,Nov,3; 2015,Jan,16; 2014,Jan,11

37187 Percutaneous transluminal mechanical thrombectomy, vein(s), including intraprocedural pharmacological thrombolytic injections and fluoroscopic guidance

INCLUDES *Secondary or subsequent intravenous injection after another initial service*
EXCLUDES *Therapeutic, prophylactic, or diagnostic injection (96375)*
11.4 55.5 **FUD** 000 [J] [J8] [50] [▣]
AMA: 2018,Jan,8; 2017,Jan,8; 2016,Jul,6; 2016,Mar,3; 2016,Jan,13; 2015,Nov,3; 2015,Jan,16; 2014,Jan,11

37188 Percutaneous transluminal mechanical thrombectomy, vein(s), including intraprocedural pharmacological thrombolytic injections and fluoroscopic guidance, repeat treatment on subsequent day during course of thrombolytic therapy

EXCLUDES *Therapeutic, prophylactic, or diagnostic injection (96375)*
8.03 46.7 **FUD** 000 [T] [62] [50] [▣]
AMA: 2018,Jan,8; 2017,Jan,8; 2016,Jul,6; 2016,Mar,3; 2016,Jan,13; 2015,Nov,3; 2015,Jan,16; 2014,Jan,11

37191-37193 Vena Cava Filters

37191 Insertion of intravascular vena cava filter, endovascular approach including vascular access, vessel selection, and radiological supervision and interpretation, intraprocedural roadmapping, and imaging guidance (ultrasound and fluoroscopy), when performed

EXCLUDES *Open ligation of inferior vena cava via laparotomy or retroperitoneal approach (37619)*
6.49 69.9 **FUD** 000 [T] [▣]
AMA: 2018,Jan,8; 2017,Feb,14; 2017,Jan,8; 2016,May,11; 2016,Jan,13; 2015,Jan,16; 2014,Jan,11

37192 Repositioning of intravascular vena cava filter, endovascular approach including vascular access, vessel selection, and radiological supervision and interpretation, intraprocedural roadmapping, and imaging guidance (ultrasound and fluoroscopy), when performed

EXCLUDES *Insertion of intravascular vena cava filter (37191)*
9.98 37.4 **FUD** 000 [T] [▣]
AMA: 2018,Jan,8; 2017,Jan,8; 2016,May,11; 2016,Jan,13; 2015,Jan,16; 2014,Jan,11

37193 Retrieval (removal) of intravascular vena cava filter, endovascular approach including vascular access, vessel selection, and radiological supervision and interpretation, intraprocedural roadmapping, and imaging guidance (ultrasound and fluoroscopy), when performed

EXCLUDES *Transcatheter retrieval, percutaneous, of intravascular foreign body (37197)*
10.1 44.0 **FUD** 000 [T] [▣]
AMA: 2018,Jan,8; 2017,Jan,8; 2016,May,11; 2016,Jan,13; 2015,Jan,16; 2014,Jan,11

37195 Intravenous Cerebral Thrombolysis

37195 **Thrombolysis, cerebral, by intravenous infusion**

🔹 0.00   🔧 0.00   **FUD** XXX   Ⓣ 80 ▭

AMA: 2014,Jan,11

37197-37214 Transcatheter Procedures: Infusions, Biopsy, Foreign Body Removal

37197 **Transcatheter retrieval, percutaneous, of intravascular foreign body (eg, fractured venous or arterial catheter), includes radiological supervision and interpretation, and imaging guidance (ultrasound or fluoroscopy), when performed**

EXCLUDES *Percutaneous vena cava filter retrieval (37193)*
Removal leadless pacemaker system ([[33275]])

🔹 8.78   🔧 43.4   **FUD** 000   Ⓣ G2 ▭

AMA: 2018,Jan,8; 2017,Feb,14; 2017,Jan,8; 2016,May,11; 2016,Jan,13; 2015,Jan,16; 2014,Jan,11

37200 **Transcatheter biopsy**

🔀 (75970)

🔹 6.30   🔧 6.30   **FUD** 000   Ⓣ G2 ▭

AMA: 2014,Jan,11

37211 **Transcatheter therapy, arterial infusion for thrombolysis other than coronary or intracranial, any method, including radiological supervision and interpretation, initial treatment day**

INCLUDES Catheter change or position change
E&M services on the day of and related to thrombolysis
First day of transcatheter thrombolytic infusion
Fluoroscopic guidance
Follow-up arteriography or venography
Radiologic supervision and interpretation

EXCLUDES *Angiography through existing catheter for follow-up study for transcatheter therapy, embolization, or infusion, other than for thrombolysis (75898)*
Catheter placement
Declotting of implanted catheter or vascular access device by thrombolytic agent (36593)
Diagnostic studies
Intracranial arterial mechanical thrombectomy or infusion (61645)
Percutaneous interventions
Procedure performed more than one time per date of service
Ultrasound guidance (76937)

Code also significant, separately identifiable E&M service on the day of thrombolysis using modifier 25

🔹 11.2   🔧 11.2   **FUD** 000   Ⓣ G2 50 ▭

AMA: 2019,Sep,6; 2018,Jan,8; 2017,Jan,8; 2016,Jul,6; 2016,Mar,3; 2016,Jan,13; 2015,Nov,3; 2015,Jan,16; 2014,Jan,11

37212 **Transcatheter therapy, venous infusion for thrombolysis, any method, including radiological supervision and interpretation, initial treatment day**

INCLUDES Catheter change or position change
E&M services on the day of and related to thrombolysis

EXCLUDES *Angiography through existing catheter for follow-up study for transcatheter therapy, embolization, or infusion, other than for thrombolysis (75898)*
Catheter placement
First day of transcatheter thrombolytic infusion
Declotting of implanted catheter or vascular access device by thrombolytic agent (36593)
Fluoroscopic guidance
Follow-up arteriography or venography
Diagnostic studies
Initiation and completion of thrombolysis on same date of service
Percutaneous interventions
Radiologic supervision and interpretation
Procedure performed more than one time per date of service
Ultrasound guidance (76937)

Code also significant, separately identifiable E&M service on the day of thrombolysis using modifier 25

🔹 9.81   🔧 9.81   **FUD** 000   Ⓣ G2 50 ▭

AMA: 2019,Sep,6; 2018,Jan,8; 2017,Jan,8; 2016,Jul,6; 2016,Mar,3; 2016,Jan,13; 2015,Nov,3; 2015,Jan,16; 2014,Jan,11

37213 **Transcatheter therapy, arterial or venous infusion for thrombolysis other than coronary, any method, including radiological supervision and interpretation, continued treatment on subsequent day during course of thrombolytic therapy, including follow-up catheter contrast injection, position change, or exchange, when performed;**

INCLUDES Continued thrombolytic infusions on subsequent days besides the initial and last days of treatment
E&M services on the day of and related to thrombolysis
Fluoroscopic guidance
Radiologic supervision and interpretation

EXCLUDES *Angiography through existing catheter for follow-up study for transcatheter therapy, embolization, or infusion, other than for thrombolysis (75898)*
Catheter placement
Declotting of implanted catheter or vascular access device by thrombolytic agent (36593)
Diagnostic studies
Percutaneous interventions
Procedure performed more than one time per date of service
Ultrasound guidance (76937)

Code also significant, separately identifiable E&M service on the day of thrombolysis using modifier 25

🔹 6.76   🔧 6.76   **FUD** 000   Ⓣ ▭

AMA: 2019,Sep,6; 2018,Jan,8; 2017,Jan,8; 2016,Jul,6; 2016,Mar,3; 2016,Jan,13; 2015,Nov,3; 2015,Jan,16; 2014,Jan,11

37214 **cessation of thrombolysis including removal of catheter and vessel closure by any method**

INCLUDES
E&M services on the day of and related to thrombolysis
Fluoroscopic guidance
Last day of transcatheter thrombolytic infusions
Radiologic supervision and interpretation

EXCLUDES
Angiography through existing catheter for follow-up study for transcatheter therapy, embolization, or infusion, other than for thrombolysis (75898)
Catheter placement
Declotting of implanted catheter or vascular access device by thrombolytic agent (36593)
Diagnostic studies
Percutaneous interventions
Procedure performed more than one time per date of service
Ultrasound guidance (76937)

Code also significant, separately identifiable E&M service on the day of thrombolysis using modifier 25

⚕ 3.57 ⚕ 3.57 **FUD** 000 T 🖥

AMA: 2019,Sep,6; 2018,Jan,8; 2017,Jan,8; 2016,Jul,6; 2016,Mar,3; 2016,Jan,13; 2015,Nov,3; 2015,Jan,16; 2014,Jan,11

37215-37216 Stenting of Cervical Carotid Artery with/without Insertion Distal Embolic Protection Device

INCLUDES
Carotid stenting, if required
Ipsilateral cerebral and cervical carotid diagnostic imaging/supervision and interpretation
Ipsilateral selective carotid catheterization

EXCLUDES
Carotid catheterization and imaging, if carotid stenting not required
Selective catheter placement, common carotid or innominate artery (36222-36224)
Transcatheter placement extracranial vertebral artery stents, open or percutaneous (0075T, 0076T)

37215 **Transcatheter placement of intravascular stent(s), cervical carotid artery, open or percutaneous, including angioplasty, when performed, and radiological supervision and interpretation; with distal embolic protection**

⚕ 29.2 ⚕ 29.2 **FUD** 090 C 80 50 🖥

AMA: 2018,Jan,8; 2017,Jul,3; 2017,Jan,8; 2016,Jan,13; 2015,Jan,16; 2014,Mar,8; 2014,Jan,11

Balloon is advanced to the affected portion of artery

Balloon is inflated, which activates the stent

The catheter is withdrawn

Clot filitering stent

Temporal artery

External carotid

Internal carotid

Common carotid (cervical)

37216 **without distal embolic protection**

⚕ 29.2 ⚕ 29.2 **FUD** 090 E 🖥

AMA: 2018,Jan,8; 2017,Jul,3; 2017,Jan,8; 2016,Jan,13; 2015,Jan,16; 2014,Mar,8; 2014,Jan,11

37217-37218 Stenting of Intrathoracic Carotid Artery/Innominate Artery

INCLUDES
Access to vessel (open)
Arteriotomy closure by suture
Catheterization of the vessel (selective)
Imaging during and after the procedure
Radiological supervision and interpretation

EXCLUDES
Transcatheter insertion extracranial vertebral artery stents, open or percutaneous (0075T-0076T)
Transcatheter insertion intracranial stents (61635)
Transcatheter insertion intravascular cervical carotid artery stents, open or percutaneous (37215-37216)

37217 **Transcatheter placement of intravascular stent(s), intrathoracic common carotid artery or innominate artery by retrograde treatment, open ipsilateral cervical carotid artery exposure, including angioplasty, when performed, and radiological supervision and interpretation**

⚕ 31.3 ⚕ 31.3 **FUD** 090 C 80 50 🖥

AMA: 2018,Jan,8; 2017,Jul,3; 2017,Jan,8; 2016,Jan,13; 2015,May,7; 2015,Jan,16; 2014,Mar,8; 2014,Jan,11

37218 **Transcatheter placement of intravascular stent(s), intrathoracic common carotid artery or innominate artery, open or percutaneous antegrade approach, including angioplasty, when performed, and radiological supervision and interpretation**

EXCLUDES
Selective catheter placement, common carotid or innominate artery (36222-36224)

⚕ 23.7 ⚕ 23.7 **FUD** 090 C 80 50 🖥

AMA: 2018,Jan,8; 2017,Jul,3; 2017,Jan,8; 2016,Jan,13; 2015,May,7

Cardiovascular, Hemic, and Lymphatic

37220 — 37231

37220-37235 Endovascular Revascularization Lower Extremities

INCLUDES Percutaneous and open interventional and associated procedures for lower extremity occlusive disease; unilateral
Accessing the vessel
Arteriotomy closure by suturing of puncture or pressure with application of arterial closure device
Atherectomy (e.g., directional, laser, rotational)
Balloon angioplasty (e.g., cryoplasty, cutting balloon, low-profile)
Catheterization of the vessel (selective)
Embolic protection
Imaging once procedure is complete
Radiological supervision and interpretation of intervention(s)
Stenting (e.g., bare metal, balloon-expandable, covered, drug-eluting, self-expanding)
Traversing the lesion
Reporting the most comprehensive treatment in a given vessel according to the following hierarchy:
1. Stent and atherectomy
2. Atherectomy
3. Stent
4. PTA
Revascularization procedures for three arterial vascular territories:
Femoral/popliteal vascular territory including the common, deep, and superficial femoral arteries, and the popliteal artery (one extremity = a single vessel) (37224-37227)
Iliac vascular territory: common iliac, external iliac, internal iliac (37220-37223)
Tibial/peroneal territory: includes anterior tibial, peroneal artery, posterior tibial (37228-37235)

EXCLUDES Assignment of more than one code from this family for each lower extremity vessel treated
Assignment of more than one code when multiple vessels are treated in the femoral/popliteal territory (report the most complex service for more than one lesion in the territory); when a contiguous lesion that spans from one territory to another can be opened with a single procedure; or when more than one stent is deployed in the same vessel
Extensive repair or replacement of artery (35226, 35286)
Mechanical thrombectomy and/or thrombolysis
Code also add-on codes for different vessels, but not different lesions in the same vessel; and for multiple territories in the same leg
Code also modifier 59 if same territory(ies) of both legs are treated during the same surgical session
Code first one primary code for the initial service in each leg

37220 Revascularization, endovascular, open or percutaneous, iliac artery, unilateral, initial vessel; with transluminal angioplasty
Code also only when transluminal angioplasty is performed outside the treatment target zone of (34701-34708, 34709, [34718], 34710-34711, 34845-34848)
11.6   83.7   **FUD** 000   J 62 80 50
AMA: 2019,Jun,14; 2018,Jan,8; 2017,Jul,3; 2017,Jan,8; 2016,Jul,8; 2016,Jan,13; 2015,Jan,16; 2014,Jan,11

37221 with transluminal stent placement(s), includes angioplasty within the same vessel, when performed
Code also only when transluminal angioplasty is performed outside the treatment target zone of (34701-34708, 34709, [34718], 34710-34711, 34845-34848)
14.4   118.   **FUD** 000   J J8 80 50
AMA: 2019,Jun,14; 2018,Jan,8; 2017,Dec,3; 2017,Jul,3; 2017,Jan,8; 2016,Jul,6; 2016,Jul,8; 2016,Jan,13; 2015,Jan,13; 2015,Jan,16; 2014,Jan,11

+ 37222 Revascularization, endovascular, open or percutaneous, iliac artery, each additional ipsilateral iliac vessel; with transluminal angioplasty (List separately in addition to code for primary procedure)
Code also only when transluminal angioplasty is performed outside the treatment target zone of (34701-34708, 34709, [34718], 34710-34711, 34845-34848)
Code first (37220-37221)
5.42   22.6   **FUD** ZZZ   N N1 80 50
AMA: 2019,Jun,14; 2018,Jan,8; 2017,Jul,3; 2017,Jan,8; 2016,Jul,8; 2016,Jan,13; 2015,Jan,16; 2014,Jan,11

+ 37223 with transluminal stent placement(s), includes angioplasty within the same vessel, when performed (List separately in addition to code for primary procedure)
Code also only when transluminal angioplasty is performed outside the treatment target zone of (34701-34708, 34709, [34718], 34710-34711, 34845-34848)
Code first (37221)
6.20   62.6   **FUD** ZZZ   N N1 80 50
AMA: 2019,Jun,14; 2018,Jan,8; 2017,Dec,3; 2017,Jul,3; 2017,Jan,8; 2016,Jul,8; 2016,Jul,6; 2016,Jan,13; 2015,Jan,16; 2014,Jan,11

37224 Revascularization, endovascular, open or percutaneous, femoral, popliteal artery(s), unilateral; with transluminal angioplasty
EXCLUDES Revascularization with intravascular stent grafts in femoral-popliteal segment (0505T)
12.9   100.   **FUD** 000   J J8 80 50
AMA: 2019,Jun,14; 2018,Jan,8; 2017,Jul,3; 2017,Jan,8; 2016,Jul,8; 2016,Jan,13; 2015,Jan,16; 2014,Jan,11

37225 with atherectomy, includes angioplasty within the same vessel, when performed
EXCLUDES Revascularization with intravascular stent grafts in femoral-popliteal segment (0505T)
17.6   345.   **FUD** 000   J J8 80 50
AMA: 2019,Jun,14; 2018,Jan,8; 2017,Jul,3; 2017,Jan,8; 2016,Jul,8; 2016,Jan,13; 2015,Jan,16; 2014,Jan,11

37226 with transluminal stent placement(s), includes angioplasty within the same vessel, when performed
EXCLUDES Revascularization with intravascular stent grafts in femoral-popliteal segment (0505T)
15.1   299.   **FUD** 000   J J8 80 50
AMA: 2019,Jun,14; 2018,Jan,8; 2017,Jul,3; 2017,Jan,8; 2016,Jul,6; 2016,Jul,8; 2016,Jan,13; 2015,Jan,16; 2014,Jan,11

37227 with transluminal stent placement(s) and atherectomy, includes angioplasty within the same vessel, when performed
EXCLUDES Revascularization with intravascular stent grafts in femoral-popliteal segment (0505T)
21.1   444.   **FUD** 000   J J8 80 50
AMA: 2019,Jun,14; 2018,Jan,8; 2017,Jul,3; 2017,Jan,8; 2016,Jul,6; 2016,Jul,8; 2016,Jan,13; 2015,Jan,16; 2014,Jan,11

37228 Revascularization, endovascular, open or percutaneous, tibial, peroneal artery, unilateral, initial vessel; with transluminal angioplasty
15.8   145.   **FUD** 000   J J8 80 50
AMA: 2019,Jun,14; 2018,Jan,8; 2017,Jul,3; 2017,Jan,8; 2016,Jul,8; 2016,Jan,13; 2015,Jan,16; 2014,Jan,11

37229 with atherectomy, includes angioplasty within the same vessel, when performed
20.5   345.   **FUD** 000   J J8 80 50
AMA: 2019,Jun,14; 2018,Jan,8; 2017,Jul,3; 2017,Jan,8; 2016,Jul,8; 2016,Jan,13; 2015,Jan,16; 2014,Jan,11

37230 with transluminal stent placement(s), includes angioplasty within the same vessel, when performed
20.3   294.   **FUD** 000   J J8 80 50
AMA: 2019,Jun,14; 2018,Jan,8; 2017,Jul,3; 2017,Jan,8; 2016,Jul,6; 2016,Jan,13; 2015,Jan,16; 2014,Jan,11

37231 with transluminal stent placement(s) and atherectomy, includes angioplasty within the same vessel, when performed
22.1   422.   **FUD** 000   J J8 80 50
AMA: 2019,Jun,14; 2018,Jan,8; 2017,Jul,3; 2017,Jan,8; 2016,Jul,8; 2016,Jul,6; 2016,Jan,13; 2015,Jan,16; 2014,Jan,11

+ **37232** **Revascularization, endovascular, open or percutaneous, tibial/peroneal artery, unilateral, each additional vessel; with transluminal angioplasty (List separately in addition to code for primary procedure)**
Code first (37228-37231)
🚗 5.85 ⚕ 31.1 **FUD** ZZZ ⬜ N N1 80 50 ▢
AMA: 2019,Jun,14; 2018,Jan,8; 2017,Jul,3; 2017,Jan,8; 2016,Jul,8; 2016,Jan,13; 2015,Jan,16; 2014,Jan,11

+ **37233** **with atherectomy, includes angioplasty within the same vessel, when performed (List separately in addition to code for primary procedure)**
Code first (37229, 37231)
🚗 9.53 ⚕ 37.9 **FUD** ZZZ N N1 80 50 ▢
AMA: 2019,Jun,14; 2018,Jan,8; 2017,Jul,3; 2017,Jan,8; 2016,Jul,8; 2016,Jan,13; 2015,Jan,16; 2014,Jan,11

+ **37234** **with transluminal stent placement(s), includes angioplasty within the same vessel, when performed (List separately in addition to code for primary procedure)**
Code first (37229-37231)
🚗 8.32 ⚕ 109. **FUD** ZZZ N N1 80 50 ▢
AMA: 2019,Jun,14; 2018,Jan,8; 2017,Jul,3; 2017,Jan,8; 2016,Jul,8; 2016,Jul,6; 2016,Jan,13; 2015,Jan,16; 2014,Jan,11

+ **37235** **with transluminal stent placement(s) and atherectomy, includes angioplasty within the same vessel, when performed (List separately in addition to code for primary procedure)**
Code first (37231)
🚗 11.6 ⚕ 119. **FUD** ZZZ N N1 80 50 ▢
AMA: 2019,Jun,14; 2018,Jan,8; 2017,Jul,3; 2017,Jan,8; 2016,Jul,6; 2016,Jul,8; 2016,Jan,13; 2015,Jan,16; 2014,Jan,11

37246-37249 [37246, 37247, 37248, 37249] Transluminal Balloon Angioplasty

INCLUDES Open and percutaneous balloon angioplasty
Radiological supervision and interpretation (37220-37235)

EXCLUDES Angioplasty of other vessels:
Aortic/visceral arteries (with endovascular repair) (34841-34848)
Coronary artery (92920-92944)
Intracranial artery (61630, 61635)
Performed in a hemodialysis circuit (36901-36909)
Percutaneous removal of thrombus/infusion of thrombolytics (37184-37188, 37211-37214)
Pulmonary artery (92997-92998)
Use of codes more than one time for all services performed in a single vessel or treatable with one angioplasty procedure

Code also angioplasty of different vessel, when performed ([37247], [37249])
Code also extensive repair or replacement of artery, when performed (35226, 35286)
Code also intravascular ultrasound, when performed (37252-37253)

\# **37246** **Transluminal balloon angioplasty (except lower extremity artery(ies) for occlusive disease, intracranial, coronary, pulmonary, or dialysis circuit), open or percutaneous, including all imaging and radiological supervision and interpretation necessary to perform the angioplasty within the same artery; initial artery**

EXCLUDES Intravascular stent placement except lower extremities (37236-37237)
Revascularization lower extremities (37220-37235)
Stent placement:
Cervical carotid artery (37215-37216)
Intrathoracic carotid or innominate artery (37217-37218)
Code first (37239)
🚗 10.1 ⚕ 59.2 **FUD** 000 J G2 50 ▢
AMA: 2018,Jan,8; 2017,Aug,10; 2017,Jul,3

+ \# **37247** **each additional artery (List separately in addition to code for primary procedure)**

EXCLUDES Intravascular stent placement except lower extremities (37236-37237)
Revascularization lower extremities (37220-37235)
Stent placement:
Cervical carotid artery (37215-37216)
Intrathoracic carotid or innominate artery (37217-37218)
Code first ([37246])
🚗 4.97 ⚕ 22.5 **FUD** ZZZ N N1 50 ▢
AMA: 2018,Jan,8; 2017,Aug,10; 2017,Jul,3

\# **37248** **Transluminal balloon angioplasty (except dialysis circuit), open or percutaneous, including all imaging and radiological supervision and interpretation necessary to perform the angioplasty within the same vein; initial vein**

EXCLUDES Placement of intravascular (venous) stent in same vein, same session as (37238-37239)
Revascularization with intravascular stent grafts in femoral-popliteal segment (0505T)
🚗 8.66 ⚕ 42.3 **FUD** 000 J G2 50 ▢
AMA: 2018,Jan,8; 2017,Aug,10; 2017,Jul,3; 2017,Mar,3

+ \# **37249** **each additional vein (List separately in addition to code for primary procedure)**

EXCLUDES Placement of intravascular (venous) stent in same vein, same session as (37238-37239)
Revascularization with intravascular stent grafts in femoral-popliteal segment (0505T)
Code first (37239)
🚗 4.22 ⚕ 16.7 **FUD** ZZZ N N1 50 ▢
AMA: 2018,Jan,8; 2017,Aug,10; 2017,Jul,3; 2017,Mar,3

Cardiovascular, Hemic, and Lymphatic *(left margin)*

37236 — 37247 *(left margin)*

37236-37239 Endovascular Revascularization Excluding Lower Extremities

INCLUDES Arteriotomy closure by suturing of a puncture, pressure or application of arterial closure device
Balloon angioplasty
  Post-dilation after stent deployment
  Predilation performed as primary or secondary angioplasty
  Treatment of lesion inside same vessel but outside of stented portion
  Treatment using different-sized balloons to accomplish the procedure
Endovascular revascularization of arteries and veins other than carotid, coronary, extracranial, intracranial, lower extremities
Imaging once procedure is complete
Radiological supervision and interpretation
Stent placement provided as the only treatment

EXCLUDES *Angioplasty in an unrelated vessel*
Extensive repair or replacement of an artery (35226, 35286)
Insertion of multiple stents in a single vessel using more than one code
Intravascular ultrasound (37252-37253)
Mechanical thrombectomy (37184-37188)
Selective and nonselective catheterization (36005, 36010-36015, 36200, 36215-36218, 36245-36248)
Stent placement in:
  Arteries of the lower extremities for occlusive disease (37221, 37223, 37226-37227, 37230-37231, 37234-37235)
  Cervical carotid artery (37215-37216)
  Extracranial vertebral (0075T-0076T)
  Hemodialysis circuit (36903, 36905, 36908)
  Intracoronary (92928-92929, 92933-92934, 92937-92938, 92941, 92943-92944)
  Intracranial (61635)
  Intrathoracic common carotid or innominate artery, retrograde or antegrade approach (37218)
  Visceral arteries with fenestrated aortic repair (34841-34848)
Thrombolytic therapy (37211-37214)
Ultrasound guidance (76937)
Code also add-on codes for different vessels treated during the same operative session

37236 **Transcatheter placement of an intravascular stent(s) (except lower extremity artery(s) for occlusive disease, cervical carotid, extracranial vertebral or intrathoracic carotid, intracranial, or coronary), open or percutaneous, including radiological supervision and interpretation and including all angioplasty within the same vessel, when performed; initial artery**

EXCLUDES *Procedures in the same target treatment zone with (34841-34848)*
12.9 101. **FUD** 000 J J8 80 50
AMA: 2018,Jan,8; 2017,Dec,3; 2017,Jul,3; 2017,Jan,8; 2016,Jul,3; 2016,Jul,6; 2016,Mar,5; 2016,Jan,13; 2015,May,7; 2015,Jan,16; 2014,Jan,11

+ 37237 **each additional artery (List separately in addition to code for primary procedure)**

EXCLUDES *Procedures in the same target treatment zone with (34841-34848)*
Code first (37236)
6.19 60.3 **FUD** ZZZ N N1 80 50
AMA: 2018,Jan,8; 2017,Dec,3; 2017,Jul,3; 2017,Jan,8; 2016,Jul,6; 2016,Mar,5; 2016,Jan,13; 2015,Jan,16; 2014,Jan,11

37238 **Transcatheter placement of an intravascular stent(s), open or percutaneous, including radiological supervision and interpretation and including angioplasty within the same vessel, when performed; initial vein**

EXCLUDES *Revascularization with intravascular stent grafts in femoral-popliteal segment (0505T)*
8.82 102. **FUD** 000 J J8 80 50
AMA: 2018,Jan,8; 2017,Jul,3; 2017,Mar,3; 2017,Jan,8; 2016,Jul,6; 2016,Jun,8; 2014,Jan,11

+ 37239 **each additional vein (List separately in addition to code for primary procedure)**

EXCLUDES *Revascularization with intravascular stent grafts in femoral-popliteal segment (0505T)*
Code first (37238)
4.42 48.9 **FUD** ZZZ N N1 80 50
AMA: 2018,Jan,8; 2017,Jul,3; 2017,Mar,3; 2017,Jan,8; 2016,Jul,6; 2014,Jan,11

37241-37249 Therapeutic Vascular Embolization/Occlusion

INCLUDES Embolization or occlusion of arteries, lymphatics, and veins except for head/neck and central nervous system
Imaging once procedure is complete
Intraprocedural guidance
Radiological supervision and interpretation
Roadmapping
Stent placement provided as support for embolization

EXCLUDES *Embolization code assigned more than once per operative field*
Head, neck, or central nervous system embolization (61624, 61626, 61710)
Multiple codes for indications that overlap, code only the indication needing the most immediate attention
Stent deployment as primary management of aneurysm, pseudoaneurysm, or vascular extravasation
Vein destruction with sclerosing solution (36468-36471)
Code also additional embolization procedure(s) and the appropriate modifiers (eg, modifier 59) when embolization procedures are performed in multiple operative fields
Code also diagnostic angiography and catheter placement using modifier 59 when appropriate

37241 **Vascular embolization or occlusion, inclusive of all radiological supervision and interpretation, intraprocedural roadmapping, and imaging guidance necessary to complete the intervention; venous, other than hemorrhage (eg, congenital or acquired venous malformations, venous and capillary hemangiomas, varices, varicoceles)**

EXCLUDES *Embolization of side branch(s) of an outflow vein from a hemodialysis access (36909)*
Procedure in same operative field with:
  Endovenous ablation therapy of incompetent vein (36475-36479)
  Injection of sclerosing solution; single vein (36470-36471)
  Transcatheter embolization procedures (75894, 75898)
  Vein destruction (36468-36479 [36465, 36466])
12.8 137. **FUD** 000 J P2
AMA: 2019,Sep,6; 2018,Mar,3; 2018,Jan,8; 2017,Mar,3; 2017,Jan,8; 2016,Nov,3; 2016,Jan,13; 2015,Nov,3; 2015,Aug,8; 2015,Apr,10; 2015,Jan,16; 2014,Oct,6; 2014,Aug,14; 2014,Jan,11

37242 **arterial, other than hemorrhage or tumor (eg, congenital or acquired arterial malformations, arteriovenous malformations, arteriovenous fistulas, aneurysms, pseudoaneurysms)**

EXCLUDES *Percutaneous treatment of pseudoaneurysm of an extremity (36002)*
13.8 211. **FUD** 000 J J8
AMA: 2019,Sep,6; 2018,Jul,14; 2018,Mar,3; 2018,Jan,8; 2017,Jan,8; 2016,Jan,13; 2015,Nov,3; 2015,Jan,16; 2014,Oct,6; 2014,Jan,11

37243 **for tumors, organ ischemia, or infarction**

INCLUDES Embolization of uterine fibroids (37244)
EXCLUDES *Procedure in same operative field:*
  Angiography (75898)
  Transcatheter embolization in same operative field (75894)
Code also chemotherapy when provided with embolization procedure (96420-96425)
Code also injection of radioisotopes when provided with embolization procedure (79445)
16.3 273. **FUD** 000 J 62
AMA: 2019,Sep,6; 2018,Mar,3; 2018,Jan,8; 2017,Jan,8; 2016,Jan,13; 2015,Nov,3; 2015,Jan,16; 2014,Oct,6; 2014,Jan,11

37244 **for arterial or venous hemorrhage or lymphatic extravasation**

INCLUDES Embolization of uterine arteries for hemorrhage
19.3 195. **FUD** 000 J
AMA: 2019,Sep,6; 2018,Jul,14; 2018,Mar,3; 2018,Jan,8; 2017,Oct,9; 2017,Jan,8; 2016,Jan,13; 2015,Nov,3; 2015,Jan,16; 2014,Oct,6; 2014,Aug,14; 2014,Jan,11

37246 **Resequenced code. See code following 37235.**

37247 **Resequenced code. See code following 37235.**

37248	Resequenced code. See code following 37235.
37249	Resequenced code. See code following 37235.

37252-37253 Intravascular Ultrasound: Noncoronary

INCLUDES Manipulation and repositioning of the transducer prior to and after therapeutic interventional procedures

EXCLUDES *Selective or non-selective catheter placement for access (36005-36248)*
Transcatheter procedures (37200, 37236-37239, 37241-37244, 61624, 61626)
Vena cava filter procedures (37191-37193, 37197)

Code first (33361-33369, 33477, 33880-33886, 34701-34708, 34709, [34718], 34710-34711, 34712, 34841-34848, 36010-36015, 36100-36218, 36221-36228, 36245-36248, 36251-36254, 36481, 36555-36571 [36572, 36573], 36578, 36580-36585, 36595, 36901-36909, 37184-37188, 37200, 37211-37218, 37220-37239 [37246, 37247, 37248, 37249], 37241-37244, 61623, 75600-75635, 75705-75774, 75805, 75807, 75810, 75820-75833, 75860-75872, 75885-75898, 75901-75902, 75956-75959, 75970, 76000, 77001, 0075T-0076T, 0234T-0238T, 0338T)

+ **37252** **Intravascular ultrasound (noncoronary vessel) during diagnostic evaluation and/or therapeutic intervention, including radiological supervision and interpretation; initial noncoronary vessel (List separately in addition to code for primary procedure)**
Code first primary procedure
🔧 2.65 ✂ 35.7 **FUD** ZZZ   N N1 80 ▭
AMA: 2018,Jan,8; 2017,Dec,3; 2017,Aug,10; 2017,Mar,3; 2017,Jan,8; 2016,Jul,6; 2016,May,11

+ **37253** **each additional noncoronary vessel (List separately in addition to code for primary procedure)**
Code first (37252)
🔧 2.13 ✂ 5.60 **FUD** ZZZ   N N1 80 ▭
AMA: 2018,Jan,8; 2017,Dec,3; 2017,Aug,10; 2017,Mar,3; 2017,Jan,8; 2016,Jul,6; 2016,May,11

37500-37501 Vascular Endoscopic Procedures

INCLUDES Diagnostic endoscopy
EXCLUDES *Open procedure (37760)*

37500 **Vascular endoscopy, surgical, with ligation of perforator veins, subfascial (SEPS)**
🔧 18.3 ✂ 18.3 **FUD** 090   T A2 50 ▭
AMA: 2018,Jan,8; 2017,Jan,8; 2016,Jan,13; 2015,Jan,16; 2014,Jan,11

37501 **Unlisted vascular endoscopy procedure**
🔧 0.00 ✂ 0.00 **FUD** YYY   T 50 ▭
AMA: 2014,Jan,11

37565-37606 Ligation Procedures: Jugular Vein, Carotid Arteries

CMS: 100-03,160.8 Electroencephalographic Monitoring During Cerebral Vasculature Surgery
EXCLUDES *Arterial balloon occlusion, endovascular, temporary (61623)*
Suture of arteries and veins (35201-35286)
Transcatheter arterial embolization/occlusion, permanent (61624-61626)
Treatment of intracranial aneurysm (61703)

37565 **Ligation, internal jugular vein**
🔧 20.7 ✂ 20.7 **FUD** 090   T 80 50 ▭
AMA: 2014,Jan,11

37600 **Ligation; external carotid artery**
🔧 21.0 ✂ 21.0 **FUD** 090   T 80 ▭
AMA: 2014,Jan,11

External carotid artery is ligated

External carotid artery

Internal carotid artery

Common carotid artery

Sternocleidomastoid muscle

37605 **internal or common carotid artery**
🔧 21.3 ✂ 21.3 **FUD** 090   T 80 ▭
AMA: 2014,Jan,11

37606 **internal or common carotid artery, with gradual occlusion, as with Selverstone or Crutchfield clamp**
🔧 20.9 ✂ 20.9 **FUD** 090   T 80 ▭
AMA: 2014,Jan,11

37607-37609 Ligation Hemodialysis Angioaccess or Temporal Artery

EXCLUDES *Suture of arteries and veins (35201-35286)*

37607 **Ligation or banding of angioaccess arteriovenous fistula**
🔧 10.8 ✂ 10.8 **FUD** 090   T A2 ▭
AMA: 2014,Jan,11

37609 **Ligation or biopsy, temporal artery**
🔧 5.94 ✂ 8.87 **FUD** 010   J A2 50 ▭
AMA: 2014,Jan,11

37615-37618 Arterial Ligation, Major Vessel, for Injury/Rupture

EXCLUDES *Suture of arteries and veins (35201-35286)*

37615 **Ligation, major artery (eg, post-traumatic, rupture); neck**
INCLUDES Touroff ligation
🔧 15.2 ✂ 15.2 **FUD** 090   T 80 ▭
AMA: 2014,Jan,11

37616 **chest**
INCLUDES Bardenheuer operation
🔧 32.0 ✂ 32.0 **FUD** 090   C 80 ▭
AMA: 2014,Jan,11

37617 **abdomen**
🔧 38.8 ✂ 38.8 **FUD** 090   C 80 ▭
AMA: 2018,Jan,8; 2017,Jan,8; 2016,Jan,13; 2015,Jan,16; 2014,Jan,11

37618 **extremity**
🔧 11.1 ✂ 11.1 **FUD** 090   C 80 ▭
AMA: 2014,Jan,11

37619 Ligation Inferior Vena Cava

EXCLUDES *Suture of arteries and veins (35201-35286)*
Endovascular delivery of inferior vena cava filter (37191)

37619 **Ligation of inferior vena cava**
🔧 50.1 ✂ 50.1 **FUD** 090   T 80 ▭
AMA: 2018,Jan,8; 2017,Jan,8; 2016,Jan,13; 2015,Jan,16; 2014,Jan,11

37650-37660 Venous Ligation, Femoral and Common Iliac

EXCLUDES Suture of arteries and veins (35201-35286)

37650 Ligation of femoral vein
🚑 13.2   ⚖ 13.2   **FUD** 090   T A2 50 ▢
AMA: 2014,Jan,11

37660 Ligation of common iliac vein
🚑 38.1   ⚖ 38.1   **FUD** 090   C 80 50 ▢
AMA: 2014,Jan,11

37700-37785 Treatment of Varicose Veins of Legs

EXCLUDES Suture of arteries and veins (35201-35286)

37700 Ligation and division of long saphenous vein at saphenofemoral junction, or distal interruptions
INCLUDES Babcock operation
EXCLUDES Ligation, division, and stripping of vein (37718, 37722)
🚑 7.07   ⚖ 7.07   **FUD** 090   T A2 50 ▢
AMA: 2018,Mar,3; 2018,Jan,8; 2017,Jan,8; 2016,Jan,13; 2015,Jan,16; 2014,Jan,11

37718 Ligation, division, and stripping, short saphenous vein
EXCLUDES Ligation, division, and stripping of vein (37700, 37735, 37780)
🚑 12.4   ⚖ 12.4   **FUD** 090   T A2 50 ▢
AMA: 2018,Mar,3; 2018,Jan,8; 2017,Jan,8; 2014,Jan,11

37722 Ligation, division, and stripping, long (greater) saphenous veins from saphenofemoral junction to knee or below
EXCLUDES Ligation, division, and stripping of vein (37700, 37718, 37735)
🚑 13.7   ⚖ 13.7   **FUD** 090   T A2 50 ▢
AMA: 2018,Mar,3; 2018,Jan,8; 2017,Jan,8; 2014,Jan,11

37735 Ligation and division and complete stripping of long or short saphenous veins with radical excision of ulcer and skin graft and/or interruption of communicating veins of lower leg, with excision of deep fascia
EXCLUDES Ligation, division, and stripping of vein (37700, 37718, 37722, 37780)
🚑 16.7   ⚖ 16.7   **FUD** 090   T A2 50 ▢
AMA: 2018,Mar,3; 2018,Jan,8; 2017,Jan,8; 2016,Jan,13; 2015,Jan,16; 2014,Jan,11

37760 Ligation of perforator veins, subfascial, radical (Linton type), including skin graft, when performed, open,1 leg
EXCLUDES Duplex scan of extremity veins (93971)
Ligation of subfascial perforator veins, endoscopic (37500)
Ultrasonic guidance (76937, 76942, 76998)
🚑 18.0   ⚖ 18.0   **FUD** 090   T A2 50 ▢
AMA: 2018,Mar,3; 2018,Jan,8; 2017,Jan,8; 2016,Jan,13; 2015,Jan,16; 2014,Jan,11

37761 Ligation of perforator vein(s), subfascial, open, including ultrasound guidance, when performed, 1 leg
EXCLUDES Duplex scan of extremity veins (93971)
Ligation of subfascial perforator veins, endoscopic (37500)
Ultrasonic guidance (76937, 76942, 76998)
🚑 15.6   ⚖ 15.6   **FUD** 090   T R2 80 50 ▢
AMA: 2018,Mar,3; 2018,Jan,8; 2017,Jan,8; 2016,Jan,13; 2015,Jan,16; 2014,Jan,11

37765 Stab phlebectomy of varicose veins, 1 extremity; 10-20 stab incisions
EXCLUDES Fewer than 10 incisions (37799)
More than 20 incisions (37766)
🚑 12.9   ⚖ 18.5   **FUD** 090   T P3 50 ▢
AMA: 2018,Mar,3; 2018,Jan,8; 2017,Jan,8; 2016,Nov,3; 2016,Jan,13; 2015,Jan,16; 2014,Oct,6; 2014,Jan,11

37766 more than 20 incisions
EXCLUDES Fewer than 10 incisions (37799)
10-20 incisions (37765)
🚑 15.8   ⚖ 22.0   **FUD** 090   T P3 50 ▢
AMA: 2018,Mar,3; 2018,Jan,8; 2017,Jan,8; 2016,Nov,3; 2016,Jan,13; 2015,Jan,16; 2014,Oct,6; 2014,Jan,11

37780 Ligation and division of short saphenous vein at saphenopopliteal junction (separate procedure)
🚑 6.75   ⚖ 6.75   **FUD** 090   T A2 50 ▢
AMA: 2018,Jan,8; 2017,Jan,8; 2016,Jan,13; 2015,Jan,16; 2014,Jan,11

37785 Ligation, division, and/or excision of varicose vein cluster(s), 1 leg
🚑 7.45   ⚖ 10.0   **FUD** 090   T A2 50 ▢
AMA: 2018,Jan,8; 2017,Jan,8; 2016,Jan,13; 2015,Jan,16; 2014,Jan,11

37788-37790 Treatment of Vascular Disease of the Penis

37788 Penile revascularization, artery, with or without vein graft ♂
🚑 36.5   ⚖ 36.5   **FUD** 090   C 80
AMA: 2014,Jan,11

37790 Penile venous occlusive procedure
🚑 14.0   ⚖ 14.0   **FUD** 090   J A2 80 ▢
AMA: 2014,Jan,11

37799 Unlisted Vascular Surgery Procedures

CMS: 100-04,32,161 Intracranial Percutaneous Transluminal Angioplasty (PTA) With Stenting; 100-04,4,180.3 Unlisted Service or Procedure

37799 Unlisted procedure, vascular surgery
🚑 0.00   ⚖ 0.00   **FUD** YYY   T 80 ▢
AMA: 2018,Nov,11; 2018,Jan,8; 2017,Jan,8; 2016,Nov,3; 2016,Jan,13; 2015,Apr,10; 2015,Jan,16; 2014,Oct,6; 2014,Aug,14; 2014,Mar,8; 2014,Jan,11

38100-38200 Splenic Procedures

38100 Splenectomy; total (separate procedure)
🚑 33.4   ⚖ 33.4   **FUD** 090   C 80 ▢
AMA: 2018,Jan,8; 2017,Jan,8; 2016,Jan,13; 2015,Jan,16; 2014,Jan,11

Short gastric vessels ligated
Ligated splenic artery
Splenic vein
Pancreas
Gastro-splenic ligament
Ruptured spleen

38101 partial (separate procedure)
🚑 33.5   ⚖ 33.5   **FUD** 090   C 80 ▢
AMA: 2018,Jan,8; 2017,Jan,8; 2016,Jan,13; 2015,Jan,16; 2014,Jan,11

+ **38102 total, en bloc for extensive disease, in conjunction with other procedure (List in addition to code for primary procedure)**
Code first primary procedure
🚑 7.65   ⚖ 7.65   **FUD** ZZZ   C 80 ▢
AMA: 2018,Jan,8; 2017,Jan,8; 2016,Jan,13; 2015,Jan,16; 2014,Jan,11

26/TC PC/TC Only   A2-Z3 ASC Payment   50 Bilateral   ♂ Male Only   ♀ Female Only   🚑 Facility RVU   ⚖ Non-Facility RVU   ▢ CCI   ✖ CLIA
FUD Follow-up Days   CMS: IOM   AMA: CPT Asst   A-Y OPPSI   80/80 Surg Assist Allowed / w/Doc   Lab Crosswalk   Radiology Crosswalk

  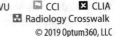

180   CPT © 2019 American Medical Association. All Rights Reserved.   © 2019 Optum360, LLC

38115 Repair of ruptured spleen (splenorrhaphy) with or without partial splenectomy

📷 37.0 ⚕ 37.0 **FUD** 090 [C] [80] [▢]

AMA: 2018,Jan,8; 2017,Jan,8; 2016,Jan,13; 2015,Jan,16; 2014,Jan,11

38120 Laparoscopy, surgical, splenectomy

INCLUDES Diagnostic laparoscopy (49320)

📷 30.5 ⚕ 30.5 **FUD** 090 [J] [80] [▢]

AMA: 2018,Jan,8; 2017,Jan,8; 2016,Jan,13; 2015,Jan,16; 2014,Jan,11

38129 Unlisted laparoscopy procedure, spleen

📷 0.00 ⚕ 0.00 **FUD** YYY [J] [80] [▢]

AMA: 2018,Jan,8; 2017,Jan,8; 2016,Jan,13; 2015,Jan,16; 2014,Jan,11

38200 Injection procedure for splenoportography

➕ (75810)

📷 3.84 ⚕ 3.84 **FUD** 000 [N] [M1] [80] [▢]

AMA: 2014,Jan,11

38204-38215 Hematopoietic Stem Cell Preparation

CMS: 100-03,110.23 Stem Cell Transplantation; 100-04,3,90.3 Stem Cell Transplantation; 100-04,3,90.3.1 Allogeneic Stem Cell Transplantation; 100-04,3,90.3.3 Billing for Allogeneic Stem Cell Transplants; 100-04,32,90 Billing for Stem Cell Transplantation; 100-04,32,90.2.1 Coding for Stem Cell Transplantation; 100-04,4,231.10 Billing for Autologous Stem Cell Transplants; 100-04,4,231.11 Billing for Allogeneic Stem Cell Transplants

INCLUDES Preservation, preparation, purification of stem cells before transplant or reinfusion

EXCLUDES *Procedure performed more than one time per day*

38204 Management of recipient hematopoietic progenitor cell donor search and cell acquisition

📷 3.03 ⚕ 3.03 **FUD** XXX [N] [M1] [▢]

AMA: 2018,Jan,8; 2017,Jan,8; 2016,Jan,13; 2015,Jan,16; 2014,Jan,11

38205 Blood-derived hematopoietic progenitor cell harvesting for transplantation, per collection; allogeneic

📷 2.38 ⚕ 2.38 **FUD** 000 [B] [80] [▢]

AMA: 2018,May,3; 2018,Jan,8; 2017,Jan,8; 2016,Jan,13; 2015,Jan,16; 2014,Jan,11

38206 autologous

📷 2.39 ⚕ 2.39 **FUD** 000 [S] [G2] [80] [▢]

AMA: 2018,May,3; 2018,Jan,8; 2017,Jan,8; 2016,Jan,13; 2015,Jan,16; 2014,Jan,11

38207 Transplant preparation of hematopoietic progenitor cells; cryopreservation and storage

EXCLUDES *Flow cytometry (88182, 88184-88189)*

🔬 (88240)

📷 1.35 ⚕ 1.35 **FUD** XXX [S] [▢]

AMA: 2018,Jan,8; 2017,Jan,8; 2016,Jan,13; 2015,Jan,16; 2014,Jan,11

38208 thawing of previously frozen harvest, without washing, per donor

EXCLUDES *Flow cytometry (88182, 88184-88189)*

🔬 (88241)

📷 0.86 ⚕ 0.86 **FUD** XXX [S] [▢]

AMA: 2018,Jan,8; 2017,Jan,8; 2016,Jan,13; 2015,Jan,16; 2014,Jan,11

38209 thawing of previously frozen harvest, with washing, per donor

EXCLUDES *Flow cytometry (88182, 88184-88189)*

📷 0.36 ⚕ 0.36 **FUD** XXX [S] [▢]

AMA: 2018,Jan,8; 2017,Jan,8; 2016,Jan,13; 2015,Jan,16; 2014,Jan,11

38210 specific cell depletion within harvest, T-cell depletion

EXCLUDES *Flow cytometry (88182, 88184-88189)*

📷 2.40 ⚕ 2.40 **FUD** XXX [S] [▢]

AMA: 2018,Jan,8; 2017,Jan,8; 2016,Jan,13; 2015,Jan,16; 2014,Jan,11

38211 tumor cell depletion

EXCLUDES *Flow cytometry (88182, 88184-88189)*

📷 2.16 ⚕ 2.16 **FUD** XXX [S] [▢]

AMA: 2018,Jan,8; 2017,Jan,8; 2016,Jan,13; 2015,Jan,16; 2014,Jan,11

38212 red blood cell removal

EXCLUDES *Flow cytometry (88182, 88184-88189)*

📷 1.43 ⚕ 1.43 **FUD** XXX [S] [▢]

AMA: 2018,Jan,8; 2017,Jan,8; 2016,Jan,13; 2015,Jan,16; 2014,Jan,11

38213 platelet depletion

EXCLUDES *Flow cytometry (88182, 88184-88189)*

📷 0.36 ⚕ 0.36 **FUD** XXX [S] [▢]

AMA: 2018,Jan,8; 2017,Jan,8; 2016,Jan,13; 2015,Jan,16; 2014,Jan,11

38214 plasma (volume) depletion

EXCLUDES *Flow cytometry (88182, 88184-88189)*

📷 1.23 ⚕ 1.23 **FUD** XXX [S] [▢]

AMA: 2018,Jan,8; 2017,Jan,8; 2016,Jan,13; 2015,Jan,16; 2014,Jan,11

38215 cell concentration in plasma, mononuclear, or buffy coat layer

EXCLUDES *Flow cytometry (88182, 88184-88189)*

📷 1.43 ⚕ 1.43 **FUD** XXX [S] [▢]

AMA: 2018,Jan,8; 2017,Jan,8; 2016,Jan,13; 2015,Jan,16; 2014,Jan,11

38220-38232 Bone Marrow Procedures

CMS: 100-03,110.23 Stem Cell Transplantation; 100-04,3,90.3 Stem Cell Transplantation; 100-04,32,90 Billing for Stem Cell Transplantation; 100-04,4,231.11 Billing for Allogeneic Stem Cell Transplants

38220 Diagnostic bone marrow; aspiration(s)

EXCLUDES *Aspiration of bone marrow for spinal graft (20939)*
Bone marrow biopsy (38221)
Bone marrow for platelet rich stem cell injection (0232T)
Code also biopsy bone marrow during same session (38222)

📷 1.99 ⚕ 4.71 **FUD** XXX [J] [P3] [80] [50] [▢]

AMA: 2018,May,3; 2018,Jan,8; 2017,Jan,8; 2016,Jan,13; 2015,Mar,9; 2015,Jan,16; 2014,Jan,11

38221 biopsy(ies)

EXCLUDES *Aspiration and biopsy during same session (38222)*
Aspiration of bone marrow (38220)

🔬 (88305)

📷 2.00 ⚕ 4.39 **FUD** XXX [J] [P3] [80] [50] [▢]

AMA: 2018,May,3; 2018,Jan,8; 2017,Jan,8; 2016,Jan,13; 2015,Mar,9; 2014,Jan,11

38222 biopsy(ies) and aspiration(s)

EXCLUDES *Aspiration of bone marrow only (38221)*
Biopsy of bone marrow only (38220)

🔬 (88305)

📷 2.24 ⚕ 4.87 **FUD** XXX [J] [P3] [80] [50] [▢]

AMA: 2018,May,3

38230 Bone marrow harvesting for transplantation; allogeneic

EXCLUDES *Aspiration of bone marrow for platelet rich stem cell injection (0232T)*
Harvesting of blood-derived hematopoietic progenitor cells for transplant (allogeneic) (38205)

📷 5.97 ⚕ 5.97 **FUD** 000 [S] [G2] [80] [▢]

AMA: 2018,Jan,8; 2017,Jan,8; 2016,Jan,13; 2015,Jan,16; 2014,Jan,11

38232 autologous

EXCLUDES *Aspiration of bone marrow (38220, 38222)*
Aspiration of bone marrow for platelet rich stem cell injection (0232T)
Aspiration of bone marrow for spinal graft (20939)
Harvesting of blood-derived peripheral stem cells for transplant (allogenic/autologous) (38205-38206)

📷 5.75 ⚕ 5.75 **FUD** 000 [S] [G2] [80] [▢]

AMA: 2018,Jan,8; 2017,Jan,8; 2016,Jan,13; 2015,Jan,16; 2014,Jan,11

● New Code ▲ Revised Code ○ Reinstated ● New Web Release ▲ Revised Web Release + Add-on Unlisted Not Covered # Resequenced
50 Optum Mod 50 Exempt ⊘ AMA Mod 51 Exempt 51 Optum Mod 51 Exempt 63 Mod 63 Exempt ⊬ Non-FDA Drug ★ Telemedicine M Maternity A Age Edit

CPT © 2019 American Medical Association. All Rights Reserved.

38240-38243 [38243] Hematopoietic Progenitor Cell Transplantation

CMS: 100-03,110.23 Stem Cell Transplantation; 100-04,3,90.3 Stem Cell Transplantation; 100-04,3,90.3.1 Allogeneic Stem Cell Transplantation; 100-04,3,90.3.2 Autologous Stem Cell Transplantation (AuSCT); 100-04,3,90.3.3 Billing for Allogeneic Stem Cell Transplants; 100-04,32,90 Billing for Stem Cell Transplantation; 100-04,32,90.2 Allogeneic Stem Cell Transplantation; 100-04,32,90.2.1 Coding for Stem Cell Transplantation; 100-04,32,90.3 Autologous Stem Cell Transplantation; 100-04,32,90.4 Edits Stem Cell Transplant; 100-04,32,90.6 Clinical Trials for Stem Cell Transplant for Myelodysplastic Syndrome (; 100-04,4,231.10 Billing for Autologous Stem Cell Transplants; 100-04,4,231.11 Billing for Allogeneic Stem Cell Transplants

INCLUDES Evaluation of patient prior to, during, and after the infusion
Management of uncomplicated adverse reactions such as hives or nausea
Monitoring of physiological parameters
Physician presence during the infusion
Supervision of clinical staff

EXCLUDES *Administration of fluids for the transplant or for incidental hydration separately*
Concurrent administration of medications with the infusion for the transplant
Cryopreservation, freezing, and storage of hematopoietic progenitor cells for transplant (38207)
Human leukocyte antigen (HLA) testing (81379-81383, 86812-86821)
Modification, treatment, processing of hematopoietic progenitor cell specimens for transplant (38210-38215)
Thawing and expansion of hematopoietic progenitor cells for transplant (38208-38209)

Code also administration of medications and/or fluids not related to the transplant with modifier 59
Code also E&M service for the treatment of more complicated adverse reactions after the infusion, as appropriate
Code also separately identifiable E&M service on the same date, using modifier 25 as appropriate (99211-99215, 99217-99220, [99224, 99225, 99226], 99221-99223, 99231-99239, 99471-99472, 99475-99476)

38240 **Hematopoietic progenitor cell (HPC); allogeneic transplantation per donor**

    EXCLUDES *Allogeneic lymphocyte infusions on same date of service with (38242)*
Hematopoietic progenitor cell (HPC); HPC boost on same date of service with ([38243])

    🏥 6.53   🔖 6.53 **FUD** XXX   J 80 ▢

    AMA: 2018,Jan,8; 2017,Jan,8; 2016,Jan,13; 2015,Jan,16; 2014,Jan,11

38241 **autologous transplantation**

    🏥 4.88   🔖 4.88 **FUD** XXX   S G2 80 ▢

    AMA: 2018,Jan,8; 2017,Jan,8; 2016,Jan,13; 2015,Jan,16; 2014,Jan,11

\# **38243** **HPC boost**

    EXCLUDES *Allogeneic lymphocyte infusions on same date of service with (38242)*
Hematopoietic progenitor cell (HPC); allogeneic transplantation per donor on same date of service with (38240)

    🏥 3.47   🔖 3.47 **FUD** 000   S R2 80 ▢

    AMA: 2018,Jan,8; 2017,Jan,8; 2016,Jan,13; 2015,Feb,10; 2015,Jan,16; 2014,Jan,11

38242 **Allogeneic lymphocyte infusions**

    EXCLUDES *Aspiration of bone marrow (38220, 38222)*
Aspiration of bone marrow for platelet rich stem cell injection (0232T)
Aspiration of bone marrow for spinal graft (20939)
Hematopoietic progenitor cell (HPC); allogeneic transplantation per donor on same date of service with (38240)
Hematopoietic progenitor cell (HPC); HPC boost on same date of service with ([38243])

    🔬 (81379-81383, 86812-86813, 86816-86817, 86821)

    🏥 3.45   🔖 3.45 **FUD** 000   S R2 80 ▢

    AMA: 2018,Jan,8; 2017,Jan,8; 2016,Jan,13; 2015,Jan,16; 2014,Jan,11

38243 **Resequenced code. See code following 38241.**

38300-38382 Incision Lymphatic Vessels

38300 **Drainage of lymph node abscess or lymphadenitis; simple**

    🏥 5.86   🔖 9.20 **FUD** 010   J A2 ▢

    AMA: 2014,Jan,11

38305 **extensive**

    🏥 14.0   🔖 14.0 **FUD** 090   J A2 ▢

    AMA: 2014,Jan,11

38308 **Lymphangiotomy or other operations on lymphatic channels**

    🏥 13.0   🔖 13.0 **FUD** 090   J A2 80 ▢

    AMA: 2014,Jan,11

38380 **Suture and/or ligation of thoracic duct; cervical approach**

    🏥 16.3   🔖 16.3 **FUD** 090   C 80 ▢

    AMA: 2014,Jan,11

38381 **thoracic approach**

    🏥 23.2   🔖 23.2 **FUD** 090   C 80 ▢

    AMA: 2014,Jan,11

38382 **abdominal approach**

    🏥 19.4   🔖 19.4 **FUD** 090   C 80 ▢

    AMA: 2014,Jan,11

38500-38555 Biopsy/Excision Lymphatic Vessels

EXCLUDES *Injection for sentinel node identification (38792)*
Percutaneous needle biopsy retroperitoneal mass (49180)

38500 **Biopsy or excision of lymph node(s); open, superficial**

    EXCLUDES *Lymphadenectomy (38700-38780)*

    🏥 7.36   🔖 9.58 **FUD** 010   J A2 50 ▢

    AMA: 2019,Feb,8; 2018,Jan,8; 2017,Jan,8; 2016,Jan,13; 2015,Jan,16; 2014,Jan,11

38505 **by needle, superficial (eg, cervical, inguinal, axillary)**

    EXCLUDES *Fine needle aspiration (10004-10012, 10021)*

    🔬 (88172-88173)

    📷 (76942, 77002, 77012, 77021)

    🏥 2.02   🔖 3.56 **FUD** 000   J A2 50 ▢

    AMA: 2019,Feb,8; 2018,Jan,8; 2017,Jan,8; 2016,Jan,13; 2015,Jan,16; 2014,Jan,11

38510 **open, deep cervical node(s)**

    🏥 12.0   🔖 14.9 **FUD** 010   J A2 50 ▢

    AMA: 2019,Feb,8; 2018,Jan,8; 2017,Jan,8; 2016,Jan,13; 2015,Jan,16; 2014,Jan,11

38520 **open, deep cervical node(s) with excision scalene fat pad**

    🏥 13.4   🔖 13.4 **FUD** 090   J A2 50 ▢

    AMA: 2019,Feb,8; 2018,Jan,8; 2017,Jan,8; 2016,Jan,13; 2015,Jan,16; 2014,Jan,11

38525 **open, deep axillary node(s)**

    🏥 12.6   🔖 12.6 **FUD** 090   J A2 50 ▢

    AMA: 2019,Feb,8; 2018,Jan,8; 2017,Jan,8; 2016,Jan,13; 2015,Mar,5; 2015,Jan,16; 2014,Apr,10; 2014,Jan,11

38530 **open, internal mammary node(s)**

    EXCLUDES *Fine needle aspiration (10005-10012)*
Lymphadenectomy (38720-38746)

    🏥 16.1   🔖 16.1 **FUD** 090   J A2 80 50 ▢

    AMA: 2019,Feb,8; 2018,Jan,8; 2017,Jan,8; 2016,Jan,13; 2015,Jan,16; 2014,Apr,10; 2014,Jan,11

38531 **open, inguinofemoral node(s)**

    🏥 12.6   🔖 12.6 **FUD** 090   80 50 ▢

    AMA: 2019,Feb,8

38542 **Dissection, deep jugular node(s)**

    EXCLUDES *Complete cervical lymphadenectomy (38720)*

    🏥 14.8   🔖 14.8 **FUD** 090   J A2 80 50 ▢

    AMA: 2019,Feb,8; 2018,Jan,8; 2017,Jan,8; 2016,Jan,13; 2015,Jan,16; 2014,Jan,11

38550 **Excision of cystic hygroma, axillary or cervical; without deep neurovascular dissection**

    🏥 14.7   🔖 14.7 **FUD** 090   J A2 80 ▢

    AMA: 2014,Jan,11

38555 **with deep neurovascular dissection**

    🏥 29.2   🔖 29.2 **FUD** 090   J A2 80 ▢

    AMA: 2014,Jan,11

38562-38564 Limited Lymphadenectomy: Staging

38562 Limited lymphadenectomy for staging (separate procedure); pelvic and para-aortic

    EXCLUDES *Prostatectomy (55812, 55842)*
        Radioactive substance inserted into prostate (55862)

    🔲 20.4   20.4   **FUD** 090   C 80 ▢

    AMA: 2019,Feb,8; 2018,Jan,8; 2017,Jan,8; 2016,Jan,13; 2015,Jan,16; 2014,Jan,11

38564 retroperitoneal (aortic and/or splenic)

    🔲 20.4   20.4   **FUD** 090   C 80 ▢

    AMA: 2019,Feb,8; 2014,Jan,11

38570-38589 Laparoscopic Lymph Node Procedures

  INCLUDES Diagnostic laparoscopy (49320)
  EXCLUDES *Laparoscopy with draining of lymphocele to peritoneal cavity (49323)*
    Limited lymphadenectomy:
      Pelvic (38562)
      Retroperitoneal (38564)

38570 Laparoscopy, surgical; with retroperitoneal lymph node sampling (biopsy), single or multiple

    🔲 14.7   14.7   **FUD** 010   J A2 80 ▢

    AMA: 2019,Feb,8; 2018,Jan,8; 2017,Jan,8; 2016,Jan,13; 2015,Jan,16; 2014,Jan,11

38571 with bilateral total pelvic lymphadenectomy

    🔲 19.1   19.1   **FUD** 010   J A2 80 ▢

    AMA: 2019,Feb,8; 2018,Jan,8; 2017,Jan,8; 2016,Jan,13; 2015,Jan,16; 2014,Jan,11

38572 with bilateral total pelvic lymphadenectomy and peri-aortic lymph node sampling (biopsy), single or multiple

    EXCLUDES *Lymphocele drainage into peritoneal cavity (49323)*

    🔲 26.7   26.7   **FUD** 010   J A2 80 ▢

    AMA: 2019,Feb,8; 2018,Jan,8; 2017,Jan,8; 2016,Jan,13; 2015,Jan,13; 2015,Jan,16; 2014,Jan,11

38573 with bilateral total pelvic lymphadenectomy and peri-aortic lymph node sampling, peritoneal washings, peritoneal biopsy(ies), omentectomy, and diaphragmatic washings, including diaphragmatic and other serosal biopsy(ies), when performed

    EXCLUDES *Laparoscopic hysterectomy procedures (58541-58554)*
      Laparoscopic omentopexy (separate procedure) (49326)
      Laparoscopy abdomen, diagnostic (separate procedure)(49320)
      Laparoscopy unlisted (38589)
      Laparoscopy without omentectomy (38570-38572)
      Lymphadenectomy for staging (38562-38564)
      Omentectomy (separate procedure) (49255)
      Pelvic lymphadenectomy of external iliac, hypogastric, and obturator nodes (38770)
      Retroperitoneal lymphadenectomy of aortic, pelvic, and renal nodes (separate procedure)(38780)

    🔲 33.7   33.7   **FUD** 010   J G2 80 ▢

    AMA: 2019,Mar,5; 2018,Apr,10

38589 Unlisted laparoscopy procedure, lymphatic system

    🔲 0.00   0.00   **FUD** YYY   J 80 50 ▢

    AMA: 2018,Apr,10; 2018,Jan,8; 2017,Jan,8; 2016,Jan,13; 2015,Jan,16; 2014,Jan,11

38700-38780 Lymphadenectomy Procedures

  INCLUDES Lymph node biopsy/excision (38500)
  EXCLUDES *Excision of lymphedematous skin and subcutaneous tissue (15004-15005)*
    Limited lymphadenectomy
      Pelvic (38562)
      Retroperitoneal (38564)
    Repair of lymphedematous skin and tissue (15570-15650)

38700 Suprahyoid lymphadenectomy

    🔲 23.1   23.1   **FUD** 090   J G2 80 50 ▢

    AMA: 2019,Feb,8; 2018,Jan,8; 2017,Jan,8; 2016,Jan,13; 2015,Jan,16; 2014,Jan,11

38720 Cervical lymphadenectomy (complete)

    🔲 38.6   38.6   **FUD** 090   J 80 50 ▢

    AMA: 2019,Feb,8; 2018,Jan,8; 2017,Jan,8; 2016,Jan,13; 2015,Jan,16; 2014,Jan,11

38724 Cervical lymphadenectomy (modified radical neck dissection)

    🔲 41.6   41.6   **FUD** 090   C 80 50 ▢

    AMA: 2019,Mar,10; 2019,Feb,8; 2018,Jan,8; 2017,Jan,8; 2016,Jan,13; 2015,Jan,16; 2014,Jan,11

38740 Axillary lymphadenectomy; superficial

    🔲 20.1   20.1   **FUD** 090   J A2 80 50 ▢

    AMA: 2019,Feb,8; 2018,Jan,8; 2017,Jan,8; 2016,Jan,13; 2015,Jan,16; 2014,Apr,10; 2014,Jan,11

38745 complete

    🔲 25.4   25.4   **FUD** 090   J A2 80 50 ▢

    AMA: 2019,Feb,8; 2014,Jan,11

+ 38746 Thoracic lymphadenectomy by thoracotomy, mediastinal and regional lymphadenectomy (List separately in addition to code for primary procedure)

    INCLUDES   Left side
        Aortopulmonary window
        Inferior pulmonary ligament
        Paraesophageal
        Subcarinal
      Right side
        Inferior pulmonary ligament
        Paraesophageal
        Paratracheal
        Subcarinal

    EXCLUDES *Thoracoscopic mediastinal and regional lymphadenectomy (32674)*

    Code first (21601, 31760, 31766, 31786, 32096-32200, 32220-32320, 32440-32491, 32503-32505, 33025, 33030, 33050-33130, 39200-39220, 39560-39561, 43101, 43112, 43117-43118, 43122-43123, 43351, 60270, 60505)

    🔲 6.23   6.23   **FUD** ZZZ   C 80 ▢

    AMA: 2019,Feb,8; 2018,Jan,8; 2017,Jan,8; 2016,Jan,13; 2015,Jan,16; 2014,May,3; 2014,Jan,11

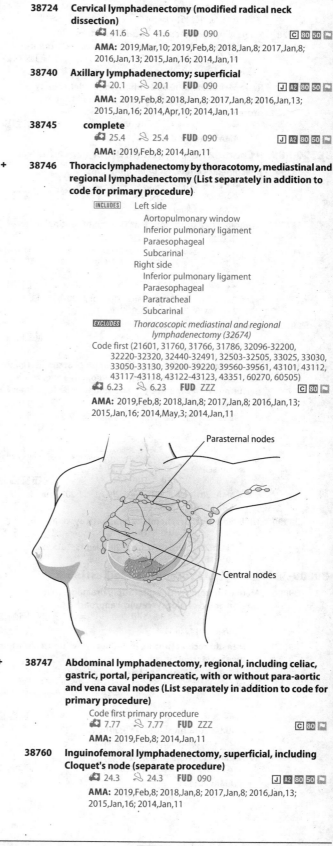

Parasternal nodes

Central nodes

+ 38747 Abdominal lymphadenectomy, regional, including celiac, gastric, portal, peripancreatic, with or without para-aortic and vena caval nodes (List separately in addition to code for primary procedure)

    Code first primary procedure

    🔲 7.77   7.77   **FUD** ZZZ   C 80 ▢

    AMA: 2019,Feb,8; 2014,Jan,11

38760 Inguinofemoral lymphadenectomy, superficial, including Cloquet's node (separate procedure)

    🔲 24.3   24.3   **FUD** 090   J A2 80 50 ▢

    AMA: 2019,Feb,8; 2018,Jan,8; 2017,Jan,8; 2016,Jan,13; 2015,Jan,16; 2014,Jan,11

38765 Inguinofemoral lymphadenectomy, superficial, in continuity with pelvic lymphadenectomy, including external iliac, hypogastric, and obturator nodes (separate procedure)

🔲 37.6   ⚕ 37.6   **FUD** 090   C 80 50 📱

AMA: 2019,Feb,8; 2018,Jan,8; 2017,Jan,8; 2016,Jan,13; 2015,Jan,16; 2014,Jan,11

38770 Pelvic lymphadenectomy, including external iliac, hypogastric, and obturator nodes (separate procedure)

🔲 23.4   ⚕ 23.4   **FUD** 090   C 80 50 📱

AMA: 2019,Feb,8; 2014,Jan,11

38780 Retroperitoneal transabdominal lymphadenectomy, extensive, including pelvic, aortic, and renal nodes (separate procedure)

🔲 29.7   ⚕ 29.7   **FUD** 090   C 80 📱

AMA: 2019,Feb,8; 2014,Jan,11

38790-38999 Cannulation/Injection/Other Procedures

38790 Injection procedure; lymphangiography

🔲 (75801-75807)

🔲 2.39   ⚕ 2.39   **FUD** 000   N N1 50 📱

AMA: 2014,Jan,11

38792 radioactive tracer for identification of sentinel node

EXCLUDES Sentinel node excision (38500-38542)
Sentinel node(s) identification (mapping) intraoperative with nonradioactive dye injection (38900)

🔲 (78195)

🔲 0.96   ⚕ 2.34   **FUD** 000   01 N1 50 📱

AMA: 2019,Feb,8; 2018,Jan,8; 2017,Jan,8; 2016,Jan,13; 2015,Mar,5; 2015,Jan,16; 2014,Jan,11

38794 Cannulation, thoracic duct

🔲 8.57   ⚕ 8.57   **FUD** 090   N N1 80 📱

AMA: 2014,Jan,11

+ **38900** Intraoperative identification (eg, mapping) of sentinel lymph node(s) includes injection of non-radioactive dye, when performed (List separately in addition to code for primary procedure)

EXCLUDES Injection of tracer for sentinel node identification (38792)
Code first (19302, 19307, 38500, 38510, 38520, 38525, 38530-38531, 38542, 38562-38564, 38570-38572, 38740, 38745, 38760, 38765, 38770, 38780, 56630-56634, 56637, 56640)

🔲 4.00   ⚕ 4.00   **FUD** ZZZ   N N1 80 50 📱

AMA: 2019,Feb,8; 2018,Jan,8; 2017,Jan,8; 2016,Jan,13; 2015,Mar,5; 2014,Jan,11

38999 Unlisted procedure, hemic or lymphatic system

🔲 0.00   ⚕ 0.00   **FUD** YYY   S 80 📱

AMA: 2018,Jan,8; 2017,Jan,8; 2016,Jan,13; 2015,Jan,16; 2014,Jan,11

39000-39499 Surgical Procedures: Mediastinum

39000 Mediastinotomy with exploration, drainage, removal of foreign body, or biopsy; cervical approach

🔲 14.3   ⚕ 14.3   **FUD** 090   C 80 📱

AMA: 2014,Jan,11

39010 transthoracic approach, including either transthoracic or median sternotomy

EXCLUDES ECMO/ECLS insertion or reposition of cannula (33955-33956, [33963, 33964])
Video-assisted thoracic surgery (VATS) pericardial biopsy (32604)

🔲 22.7   ⚕ 22.7   **FUD** 090   C 80 📱

AMA: 2018,Jan,8; 2017,Jan,8; 2016,Jan,13; 2015,Jul,3; 2015,Jan,16; 2014,Jan,11; 2014,Jan,5

39200 Resection of mediastinal cyst

🔲 25.2   ⚕ 25.2   **FUD** 090   C 80 📱

AMA: 2014,Jan,11

39220 Resection of mediastinal tumor

EXCLUDES Thymectomy (60520)
Thyroidectomy, substernal (60270)
Video-assisted thoracic surgery (VATS) resection cyst, mass, or tumor of mediastinum (32662)

🔲 32.7   ⚕ 32.7   **FUD** 090   C 80 📱

AMA: 2014,Jan,11

39401 Mediastinoscopy; includes biopsy(ies) of mediastinal mass (eg, lymphoma), when performed

🔲 8.96   ⚕ 8.96   **FUD** 090   J 📱

AMA: 2018,Jan,8; 2017,Jan,8; 2016,Jun,4

39402 with lymph node biopsy(ies) (eg, lung cancer staging)

🔲 11.7   ⚕ 11.7   **FUD** 000   J 📱

AMA: 2018,Jan,8; 2017,Jan,8; 2016,Jun,4

39499 Unlisted procedure, mediastinum

🔲 0.00   ⚕ 0.00   **FUD** YYY   C 80 📱

AMA: 2014,Jan,11

39501-39599 Surgical Procedures: Diaphragm

EXCLUDES Esophagogastric fundoplasty, with fundic patch (43325)
Repair of diaphragmatic (esophageal) hernias:
Laparoscopic with fundoplication (43280-43282)
Laparotomy (43332-43333)
Thoracoabdominal (43336-43337)
Thoracotomy (43334-43335)

39501 Repair, laceration of diaphragm, any approach

🔲 24.6   ⚕ 24.6   **FUD** 090   C 80 📱

AMA: 2018,Jan,8; 2017,Jan,8; 2016,Jan,13; 2015,Jan,16; 2014,Dec,16; 2014,Dec,16; 2014,Jan,11

39503 Repair, neonatal diaphragmatic hernia, with or without chest tube insertion and with or without creation of ventral hernia   A

🔲 173.   ⚕ 173.   **FUD** 090   63 C 80 📱

AMA: 2018,Jan,8; 2017,Jan,8; 2016,Jan,13; 2015,Jan,16; 2014,Jan,11

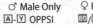

Trachea

Lungs

Diaphragm

A defect of the diaphragm can allow abdominal contents to herniate into the thoracic cavity

39540 Repair, diaphragmatic hernia (other than neonatal), traumatic; acute

🔲 25.2   ⚕ 25.2   **FUD** 090   C 80 📱

AMA: 2018,Jan,8; 2017,Jan,8; 2016,Jan,13; 2015,Jan,16; 2014,Jan,11

39541 chronic

🔲 27.2   ⚕ 27.2   **FUD** 090   C 80 📱

AMA: 2018,Jan,8; 2017,Jan,8; 2016,Jan,13; 2015,Jan,16; 2014,Jan,11

39545 Imbrication of diaphragm for eventration, transthoracic or transabdominal, paralytic or nonparalytic

🔲 25.7   ⚕ 25.7   **FUD** 090   C 80 📱

AMA: 2018,Jan,8; 2017,Jan,8; 2016,Jan,13; 2015,Jan,16; 2014,Jan,11

26/TC PC/TC Only   A2-Z3 ASC Payment   50 Bilateral   ♂ Male Only   ♀ Female Only   🔲 Facility RVU   ⚕ Non-Facility RVU   📱 CCI   ☒ CLIA
FUD Follow-up Days   **CMS:** IOM   **AMA:** CPT Asst   A-Y OPPSI   80/80 Surg Assist Allowed / w/Doc   📱 Lab Crosswalk   ☒ Radiology Crosswalk

184   CPT © 2019 American Medical Association. All Rights Reserved.   © 2019 Optum360, LLC

39560   Resection, diaphragm; with simple repair (eg, primary suture)
       23.1   23.1   **FUD** 090   C 80 ▭
       AMA: 2018,Jan,8; 2017,Jan,8; 2016,Jan,13; 2015,Jan,16; 2014,Jan,11

39561   with complex repair (eg, prosthetic material, local muscle flap)
       35.9   35.9   **FUD** 090   C 80 ▭
       AMA: 2018,Jan,8; 2017,Jan,8; 2016,Jan,13; 2015,Jan,16; 2014,Jan,11

39599   Unlisted procedure, diaphragm
       0.00   0.00   **FUD** YYY   C 80 ▭
       AMA: 2014,Jan,11

40490-40799 Resection and Repair Procedures of the Lips

EXCLUDES *Procedures on the skin of lips-see integumentary section codes*

40490 **Biopsy of lip**
🚗 2.09 ⚕ 3.59 **FUD** 000 T P3 ▱
AMA: 2019,Jan,9; 2014,Jan,11

40500 **Vermilionectomy (lip shave), with mucosal advancement**
🚗 10.4 ⚕ 14.6 **FUD** 090 J A2 ▱
AMA: 2014,Jan,11

40510 **Excision of lip; transverse wedge excision with primary closure**
EXCLUDES *Excision of mucous lesions (40810-40816)*
🚗 10.1 ⚕ 13.9 **FUD** 090 J A2 ▱
AMA: 2014,Jan,11

40520 **V-excision with primary direct linear closure**
EXCLUDES *Excision of mucous lesions (40810-40816)*
🚗 10.2 ⚕ 14.1 **FUD** 090 J A2 ▱
AMA: 2014,Jan,11

40525 **full thickness, reconstruction with local flap (eg, Estlander or fan)**
🚗 15.8 ⚕ 15.8 **FUD** 090 J A2 ▱
AMA: 2014,Jan,11

40527 **full thickness, reconstruction with cross lip flap (Abbe-Estlander)**
INCLUDES *Cleft lip repair with cross lip pedicle flap (Abbe-Estlander type), without pedicle sectioning and insertion*
EXCLUDES *Cleft lip repair with cross lip pedicle flap (Abbe-Estlander type), with pedicle sectioning and insertion (40761)*
🚗 17.7 ⚕ 17.7 **FUD** 090 J A2 80 ▱
AMA: 2014,Jan,11

40530 **Resection of lip, more than one-fourth, without reconstruction**
EXCLUDES *Reconstruction (13131-13153)*
🚗 11.5 ⚕ 15.5 **FUD** 090 J A2 ▱
AMA: 2014,Jan,11

40650 **Repair lip, full thickness; vermilion only**
🚗 8.71 ⚕ 13.0 **FUD** 090 T A2 80 ▱
AMA: 2018,Jan,8; 2017,Jan,8; 2016,Nov,7; 2016,Jan,13; 2015,Jan,16; 2014,Jan,11

40652 **up to half vertical height**
🚗 10.1 ⚕ 14.2 **FUD** 090 T A2 80 ▱
AMA: 2018,Jan,8; 2017,Jan,8; 2016,Nov,7; 2016,Jan,13; 2015,Jan,16; 2014,Jan,11

40654 **over one-half vertical height, or complex**
🚗 12.2 ⚕ 16.4 **FUD** 090 T A2 ▱
AMA: 2018,Jan,8; 2017,Jan,8; 2016,Nov,7; 2014,Jan,11

40700 **Plastic repair of cleft lip/nasal deformity; primary, partial or complete, unilateral**
EXCLUDES *Cleft lip repair with cross lip pedicle flap (Abbe-Estlander type):*
With pedicle sectioning and insertion (40761)
Without pedicle sectioning and insertion (40527)
Rhinoplasty for nasal deformity secondary to congenital cleft lip (30460, 30462)
🚗 29.0 ⚕ 29.0 **FUD** 090 J A2 80 ▱
AMA: 2018,Jan,8; 2017,Jan,8; 2016,Jan,13; 2015,Jan,16; 2014,Dec,18; 2014,Jan,11

40701 **primary bilateral, 1-stage procedure**
EXCLUDES *Cleft lip repair with cross lip pedicle flap (Abbe-Estlander type):*
With pedicle sectioning and insertion (40761)
Without pedicle sectioning and insertion (40527)
Rhinoplasty for nasal deformity secondary to congenital cleft lip (30460, 30462)
🚗 34.4 ⚕ 34.4 **FUD** 090 J A2 80 ▱
AMA: 2018,Jan,8; 2017,Jan,8; 2016,Jan,13; 2015,Jan,16; 2014,Dec,18; 2014,Jan,11

Bilateral cleft lip

Cleft margins on both sides are incised

Margins are closed, correcting cleft

40702 **primary bilateral, 1 of 2 stages**
EXCLUDES *Cleft lip repair with cross lip pedicle flap (Abbe-Estlander type):*
With pedicle sectioning and insertion (40761)
Without pedicle sectioning and insertion (40527)
Rhinoplasty for nasal deformity secondary to congenital cleft lip (30460, 30462)
🚗 28.9 ⚕ 28.9 **FUD** 090 J A2 80 ▱
AMA: 2018,Jan,8; 2017,Jan,8; 2016,Jan,13; 2015,Jan,16; 2014,Dec,18; 2014,Jan,11

40720 **secondary, by recreation of defect and reclosure**
EXCLUDES *Cleft lip repair with cross lip pedicle flap (Abbe-Estlander type):*
With pedicle sectioning and insertion (40761)
Without pedicle sectioning and insertion (40527)
Rhinoplasty for nasal deformity secondary to congenital cleft lip (30460, 30462)
🚗 29.7 ⚕ 29.7 **FUD** 090 J A2 80 50 ▱
AMA: 2018,Jan,8; 2017,Jan,8; 2016,Jan,13; 2015,Jan,16; 2014,Dec,18; 2014,Jan,11

40761 **with cross lip pedicle flap (Abbe-Estlander type), including sectioning and inserting of pedicle**
EXCLUDES *Cleft lip repair with cross lip pedicle flap (Abbe-Estlander type) without sectioning and insertion of pedicle (40527)*
Cleft palate repair (42200-42225)
Other reconstructive procedures (14060-14061, 15120-15261, 15574, 15576, 15630)
🚗 31.3 ⚕ 31.3 **FUD** 090 J A2 ▱
AMA: 2014,Jan,11

40799 **Unlisted procedure, lips**
🚗 0.00 ⚕ 0.00 **FUD** YYY T 80 ▱
AMA: 2014,Jan,11

40800-40819 Incision and Resection of Buccal Cavity

INCLUDES Mucosal/submucosal tissue of lips/cheeks
Oral cavity outside the dentoalveolar structures

40800 **Drainage of abscess, cyst, hematoma, vestibule of mouth; simple**
🚗 3.72 ⚕ 6.08 **FUD** 010 T P3 ▱
AMA: 2014,Jan,11

40801 **complicated**
🚗 6.26 ⚕ 8.86 **FUD** 010 T A2 ▱
AMA: 2014,Jan,11

40804 Removal of embedded foreign body, vestibule of mouth; simple
🔲 3.36 🔲 5.47 **FUD** 010   [Q1] [N1] [80] ▢
AMA: 2014,Jan,11

40805 complicated
🔲 6.43 🔲 8.91 **FUD** 010   [T] [P3] [80] ▢
AMA: 2014,Jan,11

40806 Incision of labial frenum (frenotomy)
🔲 0.93 🔲 2.91 **FUD** 000   [T] [P3] [80] ▢
AMA: 2014,Jan,11

40808 Biopsy, vestibule of mouth
🔲 3.06 🔲 5.37 **FUD** 010   [T] [P3] ▢
AMA: 2019,Jan,9; 2014,Jan,11

40810 Excision of lesion of mucosa and submucosa, vestibule of mouth; without repair
🔲 3.64 🔲 5.99 **FUD** 010   [J] [P3] ▢
AMA: 2014,Jan,11

40812 with simple repair
🔲 5.63 🔲 8.30 **FUD** 010   [J] [P3] ▢
AMA: 2014,Jan,11

40814 with complex repair
🔲 8.71 🔲 11.0 **FUD** 090   [J] [A2] ▢
AMA: 2014,Jan,11

40816 complex, with excision of underlying muscle
🔲 9.02 🔲 11.5 **FUD** 090   [J] [A2] ▢
AMA: 2014,Jan,11

40818 Excision of mucosa of vestibule of mouth as donor graft
🔲 7.91 🔲 10.5 **FUD** 090   [T] [A2] [80] ▢
AMA: 2014,Jan,11

40819 Excision of frenum, labial or buccal (frenumectomy, frenulectomy, frenectomy)
🔲 6.79 🔲 9.05 **FUD** 090   [T] [A2] [80] ▢
AMA: 2014,Jan,11

40820 Destruction of Lesion of Buccal Cavity

CMS: 100-03,140.5 Laser Procedures

[INCLUDES] Mucosal/submucosal tissue of lips/cheeks
Oral cavity outside the dentoalveolar structures

40820 Destruction of lesion or scar of vestibule of mouth by physical methods (eg, laser, thermal, cryo, chemical)
🔲 4.91 🔲 7.54 **FUD** 010   [J] [P3] ▢
AMA: 2014,Jan,11

40830-40899 Repair Procedures of the Buccal Cavity

[INCLUDES] Mucosal/submucosal tissue of lips/cheeks
Oral cavity outside the dentoalveolar structures
[EXCLUDES] Skin grafts (15002-15630)

40830 Closure of laceration, vestibule of mouth; 2.5 cm or less
🔲 4.79 🔲 7.78 **FUD** 010   [T] [G2] [80] ▢
AMA: 2014,Jan,11

40831 over 2.5 cm or complex
🔲 6.55 🔲 9.95 **FUD** 010   [T] [A2] [80] ▢
AMA: 2014,Jan,11

40840 Vestibuloplasty; anterior
🔲 18.0 🔲 23.5 **FUD** 090   [J] [A2] [80] ▢
AMA: 2014,Jan,11

40842 posterior, unilateral
🔲 17.7 🔲 22.8 **FUD** 090   [J] [A2] [80] ▢
AMA: 2014,Jan,11

40843 posterior, bilateral
🔲 23.6 🔲 30.1 **FUD** 090   [J] [A2] [80] ▢
AMA: 2014,Jan,11

40844 entire arch
🔲 31.8 🔲 39.2 **FUD** 090   [J] [A2] [80] ▢
AMA: 2014,Jan,11

40845 complex (including ridge extension, muscle repositioning)
🔲 35.2 🔲 42.2 **FUD** 090   [J] [A2] [80] ▢
AMA: 2014,Jan,11

40899 Unlisted procedure, vestibule of mouth
🔲 0.00 🔲 0.00 **FUD** YYY   [T] [80] ▢
AMA: 2014,Jan,11

41000-41018 Surgical Incision of Floor of Mouth or Tongue

[EXCLUDES] Frenoplasty (41520)

41000 Intraoral incision and drainage of abscess, cyst, or hematoma of tongue or floor of mouth; lingual
🔲 3.22 🔲 4.65 **FUD** 010   [T] [P3] ▢
AMA: 2014,Jan,11

A small incision is made in the floor of the mouth; the cyst is opened and the fluid is drained

Cyst and line of incision

41005 sublingual, superficial
🔲 3.54 🔲 6.34 **FUD** 010   [T] [A2] [80] ▢
AMA: 2014,Jan,11

41006 sublingual, deep, supramylohyoid
🔲 7.36 🔲 10.2 **FUD** 090   [T] [A2] [80] ▢
AMA: 2014,Jan,11

41007 submental space
🔲 7.12 🔲 10.0 **FUD** 090   [T] [A2] [80] ▢
AMA: 2014,Jan,11

41008 submandibular space
🔲 7.74 🔲 11.0 **FUD** 090   [J] [A2] [80] ▢
AMA: 2014,Jan,11

41009 masticator space
🔲 8.46 🔲 11.8 **FUD** 090   [T] [A2] [80] ▢
AMA: 2014,Jan,11

41010 Incision of lingual frenum (frenotomy)
🔲 3.11 🔲 5.90 **FUD** 010   [T] [A2] [80] ▢
AMA: 2018,Jan,8; 2017,Nov,10; 2017,Sep,14; 2014,Jan,11

41015 Extraoral incision and drainage of abscess, cyst, or hematoma of floor of mouth; sublingual
🔲 9.53 🔲 12.0 **FUD** 090   [T] [A2] [80] ▢
AMA: 2014,Jan,11

41016 submental
🔲 10.0 🔲 12.8 **FUD** 090   [J] [A2] [80] ▢
AMA: 2014,Jan,11

41017 submandibular
🔲 10.1 🔲 13.0 **FUD** 090   [J] [A2] [80] ▢
AMA: 2014,Jan,11

41018 masticator space
🔲 11.8 🔲 14.7 **FUD** 090   [T] [A2] [80] ▢
AMA: 2014,Jan,11

41019 Placement of Devices for Brachytherapy

EXCLUDES   *Application of interstitial radioelements (77770-77772, 77778)*
Intracranial brachytherapy radiation sources with stereotactic insertion (61770)

41019   **Placement of needles, catheters, or other device(s) into the head and/or neck region (percutaneous, transoral, or transnasal) for subsequent interstitial radioelement application**

(76942, 77002, 77012, 77021)

13.7   13.7   **FUD** 000   J 62 80

AMA: 2018,Jan,8; 2017,Jan,8; 2016,Jan,13; 2015,Jan,16; 2014,Jan,11

41100-41599 Resection and Repair of the Tongue

41100   **Biopsy of tongue; anterior two-thirds**

3.07   4.94   **FUD** 010   T P3

AMA: 2019,Jan,9; 2014,Jan,11

Anterior (front) two-thirds of tongue makes up most of the easily visible portions

Anterior two-thirds

Lesion and elliptical incision

41105   **posterior one-third**

3.19   5.02   **FUD** 010   J P3

AMA: 2014,Jan,11

41108   **Biopsy of floor of mouth**

2.58   4.37   **FUD** 010   J P3

AMA: 2019,Jan,9; 2014,Jan,11

41110   **Excision of lesion of tongue without closure**

3.77   6.21   **FUD** 010   J P3

AMA: 2014,Jan,11

41112   **Excision of lesion of tongue with closure; anterior two-thirds**

7.22   9.65   **FUD** 090   J A2

AMA: 2014,Jan,11

41113   **posterior one-third**

7.98   10.5   **FUD** 090   J A2

AMA: 2014,Jan,11

41114   **with local tongue flap**

INCLUDES   Excision lesion of tongue with closure anterior/posterior two-thirds (41112-41113)

18.1   18.1   **FUD** 090   J A2 80

AMA: 2014,Jan,11

41115   **Excision of lingual frenum (frenectomy)**

4.17   7.17   **FUD** 010   T P3 80

AMA: 2018,Jan,8; 2017,Nov,10; 2017,Sep,14; 2014,Jan,11

41116   **Excision, lesion of floor of mouth**

6.31   9.55   **FUD** 090   J A2

AMA: 2014,Jan,11

41120   **Glossectomy; less than one-half tongue**

30.8   30.8   **FUD** 090   J A2 80

AMA: 2018,Jan,8; 2017,Jan,8; 2016,Jan,13; 2015,Jan,16; 2014,Jan,11

41130   **hemiglossectomy**

38.0   38.0   **FUD** 090   C 80

AMA: 2018,Jan,8; 2017,Jan,8; 2016,Jan,13; 2015,Jan,16; 2014,Jan,11

41135   **partial, with unilateral radical neck dissection**

62.9   62.9   **FUD** 090   C 80

AMA: 2018,Jan,8; 2017,Jan,8; 2016,Jan,13; 2015,Jan,16; 2014,Jan,11

41140   **complete or total, with or without tracheostomy, without radical neck dissection**

INCLUDES   Regnoli's excision

63.0   63.0   **FUD** 090   C 80

AMA: 2018,Jan,8; 2017,Jan,8; 2016,Jan,13; 2015,Jan,16; 2014,Jan,11

41145   **complete or total, with or without tracheostomy, with unilateral radical neck dissection**

79.8   79.8   **FUD** 090   C 80

AMA: 2018,Jan,8; 2017,Jan,8; 2016,Jan,13; 2015,Jan,16; 2014,Jan,11

41150   **composite procedure with resection floor of mouth and mandibular resection, without radical neck dissection**

63.5   63.5   **FUD** 090   C 80

AMA: 2018,Jan,8; 2017,Jan,8; 2016,Jan,13; 2015,Jan,16; 2014,Jan,11

41153   **composite procedure with resection floor of mouth, with suprahyoid neck dissection**

68.8   68.8   **FUD** 090   C 80

AMA: 2018,Jan,8; 2017,Jan,8; 2016,Jan,13; 2015,Jan,16; 2014,Jan,11

41155   **composite procedure with resection floor of mouth, mandibular resection, and radical neck dissection (Commando type)**

87.2   87.2   **FUD** 090   C 80

AMA: 2018,Jan,8; 2017,Jan,8; 2016,Jan,13; 2015,Jan,16; 2014,Jan,11

41250   **Repair of laceration 2.5 cm or less; floor of mouth and/or anterior two-thirds of tongue**

4.42   7.84   **FUD** 010   Q1 N1 80

AMA: 2014,Jan,11

41251   **posterior one-third of tongue**

5.33   8.79   **FUD** 010   T A2 80

AMA: 2014,Jan,11

41252   **Repair of laceration of tongue, floor of mouth, over 2.6 cm or complex**

6.01   9.13   **FUD** 010   T A2 80

AMA: 2014,Jan,11

41510   **Suture of tongue to lip for micrognathia (Douglas type procedure)**

13.0   13.0   **FUD** 090   J A2 80

AMA: 2018,Jan,8; 2017,Jan,8; 2016,Jan,13; 2015,Jan,16; 2014,Jan,11

41512   **Tongue base suspension, permanent suture technique**

EXCLUDES   *Suture tongue to lip for micrognathia (41510)*

18.9   18.9   **FUD** 090   J 62 80

AMA: 2018,Jan,8; 2017,Jan,8; 2016,Jan,13; 2015,Jan,16; 2014,Jan,11

41520   **Frenoplasty (surgical revision of frenum, eg, with Z-plasty)**

EXCLUDES   *Frenotomy (40806, 41010)*

7.11   10.1   **FUD** 090   J A2 80

AMA: 2018,Jan,8; 2017,Nov,10; 2017,Sep,14; 2014,Jan,11

41530   **Submucosal ablation of the tongue base, radiofrequency, 1 or more sites, per session**

10.7   27.4   **FUD** 000   J P3 80

AMA: 2018,Jan,8; 2017,Jan,8; 2016,Jan,13; 2015,Jan,16; 2014,Jan,11

41599   **Unlisted procedure, tongue, floor of mouth**

0.00   0.00   **FUD** YYY   T 80

AMA: 2018,Jan,8; 2017,Jan,8; 2016,Jan,13; 2015,Jan,16; 2014,Jan,11

41800-41899 Procedures of the Teeth and Supporting Structures

41800 Drainage of abscess, cyst, hematoma from dentoalveolar structures

🛠 4.35   ♒ 8.29   **FUD** 010   Q1 N1 ▣

AMA: 2014,Jan,11

41805 Removal of embedded foreign body from dentoalveolar structures; soft tissues

🛠 5.44   ♒ 8.28   **FUD** 010   T P3 80 ▣

AMA: 2014,Jan,11

41806 bone

🛠 7.97   ♒ 11.3   **FUD** 010   T P3 80 ▣

AMA: 2014,Jan,11

41820 Gingivectomy, excision gingiva, each quadrant

🛠 0.00   ♒ 0.00   **FUD** 010   J R2 80 ▣

AMA: 2014,Jan,11

Gingival recession

Excessive mucosal growth

Gingivitis is an inflammatory response to bacteria on the teeth; it is characterized by tender, red, swollen gums and can lead to gingival recession

41821 Operculectomy, excision pericoronal tissues

🛠 0.00   ♒ 0.00   **FUD** 000   T G2 80 ▣

AMA: 2014,Jan,11

41822 Excision of fibrous tuberosities, dentoalveolar structures

🛠 5.08   ♒ 8.17   **FUD** 010   T P3 80 ▣

AMA: 2014,Jan,11

41823 Excision of osseous tuberosities, dentoalveolar structures

🛠 9.27   ♒ 12.6   **FUD** 090   J P3 80 ▣

AMA: 2014,Jan,11

41825 Excision of lesion or tumor (except listed above), dentoalveolar structures; without repair

> **EXCLUDES** *Lesion destruction nonexcisional (41850)*

🛠 3.53   ♒ 6.19   **FUD** 010   J P3 ▣

AMA: 2014,Jan,11

41826 with simple repair

> **EXCLUDES** *Lesion destruction nonexcisional (41850)*

🛠 6.10   ♒ 9.09   **FUD** 010   J P3 ▣

AMA: 2014,Jan,11

41827 with complex repair

> **EXCLUDES** *Lesion destruction nonexcisional (41850)*

🛠 8.85   ♒ 12.8   **FUD** 090   J A2 ▣

AMA: 2014,Jan,11

41828 Excision of hyperplastic alveolar mucosa, each quadrant (specify)

🛠 6.05   ♒ 9.02   **FUD** 010   J P3 80 ▣

AMA: 2014,Jan,11

41830 Alveolectomy, including curettage of osteitis or sequestrectomy

🛠 8.07   ♒ 11.4   **FUD** 010   J P3 80 ▣

AMA: 2014,Jan,11

41850 Destruction of lesion (except excision), dentoalveolar structures

🛠 0.00   ♒ 0.00   **FUD** 000   T R2 80 ▣

AMA: 2014,Jan,11

41870 Periodontal mucosal grafting

🛠 0.00   ♒ 0.00   **FUD** 000   J G2 80 ▣

AMA: 2014,Jan,11

41872 Gingivoplasty, each quadrant (specify)

🛠 7.69   ♒ 11.2   **FUD** 090   J P3 80 ▣

AMA: 2014,Jan,11

41874 Alveoloplasty, each quadrant (specify)

> **EXCLUDES** *Fracture reduction (21421-21490)*
> *Laceration closure (40830-40831)*
> *Maxilla osteotomy, segmental (21206)*

🛠 7.41   ♒ 11.1   **FUD** 090   J P3 80 ▣

AMA: 2014,Jan,11

41899 Unlisted procedure, dentoalveolar structures

🛠 0.00   ♒ 0.00   **FUD** YYY   T 80 ▣

AMA: 2014,Jan,11

42000-42299 Procedures of the Palate and Uvula

42000 Drainage of abscess of palate, uvula

🛠 2.98   ♒ 4.45   **FUD** 010   T A2 80 ▣

AMA: 2014,Jan,11

42100 Biopsy of palate, uvula

🛠 3.14   ♒ 4.28   **FUD** 010   T P3

AMA: 2014,Jan,11

42104 Excision, lesion of palate, uvula; without closure

🛠 3.98   ♒ 6.20   **FUD** 010   J P3

AMA: 2014,Jan,11

42106 with simple primary closure

🛠 5.06   ♒ 7.79   **FUD** 010   J P3

AMA: 2014,Jan,11

42107 with local flap closure

> **EXCLUDES** *Mucosal graft (40818)*
> *Skin graft (14040-14302)*

🛠 9.94   ♒ 13.3   **FUD** 090   J A2

AMA: 2014,Jan,11

42120 Resection of palate or extensive resection of lesion

> **EXCLUDES** *Palate reconstruction using extraoral tissue*
> *(14040-14302, 15050, 15120, 15240, 15576)*

🛠 29.1   ♒ 29.1   **FUD** 090   J A2 80 ▣

AMA: 2014,Jan,11

42140 Uvulectomy, excision of uvula

🛠 4.46   ♒ 7.67   **FUD** 090   J A2 ▣

AMA: 2014,Jan,11

42145 Palatopharyngoplasty (eg, uvulopalatopharyngoplasty, uvulopharyngoplasty)

> **EXCLUDES** *Excision of maxillary torus palatinus (21032)*
> *Excision of torus mandibularis (21031)*

🛠 19.9   ♒ 19.9   **FUD** 090   J A2 ▣

AMA: 2018,Jan,8; 2017,Jan,8; 2016,Jan,13; 2015,Jan,16; 2014,Jan,11

42160 Destruction of lesion, palate or uvula (thermal, cryo or chemical)

🛠 4.21   ♒ 6.69   **FUD** 010   J P3 80 ▣

AMA: 2018,Jan,8; 2017,Jan,8; 2016,Jan,13; 2015,Jan,16; 2014,Jan,11

42180 Repair, laceration of palate; up to 2 cm

🛠 5.28   ♒ 7.08   **FUD** 010   T A2 80 ▣

AMA: 2014,Jan,11

42182 over 2 cm or complex

🛠 7.35   ♒ 9.26   **FUD** 010   J A2 80 ▣

AMA: 2014,Jan,11

| 26/TC PC/TC Only | A2-Z3 ASC Payment | 50 Bilateral | ♂ Male Only | ♀ Female Only | 🛠 Facility RVU | ♒ Non-Facility RVU | ▣ CCI | ✖ CLIA |
| **FUD** Follow-up Days | **CMS:** IOM | **AMA:** CPT Asst | A-Y OPPSI | 80/80 Surg Assist Allowed / w/Doc | ▣ Lab Crosswalk | | ▣ Radiology Crosswalk | |

190   CPT © 2019 American Medical Association. All Rights Reserved.   © 2019 Optum360, LLC

Digestive System

41800 — 42182

42200   **Palatoplasty for cleft palate, soft and/or hard palate only**
⚙ 27.3   ⚒ 27.3   **FUD** 090   J A2 80 ▣
AMA: 2018,Jan,8; 2017,Jan,8; 2016,Jan,13; 2015,Mar,9; 2015,Jan,16; 2014,Jul,8; 2014,Jan,11

42205   **Palatoplasty for cleft palate, with closure of alveolar ridge; soft tissue only**
⚙ 28.4   ⚒ 28.4   **FUD** 090   J A2 80 ▣
AMA: 2014,Jan,11

42210   **with bone graft to alveolar ridge (includes obtaining graft)**
⚙ 31.7   ⚒ 31.7   **FUD** 090   J A2 80 ▣
AMA: 2014,Jan,11

42215   **Palatoplasty for cleft palate; major revision**
⚙ 20.7   ⚒ 20.7   **FUD** 090   J A2 80 ▣
AMA: 2014,Jan,11

42220   **secondary lengthening procedure**
⚙ 17.0   ⚒ 17.0   **FUD** 090   J A2 80 ▣
AMA: 2014,Jan,11

42225   **attachment pharyngeal flap**
⚙ 28.4   ⚒ 28.4   **FUD** 090   J G2 80 ▣
AMA: 2018,Jan,8; 2017,Jan,8; 2016,Jan,13; 2015,Jan,16; 2014,Jan,11

42226   **Lengthening of palate, and pharyngeal flap**
⚙ 25.3   ⚒ 25.3   **FUD** 090   J A2 30 ▣
AMA: 2014,Jan,11

42227   **Lengthening of palate, with island flap**
⚙ 23.8   ⚒ 23.8   **FUD** 090   J G2 80 ▣
AMA: 2014,Jan,11

42235   **Repair of anterior palate, including vomer flap**
EXCLUDES   *Oronasal fistula repair (30600)*
⚙ 20.9   ⚒ 20.9   **FUD** 090   J A2 80 ▣
AMA: 2018,Jan,8; 2017,Jan,8; 2016,Jan,13; 2015,Mar,9; 2015,Jan,16; 2014,Jul,8; 2014,Jan,11

42260   **Repair of nasolabial fistula**
EXCLUDES   *Cleft lip repair (40700-40761)*
⚙ 18.9   ⚒ 23.5   **FUD** 090   J A2 80 ▣
AMA: 2014,Jan,11

42280   **Maxillary impression for palatal prosthesis**
⚙ 3.21   ⚒ 5.10   **FUD** 010   T P3 80 ▣
AMA: 2014,Jan,11

42281   **Insertion of pin-retained palatal prosthesis**
⚙ 4.75   ⚒ 6.56   **FUD** 010   J G2 80 ▣
AMA: 2014,Jan,11

42299   **Unlisted procedure, palate, uvula**
⚙ 0.00   ⚒ 0.00   **FUD** YYY   T 80 ▣
AMA: 2018,Jan,8; 2017,Jan,8; 2016,Jan,13; 2015,Jan,16; 2014,Jul,8; 2014,Jan,11

42300-42699 Procedures of the Salivary Ducts and Glands

42300   **Drainage of abscess; parotid, simple**
⚙ 4.38   ⚒ 6.02   **FUD** 010   T A2 ▣
AMA: 2014,Jan,11

42305   **parotid, complicated**
⚙ 12.3   ⚒ 12.3   **FUD** 090   J A2 80 ▣
AMA: 2014,Jan,11

42310   **Drainage of abscess; submaxillary or sublingual, intraoral**
⚙ 3.92   ⚒ 5.08   **FUD** 010   T A2 80 ▣
AMA: 2014,Jan,11

42320   **submaxillary, external**
⚙ 5.05   ⚒ 7.24   **FUD** 010   T A2 80 ▣
AMA: 2014,Jan,11

42330   **Sialolithotomy; submandibular (submaxillary), sublingual or parotid, uncomplicated, intraoral**
⚙ 4.72   ⚒ 6.65   **FUD** 010   J P3 ▣
AMA: 2014,Jan,11

42335   **submandibular (submaxillary), complicated, intraoral**
⚙ 7.38   ⚒ 11.1   **FUD** 090   J P3 ▣
AMA: 2014,Jan,11

42340   **parotid, extraoral or complicated intraoral**
⚙ 9.73   ⚒ 13.8   **FUD** 090   J A2 80 50 ▣
AMA: 2014,Jan,11

42400   **Biopsy of salivary gland; needle**
EXCLUDES   *Fine needle aspiration (10021, [10004, 10005, 10006, 10007, 10008, 10009, 10010, 10011, 10012])*
⚙ (76942, 77002, 77012, 77021)
✄ (88172-88173)
⚙ 1.55   ⚒ 2.95   **FUD** 000   T P3 ▣
AMA: 2019,Apr,4; 2014,Jan,11

42405   **incisional**
⚙ (76942, 77002, 77012, 77021)
⚙ 6.50   ⚒ 8.59   **FUD** 010   J A2
AMA: 2014,Jan,11

42408   **Excision of sublingual salivary cyst (ranula)**
⚙ 10.2   ⚒ 14.7   **FUD** 090   J A2 80 ▣
AMA: 2014,Jan,11

42409   **Marsupialization of sublingual salivary cyst (ranula)**
⚙ 6.41   ⚒ 9.99   **FUD** 090   J A2 80 ▣
AMA: 2014,Jan,11

42410   **Excision of parotid tumor or parotid gland; lateral lobe, without nerve dissection**
EXCLUDES   *Facial nerve suture or graft (64864, 64865, 69740, 69745)*
⚙ 17.9   ⚒ 17.9   **FUD** 090   J A2 80 50 ▣
AMA: 2014,Jan,11

42415   **lateral lobe, with dissection and preservation of facial nerve**
EXCLUDES   *Facial nerve suture or graft (64864, 64865, 69740, 69745)*
⚙ 30.3   ⚒ 30.3   **FUD** 090   J A2 80 50 ▣
AMA: 2014,Jan,11

42420   **total, with dissection and preservation of facial nerve**
EXCLUDES   *Facial nerve suture or graft (64864, 64865, 69740, 69745)*
⚙ 34.0   ⚒ 34.0   **FUD** 090   J A2 80 50 ▣
AMA: 2014,Jan,11

42425   **total, en bloc removal with sacrifice of facial nerve**
EXCLUDES   *Facial nerve suture or graft (64864, 64865, 69740, 69745)*
⚙ 23.9   ⚒ 23.9   **FUD** 090   J A2 80 50 ▣
AMA: 2014,Jan,11

42426   **total, with unilateral radical neck dissection**
EXCLUDES   *Facial nerve suture or graft (64864, 64865, 69740, 69745)*
⚙ 38.8   ⚒ 38.8   **FUD** 090   C 80 50 ▣
AMA: 2018,Jan,8; 2017,Jan,8; 2016,Jan,13; 2015,Jan,16; 2014,Jan,11

42440   **Excision of submandibular (submaxillary) gland**
⚙ 11.8   ⚒ 11.8   **FUD** 090   J A2 80 50 ▣
AMA: 2014,Jan,11

42450   **Excision of sublingual gland**
⚙ 10.2   ⚒ 13.0   **FUD** 090   J A2 80 ▣
AMA: 2014,Jan,11

42500   **Plastic repair of salivary duct, sialodochoplasty; primary or simple**
⚙ 9.80   ⚒ 12.4   **FUD** 090   J A2 80 ▣
AMA: 2014,Jan,11

42505   **secondary or complicated**
⚙ 12.9   ⚒ 15.9   **FUD** 090   J A2
AMA: 2014,Jan,11

42507   **Parotid duct diversion, bilateral (Wilke type procedure);**
⚙ 14.4   ⚒ 14.4   **FUD** 090   J A2 80 ▣
AMA: 2014,Jan,11

42509 with excision of both submandibular glands
🔲 23.9   🔲 23.9   **FUD** 090   J A2 80 ▣
AMA: 2014,Jan,11

42510 with ligation of both submandibular (Wharton's) ducts
🔲 17.7   🔲 17.7   **FUD** 090   J A2 80 ▣
AMA: 2014,Jan,11

42550 Injection procedure for sialography
⚡ (70390)
🔲 1.84   🔲 4.17   **FUD** 000   N N1 ▣
AMA: 2014,Jan,11

42600 Closure salivary fistula
🔲 10.0   🔲 14.1   **FUD** 090   J A2 80 ▣
AMA: 2014,Jan,11

42650 Dilation salivary duct
🔲 1.66   🔲 2.31   **FUD** 000   T P3 ▣
AMA: 2014,Jan,11

42660 Dilation and catheterization of salivary duct, with or without injection
🔲 2.57   🔲 3.61   **FUD** 000   T P3 80 ▣
AMA: 2014,Jan,11

42665 Ligation salivary duct, intraoral
🔲 5.96   🔲 9.42   **FUD** 090   J A2 80 ▣
AMA: 2014,Jan,11

42699 Unlisted procedure, salivary glands or ducts
🔲 0.00   🔲 0.00   **FUD** YYY   T 80 ▣
AMA: 2014,Jan,11

42700-42999 Procedures of the Adenoids/Throat/Tonsils

42700 Incision and drainage abscess; peritonsillar
🔲 3.88   🔲 5.43   **FUD** 010   T A2 ▣
AMA: 2014,Jan,11

42720 retropharyngeal or parapharyngeal, intraoral approach
🔲 11.2   🔲 13.0   **FUD** 010   J A2 80 ▣
AMA: 2014,Jan,11

42725 retropharyngeal or parapharyngeal, external approach
🔲 23.5   🔲 23.5   **FUD** 090   J A2 80 ▣
AMA: 2014,Jan,11

42800 Biopsy; oropharynx
EXCLUDES *Laryngoscopy with biopsy (31510, 31535-31536, 31576)*
🔲 3.23   🔲 4.50   **FUD** 010   J P3 ▣
AMA: 2014,Jan,11

42804 nasopharynx, visible lesion, simple
EXCLUDES *Laryngoscopy with biopsy (31510, 31535-31536)*
🔲 3.28   🔲 5.65   **FUD** 010   J A2 ▣
AMA: 2014,Jan,11

42806 nasopharynx, survey for unknown primary lesion
EXCLUDES *Laryngoscopy with biopsy (31510, 31535-31536)*
🔲 3.81   🔲 6.32   **FUD** 010   J A2 ▣
AMA: 2014,Jan,11

42808 Excision or destruction of lesion of pharynx, any method
🔲 4.67   🔲 6.52   **FUD** 010   J A2 ▣
AMA: 2014,Jan,11

42809 Removal of foreign body from pharynx
🔲 3.53   🔲 5.75   **FUD** 010   01 N1 ▣
AMA: 2014,Jan,11

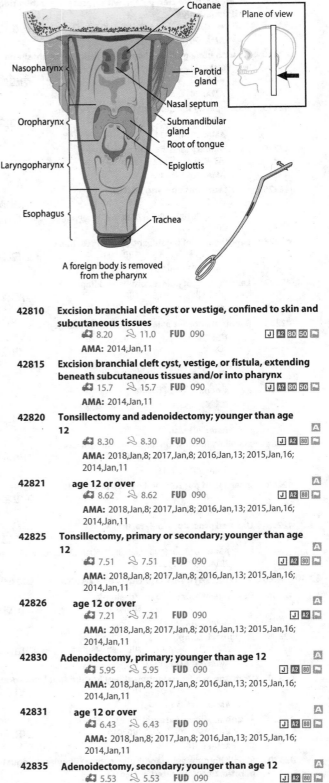

A foreign body is removed from the pharynx

42810 Excision branchial cleft cyst or vestige, confined to skin and subcutaneous tissues
🔲 8.20   🔲 11.0   **FUD** 090   J A2 80 50 ▣
AMA: 2014,Jan,11

42815 Excision branchial cleft cyst, vestige, or fistula, extending beneath subcutaneous tissues and/or into pharynx
🔲 15.7   🔲 15.7   **FUD** 090   J A2 80 50 ▣
AMA: 2014,Jan,11

42820 Tonsillectomy and adenoidectomy; younger than age 12   A
🔲 8.30   🔲 8.30   **FUD** 090   J A2 80 ▣
AMA: 2018,Jan,8; 2017,Jan,8; 2016,Jan,13; 2015,Jan,16; 2014,Jan,11

42821 age 12 or over   A
🔲 8.62   🔲 8.62   **FUD** 090   J A2 80 ▣
AMA: 2018,Jan,8; 2017,Jan,8; 2016,Jan,13; 2015,Jan,16; 2014,Jan,11

42825 Tonsillectomy, primary or secondary; younger than age 12   A
🔲 7.51   🔲 7.51   **FUD** 090   J A2 80 ▣
AMA: 2018,Jan,8; 2017,Jan,8; 2016,Jan,13; 2015,Jan,16; 2014,Jan,11

42826 age 12 or over   A
🔲 7.21   🔲 7.21   **FUD** 090   J A2 ▣
AMA: 2018,Jan,8; 2017,Jan,8; 2016,Jan,13; 2015,Jan,16; 2014,Jan,11

42830 Adenoidectomy, primary; younger than age 12   A
🔲 5.95   🔲 5.95   **FUD** 090   J A2 80 ▣
AMA: 2018,Jan,8; 2017,Jan,8; 2016,Jan,13; 2015,Jan,16; 2014,Jan,11

42831 age 12 or over   A
🔲 6.43   🔲 6.43   **FUD** 090   J A2 80 ▣
AMA: 2018,Jan,8; 2017,Jan,8; 2016,Jan,13; 2015,Jan,16; 2014,Jan,11

42835 Adenoidectomy, secondary; younger than age 12   A
🔲 5.53   🔲 5.53   **FUD** 090   J A2 80 ▣
AMA: 2018,Jan,8; 2017,Jan,8; 2016,Jan,13; 2015,Jan,16; 2014,Jan,11

26/TC PC/TC Only   A2-Z3 ASC Payment   50 Bilateral   ♂ Male Only   ♀ Female Only   🔲 Facility RVU   🔲 Non-Facility RVU   🔲 CCI   ⚡ CLIA
FUD Follow-up Days   **CMS:** IOM   **AMA:** CPT Asst   A-Y OPPSI   80/80 Surg Assist Allowed / w/Doc   🔲 Lab Crosswalk   🔲 Radiology Crosswalk

192   CPT © 2019 American Medical Association. All Rights Reserved.   © 2019 Optum360, LLC

42836   **age 12 or over**
🚗 6.90   ⚕ 6.90   **FUD** 090   `J` `A2` `80` 🖥
AMA: 2018,Jan,8; 2017,Jan,8; 2016,Jan,13; 2015,Jan,16; 2014,Jan,11

42842   **Radical resection of tonsil, tonsillar pillars, and/or retromolar trigone; without closure**
🚗 29.0   ⚕ 29.0   **FUD** 090   `J` `80` 🖥
AMA: 2018,Jan,8; 2017,Jan,8; 2016,Jan,13; 2015,Jan,16; 2014,Jan,11

42844   **closure with local flap (eg, tongue, buccal)**
🚗 39.9   ⚕ 39.9   **FUD** 090   `J` `80` 🖥
AMA: 2018,Jan,8; 2017,Jan,8; 2016,Jan,13; 2015,Jan,16; 2014,Jan,11

42845   **closure with other flap**
Code also closure with other flap(s)
Code also radical neck dissection when combined (38720)
🚗 64.3   ⚕ 64.3   **FUD** 090   `C` `80` 🖥
AMA: 2018,Jan,8; 2017,Jan,8; 2016,Jan,13; 2015,Jan,16; 2014,Jan,11

42860   **Excision of tonsil tags**
🚗 5.39   ⚕ 5.39   **FUD** 090   `J` `A2` `80` 🖥
AMA: 2014,Jan,11

Tonsillar tags or polyps are removed

42870   **Excision or destruction lingual tonsil, any method (separate procedure)**
EXCLUDES   _Nasopharynx resection (juvenile angiofibroma) by transzygomatic/bicoronal approach (61586, 61600)_
🚗 17.0   ⚕ 17.0   **FUD** 090   `J` `A2` `80` 🖥
AMA: 2014,Jan,11

42890   **Limited pharyngectomy**
Code also radical neck dissection when combined (38720)
🚗 41.2   ⚕ 41.2   **FUD** 090   `J` `A2` `80` 🖥
AMA: 2014,Jan,11

42892   **Resection of lateral pharyngeal wall or pyriform sinus, direct closure by advancement of lateral and posterior pharyngeal walls**
Code also radical neck dissection when combined (38720)
🚗 54.2   ⚕ 54.2   **FUD** 090   `J` `A2` `80` 🖥
AMA: 2018,Jan,8; 2017,Jan,8; 2016,Jan,13; 2015,Jan,16; 2014,Jan,11

42894   **Resection of pharyngeal wall requiring closure with myocutaneous or fasciocutaneous flap or free muscle, skin, or fascial flap with microvascular anastomosis**
EXCLUDES   _Flap used for reconstruction (15730, 15733-15734, 15756-15758)_
Code also radical neck dissection when combined (38720)
🚗 68.5   ⚕ 68.5   **FUD** 090   `C` `80` 🖥
AMA: 2018,Jan,8; 2017,Jan,8; 2016,Jan,13; 2015,Jan,16; 2014,Jan,11

42900   **Suture pharynx for wound or injury**
🚗 9.65   ⚕ 9.65   **FUD** 010   `T` `A2` `80` 🖥
AMA: 2014,Jan,11

42950   **Pharyngoplasty (plastic or reconstructive operation on pharynx)**
EXCLUDES   _Pharyngeal flap (42225)_
🚗 23.2   ⚕ 23.2   **FUD** 090   `J` `A2` `80` 🖥
AMA: 2018,Jan,8; 2017,Jan,8; 2016,Apr,8; 2014,Jan,11

42953   **Pharyngoesophageal repair**
Code also closure using myocutaneous or other flap
🚗 27.9   ⚕ 27.9   **FUD** 090   `C` `80` 🖥
AMA: 2014,Jan,11

42955   **Pharyngostomy (fistulization of pharynx, external for feeding)**
🚗 22.0   ⚕ 22.0   **FUD** 090   `T` `A2` `80` 🖥
AMA: 2014,Jan,11

42960   **Control oropharyngeal hemorrhage, primary or secondary (eg, post-tonsillectomy); simple**
🚗 4.83   ⚕ 4.83   **FUD** 010   `T` `A2` `80` 🖥
AMA: 2014,Jan,11

42961   **complicated, requiring hospitalization**
🚗 11.9   ⚕ 11.9   **FUD** 090   `C` `80` 🖥
AMA: 2014,Jan,11

42962   **with secondary surgical intervention**
🚗 14.8   ⚕ 14.8   **FUD** 090   `J` `A2` 🖥
AMA: 2014,Jan,11

42970   **Control of nasopharyngeal hemorrhage, primary or secondary (eg, postadenoidectomy); simple, with posterior nasal packs, with or without anterior packs and/or cautery**
🚗 11.8   ⚕ 11.8   **FUD** 090   `T` `R2` 🖥
AMA: 2014,Jan,11

42971   **complicated, requiring hospitalization**
🚗 13.0   ⚕ 13.0   **FUD** 090   `C` `80` 🖥
AMA: 2014,Jan,11

42972   **with secondary surgical intervention**
🚗 14.6   ⚕ 14.6   **FUD** 090   `J` `A2` `80` 🖥
AMA: 2014,Jan,11

42999   **Unlisted procedure, pharynx, adenoids, or tonsils**
🚗 0.00   ⚕ 0.00   **FUD** YYY   `T` `80` 🖥
AMA: 2018,Jan,8; 2017,Jan,8; 2016,Jan,13; 2015,Jan,16; 2014,Feb,11; 2014,Jan,11

43020-43135 Incision/Resection of Esophagus

EXCLUDES   _Gastrointestinal reconstruction for previous esophagectomy (43360-43361)_
Gastrotomy with intraluminal tube insertion (43510)

43020   **Esophagotomy, cervical approach, with removal of foreign body**
EXCLUDES   _Laparotomy with esophageal intubation (43510)_
🚗 16.1   ⚕ 16.1   **FUD** 090   `T` `80` 🖥
AMA: 2014,Jan,11

43030   **Cricopharyngeal myotomy**
EXCLUDES   _Laparotomy with esophageal intubation (43510)_
🚗 14.9   ⚕ 14.9   **FUD** 090   `J` `62` `80` 🖥
AMA: 2014,Jan,11

Digestive System

43045 — 43180

43045 Esophagotomy, thoracic approach, with removal of foreign body

> EXCLUDES Laparotomy with esophageal intubation (43510)
> 🖫 37.6　⚕ 37.6　**FUD** 090　　C 80 ▢
> AMA: 2014,Jan,11

43100 Excision of lesion, esophagus, with primary repair; cervical approach

> EXCLUDES Wide excision of malignant lesion of cervical esophagus, with total laryngectomy:
> With radical neck dissection (31365, 43107, 43116, 43124)
> Without radical neck dissection (31360, 43107, 43116, 43124)
> 🖫 18.0　⚕ 18.0　**FUD** 090　　C 80 ▢
> AMA: 2014,Jan,11

43101 thoracic or abdominal approach

> EXCLUDES Wide excision of malignant lesion of cervical esophagus with total laryngectomy:
> With radical neck dissection (31365, 43107, 43116, 43124)
> Without radical neck dissection (31360, 43107, 43116, 43124)
> 🖫 29.1　⚕ 29.1　**FUD** 090　　C 80 ▢
> AMA: 2018,Jan,8; 2017,Jan,8; 2016,Jan,13; 2015,Jan,16; 2014,Jan,11

43107 Total or near total esophagectomy, without thoracotomy; with pharyngogastrostomy or cervical esophagogastrostomy, with or without pyloroplasty (transhiatal)

> 🖫 86.5　⚕ 86.5　**FUD** 090　　C 80 ▢
> AMA: 2014,Jan,11

43108 with colon interposition or small intestine reconstruction, including intestine mobilization, preparation and anastomosis(es)

> 🖫 129.　⚕ 129.　**FUD** 090　　C 80 ▢
> AMA: 2014,Jan,11

43112 Total or near total esophagectomy, with thoracotomy; with pharyngogastrostomy or cervical esophagogastrostomy, with or without pyloroplasty (ie, McKeown esophagectomy or tri-incisional esophagectomy)

> 🖫 101.　⚕ 101.　**FUD** 090　　C 80 ▢
> AMA: 2018,Jul,7; 2018,Jan,8; 2017,Jan,8; 2016,Jan,13; 2015,Jan,16; 2014,Jan,11

43113 with colon interposition or small intestine reconstruction, including intestine mobilization, preparation, and anastomosis(es)

> 🖫 126.　⚕ 126.　**FUD** 090　　C 80 ▢
> AMA: 2014,Jan,11

43116 Partial esophagectomy, cervical, with free intestinal graft, including microvascular anastomosis, obtaining the graft and intestinal reconstruction

> INCLUDES Operating microscope (69990)
> EXCLUDES Free jejunal graft with microvascular anastomosis done by a different physician (43496)
> Code also modifier 52 if intestinal or free jejunal graft with microvascular anastomosis is done by another physician
> 🖫 145.　⚕ 145.　**FUD** 090　　C 80 ▢
> AMA: 2016,Feb,12; 2014,Jan,11

43117 Partial esophagectomy, distal two-thirds, with thoracotomy and separate abdominal incision, with or without proximal gastrectomy; with thoracic esophagogastrostomy, with or without pyloroplasty (Ivor Lewis)

> EXCLUDES Esophagogastrectomy (lower third) and vagotomy (43122)
> Total esophagectomy with gastropharyngostomy (43107, 43124)
> 🖫 94.3　⚕ 94.3　**FUD** 090　　C 80 ▢
> AMA: 2014,Jan,11

43118 with colon interposition or small intestine reconstruction, including intestine mobilization, preparation, and anastomosis(es)

> EXCLUDES Esophagogastrectomy (lower third) and vagotomy (43122)
> Total esophagectomy with gastropharyngostomy (43107, 43124)
> 🖫 105.　⚕ 105.　**FUD** 090　　C 80 ▢
> AMA: 2014,Jan,11

43121 Partial esophagectomy, distal two-thirds, with thoracotomy only, with or without proximal gastrectomy, with thoracic esophagogastrostomy, with or without pyloroplasty

> 🖫 83.0　⚕ 83.0　**FUD** 090　　C 80 ▢
> AMA: 2014,Jan,11

43122 Partial esophagectomy, thoracoabdominal or abdominal approach, with or without proximal gastrectomy; with esophagogastrostomy, with or without pyloroplasty

> 🖫 74.1　⚕ 74.1　**FUD** 090　　C 80 ▢
> AMA: 2014,Jan,11

43123 with colon interposition or small intestine reconstruction, including intestine mobilization, preparation, and anastomosis(es)

> 🖫 131.　⚕ 131.　**FUD** 090　　C 80 ▢
> AMA: 2014,Jan,11

43124 Total or partial esophagectomy, without reconstruction (any approach), with cervical esophagostomy

> 🖫 110.　⚕ 110.　**FUD** 090　　C 80 ▢
> AMA: 2018,Jan,8; 2017,Jan,8; 2016,Jan,13; 2015,Jan,16; 2014,Jan,11

43130 Diverticulectomy of hypopharynx or esophagus, with or without myotomy; cervical approach

> EXCLUDES Diverticulectomy hypopharynx or cervical esophagus, endoscopic (43180)
> 🖫 22.6　⚕ 22.6　**FUD** 090　　J 62 80 ▢
> AMA: 2018,Jan,8; 2017,Jan,8; 2016,Jan,13; 2015,Jan,16; 2014,Jan,11

43135 thoracic approach

> EXCLUDES Diverticulectomy hypopharynx or cervical esophagus, endoscopic (43180)
> 🖫 42.7　⚕ 42.7　**FUD** 090　　C 80 ▢
> AMA: 2018,Jan,8; 2017,Jan,8; 2016,Jan,13; 2015,Jan,16; 2014,Jan,11

43180-43233 [43211, 43212, 43213, 43214] Endoscopic Procedures: Esophagus

> INCLUDES Control of bleeding as a result of endoscopic procedure during same operative session
> Diagnostic endoscopy with surgical endoscopy
> Examination of upper esophageal sphincter (cricopharyngeus muscle) to/including the gastroesophageal junction
> Retroflexion examination of proximal region of stomach

43180 Esophagoscopy, rigid, transoral with diverticulectomy of hypopharynx or cervical esophagus (eg, Zenker's diverticulum), with cricopharyngeal myotomy, includes use of telescope or operating microscope and repair, when performed

> INCLUDES Operating microscope (69990)
> EXCLUDES Esophagogastroduodenoscopy, flexible, transoral; with esophagogastric fundoplasty (43210)
> Open diverticulectomy hypopharynx or esophagus (43130-43135)
> 🖫 15.7　⚕ 15.7　**FUD** 090　　J 62 ▢
> AMA: 2018,Jan,8; 2017,Jan,8; 2016,Feb,12; 2016,Jan,13; 2015,Nov,8

194　　　　　　　　CPT © 2019 American Medical Association. All Rights Reserved.　　　　　　© 2019 Optum360, LLC
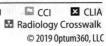

43191 Esophagoscopy, rigid, transoral; diagnostic, including collection of specimen(s) by brushing or washing when performed (separate procedure)

EXCLUDES Esophagogastroduodenoscopy, flexible, transoral; with esophagogastric fundoplasty (43210)
Esophagoscopy, flexible, transnasal (43197-43198)
Esophagoscopy. flexible, transoral (43200)
Esophagoscopy, rigid, transoral (43192-43196)

🚑 4.47 ⚕ 4.47 **FUD** 000   J G2 ▭

AMA: 2018,Jan,8; 2017,Jan,8; 2016,Jan,13; 2015,Nov,8; 2015,Jan,16; 2014,Feb,9; 2014,Jan,11

43192 with directed submucosal injection(s), any substance

EXCLUDES Esophagoscopy, flexible, transnasal; with biopsy, single or multiple (43197-43198)
Esophagoscopy, flexible, transoral (43201)
Esophagoscopy, rigid or flexible, diagnostic (43191, 43197)
Injection sclerosis of esophageal varices:
Flexible, transoral (43204)
Rigid, transoral (43499)

🚑 4.88 ⚕ 4.88 **FUD** 000   J G2 ▭

AMA: 2018,Jan,8; 2017,Jan,8; 2016,Jan,13; 2015,Jan,16; 2014,Feb,9; 2014,Jan,11

43193 with biopsy, single or multiple

EXCLUDES Esophagoscopy, flexible, transnasal; with biopsy, single or multiple (43197-43198)
Esophagoscopy, rigid or flexible, diagnostic (43191, 43197)
Flexible, transoral (43202)

🚑 4.88 ⚕ 4.88 **FUD** 000   J G2 ▭

AMA: 2018,Jan,8; 2017,Jan,8; 2016,Jan,13; 2015,Jan,16; 2014,Feb,9; 2014,Jan,11

43194 with removal of foreign body(s)

EXCLUDES Esophagoscopy, flexible, transnasal; with biopsy, single or multiple (43198)
Esophagoscopy, rigid or flexible, diagnostic (43191, 43197)
Flexible, transoral (43215)

☢ (76000)

🚑 5.58 ⚕ 5.58 **FUD** 000   J G2 ▭

AMA: 2018,Jan,8; 2017,Jan,8; 2016,Jan,13; 2015,Jan,16; 2014,Feb,9; 2014,Jan,11

43195 with balloon dilation (less than 30 mm diameter)

EXCLUDES Dilation of esophagus:
Flexible, with balloon diameter 30 mm or larger (43214, 43233)
Flexible, with balloon diameter less than 30 mm (43220)
Without endoscopic visualization (43450-43453)
Esophagoscopy, flexible, transnasal; with biopsy, single or multiple (43198)
Esophagoscopy, rigid or flexible, diagnostic (43191, 43197)

☢ (74360)

🚑 5.32 ⚕ 5.32 **FUD** 000   J G2 ▭

AMA: 2018,Jan,8; 2017,Jan,8; 2016,Jan,13; 2015,Jan,16; 2014,Feb,9; 2014,Jan,11

43196 with insertion of guide wire followed by dilation over guide wire

EXCLUDES Esophagoscopy, flexible, transnasal; with biopsy, single or multiple (43198)
Esophagoscopy, rigid or flexible, diagnostic (43191, 43197)
Flexible, transoral (43226)

☢ (74360)

🚑 5.67 ⚕ 5.67 **FUD** 000   J G2 ▭

AMA: 2018,Jan,8; 2017,Jan,8; 2016,Jan,13; 2015,Jan,16; 2014,Feb,9; 2014,Jan,11

43197 Esophagoscopy, flexible, transnasal; diagnostic, including collection of specimen(s) by brushing or washing, when performed (separate procedure)

EXCLUDES Esophagogastroduodenoscopy, flexible, transoral (43235-43259 [43233, 43266, 43270])
Esophagoscopy, flexible, transnasal; with biopsy, single or multiple (43198)
Flexible, transoral (43200-43232 [43211, 43212, 43213, 43214])
Laryngoscopy, flexible fiberoptic; diagnostic (31575)
Nasal endoscopy, diagnostic, unless different type of endoscope used (31231)
Nasopharyngoscopy with endoscope (92511)
Rigid, transoral (43191-43196)

🚑 2.40 ⚕ 5.34 **FUD** 000   T P3 ▭

AMA: 2018,Jan,8; 2017,Jul,7; 2017,Jan,8; 2016,Dec,13; 2016,Sep,6; 2016,Jan,13; 2015,Nov,8; 2015,Jan,16; 2014,Feb,9; 2014,Jan,11

43198 with biopsy, single or multiple

EXCLUDES Esophagogastroduodenoscopy, flexible, transoral (43235-43259 [43233, 43266, 43270])
Flexible, transoral (43200-43232 [43211, 43212, 43213, 43214])
Laryngoscopy, flexible fiberoptic; diagnostic (31575)
Nasal endoscopy, diagnostic, unless different type of endoscope used (31231)
Nasopharyngoscopy with endoscope (92511)
Rigid, transoral (43191-43197)

🚑 2.86 ⚕ 5.88 **FUD** 000   T P3 ▭

AMA: 2018,Jan,8; 2017,Jul,7; 2017,Jan,8; 2016,Dec,13; 2016,Sep,6; 2016,Jan,13; 2015,Jan,16; 2014,Feb,9; 2014,Jan,11

43200 Esophagoscopy, flexible, transoral; diagnostic, including collection of specimen(s) by brushing or washing, when performed (separate procedure)

EXCLUDES Esophagoscopy, flexible, transoral (43201-43232 [43211, 43212, 43213, 43214])
Flexible, transnasal (43197-43198)
Rigid, transoral (43191)
Upper gastrointestinal endoscopy (43235)

🚑 2.53 ⚕ 6.50 **FUD** 000   T A2 ▭

AMA: 2018,Jan,8; 2017,Jan,8; 2016,Jan,13; 2015,Nov,8; 2015,Jan,16; 2014,Feb,9; 2014,Jan,11

43201 with directed submucosal injection(s), any substance

EXCLUDES Esophagoscopy, flexible, transnasal (43197-43198)
Esophagoscopy, flexible, transoral on the same lesion (43200, 43204, 43211, 43227)
Injection sclerosis of esophageal varices:
Flexible, transoral (43204)
Rigid, transoral (43192, 43499)

🚑 2.99 ⚕ 6.55 **FUD** 000   J A2 ▭

AMA: 2018,Jan,8; 2017,Jan,8; 2016,Jan,13; 2015,Jan,16; 2014,Feb,9; 2014,Jan,11

43202 with biopsy, single or multiple

EXCLUDES Esophagoscopy, flexible, transoral; diagnostic (43200)
Esophagoscopy, flexible, transoral on same lesion (43211)
Flexible, transnasal (43197-43198)
Rigid, transoral (43193)

🚑 3.00 ⚕ 9.16 **FUD** 000   J A2 ▭

AMA: 2018,Jan,8; 2017,Jan,8; 2016,Jan,13; 2015,Jan,16; 2014,Feb,9; 2014,Jan,11

Digestive System

43204 — 43214

43204 **with injection sclerosis of esophageal varices**

EXCLUDES Band ligation non-variceal bleeding (43227)

Esophagoscopy, flexible, transnasal or transoral; diagnostic (43197-43198, 43200)

Esophagoscopy, flexible, transoral; with control of bleeding, any method on the same lesion (43227)

Esophagoscopy, flexible, transoral; with directed submucosal injection(s), any substance on the same lesion (43201)

Rigid, transoral (43499)

🔧 3.96   ⚕ 3.96   **FUD** 000   J A2 🖵

AMA: 2018,Jan,8; 2017,Jan,8; 2016,Jan,13; 2015,Jan,16; 2014,Feb,9; 2014,Jan,11

43205 **with band ligation of esophageal varices**

EXCLUDES Band ligation non-variceal bleeding on the same lesion (43227)

Esophagoscopy, flexible, transnasal or transoral; diagnostic (43197-43198, 43200)

🔧 4.13   ⚕ 4.13   **FUD** 000   J A2 🖵

AMA: 2018,Jan,8; 2017,Jan,8; 2016,Jan,13; 2015,Jan,16; 2014,Feb,9; 2014,Jan,11

43206 **with optical endomicroscopy**

EXCLUDES Esophagoscopy, flexible, transnasal or transoral; diagnostic (43197-43198, 43200)

Optical endomicroscopic image(s), interpretation and report (88375)

Code also contrast agent

🔧 3.90   ⚕ 7.85   **FUD** 000   J G2 🖵

AMA: 2018,Jan,8; 2017,Nov,10; 2017,Jan,8; 2016,Jan,13; 2015,Jan,16; 2014,Feb,9; 2014,Jan,11

43210 **Resequenced code. See code following 43259.**

43211 **Resequenced code. See code following 43217.**

43212 **Resequenced code. See code following 43217.**

43213 **Resequenced code. See code following 43220.**

43214 **Resequenced code. See code following 43220.**

43215 **with removal of foreign body(s)**

EXCLUDES Esophagoscopy, flexible, transnasal or transoral; diagnostic (43197-43198, 43200)

Rigid, transoral (43194)

Upper gastrointestinal endoscopy (43247)

📷 (76000)

🔧 4.14   ⚕ 10.5   **FUD** 000   J A2 🖵

AMA: 2018,Jan,8; 2017,Jan,8; 2016,Jan,13; 2015,Jan,16; 2014,Feb,9; 2014,Jan,11

43216 **with removal of tumor(s), polyp(s), or other lesion(s) by hot biopsy forceps**

EXCLUDES Esophagoscopy, flexible, transnasal or transoral; diagnostic (43197-43198, 43200)

Removal by snare technique (43217)

🔧 3.86   ⚕ 10.6   **FUD** 000   J A2 🖵

AMA: 2018,Jan,8; 2017,Jan,8; 2016,Jan,13; 2015,Jan,16; 2014,Feb,9; 2014,Jan,11

43217 **with removal of tumor(s), polyp(s), or other lesion(s) by snare technique**

EXCLUDES Esophagoscopy, flexible, transnasal or transoral; diagnostic (43197-43198, 43200)

Esophagoscopy, flexible, transoral; with endoscopic mucosal resection on the same lesion (43211)

Upper gastrointestinal endoscopy with snare technique (43251)

🔧 4.69   ⚕ 11.1   **FUD** 000   J A2 🖵

AMA: 2018,Jan,8; 2017,Jan,8; 2016,Jan,13; 2015,Jan,16; 2014,Feb,9; 2014,Jan,11

\# **43211** **with endoscopic mucosal resection**

EXCLUDES Esophagoscopy, flexible, transnasal or transoral; diagnostic (43197-43198, 43200)

Esophagoscopy, flexible, transoral; with directed submucosal injection(s) (43201-43202)

Esophagoscopy, flexible, transoral; with removal of tumor(s), polyp(s), or other lesion(s) by snare technique (43217)

🔧 6.87   ⚕ 6.87   **FUD** 000   J G2 🖵

AMA: 2018,Jan,8; 2017,Nov,10; 2017,Jan,8; 2016,Jan,13; 2015,Jan,16; 2014,Feb,9; 2014,Jan,11

\# **43212** **with placement of endoscopic stent (includes pre- and post-dilation and guide wire passage, when performed)**

EXCLUDES Esophagogastroduodenoscopy, flexible, transoral; with insertion of intraluminal tube or catheter (43241)

Esophagoscopy, flexible, transnasal or transoral; diagnostic (43197-43198, 43200)

Esophagoscopy, flexible, transoral; with insertion of guide wire followed by passage of dilator(s) over guide wire (43226)

Esophagoscopy, flexible, transoral; with transendoscopic balloon dilation (43220)

📷 (74360)

🔧 5.54   ⚕ 5.54   **FUD** 000   J J8 🖵

AMA: 2018,Jan,8; 2017,Jan,8; 2016,Jan,13; 2015,Jan,16; 2014,Feb,9; 2014,Jan,11

43220 **with transendoscopic balloon dilation (less than 30 mm diameter)**

EXCLUDES Dilation of esophagus:

Rigid, with balloon diameter 30 mm or larger (43214)

Rigid, with balloon diameter less than 30mm (43195)

Without endoscopic visualization (43450, 43453)

Esophagoscopy, flexible, transnasal; diagnostic (43197-43198)

Esophagoscopy, flexible, transoral (43200, 43212, 43226, 43229)

📷 (74360)

🔧 3.43   ⚕ 29.5   **FUD** 000   J A2 🖵

AMA: 2018,Jan,8; 2017,Jan,8; 2016,Jan,13; 2015,Jan,16; 2014,Feb,9; 2014,Jan,11

\# **43213** **with dilation of esophagus, by balloon or dilator, retrograde (includes fluoroscopic guidance, when performed)**

INCLUDES Fluoroscopy (76000)

EXCLUDES Esophagoscopy, flexible, transnasal or transoral; diagnostic (43197-43198, 43200)

Intraluminal dilation of strictures and/or obstructions (eg, esophagus), radiological supervision and interpretation (74360)

Code also each additional stricture treated in same operative session with modifier 59 and (43213)

🔧 7.56   ⚕ 33.8   **FUD** 000   J G2 🖵

AMA: 2018,Jan,8; 2017,Jan,8; 2016,Jan,13; 2015,Jan,16; 2014,Feb,9; 2014,Jan,11

\# **43214** **with dilation of esophagus with balloon (30 mm diameter or larger) (includes fluoroscopic guidance, when performed)**

INCLUDES Fluoroscopy (76000)

EXCLUDES Esophagoscopy, flexible, transnasal or transoral; diagnostic (43197-43198, 43200)

Intraluminal dilation of strictures and/or obstructions (eg, esophagus), radiological supervision and interpretation (74360)

🔧 5.61   ⚕ 5.61   **FUD** 000   J G2 🖵

AMA: 2018,Jan,8; 2017,Jan,8; 2016,Jan,13; 2015,Jan,16; 2014,Feb,9; 2014,Jan,11

26/TC PC/TC Only   A2-Z3 ASC Payment   50 Bilateral   ♂ Male Only   ♀ Female Only   🔧 Facility RVU   ⚕ Non-Facility RVU   🖵 CCI   ✖ CLIA
FUD Follow-up Days   **CMS:** IOM   **AMA:** CPT Asst   A-Y OPPSI   80/80 Surg Assist Allowed / w/Doc   📷 Lab Crosswalk   📷 Radiology Crosswalk

196   CPT © 2019 American Medical Association. All Rights Reserved.   © 2019 Optum360, LLC

43226 **with insertion of guide wire followed by passage of dilator(s) over guide wire**

> EXCLUDES *Esophagoscopy, flexible, transnasal or transoral; diagnostic (43197-43198, 43200)*
> *Esophagoscopy, flexible, transoral; with ablation of tumor(s), polyp(s), or other lesion(s) on the same lesion (43229)*
> *Esophagoscopy, flexible, transoral; with placement of endoscopic stent (43212)*
> *Esophagoscopy, flexible, transoral; with transendoscopic balloon dilation (43220)*
> *Rigid, transoral (43196)*

⬛ (74360)

🔲 3.80   ⚕ 9.59   **FUD** 000   　 J A2 ▣

AMA: 2018,Jan,8; 2017,Jan,8; 2016,Jan,13; 2015,Jan,16; 2014,Feb,9; 2014,Jan,11

43227 **with control of bleeding, any method**

> EXCLUDES *Esophagoscopy, flexible, transnasal or transoral; diagnostic (43197-43198, 43200)*
> *Esophagoscopy, flexible, transoral; with directed submucosal injection(s) on the same lesion (43201)*
> *Esophagoscopy, flexible, transoral; with injection sclerosis of esophageal varices on the same lesion (43204-43205)*

🔲 4.84   ⚕ 17.7   **FUD** 000   　 J A2 ▣

AMA: 2018,Jan,8; 2017,Jan,8; 2016,Jan,13; 2015,Jan,16; 2014,Feb,9; 2014,Feb,11; 2014,Jan,11

43229 **with ablation of tumor(s), polyp(s), or other lesion(s) (includes pre- and post-dilation and guide wire passage, when performed)**

> EXCLUDES *Esophagoscopy, flexible, transnasal or transoral; diagnostic (43197-43198, 43200)*
> *Esophagoscopy, flexible, transoral; with insertion of guide wire followed by passage of dilator(s) over guide wire on the same lesion (43226)*
> *Esophagoscopy, flexible, transoral; with transendoscopic balloon dilation on the same lesion (43220)*

Code also esophagoscopic photodynamic therapy, when performed (96570-96571)

🔲 5.77   ⚕ 19.0   **FUD** 000   　 J G2 ▣

AMA: 2018,Jan,8; 2017,Jan,8; 2016,Jan,13; 2015,Jan,16; 2014,Feb,9; 2014,Jan,11

43231 **with endoscopic ultrasound examination**

> EXCLUDES *Esophagoscopy, flexible, transnasal or transoral; diagnostic (43197-43198, 43200)*
> *Esophagoscopy, flexible, transoral; with transendoscopic ultrasound-guided intramural or transmural fine needle aspiration/biopsy(s) (43232)*
> *Gastrointestinal endoscopic ultrasound, supervision, and interpretation (76975)*
> *Procedure performed more than one time per operative session*

🔲 4.65   ⚕ 9.79   **FUD** 000   　 J A2 ▣

AMA: 2018,Jan,8; 2017,Jan,8; 2016,Jan,13; 2015,Jan,16; 2014,Feb,9; 2014,Jan,11

43232 **with transendoscopic ultrasound-guided intramural or transmural fine needle aspiration/biopsy(s)**

> EXCLUDES *Esophagoscopy, flexible, transnasal or transoral; diagnostic (43197-43198, 43200)*
> *Esophagoscopy, flexible, transoral; with endoscopic ultrasound examination (43231)*
> *Gastrointestinal endoscopic ultrasound, supervision and interpretation (76975)*
> *Procedure performed more than one time per operative session*
> *Ultrasonic guidance (76942)*

🔲 5.82   ⚕ 11.8   **FUD** 000   　 J A2 ▣

AMA: 2018,Jan,8; 2017,Jan,8; 2016,Jan,13; 2015,Jan,16; 2014,Feb,9; 2014,Jan,11

43233 **Resequenced code. See code following 43249.**

43235-43210 [43210, 43233, 43266, 43270] Endoscopic Procedures: Esophagogastroduodenoscopy (EGD)

> INCLUDES Control of bleeding as result of the endoscopic procedure during same operative session
> Diagnostic endoscopy with surgical endoscopy
> EXCLUDES *Exam of jejunum distal to the anastomosis in surgically altered stomach, including post-gastroenterostomy (Billroth II) and gastric bypass (43235-43259 [43233, 43266, 43270])*
> *Exam of upper esophageal sphincter (cricopharyngeus muscle) to/including gastroesophageal junction and/or retroflexion exam of proximal region of stomach (43197-43232 [43211, 43212, 43213, 43214])*

Code also modifier 52 when duodenum is not examined either deliberately or due to significant issues and repeat procedure will not be performed

Code also modifier 53 when duodenum is not examined either deliberately or due to significant issues and repeat procedure is planned

43235 **Esophagogastroduodenoscopy, flexible, transoral; diagnostic, including collection of specimen(s) by brushing or washing, when performed (separate procedure)**

> EXCLUDES *Endoscopy of small intestine (44360-44379)*
> *Esophagogastroduodenoscopy, flexible, transoral; with esophagogastric fundoplasty (43210)*
> *Esophagoscopy, flexible, transnasal; diagnostic (43197-43198)*
> *Procedure performed with surgical endoscopy (43236-43259 [43233, 43266, 43270])*

🔲 3.58   ⚕ 7.61   **FUD** 000   　 T A2 ▣

AMA: 2018,Jul,14; 2018,Jan,8; 2017,Jul,10; 2017,Jan,8; 2016,Jan,13; 2015,Nov,8; 2015,Jan,16; 2014,Jan,11

Examination using small diameter flexible endoscope

Esophagus

Stomach

Duodenum

43236 **with directed submucosal injection(s), any substance**

> EXCLUDES *Endoscopy of small intestine (44360-44379)*
> *Esophagogastroduodenoscopy, flexible, transoral; with control of bleeding, any method (43255)*
> *Esophagogastroduodenoscopy, flexible, transoral; with endoscopic mucosal resection on the same lesion (43254)*
> *Esophagogastroduodenoscopy, flexible, transoral; with injection sclerosis of esophageal/gastric varices on the same lesion (43243)*
> *Esophagoscopy, flexible, transnasal or transoral; diagnostic (43197-43198, 43235)*
> *Injection sclerosis of varices, esophageal/gastric (43243)*

🔲 4.05   ⚕ 10.0   **FUD** 000   　 T A2 ▣

AMA: 2018,Jan,8; 2017,Jan,8; 2016,Jan,13; 2015,Jan,16; 2014,Jan,11

Digestive System

43237 — 43245

43237 **with endoscopic ultrasound examination limited to the esophagus, stomach or duodenum, and adjacent structures**

INCLUDES Gastrointestinal endoscopic ultrasound, supervision and interpretation (76975)

EXCLUDES *Endoscopy of small intestine (44360-44379)*
Esophagogastroduodenoscopy, flexible, transoral (43235, 43238, 43242, 43253, 43259)
Esophagoscopy, flexible, transnasal; diagnostic (43197-43198)
Procedure performed more than one time per operative session

⚕ 5.73   ⚕ 5.73   **FUD** 000   J A2 ▭

AMA: 2018,Jan,8; 2017,Jan,8; 2016,Jan,13; 2016,Jan,11; 2015,Jan,16; 2014,Jan,11

43238 **with transendoscopic ultrasound-guided intramural or transmural fine needle aspiration/biopsy(s), (includes endoscopic ultrasound examination limited to the esophagus, stomach or duodenum, and adjacent structures)**

INCLUDES Gastrointestinal endoscopic ultrasound, supervision and interpretation (76975)
Ultrasonic guidance (76942)

EXCLUDES *Endoscopy of small intestine (44360-44379)*
Esophagogastroduodenoscopy, flexible, transoral (43235, 43237, 43242)
Esophagoscopy, flexible, transnasal (43197-43198)
Procedure performed more than one time per operative session

⚕ 6.81   ⚕ 6.81   **FUD** 000   J A2 ▭

AMA: 2018,Jan,8; 2017,Jan,8; 2016,Jan,13; 2015,Jan,16; 2014,Jan,11

43239 **with biopsy, single or multiple**

EXCLUDES *Endoscopy of small intestine (44360-44379)*
Esophagogastroduodenoscopy, flexible, transoral; diagnostic (43235)
Esophagogastroduodenoscopy, flexible, transoral; with endoscopic mucosal resection on the same lesion (43254)
Esophagoscopy, flexible, transnasal (43197-43198)

⚕ 4.05   ⚕ 10.1   **FUD** 000   T A2 ▭

AMA: 2018,Jul,14; 2018,Jan,8; 2017,Jan,8; 2016,Jan,13; 2015,Jan,16; 2014,Jan,11

43240 **with transmural drainage of pseudocyst (includes placement of transmural drainage catheter[s]/stent[s], when performed, and endoscopic ultrasound, when performed)**

EXCLUDES *Endoscopic pancreatic necrosectomy (48999)*
Endoscopy of small intestine (44360-44379)
Esophagogastroduodenoscopy, flexible, transoral (43235, 43242, [43266], 43259)
Esophagogastroduodenoscopy, flexible, transoral; with transendoscopic ultrasound-guided transmural injection of diagnostic or therapeutic substance(s) on the same lesion (43253)
Esophagoscopy, flexible, transnasal (43197-43198)
Procedure performed more than one time per operative session

⚕ 11.5   ⚕ 11.5   **FUD** 000   J J8 ▭

AMA: 2018,Jan,8; 2017,Jan,8; 2016,Jan,13; 2015,Jan,16; 2014,Jan,11

43241 **with insertion of intraluminal tube or catheter**

EXCLUDES *Endoscopy of small intestine (44360-44379)*
Esophagogastroduodenoscopy, flexible, transoral (43235, [43266])
Esophagoscopy, flexible, transnasal or transoral (43197-43198, 43212)
Insertion long gastrointestinal tube (44500, 74340)
Naso or oro-gastric requiring professional skill and fluoroscopic guidance (43752)

⚕ 4.17   ⚕ 4.17   **FUD** 000   J A2 ▭

AMA: 2018,Jan,8; 2017,Jan,8; 2016,Jan,13; 2015,Jan,16; 2014,Jan,11

43242 **with transendoscopic ultrasound-guided intramural or transmural fine needle aspiration/biopsy(s) (includes endoscopic ultrasound examination of the esophagus, stomach, and either the duodenum or a surgically altered stomach where the jejunum is examined distal to the anastomosis)**

INCLUDES Gastrointestinal endoscopic ultrasound, supervision and interpretation (76975)
Ultrasonic guidance (76942)

EXCLUDES *Endoscopy of small intestine (44360-44379)*
Esophagogastroduodenoscopy, flexible, transoral (43235, 43237-43238, 43240, 43259)
Esophagoscopy, flexible, transnasal (43197-43198)
Procedure performed more than one time per operative session
Transmural fine needle biopsy/aspiration with ultrasound guidance, transendoscopic, esophagus/stomach/duodenum/neighboring structure (43238)

▣ 88172-88173

⚕ 7.69   ⚕ 7.69   **FUD** 000   J A2 ▭

AMA: 2018,Jan,8; 2017,Jan,8; 2016,Jan,13; 2015,Jan,16; 2014,Jan,11

43243 **with injection sclerosis of esophageal/gastric varices**

EXCLUDES *Endoscopy of small intestine (44360-44379)*
Esophagogastroduodenoscopy, flexible, transoral; diagnostic (43235)
Esophagogastroduodenoscopy, flexible, transoral with on the same lesion (43236, 43255)
Esophagoscopy, flexible, transnasal (43197-43198)

⚕ 6.94   ⚕ 6.94   **FUD** 000   J A2 ▭

AMA: 2018,Jan,8; 2017,Jan,8; 2016,Jan,13; 2015,Jan,16; 2014,Jan,11

43244 **with band ligation of esophageal/gastric varices**

EXCLUDES *Band ligation, non-variceal bleeding (43255)*
Endoscopy of small intestine (44360-44379)
Esophagogastroduodenoscopy, flexible, transoral (43235, 43255)·
Esophagoscopy, flexible, transnasal (43197-43198)

⚕ 7.17   ⚕ 7.17   **FUD** 000   J A2 ▭

AMA: 2018,Jan,8; 2017,Jan,8; 2016,Jan,13; 2015,Jan,16; 2014,Jan,11

43245 **with dilation of gastric/duodenal stricture(s) (eg, balloon, bougie)**

EXCLUDES *Endoscopy of small intestine (44360-44379)*
Esophagogastroduodenoscopy, flexible, transoral (43235, [43266])
Esophagoscopy, flexible, transnasal (43197-43198)

▣ (74360)

⚕ 5.13   ⚕ 16.2   **FUD** 000   J A2 ▭

AMA: 2018,Jan,8; 2017,Jan,8; 2016,Jan,13; 2015,Jan,16; 2014,Jan,11

43246 **with directed placement of percutaneous gastrostomy tube**

EXCLUDES Endoscopy of small intestine (44360-44372, 44376-44379)

Esophagogastroduodenoscopy, flexible, transoral; diagnostic (43235)

Esophagoscopy, flexible, transnasal (43197-43198)

Gastrostomy tube replacement without endoscopy or imaging (43762-43763)

Percutaneous insertion of gastrostomy tube (49440)

5.86 5.86 **FUD** 000 J A2 80

AMA: 2019,Feb,5; 2018,Jan,8; 2017,Jan,8; 2016,Jan,13; 2015,Jan,16; 2014,Jan,11

Endoscope
Esophagus
Gastrostomy tube (PEG)
Stomach
Duodenum

43247 **with removal of foreign body(s)**

EXCLUDES Endoscopy of small intestine (44360-44379)

Esophagogastroduodenoscopy, flexible, transoral; diagnostic (43235)

Esophagoscopy, flexible, transnasal (43197-43198)

(76000)

5.18 10.2 **FUD** 000 T A2

AMA: 2018,Jan,8; 2017,Jan,8; 2016,Jan,13; 2015,Jan,16; 2014,Jan,11

43248 **with insertion of guide wire followed by passage of dilator(s) through esophagus over guide wire**

EXCLUDES Endoscopy of small intestine (44360-44379)

Esophagogastroduodenoscopy, flexible, transoral (43235, [43266], [43270])

Esophagoscopy, flexible, transnasal (43197-43198)

(74360)

4.86 10.5 **FUD** 000 T A2

AMA: 2018,Jan,8; 2017,Jul,10; 2017,Jan,8; 2016,Jan,13; 2015,Jan,16; 2014,Jan,11

43249 **with transendoscopic balloon dilation of esophagus (less than 30 mm diameter)**

EXCLUDES Endoscopy of small intestine (44360-44379)

Esophagogastroduodenoscopy, flexible, transoral (43235, [43266], [43270])

Esophagoscopy, flexible, transnasal (43197-43198)

(74360)

4.49 29.9 **FUD** 000 J A2

AMA: 2018,Jul,14; 2018,Jan,8; 2017,Jan,8; 2016,Jan,13; 2015,Jan,16; 2014,Jan,11

\# **43233** **with dilation of esophagus with balloon (30 mm diameter or larger) (includes fluoroscopic guidance, when performed)**

INCLUDES Fluoroscopy (76000)

EXCLUDES Endoscopy of small intestine (44360-44379)

Esophagogastroduodenoscopy, flexible, transoral (43235, [43266], [43270])

Esophagoscopy, flexible, transnasal (43197-43198)

Intraluminal dilation of strictures and/or obstructions (e.g., esophagus), radiological supervision and interpretation (74360)

6.68 6.68 **FUD** 000 J G2

AMA: 2018,Jan,8; 2017,Jan,8; 2016,Jan,13; 2015,Jan,16; 2014,Jan,11

43250 **with removal of tumor(s), polyp(s), or other lesion(s) by hot biopsy forceps**

EXCLUDES Endoscopy of small intestine (44360-44379)

Esophagogastroduodenoscopy, flexible, transoral (43235)

Esophagoscopy, flexible, transnasal (43197-43198)

4.97 11.8 **FUD** 000 J A2

AMA: 2018,Jan,8; 2017,Jan,8; 2016,Jan,13; 2015,Jan,16; 2014,Jan,11

43251 **with removal of tumor(s), polyp(s), or other lesion(s) by snare technique**

EXCLUDES Endoscopic mucosal resection when performed on same lesion (43254)

Endoscopy of small intestine (44360-44379)

Esophagogastroduodenoscopy, flexible, transoral (43235)

Esophagoscopy, flexible, transnasal (43197-43198)

5.74 13.0 **FUD** 000 J A2

AMA: 2018,Jan,8; 2017,Jan,8; 2016,Jan,13; 2015,Jan,16; 2014,Jan,11

43252 **with optical endomicroscopy**

EXCLUDES Endoscopy of small intestine (44360-44379)

Esophagogastroduodenoscopy, flexible, transoral (43235)

Esophagoscopy, flexible, transnasal (43197-43198)

Optical endomicroscopic image(s), interpretation and report (88375)

Code also contrast agent

4.95 8.96 **FUD** 000 J G2

AMA: 2018,Jan,8; 2017,Jan,8; 2016,Jan,13; 2015,Jan,16; 2014,Jan,11

43253 **with transendoscopic ultrasound-guided transmural injection of diagnostic or therapeutic substance(s) (eg, anesthetic, neurolytic agent) or fiducial marker(s) (includes endoscopic ultrasound examination of the esophagus, stomach, and either the duodenum or a surgically altered stomach where the jejunum is examined distal to the anastomosis)**

INCLUDES Gastrointestinal endoscopic ultrasound, supervision and interpretation (76975)

Ultrasonic guidance (76942)

EXCLUDES Endoscopy of small intestine (44360-44379)

Esophagogastroduodenoscopy, flexible, transoral (43235, 43237, 43259)

Esophagogastroduodenoscopy, flexible, transoral; with transmural drainage of pseudocyst on the same lesion with (43240)

Esophagoscopy, flexible, transnasal (43197-43198)

Procedure performed more than one time per operative session

Transmural fine needle biopsy/aspiration with ultrasound guidance, transendoscopic, esophagus/stomach/duodenum/neighboring structures (43238, 43242)

7.70 7.70 **FUD** 000 J G2

AMA: 2018,Apr,10; 2018,Jan,8; 2017,Jan,8; 2016,Jan,13; 2015,Jan,16; 2014,Jan,11

Digestive System

43254 — 43261

43254   **with endoscopic mucosal resection**

EXCLUDES   *Endoscopy of small intestine (44360-44379)*
            Esophagogastroduodenoscopy, flexible, transoral; diagnostic (43235)
            Esophagogastroduodenoscopy, flexible, transoral on the same lesion (43236, 43239, 43251)
            Esophagoscopy, flexible, transnasal (43197-43198)

🔧 7.91   ⚕ 7.91   **FUD** 000   J G2 ▢

AMA: 2018,Jan,8; 2017,Jan,8; 2016,Jan,13; 2015,Jan,16; 2014,Jan,11

43255   **with control of bleeding, any method**

EXCLUDES   *Endoscopy of small intestine (44360-44379)*
            Esophagogastroduodenoscopy, flexible, transoral (43235)
            Esophagogastroduodenoscopy, flexible, transoral on the same lesion (43236, 43243-43244)
            Esophagoscopy, flexible, transnasal (43197-43198)

🔧 5.87   ⚕ 18.7   **FUD** 000   J A2 ▢

AMA: 2018,Jan,8; 2017,Jan,8; 2016,Jan,13; 2015,Jan,16; 2014,Jan,11

43266   **with placement of endoscopic stent (includes pre- and post-dilation and guide wire passage, when performed)**

🔧 6.39   ⚕ 6.39   **FUD** 000   J J8 ▢

AMA: 2018,Jan,8; 2017,Jan,8; 2016,Jan,13; 2015,Jan,16; 2014,Jan,11

43257   **with delivery of thermal energy to the muscle of lower esophageal sphincter and/or gastric cardia, for treatment of gastroesophageal reflux disease**

EXCLUDES   *Endoscopy small intestine (44360-44379)*
            Esophageal lesion ablation (43229, [43270])
            Esophagogastroduodenoscopy, flexible, transoral; diagnostic (43235)
            Esophagoscopy, flexible, transnasal (43197-43198)

🔧 6.80   ⚕ 6.80   **FUD** 000   J A2 ▢

AMA: 2018,Jan,8; 2017,Jan,8; 2016,Jan,13; 2015,Jan,16; 2014,Jan,11

43270   **with ablation of tumor(s), polyp(s), or other lesion(s) (includes pre- and post-dilation and guide wire passage, when performed)**

INCLUDES   *Endoscopic dilation performed on same lesion (43248-43249)*

EXCLUDES   *Endoscopy small intestine (44360-44379)*
            Esophagogastroduodenoscopy, flexible, transoral (43235)
            Esophagoscopy, flexible, transnasal (43197-43198)

Code also photodynamic therapy, if performed (96570-96571)

🔧 6.57   ⚕ 19.6   **FUD** 000   J G2 ▢

AMA: 2018,Jan,8; 2017,Jan,8; 2016,Jan,13; 2015,Jan,16; 2014,Jan,11

43259   **with endoscopic ultrasound examination, including the esophagus, stomach, and either the duodenum or a surgically altered stomach where the jejunum is examined distal to the anastomosis**

INCLUDES   *Gastrointestinal endoscopic ultrasound, supervision and interpretation (76975)*

EXCLUDES   *Endoscopy of small intestine (44360-44379)*
            Esophagogastroduodenoscopy, flexible, transoral (43235, 43237, 43240, 43242, 43253)
            Esophagoscopy, flexible, transnasal (43197-43198)
            Procedure performed more than one time per operative session

🔧 6.62   ⚕ 6.62   **FUD** 000   J A2 ▢

AMA: 2018,Jan,8; 2017,Jan,8; 2016,Jan,13; 2016,Jan,11; 2015,Jan,16; 2014,Jan,11

43210   **with esophagogastric fundoplasty, partial or complete, includes duodenoscopy when performed**

EXCLUDES   *Esophagoscopy, flexible, transnasal (43197)*
            Esophagoscopy, flexible, transoral (43200, 43235)
            Esophagoscopy, rigid, transoral (43180, 43191)

🔧 12.5   ⚕ 12.5   **FUD** 000   J G2 ▢

AMA: 2018,Jan,8; 2017,Jan,8; 2016,Jan,13; 2015,Nov,8

43260-43278 [43274, 43275, 43276, 43278] Endoscopic Procedures: ERCP

INCLUDES   Diagnostic endoscopy with surgical endoscopy
            Pancreaticobiliary system:
                Biliary tree (right and left hepatic ducts, cystic duct/gallbladder, and common bile ducts)
                Pancreas (major and minor ducts)

EXCLUDES   *ERCP via Roux-en-Y anatomy (for instance post-gastric or bariatric bypass or post total gastrectomy) or via gastrostomy (open or laparoscopic) (47999, 48999)*
            Optical endomicroscopy of biliary tract and pancreas, report one time per session (0397T)
            Percutaneous biliary catheter procedures (47490-47544)

Code also appropriate endoscopy of each anatomic site examined
Code also sphincteroplasty or ductal stricture dilation, when performed prior to the debris/stone removal from the duct ([43277])
Code also the appropriate ERCP procedure when performed on altered postoperative anatomy (i.e. Billroth II gastroenterostomy)

☒ (74328-74330)

43260   **Endoscopic retrograde cholangiopancreatography (ERCP); diagnostic, including collection of specimen(s) by brushing or washing, when performed (separate procedure)**

EXCLUDES   *Endoscopic retrograde cholangiopancreatography (ERCP) (43261-43265, 43274-43278 [43274, 43275, 43276, 43277, 43278])*

🔧 9.45   ⚕ 9.45   **FUD** 000   J A2 ▢

AMA: 2018,Jan,8; 2017,Jan,8; 2016,Jan,13; 2015,Dec,3; 2015,Jan,16; 2014,Jan,11

43261   **with biopsy, single or multiple**

EXCLUDES   *Endoscopic retrograde cholangiopancreatography (ERCP); diagnostic (43260)*
            Percutaneous endoluminal biopsy of biliary tree (47543)

🔧 9.92   ⚕ 9.92   **FUD** 000   J A2 ▢

AMA: 2018,Jan,8; 2017,Jan,8; 2016,Jan,13; 2015,Dec,3; 2015,Jan,16; 2014,Jan,11

26/TC PC/TC Only   A2-Z3 ASC Payment   50 Bilateral   ♂ Male Only   ♀ Female Only   🔧 Facility RVU   ⚕ Non-Facility RVU   ▢ CCI   ☒ CLIA
FUD Follow-up Days   CMS: IOM   AMA: CPT Asst   A-Y OPPSI   80/80 Surg Assist Allowed / w/Doc   ▢ Lab Crosswalk   ☒ Radiology Crosswalk

200   CPT © 2019 American Medical Association. All Rights Reserved.   © 2019 Optum360, LLC

43262 **with sphincterotomy/papillotomy**

EXCLUDES *Endoscopic retrograde cholangiopancreatography (ERCP) (43260, [43277])*

Endoscopic retrograde cholangiopancreatography (ERCP) with placement or exchange of stent in the same location ([43274])

Endoscopic retrograde cholangiopancreatography (ERCP) with removal foreign body in the same location ([43276])

Esophagogastroduodenoscopy, flexible, transoral with ablation of tumor(s), polyp(s), or other lesion(s) in the same location ([43270])

Percutaneous balloon dilation biliary duct or ampulla (47542)

Code also procedure performed with sphincterotomy (43261, 43263-43265, [43275], [43278])

🔧 10.4 ⚕ 10.4 **FUD** 000 [J] [A2] 🔲

AMA: 2018,Jan,8; 2017,Jan,8; 2016,Jan,13; 2015,Dec,3; 2015,Jan,16; 2014,Jan,11

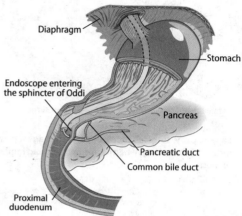

Diaphragm

Stomach

Endoscope entering the sphincter of Oddi

Pancreas

Pancreatic duct

Common bile duct

Proximal duodenum

An endoscope is fed through the stomach and into the duodenum Usually a smaller sub-scope is fed up the sphincter of Oddi and into the ducts that drain the pancreas and the gallbladder (common bile)

43263 **with pressure measurement of sphincter of Oddi**

EXCLUDES *Endoscopic retrograde cholangiopancreatography (ERCP); diagnostic (43260)*

Procedure performed more than one time per session

🔧 10.4 ⚕ 10.4 **FUD** 000 [J] [A2] 🔲

AMA: 2018,Jan,8; 2017,Jan,8; 2016,Jan,13; 2015,Jan,16; 2014,Jan,11

43264 **with removal of calculi/debris from biliary/pancreatic duct(s)**

INCLUDES Incidental dilation due to passage of instrument

EXCLUDES *Endoscopic retrograde cholangiopancreatography (ERCP) (43260, 43265)*

Findings without debris or calculi, even if balloon was used

Percutaneous calculus/debris removal (47544)

Code also sphincteroplasty when dilation is necessary in order to access the area of debris/stones ([43277])

🔧 10.6 ⚕ 10.6 **FUD** 000 [J] [A2] 🔲

AMA: 2018,Jan,8; 2017,Jan,8; 2016,Jan,13; 2015,Dec,3; 2015,Jan,16; 2014,Jan,11

43265 **with destruction of calculi, any method (eg, mechanical, electrohydraulic, lithotripsy)**

INCLUDES Incidental dilation due to passage of instrument

Stone removal when in the same ductal system

EXCLUDES *Endoscopic retrograde cholangiopancreatography (ERCP) (43260, 43264)*

Findings without debris or calculi, even if balloon was used

Percutaneous calculus/debris removal (47544)

Code also sphincteroplasty when dilation is necessary in order to access the area of debris/stones ([43277])

🔧 12.6 ⚕ 12.6 **FUD** 000 [J] [A2] 🔲

AMA: 2018,Jan,8; 2017,Jan,8; 2016,Jan,13; 2015,Dec,3; 2015,Jan,16; 2014,Jan,11

43266 Resequenced code. See code following 43255.

43270 Resequenced code. See code following 43257.

\# **43274** **with placement of endoscopic stent into biliary or pancreatic duct, including pre- and post-dilation and guide wire passage, when performed, including sphincterotomy, when performed, each stent**

INCLUDES Balloon dilation when in the same duct

Tube placement for naso-pancreatic or naso-biliary drainage

EXCLUDES *Percutaneous placement biliary stent (47538-47540)*

Procedures for stent placement or exchange in the same duct (43262, [43275], [43276], [43277])

Code also for each additional stent placement in different ducts or side by side in same duct in same session/day, using modifier 59 with ([43274])

🔧 13.5 ⚕ 13.5 **FUD** 000 [J] [G2] 🔲

AMA: 2018,Jan,8; 2017,Jan,8; 2016,Jan,13; 2015,Jan,16; 2014,Jan,11

\# **43275** **with removal of foreign body(s) or stent(s) from biliary/pancreatic duct(s)**

EXCLUDES *Endoscopic retrograde cholangiopancreatography (ERCP) (43260, [43274], [43276])*

Pancreatic or biliary duct stent removal without ERCP (43247)

Percutaneous calculus/debris removal (47544)

Procedure performed more than one time per session

🔧 11.0 ⚕ 11.0 **FUD** 000 [J] [G2] 🔲

AMA: 2018,Jan,8; 2017,Jan,8; 2016,Jan,13; 2015,Jan,16; 2014,Jan,11

\# **43276** **with removal and exchange of stent(s), biliary or pancreatic duct, including pre- and post-dilation and guide wire passage, when performed, including sphincterotomy, when performed, each stent exchanged**

INCLUDES Balloon dilation when in the same duct

Stent placement or exchange of one stent

EXCLUDES *Endoscopic retrograde cholangiopancreatography (ERCP) (43260, [43275])*

Procedures for stent insertion or exchange of stent in same duct (43262, [43274])

Code also each additional stent exchanged in same session/day, using modifier 59 with ([43276])

🔧 14.1 ⚕ 14.1 **FUD** 000 [J] [G2] 🔲

AMA: 2018,Jan,8; 2017,Jan,8; 2016,Jan,13; 2015,Jan,16; 2014,Jan,11

Digestive System

43277 — 43285

**43277** **with trans-endoscopic balloon dilation of biliary/pancreatic duct(s) or of ampulla (sphincteroplasty), including sphincterotomy, when performed, each duct**

> EXCLUDES Endoscopic retrograde cholangiopancreatography (ERCP) (43260, 43262, [43274], [43276])
> Endoscopic retrograde cholangiopancreatography (ERCP); with ablation of tumor(s), polyp(s), or other lesion(s) for the same lesion ([43278])
> Percutaneous dilation biliary duct/ampulla (47542)
> Removal of stone/debris, dilation incidental to instrument passage (43264-43265)

Code also both right and left hepatic duct (bilateral) balloon dilation, using ([43277]) and append modifier 59 to second procedure

Code also each additional balloon dilation in different ducts or side by side in same duct in same session/day, using modifier 59 with ([43277])

Code also same session sphincterotomy without sphincteroplasty in different duct, using modifier 59 with (43262)

🔲 11.0   ⚫ 11.0   **FUD** 000   [J] [62] 🔲

AMA: 2018,Jan,8; 2017,Jan,8; 2016,Jan,13; 2015,Dec,3; 2015,Jan,16; 2014,Jan,11

**43278** **with ablation of tumor(s), polyp(s), or other lesion(s), including pre- and post-dilation and guide wire passage, when performed**

> EXCLUDES Ampullectomy (43254)
> Endoscopic retrograde cholangiopancreatography (ERCP); diagnostic (43260)
> Endoscopic retrograde cholangiopancreatography (ERCP); with trans-endoscopic balloon dilation of biliary/pancreatic duct(s) or of ampulla (sphincteroplasty) on the same lesion with ([43277])

🔲 12.6   ⚫ 12.6   **FUD** 000   [J] [62] 🔲

AMA: 2018,Jan,8; 2017,Jan,8; 2016,Jan,13; 2015,Jan,16; 2014,Jan,11

+ **43273** **Endoscopic cannulation of papilla with direct visualization of pancreatic/common bile duct(s) (List separately in addition to code(s) for primary procedure)**

🔲 3.49   ⚫ 3.49   **FUD** ZZZ   [N] [N1] [80] 🔲

AMA: 2018,Jan,8; 2017,Jan,8; 2016,Jan,13; 2015,Jan,16; 2014,Jan,11

43274 **Resequenced code. See code following numeric code 43270.**

43275 **Resequenced code. See code following numeric code 43270.**

43276 **Resequenced code. See code following numeric code 43270.**

43277 **Resequenced code. See code following numeric code 43270.**

43278 **Resequenced code. See code following numeric code 43270.**

43279-43289 Laparoscopic Procedures of Esophagus

INCLUDES Diagnostic laparoscopy with surgical laparoscopy (49320)

43279 **Laparoscopy, surgical, esophagomyotomy (Heller type), with fundoplasty, when performed**

> EXCLUDES Esophagomyotomy, open method (43330-43331)
> Laparoscopy, surgical, esophagogastric fundoplasty (43280)

🔲 37.3   ⚫ 37.3   **FUD** 090   [C] [80] 🔲

AMA: 2018,Jan,8; 2017,Aug,6; 2017,Jan,8; 2016,Jan,13; 2015,Jan,16; 2014,Jan,11

43280 **Laparoscopy, surgical, esophagogastric fundoplasty (eg, Nissen, Toupet procedures)**

> EXCLUDES Esophagogastric fundoplasty, open method (43327-43328)
> Esophagogastroduodenoscopy fundoplasty, transoral (43210)
> Laparoscopy, surgical, esophageal sphincter augmentation (43284-43285)
> Laparoscopy, surgical, esophagomyotomy (43279)
> Laparoscopy, surgical, fundoplasty (43281-43282)

🔲 31.3   ⚫ 31.3   **FUD** 090   [J] [80] 🔲

AMA: 2018,Jan,8; 2017,Aug,6; 2017,Jan,8; 2016,Jan,13; 2015,Nov,8; 2015,Jan,16; 2014,Dec,16; 2014,Dec,16; 2014,Jan,11

Esophagus
Diaphragm
Fundus of stomach

Normal stomach   **After surgery**

43281 **Laparoscopy, surgical, repair of paraesophageal hernia, includes fundoplasty, when performed; without implantation of mesh**

> EXCLUDES Dilation of esophagus (43450, 43453)
> Implantation of mesh or other prosthesis (49568)
> Laparoscopy, surgical, esophagogastric fundoplasty (43280)
> Transabdominal repair of paraesophageal hiatal hernia (43332-43333)
> Transthoracic repair of diaphragmatic hernia (43334-43335)

🔲 44.7   ⚫ 44.7   **FUD** 090   [J] [80] 🔲

AMA: 2018,Nov,11; 2018,Sep,14; 2018,Jan,8; 2017,Aug,6; 2017,Jan,8; 2016,Jan,13; 2015,Jan,16; 2014,Dec,16; 2014,Dec,16; 2014,Jan,11

43282 **with implantation of mesh**

> EXCLUDES Dilation of esophagus (43450, 43453)
> Laparoscopy, surgical, esophagogastric fundoplasty (43280)
> Transabdominal paraesophageal hernia repair (43332-43333)
> Transthoracic paraesophageal hernia repair (43334-43335)

🔲 50.3   ⚫ 50.3   **FUD** 090   [J] [80] 🔲

AMA: 2018,Jan,8; 2017,Aug,6; 2017,Jan,8; 2016,Aug,9; 2016,Jan,13; 2015,Jan,16; 2014,Dec,16; 2014,Dec,16; 2014,Jan,11

+ **43283** **Laparoscopy, surgical, esophageal lengthening procedure (eg, Collis gastroplasty or wedge gastroplasty) (List separately in addition to code for primary procedure)**

Code first (43280-43282)

🔲 4.60   ⚫ 4.60   **FUD** ZZZ   [C] [80] 🔲

AMA: 2018,Jan,8; 2017,Jan,8; 2016,Jan,13; 2015,Jan,16; 2014,Jan,11

43284 **Laparoscopy, surgical, esophageal sphincter augmentation procedure, placement of sphincter augmentation device (ie, magnetic band), including cruroplasty when performed**

> EXCLUDES Performed during the same session (43279-43282)

🔲 18.6   ⚫ 18.6   **FUD** 090   [J] [J8] [80] 🔲

AMA: 2019,Apr,10; 2018,Sep,14; 2018,Jan,8; 2017,Aug,6

43285 **Removal of esophageal sphincter augmentation device**

🔲 19.0   ⚫ 19.0   **FUD** 090   [02] [62] [80] 🔲

AMA: 2018,Jan,8; 2017,Aug,6

43286 Esophagectomy, total or near total, with laparoscopic mobilization of the abdominal and mediastinal esophagus and proximal gastrectomy, with laparoscopic pyloric drainage procedure if performed, with open cervical pharyngogastrostomy or esophagogastrostomy (ie, laparoscopic transhiatal esophagectomy)
🔲 90.9   🔲 90.9   **FUD** 090   © 80 ▣
AMA: 2018,Jul,7

43287 Esophagectomy, distal two-thirds, with laparoscopic mobilization of the abdominal and lower mediastinal esophagus and proximal gastrectomy, with laparoscopic pyloric drainage procedure if performed, with separate thoracoscopic mobilization of the middle and upper mediastinal esophagus and thoracic esophagogastrostomy (ie, laparoscopic thoracoscopic esophagectomy, Ivor Lewis esophagectomy)
EXCLUDES *Right tube thoracostomy (32551)*
🔲 104.   🔲 104.   **FUD** 090   © 80 ▣
AMA: 2018,Jul,7

43288 Esophagectomy, total or near total, with thoracoscopic mobilization of the upper, middle, and lower mediastinal esophagus, with separate laparoscopic proximal gastrectomy, with laparoscopic pyloric drainage procedure if performed, with open cervical pharyngogastrostomy or esophagogastrostomy (ie, thoracoscopic, laparoscopic and cervical incision esophagectomy, McKeown esophagectomy, tri-incisional esophagectomy)
EXCLUDES *Right tube thoracostomy (32551)*
🔲 108.   🔲 108.   **FUD** 090   © 80 ▣
AMA: 2018,Jul,7

43289 Unlisted laparoscopy procedure, esophagus
🔲 0.00   🔲 0.00   **FUD** YYY   J 80 50 ▣
AMA: 2018,Jul,7; 2018,Jan,8; 2017,Jan,8; 2016,Jan,13; 2015,Jan,16; 2014,Dec,16; 2014,Dec,16; 2014,Jan,11

43300-43425 Open Esophageal Repair Procedures

43300 Esophagoplasty (plastic repair or reconstruction), cervical approach; without repair of tracheoesophageal fistula
🔲 17.6   🔲 17.6   **FUD** 090   © 80 ▣
AMA: 2014,Jan,11

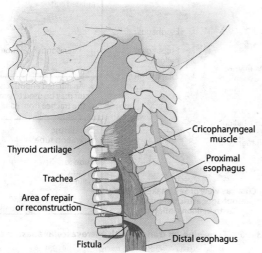

Thyroid cartilage
Cricopharyngeal muscle
Proximal esophagus
Trachea
Area of repair or reconstruction
Fistula
Distal esophagus

Example of esophageal atresia where the proximal esophagus fails to communicate with the lower portion; note that a fistula has developed from the trachea

43305 with repair of tracheoesophageal fistula
🔲 31.3   🔲 31.3   **FUD** 090   © 80 ▣
AMA: 2014,Jan,11

43310 Esophagoplasty (plastic repair or reconstruction), thoracic approach; without repair of tracheoesophageal fistula
🔲 43.0   🔲 43.0   **FUD** 090   © 80 ▣
AMA: 2014,Jan,11

43312 with repair of tracheoesophageal fistula
🔲 46.3   🔲 46.3   **FUD** 090   © 80 ▣
AMA: 2014,Jan,11

43313 Esophagoplasty for congenital defect (plastic repair or reconstruction), thoracic approach; without repair of congenital tracheoesophageal fistula
🔲 79.3   🔲 79.3   **FUD** 090   63 © 80 ▣
AMA: 2014,Jan,11

43314 with repair of congenital tracheoesophageal fistula
🔲 85.4   🔲 85.4   **FUD** 090   63 © 80 ▣
AMA: 2014,Jan,11

43320 Esophagogastrostomy (cardioplasty), with or without vagotomy and pyloroplasty, transabdominal or transthoracic approach
EXCLUDES *Laparoscopic approach (43280)*
🔲 40.5   🔲 40.5   **FUD** 090   © 80 ▣
AMA: 2014,Jan,11

43325 Esophagogastric fundoplasty, with fundic patch (Thal-Nissen procedure)
EXCLUDES *Myotomy, cricopharyngeal (43030)*
🔲 39.4   🔲 39.4   **FUD** 090   © 80 ▣
AMA: 2014,Jan,11

43327 Esophagogastric fundoplasty partial or complete; laparotomy
🔲 23.7   🔲 23.7   **FUD** 090   © 80 ▣
AMA: 2018,Jan,8; 2017,Jan,8; 2016,Jan,13; 2015,Nov,8; 2015,Jan,16; 2014,Jan,11

43328 thoracotomy
EXCLUDES *Esophagogastroduodenoscopy fundoplasty, transoral (43210)*
🔲 32.6   🔲 32.6   **FUD** 090   © 80 ▣
AMA: 2018,Jan,8; 2017,Jan,8; 2016,Jan,13; 2015,Nov,8; 2015,Jan,16; 2014,Jan,11

43330 Esophagomyotomy (Heller type); abdominal approach
EXCLUDES *Esophagomyotomy, laparoscopic method (43279)*
🔲 38.7   🔲 38.7   **FUD** 090   © 80 ▣
AMA: 2018,Jan,8; 2017,Jan,8; 2016,Jan,13; 2015,Jan,16; 2014,Jan,11

43331 thoracic approach
EXCLUDES *Thoracoscopy with esophagomyotomy (32665)*
🔲 38.7   🔲 38.7   **FUD** 090   © 80 ▣
AMA: 2018,Jan,8; 2017,Jan,8; 2016,Jan,13; 2015,Jan,16; 2014,Jan,11

43332 Repair, paraesophageal hiatal hernia (including fundoplication), via laparotomy, except neonatal; without implantation of mesh or other prosthesis
EXCLUDES *Neonatal diaphragmatic hernia repair (39503)*
🔲 33.6   🔲 33.6   **FUD** 090   © 80 ▣
AMA: 2018,Jan,8; 2017,Jan,8; 2016,Jan,13; 2015,Jan,16; 2014,Jan,11

43333 with implantation of mesh or other prosthesis
EXCLUDES *Neonatal diaphragmatic hernia repair (39503)*
🔲 36.5   🔲 36.5   **FUD** 090   © 80 ▣
AMA: 2018,Jan,8; 2017,Jan,8; 2016,Jan,13; 2015,Jan,16; 2014,Jan,11

43334 Repair, paraesophageal hiatal hernia (including fundoplication), via thoracotomy, except neonatal; without implantation of mesh or other prosthesis
EXCLUDES *Neonatal diaphragmatic hernia repair (39503)*
🔲 36.2   🔲 36.2   **FUD** 090   © 80 ▣
AMA: 2018,Jan,8; 2017,Jan,8; 2016,Jan,13; 2015,Jan,16; 2014,Jan,11

43335 with implantation of mesh or other prosthesis
  EXCLUDES *Neonatal diaphragmatic hernia repair (39503)*
  ⚙ 38.8 ⚒ 38.8 **FUD** 090 `C` `80` ▢
  AMA: 2018,Jan,8; 2017,Jan,8; 2016,Jan,13; 2015,Jan,16; 2014,Jan,11

43336 Repair, paraesophageal hiatal hernia, (including fundoplication), via thoracoabdominal incision, except neonatal; without implantation of mesh or other prosthesis
  EXCLUDES *Neonatal diaphragmatic hernia repair (39503)*
  ⚙ 43.8 ⚒ 43.8 **FUD** 090 `C` `80` ▢
  AMA: 2018,Jan,8; 2017,Jan,8; 2016,Jan,13; 2015,Jan,16; 2014,Jan,11

43337 with implantation of mesh or other prosthesis
  EXCLUDES *Neonatal diaphragmatic hernia repair (39503)*
  ⚙ 44.9 ⚒ 44.9 **FUD** 090 `C` `80` ▢
  AMA: 2018,Jan,8; 2017,Jan,8; 2016,Jan,13; 2015,Jan,16; 2014,Jan,11

+ 43338 Esophageal lengthening procedure (eg, Collis gastroplasty or wedge gastroplasty) (List separately in addition to code for primary procedure)
  Code first (43280, 43327-43337)
  ⚙ 3.37 ⚒ 3.37 **FUD** ZZZ `C` `80` ▢
  AMA: 2018,Jan,8; 2017,Jan,8; 2016,Jan,13; 2015,Jan,16; 2014,Jan,11

43340 Esophagojejunostomy (without total gastrectomy); abdominal approach
  ⚙ 40.0 ⚒ 40.0 **FUD** 090 `C` `80` ▢
  AMA: 2014,Jan,11

43341 thoracic approach
  ⚙ 40.6 ⚒ 40.6 **FUD** 090 `C` `80` ▢
  AMA: 2014,Jan,11

43351 Esophagostomy, fistulization of esophagus, external; thoracic approach
  ⚙ 38.1 ⚒ 38.1 **FUD** 090 `C` `80` ▢
  AMA: 2014,Jan,11

43352 cervical approach
  ⚙ 30.8 ⚒ 30.8 **FUD** 090 `C` `80` ▢
  AMA: 2014,Jan,11

43360 Gastrointestinal reconstruction for previous esophagectomy, for obstructing esophageal lesion or fistula, or for previous esophageal exclusion; with stomach, with or without pyloroplasty
  ⚙ 65.3 ⚒ 65.3 **FUD** 090 `C` `80` ▢
  AMA: 2014,Jan,11

43361 with colon interposition or small intestine reconstruction, including intestine mobilization, preparation, and anastomosis(es)
  ⚙ 78.3 ⚒ 78.3 **FUD** 090 `C` `80` ▢
  AMA: 2014,Jan,11

43400 Ligation, direct, esophageal varices
  ⚙ 44.2 ⚒ 44.2 **FUD** 090 `C` `80` ▢
  AMA: 2014,Jan,11

~~43401~~ ~~Transection of esophagus with repair, for esophageal varices~~

43405 Ligation or stapling at gastroesophageal junction for pre-existing esophageal perforation
  ⚙ 42.1 ⚒ 42.1 **FUD** 090 `C` `80` ▢
  AMA: 2014,Jan,11

43410 Suture of esophageal wound or injury; cervical approach
  ⚙ 29.4 ⚒ 29.4 **FUD** 090 `C` `80` ▢
  AMA: 2018,Jan,8; 2017,Jan,8; 2016,Jan,13; 2015,Jan,16; 2014,Jan,11

43415 transthoracic or transabdominal approach
  ⚙ 74.6 ⚒ 74.6 **FUD** 090 `C` `80` ▢
  AMA: 2014,Jan,11

43420 Closure of esophagostomy or fistula; cervical approach
  EXCLUDES *Paraesophageal hiatal hernia repair:*
    Transabdominal (43332-43333)
    Transthoracic (43334-43335)
  ⚙ 29.1 ⚒ 29.1 **FUD** 090 `J` `80` ▢
  AMA: 2014,Jan,11

43425 transthoracic or transabdominal approach
  EXCLUDES *Paraesophageal hiatal hernia repair:*
    Transabdominal (43332-43333)
    Transthoracic (43334-43335)
  ⚙ 41.8 ⚒ 41.8 **FUD** 090 `C` `80` ▢
  AMA: 2014,Jan,11

43450-43453 Esophageal Dilation

43450 Dilation of esophagus, by unguided sound or bougie, single or multiple passes
  ⚒ (74220, 74360)
  ⚙ 2.31 ⚒ 4.70 **FUD** 000 `T` `A2` ▢
  AMA: 2018,Jan,8; 2017,Jul,10; 2017,Jan,8; 2016,Jan,13; 2015,Jan,16; 2014,Jan,11

43453 Dilation of esophagus, over guide wire
  EXCLUDES *Dilation performed with direct visualization (43195, 43226)*
    Endoscopic dilation by dilator or balloon:
    Balloon diameter 30 mm or larger (43214, 43233)
    Balloon diameter less than 30 mm (43195, 43220, 43249)
  ⚒ (74220, 74360)
  ⚙ 2.50 ⚒ 25.4 **FUD** 000 `J` `A2` ▢
  AMA: 2018,Jan,8; 2017,Jan,8; 2016,Jan,13; 2015,Jan,16; 2014,Jan,11

43460-43499 Other/Unlisted Esophageal Procedures

43460 Esophagogastric tamponade, with balloon (Sengstaken type)
  EXCLUDES *Removal of foreign body of the esophagus with balloon catheter (43499, 74235)*
  ⚒ (74220)
  ⚙ 6.22 ⚒ 6.22 **FUD** 000 `C` ▢
  AMA: 2014,Jan,11

Cutaway view of Sengstaken-type esophagogastric tamponade with balloons inflated

An inflated endotracheal cuff may be used to protect the trachea from collapse

43496 Free jejunum transfer with microvascular anastomosis
  INCLUDES Operating microscope (69990)
  ⚙ 0.00 ⚒ 0.00 **FUD** 090 `C` `80` ▢
  AMA: 2018,Jan,8; 2017,Jan,8; 2016,Feb,12; 2016,Jan,13; 2015,Jan,16; 2014,Jan,11

43499 Unlisted procedure, esophagus
  ⚙ 0.00 ⚒ 0.00 **FUD** YYY `T` ▢
  AMA: 2018,Jul,7; 2018,Jan,8; 2017,Jan,8; 2016,Jan,13; 2015,Nov,10; 2015,Nov,8; 2015,Jan,16; 2014,Jan,11

26/TC PC/TC Only | A2-Z3 ASC Payment | 50 Bilateral | ♂ Male Only | ♀ Female Only | ⚙ Facility RVU | ⚒ Non-Facility RVU | ▢ CCI | ☒ CLIA
FUD Follow-up Days | CMS: IOM | AMA: CPT Asst | A-Y OPPSI | 80/80 Surg Assist Allowed / w/Doc | Lab Crosswalk | Radiology Crosswalk

43500-43641 Open Gastric Incisional and Resection Procedures

43500 **Gastrotomy; with exploration or foreign body removal**
    ⚕ 22.7   ⚕ 22.7   **FUD** 090   C 80 ▣
    AMA: 2014,Jan,11

43501 **with suture repair of bleeding ulcer**
    ⚕ 39.0   ⚕ 39.0   **FUD** 090   C 80 ▣
    AMA: 2014,Jan,11

43502 **with suture repair of pre-existing esophagogastric laceration (eg, Mallory-Weiss)**
    ⚕ 44.3   ⚕ 44.3   **FUD** 090   C 80 ▣
    AMA: 2014,Jan,11

43510 **with esophageal dilation and insertion of permanent intraluminal tube (eg, Celestin or Mousseaux-Barbin)**
    ⚕ 27.4   ⚕ 27.4   **FUD** 090   T 80 ▣
    AMA: 2014,Jan,11

43520 **Pyloromyotomy, cutting of pyloric muscle (Fredet-Ramstedt type operation)**
    ⚕ 19.9   ⚕ 19.9   **FUD** 090   63 C 80 ▣
    AMA: 2014,Jan,11

43605 **Biopsy of stomach, by laparotomy**
    ⚕ 24.3   ⚕ 24.3   **FUD** 090   C 80 ▣
    AMA: 2014,Jan,11

43610 **Excision, local; ulcer or benign tumor of stomach**
    ⚕ 28.5   ⚕ 28.5   **FUD** 090   C 80 ▣
    AMA: 2014,Jan,11

43611 **malignant tumor of stomach**
    ⚕ 35.5   ⚕ 35.5   **FUD** 090   C 80 ▣
    AMA: 2014,Jan,11

43620 **Gastrectomy, total; with esophagoenterostomy**
    ⚕ 57.0   ⚕ 57.0   **FUD** 090   C 80 ▣
    AMA: 2014,Jan,11

43621 **with Roux-en-Y reconstruction**
    ⚕ 65.9   ⚕ 65.9   **FUD** 090   C 80 ▣
    AMA: 2014,Jan,11

43622 **with formation of intestinal pouch, any type**
    ⚕ 67.2   ⚕ 67.2   **FUD** 090   C 80 ▣
    AMA: 2014,Jan,11

43631 **Gastrectomy, partial, distal; with gastroduodenostomy**
    INCLUDES   Billroth operation
    ⚕ 42.0   ⚕ 42.0   **FUD** 090   C 80 ▣
    AMA: 2014,Jan,11

43632 **with gastrojejunostomy**
    INCLUDES   Polya anastomosis
    ⚕ 59.0   ⚕ 59.0   **FUD** 090   C 80 ▣
    AMA: 2014,Jan,11

43633 **with Roux-en-Y reconstruction**
    ⚕ 55.8   ⚕ 55.8   **FUD** 090   C 80 ▣
    AMA: 2014,Jan,11

43634 **with formation of intestinal pouch**
    ⚕ 61.8   ⚕ 61.8   **FUD** 090   C 80 ▣
    AMA: 2014,Jan,11

+ 43635 **Vagotomy when performed with partial distal gastrectomy (List separately in addition to code[s] for primary procedure)**
    Code first as appropriate (43631-43634)
    ⚕ 3.26   ⚕ 3.26   **FUD** ZZZ   C 80 ▣
    AMA: 2014,Jan,11

43640 **Vagotomy including pyloroplasty, with or without gastrostomy; truncal or selective**
    EXCLUDES   *Pyloroplasty (43800)*
                 Vagotomy (64755, 64760)
    ⚕ 34.1   ⚕ 34.1   **FUD** 090   C 80 ▣
    AMA: 2014,Jan,11

43641 **parietal cell (highly selective)**
    EXCLUDES   *Upper gastrointestinal endoscopy (43235-43259 [43233, 43266, 43270])*
    ⚕ 34.9   ⚕ 34.9   **FUD** 090   C 80 ▣
    AMA: 2014,Jan,11

43644-43645 Laparoscopic Gastric Bypass with Small Bowel Resection

CMS: 100-03,100.1 Bariatric Surgery for Treatment Co-morbid Conditions Due to Morbid Obesity; 100-04,32,150.1 Bariatric Surgery: Treatment of Co-Morbid Conditions Due to Morbid Obesity; 100-04,32,150.2 HCPCS Procedure Codes for Bariatric Surgery; 100-04,32,150.5 ICD Diagnosis Codes for BMI ≥35; 100-04,32,150.6 Bariatric Surgery Claims Guidance

INCLUDES   Diagnostic laparoscopy (49320)
EXCLUDES   *Endoscopy, upper gastrointestinal, (esophagus/stomach/duodenum/jejunum) (43235-43259 [43233, 43266, 43270])*

43644 **Laparoscopy, surgical, gastric restrictive procedure; with gastric bypass and Roux-en-Y gastroenterostomy (roux limb 150 cm or less)**
    EXCLUDES   *Roux limb less than 150 cm (43846)*
                 Roux limb greater than 150 cm (43645)
    ⚕ 50.2   ⚕ 50.2   **FUD** 090   C 80 ▣
    AMA: 2014,Jan,11

43645 **with gastric bypass and small intestine reconstruction to limit absorption**
    EXCLUDES   *Roux limb less than 150 cm (43847)*
    ⚕ 53.7   ⚕ 53.7   **FUD** 090   C 80 ▣
    AMA: 2018,Jan,8; 2017,Jan,8; 2016,Jan,13; 2015,Jan,16; 2014,Jan,11

43647-43659 Other and Unlisted Laparoscopic Gastric Procedures

INCLUDES   Diagnostic laparoscopy (49320)
EXCLUDES   *Endoscopy, upper gastrointestinal, (esophagus/stomach/duodenum/jejunum) (43235-43259 [43233, 43266, 43270])*

43647 **Laparoscopy, surgical; implantation or replacement of gastric neurostimulator electrodes, antrum**
    EXCLUDES   *Electronic analysis/programming gastric neurostimulator (95980-95982)*
                 Insertion gastric neurostimulator pulse generator (64590)
                 Laparoscopy with implantation, removal, or revision of gastric neurostimulator electrodes on the lesser curvature of the stomach (43659)
                 Open method (43881)
                 Vagus nerve blocking pulse generator and/or neurostimulator electrode array implantation, reprogramming, replacement, revision, or removal at the esophagogastric junction performed laparoscopically (0312T-0317T)
    ⚕ 0.00   ⚕ 0.00   **FUD** YYY   J 80 ▣
    AMA: 2019,Feb,6; 2018,Jan,8; 2017,Jan,8; 2016,Jan,13; 2015,Jan,16; 2014,Jan,11

43648 **revision or removal of gastric neurostimulator electrodes, antrum**
    EXCLUDES   *Electronic analysis/programming gastric neurostimulator (95980-95982)*
                 Laparoscopy with implantation, removal, or revision of gastric neurostimulator electrodes on the lesser curvature of the stomach (43659)
                 Open method (43882)
                 Revision/removal gastric neurostimulator pulse generator (64595)
                 Vagus nerve blocking pulse generator and/or neurostimulator electrode array implantation, reprogramming, replacement, revision, or removal at the esophagogastric junction performed laparoscopically (0312T-0317T)
    ⚕ 0.00   ⚕ 0.00   **FUD** YYY   J 80 ▣
    AMA: 2019,Feb,6; 2018,Jan,8; 2017,Jan,8; 2016,Jan,13; 2015,Jan,16; 2014,Jan,11

Digestive System (left margin)

43651 — 43773 (left margin)

43651   **Laparoscopy, surgical; transection of vagus nerves, truncal**
    18.9   18.9   **FUD** 090   [J] [80]
    AMA: 2018,Jan,8; 2017,Jan,8; 2016,Jan,13; 2015,Jan,16; 2014,Jan,11

43652   **transection of vagus nerves, selective or highly selective**
    22.1   22.1   **FUD** 090   [J] [80]
    AMA: 2018,Jan,8; 2017,Jan,8; 2016,Jan,13; 2015,Jan,16; 2014,Jan,11

43653   **gastrostomy, without construction of gastric tube (eg, Stamm procedure) (separate procedure)**
    16.6   16.6   **FUD** 090   [J] [A2] [80]
    AMA: 2018,Jan,8; 2017,Jan,8; 2016,Jan,13; 2015,Jan,16; 2014,Jan,11

43659   **Unlisted laparoscopy procedure, stomach**
    0.00   0.00   **FUD** YYY   [J] [80] [50]
    AMA: 2018,Jul,7; 2018,Jan,8; 2017,Jan,8; 2016,Jan,13; 2015,Jan,16; 2014,Jan,11

43752-43763 Nonsurgical Gastric Tube Procedures

43752   **Naso- or oro-gastric tube placement, requiring physician's skill and fluoroscopic guidance (includes fluoroscopy, image documentation and report)**
    EXCLUDES   *Critical care services (99291-99292)*
      Initial inpatient neonatal/pediatric critical care, per day (99468-99469, 99471-99472)
      Insertion long gastrointestinal tube (44500, 74340)
      Percutaneous insertion of gastrostomy tube (43246, 49440)
      Subsequent intensive care, per day, for low birth weight infant (99478-99479)
    1.17   1.17   **FUD** 000   [01] [62]
    AMA: 2019,Aug,8; 2018,Mar,11; 2018,Jan,8; 2017,Jan,8; 2016,Jan,13; 2015,Jan,16; 2014,May,4; 2014,Jan,11

43753   **Gastric intubation and aspiration(s) therapeutic, necessitating physician's skill (eg, for gastrointestinal hemorrhage), including lavage if performed**
    0.63   0.63   **FUD** 000   [01] [N1] [80]
    AMA: 2019,Aug,8; 2018,Jan,8; 2017,Jan,8; 2016,Jan,13; 2015,Jan,16; 2014,May,4; 2014,Jan,11

43754   **Gastric intubation and aspiration, diagnostic; single specimen (eg, acid analysis)**
    EXCLUDES   *Analysis of gastric acid (82930)*
      Naso- or oro-gastric tube placement using fluoroscopic guidance (43752)
    1.05   4.63   **FUD** 000   [01] [N1] [80]
    AMA: 2018,Jan,8; 2017,Jan,8; 2016,Jan,13; 2015,Jan,16; 2014,Jan,11

43755   **collection of multiple fractional specimens with gastric stimulation, single or double lumen tube (gastric secretory study) (eg, histamine, insulin, pentagastrin, calcium, secretin), includes drug administration**
    EXCLUDES   *Analysis of gastric acid (82930)*
      Naso- or oro-gastric tube placement using fluoroscopic guidance (43752)
    Code also drugs or substances administered
    1.74   4.43   **FUD** 000   [S] [62] [80]
    AMA: 2018,Jan,8; 2017,Jan,8; 2016,Jan,13; 2015,Jan,16; 2014,Jan,11

43756   **Duodenal intubation and aspiration, diagnostic, includes image guidance; single specimen (eg, bile study for crystals or afferent loop culture)**
    Code also drugs or substances administered
    (89049-89240)
    1.48   6.52   **FUD** 000   [01] [62] [80]
    AMA: 2018,Jan,8; 2017,Jan,8; 2016,Jan,13; 2015,Jan,16; 2014,Jan,11

43757   **collection of multiple fractional specimens with pancreatic or gallbladder stimulation, single or double lumen tube, includes drug administration**
    Code also drugs or substances administered
    (89049-89240)
    2.23   9.08   **FUD** 000   [T] [62] [80]
    AMA: 2018,Jan,8; 2017,Jan,8; 2016,Jan,13; 2015,Jan,16; 2014,Jan,11

43761   **Repositioning of a naso- or oro-gastric feeding tube, through the duodenum for enteric nutrition**
    EXCLUDES   *Conversion of gastrostomy tube to gastro-jejunostomy tube, percutaneous (49446)*
      Gastrostomy tube converted endoscopically to jejunostomy tube (44373)
      Insertion long gastrointestinal tube (44500, 74340)
    (76000)
    2.98   3.43   **FUD** 000   [T] [A2]
    AMA: 2018,Jan,8; 2017,Jan,8; 2016,Jan,13; 2015,Jan,16; 2014,Jan,11

43762   **Replacement of gastrostomy tube, percutaneous, includes removal, when performed, without imaging or endoscopic guidance; not requiring revision of gastrostomy tract**
    1.09   6.31   **FUD** 000   [62]
    AMA: 2019,Feb,5

43763   **requiring revision of gastrostomy tract**
    EXCLUDES   *Gastrostomy tube replacement using fluoroscopy (49450)*
      Percutaneous insertion of gastrostomy tube (43246)
    2.41   9.37   **FUD** 000   [62]
    AMA: 2019,Feb,5

43770-43775 Laparoscopic Bariatric Procedures

CMS: 100-03,100.1 Bariatric Surgery for Treatment Co-morbid Conditions Due to Morbid Obesity; 100-04,32,150.1 Bariatric Surgery: Treatment of Co-Morbid Conditions Due to Morbid Obesity; 100-04,32,150.2 HCPCS Procedure Codes for Bariatric Surgery; 100-04,32,150.5 ICD Diagnosis Codes for BMI ≥35; 100-04,32,150.6 Bariatric Surgery Claims Guidance

    INCLUDES   Diagnostic laparoscopy (49320)
      Stomach/duodenum/jejunum/ileum
      Subsequent band adjustments (change of the gastric band component diameter by injection/aspiration of fluid through the subcutaneous port component) during the postoperative period

43770   **Laparoscopy, surgical, gastric restrictive procedure; placement of adjustable gastric restrictive device (eg, gastric band and subcutaneous port components)**
    Code also modifier 52 for placement of individual component
    32.5   32.5   **FUD** 090   [J] [80]
    AMA: 2018,Jan,8; 2017,Jan,8; 2016,Jan,13; 2015,Jan,16; 2014,Jan,11

43771   **revision of adjustable gastric restrictive device component only**
    36.7   36.7   **FUD** 090   [C] [80]
    AMA: 2018,Jan,8; 2017,Jan,8; 2016,Jan,13; 2015,Jan,16; 2014,Jan,11

43772   **removal of adjustable gastric restrictive device component only**
    27.4   27.4   **FUD** 090   [J] [80]
    AMA: 2018,Jan,8; 2017,Jan,8; 2016,Jan,13; 2015,Jan,16; 2014,Jan,11

43773   **removal and replacement of adjustable gastric restrictive device component only**
    EXCLUDES   *Laparoscopy, surgical, gastric restrictive procedure; removal of adjustable gastric restrictive device component only (43772)*
    37.1   37.1   **FUD** 090   [J] [80]
    AMA: 2018,Jan,8; 2017,Jan,8; 2016,Jan,13; 2015,Jan,16; 2014,Jan,11

43774 removal of adjustable gastric restrictive device and subcutaneous port components

> EXCLUDES Removal/replacement of subcutaneous port components and gastric band (43659)

> 🚑 27.8 ⚕ 27.8 **FUD** 090 J 80 ▢

> AMA: 2018,Jan,8; 2017,Jan,8; 2016,Jan,13; 2015,Jan,16; 2014,Jan,11

43775 longitudinal gastrectomy (ie, sleeve gastrectomy)

> EXCLUDES Open gastric restrictive procedure for morbid obesity, without gastric bypass, other than vertical-banded gastroplasty (43843)
> Vagus nerve blocking pulse generator and/or neurostimulator electrode array implantation, reprogramming, replacement, revision, or removal at the esophagogastric junction performed laparoscopically (0312T-0317T)

> 🚑 32.3 ⚕ 32.3 **FUD** 090 C 80 ▢

> AMA: 2014,Jan,11

Gastric "sleeve"

Pylorus

Excised stomach

43800-43840 Open Gastric Incisional/Repair/Resection Procedures

43800 Pyloroplasty

> EXCLUDES Vagotomy with pyloroplasty (43640)

> 🚑 26.9 ⚕ 26.9 **FUD** 090 C 80 ▢

> AMA: 2014,Jan,11

43810 Gastroduodenostomy

> 🚑 29.5 ⚕ 29.5 **FUD** 090 C 80 ▢

> AMA: 2014,Jan,11

43820 Gastrojejunostomy; without vagotomy

> 🚑 38.9 ⚕ 38.9 **FUD** 090 C 80 ▢

> AMA: 2014,Jan,11

43825 with vagotomy, any type

> 🚑 38.0 ⚕ 38.0 **FUD** 090 C 80 ▢

> AMA: 2014,Jan,11

43830 Gastrostomy, open; without construction of gastric tube (eg, Stamm procedure) (separate procedure)

> 🚑 20.3 ⚕ 20.3 **FUD** 090 J 80 ▢

> AMA: 2019,Feb,5; 2018,Jan,8; 2017,Jan,8; 2016,Jan,13; 2015,Jan,16; 2014,Jan,11

43831 neonatal, for feeding A

> EXCLUDES Change of gastrostomy tube (43762-43763)
> Gastrostomy tube replacement using fluoroscopy (49450)

> 🚑 17.3 ⚕ 17.3 **FUD** 090 63 T 80 ▢

> AMA: 2019,Feb,5; 2018,Jan,8; 2017,Jan,8; 2016,Jan,13; 2015,Jan,16; 2014,Jan,11

43832 with construction of gastric tube (eg, Janeway procedure)

> EXCLUDES Endoscopic placement of percutaneous gastrostomy tube (43246)

> 🚑 30.0 ⚕ 30.0 **FUD** 090 C 80 ▢

> AMA: 2018,Jan,8; 2017,Jan,8; 2016,Jan,13; 2015,Jan,16; 2014,Jan,11

43840 Gastrorrhaphy, suture of perforated duodenal or gastric ulcer, wound, or injury

> 🚑 39.4 ⚕ 39.4 **FUD** 090 C 80 ▢

> AMA: 2014,Jan,11

43842-43848 Open Bariatric Procedures for Morbid Obesity

CMS: 100-03,100.1 Bariatric Surgery for Treatment Co-morbid Conditions Due to Morbid Obesity; 100-04,32,150.1 Bariatric Surgery: Treatment of Co-Morbid Conditions Due to Morbid Obesity; 100-04,32,150.2 HCPCS Procedure Codes for Bariatric Surgery; 100-04,32,150.5 ICD Diagnosis Codes for BMI ≥35; 100-04,32,150.6 Bariatric Surgery Claims Guidance

43842 Gastric restrictive procedure, without gastric bypass, for morbid obesity; vertical-banded gastroplasty

> 🚑 34.5 ⚕ 34.5 **FUD** 090 E ▢

> AMA: 2018,Jan,8; 2017,Jan,8; 2016,Jan,13; 2015,Jan,16; 2014,Jan,11

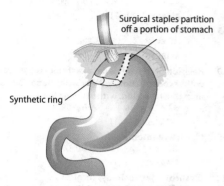

Surgical staples partition off a portion of stomach

Synthetic ring

The stomach is surgically restricted to treat morbid obesity; a vertical-banded partitioning technique gives the patient a sensation of fullness, thus decreasing daily caloric intake

43843 other than vertical-banded gastroplasty

> EXCLUDES Laparoscopic longitudinal gastrectomy (e.g., sleeve gastrectomy) (43775)

> 🚑 37.2 ⚕ 37.2 **FUD** 090 C 80 ▢

> AMA: 2018,Jan,8; 2017,Jan,8; 2016,Jan,13; 2015,Jan,16; 2014,Jan,11

43845 Gastric restrictive procedure with partial gastrectomy, pylorus-preserving duodenoileostomy and ileoileostomy (50 to 100 cm common channel) to limit absorption (biliopancreatic diversion with duodenal switch)

> EXCLUDES Enteroenterostomy, anastomosis of intestine (44130)
> Exploratory laparotomy, exploratory celiotomy (49000)
> Gastrectomy, partial, distal; with Roux-en-Y reconstruction (43633)
> Gastric restrictive procedure, with gastric bypass for morbid obesity; with small intestine reconstruction (43847)

> 🚑 56.5 ⚕ 56.5 **FUD** 090 C 80 ▢

> AMA: 2018,Jan,8; 2017,Jan,8; 2016,Jan,13; 2015,Jan,16; 2014,Jan,11

43846 Gastric restrictive procedure, with gastric bypass for morbid obesity; with short limb (150 cm or less) Roux-en-Y gastroenterostomy

> EXCLUDES Performed laparoscopically (43644)
> Roux limb more than 150 cm (43847)

> 🚑 47.0 ⚕ 47.0 **FUD** 090 C 80 ▢

> AMA: 2018,Jan,8; 2017,Jan,8; 2016,Jan,13; 2015,Jan,16; 2014,Jan,11

43847 with small intestine reconstruction to limit absorption

> EXCLUDES Performed laparoscopically (43645)

> 🚑 52.4 ⚕ 52.4 **FUD** 090 C 80 ▢

> AMA: 2018,Jan,8; 2017,Jan,8; 2016,Jan,13; 2015,Jan,16; 2014,Jan,11

Digestive System

43848 — 44010

43848 Revision, open, of gastric restrictive procedure for morbid obesity, other than adjustable gastric restrictive device (separate procedure)

> EXCLUDES Gastric restrictive port procedures (43886-43888)
> Procedures for adjustable gastric restrictive devices (43770-43774)

🚗 55.9   ⚕ 55.9   **FUD** 090   C 80 ▣

AMA: 2018,Jan,8; 2017,Jan,8; 2016,Jan,13; 2015,Jan,16; 2014,Jan,11

43850-43882 Open Gastric Procedures: Closure/Implantation/Replacement/Revision

43850 Revision of gastroduodenal anastomosis (gastroduodenostomy) with reconstruction; without vagotomy

🚗 47.3   ⚕ 47.3   **FUD** 090   C 80 ▣

AMA: 2014,Jan,11

43855 with vagotomy

🚗 49.1   ⚕ 49.1   **FUD** 090   C 80 ▣

AMA: 2014,Jan,11

43860 Revision of gastrojejunal anastomosis (gastrojejunostomy) with reconstruction, with or without partial gastrectomy or intestine resection; without vagotomy

🚗 47.4   ⚕ 47.4   **FUD** 090   C 80 ▣

AMA: 2014,Jan,11

43865 with vagotomy

🚗 49.7   ⚕ 49.7   **FUD** 090   C 80 ▣

AMA: 2014,Jan,11

43870 Closure of gastrostomy, surgical

🚗 20.6   ⚕ 20.6   **FUD** 090   J A2 80 ▣

AMA: 2018,Jul,14; 2014,Jan,11

43880 Closure of gastrocolic fistula

🚗 46.1   ⚕ 46.1   **FUD** 090   C 80 ▣

AMA: 2014,Jan,11

43881 Implantation or replacement of gastric neurostimulator electrodes, antrum, open

> EXCLUDES Electronic analysis and programming (95980-95982)
> Implantation/removal/revision gastric neurostimulator electrodes, lesser curvature or vagal trunk (EGJ):
>   Laparoscopically (43659)
>   Open, lesser curvature (43999)
> Implantation/replacement performed laparoscopically (43647)
> Insertion of gastric neurostimulator pulse generator (64590)
> Vagus nerve blocking pulse generator and/or neurostimulator electrode array implantation, reprogramming, replacement, revision, or removal at the esophagogastric junction performed laparoscopically (0312T-0317T)

🚗 0.00   ⚕ 0.00   **FUD** YYY   C 80 ▣

AMA: 2019,Feb,6; 2018,Jan,8; 2017,Jan,8; 2016,Jan,13; 2015,Jan,16; 2014,Jan,11

43882 Revision or removal of gastric neurostimulator electrodes, antrum, open

> EXCLUDES Electronic analysis and programming (95980-95982)
> Implantation/removal/revision gastric neurostimulator electrodes, lesser curvature or vagal trunk (EGJ):
>   Laparoscopic (43659)
>   Open, lesser curvature (43999)
> Revision/removal gastric neurostimulator electrodes, antrum, performed laparoscopically (43648)
> Revision/removal gastric neurostimulator pulse generator (64595)
> Vagus nerve blocking pulse generator and/or neurostimulator electrode array implantation, reprogramming, replacement, revision, or removal at the esophagogastric junction performed laparoscopically (0312T-0317T)

🚗 0.00   ⚕ 0.00   **FUD** YYY   C 80 ▣

AMA: 2019,Feb,6; 2018,Jan,8; 2017,Jan,8; 2016,Jan,13; 2015,Jan,16; 2014,Jan,11

43886-43999 Bariatric Procedures: Removal/Replacement/Revision Port Components

CMS: 100-04,32,150.1 Bariatric Surgery: Treatment of Co-Morbid Conditions Due to Morbid Obesity; 100-04,32,150.2 HCPCS Procedure Codes for Bariatric Surgery; 100-04,32,150.5 ICD Diagnosis Codes for BMI ≥35; 100-04,32,150.6 Bariatric Surgery Claims Guidance

43886 Gastric restrictive procedure, open; revision of subcutaneous port component only

🚗 10.5   ⚕ 10.5   **FUD** 090   T 62 80 ▣

AMA: 2018,Jan,8; 2017,Jan,8; 2016,Jan,13; 2015,Jan,16; 2014,Jan,11

43887 removal of subcutaneous port component only

> EXCLUDES Gastric band and subcutaneous port components:
>   Removal and replacement performed laparoscopically (43659)
>   Removal performed laparoscopically (43774)

🚗 9.48   ⚕ 9.48   **FUD** 090   02 62 80 ▣

AMA: 2018,Jan,8; 2017,Jan,8; 2016,Jan,13; 2015,Jan,16; 2014,Jan,11

43888 removal and replacement of subcutaneous port component only

> EXCLUDES Gastric band and subcutaneous port components:
>   Removal and replacement performed laparoscopically (43659)
>   Removal performed laparoscopically (43774)
> Gastric restrictive procedure, open; removal of subcutaneous port component only (43887)

🚗 13.3   ⚕ 13.3   **FUD** 090   T 62 80 ▣

AMA: 2018,Jan,8; 2017,Jan,8; 2016,Jan,13; 2015,Jan,16; 2014,Jan,11

43999 Unlisted procedure, stomach

🚗 0.00   ⚕ 0.00   **FUD** YYY   T 80 ▣

AMA: 2018,Dec,10; 2018,Dec,10; 2018,Jul,14; 2018,Jan,8; 2017,Jan,8; 2016,Jan,13; 2015,Jan,16; 2014,Jan,11

44005-44130 Incisional and Resection Procedures of Bowel

44005 Enterolysis (freeing of intestinal adhesion) (separate procedure)

> EXCLUDES Enterolysis performed laparoscopically (44180)
> Excision of ileoanal reservoir with ileostomy (45136)

🚗 31.7   ⚕ 31.7   **FUD** 090   C 80 ▣

AMA: 2018,Feb,11; 2018,Jan,8; 2017,Jan,8; 2016,Jan,13; 2015,Jan,16; 2014,Jan,11

44010 Duodenotomy, for exploration, biopsy(s), or foreign body removal

🚗 24.9   ⚕ 24.9   **FUD** 090   C 80 ▣

AMA: 2014,Jan,11

The duodenum is surgically accessed and explored A foreign body may be removed and/or a biopsy specimen taken

+ 44015 Tube or needle catheter jejunostomy for enteral alimentation, intraoperative, any method (List separately in addition to primary procedure)

Code first the primary procedure

🖐 4.13 ✂ 4.13 **FUD** ZZZ C 80 ▢

AMA: 2018,Jan,8; 2017,Jan,8; 2016,Jan,13; 2015,Jan,16; 2014,Jan,11

44020 Enterotomy, small intestine, other than duodenum; for exploration, biopsy(s), or foreign body removal

🖐 28.2 ✂ 28.2 **FUD** 090 C 80 ▢

AMA: 2014,Jan,11

44021 for decompression (eg, Baker tube)

🖐 28.3 ✂ 28.3 **FUD** 090 C 80 ▢

AMA: 2014,Jan,11

44025 Colotomy, for exploration, biopsy(s), or foreign body removal

INCLUDES Amussat's operation

EXCLUDES Intestine exteriorization (Mikulicz resection with crushing of spur) (44602-44605)

🖐 28.5 ✂ 28.5 **FUD** 090 C 80 ▢

AMA: 2014,Jan,11

44050 Reduction of volvulus, intussusception, internal hernia, by laparotomy

🖐 27.1 ✂ 27.1 **FUD** 090 C 80 ▢

AMA: 2014,Jan,11

44055 Correction of malrotation by lysis of duodenal bands and/or reduction of midgut volvulus (eg, Ladd procedure)

🖐 43.4 ✂ 43.4 **FUD** 090 63 C 80 ▢

AMA: 2014,Jan,11

44100 Biopsy of intestine by capsule, tube, peroral (1 or more specimens)

🖐 3.14 ✂ 3.14 **FUD** 000 T A2 ▢

AMA: 2014,Jan,11

44110 Excision of 1 or more lesions of small or large intestine not requiring anastomosis, exteriorization, or fistulization; single enterotomy

🖐 24.6 ✂ 24.6 **FUD** 090 C 80 ▢

AMA: 2014,Jan,11

44111 multiple enterotomies

🖐 28.5 ✂ 28.5 **FUD** 090 C 80 ▢

AMA: 2014,Jan,11

44120 Enterectomy, resection of small intestine; single resection and anastomosis

EXCLUDES Excision of ileoanal reservoir with ileostomy (45136)

🖐 35.4 ✂ 35.4 **FUD** 090 C 80 ▢

AMA: 2018,Nov,11; 2018,Jan,8; 2017,Jan,8; 2016,Jan,13; 2015,Jan,16; 2014,Jan,11

+ 44121 each additional resection and anastomosis (List separately in addition to code for primary procedure)

Code first (44120)

🖐 7.04 ✂ 7.04 **FUD** ZZZ C 80 ▢

AMA: 2014,Jan,11

44125 with enterostomy

🖐 34.2 ✂ 34.2 **FUD** 090 C 80 ▢

AMA: 2014,Jan,11

44126 Enterectomy, resection of small intestine for congenital atresia, single resection and anastomosis of proximal segment of intestine; without tapering

🖐 71.7 ✂ 71.7 **FUD** 090 63 C 80 ▢

AMA: 2014,Jan,11

44127 with tapering

🖐 82.9 ✂ 82.9 **FUD** 090 63 C 80 ▢

AMA: 2014,Jan,11

+ 44128 each additional resection and anastomosis (List separately in addition to code for primary procedure)

Code first single resection of small intestine (44126, 44127)

🖐 7.10 ✂ 7.10 **FUD** ZZZ 63 C 80 ▢

AMA: 2014,Jan,11

44130 Enteroenterostomy, anastomosis of intestine, with or without cutaneous enterostomy (separate procedure)

🖐 38.1 ✂ 38.1 **FUD** 090 C 80 ▢

AMA: 2014,Jan,11

44132-44137 Intestine Transplant Procedures

CMS: 100-03,260.5 Intestinal and Multi-Visceral Transplantation; 100-04,3,90.6 Intestinal and Multi-Visceral Transplants

44132 Donor enterectomy (including cold preservation), open; from cadaver donor

INCLUDES Graft:
Cold preservation
Harvest

EXCLUDES Preparation/reconstruction of backbench intestinal graft (44715, 44720-44721)

🖐 0.00 ✂ 0.00 **FUD** XXX C 80 ▢

AMA: 2014,Jan,11

44133 partial, from living donor

INCLUDES Donor care
Graft:
Cold preservation
Harvest

EXCLUDES Preparation/reconstruction of backbench intestinal graft (44715, 44720-44721)

🖐 0.00 ✂ 0.00 **FUD** XXX C 80 ▢

AMA: 2014,Jan,11

44135 Intestinal allotransplantation; from cadaver donor

INCLUDES Allograft transplantation
Recipient care

🖐 0.00 ✂ 0.00 **FUD** XXX C 80 ▢

AMA: 2014,Jan,11

44136 from living donor

INCLUDES Allograft transplantation
Recipient care

🖐 0.00 ✂ 0.00 **FUD** XXX C 80 ▢

AMA: 2014,Jan,11

44137 Removal of transplanted intestinal allograft, complete

EXCLUDES Partial removal of transplant allograft (44120-44121, 44140)

🖐 0.00 ✂ 0.00 **FUD** XXX C 80 ▢

AMA: 2014,Jan,11

44139-44160 Colon Resection Procedures

+ 44139 Mobilization (take-down) of splenic flexure performed in conjunction with partial colectomy (List separately in addition to primary procedure)

Code first partial colectomy (44140-44147)

🖐 3.51 ✂ 3.51 **FUD** ZZZ C 80 ▢

AMA: 2014,Jan,11

44140 Colectomy, partial; with anastomosis

EXCLUDES Laparoscopic method (44204)

🖐 38.9 ✂ 38.9 **FUD** 090 C 80 ▢

AMA: 2018,Jan,8; 2017,Jan,8; 2016,Jan,13; 2015,Jan,16; 2014,Jan,11

44141 with skin level cecostomy or colostomy

🖐 52.9 ✂ 52.9 **FUD** 090 C 80 ▢

AMA: 2018,Jan,8; 2017,Jan,8; 2016,Jan,13; 2015,Jan,16; 2014,Jan,11

44143 with end colostomy and closure of distal segment (Hartmann type procedure)

EXCLUDES Laparoscopic method (44206)

🖐 48.2 ✂ 48.2 **FUD** 090 C 80 ▢

AMA: 2018,Jan,8; 2017,Jan,8; 2016,Jan,13; 2015,Jan,16; 2014,Jan,11

Digestive System

44144 — 44208

44144   **with resection, with colostomy or ileostomy and creation of mucofistula**

     🛏 51.3   ✂ 51.3   **FUD** 090   C 80 ▭

     AMA: 2018,Jan,8; 2017,Jan,8; 2016,Jan,13; 2015,Jan,16; 2014,Jan,11

44145   **with coloproctostomy (low pelvic anastomosis)**

     EXCLUDES   *Laparoscopic method (44207)*

     🛏 48.0   ✂ 48.0   **FUD** 090   C 80 ▭

     AMA: 2014,Jan,11

44146   **with coloproctostomy (low pelvic anastomosis), with colostomy**

     EXCLUDES   *Laparoscopic method (44208)*

     🛏 61.3   ✂ 61.3   **FUD** 090   C 80 ▭

     AMA: 2018,Jun,11; 2018,Jan,8; 2017,Jan,8; 2016,Jan,13; 2015,Jan,16; 2014,Jan,11

44147   **abdominal and transanal approach**

     🛏 56.3   ✂ 56.3   **FUD** 090   C 80 ▭

     AMA: 2018,Jan,8; 2017,Jan,8; 2016,Jan,13; 2015,Jan,16; 2014,Jan,11

44150   **Colectomy, total, abdominal, without proctectomy; with ileostomy or ileoproctostomy**

     INCLUDES   Lane's operation

     EXCLUDES   *Laparoscopic method (44210)*

     🛏 54.0   ✂ 54.0   **FUD** 090   C 80 ▭

     AMA: 2014,Jan,11

44151   **with continent ileostomy**

     🛏 62.7   ✂ 62.7   **FUD** 090   C 80 ▭

     AMA: 2014,Jan,11

44155   **Colectomy, total, abdominal, with proctectomy; with ileostomy**

     INCLUDES   Miles' colectomy

     EXCLUDES   *Laparoscopic method (44212)*

     🛏 60.1   ✂ 60.1   **FUD** 090   C 80 ▭

     AMA: 2014,Jan,11

44156   **with continent ileostomy**

     🛏 67.1   ✂ 67.1   **FUD** 090   C 80 ▭

     AMA: 2014,Jan,11

44157   **with ileoanal anastomosis, includes loop ileostomy, and rectal mucosectomy, when performed**

     🛏 63.6   ✂ 63.6   **FUD** 090   C 80 ▭

     AMA: 2014,Jan,11

44158   **with ileoanal anastomosis, creation of ileal reservoir (S or J), includes loop ileostomy, and rectal mucosectomy, when performed**

     EXCLUDES   *Laparoscopic method (44211)*

     🛏 65.2   ✂ 65.2   **FUD** 090   C 80 ▭

     AMA: 2014,Jan,11

44160   **Colectomy, partial, with removal of terminal ileum with ileocolostomy**

     EXCLUDES   *Laparoscopic method (44205)*

     🛏 36.0   ✂ 36.0   **FUD** 090   C 80 ▭

     AMA: 2018,Jan,8; 2017,Jan,8; 2016,Jan,13; 2015,Jan,16; 2014,Jan,11

44180 Laparoscopic Enterolysis

INCLUDES   Diagnostic laparoscopy (49320)

EXCLUDES   *Laparoscopic salpingolysis/ovariolysis (58660)*

44180   **Laparoscopy, surgical, enterolysis (freeing of intestinal adhesion) (separate procedure)**

     🛏 26.6   ✂ 26.6   **FUD** 090   J 80 ▭

     AMA: 2018,Feb,11; 2018,Jan,8; 2017,Jan,8; 2016,Jan,13; 2015,Jan,16; 2014,Jan,11

44186-44238 Laparoscopic Enterostomy Procedures

INCLUDES   Diagnostic laparoscopy (49320)

44186   **Laparoscopy, surgical; jejunostomy (eg, for decompression or feeding)**

     🛏 18.8   ✂ 18.8   **FUD** 090   J 80 ▭

     AMA: 2018,Jan,8; 2017,Jan,8; 2016,Jan,13; 2015,Jan,16; 2014,Jan,11

44187   **ileostomy or jejunostomy, non-tube**

     EXCLUDES   *Open method (44310)*

     🛏 31.8   ✂ 31.8   **FUD** 090   C 80 ▭

     AMA: 2019,Sep,10; 2018,Jan,8; 2017,Jan,8; 2016,Jan,13; 2015,Jan,16; 2014,Jan,11

44188   **Laparoscopy, surgical, colostomy or skin level cecostomy**

     EXCLUDES   *Laparoscopy, surgical, appendectomy (44970)*

                 Open method (44320)

     🛏 35.4   ✂ 35.4   **FUD** 090   C 80 ▭

     AMA: 2018,Jan,8; 2017,Jan,8; 2016,Jan,13; 2015,Jan,16; 2014,Jan,11

44202   **Laparoscopy, surgical; enterectomy, resection of small intestine, single resection and anastomosis**

     EXCLUDES   *Open method (44120)*

     🛏 40.1   ✂ 40.1   **FUD** 090   C 80 ▭

     AMA: 2018,Jan,8; 2017,Jan,8; 2016,Jan,13; 2015,Jan,16; 2014,Jan,11

+ 44203   **each additional small intestine resection and anastomosis (List separately in addition to code for primary procedure)**

     EXCLUDES   *Open method (44121)*

     Code first single resection of small intestine (44202)

     🛏 6.96   ✂ 6.96   **FUD** ZZZ   C 80 ▭

     AMA: 2018,Jan,8; 2017,Jan,8; 2016,Jan,13; 2015,Jan,16; 2014,Jan,11

44204   **colectomy, partial, with anastomosis**

     EXCLUDES   *Open method (44140)*

     🛏 44.6   ✂ 44.6   **FUD** 090   C 80 ▭

     AMA: 2018,Jan,8; 2017,Dec,14; 2017,Jan,8; 2016,Jan,13; 2015,Jan,16; 2014,Jan,11

44205   **colectomy, partial, with removal of terminal ileum with ileocolostomy**

     EXCLUDES   *Open method (44160)*

     🛏 38.7   ✂ 38.7   **FUD** 090   C 80 ▭

     AMA: 2018,Jan,8; 2017,Jan,8; 2016,Jan,13; 2015,Jan,16; 2014,Jan,11

44206   **colectomy, partial, with end colostomy and closure of distal segment (Hartmann type procedure)**

     EXCLUDES   *Open method (44143)*

     🛏 50.6   ✂ 50.6   **FUD** 090   C 80 ▭

     AMA: 2018,Jan,8; 2017,Jan,8; 2016,Jan,13; 2015,Jan,16; 2014,Jan,11

44207   **colectomy, partial, with anastomosis, with coloproctostomy (low pelvic anastomosis)**

     EXCLUDES   *Open method (44145)*

     🛏 52.6   ✂ 52.6   **FUD** 090   C 80 ▭

     AMA: 2018,Jan,8; 2017,Jan,8; 2016,Jan,13; 2015,Jan,16; 2014,Jan,11

44208   **colectomy, partial, with anastomosis, with coloproctostomy (low pelvic anastomosis) with colostomy**

     EXCLUDES   *Open method (44146)*

     🛏 57.4   ✂ 57.4   **FUD** 090   C 80 ▭

     AMA: 2018,Jan,8; 2017,Jan,8; 2016,Jan,13; 2015,Jan,16; 2014,Jan,11

26/TC PC/TC Only   A2-Z3 ASC Payment   50 Bilateral   ♂ Male Only   ♀ Female Only   🛏 Facility RVU   ✂ Non-Facility RVU   ▭ CCI   ✖ CLIA

FUD Follow-up Days   **CMS:** IOM   **AMA:** CPT Asst   A-Y OPPSI   80/80 Surg Assist Allowed / w/Doc   Lab Crosswalk   Radiology Crosswalk

210   CPT © 2019 American Medical Association. All Rights Reserved.   © 2019 Optum360, LLC

44210 colectomy, total, abdominal, without proctectomy, with ileostomy or ileoproctostomy

    EXCLUDES   *Open method (44150)*

    🚗 51.5   ⚕ 51.5   **FUD** 090   C 80 ▣

    AMA: 2018,Jan,8; 2017,Jan,8; 2016,Jan,13; 2015,Jan,16; 2014,Jan,11

44211 colectomy, total, abdominal, with proctectomy, with ileoanal anastomosis, creation of ileal reservoir (S or J), with loop ileostomy, includes rectal mucosectomy, when performed

    EXCLUDES   *Open method (44157-44158)*

    🚗 62.9   ⚕ 62.9   **FUD** 090   C 80 ▣

    AMA: 2018,Jan,8; 2017,Jan,8; 2016,Jan,13; 2015,Jan,16; 2014,Jan,11

44212 colectomy, total, abdominal, with proctectomy, with ileostomy

    EXCLUDES   *Open method (44155)*

    🚗 59.1   ⚕ 59.1   **FUD** 090   C 80 ▣

    AMA: 2018,Jan,8; 2017,Jan,8; 2016,Jan,13; 2015,Jan,16; 2014,Jan,11

+ 44213 Laparoscopy, surgical, mobilization (take-down) of splenic flexure performed in conjunction with partial colectomy (List separately in addition to primary procedure)

    EXCLUDES   *Open method (44139)*

    Code first partial colectomy (44204-44208)

    🚗 5.45   ⚕ 5.45   **FUD** ZZZ   C 80 ▣

    AMA: 2018,Jan,8; 2017,Jan,8; 2016,Jan,13; 2015,Jan,16; 2014,Jan,11

44227 Laparoscopy, surgical, closure of enterostomy, large or small intestine, with resection and anastomosis

    EXCLUDES   *Open method (44625-44626)*

    🚗 48.2   ⚕ 48.2   **FUD** 090   C 80 ▣

    AMA: 2018,Jan,8; 2017,Jan,8; 2016,Jan,13; 2015,Jan,16; 2014,Jan,11

44238 Unlisted laparoscopy procedure, intestine (except rectum)

    🚗 0.00   ⚕ 0.00   **FUD** YYY   J 80 50 ▣

    AMA: 2018,Jan,8; 2017,Jul,10; 2017,Jan,8; 2016,Jan,13; 2015,Jan,16; 2014,Jan,11

44300-44346 Open Enterostomy Procedures

44300 Placement, enterostomy or cecostomy, tube open (eg, for feeding or decompression) (separate procedure)

    EXCLUDES   *Intraoperative lavage, colon (44701)*

    Other gastrointestinal tube(s) placed percutaneously with fluoroscopic imaging guidance (49441-49442)

    🚗 24.4   ⚕ 24.4   **FUD** 090   C 80 ▣

    AMA: 2018,Jan,8; 2017,Jan,8; 2016,Jan,13; 2015,Jan,16; 2014,Jan,11

44310 Ileostomy or jejunostomy, non-tube

    EXCLUDES   *Colectomy, partial; with resection, with colostomy or ileostomy and creation of mucofistula (44144)*

    Colectomy, total, abdominal (44150-44151, 44155-44156)

    Excision of ileoanal reservoir with ileostomy (45136)

    Laparoscopic method (44187)

    Proctectomy (45113, 45119)

    🚗 30.2   ⚕ 30.2   **FUD** 090   C 80 ▣

    AMA: 2018,Jan,8; 2017,Jan,8; 2016,Jan,13; 2015,Jan,16; 2014,Jan,11

44312 Revision of ileostomy; simple (release of superficial scar) (separate procedure)

    🚗 17.1   ⚕ 17.1   **FUD** 090   T A2 80 ▣

    AMA: 2014,Jan,11

44314 complicated (reconstruction in-depth) (separate procedure)

    🚗 29.1   ⚕ 29.1   **FUD** 090   C 80 ▣

    AMA: 2014,Jan,11

44316 Continent ileostomy (Kock procedure) (separate procedure)

    EXCLUDES   *Fiberoptic evaluation (44385)*

    🚗 41.0   ⚕ 41.0   **FUD** 090   C 80 ▣

    AMA: 2014,Jan,11

44320 Colostomy or skin level cecostomy;

    EXCLUDES   *Closure of fistula (45805, 45825, 57307)*

    Colectomy, partial (44141, 44144, 44146)

    Exploration, repair, and presacral drainage (45563)

    Laparoscopic method (44188)

    Pelvic exenteration (45126, 51597, 58240)

    Proctectomy (45110, 45119)

    Suture of large intestine (44605)

    Ureterosigmoidostomy (50810)

    🚗 34.8   ⚕ 34.8   **FUD** 090   C 80 ▣

    AMA: 2018,Jan,8; 2017,Jan,8; 2016,Jan,13; 2015,Jan,16; 2014,Jan,11

44322 with multiple biopsies (eg, for congenital megacolon) (separate procedure)

    🚗 29.0   ⚕ 29.0   **FUD** 090   C 80 ▣

    AMA: 2014,Jan,11

44340 Revision of colostomy; simple (release of superficial scar) (separate procedure)

    🚗 18.0   ⚕ 18.0   **FUD** 090   T A2 ▣

    AMA: 2014,Jan,11

44345 complicated (reconstruction in-depth) (separate procedure)

    🚗 30.4   ⚕ 30.4   **FUD** 090   C 80 ▣

    AMA: 2014,Jan,11

44346 with repair of paracolostomy hernia (separate procedure)

    🚗 34.2   ⚕ 34.2   **FUD** 090   C 80 ▣

    AMA: 2018,Jan,8; 2017,Jan,8; 2016,Jan,13; 2015,Jan,16; 2014,Jan,11

Skin

Herniations that have formed around the site of a colostomy are repaired

The colon is mobilized, trimmed if necessary, and a new stoma is often created

44360-44379 Endoscopy of Small Intestine

    INCLUDES   Control of bleeding as a result of endoscopic procedure during same operative session

    EXCLUDES   *Esophagogastroduodenoscopy, flexible, transoral (43235-43259 [43233, 43266, 43270])*

    Retrograde exam through anus/colon stoma (44799)

44360 Small intestinal endoscopy, enteroscopy beyond second portion of duodenum, not including ileum; diagnostic, including collection of specimen(s) by brushing or washing, when performed (separate procedure)

    EXCLUDES   *Small intestinal endoscopy, enteroscopy (44376-44379)*

    🚗 4.20   ⚕ 4.20   **FUD** 000   J A2 ▣

    AMA: 2018,Jan,8; 2017,Jan,8; 2016,Jan,13; 2015,Jan,16; 2014,Nov,3; 2014,Jan,11

44361 with biopsy, single or multiple

    EXCLUDES   *Small intestinal endoscopy, enteroscopy (44376-44379)*

    🚗 4.65   ⚕ 4.65   **FUD** 000   J A2 ▣

    AMA: 2014,Nov,3; 2014,Jan,11

44363 with removal of foreign body(s)

> *EXCLUDES* *Small intestinal endoscopy, enteroscopy (44376-44379)*
>
> 🔧 5.62   ⚖ 5.62   **FUD** 000   J A2 80 ▢
>
> **AMA:** 2014,Nov,3; 2014,Jan,11

44364 with removal of tumor(s), polyp(s), or other lesion(s) by snare technique

> *EXCLUDES* *Small intestinal endoscopy, enteroscopy (44376-44379)*
>
> 🔧 5.99   ⚖ 5.99   **FUD** 000   J A2 80 ▢
>
> **AMA:** 2014,Nov,3; 2014,Jan,11

44365 with removal of tumor(s), polyp(s), or other lesion(s) by hot biopsy forceps or bipolar cautery

> *EXCLUDES* *Small intestinal endoscopy, enteroscopy (44376-44379)*
>
> 🔧 5.32   ⚖ 5.32   **FUD** 000   J A2 80 ▢
>
> **AMA:** 2014,Nov,3; 2014,Jan,11

44366 with control of bleeding (eg, injection, bipolar cautery, unipolar cautery, laser, heater probe, stapler, plasma coagulator)

> *EXCLUDES* *Small intestinal endoscopy, enteroscopy (44376-44379)*
>
> 🔧 7.02   ⚖ 7.02   **FUD** 000   J A2 ▢
>
> **AMA:** 2018,Jan,8; 2017,Jan,8; 2016,Jan,13; 2015,Jan,16; 2014,Nov,3; 2014,Jan,11

44369 with ablation of tumor(s), polyp(s), or other lesion(s) not amenable to removal by hot biopsy forceps, bipolar cautery or snare technique

> *EXCLUDES* *Small intestinal endoscopy, enteroscopy (44376-44379)*
>
> 🔧 7.19   ⚖ 7.19   **FUD** 000   J A2 80 ▢
>
> **AMA:** 2014,Nov,3; 2014,Jan,11

44370 with transendoscopic stent placement (includes predilation)

> *EXCLUDES* *Small intestinal endoscopy, enteroscopy (44376-44379)*
>
> 🔧 7.80   ⚖ 7.80   **FUD** 000   J J8 80 ▢
>
> **AMA:** 2018,Jan,8; 2017,Jan,8; 2016,Jan,13; 2015,Jan,16; 2014,Nov,3; 2014,Jan,11

44372 with placement of percutaneous jejunostomy tube

> *EXCLUDES* *Small intestinal endoscopy, enteroscopy (44376-44379)*
>
> 🔧 7.02   ⚖ 7.02   **FUD** 000   J A2 ▢
>
> **AMA:** 2018,Jan,8; 2017,Jan,8; 2016,Jan,13; 2015,Jan,16; 2014,Nov,3; 2014,Jan,11

44373 with conversion of percutaneous gastrostomy tube to percutaneous jejunostomy tube

> *EXCLUDES* *Jejunostomy, fiberoptic, through stoma (43235)*
>   *Small intestinal endoscopy, enteroscopy (44376-44379)*
>
> 🔧 5.62   ⚖ 5.62   **FUD** 000   J A2 ▢
>
> **AMA:** 2018,Jan,8; 2017,Jan,8; 2016,Jan,13; 2015,Jan,16; 2014,Nov,3; 2014,Jan,11

44376 Small intestinal endoscopy, enteroscopy beyond second portion of duodenum, including ileum; diagnostic, with or without collection of specimen(s) by brushing or washing (separate procedure)

> *EXCLUDES* *Small intestinal endoscopy, enteroscopy (44360-44373)*
>
> 🔧 8.33   ⚖ 8.33   **FUD** 000   J A2 80 ▢
>
> **AMA:** 2018,Jan,8; 2017,Jan,8; 2016,Jan,13; 2015,Jan,16; 2014,Nov,3; 2014,Jan,11

44377 with biopsy, single or multiple

> *EXCLUDES* *Small intestinal endoscopy, enteroscopy (44360-44373)*
>
> 🔧 8.77   ⚖ 8.77   **FUD** 000   J A2 80 ▢
>
> **AMA:** 2018,Jan,8; 2017,Jan,8; 2016,Jan,13; 2015,Jan,16; 2014,Nov,3; 2014,Jan,11

44378 with control of bleeding (eg, injection, bipolar cautery, unipolar cautery, laser, heater probe, stapler, plasma coagulator)

> *EXCLUDES* *Small intestinal endoscopy, enteroscopy (44360-44373)*
>
> 🔧 11.2   ⚖ 11.2   **FUD** 000   J A2 80 ▢
>
> **AMA:** 2018,Jan,8; 2017,Jan,8; 2016,Jan,13; 2015,Jan,16; 2014,Nov,3; 2014,Jan,11

44379 with transendoscopic stent placement (includes predilation)

> *EXCLUDES* *Small intestinal endoscopy, enteroscopy (44360-44373)*
>
> 🔧 11.9   ⚖ 11.9   **FUD** 000   J A2 80 ▢
>
> **AMA:** 2018,Jan,8; 2017,Jan,8; 2016,Jan,13; 2015,Jan,16; 2014,Nov,3; 2014,Jan,11

44380-44384 [44381] Ileoscopy Via Stoma

> *INCLUDES* Control of bleeding as result of endoscopic procedure during same operative session
>
> *EXCLUDES* *Computed tomographic colonography (74261-74263)*
>
> Code also exam of nonfunctional distal colon/rectum, when performed, with:
>   Anoscopy (46600, 46604-46606, 46608-46615)
>   Proctosigmoidoscopy (45300-45327)
>   Sigmoidoscopy (45330-45347 [45346])

44380 Ileoscopy, through stoma; diagnostic, including collection of specimen(s) by brushing or washing, when performed (separate procedure)

> *EXCLUDES* *Ileoscopy, through stoma (44382-44384 [44381])*
>
> 🔧 1.64   ⚖ 4.97   **FUD** 000   T A2 ▢
>
> **AMA:** 2018,Jan,8; 2017,Jan,8; 2016,Jan,13; 2015,Jan,16; 2014,Dec,3; 2014,Nov,3; 2014,Jan,11

44381 **Resequenced code. See code following 44382.**

44382 with biopsy, single or multiple

> *EXCLUDES* *Ileoscopy, through stoma; diagnostic (44380)*
>
> 🔧 2.14   ⚖ 7.80   **FUD** 000   T A2 ▢
>
> **AMA:** 2018,Jan,8; 2017,Jan,8; 2016,Jan,13; 2015,Jan,16; 2014,Dec,3; 2014,Nov,3; 2014,Jan,11

**44381** with transendoscopic balloon dilation

> *EXCLUDES* *Ileoscopy, through stoma (44380, 44384)*
>
> Code also each additional stricture dilated in same session, using modifier 59 with (44381)
>
> ⚡ (74360)
>
> 🔧 2.44   ⚖ 27.0   **FUD** 000   J G2 ▢
>
> **AMA:** 2018,Jan,8; 2017,Jan,8; 2016,Jan,13; 2015,Jan,16; 2014,Dec,3; 2014,Nov,3

44384 with placement of endoscopic stent (includes pre- and post-dilation and guide wire passage, when performed)

> *EXCLUDES* *Ileoscopy, through stoma (44380-44381)*
>
> ⚡ (74360)
>
> 🔧 4.47   ⚖ 4.47   **FUD** 000   J G2 ▢
>
> **AMA:** 2018,Jan,8; 2017,Jan,8; 2016,Jan,13; 2015,Jan,16; 2014,Dec,3; 2014,Nov,3

44385-44386 Endoscopy of Small Intestinal Pouch

> *INCLUDES* Control of bleeding as result of the endoscopic procedure during same operative session
>
> *EXCLUDES* *Computed tomographic colonography (74261-74263)*

44385 Endoscopic evaluation of small intestinal pouch (eg, Kock pouch, ileal reservoir [S or J]); diagnostic, including collection of specimen(s) by brushing or washing, when performed (separate procedure)

> *EXCLUDES* *Endoscopic evaluation of small intestinal pouch (44386)*
>
> 🔧 2.09   ⚖ 5.60   **FUD** 000   T A2 ▢
>
> **AMA:** 2018,Jan,8; 2017,Jan,8; 2016,Jan,13; 2015,Jan,16; 2014,Dec,3; 2014,Nov,3; 2014,Jan,11

44386 with biopsy, single or multiple

> *EXCLUDES* *Endoscopic evaluation of small intestinal pouch (44385)*
>
> 🔧 2.60   ⚖ 8.36   **FUD** 000   T A2 ▢
>
> **AMA:** 2018,Jan,8; 2017,Jan,8; 2016,Jan,13; 2015,Jan,16; 2014,Dec,3; 2014,Nov,3; 2014,Jan,11

26/TC PC/TC Only   A2-Z3 ASC Payment   50 Bilateral   ♂ Male Only   ♀ Female Only   🔧 Facility RVU   ⚖ Non-Facility RVU   ▢ CCI   ⚡ CLIA
FUD Follow-up Days   **CMS:** IOM   **AMA:** CPT Asst   A-Y OPPSI   80/80 Surg Assist Allowed / w/Doc   ▲ Lab Crosswalk   ⚡ Radiology Crosswalk

212   CPT © 2019 American Medical Association. All Rights Reserved.   © 2019 Optum360, LLC

44388-44408 [44401] Colonoscopy Via Stoma

INCLUDES Control of bleeding as result of endoscopic procedure during same operative session

EXCLUDES *Colonoscopy via rectum (45378, 45392-45393 [45390, 45398])*
Computed tomographic colonography (74261-74263)

Code also exam of nonfunctional distal colon/rectum, when performed, with:
Anoscopy (46600, 46604-46606, 46608-46615)
Proctosigmoidoscopy (45300-45327)
Sigmoidoscopy (45330-45347 [45346])

44388 **Colonoscopy through stoma; diagnostic, including collection of specimen(s) by brushing or washing, when performed (separate procedure)**

EXCLUDES *Colonoscopy through stoma (44389-44408 [44401])*

Code also modifier 53 when planned total colonoscopy cannot be completed

⚕ 4.56 ☒ 8.42 **FUD** 000 T A2 🖵

AMA: 2018,Jan,8; 2017,Jan,8; 2016,Jan,13; 2015,Jan,16; 2014,Dec,3; 2014,Nov,3; 2014,Jan,11

44389 **with biopsy, single or multiple**

EXCLUDES *Colonoscopy through stoma; diagnostic (44388)*
Colonoscopy through stoma; with endoscopic mucosal resection on the same lesion (44403)

Code also modifier 52 when colonoscope fails to reach the junction of the small intestine

⚕ 5.02 ☒ 11.0 **FUD** 000 T A2 🖵

AMA: 2018,Jan,8; 2017,Jan,8; 2016,Jan,13; 2015,Jan,16; 2014,Dec,3; 2014,Nov,3; 2014,Jan,11

44390 **with removal of foreign body(s)**

EXCLUDES *Colonoscopy through stoma; diagnostic (44388)*

Code also modifier 52 when colonoscope fails to reach the junction of the small intestine

⚕ (76000)

⚕ 6.17 ☒ 10.9 **FUD** 000 T A2 🖵

AMA: 2018,Jan,8; 2017,Jan,8; 2016,Jan,13; 2015,Jan,16; 2014,Dec,3; 2014,Nov,3; 2014,Jan,11

44391 **with control of bleeding, any method**

EXCLUDES *Colonoscopy through stoma; diagnostic (44388)*
Colonoscopy through stoma; with directed submucosal injection(s) on the same lesion (44404)

Code also modifier 52 when colonoscope fails to reach the junction of the small intestine

⚕ 6.72 ☒ 19.3 **FUD** 000 T A2 🖵

AMA: 2018,Jan,8; 2017,Jan,8; 2016,Jan,13; 2015,Jan,16; 2014,Dec,3; 2014,Nov,3; 2014,Jan,11

44392 **with removal of tumor(s), polyp(s), or other lesion(s) by hot biopsy forceps**

EXCLUDES *Colonoscopy through stoma; diagnostic (44388)*

Code also modifier 52 when colonoscope fails to reach the junction of the small intestine

⚕ 5.82 ☒ 10.2 **FUD** 000 T A2 🖵

AMA: 2018,Jan,8; 2017,Jan,8; 2016,Jan,13; 2015,Jan,16; 2014,Dec,3; 2014,Nov,3; 2014,Jan,11

\# **44401** **with ablation of tumor(s), polyp(s), or other lesion(s) (includes pre-and post-dilation and guide wire passage, when performed)**

EXCLUDES *Colonoscopy through stoma; diagnostic (44388)*
Colonoscopy through stoma; with transendoscopic balloon dilation on the same lesion (44405)

Code also modifier 52 when colonoscope fails to reach the junction of the small intestine

⚕ 7.09 ☒ 86.2 **FUD** 000 T G2 🖵

AMA: 2018,Jan,8; 2017,Jan,8; 2016,Jan,13; 2015,Jan,16; 2014,Dec,3; 2014,Nov,3

44394 **with removal of tumor(s), polyp(s), or other lesion(s) by snare technique**

EXCLUDES *Colonoscopy through stoma; diagnostic (44388)*
Colonoscopy through stoma; with endoscopic mucosal resection on the same lesion (44403)

Code also modifier 52 when colonoscope fails to reach the junction of the small intestine

⚕ 6.60 ☒ 11.7 **FUD** 000 T A2 🖵

AMA: 2018,Jan,8; 2017,Jan,8; 2016,Jan,13; 2015,Jan,16; 2014,Dec,3; 2014,Nov,3; 2014,Jan,11

44401 **Resequenced code. See code following 44392.**

44402 **with endoscopic stent placement (including pre- and post-dilation and guide wire passage, when performed)**

EXCLUDES *Colonoscopy through stoma (44388, 44405)*

Code also modifier 52 when colonoscope fails to reach the junction of the small intestine

⚕ (74360)

⚕ 7.66 ☒ 7.66 **FUD** 000 J J8 🖵

AMA: 2018,Jan,8; 2017,Jan,8; 2016,Jan,13; 2015,Jan,16; 2014,Dec,3; 2014,Nov,3

44403 **with endoscopic mucosal resection**

EXCLUDES *Colonoscopy through stoma; diagnostic (44388)*
Colonoscopy through stoma on the same lesion (44389, 44394, 44404)

Code also modifier 52 when colonoscope fails to reach the junction of the small intestine

⚕ 8.89 ☒ 8.89 **FUD** 000 T G2 🖵

AMA: 2018,Jan,8; 2017,Jan,8; 2016,Jan,13; 2015,Jan,16; 2014,Dec,3; 2014,Nov,3

44404 **with directed submucosal injection(s), any substance**

EXCLUDES *Colonoscopy through stoma; diagnostic (44388)*
Colonoscopy through stoma on the same lesion (44391, 44403)

Code also modifier 52 when colonoscope fails to reach the junction of the small intestine

⚕ 5.03 ☒ 10.8 **FUD** 000 T G2 🖵

AMA: 2018,Jan,8; 2017,Jan,8; 2016,Jan,13; 2015,Jan,16; 2014,Dec,3; 2014,Nov,3

44405 **with transendoscopic balloon dilation**

EXCLUDES *Colonoscopy through stoma (44388, [44401], 44402)*

Code also each additional stricture dilated in same session, using modifier 59 with (44405)

Code also modifier 52 when colonoscope fails to reach the junction of the small intestine

⚕ (74360)

⚕ 5.37 ☒ 15.5 **FUD** 000 T G2 🖵

AMA: 2018,Jan,8; 2017,Jan,8; 2016,Jan,13; 2015,Jan,16; 2014,Dec,3; 2014,Nov,3

44406 **with endoscopic ultrasound examination, limited to the sigmoid, descending, transverse, or ascending colon and cecum and adjacent structures**

INCLUDES Gastrointestinal endoscopic ultrasound, supervision and interpretation (76975)

EXCLUDES *Colonoscopy through stoma (44388, 44407)*
Procedure performed more than one time per operative session

Code also modifier 52 when colonoscope fails to reach the junction of the small intestine

⚕ 6.73 ☒ 6.73 **FUD** 000 T G2 🖵

AMA: 2018,Jan,8; 2017,Jan,8; 2016,Jan,13; 2015,Jan,16; 2014,Dec,3; 2014,Nov,3

44407 with transendoscopic ultrasound guided intramural or transmural fine needle aspiration/biopsy(s), includes endoscopic ultrasound examination limited to the sigmoid, descending, transverse, or ascending colon and cecum and adjacent structures

> **INCLUDES** Gastrointestinal endoscopic ultrasound, supervision and interpretation (76975)
> Ultrasonic guidance (76942)
>
> **EXCLUDES** *Colonoscopy through stoma (44388, 44406)*
> *Procedure performed more than one time per operative session*
>
> Code also modifier 52 when colonoscope fails to reach the junction of the small intestine

🔲 8.08   🔲 8.08   **FUD** 000   T G2 🔲

AMA: 2018,Jan,8; 2017,Jan,8; 2016,Jan,13; 2015,Jan,16; 2014,Dec,3; 2014,Nov,3

44408 with decompression (for pathologic distention) (eg, volvulus, megacolon), including placement of decompression tube, when performed

> **EXCLUDES** *Colonoscopy through stoma; diagnostic (44388)*
> *Procedure performed more than one time per operative session*

🔲 6.79   🔲 6.79   **FUD** 000   T G2 🔲

AMA: 2018,Jan,8; 2017,Jan,8; 2016,Jan,13; 2015,Jan,16; 2014,Dec,3; 2014,Nov,3

44500 Gastrointestinal Intubation

44500 Introduction of long gastrointestinal tube (eg, Miller-Abbott) (separate procedure)

> **EXCLUDES** *Placement of oro- or naso-gastric tube (43752)*
>
> 🔲 (74340)

🔲 0.56   🔲 0.56   **FUD** 000   🚫 T G2 80 🔲

AMA: 2018,Jan,8; 2017,Jan,8; 2016,Sep,9; 2016,Jan,13; 2015,Jan,16; 2014,Jan,11

44602-44680 Open Repair Procedures of Intestines

44602 Suture of small intestine (enterorrhaphy) for perforated ulcer, diverticulum, wound, injury or rupture; single perforation

🔲 40.9   🔲 40.9   **FUD** 090   C 80 🔲

AMA: 2014,Jan,11

44603 multiple perforations

🔲 47.0   🔲 47.0   **FUD** 090   C 80 🔲

AMA: 2014,Jan,11

44604 Suture of large intestine (colorrhaphy) for perforated ulcer, diverticulum, wound, injury or rupture (single or multiple perforations); without colostomy

🔲 30.7   🔲 30.7   **FUD** 090   C 80 🔲

AMA: 2014,Jan,11

44605 with colostomy

🔲 37.7   🔲 37.7   **FUD** 090   C 80 🔲

AMA: 2014,Jan,11

44615 Intestinal stricturoplasty (enterotomy and enterorrhaphy) with or without dilation, for intestinal obstruction

🔲 31.1   🔲 31.1   **FUD** 090   C 80 🔲

AMA: 2014,Jan,11

44620 Closure of enterostomy, large or small intestine;

> **EXCLUDES** *Laparoscopic method (44227)*

🔲 25.1   🔲 25.1   **FUD** 090   C 80 🔲

AMA: 2014,Jan,11

44625 with resection and anastomosis other than colorectal

> **EXCLUDES** *Laparoscopic method (44227)*

🔲 29.4   🔲 29.4   **FUD** 090   C 80 🔲

AMA: 2014,Jan,11

44626 with resection and colorectal anastomosis (eg, closure of Hartmann type procedure)

> **EXCLUDES** *Laparoscopic method (44227)*

🔲 46.4   🔲 46.4   **FUD** 090   C 80 🔲

AMA: 2014,Jan,11

44640 Closure of intestinal cutaneous fistula

🔲 40.6   🔲 40.6   **FUD** 090   C 80 🔲

AMA: 2014,Jan,11

44650 Closure of enteroenteric or enterocolic fistula

🔲 41.8   🔲 41.8   **FUD** 090   C 80 🔲

AMA: 2014,Jan,11

44660 Closure of enterovesical fistula; without intestinal or bladder resection

> **EXCLUDES** *Closure of fistula:*
> *Gastrocolic (43880)*
> *Rectovesical (45800, 45805)*
> *Renocolic (50525-50526)*

🔲 38.7   🔲 38.7   **FUD** 090   C 80 🔲

AMA: 2014,Jan,11

44661 with intestine and/or bladder resection

> **EXCLUDES** *Closure of fistula:*
> *Gastrocolic (43880)*
> *Rectovesical (45800, 45805)*
> *Renocolic (50525-50526)*

🔲 44.9   🔲 44.9   **FUD** 090   C 80 🔲

AMA: 2014,Jan,11

44680 Intestinal plication (separate procedure)

> **INCLUDES** Noble intestinal plication

🔲 31.0   🔲 31.0   **FUD** 090   C 80 🔲

AMA: 2014,Jan,11

44700-44705 Other Intestinal Procedures

44700 Exclusion of small intestine from pelvis by mesh or other prosthesis, or native tissue (eg, bladder or omentum)

> **EXCLUDES** *Therapeutic radiation clinical treatment (77261-77799 [77295, 77385, 77386, 77387, 77424, 77425])*

🔲 29.1   🔲 29.1   **FUD** 090   C 80 🔲

AMA: 2014,Jan,11

+ 44701 Intraoperative colonic lavage (List separately in addition to code for primary procedure)

> **EXCLUDES** *Appendectomy (44950-44960)*
>
> Code first as appropriate (44140, 44145, 44150, 44604)

🔲 4.95   🔲 4.95   **FUD** ZZZ   N M 80 🔲

AMA: 2014,Jan,11

44705 Preparation of fecal microbiota for instillation, including assessment of donor specimen

> **EXCLUDES** *Fecal instillation by enema or oro-nasogastric tube (44799)*
> *Therapeutic enema (74283)*

🔲 2.16   🔲 3.25   **FUD** XXX   B 🔲

AMA: 2018,Jan,8; 2017,Jan,8; 2016,Jan,13; 2015,Jan,16; 2014,Jan,11

44715-44799 Backbench Transplant Procedures

CMS: 100-04,3,90.6 Intestinal and Multi-Visceral Transplants

44715 Backbench standard preparation of cadaver or living donor intestine allograft prior to transplantation, including mobilization and fashioning of the superior mesenteric artery and vein

> **INCLUDES** Mobilization/fashioning of superior mesenteric vein/artery

🔲 0.00   🔲 0.00   **FUD** XXX   C 80 🔲

AMA: 2014,Jan,11

44720 Backbench reconstruction of cadaver or living donor intestine allograft prior to transplantation; venous anastomosis, each

🔲 7.99   🔲 7.99   **FUD** XXX   C 80 🔲

AMA: 2014,Jan,11

44721 arterial anastomosis, each

🔲 11.1   🔲 11.1   **FUD** XXX   C 80 🔲

AMA: 2018,Jan,8; 2017,Jan,8; 2016,Jan,13; 2015,Jan,16; 2014,Jan,11

26/TC PC/TC Only   A2-Z3 ASC Payment   50 Bilateral   ♂ Male Only   ♀ Female Only   🔲 Facility RVU   🔲 Non-Facility RVU   🔲 CCI   ✖ CLIA
FUD Follow-up Days   **CMS:** IOM   **AMA:** CPT Asst   A-Y OPPSI   80/80 Surg Assist Allowed / w/Doc   🔲 Lab Crosswalk   🔲 Radiology Crosswalk

214   CPT © 2019 American Medical Association. All Rights Reserved.   © 2019 Optum360, LLC

44799 Unlisted procedure, small intestine

> EXCLUDES Unlisted colon procedure (45399)
> Unlisted intestinal procedure performed laparoscopically (44238)
> Unlisted rectal procedure (45499, 45999)

🚑 0.00   ⚕ 0.00   **FUD** YYY

T 🔲

AMA: 2018,Jan,8; 2017,Jan,8; 2016,Jan,13; 2015,Jan,16; 2014,Nov,3; 2014,Jan,11

44800-44899 Meckel's Diverticulum and Mesentery Procedures

44800 Excision of Meckel's diverticulum (diverticulectomy) or omphalomesenteric duct

🚑 22.2   ⚕ 22.2   **FUD** 090

C 80 🔲

AMA: 2014,Jan,11

44820 Excision of lesion of mesentery (separate procedure)

> EXCLUDES Resection of intestine (44120-44128, 44140-44160)

🚑 24.2   ⚕ 24.2   **FUD** 090

C 80 🔲

AMA: 2014,Jan,11

44850 Suture of mesentery (separate procedure)

> EXCLUDES Internal hernia repair/reduction (44050)

🚑 21.7   ⚕ 21.7   **FUD** 090

C 80 🔲

AMA: 2014,Jan,11

44899 Unlisted procedure, Meckel's diverticulum and the mesentery

🚑 0.00   ⚕ 0.00   **FUD** YYY

C 80 🔲

AMA: 2014,Jan,11

44900-44979 Open and Endoscopic Appendix Procedures

44900 Incision and drainage of appendiceal abscess, open

> EXCLUDES Image guided percutaneous catheter drainage (49406)

🚑 22.4   ⚕ 22.4   **FUD** 090

C 80 🔲

AMA: 2014,Jan,11

44950 Appendectomy;

> INCLUDES Battle's operation
> EXCLUDES Procedure performed with other intra-abdominal procedure(s) when appendectomy is incidental

🚑 18.6   ⚕ 18.6   **FUD** 090

J 80 🔲

AMA: 2018,Jan,8; 2017,Jan,8; 2016,Jan,13; 2015,Jan,16; 2014,Jan,11

Cecum

Swollen and inflamed appendix

+ **44955** when done for indicated purpose at time of other major procedure (not as separate procedure) (List separately in addition to code for primary procedure)

Code first primary procedure

🚑 2.45   ⚕ 2.45   **FUD** ZZZ

N 80 🔲

AMA: 2018,Jan,8; 2017,Jan,8; 2016,Jan,13; 2015,Jan,16; 2014,Jan,11

44960 for ruptured appendix with abscess or generalized peritonitis

> INCLUDES Battle's operation

🚑 25.4   ⚕ 25.4   **FUD** 090

C 80 🔲

AMA: 2018,Jan,8; 2017,Jan,8; 2016,Jan,13; 2015,Jan,16; 2014,Jan,11

44970 Laparoscopy, surgical, appendectomy

> INCLUDES Diagnostic laparoscopy

🚑 17.4   ⚕ 17.4   **FUD** 090

J 80 🔲

AMA: 2018,Jan,8; 2017,Jan,8; 2016,Jan,13; 2015,Mar,3; 2015,Jan,16; 2014,Jan,11

44979 Unlisted laparoscopy procedure, appendix

🚑 0.00   ⚕ 0.00   **FUD** YYY

J 80 50 🔲

AMA: 2018,Jan,8; 2017,Jan,8; 2016,Jan,13; 2015,Jan,16; 2014,Jan,11

45000-45190 Open and Transrectal Procedures of Rectum

45000 Transrectal drainage of pelvic abscess

> EXCLUDES Image guided transrectal catheter drainage (49407)

🚑 12.2   ⚕ 12.2   **FUD** 090

T A2 🔲

AMA: 2014,Jan,11

45005 Incision and drainage of submucosal abscess, rectum

🚑 4.66   ⚕ 8.14   **FUD** 010

T A2 🔲

AMA: 2014,Jan,11

45020 Incision and drainage of deep supralevator, pelvirectal, or retrorectal abscess

> EXCLUDES Incision and drainage of perianal, ischiorectal, intramural abscess (46050, 46060)

🚑 16.5   ⚕ 16.5   **FUD** 090

J A2 🔲

AMA: 2014,Jan,11

45100 Biopsy of anorectal wall, anal approach (eg, congenital megacolon)

> EXCLUDES Biopsy performed endoscopically (45305)

🚑 8.64   ⚕ 8.64   **FUD** 090

J A2 🔲

AMA: 2014,Jan,11

45108 Anorectal myomectomy

🚑 10.7   ⚕ 10.7   **FUD** 090

J A2 🔲

AMA: 2014,Jan,11

45110 Proctectomy; complete, combined abdominoperineal, with colostomy

> EXCLUDES Laparoscopic method (45395)

🚑 53.3   ⚕ 53.3   **FUD** 090

C 80 🔲

AMA: 2014,Jan,11

45111 partial resection of rectum, transabdominal approach

> INCLUDES Luschka proctectomy

🚑 31.4   ⚕ 31.4   **FUD** 090

C 80 🔲

AMA: 2014,Jan,11

45112 Proctectomy, combined abdominoperineal, pull-through procedure (eg, colo-anal anastomosis)

> EXCLUDES Proctectomy for colo-anal anastomosis with creation of colonic pouch or reservoir (45119)

🚑 54.0   ⚕ 54.0   **FUD** 090

C 80 🔲

AMA: 2014,Jan,11

45113 Proctectomy, partial, with rectal mucosectomy, ileoanal anastomosis, creation of ileal reservoir (S or J), with or without loop ileostomy

🚑 54.7   ⚕ 54.7   **FUD** 090

C 80 🔲

AMA: 2014,Jan,11

45114 Proctectomy, partial, with anastomosis; abdominal and transsacral approach

🚑 52.8   ⚕ 52.8   **FUD** 090

C 80 🔲

AMA: 2014,Jan,11

45116 transsacral approach only (Kraske type)

🚑 45.1   ⚕ 45.1   **FUD** 090

C 80 🔲

AMA: 2014,Jan,11

45119 Proctectomy, combined abdominoperineal pull-through procedure (eg, colo-anal anastomosis), with creation of colonic reservoir (eg, J-pouch), with diverting enterostomy when performed

> EXCLUDES Laparoscopic method (45397)

🚑 55.9   ⚕ 55.9   **FUD** 090

C 80 🔲

AMA: 2018,Jan,8; 2017,Jan,8; 2016,Jan,13; 2015,Jan,16; 2014,Jan,11

● New Code   ▲ Revised Code   ○ Reinstated   ● New Web Release   ▲ Revised Web Release   + Add-on   Unlisted   Not Covered   # Resequenced
50 Optum Mod 50 Exempt   ⚕ AMA Mod 51 Exempt   51 Optum Mod 51 Exempt   63 Mod 63 Exempt   ⁄ Non-FDA Drug   ★ Telemedicine   M Maternity   A Age Edit

45120 **Proctectomy, complete (for congenital megacolon), abdominal and perineal approach; with pull-through procedure and anastomosis (eg, Swenson, Duhamel, or Soave type operation)**
🔪 46.2 ⚕ 46.2 **FUD** 090 C 80 ▭
AMA: 2014,Jan,11

45121 **with subtotal or total colectomy, with multiple biopsies**
🔪 50.5 ⚕ 50.5 **FUD** 090 C 80 ▭
AMA: 2014,Jan,11

45123 **Proctectomy, partial, without anastomosis, perineal approach**
🔪 32.4 ⚕ 32.4 **FUD** 090 C 80 ▭
AMA: 2014,Jan,11

45126 **Pelvic exenteration for colorectal malignancy, with proctectomy (with or without colostomy), with removal of bladder and ureteral transplantations, and/or hysterectomy, or cervicectomy, with or without removal of tube(s), with or without removal of ovary(s), or any combination thereof**
🔪 80.5 ⚕ 80.5 **FUD** 090 C 80 ▭
AMA: 2014,Jan,11

45130 **Excision of rectal procidentia, with anastomosis; perineal approach**
INCLUDES Altemeier procedure
🔪 31.4 ⚕ 31.4 **FUD** 090 C 80 ▭
AMA: 2014,Jan,11

45135 **abdominal and perineal approach**
INCLUDES Altemeier procedure
🔪 37.6 ⚕ 37.6 **FUD** 090 C 80 ▭
AMA: 2014,Jan,11

45136 **Excision of ileoanal reservoir with ileostomy**
EXCLUDES Enterolysis (44005)
Ileostomy or jejunostomy, non-tube (44310)
🔪 53.3 ⚕ 53.3 **FUD** 090 C 80 ▭
AMA: 2014,Jan,11

45150 **Division of stricture of rectum**
🔪 12.0 ⚕ 12.0 **FUD** 090 T A2 80 ▭
AMA: 2014,Jan,11

45160 **Excision of rectal tumor by proctotomy, transsacral or transcoccygeal approach**
🔪 29.7 ⚕ 29.7 **FUD** 090 J A2 80 ▭
AMA: 2014,Jan,11

45171 **Excision of rectal tumor, transanal approach; not including muscularis propria (ie, partial thickness)**
EXCLUDES Transanal destruction of rectal tumor (45190)
Transanal endoscopic microsurgical tumor excision (TEMS) (0184T)
🔪 17.4 ⚕ 17.4 **FUD** 090 J G2 80 ▭
AMA: 2018,Jan,8; 2017,Jan,8; 2016,Jan,13; 2015,Jan,16; 2014,Jan,11

45172 **including muscularis propria (ie, full thickness)**
EXCLUDES Transanal destruction of rectal tumor (45190)
Transanal endoscopic microsurgical tumor excision (TEMS) (0184T)
🔪 23.5 ⚕ 23.5 **FUD** 090 J G2 80 ▭
AMA: 2018,Feb,11; 2018,Jan,8; 2017,Jan,8; 2016,Jan,13; 2015,Jan,16; 2014,Jan,11

45190 **Destruction of rectal tumor (eg, electrodesiccation, electrosurgery, laser ablation, laser resection, cryosurgery) transanal approach**
EXCLUDES Transanal endoscopic microsurgical tumor excision (TEMS) (0184T)
Transanal excision of rectal tumor (45171-45172)
🔪 20.1 ⚕ 20.1 **FUD** 090 J A2 ▭
AMA: 2018,Jan,8; 2017,Jan,8; 2016,Jan,13; 2015,Jan,16; 2014,Jan,11

45300-45327 Rigid Proctosigmoidoscopy Procedures

INCLUDES Control of bleeding as result of the endoscopic procedure during same operative session
Exam of:
Entire rectum
Portion of sigmoid colon
EXCLUDES Computed tomographic colonography (74261-74263)
Code also examination of colon through stoma:
Colonoscopy via stoma (44388-44408 [44401])
Ileoscopy via stoma (44380-44384 [44381])

45300 **Proctosigmoidoscopy, rigid; diagnostic, with or without collection of specimen(s) by brushing or washing (separate procedure)**
☢ (74360)
🔪 1.41 ⚕ 3.47 **FUD** 000 T P3 ▭
AMA: 2018,Jan,8; 2017,Jan,8; 2016,Jan,13; 2015,Jan,16; 2014,Jan,11

45303 **with dilation (eg, balloon, guide wire, bougie)**
☢ (74360)
🔪 2.47 ⚕ 26.3 **FUD** 000 T P2 ▭
AMA: 2018,Jan,8; 2017,Jan,8; 2016,Jan,13; 2015,Jan,16; 2014,Jan,11

45305 **with biopsy, single or multiple**
🔪 2.11 ⚕ 4.38 **FUD** 000 T A2 ▭
AMA: 2018,Jan,8; 2017,Jan,8; 2016,Jan,13; 2015,Jan,16; 2014,Jan,11

45307 **with removal of foreign body**
🔪 2.79 ⚕ 5.03 **FUD** 000 J A2 80 ▭
AMA: 2018,Jan,8; 2017,Jan,8; 2016,Jan,13; 2015,Jan,16; 2014,Jan,11

45308 **with removal of single tumor, polyp, or other lesion by hot biopsy forceps or bipolar cautery**
🔪 2.43 ⚕ 4.93 **FUD** 000 J A2 ▭
AMA: 2018,Jan,8; 2017,Jan,8; 2016,Jan,13; 2015,Jan,16; 2014,Jan,11

Hot biopsy forceps or cautery

Rectal tumor

Rectal polyp

Sigmoid flexure

Rigid scope

Sigmoid

A rigid proctosigmoid procedure of the rectum and sigmoid is performed

45309 **with removal of single tumor, polyp, or other lesion by snare technique**
🔪 2.59 ⚕ 5.11 **FUD** 000 T A2 ▭
AMA: 2018,Jan,8; 2017,Jan,8; 2016,Jan,13; 2015,Jan,16; 2014,Jan,11

45315 **with removal of multiple tumors, polyps, or other lesions by hot biopsy forceps, bipolar cautery or snare technique**
🔪 3.07 ⚕ 5.61 **FUD** 000 T A2 ▭
AMA: 2018,Jan,8; 2017,Jan,8; 2016,Jan,13; 2015,Jan,16; 2014,Jan,11

26/TC PC/TC Only   A2-Z3 ASC Payment   50 Bilateral   ♂ Male Only   ♀ Female Only   🔪 Facility RVU   ⚕ Non-Facility RVU   ▭ CCI   ☒ CLIA
FUD Follow-up Days   CMS: IOM   AMA: CPT Asst   A-Y OPPSI   80/80 Surg Assist Allowed / w/Doc   ▧ Lab Crosswalk   ☢ Radiology Crosswalk

216   CPT © 2019 American Medical Association. All Rights Reserved.   © 2019 Optum360, LLC

45317   with control of bleeding (eg, injection, bipolar cautery, unipolar cautery, laser, heater probe, stapler, plasma coagulator)

🚑 3.24   ⚖ 5.52   **FUD** 000   T A2 📖

AMA: 2018,Jan,8; 2017,Jan,8; 2016,Jan,13; 2015,Jan,16; 2014,Jan,11

45320   with ablation of tumor(s), polyp(s), or other lesion(s) not amenable to removal by hot biopsy forceps, bipolar cautery or snare technique (eg, laser)

🚑 3.04   ⚖ 5.47   **FUD** 000   J A2 📖

AMA: 2018,Jan,8; 2017,Jan,8; 2016,Jan,13; 2015,Jan,16; 2014,Jan,11

45321   with decompression of volvulus

🚑 2.99   ⚖ 2.99   **FUD** 000   J A2 📖

AMA: 2018,Jan,8; 2017,Jan,8; 2016,Jan,13; 2015,Jan,16; 2014,Jan,11

45327   with transendoscopic stent placement (includes predilation)

🚑 3.38   ⚖ 3.38   **FUD** 000   J A2 📖

AMA: 2018,Jan,8; 2017,Jan,8; 2016,Jan,13; 2015,Jan,16; 2014,Jan,11

45330-45350 [45346] Flexible Sigmoidoscopy Procedures

INCLUDES   Control of bleeding as result of the endoscopic procedure during same operative session
Exam of:
    Entire rectum
    Entire sigmoid colon
    Portion of descending colon (when performed)

EXCLUDES   *Computed tomographic colonography (74261-74263)*
Code also examination of colon through stoma when appropriate:
    Colonoscopy (44388-44408 [44401])
    Ileoscopy (44380-44384 [44381])

45330   Sigmoidoscopy, flexible; diagnostic, including collection of specimen(s) by brushing or washing, when performed (separate procedure)

EXCLUDES   *Sigmoidoscopy, flexible (45331-45350 [45346])*

🚑 1.63   ⚖ 4.88   **FUD** 000   T P3 📖

AMA: 2018,Jan,8; 2017,Jan,8; 2016,Feb,13; 2016,Jan,13; 2015,Sep,12; 2015,Jan,16; 2014,Dec,18; 2014,Dec,3; 2014,Jan,11

45331   with biopsy, single or multiple

EXCLUDES   *Sigmoidoscopy, flexible; with endoscopic mucosal resection on the same lesion (45349)*

🚑 2.08   ⚖ 7.60   **FUD** 000   T A2 📖

AMA: 2018,Jan,8; 2017,Jan,8; 2016,Feb,13; 2016,Jan,13; 2015,Jan,16; 2014,Dec,3; 2014,Dec,18; 2014,Jan,11

45332   with removal of foreign body(s)

EXCLUDES   *Sigmoidoscopy, flexible; diagnostic (45330)*
🔧 (76000)

🚑 3.06   ⚖ 7.36   **FUD** 000   T A2 📖

AMA: 2018,Jan,8; 2017,Jan,8; 2016,Feb,13; 2016,Jan,13; 2015,Jan,16; 2014,Dec,3; 2014,Dec,18; 2014,Jan,11

45333   with removal of tumor(s), polyp(s), or other lesion(s) by hot biopsy forceps

EXCLUDES   *Sigmoidoscopy, flexible; diagnostic (45330)*

🚑 2.73   ⚖ 8.67   **FUD** 000   T A2 📖

AMA: 2018,Jan,8; 2017,Jan,8; 2016,Feb,13; 2016,Jan,13; 2015,Jan,16; 2014,Dec,3; 2014,Dec,18; 2014,Jan,11

45334   with control of bleeding, any method

EXCLUDES   *Sigmoidoscopy, flexible; diagnostic (45330)*
Sigmoidoscopy, flexible; with band ligation on the same lesion (45350)
Sigmoidoscopy, flexible; with directed submucosal injection on the same lesion (45335)

🚑 3.44   ⚖ 15.3   **FUD** 000   T A2 📖

AMA: 2018,Jan,8; 2017,Jan,8; 2016,Feb,13; 2016,Jan,13; 2015,Jan,16; 2014,Dec,3; 2014,Dec,18; 2014,Jan,11

45335   with directed submucosal injection(s), any substance

EXCLUDES   *Sigmoidoscopy, flexible; diagnostic (45330)*
Sigmoidoscopy, flexible; with control of bleeding on the same lesion (45334)
Sigmoidoscopy, flexible; with endoscopic mucosal resection on the same lesion (45349)

🚑 1.93   ⚖ 7.15   **FUD** 000   T A2 📖

AMA: 2018,Jan,8; 2017,Jan,8; 2016,Feb,13; 2016,Jan,13; 2015,Jan,16; 2014,Dec,18; 2014,Dec,3; 2014,Jan,11

45337   with decompression (for pathologic distention) (eg, volvulus, megacolon), including placement of decompression tube, when performed

EXCLUDES   *Procedure performed more than one time per operative session*
Sigmoidoscopy, flexible; diagnostic (45330)

🚑 3.37   ⚖ 3.37   **FUD** 000   T A2 📖

AMA: 2018,Jan,8; 2017,Jan,8; 2016,Feb,13; 2016,Jan,13; 2015,Jan,16; 2014,Dec,3; 2014,Dec,18; 2014,Jan,11

45338   with removal of tumor(s), polyp(s), or other lesion(s) by snare technique

EXCLUDES   *Sigmoidoscopy, flexible; diagnostic (45330)*
Sigmoidoscopy, flexible; with endoscopic mucosal resection on the same lesion (45349)

🚑 3.50   ⚖ 7.89   **FUD** 000   T A2 📖

AMA: 2018,Jan,8; 2017,Jan,8; 2016,Feb,13; 2016,Jan,13; 2015,Jan,16; 2014,Dec,18; 2014,Dec,3; 2014,Jan,11

 # 45346   with ablation of tumor(s), polyp(s), or other lesion(s) (includes pre- and post-dilation and guide wire passage, when performed)

EXCLUDES   *Sigmoidoscopy, flexible; diagnostic (45330)*
Sigmoidoscopy, flexible; with transendoscopic balloon dilation on the same lesion (45340)

🚑 4.70   ⚖ 82.3   **FUD** 000   T 62 📖

AMA: 2018,Jan,8; 2017,Jan,8; 2016,Feb,13; 2016,Jan,13; 2015,Jan,16; 2014,Dec,3

45340   with transendoscopic balloon dilation

EXCLUDES   *Sigmoidoscopy, flexible (45330, [45346], 45347)*
Code also each additional stricture dilated in same session, using modifier 59 with (45340)
🔧 (74360)

🚑 2.26   ⚖ 12.6   **FUD** 000   T A2 📖

AMA: 2018,Jan,8; 2017,Jan,8; 2016,Feb,13; 2016,Jan,13; 2015,Jan,16; 2014,Dec,18; 2014,Dec,3; 2014,Jan,11

45341   with endoscopic ultrasound examination

INCLUDES   Ultrasound, transrectal (76872)

EXCLUDES   *Gastrointestinal endoscopic ultrasound, supervision and interpretation (76975)*
Procedure performed more than one time per operative session
Sigmoidoscopy, flexible (45330, 45342)

🚑 3.61   ⚖ 3.61   **FUD** 000   T A2 📖

AMA: 2018,Jan,8; 2017,Jan,8; 2016,Feb,13; 2016,Jan,13; 2015,Jan,16; 2014,Dec,3; 2014,Dec,18; 2014,Jan,11

45342   with transendoscopic ultrasound guided intramural or transmural fine needle aspiration/biopsy(s)

INCLUDES   Gastrointestinal endoscopic ultrasound, supervision and interpretation (76975)
Ultrasonic guidance (76942)
Ultrasound, transrectal (76872)

EXCLUDES   *Sigmoidoscopy, flexible (45330, 45341)*
Procedure performed more than one time per operative session

🚑 4.96   ⚖ 4.96   **FUD** 000   T A2 📖

AMA: 2018,Jan,8; 2017,Jan,8; 2016,Feb,13; 2016,Jan,13; 2015,Jan,16; 2014,Dec,3; 2014,Dec,18; 2014,Jan,11

45346   Resequenced code. See code following 45338.

45347   **with placement of endoscopic stent (includes pre- and post-dilation and guide wire passage, when performed)**
> EXCLUDES *Sigmoidoscopy, flexible (45330, 45340)*
> ⚡ (74360)
> 🔧 4.52   ⚕ 4.52   **FUD** 000   [J] [J8] 🖳
> **AMA:** 2018,Jan,8; 2017,Jan,8; 2016,Feb,13; 2016,Jan,13; 2015,Jan,16; 2014,Dec,3

45349   **with endoscopic mucosal resection**
> EXCLUDES *Procedure performed on the same lesion with (45331, 45335, 45338, 45350)*
>   *Sigmoidoscopy, flexible; diagnostic (45330)*
> 🔧 5.80   ⚕ 5.80   **FUD** 000   [T] [G2] 🖳
> **AMA:** 2018,Jan,8; 2017,Jan,8; 2016,Jan,13; 2015,Jan,16; 2014,Dec,3

45350   **with band ligation(s) (eg, hemorrhoids)**
> EXCLUDES *Hemorrhoidectomy, internal, by rubber band ligation (46221)*
>   *Procedure performed more than one time per operative session*
>   *Sigmoidoscopy, flexible; diagnostic (45330)*
>   *Sigmoidoscopy, flexible; with control of bleeding, same lesion (45334)*
>   *Sigmoidoscopy, flexible; with endoscopic mucosal resection (45349)*
> 🔧 2.94   ⚕ 16.4   **FUD** 000   [T] [G2] 🖳
> **AMA:** 2018,Jan,8; 2017,Jan,8; 2016,Jan,13; 2015,Jan,16; 2014,Dec,3

45378-45398 [45388, 45390, 45398] Flexible and Rigid Colonoscopy Procedures

> INCLUDES Control of bleeding as result of the endoscopic procedure during same operative session
>   Exam of:
>   Entire colon (rectum to cecum)
>   Terminal ileum (when performed)
> EXCLUDES *Computed tomographic colonography (74261-74263)*
> Code also modifier 53 (physician), or 73, 74 (facility) for an incomplete colonoscopy

45378   **Colonoscopy, flexible; diagnostic, including collection of specimen(s) by brushing or washing, when performed (separate procedure)**
> EXCLUDES *Colonoscopy, flexible (45379-45393 [45388, 45390, 45398])*
>   *Decompression for pathological distention (45393)*
> Code also modifier 53 (physician), or 73, 74 (facility) for an incomplete colonoscopy
> 🔧 5.41   ⚕ 9.18   **FUD** 000   [T] [A2] 🖳
> **AMA:** 2018,Jan,7; 2018,Jan,8; 2017,Sep,14; 2017,Jan,8; 2016,Jan,13; 2015,Sep,12; 2015,Jan,16; 2014,Dec,3; 2014,Nov,3; 2014,Jan,11

45379   **with removal of foreign body(s)**
> EXCLUDES *Colonoscopy, flexible; diagnostic (45378)*
> Code also modifier 52 when colonoscope fails to reach the junction of the small intestine
> ⚡ (76000)
> 🔧 7.00   ⚕ 11.8   **FUD** 000   [T] [A2] 🖳
> **AMA:** 2018,Jan,8; 2017,Jan,8; 2016,Jan,13; 2015,Jan,16; 2014,Dec,3; 2014,Jan,11

45380   **with biopsy, single or multiple**
> EXCLUDES *Colonoscopy, flexible; diagnostic (45378)*
>   *Colonoscopy, flexible; with endoscopic mucosal resection on the same lesion (45390)*
> Code also modifier 52 when colonoscope fails to reach the junction of the small intestine
> 🔧 5.87   ⚕ 11.7   **FUD** 000   [T] [A2] 🖳
> **AMA:** 2018,Jan,8; 2017,Jan,8; 2016,Jan,13; 2015,Jan,16; 2014,Dec,3; 2014,Jan,11

45381   **with directed submucosal injection(s), any substance**
> EXCLUDES *Colonoscopy, flexible; diagnostic (45378)*
>   *Colonoscopy, flexible; with control of bleeding on the same lesion (45382)*
>   *Colonoscopy, flexible; with endoscopic mucosal resection on the same lesion (45390)*
> Code also modifier 52 when colonoscope fails to reach the junction of the small intestine
> 🔧 5.87   ⚕ 11.5   **FUD** 000   [T] [A2] 🖳
> **AMA:** 2018,Jan,8; 2017,Jan,8; 2017,Jan,6; 2016,Jan,13; 2015,Jan,16; 2014,Dec,3; 2014,Jan,11

45382   **with control of bleeding, any method**
> EXCLUDES *Colonoscopy, flexible; diagnostic (45378)*
>   *Colonoscopy, flexible; with band ligation on the same lesion ([45398])*
>   *Colonoscopy, flexible; with directed submucosal injection on the same lesion (45381)*
> Code also modifier 52 when colonoscope fails to reach the junction of the small intestine
> 🔧 7.58   ⚕ 20.2   **FUD** 000   [T] [A2] 🖳
> **AMA:** 2018,Jan,8; 2017,Jan,8; 2016,Jan,13; 2015,Jan,16; 2014,Dec,3; 2014,Jan,11

\#   **45388**   **with ablation of tumor(s), polyp(s), or other lesion(s) (includes pre- and post-dilation and guide wire passage, when performed)**
> EXCLUDES *Colonoscopy, flexible (45378, 45386)*
> Code also modifier 53 (physician), or 73, 74 (facility) for an incomplete colonoscopy
> 🔧 7.92   ⚕ 86.8   **FUD** 000   [T] [G2] 🖳
> **AMA:** 2018,Jan,8; 2017,Jan,8; 2016,Jan,13; 2015,Jan,16; 2014,Dec,3

45384   **with removal of tumor(s), polyp(s), or other lesion(s) by hot biopsy forceps**
> EXCLUDES *Colonoscopy, flexible; diagnostic (45378)*
> Code also modifier 52 when colonoscope fails to reach the junction of the small intestine
> 🔧 6.68   ⚕ 13.1   **FUD** 000   [T] [A2] 🖳
> **AMA:** 2018,Jan,8; 2017,Jan,8; 2016,Jan,13; 2015,Jun,10; 2015,Jan,16; 2014,Dec,3; 2014,Jan,11

45385   **with removal of tumor(s), polyp(s), or other lesion(s) by snare technique**
> EXCLUDES *Colonoscopy, flexible; diagnostic (45378)*
>   *Colonoscopy, flexible; with endoscopic mucosal resection on the same lesion (45390)*
> 🔧 7.45   ⚕ 12.3   **FUD** 000   [T] [A2] 🖳
> **AMA:** 2018,Jan,8; 2017,Jan,8; 2017,Jan,6; 2016,Jan,13; 2015,Jan,16; 2014,Dec,3; 2014,Jan,11

45386   **with transendoscopic balloon dilation**
> EXCLUDES *Colonoscopy, flexible (45378, [45388], 45389)*
> Code also each additional stricture dilated in same operative session, using modifier 59 with (45386)
> ⚡ (74360)
> 🔧 6.20   ⚕ 17.0   **FUD** 000   [T] [A2] 🖳
> **AMA:** 2018,Jan,8; 2017,Jan,8; 2016,Jan,13; 2015,Jan,16; 2014,Dec,3; 2014,Jan,11

45388   Resequenced code. See code following 45382.

45389   **with endoscopic stent placement (includes pre- and post-dilation and guide wire passage, when performed)**
> EXCLUDES *Colonoscopy, flexible (45378, 45386)*
> ⚡ (74360)
> 🔧 8.49   ⚕ 8.49   **FUD** 000   [J] [J8] 🖳
> **AMA:** 2018,Jan,8; 2017,Jan,8; 2016,Jan,13; 2015,Jan,16; 2014,Dec,3

45390   Resequenced code. See code following 45392.

45391 with endoscopic ultrasound examination limited to the rectum, sigmoid, descending, transverse, or ascending colon and cecum, and adjacent structures

INCLUDES Gastrointestinal endoscopic ultrasound, supervision and interpretation (76975)
Ultrasound, transrectal (76872)

EXCLUDES Colonoscopy, flexible (45378, 45392)
Procedure performed more than one time per operative session

🚑 7.55 ⚖ 7.55 **FUD** 000 T A2 🖵

AMA: 2018,Jan,8; 2017,Jan,8; 2016,Jan,13; 2015,Jan,16; 2014,Dec,3; 2014,Jan,11

45392 with transendoscopic ultrasound guided intramural or transmural fine needle aspiration/biopsy(s), includes endoscopic ultrasound examination limited to the rectum, sigmoid, descending, transverse, or ascending colon and cecum, and adjacent structures

INCLUDES Gastrointestinal endoscopic ultrasound, supervision and interpretation (76975)
Ultrasonic guidance (76942)
Ultrasound, transrectal (76872)

EXCLUDES Colonoscopy, flexible (45378, 45391)
Procedure performed more than one time per operative session

🚑 8.91 ⚖ 8.91 **FUD** 000 T A2 🖵

AMA: 2018,Jan,8; 2017,Jan,8; 2016,Jan,13; 2015,Jan,16; 2014,Dec,3; 2014,Jan,11

 # 45390 with endoscopic mucosal resection

EXCLUDES Colonoscopy, flexible; diagnostic (45378)
Colonoscopy, flexible; with band ligation on the same lesion ([45398])
Colonoscopy, flexible; with biopsy on the same lesion (45380-45381)
Colonoscopy, flexible; with removal of tumor(s), polyp(s), or other lesion(s) by snare technique on the same lesion (45385)

🚑 9.74 ⚖ 9.74 **FUD** 000 T G2 🖵

AMA: 2018,Jan,8; 2017,Jan,8; 2017,Jan,6; 2016,Jan,13; 2015,Jan,16; 2014,Dec,3

45393 with decompression (for pathologic distention) (eg, volvulus, megacolon), including placement of decompression tube, when performed

EXCLUDES Colonoscopy, flexible; diagnostic (45378)
Procedure performed more than one time per operative session

🚑 7.41 ⚖ 7.41 **FUD** 000 T G2 🖵

AMA: 2018,Jan,8; 2017,Jan,8; 2016,Jan,13; 2015,Jan,16; 2014,Dec,3

 # 45398 with band ligation(s) (eg, hemorrhoids)

EXCLUDES Bleeding control by band ligation (45382)
Colonoscopy, flexible (45378, 45390)
Hemorrhoidectomy, internal, by rubber band ligation (46221)
Procedure performed more than one time per operative session
Code also modifier 52 when colonoscope fails to reach the junction of the small intestine

🚑 6.88 ⚖ 20.8 **FUD** 000 T G2 🖵

AMA: 2018,Jan,7; 2018,Jan,8; 2017,Sep,14; 2017,Jan,8; 2016,Jan,13; 2015,Jan,16; 2014,Dec,3

45395-45499 Laparoscopic Procedures of Rectum

INCLUDES Diagnostic laparoscopy

45395 Laparoscopy, surgical; proctectomy, complete, combined abdominoperineal, with colostomy

EXCLUDES Open method (45110)

🚑 57.1 ⚖ 57.1 **FUD** 090 C 80 🖵

AMA: 2018,Jan,8; 2017,Jan,8; 2016,Jan,13; 2015,Jan,16; 2014,Jan,11

45397 proctectomy, combined abdominoperineal pull-through procedure (eg, colo-anal anastomosis), with creation of colonic reservoir (eg, J-pouch), with diverting enterostomy, when performed

EXCLUDES Open method (45119)

🚑 62.1 ⚖ 62.1 **FUD** 090 C 80 🖵

AMA: 2018,Jan,8; 2017,Jan,8; 2016,Jan,13; 2015,Jan,16; 2014,Jan,11

45398 Resequenced code. See code following 45393.

45399 Resequenced code. See code before 45990.

45400 Laparoscopy, surgical; proctopexy (for prolapse)

EXCLUDES Open method (45540-45541)

🚑 32.9 ⚖ 32.9 **FUD** 090 C 80 🖵

AMA: 2018,Jan,8; 2017,Jan,8; 2016,Jan,13; 2015,Jan,16; 2014,Jan,11

45402 proctopexy (for prolapse), with sigmoid resection

EXCLUDES Open method (45550)

🚑 43.8 ⚖ 43.8 **FUD** 090 C 80 🖵

AMA: 2018,Jan,8; 2017,Jan,8; 2016,Jan,13; 2015,Jan,16; 2014,Jan,11

45499 Unlisted laparoscopy procedure, rectum

EXCLUDES Unlisted rectal procedure performed via open technique (45999)

🚑 0.00 ⚖ 0.00 **FUD** YYY J 80 🖵

AMA: 2014,Jan,11

45500-45825 Open Repairs of Rectum

45500 Proctoplasty; for stenosis

🚑 16.1 ⚖ 16.1 **FUD** 090 J A2 80 🖵

AMA: 2014,Jan,11

45505 for prolapse of mucous membrane

🚑 17.1 ⚖ 17.1 **FUD** 090 J A2

AMA: 2018,Jan,8; 2017,Jan,8; 2016,Jan,13; 2015,Mar,9; 2015,Jan,16; 2014,Jan,11

45520 Perirectal injection of sclerosing solution for prolapse

🚑 1.16 ⚖ 4.41 **FUD** 000 01 NI

AMA: 2018,Jan,8; 2017,Jan,8; 2016,Jan,13; 2015,Jan,16; 2014,Jan,11

45540 Proctopexy (eg, for prolapse); abdominal approach

EXCLUDES Laparoscopic method (45400)

🚑 30.6 ⚖ 30.6 **FUD** 090 C 80 🖵

AMA: 2014,Jan,11

45541 perineal approach

🚑 27.3 ⚖ 27.3 **FUD** 090 J G2 80 🖵

AMA: 2014,Jan,11

45550 with sigmoid resection, abdominal approach

INCLUDES Frickman proctopexy

EXCLUDES Laparoscopic method (45402)

🚑 42.4 ⚖ 42.4 **FUD** 090 C 80 🖵

AMA: 2014,Jan,11

45560 Repair of rectocele (separate procedure)

EXCLUDES Posterior colporrhaphy with rectocele repair (57250)

🔧 19.7   ✂ 19.7   **FUD** 090   J A2 80 ▣

AMA: 2014,Jan,11

The posterior wall of the vagina is opened directly over the rectocele; the walls of both structures are repaired; a rectocele is a herniated protrusion of part of the rectum into the vagina

45562 Exploration, repair, and presacral drainage for rectal injury;

🔧 32.4   ✂ 32.4   **FUD** 090   C 80 ▣

AMA: 2014,Jan,11

45563 with colostomy

INCLUDES Maydl colostomy

🔧 47.9   ✂ 47.9   **FUD** 090   C 80 ▣

AMA: 2014,Jan,11

45800 Closure of rectovesical fistula;

🔧 36.4   ✂ 36.4   **FUD** 090   C 80 ▣

AMA: 2014,Jan,11

45805 with colostomy

🔧 42.5   ✂ 42.5   **FUD** 090   C 80 ▣

AMA: 2014,Jan,11

45820 Closure of rectourethral fistula;

EXCLUDES Closure of fistula, rectovaginal (57300-57308)

🔧 36.7   ✂ 36.7   **FUD** 090   C 80 ▣

AMA: 2014,Jan,11

45825 with colostomy

EXCLUDES Closure of fistula, rectovaginal (57300-57308)

🔧 44.4   ✂ 44.4   **FUD** 090   C 80 ▣

AMA: 2014,Jan,11

45900-45999 [45399] Closed Procedures of Rectum With Anesthesia

45900 Reduction of procidentia (separate procedure) under anesthesia

🔧 5.83   ✂ 5.83   **FUD** 010   T A2 80 ▣

AMA: 2014,Jan,11

45905 Dilation of anal sphincter (separate procedure) under anesthesia other than local

🔧 4.87   ✂ 4.87   **FUD** 010   T A2 ▣

AMA: 2014,Jan,11

45910 Dilation of rectal stricture (separate procedure) under anesthesia other than local

🔧 5.53   ✂ 5.53   **FUD** 010   T A2 ▣

AMA: 2014,Jan,11

45915 Removal of fecal impaction or foreign body (separate procedure) under anesthesia

🔧 6.59   ✂ 9.70   **FUD** 010   T A2 ▣

AMA: 2018,Jan,8; 2017,Jan,8; 2016,Jan,13; 2015,Jan,16; 2014,Jan,11

\# **45399** Unlisted procedure, colon

🔧 0.00   ✂ 0.00   **FUD** YYY   T ▣

AMA: 2018,Jan,8; 2017,Jan,8; 2016,Jan,13; 2015,Jan,16; 2014,Dec,3; 2014,Nov,3

45990 Anorectal exam, surgical, requiring anesthesia (general, spinal, or epidural), diagnostic

INCLUDES Diagnostic:
    Anoscopy
    Proctoscopy, rigid
   Exam:
    Pelvic (when performed)
    Perineal, external
    Rectal, digital

EXCLUDES Anogenital examination (99170)
   Anoscopy; diagnostic (46600)
   Pelvic examination under anesthesia (57410)
   Proctosigmoidoscopy, rigid (45300-45327)

🔧 3.09   ✂ 3.09   **FUD** 000   J A2 80 ▣

AMA: 2018,Jan,8; 2017,Jan,8; 2016,Jan,13; 2015,Jan,16; 2014,Jan,11

45999 Unlisted procedure, rectum

EXCLUDES Unlisted rectal procedure performed laparoscopically (45499)

🔧 0.00   ✂ 0.00   **FUD** YYY   T 80 ▣

AMA: 2018,Jan,8; 2017,Jan,8; 2016,Jan,13; 2015,Jan,16; 2014,Jan,11

46020-46083 Surgical Incision of Anus

EXCLUDES Cryosurgical destruction of hemorrhoid(s) (46999)
Fistulotomy, subcutaneous (46270)
Hemorrhoidopexy ([46947])
Injection of hemorrhoid(s) (46500)
Thermal energy destruction of internal hemorrhoid(s) (46930)

46020 Placement of seton

EXCLUDES Anoscopy; diagnostic (46600)
   Incision and drainage of ischiorectal or intramural abscess (46060)
   Surgical anal fistula treatment (46280)

🔧 6.79   ✂ 8.00   **FUD** 010   J A2 ▣

AMA: 2014,Jan,11

46030 Removal of anal seton, other marker

🔧 2.59   ✂ 4.04   **FUD** 010   T A2 80 ▣

AMA: 2014,Jan,11

46040 Incision and drainage of ischiorectal and/or perirectal abscess (separate procedure)

🔧 12.0   ✂ 15.5   **FUD** 090   T A2 ▣

AMA: 2014,Jan,11

46045 Incision and drainage of intramural, intramuscular, or submucosal abscess, transanal, under anesthesia

🔧 12.5   ✂ 12.5   **FUD** 090   J A2 ▣

AMA: 2014,Jan,11

46050 Incision and drainage, perianal abscess, superficial

EXCLUDES Incision and drainage abscess:
   Ischiorectal/intramural (46060)
   Supralevator/pelvirectal/retrorectal (45020)

🔧 2.82   ✂ 5.98   **FUD** 010   T A2 ▣

AMA: 2014,Jan,11

46060 Incision and drainage of ischiorectal or intramural abscess, with fistulectomy or fistulotomy, submuscular, with or without placement of seton

EXCLUDES Incision and drainage abscess:
   Supralevator/pelvirectal/retrorectal (45020)
   Placement of seton (46020)

🔧 13.8   ✂ 13.8   **FUD** 090   J A2 ▣

AMA: 2014,Jan,11

46070 Incision, anal septum (infant)   A

EXCLUDES Anoplasty (46700-46705)

🔧 7.52   ✂ 7.52   **FUD** 090   63 J G2 80 ▣

AMA: 2014,Jan,11

46080 Sphincterotomy, anal, division of sphincter (separate procedure)

🔧 4.59   ✂ 7.41   **FUD** 010   J A2 ▣

AMA: 2014,Jan,11

26/TC PC/TC Only	A2-Z3 ASC Payment	50 Bilateral	♂ Male Only	♀ Female Only	🔧 Facility RVU	✂ Non-Facility RVU	▣ CCI	☒ CLIA
FUD Follow-up Days	**CMS:** IOM	**AMA:** CPT Asst	A-Y OPPSI	80/80 Surg Assist Allowed / w/Doc		◨ Lab Crosswalk	◨ Radiology Crosswalk	

220   CPT © 2019 American Medical Association. All Rights Reserved.   © 2019 Optum360, LLC

46083 **Incision of thrombosed hemorrhoid, external**
3.08 5.24 **FUD** 010 T P2
AMA: 2018,Jan,8; 2017,Jan,8; 2016,Jan,13; 2015,Jan,16; 2014,Jan,11

46200-46262 [46220, 46320, 46945, 46946, 46948] Anal Resection and Hemorrhoidectomies

EXCLUDES *Cryosurgical destruction of hemorrhoid(s) (46999)*
Hemorrhoidopexy ([46947])
Injection of hemorrhoid(s) (46500)
Thermal energy destruction of internal hemorrhoid(s) (46930)

46200 **Fissurectomy, including sphincterotomy, when performed**
9.45 13.0 **FUD** 090 J A2
AMA: 2014,Jan,11

46220 Resequenced code. See code before 46230.

46221 **Hemorrhoidectomy, internal, by rubber band ligation(s)**
EXCLUDES *Colonoscopy or sigmoidoscopy, flexible; with band ligation (45350, [45398])*
Transanal hemorrhoidal dearterialization, two or more columns/groups ([46948])
5.51 7.77 **FUD** 010 T P3
AMA: 2018,Jan,7; 2018,Jan,8; 2017,Sep,14; 2017,Jan,8; 2016,Jan,13; 2015,Apr,10; 2015,Jan,16; 2014,Dec,3; 2014,Jan,11

▲ # **46945** **Hemorrhoidectomy, internal, by ligation other than rubber band; single hemorrhoid column/group, without imaging guidance**
EXCLUDES *Transanal hemorrhoidal dearterialization, two or more columns/groups ([46948])*
Ultrasonic guidance (76942)
Ultrasonic guidance, intraoperative (76998)
Ultrasound, transrectal (76872)
6.54 9.08 **FUD** 090 J P3
AMA: 2018,Jan,8; 2017,Jan,8; 2016,Jan,13; 2015,Apr,10; 2014,Jan,11

▲ # **46946** **2 or more hemorrhoid columns/groups, without imaging guidance**
EXCLUDES *Transanal hemorrhoidal dearterialization, two or more columns/groups ([46948])*
Ultrasonic guidance (76942)
Ultrasonic guidance, intraoperative (76998)
Ultrasound, transrectal (76872)
6.50 9.17 **FUD** 090 J A2
AMA: 2018,Jan,8; 2017,Jan,8; 2016,Jan,13; 2015,Apr,10; 2014,Jan,11

● # **46948** **Hemorrhoidectomy, internal, by transanal hemorrhoidal dearterialization, 2 or more hemorrhoid columns/groups, including ultrasound guidance, with mucopexy, when performed**
0.00 0.00 **FUD** 000
EXCLUDES *Transanal hemorrhoidal dearterialization, single column/group (46999)*
Ultrasonic guidance (76942)
Ultrasonic guidance, intraoperative (76998)
Ultrasound, transrectal (76872)

46220 **Excision of single external papilla or tag, anus**
3.44 6.22 **FUD** 010 T A2
AMA: 2014,Jan,11

46230 **Excision of multiple external papillae or tags, anus**
4.99 8.11 **FUD** 010 J A2
AMA: 2014,Jan,11

46320 **Excision of thrombosed hemorrhoid, external**
3.22 5.43 **FUD** 010 T P3
AMA: 2014,Jan,11

46250 **Hemorrhoidectomy, external, 2 or more columns/groups**
EXCLUDES *Hemorrhoidectomy, external, single column/group (46999)*
Transanal hemorrhoidal dearterialization, two or more columns/groups ([46948])
9.13 13.4 **FUD** 090 J A2
AMA: 2014,Jan,11

46255 **Hemorrhoidectomy, internal and external, single column/group;**
EXCLUDES *Transanal hemorrhoidal dearterialization, two or more columns/groups ([46948])*
10.2 14.7 **FUD** 090 J A2
AMA: 2018,Jan,8; 2017,Jan,8; 2016,Jan,13; 2015,Jan,16; 2014,Oct,14; 2014,Jan,11

46257 **with fissurectomy**
EXCLUDES *Transanal hemorrhoidal dearterialization, two or more columns/groups ([46948])*
12.2 12.2 **FUD** 090 J A2
AMA: 2014,Jan,11

46258 **with fistulectomy, including fissurectomy, when performed**
EXCLUDES *Transanal hemorrhoidal dearterialization, two or more columns/groups ([46948])*
13.5 13.5 **FUD** 090 J A2 80
AMA: 2014,Jan,11

46260 **Hemorrhoidectomy, internal and external, 2 or more columns/groups;**
INCLUDES Whitehead hemorrhoidectomy
EXCLUDES *Transanal hemorrhoidal dearterialization, two or more columns/groups ([46948])*
13.7 13.7 **FUD** 090 J A2
AMA: 2014,Jan,11

46261 **with fissurectomy**
EXCLUDES *Transanal hemorrhoidal dearterialization, two or more columns/groups ([46948])*
15.0 15.0 **FUD** 090 J A2
AMA: 2014,Jan,11

46262 **with fistulectomy, including fissurectomy, when performed**
EXCLUDES *Transanal hemorrhoidal dearterialization, two or more columns/groups ([46948])*
16.0 16.0 **FUD** 090 J A2
AMA: 2018,Jan,8; 2017,Jan,8; 2016,Jan,13; 2015,Jan,16; 2014,Jan,11

46270-46320 Resection of Anal Fistula

46270 **Surgical treatment of anal fistula (fistulectomy/fistulotomy); subcutaneous**
11.3 14.8 **FUD** 090 J A2
AMA: 2014,Jan,11

46275 **intersphincteric**
11.9 15.6 **FUD** 090 J A2
AMA: 2014,Jan,11

46280 **transsphincteric, suprasphincteric, extrasphincteric or multiple, including placement of seton, when performed**
EXCLUDES *Placement of seton (46020)*
13.6 13.6 **FUD** 090 J A2
AMA: 2014,Jan,11

46285 **second stage**
11.9 15.5 **FUD** 090 J A2
AMA: 2014,Jan,11

46288 **Closure of anal fistula with rectal advancement flap**
15.8 15.8 **FUD** 090 J A2
AMA: 2014,Jan,11

46320 Resequenced code. See code following 46230.

● New Code ▲ Revised Code ○ Reinstated ● New Web Release ▲ Revised Web Release + Add-on Unlisted Not Covered # Resequenced
50 Optum Mod 50 Exempt Ⓢ AMA Mod 51 Exempt 51 Optum Mod 51 Exempt 63 Mod 63 Exempt ✗ Non-FDA Drug ★ Telemedicine Ⓜ Maternity Ⓐ Age Edit

CPT © 2019 American Medical Association. All Rights Reserved.

Digestive System

46500 — 46712

46500 Other Hemorrhoid Procedures

EXCLUDES Anoscopic injection of bulking agent, submucosal, for fecal incontinence (46999)

46500   Injection of sclerosing solution, hemorrhoids
🔹 5.12   ⚖ 8.23   **FUD** 010   T P3 🔲
AMA: 2018,Jan,8; 2017,Jan,8; 2016,Jan,13; 2015,Jan,16; 2014,Jan,11

 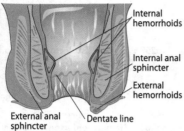

Internal hemorrhoids

Internal anal sphincter

External hemorrhoids

External anal sphincter — Dentate line

A sclerosing agent is injected into the tissues underlying hemorrhoids

46505 Chemodenervation Anal Sphincter

EXCLUDES Chemodenervation of:
Extremity muscles (64642-64645)
Muscles/facial nerve (64612)
Neck muscles (64616)
Other peripheral nerve/branch (64640)
Pudendal nerve (64630)
Trunk muscles (64646-64647)
Code also drug(s)/substance(s) given

46505   Chemodenervation of internal anal sphincter
🔹 6.93   ⚖ 8.35   **FUD** 010   T G2 50 🔲
AMA: 2019,Apr,9; 2018,Jan,8; 2017,Jan,8; 2016,Jan,13; 2015,Jan,16; 2014,Jan,11

46600-46615 Anoscopic Procedures

EXCLUDES Delivery of thermal energy via anoscope to the muscle of the anal canal (46999)
Injection of bulking agent, submucosal, for fecal incontinence (46999)

46600   Anoscopy; diagnostic, including collection of specimen(s) by brushing or washing, when performed (separate procedure)
EXCLUDES Excision of rectal tumor, transanal endoscopic microsurgical approach (ie, TEMS) (0184T)
High-resolution anoscopy (HRA), diagnostic (46601)
Surgical incision of anus (46020-46761 [46220, 46320, 46320, 46945, 46946, 46947, 46948])
🔹 1.18   ⚖ 2.72   **FUD** 000   01 N1 🔲
AMA: 2018,Jan,7; 2018,Jan,8; 2017,Jan,8; 2016,Jan,13; 2015,Jan,16; 2014,Jan,11

46601   diagnostic, with high-resolution magnification (HRA) (eg, colposcope, operating microscope) and chemical agent enhancement, including collection of specimen(s) by brushing or washing, when performed
INCLUDES   . Operating microscope (69990)
🔹 2.70   ⚖ 3.97   **FUD** 000   01 N1 🔲
AMA: 2018,Oct,11; 2016,Feb,12

46604   with dilation (eg, balloon, guide wire, bougie)
🔹 1.90   ⚖ 18.3   **FUD** 000   T P2 🔲
AMA: 2018,Jan,8; 2017,Jan,8; 2016,Jan,13; 2015,Jan,16; 2014,Jan,11

46606   with biopsy, single or multiple
EXCLUDES High resolution anoscopy (HRA) with biopsy (46607)
🔹 2.17   ⚖ 6.89   **FUD** 000   T P3 🔲
AMA: 2019,Sep,10; 2018,Jan,8; 2017,Jan,8; 2016,Jan,13; 2015,Jan,16; 2014,Jan,11

46607   with high-resolution magnification (HRA) (eg, colposcope, operating microscope) and chemical agent enhancement, with biopsy, single or multiple
INCLUDES   Operating microscope (69990)
🔹 3.64   ⚖ 5.59   **FUD** 000   T G2 🔲
AMA: 2018,Oct,11; 2016,Feb,12

46608   with removal of foreign body
🔹 2.43   ⚖ 7.26   **FUD** 000   T A2 🔲
AMA: 2018,Jan,8; 2017,Jan,8; 2016,Jan,13; 2015,Jan,16; 2014,Jan,11

46610   with removal of single tumor, polyp, or other lesion by hot biopsy forceps or bipolar cautery
🔹 2.32   ⚖ 6.89   **FUD** 000   J A2 🔲
AMA: 2018,Jan,8; 2017,Jan,8; 2016,Jan,13; 2015,Jan,16; 2014,Jan,11

46611   with removal of single tumor, polyp, or other lesion by snare technique
🔹 2.33   ⚖ 5.43   **FUD** 000   T A2 🔲
AMA: 2018,Jan,8; 2017,Jan,8; 2016,Jan,13; 2015,Jan,16; 2014,Jan,11

46612   with removal of multiple tumors, polyps, or other lesions by hot biopsy forceps, bipolar cautery or snare technique
🔹 2.75   ⚖ 8.39   **FUD** 000   J A2 🔲
AMA: 2018,Jan,8; 2017,Jan,8; 2016,Jan,13; 2015,Jan,16; 2014,Jan,11

46614   with control of bleeding (eg, injection, bipolar cautery, unipolar cautery, laser, heater probe, stapler, plasma coagulator)
🔹 1.87   ⚖ 3.97   **FUD** 000   T P3 🔲
AMA: 2018,Jan,8; 2017,Jan,8; 2016,Jan,13; 2015,Jan,16; 2014,Jan,11

46615   with ablation of tumor(s), polyp(s), or other lesion(s) not amenable to removal by hot biopsy forceps, bipolar cautery or snare technique
🔹 2.64   ⚖ 4.34   **FUD** 000   J A2 🔲
AMA: 2018,Jan,8; 2017,Jan,8; 2016,Jan,13; 2015,Jan,16; 2014,Jan,11

46700-46947 [46947] Anal Repairs and Stapled Hemorrhoidopexy

46700   Anoplasty, plastic operation for stricture; adult
🔹 18.9   ⚖ 18.9   **FUD** 090   J A2 🔲
AMA: 2014,Jan,11

46705   infant   A
EXCLUDES Anal septum incision (46070)
🔹 16.1   ⚖ 16.1   **FUD** 090   63 C 80 🔲
AMA: 2014,Jan,11

46706   Repair of anal fistula with fibrin glue
🔹 5.10   ⚖ 5.10   **FUD** 010   J A2 🔲
AMA: 2014,Jan,11

46707   Repair of anorectal fistula with plug (eg, porcine small intestine submucosa [SIS])
🔹 14.2   ⚖ 14.2   **FUD** 090   J G2 80 🔲
AMA: 2018,Jan,8; 2017,Jan,8; 2016,Jan,13; 2015,Jan,16; 2014,Jan,11

46710   Repair of ileoanal pouch fistula/sinus (eg, perineal or vaginal), pouch advancement; transperineal approach
🔹 32.1   ⚖ 32.1   **FUD** 090   C 80 🔲
AMA: 2018,Jan,8; 2017,Jan,8; 2016,Jan,13; 2015,Jan,16; 2014,Jan,11

46712   combined transperineal and transabdominal approach
🔹 64.7   ⚖ 64.7   **FUD** 090   C 80 🔲
AMA: 2018,Jan,8; 2017,Jan,8; 2016,Jan,13; 2015,Jan,16; 2014,Jan,11

46715 Repair of low imperforate anus; with anoperineal fistula (cut-back procedure)
　　　🚑 15.7　✂ 15.7　**FUD** 090　　　63 C 80 ▭
　　　AMA: 2014,Jan,11

46716 with transposition of anoperineal or anovestibular fistula
　　　🚑 35.1　✂ 35.1　**FUD** 090　　　63 C 80 ▭
　　　AMA: 2014,Jan,11

46730 Repair of high imperforate anus without fistula; perineal or sacroperineal approach
　　　🚑 57.0　✂ 57.0　**FUD** 090　　　63 C 80 ▭
　　　AMA: 2014,Jan,11

46735 combined transabdominal and sacroperineal approaches
　　　🚑 65.8　✂ 65.8　**FUD** 090　　　63 C 80 ▭
　　　AMA: 2014,Jan,11

46740 Repair of high imperforate anus with rectourethral or rectovaginal fistula; perineal or sacroperineal approach
　　　🚑 62.3　✂ 62.3　**FUD** 090　　　63 C 80 ▭
　　　AMA: 2014,Jan,11

46742 combined transabdominal and sacroperineal approaches
　　　🚑 72.2　✂ 72.2　**FUD** 090　　　63 C 80 ▭
　　　AMA: 2014,Jan,11

46744 Repair of cloacal anomaly by anorectovaginoplasty and urethroplasty, sacroperineal approach　　　♀
　　　🚑 102.　✂ 102.　**FUD** 090　　　63 C 80 ▭
　　　AMA: 2014,Jan,11

46746 Repair of cloacal anomaly by anorectovaginoplasty and urethroplasty, combined abdominal and sacroperineal approach;　　　♀
　　　🚑 113.　✂ 113.　**FUD** 090　　　C 80 ▭
　　　AMA: 2014,Jan,11

46748 with vaginal lengthening by intestinal graft or pedicle flaps　　　♀
　　　🚑 122.　✂ 122.　**FUD** 090　　　C 80 ▭
　　　AMA: 2014,Jan,11

46750 Sphincteroplasty, anal, for incontinence or prolapse; adult
　　　🚑 21.6　✂ 21.6　**FUD** 090　　　J A2 80 ▭
　　　AMA: 2014,Jan,11

46751 child　　　A
　　　🚑 19.0　✂ 19.0　**FUD** 090　　　C 80 ▭
　　　AMA: 2014,Jan,11

46753 Graft (Thiersch operation) for rectal incontinence and/or prolapse
　　　🚑 17.7　✂ 17.7　**FUD** 090　　　J A2 ▭
　　　AMA: 2014,Jan,11

46754 Removal of Thiersch wire or suture, anal canal
　　　🚑 6.75　✂ 9.03　**FUD** 010　　　J A2 80 ▭
　　　AMA: 2014,Jan,11

46760 Sphincteroplasty, anal, for incontinence, adult; muscle transplant
　　　🚑 31.7　✂ 31.7　**FUD** 090　　　J A2 80 ▭
　　　AMA: 2014,Jan,11

46761 levator muscle imbrication (Park posterior anal repair)
　　　🚑 26.4　✂ 26.4　**FUD** 090　　　J A2 80 ▭
　　　AMA: 2014,Jan,11

46947 Hemorrhoidopexy (eg, for prolapsing internal hemorrhoids) by stapling
　　　🚑 11.0　✂ 11.0　**FUD** 090　　　J A2 ▭
　　　AMA: 2018,Jan,8; 2017,Jan,8; 2016,Jan,13; 2015,Jan,16; 2014,Jan,11

46900-46999 Destruction Procedures: Anus

46900 Destruction of lesion(s), anus (eg, condyloma, papilloma, molluscum contagiosum, herpetic vesicle), simple; chemical
　　　🚑 3.92　✂ 6.76　**FUD** 010　　　T P2 ▭
　　　AMA: 2014,Jan,11

46910 electrodesiccation
　　　🚑 3.86　✂ 7.39　**FUD** 010　　　T P3 ▭
　　　AMA: 2014,Jan,11

46916 cryosurgery
　　　🚑 4.14　✂ 6.83　**FUD** 010　　　T P2 ▭
　　　AMA: 2014,Jan,11

46917 laser surgery
　　　🚑 3.73　✂ 12.2　**FUD** 010　　　J A2 ▭
　　　AMA: 2014,Jan,11

46922 surgical excision
　　　🚑 3.92　✂ 8.00　**FUD** 010　　　J A2 ▭
　　　AMA: 2014,Jan,11

46924 Destruction of lesion(s), anus (eg, condyloma, papilloma, molluscum contagiosum, herpetic vesicle), extensive (eg, laser surgery, electrosurgery, cryosurgery, chemosurgery)
　　　🚑 5.21　✂ 15.1　**FUD** 010　　　J A2 ▭
　　　AMA: 2014,Jan,11

46930 Destruction of internal hemorrhoid(s) by thermal energy (eg, infrared coagulation, cautery, radiofrequency)
　　　EXCLUDES　Other hemorrhoid procedures:
　　　　　　Cryosurgery destruction (46999)
　　　　　　Excision ([46320], 46250-46262)
　　　　　　Hemorrhoidopexy ([46947])
　　　　　　Incision (46083)
　　　　　　Injection sclerosing solution (46500)
　　　　　　Ligation (46221, [46945, 46946])
　　　🚑 4.28　✂ 6.02　**FUD** 090　　　T P3 80 ▭
　　　AMA: 2018,Jan,8; 2017,Jan,8; 2016,Jul,8; 2016,Jan,13; 2015,Apr,10; 2014,Jan,11

46940 Curettage or cautery of anal fissure, including dilation of anal sphincter (separate procedure); initial
　　　🚑 4.20　✂ 6.79　**FUD** 010　　　J P3 ▭
　　　AMA: 2014,Jan,11

46942 subsequent
　　　🚑 3.78　✂ 6.48　**FUD** 010　　　T P3 80 ▭
　　　AMA: 2014,Jan,11

46945 Resequenced code. See code following 46221.

46946 Resequenced code. See code following resequenced code 46945.

46947 Resequenced code. See code following 46761.

46948 Resequenced code. See code before resequenced code 46220.

46999 Unlisted procedure, anus
　　　🚑 0.00　✂ 0.00　**FUD** YYY　　　T 80 ▭
　　　AMA: 2018,Oct,11; 2018,Jan,8; 2017,Jan,8; 2016,Jan,13; 2015,Apr,10; 2015,Jan,16; 2014,Jan,11

47000-47001 Needle Biopsy of Liver
　EXCLUDES　Fine needle aspiration (10021, [10004, 10005, 10006, 10007, 10008, 10009, 10010, 10011, 10012])

47000 Biopsy of liver, needle; percutaneous
　　　🔬 (76942, 77002, 77012, 77021)
　　　🔬 (88172-88173)
　　　🚑 2.58　✂ 8.72　**FUD** 000　　　J A2 ▭
　　　AMA: 2019,Apr,4; 2018,Jan,8; 2017,Jan,8; 2016,Jan,13; 2015,Jan,16; 2014,Jan,11

Digestive System

+ 47001 **when done for indicated purpose at time of other major procedure (List separately in addition to code for primary procedure)**

Code first primary procedure
🔲 (76942, 77002)
🔳 (88172-88173)
🚒 3.02   ⚔ 3.02   **FUD** ZZZ   N NI ▭

AMA: 2018,Jan,8; 2017,Jan,8; 2016,Jan,13; 2015,Jan,16; 2014,Jan,11

47010-47130 Open Incisional and Resection Procedures of Liver

47010 **Hepatotomy, for open drainage of abscess or cyst, 1 or 2 stages**

EXCLUDES *Image guided percutaneous catheter drainage (49505)*
🚒 35.1   ⚔ 35.1   **FUD** 090   C 80 ▭

AMA: 2014,Jan,11

47015 **Laparotomy, with aspiration and/or injection of hepatic parasitic (eg, amoebic or echinococcal) cyst(s) or abscess(es)**
🚒 33.7   ⚔ 33.7   **FUD** 090   C 80 ▭

AMA: 2014,Jan,11

47100 **Biopsy of liver, wedge**
🚒 24.5   ⚔ 24.5   **FUD** 090   C 80 ▭

AMA: 2014,Jan,11

47120 **Hepatectomy, resection of liver; partial lobectomy**
🚒 67.7   ⚔ 67.7   **FUD** 090   C 80 ▭

AMA: 2018,Jan,8; 2017,Jan,8; 2016,Oct,11; 2016,Jan,13; 2015,Jan,16; 2014,Sep,13; 2014,Jan,11

47122 **trisegmentectomy**
🚒 99.6   ⚔ 99.6   **FUD** 090   C 80 ▭

AMA: 2014,Jan,11

47125 **total left lobectomy**
🚒 89.5   ⚔ 89.5   **FUD** 090   C 80 ▭

AMA: 2014,Jan,11

47130 **total right lobectomy**
🚒 96.2   ⚔ 96.2   **FUD** 090   C 80 ▭

AMA: 2014,Jan,11

47133-47147 Liver Transplant Procedures

CMS: 100-03,260.1 Adult Liver Transplantation; 100-03,260.2 Pediatric Liver Transplantation; 100-04,3,90.4 Liver Transplants; 100-04,3,90.4.1 Standard Liver Acquisition Charge; 100-04,3,90.4.2 Billing for Liver Transplant and Acquisition Services; 100-04,3,90.6 Intestinal and Multi-Visceral Transplants

47133 **Donor hepatectomy (including cold preservation), from cadaver donor**

INCLUDES Graft:
Cold preservation
Harvest
🚒 0.00   ⚔ 0.00   **FUD** XXX   C ▭

AMA: 2014,Jan,11

47135 **Liver allotransplantation, orthotopic, partial or whole, from cadaver or living donor, any age**

INCLUDES Partial/whole recipient hepatectomy
Partial/whole transplant of allograft
Recipient care
🚒 156.   ⚔ 156.   **FUD** 090   C 80 ▭

AMA: 2018,Jan,8; 2017,Jan,8; 2016,Jan,13; 2015,Jan,16; 2014,Jan,11

47140 **Donor hepatectomy (including cold preservation), from living donor; left lateral segment only (segments II and III)**

INCLUDES Donor care
Graft:
Cold preservation
Harvest
🚒 103.   ⚔ 103.   **FUD** 090   C 80 ▭

AMA: 2018,Jan,8; 2017,Jan,8; 2016,Jan,13; 2015,Jan,16; 2014,Jan,11

47141 **total left lobectomy (segments II, III and IV)**

INCLUDES Donor care
Graft:
Cold preservation
Harvest
🚒 124.   ⚔ 124.   **FUD** 090   C 80 ▭

AMA: 2014,Jan,11

47142 **total right lobectomy (segments V, VI, VII and VIII)**

INCLUDES Donor care
Graft:
Cold preservation
Harvest
🚒 136.   ⚔ 136.   **FUD** 090   C 80 ▭

AMA: 2014,Jan,11

47143 **Backbench standard preparation of cadaver donor whole liver graft prior to allotransplantation, including cholecystectomy, if necessary, and dissection and removal of surrounding soft tissues to prepare the vena cava, portal vein, hepatic artery, and common bile duct for implantation; without trisegment or lobe split**

EXCLUDES *Cholecystectomy (47600, 47610)*
Hepatectomy (47120-47125)
🚒 0.00   ⚔ 0.00   **FUD** XXX   C 80 ▭

AMA: 2018,Jan,8; 2017,Jan,8; 2016,Jan,13; 2015,Jan,16; 2014,Jan,11

47144 **with trisegment split of whole liver graft into 2 partial liver grafts (ie, left lateral segment [segments II and III] and right trisegment [segments I and IV through VIII])**

EXCLUDES *Cholecystectomy (47600, 47610)*
Hepatectomy (47120-47125)
🚒 0.00   ⚔ 0.00   **FUD** 090   C 80 ▭

AMA: 2014,Jan,11

47145 **with lobe split of whole liver graft into 2 partial liver grafts (ie, left lobe [segments II, III, and IV] and right lobe [segments I and V through VIII])**

EXCLUDES *Cholecystectomy (47600, 47610)*
Hepatectomy (47120-47125)
🚒 0.00   ⚔ 0.00   **FUD** XXX   C 80 ▭

AMA: 2014,Jan,11

47146 **Backbench reconstruction of cadaver or living donor liver graft prior to allotransplantation; venous anastomosis, each**

EXCLUDES *Cholecystectomy (47600, 47610)*
Hepatectomy (47120-47125)
🚒 9.43   ⚔ 9.43   **FUD** XXX   C 80 ▭

AMA: 2014,Jan,11

47147 **arterial anastomosis, each**

EXCLUDES *Cholecystectomy (47600, 47610)*
Hepatectomy (47120-47125)
🚒 11.1   ⚔ 11.1   **FUD** XXX   C 80 ▭

AMA: 2014,Jan,11

47300-47362 Open Repair of Liver

47300   **Marsupialization of cyst or abscess of liver**
32.8   32.8   **FUD** 090   C 80
AMA: 2014,Jan,11

Anterior abdominal skin   Hepatic cyst

Cutaway view of liver

Marsupialization of cyst

A liver cyst or abscess is marsupialized; this method involves surgical access to the cyst and making an incision into it; the edges of the cyst are sutured to the abdominal wall and drainage, open or closed, is placed into the cyst

47350   **Management of liver hemorrhage; simple suture of liver wound or injury**
39.7   39.7   **FUD** 090   C 80
AMA: 2014,Jan,11

47360   **complex suture of liver wound or injury, with or without hepatic artery ligation**
54.5   54.5   **FUD** 090   C 80
AMA: 2014,Jan,11

47361   **exploration of hepatic wound, extensive debridement, coagulation and/or suture, with or without packing of liver**
88.0   88.0   **FUD** 090   C 80
AMA: 2014,Jan,11

47362   **re-exploration of hepatic wound for removal of packing**
42.1   42.1   **FUD** 090   C 80
AMA: 2014,Jan,11

47370-47379 Laparoscopic Ablation Liver Tumors

INCLUDES   Diagnostic laparoscopy (49320)

47370   **Laparoscopy, surgical, ablation of 1 or more liver tumor(s); radiofrequency**
(76940)
36.2   36.2   **FUD** 090   J 80
AMA: 2018,Jan,8; 2017,Jan,8; 2016,Jan,13; 2015,Jan,16; 2014,Jan,11

47371   **cryosurgical**
(76940)
36.5   36.5   **FUD** 090   J 80
AMA: 2014,Jan,11

47379   **Unlisted laparoscopic procedure, liver**
0.00   0.00   **FUD** YYY   J 80
AMA: 2018,Aug,10; 2018,Jan,8; 2017,Jan,8; 2016,Jan,13; 2015,Jan,16; 2014,Dec,18; 2014,Jan,11

47380-47399 Open/Percutaneous Ablation Liver Tumors

47380   **Ablation, open, of 1 or more liver tumor(s); radiofrequency**
(76940)
41.8   41.8   **FUD** 090   C 80
AMA: 2018,Jan,8; 2017,Jan,8; 2016,Jan,13; 2015,Jan,16; 2014,Jan,11

47381   **cryosurgical**
(76940)
43.0   43.0   **FUD** 090   C 80
AMA: 2014,Jan,11

47382   **Ablation, 1 or more liver tumor(s), percutaneous, radiofrequency**
(76940, 77013, 77022)
21.5   130.   **FUD** 010   J 62
AMA: 2018,Jan,8; 2017,Jan,8; 2016,Jan,13; 2015,Jan,16; 2014,Jan,11

47383   **Ablation, 1 or more liver tumor(s), percutaneous, cryoablation**
(76940, 77013, 77022)
13.2   196.   **FUD** 010   J J8
AMA: 2018,Jan,8; 2017,Jan,8; 2016,Jan,13; 2015,Jan,16; 2014,Dec,18

47399   **Unlisted procedure, liver**
0.00   0.00   **FUD** YYY   T
AMA: 2018,Jan,8; 2017,Mar,10; 2017,Jan,8; 2016,Jan,13; 2015,Jan,16; 2014,Dec,18; 2014,Jan,11

47400-47490 Biliary Tract Procedures

47400   **Hepaticotomy or hepaticostomy with exploration, drainage, or removal of calculus**
62.6   62.6   **FUD** 090   C 80
AMA: 2014,Jan,11

47420   **Choledochotomy or choledochostomy with exploration, drainage, or removal of calculus, with or without cholecystotomy; without transduodenal sphincterotomy or sphincteroplasty**
38.9   38.9   **FUD** 090   C 80
AMA: 2014,Jan,11

47425   **with transduodenal sphincterotomy or sphincteroplasty**
39.7   39.7   **FUD** 090   C 80
AMA: 2014,Jan,11

47460   **Transduodenal sphincterotomy or sphincteroplasty, with or without transduodenal extraction of calculus (separate procedure)**
36.8   36.8   **FUD** 090   C 80
AMA: 2014,Jan,11

47480   **Cholecystotomy or cholecystostomy, open, with exploration, drainage, or removal of calculus (separate procedure)**
EXCLUDES   Percutaneous cholecystostomy (47490)
25.4   25.4   **FUD** 090   C 80
AMA: 2018,Jan,8; 2017,Jan,8; 2016,Jan,13; 2015,Jan,16; 2014,Jan,11

47490   **Cholecystostomy, percutaneous, complete procedure, including imaging guidance, catheter placement, cholecystogram when performed, and radiological supervision and interpretation**

> **INCLUDES** Radiological guidance (75989, 76942, 77002, 77012, 77021)
> **EXCLUDES** *Injection procedure for cholangiography (47531-47532)*
> *Open cholecystostomy (47480)*

> 🖩 9.56   ⚖ 9.56   **FUD** 010   J ▢

AMA: 2018,Jan,8; 2017,Jan,8; 2016,Jan,13; 2015,Dec,3; 2015,Jan,16; 2014,Jan,11

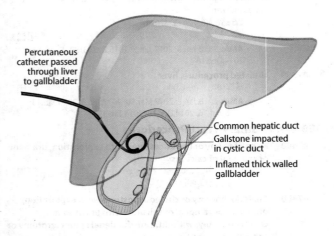

Percutaneous catheter passed through liver to gallbladder

Common hepatic duct
Gallstone impacted in cystic duct
Inflamed thick walled gallbladder

47531-47532 Injection/Insertion Procedures of Biliary Tract

> **INCLUDES** Contrast material injection
> Radiologic supervision and interpretation
> **EXCLUDES** *Intraoperative cholangiography (74300-74301)*
> *Procedures performed via the same access (47490, 47533-47541)*

47531   **Injection procedure for cholangiography, percutaneous, complete diagnostic procedure including imaging guidance (eg, ultrasound and/or fluoroscopy) and all associated radiological supervision and interpretation; existing access**

> 🖩 2.06   ⚖ 9.89   **FUD** 000   02 N1 ▢

AMA: 2018,Jan,8; 2017,Jan,8; 2015,Dec,3

47532   **new access (eg, percutaneous transhepatic cholangiogram)**

> 🖩 6.18   ⚖ 23.2   **FUD** 000   02 N1 ▢

AMA: 2018,Jan,8; 2017,Jan,8; 2015,Dec,3

47533-47544 Percutaneous Procedures of the Biliary Tract

47533   **Placement of biliary drainage catheter, percutaneous, including diagnostic cholangiography when performed, imaging guidance (eg, ultrasound and/or fluoroscopy), and all associated radiological supervision and interpretation; external**

> **EXCLUDES** *Conversion to internal-external drainage catheter (47535)*
> *Percutaneous placement stent in bile duct (47538)*
> *Placement stent into bile duct, new access (47540)*
> *Replacement existing internal drainage catheter (47536)*

> 🖩 7.74   ⚖ 35.2   **FUD** 000   J 62 ▢

AMA: 2018,Jan,8; 2017,Jan,8; 2015,Dec,3

47534   **internal-external**

> **EXCLUDES** *Conversion to external only drainage catheter (47536)*
> *Percutaneous placement stent in bile duct (47538)*
> *Placement stent into bile duct, new access (47540)*

> 🖩 10.8   ⚖ 41.0   **FUD** 000   J 62 ▢

AMA: 2018,Jan,8; 2017,Jan,8; 2015,Dec,3

47535   **Conversion of external biliary drainage catheter to internal-external biliary drainage catheter, percutaneous, including diagnostic cholangiography when performed, imaging guidance (eg, fluoroscopy), and all associated radiological supervision and interpretation**

> 🖩 5.75   ⚖ 28.4   **FUD** 000   J 62 ▢

AMA: 2018,Jan,8; 2017,Jan,8; 2015,Dec,3

47536   **Exchange of biliary drainage catheter (eg, external, internal-external, or conversion of internal-external to external only), percutaneous, including diagnostic cholangiography when performed, imaging guidance (eg, fluoroscopy), and all associated radiological supervision and interpretation**

> **INCLUDES** Exchange of one drainage catheter
> **EXCLUDES** *Placement of stent(s) into a bile duct, percutaneous (47538)*
> Code also exchange of additional catheters in same session with modifier 59 (47536)

> 🖩 3.84   ⚖ 19.5   **FUD** 000   J 62 ▢

AMA: 2018,Jan,8; 2017,Jan,8; 2015,Dec,3

47537   **Removal of biliary drainage catheter, percutaneous, requiring fluoroscopic guidance (eg, with concurrent indwelling biliary stents), including diagnostic cholangiography when performed, imaging guidance (eg, fluoroscopy), and all associated radiological supervision and interpretation**

> **EXCLUDES** *Placement of stent(s) into a bile duct via the same access (47538)*
> *Removal without use of fluoroscopic guidance; report with appropriate E&M service code*

> 🖩 2.79   ⚖ 11.5   **FUD** 000   02 62 ▢

AMA: 2018,Jan,8; 2017,Jan,8; 2015,Dec,3

47538   **Placement of stent(s) into a bile duct, percutaneous, including diagnostic cholangiography, imaging guidance (eg, fluoroscopy and/or ultrasound), balloon dilation, catheter exchange(s) and catheter removal(s) when performed, and all associated radiological supervision and interpretation; existing access**

> **EXCLUDES** *Drainage catheter inserted following stent placement (47536)*
> *Procedures performed via the same access (47536-47537)*
> *Treatment of same lesion in same operative session ([43277], 47542, 47555-47556)*
> Code also multiple stents placed during same session when: (47538-47540)
> Serial stents placed within the same bile duct;
> Stent placement via two or more percutaneous access sites or the space between two other stents
> Two or more stents inserted through the same percutaneous access

> 🖩 6.88   ⚖ 121.   **FUD** 000   J J8 ▢

AMA: 2018,Jan,8; 2017,Jan,8; 2016,Mar,10; 2015,Dec,3

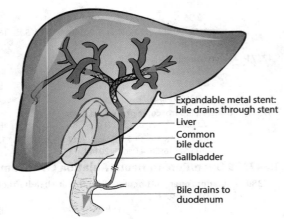

Expandable metal stent: bile drains through stent
Liver
Common bile duct
Gallbladder

Bile drains to duodenum

| 26/TC PC/TC Only | A2-Z3 ASC Payment | 50 Bilateral | ♂ Male Only | ♀ Female Only | 🖩 Facility RVU | ⚖ Non-Facility RVU | ▢ CCI | ☒ CLIA |
| FUD Follow-up Days | CMS: IOM | AMA: CPT Asst | A-Y OPPSI | 80/80 Surg Assist Allowed / w/Doc | | ▢ Lab Crosswalk | ▢ Radiology Crosswalk |

226   CPT © 2019 American Medical Association. All Rights Reserved.   © 2019 Optum360, LLC

47539 new access, without placement of separate biliary drainage catheter

> EXCLUDES *Treatment of same lesion in same session ([43277], 47542, 47555-47556)*
>
> Code also multiple stents placed during same session when: (47538-47540)
> Serial stents placed within the same bile duct
> Stent placement via two or more percutaneous access sites or the space between two other stents
> Two or more stents inserted through the same percutaneous access

🚑 12.4 ⚕ 135. **FUD** 000 [J] [J8] 🖵

AMA: 2018,Jan,8; 2017,Jan,8; 2016,Mar,10; 2015,Dec,3

47540 new access, with placement of separate biliary drainage catheter (eg, external or internal-external)

> EXCLUDES *Procedure performed via the same access (47533-47534)*
>
> *Treatment of same lesion in same session ([43277], 47542, 47555-47556)*
>
> Code also multiple stents placed during same session when: (47538-47540)
> Serial stents placed within the same bile duct;
> Stent placement via two or more percutaneous access sites or the space between two other stents;
> Two or more stents inserted through the same percutaneous access

🚑 12.8 ⚕ 137. **FUD** 000 [J] [J8] 🖵

AMA: 2018,Jan,8; 2017,Jan,8; 2016,Mar,10; 2015,Dec,3

47541 Placement of access through the biliary tree and into small bowel to assist with an endoscopic biliary procedure (eg, rendezvous procedure), percutaneous, including diagnostic cholangiography when performed, imaging guidance (eg, ultrasound and/or fluoroscopy), and all associated radiological supervision and interpretation, new access

> EXCLUDES *Access through biliary tree into small bowel for endoscopic biliary procedure (47535-47537)*
>
> *Conversion, exchange, or removal of external biliary drainage catheter (47535-47537)*
>
> *Injection procedure for cholangiography (47531-47532)*
>
> *Placement of biliary drainage catheter (47533-47534)*
>
> *Placement of stent(s) into a bile duct (47538-47540)*
>
> *Procedure performed when previous catheter access exists*

🚑 9.64 ⚕ 33.8 **FUD** 000 [J] [G2] 🖵

AMA: 2018,Jan,8; 2017,Jan,8; 2015,Dec,3

+ **47542** Balloon dilation of biliary duct(s) or of ampulla (sphincteroplasty), percutaneous, including imaging guidance (eg, fluoroscopy), and all associated radiological supervision and interpretation, each duct (List separately in addition to code for primary procedure)

> EXCLUDES *Biliary endoscopy, with dilation of biliary duct stricture (47555-47556)*
>
> *Endoscopic balloon dilation ([43277], 47555-47556)*
>
> *Endoscopic retrograde cholangiopancreatography (ERCP) (43262, [43277])*
>
> *Placement of stent(s) into a bile duct (47538-47540)*
>
> *Procedure performed with balloon used to remove calculi, debris, sludge without dilation (47544)*
>
> Code also one additional dilation code when more than one dilation performed in same session, using modifier 59 with (47542)
> Code first (47531-47537, 47541)

🚑 3.94 ⚕ 13.9 **FUD** ZZZ [N] [N1] 🖵

AMA: 2018,Jan,8; 2017,Jan,8; 2015,Dec,3

+ **47543** Endoluminal biopsy(ies) of biliary tree, percutaneous, any method(s) (eg, brush, forceps, and/or needle), including imaging guidance (eg, fluoroscopy), and all associated radiological supervision and interpretation, single or multiple (List separately in addition to code for primary procedure)

> EXCLUDES *Endoscopic biopsy (46261, 47553)*
>
> *Endoscopic brushings (43260, 47552)*
>
> *Procedure performed more than one time per session*
>
> Code first (47531-47540)

🚑 4.20 ⚕ 13.3 **FUD** ZZZ [N] [N1] 🖵

AMA: 2018,Jan,8; 2017,Jan,8; 2015,Dec,3

+ **47544** Removal of calculi/debris from biliary duct(s) and/or gallbladder, percutaneous, including destruction of calculi by any method (eg, mechanical, electrohydraulic, lithotripsy) when performed, imaging guidance (eg, fluoroscopy), and all associated radiological supervision and interpretation (List separately in addition to code for primary procedure)

> EXCLUDES *Device deployment without findings of calculi/debris*
>
> *Endoscopic calculi removal/destruction (43264-43265, 47554)*
>
> *Endoscopic retrograde cholangiopancreatography (ERCP); with removal of calculi/debris from biliary/pancreatic duct(s) (43264)*
>
> *Procedures with removal of incidental debris (47531-47543)*
>
> Code first when debris removal not incidental, as appropriate (47531-47540)

🚑 4.61 ⚕ 29.2 **FUD** ZZZ [N] [N1] 🖵

AMA: 2018,Jan,8; 2017,Jan,8; 2015,Dec,3

47550-47556 Endoscopic Procedures of the Biliary Tract

> INCLUDES Diagnostic endoscopy (49320)
>
> EXCLUDES *Endoscopic retrograde cholangiopancreatography (ERCP) (43260-43265, [43274], [43275], [43276], [43277], [43278], 74328-74330, 74363)*

+ **47550** Biliary endoscopy, intraoperative (choledochoscopy) (List separately in addition to code for primary procedure)

> Code first primary procedure

🚑 4.80 ⚕ 4.80 **FUD** ZZZ [C] [80] 🖵

AMA: 2014,Jan,11

47552 Biliary endoscopy, percutaneous via T-tube or other tract; diagnostic, with collection of specimen(s) by brushing and/or washing, when performed (separate procedure)

🚑 9.01 ⚕ 9.01 **FUD** 000 [J] [A2] 🖵

AMA: 2018,Jan,8; 2017,Jan,8; 2016,Jan,13; 2015,Dec,3; 2015,Jan,16; 2014,Jan,11

47553 with biopsy, single or multiple

🚑 8.91 ⚕ 8.91 **FUD** 000 [J] [A2] 🖵

AMA: 2018,Jan,8; 2017,Jan,8; 2016,Jan,13; 2015,Dec,3; 2015,Jan,16; 2014,Jan,11

47554 with removal of calculus/calculi

🚑 14.9 ⚕ 14.9 **FUD** 000 [J] [A2] 🖵

AMA: 2018,Jan,8; 2017,Jan,8; 2016,Jan,13; 2015,Dec,3; 2015,Jan,16; 2014,Jan,11

47555 with dilation of biliary duct stricture(s) without stent

🔲 (74363)

🚑 9.46 ⚕ 9.46 **FUD** 000 [J] [A2] 🖵

AMA: 2018,Jan,8; 2017,Jan,8; 2016,Jan,13; 2015,Dec,3; 2015,Jan,16; 2014,Jan,11

47556 with dilation of biliary duct stricture(s) with stent

🔲 (74363)

🚑 10.7 ⚕ 10.7 **FUD** 000 [J] [J8] 🖵

AMA: 2018,Jan,8; 2017,Jan,8; 2016,Jan,13; 2015,Dec,3; 2015,Jan,16; 2014,Jan,11

47562-47579 Laparoscopic Gallbladder Procedures

> INCLUDES Diagnostic laparoscopy (49320)

47562 Laparoscopy, surgical; cholecystectomy

🚑 19.0 ⚕ 19.0 **FUD** 090 [J] [G2] [80] 🖵

AMA: 2018,Jan,8; 2017,Jan,8; 2016,Jan,13; 2015,Jan,16; 2014,Jan,11

47563   **cholecystectomy with cholangiography**

EXCLUDES   *Percutaneous cholangiography (47531-47532)*

Code also intraoperative radiology supervision and interpretation (74300-74301)

🔧 20.7   🔨 20.7   **FUD** 090   J 62 80 ▭

AMA: 2019,Mar,10; 2018,Jan,8; 2017,Jan,8; 2016,Jan,13; 2015,Jan,16; 2014,Jan,11

47564   **cholecystectomy with exploration of common duct**

🔧 32.2   🔨 32.2   **FUD** 090   J 62 80 ▭

AMA: 2018,Jan,8; 2017,Jan,8; 2016,Jan,13; 2015,Jan,16; 2014,Jan,11

47570   **cholecystoenterostomy**

🔧 22.5   🔨 22.5   **FUD** 090   C 80 ▭

AMA: 2018,Jan,8; 2017,Jan,8; 2016,Jan,13; 2015,Jan,16; 2014,Jan,11

47579   **Unlisted laparoscopy procedure, biliary tract**

🔧 0.00   🔨 0.00   **FUD** YYY   J 80 50 ▭

AMA: 2018,Jan,8; 2017,Jan,8; 2016,Jan,13; 2015,Jan,16; 2014,Jan,11

47600-47620 Open Gallbladder Procedures

47600   **Cholecystectomy;**

EXCLUDES   *Laparoscopic method (47562-47564)*

🔧 30.9   🔨 30.9   **FUD** 090   C 80 ▭

AMA: 2018,Jan,8; 2017,Jan,8; 2016,Jan,13; 2015,Jan,16; 2014,Jan,11

47605   **with cholangiography**

EXCLUDES   *Laparoscopic method (47563-47564)*

🔧 32.6   🔨 32.6   **FUD** 090   C 80 ▭

AMA: 2018,Jan,8; 2017,Jan,8; 2016,Jan,13; 2015,Jan,16; 2014,Jan,11

47610   **Cholecystectomy with exploration of common duct;**

EXCLUDES   *Laparoscopic method (47564)*

Code also biliary endoscopy when performed in conjunction with cholecystectomy with exploration of common duct (47550)

🔧 36.3   🔨 36.3   **FUD** 090   C 80 ▭

AMA: 2018,Jan,8; 2017,Jan,8; 2016,Jan,13; 2015,Jan,16; 2014,Jan,11

47612   **with choledochoenterostomy**

🔧 36.6   🔨 36.6   **FUD** 090   C 80 ▭

AMA: 2014,Jan,11

47620   **with transduodenal sphincterotomy or sphincteroplasty, with or without cholangiography**

🔧 40.0   🔨 40.0   **FUD** 090   C 80 ▭

AMA: 2014,Jan,11

47700-47999 Open Resection and Repair of Biliary Tract

47700   **Exploration for congenital atresia of bile ducts, without repair, with or without liver biopsy, with or without cholangiography**

🔧 30.6   🔨 30.6   **FUD** 090   63 C 80 ▭

AMA: 2014,Jan,11

47701   **Portoenterostomy (eg, Kasai procedure)**

🔧 49.5   🔨 49.5   **FUD** 090   63 C 80 ▭

AMA: 2014,Jan,11

47711   **Excision of bile duct tumor, with or without primary repair of bile duct; extrahepatic**

EXCLUDES   *Anastomosis (47760-47800)*

🔧 45.1   🔨 45.1   **FUD** 090   C 80 ▭

AMA: 2014,Jan,11

47712   **intrahepatic**

EXCLUDES   *Anastomosis (47760-47800)*

🔧 58.1   🔨 58.1   **FUD** 090   C 80 ▭

AMA: 2014,Jan,11

47715   **Excision of choledochal cyst**

🔧 38.6   🔨 38.6   **FUD** 090   C 80 ▭

AMA: 2018,Jan,8; 2017,Jan,8; 2016,Jan,13; 2015,Jan,16; 2014,Jan,11

47720   **Cholecystoenterostomy; direct**

EXCLUDES   *Laparoscopic method (47570)*

🔧 33.4   🔨 33.4   **FUD** 090   C 80 ▭

AMA: 2018,Jan,8; 2017,Jan,8; 2016,Jan,13; 2015,Jan,16; 2014,Jan,11

47721   **with gastroenterostomy**

🔧 39.3   🔨 39.3   **FUD** 090   C 80 ▭

AMA: 2014,Jan,11

47740   **Roux-en-Y**

🔧 37.7   🔨 37.7   **FUD** 090   C 80 ▭

AMA: 2014,Jan,11

47741   **Roux-en-Y with gastroenterostomy**

🔧 42.8   🔨 42.8   **FUD** 090   C 80 ▭

AMA: 2014,Jan,11

47760   **Anastomosis, of extrahepatic biliary ducts and gastrointestinal tract**

🔧 65.4   🔨 65.4   **FUD** 090   C 80 ▭

AMA: 2014,Jan,11

47765   **Anastomosis, of intrahepatic ducts and gastrointestinal tract**

INCLUDES   Longmire anastomosis

🔧 88.4   🔨 88.4   **FUD** 090   C 80 ▭

AMA: 2014,Jan,11

47780   **Anastomosis, Roux-en-Y, of extrahepatic biliary ducts and gastrointestinal tract**

🔧 71.8   🔨 71.8   **FUD** 090   C 80 ▭

AMA: 2014,Jan,11

47785   **Anastomosis, Roux-en-Y, of intrahepatic biliary ducts and gastrointestinal tract**

🔧 94.4   🔨 94.4   **FUD** 090   C 80 ▭

AMA: 2014,Jan,11

47800   **Reconstruction, plastic, of extrahepatic biliary ducts with end-to-end anastomosis**

🔧 45.5   🔨 45.5   **FUD** 090   C 80 ▭

AMA: 2014,Jan,11

47801   **Placement of choledochal stent**

🔧 32.3   🔨 32.3   **FUD** 090   C 80 ▭

AMA: 2018,Jan,8; 2017,Jan,8; 2016,Jan,13; 2015,Jan,16; 2014,Jan,11

47802   **U-tube hepaticoenterostomy**

🔧 44.3   🔨 44.3   **FUD** 090   C 80 ▭

AMA: 2014,Jan,11

47900   **Suture of extrahepatic biliary duct for pre-existing injury (separate procedure)**

🔧 39.7   🔨 39.7   **FUD** 090   C 80 ▭

AMA: 2014,Jan,11

47999   **Unlisted procedure, biliary tract**

🔧 0.00   🔨 0.00   **FUD** YYY   T ▭

AMA: 2018,Jan,8; 2017,Jan,8; 2016,Jan,13; 2015,Jan,16; 2014,Jan,11

26/TC PC/TC Only   A2-Z3 ASC Payment   50 Bilateral   ♂ Male Only   ♀ Female Only   🔧 Facility RVU   🔨 Non-Facility RVU   ▭ CCI   ☒ CLIA
FUD Follow-up Days   CMS: IOM   AMA: CPT Asst   A-Y OPPSI   80/80 Surg Assist Allowed / w/Doc   ▭ Lab Crosswalk   ☒ Radiology Crosswalk

228   CPT © 2019 American Medical Association. All Rights Reserved.   © 2019 Optum360, LLC

48000-48548 Open Procedures of the Pancreas

EXCLUDES Peroral pancreatic procedures performed endoscopically (43260-43265, [43274], [43275], [43276], [43277], [43278])

48000 Placement of drains, peripancreatic, for acute pancreatitis;
54.6   54.6   **FUD** 090
AMA: 2014,Jan,11

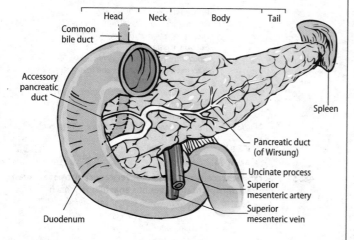

Head   Neck   Body   Tail
Common bile duct
Accessory pancreatic duct
Spleen
Pancreatic duct (of Wirsung)
Uncinate process
Superior mesenteric artery
Superior mesenteric vein
Duodenum

48001 with cholecystostomy, gastrostomy, and jejunostomy
66.6   66.6   **FUD** 090
AMA: 2014,Jan,11

48020 Removal of pancreatic calculus
34.1   34.1   **FUD** 090
AMA: 2014,Jan,11

48100 Biopsy of pancreas, open (eg, fine needle aspiration, needle core biopsy, wedge biopsy)
25.8   25.8   **FUD** 090
AMA: 2014,Jan,11

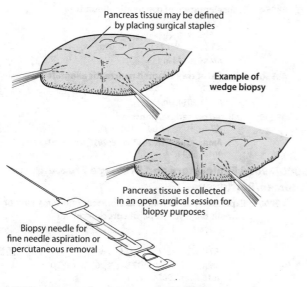

Pancreas tissue may be defined by placing surgical staples
Example of wedge biopsy
Pancreas tissue is collected in an open surgical session for biopsy purposes
Biopsy needle for fine needle aspiration or percutaneous removal

48102 Biopsy of pancreas, percutaneous needle
EXCLUDES Fine needle aspiration ([10005, 10006, 10007, 10008, 10009, 10010, 10011, 10012])
(76942, 77002, 77012, 77021)
(88172-88173)
6.95   15.2   **FUD** 010
AMA: 2019,Apr,4; 2014,Jan,11

48105 Resection or debridement of pancreas and peripancreatic tissue for acute necrotizing pancreatitis
82.4   82.4   **FUD** 090
AMA: 2014,Jan,11

48120 Excision of lesion of pancreas (eg, cyst, adenoma)
32.0   32.0   **FUD** 090
AMA: 2014,Jan,11

48140 Pancreatectomy, distal subtotal, with or without splenectomy; without pancreaticojejunostomy
45.4   45.4   **FUD** 090
AMA: 2018,Jan,8; 2017,Jul,10; 2014,Jan,11

48145 with pancreaticojejunostomy
47.4   47.4   **FUD** 090
AMA: 2014,Jan,11

48146 Pancreatectomy, distal, near-total with preservation of duodenum (Child-type procedure)
54.5   54.5   **FUD** 090
AMA: 2014,Jan,11

Gallbladder
Accessory outlet
Spleen
Major papilla for main pancreatic duct

48148 Excision of ampulla of Vater
36.2   36.2   **FUD** 090
AMA: 2014,Jan,11

48150 Pancreatectomy, proximal subtotal with total duodenectomy, partial gastrectomy, choledochoenterostomy and gastrojejunostomy (Whipple-type procedure); with pancreatojejunostomy
90.6   90.6   **FUD** 090
AMA: 2018,Jan,8; 2017,Jan,8; 2016,Jan,13; 2015,Dec,16; 2014,Jan,11

48152 without pancreatojejunostomy
84.0   84.0   **FUD** 090
AMA: 2014,Jan,11

48153 Pancreatectomy, proximal subtotal with near-total duodenectomy, choledochoenterostomy and duodenojejunostomy (pylorus-sparing, Whipple-type procedure); with pancreatojejunostomy
90.1   90.1   **FUD** 090
AMA: 2014,Jan,11

48154 without pancreatojejunostomy
84.3   84.3   **FUD** 090
AMA: 2014,Jan,11

48155 Pancreatectomy, total
52.6   52.6   **FUD** 090
AMA: 2014,Jan,11

Digestive System

48160 — 49002

48160 Pancreatectomy, total or subtotal, with autologous transplantation of pancreas or pancreatic islet cells

EXCLUDES Laparoscopic pancreatic islet cell transplantation (0585T)
Open pancreatic islet cell transplantation (0586T)
Percutaneous pancreatic islet cell transplantation (0584T)

🔾 0.00   ⚖ 0.00   **FUD** XXX   E 🖳

AMA: 2014,Jan,11

+ 48400 Injection procedure for intraoperative pancreatography (List separately in addition to code for primary procedure)

Code first primary procedure
⚕ (74300-74301)

🔾 3.07   ⚖ 3.07   **FUD** ZZZ   C 80 🖳

AMA: 2018,Jan,8; 2017,Jan,8; 2016,Jan,13; 2015,Jan,16; 2014,Jan,11

48500 Marsupialization of pancreatic cyst

🔾 33.4   ⚖ 33.4   **FUD** 090   C 80 🖳

AMA: 2014,Jan,11

48510 External drainage, pseudocyst of pancreas, open

EXCLUDES Image guided percutaneous catheter drainage (49405)

🔾 31.8   ⚖ 31.8   **FUD** 090   C 80 🖳

AMA: 2014,Jan,11

48520 Internal anastomosis of pancreatic cyst to gastrointestinal tract; direct

🔾 31.5   ⚖ 31.5   **FUD** 090   C 80 🖳

AMA: 2014,Jan,11

48540 Roux-en-Y

🔾 37.8   ⚖ 37.8   **FUD** 090   C 80 🖳

AMA: 2014,Jan,11

48545 Pancreatorrhaphy for injury

🔾 39.0   ⚖ 39.0   **FUD** 090   C 80 🖳

AMA: 2014,Jan,11

48547 Duodenal exclusion with gastrojejunostomy for pancreatic injury

🔾 51.9   ⚖ 51.9   **FUD** 090   C 80 🖳

AMA: 2014,Jan,11

48548 Pancreaticojejunostomy, side-to-side anastomosis (Puestow-type operation)

🔾 48.2   ⚖ 48.2   **FUD** 090   C 80 🖳

AMA: 2014,Jan,11

48550-48999 Pancreas Transplant Procedures

CMS: 100-03,260.3 Pancreas Transplants; 100-04,3,90.5 Pancreas Transplants with Kidney Transplants; 100-04,3,90.5.1 Pancreas Transplants Alone

48550 Donor pancreatectomy (including cold preservation), with or without duodenal segment for transplantation

INCLUDES Graft:
Cold preservation
Harvest (with or without duodenal segment)

🔾 0.00   ⚖ 0.00   **FUD** XXX   E 🖳

AMA: 2018,Jan,8; 2017,Jan,8; 2016,Jan,13; 2015,Jan,16; 2014,Jan,11

48551 Backbench standard preparation of cadaver donor pancreas allograft prior to transplantation, including dissection of allograft from surrounding soft tissues, splenectomy, duodenotomy, ligation of bile duct, ligation of mesenteric vessels, and Y-graft arterial anastomoses from iliac artery to superior mesenteric artery and to splenic artery

EXCLUDES Biopsy of pancreas (48100-48102)
Bypass graft, with vein (35531, 35563)
Duodenotomy (44010)
Endoscopic procedures of the biliary tract (47550-47556)
Excision of lesion of mesentery (44820)
Excision of lesion of pancreas (48120)
Pancreatorrhaphy for injury (48545)
Placement of vein patch or cuff at distal anastomosis of bypass graft (35685)
Resection or debridement of pancreas (48105)
Splenectomy (38100-38102)
Suture of mesentery (44850)
Transduodenal sphincterotomy, sphincteroplasty (47460)

🔾 0.00   ⚖ 0.00   **FUD** XXX   C 80 🖳

AMA: 2014,Jan,11

48552 Backbench reconstruction of cadaver donor pancreas allograft prior to transplantation, venous anastomosis, each

EXCLUDES Biopsy of pancreas (48100-48102)
Bypass graft, with vein (35531, 35563)
Duodenotomy (44010)
Endoscopic procedures of the biliary tract (47550-47556)
Excision of lesion of mesentery (44820)
Excision of lesion of pancreas (48120)
Pancreatorrhaphy for injury (48545)
Placement of vein patch or cuff at distal anastomosis of bypass graft (35685)
Resection or debridement of pancreas (48105)
Splenectomy (38100-38102)
Suture of mesentery (44850)
Transduodenal sphincterotomy, sphincteroplasty (47460)

🔾 6.87   ⚖ 6.87   **FUD** XXX   C 80 🖳

AMA: 2014,Jan,11

48554 Transplantation of pancreatic allograft

INCLUDES Allograft transplant
Recipient care

🔾 73.9   ⚖ 73.9   **FUD** 090   C 80 🖳

AMA: 2014,Jan,11

48556 Removal of transplanted pancreatic allograft

🔾 36.9   ⚖ 36.9   **FUD** 090   C 80 🖳

AMA: 2014,Jan,11

48999 Unlisted procedure, pancreas

🔾 0.00   ⚖ 0.00   **FUD** YYY   T 80 🖳

AMA: 2018,Jan,8; 2017,Jan,8; 2016,Jan,13; 2015,Jan,16; 2014,Jan,11

49000-49084 Exploratory and Drainage Procedures: Abdomen/Peritoneum

49000 Exploratory laparotomy, exploratory celiotomy with or without biopsy(s) (separate procedure)

EXCLUDES Exploration of penetrating wound without laparotomy (20102)

🔾 22.3   ⚖ 22.3   **FUD** 090   C 80 🖳

AMA: 2018,Jan,8; 2017,Dec,3; 2017,Jan,8; 2016,Jan,13; 2015,Jan,16; 2014,Jan,11

49002 Reopening of recent laparotomy

EXCLUDES Hepatic wound re-exploration for packing removal (47362)
Pelvic wound re-exploration for packing removal/repacking (49014)

🔾 30.3   ⚖ 30.3   **FUD** 090   C 80 🖳

AMA: 2018,Jan,8; 2017,Jan,8; 2016,Jan,13; 2015,Jan,16; 2014,Jan,11

49010　**Exploration, retroperitoneal area with or without biopsy(s) (separate procedure)**

EXCLUDES　*Exploration of penetrating wound without laparotomy (20102)*

🔲 26.9　⚗ 26.9　**FUD** 090　　　C 80 🔲

AMA: 2014,Jan,11

● 49013　**Preperitoneal pelvic packing for hemorrhage associated with pelvic trauma, including local exploration**

● 49014　**Re-exploration of pelvic wound with removal of preperitoneal pelvic packing, including repacking, when performed**

49020　**Drainage of peritoneal abscess or localized peritonitis, exclusive of appendiceal abscess, open**

EXCLUDES　*Appendiceal abscess (44900)*

Image guided percutaneous catheter drainage of abscess/peritonitis via catheter (49406)

Image-guided transrectal/transvaginal drainage of peritoneal abscess via catheter (49407)

🔲 46.1　⚗ 46.1　**FUD** 090　　　C 80 🔲

AMA: 2014,Jan,11

49040　**Drainage of subdiaphragmatic or subphrenic abscess, open**

EXCLUDES　*Image-guided percutaneous drainage of subdiaphragmatic/subphrenic abscess via catheter (49406)*

🔲 28.9　⚗ 28.9　**FUD** 090　　　C 80 🔲

AMA: 2014,Jan,11

49060　**Drainage of retroperitoneal abscess, open**

EXCLUDES　*Image-guided percutaneous drainage of retroperitoneal abscess via catheter (49406)*

Transrectal/transvaginal image-guided drainage of retroperitoneal abscess via catheter (49407)

🔲 31.8　⚗ 31.8　**FUD** 090　　　C 🔲

AMA: 2018,Jan,8; 2017,Jan,8; 2016,Jan,13; 2015,Jan,16; 2014,Jan,11

49062　**Drainage of extraperitoneal lymphocele to peritoneal cavity, open**

EXCLUDES　*Drainage of lymphocele to peritoneal cavity, laparoscopic (49323)*

Image-guided percutaneous drainage of retroperitoneal lymphocele via catheter (49406)

🔲 21.3　⚗ 21.3　**FUD** 090　　　C 80 🔲

AMA: 2018,Jan,8; 2017,Jan,8; 2016,Jan,13; 2015,Jan,16; 2014,Jan,11

49082　**Abdominal paracentesis (diagnostic or therapeutic); without imaging guidance**

🔲 2.12　⚗ 5.67　**FUD** 000　　　T 62 🔲

AMA: 2018,Jan,8; 2017,Jan,8; 2016,Jan,13; 2015,Jan,16; 2014,Jan,11

49083　**with imaging guidance**

INCLUDES　Radiological guidance (76942, 77002, 77012, 77021)

EXCLUDES　*Image-guided percutaneous drainage of retroperitoneal abscess via catheter (49406)*

🔲 3.11　⚗ 8.44　**FUD** 000　　　T 62 🔲

AMA: 2018,Jan,8; 2017,Jan,8; 2016,Jan,13; 2015,Jan,16; 2014,Mar,13; 2014,Jan,11

49084　**Peritoneal lavage, including imaging guidance, when performed**

INCLUDES　Radiological guidance (76942, 77002, 77012, 77021)

EXCLUDES　*Image-guided percutaneous drainage of retroperitoneal abscess via catheter (49406)*

🔲 3.13　⚗ 3.13　**FUD** 000　　　T 62 🔲

AMA: 2018,Jan,8; 2017,Jan,8; 2016,Jan,13; 2015,Jan,16; 2014,Jan,11

49180 Biopsy of Mass: Abdomen/Retroperitoneum

EXCLUDES　*Fine needle aspiration (10021, [10004, 10005, 10006, 10007, 10008, 10009, 10010, 10011, 10012])*

Lysis of intestinal adhesions (44005)

49180　**Biopsy, abdominal or retroperitoneal mass, percutaneous needle**

📷 (76942, 77002, 77012, 77021)

🔳 (88172-88173)

🔲 2.46　⚗ 4.71　**FUD** 000　　　J A2 🔲

AMA: 2019,Feb,8; 2019,Apr,4; 2018,Jan,8; 2017,Jan,8; 2016,Jan,13; 2015,Jan,16; 2014,Jan,11

49185 Sclerotherapy of a Fluid Collection

49185　**Sclerotherapy of a fluid collection (eg, lymphocele, cyst, or seroma), percutaneous, including contrast injection(s), sclerosant injection(s), diagnostic study, imaging guidance (eg, ultrasound, fluoroscopy) and radiological supervision and interpretation when performed**

INCLUDES　Multiple lesions treated via same access

EXCLUDES　*Contrast injection for assessment of abscess or cyst (49424)*

Pleurodesis (32560)

Radiologic examination, abscess, fistula or sinus tract stud (76080)

Sclerosis of veins/endovenous ablation of incompetent veins of extremity (36468, 36470-36471, 36475-36476, 36478-36479)

Sclerotherapy of lymphatic/vascular malformation (37241)

Code also access or drainage via needle or catheter (10030, 10160, 49405-49407, 50390)

Code also existing catheter exchange pre- or post-sclerosant injection (49423, 75984)

Code also modifier 59 for treatment of multiple lesions in same session via separate access

🔲 3.48　⚗ 30.2　**FUD** 000　　　T 🔲

AMA: 2018,Jan,8; 2017,Jan,8; 2016,Mar,10

49203-49205 Open Destruction or Excision: Abdominal Tumors

EXCLUDES　*Ablation, open, 1 or more renal mass lesion(s), cryosurgical*

Biopsy of kidney or ovary (50205, 58900)

Cryoablation of renal tumor (50250, 50593)

Excision of perinephric cyst (50290)

Excision of presacral or sacrococcygeal tumor (49215)

Exploration, renal or retroperitoneal area (49010, 50010)

Exploratory laparotomy (49000)

Laparotomy, for staging or restaging of ovarian, tubal, or primary peritoneal malignancy (58960)

Nephrectomy (50225, 50236)

Oophorectomy (58940-58958)

Ovarian cystectomy (58925)

Pelvic or retroperitoneal lymphadenectomy (38770, 38780)

Primary, recurrent ovarian, uterine, or tubal resection (58957-58958)

Wedge resection or bisection of ovary (58920)

Code also colectomy (44140)

Code also nephrectomy (50220, 50240)

Code also small bowel resection (44120)

Code also vena caval resection with reconstruction (37799)

49203　**Excision or destruction, open, intra-abdominal tumors, cysts or endometriomas, 1 or more peritoneal, mesenteric, or retroperitoneal primary or secondary tumors; largest tumor 5 cm diameter or less**

🔲 34.7　⚗ 34.7　**FUD** 090　　　C 80 🔲

AMA: 2018,Jan,8; 2017,Jan,8; 2016,Jan,13; 2015,Jan,16; 2014,Jan,11

49204　**largest tumor 5.1-10.0 cm diameter**

🔲 44.3　⚗ 44.3　**FUD** 090　　　C 80 🔲

AMA: 2018,Jan,8; 2017,Jan,8; 2016,Jan,13; 2015,Jan,16; 2014,Jan,11

49205　**largest tumor greater than 10.0 cm diameter**

🔲 51.0　⚗ 51.0　**FUD** 090　　　C 80 🔲

AMA: 2018,Jan,8; 2017,Jan,8; 2016,Jan,13; 2015,Jan,16; 2014,Jan,11

49215 Resection Presacral/Sacrococcygeal Tumor

49215 Excision of presacral or sacrococcygeal tumor
📷 64.2 ⚕ 64.2 **FUD** 090   63 C 80 ▥
AMA: 2014,Jan,11

49220-49255 Other Open Abdominal Procedures

EXCLUDES *Lysis of intestinal adhesions (44005)*

49220 Staging laparotomy for Hodgkins disease or lymphoma
(includes splenectomy, needle or open biopsies of both liver
lobes, possibly also removal of abdominal nodes, abdominal
node and/or bone marrow biopsies, ovarian repositioning)
📷 28.2 ⚕ 28.2 **FUD** 090   C 80 ▥
AMA: 2014,Jan,11

49250 Umbilectomy, omphalectomy, excision of umbilicus (separate
procedure)
📷 17.0 ⚕ 17.0 **FUD** 090   J A2 ▥
AMA: 2014,Jan,11

49255 Omentectomy, epiploectomy, resection of omentum (separate
procedure)
📷 22.9 ⚕ 22.9 **FUD** 090   C 80 ▥
AMA: 2018,Mar,11; 2018,Jan,8; 2017,Jan,8; 2016,Jan,13;
2015,Jan,16; 2014,Jan,11

49320-49329 Laparoscopic Procedures of the Abdomen/Peritoneum/Omentum

INCLUDES *Diagnostic laparoscopy (49320)*
EXCLUDES *Fulguration/excision of lesions of ovary/pelvic viscera/peritoneal surface,
performed laparoscopically (58662)*

49320 Laparoscopy, abdomen, peritoneum, and omentum,
diagnostic, with or without collection of specimen(s) by
brushing or washing (separate procedure)
📷 9.43 ⚕ 9.43 **FUD** 010   J A2 80 ▥
AMA: 2018,Jan,8; 2017,Apr,7; 2017,Jan,8; 2016,Jan,13;
2015,Dec,16; 2015,Jan,16; 2014,Jan,11

49321 Laparoscopy, surgical; with biopsy (single or multiple)
📷 9.97 ⚕ 9.97 **FUD** 010   J A2 80 ▥
AMA: 2018,Aug,10; 2018,Jan,8; 2017,Jan,8; 2016,Jan,13;
2015,Jan,16; 2014,Jan,11

49322 with aspiration of cavity or cyst (eg, ovarian cyst) (single
or multiple)
📷 10.7 ⚕ 10.7 **FUD** 010   J A2 80 ▥
AMA: 2018,Jan,8; 2017,Jan,8; 2016,Jan,13; 2015,Jan,16;
2014,Jan,11

49323 with drainage of lymphocele to peritoneal cavity
EXCLUDES *Open drainage of lymphocele to peritoneal cavity
(49062)*
📷 18.3 ⚕ 18.3 **FUD** 090   J 80 ▥
AMA: 2018,Jan,8; 2017,Jan,8; 2016,Jan,13; 2015,Jan,16;
2014,Jan,11

49324 with insertion of tunneled intraperitoneal catheter
EXCLUDES *Open approach (49421)*
Code also insertion of subcutaneous extension to intraperitoneal
cannula with remote chest exit site, when appropriate
(49435)
📷 11.2 ⚕ 11.2 **FUD** 010   J 62 80 ▥
AMA: 2014,Jan,11

49325 with revision of previously placed intraperitoneal cannula
or catheter, with removal of intraluminal obstructive
material if performed
📷 11.9 ⚕ 11.9 **FUD** 010   J 62 80 ▥
AMA: 2014,Jan,11

+ **49326** with omentopexy (omental tacking procedure) (List
separately in addition to code for primary procedure)
Code first laparoscopy with permanent intraperitoneal cannula
or catheter insertion or revision of previously placed
catheter/cannula (49324, 49325)
📷 5.47 ⚕ 5.47 **FUD** ZZZ   N N1 80 ▥
AMA: 2014,Jan,11

+ **49327** with placement of interstitial device(s) for radiation
therapy guidance (eg, fiducial markers, dosimeter),
intra-abdominal, intrapelvic, and/or retroperitoneum,
including imaging guidance, if performed, single or
multiple (List separately in addition to code for primary
procedure)
EXCLUDES *Open approach (49412)*
Percutaneous approach (49411)
Code first laparoscopic abdominal, pelvic or retroperitoneal
procedures
📷 3.79 ⚕ 3.79 **FUD** ZZZ   N N1 80 ▥
AMA: 2014,Jan,11

49329 Unlisted laparoscopy procedure, abdomen, peritoneum and
omentum
📷 0.00 ⚕ 0.00 **FUD** YYY   J 80 50 ▥
AMA: 2019,Mar,10; 2018,Jan,8; 2017,Jan,8; 2016,Jan,13;
2015,Jan,16; 2014,Jan,11

49400-49436 Peritoneal and Visceral Procedures: Drainage/Insertion/Modifications/Removal

49400 Injection of air or contrast into peritoneal cavity (separate
procedure)
📷 (74190)
📷 2.68 ⚕ 3.93 **FUD** 000   N N1 ▥
AMA: 2018,Jan,8; 2017,Jan,8; 2016,Jan,13; 2015,Jan,16;
2014,Jan,11

49402 Removal of peritoneal foreign body from peritoneal cavity
EXCLUDES *Enterolysis (44005)*
*Percutaneous or open drainage or lavage (49020, 49040,
49082-49084, 49406)*
*Percutaneous tunneled intraperitoneal catheter
insertion without subcutaneous port (49418)*
📷 24.8 ⚕ 24.8 **FUD** 090   J A2 ▥
AMA: 2014,Jan,11

49405 Image-guided fluid collection drainage by catheter (eg,
abscess, hematoma, seroma, lymphocele, cyst); visceral (eg,
kidney, liver, spleen, lung/mediastinum), percutaneous
INCLUDES *Radiological guidance (75989, 76942, 77002-77003,
77012, 77021)*
EXCLUDES *Open drainage (47010, 48510, 50020)*
Percutaneous cholecystostomy (47490)
Percutaneous pleural drainage (32556-32557)
Pneumonostomy (32200)
Thoracentesis (32554-32555)
Code also each individual collection drained per separate
catheter
📷 5.72 ⚕ 23.9 **FUD** 000   J ▥
AMA: 2018,Jan,8; 2017,Jan,8; 2016,Jan,13; 2015,Jan,16;
2014,May,9; 2014,Jan,11

49406 peritoneal or retroperitoneal, percutaneous
INCLUDES *Radiological guidance (75989, 76942, 77002-77003,
77012, 77021)*
EXCLUDES *Diagnostic or therapeutic percutaneous abdominal
paracentesis (49082-49083)*
*Open peritoneal/retroperitoneal drainage (44900,
49020-49062, 49084, 50020, 58805, 58822)*
Open transrectal drainage pelvic abscess (45000)
*Percutaneous tunneled intraperitoneal catheter
insertion without subcutaneous port (49418)*
*Transrectal/transvaginal image-guided
peritoneal/retroperitoneal drainage via catheter
(49407)*
Code also each individual collection drained per separate
catheter
📷 5.72 ⚕ 23.9 **FUD** 000   J 62 ▥
AMA: 2018,Jan,8; 2017,Jan,8; 2016,Jan,13; 2015,Jan,16;
2014,May,9; 2014,Jan,11

28/TC PC/TC Only   A2-Z3 ASC Payment   50 Bilateral   ♂ Male Only   ♀ Female Only   📷 Facility RVU   ⚕ Non-Facility RVU   ▥ CCI   ✖ CLIA
FUD Follow-up Days   CMS: IOM   AMA: CPT Asst   A-Y OPPSI   80/80 Surg Assist Allowed / w/Doc   ▦ Lab Crosswalk   ✚ Radiology Crosswalk

232   CPT © 2019 American Medical Association. All Rights Reserved.   © 2019 Optum360, LLC

49407 peritoneal or retroperitoneal, transvaginal or transrectal

> INCLUDES Radiological guidance (75989, 76942, 77002-77003, 77012, 77021)
>
> EXCLUDES Image guided percutaneous catheter drainage of soft tissue (eg, abdominal wall, neck, extremity) (10030)
> Open transrectal/transvaginal drainage (45000, 58800, 58820)
> Percutaneous pleural drainage (32556-32557)
> Peritoneal drainage or lavage, open or percutaneous (49020, 49040, 49060)
> Thoracentesis (32554-32555)
> Code also each individual collection drained per separate catheter

6.06   19.4   **FUD** 000   J 62 ▢

AMA: 2018,Jan,8; 2017,Jan,8; 2016,Jan,13; 2015,Jan,16; 2014,May,9; 2014,Jan,11

49411 Placement of interstitial device(s) for radiation therapy guidance (eg, fiducial markers, dosimeter), percutaneous, intra-abdominal, intra-pelvic (except prostate), and/or retroperitoneum, single or multiple

> EXCLUDES Placement (percutaneous) of interstitial device(s) for intrathoracic radiation therapy guidance (32553)
> Code also supply of device
> (76942, 77002, 77012, 77021)

5.34   13.7   **FUD** 000   S P3 80 ▢

AMA: 2018,Jan,8; 2017,Jan,8; 2016,Jun,3; 2016,Jan,13; 2015,Jan,16; 2014,Jan,11

+ **49412** Placement of interstitial device(s) for radiation therapy guidance (eg, fiducial markers, dosimeter), open, intra-abdominal, intrapelvic, and/or retroperitoneum, including image guidance, if performed, single or multiple (List separately in addition to code for primary procedure)

> EXCLUDES Laparoscopic approach (49327)
> Percutaneous approach (49411)
> Code first open abdominal, pelvic or retroperitoneal procedure(s)

2.41   2.41   **FUD** ZZZ   C 80 ▢

AMA: 2014,Jan,11

49418 Insertion of tunneled intraperitoneal catheter (eg, dialysis, intraperitoneal chemotherapy instillation, management of ascites), complete procedure, including imaging guidance, catheter placement, contrast injection when performed, and radiological supervision and interpretation, percutaneous

5.89   36.1   **FUD** 000   J 62 80 ▢

AMA: 2014,Jan,11

49419 Insertion of tunneled intraperitoneal catheter, with subcutaneous port (ie, totally implantable)

> EXCLUDES Removal of catheter/cannula (49422)

12.7   12.7   **FUD** 090   T A2 ▢

AMA: 2014,Jan,11

49421 Insertion of tunneled intraperitoneal catheter for dialysis, open

> EXCLUDES Laparoscopic approach (49324)
> Code also insertion of subcutaneous extension to intraperitoneal cannula with remote chest exit site, when appropriate (49435)

6.64   6.64   **FUD** 000   J 62 ▢

AMA: 2018,Jan,8; 2017,Jan,8; 2016,Jan,13; 2015,Jan,16; 2014,Jan,11

49422 Removal of tunneled intraperitoneal catheter

> EXCLUDES Removal temporary catheter or cannula (Use appropriate E&M code)

6.46   6.46   **FUD** 000   02 A2 ▢

AMA: 2014,Jan,11

49423 Exchange of previously placed abscess or cyst drainage catheter under radiological guidance (separate procedure)

> (75984)

2.07   16.1   **FUD** 000   J 62 80 ▢

AMA: 2018,Jan,8; 2017,Jan,8; 2016,Jan,13; 2015,Jan,16; 2014,Jan,11

49424 Contrast injection for assessment of abscess or cyst via previously placed drainage catheter or tube (separate procedure)

> (76080)

1.10   4.35   **FUD** 000   N N1 80 ▢

AMA: 2018,Jan,8; 2017,Jan,8; 2016,Jan,13; 2015,Jan,16; 2014,Jan,11

49425 Insertion of peritoneal-venous shunt

20.8   20.8   **FUD** 090   C 80 ▢

AMA: 2014,Jan,11

49426 Revision of peritoneal-venous shunt

> EXCLUDES Shunt patency test (78291)

17.8   17.8   **FUD** 090   J A2 ▢

AMA: 2014,Jan,11

49427 Injection procedure (eg, contrast media) for evaluation of previously placed peritoneal-venous shunt

> (75809, 78291)

1.32   1.32   **FUD** 000   N N1 80 ▢

AMA: 2014,Jan,11

49428 Ligation of peritoneal-venous shunt

12.5   12.5   **FUD** 010   C ▢

AMA: 2014,Jan,11

49429 Removal of peritoneal-venous shunt

13.3   13.3   **FUD** 010   02 62 ▢

AMA: 2014,Jan,11

+ **49435** Insertion of subcutaneous extension to intraperitoneal cannula or catheter with remote chest exit site (List separately in addition to code for primary procedure)

> Code first permanent insertion of intraperitoneal catheter/cannula (49324, 49421)

3.45   3.45   **FUD** ZZZ   N N1 80 ▢

AMA: 2014,Jan,11

49436 Delayed creation of exit site from embedded subcutaneous segment of intraperitoneal cannula or catheter

5.36   5.36   **FUD** 010   J 62 80 ▢

AMA: 2014,Jan,11

49440-49442 Insertion of Percutaneous Gastrointestinal Tube

> EXCLUDES Naso- or oro-gastric tube placement (43752)

49440 Insertion of gastrostomy tube, percutaneous, under fluoroscopic guidance including contrast injection(s), image documentation and report

> INCLUDES Needle placement with fluoroscopic guidance (77002)
> Code also gastrostomy to gastro-jejunostomy tube conversion with initial gastrostomy tube insertion, when performed (49446)

5.96   26.9   **FUD** 010   J 62 80 ▢

AMA: 2018,Jan,8; 2017,Jan,8; 2016,Jan,13; 2015,Jan,16; 2014,Dec,18; 2014,Sep,5; 2014,Jan,11

49441 Insertion of duodenostomy or jejunostomy tube, percutaneous, under fluoroscopic guidance including contrast injection(s), image documentation and report

> EXCLUDES Gastrostomy tube to gastrojejunostomy tube conversion (49446)

7.00   30.6   **FUD** 010   J 62 80 ▢

AMA: 2018,Jan,8; 2017,Jan,8; 2016,Jan,13; 2015,Jan,16; 2014,Dec,18; 2014,Sep,5; 2014,Jan,11

Digestive System (side tab)

49442 — 49505 (side tab)

49442   Insertion of cecostomy or other colonic tube, percutaneous, under fluoroscopic guidance including contrast injection(s), image documentation and report

     🔷 6.04   ⚕ 25.4   **FUD** 010   T 62 80 ▭

     AMA: 2018,Jan,8; 2017,Jan,8; 2016,Jan,13; 2015,Jan,16; 2014,Dec,18; 2014,Sep,5; 2014,Jan,11

49446 Percutaneous Conversion: Gastrostomy to Gastro-jejunostomy Tube

EXCLUDES   *Code also initial gastrostomy tube insertion (49440) when conversion is performed at the same time*

49446   Conversion of gastrostomy tube to gastro-jejunostomy tube, percutaneous, under fluoroscopic guidance including contrast injection(s), image documentation and report

     🔷 4.30   ⚕ 25.9   **FUD** 000   J 62 80 ▭

     AMA: 2018,Jan,8; 2017,Jan,8; 2016,Jan,13; 2015,Jan,16; 2014,Sep,5; 2014,Jan,11

49450-49452 Replacement Gastrointestinal Tube

EXCLUDES   *Placement of new tube whether gastrostomy, jejunostomy, duodenostomy, gastro-jejunostomy, or cecostomy at different percutaneous site (49440-49442)*

49450   Replacement of gastrostomy or cecostomy (or other colonic) tube, percutaneous, under fluoroscopic guidance including contrast injection(s), image documentation and report

     EXCLUDES   *Change of gastrostomy tube, percutaneous, without imaging or endoscopic guidance (43762-43763)*

     🔷 1.92   ⚕ 18.8   **FUD** 000   T 62 80 ▭

     AMA: 2019,Feb,5; 2018,Jan,8; 2017,Jan,8; 2016,Jan,13; 2015,Jan,16; 2014,Sep,5; 2014,Jan,11

49451   Replacement of duodenostomy or jejunostomy tube, percutaneous, under fluoroscopic guidance including contrast injection(s), image documentation and report

     🔷 2.62   ⚕ 20.4   **FUD** 000   T 62 80 ▭

     AMA: 2018,Jan,8; 2017,Jan,8; 2016,Jan,13; 2015,Jan,16; 2014,Dec,18; 2014,Sep,5; 2014,Jan,11

49452   Replacement of gastro-jejunostomy tube, percutaneous, under fluoroscopic guidance including contrast injection(s), image documentation and report

     🔷 4.01   ⚕ 25.1   **FUD** 000   T 62 80 ▭

     AMA: 2018,Jan,8; 2017,Jan,8; 2016,Jan,13; 2015,Jan,16; 2014,Sep,5; 2014,Jan,11

49460-49465 Removal of Obstruction/Injection for Contrast Through Gastrointestinal Tube

49460   Mechanical removal of obstructive material from gastrostomy, duodenostomy, jejunostomy, gastro-jejunostomy, or cecostomy (or other colonic) tube, any method, under fluoroscopic guidance including contrast injection(s), if performed, image documentation and report

     INCLUDES   Contrast injection (49465)

     EXCLUDES   *Replacement of gastrointestinal tube (49450-49452)*

     🔷 1.39   ⚕ 20.4   **FUD** 000   T 62 80 ▭

     AMA: 2018,Jan,8; 2017,Jan,8; 2016,Jan,13; 2015,Jan,16; 2014,Sep,5; 2014,Jan,11

49465   Contrast injection(s) for radiological evaluation of existing gastrostomy, duodenostomy, jejunostomy, gastro-jejunostomy, or cecostomy (or other colonic) tube, from a percutaneous approach including image documentation and report

     EXCLUDES   *Mechanical removal of obstructive material from gastrointestinal tube (49460)*
                      Replacement of gastrointestinal tube (49450-49452)

     🔷 0.89   ⚕ 4.48   **FUD** 000   Q1 62 80 ▭

     AMA: 2018,Jan,8; 2017,Jan,8; 2016,Jan,13; 2015,Jan,16; 2014,Sep,5; 2014,Jan,11

49491-49492 Inguinal Hernia Repair on Premature Infant

INCLUDES   Hernia repairs done on preterm infants younger than or equal to 50 weeks postconception age but younger than 6 months of age since birth
        Initial repair: no previous repair required
        Mesh or other prosthesis

EXCLUDES   *Abdominal wall debridement (11042, 11043)*
        Intra-abdominal hernia repair/reduction (44050)

Code also repair or excision of testicle(s), intestine, ovaries if performed (44120, 54520, 58940)

49491   Repair, initial inguinal hernia, preterm infant (younger than 37 weeks gestation at birth), performed from birth up to 50 weeks postconception age, with or without hydrocelectomy; reducible   A

     🔷 23.0   ⚕ 23.0   **FUD** 090   63 J 80 50 ▭

     AMA: 2018,Jan,8; 2017,Jan,8; 2016,Jan,13; 2015,Jan,16; 2014,Jan,11

49492   incarcerated or strangulated   A

     🔷 27.7   ⚕ 27.7   **FUD** 090   63 J 80 50 ▭

     AMA: 2018,Jan,8; 2017,Jan,8; 2016,Jan,13; 2015,Jan,16; 2014,Jan,11

49495-49557 Hernia Repair: Femoral/Inguinal /Lumbar

INCLUDES   Initial repair: no previous repair required
        Mesh or other prosthesis
        Recurrent repair: required previous repair(s)

EXCLUDES   *Abdominal wall debridement (11042, 11043)*
        Intra-abdominal hernia repair/reduction (44050)

Code also repair or excision of testicle(s), intestine, ovaries if performed (44120, 54520, 58940)

49495   Repair, initial inguinal hernia, full term infant younger than age 6 months, or preterm infant older than 50 weeks postconception age and younger than age 6 months at the time of surgery, with or without hydrocelectomy; reducible   A

     INCLUDES   Hernia repairs done on preterm infants older than 50 weeks postconception age and younger than 6 months

     🔷 11.8   ⚕ 11.8   **FUD** 090   63 J A2 80 50 ▭

     AMA: 2018,Jan,8; 2017,Jan,8; 2016,Jan,13; 2015,Jan,16; 2014,Jan,11

49496   incarcerated or strangulated   A

     INCLUDES   Hernia repairs done on preterm infants older than 50 weeks postconception age and younger than 6 months

     🔷 17.7   ⚕ 17.7   **FUD** 090   63 J A2 80 50 ▭

     AMA: 2018,Jan,8; 2017,Jan,8; 2016,Jan,13; 2015,Jan,16; 2014,Jan,11

49500   Repair initial inguinal hernia, age 6 months to younger than 5 years, with or without hydrocelectomy; reducible   A

     INCLUDES   Repairs performed on patients 6 months to younger than 5 years old

     🔷 11.9   ⚕ 11.9   **FUD** 090   J A2 80 50 ▭

     AMA: 2018,Jan,8; 2017,Jan,8; 2016,Jan,13; 2015,Jan,16; 2014,Nov,14; 2014,Jan,11

49501   incarcerated or strangulated   A

     INCLUDES   Repairs performed on patients 6 months to younger than 5 years old

     🔷 17.5   ⚕ 17.5   **FUD** 090   J A2 80 50 ▭

     AMA: 2018,Jan,8; 2017,Jan,8; 2016,Jan,13; 2015,Jan,16; 2014,Jan,11

49505   Repair initial inguinal hernia, age 5 years or older; reducible   A

     INCLUDES   MacEwen hernia repair
     Code also when performed:
        Excision of hydrocele (55040)
        Excision of spermatocele (54840)
        Simple orchiectomy (54520)

     🔷 15.0   ⚕ 15.0   **FUD** 090   J A2 80 50 ▭

     AMA: 2018,Jan,8; 2017,Jan,8; 2016,Jan,13; 2015,Jan,16; 2014,Jan,11

26/TC PC/TC Only   A2-Z3 ASC Payment   50 Bilateral   ♂ Male Only   ♀ Female Only   🔷 Facility RVU   ⚕ Non-Facility RVU   ▭ CCI   ✖ CLIA
FUD Follow-up Days   CMS: IOM   AMA: CPT Asst   A-Y OPPSI   80/80 Surg Assist Allowed / w/Doc   ◣ Lab Crosswalk   ▣ Radiology Crosswalk

                     CPT © 2019 American Medical Association. All Rights Reserved.   © 2019 Optum360, LLC

49507   **incarcerated or strangulated**   Ⓐ

    Code also when performed:
      Excision of hydrocele (55040)
      Excision of spermatocele (54840)
      Simple orchiectomy (54520)
    🖧 16.9   ⚕ 16.9   **FUD** 090   J A2 80 50 ▭

    AMA: 2018,Jan,8; 2017,Jan,8; 2016,Jan,13; 2015,Jan,16; 2014,Jan,11

49520   **Repair recurrent inguinal hernia, any age; reducible**

    🖧 18.3   ⚕ 18.3   **FUD** 090   J A2 80 50 ▭

    AMA: 2018,Jan,8; 2017,Jan,8; 2016,Jan,13; 2015,Jan,16; 2014,Jan,11

49521   **incarcerated or strangulated**

    🖧 20.7   ⚕ 20.7   **FUD** 090   J A2 80 50 ▭

    AMA: 2018,Jan,8; 2017,Jan,8; 2016,Jan,13; 2015,Jan,16; 2014,Jan,11

49525   **Repair inguinal hernia, sliding, any age**

    EXCLUDES   *Inguinal hernia repair, incarcerated/strangulated (49496, 49501, 49507, 49521)*
    🖧 16.6   ⚕ 16.6   **FUD** 090   J A2 80 50 ▭

    AMA: 2018,Jan,8; 2017,Jan,8; 2016,Jan,13; 2015,Jan,16; 2014,Jan,11

Peritoneal lining is forced through a defect in the inguinal wall

A peritoneal sac is created

Sliding inguinal hernia

Anterior inguinal wall

Spermatic cord

Inguinal ligament

Femoral sheath

Because the bowel is attached to the peritoneum, it is pulled through the abdominal defect as well

49540   **Repair lumbar hernia**

    🖧 19.5   ⚕ 19.5   **FUD** 090   J A2 80 50 ▭

    AMA: 2018,Jan,8; 2017,Jan,8; 2016,Jan,13; 2015,Jan,16; 2014,Jan,11

49550   **Repair initial femoral hernia, any age; reducible**

    🖧 16.6   ⚕ 16.6   **FUD** 090   J A2 80 50 ▭

    AMA: 2018,Jan,8; 2017,Jan,8; 2016,Jan,13; 2015,Jan,16; 2014,Jan,11

49553   **incarcerated or strangulated**

    🖧 18.3   ⚕ 18.3   **FUD** 090   J A2 80 50 ▭

    AMA: 2018,Jan,8; 2017,Jan,8; 2016,Jan,13; 2015,Jan,16; 2014,Jan,11

49555   **Repair recurrent femoral hernia; reducible**

    🖧 17.3   ⚕ 17.3   **FUD** 090   J A2 80 50 ▭

    AMA: 2018,Jan,8; 2017,Jan,8; 2016,Jan,13; 2015,Jan,16; 2014,Jan,11

49557   **incarcerated or strangulated**

    🖧 20.9   ⚕ 20.9   **FUD** 090   J A2 80 50 ▭

    AMA: 2018,Jan,8; 2017,Jan,8; 2016,Jan,13; 2015,Jan,16; 2014,Jan,11

49560-49568 Hernia Repair: Incisional/Ventral

INCLUDES   Initial repair: no previous repair required
            Recurrent repair: required previous repair(s)
EXCLUDES   *Abdominal wall debridement (11042, 11043)*
            Intra-abdominal hernia repair/reduction (44050)
Code also repair or excision of testicle(s), intestine, ovaries if performed (44120, 54520, 58940)

49560   **Repair initial incisional or ventral hernia; reducible**

    Code also implantation of mesh or other prosthesis if performed (49568)
    🖧 21.3   ⚕ 21.3   **FUD** 090   J A2 80 50 ▭

    AMA: 2018,Jan,8; 2017,Jan,8; 2016,Jan,13; 2015,Jan,16; 2014,Jan,11

49561   **incarcerated or strangulated**

    Code also implantation of mesh or other prosthesis if performed (49568)
    🖧 26.9   ⚕ 26.9   **FUD** 090   J A2 80 50 ▭

    AMA: 2018,Jul,14; 2018,Mar,11; 2018,Jan,8; 2017,Jan,8; 2016,Jan,13; 2015,Jan,16; 2014,Jan,11

49565   **Repair recurrent incisional or ventral hernia; reducible**

    Code also implantation of mesh or other prosthesis if performed (49568)
    🖧 22.2   ⚕ 22.2   **FUD** 090   J A2 80 50 ▭

    AMA: 2018,Jan,8; 2017,Jan,8; 2016,Jan,13; 2015,Jan,16; 2014,Jan,11

49566   **incarcerated or strangulated**

    Code also implantation of mesh or other prosthesis if performed (49568)
    🖧 27.1   ⚕ 27.1   **FUD** 090   J A2 80 50 ▭

    AMA: 2018,Jan,8; 2017,Jan,8; 2016,Jan,13; 2015,Jan,16; 2014,Jan,11

+   **49568**   **Implantation of mesh or other prosthesis for open incisional or ventral hernia repair or mesh for closure of debridement for necrotizing soft tissue infection (List separately in addition to code for the incisional or ventral hernia repair)**

    EXCLUDES   *Reporting with modifier 50. Report once for each side when performed bilaterally*
    Code first (11004-11006, 49560-49566)
    🖧 7.77   ⚕ 7.77   **FUD** ZZZ   50 N N1 80 ▭

    AMA: 2018,Jan,8; 2017,Jan,8; 2016,Jan,13; 2015,Jan,16; 2014,Jan,11

49570-49590 Hernia Repair: Epigastric/Lateral Ventral/Umbilical

INCLUDES   Mesh or other prosthesis
EXCLUDES   *Abdominal wall debridement (11042, 11043)*
            Intra-abdominal hernia repair/reduction (44050)
Code also repair or excision of testicle(s), intestine, ovaries if performed (44120, 54520, 58940)

49570   **Repair epigastric hernia (eg, preperitoneal fat); reducible (separate procedure)**

    🖧 12.0   ⚕ 12.0   **FUD** 090   J A2 80 50 ▭

    AMA: 2018,Jan,8; 2017,Jan,8; 2016,Jan,13; 2015,Jan,16; 2014,Jan,11

49572   **incarcerated or strangulated**

    🖧 14.9   ⚕ 14.9   **FUD** 090   J A2 80 50 ▭

    AMA: 2018,Jan,8; 2017,Jan,8; 2016,Jan,13; 2015,Jan,16; 2014,Jan,11

49580   **Repair umbilical hernia, younger than age 5 years; reducible**   Ⓐ

    🖧 9.63   ⚕ 9.63   **FUD** 090   J A2 80 ▭

    AMA: 2018,Jan,8; 2017,Jan,8; 2016,Jan,13; 2015,Jan,16; 2014,Jan,11

49582   **incarcerated or strangulated**   Ⓐ

    🖧 13.9   ⚕ 13.9   **FUD** 090   J A2 80 ▭

    AMA: 2018,Jan,8; 2017,Jan,8; 2016,Jan,13; 2015,Jan,16; 2014,Jan,11

49585 Repair umbilical hernia, age 5 years or older; reducible　A

INCLUDES　Mayo hernia repair

🚑 12.8　⚕ 12.8　**FUD** 090　　J A2 80 ▢

AMA: 2018,Jan,8; 2017,Jan,8; 2016,Jan,13; 2015,Jan,16; 2014,Jan,11

49587 incarcerated or strangulated　A

🚑 13.7　⚕ 13.7　**FUD** 090　　J A2 80 ▢

AMA: 2018,Jan,8; 2017,Jan,8; 2016,Jan,13; 2015,Jan,16; 2014,Jan,11

49590 Repair spigelian hernia

🚑 16.5　⚕ 16.5　**FUD** 090　　J A2 80 50 ▢

AMA: 2018,Jan,8; 2017,Jan,8; 2016,Jan,13; 2015,Jan,16; 2014,Jan,11

49600-49611 Repair Birth Defect Abdominal Wall: Omphalocele/Gastroschisis

INCLUDES　Mesh or other prosthesis

EXCLUDES　Abdominal wall debridement (11042, 11043)
Intra-abdominal hernia repair/reduction (44050)
Repair of:
　Diaphragmatic or hiatal hernia (39503, 43332-43337)
　Omentum (49999)

49600 Repair of small omphalocele, with primary closure

🚑 21.2　⚕ 21.2　**FUD** 090　　63 J A2 80 ▢

AMA: 2018,Jan,8; 2017,Jan,8; 2016,Jan,13; 2015,Jan,16; 2014,Jan,11

49605 Repair of large omphalocele or gastroschisis; with or without prosthesis

🚑 144.　⚕ 144.　**FUD** 090　　63 C 80 ▢

AMA: 2018,Jan,8; 2017,Jan,8; 2016,Jan,13; 2015,Jan,16; 2014,Jan,11

49606 with removal of prosthesis, final reduction and closure, in operating room

🚑 32.9　⚕ 32.9　**FUD** 090　　63 C 80 ▢

AMA: 2018,Jan,8; 2017,Jan,8; 2016,Jan,13; 2015,Jan,16; 2014,Jan,11

49610 Repair of omphalocele (Gross type operation); first stage

🚑 19.9　⚕ 19.9　**FUD** 090　　63 C 80 ▢

AMA: 2018,Jan,8; 2017,Jan,8; 2016,Jan,13; 2015,Jan,16; 2014,Jan,11

49611 second stage

🚑 17.6　⚕ 17.6　**FUD** 090　　63 C 80 ▢

AMA: 2018,Jan,8; 2017,Jan,8; 2016,Jan,13; 2015,Jan,16; 2014,Jan,11

49650-49659 Laparoscopic Hernia Repair

INCLUDES　Diagnostic laparoscopy (49320)

49650 Laparoscopy, surgical; repair initial inguinal hernia

🚑 12.4　⚕ 12.4　**FUD** 090　　J A2 80 50 ▢

AMA: 2018,Jan,8; 2017,Jan,8; 2016,Jan,13; 2015,Jan,16; 2014,Jul,5; 2014,Jan,11

49651 repair recurrent inguinal hernia

🚑 16.1　⚕ 16.1　**FUD** 090　　J A2 80 50 ▢

AMA: 2018,Jan,8; 2017,Jan,8; 2016,Jan,13; 2015,Jan,16; 2014,Jan,11

49652 Laparoscopy, surgical, repair, ventral, umbilical, spigelian or epigastric hernia (includes mesh insertion, when performed); reducible

INCLUDES　Laparoscopy, surgical, enterolysis (44180)

EXCLUDES　Implantation of mesh or other prosthesis (49568)

🚑 21.5　⚕ 21.5　**FUD** 090　　J 62 80 50 ▢

AMA: 2014,Jan,11

49653 incarcerated or strangulated

INCLUDES　Laparoscopy, surgical, enterolysis (44180)

EXCLUDES　Implantation of mesh or other prosthesis (49568)

🚑 26.9　⚕ 26.9　**FUD** 090　　J 62 80 50 ▢

AMA: 2014,Jan,11

49654 Laparoscopy, surgical, repair, incisional hernia (includes mesh insertion, when performed); reducible

INCLUDES　Laparoscopy, surgical, enterolysis (44180)

EXCLUDES　Implantation of mesh or other prosthesis (49568)

🚑 24.4　⚕ 24.4　**FUD** 090　　J 62 80 50 ▢

AMA: 2018,Jan,7; 2014,Jan,11

49655 incarcerated or strangulated

INCLUDES　Laparoscopy, surgical, enterolysis (44180)

EXCLUDES　Implantation of mesh or other prosthesis (49568)

🚑 29.9　⚕ 29.9　**FUD** 090　　J 62 80 50 ▢

AMA: 2018,Jan,7; 2014,Jan,11

49656 Laparoscopy, surgical, repair, recurrent incisional hernia (includes mesh insertion, when performed); reducible

INCLUDES　Laparoscopy, surgical, enterolysis (44180)

EXCLUDES　Implantation of mesh or other prosthesis (49568)

🚑 26.5　⚕ 26.5　**FUD** 090　　J 62 80 50 ▢

AMA: 2014,Jan,11

49657 incarcerated or strangulated

INCLUDES　Laparoscopy, surgical, enterolysis (44180)

EXCLUDES　Implantation of mesh or other prosthesis (49568)

🚑 38.2　⚕ 38.2　**FUD** 090　　J 62 80 50 ▢

AMA: 2014,Jan,11

49659 Unlisted laparoscopy procedure, hernioplasty, herniorrhaphy, herniotomy

🚑 0.00　⚕ 0.00　**FUD** YYY　　J 80 50 ▢

AMA: 2018,Jan,8; 2017,Jul,10; 2017,Jan,8; 2016,Jan,13; 2015,Jan,16; 2014,Dec,16; 2014,Dec,16; 2014,Jul,5; 2014,Jan,11

49900 Surgical Repair Abdominal Wall

EXCLUDES　Abdominal wall debridement (11042, 11043)
Suture of ruptured diaphragm (39540-39541)

49900 Suture, secondary, of abdominal wall for evisceration or dehiscence

🚑 23.6　⚕ 23.6　**FUD** 090　　C 80 ▢

AMA: 2018,Jan,8; 2017,Jan,8; 2016,Jan,13; 2015,Jan,16; 2014,Jan,11

49904-49999 Harvesting of Omental Flap

49904 Omental flap, extra-abdominal (eg, for reconstruction of sternal and chest wall defects)

INCLUDES　Harvest and transfer

EXCLUDES　Omental flap harvest by second surgeon: both surgeons report code with modifier 62

🚑 40.9　⚕ 40.9　**FUD** 090　　C ▢

AMA: 2014,Jan,11

+ 49905 Omental flap, intra-abdominal (List separately in addition to code for primary procedure)

EXCLUDES　Exclusion of small intestine from pelvis by mesh or other prosthesis, or native tissue (44700)

Code first primary procedure

🚑 10.2　⚕ 10.2　**FUD** ZZZ　　C 80 ▢

AMA: 2018,Jan,8; 2017,Jan,8; 2016,Jan,13; 2015,Jan,16; 2014,Jan,11

49906 Free omental flap with microvascular anastomosis

INCLUDES　Operating microscope (69990)

🚑 0.00　⚕ 0.00　**FUD** 090　　C ▢

AMA: 2018,Jan,8; 2017,Jan,8; 2016,Feb,12; 2016,Jan,13; 2015,Jan,16; 2014,Jan,11

49999 Unlisted procedure, abdomen, peritoneum and omentum

🚑 0.00　⚕ 0.00　**FUD** YYY　　T ▢

AMA: 2018,Jan,8; 2017,Jan,8; 2016,Jan,13; 2015,Jan,16; 2014,Jan,9; 2014,Jan,11

   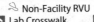

26/TC PC/TC Only　A2-Z3 ASC Payment　50 Bilateral　♂ Male Only　♀ Female Only　🚑 Facility RVU　⚕ Non-Facility RVU　▢ CCI　X CLIA
FUD Follow-up Days　CMS: IOM　AMA: CPT Asst　A-Y OPPSI　80/80 Surg Assist Allowed / w/Doc　Lab Crosswalk　Radiology Crosswalk

236　CPT © 2019 American Medical Association. All Rights Reserved.　© 2019 Optum360, LLC

50010-50045 Kidney Procedures for Exploration or Drainage

EXCLUDES Donor nephrectomy performed laparoscopically (50547)
Retroperitoneal
Abscess drainage (49060)
Exploration (49010)
Tumor/cyst excision (49203-49205)

50010 **Renal exploration, not necessitating other specific procedures**

EXCLUDES Laparoscopic ablation of mass lesions of kidney (50542)

🔧 21.2 ⚕ 21.2 **FUD** 090 C 80 50

AMA: 2014,Jan,11

Right kidney
Left kidney
Ureter
Minor calyces
Major calyces
Renal pelvis
Ureter
Medulla
Cortex

50020 **Drainage of perirenal or renal abscess, open**

EXCLUDES Image-guided percutaneous drainage of perirenal or renal abscess (49405)

🔧 29.3 ⚕ 29.3 **FUD** 090 J

AMA: 2018,Jan,8; 2017,Jan,8; 2016,Jan,13; 2015,Jan,16; 2014,May,9; 2014,Jan,11

50040 **Nephrostomy, nephrotomy with drainage**

🔧 26.8 ⚕ 26.8 **FUD** 090 C 50

AMA: 2018,Jan,8; 2017,Jan,8; 2016,Jan,13; 2015,Jan,16; 2014,Jan,11

50045 **Nephrotomy, with exploration**

EXCLUDES Renal endoscopy through nephrotomy (50570-50580)

🔧 26.9 ⚕ 26.9 **FUD** 090 C 80 50

AMA: 2018,Jan,8; 2017,Jan,8; 2016,Jan,13; 2015,Jan,16; 2014,Jan,11

50060-50081 Treatment of Kidney Stones

CMS: 100-03,230.1 NCD for Treatment of Kidney Stones

EXCLUDES Retroperitoneal:
Abscess drainage (49060)
Exploration (49010)
Tumor/cyst excision (49203-49205)

50060 **Nephrolithotomy; removal of calculus**

🔧 33.0 ⚕ 33.0 **FUD** 090 C 80 50

AMA: 2018,Jan,8; 2017,Jan,8; 2016,Jan,13; 2015,Jan,16; 2014,Jan,11

50065 **secondary surgical operation for calculus**

🔧 34.9 ⚕ 34.9 **FUD** 090 C 80 50

AMA: 2018,Jan,8; 2017,Jan,8; 2016,Jan,13; 2015,Jan,16; 2014,Jan,11

50070 **complicated by congenital kidney abnormality**

🔧 34.3 ⚕ 34.3 **FUD** 090 C 80 50

AMA: 2018,Jan,8; 2017,Jan,8; 2016,Jan,13; 2015,Jan,16; 2014,Jan,11

50075 **removal of large staghorn calculus filling renal pelvis and calyces (including anatrophic pyelolithotomy)**

🔧 42.1 ⚕ 42.1 **FUD** 090 C 80 50

AMA: 2018,Jan,8; 2017,Jan,8; 2016,Jan,13; 2015,Jan,16; 2014,Jan,11

50080 **Percutaneous nephrostolithotomy or pyelostolithotomy, with or without dilation, endoscopy, lithotripsy, stenting, or basket extraction; up to 2 cm**

EXCLUDES Dilation of existing tract by same provider ([50436, 50437])
Nephrostomy without nephrostolithotomy (50040, [50432, 50433], 52334)

📷 (76000)

🔧 25.1 ⚕ 25.1 **FUD** 090 J G2 50

AMA: 2018,Jan,8; 2017,Jan,8; 2016,Jan,13; 2015,Jan,16; 2014,Jan,11

50081 **over 2 cm**

EXCLUDES Dilation of existing tract by same provider ([50436, 50437])
Nephrostomy without nephrostolithotomy (50040, [50432, 50433], 52334)

📷 (76000)

🔧 36.9 ⚕ 36.9 **FUD** 090 J G2 80 50

AMA: 2018,Jan,8; 2017,Jan,8; 2016,Jan,13; 2015,Jan,16; 2014,Jan,11

50100 Repair of Anomalous Vessels of the Kidney

EXCLUDES Retroperitoneal:
Abscess drainage (49060)
Exploration (49010)
Tumor/cyst excision (49203-49205)

50100 **Transection or repositioning of aberrant renal vessels (separate procedure)**

🔧 31.3 ⚕ 31.3 **FUD** 090 C 80 50

AMA: 2018,Jan,8; 2017,Jan,8; 2016,Jan,13; 2015,Jan,16; 2014,Jan,11

50120-50135 Procedures of Renal Pelvis

EXCLUDES Retroperitoneal:
Abscess drainage (49060)
Exploration (49010)
Tumor/cyst excision (49203-49205)

50120 **Pyelotomy; with exploration**

INCLUDES Gol-Vernet pyelotomy

EXCLUDES Renal endoscopy through pyelotomy (50570-50580)

🔧 27.4 ⚕ 27.4 **FUD** 090 C 80 50

AMA: 2018,Jan,8; 2017,Jan,8; 2016,Jan,13; 2015,Jan,16; 2014,Jan,11

50125 **with drainage, pyelostomy**

🔧 28.4 ⚕ 28.4 **FUD** 090 C 80 50

AMA: 2018,Jan,8; 2017,Jan,8; 2016,Jan,13; 2015,Jan,16; 2014,Jan,11

50130 **with removal of calculus (pyelolithotomy, pelviolithotomy, including coagulum pyelolithotomy)**

🔧 29.9 ⚕ 29.9 **FUD** 090 C 80 50

AMA: 2018,Jan,8; 2017,Jan,8; 2016,Jan,13; 2015,Jan,16; 2014,Jan,11

50135 **complicated (eg, secondary operation, congenital kidney abnormality)**

🔧 32.4 ⚕ 32.4 **FUD** 090 C 80 50

AMA: 2018,Jan,8; 2017,Jan,8; 2016,Jan,13; 2015,Jan,16; 2014,Jan,11

50200-50205 Biopsy of Kidney

EXCLUDES Laparoscopic renal mass lesion ablation (50542)
Retroperitoneal tumor/cyst excision (49203-49205)

50200 **Renal biopsy; percutaneous, by trocar or needle**

EXCLUDES Fine needle aspiration ([10005, 10006, 10007, 10008, 10009, 10010, 10011, 10012])

📷 (76942, 77002, 77012, 77021)
🔬 (88172-88173)

🔧 3.71 ⚕ 15.2 **FUD** 000 J A2 50

AMA: 2019,Apr,4; 2018,Jan,8; 2017,Jan,8; 2016,Jan,13; 2015,Jan,16; 2014,Jan,11

50205 by surgical exposure of kidney

🔧 21.8 ⚕ 21.8 **FUD** 090 ⬜ C 80 50 ▢

AMA: 2018,Jan,8; 2017,Jan,8; 2016,Jan,13; 2015,Jan,16; 2014,Jan,11

50220-50240 Nephrectomy Procedures

EXCLUDES Laparoscopic renal mass lesion ablation (50542)
Retroperitoneal tumor/cyst excision (49203-49205)

50220 Nephrectomy, including partial ureterectomy, any open approach including rib resection;

🔧 30.3 ⚕ 30.3 **FUD** 090 ⬜ C 80 50 ▢

AMA: 2018,Jan,8; 2017,Jan,8; 2016,Jan,13; 2015,Jan,16; 2014,Jan,11

50225 complicated because of previous surgery on same kidney

🔧 34.8 ⚕ 34.8 **FUD** 090 ⬜ C 80 50 ▢

AMA: 2018,Jan,8; 2017,Jan,8; 2016,Jan,13; 2015,Jan,16; 2014,Jan,11

50230 radical, with regional lymphadenectomy and/or vena caval thrombectomy

EXCLUDES Vena caval resection with reconstruction (37799)

🔧 37.1 ⚕ 37.1 **FUD** 090 ⬜ C 80 50 ▢

AMA: 2018,Jan,8; 2017,Jan,8; 2016,Jan,13; 2015,Jan,16; 2014,Jan,11

50234 Nephrectomy with total ureterectomy and bladder cuff; through same incision

🔧 37.7 ⚕ 37.7 **FUD** 090 ⬜ C 80 50 ▢

AMA: 2018,Jan,8; 2017,Jan,8; 2016,Jan,13; 2015,Jan,16; 2014,Jan,11

50236 through separate incision

🔧 42.4 ⚕ 42.4 **FUD** 090 ⬜ C 80 50 ▢

AMA: 2018,Jan,8; 2017,Jan,8; 2016,Jan,13; 2015,Jan,16; 2014,Jan,11

50240 Nephrectomy, partial

EXCLUDES Laparoscopic partial nephrectomy (50543)

🔧 38.3 ⚕ 38.3 **FUD** 090 ⬜ C 80 50 ▢

AMA: 2018,Jan,8; 2017,Jan,8; 2016,Jan,13; 2015,Jan,16; 2014,Jan,11

50250-50290 Open Removal Kidney Lesions

EXCLUDES Open destruction or excision intra-abdominal tumors (49203-49205)

50250 Ablation, open, 1 or more renal mass lesion(s), cryosurgical, including intraoperative ultrasound guidance and monitoring, if performed

EXCLUDES Laparoscopic renal mass lesion ablation (50542)
Percutaneous renal tumor ablation (50592-50593)

🔧 35.1 ⚕ 35.1 **FUD** 090 ⬜ C 80 ▢

AMA: 2018,Jan,8; 2017,Jan,8; 2016,Jan,13; 2015,Jan,16; 2014,Jan,11

50280 Excision or unroofing of cyst(s) of kidney

EXCLUDES Renal cyst laparoscopic ablation (50541)

🔧 27.6 ⚕ 27.6 **FUD** 090 ⬜ C 80 50 ▢

AMA: 2018,Jan,8; 2017,Jan,8; 2016,Jan,13; 2015,Jan,16; 2014,Jan,11

50290 Excision of perinephric cyst

🔧 25.9 ⚕ 25.9 **FUD** 090 ⬜ C 80 ▢

AMA: 2018,Jan,8; 2017,Jan,8; 2016,Jan,13; 2015,Jan,16; 2014,Jan,11

50300-50380 Kidney Transplant Procedures

CMS: 100-04,3,90.1 Kidney Transplant - General; 100-04,3,90.1.1 Standard Kidney Acquisition Charge; 100-04,3,90.1.2 Billing for Kidney Transplant and Acquisition Services; 100-04,3,90.5 Pancreas Transplants with Kidney Transplants

EXCLUDES Dialysis procedures (90935-90999)
Lymphocele drainage to peritoneal cavity performed laparoscopically (49323)

50300 Donor nephrectomy (including cold preservation); from cadaver donor, unilateral or bilateral

INCLUDES Graft:
Cold preservation
Harvesting

EXCLUDES Donor nephrectomy performed laparoscopically (50547)

🔧 0.00 ⚕ 0.00 **FUD** XXX ⬜ C ▢

AMA: 2018,Jan,8; 2017,Jan,8; 2016,Jan,13; 2015,Jan,16; 2014,Jan,11

50320 open, from living donor

INCLUDES Donor care
Graft:
Cold preservation
Harvesting

EXCLUDES Donor nephrectomy performed laparoscopically (50547)

🔧 43.5 ⚕ 43.5 **FUD** 090 ⬜ C 80 50 ▢

AMA: 2018,Jan,8; 2017,Jan,8; 2016,Jan,13; 2015,Jan,16; 2014,Jan,11

50323 Backbench standard preparation of cadaver donor renal allograft prior to transplantation, including dissection and removal of perinephric fat, diaphragmatic and retroperitoneal attachments, excision of adrenal gland, and preparation of ureter(s), renal vein(s), and renal artery(s), ligating branches, as necessary

EXCLUDES Adrenalectomy (60540, 60545)

🔧 0.00 ⚕ 0.00 **FUD** XXX ⬜ C 80 ▢

AMA: 2018,Jan,8; 2017,Jan,8; 2016,Jan,13; 2015,Jan,16; 2014,Jan,11

50325 Backbench standard preparation of living donor renal allograft (open or laparoscopic) prior to transplantation, including dissection and removal of perinephric fat and preparation of ureter(s), renal vein(s), and renal artery(s), ligating branches, as necessary

🔧 0.00 ⚕ 0.00 **FUD** XXX ⬜ C 80 ▢

AMA: 2014,Jan,11

50327 Backbench reconstruction of cadaver or living donor renal allograft prior to transplantation; venous anastomosis, each

🔧 6.29 ⚕ 6.29 **FUD** XXX ⬜ C 80 ▢

AMA: 2014,Jan,11

50328 arterial anastomosis, each

🔧 5.51 ⚕ 5.51 **FUD** XXX ⬜ C 80 ▢

AMA: 2014,Jan,11

50329 ureteral anastomosis, each

🔧 5.24 ⚕ 5.24 **FUD** XXX ⬜ C 80 ▢

AMA: 2014,Jan,11

50340 Recipient nephrectomy (separate procedure)

🔧 27.4 ⚕ 27.4 **FUD** 090 ⬜ C 80 50 ▢

AMA: 2014,Jan,11

50360 Renal allotransplantation, implantation of graft; without recipient nephrectomy

INCLUDES Allograft transplantation
Recipient care
Code also backbench work (50323, 50325, 50327-50329)
Code also donor nephrectomy (cadaver or living donor) (50300, 50320, 50547)

🔧 70.0 ⚕ 70.0 **FUD** 090 ⬜ C 80 ▢

AMA: 2014,Jan,11

50365 with recipient nephrectomy

INCLUDES Allograft transplantation
Recipient care

⚕ 83.0 ⚕ 83.0 **FUD** 090

C 80 50 ▭

AMA: 2018,Jan,8; 2017,Jan,8; 2016,Jan,13; 2015,Jan,16;
2014,Jan,11

50370 **Removal of transplanted renal allograft**

⚕ 34.8 ⚕ 34.8 **FUD** 090

C 80 ▭

AMA: 2014,Jan,11

50380 **Renal autotransplantation, reimplantation of kidney**

INCLUDES Reimplantation of autograft
EXCLUDES Secondary procedures:
Nephrolithotomy (50060-50075)
Partial nephrectomy (50240, 50543)

⚕ 58.1 ⚕ 58.1 **FUD** 090

C 80 ▭

AMA: 2019,Sep,10; 2018,Jan,8; 2017,Jan,8; 2016,Jan,13;
2015,Jan,16; 2014,Jan,11

50382-50386 Removal With/Without Replacement Internal Ureteral Stent

INCLUDES Radiological supervision and interpretation

50382 **Removal (via snare/capture) and replacement of internally dwelling ureteral stent via percutaneous approach, including radiological supervision and interpretation**

EXCLUDES Dilation existing tract, percutaneous for endourologic
procedure ([50436, 50437])
Removal and replacement of an internally dwelling
ureteral stent using a transurethral approach
(50385)

⚕ 7.46 ⚕ 31.3 **FUD** 000

J 62 50 ▭

AMA: 2018,Jan,8; 2017,Jan,8; 2016,Jan,13; 2016,Jan,3;
2015,Jan,16; 2014,Jan,11

50384 **Removal (via snare/capture) of internally dwelling ureteral stent via percutaneous approach, including radiological supervision and interpretation**

EXCLUDES Dilation existing tract, percutaneous for endourologic
procedure ([50436, 50437])
Removal of an internally dwelling ureteral stent using
a transurethral approach (50386)

⚕ 6.68 ⚕ 25.0 **FUD** 000

02 62 50 ▭

AMA: 2018,Jan,8; 2017,Jan,8; 2016,Jan,13; 2016,Jan,3;
2015,Jan,16; 2014,Jan,11

50385 **Removal (via snare/capture) and replacement of internally dwelling ureteral stent via transurethral approach, without use of cystoscopy, including radiological supervision and interpretation**

⚕ 6.34 ⚕ 30.7 **FUD** 000

J 62 80 50 ▭

AMA: 2018,Jan,8; 2017,Jan,8; 2016,Jan,13; 2016,Jan,3;
2015,Jan,16; 2014,Jan,11

50386 **Removal (via snare/capture) of internally dwelling ureteral stent via transurethral approach, without use of cystoscopy, including radiological supervision and interpretation**

⚕ 4.70 ⚕ 20.3 **FUD** 000

02 P3 80 50 ▭

AMA: 2018,Jan,8; 2017,Jan,8; 2016,Jan,3; 2016,Jan,13;
2015,Jan,16; 2014,Jan,11

50387 Remove/Replace Accessible Ureteral Stent

EXCLUDES Removal and replacement of ureteral stent through ureterostomy tube or
ileal conduit (50688)
Removal without replacement of externally accessible ureteral stent without
fluoroscopic guidance, report with appropriate E&M code

50387 **Removal and replacement of externally accessible nephroureteral catheter (eg, external/internal stent) requiring fluoroscopic guidance, including radiological supervision and interpretation**

⚕ 2.43 ⚕ 14.6 **FUD** 000

J 62 80 50 ▭

AMA: 2018,Jan,8; 2017,Jan,8; 2016,Mar,10; 2016,Jan,13;
2016,Jan,3; 2015,Oct,5; 2015,Jan,16; 2014,Jan,11

50389-50435 [50430, 50431, 50432, 50433, 50434, 50435, 50436, 50437] Percutaneous and Injection Procedures With/Without Indwelling Tube/Catheter Access

50389 **Removal of nephrostomy tube, requiring fluoroscopic guidance (eg, with concurrent indwelling ureteral stent)**

EXCLUDES Nephrostomy tube removal without fluoroscopic
guidance, report with appropriate E&M code

⚕ 1.56 ⚕ 9.49 **FUD** 000

02 62 50 ▭

AMA: 2018,Jan,8; 2017,Jan,8; 2016,Jan,13; 2016,Jan,3;
2015,Oct,5; 2015,Jan,16; 2014,Jan,11

50390 **Aspiration and/or injection of renal cyst or pelvis by needle, percutaneous**

EXCLUDES Antegrade nephrostogram/pyelogram ([50430, 50431])
⚕ (74425, 74470, 76942, 77002, 77012, 77021)

⚕ 2.78 ⚕ 2.78 **FUD** 000

T A2 50 ▭

AMA: 2018,Jan,8; 2017,Jan,8; 2016,Jan,13; 2015,Oct,5;
2015,Jan,16; 2014,Jan,11

50391 **Instillation(s) of therapeutic agent into renal pelvis and/or ureter through established nephrostomy, pyelostomy or ureterostomy tube (eg, anticarcinogenic or antifungal agent)**

Code also therapeutic agent

⚕ 2.84 ⚕ 3.52 **FUD** 000

T P3 50 ▭

AMA: 2018,Jan,8; 2017,Jan,8; 2016,Jan,13; 2015,Oct,5;
2015,Jan,16; 2014,Jan,11

\# **50436** **Dilation of existing tract, percutaneous, for an endourologic procedure including imaging guidance (eg, ultrasound and/or fluoroscopy) and all associated radiological supervision and interpretation, with postprocedure tube placement, when performed**

⚕ 4.37 ⚕ 4.37 **FUD** 000

62 50 ▭

EXCLUDES Percutaneous nephrostolithotomy (50080-50081)
Procedure performed for same renal collecting
system/ureter ([50430, 50431, 50432, 50433],
52334, 74485)
Removal, replacement internally dwelling ureteral stent
(50382, 50384)

\# **50437** including new access into the renal collecting system

⚕ 7.29 ⚕ 7.29 **FUD** 000

62 50 ▭

EXCLUDES Percutaneous nephrostolithotomy (50080-50081)
Procedure performed for same renal collecting
system/ureter ([50430, 50431, 50432, 50433],
52334, 74485)
Removal, replacement internally dwelling ureteral stent
(50382, 50384)

50396 **Manometric studies through nephrostomy or pyelostomy tube, or indwelling ureteral catheter**

⚕ (74425)

⚕ 3.38 ⚕ 3.38 **FUD** 000

J A2 80 50 ▭

AMA: 2018,Jan,8; 2017,Jan,8; 2016,Jan,13; 2015,Jan,16;
2014,Jan,11

50365 — 50396

Urinary System *(left margin)*

50430 Injection procedure for antegrade nephrostogram and/or ureterogram, complete diagnostic procedure including imaging guidance (eg, ultrasound and fluoroscopy) and all associated radiological supervision and interpretation; new access

INCLUDES Renal pelvis and associated ureter as a single element

EXCLUDES *Procedure performed for same renal collecting system/ureter ([50432, 50433, 50434, 50435], 50693-50695, 74425)*

4.46　14.5　**FUD** 000　02 N1 80 50

AMA: 2018,Jan,8; 2017,Jan,8; 2016,Jan,3; 2016,Jan,13; 2015,Oct,5

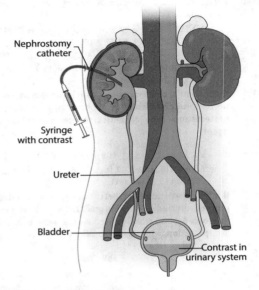

Nephrostomy catheter

Syringe with contrast

Ureter

Bladder

Contrast in urinary system

50431 existing access

INCLUDES Renal pelvis and associated ureter as a single element

EXCLUDES *Procedure performed for same renal collecting system/ureter ([50432, 50433, 50434, 50435], 50693-50695, 74425)*

1.90　6.03　**FUD** 000　02 N1 50

AMA: 2018,Jan,8; 2017,Jan,8; 2016,Jan,3; 2016,Jan,13; 2015,Oct,5

50432 Placement of nephrostomy catheter, percutaneous, including diagnostic nephrostogram and/or ureterogram when performed, imaging guidance (eg, ultrasound and/or fluoroscopy) and all associated radiological supervision and interpretation

INCLUDES Renal pelvis and associated ureter as a single element

EXCLUDES *Dilation of nephroureteral catheter tract ([50436, 50437])*
Procedure performed for same renal collecting system/ureter ([50430, 50431], [50433], 50694-50695, 74425)

5.98　23.5　**FUD** 000　J 02 50

AMA: 2018,Mar,11; 2018,Jan,8; 2017,Jan,8; 2016,Jan,3; 2016,Jan,13; 2015,Oct,5

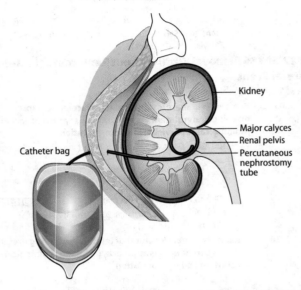

Kidney

Major calyces

Renal pelvis

Percutaneous nephrostomy tube

Catheter bag

50433 Placement of nephroureteral catheter, percutaneous, including diagnostic nephrostogram and/or ureterogram when performed, imaging guidance (eg, ultrasound and/or fluoroscopy) and all associated radiological supervision and interpretation, new access

INCLUDES Renal pelvis and associated ureter as a single element

EXCLUDES *Dilation of nephroureteral catheter tract ([50436, 50437])*
Nephroureteral catheter removal/replacement (50387)
Procedures performed for same renal collecting system/ureter ([50430, 50431, 50432], 50693-50695, 74425)

7.44　31.2　**FUD** 000　J 02 50

AMA: 2018,Mar,11; 2018,Jan,8; 2017,Jan,8; 2016,Jan,3; 2016,Jan,13; 2015,Oct,5

50434 Convert nephrostomy catheter to nephroureteral catheter, percutaneous, including diagnostic nephrostogram and/or ureterogram when performed, imaging guidance (eg, ultrasound and/or fluoroscopy) and all associated radiological supervision and interpretation, via pre-existing nephrostomy tract

INCLUDES Renal pelvis and associated ureter as a single element

EXCLUDES *Procedure performed for same renal collecting system/ureter ([50430, 50431], [50435], 50684, 50693, 74425)*

5.60　24.6　**FUD** 000　J J8 50

AMA: 2018,Jan,8; 2017,Jan,8; 2016,Jan,3; 2016,Jan,13; 2015,Oct,5

50400-50540 Open Surgical Procedures of Kidney

50435

50435 Exchange nephrostomy catheter, percutaneous, including diagnostic nephrostogram and/or ureterogram when performed, imaging guidance (eg, ultrasound and/or fluoroscopy) and all associated radiological supervision and interpretation

INCLUDES Renal pelvis and associated ureter as a single element

EXCLUDES Procedure performed for same renal collecting system/ureter ([50430, 50431], [50434], 50693, 74425)

Removal nephrostomy catheter that requires fluoroscopic guidance (50389)

2.90   14.6   **FUD** 000   J 62 50

AMA: 2018,Mar,11; 2018,Jan,8; 2017,Jan,8; 2016,Jan,3; 2016,Jan,13; 2015,Oct,5

50400-50540 Open Surgical Procedures of Kidney

50400 Pyeloplasty (Foley Y-pyeloplasty), plastic operation on renal pelvis, with or without plastic operation on ureter, nephropexy, nephrostomy, pyelostomy, or ureteral splinting; simple

EXCLUDES Laparoscopic pyeloplasty (50544)

33.5   33.5   **FUD** 090   C 80 50

AMA: 2018,Jan,8; 2017,Jan,8; 2016,Jan,13; 2015,Jan,16; 2014,Jan,11

50405 complicated (congenital kidney abnormality, secondary pyeloplasty, solitary kidney, calycoplasty)

EXCLUDES Laparoscopic pyeloplasty (50544)

40.4   40.4   **FUD** 090   C 80 50

AMA: 2018,Jan,8; 2017,Jan,8; 2016,Jan,13; 2015,Jan,16; 2014,Jan,11

50430 Resequenced code. See code following 50396.
50431 Resequenced code. See code following 50396.
50432 Resequenced code. See code following 50396.
50433 Resequenced code. See code following 50396.
50434 Resequenced code. See code following 50396.
50435 Resequenced code. See code following 50396.
50436 Resequenced code. See code following 50391.
50437 Resequenced code. See code following 50391.

50500 Nephrorrhaphy, suture of kidney wound or injury

37.3   37.3   **FUD** 090   C 80

AMA: 2014,Jan,11

Schematic of nephron

50520 Closure of nephrocutaneous or pyelocutaneous fistula

33.6   33.6   **FUD** 090   C 80

AMA: 2014,Jan,11

50525 Closure of nephrovisceral fistula (eg, renocolic), including visceral repair; abdominal approach

42.6   42.6   **FUD** 090   C 80

AMA: 2014,Jan,11

50526 thoracic approach

45.7   45.7   **FUD** 090   C 80

AMA: 2014,Jan,11

50540 Symphysiotomy for horseshoe kidney with or without pyeloplasty and/or other plastic procedure, unilateral or bilateral (1 operation)

33.2   33.2   **FUD** 090   C 80

AMA: 2014,Jan,11

50541-50549 Laparoscopic Surgical Procedures of the Kidney

INCLUDES Diagnostic laparoscopy (49320)

EXCLUDES Laparoscopic drainage of lymphocele to peritoneal cavity (49323)

50541 Laparoscopy, surgical; ablation of renal cysts

26.5   26.5   **FUD** 090   J 80 50

AMA: 2018,Jan,8; 2017,Jan,8; 2016,Jan,13; 2015,Jan,16; 2014,Jan,11

50542 ablation of renal mass lesion(s), including intraoperative ultrasound guidance and monitoring, when performed

EXCLUDES Open ablation of renal mass lesions (50250)

Percutaneous ablation of renal tumors (50592-50593)

33.7   33.7   **FUD** 090   J 80 50

AMA: 2018,Jan,8; 2017,Jan,8; 2016,Jan,13; 2015,Jan,16; 2014,Jan,11

50543 partial nephrectomy

EXCLUDES Partial nephrectomy, open approach (50240)

43.0   43.0   **FUD** 090   J 80 50

AMA: 2018,Jan,8; 2017,Jan,8; 2016,Jan,13; 2015,Jan,16; 2014,Jan,11

50544 pyeloplasty

36.0   36.0   **FUD** 090   J 80 50

AMA: 2018,Jan,8; 2017,Jan,8; 2016,Jan,13; 2015,Jan,16; 2014,Jan,11

50545 radical nephrectomy (includes removal of Gerota's fascia and surrounding fatty tissue, removal of regional lymph nodes, and adrenalectomy)

EXCLUDES Radical nephrectomy, open approach (50230)

38.7   38.7   **FUD** 090   C 80 50

AMA: 2018,Jan,8; 2017,Jan,8; 2016,Jan,13; 2015,Jan,16; 2014,Jan,11

50546 nephrectomy, including partial ureterectomy

34.8   34.8   **FUD** 090   C 80 50

AMA: 2018,Jan,8; 2017,Jan,8; 2016,Jan,13; 2015,Jan,16; 2014,Jan,11

50547 donor nephrectomy (including cold preservation), from living donor

INCLUDES Donor care

Graft:
Cold preservation
Harvesting

EXCLUDES Backbench reconstruction renal allograft prior to transplantation (50327-50329)

Backbench standard preparation of living donor renal allograft prior to transplantation (50325)

Donor nephrectomy, open approach (50320)

46.4   46.4   **FUD** 090   C 80 50

AMA: 2018,Jan,8; 2017,Jan,8; 2016,Jan,13; 2015,Jan,16; 2014,Jan,11

50548 nephrectomy with total ureterectomy

EXCLUDES Nephrectomy, open approach (50234, 50236)

38.9   38.9   **FUD** 090   C 80 50

AMA: 2018,Jan,8; 2017,Jan,8; 2016,Jan,13; 2015,Jan,16; 2014,Jan,11

50435 — 50548

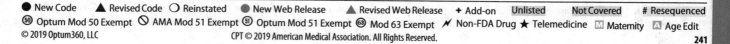

Urinary System

50549 — **50605**

50549   Unlisted laparoscopy procedure, renal
    0.00   0.00   **FUD** YYY   [J] [80] [50]
    AMA: 2018,Jan,8; 2017,Jan,8; 2016,Jan,13; 2015,Jan,16;
    2014,Jan,11

50551-50562 Endoscopic Procedures of Kidney via Established Nephrostomy/Pyelostomy Access

50551   Renal endoscopy through established nephrostomy or pyelostomy, with or without irrigation, instillation, or ureteropyelography, exclusive of radiologic service;
    8.54   10.4   **FUD** 000   [J] [A2] [80] [50]
    AMA: 2018,Jan,8; 2017,Jan,8; 2016,Jan,13; 2015,Jan,16;
    2014,Jan,11

50553   with ureteral catheterization, with or without dilation of ureter
    EXCLUDES   *Image-guided ureter dilation without endoscopic guidance (50706)*
    9.09   11.1   **FUD** 000   [J] [A2] [50]
    AMA: 2018,Jan,8; 2017,Jan,8; 2016,Jan,3; 2016,Jan,13;
    2015,Jan,16; 2014,Jan,11

50555   with biopsy
    EXCLUDES   *Image-guided biopsy ureter/renal pelvis without endoscopic guidance (50606)*
    9.88   11.9   **FUD** 000   [J] [A2] [80] [50]
    AMA: 2018,Jan,8; 2017,Jan,8; 2016,Jan,3; 2016,Jan,13;
    2015,Jan,16; 2014,Jan,11

50557   with fulguration and/or incision, with or without biopsy
    10.0   12.1   **FUD** 000   [J] [A2] [80] [50]
    AMA: 2018,Jan,8; 2017,Jan,8; 2016,Jan,13; 2015,Jan,16;
    2014,Jan,11

50561   with removal of foreign body or calculus
    11.4   13.7   **FUD** 000   [J] [A2] [80] [50]
    AMA: 2018,Jan,8; 2017,Jan,8; 2016,Jan,13; 2015,Jan,16;
    2014,Jan,11

50562   with resection of tumor
    16.8   16.8   **FUD** 090   [J] [G2] [80]
    AMA: 2018,Jan,8; 2017,Jan,8; 2016,Jan,13; 2015,Jan,16;
    2014,Jan,11

50570-50580 Endoscopic Procedures of Kidney via Nephrotomy/Pyelotomy Access

Code also if provided service is significant and identifiable (50045, 50120)

50570   Renal endoscopy through nephrotomy or pyelotomy, with or without irrigation, instillation, or ureteropyelography, exclusive of radiologic service;
    14.2   14.2   **FUD** 000   [J] [G2] [80] [50]
    AMA: 2018,Jan,8; 2017,Jan,8; 2016,Jan,13; 2015,Jan,16;
    2014,Jan,11

50572   with ureteral catheterization, with or without dilation of ureter
    EXCLUDES   *Image-guided ureter dilation without endoscopic guidance (50706)*
    15.4   15.4   **FUD** 000   [T] [G2] [80] [50]
    AMA: 2018,Jan,8; 2017,Jan,8; 2016,Jan,3; 2016,Jan,13;
    2015,Jan,16; 2014,Jan,11

50574   with biopsy
    EXCLUDES   *Image-guide ureter/renal pelvis biopsy without endoscopic guidance (50606)*
    16.3   16.3   **FUD** 000   [J] [G2] [80] [50]
    AMA: 2018,Jan,8; 2017,Jan,8; 2016,Jan,3; 2016,Jan,13;
    2015,Jan,16; 2014,Jan,11

50575   with endopyelotomy (includes cystoscopy, ureteroscopy, dilation of ureter and ureteral pelvic junction, incision of ureteral pelvic junction and insertion of endopyelotomy stent)
    20.6   20.6   **FUD** 000   [J] [G2] [50]
    AMA: 2018,Jan,8; 2017,Jan,8; 2016,Jan,13; 2015,Jan,16;
    2014,Jan,11

50576   with fulguration and/or incision, with or without biopsy
    16.3   16.3   **FUD** 000   [J] [G2] [80] [50]
    AMA: 2018,Jan,8; 2017,Jan,8; 2016,Jan,13; 2015,Jan,16;
    2014,Jan,11

50580   with removal of foreign body or calculus
    17.5   17.5   **FUD** 000   [J] [G2] [80] [50]
    AMA: 2018,Jan,8; 2017,Jan,8; 2016,Jan,13; 2015,Jan,16;
    2014,Jan,11

50590-50593 Noninvasive and Minimally Invasive Procedures of the Kidney

50590   Lithotripsy, extracorporeal shock wave
    16.4   21.0   **FUD** 090   [J] [G2] [50]
    AMA: 2018,Jan,8; 2017,Jan,8; 2016,Jan,13; 2015,Jan,16;
    2014,Jan,11

Major calyces

Medulla

Cortex

Minor calyces

Ultrasound shock waves

Renal pelvis

Calculus (kidney stone)

Ureter

50592   Ablation, 1 or more renal tumor(s), percutaneous, unilateral, radiofrequency
    (76940, 77013, 77022)
    9.93   92.3   **FUD** 010   [J] [G2] [50]
    AMA: 2014,Jan,11

50593   Ablation, renal tumor(s), unilateral, percutaneous, cryotherapy
    (76940, 77013, 77022)
    13.3   125.   **FUD** 010   [J] [J8] [80] [50]
    AMA: 2018,Jan,8; 2014,Jan,11

50600-50940 Open and Injection Procedures of Ureter

50600   Ureterotomy with exploration or drainage (separate procedure)
    Code also ureteral endoscopy through ureterotomy when procedures constitute a significant identifiable service (50970-50980)
    27.1   27.1   **FUD** 090   [C] [80] [50]
    AMA: 2014,Jan,11

50605   Ureterotomy for insertion of indwelling stent, all types
    28.6   28.6   **FUD** 090   [C] [80] [50]
    AMA: 2018,Jan,8; 2017,Jan,8; 2016,Jan,13; 2015,Jan,16;
    2014,Jan,11

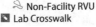

26/TC PC/TC Only   A2-Z3 ASC Payment   50 Bilateral   ♂ Male Only   ♀ Female Only   Facility RVU   Non-Facility RVU   CCI   CLIA
FUD Follow-up Days   **CMS:** IOM   **AMA:** CPT Asst   A-Y OPPSI   80/80 Surg Assist Allowed / w/Doc   Lab Crosswalk   Radiology Crosswalk

242   CPT © 2019 American Medical Association. All Rights Reserved.   © 2019 Optum360, LLC

+ 50606 Endoluminal biopsy of ureter and/or renal pelvis, non-endoscopic, including imaging guidance (eg, ultrasound and/or fluoroscopy) and all associated radiological supervision and interpretation (List separately in addition to code for primary procedure)

INCLUDES Renal pelvis and associated ureter as a single element

EXCLUDES *Procedure performed for same renal collecting system/associated ureter with (50555, 50574, 50955, 50974, 52007, 74425)*

Code first (50382-50389, [50430, 50431, 50432, 50433, 50435], 50684, 50688, 50690, 50693-50695, 51610)

🚑 4.43 ⚕ 18.8 **FUD** ZZZ N N1 50 ▱

AMA: 2018,Jan,8; 2017,Jan,8; 2016,Jan,3

50610 Ureterolithotomy; upper one-third of ureter

EXCLUDES *Cystotomy with calculus basket extraction of ureteral calculus (51065)*
Transvesical ureterolithotomy (51060)
Ureteral calculus manipulation/extraction performed endoscopically (50080-50081, 50561, 50961, 50980, 52320-52330, 52352-52353, [52356])
Ureterolithotomy performed laparoscopically (50945)

🚑 27.3 ⚕ 27.3 **FUD** 090 C 80 50 ▱

AMA: 2018,Jan,8; 2017,Jan,8; 2016,Jan,13; 2015,Jan,16; 2014,Jan,11

50620 middle one-third of ureter

EXCLUDES *Cystotomy with calculus basket extraction of ureteral calculus (51065)*
Transvesical ureterolithotomy (51060)
Ureteral calculus manipulation/extraction performed endoscopically (50080-50081, 50561, 50961, 50980, 52320-52330, 52352-52353, [52356])
Ureterolithotomy performed laparoscopically (50945)

🚑 26.1 ⚕ 26.1 **FUD** 090 C 80 50 ▱

AMA: 2018,Jan,8; 2017,Jan,8; 2016,Jan,13; 2015,Jan,16; 2014,Jan,11

50630 lower one-third of ureter

EXCLUDES *Cystotomy with calculus basket extraction of ureteral calculus (51065)*
Transvesical ureterolithotomy (51060)
Ureteral calculus manipulation/extraction performed endoscopically (50080-50081, 50561, 50961, 50980, 52320-52330, 52352-52353, [52356])
Ureterolithotomy performed laparoscopically (50945)

🚑 25.8 ⚕ 25.8 **FUD** 090 C 80 50 ▱

AMA: 2018,Jan,8; 2017,Jan,8; 2016,Jan,13; 2015,Jan,16; 2014,May,3; 2014,Jan,11

50650 Ureterectomy, with bladder cuff (separate procedure)

EXCLUDES *Ureterocele (51535, 52300)*

🚑 30.0 ⚕ 30.0 **FUD** 090 C 80 50 ▱

AMA: 2014,Jan,11

50660 Ureterectomy, total, ectopic ureter, combination abdominal, vaginal and/or perineal approach

EXCLUDES *Ureterocele (51535, 52300)*

🚑 33.1 ⚕ 33.1 **FUD** 090 C 80 ▱

AMA: 2014,Jan,11

50684 Injection procedure for ureterography or ureteropyelography through ureterostomy or indwelling ureteral catheter

EXCLUDES *Placement of nephroureteral catheter ([50433, 50434])*
Placement of ureteral stent (50693-50695)

▣ (74425)

🚑 1.45 ⚕ 3.10 **FUD** 000 N N1 50 ▱

AMA: 2018,Jan,8; 2017,Jan,8; 2016,Jan,3; 2015,Oct,5; 2014,Jan,11

50686 Manometric studies through ureterostomy or indwelling ureteral catheter

🚑 2.55 ⚕ 3.99 **FUD** 000 S P2 80 ▱

AMA: 2014,Jan,11

50688 Change of ureterostomy tube or externally accessible ureteral stent via ileal conduit

▣ (75984)

🚑 2.25 ⚕ 2.25 **FUD** 010 J A2 ▱

AMA: 2018,Jan,8; 2017,Jan,8; 2016,Jan,3; 2014,Jan,11

50690 Injection procedure for visualization of ileal conduit and/or ureteropyelography, exclusive of radiologic service

▣ (74425)

🚑 2.02 ⚕ 2.87 **FUD** 000 N N1 ▱

AMA: 2018,Jan,8; 2017,Jan,8; 2016,Jan,3; 2014,Jan,11

50693 Placement of ureteral stent, percutaneous, including diagnostic nephrostogram and/or ureterogram when performed, imaging guidance (eg, ultrasound and/or fluoroscopy), and all associated radiological supervision and interpretation; pre-existing nephrostomy tract

INCLUDES Renal pelvis and associated ureter as a single element

EXCLUDES *Procedure performed for the same renal collecting system/ureter ([50430, 50431, 50432, 50433, 50434, 50435], 50684, 74425)*

🚑 5.94 ⚕ 28.7 **FUD** 000 J 62 50 ▱

AMA: 2018,Jan,8; 2017,Jan,8; 2016,Jan,3; 2016,Jan,13; 2015,Oct,5

Proximal curl of stent in kidney

Indwelling stent

Catheter

Ureter

Distal curl of stent in bladder

Bladder

50694 new access, without separate nephrostomy catheter

INCLUDES Renal pelvis and associated ureter as a single element

EXCLUDES *Procedure performed for the same renal collecting system/ureter ([50430, 50431, 50432, 50433, 50434, 50435], 50684, 74425)*

🚑 7.77 ⚕ 31.7 **FUD** 000 J 62 50 ▱

AMA: 2018,Jan,8; 2017,Jan,8; 2016,Jan,3; 2016,Jan,13; 2015,Oct,5

50695 new access, with separate nephrostomy catheter

INCLUDES Placement of separate ureteral stent and nephrostomy catheter into a ureter/associated renal pelvis through a new access
Renal pelvis and associated ureter as a single element

EXCLUDES *Procedure performed for the same renal collecting system/ureter ([50430, 50431, 50432, 50433, 50434, 50435], 50684, 74425)*

🚑 9.95 ⚕ 38.7 **FUD** 000 J 62 50 ▱

AMA: 2018,Jan,8; 2017,Jan,8; 2016,Jan,3; 2016,Jan,13; 2015,Oct,5

50700 Ureteroplasty, plastic operation on ureter (eg, stricture)

🚑 26.7 ⚕ 26.7 **FUD** 090 C 80 50 ▱

AMA: 2014,Jan,11

+ 50705 Ureteral embolization or occlusion, including imaging guidance (eg, ultrasound and/or fluoroscopy) and all associated radiological supervision and interpretation (List separately in addition to code for primary procedure)

INCLUDES Renal pelvis and associated ureter as a single element
Code also when performed:
Additional catheter insertions
Diagnostic pyelography/ureterography
Other interventions
Code first (50382-50389, [50430, 50431, 50432, 50433, 50434, 50435], 50684, 50688, 50690, 50693-50695, 51610)
🚑 5.69 ⚕ 56.8 **FUD** ZZZ Ⓝ N1 50 📷
AMA: 2018,Jan,8; 2017,Jan,8; 2016,Jan,3

+ 50706 Balloon dilation, ureteral stricture, including imaging guidance (eg, ultrasound and/or fluoroscopy) and all associated radiological supervision and interpretation (List separately in addition to code for primary procedure)

INCLUDES Dilation of nephrostomy, ureters, or urethra (74485)
Renal pelvis and associated ureter as a single element
EXCLUDES Cystourethroscopy (52341, 52344-52345)
Renal endoscopy (50553, 50572)
Ureteral endoscopy (50953, 50972)
Code also when performed:
Additional catheter insertions
Diagnostic pyelography/ureterography
Other interventions
Code first (50382-50389, [50430, 50431, 50432, 50433, 50434, 50435], 50684, 50688, 50690, 50693-50695, 51610)
🚑 5.31 ⚕ 27.4 **FUD** ZZZ Ⓝ N1 50 📷
AMA: 2018,Jan,8; 2017,Jan,8; 2016,Jan,3

50715 Ureterolysis, with or without repositioning of ureter for retroperitoneal fibrosis
🚑 35.2 ⚕ 35.2 **FUD** 090 Ⓒ 80 50 📷
AMA: 2014,Jan,11

50722 Ureterolysis for ovarian vein syndrome ♀
🚑 29.1 ⚕ 29.1 **FUD** 090 Ⓒ 80 📷
AMA: 2014,Jan,11

50725 Ureterolysis for retrocaval ureter, with reanastomosis of upper urinary tract or vena cava
🚑 31.9 ⚕ 31.9 **FUD** 090 Ⓒ 80 📷
AMA: 2014,Jan,11

50727 Revision of urinary-cutaneous anastomosis (any type urostomy);
🚑 14.7 ⚕ 14.7 **FUD** 090 Ⓙ 62 80 📷
AMA: 2014,Jan,11

50728 with repair of fascial defect and hernia
🚑 21.2 ⚕ 21.2 **FUD** 090 Ⓒ 80 📷
AMA: 2014,Jan,11

50740 Ureteropyelostomy, anastomosis of ureter and renal pelvis
🚑 35.4 ⚕ 35.4 **FUD** 090 Ⓒ 80 50 📷
AMA: 2018,Jan,8; 2017,Jan,8; 2016,Jan,13; 2015,Jan,16; 2014,Jan,11

50750 Ureterocalycostomy, anastomosis of ureter to renal calyx
🚑 33.3 ⚕ 33.3 **FUD** 090 Ⓒ 80 50 📷
AMA: 2018,Jan,8; 2017,Jan,8; 2016,Jan,13; 2015,Jan,16; 2014,Jan,11

50760 Ureteroureterostomy
🚑 32.6 ⚕ 32.6 **FUD** 090 Ⓒ 80 50 📷
AMA: 2018,Jan,8; 2017,Jan,8; 2016,Jan,13; 2015,Jan,16; 2014,Jan,11

50770 Transureteroureterostomy, anastomosis of ureter to contralateral ureter
🚑 33.3 ⚕ 33.3 **FUD** 090 Ⓒ 80 📷
AMA: 2014,Jan,11

50780 Ureteroneocystostomy; anastomosis of single ureter to bladder

INCLUDES Minor procedures to prevent vesicoureteral reflux
EXCLUDES Cystourethroplasty with ureteroneocystostomy (51820)
🚑 31.9 ⚕ 31.9 **FUD** 090 Ⓒ 80 50 📷
AMA: 2018,Feb,11; 2018,Jan,8; 2017,Jan,8; 2016,Jan,13; 2015,Jan,16; 2014,Jan,11

50782 anastomosis of duplicated ureter to bladder
INCLUDES Minor procedures to prevent vesicoureteral reflux
🚑 31.1 ⚕ 31.1 **FUD** 090 Ⓒ 80 50 📷
AMA: 2018,Jan,8; 2017,Jan,8; 2016,Jan,13; 2015,Jan,16; 2014,Jan,11

50783 with extensive ureteral tailoring
INCLUDES Minor procedures to prevent vesicoureteral reflux
🚑 32.6 ⚕ 32.6 **FUD** 090 Ⓒ 80 50 📷
AMA: 2018,Jan,8; 2017,Jan,8; 2016,Jan,13; 2015,Jan,16; 2014,Jan,11

50785 with vesico-psoas hitch or bladder flap
INCLUDES Minor procedures to prevent vesicoureteral reflux
🚑 35.1 ⚕ 35.1 **FUD** 090 Ⓒ 80 50 📷
AMA: 2018,Jan,8; 2017,Jan,8; 2016,Jan,13; 2015,Jan,16; 2014,Jan,11

50800 Ureteroenterostomy, direct anastomosis of ureter to intestine
EXCLUDES Cystectomy with ureterosigmoidostomy/ureteroileal conduit (51580-51595)
🚑 26.8 ⚕ 26.8 **FUD** 090 Ⓒ 80 50 📷
AMA: 2018,Jan,8; 2017,Jan,8; 2016,Jan,13; 2015,Jan,16; 2014,Jan,11

50810 Ureterosigmoidostomy, with creation of sigmoid bladder and establishment of abdominal or perineal colostomy, including intestine anastomosis
EXCLUDES Cystectomy with ureterosigmoidostomy/ureteroileal conduit (51580-51595)
🚑 40.5 ⚕ 40.5 **FUD** 090 Ⓒ 80 📷
AMA: 2018,Jan,8; 2017,Jan,8; 2016,Jan,13; 2015,Jan,16; 2014,Jan,11

50815 Ureterocolon conduit, including intestine anastomosis
EXCLUDES Cystectomy with ureterosigmoidostomy/ureteroileal conduit (51580-51595)
🚑 35.3 ⚕ 35.3 **FUD** 090 Ⓒ 80 📷
AMA: 2018,Jan,8; 2017,Jan,8; 2016,Jan,13; 2015,Jan,16; 2014,Jan,11

50820 Ureteroileal conduit (ileal bladder), including intestine anastomosis (Bricker operation)
EXCLUDES Cystectomy with ureterosigmoidostomy/ureteroileal conduit (51580-51595)
🚑 38.0 ⚕ 38.0 **FUD** 090 Ⓒ 80 50 📷
AMA: 2018,Jan,8; 2017,Jan,8; 2016,Jan,13; 2015,Jan,16; 2014,Jan,11

50825 Continent diversion, including intestine anastomosis using any segment of small and/or large intestine (Kock pouch or Camey enterocystoplasty)
🚑 48.0 ⚕ 48.0 **FUD** 090 Ⓒ 80 📷
AMA: 2018,Jan,8; 2017,Jan,8; 2016,Jan,13; 2015,Jan,16; 2014,Jan,11

50830 Urinary undiversion (eg, taking down of ureteroileal conduit, ureterosigmoidostomy or ureteroenterostomy with ureteroureterostomy or ureteroneocystostomy)
🚑 52.1 ⚕ 52.1 **FUD** 090 Ⓒ 80 📷
AMA: 2018,Jan,8; 2017,Jan,8; 2016,Jan,13; 2015,Jan,16; 2014,Jan,11

50840 Replacement of all or part of ureter by intestine segment, including intestine anastomosis
🚑 35.5 ⚕ 35.5 **FUD** 090 Ⓒ 80 50 📷
AMA: 2018,Jan,8; 2017,Jan,8; 2016,Jan,13; 2015,Jan,16; 2014,Jan,11

50845 **Cutaneous appendico-vesicostomy**
INCLUDES Mitrofanoff operation
🔲 36.1 🔲 36.1 **FUD** 090
C 80 🔲
AMA: 2014,Jan,11

50860 **Ureterostomy, transplantation of ureter to skin**
🔲 27.3 🔲 27.3 **FUD** 090
C 80 50 🔲
AMA: 2014,Jan,11

50900 **Ureterorrhaphy, suture of ureter (separate procedure)**
🔲 24.3 🔲 24.3 **FUD** 090
C 80 50 🔲
AMA: 2014,Jan,11

50920 **Closure of ureterocutaneous fistula**
🔲 25.3 🔲 25.3 **FUD** 090
C 80 🔲
AMA: 2014,Jan,11

50930 **Closure of ureterovisceral fistula (including visceral repair)**
🔲 31.8 🔲 31.8 **FUD** 090
C 80 🔲
AMA: 2014,Jan,11

50940 **Deligation of ureter**
EXCLUDES Ureteroplasty/ureterolysis (50700-50860)
🔲 25.6 🔲 25.6 **FUD** 090
C 80 50 🔲
AMA: 2014,Jan,11

50945-50949 Laparoscopic Procedures of Ureter
INCLUDES Diagnostic laparoscopy (49320)
EXCLUDES Ureteroneocystostomy, open approach (50780-50785)

50945 **Laparoscopy, surgical; ureterolithotomy**
🔲 28.1 🔲 28.1 **FUD** 090
J 80 50 🔲
AMA: 2018,Jan,8; 2017,Jan,8; 2016,Jan,13; 2015,Jan,16; 2014,Jan,11

50947 **ureteroneocystostomy with cystoscopy and ureteral stent placement**
🔲 40.1 🔲 40.1 **FUD** 090
J A2 80 50 🔲
AMA: 2018,Jan,8; 2017,Jan,8; 2016,Jan,13; 2015,Jan,16; 2014,Jan,11

50948 **ureteroneocystostomy without cystoscopy and ureteral stent placement**
🔲 36.9 🔲 36.9 **FUD** 090
J A2 80 🔲
AMA: 2018,Jan,8; 2017,Jan,8; 2016,Jan,13; 2015,Jan,16; 2014,Jan,11

50949 **Unlisted laparoscopy procedure, ureter**
🔲 0.00 🔲 0.00 **FUD** YYY
J 80 50 🔲
AMA: 2018,Jan,8; 2017,Jan,8; 2016,Jan,13; 2015,Jan,16; 2014,Jan,11

50951-50961 Endoscopic Procedures of Ureter via Established Ureterostomy Access

50951 **Ureteral endoscopy through established ureterostomy, with or without irrigation, instillation, or ureteropyelography, exclusive of radiologic service;**
🔲 8.89 🔲 10.9 **FUD** 000
J A2 80 50 🔲
AMA: 2018,Jan,8; 2017,Jan,8; 2016,Jan,13; 2015,Jan,16; 2014,Jan,11

50953 **with ureteral catheterization, with or without dilation of ureter**
EXCLUDES Image-guided ureter dilation without endoscopic guidance (50706)
🔲 9.46 🔲 11.5 **FUD** 000
J A2 80 50 🔲
AMA: 2018,Jan,8; 2017,Jan,8; 2016,Jan,13; 2016,Jan,3; 2015,Jan,16; 2014,Jan,11

50955 **with biopsy**
EXCLUDES Image-guided biopsy of ureter and/or renal pelvis without endoscopic guidance (50606)
🔲 10.2 🔲 12.3 **FUD** 000
J A2 80 50 🔲
AMA: 2018,Jan,8; 2017,Jan,8; 2016,Jan,13; 2016,Jan,3; 2015,Jan,16; 2014,Jan,11

50957 **with fulguration and/or incision, with or without biopsy**
🔲 10.2 🔲 12.4 **FUD** 000
J A2 80 50 🔲
AMA: 2018,Jan,8; 2017,Jan,8; 2016,Jan,13; 2015,Jan,16; 2014,Jan,11

50961 **with removal of foreign body or calculus**
🔲 9.17 🔲 11.1 **FUD** 000
J A2 80 50 🔲
AMA: 2018,Jan,8; 2017,Jan,8; 2016,Jan,13; 2015,Jan,16; 2014,Jan,11

50970-50980 Endoscopic Procedures of Ureter via Ureterotomy
EXCLUDES Ureterotomy (50600)

50970 **Ureteral endoscopy through ureterotomy, with or without irrigation, instillation, or ureteropyelography, exclusive of radiologic service;**
🔲 10.7 🔲 10.7 **FUD** 000
J A2 80 50 🔲
AMA: 2018,Jan,8; 2017,Jan,8; 2016,Jan,13; 2015,Jan,16; 2014,Jan,11

50972 **with ureteral catheterization, with or without dilation of ureter**
EXCLUDES Image-guided ureter dilation without endoscopic guidance (50706)
🔲 10.3 🔲 10.3 **FUD** 000
J A2 80 50 🔲
AMA: 2018,Jan,8; 2017,Jan,8; 2016,Jan,3; 2016,Jan,13; 2015,Jan,16; 2014,Jan,11

50974 **with biopsy**
EXCLUDES Image-guided biopsy of ureter and/or renal pelvis without endoscopic guidance (50606)
🔲 13.6 🔲 13.6 **FUD** 000
J A2 80 50 🔲
AMA: 2018,Jan,8; 2017,Jan,8; 2016,Jan,3; 2016,Jan,13; 2015,Jan,16; 2014,Jan,11

50976 **with fulguration and/or incision, with or without biopsy**
🔲 13.5 🔲 13.5 **FUD** 000
J A2 80 50 🔲
AMA: 2018,Jan,8; 2017,Jan,8; 2016,Jan,13; 2015,Jan,16; 2014,Jan,11

50980 **with removal of foreign body or calculus**
🔲 10.3 🔲 10.3 **FUD** 000
J A2 80 50 🔲
AMA: 2018,Jan,8; 2017,Jan,8; 2016,Jan,13; 2015,Jan,16; 2014,Jan,11

51020-51080 Open Incisional Procedures of Bladder

51020 **Cystotomy or cystostomy; with fulguration and/or insertion of radioactive material**
🔲 13.5 🔲 13.5 **FUD** 090
J A2 80 🔲

51030 **with cryosurgical destruction of intravesical lesion**
🔲 13.6 🔲 13.6 **FUD** 090
J A2 80 🔲
AMA: 2014,Jan,11

51040 **Cystostomy, cystotomy with drainage**
🔲 8.36 🔲 8.36 **FUD** 090
J A2 80 🔲
AMA: 2014,Jan,11

51045 **Cystotomy, with insertion of ureteral catheter or stent (separate procedure)**
🔲 14.2 🔲 14.2 **FUD** 090
J A2 80 🔲
AMA: 2014,Jan,11

51050 **Cystolithotomy, cystotomy with removal of calculus, without vesical neck resection**
🔲 13.6 🔲 13.6 **FUD** 090
J A2 80 🔲
AMA: 2014,Jan,11

51060 **Transvesical ureterolithotomy**
🔲 16.8 🔲 16.8 **FUD** 090
J 80 🔲
AMA: 2014,Jan,11

51065 **Cystotomy, with calculus basket extraction and/or ultrasonic or electrohydraulic fragmentation of ureteral calculus**
🔲 16.7 🔲 16.7 **FUD** 090
J A2 80 🔲
AMA: 2014,Jan,11

51080 **Drainage of perivesical or prevesical space abscess**
EXCLUDES Image-guided percutaneous catheter drainage (49406)
🔲 11.8 🔲 11.8 **FUD** 090
J A2 80 🔲
AMA: 2014,Jan,11

50845 — 51080

51100-51102 Bladder Aspiration Procedures

51100   **Aspiration of bladder; by needle**
    (76942, 77002, 77012)
    1.13   1.84   **FUD** 000   T P3
    AMA: 2018,Jan,8; 2017,Jan,8; 2016,Jan,13; 2015,Jan,16; 2014,Jan,11

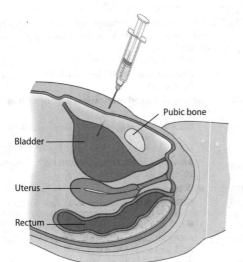

Pubic bone
Bladder
Uterus
Rectum

51101   **by trocar or intracatheter**
    (76942, 77002, 77012)
    1.50   3.79   **FUD** 000   S P3
    AMA: 2018,Jan,8; 2017,Jan,8; 2016,Jan,13; 2015,Jan,16; 2014,Jan,11

51102   **with insertion of suprapubic catheter**
    (76942, 77002, 77012)
    4.18   6.60   **FUD** 000   J A2
    AMA: 2018,Jan,8; 2017,Jan,8; 2016,Jan,13; 2015,Jan,16; 2014,Jan,11

51500-51597 Open Excisional Procedures of Bladder

51500   **Excision of urachal cyst or sinus, with or without umbilical hernia repair**
    18.4   18.4   **FUD** 090   J A2 80
    AMA: 2014,Jan,11

51520   **Cystotomy; for simple excision of vesical neck (separate procedure)**
    17.2   17.2   **FUD** 090   J A2 80
    AMA: 2014,Jan,11

51525   **for excision of bladder diverticulum, single or multiple (separate procedure)**
    EXCLUDES   Transurethral resection (52305)
    24.8   24.8   **FUD** 090   C 80
    AMA: 2014,Jan,11

51530   **for excision of bladder tumor**
    EXCLUDES   Transurethral resection (52234-52240, 52305)
    22.2   22.2   **FUD** 090   C 80
    AMA: 2014,Jan,11

51535   **Cystotomy for excision, incision, or repair of ureterocele**
    EXCLUDES   Transurethral excision (52300)
    22.5   22.5   **FUD** 090   J 62 80 50
    AMA: 2014,Jan,11

51550   **Cystectomy, partial; simple**
    27.9   27.9   **FUD** 090   C 80
    AMA: 2014,Jan,11

51555   **complicated (eg, postradiation, previous surgery, difficult location)**
    36.6   36.6   **FUD** 090   C 80
    AMA: 2014,Jan,11

51565   **Cystectomy, partial, with reimplantation of ureter(s) into bladder (ureteroneocystostomy)**
    37.5   37.5   **FUD** 090   C 80
    AMA: 2014,Jan,11

51570   **Cystectomy, complete; (separate procedure)**
    42.6   42.6   **FUD** 090   C 80
    AMA: 2014,Jan,11

51575   **with bilateral pelvic lymphadenectomy, including external iliac, hypogastric, and obturator nodes**
    52.7   52.7   **FUD** 090   C 80
    AMA: 2014,Jan,11

51580   **Cystectomy, complete, with ureterosigmoidostomy or ureterocutaneous transplantations;**
    54.7   54.7   **FUD** 090   C 80
    AMA: 2014,Jan,11

51585   **with bilateral pelvic lymphadenectomy, including external iliac, hypogastric, and obturator nodes**
    61.0   61.0   **FUD** 090   C 80
    AMA: 2014,Jan,11

51590   **Cystectomy, complete, with ureteroileal conduit or sigmoid bladder, including intestine anastomosis;**
    55.9   55.9   **FUD** 090   C 80
    AMA: 2014,Jan,11

51595   **with bilateral pelvic lymphadenectomy, including external iliac, hypogastric, and obturator nodes**
    63.3   63.3   **FUD** 090   C 80
    AMA: 2014,Jan,11

51596   **Cystectomy, complete, with continent diversion, any open technique, using any segment of small and/or large intestine to construct neobladder**
    68.1   68.1   **FUD** 090   C 80
    AMA: 2014,Jan,11

51597   **Pelvic exenteration, complete, for vesical, prostatic or urethral malignancy, with removal of bladder and ureteral transplantations, with or without hysterectomy and/or abdominoperineal resection of rectum and colon and colostomy, or any combination thereof**
    EXCLUDES   Pelvic exenteration for gynecologic malignancy (58240)
    66.3   66.3   **FUD** 090   C 80
    AMA: 2014,Jan,11

51600-51720 Injection/Insertion/Instillation Procedures of Bladder

51600   **Injection procedure for cystography or voiding urethrocystography**
    (74430, 74455)
    1.29   5.57   **FUD** 000   N N1
    AMA: 2014,Jan,11

51605   **Injection procedure and placement of chain for contrast and/or chain urethrocystography**
    (74430)
    1.11   1.11   **FUD** 000   N N1
    AMA: 2014,Jan,11

51610   **Injection procedure for retrograde urethrocystography**
    (74450)
    1.85   3.21   **FUD** 000   N N1
    AMA: 2018,Jan,8; 2017,Jan,8; 2016,Jan,3; 2014,Jan,11

51700   **Bladder irrigation, simple, lavage and/or instillation**
    0.87   2.12   **FUD** 000   T P3
    AMA: 2014,Jan,11

26/TC PC/TC Only   A2-Z3 ASC Payment   50 Bilateral   ♂ Male Only   ♀ Female Only   Facility RVU   Non-Facility RVU   CCI   CLIA
FUD Follow-up Days   **CMS:** IOM   **AMA:** CPT Asst   A-Y OPPSI   80/80 Surg Assist Allowed / w/Doc   Lab Crosswalk   Radiology Crosswalk

246   CPT © 2019 American Medical Association. All Rights Reserved.   © 2019 Optum360, LLC

51701 Insertion of non-indwelling bladder catheter (eg, straight catheterization for residual urine)

EXCLUDES Catheterization for specimen collection (P9612)
Insertion of catheter as an inclusive component of another procedure

⏱ 0.73   ⚕ 1.27   **FUD** 000   01 N1 ▭

AMA: 2018,Jan,8; 2017,Jan,8; 2016,Jan,13; 2015,Jan,16; 2014,Jan,11

51702 Insertion of temporary indwelling bladder catheter; simple (eg, Foley)

EXCLUDES Focused ultrasound ablation of uterine leiomyomata (0071T-0072T)
Insertion of catheter as an inclusive component of another procedure

⏱ 0.73   ⚕ 1.76   **FUD** 000   01 N1 ▭

AMA: 2018,Jan,8; 2017,Jan,8; 2016,Jan,13; 2015,Jan,16; 2014,May,3; 2014,Jan,11

51703 complicated (eg, altered anatomy, fractured catheter/balloon)

⏱ 2.23   ⚕ 3.78   **FUD** 000   S P2 ▭

AMA: 2018,Jan,8; 2017,Jan,8; 2016,Jan,13; 2015,Jan,16; 2014,Jan,11

51705 Change of cystostomy tube; simple

⏱ 1.50   ⚕ 2.67   **FUD** 000   T P3 ▭

AMA: 2018,Jan,8; 2017,Jan,8; 2016,Jan,13; 2015,Jan,16; 2014,Jan,11

51710 complicated

🔀 (75984)

⏱ 2.30   ⚕ 3.69   **FUD** 000   T A2 ▭

AMA: 2018,Jan,8; 2017,Jan,8; 2016,Jan,13; 2015,Jan,16; 2014,Jan,11

51715 Endoscopic injection of implant material into the submucosal tissues of the urethra and/or bladder neck

EXCLUDES Injection of bulking agent (submucosal) for fecal incontinence, via anoscope (46999)

⏱ 5.76   ⚕ 9.07   **FUD** 000   J J8 80 ▭

AMA: 2014,Jan,11

51720 Bladder instillation of anticarcinogenic agent (including retention time)

Code also bacillus Calmette-Guerin vaccine (BCG) (90586)

⏱ 1.27   ⚕ 2.40   **FUD** 000   T P3 ▭

AMA: 2018,Jan,8; 2017,Jan,8; 2016,Jan,13; 2015,Jan,16; 2014,Jan,11

51725-51798 [51797] Uroflowmetric Evaluations

INCLUDES Equipment
Fees for services of technician
Medications
Supplies
Code also modifier 26 if physician/other qualified health care professional provides only interpretation of results and/or operates the equipment

51725 Simple cystometrogram (CMG) (eg, spinal manometer)

⏱ 5.69   ⚕ 5.69   **FUD** 000   T P2 80 ▭

AMA: 2018,Jan,8; 2017,Jan,8; 2016,Jan,13; 2015,Jan,16; 2014,Jan,11

51726 Complex cystometrogram (ie, calibrated electronic equipment);

⏱ 7.94   ⚕ 7.94   **FUD** 000   T A2 ▭

AMA: 2018,Jan,8; 2017,Jan,8; 2016,Jan,13; 2015,Jan,16; 2014,Jan,11

51727 with urethral pressure profile studies (ie, urethral closure pressure profile), any technique

⏱ 9.39   ⚕ 9.39   **FUD** 000   T P3 80 ▭

AMA: 2018,Jan,8; 2017,Jan,8; 2016,Jan,13; 2015,Jan,16; 2014,Jan,11

51728 with voiding pressure studies (ie, bladder voiding pressure), any technique

⏱ 9.55   ⚕ 9.55   **FUD** 000   T P3 80 ▭

AMA: 2018,Jan,8; 2017,Jan,8; 2016,Jan,13; 2015,Jan,16; 2014,Jan,11

51729 with voiding pressure studies (ie, bladder voiding pressure) and urethral pressure profile studies (ie, urethral closure pressure profile), any technique

⏱ 10.2   ⚕ 10.2   **FUD** 000   T P3 80 ▭

AMA: 2018,Jan,8; 2017,Jan,8; 2016,Jan,13; 2015,Jan,16; 2014,Jan,11

+ # 51797 Voiding pressure studies, intra-abdominal (ie, rectal, gastric, intraperitoneal) (List separately in addition to code for primary procedure)

Code first (51728-51729)

⏱ 3.95   ⚕ 3.95   **FUD** ZZZ   N N1 80 ▭

AMA: 2018,Jan,8; 2017,Jan,8; 2016,Jan,13; 2015,Jan,16; 2014,Jan,11

51736 Simple uroflowmetry (UFR) (eg, stop-watch flow rate, mechanical uroflowmeter)

⏱ 0.40   ⚕ 0.40   **FUD** XXX   01 N1 80 ▭

AMA: 2018,Jan,8; 2017,Jan,8; 2016,Jan,13; 2015,Jan,16; 2014,Jan,11

51741 Complex uroflowmetry (eg, calibrated electronic equipment)

⏱ 0.41   ⚕ 0.41   **FUD** XXX   01 N1 ▭

AMA: 2018,Jan,8; 2017,Jan,8; 2016,Jan,13; 2015,Jan,16; 2014,Sep,13; 2014,Jan,11

51784 Electromyography studies (EMG) of anal or urethral sphincter, other than needle, any technique

EXCLUDES Stimulus evoked response (51792)

⏱ 1.93   ⚕ 1.93   **FUD** XXX   S P3 ▭

AMA: 2018,Jan,8; 2017,Jan,8; 2016,Jan,13; 2015,Jan,16; 2014,Sep,13; 2014,Feb,11; 2014,Jan,11

51785 Needle electromyography studies (EMG) of anal or urethral sphincter, any technique

⏱ 9.17   ⚕ 9.17   **FUD** XXX   T A2 80 ▭

AMA: 2018,Jan,8; 2017,Jan,8; 2016,Jan,13; 2015,Jan,16; 2014,Jan,11

51792 Stimulus evoked response (eg, measurement of bulbocavernosus reflex latency time)

EXCLUDES Electromyography studies (EMG) of anal or urethral sphincter (51784)

⏱ 6.57   ⚕ 6.57   **FUD** 000   01 N1 80 ▭

AMA: 2018,Jan,8; 2017,Jan,8; 2016,Jan,13; 2015,Jan,16; 2014,Feb,11; 2014,Jan,11

51797 Resequenced code. See code following 51729.

51798 Measurement of post-voiding residual urine and/or bladder capacity by ultrasound, non-imaging

⏱ 0.36   ⚕ 0.36   **FUD** XXX   01 N1 80 TC ▭

AMA: 2018,Jun,11; 2018,Jan,8; 2017,Jan,8; 2016,Jan,13; 2015,Jan,16; 2014,Jan,11

51800-51980 Open Repairs Urinary System

51800 Cystoplasty or cystourethroplasty, plastic operation on bladder and/or vesical neck (anterior Y-plasty, vesical fundus resection), any procedure, with or without wedge resection of posterior vesical neck

⏱ 30.3   ⚕ 30.3   **FUD** 090   C 80 ▭

AMA: 2014,Jan,11

51820 Cystourethroplasty with unilateral or bilateral ureteroneocystostomy

⏱ 31.3   ⚕ 31.3   **FUD** 090   C 80 ▭

AMA: 2014,Jan,11

51840 Anterior vesicourethropexy, or urethropexy (eg, Marshall-Marchetti-Krantz, Burch); simple

EXCLUDES Pereyra type urethropexy (57289)

⏱ 19.3   ⚕ 19.3   **FUD** 090   C 80 ▭

AMA: 2018,Jan,8; 2017,Jan,8; 2016,Jan,13; 2015,Jan,16; 2014,Jan,11

51841 complicated (eg, secondary repair)

EXCLUDES *Pereyra type urethropexy (57289)*

⚕ 22.4   ⚘ 22.4   **FUD** 090   C 80 ▭

AMA: 2018,Jan,8; 2017,Jan,8; 2016,Jan,13; 2015,Jan,16; 2014,Jan,11

51845 Abdomino-vaginal vesical neck suspension, with or without endoscopic control (eg, Stamey, Raz, modified Pereyra) ♀

⚕ 16.8   ⚘ 16.8   **FUD** 090   J 80 ▭

AMA: 2018,Jan,8; 2017,Jan,8; 2016,Jan,13; 2015,Jan,16; 2014,Jan,11

51860 Cystorrhaphy, suture of bladder wound, injury or rupture; simple

⚕ 21.5   ⚘ 21.5   **FUD** 090   J 80 ▭

AMA: 2014,Jan,11

51865 complicated

⚕ 25.9   ⚘ 25.9   **FUD** 090   C 80 ▭

AMA: 2014,Jan,11

51880 Closure of cystostomy (separate procedure)

⚕ 13.5   ⚘ 13.5   **FUD** 090   J A2 80 ▭

AMA: 2014,Jan,11

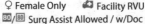

Lower ureter

Cystostomy

Bladder

Bladder

Physician removes a cystostomy tube

51900 Closure of vesicovaginal fistula, abdominal approach ♀

EXCLUDES *Vesicovaginal fistula closure, vaginal approach (57320-57330)*

⚕ 23.8   ⚘ 23.8   **FUD** 090   C 80 ▭

AMA: 2014,Jan,11

51920 Closure of vesicouterine fistula; ♀

EXCLUDES *Enterovesical fistula closure (44660-44661)*
Rectovesical fistula closure (45800-45805)

⚕ 22.0   ⚘ 22.0   **FUD** 090   C 80 ▭

AMA: 2014,Jan,11

51925 with hysterectomy ♀

EXCLUDES *Enterovesical fistula closure (44660-44661)*
Rectovesical fistula closure (45800-45805)

⚕ 29.5   ⚘ 29.5   **FUD** 090   C 80 ▭

AMA: 2014,Jan,11

51940 Closure, exstrophy of bladder

EXCLUDES *Epispadias reconstruction with exstrophy of bladder (54390)*

⚕ 47.5   ⚘ 47.5   **FUD** 090   C 80 ▭

AMA: 2014,Jan,11

51960 Enterocystoplasty, including intestinal anastomosis

⚕ 40.0   ⚘ 40.0   **FUD** 090   C 80 ▭

AMA: 2014,Jan,11

51980 Cutaneous vesicostomy

⚕ 20.6   ⚘ 20.6   **FUD** 090   C 80 ▭

AMA: 2014,Jan,11

51990-51999 Laparoscopic Procedures of Urinary System

CMS: 100-03,230.10 Incontinence Control Devices

INCLUDES   Diagnostic laparoscopy (49320)

51990 Laparoscopy, surgical; urethral suspension for stress incontinence

⚕ 21.6   ⚘ 21.6   **FUD** 090   J 80 ▭

AMA: 2019,Feb,10; 2018,Jan,8; 2017,Jan,8; 2016,Jan,13; 2015,Jan,16; 2014,Jan,11

51992 sling operation for stress incontinence (eg, fascia or synthetic)

EXCLUDES *Removal/revision of sling for stress incontinence (57287)*
Sling operation for stress incontinence, open approach (57288)

⚕ 24.0   ⚘ 24.0   **FUD** 090   J J8 80 ▭

AMA: 2019,Feb,10; 2018,Jan,8; 2017,Jan,8; 2016,Jan,13; 2015,Jan,16; 2014,Jan,11

51999 Unlisted laparoscopy procedure, bladder

⚕ 0.00   ⚘ 0.00   **FUD** YYY   J 80 ▭

AMA: 2018,Jan,8; 2017,Dec,14; 2014,Jan,11

52000-52318 Endoscopic Procedures via Urethra: Bladder and Urethra

INCLUDES   Diagnostic and therapeutic endoscopy of bowel segments utilized as replacements for native bladder

52000 Cystourethroscopy (separate procedure)

EXCLUDES *Cystourethroscopy (52001, 52320, 52325, 52327, 52330, 52332, 52334, 52341-52343, [52356], 57240, 57260, 57265)*

⚕ 2.34   ⚘ 5.39   **FUD** 000   T A2 ▭

AMA: 2019,Feb,10; 2018,Nov,10; 2018,Jan,8; 2017,Oct,9; 2017,Jan,8; 2016,Jan,13; 2015,Jan,16; 2014,May,3; 2014,Jan,11

52001 Cystourethroscopy with irrigation and evacuation of multiple obstructing clots

INCLUDES   Cystourethroscopy (separate procedure) (52000)

⚕ 8.31   ⚘ 11.3   **FUD** 000   J A2 ▭

AMA: 2014,Jan,11

52005 Cystourethroscopy, with ureteral catheterization, with or without irrigation, instillation, or ureteropyelography, exclusive of radiologic service;

INCLUDES   Howard test

⚕ 3.84   ⚘ 8.05   **FUD** 000   J A2 ▭

AMA: 2019,Mar,10; 2018,Jan,8; 2017,Jan,8; 2016,Jan,13; 2015,Jan,16; 2014,Jan,11

52007 with brush biopsy of ureter and/or renal pelvis

EXCLUDES *Image-guided ureter/renal pelvis biopsy without endoscopic guidance (50606)*

⚕ 4.80   ⚘ 13.1   **FUD** 000   J A2 50 ▭

AMA: 2018,Jan,8; 2017,Jan,8; 2016,Jan,13; 2016,Jan,3; 2015,Jan,16; 2014,Jan,11

52010 Cystourethroscopy, with ejaculatory duct catheterization, with or without irrigation, instillation, or duct radiography, exclusive of radiologic service ♂

⊠ (74440)

⚕ 4.79   ⚘ 10.9   **FUD** 000   T A2 ▭

AMA: 2018,Jan,8; 2017,Jan,8; 2016,Jan,13; 2015,Jan,16; 2014,Jan,11

52204 Cystourethroscopy, with biopsy(s)

⚕ 4.08   ⚘ 10.8   **FUD** 000   J A2 ▭

AMA: 2018,Jan,8; 2017,Jan,8; 2016,May,12; 2016,Jan,13; 2015,Jan,16; 2014,Jan,11

52214 **Cystourethroscopy, with fulguration (including cryosurgery or laser surgery) of trigone, bladder neck, prostatic fossa, urethra, or periurethral glands**

Code also modifier 78 when performed by same physician:
During postoperative period (52601, 52630)
During the postoperative period of a related surgical procedure
For postoperative bleeding

🔹 5.10   ✄ 20.0   **FUD** 000   J A2 ▣

AMA: 2018,Jan,8; 2017,Jan,8; 2016,May,12; 2016,Jan,13; 2015,Jan,16; 2014,Jan,11

52224 **Cystourethroscopy, with fulguration (including cryosurgery or laser surgery) or treatment of MINOR (less than 0.5 cm) lesion(s) with or without biopsy**

🔹 5.89   ✄ 20.9   **FUD** 000   J A2 ▣

AMA: 2018,Jan,8; 2017,Jan,8; 2016,May,12; 2016,Jan,13; 2015,Jan,16; 2014,Jan,11

52234 **Cystourethroscopy, with fulguration (including cryosurgery or laser surgery) and/or resection of; SMALL bladder tumor(s) (0.5 up to 2.0 cm)**

EXCLUDES   *Bladder tumor excision through cystotomy (51530)*

🔹 7.12   ✄ 7.12   **FUD** 000   J A2 ▣

AMA: 2018,Jan,8; 2017,Jan,8; 2016,May,12; 2016,Jan,13; 2015,Jan,16; 2014,Jan,11

52235 **MEDIUM bladder tumor(s) (2.0 to 5.0 cm)**

EXCLUDES   *Bladder tumor excision through cystotomy (51530)*

🔹 8.34   ✄ 8.34   **FUD** 000   J A2 ▣

AMA: 2018,Jan,8; 2017,Jan,8; 2016,May,12; 2016,Jan,13; 2015,Jan,16; 2014,Jan,11

52240 **LARGE bladder tumor(s)**

EXCLUDES   *Bladder tumor excision through cystotomy (51530)*

🔹 11.3   ✄ 11.3   **FUD** 000   J A2 ▣

AMA: 2018,Jan,8; 2017,Jan,8; 2016,May,12; 2016,Jan,13; 2015,Jan,16; 2014,Jan,11

52250 **Cystourethroscopy with insertion of radioactive substance, with or without biopsy or fulguration**

🔹 6.92   ✄ 6.92   **FUD** 000   J A2 ▣

AMA: 2018,Jan,8; 2017,Jan,8; 2016,Jan,13; 2015,Jan,16; 2014,Jan,11

52260 **Cystourethroscopy, with dilation of bladder for interstitial cystitis; general or conduction (spinal) anesthesia**

🔹 6.07   ✄ 6.07   **FUD** 000   J A2 ▣

AMA: 2018,Jan,8; 2017,Jan,8; 2016,Jan,13; 2015,Jan,16; 2014,Jan,11

52265 **local anesthesia**

🔹 4.67   ✄ 10.6   **FUD** 000   J P3 ▣

AMA: 2018,Jan,8; 2017,Jan,8; 2016,Jan,13; 2015,Jan,16; 2014,Jan,11

52270 **Cystourethroscopy, with internal urethrotomy; female**   ♀

🔹 5.27   ✄ 10.9   **FUD** 000   J A2 ▣

AMA: 2018,Jan,8; 2017,Jan,8; 2016,Jan,13; 2015,Jan,16; 2014,Jan,11

52275 **male**   ♂

🔹 7.19   ✄ 14.4   **FUD** 000   J A2 ▣

AMA: 2018,Jan,8; 2017,Jan,8; 2016,Jan,13; 2015,Jan,16; 2014,Jan,11

52276 **Cystourethroscopy with direct vision internal urethrotomy**

🔹 7.65   ✄ 7.65   **FUD** 000   J A2 ▣

AMA: 2019,Feb,10; 2018,Jan,8; 2017,Jan,8; 2016,Jan,13; 2015,Jan,16; 2014,Jan,11

52277 **Cystourethroscopy, with resection of external sphincter (sphincterotomy)**

🔹 9.35   ✄ 9.35   **FUD** 000   J A2 80 ▣

AMA: 2018,Jan,8; 2017,Jan,8; 2016,Jan,13; 2015,Jan,16; 2014,Jan,11

52281 **Cystourethroscopy, with calibration and/or dilation of urethral stricture or stenosis, with or without meatotomy, with or without injection procedure for cystography, male or female**

EXCLUDES   *Urethral delivery therapeutic drug (0499T)*

🔹 4.40   ✄ 8.53   **FUD** 000   J A2 ▣

AMA: 2018,Jan,8; 2017,Oct,9; 2017,Jan,8; 2016,Jan,13; 2015,Jan,16; 2014,Jan,11

52282 **Cystourethroscopy, with insertion of permanent urethral stent**

EXCLUDES   *Placement of temporary prostatic urethral stent (53855)*

🔹 9.76   ✄ 9.76   **FUD** 000   J A2 ▣

AMA: 2018,Jan,8; 2017,Jan,8; 2016,Jan,13; 2015,Jun,5; 2015,Jan,16; 2014,Jan,11

52283 **Cystourethroscopy, with steroid injection into stricture**

🔹 5.83   ✄ 8.68   **FUD** 000   J A2 ▣

AMA: 2019,Feb,10; 2018,Jan,8; 2017,Jan,8; 2016,Jan,13; 2015,Mar,9; 2015,Jan,16; 2014,Jan,11

52285 **Cystourethroscopy for treatment of the female urethral syndrome with any or all of the following: urethral meatotomy, urethral dilation, internal urethrotomy, lysis of urethrovaginal septal fibrosis, lateral incisions of the bladder neck, and fulguration of polyp(s) of urethra, bladder neck, and/or trigone**   ♀

🔹 5.66   ✄ 8.66   **FUD** 000   J A2 ▣

AMA: 2018,Jan,8; 2017,Jan,8; 2016,Jan,13; 2015,Jan,16; 2014,Jan,11

52287 **Cystourethroscopy, with injection(s) for chemodenervation of the bladder**

Code also supply of chemodenervation agent

🔹 4.89   ✄ 9.65   **FUD** 000   J G2 ▣

AMA: 2019,Apr,9; 2014,Jan,11

52290 **Cystourethroscopy; with ureteral meatotomy, unilateral or bilateral**

🔹 7.07   ✄ 7.07   **FUD** 000   J A2 ▣

AMA: 2018,Jan,8; 2017,Jan,8; 2016,Jan,13; 2015,Jan,16; 2014,Jan,11

52300 **with resection or fulguration of orthotopic ureterocele(s), unilateral or bilateral**

🔹 8.09   ✄ 8.09   **FUD** 000   J A2 80 ▣

AMA: 2018,Jan,8; 2017,Jan,8; 2016,Jan,13; 2015,Jan,16; 2014,Jan,11

52301 **with resection or fulguration of ectopic ureterocele(s), unilateral or bilateral**

🔹 8.38   ✄ 8.38   **FUD** 000   J A2 80 ▣

AMA: 2018,Jan,8; 2017,Jan,8; 2016,Jan,13; 2015,Jan,16; 2014,Jan,11

52305 **with incision or resection of orifice of bladder diverticulum, single or multiple**

🔹 8.06   ✄ 8.06   **FUD** 000   J A2 ▣

AMA: 2018,Jan,8; 2017,Jan,8; 2016,Jan,13; 2015,Jan,16; 2014,Jan,11

52310 **Cystourethroscopy, with removal of foreign body, calculus, or ureteral stent from urethra or bladder (separate procedure); simple**

Code also modifier 58 for removal of a self-retaining, indwelling ureteral stent

🔹 4.38   ✄ 7.68   **FUD** 000   J A2 ▣

AMA: 2018,Jan,8; 2017,Jan,8; 2016,Jan,13; 2015,Jun,5; 2015,Jan,16; 2014,Jan,11

52315 **complicated**

Code also modifier 58 for removal of a self-retaining, indwelling ureteral stent

🔹 7.94   ✄ 12.6   **FUD** 000   J A2 ▣

AMA: 2018,Jan,8; 2017,Jan,8; 2016,Jan,13; 2015,Jan,16; 2014,Jan,11

● New Code   ▲ Revised Code   ○ Reinstated   ● New Web Release   ▲ Revised Web Release   + Add-on   Unlisted   Not Covered   # Resequenced
50 Optum Mod 50 Exempt   ⊘ AMA Mod 51 Exempt   51 Optum Mod 51 Exempt   63 Mod 63 Exempt   ⚕ Non-FDA Drug   ★ Telemedicine   M Maternity   ▲ Age Edit

52317 Litholapaxy: crushing or fragmentation of calculus by any means in bladder and removal of fragments; simple or small (less than 2.5 cm)

🖪 10.0   ⚕ 24.1   **FUD** 000   [J] [A2] 🖴

AMA: 2018,Jan,8; 2017,Jan,8; 2016,Jan,13; 2015,Jan,16; 2014,Jan,11

52318 complicated or large (over 2.5 cm)

🖪 13.7   ⚕ 13.7   **FUD** 000   [J] [A2] 🖴

AMA: 2018,Jan,8; 2017,Jan,8; 2016,Jan,13; 2015,Jan,16; 2014,Jan,11

52320-52356 [52356] Endoscopic Procedures via Urethra: Renal Pelvis and Ureter

INCLUDES   Diagnostic cystourethroscopy when performed with therapeutic cystourethroscopy
Insertion/removal of temporary ureteral catheter (52005)

EXCLUDES   *Self-retaining/indwelling ureteral stent removal by cystourethroscope, with modifier 58 if appropriate (52310, 52315)*

Code also the insertion of an indwelling stent performed in addition to other procedures within this section (52332)

52320 Cystourethroscopy (including ureteral catheterization); with removal of ureteral calculus

INCLUDES   Cystourethroscopy (separate procedure) (52000)

🖪 7.13   ⚕ 7.13   **FUD** 000   [J] [A2] [50] 🖴

AMA: 2018,Jan,8; 2017,Jan,8; 2016,Jan,13; 2015,Jan,16; 2014,Jan,11

52325 with fragmentation of ureteral calculus (eg, ultrasonic or electro-hydraulic technique)

INCLUDES   Cystourethroscopy (separate procedure) (52000)

🖪 9.27   ⚕ 9.27   **FUD** 000   [J] [A2] [50] 🖴

AMA: 2018,Jan,8; 2017,Jan,8; 2016,Jan,13; 2015,Jan,16; 2014,Jan,11

52327 with subureteric injection of implant material

INCLUDES   Cystourethroscopy (separate procedure) (52000)

🖪 7.59   ⚕ 7.59   **FUD** 000   [J] [J8] [50] 🖴

AMA: 2018,Jan,8; 2017,Jan,8; 2016,Jan,13; 2015,Jan,16; 2014,Jan,11

52330 with manipulation, without removal of ureteral calculus

INCLUDES   Cystourethroscopy (separate procedure) (52000)

🖪 7.63   ⚕ 15.4   **FUD** 000   [J] [A2] [50] 🖴

AMA: 2018,Jan,8; 2017,Jan,8; 2016,Jan,13; 2015,Jan,16; 2014,May,3; 2014,Jan,11

52332 Cystourethroscopy, with insertion of indwelling ureteral stent (eg, Gibbons or double-J type)

INCLUDES   Cystourethroscopy (separate procedure) (52000)

EXCLUDES   *Cystourethroscopy, with ureteroscopy and/or pyeloscopy; with lithotripsy when performed on the same side with (52353, [52356])*

🖪 4.50   ⚕ 13.5   **FUD** 000   [J] [A2] [50] 🖴

AMA: 2018,Jan,8; 2017,Jan,8; 2016,Jan,13; 2015,Jan,16; 2014,May,3; 2014,Jan,11

52334 Cystourethroscopy with insertion of ureteral guide wire through kidney to establish a percutaneous nephrostomy, retrograde

INCLUDES   Cystourethroscopy (separate procedure) (52000)

EXCLUDES   *Cystourethroscopy with incision/fulguration/resection of congenital posterior urethral valves/obstructive hypertrophic mucosal folds (52400)*
Cystourethroscopy with pyeloscopy and/or ureteroscopy (52351-52353 [52356])
Dilation of nephroureteral catheter tract ([50436], [50437])
Nephrostomy tract establishment only ([50432, 50433])
Percutaneous nephrostolithotomy (50080, 50081)

🖪 5.30   ⚕ 5.30   **FUD** 000   [J] [A2] 🖴

AMA: 2018,Jan,8; 2017,Jan,8; 2016,Jan,13; 2015,Jan,16; 2014,May,3; 2014,Jan,11

52341 Cystourethroscopy; with treatment of ureteral stricture (eg, balloon dilation, laser, electrocautery, and incision)

INCLUDES   Diagnostic cystourethroscopy (52351)

EXCLUDES   *Balloon dilation with imaging guidance (50706)*
Cystourethroscopy, separate procedure (52000)

🔀 (74485)

🖪 8.21   ⚕ 8.21   **FUD** 000   [J] [A2] [50] 🖴

AMA: 2018,Jan,8; 2017,Jan,8; 2016,Jan,13; 2016,Jan,3; 2015,Jan,16; 2014,Jan,11

52342 with treatment of ureteropelvic junction stricture (eg, balloon dilation, laser, electrocautery, and incision)

INCLUDES   Diagnostic cystourethroscopy (52351)

EXCLUDES   *Balloon dilation with imaging guidance (50706)*
Cystourethroscopy (separate procedure) (52000)

🔀 (74485)

🖪 8.93   ⚕ 8.93   **FUD** 000   [J] [A2] [50] 🖴

AMA: 2018,Jan,8; 2017,Jan,8; 2016,Jan,13; 2015,Jan,16; 2014,Jan,11

52343 with treatment of intra-renal stricture (eg, balloon dilation, laser, electrocautery, and incision)

INCLUDES   Diagnostic cystourethroscopy (52351)

EXCLUDES   *Balloon dilation with imaging guidance (50706)*
Cystourethroscopy (separate procedure) (52000)

🔀 (74485)

🖪 9.96   ⚕ 9.96   **FUD** 000   [J] [A2] [50] 🖴

AMA: 2018,Jan,8; 2017,Jan,8; 2016,Jan,13; 2015,Jan,16; 2014,May,3; 2014,Jan,11

52344 Cystourethroscopy with ureteroscopy; with treatment of ureteral stricture (eg, balloon dilation, laser, electrocautery, and incision)

INCLUDES   Diagnostic cystourethroscopy (52351)

EXCLUDES   *Balloon dilation, ureteral stricture (50706)*
Cystourethroscopy with transurethral resection or incision of ejaculatory ducts (52402)

🔀 (74485)

🖪 10.6   ⚕ 10.6   **FUD** 000   [J] [A2] [50] 🖴

AMA: 2018,Jan,8; 2017,Jan,8; 2016,Jan,13; 2016,Jan,3; 2015,Jan,16; 2014,Jan,11

52345 with treatment of ureteropelvic junction stricture (eg, balloon dilation, laser, electrocautery, and incision)

INCLUDES   Diagnostic cystourethroscopy (52351)

EXCLUDES   *Balloon dilation, ureteral stricture (50706)*
Cystourethroscopy with transurethral resection or incision of ejaculatory ducts (52402)

🔀 (74485)

🖪 11.4   ⚕ 11.4   **FUD** 000   [J] [A2] [80] [50] 🖴

AMA: 2018,Jan,8; 2017,Jan,8; 2016,Jan,13; 2016,Jan,3; 2015,Jan,16; 2014,Jan,11

52346 with treatment of intra-renal stricture (eg, balloon dilation, laser, electrocautery, and incision)

INCLUDES   Diagnostic cystourethroscopy (52351)

EXCLUDES   *Balloon dilation with imaging guidance (50706)*
Cystourethroscopy with transurethral resection or incision of ejaculatory ducts (52402)

🔀 (74485)

🖪 12.9   ⚕ 12.9   **FUD** 000   [J] [A2] [80] [50] 🖴

AMA: 2018,Jan,8; 2017,Jan,8; 2016,Jan,13; 2015,Jan,16; 2014,May,3; 2014,Jan,11

52351 Cystourethroscopy, with ureteroscopy and/or pyeloscopy; diagnostic

EXCLUDES   *Cystourethroscopy (52341-52346, 52352-52353 [52356])*

🖪 8.75   ⚕ 8.75   **FUD** 000   [J] [A2]

AMA: 2018,Jan,8; 2017,Jan,8; 2016,Jan,13; 2015,Jan,16; 2014,May,3; 2014,Jan,11

| 26/TC PC/TC Only | A2-Z3 ASC Payment | 50 Bilateral | ♂ Male Only | ♀ Female Only | 🖪 Facility RVU | ⚕ Non-Facility RVU | 🖴 CCI | 🗙 CLIA |
| **FUD** Follow-up Days | **CMS:** IOM | **AMA:** CPT Asst | A-Y OPPSI | 80/80 Surg Assist Allowed / w/Doc | 🗙 Lab Crosswalk | | 🔀 Radiology Crosswalk |

250

CPT © 2019 American Medical Association. All Rights Reserved.

© 2019 Optum360, LLC

52352 with removal or manipulation of calculus (ureteral catheterization is included)

INCLUDES Diagnostic cystourethroscopy (52351)

🔧 10.2 🔪 10.2 **FUD** 000 `J` `A2` `50` 🖥

AMA: 2018,Jan,8; 2017,Jan,8; 2016,Jan,13; 2015,Jan,16; 2014,Jan,11

Right kidney
Left kidney
Stone basket
Calculus
Ureters
Bladder
Cystourethroscope

52353 with lithotripsy (ureteral catheterization is included)

INCLUDES Diagnostic cystourethroscopy (52351)

EXCLUDES Cystourethroscopy when performed on the same side (52332, [52356])

🔧 11.3 🔪 11.3 **FUD** 000 `J` `A2` `50` 🖥

AMA: 2018,Jan,8; 2017,Jan,8; 2016,Jan,13; 2015,Jan,16; 2014,May,3; 2014,Jan,11

 # 52356 with lithotripsy including insertion of indwelling ureteral stent (eg, Gibbons or double-J type)

INCLUDES Diagnostic cystourethroscopy (52351)

EXCLUDES Cystourethroscopy when performed on the same side with (52332, 52353)

Cystourethroscopy (separate procedure) (52000)

🔧 12.0 🔪 12.0 **FUD** 000 `J` `62` `50` 🖥

AMA: 2018,Jan,8; 2017,Jan,8; 2016,Jan,13; 2015,Jan,16; 2014,May,3; 2014,Jan,11

52354 with biopsy and/or fulguration of ureteral or renal pelvic lesion

INCLUDES Diagnostic cystourethroscopy (52351)

EXCLUDES Image guided biopsy without endoscopic guidance (50606)

🔧 12.0 🔪 12.0 **FUD** 000 `J` `A2` `50` 🖥

AMA: 2018,Jan,8; 2017,Jan,8; 2016,Jan,13; 2015,Jan,16; 2014,May,3; 2014,Jan,11

52355 with resection of ureteral or renal pelvic tumor

INCLUDES Diagnostic cystourethroscopy (52351)

🔧 13.5 🔪 13.5 **FUD** 000 `J` `A2` `50` 🖥

AMA: 2018,Jan,8; 2017,Jan,8; 2016,Jan,13; 2015,Jan,16; 2014,May,3; 2014,Jan,11

52356 Resequenced code. See code following 52353.

52400-52700 Endoscopic Procedures via Urethra: Prostate and Vesical Neck

52400 Cystourethroscopy with incision, fulguration, or resection of congenital posterior urethral valves, or congenital obstructive hypertrophic mucosal folds

🔧 13.8 🔪 13.8 **FUD** 090 `J` `A2` 🖥

AMA: 2018,Jan,8; 2017,Jan,8; 2016,Jan,13; 2015,Jan,16; 2014,Jan,11

52402 Cystourethroscopy with transurethral resection or incision of ejaculatory ducts ♂

🔧 7.73 🔪 7.73 **FUD** 000 `J` `A2` 🖥

AMA: 2014,Jan,11

52441 Cystourethroscopy, with insertion of permanent adjustable transprostatic implant; single implant

🔧 6.55 🔪 36.1 **FUD** 000 `B` 🖥

AMA: 2018,Jan,8; 2017,Jan,8; 2016,Jan,13; 2015,Jun,5

+ 52442 each additional permanent adjustable transprostatic implant (List separately in addition to code for primary procedure)

EXCLUDES Permanent urethral stent insertion (52282)

Removal of stent, calculus or foreign body (implant) (52310)

Temporary prostatic urethral stent insertion (53855)

Code first (52441)

🔧 1.75 🔪 27.1 **FUD** ZZZ `B` 🖥

AMA: 2018,Jan,8; 2017,Jan,8; 2016,Jan,13; 2015,Jun,5

52450 Transurethral incision of prostate ♂

🔧 13.5 🔪 13.5 **FUD** 090 `J` `A2` 🖥

AMA: 2018,Jan,8; 2017,Jan,8; 2016,Jan,13; 2015,Jun,5; 2015,Jan,16; 2014,Jan,11

52500 Transurethral resection of bladder neck (separate procedure)

🔧 14.1 🔪 14.1 **FUD** 090 `J` `A2` 🖥

AMA: 2018,Jan,8; 2017,Jan,8; 2016,Jan,13; 2015,Jan,16; 2014,Jan,11

52601 Transurethral electrosurgical resection of prostate, including control of postoperative bleeding, complete (vasectomy, meatotomy, cystourethroscopy, urethral calibration and/or dilation, and internal urethrotomy are included) ♂

INCLUDES Stage 1 of partial transurethral resection of prostate

EXCLUDES Ablation by waterjet (0421T)

Excision of prostate (55801-55845)

Transurethral fulguration of prostate (52214)

Code also modifier 58 for stage 2 partial transurethral resection of prostate

🔧 21.0 🔪 21.0 **FUD** 090 `J` `A2` 🖥

AMA: 2018,Jan,8; 2017,Jan,8; 2016,Jan,13; 2015,Jun,5; 2015,Jan,16; 2014,Jan,11

52630 Transurethral resection; residual or regrowth of obstructive prostate tissue including control of postoperative bleeding, complete (vasectomy, meatotomy, cystourethroscopy, urethral calibration and/or dilation, and internal urethrotomy are included) ♂

EXCLUDES Ablation by waterjet (0421T)

Excision of prostate (55801-55845)

Code also modifier 78 when performed by same physician within the postoperative period of a related procedure

🔧 11.5 🔪 11.5 **FUD** 090 `J` `A2` 🖥

AMA: 2018,Jan,8; 2017,Jan,8; 2016,Jan,13; 2015,Jan,16; 2014,Jan,11

52640 of postoperative bladder neck contracture

EXCLUDES Excision of prostate (55801-55845)

🔧 9.14 🔪 9.14 **FUD** 090 `J` `A2` 🖥

AMA: 2018,Jan,8; 2017,Jan,8; 2016,Jan,13; 2015,Jan,16; 2014,Jan,11

52647 Laser coagulation of prostate, including control of postoperative bleeding, complete (vasectomy, meatotomy, cystourethroscopy, urethral calibration and/or dilation, and internal urethrotomy are included if performed) ♂

🔧 18.7 🔪 46.2 **FUD** 090 `J` `A2` 🖥

AMA: 2018,Jan,8; 2017,Jan,8; 2016,Jan,13; 2015,Jan,16; 2014,Jan,11

52648 Laser vaporization of prostate, including control of postoperative bleeding, complete (vasectomy, meatotomy, cystourethroscopy, urethral calibration and/or dilation, internal urethrotomy and transurethral resection of prostate are included if performed) ♂

🔧 19.9 🔪 47.7 **FUD** 090 `J` `A2` 🖥

AMA: 2018,Jan,8; 2017,Jan,8; 2016,Jan,13; 2015,Jun,5; 2015,Jan,16; 2014,Jan,11

52649 Laser enucleation of the prostate with morcellation, including control of postoperative bleeding, complete (vasectomy, meatotomy, cystourethroscopy, urethral calibration and/or dilation, internal urethrotomy and transurethral resection of prostate are included if performed) ♂

INCLUDES Cystourethroscopy (52000, 52276, 52281)
Laser coagulation of prostate (52647-52648)
Meatotomy (53020)
Transurethral resection of prostate (52601)
Vasectomy (55250)

🖬 23.8   ⅗ 23.8   **FUD** 090   J 62 80 ▣

AMA: 2018,Jan,8; 2017,Jan,8; 2016,Jan,13; 2015,Jun,5; 2014,Jan,11

52700 Transurethral drainage of prostatic abscess ♂

EXCLUDES Litholapaxy (52317, 52318)

🖬 12.7   ⅗ 12.7   **FUD** 090   J A2 80 ▣

AMA: 2018,Jan,8; 2017,Jan,8; 2016,Jan,13; 2015,Jan,16; 2014,Jan,11

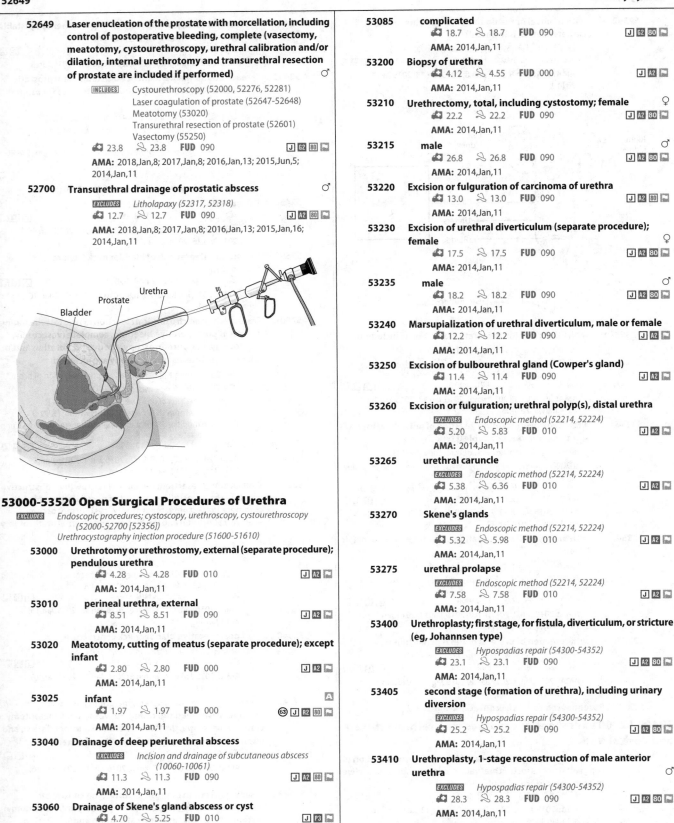

Bladder · Prostate · Urethra

53000-53520 Open Surgical Procedures of Urethra

EXCLUDES Endoscopic procedures; cystoscopy, urethroscopy, cystourethroscopy (52000-52700 [52356])
Urethrocystography injection procedure (51600-51610)

53000 Urethrotomy or urethrostomy, external (separate procedure); pendulous urethra

🖬 4.28   ⅗ 4.28   **FUD** 010   J A2 ▣

AMA: 2014,Jan,11

53010 perineal urethra, external

🖬 8.51   ⅗ 8.51   **FUD** 090   J A2 ▣

AMA: 2014,Jan,11

53020 Meatotomy, cutting of meatus (separate procedure); except infant

🖬 2.80   ⅗ 2.80   **FUD** 000   J A2 ▣

AMA: 2014,Jan,11

53025 infant   A

🖬 1.97   ⅗ 1.97   **FUD** 000   63 J R2 80 ▣

AMA: 2014,Jan,11

53040 Drainage of deep periurethral abscess

EXCLUDES Incision and drainage of subcutaneous abscess (10060-10061)

🖬 11.3   ⅗ 11.3   **FUD** 090   J A2 80 ▣

AMA: 2014,Jan,11

53060 Drainage of Skene's gland abscess or cyst

🖬 4.70   ⅗ 5.25   **FUD** 010   J P3 ▣

AMA: 2014,Jan,11

53080 Drainage of perineal urinary extravasation; uncomplicated (separate procedure)

🖬 12.1   ⅗ 12.1   **FUD** 090   J A2 ▣

AMA: 2014,Jan,11

53085 complicated

🖬 18.7   ⅗ 18.7   **FUD** 090   J 62 80 ▣

AMA: 2014,Jan,11

53200 Biopsy of urethra

🖬 4.12   ⅗ 4.55   **FUD** 000   J A2 ▣

AMA: 2014,Jan,11

53210 Urethrectomy, total, including cystostomy; female ♀

🖬 22.2   ⅗ 22.2   **FUD** 090   J A2 80 ▣

AMA: 2014,Jan,11

53215 male   ♂

🖬 26.8   ⅗ 26.8   **FUD** 090   J A2 80 ▣

AMA: 2014,Jan,11

53220 Excision or fulguration of carcinoma of urethra

🖬 13.0   ⅗ 13.0   **FUD** 090   J A2 80 ▣

AMA: 2014,Jan,11

53230 Excision of urethral diverticulum (separate procedure); female ♀

🖬 17.5   ⅗ 17.5   **FUD** 090   J A2 80 ▣

AMA: 2014,Jan,11

53235 male   ♂

🖬 18.2   ⅗ 18.2   **FUD** 090   J A2 80 ▣

AMA: 2014,Jan,11

53240 Marsupialization of urethral diverticulum, male or female

🖬 12.2   ⅗ 12.2   **FUD** 090   J A2 ▣

AMA: 2014,Jan,11

53250 Excision of bulbourethral gland (Cowper's gland)

🖬 11.4   ⅗ 11.4   **FUD** 090   J A2 ▣

AMA: 2014,Jan,11

53260 Excision or fulguration; urethral polyp(s), distal urethra

EXCLUDES Endoscopic method (52214, 52224)

🖬 5.20   ⅗ 5.83   **FUD** 010   J A2 ▣

AMA: 2014,Jan,11

53265 urethral caruncle

EXCLUDES Endoscopic method (52214, 52224)

🖬 5.38   ⅗ 6.36   **FUD** 010   J A2 ▣

AMA: 2014,Jan,11

53270 Skene's glands

EXCLUDES Endoscopic method (52214, 52224)

🖬 5.32   ⅗ 5.98   **FUD** 010   J A2 ▣

AMA: 2014,Jan,11

53275 urethral prolapse

EXCLUDES Endoscopic method (52214, 52224)

🖬 7.58   ⅗ 7.58   **FUD** 010   J A2 ▣

AMA: 2014,Jan,11

53400 Urethroplasty; first stage, for fistula, diverticulum, or stricture (eg, Johannsen type)

EXCLUDES Hypospadias repair (54300-54352)

🖬 23.1   ⅗ 23.1   **FUD** 090   J A2 80 ▣

AMA: 2014,Jan,11

53405 second stage (formation of urethra), including urinary diversion

EXCLUDES Hypospadias repair (54300-54352)

🖬 25.2   ⅗ 25.2   **FUD** 090   J A2 80 ▣

AMA: 2014,Jan,11

53410 Urethroplasty, 1-stage reconstruction of male anterior urethra ♂

EXCLUDES Hypospadias repair (54300-54352)

🖬 28.3   ⅗ 28.3   **FUD** 090   J A2 80 ▣

AMA: 2014,Jan,11

53415 Urethroplasty, transpubic or perineal, 1-stage, for reconstruction or repair of prostatic or membranous urethra ♂

🖬 32.7   ⅗ 32.7   **FUD** 090   C 80 ▣

AMA: 2014,Jan,11

26/TC PC/TC Only   A2-Z3 ASC Payment   50 Bilateral   ♂ Male Only   ♀ Female Only   🖬 Facility RVU   ⅗ Non-Facility RVU   ▣ CCI   ✖ CLIA
FUD Follow-up Days   CMS: IOM   AMA: CPT Asst   A-Y OPPSI   80/80 Surg Assist Allowed / w/Doc   Lab Crosswalk   Radiology Crosswalk

252   CPT © 2019 American Medical Association. All Rights Reserved.   © 2019 Optum360, LLC

53420	Urethroplasty, 2-stage reconstruction or repair of prostatic or membranous urethra; first stage ♂
	24.3 24.3 **FUD** 090 J A2
	AMA: 2014,Jan,11

53425	second stage ♂
	27.1 27.1 **FUD** 090 J A2 80
	AMA: 2014,Jan,11

53430	Urethroplasty, reconstruction of female urethra ♀
	27.9 27.9 **FUD** 090 J A2 80
	AMA: 2014,Jan,11

53431	Urethroplasty with tubularization of posterior urethra and/or lower bladder for incontinence (eg, Tenago, Leadbetter procedure)
	33.4 33.4 **FUD** 090 J A2 80
	AMA: 2014,Jan,11

53440	Sling operation for correction of male urinary incontinence (eg, fascia or synthetic) ♂
	21.7 21.7 **FUD** 090 J J8 80
	AMA: 2014,Jan,11

53442	Removal or revision of sling for male urinary incontinence (eg, fascia or synthetic) ♂
	22.6 22.6 **FUD** 090 J A2 80
	AMA: 2014,Jan,11

53444	Insertion of tandem cuff (dual cuff)
	22.9 22.9 **FUD** 090 J J8 80
	AMA: 2014,Jan,11

53445	Insertion of inflatable urethral/bladder neck sphincter, including placement of pump, reservoir, and cuff
	21.7 21.7 **FUD** 090 J J8 80
	AMA: 2014,Jan,11

53446	Removal of inflatable urethral/bladder neck sphincter, including pump, reservoir, and cuff
	18.5 18.5 **FUD** 090 02 A2 80
	AMA: 2014,Jan,11

53447	Removal and replacement of inflatable urethral/bladder neck sphincter including pump, reservoir, and cuff at the same operative session
	23.3 23.3 **FUD** 090 J J8 80
	AMA: 2014,Jan,11

53448	Removal and replacement of inflatable urethral/bladder neck sphincter including pump, reservoir, and cuff through an infected field at the same operative session including irrigation and debridement of infected tissue
	INCLUDES Debridement (11042, 11043)
	37.0 37.0 **FUD** 090 C 80
	AMA: 2014,Jan,11

53449	Repair of inflatable urethral/bladder neck sphincter, including pump, reservoir, and cuff
	17.6 17.6 **FUD** 090 J A2 80
	AMA: 2014,Jan,11

53450	Urethromeatoplasty, with mucosal advancement
	EXCLUDES Meatotomy (53020, 53025)
	11.8 11.8 **FUD** 090 J A2
	AMA: 2018,Jan,8; 2017,Jan,8; 2016,Jan,13; 2015,Jan,16; 2014,Jan,11

53460	Urethromeatoplasty, with partial excision of distal urethral segment (Richardson type procedure)
	13.2 13.2 **FUD** 090 J A2 80
	AMA: 2014,Jan,11

53500	Urethrolysis, transvaginal, secondary, open, including cystourethroscopy (eg, postsurgical obstruction, scarring)
	INCLUDES Cystourethroscopy (separate procedure) (52000)
	EXCLUDES Retropubic approach (53899)
	21.5 21.5 **FUD** 090 J 80
	AMA: 2018,Jan,8; 2017,Jan,8; 2016,Jan,13; 2015,Jan,16; 2014,Jan,11

53502	Urethrorrhaphy, suture of urethral wound or injury, female ♀
	14.0 14.0 **FUD** 090 J A2
	AMA: 2014,Jan,11

53505	Urethrorrhaphy, suture of urethral wound or injury; penile ♂
	14.0 14.0 **FUD** 090 J A2 80
	AMA: 2014,Jan,11

53510	perineal ♂
	18.2 18.2 **FUD** 090 J A2 80
	AMA: 2014,Jan,11

53515	prostatomembranous ♂
	23.0 23.0 **FUD** 090 J A2 80
	AMA: 2014,Jan,11

53520	Closure of urethrostomy or urethrocutaneous fistula, male (separate procedure) ♂
	EXCLUDES Closure of fistula:
	Urethrorectal (45820, 45825)
	Urethrovaginal (57310)
	16.1 16.1 **FUD** 090 J A2
	AMA: 2014,Jan,11

53600-53665 Urethral Dilation

EXCLUDES Endoscopic procedures; cystoscopy, urethroscopy, cystourethroscopy (52000-52700 [52356])
Urethral catheterization (51701-51703)
Urethrocystography injection procedure (51600-51610)
(74485)

53600	Dilation of urethral stricture by passage of sound or urethral dilator, male; initial ♂
	1.84 2.39 **FUD** 000 T P3
	AMA: 2014,Jan,11

53601	subsequent ♂
	1.55 2.29 **FUD** 000 Q1 N1
	AMA: 2014,Jan,11

53605	Dilation of urethral stricture or vesical neck by passage of sound or urethral dilator, male, general or conduction (spinal) anesthesia ♂
	EXCLUDES Procedure performed under local anesthesia (53600-53601, 53620-53621)
	1.87 1.87 **FUD** 000 J A2
	AMA: 2014,Jan,11

53620	Dilation of urethral stricture by passage of filiform and follower, male; initial ♂
	2.52 3.79 **FUD** 000 T P3
	AMA: 2014,Jan,11

53621	subsequent ♂
	2.09 3.56 **FUD** 000 T P3
	AMA: 2014,Jan,11

● New Code ▲ Revised Code ○ Reinstated ● New Web Release ▲ Revised Web Release + Add-on Unlisted Not Covered # Resequenced
50 Optum Mod 50 Exempt ⊘ AMA Mod 51 Exempt 51 Optum Mod 51 Exempt 63 Mod 63 Exempt ✂ Non-FDA Drug ★ Telemedicine M Maternity A Age Edit

CPT © 2019 American Medical Association. All Rights Reserved.

53660 Dilation of female urethra including suppository and/or instillation; initial ♀

⚕ 1.20   ✂ 1.99   **FUD** 000   [S] [P3] [CCI]

AMA: 2014,Jan,11

Urethra
Sound
Detail
Urethra
Stricture

Physician passes a dilator through a stricture in the urethra

53661 subsequent ♀

⚕ 1.17   ✂ 1.96   **FUD** 000   [01] [N1] [CCI]

AMA: 2014,Jan,11

53665 Dilation of female urethra, general or conduction (spinal) anesthesia ♀

EXCLUDES Procedure performed under local anesthesia (53660-53661)

⚕ 1.12   ✂ 1.12   **FUD** 000   [J] [A2] [CCI]

AMA: 2014,Jan,11

53850-53899 Transurethral Procedures

EXCLUDES Endoscopic procedures; cystoscopy, urethroscopy, cystourethroscopy (52000-52700 [52356])

53850 Transurethral destruction of prostate tissue; by microwave thermotherapy ♂

🔬 (81020)

⚕ 10.1   ✂ 45.4   **FUD** 090   [J] [P2] [CCI]

AMA: 2018,Nov,10; 2018,Jan,8; 2017,Jan,8; 2016,Jan,13; 2015,Jun,5; 2015,Jan,16; 2014,Jan,11

53852 by radiofrequency thermotherapy ♂

🔬 (81020)

⚕ 10.8   ✂ 43.9   **FUD** 090   [J] [P3] [CCI]

AMA: 2018,Nov,10; 2018,Jan,8; 2017,Jan,8; 2016,Jan,13; 2015,Jun,5; 2015,Jan,16; 2014,Jan,11

53854 by radiofrequency generated water vapor thermotherapy

EXCLUDES High-energy water vapor thermotherapy for transurethral ablation of malignant prostate tissue (0582T)

⚕ 10.8   ✂ 52.0   **FUD** 090   [G2] [CCI]

AMA: 2018,Nov,10

53855 Insertion of a temporary prostatic urethral stent, including urethral measurement ♂

EXCLUDES Permanent urethral stent insertion (52282)

⚕ 2.39   ✂ 21.7   **FUD** 000   [J] [P3] [80] [CCI]

AMA: 2018,Nov,10; 2018,Jan,8; 2017,Jan,8; 2016,Jan,13; 2015,Jun,5; 2015,Jan,16; 2014,Jan,11

53860 Transurethral radiofrequency micro-remodeling of the female bladder neck and proximal urethra for stress urinary incontinence ♀

⚕ 6.48   ✂ 52.7   **FUD** 090   [J] [P2] [80] [CCI]

AMA: 2014,Jan,11

53899 Unlisted procedure, urinary system

⚕ 0.00   ✂ 0.00   **FUD** YYY   [T] [80] [CCI]

AMA: 2019,Aug,10; 2018,Jan,8; 2017,Jan,8; 2016,Jan,13; 2015,Jun,5; 2015,Mar,9; 2015,Jan,16; 2014,Jan,11

26/[TC] PC/TC Only   [A2-Z3] ASC Payment   [50] Bilateral   ♂ Male Only   ♀ Female Only   ⚕ Facility RVU   ✂ Non-Facility RVU   [CCI] CCI   [X] CLIA
FUD Follow-up Days   **CMS:** IOM   **AMA:** CPT Asst   [A]-[Y] OPPSI   80/80 Surg Assist Allowed / w/Doc   🔬 Lab Crosswalk   Radiology Crosswalk

254   CPT © 2019 American Medical Association. All Rights Reserved.   © 2019 Optum360, LLC

54000-54015 Procedures of Penis: Incisional

EXCLUDES   *Debridement of abdominal perineal gangrene (11004-11006)*

54000   **Slitting of prepuce, dorsal or lateral (separate procedure); newborn**   A ♂

🔧 3.14   ⚕ 4.40   **FUD** 010   ⓺ J A2 80 ▭

AMA: 2014,Jan,11

54001   **except newborn**   ♂

🔧 4.02   ⚕ 5.44   **FUD** 010   J A2 ▭

AMA: 2014,Jan,11

54015   **Incision and drainage of penis, deep**   ♂

EXCLUDES   *Abscess, skin/subcutaneous (10060-10160)*

🔧 8.92   ⚕ 8.92   **FUD** 010   J A2 80 ▭

AMA: 2014,Jan,11

Urethra

Hematoma or abscess

Hematoma or abscess

A postoperative drain may be placed. Sutures are required to repair the operative site

The physician incises the penis to drain an abscess or hematoma

54050-54065 Destruction of Penis Lesions: Multiple Methods

EXCLUDES   *Excision/destruction other lesions (11420-11426, 11620-11626, 17000-17250, 17270-17276)*

54050   **Destruction of lesion(s), penis (eg, condyloma, papilloma, molluscum contagiosum, herpetic vesicle), simple; chemical**   ♂

🔧 3.05   ⚕ 3.80   **FUD** 010   Q1 N1 ▭

AMA: 2014,Jan,11

54055   **electrodesiccation**   ♂

🔧 2.69   ⚕ 3.49   **FUD** 010   T P3 ▭

AMA: 2014,Jan,11

54056   **cryosurgery**   ♂

🔧 3.18   ⚕ 4.03   **FUD** 010   Q1 N1 ▭

AMA: 2014,Jan,11

54057   **laser surgery**   ♂

🔧 2.76   ⚕ 3.97   **FUD** 010   T A2 ▭

AMA: 2014,Jan,11

54060   **surgical excision**   ♂

🔧 3.76   ⚕ 5.29   **FUD** 010   T A2 ▭

AMA: 2014,Jan,11

54065   **Destruction of lesion(s), penis (eg, condyloma, papilloma, molluscum contagiosum, herpetic vesicle), extensive (eg, laser surgery, electrosurgery, cryosurgery, chemosurgery)**   ♂

🔧 4.97   ⚕ 6.31   **FUD** 010   T A2 ▭

AMA: 2014,Jan,11

54100-54115 Procedures of Penis: Excisional

54100   **Biopsy of penis; (separate procedure)**   ♂

🔧 3.59   ⚕ 5.64   **FUD** 000   J A2 ▭

AMA: 2019,Jan,9; 2018,Jan,8; 2017,Jan,8; 2016,Jan,13; 2015,Jan,16; 2014,Jan,11

54105   **deep structures**   ♂

🔧 6.16   ⚕ 7.68   **FUD** 010   J A2 ▭

AMA: 2014,Jan,11

54110   **Excision of penile plaque (Peyronie disease);**   ♂

🔧 18.0   ⚕ 18.0   **FUD** 090   J A2 80 ▭

AMA: 2014,Jan,11

54111   **with graft to 5 cm in length**   ♂

🔧 23.1   ⚕ 23.1   **FUD** 090   J A2 80 ▭

AMA: 2018,Jan,8; 2017,Jan,8; 2016,Jan,13; 2015,Jan,16; 2014,Jan,11

54112   **with graft greater than 5 cm in length**   ♂

🔧 27.1   ⚕ 27.1   **FUD** 090   J A2 80 ▭

AMA: 2014,Jan,11

54115   **Removal foreign body from deep penile tissue (eg, plastic implant)**   ♂

🔧 12.2   ⚕ 13.0   **FUD** 090   J A2 80 ▭

AMA: 2014,Jan,11

54120-54135 Amputation of Penis

EXCLUDES   *Lymphadenectomy (separate procedure) (38760-38770)*

54120   **Amputation of penis; partial**   ♂

🔧 18.2   ⚕ 18.2   **FUD** 090   J A2 80 ▭

AMA: 2014,Jan,11

54125   **complete**   ♂

🔧 23.5   ⚕ 23.5   **FUD** 090   C 80 ▭

AMA: 2014,Jan,11

54130   **Amputation of penis, radical; with bilateral inguinofemoral lymphadenectomy**   ♂

🔧 34.5   ⚕ 34.5   **FUD** 090   C 80 ▭

AMA: 2014,Jan,11

54135   **in continuity with bilateral pelvic lymphadenectomy, including external iliac, hypogastric and obturator nodes**   ♂

🔧 43.7   ⚕ 43.7   **FUD** 090   C 80 ▭

AMA: 2014,Jan,11

54150-54164 Circumcision Procedures

54150   **Circumcision, using clamp or other device with regional dorsal penile or ring block**   ♂

Code also modifier 52 when performed without dorsal penile or ring block

🔧 2.83   ⚕ 4.42   **FUD** 000   ⓺ J A2 80 ▭

AMA: 2018,Jan,8; 2017,Jan,8; 2016,Jan,13; 2015,Jan,16; 2014,Jan,11

54160   **Circumcision, surgical excision other than clamp, device, or dorsal slit; neonate (28 days of age or less)**   A ♂

🔧 4.17   ⚕ 6.32   **FUD** 010   ⓺ J A2 ▭

AMA: 2018,Jan,8; 2017,Jan,8; 2016,Jan,13; 2015,Jan,16; 2014,Jan,11

54161   **older than 28 days of age**   A ♂

🔧 5.70   ⚕ 5.70   **FUD** 010   J A2 ▭

AMA: 2018,Jan,8; 2017,Jan,8; 2016,Jan,13; 2015,Jan,16; 2014,Jan,11

54162   **Lysis or excision of penile post-circumcision adhesions**   ♂

🔧 5.77   ⚕ 7.42   **FUD** 010   J A2 ▭

AMA: 2014,Jan,11

54163   **Repair incomplete circumcision**   ♂

🔧 6.31   ⚕ 6.31   **FUD** 010   J A2 ▭

AMA: 2014,Jan,11

54164   **Frenulotomy of penis**   ♂

EXCLUDES   *Circumcision (54150-54163)*

🔧 5.60   ⚕ 5.60   **FUD** 010   J A2 ▭

AMA: 2014,Jan,11

● New Code   ▲ Revised Code   ○ Reinstated   ● New Web Release   ▲ Revised Web Release   + Add-on   Unlisted   Not Covered   # Resequenced
㊿ Optum Mod 50 Exempt   Ⓢ AMA Mod 51 Exempt   ⑤ Optum Mod 51 Exempt   ⓺ Mod 63 Exempt   ✗ Non-FDA Drug   ★ Telemedicine   M Maternity   A Age Edit

54200-54250 Evaluation and Treatment of Erectile Abnormalities

54200   **Injection procedure for Peyronie disease;**   ♂
   🔲 2.42   📊 3.13   **FUD** 010   T P3 🔲
   AMA: 2014,Jan,11

54205   **with surgical exposure of plaque**   ♂
   🔲 15.4   📊 15.4   **FUD** 090   J A2 80 🔲
   AMA: 2014,Jan,11

54220   **Irrigation of corpora cavernosa for priapism**   ♂
   🔲 3.87   📊 5.97   **FUD** 000   T A2 🔲
   AMA: 2014,Jan,11

54230   **Injection procedure for corpora cavernosography**   ♂
   🔲 (74445)
   🔲 2.30   📊 2.82   **FUD** 000   N N1 🔲
   AMA: 2014,Jan,11

54231   **Dynamic cavernosometry, including intracavernosal injection of vasoactive drugs (eg, papaverine, phentolamine)**   ♂
   🔲 3.36   📊 4.08   **FUD** 000   J P3 🔲
   AMA: 2014,Jan,11

54235   **Injection of corpora cavernosa with pharmacologic agent(s) (eg, papaverine, phentolamine)**   ♂
   🔲 2.11   📊 2.56   **FUD** 000   T P3 🔲
   AMA: 2018,Jan,8; 2017,Jan,8; 2016,Jan,13; 2015,Jan,16; 2014,Jan,11

54240   **Penile plethysmography**   ♂
   🔲 2.97   📊 2.97   **FUD** 000   S P3 80 🔲
   AMA: 2014,Jan,11

54250   **Nocturnal penile tumescence and/or rigidity test**   ♂
   🔲 3.50   📊 3.50   **FUD** 000   T P3 80 🔲
   AMA: 2014,Jan,11

54300-54390 Hypospadias Repair and Related Procedures

EXCLUDES   *Other urethroplasties (53400-53430)*
     Revascularization of penis (37788)

54300   **Plastic operation of penis for straightening of chordee (eg, hypospadias), with or without mobilization of urethra**   ♂
   🔲 18.6   📊 18.6   **FUD** 090   J A2 80 🔲
   AMA: 2018,Jan,8; 2017,Jan,8; 2016,Jan,13; 2015,Jan,16; 2014,Dec,16; 2014,Dec,16; 2014,Jan,11

54304   **Plastic operation on penis for correction of chordee or for first stage hypospadias repair with or without transplantation of prepuce and/or skin flaps**   ♂
   🔲 21.6   📊 21.6   **FUD** 090   J A2 80 🔲
   AMA: 2014,Jan,11

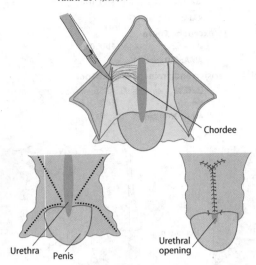

Chordee

Urethra   Penis   Urethral opening

The foreskin is used in either a free graft or a flap graft to cover the ventral skin defects created to correct the chordee

54308   **Urethroplasty for second stage hypospadias repair (including urinary diversion); less than 3 cm**   ♂
   🔲 20.6   📊 20.6   **FUD** 090   J A2 80 🔲
   AMA: 2014,Jan,11

54312   **greater than 3 cm**   ♂
   🔲 23.6   📊 23.6   **FUD** 090   J A2 80 🔲
   AMA: 2014,Jan,11

54316   **Urethroplasty for second stage hypospadias repair (including urinary diversion) with free skin graft obtained from site other than genitalia**   ♂
   🔲 28.8   📊 28.8   **FUD** 090   J A2 80 🔲
   AMA: 2014,Jan,11

54318   **Urethroplasty for third stage hypospadias repair to release penis from scrotum (eg, third stage Cecil repair)**   ♂
   🔲 20.5   📊 20.5   **FUD** 090   J A2 80 🔲
   AMA: 2014,Jan,11

54322   **1-stage distal hypospadias repair (with or without chordee or circumcision); with simple meatal advancement (eg, Magpi, V-flap)**   ♂
   🔲 22.6   📊 22.6   **FUD** 090   J A2 80 🔲
   AMA: 2014,Jan,11

54324   **with urethroplasty by local skin flaps (eg, flip-flap, prepucial flap)**   ♂
   INCLUDES   Browne's operation
   🔲 28.0   📊 28.0   **FUD** 090   J A2 80 🔲
   AMA: 2014,Jan,11

54326   **with urethroplasty by local skin flaps and mobilization of urethra**   ♂
   🔲 27.3   📊 27.3   **FUD** 090   J A2 80 🔲
   AMA: 2014,Jan,11

54328   **with extensive dissection to correct chordee and urethroplasty with local skin flaps, skin graft patch, and/or island flap**   ♂
   EXCLUDES   *Urethroplasty/straightening of chordee (54308)*
   🔲 27.1   📊 27.1   **FUD** 090   J A2 80 🔲
   AMA: 2018,Jan,8; 2017,Jan,8; 2016,Jan,13; 2015,Jan,16; 2014,Jan,11

54332 1-stage proximal penile or penoscrotal hypospadias repair requiring extensive dissection to correct chordee and urethroplasty by use of skin graft tube and/or island flap ♂
    29.3   29.3   **FUD** 090   J 80
    AMA: 2018,Jan,8; 2017,Jan,8; 2016,Jan,13; 2015,Jan,16; 2014,Jan,11

54336 1-stage perineal hypospadias repair requiring extensive dissection to correct chordee and urethroplasty by use of skin graft tube and/or island flap ♂
    34.4   34.4   **FUD** 090   J 80
    AMA: 2018,Jan,8; 2017,Jan,8; 2016,Jan,13; 2015,Jan,16; 2014,Jan,11

54340 Repair of hypospadias complications (ie, fistula, stricture, diverticula); by closure, incision, or excision, simple ♂
    16.4   16.4   **FUD** 090   J A2 80
    AMA: 2014,Jan,11

54344 requiring mobilization of skin flaps and urethroplasty with flap or patch graft ♂
    27.4   27.4   **FUD** 090   J A2 80
    AMA: 2014,Jan,11

54348 requiring extensive dissection and urethroplasty with flap, patch or tubed graft (includes urinary diversion) ♂
    29.3   29.3   **FUD** 090   J A2 80
    AMA: 2014,Jan,11

54352 Repair of hypospadias cripple requiring extensive dissection and excision of previously constructed structures including re-release of chordee and reconstruction of urethra and penis by use of local skin as grafts and island flaps and skin brought in as flaps or grafts ♂
    41.0   41.0   **FUD** 090   J A2 80
    AMA: 2014,Jan,11

54360 Plastic operation on penis to correct angulation ♂
    20.8   20.8   **FUD** 090   J A2 80
    AMA: 2014,Jan,11

54380 Plastic operation on penis for epispadias distal to external sphincter; ♂
    INCLUDES   Lowsley's operation
    23.1   23.1   **FUD** 090   J A2 80
    AMA: 2014,Jan,11

54385 with incontinence
    26.8   26.8   **FUD** 090   J A2 80
    AMA: 2014,Jan,11

54390 with exstrophy of bladder ♂
    35.9   35.9   **FUD** 090   C 80
    AMA: 2014,Jan,11

54400-54417 Procedures to Treat Impotence

CMS: 100-03,230.4 Diagnosis and Treatment of Impotence
EXCLUDES   *Other urethroplasties (53400-53430)*
         Revascularization of penis (37788)

54400 Insertion of penile prosthesis; non-inflatable (semi-rigid) ♂
    EXCLUDES   *Replacement/removal penile prosthesis (54415, 54416)*
    15.3   15.3   **FUD** 090   J J8
    AMA: 2014,Jan,11

54401 inflatable (self-contained) ♂
    EXCLUDES   *Replacement/removal penile prosthesis (54415, 54416)*
    18.9   18.9   **FUD** 090   J J8
    AMA: 2014,Jan,11

54405 Insertion of multi-component, inflatable penile prosthesis, including placement of pump, cylinders, and reservoir ♂
    Code also modifier 52 for reduced services
    23.4   23.4   **FUD** 090   J J8 80
    AMA: 2014,Jan,11

54406 Removal of all components of a multi-component, inflatable penile prosthesis without replacement of prosthesis ♂
    Code also modifier 52 for reduced services
    21.1   21.1   **FUD** 090   02 A2 80
    AMA: 2014,Jan,11

54408 Repair of component(s) of a multi-component, inflatable penile prosthesis ♂
    22.8   22.8   **FUD** 090   J A2 80
    AMA: 2014,Jan,11

54410 Removal and replacement of all component(s) of a multi-component, inflatable penile prosthesis at the same operative session ♂
    24.8   24.8   **FUD** 090   J J8 80
    AMA: 2014,Jan,11

54411 Removal and replacement of all components of a multi-component inflatable penile prosthesis through an infected field at the same operative session, including irrigation and debridement of infected tissue ♂
    INCLUDES   Debridement (11042, 11043)
    Code also modifier 52 for reduced services
    29.7   29.7   **FUD** 090   J 80
    AMA: 2014,Jan,11

54415 Removal of non-inflatable (semi-rigid) or inflatable (self-contained) penile prosthesis, without replacement of prosthesis ♂
    15.3   15.3   **FUD** 090   02 A2 80
    AMA: 2014,Jan,11

54416 Removal and replacement of non-inflatable (semi-rigid) or inflatable (self-contained) penile prosthesis at the same operative session ♂
    20.5   20.5   **FUD** 090   J J8 80
    AMA: 2014,Jan,11

54417 Removal and replacement of non-inflatable (semi-rigid) or inflatable (self-contained) penile prosthesis through an infected field at the same operative session, including irrigation and debridement of infected tissue ♂
    INCLUDES   Debridement (11042, 11043)
    25.9   25.9   **FUD** 090   J 80
    AMA: 2014,Jan,11

54420-54450 Other Procedures of the Penis

EXCLUDES   *Other urethroplasties (53400-53430)*
         Revascularization of penis (37788)

54420 Corpora cavernosa-saphenous vein shunt (priapism operation), unilateral or bilateral ♂
    20.3   20.3   **FUD** 090   J A2 80
    AMA: 2014,Jan,11

Genital System

54430 **Corpora cavernosa-corpus spongiosum shunt (priapism operation), unilateral or bilateral** ♂
📋 18.5 ⚖ 18.5 **FUD** 090 [C] [80] ⬜
AMA: 2014,Jan,11

Cross section of penis

The physician creates a communication between the corpus cavernosum and the corpus spongiosum

54435 **Corpora cavernosa-glans penis fistulization (eg, biopsy needle, Winter procedure, rongeur, or punch) for priapism** ♂
📋 12.0 ⚖ 12.0 **FUD** 090 [J] [A2] ⬜
AMA: 2014,Jan,11

54437 **Repair of traumatic corporeal tear(s)** ♂
📋 19.4 ⚖ 19.4 **FUD** 090 [J] [62] [80] ⬜
EXCLUDES Urethral repair (53410, 53415)

54438 **Replantation, penis, complete amputation including urethral repair** ♂
📋 38.7 ⚖ 38.7 **FUD** 090 [C] [80] ⬜
EXCLUDES Replantation/repair of corporeal tear in incomplete amputation penis (54437)
Replantation/urethral repair in incomplete amputation penis (53410-53415)

54440 **Plastic operation of penis for injury** ♂
📋 0.00 ⚖ 0.00 **FUD** 090 [J] [A2] [80] ⬜
AMA: 2014,Jan,11

54450 **Foreskin manipulation including lysis of preputial adhesions and stretching** ♂
📋 1.67 ⚖ 1.99 **FUD** 000 [T] [A2] ⬜
AMA: 2014,Jan,11

54500-54560 Testicular Procedures: Incisional
EXCLUDES Debridement of abdominal perineal gangrene (11004-11006)

54500 **Biopsy of testis, needle (separate procedure)** ♂
EXCLUDES Fine needle aspiration (10021, [10004, 10005, 10006, 10007, 10008, 10009, 10010, 10011, 10012])
(88172-88173)
📋 2.15 ⚖ 2.15 **FUD** 000 [J] [A2] [80] [50] ⬜
AMA: 2019,Apr,4; 2014,Jan,11

54505 **Biopsy of testis, incisional (separate procedure)** ♂
Code also when combined with epididymogram, seminal vesiculogram or vasogram (55300)
📋 6.07 ⚖ 6.07 **FUD** 010 [J] [A2] [80] [50] ⬜
AMA: 2018,Jan,8; 2017,Jan,8; 2016,Jan,13; 2014,Jan,11

54512 **Excision of extraparenchymal lesion of testis** ♂
📋 15.6 ⚖ 15.6 **FUD** 090 [J] [A2] [50] ⬜
AMA: 2018,Jan,8; 2017,Jan,8; 2016,Jan,13; 2014,Jan,11

54520 **Orchiectomy, simple (including subcapsular), with or without testicular prosthesis, scrotal or inguinal approach** ♂
INCLUDES Huggins' orchiectomy
EXCLUDES Lymphadenectomy, radical retroperitoneal (38780)
Code also hernia repair if performed (49505, 49507)
📋 9.45 ⚖ 9.45 **FUD** 090 [J] [A2] [50] ⬜
AMA: 2018,Jan,8; 2017,Jan,8; 2016,Jan,13; 2015,Jan,16; 2014,Jan,11

54522 **Orchiectomy, partial** ♂
EXCLUDES Lymphadenectomy, radical retroperitoneal (38780)
📋 17.0 ⚖ 17.0 **FUD** 090 [J] [A2] [80] [50] ⬜
AMA: 2018,Jan,8; 2017,Jan,8; 2016,Jan,13; 2015,Jan,16; 2014,Jan,11

54530 **Orchiectomy, radical, for tumor; inguinal approach** ♂
EXCLUDES Lymphadenectomy, radical retroperitoneal (38780)
📋 14.6 ⚖ 14.6 **FUD** 090 [J] [A2] [80] [50] ⬜
AMA: 2018,Jan,8; 2017,Jan,8; 2016,Jan,13; 2015,Jan,16; 2014,Jan,11

54535 **with abdominal exploration** ♂
EXCLUDES Lymphadenectomy, radical retroperitoneal (38780)
📋 21.5 ⚖ 21.5 **FUD** 090 [J] [80] [50] ⬜
AMA: 2018,Jan,8; 2017,Jan,8; 2016,Jan,13; 2015,Jan,16; 2014,Jan,11

54550 **Exploration for undescended testis (inguinal or scrotal area)** ♂
📋 14.2 ⚖ 14.2 **FUD** 090 [J] [A2] [80] [50] ⬜
AMA: 2018,Jan,8; 2017,Mar,10; 2017,Jan,8; 2016,Jan,13; 2015,Jan,16; 2014,Jan,11

54560 **Exploration for undescended testis with abdominal exploration** ♂
📋 19.8 ⚖ 19.8 **FUD** 090 [J] [62] [80] [50] ⬜
AMA: 2018,Jan,8; 2017,Jan,8; 2016,Jan,13; 2015,Jan,16; 2014,Jan,11

54600-54699 Open and Laparoscopic Testicular Procedures

54600 **Reduction of torsion of testis, surgical, with or without fixation of contralateral testis** ♂
📋 13.1 ⚖ 13.1 **FUD** 090 [J] [A2] [50] ⬜
AMA: 2018,Jan,8; 2017,Jan,8; 2016,Jan,13; 2015,Jan,16; 2014,Jan,11

Normal testes   Torsion of testis

54620 **Fixation of contralateral testis (separate procedure)** ♂
📋 8.66 ⚖ 8.66 **FUD** 010 [J] [A2] [50] ⬜
AMA: 2014,Jan,11

▲ **54640** **Orchiopexy, inguinal or scrotal approach** ♂
INCLUDES Bevan's operation
Koop inguinal orchiopexy
Prentice orchiopexy
EXCLUDES Repair inguinal hernia with inguinal orchiopexy (49495-49525)
📋 13.8 ⚖ 13.8 **FUD** 090 [J] [A2] [80] [50] ⬜
AMA: 2018,Jan,8; 2017,Mar,10; 2017,Jan,8; 2016,Jan,13; 2015,Jan,16; 2014,Jan,11

54650 Orchiopexy, abdominal approach, for intra-abdominal testis (eg, Fowler-Stephens) ♂
EXCLUDES *Laparoscopic orchiopexy (54692)*
20.5 20.5 **FUD** 090 [J] [80] [50] ▭
AMA: 2018,Jan,8; 2017,Jan,8; 2016,Jan,13; 2015,Jan,16; 2014,Jan,11

54660 Insertion of testicular prosthesis (separate procedure) ♂
10.3 10.3 **FUD** 090 [J] [J8] [80] [50] ▭
AMA: 2018,Jan,8; 2017,Jan,8; 2016,Jan,13; 2015,Jan,16; 2014,Jan,11

54670 Suture or repair of testicular injury ♂
11.7 11.7 **FUD** 090 [J] [A2] [80] [50] ▭
AMA: 2018,Jan,8; 2017,Jan,8; 2016,Jan,13; 2015,Jan,16; 2014,Jan,11

54680 Transplantation of testis(es) to thigh (because of scrotal destruction)
22.7 22.7 **FUD** 090 [J] [A2] [80] [50] ▭
AMA: 2018,Jan,8; 2017,Jan,8; 2016,Jan,13; 2015,Jan,16; 2014,Jan,11

54690 Laparoscopy, surgical; orchiectomy
INCLUDES Diagnostic laparoscopy (49320)
18.9 18.9 **FUD** 090 [J] [A2] [80] [50] ▭
AMA: 2019,Feb,10; 2018,Jan,8; 2017,Jan,8; 2016,Jan,13; 2015,Jan,16; 2014,Jan,11

54692 orchiopexy for intra-abdominal testis ♂
INCLUDES Diagnostic laparoscopy (49320)
21.9 21.9 **FUD** 090 [J] [G2] [50] ▭
AMA: 2018,Jan,8; 2017,Jan,8; 2016,Jan,13; 2015,Jan,16; 2014,Jan,11

54699 Unlisted laparoscopy procedure, testis ♂
0.00 0.00 **FUD** YYY [J] [80] [50] ▭
AMA: 2018,Jan,8; 2017,Jan,8; 2016,Jan,13; 2015,Jan,16; 2014,Jan,11

54700-54901 Open Procedures of the Epididymis

54700 Incision and drainage of epididymis, testis and/or scrotal space (eg, abscess or hematoma) ♂
EXCLUDES *Debridement of genitalia for necrotizing soft tissue infection (11004-11006)*
6.16 6.16 **FUD** 010 [J] [A2] [50] ▭
AMA: 2018,Jan,8; 2017,Jan,8; 2016,Jan,13; 2015,Jan,16; 2014,Jan,11

54800 Biopsy of epididymis, needle ♂
EXCLUDES *Fine needle aspiration (10021, [10004, 10005, 10006, 10007, 10008, 10009, 10010, 10011, 10012])*
88172-88173
3.64 3.64 **FUD** 000 [J] [A2] [80] [50] ▭
AMA: 2019,Apr,4; 2018,Jan,8; 2017,Jan,8; 2016,Jan,13; 2015,Jan,16; 2014,Jan,11

54830 Excision of local lesion of epididymis ♂
10.7 10.7 **FUD** 090 [J] [A2] [80] [50] ▭
AMA: 2018,Jan,8; 2017,Jan,8; 2016,Jan,13; 2015,Jan,16; 2014,Jan,11

54840 Excision of spermatocele, with or without epididymectomy ♂
9.29 9.29 **FUD** 090 [J] [A2] [50] ▭
AMA: 2018,Jan,8; 2017,Jan,8; 2016,Jan,13; 2015,Jan,16; 2014,Jan,11

54860 Epididymectomy; unilateral ♂
12.1 12.1 **FUD** 090 [J] [A2] ▭
AMA: 2014,Jan,11

54861 bilateral ♂
16.3 16.3 **FUD** 090 [J] [A2] [80] ▭
AMA: 2014,Jan,11

54865 Exploration of epididymis, with or without biopsy ♂
10.3 10.3 **FUD** 090 [J] [A2] [80] ▭
AMA: 2014,Jan,11

54900 Epididymovasostomy, anastomosis of epididymis to vas deferens; unilateral ♂
EXCLUDES *Operating microscope (69990)*
23.1 23.1 **FUD** 090 [J] [A2] [80] ▭
AMA: 2018,Jan,8; 2017,Jan,8; 2016,Jan,13; 2015,Jan,16; 2014,Jan,11

54901 bilateral ♂
EXCLUDES *Operating microscope (69990)*
30.5 30.5 **FUD** 090 [J] [A2] [80] ▭
AMA: 2018,Jan,8; 2017,Jan,8; 2016,Jan,13; 2015,Jan,16; 2014,Jan,11

55000-55180 Procedures of the Tunica Vaginalis and Scrotum

55000 Puncture aspiration of hydrocele, tunica vaginalis, with or without injection of medication ♂
2.45 3.34 **FUD** 000 [T] [P3] [50] ▭
AMA: 2014,Jan,11

Normal Noncommunicating hydrocele Communicating hydrocele Hydrocele of the cord

55040 Excision of hydrocele; unilateral ♂
EXCLUDES *Repair of hernia with hydrocelectomy (49495-49501)*
9.77 9.77 **FUD** 090 [J] [A2]
AMA: 2018,Jan,8; 2017,Nov,10; 2017,Jan,8; 2016,Jan,13; 2015,Jan,16; 2014,Jan,11

55041 bilateral ♂
EXCLUDES *Repair of hernia with hydrocelectomy (49495-49501)*
14.7 14.7 **FUD** 090 [J] [A2]
AMA: 2014,Jan,11

55060 Repair of tunica vaginalis hydrocele (Bottle type) ♂
11.0 11.0 **FUD** 090 [J] [A2] [80] [50] ▭
AMA: 2018,Jan,8; 2017,Jan,8; 2016,Jan,13; 2015,Jan,16; 2014,Nov,14; 2014,Jan,11

55100 Drainage of scrotal wall abscess ♂
EXCLUDES *Debridement of genitalia for necrotizing soft tissue infection (11004-11006)*
Incision and drainage of scrotal space (54700)
4.80 6.28 **FUD** 010 [J] [A2]
AMA: 2014,Jan,11

55110 Scrotal exploration ♂
11.2 11.2 **FUD** 090 [J] [A2]
AMA: 2014,Jan,11

55120 Removal of foreign body in scrotum ♂
10.2 10.2 **FUD** 090 [J] [A2] [80]
AMA: 2014,Jan,11

55150 Resection of scrotum ♂
EXCLUDES *Lesion excision of skin of scrotum (11420-11426, 11620-11626)*
14.2 14.2 **FUD** 090 [J] [A2] [80] ▭
AMA: 2014,Jan,11

55175 Scrotoplasty; simple ♂
    📖 10.5   ⅀ 10.5   **FUD** 090   [J] [A2] [80] ▭
    AMA: 2018,Jan,8; 2017,Jan,8; 2016,Jan,13; 2015,Jan,16; 2014,Dec,16; 2014,Dec,16; 2014,Jan,11

55180 complicated ♂
    📖 19.9   ⅀ 19.9   **FUD** 090   [J] [A2] [80] ▭
    AMA: 2014,Jan,11

55200-55680 Procedures of Other Male Genital Ducts and Glands

55200 Vasotomy, cannulization with or without incision of vas, unilateral or bilateral (separate procedure) ♂
    📖 8.04   ⅀ 12.1   **FUD** 090   [J] [A2] [80] ▭
    AMA: 2014,Jan,11

55250 Vasectomy, unilateral or bilateral (separate procedure), including postoperative semen examination(s) ♂
    📖 6.58   ⅀ 10.6   **FUD** 090   [J] [A2]
    AMA: 2018,Jan,8; 2017,Jan,8; 2016,Jan,13; 2015,Jan,16; 2014,Jan,11

55300 Vasotomy for vasograms, seminal vesiculograms, or epididymograms, unilateral or bilateral ♂
    Code also biopsy of testis and modifier 51 when combined (54505)
    ☢ (74440)
    📖 5.42   ⅀ 5.42   **FUD** 000   [N] [N1] [80] ▭
    AMA: 2014,Jan,11

55400 Vasovasostomy, vasovasorrhaphy ♂
    EXCLUDES   Operating microscope (69990)
    📖 14.4   ⅀ 14.4   **FUD** 090   [J] [A2] [80] [50] ▭
    AMA: 2018,Jan,8; 2017,Jan,8; 2016,Jan,13; 2015,Jan,16; 2014,Jan,11

55500 Excision of hydrocele of spermatic cord, unilateral (separate procedure) ♂
    📖 11.4   ⅀ 11.4   **FUD** 090   [J] [A2] [80] [50] ▭
    AMA: 2018,Jan,8; 2017,Jan,8; 2016,Jan,13; 2015,Jan,16; 2014,Jan,11

55520 Excision of lesion of spermatic cord (separate procedure) ♂
    📖 13.1   ⅀ 13.1   **FUD** 090   [J] [A2] [80] [50] ▭
    AMA: 2018,Jan,8; 2017,Jan,8; 2016,Jan,13; 2015,Jan,16; 2014,Jan,11

55530 Excision of varicocele or ligation of spermatic veins for varicocele; (separate procedure) ♂
    📖 10.1   ⅀ 10.1   **FUD** 090   [J] [A2] [50] ▭
    AMA: 2018,Jan,8; 2017,Jan,8; 2016,Jan,13; 2015,Jan,16; 2014,Jan,11

55535 abdominal approach ♂
    📖 12.4   ⅀ 12.4   **FUD** 090   [J] [A2] [80] [50] ▭
    AMA: 2018,Jan,8; 2017,Jan,8; 2016,Jan,13; 2015,Jan,16; 2014,Jan,11

55540 with hernia repair ♂
    📖 16.0   ⅀ 16.0   **FUD** 090   [J] [A2] [50] ▭
    AMA: 2018,Jan,8; 2017,Jan,8; 2016,Jan,13; 2015,Jan,16; 2014,Jan,11

55550 Laparoscopy, surgical, with ligation of spermatic veins for varicocele ♂
    INCLUDES   Diagnostic laparoscopy (49320)
    📖 12.4   ⅀ 12.4   **FUD** 090   [J] [A2] [80] [50] ▭
    AMA: 2018,Jan,8; 2017,Jan,8; 2016,Jan,13; 2015,Jan,16; 2014,Jan,11

55559 Unlisted laparoscopy procedure, spermatic cord ♂
    📖 0.00   ⅀ 0.00   **FUD** YYY   [J] [80] [50] ▭
    AMA: 2018,Jan,8; 2017,Jan,8; 2016,Jan,13; 2015,Jan,16; 2014,Jan,11

55600 Vesiculotomy; ♂
    📖 12.1   ⅀ 12.1   **FUD** 090   [J] [R2] [80] [50] ▭
    AMA: 2014,Jan,11

55605 complicated ♂
    📖 15.1   ⅀ 15.1   **FUD** 090   [C] [80] [50] ▭
    AMA: 2014,Jan,11

55650 Vesiculectomy, any approach ♂
    📖 20.7   ⅀ 20.7   **FUD** 090   [C] [80] [50] ▭
    AMA: 2014,Jan,11

55680 Excision of Mullerian duct cyst ♂
    EXCLUDES   Injection procedure (52010, 55300)
    📖 10.0   ⅀ 10.0   **FUD** 090   [J] [A2] [80] [50] ▭
    AMA: 2014,Jan,11

55700-55725 Procedures of Prostate: Incisional

55700 Biopsy, prostate; needle or punch, single or multiple, any approach
    EXCLUDES   Fine needle aspiration (10021, [10004, 10005, 10006, 10007, 10008, 10009, 10010, 10011, 10012])
             Needle biopsy of prostate, saturation sampling for prostate mapping (55706)
    ☢ (76942, 77002, 77012, 77021)
    ✎ (88172-88173)
    📖 3.77   ⅀ 7.12   **FUD** 000   [J] [A2] ▭
    AMA: 2018,Jul,11; 2018,Jan,8; 2017,Jan,8; 2016,Jan,13; 2015,Jan,16; 2014,Jan,11

Vas deferens
Bladder
Seminal vesicle
Ductus deferens
Pubic bone
Rectum
Prostate gland
Urethra
Penis
Epididymis
Testis

55705 incisional, any approach ♂
    📖 7.68   ⅀ 7.68   **FUD** 010   [J] [A2] ▭
    AMA: 2014,Jan,11

55706 Biopsies, prostate, needle, transperineal, stereotactic template guided saturation sampling, including imaging guidance ♂
    EXCLUDES   Biopsy, prostate; needle or punch (55700)
    📖 10.7   ⅀ 10.7   **FUD** 010   [J] [G2] [80] ▭
    AMA: 2018,Jan,8; 2017,Jan,8; 2016,Jan,13; 2015,Jan,16; 2014,Jan,11

55720 Prostatotomy, external drainage of prostatic abscess, any approach; simple ♂
    EXCLUDES   Drainage of prostatic abscess, transurethral (52700)
    📖 13.0   ⅀ 13.0   **FUD** 090   [J] [A2] [80] ▭
    AMA: 2014,Jan,11

55725 complicated ♂
    EXCLUDES   Drainage of prostatic abscess, transurethral (52700)
    📖 17.1   ⅀ 17.1   **FUD** 090   [J] [A2] [80] ▭
    AMA: 2014,Jan,11

26/TC PC/TC Only   A2-Z3 ASC Payment   50 Bilateral   ♂ Male Only   ♀ Female Only   📖 Facility RVU   ⅀ Non-Facility RVU   ▭ CCI   ☒ CLIA
FUD Follow-up Days   CMS: IOM   AMA: CPT Asst   A-Y OPPSI   80/80 Surg Assist Allowed / w/Doc   ✎ Lab Crosswalk   ☢ Radiology Crosswalk

260   CPT © 2019 American Medical Association. All Rights Reserved.   © 2019 Optum360, LLC

55801-55845 Open Prostatectomy

EXCLUDES   *Limited pelvic lymphadenectomy for staging (separate procedure) (38562)*
Node dissection, independent (38770-38780)
Transurethral prostate
  Destruction (53850-53852)
  Resection (52601-52640)

55801   **Prostatectomy, perineal, subtotal (including control of postoperative bleeding, vasectomy, meatotomy, urethral calibration and/or dilation, and internal urethrotomy)** ♂
  🚑 31.6   ✂ 31.6   **FUD** 090   C 80 ▭
  AMA: 2014,Jan,11

55810   **Prostatectomy, perineal radical;** ♂
  INCLUDES   Walsh modified radical prostatectomy
  🚑 38.0   ✂ 38.0   **FUD** 090   C 80 ▭
  AMA: 2014,Jan,11

55812   **with lymph node biopsy(s) (limited pelvic lymphadenectomy)** ♂
  🚑 46.5   ✂ 46.5   **FUD** 090   C 80 ▭
  AMA: 2014,Jan,11

55815   **with bilateral pelvic lymphadenectomy, including external iliac, hypogastric and obturator nodes** ♂
  EXCLUDES   *When performed on separate days, report: (38770, 55810)*
  Pelvic lymphadenectomy, bilateral, and append modifier 50 (38770)
  Perineal radical prostatectomy (55810)
  🚑 51.0   ✂ 51.0   **FUD** 090   C 80 ▭
  AMA: 2014,Jan,11

55821   **Prostatectomy (including control of postoperative bleeding, vasectomy, meatotomy, urethral calibration and/or dilation, and internal urethrotomy); suprapubic, subtotal, 1 or 2 stages** ♂
  🚑 25.2   ✂ 25.2   **FUD** 090   C 80 ▭
  AMA: 2014,Jan,11

55831   **retropubic, subtotal** ♂
  🚑 27.3   ✂ 27.3   **FUD** 090   C 80 ▭
  AMA: 2014,Jan,11

55840   **Prostatectomy, retropubic radical, with or without nerve sparing;** ♂
  EXCLUDES   *Prostatectomy, radical retropubic, performed laparoscopically (55866)*
  🚑 33.9   ✂ 33.9   **FUD** 090   C 80 ▭
  AMA: 2014,Jan,11

55842   **with lymph node biopsy(s) (limited pelvic lymphadenectomy)** ♂
  EXCLUDES   *Prostatectomy, retropubic radical, performed laparoscopically (55866)*
  🚑 33.9   ✂ 33.9   **FUD** 090   C 80 ▭
  AMA: 2014,Jan,11

55845   **with bilateral pelvic lymphadenectomy, including external iliac, hypogastric, and obturator nodes** ♂
  EXCLUDES   *Prostatectomy, retropubic radical, performed laparoscopically (55866)*
  When performed on separate days, report: (38770, 55840)
  Pelvic lymphadenectomy, bilateral, and append modifier 50 (38770)
  Radical prostatectomy, retropubic, with or without nerve sparing (55840)
  🚑 39.4   ✂ 39.4   **FUD** 090   C 80 ▭
  AMA: 2014,Jan,11

55860-55865 Prostate Exposure for Radiation Source Application

55860   **Exposure of prostate, any approach, for insertion of radioactive substance;** ♂
  EXCLUDES   *Interstitial radioelement application (77770-77772, 77778)*
  🚑 25.3   ✂ 25.3   **FUD** 090   J 62 ▭
  AMA: 2014,Jan,11

55862   **with lymph node biopsy(s) (limited pelvic lymphadenectomy)** ♂
  🚑 31.7   ✂ 31.7   **FUD** 090   C 80 ▭
  AMA: 2014,Jan,11

55865   **with bilateral pelvic lymphadenectomy, including external iliac, hypogastric and obturator nodes** ♂
  🚑 38.6   ✂ 38.6   **FUD** 090   C 80 ▭
  AMA: 2014,Jan,11

55866 Laparoscopic Prostatectomy

55866   **Laparoscopy, surgical prostatectomy, retropubic radical, including nerve sparing, includes robotic assistance, when performed** ♂
  INCLUDES   Diagnostic laparoscopy (49320)
  EXCLUDES   *Open method (55840)*
  🚑 41.7   ✂ 41.7   **FUD** 090   J 80 ▭
  AMA: 2018,Jan,8; 2017,Jan,8; 2016,Jan,13; 2015,Jan,16; 2014,Jan,11

55870-55899 Miscellaneous Prostate Procedures

55870   **Electroejaculation** ♂
  EXCLUDES   *Artificial insemination (58321-58322)*
  🚑 4.10   ✂ 5.04   **FUD** 000   T P3 ▭
  AMA: 2014,Jan,11

55873   **Cryosurgical ablation of the prostate (includes ultrasonic guidance and monitoring)** ♂
  🚑 22.1   ✂ 176.   **FUD** 090   J J8 ▭
  AMA: 2019,Sep,10; 2018,Jan,8; 2017,Jan,8; 2016,Jan,13; 2015,Sep,12; 2015,Jan,16; 2014,Jan,11

55874   **Transperineal placement of biodegradable material, peri-prostatic, single or multiple injection(s), including image guidance, when performed** ♂
  🚑 4.80   ✂ 98.6   **FUD** 000   T 62 ▭
  INCLUDES   Ultrasound guidance (76942)

55875   **Transperineal placement of needles or catheters into prostate for interstitial radioelement application, with or without cystoscopy** ♂
  Code also interstitial radioelement application (77770-77772, 77778)
  ⚡ (76965)
  🚑 22.1   ✂ 22.1   **FUD** 090   J A2 80 ▭
  AMA: 2018,Jan,8; 2017,Jan,8; 2016,Jan,13; 2015,Jan,16; 2014,Jan,11

55876   **Placement of interstitial device(s) for radiation therapy guidance (eg, fiducial markers, dosimeter), prostate (via needle, any approach), single or multiple** ♂
  Code also supply of device
  ⚡ (76942, 77002, 77012, 77021)
  🚑 2.91   ✂ 4.05   **FUD** 000   S P3 ▭
  AMA: 2018,Jan,8; 2017,Jan,8; 2016,Jun,3; 2016,Jan,13; 2015,Jan,16; 2014,Jan,11

55899   **Unlisted procedure, male genital system** ♂
  🚑 0.00   ✂ 0.00   **FUD** YYY   T 80 ▭
  AMA: 2019,Jun,14; 2018,Jan,8; 2017,Jan,8; 2017,Jan,6; 2016,Jan,13; 2015,Jun,5; 2015,Jan,16; 2014,Jan,11

55920 Insertion Brachytherapy Catheters/Needles Pelvis/Genitalia, Male/Female

55920 Placement of needles or catheters into pelvic organs and/or genitalia (except prostate) for subsequent interstitial radioelement application

> *EXCLUDES* *Insertion of Heyman capsules for purposes of brachytherapy (58346)*
> *Insertion of vaginal ovoids and/or uterine tandems for purposes of brachytherapy (57155)*
> *Placement of catheters or needles, prostate (55875)*

 13.0   13.0   **FUD** 000   J G2 80 ▢

AMA: 2018,Jan,8; 2017,Jan,8; 2016,Jan,13; 2015,Jan,16; 2014,Jan,11

55970-55980 Transsexual Surgery

CMS: 100-02,16,10 Exclusions from Coverage; 100-02,16,180 Services Related to Noncovered Procedures

55970 Intersex surgery; male to female   ♂

 0.00   0.00   **FUD** YYY   J ▢

AMA: 2014,Jan,11

55980 female to male   ♀

 0.00   0.00   **FUD** YYY   J ▢

AMA: 2014,Jan,11

56405-56420 Incision and Drainage of Abscess

> *EXCLUDES* *Incision and drainage Skene's gland cyst/abscess (53060)*
> *Incision and drainage subcutaneous abscess/cyst/furuncle (10040, 10060, 10061)*

56405 Incision and drainage of vulva or perineal abscess   ♀

 3.22   3.25   **FUD** 010   T P3 ▢

AMA: 2019,Jul,6; 2014,Jan,11

56420 Incision and drainage of Bartholin's gland abscess   ♀

 2.75   3.86   **FUD** 010   T P3 ▢

AMA: 2019,Jul,6; 2014,Jan,11

56440-56442 Other Female Genital Incisional Procedures

> *EXCLUDES* *Incision and drainage subcutaneous abscess/cyst/furuncle (10040, 10060, 10061)*

56440 Marsupialization of Bartholin's gland cyst   ♀

 5.15   5.15   **FUD** 010   J A2 ▢

AMA: 2019,Jul,6; 2014,Jan,11

Vaginal orifice

Bartholin's gland abscess

Perineum

Anus

56441 Lysis of labial adhesions   ♀

 4.09   4.33   **FUD** 010   J A2 80 ▢

AMA: 2019,Jul,6; 2014,Jan,11

56442 Hymenotomy, simple incision   ♀

 1.34   1.34   **FUD** 000   J A2 80 ▢

AMA: 2019,Jul,6; 2014,Jan,11

56501-56515 Destruction of Vulvar Lesions, Any Method

> *EXCLUDES* *Excision/fulguration/destruction*
> *Skene's glands (53270)*
> *Urethral caruncle (53265)*

56501 Destruction of lesion(s), vulva; simple (eg, laser surgery, electrosurgery, cryosurgery, chemosurgery)   ♀

 3.41   4.10   **FUD** 010   T P3 ▢

AMA: 2019,Aug,10; 2019,Jul,6; 2014,Jan,11

56515 extensive (eg, laser surgery, electrosurgery, cryosurgery, chemosurgery)   ♀

 5.80   6.72   **FUD** 010   T A2 ▢

AMA: 2019,Aug,10; 2019,Jul,6; 2014,Jan,11

56605-56606 Vulvar and Perineal Biopsies

> *EXCLUDES* *Excision local lesion (11420-11426, 11620-11626)*

56605 Biopsy of vulva or perineum (separate procedure); 1 lesion   ♀

 1.71   2.43   **FUD** 000   T P3 ▢

AMA: 2019,Jul,6; 2019,Jan,9; 2018,Jan,8; 2017,Jan,8; 2016,Jan,13; 2015,Jan,16; 2014,Jan,11

+ **56606** each separate additional lesion (List separately in addition to code for primary procedure)   ♀

Code first (56605)

 0.85   1.09   **FUD** ZZZ   N N1 ▢

AMA: 2019,Jul,6; 2019,Jan,9; 2014,Jan,11

56620-56640 Vulvectomy Procedures

> *INCLUDES* Removal of:
> Greater than 80% of the vulvar area - complete procedure
> Less than 80% of the vulvar area - partial procedure
> Skin and deep subcutaneous tissue - radical procedure
> Skin and superficial subcutaneous tissues - simple procedure
>
> *EXCLUDES* *Skin graft (15004-15005, 15120-15121, 15240-15241)*

56620 Vulvectomy simple; partial   ♀

 15.5   15.5   **FUD** 090   J A2 80 ▢

AMA: 2019,Jul,6; 2019,Jan,14; 2018,Jan,8; 2017,Jan,8; 2016,Jan,13; 2015,Jan,16; 2014,Jan,11

56625 complete   ♀

 18.5   18.5   **FUD** 090   J A2 80 ▢

AMA: 2019,Jul,6; 2014,Jan,11

56630 Vulvectomy, radical, partial;   ♀

Code also lymph node biopsy/excision when partial radical vulvectomy with inguinofemoral lymph node biopsy without inguinofemoral lymphadenectomy is performed (38531)

 27.2   27.2   **FUD** 090   C 80 ▢

AMA: 2019,Jul,6; 2019,Feb,8; 2014,Jan,11

56631 with unilateral inguinofemoral lymphadenectomy   ♀

> *INCLUDES* Bassett's operation

 34.4   34.4   **FUD** 090   C 80 ▢

AMA: 2019,Jul,6; 2019,Feb,8; 2014,Jan,11

56632 with bilateral inguinofemoral lymphadenectomy   ♀

> *INCLUDES* Bassett's operation

 40.6   40.6   **FUD** 090   C 80 ▢

AMA: 2019,Jul,6; 2019,Feb,8; 2014,Jan,11

56633 Vulvectomy, radical, complete;   ♀

> *INCLUDES* Bassett's operation

 35.3   35.3   **FUD** 090   C 80 ▢

AMA: 2019,Jul,6; 2019,Feb,8; 2014,Jan,11

56634 with unilateral inguinofemoral lymphadenectomy   ♀

> *INCLUDES* Bassett's operation

 38.1   38.1   **FUD** 090   C 80 ▢

AMA: 2019,Jul,6; 2019,Feb,8; 2014,Jan,11

56637   **with bilateral inguinofemoral lymphadenectomy** ♀
INCLUDES   Bassett's operation
Code also lymph node biopsy/excision when complete radical vulvectomy with inguinofemoral lymph node biopsy without inguinofemoral lymphadenectomy is performed (38531)
🔧 43.9   ⚕ 43.9   **FUD** 090   C 80 ▣
AMA: 2019,Jul,6; 2019,Feb,8; 2014,Jan,11

56640   **Vulvectomy, radical, complete, with inguinofemoral, iliac, and pelvic lymphadenectomy** ♀
INCLUDES   Bassett's operation
EXCLUDES   *Lymphadenectomy (38760-38780)*
🔧 44.8   ⚕ 44.8   **FUD** 090   C 80 50 ▣
AMA: 2019,Jul,6; 2019,Feb,8; 2014,Jan,11

56700-56740 Other Excisional Procedures: External Female Genitalia

56700   **Partial hymenectomy or revision of hymenal ring** ♀
🔧 5.38   ⚕ 5.38   **FUD** 010   J A2 80 ▣
AMA: 2019,Jul,6; 2014,Jan,11

56740   **Excision of Bartholin's gland or cyst** ♀
EXCLUDES   *Excision/fulguration/marsupialization:*
Skene's glands (53270)
Urethral carcinoma (53220)
Urethral caruncle (53265)
Urethral diverticulum (53230, 53240)
🔧 8.66   ⚕ 8.66   **FUD** 010   J A2 50 ▣
AMA: 2019,Jul,6; 2014,Jan,11

56800-56810 Repair/Reconstruction External Female Genitalia

EXCLUDES   *Repair of urethra for mucosal prolapse (53275)*

56800   **Plastic repair of introitus** ♀
INCLUDES   Emmet's operation
🔧 6.92   ⚕ 6.92   **FUD** 010   J A2 80 ▣
AMA: 2019,Jul,6; 2014,Jan,11

56805   **Clitoroplasty for intersex state** ♀
🔧 32.5   ⚕ 32.5   **FUD** 090   J G2 80 ▣
AMA: 2019,Jul,6; 2014,Jan,11

56810   **Perineoplasty, repair of perineum, nonobstetrical (separate procedure)** ♀
INCLUDES   Emmet's operation
EXCLUDES   *Genitalia wound repair (12001-12007, 12041-12047, 13131-13133)*
Introitus plastic repair (56800)
Sphincteroplasty, anal (46750-46751)
Vaginal/perineum recent injury repair, nonobstetrical (57210)
🔧 7.49   ⚕ 7.49   **FUD** 010   J A2 80 ▣
AMA: 2019,Jul,6; 2014,Jan,11

56820-56821 Vulvar Colposcopy with/without Biopsy

EXCLUDES   *Colposcopic procedures and/or examinations:*
Cervix (57452-57461)
Vagina (57420-57421)

56820   **Colposcopy of the vulva;** ♀
🔧 2.46   ⚕ 3.28   **FUD** 000   T P3 ▣
AMA: 2019,Jul,6; 2018,Jan,8; 2017,Jan,8; 2016,Jan,13; 2015,Jan,16; 2014,Jan,11

56821   **with biopsy(s)** ♀
🔧 3.28   ⚕ 4.36   **FUD** 000   T P3 ▣
AMA: 2019,Jul,6; 2018,Jan,8; 2017,Jan,8; 2016,Jan,13; 2015,Jan,16; 2014,Jan,11

57000-57023 Incisional Procedures: Vagina

57000   **Colpotomy; with exploration** ♀
🔧 5.44   ⚕ 5.44   **FUD** 010   J A2 80 ▣
AMA: 2019,Jul,6; 2018,Jan,8; 2017,Jan,8; 2016,Jan,13; 2015,Jan,16; 2014,Jan,11

57010   **with drainage of pelvic abscess** ♀
INCLUDES   Laroyenne operation
🔧 12.4   ⚕ 12.4   **FUD** 090   J A2 80 ▣
AMA: 2019,Jul,6; 2014,Jan,11

57020   **Colpocentesis (separate procedure)** ♀
🔧 2.29   ⚕ 2.77   **FUD** 000   J A2 80 ▣
AMA: 2019,Jul,6; 2014,Jan,11

Speculum   Bladder   Fluid in pelvis   Vagina   Rectum

The physician aspirates matter from the pelvis through a needle inserted through the vaginal wall

57022   **Incision and drainage of vaginal hematoma; obstetrical/postpartum** ♀
🔧 4.86   ⚕ 4.86   **FUD** 010   J R2 80 ▣
AMA: 2019,Jul,6; 2014,Jan,11

57023   **non-obstetrical (eg, post-trauma, spontaneous bleeding)** ♀
🔧 8.83   ⚕ 8.83   **FUD** 010   J A2 80 ▣
AMA: 2019,Jul,6; 2014,Jan,11

57061-57065 Destruction of Vaginal Lesions, Any Method

CMS: 100-03,140.5 Laser Procedures

57061   **Destruction of vaginal lesion(s); simple (eg, laser surgery, electrosurgery, cryosurgery, chemosurgery)** ♀
🔧 2.92   ⚕ 3.52   **FUD** 010   J P3 ▣
AMA: 2019,Jul,6; 2018,Jan,8; 2017,Jan,8; 2016,Jan,13; 2015,Jan,16; 2014,Jan,11

57065   **extensive (eg, laser surgery, electrosurgery, cryosurgery, chemosurgery)** ♀
🔧 5.08   ⚕ 5.88   **FUD** 010   J A2 ▣
AMA: 2019,Jul,6; 2018,Jan,8; 2017,Jan,8; 2016,Jan,13; 2015,Jan,16; 2014,Jan,11

57100-57135 Excisional Procedures: Vagina

57100   **Biopsy of vaginal mucosa; simple (separate procedure)** ♀
🔧 1.91   ⚕ 2.64   **FUD** 000   T P3 ▣
AMA: 2019,Jul,6; 2014,Jan,11

57105   **extensive, requiring suture (including cysts)** ♀
🔧 3.75   ⚕ 4.19   **FUD** 010   J A2 ▣
AMA: 2019,Jul,6; 2014,Jan,11

57106   **Vaginectomy, partial removal of vaginal wall;** ♀
🔧 14.5   ⚕ 14.5   **FUD** 090   J 80 ▣
AMA: 2019,Jul,6; 2018,Jan,8; 2017,Jan,8; 2016,Jan,13; 2015,Jan,16; 2014,Jan,11

57107   **with removal of paravaginal tissue (radical vaginectomy)** ♀
🔧 41.9   ⚕ 41.9   **FUD** 090   J 80 ▣
AMA: 2019,Jul,6; 2018,Jan,8; 2017,Jan,8; 2016,Jan,13; 2015,Jan,16; 2014,Jan,11

57109 **with removal of paravaginal tissue (radical vaginectomy) with bilateral total pelvic lymphadenectomy and para-aortic lymph node sampling (biopsy)** ♀

🗘 50.8   ⚕ 50.8   **FUD** 090   J 80 ▣

AMA: 2019,Jul,6; 2018,Jan,8; 2017,Jan,8; 2016,Jan,13; 2015,Jan,16; 2014,Jan,11

57110 **Vaginectomy, complete removal of vaginal wall;** ♀

🗘 25.3   ⚕ 25.3   **FUD** 090   C 80 ▣

AMA: 2019,Jul,6; 2018,Jan,8; 2017,Jan,8; 2016,Jan,13; 2015,Jan,16; 2014,Jan,11

57111 **with removal of paravaginal tissue (radical vaginectomy)** ♀

🗘 51.1   ⚕ 51.1   **FUD** 090   C 80 ▣

AMA: 2019,Jul,6; 2018,Jan,8; 2017,Jan,8; 2016,Jan,13; 2015,Jan,16; 2014,Jan,11

57112 **with removal of paravaginal tissue (radical vaginectomy) with bilateral total pelvic lymphadenectomy and para-aortic lymph node sampling (biopsy)** ♀

🗘 54.7   ⚕ 54.7   **FUD** 090   C 80 ▣

AMA: 2019,Jul,6; 2018,Jan,8; 2017,Jan,8; 2016,Jan,13; 2015,Jan,16; 2014,Jan,11

57120 **Colpocleisis (Le Fort type)** ♀

🗘 14.6   ⚕ 14.6   **FUD** 090   J 62 80 ▣

AMA: 2019,Jul,6; 2014,Jan,11

57130 **Excision of vaginal septum** ♀

🗘 4.60   ⚕ 5.32   **FUD** 010   J A2 80 ▣

AMA: 2019,Jul,6; 2014,Jan,11

57135 **Excision of vaginal cyst or tumor** ♀

🗘 5.05   ⚕ 5.80   **FUD** 010   J A2

AMA: 2019,Jul,6; 2014,Jan,11

57150-57180 Irrigation/Insertion/Introduction Vaginal Medication or Supply

57150 **Irrigation of vagina and/or application of medicament for treatment of bacterial, parasitic, or fungoid disease** ♀

🗘 0.75   ⚕ 1.38   **FUD** 000   01 N1 ▣

AMA: 2019,Jul,6; 2014,Jan,11

57155 **Insertion of uterine tandem and/or vaginal ovoids for clinical brachytherapy** ♀

      EXCLUDES   *Insertion of radioelement sources or ribbons (77761-77763, 77770-77772)*
                          The placement of needles or catheters into the pelvic organs and/or genitalia (except for the prostate) for interstitial radioelement application (55920)

🗘 8.09   ⚕ 10.6   **FUD** 000   J A2

AMA: 2019,Jul,6; 2018,Jan,8; 2017,Jan,8; 2016,Jan,13; 2015,Jan,16; 2014,Jan,11

57156 **Insertion of a vaginal radiation afterloading apparatus for clinical brachytherapy** ♀

🗘 4.27   ⚕ 5.92   **FUD** 000   T 62 80 ▣

AMA: 2019,Jul,6; 2014,Jan,11

57160 **Fitting and insertion of pessary or other intravaginal support device** ♀

🗘 1.33   ⚕ 1.79   **FUD** 000   T P3 ▣

AMA: 2019,Jul,6; 2018,Jan,8; 2017,Jan,8; 2016,Jan,13; 2015,Jan,16; 2014,Jan,11

57170 **Diaphragm or cervical cap fitting with instructions** ♀

🗘 1.37   ⚕ 1.85   **FUD** 000   T P3 80 ▣

AMA: 2019,Jul,6; 2014,Jan,11

57180 **Introduction of any hemostatic agent or pack for spontaneous or traumatic nonobstetrical vaginal hemorrhage (separate procedure)** ♀

🗘 3.11   ⚕ 4.37   **FUD** 010   T A2 ▣

AMA: 2019,Jul,6; 2018,Jan,8; 2017,Jan,8; 2016,Jan,13; 2015,Jan,16; 2014,Jan,11

57200-57335 Vaginal Repair and Reconstruction

      EXCLUDES   *Marshall-Marchetti-Kranz type urethral suspension, abdominal approach (51840-51841)*
                        Urethral suspension performed laparoscopically (51990)

57200 **Colporrhaphy, suture of injury of vagina (nonobstetrical)** ♀

🗘 8.87   ⚕ 8.87   **FUD** 090   J A2 80 ▣

AMA: 2019,Jul,6; 2014,Jan,11

57210 **Colpoperineorrhaphy, suture of injury of vagina and/or perineum (nonobstetrical)** ♀

🗘 10.6   ⚕ 10.6   **FUD** 090   J A2 80 ▣

AMA: 2019,Jul,6; 2014,Jan,11

57220 **Plastic operation on urethral sphincter, vaginal approach (eg, Kelly urethral plication)** ♀

🗘 9.24   ⚕ 9.24   **FUD** 090   J A2 80 ▣

AMA: 2019,Jul,6; 2014,Jan,11

57230 **Plastic repair of urethrocele** ♀

🗘 11.3   ⚕ 11.3   **FUD** 090   J A2 80 ▣

AMA: 2019,Jul,6; 2014,Jan,11

57240 **Anterior colporrhaphy, repair of cystocele with or without repair of urethrocele, including cystourethroscopy, when performed** ♀

      INCLUDES   Cystourethroscopy (52000)

🗘 17.0   ⚕ 17.0   **FUD** 090   J A2 80 ▣

AMA: 2019,Jul,6; 2018,Jan,8; 2017,Jan,8; 2016,Jan,13; 2015,Jan,16; 2014,Jan,11

57250 **Posterior colporrhaphy, repair of rectocele with or without perineorrhaphy** ♀

      INCLUDES   Rectocele repair (separate procedure) without posterior colporrhaphy (45560)

🗘 17.0   ⚕ 17.0   **FUD** 090   J A2 80 ▣

AMA: 2019,Jul,6; 2018,Jan,8; 2017,Jan,8; 2016,Jan,13; 2015,Jan,16; 2014,Jan,11

57260 **Combined anteroposterior colporrhaphy, including cystourethroscopy, when performed;** ♀

      INCLUDES   Cystourethroscopy (52000)

🗘 21.7   ⚕ 21.7   **FUD** 090   J A2 80 ▣

AMA: 2019,Jul,6; 2018,Jan,8; 2017,Jan,8; 2016,Jan,13; 2015,Jan,16; 2014,Jan,11

57265 **with enterocele repair** ♀

      INCLUDES   Cystourethroscopy (52000)

🗘 24.4   ⚕ 24.4   **FUD** 090   J A2 80 ▣

AMA: 2019,Jul,6; 2018,Jan,8; 2017,Jan,8; 2016,Jan,13; 2015,Jan,16; 2014,Jan,11

\+ **57267** **Insertion of mesh or other prosthesis for repair of pelvic floor defect, each site (anterior, posterior compartment), vaginal approach (List separately in addition to code for primary procedure)** ♀

      Code first (45560, 57240-57265, 57285)

🗘 7.25   ⚕ 7.25   **FUD** ZZZ   N N1 80 ▣

AMA: 2019,Jul,6; 2018,Jan,8; 2017,Jan,8; 2016,Jan,13; 2015,Jan,16; 2014,Jan,11

57268 **Repair of enterocele, vaginal approach (separate procedure)** ♀

🗘 13.9   ⚕ 13.9   **FUD** 090   J A2 80 ▣

AMA: 2019,Jul,6; 2018,Jan,8; 2017,Jan,8; 2016,Jan,13; 2015,Jan,16; 2014,Jan,11

57270 **Repair of enterocele, abdominal approach (separate procedure)** ♀

🗘 23.0   ⚕ 23.0   **FUD** 090   C 80 ▣

AMA: 2019,Jul,6; 2018,Jan,8; 2017,Jan,8; 2016,Jan,13; 2015,Jan,16; 2014,Jan,11

57280 **Colpopexy, abdominal approach** ♀

🗘 27.2   ⚕ 27.2   **FUD** 090   C 80 ▣

AMA: 2019,Jul,6; 2018,Jan,8; 2017,Jan,8; 2016,Jan,13; 2015,Jan,16; 2014,Jan,11

26/TC PC/TC Only   A2-Z3 ASC Payment   50 Bilateral   ♂ Male Only   ♀ Female Only   🗘 Facility RVU   ⚕ Non-Facility RVU   ▣ CCI   ✖ CLIA

FUD Follow-up Days   **CMS:** IOM   **AMA:** CPT Asst   A-Y OPPSI   80/80 Surg Assist Allowed / w/Doc   Lab Crosswalk   Radiology Crosswalk

264   CPT © 2019 American Medical Association. All Rights Reserved.   © 2019 Optum360, LLC

57282 Colpopexy, vaginal; extra-peritoneal approach (sacrospinous, iliococcygeus) ♀
🚑 14.5   ⚕ 14.5   **FUD** 090   J 80 ▣
AMA: 2019,Jul,6; 2018,Jan,8; 2017,Jan,8; 2016,Jan,13; 2015,Jan,16; 2014,Jan,11

57283 intra-peritoneal approach (uterosacral, levator myorrhaphy) ♀
EXCLUDES   *Excision of cervical stump (57556)*
Vaginal hysterectomy (58263, 58270, 58280, 58292, 58294)
🚑 19.6   ⚕ 19.6   **FUD** 090   J 80 ▣
AMA: 2019,Jul,6; 2018,Jan,8; 2017,Jan,8; 2016,Jan,13; 2015,Jan,16; 2014,Jan,11

57284 Paravaginal defect repair (including repair of cystocele, if performed); open abdominal approach ♀
EXCLUDES   *Anterior colporrhaphy (57240)*
Anterior vesicourethropexy (51840-51841)
Combined anteroposterior colporrhaphy (57260-57265)
Hysterectomy (58152, 58267)
Laparoscopy, surgical; urethral suspension for stress incontinence (51990)
🚑 23.3   ⚕ 23.3   **FUD** 090   J 80 ▣
AMA: 2019,Jul,6; 2018,Jan,8; 2017,Jan,8; 2016,Jan,13; 2015,Jan,16; 2014,Jan,11

57285 vaginal approach ♀
EXCLUDES   *Anterior colporrhaphy (57240)*
Combined anteroposterior colporrhaphy (57260-57265)
Laparoscopy, surgical; urethral suspension for stress incontinence (51990)
Vaginal hysterectomy (58267)
🚑 19.2   ⚕ 19.2   **FUD** 090   J 80 ▣
AMA: 2019,Jul,6; 2018,Jan,8; 2017,Jan,8; 2016,Jan,13; 2015,Jan,16; 2014,Jan,11

57287 Removal or revision of sling for stress incontinence (eg, fascia or synthetic) ♀
🚑 19.9   ⚕ 19.9   **FUD** 090   02 62 80 ▣
AMA: 2019,Jul,6; 2018,Jan,8; 2017,Jan,8; 2016,Jan,13; 2015,Jan,16; 2014,Jan,11

57288 Sling operation for stress incontinence (eg, fascia or synthetic) ♀
INCLUDES   Millin-Read operation
EXCLUDES   *Sling operation for stress incontinence performed laparoscopically (51992)*
🚑 20.6   ⚕ 20.6   **FUD** 090   J J8 80 ▣
AMA: 2019,Jul,6; 2019,Feb,10; 2018,Jan,8; 2017,Jan,8; 2016,Jan,13; 2015,Jan,16; 2014,Jan,11

57289 Pereyra procedure, including anterior colporrhaphy ♀
🚑 21.7   ⚕ 21.7   **FUD** 090   J A2 80 ▣
AMA: 2019,Jul,6; 2018,Jan,8; 2017,Jan,8; 2016,Jan,13; 2015,Jan,16; 2014,Jan,11

57291 Construction of artificial vagina; without graft ♀
INCLUDES   McIndoe vaginal construction
🚑 15.1   ⚕ 15.1   **FUD** 090   J A2 80 ▣
AMA: 2019,Jul,6; 2014,Jan,11

57292 with graft ♀
🚑 23.1   ⚕ 23.1   **FUD** 090   J 80 ▣
AMA: 2019,Jul,6; 2014,Jan,11

57295 Revision (including removal) of prosthetic vaginal graft; vaginal approach ♀
EXCLUDES   *Laparoscopic approach (57426)*
🚑 13.7   ⚕ 13.7   **FUD** 090   J 62 80 ▣
AMA: 2019,Jul,6; 2014,Jan,11

57296 open abdominal approach ♀
EXCLUDES   *Laparoscopic approach (57426)*
🚑 26.9   ⚕ 26.9   **FUD** 090   C 80 ▣
AMA: 2019,Jul,6; 2014,Jan,11

57300 Closure of rectovaginal fistula; vaginal or transanal approach ♀
🚑 16.4   ⚕ 16.4   **FUD** 090   J A2 80 ▣
AMA: 2019,Jul,6; 2014,Jan,11

57305 abdominal approach ♀
🚑 27.3   ⚕ 27.3   **FUD** 090   C 80 ▣
AMA: 2019,Jul,6; 2014,Jan,11

57307 abdominal approach, with concomitant colostomy ♀
🚑 29.9   ⚕ 29.9   **FUD** 090   C 80 ▣
AMA: 2019,Jul,6; 2014,Jan,11

57308 transperineal approach, with perineal body reconstruction, with or without levator plication ♀
🚑 19.0   ⚕ 19.0   **FUD** 090   C 80 ▣
AMA: 2019,Jul,6; 2014,Jan,11

57310 Closure of urethrovaginal fistula; ♀
🚑 13.5   ⚕ 13.5   **FUD** 090   J 62 80 ▣
AMA: 2019,Jul,6; 2014,Jan,11

57311 with bulbocavernosus transplant ♀
🚑 15.4   ⚕ 15.4   **FUD** 090   C 80 ▣
AMA: 2019,Jul,6; 2014,Jan,11

57320 Closure of vesicovaginal fistula; vaginal approach ♀
EXCLUDES   *Cystostomy, concomitant (51020-51040, 51101-51102)*
🚑 15.5   ⚕ 15.5   **FUD** 090   J 62 80 ▣
AMA: 2019,Jul,6; 2014,Jan,11

57330 transvesical and vaginal approach ♀
EXCLUDES   *Vesicovaginal fistula closure, abdominal approach (51900)*
🚑 21.6   ⚕ 21.6   **FUD** 090   J 80 ▣
AMA: 2019,Jul,6; 2014,Jan,11

57335 Vaginoplasty for intersex state ♀
🚑 32.8   ⚕ 32.8   **FUD** 090   J 80 ▣
AMA: 2019,Jul,6; 2014,Jan,11

57400-57415 Treatment of Vaginal Disorders Under Anesthesia

57400 Dilation of vagina under anesthesia (other than local) ♀
🚑 3.81   ⚕ 3.81   **FUD** 000   J A2 80 ▣
AMA: 2019,Jul,6; 2014,Jan,11

57410 Pelvic examination under anesthesia (other than local) ♀
🚑 3.05   ⚕ 3.05   **FUD** 000   J A2 ▣
AMA: 2019,Jul,6; 2018,Jan,8; 2017,Jan,8; 2016,Jan,13; 2015,Jan,16; 2014,Jan,11

57415 Removal of impacted vaginal foreign body (separate procedure) under anesthesia (other than local) ♀
EXCLUDES   *Removal of impacted vaginal foreign body without anesthesia, report with appropriate E&M code*
🚑 4.70   ⚕ 4.70   **FUD** 010   J A2 80 ▣
AMA: 2019,Jul,6; 2014,Jan,11

57420-57426 Endoscopic Vaginal Procedures

57420 Colposcopy of the entire vagina, with cervix if present; ♀
EXCLUDES   *Colposcopic procedures and/or examinations:*
   Cervix (57452-57461)
   Vulva (56820-56821)
Code also endometrial sampling (biopsy) performed at the same time as colposcopy (58110)
Code also modifier 51 for colposcopic procedures of different sites, as appropriate
🚑 2.62   ⚕ 3.45   **FUD** 000   T P3 ▣
AMA: 2019,Jul,6; 2018,Jan,8; 2017,Jan,8; 2016,Jan,13; 2015,Jan,16; 2014,Jan,11

● New Code   ▲ Revised Code   ○ Reinstated   ● New Web Release   ▲ Revised Web Release   + Add-on   Unlisted   Not Covered   # Resequenced
50 Optum Mod 50 Exempt   ⊘ AMA Mod 51 Exempt   51 Optum Mod 51 Exempt   63 Mod 63 Exempt   ∕ Non-FDA Drug   ★ Telemedicine   M Maternity   A Age Edit

57421 **with biopsy(s) of vagina/cervix** ♀

EXCLUDES *Colposcopic procedures and/or examinations:*
Cervix (57452-57461)
Vulva (56820-56821)
Code also endometrial sampling (biopsy) performed at the same
time as colposcopy (58110)
Code also modifier 51 for colposcopic procedures of multiple
sites, as appropriate

🔷 3.52 ⚖ 4.62 **FUD** 000 T P3 ▭

AMA: 2019,Jul,6; 2018,Jan,8; 2017,Jan,8; 2016,Jan,13;
2015,Jan,16; 2014,Jan,11

57423 **Paravaginal defect repair (including repair of cystocele, if
performed), laparoscopic approach** ♀

EXCLUDES *Anterior colporrhaphy (57240)*
Anterior vesicourethropexy (51840-51841)
Combined anteroposterior colporrhaphy (57260)
Diagnostic laparoscopy (49320)
Hysterectomy (58152, 58267)
*Laparoscopy, surgical; urethral suspension for stress
incontinence (51990)*

🔷 26.1 ⚖ 26.1 **FUD** 090 J 80 ▭

AMA: 2019,Jul,6; 2018,Jan,8; 2017,Jan,8; 2016,Jan,13;
2015,Jan,16; 2014,Jan,11

57425 **Laparoscopy, surgical, colpopexy (suspension of vaginal
apex)** ♀

🔷 27.6 ⚖ 27.6 **FUD** 090 J 80 ▭

AMA: 2019,Jul,6; 2014,Jan,11

57426 **Revision (including removal) of prosthetic vaginal graft,
laparoscopic approach** ♀

EXCLUDES *Open abdominal approach (57296)*
Vaginal approach (57295)

🔷 24.2 ⚖ 24.2 **FUD** 090 J G2 80 ▭

AMA: 2019,Jul,6; 2014,Jan,11

57452-57461 Endoscopic Cervical Procedures

EXCLUDES *Colposcopic procedures and/or examinations:*
Vagina (57420-57421)
Vulva (56820-56821)
Code also endometrial sampling (biopsy) performed at the same time as colposcopy
(58110)

57452 **Colposcopy of the cervix including upper/adjacent
vagina;** ♀

🔷 2.62 ⚖ 3.25 **FUD** 000 T P3 ▭

AMA: 2019,Jul,6; 2018,Jan,8; 2017,Jan,8; 2016,Jan,13;
2015,Jan,16; 2014,Jan,11

Speculum
Light beam
Uterus
Cervix
Vagina
Colposcope

57454 **with biopsy(s) of the cervix and endocervical
curettage** ♀

INCLUDES Colposcopy of the cervix (57452)

🔷 3.81 ⚖ 4.45 **FUD** 000 T P3 ▭

AMA: 2019,Jul,6; 2018,Jan,8; 2017,Jan,8; 2016,Jan,13;
2015,Jan,16; 2014,Jan,11

57455 **with biopsy(s) of the cervix** ♀

INCLUDES Colposcopy of the cervix (57452)

🔷 3.12 ⚖ 4.20 **FUD** 000 T P3 ▭

AMA: 2019,Jul,6; 2018,Jan,8; 2017,Jan,8; 2016,Jan,13;
2015,Jan,16; 2014,Jan,11

57456 **with endocervical curettage** ♀

INCLUDES Colposcopy of the cervix (57452)

EXCLUDES *Colposcopy of the cervix including upper/adjacent
vagina; with loop electrode conization of the cervix
(57461)*

🔷 2.90 ⚖ 3.95 **FUD** 000 T P3 ▭

AMA: 2019,Jul,6; 2018,Jan,8; 2017,Jan,8; 2016,Jan,13;
2015,Jan,16; 2014,Jan,11

57460 **with loop electrode biopsy(s) of the cervix** ♀

INCLUDES Colposcopy of the cervix (57452)

🔷 4.58 ⚖ 8.30 **FUD** 000 J P3 ▭

AMA: 2019,Jul,6; 2018,Jan,8; 2017,Jan,8; 2016,Jan,13;
2015,Jan,16; 2014,Jan,11

57461 **with loop electrode conization of the cervix** ♀

INCLUDES Colposcopy of the cervix (57452)

EXCLUDES *Colposcopy of the cervix including upper/adjacent
vagina; with endocervical curettage (57456)*

🔷 5.28 ⚖ 9.34 **FUD** 000 J P3 ▭

AMA: 2019,Jul,6; 2018,Jan,8; 2017,Jan,8; 2016,Jan,13;
2015,Jan,16; 2014,Jan,11

57500-57556 Cervical Procedures: Multiple Techniques

EXCLUDES *Radical surgical procedures (58200-58240)*

57500 **Biopsy of cervix, single or multiple, or local excision of lesion,
with or without fulguration (separate procedure)** ♀

🔷 2.13 ⚖ 3.80 **FUD** 000 T P3 ▭

AMA: 2019,Jul,6; 2014,Jan,11

57505 **Endocervical curettage (not done as part of a dilation and
curettage)** ♀

🔷 2.75 ⚖ 3.19 **FUD** 010 T P3 ▭

AMA: 2019,Jul,6; 2018,Jan,8; 2017,Jan,8; 2016,Jan,13;
2015,Jan,16; 2014,Jan,11

57510 **Cautery of cervix; electro or thermal** ♀

🔷 3.24 ⚖ 3.90 **FUD** 010 J P3 ▭

AMA: 2019,Jul,6; 2014,Jan,11

57511 **cryocautery, initial or repeat** ♀

🔷 3.86 ⚖ 4.43 **FUD** 010 T P3 ▭

AMA: 2019,Jul,6; 2014,Jan,11

57513 **laser ablation** ♀

🔷 3.99 ⚖ 4.61 **FUD** 010 J A2 ▭

AMA: 2019,Jul,6; 2014,Jan,11

57520 **Conization of cervix, with or without fulguration, with or
without dilation and curettage, with or without repair; cold
knife or laser** ♀

EXCLUDES *Dilation and curettage, diagnostic/therapeutic,
nonobstetrical (58120)*

🔷 8.02 ⚖ 9.16 **FUD** 090 J A2 ▭

AMA: 2019,Jul,6; 2018,Jan,8; 2017,Jan,8; 2016,Jan,13;
2015,Jan,16; 2014,Jan,11

57522 **loop electrode excision** ♀

🔷 6.98 ⚖ 7.79 **FUD** 090 J A2 ▭

AMA: 2019,Jul,6; 2018,Jan,8; 2017,Jan,8; 2016,Jan,13;
2015,Jan,16; 2014,Jan,11

57530 **Trachelectomy (cervicectomy), amputation of cervix (separate
procedure)** ♀

🔷 10.0 ⚖ 10.0 **FUD** 090 J A2 80 ▭

AMA: 2019,Jul,6; 2014,Jan,11

26/TC PC/TC Only   A2-Z3 ASC Payment   50 Bilateral   ♂ Male Only   ♀ Female Only   🔷 Facility RVU   ⚖ Non-Facility RVU   ▭ CCI   ✖ CLIA
FUD Follow-up Days   CMS: IOM   AMA: CPT Asst   A-Y OPPSI   80/80 Surg Assist Allowed / w/Doc   Lab Crosswalk   Radiology Crosswalk

266   CPT © 2019 American Medical Association. All Rights Reserved.   © 2019 Optum360, LLC

57531 Radical trachelectomy, with bilateral total pelvic lymphadenectomy and para-aortic lymph node sampling biopsy, with or without removal of tube(s), with or without removal of ovary(s) ♀

   EXCLUDES *Radical hysterectomy (58210)*
   🚗 47.8 ✂ 47.8 **FUD** 090   C 80 ▱
   AMA: 2019,Jul,6; 2014,Jan,11

57540 Excision of cervical stump, abdominal approach; ♀
   🚗 22.0 ✂ 22.0 **FUD** 090   C 80 ▱
   AMA: 2019,Jul,6; 2014,Jan,11

57545 with pelvic floor repair ♀
   🚗 23.3 ✂ 23.3 **FUD** 090   C 80 ▱
   AMA: 2019,Jul,6; 2014,Jan,11

57550 Excision of cervical stump, vaginal approach; ♀
   🚗 11.6 ✂ 11.6 **FUD** 090   J A2 80 ▱
   AMA: 2019,Jul,6; 2014,Jan,11

57555 with anterior and/or posterior repair ♀
   🚗 17.1 ✂ 17.1 **FUD** 090   J 80 ▱
   AMA: 2019,Jul,6; 2014,Jan,11

57556 with repair of enterocele ♀
   EXCLUDES *Insertion of hemostatic agent/pack for spontaneous/traumatic nonobstetrical vaginal hemorrhage (57180)*
   Intrauterine device insertion (58300)
   🚗 16.2 ✂ 16.2 **FUD** 090   J A2 80 ▱
   AMA: 2019,Jul,6; 2014,Jan,11

57558-57800 Cervical Procedures: Dilation, Suturing, or Instrumentation

57558 Dilation and curettage of cervical stump ♀
   EXCLUDES *Radical surgical procedures (58200-58240)*
   🚗 3.33 ✂ 3.80 **FUD** 010   J A2
   AMA: 2019,Jul,6; 2014,Jan,11

57700 Cerclage of uterine cervix, nonobstetrical ♀
   INCLUDES McDonald cerclage
   Shirodker operation
   🚗 9.13 ✂ 9.13 **FUD** 090   J A2 ▱
   AMA: 2019,Jul,6; 2014,Jan,11

57720 Trachelorrhaphy, plastic repair of uterine cervix, vaginal approach ♀
   INCLUDES Emmet operation
   🚗 8.89 ✂ 8.89 **FUD** 090   J A2 80 ▱
   AMA: 2019,Jul,6; 2014,Jan,11

57800 Dilation of cervical canal, instrumental (separate procedure) ♀
   🚗 1.37 ✂ 1.85 **FUD** 000   J P3 ▱
   AMA: 2019,Jul,6; 2014,Jan,11

58100-58120 Procedures Involving the Endometrium

58100 Endometrial sampling (biopsy) with or without endocervical sampling (biopsy), without cervical dilation, any method (separate procedure) ♀
   EXCLUDES *Endocervical curettage only (57505)*
   Endometrial sampling (biopsy) performed in conjunction with colposcopy (58110)
   🚗 2.01 ✂ 2.64 **FUD** 000   T P3 ▱
   AMA: 2019,Jul,6; 2014,Jan,11

+ **58110** Endometrial sampling (biopsy) performed in conjunction with colposcopy (List separately in addition to code for primary procedure) ♀
   Code first colposcopy (57420-57421, 57452-57461)
   🚗 1.17 ✂ 1.44 **FUD** ZZZ   N N1 80 ▱
   AMA: 2019,Jul,6; 2018,Jan,8; 2017,Jan,8; 2016,Jan,13; 2015,Jan,16; 2014,Jan,11

58120 Dilation and curettage, diagnostic and/or therapeutic (nonobstetrical) ♀
   EXCLUDES *Postpartum hemorrhage (59160)*
   🚗 6.35 ✂ 7.66 **FUD** 010   J A2 ▱
   AMA: 2019,Jul,6; 2018,Jan,8; 2017,Jan,8; 2016,Jan,13; 2015,Jan,16; 2014,Jan,11

Uterus
Endometrial lining
Cervix and cervical canal
Curette
Vaginal canal
Dilator expands cervical opening

58140-58146 Myomectomy Procedures

58140 Myomectomy, excision of fibroid tumor(s) of uterus, 1 to 4 intramural myoma(s) with total weight of 250 g or less and/or removal of surface myomas; abdominal approach ♀
   🚗 26.1 ✂ 26.1 **FUD** 090   C 80 ▱
   AMA: 2019,Jul,6; 2018,Jan,8; 2017,Jan,8; 2016,Jan,13; 2015,Jan,16; 2014,Jan,11

58145 vaginal approach ♀
   🚗 15.7 ✂ 15.7 **FUD** 090   J A2 80 ▱
   AMA: 2019,Jul,6; 2014,Jan,11

58146 Myomectomy, excision of fibroid tumor(s) of uterus, 5 or more intramural myomas and/or intramural myomas with total weight greater than 250 g, abdominal approach ♀
   EXCLUDES *Hysterectomy (58150-58240)*
   Myomectomy procedures (58140-58145)
   🚗 32.5 ✂ 32.5 **FUD** 090   C 80 ▱
   AMA: 2019,Jul,6; 2018,Jan,8; 2017,Jan,8; 2016,Jan,13; 2015,Jan,16; 2014,Jan,11

58150-58294 Abdominal and Vaginal Hysterectomies

CMS: 100-03,230.3 Sterilization

   EXCLUDES *Destruction/excision of endometriomas, open method (49203-49205, 58957-58958)*
   Paracentesis (49082-49083)
   Pelvic laparotomy (49000)
   Secondary closure disruption or evisceration of abdominal wall (49900)

58150 Total abdominal hysterectomy (corpus and cervix), with or without removal of tube(s), with or without removal of ovary(s); ♀
   🚗 29.1 ✂ 29.1 **FUD** 090   C 80 ▱
   AMA: 2019,Jul,6; 2018,Jan,8; 2017,Jan,8; 2016,Jan,13; 2015,Jan,16; 2014,Jan,11

58152 with colpo-urethrocystopexy (eg, Marshall-Marchetti-Krantz, Burch) ♀
   EXCLUDES *Urethrocystopexy without hysterectomy (51840-51841)*
   🚗 35.5 ✂ 35.5 **FUD** 090   C 80 ▱
   AMA: 2019,Jul,6; 2018,Jan,8; 2017,Jan,8; 2016,Jan,13; 2015,Jan,16; 2014,Jan,11

58180 Supracervical abdominal hysterectomy (subtotal hysterectomy), with or without removal of tube(s), with or without removal of ovary(s) ♀
   🚗 27.3 ✂ 27.3 **FUD** 090   C 80 ▱
   AMA: 2019,Jul,6; 2014,Jan,11

58200 **Total abdominal hysterectomy, including partial vaginectomy, with para-aortic and pelvic lymph node sampling, with or without removal of tube(s), with or without removal of ovary(s)** ♀

    🚑 39.7   ⚕ 39.7   **FUD** 090   C 80 ▭

    AMA: 2019,Jul,6; 2014,Jan,11

58210 **Radical abdominal hysterectomy, with bilateral total pelvic lymphadenectomy and para-aortic lymph node sampling (biopsy), with or without removal of tube(s), with or without removal of ovary(s)** ♀

    INCLUDES Wertheim hysterectomy

    EXCLUDES *Chemotherapy (96401-96549)*

             Hysterectomy, radical, with transposition of ovary(s) (58825)

    🚑 53.4   ⚕ 53.4   **FUD** 090   C 80 ▭

    AMA: 2019,Jul,6; 2018,Jan,8; 2017,Jan,8; 2016,Jan,13; 2015,Jan,16; 2014,Jan,11

58240 **Pelvic exenteration for gynecologic malignancy, with total abdominal hysterectomy or cervicectomy, with or without removal of tube(s), with or without removal of ovary(s), with removal of bladder and ureteral transplantations, and/or abdominoperineal resection of rectum and colon and colostomy, or any combination thereof** ♀

    EXCLUDES *Chemotherapy (96401-96549)*

             Pelvic exenteration for male genital malignancy or lower urinary tract (51597)

    🚑 84.8   ⚕ 84.8   **FUD** 090   C 80 ▭

    AMA: 2019,Jul,6; 2014,Jan,11

58260 **Vaginal hysterectomy, for uterus 250 g or less;** ♀

    🚑 23.4   ⚕ 23.4   **FUD** 090   J G2 80 ▭

    AMA: 2019,Jul,6; 2018,Jan,8; 2017,Jan,8; 2016,Jan,13; 2015,Jan,16; 2014,Jan,11

58262 **with removal of tube(s), and/or ovary(s)** ♀

    🚑 26.1   ⚕ 26.1   **FUD** 090   J G2 80 ▭

    AMA: 2019,Jul,6; 2014,Jan,11

58263 **with removal of tube(s), and/or ovary(s), with repair of enterocele** ♀

    🚑 28.0   ⚕ 28.0   **FUD** 090   J 80 ▭

    AMA: 2019,Jul,6; 2014,Jan,11

58267 **with colpo-urethrocystopexy (Marshall-Marchetti-Krantz type, Pereyra type) with or without endoscopic control** ♀

    🚑 29.8   ⚕ 29.8   **FUD** 090   C 80 ▭

    AMA: 2019,Jul,6; 2018,Jan,8; 2017,Jan,8; 2016,Jan,13; 2015,Jan,16; 2014,Jan,11

58270 **with repair of enterocele** ♀

    EXCLUDES *Vaginal hysterectomy with repair of enterocele and removal of tubes and/or ovaries (58263)*

    🚑 25.0   ⚕ 25.0   **FUD** 090   J 80 ▭

    AMA: 2019,Jul,6; 2014,Jan,11

Uterus is removed vaginally

Excision around cervix

Ovary

Round ligament

Broad ligament

Cervix

Protruding intestine (enterocele)

Posterior wall of vagina (site of protrusion)

Repair of enterocele

Posterior vaginal wall

58275 **Vaginal hysterectomy, with total or partial vaginectomy;** ♀

    🚑 27.9   ⚕ 27.9   **FUD** 090   C 80 ▭

    AMA: 2019,Jul,6; 2014,Jan,11

58280 **with repair of enterocele** ♀

    🚑 29.7   ⚕ 29.7   **FUD** 090   C 80 ▭

    AMA: 2019,Jul,6; 2014,Jan,11

58285 **Vaginal hysterectomy, radical (Schauta type operation)** ♀

    🚑 41.8   ⚕ 41.8   **FUD** 090   C 80 ▭

    AMA: 2019,Jul,6; 2018,Jan,8; 2017,Jan,8; 2016,Jan,13; 2015,Jan,16; 2014,Jan,11

58290 **Vaginal hysterectomy, for uterus greater than 250 g;** ♀

    🚑 32.5   ⚕ 32.5   **FUD** 090   J 80 ▭

    AMA: 2019,Jul,6; 2014,Jan,11

58291 **with removal of tube(s) and/or ovary(s)** ♀

    🚑 35.6   ⚕ 35.6   **FUD** 090   J 80 ▭

    AMA: 2019,Jul,6; 2014,Jan,11

58292 **with removal of tube(s) and/or ovary(s), with repair of enterocele** ♀

    🚑 37.0   ⚕ 37.0   **FUD** 090   J 80 ▭

    AMA: 2019,Jul,6; 2014,Jan,11

58293 **with colpo-urethrocystopexy (Marshall-Marchetti-Krantz type, Pereyra type) with or without endoscopic control** ♀

    🚑 38.5   ⚕ 38.5   **FUD** 090   C 80 ▭

    AMA: 2019,Jul,6; 2014,Jan,11

58294 **with repair of enterocele** ♀

    🚑 34.3   ⚕ 34.3   **FUD** 090   J 80 ▭

    AMA: 2019,Jul,6; 2014,Jan,11

58300-58323 Contraception and Reproduction Procedures

58300 Insertion of intrauterine device (IUD) ♀

EXCLUDES Insertion and/or removal of implantable contraceptive capsules (11976, 11981-11983)

🔧 1.54 ⚗ 2.28 **FUD** XXX   E 🖥

AMA: 2019,Jul,6; 2018,Jan,8; 2017,Jan,8; 2016,Jan,13; 2015,Jan,16; 2014,Jan,11

58301 Removal of intrauterine device (IUD) ♀

EXCLUDES Insertion and/or removal of implantable contraceptive capsules (11976, 11981-11983)

🔧 1.91 ⚗ 2.70 **FUD** 000   Q2 P3 80 🖥

AMA: 2019,Jul,6; 2018,Jan,8; 2017,Jan,8; 2016,Jan,13; 2015,Jan,16; 2014,Jan,11

58321 Artificial insemination; intra-cervical ♀

🔧 1.38 ⚗ 2.20 **FUD** 000   T P3 80 🖥

AMA: 2019,Jul,6; 2014,Jan,11

58322 intra-uterine ♀

🔧 1.65 ⚗ 2.47 **FUD** 000   T P3 80 🖥

AMA: 2019,Jul,6; 2014,Jan,11

58323 Sperm washing for artificial insemination ♀

🔧 0.35 ⚗ 0.43 **FUD** 000   T P3 80 🖥

AMA: 2019,Jul,6; 2014,Jan,11

58340-58350 Fallopian Tube Patency and Brachytherapy Procedures

58340 Catheterization and introduction of saline or contrast material for saline infusion sonohysterography (SIS) or hysterosalpingography ♀

🔄 (74740, 76831)

🔧 1.64 ⚗ 4.47 **FUD** 000   N N1 🖥

AMA: 2019,Jul,6; 2018,Jan,8; 2017,Jan,8; 2016,Jan,13; 2015,Jan,16; 2014,Jan,11

58345 Transcervical introduction of fallopian tube catheter for diagnosis and/or re-establishing patency (any method), with or without hysterosalpingography ♀

🔄 (74742)

🔧 7.94 ⚗ 7.94 **FUD** 010   J R2 80 50 🖥

AMA: 2019,Jul,6; 2018,Jan,8; 2017,Jan,8; 2016,Jan,13; 2015,Jan,16; 2014,Jan,11

58346 Insertion of Heyman capsules for clinical brachytherapy ♀

EXCLUDES Insertion of radioelement sources or ribbons (77761-77763, 77770-77772)
The placement of needles or catheters into the pelvic organs and/or genitalia (except for the prostate) for interstitial radioelement application (55920)

🔧 13.2 ⚗ 13.2 **FUD** 090   J A2 🖥

AMA: 2019,Jul,6; 2018,Jan,8; 2017,Jan,8; 2016,Jan,13; 2015,Jan,16; 2014,Jan,11

58350 Chromotubation of oviduct, including materials ♀

🔧 2.34 ⚗ 3.07 **FUD** 010   J A2 50 🖥

AMA: 2019,Jul,6; 2018,Jan,8; 2017,Jan,8; 2016,Jan,13; 2015,Jan,16; 2014,Jan,11

58353-58356 Ablation of Endometrium

EXCLUDES Destruction/excision of endometriomas, open method (49203-49205)

58353 Endometrial ablation, thermal, without hysteroscopic guidance ♀

EXCLUDES Endometrial ablation performed hysteroscopically (58563)

🔧 6.27 ⚗ 28.0 **FUD** 010   J A2 🖥

AMA: 2019,Jul,6; 2018,Jan,8; 2017,Jan,8; 2016,Jan,13; 2015,Jan,16; 2014,Jan,11

58356 Endometrial cryoablation with ultrasonic guidance, including endometrial curettage, when performed ♀

EXCLUDES Dilation and curettage (58120)
Endometrial biopsy (58100)
Hysterosalpingography (58340)
Ultrasound (76700, 76856)

🔧 9.84 ⚗ 52.1 **FUD** 010   J P3 80 🖥

AMA: 2019,Jul,6; 2014,Jan,11

58400-58540 Uterine Repairs: Vaginal and Abdominal

58400 Uterine suspension, with or without shortening of round ligaments, with or without shortening of sacrouterine ligaments; (separate procedure) ♀

INCLUDES Alexander's operation
Baldy-Webster operation
Manchester colporrhaphy

EXCLUDES Anastomosis of tubes to uterus (58752)

🔧 12.7 ⚗ 12.7 **FUD** 090   C 80 🖥

AMA: 2019,Jul,6; 2014,Jan,11

58410 with presacral sympathectomy ♀

INCLUDES Alexander's operation

EXCLUDES Anastomosis of tubes to uterus (58752)

🔧 22.7 ⚗ 22.7 **FUD** 090   C 80 🖥

AMA: 2019,Jul,6; 2018,Jan,8; 2017,Jan,8; 2016,Jan,13; 2015,Jan,16; 2014,Jan,11

58520 Hysterorrhaphy, repair of ruptured uterus (nonobstetrical) ♀

🔧 22.3 ⚗ 22.3 **FUD** 090   C 80 🖥

AMA: 2019,Jul,6; 2014,Jan,11

58540 Hysteroplasty, repair of uterine anomaly (Strassman type) ♀

INCLUDES Strassman type

EXCLUDES Vesicouterine fistula closure (51920)

🔧 25.7 ⚗ 25.7 **FUD** 090   C 80 🖥

AMA: 2019,Jul,6; 2014,Jan,11

58674-58554 [58674] Laparoscopic Procedures of the Uterus

INCLUDES Diagnostic laparoscopy
EXCLUDES Hysteroscopy (58555-58565)

\# **58674** Laparoscopy, surgical, ablation of uterine fibroid(s) including intraoperative ultrasound guidance and monitoring, radiofrequency ♀

INCLUDES Intraoperative ultrasound (76998)

EXCLUDES Laparoscopy (49320, 58541-58554, 58570-58573)

🔧 23.0 ⚗ 23.0 **FUD** 090   J G2 80 🖥

AMA: 2019,Jul,6; 2018,Jan,8; 2017,Apr,7; 2017,Feb,14

58541 Laparoscopy, surgical, supracervical hysterectomy, for uterus 250 g or less; ♀

EXCLUDES Colpotomy (57000)
Hysteroscopy (58561)
Laparoscopy (49320, 58545-58546, 58661, 58670-58671)
Myomectomy procedures (58140-58146)
Pelvic examination under anesthesia (57410)
Treatment of nonobstetrical vaginal hemorrhage (57180)

🔧 20.3 ⚗ 20.3 **FUD** 090   J G2 80 🖥

AMA: 2019,Jul,6; 2018,Jan,8; 2017,Apr,7; 2017,Jan,8; 2016,Jan,13; 2015,Jan,16; 2014,Jan,11

58542 with removal of tube(s) and/or ovary(s) ♀

> EXCLUDES Colpotomy (57000)
> Hysteroscopy (58561)
> Laparoscopy (49320, 58545-58546, 58661,
>   58670-58671)
> Myomectomy procedures (58140-58146)
> Pelvic examination under anesthesia (57410)
> Treatment of nonobstetrical vaginal hemorrhage
>   (57180)

🛢 23.2 ⚕ 23.2 **FUD** 090 [J][G2][80][⊡]
AMA: 2019,Jul,6; 2018,Jan,8; 2017,Apr,7; 2017,Jan,8; 2016,Jan,13;
2015,Jan,16; 2014,Jan,11

58543 Laparoscopy, surgical, supracervical hysterectomy, for uterus
greater than 250 g; ♀

> EXCLUDES Colpotomy (57000)
> Hysteroscopy (58561)
> Laparoscopy (49320, 58545-58546, 58661,
>   58670-58671)
> Myomectomy procedures (58140-58146)
> Pelvic examination under anesthesia (57410)
> Treatment of nonobstetrical vaginal hemorrhage
>   (57180)

🛢 23.5 ⚕ 23.5 **FUD** 090 [J][G2][80][⊡]
AMA: 2019,Jul,6; 2018,Jan,8; 2017,Apr,7; 2017,Jan,8; 2016,Jan,13;
2015,Jan,16; 2014,Jan,11

58544 with removal of tube(s) and/or ovary(s) ♀

> EXCLUDES Colpotomy (57000)
> Hysteroscopy (58561)
> Laparoscopy (49320, 58545-58546, 58661,
>   58670-58671)
> Myomectomy procedures (58140-58146)
> Pelvic examination under anesthesia (57410)
> Treatment of nonobstetrical vaginal hemorrhage
>   (57180)

🛢 25.5 ⚕ 25.5 **FUD** 090 [J][G2][80][⊡]
AMA: 2019,Jul,6; 2018,Jan,8; 2017,Apr,7; 2017,Jan,8; 2016,Jan,13;
2015,Jan,16; 2014,Jan,11

58545 Laparoscopy, surgical, myomectomy, excision; 1 to 4
intramural myomas with total weight of 250 g or less and/or
removal of surface myomas ♀

🛢 25.6 ⚕ 25.6 **FUD** 090 [J][A2][80][⊡]
AMA: 2019,Jul,6; 2017,Apr,7; 2014,Jan,11

58546 5 or more intramural myomas and/or intramural myomas
with total weight greater than 250 g ♀

🛢 31.6 ⚕ 31.6 **FUD** 090 [J][A2][80][⊡]
AMA: 2019,Jul,6; 2018,Jan,8; 2017,Apr,7; 2017,Jan,8; 2016,Jan,13;
2015,Jan,16; 2014,Jan,11

58548 Laparoscopy, surgical, with radical hysterectomy, with
bilateral total pelvic lymphadenectomy and para-aortic lymph
node sampling (biopsy), with removal of tube(s) and ovary(s),
if performed ♀

> EXCLUDES Laparoscopy (38570-38572, 58550-58554)
> Radical hysterectomy (58210, 58285)

🛢 55.0 ⚕ 55.0 **FUD** 090 [C][80][⊡]
AMA: 2019,Jul,6; 2019,Mar,5; 2018,Jan,8; 2017,Apr,7; 2017,Jan,8;
2016,Jan,13; 2015,Sep,12; 2015,Jan,16; 2014,Jan,11

58550 Laparoscopy, surgical, with vaginal hysterectomy, for uterus
250 g or less; ♀

> EXCLUDES Colpotomy (57000)
> Hysteroscopy (58561)
> Laparoscopy (49320, 58545-58546, 58661,
>   58670-58671)
> Myomectomy procedures (58140-58146)
> Pelvic examination under anesthesia (57410)
> Treatment of nonobstetrical vaginal hemorrhage
>   (57180)

🛢 24.9 ⚕ 24.9 **FUD** 090 [J][A2][80][⊡]
AMA: 2019,Jul,6; 2018,Jan,8; 2017,Apr,7; 2017,Jan,8; 2016,Jan,13;
2015,Jan,16; 2014,Jan,11

58552 with removal of tube(s) and/or ovary(s) ♀

> EXCLUDES Colpotomy (57000)
> Hysteroscopy (58561)
> Laparoscopy (49320, 58545-58546, 58661,
>   58670-58671)
> Myomectomy procedures (58140-58146)
> Pelvic examination under anesthesia (57410)
> Treatment of nonobstetrical vaginal hemorrhage
>   (57180)

🛢 28.0 ⚕ 28.0 **FUD** 090 [J][G2][80][⊡]
AMA: 2019,Jul,6; 2018,Jan,8; 2017,Apr,7; 2017,Jan,8; 2016,Jan,13;
2015,Jan,16; 2014,Jan,11

58553 Laparoscopy, surgical, with vaginal hysterectomy, for uterus
greater than 250 g; ♀

> EXCLUDES Colpotomy (57000)
> Hysteroscopy (58561)
> Laparoscopy (49320, 58545-58546, 58661,
>   58670-58671)
> Myomectomy procedures (58140-58146)
> Pelvic examination under anesthesia (57410)
> Treatment of nonobstetrical vaginal hemorrhage
>   (57180)

🛢 31.8 ⚕ 31.8 **FUD** 090 [J][G2][80][⊡]
AMA: 2019,Jul,6; 2018,Jan,8; 2017,Apr,7; 2014,Jan,11

58554 with removal of tube(s) and/or ovary(s) ♀

> EXCLUDES Colpotomy (57000)
> Hysteroscopy (58561)
> Laparoscopy (49320, 58545-58546, 58661,
>   58670-58671)
> Myomectomy procedures (58140-58146)
> Pelvic examination under anesthesia (57410)
> Treatment of nonobstetrical vaginal hemorrhage
>   (57180)

🛢 37.6 ⚕ 37.6 **FUD** 090 [J][G2][80][⊡]
AMA: 2019,Jul,6; 2018,Jan,8; 2017,Apr,7; 2014,Jan,11

58555-58565 Hysteroscopy

> INCLUDES Diagnostic hysteroscopy (58555)
> EXCLUDES Laparoscopy (58541-58554, 58570-58578)

58555 Hysteroscopy, diagnostic (separate procedure) ♀

🛢 4.35 ⚕ 8.40 **FUD** 000 [J][A2][80][⊡]
AMA: 2019,Jul,6; 2018,Jan,8; 2017,Jan,8; 2016,Jan,13;
2015,Jan,16; 2014,Jan,11

Hysteroscope — Bladder — Uterus — Ovary — Spine — Vagina — Cervix

58558 Hysteroscopy, surgical; with sampling (biopsy) of
endometrium and/or polypectomy, with or without D &
C ♀

🛢 6.63 ⚕ 38.8 **FUD** 000 [J][A2][⊡]
AMA: 2019,Jul,6; 2018,Jan,8; 2017,Jan,8; 2016,Jan,13;
2015,Jan,16; 2014,Jan,11

58559 with lysis of intrauterine adhesions (any method) ♀
🛢 8.20 ⚕ 8.20 **FUD** 000 [J][A2][⊡]
AMA: 2019,Jul,6; 2018,Jan,8; 2017,Jan,8; 2016,Jan,13;
2015,Jan,16; 2014,Jan,11

58560   with division or resection of intrauterine septum (any method) ♀

    8.95   8.95   **FUD** 000   J A2 80 🖃

AMA: 2019,Jul,6; 2018,Jan,8; 2017,Jan,8; 2016,Jan,13; 2015,Jan,16; 2014,Jan,11

58561   with removal of leiomyomata ♀

    10.2   10.2   **FUD** 000   J A2 80 🖃

AMA: 2019,Jul,6; 2018,Jan,8; 2017,Jan,8; 2016,Jan,13; 2015,Jan,16; 2014,Jan,11

58562   with removal of impacted foreign body ♀

    6.34   10.3   **FUD** 000   J A2 🖃

AMA: 2019,Jul,6; 2018,Jan,8; 2017,Jan,8; 2016,Jan,13; 2015,Jan,16; 2014,Jan,11

58563   with endometrial ablation (eg, endometrial resection, electrosurgical ablation, thermoablation) ♀

    7.05   50.2   **FUD** 000   J A2 80 🖃

AMA: 2019,Jul,6; 2018,Jan,8; 2017,Jan,8; 2016,Jan,13; 2015,Jan,16; 2015,Jan,13; 2014,Jan,11

58565   with bilateral fallopian tube cannulation to induce occlusion by placement of permanent implants ♀

    EXCLUDES   *Diagnostic hysteroscopy (58555)*
                   Dilation of cervical canal (57800)
                   Code also modifier 52 when a unilateral procedure is performed

    12.4   51.8   **FUD** 090   J J8 🖃

AMA: 2019,Jul,6; 2018,Jan,8; 2017,Jan,8; 2016,Jan,13; 2015,Jan,16; 2014,Jan,11

58570-58579 Other Uterine Endoscopy

INCLUDES   Diagnostic laparoscopy
EXCLUDES   *Hysteroscopy (58555-58565)*

58570   Laparoscopy, surgical, with total hysterectomy, for uterus 250 g or less; ♀

    EXCLUDES   *Colpotomy (57000)*
                   Hysteroscopy (58561)
                   Laparoscopy (49320, 58545-58546, 58661, 58670-58671)
                   Myomectomy procedures (58140-58146)
                   Pelvic examination under anesthesia (57410)
                   Total abdominal hysterectomy (58150)
                   Treatment of nonobstetrical vaginal hemorrhage (57180)

    22.4   22.4   **FUD** 090   J G2 80 🖃

AMA: 2019,Jul,6; 2018,Jan,8; 2017,Apr,7; 2014,Jan,11

58571   with removal of tube(s) and/or ovary(s) ♀

    EXCLUDES   *Colpotomy (57000)*
                   Hysteroscopy (58561)
                   Laparoscopy (49320, 58545-58546, 58661, 58670-58671)
                   Myomectomy procedures (58140-58146)
                   Pelvic examination under anesthesia (57410)
                   Total abdominal hysterectomy (58150)
                   Treatment of nonobstetrical vaginal hemorrhage (57180)

    25.8   25.8   **FUD** 090   J G2 80 🖃

AMA: 2019,Jul,6; 2018,Feb,11; 2018,Jan,8; 2017,Apr,7; 2017,Jan,8; 2016,Jan,13; 2015,Jan,16; 2014,Jan,11

58572   Laparoscopy, surgical, with total hysterectomy, for uterus greater than 250 g; ♀

    EXCLUDES   *Colpotomy (57000)*
                   Hysteroscopy (58561)
                   Laparoscopy (49320, 58545-58546, 58661, 58670-58671)
                   Myomectomy procedures (58140-58146)
                   Pelvic examination under anesthesia (57410)
                   Total abdominal hysterectomy (58150)
                   Treatment of nonobstetrical vaginal hemorrhage (57180)

    29.3   29.3   **FUD** 090   J G2 80 🖃

AMA: 2019,Jul,6; 2018,Jan,8; 2017,Apr,7; 2014,Jan,11

58573   with removal of tube(s) and/or ovary(s) ♀

    EXCLUDES   *Colpotomy (57000)*
                   Hysteroscopy (58561)
                   Laparoscopy (49320, 58545-58546, 58661, 58670-58671)
                   Myomectomy procedures (58140-58146)
                   Pelvic examination under anesthesia (57410)
                   Total abdominal hysterectomy (58150)
                   Treatment of nonobstetrical vaginal hemorrhage (57180)

    35.0   35.0   **FUD** 090   J G2 80 🖃

AMA: 2019,Jul,6; 2019,Mar,5; 2018,Apr,10; 2018,Feb,11; 2018,Jan,8; 2017,Apr,7; 2017,Jan,8; 2016,Jan,13; 2015,Jan,16; 2014,Jan,11

58575   Laparoscopy, surgical, total hysterectomy for resection of malignancy (tumor debulking), with omentectomy including salpingo-oophorectomy, unilateral or bilateral, when performed ♀

    EXCLUDES   *Laparoscopy (49320-49321, 58570-58573, 58661)*
                   Omentectomy (49255)

    54.4   54.4   **FUD** 090   C 80 🖃

AMA: 2019,Jul,6; 2019,Mar,5

58578   Unlisted laparoscopy procedure, uterus ♀

    0.00   0.00   **FUD** YYY   J 80 50 🖃

AMA: 2019,Jul,6; 2018,Jan,8; 2017,Jan,8; 2016,Jan,13; 2015,Jan,16; 2014,Jan,11

58579   Unlisted hysteroscopy procedure, uterus ♀

    0.00   0.00   **FUD** YYY   T 80 50 🖃

AMA: 2019,Jul,6; 2018,Jan,8; 2017,Jan,8; 2016,Jan,13; 2015,Jan,16; 2014,Jan,11

58600-58615 Sterilization by Tubal Interruption

CMS: 100-03,230.3 Sterilization
EXCLUDES   *Destruction/excision of endometriomas, open method (49203-49205)*

58600   Ligation or transection of fallopian tube(s), abdominal or vaginal approach, unilateral or bilateral ♀

    INCLUDES   Madlener operation

    10.3   10.3   **FUD** 090   J G2 80 🖃

AMA: 2019,Jul,6; 2018,Jan,8; 2017,Jan,8; 2016,Jan,13; 2015,Jan,16; 2014,Jan,11

58605   Ligation or transection of fallopian tube(s), abdominal or vaginal approach, postpartum, unilateral or bilateral, during same hospitalization (separate procedure) ♀

    EXCLUDES   *Laparoscopic methods (58670-58671)*

    9.35   9.35   **FUD** 090   C 80 🖃

AMA: 2019,Jul,6; 2018,Jan,8; 2017,Jan,8; 2016,Jan,13; 2015,Jan,16; 2014,Jan,11

+ **58611**   Ligation or transection of fallopian tube(s) when done at the time of cesarean delivery or intra-abdominal surgery (not a separate procedure) (List separately in addition to code for primary procedure) ♀

    Code first primary procedure

    2.17   2.17   **FUD** ZZZ   C 80 🖃

AMA: 2019,Jul,6; 2014,Jan,11

58615   Occlusion of fallopian tube(s) by device (eg, band, clip, Falope ring) vaginal or suprapubic approach ♀

    EXCLUDES   *Laparoscopic method (58671)*
                   Lysis of adnexal adhesions (58740)

    6.95   6.95   **FUD** 010   J G2 80 🖃

AMA: 2019,Jul,6; 2018,Jan,8; 2017,Jan,8; 2016,Jan,13; 2015,Jan,16; 2014,Jan,11

58660-58679 Endoscopic Procedures Fallopian Tubes and/or Ovaries

CMS: 100-03,230.3 Sterilization

INCLUDES   Diagnostic laparoscopy (49320)

EXCLUDES   Laparoscopy with biopsy of fallopian tube or ovary (49321)
Laparoscopy with ovarian cyst aspiration (49322)

58660   Laparoscopy, surgical; with lysis of adhesions (salpingolysis, ovariolysis) (separate procedure) ♀
🔧 19.2   ⚕ 19.2   **FUD** 090   J A2 80 ▣
AMA: 2019,Jul,6; 2018,Jan,8; 2017,Jan,8; 2016,Jan,13; 2015,Jan,16; 2014,Jan,11

58661   with removal of adnexal structures (partial or total oophorectomy and/or salpingectomy) ♀
🔧 18.5   ⚕ 18.5   **FUD** 010   J A2 80 50 ▣
AMA: 2019,Jul,6; 2018,Jan,8; 2017,Jan,8; 2016,Jan,13; 2015,Jan,16; 2014,Jan,11

58662   with fulguration or excision of lesions of the ovary, pelvic viscera, or peritoneal surface by any method ♀
🔧 20.2   ⚕ 20.2   **FUD** 090   J A2 80 ▣
AMA: 2019,Jul,6; 2018,Jan,8; 2017,Dec,14; 2017,Jan,8; 2016,Jan,13; 2015,Jan,16; 2014,Jan,11

58670   with fulguration of oviducts (with or without transection) ♀
🔧 10.3   ⚕ 10.3   **FUD** 090   J A2 ▣
AMA: 2019,Jul,6; 2018,Jan,8; 2017,Jan,8; 2016,Jan,13; 2015,Jan,16; 2014,Jan,11

58671   with occlusion of oviducts by device (eg, band, clip, or Falope ring) ♀
🔧 10.3   ⚕ 10.3   **FUD** 090   J A2 ▣
AMA: 2019,Jul,6; 2018,Jan,8; 2017,Jan,8; 2016,Jan,13; 2015,Jan,16; 2014,Jan,11

58672   with fimbrioplasty ♀
🔧 20.7   ⚕ 20.7   **FUD** 090   J A2 80 50 ▣
AMA: 2019,Jul,6; 2018,Jan,8; 2017,Jan,8; 2016,Jan,13; 2015,Jan,16; 2014,Jan,11

58673   with salpingostomy (salpingoneostomy) ♀
🔧 22.5   ⚕ 22.5   **FUD** 090   J A2 80 50 ▣
AMA: 2019,Jul,6; 2018,Jan,8; 2017,Jan,8; 2016,Jan,13; 2015,Jan,16; 2014,Jan,11

58674   Resequenced code. See code before 58541.

58679   Unlisted laparoscopy procedure, oviduct, ovary ♀
🔧 0.00   ⚕ 0.00   **FUD** YYY   J 80 50 ▣
AMA: 2019,Jul,6; 2018,Jan,8; 2017,Jan,8; 2016,Jan,13; 2015,Jan,16; 2014,Jan,11

58700-58770 Open Procedures Fallopian Tubes, with/without Ovaries

EXCLUDES   Destruction/excision of endometriomas, open method (49203-49205, 58957-58958)

58700   Salpingectomy, complete or partial, unilateral or bilateral (separate procedure) ♀
🔧 22.3   ⚕ 22.3   **FUD** 090   C 80 ▣
AMA: 2019,Jul,6; 2018,Sep,14; 2014,Jan,11

58720   Salpingo-oophorectomy, complete or partial, unilateral or bilateral (separate procedure) ♀
🔧 21.3   ⚕ 21.3   **FUD** 090   C 80 ▣
AMA: 2019,Jul,6; 2018,Jan,8; 2017,Jan,8; 2016,Jan,13; 2015,Jan,16; 2014,Jan,11

58740   Lysis of adhesions (salpingolysis, ovariolysis) ♀
EXCLUDES   Excision/fulguration of lesions performed laparoscopically (58662)
Laparoscopic method (58660)
🔧 25.5   ⚕ 25.5   **FUD** 090   C 80 ▣
AMA: 2019,Jul,6; 2018,Jan,8; 2017,Jan,8; 2016,Jan,13; 2015,Jan,16; 2014,Jan,11

58750   Tubotubal anastomosis ♀
🔧 25.5   ⚕ 25.5   **FUD** 090   C 80 50 ▣
AMA: 2019,Jul,6; 2014,Jan,11

Occluded section of tube is excised

Ovary

Tube ends are sutured

58752   Tubouterine implantation ♀
🔧 25.4   ⚕ 25.4   **FUD** 090   C 80 50 ▣
AMA: 2019,Jul,6; 2014,Jan,11

58760   Fimbrioplasty ♀
EXCLUDES   Laparoscopic method (58672)
🔧 22.9   ⚕ 22.9   **FUD** 090   C 80 50 ▣
AMA: 2019,Jul,6; 2018,Jan,8; 2017,Jan,8; 2016,Jan,13; 2015,Jan,16; 2014,Jan,11

58770   Salpingostomy (salpingoneostomy) ♀
EXCLUDES   Laparoscopic method (58673)
🔧 24.1   ⚕ 24.1   **FUD** 090   J 80 50 ▣
AMA: 2019,Jul,6; 2018,Jan,8; 2017,Jan,8; 2016,Jan,13; 2015,Jan,16; 2014,Jan,11

58800-58925 Open Procedures: Ovary

CMS: 100-03,230.3 Sterilization

EXCLUDES   Destruction/excision of endometriomas, open method (49203-49205, 58957-58958)

58800   Drainage of ovarian cyst(s), unilateral or bilateral (separate procedure); vaginal approach ♀
🔧 8.55   ⚕ 9.35   **FUD** 090   J A2
AMA: 2019,Jul,6; 2014,Jan,11

58805   abdominal approach ♀
🔧 11.6   ⚕ 11.6   **FUD** 090   J G2 80 ▣
AMA: 2019,Jul,6; 2014,Jan,11

58820   Drainage of ovarian abscess; vaginal approach, open ♀
EXCLUDES   Transrectal fluid drainage using catheter, image guided (49407)
🔧 9.02   ⚕ 9.02   **FUD** 090   J A2 80 50 ▣
AMA: 2019,Jul,6; 2014,Jan,11

58822   abdominal approach ♀
EXCLUDES   Transrectal fluid drainage using catheter, image guided (49407)
🔧 19.8   ⚕ 19.8   **FUD** 090   C 80 50 ▣
AMA: 2019,Jul,6; 2014,Jan,11

58825   Transposition, ovary(s) ♀
🔧 19.7   ⚕ 19.7   **FUD** 090   C 80 ▣
AMA: 2019,Jul,6; 2014,Jan,11

58900   Biopsy of ovary, unilateral or bilateral (separate procedure) ♀
EXCLUDES   Laparoscopy with biopsy of fallopian tube or ovary (49321)
🔧 11.8   ⚕ 11.8   **FUD** 090   J A2 80 ▣
AMA: 2019,Jul,6; 2018,Jan,8; 2017,Jan,8; 2016,Jan,13; 2015,Jan,16; 2014,Jan,11

58920	Wedge resection or bisection of ovary, unilateral or bilateral ♀

    ⚕ 19.8   🔪 19.8   **FUD** 090   J 80 ▢

    AMA: 2019,Jul,6; 2014,Jan,11

58925	Ovarian cystectomy, unilateral or bilateral ♀

    ⚕ 21.4   🔪 21.4   **FUD** 090   J 80 ▢

    AMA: 2019,Jul,6; 2014,Jan,11

58940-58960 Removal Ovary(s) with/without Multiple Procedures for Malignancy

CMS: 100-03,230.3 Sterilization

EXCLUDES   Chemotherapy (96401-96549)
         Destruction/excision of tumors, cysts, or endometriomas, open method
         (49203-49205)

58940	Oophorectomy, partial or total, unilateral or bilateral; ♀

     EXCLUDES   Oophorectomy with tumor debulking for ovarian
             malignancy (58952)

    ⚕ 15.3   🔪 15.3   **FUD** 090   C 80 ▢

    AMA: 2019,Jul,6; 2018,Jan,8; 2017,Jan,8; 2016,Jan,13;
    2015,Jan,16; 2014,Jan,11

58943	for ovarian, tubal or primary peritoneal malignancy, with para-aortic and pelvic lymph node biopsies, peritoneal washings, peritoneal biopsies, diaphragmatic assessments, with or without salpingectomy(s), with or without omentectomy ♀

    ⚕ 34.1   🔪 34.1   **FUD** 090   C 80 ▢

    AMA: 2019,Jul,6; 2014,Jan,11

58950	Resection (initial) of ovarian, tubal or primary peritoneal malignancy with bilateral salpingo-oophorectomy and omentectomy; ♀

     EXCLUDES   Resection/tumor debulking of recurrent
             ovarian/tubal/primary peritoneal/uterine
             malignancy (58957-58958)

    ⚕ 32.9   🔪 32.9   **FUD** 090   C 80 ▢

    AMA: 2019,Jul,6; 2014,Jan,11

58951	with total abdominal hysterectomy, pelvic and limited para-aortic lymphadenectomy ♀

     EXCLUDES   Resection/tumor debulking of recurrent
             ovarian/tubal/primary peritoneal/uterine
             malignancy (58957-58958)

    ⚕ 42.1   🔪 42.1   **FUD** 090   C 80 ▢

    AMA: 2019,Jul,6; 2018,Jan,8; 2017,Jan,8; 2016,Jan,13;
    2015,Jan,16; 2014,Jan,11

58952	with radical dissection for debulking (ie, radical excision or destruction, intra-abdominal or retroperitoneal tumors) ♀

     EXCLUDES   Resection/tumor debulking of recurrent
             ovarian/tubal/primary peritoneal/uterine
             malignancy (58957-58958)

    ⚕ 47.8   🔪 47.8   **FUD** 090   C 80 ▢

    AMA: 2019,Jul,6; 2018,Jan,8; 2017,Jan,8; 2016,Jan,13;
    2015,Jan,16; 2014,Jan,11

58953	Bilateral salpingo-oophorectomy with omentectomy, total abdominal hysterectomy and radical dissection for debulking; ♀

    ⚕ 58.9   🔪 58.9   **FUD** 090   C 80 ▢

    AMA: 2019,Jul,6; 2018,Jan,8; 2017,Jan,8; 2016,Jan,13;
    2015,Jan,16; 2014,May,10; 2014,Jan,11

58954	with pelvic lymphadenectomy and limited para-aortic lymphadenectomy ♀

    ⚕ 63.9   🔪 63.9   **FUD** 090   C 80 ▢

    AMA: 2019,Jul,6; 2018,Jan,8; 2017,Jan,8; 2016,Jan,13;
    2015,Jan,16; 2014,Jan,11

58956	Bilateral salpingo-oophorectomy with total omentectomy, total abdominal hysterectomy for malignancy ♀

     EXCLUDES   Biopsy of ovary (58900)
             Hysterectomy (58150, 58180, 58262-58263)
             Laparoscopy (58550, 58661)
             Omentectomy (49255)
             Oophorectomy (58940)
             Ovarian cystectomy (58925)
             Resection of malignancy (58957-58958)
             Salpingectomy salpingo-oophorectomy, (58700, 58720)

    ⚕ 39.9   🔪 39.9   **FUD** 090   C 80 ▢

    AMA: 2019,Jul,6; 2018,Jan,8; 2017,Jan,8; 2016,Jan,13;
    2015,Jan,16; 2014,May,10; 2014,Jan,11

58957	Resection (tumor debulking) of recurrent ovarian, tubal, primary peritoneal, uterine malignancy (intra-abdominal, retroperitoneal tumors), with omentectomy, if performed; ♀

     EXCLUDES   Biopsy of ovary (58900-58960)
             Destruction, excision cysts, endometriomas, or tumors
               (49203-49215)
             Enterolysis (44005)
             Exploratory laparotomy (49000)
             Lymphadenectomy (38770, 38780)
             Omentectomy (49255)

    ⚕ 46.2   🔪 46.2   **FUD** 090   C 80 ▢

    AMA: 2019,Jul,6; 2014,Jan,11

58958	with pelvic lymphadenectomy and limited para-aortic lymphadenectomy ♀

     EXCLUDES   Biopsy of ovary (58900-58960)
             Destruction, excision cysts, endometriomas, or tumors
               (49203-49215)
             Enterolysis (44005)
             Exploratory laparotomy (49000)
             Lymphadenectomy (38770, 38780)
             Omentectomy (49255)

    ⚕ 51.2   🔪 51.2   **FUD** 090   C 80 ▢

    AMA: 2019,Jul,6; 2014,Jan,11

58960	Laparotomy, for staging or restaging of ovarian, tubal, or primary peritoneal malignancy (second look), with or without omentectomy, peritoneal washing, biopsy of abdominal and pelvic peritoneum, diaphragmatic assessment with pelvic and limited para-aortic lymphadenectomy ♀

     EXCLUDES   Resection of malignancy (58957-58958)

    ⚕ 28.2   🔪 28.2   **FUD** 090   C 80 ▢

    AMA: 2019,Jul,6; 2014,Jan,11

58970-58999 Procedural Components: In Vitro Fertilization

58970	Follicle puncture for oocyte retrieval, any method M ♀

    📷 (76948)

    ⚕ 5.62   🔪 6.43   **FUD** 000   T A2 80 ▢

    AMA: 2019,Jul,6; 2014,Jan,11

58974	Embryo transfer, intrauterine M ♀

    ⚕ 0.00   🔪 0.00   **FUD** 000   T A2 80 ▢

    AMA: 2019,Jul,6; 2014,Jan,11

58976	Gamete, zygote, or embryo intrafallopian transfer, any method M ♀

     EXCLUDES   Adnexal procedures performed laparoscopically
             (58660-58673)

    ⚕ 6.06   🔪 7.05   **FUD** 000   T A2 80 ▢

    AMA: 2019,Jul,6; 2018,Jan,8; 2017,Jan,8; 2016,Jan,13;
    2015,Jan,16; 2014,Jan,11

58999	Unlisted procedure, female genital system (nonobstetrical) ♀

    ⚕ 0.00   🔪 0.00   **FUD** YYY   T ▢

    AMA: 2019,Jul,6; 2018,Jan,8; 2017,Jan,8; 2016,Jan,13;
    2015,Jan,16; 2014,Jan,11

● New Code   ▲ Revised Code   ○ Reinstated   ● New Web Release   ▲ Revised Web Release   + Add-on   Unlisted   Not Covered   # Resequenced
50 Optum Mod 50 Exempt   △ AMA Mod 51 Exempt   51 Optum Mod 51 Exempt   63 Mod 63 Exempt   ✗ Non-FDA Drug   ★ Telemedicine   M Maternity   A Age Edit

59000-59001 Aspiration of Amniotic Fluid

EXCLUDES *Intrauterine fetal transfusion (36460)*
Unlisted fetal invasive procedure (59897)

59000   Amniocentesis; diagnostic   M ♀
   ⚕ (76946)
   ⚐ 2.33   ⚖ 3.53   **FUD** 000   T P3 ▭
   AMA: 2019,Jul,6; 2018,Jan,8; 2017,Jan,8; 2016,Jan,13;
   2015,Jan,16; 2014,Jan,11

**59001   therapeutic amniotic fluid reduction (includes ultrasound
                guidance)**   M ♀
   ⚐ 5.15   ⚖ 5.15   **FUD** 000   T R2 ▭
   AMA: 2019,Jul,6; 2018,Jan,8; 2017,Jan,8; 2016,Jan,13;
   2015,Jan,16; 2014,Jan,11

59012-59076 Fetal Testing and Treatment

EXCLUDES *Intrauterine fetal transfusion (36460)*
Unlisted fetal invasive procedures (59897)

59012   Cordocentesis (intrauterine), any method   M ♀
   ⚕ (76941)
   ⚐ 5.82   ⚖ 5.82   **FUD** 000   T G2 80 ▭
   AMA: 2019,Jul,6; 2014,Jan,11

59015   Chorionic villus sampling, any method   M ♀
   ⚕ (76945)
   ⚐ 3.78   ⚖ 4.47   **FUD** 000   T P3 80 ▭
   AMA: 2019,Jul,6; 2018,Jan,8; 2017,Jan,8; 2016,Jan,13;
   2015,Jan,16; 2014,Jan,11

59020   Fetal contraction stress test   M ♀
   ⚐ 1.99   ⚖ 1.99   **FUD** 000   T P3 80 ▭
   AMA: 2019,Jul,6; 2018,Jan,8; 2017,Jan,8; 2016,Jan,13;
   2015,Jan,16; 2014,Jan,11

59025   Fetal non-stress test   M ♀
   ⚐ 1.37   ⚖ 1.37   **FUD** 000   T P3 80 ▭
   AMA: 2019,Jul,6; 2018,Jan,8; 2017,Jan,8; 2016,Jan,13;
   2015,Jan,16; 2014,Jan,11

59030   Fetal scalp blood sampling   M ♀
   Code also modifier 76 or 77, as appropriate, for repeat fetal scalp
   blood sampling
   ⚐ 3.25   ⚖ 3.25   **FUD** 000   T 80 ▭
   AMA: 2019,Jul,6; 2014,Jan,11

**59050   Fetal monitoring during labor by consulting physician (ie,
           non-attending physician) with written report; supervision
           and interpretation**   M ♀
   ⚐ 1.46   ⚖ 1.46   **FUD** XXX   M 80 ▭
   AMA: 2019,Jul,6; 2014,Jan,11

59051   interpretation only   M ♀
   ⚐ 1.21   ⚖ 1.21   **FUD** XXX   B 80 ▭
   AMA: 2019,Jul,6; 2014,Jan,11

**59070   Transabdominal amnioinfusion, including ultrasound
           guidance**   M ♀
   ⚐ 8.92   ⚖ 11.5   **FUD** 000   T G2 80 ▭
   AMA: 2019,Jul,6; 2018,Jan,8; 2017,Jan,8; 2016,Jan,13;
   2015,Jan,16; 2014,Jan,11

**59072   Fetal umbilical cord occlusion, including ultrasound
           guidance**   M ♀
   ⚐ 15.0   ⚖ 15.0   **FUD** 000   T G2 ▭
   AMA: 2019,Jul,6; 2018,Jan,8; 2017,Jan,8; 2016,Jan,13;
   2015,Jan,16; 2014,Jan,11

**59074   Fetal fluid drainage (eg, vesicocentesis, thoracocentesis,
           paracentesis), including ultrasound guidance**   M ♀
   ⚐ 8.92   ⚖ 11.1   **FUD** 000   T G2 80 ▭
   AMA: 2019,Jul,6; 2018,Jan,8; 2017,Jan,8; 2016,Jan,13;
   2015,Jan,16; 2014,Jan,11

**59076   Fetal shunt placement, including ultrasound
           guidance**   M ♀
   ⚐ 15.0   ⚖ 15.0   **FUD** 000   T G2 80 ▭
   AMA: 2019,Jul,6; 2018,Jan,8; 2017,Jan,8; 2016,Jan,13;
   2015,Jan,16; 2014,Jan,11

59100-59151 Tubal Pregnancy/Hysterotomy Procedures

CMS: 100-03,230.3 Sterilization

**59100   Hysterotomy, abdominal (eg, for hydatidiform mole,
           abortion)**   M ♀
   Code also ligation of fallopian tubes when performed at the
   same time as hysterotomy (58611)
   ⚐ 24.1   ⚖ 24.1   **FUD** 090   J R2 80 ▭
   AMA: 2019,Jul,6; 2014,Jan,11

**59120   Surgical treatment of ectopic pregnancy; tubal or ovarian,
           requiring salpingectomy and/or oophorectomy, abdominal
           or vaginal approach**   M ♀
   ⚐ 23.0   ⚖ 23.0   **FUD** 090   C 80 ▭
   AMA: 2019,Jul,6; 2014,Jan,11

**59121   tubal or ovarian, without salpingectomy and/or
                oophorectomy**   M ♀
   ⚐ 23.0   ⚖ 23.0   **FUD** 090   C 80 ▭
   AMA: 2019,Jul,6; 2014,Jan,11

59130   abdominal pregnancy   M ♀
   ⚐ 26.8   ⚖ 26.8   **FUD** 090   C 80 ▭
   AMA: 2019,Jul,6; 2014,Jan,11

**59135   interstitial, uterine pregnancy requiring total
                hysterectomy**   M ♀
   ⚐ 26.5   ⚖ 26.5   **FUD** 090   C 80 ▭
   AMA: 2019,Jul,6; 2014,Jan,11

**59136   interstitial, uterine pregnancy with partial resection of
                uterus**   M ♀
   ⚐ 25.4   ⚖ 25.4   **FUD** 090   C 80 ▭
   AMA: 2019,Jul,6; 2014,Jan,11

59140   cervical, with evacuation   M ♀
   ⚐ 11.6   ⚖ 11.6   **FUD** 090   C 80 ▭
   AMA: 2019,Jul,6; 2014,Jan,11

**59150   Laparoscopic treatment of ectopic pregnancy; without
           salpingectomy and/or oophorectomy**   M ♀
   ⚐ 22.3   ⚖ 22.3   **FUD** 090   J G2 80 ▭
   AMA: 2019,Jul,6; 2018,Jan,8; 2017,Jan,8; 2016,Jan,13;
   2015,Jan,16; 2014,Jan,11

59151   with salpingectomy and/or oophorectomy   M ♀
   ⚐ 21.7   ⚖ 21.7   **FUD** 090   J G2 80 ▭
   AMA: 2019,Jul,6; 2014,Jan,11

59160-59200 Procedures of Uterus Prior To/After Delivery

59160   Curettage, postpartum   M ♀
   ⚐ 5.11   ⚖ 6.21   **FUD** 010   J A2 80 ▭
   AMA: 2019,Jul,6; 2018,Jan,8; 2017,Jan,8; 2016,Jan,13;
   2015,Jan,16; 2014,Jan,11

**59200   Insertion of cervical dilator (eg, laminaria, prostaglandin)
           (separate procedure)**   M ♀
   EXCLUDES *Fetal transfusion, intrauterine (36460)*
            *Hypertonic solution/prostaglandin introduction for
             labor initiation (59850-59857)*
   ⚐ 1.29   ⚖ 2.23   **FUD** 000   T P3 ▭
   AMA: 2019,Jul,6; 2018,Jan,8; 2017,Dec,14; 2017,Jan,8;
   2016,Jan,13; 2015,Jan,16; 2014,Jan,11

59300-59350 Postpartum Vaginal/Cervical/Uterine Repairs

EXCLUDES *Nonpregnancy-related cerclage (57700)*

59300   Episiotomy or vaginal repair, by other than attending   M ♀
   ⚐ 4.26   ⚖ 5.77   **FUD** 000   J P3 80 ▭
   AMA: 2019,Jul,6; 2014,Jan,11

26/TC PC/TC Only   A2-Z3 ASC Payment   50 Bilateral   ♂ Male Only   ♀ Female Only   ⚐ Facility RVU   ⚖ Non-Facility RVU   ▭ CCI   ✖ CLIA
FUD Follow-up Days   **CMS:** IOM   **AMA:** CPT Asst   A-Y OPPSI   80/80 Surg Assist Allowed / w/Doc   ▪ Lab Crosswalk   ⚕ Radiology Crosswalk

274   CPT © 2019 American Medical Association. All Rights Reserved.   © 2019 Optum360, LLC

59320 Cerclage of cervix, during pregnancy; vaginal

🚑 4.37 ⚕ 4.37 **FUD** 000 Ⓜ ♀

[J] [A2] [80] 🖵

AMA: 2019,Jul,6; 2018,Jan,8; 2017,Jan,8; 2016,Jan,13; 2015,Jan,16; 2014,Jan,11

- Uterine cavity
- Amniotic sac
- Uterus at term
- Cervix
- Cervix
- Vagina
- Cerclage sutures
- Vaginal canal
- Pubic bone

59325 abdominal

🚑 6.96 ⚕ 6.96 **FUD** 000 Ⓜ ♀

[C] [80] 🖵

AMA: 2019,Jul,6; 2018,Jan,8; 2017,Jan,8; 2016,Jan,13; 2015,Jan,16; 2014,Jan,11

59350 Hysterorrhaphy of ruptured uterus

🚑 8.08 ⚕ 8.08 **FUD** 000 Ⓜ ♀

[C] [80] 🖵

AMA: 2019,Jul,6; 2014,Jan,11

59400-59410 Vaginal Delivery: Comprehensive and Component Services

CMS: 100-02,15,180 Nurse-Midwife (CNM) Services; 100-02,15,20.1 Physician Expense for Surgery, Childbirth, and Treatment for Infertility

INCLUDES Care provided for an uncomplicated pregnancy including delivery as well as antepartum and postpartum care:
- Admission history
- Admission to hospital
- Artificial rupture of membranes
- Management of uncomplicated labor
- Physical exam
- Vaginal delivery with or without episiotomy or forceps

EXCLUDES *Medical complications of pregnancy, labor, and delivery:*
- *Cardiac problems*
- *Diabetes*
- *Hyperemesis*
- *Hypertension*
- *Neurological problems*
- *Premature rupture of membranes*
- *Pre-term labor*
- *Toxemia*
- *Trauma*
- *Newborn circumcision (54150, 54160)*
- *Services incidental to or unrelated to the pregnancy*

59400 Routine obstetric care including antepartum care, vaginal delivery (with or without episiotomy, and/or forceps) and postpartum care

Ⓜ ♀

INCLUDES Fetal heart tones

Hospital/office visits following cesarean section or vaginal delivery

Initial/subsequent history

Physical exams

Recording of weight/blood pressures

Routine chemical urinalysis

Routine prenatal visits:
- Each month up to 28 weeks gestation
- Every other week from 29 to 36 weeks gestation
- Weekly from 36 weeks until delivery

🚑 60.4 ⚕ 60.4 **FUD** MMM [B] 🖵

AMA: 2019,Jul,6; 2018,Jan,8; 2017,Jan,8; 2016,Jan,13; 2015,Jan,16; 2014,Jan,11

59409 Vaginal delivery only (with or without episiotomy and/or forceps);

Ⓜ ♀

Code also inpatient management after delivery/discharge services (99217-99239 [99224, 99225, 99226])

🚑 23.3 ⚕ 23.3 **FUD** MMM [J] [80] 🖵

AMA: 2019,Jul,6; 2018,Jan,8; 2017,Jan,8; 2016,Jan,13; 2015,Jan,16; 2014,Jan,11

59410 including postpartum care

Ⓜ ♀

INCLUDES Hospital/office visits following cesarean section or vaginal delivery

🚑 29.9 ⚕ 29.9 **FUD** MMM [B] 🖵

AMA: 2019,Jul,6; 2014,Jan,11

59412-59414 Other Maternity Services

CMS: 100-02,15,180 Nurse-Midwife (CNM) Services; 100-02,15,20.1 Physician Expense for Surgery, Childbirth, and Treatment for Infertility

59412 External cephalic version, with or without tocolysis

Ⓜ ♀

Code also delivery code(s)

🚑 2.95 ⚕ 2.95 **FUD** MMM [J] [62] [80] 🖵

AMA: 2019,Jul,6; 2014,Jan,11

Complete breech presentation at term

The physician feels for the baby's head and bottom externally

Turning the baby by applying external pressure

Baby is in cephalic presentation, engaged for normal delivery

59414 Delivery of placenta (separate procedure)

Ⓜ ♀

🚑 2.65 ⚕ 2.65 **FUD** MMM [J] [62] [80] 🖵

AMA: 2019,Jul,6; 2018,Jan,8; 2017,Jan,8; 2016,Jan,13; 2015,Jan,16; 2014,Jan,11

59425-59430 Prenatal and Postpartum Visits

CMS: 100-02,15,180 Nurse-Midwife (CNM) Services; 100-02,15,20.1 Physician Expense for Surgery, Childbirth, and Treatment for Infertility

INCLUDES Physician/other qualified health care professional providing all or a portion of antepartum/postpartum care, but no delivery due to:
Referral to another physician for delivery
Termination of pregnancy by abortion

EXCLUDES *Antepartum care, 1-3 visits, report with appropriate E&M service code*
Medical complications of pregnancy, labor, and delivery:
Cardiac problems
Diabetes
Hyperemesis
Hypertension
Neurological problems
Premature rupture of membranes
Pre-term labor
Toxemia
Trauma
Newborn circumcision (54150, 54160)
Services incidental to or unrelated to the pregnancy

59425   Antepartum care only; 4-6 visits   M ♀

INCLUDES Fetal heart tones
Initial/subsequent history
Physical exams
Recording of weight/blood pressures
Routine chemical urinalysis
Routine prenatal visits:
Each month up to 28 weeks gestation
Every other week from 29 to 36 weeks gestation
Weekly from 36 weeks until delivery

🔷 10.2   ⚖ 13.1   **FUD** MMM   B 80 🖥

AMA: 2019,Jul,6; 2018,Jan,8; 2017,Jan,8; 2016,Jan,13; 2015,Jan,16; 2014,Jan,11

59426   7 or more visits   M ♀

INCLUDES Biweekly visits to 36 weeks gestation
Fetal heart tones
Initial/subsequent history
Monthly visits up to 28 weeks gestation
Physical exams
Recording of weight/blood pressures
Routine chemical urinalysis
Weekly visits until delivery

🔷 17.9   ⚖ 23.5   **FUD** MMM   B 80 🖥

AMA: 2019,Jul,6; 2018,Jan,8; 2017,Jan,8; 2016,Jan,13; 2015,Jan,16; 2014,Jan,11

59430   Postpartum care only (separate procedure)   M ♀

INCLUDES Office/other outpatient visits following cesarean section or vaginal delivery

🔷 3.97   ⚖ 5.57   **FUD** MMM   B 🖥

AMA: 2019,Jul,6; 2018,Jan,8; 2017,Jan,8; 2016,Jan,13; 2015,Jan,16; 2014,Jan,11

59510-59525 Cesarean Section Delivery: Comprehensive and Components of Care

CMS: 100-02,15,20.1 Physician Expense for Surgery, Childbirth, and Treatment for Infertility

INCLUDES Classic cesarean section
Low cervical cesarean section

EXCLUDES *Infant standby attendance (99360)*
Medical complications of pregnancy, labor, and delivery:
Cardiac problems
Diabetes
Hyperemesis
Hypertension
Neurological problems
Premature rupture of membranes
Pre-term labor
Toxemia
Trauma
Newborn circumcision (54150, 54160)
Services incidental to or unrelated to the pregnancy
Vaginal delivery after prior cesarean section (59610-59614)

59510   Routine obstetric care including antepartum care, cesarean delivery, and postpartum care   M ♀

INCLUDES Admission history
Admission to hospital
Cesarean delivery
Fetal heart tones
Hospital/office visits following cesarean section
Initial/subsequent history
Management of uncomplicated labor
Physical exam
Recording of weight/blood pressures
Routine chemical urinalysis
Routine prenatal visits:
Each month up to 28 weeks gestation
Every other week 29 to 36 weeks gestation
Weekly from 36 weeks until delivery

EXCLUDES *Medical problems complicating labor and delivery*

🔷 67.0   ⚖ 67.0   **FUD** MMM   B 🖥

AMA: 2019,Jul,6; 2018,Jan,8; 2017,Jan,8; 2016,Jan,13; 2015,Jan,16; 2014,Jan,11

Body of uterus
Tube
Classical
Low vertical
Low transverse
Amniotic sac
Uterus at term
Cervix
Vagina
Pubic bone

Types of Cesarean section are classified by uterine incision

59514   Cesarean delivery only;   M ♀

INCLUDES Admission history
Admission to hospital
Cesarean delivery
Management of uncomplicated labor
Physical exam

EXCLUDES *Medical problems complicating labor and delivery*

Code also inpatient management after delivery/discharge services (99217-99239 [99224, 99225, 99226])

🔷 26.3   ⚖ 26.3   **FUD** MMM   C 80 🖥

AMA: 2019,Jul,6; 2018,Jan,8; 2017,Jan,8; 2016,Jan,13; 2015,Jan,16; 2014,Jan,11

26/TC PC/TC Only   A2-Z3 ASC Payment   50 Bilateral   ♂ Male Only   ♀ Female Only   🔷 Facility RVU   ⚖ Non-Facility RVU   🖥 CCI   ❌ CLIA
FUD Follow-up Days   **CMS:** IOM   **AMA:** CPT Asst   A-Y OPPSI   80/80 Surg Assist Allowed / w/Doc   Lab Crosswalk   Radiology Crosswalk

276   CPT © 2019 American Medical Association. All Rights Reserved.   © 2019 Optum360, LLC

59515   **including postpartum care** Ⓜ ♀
    INCLUDES   Admission history
            Admission to hospital
            Cesarean delivery
            Hospital/office visits following cesarean section or
                vaginal delivery
            Management of uncomplicated labor
            Physical exam
    EXCLUDES   Medical problems complicating labor and delivery
    📠 36.4   ⚕ 36.4   **FUD** MMM   Ⓑ 🖿
    AMA: 2019,Jul,6; 2018,Jan,8; 2017,Jan,8; 2016,Jan,13;
    2015,Jan,16; 2014,Jan,11

+ 59525   **Subtotal or total hysterectomy after cesarean delivery (List
    separately in addition to code for primary procedure)** Ⓜ ♀
            Code first cesarean delivery (59510, 59514, 59515, 59618, 59620,
            59622)
    📠 13.9   ⚕ 13.9   **FUD** ZZZ   Ⓒ 80 🖿
    AMA: 2019,Jul,6; 2014,Jan,11

59610-59614 Vaginal Delivery After Prior Cesarean Section: Comprehensive and Components of Care

CMS: 100-02,15,180 Nurse-Midwife (CNM) Services; 100-02,15,20.1 Physician Expense for Surgery, Childbirth, and Treatment for Infertility
    INCLUDES   Admission history
            Admission to hospital
            Management of uncomplicated labor
            Patients with previous cesarean delivery who present with the expectation
                of a vaginal delivery
            Physical exam
            Successful vaginal delivery after previous cesarean delivery (VBAC)
            Vaginal delivery with or without episiotomy or forceps
    EXCLUDES   Elective cesarean delivery (59510, 59514, 59515)
            Medical complications of pregnancy, labor, and delivery:
                Cardiac problems
                Diabetes
                Hyperemesis
                Hypertension
                Neurological problems
                Premature rupture of membranes
                Pre-term labor
                Toxemia
                Trauma
            Newborn circumcision (54150, 54160)
            Services incidental to or unrelated to the pregnancy

59610   **Routine obstetric care including antepartum care, vaginal
    delivery (with or without episiotomy, and/or forceps) and
    postpartum care, after previous cesarean delivery** Ⓜ ♀
    INCLUDES   Fetal heart tones
            Hospital/office visits following cesarean section or
                vaginal delivery
            Initial/subsequent history
            Physical exams
            Recording of weight/blood pressures
            Routine chemical urinalysis
            Routine prenatal visits:
                Each month up to 28 weeks gestation
                Every other week 29 to 36 weeks gestation
                Weekly from 36 weeks until delivery
    📠 63.4   ⚕ 63.4   **FUD** MMM   Ⓑ 80 🖿
    AMA: 2019,Jul,6; 2018,Jan,8; 2017,Jan,8; 2016,Jan,13;
    2015,Jan,16; 2014,Jan,11

59612   **Vaginal delivery only, after previous cesarean delivery (with
    or without episiotomy and/or forceps);** Ⓜ ♀
            Code also inpatient management after delivery/discharge
            services (99217-99239 [99224, 99225, 99226])
    📠 26.3   ⚕ 26.3   **FUD** MMM   Ⓙ 80 🖿
    AMA: 2019,Jul,6; 2018,Jan,8; 2017,Jan,8; 2016,Jan,13;
    2015,Jan,16; 2014,Jan,11

59614   **including postpartum care** Ⓜ ♀
    INCLUDES   Hospital/office visits following cesarean section or
                vaginal delivery
    📠 32.6   ⚕ 32.6   **FUD** MMM   Ⓑ 80 🖿
    AMA: 2019,Jul,6; 2018,Jan,8; 2017,Jan,8; 2016,Jan,13;
    2015,Jan,16; 2014,Jan,11

59618-59622 Cesarean Section After Attempted Vaginal Birth/Prior C-Section

CMS: 100-02,15,20.1 Physician Expense for Surgery, Childbirth, and Treatment for Infertility
    INCLUDES   Admission history
            Admission to hospital
            Cesarean delivery
            Cesarean delivery following an unsuccessful vaginal delivery attempt after
                previous cesarean delivery
            Management of uncomplicated labor
            Patients with previous cesarean delivery who present with the expectation
                of a vaginal delivery
            Physical exam
    EXCLUDES   Elective cesarean delivery (59510, 59514, 59515)
            Medical complications of pregnancy, labor, and delivery:
                Cardiac problems
                Diabetes
                Hyperemesis
                Hypertension
                Neurological problems
                Premature rupture of membranes
                Pre-term labor
                Toxemia
                Trauma
            Newborn circumcision (54150, 54160)
            Services incidental to or unrelated to the pregnancy

59618   **Routine obstetric care including antepartum care, cesarean
    delivery, and postpartum care, following attempted vaginal
    delivery after previous cesarean delivery** Ⓜ ♀
    INCLUDES   Fetal heart tones
            Hospital/office visits following cesarean section or
                vaginal delivery
            Initial/subsequent history
            Physical exams
            Recording of weight/blood pressures
            Routine chemical urinalysis
            Routine prenatal visits:
                Each month up to 28 weeks gestation
                Every two weeks 29 to 36 weeks gestation
                Weekly from 36 weeks until delivery
    📠 67.8   ⚕ 67.8   **FUD** MMM   Ⓑ 80 🖿
    AMA: 2019,Jul,6; 2018,Jan,8; 2017,Jan,8; 2016,Jan,13;
    2015,Jan,16; 2014,Jan,11

59620   **Cesarean delivery only, following attempted vaginal delivery
    after previous cesarean delivery;** Ⓜ ♀
            Code also inpatient management after delivery/discharge
            services (99217-99239 [99224, 99225, 99226])
    📠 27.0   ⚕ 27.0   **FUD** MMM   Ⓒ 80 🖿
    AMA: 2019,Jul,6; 2018,Jan,8; 2017,Jan,8; 2016,Jan,13;
    2015,Jan,16; 2014,Jan,11

59622   **including postpartum care** Ⓜ ♀
    INCLUDES   Hospital/office visits following cesarean section or
                vaginal delivery
    📠 37.4   ⚕ 37.4   **FUD** MMM   Ⓑ 80 🖿
    AMA: 2019,Jul,6; 2018,Jan,8; 2017,Jan,8; 2016,Jan,13;
    2015,Jan,16; 2014,Jan,11

59812-59830 Treatment of Miscarriage

CMS: 100-02,15,20.1 Physician Expense for Surgery, Childbirth, and Treatment for Infertility
    EXCLUDES   Medical treatment of spontaneous complete abortion, any trimester
                (99201-99233 [99224, 99225, 99226])

59812   **Treatment of incomplete abortion, any trimester, completed
    surgically** Ⓜ ♀
    INCLUDES   Surgical treatment of spontaneous abortion
    📠 8.59   ⚕ 9.37   **FUD** 090   Ⓙ A2 🖿
    AMA: 2019,Jul,6; 2018,Jan,8; 2017,Jan,8; 2016,Jan,13;
    2015,Jan,16; 2014,Jan,11

59820   **Treatment of missed abortion, completed surgically; first
    trimester** Ⓜ ♀
    📠 10.4   ⚕ 11.2   **FUD** 090   Ⓙ A2 🖿
    AMA: 2019,Jul,6; 2018,Jan,8; 2017,Jan,8; 2016,Jan,13;
    2015,Jan,16; 2014,Jan,11

59821 second trimester ▢M ♀
🚗 10.3 ⚕ 11.2 **FUD** 090 ▢J ▢A2 ▢80 ▢
AMA: 2019,Jul,6; 2018,Jan,8; 2017,Jan,8; 2016,Jan,13;
2015,Jan,16; 2014,Jan,11

59830 Treatment of septic abortion, completed surgically ▢M ♀
🚗 12.7 ⚕ 12.7 **FUD** 090 ▢C ▢80 ▢
AMA: 2019,Jul,6; 2018,Jan,8; 2017,Jan,8; 2016,Jan,13;
2015,Jan,16; 2014,Jan,11

59840-59866 Elective Abortions

CMS: 100-02,1,90 Termination of Pregnancy; 100-02,15,20.1 Physician Expense for Surgery, Childbirth, and Treatment for Infertility; 100-03,140.1 Abortion; 100-04,3,100.1 Billing for Abortion Services

59840 Induced abortion, by dilation and curettage ▢M ♀
🚗 6.08 ⚕ 6.50 **FUD** 010 ▢J ▢A2 ▢80 ▢
AMA: 2019,Jul,6; 2018,Jan,8; 2017,Jan,8; 2016,Jan,13;
2015,Jan,16; 2014,Jan,11

59841 Induced abortion, by dilation and evacuation ▢M ♀
🚗 10.4 ⚕ 11.2 **FUD** 010 ▢J ▢A2 ▢80 ▢
AMA: 2019,Jul,6; 2018,Jan,8; 2017,Jan,8; 2016,Jan,13;
2015,Jan,16; 2014,Jan,11

59850 Induced abortion, by 1 or more intra-amniotic injections (amniocentesis-injections), including hospital admission and visits, delivery of fetus and secundines; ▢M ♀
EXCLUDES Cervical dilator insertion (59200)
🚗 10.1 ⚕ 10.1 **FUD** 090 ▢C ▢80 ▢
AMA: 2019,Jul,6; 2018,Jan,8; 2017,Jan,8; 2016,Jan,13;
2015,Jan,16; 2014,Jan,11

59851 with dilation and curettage and/or evacuation ▢M ♀
EXCLUDES Cervical dilator insertion (59200)
🚗 10.9 ⚕ 10.9 **FUD** 090 ▢C ▢80 ▢
AMA: 2019,Jul,6; 2018,Jan,8; 2017,Jan,8; 2016,Jan,13;
2015,Jan,16; 2014,Jan,11

59852 with hysterotomy (failed intra-amniotic injection) ▢M ♀
EXCLUDES Cervical dilator insertion (59200)
🚗 15.0 ⚕ 15.0 **FUD** 090 ▢C ▢80 ▢
AMA: 2019,Jul,6; 2018,Jan,8; 2017,Jan,8; 2016,Jan,13;
2015,Jan,16; 2014,Jan,11

59855 Induced abortion, by 1 or more vaginal suppositories (eg, prostaglandin) with or without cervical dilation (eg, laminaria), including hospital admission and visits, delivery of fetus and secundines; ▢M ♀
🚗 12.0 ⚕ 12.0 **FUD** 090 ▢C ▢80 ▢
AMA: 2019,Jul,6; 2014,Jan,11

59856 with dilation and curettage and/or evacuation ▢M ♀
🚗 14.1 ⚕ 14.1 **FUD** 090 ▢C ▢80 ▢
AMA: 2019,Jul,6; 2014,Jan,11

59857 with hysterotomy (failed medical evacuation) ▢M ♀
🚗 15.0 ⚕ 15.0 **FUD** 090 ▢C ▢80 ▢
AMA: 2019,Jul,6; 2014,Jan,11

59866 Multifetal pregnancy reduction(s) (MPR) ▢M ♀
🚗 6.22 ⚕ 6.22 **FUD** 000 ▢T ▢62 ▢80 ▢
AMA: 2019,Jul,6; 2014,Jan,11

59870-59899 Miscellaneous Obstetrical Procedures

CMS: 100-02,15,20.1 Physician Expense for Surgery, Childbirth, and Treatment for Infertility

59870 Uterine evacuation and curettage for hydatidiform mole ▢M ♀
🚗 14.0 ⚕ 14.0 **FUD** 090 ▢J ▢A2 ▢80 ▢
AMA: 2019,Jul,6; 2018,Jan,8; 2017,Jan,8; 2016,Jan,13;
2015,Jan,16; 2014,Jan,11

59871 Removal of cerclage suture under anesthesia (other than local) ▢M ♀
🚗 3.83 ⚕ 3.83 **FUD** 000 ▢Q2 ▢A2 ▢80 ▢
AMA: 2019,Jul,6; 2018,Jan,8; 2017,Jan,8; 2016,Jan,13;
2015,Jan,16; 2014,Jan,11

59897 Unlisted fetal invasive procedure, including ultrasound guidance, when performed ▢M ♀
🚗 0.00 ⚕ 0.00 **FUD** YYY ▢T ▢
AMA: 2019,Jul,6; 2014,Jan,11

59898 Unlisted laparoscopy procedure, maternity care and delivery ▢M ♀
🚗 0.00 ⚕ 0.00 **FUD** YYY ▢J ▢80 ▢50 ▢
AMA: 2019,Jul,6; 2018,Jan,8; 2017,Jan,8; 2016,Jan,13;
2015,Jan,16; 2014,Jan,11

59899 Unlisted procedure, maternity care and delivery ▢M ♀
🚗 0.00 ⚕ 0.00 **FUD** YYY ▢T ▢80 ▢
AMA: 2019,Jul,6; 2018,Jan,8; 2017,Jan,8; 2016,Jan,13;
2015,Jan,16; 2014,Jan,11

26/TC PC/TC Only **A2-Z3** ASC Payment **50** Bilateral ♂ Male Only ♀ Female Only 🚗 Facility RVU ⚕ Non-Facility RVU ▢ CCI ▢ CLIA
FUD Follow-up Days **CMS:** IOM **AMA:** CPT Asst **A-Y** OPPSI **80/80** Surg Assist Allowed / w/Doc ▢ Lab Crosswalk ▢ Radiology Crosswalk

278   CPT © 2019 American Medical Association. All Rights Reserved.   © 2019 Optum360, LLC

60000 I&D of Infected Thyroglossal Cyst

60000   **Incision and drainage of thyroglossal duct cyst, infected**
🔧 4.36   ✂ 4.88   **FUD** 010   ⬚T ⬚A2 ⬚80 🖼
AMA: 2014,Jan,11

60100 Core Needle Biopsy: Thyroid

EXCLUDES   *Fine needle aspiration (10021, [10004, 10005, 10006, 10007, 10008, 10009, 10010, 10011, 10012])*

60100   **Biopsy thyroid, percutaneous core needle**
📷 (76942, 77002, 77012, 77021)
📷 (88172-88173)
🔧 2.27   ✂ 3.20   **FUD** 000   ⬚T ⬚P3 🖼
AMA: 2019,Apr,4; 2018,Jan,8; 2017,Jan,8; 2016,Jan,13; 2015,Jan,16; 2014,Jan,11

60200 Surgical Removal Thyroid Cyst or Mass; Division of Isthmus

60200   **Excision of cyst or adenoma of thyroid, or transection of isthmus**
🔧 19.0   ✂ 19.0   **FUD** 090   ⬚J ⬚A2 ⬚80 🖼
AMA: 2018,Jan,8; 2017,Jan,8; 2016,Jan,13; 2015,Jan,16; 2014,Jan,11

Lateral view

Thyroglossal duct (dotted line)   Hyoid bone
Cricothyroid muscle
Anterior view
Thyroid cartilage
Cricoid cartilage
Thyroid gland
Trachea
Esophagus
Crico-thyroid ligament
Epiglottis
Hyoid bone
Pyramid lobe
Thyroid cartilage
Right lobe
Cricoid cartilage
Left lobe
Isthmus
Thyroid gland

60210-60225 Subtotal Thyroidectomy

60210   **Partial thyroid lobectomy, unilateral; with or without isthmusectomy**
🔧 20.3   ✂ 20.3   **FUD** 090   ⬚J ⬚62 ⬚80 🖼
AMA: 2018,Jan,8; 2017,Jan,8; 2016,Jan,13; 2015,Jan,16; 2014,Jan,11

60212   **with contralateral subtotal lobectomy, including isthmusectomy**
🔧 29.0   ✂ 29.0   **FUD** 090   ⬚J ⬚62 ⬚80 🖼
AMA: 2018,Jan,8; 2017,Jan,8; 2016,Jan,13; 2015,Jan,16; 2014,Jan,11

60220   **Total thyroid lobectomy, unilateral; with or without isthmusectomy**
🔧 20.3   ✂ 20.3   **FUD** 090   ⬚J ⬚62 ⬚80 🖼
AMA: 2018,Jan,8; 2017,Jan,8; 2016,Jan,13; 2015,Jan,16; 2014,Jan,11

60225   **with contralateral subtotal lobectomy, including isthmusectomy**
🔧 26.7   ✂ 26.7   **FUD** 090   ⬚J ⬚62 ⬚80 🖼
AMA: 2018,Jan,8; 2017,Jan,8; 2016,Jan,13; 2015,Jan,16; 2014,Jan,11

60240-60271 Complete Thyroidectomy Procedures

60240   **Thyroidectomy, total or complete**
EXCLUDES   *Subtotal or partial thyroidectomy (60271)*
🔧 26.4   ✂ 26.4   **FUD** 090   ⬚J ⬚62 ⬚80 🖼
AMA: 2018,Jan,8; 2017,Jan,8; 2016,Jan,13; 2015,Jan,16; 2014,Jan,11

60252   **Thyroidectomy, total or subtotal for malignancy; with limited neck dissection**
🔧 38.0   ✂ 38.0   **FUD** 090   ⬚80 🖼
AMA: 2018,Jan,8; 2017,Jan,8; 2016,Jan,13; 2015,Jan,16; 2014,Jan,11

60254   **with radical neck dissection**
🔧 48.1   ✂ 48.1   **FUD** 090   ⬚C ⬚80 🖼
AMA: 2018,Jan,8; 2017,Jan,8; 2016,Jan,13; 2015,Jan,16; 2014,Jan,11

60260   **Thyroidectomy, removal of all remaining thyroid tissue following previous removal of a portion of thyroid**
🔧 31.4   ✂ 31.4   **FUD** 090   ⬚J ⬚80 ⬚50 🖼
AMA: 2018,Jan,8; 2017,Jan,8; 2016,Jan,13; 2015,Jan,16; 2014,Jan,11

60270   **Thyroidectomy, including substernal thyroid; sternal split or transthoracic approach**
🔧 39.4   ✂ 39.4   **FUD** 090   ⬚C ⬚80 🖼
AMA: 2018,Jan,8; 2017,Jan,8; 2016,Jan,13; 2015,Jan,16; 2014,Jan,11

60271   **cervical approach**
🔧 30.4   ✂ 30.4   **FUD** 090   ⬚J ⬚80 🖼
AMA: 2018,Jan,8; 2017,Jan,8; 2016,Jan,13; 2015,Jan,16; 2014,Jan,11

60280-60300 Treatment of Cyst/Sinus of Thyroid

60280   **Excision of thyroglossal duct cyst or sinus;**
EXCLUDES   *Thyroid ultrasound (76536)*
🔧 12.6   ✂ 12.6   **FUD** 090   ⬚J ⬚A2 ⬚80 🖼
AMA: 2014,Jan,11

60281   **recurrent**
EXCLUDES   *Thyroid ultrasound (76536)*
🔧 16.8   ✂ 16.8   **FUD** 090   ⬚J ⬚A2 ⬚80 🖼
AMA: 2014,Jan,11

60300   **Aspiration and/or injection, thyroid cyst**
EXCLUDES   *Fine needle aspiration (10021, [10004, 10005, 10006, 10007, 10008, 10009, 10010, 10011, 10012])*
📷 (76942, 77012)
🔧 1.44   ✂ 3.27   **FUD** 000   ⬚T ⬚P3 🖼
AMA: 2014,Jan,11

60500-60512 Parathyroid Procedures

60500   **Parathyroidectomy or exploration of parathyroid(s);**
🔧 27.8   ✂ 27.8   **FUD** 090   ⬚J ⬚62 ⬚80 🖼
AMA: 2018,Jan,8; 2017,Jan,8; 2016,Jan,13; 2015,Jan,16; 2014,Jan,11

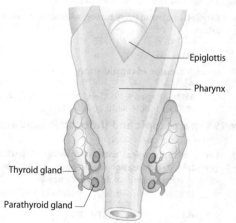

Epiglottis
Pharynx
Thyroid gland
Parathyroid gland

Posterior view of pharynx, thyroid glands, and parathyroid glands

Endocrine System

60502 re-exploration
🔹 37.2 ⚸ 37.2 **FUD** 090   J 80 ▢
AMA: 2018,Jan,8; 2017,Jan,8; 2016,Jan,13; 2015,Jan,16; 2014,Jan,11

60505 with mediastinal exploration, sternal split or transthoracic approach
🔹 40.1 ⚸ 40.1 **FUD** 090   C 80 ▢
AMA: 2018,Jan,8; 2017,Jan,8; 2016,Jan,13; 2015,Jan,16; 2014,Jan,11

+ **60512** Parathyroid autotransplantation (List separately in addition to code for primary procedure)
Code first (60212, 60225, 60240, 60252, 60254, 60260, 60270-60271, 60500, 60502, 60505)
🔹 7.03 ⚸ 7.03 **FUD** ZZZ   N 80 ▢
AMA: 2018,Jan,8; 2017,Jan,8; 2017,Jan,6; 2016,Jan,13; 2015,Jan,16; 2014,Jan,11

60520-60522 Thymus Procedures

EXCLUDES Surgical thoracoscopy (video-assisted thoracic surgery (VATS) thymectomy (32673)

60520 Thymectomy, partial or total; transcervical approach (separate procedure)
🔹 30.2 ⚸ 30.2 **FUD** 090   J 80 ▢
AMA: 2019,Mar,10; 2014,Jan,11

60521 sternal split or transthoracic approach, without radical mediastinal dissection (separate procedure)
🔹 32.4 ⚸ 32.4 **FUD** 090   C 80 ▢
AMA: 2018,Jan,8; 2017,Jan,8; 2016,Jan,13; 2015,Jan,16; 2014,Jan,11

60522 sternal split or transthoracic approach, with radical mediastinal dissection (separate procedure)
🔹 39.5 ⚸ 39.5 **FUD** 090   C 80 ▢
AMA: 2014,Jan,11

60540-60545 Adrenal Gland Procedures

EXCLUDES Laparoscopic approach (60650)
Removal of remote or disseminated pheochromocytoma (49203-49205)
Standard backbench preparation of cadaver donor (50323)

60540 Adrenalectomy, partial or complete, or exploration of adrenal gland with or without biopsy, transabdominal, lumbar or dorsal (separate procedure);
🔹 30.8 ⚸ 30.8 **FUD** 090   C 80 50 ▢
AMA: 2014,Jan,11

60545 with excision of adjacent retroperitoneal tumor
🔹 35.3 ⚸ 35.3 **FUD** 090   C 80 50 ▢
AMA: 2014,Jan,11

60600-60605 Carotid Body Procedures

60600 Excision of carotid body tumor; without excision of carotid artery
🔹 39.6 ⚸ 39.6 **FUD** 090   C 80 ▢
AMA: 2014,Jan,11

60605 with excision of carotid artery
🔹 47.9 ⚸ 47.9 **FUD** 090   C 80 ▢
AMA: 2018,Sep,9; 2017,Sep,13; 2016,Nov,8; 2016,Oct,10; 2016,Sep,8; 2016,Jul,10; 2014,Jan,11

60650-60699 Laparoscopic and Unlisted Procedures

INCLUDES Diagnostic laparoscopy (49320)

60650 Laparoscopy, surgical, with adrenalectomy, partial or complete, or exploration of adrenal gland with or without biopsy, transabdominal, lumbar or dorsal
EXCLUDES Peritoneoscopy performed as separate procedure (49320)
🔹 34.5 ⚸ 34.5 **FUD** 090   C 80 50 ▢
AMA: 2018,Jan,8; 2017,Jan,8; 2016,Jan,13; 2015,Jan,16; 2014,Jan,11

60659 Unlisted laparoscopy procedure, endocrine system
🔹 0.00 ⚸ 0.00 **FUD** YYY   J 80 50 ▢
AMA: 2018,Jan,8; 2017,Jan,8; 2016,Jan,13; 2015,Jan,16; 2014,Jan,11

60699 Unlisted procedure, endocrine system
🔹 0.00 ⚸ 0.00 **FUD** YYY   J 80 ▢
AMA: 2018,Jan,8; 2017,Jan,8; 2016,Jan,13; 2015,Jan,16; 2014,Jan,11

61000-61253 Transcranial Access via Puncture, Burr Hole, Twist Hole, or Trephine

EXCLUDES Injection for:
Cerebral angiography (36100-36218)

61000 Subdural tap through fontanelle, or suture, infant, unilateral or bilateral; initial **A**

EXCLUDES Injection for:
Pneumoencephalography (61055)
Ventriculography (61026, 61120)

🚑 3.19   3.19 **FUD** 000 **T R2**

AMA: 2014,Jan,11

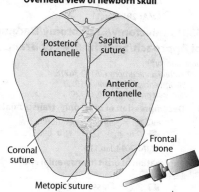

Overhead view of newborn skull

Posterior fontanelle
Sagittal suture
Anterior fontanelle
Coronal suture
Frontal bone
Metopic suture

An initial tap through to the subdural level is performed on an infant via a fontanelle or suture, either unilateral or bilateral

61001 subsequent taps **A**
🚑 3.16   3.16 **FUD** 000 **T R2**
AMA: 2014,Jan,11

61020 Ventricular puncture through previous burr hole, fontanelle, suture, or implanted ventricular catheter/reservoir; without injection
🚑 2.87   2.87 **FUD** 000 **T A2**
AMA: 2014,Jan,11

61026 with injection of medication or other substance for diagnosis or treatment
INCLUDES Injection for ventriculography
🚑 3.05   3.05 **FUD** 000 **T A2**
AMA: 2014,Jan,11

61050 Cisternal or lateral cervical (C1-C2) puncture; without injection (separate procedure)
🚑 2.45   2.45 **FUD** 000 **T A2 80**
AMA: 2014,Jan,11

61055 with injection of medication or other substance for diagnosis or treatment
INCLUDES Injection for pneumoencephalography
EXCLUDES Myelography via lumbar injection (62302-62305)
Radiology procedures except when furnished by a different provider
🚑 3.62   3.62 **FUD** 000 **T A2**
AMA: 2014,Sep,3; 2014,Jan,11

61070 Puncture of shunt tubing or reservoir for aspiration or injection procedure
🔳 (75809)
🚑 1.64   1.64 **FUD** 000 **T A2**
AMA: 2018,Jan,8; 2017,Jan,8; 2016,Jan,13; 2015,Jan,16; 2014,Jan,11

61105 Twist drill hole for subdural or ventricular puncture
🚑 13.5   13.5 **FUD** 090 **C 80**
AMA: 2014,Jan,11

61107 Twist drill hole(s) for subdural, intracerebral, or ventricular puncture; for implanting ventricular catheter, pressure recording device, or other intracerebral monitoring device
Code also intracranial neuroendoscopic ventricular catheter insertion or reinsertion, when performed (62160)
🚑 9.20   9.20 **FUD** 000 **⊘ C**
AMA: 2014,Jan,11

61108 for evacuation and/or drainage of subdural hematoma
🚑 26.0   26.0 **FUD** 090 **C**
AMA: 2014,Jan,11

61120 Burr hole(s) for ventricular puncture (including injection of gas, contrast media, dye, or radioactive material)
INCLUDES Includes: Injection for ventriculography
🚑 21.8   21.8 **FUD** 090 **C 80**
AMA: 2014,Jan,11

61140 Burr hole(s) or trephine; with biopsy of brain or intracranial lesion
🚑 36.9   36.9 **FUD** 090 **C 80**
AMA: 2014,Jan,11

61150 with drainage of brain abscess or cyst
🚑 39.8   39.8 **FUD** 090 **C**
AMA: 2014,Jan,11

61151 with subsequent tapping (aspiration) of intracranial abscess or cyst
🚑 29.1   29.1 **FUD** 090 **C**
AMA: 2014,Jan,11

61154 Burr hole(s) with evacuation and/or drainage of hematoma, extradural or subdural
🚑 37.1   37.1 **FUD** 090 **C 80 50**
AMA: 2014,Jan,11

61156 Burr hole(s); with aspiration of hematoma or cyst, intracerebral
🚑 36.5   36.5 **FUD** 090 **C 80**
AMA: 2014,Jan,11

61210 for implanting ventricular catheter, reservoir, EEG electrode(s), pressure recording device, or other cerebral monitoring device (separate procedure)
Code also intracranial neuroendoscopic ventricular catheter insertion or reinsertion, when performed (62160)
🚑 10.8   10.8 **FUD** 000 **C**
AMA: 2018,Jan,8; 2017,Jan,8; 2016,Jan,13; 2015,Jan,16; 2014,Jan,11

61215 Insertion of subcutaneous reservoir, pump or continuous infusion system for connection to ventricular catheter
EXCLUDES Chemotherapy (96450)
Refilling and maintenance of implantable infusion pump (95990)
🚑 14.8   14.8 **FUD** 090 **J A2**
AMA: 2018,Jan,8; 2017,Jan,8; 2016,Jan,13; 2015,Jan,16; 2014,Jan,11

61250 Burr hole(s) or trephine, supratentorial, exploratory, not followed by other surgery
EXCLUDES Burr hole or trephine followed by craniotomy at same operative session (61304-61321)
🚑 25.4   25.4 **FUD** 090 **C 80 50**
AMA: 2014,Jan,11

61253 Burr hole(s) or trephine, infratentorial, unilateral or bilateral
EXCLUDES Burr hole or trephine followed by craniotomy at same operative session (61304-61321)
🚑 29.1   29.1 **FUD** 090 **C 80**
AMA: 2018,Jan,8; 2017,Jan,8; 2016,Jan,13; 2015,Jan,16; 2014,Jan,11

61304-61323 Craniectomy/Craniotomy: By Indication/Specific Area of Brain

EXCLUDES Injection for:
Cerebral angiography (36100-36218)
Pneumoencephalography (61055)
Ventriculography (61026, 61120)

61304 Craniectomy or craniotomy, exploratory; supratentorial

EXCLUDES Other craniectomy/craniotomy procedures when performed at the same anatomical site and during the same surgical encounter

🚑 48.1 ⚕ 48.1 **FUD** 090 C 80 ▭

AMA: 2014,Jan,11

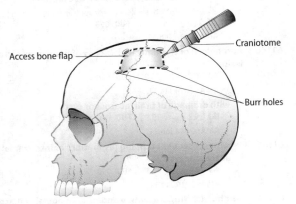

Access bone flap
Craniotome
Burr holes

61305 infratentorial (posterior fossa)

EXCLUDES Other craniectomy/craniotomy procedures when performed at the same anatomical site and during the same surgical encounter

🚑 58.6 ⚕ 58.6 **FUD** 090 C 80 ▭

AMA: 2014,Jan,11

61312 Craniectomy or craniotomy for evacuation of hematoma, supratentorial; extradural or subdural

🚑 60.8 ⚕ 60.8 **FUD** 090 C 80 ▭

AMA: 2018,Jan,8; 2017,Jan,8; 2016,Jan,13; 2015,Jan,16; 2014,Jan,11

61313 intracerebral

🚑 58.0 ⚕ 58.0 **FUD** 090 C 80 ▭

AMA: 2014,Jan,11

61314 Craniectomy or craniotomy for evacuation of hematoma, infratentorial; extradural or subdural

🚑 53.2 ⚕ 53.2 **FUD** 090 C 80 ▭

AMA: 2014,Jan,11

61315 intracerebellar

🚑 60.4 ⚕ 60.4 **FUD** 090 C 80 ▭

AMA: 2014,Jan,11

+ 61316 Incision and subcutaneous placement of cranial bone graft (List separately in addition to code for primary procedure)

Code first (61304, 61312-61313, 61322-61323, 61340, 61570-61571, 61680-61705)

🚑 2.60 ⚕ 2.60 **FUD** ZZZ C ▭

AMA: 2014,Jan,11

61320 Craniectomy or craniotomy, drainage of intracranial abscess; supratentorial

🚑 55.5 ⚕ 55.5 **FUD** 090 C 80 ▭

AMA: 2014,Jan,11

61321 infratentorial

🚑 62.7 ⚕ 62.7 **FUD** 090 C 80 ▭

AMA: 2014,Jan,11

61322 Craniectomy or craniotomy, decompressive, with or without duraplasty, for treatment of intracranial hypertension, without evacuation of associated intraparenchymal hematoma; without lobectomy

EXCLUDES Craniectomy or craniotomy for evacuation of hematoma (61313)
Subtemporal decompression (61340)

🚑 69.7 ⚕ 69.7 **FUD** 090 C 80 ▭

AMA: 2018,Aug,10; 2014,Jan,11

61323 with lobectomy

EXCLUDES Craniectomy or craniotomy for evacuation of hematoma (61313)
Subtemporal decompression (61340)

🚑 69.8 ⚕ 69.8 **FUD** 090 C 80 ▭

AMA: 2014,Jan,11

61330-61530 Craniectomy/Craniotomy/Decompression Brain By Surgical Approach/Specific Area of Brain

EXCLUDES Injection for:
Cerebral angiography (36100-36218)
Pneumoencephalography (61055)
Ventriculography (61026, 61120)

61330 Decompression of orbit only, transcranial approach

INCLUDES Naffziger operation

🚑 52.8 ⚕ 52.8 **FUD** 090 J 62 80 50 ▭

AMA: 2014,Jan,11

61333 Exploration of orbit (transcranial approach); with removal of lesion

🚑 59.6 ⚕ 59.6 **FUD** 090 C 80 50 ▭

AMA: 2014,Jan,11

61340 Subtemporal cranial decompression (pseudotumor cerebri, slit ventricle syndrome)

EXCLUDES Decompression craniotomy or craniectomy for intracranial hypertension, without hematoma removal (61322-61323)

🚑 42.4 ⚕ 42.4 **FUD** 090 C 80 50 ▭

AMA: 2014,Jan,11

61343 Craniectomy, suboccipital with cervical laminectomy for decompression of medulla and spinal cord, with or without dural graft (eg, Arnold-Chiari malformation)

🚑 64.0 ⚕ 64.0 **FUD** 090 C 80 ▭

AMA: 2014,Jan,11

61345 Other cranial decompression, posterior fossa

EXCLUDES Kroenlein procedure (67445)
Orbital decompression using a lateral wall approach (67445)

🚑 60.1 ⚕ 60.1 **FUD** 090 C 80 ▭

AMA: 2014,Jan,11

61450 Craniectomy, subtemporal, for section, compression, or decompression of sensory root of gasserian ganglion

INCLUDES Frazier-Spiller procedure
Hartley-Krause
Krause decompression
Taarnhoj procedure

🚑 56.6 ⚕ 56.6 **FUD** 090 C 80 ▭

AMA: 2014,Jan,11

61458 Craniectomy, suboccipital; for exploration or decompression of cranial nerves

INCLUDES Jannetta decompression

🚑 58.8 ⚕ 58.8 **FUD** 090 C 80 ▭

AMA: 2014,Jan,11

61460   **for section of 1 or more cranial nerves**
    🚑 61.7   ✂ 61.7   **FUD** 090   C 80 ▣
    AMA: 2014,Jan,11

Olfactory nerve (I)
Optic nerve (II)
Oculomotor nerve (III)
Trochlear nerve (IV)
Trigeminal nerve (V)
Abducens nerve (VI)
Facial nerve (VII)
Vestibulocochlear nerve (VIII)
Glossopharyngeal nerve (IX)
Vagus nerve (X)
Hypoglossal nerve (XII)
Accessory nerve (XI)
Pons

61500   **Craniectomy; with excision of tumor or other bone lesion of skull**
    🚑 38.2   ✂ 38.2   **FUD** 090   C 80 ▣
    AMA: 2018,Jan,8; 2017,Jan,8; 2016,Jan,13; 2015,Jan,16; 2014,Jan,11; 2014,Jan,9

61501   **for osteomyelitis**
    🚑 33.1   ✂ 33.1   **FUD** 090   C 80 ▣
    AMA: 2018,Jan,8; 2017,Jan,8; 2016,Jan,13; 2015,Jan,16; 2014,Jan,11; 2014,Jan,9

61510   **Craniectomy, trephination, bone flap craniotomy; for excision of brain tumor, supratentorial, except meningioma**
    🚑 64.0   ✂ 64.0   **FUD** 090   C 80 ▣
    AMA: 2014,Jan,11

61512   **for excision of meningioma, supratentorial**
    🚑 74.8   ✂ 74.8   **FUD** 090   C 80 ▣
    AMA: 2014,Jan,11

61514   **for excision of brain abscess, supratentorial**
    🚑 55.9   ✂ 55.9   **FUD** 090   C 80 ▣
    AMA: 2014,Jan,11

61516   **for excision or fenestration of cyst, supratentorial**
    EXCLUDES   *Craniopharyngioma (61545)*
            Pituitary tumor removal (61546, 61548)
    🚑 54.4   ✂ 54.4   **FUD** 090   C 80 ▣
    AMA: 2014,Jan,11

+ 61517   **Implantation of brain intracavitary chemotherapy agent (List separately in addition to code for primary procedure)**
    EXCLUDES   *Intracavity radioelement source or ribbon implantation (77770-77772)*
    Code first (61510, 61518)
    🚑 2.59   ✂ 2.59   **FUD** ZZZ   C ▣
    AMA: 2014,Jan,11

61518   **Craniectomy for excision of brain tumor, infratentorial or posterior fossa; except meningioma, cerebellopontine angle tumor, or midline tumor at base of skull**
    🚑 81.0   ✂ 81.0   **FUD** 090   C 80 ▣
    AMA: 2014,Jan,11

61519   **meningioma**
    🚑 86.7   ✂ 86.7   **FUD** 090   C 80 ▣
    AMA: 2014,Jan,11

61520   **cerebellopontine angle tumor**
    🚑 110.   ✂ 110.   **FUD** 090   C 80 ▣
    AMA: 2014,Jan,11

Central sulcus
Parietal lobe
Frontal lobe
Occipital lobe
Lateral sulcus
Temporal lobe
Cerebellum
Pons
Medulla oblongata

61521   **midline tumor at base of skull**
    🚑 93.7   ✂ 93.7   **FUD** 090   C 80 ▣
    AMA: 2018,Jan,8; 2017,Jan,8; 2016,Jan,13; 2015,Jan,16; 2014,Jan,11

61522   **Craniectomy, infratentorial or posterior fossa; for excision of brain abscess**
    🚑 62.9   ✂ 62.9   **FUD** 090   C 80 ▣
    AMA: 2014,Jan,11

61524   **for excision or fenestration of cyst**
    🚑 60.8   ✂ 60.8   **FUD** 090   C 80 ▣
    AMA: 2014,Jan,11

61526   **Craniectomy, bone flap craniotomy, transtemporal (mastoid) for excision of cerebellopontine angle tumor;**
    🚑 97.9   ✂ 97.9   **FUD** 090   C ▣
    AMA: 2018,Mar,11; 2018,Jan,8; 2017,Jan,8; 2016,Jan,13; 2015,Jan,16; 2014,Jan,11

61530   **combined with middle/posterior fossa craniotomy/craniectomy**
    🚑 91.0   ✂ 91.0   **FUD** 090   C ▣
    AMA: 2014,Jan,11

61531-61545 Procedures for Seizures/Implanted Electrodes/Choroid Plexus/Craniopharyngioma

    EXCLUDES   *Craniotomy for:*
            Multiple subpial transections during procedure (61567)
            Selective amygdalohippocampectomy (61566)
        Injection for:
            Cerebral angiography (36100-36218)
            Pneumoencephalography (61055)
            Ventriculography (61026, 61120)

61531   **Subdural implantation of strip electrodes through 1 or more burr or trephine hole(s) for long-term seizure monitoring**
    EXCLUDES   *Continuous EEG observation ([95700, 95705, 95706, 95707, 95708, 95709, 95710, 95711, 95712, 95713, 95714, 95715, 95716, 95717, 95718, 95719, 95720, 95721, 95722, 95723, 95724, 95725, 95726])*
            Craniotomy for intracranial arteriovenous malformation removal (61680-61692)
            Stereotactic insertion of electrodes (61760)
    🚑 35.2   ✂ 35.2   **FUD** 090   C 80 ▣
    AMA: 2019,Jul,10; 2014,Jan,11

Nervous System

61533 — 61567

61533   **Craniotomy with elevation of bone flap; for subdural implantation of an electrode array, for long-term seizure monitoring**

> EXCLUDES   Continuous EEG monitoring ([95700, 95705, 95706, 95707, 95708, 95709, 95710, 95711, 95712, 95713, 95714, 95715, 95716, 95717, 95718, 95719, 95720, 95721, 95722, 95723, 95724, 95725, 95726])

44.4   44.4   **FUD** 090   C 80

AMA: 2014,Jan,11

61534   **for excision of epileptogenic focus without electrocorticography during surgery**

47.4   47.4   **FUD** 090   C 80

AMA: 2014,Jan,11

61535   **for removal of epidural or subdural electrode array, without excision of cerebral tissue (separate procedure)**

29.1   29.1   **FUD** 090   C 80

AMA: 2019,Jul,10; 2014,Jan,11

61536   **for excision of cerebral epileptogenic focus, with electrocorticography during surgery (includes removal of electrode array)**

76.1   76.1   **FUD** 090   C 80

AMA: 2014,Jan,11

61537   **for lobectomy, temporal lobe, without electrocorticography during surgery**

72.4   72.4   **FUD** 090   C 80

AMA: 2014,Jan,11

61538   **for lobectomy, temporal lobe, with electrocorticography during surgery**

78.2   78.2   **FUD** 090   C 80

AMA: 2019,Mar,6; 2014,Jan,11

61539   **for lobectomy, other than temporal lobe, partial or total, with electrocorticography during surgery**

69.6   69.6   **FUD** 090   C 80

AMA: 2019,Mar,6; 2014,Jan,11

61540   **for lobectomy, other than temporal lobe, partial or total, without electrocorticography during surgery**

64.2   64.2   **FUD** 090   C 80

AMA: 2014,Jan,11

61541   **for transection of corpus callosum**

63.3   63.3   **FUD** 090   C 80

AMA: 2014,Jan,11

61543   **for partial or subtotal (functional) hemispherectomy**

61.7   61.7   **FUD** 090   C 80

AMA: 2014,Jan,11

61544   **for excision or coagulation of choroid plexus**

56.0   56.0   **FUD** 090   C 80

AMA: 2014,Jan,11

61545   **for excision of craniopharyngioma**

93.0   93.0   **FUD** 090   C 80

AMA: 2014,Jan,11

61546-61548 Removal Pituitary Gland/Tumor

> EXCLUDES   Injection for:
> Cerebral angiography (36100-36218)
> Pneumoencephalography (61055)
> Ventriculography (61026, 61120)

61546   **Craniotomy for hypophysectomy or excision of pituitary tumor, intracranial approach**

68.0   68.0   **FUD** 090   C 80

AMA: 2014,Jan,11

61548   **Hypophysectomy or excision of pituitary tumor, transnasal or transseptal approach, nonstereotactic**

> INCLUDES   Operating microscope (69990)

45.8   45.8   **FUD** 090   C 80

AMA: 2016,Feb,12; 2014,Jan,11

61550-61559 Craniosynostosis Procedures

> EXCLUDES   Injection for:
> Cerebral angiography (36100-36218)
> Pneumoencephalography (61055)
> Ventriculography (61026, 61120)
> Orbital hypertelorism reconstruction (21260-21263)
> Reconstruction (21172-21180)

61550   **Craniectomy for craniosynostosis; single cranial suture**

32.1   32.1   **FUD** 090   C 80

AMA: 2018,Jan,8; 2017,Jan,8; 2016,Jan,13; 2015,Jan,16; 2014,Jan,11

61552   **multiple cranial sutures**

43.5   43.5   **FUD** 090   C 80

AMA: 2018,Jan,8; 2017,Jan,8; 2016,Jan,13; 2015,Jan,16; 2014,Jan,11

61556   **Craniotomy for craniosynostosis; frontal or parietal bone flap**

50.1   50.1   **FUD** 090   C 80

AMA: 2018,Jan,8; 2017,Jan,8; 2016,Jan,13; 2015,Jan,16; 2014,Jan,11

61557   **bifrontal bone flap**

49.4   49.4   **FUD** 090   C 80

AMA: 2018,Jan,8; 2017,Jan,8; 2016,Jan,13; 2015,Jan,16; 2014,Jan,11

61558   **Extensive craniectomy for multiple cranial suture craniosynostosis (eg, cloverleaf skull); not requiring bone grafts**

55.2   55.2   **FUD** 090   C 80

AMA: 2018,Jan,8; 2017,Jan,8; 2016,Jan,13; 2015,Jan,16; 2014,Jan,11

61559   **recontouring with multiple osteotomies and bone autografts (eg, barrel-stave procedure) (includes obtaining grafts)**

70.5   70.5   **FUD** 090   C 80

AMA: 2018,Jan,8; 2017,Jan,8; 2016,Jan,13; 2015,Jan,16; 2014,Jan,11

61563-61564 Removal Cranial Bone Tumor With/Without Optic Nerve Decompression

> EXCLUDES   Injection for:
> Cerebral angiography (36100-36218)
> Pneumoencephalography (61055)
> Ventriculography (61026, 61120)
> Reconstruction (21181-21183)

61563   **Excision, intra and extracranial, benign tumor of cranial bone (eg, fibrous dysplasia); without optic nerve decompression**

57.5   57.5   **FUD** 090   C 80

AMA: 2014,Jan,11

61564   **with optic nerve decompression**

70.9   70.9   **FUD** 090   C 80 50

AMA: 2014,Jan,11

61566-61567 Craniotomy for Seizures

> EXCLUDES   Injection for:
> Cerebral angiography (36100-36218)
> Pneumoencephalography (61055)
> Ventriculography (61026, 61120)

61566   **Craniotomy with elevation of bone flap; for selective amygdalohippocampectomy**

66.1   66.1   **FUD** 090   C 80

AMA: 2018,Nov,7; 2014,Jan,11

61567   **for multiple subpial transections, with electrocorticography during surgery**

75.5   75.5   **FUD** 090   C 80

AMA: 2014,Jan,11

26/TC PC/TC Only   A2-Z3 ASC Payment   50 Bilateral   ♂ Male Only   ♀ Female Only   Facility RVU   Non-Facility RVU   CCI   CLIA
FUD Follow-up Days   CMS: IOM   AMA: CPT Asst   A-Y OPPSI   80/80 Surg Assist Allowed / w/Doc   Lab Crosswalk   Radiology Crosswalk

284   CPT © 2019 American Medical Association. All Rights Reserved.   © 2019 Optum360, LLC

61570-61571 Removal of Foreign Body from Brain

EXCLUDES Injection for:
Cerebral angiography (36100-36218)
Pneumoencephalography (61055)
Ventriculography (61026, 61120)
Sequestrectomy for osteomyelitis (61501)

61570 **Craniectomy or craniotomy; with excision of foreign body from brain**

📷 54.5 ⚕ 54.5 **FUD** 090   C 80 ▢

AMA: 2014,Jan,11

61571 **with treatment of penetrating wound of brain**

📷 57.3 ⚕ 57.3 **FUD** 090   C 80 ▢

AMA: 2014,Jan,11

61575-61576 Transoral Approach Posterior Cranial Fossa/Upper Cervical Cord

EXCLUDES Arthrodesis (22548)
Injection for:
Cerebral angiography (36100-36218)
Pneumoencephalography (61055)
Ventriculography (61026, 61120)

61575 **Transoral approach to skull base, brain stem or upper spinal cord for biopsy, decompression or excision of lesion;**

📷 73.6 ⚕ 73.6 **FUD** 090   C 80 ▢

AMA: 2014,Jan,11

61576 **requiring splitting of tongue and/or mandible (including tracheostomy)**

📷 121. ⚕ 121. **FUD** 090   C 80 ▢

AMA: 2014,Jan,11

61580-61598 Surgical Approach: Cranial Fossae

EXCLUDES Definitive surgery (61600-61616)
Dural repair and/or reconstruction (61618-61619)
Injection for:
Cerebral angiography (36100-36218)
Pneumoencephalography (61055)
Ventriculography (61026, 61120)
Primary closure (15730, 15733, 15756-15758)

61580 **Craniofacial approach to anterior cranial fossa; extradural, including lateral rhinotomy, ethmoidectomy, sphenoidectomy, without maxillectomy or orbital exenteration**

📷 70.3 ⚕ 70.3 **FUD** 090   C 50 ▢

AMA: 2018,Jan,8; 2017,Jan,8; 2016,Jan,13; 2015,Jan,16; 2014,Jan,11

61581 **extradural, including lateral rhinotomy, orbital exenteration, ethmoidectomy, sphenoidectomy and/or maxillectomy**

📷 76.1 ⚕ 76.1 **FUD** 090   C 50 ▢

AMA: 2018,Jan,8; 2017,Jan,8; 2016,Jan,13; 2015,Jan,16; 2014,Jan,11

61582 **extradural, including unilateral or bifrontal craniotomy, elevation of frontal lobe(s), osteotomy of base of anterior cranial fossa**

📷 88.5 ⚕ 88.5 **FUD** 090   C 80 ▢

AMA: 2018,Jan,8; 2017,Jan,8; 2016,Jan,13; 2015,Jan,16; 2014,Jan,11

61583 **intradural, including unilateral or bifrontal craniotomy, elevation or resection of frontal lobe, osteotomy of base of anterior cranial fossa**

📷 84.2 ⚕ 84.2 **FUD** 090   C 80 ▢

AMA: 2018,Jan,8; 2017,Dec,13; 2017,Jan,8; 2016,Jan,13; 2015,Jan,16; 2014,Jan,11

61584 **Orbitocranial approach to anterior cranial fossa, extradural, including supraorbital ridge osteotomy and elevation of frontal and/or temporal lobe(s); without orbital exenteration**

📷 83.7 ⚕ 83.7 **FUD** 090   C 80 50 ▢

AMA: 2018,Jan,8; 2017,Jan,8; 2016,Jan,13; 2015,Jan,16; 2014,Jan,11

61585 **with orbital exenteration**

📷 95.1 ⚕ 95.1 **FUD** 090   C 80 50 ▢

AMA: 2018,Jan,8; 2017,Jan,8; 2016,Jan,13; 2015,Jan,16; 2014,Jan,11

61586 **Bicoronal, transzygomatic and/or LeFort I osteotomy approach to anterior cranial fossa with or without internal fixation, without bone graft**

📷 70.5 ⚕ 70.5 **FUD** 090   C 80 ▢

AMA: 2014,Jan,11

61590 **Infratemporal pre-auricular approach to middle cranial fossa (parapharyngeal space, infratemporal and midline skull base, nasopharynx), with or without disarticulation of the mandible, including parotidectomy, craniotomy, decompression and/or mobilization of the facial nerve and/or petrous carotid artery**

📷 88.1 ⚕ 88.1 **FUD** 090   C 80 50 ▢

AMA: 2018,Jan,8; 2017,Jan,8; 2016,Jan,13; 2015,Jan,16; 2014,Jan,11

61591 **Infratemporal post-auricular approach to middle cranial fossa (internal auditory meatus, petrous apex, tentorium, cavernous sinus, parasellar area, infratemporal fossa) including mastoidectomy, resection of sigmoid sinus, with or without decompression and/or mobilization of contents of auditory canal or petrous carotid artery**

📷 89.1 ⚕ 89.1 **FUD** 090   C 80 50 ▢

AMA: 2018,Jan,8; 2017,Jan,8; 2016,Jan,13; 2015,Jan,16; 2014,Jan,11

61592 **Orbitocranial zygomatic approach to middle cranial fossa (cavernous sinus and carotid artery, clivus, basilar artery or petrous apex) including osteotomy of zygoma, craniotomy, extra- or intradural elevation of temporal lobe**

📷 92.5 ⚕ 92.5 **FUD** 090   C 80 50 ▢

AMA: 2018,Jan,8; 2017,Jan,8; 2016,Jan,13; 2015,Jan,16; 2014,Jan,11

61595 **Transtemporal approach to posterior cranial fossa, jugular foramen or midline skull base, including mastoidectomy, decompression of sigmoid sinus and/or facial nerve, with or without mobilization**

📷 68.1 ⚕ 68.1 **FUD** 090   C 50 ▢

AMA: 2018,Mar,11; 2018,Jan,8; 2017,Jan,8; 2016,Jan,13; 2015,Jan,16; 2014,Jan,11

61596 **Transcochlear approach to posterior cranial fossa, jugular foramen or midline skull base, including labyrinthectomy, decompression, with or without mobilization of facial nerve and/or petrous carotid artery**

📷 70.1 ⚕ 70.1 **FUD** 090   C 80 50 ▢

AMA: 2018,Jan,8; 2017,Jan,8; 2016,Jan,13; 2015,Jan,16; 2014,Jan,11

61597 **Transcondylar (far lateral) approach to posterior cranial fossa, jugular foramen or midline skull base, including occipital condylectomy, mastoidectomy, resection of C1-C3 vertebral body(s), decompression of vertebral artery, with or without mobilization**

📷 85.5 ⚕ 85.5 **FUD** 090   C 80 50 ▢

AMA: 2018,Jan,8; 2017,Jan,8; 2016,Jan,13; 2015,Jan,16; 2014,Jan,11

61598 **Transpetrosal approach to posterior cranial fossa, clivus or foramen magnum, including ligation of superior petrosal sinus and/or sigmoid sinus**

📷 82.9 ⚕ 82.9 **FUD** 090   C 80 ▢

AMA: 2018,Jan,8; 2017,Jan,8; 2016,Jan,13; 2015,Jan,16; 2014,Jan,11

61600-61616 Definitive Procedures: Cranial Fossae

EXCLUDES   Dural repair and/or reconstruction (61618-61619)
            Injection for:
               Cerebral angiography (36100-36218)
               Pneumoencephalography (61055)
               Ventriculography (61026, 61120)
            Primary closure (15730, 15733, 15756-15758)
            Surgical approach (61580-61598)

61600   Resection or excision of neoplastic, vascular or infectious lesion of base of anterior cranial fossa; extradural
            🔧 61.5   ⚕ 61.5   **FUD** 090   C 80 ▭
            AMA: 2018,Jan,8; 2017,Jan,8; 2016,Jan,13; 2015,Jan,16; 2014,Jan,11

61601   intradural, including dural repair, with or without graft
            🔧 70.1   ⚕ 70.1   **FUD** 090   C 80 ▭
            AMA: 2018,Jan,8; 2017,Jan,8; 2016,Jan,13; 2015,Jan,16; 2014,Jan,11

61605   Resection or excision of neoplastic, vascular or infectious lesion of infratemporal fossa, parapharyngeal space, petrous apex; extradural
            🔧 62.1   ⚕ 62.1   **FUD** 090   C 80 ▭
            AMA: 2018,Jan,8; 2017,Jan,8; 2016,Jan,13; 2015,Jan,16; 2014,Jan,11

61606   intradural, including dural repair, with or without graft
            🔧 85.7   ⚕ 85.7   **FUD** 090   C 80 ▭
            AMA: 2018,Jan,8; 2017,Jan,8; 2016,Jan,13; 2015,Jan,16; 2014,Jan,11

61607   Resection or excision of neoplastic, vascular or infectious lesion of parasellar area, cavernous sinus, clivus or midline skull base; extradural
            🔧 77.8   ⚕ 77.8   **FUD** 090   C 80 ▭
            AMA: 2018,Jan,8; 2017,Jan,8; 2016,Jan,13; 2015,Jan,16; 2014,Jan,11

61608   intradural, including dural repair, with or without graft
            🔧 95.7   ⚕ 95.7   **FUD** 090   C 80 ▭
            AMA: 2018,Jan,8; 2017,Jan,8; 2016,Jan,13; 2015,Jan,16; 2014,Jan,11

+ **61611** Transection or ligation, carotid artery in petrous canal; without repair (List separately in addition to code for primary procedure)
            Code first (61605-61608)
            🔧 13.8   ⚕ 13.8   **FUD** ZZZ   C 80 ▭
            AMA: 2018,Jan,8; 2017,Jan,8; 2016,Jan,13; 2015,Jan,16; 2014,Jan,11

61613   Obliteration of carotid aneurysm, arteriovenous malformation, or carotid-cavernous fistula by dissection within cavernous sinus
            🔧 96.9   ⚕ 96.9   **FUD** 090   C 80 50 ▭
            AMA: 2018,Jan,8; 2017,Jan,8; 2016,Jan,13; 2015,Jan,16; 2014,Jan,11

61615   Resection or excision of neoplastic, vascular or infectious lesion of base of posterior cranial fossa, jugular foramen, foramen magnum, or C1-C3 vertebral bodies; extradural
            🔧 81.9   ⚕ 81.9   **FUD** 090   C 80 ▭
            AMA: 2018,Jan,8; 2017,Jan,8; 2016,Jan,13; 2015,Jan,16; 2014,Jan,11

61616   intradural, including dural repair, with or without graft
            🔧 97.3   ⚕ 97.3   **FUD** 090   C 80 ▭
            AMA: 2018,Mar,11; 2018,Jan,8; 2017,Jan,8; 2016,Jan,13; 2015,Jan,16; 2014,Jan,11

61618-61619 Reconstruction Post-Surgical Cranial Fossae Defects

EXCLUDES   Definitive surgery (61600-61616)
            Injection for:
               Cerebral angiography (36100-36218)
               Pneumoencephalography (61055)
               Ventriculography (61026, 61120)
            Primary closure (15730, 15733, 15756-15758)
            Surgical approach (61580-61598)

61618   Secondary repair of dura for cerebrospinal fluid leak, anterior, middle or posterior cranial fossa following surgery of the skull base; by free tissue graft (eg, pericranium, fascia, tensor fascia lata, adipose tissue, homologous or synthetic grafts)
            🔧 37.5   ⚕ 37.5   **FUD** 090   C 80 ▭
            AMA: 2018,Jan,8; 2017,Jan,8; 2016,Jan,13; 2015,Jan,16; 2014,Jan,11

61619   by local or regionalized vascularized pedicle flap or myocutaneous flap (including galea, temporalis, frontalis or occipitalis muscle)
            🔧 41.3   ⚕ 41.3   **FUD** 090   C 80 ▭
            AMA: 2018,Jan,8; 2017,Jan,8; 2016,Jan,13; 2015,Jan,16; 2014,Jan,11

61623-61651 Neurovascular Interventional Procedures

61623   Endovascular temporary balloon arterial occlusion, head or neck (extracranial/intracranial) including selective catheterization of vessel to be occluded, positioning and inflation of occlusion balloon, concomitant neurological monitoring, and radiologic supervision and interpretation of all angiography required for balloon occlusion and to exclude vascular injury post occlusion

            EXCLUDES   Diagnostic angiography of target artery just before temporary occlusion; report only radiological supervision and interpretation
                        Selective catheterization and angiography of artery besides the target artery; report catheterization and radiological supervision and interpretation codes as appropriate
            🔧 16.6   ⚕ 16.6   **FUD** 000   J ▭
            AMA: 2018,Jan,8; 2017,Jan,8; 2016,Jan,13; 2015,Jan,16; 2014,Jan,11

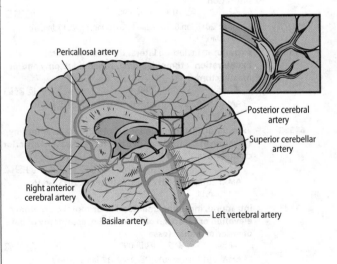

Pericallosal artery
Posterior cerebral artery
Superior cerebellar artery
Right anterior cerebral artery
Basilar artery
Left vertebral artery

61600 — 61623

61624 Transcatheter permanent occlusion or embolization (eg, for tumor destruction, to achieve hemostasis, to occlude a vascular malformation), percutaneous, any method; central nervous system (intracranial, spinal cord)

> EXCLUDES Non-central nervous system transcatheter occlusion or embolization other than head or neck (37241-37244)

> (75894)

> 33.7 33.7 **FUD** 000 C ▢

> AMA: 2019,Sep,6; 2018,Jan,8; 2017,Jan,8; 2016,Jan,13; 2015,Jan,16; 2014,Jan,11

61626 non-central nervous system, head or neck (extracranial, brachiocephalic branch)

> EXCLUDES Non-central nervous system transcatheter occlusion or embolization other than head or neck (37241-37244)

> (75894)

> 25.5 25.5 **FUD** 000 J ▢

> AMA: 2019,Sep,6; 2018,Jan,8; 2017,Jan,8; 2016,Jan,13; 2015,Jan,16; 2014,Jan,11

61630 Balloon angioplasty, intracranial (eg, atherosclerotic stenosis), percutaneous

> INCLUDES Diagnostic arteriogram if stent or angioplasty is necessary
> Radiology services for arteriography of target vascular territory
> Selective catheterization of the target vascular territory

> EXCLUDES Diagnostic arteriogram if stent or angioplasty is not necessary (use applicable code for selective catheterization and radiology services)
> Percutaneous arterial transluminal mechanical thrombectomy and/or infusion for thrombolysis performed in the same vascular territory (61645)

> 40.6 40.6 **FUD** XXX C 80 ▢

> AMA: 2018,Jan,8; 2017,Jul,3; 2017,Apr,9; 2017,Jan,8; 2016,Mar,3; 2016,Jan,13; 2015,Nov,3; 2015,Jan,16; 2014,Jan,11

61635 Transcatheter placement of intravascular stent(s), intracranial (eg, atherosclerotic stenosis), including balloon angioplasty, if performed

> INCLUDES Diagnostic arteriogram if stent or angioplasty is necessary
> Radiology services for arteriography of target vascular territory
> Selective catheterization of the target vascular territory

> EXCLUDES Diagnostic arteriogram if stent or angioplasty is not necessary (use applicable code for selective catheterization and radiology services)
> Percutaneous arterial transluminal thrombectomy in same vascular territory (61645)

> 42.6 42.6 **FUD** XXX C 80 ▢

> AMA: 2018,Jan,8; 2017,Jul,3; 2017,Jan,8; 2016,Mar,3; 2016,Jan,13; 2015,Nov,3; 2015,Jan,16; 2014,Mar,8; 2014,Jan,11

61640 Balloon dilatation of intracranial vasospasm, percutaneous; initial vessel

> INCLUDES Angiography after dilation of vessel
> Fluoroscopic guidance
> Injection of contrast material
> Roadmapping
> Selective catheterization of target vessel
> Vessel analysis

> EXCLUDES Endovascular intracranial prolonged administration of pharmacologic agent performed in the same vascular territory (61650-61651)

> 14.0 14.0 **FUD** 000 E ▢

> AMA: 2018,Jan,8; 2017,Jan,8; 2016,Mar,3; 2016,Jan,13; 2015,Nov,3; 2015,Jan,16; 2014,May,10; 2014,Jan,11

+ 61641 each additional vessel in same vascular territory (List separately in addition to code for primary procedure)

> INCLUDES Angiography after dilation of vessel
> Fluoroscopic guidance
> Injection of contrast material
> Roadmapping
> Selective catheterization of target vessel
> Vessel analysis
> Code first (61640)

> 4.92 4.92 **FUD** ZZZ E ▢

> AMA: 2018,Jan,8; 2017,Jan,8; 2016,Mar,3; 2016,Jan,13; 2015,Nov,3; 2015,Jan,16; 2014,May,10; 2014,Jan,11

+ 61642 each additional vessel in different vascular territory (List separately in addition to code for primary procedure))

> INCLUDES Angiography after dilation of vessel
> Fluoroscopic guidance
> Injection of contrast material
> Roadmapping
> Selective catheterization of target vessel
> Vessel analysis

> EXCLUDES Endovascular intracranial prolonged administration of pharmacologic agent performed in the same vascular territory (61650-61651)
> Code first (61640)

> 9.84 9.84 **FUD** ZZZ E ▢

> AMA: 2018,Jan,8; 2017,Jan,8; 2016,Mar,3; 2016,Jan,13; 2015,Nov,3; 2015,Jan,16; 2014,May,10; 2014,Jan,11

61645 Percutaneous arterial transluminal mechanical thrombectomy and/or infusion for thrombolysis, intracranial, any method, including diagnostic angiography, fluoroscopic guidance, catheter placement, and intraprocedural pharmacological thrombolytic injection(s)

> INCLUDES Interventions performed in an intracranial artery including:
> Angiography with radiologic supervision and interpretation (diagnostic and subsequent)
> Closure of arteriotomy by any method
> Fluoroscopy
> Patient monitoring
> Procedures performed in vascular territories:
> Left carotid
> Right carotid
> Vertebro-basilar

> EXCLUDES Procedure performed in the same vascular target area:
> Balloon angioplasty, intracranial (61630)
> Diagnostic studies: aortic arch, carotid, and vertebral arteries (36221-36228)
> Endovascular intracranial prolonged administration of pharmacologic agent (61650-61651)
> Transcatheter placement of intravascular stent (61635)
> Transluminal thrombectomy (37184, 37186)
> Use of code more than one time for treatment of each intracranial vascular territory
> Venous thrombectomy or thrombolysis (37187-37188, 37212, 37214)

> 24.3 24.3 **FUD** 000 C 80 50 ▢

> AMA: 2019,Sep,6; 2019,Sep,5; 2018,Jan,8; 2017,Jan,8; 2016,Mar,3; 2016,Jan,13; 2015,Dec,18; 2015,Nov,3

61650 Endovascular intracranial prolonged administration of pharmacologic agent(s) other than for thrombolysis, arterial, including catheter placement, diagnostic angiography, and imaging guidance; initial vascular territory

INCLUDES Interventions performed in an intracranial artery, including:
Angiography with radiologic supervision and interpretation (diagnostic and subsequent)
Closure of arteriotomy by any method
Fluoroscopy
Patient monitoring
Procedures performed in vascular territories:
Left carotid
Right carotid
Vertebro-basilar
Prolonged (at least 10 minutes) arterial administration of non-thrombolytic agents

EXCLUDES *Procedure performed in the same vascular target area:*
Balloon dilatation of intracranial vasospasm (61640-61642)
Chemotherapy administration (96420-96425)
Diagnostic studies: aortic arch, carotid, and vertebral arteries (36221-36228)
Transluminal thrombectomy (37184, 37186, 61645)
Treatment of an iatrogenic condition
Use of code more than one time for treatment of each intracranial vascular territory
Venous thrombectomy or thrombolysis

🚑 16.1 ⚖ 16.1 **FUD** 000 C 🖿

AMA: 2019,Sep,6; 2018,Jan,8; 2017,Jan,8; 2016,Mar,3; 2016,Jan,13; 2015,Nov,3

+ 61651 each additional vascular territory (List separately in addition to code for primary procedure)

INCLUDES Interventions performed in an intracranial artery including:
Angiography with radiologic supervision and interpretation (diagnostic and subsequent)
Closure of arteriotomy by any method
Fluoroscopy
Patient monitoring
Procedures performed in vascular territories:
Left carotid
Right carotid
Vertebro-basilar
Prolonged (at least 10 minutes) arterial administration of non-thrombolytic agents

EXCLUDES *Procedure performed in the same vascular target area:*
Balloon dilatation of intracranial vasospasm . (61640-61642)
Chemotherapy administration (96420-96425)
Diagnostic studies: aortic arch, carotid, and vertebral arteries (36221-36228)
Transluminal thrombectomy (37184, 37186, 61645)
Treatment of an iatrogenic condition
Use of code more than two times for treatment of the two remaining intracranial vascular territory(ies)
Venous thrombectomy or thrombolysis
Code first (61650)

🚑 7.01 ⚖ 7.01 **FUD** ZZZ C 🖿

AMA: 2019,Sep,6; 2018,Jan,8; 2017,Jan,8; 2016,Mar,3; 2016,Jan,13; 2015,Nov,3

61680-61692 Surgical Treatment of Arteriovenous Malformation of the Brain

INCLUDES Craniotomy

61680 Surgery of intracranial arteriovenous malformation; supratentorial, simple

🚑 66.1 ⚖ 66.1 **FUD** 090 C 80 🖿

AMA: 2014,Jan,11

61682 supratentorial, complex

🚑 123. ⚖ 123. **FUD** 090 C 80 🖿

AMA: 2018,Jan,8; 2017,Jan,8; 2016,Jan,13; 2015,Jan,16; 2014,Jan,11

61684 infratentorial, simple

🚑 84.0 ⚖ 84.0 **FUD** 090 C 80 🖿

AMA: 2014,Jan,11

61686 infratentorial, complex

🚑 136. ⚖ 136. **FUD** 090 C 80 🖿

AMA: 2018,Jan,8; 2017,Jan,8; 2016,Jan,13; 2015,Jan,16; 2014,Jan,11

61690 dural, simple

🚑 63.6 ⚖ 63.6 **FUD** 090 C 80 🖿

AMA: 2014,Jan,11

61692 dural, complex

🚑 108. ⚖ 108. **FUD** 090 C 80 🖿

AMA: 2018,Jan,8; 2017,Jan,8; 2016,Jan,13; 2015,Jan,16; 2014,Jan,11

61697-61703 Surgical Treatment Brain Aneurysm

INCLUDES Craniotomy

61697 Surgery of complex intracranial aneurysm, intracranial approach; carotid circulation

INCLUDES Aneurysms bigger than 15 mm
Calcification of the aneurysm neck
Inclusion of normal vessels in aneurysm neck
Surgery needing temporary vessel occlusion, trapping, or cardiopulmonary bypass to treat aneurysm

🚑 125. ⚖ 125. **FUD** 090 C 80 🖿

AMA: 2018,Jan,8; 2017,Dec,13; 2014,Jan,11

61698 vertebrobasilar circulation

INCLUDES Aneurysm bigger than 15 mm
Calcification of aneurysm neck
Inclusion of normal vessels into aneurysm neck
Surgery needing temporary vessel occlusion, trapping, or cardiopulmonary bypass to treat aneurysm

🚑 140. ⚖ 140. **FUD** 090 C 80 🖿

AMA: 2014,Jan,11

61700 Surgery of simple intracranial aneurysm, intracranial approach; carotid circulation

🚑 100. ⚖ 100. **FUD** 090 C 80 🖿

AMA: 2018,Jan,8; 2017,Dec,13; 2017,Jan,8; 2016,Jan,13; 2015,Jan,16; 2014,Jan,11

61702 vertebrobasilar circulation

🚑 118. ⚖ 118. **FUD** 090 C 80 🖿

AMA: 2014,Jan,11

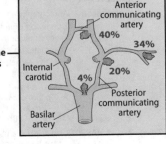

Berry aneurysm

Berry aneurysms form at the site of a weakness in an arterial wall, often at a junction

Common sites of berry aneurysms in the circle of Willis arteries

Anterior communicating artery 40%
34%
Internal carotid
20%
4%
Posterior communicating artery
Basilar artery

26/TC PC/TC Only A2-Z3 ASC Payment 50 Bilateral ♂ Male Only ♀ Female Only 🚑 Facility RVU ⚖ Non-Facility RVU CCI CLIA
FUD Follow-up Days CMS: IOM AMA: CPT Asst A-Y OPPSI 80/80 Surg Assist Allowed / w/Doc Lab Crosswalk Radiology Crosswalk

288 CPT © 2019 American Medical Association. All Rights Reserved. © 2019 Optum360, LLC

61703 Surgery of intracranial aneurysm, cervical approach by application of occluding clamp to cervical carotid artery (Selverstone-Crutchfield type)

EXCLUDES Cervical approach for direct ligation of carotid artery (37600-37606)

39.9   39.9   **FUD** 090   C 80

AMA: 2014,Jan,11

61705-61710 Other Procedures for Aneurysm, Arteriovenous Malformation, and Carotid-Cavernous Fistula

INCLUDES Craniotomy

61705 Surgery of aneurysm, vascular malformation or carotid-cavernous fistula; by intracranial and cervical occlusion of carotid artery

73.6   73.6   **FUD** 090   C 80

AMA: 2014,Jan,11

61708 by intracranial electrothrombosis

EXCLUDES Ligation or gradual occlusion of internal or common carotid artery (37605-37606)

75.1   75.1   **FUD** 090   C 80

AMA: 2014,Jan,11

61710 by intra-arterial embolization, injection procedure, or balloon catheter

63.3   63.3   **FUD** 090   C 80

AMA: 2018,Jan,8; 2017,Jan,8; 2016,Jan,13; 2015,Jan,16; 2014,Jan,11

61711 Extracranial-Intracranial Bypass

CMS: 100-02,16,10 Exclusions from Coverage; 100-03,20.2 Extracranial-intracranial (EC-IC) Arterial Bypass Surgery

INCLUDES Craniotomy

EXCLUDES Carotid or vertebral thromboendarterectomy (35301)

Code also operating microscope when appropriate (69990)

61711 Anastomosis, arterial, extracranial-intracranial (eg, middle cerebral/cortical) arteries

75.8   75.8   **FUD** 090   C 80

AMA: 2014,Jan,11

61720-61791 Stereotactic Procedures of the Brain

61720 Creation of lesion by stereotactic method, including burr hole(s) and localizing and recording techniques, single or multiple stages; globus pallidus or thalamus

37.3   37.3   **FUD** 090   J

AMA: 2018,Jan,8; 2017,Jan,8; 2016,Jan,13; 2015,Jan,16; 2014,Jul,8; 2014,Jan,11

61735 subcortical structure(s) other than globus pallidus or thalamus

46.8   46.8   **FUD** 090   C

AMA: 2014,Jul,8; 2014,Jan,11

61750 Stereotactic biopsy, aspiration, or excision, including burr hole(s), for intracranial lesion;

41.4   41.4   **FUD** 090   C

AMA: 2018,Jan,8; 2017,Jan,8; 2016,Jan,13; 2015,Jan,16; 2014,Jul,8; 2014,Jan,11

61751 with computed tomography and/or magnetic resonance guidance

(70450, 70460, 70470, 70551-70553)

40.4   40.4   **FUD** 090   C

AMA: 2018,Jan,8; 2017,Jan,8; 2016,Jan,13; 2015,Jan,16; 2014,Jul,8; 2014,Jan,11

61760 Stereotactic implantation of depth electrodes into the cerebrum for long-term seizure monitoring

46.0   46.0   **FUD** 090   C

AMA: 2014,Jul,8; 2014,Jan,11

61770 Stereotactic localization, including burr hole(s), with insertion of catheter(s) or probe(s) for placement of radiation source

47.7   47.7   **FUD** 090   J 02

AMA: 2018,Jan,8; 2017,Jan,8; 2016,Jan,13; 2015,Jan,16; 2014,Jul,8; 2014,Jan,11

+ **61781** Stereotactic computer-assisted (navigational) procedure; cranial, intradural (List separately in addition to code for primary procedure)

EXCLUDES Creation of lesion by stereotactic method (61720-61791)

Extradural stereotactic computer-assisted procedure for same surgical session by same individual (61782)

Radiation treatment delivery, stereotactic radiosurgery (SRS) (77371-77373)

Stereotactic implantation of neurostimulator electrode array (61863-61868)

Stereotactic radiation treatment management (77432)

Stereotactic radiosurgery (61796-61799)

Ventriculocisternostomy (62201)

Code first primary procedure

6.94   6.94   **FUD** ZZZ   N N1 80

AMA: 2018,Jan,8; 2017,Jan,8; 2016,Jan,13; 2015,Jan,16; 2014,Sep,13; 2014,Jul,8; 2014,Jan,11

Stereotactic guide in place

Computer assistance determines precise coordinates for a stereotactic intracranial procedure

CT or MRI scan

+ **61782** cranial, extradural (List separately in addition to code for primary procedure)

EXCLUDES Intradural stereotactic computer-assisted procedure for same surgical session by same individual (61781)

Stereotactic radiosurgery (61796-61799)

Code first primary procedure

5.02   5.02   **FUD** ZZZ   N N1 80

AMA: 2018,Apr,3; 2018,Jan,8; 2017,Jan,8; 2016,Jan,13; 2015,Jan,16; 2014,Jul,8; 2014,Jan,11

+ **61783** spinal (List separately in addition to code for primary procedure)

EXCLUDES Stereotactic radiosurgery (61796-61799, 63620-63621)

Code first primary procedure

6.80   6.80   **FUD** ZZZ   N N1 80

AMA: 2018,Jan,8; 2017,Jan,8; 2016,Jan,13; 2015,Jan,16; 2014,Jul,8; 2014,Jan,11

61790 Creation of lesion by stereotactic method, percutaneous, by neurolytic agent (eg, alcohol, thermal, electrical, radiofrequency); gasserian ganglion

25.7   25.7   **FUD** 090   J A2 50

AMA: 2014,Jul,8; 2014,Jan,11

61791 trigeminal medullary tract

33.0   33.0   **FUD** 090   J A2 80 50

AMA: 2018,Jan,8; 2017,Jan,8; 2016,Jan,13; 2015,Jan,16; 2014,Jul,8; 2014,Jan,11

● New Code   ▲ Revised Code   ○ Reinstated   ● New Web Release   ▲ Revised Web Release   + Add-on   Unlisted   Not Covered   # Resequenced

50 Optum Mod 50 Exempt   51 AMA Mod 51 Exempt   51 Optum Mod 51 Exempt   63 Mod 63 Exempt   Non-FDA Drug   ★ Telemedicine   M Maternity   A Age Edit

© 2019 Optum360, LLC   CPT © 2019 American Medical Association. All Rights Reserved.   289

61796-61800 Stereotactic Radiosurgery (SRS): Brain

INCLUDES Planning, dosimetry, targeting, positioning or blocking performed by the neurosurgeon

EXCLUDES *Application of cranial tongs, caliper, or stereotactic frame (20660)*
Intensity modulated beam delivery plan and treatment (77301, 77385-77386)
Radiation treatment management and radiosurgery by the same provider (77427-77435)
Stereotactic body radiation therapy (77373, 77435)
Stereotactic radiosurgery more than once per lesion per treatment course
Treatment planning, physics and dosimetry, and treatment delivery performed by the radiation oncologist

61796 **Stereotactic radiosurgery (particle beam, gamma ray, or linear accelerator); 1 simple cranial lesion**

INCLUDES Lesions < 3.5 cm

EXCLUDES *Stereotactic computer-assisted procedures (61781-61783)*
Stereotactic radiosurgery (61798)
Treatment of complex lesions: (61798-61799)
Arteriovenous malformations (AVM)
Brainstem lesions
Cavernous sinus/parasellar/petroclival tumors, glomus tumors, pituitary tumors, and tumors of pineal region
Lesions located <= 5 mm from the optic nerve, chasm, or tract
Schwannomas
Use of code more than one time per treatment course
Code also stereotactic headframe application, when performed (61800)

🖥 29.7   ⚕ 29.7   **FUD** 090   Ⓑ 80 ▣

AMA: 2018,Jan,8; 2017,Jan,8; 2016,Jan,13; 2015,Jun,6; 2015,Jan,16; 2014,Jul,8; 2014,Jan,11

+ 61797 **each additional cranial lesion, simple (List separately in addition to code for primary procedure)**

INCLUDES Lesions < 3.5 cm

EXCLUDES *Stereotactic computer-assisted procedures (61781-61783)*
Treatment of complex lesions: (61798-61799)
Arteriovenous malformations (AVM)
Brainstem lesion
Cavernous sinus/parasellar/petroclival tumors, glomus tumors, pituitary tumor, tumors of pineal region
Lesions located <= 5 mm from the optic nerve, chasm, or tract
Schwannomas
Use of code for additional stereotactic radiosurgery more than four times in total per treatment course when used alone or in combination with (61799)
Code first (61796, 61798)

🖥 6.48   ⚕ 6.48   **FUD** ZZZ   Ⓑ 80 ▣

AMA: 2018,Jan,8; 2017,Jan,8; 2016,Jan,13; 2015,Jun,6; 2015,Jan,16; 2014,Jul,8; 2014,Jan,11

61798 **1 complex cranial lesion**

INCLUDES All therapeutic lesion creation procedures
Treatment of complex lesions:
Arteriovenous malformations (AVM)
Brainstem lesions
Cavernous sinus, parasellar, petroclival, glomus, pineal region, and pituitary tumors
Lesions located <= 5 mm from the optic nerve, chasm, or tract
Lesions >= 3.5 cm
Schwannomas
Treatment of multiple lesions as long as one is complex

EXCLUDES *Stereotactic computer-assisted procedures (61781-61783)*
Stereotactic radiosurgery (61796)
Use of code more than one time per treatment course
Code also stereotactic headframe application, when performed (61800)

🖥 40.5   ⚕ 40.5   **FUD** 090   Ⓑ 80 ▣

AMA: 2018,Jan,8; 2017,Jan,8; 2016,Jan,13; 2015,Jun,6; 2015,Jan,16; 2014,Jul,8; 2014,Jan,11

+ 61799 **each additional cranial lesion, complex (List separately in addition to code for primary procedure)**

INCLUDES All therapeutic lesion creation procedures
Treatment of complex lesions:
Arteriovenous malformations (AVM)
Brainstem lesions
Cavernous sinus, parasellar, petroclival, glomus, pineal region, and pituitary tumors
Lesions located <= 5 mm from the optic nerve, chasm, or tract
Lesions >= 3.5 cm
Schwannomas

EXCLUDES *Stereotactic computer-assisted procedures (61781-61783)*
Use of code for additional stereotactic radiosurgery more than four times in total per treatment course when used alone or in combination with (61797)
Code first (61798)

🖥 8.98   ⚕ 8.98   **FUD** ZZZ   Ⓑ 80 ▣

AMA: 2018,Jan,8; 2017,Jan,8; 2016,Jan,13; 2015,Jun,6; 2015,Jan,16; 2014,Jul,8; 2014,Jan,11

+ 61800 **Application of stereotactic headframe for stereotactic radiosurgery (List separately in addition to code for primary procedure)**
Code first (61796, 61798)

🖥 4.52   ⚕ 4.52   **FUD** ZZZ   Ⓑ 80 ▣

AMA: 2018,Jan,8; 2017,Jan,8; 2016,Jan,13; 2015,Jun,6; 2015,Jan,16; 2014,Jan,11

61850-61888 Intracranial Neurostimulation

INCLUDES Analysis of system at time of implantation (95970)
Microelectrode recording by operating surgeon

EXCLUDES *Electronic analysis and reprogramming of neurostimulator pulse generator (95970, 95976-95977, [95983, 95984])*
Neurophysiological mapping by another physician/qualified health care professional (95961-95962)

61850 **Twist drill or burr hole(s) for implantation of neurostimulator electrodes, cortical**

🖥 28.1   ⚕ 28.1   **FUD** 090   Ⓒ 80 ▣

AMA: 2019,Feb,6; 2018,Jan,8; 2017,Jan,8; 2016,Jan,13; 2015,Jan,16; 2014,Jan,11

61860 **Craniectomy or craniotomy for implantation of neurostimulator electrodes, cerebral, cortical**

🖥 46.0   ⚕ 46.0   **FUD** 090   Ⓒ 80 ▣

AMA: 2019,Feb,6; 2018,Jan,8; 2017,Jan,8; 2016,Jan,13; 2015,Jan,16; 2014,Jan,11

61863 **Twist drill, burr hole, craniotomy, or craniectomy with stereotactic implantation of neurostimulator electrode array in subcortical site (eg, thalamus, globus pallidus, subthalamic nucleus, periventricular, periaqueductal gray), without use of intraoperative microelectrode recording; first array**

🖥 43.9   ⚕ 43.9   **FUD** 090   Ⓒ 80 50 ▣

AMA: 2019,Feb,6; 2018,Jan,8; 2017,Jan,8; 2016,Jan,13; 2015,Jan,16; 2014,Jul,8; 2014,Jan,11

+ 61864 **each additional array (List separately in addition to primary procedure)**
Code first (61863)

🖥 8.36   ⚕ 8.36   **FUD** ZZZ   Ⓒ 80 ▣

AMA: 2019,Feb,6; 2014,Jul,8; 2014,Jan,11

61867 **Twist drill, burr hole, craniotomy, or craniectomy with stereotactic implantation of neurostimulator electrode array in subcortical site (eg, thalamus, globus pallidus, subthalamic nucleus, periventricular, periaqueductal gray), with use of intraoperative microelectrode recording; first array**

🖥 66.8   ⚕ 66.8   **FUD** 090   Ⓒ 80 50 ▣

AMA: 2019,Feb,6; 2014,Jul,8; 2014,Jan,11

+ 61868 **each additional array (List separately in addition to primary procedure)**
Code first (61867)

🖥 14.7   ⚕ 14.7   **FUD** ZZZ   Ⓒ 80 ▣

AMA: 2019,Feb,6; 2018,Jan,8; 2017,Jan,8; 2016,Jan,13; 2015,Jan,16; 2014,Jul,8; 2014,Jan,11

26/TC PC/TC Only   A2-Z3 ASC Payment   50 Bilateral   ♂ Male Only   ♀ Female Only   🖥 Facility RVU   ⚕ Non-Facility RVU   ▣ CCI   ✖ CLIA
FUD Follow-up Days   CMS: IOM   AMA: CPT Asst   A-Y OPPSI   80/80 Surg Assist Allowed / w/Doc   ▣ Lab Crosswalk   ▣ Radiology Crosswalk

61870 Craniectomy for implantation of neurostimulator electrodes, cerebellar, cortical
🚑 34.7 ✂ 34.7 **FUD** 090 [C] [80] [▭]
AMA: 2019,Feb,6; 2014,Jan,11

61880 Revision or removal of intracranial neurostimulator electrodes
🚑 16.6 ✂ 16.6 **FUD** 090 [02] [62] [80] [50] [▭]
AMA: 2019,Feb,6; 2014,Jan,11

61885 Insertion or replacement of cranial neurostimulator pulse generator or receiver, direct or inductive coupling; with connection to a single electrode array
EXCLUDES *Percutaneous procedure to place cranial nerve neurostimulator electrode(s) (64553)*
Revision or replacement cranial nerve neurostimulator electrode array (64569)
🚑 14.9 ✂ 14.9 **FUD** 090 [J] [J8] [80] [50] [▭]
AMA: 2019,Feb,6; 2018,Jan,8; 2017,Jan,8; 2016,Jan,13; 2015,Jan,16; 2014,Jan,11

61886 with connection to 2 or more electrode arrays
EXCLUDES *Percutaneous procedure to place cranial nerve neurostimulator electrode(s) (64553)*
Revision or replacement cranial nerve neurostimulator electrode array (64569)
🚑 24.7 ✂ 24.7 **FUD** 090 [J] [J8] [80] [▭]
AMA: 2019,Feb,6; 2018,Jan,8; 2017,Jan,8; 2016,Jan,13; 2015,Jan,16; 2014,Jan,11

61888 Revision or removal of cranial neurostimulator pulse generator or receiver
EXCLUDES *Insertion or replacement of cranial neurostimulator pulse generator or receiver (61885-61886)*
🚑 11.5 ✂ 11.5 **FUD** 010 [J] [J8] [50] [▭]
AMA: 2019,Feb,6; 2018,Jan,8; 2017,Jan,8; 2016,Jan,13; 2015,Jan,16; 2014,Jan,11

62000-62148 Repair of Skull and/or Cerebrospinal Fluid Leaks

62000 Elevation of depressed skull fracture; simple, extradural
🚑 30.2 ✂ 30.2 **FUD** 090 [J] [▭]
AMA: 2014,Jan,11

62005 compound or comminuted, extradural
🚑 36.6 ✂ 36.6 **FUD** 090 [C] [80] [▭]
AMA: 2014,Jan,11

62010 with repair of dura and/or debridement of brain
🚑 45.0 ✂ 45.0 **FUD** 090 [C] [80] [▭]
AMA: 2014,Jan,11

62100 Craniotomy for repair of dural/cerebrospinal fluid leak, including surgery for rhinorrhea/otorrhea
EXCLUDES *Repair of spinal fluid leak (63707, 63709)*
🚑 46.4 ✂ 46.4 **FUD** 090 [C] [80] [▭]
AMA: 2014,Jan,11

62115 Reduction of craniomegalic skull (eg, treated hydrocephalus); not requiring bone grafts or cranioplasty
🚑 49.2 ✂ 49.2 **FUD** 090 [C] [80] [▭]
AMA: 2014,Jan,11

62117 requiring craniotomy and reconstruction with or without bone graft (includes obtaining grafts)
🚑 57.8 ✂ 57.8 **FUD** 090 [C] [80] [▭]
AMA: 2014,Jan,11

62120 Repair of encephalocele, skull vault, including cranioplasty
🚑 61.9 ✂ 61.9 **FUD** 090 [C] [80] [▭]
AMA: 2014,Jan,11

62121 Craniotomy for repair of encephalocele, skull base
🚑 45.7 ✂ 45.7 **FUD** 090 [C] [80] [▭]
AMA: 2014,Jan,11

62140 Cranioplasty for skull defect; up to 5 cm diameter
🚑 29.9 ✂ 29.9 **FUD** 090 [C] [80] [▭]
AMA: 2018,Jan,8; 2017,Jan,8; 2016,Jan,13; 2015,Jan,16; 2014,Jan,11; 2014,Jan,9

62141 larger than 5 cm diameter
🚑 33.1 ✂ 33.1 **FUD** 090 [C] [80] [▭]
AMA: 2018,Jan,8; 2017,Jan,8; 2016,Jan,13; 2015,Jan,16; 2014,Jan,11; 2014,Jan,9

62142 Removal of bone flap or prosthetic plate of skull
🚑 25.8 ✂ 25.8 **FUD** 090 [C] [80] [▭]
AMA: 2018,Jan,8; 2017,Jan,8; 2016,Jan,13; 2015,Jan,16; 2014,Jan,11; 2014,Jan,9

62143 Replacement of bone flap or prosthetic plate of skull
🚑 30.3 ✂ 30.3 **FUD** 090 [C] [80] [▭]
AMA: 2018,Jan,8; 2017,Jan,8; 2016,Jan,13; 2015,Jan,16; 2014,Jan,11; 2014,Jan,9

62145 Cranioplasty for skull defect with reparative brain surgery
🚑 41.0 ✂ 41.0 **FUD** 090 [C] [80] [▭]
AMA: 2018,Jan,8; 2017,Jan,8; 2016,Jan,13; 2015,Jan,16; 2014,Jan,11; 2014,Jan,9

62146 Cranioplasty with autograft (includes obtaining bone grafts); up to 5 cm diameter
🚑 34.2 ✂ 34.2 **FUD** 090 [C] [80] [▭]
AMA: 2018,Jan,8; 2017,Jan,8; 2016,Jan,13; 2015,Jan,16; 2014,Jan,11; 2014,Jan,9

62147 larger than 5 cm diameter
🚑 41.9 ✂ 41.9 **FUD** 090 [C] [80] [▭]
AMA: 2018,Jan,8; 2017,Jan,8; 2016,Jan,13; 2015,Jan,16; 2014,Jan,11; 2014,Jan,9

+ 62148 Incision and retrieval of subcutaneous cranial bone graft for cranioplasty (List separately in addition to code for primary procedure)
Code first (62140-62147)
🚑 3.73 ✂ 3.73 **FUD** ZZZ [C] [▭]
AMA: 2014,Jan,11

62160-62165 Neuroendoscopic Brain Procedures
INCLUDES Diagnostic endoscopy

+ 62160 Neuroendoscopy, intracranial, for placement or replacement of ventricular catheter and attachment to shunt system or external drainage (List separately in addition to code for primary procedure)
Code first (61107, 61210, 62220-62230, 62258)
🚑 5.61 ✂ 5.61 **FUD** ZZZ [N] [N1] [▭]
AMA: 2018,Jan,8; 2017,Jan,8; 2016,Jan,13; 2015,Jan,16; 2014,Jan,11

62161 Neuroendoscopy, intracranial; with dissection of adhesions, fenestration of septum pellucidum or intraventricular cysts (including placement, replacement, or removal of ventricular catheter)
🚑 44.1 ✂ 44.1 **FUD** 090 [C] [80] [▭]
AMA: 2014,Jan,11

62162 with fenestration or excision of colloid cyst, including placement of external ventricular catheter for drainage
🚑 55.3 ✂ 55.3 **FUD** 090 [C] [80] [▭]
AMA: 2014,Jan,11

62163 with retrieval of foreign body
🚑 34.4 ✂ 34.4 **FUD** 090 [C] [80] [▭]
AMA: 2014,Jan,11

62164 with excision of brain tumor, including placement of external ventricular catheter for drainage
🚑 61.5 ✂ 61.5 **FUD** 090 [C] [80] [▭]
AMA: 2014,Jan,11

62165 with excision of pituitary tumor, transnasal or trans-sphenoidal approach
🚑 44.6 ✂ 44.6 **FUD** 090 [C] [80] [▭]
AMA: 2018,Jan,8; 2017,Dec,14; 2014,Jan,11

62180-62258 Cerebrospinal Fluid Diversion Procedures

62180 Ventriculocisternostomy (Torkildsen type operation)
🚑 47.0 ✂ 47.0 **FUD** 090 [C] [80] [▭]
AMA: 2014,Jan,11

Nervous System

62190 — 62267

62190   Creation of shunt; subarachnoid/subdural-atrial, -jugular, -auricular
      🏥 27.1   ✂ 27.1   **FUD** 090   C 🖵
      AMA: 2014,Jan,11

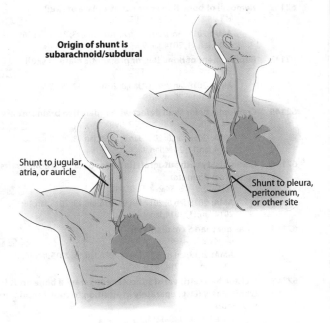

Origin of shunt is subarachnoid/subdural

Shunt to jugular, atria, or auricle

Shunt to pleura, peritoneum, or other site

62192   subarachnoid/subdural-peritoneal, -pleural, other terminus
      🏥 28.5   ✂ 28.5   **FUD** 090   C 80 🖵
      AMA: 2014,Jan,11

62194   Replacement or irrigation, subarachnoid/subdural catheter
      🏥 14.2   ✂ 14.2   **FUD** 010   J A2 80 🖵
      AMA: 2018,Jan,8; 2017,Jan,8; 2016,Jan,13; 2015,Jan,16; 2014,Jan,11

62200   Ventriculocisternostomy, third ventricle;
      INCLUDES   Dandy ventriculocisternostomy
      🏥 40.4   ✂ 40.4   **FUD** 090   C 80 🖵
      AMA: 2014,Jan,11

62201   stereotactic, neuroendoscopic method
      EXCLUDES   *Intracranial neuroendoscopic surgery (62161-62165)*
      🏥 35.3   ✂ 35.3   **FUD** 090   C 🖵
      AMA: 2018,Jan,8; 2017,Jan,8; 2016,Jan,13; 2015,Jan,16; 2014,Jul,8; 2014,Jan,11

62220   Creation of shunt; ventriculo-atrial, -jugular, -auricular
      Code also intracranial neuroendoscopic ventricular catheter insertion, when performed (62160)
      🏥 29.2   ✂ 29.2   **FUD** 090   C 80 🖵
      AMA: 2014,Jan,11

62223   ventriculo-peritoneal, -pleural, other terminus
      Code also intracranial neuroendoscopic ventricular catheter insertion, when performed (62160)
      🏥 30.3   ✂ 30.3   **FUD** 090   C 80 🖵
      AMA: 2014,Jan,11

62225   Replacement or irrigation, ventricular catheter
      Code also intracranial neuroendoscopic ventricular catheter insertion, when performed (62160)
      🏥 15.3   ✂ 15.3   **FUD** 090   J A2 🖵
      AMA: 2018,Jan,8; 2017,Jan,8; 2016,Jan,13; 2015,Jan,16; 2014,Jan,11

62230   Replacement or revision of cerebrospinal fluid shunt, obstructed valve, or distal catheter in shunt system
      Code also intracranial neuroendoscopic ventricular catheter insertion, when performed (62160)
      Code also when proximal catheter and valve are replaced (62225)
      🏥 24.5   ✂ 24.5   **FUD** 090   J A2 80 🖵
      AMA: 2018,Jan,8; 2017,Jan,8; 2016,Jan,13; 2015,Jan,16; 2014,Jan,11

62252   Reprogramming of programmable cerebrospinal shunt
      🏥 2.34   ✂ 2.34   **FUD** XXX   S P3 80 🖵
      AMA: 2014,Jan,11

62256   Removal of complete cerebrospinal fluid shunt system; without replacement
      EXCLUDES   *Reprogramming cerebrospinal fluid (CSF) shunt (62252)*
      🏥 17.5   ✂ 17.5   **FUD** 090   C 80 🖵
      AMA: 2014,Jan,11

62258   with replacement by similar or other shunt at same operation
      EXCLUDES   *Aspiration or irrigation of shunt reservoir (61070)*
               Reprogramming of a cerebrospinal fluid (CSF) shunt (62252)
      Code also intracranial neuroendoscopic ventricular catheter insertion, when performed (62160)
      🏥 32.5   ✂ 32.5   **FUD** 090   C 80 🖵
      AMA: 2018,Jan,8; 2017,Jan,8; 2016,Jan,13; 2015,Jan,16; 2014,Jan,11

62263-62264 Lysis of Epidural Lesions with Injection of Solution/Mechanical Methods

INCLUDES   Epidurography (72275)
            Fluoroscopic guidance (77003)
            Percutaneous mechanical lysis

62263   Percutaneous lysis of epidural adhesions using solution injection (eg, hypertonic saline, enzyme) or mechanical means (eg, catheter) including radiologic localization (includes contrast when administered), multiple adhesiolysis sessions; 2 or more days
      INCLUDES   All adhesiolysis treatments, injections, and infusions during course of treatment
            Percutaneous epidural catheter insertion and removal for neurolytic agent injections during a series of treatment sessions
      EXCLUDES   *Procedure performed more than one time for the complete series spanning two or more treatment days*
      🏥 8.92   ✂ 17.1   **FUD** 010   T A2 🖵
      AMA: 2018,Jan,8; 2017,Jan,8; 2016,Jan,13; 2015,Jan,16; 2014,Jan,11

62264   1 day
      INCLUDES   Multiple treatment sessions performed on the same day
      EXCLUDES   *Percutaneous lysis of epidural adhesions using solution injection, 2 or more days (62263)*
      🏥 6.89   ✂ 12.2   **FUD** 010   T A2 🖵
      AMA: 2018,Jan,8; 2017,Jan,8; 2016,Jan,13; 2015,Jan,16; 2014,Jan,11

62267-62269 Percutaneous Procedures of Spinal Cord

62267   Percutaneous aspiration within the nucleus pulposus, intervertebral disc, or paravertebral tissue for diagnostic purposes
      EXCLUDES   *Bone biopsy (20225)*
            Decompression of intervertebral disc (62287)
            Fine needle aspiration ([10005, 10006, 10007, 10008, 10009, 10010, 10011, 10012]
            Injection for discography (62290-62291)
      Code also fluoroscopic guidance (77003)
      🏥 4.55   ✂ 7.34   **FUD** 000   T G2 80 🖵
      AMA: 2019,Apr,4; 2018,Jan,8; 2017,Feb,12; 2017,Jan,8; 2016,Jan,13; 2015,Jan,16; 2014,Jan,11

26/TC PC/TC Only   A2-Z3 ASC Payment   50 Bilateral   ♂ Male Only   ♀ Female Only   🏥 Facility RVU   ✂ Non-Facility RVU   🖵 CCI   ❌ CLIA
FUD Follow-up Days   **CMS:** IOM   **AMA:** CPT Asst   A-Y OPPSI   80/80 Surg Assist Allowed / w/Doc   Lab Crosswalk   Radiology Crosswalk

292   CPT © 2019 American Medical Association. All Rights Reserved.   © 2019 Optum360, LLC

62268   **Percutaneous aspiration, spinal cord cyst or syrinx**

     (76942, 77002, 77012)

     7.40   7.40   **FUD** 000   T A2

     AMA: 2018,Jan,8; 2017,Dec,13; 2014,Jan,11

62269   **Biopsy of spinal cord, percutaneous needle**

     EXCLUDES   *Fine needle aspiration [(10005, 1006, 1007, 1008, 1009, 10010, 10011, 10012)]*

     (76942, 77002, 77012)

     (88172-88173)

     7.66   7.66   **FUD** 000   J A2 80

     AMA: 2019,Apr,4; 2014,Jan,11

62270-62329 [62328, 62329] Spinal Puncture, Subarachnoid Space, Diagnostic/Therapeutic

Code also fluoroscopic guidance (77003)

▲   **62270**   **Spinal puncture, lumbar, diagnostic;**

     EXCLUDES   *Radiological guidance (77003, 77012)*

              Ultrasound or MRI guidance (76942, 77021)

     2.23   4.22   **FUD** 000   T A2

     AMA: 2018,Jan,8; 2017,Jan,8; 2016,Jan,13; 2015,Jan,16; 2014,Sep,3; 2014,Jan,11

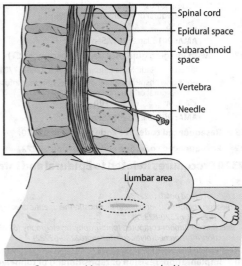

Spinal cord
Epidural space
Subarachnoid space
Vertebra
Needle

Lumbar area

Common position to access vertebral interspace

● #   **62328**   **with fluoroscopic or CT guidance**

     0.00   0.00   **FUD** 000

     EXCLUDES   *Radiological guidance (77003, 77012)*

              Ultrasound or MRI guidance (76942, 77021)

▲   **62272**   **Spinal puncture, therapeutic, for drainage of cerebrospinal fluid (by needle or catheter);**

     EXCLUDES   *Radiological guidance (77003, 77012)*

              Ultrasound or MRI guidance (76942, 77021)

     2.41   5.57   **FUD** 000   T A2

     AMA: 2018,Jan,8; 2017,Jan,8; 2016,Jan,13; 2015,Jan,16; 2014,Jan,11

● #   **62329**   **with fluoroscopic or CT guidance**

     0.00   0.00   **FUD** 000

     EXCLUDES   *Radiological guidance (77003, 77012)*

              Ultrasound or MRI guidance (76942, 77021)

62273 Epidural Blood Patch

CMS: 100-03,10.5 NCD for Autogenous Epidural Blood Graft (10.5)

     EXCLUDES   *Injection of diagnostic or therapeutic material (62320-62327)*

Code also fluoroscopic guidance (77003)

   62273   **Injection, epidural, of blood or clot patch**

     3.26   4.93   **FUD** 000   T A2

     AMA: 2018,Jan,8; 2017,Jan,8; 2016,Jan,13; 2015,Jan,16; 2014,Jan,11

62280-62282 Neurolysis

   INCLUDES   Contrast injection during fluoroscopic guidance/localization

   EXCLUDES   *Injection of diagnostic or therapeutic material only (62320-62327)*

Code also fluoroscopic guidance and localization unless a formal contrast study is performed (77003)

   62280   **Injection/infusion of neurolytic substance (eg, alcohol, phenol, iced saline solutions), with or without other therapeutic substance; subarachnoid**

     4.76   9.45   **FUD** 010   T A2

     AMA: 2018,Jan,8; 2017,Jan,8; 2016,Jan,13; 2015,Jan,16; 2014,Jan,11

   62281   **epidural, cervical or thoracic**

     4.58   6.94   **FUD** 010   T A2

     AMA: 2018,Jan,8; 2017,Jan,8; 2016,Jan,13; 2015,Jan,16; 2014,Jan,11

   62282   **epidural, lumbar, sacral (caudal)**

     4.16   8.63   **FUD** 010   T A2

     AMA: 2018,Jan,8; 2017,Jan,8; 2016,Jan,13; 2015,Jan,16; 2014,Jan,11

62284-62294 Injection/Aspiration of Spine, Diagnostic/Therapeutic

   62284   **Injection procedure for myelography and/or computed tomography, lumbar**

     EXCLUDES   *Injection at C1-C2 (61055)*

              Myelography (62302-62305, 72240, 72255, 72265, 72270)

Code also fluoroscopic guidance (77003)

     2.54   5.61   **FUD** 000   N N1

     AMA: 2018,Jan,8; 2017,Jan,8; 2016,Jan,13; 2015,Jan,16; 2014,Sep,3; 2014,Jan,11

   62287   **Decompression procedure, percutaneous, of nucleus pulposus of intervertebral disc, any method utilizing needle based technique to remove disc material under fluoroscopic imaging or other form of indirect visualization, with discography and/or epidural injection(s) at the treated level(s), when performed, single or multiple levels, lumbar**

     INCLUDES   Endoscopic approach

     EXCLUDES   *Injection for discography (62290)*

              Injection of diagnostic or therapeutic substance(s) (62322)

              Lumbar discography (72295)

              Percutaneous aspiration, diagnostic (62267)

              Percutaneous decompression of nucleus pulposus of an intervertebral disc, non-needle based technique (0274T-0275T)

              Radiological guidance (77003, 77012)

     16.7   16.7   **FUD** 090   J A2

     AMA: 2018,Jan,8; 2017,Feb,12; 2017,Jan,8; 2016,Jan,13; 2015,Mar,9; 2015,Jan,16; 2014,Apr,10; 2014,Jan,11

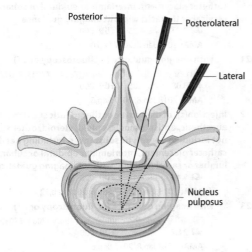

Posterior
Posterolateral
Lateral
Nucleus pulposus

62290 Injection procedure for discography, each level; lumbar

⬛ (72295)

🔷 4.81   🔶 9.62   **FUD** 000   N N1 ▭

AMA: 2018,Jan,8; 2017,Feb,12; 2017,Jan,8; 2016,Jan,13; 2015,Jan,16; 2014,Jan,11

62291 cervical or thoracic

⬛ (72285)

🔷 4.65   🔶 9.28   **FUD** 000   N N1 ▭

AMA: 2018,Jan,8; 2017,Jan,8; 2016,Jan,13; 2015,Jan,16; 2014,Jan,11

62292 Injection procedure for chemonucleolysis, including discography, intervertebral disc, single or multiple levels, lumbar

🔷 16.4   🔶 16.4   **FUD** 090   J R2 80 ▭

AMA: 2018,Jan,8; 2017,Jan,8; 2016,Jan,13; 2015,Jan,16; 2014,Jan,11

62294 Injection procedure, arterial, for occlusion of arteriovenous malformation, spinal

🔷 27.8   🔶 27.8   **FUD** 090   T A2 ▭

AMA: 2014,Jan,11

62302-62305 Myelography

EXCLUDES   C1-C2 injection (61055)
Lumbar myelogram furnished by other providers (62284, 72240, 72255, 72265, 72270)

62302 Myelography via lumbar injection, including radiological supervision and interpretation; cervical

🔷 3.51   🔶 7.13   **FUD** 000   Q2 N1 ▭

EXCLUDES   Myelography (62303-62305)

62303 thoracic

🔷 3.51   🔶 7.29   **FUD** 000   Q2 N1 ▭

EXCLUDES   Myelography (62302, 62304-62305)

62304 lumbosacral

🔷 3.45   🔶 7.04   **FUD** 000   Q2 N1 ▭

EXCLUDES   Myelography (62302-62303, 62305)

62305 2 or more regions (eg, lumbar/thoracic, cervical/thoracic, lumbar/cervical, lumbar/thoracic/cervical)

🔷 3.60   🔶 7.65   **FUD** 000   Q2 N1 ▭

EXCLUDES   Myelography (62302-62305)

62320-62329 Injection/Infusion Diagnostic/Therapeutic Material

EXCLUDES   Epidurography (72275)
Transforaminal epidural injection (64479-64484)
Use of code more than one time even when catheter tip or injected drug travels into a different area of the spine

62320 Injection(s), of diagnostic or therapeutic substance(s) (eg, anesthetic, antispasmodic, opioid, steroid, other solution), not including neurolytic substances, including needle or catheter placement, interlaminar epidural or subarachnoid, cervical or thoracic; without imaging guidance

🔷 2.87   🔶 4.73   **FUD** 000   T G2 ▭

AMA: 2018,Jan,8; 2017,Sep,6

62321 with imaging guidance (ie, fluoroscopy or CT)

INCLUDES   Radiologic guidance (76942, 77003, 77012)

🔷 3.08   🔶 7.05   **FUD** 000   T G2 ▭

AMA: 2018,Jan,8; 2017,Sep,6

62322 Injection(s), of diagnostic or therapeutic substance(s) (eg, anesthetic, antispasmodic, opioid, steroid, other solution), not including neurolytic substances, including needle or catheter placement, interlaminar epidural or subarachnoid, lumbar or sacral (caudal); without imaging guidance

🔷 2.49   🔶 4.44   **FUD** 000   T G2 ▭

AMA: 2018,Jan,8; 2017,Sep,6; 2017,Feb,12

62323 with imaging guidance (ie, fluoroscopy or CT)

INCLUDES   Radiologic guidance (76942, 77003, 77012)

🔷 2.85   🔶 6.96   **FUD** 000   T G2 ▭

AMA: 2018,Jan,8; 2017,Sep,6

62324 Injection(s), including indwelling catheter placement, continuous infusion or intermittent bolus, of diagnostic or therapeutic substance(s) (eg, anesthetic, antispasmodic, opioid, steroid, other solution), not including neurolytic substances, interlaminar epidural or subarachnoid, cervical or thoracic; without imaging guidance

Code also hospital management of continuous infusion of drug, epidural or subarachnoid (01996)

🔷 2.60   🔶 4.14   **FUD** 000   T G2 ▭

AMA: 2018,Jan,8; 2017,Sep,6

62325 with imaging guidance (ie, fluoroscopy or CT)

INCLUDES   Radiologic guidance (76942, 77003, 77012)

Code also hospital management of continuous infusion of drug, epidural or subarachnoid (01996)

🔷 3.00   🔶 6.27   **FUD** 000   T G2 ▭

AMA: 2018,Jan,8; 2017,Sep,6

62326 Injection(s), including indwelling catheter placement, continuous infusion or intermittent bolus, of diagnostic or therapeutic substance(s) (eg, anesthetic, antispasmodic, opioid, steroid, other solution), not including neurolytic substances, interlaminar epidural or subarachnoid, lumbar or sacral (caudal); without imaging guidance

Code also hospital management of continuous infusion of drug, epidural or subarachnoid (01996)

🔷 2.58   🔶 4.36   **FUD** 000   T G2 ▭

AMA: 2018,Jan,8; 2017,Sep,6

62327 with imaging guidance (ie, fluoroscopy or CT)

INCLUDES   Radiologic guidance (76942, 77003, 77012)

Code also hospital management of continuous infusion of drug, epidural or subarachnoid (01996)

🔷 2.74   🔶 6.39   **FUD** 000   T G2 ▭

AMA: 2018,Jan,8; 2017,Sep,6

62328   **Resequenced code. See code following 62270.**

62329   **Resequenced code. See code following 62272.**

62350-62370 Procedures Related to Epidural and Intrathecal Catheters

EXCLUDES   Epidural blood patch (62273)
Injection epidural/subarachnoid diagnostic/therapeutic drugs ([62328], [62329], 62320-62327)
Injection for lumbar computed tomography/myelography (62284)
Injection/infusion neurolytic substances (62280-62282)
Spinal puncture (62270-62272)

62350 Implantation, revision or repositioning of tunneled intrathecal or epidural catheter, for long-term medication administration via an external pump or implantable reservoir/infusion pump; without laminectomy

EXCLUDES   Maintenance and refilling of infusion pumps for CNS drug therapy (95990-95991)

🔷 11.5   🔶 11.5   **FUD** 010   J J8 ▭

AMA: 2018,Jan,8; 2017,Jan,8; 2016,Jan,13; 2015,Jan,16; 2014,Jan,11

62351 with laminectomy

EXCLUDES   Maintenance and refilling of infusion pumps for CNS drug therapy (95990-95991)

🔷 24.8   🔶 24.8   **FUD** 090   J 80 ▭

AMA: 2018,Jan,8; 2017,Jan,8; 2016,Jan,13; 2015,Jan,16; 2014,Jan,11

62355 Removal of previously implanted intrathecal or epidural catheter

🔷 7.73   🔶 7.73   **FUD** 010   Q2 A2 80 ▭

AMA: 2014,Jan,11

62360 Implantation or replacement of device for intrathecal or epidural drug infusion; subcutaneous reservoir

🔷 9.13   🔶 9.13   **FUD** 010   J J8 80 ▭

AMA: 2014,Jan,11

62361 nonprogrammable pump

🔷 12.5   🔶 12.5   **FUD** 010   J J8 80 ▭

AMA: 2014,Jan,11

26/TC PC/TC Only   A2-Z3 ASC Payment   50 Bilateral   ♂ Male Only   ♀ Female Only   🔷 Facility RVU   🔶 Non-Facility RVU   ▭ CCI   ✖ CLIA
FUD Follow-up Days   **CMS:** IOM   **AMA:** CPT Asst   A-Y OPPSI   80/80 Surg Assist Allowed / w/Doc   ▪ Lab Crosswalk   ▪ Radiology Crosswalk

294   CPT © 2019 American Medical Association. All Rights Reserved.   © 2019 Optum360, LLC

62362   programmable pump, including preparation of pump, with or without programming

11.0   11.0   **FUD** 010

[J] [J8] [80] [⬜]

AMA: 2018,Jan,8; 2017,Jan,8; 2016,Jan,13; 2015,Jan,16; 2014,Jan,11

62365   Removal of subcutaneous reservoir or pump, previously implanted for intrathecal or epidural infusion

8.52   8.52   **FUD** 010

[Q2] [A2] [80] [⬜]

AMA: 2014,Jan,11

62367   Electronic analysis of programmable, implanted pump for intrathecal or epidural drug infusion (includes evaluation of reservoir status, alarm status, drug prescription status); without reprogramming or refill

EXCLUDES   *Maintenance and refilling of infusion pumps for CNS drug therapy (95990-95991)*

0.72   1.14   **FUD** XXX

[S] [P3] [⬜]

AMA: 2018,Jan,8; 2017,Jan,8; 2016,Jan,13; 2015,Jan,16; 2014,Jan,11

62368   with reprogramming

EXCLUDES   *Maintenance and refilling of infusion pumps for CNS drug therapy (95990-95991)*

1.01   1.57   **FUD** XXX

[S] [P3] [⬜]

AMA: 2018,Jan,8; 2017,Jan,8; 2016,Jan,13; 2015,Jan,16; 2014,Jan,11

62369   with reprogramming and refill

EXCLUDES   *Maintenance and refilling of infusion pumps for CNS drug therapy (95990-95991)*

1.01   3.34   **FUD** XXX

[S] [P3] [⬜]

AMA: 2018,Jan,8; 2017,Jan,8; 2016,Jan,13; 2015,Jan,16; 2014,Jan,11

62370   with reprogramming and refill (requiring skill of a physician or other qualified health care professional)

EXCLUDES   *Maintenance and refilling of infusion pumps for CNS drug therapy (95990-95991)*

1.33   3.47   **FUD** XXX

[S] [P3] [⬜]

AMA: 2018,Jan,8; 2017,Jan,8; 2016,Jan,13; 2015,Jan,16; 2014,Jan,11

62380 Endoscopic Decompression/Laminectomy/Laminotomy

EXCLUDES   *Open decompression (63030, 63056)*
Percutaneous decompression (62267, 0274T-0275T)
Code also operating microscope, when applicable (69990)

62380   Endoscopic decompression of spinal cord, nerve root(s), including laminotomy, partial facetectomy, foraminotomy, discectomy and/or excision of herniated intervertebral disc, 1 interspace, lumbar

0.00   0.00   **FUD** 090

[J] [62] [80] [50] [⬜]

AMA: 2018,Jan,8; 2017,Feb,12

63001-63048 Posterior Midline Approach: Laminectomy/Laminotomy/Decompression

INCLUDES   Endoscopic assistance through open and direct visualization
EXCLUDES   *Arthrodesis (22590-22614)*
Percutaneous decompression (62287, 0274T, 0275T)
Code also operating microscope, when applicable (69990)

63001   Laminectomy with exploration and/or decompression of spinal cord and/or cauda equina, without facetectomy, foraminotomy or discectomy (eg, spinal stenosis), 1 or 2 vertebral segments; cervical

36.0   36.0   **FUD** 090

[J] [62] [80] [⬜]

AMA: 2018,Jan,8; 2017,Mar,7; 2017,Jan,8; 2016,Jan,13; 2015,Jan,16; 2014,Jan,11

63003   thoracic

36.0   36.0   **FUD** 090

[J] [62] [80] [⬜]

AMA: 2018,Jan,8; 2017,Mar,7; 2017,Jan,8; 2016,Jan,13; 2015,Jan,16; 2014,Jan,11

63005   lumbar, except for spondylolisthesis

34.4   34.4   **FUD** 090

[J] [62] [80] [⬜]

AMA: 2018,Jan,8; 2017,Mar,7; 2017,Feb,9; 2017,Jan,8; 2016,Jan,13; 2015,Jan,16; 2014,Jan,11

63011   sacral

31.6   31.6   **FUD** 090

[J] [80] [⬜]

AMA: 2018,Jan,8; 2017,Mar,7; 2017,Jan,8; 2016,Jan,13; 2015,Jan,16; 2014,Jan,11

63012   Laminectomy with removal of abnormal facets and/or pars inter-articularis with decompression of cauda equina and nerve roots for spondylolisthesis, lumbar (Gill type procedure)

34.6   34.6   **FUD** 090

[J] [80] [⬜]

AMA: 2018,Jan,8; 2017,Mar,7; 2017,Feb,9; 2017,Jan,8; 2016,Jan,13; 2015,Jan,16; 2014,Jan,11

63015   Laminectomy with exploration and/or decompression of spinal cord and/or cauda equina, without facetectomy, foraminotomy or discectomy (eg, spinal stenosis), more than 2 vertebral segments; cervical

43.2   43.2   **FUD** 090

[J] [80] [⬜]

AMA: 2018,Jan,8; 2017,Mar,7; 2017,Jan,8; 2016,Jan,13; 2015,Jan,16; 2014,Jan,11

63016   thoracic

44.3   44.3   **FUD** 090

[J] [80] [⬜]

AMA: 2018,Jan,8; 2017,Mar,7; 2017,Jan,8; 2016,Jan,13; 2015,Jan,16; 2014,Jan,11

63017   lumbar

36.7   36.7   **FUD** 090

[J] [80] [⬜]

AMA: 2018,Jan,8; 2017,Mar,7; 2017,Feb,9; 2017,Jan,8; 2016,Jan,13; 2015,Jan,16; 2014,Jan,11

Nerve root problems in C5 through C7 cause paralysis of the upper limb

C1 to C4
C5 to C7

Atlas (C1)
Axis (C2)

The specialized atlas allows for rotary motion, which turns the head

63020   Laminotomy (hemilaminectomy), with decompression of nerve root(s), including partial facetectomy, foraminotomy and/or excision of herniated intervertebral disc; 1 interspace, cervical

33.6   33.6   **FUD** 090

[J] [62] [80] [50] [⬜]

AMA: 2018,Jan,8; 2017,Mar,7; 2017,Jan,8; 2016,Jan,13; 2015,Jan,16; 2014,Jan,11

63030   1 interspace, lumbar

28.2   28.2   **FUD** 090

[J] [62] [80] [50] [⬜]

AMA: 2018,Jan,8; 2017,Mar,7; 2017,Feb,9; 2017,Feb,12; 2017,Jan,8; 2016,May,13; 2016,Jan,13; 2015,Jan,16; 2014,Jan,11

+ 63035 each additional interspace, cervical or lumbar (List separately in addition to code for primary procedure)

EXCLUDES *Reporting with modifier 50. Report once for each side when performed bilaterally*

Code first (63020-63030)

🔧 5.58 ⚖ 5.58 **FUD** ZZZ [50] [N] [80] 🔲

AMA: 2018,Jan,8; 2017,Feb,9; 2017,Jan,8; 2016,Jan,13; 2015,Jan,16; 2014,Jan,11

63040 Laminotomy (hemilaminectomy), with decompression of nerve root(s), including partial facetectomy, foraminotomy and/or excision of herniated intervertebral disc, reexploration, single interspace; cervical

🔧 40.4 ⚖ 40.4 **FUD** 090 [J] [80] [50] 🔲

AMA: 2018,Jan,8; 2017,Mar,7; 2017,Jan,8; 2016,Jan,13; 2015,Jan,16; 2014,Jan,11

63042 lumbar

🔧 37.6 ⚖ 37.6 **FUD** 090 [J] [62] [80] [50] 🔲

AMA: 2018,Jan,8; 2017,Mar,7; 2017,Feb,9; 2017,Jan,8; 2016,Jan,13; 2015,Jan,16; 2014,Jan,11

+ 63043 each additional cervical interspace (List separately in addition to code for primary procedure)

EXCLUDES *Reporting with modifier 50. Report once for each side when performed bilaterally*

Code first (63040)

🔧 0.00 ⚖ 0.00 **FUD** ZZZ [50] [N] [80] 🔲

AMA: 2018,Jan,8; 2017,Jan,8; 2016,Jan,13; 2015,Jan,16; 2014,Jan,11

+ 63044 each additional lumbar interspace (List separately in addition to code for primary procedure)

EXCLUDES *Reporting with modifier 50. Report once for each side when performed bilaterally*

Code first (63042)

🔧 0.00 ⚖ 0.00 **FUD** ZZZ [50] [N] [N1] [80] 🔲

AMA: 2018,Jan,8; 2017,Feb,9; 2017,Jan,8; 2016,Jan,13; 2015,Jan,16; 2014,Jan,11

63045 Laminectomy, facetectomy and foraminotomy (unilateral or bilateral with decompression of spinal cord, cauda equina and/or nerve root[s], [eg, spinal or lateral recess stenosis]), single vertebral segment; cervical

🔧 37.3 ⚖ 37.3 **FUD** 090 [J] [62] [80] 🔲

AMA: 2018,Jan,8; 2017,Mar,7; 2017,Jan,8; 2016,Jan,13; 2015,Jan,16; 2014,Jan,11

63046 thoracic

🔧 35.6 ⚖ 35.6 **FUD** 090 [J] [62] [80] 🔲

AMA: 2018,Jan,8; 2017,Mar,7; 2017,Jan,8; 2016,Jan,13; 2015,Jan,16; 2014,Jan,11

63047 lumbar

🔧 31.9 ⚖ 31.9 **FUD** 090 [J] [62] [80] 🔲

AMA: 2018,May,10; 2018,May,9; 2018,Jan,8; 2017,Mar,7; 2017,Feb,9; 2017,Feb,12; 2017,Jan,8; 2016,Oct,11; 2016,Jan,13; 2015,Jan,16; 2014,Dec,16; 2014,Dec,16; 2014,Jan,11

+ 63048 each additional segment, cervical, thoracic, or lumbar (List separately in addition to code for primary procedure)

Code first (63045-63047)

🔧 6.17 ⚖ 6.17 **FUD** ZZZ [N] [80] 🔲

AMA: 2018,Jan,8; 2017,Feb,9; 2017,Jan,8; 2016,Jan,13; 2015,Jan,16; 2014,Jan,11

63050-63051 Cervical Laminoplasty: Posterior Midline Approach

EXCLUDES *Procedure performed on the same vertebral segment(s) (22600, 22614, 22840-22842, 63001, 63015, 63045, 63048, 63295)*

63050 Laminoplasty, cervical, with decompression of the spinal cord, 2 or more vertebral segments;

🔧 43.5 ⚖ 43.5 **FUD** 090 [C] [80] 🔲

AMA: 2018,Jan,8; 2017,Mar,7; 2017,Jan,8; 2016,Jan,13; 2015,Jan,16; 2014,Jan,11

63051 with reconstruction of the posterior bony elements (including the application of bridging bone graft and non-segmental fixation devices [eg, wire, suture, mini-plates], when performed)

🔧 49.7 ⚖ 49.7 **FUD** 090 [C] [80] 🔲

AMA: 2018,Jan,8; 2017,Mar,7; 2017,Jan,8; 2016,Jan,13; 2015,Jan,16; 2014,Jan,11

63055-63066 Spinal Cord/Nerve Root Decompression: Costovertebral or Transpedicular Approach

63055 Transpedicular approach with decompression of spinal cord, equina and/or nerve root(s) (eg, herniated intervertebral disc), single segment; thoracic

🔧 47.4 ⚖ 47.4 **FUD** 090 [J] [62] [80] 🔲

AMA: 2018,Jan,8; 2017,Mar,7; 2017,Jan,8; 2016,Jan,13; 2015,Jan,16; 2014,Jan,11

63056 lumbar (including transfacet, or lateral extraforaminal approach) (eg, far lateral herniated intervertebral disc)

🔧 43.2 ⚖ 43.2 **FUD** 090 [J] [62] [80] 🔲

AMA: 2018,Jan,8; 2017,Mar,7; 2017,Feb,12; 2017,Jan,8; 2016,Jan,13; 2015,Jan,16; 2014,Jan,11; 2014,Jan,9

+ 63057 each additional segment, thoracic or lumbar (List separately in addition to code for primary procedure)

Code first (63055-63056)

🔧 9.32 ⚖ 9.32 **FUD** ZZZ [N] [80] 🔲

AMA: 2018,Jan,8; 2017,Jan,8; 2016,Jan,13; 2015,Jan,16; 2014,Jan,11

63064 Costovertebral approach with decompression of spinal cord or nerve root(s) (eg, herniated intervertebral disc), thoracic; single segment

EXCLUDES *Laminectomy with intraspinal thoracic lesion removal (63266, 63271, 63276, 63281, 63286)*

🔧 51.9 ⚖ 51.9 **FUD** 090 [J] [80] 🔲

AMA: 2018,Jan,8; 2017,Mar,7; 2017,Jan,8; 2016,Jan,13; 2015,Jan,16; 2014,Jan,11

+ 63066 each additional segment (List separately in addition to code for primary procedure)

EXCLUDES *Laminectomy with intraspinal thoracic lesion removal (63266, 63271, 63276, 63281, 63286)*

Code first (63064)

🔧 6.09 ⚖ 6.09 **FUD** ZZZ [N] [80] 🔲

AMA: 2014,Jan,11

63075-63078 Discectomy: Anterior or Anterolateral Approach

INCLUDES Operating microscope (69990)

63075 Discectomy, anterior, with decompression of spinal cord and/or nerve root(s), including osteophytectomy; cervical, single interspace

EXCLUDES *Anterior cervical discectomy and anterior interbody fusion at same level during same operative session (22551)*

Anterior interbody arthrodesis (even by another provider) (22554)

🔧 39.2 ⚖ 39.2 **FUD** 090 [J] [80] 🔲

AMA: 2018,Jan,8; 2017,Mar,7; 2017,Jan,8; 2016,Feb,12; 2016,Jan,13; 2015,Apr,7; 2015,Jan,16; 2014,Jan,11

+ 63076 cervical, each additional interspace (List separately in addition to code for primary procedure)

EXCLUDES *Anterior cervical discectomy and anterior interbody fusion at same level during same operative session (22552)*

Anterior interbody arthrodesis (even by another provider) (22554)

Code first (63075)

🔧 7.20 ⚖ 7.20 **FUD** ZZZ [N] [80] 🔲

AMA: 2018,Jan,8; 2017,Jan,8; 2016,Feb,12; 2016,Jan,13; 2015,Jan,16; 2014,Jan,11

63077 thoracic, single interspace
44.2 ⚕ 44.2 **FUD** 090 C 80 ▢
AMA: 2018,Jan,8; 2017,Mar,7; 2017,Jan,8; 2016,Feb,12; 2016,Jan,13; 2015,Jan,16; 2014,Jan,11

+ 63078 thoracic, each additional interspace (List separately in addition to code for primary procedure)
Code first (63077)
6.13 ⚕ 6.13 **FUD** ZZZ C 80 ▢
AMA: 2018,Jan,8; 2017,Jan,8; 2016,Feb,12; 2016,Jan,13; 2015,Jan,16; 2014,Jan,11

63081-63091 Vertebral Corpectomy, All Levels, Anterior Approach

INCLUDES Disc removal at the level below and/or above vertebral segment
Partial removal:
Cervical: Removal of ≥ 1/2 of vertebral body
Lumbar: Removal of ≥ 1/3 of vertebral body
Thoracic: Removal of ≥ 1/3 of vertebral body
EXCLUDES *Arthrodesis (22548-22812)*
Code also reconstruction (20930-20938, 22548-22812, 22840-22855 [22859])

63081 Vertebral corpectomy (vertebral body resection), partial or complete, anterior approach with decompression of spinal cord and/or nerve root(s); cervical, single segment
EXCLUDES *Transoral approach (61575-61576)*
51.1 ⚕ 51.1 **FUD** 090 C 80 ▢
AMA: 2018,Jan,8; 2017,Mar,7; 2017,Jan,8; 2016,Apr,8; 2016,Jan,13; 2015,Jun,10; 2015,Jan,16; 2014,Jan,11

+ 63082 cervical, each additional segment (List separately in addition to code for primary procedure)
EXCLUDES *Transoral approach (61575-61576)*
Code first (63081)
7.77 ⚕ 7.77 **FUD** ZZZ C 80 ▢
AMA: 2018,Jan,8; 2017,Jan,8; 2016,Apr,8; 2016,Jan,13; 2015,Jan,16; 2014,Jan,11

63085 Vertebral corpectomy (vertebral body resection), partial or complete, transthoracic approach with decompression of spinal cord and/or nerve root(s); thoracic, single segment
55.9 ⚕ 55.9 **FUD** 090 C 80 ▢
AMA: 2018,Jan,8; 2017,Mar,7; 2017,Jan,8; 2016,Apr,8; 2016,Jan,13; 2015,Jan,16; 2014,Jan,11

+ 63086 thoracic, each additional segment (List separately in addition to code for primary procedure)
Code first (63085)
5.58 ⚕ 5.58 **FUD** ZZZ C 80 ▢
AMA: 2018,Jan,8; 2017,Jan,8; 2016,Apr,8; 2016,Jan,13; 2015,Jan,16; 2014,Jan,11

63087 Vertebral corpectomy (vertebral body resection), partial or complete, combined thoracolumbar approach with decompression of spinal cord, cauda equina or nerve root(s), lower thoracic or lumbar; single segment
70.3 ⚕ 70.3 **FUD** 090 C 80 ▢
AMA: 2018,Jan,8; 2017,Mar,7; 2017,Jan,8; 2016,Apr,8; 2016,Jan,13; 2015,Jan,16; 2014,Jan,11

+ 63088 each additional segment (List separately in addition to code for primary procedure)
Code first (63087)
7.53 ⚕ 7.53 **FUD** ZZZ C 80 ▢
AMA: 2018,Jan,8; 2017,Jan,8; 2016,Apr,8; 2016,Jan,13; 2015,Jan,16; 2014,Jan,11

63090 Vertebral corpectomy (vertebral body resection), partial or complete, transperitoneal or retroperitoneal approach with decompression of spinal cord, cauda equina or nerve root(s), lower thoracic, lumbar, or sacral; single segment
56.9 ⚕ 56.9 **FUD** 090 C 80 ▢
AMA: 2018,Jan,8; 2017,Mar,7; 2017,Jan,8; 2016,Apr,8; 2016,Jan,13; 2015,Jan,16; 2014,Jan,11

+ 63091 each additional segment (List separately in addition to code for primary procedure)
Code first (63090)
5.18 ⚕ 5.18 **FUD** ZZZ C 80 ▢
AMA: 2018,Jan,8; 2017,Jan,8; 2016,Apr,8; 2016,Jan,13; 2015,Jan,16; 2014,Jan,11

63101-63103 Corpectomy: Lateral Extracavitary Approach

INCLUDES Partial removal:
Cervical: Removal of ≥ 1/2 of vertebral body
Lumbar: Removal of ≥ 1/3 of vertebral body
Thoracic: Removal of ≥ 1/3 of vertebral body

63101 Vertebral corpectomy (vertebral body resection), partial or complete, lateral extracavitary approach with decompression of spinal cord and/or nerve root(s) (eg, for tumor or retropulsed bone fragments); thoracic, single segment
67.8 ⚕ 67.8 **FUD** 090 C 80 ▢
AMA: 2018,Jan,8; 2017,Mar,7; 2017,Jan,8; 2016,Jan,13; 2015,Jan,16; 2014,Jan,11

63102 lumbar, single segment
66.0 ⚕ 66.0 **FUD** 090 C 80 ▢
AMA: 2018,Jan,8; 2017,Mar,7; 2017,Jan,8; 2016,Jan,13; 2015,Jan,16; 2014,Jan,11

+ 63103 thoracic or lumbar, each additional segment (List separately in addition to code for primary procedure)
Code first (63101-63102)
8.60 ⚕ 8.60 **FUD** ZZZ C 80 ▢
AMA: 2014,Jan,11

63170-63295 Laminectomies

63170 Laminectomy with myelotomy (eg, Bischof or DREZ type), cervical, thoracic, or thoracolumbar
46.8 ⚕ 46.8 **FUD** 090 C 80 ▢
AMA: 2018,Jan,8; 2017,Mar,7; 2017,Jan,8; 2016,Jan,13; 2015,Jan,16; 2014,Jan,11

63172 Laminectomy with drainage of intramedullary cyst/syrinx; to subarachnoid space
40.4 ⚕ 40.4 **FUD** 090 C 80 ▢
AMA: 2018,Jan,8; 2017,Mar,7; 2017,Jan,8; 2016,Jan,13; 2015,Jan,16; 2014,Jan,11

63173 to peritoneal or pleural space
50.7 ⚕ 50.7 **FUD** 090 C 80 ▢
AMA: 2018,Jan,8; 2017,Mar,7; 2017,Jan,8; 2016,Jan,13; 2015,Jan,16; 2014,Jan,11

63180 Laminectomy and section of dentate ligaments, with or without dural graft, cervical; 1 or 2 segments
43.6 ⚕ 43.6 **FUD** 090 C 80 ▢
AMA: 2018,Jan,8; 2017,Mar,7; 2017,Jan,8; 2016,Jan,13; 2015,Jan,16; 2014,Jan,11

63182 more than 2 segments
47.9 ⚕ 47.9 **FUD** 090 C 80 ▢
AMA: 2018,Jan,8; 2017,Mar,7; 2017,Jan,8; 2016,Jan,13; 2015,Jan,16; 2014,Jan,11

63185 Laminectomy with rhizotomy; 1 or 2 segments
INCLUDES Dana rhizotomy
Stoffel rhizotomy
33.2 ⚕ 33.2 **FUD** 090 C 80 ▢
AMA: 2018,Jan,8; 2017,Mar,7; 2017,Jan,8; 2016,Jan,13; 2015,Jan,16; 2014,Jan,11

63190 more than 2 segments
36.1 ⚕ 36.1 **FUD** 090 C 80 ▢
AMA: 2018,Jan,8; 2017,Mar,7; 2017,Jan,8; 2016,Jan,13; 2015,Jan,16; 2014,Jan,11

63191 Laminectomy with section of spinal accessory nerve
EXCLUDES *Division of sternocleidomastoid muscle for torticollis (21720)*
40.5 ⚕ 40.5 **FUD** 090 C 80 50 ▢
AMA: 2018,Jan,8; 2017,Mar,7; 2017,Jan,8; 2016,Jan,13; 2015,Jan,16; 2014,Jan,11

63194 **Laminectomy with cordotomy, with section of 1 spinothalamic tract, 1 stage; cervical**
　🔹 46.9　　✂ 46.9　　**FUD** 090　　🅒 80 ▢
AMA: 2018,Jan,8; 2017,Mar,7; 2017,Jan,8; 2016,Jan,13; 2015,Jan,16; 2014,Jan,11

63195 **thoracic**
　🔹 45.1　　✂ 45.1　　**FUD** 090　　🅒 80 ▢
AMA: 2018,Jan,8; 2017,Mar,7; 2017,Jan,8; 2016,Jan,13; 2015,Jan,16; 2014,Jan,11

63196 **Laminectomy with cordotomy, with section of both spinothalamic tracts, 1 stage; cervical**
　🔹 52.4　　✂ 52.4　　**FUD** 090　　🅒 80 ▢
AMA: 2018,Jan,8; 2017,Mar,7; 2017,Jan,8; 2016,Jan,13; 2015,Jan,16; 2014,Jan,11

63197 **thoracic**
　🔹 50.3　　✂ 50.3　　**FUD** 090　　🅒 80 ▢
AMA: 2018,Jan,8; 2017,Mar,7; 2017,Jan,8; 2016,Jan,13; 2015,Jan,16; 2014,Jan,11

63198 **Laminectomy with cordotomy with section of both spinothalamic tracts, 2 stages within 14 days; cervical**
　INCLUDES　Keen laminectomy
　🔹 61.5　　✂ 61.5　　**FUD** 090　　🅒 80 ▢
AMA: 2018,Jan,8; 2017,Mar,7; 2017,Jan,8; 2016,Jan,13; 2015,Jan,16; 2014,Jan,11

63199 **thoracic**
　🔹 64.5　　✂ 64.5　　**FUD** 090　　🅒 80 ▢
AMA: 2018,Jan,8; 2017,Mar,7; 2017,Jan,8; 2016,Jan,13; 2015,Jan,16; 2014,Jan,11

63200 **Laminectomy, with release of tethered spinal cord, lumbar**
　🔹 44.7　　✂ 44.7　　**FUD** 090　　🅒 80 ▢
AMA: 2018,Jan,8; 2017,Mar,7; 2017,Jan,8; 2016,Jan,13; 2015,Jan,16; 2014,Jan,11

63250 **Laminectomy for excision or occlusion of arteriovenous malformation of spinal cord; cervical**
　🔹 87.8　　✂ 87.8　　**FUD** 090　　🅒 80 ▢
AMA: 2018,Jan,8; 2017,Mar,7; 2017,Jan,8; 2016,Jan,13; 2015,Jan,16; 2014,Jan,11

Cervical C1 to C7 / Thoracic T1 to T12 / Lumbar L1 to L5 / Sacrum
Dura mater / Nerve roots / Pia mater / Arachnoid / White matter / Gray matter

Schematic of spinal cord layers

63251 **thoracic**
　🔹 89.7　　✂ 89.7　　**FUD** 090　　🅒 80 ▢
AMA: 2018,Jan,8; 2017,Mar,7; 2017,Jan,8; 2016,Jan,13; 2015,Jan,16; 2014,Jan,11

63252 **thoracolumbar**
　🔹 89.7　　✂ 89.7　　**FUD** 090　　🅒 80 ▢
AMA: 2018,Jan,8; 2017,Mar,7; 2017,Jan,8; 2016,Jan,13; 2015,Jan,16; 2014,Jan,11

63265 **Laminectomy for excision or evacuation of intraspinal lesion other than neoplasm, extradural; cervical**
　🔹 48.6　　✂ 48.6　　**FUD** 090　　🅒 80 ▢
AMA: 2018,Jan,8; 2017,Mar,7; 2017,Jan,8; 2016,Jan,13; 2015,Jan,16; 2014,Jan,11

63266 **thoracic**
　🔹 50.2　　✂ 50.2　　**FUD** 090　　🅒 80 ▢
AMA: 2017,Mar,7; 2014,Jan,11

63267 **lumbar**
　🔹 39.8　　✂ 39.8　　**FUD** 090　　🅒 80 ▢
AMA: 2018,Jan,8; 2017,Mar,7; 2017,Jan,8; 2016,Jan,13; 2015,Jan,16; 2014,Jan,11

63268 **sacral**
　🔹 41.2　　✂ 41.2　　**FUD** 090　　🅒 80 ▢
AMA: 2018,Jan,8; 2017,Mar,7; 2017,Jan,8; 2016,Jan,13; 2015,Jan,16; 2014,Jan,11

63270 **Laminectomy for excision of intraspinal lesion other than neoplasm, intradural; cervical**
　🔹 61.1　　✂ 61.1　　**FUD** 090　　🅒 80 ▢
AMA: 2018,Jan,8; 2017,Mar,7; 2017,Jan,8; 2016,Jan,13; 2015,Jan,16; 2014,Jan,11

63271 **thoracic**
　🔹 60.4　　✂ 60.4　　**FUD** 090　　🅒 80 ▢
AMA: 2018,Jan,8; 2017,Mar,7; 2017,Jan,8; 2016,Jan,13; 2015,Jan,16; 2014,Jan,11

63272 **lumbar**
　🔹 55.1　　✂ 55.1　　**FUD** 090　　🅒 80 ▢
AMA: 2018,Jan,8; 2017,Mar,7; 2017,Jan,8; 2016,Jan,13; 2015,Jan,16; 2014,Jan,11

63273 **sacral**
　🔹 54.9　　✂ 54.9　　**FUD** 090　　🅒 80 ▢
AMA: 2018,Jan,8; 2017,Mar,7; 2017,Jan,8; 2016,Jan,13; 2015,Jan,16; 2014,Jan,11

63275 **Laminectomy for biopsy/excision of intraspinal neoplasm; extradural, cervical**
　🔹 52.6　　✂ 52.6　　**FUD** 090　　🅒 80 ▢
AMA: 2018,Jan,8; 2017,Mar,7; 2017,Jan,8; 2016,Jan,13; 2015,Jan,16; 2014,Jan,11

63276 **extradural, thoracic**
　🔹 52.2　　✂ 52.2　　**FUD** 090　　🅒 80 ▢
AMA: 2018,Jan,8; 2017,Mar,7; 2017,Jan,8; 2016,Jan,13; 2015,Jan,16; 2014,Jan,11

63277 **extradural, lumbar**
　🔹 45.3　　✂ 45.3　　**FUD** 090　　🅒 80 ▢
AMA: 2018,Jan,8; 2017,Mar,7; 2017,Jan,8; 2016,Jan,13; 2015,Jan,16; 2014,Jan,11

63278 **extradural, sacral**
　🔹 46.7　　✂ 46.7　　**FUD** 090　　🅒 80 ▢
AMA: 2018,Jan,8; 2017,Mar,7; 2017,Jan,8; 2016,Jan,13; 2015,Jan,16; 2014,Jan,11

63280 **intradural, extramedullary, cervical**
　🔹 61.9　　✂ 61.9　　**FUD** 090　　🅒 80 ▢
AMA: 2018,Jan,8; 2017,Mar,7; 2017,Jan,8; 2016,Jan,13; 2015,Jan,16; 2014,Jan,11

63281 **intradural, extramedullary, thoracic**
　🔹 61.2　　✂ 61.2　　**FUD** 090　　🅒 80 ▢
AMA: 2018,Jan,8; 2017,Mar,7; 2017,Jan,8; 2016,Jan,13; 2015,Jan,16; 2014,Jan,11

63282 **intradural, extramedullary, lumbar**
　🔹 57.7　　✂ 57.7　　**FUD** 090　　🅒 80 ▢
AMA: 2018,Jan,8; 2017,Mar,7; 2017,Jan,8; 2016,Jan,13; 2015,Jan,16; 2014,Jan,11

63283 **intradural, sacral**
　🔹 55.3　　✂ 55.3　　**FUD** 090　　🅒 80 ▢
AMA: 2018,Jan,8; 2017,Mar,7; 2017,Jan,8; 2016,Jan,13; 2015,Jan,16; 2014,Jan,11

26/TC PC/TC Only　　A2-Z3 ASC Payment　　50 Bilateral　　♂ Male Only　　♀ Female Only　　🔹 Facility RVU　　✂ Non-Facility RVU　　▢ CCI　　✖ CLIA
FUD Follow-up Days　　CMS: IOM　　AMA: CPT Asst　　A-Y OPPSI　　80/80 Surg Assist Allowed / w/Doc　　Lab Crosswalk　　Radiology Crosswalk

298　　　　　　　　　CPT © 2019 American Medical Association. All Rights Reserved.　　　　　　© 2019 Optum360, LLC

63285 **intradural, intramedullary, cervical**
🚗 77.2   ⚕ 77.2   **FUD** 090   C 80 ▣
AMA: 2018,Jan,8; 2017,Mar,7; 2017,Jan,8; 2016,Jan,13; 2015,Jan,16; 2014,Jan,11

63286 **intradural, intramedullary, thoracic**
🚗 75.6   ⚕ 75.6   **FUD** 090   C 80 ▣
AMA: 2018,Jan,8; 2017,Mar,7; 2017,Jan,8; 2016,Jan,13; 2015,Jan,16; 2014,Jan,11

63287 **intradural, intramedullary, thoracolumbar**
🚗 81.0   ⚕ 81.0   **FUD** 090   C 80 ▣
AMA: 2018,Jan,8; 2017,Mar,7; 2017,Jan,8; 2016,Jan,13; 2015,Jan,16; 2014,Jan,11

63290 **combined extradural-intradural lesion, any level**
EXCLUDES *Drainage intramedullary cyst or syrinx (63172-63173)*
🚗 82.4   ⚕ 82.4   **FUD** 090   C 80 ▣
AMA: 2018,Jan,8; 2017,Mar,7; 2017,Jan,8; 2016,Jan,13; 2015,Jan,16; 2014,Jan,11

+ **63295** **Osteoplastic reconstruction of dorsal spinal elements, following primary intraspinal procedure (List separately in addition to code for primary procedure)**
EXCLUDES *Procedure performed at the same vertebral segment(s) (22590-22614, 22840-22844, 63050-63051)*
Code first (63172-63173, 63185, 63190, 63200-63290)
🚗 9.76   ⚕ 9.76   **FUD** ZZZ   C 80 ▣
AMA: 2014,Jan,11

63300-63308 Vertebral Corpectomy for Intraspinal Lesion: Anterior/Anterolateral Approach

INCLUDES Partial removal:
Cervical: Removal of ≥ 1/2 of vertebral body
Lumbar: Removal of ≥ 1/3 of vertebral body
Thoracic: Removal of ≥ 1/3 of vertebral body
EXCLUDES *Arthrodesis (22548-22585)*
Spinal reconstruction (20930-20938)

63300 **Vertebral corpectomy (vertebral body resection), partial or complete, for excision of intraspinal lesion, single segment; extradural, cervical**
🚗 53.6   ⚕ 53.6   **FUD** 090   C 80 ▣
AMA: 2018,Jan,8; 2017,Mar,7; 2017,Jan,8; 2016,Jan,13; 2015,Jan,16; 2014,Jan,11

63301 **extradural, thoracic by transthoracic approach**
🚗 64.9   ⚕ 64.9   **FUD** 090   C 80 ▣
AMA: 2018,Jan,8; 2017,Mar,7; 2017,Jan,8; 2016,Jan,13; 2015,Jan,16; 2014,Jan,11

63302 **extradural, thoracic by thoracolumbar approach**
🚗 64.1   ⚕ 64.1   **FUD** 090   C 80 ▣
AMA: 2018,Jan,8; 2017,Mar,7; 2017,Jan,8; 2016,Jan,13; 2015,Jan,16; 2014,Jan,11

63303 **extradural, lumbar or sacral by transperitoneal or retroperitoneal approach**
🚗 63.1   ⚕ 63.1   **FUD** 090   C 80 ▣
AMA: 2018,Jan,8; 2017,Mar,7; 2017,Jan,8; 2016,Jan,13; 2015,Jan,16; 2014,Jan,11

63304 **intradural, cervical**
🚗 69.2   ⚕ 69.2   **FUD** 090   C 80 ▣
AMA: 2018,Jan,8; 2017,Mar,7; 2017,Jan,8; 2016,Jan,13; 2015,Jan,16; 2014,Jan,11

63305 **intradural, thoracic by transthoracic approach**
🚗 73.7   ⚕ 73.7   **FUD** 090   C 80 ▣
AMA: 2018,Jan,8; 2017,Mar,7; 2017,Jan,8; 2016,Jan,13; 2015,Jan,16; 2014,Jan,11

63306 **intradural, thoracic by thoracolumbar approach**
🚗 72.4   ⚕ 72.4   **FUD** 090   C 80 ▣
AMA: 2018,Jan,8; 2017,Mar,7; 2017,Jan,8; 2016,Jan,13; 2015,Jan,16; 2014,Jan,11

63307 **intradural, lumbar or sacral by transperitoneal or retroperitoneal approach**
🚗 71.0   ⚕ 71.0   **FUD** 090   C 80 ▣
AMA: 2018,Jan,8; 2017,Mar,7; 2017,Jan,8; 2016,Jan,13; 2015,Jan,16; 2014,Jan,11

+ **63308** **each additional segment (List separately in addition to codes for single segment)**
Code first (63300-63307)
🚗 9.46   ⚕ 9.46   **FUD** ZZZ   C 80 ▣
AMA: 2014,Jan,11

63600-63610 Stereotactic Procedures of the Spinal Cord

63600 **Creation of lesion of spinal cord by stereotactic method, percutaneous, any modality (including stimulation and/or recording)**
🚗 32.0   ⚕ 32.0   **FUD** 090   J A2 80 ▣
AMA: 2014,Jan,11

63610 **Stereotactic stimulation of spinal cord, percutaneous, separate procedure not followed by other surgery**
🚗 17.1   ⚕ 17.1   **FUD** 000   J J8 80 ▣
AMA: 2014,Jan,11

63620-63621 Stereotactic Radiosurgery (SRS): Spine

INCLUDES Computer assisted planning
Planning dosimetry, targeting, positioning, or blocking by neurosurgeon
EXCLUDES *Arteriovenous malformations (see Radiation Oncology Section)*
Intensity modulated beam delivery plan and treatment (77301, 77385-77386)
Radiation treatment management by the same provider (77427-77432)
Stereotactic body radiation therapy (77373, 77435)
Stereotactic computer-assisted procedures (61781-61783)
Treatment planning, physics, dosimetry, treatment delivery and management provided by the radiation oncologist (77261-77790 [77295, 77385, 77386, 77387, 77424, 77425])

63620 **Stereotactic radiosurgery (particle beam, gamma ray, or linear accelerator); 1 spinal lesion**
EXCLUDES *Use of code more than one time per treatment course*
🚗 32.8   ⚕ 32.8   **FUD** 090   B 80 ▣
AMA: 2018,Jan,8; 2017,Jan,8; 2016,Jan,13; 2015,Jun,6; 2015,Jan,16; 2014,Jan,11

+ **63621** **each additional spinal lesion (List separately in addition to code for primary procedure)**
EXCLUDES *Use of code more than one time per lesion*
Use of code more than two times per entire treatment course
Code first (63620)
🚗 7.48   ⚕ 7.48   **FUD** ZZZ   B 80 ▣
AMA: 2018,Jan,8; 2017,Jan,8; 2016,Jan,13; 2015,Jun,6; 2015,Jan,16; 2014,Jan,11

63650-63688 Spinal Neurostimulation

INCLUDES Analysis of system at time of implantation (95970)
Complex and simple neurostimulators
EXCLUDES *Analysis and programming of neurostimulator pulse generator (95970-95972)*

63650 **Percutaneous implantation of neurostimulator electrode array, epidural**
INCLUDES The following are components of a neurostimulator system:
Collection of contacts of which four or more provide the electrical stimulation in the epidural space
Contacts on a catheter-type lead (array)
Extension
External controller
Implanted neurostimulator
🚗 11.8   ⚕ 45.9   **FUD** 010   J J8 ▣
AMA: 2019,Feb,6; 2018,Oct,11; 2018,Jan,8; 2017,Dec,13; 2017,Jan,8; 2016,Jan,13; 2016,Jan,11; 2015,Dec,18; 2015,Jan,16; 2014,Jan,11

63655 **Laminectomy for implantation of neurostimulator electrodes, plate/paddle, epidural**

INCLUDES The following are components of a neurostimulator system:
Collection of contacts of which four or more provide the electrical stimulation in the epidural space
Contacts on a plate or paddle-shaped surface for systems placed by open exposure
Extension
External controller
Implanted neurostimulator

🔁 24.1   ⚕ 24.1   **FUD** 090   J J8 80 ▭

AMA: 2019,Feb,6; 2018,Jan,8; 2017,Jan,8; 2016,Jan,13; 2015,Jan,16; 2014,Jan,11

63661 **Removal of spinal neurostimulator electrode percutaneous array(s), including fluoroscopy, when performed**

INCLUDES The following are components of a neurostimulator system:
Collection of contacts of which four or more provide the electrical stimulation in the epidural space
Contacts on a catheter-type lead (array)
Extension
External controller
Implanted neurostimulator

EXCLUDES Use of code when removing or replacing a temporary array placed percutaneously for an external generator

🔁 9.32   ⚕ 17.5   **FUD** 010   02 G2 80 ▭

AMA: 2019,Feb,6; 2018,Jan,8; 2017,Jan,8; 2016,Jan,13; 2015,Jan,16; 2014,Jan,11

63662 **Removal of spinal neurostimulator electrode plate/paddle(s) placed via laminotomy or laminectomy, including fluoroscopy, when performed**

INCLUDES The following are components of a neurostimulator system:
Collection of contacts of which four or more provide the electrical stimulation in the epidural space
Contacts on a plate or paddle-shaped surface for systems placed by open exposure
Extension
External controller
Implanted neurostimulator

🔁 24.4   ⚕ 24.4   **FUD** 090   02 G2 80 ▭

AMA: 2019,Feb,6; 2018,Jan,8; 2017,Jan,8; 2016,Jan,13; 2015,Jan,16; 2014,Jan,11

63663 **Revision including replacement, when performed, of spinal neurostimulator electrode percutaneous array(s), including fluoroscopy, when performed**

INCLUDES The following are components of a neurostimulator system:
Collection of contacts of which four or more provide the electrical stimulation in the epidural space
Contacts on a catheter-type lead (array)
Extension
External controller
Implanted neurostimulator

EXCLUDES Removal of spinal neurostimulator electrode percutaneous array(s), plate/paddle(s) at same level (63661-63662)
Use of code when removing or replacing a temporary array placed percutaneously for an external generator

🔁 12.9   ⚕ 23.4   **FUD** 010   J J8 80 ▭

AMA: 2019,Feb,6; 2018,Jan,8; 2017,Jan,8; 2016,Jan,13; 2015,Jan,16; 2014,Jan,11

63664 **Revision including replacement, when performed, of spinal neurostimulator electrode plate/paddle(s) placed via laminotomy or laminectomy, including fluoroscopy, when performed**

INCLUDES The following are components of a neurostimulator system:
Collection of contacts of which four or more provide the electrical stimulation in the epidural space
Contacts on a plate or paddle-shaped surface for systems placed by open exposure
Extension
External controller
Implanted neurostimulator

EXCLUDES Removal of spinal neurostimulator electrode percutaneous array(s), plate/paddle(s) at same level (63661-63662)

🔁 25.2   ⚕ 25.2   **FUD** 090   J J8 80 ▭

AMA: 2019,Feb,6; 2018,Jan,8; 2017,Jan,8; 2016,Jan,13; 2015,Jan,16; 2014,Jan,11

63685 **Insertion or replacement of spinal neurostimulator pulse generator or receiver, direct or inductive coupling**

EXCLUDES Use of code for insertion/replacement with code for revision/removal (63688)

🔁 10.4   ⚕ 10.4   **FUD** 010   J J8 80 ▭

AMA: 2019,Feb,6; 2018,Jan,8; 2017,Dec,13; 2017,Jan,8; 2016,Jan,13; 2015,Jan,16; 2014,Jan,11

63688 **Revision or removal of implanted spinal neurostimulator pulse generator or receiver**

EXCLUDES Use of code for revision/removal with code for insertion/replacement (63685)

🔁 10.7   ⚕ 10.7   **FUD** 010   02 A2 ▭

AMA: 2019,Feb,6; 2018,Jan,8; 2017,Jan,8; 2016,Jan,13; 2015,Jan,16; 2014,Jan,11

63700-63706 Repair Congenital Neural Tube Defects

EXCLUDES Complex skin repair (see appropriate integumentary closure code)

63700 **Repair of meningocele; less than 5 cm diameter**

🔁 38.2   ⚕ 38.2   **FUD** 090   63 C 80 ▭

AMA: 2014,Jan,11

Most children with severe spina bifida also have hydrocephalus, which is excessive fluid in the skull

Cervical

Thoracic

Lumbar

A fluid-filled herniation that protrudes is spina bifida cystica, or meningocele

If nerves protrude into the defect, it is called rachischisis, or meningomyelocele

Dura mater

Spinal cord

Vertebra

63702 **larger than 5 cm diameter**

🔁 41.8   ⚕ 41.8   **FUD** 090   63 C 80 ▭

AMA: 2014,Jan,11

63704 **Repair of myelomeningocele; less than 5 cm diameter**

🔁 48.5   ⚕ 48.5   **FUD** 090   63 C 80 ▭

AMA: 2014,Jan,11

26/TC PC/TC Only   A2-Z3 ASC Payment   50 Bilateral   ♂ Male Only   ♀ Female Only   🔁 Facility RVU   ⚕ Non-Facility RVU   ▭ CCI   ✖ CLIA
FUD Follow-up Days   **CMS:** IOM   **AMA:** CPT Asst   A-Y OPPSI   80/80 Surg Assist Allowed / w/Doc   ▧ Lab Crosswalk   ▦ Radiology Crosswalk

© 2019 Optum360, LLC

63706 larger than 5 cm diameter
54.0 ⚗ 54.0 **FUD** 090   63 C 80 ▢
AMA: 2014,Jan,11

63707-63710 Repair Dural Cerebrospinal Fluid Leak

63707 Repair of dural/cerebrospinal fluid leak, not requiring laminectomy
26.9 ⚗ 26.9 **FUD** 090   C 80 ▢
AMA: 2014,Jan,11

63709 Repair of dural/cerebrospinal fluid leak or pseudomeningocele, with laminectomy
32.0 ⚗ 32.0 **FUD** 090   C 80 ▢
AMA: 2014,Jan,11

63710 Dural graft, spinal
EXCLUDES *Laminectomy and section of dentate ligament (63180, 63182)*
31.6 ⚗ 31.6 **FUD** 090   C 80 ▢
AMA: 2014,Jan,11

63740-63746 Cerebrospinal Fluid (CSF) Shunt: Lumbar

EXCLUDES *Placement of subarachnoid catheter with reservoir and/or pump:*
Not requiring laminectomy (62350, 62360-62362)
With laminectomy (62351, 62360-62362)

63740 Creation of shunt, lumbar, subarachnoid-peritoneal, -pleural, or other; including laminectomy
28.5 ⚗ 28.5 **FUD** 090   C 80 ▢
AMA: 2014,Jan,11

63741 percutaneous, not requiring laminectomy
19.7 ⚗ 19.7 **FUD** 090   J 80 ▢
AMA: 2014,Jan,11

63744 Replacement, irrigation or revision of lumbosubarachnoid shunt
19.5 ⚗ 19.5 **FUD** 090   J J8 80 ▢
AMA: 2014,Jan,11

63746 Removal of entire lumbosubarachnoid shunt system without replacement
17.6 ⚗ 17.6 **FUD** 090   Q2 A2 80 ▢
AMA: 2014,Jan,11

64400-64463 Nerve Blocks

EXCLUDES *Epidural or subarachnoid injection (62320-62327)*
Nerve destruction (62280-62282, 64600-64681 [64633, 64634, 64635, 64636])

▲ **64400** Injection(s), anesthetic agent(s) and/or steroid; trigeminal nerve, each branch (ie, ophthalmic, maxillary, mandibular)
EXCLUDES *Destruction of genicular nerve branches ([64624])*
Imaging guidance and localization
Injection of genicular nerve branches (64454)
Use of code more than one time per encounter when multiple injections are required to block nerve and branches
2.08 ⚗ 3.88 **FUD** 000   T P3 50 ▢
AMA: 2018,Jan,8; 2017,Jan,8; 2016,Jan,13; 2015,Jan,16; 2014,Jan,11

64402 facial nerve
To report, see (64999)

▲ **64405** greater occipital nerve
EXCLUDES *Destruction of genicular nerve branches ([64624])*
Imaging guidance and localization
Injection of genicular nerve branches (64454)
Use of code more than one time per encounter when multiple injections are required to block nerve and branches
1.54 ⚗ 2.37 **FUD** 000   T P3 50 ▢
AMA: 2018,Jan,8; 2017,Jan,8; 2016,Oct,11; 2016,Jan,13; 2015,Jan,16; 2014,Jan,11

▲ **64408** vagus nerve
EXCLUDES *Destruction of genicular nerve branches ([64624])*
Imaging guidance and localization
Injection of genicular nerve branches (64454)
Use of code more than one time per encounter when multiple injections are required to block nerve and branches
2.44 ⚗ 3.35 **FUD** 000   T P3 80 50 ▢
AMA: 2018,Jan,8; 2017,Jan,8; 2016,Jan,13; 2015,Jan,16; 2014,Jan,11

64410 phrenic nerve
To report, see (64999)

64413 cervical plexus
To report, see (64999)

▲ **64415** brachial plexus
EXCLUDES *Destruction of genicular nerve branches ([64624])*
Imaging guidance and localization
Injection of genicular nerve branches (64454)
Use of code more than one time per encounter when multiple injections are required to block nerve and branches
1.87 ⚗ 3.38 **FUD** 000   T A2 50 ▢
AMA: 2018,Jan,8; 2017,Jan,8; 2016,Jan,13; 2015,Jan,16; 2014,Jan,11

▲ **64416** brachial plexus, continuous infusion by catheter (including catheter placement)
EXCLUDES *Destruction of genicular nerve branches ([64624])*
Imaging guidance and localization
Injection of genicular nerve branches (64454)
Management of epidural or subarachnoid continuous drug administration (01996)
Use of code more than one time per encounter when multiple injections are required to block nerve and branches
2.28 ⚗ 2.28 **FUD** 000   T G2 50 ▢
AMA: 2018,Jan,8; 2017,Jan,8; 2016,Jan,13; 2015,Jan,16; 2014,Jan,11

▲ **64417** axillary nerve
EXCLUDES *Destruction of genicular nerve branches ([64624])*
Imaging guidance and localization
Injection of genicular nerve branches (64454)
Use of code more than one time per encounter when multiple injections are required to block nerve and branches
2.02 ⚗ 3.76 **FUD** 000   T A2 50 ▢
AMA: 2018,Jan,8; 2017,Jan,8; 2016,Jan,13; 2015,Jan,16; 2014,Jan,11

▲ **64418** suprascapular nerve
EXCLUDES *Destruction of genicular nerve branches ([64624])*
Imaging guidance and localization
Injection of genicular nerve branches (64454)
Use of code more than one time per encounter when multiple injections are required to block nerve and branches
1.64 ⚗ 2.71 **FUD** 000   T P3 50 ▢
AMA: 2018,Jan,8; 2017,Jan,8; 2016,Jan,13; 2015,Jan,16; 2014,Jan,11

▲ **64420** intercostal nerve, single level
EXCLUDES *Destruction of genicular nerve branches ([64624])*
Imaging guidance and localization
Injection of genicular nerve branches (64454)
Use of code more than one time per encounter when multiple injections are required to block nerve and branches
1.92 ⚗ 3.15 **FUD** 000   T A2 ▢
AMA: 2018,Jan,8; 2017,Jan,8; 2016,Jan,9; 2016,Jan,13; 2015,Jun,3; 2015,Jan,16; 2014,Jan,11

▲ + **64421** **intercostal nerve, each additional level (List separately in addition to code for primary procedure)**

EXCLUDES *Destruction of genicular nerve branches ([64624])*
Imaging guidance and localization
Injection of genicular nerve branches (64454)
Reporting with modifier 50. Report once for each side when performed bilaterally
Use of code more than one time per encounter when multiple injections are required to block nerve and branches

🔹 2.64   ⚕ 4.46   **FUD** 000   50 T A2 ▢

AMA: 2018,Jan,8; 2017,Jan,8; 2016,Jan,9; 2016,Jan,13; 2015,Jun,3; 2015,Jan,16; 2014,Jan,11

▲ **64425** **ilioinguinal, iliohypogastric nerves**

EXCLUDES *Destruction of genicular nerve branches ([64624])*
Imaging guidance and localization
Injection of genicular nerve branches (64454)
Use of code more than one time per encounter when multiple injections are required to block nerve and branches

🔹 2.72   ⚕ 3.93   **FUD** 000   T P3 50 ▢

AMA: 2018,Jan,8; 2017,Jan,8; 2016,Jan,13; 2015,Jun,3; 2015,Jan,16; 2014,Jan,11

▲ **64430** **pudendal nerve**

EXCLUDES *Destruction of genicular nerve branches ([64624])*
Imaging guidance and localization
Injection of genicular nerve branches (64454)
Use of code more than one time per encounter when multiple injections are required to block nerve and branches

🔹 2.30   ⚕ 4.14   **FUD** 000   T A2 50 ▢

AMA: 2018,Jan,8; 2017,Jan,8; 2016,Jan,13; 2015,Jan,16; 2014,Jan,11

▲ **64435** **paracervical (uterine) nerve**   ♀

EXCLUDES *Destruction of genicular nerve branches ([64624])*
Imaging guidance and localization
Injection of genicular nerve branches (64454)
Use of code more than one time per encounter when multiple injections are required to block nerve and branches

🔹 2.35   ⚕ 4.00   **FUD** 000   T P3 50 ▢

AMA: 2018,Jan,8; 2017,Jan,8; 2016,Jan,13; 2015,Jan,16; 2014,Jan,11

▲ **64445** **sciatic nerve**

EXCLUDES *Destruction of genicular nerve branches ([64624])*
Imaging guidance and localization
Injection of genicular nerve branches (64454)
Use of code more than one time per encounter when multiple injections are required to block nerve and branches

🔹 2.09   ⚕ 3.89   **FUD** 000   T P3 50 ▢

AMA: 2018,Jan,8; 2017,Jan,8; 2016,Jan,13; 2015,Jan,16; 2014,Jan,11

▲ **64446** **sciatic nerve, continuous infusion by catheter (including catheter placement)**

EXCLUDES *Destruction of genicular nerve branches ([64624])*
Imaging guidance and localization
Injection of genicular nerve branches (64454)
Management of epidural or subarachnoid continuous drug administration (01996)
Use of code more than one time per encounter when multiple injections are required to block nerve and branches

🔹 2.28   ⚕ 2.28   **FUD** 000   T G2 50 ▢

AMA: 2018,Jan,8; 2017,Jan,8; 2016,Jan,13; 2015,Jan,16; 2014,Jan,11

▲ **64447** **femoral nerve**

EXCLUDES *Destruction of genicular nerve branches ([64624])*
Imaging guidance and localization
Injection of genicular nerve branches (64454)
Management of epidural or subarachnoid continuous drug administration (01996)
Use of code more than one time per encounter when multiple injections are required to block nerve and branches

🔹 1.91   ⚕ 3.46   **FUD** 000   T P3 50 ▢

AMA: 2018,Jan,8; 2017,Jan,8; 2016,Jan,13; 2015,Sep,12; 2015,Jan,16; 2014,Dec,16; 2014,Dec,16; 2014,Nov,14; 2014,Jan,11

▲ **64448** **femoral nerve, continuous infusion by catheter (including catheter placement)**

EXCLUDES *Destruction of genicular nerve branches ([64624])*
Imaging guidance and localization
Injection of genicular nerve branches (64454)
Management of epidural or subarachnoid continuous drug administration (01996)
Use of code more than one time per encounter when multiple injections are required to block nerve and branches

🔹 2.05   ⚕ 2.05   **FUD** 000   T G2 50 ▢

AMA: 2018,Jan,8; 2017,Jan,8; 2016,Jan,13; 2015,Sep,12; 2015,Jan,16; 2014,Dec,16; 2014,Dec,16; 2014,Nov,14; 2014,Jan,11

▲ **64449** **lumbar plexus, posterior approach, continuous infusion by catheter (including catheter placement)**

EXCLUDES *Destruction of genicular nerve branches ([64624])*
Imaging guidance and localization
Injection of genicular nerve branches (64454)
Management of epidural or subarachnoid continuous drug administration (01996)
Use of code more than one time per encounter when multiple injections are required to block nerve and branches

🔹 2.44   ⚕ 2.44   **FUD** 000   T G2 50 ▢

AMA: 2018,Jan,8; 2017,Jan,8; 2016,Jan,13; 2015,Jan,16; 2014,Jan,11

▲ **64450** **other peripheral nerve or branch**

EXCLUDES *Destruction of genicular nerve branches ([64624])*
Imaging guidance and localization
Injection of genicular nerve branches (64454)
Injection of nerves innervating the sacroiliac joint (64451)
Use of code more than one time per encounter when multiple injections are required to block nerve and branches

🔹 1.28   ⚕ 2.19   **FUD** 000   T P3 50 ▢

AMA: 2018,Nov,10; 2018,Jan,8; 2017,Jan,8; 2016,Oct,11; 2016,Jan,13; 2015,Nov,10; 2015,Sep,12; 2015,Jun,3; 2015,Jan,16; 2014,Jan,11

● **64451** **nerves innervating the sacroiliac joint, with image guidance (ie, fluoroscopy or computed tomography)**

INCLUDES *Imaging guidance and any contrast injection*

EXCLUDES *Destruction of genicular nerve branches ([64624])*
Injection of genicular nerve branches (64454)
Use of code more than one time per encounter when multiple injections are required to block nerve and branches

● **64454** **genicular nerve branches, including imaging guidance, when performed**

INCLUDES *Imaging guidance and any contrast injection*

EXCLUDES *Destruction of genicular nerve branches ([64624])*
Injection of genicular nerve branches (64454)
Use of code more than one time per encounter when multiple injections are required to block nerve and branches

Modifier 52 for injection of fewer than all of the following genicular nerve branches: superolateral, superomedial, and inferomedial

64455 Injection(s), anesthetic agent and/or steroid, plantar common digital nerve(s) (eg, Morton's neuroma)

> INCLUDES Single or multiple injections on the same site
> EXCLUDES *Destruction by neurolytic agent; plantar common digital nerve (64632)*
> *·Destruction of genicular nerve branches ([64624])*
> *Imaging guidance and localization*
> *Injection of genicular nerve branches (64454)*
> *Use of code more than one time per encounter when multiple injections are required to block nerve and branches*

> 🔧 1.00 ⚕ 1.36 **FUD** 000 T P3 80 50 ▣

> **AMA:** 2018,Jan,8; 2017,Jan,8; 2016,Jan,13; 2015,Jan,16; 2014,Jan,11

64461 Resequenced code. See code following 64484.

64462 Resequenced code. See code following 64484.

64463 Resequenced code. See code following 64484.

64479-64484 Transforaminal Injection

> INCLUDES Imaging guidance (fluoroscopy or CT) and contrast injection
> EXCLUDES *Epidural or subarachnoid injection (62320-62327)*
> *Nerve destruction (62280-62282, 64600-64681 [64633, 64634, 64635, 64636])*

64479 Injection(s), anesthetic agent and/or steroid, transforaminal epidural, with imaging guidance (fluoroscopy or CT); cervical or thoracic, single level

> INCLUDES Imaging guidance and any contrast injection
> Single or multiple injections on the same site
> Transforaminal epidural injection at T12-L1 level
> EXCLUDES *Transforaminal epidural injection using ultrasonic guidance (0228T)*

> 🔧 3.76 ⚕ 6.95 **FUD** 000 T A2 50 ▣

> **AMA:** 2018,Jan,8; 2017,Jan,8; 2016,Jan,13; 2016,Jan,9; 2015,Jan,16; 2014,Jan,11

Thoracic vertebra (superior view)

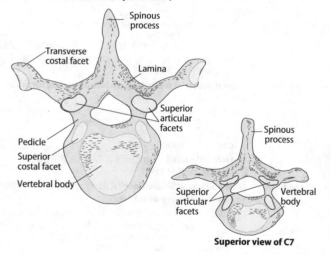

Superior view of C7

+ 64480 cervical or thoracic, each additional level (List separately in addition to code for primary procedure)

> INCLUDES Imaging guidance and any contrast injection
> Single or multiple injections on the same site
> EXCLUDES *Destruction of genicular nerve branches ([64624])*
> *Injection of genicular nerve branches (64454)*
> *Reporting with modifier 50. Report once for each side when performed bilaterally*
> *Transforaminal epidural injection at T12-L1 level*
> *Transforaminal epidural injection using ultrasonic guidance (0229T)*
> *Use of code more than one time per encounter when multiple injections are required to block nerve and branches*
> Code first (64479)

> 🔧 1.80 ⚕ 3.42 **FUD** ZZZ 50 N N1 ▣

> **AMA:** 2018,Jan,8; 2017,Jan,8; 2016,Jan,9; 2016,Jan,13; 2015,Jan,16; 2014,Jan,11

64483 lumbar or sacral, single level

> INCLUDES Imaging guidance and any contrast injection
> Single or multiple injections on the same site
> EXCLUDES *Destruction of genicular nerve branches ([64624])*
> *Injection of genicular nerve branches (64454)*
> *Transforaminal epidural injection using ultrasonic guidance (0230T)*
> *Use of code more than one time per encounter when multiple injections are required to block nerve and branches*

> 🔧 3.19 ⚕ 6.44 **FUD** 000 T A2 50 ▣

> **AMA:** 2018,Jan,8; 2017,Jan,8; 2016,Oct,11; 2016,Jan,13; 2016,Jan,9; 2015,Jan,16; 2014,Jan,11

+ 64484 lumbar or sacral, each additional level (List separately in addition to code for primary procedure)

> INCLUDES Imaging guidance and any contrast injection
> Single or multiple injections on the same site
> EXCLUDES *Destruction of genicular nerve branches ([64624])*
> *Injection of genicular nerve branches (64454)*
> *Reporting with modifier 50. Report once for each side when performed bilaterally*
> *Transforaminal epidural injection using ultrasonic guidance (0231T)*
> *Use of code more than one time per encounter when multiple injections are required to block nerve and branches*
> Code first (64483)

> 🔧 1.49 ⚕ 2.79 **FUD** ZZZ 50 N N1 ▣

> **AMA:** 2018,Jan,8; 2017,Jan,8; 2016,Jan,9; 2016,Jan,13; 2015,Jan,16; 2014,Jan,11

64461-64463 [64461, 64462, 64463] Paravertebral Blocks

> INCLUDES Radiological guidance (76942, 77002-77003)
> EXCLUDES *Injection of:*
> *Anesthetic agent (64420-64421, 64479-64480)*
> *Diagnostic or therapeutic substance (62320, 62324, 64490-64492)*

 # 64461 Paravertebral block (PVB) (paraspinous block), thoracic; single injection site (includes imaging guidance, when performed)

> INCLUDES Imaging guidance and any contrast injection
> EXCLUDES *Destruction of genicular nerve branches ([64624])*
> *Injection of genicular nerve branches (64454)*
> *Use of code more than one time per encounter when multiple injections are required to block nerve and branches*

> 🔧 2.33 ⚕ 3.96 **FUD** 000 T G2 50 ▣

> **AMA:** 2018,Dec,8; 2018,Dec,8; 2018,Jan,8; 2017,Jan,8; 2016,Jan,9

Nervous System

64462 — 64510

+ # 64462 **second and any additional injection site(s) (includes imaging guidance, when performed) (List separately in addition to code for primary procedure)**

INCLUDES Imaging guidance and any contrast injection

EXCLUDES *Destruction of genicular nerve branches ([64624])*
Injection of genicular nerve branches (64454)
Procedure performed more than one time per day
Reporting with modifier 50. Report once for each side when performed bilaterally

Code first (64461)

🔒 1.47 ⚕ 2.20 **FUD** ZZZ   ⑤⓪ Ⓝ Ⓝ1 ▭

AMA: 2018,Dec,8; 2018,Dec,8; 2018,Jan,8; 2017,Jan,8; 2016,Jan,9

 # 64463 **continuous infusion by catheter (includes imaging guidance, when performed)**

INCLUDES Imaging guidance and any contrast injection

EXCLUDES *Destruction of genicular nerve branches ([64624])*
Injection of genicular nerve branches (64454)
Use of code more than one time per encounter when multiple injections are required to block nerve and branches

🔒 2.42 ⚕ 5.13 **FUD** 000   Ⓣ ⑥2 ⑤⓪ ▭

AMA: 2018,Dec,8; 2018,Dec,8; 2018,Jan,8; 2017,Jan,8; 2016,Jan,9

64486-64489 Transversus Abdominis Plane (TAP) Block

64486 **Transversus abdominis plane (TAP) block (abdominal plane block, rectus sheath block) unilateral; by injection(s) (includes imaging guidance, when performed)**

INCLUDES Imaging guidance and any contrast injection

EXCLUDES *Destruction of genicular nerve branches ([64624])*
Injection of genicular nerve branches (64454)
Use of code more than one time per encounter when multiple injections are required to block nerve and branches

🔒 1.61 ⚕ 3.12 **FUD** 000   Ⓝ Ⓝ1 ⑤⓪ ▭

AMA: 2018,Jan,8; 2017,Jan,8; 2016,Jan,13; 2015,Jun,3

64487 **by continuous infusion(s) (includes imaging guidance, when performed)**

INCLUDES Imaging guidance and any contrast injection

EXCLUDES *Destruction of genicular nerve branches ([64624])*
Injection of genicular nerve branches (64454)
Use of code more than one time per encounter when multiple injections are required to block nerve and branches

🔒 1.87 ⚕ 4.49 **FUD** 000   Ⓝ Ⓝ1 ⑤⓪ ▭

AMA: 2018,Jan,8; 2017,Jan,8; 2016,Jan,13; 2015,Jun,3

64488 **Transversus abdominis plane (TAP) block (abdominal plane block, rectus sheath block) bilateral; by injections (includes imaging guidance, when performed)**

INCLUDES Imaging guidance and any contrast injection

EXCLUDES *Destruction of genicular nerve branches ([64624])*
Injection of genicular nerve branches (64454)
Use of code more than one time per encounter when multiple injections are required to block nerve and branches

🔒 2.02 ⚕ 3.83 **FUD** 000   Ⓝ Ⓝ1 ▭

AMA: 2018,Jan,8; 2017,Jan,8; 2016,Jan,13; 2015,Jun,3

64489 **by continuous infusions (includes imaging guidance, when performed)**

INCLUDES Imaging guidance and any contrast injection

EXCLUDES *Destruction of genicular nerve branches ([64624])*
Injection of genicular nerve branches (64454)
Use of code more than one time per encounter when multiple injections are required to block nerve and branches

🔒 2.27 ⚕ 6.65 **FUD** 000   Ⓝ Ⓝ1 ▭

AMA: 2018,Jan,8; 2017,Jan,8; 2016,Jan,13; 2015,Jun,3

64490-64495 Paraspinal Nerve Injections

INCLUDES Image guidance (CT or fluoroscopy) and any contrast injection

EXCLUDES *Injection without imaging (20552-20553)*
Ultrasonic guidance (0213T-0218T)

64490 **Injection(s), diagnostic or therapeutic agent, paravertebral facet (zygapophyseal) joint (or nerves innervating that joint) with image guidance (fluoroscopy or CT), cervical or thoracic; single level**

INCLUDES Injection of T12-L1 joint and nerves that innervate that joint

🔒 3.03 ⚕ 5.39 **FUD** 000   Ⓣ ⑥2 ⑧0 ⑤⓪ ▭

AMA: 2018,Jan,8; 2017,Jan,8; 2016,Jan,9; 2016,Jan,13; 2015,Jan,16; 2014,Jan,11

+ 64491 **second level (List separately in addition to code for primary procedure)**

EXCLUDES *Reporting with modifier 50. Report once for each side when performed bilaterally*

Code first (64490)

🔒 1.72 ⚕ 2.68 **FUD** ZZZ   ⑤⓪ Ⓝ Ⓝ1 ⑧0 ▭

AMA: 2018,Jan,8; 2017,Jan,8; 2016,Jan,9; 2016,Jan,13; 2015,Jan,16; 2014,Jan,11

+ 64492 **third and any additional level(s) (List separately in addition to code for primary procedure)**

EXCLUDES *Procedure performed more than one time per day*
Reporting with modifier 50. Report once for each side when performed bilaterally

Code also when appropriate (64491)
Code first (64490)

🔒 1.74 ⚕ 2.70 **FUD** ZZZ   ⑤⓪ Ⓝ Ⓝ1 ⑧0 ▭

AMA: 2018,Jan,8; 2017,Jan,8; 2016,Jan,9; 2016,Jan,13; 2015,Jan,16; 2014,Jan,11

64493 **Injection(s), diagnostic or therapeutic agent, paravertebral facet (zygapophyseal) joint (or nerves innervating that joint) with image guidance (fluoroscopy or CT), lumbar or sacral; single level**

EXCLUDES *Injection of nerves innervating the sacroiliac joint (64451)*

🔒 2.58 ⚕ 4.91 **FUD** 000   Ⓣ ⑥2 ⑧0 ⑤⓪ ▭

AMA: 2018,May,10; 2018,Jan,8; 2017,Jan,8; 2016,Jan,13; 2015,Jan,16; 2014,Jan,11

+ 64494 **second level (List separately in addition to code for primary procedure)**

EXCLUDES *Reporting with modifier 50. Report once for each side when performed bilaterally*

Code first (64493)

🔒 1.49 ⚕ 2.49 **FUD** ZZZ   ⑤⓪ Ⓝ Ⓝ1 ⑧0 ▭

AMA: 2018,May,10; 2018,Jan,8; 2017,Jan,8; 2016,Jan,13; 2015,Jan,16; 2014,Jan,11

+ 64495 **third and any additional level(s) (List separately in addition to code for primary procedure)**

EXCLUDES *Procedure performed more than one time per day*
Reporting with modifier 50. Report once for each side when performed bilaterally

Code also when appropriate (64494)
Code first (64493)

🔒 1.51 ⚕ 2.49 **FUD** ZZZ   ⑤⓪ Ⓝ Ⓝ1 ⑧0 ▭

AMA: 2018,May,10; 2018,Jan,8; 2017,Jan,8; 2016,Jan,13; 2015,Jan,16; 2014,Jan,11

64505-64530 Sympathetic Nerve Blocks

64505 **Injection, anesthetic agent; sphenopalatine ganglion**

🔒 2.69 ⚕ 3.36 **FUD** 000   Ⓣ P3 ⑤⓪ ▭

AMA: 2018,Jan,8; 2017,Jan,8; 2016,Jan,13; 2015,Jan,16; 2014,Jul,8; 2014,Jan,11

64510 **stellate ganglion (cervical sympathetic)**

🔒 2.13 ⚕ 3.78 **FUD** 000   Ⓣ A2 ⑤⓪ ▭

AMA: 2018,Jan,8; 2017,Jan,8; 2016,Jan,13; 2015,Jan,16; 2014,Jan,11

64517   **superior hypogastric plexus**
   📋 3.60   ⚲ 5.43   **FUD** 000   [T] [A2] 🔲
   AMA: 2018,Jan,8; 2017,Jan,8; 2016,Jan,13; 2015,Jan,16;
   2014,Jan,11

64520   **lumbar or thoracic (paravertebral sympathetic)**
   📋 2.34   ⚲ 5.75   **FUD** 000   [T] [A2] [50] 🔲
   AMA: 2018,Jan,8; 2017,Jan,8; 2016,Jan,13; 2015,Jan,16;
   2014,Jan,11

64530   **celiac plexus, with or without radiologic monitoring**
   EXCLUDES   *Transmural anesthetic injection with transendoscopic*
              ultrasound-guidance (43253)
   📋 2.63   ⚲ 5.73   **FUD** 000   [T] [A2] 🔲
   AMA: 2018,Jan,8; 2017,Jan,8; 2016,Jan,13; 2015,Jan,16;
   2014,Jan,11

64553-64570 Electrical Nerve Stimulation: Insertion/Replacement/Removal/Revision

INCLUDES   Analysis of system at time of implantation (95970)
           Simple and complex neurostimulators
EXCLUDES   *Analysis and programming of neurostimulator pulse generator (95970-95972)*
           TENS therapy (97014, 97032)

64553   **Percutaneous implantation of neurostimulator electrode array; cranial nerve**
   INCLUDES   Temporary and permanent percutaneous array
              placement
   EXCLUDES   *Open procedure (61885-61886)*
              Percutaneous electrical stimulation of peripheral nerve
              with needle or needle electrodes (64999)
   📋 10.1   ⚲ 48.8   **FUD** 010   [J] [J8] [80] 🔲
   AMA: 2019,Feb,6; 2018,Oct,8; 2018,Jan,8; 2017,Jan,8;
   2016,Jan,13; 2015,Jan,16; 2014,Jan,11

64555   **peripheral nerve (excludes sacral nerve)**
   INCLUDES   Temporary and permanent percutaneous array
              placement
   EXCLUDES   *Percutaneous electrical stimulation of a cranial nerve*
              with needle or needle electrodes (64999)
              Posterior tibial neurostimulation (64566)
   📋 9.85   ⚲ 44.3   **FUD** 010   [J] [J8] 🔲
   AMA: 2019,Feb,6; 2018,Oct,8; 2018,Aug,10; 2018,Jan,8;
   2017,Dec,13; 2017,Jan,8; 2016,Feb,13; 2016,Jan,13; 2015,Jan,16;
   2015,Jan,13; 2014,Jan,11

64561   **sacral nerve (transforaminal placement) including image guidance, if performed**
   INCLUDES   Temporary and permanent percutaneous array
              placement
   EXCLUDES   *Percutaneous electrical stimulation or neuromodulation*
              with needle or needle electrodes (64999)
   📋 8.75   ⚲ 20.9   **FUD** 010   [J] [J8] [50] 🔲
   AMA: 2019,Feb,6; 2018,Oct,8; 2018,Jan,8; 2017,Jan,8;
   2016,Jan,13; 2015,Jan,16; 2014,Sep,5; 2014,Jan,11

64566   **Posterior tibial neurostimulation, percutaneous needle electrode, single treatment, includes programming**
   EXCLUDES   *Electronic analysis of implanted neurostimulator pulse*
              generator system (95970-95972)
              Percutaneous implantation of neurostimulator electrode
              array; peripheral nerve (64555)
   📋 0.87   ⚲ 3.62   **FUD** 000   [T] [P3] [80] 🔲
   AMA: 2019,Feb,6; 2018,Oct,8; 2018,Jan,8; 2017,Jan,8;
   2016,Jan,13; 2015,Jan,16; 2014,Jan,11

64568   **Incision for implantation of cranial nerve (eg, vagus nerve) neurostimulator electrode array and pulse generator**
   EXCLUDES   *Insertion chest wall respiratory sensor electrode or array*
              with pulse generator connection (0466T)
              Insertion, replacement of cranial neurostimulator pulse
              generator or receiver (61885-61886)
              Removal of neurostimulator electrode array and pulse
              generator (64570)
   📋 18.4   ⚲ 18.4   **FUD** 090   [J] [J8] [80] [50] 🔲
   AMA: 2019,Feb,6; 2018,Mar,9; 2018,Jan,8; 2017,Jan,8;
   2016,Nov,6; 2016,Jan,13; 2015,Jan,16; 2014,Jan,11

64569   **Revision or replacement of cranial nerve (eg, vagus nerve) neurostimulator electrode array, including connection to existing pulse generator**
   EXCLUDES   *Removal of neurostimulator electrode array and pulse*
              generator (64570)
              Replacement of pulse generator (61885)
              Revision or replacement chest wall respiratory sensor
              electrode with pulse generator connection (0467T)
              Revision, removal pulse generator (61888)
   📋 22.1   ⚲ 22.1   **FUD** 090   [J] [J8] [80] [50] 🔲
   AMA: 2019,Feb,6; 2018,Mar,9; 2018,Jan,8; 2017,Jan,8;
   2016,Nov,6; 2016,Jan,13; 2015,Jan,16; 2014,Jan,11

64570   **Removal of cranial nerve (eg, vagus nerve) neurostimulator electrode array and pulse generator**
   EXCLUDES   *Laparoscopic revision, replacement, removal, or*
              implantation of vagus nerve blocking
              neurostimulator pulse generator and/or electrode
              array at the esophagogastric junction
              (0312T-0317T)
              Removal of chest wall respiratory sensor electrode or
              array (0468T)
              Revision, removal pulse generator (61888)
   📋 21.4   ⚲ 21.4   **FUD** 090   [02] [G2] [80] [50] 🔲
   AMA: 2019,Feb,6; 2018,Mar,9; 2018,Jan,8; 2017,Jan,8;
   2016,Nov,6; 2016,Jan,13; 2015,Jan,16; 2014,Jan,11

64575-64595 Implantation/Revision/Removal Neurostimulators: Incisional

INCLUDES   Simple and complex neurostimulators
EXCLUDES   *Analysis and programming of neurostimulator pulse generator (95970-95972)*

64575   **Incision for implantation of neurostimulator electrode array; peripheral nerve (excludes sacral nerve)**
   📋 9.60   ⚲ 9.60   **FUD** 090   [J] [J8] 🔲
   AMA: 2019,Feb,6; 2014,Jan,11

64580   **neuromuscular**
   📋 8.88   ⚲ 8.88   **FUD** 090   [J] [G2] [80] 🔲
   AMA: 2019,Feb,6; 2014,Jan,11

64581   **sacral nerve (transforaminal placement)**
   📋 19.0   ⚲ 19.0   **FUD** 090   [J] [J8] 🔲
   AMA: 2019,Feb,6; 2018,Jan,8; 2017,Jan,8; 2016,Jan,13;
   2015,Jan,16; 2014,Sep,5; 2014,Jan,11

64585   **Revision or removal of peripheral neurostimulator electrode array**
   📋 4.14   ⚲ 7.03   **FUD** 010   [02] [A2] 🔲
   AMA: 2019,Feb,6; 2014,Jan,11

64590   **Insertion or replacement of peripheral or gastric neurostimulator pulse generator or receiver, direct or inductive coupling**
   EXCLUDES   *Revision, removal of neurostimulator pulse generator*
              (64595)
   📋 4.64   ⚲ 7.60   **FUD** 010   [J] [J8] 🔲
   AMA: 2019,Feb,6; 2018,Aug,10; 2018,Jan,8; 2017,Dec,13;
   2017,Jan,8; 2016,Jan,13; 2015,Jan,13; 2015,Jan,16; 2014,Jan,11

64595   **Revision or removal of peripheral or gastric neurostimulator pulse generator or receiver**
   EXCLUDES   *Insertion, replacement of neurostimulator pulse*
              generator (64590)
   📋 3.63   ⚲ 6.89   **FUD** 010   [02] [J8] 🔲
   AMA: 2019,Feb,6; 2018,Jan,8; 2017,Jan,8; 2016,Jan,13;
   2015,Jan,16; 2014,Jan,11

64600-64610 Chemical Denervation Trigeminal Nerve

INCLUDES   Injection of therapeutic medication

EXCLUDES   *Electromyography or muscle electric stimulation guidance (95873-95874)*
Nerve destruction of:
Anal sphincter (46505)
Bladder (52287)
Strabismus that involves the extraocular muscles (67345)
Treatments that do not destroy the target nerve (64999)
Code also chemodenervation agent

64600   Destruction by neurolytic agent, trigeminal nerve; supraorbital, infraorbital, mental, or inferior alveolar branch

  6.66   12.3   **FUD** 010   T A2

AMA: 2019,Apr,9; 2018,Jan,8; 2017,Jan,8; 2016,Jan,13; 2015,Jan,16; 2014,Jan,11

Supratrochlear nerve
Supraorbital nerve
Trigeminal nerve (CN V) branches in infratemporal fossa
V2 branch
V1 branch
Infraorbital nerve
V3 branch
Temporal
Zygomatic
Mental nerve
Mental foramen
Cervical

64605   second and third division branches at foramen ovale

  10.0   16.8   **FUD** 010   J A2 80 50

AMA: 2019,Apr,9; 2018,Jan,8; 2017,Jan,8; 2016,Jan,13; 2015,Jan,16; 2014,Jan,11

64610   second and third division branches at foramen ovale under radiologic monitoring

  14.2   22.0   **FUD** 010   J A2 50

AMA: 2019,Apr,9; 2018,Jan,8; 2017,Apr,9; 2017,Jan,8; 2016,Jan,13; 2015,Jan,16; 2014,Jan,11

64624 [64624] Chemical Denervation Genicular Nerve Branches

● #   **64624   Destruction by neurolytic agent, genicular nerve branches including imaging guidance, when performed**

  0.00   0.00   **FUD** 000

EXCLUDES   *Injection of genicular nerve branches (64454)*
Code also modifier 52 for destruction of fewer than all of the following genicular nerve branches: superolateral, superomedial, and inferomedial

64625 [64625] Radiofrequency Ablation Sacroiliac Joint Nerves

● #   **64625   Radiofrequency ablation, nerves innervating the sacroiliac joint, with image guidance (ie, fluoroscopy or computed tomography)**

  0.00   0.00   **FUD** 000

INCLUDES   CT needle guidance (77012)
Electrical stimulation or needle electromyelograph for guidance (95873-95874)
Fluoroscopic needle guidance or localization (77002-77003)

EXCLUDES   *Destruction by neurolytic agent, paravertebral facet joint nerve ([64624])*
Radiofrequency ablation with ultrasound (76999)

64611-64617 Chemical Denervation Procedures Head and Neck

INCLUDES   Injection of therapeutic medication

EXCLUDES   *Electromyography or muscle electric stimulation guidance (95873-95874)*
Nerve destruction of:
Anal sphincter (46505)
Bladder (52287)
Extraocular muscles to treat strabismus (67345)
Treatments that do not destroy the target nerve (64999)

64611   Chemodenervation of parotid and submandibular salivary glands, bilateral

Code also modifier 52 for injection of fewer than four salivary glands

  3.03   3.45   **FUD** 010   T P3 80

AMA: 2019,Apr,9; 2018,Jan,8; 2017,Jan,8; 2016,Jan,13; 2015,Jan,16; 2014,Jan,11

64612   Chemodenervation of muscle(s); muscle(s) innervated by facial nerve, unilateral (eg, for blepharospasm, hemifacial spasm)

  3.39   3.83   **FUD** 010   T P3 50

AMA: 2019,Apr,9; 2018,Jan,8; 2017,Jan,8; 2016,Jan,13; 2015,Jan,16; 2014,May,5; 2014,Jan,11; 2014,Jan,6

64615   muscle(s) innervated by facial, trigeminal, cervical spinal and accessory nerves, bilateral (eg, for chronic migraine)

EXCLUDES   *Chemodenervation (64612, 64616-64617, 64642-64647)*
Procedure performed more than one time per session
Code also any guidance by muscle electrical stimulation or needle electromyography but report only once (95873-95874)

  3.58   4.27   **FUD** 010   T P3

AMA: 2019,Apr,9; 2018,Jan,8; 2017,Jan,8; 2016,Jan,13; 2015,Jan,16; 2014,Jan,11; 2014,Jan,6

64616   neck muscle(s), excluding muscles of the larynx, unilateral (eg, for cervical dystonia, spasmodic torticollis)

Code also guidance by muscle electrical stimulation or needle electromyography, but report only once (95873-95874)

  3.18   3.80   **FUD** 010   T P3 50

AMA: 2019,Apr,9; 2018,Jan,8; 2017,Jan,8; 2016,Jan,13; 2015,Jan,16; 2014,May,5; 2014,Jan,6; 2014,Jan,11

64617   larynx, unilateral, percutaneous (eg, for spasmodic dysphonia), includes guidance by needle electromyography, when performed

EXCLUDES   *Chemodenervation of larynx via direct laryngoscopy (31570-31571)*
Diagnostic needle electromyography of larynx (95865)
Electrical stimulation guidance for chemodenervation (95873-95874)

  3.14   4.62   **FUD** 010   T P3 50

AMA: 2019,Apr,9; 2018,Jan,8; 2017,Jan,8; 2016,Jan,13; 2015,Jan,16; 2014,Jan,6; 2014,Jan,11

64620-64640 [64633, 64634, 64635, 64636] Chemical Denervation Intercostal, Facet Joint, Plantar, and Pudendal Nerve(s)

INCLUDES   Injection of therapeutic medication

64620   Destruction by neurolytic agent, intercostal nerve

  5.00   5.91   **FUD** 010   T A2

AMA: 2019,Apr,9; 2018,Jan,8; 2017,Jan,8; 2016,Jan,13; 2015,Jan,16; 2014,Jan,6; 2014,Jan,11

64624   **Resequenced code. See code following 64610.**

64625   **Resequenced code. See code before 64611.**

| 26/TC PC/TC Only | A2-Z3 ASC Payment | 50 Bilateral | ♂ Male Only | ♀ Female Only | Facility RVU | Non-Facility RVU | CCI | CLIA |
| FUD Follow-up Days | CMS: IOM | AMA: CPT Asst | A-Y OPPSI | 80/80 Surg Assist Allowed / w/Doc | Lab Crosswalk | Radiology Crosswalk | | |

306

CPT © 2019 American Medical Association. All Rights Reserved.

© 2019 Optum360, LLC

Nervous System

64600 — 64625

**64633** **Destruction by neurolytic agent, paravertebral facet joint nerve(s), with imaging guidance (fluoroscopy or CT); cervical or thoracic, single facet joint**

INCLUDES Paravertebral facet destruction of T12-L1 joint or nerve(s) that innervate that joint
Radiological guidance (77003, 77012)

EXCLUDES *Denervation performed using chemical, low grade thermal, or pulsed radiofrequency methods (64999)*
Destruction of paravertebral facet joint nerve(s) without imaging guidance (64999)

6.43 ⚕ 11.8 **FUD** 010 J 62 50 🖪

AMA: 2019,Apr,9; 2018,Jan,8; 2017,Jan,8; 2016,Jan,13; 2015,Feb,9; 2015,Jan,16; 2014,Jan,11

+ # **64634** **cervical or thoracic, each additional facet joint (List separately in addition to code for primary procedure)**

INCLUDES Radiological guidance (77003, 77012)

EXCLUDES *Denervation performed using chemical, low grade thermal, or pulsed radiofrequency methods (64999)*
Destruction of paravertebral facet joint nerve(s) without imaging guidance (64999)
Reporting with modifier 50. Report once for each side when performed bilaterally

Code first ([64633])

1.95 ⚕ 5.34 **FUD** ZZZ 50 N N1 🖪

AMA: 2019,Apr,9; 2018,Jan,8; 2017,Jan,8; 2016,Jan,13; 2015,Feb,9; 2015,Jan,16; 2014,Jan,11

**64635** **lumbar or sacral, single facet joint**

INCLUDES Radiological guidance (77003, 77012)

EXCLUDES *Denervation performed using chemical, low grade thermal, or pulsed radiofrequency methods (64999)*
Destruction of individual nerves, sacroiliac joint, by neurolytic agent (64640)
Destruction of paravertebral facet joint nerve(s) without imaging guidance (64999)

6.34 ⚕ 11.7 **FUD** 010 J 62 50 🖪

AMA: 2019,Apr,9; 2018,Jan,8; 2017,Jan,8; 2016,Jan,13; 2015,Feb,9; 2015,Jan,16; 2014,Jan,11

+ # **64636** **lumbar or sacral, each additional facet joint (List separately in addition to code for primary procedure)**

INCLUDES Radiological guidance (77003, 77012)

EXCLUDES *Denervation performed using chemical, low grade thermal, or pulsed radiofrequency methods (64999)*
Destruction of individual nerves, sacroiliac joint, by neurolytic agent (64640)
Destruction of paravertebral facet joint nerve(s) without imaging guidance (64999)
Reporting with modifier 50. Report once for each side when performed bilaterally

Code first ([64635])

1.71 ⚕ 4.85 **FUD** ZZZ 50 N N1 🖪

AMA: 2019,Apr,9; 2018,Jan,8; 2017,Jan,8; 2016,Jan,13; 2015,Feb,9; 2015,Jan,16; 2014,Jan,11

64630 **Destruction by neurolytic agent; pudendal nerve**

5.47 ⚕ 6.77 **FUD** 010 T A2 80 🖪

AMA: 2019,Apr,9; 2018,Jan,8; 2017,Oct,9; 2017,Jan,8; 2016,Jan,13; 2015,Jan,16; 2014,Jan,11

64632 **plantar common digital nerve**

EXCLUDES *Injection(s), anesthetic agent and/or steroid (64455)*

1.96 ⚕ 2.45 **FUD** 010 T P3 80 50 🖪

AMA: 2019,Apr,9; 2018,Jan,8; 2017,Oct,9; 2017,Jan,8; 2016,Jan,13; 2015,Jul,10; 2015,Jan,16; 2014,Jan,11

64633 **Resequenced code. See code following 64620.**

64634 **Resequenced code. See code following 64620.**

64635 **Resequenced code. See code following 64620.**

64636 **Resequenced code. See code before 64630.**

64640 **other peripheral nerve or branch**

INCLUDES Neurolytic destruction of nerves of sacroiliac joint

2.69 ⚕ 3.86 **FUD** 010 T P3 50 🖪

AMA: 2019,Apr,9; 2018,Jan,8; 2018,Jan,7; 2017,Oct,9; 2017,Jan,8; 2016,Jan,13; 2015,Jan,16; 2014,Jan,11

64642-64645 Chemical Denervation Extremity Muscles

INCLUDES Trunk muscles include erector spine, obliques, paraspinal, and rectus abdominus. The rest of the muscles are considered neck, head or extremity muscles

EXCLUDES *Chemodenervation with needle-guided electromyography or with guidance provided by muscle electrical stimulation (95873-95874)*
Procedure performed more than once per extremity
Code also other extremities when appropriate, up to a total of 4 units per patient (if all extremities are injected) (64642-64645)

64642 **Chemodenervation of one extremity; 1-4 muscle(s)**

EXCLUDES *Use of more than one base code per session (64642)*

3.12 ⚕ 4.15 **FUD** 000 T P3

AMA: 2019,Aug,10; 2019,Apr,9; 2018,Jan,8; 2017,Jan,8; 2016,Jan,13; 2015,Jan,16; 2014,Oct,14; 2014,Jan,6; 2014,Jan,11

+ **64643** **each additional extremity, 1-4 muscle(s) (List separately in addition to code for primary procedure)**

Code first (64642, 64644)

2.08 ⚕ 2.65 **FUD** ZZZ N N1 🖪

AMA: 2019,Aug,10; 2019,Apr,9; 2018,Jan,8; 2017,Jan,8; 2016,Jan,13; 2015,Jan,16; 2014,Oct,14; 2014,Jan,6; 2014,Jan,11

64644 **Chemodenervation of one extremity; 5 or more muscles**

3.42 ⚕ 4.82 **FUD** 000 T P3 🖪

AMA: 2019,Aug,10; 2019,Apr,9; 2018,Jan,8; 2017,Jan,8; 2016,Jan,13; 2015,Jan,16; 2014,Oct,14; 2014,Jan,6; 2014,Jan,11

+ **64645** **each additional extremity, 5 or more muscles (List separately in addition to code for primary procedure)**

Code first (64644)

2.40 ⚕ 3.33 **FUD** ZZZ N N1 🖪

AMA: 2019,Aug,10; 2019,Apr,9; 2018,Jan,8; 2017,Jan,8; 2016,Jan,13; 2015,Jan,16; 2014,Oct,14; 2014,Jan,6; 2014,Jan,11

64646-64647 Chemical Denervation Trunk Muscles

EXCLUDES *Procedure performed more than once per session*

64646 **Chemodenervation of trunk muscle(s); 1-5 muscle(s)**

3.34 ⚕ 4.35 **FUD** 000 T P3 🖪

AMA: 2019,Apr,9; 2018,Jan,8; 2017,Jan,8; 2016,Jan,13; 2015,Jan,16; 2014,Jan,6; 2014,Jan,11

64647 **6 or more muscles**

3.96 ⚕ 5.12 **FUD** 000 T P3 🖪

AMA: 2019,Apr,9; 2018,Jan,8; 2017,Jan,8; 2016,Jan,13; 2015,Jan,16; 2014,Jan,6; 2014,Jan,11

64650-64653 Chemical Denervation Eccrine Glands

INCLUDES Injection of therapeutic medication

EXCLUDES *Bladder chemodenervation (52287)*
Chemodenervation of extremities (64999)
Code also drugs or other substances used

64650 **Chemodenervation of eccrine glands; both axillae**

1.21 ⚕ 2.25 **FUD** 000 T P3 80 🖪

AMA: 2019,Apr,9; 2018,Jan,8; 2017,Jan,8; 2016,Jan,13; 2015,Jan,16; 2014,Jan,11

64653 **other area(s) (eg, scalp, face, neck), per day**

1.55 ⚕ 2.76 **FUD** 000 T P3 80 🖪

AMA: 2019,Apr,9; 2018,Jan,8; 2017,Jan,8; 2016,Jan,13; 2015,Jan,16; 2014,Jan,11

64680-64681 Neurolysis: Celiac Plexus, Superior Hypogastric Plexus

INCLUDES Injection of therapeutic medication

64680 **Destruction by neurolytic agent, with or without radiologic monitoring; celiac plexus**

EXCLUDES *Transmural neurolytic agent injection with transendoscopic ultrasound guidance (43253)*

4.66 ⚕ 9.07 **FUD** 010 T A2 🖪

AMA: 2019,Apr,9; 2018,Jan,8; 2017,Jan,8; 2016,Jan,13; 2015,Jan,16; 2014,Jan,11

● New Code   ▲ Revised Code   ○ Reinstated   ● New Web Release   ▲ Revised Web Release   + Add-on   Unlisted   Not Covered   # Resequenced
50 Optum Mod 50 Exempt   Ⓢ AMA Mod 51 Exempt   51 Optum Mod 51 Exempt   63 Mod 63 Exempt   ✗ Non-FDA Drug   ★ Telemedicine   M Maternity   A Age Edit

CPT © 2019 American Medical Association. All Rights Reserved.

Nervous System

64681 — 64776

64681	**superior hypogastric plexus**

📖 7.87   ⚗ 16.4   **FUD** 010   T A2

AMA: 2019,Apr,9; 2018,Jan,8; 2017,Jan,8; 2016,Jan,13; 2015,Jan,16; 2014,Jan,11

64702-64727 Decompression and/or Transposition of Nerve

INCLUDES   External neurolysis and/or transposition to repair or restore a nerve
Neuroplasty with nerve wrapping
Surgical decompression/freeing of nerve from scar tissue

EXCLUDES   *Facial nerve decompression (69720)*
Percutaneous neurolysis (62263-62264, 62280-62282)

64702	**Neuroplasty; digital, 1 or both, same digit**

📖 14.4   ⚗ 14.4   **FUD** 090   J A2

AMA: 2018,Jan,8; 2017,Jan,8; 2016,Jan,13; 2015,Jan,16; 2014,Jan,11

64704	**nerve of hand or foot**

📖 9.23   ⚗ 9.23   **FUD** 090   J A2 80

AMA: 2018,Jan,8; 2017,Jan,8; 2016,Jan,13; 2015,Jan,16; 2014,Jan,11

64708	**Neuroplasty, major peripheral nerve, arm or leg, open; other than specified**

📖 14.4   ⚗ 14.4   **FUD** 090   J G2 80

AMA: 2018,Jan,8; 2017,Nov,10; 2017,Jan,8; 2016,Jan,13; 2015,Jan,16; 2014,Jan,11

64712	**sciatic nerve**

📖 16.7   ⚗ 16.7   **FUD** 090   J G2 80 50

AMA: 2018,Jan,8; 2017,Jan,8; 2016,Jan,13; 2015,Jan,16; 2014,Jan,11

64713	**brachial plexus**

📖 22.4   ⚗ 22.4   **FUD** 090   J G2 80 50

AMA: 2018,Jan,8; 2017,Jan,8; 2016,Jan,13; 2015,Jan,16; 2014,Jan,11

64714	**lumbar plexus**

📖 20.8   ⚗ 20.8   **FUD** 090   J G2 80 50

AMA: 2018,Jan,8; 2017,Jan,8; 2016,Jan,13; 2015,Jan,16; 2014,Jan,11

64716	**Neuroplasty and/or transposition; cranial nerve (specify)**

📖 15.0   ⚗ 15.0   **FUD** 090   J A2 80

AMA: 2018,Jan,8; 2017,Jan,8; 2016,Jan,13; 2015,Jan,16; 2014,Jan,11

64718	**ulnar nerve at elbow**

📖 17.0   ⚗ 17.0   **FUD** 090   J A2 80 50

AMA: 2018,Jan,8; 2017,Jan,8; 2016,Jan,13; 2015,Jan,16; 2014,Jan,11

64719	**ulnar nerve at wrist**

📖 11.5   ⚗ 11.5   **FUD** 090   J A2 50

AMA: 2018,Jan,8; 2017,Jan,8; 2016,Jan,13; 2015,Jan,16; 2014,Jan,11

64721	**median nerve at carpal tunnel**

EXCLUDES   *Arthroscopic procedure (29848)*

📖 12.3   ⚗ 12.4   **FUD** 090   J A2 50

AMA: 2018,Jan,8; 2017,Jan,8; 2016,Jan,13; 2015,Jul,10; 2015,Jan,16; 2014,Jan,11

64722	**Decompression; unspecified nerve(s) (specify)**

📖 10.2   ⚗ 10.2   **FUD** 090   J A2 80

AMA: 2018,Jan,8; 2017,Jan,8; 2016,Jan,13; 2015,Jan,16; 2014,Jan,11

64726	**plantar digital nerve**

📖 7.80   ⚗ 7.80   **FUD** 090   J A2

AMA: 2018,Jan,8; 2017,Jan,8; 2016,Jan,13; 2015,Jan,16; 2014,Jan,11

+	64727	**Internal neurolysis, requiring use of operating microscope (List separately in addition to code for neuroplasty) (Neuroplasty includes external neurolysis)**

INCLUDES   Operating microscope (69990)
Code first neuroplasty (64702-64721)

📖 5.31   ⚗ 5.31   **FUD** ZZZ   N N1

AMA: 2018,Jan,8; 2017,Jan,8; 2016,Feb,12; 2016,Jan,13; 2015,Jan,16; 2014,Jan,11

64732-64772 Surgical Avulsion/Transection of Nerve

EXCLUDES   *Stereotactic lesion of gasserian ganglion (61790)*

64732	**Transection or avulsion of; supraorbital nerve**

📖 12.8   ⚗ 12.8   **FUD** 090   J A2 80 50

AMA: 2018,Jan,8; 2017,Jan,8; 2016,Jan,13; 2015,Jan,16; 2014,Jan,11

64734	**infraorbital nerve**

📖 14.5   ⚗ 14.5   **FUD** 090   J A2 80 50

AMA: 2014,Jan,11

64736	**mental nerve**

📖 10.7   ⚗ 10.7   **FUD** 090   J A2 80 50

AMA: 2014,Jan,11

64738	**inferior alveolar nerve by osteotomy**

📖 13.3   ⚗ 13.3   **FUD** 090   J A2 80 50

AMA: 2014,Jan,11

64740	**lingual nerve**

📖 14.0   ⚗ 14.0   **FUD** 090   J A2 80 50

AMA: 2014,Jan,11

64742	**facial nerve, differential or complete**

📖 14.1   ⚗ 14.1   **FUD** 090   J A2 80 50

AMA: 2014,Jan,11

64744	**greater occipital nerve**

📖 14.2   ⚗ 14.2   **FUD** 090   J A2 80 50

AMA: 2014,Jan,11

64746	**phrenic nerve**

📖 12.4   ⚗ 12.4   **FUD** 090   J A2 80 50

AMA: 2014,Jan,11

64755	**vagus nerves limited to proximal stomach (selective proximal vagotomy, proximal gastric vagotomy, parietal cell vagotomy, supra- or highly selective vagotomy)**

EXCLUDES   *Laparoscopic procedure (43652)*

📖 26.6   ⚗ 26.6   **FUD** 090   C 80

AMA: 2018,Jan,8; 2017,Jan,8; 2016,Jan,13; 2015,Jan,16; 2014,Jan,11

64760	**vagus nerve (vagotomy), abdominal**

EXCLUDES   *Laparoscopic procedure (43651)*

📖 14.9   ⚗ 14.9   **FUD** 090   C 80

AMA: 2018,Jan,8; 2017,Jan,8; 2016,Jan,13; 2015,Jan,16; 2014,Jan,11

64763	**Transection or avulsion of obturator nerve, extrapelvic, with or without adductor tenotomy**

📖 14.7   ⚗ 14.7   **FUD** 090   J G2 80 50

AMA: 2014,Jan,11

64766	**Transection or avulsion of obturator nerve, intrapelvic, with or without adductor tenotomy**

📖 18.2   ⚗ 18.2   **FUD** 090   J G2 80 50

AMA: 2014,Jan,11

64771	**Transection or avulsion of other cranial nerve, extradural**

📖 17.0   ⚗ 17.0   **FUD** 090   J A2 80

AMA: 2014,Jan,11

64772	**Transection or avulsion of other spinal nerve, extradural**

EXCLUDES   *Removal of tender scar and soft tissue including neuroma if necessary (11400-11446, 13100-13153)*

📖 16.2   ⚗ 16.2   **FUD** 090   J A2 80

AMA: 2018,Jan,8; 2017,Jan,8; 2016,Jan,13; 2015,Apr,10; 2014,Jan,11

64774-64823 Excisional Nerve Procedures

EXCLUDES   *Morton neuroma excision (28080)*

64774	**Excision of neuroma; cutaneous nerve, surgically identifiable**

📖 11.7   ⚗ 11.7   **FUD** 090   J A2

AMA: 2014,Jan,11

64776	**digital nerve, 1 or both, same digit**

📖 11.1   ⚗ 11.1   **FUD** 090   J A2 80

AMA: 2014,Jan,11

26/TC PC/TC Only   A2-Z3 ASC Payment   50 Bilateral   ♂ Male Only   ♀ Female Only   📖 Facility RVU   ⚗ Non-Facility RVU   CCI   CLIA
FUD Follow-up Days   CMS: IOM   AMA: CPT Asst   A-Y OPPSI   80/80 Surg Assist Allowed / w/Doc   Lab Crosswalk   Radiology Crosswalk

308   CPT © 2019 American Medical Association. All Rights Reserved.   © 2019 Optum360, LLC

+ **64778** **digital nerve, each additional digit (List separately in addition to code for primary procedure)**
Code first (64776)
⏱ 5.30   ⚕ 5.30   **FUD** ZZZ   N N1 ▭
AMA: 2014,Jan,11

64782 **hand or foot, except digital nerve**
⏱ 13.2   ⚕ 13.2   **FUD** 090   J A2 ▭
AMA: 2014,Jan,11

+ **64783** **hand or foot, each additional nerve, except same digit (List separately in addition to code for primary procedure)**
Code first (64782)
⏱ 6.33   ⚕ 6.33   **FUD** ZZZ   N N1 ▭
AMA: 2014,Jan,11

64784 **major peripheral nerve, except sciatic**
⏱ 20.9   ⚕ 20.9   **FUD** 090   J A2 80 ▭
AMA: 2014,Jan,11

64786 **sciatic nerve**
⏱ 29.0   ⚕ 29.0   **FUD** 090   J A2 80 50 ▭
AMA: 2014,Jan,11

+ **64787** **Implantation of nerve end into bone or muscle (List separately in addition to neuroma excision)**
Code also, when appropriate (64774-64786)
⏱ 6.96   ⚕ 6.96   **FUD** ZZZ   N N1 80 ▭
AMA: 2014,Jan,11

64788 **Excision of neurofibroma or neurolemmoma; cutaneous nerve**
⏱ 11.5   ⚕ 11.5   **FUD** 090   J A2 ▭
AMA: 2018,Jan,8; 2017,Jan,8; 2016,Apr,3; 2014,Jan,11

64790 **major peripheral nerve**
⏱ 24.1   ⚕ 24.1   **FUD** 090   J A2 80 ▭
AMA: 2018,Jan,8; 2017,Jan,8; 2016,Apr,3; 2014,Jan,11

64792 **extensive (including malignant type)**
EXCLUDES Destruction neurofibroma of skin (0419T-0420T)
⏱ 31.4   ⚕ 31.4   **FUD** 090   J A2 80 ▭
AMA: 2018,Jan,8; 2017,Jan,8; 2016,Apr,3; 2014,Jan,11

64795 **Biopsy of nerve**
⏱ 5.64   ⚕ 5.64   **FUD** 000   J A2 ▭
AMA: 2014,Jan,11

64802 **Sympathectomy, cervical**
⏱ 24.3   ⚕ 24.3   **FUD** 090   J A2 80 50 ▭
AMA: 2014,Jan,11

64804 **Sympathectomy, cervicothoracic**
⏱ 34.7   ⚕ 34.7   **FUD** 090   J 80 50 ▭
AMA: 2014,Jan,11

64809 **Sympathectomy, thoracolumbar**
INCLUDES Leriche sympathectomy
⏱ 31.8   ⚕ 31.8   **FUD** 090   C 80 50 ▭
AMA: 2014,Jan,11

64818 **Sympathectomy, lumbar**
⏱ 22.5   ⚕ 22.5   **FUD** 090   C 80 50 ▭
AMA: 2014,Jan,11

64820 **Sympathectomy; digital arteries, each digit**
INCLUDES Operating microscope (69990)
⏱ 20.5   ⚕ 20.5   **FUD** 090   J G2 ▭
AMA: 2018,Jan,8; 2017,Jan,8; 2016,Feb,12; 2016,Jan,13; 2015,Jan,16; 2014,Jan,11

64821 **radial artery**
INCLUDES Operating microscope (69990)
⏱ 20.0   ⚕ 20.0   **FUD** 090   J A2 50 ▭
AMA: 2016,Feb,12; 2014,Jan,11

64822 **ulnar artery**
INCLUDES Operating microscope (69990)
⏱ 20.0   ⚕ 20.0   **FUD** 090   J G2 50 ▭
AMA: 2016,Feb,12; 2014,Jan,11

64823 **superficial palmar arch**
INCLUDES Operating microscope (69990)
⏱ 22.7   ⚕ 22.7   **FUD** 090   J G2 50 ▭
AMA: 2016,Feb,12; 2014,Jan,11

64831-64907 Nerve Repair: Suture and Nerve Grafts

64831 **Suture of digital nerve, hand or foot; 1 nerve**
⏱ 19.7   ⚕ 19.7   **FUD** 090   J A2 50 ▭
AMA: 2018,Jan,8; 2017,Jan,8; 2016,Jan,13; 2015,Jan,16; 2014,Sep,13; 2014,Jan,11

+ **64832** **each additional digital nerve (List separately in addition to code for primary procedure)**
Code first (64831)
⏱ 9.73   ⚕ 9.73   **FUD** ZZZ   N N1 80 ▭
AMA: 2018,Jan,8; 2017,Jan,8; 2016,Jan,13; 2015,Jan,16; 2014,Jan,11

64834 **Suture of 1 nerve; hand or foot, common sensory nerve**
⏱ 21.3   ⚕ 21.3   **FUD** 090   J A2 80 50 ▭
AMA: 2014,Jan,11

64835 **median motor thenar**
⏱ 23.4   ⚕ 23.4   **FUD** 090   J A2 80 50 ▭
AMA: 2014,Jan,11

64836 **ulnar motor**
⏱ 23.5   ⚕ 23.5   **FUD** 090   J A2 80 50 ▭
AMA: 2014,Jan,11

+ **64837** **Suture of each additional nerve, hand or foot (List separately in addition to code for primary procedure)**
Code first (64834-64836)
⏱ 10.6   ⚕ 10.6   **FUD** ZZZ   N N1 80 ▭
AMA: 2014,Jan,11

64840 **Suture of posterior tibial nerve**
⏱ 27.8   ⚕ 27.8   **FUD** 090   J A2 80 50 ▭
AMA: 2014,Jan,11

64856 **Suture of major peripheral nerve, arm or leg, except sciatic; including transposition**
⏱ 29.2   ⚕ 29.2   **FUD** 090   J A2 ▭
AMA: 2014,Jan,11

64857 **without transposition**
⏱ 30.4   ⚕ 30.4   **FUD** 090   J A2 80 ▭
AMA: 2014,Jan,11

64858 **Suture of sciatic nerve**
⏱ 34.0   ⚕ 34.0   **FUD** 090   J A2 80 50 ▭
AMA: 2014,Jan,11

+ **64859** **Suture of each additional major peripheral nerve (List separately in addition to code for primary procedure)**
Code first (64856-64857)
⏱ 7.24   ⚕ 7.24   **FUD** ZZZ   N N1 80 ▭
AMA: 2014,Jan,11

64861 **Suture of; brachial plexus**
⏱ 44.5   ⚕ 44.5   **FUD** 090   J A2 80 50 ▭
AMA: 2014,Jan,11

64862 **lumbar plexus**
⏱ 39.3   ⚕ 39.3   **FUD** 090   J A2 80 50 ▭
AMA: 2014,Jan,11

64864 **Suture of facial nerve; extracranial**
⏱ 24.9   ⚕ 24.9   **FUD** 090   J A2 80 ▭
AMA: 2014,Jan,11

64865 **infratemporal, with or without grafting**
⏱ 31.4   ⚕ 31.4   **FUD** 090   J A2 80 ▭
AMA: 2014,Jan,11

64866 **Anastomosis; facial-spinal accessory**
⏱ 36.7   ⚕ 36.7   **FUD** 090   C 80 ▭
AMA: 2014,Jan,11

64868 **facial-hypoglossal**
INCLUDES Korte-Ballance anastomosis
⏱ 28.8   ⚕ 28.8   **FUD** 090   C 80 ▭
AMA: 2014,Jan,11

● New Code   ▲ Revised Code   ○ Reinstated   ● New Web Release   ▲ Revised Web Release   + Add-on   Unlisted   Not Covered   # Resequenced
50 Optum Mod 50 Exempt   ⊘ AMA Mod 51 Exempt   51 Optum Mod 51 Exempt   63 Mod 63 Exempt   ✗ Non-FDA Drug   ★ Telemedicine   M Maternity   A Age Edit

CPT © 2019 American Medical Association. All Rights Reserved.

+ 64872   Suture of nerve; requiring secondary or delayed suture (List separately in addition to code for primary neurorrhaphy)
Code first (64831-64865)
🔧 3.39   ✂ 3.39   **FUD** ZZZ   N N1 80 ▢
AMA: 2014,Jan,11

+ 64874   requiring extensive mobilization, or transposition of nerve (List separately in addition to code for nerve suture)
Code first (64831-64865)
🔧 5.06   ✂ 5.06   **FUD** ZZZ   N N1 80 ▢
AMA: 2014,Jan,11

+ 64876   requiring shortening of bone of extremity (List separately in addition to code for nerve suture)
Code first (64831-64865)
🔧 5.75   ✂ 5.75   **FUD** ZZZ   N N1 80 ▢
AMA: 2014,Jan,11

64885   Nerve graft (includes obtaining graft), head or neck; up to 4 cm in length
🔧 32.1   ✂ 32.1   **FUD** 090   J J8 80 ▢
AMA: 2018,Jan,8; 2017,Dec,12; 2017,Jan,8; 2016,Jan,13; 2015,Jan,16; 2014,Jan,11

64886   more than 4 cm length
🔧 37.2   ✂ 37.2   **FUD** 090   J J8 80 ▢
AMA: 2018,Jan,8; 2017,Dec,12; 2017,Jan,8; 2016,Jan,13; 2015,Jan,16; 2014,Jan,11

64890   Nerve graft (includes obtaining graft), single strand, hand or foot; up to 4 cm length
🔧 31.2   ✂ 31.2   **FUD** 090   J J8 80 ▢
AMA: 2018,Jan,8; 2017,Dec,12; 2017,Jan,8; 2016,Jan,13; 2015,Aug,8; 2015,Apr,10; 2014,Jan,11

64891   more than 4 cm length
🔧 33.2   ✂ 33.2   **FUD** 090   J G2 80 ▢
AMA: 2018,Jan,8; 2017,Dec,12; 2014,Jan,11

64892   Nerve graft (includes obtaining graft), single strand, arm or leg; up to 4 cm length
🔧 30.1   ✂ 30.1   **FUD** 090   J A2 80 ▢
AMA: 2018,Jan,8; 2017,Dec,12; 2014,Jan,11

64893   more than 4 cm length
🔧 32.4   ✂ 32.4   **FUD** 090   J G2 80 ▢
AMA: 2018,Jan,8; 2017,Dec,12; 2014,Jan,11

64895   Nerve graft (includes obtaining graft), multiple strands (cable), hand or foot; up to 4 cm length
🔧 38.4   ✂ 38.4   **FUD** 090   J A2 80 ▢
AMA: 2018,Jan,8; 2017,Dec,12; 2017,Jan,8; 2016,Jan,13; 2015,Jan,16; 2014,Jan,11

64896   more than 4 cm length
🔧 41.4   ✂ 41.4   **FUD** 090   J A2 80 ▢
AMA: 2018,Jan,8; 2017,Dec,12; 2017,Jan,8; 2016,Jan,13; 2015,Jan,16; 2014,Jan,11

64897   Nerve graft (includes obtaining graft), multiple strands (cable), arm or leg; up to 4 cm length
🔧 36.4   ✂ 36.4   **FUD** 090   J G2 80 ▢
AMA: 2018,Jan,8; 2017,Dec,12; 2017,Jan,8; 2016,Jan,13; 2015,Jan,16; 2014,Jan,11

64898   more than 4 cm length
🔧 39.7   ✂ 39.7   **FUD** 090   J A2 80 ▢
AMA: 2018,Jan,8; 2017,Dec,12; 2017,Jan,8; 2016,Jan,13; 2015,Jan,16; 2014,Jan,11

+ 64901   Nerve graft, each additional nerve; single strand (List separately in addition to code for primary procedure)
Code first (64885-64893)
🔧 17.4   ✂ 17.4   **FUD** ZZZ   N N1 80 ▢
AMA: 2018,Jan,8; 2017,Dec,12; 2017,Jan,8; 2016,Jan,13; 2015,Jan,16; 2014,Jan,11

+ 64902   multiple strands (cable) (List separately in addition to code for primary procedure)
Code first (64885-64886, 64895-64898)
🔧 20.1   ✂ 20.1   **FUD** ZZZ   N N1 80 ▢
AMA: 2018,Jan,8; 2017,Dec,12; 2017,Jan,8; 2016,Jan,13; 2015,Jan,16; 2014,Jan,11

64905   Nerve pedicle transfer; first stage
🔧 29.4   ✂ 29.4   **FUD** 090   J A2 80 ▢
AMA: 2018,Jan,8; 2017,Dec,12; 2014,Jan,11

64907   second stage
🔧 37.7   ✂ 37.7   **FUD** 090   J A2 80 ▢
AMA: 2018,Jan,8; 2017,Dec,12; 2014,Jan,11

64910-64999 Nerve Repair: Synthetic and Vein Grafts

64910   Nerve repair; with synthetic conduit or vein allograft (eg, nerve tube), each nerve
INCLUDES   Operating microscope (69990)
🔧 22.8   ✂ 22.8   **FUD** 090   J J8 80 ▢
AMA: 2018,Jan,8; 2017,Dec,12; 2017,Jan,8; 2016,Jan,13; 2015,Aug,8; 2015,Apr,10; 2015,Jan,16; 2014,Jan,11

Damaged nerve

Healthy nerve

Artificial nerve conduit

A synthetic "bridge" is affixed to each end of a severed nerve with sutures
The procedure is performed using an operating microscope

64911   with autogenous vein graft (includes harvest of vein graft), each nerve
INCLUDES   Operating microscope (69990)
🔧 29.6   ✂ 29.6   **FUD** 090   J 80 ▢
AMA: 2018,Jan,8; 2017,Dec,12; 2017,Jan,8; 2016,Jan,13; 2015,Jan,16; 2014,Jan,11

64912   with nerve allograft, each nerve, first strand (cable)
INCLUDES   Operating microscope (69990)
🔧 22.3   ✂ 22.3   **FUD** 090   J G2 80 ▢
AMA: 2018,Jan,8; 2017,Dec,12

+ 64913   with nerve allograft, each additional strand (List separately in addition to code for primary procedure)
INCLUDES   Operating microscope (69990)
Code first (64912)
🔧 4.50   ✂ 4.50   **FUD** ZZZ   N N1 80 ▢
AMA: 2018,Jan,8; 2017,Dec,12

64999 **Unlisted procedure, nervous system**
🔧 0.00   ✂ 0.00   **FUD** YYY   T 80

AMA: 2019,Jul,10; 2019,May,10; 2019,Apr,9; 2018,Dec,8;
2018,Dec,8; 2018,Oct,8; 2018,Oct,11; 2018,Aug,10; 2018,Mar,9;
2018,Jan,7; 2018,Jan,8; 2017,Dec,13; 2017,Dec,14; 2017,Dec,12;
2017,Jan,8; 2016,Nov,6; 2016,Oct,11; 2016,Feb,13; 2016,Jan,13;
2015,Oct,9; 2015,Aug,8; 2015,Jul,10; 2015,Apr,10; 2015,Feb,9;
2015,Jan,16; 2014,Jul,8; 2014,Feb,11; 2014,Jan,11; 2014,Jan,9;
2014,Jan,8

65091-65093 Surgical Removal of Eyeball Contents

INCLUDES   Operating microscope (69990)

65091   Evisceration of ocular contents; without implant
📅 18.4   ⚖ 18.4   **FUD** 090   J A2 80 50 ▣
AMA: 2016,Feb,12; 2014,Jan,11

Conjunctiva
Sclera

Muscles are severed at their attachment to the eyeball

Evisceration involves removal of the contents of the eyeball: the vitreous; retina; choroid; lens; iris; and ciliary muscle. Only the scleral shell remains. A temporary or permanent implant is usually inserted

Enucleation involves severing the extraorbital muscles and optic nerve with removal of the eyeball. An implant is usually inserted and, if permanent, may involve attachment to the severed extraorbital muscles

65093   with implant
📅 18.2   ⚖ 18.2   **FUD** 090   J A2 50 ▣
AMA: 2016,Feb,12; 2014,Jan,11

65101-65105 Surgical Removal of Eyeball

INCLUDES   Operating microscope (69990)
EXCLUDES   Conjunctivoplasty following enucleation (68320-68328)

65101   Enucleation of eye; without implant
📅 21.3   ⚖ 21.3   **FUD** 090   J A2 50 ▣
AMA: 2016,Feb,12; 2014,Jan,11

65103   with implant, muscles not attached to implant
📅 22.2   ⚖ 22.2   **FUD** 090   J A2 50 ▣
AMA: 2016,Feb,12; 2014,Jan,11

65105   with implant, muscles attached to implant
📅 24.4   ⚖ 24.4   **FUD** 090   J A2 80 50 ▣
AMA: 2016,Feb,12; 2014,Jan,11

65110-65114 Surgical Removal of Orbital Contents

INCLUDES   Operating microscope (69990)
EXCLUDES   Free full thickness graft (15260-15261)
Repair more extensive than skin (67930-67975)
Skin graft (15120-15121)

65110   Exenteration of orbit (does not include skin graft), removal of orbital contents; only
📅 35.0   ⚖ 35.0   **FUD** 090   J A2 80 50 ▣
AMA: 2016,Feb,12; 2014,Jan,11

65112   with therapeutic removal of bone
📅 40.5   ⚖ 40.5   **FUD** 090   J A2 80 50 ▣
AMA: 2016,Feb,12; 2014,Jan,11

65114   with muscle or myocutaneous flap
📅 42.5   ⚖ 42.5   **FUD** 090   J A2 80 50 ▣
AMA: 2016,Feb,12; 2014,Jan,11

65125-65175 Implant Procedures: Insertion, Removal, and Revision

INCLUDES   Operating microscope (69990)
EXCLUDES   Orbital implant insertion outside muscle cone (67550)
Orbital implant removal or revision outside muscle cone (67560)

65125   Modification of ocular implant with placement or replacement of pegs (eg, drilling receptacle for prosthesis appendage) (separate procedure)
📅 8.32   ⚖ 13.0   **FUD** 090   J 02 50 ▣
AMA: 2016,Feb,12; 2014,Jan,11

65130   Insertion of ocular implant secondary; after evisceration, in scleral shell
📅 21.1   ⚖ 21.1   **FUD** 090   J A2 50 ▣
AMA: 2016,Feb,12; 2014,Jan,11

65135   after enucleation, muscles not attached to implant
📅 21.4   ⚖ 21.4   **FUD** 090   J A2 50 ▣
AMA: 2016,Feb,12; 2014,Jan,11

65140   after enucleation, muscles attached to implant
📅 23.3   ⚖ 23.3   **FUD** 090   J A2 50 ▣
AMA: 2016,Feb,12; 2014,Jan,11

65150   Reinsertion of ocular implant; with or without conjunctival graft
📅 16.8   ⚖ 16.8   **FUD** 090   J A2 80 50 ▣
AMA: 2016,Feb,12; 2014,Jan,11

65155   with use of foreign material for reinforcement and/or attachment of muscles to implant
📅 24.4   ⚖ 24.4   **FUD** 090   J A2 50 ▣
AMA: 2016,Feb,12; 2014,Jan,11

65175   Removal of ocular implant
📅 19.0   ⚖ 19.0   **FUD** 090   J A2 50 ▣
AMA: 2016,Feb,12; 2014,Jan,11

65205-65265 Foreign Body Removal By Area of Eye

INCLUDES   Operating microscope (69990)
EXCLUDES   Removal:
Anterior segment implant (65920)
Ocular implant (65175)
Orbital implant outside muscle cone (67560)
Posterior segment implant (67120)
Removal of foreign body:
Eyelid (67938)
Lacrimal system (68530)
Orbit:
Frontal approach (67413)
Lateral approach (67430)

65205   Removal of foreign body, external eye; conjunctival superficial
🔲 (70030, 76529)
📅 1.02   ⚖ 1.31   **FUD** 000   01 N1 50 ▣
AMA: 2018,Jan,8; 2017,Jan,8; 2016,Feb,12; 2016,Jan,13; 2015,Jan,16; 2014,Jan,11

65210   conjunctival embedded (includes concretions), subconjunctival, or scleral nonperforating
🔲 (70030, 76529)
📅 1.22   ⚖ 1.60   **FUD** 000   01 N1 50 ▣
AMA: 2016,Feb,12; 2014,Jan,11

65220   corneal, without slit lamp
EXCLUDES   Repair of corneal wound with foreign body (65275)
🔲 (70030, 76529)
📅 1.19   ⚖ 1.68   **FUD** 000   01 N1 50 ▣
AMA: 2018,Jan,8; 2017,Jan,8; 2016,Feb,12; 2016,Jan,13; 2015,Jan,16; 2014,Jan,11

65222   corneal, with slit lamp
EXCLUDES   Repair of corneal wound with foreign body (65275)
🔲 (70030, 76529)
📅 1.48   ⚖ 1.93   **FUD** 000   01 N1 50 ▣
AMA: 2018,Jan,8; 2017,Jan,8; 2016,Feb,12; 2016,Jan,13; 2015,Jan,16; 2014,Jan,11

65235   Removal of foreign body, intraocular; from anterior chamber of eye or lens
🔲 (70030, 76529)
📅 20.2   ⚖ 20.2   **FUD** 090   J A2 80 50 ▣
AMA: 2018,Jan,8; 2017,Jan,8; 2016,Feb,12; 2016,Jan,13; 2015,Jan,16; 2014,Jan,11

65260   from posterior segment, magnetic extraction, anterior or posterior route
🔲 (70030, 76529)
📅 27.4   ⚖ 27.4   **FUD** 090   J A2 80 50 ▣
AMA: 2016,Feb,12; 2014,Jan,11

65265 from posterior segment, nonmagnetic extraction
📷 (70030, 76529)
📷 30.7 ⚖ 30.7 **FUD** 090 [J] [A2] [80] [50] [▭]
AMA: 2016,Feb,12; 2014,Jan,11

65270-65290 Laceration Repair External Eye

INCLUDES Conjunctival flap
Operating microscope (69990)
Restoration of anterior chamber with air or saline injection

EXCLUDES Repair:
Ciliary body or iris (66680)
Eyelid laceration (12011-12018, 12051-12057, 13151-13160, 67930, 67935)
Lacrimal system injury (68700)
Surgical wound (66250)
Treatment of orbit fracture (21385-21408)

65270 Repair of laceration; conjunctiva, with or without nonperforating laceration sclera, direct closure
📷 4.01 ⚖ 7.79 **FUD** 010 [J] [A2] [80] [50] [▭]
AMA: 2018,Jan,8; 2017,Jan,8; 2016,Feb,12; 2016,Jan,13; 2015,Jan,16; 2014,Jan,11

65272 conjunctiva, by mobilization and rearrangement, without hospitalization
📷 10.0 ⚖ 14.5 **FUD** 090 [J] [A2] [50] [▭]
AMA: 2016,Feb,12; 2014,Jan,11

65273 conjunctiva, by mobilization and rearrangement, with hospitalization
📷 10.8 ⚖ 10.8 **FUD** 090 [C] [50] [▭]
AMA: 2016,Feb,12; 2014,Jan,11

65275 cornea, nonperforating, with or without removal foreign body
📷 13.1 ⚖ 16.5 **FUD** 090 [J] [A2] [80] [50] [▭]
AMA: 2016,Feb,12; 2014,Jan,11

65280 cornea and/or sclera, perforating, not involving uveal tissue
EXCLUDES Procedure performed for surgical wound repair
📷 19.1 ⚖ 19.1 **FUD** 090 [J] [A2] [80] [50] [▭]
AMA: 2018,Jan,8; 2017,Jan,8; 2016,Feb,12; 2016,Jan,13; 2015,Jan,16; 2014,Jan,11

65285 cornea and/or sclera, perforating, with reposition or resection of uveal tissue
EXCLUDES Procedure performed for surgical wound repair
📷 31.5 ⚖ 31.5 **FUD** 090 [J] [A2] [50] [▭]
AMA: 2018,Jan,8; 2017,Jan,8; 2016,Feb,12; 2016,Jan,13; 2015,Jan,16; 2014,Jan,11

65286 application of tissue glue, wounds of cornea and/or sclera
📷 14.1 ⚖ 20.0 **FUD** 090 [J] [P3] [50] [▭]
AMA: 2018,Jan,8; 2017,Jan,8; 2016,Feb,12; 2016,Jan,13; 2015,Jan,16; 2014,Jan,11

65290 Repair of wound, extraocular muscle, tendon and/or Tenon's capsule
📷 13.9 ⚖ 13.9 **FUD** 090 [J] [A2] [50] [▭]
AMA: 2016,Feb,12; 2014,Jan,11

65400-65600 Removal Corneal Lesions

INCLUDES Operating microscope (69990)

65400 Excision of lesion, cornea (keratectomy, lamellar, partial), except pterygium
📷 17.1 ⚖ 19.4 **FUD** 090 [T] [A2] [50] [▭]
AMA: 2018,Jan,8; 2017,Jan,8; 2016,Feb,12; 2016,Jan,13; 2015,Jan,16; 2014,Jan,11

65410 Biopsy of cornea
📷 2.96 ⚖ 4.11 **FUD** 000 [J] [A2] [80] [50] [▭]
AMA: 2018,Jan,8; 2017,Jan,8; 2016,Feb,12; 2016,Jan,13; 2015,Jan,16; 2014,Jan,11

65420 Excision or transposition of pterygium; without graft
📷 10.7 ⚖ 14.9 **FUD** 090 [J] [A2] [50] [▭]
AMA: 2018,Jan,8; 2017,Jan,8; 2016,Feb,12; 2016,Jan,13; 2015,Jan,16; 2014,Jan,11

Conjunctiva

The conjunctiva is subject to numerous acute and chronic irritations and disorders

Cornea

Lens

Posterior chamber

Iris

Pterygium

Anterior chamber

65426 with graft
📷 13.6 ⚖ 18.7 **FUD** 090 [J] [A2] [50] [▭]
AMA: 2018,May,10; 2018,Jan,8; 2017,Jan,8; 2016,Feb,12; 2016,Jan,13; 2015,Jan,16; 2014,Jan,11

65430 Scraping of cornea, diagnostic, for smear and/or culture
📷 2.94 ⚖ 3.31 **FUD** 000 [01] [N1] [50] [▭]
AMA: 2016,Feb,12; 2014,Jan,11

65435 Removal of corneal epithelium; with or without chemocauterization (abrasion, curettage)
EXCLUDES Collagen cross-linking of cornea (0402T)
📷 1.98 ⚖ 2.32 **FUD** 000 [T] [P3] [50] [▭]
AMA: 2018,Jan,8; 2017,Jan,8; 2016,Feb,12; 2016,Jan,13; 2015,Jan,16; 2014,Jan,11

65436 with application of chelating agent (eg, EDTA)
📷 10.5 ⚖ 11.0 **FUD** 090 [J] [P3] [50] [▭]
AMA: 2016,Feb,12; 2014,Jan,11

65450 Destruction of lesion of cornea by cryotherapy, photocoagulation or thermocauterization
📷 9.15 ⚖ 9.30 **FUD** 090 [T] [G2] [50] [▭]
AMA: 2016,Feb,12; 2014,Jan,11

65600 Multiple punctures of anterior cornea (eg, for corneal erosion, tattoo)
📷 9.74 ⚖ 11.3 **FUD** 090 [J] [P3] [50] [▭]
AMA: 2016,Feb,12; 2014,Jan,11

65710-65757 Corneal Transplants

CMS: 100-03,80.7 Refractive Keratoplasty
INCLUDES Operating microscope (69990)
EXCLUDES Computerized corneal topography (92025)
Processing, preserving, and transporting corneal tissue (V2785)

65710 Keratoplasty (corneal transplant); anterior lamellar
INCLUDES Use and preparation of fresh or preserved graft
EXCLUDES Refractive keratoplasty surgery (65760-65767)
📷 31.7 ⚖ 31.7 **FUD** 090 [J] [A2] [80] [50] [▭]
AMA: 2018,Jan,8; 2017,Jan,8; 2016,Feb,12; 2016,Jan,13; 2015,Jan,16; 2014,Jan,11

65730 penetrating (except in aphakia or pseudophakia)
INCLUDES Use and preparation of fresh or preserved graft
EXCLUDES Refractive keratoplasty surgery (65760-65767)
📷 35.1 ⚖ 35.1 **FUD** 090 [J] [A2] [80] [50] [▭]
AMA: 2018,Jan,8; 2017,Jan,8; 2016,Feb,12; 2016,Jan,13; 2015,Jan,16; 2014,Jan,11

65750 penetrating (in aphakia)
INCLUDES Use and preparation of fresh or preserved graft
EXCLUDES Refractive keratoplasty surgery (65760-65767)
📷 35.3 ⚖ 35.3 **FUD** 090 [J] [A2] [80] [50] [▭]
AMA: 2018,Jan,8; 2017,Jan,8; 2016,Feb,12; 2016,Jan,13; 2015,Jan,16; 2014,Jan,11

65755 penetrating (in pseudophakia)

INCLUDES Use and preparation of fresh or preserved graft

EXCLUDES Refractive keratoplasty surgery (65760-65767)

📷 35.1 ✂ 35.1 **FUD** 090   J A2 80 50 🖵

AMA: 2018,Jan,8; 2017,Jan,8; 2016,Feb,12; 2016,Jan,13; 2015,Jan,16; 2014,Jan,11

65756 endothelial

EXCLUDES Refractive keratoplasty surgery (65760-65767)

Code also donor material

Code also if appropriate (65757)

📷 33.6 ✂ 33.6 **FUD** 090   J 62 80 50 🖵

AMA: 2018,Jan,8; 2017,Jan,8; 2016,Feb,12; 2016,Jan,13; 2015,Jan,16; 2014,Jan,11

+ 65757 Backbench preparation of corneal endothelial allograft prior to transplantation (List separately in addition to code for primary procedure)

Code first (65756)

📷 0.00 ✂ 0.00 **FUD** ZZZ   N N1 80 🖵

AMA: 2018,Jan,8; 2017,Jan,8; 2016,Feb,12; 2016,Jan,13; 2015,Jan,16; 2014,Aug,14; 2014,Jan,11

65760-65785 Corneal Refractive Procedures

CMS: 100-03,80.7 Refractive Keratoplasty

INCLUDES Operating microscope (69990)

EXCLUDES Unlisted corneal procedures (66999)

65760 Keratomileusis

EXCLUDES Computerized corneal topography (92025)

📷 0.00 ✂ 0.00 **FUD** XXX   E 🖵

AMA: 2016,Feb,12; 2014,Jan,11

65765 Keratophakia

EXCLUDES Computerized corneal topography (92025)

📷 0.00 ✂ 0.00 **FUD** XXX   E 🖵

AMA: 2016,Feb,12; 2014,Jan,11

65767 Epikeratoplasty

EXCLUDES Computerized corneal topography (92025)

📷 0.00 ✂ 0.00 **FUD** XXX   E 🖵

AMA: 2016,Feb,12; 2014,Jan,11

65770 Keratoprosthesis

EXCLUDES Computerized corneal topography (92025)

📷 39.6 ✂ 39.6 **FUD** 090   J J8 80 50 🖵

AMA: 2016,Feb,12; 2014,Jan,11

65771 Radial keratotomy

EXCLUDES Computerized corneal topography (92025)

📷 0.00 ✂ 0.00 **FUD** XXX   E 🖵

AMA: 2016,Feb,12; 2014,Jan,11

65772 Corneal relaxing incision for correction of surgically induced astigmatism

📷 11.5 ✂ 12.8 **FUD** 090   T A2 50 🖵

AMA: 2016,Feb,12; 2014,Jan,11

65775 Corneal wedge resection for correction of surgically induced astigmatism

EXCLUDES Fitting of contact lens to treat disease (92071-92072)

📷 15.8 ✂ 15.8 **FUD** 090   J A2 50 🖵

AMA: 2018,Jan,8; 2017,Jan,8; 2016,Feb,12; 2016,Jan,13; 2015,Jan,16; 2014,Jan,11

65778 Placement of amniotic membrane on the ocular surface; without sutures

EXCLUDES Ocular surface reconstruction (65780)

Removal of corneal epithelium (65435)

Scraping of cornea, diagnostic (65430)

Use of tissue glue to place amniotic membrane (66999)

📷 1.58 ✂ 40.0 **FUD** 000   02 N1 80 50 🖵

AMA: 2018,Feb,11; 2018,Jan,8; 2017,Jan,8; 2016,Feb,12; 2016,Jan,13; 2015,Jan,16; 2014,May,5; 2014,Jan,11

65779 single layer, sutured

EXCLUDES Ocular surface reconstruction (65780)

Removal of corneal epithelium (65435)

Scraping of cornea, diagnostic (65430)

Use of tissue glue to place amniotic membrane (66999)

📷 4.32 ✂ 34.5 **FUD** 000   02 N1 80 50 🖵

AMA: 2018,Feb,11; 2018,Jan,8; 2017,Jan,8; 2016,Feb,12; 2016,Jan,13; 2015,Jan,16; 2014,May,5; 2014,Jan,11

65780 Ocular surface reconstruction; amniotic membrane transplantation, multiple layers

EXCLUDES Placement amniotic membrane without reconstruction without sutures or single layer sutures (65778-65779)

📷 18.9 ✂ 18.9 **FUD** 090   J A2 50 🖵

AMA: 2018,Feb,11; 2018,Jan,8; 2017,Jan,8; 2016,Feb,12; 2016,Jan,13; 2015,Jan,16; 2014,May,5; 2014,Jan,11

65781 limbal stem cell allograft (eg, cadaveric or living donor)

📷 37.9 ✂ 37.9 **FUD** 090   J A2 80 50 🖵

AMA: 2018,Jan,8; 2017,Jan,8; 2016,Feb,12; 2016,Jan,13; 2015,Jan,16; 2014,Jan,11

65782 limbal conjunctival autograft (includes obtaining graft)

EXCLUDES Conjunctival allograft harvest from a living donor (68371)

📷 32.6 ✂ 32.6 **FUD** 090   J A2 50 🖵

AMA: 2018,Jan,8; 2017,Jan,8; 2016,Feb,12; 2016,Jan,13; 2015,Jan,16; 2014,Jan,11

65785 Implantation of intrastromal corneal ring segments

📷 12.5 ✂ 69.5 **FUD** 090   J P2 50 🖵

AMA: 2016,Feb,12

65800-66030 Anterior Segment Procedures

INCLUDES Operating microscope (69990)

EXCLUDES Unlisted procedures of anterior segment (66999)

65800 Paracentesis of anterior chamber of eye (separate procedure); with removal of aqueous

EXCLUDES Insertion of ocular telescope prosthesis (0308T)

📷 2.59 ✂ 3.42 **FUD** 000   J A2 50 🖵

AMA: 2018,Jan,8; 2017,Jan,8; 2016,Feb,12; 2016,Jan,13; 2015,Jan,16; 2014,Jan,11

65810 with removal of vitreous and/or discission of anterior hyaloid membrane, with or without air injection

EXCLUDES Insertion of ocular telescope prosthesis (0308T)

📷 13.2 ✂ 13.2 **FUD** 090   J A2 50 🖵

AMA: 2018,Jan,8; 2017,Jan,8; 2016,Feb,12; 2016,Jan,13; 2015,Jan,16; 2014,Jan,11

65815 with removal of blood, with or without irrigation and/or air injection

EXCLUDES Injection only (66020-66030)

Insertion of ocular telescope prosthesis (0308T)

Removal of blood clot only (65930)

📷 13.5 ✂ 18.2 **FUD** 090   J A2 50 🖵

AMA: 2018,Jan,8; 2017,Jan,8; 2016,Feb,12; 2016,Jan,13; 2015,Jan,16; 2014,Jan,11

65820 Goniotomy

INCLUDES Barkan's operation

Code also ophthalmic endoscope if used (69990)

📷 21.5 ✂ 21.5 **FUD** 090   63 J A2 80 50 🖵

AMA: 2019,Sep,10; 2018,Dec,8; 2018,Dec,8; 2018,Jul,3; 2018,Jan,8; 2017,Jan,8; 2016,Feb,12; 2016,Jan,13; 2015,Jan,16; 2014,Jan,11

65850 Trabeculotomy ab externo

📷 23.8 ✂ 23.8 **FUD** 090   J A2 50 🖵

AMA: 2016,Feb,12; 2014,Jan,11

65855 Trabeculoplasty by laser surgery

EXCLUDES Severing adhesions of anterior segment (65860-65880)

Trabeculectomy ab externo (66170)

📷 5.91 ✂ 7.01 **FUD** 010   T P3 50 🖵

AMA: 2018,Jan,8; 2017,Jan,8; 2016,Feb,12; 2016,Jan,13; 2015,Jan,16; 2014,Jan,11

● New Code ▲ Revised Code ○ Reinstated ● New Web Release ▲ Revised Web Release + Add-on Unlisted Not Covered # Resequenced

50 Optum Mod 50 Exempt ⊘ AMA Mod 51 Exempt 51 Optum Mod 51 Exempt 63 Mod 63 Exempt ∕ Non-FDA Drug ★ Telemedicine M Maternity A Age Edit

© 2019 Optum360, LLC   CPT © 2019 American Medical Association. All Rights Reserved.

315

65860 Severing adhesions of anterior segment, laser technique (separate procedure)
🔲 7.18   ⚖ 8.81   **FUD** 090   T P3 80 50 ▢
AMA: 2016,Feb,12; 2014,Jan,11

65865 Severing adhesions of anterior segment of eye, incisional technique (with or without injection of air or liquid) (separate procedure); goniosynechiae
> *EXCLUDES* Laser trabeculectomy (65855)

🔲 13.4   ⚖ 13.4   **FUD** 090   J A2 50 ▢
AMA: 2016,Feb,12; 2014,Jan,11

65870 anterior synechiae, except goniosynechiae
🔲 16.7   ⚖ 16.7   **FUD** 090   J A2 50 ▢
AMA: 2016,Feb,12; 2014,Jan,11

65875 posterior synechiae
Code also ophthalmic endoscope if used (66990)
🔲 17.9   ⚖ 17.9   **FUD** 090   J A2 50 ▢
AMA: 2018,Jan,8; 2017,Jan,8; 2016,Feb,12; 2016,Jan,13; 2015,Jan,16; 2014,Jan,11

65880 corneovitreal adhesions
> *EXCLUDES* Laser procedure (66821)

🔲 18.8   ⚖ 18.8   **FUD** 090   J A2 50 ▢
AMA: 2016,Feb,12; 2014,Jan,11

65900 Removal of epithelial downgrowth, anterior chamber of eye
🔲 27.6   ⚖ 27.6   **FUD** 090   J A2 80 50 ▢
AMA: 2016,Feb,12; 2014,Jan,11

65920 Removal of implanted material, anterior segment of eye
Code also ophthalmic endoscope if used (66990)
🔲 22.4   ⚖ 22.4   **FUD** 090   J A2 50 ▢
AMA: 2018,Jan,8; 2017,Jan,8; 2016,Feb,12; 2016,Jan,13; 2015,Jan,16; 2014,Jan,11

65930 Removal of blood clot, anterior segment of eye
🔲 18.0   ⚖ 18.0   **FUD** 090   J A2 50 ▢
AMA: 2016,Feb,12; 2014,Jan,11

66020 Injection, anterior chamber of eye (separate procedure); air or liquid
> *EXCLUDES* Insertion of ocular telescope prosthesis (0308T)

🔲 3.74   ⚖ 5.43   **FUD** 010   J A2 50 ▢
AMA: 2018,Jan,8; 2017,Jan,8; 2016,Feb,12; 2016,Jan,13; 2015,Jan,16; 2014,Jan,11

66030 medication
> *EXCLUDES* Insertion of ocular telescope prosthesis (0308T)

🔲 3.16   ⚖ 4.87   **FUD** 010   J A2 50 ▢
AMA: 2016,Feb,12; 2014,Jan,11

66130 Excision Scleral Lesion
> *INCLUDES* Operating microscope (69990)
> *EXCLUDES* Intraocular foreign body removal (65235)
> Surgery on posterior sclera (67250, 67255)

66130 Excision of lesion, sclera
🔲 16.1   ⚖ 19.9   **FUD** 090   J A2 80 50 ▢
AMA: 2016,Feb,12; 2014,Jan,11

66150-66185 Procedures for Glaucoma
> *INCLUDES* Operating microscope (69990)
> *EXCLUDES* Intraocular foreign body removal (65235)
> Surgery on posterior sclera (67250, 67255)

66150 Fistulization of sclera for glaucoma; trephination with iridectomy
🔲 24.9   ⚖ 24.9   **FUD** 090   J A2 50 ▢
AMA: 2018,Jul,3; 2016,Feb,12; 2014,Jan,11

66155 thermocauterization with iridectomy
🔲 24.9   ⚖ 24.9   **FUD** 090   J A2 50 ▢
AMA: 2018,Jul,3; 2016,Feb,12; 2014,Jan,11

66160 sclerectomy with punch or scissors, with iridectomy
> *INCLUDES* Knapp's operation

🔲 28.1   ⚖ 28.1   **FUD** 090   J A2 50 ▢
AMA: 2018,Jul,3; 2016,Feb,12; 2014,Jan,11

66170 trabeculectomy ab externo in absence of previous surgery
> *EXCLUDES* Repair of surgical wound (66250)
> Trabeculectomy ab externo (65850)

🔲 31.1   ⚖ 31.1   **FUD** 090   J A2 80 50 ▢
AMA: 2018,Dec,8; 2018,Dec,10; 2018,Dec,8; 2018,Dec,10; 2018,Jul,3; 2018,Jan,8; 2017,Jan,8; 2016,Feb,12; 2016,Jan,13; 2015,Jan,16; 2014,Jan,11

66172 trabeculectomy ab externo with scarring from previous ocular surgery or trauma (includes injection of antifibrotic agents)
🔲 33.9   ⚖ 33.9   **FUD** 090   J A2 80 50 ▢
AMA: 2019,Apr,7; 2018,Dec,10; 2018,Dec,10; 2018,Jul,3; 2018,Jan,8; 2017,Jan,8; 2016,Feb,12; 2016,Jan,13; 2015,Jan,16; 2014,Jan,11

66174 Transluminal dilation of aqueous outflow canal; without retention of device or stent
🔲 26.9   ⚖ 26.9   **FUD** 090   J A2 80 50 ▢
AMA: 2019,Sep,10; 2018,Dec,8; 2018,Dec,8; 2016,Feb,12; 2014,Jan,11

66175 with retention of device or stent
🔲 28.2   ⚖ 28.2   **FUD** 090   J A2 80 50 ▢
AMA: 2016,Feb,12; 2014,Jan,11

66179 Aqueous shunt to extraocular equatorial plate reservoir, external approach; without graft
🔲 30.6   ⚖ 30.6   **FUD** 090   J G2 80 50 ▢
AMA: 2018,Jul,3; 2018,Jan,8; 2017,Jan,8; 2016,Feb,12; 2016,Jan,13; 2015,Jan,10

66180 with graft
> *EXCLUDES* Scleral reinforcement (67255)

🔲 32.3   ⚖ 32.3   **FUD** 090   J J8 80 50 ▢
AMA: 2018,Jul,3; 2018,Jan,8; 2017,Jan,8; 2016,Feb,12; 2016,Jan,13; 2015,Jan,16; 2015,Jan,10; 2014,Jan,11

66183 Insertion of anterior segment aqueous drainage device, without extraocular reservoir, external approach
🔲 29.2   ⚖ 29.2   **FUD** 090   J J8 80 50 ▢
AMA: 2018,Jul,3; 2018,Jan,8; 2017,Jan,8; 2016,Feb,12; 2016,Jan,13; 2015,Jan,16; 2014,May,5; 2014,Jan,11

66184 Revision of aqueous shunt to extraocular equatorial plate reservoir; without graft
🔲 22.3   ⚖ 22.3   **FUD** 090   J G2 80 50 ▢
AMA: 2018,Jan,8; 2017,Jan,8; 2016,Feb,12; 2016,Jan,13; 2015,Jan,10

66185 with graft
> *EXCLUDES* Implanted shunt removal (67120)
> Scleral reinforcement (67255)

🔲 24.0   ⚖ 24.0   **FUD** 090   J A2 80 50 ▢
AMA: 2018,Jan,8; 2017,Jan,8; 2016,Feb,12; 2016,Jan,13; 2015,Jan,10; 2014,Jan,11

66225 Staphyloma Repair
> *INCLUDES* Operating microscope (69990)
> *EXCLUDES* Scleral procedures with retinal procedures (67101-67228)
> Scleral reinforcement (67250, 67255)

66225 Repair of scleral staphyloma; with graft
🔲 26.4   ⚖ 26.4   **FUD** 090   J A2 50 ▢
AMA: 2016,Feb,12; 2014,Jan,11

66250 Anterior Segment Operative Wound Revision or Repair
> *INCLUDES* Operating microscope (69990)
> *EXCLUDES* Unlisted procedures of anterior sclera (66999)

66250 Revision or repair of operative wound of anterior segment, any type, early or late, major or minor procedure
🔲 15.8   ⚖ 21.4   **FUD** 090   J A2 50 ▢
AMA: 2018,Dec,8; 2018,Dec,8; 2018,Jan,8; 2017,Jan,8; 2016,Feb,12; 2016,Jan,13; 2015,Jan,16; 2014,Jan,11

26/TC PC/TC Only   A2-Z3 ASC Payment   50 Bilateral   ♂ Male Only   ♀ Female Only   🔲 Facility RVU   ⚖ Non-Facility RVU   ▢ CCI   ✖ CLIA
FUD Follow-up Days   CMS: IOM   AMA: CPT Asst   A-Y OPPSI   80/80 Surg Assist Allowed / w/Doc   ⚖ Lab crosswalk   Radiology crosswalk

316   CPT © 2019 American Medical Association. All Rights Reserved.   © 2019 Optum360, LLC

66500-66505 Iridotomy With/Without Transfixion

INCLUDES   Operating microscope (69990)
EXCLUDES   *Photocoagulation iridotomy (66761)*

66500   **Iridotomy by stab incision (separate procedure); except transfixion**
🚑 10.2   ✂ 10.2   **FUD** 090   J A2 50 ▢
AMA: 2016,Feb,12; 2014,Jan,11

66505   **with transfixion as for iris bombe**
🚑 11.1   ✂ 11.1   **FUD** 090   J A2 50 ▢
AMA: 2016,Feb,12; 2014,Jan,11

66600-66635 Iridectomy Procedures

INCLUDES   Operating microscope (69990)
EXCLUDES   *Insertion of ocular telescope prosthesis (0308T)*
           Photocoagulation coreoplasty (66762)

66600   **Iridectomy, with corneoscleral or corneal section; for removal of lesion**
🚑 23.9   ✂ 23.9   **FUD** 090   J A2 50 ▢
AMA: 2016,Feb,12; 2014,Jan,11

66605   **with cyclectomy**
🚑 30.3   ✂ 30.3   **FUD** 090   J A2 50 ▢
AMA: 2016,Feb,12; 2014,Jan,11

66625   **peripheral for glaucoma (separate procedure)**
🚑 12.2   ✂ 12.2   **FUD** 090   J A2 50 ▢
AMA: 2016,Feb,12; 2014,Jan,11

66630   **sector for glaucoma (separate procedure)**
🚑 16.1   ✂ 16.1   **FUD** 090   J A2 50 ▢
AMA: 2016,Feb,12; 2014,Jan,11

66635   **optical (separate procedure)**
🚑 16.3   ✂ 16.3   **FUD** 090   J A2 50 ▢
AMA: 2016,Feb,12; 2014,Jan,11

66680-66770 Other Procedures of the Uveal Tract

INCLUDES   Operating microscope (69990)
EXCLUDES   *Unlisted procedures of ciliary body or iris (66999)*

66680   **Repair of iris, ciliary body (as for iridodialysis)**
EXCLUDES   *Resection or repositioning of uveal tissue for perforating laceration of cornea and/or sclera (65285)*
🚑 14.7   ✂ 14.7   **FUD** 090   J A2 50 ▢
AMA: 2016,Feb,12; 2014,Jan,11

66682   **Suture of iris, ciliary body (separate procedure) with retrieval of suture through small incision (eg, McCannel suture)**
🚑 18.3   ✂ 18.3   **FUD** 090   J A2 50 ▢
AMA: 2016,Feb,12; 2014,Jan,11

66700   **Ciliary body destruction; diathermy**
INCLUDES   Heine's operation
🚑 11.1   ✂ 12.8   **FUD** 090   J A2 80 50 ▢
AMA: 2016,Feb,12; 2014,Jan,11

66710   **cyclophotocoagulation, transscleral**
🚑 11.1   ✂ 12.6   **FUD** 090   J A2 50 ▢
AMA: 2018,Jan,8; 2017,Jan,8; 2016,Feb,12; 2016,Jan,13; 2015,Jan,16; 2014,Jan,11

▲ **66711**   **cyclophotocoagulation, endoscopic, without concomitant removal of crystalline lens**
EXCLUDES   *Endoscopic cyclophotocoagulation performed in conjunction with extracapsular cataract removal with insertion of lens ([66987], [66988])*
🚑 18.2   ✂ 18.2   **FUD** 090   J A2 50 ▢
AMA: 2018,Jan,8; 2017,Jan,8; 2016,Feb,12; 2016,Jan,13; 2015,Jan,16; 2014,Jan,11

66720   **cryotherapy**
🚑 11.6   ✂ 13.1   **FUD** 090   J A2 50 ▢
AMA: 2016,Feb,12; 2014,Jan,11

66740   **cyclodialysis**
🚑 11.1   ✂ 12.5   **FUD** 090   J A2 50 ▢
AMA: 2016,Feb,12; 2014,Jan,11

66761   **Iridotomy/iridectomy by laser surgery (eg, for glaucoma) (per session)**
EXCLUDES   *Insertion of ocular telescope prosthesis (0308T)*
🚑 6.71   ✂ 8.50   **FUD** 010   T P3 50 ▢
AMA: 2018,Jan,8; 2017,Jan,8; 2016,Feb,12; 2016,Jan,13; 2015,Jan,16; 2014,Jan,11

66762   **Iridoplasty by photocoagulation (1 or more sessions) (eg, for improvement of vision, for widening of anterior chamber angle)**
🚑 12.0   ✂ 13.5   **FUD** 090   T P2 50 ▢
AMA: 2018,Jan,8; 2017,Jan,8; 2016,Feb,12; 2016,Jan,13; 2015,Jan,16; 2014,Jan,11

66770   **Destruction of cyst or lesion iris or ciliary body (nonexcisional procedure)**
EXCLUDES   *Excision:*
           Epithelial downgrowth (65900)
           Iris, ciliary body lesion (66600-66605)
🚑 13.7   ✂ 15.0   **FUD** 090   T P2 50 ▢
AMA: 2016,Feb,12; 2014,Jan,11

66820-66825 Post-Cataract Surgery Procedures

INCLUDES   Operating microscope (69990)

66820   **Discission of secondary membranous cataract (opacified posterior lens capsule and/or anterior hyaloid); stab incision technique (Ziegler or Wheeler knife)**
🚑 11.4   ✂ 11.4   **FUD** 090   J 02 50 ▢
AMA: 2016,Feb,12; 2014,Jan,11

Cataract — Iris — Lens
Artificial lens — Cornea — Opaque lens capsule — Iris

An after-cataract is a cataract that develops in a lens tissue that remains after most of the lens has already been removed

66821   **laser surgery (eg, YAG laser) (1 or more stages)**
🚑 8.85   ✂ 9.42   **FUD** 090   T A2 50 ▢
AMA: 2016,Feb,12; 2014,Jan,11

66825   **Repositioning of intraocular lens prosthesis, requiring an incision (separate procedure)**
EXCLUDES   *Insertion of ocular telescope prosthesis (0308T)*
🚑 21.8   ✂ 21.8   **FUD** 090   J A2 80 50 ▢
AMA: 2016,Feb,12; 2014,Jan,11

66830-66940 Cataract Extraction; Without Insertion Intraocular Lens

CMS: 100-03,80.10 Phacoemulsification Procedure--Cataract Extraction

INCLUDES Anterior and/or posterior capsulotomy
Enzymatic zonulysis
Iridectomy/iridotomy
Lateral canthotomy
Medications
Operating microscope (69990)
Subconjunctival injection
Subtenon injection
Use of viscoelastic material

EXCLUDES *Removal of intralenticular foreign body without lens excision (65235)*
Repair of surgical laceration (66250)

66830 **Removal of secondary membranous cataract (opacified posterior lens capsule and/or anterior hyaloid) with corneo-scleral section, with or without iridectomy (iridocapsulotomy, iridocapsulectomy)**

INCLUDES Graefe's operation

⚕ 20.1   ⚕ 20.1   **FUD** 090   J A2 50 ▭

AMA: 2016,Feb,12; 2014,Jan,11

A congenital keyhole pupil is also called a coloboma of the iris

66840 **Removal of lens material; aspiration technique, 1 or more stages**

INCLUDES Fukala's operation

⚕ 19.7   ⚕ 19.7   **FUD** 090   J A2 50 ▭

AMA: 2018,Jan,8; 2017,Jan,8; 2016,Sep,9; 2016,Jun,6; 2016,Apr,8; 2016,Feb,12; 2016,Jan,13; 2015,Jan,16; 2014,Jan,11

66850 **phacofragmentation technique (mechanical or ultrasonic) (eg, phacoemulsification), with aspiration**

⚕ 22.5   ⚕ 22.5   **FUD** 090   J A2 50 ▭

AMA: 2018,Jan,8; 2017,Jan,8; 2016,Jun,6; 2016,Feb,12; 2016,Jan,13; 2015,Jan,16; 2014,Jan,11

66852 **pars plana approach, with or without vitrectomy**

⚕ 23.9   ⚕ 23.9   **FUD** 090   J A2 80 50 ▭

AMA: 2018,Jan,8; 2017,Jan,8; 2016,Jun,6; 2016,Feb,12; 2016,Jan,13; 2015,Jan,16; 2014,Jan,11

66920 **intracapsular**

⚕ 21.4   ⚕ 21.4   **FUD** 090   J A2 80 50 ▭

AMA: 2018,Jan,8; 2017,Jan,8; 2016,Feb,12; 2016,Jan,13; 2015,Jan,16; 2014,Jan,11

66930 **intracapsular, for dislocated lens**

⚕ 24.3   ⚕ 24.3   **FUD** 090   J A2 80 50 ▭

AMA: 2018,Jan,8; 2017,Jan,8; 2016,Feb,12; 2016,Jan,13; 2015,Jan,16; 2014,Jan,11

66940 **extracapsular (other than 66840, 66850, 66852)**

⚕ 22.2   ⚕ 22.2   **FUD** 090   J A2 80 50 ▭

AMA: 2018,Jan,8; 2017,Jan,8; 2016,Jun,6; 2016,Feb,12; 2016,Jan,13; 2015,Jan,16; 2014,Jan,11

66982-66988 [66987, 66988] Cataract Extraction: With Insertion Intraocular Lens

INCLUDES Anterior or posterior capsulotomy
Enzymatic zonulysis
Iridectomy/iridotomy
Lateral canthotomy
Medications
Operating microscope (69990)
Subconjunctival injection
Subtenon injection
Use of viscoelastic material

EXCLUDES *Implanted material removal from the anterior segment (65920)*
Insertion of ocular telescope prosthesis (0308T)
Secondary fixation (66682)
Supply of intraocular lens

▲ **66982** **Extracapsular cataract removal with insertion of intraocular lens prosthesis (1-stage procedure), manual or mechanical technique (eg, irrigation and aspiration or phacoemulsification), complex, requiring devices or techniques not generally used in routine cataract surgery (eg, iris expansion device, suture support for intraocular lens, or primary posterior capsulorrhexis) or performed on patients in the amblyogenic developmental stage; without endoscopic cyclophotocoagulation**

EXCLUDES *Complex extracapsular cataract removal in conjunction with endoscopic cyclophotocoagulation ([66987])*
Insertion of ocular telescope prosthesis (0308T)

☢ (76519)

⚕ 22.5   ⚕ 22.5   **FUD** 090   J A2 50 ▭

AMA: 2018,Dec,6; 2018,Dec,6; 2018,Jan,8; 2017,Dec,14; 2017,Jan,8; 2016,Mar,10; 2016,Feb,12; 2016,Jan,13; 2015,Jan,16; 2014,Jan,11

● # **66987** **with endoscopic cyclophotocoagulation**

⚕ 0.00   ⚕ 0.00   **FUD** 000

EXCLUDES *Complex extracapsular cataract removal without endoscopic cyclophotocoagulation (66982)*
Insertion of ocular telescope prosthesis (0308T)

66983 **Intracapsular cataract extraction with insertion of intraocular lens prosthesis (1 stage procedure)**

☢ (76519)

⚕ 21.0   ⚕ 21.0   **FUD** 090   J A2 50 ▭

AMA: 2018,Jan,8; 2017,Jan,8; 2016,Feb,12; 2016,Jan,13; 2015,Jan,16; 2014,Jan,11

▲ **66984** **Extracapsular cataract removal with insertion of intraocular lens prosthesis (1 stage procedure), manual or mechanical technique (eg, irrigation and aspiration or phacoemulsification); without endoscopic cyclophotocoagulation**

EXCLUDES *Complex extracapsular cataract removal (66982)*
Extracapsular cataract removal in conjunction with endoscopic cyclophotocoagulation ([66988])
Insertion of ocular telescope prosthesis (0308T)

☢ (76519)

⚕ 18.1   ⚕ 18.1   **FUD** 090   J A2 50 ▭

AMA: 2018,Dec,6; 2018,Dec,6; 2018,Jan,8; 2017,Jan,8; 2016,Feb,12; 2016,Jan,13; 2015,Jan,16; 2014,Jan,11

● # **66988** **with endoscopic cyclophotocoagulation**

⚕ 0.00   ⚕ 0.00   **FUD** 000

EXCLUDES *Complex extracapsular cataract removal in conjunction with endoscopic cyclophotocoagulation ([66987])*
Extracapsular cataract removal without endoscopic cyclophotocoagulation (66984)
Insertion of ocular telescope prosthesis (0308T)

26/TC PC/TC Only   A2-Z3 ASC Payment   50 Bilateral   ♂ Male Only   ♀ Female Only   ⚕ Facility RVU   ⚕ Non-Facility RVU   ▭ CCI   ☒ CLIA
FUD Follow-up Days   CMS: IOM   AMA: CPT Asst   A-Y OPPSI   80/80 Surg Assist Allowed / w/Doc   ☒ Lab crosswalk   ☢ Radiology crosswalk

318   CPT © 2019 American Medical Association. All Rights Reserved.   © 2019 Optum360, LLC

66985-66988 Secondary Insertion or Replacement of Intraocular Lens

INCLUDES Operating microscope (69990)

EXCLUDES *Implanted material removal from the anterior segment (65920)*
Insertion of ocular telescope prosthesis (0308T)
Secondary fixation (66682)
Supply of intraocular lens

Code also ophthalmic endoscope if used (66990)

66985 Insertion of intraocular lens prosthesis (secondary implant), not associated with concurrent cataract removal

EXCLUDES *Insertion of lens at the time of cataract procedure (66982-66984)*

🔲 (76519)

🚑 21.8   ⚕ 21.8   **FUD** 090   J A2 50 ▣

AMA: 2018,Jan,8; 2017,Jan,8; 2016,Feb,12; 2016,Jan,13; 2015,Jan,16; 2014,Jan,11

66986 Exchange of intraocular lens

🔲 (76519)

🚑 25.8   ⚕ 25.8   **FUD** 090   J A2 50 ▣

AMA: 2018,Jan,8; 2017,Jan,8; 2016,Feb,12; 2016,Jan,13; 2015,Jan,16; 2014,Jan,11

66987 Resequenced code. See code following 66982.

66988 Resequenced code. See code following 66984.

66990-66999 Ophthalmic Endoscopy

INCLUDES Operating microscope (69990)

+ 66990 Use of ophthalmic endoscope (List separately in addition to code for primary procedure)

Code first (65820, 65875, 65920, 66985-66986, 67036, 67039-67043, 67113)

🚑 2.56   ⚕ 2.56   **FUD** ZZZ   N N1 ▣

AMA: 2018,Jul,3; 2018,Jan,8; 2017,Jan,8; 2016,Sep,5; 2016,Feb,12; 2016,Jan,13; 2015,Jan,16; 2014,Jan,11

66999 Unlisted procedure, anterior segment of eye

🚑 0.00   ⚕ 0.00   **FUD** YYY   J 80 50 ▣

AMA: 2018,Jan,8; 2017,Jan,8; 2016,Apr,8; 2016,Feb,12; 2016,Jan,13; 2015,Jan,16; 2014,Jan,11

67005-67015 Vitrectomy: Partial and Subtotal

INCLUDES Operating microscope (69990)

67005 Removal of vitreous, anterior approach (open sky technique or limbal incision); partial removal

EXCLUDES *Anterior chamber vitrectomy by paracentesis (65810)*
Severing of corneovitreal adhesions (65880)

🚑 13.4   ⚕ 13.4   **FUD** 090   J A2 50 ▣

AMA: 2018,Jan,8; 2017,Jan,8; 2016,Feb,12; 2016,Jan,13; 2015,Jan,16; 2014,Jan,11

67010 subtotal removal with mechanical vitrectomy

EXCLUDES *Anterior chamber vitrectomy by paracentesis (65810)*
Severing of corneovitreal adhesions (65880)

🚑 15.4   ⚕ 15.4   **FUD** 090   J A2 50 ▣

AMA: 2018,Jan,8; 2017,Jan,8; 2016,Feb,12; 2016,Jan,13; 2015,Jan,16; 2014,Jan,11

67015 Aspiration or release of vitreous, subretinal or choroidal fluid, pars plana approach (posterior sclerotomy)

🚑 16.5   ⚕ 16.5   **FUD** 090   J A2 50 ▣

AMA: 2018,Jan,8; 2017,Jan,8; 2016,Sep,5; 2016,Jun,6; 2016,Feb,12; 2014,Jan,11

67025-67028 Intravitreal Injection/Implantation

INCLUDES Operating microscope (69990)

67025 Injection of vitreous substitute, pars plana or limbal approach (fluid-gas exchange), with or without aspiration (separate procedure)

🚑 17.9   ⚕ 20.8   **FUD** 090   J A2 50 ▣

AMA: 2019,Aug,10; 2018,Feb,3; 2016,Feb,12; 2014,Jan,11

67027 Implantation of intravitreal drug delivery system (eg, ganciclovir implant), includes concomitant removal of vitreous

EXCLUDES *Removal of drug delivery system (67121)*

🚑 24.2   ⚕ 24.2   **FUD** 090   J A2 80 50 ▣

AMA: 2018,Feb,3; 2018,Jan,8; 2017,Jan,8; 2016,Feb,12; 2016,Jan,13; 2015,Jan,16; 2014,Jan,11

67028 Intravitreal injection of a pharmacologic agent (separate procedure)

🚑 2.83   ⚕ 2.89   **FUD** 000   S P3 50 ▣

AMA: 2018,Feb,3; 2018,Jan,8; 2017,Jan,8; 2016,Feb,12; 2016,Jan,13; 2015,Jan,16; 2014,Jan,11

67030-67031 Incision of Vitreous Strands/Membranes

INCLUDES Operating microscope (69990)

67030 Discission of vitreous strands (without removal), pars plana approach

🚑 15.2   ⚕ 15.2   **FUD** 090   J A2 50 ▣

AMA: 2016,Feb,12; 2014,Jan,11

67031 Severing of vitreous strands, vitreous face adhesions, sheets, membranes or opacities, laser surgery (1 or more stages)

🚑 10.1   ⚕ 11.1   **FUD** 090   T A2 50 ▣

AMA: 2016,Feb,12; 2014,Jan,11

67036-67043 Pars Plana Mechanical Vitrectomy

INCLUDES Operating microscope (69990)

EXCLUDES *Foreign body removal (65260, 65265)*
Lens removal (66850)
Unlisted vitreal procedures (67299)
Vitrectomy in retinal detachment (67108, 67113)

Code also ophthalmic endoscope if used (66990)

67036 Vitrectomy, mechanical, pars plana approach;

🚑 25.6   ⚕ 25.6   **FUD** 090   J A2 80 50 ▣

AMA: 2018,Jan,8; 2017,Jan,8; 2016,Sep,5; 2016,Feb,12; 2016,Jan,13; 2015,Jan,16; 2014,Jan,11

67039 with focal endolaser photocoagulation

🚑 27.4   ⚕ 27.4   **FUD** 090   J A2 80 50 ▣

AMA: 2018,Jan,8; 2017,Jan,8; 2016,Sep,5; 2016,Feb,12; 2016,Jan,13; 2015,Jan,16; 2014,Jan,11

67040 with endolaser panretinal photocoagulation

🚑 29.6   ⚕ 29.6   **FUD** 090   J A2 80 50 ▣

AMA: 2018,Jan,8; 2017,Jan,8; 2016,Sep,5; 2016,Feb,12; 2016,Jan,13; 2015,Jan,16; 2014,Jan,11

67041 with removal of preretinal cellular membrane (eg, macular pucker)

🚑 32.7   ⚕ 32.7   **FUD** 090   J G2 80 50 ▣

AMA: 2018,Jan,8; 2017,Jan,8; 2016,Sep,5; 2016,Feb,12; 2016,Jan,13; 2015,Jan,16; 2014,Jan,11

67042 with removal of internal limiting membrane of retina (eg, for repair of macular hole, diabetic macular edema), includes, if performed, intraocular tamponade (ie, air, gas or silicone oil)

🚑 32.7   ⚕ 32.7   **FUD** 090   J G2 80 50 ▣

AMA: 2018,Jan,8; 2017,Jan,8; 2016,Sep,5; 2016,Feb,12; 2016,Jan,13; 2015,Jan,16; 2014,Jan,11

67043 with removal of subretinal membrane (eg, choroidal neovascularization), includes, if performed, intraocular tamponade (ie, air, gas or silicone oil) and laser photocoagulation

🚑 34.5   ⚕ 34.5   **FUD** 090   J G2 80 50 ▣

AMA: 2018,Jan,8; 2017,Jan,8; 2016,Sep,5; 2016,Feb,12; 2016,Jan,13; 2015,Jan,16; 2014,Jan,11

67101-67115 Detached Retina Repair

INCLUDES Operating microscope (69990)
Primary technique when cryotherapy and/or diathermy and/or photocoagulation are used in combination

67101 **Repair of retinal detachment, including drainage of subretinal fluid when performed; cryotherapy**
🔲 8.10 ✄ 9.40 **FUD** 010 J P3 50 ▭
AMA: 2018,Jan,8; 2017,Feb,14; 2017,Jan,8; 2016,Sep,5; 2016,Jun,6; 2016,Feb,12; 2016,Jan,13; 2015,Jan,16; 2014,Jan,11

Optic nerve
Vitreous
Optic disc
Choroid
Sclera
Retina
Posterior chamber Pars plana

67105 **photocoagulation**
🔲 7.82 ✄ 8.45 **FUD** 010 T P3 50 ▭
AMA: 2018,Jan,8; 2017,Feb,14; 2017,Jan,8; 2016,Sep,5; 2016,Jun,6; 2016,Feb,12; 2016,Jan,13; 2015,Jan,16; 2014,Jan,11

67107 **Repair of retinal detachment; scleral buckling (such as lamellar scleral dissection, imbrication or encircling procedure), including, when performed, implant, cryotherapy, photocoagulation, and drainage of subretinal fluid**
INCLUDES Gonin's operation
🔲 32.1 ✄ 32.1 **FUD** 090 J G2 80 50 ▭
AMA: 2019,Aug,10; 2018,Jan,8; 2017,Jan,8; 2016,Sep,5; 2016,Jun,6; 2016,Feb,12; 2014,Jan,11

67108 **with vitrectomy, any method, including, when performed, air or gas tamponade, focal endolaser photocoagulation, cryotherapy, drainage of subretinal fluid, scleral buckling, and/or removal of lens by same technique**
🔲 34.1 ✄ 34.1 **FUD** 090 J G2 80 50 ▭
AMA: 2018,Jan,8; 2017,Jan,8; 2016,Sep,5; 2016,Jun,6; 2016,Feb,12; 2016,Jan,13; 2015,Jan,16; 2014,Jan,11

67110 **by injection of air or other gas (eg, pneumatic retinopexy)**
🔲 23.1 ✄ 25.0 **FUD** 090 J P3 50 ▭
AMA: 2018,Jan,8; 2017,Jan,8; 2016,Sep,5; 2016,Jun,6; 2016,Feb,12; 2014,Jan,11

67113 **Repair of complex retinal detachment (eg, proliferative vitreoretinopathy, stage C-1 or greater, diabetic traction retinal detachment, retinopathy of prematurity, retinal tear of greater than 90 degrees), with vitrectomy and membrane peeling, including, when performed, air, gas, or silicone oil tamponade, cryotherapy, endolaser photocoagulation, drainage of subretinal fluid, scleral buckling, and/or removal of lens**
EXCLUDES Vitrectomy for other than retinal detachment, pars plana approach (67036-67043)
Code also ophthalmic endoscope if used (66990)
🔲 38.0 ✄ 38.0 **FUD** 090 J G2 80 50 ▭
AMA: 2018,Jan,8; 2017,Jan,8; 2016,Sep,5; 2016,Jun,6; 2016,Feb,12; 2016,Jan,13; 2015,Jan,16; 2014,Jan,11

67115 **Release of encircling material (posterior segment)**
🔲 14.1 ✄ 14.1 **FUD** 090 J A2 50 ▭
AMA: 2016,Feb,12; 2014,Jan,11

67120-67121 Removal of Previously Implanted Prosthetic Device

INCLUDES Operating microscope (69990)
EXCLUDES Foreign body removal (65260, 65265)
Removal of implanted material anterior segment (65920)

67120 **Removal of implanted material, posterior segment; extraocular**
🔲 15.8 ✄ 18.8 **FUD** 090 J A2 50 ▭
AMA: 2016,Feb,12; 2014,Jan,11

67121 **intraocular**
🔲 25.8 ✄ 25.8 **FUD** 090 J A2 80 50 ▭
AMA: 2016,Feb,12; 2014,Jan,11

67141-67145 Retinal Detachment: Preventative Procedures

INCLUDES Operating microscope (69990)
Treatment at one or more sessions that may occur at different encounters
EXCLUDES Procedure performed more than one time during a defined period of treatment

67141 **Prophylaxis of retinal detachment (eg, retinal break, lattice degeneration) without drainage, 1 or more sessions; cryotherapy, diathermy**
🔲 13.8 ✄ 14.9 **FUD** 090 T A2 50 ▭
AMA: 2018,Jan,8; 2017,Jan,8; 2016,Sep,5; 2016,Feb,12; 2016,Jan,13; 2015,Jan,16; 2014,Jan,11

67145 **photocoagulation (laser or xenon arc)**
🔲 14.1 ✄ 15.0 **FUD** 090 T P2 50 ▭
AMA: 2018,Jan,8; 2017,Jan,8; 2016,Sep,5; 2016,Feb,12; 2016,Jan,13; 2015,Jan,16; 2014,Jan,11

67208-67218 Destruction of Retinal Lesions

INCLUDES Operating microscope (69990)
Treatment at one or more sessions that may occur at different encounters
EXCLUDES Procedure performed more than one time during a defined period of treatment
Unlisted retinal procedures (67299)

67208 **Destruction of localized lesion of retina (eg, macular edema, tumors), 1 or more sessions; cryotherapy, diathermy**
🔲 16.4 ✄ 17.0 **FUD** 090 T P2 50 ▭
AMA: 2018,Jan,8; 2017,Jan,8; 2016,Feb,12; 2016,Jan,13; 2015,Jan,16; 2014,Jan,11

67210 **photocoagulation**
🔲 14.2 ✄ 14.7 **FUD** 090 T P2 50 ▭
AMA: 2018,Jan,8; 2017,Jan,8; 2016,Feb,12; 2016,Jan,13; 2015,Jan,16; 2014,Jan,11

67218 **radiation by implantation of source (includes removal of source)**
🔲 39.3 ✄ 39.3 **FUD** 090 J A2 50 ▭
AMA: 2018,Jan,8; 2017,Jan,8; 2016,Feb,12; 2016,Jan,13; 2015,Jan,16; 2014,Jan,11

67220-67225 Destruction of Choroidal Lesions

INCLUDES Operating microscope (69990)

67220 **Destruction of localized lesion of choroid (eg, choroidal neovascularization); photocoagulation (eg, laser), 1 or more sessions**
INCLUDES Treatment at one or more sessions that may occur at different encounters
EXCLUDES Procedure performed more than one time during a defined period of treatment
🔲 14.2 ✄ 15.1 **FUD** 090 T P2 50 ▭
AMA: 2018,Jan,8; 2017,Jan,8; 2016,Feb,12; 2016,Jan,13; 2015,Jan,16; 2014,Jan,11

67221 **photodynamic therapy (includes intravenous infusion)**
🔲 6.05 ✄ 8.07 **FUD** 000 T P3 ▭
AMA: 2018,Feb,10; 2018,Jan,8; 2017,Jan,8; 2016,Feb,12; 2016,Jan,13; 2015,Jan,16; 2014,Jan,11

+ 67225 photodynamic therapy, second eye, at single session (List separately in addition to code for primary eye treatment)

Code first (67221)

⚕ 0.80   ⚕ 0.84   **FUD** ZZZ   N M1 ▢

AMA: 2018,Jan,8; 2017,Jan,8; 2016,Feb,12; 2016,Jan,13; 2015,Jan,16; 2014,Jan,11

67227-67229 Destruction Retinopathy

INCLUDES Operating microscope (69990)
EXCLUDES Unlisted retinal procedures (67299)

67227 Destruction of extensive or progressive retinopathy (eg, diabetic retinopathy), cryotherapy, diathermy

⚕ 7.30   ⚕ 8.34   **FUD** 010   J P3 50 ▢

AMA: 2018,Jan,8; 2017,Jan,8; 2016,Feb,12; 2016,Jan,13; 2015,Jan,16; 2014,Jan,11

67228 Treatment of extensive or progressive retinopathy (eg, diabetic retinopathy), photocoagulation

⚕ 8.72   ⚕ 9.73   **FUD** 010   T P3 50 ▢

AMA: 2018,Jan,8; 2017,Jan,8; 2016,Feb,12; 2016,Jan,13; 2015,Jan,16; 2014,Jan,11

67229 Treatment of extensive or progressive retinopathy, 1 or more sessions, preterm infant (less than 37 weeks gestation at birth), performed from birth up to 1 year of age (eg, retinopathy of prematurity), photocoagulation or cryotherapy

INCLUDES Treatment at one or more sessions that may occur at different encounters
EXCLUDES Procedure performed more than one time during a defined period of treatment

⚕ 33.1   ⚕ 33.1   **FUD** 090   T R2 50 ▢

AMA: 2018,Jan,8; 2017,Jan,8; 2016,Feb,12; 2016,Jan,13; 2015,Jan,16; 2014,Jan,11

67250-67255 Reinforcement of Posterior Sclera

INCLUDES Operating microscope (69990)
EXCLUDES Removal of lesion of sclera (66130)
Repair scleral staphyloma (66225)

67250 Scleral reinforcement (separate procedure); without graft

⚕ 22.6   ⚕ 22.6   **FUD** 090   J A2 50 ▢

AMA: 2016,Feb,12; 2014,Jan,11

67255 with graft

EXCLUDES Aqueous shunt to extraocular equatorial plate reservoir (66180)
Revision of aqueous shunt to extraocular equatorial plate reservoir; with graft (66185)

⚕ 19.4   ⚕ 19.4   **FUD** 090   J A2 80 50 ▢

AMA: 2018,Jan,8; 2017,Jan,8; 2016,Feb,12; 2016,Jan,13; 2015,Jan,16; 2015,Jan,10; 2014,Jan,11

67299 Unlisted Posterior Segment Procedure

CMS: 100-04,4,180.3 Unlisted Service or Procedure
INCLUDES Operating microscope (69990)

67299 Unlisted procedure, posterior segment

⚕ 0.00   ⚕ 0.00   **FUD** YYY   J 80 50 ▢

AMA: 2018,Jan,8; 2017,Jan,8; 2016,Feb,12; 2016,Jan,13; 2015,Jan,16; 2014,Jan,11

67311-67334 Strabismus Procedures on Extraocular Muscles

INCLUDES Operating microscope (69990)
Code also adjustable sutures (67335)

67311 Strabismus surgery, recession or resection procedure; 1 horizontal muscle

⚕ 16.9   ⚕ 16.9   **FUD** 090   J A2 50 ▢

AMA: 2018,Jan,8; 2017,Jan,8; 2017,Jan,6; 2016,Feb,12; 2016,Jan,13; 2015,Jan,16; 2014,Jan,11

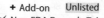

Superior rectus
Superior oblique
Lateral rectus
Inferior oblique
Inferior rectus
Medial rectus (not shown)

Muscles of the eyeball (right eye shown)

67312 2 horizontal muscles

⚕ 20.2   ⚕ 20.2   **FUD** 090   J A2 50 ▢

AMA: 2018,Jan,8; 2017,Jan,8; 2016,Feb,12; 2016,Jan,13; 2015,Jan,16; 2014,Jan,11

67314 1 vertical muscle (excluding superior oblique)

⚕ 19.1   ⚕ 19.1   **FUD** 090   J A2 50 ▢

AMA: 2018,Jan,8; 2017,Jan,8; 2016,Feb,12; 2016,Jan,13; 2015,Jan,16; 2014,Jan,11

67316 2 or more vertical muscles (excluding superior oblique)

⚕ 22.7   ⚕ 22.7   **FUD** 090   J A2 80 50 ▢

AMA: 2018,Jan,8; 2017,Jan,8; 2016,Feb,12; 2016,Jan,13; 2015,Jan,16; 2014,Jan,11

67318 Strabismus surgery, any procedure, superior oblique muscle

⚕ 19.9   ⚕ 19.9   **FUD** 090   J A2 50 ▢

AMA: 2018,Jan,8; 2017,Jan,8; 2016,Feb,12; 2016,Jan,13; 2015,Jan,16; 2014,Jan,11

+ 67320 Transposition procedure (eg, for paretic extraocular muscle), any extraocular muscle (specify) (List separately in addition to code for primary procedure)

Code first (67311-67318)

⚕ 9.17   ⚕ 9.17   **FUD** ZZZ   N M1 ▢

AMA: 2018,Jan,8; 2017,Jan,8; 2016,Feb,12; 2016,Jan,13; 2015,Jan,16; 2014,Jan,11

+ 67331 Strabismus surgery on patient with previous eye surgery or injury that did not involve the extraocular muscles (List separately in addition to code for primary procedure)

Code first (67311-67318)

⚕ 8.70   ⚕ 8.70   **FUD** ZZZ   N M1 50 ▢

AMA: 2018,Jan,8; 2017,Jan,8; 2016,Feb,12; 2016,Jan,13; 2015,Jan,16; 2014,Jan,11

+ 67332 Strabismus surgery on patient with scarring of extraocular muscles (eg, prior ocular injury, strabismus or retinal detachment surgery) or restrictive myopathy (eg, dysthyroid ophthalmopathy) (List separately in addition to code for primary procedure)

Code first (67311-67318)

⚕ 9.44   ⚕ 9.44   **FUD** ZZZ   N M1 50 ▢

AMA: 2018,Jan,8; 2017,Jan,8; 2016,Feb,12; 2016,Jan,13; 2015,Jan,16; 2014,Jan,11

+ **67334** Strabismus surgery by posterior fixation suture technique, with or without muscle recession (List separately in addition to code for primary procedure)
Code first (67311-67318)
🔧 8.59 ⚕ 8.59 **FUD** ZZZ N M1 50 ▢
AMA: 2018,Jan,8; 2017,Jan,8; 2016,Feb,12; 2016,Jan,13; 2015,Jan,16; 2014,Jan,11

67335-67399 Other Procedures of Extraocular Muscles
INCLUDES Operating microscope (69990)

+ **67335** Placement of adjustable suture(s) during strabismus surgery, including postoperative adjustment(s) of suture(s) (List separately in addition to code for specific strabismus surgery)
Code first (67311-67334)
🔧 4.21 ⚕ 4.21 **FUD** ZZZ N M1 50 ▢
AMA: 2018,Jan,8; 2017,Jan,8; 2016,Feb,12; 2016,Jan,13; 2015,Jan,16; 2014,Jan,11

+ **67340** Strabismus surgery involving exploration and/or repair of detached extraocular muscle(s) (List separately in addition to code for primary procedure)
INCLUDES Hummelsheim operation
Code first (67311-67334)
🔧 10.1 ⚕ 10.1 **FUD** ZZZ N M1 80 ▢
AMA: 2018,Jan,8; 2017,Jan,8; 2016,Feb,12; 2016,Jan,13; 2015,Jan,16; 2014,Jan,11

67343 Release of extensive scar tissue without detaching extraocular muscle (separate procedure)
Code also if these procedures are performed on other than the affected muscle (67311-67340)
🔧 18.5 ⚕ 18.5 **FUD** 090 J A2 50 ▢
AMA: 2018,Jan,8; 2017,Jan,8; 2016,Feb,12; 2016,Jan,13; 2015,Jan,16; 2014,Jan,11

67345 Chemodenervation of extraocular muscle
EXCLUDES Nerve destruction for blepharospasm and other neurological disorders (64612, 64616)
🔧 6.22 ⚕ 6.96 **FUD** 010 T P3 50 ▢
AMA: 2019,Apr,9; 2018,Jan,8; 2017,Jan,8; 2016,Feb,12; 2016,Jan,13; 2015,Jan,16; 2014,May,5; 2014,Jan,11

67346 Biopsy of extraocular muscle
EXCLUDES Repair laceration extraocular muscle, tendon, or Tenon's capsule (65290)
🔧 5.50 ⚕ 5.50 **FUD** 000 J A2 80 50 ▢
AMA: 2016,Feb,12; 2014,Jan,11

67399 Unlisted procedure, extraocular muscle
🔧 0.00 ⚕ 0.00 **FUD** YYY T 80 50 ▢
AMA: 2018,Jan,8; 2017,Jul,10; 2016,Feb,12; 2014,Jan,11

67400-67415 Frontal Orbitotomy
INCLUDES Operating microscope (69990)

67400 Orbitotomy without bone flap (frontal or transconjunctival approach); for exploration, with or without biopsy
🔧 26.7 ⚕ 26.7 **FUD** 090 J A2 50 ▢
AMA: 2016,Feb,12; 2014,Jan,11

67405 with drainage only
🔧 22.8 ⚕ 22.8 **FUD** 090 J A2 50 ▢
AMA: 2018,Jan,8; 2017,Jan,8; 2016,Feb,12; 2016,Jan,13; 2015,Jan,16; 2014,Jan,11

67412 with removal of lesion
🔧 24.6 ⚕ 24.6 **FUD** 090 J A2 50 ▢
AMA: 2016,Feb,12; 2014,Jan,11

67413 with removal of foreign body
🔧 24.7 ⚕ 24.7 **FUD** 090 J A2 80 50 ▢
AMA: 2016,Feb,12; 2014,Jan,11

67414 with removal of bone for decompression
🔧 38.1 ⚕ 38.1 **FUD** 090 J G2 80 50 ▢
AMA: 2018,Jan,8; 2017,Jan,8; 2016,Feb,12; 2016,Jan,13; 2015,Jan,16; 2014,Jan,11

67415 Fine needle aspiration of orbital contents
EXCLUDES Decompression optic nerve (67570)
Exenteration, enucleation, and repair (65101-65175)
🔧 2.97 ⚕ 2.97 **FUD** 000 J A2 80 50 ▢
AMA: 2016,Feb,12; 2014,Jan,11

67420-67450 Lateral Orbitotomy
INCLUDES Operating microscope (69990)
EXCLUDES Orbital implant (67550, 67560)
Surgical removal of all or some of the orbital contents or repair after removal (65091-65175)
Transcranial approach orbitotomy (61330, 61333)

67420 Orbitotomy with bone flap or window, lateral approach (eg, Kroenlein); with removal of lesion
🔧 46.2 ⚕ 46.2 **FUD** 090 J A2 80 50 ▢
AMA: 2016,Feb,12; 2014,Jan,11

67430 with removal of foreign body
🔧 35.9 ⚕ 35.9 **FUD** 090 J A2 80 50 ▢
AMA: 2016,Feb,12; 2014,Jan,11

67440 with drainage
🔧 34.7 ⚕ 34.7 **FUD** 090 J A2 80 50 ▢
AMA: 2016,Feb,12; 2014,Jan,11

67445 with removal of bone for decompression
EXCLUDES Decompression optic nerve sheath (67570)
🔧 40.3 ⚕ 40.3 **FUD** 090 J A2 80 50 ▢
AMA: 2016,Feb,12; 2014,Jan,11

67450 for exploration, with or without biopsy
🔧 36.1 ⚕ 36.1 **FUD** 090 J A2 80 50 ▢
AMA: 2016,Feb,12; 2014,Jan,11

67500-67515 Eye Injections
INCLUDES Operating microscope (69990)

67500 Retrobulbar injection; medication (separate procedure, does not include supply of medication)
🔧 1.73 ⚕ 2.02 **FUD** 000 T G2 50 ▢
AMA: 2018,Jan,8; 2017,Jan,8; 2016,Feb,12; 2016,Jan,13; 2015,Jan,16; 2014,Jan,11

67505 alcohol
🔧 2.03 ⚕ 2.38 **FUD** 000 T P3 50 ▢
AMA: 2016,Feb,12; 2014,Jan,11

67515 Injection of medication or other substance into Tenon's capsule
EXCLUDES Subconjunctival injection (68200)
🔧 2.06 ⚕ 2.24 **FUD** 000 T P3 50 ▢
AMA: 2018,Jan,8; 2017,Jan,8; 2016,Feb,12; 2016,Jan,13; 2015,Jan,16; 2014,Jan,11

67550-67560 Orbital Implant
INCLUDES Operating microscope (69990)
EXCLUDES Fracture repair malar area, orbit (21355-21408)
Ocular implant inside muscle cone (65093-65105, 65130-65175)

67550 Orbital implant (implant outside muscle cone); insertion
🔧 27.8 ⚕ 27.8 **FUD** 090 J A2 50 ▢
AMA: 2016,Feb,12; 2014,Jan,11

67560 removal or revision
🔧 28.5 ⚕ 28.5 **FUD** 090 J A2 80 50 ▢
AMA: 2016,Feb,12; 2014,Jan,11

67570-67599 Other and Unlisted Orbital Procedures
INCLUDES Operating microscope (69990)

67570 Optic nerve decompression (eg, incision or fenestration of optic nerve sheath)
🔧 33.9 ⚕ 33.9 **FUD** 090 J A2 80 50 ▢
AMA: 2016,Feb,12; 2014,Jan,11

67599 Unlisted procedure, orbit
🔧 0.00 ⚕ 0.00 **FUD** YYY T 80 50 ▢
AMA: 2016,Feb,12; 2014,Jan,11

67700-67810 [67810] Incisional Procedures of Eyelids

INCLUDES   Operating microscope (69990)

67700   Blepharotomy, drainage of abscess, eyelid
🔪 3.31   ✂ 7.82   **FUD** 010   T P2 50 ▣
AMA: 2018,Jan,8; 2017,Jan,8; 2016,Feb,12; 2016,Jan,13; 2015,Jan,16; 2014,Jan,11

67710   Severing of tarsorrhaphy
🔪 2.77   ✂ 6.56   **FUD** 010   T P3 50 ▣
AMA: 2018,Jan,8; 2017,Jan,8; 2016,Feb,12; 2016,Jan,13; 2015,Jan,16; 2014,Jan,11

67715   Canthotomy (separate procedure)
EXCLUDES   Canthoplasty (67950)
Symblepharon division (68340)
🔪 3.08   ✂ 7.07   **FUD** 010   J A2 50 ▣
AMA: 2018,Jan,8; 2017,Jan,8; 2016,Feb,12; 2016,Jan,13; 2015,Jan,16; 2014,Jan,11

 #   67810   Incisional biopsy of eyelid skin including lid margin
EXCLUDES   Biopsy of eyelid skin (11102-11107)
🔪 2.03   ✂ 4.99   **FUD** 000   T P3 50 ▣
AMA: 2019,Jan,9; 2018,Jan,8; 2017,Jan,8; 2016,Feb,12; 2016,Jan,13; 2015,Jan,16; 2014,Jan,11

67800-67808 Excision of Chalazion (Meibomian Cyst)

INCLUDES   Lesion removal requiring more than skin:
Lid margin
Palpebral conjunctiva
Tarsus
Operating microscope (69990)
EXCLUDES   Blepharoplasty, graft, or reconstructive procedures (67930-67975)
Excision/destruction skin lesion of eyelid (11310-11313, 11440-11446, 11640-11646, 17000-17004)

67800   Excision of chalazion; single
🔪 2.93   ✂ 3.64   **FUD** 010   T P3 ▣
AMA: 2018,Jan,8; 2017,Jan,8; 2016,Feb,12; 2016,Jan,13; 2015,Jan,16; 2014,Jan,11

67801   multiple, same lid
🔪 3.79   ✂ 4.64   **FUD** 010   T P3 ▣
AMA: 2016,Feb,12; 2014,Jan,11

67805   multiple, different lids
🔪 4.67   ✂ 5.76   **FUD** 010   T P3 ▣
AMA: 2018,Jan,8; 2017,Jan,8; 2016,Feb,12; 2016,Jan,13; 2015,Jan,16; 2014,Jan,11

67808   under general anesthesia and/or requiring hospitalization, single or multiple
🔪 10.4   ✂ 10.4   **FUD** 090   J A2 ▣
AMA: 2016,Feb,12; 2014,Jan,11

67810-67850 Other Eyelid Procedures

INCLUDES   Operating microscope (69990)

67810   Resequenced code. See code following 67715.

67820   Correction of trichiasis; epilation, by forceps only
🔪 0.99   ✂ 0.93   **FUD** 000   01 N1 50 ▣
AMA: 2018,Jan,8; 2017,Jan,8; 2016,Feb,12; 2016,Jan,13; 2015,Jan,16; 2014,Jan,11

67825   epilation by other than forceps (eg, by electrosurgery, cryotherapy, laser surgery)
🔪 3.46   ✂ 3.71   **FUD** 010   T P3 50 ▣
AMA: 2018,Jan,8; 2017,Jan,8; 2016,Feb,12; 2016,Jan,13; 2015,Jan,16; 2014,Jan,11

67830   incision of lid margin
🔪 3.92   ✂ 7.64   **FUD** 010   T A2 50 ▣
AMA: 2016,Feb,12; 2014,Jan,11

67835   incision of lid margin, with free mucous membrane graft
🔪 12.4   ✂ 12.4   **FUD** 090   J A2 80 50 ▣
AMA: 2016,Feb,12; 2014,Jan,11

67840   Excision of lesion of eyelid (except chalazion) without closure or with simple direct closure
EXCLUDES   Eyelid resection and reconstruction (67961, 67966)
🔪 4.49   ✂ 7.91   **FUD** 010   T P3 50 ▣
AMA: 2019,Jan,14; 2016,Feb,12; 2014,Jan,11

67850   Destruction of lesion of lid margin (up to 1 cm)
EXCLUDES   Mohs micro procedures (17311-17315)
Topical chemotherapy (99201-99215)
🔪 3.84   ✂ 6.13   **FUD** 010   T P3 50 ▣
AMA: 2016,Feb,12; 2014,Jan,11

67875-67882 Suturing of the Eyelids

INCLUDES   Operating microscope (69990)
EXCLUDES   Canthoplasty (67950)
Canthotomy (67715)
Severing of tarsorrhaphy (67710)

67875   Temporary closure of eyelids by suture (eg, Frost suture)
🔪 2.75   ✂ 4.96   **FUD** 000   T G2 50 ▣
AMA: 2016,Feb,12; 2014,Jan,11

67880   Construction of intermarginal adhesions, median tarsorrhaphy, or canthorrhaphy;
🔪 10.4   ✂ 13.1   **FUD** 090   J A2 50 ▣
AMA: 2016,Feb,12; 2014,Jan,11

67882   with transposition of tarsal plate
🔪 13.4   ✂ 16.1   **FUD** 090   J A2 50 ▣
AMA: 2016,Feb,12; 2014,Jan,11

67900-67912 Repair of Ptosis/Retraction Eyelids, Eyebrows

INCLUDES   Operating microscope (69990)

67900   Repair of brow ptosis (supraciliary, mid-forehead or coronal approach)
EXCLUDES   Forehead rhytidectomy (15824)
🔪 14.4   ✂ 18.2   **FUD** 090   J A2 50 ▣
AMA: 2018,Jan,8; 2017,Jan,8; 2016,Feb,12; 2016,Jan,13; 2015,Jan,16; 2014,Jan,11

67901   Repair of blepharoptosis; frontalis muscle technique with suture or other material (eg, banked fascia)
🔪 16.5   ✂ 21.9   **FUD** 090   J A2 50 ▣
AMA: 2018,Jan,8; 2017,Jul,10; 2017,Jan,8; 2016,Feb,12; 2016,Jan,13; 2015,Jan,16; 2014,Jan,11

67902   frontalis muscle technique with autologous fascial sling (includes obtaining fascia)
🔪 20.5   ✂ 20.5   **FUD** 090   J A2 50 ▣
AMA: 2018,Jan,8; 2017,Jan,8; 2016,Feb,12; 2016,Jan,13; 2015,Jan,16; 2014,Jan,11

67903   (tarso) levator resection or advancement, internal approach
🔪 13.7   ✂ 16.9   **FUD** 090   J A2 50 ▣
AMA: 2018,Jan,8; 2017,Jan,8; 2016,Feb,12; 2016,Jan,13; 2015,Jan,16; 2014,Jan,11

67904   **(tarso) levator resection or advancement, external approach**

INCLUDES   Everbusch's operation

🔧 16.9   ⚕ 20.9   **FUD** 090   J A2 50 ▭

AMA: 2018,Jan,8; 2017,Jan,8; 2016,Feb,12; 2016,Jan,13; 2015,Jan,16; 2014,Jan,11

67906   **superior rectus technique with fascial sling (includes obtaining fascia)**

🔧 14.4   ⚕ 14.4   **FUD** 090   J A2 50 ▭

AMA: 2018,Jan,8; 2017,Jan,8; 2016,Feb,12; 2016,Jan,13; 2015,Jan,16; 2014,Jan,11

67908   **conjunctivo-tarso-Muller's muscle-levator resection (eg, Fasanella-Servat type)**

🔧 12.1   ⚕ 14.1   **FUD** 090   J A2 50 ▭

AMA: 2018,Jan,8; 2017,Jan,8; 2016,Feb,12; 2016,Jan,13; 2015,Jan,16; 2014,Jan,11

67909   **Reduction of overcorrection of ptosis**

🔧 12.4   ⚕ 15.3   **FUD** 090   J A2 50 ▭

AMA: 2018,Jan,8; 2017,Jan,8; 2016,Feb,12; 2016,Jan,13; 2015,Jan,16; 2014,Jan,11

67911   **Correction of lid retraction**

EXCLUDES   Autologous graft harvest ([15769], 20920, 20922)
Lid defect correction using fat obtained via liposuction (15773-15774)
Mucous membrane graft repair of trichiasis (67835)

🔧 15.9   ⚕ 15.9   **FUD** 090   J A2 50 ▭

AMA: 2018,Jan,8; 2017,Jan,8; 2016,Feb,12; 2016,Jan,13; 2015,Jan,16; 2014,Jan,11

67912   **Correction of lagophthalmos, with implantation of upper eyelid lid load (eg, gold weight)**

🔧 13.8   ⚕ 25.4   **FUD** 090   J A2 50 ▭

AMA: 2018,Jan,8; 2017,Jan,8; 2016,Feb,12; 2016,Jan,13; 2015,Jan,16; 2014,Jan,11

67914-67924 Repair Ectropion/Entropion

INCLUDES   Operating microscope (69990)
EXCLUDES   Cicatricial ectropion or entropion with scar excision or graft (67961-67966)

67914   **Repair of ectropion; suture**

INCLUDES   Canthoplasty (67950)

🔧 9.29   ⚕ 13.5   **FUD** 090   J A2 50 ▭

AMA: 2018,Jan,8; 2017,Jan,8; 2016,Feb,12; 2016,Jan,13; 2015,Jan,16; 2014,Jan,11

67915   **thermocauterization**

🔧 5.62   ⚕ 8.52   **FUD** 090   J P3 50 ▭

AMA: 2018,Jan,8; 2017,Jan,8; 2016,Feb,12; 2016,Jan,13; 2015,Jan,16; 2014,Jan,11

67916   **excision tarsal wedge**

🔧 12.2   ⚕ 17.0   **FUD** 090   J A2 50 ▭

AMA: 2018,Jan,8; 2017,Jan,8; 2016,Feb,12; 2016,Jan,13; 2015,Jan,16; 2014,Jan,11

67917   **extensive (eg, tarsal strip operations)**

EXCLUDES   Repair of everted punctum (68705)

🔧 13.0   ⚕ 17.3   **FUD** 090   J A2 50 ▭

AMA: 2018,Jan,8; 2017,Jan,8; 2016,Feb,12; 2016,Jan,13; 2015,Jan,16; 2014,Jan,11

67921   **Repair of entropion; suture**

🔧 8.82   ⚕ 13.2   **FUD** 090   J A2 50 ▭

AMA: 2018,Jan,8; 2017,Jan,8; 2016,Feb,12; 2016,Jan,13; 2015,Jan,16; 2014,Jan,11

67922   **thermocauterization**

🔧 5.60   ⚕ 8.37   **FUD** 090   J P3 50 ▭

AMA: 2018,Jan,8; 2017,Jan,8; 2016,Feb,12; 2016,Jan,13; 2015,Jan,16; 2014,Jan,11

67923   **excision tarsal wedge**

🔧 12.2   ⚕ 17.0   **FUD** 090   J A2 50 ▭

AMA: 2018,Jan,8; 2017,Jan,8; 2016,Feb,12; 2016,Jan,13; 2015,Jan,16; 2014,Jan,11

67924   **extensive (eg, tarsal strip or capsulopalpebral fascia repairs operation)**

INCLUDES   Canthoplasty (67950)

🔧 13.0   ⚕ 18.1   **FUD** 090   J A2 50 ▭

AMA: 2018,Jan,8; 2017,Jan,8; 2016,Feb,12; 2016,Jan,13; 2015,Jan,16; 2014,Jan,11

67930-67935 Repair Eyelid Wound

INCLUDES   Operating microscope (69990)
Repairs involving more than skin:
    Lid margin
    Palpebral conjunctiva
    Tarsus
EXCLUDES   Blepharoplasty for entropion or ectropion (67916-67917, 67923-67924)
Correction of lid retraction and blepharoptosis (67901-67911)
Free graft (15120-15121, 15260-15261)
Graft preparation (15004)
Plastic repair of lacrimal canaliculi (68700)
Removal of eyelid lesion (67800 [67810], 67840-67850)
Repair involving skin of eyelid (12011-12018, 12051-12057, 13151-13153)
Repair of blepharochalasis (15820-15823)
Skin adjacent tissue transfer (14060-14061)
Tarsorrhaphy, canthorrhaphy (67880, 67882)

67930   **Suture of recent wound, eyelid, involving lid margin, tarsus, and/or palpebral conjunctiva direct closure; partial thickness**

🔧 6.82   ⚕ 10.4   **FUD** 010   J P3 50 ▭

AMA: 2016,Feb,12; 2014,Jan,11

67935   **full thickness**

🔧 12.6   ⚕ 16.9   **FUD** 090   J A2 50 ▭

AMA: 2016,Feb,12; 2014,Jan,11

67938-67999 Eyelid Reconstruction/Repair/Removal Deep Foreign Body

INCLUDES   Operating microscope (69990)
EXCLUDES   Blepharoplasty for entropion or ectropion (67916-67917, 67923-67924)
Correction of lid retraction and blepharoptosis (67901-67911)
Free graft (15120-15121, 15260-15261)
Graft preparation (15004)
Plastic repair of lacrimal canaliculi (68700)
Removal of eyelid lesion (67800-67808, 67840-67850)
Repair involving skin of eyelid (12011-12018, 12051-12057, 13151-13153)
Repair of blepharochalasis (15820-15823)
Skin adjacent tissue transfer (14060-14061)
Tarsorrhaphy, canthorrhaphy (67880, 67882)

67938   **Removal of embedded foreign body, eyelid**

🔧 3.31   ⚕ 7.19   **FUD** 010   T P2 50 ▭

AMA: 2018,Jan,8; 2017,Jan,8; 2016,Feb,12; 2016,Jan,13; 2015,Jan,16; 2014,May,5; 2014,Jan,11

67950   **Canthoplasty (reconstruction of canthus)**

🔧 13.1   ⚕ 16.3   **FUD** 090   J A2 50 ▭

AMA: 2016,Feb,12; 2014,Jan,11

67961   **Excision and repair of eyelid, involving lid margin, tarsus, conjunctiva, canthus, or full thickness, may include preparation for skin graft or pedicle flap with adjacent tissue transfer or rearrangement; up to one-fourth of lid margin**

INCLUDES   Canthoplasty (67950)
EXCLUDES   Delay flap (15630)
Flap attachment (15650)
Free skin grafts (15120-15121, 15260-15261)
Tubed pedicle flap preparation (15576)

🔧 12.9   ⚕ 16.4   **FUD** 090   J A2 80 50 ▭

AMA: 2018,Jan,8; 2017,Jan,8; 2016,Feb,12; 2016,Jan,13; 2015,Jan,16; 2014,Jan,11

67966   **over one-fourth of lid margin**

INCLUDES   Canthoplasty (67950)
EXCLUDES   Delay flap (15630)
Flap attachment (15650)
Free skin grafts (15120-15121, 15260-15261)
Tubed pedicle flap preparation (15576)

🔧 18.7   ⚕ 21.9   **FUD** 090   J A2 50 ▭

AMA: 2018,Jan,8; 2017,Jan,8; 2016,Feb,12; 2016,Jan,13; 2015,Jan,16; 2014,Jan,11

26/TC PC/TC Only   A2-Z3 ASC Payment   50 Bilateral   ♂ Male Only   ♀ Female Only   🔧 Facility RVU   ⚕ Non-Facility RVU   ▭ CCI   ☒ CLIA
FUD Follow-up Days   CMS: IOM   AMA: CPT Asst   A-Y OPPSI   80/80 Surg Assist Allowed / w/Doc   Lab crosswalk   Radiology crosswalk

324   CPT © 2019 American Medical Association. All Rights Reserved.   © 2019 Optum360, LLC

67971 Reconstruction of eyelid, full thickness by transfer of tarsoconjunctival flap from opposing eyelid; up to two-thirds of eyelid, 1 stage or first stage

 INCLUDES Dupuy-Dutemp reconstruction
    Landboldt's operation
  🔲 20.5 ⚕ 20.5 **FUD** 090   J A2 50 ▢
  AMA: 2016,Feb,12; 2014,Jan,11

67973 total eyelid, lower, 1 stage or first stage

 INCLUDES Landboldt's operation
  🔲 26.4 ⚕ 26.4 **FUD** 090 J A2 80 50 ▢
  AMA: 2016,Feb,12; 2014,Jan,11

67974 total eyelid, upper, 1 stage or first stage

 INCLUDES Landboldt's operation
  🔲 26.4 ⚕ 26.4 **FUD** 090 J A2 80 50 ▢
  AMA: 2016,Feb,12; 2014,Jan,11

67975 second stage

 INCLUDES Landboldt's operation
  🔲 19.4 ⚕ 19.4 **FUD** 090 J A2 50 ▢
  AMA: 2016,Feb,12; 2014,Jan,11

67999 Unlisted procedure, eyelids

  🔲 0.00 ⚕ 0.00 **FUD** YYY T 80 50 ▢
  AMA: 2018,Jan,8; 2017,Jul,10; 2017,Jan,8; 2016,Feb,12; 2016,Jan,13; 2015,Jan,16; 2014,Jan,11

68020-68200 Conjunctival Biopsy/Injection/Treatment of Lesions

 INCLUDES Operating microscope (69990)
 EXCLUDES *Foreign body removal (65205-65265)*

68020 Incision of conjunctiva, drainage of cyst

  🔲 3.15 ⚕ 3.44 **FUD** 010 T P3 50 ▢
  AMA: 2016,Feb,12; 2014,Jan,11

68040 Expression of conjunctival follicles (eg, for trachoma)

 EXCLUDES *Automated evacuation meibomian glands with heat/pressure (0207T)*
    Manual evacuation of meibomian glands ([0563T])
  🔲 1.41 ⚕ 1.78 **FUD** 000 T P3 50 ▢
  AMA: 2018,Jan,8; 2017,Jan,8; 2016,Feb,12; 2016,Jan,13; 2015,Jan,16; 2014,May,5; 2014,Jan,11

68100 Biopsy of conjunctiva

  🔲 2.75 ⚕ 4.97 **FUD** 000 J P3 50 ▢
  AMA: 2019,Jan,9; 2016,Feb,12; 2014,Jan,11

68110 Excision of lesion, conjunctiva; up to 1 cm

  🔲 4.22 ⚕ 6.56 **FUD** 010 J P3 50 ▢
  AMA: 2018,Feb,11; 2018,Jan,8; 2017,Jan,6; 2016,Feb,12; 2014,Jan,11

68115 over 1 cm

  🔲 5.23 ⚕ 9.07 **FUD** 010 J A2 50 ▢
  AMA: 2018,Feb,11; 2016,Feb,12; 2014,Jan,11

68130 with adjacent sclera

  🔲 11.7 ⚕ 15.4 **FUD** 090 J A2 50 ▢
  AMA: 2016,Feb,12; 2014,Jan,11

68135 Destruction of lesion, conjunctiva

  🔲 4.28 ⚕ 4.49 **FUD** 010 J P3 50 ▢
  AMA: 2016,Feb,12; 2014,Jan,11

68200 Subconjunctival injection

 EXCLUDES *Retrobulbar or Tenon's capsule injection (67500-67515)*
  🔲 0.99 ⚕ 1.18 **FUD** 000 01 N1 50 ▢
  AMA: 2018,Jan,8; 2017,Jan,8; 2016,Feb,12; 2016,Jan,13; 2015,Jan,16; 2014,Jan,11

68320-68340 Conjunctivoplasty Procedures

 INCLUDES Operating microscope (69990)
 EXCLUDES *Conjunctival foreign body removal (65205, 65210)*
    Laceration repair (65270-65273)

68320 Conjunctivoplasty; with conjunctival graft or extensive rearrangement

  🔲 15.3 ⚕ 20.8 **FUD** 090 J A2 50 ▢
  AMA: 2018,Jan,8; 2017,Jan,8; 2016,Feb,12; 2016,Jan,13; 2015,Jan,16; 2014,Jan,11

68325 with buccal mucous membrane graft (includes obtaining graft)

  🔲 18.6 ⚕ 18.6 **FUD** 090 J A2 50 ▢
  AMA: 2016,Feb,12; 2014,Jan,11

68326 Conjunctivoplasty, reconstruction cul-de-sac; with conjunctival graft or extensive rearrangement

  🔲 18.3 ⚕ 18.3 **FUD** 090 J A2 50 ▢
  AMA: 2016,Feb,12; 2014,Jan,11

68328 with buccal mucous membrane graft (includes obtaining graft)

  🔲 20.1 ⚕ 20.1 **FUD** 090 J A2 80 50 ▢
  AMA: 2016,Feb,12; 2014,Jan,11

68330 Repair of symblepharon; conjunctivoplasty, without graft

  🔲 13.1 ⚕ 17.3 **FUD** 090 J A2 80 50 ▢
  AMA: 2016,Feb,12; 2014,Jan,11

68335 with free graft conjunctiva or buccal mucous membrane (includes obtaining graft)

  🔲 18.4 ⚕ 18.4 **FUD** 090 J A2 50 ▢
  AMA: 2016,Feb,12; 2014,Jan,11

68340 division of symblepharon, with or without insertion of conformer or contact lens

  🔲 11.3 ⚕ 16.0 **FUD** 090 J A2 80 50 ▢
  AMA: 2016,Feb,12; 2014,Jan,11

68360-68399 Conjunctival Flaps and Unlisted Procedures

 INCLUDES Operating microscope (69990)

68360 Conjunctival flap; bridge or partial (separate procedure)

 EXCLUDES *Conjunctival flap for injury (65280, 65285)*
    Conjunctival foreign body removal (65205, 65210)
    Surgical wound repair (66250)
  🔲 11.7 ⚕ 15.3 **FUD** 090 J A2 50 ▢
  AMA: 2016,Feb,12; 2014,Jan,11

68362 total (such as Gunderson thin flap or purse string flap)

 EXCLUDES *Conjunctival flap for injury (65280, 65285)*
    Conjunctival foreign body removal (65205, 65210)
    Surgical wound repair (66250)
  🔲 18.6 ⚕ 18.6 **FUD** 090 J A2 50 ▢
  AMA: 2018,Jan,8; 2017,Jan,8; 2016,Feb,12; 2016,Jan,13; 2015,Jan,16; 2014,Jan,11

68371 Harvesting conjunctival allograft, living donor

  🔲 11.7 ⚕ 11.7 **FUD** 010 J A2 50 ▢
  AMA: 2018,Jan,8; 2017,Jan,8; 2016,Feb,12; 2016,Jan,13; 2015,Jan,16; 2014,Jan,11

68399 Unlisted procedure, conjunctiva

  🔲 0.00 ⚕ 0.00 **FUD** YYY T 80 50 ▢
  AMA: 2018,Jan,8; 2017,Jan,8; 2016,Feb,12; 2016,Jan,13; 2015,Jan,16; 2014,Jan,11

68400-68899 Nasolacrimal System Procedures

INCLUDES   Operating microscope (69990)

68400   Incision, drainage of lacrimal gland
🔲 3.76   ⚖ 8.24   **FUD** 010   T P3 50 ▭
AMA: 2016,Feb,12; 2014,Jan,11

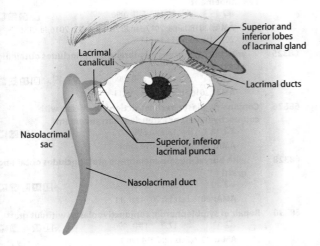

Superior and inferior lobes of lacrimal gland

Lacrimal canaliculi

Lacrimal ducts

Nasolacrimal sac

Superior, inferior lacrimal puncta

Nasolacrimal duct

68420   Incision, drainage of lacrimal sac (dacryocystotomy or dacryocystostomy)
🔲 4.78   ⚖ 9.28   **FUD** 010   J P3 50 ▭
AMA: 2016,Feb,12; 2014,Jan,11

68440   Snip incision of lacrimal punctum
🔲 2.81   ⚖ 2.92   **FUD** 010   T P3 50 ▭
AMA: 2016,Feb,12; 2014,Jan,11

68500   Excision of lacrimal gland (dacryoadenectomy), except for tumor; total
🔲 27.8   ⚖ 27.8   **FUD** 090   J A2 50 ▭
AMA: 2016,Feb,12; 2014,Jan,11

68505   partial
🔲 27.7   ⚖ 27.7   **FUD** 090   J A2 50 ▭
AMA: 2016,Feb,12; 2014,Jan,11

68510   Biopsy of lacrimal gland
🔲 8.33   ⚖ 12.8   **FUD** 000   J A2 80 50 ▭
AMA: 2016,Feb,12; 2014,Jan,11

68520   Excision of lacrimal sac (dacryocystectomy)
🔲 19.6   ⚖ 19.6   **FUD** 090   J A2 80 50 ▭
AMA: 2016,Feb,12; 2014,Jan,11

68525   Biopsy of lacrimal sac
🔲 7.52   ⚖ 7.52   **FUD** 000   J A2 50 ▭
AMA: 2016,Feb,12; 2014,Jan,11

68530   Removal of foreign body or dacryolith, lacrimal passages
INCLUDES   Meller's excision
🔲 7.29   ⚖ 12.2   **FUD** 010   T P2 50 ▭
AMA: 2016,Feb,12; 2014,Jan,11

68540   Excision of lacrimal gland tumor; frontal approach
🔲 26.5   ⚖ 26.5   **FUD** 090   J A2 50 ▭
AMA: 2016,Feb,12; 2014,Jan,11

68550   involving osteotomy
🔲 32.5   ⚖ 32.5   **FUD** 090   J A2 50 ▭
AMA: 2016,Feb,12; 2014,Jan,11

68700   Plastic repair of canaliculi
🔲 17.1   ⚖ 17.1   **FUD** 090   J A2 50 ▭
AMA: 2016,Feb,12; 2014,Jan,11

68705   Correction of everted punctum, cautery
🔲 4.72   ⚖ 6.99   **FUD** 010   T P2 50 ▭
AMA: 2018,Jan,8; 2017,Jan,8; 2016,Feb,12; 2016,Jan,13; 2015,Jan,16; 2014,Jan,11

68720   Dacryocystorhinostomy (fistulization of lacrimal sac to nasal cavity)
🔲 21.6   ⚖ 21.6   **FUD** 090   J A2 80 50 ▭
AMA: 2018,Jan,8; 2017,Jan,8; 2016,Feb,12; 2016,Jan,13; 2015,Jan,16; 2014,Jan,11

68745   Conjunctivorhinostomy (fistulization of conjunctiva to nasal cavity); without tube
🔲 21.6   ⚖ 21.6   **FUD** 090   J A2 80 50 ▭
AMA: 2016,Feb,12; 2014,Jan,11

68750   with insertion of tube or stent
🔲 22.4   ⚖ 22.4   **FUD** 090   J A2 80 50 ▭
AMA: 2018,Jan,8; 2017,Jan,8; 2016,Feb,12; 2016,Jan,13; 2015,Jan,16; 2014,Jan,11

68760   Closure of the lacrimal punctum; by thermocauterization, ligation, or laser surgery
🔲 4.15   ⚖ 5.92   **FUD** 010   T P3 50 ▭
AMA: 2016,Feb,12; 2014,Jan,11

68761   by plug, each
EXCLUDES   Drug-eluting lacrimal implant (0356T)
              Drug-eluting ocular insert (0444T-0445T)
🔲 3.36   ⚖ 4.22   **FUD** 010   T P3 80 50 ▭
AMA: 2018,Jan,8; 2017,Jan,8; 2016,Feb,12; 2016,Jan,13; 2015,Jan,16; 2014,Jan,11

68770   Closure of lacrimal fistula (separate procedure)
🔲 17.8   ⚖ 17.8   **FUD** 090   J A2 80 50 ▭
AMA: 2016,Feb,12; 2014,Jan,11

68801   Dilation of lacrimal punctum, with or without irrigation
🔲 2.22   ⚖ 2.57   **FUD** 010   01 N1 50 ▭
AMA: 2016,Feb,12; 2014,Jan,11

68810   Probing of nasolacrimal duct, with or without irrigation;
EXCLUDES   Ophthalmological exam under anesthesia (92018)
🔲 3.64   ⚖ 4.47   **FUD** 010   T A2 50 ▭
AMA: 2018,Jan,8; 2017,Jan,8; 2016,Feb,12; 2016,Jan,13; 2015,Jan,16; 2014,Jan,11

68811   requiring general anesthesia
EXCLUDES   Ophthalmological exam under anesthesia (92018)
🔲 3.87   ⚖ 3.87   **FUD** 010   J A2 50 ▭
AMA: 2018,Jan,8; 2017,Jan,8; 2016,Feb,12; 2016,Jan,13; 2015,Jan,16; 2014,Jan,11

68815   with insertion of tube or stent
EXCLUDES   Drug eluting ocular insert (0444T-0445T)
              Drug eluting lacrimal implant (0356T)
              Ophthalmological exam under anesthesia (92018)
🔲 6.31   ⚖ 11.2   **FUD** 010   J A2 50 ▭
AMA: 2018,Jan,8; 2017,Jan,8; 2016,Feb,12; 2016,Jan,13; 2015,Jan,16; 2014,Jan,11

68816   with transluminal balloon catheter dilation
EXCLUDES   Probing of nasolacrimal duct (68810-68811, 68815)
🔲 4.49   ⚖ 20.5   **FUD** 010   J 02 50 ▭
AMA: 2018,Jan,8; 2017,Jan,8; 2016,Feb,12; 2016,Jan,13; 2015,Jan,16; 2014,Jan,11

68840   Probing of lacrimal canaliculi, with or without irrigation
🔲 3.31   ⚖ 3.67   **FUD** 010   T P3 50 ▭
AMA: 2016,Feb,12; 2014,Jan,11

68850   Injection of contrast medium for dacryocystography
🔀 (70170, 78660)
🔲 1.59   ⚖ 1.79   **FUD** 000   N N1 50 ▭
AMA: 2018,Jan,8; 2017,Jan,8; 2016,Feb,12; 2016,Jan,13; 2015,Jan,16; 2014,Jan,11

68899   Unlisted procedure, lacrimal system
🔲 0.00   ⚖ 0.00   **FUD** YYY   T 80 50 ▭
AMA: 2014,Jan,11

69000-69020 Treatment External Abscess/Hematoma

69000   **Drainage external ear, abscess or hematoma; simple**
🖐 3.42   ✄ 5.29   **FUD** 010   T P3 50
AMA: 2018,Jan,8; 2017,Jan,8; 2016,Jan,13; 2015,Jan,16; 2014,Jan,11

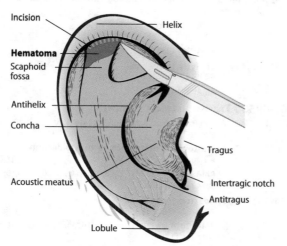

Incision
Helix
Hematoma
Scaphoid fossa
Antihelix
Concha
Tragus
Acoustic meatus
Intertragic notch
Antitragus
Lobule

An incision is made to drain the contents of an abscess or hematoma

69005   **complicated**
🖐 4.50   ✄ 6.13   **FUD** 010   J P3 50
AMA: 2014,Jan,11

69020   **Drainage external auditory canal, abscess**
🖐 4.03   ✄ 6.57   **FUD** 010   T P3 50
AMA: 2018,Jan,8; 2017,Jan,8; 2016,Jan,13; 2015,Jan,16; 2014,Jan,11

69090 Cosmetic Ear Piercing

CMS: 100-02,16,10 Exclusions from Coverage; 100-02,16,120 Cosmetic Procedures

69090   **Ear piercing**
🖐 0.00   ✄ 0.00   **FUD** XXX   E
AMA: 2014,Jan,11

69100-69222 External Ear/Auditory Canal Procedures

EXCLUDES   Reconstruction of ear (see integumentary section codes)

69100   **Biopsy external ear**
🖐 1.40   ✄ 2.79   **FUD** 000   T P3
AMA: 2019,Jan,9; 2014,Jan,11

69105   **Biopsy external auditory canal**
🖐 1.79   ✄ 3.99   **FUD** 000   T P3 50
AMA: 2014,Jan,11

69110   **Excision external ear; partial, simple repair**
🖐 9.21   ✄ 13.0   **FUD** 090   J A2 50
AMA: 2014,Jan,11

69120   **complete amputation**
🖐 11.3   ✄ 11.3   **FUD** 090   J A2
AMA: 2014,Jan,11

69140   **Excision exostosis(es), external auditory canal**
🖐 25.0   ✄ 25.0   **FUD** 090   J A2 80 50
AMA: 2014,Jan,11

69145   **Excision soft tissue lesion, external auditory canal**
🖐 7.04   ✄ 11.1   **FUD** 090   J A2 50
AMA: 2014,Jan,11

69150   **Radical excision external auditory canal lesion; without neck dissection**
EXCLUDES   Skin graft (15004-15261)
Temporal bone resection (69535)
🖐 29.5   ✄ 29.5   **FUD** 090   J A2
AMA: 2014,Jan,11

69155   **with neck dissection**
EXCLUDES   Skin graft (15004-15261)
Temporal bone resection (69535)
🖐 47.0   ✄ 47.0   **FUD** 090   C 80
AMA: 2014,Jan,11

69200   **Removal foreign body from external auditory canal; without general anesthesia**
🖐 1.35   ✄ 2.32   **FUD** 000   Q1 N1 50
AMA: 2014,Jan,11

69205   **with general anesthesia**
🖐 2.82   ✄ 2.82   **FUD** 010   J A2 50
AMA: 2018,Jan,8; 2017,Jan,8; 2016,Jan,13; 2015,Jan,16; 2014,Jan,11

69209   **Removal impacted cerumen using irrigation/lavage, unilateral**
EXCLUDES   Removal impacted cerumen using instrumentation (69210)
Removal of nonimpacted cerumen (see appropriate E&M code(s)) (99201-99233 [99224, 99225, 99226], 99241-99255, 99281-99285, 99304-99318, 99324-99337, 99341-99350)
🖐 0.40   ✄ 0.40   **FUD** 000   Q1 N1 50
AMA: 2018,Jan,8; 2017,Jan,8; 2016,Mar,10; 2016,Feb,13; 2016,Jan,7

69210   **Removal impacted cerumen requiring instrumentation, unilateral**
EXCLUDES   Removal of impacted cerumen using irrigation or lavage (69209)
Removal of nonimpacted cerumen (see appropriate E&M code(s)) (99201-99233 [99224, 99225, 99226], 99241-99255, 99281-99285, 99304-99318, 99324-99337, 99341-99350)
🖐 0.94   ✄ 1.34   **FUD** 000   Q1 N1
AMA: 2018,Jan,8; 2017,Jan,8; 2016,Mar,10; 2016,Feb,13; 2016,Jan,13; 2016,Jan,7; 2015,Jan,16; 2014,Nov,14; 2014,Jan,11

69220   **Debridement, mastoidectomy cavity, simple (eg, routine cleaning)**
🖐 1.47   ✄ 2.29   **FUD** 000   Q1 N1 50
AMA: 2014,Jan,11

69222   **Debridement, mastoidectomy cavity, complex (eg, with anesthesia or more than routine cleaning)**
🖐 3.84   ✄ 6.12   **FUD** 010   T P3 50
AMA: 2014,Jan,11

69300 Plastic Surgery for Prominent Ears

CMS: 100-02,16,120 Cosmetic Procedures; 100-02,16,180 Services Related to Noncovered Procedures

EXCLUDES   Suture of laceration of external ear (12011-14302)

69300   **Otoplasty, protruding ear, with or without size reduction**
🖐 13.8   ✄ 18.1   **FUD** YYY   J A2 80 50
AMA: 2014,Jan,11

69310-69399 Reconstruction Auditory Canal: Postaural Approach

EXCLUDES   Suture of laceration of external ear (12011-14302)

69310   **Reconstruction of external auditory canal (meatoplasty) (eg, for stenosis due to injury, infection) (separate procedure)**
🖐 31.0   ✄ 31.0   **FUD** 090   J A2 50
AMA: 2018,Jan,8; 2017,Jan,8; 2016,Jan,13; 2015,Jan,16; 2014,Jul,8; 2014,Jan,11; 2014,Jan,9

69320   **Reconstruction external auditory canal for congenital atresia, single stage**
EXCLUDES   Other reconstruction surgery with graft (13151-15760, 21230-21235)
Tympanoplasty (69631, 69641)
🖐 43.5   ✄ 43.5   **FUD** 090   J A2 80 50
AMA: 2014,Jan,11

69399   **Unlisted procedure, external ear**
EXCLUDES   Otoscopy under general anesthesia (92502)
🖐 0.00   ✄ 0.00   **FUD** YYY   T 80
AMA: 2014,Jan,11

69420-69450 Ear Drum Procedures

69420 **Myringotomy including aspiration and/or eustachian tube inflation**
🔲 3.41   🔲 5.36   **FUD** 010   T P2 50

AMA: 2018,Jan,8; 2017,Jan,8; 2016,Jan,13; 2015,Jan,16; 2014,Jan,11

69421 **Myringotomy including aspiration and/or eustachian tube inflation requiring general anesthesia**
🔲 4.22   🔲 4.22   **FUD** 010   J A2 50

AMA: 2018,Jan,8; 2017,Jan,8; 2016,Jan,13; 2015,Jan,16; 2014,Jan,11

69424 **Ventilating tube removal requiring general anesthesia**

EXCLUDES Cochlear device implantation (69930)
Eardrum repair (69610-69646)
Foreign body removal (69205)
Implantation, replacement of electromagnetic bone conduction hearing device in temporal bone (69710-69745)
Labyrinth procedures (69801-69915)
Mastoid obliteration (69670)
Myringotomy (69420-69421)
Polyp, glomus tumor removal (69535-69554)
Removal impacted cerumen requiring instrumentation (69210)
Repair of window (69666-69667)
Revised mastoidectomy (69601-69605)
Stapes procedures (69650-69662)
Transmastoid excision (69501-69530)
Tympanic neurectomy (69676)
Tympanostomy, tympanolysis (69433-69450)

🔲 1.75   🔲 3.63   **FUD** 000   Q2 P3 50

AMA: 2018,Jan,8; 2017,Jan,8; 2016,Jan,13; 2015,Jan,16; 2014,Jan,11

69433 **Tympanostomy (requiring insertion of ventilating tube), local or topical anesthesia**

EXCLUDES Tympanostomy with tube insertion using iontophoresis and automated tube delivery system (0583T)

🔲 3.75   🔲 5.67   **FUD** 010   T P3 50

AMA: 2018,Feb,11; 2018,Jan,8; 2017,Jan,8; 2016,Jan,13; 2015,Jan,16; 2014,Jan,11

Tympanic membrane

External auditory canal

Tympanic membrane

Tube

69436 **Tympanostomy (requiring insertion of ventilating tube), general anesthesia**
🔲 4.51   🔲 4.51   **FUD** 010   T A2 50

AMA: 2018,Feb,11; 2018,Jan,8; 2017,Jan,8; 2016,Jan,13; 2015,Jan,16; 2014,Jan,11

69440 **Middle ear exploration through postauricular or ear canal incision**

EXCLUDES Atticotomy (69601-69605)

🔲 19.5   🔲 19.5   **FUD** 090   J A2 50

AMA: 2014,Jan,11

69450 **Tympanolysis, transcanal**
🔲 15.4   🔲 15.4   **FUD** 090   J A2 80 50

AMA: 2014,Jan,11

69501-69530 Transmastoid Excision

EXCLUDES Mastoidectomy cavity debridement (69220, 69222)
Skin graft (15004-15770)

69501 **Transmastoid antrotomy (simple mastoidectomy)**
🔲 20.6   🔲 20.6   **FUD** 090   J A2 50

AMA: 2018,Jan,8; 2017,Jan,8; 2016,Jan,13; 2015,Jan,16; 2014,Jan,11

69502 **Mastoidectomy; complete**
🔲 27.3   🔲 27.3   **FUD** 090   J A2 80 50

AMA: 2018,Jan,8; 2017,Jan,8; 2016,Jan,13; 2015,Jan,16; 2014,Jan,11

69505 **modified radical**
🔲 34.2   🔲 34.2   **FUD** 090   J A2 80 50

AMA: 2018,Jan,8; 2017,Jan,8; 2016,Jan,13; 2015,Jan,16; 2014,Jan,11

69511 **radical**
🔲 35.1   🔲 35.1   **FUD** 090   J A2 80 50

AMA: 2018,Jan,8; 2017,Jan,8; 2016,Jan,13; 2015,Jan,16; 2014,Jan,11

69530 **Petrous apicectomy including radical mastoidectomy**
🔲 47.1   🔲 47.1   **FUD** 090   J A2 80 50

AMA: 2014,Jan,11

69535-69554 Polyp and Glomus Tumor Removal

69535 **Resection temporal bone, external approach**

EXCLUDES Middle fossa approach (69950-69970)

🔲 76.7   🔲 76.7   **FUD** 090   C 50

AMA: 2014,Jan,11

69540 **Excision aural polyp**
🔲 3.59   🔲 5.87   **FUD** 010   T P3 50

AMA: 2014,Jan,11

69550 **Excision aural glomus tumor; transcanal**
🔲 29.6   🔲 29.6   **FUD** 090   J A2 80 50

AMA: 2014,Jan,11

69552 **transmastoid**
🔲 44.7   🔲 44.7   **FUD** 090   J A2 80 50

AMA: 2014,Jan,11

69554 **extended (extratemporal)**
🔲 71.8   🔲 71.8   **FUD** 090   C 80 50

AMA: 2014,Jan,11

69601-69605 Revised Mastoidectomy

EXCLUDES Skin graft (15120-15121, 15260-15261)

69601 **Revision mastoidectomy; resulting in complete mastoidectomy**
🔲 29.5   🔲 29.5   **FUD** 090   J A2 80 50

AMA: 2018,Jan,8; 2017,Jan,8; 2016,Jan,13; 2015,Jan,16; 2014,Jan,11

69602 **resulting in modified radical mastoidectomy**
🔲 30.9   🔲 30.9   **FUD** 090   J A2 80 50

AMA: 2018,Jan,8; 2017,Jan,8; 2016,Jan,13; 2015,Jan,16; 2014,Jan,11

69603 resulting in radical mastoidectomy
🔪 35.9 ✂ 35.9 **FUD** 090 [J] [A2] [80] [50] [□]
AMA: 2018,Jan,8; 2017,Jan,8; 2016,Jan,13; 2015,Jan,16; 2014,Jan,11

69604 resulting in tympanoplasty
EXCLUDES Secondary tympanoplasty following mastoidectomy (69631-69632)
🔪 31.6 ✂ 31.6 **FUD** 090 [J] [A2] [50] [□]
AMA: 2018,Jan,8; 2017,Jan,8; 2016,Jan,13; 2015,Jan,16; 2014,Jan,11

69605 with apicectomy
🔪 44.4 ✂ 44.4 **FUD** 090 [J] [A2] [80] [50] [□]
AMA: 2014,Jan,11

69610-69646 Eardrum Repair with/without Other Procedures

69610 Tympanic membrane repair, with or without site preparation of perforation for closure, with or without patch
🔪 8.27 ✂ 10.8 **FUD** 010 [J] [P3] [50] [□]
AMA: 2018,Jan,8; 2017,Jan,8; 2016,Jan,13; 2015,May,10; 2015,Apr,10; 2015,Jan,16; 2014,Jan,11

69620 Myringoplasty (surgery confined to drumhead and donor area)
🔪 13.8 ✂ 19.8 **FUD** 090 [J] [A2] [50] [□]
AMA: 2018,Jan,8; 2017,Jan,8; 2016,Jan,13; 2015,May,10; 2015,Apr,10; 2015,Jan,16; 2014,Jan,11

69631 Tympanoplasty without mastoidectomy (including canalplasty, atticotomy and/or middle ear surgery), initial or revision; without ossicular chain reconstruction
🔪 25.1 ✂ 25.1 **FUD** 090 [J] [A2] [50] [□]
AMA: 2018,Jan,8; 2017,Jan,8; 2016,Jan,13; 2015,Jan,16; 2014,Jan,11

69632 with ossicular chain reconstruction (eg, postfenestration)
🔪 30.6 ✂ 30.6 **FUD** 090 [J] [A2] [50] [□]
AMA: 2018,Jan,8; 2017,Jan,8; 2016,Jan,13; 2015,Jan,16; 2014,Jan,11

69633 with ossicular chain reconstruction and synthetic prosthesis (eg, partial ossicular replacement prosthesis [PORP], total ossicular replacement prosthesis [TORP])
🔪 29.7 ✂ 29.7 **FUD** 090 [J] [A2] [50] [□]
AMA: 2018,Jan,8; 2017,Jan,8; 2016,Jan,13; 2015,Jan,16; 2014,Jan,11

69635 Tympanoplasty with antrotomy or mastoidotomy (including canalplasty, atticotomy, middle ear surgery, and/or tympanic membrane repair); without ossicular chain reconstruction
🔪 35.3 ✂ 35.3 **FUD** 090 [J] [A2] [50] [□]
AMA: 2018,Jan,8; 2017,Jan,8; 2016,Jan,13; 2015,Jan,16; 2014,Jan,11

Helix, Scaphoid fossa, Ossicular chain, Semicircular canals, Cochlear nerve, Malleus, Incus, Stapes, External acoustic canal, Concha, Tympanic membrane (eardrum), Cochlea, Lobule, Detail of ossicular chain

69636 with ossicular chain reconstruction
🔪 39.3 ✂ 39.3 **FUD** 090 [J] [A2] [80] [50] [□]
AMA: 2018,Jan,8; 2017,Jan,8; 2016,Jan,13; 2015,Jan,16; 2014,Jan,11

69637 with ossicular chain reconstruction and synthetic prosthesis (eg, partial ossicular replacement prosthesis [PORP], total ossicular replacement prosthesis [TORP])
🔪 39.9 ✂ 39.9 **FUD** 090 [J] [A2] [80] [50] [□]
AMA: 2018,Jan,8; 2017,Jan,8; 2016,Jan,13; 2015,Jan,16; 2014,Jan,11

69641 Tympanoplasty with mastoidectomy (including canalplasty, middle ear surgery, tympanic membrane repair); without ossicular chain reconstruction
🔪 29.6 ✂ 29.6 **FUD** 090 [J] [A2] [50] [□]
AMA: 2018,Jan,8; 2017,Jan,8; 2016,Jan,13; 2015,Jan,16; 2014,Jan,11

69642 with ossicular chain reconstruction
🔪 38.0 ✂ 38.0 **FUD** 090 [J] [A2] [50] [□]
AMA: 2018,Jan,8; 2017,Jan,8; 2016,Jan,13; 2015,Jan,16; 2014,Jan,11

69643 with intact or reconstructed wall, without ossicular chain reconstruction
🔪 34.7 ✂ 34.7 **FUD** 090 [J] [A2] [50] [□]
AMA: 2018,Jan,8; 2017,Jan,8; 2016,Jan,13; 2015,Jan,16; 2014,Jan,11

69644 with intact or reconstructed canal wall, with ossicular chain reconstruction
🔪 42.1 ✂ 42.1 **FUD** 090 [J] [A2] [50] [□]
AMA: 2018,Jan,8; 2017,Jan,8; 2016,Jan,13; 2015,Jan,16; 2014,Jan,11

69645 radical or complete, without ossicular chain reconstruction
🔪 41.4 ✂ 41.4 **FUD** 090 [J] [A2] [50] [□]
AMA: 2018,Jan,8; 2017,Jan,8; 2016,Jan,13; 2015,Jan,16; 2014,Jan,11

69646 radical or complete, with ossicular chain reconstruction
🔪 44.1 ✂ 44.1 **FUD** 090 [J] [A2] [80] [50] [□]
AMA: 2018,Jan,8; 2017,Jan,8; 2016,Jan,13; 2015,Jan,16; 2014,Jan,11

69650-69662 Stapes Procedures

69650 Stapes mobilization
🔪 22.8 ✂ 22.8 **FUD** 090 [J] [A2] [50] [□]
AMA: 2014,Jan,11

69660 Stapedectomy or stapedotomy with reestablishment of ossicular continuity, with or without use of foreign material;
🔪 26.3 ✂ 26.3 **FUD** 090 [J] [A2] [50] [□]
AMA: 2014,Jan,11

69661 with footplate drill out
🔪 34.3 ✂ 34.3 **FUD** 090 [J] [A2] [80] [50] [□]
AMA: 2014,Jan,11

69662 Revision of stapedectomy or stapedotomy
🔪 32.9 ✂ 32.9 **FUD** 090 [J] [A2] [50] [□]
AMA: 2014,Jan,11

69666-69700 Other Inner Ear Procedures

69666 Repair oval window fistula
🔪 22.9 ✂ 22.9 **FUD** 090 [J] [A2] [80] [50] [□]
AMA: 2014,Jan,11

69667 Repair round window fistula
🔪 23.0 ✂ 23.0 **FUD** 090 [J] [A2] [80] [50] [□]
AMA: 2014,Jan,11

69670 Mastoid obliteration (separate procedure)
🔪 26.8 ✂ 26.8 **FUD** 090 [J] [A2] [80] [50] [□]
AMA: 2014,Jan,11

69676 Tympanic neurectomy
🔪 23.6 ✂ 23.6 **FUD** 090 [J] [A2] [50] [□]
AMA: 2014,Jan,11

69700 Closure postauricular fistula, mastoid (separate procedure)
🔧 19.3 ✂ 19.3 **FUD** 090   T A2 50 ▭
AMA: 2014,Jan,11

69710-69718 Procedures Related to Hearing Aids/Auditory Implants
CMS: 100-02,16,100 Hearing Devices

69710 Implantation or replacement of electromagnetic bone conduction hearing device in temporal bone
INCLUDES Removal of existing device when performing replacement procedure
🔧 0.00 ✂ 0.00 **FUD** XXX   E ▭
AMA: 2014,Jan,11

69711 Removal or repair of electromagnetic bone conduction hearing device in temporal bone
🔧 24.2 ✂ 24.2 **FUD** 090   J A2 80 50 ▭
AMA: 2014,Jan,11

69714 Implantation, osseointegrated implant, temporal bone, with percutaneous attachment to external speech processor/cochlear stimulator; without mastoidectomy
🔧 30.4 ✂ 30.4 **FUD** 090   J J8 50 ▭
AMA: 2018,Jan,8; 2017,Jan,8; 2016,Jan,13; 2015,Jan,16; 2014,Jan,11

69715 with mastoidectomy
🔧 37.6 ✂ 37.6 **FUD** 090   J J8 50 ▭
AMA: 2014,Jan,11

69717 Replacement (including removal of existing device), osseointegrated implant, temporal bone, with percutaneous attachment to external speech processor/cochlear stimulator; without mastoidectomy
🔧 31.9 ✂ 31.9 **FUD** 090   J J8 50 ▭
AMA: 2014,Jan,11

69718 with mastoidectomy
🔧 38.0 ✂ 38.0 **FUD** 090   J G2 50 ▭
AMA: 2014,Jan,11

69720-69799 Procedures of the Facial Nerve
EXCLUDES Extracranial suture of facial nerve (64864)

69720 Decompression facial nerve, intratemporal; lateral to geniculate ganglion
🔧 34.1 ✂ 34.1 **FUD** 090   J A2 80 50 ▭
AMA: 2014,Jan,11

69725 including medial to geniculate ganglion
🔧 53.5 ✂ 53.5 **FUD** 090   J 80 50 ▭
AMA: 2014,Jan,11

69740 Suture facial nerve, intratemporal, with or without graft or decompression; lateral to geniculate ganglion
🔧 33.2 ✂ 33.2 **FUD** 090   J A2 80 50 ▭
AMA: 2014,Jan,11

69745 including medial to geniculate ganglion
🔧 35.3 ✂ 35.3 **FUD** 090   J A2 80 50 ▭
AMA: 2014,Jan,11

69799 Unlisted procedure, middle ear
🔧 0.00 ✂ 0.00 **FUD** YYY   T 80 50 ▭
AMA: 2019,Jan,14; 2018,Jan,8; 2017,Jan,8; 2016,Jan,13; 2015,Jan,16; 2014,Jan,11

69801-69915 Procedures of the Labyrinth

69801 Labyrinthotomy, with perfusion of vestibuloactive drug(s), transcanal
EXCLUDES Myringotomy, tympanostomy on the same ear (69420-69421, 69433, 69436)
Procedure performed more than one time per day
🔧 3.58 ✂ 5.83 **FUD** 000   T P3 80 50 ▭
AMA: 2018,Jan,8; 2017,Jan,8; 2016,Jan,13; 2015,Jan,16; 2014,Jan,11

69805 Endolymphatic sac operation; without shunt
🔧 29.8 ✂ 29.8 **FUD** 090   J A2 80 50 ▭
AMA: 2014,Jan,11

69806 with shunt
🔧 26.6 ✂ 26.6 **FUD** 090   J A2 50 ▭
AMA: 2014,Jan,11

69905 Labyrinthectomy; transcanal
🔧 26.0 ✂ 26.0 **FUD** 090   J A2 50 ▭
AMA: 2014,Jan,11

69910 with mastoidectomy
🔧 28.7 ✂ 28.7 **FUD** 090   J A2 80 50 ▭
AMA: 2014,Jan,11

69915 Vestibular nerve section, translabyrinthine approach
EXCLUDES Transcranial approach (69950)
🔧 43.6 ✂ 43.6 **FUD** 090   J A2 80 50 ▭
AMA: 2014,Jan,11

69930-69949 Cochlear Implantation
CMS: 100-02,16,100 Hearing Devices

69930 Cochlear device implantation, with or without mastoidectomy
🔧 34.8 ✂ 34.8 **FUD** 090   J J8 80 50 ▭
AMA: 2014,Jan,11

The internal coil is secured to the temporal bone and an electrode is fed through the round window into the cochlea

69949 Unlisted procedure, inner ear
🔧 0.00 ✂ 0.00 **FUD** YYY   T 80 50 ▭
AMA: 2014,Jan,11

69950-69979 Inner Ear Procedures via Craniotomy
EXCLUDES External approach (69535)

69950 Vestibular nerve section, transcranial approach
🔧 50.6 ✂ 50.6 **FUD** 090   C 80 50 ▭
AMA: 2014,Jan,11

69955 Total facial nerve decompression and/or repair (may include graft)
🔧 56.2 ✂ 56.2 **FUD** 090   J 80 50 ▭
AMA: 2014,Jan,11

69960 Decompression internal auditory canal
🔧 54.6 ✂ 54.6 **FUD** 090   J 80 50 ▭
AMA: 2014,Jan,11

69970 Removal of tumor, temporal bone
🔧 61.0 ✂ 61.0 **FUD** 090   J 80 50 ▭
AMA: 2014,Jan,11

69979 Unlisted procedure, temporal bone, middle fossa approach
🔧 0.00 ✂ 0.00 **FUD** YYY   T 80 50 ▭
AMA: 2018,Jan,8; 2017,Jan,8; 2016,Jan,13; 2015,Jan,16; 2014,Sep,13; 2014,Jan,11

26/TC PC/TC Only   A2-Z3 ASC Payment   50 Bilateral   ♂ Male Only   ♀ Female Only   🔧 Facility RVU   ✂ Non-Facility RVU   ▭ CCI   ✖ CLIA
FUD Follow-up Days   CMS: IOM   AMA: CPT Asst   A-Y OPPSI   80/80 Surg Assist Allowed / w/Doc   Lab crosswalk   Radiology crosswalk

330   CPT © 2019 American Medical Association. All Rights Reserved.   © 2019 Optum360, LLC

69990 Operating Microscope

EXCLUDES *Magnifying loupes*
*Use of code with (15756-15758, 15842, 19364, 19368, 20955-20962,
20969-20973, 22551-22552, 22856-22857 [22858], 22861, 26551-26554,
26556, 31526, 31531, 31536, 31541-31546, 31561, 31571, 43116, 43180,
43496, 46601, 46607, 49906, 61548, 63075-63078, 64727, 64820-64823,
64912-64913, 65091-68850 [66987, 66988, 67810], 0184T, 0308T, 0402T,
0583T)*

+   69990   **Microsurgical techniques, requiring use of operating
microscope (List separately in addition to code for primary
procedure)**
Code first primary procedure
⚙ 6.40 ⚖ 6.40 **FUD** ZZZ   N NI 80 ▱
AMA: 2018,Feb,11; 2018,Jan,8; 2017,Dec,12; 2017,Dec,13;
2017,Dec,14; 2017,Jan,8; 2016,Feb,12; 2016,Jan,13; 2015,Jan,16;
2014,Sep,13; 2014,Apr,10; 2014,Jan,11; 2014,Jan,8

70010-70015 Radiography: Neurodiagnostic

70010 **Myelography, posterior fossa, radiological supervision and interpretation**
🖬 1.73 ⚲ 1.73 **FUD** XXX [02] [N1] [80] ▭
AMA: 2018,Jan,8; 2017,Jan,8; 2016,Jan,13; 2015,Jan,16; 2014,Jan,11

70015 **Cisternography, positive contrast, radiological supervision and interpretation**
🖬 4.35 ⚲ 4.35 **FUD** XXX [02] [N1] [80] ▭
AMA: 2014,Jan,11

70030-70390 Radiography: Head, Neck, Orofacial Structures

INCLUDES Minimum number of views or more views when needed to adequately complete the study
Radiographs that have to be repeated during the encounter due to substandard quality; only one unit of service is reported

EXCLUDES Obtaining more films after review of initial films, based on the discretion of the radiologist, an order for the test, and a change in the patient's condition

70030 **Radiologic examination, eye, for detection of foreign body**
🖬 0.83 ⚲ 0.83 **FUD** XXX [01] [N1] [80] ▭
AMA: 2014,Jan,11

70100 **Radiologic examination, mandible; partial, less than 4 views**
🖬 0.97 ⚲ 0.97 **FUD** XXX [01] [N1] [80] ▭
AMA: 2014,Jan,11

70110 **complete, minimum of 4 views**
🖬 1.13 ⚲ 1.13 **FUD** XXX [01] [N1] [80] ▭
AMA: 2014,Jan,11

70120 **Radiologic examination, mastoids; less than 3 views per side**
🖬 0.97 ⚲ 0.97 **FUD** XXX [01] [N1] [80] ▭
AMA: 2014,Jan,11

70130 **complete, minimum of 3 views per side**
🖬 1.61 ⚲ 1.61 **FUD** XXX [01] [N1] [80] ▭
AMA: 2014,Jan,11

70134 **Radiologic examination, internal auditory meati, complete**
🖬 1.51 ⚲ 1.51 **FUD** XXX [01] [N1] [80] ▭
AMA: 2014,Jan,11

70140 **Radiologic examination, facial bones; less than 3 views**
🖬 0.86 ⚲ 0.86 **FUD** XXX [01] [N1] [80] ▭
AMA: 2014,Jan,11

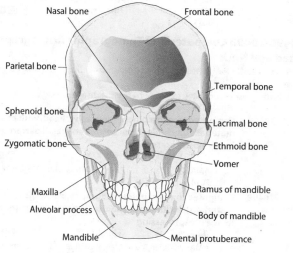

70150 **complete, minimum of 3 views**
🖬 1.23 ⚲ 1.23 **FUD** XXX [01] [N1] [80] ▭
AMA: 2014,Jan,11

70160 **Radiologic examination, nasal bones, complete, minimum of 3 views**
🖬 0.97 ⚲ 0.97 **FUD** XXX [01] [N1] [80] ▭
AMA: 2014,Jan,11

70170 **Dacryocystography, nasolacrimal duct, radiological supervision and interpretation**
EXCLUDES Injection of contrast (68850)
🖬 0.00 ⚲ 0.00 **FUD** XXX [02] [N1] [80] ▭
AMA: 2014,Jan,11

70190 **Radiologic examination; optic foramina**
🖬 1.03 ⚲ 1.03 **FUD** XXX [01] [N1] [80] ▭
AMA: 2014,Jan,11

70200 **orbits, complete, minimum of 4 views**
🖬 1.24 ⚲ 1.24 **FUD** XXX [01] [N1] [80] ▭
AMA: 2014,Jan,11

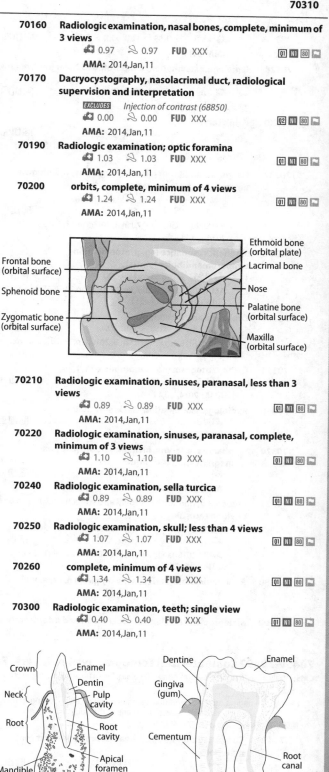

70210 **Radiologic examination, sinuses, paranasal, less than 3 views**
🖬 0.89 ⚲ 0.89 **FUD** XXX [01] [N1] [80] ▭
AMA: 2014,Jan,11

70220 **Radiologic examination, sinuses, paranasal, complete, minimum of 3 views**
🖬 1.10 ⚲ 1.10 **FUD** XXX [01] [N1] [80] ▭
AMA: 2014,Jan,11

70240 **Radiologic examination, sella turcica**
🖬 0.89 ⚲ 0.89 **FUD** XXX [01] [N1] [80] ▭
AMA: 2014,Jan,11

70250 **Radiologic examination, skull; less than 4 views**
🖬 1.07 ⚲ 1.07 **FUD** XXX [01] [N1] [80] ▭
AMA: 2014,Jan,11

70260 **complete, minimum of 4 views**
🖬 1.34 ⚲ 1.34 **FUD** XXX [01] [N1] [80] ▭
AMA: 2014,Jan,11

70300 **Radiologic examination, teeth; single view**
🖬 0.40 ⚲ 0.40 **FUD** XXX [01] [N1] [80] ▭
AMA: 2014,Jan,11

Section of incisor   Section of molar

70310 **partial examination, less than full mouth**
🖬 1.06 ⚲ 1.06 **FUD** XXX [01] [N1] [80] ▭
AMA: 2014,Jan,11

70320 — 70498

70320 **complete, full mouth**
🔲 1.53　✂ 1.53　**FUD** XXX　[01] [N1] [80] 🖵
AMA: 2014,Jan,11

70328 **Radiologic examination, temporomandibular joint, open and closed mouth; unilateral**
🔲 0.89　✂ 0.89　**FUD** XXX　[01] [N1] [80] 🖵
AMA: 2014,Jan,11

70330 **bilateral**
🔲 1.39　✂ 1.39　**FUD** XXX　[01] [N1] [80] 🖵
AMA: 2018,Jan,8; 2017,Jan,8; 2016,Jan,13; 2015,Jan,16; 2014,Jan,11

70332 **Temporomandibular joint arthrography, radiological supervision and interpretation**
INCLUDES　Fluoroscopic guidance (77002)
🔲 2.15　✂ 2.15　**FUD** XXX　[02] [N1] [80] 🖵
AMA: 2018,Jan,8; 2017,Jan,8; 2016,Jan,13; 2015,Jan,16; 2014,Jan,11

70336 **Magnetic resonance (eg, proton) imaging, temporomandibular joint(s)**
🔲 8.86　✂ 8.86　**FUD** XXX　[03] [Z2] [80] 🖵
AMA: 2018,Jan,8; 2017,Jan,8; 2016,Jan,13; 2015,Aug,6; 2015,Jan,16; 2014,Jan,11

70350 **Cephalogram, orthodontic**
🔲 0.53　✂ 0.53　**FUD** XXX　[01] [N1] [80] 🖵
AMA: 2018,Jan,8; 2017,Jan,8; 2016,Jan,13; 2015,Jan,16; 2014,Jan,11

70355 **Orthopantogram (eg, panoramic x-ray)**
🔲 0.56　✂ 0.56　**FUD** XXX　[01] [N1] [80] 🖵
AMA: 2014,Jan,11

70360 **Radiologic examination; neck, soft tissue**
🔲 0.85　✂ 0.85　**FUD** XXX　[01] [N1] [80] 🖵
AMA: 2014,Jan,11

70370 **pharynx or larynx, including fluoroscopy and/or magnification technique**
🔲 2.27　✂ 2.27　**FUD** XXX　[01] [N1] [80] 🖵
AMA: 2014,Jan,11

70371 **Complex dynamic pharyngeal and speech evaluation by cine or video recording**
EXCLUDES　Laryngeal computed tomography (70490-70492)
🔲 2.77　✂ 2.77　**FUD** XXX　[01] [N1] [80] 🖵
AMA: 2018,Jan,8; 2017,Jan,8; 2016,Jan,13; 2015,Jan,16; 2014,Jul,5; 2014,Jan,11

70380 **Radiologic examination, salivary gland for calculus**
🔲 0.95　✂ 0.95　**FUD** XXX　[01] [N1] [80] 🖵
AMA: 2014,Jan,11

70390 **Sialography, radiological supervision and interpretation**
🔲 2.90　✂ 2.90　**FUD** XXX　[02] [N1] [80] 🖵
AMA: 2014,Jan,11

70450-70492 Computerized Tomography: Head, Neck, Face

CMS: 100-04,4,250.16 Multiple Procedure Payment Reduction: Certain Diagnostic Imaging Procedures Rendered by Physicians

INCLUDES　Imaging using tomographic technique enhanced by computer imaging to create a cross-sectional plane of the body
EXCLUDES　3D rendering (76376-76377)

70450 **Computed tomography, head or brain; without contrast material**
🔲 3.26　✂ 3.26　**FUD** XXX　[03] [Z2] [80] 🖵
AMA: 2018,Jan,8; 2017,Jan,8; 2016,Jan,13; 2015,Jan,16; 2014,Jan,11

70460 **with contrast material(s)**
🔲 4.61　✂ 4.61　**FUD** XXX　[03] [Z2] [80] 🖵
AMA: 2018,Jan,8; 2017,Jan,8; 2016,Jan,13; 2015,Jan,16; 2014,Jan,11

70470 **without contrast material, followed by contrast material(s) and further sections**
🔲 5.39　✂ 5.39　**FUD** XXX　[03] [Z2] [80] 🖵
AMA: 2018,Jan,8; 2017,Jan,8; 2016,Jan,13; 2015,Jan,16; 2014,Jan,11

70480 **Computed tomography, orbit, sella, or posterior fossa or outer, middle, or inner ear; without contrast material**
🔲 6.55　✂ 6.55　**FUD** XXX　[03] [Z2] [80] 🖵
AMA: 2018,Jan,8; 2017,Jan,8; 2016,Jan,13; 2015,Jan,16; 2014,Jan,11

70481 **with contrast material(s)**
🔲 7.76　✂ 7.76　**FUD** XXX　[03] [Z2] [80] 🖵
AMA: 2018,Jan,8; 2017,Jan,8; 2016,Jan,13; 2015,Jan,16; 2014,Jan,11

70482 **without contrast material, followed by contrast material(s) and further sections**
🔲 8.45　✂ 8.45　**FUD** XXX　[03] [Z2] [80] 🖵
AMA: 2014,Jan,11

70486 **Computed tomography, maxillofacial area; without contrast material**
🔲 3.92　✂ 3.92　**FUD** XXX　[03] [Z2] [80] 🖵
AMA: 2018,Jan,8; 2017,Jan,8; 2016,Jan,13; 2015,Jan,16; 2014,Jan,11

70487 **with contrast material(s)**
🔲 4.71　✂ 4.71　**FUD** XXX　[03] [Z2] [80] 🖵
AMA: 2014,Jan,11

70488 **without contrast material, followed by contrast material(s) and further sections**
🔲 5.74　✂ 5.74　**FUD** XXX　[03] [Z2] [80] 🖵
AMA: 2014,Jan,11

70490 **Computed tomography, soft tissue neck; without contrast material**
EXCLUDES　CT of the cervical spine (72125)
🔲 4.63　✂ 4.63　**FUD** XXX　[03] [Z2] [80] 🖵
AMA: 2014,Jan,11

70491 **with contrast material(s)**
EXCLUDES　CT of the cervical spine (72126)
🔲 5.71　✂ 5.71　**FUD** XXX　[03] [Z2] [80] 🖵
AMA: 2014,Jan,11

70492 **without contrast material followed by contrast material(s) and further sections**
EXCLUDES　CT of the cervical spine (72125-72127)
🔲 6.88　✂ 6.88　**FUD** XXX　[03] [Z2] [80] 🖵
AMA: 2014,Jan,11

70496-70498 Computerized Tomographic Angiography: Head and Neck

CMS: 100-04,4,250.16 Multiple Procedure Payment Reduction: Certain Diagnostic Imaging Procedures Rendered by Physicians

INCLUDES　Use of computed tomography to visualize arterial and venous vessels of the body

70496 **Computed tomographic angiography, head, with contrast material(s), including noncontrast images, if performed, and image postprocessing**
🔲 8.31　✂ 8.31　**FUD** XXX　[03] [Z2] [80] 🖵
AMA: 2018,Jan,8; 2017,Jan,8; 2016,Jan,13; 2015,Jan,16; 2014,Jan,11

70498 **Computed tomographic angiography, neck, with contrast material(s), including noncontrast images, if performed, and image postprocessing**
🔲 8.29　✂ 8.29　**FUD** XXX　[03] [Z2] [80] 🖵
AMA: 2018,Jan,8; 2017,Jan,8; 2016,Jan,13; 2015,Jan,16; 2014,Jan,11

| 26/TC PC/TC Only | A2-Z3 ASC Payment | 50 Bilateral | ♂ Male Only | ♀ Female Only | 🔲 Facility RVU | ✂ Non-Facility RVU | 🖵 CCI | ☒ CLIA |
| **FUD** Follow-up Days | **CMS:** IOM | **AMA:** CPT Asst | A-Y OPPSI | 80/80 Surg Assist Allowed / w/Doc | 🔲 Lab Crosswalk | | 🔲 Radiology Crosswalk | |

334

70540-70543 Magnetic Resonance Imaging: Face, Neck, Orbits

CMS: 100-04,4,250.16 Multiple Procedure Payment Reduction: Certain Diagnostic Imaging Procedures Rendered by Physicians

INCLUDES Application of an external magnetic field that forces alignment of hydrogen atom nuclei in soft tissues which converts to sets of tomographic images that can be displayed as three-dimensional images

EXCLUDES *Magnetic resonance angiography head/neck (70544-70549)*
Procedure performed more than one time per session

70540 **Magnetic resonance (eg, proton) imaging, orbit, face, and/or neck; without contrast material(s)**
7.48   7.48   **FUD** XXX   03 Z2 80

AMA: 2018,Jan,8; 2017,Jan,8; 2016,Jan,13; 2015,Jan,16; 2014,Jan,11

70542 **with contrast material(s)**
8.89   8.89   **FUD** XXX   03 Z2 80

AMA: 2018,Jan,8; 2017,Jan,8; 2016,Jan,13; 2015,Jan,16; 2014,Jan,11

70543 **without contrast material(s), followed by contrast material(s) and further sequences**
11.1   11.1   **FUD** XXX   03 Z2 80

AMA: 2018,Jan,8; 2017,Jan,8; 2016,Jan,13; 2015,Jan,16; 2014,Jan,11

70544-70549 Magnetic Resonance Angiography: Head and Neck

CMS: 100-04,13,40.1.1 Magnetic Resonance Angiography; 100-04,13,40.1.2 HCPCS Coding Requirements; 100-04,4,250.16 Multiple Procedure Payment Reduction: Certain Diagnostic Imaging Procedures Rendered by Physicians

INCLUDES Use of magnetic fields and radio waves to produce detailed cross-sectional images of internal body structures

EXCLUDES *Use of code with the following unless a separate diagnostic MRI is performed (70551-70553)*

70544 **Magnetic resonance angiography, head; without contrast material(s)**
7.84   7.84   **FUD** XXX   03 Z2 80

AMA: 2018,Jan,8; 2017,Jan,8; 2016,Jan,13; 2015,Jan,16; 2014,Jan,11

70545 **with contrast material(s)**
7.78   7.78   **FUD** XXX   03 Z2 80

AMA: 2018,Jan,8; 2017,Jan,8; 2016,Jan,13; 2015,Jan,16; 2014,Jan,11

70546 **without contrast material(s), followed by contrast material(s) and further sequences**
11.5   11.5   **FUD** XXX   03 Z2 80

AMA: 2018,Jan,8; 2017,Jan,8; 2016,Jan,13; 2015,Jan,16; 2014,Jan,11

70547 **Magnetic resonance angiography, neck; without contrast material(s)**
7.87   7.87   **FUD** XXX   03 Z2 80

AMA: 2018,Jan,8; 2017,Jan,8; 2016,Jan,13; 2015,Jan,16; 2014,Jan,11

70548 **with contrast material(s)**
8.66   8.66   **FUD** XXX   03 Z2 80

AMA: 2018,Jan,8; 2017,Jan,8; 2016,Jan,13; 2015,Jan,16; 2014,Jan,11

70549 **without contrast material(s), followed by contrast material(s) and further sequences**
12.0   12.0   **FUD** XXX   03 Z2 80

AMA: 2018,Jan,8; 2017,Jan,8; 2016,Jan,13; 2015,Jan,16; 2014,Jan,11

70551-70553 Magnetic Resonance Imaging: Brain and Brain Stem

CMS: 100-04,4,200.3.2 Multi-Source Photon Stereotactic Radiosurgery Planning and Delivery; 100-04,4,250.16 Multiple Procedure Payment Reduction: Certain Diagnostic Imaging Procedures Rendered by Physicians

INCLUDES Application of an external magnetic field that forces alignment of hydrogen atom nuclei in soft tissues which converts to sets of tomographic images that can be displayed as three-dimensional images

EXCLUDES *Magnetic spectroscopy (76390)*

70551 **Magnetic resonance (eg, proton) imaging, brain (including brain stem); without contrast material**
6.38   6.38   **FUD** XXX   03 Z2 80

AMA: 2018,Jan,8; 2017,Jan,8; 2016,Jan,13; 2015,Jan,16; 2014,Jan,11

70552 **with contrast material(s)**
8.86   8.86   **FUD** XXX   03 Z2 80

AMA: 2018,Jan,8; 2017,Jan,8; 2016,Jan,13; 2015,Jan,16; 2014,Jan,11

70553 **without contrast material, followed by contrast material(s) and further sequences**
10.4   10.4   **FUD** XXX   03 Z2 80

AMA: 2018,Jan,8; 2017,Jan,8; 2016,Jan,13; 2015,Jan,16; 2014,Jan,11

70554-70555 Magnetic Resonance Imaging: Brain Mapping

INCLUDES Neuroimaging technique using MRI to identify and map signals related to brain activity

EXCLUDES *Use of code with the following unless a separate diagnostic MRI is performed (70551-70553)*

70554 **Magnetic resonance imaging, brain, functional MRI; including test selection and administration of repetitive body part movement and/or visual stimulation, not requiring physician or psychologist administration**

EXCLUDES *Functional brain mapping (96020)*
Testing performed by a physician or psychologist (70555)

12.4   12.4   **FUD** XXX   03 Z2 80

AMA: 2018,Jan,8; 2017,Jan,8; 2016,Jan,13; 2015,Jan,16; 2014,Jan,11

70555 **requiring physician or psychologist administration of entire neurofunctional testing**

EXCLUDES *Testing performed by a technologist, nonphysician, or nonpsychologist (70554)*

Code also (96020)
0.00   0.00   **FUD** XXX   S Z2 80

AMA: 2018,Jan,8; 2017,Jan,8; 2016,Jan,13; 2015,Jan,16; 2014,Jan,11

70557-70559 Magnetic Resonance Imaging: Intraoperative

EXCLUDES *Intracranial lesion stereotaxic biopsy with magnetic resonance guidance (61751, 77021-77022)*
Procedures performed more than one time per surgical encounter
Use of codes unless a separate report is generated

Code also stereotactic biopsy, aspiration, or excision, when performed with magnetic resonance imaging (61751)

70557 **Magnetic resonance (eg, proton) imaging, brain (including brain stem and skull base), during open intracranial procedure (eg, to assess for residual tumor or residual vascular malformation); without contrast material**
0.00   0.00   **FUD** XXX   S Z2 80

AMA: 2014,Jan,11

70558 **with contrast material(s)**
0.00   0.00   **FUD** XXX   S Z2 80

AMA: 2014,Jan,11

70559 **without contrast material(s), followed by contrast material(s) and further sequences**
0.00   0.00   **FUD** XXX   S Z2 80

AMA: 2014,Jan,11

71045-71130 Radiography: Thorax

71045 Radiologic examination, chest; single view

> EXCLUDES Acute abdomen series, complete (2 or more views) including a view of the chest (74022)
> Remotely performed CAD (0175T)
> Code also concurrent computer-aided detection (CAD) (0174T)

📷 0.70 🔾 0.70 **FUD** XXX 03 Z3 80 🖵

AMA: 2019,Aug,8; 2019,May,10; 2019,Mar,10; 2018,Apr,7

71046 2 views

> EXCLUDES Acute abdomen series, complete (2 or more views) including a view of the chest (74022)
> Remotely performed CAD (0175T)
> Code also concurrent computer-aided detection (CAD) (0174T)

📷 0.89 🔾 0.89 **FUD** XXX 03 Z3 80 🖵

AMA: 2019,Aug,8; 2019,Mar,10; 2018,Apr,7

71047 3 views

> EXCLUDES Complete acute abdomen series (2 or more views) that includes a view of the chest (74022)
> Remotely performed CAD (0175T)
> Code also concurrent computer-aided detection (CAD) (0174T)

📷 1.12 🔾 1.12 **FUD** XXX 01 N1 80 🖵

AMA: 2019,Mar,10; 2018,Apr,7

71048 4 or more views

> EXCLUDES Acute abdomen series, complete (2 or more views) including a view of the chest (74022)
> Remotely performed CAD (0175T)
> Code also concurrent computer-aided detection (CAD) (0174T)

📷 1.21 🔾 1.21 **FUD** XXX 01 N1 80 🖵

AMA: 2019,Mar,10; 2018,Apr,7

71100 Radiologic examination, ribs, unilateral; 2 views

📷 0.97 🔾 0.97 **FUD** XXX 01 N1 80 🖵

AMA: 2014,Jan,11

Hyoid bone
Manubrium of sternum
Trachea
Sternum
Xiphoid process

71101 including posteroanterior chest, minimum of 3 views

📷 1.11 🔾 1.11 **FUD** XXX 01 N1 80 🖵

AMA: 2014,Jan,11

71110 Radiologic examination, ribs, bilateral; 3 views

📷 1.16 🔾 1.16 **FUD** XXX 01 N1 80 🖵

AMA: 2014,Jan,11

71111 including posteroanterior chest, minimum of 4 views

📷 1.38 🔾 1.38 **FUD** XXX 01 N1 80 🖵

AMA: 2014,Jan,11

71120 Radiologic examination; sternum, minimum of 2 views

📷 0.88 🔾 0.88 **FUD** XXX 01 N1 80 🖵

AMA: 2014,Jan,11

71130 sternoclavicular joint or joints, minimum of 3 views

📷 1.05 🔾 1.05 **FUD** XXX 01 N1 80 🖵

AMA: 2014,Jan,11

71250-71270 Computerized Tomography: Thorax

CMS: 100-04,4,250.16 Multiple Procedure Payment Reduction: Certain Diagnostic Imaging Procedures Rendered by Physicians

> INCLUDES Imaging using tomographic technique enhanced by computer imaging to create a cross-sectional plane of the body
> EXCLUDES 3D rendering (76376-76377)
> CT of the heart (75571-75574)

71250 Computed tomography, thorax; without contrast material

📷 4.47 🔾 4.47 **FUD** XXX 03 Z2 80 🖵

AMA: 2018,Jan,8; 2017,Jan,8; 2016,Jan,13; 2015,Jan,16; 2014,Jan,11

71260 with contrast material(s)

📷 5.53 🔾 5.53 **FUD** XXX 03 Z2 80 🖵

AMA: 2018,Jan,8; 2017,Jan,8; 2016,Jan,13; 2015,Jan,16; 2014,Jan,11

71270 without contrast material, followed by contrast material(s) and further sections

📷 6.56 🔾 6.56 **FUD** XXX 03 Z2 80 🖵

AMA: 2018,Jan,8; 2017,Jan,8; 2016,Jan,13; 2015,Jan,16; 2014,Jan,11

71275 Computerized Tomographic Angiography: Thorax

CMS: 100-04,4,250.16 Multiple Procedure Payment Reduction: Certain Diagnostic Imaging Procedures Rendered by Physicians

> INCLUDES Multiple rapid thin section CT scans to create cross-sectional images of bones, organs and tissues
> EXCLUDES CT angiography of coronary arteries that includes calcification score and/or cardiac morphology (75574)

71275 Computed tomographic angiography, chest (noncoronary), with contrast material(s), including noncontrast images, if performed, and image postprocessing

📷 8.50 🔾 8.50 **FUD** XXX 03 Z2 80 🖵

AMA: 2018,Jan,8; 2017,Jan,8; 2016,Jan,13; 2015,Jan,16; 2014,Jan,11

71550-71552 Magnetic Resonance Imaging: Thorax

CMS: 100-04,4,250.16 Multiple Procedure Payment Reduction: Certain Diagnostic Imaging Procedures Rendered by Physicians

> INCLUDES Application of an external magnetic field that forces alignment of hydrogen atom nuclei in soft tissues which converts to sets of tomographic images that can be displayed as three-dimensional images
> EXCLUDES MRI of the breast (77046-77049)

71550 Magnetic resonance (eg, proton) imaging, chest (eg, for evaluation of hilar and mediastinal lymphadenopathy); without contrast material(s)

📷 11.4 🔾 11.4 **FUD** XXX 03 Z2 80 🖵

AMA: 2018,Jan,8; 2017,Jan,8; 2016,Jan,13; 2015,Jan,16; 2014,Jan,11

71551 with contrast material(s)

📷 12.6 🔾 12.6 **FUD** XXX 03 Z2 80 🖵

AMA: 2018,Jan,8; 2017,Jan,8; 2016,Jan,13; 2015,Jan,16; 2014,Jan,11

71552 without contrast material(s), followed by contrast material(s) and further sequences

📷 15.9 🔾 15.9 **FUD** XXX 03 Z2 80 🖵

AMA: 2018,Jan,8; 2017,Jan,8; 2016,Jan,13; 2015,Jan,16; 2014,Jan,11

71555 Magnetic Resonance Angiography: Thorax

CMS: 100-04,13,40.1.1 Magnetic Resonance Angiography; 100-04,13,40.1.2 HCPCS Coding Requirements; 100-04,4,250.16 Multiple Procedure Payment Reduction: Certain Diagnostic Imaging Procedures Rendered by Physicians

71555 Magnetic resonance angiography, chest (excluding myocardium), with or without contrast material(s)

📷 11.0 🔾 11.0 **FUD** XXX B 80 🖵

AMA: 2018,Jan,8; 2017,Jan,8; 2016,Jan,13; 2015,Jan,16; 2014,Jan,11

26/TC PC/TC Only A2-Z3 ASC Payment 50 Bilateral ♂ Male Only ♀ Female Only 📷 Facility RVU 🔾 Non-Facility RVU 🖵 CCI ☒ CLIA
FUD Follow-up Days **CMS:** IOM **AMA:** CPT Asst A-Y OPPSI 80/80 Surg Assist Allowed / w/Doc 🔳 Lab Crosswalk Radiology Crosswalk

72020-72120 Radiography: Spine

INCLUDES Minimum number of views or more views when needed to adequately complete the study
Radiographs that have to be repeated during the encounter due to substandard quality; only one unit of service is reported

EXCLUDES *Obtaining more films after review of initial films, based on the discretion of the radiologist, an order for the test, and a change in the patient's condition*

72020 **Radiologic examination, spine, single view, specify level**
EXCLUDES *Single view of entire thoracic and lumbar spine (72081)*
🚑 0.65 🔬 0.65 **FUD** XXX [01] [N1] [80] 🖥
AMA: 2018,Jan,8; 2017,Jan,8; 2016,Sep,4; 2016,Jan,13; 2015,Oct,9; 2015,Jan,16; 2014,Jan,11

72040 **Radiologic examination, spine, cervical; 2 or 3 views**
🚑 1.03 🔬 1.03 **FUD** XXX [01] [N1] [80] 🖥
AMA: 2018,Aug,10; 2018,Jan,8; 2017,Jan,8; 2016,Jan,13; 2015,Jan,16; 2014,Jan,11

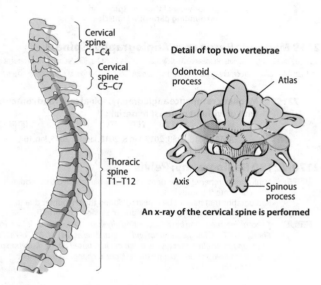

Cervical spine C1–C4
Cervical spine C5–C7
Thoracic spine T1–T12

Detail of top two vertebrae
Odontoid process
Atlas
Axis
Spinous process

An x-ray of the cervical spine is performed

72050 **4 or 5 views**
🚑 1.42 🔬 1.42 **FUD** XXX [01] [N1] [80] 🖥
AMA: 2014,Jan,11

72052 **6 or more views**
🚑 1.69 🔬 1.69 **FUD** XXX [01] [N1] [80] 🖥
AMA: 2014,Jan,11

72070 **Radiologic examination, spine; thoracic, 2 views**
🚑 0.96 🔬 0.96 **FUD** XXX [01] [N1] [80] 🖥
AMA: 2018,Jan,8; 2017,Jan,8; 2016,Jan,13; 2015,Jan,16; 2014,Jan,11

72072 **thoracic, 3 views**
🚑 1.02 🔬 1.02 **FUD** XXX [01] [N1] [80] 🖥
AMA: 2018,Jan,8; 2017,Jan,8; 2016,Jan,13; 2015,Jan,16; 2014,Jan,11

72074 **thoracic, minimum of 4 views**
🚑 1.12 🔬 1.12 **FUD** XXX [01] [N1] [80] 🖥
AMA: 2018,Jan,8; 2017,Jan,8; 2016,Jan,13; 2015,Jan,16; 2014,Jan,11

72080 **thoracolumbar junction, minimum of 2 views**
EXCLUDES *Single view of thoracolumbar junction (72020)*
🚑 0.95 🔬 0.95 **FUD** XXX [01] [N1] [80] 🖥
AMA: 2018,Jan,8; 2017,Jan,8; 2016,Sep,4; 2016,Jan,13; 2015,Oct,9; 2015,Jan,16; 2014,Jan,11

72081 **Radiologic examination, spine, entire thoracic and lumbar, including skull, cervical and sacral spine if performed (eg, scoliosis evaluation); one view**
🚑 1.14 🔬 1.14 **FUD** XXX [01] [N1] [80] 🖥
AMA: 2018,Jan,8; 2017,Jan,8; 2016,Sep,4

72082 **2 or 3 views**
🚑 1.83 🔬 1.83 **FUD** XXX [01] [N1] [80] 🖥
AMA: 2018,Jan,8; 2017,Jan,8; 2016,Sep,4

72083 **4 or 5 views**
🚑 2.16 🔬 2.16 **FUD** XXX [S] [Z2] [80] 🖥
AMA: 2018,Jan,8; 2017,Jan,8; 2016,Sep,4

72084 **minimum of 6 views**
🚑 2.52 🔬 2.52 **FUD** XXX [S] [Z2] [80] 🖥
AMA: 2018,Jan,8; 2017,Jan,8; 2016,Sep,4

72100 **Radiologic examination, spine, lumbosacral; 2 or 3 views**
🚑 1.03 🔬 1.03 **FUD** XXX [01] [N1] [80] 🖥
AMA: 2018,Jan,8; 2017,Jan,8; 2016,Jan,13; 2015,Jan,16; 2014,Jan,11

72110 **minimum of 4 views**
🚑 1.44 🔬 1.44 **FUD** XXX [01] [N1] [80] 🖥
AMA: 2018,Jan,8; 2017,Jan,8; 2016,Jan,13; 2015,Jan,16; 2014,Jan,11

72114 **complete, including bending views, minimum of 6 views**
🚑 1.64 🔬 1.64 **FUD** XXX [01] [N1] [80] 🖥
AMA: 2014,Jan,11

72120 **bending views only, 2 or 3 views**
🚑 1.21 🔬 1.21 **FUD** XXX [01] [N1] [80] 🖥
AMA: 2018,Jan,8; 2017,Jan,8; 2016,Aug,7; 2014,Jan,11

72125-72133 Computerized Tomography: Spine

CMS: 100-04,12,20.4.7 Services Not Meeting National Electrical Manufacturers Association (NEMA) Standard; 100-04,4,20.6.12 Use of HCPCS Modifier – CT; 100-04,4,250.16 Multiple Procedure Payment Reduction: Certain Diagnostic Imaging Procedures Rendered by Physicians

INCLUDES Imaging using tomographic technique enhanced by computer imaging to create a cross-sectional plane of the body
EXCLUDES *3D rendering (76376-76377)*
Code also intrathecal injection procedure when performed (61055, 62284)

72125 **Computed tomography, cervical spine; without contrast material**
🚑 5.18 🔬 5.18 **FUD** XXX [03] [Z2] [80] 🖥
AMA: 2014,Jan,11

72126 **with contrast material**
🚑 6.40 🔬 6.40 **FUD** XXX [03] [Z3] [80] 🖥
AMA: 2018,Jan,8; 2017,Jan,8; 2016,Jan,13; 2015,Jan,16; 2014,Jan,11

72127 **without contrast material, followed by contrast material(s) and further sections**
🚑 7.58 🔬 7.58 **FUD** XXX [03] [Z2] [80] 🖥
AMA: 2014,Jan,11

72128 **Computed tomography, thoracic spine; without contrast material**
🚑 5.08 🔬 5.08 **FUD** XXX [03] [Z2] [80] 🖥
AMA: 2014,Jan,11

72129 **with contrast material**
🚑 6.44 🔬 6.44 **FUD** XXX [03] [Z2] [80] 🖥
AMA: 2019,Jan,14; 2018,Jan,8; 2017,Jan,8; 2016,Jan,13; 2015,Jan,16; 2014,Jan,11

72130 **without contrast material, followed by contrast material(s) and further sections**
🚑 7.59 🔬 7.59 **FUD** XXX [03] [Z2] [80] 🖥
AMA: 2014,Jan,11

72131 **Computed tomography, lumbar spine; without contrast material**
🚑 5.06 🔬 5.06 **FUD** XXX [03] [Z2] [80] 🖥
AMA: 2014,Jan,11

72132 **with contrast material**
🚑 6.41 🔬 6.41 **FUD** XXX [03] [Z3] [80] 🖥
AMA: 2019,Jan,14; 2018,Jan,8; 2017,Jan,8; 2016,Jan,13; 2015,Jan,16; 2014,Jan,11

Radiology *(side margin)*

72133 — 72192 *(side margin)*

72133   **without contrast material, followed by contrast material(s) and further sections**

     7.56   7.56   **FUD** XXX   03 Z2 80

     AMA: 2014,Jan,11

72141-72158 Magnetic Resonance Imaging: Spine

CMS: 100-04,4,250.16 Multiple Procedure Payment Reduction: Certain Diagnostic Imaging Procedures Rendered by Physicians

INCLUDES   Application of an external magnetic field that forces alignment of hydrogen atom nuclei in soft tissues which converts to sets of tomographic images that can be displayed as three-dimensional images

Code also intrathecal injection procedure when performed (61055, 62284)

72141   **Magnetic resonance (eg, proton) imaging, spinal canal and contents, cervical; without contrast material**

     6.22   6.22   **FUD** XXX   03 Z2 80

     AMA: 2018,Jan,8; 2017,Jan,8; 2016,Jan,13; 2015,Jan,16; 2014,Jun,14; 2014,Jan,11

72142   **with contrast material(s)**

     EXCLUDES   *MRI of cervical spinal canal performed without contrast followed by repeating the study with contrast (72156)*

     9.03   9.03   **FUD** XXX   03 Z2 80

     AMA: 2018,Jan,8; 2017,Jan,8; 2016,Jan,13; 2015,Jan,16; 2014,Jan,11

72146   **Magnetic resonance (eg, proton) imaging, spinal canal and contents, thoracic; without contrast material**

     6.23   6.23   **FUD** XXX   03 Z2 80

     AMA: 2018,Jan,8; 2017,Jan,8; 2016,Jan,13; 2015,Jan,16; 2014,Jun,14; 2014,Jan,11

72147   **with contrast material(s)**

     EXCLUDES   *MRI of thoracic spinal canal performed without contrast followed by repeating the study with contrast (72157)*

     8.98   8.98   **FUD** XXX   03 Z2 80

     AMA: 2018,Jan,8; 2017,Jan,8; 2016,Jan,13; 2015,Jan,16; 2014,Jan,11

72148   **Magnetic resonance (eg, proton) imaging, spinal canal and contents, lumbar; without contrast material**

     6.23   6.23   **FUD** XXX   03 Z2 80

     AMA: 2018,Jan,8; 2017,Jan,8; 2016,Jan,13; 2015,Jan,16; 2014,Jun,14; 2014,Jan,11

72149   **with contrast material(s)**

     EXCLUDES   *MRI of lumbar spinal canal performed without contrast followed by repeating the study with contrast . (72158)*

     8.92   8.92   **FUD** XXX   03 Z2 80

     AMA: 2014,Jan,11

72156   **Magnetic resonance (eg, proton) imaging, spinal canal and contents, without contrast material, followed by contrast material(s) and further sequences; cervical**

     10.5   10.5   **FUD** XXX   03 Z2 80

     AMA: 2014,Jan,11

72157   **thoracic**

     10.5   10.5   **FUD** XXX   03 Z2 80

     AMA: 2014,Jan,11

72158   **lumbar**

     10.5   10.5   **FUD** XXX   03 Z2 80

     AMA: 2014,Jan,11

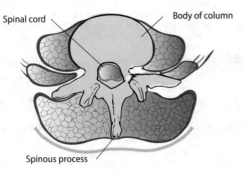

Superior view of thoracic spine and surrounding paraspinal muscles

(labels: Spinal cord, Body of column, Spinous process)

72159 Magnetic Resonance Angiography: Spine

CMS: 100-04,13,40.1.1 Magnetic Resonance Angiography; 100-04,13,40.1.2 HCPCS Coding Requirements; 100-04,4,250.16 Multiple Procedure Payment Reduction: Certain Diagnostic Imaging Procedures Rendered by Physicians

72159   **Magnetic resonance angiography, spinal canal and contents, with or without contrast material(s)**

     11.4   11.4   **FUD** XXX   B 80

     AMA: 2018,Jan,8; 2017,Jan,8; 2016,Jan,13; 2015,Jan,16; 2014,Jan,11

72170-72190 Radiography: Pelvis

INCLUDES   Minimum number of views or more views when needed to adequately complete the study

     Radiographs that have to be repeated during the encounter due to substandard quality; only one unit of service is reported

EXCLUDES   *A second interpretation by the requesting physician (included in E&M service)*

Combined CT or CT angiography of abdomen and pelvis (74174, 74176-74178)

Obtaining more films after review of initial films, based on the discretion of the radiologist, an order for the test, and a change in the patient's condition

Pelvimetry (74710)

72170   **Radiologic examination, pelvis; 1 or 2 views**

     0.93   0.93   **FUD** XXX   01 N1 80

     AMA: 2018,Jan,8; 2017,Jan,8; 2016,Aug,7; 2016,Jun,5; 2016,Jan,13; 2015,Jan,16; 2014,Jan,11

72190   **complete, minimum of 3 views**

     1.12   1.12   **FUD** XXX   01 N1 80

     AMA: 2016,Jun,5; 2014,Jan,11

72191 Computerized Tomographic Angiography: Pelvis

CMS: 100-04,4,250.16 Multiple Procedure Payment Reduction: Certain Diagnostic Imaging Procedures Rendered by Physicians

EXCLUDES   *Computed tomographic angiography (73706, 74174-74175, 75635)*

72191   **Computed tomographic angiography, pelvis, with contrast material(s), including noncontrast images, if performed, and image postprocessing**

     8.85   8.85   **FUD** XXX   03 Z2 80

     AMA: 2018,Jan,8; 2017,Jan,8; 2016,Jan,13; 2015,Jan,16; 2014,Jan,11

72192-72194 Computerized Tomography: Pelvis

CMS: 100-04,4,250.16 Multiple Procedure Payment Reduction: Certain Diagnostic Imaging Procedures Rendered by Physicians

EXCLUDES   *3D rendering (76376-76377)*

Combined CT of abdomen and pelvis (74176-74178)

CT colonography, diagnostic (74261-74262)

CT colonography, screening (74263)

72192   **Computed tomography, pelvis; without contrast material**

     4.10   4.10   **FUD** XXX   03 Z2 80

     AMA: 2018,Jan,8; 2017,Jan,8; 2016,Jan,13; 2015,Jan,16; 2014,Jan,11

26/TC PC/TC Only	A2-Z3 ASC Payment	50 Bilateral	♂ Male Only	♀ Female Only	Facility RVU	Non-Facility RVU	CCI	CLIA

FUD Follow-up Days   **CMS:** IOM   **AMA:** CPT Asst   A-Y OPPSI   80/80 Surg Assist Allowed / w/Doc   Lab Crosswalk   Radiology Crosswalk

338   CPT © 2019 American Medical Association. All Rights Reserved.   © 2019 Optum360, LLC

72193   **with contrast material(s)**
     6.59   6.59   **FUD** XXX   03 Z2 80 ▣

     AMA: 2018,Jan,8; 2017,Jan,8; 2016,Jan,13; 2015,Jan,16; 2014,Jan,11

72194   **without contrast material, followed by contrast material(s) and further sections**
     7.48   7.48   **FUD** XXX   03 Z2 80 ▣

     AMA: 2018,Jan,8; 2017,Jan,8; 2016,Jan,13; 2015,Jan,16; 2014,Jan,11

72195-72197 Magnetic Resonance Imaging: Pelvis

CMS: 100-04,4,250.16 Multiple Procedure Payment Reduction: Certain Diagnostic Imaging Procedures Rendered by Physicians

INCLUDES   Application of an external magnetic field that forces alignment of hydrogen atom nuclei in soft tissues which converts to sets of tomographic images that can be displayed as three-dimensional images

EXCLUDES   *Magnetic resonance imaging of fetus(es) (74712-74713)*

72195   **Magnetic resonance (eg, proton) imaging, pelvis; without contrast material(s)**
     7.62   7.62   **FUD** XXX   03 Z2 80 ▣

     AMA: 2018,Jul,11; 2018,Jan,8; 2017,Jan,8; 2016,Jun,5; 2016,Jan,13; 2015,Jan,16; 2014,Jun,14; 2014,Jan,11

72196   **with contrast material(s)**
     8.90   8.90   **FUD** XXX   03 Z2 80 ▣

     AMA: 2018,Jul,11; 2018,Jan,8; 2017,Jan,8; 2016,Jun,5; 2016,Jan,13; 2015,Jan,16; 2014,Jan,11

72197   **without contrast material(s), followed by contrast material(s) and further sequences**
     11.2   11.2   **FUD** XXX   03 Z2 80 ▣

     AMA: 2018,Jul,11; 2018,Jan,8; 2017,Jan,8; 2016,Jun,5; 2016,Jan,13; 2015,Jan,16; 2014,Jan,11

72198 Magnetic Resonance Angiography: Pelvis

CMS: 100-04,13,40.1.1 Magnetic Resonance Angiography; 100-04,13,40.1.2 HCPCS Coding Requirements; 100-04,4,250.16 Multiple Procedure Payment Reduction: Certain Diagnostic Imaging Procedures Rendered by Physicians

INCLUDES   Use of magnetic fields and radio waves to produce detailed cross-sectional images of the arteries and veins

72198   **Magnetic resonance angiography, pelvis, with or without contrast material(s)**
     11.0   11.0   **FUD** XXX   B 80 ▣

     AMA: 2018,Jan,8; 2017,Jan,8; 2016,Jan,13; 2015,Jan,16; 2014,Jan,11

72200-72220 Radiography: Pelvisacral

INCLUDES   Minimum number of views or more views when needed to adequately complete the study
     Radiographs that have to be repeated during the encounter due to substandard quality; only one unit of service is reported

EXCLUDES   *Obtaining more films after review of initial films, based on the discretion of the radiologist, an order for the test, and a change in the patient's condition*
     Second interpretation by the requesting physician (included in E&M service)

72200   **Radiologic examination, sacroiliac joints; less than 3 views**
     0.87   0.87   **FUD** XXX   01 N1 80 ▣

     AMA: 2014,Jan,11

72202   **3 or more views**
     0.98   0.98   **FUD** XXX   01 N1 80 ▣

     AMA: 2014,Jan,11

72220   **Radiologic examination, sacrum and coccyx, minimum of 2 views**
     0.86   0.86   **FUD** XXX   01 N1 80 ▣

     AMA: 2014,Jan,11

72240-72270 Myelography with Contrast: Spinal Cord

CMS: 100-04,13,30.1.3.1 Payment for Low Osmolar Contrast Material

EXCLUDES   *Injection procedure for myelography (62284)*
     Myelography (62302-62305)
Code also injection at C1-C2 for complete myelography (61055)

72240   **Myelography, cervical, radiological supervision and interpretation**
     2.94   2.94   **FUD** XXX   02 N1 80 ▣

     AMA: 2018,Jan,8; 2017,Jan,8; 2016,Jan,13; 2015,Jan,16; 2014,Sep,3; 2014,Jan,11

72255   **Myelography, thoracic, radiological supervision and interpretation**
     2.99   2.99   **FUD** XXX   02 N1 80 ▣

     AMA: 2018,Jan,8; 2017,Jan,8; 2016,Jan,13; 2015,Jan,16; 2014,Sep,3; 2014,Jan,11

72265   **Myelography, lumbosacral, radiological supervision and interpretation**
     2.75   2.75   **FUD** XXX   02 N1 80 ▣

     AMA: 2018,Jan,8; 2017,Jan,8; 2016,Jan,13; 2015,Jan,16; 2014,Sep,3; 2014,Jan,11

72270   **Myelography, 2 or more regions (eg, lumbar/thoracic, cervical/thoracic, lumbar/cervical, lumbar/thoracic/cervical), radiological supervision and interpretation**
     3.82   3.82   **FUD** XXX   02 N1 80 ▣

     AMA: 2018,Jan,8; 2017,Jan,8; 2016,Jan,13; 2015,Jan,16; 2014,Sep,3; 2014,Jan,11

72275 Radiography: Epidural Space

INCLUDES   Epidurogram, documentation of images, formal written report
     Fluoroscopic guidance (77003)

EXCLUDES   *Arthrodesis (22586)*
     Second interpretation by the requesting physician (included in E&M service)
Code also injection procedure as appropriate (62280-62282, 62320-62327, 64479-64480, 64483-64484)

72275   **Epidurography, radiological supervision and interpretation**
     3.48   3.48   **FUD** XXX   N N1 80 ▣

     AMA: 2018,Jan,8; 2017,Jan,8; 2016,Jan,13; 2015,Jan,16; 2014,Jan,11

72285 Radiography: Intervertebral Disc (Cervical/Thoracic)

CMS: 100-04,13,30.1.3.1 Payment for Low Osmolar Contrast Material
Code also discography injection procedure (62291)

72285   **Discography, cervical or thoracic, radiological supervision and interpretation**
     3.32   3.32   **FUD** XXX   02 N1 80 ▣

     AMA: 2018,Jan,8; 2017,Jan,8; 2016,Jan,13; 2015,Jan,16; 2014,Jan,11

72295 Radiography: Intervertebral Disc (Lumbar)

CMS: 100-04,13,30.1.3.1 Payment for Low Osmolar Contrast Material
Code also discography injection procedure (62290)

72295   **Discography, lumbar, radiological supervision and interpretation**
     2.90   2.90   **FUD** XXX   02 N1 80 ▣

     AMA: 2018,Jan,8; 2017,Feb,12; 2017,Jan,8; 2016,Jan,13; 2015,Jan,16; 2014,Jan,11

Radiology

73000 — 73201

73000-73085 Radiography: Shoulder and Upper Arm

INCLUDES Minimum number of views or more views when needed to adequately complete the study
Radiographs that have to be repeated during the encounter due to substandard quality; only one unit of service is reported

EXCLUDES *Obtaining more films after review of initial films, based on the discretion of the radiologist, an order for the test, and a change in the patient's condition*
Second interpretation by the requesting physician (included in E&M service)
Stress views of upper body joint(s), when performed (77071)

73000 **Radiologic examination; clavicle, complete**
🔲 0.82 ⚕ 0.82 **FUD** XXX [01] [N1] [80] [▭]
AMA: 2014,Jan,11

Radiograph

Gold wedding band absorbs all x-rays (white)

Air allows all rays to reach film (black)

Soft tissues absorb part of rays and will vary in gray intensity

Calcium in bone absorbs most of rays and is nearly white

X-ray beam

Film

Posterioranterior (PA) chest study; lateral views also common

73010 **scapula, complete**
🔲 0.90 ⚕ 0.90 **FUD** XXX [01] [N1] [80] [▭]
AMA: 2014,Jan,11

73020 **Radiologic examination, shoulder; 1 view**
🔲 0.67 ⚕ 0.67 **FUD** XXX [01] [N1] [80] [▭]
AMA: 2014,Jan,11

73030 **complete, minimum of 2 views**
🔲 0.85 ⚕ 0.85 **FUD** XXX [01] [N1] [80] [▭]
AMA: 2014,Jan,11

73040 **Radiologic examination, shoulder, arthrography, radiological supervision and interpretation**
INCLUDES Fluoroscopic guidance (77002)
Code also arthrography injection procedure (23350)
🔲 3.12 ⚕ 3.12 **FUD** XXX [02] [N1] [80] [▭]
AMA: 2018,Jan,8; 2017,Jan,8; 2016,Jan,13; 2015,Jan,16; 2014,Jan,11

73050 **Radiologic examination; acromioclavicular joints, bilateral, with or without weighted distraction**
🔲 1.05 ⚕ 1.05 **FUD** XXX [01] [N1] [80] [▭]
AMA: 2014,Jan,11

73060 **humerus, minimum of 2 views**
🔲 0.85 ⚕ 0.85 **FUD** XXX [01] [N1] [80] [▭]
AMA: 2014,Jan,11

73070 **Radiologic examination, elbow; 2 views**
🔲 0.76 ⚕ 0.76 **FUD** XXX [01] [N1] [80] [▭]
AMA: 2018,Jan,8; 2017,Jan,8; 2016,Jan,13; 2015,Jan,16; 2014,Jan,11

73080 **complete, minimum of 3 views**
🔲 0.84 ⚕ 0.84 **FUD** XXX [01] [N1] [80] [▭]
AMA: 2014,Jan,11

73085 **Radiologic examination, elbow, arthrography, radiological supervision and interpretation**
INCLUDES Fluoroscopic guidance (77002)
Code also arthrography injection procedure (24220)
🔲 2.99 ⚕ 2.99 **FUD** XXX [02] [N1] [80] [▭]
AMA: 2018,Jan,8; 2017,Jan,8; 2016,Jan,13; 2015,Jan,16; 2014,Jan,11

73090-73140 Radiography: Forearm and Hand

INCLUDES Minimum number of views or more views when needed to adequately complete the study
Radiographs that have to be repeated during the encounter due to substandard quality; only one unit of service is reported

EXCLUDES *Obtaining more films after review of initial films, based on the discretion of the radiologist, an order for the test, and a change in the patient's condition*
Second interpretation by the requesting physician (included in E&M service)
Stress views of upper body joint(s), when performed (77071)

73090 **Radiologic examination; forearm, 2 views**
🔲 0.79 ⚕ 0.79 **FUD** XXX [01] [N1] [80] [▭]
AMA: 2018,Jan,8; 2017,Jan,8; 2016,Jan,13; 2015,Jan,16; 2014,Jan,11

73092 **upper extremity, infant, minimum of 2 views** [A]
🔲 0.81 ⚕ 0.81 **FUD** XXX [01] [N1] [80] [▭]
AMA: 2014,Jan,11

73100 **Radiologic examination, wrist; 2 views**
🔲 0.90 ⚕ 0.90 **FUD** XXX [01] [N1] [80] [▭]
AMA: 2018,Oct,11; 2018,Jan,8; 2017,Jan,8; 2016,Jan,13; 2015,Jan,16; 2014,Jan,11

73110 **complete, minimum of 3 views**
🔲 1.03 ⚕ 1.03 **FUD** XXX [01] [N1] [80] [▭]
AMA: 2018,Oct,11; 2018,Jan,8; 2017,Jan,8; 2016,Jan,13; 2015,Jan,16; 2014,Jan,11

73115 **Radiologic examination, wrist, arthrography, radiological supervision and interpretation**
INCLUDES Fluoroscopic guidance (77002)
Code also arthrography injection procedure (25246)
🔲 3.33 ⚕ 3.33 **FUD** XXX [02] [N1] [80] [▭]
AMA: 2018,Jan,8; 2017,Jan,8; 2016,Jan,13; 2015,Jan,16; 2014,Jan,11

73120 **Radiologic examination, hand; 2 views**
🔲 0.82 ⚕ 0.82 **FUD** XXX [01] [N1] [80] [▭]
AMA: 2018,Oct,11; 2014,Jan,11

73130 **minimum of 3 views**
🔲 0.94 ⚕ 0.94 **FUD** XXX [01] [N1] [80] [▭]
AMA: 2014,Jan,11

73140 **Radiologic examination, finger(s), minimum of 2 views**
🔲 0.95 ⚕ 0.95 **FUD** XXX [01] [N1] [80] [▭]
AMA: 2018,Jan,8; 2017,Jan,8; 2016,Jan,13; 2015,Jan,16; 2014,Jan,11

73200-73202 Computerized Tomography: Shoulder, Arm, Hand

CMS: 100-04,4,250.16 Multiple Procedure Payment Reduction: Certain Diagnostic Imaging Procedures Rendered by Physicians

INCLUDES Imaging using tomographic technique enhanced by computer imaging to create a cross-sectional plane of the body
Intravascular, intrathecal, or intra-articular contrast materials when noted in code descriptor

EXCLUDES *3D rendering (76376-76377)*

73200 **Computed tomography, upper extremity; without contrast material**
🔲 5.05 ⚕ 5.05 **FUD** XXX [03] [Z2] [80] [▭]
AMA: 2018,Jan,8; 2017,Jan,8; 2016,Jan,13; 2015,Jan,16; 2014,Jan,11

73201 **with contrast material(s)**
🔲 6.28 ⚕ 6.28 **FUD** XXX [03] [Z3] [80] [▭]
AMA: 2018,Jan,8; 2017,Jan,8; 2016,Jan,13; 2015,Aug,6; 2015,Jan,16; 2014,Jan,11

73202 without contrast material, followed by contrast material(s) and further sections

🚑 7.82   ⚕ 7.82   **FUD** XXX   03 Z2 80 ▣

AMA: 2014,Jan,11

73206 Computerized Tomographic Angiography: Shoulder, Arm, and Hand

CMS: 100-04,4,250.16 Multiple Procedure Payment Reduction: Certain Diagnostic Imaging Procedures Rendered by Physicians

INCLUDES   Intravascular, intrathecal, or intra-articular contrast materials when noted in code descriptor
Multiple rapid thin section CT scans to create cross-sectional images of the arteries and veins

73206 Computed tomographic angiography, upper extremity, with contrast material(s), including noncontrast images, if performed, and image postprocessing

🚑 9.24   ⚕ 9.24   **FUD** XXX   03 Z2 80 ▣

AMA: 2018,Jan,8; 2017,Jan,8; 2016,Jan,13; 2015,Jan,16; 2014,Jan,11

73218-73223 Magnetic Resonance Imaging: Shoulder, Arm, Hand

CMS: 100-04,4,250.16 Multiple Procedure Payment Reduction: Certain Diagnostic Imaging Procedures Rendered by Physicians

INCLUDES   Application of an external magnetic field that forces alignment of hydrogen atom nuclei in soft tissues which converts to sets of tomographic images that can be displayed as three-dimensional images
Intravascular, intrathecal, or intra-articular contrast materials when noted in code descriptor

73218 Magnetic resonance (eg, proton) imaging, upper extremity, other than joint; without contrast material(s)

🚑 10.1   ⚕ 10.1   **FUD** XXX   03 Z2 80 ▣

AMA: 2018,Jan,8; 2017,Jan,8; 2016,Jan,13; 2015,Jan,16; 2014,Jan,11

73219 with contrast material(s)

🚑 11.1   ⚕ 11.1   **FUD** XXX   03 Z2 80 ▣

AMA: 2018,Jan,8; 2017,Jan,8; 2016,Jan,13; 2015,Jan,16; 2014,Jan,11

73220 without contrast material(s), followed by contrast material(s) and further sequences

🚑 13.7   ⚕ 13.7   **FUD** XXX   03 Z2 80 ▣

AMA: 2018,Jan,8; 2017,Jan,8; 2016,Jan,13; 2015,Jan,16; 2014,Jan,11

73221 Magnetic resonance (eg, proton) imaging, any joint of upper extremity; without contrast material(s)

🚑 6.57   ⚕ 6.57   **FUD** XXX   03 Z2 80 ▣

AMA: 2018,Jan,8; 2017,Jan,8; 2016,Jan,13; 2015,Jan,16; 2014,Jan,11

73222 with contrast material(s)

🚑 10.4   ⚕ 10.4   **FUD** XXX   03 Z3 80 ▣

AMA: 2018,Jan,8; 2017,Jan,8; 2016,Jan,13; 2015,Aug,6; 2015,Jan,16; 2014,Jan,11

73223 without contrast material(s), followed by contrast material(s) and further sequences

🚑 12.9   ⚕ 12.9   **FUD** XXX   03 Z2 80 ▣

AMA: 2018,Jan,8; 2017,Jan,8; 2016,Jan,13; 2015,Jan,16; 2014,Jan,11

73225 Magnetic Resonance Angiography: Shoulder, Arm, Hand

CMS: 100-04,13,40.1.1 Magnetic Resonance Angiography; 100-04,4,250.16 Multiple Procedure Payment Reduction: Certain Diagnostic Imaging Procedures Rendered by Physicians

INCLUDES   Intravascular, intrathecal, or intra-articular contrast materials when noted in code descriptor
Use of magnetic fields and radio waves to produce detailed cross-sectional images of the arteries and veins

73225 Magnetic resonance angiography, upper extremity, with or without contrast material(s)

🚑 10.9   ⚕ 10.9   **FUD** XXX   B 80 ▣

AMA: 2018,Jan,8; 2017,Jan,8; 2016,Jan,13; 2015,Jan,16; 2014,Jan,11

73501-73552 Radiography: Pelvic Region and Thigh

EXCLUDES   *Stress views of lower body joint(s), when performed (77071)*

73501 Radiologic examination, hip, unilateral, with pelvis when performed; 1 view

🚑 0.87   ⚕ 0.87   **FUD** XXX   01 N1 80 ▣

AMA: 2018,Jan,8; 2017,Jan,8; 2016,Aug,7; 2016,Jun,8; 2016,Jan,13; 2015,Oct,9

73502 2-3 views

🚑 1.21   ⚕ 1.21   **FUD** XXX   01 N1 80 ▣

AMA: 2018,Jan,8; 2017,Jan,8; 2016,Aug,7; 2016,Jun,8; 2016,Jan,13; 2015,Oct,9

73503 minimum of 4 views

🚑 1.51   ⚕ 1.51   **FUD** XXX   01 N1 80 ▣

AMA: 2018,Jan,8; 2017,Jan,8; 2016,Aug,7; 2016,Jun,8; 2016,Jan,13; 2015,Oct,9

73521 Radiologic examination, hips, bilateral, with pelvis when performed; 2 views

🚑 1.08   ⚕ 1.08   **FUD** XXX   01 N1 80 ▣

AMA: 2018,Jan,8; 2017,Jan,8; 2016,Aug,7; 2016,Jun,8; 2016,Jan,13; 2015,Oct,9

73522 3-4 views

🚑 1.41   ⚕ 1.41   **FUD** XXX   01 N1 80 ▣

AMA: 2018,Jan,8; 2017,Jan,8; 2016,Aug,7; 2016,Jun,8; 2016,Jan,13; 2015,Oct,9

73523 minimum of 5 views

🚑 1.65   ⚕ 1.65   **FUD** XXX   S N1 80 ▣

AMA: 2018,Jan,8; 2017,Jan,8; 2016,Aug,7; 2016,Jun,8; 2016,Jan,13; 2015,Oct,9

73525 Radiologic examination, hip, arthrography, radiological supervision and interpretation

INCLUDES   Fluoroscopic guidance (77002)

🚑 3.18   ⚕ 3.18   **FUD** XXX   02 N1 80 ▣

AMA: 2018,Jan,8; 2017,Jan,8; 2016,Nov,10; 2016,Aug,7; 2016,Jan,13; 2016,Jan,16; 2014,Jan,11

73551 Radiologic examination, femur; 1 view

🚑 0.80   ⚕ 0.80   **FUD** XXX   01 N1 80 ▣

AMA: 2018,Jan,8; 2017,Jan,8; 2016,Aug,7

73552 minimum 2 views

🚑 0.94   ⚕ 0.94   **FUD** XXX   01 N1 80 ▣

AMA: 2018,Jan,8; 2017,Nov,10; 2017,Jan,8; 2016,Aug,7

73560-73660 Radiography: Lower Leg, Ankle, and Foot

EXCLUDES   *Stress views of lower body joint(s), when performed (77071)*

73560 Radiologic examination, knee; 1 or 2 views

🚑 0.91   ⚕ 0.91   **FUD** XXX   01 N1 80 ▣

AMA: 2018,Jan,8; 2017,Jan,8; 2016,Jan,13; 2015,May,10; 2015,Feb,10; 2014,Jan,11

73562 3 views

🚑 1.05   ⚕ 1.05   **FUD** XXX   01 N1 80 ▣

AMA: 2014,Jan,11

73564 complete, 4 or more views

🚑 1.17   ⚕ 1.17   **FUD** XXX   01 N1 80 ▣

AMA: 2018,Jan,8; 2017,Jan,8; 2016,Jan,13; 2015,May,10; 2015,Feb,10; 2015,Jan,16; 2014,Jan,11

73565 both knees, standing, anteroposterior

🚑 1.05   ⚕ 1.05   **FUD** XXX   01 N1 80 ▣

AMA: 2018,Jan,8; 2017,Jan,8; 2016,Jan,13; 2015,May,10; 2015,Feb,10; 2014,Jan,11

73580 Radiologic examination, knee, arthrography, radiological supervision and interpretation

INCLUDES   Fluoroscopic guidance (77002)

🚑 3.59   ⚕ 3.59   **FUD** XXX   02 N1 80 ▣

AMA: 2019,Aug,7; 2018,Jan,8; 2017,Jan,8; 2016,Jan,13; 2015,Aug,6; 2015,Jan,16; 2014,Jan,11

73590 Radiologic examination; tibia and fibula, 2 views
  🎥 0.83 ⚖ 0.83 **FUD** XXX   01 N1 80 ▭
  AMA: 2018,Jan,8; 2017,Nov,10; 2017,Jan,8; 2016,Jan,13; 2015,Jan,16; 2014,Jan,11

73592 lower extremity, infant, minimum of 2 views   A
  🎥 0.81 ⚖ 0.81 **FUD** XXX   01 N1 80 ▭
  AMA: 2018,Jan,8; 2017,Nov,10; 2014,Jan,11

73600 Radiologic examination, ankle; 2 views
  🎥 0.87 ⚖ 0.87 **FUD** XXX   01 N1 80 ▭
  AMA: 2018,Jan,8; 2017,Jan,8; 2016,Jan,13; 2015,Jan,16; 2014,Jan,11

73610 complete, minimum of 3 views
  🎥 0.94 ⚖ 0.94 **FUD** XXX   01 N1 80 ▭
  AMA: 2018,Jan,8; 2017,Jan,8; 2016,Jan,13; 2015,Jan,16; 2014,Jan,11

73615 Radiologic examination, ankle, arthrography, radiological supervision and interpretation
  INCLUDES Fluoroscopic guidance (77002)
  🎥 3.34 ⚖ 3.34 **FUD** XXX   02 N1 80 ▭
  AMA: 2018,Jan,8; 2017,Jan,8; 2016,Jan,13; 2015,Jan,16; 2014,Jan,11

73620 Radiologic examination, foot; 2 views
  🎥 0.76 ⚖ 0.76 **FUD** XXX   01 N1 80 ▭
  AMA: 2018,Jan,8; 2017,Jan,8; 2016,Jan,13; 2015,Jan,16; 2014,Jan,11

73630 complete, minimum of 3 views
  🎥 0.88 ⚖ 0.88 **FUD** XXX   01 N1 80 ▭
  AMA: 2014,Jan,11

73650 Radiologic examination; calcaneus, minimum of 2 views
  🎥 0.76 ⚖ 0.76 **FUD** XXX   01 N1 80 ▭
  AMA: 2014,Jan,11

73660 toe(s), minimum of 2 views
  🎥 0.81 ⚖ 0.81 **FUD** XXX   01 N1 80 ▭
  AMA: 2014,Jan,11

73700-73702 Computerized Tomography: Leg, Ankle, and Foot

CMS: 100-04,4,250.16 Multiple Procedure Payment Reduction: Certain Diagnostic Imaging Procedures Rendered by Physicians

  EXCLUDES 3D rendering (76376-76377)

73700 Computed tomography, lower extremity; without contrast material
  🎥 5.06 ⚖ 5.06 **FUD** XXX   03 Z2 80 ▭
  AMA: 2018,Jan,8; 2017,Jan,8; 2016,Jan,13; 2015,Jan,16; 2014,Jan,11

73701 with contrast material(s)
  🎥 6.36 ⚖ 6.36 **FUD** XXX   03 Z2 80 ▭
  AMA: 2019,Aug,7; 2018,Jan,8; 2017,Jan,8; 2016,Jan,13; 2015,Jan,16; 2014,Jan,11

73702 without contrast material, followed by contrast material(s) and further sections
  🎥 7.70 ⚖ 7.70 **FUD** XXX   03 Z2 80 ▭
  AMA: 2019,Aug,7; 2018,Jan,8; 2017,Jan,8; 2016,Jan,13; 2015,Jan,16; 2014,Jan,11

73706 Computerized Tomographic Angiography: Leg, Ankle, and Foot

CMS: 100-04,4,250.16 Multiple Procedure Payment Reduction: Certain Diagnostic Imaging Procedures Rendered by Physicians

  EXCLUDES CT angiography for aorto-iliofemoral runoff (75635)

73706 Computed tomographic angiography, lower extremity, with contrast material(s), including noncontrast images, if performed, and image postprocessing
  🎥 10.0 ⚖ 10.0 **FUD** XXX   03 Z2 80 ▭
  AMA: 2018,Jan,8; 2017,Jan,8; 2016,Jan,13; 2015,Jan,16; 2014,Jan,11

73718-73723 Magnetic Resonance Imaging: Leg, Ankle, and Foot

CMS: 100-04,4,250.16 Multiple Procedure Payment Reduction: Certain Diagnostic Imaging Procedures Rendered by Physicians

73718 Magnetic resonance (eg, proton) imaging, lower extremity other than joint; without contrast material(s)
  🎥 7.39 ⚖ 7.39 **FUD** XXX   03 Z2 80 ▭
  AMA: 2018,Jan,8; 2017,Jan,8; 2016,Jan,13; 2015,Jan,16; 2014,Jan,11

73719 with contrast material(s)
  🎥 8.74 ⚖ 8.74 **FUD** XXX   03 Z2 80 ▭
  AMA: 2019,Aug,7; 2018,Jan,8; 2017,Jan,8; 2016,Jan,13; 2015,Jan,16; 2014,Jan,11

73720 without contrast material(s), followed by contrast material(s) and further sequences
  🎥 11.2 ⚖ 11.2 **FUD** XXX   03 Z2 80 ▭
  AMA: 2019,Aug,7; 2018,Jan,8; 2017,Jan,8; 2016,Jan,13; 2015,Jan,16; 2014,Jan,11

73721 Magnetic resonance (eg, proton) imaging, any joint of lower extremity; without contrast material
  🎥 6.57 ⚖ 6.57 **FUD** XXX   03 Z2 80 ▭
  AMA: 2018,Jan,8; 2017,Jan,8; 2016,Jan,13; 2015,Jan,16; 2014,Jan,11

73722 with contrast material(s)
  🎥 10.5 ⚖ 10.5 **FUD** XXX   03 Z3 80 ▭
  AMA: 2019,Aug,7; 2018,Jan,8; 2017,Jan,8; 2016,Jan,13; 2015,Aug,6; 2015,Jan,16; 2014,Jan,11

73723 without contrast material(s), followed by contrast material(s) and further sequences
  🎥 12.9 ⚖ 12.9 **FUD** XXX   03 Z2 80 ▭
  AMA: 2019,Aug,7; 2018,Jan,8; 2017,Jan,8; 2016,Jan,13; 2015,Jan,16; 2014,Jan,11

73725 Magnetic Resonance Angiography: Leg, Ankle, and Foot

CMS: 100-04,13,40.1.2 HCPCS Coding Requirements; 100-04,4,250.16 Multiple Procedure Payment Reduction: Certain Diagnostic Imaging Procedures Rendered by Physicians

73725 Magnetic resonance angiography, lower extremity, with or without contrast material(s)
  🎥 11.1 ⚖ 11.1 **FUD** XXX   B 80 ▭
  AMA: 2018,Jan,8; 2017,Jan,8; 2016,Jan,13; 2015,Jan,16; 2014,Jan,11

74018-74022 Radiography: Abdomen--General

74018 Radiologic examination, abdomen; 1 view
  🎥 0.80 ⚖ 0.80 **FUD** XXX   01 N1 80 ▭
  AMA: 2019,May,10; 2018,Apr,7

74019 2 views
  🎥 0.98 ⚖ 0.98 **FUD** XXX   01 N1 80 ▭
  AMA: 2018,Apr,7

74021 3 or more views
  🎥 1.13 ⚖ 1.13 **FUD** XXX   01 N1 80 ▭
  AMA: 2018,Apr,7

26/TC PC/TC Only   A2-Z3 ASC Payment   50 Bilateral   ♂ Male Only   ♀ Female Only   🎥 Facility RVU   ⚖ Non-Facility RVU   ▭ CCI   ❎ CLIA
FUD Follow-up Days   CMS: IOM   AMA: CPT Asst   A-Y OPPSI   80/80 Surg Assist Allowed / w/Doc   🔲 Lab Crosswalk   🔄 Radiology Crosswalk

▲ **74022** **Radiologic examination, complete acute abdomen series, including 2 or more views of the abdomen (eg, supine, erect, decubitus), and a single view chest**

🚑 1.31　🔧 1.31　**FUD** XXX　`01` `N1` `80` 🖥

AMA: 2019,May,10; 2018,Apr,7; 2016,Jun,5; 2014,Jan,11

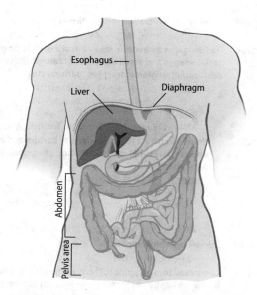

Esophagus

Liver　　Diaphragm

Abdomen

Pelvis area

74150-74170 Computerized Tomography: Abdomen–General

CMS: 100-04,4,250.16 Multiple Procedure Payment Reduction: Certain Diagnostic Imaging Procedures Rendered by Physicians

> EXCLUDES　3D rendering (76376-76377)
> Combined CT of abdomen and pelvis (74176-74178)
> CT colonography, diagnostic (74261-74262)
> CT colonography, screening (74263)

74150 **Computed tomography, abdomen; without contrast material**

🚑 4.22　🔧 4.22　**FUD** XXX　`03` `Z2` `80` 🖥

AMA: 2018,Jan,8; 2017,Jan,8; 2016,Jun,5; 2016,Jan,13; 2015,Jan,16; 2014,Jan,11

74160 **with contrast material(s)**

🚑 6.72　🔧 6.72　**FUD** XXX　`03` `Z2` `80` 🖥

AMA: 2018,Jan,8; 2017,Jan,8; 2016,Jun,5; 2016,Jan,13; 2015,Jan,16; 2014,Jan,11

74170 **without contrast material, followed by contrast material(s) and further sections**

🚑 7.62　🔧 7.62　**FUD** XXX　`03` `Z2` `80` 🖥

AMA: 2018,Jan,8; 2017,Jan,8; 2016,Jun,5; 2016,Jan,13; 2015,Jan,16; 2014,Jan,11

74174-74175 Computerized Tomographic Angiography: Abdomen and Pelvis

CMS: 100-04,4,250.16 Multiple Procedure Payment Reduction: Certain Diagnostic Imaging Procedures Rendered by Physicians

> EXCLUDES　CT angiography for aorto-iliofemoral runoff (75635)
> CT angiography, lower extremity (73706)
> CT angiography, pelvis (72191)

74174 **Computed tomographic angiography, abdomen and pelvis, with contrast material(s), including noncontrast images, if performed, and image postprocessing**

> EXCLUDES　3D rendering (76376-76377)
> Computed tomographic angiography abdomen (74175)

🚑 11.1　🔧 11.1　**FUD** XXX　`S` `Z2` `80` 🖥

AMA: 2014,Jan,11

74175 **Computed tomographic angiography, abdomen, with contrast material(s), including noncontrast images, if performed, and image postprocessing**

🚑 8.87　🔧 8.87　**FUD** XXX　`03` `Z2` `80` 🖥

AMA: 2018,Jan,8; 2017,Jan,8; 2016,Jan,13; 2015,Jan,16; 2014,Jan,11

74176-74178 Computerized Tomography: Abdomen and Pelvis

CMS: 100-04,4,250.16 Multiple Procedure Payment Reduction: Certain Diagnostic Imaging Procedures Rendered by Physicians

> EXCLUDES　Computed tomography of abdomen or pelvis alone (72192-72194, 74150-74170)
> Procedure performed more than one time for each combined examination of the abdomen and pelvis

74176 **Computed tomography, abdomen and pelvis; without contrast material**

🚑 5.65　🔧 5.65　**FUD** XXX　`03` `Z3` 🖥

AMA: 2018,Jan,8; 2017,Jan,8; 2016,Jan,13; 2015,Jan,16; 2014,Jan,11

74177 **with contrast material(s)**

🚑 8.99　🔧 8.99　**FUD** XXX　`03` `Z2` 🖥

AMA: 2018,Jan,8; 2017,Jan,8; 2016,Jan,13; 2015,Jan,16; 2014,Jan,11

74178 **without contrast material in one or both body regions, followed by contrast material(s) and further sections in one or both body regions**

🚑 10.1　🔧 10.1　**FUD** XXX　`03` `Z2` 🖥

AMA: 2018,Jan,8; 2017,Jan,8; 2016,Jan,13; 2015,Jan,16; 2014,Jan,11

74181-74183 Magnetic Resonance Imaging: Abdomen–General

CMS: 100-04,4,250.16 Multiple Procedure Payment Reduction: Certain Diagnostic Imaging Procedures Rendered by Physicians

74181 **Magnetic resonance (eg, proton) imaging, abdomen; without contrast material(s)**

🚑 6.88　🔧 6.88　**FUD** XXX　`03` `Z2` `80` 🖥

AMA: 2018,Mar,11; 2018,Jan,8; 2017,Jan,8; 2016,Jan,13; 2015,Jan,16; 2014,Jan,11

74182 **with contrast material(s)**

🚑 10.1　🔧 10.1　**FUD** XXX　`03` `Z2` `80` 🖥

AMA: 2018,Mar,11; 2018,Jan,8; 2017,Jan,8; 2016,Jan,13; 2015,Jan,16; 2014,Jan,11

74183 **without contrast material(s), followed by with contrast material(s) and further sequences**

🚑 11.2　🔧 11.2　**FUD** XXX　`03` `Z2` `80` 🖥

AMA: 2018,Mar,11; 2018,Jan,8; 2017,Jan,8; 2016,Jan,13; 2015,Jan,16; 2014,Jan,11

74185 Magnetic Resonance Angiography: Abdomen–General

CMS: 100-04,13,40.1.1 Magnetic Resonance Angiography; 100-04,13,40.1.2 HCPCS Coding Requirements; 100-04,4,250.16 Multiple Procedure Payment Reduction: Certain Diagnostic Imaging Procedures Rendered by Physicians

74185 **Magnetic resonance angiography, abdomen, with or without contrast material(s)**

🚑 11.1　🔧 11.1　**FUD** XXX　`B` `80` 🖥

AMA: 2018,Jan,8; 2017,Jan,8; 2016,Jan,13; 2015,Jan,16; 2014,Jan,11

74190 Peritoneography

74190 **Peritoneogram (eg, after injection of air or contrast), radiological supervision and interpretation**

> EXCLUDES　Computed tomography, pelvis or abdomen (72192, 74150)
> Code also injection procedure (49400)

🚑 0.00　🔧 0.00　**FUD** XXX　`02` `N1` `80` 🖥

AMA: 2018,Jan,8; 2017,Jan,8; 2016,Jan,13; 2015,Jan,16; 2014,Jan,11

● New Code　▲ Revised Code　○ Reinstated　● New Web Release　▲ Revised Web Release　＋ Add-on　Unlisted　Not Covered　# Resequenced
㊿ Optum Mod 50 Exempt　⊘ AMA Mod 51 Exempt　⑤ Optum Mod 51 Exempt　㊿ Mod 63 Exempt　✗ Non-FDA Drug　★ Telemedicine　Ⓜ Maternity　Ⓐ Age Edit

74210-74235 Radiography: Throat and Esophagus

EXCLUDES *Percutaneous placement of gastrostomy tube, endoscopic (43246)*
Percutaneous placement of gastrostomy tube, fluoroscopic guidance (49440)

▲ 74210 **Radiologic examination, pharynx and/or cervical esophagus, including scout neck radiograph(s) and delayed image(s), when performed, contrast (eg, barium) study**

🔲 2.49 🔲 2.49 **FUD** XXX 〔01〕〔N1〕〔80〕🔲

AMA: 2014,Jan,11

▲ 74220 **Radiologic examination, esophagus, including scout chest radiograph(s) and delayed image(s), when performed; single-contrast (eg, barium) study**

EXCLUDES *Double-contrast study (74221)*
Small bowel follow-through (74248)
Upper GI tract studies (74240-74246)

🔲 2.73 🔲 2.73 **FUD** XXX 〔01〕〔N1〕〔80〕🔲

AMA: 2014,Jan,11

● 74221 **double-contrast (eg, high-density barium and effervescent agent) study**

EXCLUDES *Single-contrast study (74220)*
Small bowel follow-through (74248)
Upper GI tract studies (74240-74246)

▲ 74230 **Radiologic examination, swallowing function, with cineradiography/videoradiography, including scout neck radiograph(s) and delayed image(s), when performed, contrast (eg, barium) study**

EXCLUDES *Swallowing function motion fluoroscopic examination (92611)*

🔲 3.59 🔲 3.59 **FUD** XXX 〔01〕〔N1〕〔80〕🔲

AMA: 2018,Jan,8; 2017,Jan,8; 2016,Jan,13; 2015,Jan,16; 2014,Jul,5; 2014,Jan,11

74235 **Removal of foreign body(s), esophageal, with use of balloon catheter, radiological supervision and interpretation**

Code also procedure (43499)

🔲 0.00 🔲 0.00 **FUD** XXX 〔N〕〔N1〕〔80〕🔲

AMA: 2014,Jan,11

74240-74283 Radiography: Intestines

EXCLUDES *Percutaneous placement of gastrostomy tube, endoscopic (43246)*
Percutaneous placement of gastrostomy tube, fluoroscopic guidance (49440)

▲ 74240 **Radiologic examination, upper gastrointestinal tract, including scout abdominal radiograph(s) and delayed image(s), when performed; single-contrast (eg, barium) study**

INCLUDES Upper GI with KUB

EXCLUDES *Double-contrast study (74246)*
Esophagus studies (74220-74221)
Small bowel follow-through when performed (74248)

🔲 3.45 🔲 3.45 **FUD** XXX 〔01〕〔Z3〕〔80〕🔲

AMA: 2018,Jan,8; 2017,Jan,8; 2016,Sep,7; 2014,Jan,11

~~74241~~ ~~with or without delayed images, with KUB~~

To report, see (74240)

~~74245~~ ~~with small intestine, includes multiple serial images~~

To report, see (74240, 74248)

▲ 74246 **double-contrast (eg, high-density barium and effervescent agent) study, including glucagon, when administered**

INCLUDES Upper GI with KUB

EXCLUDES *Esophagus studies (74220-74221)*
Single-contrast study (74240)

🔲 3.84 🔲 3.84 **FUD** XXX 〔01〕〔Z2〕〔80〕🔲

AMA: 2018,Jan,8; 2017,Jan,8; 2016,Sep,7; 2014,Jan,11

~~74247~~ ~~with or without delayed images, with KUB~~

To report, see (74246)

● + 74248 **Radiologic small intestine follow-through study, including multiple serial images (List separately in addition to code for primary procedure for upper GI radiologic examination)**

🔲 0.00 🔲 0.00 **FUD** 000

EXCLUDES *Single- or double-contrast small intestine studies (74250-74251)*

Code first (74240, 74246)

~~74249~~ ~~with small intestine follow-through~~

To report, see (74246, 74248)

▲ 74250 **Radiologic examination, small intestine, including multiple serial images and scout abdominal radiograph(s), when performed; single-contrast (eg, barium) study**

EXCLUDES *Double-contrast study (74251)*
Small bowel follow-through (74248)

🔲 3.18 🔲 3.18 **FUD** XXX 〔01〕〔Z2〕〔80〕🔲

AMA: 2018,Jan,8; 2017,Jan,8; 2016,Sep,7; 2014,Jan,11

▲ 74251 **double-contrast (eg, high-density barium and air via enteroclysis tube) study, including glucagon, when administered**

EXCLUDES *Single-contrast study (74250)*
Small bowel follow-through (74248)

Insertion long gastrointestinal tube (44500, 74340)

🔲 12.1 🔲 12.1 **FUD** XXX 〔S〕〔Z2〕〔80〕🔲

AMA: 2018,Jan,8; 2017,Jan,8; 2016,Sep,7; 2014,Jan,11

~~74260~~ ~~Duodenography, hypotonic~~

To report, see (74251)

74261 **Computed tomographic (CT) colonography, diagnostic, including image postprocessing; without contrast material**

EXCLUDES *3D rendering (76376-76377)*
Computed tomography of abdomen or pelvis alone (72192-72194, 74150-74170)
Screening computed tomographic (CT) colonography (74263)

🔲 13.5 🔲 13.5 **FUD** XXX 〔03〕〔Z2〕〔80〕🔲

AMA: 2018,Jan,8; 2017,Jan,8; 2016,Jan,13; 2015,Jan,16; 2014,Jan,11

74262 **with contrast material(s) including non-contrast images, if performed**

EXCLUDES *3D rendering (76376-76377)*
Computed tomography of abdomen or pelvis alone (72192-72194, 74150-74170)
Screening computed tomographic (CT) colonography (74263)

🔲 15.2 🔲 15.2 **FUD** XXX 〔03〕〔Z2〕〔80〕🔲

AMA: 2018,Jan,8; 2017,Jan,8; 2016,Jan,13; 2015,Jan,16; 2014,Jan,11

74263 **Computed tomographic (CT) colonography, screening, including image postprocessing**

EXCLUDES *3D rendering (76376-76377)*
Computed tomographic (CT) colonography (74261-74262)
Computed tomography of abdomen or pelvis alone (72192-72194, 74150-74170)

🔲 21.3 🔲 21.3 **FUD** XXX 〔E〕🔲

AMA: 2018,Jan,8; 2017,Jan,8; 2016,Jan,13; 2015,Jan,16; 2014,Jan,11

▲ 74270 **Radiologic examination, colon, including scout abdominal radiograph(s) and delayed image(s), when performed; single-contrast (eg, barium) study**

EXCLUDES *Double-contrast study (74280)*

🔲 4.54 🔲 4.54 **FUD** XXX 〔01〕〔N1〕〔80〕🔲

AMA: 2018,Jan,8; 2017,Jan,8; 2016,Jan,13; 2015,Jan,16; 2014,Jan,11

▲ 74280 **double-contrast (eg, high density barium and air) study, including glucagon, when administered**

EXCLUDES *Single-contrast study (74270)*

🔲 6.41 🔲 6.41 **FUD** XXX 〔S〕〔Z2〕〔80〕🔲

AMA: 2014,Jan,11

74283 Therapeutic enema, contrast or air, for reduction of intussusception or other intraluminal obstruction (eg, meconium ileus)
6.61 6.61 **FUD** XXX [S] [Z2] [80] [▭]
AMA: 2014,Jan,11

74290-74330 Radiography: Biliary Tract

74290 Cholecystography, oral contrast
2.15 2.15 **FUD** XXX [01] [N1] [80] [▭]
AMA: 2014,Jan,11

74300 Cholangiography and/or pancreatography; intraoperative, radiological supervision and interpretation
0.00 0.00 **FUD** XXX [N] [N1] [80] [▭]
AMA: 2018,Jan,8; 2017,Jan,8; 2016,Jan,13; 2015,Dec,3; 2015,Jan,16; 2014,Jan,11

+ 74301 additional set intraoperative, radiological supervision and interpretation (List separately in addition to code for primary procedure)
Code first (74300)
0.00 0.00 **FUD** ZZZ [N] [N1] [80] [▭]
AMA: 2015,Dec,3; 2014,Jan,11

74328 Endoscopic catheterization of the biliary ductal system, radiological supervision and interpretation
Code also ERCP(~43261-43265, 43274-43278 [43274, 43275, 43276, 43277,43278])
0.00 0.00 **FUD** XXX [N] [N1] [80] [▭]
AMA: 2018,Jan,8; 2017,Jan,8; 2016,Jan,13; 2015,Jan,16; 2014,Jan,11

74329 Endoscopic catheterization of the pancreatic ductal system, radiological supervision and interpretation
Code also ERCP (~43261-43265, 43274-43278 [43274, 43275, 43276, 43277, 43278])
0.00 0.00 **FUD** XXX [N] [N1] [80] [▭]
AMA: 2014,Jan,11

74330 Combined endoscopic catheterization of the biliary and pancreatic ductal systems, radiological supervision and interpretation
Code also ERCP (~43261-43265, 43274-43278 [43274, 43275, 43276, 43277, 43278])
0.00 0.00 **FUD** XXX [N] [N1] [80] [▭]
AMA: 2014,Jan,11

74340-74363 Radiography: Bilidigestive Intubation

EXCLUDES Percutaneous insertion of gastrostomy tube, endoscopic (43246)
Percutaneous placement of gastrotomy tube, fluoroscopic guidance (49440)

74340 Introduction of long gastrointestinal tube (eg, Miller-Abbott), including multiple fluoroscopies and images, radiological supervision and interpretation
Code also placement of tube (44500)
0.00 0.00 **FUD** XXX [N] [N1] [80] [▭]
AMA: 2018,Jan,8; 2017,Jan,8; 2016,Sep,9; 2014,Jan,11

74355 Percutaneous placement of enteroclysis tube, radiological supervision and interpretation
INCLUDES Fluoroscopic guidance (77002)
0.00 0.00 **FUD** XXX [N] [N1] [80] [▭]
AMA: 2018,Jan,8; 2017,Jan,8; 2016,Jan,13; 2015,Jan,16; 2014,Jan,11

74360 Intraluminal dilation of strictures and/or obstructions (eg, esophagus), radiological supervision and interpretation
EXCLUDES Esophagogastroduodenoscopy, flexible, transoral; with dilation of esophagus (43233)
Esophagoscopy, flexible, transoral; with dilation of esophagus (43213-43214)
0.00 0.00 **FUD** XXX [N] [N1] [80] [▭]
AMA: 2018,Jan,8; 2017,Jan,8; 2016,Jan,13; 2015,Jan,16; 2014,Jan,11

74363 Percutaneous transhepatic dilation of biliary duct stricture with or without placement of stent, radiological supervision and interpretation
EXCLUDES Surgical procedure (47555-47556)
0.00 0.00 **FUD** XXX [N] [N1] [80] [▭]
AMA: 2014,Jan,11

74400-74775 Radiography: Urogenital

74400 Urography (pyelography), intravenous, with or without KUB, with or without tomography
3.36 3.36 **FUD** XXX [S] [Z2] [80] [▭]
AMA: 2014,Jan,11

74410 Urography, infusion, drip technique and/or bolus technique;
3.41 3.41 **FUD** XXX [S] [Z2] [80] [▭]
AMA: 2014,Jan,11

74415 with nephrotomography
4.07 4.07 **FUD** XXX [S] [Z2] [80] [▭]
AMA: 2014,Jan,11

74420 Urography, retrograde, with or without KUB
2.02 2.02 **FUD** XXX [S] [Z2] [80] [▭]
AMA: 2018,Jan,8; 2017,Jan,8; 2016,Jan,13; 2015,Jan,16; 2014,Jan,11

74425 Urography, antegrade (pyelostogram, nephrostogram, loopogram), radiological supervision and interpretation
EXCLUDES Injection for antegrade nephrostogram and/or ureterogram ([50430, 50431, 50432, 50433, 50434, 50435])
Ureteral stent placement (50693-50695)
0.00 0.00 **FUD** XXX [02] [N1] [80] [▭]
AMA: 2018,Jan,8; 2017,Jan,8; 2016,Jan,13; 2016,Jan,3; 2015,Oct,5; 2015,Jan,16; 2014,Jan,11

Nephrostomy catheter
Syringe with contrast
Ureter
Bladder
Contrast in urinary system
Nephrostogram

74430 Cystography, minimum of 3 views, radiological supervision and interpretation
1.11 1.11 **FUD** XXX [02] [N1] [80] [▭]
AMA: 2014,Jan,11

74440 Vasography, vesiculography, or epididymography, radiological supervision and interpretation ♂
2.44 2.44 **FUD** XXX [02] [N1] [80] [▭]
AMA: 2014,Jan,11

74445 **Corpora cavernosography, radiological supervision and interpretation** ♂

    INCLUDES   Needle placement with fluoroscopic guidance (77002)

    🔲 0.00   ⚖ 0.00   **FUD** XXX   02 N1 80 🔲

    AMA: 2018,Jan,8; 2017,Jan,8; 2016,Jan,13; 2015,Jan,16; 2014,Jan,11

74450 **Urethrocystography, retrograde, radiological supervision and interpretation**

    🔲 0.00   ⚖ 0.00   **FUD** XXX   02 N1 80 🔲

    AMA: 2014,Jan,11

74455 **Urethrocystography, voiding, radiological supervision and interpretation**

    🔲 2.55   ⚖ 2.55   **FUD** XXX   02 N1 80 🔲

    AMA: 2014,Jan,11

74470 **Radiologic examination, renal cyst study, translumbar, contrast visualization, radiological supervision and interpretation**

    INCLUDES   Needle placement with fluoroscopic guidance (77002)

    🔲 0.00   ⚖ 0.00   **FUD** XXX   02 N1 80 🔲

    AMA: 2018,Jan,8; 2017,Jan,8; 2016,Jan,13; 2015,Jan,16; 2014,Jan,11

74485 **Dilation of ureter(s) or urethra, radiological supervision and interpretation**

    EXCLUDES   *Change of pyelostomy/nephrostomy tube ([50435])*

           Nephrostomy tract dilation for procedure ([50436, 50437])

           Ureter dilation without radiologic guidance (52341, 52344)

    🔲 3.02   ⚖ 3.02   **FUD** XXX   02 N1 80 🔲

    AMA: 2018,Jan,8; 2017,Jan,8; 2016,Jan,13; 2016,Jan,3; 2015,Oct,5; 2015,Jan,16; 2014,Jan,11

74710 **Pelvimetry, with or without placental localization** ♀

    EXCLUDES   *Imaging procedures on abdomen and pelvis (72170-72190, 74018-74019, 74021-74022, 74150-74170)*

    🔲 1.08   ⚖ 1.08   **FUD** XXX   01 N1 80 🔲

    AMA: 2014,Jan,11

74712 **Magnetic resonance (eg, proton) imaging, fetal, including placental and maternal pelvic imaging when performed; single or first gestation** ♀

    EXCLUDES   *Imaging of maternal pelvis or placenta without fetal imaging (72195-72197)*

    🔲 13.5   ⚖ 13.5   **FUD** XXX   S Z2 80 🔲

    AMA: 2018,Jan,8; 2017,Jan,8; 2016,Jun,5

+ 74713 **each additional gestation (List separately in addition to code for primary procedure)** ♀

    EXCLUDES   *Imaging of maternal pelvis or placenta without fetal imaging (72195-72197)*

    Code first (74712)

    🔲 6.60   ⚖ 6.60   **FUD** ZZZ   N N1 80 🔲

    AMA: 2018,Jan,8; 2017,Jan,8; 2016,Jun,5

74740 **Hysterosalpingography, radiological supervision and interpretation** ♀

    EXCLUDES   *Imaging procedures on abdomen and pelvis (72170-72190, 74018-74019, 74021-74022, 74150-74170)*

    Code also injection of saline/contrast (58340)

    🔲 2.32   ⚖ 2.32   **FUD** XXX   02 N1 80 🔲

    AMA: 2018,Jan,8; 2017,Jan,8; 2016,Jan,13; 2015,Jan,16; 2014,Jan,11

Tube

Ovary

Uterus

Delivery apparatus

Cervix

Vaginal canal

Hysterosalpingography (imaging of the uterus and tubes) is performed. Report for radiological supervision and interpretation

74742 **Transcervical catheterization of fallopian tube, radiological supervision and interpretation** ♀

    EXCLUDES   *Imaging procedures on abdomen and pelvis (72170-72190, 74018-74019, 74021-74022, 74150-74170)*

    Code also (58345)

    🔲 0.00   ⚖ 0.00   **FUD** XXX   N N1 80 🔲

    AMA: 2018,Jan,8; 2017,Jan,8; 2016,Jan,13; 2015,Jan,16; 2014,Jan,11

74775 **Perineogram (eg, vaginogram, for sex determination or extent of anomalies)** M ♀

    EXCLUDES   *Imaging procedures on abdomen and pelvis (72170-72190, 74018-74019, 74021-74022, 74150-74170)*

    🔲 0.00   ⚖ 0.00   **FUD** XXX   S Z2 80 🔲

    AMA: 2014,Jan,11

75557-75565 Magnetic Resonance Imaging: Heart Structure and Physiology

    INCLUDES   Physiologic evaluation of cardiac function

    EXCLUDES   *3D rendering (76376-76377)*

           Cardiac catheterization procedures (93451-93572)

           Use of more than one code in this group per session

    Code also separate vascular injection (36000-36299)

75557 **Cardiac magnetic resonance imaging for morphology and function without contrast material;**

    🔲 9.16   ⚖ 9.16   **FUD** XXX   03 Z2 80 🔲

    AMA: 2018,Jan,8; 2017,Jan,8; 2016,Jan,13; 2015,Jan,16; 2014,Jan,11

75559 **with stress imaging**

    INCLUDES   Pharmacologic wall motion stress evaluation without contrast

    Code also stress testing when performed (93015-93018)

    🔲 12.7   ⚖ 12.7   **FUD** XXX   03 Z2 80 🔲

    AMA: 2018,Jan,8; 2017,Jan,8; 2016,Jan,13; 2015,Jan,16; 2014,Jan,11

26/TC PC/TC Only   A2-Z3 ASC Payment   50 Bilateral   ♂ Male Only   ♀ Female Only   🔲 Facility RVU   ⚖ Non-Facility RVU   🔲 CCI   ✖ CLIA

FUD Follow-up Days   **CMS:** IOM   **AMA:** CPT Asst   A-Y OPPSI   80/80 Surg Assist Allowed / w/Doc   Lab Crosswalk   Radiology Crosswalk

346   CPT © 2019 American Medical Association. All Rights Reserved.   © 2019 Optum360, LLC

75561 Cardiac magnetic resonance imaging for morphology and function without contrast material(s), followed by contrast material(s) and further sequences;

🔧 12.0 ⚖ 12.0 **FUD** XXX   `03` `Z2` `80` 🖵

AMA: 2018,Jan,8; 2017,Jan,8; 2016,Jan,13; 2015,Jan,16; 2014,Jan,11

75563 with stress imaging

INCLUDES Pharmacologic perfusion stress evaluation with contrast
Code also stress testing when performed (93015-93018)

🔧 14.2 ⚖ 14.2 **FUD** XXX   `03` `Z2` `80` 🖵

AMA: 2018,Jan,8; 2017,Jan,8; 2016,Jan,13; 2015,Jan,16; 2014,Jan,11

+ **75565** Cardiac magnetic resonance imaging for velocity flow mapping (List separately in addition to code for primary procedure)

Code first (75557, 75559, 75561, 75563)

🔧 1.51 ⚖ 1.51 **FUD** ZZZ   `N` `N1` `80` 🖵

AMA: 2018,Jan,8; 2017,Jan,8; 2016,Jan,13; 2015,Jan,16; 2014,Jan,11

75571-75574 Computed Tomographic Imaging: Heart

CMS: 100-04,12,20.4.7 Services Not Meeting National Electrical Manufacturers Association (NEMA) Standard; 100-04,4,20.6.12 Use of HCPCS Modifier – CT; 100-04,4,250.16 Multiple Procedure Payment Reduction: Certain Diagnostic Imaging Procedures Rendered by Physicians

EXCLUDES 3D rendering (76376-76377)
Use of more than one code in this group per session

75571 Computed tomography, heart, without contrast material, with quantitative evaluation of coronary calcium

🔧 2.92 ⚖ 2.92 **FUD** XXX   `01` `N1` `80` 🖵

AMA: 2018,Jan,8; 2017,Jan,8; 2016,Jan,13; 2015,Jan,16; 2014,Jan,11

75572 Computed tomography, heart, with contrast material, for evaluation of cardiac structure and morphology (including 3D image postprocessing, assessment of cardiac function, and evaluation of venous structures, if performed)

🔧 7.52 ⚖ 7.52 **FUD** XXX   `S` `Z2` `80` 🖵

AMA: 2018,Jan,8; 2017,Jan,8; 2016,Jan,13; 2015,Jan,16; 2014,Jan,11

75573 Computed tomography, heart, with contrast material, for evaluation of cardiac structure and morphology in the setting of congenital heart disease (including 3D image postprocessing, assessment of LV cardiac function, RV structure and function and evaluation of venous structures, if performed)

🔧 10.1 ⚖ 10.1 **FUD** XXX   `S` `Z2` `80` 🖵

AMA: 2018,Jan,8; 2017,Jan,8; 2016,Jan,13; 2015,Jan,16; 2014,Jan,11

75574 Computed tomographic angiography, heart, coronary arteries and bypass grafts (when present), with contrast material, including 3D image postprocessing (including evaluation of cardiac structure and morphology, assessment of cardiac function, and evaluation of venous structures, if performed)

🔧 11.0 ⚖ 11.0 **FUD** XXX   `S` `Z2` `80` 🖵

AMA: 2018,Jan,8; 2017,Jan,8; 2016,Jan,13; 2015,Jan,16; 2014,Jan,11

75600-75774 Radiography: Arterial

INCLUDES Diagnostic angiography specifically included in the interventional code description
The following diagnostic procedures with interventional supervision and interpretation:
Angiography
Contrast injection
Fluoroscopic guidance for intervention
Post-angioplasty/atherectomy/stent angiography
Roadmapping
Vessel measurement

EXCLUDES Catheterization codes for diagnostic angiography of lower extremity when an access site other than the site used for the therapy is required
Diagnostic angiogram during a separate encounter from the interventional procedure
Diagnostic angiography with interventional procedure if:
1. No previous catheter-based angiogram is accessible and a complete diagnostic procedure is performed and the decision to proceed with an interventional procedure is based on the diagnostic service, OR
2. The previous diagnostic angiogram is accessible but the documentation in the medical record specifies that:
   A. the patient's condition has changed
   B. there is insufficient imaging of the patient's anatomy and/or disease, OR
   C. there is a clinical change during the procedure that necessitates a new examination away from the site of the intervention
3. Modifier 59 is appended to the code(s) for the diagnostic radiological supervision and interpretation service to indicate the guidelines were met
Intra-arterial procedures (36100-36248)
Intravenous procedures (36000, 36005-36015)

75600 Aortography, thoracic, without serialography, radiological supervision and interpretation

EXCLUDES Supravalvular aortography (93567)

🔧 5.63 ⚖ 5.63 **FUD** XXX   `02` `N1` `80` 🖵

AMA: 2014,Jan,11

75605 Aortography, thoracic, by serialography, radiological supervision and interpretation

EXCLUDES Supravalvular aortography (93567)

🔧 3.78 ⚖ 3.78 **FUD** XXX   `02` `N1` `80` 🖵

AMA: 2018,Jan,8; 2017,Jan,8; 2016,Jan,13; 2015,Jan,16; 2014,Jan,11

75625 Aortography, abdominal, by serialography, radiological supervision and interpretation

EXCLUDES Supravalvular aortography (93567)

🔧 3.73 ⚖ 3.73 **FUD** XXX   `02` `N1` `80` 🖵

AMA: 2018,Jan,8; 2017,Jan,8; 2016,Jan,13; 2015,Jan,16; 2014,Jan,11

75630 Aortography, abdominal plus bilateral iliofemoral lower extremity, catheter, by serialography, radiological supervision and interpretation

EXCLUDES Supravalvular aortography (93567)

🔧 4.68 ⚖ 4.68 **FUD** XXX   `02` `N1` `80` 🖵

AMA: 2018,Jan,8; 2017,Jan,8; 2016,Jan,13; 2015,Jan,16; 2014,Jan,11

75635 Computed tomographic angiography, abdominal aorta and bilateral iliofemoral lower extremity runoff, with contrast material(s), including noncontrast images, if performed, and image postprocessing

EXCLUDES 3D rendering (76376-76377)
Computed tomographic angiography, abdomen, lower extremity, pelvis (72191, 73706, 74174-74175)

🔧 12.4 ⚖ 12.4 **FUD** XXX   `02` `N1` `80` 🖵

AMA: 2018,Jan,8; 2017,Jan,8; 2016,Jan,13; 2015,Jan,16; 2014,Jan,11

75705 Angiography, spinal, selective, radiological supervision and interpretation

🔧 7.13 ⚖ 7.13 **FUD** XXX   `02` `N1` `80` 🖵

AMA: 2014,Jan,11

75710 Angiography, extremity, unilateral, radiological supervision and interpretation

    📷 4.73   ⚖ 4.73   **FUD** XXX   02 N1 80 ▭

    AMA: 2018,Jan,8; 2017,Mar,3; 2017,Jan,8; 2016,Jan,13; 2015,Jan,16; 2014,Jan,11

75716 Angiography, extremity, bilateral, radiological supervision and interpretation

    📷 5.04   ⚖ 5.04   **FUD** XXX   02 N1 80 ▭

    AMA: 2018,Jan,8; 2017,Jan,8; 2016,Jan,13; 2015,Jan,16; 2014,Jan,11

75726 Angiography, visceral, selective or supraselective (with or without flush aortogram), radiological supervision and interpretation

    EXCLUDES   *Selective angiography, each additional visceral vessel examined after basic examination (75774)*

    📷 4.08   ⚖ 4.08   **FUD** XXX   02 N1 80 ▭

    AMA: 2014,Jan,11

75731 Angiography, adrenal, unilateral, selective, radiological supervision and interpretation

    📷 4.73   ⚖ 4.73   **FUD** XXX   02 N1 80 ▭

    AMA: 2014,Jan,11

75733 Angiography, adrenal, bilateral, selective, radiological supervision and interpretation

    📷 5.09   ⚖ 5.09   **FUD** XXX   02 N1 80 ▭

    AMA: 2014,Jan,11

75736 Angiography, pelvic, selective or supraselective, radiological supervision and interpretation

    📷 4.38   ⚖ 4.38   **FUD** XXX   02 N1 80 ▭

    AMA: 2014,Jan,11

75741 Angiography, pulmonary, unilateral, selective, radiological supervision and interpretation

    📷 4.13   ⚖ 4.13   **FUD** XXX   02 N1 80 ▭

    AMA: 2019,Jun,3; 2018,Jan,8; 2017,Jan,8; 2016,Jan,13; 2015,Jan,16; 2014,Jan,11

75743 Angiography, pulmonary, bilateral, selective, radiological supervision and interpretation

    📷 4.64   ⚖ 4.64   **FUD** XXX   02 N1 80 ▭

    AMA: 2019,Jun,3; 2018,Jan,8; 2017,Jan,8; 2016,Jan,13; 2015,Jan,16; 2014,Jan,11

75746 Angiography, pulmonary, by nonselective catheter or venous injection, radiological supervision and interpretation

    EXCLUDES   *Nonselective injection procedure or catheter introduction with cardiac cath (93568)*

    📷 4.16   ⚖ 4.16   **FUD** XXX   02 N1 80 ▭

    AMA: 2019,Jun,3; 2014,Jan,11

75756 Angiography, internal mammary, radiological supervision and interpretation

    EXCLUDES   *Internal mammary angiography with cardiac cath (93455, 93457, 93459, 93461, 93564)*

    📷 4.79   ⚖ 4.79   **FUD** XXX   02 N1 80 ▭

    AMA: 2018,Jan,8; 2017,Jan,8; 2016,Jan,13; 2015,Jan,16; 2014,Jan,11

+ 75774 Angiography, selective, each additional vessel studied after basic examination, radiological supervision and interpretation (List separately in addition to code for primary procedure)

    EXCLUDES   *Angiography (75600-75756)*
         Cardiac cath procedures (93452-93462, 93531-93533, 93563-93568)
         Catheterizations (36215-36248)
         Dialysis circuit angiography (current access), use modifier 52 with (36901)
         Nonselective catheter placement, thoracic aorta (36221-36228)

    Code also diagnostic angiography of upper extremities and other vascular beds (except cervicocerebral vessels), when appropriate
    Code first initial vessel

    📷 2.33   ⚖ 2.33   **FUD** ZZZ   N N1 80 ▭

    AMA: 2018,Jan,8; 2017,Jan,8; 2016,Jan,13; 2015,Jan,16; 2014,Jan,11

75801-75893 Radiography: Lymphatic and Venous

INCLUDES   Diagnostic venography specifically included in the interventional code description
The following diagnostic procedures with interventional supervision and interpretation:
    Contrast injection
    Fluoroscopic guidance for intervention
    Post-angioplasty/venography
    Roadmapping
    Venography
    Vessel measurement

EXCLUDES   *Diagnostic venogram during a separate encounter from the interventional procedure*
Diagnostic venography with interventional procedure if:
1. No previous catheter-based venogram is accessible and a complete diagnostic procedure is performed and the decision to proceed with an interventional procedure is based on the diagnostic service, OR
2. The previous diagnostic venogram is accessible but the documentation in the medical record specifies that:
    A. The patient's condition has changed
    B. There is insufficient imaging of the patient's anatomy and/or disease, OR
    C. There is a clinical change during the procedure that necessitates a new examination away from the site of the intervention
Intravenous procedures (36000-36015, 36400-36510 [36465, 36466, 36482, 36483])
Lymphatic injection procedures (38790)

75801 Lymphangiography, extremity only, unilateral, radiological supervision and interpretation

    📷 0.00   ⚖ 0.00   **FUD** XXX   02 N1 80 ▭

    AMA: 2014,Jan,11

75803 Lymphangiography, extremity only, bilateral, radiological supervision and interpretation

    📷 0.00   ⚖ 0.00   **FUD** XXX   02 N1 80 ▭

    AMA: 2014,Jan,11

75805 Lymphangiography, pelvic/abdominal, unilateral, radiological supervision and interpretation

    📷 0.00   ⚖ 0.00   **FUD** XXX   02 N1 80 ▭

    AMA: 2014,Jan,11

75807 Lymphangiography, pelvic/abdominal, bilateral, radiological supervision and interpretation

    📷 0.00   ⚖ 0.00   **FUD** XXX   02 N1 80 ▭

    AMA: 2014,Jan,11

75809 Shuntogram for investigation of previously placed indwelling nonvascular shunt (eg, LeVeen shunt, ventriculoperitoneal shunt, indwelling infusion pump), radiological supervision and interpretation

    Code also surgical procedure (49427, 61070)

    📷 2.69   ⚖ 2.69   **FUD** XXX   02 N1 80 ▭

    AMA: 2018,Jan,8; 2017,Jan,8; 2016,Jan,13; 2015,Jan,16; 2014,Jan,11

75810 Splenoportography, radiological supervision and interpretation

    📷 0.00   ⚖ 0.00   **FUD** XXX   02 N1 80 ▭

    AMA: 2018,Jan,8; 2017,Jan,8; 2016,Jan,13; 2015,Jan,16; 2014,Jan,11

75820 Venography, extremity, unilateral, radiological supervision and interpretation

    📷 3.15   ⚖ 3.15   **FUD** XXX   02 N1 80 ▭

    AMA: 2019,Mar,6; 2018,Jan,8; 2017,Jan,8; 2016,May,5; 2016,Jan,13; 2015,May,3; 2015,Jan,16; 2014,Jan,11

75822 Venography, extremity, bilateral, radiological supervision and interpretation

    📷 3.68   ⚖ 3.68   **FUD** XXX   02 N1 80 ▭

    AMA: 2014,Jan,11

75825 Venography, caval, inferior, with serialography, radiological supervision and interpretation

    📷 3.68   ⚖ 3.68   **FUD** XXX   02 N1 80 ▭

    AMA: 2018,Jan,8; 2017,Feb,14; 2017,Jan,8; 2016,Jan,13; 2015,Jan,16; 2014,Jan,11

26/TC	PC/TC Only	A2-Z3	ASC Payment	50	Bilateral	♂ Male Only	♀ Female Only	📷 Facility RVU	⚖ Non-Facility RVU	▭ CCI	✕ CLIA
FUD	Follow-up Days	**CMS:** IOM		**AMA:** CPT Asst		A-Y OPPSI		80/80 Surg Assist Allowed / w/Doc	✕ Lab Crosswalk		✕ Radiology Crosswalk

348   CPT © 2019 American Medical Association. All Rights Reserved.   © 2019 Optum360, LLC

75827 Venography, caval, superior, with serialography, radiological supervision and interpretation
🚗 3.82   3.82 **FUD** XXX   02 N1 80
AMA: 2018,Jan,8; 2017,Jan,8; 2016,Jan,13; 2015,Jan,16; 2014,Jan,11

75831 Venography, renal, unilateral, selective, radiological supervision and interpretation
🚗 3.84   3.84 **FUD** XXX   02 N1 80
AMA: 2014,Jan,11

75833 Venography, renal, bilateral, selective, radiological supervision and interpretation
🚗 4.55   4.55 **FUD** XXX   02 N1 80
AMA: 2014,Jan,11

75840 Venography, adrenal, unilateral, selective, radiological supervision and interpretation
🚗 4.08   4.08 **FUD** XXX   02 N1 80
AMA: 2014,Jan,11

75842 Venography, adrenal, bilateral, selective, radiological supervision and interpretation
🚗 4.95   4.95 **FUD** XXX   02 N1 80
AMA: 2014,Jan,11

75860 Venography, venous sinus (eg, petrosal and inferior sagittal) or jugular, catheter, radiological supervision and interpretation
🚗 3.99   3.99 **FUD** XXX   02 N1 80
AMA: 2014,Jan,11

75870 Venography, superior sagittal sinus, radiological supervision and interpretation
🚗 5.30   5.30 **FUD** XXX   02 N1 80
AMA: 2014,Jan,11

75872 Venography, epidural, radiological supervision and interpretation
🚗 4.08   4.08 **FUD** XXX   02 N1 80
AMA: 2014,Jan,11

75880 Venography, orbital, radiological supervision and interpretation
🚗 3.44   3.44 **FUD** XXX   02 N1 80
AMA: 2014,Jan,11

75885 Percutaneous transhepatic portography with hemodynamic evaluation, radiological supervision and interpretation
🚗 4.29   4.29 **FUD** XXX   02 N1 80
AMA: 2018,Jan,8; 2017,Jan,8; 2016,Jan,13; 2015,Jan,16; 2014,Jan,11

Inferior vena cava, Liver, Stomach, Portal vein, Spleen, Splenic vein, Superior mesenteric, Inferior mesenteric, Left colic

Schematic showing the portal vein

75887 Percutaneous transhepatic portography without hemodynamic evaluation, radiological supervision and interpretation
🚗 4.31   4.31 **FUD** XXX   02 N1 80
AMA: 2018,Jan,8; 2017,Jan,8; 2016,Jan,13; 2015,Jan,16; 2014,Jan,11

75889 Hepatic venography, wedged or free, with hemodynamic evaluation, radiological supervision and interpretation
🚗 3.93   3.93 **FUD** XXX   02 N1 80
AMA: 2014,Jan,11

75891 Hepatic venography, wedged or free, without hemodynamic evaluation, radiological supervision and interpretation
🚗 3.98   3.98 **FUD** XXX   02 N1 80
AMA: 2014,Jan,11

75893 Venous sampling through catheter, with or without angiography (eg, for parathyroid hormone, renin), radiological supervision and interpretation
Code also surgical procedure (36500)
🚗 3.32   3.32 **FUD** XXX   02 N1 80
AMA: 2014,Jan,11

75894-75902 Transcatheter Procedures

INCLUDES The following diagnostic procedures with interventional supervision and interpretation:
Angiography/venography
Completion angiography/venography except for those services allowed by (75898)
Contrast injection
Fluoroscopic guidance for intervention
Roadmapping
Vessel measurement

EXCLUDES *Diagnostic angiography/venography performed at the same session as transcatheter therapy unless it is specifically included in the code descriptor or is excluded in the venography/angiography notes (75600-75893)*

75894 Transcatheter therapy, embolization, any method, radiological supervision and interpretation
EXCLUDES *Endovenous ablation therapy of incompetent vein (36478-36479)*
Transluminal balloon angioplasty (36475-36476)
Vascular embolization or occlusion (37241-37244)
🚗 0.00   0.00 **FUD** XXX   N N1 80
AMA: 2018,Mar,3; 2018,Jan,8; 2017,Jan,8; 2016,Nov,3; 2016,Jan,13; 2015,Jan,16; 2014,Oct,6; 2014,Jan,11

75898 Angiography through existing catheter for follow-up study for transcatheter therapy, embolization or infusion, other than for thrombolysis
EXCLUDES *Percutaneous arterial transluminal mechanical thrombectomy (61645)*
Prolonged endovascular intracranial administration of pharmacologic agent(s) (61650-61651)
Transcatheter therapy, arterial infusion for thrombolysis (37211-37214)
Vascular embolization or occlusion (37241-37244)
🚗 0.00   0.00 **FUD** XXX   02 N1 80
AMA: 2019,Sep,6; 2018,Jan,8; 2017,Jan,8; 2016,Jan,13; 2015,Nov,3; 2015,Jan,16; 2014,Oct,6; 2014,Jan,11

75901 Mechanical removal of pericatheter obstructive material (eg, fibrin sheath) from central venous device via separate venous access, radiologic supervision and interpretation
EXCLUDES *Venous catheterization (36010-36012)*
Code also surgical procedure (36595)
🚗 5.62   5.62 **FUD** XXX   N N1 80
AMA: 2018,Jan,8; 2017,Jan,8; 2016,Jan,13; 2015,Jan,16; 2014,Jan,11

75902 Mechanical removal of intraluminal (intracatheter) obstructive material from central venous device through device lumen, radiologic supervision and interpretation

EXCLUDES *Venous catheterization (36010-36012)*

Code also surgical procedure (36596)

🔲 2.22 ⚖ 2.22 **FUD** XXX N NI 80 ▢

AMA: 2018,Jan,8; 2017,Jan,8; 2016,Jan,13; 2015,Jan,16; 2014,Jan,11

75956-75959 Endovascular Aneurysm Repair

INCLUDES The following diagnostic procedures with interventional supervision and interpretation:
Angiography/venography
Completion angiography/venography except for those services allowed by (75898)
Contrast injection
Fluoroscopic guidance for intervention
Injection procedure only for transcatheter therapy or biopsy (36100-36299)
Percutaneous needle biopsy
Pancreas (48102)
Retroperitoneal lymph node/mass (49180)
Roadmapping
Vessel measurement

EXCLUDES *Diagnostic angiography/venography performed at the same session as transcatheter therapy unless it is specifically included in the code descriptor (75600-75893)*
Radiological supervision and interpretation for transluminal angioplasty in:
Femoral/popliteal arteries (37224-37227)
Iliac artery (37220-37223)
Tibial/peroneal artery (37228-37235)

75956 Endovascular repair of descending thoracic aorta (eg, aneurysm, pseudoaneurysm, dissection, penetrating ulcer, intramural hematoma, or traumatic disruption); involving coverage of left subclavian artery origin, initial endoprosthesis plus descending thoracic aortic extension(s), if required, to level of celiac artery origin, radiological supervision and interpretation

Code also endovascular graft implantation (33880)

🔲 0.00 ⚖ 0.00 **FUD** XXX C 80 ▢

AMA: 2018,Jan,8; 2017,Jan,8; 2016,Jan,13; 2015,Jan,16; 2014,Jan,11

75957 not involving coverage of left subclavian artery origin, initial endoprosthesis plus descending thoracic aortic extension(s), if required, to level of celiac artery origin, radiological supervision and interpretation

Code also endovascular graft implantation (33881)

🔲 0.00 ⚖ 0.00 **FUD** XXX C 80 ▢

AMA: 2018,Jan,8; 2017,Jan,8; 2016,Jan,13; 2015,Jan,16; 2014,Jan,11

75958 Placement of proximal extension prosthesis for endovascular repair of descending thoracic aorta (eg, aneurysm, pseudoaneurysm, dissection, penetrating ulcer, intramural hematoma, or traumatic disruption), radiological supervision and interpretation

Code also placement of each additional proximal extension(s) (75958)
Code also proximal endovascular extension implantation (33883-33884)

🔲 0.00 ⚖ 0.00 **FUD** XXX C 80 ▢

AMA: 2018,Jan,8; 2017,Jan,8; 2016,Jan,13; 2015,Jan,16; 2014,Jan,11

75959 Placement of distal extension prosthesis(s) (delayed) after endovascular repair of descending thoracic aorta, as needed, to level of celiac origin, radiological supervision and interpretation

INCLUDES Corresponding services for placement of distal thoracic endovascular extension(s) placed during procedure following the principal procedure

EXCLUDES *Endovascular repair of descending thoracic aorta (75956-75957)*
Use of code more than one time no matter how many modules are deployed

Code also placement of distal endovascular extension (33886)

🔲 0.00 ⚖ 0.00 **FUD** XXX C 80 ▢

AMA: 2018,Jan,8; 2017,Jan,8; 2016,Jan,13; 2015,Jan,16; 2014,Jan,11

75970 Percutaneous Transluminal Angioplasty

INCLUDES The following diagnostic procedures with interventional supervision and interpretation:
Angiography/venography
Completion angiography/venography except for those services allowed by (75898)
Contrast injection
Fluoroscopic guidance for intervention
Roadmapping
Vessel measurement

EXCLUDES *Diagnostic angiography/venography performed at the same session as transcatheter therapy unless it is specifically included in the code descriptor (75600-75893)*
Injection procedure only for transcatheter therapy or biopsy (36100-36299)
Percutaneous needle biopsy (48102)
Pancreas (48102)
Retroperitoneal lymph node/mass (49180)
Radiological supervision and interpretation for transluminal balloon angioplasty in:
Femoral/popliteal arteries (37224-37227)
Iliac artery (37220-37223)
Tibial/peroneal artery (37228-37235)
Transcatheter renal/ureteral biopsy (52007)

75970 Transcatheter biopsy, radiological supervision and interpretation

🔲 0.00 ⚖ 0.00 **FUD** XXX N NI 80 ▢

AMA: 2018,Jan,8; 2014,Jan,11

75984-75989 Percutaneous Drainage

75984 Change of percutaneous tube or drainage catheter with contrast monitoring (eg, genitourinary system, abscess), radiological supervision and interpretation

EXCLUDES *Change only of nephrostomy/pyelostomy tube ([50435])*
Cholecystostomy, percutaneous (47490)
Introduction procedure only for percutaneous biliary drainage (47531-47544)
Nephrostolithotomy/pyelostolithotomy, percutaneous (50080-50081)
Percutaneous replacement of gastrointestinal tube using fluoroscopic guidance (49450-49452)
Removal and/or replacement of internal ureteral stent using transurethral approach (50385-50386)

🔲 2.89 ⚖ 2.89 **FUD** XXX N NI 80 ▢

AMA: 2014,Jan,11

75989 Radiological guidance (ie, fluoroscopy, ultrasound, or computed tomography), for percutaneous drainage (eg, abscess, specimen collection), with placement of catheter, radiological supervision and interpretation

INCLUDES Imaging guidance

EXCLUDES *Cholecystostomy (47490)*
Image-guided fluid collection drainage by catheter (10030, 49405-49407)
Pericardial drainage (33017-33019)
Thoracentesis (32554-32557)

🔲 3.42 ⚖ 3.42 **FUD** XXX N NI 80 ▢

AMA: 2018,Jan,8; 2017,Jan,8; 2016,Jan,13; 2015,Dec,3; 2015,Jan,16; 2014,May,9; 2014,Jan,11

26/TC PC/TC Only   A2-Z3 ASC Payment   50 Bilateral   ♂ Male Only   ♀ Female Only   🔲 Facility RVU   ⚖ Non-Facility RVU   ▢ CCI   ✖ CLIA
FUD Follow-up Days   CMS: IOM   AMA: CPT Asst   A-Y OPPSI   80/80 Surg Assist Allowed / w/Doc   ◣ Lab Crosswalk   ✚ Radiology Crosswalk

350   CPT © 2019 American Medical Association. All Rights Reserved.   © 2019 Optum360, LLC

76000-76140 Miscellaneous Techniques

EXCLUDES Arthrography:
Ankle (73615)
Elbow (73085)
Hip (73525)
Knee (73580)
Shoulder (73040)
Wrist (73115)
CT cerebral perfusion test (0042T)

76000 **Fluoroscopy (separate procedure), up to 1 hour physician or other qualified health care professional time**

EXCLUDES Extracorporeal membrane oxygenation (ECMO)/extracorporeal life support (ECLS) (33957-33959, [33962, 33963, 33964])
Insertion/removal/replacement wireless cardiac stimulator (0515T-0520T)
Insertion/replacement/removal leadless pacemaker ([33274, 33275])

🔲 1.33   ⚖ 1.33   **FUD** XXX   Ⓢ Ⓩ3 80 ⊡

AMA: 2019,Sep,10; 2019,Sep,5; 2019,Jun,3; 2019,Mar,6; 2018,Apr,7; 2018,Mar,3; 2018,Jan,8; 2017,Jan,8; 2016,Nov,3; 2016,Aug,5; 2016,May,13; 2016,May,5; 2016,Mar,5; 2016,Jan,11; 2016,Jan,13; 2015,Nov,3; 2015,Sep,3; 2015,May,3; 2015,Jan,16; 2014,Dec,3; 2014,Nov,5; 2014,Oct,6; 2014,Sep,5; 2014,Jan,11

76010 **Radiologic examination from nose to rectum for foreign body, single view, child** Ⓐ

🔲 0.77   ⚖ 0.77   **FUD** XXX   01 N1 80 ⊡

AMA: 2018,Jan,8; 2017,Jan,8; 2016,Jan,13; 2015,Jan,16; 2014,Jan,11

76080 **Radiologic examination, abscess, fistula or sinus tract study, radiological supervision and interpretation**

EXCLUDES Contrast injections, radiology evaluation, and guidance via fluoroscopy of gastrostomy, duodenostomy, jejunostomy, gastro-jejunostomy, or cecostomy tube (49465)

🔲 1.61   ⚖ 1.61   **FUD** XXX   02 N1 80 ⊡

AMA: 2018,Jan,8; 2017,Jan,8; 2016,Jan,13; 2015,Jan,16; 2014,Jan,11

76098 **Radiological examination, surgical specimen**

EXCLUDES Breast biopsy with placement of breast localization device(s) (19081-19086)

🔲 0.47   ⚖ 0.47   **FUD** XXX   02 N1 80 ⊡

AMA: 2012,Feb,9-10; 1997,Nov,1

76100 **Radiologic examination, single plane body section (eg, tomography), other than with urography**

🔲 2.67   ⚖ 2.67   **FUD** XXX   01 N1 80 ⊡

AMA: 2012,Feb,9-10; 1997,Nov,1

76101 **Radiologic examination, complex motion (ie, hypercycloidal) body section (eg, mastoid polytomography), other than with urography; unilateral**

EXCLUDES Nephrotomography (74415)
Panoramic x-ray (70355)
Procedure performed more than one time per day

🔲 2.65   ⚖ 2.65   **FUD** XXX   01 Z2 80 ⊡

AMA: 2012,Feb,9-10; 1997,Nov,1

76102 **bilateral**

EXCLUDES Nephrotomography (74415)
Panoramic x-ray (70355)
Procedure performed more than one time per day

🔲 4.88   ⚖ 4.88   **FUD** XXX   Ⓢ Z2 80 ⊡

AMA: 2012,Feb,9-10; 1997,Nov,1

76120 **Cineradiography/videoradiography, except where specifically included**

🔲 2.87   ⚖ 2.87   **FUD** XXX   01 N1 80 ⊡

AMA: 2018,Jan,8; 2017,Jan,8; 2016,Jan,13; 2015,Jan,16; 2014,Jan,11

+ 76125 **Cineradiography/videoradiography to complement routine examination (List separately in addition to code for primary procedure)**

Code first primary procedure

🔲 0.00   ⚖ 0.00   **FUD** ZZZ   N N1 80 ⊡

AMA: 2018,Jan,8; 2017,Jan,8; 2016,Jan,13; 2015,Jan,16; 2014,Jan,11

76140 **Consultation on X-ray examination made elsewhere, written report**

🔲 0.00   ⚖ 0.00   **FUD** XXX   Ⓔ ⊡

AMA: 2018,Jan,8; 2017,Jan,8; 2016,Jan,13; 2015,Jan,16; 2014,Jan,11

76376-76377 Three-dimensional Manipulation

INCLUDES Concurrent physician supervision of image postprocessing
3D manipulation of volumetric data set
Rendering of image

EXCLUDES Anatomic guide 3D-printed and designed from image data set (0561T-0562T)
Anatomic model 3D-printed from image data set (0559T-0560T)
Arthrography:
Ankle (73615)
Elbow (73085)
Hip (73525)
Knee (73580)
Shoulder (73040)
Wrist (73115)
Cardiac magnetic resonance imaging (75557, 75559, 75561, 75563, 75565)
Computed tomographic angiography (70496, 70498, 71275, 72191, 73206, 73706, 74174-74175, 74261-74263, 75571-75574, 75635)
Computer-aided detection of MRI data for lesion, breast MRI (77046-77049)
CT cerebral perfusion test (0042T)
Digital breast tomosynthesis (77061-77063)
Echocardiography, transesophageal (TEE) for guidance (93355)
Magnetic resonance angiography (70544-70549, 71555, 72198, 73225, 73725, 74185)
Nuclear radiology procedures (78012-78999)
Physician planning of a patient-specific fenestrated visceral aortic endograft (34839)

Code also base imaging procedure(s)

76376 **3D rendering with interpretation and reporting of computed tomography, magnetic resonance imaging, ultrasound, or other tomographic modality with image postprocessing under concurrent supervision; not requiring image postprocessing on an independent workstation**

EXCLUDES 3D rendering (76377)
Bronchoscopy, with computer-assisted, image-guided navigation (31627)

🔲 0.65   ⚖ 0.65   **FUD** XXX   N N1 80 ⊡

AMA: 2019,Aug,5; 2019,Sep,10; 2018,Jul,11; 2018,Jan,8; 2017,Jan,8; 2016,Apr,8; 2016,Jan,13; 2015,Jan,16; 2014,Jan,11

76377 **requiring image postprocessing on an independent workstation**

EXCLUDES 3D rendering (76376)

🔲 2.01   ⚖ 2.01   **FUD** XXX   N N1 80 ⊡

AMA: 2019,Aug,5; 2019,Sep,10; 2018,Jul,11; 2018,Jan,8; 2017,Jan,8; 2016,Apr,8; 2016,Jan,13; 2015,Jan,16; 2014,Jan,11

76380 Computerized Tomography: Delimited

EXCLUDES Arthrography:
Ankle (73615)
Elbow (73085)
Hip (73525)
Knee (73580)
Shoulder (73040)
Wrist (73115)
CT cerebral perfusion test (0042T)

76380 **Computed tomography, limited or localized follow-up study**

🔲 4.07   ⚖ 4.07   **FUD** XXX   01 N1 80 ⊡

AMA: 2019,Mar,10; 2018,Jan,8; 2017,Jan,8; 2016,Jan,13; 2015,Jan,16; 2014,Jan,11

76390-76391 Magnetic Resonance Spectroscopy

EXCLUDES Arthrography:
    Ankle (73615)
    Elbow (73085)
    Hip (73525)
    Knee (73580)
    Shoulder (73040)
    Wrist (73115)
    CT cerebral perfusion test (0042T)

76390   **Magnetic resonance spectroscopy**
      EXCLUDES   MRI
      🔲 12.3   🔲 12.3   **FUD** XXX   E 🔲
      AMA: 2012,Feb,9-10; 1997,Nov,1

76391   **Magnetic resonance (eg, vibration) elastography**
      🔲 6.66   🔲 6.66   **FUD** XXX   Z2 80 🔲
      AMA: 2019,Aug,3

76496-76499 Unlisted Radiology Procedures

76496   **Unlisted fluoroscopic procedure (eg, diagnostic, interventional)**
      🔲 0.00   🔲 0.00   **FUD** XXX   01 N1 80 🔲
      AMA: 2012,Feb,9-10; 1997,Nov,1

76497   **Unlisted computed tomography procedure (eg, diagnostic, interventional)**
      🔲 0.00   🔲 0.00   **FUD** XXX   01 N1 80 🔲
      AMA: 2018,Sep,10; 2018,Jan,8; 2017,Jan,8; 2016,Jan,13; 2015,Jan,16; 2014,Jan,11

76498   **Unlisted magnetic resonance procedure (eg, diagnostic, interventional)**
      🔲 0.00   🔲 0.00   **FUD** XXX   S Z2 80 🔲
      AMA: 2019,Aug,5; 2018,Jul,11; 2018,Jan,8; 2017,Jan,8; 2016,Jan,13; 2015,Jan,16; 2014,Jan,11

76499   **Unlisted diagnostic radiographic procedure**
      🔲 0.00   🔲 0.00   **FUD** XXX   01 N1 80 🔲
      AMA: 2018,Jan,8; 2017,Jan,8; 2016,Dec,15; 2016,Jul,8; 2016,Jan,13; 2015,Jan,16; 2014,Jan,11

76506 Ultrasound: Brain

INCLUDES Required permanent documentation of ultrasound images except when diagnostic purpose is biometric measurement
          Written documentation
EXCLUDES Noninvasive vascular studies, diagnostic (93880-93990)
          Ultrasound exam that does not include thorough assessment of organ or site, recorded image, and written report

76506   **Echoencephalography, real time with image documentation (gray scale) (for determination of ventricular size, delineation of cerebral contents, and detection of fluid masses or other intracranial abnormalities), including A-mode encephalography as secondary component where indicated**
      🔲 3.26   🔲 3.26   **FUD** XXX   01 N1 80 🔲
      AMA: 2018,Jan,8; 2017,Jan,8; 2016,Jan,13; 2015,Jan,16; 2014,Jan,11

76510-76529 Ultrasound: Eyes

INCLUDES Required permanent documentation of ultrasound images except when diagnostic purpose is biometric measurement
          Written documentation

76510   **Ophthalmic ultrasound, diagnostic; B-scan and quantitative A-scan performed during the same patient encounter**
      🔲 3.15   🔲 3.15   **FUD** XXX   01 N1 80 🔲
      AMA: 2018,Jan,8; 2017,Jan,8; 2016,Jan,13; 2015,Jan,16; 2014,Jan,11

76511   **quantitative A-scan only**
      🔲 1.93   🔲 1.93   **FUD** XXX   01 N1 80 🔲
      AMA: 2019,Jan,12; 2018,Jan,8; 2017,Jan,8; 2016,Jan,13; 2015,Jan,16; 2014,Jan,11

76512   **B-scan (with or without superimposed non-quantitative A-scan)**
      🔲 1.73   🔲 1.73   **FUD** XXX   01 N1 80 🔲
      AMA: 2019,Jan,12; 2018,Jan,8; 2017,Jan,8; 2016,Jan,13; 2015,Jan,16; 2014,Jan,11

76513   **anterior segment ultrasound, immersion (water bath) B-scan or high resolution biomicroscopy**
      EXCLUDES Computerized ophthalmic testing other than by ultrasound (92132-92134)
      🔲 2.78   🔲 2.78   **FUD** XXX   01 N1 80 🔲
      AMA: 2019,Jan,12; 2018,Jan,8; 2017,Jan,8; 2016,Jan,13; 2015,Jan,16; 2014,Jan,11

76514   **corneal pachymetry, unilateral or bilateral (determination of corneal thickness)**
      INCLUDES Biometric measurement for which permanent documentation of images is not required
      EXCLUDES Collagen cross-linking of cornea (0402T)
      🔲 0.36   🔲 0.36   **FUD** XXX   01 N1 80 🔲
      AMA: 2019,Jan,12; 2018,Jan,8; 2017,Jan,8; 2016,Feb,12; 2016,Jan,13; 2015,Jan,16; 2014,Jan,11

76516   **Ophthalmic biometry by ultrasound echography, A-scan;**
      INCLUDES Biometric measurement for which permanent documentation of images is not required
      🔲 1.53   🔲 1.53   **FUD** XXX   01 N1 80 🔲
      AMA: 2019,Jan,12; 2018,Jan,8; 2017,Jan,8; 2016,Jan,13; 2015,Jan,16; 2014,Jan,11

76519   **with intraocular lens power calculation**
      INCLUDES Biometric measurement for which permanent documentation of images is not required
           Written prescription that satisfies requirement for written report
      EXCLUDES Partial coherence interferometry (92136)
      🔲 1.87   🔲 1.87   **FUD** XXX   01 N1 80 🔲
      AMA: 2019,Jan,12; 2018,Jan,8; 2017,Jan,8; 2016,Jan,13; 2015,Jan,16; 2014,Jan,11

76529   **Ophthalmic ultrasonic foreign body localization**
      🔲 2.33   🔲 2.33   **FUD** XXX   01 N1 80 🔲
      AMA: 2019,Jan,12; 2018,Jan,8; 2017,Jan,8; 2016,Jan,13; 2015,Jan,16; 2014,Jan,11

76536-76800 Ultrasound: Neck, Thorax, Abdomen, and Spine

INCLUDES Required permanent documentation of ultrasound images except when diagnostic purpose is biometric measurement
          Written documentation
EXCLUDES Focused ultrasound ablation of uterine leiomyomata (0071T-0072T)
          Ultrasound exam that does not include thorough assessment of organ or site, recorded image, and written report

76536   **Ultrasound, soft tissues of head and neck (eg, thyroid, parathyroid, parotid), real time with image documentation**
      🔲 3.25   🔲 3.25   **FUD** XXX   01 N1 80 🔲
      AMA: 2018,Jan,8; 2017,Oct,9; 2017,Jan,8; 2016,Jan,13; 2015,Jan,16; 2014,Jan,11

76604   **Ultrasound, chest (includes mediastinum), real time with image documentation**
      🔲 2.51   🔲 2.51   **FUD** XXX   01 N1 80 🔲
      AMA: 2018,Jan,8; 2017,Oct,9; 2017,Jan,8; 2016,Jan,13; 2015,Jan,16; 2014,Jan,11

76641   **Ultrasound, breast, unilateral, real time with image documentation, including axilla when performed; complete**
      INCLUDES Complete examination of all four quadrants, retroareolar region, and axilla when performed
      EXCLUDES Procedure performed more than one time per breast per session
      🔲 3.02   🔲 3.02   **FUD** XXX   01 N1 80 50 🔲
      AMA: 2018,Jan,8; 2017,Oct,9; 2017,Jan,8; 2016,Jan,13; 2015,Aug,8

76642   **limited**
      INCLUDES Examination not including all of the elements in complete examination
      EXCLUDES Procedure performed more than one time per breast per session
      🔲 2.47   🔲 2.47   **FUD** XXX   01 N1 80 50 🔲
      AMA: 2018,Jan,8; 2017,Oct,9

26/TC PC/TC Only   A2-Z3 ASC Payment   50 Bilateral   ♂ Male Only   ♀ Female Only   🔲 Facility RVU   🔲 Non-Facility RVU   🔲 CCI   ❌ CLIA
FUD Follow-up Days   **CMS:** IOM   **AMA:** CPT Asst   A-Y OPPSI   80/80 Surg Assist Allowed / w/Doc   🔲 Lab Crosswalk   🔲 Radiology Crosswalk

352   CPT © 2019 American Medical Association. All Rights Reserved.   © 2019 Optum360, LLC

76700 **Ultrasound, abdominal, real time with image documentation; complete**

INCLUDES Real time scans of:
Common bile duct
Gall bladder
Inferior vena cava
Kidneys
Liver
Pancreas
Spleen
Upper abdominal aorta

🚑 3.43   ♨ 3.43   **FUD** XXX   Q3 Z2 80 ▭

AMA: 2018,Jan,8; 2017,Oct,9; 2017,Jan,8; 2016,Jan,13; 2015,Jan,16; 2014,Jan,11

76705 **limited (eg, single organ, quadrant, follow-up)**

🚑 2.56   ♨ 2.56   **FUD** XXX   Q3 Z2 80 ▭

AMA: 2018,Jan,8; 2017,Oct,9; 2017,Jan,8; 2016,Jan,13; 2015,Jan,16; 2014,Jan,11

76706 **Ultrasound, abdominal aorta, real time with image documentation, screening study for abdominal aortic aneurysm (AAA)**

EXCLUDES Diagnostic ultrasound of aorta (76770-76775)
Duplex scan of aorta (93978-93979)

🚑 3.20   ♨ 3.20   **FUD** XXX   S 80 ▭

AMA: 2018,Jan,8; 2017,Sep,11

76770 **Ultrasound, retroperitoneal (eg, renal, aorta, nodes), real time with image documentation; complete**

INCLUDES Complete assessment of kidneys and bladder if history indicates urinary pathology
Real time scans of:
Abdominal aorta
Common iliac artery origins
Inferior vena cava
Kidneys

🚑 3.18   ♨ 3.18   **FUD** XXX   Q3 Z2 80 ▭

AMA: 2018,Jan,8; 2017,Oct,9; 2017,Jan,8; 2016,Jan,13; 2015,Jan,16; 2014,Jan,11

76775 **limited**

🚑 1.65   ♨ 1.65   **FUD** XXX   Q1 N1 80 ▭

AMA: 2018,Jan,8; 2017,Oct,9; 2017,Jan,8; 2016,Jan,13; 2015,Jan,16; 2014,Jan,11

76776 **Ultrasound, transplanted kidney, real time and duplex Doppler with image documentation**

EXCLUDES Abdominal/pelvic/scrotal contents/retroperitoneal duplex scan (93975-93976)
Transplanted kidney ultrasound without duplex doppler (76775)

🚑 4.38   ♨ 4.38   **FUD** XXX   Q3 Z2 80 ▭

AMA: 2018,Jan,8; 2017,Jan,8; 2016,Jan,13; 2015,Jan,16; 2014,Jan,11

76800 **Ultrasound, spinal canal and contents**

🚑 4.04   ♨ 4.04   **FUD** XXX   Q1 N1 80 ▭

AMA: 2018,Jan,8; 2017,Jan,8; 2016,Jan,13; 2015,Jan,16; 2014,Jan,11

76801-76802 Ultrasound: Pregnancy Less Than 14 Weeks

INCLUDES Determination of the number of gestational sacs and fetuses
Gestational sac/fetal measurement appropriate for gestational age (younger than 14 weeks 0 days)
Inspection of the maternal uterus and adnexa
Quality analysis of amniotic fluid volume/gestational sac shape
Visualization of fetal and placental anatomic formation
Written documentation of each component of exam
EXCLUDES Focused ultrasound ablation of uterine leiomyomata (0071T-0072T)
Ultrasound exam that does not include thorough assessment of organ or site, recorded image, and written report

76801 **Ultrasound, pregnant uterus, real time with image documentation, fetal and maternal evaluation, first trimester (< 14 weeks 0 days), transabdominal approach; single or first gestation**   M ♀

EXCLUDES Fetal nuchal translucency measurement, first trimester (76813)

🚑 3.46   ♨ 3.46   **FUD** XXX   S Z2 80 ▭

AMA: 2018,Jan,8; 2017,Jan,8; 2016,Jan,13; 2015,Jan,16; 2014,Jan,11

+ **76802** **each additional gestation (List separately in addition to code for primary procedure)**   M ♀

EXCLUDES Fetal nuchal translucency measurement, first trimester (76814)
Code first (76801)

🚑 1.81   ♨ 1.81   **FUD** ZZZ   N N1 80 ▭

AMA: 2018,Jan,8; 2017,Jan,8; 2016,Jan,13; 2015,Jan,16; 2014,Jan,11

76805-76810 Ultrasound: Pregnancy of 14 Weeks or More

INCLUDES Determination of the number of gestational/chorionic sacs and fetuses
Evaluation of:
Amniotic fluid
Four chambered heart
Intracranial, spinal, abdominal anatomy
Placenta location
Umbilical cord insertion site
Examination of maternal adnexa if visible
Gestational sac/fetal measurement appropriate for gestational age (older than or equal to 14 weeks 0 days)
Written documentation of each component of exam
EXCLUDES Focused ultrasound ablation of uterine leiomyomata (0071T-0072T)
Ultrasound exam that does not include thorough assessment of organ or site, recorded image, and written report

76805 **Ultrasound, pregnant uterus, real time with image documentation, fetal and maternal evaluation, after first trimester (> or = 14 weeks 0 days), transabdominal approach; single or first gestation**   M ♀

🚑 3.97   ♨ 3.97   **FUD** XXX   S Z2 80 ▭

AMA: 2018,Jan,8; 2017,Jan,8; 2016,Jan,13; 2015,Jan,16; 2014,Jan,11

+ **76810** **each additional gestation (List separately in addition to code for primary procedure)**   M ♀

Code first (76805)

🚑 2.63   ♨ 2.63   **FUD** ZZZ   N N1 80 ▭

AMA: 2018,Jan,8; 2017,Jan,8; 2016,Jan,13; 2015,Jan,16; 2014,Jan,11

76811-76812 Ultrasound: Pregnancy, with Additional Studies of Fetus

INCLUDES Determination of the number of gestational/chorionic sacs and fetuses
Evaluation of:
    Abdominal organ specific anatomy
    Amniotic fluid
    Chest anatomy
    Face
    Fetal brain/ventricles
    Four chambered heart
    Heart/outflow tracts and chest anatomy
    Intracranial, spinal, abdominal anatomy
    Limbs including number, length, and architecture
    Other fetal anatomy as indicated
    Placenta location
    Umbilical cord insertion site
Examination of maternal adnexa if visible
Gestational sac/fetal measurement appropriate for gestational age (older than or equal to 14 weeks 0 days)
Written documentation of each component of exam, including reason for nonvisualization, when applicable

EXCLUDES *Focused ultrasound ablation of uterine leiomyomata (0071T-0072T)*
Ultrasound exam that does not include thorough assessment organ or site, recorded image, and written report

76811 Ultrasound, pregnant uterus, real time with image documentation, fetal and maternal evaluation plus detailed fetal anatomic examination, transabdominal approach; single or first gestation   M ♀
    ⊞ 5.12   ⚕ 5.12   **FUD** XXX   S Z3 80 ▭
    AMA: 2018,Jan,8; 2017,Jan,8; 2016,Jan,13; 2015,Jan,16; 2014,Jan,11

+ 76812 each additional gestation (List separately in addition to code for primary procedure)   M ♀
    Code first (76811)
    ⊞ 5.72   ⚕ 5.72   **FUD** ZZZ   N N1 80 ▭
    AMA: 2018,Jan,8; 2017,Jan,8; 2016,Jan,13; 2015,Jan,16; 2014,Jan,11

76813-76828 Ultrasound: Other Fetal Evaluations

INCLUDES Required permanent documentation of ultrasound images except when diagnostic purpose is biometric measurement
Written documentation

EXCLUDES *Focused ultrasound ablation of uterine leiomyomata (0071T-0072T)*
Ultrasound exam that does not include thorough assessment of organ or site, recorded image, and written report

76813 Ultrasound, pregnant uterus, real time with image documentation, first trimester fetal nuchal translucency measurement, transabdominal or transvaginal approach; single or first gestation   M ♀
    ⊞ 3.45   ⚕ 3.45   **FUD** XXX   Q1 N1 80 ▭
    AMA: 2018,Jan,8; 2017,Jan,8; 2016,Jan,13; 2015,Jan,16; 2014,Jan,11

+ 76814 each additional gestation (List separately in addition to code for primary procedure)   M ♀
    Code first (76813)
    ⊞ 2.27   ⚕ 2.27   **FUD** XXX   N N1 80 ▭
    AMA: 2018,Jan,8; 2017,Jan,8; 2016,Jan,13; 2015,Jan,16; 2014,Jan,11

76815 Ultrasound, pregnant uterus, real time with image documentation, limited (eg, fetal heart beat, placental location, fetal position and/or qualitative amniotic fluid volume), 1 or more fetuses   M ♀
    INCLUDES Exam concentrating on one or more elements
    Reporting only one time per exam, instead of per element
    EXCLUDES *Fetal nuchal translucency measurement, first trimester (76813-76814)*
    ⊞ 2.38   ⚕ 2.38   **FUD** XXX   Q1 N1 80 ▭
    AMA: 2018,Jan,8; 2017,Jan,8; 2016,Jan,13; 2015,Jan,16; 2014,Jan,11

76816 Ultrasound, pregnant uterus, real time with image documentation, follow-up (eg, re-evaluation of fetal size by measuring standard growth parameters and amniotic fluid volume, re-evaluation of organ system(s) suspected or confirmed to be abnormal on a previous scan), transabdominal approach, per fetus   M ♀
    INCLUDES Re-evaluation of fetal size, interval growth, or aberrancies noted on a prior ultrasound
    Code also modifier 59 for examination of each additional fetus in a multiple pregnancy
    ⊞ 3.23   ⚕ 3.23   **FUD** XXX   Q1 N1 80 ▭
    AMA: 2018,Jan,8; 2017,Jan,8; 2016,Jan,13; 2015,Jan,16; 2014,Jan,11

76817 Ultrasound, pregnant uterus, real time with image documentation, transvaginal   M ♀
    EXCLUDES *Transvaginal ultrasound, non-obstetrical (76830)*
    Code also transabdominal obstetrical ultrasound, if performed
    ⊞ 2.73   ⚕ 2.73   **FUD** XXX   Q1 N1 80 ▭
    AMA: 2018,Jan,8; 2017,Jan,8; 2016,Jan,13; 2015,Jan,16; 2014,Jan,11

76818 Fetal biophysical profile; with non-stress testing   M ♀
    Code also modifier 59 for each additional fetus
    ⊞ 3.44   ⚕ 3.44   **FUD** XXX   S Z2 80 ▭
    AMA: 2018,Jan,8; 2017,Jan,8; 2016,Jan,13; 2015,Jan,16; 2014,Jan,11

76819 without non-stress testing   M ♀
    EXCLUDES *Amniotic fluid index without non-stress test (76815)*
    Code also modifier 59 for each additional fetus
    ⊞ 2.52   ⚕ 2.52   **FUD** XXX   S Z3 80 ▭
    AMA: 2018,Jan,8; 2017,Jan,8; 2016,Jan,13; 2015,Jan,16; 2014,Jan,11

76820 Doppler velocimetry, fetal; umbilical artery   M
    ⊞ 1.35   ⚕ 1.35   **FUD** XXX   Q1 N1 80 ▭
    AMA: 2018,Jan,8; 2017,Jan,8; 2016,Jul,8; 2016,Jan,13; 2015,Jan,16; 2014,Jan,11

76821 middle cerebral artery   M
    ⊞ 2.61   ⚕ 2.61   **FUD** XXX   Q1 N1 80 ▭
    AMA: 2018,Jan,8; 2017,Jan,8; 2016,Jan,13; 2015,Jan,16; 2014,Jan,11

76825 Echocardiography, fetal, cardiovascular system, real time with image documentation (2D), with or without M-mode recording;   M ♀
    ⊞ 7.79   ⚕ 7.79   **FUD** XXX   S Z3 80 ▭
    AMA: 2018,Jan,8; 2017,Sep,14; 2017,Jan,8; 2016,Jan,13; 2015,Jan,16; 2014,Jan,11

76826 follow-up or repeat study   M ♀
    ⊞ 4.62   ⚕ 4.62   **FUD** XXX   S Z2 80 ▭
    AMA: 2018,Jan,8; 2017,Sep,14

76827 Doppler echocardiography, fetal, pulsed wave and/or continuous wave with spectral display; complete   M ♀
    ⊞ 2.11   ⚕ 2.11   **FUD** XXX   Q1 N1 80 ▭
    AMA: 2018,Jan,8; 2017,Jan,8; 2016,Jan,13; 2015,Jan,16; 2014,Jan,11

76828 follow-up or repeat study   M ♀
    EXCLUDES *Color mapping (93325)*
    ⊞ 1.51   ⚕ 1.51   **FUD** XXX   Q1 N1 80 ▭
    AMA: 2018,Jan,8; 2017,Jan,8; 2016,Jan,13; 2015,Jan,16; 2014,Jan,11

76830-76873 Ultrasound: Male and Female Genitalia

INCLUDES Required permanent documentation of ultrasound images except when diagnostic purpose is biometric measurement
Written documentation

EXCLUDES Focused ultrasound ablation of uterine leiomyomata (0071T-0072T)
Ultrasound exam that does not include thorough assessment of organ or site, recorded image, and written report

76830 Ultrasound, transvaginal ♀

EXCLUDES Transvaginal ultrasound, obstetric (76817)

Code also transabdominal non-obstetrical ultrasound, if performed

🚑 3.44 ⚕ 3.44 **FUD** XXX [S] [Z2] [80] [⊡]

AMA: 2018,Jan,8; 2017,Oct,9; 2017,Jan,8; 2016,Jan,13; 2015,Jan,16; 2014,Jan,11

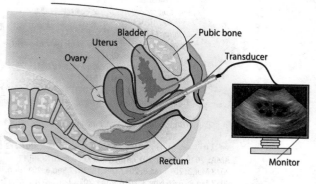

Ultrasound is performed in real time with image documentation by a transvaginal approach

76831 Saline infusion sonohysterography (SIS), including color flow Doppler, when performed ♀

Code also saline introduction for saline infusion sonohysterography (58340)

🚑 3.35 ⚕ 3.35 **FUD** XXX [03] [Z3] [80] [⊡]

AMA: 2018,Jan,8; 2017,Jan,8; 2016,Jan,13; 2015,Jan,16; 2014,Jan,11

76856 Ultrasound, pelvic (nonobstetric), real time with image documentation; complete

INCLUDES Total examination of the female pelvic anatomy which includes:
  Bladder measurement
  Description and measurement of the uterus and adnexa
  Description of any pelvic pathology
  Measurement of the endometrium
Total examination of the male pelvis which includes:
  Bladder measurement
  Description of any pelvic pathology
  Evaluation of prostate and seminal vesicles

🚑 3.09 ⚕ 3.09 **FUD** XXX [03] [Z2] [80] [⊡]

AMA: 2018,Jan,8; 2017,Oct,9; 2017,Jan,8; 2016,Aug,9; 2016,Jan,13; 2015,Jan,16; 2014,Jan,11

76857 limited or follow-up (eg, for follicles)

INCLUDES Focused evaluation limited to:
  Evaluation of one or more elements listed in 76856 and/or
  Reevaluation of one or more pelvic aberrancies noted on a prior ultrasound
  Urinary bladder alone

EXCLUDES Bladder volume or post-voided residual measurement without imaging the bladder (51798)
Urinary bladder and kidneys (76770)

🚑 1.38 ⚕ 1.38 **FUD** XXX [03] [Z3] [80] [⊡]

AMA: 2018,Jan,8; 2017,Oct,9; 2017,Jan,8; 2016,Jan,13; 2015,Jan,16; 2014,Jan,11

76870 Ultrasound, scrotum and contents ♂

🚑 2.97 ⚕ 2.97 **FUD** XXX [01] [N1] [80] [⊡]

AMA: 2018,Jan,8; 2017,Oct,9

76872 Ultrasound, transrectal;

EXCLUDES Colonoscopy (45391-45392)
Hemorrhoidectomy by transanal hemorrhoidal dearterialization ([46948])
Sigmoidoscopy (45341-45342)
Transurethral prostate ablation (0421T)

🚑 3.62 ⚕ 3.62 **FUD** XXX [S] [Z2] [80] [⊡]

AMA: 2018,Nov,10; 2018,Jul,11; 2018,Jan,8; 2017,Oct,9; 2017,Jan,8; 2016,Jan,13; 2015,Jan,16; 2014,Jan,11

76873 prostate volume study for brachytherapy treatment planning (separate procedure) ♂

🚑 4.91 ⚕ 4.91 **FUD** XXX [S] [Z2] [80] [⊡]

AMA: 2018,Jan,8; 2017,Jan,8; 2016,Jan,13; 2015,Jan,16; 2014,Jan,11

76881-76886 Ultrasound: Extremities

EXCLUDES Doppler studies of the extremities (93925-93926, 93930-93931, 93970-93971)

76881 Ultrasound, complete joint (ie, joint space and peri-articular soft tissue structures) real-time with image documentation

INCLUDES Real time scans of a specific joint including assessment of:
  Joint space
  Muscles
  Other soft tissue
  Tendons
Required permanent documentation of images
Stress manipulations and dynamic imaging when performed
Written documentation including an explanation of any components of the joint that cannot be visualized

🚑 2.51 ⚕ 2.51 **FUD** XXX [S] [Z3] [80] [⊡]

AMA: 2018,Jan,8; 2017,Oct,9; 2017,Jan,8; 2016,Sep,9

76882 Ultrasound, limited, joint or other nonvascular extremity structure(s) (eg, joint space, peri-articular tendon[s], muscle[s], nerve[s], other soft tissue structure[s], or soft tissue mass[es]), real-time with image documentation

INCLUDES Limited examination of a joint or for evaluation of an extremity for a mass or other abnormality not requiring all of the components of a complete joint evaluation (76881)
Real time scans of a specific joint including assessment of:
  Joint space
  Muscles
  Other soft tissue
  Tendons
Required permanent documentation of images
Written documentation containing a description of all of the components of the joint visualized

🚑 1.62 ⚕ 1.62 **FUD** XXX [01] [N1] [80] [⊡]

AMA: 2018,Jan,8; 2017,Oct,9; 2017,Jan,8; 2016,Sep,9

76885 Ultrasound, infant hips, real time with imaging documentation; dynamic (requiring physician or other qualified health care professional manipulation) [A]

🚑 4.05 ⚕ 4.05 **FUD** XXX [01] [N1] [80] [⊡]

AMA: 2012,Feb,9-10; 2002,May,7

76886 limited, static (not requiring physician or other qualified health care professional manipulation) [A]

🚑 2.97 ⚕ 2.97 **FUD** XXX [01] [N1] [80] [⊡]

AMA: 2012,Feb,9-10; 2002,May,7

76930-76970 Imaging Guidance: Ultrasound

INCLUDES Required permanent documentation of ultrasound images except when diagnostic purpose is biometric measurement
Written documentation

EXCLUDES Focused ultrasound ablation of uterine leiomyomata (0071T-0072T)
Ultrasound exam that does not include thorough assessment of organ or site, recorded image, and written report

76930 ~~Ultrasonic guidance for pericardiocentesis, imaging supervision and interpretation~~

To report, see (33016-33018)

76932 **Ultrasonic guidance for endomyocardial biopsy, imaging supervision and interpretation**
    🔲 0.00   ⚕ 0.00   **FUD** YYY   N N1 80 🖵
    AMA: 2012,Feb,9-10; 2001,Sep,4

76936 **Ultrasound guided compression repair of arterial pseudoaneurysm or arteriovenous fistulae (includes diagnostic ultrasound evaluation, compression of lesion and imaging)**
    🔲 7.60   ⚕ 7.60   **FUD** XXX   S Z2 80 🖵
    AMA: 2012,Feb,9-10; 2002,May,7

+ 76937 **Ultrasound guidance for vascular access requiring ultrasound evaluation of potential access sites, documentation of selected vessel patency, concurrent realtime ultrasound visualization of vascular needle entry, with permanent recording and reporting (List separately in addition to code for primary procedure)**
    INCLUDES   Ultrasonic guidance (76942)
    EXCLUDES   *Extremity venous noninvasive vascular diagnostic study performed separately from venous access guidance (93970-93971)*
          Insertion of intravascular vena cava filter (37191-37193)
          Insertion/replacement leadless pacemaker ([33274])
          Ligation perforator veins (37760-37761)
          Removal leadless pacemaker ([33275])
          Revascularization with intravascular stent grafts in femoral-popliteal segment (0505T)
    Code first primary procedure
    🔲 0.96   ⚕ 0.96   **FUD** ZZZ   N N1 60 🖵
    AMA: 2019,May,3; 2019,Mar,6; 2018,Mar,3; 2018,Jan,8; 2017,Dec,3; 2017,Aug,10; 2017,Jul,3; 2017,Mar,3; 2017,Jan,8; 2016,Nov,3; 2016,Jul,6; 2016,Jan,13; 2015,Jul,10; 2015,Jan,16; 2014,Oct,6; 2014,Jan,11

76940 **Ultrasound guidance for, and monitoring of, parenchymal tissue ablation**
    EXCLUDES   *Ablation (20982-20983, [32994], 32998, 47370-47383, 50250, 50542, 50592-50593, 0582T)*
          Ultrasound guidance:
          Intraoperative (76998)
          Needle placement (76942)
    🔲 0.00   ⚕ 0.00   **FUD** YYY   N N1 80 🖵
    AMA: 2018,Jan,8; 2017,Nov,8; 2017,Jan,8; 2016,Jan,13; 2015,Jul,8; 2015,Jan,16; 2014,Jan,11

76941 **Ultrasonic guidance for intrauterine fetal transfusion or cordocentesis, imaging supervision and interpretation**   M ♀
    Code also surgical procedure (36460, 59012)
    🔲 0.00   ⚕ 0.00   **FUD** XXX   N N1 80 🖵
    AMA: 2012,Feb,9-10; 2001,Sep,4

76942 **Ultrasonic guidance for needle placement (eg, biopsy, aspiration, injection, localization device), imaging supervision and interpretation**
    EXCLUDES   *Arthrocentesis (20604, 20606, 20611)*
          Autologous WBC injection (0481T)
          Breast biopsy with placement of localization device(s) (19083)
          Esophagogastroduodenoscopy (43237, 43242)
          Esophagoscopy (43232)
          Fine needle aspiration biopsy ([10004], [10005], [10006], 10021)
          Gastrointestinal endoscopic ultrasound (76975)
          Hemorrhoidectomy by transanal hemorrhoidal dearterialization ([46948])
          Image-guided fluid collection drainage by catheter (10030)
          Injection procedures (27096, 64479-64484, 0228T-0232T)
          Ligation (37760-37761)
          Paravertebral facet joint injections (64490-64491, 64493-64495, 0213T-0218T)
          Placement of breast localization device(s) (19285)
          Sigmoidoscopy (45341-45342)
          Thoracentesis (32554-32557)
          Transperineal placement, periprostatic biodegradable material (55874)
          Transurethral ablation, malignant prostate tissue (0582T)
    🔲 1.61   ⚕ 1.61   **FUD** XXX   N N1 80 🖵
    AMA: 2019,Aug,10; 2019,Apr,4; 2019,Feb,8; 2018,Jul,11; 2018,Mar,3; 2018,Jan,8; 2017,Dec,13; 2017,Sep,6; 2017,Jun,10; 2017,Jan,8; 2016,Nov,3; 2016,Jun,3; 2016,Jan,9; 2016,Jan,13; 2015,Dec,3; 2015,Nov,10; 2015,Aug,8; 2015,Feb,6; 2015,Jan,16; 2014,Oct,6; 2014,Jan,11

76945 **Ultrasonic guidance for chorionic villus sampling, imaging supervision and interpretation**   M ♀
    Code also surgical procedure (59015)
    🔲 0.00   ⚕ 0.00   **FUD** XXX   N N1 80 🖵
    AMA: 2012,Feb,9-10; 2001,Sep,4

76946 **Ultrasonic guidance for amniocentesis, imaging supervision and interpretation**   M ♀
    🔲 0.92   ⚕ 0.92   **FUD** XXX   N N1 80 🖵
    AMA: 2012,Feb,9-10; 2001,Sep,4

76948 **Ultrasonic guidance for aspiration of ova, imaging supervision and interpretation**   M ♀
    🔲 2.12   ⚕ 2.12   **FUD** XXX   N N1 80 🖵
    AMA: 2012,Feb,9-10; 2001,Sep,4

76965 **Ultrasonic guidance for interstitial radioelement application**
    🔲 2.62   ⚕ 2.62   **FUD** XXX   N N1 80 🖵
    AMA: 2012,Feb,9-10; 1997,Nov,1

76970 **Ultrasound study follow-up (specify)**
    🔲 2.54   ⚕ 2.54   **FUD** XXX   01 N1 80 🖵
    AMA: 2012,Feb,9-10; 1997,Nov,1

76975 Endoscopic Ultrasound

    INCLUDES   Required permanent documentation of ultrasound images except when diagnostic purpose is biometric measurement
          Written documentation
    EXCLUDES   *Focused ultrasound ablation of uterine leiomyomata (0071T-0072T)*
          Ultrasound exam that does not include thorough assessment of organ or site, recorded image, and written report

76975 **Gastrointestinal endoscopic ultrasound, supervision and interpretation**
    INCLUDES   Ultrasonic guidance (76942)
    EXCLUDES   *Colonoscopy (44406-44407, 45391-45392)*
          Esophagogastroduodenoscopy (43237-43238, 43240, 43242, 43259)
          Esophagoscopy (43231-43232)
          Sigmoidoscopy (45341-45342)
    🔲 0.00   ⚕ 0.00   **FUD** XXX   02 N1 80 🖵
    AMA: 2018,Jan,8; 2017,Jan,8; 2016,Jan,13; 2015,Jan,16; 2014,Jan,11

*Left margin: Radiology   76932 — 76975*

76977 Bone Density Measurements: Ultrasound

CMS: 100-02,15,80.5.5 Frequency Standards

INCLUDES   Required permanent documentation of ultrasound images except when diagnostic purpose is biometric measurement
Written documentation

EXCLUDES   *Ultrasound exam that does not include thorough assessment of organ or site, recorded image, and written report*

76977   **Ultrasound bone density measurement and interpretation, peripheral site(s), any method**
0.21 0.21 **FUD** XXX   S Z3 80 ▭
AMA: 2012,Feb,9-10; 1998,Nov,1

76978-76979 Targeted Dynamic Microbubble Sonographic Contrast Characterization: Ultrasound

INCLUDES   Intravenous injection (96374)

76978   **Ultrasound, targeted dynamic microbubble sonographic contrast characterization (non-cardiac); initial lesion**
9.18 9.18 **FUD** XXX · Z2 80 ▭
AMA: 2019,Jun,9

+ **76979**   **each additional lesion with separate injection (List separately in addition to code for primary procedure)**
Code first (76978)
6.23 6.23 **FUD** ZZZ   N1 80 ▭
AMA: 2019,Jun,9

76981-76983 Elastography: Ultrasound

EXCLUDES   *Shear wave liver elastography (91200)*

76981   **Ultrasound, elastography; parenchyma (eg, organ)**
EXCLUDES   *Use of code more than one time in each session for the same parenchymal organ and/or parenchymal organ and lesion*
3.04 3.04 **FUD** XXX   Z2 80 ▭
AMA: 2019,Aug,3

76982   **first target lesion**
2.72 2.72 **FUD** XXX   Z2 80 ▭
AMA: 2019,Aug,3

+ **76983**   **each additional target lesion (List separately in addition to code for primary procedure)**
EXCLUDES   *Use of code more than two times for each organ*
Code first (76982)
1.67 1.67 **FUD** ZZZ   N1 80 ▭
AMA: 2019,Aug,3

76998-76999 Imaging Guidance During Surgery: Ultrasound

INCLUDES   Required permanent documentation of ultrasound images except when diagnostic purpose is biometric measurement
Written documentation

EXCLUDES   *Focused ultrasound ablation of uterine leiomyomata (0071T-0072T)*
Ultrasound exam that does not include thorough assessment of organ or site, recorded image, and written report

76998   **Ultrasonic guidance, intraoperative**
EXCLUDES   *Ablation (47370-47371, 47380-47382)*
Endovenous ablation therapy of incompetent vein (36475, 36479)
Hemorrhoidectomy by transanal hemorrhoidal dearterialization ([46948])
Ligation (37760-37761)
Wireless cardiac stimulator (0515T-0520T)
0.00 0.00 **FUD** XXX   N N1 80 ▭
AMA: 2018,Mar,3; 2018,Jan,8; 2017,Apr,7; 2017,Jan,8; 2016,Nov,3; 2016,Jan,13; 2015,Aug,8; 2015,Jan,16; 2014,Oct,6; 2014,Jan,5; 2014,Jan,11

76999   **Unlisted ultrasound procedure (eg, diagnostic, interventional)**
0.00 0.00 **FUD** XXX   01 N1 80 ▭
AMA: 2018,Jul,11; 2018,Jan,8; 2017,Jan,8; 2016,Jan,13; 2015,Jan,16; 2014,Jan,11

77001-77022 Imaging Guidance Techniques

+ **77001**   **Fluoroscopic guidance for central venous access device placement, replacement (catheter only or complete), or removal (includes fluoroscopic guidance for vascular access and catheter manipulation, any necessary contrast injections through access site or catheter with related venography radiologic supervision and interpretation, and radiographic documentation of final catheter position) (List separately in addition to code for primary procedure)**

INCLUDES   Fluoroscopic guidance for needle placement (77002)

EXCLUDES   *Any procedure codes that include fluoroscopic guidance in the code descriptor*
Extracorporeal membrane oxygenation (ECMO)/extracorporeal life support (ECLS) (33957-33959, [33962, 33963, 33964])
Formal extremity venography performed separately from venous access and interpreted separately (36005, 75820, 75822, 75825, 75827)
Insertion peripherally inserted central venous catheter (PICC) (36568-36569, [36572, 36573])
Replacement of peripherally inserted central venous catheter (PICC) (36584)

Code first primary procedure
2.55 2.55 **FUD** ZZZ   N N1 80 ▭
AMA: 2019,May,3; 2018,Jan,8; 2017,Jan,8; 2016,Jan,13; 2015,Jan,16; 2014,Jan,11

+ **77002**   **Fluoroscopic guidance for needle placement (eg, biopsy, aspiration, injection, localization device) (List separately in addition to code for primary procedure)**

EXCLUDES   *Ablation therapy (20982-20983)*
Any procedure codes that include fluoroscopic guidance in the code descriptor:
Radiological guidance for percutaneous drainage by catheter (75989)
Transhepatic portography (75885, 75887)
Arthrography procedure(s) (70332, 73040, 73085, 73115, 73525, 73580, 73615)
Biopsy, breast, with placement of breast localization device(s) (19081-19086)
Image-guided fluid collection drainage by catheter (10030)
Placement of breast localization device(s) (19281-19288)
Platelet rich plasma injection(s) (0232T)
Thoracentesis (32554-32557)

Code first surgical procedure (10160, 20206, 20220, 20225, 20520, 20525-20526, 20550-20555, 20600, 20605, 20610, 20612, 20615, 21116, 21550, 23350, 24220, 25246, 27093-27095, 27369, 27648, 32400-32405, 32553, 36002, 38220-38222, 38505, 38794, 41019, 42400-42405, 47000-47001, 48102, 49180, 49411, 50200, 50390, 51100-51102, 55700, 55876, 60100, 62268-62269, 64505, 64600-64605)
2.86 2.86 **FUD** ZZZ   N N1 80 ▭
AMA: 2019,Aug,7; 2019,Mar,6; 2019,Apr,4; 2019,Feb,8; 2018,Dec,10; 2018,Dec,10; 2018,Jan,8; 2017,Jun,10; 2017,Jan,8; 2016,Sep,9; 2016,Aug,7; 2016,Jun,3; 2016,Jan,13; 2016,Jan,9; 2015,Dec,3; 2015,Aug,6; 2015,Jul,8; 2015,Feb,10; 2015,Feb,6; 2015,Jan,16; 2014,Jan,11

Radiology

77003 — 77061

+ 77003 Fluoroscopic guidance and localization of needle or catheter tip for spine or paraspinous diagnostic or therapeutic injection procedures (epidural or subarachnoid) (List separately in addition to code for primary procedure)

EXCLUDES Any procedure codes that include fluoroscopic guidance in the code descriptor
Arthrodesis (22586)
Image-guided fluid collection drainage by catheter (10030)
Injection of medication (subarachnoid/interlaminar epidural) (62320, 62321, 62322, 62323, 62324, 62325, 62326, 62327)
Spinal puncture (62270, [62328], 62272, [62329])
Code first (61050-61055, 62267, 62273, 62280-62284, 64510, 64517, 64520, 64610, 96450)

🖩 2.77 🔾 2.77 **FUD** ZZZ N N1 80 ▭

AMA: 2018,Jan,8; 2017,Dec,13; 2017,Sep,6; 2017,Feb,9; 2017,Feb,12; 2017,Jan,8; 2016,Jan,9; 2016,Jan,13; 2016,Jan,11; 2015,Jan,16; 2014,Jan,11

77011 Computed tomography guidance for stereotactic localization

EXCLUDES Arthrodesis (22586)

🖩 6.47 🔾 6.47 **FUD** XXX N N1 ▭

AMA: 2018,Jan,8; 2017,Jan,8; 2016,Jan,13; 2015,Jan,16; 2014,Jan,11

77012 Computed tomography guidance for needle placement (eg, biopsy, aspiration, injection, localization device), radiological supervision and interpretation

EXCLUDES Arthrodesis (22586)
Autologous white blood cell concentrate (0481T)
Destruction of paravertebral facet joint nerve by neurolysis ([64633, 64634, 64635, 64636])
Fine needle aspiration biopsy using CT guidance ([10009, 10010])
Image-guided fluid collection drainage by catheter (10030)
Injection, paravertebral facet joint (64490-64495)
Platelet rich plasma injection(s) (0232T)
Sacroiliac joint arthrography (27096)
Spinal puncture (62270, [62328], 62272, [62329])
Thoracentesis (32554-32557)
Transforaminal epidural needle placement/injection (64479-64480, 64483-64484)

🖩 4.27 🔾 4.27 **FUD** XXX N N1 ▭

AMA: 2019,Feb,8; 2019,Apr,4; 2018,Jan,8; 2017,Sep,6; 2017,Feb,12; 2017,Jan,8; 2016,Jun,3; 2016,Jan,13; 2015,Dec,3; 2015,Feb,6; 2015,Jan,16; 2014,Jan,11

77013 Computed tomography guidance for, and monitoring of, parenchymal tissue ablation

EXCLUDES Ablation therapy (20982-20983, 32994, 32998, 47382-47383, 50592-50593)

🖩 0.00 🔾 0.00 **FUD** XXX N N1 80 ▭

AMA: 2018,Jan,8; 2017,Nov,8; 2017,Jan,8; 2016,Jan,13; 2015,Jul,8; 2015,Jan,16; 2014,Jan,11

77014 Computed tomography guidance for placement of radiation therapy fields

Code also placement of interstitial device(s) for radiation therapy guidance (31627, 32553, 49411, 55876)

🖩 3.41 🔾 3.41 **FUD** XXX N N1 ▭

AMA: 2018,Jan,8; 2017,Jan,8; 2016,Feb,3; 2016,Jan,13; 2015,Apr,10; 2015,Jan,16; 2014,Jan,11

77021 Magnetic resonance imaging guidance for needle placement (eg, for biopsy, needle aspiration, injection, or placement of localization device) radiological supervision and interpretation

EXCLUDES Autologous white blood cell concentrate (0481T)
Biopsy, breast, with placement of breast localization device(s) (19085)
Fine needle aspiration biopsy using MR guidance ([10011, 10012])
Image-guided fluid collection drainage by catheter (10030)
Placement of breast localization device(s) (19287)
Platelet rich plasma injection(s) (0232T)
Surgical procedure
Thoracentesis (32554-32557)

🖩 13.4 🔾 13.4 **FUD** XXX N N1 ▭

AMA: 2019,Feb,8; 2019,Apr,4; 2018,Jul,11; 2018,Jan,8; 2017,Jun,10; 2017,Jan,8; 2016,Jun,3; 2016,Jan,13; 2015,Dec,3; 2015,Feb,6; 2015,Jan,16; 2014,Jan,11

77022 Magnetic resonance imaging guidance for, and monitoring of, parenchymal tissue ablation

EXCLUDES Ablation:
Percutaneous radiofrequency (32994, 32998, 47382-47383, 50592-50593)
Reduction or eradication of 1 or more bone tumors (20982-20983)
Uterine leiomyomata by focused ablation (0071T-0072T)

🖩 0.00 🔾 0.00 **FUD** XXX N N1 80 ▭

AMA: 2019,Sep,10; 2018,Mar,3; 2018,Jan,8; 2017,Nov,8; 2017,Jan,8; 2016,Nov,3; 2016,Jan,13; 2015,Jul,8; 2015,Jan,16; 2014,Oct,6; 2014,Jan,11

77046-77067 Radiography: Breast

77046 Magnetic resonance imaging, breast, without contrast material; unilateral

🖩 7.02 🔾 7.02 **FUD** XXX Z2 80 ▭

AMA: 2019,Aug,5

77047 bilateral

🖩 7.21 🔾 7.21 **FUD** XXX Z2 80 ▭

AMA: 2019,Aug,5

77048 Magnetic resonance imaging, breast, without and with contrast material(s), including computer-aided detection (CAD real-time lesion detection, characterization and pharmacokinetic analysis), when performed; unilateral

🖩 11.1 🔾 11.1 **FUD** XXX 80 ▭

AMA: 2019,Aug,5

77049 bilateral

🖩 11.3 🔾 11.3 **FUD** XXX 80 ▭

AMA: 2019,Aug,5

77053 Mammary ductogram or galactogram, single duct, radiological supervision and interpretation

Code also injection procedure (19030)

🖩 1.62 🔾 1.62 **FUD** XXX Q2 N1 ▭

AMA: 2018,Jan,8; 2017,Jan,8; 2016,Jan,13; 2015,Jan,16; 2014,Jan,11

77054 Mammary ductogram or galactogram, multiple ducts, radiological supervision and interpretation

🖩 2.12 🔾 2.12 **FUD** XXX Q2 N1 ▭

AMA: 2018,Jan,8; 2017,Jan,8; 2016,Jan,13; 2015,Jan,16; 2014,Jan,11

77061 Diagnostic digital breast tomosynthesis; unilateral

EXCLUDES 3D rendering (76376-76377)
Screening mammography (77067)

🖩 0.00 🔾 0.00 **FUD** XXX E ▭

AMA: 2018,Jan,8

| 26/TC PC/TC Only | A2-Z3 ASC Payment | 50 Bilateral | ♂ Male Only | ♀ Female Only | 🖩 Facility RVU | 🔾 Non-Facility RVU | ▭ CCI | ✖ CLIA |
| FUD Follow-up Days | CMS: IOM | AMA: CPT Asst | A-Y OPPSI | 80/80 Surg Assist Allowed / w/Doc | | 🔾 Lab Crosswalk | 🔄 Radiology Crosswalk | |

358

CPT © 2019 American Medical Association. All Rights Reserved.

© 2019 Optum360, LLC

77062 **bilateral**

> EXCLUDES 3D rendering (76376-76377)
> Screening mammography (77067)
>
> 🚑 0.00   ⚕ 0.00   **FUD** XXX   E ▢
>
> **AMA:** 2018,Jan,8; 2017,Jan,8; 2016,Dec,15

+ **77063** **Screening digital breast tomosynthesis, bilateral (List separately in addition to code for primary procedure)**

> EXCLUDES 3D rendering (76376-76377)
> Diagnostic mammography (77065-77066)
> Code first (77067)
>
> 🚑 1.55   ⚕ 1.55   **FUD** ZZZ   A ▢
>
> **AMA:** 2018,Jan,8; 2017,Jan,8; 2016,Dec,15

77065 **Diagnostic mammography, including computer-aided detection (CAD) when performed; unilateral**

> 🚑 3.77   ⚕ 3.77   **FUD** XXX   A 80 ▢
>
> **AMA:** 2019,Aug,5; 2018,Jan,8; 2017,Jan,8; 2016,Dec,15

77066 **bilateral**

> 🚑 4.77   ⚕ 4.77   **FUD** XXX   A 80 ▢
>
> **AMA:** 2019,Aug,5; 2018,Jan,8; 2017,Jan,8; 2016,Dec,15

77067 **Screening mammography, bilateral (2-view study of each breast), including computer-aided detection (CAD) when performed**

> EXCLUDES Breast scan, electrical impedance (76499)
>
> 🚑 3.84   ⚕ 3.84   **FUD** XXX   A 80 ▢
>
> **AMA:** 2019,Aug,5; 2018,Jan,8; 2017,Jan,8; 2016,Dec,15

77071-77086 [77085, 77086] Additional Evaluations of Bones and Joints

77071 **Manual application of stress performed by physician or other qualified health care professional for joint radiography, including contralateral joint if indicated**

> Code also interpretation of stressed images according to anatomical site and number of views
>
> 🚑 1.43   ⚕ 1.43   **FUD** XXX   01 N1 80 26 ▢
>
> **AMA:** 2018,Jan,8; 2017,Jan,8; 2016,Jan,13; 2015,Jan,16; 2014,Jan,11

77072 **Bone age studies**

> 🚑 0.68   ⚕ 0.68   **FUD** XXX   01 N1 80 ▢
>
> **AMA:** 2018,Jan,8; 2017,Jan,8; 2016,Jan,13; 2015,Jan,16; 2014,Jan,11

77073 **Bone length studies (orthoroentgenogram, scanogram)**

> 🚑 1.06   ⚕ 1.06   **FUD** XXX   01 N1 80 ▢
>
> **AMA:** 2018,Jan,8; 2017,Jan,8; 2016,Jan,13; 2015,Jan,16; 2014,Jan,11

77074 **Radiologic examination, osseous survey; limited (eg, for metastases)**

> 🚑 1.91   ⚕ 1.91   **FUD** XXX   01 N1 80 ▢
>
> **AMA:** 2018,Jan,8; 2017,Jan,8; 2016,Jan,13; 2015,Jan,16; 2014,Jan,11

77075 **complete (axial and appendicular skeleton)**

> 🚑 2.60   ⚕ 2.60   **FUD** XXX   01 N1 80 ▢
>
> **AMA:** 2018,Jan,8; 2017,Jan,8; 2016,Jan,13; 2015,Jan,16; 2014,Jan,11

77076 **Radiologic examination, osseous survey, infant**

> 🚑 2.85   ⚕ 2.85   **FUD** XXX   01 N1 80 ▢
>
> **AMA:** 2018,Jan,8; 2017,Jan,8; 2016,Jan,13; 2015,Jan,16; 2014,Jan,11

77077 **Joint survey, single view, 2 or more joints (specify)**

> 🚑 1.09   ⚕ 1.09   **FUD** XXX   01 N1 80 ▢
>
> **AMA:** 2018,Jan,8; 2017,Jan,8; 2016,Jan,13; 2015,Jan,16; 2014,Jan,11

77078 **Computed tomography, bone mineral density study, 1 or more sites, axial skeleton (eg, hips, pelvis, spine)**

> 🚑 3.24   ⚕ 3.24   **FUD** XXX   S Z2 80 ▢
>
> **AMA:** 2018,Jan,8; 2017,Jan,8; 2016,Jan,13; 2015,Jan,16; 2014,Jan,11

77080 **Dual-energy X-ray absorptiometry (DXA), bone density study, 1 or more sites; axial skeleton (eg, hips, pelvis, spine)**

> EXCLUDES Dual-energy x-ray absorptiometry (DXA), bone density study ([77085])
> Vertebral fracture assessment via dual-energy x-ray absorptiometry (DXA) ([77086])
>
> 🚑 1.13   ⚕ 1.13   **FUD** XXX   S Z3 80 ▢
>
> **AMA:** 2018,Jan,8; 2017,Jan,8; 2016,Jan,13; 2015,Jan,16; 2014,Jan,11

77081 **appendicular skeleton (peripheral) (eg, radius, wrist, heel)**

> 🚑 0.94   ⚕ 0.94   **FUD** XXX   S Z3 80 ▢
>
> **AMA:** 2018,Jan,8; 2017,Jan,8; 2016,Jan,13; 2015,Jan,16; 2014,Jan,11

\# **77085** **axial skeleton (eg, hips, pelvis, spine), including vertebral fracture assessment**

> 🚑 1.54   ⚕ 1.54   **FUD** XXX   01 N1 80 ▢
>
> EXCLUDES Dual-energy x-ray absorptiometry (DXA), bone density study (77080)
> Vertebral fracture assessment via dual-energy x-ray absorptiometry (DXA) ([77086])

\# **77086** **Vertebral fracture assessment via dual-energy X-ray absorptiometry (DXA)**

> 🚑 0.99   ⚕ 0.99   **FUD** XXX   01 N1 80 ▢
>
> EXCLUDES Dual-energy x-ray absorptiometry (DXA), bone density study (77080)
> Therapy performed more than one time for treatment to a specific area
> Vertebral fracture assessment via dual-energy x-ray absorptiometry (DXA) ([77085])

77084 **Magnetic resonance (eg, proton) imaging, bone marrow blood supply**

> 🚑 10.7   ⚕ 10.7   **FUD** XXX   S Z2 80 ▢
>
> **AMA:** 2018,Jan,8; 2017,Jan,8; 2016,Jan,13; 2015,Jan,16; 2014,Jan,11

77085 **Resequenced code. See code following 77081.**

77086 **Resequenced code. See code before 77084.**

77261-77263 Therapeutic Radiology: Treatment Planning

> INCLUDES Determination of:
> Appropriate treatment devices
> Number and size of treatment ports
> Treatment method
> Treatment time/dosage
> Treatment volume
> Interpretation of special testing
> Tumor localization
>
> EXCLUDES Brachytherapy (0394T-0395T)
> Radiation treatment delivery, superficial (77401)

77261 **Therapeutic radiology treatment planning; simple**

> INCLUDES Planning for single treatment area included in a single port or simple parallel opposed ports with simple or no blocking
>
> 🚑 2.03   ⚕ 2.03   **FUD** XXX   B 80 26 ▢
>
> **AMA:** 2018,Jan,8; 2017,Jan,8; 2016,Feb,3; 2016,Jan,13; 2015,Jan,16; 2014,Jan,11

77262 **intermediate**

> INCLUDES Planning for three or more converging ports, two separate treatment sites, multiple blocks, or special time dose constraints
>
> 🚑 3.06   ⚕ 3.06   **FUD** XXX   B 80 26 ▢
>
> **AMA:** 2018,Jan,8; 2017,Jan,8; 2016,Feb,3; 2016,Jan,13; 2015,Jan,16; 2014,Jan,11

77263 **complex**

> INCLUDES Planning for very complex blocking, custom shielding blocks, tangential ports, special wedges or compensators, three or more separate treatment areas, rotational or special beam considerations, combination of treatment modalities
>
> 🚑 4.78   ⚕ 4.78   **FUD** XXX   B 80 26 ▢
>
> **AMA:** 2018,Jan,8; 2017,Jan,8; 2016,Feb,3; 2016,Jan,13; 2015,Jan,16; 2014,Jan,11

77280-77299 Radiation Therapy Simulation

77280 **Therapeutic radiology simulation-aided field setting; simple**

INCLUDES Simulation of a single treatment site

🔲 7.84 🔲 7.84 **FUD** XXX S Z2 80 ▭

AMA: 2018,Jan,8; 2017,Jan,8; 2016,Jan,13; 2015,Apr,10; 2015,Jan,16; 2014,Jan,11

77285 **intermediate**

INCLUDES Two different treatment sites

🔲 12.9 🔲 12.9 **FUD** XXX S Z2 80 ▭

AMA: 2018,Jan,8; 2017,Jan,8; 2016,Jan,13; 2015,Apr,10; 2015,Jan,16; 2014,Jan,11

77290 **complex**

INCLUDES Brachytherapy
Complex blocking
Contrast material
Custom shielding blocks
Hyperthermia probe verification
Rotation, arc or particle therapy
Simulation to ≥ 3 treatment sites

🔲 14.4 🔲 14.4 **FUD** XXX S Z2 80 ▭

AMA: 2018,Jan,8; 2017,Jan,8; 2016,Sep,9; 2016,Jan,13; 2015,Apr,10; 2015,Jan,16; 2014,Jan,11

+ 77293 **Respiratory motion management simulation (List separately in addition to code for primary procedure)**

Code first (77295, 77301)

🔲 13.0 🔲 13.0 **FUD** ZZZ N N1 80 ▭

AMA: 2018,Jan,8; 2017,Jan,8; 2016,Jan,13; 2015,Dec,16

77295 **Resequenced code. See code before 77300.**

77299 **Unlisted procedure, therapeutic radiology clinical treatment planning**

🔲 0.00 🔲 0.00 **FUD** XXX S Z2 80 ▭

AMA: 2018,Jan,8; 2017,Jan,8; 2016,Jan,13; 2015,Jan,16; 2014,Jan,11

77295-77370 [77295] Radiation Physics Services

 # 77295 **3-dimensional radiotherapy plan, including dose-volume histograms**

🔲 13.9 🔲 13.9 **FUD** XXX S Z3 80 ▭

AMA: 2018,Jan,8; 2017,Jan,8; 2016,Jan,13; 2015,Dec,16; 2015,Jun,6; 2015,Jan,16; 2014,Jan,11

77300 **Basic radiation dosimetry calculation, central axis depth dose calculation, TDF, NSD, gap calculation, off axis factor, tissue inhomogeneity factors, calculation of non-ionizing radiation surface and depth dose, as required during course of treatment, only when prescribed by the treating physician**

EXCLUDES Brachytherapy (77316-77318, 77767-77772, 0394T-0395T)
Teletherapy plan (77306-77307, 77321)

🔲 1.89 🔲 1.89 **FUD** XXX S Z3 80 ▭

AMA: 2018,Jan,8; 2017,Jan,8; 2016,Jan,13; 2015,Jan,16; 2014,Jan,11

77301 **Intensity modulated radiotherapy plan, including dose-volume histograms for target and critical structure partial tolerance specifications**

🔲 55.0 🔲 55.0 **FUD** XXX S Z2 80 ▭

AMA: 2018,Jan,8; 2017,Jan,8; 2016,Jan,13; 2015,Jan,16; 2014,Jan,11

77306 **Teletherapy isodose plan; simple (1 or 2 unmodified ports directed to a single area of interest), includes basic dosimetry calculation(s)**

EXCLUDES Brachytherapy (0394T-0395T)
Radiation dosimetry calculation (77300)
Radiation treatment delivery (77401)
Therapy performed more than one time for treatment to a specific area

🔲 4.25 🔲 4.25 **FUD** XXX S Z3 80 ▭

AMA: 2018,Jan,8; 2017,Jan,8; 2016,Feb,3

77307 **complex (multiple treatment areas, tangential ports, the use of wedges, blocking, rotational beam, or special beam considerations), includes basic dosimetry calculation(s)**

EXCLUDES Brachytherapy (0394T-0395T)
Radiation dosimetry calculation (77300)
Radiation treatment delivery (77401)
Therapy performed more than one time for treatment to a specific area

🔲 8.22 🔲 8.22 **FUD** XXX S Z3 80 ▭

AMA: 2018,Jan,8; 2017,Jan,8; 2016,Feb,3

77316 **Brachytherapy isodose plan; simple (calculation[s] made from 1 to 4 sources, or remote afterloading brachytherapy, 1 channel), includes basic dosimetry calculation(s)**

EXCLUDES Brachytherapy (0394T-0395T)
Radiation dosimetry calculation (77300)
Radiation treatment delivery (77401)

🔲 5.78 🔲 5.78 **FUD** XXX S Z3 80 ▭

AMA: 2018,Jan,8; 2017,Jan,8; 2016,Feb,3

77317 **intermediate (calculation[s] made from 5 to 10 sources, or remote afterloading brachytherapy, 2-12 channels), includes basic dosimetry calculation(s)**

EXCLUDES Brachytherapy (0394T-0395T)
Radiation dosimetry calculation (77300)
Radiation treatment delivery (77401)

🔲 7.57 🔲 7.57 **FUD** XXX S Z2 80 ▭

AMA: 2018,Jan,8; 2017,Jan,8

77318 **complex (calculation[s] made from over 10 sources, or remote afterloading brachytherapy, over 12 channels), includes basic dosimetry calculation(s)**

EXCLUDES Brachytherapy (0394T-0395T)
Radiation dosimetry calculation (77300)
Radiation treatment delivery (77401)

🔲 10.8 🔲 10.8 **FUD** XXX S Z2 80 ▭

AMA: 2018,Jan,8; 2017,Jan,8; 2016,Feb,3

77321 **Special teletherapy port plan, particles, hemibody, total body**

🔲 2.66 🔲 2.66 **FUD** XXX S Z3 80 ▭

AMA: 2018,Jan,8; 2017,Jan,8; 2016,Jan,13; 2015,Jan,16; 2014,Jan,11

77331 **Special dosimetry (eg, TLD, microdosimetry) (specify), only when prescribed by the treating physician**

🔲 1.84 🔲 1.84 **FUD** XXX S Z3 80 ▭

AMA: 2018,Jan,8; 2017,Jan,8; 2016,Jan,13; 2015,Jun,6; 2015,Jan,16; 2014,Jan,11

77332 **Treatment devices, design and construction; simple (simple block, simple bolus)**

EXCLUDES Brachytherapy (0394T-0395T)
Radiation treatment delivery (77401)

🔲 1.49 🔲 1.49 **FUD** XXX S Z3 80 ▭

AMA: 2018,Jan,8; 2017,Jan,8; 2016,Feb,3; 2016,Jan,13; 2015,Jan,16; 2014,Jan,11

77333 **intermediate (multiple blocks, stents, bite blocks, special bolus)**

EXCLUDES Brachytherapy (0394T-0395T)
Radiation treatment delivery (77401)

🔲 3.10 🔲 3.10 **FUD** XXX S Z2 80 ▭

AMA: 2018,Jan,8; 2017,Jan,8; 2016,Feb,3; 2016,Jan,13; 2015,Jan,16; 2014,Jan,11

77334 **complex (irregular blocks, special shields, compensators, wedges, molds or casts)**

EXCLUDES Brachytherapy (0394T-0395T)
Radiation treatment delivery (77401)

🔲 3.64 🔲 3.64 **FUD** XXX S Z3 80 ▭

AMA: 2018,Jan,8; 2017,Jan,8; 2016,Sep,9; 2016,Feb,3; 2016,Jan,13; 2015,Dec,16; 2015,Jan,16; 2014,Jan,11

77336 Continuing medical physics consultation, including assessment of treatment parameters, quality assurance of dose delivery, and review of patient treatment documentation in support of the radiation oncologist, reported per week of therapy

EXCLUDES Brachytherapy (0394T-0395T)
Radiation treatment delivery (77401)

2.26   2.26   FUD XXX   S Z2 80 TC

AMA: 2018,Jan,8; 2017,Jan,8; 2016,Feb,3; 2016,Jan,13; 2015,Jan,16; 2014,Jan,11

77338 Multi-leaf collimator (MLC) device(s) for intensity modulated radiation therapy (IMRT), design and construction per IMRT plan

EXCLUDES Immobilization in IMRT treatment (77332-77334)
Intensity modulated radiation treatment delivery (IMRT) (77385)
Use of code more than one time per IMRT plan

14.1   14.1   FUD XXX   S Z2 80

AMA: 2018,Jan,8; 2017,Jan,8; 2016,Jan,13; 2015,Jan,16; 2014,Jan,11

77370 Special medical radiation physics consultation

3.52   3.52   FUD XXX   S Z2 80 TC

AMA: 2018,Jan,8; 2017,Jan,8; 2016,Feb,3; 2016,Jan,13; 2015,Jun,6; 2015,Jan,16; 2014,Jan,11

77371-77399 Stereotactic Radiosurgery (SRS) Planning and Delivery

77371 Radiation treatment delivery, stereotactic radiosurgery (SRS), complete course of treatment of cranial lesion(s) consisting of 1 session; multi-source Cobalt 60 based

EXCLUDES Guidance with computed tomography for radiation therapy field placement (77014)

0.00   0.00   FUD XXX   J 80 TC

AMA: 2018,Jan,8; 2017,Jan,8; 2016,Jan,13; 2015,Jan,16; 2014,Jul,8; 2014,Jan,11

77372 linear accelerator based

EXCLUDES Guidance with computed tomography for radiation therapy field placement (77014)
Radiation treatment supervision (77432)

30.2   30.2   FUD XXX   J 80 TC

AMA: 2018,Jan,8; 2017,Jan,8; 2016,Jan,13; 2015,Jan,16; 2014,Jul,8; 2014,Jan,11

77373 Stereotactic body radiation therapy, treatment delivery, per fraction to 1 or more lesions, including image guidance, entire course not to exceed 5 fractions

EXCLUDES Guidance with computed tomography for radiation therapy field placement (77014)
Intensity modulated radiation treatment delivery (IMRT) (77385-77386)
Radiation treatment delivery (77401-77402, 77407, 77412)
Single fraction cranial lesion(s) (77371-77372)

36.6   36.6   FUD XXX   S 80 TC

AMA: 2018,Jan,8; 2017,Jan,8; 2016,Jan,13; 2015,Jun,6; 2015,Jan,16; 2014,Jul,8; 2014,Jan,11

77385 Resequenced code. See code following 77417.

77386 Resequenced code. See code following 77417.

77387 Resequenced code. See code following 77417.

77399 Unlisted procedure, medical radiation physics, dosimetry and treatment devices, and special services

0.00   0.00   FUD XXX   S Z2 80

AMA: 2018,Jan,8; 2017,Jan,8; 2016,Jan,13; 2015,Jan,16; 2014,Jan,11

77401-77425 [77385, 77386, 77387, 77424, 77425] Radiation Treatment

INCLUDES Technical component and assorted energy levels

77401 Radiation treatment delivery, superficial and/or ortho voltage, per day

EXCLUDES Continuing medical physics consultation (77336)
Isodose plan:
Brachytherapy (77316-77318)
Teletherapy (77306-77307)
Management of:
Intraoperative radiation treatment (77469-77470)
Radiation therapy (77431-77432)
Radiation treatment (77427)
Stereotactic body radiation therapy (77435)
Stereotactic body radiation therapy, treatment delivery (77373)
Unlisted procedure, therapeutic radiology treatment management (77499)
Therapeutic radiology treatment planning (77261-77263)
Treatment devices, design and construction (77332-77334)
Code also E&M services when performed alone, as appropriate

0.70   0.70   FUD XXX   S Z3 80 TC

AMA: 2018,Jan,8; 2017,Jan,8; 2016,Feb,3; 2016,Jan,13; 2015,Dec,14; 2015,Jan,16; 2014,Jan,11

77402 Radiation treatment delivery, ≥1 MeV; simple

EXCLUDES Stereotactic body radiation therapy, treatment delivery (77373)

0.00   0.00   FUD XXX   S Z2 80 TC

AMA: 2018,Jan,8; 2017,Jan,8; 2016,Jun,9; 2016,Mar,7; 2016,Feb,3; 2016,Jan,13; 2015,Dec,14; 2015,Jan,16; 2014,Jan,11

77407 intermediate

EXCLUDES Stereotactic body radiation therapy, treatment delivery (77373)

0.00   0.00   FUD XXX   S Z2 80 TC

AMA: 2018,Jan,8; 2017,Jan,8; 2016,Jun,9; 2016,Mar,7; 2016,Feb,3; 2016,Jan,13; 2015,Dec,14; 2015,Jan,16; 2014,Jan,11

77412 complex

0.00   0.00   FUD XXX   S Z2 80 TC

AMA: 2018,Jan,8; 2017,Jan,8; 2016,Jun,9; 2016,Mar,7; 2016,Feb,3; 2016,Jan,13; 2015,Dec,14; 2015,Jan,16; 2014,Jan,11

77417 Therapeutic radiology port image(s)

0.32   0.32   FUD XXX   N NI 80 TC

AMA: 2018,Jan,8; 2017,Dec,14; 2017,Jan,8; 2016,Jan,13; 2015,Dec,14; 2015,Jan,16; 2014,Jan,11

\# **77385** Intensity modulated radiation treatment delivery (IMRT), includes guidance and tracking, when performed; simple

0.00   0.00   FUD XXX   S Z2 80 TC

AMA: 2018,Jan,8; 2017,Jan,8; 2016,Feb,3

\# **77386** complex

0.00   0.00   FUD XXX   S Z2 80 TC

AMA: 2018,Jan,8; 2017,Jan,8; 2016,Feb,3

\# **77387** Guidance for localization of target volume for delivery of radiation treatment, includes intrafraction tracking, when performed

0.00   0.00   FUD XXX   N NI 80

AMA: 2018,Jan,8; 2017,Jan,8; 2016,Feb,3; 2016,Jan,13; 2015,Dec,16; 2015,Dec,14

\# **77424** Intraoperative radiation treatment delivery, x-ray, single treatment session

0.00   0.00   FUD XXX   J Z2

AMA: 2018,Jan,8; 2017,Jan,8; 2016,Jan,13; 2015,Dec,14

\# **77425** Intraoperative radiation treatment delivery, electrons, single treatment session

0.00   0.00   FUD XXX   J Z2

AMA: 2018,Jan,8; 2017,Jan,8; 2016,Jan,13; 2015,Dec,14; 2015,Jan,16; 2014,Jan,11

77336 — 77425

77423-77425 Neutron Therapy

77423   **High energy neutron radiation treatment delivery, 1 or more isocenter(s) with coplanar or non-coplanar geometry with blocking and/or wedge, and/or compensator(s)**

🚗 0.00   🔧 0.00   **FUD** XXX   [S] [Z3] [80] [TC] [▭]

AMA: 2018,Jan,8; 2017,Jan,8; 2016,Jan,13; 2015,Dec,14; 2015,Jan,16; 2014,Jan,11

77424   **Resequenced code. See code following 77417.**

77425   **Resequenced code. See code following 77417.**

77427-77499 Radiation Therapy Management

INCLUDES   Assessment of patient for medical evaluation and management (at least one per treatment management service) that includes:
Coordination of care/treatment
Evaluation of patient's response to treatment
Review of:
Dose delivery
Dosimetry
Lab tests
Patient treatment set-up
Port film
Treatment parameters
X-rays
Units of five fractions or treatment sessions regardless of time. Two or more fractions performed on the same day can be counted separately provided there is a distinct break in service between sessions and the fractions are of the character usually furnished on different days.

EXCLUDES   *High dose rate electronic brachytherapy (0394T-0395T)*
Radiation treatment delivery (77401)

77427   **Radiation treatment management, 5 treatments**

🚗 5.37   🔧 5.37   **FUD** XXX   [B] [26] [▭]

AMA: 2018,Jan,8; 2017,Jan,8; 2016,Feb,3; 2016,Jan,13; 2015,Jun,6; 2015,Jan,16; 2014,Jan,11

77431   **Radiation therapy management with complete course of therapy consisting of 1 or 2 fractions only**

🚗 2.96   🔧 2.96   **FUD** XXX   [B] [80] [26] [▭]

AMA: 2018,Jan,8; 2017,Jan,8; 2016,Feb,3; 2016,Jan,13; 2015,Jun,6; 2015,Jan,16; 2014,Jan,11

77432   **Stereotactic radiation treatment management of cranial lesion(s) (complete course of treatment consisting of 1 session)**

🚗 12.0   🔧 12.0   **FUD** XXX   [B] [80] [26] [▭]

AMA: 2018,Jan,8; 2017,Jan,8; 2016,Feb,3; 2016,Jan,13; 2015,Dec,14; 2015,Dec,16; 2015,Jun,6; 2015,Jan,16; 2014,Jul,8; 2014,Jan,11

77435   **Stereotactic body radiation therapy, treatment management, per treatment course, to 1 or more lesions, including image guidance, entire course not to exceed 5 fractions**

🚗 18.1   🔧 18.1   **FUD** XXX   [N] [N1] [80] [26] [▭]

AMA: 2018,Jan,8; 2017,Jan,8; 2016,Feb,3; 2016,Jan,13; 2015,Dec,14; 2015,Jun,6; 2015,Jan,16; 2014,Jan,11

77469   **Intraoperative radiation treatment management**

🚗 9.00   🔧 9.00   **FUD** XXX   [B] [80] [▭]

AMA: 2018,Jan,8; 2017,Jan,8; 2016,Feb,3; 2015,Jun,6

77470   **Special treatment procedure (eg, total body irradiation, hemibody radiation, per oral or endocavitary irradiation)**

🚗 3.75   🔧 3.75   **FUD** XXX   [S] [Z3] [80] [▭]

AMA: 2018,Jan,8; 2017,Jan,8; 2016,Feb,3; 2016,Jan,13; 2015,Jun,6; 2015,Jan,16; 2014,Jan,11

77499   **Unlisted procedure, therapeutic radiology treatment management**

🚗 0.00   🔧 0.00   **FUD** XXX   [B] [80] [▭]

AMA: 2018,Jan,8; 2017,Jan,8; 2016,Feb,3; 2016,Jan,13; 2015,Jun,6; 2015,Jan,16; 2014,Jan,11

77520-77525 Proton Therapy

EXCLUDES   *High dose rate electronic brachytherapy, per fraction (0394T-0395T)*

77520   **Proton treatment delivery; simple, without compensation**

🚗 0.00   🔧 0.00   **FUD** XXX   [S] [Z2] [80] [TC] [▭]

AMA: 2018,Jan,8; 2017,Jan,8; 2016,Jan,13; 2015,Jan,16; 2014,Jan,11

77522   **simple, with compensation**

🚗 0.00   🔧 0.00   **FUD** XXX   [S] [Z2] [80] [TC] [▭]

AMA: 2012,Feb,9-10; 2010,Oct,3-4

77523   **intermediate**

🚗 0.00   🔧 0.00   **FUD** XXX   [S] [Z2] [80] [TC] [▭]

AMA: 2018,Jan,8; 2017,Jan,8; 2016,Jan,13; 2015,Jan,16; 2014,Jan,11

77525   **complex**

🚗 0.00   🔧 0.00   **FUD** XXX   [S] [Z2] [80] [TC] [▭]

AMA: 2012,Feb,9-10; 2010,Oct,3-4

77600-77620 Hyperthermia Treatment

CMS: 100-03,110.1 Hyperthermia for Treatment of Cancer

INCLUDES   Interstitial insertion of temperature sensors
Management during the course of therapy
Normal follow-up care for three months after completion
Physics planning
Use of heat generating devices

EXCLUDES   *Initial E&M service*
Radiation therapy treatment (77371-77373, 77401-77412, 77423)

77600   **Hyperthermia, externally generated; superficial (ie, heating to a depth of 4 cm or less)**

🚗 12.7   🔧 12.7   **FUD** XXX   [S] [Z2] [80] [▭]

AMA: 2018,Jan,8; 2017,Jan,8; 2016,Jan,13; 2015,Jan,16; 2014,Jan,11

77605   **deep (ie, heating to depths greater than 4 cm)**

🚗 22.0   🔧 22.0   **FUD** XXX   [S] [Z2] [80] [▭]

AMA: 2018,Jan,8; 2017,Jan,8; 2016,Jan,13; 2015,Jan,16; 2014,Jan,11

77610   **Hyperthermia generated by interstitial probe(s); 5 or fewer interstitial applicators**

🚗 19.6   🔧 19.6   **FUD** XXX   [S] [Z2] [80] [▭]

AMA: 2018,Jan,8; 2017,Jan,8; 2016,Jan,13; 2015,Jan,16; 2014,Jan,11

77615   **more than 5 interstitial applicators**

🚗 30.0   🔧 30.0   **FUD** XXX   [S] [Z2] [80] [▭]

AMA: 2018,Jan,8; 2017,Jan,8; 2016,Jan,13; 2015,Jan,16; 2014,Jan,11

77620   **Hyperthermia generated by intracavitary probe(s)**

🚗 14.6   🔧 14.6   **FUD** XXX   [S] [Z2] [80] [▭]

AMA: 2018,Jan,8; 2017,Jan,8; 2016,Jan,13; 2015,Jan,16; 2014,Jan,11

77750-77799 Brachytherapy

CMS: 100-04,13,70.4 Clinical Brachytherapy; 100-04,13,70.5 Radiation Physics Services; 100-04,4,61.4.4 Billing for Brachytherapy Source Supervision, Handling and Loading Costs

INCLUDES   Hospital admission and daily visits

EXCLUDES   *Placement of:*
Heyman capsules (58346)
Ovoids and tandems (57155)

77750   **Infusion or instillation of radioelement solution (includes 3-month follow-up care)**

🚗 10.7   🔧 10.7   **FUD** 090   [S] [Z2] [80] [▭]

AMA: 2018,Jan,8; 2017,Jan,8; 2016,Jan,13; 2015,Jan,16; 2014,Jan,11

77761   **Intracavitary radiation source application; simple**

🚗 11.3   🔧 11.3   **FUD** 090   [S] [Z3] [80] [▭]

AMA: 2018,Jan,8; 2017,Jan,8; 2016,Jan,13; 2015,Jan,16; 2014,Jan,11

77762   **intermediate**

🚗 15.0   🔧 15.0   **FUD** 090   [S] [Z3] [80] [▭]

AMA: 2018,Jan,8; 2017,Jan,8; 2016,Jan,13; 2015,Jan,16; 2014,Jan,11

77763   **complex**

🚗 21.3   🔧 21.3   **FUD** 090   [S] [Z3] [80] [▭]

AMA: 2018,Jan,8; 2017,Jan,8; 2016,Jan,13; 2015,Jan,16; 2014,Jan,11

26/TC PC/TC Only   A2-Z3 ASC Payment   50 Bilateral   ♂ Male Only   ♀ Female Only   🚗 Facility RVU   🔧 Non-Facility RVU   ▭ CCI   ✖ CLIA
FUD Follow-up Days   CMS: IOM   AMA: CPT Asst   A-Y OPPSI   80/80 Surg Assist Allowed / w/Doc   Lab Crosswalk   Radiology Crosswalk

362   CPT © 2019 American Medical Association. All Rights Reserved.   © 2019 Optum360, LLC

77767 Remote afterloading high dose rate radionuclide skin surface brachytherapy, includes basic dosimetry, when performed; lesion diameter up to 2.0 cm or 1 channel
6.60 6.60 **FUD** XXX S Z2 80 ▢

77768 lesion diameter over 2.0 cm and 2 or more channels, or multiple lesions
10.1 10.1 **FUD** XXX S Z2 80 ▢

77770 Remote afterloading high dose rate radionuclide interstitial or intracavitary brachytherapy, includes basic dosimetry, when performed; 1 channel
9.36 9.36 **FUD** XXX S Z4 80 ▢

77771 2-12 channels
17.0 17.0 **FUD** XXX S Z2 80 ▢

77772 over 12 channels
25.8 25.8 **FUD** XXX S Z2 80 ▢

77778 Interstitial radiation source application, complex, includes supervision, handling, loading of radiation source, when performed
24.0 24.0 **FUD** 000 S Z2 80 ▢
AMA: 2018,Jan,8; 2017,Jan,8; 2016,Jan,13; 2015,Jan,16; 2014,Jan,11

77789 Surface application of low dose rate radionuclide source
3.49 3.49 **FUD** 000 S Z2 80 ▢
AMA: 2018,Jan,8; 2017,Jan,8; 2016,Jan,13; 2015,Jan,16; 2014,Jan,11

77790 Supervision, handling, loading of radiation source
0.43 0.43 **FUD** XXX N N1 80 TC ▢
AMA: 2018,Jan,8; 2017,Jan,8; 2016,Jan,13; 2015,Jan,16; 2014,Jan,11

77799 Unlisted procedure, clinical brachytherapy
0.00 0.00 **FUD** XXX S Z2 80 ▢
AMA: 2018,Jan,8; 2017,Jan,8; 2016,Jan,13; 2015,Jan,16; 2014,Jan,11

78012-78099 Nuclear Radiology: Thyroid, Parathyroid, Adrenal
EXCLUDES Diagnostic services (see appropriate sections)
Follow-up care (see appropriate section)
Code also radiopharmaceutical(s) and/or drug(s) supplied

78012 Thyroid uptake, single or multiple quantitative measurement(s) (including stimulation, suppression, or discharge, when performed)
2.34 2.34 **FUD** XXX S Z2 ▢
AMA: 2018,Jan,8; 2017,Jan,8; 2016,Jan,13; 2015,Jan,16

78013 Thyroid imaging (including vascular flow, when performed);
5.54 5.54 **FUD** XXX S Z2 ▢
AMA: 2018,Jan,8; 2017,Jan,8; 2016,Jan,13; 2015,Jan,16

78014 with single or multiple uptake(s) quantitative measurement(s) (including stimulation, suppression, or discharge, when performed)
6.95 6.95 **FUD** XXX S Z2 80 ▢
AMA: 2018,Jan,8; 2017,Jan,8; 2016,Jan,13; 2015,Jan,16

78015 Thyroid carcinoma metastases imaging; limited area (eg, neck and chest only)
6.47 6.47 **FUD** XXX S Z2 80 ▢
AMA: 2018,Jan,8; 2017,Jan,8; 2016,Jan,13; 2015,Jan,16; 2014,Jan,11

78016 with additional studies (eg, urinary recovery)
8.12 8.12 **FUD** XXX S Z2 80 ▢
AMA: 2018,Jan,8; 2017,Jan,8; 2016,Jan,13; 2015,Jan,16; 2014,Jan,11

78018 whole body
9.03 9.03 **FUD** XXX S Z2 80 ▢
AMA: 2018,Jan,8; 2017,Jan,8; 2016,Jan,13; 2015,Jan,16; 2014,Jan,11

+ **78020** Thyroid carcinoma metastases uptake (List separately in addition to code for primary procedure)
2.41 2.41 **FUD** ZZZ N N1 80 ▢
AMA: 2018,Jan,8; 2017,Jan,8; 2016,Jan,13; 2015,Jan,16; 2014,Jan,11

78070 Parathyroid planar imaging (including subtraction, when performed);
EXCLUDES Distribution of radiopharmaceutical agents or tumor localization (78800-78802, [78804], 78803)
Radiopharmaceutical quantification measurements ([78835])
SPECT with concurrently acquired CT transmission scan ([78830, 78831, 78832])
8.61 8.61 **FUD** XXX S Z2 80 ▢
AMA: 2018,Jan,8; 2017,Jan,8; 2016,Dec,9; 2016,Dec,16; 2016,Jan,13; 2015,Jan,16; 2014,Jan,11

78071 with tomographic (SPECT)
EXCLUDES Distribution of radiopharmaceutical agents or tumor localization (78800-78802, [78804], 78803)
Radiopharmaceutical quantification measurements ([78835])
SPECT with concurrently acquired CT transmission scan ([78830, 78831, 78832])
10.2 10.2 **FUD** XXX S Z2 80 ▢
AMA: 2018,Jan,8; 2017,Jan,8; 2016,Dec,16; 2016,Dec,9

78072 with tomographic (SPECT), and concurrently acquired computed tomography (CT) for anatomical localization
EXCLUDES Distribution of radiopharmaceutical agents or tumor localization (78800-78802, [78804], 78803)
Radiopharmaceutical quantification measurements ([78835])
SPECT with concurrently acquired CT transmission scan ([78830, 78831, 78832])
11.2 11.2 **FUD** XXX S Z2 80 ▢
AMA: 2018,Jan,8; 2017,Jan,8; 2016,Dec,16; 2016,Dec,9

78075 Adrenal imaging, cortex and/or medulla
13.0 13.0 **FUD** XXX S Z2 80 ▢
AMA: 2018,Jan,8; 2017,Jan,8; 2016,Jan,13; 2015,Jan,16; 2014,Jan,11

78099 Unlisted endocrine procedure, diagnostic nuclear medicine
0.00 0.00 **FUD** XXX S Z2 80 ▢
AMA: 2018,Jan,8; 2017,Jan,8; 2016,Dec,9; 2016,Jan,13; 2015,Jan,16; 2014,Jan,11

Lateral view / Anterior view — Thyroglossal duct (dotted line), Hyoid bone, Thyroid cartilage, Cricoid cartilage, Crico-thyroid muscle, Thyroid gland, Trachea, Esophagus, Epiglottis, Pyramid lobe, Isthmus

Radiology *(side margin)*

78102 — 78267 *(side margin)*

78102-78199 Nuclear Radiology: Blood Forming Organs

EXCLUDES Diagnostic services (see appropriate sections)
Follow-up care (see appropriate section)
Radioimmunoassays (82009-84999 [82042, 82652])
Code also radiopharmaceutical(s) and/or drug(s) supplied

78102 Bone marrow imaging; limited area
4.89 4.89 FUD XXX S Z2 80
AMA: 2018,Jan,8; 2017,Jan,8; 2016,Jan,13; 2015,Jan,16; 2014,Jan,11

78103 multiple areas
6.27 6.27 FUD XXX S Z2 80
AMA: 2012,Feb,9-10; 2007,Jan,28-31

78104 whole body
7.15 7.15 FUD XXX S Z2 80
AMA: 2012,Feb,9-10; 2007,Jan,28-31

78110 Plasma volume, radiopharmaceutical volume-dilution technique (separate procedure); single sampling
1.99 1.99 FUD XXX S Z2 80
AMA: 2012,Feb,9-10; 2007,Jan,28-31

78111 multiple samplings
2.11 2.11 FUD XXX S Z2 80
AMA: 2012,Feb,9-10; 2007,Jan,28-31

78120 Red cell volume determination (separate procedure); single sampling
2.04 2.04 FUD XXX S Z2 80
AMA: 2012,Feb,9-10; 2007,Jan,28-31

78121 multiple samplings
2.23 2.23 FUD XXX S Z2 80
AMA: 2012,Feb,9-10; 2007,Jan,28-31

78122 Whole blood volume determination, including separate measurement of plasma volume and red cell volume (radiopharmaceutical volume-dilution technique)
2.73 2.73 FUD XXX S Z2 80
AMA: 2012,Feb,9-10; 2007,Jan,28-31

78130 Red cell survival study;
3.56 3.56 FUD XXX S Z2 80
AMA: 2012,Feb,9-10; 2007,Jan,28-31

78135 differential organ/tissue kinetics (eg, splenic and/or hepatic sequestration)
8.02 8.02 FUD XXX S Z2 80
AMA: 2012,Feb,9-10; 2007,Jan,28-31

78140 Labeled red cell sequestration, differential organ/tissue (eg, splenic and/or hepatic)
3.14 3.14 FUD XXX S Z2 80
AMA: 2012,Feb,9-10; 2007,Jan,28-31

78185 Spleen imaging only, with or without vascular flow
EXCLUDES Liver imaging (78215-78216)
4.87 4.87 FUD XXX S Z2 80
AMA: 2012,Feb,9-10; 2007,Jan,28-31

78191 Platelet survival study
3.56 3.56 FUD XXX S Z2 80
AMA: 2012,Feb,9-10; 2007,Jan,28-31

78195 Lymphatics and lymph nodes imaging
EXCLUDES Sentinel node identification without scintigraphy (38792)
Sentinel node removal (38500-38542)
10.2 10.2 FUD XXX S Z2 80
AMA: 2018,Jan,8; 2017,Jan,8; 2016,Jan,13; 2015,Jan,16; 2014,Jan,11

78199 Unlisted hematopoietic, reticuloendothelial and lymphatic procedure, diagnostic nuclear medicine
0.00 0.00 FUD XXX S Z2 80
AMA: 2018,Jan,8; 2017,Jan,8; 2016,Jan,13; 2015,Jan,16; 2014,Jan,11

78201-78299 Nuclear Radiology: Digestive System

EXCLUDES Diagnostic services (see appropriate sections)
Follow-up care (see appropriate section)
Code also radiopharmaceutical(s) and/or drug(s) supplied

78201 Liver imaging; static only
EXCLUDES Spleen imaging only (78185)
5.49 5.49 FUD XXX S Z2 80
AMA: 2018,Jan,8; 2017,Jan,8; 2016,Jan,13; 2015,Jan,16; 2014,Jan,11

78202 with vascular flow
EXCLUDES Spleen imaging only (78185)
5.82 5.82 FUD XXX S Z2 80
AMA: 2012,Feb,9-10; 2007,Jan,28-31

78205 Liver imaging (SPECT);
To report, see (78803)

78206 with vascular flow
To report, see (78803)

78215 Liver and spleen imaging; static only
5.61 5.61 FUD XXX S Z2 80
AMA: 2012,Feb,9-10; 2007,Jan,28-31

78216 with vascular flow
3.68 3.68 FUD XXX S Z2 80
AMA: 2012,Feb,9-10; 2007,Jan,28-31

78226 Hepatobiliary system imaging, including gallbladder when present;
9.52 9.52 FUD XXX S Z2 80
AMA: 2012,Feb,9-10

78227 with pharmacologic intervention, including quantitative measurement(s) when performed
12.8 12.8 FUD XXX S Z2 80
AMA: 2012,Feb,9-10

78230 Salivary gland imaging;
5.03 5.03 FUD XXX S Z2 80
AMA: 2012,Feb,9-10; 2007,Jan,28-31

78231 with serial images
2.98 2.98 FUD XXX S Z2 80
AMA: 2012,Feb,9-10; 2007,Jan,28-31

78232 Salivary gland function study
2.92 2.92 FUD XXX S Z2 80
AMA: 2012,Feb,9-10; 2007,Jan,28-31

78258 Esophageal motility
6.31 6.31 FUD XXX S Z2 80
AMA: 2012,Feb,9-10; 2007,Jan,28-31

78261 Gastric mucosa imaging
5.83 5.83 FUD XXX S Z2 80
AMA: 2012,Feb,9-10; 2007,Jan,28-31

78262 Gastroesophageal reflux study
6.95 6.95 FUD XXX S Z2 80
AMA: 2018,Jan,8; 2017,Jan,8; 2016,Jan,13; 2015,Dec,11

78264 Gastric emptying imaging study (eg, solid, liquid, or both);
EXCLUDES Procedure performed more than one time per study
9.65 9.65 FUD XXX S Z2 80
AMA: 2018,Jan,8; 2017,Jan,8; 2016,Jan,13; 2015,Dec,11

78265 with small bowel transit
EXCLUDES Procedure performed more than one time per study
11.4 11.4 FUD XXX S Z2 80
AMA: 2018,Jan,8; 2017,Jan,8; 2015,Dec,11

78266 with small bowel and colon transit, multiple days
EXCLUDES Procedure performed more than one time per study
13.5 13.5 FUD XXX S Z2 80
AMA: 2018,Jan,8; 2017,Jan,8; 2015,Dec,11

78267 Urea breath test, C-14 (isotopic); acquisition for analysis
EXCLUDES Breath hydrogen/methane test (91065)
0.00 0.00 FUD XXX A
AMA: 2018,Jan,8; 2017,Jan,8; 2016,Jan,13; 2015,Jan,16; 2014,Jan,11

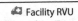

78268   analysis

EXCLUDES   *Breath hydrogen/methane test (91065)*

🚑 0.00   🔧 0.00   **FUD** XXX   [A][🖥]

AMA: 2018,Jan,8; 2017,Jan,8; 2016,Jan,13; 2015,Jan,16; 2014,Jan,11

78278   **Acute gastrointestinal blood loss imaging**

🚑 10.0   🔧 10.0   **FUD** XXX   [S][Z2][80][🖥]

AMA: 2012,Feb,9-10; 2007,Jan,28-31

78282   **Gastrointestinal protein loss**

🚑 0.00   🔧 0.00   **FUD** XXX   [S][Z2][80][🖥]

AMA: 2018,Jul,14

78290   **Intestine imaging (eg, ectopic gastric mucosa, Meckel's localization, volvulus)**

🚑 9.53   🔧 9.53   **FUD** XXX   [S][Z2][80][🖥]

AMA: 2012,Feb,9-10; 2007,Jan,28-31

78291   **Peritoneal-venous shunt patency test (eg, for LeVeen, Denver shunt)**

Code also (49427)

🚑 7.39   🔧 7.39   **FUD** XXX   [S][Z2][80][🖥]

AMA: 2012,Feb,9-10; 2007,Jan,28-31

78299   **Unlisted gastrointestinal procedure, diagnostic nuclear medicine**

🚑 0.00   🔧 0.00   **FUD** XXX   [S][Z2][80][🖥]

AMA: 2018,Jan,8; 2017,Jan,8; 2016,Jan,13; 2015,Jan,16; 2014,Jan,11

78300-78399 Nuclear Radiology: Bones and Joints

EXCLUDES   *Diagnostic services (see appropriate sections)*
Follow-up care (see appropriate section)
Code also radiopharmaceutical(s) and/or drug(s) supplied

78300   **Bone and/or joint imaging; limited area**

🚑 6.63   🔧 6.63   **FUD** XXX   [S][Z2][80][🖥]

AMA: 2018,Jan,8; 2017,Jan,8; 2016,Jan,13; 2015,Jan,16; 2014,Jan,11

78305   **multiple areas**

🚑 8.08   🔧 8.08   **FUD** XXX   [S][Z2][80][🖥]

AMA: 2018,Jan,8; 2017,Jan,8; 2016,Jan,13; 2015,Jan,16; 2014,Jan,11

78306   **whole body**

🚑 8.71   🔧 8.71   **FUD** XXX   [S][Z2][80][🖥]

AMA: 2018,Jan,8; 2017,Jan,8; 2016,Jan,13; 2015,Jan,16; 2014,Jan,11

78315   **3 phase study**

🚑 9.98   🔧 9.98   **FUD** XXX   [S][Z2][80][🖥]

AMA: 2018,Jan,8; 2017,Jan,8; 2016,Jan,13; 2015,Jan,16; 2014,Jan,11

78320   ~~tomographic (SPECT)~~

To report, see (78803)

78350   **Bone density (bone mineral content) study, 1 or more sites; single photon absorptiometry**

🚑 0.93   🔧 0.93   **FUD** XXX   [E][🖥]

AMA: 2012,Feb,9-10; 2007,Jan,28-31

78351   **dual photon absorptiometry, 1 or more sites**

🚑 0.44   🔧 0.44   **FUD** XXX   [E][🖥]

AMA: 2012,Feb,9-10; 2007,Jan,28-31

78399   **Unlisted musculoskeletal procedure, diagnostic nuclear medicine**

🚑 0.00   🔧 0.00   **FUD** XXX   [S][Z2][80][🖥]

AMA: 2018,Jan,8; 2017,Jan,8; 2016,Jan,13; 2015,Jan,16; 2014,Jan,11

78414-78499 [78429, 78430, 78431, 78432, 78433, 78434] Nuclear Radiology: Heart and Vascular

EXCLUDES   *Diagnostic services (see appropriate sections)*
Follow-up care (see appropriate section)
Code also radiopharmaceutical(s) and/or drug(s) supplied

78414   **Determination of central c-v hemodynamics (non-imaging) (eg, ejection fraction with probe technique) with or without pharmacologic intervention or exercise, single or multiple determinations**

🚑 0.00   🔧 0.00   **FUD** XXX   [S][Z2][80][🖥]

AMA: 2018,Jan,8; 2017,Jan,8; 2016,Jan,13; 2015,Jan,16; 2014,Jan,11

78428   **Cardiac shunt detection**

🚑 5.29   🔧 5.29   **FUD** XXX   [S][Z2][80][🖥]

AMA: 2018,Jan,8; 2017,Jan,8; 2016,Jan,13; 2015,Jan,16; 2014,Jan,11

78429   **Resequenced code. See code following 78459.**

78430   **Resequenced code. See code following 78491.**

78431   **Resequenced code. See code following 78492.**

78432   **Resequenced code. See code following 78492.**

78433   **Resequenced code. See code following 78492.**

78434   **Resequenced code. See code following 78492.**

78445   **Non-cardiac vascular flow imaging (ie, angiography, venography)**

🚑 5.38   🔧 5.38   **FUD** XXX   [S][Z2][80][🖥]

AMA: 2018,Jan,8; 2017,Jan,8; 2016,Jan,13; 2015,Jan,16; 2014,Jan,11

78451   **Myocardial perfusion imaging, tomographic (SPECT) (including attenuation correction, qualitative or quantitative wall motion, ejection fraction by first pass or gated technique, additional quantification, when performed); single study, at rest or stress (exercise or pharmacologic)**

EXCLUDES   *Distribution of radiopharmaceutical agents or tumor localization (78800-78802, [78804], 78803)*
Radiopharmaceutical quantification measurements ([78835])
SPECT with concurrently acquired CT transmission scan ([78830, 78831, 78832])

Code also stress testing when performed (93015-93018)

🚑 9.77   🔧 9.77   **FUD** XXX   [S][Z2][80][🖥]

AMA: 2018,Jan,8; 2017,Jan,8; 2016,Jan,13; 2015,Jan,16; 2014,Jan,11

78452   **multiple studies, at rest and/or stress (exercise or pharmacologic) and/or redistribution and/or rest reinjection**

EXCLUDES   *Distribution of radiopharmaceutical agents or tumor localization (78800-78802, [78804], 78803)*
Radiopharmaceutical quantification measurements ([78835])
SPECT with concurrently acquired CT transmission scan ([78830, 78831, 78832])

Code also stress testing when performed (93015-93018)

🚑 13.6   🔧 13.6   **FUD** XXX   [S][Z2][80][🖥]

AMA: 2018,Jan,8; 2017,Jan,8; 2016,Jan,13; 2015,Jan,16; 2014,Jan,11

78453   **Myocardial perfusion imaging, planar (including qualitative or quantitative wall motion, ejection fraction by first pass or gated technique, additional quantification, when performed); single study, at rest or stress (exercise or pharmacologic)**

Code also stress testing when performed (93015-93018)

🚑 8.78   🔧 8.78   **FUD** XXX   [S][Z2][80][🖥]

AMA: 2018,Jan,8; 2017,Jan,8; 2016,Jan,13; 2015,Jan,16; 2014,Jan,11

78454   multiple studies, at rest and/or stress (exercise or pharmacologic) and/or redistribution and/or rest reinjection

Code also stress testing when performed (93015-93018)

🔲 12.5   🔲 12.5   **FUD** XXX   S Z2 80 🔲

AMA: 2018,Jan,8; 2017,Jan,8; 2016,Jan,13; 2015,Jan,16; 2014,Jan,11

78456   **Acute venous thrombosis imaging, peptide**

🔲 8.93   🔲 8.93   **FUD** XXX   S Z2 🔲

AMA: 2018,Jan,8; 2017,Jan,8; 2016,Jan,13; 2015,Jan,16; 2014,Jan,11

78457   **Venous thrombosis imaging, venogram; unilateral**

🔲 5.52   🔲 5.52   **FUD** XXX   S Z2 80 🔲

AMA: 2018,Jan,8; 2017,Jan,8; 2016,Jan,13; 2015,Jan,16; 2014,Jan,11

78458   **bilateral**

🔲 5.92   🔲 5.92   **FUD** XXX   S Z2 80 🔲

AMA: 2018,Jan,8; 2017,Jan,8; 2016,Jan,13; 2015,Jan,16; 2014,Jan,11

▲ **78459**   **Myocardial imaging, positron emission tomography (PET), metabolic evaluation study (including ventricular wall motion[s] and/or ejection fraction[s], when performed), single study;**

INCLUDES   Examination of CT transmission images for field of view anatomy review

EXCLUDES   CT coronary calcium scoring (75571)

CT for other than attenuation correction/anatomical localization; use site-specific CT code with modifier 59

Myocardial perfusion studies (78491-78492)

🔲 0.00   🔲 0.00   **FUD** XXX   S Z2 80 🔲

AMA: 2018,Jan,8; 2017,Jan,8; 2016,Jan,13; 2015,Jan,16; 2014,Jan,11

● # **78429**   **with concurrently acquired computed tomography transmission scan**

🔲 0.00   🔲 0.00   **FUD** 000

INCLUDES   Examination of CT transmission images for field of view anatomy review

EXCLUDES   CT coronary calcium scoring (75571)

CT for other than attenuation correction/anatomical localization; use site-specific CT code with modifier 59

78466   **Myocardial imaging, infarct avid, planar; qualitative or quantitative**

🔲 5.67   🔲 5.67   **FUD** XXX   S Z2 80 🔲

AMA: 2012,Feb,9-10; 2010,May,5-6

78468   **with ejection fraction by first pass technique**

🔲 5.88   🔲 5.88   **FUD** XXX   S Z2 80 🔲

AMA: 2018,Jan,8; 2017,Jan,8; 2016,Jan,13; 2015,Jan,16; 2014,Jan,11

78469   **tomographic SPECT with or without quantification**

EXCLUDES   Distribution of radiopharmaceutical agents or tumor localization (78800-78802, [78804], 78803)

Myocardial sympathetic innervation imaging (0331T-0332T)

Radiopharmaceutical quantification measurements ([78835])

SPECT with concurrently acquired CT transmission scan ([78830, 78831, 78832])

🔲 6.50   🔲 6.50   **FUD** XXX   S Z2 80 🔲

AMA: 2018,Nov,11; 2018,Jan,8; 2017,Jan,8; 2016,Jan,13; 2015,Jan,16; 2014,Jan,11

78472   **Cardiac blood pool imaging, gated equilibrium; planar, single study at rest or stress (exercise and/or pharmacologic), wall motion study plus ejection fraction, with or without additional quantitative processing**

EXCLUDES   Cardiac blood pool imaging (78481, 78483, 78494)

Myocardial perfusion imaging (78451-78454)

Right ventricular ejection fraction by first pass technique (78496)

Code also stress testing when performed (93015-93018)

🔲 6.59   🔲 6.59   **FUD** XXX   S Z2 80 🔲

AMA: 2018,Jan,8; 2017,Jan,8; 2016,Jan,13; 2015,Jan,16; 2014,Jan,11

78473   **multiple studies, wall motion study plus ejection fraction, at rest and stress (exercise and/or pharmacologic), with or without additional quantification**

EXCLUDES   Cardiac blood pool imaging (78481, 78483, 78494)

Myocardial perfusion imaging (78451-78454)

Code also stress testing when performed (93015-93018)

🔲 8.32   🔲 8.32   **FUD** XXX   S Z2 80 🔲

AMA: 2018,Jan,8; 2017,Jan,8; 2016,Jan,13; 2015,Jan,16; 2014,Jan,11

78481   **Cardiac blood pool imaging (planar), first pass technique; single study, at rest or with stress (exercise and/or pharmacologic), wall motion study plus ejection fraction, with or without quantification**

EXCLUDES   Myocardial perfusion imaging (78451-78454)

Code also stress testing when performed (93015-93018)

🔲 5.06   🔲 5.06   **FUD** XXX   S Z2 80 🔲

AMA: 2018,Jan,8; 2017,Jan,8; 2016,Jan,13; 2015,Jan,16; 2014,Jan,11

78483   **multiple studies, at rest and with stress (exercise and/or pharmacologic), wall motion study plus ejection fraction, with or without quantification**

EXCLUDES   Blood flow studies of the brain (78610)

Myocardial perfusion imaging (78451-78454)

Code also stress testing when performed (93015-93018)

🔲 6.83   🔲 6.83   **FUD** XXX   S Z2 80 🔲

AMA: 2018,Jan,8; 2017,Jan,8; 2016,Jan,13; 2015,Jan,16; 2014,Jan,11

▲ **78491**   **Myocardial imaging, positron emission tomography (PET), perfusion study (including ventricular wall motion[s] and/or ejection fraction[s], when performed); single study, at rest or stress (exercise or pharmacologic)**

Code also stress testing when performed (93015-93018)

🔲 0.00   🔲 0.00   **FUD** XXX   S Z2 80 🔲

AMA: 2018,Jan,8; 2017,Jan,8; 2016,Jan,13; 2015,Jan,16; 2014,Jan,11

● # **78430**   **single study, at rest or stress (exercise or pharmacologic), with concurrently acquired computed tomography transmission scan**

🔲 0.00   🔲 0.00   **FUD** 000

INCLUDES   Examination of CT transmission images for field of view anatomy review

Code also stress testing when performed (93015-93018)

▲ **78492**   **multiple studies at rest and stress (exercise or pharmacologic)**

Code also stress testing when performed (93015-93018)

🔲 0.00   🔲 0.00   **FUD** XXX   S Z2 80 🔲

AMA: 2018,Jan,8; 2017,Jan,8; 2016,Jan,13; 2015,Jan,16; 2014,Jan,11

● # **78431**   **multiple studies at rest and stress (exercise or pharmacologic), with concurrently acquired computed tomography transmission scan**

🔲 0.00   🔲 0.00   **FUD** 000

INCLUDES   Examination of CT transmission images for field of view anatomy review

Code also stress testing when performed (93015-93018)

26/TC PC/TC Only   A2-Z3 ASC Payment   50 Bilateral   ♂ Male Only   ♀ Female Only   🔲 Facility RVU   🔲 Non-Facility RVU   🔲 CCI   ☒ CLIA

FUD Follow-up Days   CMS: IOM   AMA: CPT Asst   A-Y OPPSI   80/80 Surg Assist Allowed / w/Doc   🔲 Lab Crosswalk   🔲 Radiology Crosswalk

366   CPT © 2019 American Medical Association. All Rights Reserved.   © 2019 Optum360, LLC

● # **78432** **Myocardial imaging, positron emission tomography (PET), combined perfusion with metabolic evaluation study (including ventricular wall motion[s] and/or ejection fraction[s], when performed), dual radiotracer (eg, myocardial viability);**

🚑 0.00   ⚕ 0.00   **FUD** 000

Code also stress testing when performed (93015-93018)

● # **78433** **with concurrently acquired computed tomography transmission scan**

🚑 0.00   ⚕ 0.00   **FUD** 000

INCLUDES Examination of CT transmission images for field of view anatomy review

EXCLUDES CT for other than attenuation correction/anatomical localization; use site-specific CT code with modifier 59

Code also stress testing when performed (93015-93018)

● + # **78434** **Absolute quantitation of myocardial blood flow (AQMBF), positron emission tomography (PET), rest and pharmacologic stress (List separately in addition to code for primary procedure)**

🚑 0.00   ⚕ 0.00   **FUD** 000

EXCLUDES CT coronary calcium scoring (75571)
Myocardial imaging by planar or SPECT (78451-78454)
Code first ([78431], 78492)

78494 **Cardiac blood pool imaging, gated equilibrium, SPECT, at rest, wall motion study plus ejection fraction, with or without quantitative processing**

EXCLUDES Distribution of radiopharmaceutical agents or tumor localization (78800-78802, [78804], 78803)
Radiopharmaceutical quantification measurements ([78835])
SPECT with concurrently acquired CT transmission scan ([78830, 78831, 78832])

🚑 6.51   ⚕ 6.51   **FUD** XXX   S Z2 80 ▣

AMA: 2018,Jan,8; 2017,Jan,8; 2016,Jan,13; 2015,Jan,16; 2014,Jan,11

+ **78496** **Cardiac blood pool imaging, gated equilibrium, single study, at rest, with right ventricular ejection fraction by first pass technique (List separately in addition to code for primary procedure)**

Code first (78472)

🚑 1.25   ⚕ 1.25   **FUD** ZZZ   N N1 80 ▣

AMA: 2018,Jan,8; 2017,Jan,8; 2016,Jan,13; 2015,Jan,16; 2014,Jan,11

78499 **Unlisted cardiovascular procedure, diagnostic nuclear medicine**

🚑 0.00   ⚕ 0.00   **FUD** XXX   S Z2 80 ▣

AMA: 2018,Jan,8; 2017,Jan,8; 2016,Jan,13; 2015,Jan,16; 2014,Jan,11

78579-78599 Nuclear Radiology: Lungs

EXCLUDES Diagnostic services (see appropriate sections)
Follow-up care (see appropriate sections)
Code also radiopharmaceutical(s) and/or drug(s) supplied

78579 **Pulmonary ventilation imaging (eg, aerosol or gas)**

EXCLUDES Procedure performed more than one time per imaging session

🚑 5.36   ⚕ 5.36   **FUD** XXX   S Z2 80 ▣

AMA: 2012,Feb,9-10

78580 **Pulmonary perfusion imaging (eg, particulate)**

EXCLUDES Myocardial perfusion imaging (78451-78454)
Procedure performed more than one time per imaging session

🚑 6.87   ⚕ 6.87   **FUD** XXX   S Z2 80 ▣

AMA: 2018,Jan,8; 2017,Jan,8; 2016,Jan,13; 2015,Jan,16; 2014,Jan,11

78582 **Pulmonary ventilation (eg, aerosol or gas) and perfusion imaging**

EXCLUDES Myocardial perfusion imaging (78451-78454)
Procedure performed more than one time per imaging session

🚑 9.64   ⚕ 9.64   **FUD** XXX   S Z2 80 ▣

AMA: 2012,Feb,9-10

78597 **Quantitative differential pulmonary perfusion, including imaging when performed**

EXCLUDES Myocardial perfusion imaging (78451-78454)
Procedure performed more than one time per imaging session

🚑 5.79   ⚕ 5.79   **FUD** XXX   S Z2 80 ▣

AMA: 2012,Feb,9-10

78598 **Quantitative differential pulmonary perfusion and ventilation (eg, aerosol or gas), including imaging when performed**

EXCLUDES Myocardial perfusion imaging (78451-78454)
Procedure performed more than one time per imaging session

🚑 8.80   ⚕ 8.80   **FUD** XXX   S Z2 80 ▣

AMA: 2012,Feb,9-10

78599 **Unlisted respiratory procedure, diagnostic nuclear medicine**

🚑 0.00   ⚕ 0.00   **FUD** XXX   S Z2 80 ▣

AMA: 2018,Jan,8; 2017,Jan,8; 2016,Jan,13; 2015,Jan,16; 2014,Jan,11

78600-78650 Nuclear Radiology: Brain/Cerebrospinal Fluid

EXCLUDES Diagnostic services (see appropriate sections)
Follow-up care (see appropriate section)
Code also radiopharmaceutical(s) and/or drug(s) supplied

78600 **Brain imaging, less than 4 static views;**

🚑 5.32   ⚕ 5.32   **FUD** XXX   S Z2 80 ▣

AMA: 2018,Jan,8; 2017,Jan,8; 2016,Jan,13; 2015,Jan,16; 2014,Jan,11

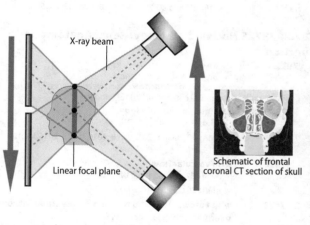

X-ray beam

Linear focal plane

Schematic of frontal coronal CT section of skull

78601 **with vascular flow**

🚑 6.25   ⚕ 6.25   **FUD** XXX   S Z2 80 ▣

AMA: 2012,Feb,9-10; 2007,Jan,28-31

78605 **Brain imaging, minimum 4 static views;**

🚑 5.74   ⚕ 5.74   **FUD** XXX   S Z2 80 ▣

AMA: 2012,Feb,9-10; 2007,Jan,28-31

78606 **with vascular flow**

🚑 9.50   ⚕ 9.50   **FUD** XXX   S Z2 80 ▣

AMA: 2012,Feb,9-10; 2007,Jan,28-31

~~78607~~ **~~Brain imaging, tomographic (SPECT)~~**

To report, see (78803)

78608 **Brain imaging, positron emission tomography (PET); metabolic evaluation**

🚑 0.00   ⚕ 0.00   **FUD** XXX   S Z2 80 ▣

AMA: 2012,Feb,9-10; 2007,Jan,28-31

78609 perfusion evaluation
2.12 — 2.12 **FUD** XXX E
AMA: 2012,Feb,9-10; 2007,Jan,28-31

78610 Brain imaging, vascular flow only
5.04 — 5.04 **FUD** XXX S Z2 80
AMA: 2012,Feb,9-10; 2007,Jan,28-31

78630 Cerebrospinal fluid flow, imaging (not including introduction of material); cisternography
Code also injection procedure (61000-61070, 62270-62327)
9.74 — 9.74 **FUD** XXX S Z2 80
AMA: 2018,Jan,8

78635 ventriculography
Code also injection procedure (61000-61070, 62270-62294)
9.77 — 9.77 **FUD** XXX S Z2 80
AMA: 2012,Feb,9-10; 2007,Jan,28-31

78645 shunt evaluation
Code also injection procedure (61000-61070, 62270-62294)
9.37 — 9.37 **FUD** XXX S Z2 80
AMA: 2012,Feb,9-10; 2007,Jan,28-31

78647 tomographic (SPECT)
To report, see (78803)

78650 Cerebrospinal fluid leakage detection and localization
Code also injection procedure (61000-61070, 62270-62294)
7.89 — 7.89 **FUD** XXX S Z2 80
AMA: 2012,Feb,9-10; 2007,Jan,28-31

78660-78699 Nuclear Radiology: Lacrimal Duct System
Code also radiopharmaceutical(s) and/or drug(s) supplied

78660 Radiopharmaceutical dacryocystography
5.26 — 5.26 **FUD** XXX S Z2 80
AMA: 2012,Feb,9-10; 2007,Jan,28-31

78699 Unlisted nervous system procedure, diagnostic nuclear medicine
0.00 — 0.00 **FUD** XXX S Z2 80
AMA: 2018,Jan,8; 2017,Jan,8; 2016,Jan,13; 2015,Jan,16; 2014,Jan,11

78700-78725 Nuclear Radiology: Renal Anatomy and Function
EXCLUDES Diagnostic services (see appropriate sections)
Follow-up care (see appropriate section)
Renal endoscopy with insertion of radioactive substances (77778)
Code also radiopharmaceutical(s) and/or drug(s) supplied

78700 Kidney imaging morphology;
4.92 — 4.92 **FUD** XXX S Z2 80
AMA: 2018,Jan,8; 2017,Jan,8; 2016,Jan,13; 2015,Jan,16; 2014,Jan,11

78701 with vascular flow
6.26 — 6.26 **FUD** XXX S Z2 80
AMA: 2012,Feb,9-10; 2007,Mar,7-8

78707 with vascular flow and function, single study without pharmacological intervention
6.69 — 6.69 **FUD** XXX S Z2 80
AMA: 2018,Jan,8; 2017,Jan,8; 2016,Jan,13; 2015,Jan,16; 2014,Jan,11

78708 with vascular flow and function, single study, with pharmacological intervention (eg, angiotensin converting enzyme inhibitor and/or diuretic)
5.09 — 5.09 **FUD** XXX S Z2 80
AMA: 2018,Jan,8; 2017,Jan,8; 2016,Jan,13; 2015,Jan,16; 2014,Jan,11

78709 with vascular flow and function, multiple studies, with and without pharmacological intervention (eg, angiotensin converting enzyme inhibitor and/or diuretic)
10.6 — 10.6 **FUD** XXX S Z2 80
AMA: 2018,Jan,8; 2017,Jan,8; 2016,Jan,13; 2015,Jan,16; 2014,Jan,11

78710 tomographic (SPECT)
To report, see (78803)

78725 Kidney function study, non-imaging radioisotopic study
3.11 — 3.11 **FUD** XXX S Z2 80
AMA: 2012,Feb,9-10; 2007,Jan,28-31

78730-78799 Nuclear Radiology: Urogenital
EXCLUDES Diagnostic services (see appropriate sections)
Follow-up care (see appropriate section)
Code also radiopharmaceutical(s) and/or drug(s) supplied

+ **78730** Urinary bladder residual study (List separately in addition to code for primary procedure)
EXCLUDES Measurement of postvoid residual urine and/or bladder capacity using ultrasound (51798)
Ultrasound imaging of the bladder only with measurement of postvoid residual urine (76857)
Code first (78740)
2.22 — 2.22 **FUD** ZZZ N N1 80
AMA: 2018,Jan,8; 2017,Jan,8; 2016,Jan,13; 2015,Jan,16; 2014,Jan,11

78740 Ureteral reflux study (radiopharmaceutical voiding cystogram)
EXCLUDES Catheterization (51701-51703)
Code also urinary bladder residual study (78730)
6.29 — 6.29 **FUD** XXX S Z2 80
AMA: 2012,Feb,9-10; 2007,Jan,28-31

78761 Testicular imaging with vascular flow ♂
6.08 — 6.08 **FUD** XXX S Z2 80
AMA: 2018,Jan,8; 2017,Jan,8; 2016,Jan,13; 2015,Jan,16; 2014,Jan,11

78799 Unlisted genitourinary procedure, diagnostic nuclear medicine
0.00 — 0.00 **FUD** XXX S Z2 80
AMA: 2018,Jan,8; 2017,Jan,8; 2016,Jan,13; 2015,Jan,16; 2014,Jan,11

78800-78835 [78804, 78830, 78831, 78832, 78835] Nuclear Radiology: Tumor Localization
EXCLUDES CSF studies requiring injection procedure (61055, 61070, 62320-62323)
Code also radiopharmaceutical(s) and/or drug(s) supplied

▲ **78800** Radiopharmaceutical localization of tumor, inflammatory process or distribution of radiopharmaceutical agent(s) (includes vascular flow and blood pool imaging, when performed); planar, single area (eg, head, neck, chest, pelvis), single day imaging
INCLUDES Ocular radiophosphorus tumor identification
EXCLUDES Specific organ (see appropriate site)
5.61 — 5.61 **FUD** XXX S Z2 80
AMA: 2018,Nov,11; 2018,Jan,8; 2017,Jan,8; 2016,Jan,13; 2015,Jan,16; 2014,Jan,11

▲ **78801** planar, 2 or more areas (eg, abdomen and pelvis, head and chest), 1 or more days imaging or single area imaging over 2 or more days
7.42 — 7.42 **FUD** XXX S Z2 80
AMA: 2018,Jan,8; 2017,Jan,8; 2016,Jan,13; 2015,Jan,16; 2014,Jan,11

▲ **78802** planar, whole body, single day imaging
9.29 — 9.29 **FUD** XXX S Z2 80
AMA: 2012,Feb,9-10; 2007,Jan,28-31

▲ # **78804** planar, whole body, requiring 2 or more days imaging
16.3 — 16.3 **FUD** XXX S Z2 80
AMA: 2012,Feb,9-10; 2007,Jan,28-31

▲ **78803** tomographic (SPECT), single area (eg, head, neck, chest, pelvis), single day imaging
9.81 — 9.81 **FUD** XXX S Z2 80
AMA: 2018,Nov,11; 2018,Jan,8; 2017,Jan,8; 2016,Dec,9; 2016,Dec,16; 2016,Jan,13; 2015,Oct,9

78804 Resequenced code. See code following 78802.

 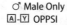

~~**78805**~~ ~~Radiopharmaceutical localization of inflammatory process; limited area~~

> To report, see (78300, 78305-78306, 78315, 78800-78803, 78830-78832)

~~**78806**~~ ~~whole body~~

> To report, see (78300, 78305-78306, 78315, 78800-78803, 78830-78832)

~~**78807**~~ ~~tomographic (SPECT)~~

> To report, see (78300, 78305-78306, 78315, 78800-78803, 78830-78832)

● # **78830** **tomographic (SPECT) with concurrently acquired computed tomography (CT) transmission scan for anatomical review, localization and determination/detection of pathology, single area (eg, head, neck, chest, pelvis), single day imaging**
  📷 0.00   ⚕ 0.00   **FUD** 000

● # **78831** **tomographic (SPECT), minimum 2 areas (eg, pelvis and knees, abdomen and pelvis), single day imaging, or single area imaging over 2 or more days**
  📷 0.00   ⚕ 0.00   **FUD** 000

● # **78832** **tomographic (SPECT) with concurrently acquired computed tomography (CT) transmission scan for anatomical review, localization and determination/detection of pathology, minimum 2 areas (eg, pelvis and knees, abdomen and pelvis), single day imaging, or single area imaging over 2 or more days**
  📷 0.00   ⚕ 0.00   **FUD** 000

● + # **78835** **Radiopharmaceutical quantification measurement(s) single area (List separately in addition to code for primary procedure)**
  📷 0.00   ⚕ 0.00   **FUD** 000

78808 Intravenous Injection for Radiopharmaceutical Localization

Code also radiopharmaceutical(s) and/or drug(s) supplied

78808 **Injection procedure for radiopharmaceutical localization by non-imaging probe study, intravenous (eg, parathyroid adenoma)**
  📷 1.12   ⚕ 1.12   **FUD** XXX   [Q1] [N1] [80] [▭]
  AMA: 2018,Jan,8; 2017,Jan,8; 2016,Dec,9

78811-78999 Nuclear Radiology: Diagnosis, Staging, Restaging or Monitoring Cancer

CMS: 100-03,220.6.17 Positron Emission Tomography (FDG) for Oncologic Conditions; 100-03,220.6.19 NaF-18 PET to Identify Bone Metastasis of Cancer; 100-03,220.6.9 FDG PET for Refractory Seizures; 100-04,13,60 Positron Emission Tomography (PET) Scans - General Information; 100-04,13,60.13 Billing for PET Scans for Specific Indications of Cervical Cancer; 100-04,13,60.15 Billing for CMS-Approved Clinical Trials for PET Scans; 100-04,13,60.16 Billing and Coverage for PET Scans; 100-04,13,60.17 Billing and Coverage Changes for PET Scans for Cervical Cancer; 100-04,13,60.18 Billing and Coverage for PET (NaF-18) Scans to Identify Bone Metastasis; 100-04,13,60.2 Use of Gamma Cameras, Full and Partial Ring PET Scanners; 100-04,13,60.3 PET Scan Qualifying Conditions; 100-04,13,60.3.1 Appropriate Codes for PET Scans; 100-04,13,60.3.2 Tracer Codes Required for Positron Emission Tomography (PET) Scans

> EXCLUDES   CT scan performed for other than attenuation correction and anatomical localization (report with the appropriate site-specific CT code and modifier 59)
> Ocular radiophosphorus tumor identification (78800)
> PET brain scan (78608-78609)
> PET myocardial imaging (78459, 78491-78492)
> Procedure performed more than one time per imaging session

Code also radiopharmaceutical(s) and/or drug(s) supplied

78811 **Positron emission tomography (PET) imaging; limited area (eg, chest, head/neck)**
  📷 0.00   ⚕ 0.00   **FUD** XXX   [S] [Z2] [80] [▭]
  AMA: 2018,Jan,8; 2017,Jan,8; 2016,Jan,13; 2015,Jan,16; 2014,Jan,11

78812 **skull base to mid-thigh**
  📷 0.00   ⚕ 0.00   **FUD** XXX   [S] [Z2] [80] [▭]
  AMA: 2018,Jan,8; 2017,Jan,8; 2016,Jan,13; 2015,Jan,16; 2014,Jan,11

78813 **whole body**
  📷 0.00   ⚕ 0.00   **FUD** XXX   [S] [Z2] [80] [▭]
  AMA: 2018,Jan,8; 2017,Jan,8; 2016,Jan,13; 2015,Jan,16; 2014,Jan,11

78814 **Positron emission tomography (PET) with concurrently acquired computed tomography (CT) for attenuation correction and anatomical localization imaging; limited area (eg, chest, head/neck)**
  📷 0.00   ⚕ 0.00   **FUD** XXX   [S] [Z2] [80] [▭]
  AMA: 2018,Jan,8; 2017,Jan,8; 2016,Jan,13; 2015,Jan,16; 2014,Jan,11

78815 **skull base to mid-thigh**
  📷 0.00   ⚕ 0.00   **FUD** XXX   [S] [Z2] [80] [▭]
  AMA: 2018,Jan,8; 2017,Jan,8; 2016,Jan,13; 2015,Jan,16; 2014,Jan,11

78816 **whole body**
  📷 0.00   ⚕ 0.00   **FUD** XXX   [S] [Z2] [80] [▭]
  AMA: 2018,Jan,8; 2017,Jan,8; 2016,Jan,13; 2015,Jan,16; 2014,Jan,11

78830 Resequenced code. See code following resequenced numeric code 78804.

78831 Resequenced code. See code following resequenced numeric code 78804.

78832 Resequenced code. See code following resequenced numeric code 78804.

78835 Resequenced code. See code following resequenced numeric code 78804.

78999 **Unlisted miscellaneous procedure, diagnostic nuclear medicine**
  📷 0.00   ⚕ 0.00   **FUD** XXX   [S] [Z2] [80] [▭]
  AMA: 2018,Jan,8; 2017,Jan,8; 2016,Dec,9; 2016,Dec,16; 2016,Jan,13; 2015,Oct,9; 2015,Jan,16; 2014,Jan,11

79005-79999 Systemic Radiopharmaceutical Therapy

> EXCLUDES   Imaging guidance
> Injection into artery, body cavity, or joint (see appropriate injection codes)
> Radiological supervision and interpretation

79005 **Radiopharmaceutical therapy, by oral administration**
  > EXCLUDES   Monoclonal antibody treatment (79403)
  📷 3.91   ⚕ 3.91   **FUD** XXX   [S] [Z3] [80] [▭]
  AMA: 2018,Jan,8; 2017,Jan,8; 2016,Jan,13; 2015,Jan,16; 2014,Jan,11

79101 **Radiopharmaceutical therapy, by intravenous administration**
  > EXCLUDES   Administration of nonantibody radioelement solution including follow-up care (77750)
  > Hydration infusion (96360)
  > Intravenous injection, IV push (96374-96375, 96409)
  > Radiolabeled monoclonal antibody IV infusion (79403)
  > Venipuncture (36400, 36410)
  📷 4.18   ⚕ 4.18   **FUD** XXX   [S] [Z3] [80] [▭]
  AMA: 2018,Jan,8; 2017,Jan,8; 2016,Jan,13; 2015,Jan,16; 2014,Jan,11

79200 **Radiopharmaceutical therapy, by intracavitary administration**
  📷 3.83   ⚕ 3.83   **FUD** XXX   [S] [Z3] [80] [▭]
  AMA: 2018,Jan,8; 2017,Jan,8; 2016,Jan,13; 2015,Jan,16; 2014,Jan,11

79300 **Radiopharmaceutical therapy, by interstitial radioactive colloid administration**
  📷 0.00   ⚕ 0.00   **FUD** XXX   [S] [Z2] [80] [▭]
  AMA: 2018,Jan,8; 2017,Jan,8; 2016,Jan,13; 2015,Jan,16; 2014,Jan,11

● New Code   ▲ Revised Code   ○ Reinstated   ● New Web Release   ▲ Revised Web Release   + Add-on   Unlisted   Not Covered   # Resequenced
㊿ Optum Mod 50 Exempt   Ⓝ AMA Mod 51 Exempt   ⑤ Optum Mod 51 Exempt   ⑥ Mod 63 Exempt   ⩊ Non-FDA Drug   ★ Telemedicine   Ⓜ Maternity   Ⓐ Age Edit

CPT © 2019 American Medical Association. All Rights Reserved.

79403   Radiopharmaceutical therapy, radiolabeled monoclonal antibody by intravenous infusion

    EXCLUDES *Intravenous radiopharmaceutical therapy (79101)*

    🚗 5.44   ⚖ 5.44   **FUD** XXX   S Z3 80 🖳

    AMA: 2018,Jan,8; 2017,Jan,8; 2016,Jan,13; 2015,Jan,16; 2014,Jan,11

79440   Radiopharmaceutical therapy, by intra-articular administration

    🚗 3.45   ⚖ 3.45   **FUD** XXX   S Z3 80 🖳

    AMA: 2018,Jan,8; 2017,Jan,8; 2016,Jan,13; 2015,Jan,16; 2014,Jan,11

79445   Radiopharmaceutical therapy, by intra-arterial particulate administration

    EXCLUDES *Intra-arterial injections (96373, 96420)*

               Procedural and radiological supervision and interpretation for angiographic and interventional procedures before intra-arterial radiopharmaceutical therapy

    🚗 0.00   ⚖ 0.00   **FUD** XXX   S Z2 80 🖳

    AMA: 2018,Jan,8; 2017,Jan,8; 2016,Jan,13; 2015,Jan,16; 2014,Jan,11

79999   Radiopharmaceutical therapy, unlisted procedure

    🚗 0.00   ⚖ 0.00   **FUD** XXX   S Z2 80 🖳

    AMA: 2018,Jan,8; 2017,Jan,8; 2016,Jan,13; 2015,Jan,16; 2014,Jan,11

26/TC PC/TC Only   A2-Z3 ASC Payment   50 Bilateral   ♂ Male Only   ♀ Female Only   🚗 Facility RVU   ⚖ Non-Facility RVU   🖳 CCI   ✖ CLIA

FUD Follow-up Days   **CMS:** IOM   **AMA:** CPT Asst   A-Y OPPSI   80/80 Surg Assist Allowed / w/Doc   🔲 Lab Crosswalk   🔲 Radiology Crosswalk

370   CPT © 2019 American Medical Association. All Rights Reserved.   © 2019 Optum360, LLC

80047-80081 [80081] Multi-test Laboratory Panels

INCLUDES Groups of specified tests that may be reported as a panel

EXCLUDES *Reporting two or more panel codes that include the same tests; report the panel with the highest number of tests in common to meet the definition of the panel code*

Code also individual tests that are not part of the panel, when appropriate

80047 Basic metabolic panel (Calcium, ionized)

INCLUDES Calcium, ionized (82330)
Carbon dioxide (bicarbonate) (82374)
Chloride (82435)
Creatinine (82565)
Glucose (82947)
Potassium (84132)
Sodium (84295)
Urea nitrogen (BUN) (84520)

🚑 0.00   ✂ 0.00   **FUD** XXX   ☒ ⓠ ▭

AMA: 2018,Jan,8; 2017,Jan,8; 2016,Jan,13; 2015,Jan,16; 2014,Jan,11

80048 Basic metabolic panel (Calcium, total)

INCLUDES Calcium, total (82310)
Carbon dioxide (bicarbonate) (82374)
Chloride (82435)
Creatinine (82565)
Glucose (82947)
Potassium (84132)
Sodium (84295)
Urea nitrogen (BUN) (84520)

🚑 0.00   ✂ 0.00   **FUD** XXX   ☒ ⓠ ▭

AMA: 2018,Jan,8; 2017,Jan,8; 2016,Jan,13; 2015,Jan,16; 2014,Jan,11

80050 General health panel

INCLUDES Complete blood count (CBC), automated, with:
Manual differential WBC count
Blood smear with manual differential AND complete (CBC), automated (85007, 85027)
Manual differential WBC count, buffy coat AND complete (CBC), automated (85009, 85027)
OR
Automated differential WBC count
Automated differential WBC count AND complete (CBC), automated/automated differential WBC count (85004, 85025)
Automated differential WBC count AND complete (CBC), automated (85004, 85027)
Comprehensive metabolic profile (80053)
Thyroid stimulating hormone (84443)

🚑 0.00   ✂ 0.00   **FUD** XXX   Ⓔ ▭

AMA: 2018,Jan,8; 2017,Jan,8; 2016,Jan,13; 2015,Jan,16; 2014,Jan,11

80051 Electrolyte panel

INCLUDES Carbon dioxide (bicarbonate) (82374)
Chloride (82435)
Potassium (84132)
Sodium (84295)

🚑 0.00   ✂ 0.00   **FUD** XXX   ☒ ⓠ ▭

AMA: 2018,Jan,8; 2017,Jan,8; 2016,Jan,13; 2015,Jan,16; 2014,Jan,11

80053 Comprehensive metabolic panel

INCLUDES Albumin (82040)
Bilirubin, total (82247)
Calcium, total (82310)
Carbon dioxide (bicarbonate) (82374)
Chloride (82435)
Creatinine (82565)
Glucose (82947)
Phosphatase, alkaline (84075)
Potassium (84132)
Protein, total (84155)
Sodium (84295)
Transferase, alanine amino (ALT) (SGPT) (84460)
Transferase, aspartate amino (AST) (SGOT) (84450)
Urea nitrogen (BUN) (84520)

🚑 0.00   ✂ 0.00   **FUD** XXX   ☒ ⓠ ▭

AMA: 2018,Jan,8; 2017,Jan,8; 2016,Jan,13; 2015,Jan,16; 2014,Jan,11

80055 Obstetric panel Ⓜ ♀

INCLUDES Complete blood count (CBC), automated, with:
Manual differential WBC count
Blood smear with manual differential AND complete (CBC), automated (85007, 85027)
Manual differential WBC count, buffy coat AND complete (CBC), automated (85009, 85027)
OR
Automated differential WBC count
Automated differential WBC count AND complete (CBC), automated/automated differential WBC count (85004, 85025)
Automated differential WBC count AND complete (CBC), automated (85004, 85027)
Blood typing, ABO and Rh (86900-86901)
Hepatitis B surface antigen (HBsAg) (87340)
RBC antibody screen, each serum technique (86850)
Rubella antibody (86762)
Syphilis test, non-treponemal antibody qualitative (86592)

EXCLUDES *Use of code when syphilis screening is provided using a treponemal antibody approach. Instead, assign individual codes for tests performed in the OB panel (86780)*

🚑 0.00   ✂ 0.00   **FUD** XXX   ⓠ ▭

AMA: 2018,Jan,8; 2017,Jan,8; 2016,Jan,13; 2015,Jan,16; 2014,Jan,11

80081 Obstetric panel (includes HIV testing) Ⓜ ♀

INCLUDES Complete blood count (CBC), automated, with:
Manual differential WBC count
Blood smear with manual differential AND complete (CBC), automated (85007, 85027)
Manual differential WBC count, buffy count AND complete (CBC), automated (85009, 85027)
OR
Automated differential WBC count
Automated differential WBC count AND complete (CBC), automated/automated differential WBC count (85004, 85025)
Automated differential WBC count AND complete (CBC), automated (85004, 85027)
Blood typing, ABO and Rh (86900-86901)
Hepatitis B surface antigen (HBsAg) (87340)
HIV-1 antigens, with HIV-1 and HIV-2 antibodies, single result (87389)
RBC antibody screen, each serum technique (86850)
Rubella antibody (86762)
Syphilis test, non-treponemal antibody qualitative (86592)

EXCLUDES *Use of code when syphilis screening is provided using a treponemal antibody approach. Instead, assign individual codes for tests performed in the OB panel (86780)*

🚑 0.00   ✂ 0.00   **FUD** XXX   ⓠ ▭

AMA: 2018,Jan,8; 2017,Jan,8; 2016,Jan,13

● New Code   ▲ Revised Code   ○ Reinstated   ● New Web Release   ▲ Revised Web Release   + Add-on   Unlisted   Not Covered   # Resequenced
㊿ Optum Mod 50 Exempt   ⊘ AMA Mod 51 Exempt   ㋼ Optum Mod 51 Exempt   ㊿ Mod 63 Exempt   ✗ Non-FDA Drug   ★ Telemedicine   Ⓜ Maternity   Ⓐ Age Edit

CPT © 2019 American Medical Association. All Rights Reserved.

80061	**Lipid panel**
	INCLUDES
	Cholesterol, serum, total (82465)
	Lipoprotein, direct measurement, high density cholesterol (HDL cholesterol) (83718)
	Triglycerides (84478)

🖐 0.00 ⚕ 0.00 **FUD** XXX ☒ Ⓐ ▱

AMA: 2018,Jan,8; 2017,Sep,11; 2017,Jan,8; 2016,Jan,13; 2015,Jan,16; 2014,Jan,11

80069 Renal function panel

INCLUDES
Albumin (82040)
Calcium, total (82310)
Carbon dioxide (bicarbonate) (82374)
Chloride (82435)
Creatinine (82565)
Glucose (82947)
Phosphorus inorganic (phosphate) (84100)
Potassium (84132)
Sodium (84295)
Urea nitrogen (BUN) (84520)

🖐 0.00 ⚕ 0.00 **FUD** XXX ☒ Ⓠ ▱

AMA: 2018,Jan,8; 2017,Jan,8; 2016,Jan,13; 2015,Jan,16; 2014,Jan,11

80074 Acute hepatitis panel

INCLUDES
Hepatitis A antibody (HAAb) IgM (86709)
Hepatitis B core antibody (HBcAb), IgM (86705)
Hepatitis B surface antigen (HBsAg) (87340)
Hepatitis C antibody (86803)

🖐 0.00 ⚕ 0.00 **FUD** XXX Ⓠ ▱

AMA: 2018,Jan,8; 2017,Jan,8; 2016,Jan,13; 2015,Jan,16; 2014,Jan,11

80076 Hepatic function panel

INCLUDES
Albumin (82040)
Bilirubin, direct (82248)
Bilirubin, total (82247)
Phosphatase, alkaline (84075)
Protein, total (84155)
Transferase, alanine amino (ALT) (SGPT) (84460)
Transferase, aspartate amino (AST) (SGOT) (84450)

🖐 0.00 ⚕ 0.00 **FUD** XXX Ⓠ ▱

AMA: 2018,Jan,8; 2017,Jan,8; 2016,Jan,13; 2015,Jan,16; 2014,Jan,11

80081 **Resequenced code. See code following 80055.**

80305-80307 [80305, 80306, 80307] Nonspecific Drug Screening

INCLUDES
All testing procedures provided despite the number of tests performed per modality

EXCLUDES
Confirmatory drug testing ([80320, 80321, 80322, 80323, 80324, 80325, 80326, 80327, 80328, 80329, 80330, 80331, 80332, 80333, 80334, 80335, 80336, 80337, 80338, 80339, 80340, 80341, 80342, 80343, 80344, 80345, 80346, 80347, 80348, 80349, 80350, 80351, 80352, 80353, 80354, 80355, 80356, 80357, 80358, 80359, 80360, 80361, 80362, 80363, 80364, 80365, 80366, 80367, 80368, 80369, 80370, 80371, 80372, 80373, 80374, 80375, 80376, 80377, 83992], [83992])
Validation testing

\# **80305 Drug test(s), presumptive, any number of drug classes, any number of devices or procedures; capable of being read by direct optical observation only (eg, utilizing immunoassay [eg, dipsticks, cups, cards, or cartridges]), includes sample validation when performed, per date of service**

🖐 0.00 ⚕ 0.00 **FUD** XXX ☒ Ⓠ ▱

AMA: 2018,Jul,14; 2018,Jan,8; 2017,Mar,6

\# **80306 read by instrument assisted direct optical observation (eg, utilizing immunoassay [eg, dipsticks, cups, cards, or cartridges]), includes sample validation when performed, per date of service**

🖐 0.00 ⚕ 0.00 **FUD** XXX Ⓠ ▱

AMA: 2018,Jan,8; 2017,Mar,6

\# **80307 by instrument chemistry analyzers (eg, utilizing immunoassay [eg, EIA, ELISA, EMIT, FPIA, IA, KIMS, RIA]), chromatography (eg, GC, HPLC), and mass spectrometry either with or without chromatography, (eg, DART, DESI, GC-MS, GC-MS/MS, LC-MS, LC-MS/MS, LDTD, MALDI, TOF) includes sample validation when performed, per date of service**

🖐 0.00 ⚕ 0.00 **FUD** XXX Ⓠ ▱

AMA: 2018,Jan,8; 2017,Mar,6

80320-80377 [80320, 80321, 80322, 80323, 80324, 80325, 80326, 80327, 80328, 80329, 80330, 80331, 80332, 80333, 80334, 80335, 80336, 80337, 80338, 80339, 80340, 80341, 80342, 80343, 80344, 80345, 80346, 80347, 80348, 80349, 80350, 80351, 80352, 80353, 80354, 80355, 80356, 80357, 80358, 80359, 80360, 80361, 80362, 80363, 80364, 80365, 80366, 80367, 80368, 80369, 80370, 80371, 80372, 80373, 80374, 80375, 80376, 80377, 83992] Confirmatory Drug Testing

INCLUDES
Antihistamine drug tests ([80375, 80376, 80377])
Detection of specific drugs using methods other than immunoassay or enzymatic technique

EXCLUDES
Metabolites separate from the code for the drug except when a distinct code is available

\# **80320 Alcohols**

🖐 0.00 ⚕ 0.00 **FUD** XXX Ⓑ ▱

AMA: 2018,Jan,8; 2017,Jan,8; 2016,Jan,13; 2015,Apr,3

\# **80321 Alcohol biomarkers; 1 or 2**

🖐 0.00 ⚕ 0.00 **FUD** XXX Ⓑ ▱

AMA: 2015,Apr,3

\# **80322 3 or more**

🖐 0.00 ⚕ 0.00 **FUD** XXX Ⓑ ▱

AMA: 2015,Apr,3

\# **80323 Alkaloids, not otherwise specified**

🖐 0.00 ⚕ 0.00 **FUD** XXX Ⓑ ▱

AMA: 2015,Apr,3

\# **80324 Amphetamines; 1 or 2**

🖐 0.00 ⚕ 0.00 **FUD** XXX Ⓑ ▱

AMA: 2015,Apr,3

\# **80325 3 or 4**

🖐 0.00 ⚕ 0.00 **FUD** XXX Ⓑ ▱

AMA: 2015,Apr,3

\# **80326 5 or more**

🖐 0.00 ⚕ 0.00 **FUD** XXX Ⓑ ▱

AMA: 2015,Apr,3

\# **80327 Anabolic steroids; 1 or 2**

🖐 0.00 ⚕ 0.00 **FUD** XXX Ⓑ ▱

AMA: 2015,Apr,3

\# **80328 3 or more**

EXCLUDES
Analysis dihydrotestosterone for monitoring, endogenous levels of hormone (82642)

🖐 0.00 ⚕ 0.00 **FUD** XXX Ⓑ ▱

AMA: 2015,Apr,3

\# **80329 Analgesics, non-opioid; 1 or 2**

🖐 0.00 ⚕ 0.00 **FUD** XXX Ⓑ ▱

AMA: 2015,Apr,3

\# **80330 3-5**

🖐 0.00 ⚕ 0.00 **FUD** XXX Ⓑ ▱

AMA: 2015,Apr,3

\# **80331 6 or more**

🖐 0.00 ⚕ 0.00 **FUD** XXX Ⓑ ▱

AMA: 2015,Apr,3

\# **80332 Antidepressants, serotonergic class; 1 or 2**

🖐 0.00 ⚕ 0.00 **FUD** XXX Ⓑ ▱

AMA: 2015,Apr,3

26/TC PC/TC Only A2-Z3 ASC Payment -50 Bilateral ♂ Male Only ♀ Female Only 🖐 Facility RVU ⚕ Non-Facility RVU ▱ CCI ☒ CLIA
FUD Follow-up Days CMS: IOM AMA: CPT Asst A-Y OPPSI 80/80 Surg Assist Allowed / w/Doc Lab Crosswalk Radiology Crosswalk

CPT © 2019 American Medical Association. All Rights Reserved.
© 2019 Optum360, LLC

80333 — 80371 Pathology and Laboratory

| # | 80333 | **3-5** |
| # | 80334 | **6 or more** |

 # 80333 **3-5**
🚑 0.00   🔪 0.00   **FUD** XXX   B 🔲
AMA: 2015,Apr,3

 # 80334 **6 or more**
🚑 0.00   🔪 0.00   **FUD** XXX   B 🔲
AMA: 2015,Apr,3

 # 80335 **Antidepressants, tricyclic and other cyclicals; 1 or 2**
🚑 0.00   🔪 0.00   **FUD** XXX   B 🔲
AMA: 2015,Apr,3

 # 80336 **3-5**
🚑 0.00   🔪 0.00   **FUD** XXX   B 🔲
AMA: 2015,Apr,3

 # 80337 **6 or more**
🚑 0.00   🔪 0.00   **FUD** XXX   B 🔲
AMA: 2015,Apr,3

 # 80338 **Antidepressants, not otherwise specified**
🚑 0.00   🔪 0.00   **FUD** XXX   B 🔲
AMA: 2015,Apr,3

 # 80339 **Antiepileptics, not otherwise specified; 1-3**
🚑 0.00   🔪 0.00   **FUD** XXX   B 🔲
AMA: 2015,Apr,3

 # 80340 **4-6**
🚑 0.00   🔪 0.00   **FUD** XXX   B 🔲
AMA: 2015,Apr,3

 # 80341 **7 or more**
EXCLUDES *Definitive drug testing for antihistamines ([80375, 80376, 80377])*
🚑 0.00   🔪 0.00   **FUD** XXX   B 🔲
AMA: 2015,Apr,3

 # 80342 **Antipsychotics, not otherwise specified; 1-3**
🚑 0.00   🔪 0.00   **FUD** XXX   B 🔲
AMA: 2015,Apr,3

 # 80343 **4-6**
🚑 0.00   🔪 0.00   **FUD** XXX   B 🔲
AMA: 2015,Apr,3

 # 80344 **7 or more**
🚑 0.00   🔪 0.00   **FUD** XXX   B 🔲
AMA: 2015,Apr,3

 # 80345 **Barbiturates**
🚑 0.00   🔪 0.00   **FUD** XXX   B 🔲
AMA: 2015,Apr,3

 # 80346 **Benzodiazepines; 1-12**
🚑 0.00   🔪 0.00   **FUD** XXX   B 🔲
AMA: 2015,Apr,3

 # 80347 **13 or more**
🚑 0.00   🔪 0.00   **FUD** XXX   B 🔲
AMA: 2015,Apr,3

 # 80348 **Buprenorphine**
🚑 0.00   🔪 0.00   **FUD** XXX   B 🔲
AMA: 2015,Apr,3

 # 80349 **Cannabinoids, natural**
🚑 0.00   🔪 0.00   **FUD** XXX   B 🔲
AMA: 2015,Apr,3

 # 80350 **Cannabinoids, synthetic; 1-3**
🚑 0.00   🔪 0.00   **FUD** XXX   B 🔲
AMA: 2015,Apr,3

 # 80351 **4-6**
🚑 0.00   🔪 0.00   **FUD** XXX   B 🔲
AMA: 2015,Apr,3

 # 80352 **7 or more**
🚑 0.00   🔪 0.00   **FUD** XXX   B 🔲
AMA: 2015,Apr,3

 # 80353 **Cocaine**
🚑 0.00   🔪 0.00   **FUD** XXX   B 🔲
AMA: 2015,Apr,3

 # 80354 **Fentanyl**
🚑 0.00   🔪 0.00   **FUD** XXX   B 🔲
AMA: 2015,Apr,3

 # 80355 **Gabapentin, non-blood**
EXCLUDES *Therapeutic drug assay ([80171])*
🚑 0.00   🔪 0.00   **FUD** XXX   B 🔲
AMA: 2018,Jan,8; 2017,Jan,8; 2016,Jan,13; 2015,Apr,3

 # 80356 **Heroin metabolite**
🚑 0.00   🔪 0.00   **FUD** XXX   B 🔲
AMA: 2015,Apr,3

 # 80357 **Ketamine and norketamine**
🚑 0.00   🔪 0.00   **FUD** XXX   B 🔲
AMA: 2015,Apr,3

 # 80358 **Methadone**
🚑 0.00   🔪 0.00   **FUD** XXX   B 🔲
AMA: 2015,Apr,3

 # 80359 **Methylenedioxyamphetamines (MDA, MDEA, MDMA)**
🚑 0.00   🔪 0.00   **FUD** XXX   B 🔲
AMA: 2015,Apr,3

 # 80360 **Methylphenidate**
🚑 0.00   🔪 0.00   **FUD** XXX   B 🔲
AMA: 2015,Apr,3

 # 80361 **Opiates, 1 or more**
🚑 0.00   🔪 0.00   **FUD** XXX   B 🔲
AMA: 2015,Apr,3

 # 80362 **Opioids and opiate analogs; 1 or 2**
🚑 0.00   🔪 0.00   **FUD** XXX   B 🔲
AMA: 2015,Apr,3

 # 80363 **3 or 4**
🚑 0.00   🔪 0.00   **FUD** XXX   B 🔲
AMA: 2015,Apr,3

 # 80364 **5 or more**
🚑 0.00   🔪 0.00   **FUD** XXX   B 🔲
AMA: 2015,Apr,3

 # 80365 **Oxycodone**
🚑 0.00   🔪 0.00   **FUD** XXX   B 🔲
AMA: 2015,Apr,3

 # 83992 **Phencyclidine (PCP)**
🚑 0.00   🔪 0.00   **FUD** XXX   E 🔲
AMA: 2018,Jan,8; 2017,Jan,8; 2016,Jan,13; 2015,Jun,10; 2015,Apr,3

 # 80366 **Pregabalin**
🚑 0.00   🔪 0.00   **FUD** XXX   B 🔲
AMA: 2015,Apr,3

 # 80367 **Propoxyphene**
🚑 0.00   🔪 0.00   **FUD** XXX   B 🔲
AMA: 2015,Apr,3

 # 80368 **Sedative hypnotics (non-benzodiazepines)**
🚑 0.00   🔪 0.00   **FUD** XXX   B 🔲
AMA: 2015,Apr,3

 # 80369 **Skeletal muscle relaxants; 1 or 2**
🚑 0.00   🔪 0.00   **FUD** XXX   B 🔲
AMA: 2015,Apr,3

 # 80370 **3 or more**
🚑 0.00   🔪 0.00   **FUD** XXX   B 🔲
AMA: 2015,Apr,3

 # 80371 **Stimulants, synthetic**
🚑 0.00   🔪 0.00   **FUD** XXX   B 🔲
AMA: 2015,Apr,3

\# | **80372** | **Tapentadol**
🚘 0.00   ⚕ 0.00   **FUD** XXX   B ▣
AMA: 2015,Apr,3

\# | **80373** | **Tramadol**
🚘 0.00   ⚕ 0.00   **FUD** XXX   B ▣
AMA: 2015,Apr,3

\# | **80374** | **Stereoisomer (enantiomer) analysis, single drug class**
Code also index drug analysis if appropriate
🚘 0.00   ⚕ 0.00   **FUD** XXX   B ▣
AMA: 2015,Apr,3

\# | **80375** | **Drug(s) or substance(s), definitive, qualitative or quantitative, not otherwise specified; 1-3**
🚘 0.00   ⚕ 0.00   **FUD** XXX   B ▣
AMA: 2018,Jan,8; 2017,Jan,8; 2016,Jan,13; 2015,Apr,3

\# | **80376** | **4-6**
🚘 0.00   ⚕ 0.00   **FUD** XXX   B ▣
AMA: 2018,Jan,8; 2017,Jan,8; 2016,Jan,13; 2015,Apr,3

\# | **80377** | **7 or more**
EXCLUDES   *Definitive drug testing for antihistamines ([80375, 80376, 80377])*
🚘 0.00   ⚕ 0.00   **FUD** XXX   B ▣
AMA: 2018,Jan,8; 2017,Jan,8; 2016,Jan,13; 2015,Apr,3

80145-80377 [80164, 80165, 80171, 80230, 80235, 80280, 80285] Therapeutic Drug Levels

INCLUDES   Testing of drug and metabolite(s) in primary code
Tests on specimens from blood and blood components, and spinal fluid

● | 80145 | **Adalimumab**

80150 | **Amikacin**
🚘 0.00   ⚕ 0.00   **FUD** XXX   Q ▣
AMA: 2018,Jan,8; 2017,Jan,8; 2016,Jan,13; 2015,Apr,3; 2015,Jan,16; 2014,Jan,11

80155 | **Caffeine**
🚘 0.00   ⚕ 0.00   **FUD** XXX   Q ▣
AMA: 2015,Apr,3; 2014,Jan,11

80156 | **Carbamazepine; total**
🚘 0.00   ⚕ 0.00   **FUD** XXX   Q ▣
AMA: 2018,Jan,8; 2017,Jan,8; 2016,Jan,13; 2015,Apr,3; 2015,Jan,16; 2014,Jan,11

80157 | **free**
🚘 0.00   ⚕ 0.00   **FUD** XXX   Q ▣
AMA: 2018,Jan,8; 2017,Jan,8; 2016,Jan,13; 2015,Apr,3; 2015,Jan,16; 2014,Jan,11

80158 | **Cyclosporine**
🚘 0.00   ⚕ 0.00   **FUD** XXX   Q ▣
AMA: 2018,Jan,8; 2017,Jan,8; 2016,Jan,13; 2015,Apr,3; 2015,Jan,16; 2014,Jan,11

80159 | **Clozapine**
🚘 0.00   ⚕ 0.00   **FUD** XXX   Q ▣
AMA: 2015,Apr,3; 2014,Jan,11

80162 | **Digoxin; total**
🚘 0.00   ⚕ 0.00   **FUD** XXX   Q ▣
AMA: 2018,Jan,8; 2017,Jan,8; 2016,Jan,13; 2015,Apr,3; 2015,Jan,16; 2014,Jan,11

80163 | **free**
🚘 0.00   ⚕ 0.00   **FUD** XXX   Q ▣
AMA: 2018,Jan,8; 2017,Jan,8; 2016,Jan,13; 2015,Apr,3

80164 | **Resequenced code. See code following 80201.**

80165 | **Resequenced code. See code following 80201.**

80168 | **Ethosuximide**
🚘 0.00   ⚕ 0.00   **FUD** XXX   Q ▣
AMA: 2018,Jan,8; 2017,Jan,8; 2016,Jan,13; 2015,Apr,3; 2015,Jan,16; 2014,Jan,11

80169 | **Everolimus**
🚘 0.00   ⚕ 0.00   **FUD** XXX   Q ▣
AMA: 2015,Apr,3; 2014,Jan,11

\# | 80171 | **Gabapentin, whole blood, serum, or plasma**
🚘 0.00   ⚕ 0.00   **FUD** XXX   Q ▣
AMA: 2018,Jan,8; 2017,Jan,8; 2016,Jan,13; 2015,Apr,3; 2014,Jan,11

80170 | **Gentamicin**
🚘 0.00   ⚕ 0.00   **FUD** XXX   Q ▣
AMA: 2018,Jan,8; 2017,Jan,8; 2016,Jan,13; 2015,Apr,3; 2015,Jan,16; 2014,Jan,11

80171 | **Resequenced code. See code following 80169.**

80173 | **Haloperidol**
🚘 0.00   ⚕ 0.00   **FUD** XXX   Q ▣
AMA: 2018,Jan,8; 2017,Jan,8; 2016,Jan,13; 2015,Apr,3; 2015,Jan,16; 2014,Jan,11

● \# | 80230 | **Infliximab**
🚘 0.00   ⚕ 0.00   **FUD** 000

● \# | 80235 | **Lacosamide**
🚘 0.00   ⚕ 0.00   **FUD** 000

80175 | **Lamotrigine**
🚘 0.00   ⚕ 0.00   **FUD** XXX   Q ▣
AMA: 2015,Apr,3; 2014,Jan,11

80176 | **Lidocaine**
🚘 0.00   ⚕ 0.00   **FUD** XXX   Q ▣
AMA: 2018,Jan,8; 2017,Jan,8; 2016,Jan,13; 2015,Apr,3; 2015,Jan,16; 2014,Jan,11

80177 | **Levetiracetam**
🚘 0.00   ⚕ 0.00   **FUD** XXX   Q ▣
AMA: 2015,Apr,3; 2014,Jan,11

80178 | **Lithium**
🚘 0.00   ⚕ 0.00   **FUD** XXX   ✖ Q ▣
AMA: 2018,Jan,8; 2017,Jan,8; 2016,Jan,13; 2015,Apr,3; 2015,Jan,16; 2014,Jan,11

80180 | **Mycophenolate (mycophenolic acid)**
🚘 0.00   ⚕ 0.00   **FUD** XXX   Q ▣
AMA: 2015,Apr,3; 2014,Jan,11

80183 | **Oxcarbazepine**
🚘 0.00   ⚕ 0.00   **FUD** XXX   Q ▣
AMA: 2015,Apr,3; 2014,Jan,11

80184 | **Phenobarbital**
🚘 0.00   ⚕ 0.00   **FUD** XXX   Q ▣
AMA: 2018,Jan,8; 2017,Jan,8; 2016,Jan,13; 2015,Apr,3; 2015,Jan,16; 2014,Jan,11

80185 | **Phenytoin; total**
🚘 0.00   ⚕ 0.00   **FUD** XXX   Q ▣
AMA: 2018,Jan,8; 2017,Jan,8; 2016,Jan,13; 2015,Apr,3; 2015,Jan,16; 2014,Jan,11

80186 | **free**
🚘 0.00   ⚕ 0.00   **FUD** XXX   Q ▣
AMA: 2018,Jan,8; 2017,Jan,8; 2016,Jan,13; 2015,Apr,3; 2015,Jan,16; 2014,Jan,11

● | 80187 | **Posaconazole**

80188 | **Primidone**
🚘 0.00   ⚕ 0.00   **FUD** XXX   Q ▣
AMA: 2018,Jan,8; 2017,Jan,8; 2016,Jan,13; 2015,Apr,3; 2015,Jan,16; 2014,Jan,11

26/TC PC/TC Only   A2-Z3 ASC Payment   50 Bilateral   ♂ Male Only   ♀ Female Only   🚘 Facility RVU   ⚕ Non-Facility RVU   ▣ CCI   ✖ CLIA
FUD Follow-up Days   **CMS:** IOM   **AMA:** CPT Asst   A-Y OPPSI   80/80 Surg Assist Allowed / w/Doc   Lab Crosswalk   Radiology Crosswalk

CPT © 2019 American Medical Association. All Rights Reserved.

374   © 2019 Optum360, LLC

80190	**Procainamide;**	
	�100 0.00 ✂ 0.00 **FUD** XXX	🔲🔳
	AMA: 2018,Jan,8; 2017,Jan,8; 2016,Jan,13; 2015,Apr,3; 2015,Jan,16; 2014,Jan,11	
80192	**with metabolites (eg, n-acetyl procainamide)**	
	🚚 0.00 ✂ 0.00 **FUD** XXX	🔲🔳
	AMA: 2018,Jan,8; 2017,Jan,8; 2016,Jan,13; 2015,Apr,3; 2015,Jan,16; 2014,Jan,11	
80194	**Quinidine**	
	🚚 0.00 ✂ 0.00 **FUD** XXX	🔲🔳
	AMA: 2018,Jan,8; 2017,Jan,8; 2016,Jan,13; 2015,Apr,3; 2015,Jan,16; 2014,Jan,11	
80195	**Sirolimus**	
	🚚 0.00 ✂ 0.00 **FUD** XXX	🔲🔳
	AMA: 2018,Jan,8; 2017,Jan,8; 2016,Jan,13; 2015,Apr,3; 2015,Jan,16; 2014,Jan,11	
80197	**Tacrolimus**	
	🚚 0.00 ✂ 0.00 **FUD** XXX	🔲🔳
	AMA: 2018,Jan,8; 2017,Jan,8; 2016,Jan,13; 2015,Apr,3; 2015,Jan,16; 2014,Jan,11	
80198	**Theophylline**	
	🚚 0.00 ✂ 0.00 **FUD** XXX	🔲🔳
	AMA: 2018,Jan,8; 2017,Jan,8; 2016,Jan,13; 2015,Apr,3; 2015,Jan,16; 2014,Jan,11	
80199	**Tiagabine**	
	🚚 0.00 ✂ 0.00 **FUD** XXX	🔲🔳
	AMA: 2015,Apr,3; 2014,Jan,11	
80200	**Tobramycin**	
	🚚 0.00 ✂ 0.00 **FUD** XXX	🔲🔳
	AMA: 2018,Jan,8; 2017,Jan,8; 2016,Jan,13; 2015,Apr,3; 2015,Jan,16; 2014,Jan,11	
80201	**Topiramate**	
	🚚 0.00 ✂ 0.00 **FUD** XXX	🔲🔳
	AMA: 2018,Jan,8; 2017,Jan,8; 2016,Jan,13; 2015,Apr,3; 2015,Jan,16; 2014,Jan,11	
# **80164**	**Valproic acid (dipropylacetic acid); total**	
	🚚 0.00 ✂ 0.00 **FUD** XXX	🔲🔳
	AMA: 2018,Jan,8; 2017,Jan,8; 2016,Jan,13; 2015,Apr,3; 2015,Jan,16; 2014,Jan,11	
# **80165**	**free**	
	🚚 0.00 ✂ 0.00 **FUD** XXX	🔲🔳
	AMA: 2018,Jan,8; 2017,Jan,8; 2016,Jan,13; 2015,Apr,3	
80202	**Vancomycin**	
	🚚 0.00 ✂ 0.00 **FUD** XXX	🔲🔳
	AMA: 2018,Jan,8; 2017,Jan,8; 2016,Jan,13; 2015,Apr,3; 2015,Jan,16; 2014,Jan,11	
● # **80280**	**Vedolizumab**	
	🚚 0.00 ✂ 0.00 **FUD** 000	
● # **80285**	**Voriconazole**	
	🚚 0.00 ✂ 0.00 **FUD** 000	
80203	**Zonisamide**	
	🚚 0.00 ✂ 0.00 **FUD** XXX	🔲🔳
	AMA: 2015,Apr,3; 2014,Jan,11	
80230	**Resequenced code. See code following 80173.**	
80235	**Resequenced code. See code before 80175.**	
80280	**Resequenced code. See code following 80202.**	
80285	**Resequenced code. See code before 80203.**	
80299	**Quantitation of therapeutic drug, not elsewhere specified**	
	🚚 0.00 ✂ 0.00 **FUD** XXX	🔲🔳
	AMA: 2018,Jan,8; 2017,Jan,8; 2016,Jan,13; 2015,Apr,3; 2015,Jan,16; 2014,Jan,11	
80305	**Resequenced code. See code before 80145.**	
80306	**Resequenced code. See code before 80145.**	
80307	**Resequenced code. See code before 80145.**	

80320	Resequenced code. See code before 80145.
80321	Resequenced code. See code before 80145.
80322	Resequenced code. See code before 80145.
80323	Resequenced code. See code before 80145.
80324	Resequenced code. See code before 80145.
80325	Resequenced code. See code before 80145.
80326	Resequenced code. See code before 80145.
80327	Resequenced code. See code before 80145.
80328	Resequenced code. See code before 80145.
80329	Resequenced code. See code before 80145.
80330	Resequenced code. See code before 80145.
80331	Resequenced code. See code before 80145.
80332	Resequenced code. See code before 80145.
80333	Resequenced code. See code before 80145.
80334	Resequenced code. See code before 80145.
80335	Resequenced code. See code before 80145.
80336	Resequenced code. See code before 80145.
80337	Resequenced code. See code before 80145.
80338	Resequenced code. See code before 80145.
80339	Resequenced code. See code before 80145.
80340	Resequenced code. See code before 80145.
80341	Resequenced code. See code before 80145.
80342	Resequenced code. See code before 80145.
80343	Resequenced code. See code before 80145.
80344	Resequenced code. See code before 80145.
80345	Resequenced code. See code before 80145.
80346	Resequenced code. See code before 80145.
80347	Resequenced code. See code before 80145.
80348	Resequenced code. See code before 80145.
80349	Resequenced code. See code before 80145.
80350	Resequenced code. See code before 80145.
80351	Resequenced code. See code before 80145.
80352	Resequenced code. See code before 80145.
80353	Resequenced code. See code before 80145.
80354	Resequenced code. See code before 80145.
80355	Resequenced code. See code before 80145.
80356	Resequenced code. See code before 80145.
80357	Resequenced code. See code before 80145.
80358	Resequenced code. See code before 80145.
80359	Resequenced code. See code before 80145.
80360	Resequenced code. See code before 80145.
80361	Resequenced code. See code before 80145.
80362	Resequenced code. See code before 80145.
80363	Resequenced code. See code before 80145.
80364	Resequenced code. See code before 80145.
80365	Resequenced code. See code before 80145.
80366	Resequenced code. See code before 80145.
80367	Resequenced code. See code before 80145.
80368	Resequenced code. See code before 80145.
80369	Resequenced code. See code before 80145.
80370	Resequenced code. See code before 80145.
80371	Resequenced code. See code before 80145.
80372	Resequenced code. See code before 80145.
80373	Resequenced code. See code before 80145.

80374	Resequenced code. See code before 80145.
80375	Resequenced code. See code before 80145.
80376	Resequenced code. See code before 80145.
80377	Resequenced code. See code before 80145.

80400-80439 Stimulation and Suppression Test Panels

EXCLUDES Administration of evocative or suppressive material (96365-96368, 96372, 96374-96376, C8957)
Evocative or suppression test substances, as applicable
Physician monitoring and attendance during test (see E&M services)

80400   ACTH stimulation panel; for adrenal insufficiency
INCLUDES Cortisol x 2 (82533)
0.00   0.00   FUD XXX
AMA: 2018,Jan,8; 2017,Jan,8; 2016,Jan,13; 2015,Jan,16; 2014,Jan,11

80402   for 21 hydroxylase deficiency
INCLUDES 17 hydroxyprogesterone X 2 (83498)
Cortisol x 2 (82533)
0.00   0.00   FUD XXX
AMA: 2014,Jan,11

80406   for 3 beta-hydroxydehydrogenase deficiency
INCLUDES 17 hydroxypregnenolone x 2 (84143)
Cortisol x 2 (82533)
0.00   0.00   FUD XXX
AMA: 2014,Jan,11

80408   Aldosterone suppression evaluation panel (eg, saline infusion)
INCLUDES Aldosterone x 2 (82088)
Renin x 2 (84244)
0.00   0.00   FUD XXX
AMA: 2014,Jan,11

80410   Calcitonin stimulation panel (eg, calcium, pentagastrin)
INCLUDES Calcitonin x 3 (82308)
0.00   0.00   FUD XXX
AMA: 2014,Jan,11

80412   Corticotropic releasing hormone (CRH) stimulation panel
INCLUDES Adrenocorticotropic hormone (ACTH) x 6 (82024)
Cortisol x 6 (82533)
0.00   0.00   FUD XXX
AMA: 2014,Jan,11

80414   Chorionic gonadotropin stimulation panel; testosterone response
INCLUDES Testosterone x 2 on three pooled blood samples (84403)
0.00   0.00   FUD XXX
AMA: 2014,Jan,11

80415   estradiol response
INCLUDES Estradiol x 2 on three pooled blood samples (82670)
0.00   0.00   FUD XXX
AMA: 2014,Jan,11

80416   Renal vein renin stimulation panel (eg, captopril)
INCLUDES Renin x 6 (84244)
0.00   0.00   FUD XXX
AMA: 2014,Jan,11

80417   Peripheral vein renin stimulation panel (eg, captopril)
INCLUDES Renin x 2 (84244)
0.00   0.00   FUD XXX
AMA: 2014,Jan,11

80418   Combined rapid anterior pituitary evaluation panel
INCLUDES Adrenocorticotropic hormone (ACTH) x 4 (82024)
Cortisol x 4 (82533)
Follicle stimulating hormone (FSH) x 4 (83001)
Human growth hormone x 4 (83003)
Luteinizing hormone (LH) x 4 (83002)
Prolactin x 4 (84146)
Thyroid stimulating hormone (TSH) x 4 (84443)
0.00   0.00   FUD XXX
AMA: 2014,Jan,11

80420   Dexamethasone suppression panel, 48 hour
INCLUDES Cortisol x 2 (82533)
Free cortisol, urine x 2 (82530)
Volume measurement for timed collection x 2 (81050)
EXCLUDES Single dose dexamethasone (82533)
0.00   0.00   FUD XXX
AMA: 2014,Jan,11

80422   Glucagon tolerance panel; for insulinoma
INCLUDES Glucose x 3 (82947)
Insulin x 3 (83525)
0.00   0.00   FUD XXX
AMA: 2014,Jan,11

80424   for pheochromocytoma
INCLUDES Catecholamines, fractionated x 2 (82384)
0.00   0.00   FUD XXX
AMA: 2014,Jan,11

80426   Gonadotropin releasing hormone stimulation panel
INCLUDES Follicle stimulating hormone (FSH) x 4 (83001)
Luteinizing hormone (LH) x 4 (83002)
0.00   0.00   FUD XXX
AMA: 2014,Jan,11

80428   Growth hormone stimulation panel (eg, arginine infusion, l-dopa administration)
INCLUDES Human growth hormone (HGH) x 4 (83003)
0.00   0.00   FUD XXX
AMA: 2014,Jan,11

80430   Growth hormone suppression panel (glucose administration)
INCLUDES Glucose x 3 (82947)
Human growth hormone (HGH) x 4 (83003)
0.00   0.00   FUD XXX
AMA: 2014,Jan,11

80432   Insulin-induced C-peptide suppression panel
INCLUDES C-peptide x 5 (84681)
Glucose x 5 (82947)
Insulin (83525)
0.00   0.00   FUD XXX
AMA: 2014,Jan,11

80434   Insulin tolerance panel; for ACTH insufficiency
INCLUDES Cortisol x 5 (82533)
Glucose x 5 (82947)
0.00   0.00   FUD XXX
AMA: 2014,Jan,11

80435   for growth hormone deficiency
INCLUDES Glucose x 5 (82947)
Human growth hormone (HGH) x 5 (83003)
0.00   0.00   FUD XXX
AMA: 2014,Jan,11

80436   Metyrapone panel
INCLUDES 11 deoxycortisol x 2 (82634)
Cortisol x 2 (82533)
0.00   0.00   FUD XXX
AMA: 2014,Jan,11

CPT © 2019 American Medical Association. All Rights Reserved.

80438 Thyrotropin releasing hormone (TRH) stimulation panel; 1 hour

INCLUDES Thyroid stimulating hormone (TSH) x 3 (84443)

🚗 0.00   ⚕ 0.00   **FUD** XXX

AMA: 2014,Jan,11

80439 2 hour

INCLUDES Thyroid stimulating hormone (TSH) x 4 (84443)

🚗 0.00   ⚕ 0.00   **FUD** XXX

AMA: 2014,Jan,11

80500-80502 Consultation By Clinical Pathologist

INCLUDES Pharmacokinetic consultations
Written report by pathologist for tests requiring additional medical judgment and requested by a physician or other qualified health care professional

EXCLUDES *Consultations that include patient examination*
Use of code when a medical interpretive assessment is not provided

80500 Clinical pathology consultation; limited, without review of patient's history and medical records

🚗 0.56   ⚕ 0.65   **FUD** XXX

AMA: 2018,Jan,8; 2017,Jan,8; 2016,Jan,13; 2015,Jan,16; 2014,Jan,11

80502 comprehensive, for a complex diagnostic problem, with review of patient's history and medical records

🚗 2.01   ⚕ 2.10   **FUD** XXX

AMA: 2018,Jan,8; 2017,Jan,8; 2016,Jan,13; 2015,Jan,16; 2014,Jan,11

81000-81099 Urine Tests

81000 Urinalysis, by dip stick or tablet reagent for bilirubin, glucose, hemoglobin, ketones, leukocytes, nitrite, pH, protein, specific gravity, urobilinogen, any number of these constituents; non-automated, with microscopy

🚗 0.00   ⚕ 0.00   **FUD** XXX

AMA: 2018,Jul,14; 2018,Jan,8; 2017,Jan,8; 2016,Jan,13; 2015,Jan,16; 2014,Jan,11

81001 automated, with microscopy

🚗 0.00   ⚕ 0.00   **FUD** XXX

AMA: 2014,Jan,11

81002 non-automated, without microscopy

INCLUDES Mosenthal test

🚗 0.00   ⚕ 0.00   **FUD** XXX

AMA: 2018,Jan,8; 2017,Jan,8; 2016,Jan,13; 2015,Jan,16; 2014,Jan,11

81003 automated, without microscopy

🚗 0.00   ⚕ 0.00   **FUD** XXX

AMA: 2018,Jan,8; 2017,Jan,8; 2016,Jan,13; 2015,Jan,16; 2014,Jan,11

81005 Urinalysis; qualitative or semiquantitative, except immunoassays

INCLUDES Benedict test for dextrose

EXCLUDES *Immunoassay, qualitative or semiquantitative (83518)*
Microalbumin (82043-82044)
Nonimmunoassay reagent strip analysis (81000, 81002)

🚗 0.00   ⚕ 0.00   **FUD** XXX

AMA: 2018,Jan,8; 2017,Jan,8; 2016,Jan,13; 2015,Jan,16; 2014,Jan,11

81007 bacteriuria screen, except by culture or dipstick

EXCLUDES *Culture (87086-87088)*
Dipstick (81000, 81002)

🚗 0.00   ⚕ 0.00   **FUD** XXX

AMA: 2014,Jan,11

81015 microscopic only

EXCLUDES *Sperm evaluation for retrograde ejaculation (89331)*

🚗 0.00   ⚕ 0.00   **FUD** XXX

AMA: 2018,Jan,8; 2017,Nov,10; 2014,Jan,11

81020 2 or 3 glass test

INCLUDES Valentine's test

🚗 0.00   ⚕ 0.00   **FUD** XXX

AMA: 2014,Jan,11

81025 Urine pregnancy test, by visual color comparison methods

🚗 0.00   ⚕ 0.00   **FUD** XXX

AMA: 2018,Jan,8; 2017,Jan,8; 2016,Jan,13; 2015,Jan,16; 2014,Jan,11

81050 Volume measurement for timed collection, each

🚗 0.00   ⚕ 0.00   **FUD** XXX

AMA: 2014,Jan,11

81099 Unlisted urinalysis procedure

🚗 0.00   ⚕ 0.00   **FUD** XXX

AMA: 2018,Jan,8; 2017,Jan,8; 2016,Jan,13; 2015,Jan,16; 2014,Jan,11

81105-81364 [81105, 81106, 81107, 81108, 81109, 81110, 81111, 81112, 81120, 81121, 81161, 81162, 81163, 81164, 81165, 81166, 81167, 81173, 81174, 81184, 81185, 81186, 81187, 81188, 81189, 81190, 81200, 81201, 81202, 81203, 81204, 81205, 81206, 81207, 81208, 81209, 81210, 81219, 81227, 81230, 81231, 81233, 81234, 81238, 81239, 81245, 81246, 81250, 81257, 81258, 81259, 81261, 81262, 81263, 81264, 81265, 81266, 81267, 81268, 81269, 81271, 81274, 81277, 81283, 81284, 81285, 81286, 81287, 81288, 81289, 81291, 81292, 81293, 81294, 81295, 81301, 81302, 81303, 81304, 81306, 81307, 81308, 81309, 81312, 81320, 81324, 81325, 81326, 81332, 81334, 81336, 81337, 81343, 81344, 81345, 81361, 81362, 81363, 81364] Gene Analysis: Tier 1 Procedures

INCLUDES All analytical procedures in the evaluation such as:
Amplification
Cell lysis
Detection
Digestion
Extraction
Nucleic acid stabilization
Code selection based on specific gene being reviewed
Evaluation of constitutional or somatic gene variations
Evaluation of the presence of gene variants using the common gene variant name
Examples of proteins or diseases in the code description that are not all inclusive
Gene specific and genomic testing
Generally all the listed gene variants in the code description would be tested but lists are not all inclusive
Genes described using Human Genome Organization (HUGO) approved names
Qualitative results unless otherwise stated
Tier 1 molecular pathology codes (81105-81254 [81161, 81162, 81163, 81164, 81165, 81166, 81167, 81173, 81174, 81184, 81185, 81186, 81187, 81188, 81189, 81190, 81200, 81201, 81202, 81203, 81204, 81205, 81206, 81207, 81208, 81209, 81210, 81219, 81227, 81230, 81231, 81233, 81234, 81238, 81239, 81245, 81246, 81250, 81257, 81258, 81259, 81265, 81266, 81267, 81268, 81269, 81284, 81285, 81286, 81289, 81361, 81362, 81363, 81364])

EXCLUDES *Full gene sequencing using separate gene variant assessment codes unless it is specifically stated in the code description*
In situ hybridization analyses (88271-88275, 88365-88368 [88364, 88373, 88374])
Microbial identification (87149-87153, 87471-87801 [87623, 87624, 87625], 87900-87904 [87906, 87910, 87912])
Other related gene variants not listed in code
Tier 1 molecular pathology codes (81370-81383)
Tier 2 codes (81400-81408)
Unlisted molecular pathology procedures ([81479])

Code also modifier 26 when only interpretation and report are performed
Code also services required before cell lysis

81105 Resequenced code. See code before 81260.

81106 Resequenced code. See code before 81260.

81107 Resequenced code. See code before 81260.

81108	Resequenced code. See code before 81260.
81109	Resequenced code. See code before 81260.
81110	Resequenced code. See code before 81260.
81111	Resequenced code. See code before 81260.
81112	Resequenced code. See code before 81260.
81120	Resequenced code. See code before 81260.
81121	Resequenced code. See code before 81260.
81161	Resequenced code. See code following numeric code 81231.
81162	Resequenced code. See code following resequenced code 81210.
81163	Resequenced code. See code following resequenced code 81210.
81164	Resequenced code. See code following resequenced code 81210.
81165	Resequenced code. See code following 81212.
81166	Resequenced code. See code following 81212.
81167	Resequenced code. See code following 81216.

81170 *ABL1 (ABL proto-oncogene 1, non-receptor tyrosine kinase)* (eg, acquired imatinib tyrosine kinase inhibitor resistance), gene analysis, variants in the kinase domain
📦 0.00 📛 0.00 **FUD** XXX Ⓐ 🖾
AMA: 2018,Jan,8; 2017,Jan,8; 2016,Aug,9

81171 *AFF2 (AF4/FMR2 family, member 2 [FMR2])* (eg, fragile X mental retardation 2 [FRAXE]) gene analysis; evaluation to detect abnormal (eg, expanded) alleles
📦 0.00 📛 0.00 **FUD** XXX 🖾

81172   characterization of alleles (eg, expanded size and methylation status)
📦 0.00 📛 0.00 **FUD** XXX 🖾

| 81173 | Resequenced code. See code following resequenced code 81204. |
| 81174 | Resequenced code. See code following resequenced code 81204. |

\# 81201 *APC (adenomatous polyposis coli)* (eg, familial adenomatosis polyposis [FAP], attenuated FAP) gene analysis; full gene sequence
📦 0.00 📛 0.00 **FUD** XXX Ⓐ 🖾
AMA: 2018,Nov,9; 2018,Jan,8; 2017,Jan,8; 2016,Aug,9; 2016,Jan,13; 2015,Jan,16; 2014,Jan,11

\# 81202   known familial variants
📦 0.00 📛 0.00 **FUD** XXX Ⓐ 🖾
AMA: 2018,Nov,9; 2018,Jan,8; 2017,Jan,8; 2016,Aug,9; 2016,Jan,13; 2015,Jan,16; 2014,Jan,11

\# 81203   duplication/deletion variants
📦 0.00 📛 0.00 **FUD** XXX Ⓐ 🖾
AMA: 2018,Nov,9; 2018,Jan,8; 2017,Jan,8; 2016,Aug,9; 2016,Jan,13; 2015,Jan,16; 2014,Jan,11

\# 81204 *AR (androgen receptor)* (eg, spinal and bulbar muscular atrophy, Kennedy disease, X chromosome inactivation) gene analysis; characterization of alleles (eg, expanded size or methylation status)
📦 0.00 📛 0.00 **FUD** XXX 🖾
AMA: 2018,Nov,9

\# 81173   full gene sequence
📦 0.00 📛 0.00 **FUD** XXX 🖾

\# 81174   known familial variant
📦 0.00 📛 0.00 **FUD** XXX 🖾

\# 81200 *ASPA (aspartoacylase)* (eg, Canavan disease) gene analysis, common variants (eg, E285A, Y231X)
📦 0.00 📛 0.00 **FUD** XXX Ⓐ 🖾
AMA: 2018,Nov,9; 2018,Jan,8; 2017,Jan,8; 2016,Aug,9; 2016,Jan,13; 2015,Jan,16; 2014,Jan,11

81175 *ASXL1 (additional sex combs like 1, transcriptional regulator)* (eg, myelodysplastic syndrome, myeloproliferative neoplasms, chronic myelomonocytic leukemia), gene analysis; full gene sequence
📦 0.00 📛 0.00 **FUD** XXX Ⓐ 🖾

81176   targeted sequence analysis (eg, exon 12)
📦 0.00 📛 0.00 **FUD** XXX Ⓐ 🖾

81177 *ATN1 (atrophin 1)* (eg, dentatorubral-pallidoluysian atrophy) gene analysis, evaluation to detect abnormal (eg, expanded) alleles
📦 0.00 📛 0.00 **FUD** XXX 🖾

81178 *ATXN1 (ataxin 1)* (eg, spinocerebellar ataxia) gene analysis, evaluation to detect abnormal (eg, expanded) alleles
📦 0.00 📛 0.00 **FUD** XXX
AMA: 2019,Sep,7

81179 *ATXN2 (ataxin 2)* (eg, spinocerebellar ataxia) gene analysis, evaluation to detect abnormal (eg, expanded) alleles
📦 0.00 📛 0.00 **FUD** XXX 🖾
AMA: 2019,Sep,7

81180 *ATXN3 (ataxin 3)* (eg, spinocerebellar ataxia, Machado-Joseph disease) gene analysis, evaluation to detect abnormal (eg, expanded) alleles
📦 0.00 📛 0.00 **FUD** XXX 🖾
AMA: 2019,Sep,7

81181 *ATXN7 (ataxin 7)* (eg, spinocerebellar ataxia) gene analysis, evaluation to detect abnormal (eg, expanded) alleles
📦 0.00 📛 0.00 **FUD** XXX 🖾
AMA: 2019,Sep,7

81182 *ATXN8OS (ATXN8 opposite strand [non-protein coding])* (eg, spinocerebellar ataxia) gene analysis, evaluation to detect abnormal (eg, expanded) alleles
📦 0.00 📛 0.00 **FUD** XXX 🖾
AMA: 2019,Sep,7

81183 *ATXN10 (ataxin 10)* (eg, spinocerebellar ataxia) gene analysis, evaluation to detect abnormal (eg, expanded) alleles
📦 0.00 📛 0.00 **FUD** XXX 🖾
AMA: 2019,Sep,7

81184	Resequenced code. See code following resequenced code 81233.
81185	Resequenced code. See code following resequenced code 81233.
81186	Resequenced code. See code following resequenced code 81233.
81187	Resequenced code. See code following resequenced code 81268.
81188	Resequenced code. See code following resequenced code 81266.
81189	Resequenced code. See code following resequenced code 81266.
81190	Resequenced code. See code following resequenced code 81266.
81200	Resequenced code. See code before 81175.
81201	Resequenced code. See code following numeric code 81174.
81202	Resequenced code. See code following numeric code 81174.
81203	Resequenced code. See code following numeric code 81174.
81204	Resequenced code. See code following numeric code 81174.
81205	Resequenced code. See code following numeric code 81210.
81206	Resequenced code. See code following numeric code 81210.

81207 Resequenced code. See code following numeric code 81210.

81208 Resequenced code. See code following numeric code 81210.

81209 Resequenced code. See code following numeric code 81210.

81210 Resequenced code. See code following resequenced code 81209.

\# **81205** *BCKDHB (branched-chain keto acid dehydrogenase E1, beta polypeptide) (eg, maple syrup urine disease) gene analysis, common variants (eg, R183P, G278S, E422X)*

    🚑 0.00   ✂ 0.00   **FUD** XXX   Ⓐ 🔲

    AMA: 2018,Nov,9; 2018,Jan,8; 2017,Jan,8; 2016,Aug,9; 2016,Jan,13; 2015,Jan,16; 2014,Jan,11

\# **81206** *BCR/ABL1 (t(9;22)) (eg, chronic myelogenous leukemia) translocation analysis; major breakpoint, qualitative or quantitative*

    🚑 0.00   ✂ 0.00   **FUD** XXX   Ⓐ 🔲

    AMA: 2018,Nov,9; 2018,Jan,8; 2017,Jan,8; 2016,Aug,9; 2016,Jan,13; 2015,Jan,16; 2014,Jan,11

\# **81207** minor breakpoint, qualitative or quantitative

    🚑 0.00   ✂ 0.00   **FUD** XXX   Ⓐ 🔲

    AMA: 2018,Nov,9; 2018,Jan,8; 2017,Jan,8; 2016,Aug,9; 2016,Jan,13; 2015,Jan,16; 2014,Jan,11

\# **81208** other breakpoint, qualitative or quantitative

    🚑 0.00   ✂ 0.00   **FUD** XXX   Ⓐ 🔲

    AMA: 2018,Nov,9; 2018,Jan,8; 2017,Jan,8; 2016,Aug,9; 2016,Jan,13; 2015,Jan,16; 2014,Jan,11

\# **81209** *BLM (Bloom syndrome, RecQ helicase-like) (eg, Bloom syndrome) gene analysis, 2281del6ins7 variant*

    🚑 0.00   ✂ 0.00   **FUD** XXX   Ⓐ 🔲

    AMA: 2018,Nov,9; 2018,Jan,8; 2017,Jan,8; 2016,Aug,9; 2016,Jan,13; 2015,Jan,16; 2014,Jan,11

\# **81210** *BRAF (B-Raf proto-oncogene, serine/threonine kinase) (eg, colon cancer, melanoma), gene analysis, V600 variant(s)*

    🚑 0.00   ✂ 0.00   **FUD** XXX   Ⓐ 🔲

    AMA: 2018,Nov,9; 2018,Jan,8; 2017,Jan,8; 2016,Aug,9; 2016,Jan,13; 2015,Jan,16; 2014,Jan,11

\# **81162** *BRCA1 (BRCA1, DNA repair associated), BRCA2 (BRCA2, DNA repair associated) (eg, hereditary breast and ovarian cancer) gene analysis; full sequence analysis and full duplication/deletion analysis (ie, detection of large gene rearrangements)*

    EXCLUDES *BRCA1 common duplication/deletion variant ([81479])*
        BRCA1, BRCA2 full duplication/deletion analysis only (81164, 81166-81167, 81216)
        BRCA1, BRCA2 full sequence analysis only (81163, 81165)
        BRCA1, BRCA2 known familial variant only (81217)
        Hereditary breast cancer genomic sequence analysis panel (81432)

    🚑 0.00   ✂ 0.00   **FUD** XXX   Ⓐ 🔲

    AMA: 2019,May,5; 2018,Jan,8; 2017,Jan,8; 2016,Aug,9

\# **81163** full sequence analysis

    EXCLUDES *BRCA1 common duplication/deletion variant ([81479])*
        BRCA1, BRCA2 full duplication/deletion analysis only (81164, 81216)
        BRCA1, BRCA2 full sequence analysis and full duplication/deletion analysis (81162)
        BRCA1, BRCA2 full sequence analysis only (81165)
        Hereditary breast cancer genomic sequence analysis panel (81432)

    🚑 0.00   ✂ 0.00   **FUD** XXX   🔲

    AMA: 2019,May,5

\# **81164** full duplication/deletion analysis (ie, detection of large gene rearrangements)

    EXCLUDES *BRCA1 common duplication/deletion variant ([81479])*
        BRCA1, BRCA2 full sequence analysis and full duplication/deletion analysis (81162)
        BRCA1, BRCA2 full sequence analysis only (81163)
        BRCA1, BRCA2 full duplication/deletion analysis only (81166-81167)
        BRCA1, BRCA2 known familial variant only (81217)

    🚑 0.00   ✂ 0.00   **FUD** XXX   Ⓐ 🔲

    AMA: 2019,May,5

81212 185delAG, 5385insC, 6174delT variants

    🚑 0.00   ✂ 0.00   **FUD** XXX   Ⓐ 🔲

    AMA: 2019,May,5; 2018,Nov,9; 2018,Jan,8; 2017,Jan,8; 2016,Aug,9; 2016,Jan,13; 2015,Jan,16; 2014,Jan,11

\# **81165** *BRCA1 (BRCA1, DNA repair associated) (eg, hereditary breast and ovarian cancer) gene analysis; full sequence analysis*

    EXCLUDES *BRCA1 common duplication/deletion variant ([81479])*
        BRCA1, BRCA2 full sequence analysis and full duplication/deletion analysis (81162)
        BRCA1, BRCA2 full sequence analysis only (81163)
        Hereditary breast cancer genomic sequence analysis panel (81432)

    🚑 0.00   ✂ 0.00   **FUD** XXX   🔲

    AMA: 2019,May,5

\# **81166** full duplication/deletion analysis (ie, detection of large gene rearrangements)

    EXCLUDES *BRCA1 common duplication/deletion variant ([81479])*
        BRCA1, BRCA2 full duplication/deletion analysis only (81164)
        BRCA1, BRCA2 full sequence analysis and full duplication/deletion analysis (81162)

    🚑 0.00   ✂ 0.00   **FUD** XXX

    AMA: 2019,May,5

81215 known familial variant

    EXCLUDES *BRCA1 common duplication/deletion variant ([81479])*

    🚑 0.00   ✂ 0.00   **FUD** XXX   Ⓐ 🔲

    AMA: 2019,May,5; 2018,Nov,9; 2018,Jan,8; 2017,Jan,8; 2016,Aug,9; 2016,Jan,13; 2015,Jan,16; 2014,Jan,11

81216 *BRCA2 (BRCA2, DNA repair associated) (eg, hereditary breast and ovarian cancer) gene analysis; full sequence analysis*

    EXCLUDES *BRCA1, BRCA2 full sequence analysis only (81163)*
        BRCA1, BRCA2 full sequence analysis and full duplication/deletion analysis (81162)
        Hereditary breast cancer genomic sequence analysis panel (81432)

    🚑 0.00   ✂ 0.00   **FUD** XXX   Ⓐ 🔲

    AMA: 2019,May,5; 2018,Nov,9; 2018,Jan,8; 2017,Jan,8; 2016,Aug,9; 2016,Jan,13; 2015,Jan,16; 2014,Jan,11

\# **81167** full duplication/deletion analysis (ie, detection of large gene rearrangements)

    EXCLUDES *BRCA1, BRCA2 full duplication/deletion analysis only (81164, 81167)*
        BRCA1, BRCA2 full sequence analysis and full duplication/deletion analysis (81162)

    🚑 0.00   ✂ 0.00   **FUD** XXX   🔲

    AMA: 2019,May,5

81217 known familial variant

    EXCLUDES *BRCA1, BRCA2 full duplication/deletion analysis only (81164, 81167)*
        BRCA1, BRCA2 full sequence analysis and full duplication/deletion analysis (81162)

    🚑 0.00   ✂ 0.00   **FUD** XXX   Ⓐ 🔲

    AMA: 2019,May,5; 2018,Nov,9; 2018,Jan,8; 2017,Jan,8; 2016,Aug,9; 2016,Jan,13; 2015,Jan,16; 2014,Jan,11

\# **81233** *BTK (Bruton's tyrosine kinase) (eg, chronic lymphocytic leukemia) gene analysis, common variants (eg, C481S, C481R, C481F)*

    🚑 0.00   ✂ 0.00   **FUD** XXX   🔲

    AMA: 2018,Nov,9

● New Code ▲ Revised Code ○ Reinstated ● New Web Release ▲ Revised Web Release + Add-on Unlisted Not Covered \# Resequenced
㊿ Optum Mod 50 Exempt △ AMA Mod 51 Exempt ⑤ Optum Mod 51 Exempt ㊿ Mod 63 Exempt ✗ Non-FDA Drug ★ Telemedicine Ⓜ Maternity Ⓐ Age Edit

81184 CACNA1A (calcium voltage-gated channel subunit alpha1 A) (eg, spinocerebellar ataxia) gene analysis; evaluation to detect abnormal (eg, expanded) alleles

📠 0.00 ✂ 0.00 **FUD** XXX A ▣

81185 full gene sequence

📠 0.00 ✂ 0.00 **FUD** XXX ▣

81186 known familial variant

📠 0.00 ✂ 0.00 **FUD** XXX ▣

81219 CALR (calreticulin) (eg, myeloproliferative disorders), gene analysis, common variants in exon 9

📠 0.00 ✂ 0.00 **FUD** XXX A ▣

AMA: 2018,Nov,9; 2018,Jan,8; 2017,Jan,8; 2016,Aug,9

81218 CEBPA (CCAAT/enhancer binding protein [C/EBP], alpha) (eg, acute myeloid leukemia), gene analysis, full gene sequence

📠 0.00 ✂ 0.00 **FUD** XXX A ▣

AMA: 2018,Nov,9; 2018,Jan,8; 2017,Jan,8; 2016,Aug,9

81219 Resequenced code. See code before 81218.

81220 CFTR (cystic fibrosis transmembrane conductance regulator) (eg, cystic fibrosis) gene analysis; common variants (eg, ACMG/ACOG guidelines)

EXCLUDES *Excludes Intron 8 poly-T analysis performed in conjunction with 81220 in a R117H positive patient*

📠 0.00 ✂ 0.00 **FUD** XXX A ▣

AMA: 2018,Nov,9; 2018,Jan,8; 2017,Jan,8; 2016,Aug,9; 2016,Jan,13; 2015,Jan,16; 2014,Jan,11

81221 known familial variants

📠 0.00 ✂ 0.00 **FUD** XXX A ▣

AMA: 2018,Nov,9; 2018,Jan,8; 2017,Jan,8; 2016,Aug,9; 2016,Jan,13; 2015,Jan,16; 2014,Jan,11

81222 duplication/deletion variants

📠 0.00 ✂ 0.00 **FUD** XXX A ▣

AMA: 2018,Nov,9; 2018,Jan,8; 2017,Jan,8; 2016,Aug,9; 2016,Jan,13; 2015,Jan,16; 2014,Jan,11

81223 full gene sequence

📠 0.00 ✂ 0.00 **FUD** XXX A ▣

AMA: 2018,Nov,9; 2018,Jan,8; 2017,Jan,8; 2016,Aug,9; 2016,Jan,13; 2015,Jan,16; 2014,Jan,11

81224 intron 8 poly-T analysis (eg, male infertility)

📠 0.00 ✂ 0.00 **FUD** XXX A ▣

AMA: 2018,Nov,9; 2018,Jan,8; 2017,Jan,8; 2016,Aug,9; 2016,Jan,13; 2015,Jan,16; 2014,Jan,11

81267 Chimerism (engraftment) analysis, post transplantation specimen (eg, hematopoietic stem cell), includes comparison to previously performed baseline analyses; without cell selection

📠 0.00 ✂ 0.00 **FUD** XXX A ▣

AMA: 2018,Nov,9; 2018,Jan,8; 2017,Jan,8; 2016,Aug,9; 2016,Jan,13; 2015,Jan,16; 2014,Jan,11

81268 with cell selection (eg, CD3, CD33), each cell type

📠 0.00 ✂ 0.00 **FUD** XXX A ▣

AMA: 2018,Nov,9; 2018,Jan,8; 2017,Jan,8; 2016,Aug,9; 2016,Jan,13; 2015,Jan,16; 2014,Jan,11

81187 CNBP (CCHC-type zinc finger nucleic acid binding protein) (eg, myotonic dystrophy type 2) gene analysis, evaluation to detect abnormal (eg, expanded) alleles

📠 0.00 ✂ 0.00 **FUD** XXX ▣

81265 Comparative analysis using Short Tandem Repeat (STR) markers; patient and comparative specimen (eg, pre-transplant recipient and donor germline testing, post-transplant non-hematopoietic recipient germline [eg, buccal swab or other germline tissue sample] and donor testing, twin zygosity testing, or maternal cell contamination of fetal cells)

📠 0.00 ✂ 0.00 **FUD** XXX A ▣

AMA: 2018,Nov,9; 2018,Jan,8; 2017,Jan,8; 2016,Aug,9; 2016,Jan,13; 2015,Jan,16; 2014,Jan,11

+ # 81266 each additional specimen (eg, additional cord blood donor, additional fetal samples from different cultures, or additional zygosity in multiple birth pregnancies) (List separately in addition to code for primary procedure)

📠 0.00 ✂ 0.00 **FUD** XXX A ▣

AMA: 2018,Nov,9; 2018,Jan,8; 2017,Jan,8; 2016,Aug,9; 2016,Jan,13; 2015,Jan,16; 2014,Jan,11

81188 CSTB (cystatin B) (eg, Unverricht-Lundborg disease) gene analysis; evaluation to detect abnormal (eg, expanded) alleles

📠 0.00 ✂ 0.00 **FUD** XXX ▣

81189 full gene sequence

📠 0.00 ✂ 0.00 **FUD** XXX ▣

81190 known familial variant(s)

📠 0.00 ✂ 0.00 **FUD** XXX ▣

81227 CYP2C9 (cytochrome P450, family 2, subfamily C, polypeptide 9) (eg, drug metabolism), gene analysis, common variants (eg, *2, *3, *5, *6)

📠 0.00 ✂ 0.00 **FUD** XXX A ▣

AMA: 2018,Nov,9; 2018,Jan,8; 2017,Jan,8; 2016,Aug,9; 2016,Jan,13; 2015,Jan,16; 2014,Jan,11

81225 CYP2C19 (cytochrome P450, family 2, subfamily C, polypeptide 19) (eg, drug metabolism), gene analysis, common variants (eg, *2, *3, *4, *8, *17)

📠 0.00 ✂ 0.00 **FUD** XXX A ▣

AMA: 2018,Nov,9; 2018,Jan,8; 2017,Jan,8; 2016,Aug,9; 2016,Jan,13; 2015,Jan,16; 2014,Jan,11

81226 CYP2D6 (cytochrome P450, family 2, subfamily D, polypeptide 6) (eg, drug metabolism), gene analysis, common variants (eg, *2, *3, *4, *5, *6, *9, *10, *17, *19, *29, *35, *41, *1XN, *2XN, *4XN)

📠 0.00 ✂ 0.00 **FUD** XXX A ▣

AMA: 2018,Nov,9; 2018,Jan,8; 2017,Jan,8; 2016,Aug,9; 2016,Jan,13; 2015,Jan,16; 2014,Jan,11

81227 Resequenced code. See code before 81225.

81230 CYP3A4 (cytochrome P450 family 3 subfamily A member 4) (eg, drug metabolism), gene analysis, common variant(s) (eg, *2, *22)

📠 0.00 ✂ 0.00 **FUD** XXX A ▣

AMA: 2018,Nov,9

81231 CYP3A5 (cytochrome P450 family 3 subfamily A member 5) (eg, drug metabolism), gene analysis, common variants (eg, *2, *3, *4, *5, *6, *7)

📠 0.00 ✂ 0.00 **FUD** XXX A ▣

AMA: 2018,Nov,9

81228 Cytogenomic constitutional (genome-wide) microarray analysis; interrogation of genomic regions for copy number variants (eg, bacterial artificial chromosome [BAC] or oligo-based comparative genomic hybridization [CGH] microarray analysis)

EXCLUDES *Analyte-specific molecular pathology procedures included in microarray analysis*
When performed in conjunction with single nucleotide polymorphism interrogation (81229)

📠 0.00 ✂ 0.00 **FUD** XXX A ▣

AMA: 2018,Nov,9; 2018,Jan,8; 2017,Apr,3; 2017,Jan,8; 2016,Aug,9; 2016,Jan,13; 2015,Jan,16; 2014,Jan,11

81229 **interrogation of genomic regions for copy number and single nucleotide polymorphism (SNP) variants for chromosomal abnormalities**

EXCLUDES *Analyte-specific molecular pathology procedures included in microarray analysis*
Copy number variant detection using oligonucleotide interrogation only (81228)
Fetal genomic sequencing or other molecular multianalyte assays using circulating cell-free DNA in maternal blood ([81479], 81420, 81422)
Molecular cytogenetics; DNA probe (88271)
Specific code for targeted cytogenomic constitutional microarray analysis
Unlisted molecular pathology procedures ([81479])

⚕ 0.00 ✂ 0.00 **FUD** XXX [A][☐]

AMA: 2018,Nov,9; 2018,Jan,8; 2017,Apr,3; 2017,Jan,8; 2016,Aug,9; 2016,Jan,13; 2015,Jan,16; 2014,Jan,11

● # 81277 **Cytogenomic neoplasia (genome-wide) microarray analysis, interrogation of genomic regions for copy number and loss-of-heterozygosity variants for chromosomal abnormalities**

⚕ 0.00 ✂ 0.00 **FUD** 000

EXCLUDES *Analyte-specific molecular pathology procedures included in microarray analysis for neoplasia*
Molecular cytogenetics; DNA probe (88271)

81230 **Resequenced code. See code following numeric code 81227.**

81231 **Resequenced code. See code following numeric code 81227.**

81161 *DMD (dystrophin)* **(eg, Duchenne/Becker muscular dystrophy) deletion analysis, and duplication analysis, if performed**

⚕ 0.00 ✂ 0.00 **FUD** XXX [A][☐]

AMA: 2018,Nov,9; 2018,Jan,8; 2017,Jan,8; 2016,Aug,9; 2014,Jan,11

81234 *DMPK (DM1 protein kinase)* **(eg, myotonic dystrophy type 1) gene analysis; evaluation to detect abnormal (expanded) alleles**

⚕ 0.00 ✂ 0.00 **FUD** XXX [☐]

AMA: 2018,Nov,9

81239 **characterization of alleles (eg, expanded size)**

⚕ 0.00 ✂ 0.00 **FUD** XXX [☐]

AMA: 2018,Nov,9

81232 *DPYD (dihydropyrimidine dehydrogenase)* **(eg, 5-fluorouracil/5-FU and capecitabine drug metabolism), gene analysis, common variant(s) (eg, *2A, *4, *5, *6)**

⚕ 0.00 ✂ 0.00 **FUD** XXX [A][☐]

AMA: 2018,Nov,9

81233 **Resequenced code. See code following 81217.**

81234 **Resequenced code. See code following numeric code 81231.**

81235 *EGFR (epidermal growth factor receptor)* **(eg, non-small cell lung cancer) gene analysis, common variants (eg, exon 19 LREA deletion, L858R, T790M, G719A, G719S, L861Q)**

⚕ 0.00 ✂ 0.00 **FUD** XXX [A][☐]

AMA: 2018,Nov,9; 2018,Jan,8; 2017,Jan,8; 2016,Aug,9; 2016,Jan,13; 2015,Jan,16; 2014,Jan,11

81236 *EZH2 (enhancer of zeste 2 polycomb repressive complex 2 subunit)* **(eg, myelodysplastic syndrome, myeloproliferative neoplasms) gene analysis, full gene sequence**

⚕ 0.00 ✂ 0.00 **FUD** XXX [☐]

AMA: 2019,Jul,3; 2018,Nov,9

81237 *EZH2 (enhancer of zeste 2 polycomb repressive complex 2 subunit)* **(eg, diffuse large B-cell lymphoma) gene analysis, common variant(s) (eg, codon 646)**

⚕ 0.00 ✂ 0.00 **FUD** XXX [☐]

AMA: 2019,Jul,3; 2018,Nov,9

81238 **Resequenced code. See code following 81241.**

81239 **Resequenced code. See code before 81232.**

81240 *F2 (prothrombin, coagulation factor II)* **(eg, hereditary hypercoagulability) gene analysis, 20210G>A variant**

⚕ 0.00 ✂ 0.00 **FUD** XXX [A][☐]

AMA: 2018,Nov,9; 2018,Jan,8; 2017,Jan,8; 2016,Aug,9; 2016,Jan,13; 2015,Jan,16; 2014,Jan,11

81241 *F5 (coagulation factor V)* **(eg, hereditary hypercoagulability) gene analysis, Leiden variant**

⚕ 0.00 ✂ 0.00 **FUD** XXX [A][☐]

AMA: 2018,Nov,9; 2018,Jan,8; 2017,Jan,8; 2016,Aug,9; 2016,Jan,13; 2015,Jan,16; 2014,Jan,11

81238 *F9 (coagulation factor IX)* **(eg, hemophilia B), full gene sequence**

⚕ 0.00 ✂ 0.00 **FUD** XXX [A][☐]

AMA: 2018,Nov,9

81242 *FANCC (Fanconi anemia, complementation group C)* **(eg, Fanconi anemia, type C) gene analysis, common variant (eg, IVS4+4A>T)**

⚕ 0.00 ✂ 0.00 **FUD** XXX [A][☐]

AMA: 2018,Nov,9; 2018,Jan,8; 2017,Jan,8; 2016,Aug,9; 2016,Jan,13; 2015,Jan,16; 2014,Jan,11

81245 *FLT3 (fms-related tyrosine kinase 3)* **(eg, acute myeloid leukemia), gene analysis; internal tandem duplication (ITD) variants (ie, exons 14, 15)**

⚕ 0.00 ✂ 0.00 **FUD** XXX [A][☐]

AMA: 2018,Nov,9; 2018,Jan,8; 2017,Jan,8; 2016,Aug,9; 2016,Jan,13; 2015,Jan,16; 2015,Jan,3; 2014,Jan,11

81246 **tyrosine kinase domain (TKD) variants (eg, D835, I836)**

⚕ 0.00 ✂ 0.00 **FUD** XXX [A][☐]

AMA: 2018,Nov,9; 2018,Jan,8; 2017,Jan,8; 2016,Aug,9; 2016,Jan,13; 2015,Jan,3

81243 *FMR1 (fragile X mental retardation 1)* **(eg, fragile X mental retardation) gene analysis; evaluation to detect abnormal (eg, expanded) alleles**

INCLUDES Evaluation to detect and characterize abnormal alleles using a single assay [eg, PCR]

EXCLUDES *Evaluation to detect and characterize abnormal alleles (81244)*

⚕ 0.00 ✂ 0.00 **FUD** XXX [A][☐]

AMA: 2019,Jul,3; 2018,Nov,9; 2018,Jan,8; 2017,Jan,8; 2016,Aug,9; 2016,Jan,13; 2015,Jan,16; 2014,Jan,11

81244 **characterization of alleles (eg, expanded size and promoter methylation status)**

EXCLUDES *Evaluation to detect and characterize abnormal alleles using a single assay [eg, PCR] (81243)*

⚕ 0.00 ✂ 0.00 **FUD** XXX [A][☐]

AMA: 2019,Jul,3; 2018,Nov,9; 2018,Jan,8; 2017,Jan,8; 2016,Aug,9; 2016,Jan,13; 2015,Jan,16; 2014,Jan,11

81245 **Resequenced code. See code following 81242.**

81246 **Resequenced code. See code following 81242.**

81284 *FXN (frataxin)* **(eg, Friedreich ataxia) gene analysis; evaluation to detect abnormal (expanded) alleles**

⚕ 0.00 ✂ 0.00 **FUD** XXX [☐]

AMA: 2018,Nov,9

81285 **characterization of alleles (eg, expanded size)**

⚕ 0.00 ✂ 0.00 **FUD** XXX [☐]

AMA: 2018,Nov,9

81286 **full gene sequence**

⚕ 0.00 ✂ 0.00 **FUD** XXX [☐]

AMA: 2018,Nov,9

81289 **known familial variant(s)**

⚕ 0.00 ✂ 0.00 **FUD** XXX [☐]

AMA: 2018,Nov,9

\# **81250** *G6PC (glucose-6-phosphatase, catalytic subunit) (eg, Glycogen storage disease, type 1a, von Gierke disease) gene analysis, common variants (eg, R83C, Q347X)*
0.00 ⚕ 0.00 **FUD** XXX A 🖾
AMA: 2018,Nov,9; 2018,Jan,8; 2017,Jan,8; 2016,Aug,9; 2016,Jan,13; 2015,Jan,16; 2014,Jan,11

81247 *G6PD (glucose-6-phosphate dehydrogenase) (eg, hemolytic anemia, jaundice), gene analysis; common variant(s) (eg, A, A-)*
0.00 ⚕ 0.00 **FUD** XXX A 🖾
AMA: 2018,Nov,9

81248 **known familial variant(s)**
0.00 ⚕ 0.00 **FUD** XXX A 🖾
AMA: 2018,Nov,9

81249 **full gene sequence**
0.00 ⚕ 0.00 **FUD** XXX A 🖾
AMA: 2018,Nov,9

81250 **Resequenced code. See code before 81247.**

81251 *GBA (glucosidase, beta, acid) (eg, Gaucher disease) gene analysis, common variants (eg, N370S, 84GG, L444P, IVS2+1G>A)*
0.00 ⚕ 0.00 **FUD** XXX A 🖾
AMA: 2018,Nov,9; 2018,Jan,8; 2017,Jan,8; 2016,Aug,9; 2016,Jan,13; 2015,Jan,16; 2014,Jan,11

81252 *GJB2 (gap junction protein, beta 2, 26kDa, connexin 26) (eg, nonsyndromic hearing loss) gene analysis; full gene sequence*
0.00 ⚕ 0.00 **FUD** XXX A 🖾
AMA: 2018,Nov,9; 2018,Jan,8; 2017,Jan,8; 2016,Aug,9; 2016,Jan,13; 2015,Jan,16; 2014,Jan,11

81253 **known familial variants**
0.00 ⚕ 0.00 **FUD** XXX A 🖾
AMA: 2018,Nov,9; 2018,Jan,8; 2017,Jan,8; 2016,Aug,9; 2016,Jan,13; 2015,Jan,16; 2014,Jan,11

81254 *GJB6 (gap junction protein, beta 6, 30kDa, connexin 30) (eg, nonsyndromic hearing loss) gene analysis, common variants (eg, 309kb [del(GJB6-D13S1830)] and 232kb [del(GJB6-D13S1854)])*
0.00 ⚕ 0.00 **FUD** XXX A 🖾
AMA: 2018,Nov,9; 2018,Jan,8; 2017,Jan,8; 2016,Aug,9; 2016,Jan,13; 2015,Jan,16; 2014,Jan,11

\# **81257** *HBA1/HBA2 (alpha globin 1 and alpha globin 2) (eg, alpha thalassemia, Hb Bart hydrops fetalis syndrome, HbH disease), gene analysis; common deletions or variant (eg, Southeast Asian, Thai, Filipino, Mediterranean, alpha3.7, alpha4.2, alpha20.5, Constant Spring)*
0.00 ⚕ 0.00 **FUD** XXX A 🖾
AMA: 2018,Nov,9; 2018,Jan,8; 2017,Jan,8; 2016,Aug,9; 2016,Jan,13; 2015,Jan,16; 2014,Jan,11

\# **81258** **known familial variant**
0.00 ⚕ 0.00 **FUD** XXX A 🖾
AMA: 2018,Nov,9

\# **81259** **full gene sequence**
0.00 ⚕ 0.00 **FUD** XXX A 🖾
AMA: 2018,Nov,9

\# **81269** **duplication/deletion variants**
0.00 ⚕ 0.00 **FUD** XXX A 🖾
AMA: 2018,Nov,9

\# **81361** *HBB (hemoglobin, subunit beta) (eg, sickle cell anemia, beta thalassemia, hemoglobinopathy); common variant(s) (eg, HbS, HbC, HbE)*
0.00 ⚕ 0.00 **FUD** XXX A 🖾
AMA: 2018,Nov,9

\# **81362** **known familial variant(s)**
0.00 ⚕ 0.00 **FUD** XXX A 🖾
AMA: 2018,Nov,9

\# **81363** **duplication/deletion variant(s)**
0.00 ⚕ 0.00 **FUD** XXX A 🖾
AMA: 2018,Nov,9; 2018,Sep,14

\# **81364** **full gene sequence**
0.00 ⚕ 0.00 **FUD** XXX A 🖾
AMA: 2018,Nov,9; 2018,Sep,14

81255 *HEXA (hexosaminidase A [alpha polypeptide]) (eg, Tay-Sachs disease) gene analysis, common variants (eg, 1278insTATC, 1421+1G>C, G269S)*
0.00 ⚕ 0.00 **FUD** XXX A 🖾
AMA: 2018,Nov,9; 2018,Jan,8; 2017,Jan,8; 2016,Aug,9; 2016,Jan,13; 2015,Jan,16; 2014,Jan,11

81256 *HFE (hemochromatosis) (eg, hereditary hemochromatosis) gene analysis, common variants (eg, C282Y, H63D)*
0.00 ⚕ 0.00 **FUD** XXX A 🖾
AMA: 2018,Nov,9; 2018,Jan,8; 2017,Jan,8; 2016,Aug,9; 2016,Jan,13; 2015,Jan,16; 2014,Jan,11

81257 **Resequenced code. See code following 81254.**

81258 **Resequenced code. See code following 81254.**

81259 **Resequenced code. See code following 81254.**

\# **81271** *HTT (huntingtin) (eg, Huntington disease) gene analysis; evaluation to detect abnormal (eg, expanded) alleles*
0.00 ⚕ 0.00 **FUD** XXX 🖾
AMA: 2018,Nov,9

\# **81274** **characterization of alleles (eg, expanded size)**
0.00 ⚕ 0.00 **FUD** XXX A 🖾
AMA: 2018,Nov,9

\# **81105** *Human Platelet Antigen 1 genotyping (HPA-1), ITGB3 (integrin, beta 3 [platelet glycoprotein IIIa], antigen CD61 [GPIIIa]) (eg, neonatal alloimmune thrombocytopenia [NAIT], post-transfusion purpura), gene analysis, common variant, HPA-1a/b (L33P)*
0.00 ⚕ 0.00 **FUD** XXX A 🖾

\# **81106** *Human Platelet Antigen 2 genotyping (HPA-2), GP1BA (glycoprotein Ib [platelet], alpha polypeptide [GPIba]) (eg, neonatal alloimmune thrombocytopenia [NAIT], post-transfusion purpura), gene analysis, common variant, HPA-2a/b (T145M)*
0.00 ⚕ 0.00 **FUD** XXX A 🖾

\# **81107** *Human Platelet Antigen 3 genotyping (HPA-3), ITGA2B (integrin, alpha 2b [platelet glycoprotein IIb of IIb/IIIa complex], antigen CD41 [GPIIb]) (eg, neonatal alloimmune thrombocytopenia [NAIT], post-transfusion purpura), gene analysis, common variant, HPA-3a/b (I843S)*
0.00 ⚕ 0.00 **FUD** XXX A 🖾

\# **81108** *Human Platelet Antigen 4 genotyping (HPA-4), ITGB3 (integrin, beta 3 [platelet glycoprotein IIIa], antigen CD61 [GPIIIa]) (eg, neonatal alloimmune thrombocytopenia [NAIT], post-transfusion purpura), gene analysis, common variant, HPA-4a/b (R143Q)*
0.00 ⚕ 0.00 **FUD** XXX A 🖾

\# **81109** *Human Platelet Antigen 5 genotyping (HPA-5), ITGA2 (integrin, alpha 2 [CD49B, alpha 2 subunit of VLA-2 receptor] [GPIa]) (eg, neonatal alloimmune thrombocytopenia [NAIT], post-transfusion purpura), gene analysis, common variant (eg, HPA-5a/b (K505E))*
0.00 ⚕ 0.00 **FUD** XXX A 🖾

\# **81110** *Human Platelet Antigen 6 genotyping (HPA-6w), ITGB3 (integrin, beta 3 [platelet glycoprotein IIIa, antigen CD61] [GPIIIa]) (eg, neonatal alloimmune thrombocytopenia [NAIT], post-transfusion purpura), gene analysis, common variant, HPA-6a/b (R489Q)*
0.00 ⚕ 0.00 **FUD** XXX A 🖾

26/TC PC/TC Only   N2-N3 ASC Payment   50 Bilateral   ♂ Male Only   ♀ Female Only   🏥 Facility RVU   ⚕ Non-Facility RVU   🖵 CCI   ❌ CLIA
FUD Follow-up Days   CMS: IOM   AMA: CPT Asst   A-Y OPPSI   80/80 Surg Assist Allowed / w/Doc   🖾 Lab Crosswalk   🖾 Radiology Crosswalk

382

Pathology and Laboratory

\# **81111** _Human Platelet Antigen 9 genotyping (HPA-9w), ITGA2B (integrin, alpha 2b [platelet glycoprotein IIb of IIb/IIIa complex, antigen CD41] [GPIIb]) (eg, neonatal alloimmune thrombocytopenia [NAIT], post-transfusion purpura), gene analysis, common variant, HPA-9a/b (V837M)_
🚗 0.00   ⚕ 0.00   **FUD** XXX   Ⓐ ▱

\# **81112** _Human Platelet Antigen 15 genotyping (HPA-15), CD109 (CD109 molecule) (eg, neonatal alloimmune thrombocytopenia [NAIT], post-transfusion purpura), gene analysis, common variant, HPA-15a/b (S682Y)_
Ⓐ ▱

\# **81120** _IDH1 (isocitrate dehydrogenase 1 [NADP+], soluble) (eg, glioma), common variants (eg, R132H, R132C)_
FUD XXX   Ⓐ ▱

\# **81121** _IDH2 (isocitrate dehydrogenase 2 [NADP+], mitochondrial) (eg, glioma), common variants (eg, R140W, R172M)_
FUD XXX   Ⓐ ▱

\# **81283** _IFNL3 (interferon, lambda 3) (eg, drug response), gene analysis, rs12979860 variant_
FUD XXX   Ⓐ ▱
AMA: 2018,Nov,9

\# **81261** _IGH@ (Immunoglobulin heavy chain locus) (eg, leukemias and lymphomas, B-cell), gene rearrangement analysis to detect abnormal clonal population(s); amplified methodology (eg, polymerase chain reaction)_
🚗 0.00   ⚕ 0.00   **FUD** XXX   Ⓐ ▱
AMA: 2018,Nov,9; 2018,Jan,8; 2017,Jan,8; 2016,Aug,9; 2016,Jan,13; 2015,Jan,16; 2014,Jan,11

\# **81262** **direct probe methodology (eg, Southern blot)**
🚗 0.00   ⚕ 0.00   **FUD** XXX   Ⓐ ▱
AMA: 2018,Nov,9; 2018,Jan,8; 2017,Jan,8; 2016,Aug,9; 2016,Jan,13; 2015,Jan,16; 2014,Jan,11

\# **81263** _IGH@ (Immunoglobulin heavy chain locus) (eg, leukemia and lymphoma, B-cell), variable region somatic mutation analysis_
🚗 0.00   ⚕ 0.00   **FUD** XXX   Ⓐ ▱
AMA: 2018,Nov,9; 2018,Jan,8; 2017,Jan,8; 2016,Aug,9; 2016,Jan,13; 2015,Jan,16; 2014,Jan,11

\# **81264** _IGK@ (Immunoglobulin kappa light chain locus) (eg, leukemia and lymphoma, B-cell), gene rearrangement analysis, evaluation to detect abnormal clonal population(s)_
🚗 0.00   ⚕ 0.00   **FUD** XXX   Ⓐ ▱
AMA: 2018,Nov,9; 2018,Jan,8; 2017,Jan,8; 2016,Aug,9; 2016,Jan,13; 2015,Jan,16; 2014,Jan,11

81260 _IKBKAP (inhibitor of kappa light polypeptide gene enhancer in B-cells, kinase complex-associated protein) (eg, familial dysautonomia) gene analysis, common variants (eg, 2507+6T>C, R696P)_
FUD XXX   Ⓐ ▱
AMA: 2018,Nov,9; 2018,Jan,8; 2017,Jan,8; 2016,Aug,9; 2016,Jan,13; 2015,Jan,16; 2014,Jan,11

81261 Resequenced code. See code before 81260.

81262 Resequenced code. See code before 81260.

81263 Resequenced code. See code following resequenced code 81262.

81264 Resequenced code. See code before 81260.

81265 Resequenced code. See code following resequenced code 81187.

81266 Resequenced code. See code following resequenced code 81265.

81267 Resequenced code. See code following 81224.

81268 Resequenced code. See code following 81224.

81269 Resequenced code. See code following resequenced code 81259.

81270 _JAK2 (Janus kinase 2) (eg, myeloproliferative disorder) gene analysis, p.Val617Phe (V617F) variant_
Ⓐ ▱
AMA: 2018,Nov,9; 2018,Jan,8; 2017,Jan,8; 2016,Aug,9; 2016,Jan,13; 2015,Jan,16; 2014,Jan,11

81271 Resequenced code. See code following numeric code 81259.

81272 _KIT (v-kit Hardy-Zuckerman 4 feline sarcoma viral oncogene homolog) (eg, gastrointestinal stromal tumor [GIST], acute myeloid leukemia, melanoma), gene analysis, targeted sequence analysis (eg, exons 8, 11, 13, 17, 18)_
🚗 0.00   ⚕ 0.00   **FUD** XXX   Ⓐ ▱
AMA: 2018,Nov,9; 2018,Jan,8; 2017,Jan,8; 2016,Aug,9

81273 _KIT (v-kit Hardy-Zuckerman 4 feline sarcoma viral oncogene homolog) (eg, mastocytosis), gene analysis, D816 variant_
🚗 0.00   ⚕ 0.00   **FUD** XXX   Ⓐ ▱
AMA: 2018,Nov,9; 2018,Jan,8; 2017,Jan,8; 2016,Aug,9

81274 Resequenced code. See code following resequenced code 81271.

81275 _KRAS (Kirsten rat sarcoma viral oncogene homolog) (eg, carcinoma) gene analysis; variants in exon 2 (eg, codons 12 and 13)_
🚗 0.00   ⚕ 0.00   **FUD** XXX   Ⓐ ▱
AMA: 2018,Nov,9; 2018,Jan,8; 2017,Jan,8; 2016,Aug,9; 2016,Jan,13; 2015,Jan,16; 2014,Jan,11

81276 **additional variant(s) (eg, codon 61, codon 146)**
🚗 0.00   ⚕ 0.00   **FUD** XXX   Ⓐ ▱
AMA: 2018,Nov,9; 2018,Jan,8; 2017,Jan,8; 2016,Aug,9

81277 Resequenced code. See code following 81229.

81283 Resequenced code. See code following resequenced code 81121.

81284 Resequenced code. See code following numeric code 81246.

81285 Resequenced code. See code following numeric code 81246.

81286 Resequenced code. See code following numeric code 81246.

81287 Resequenced code. See code following resequenced code 81304.

81288 Resequenced code. See code following resequenced code 81292.

81289 Resequenced code. See code following numeric code 81246.

81290 _MCOLN1 (mucolipin 1) (eg, Mucolipidosis, type IV) gene analysis, common variants (eg, IVS3-2A>G, del6.4kb)_
🚗 0.00   ⚕ 0.00   **FUD** XXX   Ⓐ ▱
AMA: 2018,Nov,9; 2018,Jan,8; 2017,Jan,8; 2016,Aug,9; 2016,Jan,13; 2015,Jan,16; 2014,Jan,11

\# **81302** _MECP2 (methyl CpG binding protein 2) (eg, Rett syndrome) gene analysis; full sequence analysis_
🚗 0.00   ⚕ 0.00   **FUD** XXX   Ⓐ ▱
AMA: 2018,Nov,9; 2018,Jan,8; 2017,Jan,8; 2016,Aug,9; 2016,Jan,13; 2015,Jan,16; 2014,Jan,11

\# **81303** **known familial variant**
🚗 0.00   ⚕ 0.00   **FUD** XXX   Ⓐ ▱
AMA: 2018,Nov,9; 2018,Jan,8; 2017,Jan,8; 2016,Aug,9; 2016,Jan,13; 2015,Jan,16; 2014,Jan,11

\# **81304** **duplication/deletion variants**
🚗 0.00   ⚕ 0.00   **FUD** XXX   Ⓐ ▱
AMA: 2018,Nov,9; 2018,Jan,8; 2017,Jan,8; 2016,Aug,9; 2016,Jan,13; 2015,Jan,16; 2014,Jan,11

● New Code   ▲ Revised Code   ○ Reinstated   ● New Web Release   ▲ Revised Web Release   + Add-on   Unlisted   Not Covered   \# Resequenced
㊿ Optum Mod 50 Exempt   Ⓢ AMA Mod 51 Exempt   �51 Optum Mod 51 Exempt   ㊶ Mod 63 Exempt   ⁄ Non-FDA Drug   ★ Telemedicine   Ⓜ Maternity   Ⓐ Age Edit

\# 81287 **MGMT (O-6-methylguanine-DNA methyltransferase) (eg, glioblastoma multiforme), promoter methylation analysis**
🚗 0.00 ✂ 0.00 **FUD** XXX   [A] [▣]
AMA: 2019,Jul,3; 2018,Dec,10; 2018,Dec,10; 2018,Nov,9; 2018,Jan,8; 2017,Jan,8; 2016,Aug,9; 2014,Jan,11

\# 81301 **Microsatellite instability analysis (eg, hereditary non-polyposis colorectal cancer, Lynch syndrome) of markers for mismatch repair deficiency (eg, BAT25, BAT26), includes comparison of neoplastic and normal tissue, if performed**
🚗 0.00 ✂ 0.00 **FUD** XXX   [A] [▣]
AMA: 2018,Nov,9; 2018,Jan,8; 2017,Jan,8; 2016,Aug,9; 2016,Jan,13; 2015,Jan,16; 2014,Jan,11

\# 81292 **MLH1 (mutL homolog 1, colon cancer, nonpolyposis type 2) (eg, hereditary non-polyposis colorectal cancer, Lynch syndrome) gene analysis; full sequence analysis**
🚗 0.00 ✂ 0.00 **FUD** XXX   [A] [▣]
AMA: 2018,Nov,9; 2018,Jan,8; 2017,Jan,8; 2016,Aug,9; 2016,Jan,13; 2015,Jan,16; 2015,Jan,3; 2014,Jan,11

\# 81288 **promoter methylation analysis**
🚗 0.00 ✂ 0.00 **FUD** XXX   [A] [▣]
AMA: 2018,Nov,9; 2018,Jan,8; 2017,Jan,8; 2016,Aug,9; 2016,Jan,13; 2015,Jan,3

\# 81293 **known familial variants**
🚗 0.00 ✂ 0.00 **FUD** XXX   [A] [▣]
AMA: 2018,Nov,9; 2018,Jan,8; 2017,Jan,8; 2016,Aug,9; 2016,Jan,13; 2015,Jan,16; 2014,Jan,11

\# 81294 **duplication/deletion variants**
🚗 0.00 ✂ 0.00 **FUD** XXX   [A] [▣]
AMA: 2018,Nov,9; 2018,Jan,8; 2017,Jan,8; 2016,Aug,9; 2016,Jan,13; 2015,Jan,16; 2014,Jan,11

\# 81295 **MSH2 (mutS homolog 2, colon cancer, nonpolyposis type 1) (eg, hereditary non-polyposis colorectal cancer, Lynch syndrome) gene analysis; full sequence analysis**
🚗 0.00 ✂ 0.00 **FUD** XXX   [A] [▣]
AMA: 2018,Nov,9; 2018,Jan,8; 2017,Jan,8; 2016,Aug,9; 2016,Jan,13; 2015,Jan,16; 2014,Jan,11

81291 Resequenced code. See code before 81305.

81292 Resequenced code. See code before numeric code 81291.

81293 Resequenced code. See code before numeric code 81291.

81294 Resequenced code. See code before numeric code 81291.

81295 Resequenced code. See code before numeric code 81291.

81296 **known familial variants**
🚗 0.00 ✂ 0.00 **FUD** XXX   [A] [▣]
AMA: 2018,Nov,9; 2018,Jan,8; 2017,Jan,8; 2016,Aug,9; 2016,Jan,13; 2015,Jan,16; 2014,Jan,11

81297 **duplication/deletion variants**
🚗 0.00 ✂ 0.00 **FUD** XXX   [A] [▣]
AMA: 2018,Nov,9; 2018,Jan,8; 2017,Jan,8; 2016,Aug,9; 2016,Jan,13; 2015,Jan,16; 2014,Jan,11

81298 **MSH6 (mutS homolog 6 [E. coli]) (eg, hereditary non-polyposis colorectal cancer, Lynch syndrome) gene analysis; full sequence analysis**
🚗 0.00 ✂ 0.00 **FUD** XXX   [A] [▣]
AMA: 2018,Nov,9; 2018,Jan,8; 2017,Jan,8; 2016,Aug,9; 2016,Jan,13; 2015,Jan,16; 2014,Jan,11

81299 **known familial variants**
🚗 0.00 ✂ 0.00 **FUD** XXX   [A] [▣]
AMA: 2018,Nov,9; 2018,Jan,8; 2017,Jan,8; 2016,Aug,9; 2016,Jan,13; 2015,Jan,16; 2014,Jan,11

81300 **duplication/deletion variants**
🚗 0.00 ✂ 0.00 **FUD** XXX   [A] [▣]
AMA: 2018,Nov,9; 2018,Jan,8; 2017,Jan,8; 2016,Aug,9; 2016,Jan,13; 2015,Jan,16; 2014,Jan,11

81301 Resequenced code. See code following resequenced code 81287.

81302 Resequenced code. See code following 81290.

81303 Resequenced code. See code following 81290.

81304 Resequenced code. See code following 81290.

\# 81291 **MTHFR (5,10-methylenetetrahydrofolate reductase) (eg, hereditary hypercoagulability) gene analysis, common variants (eg, 677T, 1298C)**
🚗 0.00 ✂ 0.00 **FUD** XXX   [A] [▣]
AMA: 2018,Nov,9; 2018,Jan,8; 2017,Jan,8; 2016,Aug,9; 2016,Jan,13; 2015,Jan,16; 2014,Jan,11

81305 **MYD88 (myeloid differentiation primary response 88) (eg, Waldenstrom's macroglobulinemia, lymphoplasmacytic leukemia) gene analysis, p.Leu265Pro (L265P) variant**
🚗 0.00 ✂ 0.00 **FUD** XXX   [▣]
AMA: 2019,Jul,3; 2018,Nov,9

81306 Resequenced code. See code following numeric code 81312.

81307 Resequenced code. See code before 81313.

81308 Resequenced code. See code before 81313.

81309 Resequenced code. See code following 81314.

81310 **NPM1 (nucleophosmin) (eg, acute myeloid leukemia) gene analysis, exon 12 variants**
🚗 0.00 ✂ 0.00 **FUD** XXX   [A] [▣]
AMA: 2018,Nov,9; 2018,Jan,8; 2017,Jan,8; 2016,Aug,9; 2016,Jan,13; 2015,Jan,16; 2014,Jan,11

81311 **NRAS (neuroblastoma RAS viral [v-ras] oncogene homolog) (eg, colorectal carcinoma), gene analysis, variants in exon 2 (eg, codons 12 and 13) and exon 3 (eg, codon 61)**
🚗 0.00 ✂ 0.00 **FUD** XXX   [A] [▣]
AMA: 2018,Nov,9; 2018,Jan,8; 2017,Jan,8; 2016,Aug,9

81312 Resequenced code. See code following resequenced code 81306.

\# 81306 **NUDT15 (nudix hydrolase 15) (eg, drug metabolism) gene analysis, common variant(s) (eg, *2, *3, *4, *5, *6)**
🚗 0.00 ✂ 0.00 **FUD** XXX   [A] [▣]
AMA: 2019,Jul,3; 2018,Nov,9

\# 81312 **PABPN1 (poly[A] binding protein nuclear 1) (eg, oculopharyngeal muscular dystrophy) gene analysis, evaluation to detect abnormal (eg, expanded) alleles**
🚗 0.00 ✂ 0.00 **FUD** XXX   [▣]
AMA: 2018,Nov,9

● \# 81307 **PALB2 (partner and localizer of BRCA2) (eg, breast and pancreatic cancer) gene analysis; full gene sequence**
🚗 0.00 ✂ 0.00 **FUD** 000

● \# 81308 **known familial variant**
🚗 0.00 ✂ 0.00 **FUD** 000

81313 **PCA3/KLK3 (prostate cancer antigen 3 [non-protein coding]/kallikrein-related peptidase 3 [prostate specific antigen]) ratio (eg, prostate cancer)**
🚗 0.00 ✂ 0.00 **FUD** XXX   [A] [▣]
AMA: 2018,Nov,9; 2018,Jan,8; 2017,Jan,8; 2016,Aug,9; 2016,Jan,13; 2015,Jan,3

81314 **PDGFRA (platelet-derived growth factor receptor, alpha polypeptide) (eg, gastrointestinal stromal tumor [GIST]), gene analysis, targeted sequence analysis (eg, exons 12, 18)**
🚗 0.00 ✂ 0.00 **FUD** XXX   [A] [▣]
AMA: 2018,Nov,9; 2018,Jan,8; 2017,Jan,8; 2016,Aug,9

● \# 81309 **PIK3CA (phosphatidylinositol-4, 5-biphosphate 3-kinase, catalytic subunit alpha) (eg, colorectal and breast cancer) gene analysis, targeted sequence analysis (eg, exons 7, 9, 20)**
🚗 0.00 ✂ 0.00 **FUD** 000

\# 81320 **PLCG2 (phospholipase C gamma 2) (eg, chronic lymphocytic leukemia) gene analysis, common variants (eg, R665W, S707F, L845F)**
🚗 0.00 ✂ 0.00 **FUD** XXX   [▣]
AMA: 2019,Jul,3; 2018,Nov,9

26/TC PC/TC Only   A2-Z3 **ASC Payment**   50 **Bilateral**   ♂ **Male Only**   ♀ **Female Only**   🚗 **Facility RVU**   ✂ **Non-Facility RVU**   ▢ **CCI**   ✗ **CLIA**
FUD Follow-up Days   **CMS:** IOM   **AMA:** CPT Asst   A-Y **OPPSI**   80/80 **Surg Assist Allowed / w/Doc**   **Lab Crosswalk**   **Radiology Crosswalk**

81315 *PML/RARalpha, (t(15;17)), (promyelocytic leukemia/retinoic acid receptor alpha) (eg, promyelocytic leukemia) translocation analysis; common breakpoints (eg, intron 3 and intron 6), qualitative or quantitative*

🔧 0.00 ✂ 0.00 **FUD** XXX 🅰🖳

AMA: 2018,Nov,9; 2018,Jan,8; 2017,Jan,8; 2016,Aug,9; 2016,Jan,13; 2015,Jan,16; 2014,Jan,11

81316 **single breakpoint (eg, intron 3, intron 6 or exon 6), qualitative or quantitative**

🔧 0.00 ✂ 0.00 **FUD** XXX 🅰🖳

AMA: 2018,Nov,9; 2018,Jan,8; 2017,Jan,8; 2016,Aug,9; 2016,Jan,13; 2015,Jan,16; 2014,Jan,11

\# **81324** *PMP22 (peripheral myelin protein 22) (eg, Charcot-Marie-Tooth, hereditary neuropathy with liability to pressure palsies) gene analysis; duplication/deletion analysis*

🔧 0.00 ✂ 0.00 **FUD** XXX 🅰🖳

AMA: 2018,Nov,9; 2018,Jan,8; 2017,Jan,8; 2016,Aug,9; 2016,Jan,13; 2015,Jan,16; 2014,Jan,11

\# **81325** **full sequence analysis**

🔧 0.00 ✂ 0.00 **FUD** XXX 🅰🖳

AMA: 2018,Nov,9; 2018,May,6; 2018,Jan,8; 2017,Jan,8; 2016,Aug,9; 2016,Jan,13; 2015,Jan,16; 2014,Jan,11

\# **81326** **known familial variant**

🔧 0.00 ✂ 0.00 **FUD** XXX 🅰🖳

AMA: 2018,Nov,9; 2018,Jan,8; 2017,Jan,8; 2016,Aug,9; 2016,Jan,13; 2015,Jan,16; 2014,Jan,11

81317 *PMS2 (postmeiotic segregation increased 2 [S. cerevisiae]) (eg, hereditary non-polyposis colorectal cancer, Lynch syndrome) gene analysis; full sequence analysis*

🔧 0.00 ✂ 0.00 **FUD** XXX 🅰🖳

AMA: 2018,Nov,9; 2018,Jan,8; 2017,Jan,8; 2016,Aug,9; 2016,Jan,13; 2015,Jan,16; 2014,Jan,11

81318 **known familial variants**

🔧 0.00 ✂ 0.00 **FUD** XXX 🅰🖳

AMA: 2018,Nov,9; 2018,Jan,8; 2017,Jan,8; 2016,Aug,9; 2016,Jan,13; 2015,Jan,16; 2014,Jan,11

81319 **duplication/deletion variants**

🔧 0.00 ✂ 0.00 **FUD** XXX 🅰🖳

AMA: 2018,Nov,9; 2018,Jan,8; 2017,Jan,8; 2016,Aug,9; 2016,Jan,13; 2015,Jan,16; 2014,Jan,11

81320 Resequenced code. See code before 81315.

\# **81343** *PPP2R2B (protein phosphatase 2 regulatory subunit Bbeta) (eg, spinocerebellar ataxia) gene analysis, evaluation to detect abnormal (eg, expanded) alleles*

🔧 0.00 ✂ 0.00 **FUD** XXX 🖳

AMA: 2018,Nov,9

81321 *PTEN (phosphatase and tensin homolog) (eg, Cowden syndrome, PTEN hamartoma tumor syndrome) gene analysis; full sequence analysis*

🔧 0.00 ✂ 0.00 **FUD** XXX 🅰🖳

AMA: 2018,Nov,9; 2018,Jan,8; 2017,Jan,8; 2016,Aug,9; 2016,Jan,13; 2015,Jan,16; 2014,Jan,11

81322 **known familial variant**

🔧 0.00 ✂ 0.00 **FUD** XXX 🅰🖳

AMA: 2018,Nov,9; 2018,Jan,8; 2017,Jan,8; 2016,Aug,9; 2016,Jan,13; 2015,Jan,16; 2014,Jan,11

81323 **duplication/deletion variant**

🔧 0.00 ✂ 0.00 **FUD** XXX 🅰🖳

AMA: 2018,Nov,9; 2018,Jan,8; 2017,Jan,8; 2016,Aug,9; 2016,Jan,13; 2015,Jan,16; 2014,Jan,11

81324 Resequenced code. See code following 81316.

81325 Resequenced code. See code following 81316.

81326 Resequenced code. See code following 81316.

\# **81334** *RUNX1 (runt related transcription factor 1) (eg, acute myeloid leukemia, familial platelet disorder with associated myeloid malignancy) gene analysis, targeted sequence analysis (eg, exons 3-8)*

🔧 0.00 ✂ 0.00 **FUD** XXX 🅰🖳

AMA: 2018,Nov,9

81327 *SEPT9 (Septin9) (eg, colorectal cancer) promoter methylation analysis*

🔧 0.00 ✂ 0.00 **FUD** XXX 🅰🖳

AMA: 2019,Jul,3; 2018,Nov,9

\# **81332** *SERPINA1 (serpin peptidase inhibitor, clade A, alpha-1 antiproteinase, antitrypsin, member 1) (eg, alpha-1-antitrypsin deficiency), gene analysis, common variants (eg, *S and *Z)*

🔧 0.00 ✂ 0.00 **FUD** XXX 🅰🖳

AMA: 2018,Nov,9; 2018,Jan,8; 2017,Jan,8; 2016,Aug,9; 2016,Jan,13; 2015,Jan,16; 2014,Jan,11

81328 *SLCO1B1 (solute carrier organic anion transporter family, member 1B1) (eg, adverse drug reaction), gene analysis, common variant(s) (eg, *5)*

🔧 0.00 ✂ 0.00 **FUD** XXX 🅰🖳

AMA: 2018,Nov,9

81329 *SMN1 (survival of motor neuron 1, telomeric) (eg, spinal muscular atrophy) gene analysis; dosage/deletion analysis (eg, carrier testing), includes SMN2 (survival of motor neuron 2, centromeric) analysis, if performed*

🔧 0.00 ✂ 0.00 **FUD** XXX 🖳

AMA: 2019,Jul,3; 2018,Nov,9

\# **81336** **full gene sequence**

🔧 0.00 ✂ 0.00 **FUD** XXX 🖳

AMA: 2019,Jul,3; 2018,Nov,9

\# **81337** **known familial sequence variant(s)**

🔧 0.00 ✂ 0.00 **FUD** XXX 🖳

AMA: 2019,Jul,3; 2018,Nov,9

81330 *SMPD1(sphingomyelin phosphodiesterase 1, acid lysosomal) (eg, Niemann-Pick disease, Type A) gene analysis, common variants (eg, R496L, L302P, fsP330)*

🔧 0.00 ✂ 0.00 **FUD** XXX 🅰🖳

AMA: 2018,Nov,9; 2018,Jan,8; 2017,Jan,8; 2016,Aug,9; 2016,Jan,13; 2015,Jan,16; 2014,Jan,11

81331 *SNRPN/UBE3A (small nuclear ribonucleoprotein polypeptide N and ubiquitin protein ligase E3A) (eg, Prader-Willi syndrome and/or Angelman syndrome), methylation analysis*

🔧 0.00 ✂ 0.00 **FUD** XXX 🅰🖳

AMA: 2018,Nov,9; 2018,Jan,8; 2017,Jan,8; 2016,Aug,9; 2016,Jan,13; 2015,Jan,16; 2014,Jan,11

81332 Resequenced code. See code following 81327.

\# **81344** *TBP (TATA box binding protein) (eg, spinocerebellar ataxia) gene analysis, evaluation to detect abnormal (eg, expanded) alleles*

🔧 0.00 ✂ 0.00 **FUD** XXX 🖳

AMA: 2018,Nov,9

\# **81345** *TERT (telomerase reverse transcriptase) (eg, thyroid carcinoma, glioblastoma multiforme) gene analysis, targeted sequence analysis (eg, promoter region)*

🔧 0.00 ✂ 0.00 **FUD** XXX 🖳

AMA: 2019,Jul,3; 2018,Nov,9

81333 *TGFBI (transforming growth factor beta-induced) (eg, corneal dystrophy) gene analysis, common variants (eg, R124H, R124C, R124L, R555W, R555Q)*

🔧 0.00 ✂ 0.00 **FUD** XXX 🖳

AMA: 2019,Jul,3; 2018,Nov,9

81334 Resequenced code. See code following numeric code 81326.

81335 *TPMT (thiopurine S-methyltransferase) (eg, drug metabolism), gene analysis, common variants (eg, *2, *3)*

🔧 0.00 ✂ 0.00 **FUD** XXX 🅰🖳

AMA: 2018,Nov,9

81336	Resequenced code. See code following 81329.
81337	Resequenced code. See code following 81329.

81340 *TRB@ (T cell antigen receptor, beta)* **(eg, leukemia and lymphoma), gene rearrangement analysis to detect abnormal clonal population(s); using amplification methodology (eg, polymerase chain reaction)**

    🔧 0.00   ✂ 0.00   **FUD** XXX   [A][□]

    AMA: 2018,Nov,9; 2018,Jan,8; 2017,Jan,8; 2016,Aug,9; 2016,Jan,13; 2015,Jan,16; 2014,Jan,11

81341 **using direct probe methodology (eg, Southern blot)**

    🔧 0.00   ✂ 0.00   **FUD** XXX   [A][□]

    AMA: 2018,Nov,9; 2018,Jan,8; 2017,Jan,8; 2016,Aug,9; 2016,Jan,13; 2015,Jan,16; 2014,Jan,11

81342 *TRG@ (T cell antigen receptor, gamma)* **(eg, leukemia and lymphoma), gene rearrangement analysis, evaluation to detect abnormal clonal population(s)**

    🔧 0.00   ✂ 0.00   **FUD** XXX   [A][□]

    AMA: 2018,Nov,9; 2018,Jan,8; 2017,Jan,8; 2016,Aug,9; 2016,Jan,13; 2015,Jan,16; 2014,Jan,11

81343	Resequenced code. See code following numeric code 81320.
81344	Resequenced code. See code following numeric code 81332.
81345	Resequenced code. See code following numeric code 81332.

81346 *TYMS (thymidylate synthetase)* **(eg, 5-fluorouracil/5-FU drug metabolism), gene analysis, common variant(s) (eg, tandem repeat variant)**

    🔧 0.00   ✂ 0.00   **FUD** XXX   [A][□]

    AMA: 2018,Nov,9

▲ **81350** *UGT1A1 (UDP glucuronosyltransferase 1 family, polypeptide A1)* **(eg, drug metabolism, hereditary unconjugated hyperbilirubinemia [Gilbert syndrome]) gene analysis, common variants (eg, *28, *36, *37)**

    🔧 0.00   ✂ 0.00   **FUD** XXX   [A][□]

    AMA: 2018,Nov,9; 2018,Jan,8; 2017,Jan,8; 2016,Aug,9; 2016,Jan,13; 2015,Jan,16; 2014,Jan,11

81355 *VKORC1 (vitamin K epoxide reductase complex, subunit 1)* **(eg, warfarin metabolism), gene analysis, common variant(s) (eg, -1639G>A, c.173+1000C>T)**

    🔧 0.00   ✂ 0.00   **FUD** XXX   [A][□]

    AMA: 2018,Nov,9; 2018,Jan,8; 2017,Jan,8; 2016,Aug,9; 2016,Jan,13; 2015,Jan,16; 2014,Jan,11

81361	Resequenced code. See code following 81254.
81362	Resequenced code. See code following 81254.
81363	Resequenced code. See code following 81254.
81364	Resequenced code. See code following 81254.

81370-81383 Human Leukocyte Antigen (HLA) Testing

INCLUDES Additional testing that must be performed to resolve ambiguous allele combinations for high-resolution typing
All analytical procedures in the evaluation such as:
   Amplification
   Cell lysis
   Detection
   Digestion
   Extraction
   Nucleic acid stabilization
Analysis to identify human leukocyte antigen (HLA) alleles and allele groups connected to specific diseases and individual response to drug therapy in addition to other clinical uses
Code selection based on specific gene being reviewed
Evaluation of the presence of gene variants using the common gene variant name
Examples of proteins or diseases in the code description that are not all inclusive
Generally all the listed gene variants in the code description would be tested but lists are not all inclusive
Genes described using Human Genome Organization (HUGO) approved names
High-resolution typing resolves the common well-defined (CWD) alleles and is usually identified by at least four-digits. There are some instances when high-resolution typing may include some ambiguities for rare alleles, and those may be reported as a string of alleles or an NMDP code
Histocompatibility antigen testing
Intermediate resolution HLA testing is identified by a string of alleles or a National Marrow Donor Program (NMDP) code
Low and intermediate resolution are considered low resolution for code assignment
Low-resolution HLA type reporting is identified by two-digit HLA name
Multiple variant alleles or allele groups that can be identified by typing
One or more HLA genes in specific clinical circumstances
Qualitative results unless otherwise stated
Typing performed to determine the compatibility of recipients and potential donors undergoing solid organ or hematopoietic stem cell pretransplantation testing

EXCLUDES Full gene sequencing using separate gene variant assessment codes unless it is specifically stated in the code description
HLA antigen typing by nonmolecular pathology methods (86812-86821)
In situ hybridization analyses (88271-88275, 88368-88375 [88377])
Microbial identification (87149-87153, 87471-87801 [87623, 87624, 87625], 87900-87904 [87906, 87910, 87912])
Other related gene variants not listed in code
Tier 1 molecular pathology codes (81105-81254 [81161, 81162, 81163, 81164, 81165, 81166, 81167, 81173, 81174, 81184, 81185, 81186, 81187, 81188, 81189, 81190, 81200, 81201, 81202, 81203, 81204, 81205, 81206, 81207, 81208, 81209, 81210, 81219, 81227, 81230, 81231, 81233, 81234, 81238, 81239, 81245, 81246, 81250, 81257, 81258, 81259, 81265, 81266, 81267, 81268, 81269, 81284, 81285, 81286, 81289, 81361, 81362, 81363, 81364])
Tier 2 and unlisted molecular pathology procedures (81400-81408, [81479])
Code also modifier 26 when only interpretation and report are performed
Code also services required before cell lysis

81370 **HLA Class I and II typing, low resolution (eg, antigen equivalents);** *HLA-A, -B, -C, -DRB1/3/4/5, and -DQB1*

    🔧 0.00   ✂ 0.00   **FUD** XXX   [A][□]

    AMA: 2018,Nov,9; 2018,Jan,8; 2017,Jan,8; 2016,Aug,9; 2016,Jan,13; 2015,Jan,16; 2014,Jan,11

81371 *HLA-A, -B, and -DRB1* **(eg, verification typing)**

    🔧 0.00   ✂ 0.00   **FUD** XXX   [A][□]

    AMA: 2018,Nov,9; 2018,Jan,8; 2017,Jan,8; 2016,Aug,9; 2016,Jan,13; 2015,Jan,16; 2014,Jan,11

81372 **HLA Class I typing, low resolution (eg, antigen equivalents); complete** *(ie, HLA-A, -B, and -C)*

    EXCLUDES *Class I and II low-resolution HLA typing for HLA-A, -B, -C, -DRB1/3/4/5, and -DQB1 (81370)*

    🔧 0.00   ✂ 0.00   **FUD** XXX   [A][□]

    AMA: 2018,Nov,9; 2018,Jan,8; 2017,Jan,8; 2016,Aug,9; 2016,Jan,13; 2015,Jan,16; 2014,Jan,11

81373 **one locus *(eg, HLA-A, -B, or -C)*, each**

EXCLUDES A complete Class 1 (HLA-A, -B, and -C) low-resolution typing (81372)

Reporting the presence or absence of a single antigen equivalent using low-resolution methodology (81374)

🖥 0.00 ⚖ 0.00 **FUD** XXX 🅰 ▢

AMA: 2018,Nov,9; 2018,Jan,8; 2017,Jan,8; 2016,Aug,9; 2016,Jan,13; 2015,Jan,16; 2014,Jan,11

81374 **one antigen equivalent *(eg, B*27)*, each**

EXCLUDES Testing for the presence or absence of more than 2 antigen equivalents at a locus, use the following code for each locus test (81373)

🖥 0.00 ⚖ 0.00 **FUD** XXX 🅰 ▢

AMA: 2018,Nov,9; 2018,Jan,8; 2017,Jan,8; 2016,Aug,9; 2016,Jan,13; 2015,Jan,16; 2014,Jan,11

81375 **HLA Class II typing, low resolution (eg, antigen equivalents); HLA-DRB1/3/4/5 and -DQB1**

EXCLUDES Class I and II low-resolution HLA typing for HLA-A, -B, -C, -DRB 1/3/4/5, and DQB1 (81370)

🖥 0.00 ⚖ 0.00 **FUD** XXX 🅰 ▢

AMA: 2018,Nov,9; 2018,Jan,8; 2017,Jan,8; 2016,Aug,9; 2016,Jan,13; 2015,Jan,16; 2014,Jan,11

81376 **one locus *(eg, HLA-DRB1, -DRB3/4/5, -DQB1, -DQA1, -DPB1, or -DPA1)*, each**

INCLUDES Low-resolution typing, HLA-DRB1/3/4/5 reported as a single locus

EXCLUDES Low-resolution typing for HLA-DRB1/3/4/5 and -DQB1 (81375)

🖥 0.00 ⚖ 0.00 **FUD** XXX 🅰 ▢

AMA: 2018,Nov,9; 2018,Jan,8; 2017,Jan,8; 2016,Aug,9; 2016,Jan,13; 2015,Jan,16; 2014,Jan,11

81377 **one antigen equivalent, each**

EXCLUDES Testing for presence or absence of more than two antigen equivalents at a locus (81376)

🖥 0.00 ⚖ 0.00 **FUD** XXX 🅰 ▢

AMA: 2018,Nov,9; 2018,Jan,8; 2017,Jan,8; 2016,Aug,9; 2016,Jan,13; 2015,Jan,16; 2014,Jan,11

81378 **HLA Class I and II typing, high resolution (ie, alleles or allele groups), HLA-A, -B, -C, and -DRB1**

🖥 0.00 ⚖ 0.00 **FUD** XXX 🅰 ▢

AMA: 2018,Nov,9; 2018,Jan,8; 2017,Jan,8; 2016,Aug,9; 2016,Jan,13; 2015,Jan,16; 2014,Jan,11

81379 **HLA Class I typing, high resolution (ie, alleles or allele groups); complete (ie, HLA-A, -B, and -C)**

🖥 0.00 ⚖ 0.00 **FUD** XXX 🅰 ▢

AMA: 2018,Nov,9; 2018,Jan,8; 2017,Jan,8; 2016,Aug,9; 2016,Jan,13; 2015,Jan,16; 2014,Jan,11

81380 **one locus *(eg, HLA-A, -B, or -C)*, each**

EXCLUDES Complete Class I high-resolution typing for HLA-A, -B, and -C (81379)

Testing for presence or absence of a single allele or allele group using high-resolution methodology (81381)

🖥 0.00 ⚖ 0.00 **FUD** XXX 🅰 ▢

AMA: 2018,Nov,9; 2018,Jan,8; 2017,Jan,8; 2016,Aug,9; 2016,Jan,13; 2015,Jan,16; 2014,Jan,11

81381 **one allele or allele group *(eg, B*57:01P)*, each**

EXCLUDES Testing for the presence or absence of more than two alleles or allele groups of locus, report the following code for each locus (81380)

🖥 0.00 ⚖ 0.00 **FUD** XXX 🅰 ▢

AMA: 2018,Nov,9; 2018,Jan,8; 2017,Jan,8; 2016,Aug,9; 2016,Jan,13; 2015,Jan,16; 2014,Jan,11

81382 **HLA Class II typing, high resolution (ie, alleles or allele groups); one locus *(eg, HLA-DRB1, -DRB3/4/5, -DQB1, -DQA1, -DPB1, or -DPA1)*, each**

INCLUDES Typing of one or all of the DRB3/4/5 genes is regarded as one locus

EXCLUDES Testing for just the presence or absence of a single allele or allele group using high-resolution methodology (81383)

🖥 0.00 ⚖ 0.00 **FUD** XXX 🅰 ▢

AMA: 2018,Nov,9; 2018,Jan,8; 2017,Jan,8; 2016,Jan,13; 2015,Jan,16; 2014,Jan,11

81383 **one allele or allele group *(eg, HLA-DQB1*06:02P)*, each**

EXCLUDES For testing for the presence or absence of more than two alleles or allele groups at a locus, report the following code for each locus (81382)

🖥 0.00 ⚖ 0.00 **FUD** XXX 🅰 ▢

AMA: 2018,Nov,9; 2018,Jan,8; 2017,Jan,8; 2016,Jan,13; 2015,Jan,16; 2014,Jan,11

81400-81479 [81479] Molecular Pathology Tier 2 Procedures

INCLUDES All analytical procedures in the evaluation such as:
Amplification
Cell lysis
Detection
Digestion
Extraction
Nucleic acid stabilization
Code selection based on specific gene being reviewed
Codes that are arranged by level of technical resources and work involved
Evaluation of the presence of a gene variant using the common gene variant name
Examples of proteins or diseases in the code description (not all inclusive)
Generally all the listed gene variants in the code description would be tested but lists are not all inclusive
Genes described using the Human Genome Organization (HUGO) approved names
Histocompatibility testing
Qualitative results unless otherwise stated
Specific analytes listed after the code description to use for selecting the appropriate molecular pathology procedure
Targeted genomic testing (81410-81471 [81448])
Testing for diseases that are more rare

EXCLUDES Full gene sequencing using separate gene variant assessment codes unless it is specifically stated in the code description
In situ hybridization analyses (88271-88275, 88365-88368 [88364, 88373, 88374])
Microbial identification (87149-87153, 87471-87801 [87623, 87624, 87625], 87900-87904 [87906, 87910, 87912])
Other related gene variants not listed in code
Tier 1 molecular pathology (81105-81254 [81161, 81162, 81163, 81164, 81165, 81166, 81167, 81173, 81174, 81184, 81185, 81186, 81187, 81188, 81189, 81190, 81200, 81201, 81202, 81203, 81204, 81205, 81206, 81207, 81208, 81209, 81210, 81219, 81227, 81230, 81231, 81233, 81234, 81238, 81239, 81245, 81246, 81250, 81257, 81258, 81259, 81265, 81266, 81267, 81268, 81269, 81284, 81285, 81286, 81289, 81361, 81362, 81363, 81364])
Unlisted molecular pathology procedures ([81479])
Code also modifier 26 when only interpretation and report are performed
Code also services required before cell lysis

81400 **Molecular pathology procedure, Level 1 (eg, identification of single germline variant [eg, SNP] by techniques such as restriction enzyme digestion or melt curve analysis)**

ACADM (acyl-CoA dehydrogenase, C-4 to C-12 straight chain, MCAD) (eg, medium chain acyl dehydrogenase deficiency), K304E variant

ACE (angiotensin converting enzyme) (eg, hereditary blood pressure regulation), insertion/deletion variant

AGTR1 (angiotensin II receptor, type 1) (eg, essential hypertension), 1166A>C variant

BCKDHA (branched chain keto acid dehydrogenase E1, alpha polypeptide) (eg, maple syrup urine disease, type 1A), Y438N variant

CCR5 (chemokine C-C motif receptor 5) (eg, HIV resistance), 32-bp deletion mutation/794 825del32 deletion

CLRN1 (clarin 1) (eg, Usher syndrome, type 3), N48K variant

F2 (coagulation factor 2) (eg, hereditary hypercoagulability), 1199G>A variant

F5 (coagulation factor V) (eg, hereditary hypercoagulability), HR2 variant

F7 (coagulation factor VII [serum prothrombin conversion accelerator]) (eg, hereditary hypercoagulability), R353Q variant

F13B (coagulation factor XIII, B polypeptide) (eg, hereditary hypercoagulability), V34L variant

FGB (fibrinogen beta chain) (eg, hereditary ischemic heart disease), -455G>A variant

FGFR1 (fibroblast growth factor receptor 1) (eg, Pfeiffer syndrome type 1, craniosynostosis), P252R variant

FGFR3 (fibroblast growth factor receptor 3) (eg, Muenke syndrome), P250R variant

FKTN (fukutin) (eg, Fukuyama congenital muscular dystrophy), retrotransposon insertion variant

GNE (glucosamine [UDP-N-acetyl]-2 -epimerase/N-acetylmannosamine kinase) (eg, inclusion body myopathy 2 [IBM2], Nonaka myopathy), M712T variant

IVD (isovaleryl-CoA dehydrogenase) (eg, isovaleric acidemia), A282V variant

LCT (lactase-phlorizin hydrolase) (eg, lactose intolerance), 13910 C>T variant

NEB (nebulin) (eg, nemaline myopathy 2), exon 55 deletion variant

PCDH15 (protocadherin-related 15) (eg, Usher syndrome type 1F), R245X variant

SERPINE1 (serpine peptidase inhibitor clade E, member 1, plasminogen activator inhibitor -1, PAI-1) (eg, thrombophilia), 4G variant

SHOC2 (soc-2 suppressor of clear homolog) (eg, Noonan-like syndrome with loose anagen hair), S2G variant

SRY (sex determining region Y) (eg, 46,XX testicular disorder of sex development, gonadal dysgenesis), gene analysis

TOR1A (torsin family 1, member A [torsin A]) (eg, early-onset primary dystonia [DYT1]), 907_909delGAG (904_906delGAG) variant

🔷 0.00 ⚕ 0.00 **FUD** XXX   🅐 ▢

AMA: 2019,Jul,3; 2018,Nov,9; 2018,Jan,8; 2017,Jan,8; 2016,Aug,9; 2016,Jan,13; 2015,Jan,16; 2015,Jan,3; 2014,Jan,11

81401 **Molecular pathology procedure, Level 2 (eg, 2-10 SNPs, 1 methylated variant, or 1 somatic variant [typically using nonsequencing target variant analysis], or detection of a dynamic mutation disorder/triplet repeat)**

ABCC8 (ATP-binding cassette, sub-family C [CFTR/MRP], member 8) (eg, familial hyperinsulinism), common variants (eg, c.3898-9G>A [c.3992-9G>A], F1388del)

ABL1 (ABL proto oncogene 1, non-receptor tyrosine kinase) (eg, acquired imatinib resistance), T315I variant

ACADM (acyl-CoA dehydrogenase, C-4 to C-12 straight chain, MCAD) (eg, medium chain acyl dehydrogenase deficiency), common variants (eg, K304E, Y42H)

ADRB2 (adrenergic beta-2 receptor surface) (eg, drug metabolism), common variants (eg, G16R, Q27E)

APOB (apolipoprotein B) (eg, familial hypercholesterolemia type B), common variants (eg, R3500Q, R3500W)

*APOE (apolipoprotein E) (eg, hyperlipoproteinemia type III, cardiovascular disease, Alzheimer disease), common variants (eg, *2, *3, *4)*

CBFB/MYH11 (inv(16)) (eg, acute myeloid leukemia), qualitative, and quantitative, if performed

CBS (cystathionine-beta-synthase) (eg, homocystinuria, cystathionine beta-synthase deficiency), common variants (eg, I278T, G307S)

CCND1/IGH (BCL1/IgH, t(11;14)) (eg, mantle cell lymphoma) translocation analysis, major breakpoint, qualitative and quantitative, if performed

CFH/ARMS2 (complement factor H/age-related maculopathy susceptibility 2) (eg, macular degeneration), common variants (eg, Y402H [CFH], A69S [ARMS2])

DEK/NUP214 (t(6;9))(eg, acute myeloid leukemia), translocation analysis, qualitative, and quantitative, if performed

E2A/PBX1 (t(1;19)) (eg, acute lymphocytic leukemia), translocation analysis, qualitative, and quantitative, if performed

EML4/ALK (inv(2)) (eg, non-small cell lung cancer), translocation or inversion analysis

ETV6/NTRK3 (t(12;15)) (eg, congenital/infantile fibrosarcoma), translocation analysis, qualitative, and quantitative, if performed

ETV6/RUNX1 (t(12;21)) (eg, acute lymphocytic leukemia), translocation analysis, qualitative and quantitative, if performed

EWSR1/ATF1 (t(12;22)) (eg, clear cell sarcoma), translocation analysis, qualitative, and quantitative, if performed

EWSR1/ERG (t(21;22)) (eg, Ewing sarcoma/peripheral neuroectodermal tumor), translocation analysis, qualitative and quantitative, if performed

EWSR1/FLI1 (t(11;22)) (eg, Ewing sarcoma/peripheral neuroectodermal tumor), translocation analysis, qualitative and quantitative, if performed

EWSR1/WT1 (t(11;22)) (eg, desmoplastic small round cell tumor), translocation analysis, qualitative and quantitative, if performed

F11 (coagulation factor XI) (eg, coagulation disorder), common variants (eg, E117X [Type II], F283L [Type III], IVS14del14, and IVS14+1G>A [Type I])

FGFR3 (fibroblast growth factor receptor 3) (eg, achondroplasia, hypochondroplasia), common variants (eg, 1138G>A, 1138G>C, 1620C>A, 1620C>G)

FIP1L1/PDGFRA (del[4q12]) (eg, imatinib-sensitive chronic eosinophilic leukemia), qualitative and quantitative, if performed

FLG (filaggrin) (eg, ichthyosis vulgaris), common variants (eg, R501X, 2282del4, R2447X, S3247X, 3702delG)

FOXO1/PAX3 (t(2;13)) (eg, alveolar rhabdomyosarcoma), translocation analysis, qualitative and quantitative, if performed

FOXO1/PAX7 (t(1;13)) (eg, alveolar rhabdomyosarcoma), translocation analysis, qualitative and quantitative, if performed

FUS/DDIT3 (t(12;16)) (eg, myxoid liposarcoma), translocation analysis, qualitative, and quantitative, if performed

GALC (galactosylceramidase) (eg, Krabbe disease), common variants (eg, c.857G>A, 30-kb deletion)

GALT (galactose-1-phosphate uridylyltransferase) (eg, galactosemia), common variants (eg, Q188R, S135L, K285N, T138M, L195P, Y209C, IVS2-2A>G, P171S, del5kb, N314D, L218L/N314D)

H19 (imprinted maternally expressed transcript [non-protein coding]) (eg, Beckwith-Wiedemann syndrome), methylation analysis

IGH@/BCL2 (t(14;18)) (eg, follicular lymphoma), translocation and analysis; single breakpoint (eg) major breakpoint region [MBR] or minor cluster region [mcr]), qualitative or quantitative(When both MBR and mcr breakpoints are performed, use 81402)

KCNQ1OT1 (KCNQ1 overlapping transcript 1 [non-protein coding]) (e.g. Beckwith-Wiedemann syndrome), methylation analysis

LINC00518 (long intergenic non-protein coding RNA 518) (eg, melanoma), expression analysis

LRRK2 (leucine-rich repeat kinase 2) (eg, Parkinson disease), common variants (eg, R1441G, G2019S, I2020T)

MED12 (mediator complex subunit 12) (eg, FG syndrome type 1, Lujan syndrome), common variants (eg, R961W, N1007S)

MEG3/DLK1 (maternally expressed 3 [non-protein coding]/delta-like 1 homolog [Drosophila]) (eg, intrauterine growth retardation), methylation analysis

MLL/AFF1 (t(4;11)) (eg acute lymphoblastic leukemia), translocation analysis, qualitative and quantitative, if performed

MLL/MLLT3 (t(9;11)) (eg, acute myeloid leukemia) translocation analysis, qualitative and quantitative, if performed

MT-RNR1 (mitochondrially encoded 12S RNA) (eg, nonsyndromic hearing loss), common variants (eg, m.1555>G, m1494C>T)

MUTYH (mutY homolog [E.coli]) (eg, MYH–associated polyposis), common variants (eg, Y165C, G382D)

MT-ATP6 (mitochondrially encoded ATP synthase 6) (eg, neuropathy with ataxia and retinitis pigmentosa [NARP], Leigh syndrome), common variants (eg, m.8993T>G, m.8993T>C)

MT-ND4, MT-ND6 (mitochondrially encoded NADH dehydrogenase 4, mitochondrially encoded NADH dehydrogenase 6) (eg, Leber hereditary optic neuropathy [LHON]), common variants (eg m.11778G>A, m3460G>A, m14484T>C)

MT-ND5 (mitochondrially encoded tRNA leucine 1 [UUA/G], mitochondrially encoded NADH dehydrogenase 5) (eg, mitochondrial encephalopathy with lactic acidosis and stroke-like episodes [MELAS]), common variants (eg, m.3243A>G, m.3271T>C, m.3252A>G, m.13513G>A)

MT-TK (mitochondrially encoded tRNA lysine) (eg, myoclonic epilepsy with ragged-red fibers [MERRF]), common variants (eg, m8344A>G, m.8356T>C)

MT-TL1 (mitochondrially encoded tRNA leucine 1[UUA/G]) (eg, diabetes and hearing loss), common variants (eg, m.3243A>G, m.14709 T>C) MT-TL1

MT-TS1, MT-RNR1 (mitochondrially encoded tRNA serine 1 [UCN], mitochondrially encoded 12S RNA) (eg, nonsyndromic sensorineural deafness [including aminoglycoside-induced nonsyndromic deafness]) common variants (eg, m.7445A>G, m.1555A>G)

NOD2 (nucleotide-binding oligomerization domain containing 2) (eg, Crohn's disease, Blau syndrome), common variants (eg, SNP 8, SNP 12, SNP 13)

NPM/ALK (t(2;5)) (eg, anaplastic large cell lymphoma), translocation analysis

PAX8/PPARG (t(2;3) (q13;p25)) (eg, follicular thyroid carcinoma), translocation analysis

PRAME (preferentially expressed antigen in melanoma)(eg, melanoma), expression analysis

PRSS1 (protease, serine, 1 [trypsin 1]) (eg, hereditary pancreatitis), common variants (eg, N29I, A16V, R122H)

PYGM (phosphorylase, glycogen, muscle) (eg, glycogen storage disease type V, McArdle disease), common variants (eg, R50X, G205S)

RUNX1/RUNX1T1 (t(8;21)) (eg, acute myeloid leukemia) translocation analysis, qualitative and quantitative, if performed

SS18/SSX1 (t(X;18)) (eg, synovial sarcoma), translocation analysis, qualitative and quantitative, if performed

SS18/SSX2 (t(X;18)) (eg, synovial sarcoma), translocation analysis, qualitative and quantitative, if performed

VWF (von Willebrand factor) (eg, von Willebrand disease type 2N), common variants (eg, T791M, R816W, R854Q)

🔲 0.00   ✂ 0.00   **FUD** XXX   Ⓐ▣

AMA: 2019,Sep,7; 2019,Jul,3; 2018,Nov,9; 2018,Jan,8; 2017,Jan,8; 2016,Aug,9; 2016,Jan,13; 2015,Jan,16; 2015,Jan,3; 2014,Jan,11

81402 **Molecular pathology procedure, Level 3 (eg, >10 SNPs, 2-10 methylated variants, or 2-10 somatic variants [typically using non-sequencing target variant analysis], immunoglobulin and T-cell receptor gene rearrangements, duplication/deletion variants of 1 exon, loss of heterozygosity [LOH], uniparental disomy [UPD])**

Chromosome 1p-/19q- (eg, glial tumors), deletion analysis

Chromosome 18q- (eg, D18S55, D18S58, D18S61, D18S64, and D18S69) (eg, colon cancer), allelic imbalance assessment (ie, loss of heterozygosity)

COL1A1/PDGFB (t(17;22)) (eg, dermatofibrosarcoma protuberans), translocation analysis, multiple breakpoints, qualitative, and quantitative, if performed

CYP21A2 (cytochrome P450, family 21, subfamily A, polypeptide 2) (eg, congenital adrenal hyperplasia, 21-hydroxylase deficiency), common variants (eg, IVS2-13G, P30L, I172N, exon 6 mutation cluster [I235N, V236E, M238K], V281L, L307FfsX6, Q318X, R356W, P453S, G110VfsX21, 30-kb deletion variant)

ESR1/PGR (receptor 1/progesterone receptor) ratio (eg, breast cancer)

IGH@/BCL2 (t(14;18)) (eg, follicular lymphoma), translocation analysis; major breakpoint region (MBR) and minor cluster region (mcr) breakpoints, qualitative or quantitative

MEFV (Mediterranean fever) (eg, familial Mediterranean fever), common variants (eg, E148Q, P369S, F479L, M680I, I692del, M694V, M694I, K695R, V726A, A744S, R761H)

MPL (myeloproliferative leukemia virus oncogene, thrombopoietin receptor, TPOR) (eg, myeloproliferative disorder), common variants (eg, W515A, W515K, W515L, W515R)

TRD@ (T cell antigen receptor, delta) (eg, leukemia and lymphoma), gene rearrangement analysis, evaluation to detect abnormal clonal population

Uniparental disomy (UPD) (eg, Russell-Silver syndrome, Prader-Willi/Angelman syndrome), short tandem repeat (STR) analysis

🔲 0.00   ✂ 0.00   **FUD** XXX   Ⓐ▣

AMA: 2018,Nov,9; 2018,Jan,8; 2017,Jan,8; 2016,Aug,9; 2016,Jan,13; 2015,Jan,16; 2015,Jan,3; 2014,Jan,11

81403 **Molecular pathology procedure, Level 4 (eg, analysis of single exon by DNA sequence analysis, analysis of >10 amplicons using multiplex PCR in 2 or more independent reactions, mutation scanning or duplication/deletion variants of 2-5 exons)**

ANG (angiogenin, ribonuclease, RNase A family, 5) (eg, amyotrophic lateral sclerosis), full gene sequence

ARX (aristaless-related homeobox) (eg, X-linked lissencephaly with ambiguous genitalia, X-linked mental retardation), duplication/deletion analysis

CEL (carboxyl ester lipase [bile salt-stimulated lipase]) (eg, maturity-onset diabetes of the young [MODY]), targeted sequence analysis of exon 11 (eg, c.1785delC, c.1686delT)

CTNNB1 (catenin [cadherin-associated protein], beta 1, 88kDa) (eg, desmoid tumors), targeted sequence analysis (eg, exon 3)

DAZ/SRY (deleted in azoospermia and sex determining region Y) (eg, male infertility), common deletions (eg, AZFa, AZFb, AZFc, AZFd)

DNMT3A (DNA [cytosine-5-]-methyltransferase 3 alpha) (eg, acute myeloid leukemia), targeted sequence analysis (eg, exon 23)

EPCAM (epithelial cell adhesion molecule) (eg, Lynch syndrome), duplication/deletion analysis

F8 (coagulation factor VIII) (eg, hemophilia A), inversion analysis, intron 1 and intron 22A

F12 (coagulation factor XII [Hageman factor]) (eg, angioedema, hereditary, type III; factor XII deficiency), targeted sequence analysis of exon 9

FGFR3 (fibroblast growth factor receptor 3) (eg, isolated craniosynostosis), targeted sequence analysis (eg, exon 7)

(For targeted sequence analysis of multiple FGFR3 exons, use 81404) (81404)

GJB1 (gap junction protein, beta 1) (eg, Charcot-Marie-Tooth X-linked), full gene sequence

GNAQ (guanine nucleotide-binding protein G[q] subunit alpha) (eg, uveal melanoma), common variants (eg, R183, Q209)

HRAS (v-Ha-ras Harvey rat sarcoma viral oncogene homolog) (eg, Costello syndrome), exon 2 sequence

Human erythrocyte antigen gene analyses (eg, SLC14A1 [Kidd blood group], BCAM [Lutheran blood group], ICAM4 [Landsteiner-Wiener blood group], SLC4A1 [Diego blood group], AQP1 [Colton blood group], ERMAP [Scianna blood group], RHCE [Rh blood group, CcEe antigens], KEL [Kell blood group], DARC [Duffy blood group], GYPA, GYPB, GYPE [MNS blood group], ART4 [Dombrock blood group]) (eg, sickle-cell disease, thalassemia, hemolytic transfusion reactions, hemolytic disease of the fetus or newborn), common variants

JAK2 (Janus kinase 2) (eg, myeloproliferative disorder), exon 12 sequence and exon 13 sequence, if performed

KCNC3 (potassium voltage-gated channel, Shaw-related subfamily, member 3) (eg, spinocerebellar ataxia), targeted sequence analysis (eg, exon 2)

KCNJ2 (potassium inwardly-rectifying channel, subfamily J, member 2) (eg, Andersen-Tawil syndrome), full gene sequence

KCNJ11 (potassium inwardly-rectifying channel, subfamily J, member 11) (eg, familial hyperinsulinism), full gene sequence

Killer cell immunoglobulin-like receptor (KIR) gene family (eg, hematopoietic stem cell transplantation), genotyping of KIR family genes

Known familial variant, not otherwise specified, for gene listed in Tier 1 or Tier 2, or identified during a genomic sequencing procedure, DNA sequence analysis, each variant exon

(For a known familial variant that is considered a common variant, use specific common variant Tier 1 or Tier 2 code)

MC4R (melanocortin 4 receptor) (eg, obesity), full gene sequence

MICA (MHC class I polypeptide-related sequence A) (eg, solid organ transplantation), common variants (eg, *001, *002)

MPL (myeloproliferative leukemia virus oncogene, thrombopoietin receptor, TPOR) (eg, myeloproliferative disorder), exon 10 sequence

MT-RNR1 (mitochondrially encoded 12S RNA) (eg, nonsyndromic hearing loss), full gene sequence

MT-TS1 (mitochondrially encoded tRNA serine 1) (eg, nonsyndromic hearing loss), full gene sequence

NDP (Norrie disease [pseudoglioma]) (eg, Norrie disease), duplication/deletion analysis

NHLRC1 (NHL repeat containing 1) (eg, progressive myoclonus epilepsy), full gene sequence

PHOX2B (paired-like homeobox 2b) (eg, congenital central hypoventilation syndrome), duplication/deletion analysis

PLN (phospholamban) (eg, dilated cardiomyopathy, hypertrophic cardiomyopathy), full gene sequence

RHD (Rh blood group, D antigen) (eg, hemolytic disease of the fetus and newborn, Rh maternal/fetal compatibility), deletion analysis (eg, exons 4, 5, and 7, pseudogene)

RHD (Rh blood group, D antigen) (eg, hemolytic disease of the fetus and newborn, Rh maternal/fetal compatibility), deletion analysis (eg, exons 4, 5, and 7, pseudogene), performed on cell-free fetal DNA in maternal blood

(For human erythrocyte gene analysis of RHD, use a separate unit of 81403)

SH2D1A (SH2 domain containing 1A) (eg, X-linked lymphoproliferative syndrome), duplication/deletion analysis

TWIST1 (twist homolog 1 [Drosophila]) (eg, Saethre-Chotzen syndrome), duplication/deletion analysis

UBA1 (ubiquitin-like modifier activating enzyme 1) (eg, spinal muscular atrophy, X-linked), targeted sequence analysis (eg, exon 15)

VHL (von Hippel-Lindau tumor suppressor) (eg, von Hippel-Lindau familial cancer syndrome), deletion/duplication analysis

VWF (von Willebrand factor) (eg, von Willebrand disease types 2A, 2B, 2M), targeted sequence analysis (eg, exon 28)

◻ 0.00 ◻ 0.00 **FUD** XXX Ⓐ ◻

AMA: 2019,Jul,3; 2018,Nov,9; 2018,May,6; 2018,Jan,8; 2017,Jan,8; 2016,Aug,9; 2016,Jan,13; 2015,Jan,16; 2015,Jan,3; 2014,Jan,11

▲ 81404 **Molecular pathology procedure, Level 5 (eg, analysis of 2-5 exons by DNA sequence analysis, mutation scanning or duplication/deletion variants of 6-10 exons, or characterization of a dynamic mutation disorder/triplet repeat by Southern blot analysis)**

ACADS (acyl-CoA dehydrogenase, C-2 to C-3 short chain) (eg, short chain acyl-CoA dehydrogenase deficiency), targeted sequence analysis (eg, exons 5 and 6)

AQP2 (aquaporin 2 [collecting duct]) (eg, nephrogenic diabetes insipidus), full gene sequence

ARX (aristaless related homeobox) (eg, X-linked lissencephaly with ambiguous genitalia, X-linked mental retardation), full gene sequence

AVPR2 (arginine vasopressin receptor 2) (eg, nephrogenic diabetes insipidus), full gene sequence

BBS10 (Bardet-Biedl syndrome 10) (eg, Bardet-Biedl syndrome), full gene sequence

BTD (biotinidase) (eg, biotinidase deficiency), full gene sequence

C10orf2 (chromosome 10 open reading frame 2) (eg, mitochondrial DNA depletion syndrome), full gene sequence

CAV3 (caveolin 3) (eg, CAV3-related distal myopathy, limb-girdle muscular dystrophy type 1C), full gene sequence

CD40LG (CD40 ligand) (eg, X-linked hyper IgM syndrome), full gene sequence

CDKN2A (cyclin-dependent kinase inhibitor 2A) (eg, CDKN2A-related cutaneous malignant melanoma, familial atypical mole-malignant melanoma syndrome), full gene sequence

CLRN1 (clarin 1) (eg, Usher syndrome, type 3), full gene sequence

COX6B1 (cytochrome c oxidase subunit VIb polypeptide 1) (eg, mitochondrial respiratory chain complex IV deficiency), full gene sequence

CPT2 (carnitine palmitoyltransferase 2) (eg, carnitine palmitoyltransferase II deficiency), full gene sequence

CRX (cone-rod homeobox) (eg, cone-rod dystrophy 2, Leber congenital amaurosis), full gene sequence

CYP1B1 (cytochrome P450, family 1, subfamily B, polypeptide 1) (eg, primary congenital glaucoma), full gene sequence

EGR2 (early growth response 2) (eg, Charcot-Marie-Tooth), full gene sequence

EMD (emerin) (eg, Emery-Dreifuss muscular dystrophy), duplication/deletion analysis

EPM2A (epilepsy, progressive myoclonus type 2A, Lafora disease [laforin]) (eg, progressive myoclonus epilepsy), full gene sequence

FGF23 (fibroblast growth factor 23) (eg, hypophosphatemic rickets), full gene sequence

FGFR2 (fibroblast growth factor receptor 2) (eg, craniosynostosis, Apert syndrome, Crouzon syndrome), targeted sequence analysis (eg, exons 8, 10)

FGFR3 (fibroblast growth factor receptor 3) (eg, achondroplasia, hypochondroplasia), targeted sequence analysis (eg, exons 8, 11, 12, 13)

FHL1 (four and a half LIM domains 1) (eg, Emery-Dreifuss muscular dystrophy), full gene sequence

FKRP (Fukutin related protein) (eg, congenital muscular dystrophy type 1C [MDC1C], limb-girdle muscular dystrophy [LGMD] type 2I), full gene sequence

FOXG1 (forkhead box G1) (eg, Rett syndrome), full gene sequence

FSHMD1A (facioscapulohumeral muscular dystrophy 1A) (eg, facioscapulohumeral muscular dystrophy), evaluation to detect abnormal (eg, deleted) alleles

FSHMD1A (facioscapulohumeral muscular dystrophy 1A) (eg, facioscapulohumeral muscular dystrophy), characterization of haplotype(s) (ie, chromosome 4A and 4B haplotypes)

GH1 (growth hormone 1) (eg, growth hormone deficiency), full gene sequence

GP1BB (glycoprotein Ib [platelet], beta polypeptide) (eg, Bernard-Soulier syndrome type B), full gene sequence

(For common deletion variants of alpha globin 1 and alpha globin 2 genes, use 81257)

HNF1B (HNF1 homeobox B) (eg, maturity-onset diabetes of the young [MODY]), duplication/deletion analysis

HRAS (v-Ha-ras Harvey rat sarcoma viral oncogene homolog) (eg, Costello syndrome), full gene sequence

HSD3B2 (hydroxy-delta-5-steroid dehydrogenase, 3 beta- and steroid delta-isomerase 2) (eg, 3-beta-hydroxysteroid dehydrogenase type II deficiency), full gene sequence

HSD11B2 (hydroxysteroid [11-beta] dehydrogenase 2) (eg, mineralocorticoid excess syndrome), full gene sequence

HSPB1 (heat shock 27kDa protein 1) (eg, Charcot-Marie-Tooth disease), full gene sequence

INS (insulin) (eg, diabetes mellitus), full gene sequence

KCNJ1 (potassium inwardly-rectifying channel, subfamily J, member 1) (eg, Bartter syndrome), full gene sequence

KCNJ10 (potassium inwardly-rectifying channel, subfamily J, member 10) (eg, SeSAME syndrome, EAST syndrome, sensorineural hearing loss), full gene sequence

LITAF (lipopolysaccharide-induced TNF factor) (eg, Charcot-Marie-Tooth), full gene sequence

MEFV (Mediterranean fever) (eg, familial Mediterranean fever), full gene sequence

MEN1 (multiple endocrine neoplasia I) (eg, multiple endocrine neoplasia type 1, Wermer syndrome), duplication/deletion analysis

MMACHC (methylmalonic aciduria [cobalamin deficiency] cblC type, with homocystinuria) (eg, methylmalonic acidemia and homocystinuria), full gene sequence

MPV17 (MpV17 mitochondrial inner membrane protein) (eg, mitochondrial DNA depletion syndrome), duplication/deletion analysis

NDP (Norrie disease [pseudoglioma]) (eg, Norrie disease), full gene sequence

NDUFA1 (NADH dehydrogenase [ubiquinone] 1 alpha subcomplex, 1, 7.5kDa) (eg, Leigh syndrome, mitochondrial complex I deficiency), full gene sequence

NDUFAF2 (NADH dehydrogenase [ubiquinone] 1 alpha subcomplex, assembly factor 2) (eg, Leigh syndrome, mitochondrial complex I deficiency), full gene sequence

NDUFS4 (NADH dehydrogenase [ubiquinone] Fe-S protein 4, 18kDa [NADH-coenzyme Q reductase]) (eg, Leigh syndrome, mitochondrial complex I deficiency), full gene sequence

NIPA1 (non-imprinted in Prader-Willi/Angelman syndrome 1) (eg, spastic paraplegia), full gene sequence

NLGN4X (neuroligin 4, X-linked) (eg, autism spectrum disorders), duplication/deletion analysis

NPC2 (Niemann-Pick disease, type C2 [epididymal secretory protein E1]) (eg, Niemann-Pick disease type C2), full gene sequence

NR0B1 (nuclear receptor subfamily 0, group B, member 1) (eg, congenital adrenal hypoplasia), full gene sequence

PDX1 (pancreatic and duodenal homeobox 1) (eg, maturity-onset diabetes of the young [MODY]), full gene sequence

PHOX2B (paired-like homeobox 2b) (eg, congenital central hypoventilation syndrome), full gene sequence

PIK3CA (phosphatidylinositol-4,5-bisphosphate 3-kinase, catalytic subunit alpha) (eg, colorectal cancer), targeted sequence analysis (eg, exons 9 and 20)

PLP1 (proteolipid protein 1) (eg, Pelizaeus-Merzbacher disease, spastic paraplegia), duplication/deletion analysis

PQBP1 (polyglutamine binding protein 1) (eg, Renpenning syndrome), duplication/deletion analysis

PRNP (prion protein) (eg, genetic prion disease), full gene sequence

PROP1 (PROP paired-like homeobox 1) (eg, combined pituitary hormone deficiency), full gene sequence

PRPH2 (peripherin 2 [retinal degeneration, slow]) (eg, retinitis pigmentosa), full gene sequence

PRSS1 (protease, serine, 1 [trypsin 1]) (eg, hereditary pancreatitis), full gene sequence

RAF1 (v-raf-1 murine leukemia viral oncogene homolog 1) (eg, LEOPARD syndrome), targeted sequence analysis (eg, exons 7, 12, 14, 17)

RET (ret proto-oncogene) (eg, multiple endocrine neoplasia, type 2B and familial medullary thyroid carcinoma), common variants (eg, M918T, 2647_2648delinsTT, A883F)

RHO (rhodopsin) (eg, retinitis pigmentosa), full gene sequence

RP1 (retinitis pigmentosa 1) (eg, retinitis pigmentosa), full gene sequence

SCN1B (sodium channel, voltage-gated, type I, beta) (eg, Brugada syndrome), full gene sequence

SCO2 (SCO cytochrome oxidase deficient homolog 2 [SCO1L]) (eg, mitochondrial respiratory chain complex IV deficiency), full gene sequence

SDHC (succinate dehydrogenase complex, subunit C, integral membrane protein, 15kDa) (eg, hereditary paraganglioma-pheochromocytoma syndrome), duplication/deletion analysis

SDHD (succinate dehydrogenase complex, subunit D, integral membrane protein) (eg, hereditary paraganglioma), full gene sequence

SGCG (sarcoglycan, gamma [35kDa dystrophin-associated glycoprotein]) (eg, limb-girdle muscular dystrophy), duplication/deletion analysis

SH2D1A (SH2 domain containing 1A) (eg, X-linked lymphoproliferative syndrome), full gene sequence

SLC16A2 (solute carrier family 16, member 2 [thyroid hormone transporter]) (eg, specific thyroid hormone cell transporter deficiency, Allan-Herndon-Dudley syndrome), duplication/deletion analysis

SLC25A20 (solute carrier family 25 [carnitine/acylcarnitine translocase], member 20) (eg, carnitine-acylcarnitine translocase deficiency), duplication/deletion analysis

SLC25A4 (solute carrier family 25 [mitochondrial carrier; adenine nucleotide translocation], member 4) (eg, progressive external ophthalmoplegia), full gene sequence

SOD1 (superoxide dismutase 1, soluble) (eg, amyotrophic lateral sclerosis), full gene sequence

SPINK1 (serine peptidase inhibitor, Kazal type 1) (eg, hereditary pancreatitis), full gene sequence

STK11 (serine/threonine kinase 11) (eg, Peutz-Jeghers syndrome), duplication/deletion analysis

TACO1 (translational activator of mitochondrial encoded cytochrome c oxidase I) (eg, mitochondrial respiratory chain complex IV deficiency), full gene sequence

THAP1 (THAP domain containing, apoptosis associated protein 1) (eg, torsion dystonia), full gene sequence

TOR1A (torsin family 1, member A [torsin A]) (eg, torsion dystonia), full gene sequence

TP53 (tumor protein 53) (eg, tumor samples), targeted sequence analysis of 2-5 exons

TTPA (tocopherol [alpha] transfer protein) (eg, ataxia), full gene sequence

TTR (transthyretin) (eg, familial transthyretin amyloidosis), full gene sequence

TWIST1 (twist homolog 1 [Drosophila]) (eg, Saethre-Chotzen syndrome), full gene sequence

TYR (tyrosinase [oculocutaneous albinism IA]) (eg, oculocutaneous albinism IA), full gene sequence

USH1G (Usher syndrome 1G [autosomal recessive]) (eg, Usher syndrome, type 1), full gene sequence

VWF (von Willebrand factor) (eg, von Willebrand disease type 1C), targeted sequence analysis (eg, exons 26, 27, 37)

VHL (von Hippel-Lindau tumor suppressor) (eg, von Hippel-Lindau familial cancer syndrome), full gene sequence

ZEB2 (zinc finger E-box binding homeobox 2) (eg, Mowat-Wilson syndrome), duplication/deletion analysis

ZNF41 (zinc finger protein 41) (eg, X-linked mental retardation 89), full gene sequence

    🚗 0.00   ⚖ 0.00   **FUD** XXX   A ☐

AMA: 2019,Jul,3; 2018,Nov,9; 2018,May,6; 2018,Jan,8; 2017,Jan,8; 2016,Aug,9; 2016,Jan,13; 2015,Jan,16; 2015,Jan,3; 2014,Jan,11

81405   **Molecular pathology procedure, Level 6 (eg, analysis of 6-10 exons by DNA sequence analysis, mutation scanning or duplication/deletion variants of 11-25 exons, regionally targeted cytogenomic array analysis)**

ABCD1 (ATP-binding cassette, sub-family D [ALD], member 1) (eg, adrenoleukodystrophy), full gene sequence

ACADS (acyl-CoA dehydrogenase, C-2 to C-3 short chain) (eg, short chain acyl-CoA dehydrogenase deficiency), full gene sequence

ACTA2 (actin, alpha 2, smooth muscle, aorta) (eg, thoracic aortic aneurysms and aortic dissections), full gene sequence

ACTC1 (actin, alpha, cardiac muscle 1) (eg, familial hypertrophic cardiomyopathy), full gene sequence

ANKRD1 (ankyrin repeat domain 1) (eg, dilated cardiomyopathy), full gene sequence

APTX (aprataxin) (eg, ataxia with oculomotor apraxia 1), full gene sequence

ARSA (arylsulfatase A) (eg, arylsulfatase A deficiency), full gene sequence

BCKDHA (branched chain keto acid dehydrogenase E1, alpha polypeptide) (eg, maple syrup urine disease, type 1A), full gene sequence

BCS1L (BCS1-like [S. cerevisiae]) (eg, Leigh syndrome, mitochondrial complex III deficiency, GRACILE syndrome), full gene sequence

BMPR2 (bone morphogenetic protein receptor, type II [serine/threonine kinase]) (eg, heritable pulmonary arterial hypertension), duplication/deletion analysis

CASQ2 (calsequestrin 2 [cardiac muscle]) (eg, catecholaminergic polymorphic ventricular tachycardia), full gene sequence

CASR (calcium-sensing receptor) (eg, hypocalcemia), full gene sequence

CDKL5 (cyclin-dependent kinase-like 5) (eg, early infantile epileptic encephalopathy), duplication/deletion analysis

CHRNA4 (cholinergic receptor, nicotinic, alpha 4) (eg, nocturnal frontal lobe epilepsy), full gene sequence

CHRNB2 (cholinergic receptor, nicotinic, beta 2 [neuronal]) (eg, nocturnal frontal lobe epilepsy), full gene sequence

COX10 (COX10 homolog, cytochrome c oxidase assembly protein) (eg, mitochondrial respiratory chain complex IV deficiency), full gene sequence

COX15 (COX15 homolog, cytochrome c oxidase assembly protein) (eg, mitochondrial respiratory chain complex IV deficiency), full gene sequence

CPOX (coproporphyrinogen oxidase) (eg, hereditary coproporphyria), full gene sequence

CTRC (chymotrypsin C) (eg, hereditary pancreatitis), full gene sequence

CYP11B1 (cytochrome P450, family 11, subfamily B, polypeptide 1) (eg, congenital adrenal hyperplasia), full gene sequence

CYP17A1 (cytochrome P450, family 17, subfamily A, polypeptide 1) (eg, congenital adrenal hyperplasia), full gene sequence

CYP21A2 (cytochrome P450, family 21, subfamily A, polypeptide2) (eg, steroid 21-hydroxylase isoform, congenital adrenal hyperplasia), full gene sequence

Cytogenomic constitutional targeted microarray analysis of chromosome 22q13 by interrogation of genomic regions for copy number and single nucleotide polymorphism (SNP) variants for chromosomal abnormalities

(When performing genome-wide cytogenomic constitutional microarray analysis, see 81228, 81229) (81228-81229)

(Do not report analyte-specific molecular pathology procedures separately when the specific analytes are included as part of the microarray analysis of chromosome 22q13)

(Do not report 88271 when performing cytogenomic microarray analysis)

DBT (dihydrolipoamide branched chain transacylase E2) (eg, maple syrup urine disease, type 2), duplication/deletion analysis

DCX (doublecortin) (eg, X-linked lissencephaly), full gene sequence

DES (desmin) (eg, myofibrillar myopathy), full gene sequence

DFNB59 (deafness, autosomal recessive 59) (eg, autosomal recessive nonsyndromic hearing impairment), full gene sequence

DGUOK (deoxyguanosine kinase) (eg, hepatocerebral mitochondrial DNA depletion syndrome), full gene sequence

DHCR7 (7-dehydrocholesterol reductase) (eg, Smith-Lemli-Opitz syndrome), full gene sequence

EIF2B2 (eukaryotic translation initiation factor 2B, subunit 2 beta, 39kDa) (eg, leukoencephalopathy with vanishing white matter), full gene sequence

EMD (emerin) (eg, Emery-Dreifuss muscular dystrophy), full gene sequence

ENG (endoglin) (eg, hereditary hemorrhagic telangiectasia, type 1), duplication/deletion analysis

EYA1 (eyes absent homolog 1 [Drosophila]) (eg, branchio-oto-renal [BOR] spectrum disorders), duplication/deletion analysis

FGFR1 (fibroblast growth factor receptor 1) (eg, Kallmann syndrome 2), full gene sequence

FH (fumarate hydratase) (eg, fumarate hydratase deficiency, hereditary leiomyomatosis with renal cell cancer), full gene sequence

FKTN (fukutin) (eg, limb-girdle muscular dystrophy [LGMD] type 2M or 2L), full gene sequence

FTSJ1 (FtsJ RNA methyltransferase homolog 1 [E. coli]) (eg, X-linked mental retardation 9), duplication/deletion analysis

GABRG2 (gamma-aminobutyric acid [GABA] A receptor, gamma 2) (eg, generalized epilepsy with febrile seizures), full gene sequence

GCH1 (GTP cyclohydrolase 1) (eg, autosomal dominant dopa-responsive dystonia), full gene sequence

GDAP1 (ganglioside-induced differentiation-associated protein 1) (eg, Charcot-Marie-Tooth disease), full gene sequence

GFAP (glial fibrillary acidic protein) (eg, Alexander disease), full gene sequence

GHR (growth hormone receptor) (eg, Laron syndrome), full gene sequence

GHRHR (growth hormone releasing hormone receptor) (eg, growth hormone deficiency), full gene sequence

GLA (galactosidase, alpha) (eg, Fabry disease), full gene sequence

HNF1A (HNF1 homeobox A) (eg, maturity-onset diabetes of the young [MODY]), full gene sequence

HNF1B (HNF1 homeobox B) (eg, maturity-onset diabetes of the young [MODY]), full gene sequence

HTRA1 (HtrA serine peptidase 1) (eg, macular degeneration), full gene sequence

IDS (iduronate 2-sulfatase) (eg, mucopolysaccharidosis, type II), full gene sequence

IL2RG (interleukin 2 receptor, gamma) (eg, X-linked severe combined immunodeficiency), full gene sequence

ISPD (isoprenoid synthase domain containing) (eg, muscle-eye-brain disease, Walker-Warburg syndrome), full gene sequence

KRAS (Kirsten rat sarcoma viral oncogene homolog) (eg, Noonan syndrome), full gene sequence

LAMP2 (lysosomal-associated membrane protein 2) (eg, Danon disease), full gene sequence

LDLR (low density lipoprotein receptor) (eg, familial hypercholesterolemia), duplication/deletion analysis

MEN1 (multiple endocrine neoplasia I) (eg, multiple endocrine neoplasia type 1, Wermer syndrome), full gene sequence

MMAA (methylmalonic aciduria [cobalamine deficiency] type A) (eg, MMAA-related methylmalonic acidemia), full gene sequence

MMAB (methylmalonic aciduria [cobalamine deficiency] type B) (eg, MMAA-related methylmalonic acidemia), full gene sequence

MPI (mannose phosphate isomerase) (eg, congenital disorder of glycosylation 1b), full gene sequence

MPV17 (MpV17 mitochondrial inner membrane protein) (eg, mitochondrial DNA depletion syndrome), full gene sequence

MPZ (myelin protein zero) (eg, Charcot-Marie-Tooth), full gene sequence

MTM1 (myotubularin 1) (eg, X-linked centronuclear myopathy), duplication/deletion analysis

MYL2 (myosin, light chain 2, regulatory, cardiac, slow) (eg, familial hypertrophic cardiomyopathy), full gene sequence

MYL3 (myosin, light chain 3, alkali, ventricular, skeletal, slow) (eg, familial hypertrophic cardiomyopathy), full gene sequence

MYOT (myotilin) (eg, limb-girdle muscular dystrophy), full gene sequence

NDUFS7 (NADH dehydrogenase [ubiquinone] Fe-S protein 7, 20kDa [NADH-coenzyme Q reductase]) (eg, Leigh syndrome, mitochondrial complex I deficiency), full gene sequence

NDUFS8 (NADH dehydrogenase [ubiquinone] Fe-S protein 8, 23kDa [NADH-coenzyme Q reductase]) (eg, Leigh syndrome, mitochondrial complex I deficiency), full gene sequence

NDUFV1 (NADH dehydrogenase [ubiquinone] flavoprotein 1, 51kDa) (eg, Leigh syndrome, mitochondrial complex I deficiency), full gene sequence

NEFL (neurofilament, light polypeptide) (eg, Charcot-Marie-Tooth), full gene sequence

NF2 (neurofibromin 2 [merlin]) (eg, neurofibromatosis, type 2), duplication/deletion analysis

NLGN3 (neuroligin 3) (eg, autism spectrum disorders), full gene sequence

NLGN4X (neuroligin 4, X-linked) (eg, autism spectrum disorders), full gene sequence

NPHP1 (nephronophthisis 1 [juvenile]) (eg, Joubert syndrome), deletion analysis, and duplication analysis, if performed

NPHS2 (nephrosis 2, idiopathic, steroid-resistant [podocin]) (eg, steroid-resistant nephrotic syndrome), full gene sequence

NSD1 (nuclear receptor binding SET domain protein 1) (eg, Sotos syndrome), duplication/deletion analysis

OTC (ornithine carbamoyltransferase) (eg, ornithine transcarbamylase deficiency), full gene sequence

PAFAH1B1 (platelet-activating factor acetylhydrolase 1b, regulatory subunit 1 [45kDa]) (eg, lissencephaly, Miller-Dieker syndrome), duplication/deletion analysis

PARK2 (Parkinson protein 2, E3 ubiquitin protein ligase [parkin]) (eg, Parkinson disease), duplication/deletion analysis

PCCA (propionyl CoA carboxylase, alpha polypeptide) (eg, propionic acidemia, type 1), duplication/deletion analysis

PCDH19 (protocadherin 19) (eg, epileptic encephalopathy), full gene sequence

PDHA1 (pyruvate dehydrogenase [lipoamide] alpha 1) (eg, lactic acidosis), duplication/deletion analysis

PDHB (pyruvate dehydrogenase [lipoamide] beta) (eg, lactic acidosis), full gene sequence

PINK1 (PTEN induced putative kinase 1) (eg, Parkinson disease), full gene sequence

PKLR (pyruvate kinase, liver and RBC) (eg, pyruvate kinase deficiency), full gene sequence

PLP1 (proteolipid protein 1) (eg, Pelizaeus-Merzbacher disease, spastic paraplegia), full gene sequence

POU1F1 (POU class 1 homeobox 1) (eg, combined pituitary hormone deficiency), full gene sequence

PQBP1 (polyglutamine binding protein 1) (eg, Renpenning syndrome), full gene sequence

PRX (periaxin) (eg, Charcot-Marie-Tooth disease), full gene sequence

PSEN1 (presenilin 1) (eg, Alzheimer's disease), full gene sequence

RAB7A (RAB7A, member RAS oncogene family) (eg, Charcot-Marie-Tooth disease), full gene sequence

RAI1 (retinoic acid induced 1) (eg, Smith-Magenis syndrome), full gene sequence

REEP1 (receptor accessory protein 1) (eg, spastic paraplegia), full gene sequence

RET (ret proto-oncogene) (eg, multiple endocrine neoplasia, type 2A and familial medullary thyroid carcinoma), targeted sequence analysis (eg, exons 10, 11, 13-16)

RPS19 (ribosomal protein S19) (eg, Diamond-Blackfan anemia), full gene sequence

RRM2B (ribonucleotide reductase M2 B [TP53 inducible]) (eg, mitochondrial DNA depletion), full gene sequence

SCO1 (SCO cytochrome oxidase deficient homolog 1) (eg, mitochondrial respiratory chain complex IV deficiency), full gene sequence

SDHB (succinate dehydrogenase complex, subunit B, iron sulfur) (eg, hereditary paraganglioma), full gene sequence

SDHC (succinate dehydrogenase complex, subunit C, integral membrane protein, 15kDa) (eg, hereditary paraganglioma-pheochromocytoma syndrome), full gene sequence

SGCA (sarcoglycan, alpha [50kDa dystrophin-associated glycoprotein]) (eg, limb-girdle muscular dystrophy), full gene sequence

SGCB (sarcoglycan, beta [43kDa dystrophin-associated glycoprotein]) (eg, limb-girdle muscular dystrophy), full gene sequence

SGCD (sarcoglycan, delta [35kDa dystrophin-associated glycoprotein]) (eg, limb-girdle muscular dystrophy), full gene sequence

SGCE (sarcoglycan, epsilon) (eg, myoclonic dystonia), duplication/deletion analysis

SGCG (sarcoglycan, gamma [35kDa dystrophin-associated glycoprotein]) (eg, limb-girdle muscular dystrophy), full gene sequence

SHOC2 (soc-2 suppressor of clear homolog) (eg, Noonan-like syndrome with loose anagen hair), full gene sequence

SHOX (short stature homeobox) (eg, Langer mesomelic dysplasia), full gene sequence

SIL1 (SIL1 homolog, endoplasmic reticulum chaperone [S. cerevisiae]) (eg, ataxia), full gene sequence

● New Code ▲ Revised Code ○ Reinstated ● New Web Release ▲ Revised Web Release + Add-on Unlisted Not Covered # Resequenced
㊿ Optum Mod 50 Exempt Ⓢ AMA Mod 51 Exempt �51 Optum Mod 51 Exempt �63 Mod 63 Exempt ✎ Non-FDA Drug ★ Telemedicine Ⓜ Maternity Ⓐ Age Edit

CPT © 2019 American Medical Association. All Rights Reserved.

SLC2A1 (solute carrier family 2 [facilitated glucose transporter], member 1) (eg, glucose transporter type 1 [GLUT 1] deficiency syndrome), full gene sequence

SLC16A2 (solute carrier family 16, member 2 [thyroid hormone transporter]) (eg, specific thyroid hormone cell transporter deficiency, Allan-Herndon-Dudley syndrome), full gene sequence

SLC22A5 (solute carrier family 22 [organic cation/carnitine transporter], member 5) (eg, systemic primary carnitine deficiency), full gene sequence

SLC25A20 (solute carrier family 25 [carnitine/acylcarnitine translocase], member 20) (eg, carnitine-acylcarnitine translocase deficiency), full gene sequence

SMAD4 (SMAD family member 4) (eg, hemorrhagic telangiectasia syndrome, juvenile polyposis), duplication/deletion analysis

SPAST (spastin) (eg, spastic paraplegia), duplication/deletion analysis

SPG7 (spastic paraplegia 7 [pure and complicated autosomal recessive]) (eg, spastic paraplegia), duplication/deletion analysis

SPRED1 (sprouty-related, EVH1 domain containing 1) (eg, Legius syndrome), full gene sequence

STAT3 (signal transducer and activator of transcription 3 [acute-phase response factor]) (eg, autosomal dominant hyper-IgE syndrome), targeted sequence analysis (eg, exons 12, 13, 14, 16, 17, 20, 21)

STK11 (serine/threonine kinase 11) (eg, Peutz-Jeghers syndrome), full gene sequence

SURF1 (surfeit 1) (eg, mitochondrial respiratory chain complex IV deficiency), full gene sequence

TARDBP (TAR DNA binding protein) (eg, amyotrophic lateral sclerosis), full gene sequence

TBX5 (T-box 5) (eg, Holt-Oram syndrome), full gene sequence

TCF4 (transcription factor 4) (eg, Pitt-Hopkins syndrome), duplication/deletion analysis

TGFBR1 (transforming growth factor, beta receptor 1) (eg, Marfan syndrome), full gene sequence

TGFBR2 (transforming growth factor, beta receptor 2) (eg, Marfan syndrome), full gene sequence

THRB (thyroid hormone receptor, beta) (eg, thyroid hormone resistance, thyroid hormone beta receptor deficiency), full gene sequence or targeted sequence analysis of >5 exons

TK2 (thymidine kinase 2, mitochondrial) (eg, mitochondrial DNA depletion syndrome), full gene sequence

TNNC1 (troponin C type 1 [slow]) (eg, hypertrophic cardiomyopathy or dilated cardiomyopathy), full gene sequence

TNNI3 (troponin 1, type 3 [cardiac]) (eg, familial hypertrophic cardiomyopathy), full gene sequence

TP53 (tumor protein 53) (eg, Li-Fraumeni syndrome, tumor samples), full gene sequence or targeted sequence analysis of >5 exons

TPM1 (tropomyosin 1 [alpha]) (eg, familial hypertrophic cardiomyopathy), full gene sequence

TSC1 (tuberous sclerosis 1) (eg, tuberous sclerosis), duplication/deletion analysis

TYMP (thymidine phosphorylase) (eg, mitochondrial DNA depletion syndrome), full gene sequence

VWF (von Willebrand factor) (eg, von Willebrand disease type 2N), targeted sequence analysis (eg, exons 18-20, 23-25)

WT1 (Wilms tumor 1) (eg, Denys-Drash syndrome, familial Wilms tumor), full gene sequence

ZEB2 (zinc finger E-box binding homeobox 2) (eg, Mowat-Wilson syndrome), full gene sequence

🖫 0.00   🖫 0.00   **FUD** XXX   Ⓐ ▢

AMA: 2019,Jul,3; 2018,Nov,9; 2018,Sep,14; 2018,May,6; 2018,Jan,8; 2017,Jan,8; 2016,Aug,9; 2016,Jan,13; 2015,Jan,16; 2015,Jan,3; 2014,Jan,11

▲ 81406   **Molecular pathology procedure, Level 7 (eg, analysis of 11-25 exons by DNA sequence analysis, mutation scanning or duplication/deletion variants of 26-50 exons)**

ACADVL (acyl-CoA dehydrogenase, very long chain) (eg, very long chain acyl-coenzyme A dehydrogenase deficiency), full gene sequence

ACTN4 (actinin, alpha 4) (eg, focal segmental glomerulosclerosis), full gene sequence

AFG3L2 (AFG3 ATPase family gene 3-like 2 [S. cerevisiae]) (eg, spinocerebellar ataxia), full gene sequence

AIRE (autoimmune regulator) (eg, autoimmune polyendocrinopathy syndrome type 1), full gene sequence

ALDH7A1 (aldehyde dehydrogenase 7 family, member A1) (eg, pyridoxine-dependent epilepsy), full gene sequence

ANO5 (anoctamin 5) (eg, limb-girdle muscular dystrophy), full gene sequence

ANOS1 (anosim-1) (eg, Kallmann syndrome 1), full gene sequence

APP (amyloid beta [A4] precursor protein) (eg, Alzheimer's disease), full gene sequence

ASS1 (argininosuccinate synthase 1) (eg, citrullinemia type I), full gene sequence

ATL1 (atlastin GTPase 1) (eg, spastic paraplegia), full gene sequence

ATP1A2 (ATPase, Na+/K+ transporting, alpha 2 polypeptide) (eg, familial hemiplegic migraine), full gene sequence

ATP7B (ATPase, Cu++ transporting, beta polypeptide) (eg, Wilson disease), full gene sequence

BBS1 (Bardet-Biedl syndrome 1) (eg, Bardet-Biedl syndrome), full gene sequence

BBS2 (Bardet-Biedl syndrome 2) (eg, Bardet-Biedl syndrome), full gene sequence

BCKDHB (branched-chain keto acid dehydrogenase E1, beta polypeptide) (eg, maple syrup urine disease, type 1B), full gene sequence

BEST1 (bestrophin 1) (eg, vitelliform macular dystrophy), full gene sequence

BMPR2 (bone morphogenetic protein receptor, type II [serine/threonine kinase]) (eg, heritable pulmonary arterial hypertension), full gene sequence

BRAF (B-Raf proto-oncogene, serine/threonine kinase) (eg, Noonan syndrome), full gene sequence

BSCL2 (Berardinelli-Seip congenital lipodystrophy 2 [seipin]) (eg, Berardinelli-Seip congenital lipodystrophy), full gene sequence

BTK (Bruton agammaglobulinemia tyrosine kinase) (eg, X-linked agammaglobulinemia), full gene sequence

CACNB2 (calcium channel, voltage-dependent, beta 2 subunit) (eg, Brugada syndrome), full gene sequence

CAPN3 (calpain 3) (eg, limb-girdle muscular dystrophy [LGMD] type 2A, calpainopathy), full gene sequence

CBS (cystathionine-beta-synthase) (eg, homocystinuria, cystathionine beta-synthase deficiency), full gene sequence

CDH1 (cadherin 1, type 1, E-cadherin [epithelial]) (eg, hereditary diffuse gastric cancer), full gene sequence

CDKL5 (cyclin-dependent kinase-like 5) (eg, early infantile epileptic encephalopathy), full gene sequence

CLCN1 (chloride channel 1, skeletal muscle) (eg, myotonia congenita), full gene sequence

CLCNKB (chloride channel, voltage-sensitive Kb) (eg, Bartter syndrome 3 and 4b), full gene sequence

CNTNAP2 (contactin-associated protein-like 2) (eg, Pitt-Hopkins-like syndrome 1), full gene sequence

COL6A2 (collagen, type VI, alpha 2) (eg, collagen type VI-related disorders), duplication/deletion analysis

| 26/TC PC/TC Only | A2-Z3 ASC Payment | 50 Bilateral | ♂ Male Only | ♀ Female Only | 🖫 Facility RVU | 🖫 Non-Facility RVU | CCI | CLIA |
| FUD Follow-up Days | CMS: IOM | AMA: CPT Asst | A-Y OPPSI | 80/80 Surg Assist Allowed / w/Doc | Lab Crosswalk | Radiology Crosswalk |

394   CPT © 2019 American Medical Association. All Rights Reserved.   © 2019 Optum360, LLC

CPT1A (carnitine palmitoyltransferase 1A [liver]) (eg, carnitine palmitoyltransferase 1A [CPT1A] deficiency), full gene sequence

CRB1 (crumbs homolog 1 [Drosophila]) (eg, Leber congenital amaurosis), full gene sequence

CREBBP (CREB binding protein) (eg, Rubinstein-Taybi syndrome), duplication/deletion analysis

DBT (dihydrolipoamide branched chain transacylase E2) (eg, maple syrup urine disease, type 2), full gene sequence

DLAT (dihydrolipoamide S-acetyltransferase) (eg, pyruvate dehydrogenase E2 deficiency), full gene sequence

DLD (dihydrolipoamide dehydrogenase) (eg, maple syrup urine disease, type III), full gene sequence

DSC2 (desmocollin) (eg, arrhythmogenic right ventricular dysplasia/cardiomyopathy 11), full gene sequence

DSG2 (desmoglein 2) (eg, arrhythmogenic right ventricular dysplasia/cardiomyopathy 10), full gene sequence

DSP (desmoplakin) (eg, arrhythmogenic right ventricular dysplasia/cardiomyopathy 8), full gene sequence

EFHC1 (EF-hand domain [C-terminal] containing 1) (eg, juvenile myoclonic epilepsy), full gene sequence

EIF2B3 (eukaryotic translation initiation factor 2B, subunit 3 gamma, 58kDa) (eg, leukoencephalopathy with vanishing white matter), full gene sequence

EIF2B4 (eukaryotic translation initiation factor 2B, subunit 4 delta, 67kDa) (eg, leukoencephalopathy with vanishing white matter), full gene sequence

EIF2B5 (eukaryotic translation initiation factor 2B, subunit 5 epsilon, 82kDa) (eg, childhood ataxia with central nervous system hypomyelination/vanishing white matter), full gene sequence

ENG (endoglin) (eg, hereditary hemorrhagic telangiectasia, type 1), full gene sequence

EYA1 (eyes absent homolog 1 [Drosophila]) (eg, branchio-oto-renal [BOR] spectrum disorders), full gene sequence

F8 (coagulation factor VIII) (eg, hemophilia A), duplication/deletion analysis

FAH (fumarylacetoacetate hydrolase [fumarylacetoacetase]) (eg, tyrosinemia, type 1), full gene sequence

FASTKD2 (FAST kinase domains 2) (eg, mitochondrial respiratory chain complex IV deficiency), full gene sequence

FIG4 (FIG4 homolog, SAC1 lipid phosphatase domain containing [S. cerevisiae]) (eg, Charcot-Marie-Tooth disease), full gene sequence

FTSJ1 (FtsJ RNA methyltransferase homolog 1 [E. coli]) (eg, X-linked mental retardation 9), full gene sequence

FUS (fused in sarcoma) (eg, amyotrophic lateral sclerosis), full gene sequence

GAA (glucosidase, alpha; acid) (eg, glycogen storage disease type II [Pompe disease]), full gene sequence

GALC (galactosylceramidase) (eg, Krabbe disease), full gene sequence

GALT (galactose-1-phosphate uridylyltransferase) (eg, galactosemia), full gene sequence

GARS (glycyl-tRNA synthetase) (eg, Charcot-Marie-Tooth disease), full gene sequence

GCDH (glutaryl-CoA dehydrogenase) (eg, glutaricacidemia type 1), full gene sequence

GCK (glucokinase [hexokinase 4]) (eg, maturity-onset diabetes of the young [MODY]), full gene sequence

GLUD1 (glutamate dehydrogenase 1) (eg, familial hyperinsulinism), full gene sequence

GNE (glucosamine [UDP-N-acetyl]-2-epimerase/N-acetylmannosamine kinase) (eg, inclusion body myopathy 2 [IBM2], Nonaka myopathy), full gene sequence

GRN (granulin) (eg, frontotemporal dementia), full gene sequence

HADHA (hydroxyacyl-CoA dehydrogenase/3-ketoacyl-CoA thiolase/enoyl-CoA hydratase [trifunctional protein] alpha subunit) (eg, long chain acyl-coenzyme A dehydrogenase deficiency), full gene sequence

HADHB (hydroxyacyl-CoA dehydrogenase/3-ketoacyl-CoA thiolase/enoyl-CoA hydratase [trifunctional protein], beta subunit) (eg, trifunctional protein deficiency), full gene sequence

HEXA (hexosaminidase A, alpha polypeptide) (eg, Tay-Sachs disease), full gene sequence

HLCS (HLCS holocarboxylase synthetase) (eg, holocarboxylase synthetase deficiency), full gene sequence

HMBS (hydroxymethylbilane synthase) (eg, acute intermittent porphyria), full gene sequence

HNF4A (hepatocyte nuclear factor 4, alpha) (eg, maturity-onset diabetes of the young [MODY]), full gene sequence

IDUA (iduronidase, alpha-L-) (eg, mucopolysaccharidosis type I), full gene sequence

INF2 (inverted formin, FH2 and WH2 domain containing) (eg, focal segmental glomerulosclerosis), full gene sequence

IVD (isovaleryl-CoA dehydrogenase) (eg, isovaleric acidemia), full gene sequence

JAG1 (jagged 1) (eg, Alagille syndrome), duplication/deletion analysis

JUP (junction plakoglobin) (eg, arrhythmogenic right ventricular dysplasia/cardiomyopathy 11), full gene sequence

KCNH2 (potassium voltage-gated channel, subfamily H [eag-related], member 2) (eg, short QT syndrome, long QT syndrome), full gene sequence

KCNQ1 (potassium voltage-gated channel, KQT-like subfamily, member 1) (eg, short QT syndrome, long QT syndrome), full gene sequence

KCNQ2 (potassium voltage-gated channel, KQT-like subfamily, member 2) (eg, epileptic encephalopathy), full gene sequence

LDB3 (LIM domain binding 3) (eg, familial dilated cardiomyopathy, myofibrillar myopathy), full gene sequence

LDLR (low density lipoprotein receptor) (eg, familial hypercholesterolemia), full gene sequence

LEPR (leptin receptor(eg, obesity with hypogonadism), full gene sequence

LHCGR (luteinizing hormone/choriogonadotropin receptor) (eg, precocious male puberty), full gene sequence

LMNA (lamin A/C) (eg, Emery-Dreifuss muscular dystrophy [EDMD1, 2 and 3] limb-girdle muscular dystrophy [LGMD] type 1B, dilated cardiomyopathy [CMD1A], familial partial lipodystrophy [FPLD2]), full gene sequence

LRP5 (low density lipoprotein receptor-related protein 5) (eg, osteopetrosis), full gene sequence

MAP2K1 (mitogen-activated protein kinase 1) (eg, cardiofaciocutaneous syndrome), full gene sequence

MAP2K2 (mitogen-activated protein kinase 2) (eg, cardiofaciocutaneous syndrome), full gene sequence

MAPT (microtubule-associated protein tau) (eg, frontotemporal dementia), full gene sequence

MCCC1 (methylcrotonoyl-CoA carboxylase 1 [alpha]) (eg, 3-methylcrotonyl-CoA carboxylase deficiency), full gene sequence

MCCC2 (methylcrotonoyl-CoA carboxylase 2 [beta]) (eg, 3-methylcrotonyl carboxylase deficiency), full gene sequence

MFN2 (mitofusin 2) (eg, Charcot-Marie-Tooth disease), full gene sequence

MTM1 (myotubularin 1) (eg, X-linked centronuclear myopathy), full gene sequence

---

● New Code ▲ Revised Code ○ Reinstated ● New Web Release ▲ Revised Web Release + Add-on Unlisted Not Covered # Resequenced
⑤⓪ Optum Mod 50 Exempt ⊘ AMA Mod 51 Exempt ⑤① Optum Mod 51 Exempt ⑥③ Mod 63 Exempt ℂ Non-FDA Drug ★ Telemedicine Ⓜ Maternity Ⓐ Age Edit

MUT (methylmalonyl CoA mutase) (eg, methylmalonic acidemia), full gene sequence

MUTYH (mutY homolog [E. coli]) (eg, MYH-associated polyposis), full gene sequence

NDUFS1 (NADH dehydrogenase [ubiquinone] Fe-S protein 1, 75kDa [NADH-coenzyme Q reductase]) (eg, Leigh syndrome, mitochondrial complex I deficiency), full gene sequence

NF2 (neurofibromin 2 [merlin]) (eg, neurofibromatosis, type 2), full gene sequence

NOTCH3 (notch 3) (eg, cerebral autosomal dominant arteriopathy with subcortical infarcts and leukoencephalopathy [CADASIL]), targeted sequence analysis (eg, exons 1-23)

NPC1 (Niemann-Pick disease, type C1) (eg, Niemann-Pick disease), full gene sequence

NPHP1 (nephronophthisis 1 [juvenile]) (eg, Joubert syndrome), full gene sequence

NSD1 (nuclear receptor binding SET domain protein 1) (eg, Sotos syndrome, full gene sequence

OPA1 (optic atrophy 1) (eg, optic atrophy), duplication/deletion analysis

OPTN (optineurin) (eg, amyotrophic lateral sclerosis), full gene sequence

PAFAH1B1 (platelet-activating factor acetylhydrolase 1b, regulatory subunit 1 [45kDa]) (eg, lissencephaly, Miller-Dieker syndrome), full gene sequence

PAH (phenylalanine hydroxylase) (eg, phenylketonuria), full gene sequence

PALB2 (partner and localizer of BRCA2) (eg, breast and pancreatic cancer), full gene sequence

PARK2 (Parkinson protein 2, E3 ubiquitin protein ligase [parkin]) (eg, Parkinson disease), full gene sequence

PAX2 (paired box 2) (eg, renal coloboma syndrome), full gene sequence

PC (pyruvate carboxylase) (eg, pyruvate carboxylase deficiency), full gene sequence

PCCA (propionyl CoA carboxylase, alpha polypeptide) (eg, propionic acidemia, type 1), full gene sequence

PCCB (propionyl CoA carboxylase, beta polypeptide) (eg, propionic acidemia), full gene sequence

PCDH15 (protocadherin-related 15) (eg, Usher syndrome type 1F), duplication/deletion analysis

PCSK9 (proprotein convertase subtilisin/kexin type 9) (eg familial hypercholesterolemia), full gene sequence

PDHA1 (pyruvate dehydrogenase [lipoamide] alpha 1) (eg, lactic acidosis), full gene sequence

PDHX (pyruvate dehydrogenase complex, component X) (eg, lactic acidosis), full gene sequence

PHEX (phosphate-regulating endopeptidase homolog, X-linked) (eg, hypophosphatemic rickets), full gene sequence

PKD2 (polycystic kidney disease 2 [autosomal dominant]) (eg, polycystic kidney disease), full gene sequence

PKP2 (plakophilin 2) (eg, arrhythmogenic right ventricular dysplasia/cardiomyopathy 9), full gene sequence

PNKD (eg, paroxysmal nonkinesigenic dyskinesia), full gene sequence

POLG (polymerase [DNA directed], gamma) (eg, Alpers-Huttenlocher syndrome, autosomal dominant progressive external ophthalmoplegia), full gene sequence

POMGNT1 (protein O-linked mannose beta1, 2-N acetylglucosaminyltransferase) (eg, muscle-eye-brain disease, Walker-Warburg syndrome), full gene sequence

POMT1 (protein-O-mannosyltransferase 1) (eg, limb-girdle muscular dystrophy [LGMD] type 2K, Walker-Warburg syndrome), full gene sequence

POMT2 (protein-O-mannosyltransferase 2) (eg, limb-girdle muscular dystrophy [LGMD] type 2N, Walker-Warburg syndrome), full gene sequence

PPOX (protoporphyrinogen oxidase) (eg, variegate porphyria), full gene sequence

PRKAG2 (protein kinase, AMP-activated, gamma 2 non-catalytic subunit) (eg, familial hypertrophic cardiomyopathy with Wolff-Parkinson-White syndrome, lethal congenital glycogen storage disease of heart), full gene sequence

PRKCG (protein kinase C, gamma) (eg, spinocerebellar ataxia), full gene sequence

PSEN2 (presenilin 2[Alzheimer's disease 4]) (eg, Alzheimer's disease), full gene sequence

PTPN11 (protein tyrosine phosphatase, non-receptor type 11) (eg, Noonan syndrome, LEOPARD syndrome), full gene sequence

PYGM (phosphorylase, glycogen, muscle) (eg, glycogen storage disease type V, McArdle disease), full gene sequence

RAF1 (v-raf-1 murine leukemia viral oncogene homolog 1) (eg, LEOPARD syndrome), full gene sequence

RET (ret proto-oncogene) (eg, Hirschsprung disease), full gene sequence

RPE65 (retinal pigment epithelium-specific protein 65kDa) (eg, retinitis pigmentosa, Leber congenital amaurosis), full gene sequence

RYR1 (ryanodine receptor 1, skeletal) (eg, malignant hyperthermia), targeted sequence analysis of exons with functionally-confirmed mutations

SCN4A (sodium channel, voltage-gated, type IV, alpha subunit) (eg, hyperkalemic periodic paralysis), full gene sequence

SCNN1A (sodium channel, nonvoltage-gated 1 alpha) (eg, pseudohypoaldosteronism), full gene sequence

SCNN1B (sodium channel, nonvoltage-gated 1, beta) (eg, Liddle syndrome, pseudohypoaldosteronism), full gene sequence

SCNN1G (sodium channel, nonvoltage-gated 1, gamma) (eg, Liddle syndrome, pseudohypoaldosteronism), full gene sequence

SDHA (succinate dehydrogenase complex, subunit A, flavoprotein [Fp]) (eg, Leigh syndrome, mitochondrial complex II deficiency), full gene sequence

SETX (senataxin) (eg, ataxia), full gene sequence

SGCE (sarcoglycan, epsilon) (eg, myoclonic dystonia), full gene sequence

SH3TC2 (SH3 domain and tetratricopeptide repeats 2) (eg, Charcot-Marie-Tooth disease), full gene sequence

SLC9A6 (solute carrier family 9 [sodium/hydrogen exchanger], member 6) (eg, Christianson syndrome), full gene sequence

SLC26A4 (solute carrier family 26, member 4) (eg, Pendred syndrome), full gene sequence

SLC37A4 (solute carrier family 37 [glucose-6-phosphate transporter], member 4) (eg, glycogen storage disease type Ib), full gene sequence

SMAD4 (SMAD family member 4) (eg, hemorrhagic telangiectasia syndrome, juvenile polyposis), full gene sequence

SOS1 (son of sevenless homolog 1) (eg, Noonan syndrome, gingival fibromatosis), full gene sequence

SPAST (spastin) (eg, spastic paraplegia), full gene sequence

SPG7 (spastic paraplegia 7 [pure and complicated autosomal recessive]) (eg, spastic paraplegia), full gene sequence

STXBP1 (syntaxin-binding protein 1) (eg, epileptic encephalopathy), full gene sequence

TAZ (tafazzin) (eg, methylglutaconic aciduria type 2, Barth syndrome), full gene sequence

| 26/TC PC/TC Only | A2-Z3 ASC Payment | 50 Bilateral | ♂ Male Only | ♀ Female Only | Facility RVU | Non-Facility RVU | CCI | CLIA |
| FUD Follow-up Days | CMS: IOM | AMA: CPT Asst | A-Y OPPSI | 80/80 Surg Assist Allowed / w/Doc | Lab Crosswalk | Radiology Crosswalk |

396
CPT © 2019 American Medical Association. All Rights Reserved.
© 2019 Optum360, LLC

TCF4 (transcription factor 4) (eg, Pitt-Hopkins syndrome), full gene sequence

TH (tyrosine hydroxylase) (eg, Segawa syndrome), full gene sequence

TMEM43 (transmembrane protein 43) (eg, arrhythmogenic right ventricular cardiomyopathy), full gene sequence

TNNT2 (troponin T, type 2 [cardiac]) (eg, familial hypertrophic cardiomyopathy), full gene sequence

TRPC6 (transient receptor potential cation channel, subfamily C, member 6) (eg, focal segmental glomerulosclerosis), full gene sequence

TSC1 (tuberous sclerosis 1) (eg, tuberous sclerosis), full gene sequence

TSC2 (tuberous sclerosis 2) (eg, tuberous sclerosis), duplication/deletion analysis

UBE3A (ubiquitin protein ligase E3A) (eg, Angelman syndrome) full gene sequence

UMOD (uromodulin) (eg, glomerulocystic kidney disease with hyperuricemia and isosthenuria), full gene sequence

VWF (von Willebrand factor) (von Willebrand disease type 2A), extended targeted sequence analysis (eg, exons 11-16, 24-26, 51, 52)

WAS (Wiskott-Aldrich syndrome [eczema-thrombocytopenia]) (eg, Wiskott-Aldrich syndrome), full gene sequence

 📖 0.00   ⅗ 0.00   **FUD** XXX   Ⓐ ▭

AMA: 2018,Nov,9; 2018,May,6; 2018,Jan,8; 2017,Apr,9; 2017,Jan,8; 2016,Aug,9; 2016,Jan,13; 2015,Jan,16; 2015,Jan,3; 2014,Jan,11

▲ **81407 Molecular pathology procedure, Level 8 (eg, analysis of 26-50 exons by DNA sequence analysis, mutation scanning or duplication/deletion variants of >50 exons, sequence analysis of multiple genes on one platform)**

ABCC8 (ATP-binding cassette, sub-family C [CFTR/MRP], member 8) (eg, familial hyperinsulinism), full gene sequence

AGL (amylo-alpha-1, 6-glucosidase, 4-alpha-glucanotransferase) (eg, glycogen storage disease type III), full gene sequence

AHI1 (Abelson helper integration site 1) (eg, Joubert syndrome), full gene sequence

APOB (apolipoprotein B) (eg, familial hypercholesterolemia type B) full gene sequence

ASPM (asp [abnormal spindle] homolog, microcephaly associated [Drosophila]) (eg, primary microcephaly), full gene sequence

CHD7 (chromodomain helicase DNA binding protein 7) (eg, CHARGE syndrome), full gene sequence

COL4A4 (collagen, type IV, alpha 4) (eg, Alport syndrome), full gene sequence

COL4A5 (collagen, type IV, alpha 5) (eg, Alport syndrome), duplication/deletion analysis

COL6A1 (collagen, type VI, alpha 1) (eg, collagen type VI-related disorders), full gene sequence

COL6A2 (collagen, type VI, alpha 2) (eg, collagen type VI-related disorders), full gene sequence

COL6A3 (collagen, type VI, alpha 3) (eg, collagen type VI-related disorders), full gene sequence

CREBBP (CREB binding protein) (eg, Rubinstein-Taybi syndrome), full gene sequence

F8 (coagulation factor VIII) (eg, hemophilia A), full gene sequence

JAG1 (jagged 1) (eg, Alagille syndrome), full gene sequence

KDM5C (lysine [K]-specific demethylase 5C) (eg, X-linked mental retardation), full gene sequence

KIAA0196 (KIAA0196) (eg, spastic paraplegia), full gene sequence

L1CAM (L1 cell adhesion molecule) (eg, MASA syndrome, X-linked hydrocephaly), full gene sequence

LAMB2 (laminin, beta 2 [laminin S]) (eg, Pierson syndrome), full gene sequence

MYBPC3 (myosin binding protein C, cardiac) (eg, familial hypertrophic cardiomyopathy), full gene sequence

MYH6 (myosin, heavy chain 6, cardiac muscle, alpha) (eg, familial dilated cardiomyopathy), full gene sequence

MYH7 (myosin, heavy chain 7, cardiac muscle, beta) (eg, familial hypertrophic cardiomyopathy, Liang distal myopathy), full gene sequence

MYO7A (myosin VIIA) (eg, Usher syndrome, type 1), full gene sequence

NOTCH1 (notch 1) (eg, aortic valve disease), full gene sequence

NPHS1 (nephrosis 1, congenital, Finnish type [nephrin]) (eg, congenital Finnish nephrosis), full gene sequence

OPA1 (optic atrophy 1) (eg, optic atrophy), full gene sequence

PCDH15 (protocadherin-related 15) (eg, Usher syndrome, type 1), full gene sequence

PKD1 (polycystic kidney disease 1 [autosomal dominant]) (eg, polycystic kidney disease), full gene sequence

PLCE1 (phospholipase C, epsilon 1) (eg, nephrotic syndrome type 3), full gene sequence

SCN1A (sodium channel, voltage-gated, type 1, alpha subunit) (eg, generalized epilepsy with febrile seizures), full gene sequence

SCN5A (sodium channel, voltage-gated, type V, alpha subunit) (eg, familial dilated cardiomyopathy), full gene sequence

SLC12A1 (solute carrier family 12 [sodium/potassium/chloride transporters], member 1) (eg, Bartter syndrome), full gene sequence

SLC12A3 (solute carrier family 12 [sodium/chloride transporters], member 3) (eg, Gitelman syndrome), full gene sequence

SPG11 (spastic paraplegia 11 [autosomal recessive]) (eg, spastic paraplegia), full gene sequence

SPTBN2 (spectrin, beta, non-erythrocytic 2) (eg, spinocerebellar ataxia), full gene sequence

TMEM67 (transmembrane protein 67) (eg, Joubert syndrome), full gene sequence

TSC2 (tuberous sclerosis 2) (eg, tuberous sclerosis), full gene sequence

USH1C (Usher syndrome 1C [autosomal recessive, severe]) (eg, Usher syndrome, type 1), full gene sequence

VPS13B (vacuolar protein sorting 13 homolog B [yeast]) (eg, Cohen syndrome), duplication/deletion analysis

WDR62 (WD repeat domain 62) (eg, primary autosomal recessive microcephaly), full gene sequence

 📖 0.00   ⅗ 0.00   **FUD** XXX   Ⓐ ▭

AMA: 2019,Jul,3; 2018,Nov,9; 2018,May,6; 2018,Jan,8; 2017,Jan,8; 2016,Aug,9; 2016,Jan,13; 2015,Jan,16; 2015,Jan,3; 2014,Jan,11

81408 Molecular pathology procedure, Level 9 (eg, analysis of >50 exons in a single gene by DNA sequence analysis)

ABCA4 (ATP-binding cassette, sub-family A [ABC1], member 4) (eg, Stargardt disease, age-related macular degeneration), full gene sequence

ATM (ataxia telangiectasia mutated) (eg, ataxia telangiectasia), full gene sequence

CDH23 (cadherin-related 23) (eg, Usher syndrome, type 1), full gene sequence

CEP290 (centrosomal protein 290kDa) (eg, Joubert syndrome), full gene sequence

COL1A1 (collagen, type I, alpha 1) (eg, osteogenesis imperfecta, type I), full gene sequence

COL1A2 (collagen, type I, alpha 2) (eg, osteogenesis imperfecta, type I), full gene sequence

COL4A1 (collagen, type IV, alpha 1) (eg, brain small-vessel disease with hemorrhage), full gene sequence

COL4A3 (collagen, type IV, alpha 3 [Goodpasture antigen]) (eg, Alport syndrome), full gene sequence

COL4A5 (collagen, type IV, alpha 5) (eg, Alport syndrome), full gene sequence

DMD (dystrophin) (eg, Duchenne/Becker muscular dystrophy), full gene sequence

DYSF (dysferlin, limb girdle muscular dystrophy 2B [autosomal recessive]) (eg, limb-girdle muscular dystrophy), full gene sequence

FBN1 (fibrillin 1) (eg, Marfan syndrome), full gene sequence

ITPR1 (inositol 1,4,5-trisphosphate receptor, type 1) (eg, spinocerebellar ataxia), full gene sequence

LAMA2 (laminin, alpha 2) (eg, congenital muscular dystrophy), full gene sequence

LRRK2 (leucine-rich repeat kinase 2) (eg, Parkinson disease), full gene sequence

MYH11 (myosin, heavy chain 11, smooth muscle) (eg, thoracic aortic aneurysms and aortic dissections), full gene sequence

NEB (nebulin) (eg, nemaline myopathy 2), full gene sequence

NF1 (neurofibromin 1) (eg, neurofibromatosis, type 1), full gene sequence

PKHD1 (polycystic kidney and hepatic disease 1) (eg, autosomal recessive polycystic kidney disease), full gene sequence

RYR1 (ryanodine receptor 1, skeletal) (eg, malignant hyperthermia), full gene sequence

RYR2 (ryanodine receptor 2 [cardiac]) (eg, catecholaminergic polymorphic ventricular tachycardia, arrhythmogenic right ventricular dysplasia), full gene sequence or targeted sequence analysis of > 50 exons

USH2A (Usher syndrome 2A [autosomal recessive, mild]) (eg, Usher syndrome, type 2), full gene sequence

VPS13B (vacuolar protein sorting 13 homolog B [yeast]) (eg, Cohen syndrome), full gene sequence

VWF (von Willebrand factor) (eg, von Willebrand disease types 1 and 3), full gene sequence

  0.00   0.00   **FUD** XXX   A ▢

  AMA: 2018,Nov,9; 2018,May,6; 2018,Jan,8; 2017,Jan,8; 2016,Aug,9; 2016,Jan,13; 2015,Jan,16; 2015,Jan,3; 2014,Jan,11

\# **81479**   **Unlisted molecular pathology procedure**   A ▢

  AMA: 2019,Jun,11; 2019,May,5; 2018,Dec,10; 2018,Dec,10; 2018,Nov,9; 2018,Sep,14; 2018,Jun,8; 2018,May,6; 2018,Jan,8; 2017,Apr,9; 2017,Jan,8; 2016,Sep,9; 2016,Aug,9; 2016,Apr,4; 2016,Jan,13; 2015,Jan,3; 2015,Jan,16; 2014,Jan,11

81410-81479 [81443, 81448] Genomic Sequencing

EXCLUDES *In situ hybridization analyses (88271-88275, 88365-88368 [88364, 88373, 88374])*
Microbial identification (87149-87153, 87471-87801 [87623, 87624, 87625], 87900-87904 [87906, 87910, 87912])

81410   **Aortic dysfunction or dilation (eg, Marfan syndrome, Loeys Dietz syndrome, Ehler Danlos syndrome type IV, arterial tortuosity syndrome); genomic sequence analysis panel, must include sequencing of at least 9 genes, including *FBN1, TGFBR1, TGFBR2, COL3A1, MYH11, ACTA2, SLC2A10, SMAD3, and MYLK***   A ▢

  0.00   0.00   **FUD** XXX

  AMA: 2018,Jan,8; 2017,Jan,8; 2016,Jan,13; 2015,Jan,3

81411   **duplication/deletion analysis panel, must include analyses for *TGFBR1, TGFBR2, MYH11, and COL3A1***   A ▢

  0.00   0.00   **FUD** XXX

  AMA: 2018,Jan,8; 2017,Jan,8; 2016,Jan,13; 2015,Jan,3

81412   **Ashkenazi Jewish associated disorders (eg, Bloom syndrome, Canavan disease, cystic fibrosis, familial dysautonomia, Fanconi anemia group C, Gaucher disease, Tay-Sachs disease), genomic sequence analysis panel, must include sequencing of at least 9 genes, including *ASPA, BLM, CFTR, FANCC, GBA, HEXA, IKBKAP, MCOLN1, and SMPD1***   A ▢

  0.00   0.00   **FUD** XXX

  AMA: 2018,Nov,9; 2018,Jan,8; 2017,Jan,8; 2016,Apr,4

81413   **Cardiac ion channelopathies (eg, Brugada syndrome, long QT syndrome, short QT syndrome, catecholaminergic polymorphic ventricular tachycardia); genomic sequence analysis panel, must include sequencing of at least 10 genes, including ANK2, CASQ2, CAV3, KCNE1, KCNE2, KCNH2, KCNJ2, KCNQ1, RYR2, and SCN5A**

  EXCLUDES *Evaluation of cardiomyopathy (81439)*

  0.00   0.00   **FUD** XXX   A ▢

  AMA: 2018,Jan,8; 2017,Apr,3

81414   **duplication/deletion gene analysis panel, must include analysis of at least 2 genes, including KCNH2 and KCNQ1**

  EXCLUDES *Evaluation of cardiomyopathy (81439)*

  0.00   0.00   **FUD** XXX   A ▢

  AMA: 2018,Jan,8; 2017,Apr,3

81415   **Exome (eg, unexplained constitutional or heritable disorder or syndrome); sequence analysis**

  0.00   0.00   **FUD** XXX   A ▢

  AMA: 2018,Jan,8; 2017,Jan,8; 2016,Jan,13; 2015,Jan,3

+   **81416**   **sequence analysis, each comparator exome (eg, parents, siblings) (List separately in addition to code for primary procedure)**

  Code first (81415)

  0.00   0.00   **FUD** XXX   A ▢

  AMA: 2018,Jan,8; 2017,Jan,8; 2016,Jan,13; 2015,Jan,3

81417   **re-evaluation of previously obtained exome sequence (eg, updated knowledge or unrelated condition/syndrome)**

  EXCLUDES *Microarray assessment (81228-81229)*
   Results that are incidental

  0.00   0.00   **FUD** XXX   A ▢

  AMA: 2018,Jan,8; 2017,Jan,8; 2016,Jan,13; 2015,Jan,3

81420   **Fetal chromosomal aneuploidy (eg, trisomy 21, monosomy X) genomic sequence analysis panel, circulating cell-free fetal DNA in maternal blood, must include analysis of chromosomes 13, 18, and 21**   M

  EXCLUDES *Genome-wide microarray analysis (81228-81229)*
   Molecular cytogenetics (88271)

  0.00   0.00   **FUD** XXX   A ▢

  AMA: 2018,Apr,10; 2018,Jan,8; 2017,Jan,8; 2016,Jan,13; 2015,Dec,18; 2015,Jan,3

81422   **Fetal chromosomal microdeletion(s) genomic sequence analysis (eg, DiGeorge syndrome, Cri-du-chat syndrome), circulating cell-free fetal DNA in maternal blood**

  EXCLUDES *Genome-wide microarray analysis (81228-81229)*
   Molecular cytogenetics (88271)

  0.00   0.00   **FUD** XXX   A ▢

  AMA: 2018,Jan,8; 2017,Apr,3

\#   **81443**   **Genetic testing for severe inherited conditions (eg, cystic fibrosis, Ashkenazi Jewish-associated disorders [eg, Bloom syndrome, Canavan disease, Fanconi anemia type C, mucolipidosis type VI, Gaucher disease, Tay-Sachs disease], beta hemoglobinopathies, phenylketonuria, galactosemia), genomic sequence analysis panel, must include sequencing of at least 15 genes (eg, *ACADM, ARSA, ASPA, ATP7B, BCKDHA, BCKDHB, BLM, CFTR, DHCR7, FANCC, G6PC, GAA, GALT, GBA, GBE1, HBB, HEXA, IKBKAP, MCOLN1, PAH*)**   ▢

  0.00   0.00   **FUD** XXX

  AMA: 2019,Jul,3; 2018,Nov,9

81425 Genome (eg, unexplained constitutional or heritable disorder or syndrome); sequence analysis

🔬 0.00   ✂ 0.00   **FUD** XXX   A ▣

AMA: 2018,Jan,8; 2017,Jan,8; 2016,Jan,13; 2015,Jan,3

+ **81426** sequence analysis, each comparator genome (eg, parents, siblings) (List separately in addition to code for primary procedure)

Code first (81425)

🔬 0.00   ✂ 0.00   **FUD** XXX   A ▣

AMA: 2018,Jan,8; 2017,Jan,8; 2016,Jan,13; 2015,Jan,3

81427 re-evaluation of previously obtained genome sequence (eg, updated knowledge or unrelated condition/syndrome)

EXCLUDES   Genome-wide microarray analysis (81228-81229)
           Results that are incidental

🔬 0.00   ✂ 0.00   **FUD** XXX   A ▣

AMA: 2018,Jan,8; 2017,Jan,8; 2016,Jan,13; 2015,Jan,3

81430 Hearing loss (eg, nonsyndromic hearing loss, Usher syndrome, Pendred syndrome); genomic sequence analysis panel, must include sequencing of at least 60 genes, including *CDH23, CLRN1, GJB2, GPR98, MTRNR1, MYO7A, MYO15A, PCDH15, OTOF, SLC26A4, TMC1, TMPRSS3, USH1C, USH1G, USH2A,* and *WFS1*

🔬 0.00   ✂ 0.00   **FUD** XXX   A ▣

AMA: 2018,Jan,8; 2017,Jan,8; 2016,Jan,13; 2015,Jan,3

81431 duplication/deletion analysis panel, must include copy number analyses for *STRC* and *DFNB1* deletions in *GJB2* and *GJB6* genes

🔬 0.00   ✂ 0.00   **FUD** XXX   A ▣

AMA: 2018,Jan,8; 2017,Jan,8; 2016,Jan,13; 2015,Jan,3

81432 Hereditary breast cancer-related disorders (eg, hereditary breast cancer, hereditary ovarian cancer, hereditary endometrial cancer); genomic sequence analysis panel, must include sequencing of at least 10 genes, always including *BRCA1, BRCA2, CDH1, MLH1, MSH2, MSH6, PALB2, PTEN, STK11,* and *TP53*

🔬 0.00   ✂ 0.00   **FUD** XXX   A ▣

AMA: 2019,May,5; 2018,Jan,8; 2017,Jan,8; 2016,Apr,4

81433 duplication/deletion analysis panel, must include analyses for *BRCA1, BRCA2, MLH1, MSH2,* and *STK11*

🔬 0.00   ✂ 0.00   **FUD** XXX   A ▣

AMA: 2018,Jan,8; 2017,Jan,8; 2016,Apr,4

81434 Hereditary retinal disorders (eg, retinitis pigmentosa, Leber congenital amaurosis, cone-rod dystrophy), genomic sequence analysis panel, must include sequencing of at least 15 genes, including *ABCA4, CNGA1, CRB1, EYS, PDE6A, PDE6B, PRPF31, PRPH2, RDH12, RHO, RP1, RP2, RPE65, RPGR,* and *USH2A*

🔬 0.00   ✂ 0.00   **FUD** XXX   A ▣

AMA: 2018,Jan,8; 2017,Jan,8; 2016,Apr,4

81435 Hereditary colon cancer disorders (eg, Lynch syndrome, PTEN hamartoma syndrome, Cowden syndrome, familial adenomatosis polyposis); genomic sequence analysis panel, must include sequencing of at least 10 genes, including *APC, BMPR1A, CDH1, MLH1, MSH2, MSH6, MUTYH, PTEN, SMAD4,* and *STK11*

🔬 0.00   ✂ 0.00   **FUD** XXX   A ▣

AMA: 2018,Jan,8; 2017,Jan,8; 2016,Apr,4; 2016,Jan,13; 2015,Jan,3

81436 duplication/deletion analysis panel, must include analysis of at least 5 genes, including *MLH1, MSH2, EPCAM, SMAD4,* and *STK11*

🔬 0.00   ✂ 0.00   **FUD** XXX   A ▣

AMA: 2018,Jan,8; 2017,Jan,8; 2016,Apr,4; 2016,Jan,13; 2015,Jan,3

81437 Hereditary neuroendocrine tumor disorders (eg, medullary thyroid carcinoma, parathyroid carcinoma, malignant pheochromocytoma or paraganglioma); genomic sequence analysis panel, must include sequencing of at least 6 genes, including *MAX, SDHB, SDHC, SDHD, TMEM127,* and *VHL*

🔬 0.00   ✂ 0.00   **FUD** XXX   A ▣

AMA: 2018,Jan,8; 2017,Jan,8; 2016,Apr,4

81438 duplication/deletion analysis panel, must include analyses for *SDHB, SDHC, SDHD,* and *VHL*

🔬 0.00   ✂ 0.00   **FUD** XXX   A ▣

AMA: 2018,Jan,8; 2017,Jan,8; 2016,Apr,4

81448 Hereditary peripheral neuropathies (eg, Charcot-Marie-Tooth, spastic paraplegia), genomic sequence analysis panel, must include sequencing of at least 5 peripheral neuropathy-related genes (eg, *BSCL2, GJB1, MFN2, MPZ, REEP1, SPAST, SPG11, SPTLC1*)

🔬 0.00   ✂ 0.00   **FUD** XXX   A ▣

AMA: 2018,May,6

81439 Hereditary cardiomyopathy (eg, hypertrophic cardiomyopathy, dilated cardiomyopathy, arrhythmogenic right ventricular cardiomyopathy), genomic sequence analysis panel, must include sequencing of at least 5 cardiomyopathy-related genes (eg, *DSG2, MYBPC3, MYH7, PKP2, TTN*)

EXCLUDES   Genetic tests of cardiac ion channelopathies
           (81413-81414)

🔬 0.00   ✂ 0.00   **FUD** XXX   A ▣

AMA: 2018,Sep,14; 2018,Jan,8; 2017,Apr,3

81440 Nuclear encoded mitochondrial genes (eg, neurologic or myopathic phenotypes), genomic sequence panel, must include analysis of at least 100 genes, including *BCS1L, C10orf2, COQ2, COX10, DGUOK, MPV17, OPA1, PDSS2, POLG, POLG2, RRM2B, SCO1, SCO2, SLC25A4, SUCLA2, SUCLG1, TAZ, TK2,* and *TYMP*

🔬 0.00   ✂ 0.00   **FUD** XXX   A ▣

AMA: 2018,Jan,8; 2017,Jan,8; 2016,Jan,13; 2015,Jan,3

81442 Noonan spectrum disorders (eg, Noonan syndrome, cardio-facio-cutaneous syndrome, Costello syndrome, LEOPARD syndrome, Noonan-like syndrome), genomic sequence analysis panel, must include sequencing of at least 12 genes, including *BRAF, CBL, HRAS, KRAS, MAP2K1, MAP2K2, NRAS, PTPN11, RAF1, RIT1, SHOC2,* and *SOS1*

🔬 0.00   ✂ 0.00   **FUD** XXX   A ▣

AMA: 2018,Jan,8; 2017,Jan,8; 2016,Apr,4

81443 Resequenced code. See code following 81422.

81445 Targeted genomic sequence analysis panel, solid organ neoplasm, DNA analysis, and RNA analysis when performed, 5-50 genes (eg, *ALK, BRAF, CDKN2A, EGFR, ERBB2, KIT, KRAS, NRAS, MET, PDGFRA, PDGFRB, PGR, PIK3CA, PTEN, RET*), interrogation for sequence variants and copy number variants or rearrangements, if performed

EXCLUDES   Microarray copy number assessment (81406)

🔬 0.00   ✂ 0.00   **FUD** XXX   A ▣

AMA: 2018,Jan,8; 2017,Jan,8; 2016,Apr,4; 2016,Jan,13; 2015,Jan,3

81448 Resequenced code. See code following 81438.

81450 Targeted genomic sequence analysis panel, hematolymphoid neoplasm or disorder, DNA analysis, and RNA analysis when performed, 5-50 genes (eg, *BRAF, CEBPA, DNMT3A, EZH2, FLT3, IDH1, IDH2, JAK2, KRAS, KIT, MLL, NRAS, NPM1, NOTCH1*), interrogation for sequence variants, and copy number variants or rearrangements, or isoform expression or mRNA expression levels, if performed

EXCLUDES   Microarray copy number assessment (81406)

🔬 0.00   ✂ 0.00   **FUD** XXX   A ▣

AMA: 2018,Jan,8; 2017,Jan,8; 2016,Apr,4; 2016,Jan,13; 2015,Jan,3

● New Code   ▲ Revised Code   ○ Reinstated   ● New Web Release   ▲ Revised Web Release   + Add-on   Unlisted   Not Covered   # Resequenced
50 Optum Mod 50 Exempt   Ⓢ AMA Mod 51 Exempt   51 Optum Mod 51 Exempt   63 Mod 63 Exempt   ✗ Non-FDA Drug   ★ Telemedicine   M Maternity   A Age Edit

81455 Targeted genomic sequence analysis panel, solid organ or hematolymphoid neoplasm, DNA analysis, and RNA analysis when performed, 51 or greater genes (eg, *ALK, BRAF, CDKN2A, CEBPA, DNMT3A, EGFR, ERBB2, EZH2, FLT3, IDH1, IDH2, JAK2, KIT, KRAS, MLL, NPM1, NRAS, MET, NOTCH1, PDGFRA, PDGFRB, PGR, PIK3CA, PTEN, RET*), interrogation for sequence variants and copy number variants or rearrangements, if performed

> EXCLUDES *Microarray copy number assessment (81406)*
> 📇 0.00 ⚕ 0.00 **FUD** XXX   Ⓐ ▯
> **AMA:** 2018,Jan,8; 2017,Jan,8; 2016,Apr,4; 2016,Jan,13; 2015,Jan,3

81460 Whole mitochondrial genome (eg, Leigh syndrome, mitochondrial encephalomyopathy, lactic acidosis, and stroke-like episodes [MELAS], myoclonic epilepsy with ragged-red fibers [MERFF], neuropathy, ataxia, and retinitis pigmentosa [NARP], Leber hereditary optic neuropathy [LHON]), genomic sequence, must include sequence analysis of entire mitochondrial genome with heteroplasmy detection

> 📇 0.00 ⚕ 0.00 **FUD** XXX   Ⓐ ▯
> **AMA:** 2018,Jan,8; 2017,Jan,8; 2016,Jan,13; 2015,Jan,3

81465 Whole mitochondrial genome large deletion analysis panel (eg, Kearns-Sayre syndrome, chronic progressive external ophthalmoplegia), including heteroplasmy detection, if performed

> 📇 0.00 ⚕ 0.00 **FUD** XXX   Ⓐ ▯
> **AMA:** 2018,Jan,8; 2017,Jan,8; 2016,Jan,13; 2015,Jan,3

81470 X-linked intellectual disability (XLID) (eg, syndromic and non-syndromic XLID); genomic sequence analysis panel, must include sequencing of at least 60 genes, including *ARX, ATRX, CDKL5, FGD1, FMR1, HUWE1, IL1RAPL, KDM5C, L1CAM, MECP2, MED12, MID1, OCRL, RPS6KA3,* and *SLC16A2*

> 📇 0.00 ⚕ 0.00 **FUD** XXX   Ⓐ ▯
> **AMA:** 2018,Jan,8; 2017,Jan,8; 2016,Jan,13; 2015,Jan,3

81471 duplication/deletion gene analysis, must include analysis of at least 60 genes, including *ARX, ATRX, CDKL5, FGD1, FMR1, HUWE1, IL1RAPL, KDM5C, L1CAM, MECP2, MED12, MID1, OCRL, RPS6KA3,* and *SLC16A2*

> 📇 0.00 ⚕ 0.00 **FUD** XXX   Ⓐ ▯
> **AMA:** 2018,Jan,8; 2017,Jan,8; 2016,Jan,13; 2015,Jan,3

81479 Resequenced code. See code following 81408.

81490-81599 [81522] Multianalyte Assays

INCLUDES Procedures using results of multiple assay panels (eg, molecular pathology, fluorescent in situ hybridization, non-nucleic acid-based) and other patient information to perform algorithmic analysis

Required analytical services (eg, amplification, cell lysis, detection, digestion, extraction, hybridization, nucleic acid stabilization) and algorithmic analysis

EXCLUDES *Genomic resequencing tests (81410-81471 [81448])*
In situ hybridization analyses (88271-88275, 88365-88368 [88364, 88373, 88374])
Microbial identification (87149-87153, 87471-87801 [87623, 87624, 87625], 87900-87904 [87906, 87910, 87912])
Multianalyte assays with algorithmic analyses without a Category I code (0002M-0007M, 0011M-0013M)

Code also procedures performed prior to cell lysis (eg, microdissection) (88380-88381)

81490 Autoimmune (rheumatoid arthritis), analysis of 12 biomarkers using immunoassays, utilizing serum, prognostic algorithm reported as a disease activity score

> 📇 0.00 ⚕ 0.00 **FUD** XXX   Ⓠ ▯
> EXCLUDES *C-reactive protein (86140)*

81493 Coronary artery disease, mRNA, gene expression profiling by real-time RT-PCR of 23 genes, utilizing whole peripheral blood, algorithm reported as a risk score

> 📇 0.00 ⚕ 0.00 **FUD** XXX   Ⓐ ▯

81500 Oncology (ovarian), biochemical assays of two proteins (CA-125 and HE4), utilizing serum, with menopausal status, algorithm reported as a risk score   ♀

> EXCLUDES *Human epididymis protein 4 (HE4) (86305)*
> *Immunoassay for tumor antigen, quantitative; CA 125 (86304)*
> 📇 0.00 ⚕ 0.00 **FUD** XXX   Ⓔ ▯
> **AMA:** 2019,Jun,11; 2015,Jan,3; 2014,Jan,11

81503 Oncology (ovarian), biochemical assays of five proteins (CA-125, apolipoprotein A1, beta-2 microglobulin, transferrin, and pre-albumin), utilizing serum, algorithm reported as a risk score   ♀

> EXCLUDES *Apolipoprotein (82172)*
> *Beta-2 microglobulin (82232)*
> *Immunoassay for tumor antigen, quantitative; CA 125 (86304)*
> *Prealbumin (84134)*
> *Transferrin (84466)*
> 📇 0.00 ⚕ 0.00 **FUD** XXX   Ⓠ ▯
> **AMA:** 2019,Jun,11; 2015,Jan,3; 2014,Jan,11

81504 Oncology (tissue of origin), microarray gene expression profiling of > 2000 genes, utilizing formalin-fixed paraffin-embedded tissue, algorithm reported as tissue similarity scores

> 📇 0.00 ⚕ 0.00 **FUD** XXX   Ⓐ ▯
> **AMA:** 2019,Jun,11; 2015,Jan,3; 2014,Jan,11

81506 Endocrinology (type 2 diabetes), biochemical assays of seven analytes (glucose, HbA1c, insulin, hs-CRP, adiponectin, ferritin, interleukin 2-receptor alpha), utilizing serum or plasma, algorithm reporting a risk score

> EXCLUDES *C-reactive protein; high sensitivity (hsCRP) (86141)*
> *Ferritin (82728)*
> *Glucose (82947)*
> *Hemoglobin; glycosylated (A1C) (83036)*
> *Immunoassay for analyte other than infectious agent antibody or infectious agent antigen (83520)*
> *Insulin; total (83525)*
> *Unlisted chemistry procedure (84999)*
> 📇 0.00 ⚕ 0.00 **FUD** XXX   Ⓔ ▯
> **AMA:** 2019,Jun,11; 2015,Jan,3; 2014,Jan,11

81507 Fetal aneuploidy (trisomy 21, 18, and 13) DNA sequence analysis of selected regions using maternal plasma, algorithm reported as a risk score for each trisomy   ♀

> EXCLUDES *Genome-wide microarray analysis (81228-81229)*
> *Molecular cytogenetics (88271)*
> 📇 0.00 ⚕ 0.00 **FUD** XXX   Ⓐ ▯
> **AMA:** 2019,Jun,11; 2018,Apr,10; 2015,Jan,3; 2014,Jan,11

81508 Fetal congenital abnormalities, biochemical assays of two proteins (PAPP-A, hCG [any form]), utilizing maternal serum, algorithm reported as a risk score   ♀

> EXCLUDES *Gonadotropin, chorionic (hCG) (84702)*
> *Pregnancy-associated plasma protein-A (PAPP-A) (84163)*
> 📇 0.00 ⚕ 0.00 **FUD** XXX   Ⓔ ▯
> **AMA:** 2019,Jun,11; 2015,Jan,3; 2014,Jan,11

81509 Fetal congenital abnormalities, biochemical assays of three proteins (PAPP-A, hCG [any form], DIA), utilizing maternal serum, algorithm reported as a risk score   ♀

> EXCLUDES *Gonadotropin, chorionic (hCG) (84702)*
> *Inhibin A (86336)*
> *Pregnancy-associated plasma protein-A (PAPP-A) (84163)*
> 📇 0.00 ⚕ 0.00 **FUD** XXX   Ⓔ ▯
> **AMA:** 2019,Jun,11; 2015,Jan,3; 2014,Jan,11

26/Ⓒ PC/TC Only   A2-Z3 ASC Payment   50 Bilateral   ♂ Male Only   ♀ Female Only   📇 Facility RVU   ⚕ Non-Facility RVU   ▯ CCI   ✖ CLIA
FUD Follow-up Days   **CMS:** IOM   **AMA:** CPT Asst   Ⓐ-Ⓨ OPPSI   80/80 Surg Assist Allowed / w/Doc   ▮ Lab Crosswalk   ▦ Radiology Crosswalk

400

81510 Fetal congenital abnormalities, biochemical assays of three analytes (AFP, uE3, hCG [any form]), utilizing maternal serum, algorithm reported as a risk score ♀

EXCLUDES Alpha-fetoprotein (AFP) (82105)
Estriol (82677)
Gonadotropin, chorionic (hCG) (84702)

🔲 0.00 🔲 0.00 **FUD** XXX E 🔲

AMA: 2019,Jun,11; 2015,Jan,3; 2014,Jan,11

81511 Fetal congenital abnormalities, biochemical assays of four analytes (AFP, uE3, hCG [any form], DIA) utilizing maternal serum, algorithm reported as a risk score (may include additional results from previous biochemical testing) ♀

EXCLUDES Alpha-fetoprotein (AFP) (82105)
Estriol (82677)
Gonadotropin, chorionic (hCG) (84702)
Inhibin A (86336)

🔲 0.00 🔲 0.00 **FUD** XXX E 🔲

AMA: 2019,Jun,11; 2015,Jan,3; 2014,Jan,11

81512 Fetal congenital abnormalities, biochemical assays of five analytes (AFP, uE3, total hCG, hyperglycosylated hCG, DIA) utilizing maternal serum, algorithm reported as a risk score ♀

EXCLUDES Alpha-fetoprotein (AFP) (82105)
Estriol (82677)
Gonadotropin, chorionic (hCG) (84702)
Inhibin A (86336)

🔲 0.00 🔲 0.00 **FUD** XXX E 🔲

AMA: 2019,Jun,11; 2015,Jan,3; 2014,Jan,11

81518 Oncology (breast), mRNA, gene expression profiling by real-time RT-PCR of 11 genes (7 content and 4 housekeeping), utilizing formalin-fixed paraffin-embedded tissue, algorithms reported as percentage risk for metastatic recurrence and likelihood of benefit from extended endocrine therapy

🔲 0.00 🔲 0.00 **FUD** XXX

AMA: 2019,Jun,11; 2019,Jul,3

● # **81522** Oncology (breast), mRNA, gene expression profiling by RT-PCR of 12 genes (8 content and 4 housekeeping), utilizing formalin-fixed paraffin-embedded tissue, algorithm reported as recurrence risk score

🔲 0.00 🔲 0.00 **FUD** 000

81519 Oncology (breast), mRNA, gene expression profiling by real-time RT-PCR of 21 genes, utilizing formalin-fixed paraffin embedded tissue, algorithm reported as recurrence score

🔲 0.00 🔲 0.00 **FUD** XXX A 🔲

AMA: 2019,Jun,11; 2018,Jan,8; 2017,Jan,8; 2016,Jan,13; 2015,Jan,3

81520 Oncology (breast), mRNA gene expression profiling by hybrid capture of 58 genes (50 content and 8 housekeeping), utilizing formalin-fixed paraffin-embedded tissue, algorithm reported as a recurrence risk score

🔲 0.00 🔲 0.00 **FUD** XXX A 🔲

AMA: 2019,Jun,11; 2018,Jun,8

81521 Oncology (breast), mRNA, microarray gene expression profiling of 70 content genes and 465 housekeeping genes, utilizing fresh frozen or formalin-fixed paraffin-embedded tissue, algorithm reported as index related to risk of distant metastasis

🔲 0.00 🔲 0.00 **FUD** XXX A 🔲

AMA: 2019,Jun,11; 2018,Jun,8

81522 Resequenced code. See code following 81518.

81525 Oncology (colon), mRNA, gene expression profiling by real-time RT-PCR of 12 genes (7 content and 5 housekeeping), utilizing formalin-fixed paraffin-embedded tissue, algorithm reported as a recurrence score

🔲 0.00 🔲 0.00 **FUD** XXX A 🔲

AMA: 2019,Jun,11

81528 Oncology (colorectal) screening, quantitative real-time target and signal amplification of 10 DNA markers (*KRAS* mutations, promoter methylation of *NDRG4* and *BMP3*) and fecal hemoglobin, utilizing stool, algorithm reported as a positive or negative result

EXCLUDES Blood, occult, by fecal hemoglobin (82274)
KRAS (Kirsten rat sarcoma viral oncogene homolog) (81275)

🔲 0.00 🔲 0.00 **FUD** XXX A 🔲

AMA: 2019,Jun,11

81535 Oncology (gynecologic), live tumor cell culture and chemotherapeutic response by DAPI stain and morphology, predictive algorithm reported as a drug response score; first single drug or drug combination

🔲 0.00 🔲 0.00 **FUD** XXX Q 🔲

AMA: 2019,Jun,11

+ **81536** each additional single drug or drug combination (List separately in addition to code for primary procedure)

Code first (81535)

🔲 0.00 🔲 0.00 **FUD** XXX Q 🔲

AMA: 2019,Jun,11

81538 Oncology (lung), mass spectrometric 8-protein signature, including amyloid A, utilizing serum, prognostic and predictive algorithm reported as good versus poor overall survival

🔲 0.00 🔲 0.00 **FUD** XXX Q 🔲

AMA: 2019,Jun,11

81539 Oncology (high-grade prostate cancer), biochemical assay of four proteins (Total PSA, Free PSA, Intact PSA, and human kallikrein-2 [hK2]), utilizing plasma or serum, prognostic algorithm reported as a probability score ♂

🔲 0.00 🔲 0.00 **FUD** XXX Q 🔲

AMA: 2019,Jun,11; 2018,Jan,8; 2017,Apr,3

81540 Oncology (tumor of unknown origin), mRNA, gene expression profiling by real-time RT-PCR of 92 genes (87 content and 5 housekeeping) to classify tumor into main cancer type and subtype, utilizing formalin-fixed paraffin-embedded tissue, algorithm reported as a probability of a predicted main cancer type and subtype

🔲 0.00 🔲 0.00 **FUD** XXX A 🔲

AMA: 2019,Jun,11

81541 Oncology (prostate), mRNA gene expression profiling by real-time RT-PCR of 46 genes (31 content and 15 housekeeping), utilizing formalin-fixed paraffin-embedded tissue, algorithm reported as a disease-specific mortality risk score

🔲 0.00 🔲 0.00 **FUD** XXX A 🔲

AMA: 2019,Jun,11; 2018,Aug,8

● **81542** Oncology (prostate), mRNA, microarray gene expression profiling of 22 content genes, utilizing formalin-fixed paraffin-embedded tissue, algorithm reported as metastasis risk score

81545 Oncology (thyroid), gene expression analysis of 142 genes, utilizing fine needle aspirate, algorithm reported as a categorical result (eg, benign or suspicious)

🔲 0.00 🔲 0.00 **FUD** XXX A 🔲

AMA: 2019,Jun,11

81551 Oncology (prostate), promoter methylation profiling by real-time PCR of 3 genes (*GSTP1, APC, RASSF1*), utilizing formalin-fixed paraffin-embedded tissue, algorithm reported as a likelihood of prostate cancer detection on repeat biopsy

🔲 0.00 🔲 0.00 **FUD** XXX A 🔲

AMA: 2019,Jun,11; 2018,Aug,8

● 81552 Oncology (uveal melanoma), mRNA, gene expression profiling by real-time RT-PCR of 15 genes (12 content and 3 housekeeping), utilizing fine needle aspirate or formalin-fixed paraffin-embedded tissue, algorithm reported as risk of metastasis

81595 Cardiology (heart transplant), mRNA, gene expression profiling by real-time quantitative PCR of 20 genes (11 content and 9 housekeeping), utilizing subfraction of peripheral blood, algorithm reported as a rejection risk score

🛠 0.00 ♒ 0.00 **FUD** XXX [A] ▢

AMA: 2019,Jun,11

81596 Infectious disease, chronic hepatitis C virus (HCV) infection, six biochemical assays (ALT, A2-macroglobulin, apolipoprotein A-1, total bilirubin, GGT, and haptoglobin) utilizing serum, prognostic algorithm reported as scores for fibrosis and necroinflammatory activity in liver

🛠 0.00 ♒ 0.00 **FUD** XXX ▢

AMA: 2019,Jun,11; 2019,Jul,3

81599 Unlisted multianalyte assay with algorithmic analysis

🛠 0.00 ♒ 0.00 **FUD** XXX [E] ▢

AMA: 2019,Jun,11; 2018,Jun,8; 2018,Apr,10; 2015,Jan,3; 2014,Jan,11

82009-82030 Chemistry: Acetaldehyde—Adenosine

INCLUDES Clinical information not requested by the ordering physician
Mathematically calculated results
Quantitative analysis unless otherwise specified
Specimens from any source unless otherwise specified

EXCLUDES *Analytes from nonrequested laboratory analysis*
Calculated results that represent a score or probability that was derived by algorithm
Drug testing ([80305, 80306, 80307], [80324, 80325, 80326, 80327, 80328, 80329, 80330, 80331, 80332, 80333, 80334, 80335, 80336, 80337, 80338, 80339, 80340, 80341, 80342, 80343, 80344, 80345, 80346, 80347, 80348, 80349, 80350, 80351, 80352, 80353, 80354, 80355, 80356, 80357, 80358, 80359, 80360, 80361, 80362, 80363, 80364, 80365, 80366, 80367, 80368, 80369, 80370, 80371, 80372, 80373, 80374, 80375, 80376, 80377, 83992])
Organ or disease panels (80048-80076 [80081])
Therapeutic drug assays (80150-80299 [80164, 80165, 80171])

82009 Ketone body(s) (eg, acetone, acetoacetic acid, beta-hydroxybutyrate); qualitative

🛠 0.00 ♒ 0.00 **FUD** XXX ▢ ▢

AMA: 2018,Jan,8; 2017,Jan,8; 2016,Jan,13; 2015,Jun,10; 2015,Apr,3; 2015,Jan,16; 2014,Jan,11

82010 quantitative

🛠 0.00 ♒ 0.00 **FUD** XXX [X] ▢ ▢

AMA: 2018,Jan,8; 2017,Jan,8; 2016,Jan,13; 2015,Jun,10; 2015,Apr,3; 2015,Jan,16; 2014,Jan,11

82013 Acetylcholinesterase

EXCLUDES *Acid phosphatase (84060-84066)*
Gastric acid analysis (82930)

🛠 0.00 ♒ 0.00 **FUD** XXX ▢ ▢

AMA: 2015,Jun,10; 2015,Apr,3; 2014,Jan,11

82016 Acylcarnitines; qualitative, each specimen

🛠 0.00 ♒ 0.00 **FUD** XXX ▢ ▢

AMA: 2015,Jun,10; 2015,Apr,3; 2014,Jan,11

82017 quantitative, each specimen

EXCLUDES *Carnitine (82379)*

🛠 0.00 ♒ 0.00 **FUD** XXX ▢ ▢

AMA: 2015,Jun,10; 2015,Apr,3; 2014,Jan,11

82024 Adrenocorticotropic hormone (ACTH)

🛠 0.00 ♒ 0.00 **FUD** XXX ▢ ▢

AMA: 2015,Jun,10; 2015,Apr,3; 2014,Jan,11

82030 Adenosine, 5-monophosphate, cyclic (cyclic AMP)

🛠 0.00 ♒ 0.00 **FUD** XXX ▢ ▢

AMA: 2015,Jun,10; 2015,Apr,3; 2014,Jan,11

82040-82045 [82042] Chemistry: Albumin

INCLUDES Clinical information not requested by the ordering physician
Mathematically calculated results
Quantitative analysis unless otherwise specified
Specimens from any other sources unless otherwise specified

EXCLUDES *Analytes from nonrequested laboratory analysis*
Calculated results that represent a score or probability that was derived by algorithm
Drug testing ([80305, 80306, 80307], [80324, 80325, 80326, 80327, 80328, 80329, 80330, 80331, 80332, 80333, 80334, 80335, 80336, 80337, 80338, 80339, 80340, 80341, 80342, 80343, 80344, 80345, 80346, 80347, 80348, 80349, 80350, 80351, 80352, 80353, 80354, 80355, 80356, 80357, 80358, 80359, 80360, 80361, 80362, 80363, 80364, 80365, 80366, 80367, 80368, 80369, 80370, 80371, 80372, 80373, 80374, 80375, 80376, 80377, 83992])
Organ or disease panels (80048-80076 [80081])
Therapeutic drug assays (80150-80299 [80164, 80165, 80171])

82040 Albumin; serum, plasma or whole blood

🛠 0.00 ♒ 0.00 **FUD** XXX [X] ▢ ▢

AMA: 2018,Jan,8; 2017,Jan,8; 2016,Jan,13; 2015,Jun,10; 2015,Apr,3; 2015,Jan,16; 2014,Jan,11

82042 **Resequenced code. See code following 82045.**

82043 urine (eg, microalbumin), quantitative

🛠 0.00 ♒ 0.00 **FUD** XXX [X] ▢ ▢

AMA: 2018,Jan,8; 2017,Jan,8; 2016,Jan,13; 2015,Jun,10; 2015,Apr,3; 2015,Jan,16; 2014,Jan,11

82044 urine (eg, microalbumin), semiquantitative (eg, reagent strip assay)

EXCLUDES *Prealbumin (84134)*

🛠 0.00 ♒ 0.00 **FUD** XXX [X] ▢ ▢

AMA: 2018,Jan,8; 2017,Jan,8; 2016,Jan,13; 2015,Jun,10; 2015,Apr,3; 2015,Jan,16; 2014,Jan,11

82045 ischemia modified

🛠 0.00 ♒ 0.00 **FUD** XXX ▢ ▢

AMA: 2015,Jun,10; 2015,Apr,3

\# 82042 other source, quantitative, each specimen

EXCLUDES *Total protein (84155-84157, 84160)*

🛠 0.00 ♒ 0.00 **FUD** XXX ▢ ▢

AMA: 2015,Jun,10; 2015,Apr,3; 2014,Jan,11

82075-82107 Chemistry: Alcohol—Alpha-fetoprotein (AFP)

INCLUDES Clinical information not requested by the ordering physician
Mathematically calculated results
Quantitative analysis unless otherwise specified
Specimens from any source unless otherwise specified

EXCLUDES *Analytes from nonrequested laboratory analysis*
Calculated results that represent a score or probability that was derived by algorithm
Drug testing ([80305, 80306, 80307], [80324, 80325, 80326, 80327, 80328, 80329, 80330, 80331, 80332, 80333, 80334, 80335, 80336, 80337, 80338, 80339, 80340, 80341, 80342, 80343, 80344, 80345, 80346, 80347, 80348, 80349, 80350, 80351, 80352, 80353, 80354, 80355, 80356, 80357, 80358, 80359, 80360, 80361, 80362, 80363, 80364, 80365, 80366, 80367, 80368, 80369, 80370, 80371, 80372, 80373, 80374, 80375, 80376, 80377, 83992])
Organ or disease panels (80048-80076 [80081])
Therapeutic drug assays (80150-80299 [80164, 80165, 80171])

82075 Alcohol (ethanol), breath

🛠 0.00 ♒ 0.00 **FUD** XXX ▢ ▢

AMA: 2015,Jun,10; 2015,Apr,3

82085 Aldolase

🛠 0.00 ♒ 0.00 **FUD** XXX ▢ ▢

AMA: 2015,Jun,10; 2015,Apr,3

82088 Aldosterone

EXCLUDES *Alkaline phosphatase (84075, 84080)*
Alphaketoglutarate (82009-82010)
Alphatocopherol (VitaminE) (84446)

🛠 0.00 ♒ 0.00 **FUD** XXX ▢ ▢

AMA: 2015,Jun,10; 2015,Apr,3

82103 Alpha-1-antitrypsin; total

🛠 0.00 ♒ 0.00 **FUD** XXX ▢ ▢

AMA: 2015,Jun,10; 2015,Apr,3

26/TC PC/TC Only   A2-Z3 ASC Payment   50 Bilateral   ♂ Male Only   ♀ Female Only   🛠 Facility RVU   ♒ Non-Facility RVU   ▢ CCI   [X] CLIA
FUD Follow-up Days   **CMS:** IOM   **AMA:** CPT Asst   A-Y OPPSI   80/80 Surg Assist Allowed / w/Doc   ▣ Lab Crosswalk   ▣ Radiology Crosswalk

82104	**phenotype**

⚕ 0.00 ✂ 0.00 **FUD** XXX 🔲🖥

AMA: 2015,Jun,10; 2015,Apr,3

82105	**Alpha-fetoprotein (AFP); serum**

⚕ 0.00 ✂ 0.00 **FUD** XXX 🔲🖥

AMA: 2015,Jun,10; 2015,Apr,3

82106	**amniotic fluid**	Ⓜ

⚕ 0.00 ✂ 0.00 **FUD** XXX 🔲🖥

AMA: 2015,Jun,10; 2015,Apr,3

82107	**AFP-L3 fraction isoform and total AFP (including ratio)**

⚕ 0.00 ✂ 0.00 **FUD** XXX 🔲🖥

AMA: 2015,Jun,10; 2015,Apr,3

82108 Chemistry: Aluminum

CMS: 100-02,11,20.2 ESRD Laboratory Services

INCLUDES Clinical information not requested by the ordering physician
Mathematically calculated results
Quantitative analysis unless otherwise specified
Specimens from any source unless otherwise specified

EXCLUDES *Analytes from nonrequested laboratory analysis*
Calculated results that represent a score or probability that was derived by algorithm
Drug testing ([80305, 80306, 80307], [80324, 80325, 80326, 80327, 80328, 80329, 80330, 80331, 80332, 80333, 80334, 80335, 80336, 80337, 80338, 80339, 80340, 80341, 80342, 80343, 80344, 80345, 80346, 80347, 80348, 80349, 80350, 80351, 80352, 80353, 80354, 80355, 80356, 80357, 80358, 80359, 80360, 80361, 80362, 80363, 80364, 80365, 80366, 80367, 80368, 80369, 80370, 80371, 80372, 80373, 80374, 80375, 80376, 80377, 83992])
Organ or disease panels (80048-80076 [80081])
Therapeutic drug assays (80150-80299 [80164, 80165, 80171])

82108	**Aluminum**

⚕ 0.00 ✂ 0.00 **FUD** XXX 🔲🖥

AMA: 2015,Jun,10; 2015,Apr,3

82120-82261 Chemistry: Amines—Biotinidase

INCLUDES Clinical information not requested by the ordering physician
Mathematically calculated results
Quantitative analysis unless otherwise specified
Specimens from any source unless otherwise specified

EXCLUDES *Analytes from nonrequested laboratory analysis*
Calculated results that represent a score or probability that was derived by algorithm
Drug testing ([80305, 80306, 80307], [80324, 80325, 80326, 80327, 80328, 80329, 80330, 80331, 80332, 80333, 80334, 80335, 80336, 80337, 80338, 80339, 80340, 80341, 80342, 80343, 80344, 80345, 80346, 80347, 80348, 80349, 80350, 80351, 80352, 80353, 80354, 80355, 80356, 80357, 80358, 80359, 80360, 80361, 80362, 80363, 80364, 80365, 80366, 80367, 80368, 80369, 80370, 80371, 80372, 80373, 80374, 80375, 80376, 80377, 83992])
Organ or disease panels (80048-80076 [80081])
Therapeutic drug assays (80150-80299 [80164, 80165, 80171])

82120	**Amines, vaginal fluid, qualitative**	♀

EXCLUDES *Combined pH and amines test for vaginitis (82120, 83986)*

❌ ⚕ 0.00 ✂ 0.00 **FUD** XXX 🔲🖥

AMA: 2018,Jan,8; 2017,Jan,8; 2016,Jan,13; 2015,Jun,10; 2015,Apr,3; 2015,Jan,16; 2014,Jan,11

82127	**Amino acids; single, qualitative, each specimen**

⚕ 0.00 ✂ 0.00 **FUD** XXX 🔲🖥

AMA: 2015,Jun,10; 2015,Apr,3

82128	**multiple, qualitative, each specimen**

⚕ 0.00 ✂ 0.00 **FUD** XXX 🔲🖥

AMA: 2015,Jun,10; 2015,Apr,3

82131	**single, quantitative, each specimen**

INCLUDES Van Slyke method

⚕ 0.00 ✂ 0.00 **FUD** XXX 🔲🖥

AMA: 2018,Jan,8; 2017,Jan,8; 2016,Jan,13; 2015,Jun,10; 2015,Apr,3; 2015,Jan,16; 2014,Jan,11

82135	**Aminolevulinic acid, delta (ALA)**

⚕ 0.00 ✂ 0.00 **FUD** XXX 🔲🖥

AMA: 2015,Jun,10; 2015,Apr,3

82136	**Amino acids, 2 to 5 amino acids, quantitative, each specimen**

⚕ 0.00 ✂ 0.00 **FUD** XXX 🔲🖥

AMA: 2015,Jun,10; 2015,Apr,3

82139	**Amino acids, 6 or more amino acids, quantitative, each specimen**

⚕ 0.00 ✂ 0.00 **FUD** XXX 🔲🖥

AMA: 2015,Jun,10; 2015,Apr,3

82140	**Ammonia**

⚕ 0.00 ✂ 0.00 **FUD** XXX 🔲🖥

AMA: 2015,Jun,10; 2015,Apr,3

82143	**Amniotic fluid scan (spectrophotometric)**	Ⓜ ♀

EXCLUDES *Amobarbital ([80345])*
L/S ratio (83661)

⚕ 0.00 ✂ 0.00 **FUD** XXX 🔲🖥

AMA: 2015,Jun,10; 2015,Apr,3

82150	**Amylase**

⚕ 0.00 ✂ 0.00 **FUD** XXX ❌🔲🖥

AMA: 2015,Jun,10; 2015,Apr,3

82154	**Androstanediol glucuronide**

⚕ 0.00 ✂ 0.00 **FUD** XXX 🔲🖥

AMA: 2018,Jan,8; 2017,Jan,8; 2016,Jan,13; 2015,Jun,10; 2015,Apr,3; 2015,Jan,16; 2014,Jan,11

82157	**Androstenedione**

⚕ 0.00 ✂ 0.00 **FUD** XXX 🔲🖥

AMA: 2015,Jun,10; 2015,Apr,3

82160	**Androsterone**

⚕ 0.00 ✂ 0.00 **FUD** XXX 🔲🖥

AMA: 2015,Jun,10; 2015,Apr,3

82163	**Angiotensin II**

⚕ 0.00 ✂ 0.00 **FUD** XXX 🔲🖥

AMA: 2015,Jun,10; 2015,Apr,3

82164	**Angiotensin I - converting enzyme (ACE)**

EXCLUDES *Antidiuretic hormone (ADH) (84588)*
Antimony (83015)
Antitrypsin, alpha-1- (82103-82104)

⚕ 0.00 ✂ 0.00 **FUD** XXX 🔲🖥

AMA: 2015,Jun,10; 2015,Apr,3

82172	**Apolipoprotein, each**

⚕ 0.00 ✂ 0.00 **FUD** XXX 🔲🖥

AMA: 2015,Jun,10; 2015,Apr,3

82175	**Arsenic**

EXCLUDES *Heavy metal screening (83015)*

⚕ 0.00 ✂ 0.00 **FUD** XXX 🔲🖥

AMA: 2015,Jun,10; 2015,Apr,3

82180	**Ascorbic acid (Vitamin C), blood**

EXCLUDES *Aspirin (acetylsalicylic acid) ([80329, 80330, 80331])*
Atherogenic index, blood, ultracentrifugation, quantitative (83701)

⚕ 0.00 ✂ 0.00 **FUD** XXX 🔲🖥

AMA: 2015,Jun,10; 2015,Apr,3

82190	**Atomic absorption spectroscopy, each analyte**

⚕ 0.00 ✂ 0.00 **FUD** XXX 🔲🖥

AMA: 2015,Jun,10; 2015,Apr,3

82232	**Beta-2 microglobulin**

⚕ 0.00 ✂ 0.00 **FUD** XXX 🔲🖥

AMA: 2015,Jun,10; 2015,Apr,3

82239	**Bile acids; total**

⚕ 0.00 ✂ 0.00 **FUD** XXX 🔲🖥

AMA: 2015,Jun,10; 2015,Apr,3

82240	**cholylglycine**

EXCLUDES *Bile pigments, urine (81000-81005)*

⚕ 0.00 ✂ 0.00 **FUD** XXX 🔲🖥

AMA: 2015,Jun,10; 2015,Apr,3

● New Code ▲ Revised Code ○ Reinstated ● New Web Release ▲ Revised Web Release + Add-on Unlisted Not Covered # Resequenced
50 Optum Mod 50 Exempt Ⓢ AMA Mod 51 Exempt Ⓢ Optum Mod 51 Exempt 63 Mod 63 Exempt ✗ Non-FDA Drug ★ Telemedicine Ⓜ Maternity Ⓐ Age Edit

Pathology and Laboratory (sidebar)

82247 — 82360 (sidebar)

82247 **Bilirubin; total**
INCLUDES Van Den Bergh test
🔧 0.00 ⚕ 0.00 **FUD** XXX   ☒ 🔲 🔲
AMA: 2018,Jan,8; 2017,Jan,8; 2016,Jan,13; 2015,Jun,10;
2015,Apr,3; 2015,Jan,16; 2014,Jan,11

82248 **direct**
🔧 0.00 ⚕ 0.00 **FUD** XXX   🔲 🔲
AMA: 2018,Jan,8; 2017,Jan,8; 2016,Jan,13; 2015,Jun,10;
2015,Apr,3; 2015,Jan,16; 2014,Jan,11

82252 **feces, qualitative**
🔧 0.00 ⚕ 0.00 **FUD** XXX   🔲 🔲
AMA: 2015,Jun,10; 2015,Apr,3

82261 **Biotinidase, each specimen**
🔧 0.00 ⚕ 0.00 **FUD** XXX   🔲 🔲
AMA: 2015,Jun,10; 2015,Apr,3

82270-82274 Chemistry: Occult Blood

CMS: 100-04,16,70.8 CLIA Waived Tests; 100-04,18,60 Colorectal Cancer Screening

INCLUDES Clinical information not requested by the ordering physician
Mathematically calculated results
Quantitative analysis unless otherwise specified
Specimens from any source unless otherwise specified
EXCLUDES Analytes from nonrequested laboratory analysis
Calculated results that represent a score or probability that was derived by
    algorithm
Drug testing ([80305, 80306, 80307], [80324, 80325, 80326, 80327, 80328,
    80329, 80330, 80331, 80332, 80333, 80334, 80335, 80336, 80337, 80338,
    80339, 80340, 80341, 80342, 80343, 80344, 80345, 80346, 80347, 80348,
    80349, 80350, 80351, 80352, 80353, 80354, 80355, 80356, 80357, 80358,
    80359, 80360, 80361, 80362, 80363, 80364, 80365, 80366, 80367, 80368,
    80369, 80370, 80371, 80372, 80373, 80374, 80375, 80376, 80377, 83992])
Organ or disease panels (80048-80076 [80081])
Therapeutic drug assays (80150-80299 [80164, 80165, 80171])

82270 **Blood, occult, by peroxidase activity (eg, guaiac), qualitative;
feces, consecutive collected specimens with single
determination, for colorectal neoplasm screening (ie, patient
was provided 3 cards or single triple card for consecutive
collection)**
INCLUDES Day test
🔧 0.00 ⚕ 0.00 **FUD** XXX   ☒ 🅰 🔲
AMA: 2018,Jan,8; 2017,Jan,8; 2016,Jan,13; 2015,Jun,10;
2015,Apr,3; 2015,Jan,16; 2014,Jan,11

82271 **other sources**
🔧 0.00 ⚕ 0.00 **FUD** XXX   ☒ 🔲 🔲
AMA: 2015,Jun,10; 2015,Apr,3

82272 **Blood, occult, by peroxidase activity (eg, guaiac), qualitative,
feces, 1-3 simultaneous determinations, performed for other
than colorectal neoplasm screening**
🔧 0.00 ⚕ 0.00 **FUD** XXX   ☒ 🔲 🔲
AMA: 2018,Jan,8; 2017,Jan,8; 2016,Jan,13; 2015,Jun,10;
2015,Apr,3; 2015,Jan,16; 2014,Jan,11

82274 **Blood, occult, by fecal hemoglobin determination by
immunoassay, qualitative, feces, 1-3 simultaneous
determinations**
🔧 0.00 ⚕ 0.00 **FUD** XXX   ☒ 🔲 🔲
AMA: 2015,Jun,10; 2015,Apr,3

82286-82308 [82652] Chemistry: Bradykinin—Calcitonin

INCLUDES Clinical information not requested by the ordering physician
Mathematically calculated results
Quantitative analysis unless otherwise specified
Specimens from any source unless otherwise specified
EXCLUDES Analytes from nonrequested laboratory analysis
Calculated results that represent a score or probability that was derived by
    algorithm
Drug testing ([80305, 80306, 80307], [80324, 80325, 80326, 80327, 80328,
    80329, 80330, 80331, 80332, 80333, 80334, 80335, 80336, 80337, 80338,
    80339, 80340, 80341, 80342, 80343, 80344, 80345, 80346, 80347, 80348,
    80349, 80350, 80351, 80352, 80353, 80354, 80355, 80356, 80357, 80358,
    80359, 80360, 80361, 80362, 80363, 80364, 80365, 80366, 80367, 80368,
    80369, 80370, 80371, 80372, 80373, 80374, 80375, 80376, 80377, 83992])
Organ or disease panels (80048-80076 [80081])
Therapeutic drug assays (80150-80299 [80164, 80165, 80171])

82286 **Bradykinin**
🔧 0.00 ⚕ 0.00 **FUD** XXX   🔲 🔲
AMA: 2015,Jun,10; 2015,Apr,3

82300 **Cadmium**
🔧 0.00 ⚕ 0.00 **FUD** XXX   🔲 🔲
AMA: 2015,Jun,10; 2015,Apr,3

82306 **Vitamin D; 25 hydroxy, includes fraction(s), if performed**
🔧 0.00 ⚕ 0.00 **FUD** XXX   🔲 🔲
AMA: 2015,Jun,10; 2015,Apr,3

\# **82652** **1, 25 dihydroxy, includes fraction(s), if performed**
🔧 0.00 ⚕ 0.00 **FUD** XXX   🔲 🔲
AMA: 2015,Jun,10; 2015,Apr,3

82308 **Calcitonin**
🔧 0.00 ⚕ 0.00 **FUD** XXX   🔲 🔲
AMA: 2015,Jun,10; 2015,Apr,3

82310-82373 Chemistry: Calcium, total; Carbohydrate Deficient Transferrin

INCLUDES Clinical information not requested by the ordering physician
Mathematically calculated results
Quantitative analysis unless otherwise specified
Specimens from any source unless otherwise specified
EXCLUDES Analytes from nonrequested laboratory analysis
Calculated results that represent a score or probability that was derived by
    algorithm
Drug testing ([80305, 80306, 80307], [80324, 80325, 80326, 80327, 80328,
    80329, 80330, 80331, 80332, 80333, 80334, 80335, 80336, 80337, 80338,
    80339, 80340, 80341, 80342, 80343, 80344, 80345, 80346, 80347, 80348,
    80349, 80350, 80351, 80352, 80353, 80354, 80355, 80356, 80357, 80358,
    80359, 80360, 80361, 80362, 80363, 80364, 80365, 80366, 80367, 80368,
    80369, 80370, 80371, 80372, 80373, 80374, 80375, 80376, 80377, 83992])
Organ or disease panels (80048-80076 [80081])
Therapeutic drug assays (80150-80299 [80164, 80165, 80171])

82310 **Calcium; total**
🔧 0.00 ⚕ 0.00 **FUD** XXX   ☒ 🔲 🔲
AMA: 2018,Jan,8; 2017,Jan,8; 2016,Jan,13; 2015,Jun,10;
2015,Apr,3; 2015,Jan,16; 2014,Jan,11

82330 **ionized**
🔧 0.00 ⚕ 0.00 **FUD** XXX   ☒ 🔲 🔲
AMA: 2018,Jan,8; 2017,Jan,8; 2016,Jan,13; 2015,Jun,10;
2015,Apr,3; 2015,Jan,16; 2014,Jan,11

82331 **after calcium infusion test**
🔧 0.00 ⚕ 0.00 **FUD** XXX   🔲 🔲
AMA: 2015,Jun,10; 2015,Apr,3

82340 **urine quantitative, timed specimen**
🔧 0.00 ⚕ 0.00 **FUD** XXX   🔲 🔲
AMA: 2015,Jun,10; 2015,Apr,3

82355 **Calculus; qualitative analysis**
🔧 0.00 ⚕ 0.00 **FUD** XXX   🔲 🔲
AMA: 2015,Jun,10; 2015,Apr,3

82360 **quantitative analysis, chemical**
🔧 0.00 ⚕ 0.00 **FUD** XXX   🔲 🔲
AMA: 2015,Jun,10; 2015,Apr,3

82365   **infrared spectroscopy**
0.00   0.00   **FUD** XXX
AMA: 2015,Jun,10; 2015,Apr,3

82370   **X-ray diffraction**
0.00   0.00   **FUD** XXX
AMA: 2015,Jun,10; 2015,Apr,3

82373   **Carbohydrate deficient transferrin**
0.00   0.00   **FUD** XXX
AMA: 2015,Jun,10; 2015,Apr,3

82374 Chemistry: Carbon Dioxide

CMS: 100-02,11,20.2 ESRD Laboratory Services; 100-02,11,30.2.2 Automated Multi-Channel Chemistry (AMCC) Tests; 100-04,16,40.6.1 Automated Multi-Channel Chemistry (AMCC) Tests for ESRD Beneficiaries; 100-04,16,70.8 CLIA Waived Tests; 100-04,16,90.2 Organ or Disease Oriented Panels

INCLUDES   Clinical information not requested by the ordering physician
Mathematically calculated results
Quantitative analysis unless otherwise specified
Specimens from any source unless otherwise specified

EXCLUDES   *Analytes from nonrequested laboratory analysis*
Calculated results that represent a score or probability that was derived by algorithm
Drug testing ([80305, 80306, 80307], [80324, 80325, 80326, 80327, 80328, 80329, 80330, 80331, 80332, 80333, 80334, 80335, 80336, 80337, 80338, 80339, 80340, 80341, 80342, 80343, 80344, 80345, 80346, 80347, 80348, 80349, 80350, 80351, 80352, 80353, 80354, 80355, 80356, 80357, 80358, 80359, 80360, 80361, 80362, 80363, 80364, 80365, 80366, 80367, 80368, 80369, 80370, 80371, 80372, 80373, 80374, 80375, 80376, 80377, 83992])
Organ or disease panels (80048-80076 [80081])
Therapeutic drug assays (80150-80299 [80164, 80165, 80171])

82374   **Carbon dioxide (bicarbonate)**
EXCLUDES   *Blood gases (82803)*
0.00   0.00   **FUD** XXX
AMA: 2018,Jan,8; 2017,Jan,8; 2016,Jan,13; 2015,Jun,10; 2015,Apr,3; 2015,Jan,16; 2014,Jan,11

82375-82376 Chemistry: Carboxyhemoglobin (Carbon Monoxide)

INCLUDES   Clinical information not requested by the ordering physician
Mathematically calculated results
Specimens from any source unless otherwise specified

EXCLUDES   *Analytes from nonrequested laboratory analysis*
Calculated results that represent a score or probability that was derived by algorithm
Drug testing ([80305, 80306, 80307], [80324, 80325, 80326, 80327, 80328, 80329, 80330, 80331, 80332, 80333, 80334, 80335, 80336, 80337, 80338, 80339, 80340, 80341, 80342, 80343, 80344, 80345, 80346, 80347, 80348, 80349, 80350, 80351, 80352, 80353, 80354, 80355, 80356, 80357, 80358, 80359, 80360, 80361, 80362, 80363, 80364, 80365, 80366, 80367, 80368, 80369, 80370, 80371, 80372, 80373, 80374, 80375, 80376, 80377, 83992])
Organ or disease panels (80048-80076 [80081])
Transcutaneous measurement of carboxyhemoglobin (88740)

82375   **Carboxyhemoglobin; quantitative**
0.00   0.00   **FUD** XXX
AMA: 2018,Jan,8; 2017,Jan,8; 2016,Jan,13; 2015,Jun,10; 2015,Apr,3; 2015,Jan,16; 2014,Jan,11

82376   **qualitative**
0.00   0.00   **FUD** XXX
AMA: 2015,Jun,10; 2015,Apr,3

82378 Chemistry: Carcinoembryonic Antigen (CEA)

CMS: 100-03,190.26 Carcinoembryonic Antigen (CEA)

INCLUDES   Clinical information not requested by the ordering physician
EXCLUDES   *Analytes from nonrequested laboratory analysis*
Calculated results that represent a score or probability that was derived by algorithm

82378   **Carcinoembryonic antigen (CEA)**
0.00   0.00   **FUD** XXX
AMA: 2018,Jan,8; 2017,Jan,8; 2016,Jan,13; 2015,Jun,10; 2015,Apr,3; 2015,Jan,16; 2014,Jan,11

82379-82415 Chemistry: Carnitine—Chloramphenicol

INCLUDES   Clinical information not requested by the ordering physician
Mathematically calculated results
Quantitative analysis unless otherwise specified
Specimens from any source unless otherwise specified

EXCLUDES   *Analytes from nonrequested laboratory analysis*
Calculated results that represent a score or probability that was derived by algorithm
Drug testing ([80305, 80306, 80307], [80324, 80325, 80326, 80327, 80328, 80329, 80330, 80331, 80332, 80333, 80334, 80335, 80336, 80337, 80338, 80339, 80340, 80341, 80342, 80343, 80344, 80345, 80346, 80347, 80348, 80349, 80350, 80351, 80352, 80353, 80354, 80355, 80356, 80357, 80358, 80359, 80360, 80361, 80362, 80363, 80364, 80365, 80366, 80367, 80368, 80369, 80370, 80371, 80372, 80373, 80374, 80375, 80376, 80377, 83992])
Organ or disease panels (80048-80076 [80081])
Therapeutic drug assays (80150-80299 [80164, 80165, 80171])

82379   **Carnitine (total and free), quantitative, each specimen**
EXCLUDES   *Acylcarnitine (82016-82017)*
0.00   0.00   **FUD** XXX
AMA: 2015,Jun,10; 2015,Apr,3

82380   **Carotene**
0.00   0.00   **FUD** XXX
AMA: 2015,Jun,10; 2015,Apr,3

82382   **Catecholamines; total urine**
0.00   0.00   **FUD** XXX
AMA: 2015,Jun,10; 2015,Apr,3

82383   **blood**
0.00   0.00   **FUD** XXX
AMA: 2015,Jun,10; 2015,Apr,3

82384   **fractionated**
EXCLUDES   *Urine metabolites (83835, 84585)*
0.00   0.00   **FUD** XXX
AMA: 2015,Jun,10; 2015,Apr,3

82387   **Cathepsin-D**
0.00   0.00   **FUD** XXX
AMA: 2015,Jun,10; 2015,Apr,3

82390   **Ceruloplasmin**
0.00   0.00   **FUD** XXX
AMA: 2015,Jun,10; 2015,Apr,3

82397   **Chemiluminescent assay**
0.00   0.00   **FUD** XXX
AMA: 2018,Jan,8; 2017,Jan,8; 2016,Jan,13; 2015,Jun,10; 2015,Apr,3; 2015,Jan,16; 2014,Jan,11

82415   **Chloramphenicol**
0.00   0.00   **FUD** XXX
AMA: 2015,Jun,10; 2015,Apr,3

82435-82438 Chemistry: Chloride

INCLUDES   Clinical information not requested by the ordering physician
Mathematically calculated results
Quantitative analysis unless otherwise specified
Specimens from any source unless otherwise specified

EXCLUDES   *Analytes from nonrequested laboratory analysis*
Calculated results that represent a score or probability that was derived by algorithm
Organ or disease panels (80048-80076 [80081])
Therapeutic drug assays (80150-80299 [80164, 80165, 80171])

82435   **Chloride; blood**
0.00   0.00   **FUD** XXX
AMA: 2018,Jan,8; 2017,Jan,8; 2016,Jan,13; 2015,Jun,10; 2015,Apr,3; 2015,Jan,16; 2014,Jan,11

82436   **urine**
0.00   0.00   **FUD** XXX
AMA: 2015,Jun,10; 2015,Apr,3

82438   **other source**
EXCLUDES   *Sweat collections by iontophoresis (89230)*
0.00   0.00   **FUD** XXX
AMA: 2018,Jan,8; 2017,Jan,8; 2016,Jan,13; 2015,Jun,10; 2015,Apr,3; 2015,Jan,16; 2014,Jan,11

● New Code   ▲ Revised Code   ○ Reinstated   ● New Web Release   ▲ Revised Web Release   + Add-on   Unlisted   Not Covered   # Resequenced
50 Optum Mod 50 Exempt   ⊘ AMA Mod 51 Exempt   51 Optum Mod 51 Exempt   63 Mod 63 Exempt   ✗ Non-FDA Drug   ★ Telemedicine   M Maternity   A Age Edit

82441 Chemistry: Chlorinated Hydrocarbons

INCLUDES Clinical information not requested by the ordering physician
Mathematically calculated results
Quantitative analysis unless otherwise specified
Specimens from any source unless otherwise specified

EXCLUDES *Analytes from nonrequested laboratory analysis*
Calculated results that represent a score or probability that was derived by algorithm

82441 **Chlorinated hydrocarbons, screen**

EXCLUDES *Cholecalciferol (Vitamin D) (82306)*

🚑 0.00   ⚕ 0.00   **FUD** XXX   ▣ ▤

AMA: 2015,Jun,10; 2015,Apr,3

82465 Chemistry: Cholesterol, Total

CMS: 100-03,190.23 Lipid Testing; 100-04,16,40.6.1 Automated Multi-Channel Chemistry (AMCC) Tests for ESRD Beneficiaries; 100-04,16,70.8 CLIA Waived Tests; 100-04,16,90.2 Organ or Disease Oriented Panels

INCLUDES Clinical information not requested by the ordering physician
Mathematically calculated results
Quantitative analysis unless otherwise specified

EXCLUDES *Analytes from nonrequested laboratory analysis*
Calculated results that represent a score or probability that was derived by algorithm
Organ or disease panels (80048-80076 [80081])

82465 **Cholesterol, serum or whole blood, total**

EXCLUDES *High density lipoprotein (HDL) (83718)*

🚑 0.00   ⚕ 0.00   **FUD** XXX   ✖ Ⓐ ▤

AMA: 2018,Jan,8; 2017,Jan,8; 2016,Jan,13; 2015,Jun,10;
2015,Apr,3; 2015,Jan,16; 2014,Jan,11

82480-82507 Chemistry: Cholinesterase—Citrate

INCLUDES Clinical information not requested by the ordering physician
Mathematically calculated results
Quantitative analysis unless otherwise specified
Specimens from any source unless otherwise specified

EXCLUDES *Analytes from nonrequested laboratory analysis*
Calculated results that represent a score or probability that was derived by algorithm
Drug testing ([80305, 80306, 80307], [80324, 80325, 80326, 80327, 80328, 80329, 80330, 80331, 80332, 80333, 80334, 80335, 80336, 80337, 80338, 80339, 80340, 80341, 80342, 80343, 80344, 80345, 80346, 80347, 80348, 80349, 80350, 80351, 80352, 80353, 80354, 80355, 80356, 80357, 80358, 80359, 80360, 80361, 80362, 80363, 80364, 80365, 80366, 80367, 80368, 80369, 80370, 80371, 80372, 80373, 80374, 80375, 80376, 80377, 83992])
Organ or disease panels (80048-80076 [80081])
Therapeutic drug assays (80150-80299 [80164, 80165, 80171])

82480 **Cholinesterase; serum**

🚑 0.00   ⚕ 0.00   **FUD** XXX   ▣ ▤

AMA: 2015,Jun,10; 2015,Apr,3

82482 **RBC**

🚑 0.00   ⚕ 0.00   **FUD** XXX   ▣ ▤

AMA: 2015,Jun,10; 2015,Apr,3

82485 **Chondroitin B sulfate, quantitative**

EXCLUDES *Chorionic gonadotropin (84702-84703)*

🚑 0.00   ⚕ 0.00   **FUD** XXX   ▣ ▤

AMA: 2015,Jun,10; 2015,Apr,3

82495 **Chromium**

🚑 0.00   ⚕ 0.00   **FUD** XXX   ▣ ▤

AMA: 2015,Jun,10; 2015,Apr,3

82507 **Citrate**

EXCLUDES *Cocaine, qualitative analysis ([80353])*
Codeine, qualitative analysis ([80361])
Complement (86160-86162)

🚑 0.00   ⚕ 0.00   **FUD** XXX   ▣ ▤

AMA: 2015,Jun,10; 2015,Apr,3

82523 Chemistry: Collagen Crosslinks, Any Method

CMS: 100-03,190.19 NCD for Collagen Crosslinks, Any Method; 100-04,16,70.8 CLIA Waived Tests

INCLUDES Clinical information not requested by the ordering physician
Mathematically calculated results
Quantitative analysis unless otherwise specified
Specimens from any source unless otherwise specified

EXCLUDES *Analytes from nonrequested laboratory analysis*
Calculated results that represent a score or probability that was derived by algorithm
Organ or disease panels (80048-80076 [80081])
Therapeutic drug assays (80150-80299 [80164, 80165, 80171])

82523 **Collagen cross links, any method**

🚑 0.00   ⚕ 0.00   **FUD** XXX   ✖ ▣ ▤

AMA: 2015,Jun,10; 2015,Apr,3

82525-82735 Chemistry: Copper—Fluoride

INCLUDES Clinical information not requested by the ordering physician
Mathematically calculated results
Quantitative analysis unless otherwise specified
Specimens from any source unless otherwise specified

EXCLUDES *Analytes from nonrequested laboratory analysis*
Calculated results that represent a score or probability that was derived by algorithm
Drug testing ([80305, 80306, 80307], [80324, 80325, 80326, 80327, 80328, 80329, 80330, 80331, 80332, 80333, 80334, 80335, 80336, 80337, 80338, 80339, 80340, 80341, 80342, 80343, 80344, 80345, 80346, 80347, 80348, 80349, 80350, 80351, 80352, 80353, 80354, 80355, 80356, 80357, 80358, 80359, 80360, 80361, 80362, 80363, 80364, 80365, 80366, 80367, 80368, 80369, 80370, 80371, 80372, 80373, 80374, 80375, 80376, 80377, 83992])
Organ or disease panels (80048-80076 [80081])
Therapeutic drug assays (80150-80299 [80164, 80165, 80171])

82525 **Copper**

EXCLUDES *Coproporphyrin (84119-84120)*
Corticosteroids (83491)

🚑 0.00   ⚕ 0.00   **FUD** XXX   ▣ ▤

AMA: 2015,Jun,10; 2015,Apr,3

82528 **Corticosterone**

INCLUDES Porter-Silber test

🚑 0.00   ⚕ 0.00   **FUD** XXX   ▣ ▤

AMA: 2015,Jun,10; 2015,Apr,3

82530 **Cortisol; free**

🚑 0.00   ⚕ 0.00   **FUD** XXX   ▣ ▤

AMA: 2018,Jan,8; 2017,Jan,8; 2016,Jan,13; 2015,Jun,10;
2015,Apr,3; 2015,Jan,16; 2014,Jan,11

82533 **total**

🚑 0.00   ⚕ 0.00   **FUD** XXX   ▣ ▤

AMA: 2018,Jan,8; 2017,Jan,8; 2016,Jan,13; 2015,Jun,10;
2015,Apr,3; 2015,Jan,16; 2014,Jan,11

82540 **Creatine**

🚑 0.00   ⚕ 0.00   **FUD** XXX   ▣ ▤

AMA: 2015,Jun,10; 2015,Apr,3

82542 **Column chromatography, includes mass spectrometry, if performed (eg, HPLC, LC, LC/MS, LC/MS-MS, GC, GC/MS-MS, GC/MS, HPLC/MS), non-drug analyte(s) not elsewhere specified, qualitative or quantitative, each specimen**

EXCLUDES *Column chromatography/mass spectrometry of drugs/substances ([80305, 80306, 80307], [80320, 80321, 80322, 80323, 80324, 80325, 80326, 80327, 80328, 80329, 80330, 80331, 80332, 80333, 80334, 80335, 80336, 80337, 80338, 80339, 80340, 80341, 80342, 80343, 80344, 80345, 80346, 80347, 80348, 80349, 80350, 80351, 80352, 80353, 80354, 80355, 80356, 80357, 80358, 80359, 80360, 80361, 80362, 80363, 80364, 80365, 80366, 80367, 80368, 80369, 80370, 80371, 80372, 80373, 80374, 80375, 80376, 80377, 83992])*

Procedure performed more than one time per specimen

🚑 0.00   ⚕ 0.00   **FUD** XXX   ▣ ▤

AMA: 2018,Jan,8; 2017,Jan,8; 2016,Jan,13; 2015,Jun,10;
2015,Apr,3

82550 **Creatine kinase (CK), (CPK); total**

🚑 0.00   ⚕ 0.00   **FUD** XXX   ✖ ▣ ▤

AMA: 2018,Jan,8; 2017,Jan,8; 2016,Jan,13; 2015,Jun,10;
2015,Apr,3; 2015,Jan,16; 2014,Jan,11

26/TC PC/TC Only	A2-Z3 ASC Payment	50 Bilateral	♂ Male Only	♀ Female Only	🚑 Facility RVU	⚕ Non-Facility RVU	▣ CCI	✖ CLIA
FUD Follow-up Days	**CMS:** IOM	**AMA:** CPT Asst	A-Y OPPSI	80/80 Surg Assist Allowed / w/Doc		▤ Lab Crosswalk		▦ Radiology Crosswalk

406   CPT © 2019 American Medical Association. All Rights Reserved.   © 2019 Optum360, LLC

82552 **isoenzymes**
🔲 0.00 ⚬ 0.00 **FUD** XXX ▣ ▢
AMA: 2018,Jan,8; 2017,Jan,8; 2016,Jan,13; 2015,Jun,10; 2015,Apr,3; 2015,Jan,16; 2014,Jan,11

82553 **MB fraction only**
🔲 0.00 ⚬ 0.00 **FUD** XXX ▣ ▢
AMA: 2018,Jan,8; 2017,Jan,8; 2016,Jan,13; 2015,Jun,10; 2015,Apr,3; 2015,Jan,16; 2014,Jan,11

82554 **isoforms**
🔲 0.00 ⚬ 0.00 **FUD** XXX ▣ ▢
AMA: 2018,Jan,8; 2017,Jan,8; 2016,Jan,13; 2015,Jun,10; 2015,Apr,3; 2015,Jan,16; 2014,Jan,11

82565 **Creatinine; blood**
🔲 0.00 ⚬ 0.00 **FUD** XXX ✖ ▣ ▢
AMA: 2018,Jan,8; 2017,Jan,8; 2016,Jan,13; 2015,Jun,10; 2015,Apr,3; 2015,Jan,16; 2014,Jan,11

82570 **other source**
🔲 0.00 ⚬ 0.00 **FUD** XXX ✖ ▣ ▢
AMA: 2015,Jun,10; 2015,Apr,3

82575 **clearance**
INCLUDES Holten test
🔲 0.00 ⚬ 0.00 **FUD** XXX ▣ ▢
AMA: 2015,Jun,10; 2015,Apr,3

82585 **Cryofibrinogen**
🔲 0.00 ⚬ 0.00 **FUD** XXX ▢
AMA: 2015,Jun,10; 2015,Apr,3

82595 **Cryoglobulin, qualitative or semi-quantitative (eg, cryocrit)**
EXCLUDES Crystals, pyrophosphate vs urate (89060)
Quantitative, cryoglobulin (82784-82785)
🔲 0.00 ⚬ 0.00 **FUD** XXX ▣ ▢
AMA: 2015,Jun,10; 2015,Apr,3

82600 **Cyanide**
🔲 0.00 ⚬ 0.00 **FUD** XXX ▣ ▢
AMA: 2015,Jun,10; 2015,Apr,3

82607 **Cyanocobalamin (Vitamin B-12);**
EXCLUDES Cyclic AMP (82030)
Cyclosporine (80158)
🔲 0.00 ⚬ 0.00 **FUD** XXX ▣ ▢
AMA: 2015,Jun,10; 2015,Apr,3

82608 **unsaturated binding capacity**
EXCLUDES Cyclic AMP (82030)
Cyclosporine (80158)
🔲 0.00 ⚬ 0.00 **FUD** XXX ▢
AMA: 2015,Jun,10; 2015,Apr,3

82610 **Cystatin C**
🔲 0.00 ⚬ 0.00 **FUD** XXX ▣ ▢
AMA: 2018,Jan,8; 2017,Jan,8; 2016,Jan,13; 2015,Jun,10; 2015,Apr,3; 2015,Jan,16; 2014,Jan,11

82615 **Cystine and homocystine, urine, qualitative**
🔲 0.00 ⚬ 0.00 **FUD** XXX ▣ ▢
AMA: 2015,Jun,10; 2015,Apr,3

82626 **Dehydroepiandrosterone (DHEA)**
EXCLUDES Anabolic steroids ([80327, 80328])
🔲 0.00 ⚬ 0.00 **FUD** XXX ▣ ▢
AMA: 2018,Jan,8; 2017,Jan,8; 2016,Jan,13; 2015,Jun,10; 2015,Apr,3; 2015,Jan,16; 2014,Jan,11

82627 **Dehydroepiandrosterone-sulfate (DHEA-S)**
EXCLUDES Delta-aminolevulinicacid (ALA) (82135)
🔲 0.00 ⚬ 0.00 **FUD** XXX ▣ ▢
AMA: 2018,Jan,8; 2017,Jan,8; 2016,Jan,13; 2015,Jun,10; 2015,Apr,3; 2015,Jan,16; 2014,Jan,11

82633 **Desoxycorticosterone, 11-**
🔲 0.00 ⚬ 0.00 **FUD** XXX ▣ ▢
AMA: 2015,Jun,10; 2015,Apr,3

82634 **Deoxycortisol, 11-**
EXCLUDES Dexamethasone suppression test (80420)
Diastase, urine (82150)
🔲 0.00 ⚬ 0.00 **FUD** XXX ▣ ▢
AMA: 2015,Jun,10; 2015,Apr,3

82638 **Dibucaine number**
EXCLUDES Dichloroethane (82441)
Dichloromethane (82441)
Diethylether (84600)
🔲 0.00 ⚬ 0.00 **FUD** XXX ▣ ▢
AMA: 2015,Jun,10; 2015,Apr,3

82642 **Dihydrotestosterone (DHT)**
🔲 0.00 ⚬ 0.00 **FUD** XXX ▢
EXCLUDES Anabolic drug testing analysis of dihydrotestosterone ([80327, 80328])
Dipropylaceticacid ([80164])
Dopamine (82382)
Duodenal contents, individual enzymes for intubation and collection (43756-43757)

82652 **Resequenced code. See code following 82306.**

82656 **Elastase, pancreatic (EL-1), fecal, qualitative or semi-quantitative**
🔲 0.00 ⚬ 0.00 **FUD** XXX ▣ ▢
AMA: 2018,Jan,8; 2017,Jan,8; 2016,Jan,13; 2015,Jun,10; 2015,Apr,3; 2015,Jan,16; 2014,Jan,11

82657 **Enzyme activity in blood cells, cultured cells, or tissue, not elsewhere specified; nonradioactive substrate, each specimen**
🔲 0.00 ⚬ 0.00 **FUD** XXX ▣ ▢
AMA: 2015,Jun,10; 2015,Apr,3

82658 **radioactive substrate, each specimen**
🔲 0.00 ⚬ 0.00 **FUD** XXX ▣ ▢
AMA: 2015,Jun,10; 2015,Apr,3

82664 **Electrophoretic technique, not elsewhere specified**
EXCLUDES Endocrine receptor assays (84233-84235)
🔲 0.00 ⚬ 0.00 **FUD** XXX ▣ ▢
AMA: 2015,Jun,10; 2015,Apr,3

82668 **Erythropoietin**
🔲 0.00 ⚬ 0.00 **FUD** XXX ▣ ▢
AMA: 2015,Jun,10; 2015,Apr,3

82670 **Estradiol**
🔲 0.00 ⚬ 0.00 **FUD** XXX ▣ ▢
AMA: 2015,Jun,10; 2015,Apr,3

82671 **Estrogens; fractionated**
EXCLUDES Estrogen receptor assay (84233)
🔲 0.00 ⚬ 0.00 **FUD** XXX ▣ ▢
AMA: 2015,Jun,10; 2015,Apr,3

82672 **total**
EXCLUDES Estrogen receptor assay (84233)
🔲 0.00 ⚬ 0.00 **FUD** XXX ▣ ▢
AMA: 2015,Jun,10; 2015,Apr,3

82677 **Estriol**
🔲 0.00 ⚬ 0.00 **FUD** XXX ▣ ▢
AMA: 2015,Jun,10; 2015,Apr,3

82679 **Estrone**
EXCLUDES Ethanol ([80320])
🔲 0.00 ⚬ 0.00 **FUD** XXX ✖ ▣ ▢
AMA: 2015,Jun,10; 2015,Apr,3

82693 **Ethylene glycol**
🔲 0.00 ⚬ 0.00 **FUD** XXX ▣ ▢
AMA: 2015,Jun,10; 2015,Apr,3

82696 **Etiocholanolone**
EXCLUDES Fractionation of ketosteroids (83593)
🔲 0.00 ⚬ 0.00 **FUD** XXX ▣ ▢
AMA: 2015,Jun,10; 2015,Apr,3

● New Code ▲ Revised Code ○ Reinstated ● New Web Release ▲ Revised Web Release + Add-on Unlisted Not Covered # Resequenced
50 Optum Mod 50 Exempt ⊘ AMA Mod 51 Exempt 51 Optum Mod 51 Exempt 63 Mod 63 Exempt ✗ Non-FDA Drug ★ Telemedicine M Maternity A Age Edit

82705   **Fat or lipids, feces; qualitative**
      🔧 0.00   ⚕ 0.00   **FUD** XXX   🔲 ▣
      AMA: 2015,Jun,10; 2015,Apr,3

82710   **quantitative**
      🔧 0.00   ⚕ 0.00   **FUD** XXX   🔲 ▣
      AMA: 2015,Jun,10; 2015,Apr,3

82715   **Fat differential, feces, quantitative**
      🔧 0.00   ⚕ 0.00   **FUD** XXX   🔲 ▣
      AMA: 2015,Jun,10; 2015,Apr,3

82725   **Fatty acids, nonesterified**
      🔧 0.00   ⚕ 0.00   **FUD** XXX   🔲 ▣
      AMA: 2015,Jun,10; 2015,Apr,3

82726   **Very long chain fatty acids**
      EXCLUDES   *Long-chain (C20-22) omega-3 fatty acids in red blood cell (RBC) membranes (0111T)*
      🔧 0.00   ⚕ 0.00   **FUD** XXX   🔲 ▣
      AMA: 2015,Jun,10; 2015,Apr,3

82728   **Ferritin**
      EXCLUDES   *Fetal hemoglobin (83030, 83033, 85460)*
                Fetoprotein, alpha-1 (82105-82106)
      🔧 0.00   ⚕ 0.00   **FUD** XXX   🔲 ▣
      AMA: 2015,Jun,10; 2015,Apr,3

82731   **Fetal fibronectin, cervicovaginal secretions, semi-quantitative**   Ⓜ ♀
      🔧 0.00   ⚕ 0.00   **FUD** XXX   🔲 ▣
      AMA: 2015,Jun,10; 2015,Apr,3

82735   **Fluoride**
      EXCLUDES   *Foam stability test (83662)*
      🔧 0.00   ⚕ 0.00   **FUD** XXX   🔲 ▣
      AMA: 2015,Jun,10; 2015,Apr,3

82746-82941 Chemistry: Folic Acid—Gastrin

INCLUDES   Clinical information not requested by the ordering physician
      Mathematically calculated results
      Quantitative analysis unless otherwise specified
      Specimens from any source unless otherwise specified

EXCLUDES   *Analytes from nonrequested laboratory analysis*
      Calculated results that represent a score or probability that was derived by algorithm
      Drug testing ([80305, 80306, 80307], [80324, 80325, 80326, 80327, 80328, 80329, 80330, 80331, 80332, 80333, 80334, 80335, 80336, 80337, 80338, 80339, 80340, 80341, 80342, 80343, 80344, 80345, 80346, 80347, 80348, 80349, 80350, 80351, 80352, 80353, 80354, 80355, 80356, 80357, 80358, 80359, 80360, 80361, 80362, 80363, 80364, 80365, 80366, 80367, 80368, 80369, 80370, 80371, 80372, 80373, 80374, 80375, 80376, 80377, 83992])
      Organ or disease panels (80048-80076 [80081])
      Therapeutic drug assays (80150-80299 [80164, 80165, 80171])

82746   **Folic acid; serum**
      🔧 0.00   ⚕ 0.00   **FUD** XXX   🔲 ▣
      AMA: 2015,Jun,10; 2015,Apr,3

82747   **RBC**
      EXCLUDES   *Follicle stimulating hormone (FSH) (83001)*
      🔧 0.00   ⚕ 0.00   **FUD** XXX   🔲 ▣
      AMA: 2015,Jun,10; 2015,Apr,3

82757   **Fructose, semen**
      EXCLUDES   *Fructosamine (82985)*
                 Fructose, TLC screen (84375)
      🔧 0.00   ⚕ 0.00   **FUD** XXX   🔲 ▣
      AMA: 2015,Jun,10; 2015,Apr,3

82759   **Galactokinase, RBC**
      🔧 0.00   ⚕ 0.00   **FUD** XXX   🔲 ▣
      AMA: 2015,Jun,10; 2015,Apr,3

82760   **Galactose**
      🔧 0.00   ⚕ 0.00   **FUD** XXX   🔲 ▣
      AMA: 2015,Jun,10; 2015,Apr,3

82775   **Galactose-1-phosphate uridyl transferase; quantitative**
      🔧 0.00   ⚕ 0.00   **FUD** XXX   🔲 ▣
      AMA: 2015,Jun,10; 2015,Apr,3

82776   **screen**
      🔧 0.00   ⚕ 0.00   **FUD** XXX   🔲 ▣
      AMA: 2015,Jun,10; 2015,Apr,3

82777   **Galectin-3**
      🔧 0.00   ⚕ 0.00   **FUD** XXX   🔲 ▣
      AMA: 2015,Jun,10; 2015,Apr,3

82784   **Gammaglobulin (immunoglobulin); IgA, IgD, IgG, IgM, each**
      INCLUDES   Farr test
      🔧 0.00   ⚕ 0.00   **FUD** XXX   🔲 ▣
      AMA: 2018,Jan,8; 2017,Jan,8; 2016,Jan,13; 2015,Jun,10; 2015,Apr,3; 2015,Jan,16; 2014,Jan,11

82785   **IgE**
      INCLUDES   Farr test
      EXCLUDES   *Allergen specific, IgE (86003, 86005)*
      🔧 0.00   ⚕ 0.00   **FUD** XXX   🔲 ▣
      AMA: 2018,Jan,8; 2017,Jan,8; 2016,Jan,13; 2015,Jun,10; 2015,Apr,3; 2015,Jan,16; 2014,Jan,11

82787   **immunoglobulin subclasses (eg, IgG1, 2, 3, or 4), each**
      EXCLUDES   *Gamma-glutamyltransferase (GGT) (82977)*
      🔧 0.00   ⚕ 0.00   **FUD** XXX   🔲 ▣
      AMA: 2015,Jun,10; 2015,Apr,3

82800   **Gases, blood, pH only**
      🔧 0.00   ⚕ 0.00   **FUD** XXX   🔲 ▣
      AMA: 2015,Jun,10; 2015,Apr,3

82803   **Gases, blood, any combination of pH, pCO2, pO2, CO2, HCO3 (including calculated O2 saturation);**
      INCLUDES   Two or more of the listed analytes
      🔧 0.00   ⚕ 0.00   **FUD** XXX   🔲 ▣
      AMA: 2015,Jun,10; 2015,Apr,3

82805   **with O2 saturation, by direct measurement, except pulse oximetry**
      🔧 0.00   ⚕ 0.00   **FUD** XXX   🔲 ▣
      AMA: 2015,Jun,10; 2015,Apr,3

82810   **Gases, blood, O2 saturation only, by direct measurement, except pulse oximetry**
      EXCLUDES   *Pulse oximetry (94760)*
      🔧 0.00   ⚕ 0.00   **FUD** XXX   🔲 ▣
      AMA: 2015,Jun,10; 2015,Apr,3

82820   **Hemoglobin-oxygen affinity (pO2 for 50% hemoglobin saturation with oxygen)**
      EXCLUDES   *Gastric acid analysis (82930)*
      🔧 0.00   ⚕ 0.00   **FUD** XXX   🔲 ▣
      AMA: 2015,Jun,10; 2015,Apr,3

82930   **Gastric acid analysis, includes pH if performed, each specimen**
      🔧 0.00   ⚕ 0.00   **FUD** XXX   🔲 ▣
      AMA: 2018,Jan,8; 2017,Jan,8; 2016,Jan,13; 2015,Jun,10; 2015,Apr,3; 2015,Jan,16; 2014,Jan,11

82938   **Gastrin after secretin stimulation**
      🔧 0.00   ⚕ 0.00   **FUD** XXX   🔲 ▣
      AMA: 2015,Jun,10; 2015,Apr,3

82941   **Gastrin**
      EXCLUDES   *Gentamicin (80170)*
                 GGT (82977)
                 Qualitative column chromatography report specific analyte or (82542)
      🔧 0.00   ⚕ 0.00   **FUD** XXX   🔲 ▣
      AMA: 2015,Jun,10; 2015,Apr,3

82943-82962 Chemistry: Glucagon—Glucose Testing

CMS: 100-03,190.20 Blood Glucose Testing

INCLUDES Clinical information not requested by the ordering physician
Mathematically calculated results
Quantitative analysis unless otherwise specified
Specimens from any source unless otherwise specified

EXCLUDES *Analytes from nonrequested laboratory analysis*
Calculated results that represent a score or probability that was derived by algorithm
Organ or disease panels (80048-80076 [80081])
Therapeutic drug assays (80150-80299 [80164, 80165, 80171])

Code also glucose administration injection (96374)

82943 **Glucagon**
🔧 0.00   ✂ 0.00   **FUD** XXX
AMA: 2015,Jun,10; 2015,Apr,3

82945 **Glucose, body fluid, other than blood**
🔧 0.00   ✂ 0.00   **FUD** XXX
AMA: 2015,Jun,10; 2015,Apr,3

82946 **Glucagon tolerance test**
🔧 0.00   ✂ 0.00   **FUD** XXX
AMA: 2015,Jun,10; 2015,Apr,3

82947 **Glucose; quantitative, blood (except reagent strip)**
🔧 0.00   ✂ 0.00   **FUD** XXX
AMA: 2018,Jan,8; 2017,Jan,8; 2016,Jan,13; 2015,Jun,10; 2015,Apr,3; 2015,Jan,16; 2014,Jan,11

82948 **blood, reagent strip**
🔧 0.00   ✂ 0.00   **FUD** XXX
AMA: 2018,Jan,8; 2017,Jan,8; 2016,Jan,13; 2015,Jun,10; 2015,Apr,3; 2015,Jan,16; 2014,Jan,11

82950 **post glucose dose (includes glucose)**
🔧 0.00   ✂ 0.00   **FUD** XXX
AMA: 2018,Jan,8; 2017,Jan,8; 2016,Jan,13; 2015,Jun,10; 2015,Apr,3; 2015,Jan,16; 2014,Jan,11

82951 **tolerance test (GTT), 3 specimens (includes glucose)**
🔧 0.00   ✂ 0.00   **FUD** XXX
AMA: 2018,Jan,8; 2017,Jan,8; 2016,Jan,13; 2015,Jun,10; 2015,Apr,3; 2015,Jan,16; 2014,Jan,11

+ **82952** **tolerance test, each additional beyond 3 specimens (List separately in addition to code for primary procedure)**
EXCLUDES *Insulin tolerance test (80434-80435)*
Leucine tolerance test (80428)
Semiquantitative urine glucose (81000, 81002, 81005, 81099)
Code first (82951)
🔧 0.00   ✂ 0.00   **FUD** XXX
AMA: 2018,Jan,8; 2017,Jan,8; 2016,Jan,13; 2015,Jun,10; 2015,Apr,3; 2015,Jan,16; 2014,Jan,11

82955 **Glucose-6-phosphate dehydrogenase (G6PD); quantitative**
Code also glucose tolerance test with medication, when performed (96374)
🔧 0.00   ✂ 0.00   **FUD** XXX
AMA: 2015,Jun,10; 2015,Apr,3

82960 **screen**
Code also glucose tolerance test with medication, when performed (96374)
🔧 0.00   ✂ 0.00   **FUD** XXX
AMA: 2015,Jun,10; 2015,Apr,3

82962 **Glucose, blood by glucose monitoring device(s) cleared by the FDA specifically for home use**
🔧 0.00   ✂ 0.00   **FUD** XXX
AMA: 2018,Jan,8; 2017,Jan,8; 2016,Jan,13; 2015,Jun,10; 2015,Apr,3; 2015,Jan,16; 2014,Jan,11

82963-83690 Chemistry: Glucosidase—Lipase

INCLUDES Clinical information not requested by the ordering physician
Mathematically calculated results
Quantitative analysis unless otherwise specified
Specimens from any source unless otherwise specified

EXCLUDES *Analytes from nonrequested laboratory analysis*
Calculated results that represent a score or probability that was derived by algorithm
Drug testing ([80305, 80306, 80307], [80324, 80325, 80326, 80327, 80328, 80329, 80330, 80331, 80332, 80333, 80334, 80335, 80336, 80337, 80338, 80339, 80340, 80341, 80342, 80343, 80344, 80345, 80346, 80347, 80348, 80349, 80350, 80351, 80352, 80353, 80354, 80355, 80356, 80357, 80358, 80359, 80360, 80361, 80362, 80363, 80364, 80365, 80366, 80367, 80368, 80369, 80370, 80371, 80372, 80373, 80374, 80375, 80376, 80377, 83992])
Organ or disease panels (80048-80076 [80081])
Therapeutic drug assays (80150-80299 [80164, 80165, 80171])

82963 **Glucosidase, beta**
🔧 0.00   ✂ 0.00   **FUD** XXX
AMA: 2015,Jun,10; 2015,Apr,3

82965 **Glutamate dehydrogenase**
🔧 0.00   ✂ 0.00   **FUD** XXX
AMA: 2015,Jun,10; 2015,Apr,3

82977 **Glutamyltransferase, gamma (GGT)**
🔧 0.00   ✂ 0.00   **FUD** XXX
AMA: 2018,Jan,8; 2017,Jan,8; 2016,Jan,13; 2015,Jun,10; 2015,Apr,3; 2015,Jan,16; 2014,Jan,11

82978 **Glutathione**
🔧 0.00   ✂ 0.00   **FUD** XXX
AMA: 2015,Jun,10; 2015,Apr,3

82979 **Glutathione reductase, RBC**
EXCLUDES *Glycohemoglobin (83036)*
🔧 0.00   ✂ 0.00   **FUD** XXX
AMA: 2015,Jun,10; 2015,Apr,3

82985 **Glycated protein**
EXCLUDES *Gonadotropin chorionic (hCG) (84702-84703)*
🔧 0.00   ✂ 0.00   **FUD** XXX
AMA: 2018,Jan,8; 2017,Jan,8; 2016,Jan,13; 2015,Jun,10; 2015,Apr,3; 2015,Jan,16; 2014,Jan,11

83001 **Gonadotropin; follicle stimulating hormone (FSH)**
🔧 0.00   ✂ 0.00   **FUD** XXX
AMA: 2015,Jun,10; 2015,Apr,3

83002 **luteinizing hormone (LH)**
EXCLUDES *Luteinizing releasing factor (LRH) (83727)*
🔧 0.00   ✂ 0.00   **FUD** XXX
AMA: 2015,Jun,10; 2015,Apr,3

83003 **Growth hormone, human (HGH) (somatotropin)**
EXCLUDES *Antibody to human growth hormone (86277)*
🔧 0.00   ✂ 0.00   **FUD** XXX
AMA: 2015,Jun,10; 2015,Apr,3

83006 **Growth stimulation expressed gene 2 (ST2, Interleukin 1 receptor like-1)**
🔧 0.00   ✂ 0.00   **FUD** XXX
AMA: 2015,Jun,10; 2015,Apr,3

83009 **Helicobacter pylori, blood test analysis for urease activity, non-radioactive isotope (eg, C-13)**
EXCLUDES *H. pylori, breath test analysis for urease activity (83013-83014)*
🔧 0.00   ✂ 0.00   **FUD** XXX
AMA: 2015,Jun,10; 2015,Apr,3

83010 **Haptoglobin; quantitative**
🔧 0.00   ✂ 0.00   **FUD** XXX
AMA: 2015,Jun,10; 2015,Apr,3

83012 **phenotypes**
🔧 0.00   ✂ 0.00   **FUD** XXX
AMA: 2015,Jun,10; 2015,Apr,3

83013 Helicobacter pylori; breath test analysis for urease activity, non-radioactive isotope (eg, C-13)
📁 0.00　　🔬 0.00　　**FUD** XXX　　🔲 🔳

AMA: 2018,Jan,8; 2017,Jan,8; 2016,Jan,13; 2015,Jun,10; 2015,Apr,3; 2015,Jan,16; 2014,Jan,11

83014 drug administration
EXCLUDES *H. pylori:*
Blood test analysis for urease activity (83009)
Enzyme immunoassay (87339)
Liquid scintillation counter (78267-78268)
Stool (87338)
📁 0.00　　🔬 0.00　　**FUD** XXX　　🔲 🔳

AMA: 2018,Jan,8; 2017,Jan,8; 2016,Jan,13; 2015,Jun,10; 2015,Apr,3; 2015,Jan,16; 2014,Jan,11

83015 Heavy metal (eg, arsenic, barium, beryllium, bismuth, antimony, mercury); qualitative, any number of analytes
INCLUDES Reinsch test
📁 0.00　　🔬 0.00　　**FUD** XXX　　🔲 🔳

AMA: 2015,Jun,10; 2015,Apr,3

83018 quantitative, each, not elsewhere specified
EXCLUDES *Evaluation of a known heavy metal with a specific code*
📁 0.00　　🔬 0.00　　**FUD** XXX　　🔲 🔳

AMA: 2015,Jun,10; 2015,Apr,3

83020 Hemoglobin fractionation and quantitation; electrophoresis (eg, A2, S, C, and/or F)
📁 0.00　　🔬 0.00　　**FUD** XXX　　🔲 80 🔳

AMA: 2015,Jun,10; 2015,Apr,3

83021 chromatography (eg, A2, S, C, and/or F)
EXCLUDES *Analysis of glycosylated (A1c) hemoglobin by chromatography or electrophoresis without an identified hemoglobin variant (83036)*
📁 0.00　　🔬 0.00　　**FUD** XXX　　🔲 🔳

AMA: 2018,Jan,8; 2017,Jan,8; 2016,Jan,13; 2015,Jun,10; 2015,Apr,3; 2015,Jan,16; 2014,Jan,11

83026 Hemoglobin; by copper sulfate method, non-automated
📁 0.00　　🔬 0.00　　**FUD** XXX　　✖ 🔲 🔳

AMA: 2015,Jun,10; 2015,Apr,3

83030 F (fetal), chemical
📁 0.00　　🔬 0.00　　**FUD** XXX　　🔲 🔳

AMA: 2015,Jun,10; 2015,Apr,3

83033 F (fetal), qualitative
📁 0.00　　🔬 0.00　　**FUD** XXX　　🔲 🔳

AMA: 2015,Jun,10; 2015,Apr,3

83036 glycosylated (A1C)
EXCLUDES *Analysis of glycosylated (A1c) hemoglobin by chromatography or electrophoresis without an identified hemoglobin variant (83020-83021)*
Detection of hemoglobin, fecal, by immunoassay (82274)
📁 0.00　　🔬 0.00　　**FUD** XXX　　✖ 🔲 🔳

AMA: 2018,Jan,8; 2017,Jan,8; 2016,Jan,13; 2015,Jun,10; 2015,Apr,3; 2015,Jan,16; 2014,Jan,11

83037 glycosylated (A1C) by device cleared by FDA for home use
📁 0.00　　🔬 0.00　　**FUD** XXX　　✖ 🔲 🔳

AMA: 2018,Jan,8; 2017,Jan,8; 2016,Jan,13; 2015,Jun,10; 2015,Apr,3; 2015,Jan,16; 2014,Jan,11

83045 methemoglobin, qualitative
📁 0.00　　🔬 0.00　　**FUD** XXX　　🔲 🔳

AMA: 2015,Jun,10; 2015,Apr,3

83050 methemoglobin, quantitative
EXCLUDES *Transcutaneous methemoglobin test (88741)*
📁 0.00　　🔬 0.00　　**FUD** XXX　　🔲 🔳

AMA: 2018,Jan,8; 2017,Jan,8; 2016,Jan,13; 2015,Jun,10; 2015,Apr,3; 2015,Jan,16; 2014,Jan,11

83051 plasma
📁 0.00　　🔬 0.00　　**FUD** XXX　　🔲 🔳

AMA: 2015,Jun,10; 2015,Apr,3

83060 sulfhemoglobin, quantitative
📁 0.00　　🔬 0.00　　**FUD** XXX　　🔲 🔳

AMA: 2015,Jun,10; 2015,Apr,3

83065 thermolabile
📁 0.00　　🔬 0.00　　**FUD** XXX　　🔲 🔳

AMA: 2015,Jun,10; 2015,Apr,3

83068 unstable, screen
📁 0.00　　🔬 0.00　　**FUD** XXX　　🔲 🔳

AMA: 2015,Jun,10; 2015,Apr,3

83069 urine
📁 0.00　　🔬 0.00　　**FUD** XXX　　🔲 🔳

AMA: 2015,Jun,10; 2015,Apr,3

83070 Hemosiderin, qualitative
EXCLUDES *HIAA (83497)*
Qualitative column chromatography report specific analyte or (82542)
📁 0.00　　🔬 0.00　　**FUD** XXX　　🔲 🔳

AMA: 2015,Jun,10; 2015,Apr,3

83080 b-Hexosaminidase, each assay
📁 0.00　　🔬 0.00　　**FUD** XXX　　🔲 🔳

AMA: 2015,Jun,10; 2015,Apr,3

83088 Histamine
EXCLUDES *Hollander test (43754-43755)*
📁 0.00　　🔬 0.00　　**FUD** XXX　　🔲 🔳

AMA: 2015,Jun,10; 2015,Apr,3

83090 Homocysteine
📁 0.00　　🔬 0.00　　**FUD** XXX　　🔲 🔳

AMA: 2018,Jan,8; 2017,Jan,8; 2016,Jan,13; 2015,Jun,10; 2015,Apr,3; 2015,Jan,16; 2014,Jan,11

83150 Homovanillic acid (HVA)
EXCLUDES *Hormone testing report from alphabetic list in Chemistry section*
Hydrogen/methane breath test (91065)
📁 0.00　　🔬 0.00　　**FUD** XXX　　🔲 🔳

AMA: 2015,Jun,10; 2015,Apr,3

83491 Hydroxycorticosteroids, 17- (17-OHCS)
EXCLUDES *Cortisol (82530, 82533)*
Deoxycortisol (82634)
📁 0.00　　🔬 0.00　　**FUD** XXX　　🔲 🔳

AMA: 2015,Jun,10; 2015,Apr,3

83497 Hydroxyindolacetic acid, 5-(HIAA)
EXCLUDES *5-Hydroxytryptamine (84260)*
Urine qualitative test (81005)
📁 0.00　　🔬 0.00　　**FUD** XXX　　🔲 🔳

AMA: 2015,Jun,10; 2015,Apr,3

83498 Hydroxyprogesterone, 17-d
📁 0.00　　🔬 0.00　　**FUD** XXX　　🔲 🔳

AMA: 2015,Jun,10; 2015,Apr,3

83500 Hydroxyproline; free
📁 0.00　　🔬 0.00　　**FUD** XXX　　🔲 🔳

AMA: 2015,Jun,10; 2015,Apr,3

83505 total
📁 0.00　　🔬 0.00　　**FUD** XXX　　🔲 🔳

AMA: 2015,Jun,10; 2015,Apr,3

83516 Immunoassay for analyte other than infectious agent antibody or infectious agent antigen; qualitative or semiquantitative, multiple step method
📁 0.00　　🔬 0.00　　**FUD** XXX　　✖ 🔲 🔳

AMA: 2015,Jun,10; 2015,Apr,3

83518 qualitative or semiquantitative, single step method (eg, reagent strip)
📁 0.00　　🔬 0.00　　**FUD** XXX　　🔲 🔳

AMA: 2015,Jun,10; 2015,Apr,3

83519 quantitative, by radioimmunoassay (eg, RIA)

📖 0.00   ⚕ 0.00   **FUD** XXX   🔲 🖥

AMA: 2018,Jan,8; 2017,Jan,8; 2016,Jan,13; 2015,Jun,10; 2015,Apr,3; 2015,Jan,16; 2014,Jan,11

83520 quantitative, not otherwise specified

EXCLUDES   Immunoassays for antibodies to infectious agent antigen report specific analyte/method from Immunology

Immunoassay of tumor antigens not elsewhere specified (86316)

Immunoglobulins (82784, 82785)

📖 0.00   ⚕ 0.00   **FUD** XXX   🔲 🖥

AMA: 2015,Jun,10; 2015,Apr,3

83525 Insulin; total

EXCLUDES   Proinsulin (84206)

📖 0.00   ⚕ 0.00   **FUD** XXX   🔲 🖥

AMA: 2015,Jun,10; 2015,Apr,3

83527 free

📖 0.00   ⚕ 0.00   **FUD** XXX   🔲 🖥

AMA: 2018,Jan,8; 2017,Jan,8; 2016,Jan,13; 2015,Jun,10; 2015,Apr,3; 2015,Jan,16; 2014,Jan,11

83528 Intrinsic factor

EXCLUDES   Intrinsic factor antibodies (86340)

📖 0.00   ⚕ 0.00   **FUD** XXX   🔲 🖥

AMA: 2015,Jun,10; 2015,Apr,3

83540 Iron

📖 0.00   ⚕ 0.00   **FUD** XXX   🔲 🖥

AMA: 2018,Jan,8; 2017,Jan,8; 2016,Jan,13; 2015,Jun,10; 2015,Apr,3; 2015,Jan,16; 2014,Jan,11

83550 Iron binding capacity

📖 0.00   ⚕ 0.00   **FUD** XXX   🔲 🖥

AMA: 2015,Jun,10; 2015,Apr,3

83570 Isocitric dehydrogenase (IDH)

EXCLUDES   Isonicotinic acid hydrazide, INH, report specific method

Isopropyl alcohol ([80320])

📖 0.00   ⚕ 0.00   **FUD** XXX   🔲 🖥

AMA: 2015,Jun,10; 2015,Apr,3

83582 Ketogenic steroids, fractionation

EXCLUDES   Ketone bodies:

Serum (82009, 82010)

Urine (81000-81003)

📖 0.00   ⚕ 0.00   **FUD** XXX   🔲 🖥

AMA: 2015,Jun,10; 2015,Apr,3

83586 Ketosteroids, 17- (17-KS); total

📖 0.00   ⚕ 0.00   **FUD** XXX   🔲 🖥

AMA: 2015,Jun,10; 2015,Apr,3

83593 fractionation

📖 0.00   ⚕ 0.00   **FUD** XXX   🔲 🖥

AMA: 2015,Jun,10; 2015,Apr,3

83605 Lactate (lactic acid)

📖 0.00   ⚕ 0.00   **FUD** XXX   ☒ 🔲 🖥

AMA: 2015,Jun,10; 2015,Apr,3

83615 Lactate dehydrogenase (LD), (LDH);

📖 0.00   ⚕ 0.00   **FUD** XXX   🔲 🖥

AMA: 2018,Jan,8; 2017,Jan,8; 2016,Jan,13; 2015,Jun,10; 2015,Apr,3; 2015,Jan,16; 2014,Jan,11

83625 isoenzymes, separation and quantitation

📖 0.00   ⚕ 0.00   **FUD** XXX   🔲 🖥

AMA: 2018,Jan,8; 2017,Jan,8; 2016,Jan,13; 2015,Jun,10; 2015,Apr,3; 2015,Jan,16; 2014,Jan,11

83630 Lactoferrin, fecal; qualitative

📖 0.00   ⚕ 0.00   **FUD** XXX   🔲 🖥

AMA: 2018,Jan,8; 2017,Jan,8; 2016,Jan,13; 2015,Jun,10; 2015,Apr,3; 2015,Jan,16; 2014,Jan,11

83631 quantitative

📖 0.00   ⚕ 0.00   **FUD** XXX   🔲 🖥

AMA: 2018,Jan,8; 2017,Jan,8; 2016,Jan,13; 2015,Jun,10; 2015,Apr,3; 2015,Jan,16; 2014,Jan,11

83632 Lactogen, human placental (HPL) human chorionic somatomammotropin   Ⓜ

📖 0.00   ⚕ 0.00   **FUD** XXX   🔲 🖥

AMA: 2015,Jun,10; 2015,Apr,3

83633 Lactose, urine, qualitative

EXCLUDES   Lactase deficiency breath hydrogen/methane test (91065)

Lactose tolerance test (82951, 82952)

📖 0.00   ⚕ 0.00   **FUD** XXX   🔲 🖥

AMA: 2015,Jun,10; 2015,Apr,3

83655 Lead

📖 0.00   ⚕ 0.00   **FUD** XXX   ☒ 🔲 🖥

AMA: 2015,Jun,10; 2015,Apr,3

83661 Fetal lung maturity assessment; lecithin sphingomyelin (L/S) ratio   Ⓜ

📖 0.00   ⚕ 0.00   **FUD** XXX   🔲 🖥

AMA: 2018,Jan,8; 2017,Jan,8; 2016,Jan,13; 2015,Jun,10; 2015,Apr,3; 2015,Jan,16; 2014,Jan,11

83662 foam stability test   Ⓜ

📖 0.00   ⚕ 0.00   **FUD** XXX   🔲 🖥

AMA: 2015,Jun,10; 2015,Apr,3

83663 fluorescence polarization   Ⓜ

📖 0.00   ⚕ 0.00   **FUD** XXX   🔲 🖥

AMA: 2015,Jun,10; 2015,Apr,3

83664 lamellar body density   Ⓜ

EXCLUDES   Phosphatidylglycerol (84081)

📖 0.00   ⚕ 0.00   **FUD** XXX   🔲 🖥

AMA: 2015,Jun,10; 2015,Apr,3

83670 Leucine aminopeptidase (LAP)

📖 0.00   ⚕ 0.00   **FUD** XXX   🔲 🖥

AMA: 2015,Jun,10; 2015,Apr,3

83690 Lipase

📖 0.00   ⚕ 0.00   **FUD** XXX   🔲 🖥

AMA: 2015,Jun,10; 2015,Apr,3

83695-83727 Chemistry: Lipoprotein—Luteinizing Releasing Factor

INCLUDES   Clinical information not requested by the ordering physician

Mathematically calculated results

Quantitative analysis unless otherwise specified

Specimens from any source unless otherwise specified

EXCLUDES   Analytes from nonrequested laboratory analysis

Calculated results that represent a score or probability that was derived by algorithm

Organ or disease panels (80048-80076 [80081])

Therapeutic drug assays (80150-80299 [80164, 80165, 80171])

83695 Lipoprotein (a)

📖 0.00   ⚕ 0.00   **FUD** XXX   🔲 🖥

AMA: 2018,Jan,8; 2017,Jan,8; 2016,Jan,13; 2015,Jun,10; 2015,Apr,3; 2015,Jan,16; 2014,Jan,11

83698 Lipoprotein-associated phospholipase A2 (Lp-PLA2)

EXCLUDES   Secretory type II phospholipase A2 (sPLA2-IIA) (0423T)

📖 0.00   ⚕ 0.00   **FUD** XXX   🔲 🖥

AMA: 2015,Jun,10; 2015,Apr,3

83700 Lipoprotein, blood; electrophoretic separation and quantitation

📖 0.00   ⚕ 0.00   **FUD** XXX   🔲 🖥

AMA: 2018,Jan,8; 2017,Jan,8; 2016,Jan,13; 2015,Jun,10; 2015,Apr,3; 2015,Jan,16; 2014,Jan,11

Pathology and Laboratory

83701 — 83883

83701 high resolution fractionation and quantitation of lipoproteins including lipoprotein subclasses when performed (eg, electrophoresis, ultracentrifugation)

🔧 0.00   🔖 0.00   **FUD** XXX   Ⓠ▣

AMA: 2018,Jan,8; 2017,Jan,8; 2016,Jan,13; 2015,Jun,10; 2015,Apr,3; 2015,Jan,16; 2014,Jan,11

83704 quantitation of lipoprotein particle number(s) (eg, by nuclear magnetic resonance spectroscopy), includes lipoprotein particle subclass(es), when performed

🔧 0.00   🔖 0.00   **FUD** XXX   Ⓠ▣

AMA: 2018,Jan,8; 2017,Jan,8; 2016,Jan,13; 2015,Jun,10; 2015,Apr,3; 2015,Jan,16; 2014,Jan,11

83718 Lipoprotein, direct measurement; high density cholesterol (HDL cholesterol)

🔧 0.00   🔖 0.00   **FUD** XXX   ✖Ⓐ▣

AMA: 2018,Jan,8; 2017,Jan,8; 2016,Jan,13; 2015,Jun,10; 2015,Apr,3; 2015,Jan,16; 2014,Jan,11

83719 VLDL cholesterol

🔧 0.00   🔖 0.00   **FUD** XXX   Ⓠ▣

AMA: 2018,Jan,8; 2017,Jan,8; 2016,Jan,13; 2015,Jun,10; 2015,Apr,3; 2015,Jan,16; 2014,Jan,11

83721 LDL cholesterol

EXCLUDES   Fractionation by high resolution electrophoresis or ultracentrifugation (83701)
Lipoprotein particle numbers and subclasses analysis by nuclear magnetic resonance spectroscopy (83704)

🔧 0.00   🔖 0.00   **FUD** XXX   ✖Ⓠ▣

AMA: 2018,Jan,8; 2017,Jan,8; 2016,Jan,13; 2015,Jun,10; 2015,Apr,3; 2015,Jan,16; 2014,Jan,11

83722 small dense LDL cholesterol

🔧 0.00   🔖 0.00   **FUD** XXX   ▣

EXCLUDES   Fractionation by high resolution electrophoresis or ultracentrifugation (83701)
Lipoprotein particle numbers/subclass analysis by nuclear magnetic resonance spectroscopy (83704)

83727 Luteinizing releasing factor (LRH)

EXCLUDES   alpha-2-Macroglobulin (86329)
Luteinizing hormone (LH) (83002)

🔧 0.00   🔖 0.00   **FUD** XXX   Ⓠ▣

AMA: 2015,Jun,10; 2015,Apr,3

83735-83885 Chemistry: Magnesium—Nickel

INCLUDES   Clinical information not requested by the ordering physician
Mathematically calculated results
Quantitative analysis unless otherwise specified
Specimens from any source unless otherwise specified

EXCLUDES   Analytes from nonrequested laboratory analysis
Calculated results that represent a score or probability that was derived by algorithm
Organ or disease panels (80048-80076 [80081])
Therapeutic drug assays (80150-80299 [80164, 80165, 80171])

83735 Magnesium

🔧 0.00   🔖 0.00   **FUD** XXX   Ⓠ▣

AMA: 2015,Jun,10; 2015,Apr,3

83775 Malate dehydrogenase

EXCLUDES   Maltose tolerance (82951, 82952)
Mammotropin (84146)

🔧 0.00   🔖 0.00   **FUD** XXX   Ⓠ▣

AMA: 2015,Jun,10; 2015,Apr,3

83785 Manganese

🔧 0.00   🔖 0.00   **FUD** XXX   Ⓠ▣

AMA: 2015,Jun,10; 2015,Apr,3

83789 Mass spectrometry and tandem mass spectrometry (eg, MS, MS/MS, MALDI, MS-TOF, QTOF), non-drug analyte(s) not elsewhere specified, qualitative or quantitative, each specimen

EXCLUDES   Column chromatography/mass spectrometry of drugs or substances ([80305], [80306], [80307], [80320, 80321, 80322, 80323, 80324, 80325, 80326, 80327, 80328, 80329, 80330, 80331, 80332, 80333, 80334, 80335, 80336, 80337, 80338, 80339, 80340, 80341, 80342, 80343, 80344, 80345, 80346, 80347, 80348, 80349, 80350, 80351, 80352, 80353, 80354, 80355, 80356, 80357, 80358, 80359, 80360, 80361, 80362, 80363, 80364, 80365, 80366, 80367, 80368, 80369, 80370, 80371, 80372, 80373, 80374, 80375, 80376, 80377, 83992])
Procedure performed more than one time per specimen
Report specific analyte testing with code(s) from Chemistry section

🔧 0.00   🔖 0.00   **FUD** XXX   Ⓠ▣

AMA: 2015,Jun,10; 2015,Apr,3

83825 Mercury, quantitative

EXCLUDES   Mercury screen (83015)

🔧 0.00   🔖 0.00   **FUD** XXX   Ⓠ▣

AMA: 2015,Jun,10; 2015,Apr,3

83835 Metanephrines

EXCLUDES   Catecholamines (82382-82384)
Methamphetamine ([80324], [80325], [80326])
Methane breath test (91065)

🔧 0.00   🔖 0.00   **FUD** XXX   Ⓠ▣

AMA: 2015,Jun,10; 2015,Apr,3

83857 Methemalbumin

EXCLUDES   Methemoglobin (83045, 83050)
Methyl alcohol ([80320])
Microalbumin
    Quantitative (82043)
    Semiquantitative (82044)

🔧 0.00   🔖 0.00   **FUD** XXX   Ⓠ▣

AMA: 2015,Jun,10; 2015,Apr,3

83861 Microfluidic analysis utilizing an integrated collection and analysis device, tear osmolarity

EXCLUDES   beta-2 Microglobulin (82232)
Code also when performed on both eyes 83861 X 2

🔧 0.00   🔖 0.00   **FUD** XXX   ✖Ⓠ▣

AMA: 2015,Jun,10; 2015,Apr,3

83864 Mucopolysaccharides, acid, quantitative   Ⓠ▣

🔧 0.00   🔖 0.00   **FUD** XXX

AMA: 2015,Jun,10; 2015,Apr,3

83872 Mucin, synovial fluid (Ropes test)

🔧 0.00   🔖 0.00   **FUD** XXX   Ⓠ▣

AMA: 2015,Jun,10; 2015,Apr,3

83873 Myelin basic protein, cerebrospinal fluid

EXCLUDES   Oligoclonal bands (83916)

🔧 0.00   🔖 0.00   **FUD** XXX   Ⓠ▣

AMA: 2015,Jun,10; 2015,Apr,3

83874 Myoglobin

🔧 0.00   🔖 0.00   **FUD** XXX   Ⓠ▣

AMA: 2018,Jan,8; 2017,Jan,8; 2016,Jan,13; 2015,Jun,10; 2015,Apr,3; 2015,Jan,16; 2014,Jan,11

83876 Myeloperoxidase (MPO)

🔧 0.00   🔖 0.00   **FUD** XXX   Ⓠ▣

AMA: 2015,Jun,10; 2015,Apr,3

83880 Natriuretic peptide

🔧 0.00   🔖 0.00   **FUD** XXX   ✖Ⓠ▣

AMA: 2018,Jan,8; 2017,Jan,8; 2016,Jan,13; 2015,Jun,10; 2015,Apr,3; 2015,Jan,16; 2014,Jan,11

83883 Nephelometry, each analyte not elsewhere specified   Ⓠ▣

🔧 0.00   🔖 0.00   **FUD** XXX

AMA: 2015,Jun,10; 2015,Apr,3

| 26/TC PC/TC Only | 82-Z3 ASC Payment | 50 Bilateral | ♂ Male Only | ♀ Female Only | 🔧 Facility RVU | 🔖 Non-Facility RVU | ▣ CCI | ✖ CLIA |
| **FUD** Follow-up Days | **CMS:** IOM | **AMA:** CPT Asst | A-Y OPPSI | 80/80 Surg Assist Allowed / w/Doc | ◼ Lab Crosswalk | | ✖ Radiology Crosswalk |

83885   **Nickel**

    0.00   0.00   **FUD** XXX

AMA: 2015,Jun,10; 2015,Apr,3

83915-84066 Chemistry: Nucleotidase 5'- —Phosphatase (Acid)

INCLUDES   Clinical information not requested by the ordering physician
Mathematically calculated results
Quantitative analysis unless otherwise specified
Specimens from any source unless otherwise specified

EXCLUDES   *Analytes from nonrequested laboratory analysis*
Calculated results that represent a score or probability that was derived by algorithm
Drug testing ([80305, 80306, 80307], [80324, 80325, 80326, 80327, 80328, 80329, 80330, 80331, 80332, 80333, 80334, 80335, 80336, 80337, 80338, 80339, 80340, 80341, 80342, 80343, 80344, 80345, 80346, 80347, 80348, 80349, 80350, 80351, 80352, 80353, 80354, 80355, 80356, 80357, 80358, 80359, 80360, 80361, 80362, 80363, 80364, 80365, 80366, 80367, 80368, 80369, 80370, 80371, 80372, 80373, 80374, 80375, 80376, 80377, 83992])
Organ or disease panels (80048-80076 [80081])
Therapeutic drug assays (80150-80299 [80164, 80165, 80171])

83915   **Nucleotidase 5'-**

    0.00   0.00   **FUD** XXX

AMA: 2015,Jun,10; 2015,Apr,3

83916   **Oligoclonal immune (oligoclonal bands)**

    0.00   0.00   **FUD** XXX

AMA: 2015,Jun,10; 2015,Apr,3

83918   **Organic acids; total, quantitative, each specimen**

    0.00   0.00   **FUD** XXX

AMA: 2018,Jan,8; 2017,Jan,8; 2016,Jan,13; 2015,Jun,10; 2015,Apr,3; 2015,Jan,16; 2014,Jan,11

83919   **qualitative, each specimen**

    0.00   0.00   **FUD** XXX

AMA: 2015,Jun,10; 2015,Apr,3

83921   **Organic acid, single, quantitative**

    0.00   0.00   **FUD** XXX

AMA: 2015,Jun,10; 2015,Apr,3

83930   **Osmolality; blood**

EXCLUDES   *Tear osmolarity (83861)*

    0.00   0.00   **FUD** XXX

AMA: 2015,Jun,10; 2015,Apr,3

83935   **urine**

EXCLUDES   *Tear osmolarity (83861)*

    0.00   0.00   **FUD** XXX

AMA: 2015,Jun,10; 2015,Apr,3

83937   **Osteocalcin (bone g1a protein)**

    0.00   0.00   **FUD** XXX

AMA: 2018,Jan,8; 2017,Jan,8; 2016,Jan,13; 2015,Jun,10; 2015,Apr,3; 2015,Jan,16; 2014,Jan,11

83945   **Oxalate**

    0.00   0.00   **FUD** XXX

AMA: 2015,Jun,10; 2015,Apr,3

83950   **Oncoprotein; HER-2/neu**

EXCLUDES   *Tissue (88342, 88365)*

    0.00   0.00   **FUD** XXX

AMA: 2015,Jun,10; 2015,Apr,3

83951   **des-gamma-carboxy-prothrombin (DCP)**

    0.00   0.00   **FUD** XXX

AMA: 2015,Jun,10; 2015,Apr,3

83970   **Parathormone (parathyroid hormone)**

EXCLUDES   *Chlorinated hydrocarbon screen (82441)*
Quantitative pesticide report code for specific method

    0.00   0.00   **FUD** XXX

AMA: 2015,Jun,10; 2015,Apr,3

83986   **pH; body fluid, not otherwise specified**

EXCLUDES   *Blood pH (82800, 82803)*

    0.00   0.00   **FUD** XXX

AMA: 2018,Jan,8; 2017,Jan,8; 2016,May,13; 2016,Jan,13; 2015,Jun,10; 2015,Apr,3; 2015,Jan,16

83987   **exhaled breath condensate**

EXCLUDES   *Blood pH (82800, 82803)*
Phenobarbital ([80345])

    0.00   0.00   **FUD** XXX

AMA: 2015,Jun,10; 2015,Apr,3

83992   **Resequenced code. See code following resequenced code 80365.**

83993   **Calprotectin, fecal**

    0.00   0.00   **FUD** XXX

AMA: 2018,Jan,8; 2017,Jan,8; 2016,Jan,13; 2015,Jun,10; 2015,Apr,3; 2015,Jan,16; 2014,Jan,11

84030   **Phenylalanine (PKU), blood**

INCLUDES   Guthrie test

EXCLUDES   *Phenylalanine-tyrosine ratio (84030, 84510)*

    0.00   0.00   **FUD** XXX

AMA: 2015,Jun,10; 2015,Apr,3

84035   **Phenylketones, qualitative**

    0.00   0.00   **FUD** XXX

AMA: 2015,Jun,10; 2015,Apr,3

84060   **Phosphatase, acid; total**

    0.00   0.00   **FUD** XXX

AMA: 2015,Jun,10; 2015,Apr,3

84066   **prostatic**

    0.00   0.00   **FUD** XXX

AMA: 2015,Jun,10; 2015,Apr,3

84075-84080 Chemistry: Phosphatase (Alkaline)

CMS: 100-03,160.17 Payment for L-Dopa /Associated Inpatient Hospital Services

INCLUDES   Clinical information not requested by the ordering physician
Mathematically calculated results
Quantitative analysis unless otherwise specified
Specimens from any source unless otherwise specified

EXCLUDES   *Analytes from nonrequested laboratory analysis*
Calculated results that represent a score or probability that was derived by algorithm
Organ or disease panels (80048-80076 [80081])

84075   **Phosphatase, alkaline;**

    0.00   0.00   **FUD** XXX

AMA: 2018,Jan,8; 2017,Jan,8; 2016,Jan,13; 2015,Jun,10; 2015,Apr,3; 2015,Jan,16; 2014,Jan,11

84078   **heat stable (total not included)**

    0.00   0.00   **FUD** XXX

AMA: 2015,Jun,10; 2015,Apr,3

84080   **isoenzymes**

    0.00   0.00   **FUD** XXX

AMA: 2015,Jun,10; 2015,Apr,3

84081-84150 Chemistry: Phosphatidylglycerol—Prostaglandin

INCLUDES   Clinical information not requested by the ordering physician
Mathematically calculated results
Quantitative analysis unless otherwise specified
Specimens from any source unless otherwise specified

EXCLUDES   *Analytes from nonrequested laboratory analysis*
Calculated results that represent a score or probability that was derived by algorithm
Organ or disease panels (80048-80076 [80081])
Therapeutic drug assays (80150-80299 [80164, 80165, 80171])

84081   **Phosphatidylglycerol**

EXCLUDES   *Cholinesterase (82480, 82482)*
Inorganic phosphates (84100)
Organic phosphates, report code for specific method

    0.00   0.00   **FUD** XXX

AMA: 2015,Jun,10; 2015,Apr,3

84085   **Phosphogluconate, 6-, dehydrogenase, RBC**

    0.00   0.00   **FUD** XXX

AMA: 2015,Jun,10; 2015,Apr,3

84087   **Phosphohexose isomerase**

    0.00   0.00   **FUD** XXX

AMA: 2015,Jun,10; 2015,Apr,3

84100 Phosphorus inorganic (phosphate);
🚑 0.00 ⚖ 0.00 **FUD** XXX ⬜⬜
AMA: 2018,Jan,8; 2017,Jan,8; 2016,Jan,13; 2015,Jun,10; 2015,Apr,3; 2015,Jan,16; 2014,Jan,11

84105 urine
EXCLUDES Pituitary gonadotropins (83001-83002)
PKU (84030, 84035)
🚑 0.00 ⚖ 0.00 **FUD** XXX ⬜⬜
AMA: 2015,Jun,10; 2015,Apr,3

84106 Porphobilinogen, urine; qualitative
🚑 0.00 ⚖ 0.00 **FUD** XXX ⬜⬜
AMA: 2015,Jun,10; 2015,Apr,3

84110 quantitative
🚑 0.00 ⚖ 0.00 **FUD** XXX ⬜⬜
AMA: 2015,Jun,10; 2015,Apr,3

84112 Evaluation of cervicovaginal fluid for specific amniotic fluid protein(s) (eg, placental alpha microglobulin-1 [PAMG-1], placental protein 12 [PP12], alpha-fetoprotein), qualitative, each specimen ♀
🚑 0.00 ⚖ 0.00 **FUD** XXX ⬜⬜
AMA: 2015,Jun,10; 2015,Apr,3

84119 Porphyrins, urine; qualitative
🚑 0.00 ⚖ 0.00 **FUD** XXX ⬜⬜
AMA: 2015,Jun,10; 2015,Apr,3

84120 quantitation and fractionation
🚑 0.00 ⚖ 0.00 **FUD** XXX ⬜⬜
AMA: 2015,Jun,10; 2015,Apr,3

84126 Porphyrins, feces, quantitative
EXCLUDES Porphyrin precursors (82135, 84106, 84110)
Protoporphyrin, RBC (84202, 84203)
🚑 0.00 ⚖ 0.00 **FUD** XXX ⬜⬜
AMA: 2015,Jun,10; 2015,Apr,3

84132 Potassium; serum, plasma or whole blood
🚑 0.00 ⚖ 0.00 **FUD** XXX ❎⬜⬜
AMA: 2018,Jan,8; 2017,Jan,8; 2016,Jan,13; 2015,Jun,10; 2015,Apr,3; 2015,Jan,16; 2014,Jan,11

84133 urine
🚑 0.00 ⚖ 0.00 **FUD** XXX ⬜⬜
AMA: 2015,Jun,10; 2015,Apr,3

84134 Prealbumin
EXCLUDES Microalbumin (82043-82044)
🚑 0.00 ⚖ 0.00 **FUD** XXX ⬜⬜
AMA: 2015,Jun,10; 2015,Apr,3

84135 Pregnanediol ♀
🚑 0.00 ⚖ 0.00 **FUD** XXX ⬜⬜
AMA: 2015,Jun,10; 2015,Apr,3

84138 Pregnanetriol ♀
🚑 0.00 ⚖ 0.00 **FUD** XXX ⬜⬜
AMA: 2015,Jun,10; 2015,Apr,3

84140 Pregnenolone
🚑 0.00 ⚖ 0.00 **FUD** XXX ⬜⬜
AMA: 2018,Jan,8; 2017,Jan,8; 2016,Jan,13; 2015,Jun,10; 2015,Apr,3; 2015,Jan,16; 2014,Jan,11

84143 17-hydroxypregnenolone
🚑 0.00 ⚖ 0.00 **FUD** XXX ⬜⬜
AMA: 2018,Jan,8; 2017,Jan,8; 2016,Jan,13; 2015,Jun,10; 2015,Apr,3; 2015,Jan,16; 2014,Jan,11

84144 Progesterone
EXCLUDES Progesterone receptor assay (84234)
Proinsulin (84206)
🚑 0.00 ⚖ 0.00 **FUD** XXX ⬜⬜
AMA: 2015,Jun,10; 2015,Apr,3

84145 Procalcitonin (PCT)
🚑 0.00 ⚖ 0.00 **FUD** XXX ⬜⬜
AMA: 2015,Jun,10; 2015,Apr,3

84146 Prolactin
🚑 0.00 ⚖ 0.00 **FUD** XXX ⬜⬜
AMA: 2015,Jun,10; 2015,Apr,3

84150 Prostaglandin, each
🚑 0.00 ⚖ 0.00 **FUD** XXX ⬜⬜
AMA: 2015,Jun,10; 2015,Apr,3

84152-84154 Chemistry: Prostate Specific Antigen

CMS: 100-03,190.31 Prostate Specific Antigen (PSA); 100-03,210.1 Prostate Cancer Screening Tests
INCLUDES Clinical information not requested by the ordering physician
Mathematically calculated results
Quantitative analysis unless otherwise specified
EXCLUDES Analytes from nonrequested laboratory analysis
Calculated results that represent a score or probability that was derived by algorithm

84152 Prostate specific antigen (PSA); complexed (direct measurement) ♂
🚑 0.00 ⚖ 0.00 **FUD** XXX ⬜⬜
AMA: 2015,Jun,10; 2015,Apr,3

84153 total ♂
🚑 0.00 ⚖ 0.00 **FUD** XXX ⬜⬜
AMA: 2018,Jan,8; 2017,Jan,8; 2016,Jan,13; 2015,Jun,10; 2015,Apr,3; 2015,Jan,16; 2014,Jan,11

84154 free ♂
🚑 0.00 ⚖ 0.00 **FUD** XXX ⬜⬜
AMA: 2018,Jan,8; 2017,Jan,8; 2016,Jan,13; 2015,Jun,10; 2015,Apr,3; 2015,Jan,16; 2014,Jan,11

84155-84157 Chemistry: Protein, Total (Not by Refractometry)

INCLUDES Clinical information not requested by the ordering physician
Mathematically calculated results
EXCLUDES Analytes from nonrequested laboratory analysis
Calculated results that represent a score or probability that was derived by algorithm
Organ or disease panels (80048-80076 [80081])

84155 Protein, total, except by refractometry; serum, plasma or whole blood
🚑 0.00 ⚖ 0.00 **FUD** XXX ❎⬜⬜
AMA: 2018,Jan,8; 2017,Jan,8; 2016,Jan,13; 2015,Jun,10; 2015,Apr,3; 2015,Jan,16; 2014,Jan,11

84156 urine
🚑 0.00 ⚖ 0.00 **FUD** XXX ⬜⬜
AMA: 2015,Jun,10; 2015,Apr,3

84157 other source (eg, synovial fluid, cerebrospinal fluid)
🚑 0.00 ⚖ 0.00 **FUD** XXX ⬜⬜
AMA: 2015,Jun,10; 2015,Apr,3

84160-84432 Chemistry: Protein, Total (Refractometry)—Thyroglobulin

INCLUDES Clinical information not requested by the ordering physician
Mathematically calculated results
Quantitative analysis unless otherwise specified
Specimens from any source unless otherwise specified
EXCLUDES Analytes from nonrequested laboratory analysis
Calculated results that represent a score or probability that was derived by algorithm
Drug testing ([80305, 80306, 80307], [80324, 80325, 80326, 80327, 80328, 80329, 80330, 80331, 80332, 80333, 80334, 80335, 80336, 80337, 80338, 80339, 80340, 80341, 80342, 80343, 80344, 80345, 80346, 80347, 80348, 80349, 80350, 80351, 80352, 80353, 80354, 80355, 80356, 80357, 80358, 80359, 80360, 80361, 80362, 80363, 80364, 80365, 80366, 80367, 80368, 80369, 80370, 80371, 80372, 80373, 80374, 80375, 80376, 80377, 83992])
Organ or disease panels (80048-80076 [80081])
Therapeutic drug assays (80150-80299 [80164, 80165, 80171])

84160 Protein, total, by refractometry, any source
EXCLUDES Urine total protein, dipstick method (81000-81003)
🚑 0.00 ⚖ 0.00 **FUD** XXX ⬜⬜
AMA: 2015,Jun,10; 2015,Apr,3

84163 Pregnancy-associated plasma protein-A (PAPP-A) ♀
🚑 0.00 ⚖ 0.00 **FUD** XXX ⬜⬜
AMA: 2015,Jun,10; 2015,Apr,3

26/TC PC/TC Only A2-Z3 ASC Payment 50 Bilateral ♂ Male Only ♀ Female Only 🚑 Facility RVU ⚖ Non-Facility RVU ⬜ CCI ❎ CLIA
FUD Follow-up Days **CMS:** IOM **AMA:** CPT Asst A-Y OPPSI 80/80 Surg Assist Allowed / w/Doc Lab Crosswalk Radiology Crosswalk

84165 Protein; electrophoretic fractionation and quantitation, serum

    0.00   0.00   **FUD** XXX   Q 80

    AMA: 2015,Jun,10; 2015,Apr,3

84166 electrophoretic fractionation and quantitation, other fluids with concentration (eg, urine, CSF)

    0.00   0.00   **FUD** XXX   Q 80

    AMA: 2015,Jun,10; 2015,Apr,3

84181 Western Blot, with interpretation and report, blood or other body fluid

    0.00   0.00   **FUD** XXX   Q 80

    AMA: 2015,Jun,10; 2015,Apr,3

84182 Western Blot, with interpretation and report, blood or other body fluid, immunological probe for band identification, each

    EXCLUDES   *Western Blot tissue analysis (88371)*

    0.00   0.00   **FUD** XXX   Q 80

    AMA: 2015,Jun,10; 2015,Apr,3

84202 Protoporphyrin, RBC; quantitative

    0.00   0.00   **FUD** XXX   Q

    AMA: 2015,Jun,10; 2015,Apr,3

84203 screen

    0.00   0.00   **FUD** XXX   Q

    AMA: 2015,Jun,10; 2015,Apr,3

84206 Proinsulin

    EXCLUDES   *Pseudocholinesterase (82480)*

    0.00   0.00   **FUD** XXX   Q

    AMA: 2015,Jun,10; 2015,Apr,3

84207 Pyridoxal phosphate (Vitamin B-6)

    0.00   0.00   **FUD** XXX   Q

    AMA: 2015,Jun,10; 2015,Apr,3

84210 Pyruvate

    0.00   0.00   **FUD** XXX   Q

    AMA: 2015,Jun,10; 2015,Apr,3

84220 Pyruvate kinase

    0.00   0.00   **FUD** XXX   Q

    AMA: 2015,Jun,10; 2015,Apr,3

84228 Quinine

    0.00   0.00   **FUD** XXX   Q

    AMA: 2018,Jan,8; 2017,Jan,8; 2016,Jan,13; 2015,Jun,10; 2015,Apr,3

84233 Receptor assay; estrogen

    0.00   0.00   **FUD** XXX   Q

    AMA: 2015,Jun,10; 2015,Apr,3

84234 progesterone

    0.00   0.00   **FUD** XXX   Q

    AMA: 2015,Jun,10; 2015,Apr,3

84235 endocrine, other than estrogen or progesterone (specify hormone)

    0.00   0.00   **FUD** XXX   Q

    AMA: 2015,Jun,10; 2015,Apr,3

84238 non-endocrine (specify receptor)

    0.00   0.00   **FUD** XXX   Q

    AMA: 2018,Jan,8; 2017,Jan,8; 2016,Jan,13; 2015,Jun,10; 2015,Apr,3; 2015,Jan,16; 2014,Jan,11

84244 Renin

    0.00   0.00   **FUD** XXX   Q

    AMA: 2015,Jun,10; 2015,Apr,3

84252 Riboflavin (Vitamin B-2)

    EXCLUDES   *Salicylates ([80329], [80330], [80331])*
        Secretin test reported with appropriate analyses (43756, 43757, 99070)

    0.00   0.00   **FUD** XXX   Q

    AMA: 2015,Jun,10; 2015,Apr,3

84255 Selenium

    0.00   0.00   **FUD** XXX   Q

    AMA: 2015,Jun,10; 2015,Apr,3

84260 Serotonin

    EXCLUDES   *Urine metabolites (HIAA) (83497)*

    0.00   0.00   **FUD** XXX   Q

    AMA: 2015,Jun,10; 2015,Apr,3

84270 Sex hormone binding globulin (SHBG)

    0.00   0.00   **FUD** XXX   Q

    AMA: 2018,Jan,8; 2017,Jan,8; 2016,Jan,13; 2015,Jun,10; 2015,Apr,3; 2015,Jan,16; 2014,Jan,11

84275 Sialic acid

    EXCLUDES   *Sickle hemoglobin (85660)*

    0.00   0.00   **FUD** XXX   Q

    AMA: 2015,Jun,10; 2015,Apr,3

84285 Silica

    0.00   0.00   **FUD** XXX   Q

    AMA: 2015,Jun,10; 2015,Apr,3

84295 Sodium; serum, plasma or whole blood

    0.00   0.00   **FUD** XXX   X Q

    AMA: 2018,Jan,8; 2017,Jan,8; 2016,Jan,13; 2015,Jun,10; 2015,Apr,3; 2015,Jan,16; 2014,Jan,11

84300 urine

    0.00   0.00   **FUD** XXX   Q

    AMA: 2015,Jun,10; 2015,Apr,3

84302 other source

    EXCLUDES   *Somatomammotropin (83632)*
        Somatotropin (83003)

    0.00   0.00   **FUD** XXX   Q

    AMA: 2018,Jan,8; 2017,Jan,8; 2016,Jan,13; 2015,Jun,10; 2015,Apr,3; 2015,Jan,16; 2014,Jan,11

84305 Somatomedin

    0.00   0.00   **FUD** XXX   Q

    AMA: 2018,Jan,8; 2017,Jan,8; 2016,Jan,13; 2015,Jun,10; 2015,Apr,3; 2015,Jan,16; 2014,Jan,11

84307 Somatostatin

    0.00   0.00   **FUD** XXX   Q

    AMA: 2018,Jan,8; 2017,Jan,8; 2016,Jan,13; 2015,Jun,10; 2015,Apr,3; 2015,Jan,16; 2014,Jan,11

84311 Spectrophotometry, analyte not elsewhere specified

    0.00   0.00   **FUD** XXX   Q

    AMA: 2015,Jun,10; 2015,Apr,3

84315 Specific gravity (except urine)

    EXCLUDES   *Stone analysis (82355-82370)*
        Suppression of growth stimulation expressed gene 2 [ST2] testing (83006)
        Urine specific gravity (81000-81003)

    0.00   0.00   **FUD** XXX   Q

    AMA: 2015,Jun,10; 2015,Apr,3

84375 Sugars, chromatographic, TLC or paper chromatography

    0.00   0.00   **FUD** XXX   Q

    AMA: 2015,Jun,10; 2015,Apr,3

84376 Sugars (mono-, di-, and oligosaccharides); single qualitative, each specimen

    0.00   0.00   **FUD** XXX   Q

    AMA: 2018,Jan,8; 2017,Jan,8; 2016,Jan,13; 2015,Jun,10; 2015,Apr,3; 2015,Jan,16; 2014,Jan,11

84377 multiple qualitative, each specimen

    0.00   0.00   **FUD** XXX   Q

    AMA: 2018,Jan,8; 2017,Jan,8; 2016,Jan,13; 2015,Jun,10; 2015,Apr,3; 2015,Jan,16; 2014,Jan,11

84378 single quantitative, each specimen

    0.00   0.00   **FUD** XXX   Q

    AMA: 2015,Jun,10; 2015,Apr,3

Pathology and Laboratory *(left margin)*

84379 — 84478 *(left margin)*

84379 multiple quantitative, each specimen
🚑 0.00   ⚕ 0.00   **FUD** XXX   🔲🔳
AMA: 2018,Jan,8; 2017,Jan,8; 2016,Jan,13; 2015,Jun,10; 2015,Apr,3; 2015,Jan,16; 2014,Jan,11

84392 **Sulfate, urine**
EXCLUDES   *Sulfhemoglobin (83060)*
T-3 (84479-84481)
T-4 (84436-84439)
🚑 0.00   ⚕ 0.00   **FUD** XXX   🔲🔳
AMA: 2015,Jun,10; 2015,Apr,3

84402 **Testosterone; free**
EXCLUDES   *Anabolic steroids ([80327, 80328])*
🚑 0.00   ⚕ 0.00   **FUD** XXX   🔲🔳
AMA: 2015,Jun,10; 2015,Apr,3

84403 total
EXCLUDES   *Anabolic steroids ([80327, 80328])*
🚑 0.00   ⚕ 0.00   **FUD** XXX   🔲🔳
AMA: 2015,Jun,10; 2015,Apr,3

84410 bioavailable, direct measurement (eg, differential precipitation)
🚑 0.00   ⚕ 0.00   **FUD** XXX   🔲🔳

84425 **Thiamine (Vitamin B-1)**
🚑 0.00   ⚕ 0.00   **FUD** XXX   🔲🔳
AMA: 2015,Jun,10; 2015,Apr,3

84430 **Thiocyanate**
🚑 0.00   ⚕ 0.00   **FUD** XXX   🔲🔳
AMA: 2015,Jun,10; 2015,Apr,3

84431 **Thromboxane metabolite(s), including thromboxane if performed, urine**
Code also for determination of concurrent urine creatinine (82570)
🚑 0.00   ⚕ 0.00   **FUD** XXX   🔲🔳
AMA: 2015,Jun,10; 2015,Apr,3

84432 **Thyroglobulin**
EXCLUDES   *Thyroglobulin antibody (86800)*
Thyrotropin releasing hormone (TRH) (80438, 80439)
🚑 0.00   ⚕ 0.00   **FUD** XXX   🔲🔳
AMA: 2018,Jan,8; 2017,Jan,8; 2016,Jan,13; 2015,Jun,10; 2015,Apr,3; 2015,Jan,16; 2014,Jan,11

84436-84445 Chemistry: Thyroid Tests

CMS: 100-03,190.22 Thyroid Testing
INCLUDES   Clinical information not requested by the ordering physician
Mathematically calculated results
Quantitative analysis unless otherwise specified
Specimens from any source unless otherwise specified
EXCLUDES   *Analytes from nonrequested laboratory analysis*
Calculated results that represent a score or probability that was derived by algorithm
Organ or disease panels (80048-80076 [80081])
Therapeutic drug assays (80150-80299 [80164, 80165, 80171])

84436 **Thyroxine; total**
🚑 0.00   ⚕ 0.00   **FUD** XXX   🔲🔳
AMA: 2018,Jan,8; 2017,Jan,8; 2016,Jan,13; 2015,Jun,10; 2015,Apr,3; 2015,Jan,16; 2014,Jan,11

84437 requiring elution (eg, neonatal)
🚑 0.00   ⚕ 0.00   **FUD** XXX   🔲🔳
AMA: 2015,Jun,10; 2015,Apr,3

84439 free
🚑 0.00   ⚕ 0.00   **FUD** XXX   🔲🔳
AMA: 2015,Jun,10; 2015,Apr,3

84442 **Thyroxine binding globulin (TBG)**
🚑 0.00   ⚕ 0.00   **FUD** XXX   🔲🔳
AMA: 2015,Jun,10; 2015,Apr,3

84443 **Thyroid stimulating hormone (TSH)**
🚑 0.00   ⚕ 0.00   **FUD** XXX   ❌🔲🔳
AMA: 2015,Jun,10; 2015,Apr,3

84445 **Thyroid stimulating immune globulins (TSI)**
EXCLUDES   *Tobramycin (80200)*
🚑 0.00   ⚕ 0.00   **FUD** XXX   🔲🔳
AMA: 2018,Jan,8; 2017,Jan,8; 2016,Jan,13; 2015,Jun,10; 2015,Apr,3; 2015,Jan,16; 2014,Jan,11

84446-84449 Chemistry: Tocopherol Alpha—Transcortin

INCLUDES   Clinical information not requested by the ordering physician
Mathematically calculated results
Quantitative analysis unless otherwise specified
Specimens from any source unless otherwise specified
EXCLUDES   *Analytes from nonrequested laboratory analysis*
Calculated results that represent a score or probability that was derived by algorithm
Organ or disease panels (80048-80076 [80081])
Therapeutic drug assays (80150-80299 [80164, 80165, 80171])

84446 **Tocopherol alpha (Vitamin E)**
🚑 0.00   ⚕ 0.00   **FUD** XXX   🔲🔳
AMA: 2015,Jun,10; 2015,Apr,3

84449 **Transcortin (cortisol binding globulin)**
🚑 0.00   ⚕ 0.00   **FUD** XXX   🔲🔳
AMA: 2018,Jan,8; 2017,Jan,8; 2016,Jan,13; 2015,Jun,10; 2015,Apr,3; 2015,Jan,16; 2014,Jan,11

84450-84460 Chemistry: Transferase

CMS: 100-02,11,30.2.2 Automated Multi-Channel Chemistry (AMCC) Tests; 100-03,160.17 Payment for L-Dopa /Associated Inpatient Hospital Services; 100-04,16,40.6.1 Automated Multi-Channel Chemistry (AMCC) Tests for ESRD Beneficiaries; 100-04,16,70.8 CLIA Waived Tests
INCLUDES   Clinical information not requested by the ordering physician
Mathematically calculated results
Quantitative analysis unless otherwise specified
EXCLUDES   *Analytes from nonrequested laboratory analysis*
Calculated results that represent a score or probability that was derived by algorithm

84450 **Transferase; aspartate amino (AST) (SGOT)**
🚑 0.00   ⚕ 0.00   **FUD** XXX   ❌🔲🔳
AMA: 2018,Jan,8; 2017,Jan,8; 2016,Jan,13; 2015,Jun,10; 2015,Apr,3; 2015,Jan,16; 2014,Jan,11

84460 alanine amino (ALT) (SGPT)
🚑 0.00   ⚕ 0.00   **FUD** XXX   ❌🔲🔳
AMA: 2018,Jan,8; 2017,Jan,8; 2016,Jan,13; 2015,Jun,10; 2015,Apr,3; 2015,Jan,16; 2014,Jan,11

84466 Chemistry: Transferrin

CMS: 100-02,11,20.2 ESRD Laboratory Services; 100-03,190.18 Serum Iron Studies
INCLUDES   Clinical information not requested by the ordering physician
Mathematically calculated results
Quantitative analysis unless otherwise specified
EXCLUDES   *Analytes from nonrequested laboratory analysis*
Calculated results that represent a score or probability that was derived by algorithm

84466 **Transferrin**
EXCLUDES   *Iron binding capacity (83550)*
🚑 0.00   ⚕ 0.00   **FUD** XXX   🔲🔳
AMA: 2018,Jan,8; 2017,Jan,8; 2016,Jan,13; 2015,Jun,10; 2015,Apr,3; 2015,Jan,16; 2014,Jan,11

84478 Chemistry: Triglycerides

CMS: 100-02,11,30.2.2 Automated Multi-Channel Chemistry (AMCC) Tests; 100-03,190.23 Lipid Testing; 100-04,16,70.8 CLIA Waived Tests; 100-04,16,90.2 Organ or Disease Oriented Panels
INCLUDES   Clinical information not requested by the ordering physician
Mathematically calculated results
EXCLUDES   *Analytes from nonrequested laboratory analysis*
Calculated results that represent a score or probability that was derived by algorithm
Organ or disease panels (80048-80076 [80081])

84478 **Triglycerides**
🚑 0.00   ⚕ 0.00   **FUD** XXX   ❌🅰🔳
AMA: 2018,Jan,8; 2017,Jan,8; 2016,Jan,13; 2015,Jun,10; 2015,Apr,3; 2015,Jan,16; 2014,Jan,11

  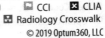

26/TC PC/TC Only   A2-Z3 ASC Payment   50 Bilateral   ♂ Male Only   ♀ Female Only   🚑 Facility RVU   ⚕ Non-Facility RVU   🔳 CCI   ❌ CLIA
FUD Follow-up Days   **CMS:** IOM   **AMA:** CPT Asst   A-Y OPPSI   80/80 Surg Assist Allowed / w/Doc   Lab Crosswalk   Radiology Crosswalk

CPT © 2019 American Medical Association. All Rights Reserved.

416   © 2019 Optum360, LLC

84479-84482 Chemistry: Thyroid Hormone—Triiodothyronine

CMS: 100-03,190.22 Thyroid Testing

INCLUDES Clinical information not requested by the ordering physician
Mathematically calculated results
Quantitative analysis unless otherwise specified
Specimens from any source unless otherwise specified

EXCLUDES Analytes from nonrequested laboratory analysis
Calculated results that represent a score or probability that was derived by algorithm
Organ or disease panels (80048-80076 [80081])

84479 **Thyroid hormone (T3 or T4) uptake or thyroid hormone binding ratio (THBR)**

0.00   0.00   **FUD** XXX

AMA: 2018,Jan,8; 2017,Jan,8; 2016,Jan,13; 2015,Jun,10; 2015,Apr,3; 2015,Jan,16; 2014,Jan,11

84480 **Triiodothyronine T3; total (TT-3)**

0.00   0.00   **FUD** XXX

AMA: 2015,Jun,10; 2015,Apr,3

84481 **free**

0.00   0.00   **FUD** XXX

AMA: 2015,Jun,10; 2015,Apr,3

84482 **reverse**

0.00   0.00   **FUD** XXX

AMA: 2018,Jan,8; 2017,Jan,8; 2016,Jan,13; 2015,Jun,10; 2015,Apr,3; 2015,Jan,16; 2014,Jan,11

84484-84512 Chemistry: Troponin (Quantitative)—Troponin (Qualitative)

INCLUDES Clinical information not requested by the ordering physician
Mathematically calculated results
Specimens from any source unless otherwise specified

EXCLUDES Analytes from nonrequested laboratory analysis
Calculated results that represent a score or probability that was derived by algorithm
Organ or disease panels

84484 **Troponin, quantitative**

EXCLUDES Qualitative troponin assay (84512)

0.00   0.00   **FUD** XXX

AMA: 2018,Jan,8; 2017,Jan,8; 2016,Jan,13; 2015,Jun,10; 2015,Apr,3; 2015,Jan,16; 2014,Jan,11

84485 **Trypsin; duodenal fluid**

0.00   0.00   **FUD** XXX

AMA: 2015,Jun,10; 2015,Apr,3

84488 **feces, qualitative**

0.00   0.00   **FUD** XXX

AMA: 2015,Jun,10; 2015,Apr,3

84490 **feces, quantitative, 24-hour collection**

0.00   0.00   **FUD** XXX

AMA: 2015,Jun,10; 2015,Apr,3

84510 **Tyrosine**

EXCLUDES Urate crystal identification (89060)

0.00   0.00   **FUD** XXX

AMA: 2015,Jun,10; 2015,Apr,3

84512 **Troponin, qualitative**

EXCLUDES Quantitative troponin assay (84484)

0.00   0.00   **FUD** XXX

AMA: 2018,Jan,8; 2017,Jan,8; 2016,Jan,13; 2015,Jun,10; 2015,Apr,3; 2015,Jan,16; 2014,Jan,11

84520-84525 Chemistry: Urea Nitrogen (Blood)

CMS: 100-03,160.17 Payment for L-Dopa /Associated Inpatient Hospital Services

INCLUDES Clinical information not requested by the ordering physician
Mathematically calculated results

EXCLUDES Analytes from nonrequested laboratory analysis
Calculated results that represent a score or probability that was derived by algorithm
Organ or disease panels (80048-80076 [80081])

84520 **Urea nitrogen; quantitative**

0.00   0.00

AMA: 2018,Jan,8; 2017,Jan,8; 2016,Jan,13; 2015,Jun,10; 2015,Apr,3; 2015,Jan,16; 2014,Jan,11

84525 **semiquantitative (eg, reagent strip test)**

INCLUDES Patterson's test

0.00   0.00   **FUD** XXX

AMA: 2018,Jan,8; 2017,Jan,8; 2016,Jan,13; 2015,Jun,10; 2015,Apr,3; 2015,Jan,16; 2014,Jan,11

84540-84630 Chemistry: Urea Nitrogen (Urine)—Zinc

INCLUDES Clinical information not requested by the ordering physician
Mathematically calculated results
Quantitative analysis unless otherwise specified
Specimens from any source unless otherwise specified

EXCLUDES Analytes from nonrequested laboratory analysis
Calculated results that represent a score or probability that was derived by algorithm
Organ or disease panels (80048-80076 [80081])
Therapeutic drug assays (80150-80299 [80164, 80165, 80171])

84540 **Urea nitrogen, urine**

0.00   0.00   **FUD** XXX

AMA: 2015,Jun,10; 2015,Apr,3

84545 **Urea nitrogen, clearance**

0.00   0.00   **FUD** XXX

AMA: 2015,Jun,10; 2015,Apr,3

84550 **Uric acid; blood**

0.00   0.00   **FUD** XXX

AMA: 2018,Jan,8; 2017,Jan,8; 2016,Jan,13; 2015,Jun,10; 2015,Apr,3; 2015,Jan,16; 2014,Jan,11

84560 **other source**

0.00   0.00   **FUD** XXX

AMA: 2015,Jun,10; 2015,Apr,3

84577 **Urobilinogen, feces, quantitative**

0.00   0.00   **FUD** XXX

AMA: 2015,Jun,10; 2015,Apr,3

84578 **Urobilinogen, urine; qualitative**

0.00   0.00   **FUD** XXX

AMA: 2015,Jun,10; 2015,Apr,3

84580 **quantitative, timed specimen**

0.00   0.00   **FUD** XXX

AMA: 2015,Jun,10; 2015,Apr,3

84583 **semiquantitative**

EXCLUDES Uroporphyrins (84120)
Valproic acid (dipropylacetic acid) ([80164])

0.00   0.00   **FUD** XXX

AMA: 2015,Jun,10; 2015,Apr,3

84585 **Vanillylmandelic acid (VMA), urine**

0.00   0.00   **FUD** XXX

AMA: 2015,Jun,10; 2015,Apr,3

84586 **Vasoactive intestinal peptide (VIP)**

0.00   0.00   **FUD** XXX

AMA: 2018,Jan,8; 2017,Jan,8; 2016,Jan,13; 2015,Jun,10; 2015,Apr,3; 2015,Jan,16; 2014,Jan,11

84588 **Vasopressin (antidiuretic hormone, ADH)**

0.00   0.00   **FUD** XXX

AMA: 2018,Jan,7; 2015,Jun,10; 2015,Apr,3

84590   Vitamin A
         EXCLUDES   Vitamin B-1 (84425)
                     Vitamin B-2 (84252)
                     Vitamin B-6 (84207)
                     Vitamin B-12 (82607)
                     Vitamin C (82180)
                     Vitamin D (82306, [82652])
                     Vitamin E (84446)
         ⚕ 0.00   ⚕ 0.00   FUD XXX   🔲🔲
         AMA: 2015,Jun,10; 2015,Apr,3

84591   Vitamin, not otherwise specified
         ⚕ 0.00   ⚕ 0.00   FUD XXX   🔲🔲
         AMA: 2015,Jun,10; 2015,Apr,3

84597   Vitamin K
         EXCLUDES   Vanillylmandelic acid (VMA) (84585)
         ⚕ 0.00   ⚕ 0.00   FUD XXX   🔲🔲
         AMA: 2015,Jun,10; 2015,Apr,3

84600   Volatiles (eg, acetic anhydride, diethylether)
         EXCLUDES   Carbon tetrachloride, dichloroethane, dichloromethane
                     (82441)
                     Isopropyl alcohol and methanol ([80320])
                     Volume, blood, RISA, or Cr-51 (78110, 78111)
         ⚕ 0.00   ⚕ 0.00   FUD XXX   🔲🔲
         AMA: 2015,Jun,10; 2015,Apr,3

84620   Xylose absorption test, blood and/or urine
         EXCLUDES   Administration (99070)
         ⚕ 0.00   ⚕ 0.00   FUD XXX   🔲🔲
         AMA: 2015,Jun,10; 2015,Apr,3

84630   Zinc
         ⚕ 0.00   ⚕ 0.00   FUD XXX   🔲🔲
         AMA: 2015,Jun,10; 2015,Apr,3

84681-84999 Other and Unlisted Chemistry Tests

INCLUDES   Clinical information not requested by the ordering physician
            Mathematically calculated results
            Quantitative analysis unless otherwise specified
            Specimens from any source unless otherwise specified
EXCLUDES   Analytes from nonrequested laboratory analysis
            Calculated results that represent a score or probability that was derived by
               algorithm
            Confirmatory testing of a not otherwise specified drug ([80375, 80376,
               80377], 80299)
            Organ or disease panels (80048-80076 [80081])

84681   C-peptide
         ⚕ 0.00   ⚕ 0.00   FUD XXX   🔲🔲
         AMA: 2015,Jun,10; 2015,Apr,3

84702   Gonadotropin, chorionic (hCG); quantitative
         ⚕ 0.00   ⚕ 0.00   FUD XXX   🔲🔲
         AMA: 2015,Jun,10; 2015,Apr,3

84703   qualitative
         EXCLUDES   Urine pregnancy test by visual color comparison (81025)
         ⚕ 0.00   ⚕ 0.00   FUD XXX   ✖🔲🔲
         AMA: 2015,Jun,10; 2015,Apr,3

84704   free beta chain
         ⚕ 0.00   ⚕ 0.00   FUD XXX   🔲🔲
         AMA: 2018,Jan,8; 2017,Jan,8; 2016,Jan,13; 2015,Jun,10;
         2015,Apr,3; 2015,Jan,16; 2014,Jan,11

84830   Ovulation tests, by visual color comparison methods for
         human luteinizing hormone   ♀
         ⚕ 0.00   ⚕ 0.00   FUD XXX   ✖🔲🔲
         AMA: 2018,Jan,8; 2017,Jan,8; 2016,Jan,13; 2015,Jun,10;
         2015,Apr,3

84999   Unlisted chemistry procedure
         EXCLUDES   Definitive drug testing, not otherwise specified ([80375],
                     [80376], [80377], 80299)
         ⚕ 0.00   ⚕ 0.00   FUD XXX   🔲🔲
         AMA: 2018,Jan,8; 2017,Jan,8; 2016,Jan,13; 2015,Apr,3;
         2015,Jan,16; 2014,Jan,11

85002 Bleeding Time Test

EXCLUDES   Agglutinins (86000, 86156, 86157)
            Antiplasmin (85410)
            Antithrombin III (85300, 85301)
            Blood banking procedures (86077-86079)

85002   Bleeding time
         ⚕ 0.00   ⚕ 0.00   FUD XXX   🔲🔲
         AMA: 2018,Jan,8; 2017,Jan,8; 2016,Jan,13; 2015,Jan,16;
         2014,Jan,11

85004-85049 Blood Counts

CMS: 100-03,190.15 Blood Counts
EXCLUDES   Agglutinins (86000, 86156-86157)
            Antiplasmin (85410)
            Antithrombin III (85300-85301)
            Blood banking procedures (86850-86999)

85004   Blood count; automated differential WBC count
         ⚕ 0.00   ⚕ 0.00   FUD XXX   🔲🔲
         AMA: 2018,Jan,8; 2017,Jan,8; 2016,Jan,13; 2015,Jan,16;
         2014,Jan,11

85007   blood smear, microscopic examination with manual
         differential WBC count
         ⚕ 0.00   ⚕ 0.00   FUD XXX   🔲🔲
         AMA: 2018,Jan,8; 2017,Jan,8; 2016,Jan,13; 2015,Jan,16;
         2014,Jan,11

85008   blood smear, microscopic examination without manual
         differential WBC count
         EXCLUDES   Cell count other fluids (eg, CSF) (89050-89051)
         ⚕ 0.00   ⚕ 0.00   FUD XXX   🔲🔲
         AMA: 2018,Jan,8; 2017,Jan,8; 2016,Jan,13; 2015,Jan,16;
         2014,Jan,11

85009   manual differential WBC count, buffy coat
         EXCLUDES   Eosinophils, nasal smear (89190)
         ⚕ 0.00   ⚕ 0.00   FUD XXX   🔲🔲
         AMA: 2018,Jan,8; 2017,Jan,8; 2016,Jan,13; 2015,Jan,16;
         2014,Jan,11

85013   spun microhematocrit
         ⚕ 0.00   ⚕ 0.00   FUD XXX   ✖🔲🔲
         AMA: 2005,Aug,7-8; 2005,Jul,11-12

85014   hematocrit (Hct)
         ⚕ 0.00   ⚕ 0.00   FUD XXX   ✖🔲🔲
         AMA: 2018,Jan,8; 2017,Jan,8; 2016,Jan,13; 2015,Jan,16;
         2014,Jan,11

85018   hemoglobin (Hgb)
         EXCLUDES   Immunoassay, hemoglobin, fecal (82274)
                     Other hemoglobin determination (83020-83069)
                     Transcutaneous hemoglobin measurement (88738)
         ⚕ 0.00   ⚕ 0.00   FUD XXX   ✖🔲🔲
         AMA: 2018,Jan,8; 2017,Jan,8; 2016,Jan,13; 2015,Jan,16;
         2014,Jan,11

85025   complete (CBC), automated (Hgb, Hct, RBC, WBC and
         platelet count) and automated differential WBC count
         ⚕ 0.00   ⚕ 0.00   FUD XXX   ✖🔲🔲
         AMA: 2018,Jan,8; 2017,Jan,8; 2016,Jan,13; 2015,Jan,16;
         2014,Jan,11

85027   complete (CBC), automated (Hgb, Hct, RBC, WBC and
         platelet count)
         ⚕ 0.00   ⚕ 0.00   FUD XXX   🔲🔲
         AMA: 2018,Jan,8; 2017,Jan,8; 2016,Jan,13; 2015,Jan,16;
         2014,Jan,11

85032   manual cell count (erythrocyte, leukocyte, or platelet)
         each
         ⚕ 0.00   ⚕ 0.00   FUD XXX   🔲🔲
         AMA: 2018,Jan,8; 2017,Jan,8; 2016,Jan,13; 2015,Jan,16;
         2014,Jan,11

26/TC PC/TC Only	A2-Z3 ASC Payment	50 Bilateral	♂ Male Only	♀ Female Only	⚕ Facility RVU	⚕ Non-Facility RVU	🔲 CCI	✖ CLIA
FUD Follow-up Days	CMS: IOM	AMA: CPT Asst	A-Y OPPSI	80/80 Surg Assist Allowed / w/Doc	🔲 Lab Crosswalk	🔲 Radiology Crosswalk		

418   CPT © 2019 American Medical Association. All Rights Reserved.   © 2019 Optum360, LLC

| 85041 | **red blood cell (RBC), automated** | | |

EXCLUDES *Complete blood count (85025, 85027)*

🚑 0.00 ⚕ 0.00 **FUD** XXX

AMA: 2018,Jan,8; 2017,Jan,8; 2016,Jan,13; 2015,Jan,16; 2014,Jan,11

| 85044 | **reticulocyte, manual** |

🚑 0.00 ⚕ 0.00 **FUD** XXX

AMA: 2018,Jan,8; 2017,Jan,8; 2016,Jan,13; 2015,Jan,16; 2014,Jan,11

| 85045 | **reticulocyte, automated** |

🚑 0.00 ⚕ 0.00 **FUD** XXX

AMA: 2018,Jan,8; 2017,Jan,8; 2016,Jan,13; 2015,Jan,16; 2014,Jan,11

| 85046 | **reticulocytes, automated, including 1 or more cellular parameters (eg, reticulocyte hemoglobin content [CHr], immature reticulocyte fraction [IRF], reticulocyte volume [MRV], RNA content), direct measurement** |

🚑 0.00 ⚕ 0.00 **FUD** XXX

AMA: 2005,Aug,7-8; 2005,Jul,11-12

| 85048 | **leukocyte (WBC), automated** |

🚑 0.00 ⚕ 0.00 **FUD** XXX

AMA: 2018,Jan,8; 2017,Jan,8; 2016,Jan,13; 2015,Jan,16; 2014,Jan,11

| 85049 | **platelet, automated** |

🚑 0.00 ⚕ 0.00 **FUD** XXX

AMA: 2005,Aug,7-8; 2005,Jul,11-12

85055-85705 Coagulopathy Testing

EXCLUDES *Agglutinins (86000, 86156-86157)*
Antiplasmin (85410)
Antithrombin III (85300-85301)
Blood banking procedures (86850-86999)

| 85055 | **Reticulated platelet assay** |

🚑 0.00 ⚕ 0.00 **FUD** XXX

AMA: 2005,Aug,7-8; 2005,Jul,11-12

| 85060 | **Blood smear, peripheral, interpretation by physician with written report** |

🚑 0.70 ⚕ 0.70 **FUD** XXX

AMA: 2005,Aug,7-8; 2005,Jul,11-12

| 85097 | **Bone marrow, smear interpretation** |

EXCLUDES *Bone biopsy (20220, 20225, 20240, 20245, 20250-20251)*
Special stains (88312-88313)

🚑 1.42 ⚕ 2.11 **FUD** XXX

AMA: 2018,Jan,8; 2017,Jan,8; 2016,Jan,13; 2015,Jan,16; 2014,Jan,11

| 85130 | **Chromogenic substrate assay** |

EXCLUDES *Circulating anticoagulant screen (mixing studies) (85611, 85732)*

🚑 0.00 ⚕ 0.00 **FUD** XXX

AMA: 2005,Aug,7-8; 2005,Jul,11-12

| 85170 | **Clot retraction** |

🚑 0.00 ⚕ 0.00 **FUD** XXX

AMA: 2005,Aug,7-8; 2005,Jul,11-12

| 85175 | **Clot lysis time, whole blood dilution** |

EXCLUDES *Clotting factor I (fibrinogen) (85384, 85385)*

🚑 0.00 ⚕ 0.00 **FUD** XXX

AMA: 2005,Aug,7-8; 2005,Jul,11-12

| 85210 | **Clotting; factor II, prothrombin, specific** |

EXCLUDES *Prothrombin time (85610-85611)*
Russell viper venom time (85612-85613)

🚑 0.00 ⚕ 0.00 **FUD** XXX

AMA: 2005,Aug,7-8; 2005,Jul,11-12

| 85220 | **factor V (AcG or proaccelerin), labile factor** |

🚑 0.00 ⚕ 0.00 **FUD** XXX

AMA: 2005,Aug,7-8; 2005,Jul,11-12

| 85230 | **factor VII (proconvertin, stable factor)** |

🚑 0.00 ⚕ 0.00 **FUD** XXX

AMA: 2005,Aug,7-8; 2005,Jul,11-12

| 85240 | **factor VIII (AHG), 1-stage** |

🚑 0.00 ⚕ 0.00 **FUD** XXX

AMA: 2005,Aug,7-8; 2005,Jul,11-12

| 85244 | **factor VIII related antigen** |

🚑 0.00 ⚕ 0.00 **FUD** XXX

AMA: 2005,Aug,7-8; 2005,Jul,11-12

| 85245 | **factor VIII, VW factor, ristocetin cofactor** |

🚑 0.00 ⚕ 0.00 **FUD** XXX

AMA: 2005,Aug,7-8; 2005,Jul,11-12

| 85246 | **factor VIII, VW factor antigen** |

🚑 0.00 ⚕ 0.00 **FUD** XXX

AMA: 2005,Aug,7-8; 2005,Jul,11-12

| 85247 | **factor VIII, von Willebrand factor, multimetric analysis** |

🚑 0.00 ⚕ 0.00 **FUD** XXX

AMA: 2005,Aug,7-8; 2005,Jul,11-12

| 85250 | **factor IX (PTC or Christmas)** |

🚑 0.00 ⚕ 0.00 **FUD** XXX

AMA: 2005,Aug,7-8; 2005,Jul,11-12

| 85260 | **factor X (Stuart-Prower)** |

🚑 0.00 ⚕ 0.00 **FUD** XXX

AMA: 2005,Aug,7-8; 2005,Jul,11-12

| 85270 | **factor XI (PTA)** |

🚑 0.00 ⚕ 0.00 **FUD** XXX

AMA: 2005,Aug,7-8; 2005,Jul,11-12

| 85280 | **factor XII (Hageman)** |

🚑 0.00 ⚕ 0.00 **FUD** XXX

AMA: 2005,Aug,7-8; 2005,Jul,11-12

| 85290 | **factor XIII (fibrin stabilizing)** |

🚑 0.00 ⚕ 0.00 **FUD** XXX

AMA: 2005,Aug,7-8; 2005,Jul,11-12

| 85291 | **factor XIII (fibrin stabilizing), screen solubility** |

🚑 0.00 ⚕ 0.00 **FUD** XXX

AMA: 2005,Aug,7-8; 2005,Jul,11-12

| 85292 | **prekallikrein assay (Fletcher factor assay)** |

🚑 0.00 ⚕ 0.00 **FUD** XXX

AMA: 2005,Aug,7-8; 2005,Jul,11-12

| 85293 | **high molecular weight kininogen assay (Fitzgerald factor assay)** |

🚑 0.00 ⚕ 0.00 **FUD** XXX

AMA: 2005,Aug,7-8; 2005,Jul,11-12

| 85300 | **Clotting inhibitors or anticoagulants; antithrombin III, activity** |

🚑 0.00 ⚕ 0.00 **FUD** XXX

AMA: 2005,Aug,7-8; 2005,Jul,11-12

| 85301 | **antithrombin III, antigen assay** |

🚑 0.00 ⚕ 0.00 **FUD** XXX

AMA: 2005,Aug,7-8; 2005,Jul,11-12

| 85302 | **protein C, antigen** |

🚑 0.00 ⚕ 0.00 **FUD** XXX

AMA: 2005,Aug,7-8; 2005,Jul,11-12

| 85303 | **protein C, activity** |

🚑 0.00 ⚕ 0.00 **FUD** XXX

AMA: 2005,Aug,7-8; 2005,Jul,11-12

| 85305 | **protein S, total** |

🚑 0.00 ⚕ 0.00 **FUD** XXX

AMA: 2005,Jul,11-12; 2005,Aug,7-8

| 85306 | **protein S, free** |

🚑 0.00 ⚕ 0.00 **FUD** XXX

AMA: 2005,Aug,7-8; 2005,Jul,11-12

| 85307 | **Activated Protein C (APC) resistance assay** |

🚑 0.00 ⚕ 0.00 **FUD** XXX

AMA: 2005,Aug,7-8; 2005,Jul,11-12

| 85335 | **Factor inhibitor test** |

🚑 0.00 ⚕ 0.00 **FUD** XXX

AMA: 2005,Aug,7-8; 2005,Jul,11-12

● New Code ▲ Revised Code ○ Reinstated ● New Web Release ▲ Revised Web Release + Add-on Unlisted Not Covered # Resequenced
⑤⓪ Optum Mod 50 Exempt ⊘ AMA Mod 51 Exempt ⑤① Optum Mod 51 Exempt ⑥③ Mod 63 Exempt ⩘ Non-FDA Drug ★ Telemedicine Ⓜ Maternity Ⓐ Age Edit

85337 **Thrombomodulin**
> EXCLUDES Mixing studies for inhibitors (85732)
> 🔹 0.00   ⚕ 0.00   **FUD** XXX   ◻◻
> AMA: 2005,Aug,7-8; 2005,Jul,11-12

85345 **Coagulation time; Lee and White**
> 🔹 0.00   ⚕ 0.00   **FUD** XXX   ◻◻
> AMA: 2005,Aug,7-8; 2005,Jul,11-12

85347 **activated**
> 🔹 0.00   ⚕ 0.00   **FUD** XXX   ◻◻
> AMA: 2019,Apr,10

85348 **other methods**
> EXCLUDES Differential count (85007-85009, 85025)
>   Duke bleeding time (85002)
>   Eosinophils, nasal smear (89190)
> 🔹 0.00   ⚕ 0.00   **FUD** XXX   ◻◻
> AMA: 2005,Aug,7-8; 2005,Jul,11-12

85360 **Euglobulin lysis**
> EXCLUDES Fetal hemoglobin (83030, 83033, 85460)
> 🔹 0.00   ⚕ 0.00   **FUD** XXX   ◻◻
> AMA: 2005,Aug,7-8; 2005,Jul,11-12

85362 **Fibrin(ogen) degradation (split) products (FDP) (FSP); agglutination slide, semiquantitative**
> EXCLUDES Immunoelectrophoresis (86320)
> 🔹 0.00   ⚕ 0.00   **FUD** XXX   ◻◻
> AMA: 2005,Aug,7-8; 2005,Jul,11-12

85366 **paracoagulation**
> 🔹 0.00   ⚕ 0.00   **FUD** XXX   ◻◻
> AMA: 2005,Aug,7-8; 2005,Jul,11-12

85370 **quantitative**
> 🔹 0.00   ⚕ 0.00   **FUD** XXX   ◻◻
> AMA: 2005,Aug,7-8; 2005,Jul,11-12

85378 **Fibrin degradation products, D-dimer; qualitative or semiquantitative**
> 🔹 0.00   ⚕ 0.00   **FUD** XXX   ◻◻
> AMA: 2018,Jan,8; 2017,Jan,8; 2016,Jan,13; 2015,Jan,16; 2014,Jan,11

85379 **quantitative**
> INCLUDES Ultrasensitive and standard sensitivity quantitative
>   D-dimer (85379)
> 🔹 0.00   ⚕ 0.00   **FUD** XXX   ◻◻
> AMA: 2005,Aug,7-8; 2005,Jul,11-12

85380 **ultrasensitive (eg, for evaluation for venous thromboembolism), qualitative or semiquantitative**
> 🔹 0.00   ⚕ 0.00   **FUD** XXX   ◻◻
> AMA: 2018,Jan,8; 2017,Jan,8; 2016,Jan,13; 2015,Jan,16; 2014,Jan,11

85384 **Fibrinogen; activity**
> 🔹 0.00   ⚕ 0.00   **FUD** XXX   ◻◻
> AMA: 2019,Apr,10

85385 **antigen**
> 🔹 0.00   ⚕ 0.00   **FUD** XXX   ◻◻
> AMA: 2005,Jul,11-12; 2005,Aug,7-8

85390 **Fibrinolysins or coagulopathy screen, interpretation and report**
> 🔹 0.00   ⚕ 0.00   **FUD** XXX   ◻80◻
> AMA: 2019,Apr,10

85396 **Coagulation/fibrinolysis assay, whole blood (eg, viscoelastic clot assessment), including use of any pharmacologic additive(s), as indicated, including interpretation and written report, per day**
> 🔹 0.58   ⚕ 0.58   **FUD** XXX   N 80 ◻
> AMA: 2019,Apr,10

85397 **Coagulation and fibrinolysis, functional activity, not otherwise specified (eg, ADAMTS-13), each analyte**
> 🔹 0.00   ⚕ 0.00   **FUD** XXX   ◻◻

85400 **Fibrinolytic factors and inhibitors; plasmin**
> 🔹 0.00   ⚕ 0.00   **FUD** XXX   ◻◻
> AMA: 2005,Aug,7-8; 2005,Jul,11-12

85410 **alpha-2 antiplasmin**
> 🔹 0.00   ⚕ 0.00   **FUD** XXX   ◻◻
> AMA: 2005,Aug,7-8; 2005,Jul,11-12

85415 **plasminogen activator**
> 🔹 0.00   ⚕ 0.00   **FUD** XXX   ◻◻
> AMA: 2005,Aug,7-8; 2005,Jul,11-12

85420 **plasminogen, except antigenic assay**
> 🔹 0.00   ⚕ 0.00   **FUD** XXX   ◻◻
> AMA: 2005,Aug,7-8; 2005,Jul,11-12

85421 **plasminogen, antigenic assay**
> EXCLUDES Fragility, red blood cell (85547, 85555-85557)
> 🔹 0.00   ⚕ 0.00   **FUD** XXX   ◻◻
> AMA: 2005,Aug,7-8; 2005,Jul,11-12

85441 **Heinz bodies; direct**
> 🔹 0.00   ⚕ 0.00   **FUD** XXX   ◻◻
> AMA: 2005,Aug,7-8; 2005,Jul,11-12

85445 **induced, acetyl phenylhydrazine**
> EXCLUDES Hematocrit (PCV) (85014, 85025, 85027)
>   Hemoglobin (83020-83068, 85018, 85025, 85027)
> 🔹 0.00   ⚕ 0.00   **FUD** XXX   ◻◻
> AMA: 2005,Aug,7-8; 2005,Jul,11-12

85460 **Hemoglobin or RBCs, fetal, for fetomaternal hemorrhage; differential lysis (Kleihauer-Betke)**   M ♀
> EXCLUDES Hemoglobin F (83030, 83033)
>   Hemolysins (86940-86941)
> 🔹 0.00   ⚕ 0.00   **FUD** XXX   ◻◻
> AMA: 2018,Jan,8; 2017,Jan,8; 2016,Jan,13; 2015,Jan,16; 2014,Jan,11

85461 **rosette**   M ♀
> 🔹 0.00   ⚕ 0.00   **FUD** XXX   ◻◻
> AMA: 2005,Jul,11-12; 2005,Aug,7-8

85475 **Hemolysin, acid**
> INCLUDES Ham test
> EXCLUDES Hemolysins and agglutinins (86940-86941)
> 🔹 0.00   ⚕ 0.00   **FUD** XXX   ◻◻
> AMA: 2005,Aug,7-8; 2005,Jul,11-12

85520 **Heparin assay**
> 🔹 0.00   ⚕ 0.00   **FUD** XXX   ◻◻
> AMA: 2005,Aug,7-8; 2005,Jul,11-12

85525 **Heparin neutralization**
> 🔹 0.00   ⚕ 0.00   **FUD** XXX   ◻◻
> AMA: 2018,Jan,8; 2017,Aug,9

85530 **Heparin-protamine tolerance test**
> 🔹 0.00   ⚕ 0.00   **FUD** XXX   ◻◻
> AMA: 2005,Aug,7-8; 2005,Jul,11-12

85536 **Iron stain, peripheral blood**
> EXCLUDES Iron stains on bone marrow or other tissues with
>   physician evaluation (88313)
> 🔹 0.00   ⚕ 0.00   **FUD** XXX   ◻◻
> AMA: 2005,Aug,7-8; 2005,Jul,11-12

85540 **Leukocyte alkaline phosphatase with count**
> 🔹 0.00   ⚕ 0.00   **FUD** XXX   ◻◻
> AMA: 2005,Aug,7-8; 2005,Jul,11-12

85547 **Mechanical fragility, RBC**
> 🔹 0.00   ⚕ 0.00   **FUD** XXX   ◻◻
> AMA: 2005,Aug,7-8; 2005,Jul,11-12

85549 **Muramidase**
> EXCLUDES Nitroblue tetrazolium dye test (86384)
> 🔹 0.00   ⚕ 0.00   **FUD** XXX   ◻◻
> AMA: 2005,Aug,7-8; 2005,Jul,11-12

| 26/TC PC/TC Only | A2-Z3 ASC Payment | 50 Bilateral | ♂ Male Only | ♀ Female Only | 🔹 Facility RVU | ⚕ Non-Facility RVU | ◻ CCI | ❌ CLIA |
| FUD Follow-up Days | CMS: IOM | AMA: CPT Asst | A-Y OPPSI | 80/80 Surg Assist Allowed / w/Doc | | 📖 Lab Crosswalk | | 📖 Radiology Crosswalk |

420   CPT © 2019 American Medical Association. All Rights Reserved.   © 2019 Optum360, LLC

85555 Osmotic fragility, RBC; unincubated
🏷 0.00 ⚕ 0.00 **FUD** XXX [Q][▯]
AMA: 2005,Aug,7-8; 2005,Jul,11-12

85557 incubated
EXCLUDES *Packed cell volume (85013)*
Parasites, blood (eg, malaria smears) (87207)
Partial thromboplastin time (85730, 85732)
Plasmin (85400)
Plasminogen (85420)
Plasminogen activator (85415)
🏷 0.00 ⚕ 0.00 **FUD** XXX [Q][▯]
AMA: 2005,Aug,7-8; 2005,Jul,11-12

85576 Platelet, aggregation (in vitro), each agent
EXCLUDES *Thromboxane metabolite(s), including thromboxane,*
when performed, in urine (84431)
🏷 0.00 ⚕ 0.00 **FUD** XXX [X][Q][80][▯]
AMA: 2019,Apr,10; 2018,Jan,8; 2017,Jan,8; 2016,Jan,13;
2015,Jan,16; 2014,Jan,11

85597 Phospholipid neutralization; platelet
🏷 0.00 ⚕ 0.00 **FUD** XXX [Q][▯]
AMA: 2018,Jan,8; 2017,Jan,8; 2016,Jan,13; 2015,Jan,16;
2014,Jan,11

85598 hexagonal phospholipid
🏷 0.00 ⚕ 0.00 **FUD** XXX [Q][▯]
AMA: 2018,Jan,8; 2017,Jan,8; 2016,Jan,13; 2015,Jan,16;
2014,Jan,11

85610 Prothrombin time;
🏷 0.00 ⚕ 0.00 **FUD** XXX [X][Q][▯]
AMA: 2005,Aug,7-8; 2005,Jul,11-12

85611 substitution, plasma fractions, each
🏷 0.00 ⚕ 0.00 **FUD** XXX [Q][▯]
AMA: 2005,Aug,7-8; 2005,Jul,11-12

85612 Russell viper venom time (includes venom); undiluted
🏷 0.00 ⚕ 0.00 **FUD** XXX [Q][▯]
AMA: 2005,Aug,7-8; 2005,Jul,11-12

85613 diluted
EXCLUDES *Red blood cell count (85025, 85027, 85041)*
🏷 0.00 ⚕ 0.00 **FUD** XXX [Q][▯]
AMA: 2005,Aug,7-8; 2005,Jul,11-12

85635 Reptilase test
EXCLUDES *Reticulocyte count (85044-85045)*
🏷 0.00 ⚕ 0.00 **FUD** XXX [Q][▯]
AMA: 2005,Aug,7-8; 2005,Jul,11-12

85651 Sedimentation rate, erythrocyte; non-automated
🏷 0.00 ⚕ 0.00 **FUD** XXX [X][▯]
AMA: 2005,Aug,7-8; 2005,Jul,11-12

85652 automated
INCLUDES *Westergren test*
🏷 0.00 ⚕ 0.00 **FUD** XXX [Q][▯]
AMA: 2005,Aug,7-8; 2005,Jul,11-12

85660 Sickling of RBC, reduction
EXCLUDES *Hemoglobin electrophoresis (83020)*
Smears (87207)
🏷 0.00 ⚕ 0.00 **FUD** XXX [Q][▯]
AMA: 2005,Aug,7-8; 2005,Jul,11-12

85670 Thrombin time; plasma
🏷 0.00 ⚕ 0.00 **FUD** XXX [Q][▯]
AMA: 2005,Jul,11-12; 2005,Aug,7-8

85675 titer
🏷 0.00 ⚕ 0.00 **FUD** XXX [Q][▯]
AMA: 2005,Jul,11-12; 2005,Aug,7-8

85705 Thromboplastin inhibition, tissue
EXCLUDES *Individual clotting factors (85245-85247)*
🏷 0.00 ⚕ 0.00 **FUD** XXX [Q][▯]
AMA: 2005,Aug,7-8; 2005,Jul,11-12

85730-85732 Partial Thromboplastin Time (PTT)

EXCLUDES *Agglutinins (86000, 86156-86157)*
Antiplasmin (85410)
Antithrombin III (85300-85301)
Blood banking procedures (86850-86999)

85730 Thromboplastin time, partial (PTT); plasma or whole blood
INCLUDES Hicks-Pitney test
🏷 0.00 ⚕ 0.00 **FUD** XXX [Q][▯]
AMA: 2005,Aug,7-8; 2005,Jul,11-12

85732 substitution, plasma fractions, each
🏷 0.00 ⚕ 0.00 **FUD** XXX [Q][▯]
AMA: 2018,Jan,8; 2017,Jan,8; 2016,Jan,13; 2015,Jan,16;
2014,Jan,11

85810-85999 Blood Viscosity and Unlisted Hematology Procedures

85810 Viscosity
EXCLUDES *von Willebrand factor assay (85245-85247)*
WBC count (85025, 85027, 85048, 89050)
🏷 0.00 ⚕ 0.00 **FUD** XXX [Q][▯]
AMA: 2018,Jan,8; 2017,Jan,8; 2016,Jan,13; 2015,Jan,16;
2014,Jan,11

85999 Unlisted hematology and coagulation procedure
🏷 0.00 ⚕ 0.00 **FUD** XXX [Q][▯]
AMA: 2018,Jan,8; 2017,Aug,9; 2017,Jan,8; 2016,Jan,13;
2015,Jan,16; 2014,Jan,11

86000-86063 Antibody Testing

86000 Agglutinins, febrile (eg, Brucella, Francisella, Murine typhus, Q fever, Rocky Mountain spotted fever, scrub typhus), each antigen
EXCLUDES *Infectious agent antibodies (86602-86804)*
🏷 0.00 ⚕ 0.00 **FUD** XXX [Q][▯]
AMA: 2018,Jan,8; 2017,Jan,8; 2016,Jan,13; 2015,Jan,16;
2014,Jan,11

86001 Allergen specific IgG quantitative or semiquantitative, each allergen
EXCLUDES *Agglutinins and autohemolysins (86940-86941)*
🏷 0.00 ⚕ 0.00 **FUD** XXX [Q][▯]
AMA: 2005,Aug,7-8; 2005,Jul,11-12

86003 Allergen specific IgE; quantitative or semiquantitative, crude allergen extract, each
EXCLUDES *Total quantitative IgE (82785)*
🏷 0.00 ⚕ 0.00 **FUD** XXX [Q][▯]
AMA: 2018,Jan,8; 2017,Jan,8; 2016,Jan,13; 2015,Jan,16;
2014,Jan,11

86005 qualitative, multiallergen screen (eg, disk, sponge, card)
EXCLUDES *Total qualitative IgE (83518)*
🏷 0.00 ⚕ 0.00 **FUD** XXX [Q][▯]
AMA: 2018,Jan,8; 2017,Jan,8; 2016,Jan,13; 2015,Jan,16;
2014,Jan,11

86008 quantitative or semiquantitative, recombinant or purified component, each
🏷 0.00 ⚕ 0.00 **FUD** XXX [Q][▯]
EXCLUDES *Alpha-1 antitrypsin (82103, 82104)*
Alpha-1 feto-protein (82105, 82106)
Anti-AChR (acetylcholine receptor) antibody titer (86255, 86256)
Anticardiolipin antibody (86147)
Anti-deoxyribonuclease titer (86215)
Anti-DNA (86225)

86021 Antibody identification; leukocyte antibodies
🏷 0.00 ⚕ 0.00 **FUD** XXX [Q][▯]
AMA: 2005,Jul,11-12; 2005,Aug,7-8

86022 platelet antibodies
🏷 0.00 ⚕ 0.00 **FUD** XXX [Q][▯]
AMA: 2005,Jul,11-12; 2005,Aug,7-8

85555 — 86022

86023 platelet associated immunoglobulin assay
🔹 0.00 ✎ 0.00 **FUD** XXX ▣ ▢

AMA: 2005,Jul,11-12; 2005,Aug,7-8

86038 **Antinuclear antibodies (ANA);**
🔹 0.00 ✎ 0.00 **FUD** XXX ▣ ▢

AMA: 2005,Aug,7-8; 2005,Jul,11-12

86039 titer
EXCLUDES *Antistreptococcal antibody, ie, anti-DNAse (86215)*
Antistreptokinase titer (86590)
🔹 0.00 ✎ 0.00 **FUD** XXX ▣ ▢

AMA: 2005,Aug,7-8; 2005,Jul,11-12

86060 **Antistreptolysin 0; titer**
EXCLUDES *Antibodies, infectious agents (86602-86804)*
🔹 0.00 ✎ 0.00 **FUD** XXX ▣ ▢

AMA: 2005,Jul,11-12; 2005,Aug,7-8

86063 screen
EXCLUDES *Antibodies to blastomyces (86612)*
Antibodies, infectious agents (86602-86804)
🔹 0.00 ✎ 0.00 **FUD** XXX ▣ ▢

AMA: 2005,Jul,11-12; 2005,Aug,7-8

86077-86079 Blood Bank Services

86077 **Blood bank physician services; difficult cross match and/or evaluation of irregular antibody(s), interpretation and written report**
🔹 1.46 ✎ 1.57 **FUD** XXX ▣ 80 ▢

AMA: 2005,Aug,7-8; 2005,Jul,11-12

86078 **investigation of transfusion reaction including suspicion of transmissible disease, interpretation and written report**
🔹 1.46 ✎ 1.57 **FUD** XXX ▣ 80 ▢

AMA: 2005,Aug,7-8; 2005,Jul,11-12

86079 **authorization for deviation from standard blood banking procedures (eg, use of outdated blood, transfusion of Rh incompatible units), with written report**
EXCLUDES *Brucella antibodies (86622)*
Candida antibodies (86628)
Candida skin test (86485)
🔹 1.46 ✎ 1.56 **FUD** XXX ▣ 80 ▢

AMA: 2005,Aug,7-8; 2005,Jul,11-12

86140-86344 [86152, 86153] Diagnostic Immunology Testing

86140 **C-reactive protein;**
EXCLUDES *Candidiasis (86628)*
🔹 0.00 ✎ 0.00 **FUD** XXX ▣ ▢

AMA: 2005,Aug,7-8; 2005,Jul,11-12

86141 high sensitivity (hsCRP)
🔹 0.00 ✎ 0.00 **FUD** XXX ▣ ▢

AMA: 2005,Aug,7-8; 2005,Jul,11-12

86146 **Beta 2 Glycoprotein I antibody, each**
🔹 0.00 ✎ 0.00 **FUD** XXX ▣ ▢

AMA: 2005,Aug,7-8; 2005,Jul,11-12

86147 **Cardiolipin (phospholipid) antibody, each Ig class**
🔹 0.00 ✎ 0.00 **FUD** XXX ▣ ▢

AMA: 2005,Aug,7-8; 2005,Jul,11-12

\# **86152** **Cell enumeration using immunologic selection and identification in fluid specimen (eg, circulating tumor cells in blood);**
🔹 0.00 ✎ 0.00 **FUD** XXX ▢

EXCLUDES *Flow cytometric immunophenotyping (88184-88189)*
Flow cytometric quantitation (86355-86357,
86359-86361, 86367)
Code also physician interpretation/report when performed
([86153])

\# **86153** **physician interpretation and report, when required**
🔹 0.00 ✎ 0.00 **FUD** 000 B 80 ▢

EXCLUDES *Flow cytometric immunophenotyping (88184-88189)*
Flow cytometric quantitation (86355-86357,
86359-86361, 86367)
Code first cell enumeration, when performed ([86152])

86148 **Anti-phosphatidylserine (phospholipid) antibody**
EXCLUDES *Antiprothrombin (phospholipid cofactor) antibody*
(86849)
🔹 0.00 ✎ 0.00 **FUD** XXX ▣ ▢

AMA: 2018,Jan,8; 2017,Jan,8; 2016,Jan,13; 2015,Jan,16;
2014,Jan,11

86152 **Resequenced code. See code following 86147.**

86153 **Resequenced code. See code before 86148.**

86155 **Chemotaxis assay, specify method**
EXCLUDES *Antibodies, coccidioides (86635)*
Clostridium difficile toxin (87230)
Skin test, coccidioides (86490)
🔹 0.00 ✎ 0.00 **FUD** XXX ▣ ▢

AMA: 2005,Aug,7-8; 2005,Jul,11-12

86156 **Cold agglutinin; screen**
🔹 0.00 ✎ 0.00 **FUD** XXX ▣ ▢

AMA: 2005,Aug,7-8; 2005,Jul,11-12

86157 titer
🔹 0.00 ✎ 0.00 **FUD** XXX ▣ ▢

AMA: 2005,Aug,7-8; 2005,Jul,11-12

86160 **Complement; antigen, each component**
🔹 0.00 ✎ 0.00 **FUD** XXX ▣ ▢

AMA: 2005,Aug,7-8; 2005,Jul,11-12

86161 functional activity, each component
🔹 0.00 ✎ 0.00 **FUD** XXX ▣ ▢

AMA: 2005,Aug,7-8; 2005,Jul,11-12

86162 total hemolytic (CH50)
🔹 0.00 ✎ 0.00 **FUD** XXX ▣ ▢

AMA: 2005,Aug,7-8; 2005,Jul,11-12

86171 **Complement fixation tests, each antigen**
EXCLUDES *Coombs test*
🔹 0.00 ✎ 0.00 **FUD** XXX ▣ ▢

AMA: 2005,Aug,7-8; 2005,Jul,11-12

86200 **Cyclic citrullinated peptide (CCP), antibody**
🔹 0.00 ✎ 0.00 **FUD** XXX ▣ ▢

AMA: 2018,Jan,8; 2017,Jan,8; 2016,Jan,13; 2015,Jan,16;
2014,Jan,11

86215 **Deoxyribonuclease, antibody**
🔹 0.00 ✎ 0.00 **FUD** XXX ▣ ▢

AMA: 2005,Aug,7-8; 2005,Jul,11-12

86225 **Deoxyribonucleic acid (DNA) antibody; native or double stranded**
EXCLUDES *Echinococcus antibodies, report code for specific method*
HIV antibody tests (86701-86703)
🔹 0.00 ✎ 0.00 **FUD** XXX ▣ ▢

AMA: 2005,Aug,7-8; 2005,Jul,11-12

86226 single stranded
EXCLUDES *Anti D.S, DNA, IFA, eg, using C. Lucilae (86255-86256)*
🔹 0.00 ✎ 0.00 **FUD** XXX ▣ ▢

AMA: 2005,Aug,7-8; 2005,Jul,11-12

86235 **Extractable nuclear antigen, antibody to, any method (eg, nRNP, SS-A, SS-B, Sm, RNP, Sc170, J01), each antibody**
🔹 0.00 ✎ 0.00 **FUD** XXX ▢

AMA: 2005,Aug,7-8; 2005,Jul,11-12

86255 **Fluorescent noninfectious agent antibody; screen, each antibody**
🔹 0.00 ✎ 0.00 **FUD** XXX ▣ 80 ▢

AMA: 2005,Aug,9-10; 2005,Aug,7-8

26/TC PC/TC Only A2-Z3 ASC Payment 50 Bilateral ♂ Male Only ♀ Female Only 🔹 Facility RVU ✎ Non-Facility RVU ▢ CCI ✖ CLIA
FUD Follow-up Days CMS: IOM AMA: CPT Asst A-Y OPPSI 80/80 Surg Assist Allowed / w/Doc ▲ Lab Crosswalk ▣ Radiology Crosswalk

422 CPT © 2019 American Medical Association. All Rights Reserved. © 2019 Optum360, LLC

86256   **titer, each antibody**

EXCLUDES   *Fluorescent technique for antigen identification in tissue (88346, [88350])*
FTA (86780)
Gel (agar) diffusion tests (86331)
Indirect fluorescence (88346, [88350])

⚕ 0.00   ⚕ 0.00   **FUD** XXX   Q 80 ▭

AMA: 2005,Aug,9-10; 2005,Aug,7-8

86277   **Growth hormone, human (HGH), antibody**

⚕ 0.00   ⚕ 0.00   **FUD** XXX   Q ▭

AMA: 2005,Aug,7-8; 2005,Jul,11-12

86280   **Hemagglutination inhibition test (HAI)**

EXCLUDES   *Antibodies to infectious agents (86602-86804)*
Rubella (86762)

⚕ 0.00   ⚕ 0.00   **FUD** XXX   Q ▭

AMA: 2005,Aug,7-8; 2005,Jul,11-12

86294   **Immunoassay for tumor antigen, qualitative or semiquantitative (eg, bladder tumor antigen)**

EXCLUDES   *Qualitative NMP22 protein (86386)*

⚕ 0.00   ⚕ 0.00   **FUD** XXX   ✗ Q ▭

AMA: 2005,Aug,7-8; 2005,Jul,11-12

86300   **Immunoassay for tumor antigen, quantitative; CA 15-3 (27.29)**

⚕ 0.00   ⚕ 0.00   **FUD** XXX   Q ▭

AMA: 2005,Aug,7-8; 2005,Jul,11-12

86301   **CA 19-9**

⚕ 0.00   ⚕ 0.00   Q ▭

AMA: 2005,Aug,7-8; 2005,Jul,11-12

86304   **CA 125**

EXCLUDES   *Antibody, hepatitis delta agent (86692)*
Measurement of serum HER-2/neu oncoprotein (83950)

⚕ 0.00   ⚕ 0.00   **FUD** XXX   Q ▭

AMA: 2005,Aug,7-8; 2005,Jul,11-12

86305   **Human epididymis protein 4 (HE4)**

⚕ 0.00   ⚕ 0.00   **FUD** XXX   Q ▭

86308   **Heterophile antibodies; screening**

EXCLUDES   *Antibodies to infectious agents (86602-86804)*

⚕ 0.00   ⚕ 0.00   **FUD** XXX   ✗ Q ▭

AMA: 2005,Jul,11-12; 2005,Aug,7-8

86309   **titer**

EXCLUDES   *Antibodies to infectious agents (86602-86804)*

⚕ 0.00   ⚕ 0.00   **FUD** XXX   Q ▭

AMA: 2005,Jul,11-12; 2005,Aug,7-8

86310   **titers after absorption with beef cells and guinea pig kidney**

EXCLUDES   *Antibodies, infectious agents (86602-86804)*
Histoplasma antibodies (86698)
Histoplasmosis skin test (86510)
Human growth hormone antibody (86277)

⚕ 0.00   ⚕ 0.00   **FUD** XXX   Q ▭

AMA: 2005,Jul,11-12; 2005,Aug,7-8

86316   **Immunoassay for tumor antigen, other antigen, quantitative (eg, CA 50, 72-4, 549), each**

⚕ 0.00   ⚕ 0.00   **FUD** XXX   Q ▭

AMA: 2018,Jan,8; 2017,Jan,8; 2016,Jan,13; 2015,Jan,16; 2014,Jan,11

86317   **Immunoassay for infectious agent antibody, quantitative, not otherwise specified**

EXCLUDES   *Immunoassay techniques for antigens (83516, 83518-83520, 87301-87450, 87810-87899)*
Particle agglutination test (86403)

⚕ 0.00   ⚕ 0.00   **FUD** XXX   Q ▭

AMA: 2005,Jul,11-12; 2005,Aug,7-8

86318   **Immunoassay for infectious agent antibody, qualitative or semiquantitative, single step method (eg, reagent strip)**

⚕ 0.00   ⚕ 0.00   **FUD** XXX   ✗ Q ▭

AMA: 2018,Jan,8; 2017,Jan,8; 2016,Jan,13; 2015,Jan,16; 2014,Jan,11

86320   **Immunoelectrophoresis; serum**

⚕ 0.00   ⚕ 0.00   **FUD** XXX   Q 80 ▭

AMA: 2005,Jul,11-12; 2005,Aug,7-8

86325   **other fluids (eg, urine, cerebrospinal fluid) with concentration**

⚕ 0.00   ⚕ 0.00   **FUD** XXX   Q 80 ▭

AMA: 2005,Jul,11-12; 2005,Aug,7-8

86327   **crossed (2-dimensional assay)**

⚕ 0.00   ⚕ 0.00   **FUD** XXX   Q 80 ▭

AMA: 2005,Jul,11-12; 2005,Aug,7-8

86329   **Immunodiffusion; not elsewhere specified**

⚕ 0.00   ⚕ 0.00   **FUD** XXX   Q ▭

AMA: 2018,Jan,8; 2017,Jan,8; 2016,Jan,13; 2015,Jan,16; 2014,Jan,11

86331   **gel diffusion, qualitative (Ouchterlony), each antigen or antibody**

⚕ 0.00   ⚕ 0.00   **FUD** XXX   Q ▭

AMA: 2005,Aug,7-8; 2005,Jul,11-12

86332   **Immune complex assay**

⚕ 0.00   ⚕ 0.00   **FUD** XXX   Q ▭

AMA: 2005,Aug,7-8; 2005,Jul,11-12

86334   **Immunofixation electrophoresis; serum**

⚕ 0.00   ⚕ 0.00   **FUD** XXX   Q 80 ▭

AMA: 2005,Jul,11-12; 2005,Aug,7-8

86335   **other fluids with concentration (eg, urine, CSF)**

⚕ 0.00   ⚕ 0.00   **FUD** XXX   Q 80 ▭

AMA: 2005,Aug,7-8; 2005,Jul,11-12

86336   **Inhibin A**

⚕ 0.00   ⚕ 0.00   **FUD** XXX   Q ▭

AMA: 2005,Aug,7-8; 2005,Jul,11-12

86337   **Insulin antibodies**

⚕ 0.00   ⚕ 0.00   **FUD** XXX   Q ▭

AMA: 2005,Aug,7-8; 2005,Jul,11-12

86340   **Intrinsic factor antibodies**

EXCLUDES   *Antibodies, leptospira (86720)*
Leukoagglutinins (86021)

⚕ 0.00   ⚕ 0.00   **FUD** XXX   Q ▭

AMA: 2005,Jul,11-12; 2005,Aug,7-8

86341   **Islet cell antibody**

⚕ 0.00   ⚕ 0.00   **FUD** XXX   Q ▭

AMA: 2018,Jan,8; 2017,Jan,8; 2016,Jan,13; 2015,Jan,16; 2014,Jan,11

86343   **Leukocyte histamine release test (LHR)**

⚕ 0.00   ⚕ 0.00   **FUD** XXX   Q ▭

AMA: 2005,Aug,7-8; 2005,Jul,11-12

86344   **Leukocyte phagocytosis**

⚕ 0.00   ⚕ 0.00   **FUD** XXX   Q ▭

AMA: 2005,Aug,7-8; 2005,Jul,11-12

86352 Assay Cellular Function

86352   **Cellular function assay involving stimulation (eg, mitogen or antigen) and detection of biomarker (eg, ATP)**

⚕ 0.00   ⚕ 0.00   **FUD** XXX   Q ▭

86353 Lymphocyte Mitogen Response Assay

CMS: 100-03,190.8 Lymphocyte Mitogen Response Assays

86353   **Lymphocyte transformation, mitogen (phytomitogen) or antigen induced blastogenesis**

EXCLUDES   *Cellular function assay with stimulation and detection of biomarker (86352)*
Malaria antibodies (86750)

⚕ 0.00   ⚕ 0.00   **FUD** XXX   Q ▭

AMA: 2005,Aug,7-8; 2005,Jul,11-12

86355-86593 Additional Diagnostic Immunology Testing

86355 **B cells, total count**

> *EXCLUDES* *Flow cytometry interpretation (88187-88189)*
> ⚕ 0.00 ✂ 0.00 **FUD** XXX ▣ ▭
>
> **AMA:** 2018,Jan,8; 2017,Jan,8; 2016,Jan,13; 2015,Jan,16; 2014,Jan,11

86356 **Mononuclear cell antigen, quantitative (eg, flow cytometry), not otherwise specified, each antigen**

> *EXCLUDES* *Flow cytometry interpretation (88187-88189)*
> ⚕ 0.00 ✂ 0.00 **FUD** XXX ▣ ▭
>
> **AMA:** 2018,Jan,8; 2017,Jan,8; 2016,Jan,13; 2015,Jan,16; 2014,Jan,11

86357 **Natural killer (NK) cells, total count**

> *EXCLUDES* *Flow cytometry interpretation (88187-88189)*
> ⚕ 0.00 ✂ 0.00 **FUD** XXX ▣ ▭
>
> **AMA:** 2018,Jan,8; 2017,Jan,8; 2016,Jan,13; 2015,Jan,16; 2014,Jan,11

86359 **T cells; total count**

> *EXCLUDES* *Flow cytometry interpretation (88187-88189)*
> ⚕ 0.00 ✂ 0.00 **FUD** XXX ▣ ▭
>
> **AMA:** 2018,Jan,8; 2017,Jan,8; 2016,Jan,13; 2015,Jan,16; 2014,Jan,11

86360 **absolute CD4 and CD8 count, including ratio**

> *EXCLUDES* *Flow cytometry interpretation (88187-88189)*
> ⚕ 0.00 ✂ 0.00 **FUD** XXX ▣ ▭
>
> **AMA:** 2018,Jan,8; 2017,Jan,8; 2016,Jan,13; 2015,Jan,16; 2014,Jan,11

86361 **absolute CD4 count**

> *EXCLUDES* *Flow cytometry interpretation (88187-88189)*
> ⚕ 0.00 ✂ 0.00 **FUD** XXX ▣ ▭
>
> **AMA:** 2018,Jan,8; 2017,Jan,8; 2016,Jan,13; 2015,Jan,16; 2014,Jan,11

86367 **Stem cells (ie, CD34), total count**

> *EXCLUDES* *Flow cytometric immunophenotyping, potential hematolymphoid neoplasia assessment (88184-88189)*
> *Flow cytometry interpretation (88187-88189)*
> ⚕ 0.00 ✂ 0.00 **FUD** XXX ▣ ▭
>
> **AMA:** 2018,Jan,8; 2017,Jan,8; 2016,Jan,13; 2015,Jan,16; 2014,Jan,11

86376 **Microsomal antibodies (eg, thyroid or liver-kidney), each**

> ⚕ 0.00 ✂ 0.00 **FUD** XXX ▣ ▭
>
> **AMA:** 2005,Jul,11-12; 2005,Aug,7-8

86382 **Neutralization test, viral**

> ⚕ 0.00 ✂ 0.00 **FUD** XXX ▣ ▭
>
> **AMA:** 2005,Aug,7-8; 2005,Jul,11-12

86384 **Nitroblue tetrazolium dye test (NTD)**

> ⚕ 0.00 ✂ 0.00 **FUD** XXX ▣ ▭
>
> **AMA:** 2005,Aug,7-8; 2005,Jul,11-12

86386 **Nuclear Matrix Protein 22 (NMP22), qualitative**

> ⚕ 0.00 ✂ 0.00 **FUD** XXX ☒ ▣ ▭
>
> *EXCLUDES* *Ouchterlony diffusion (86331)*
> *Platelet antibodies (86022, 86023)*

86403 **Particle agglutination; screen, each antibody**

> ⚕ 0.00 ✂ 0.00 **FUD** XXX ▣ ▭
>
> **AMA:** 2005,Jul,11-12; 2005,Aug,7-8

86406 **titer, each antibody**

> *EXCLUDES* *Pregnancy test (84702, 84703)*
> *Rapid plasma reagin test (RPR) (86592, 86593)*
> ⚕ 0.00 ✂ 0.00 **FUD** XXX ▣ ▭
>
> **AMA:** 2005,Jul,11-12; 2005,Aug,7-8

86430 **Rheumatoid factor; qualitative**

> ⚕ 0.00 ✂ 0.00 **FUD** XXX ▣ ▭
>
> **AMA:** 2005,Aug,7-8; 2005,Jul,11-12

86431 **quantitative**

> *EXCLUDES* *Serologic syphilis testing (86592, 86593)*
> ⚕ 0.00 ✂ 0.00 **FUD** XXX ▣ ▭
>
> **AMA:** 2005,Aug,7-8; 2005,Jul,11-12

86480 **Tuberculosis test, cell mediated immunity antigen response measurement; gamma interferon**

> ⚕ 0.00 ✂ 0.00 **FUD** XXX ▣ ▭
>
> **AMA:** 2018,Jan,8; 2017,Jan,8; 2016,Jan,13; 2015,Jan,16; 2014,Jan,11

86481 **enumeration of gamma interferon-producing T-cells in cell suspension**

> ⚕ 0.00 ✂ 0.00 **FUD** XXX ▣ ▭
>
> **AMA:** 2010,Dec,7-10

86485 **Skin test; candida**

> *EXCLUDES* *Candida antibody (86628)*
> ⚕ 0.00 ✂ 0.00 **FUD** XXX ▣① 80 TC ▭
>
> **AMA:** 2005,Jul,11-12; 2005,Aug,7-8

86486 **unlisted antigen, each**

> ⚕ 0.15 ✂ 0.15 **FUD** XXX ▣① 80 TC ▭
>
> **AMA:** 2008,Apr,5-7

86490 **coccidioidomycosis**

> ⚕ 2.49 ✂ 2.49 **FUD** XXX ▣① 80 TC ▭
>
> **AMA:** 2005,Aug,7-8; 2005,Jul,11-12

86510 **histoplasmosis**

> *EXCLUDES* *Histoplasma antibody (86698)*
> ⚕ 0.19 ✂ 0.19 **FUD** XXX ▣① 80 TC ▭
>
> **AMA:** 2005,Aug,7-8; 2005,Jul,11-12

86580 **tuberculosis, intradermal**

> *INCLUDES* Heaf test
> Intradermal Mantoux test
> *EXCLUDES* *Antibodies to sporothrix, report code for specific method*
> *Skin test for allergy (95012-95199)*
> *Smooth muscle antibody (86255-86256)*
> *Tuberculosis test, cell mediated immunity measurement of gamma interferon antigen response (86480)*
> ⚕ 0.24 ✂ 0.24 **FUD** XXX ▣① 80 TC ▭
>
> **AMA:** 2005,Aug,7-8; 2005,Jul,11-12

86590 **Streptokinase, antibody**

> *EXCLUDES* *Antibodies, infectious agents (86602-86804)*
> *Streptolysin O antibody, antistreptolysin O (86060, 86063)*
> ⚕ 0.00 ✂ 0.00 **FUD** XXX ▣ ▭
>
> **AMA:** 2005,Jul,11-12; 2005,Aug,7-8

86592 **Syphilis test, non-treponemal antibody; qualitative (eg, VDRL, RPR, ART)**

> *INCLUDES* Wasserman test
> *EXCLUDES* *Antibodies to infectious agents (86602-86804)*
> ⚕ 0.00 ✂ 0.00 **FUD** XXX Ⓐ ▭
>
> **AMA:** 2005,Jul,11-12; 2005,Aug,7-8

86593 **quantitative**

> *EXCLUDES* *Antibodies, infectious agents (86602-86804)*
> *Tetanus antibody (86774)*
> *Thyroglobulin (84432)*
> *Thyroglobulin antibody (86800)*
> *Thyroid microsomal antibody (86376)*
> *Toxoplasma antibody (86777-86778)*
> ⚕ 0.00 ✂ 0.00 **FUD** XXX Ⓐ ▭
>
> **AMA:** 2005,Jul,11-12; 2005,Aug,7-8

26/TC PC/TC Only **A2-Z3** ASC Payment **50** Bilateral ♂ Male Only ♀ Female Only ⚕ Facility RVU ✂ Non-Facility RVU ▭ CCI ☒ CLIA
FUD Follow-up Days **CMS:** IOM **AMA:** CPT Asst **A-Y** OPPSI **80/80** Surg Assist Allowed / w/Doc Lab Crosswalk Radiology Crosswalk

424

86602-86698 Testing for Antibodies to Infectious Agents: Actinomyces- Histoplasma

INCLUDES Qualitative or semiquantitative immunoassays performed by multiple-step methods for the detection of antibodies to infectious agents

EXCLUDES Detection of:
Antibodies other than those to infectious agents, see specific antibody or method
Infectious agent/antigen (87260-87899 [87623, 87624, 87625, 87806])
Immunoassays by single-step method (86318)

86602 Antibody; actinomyces
0.00 0.00 FUD XXX
AMA: 2018,Jan,8; 2017,Jan,8; 2016,Jan,13; 2015,Jan,16; 2014,Jan,11

86603 adenovirus
0.00 0.00 FUD XXX
AMA: 2005,Jul,11-12; 2005,Aug,7-8

86606 Aspergillus
0.00 0.00 FUD XXX
AMA: 2005,Jul,11-12; 2005,Aug,7-8

86609 bacterium, not elsewhere specified
0.00 0.00 FUD XXX
AMA: 2005,Jul,11-12; 2005,Aug,7-8

86611 Bartonella
0.00 0.00 FUD XXX
AMA: 2005,Jul,11-12; 2005,Aug,7-8

86612 Blastomyces
0.00 0.00 FUD XXX
AMA: 2005,Jul,11-12; 2005,Aug,7-8

86615 Bordetella
0.00 0.00 FUD XXX
AMA: 2005,Jul,11-12; 2005,Aug,7-8

86617 Borrelia burgdorferi (Lyme disease) confirmatory test (eg, Western Blot or immunoblot)
0.00 0.00 FUD XXX
AMA: 2005,Jul,11-12; 2005,Aug,7-8

86618 Borrelia burgdorferi (Lyme disease)
0.00 0.00 FUD XXX
AMA: 2005,Jul,11-12; 2005,Aug,7-8

86619 Borrelia (relapsing fever)
0.00 0.00 FUD XXX
AMA: 2005,Jul,11-12; 2005,Aug,7-8

86622 Brucella
0.00 0.00 FUD XXX
AMA: 2005,Jul,11-12; 2005,Aug,7-8

86625 Campylobacter
0.00 0.00 FUD XXX
AMA: 2005,Jul,11-12; 2005,Aug,7-8

86628 Candida
EXCLUDES Candida skin test (86485)
0.00 0.00 FUD XXX
AMA: 2005,Jul,11-12; 2005,Aug,7-8

86631 Chlamydia
0.00 0.00 FUD XXX
AMA: 2005,Jul,11-12; 2005,Aug,7-8

86632 Chlamydia, IgM
EXCLUDES Chlamydia antigen (87270, 87320)
Fluorescent antibody technique (86255-86256)
0.00 0.00 FUD XXX
AMA: 2005,Jul,11-12; 2005,Aug,7-8

86635 Coccidioides
0.00 0.00 FUD XXX
AMA: 2005,Jul,11-12; 2005,Aug,7-8

86638 Coxiella burnetii (Q fever)
0.00 0.00 FUD XXX
AMA: 2005,Jul,11-12; 2005,Aug,7-8

86641 Cryptococcus
0.00 0.00 FUD XXX
AMA: 2005,Jul,11-12; 2005,Aug,7-8

86644 cytomegalovirus (CMV)
0.00 0.00 FUD XXX
AMA: 2005,Jul,11-12; 2005,Aug,7-8

86645 cytomegalovirus (CMV), IgM
0.00 0.00 FUD XXX
AMA: 2018,Jan,8; 2017,Jan,8; 2016,Jan,13; 2015,Jan,16; 2014,Jan,11

86648 Diphtheria
0.00 0.00 FUD XXX
AMA: 2005,Jul,11-12; 2005,Aug,7-8

86651 encephalitis, California (La Crosse)
0.00 0.00 FUD XXX
AMA: 2005,Jul,11-12; 2005,Aug,7-8

86652 encephalitis, Eastern equine
0.00 0.00 FUD XXX
AMA: 2005,Jul,11-12; 2005,Aug,7-8

86653 encephalitis, St. Louis
0.00 0.00 FUD XXX
AMA: 2005,Jul,11-12; 2005,Aug,7-8

86654 encephalitis, Western equine
0.00 0.00 FUD XXX
AMA: 2005,Jul,11-12; 2005,Aug,7-8

86658 enterovirus (eg, coxsackie, echo, polio)
EXCLUDES Antibodies to:
Trichinella (86784)
Trypanosoma—see code for specific methodology
Tuberculosis (86580)
Viral—see code for specific methodology
0.00 0.00 FUD XXX
AMA: 2005,Jul,11-12; 2005,Aug,7-8

86663 Epstein-Barr (EB) virus, early antigen (EA)
0.00 0.00 FUD XXX
AMA: 2005,Jul,11-12; 2005,Aug,7-8

86664 Epstein-Barr (EB) virus, nuclear antigen (EBNA)
0.00 0.00 FUD XXX
AMA: 2005,Jul,11-12; 2005,Aug,7-8

86665 Epstein-Barr (EB) virus, viral capsid (VCA)
0.00 0.00 FUD XXX
AMA: 2005,Jul,11-12; 2005,Aug,7-8

86666 Ehrlichia
0.00 0.00 FUD XXX
AMA: 2005,Jul,11-12; 2005,Aug,7-8

86668 Francisella tularensis
0.00 0.00 FUD XXX
AMA: 2005,Jul,11-12; 2005,Aug,7-8

86671 fungus, not elsewhere specified
0.00 0.00 FUD XXX
AMA: 2005,Jul,11-12; 2005,Aug,7-8

86674 Giardia lamblia
0.00 0.00 FUD XXX
AMA: 2005,Jul,11-12; 2005,Aug,7-8

86677 Helicobacter pylori
0.00 0.00 FUD XXX
AMA: 2018,Jan,8; 2017,Jan,8; 2016,Jan,13; 2015,Jan,16; 2014,Jan,11

86682 helminth, not elsewhere specified
0.00 0.00 FUD XXX
AMA: 2005,Jul,11-12; 2005,Aug,7-8

86684 Haemophilus influenza
0.00 0.00 FUD XXX
AMA: 2005,Jul,11-12; 2005,Aug,7-8

86687	**HTLV-I**		
	0.00 0.00 **FUD** XXX		🔲 🖼
	AMA: 2005,Jul,11-12; 2005,Aug,7-8		
86688	**HTLV-II**		
	0.00 0.00 **FUD** XXX		🔲 🖼
	AMA: 2005,Jul,11-12; 2005,Aug,7-8		
86689	**HTLV or HIV antibody, confirmatory test (eg, Western Blot)**		
	0.00 0.00 **FUD** XXX		🔲 🖼
	AMA: 2018,Jan,8; 2017,Jan,8; 2016,Jan,13; 2015,Jan,16; 2014,Jan,11		
86692	**hepatitis, delta agent**		
	EXCLUDES *Hepatitis delta agent, antigen (87380)*		
	0.00 0.00 **FUD** XXX		🔲 🖼
	AMA: 2005,Jul,11-12; 2005,Aug,7-8		
86694	**herpes simplex, non-specific type test**		
	0.00 0.00 **FUD** XXX		🔲 🖼
	AMA: 2005,Jul,11-12; 2005,Aug,7-8		
86695	**herpes simplex, type 1**		
	0.00 0.00 **FUD** XXX		🔲 🖼
	AMA: 2018,Jan,8; 2017,Jan,8; 2016,Jan,13; 2015,Jan,16; 2014,Jan,11		
86696	**herpes simplex, type 2**		
	0.00 0.00 **FUD** XXX		🔲 🖼
	AMA: 2005,Jul,11-12; 2005,Aug,7-8		
86698	**histoplasma**		
	0.00 0.00 **FUD** XXX		🔲 🖼
	AMA: 2005,Jul,11-12; 2005,Aug,7-8		

86701-86703 Testing for HIV Antibodies

CMS: 100-03,190.14 Human Immunodeficiency Virus Testing (Diagnosis); 100-03,190.9 Serologic Testing for Acquired Immunodeficiency Syndrome (AIDS)

INCLUDES Qualitative or semiquantitative immunoassays performed by multiple-step methods for the detection of antibodies to infectious agents

EXCLUDES *Confirmatory test for HIV antibody (86689)*
HIV-1 antigen (87390)
HIV-1 antigen(s) with HIV 1 and 2 antibodies, single result (87389)
HIV-2 antigen (87391)
Immunoassays by single-step method (86318)

Code also modifier 92 for test performed using a kit or transportable instrument comprising all or part of a single-use, disposable analytical chamber

86701	**Antibody; HIV-1**		
	0.00 0.00 **FUD** XXX		❌ 🔲 🖼
	AMA: 2018,Jan,8; 2017,Jan,8; 2016,Jan,13; 2015,Jan,16; 2014,Jan,11		
86702	**HIV-2**		
	0.00 0.00 **FUD** XXX		🔲 🖼
	AMA: 2018,Jan,8; 2017,Jan,8; 2016,Jan,13; 2015,Jan,16; 2014,Jan,11		
86703	**HIV-1 and HIV-2, single result**		
	0.00 0.00 **FUD** XXX		🔲 🖼
	AMA: 2018,Jan,8; 2017,Jan,8; 2016,Jan,13; 2015,Jan,16; 2014,Jan,11		

86704-86804 Testing for Infectious Disease Antibodies: Hepatitis—Yersinia

INCLUDES Qualitative or semiquantitative immunoassays performed by multiple-step methods for the detection of antibodies to infectious agents

EXCLUDES *Detection of:*
Antibodies other than those to infectious agents, see specific antibody or method
Infectious agent/antigen (87260-87899 [87623, 87624, 87625, 87806])
Immunoassays by single-step method (86318)

86704	**Hepatitis B core antibody (HBcAb); total**		
	0.00 0.00 **FUD** XXX		🔲 🖼
	AMA: 2018,Jan,8; 2017,Jan,8; 2016,Jan,13; 2015,Jan,16; 2014,Jan,11		
86705	**IgM antibody**		
	0.00 0.00 **FUD** XXX		🔲 🖼
	AMA: 2018,Jan,8; 2017,Jan,8; 2016,Jan,13; 2015,Jan,16; 2014,Jan,11		

86706	**Hepatitis B surface antibody (HBsAb)**		
	0.00 0.00 **FUD** XXX		🔲 🖼
	AMA: 2005,Jul,11-12; 2005,Aug,7-8		
86707	**Hepatitis Be antibody (HBeAb)**		
	0.00 0.00 **FUD** XXX		🔲 🖼
	AMA: 2005,Jul,11-12; 2005,Aug,7-8		
86708	**Hepatitis A antibody (HAAb)**		
	0.00 0.00 **FUD** XXX		🔲 🖼
	AMA: 2018,Jan,8; 2017,Jan,8; 2016,Jan,13; 2015,Jan,16; 2014,Jan,11		
86709	**Hepatitis A antibody (HAAb), IgM antibody**		
	0.00 0.00 **FUD** XXX		🔲 🖼
	AMA: 2018,Jan,8; 2017,Jan,8; 2016,Jan,13; 2015,Jan,16; 2014,Jan,11		
86710	**Antibody; influenza virus**		
	0.00 0.00 **FUD** XXX		🔲 🖼
	AMA: 2018,Jan,8; 2017,Jan,8; 2016,Jan,13; 2015,Jan,16; 2014,Jan,11		
86711	**JC (John Cunningham) virus**		
	0.00 0.00 **FUD** XXX		🔲 🖼
86713	**Legionella**		
	0.00 0.00 **FUD** XXX		🔲 🖼
86717	**Leishmania**		
	0.00 0.00 **FUD** XXX		🖼
	AMA: 2005,Jul,11-12; 2005,Aug,7-8		
86720	**Leptospira**		
	0.00 0.00 **FUD** XXX		🔲 🖼
	AMA: 2005,Jul,11-12; 2005,Aug,7-8		
86723	**Listeria monocytogenes**		
	0.00 0.00 **FUD** XXX		🔲 🖼
	AMA: 2005,Jul,11-12; 2005,Aug,7-8		
86727	**lymphocytic choriomeningitis**		
	0.00 0.00 **FUD** XXX		🔲 🖼
	AMA: 2005,Jul,11-12; 2005,Aug,7-8		
86732	**mucormycosis**		
	0.00 0.00 **FUD** XXX		🔲 🖼
	AMA: 2005,Jul,11-12; 2005,Aug,7-8		
86735	**mumps**		
	0.00 0.00 **FUD** XXX		🔲 🖼
	AMA: 2018,Jan,8; 2017,Jan,8; 2016,Jan,13; 2015,Jan,16; 2014,Jan,11		
86738	**mycoplasma**		
	0.00 0.00 **FUD** XXX		🔲 🖼
	AMA: 2005,Jul,11-12; 2005,Aug,7-8		
86741	**Neisseria meningitidis**		
	0.00 0.00 **FUD** XXX		🔲 🖼
	. **AMA:** 2005,Jul,11-12; 2005,Aug,7-8		
86744	**Nocardia**		
	0.00 0.00 **FUD** XXX		🔲 🖼
	AMA: 2005,Jul,11-12; 2005,Aug,7-8		
86747	**parvovirus**		
	0.00 0.00 **FUD** XXX		🔲 🖼
	AMA: 2005,Jul,11-12; 2005,Aug,7-8		
86750	**Plasmodium (malaria)**		
	0.00 0.00 **FUD** XXX		🔲 🖼
	AMA: 2005,Jul,11-12; 2005,Aug,7-8		
86753	**protozoa, not elsewhere specified**		
	0.00 0.00 **FUD** XXX		🔲 🖼
	AMA: 2005,Jul,11-12; 2005,Aug,7-8		
86756	**respiratory syncytial virus**		
	0.00 0.00 **FUD** XXX		🔲 🖼
	AMA: 2005,Jul,11-12; 2005,Aug,7-8		

26/TC PC/TC Only	A2-Z3 ASC Payment	50 Bilateral	♂ Male Only	♀ Female Only	🚑 Facility RVU	🔧 Non-Facility RVU	🔲 CCI	❌ CLIA
FUD Follow-up Days	**CMS:** IOM	**AMA:** CPT Asst	A-Y OPPSI	80/80 Surg Assist Allowed / w/Doc		🖼 Lab Crosswalk	🔴 Radiology Crosswalk	

CPT © 2019 American Medical Association. All Rights Reserved.

© 2019 Optum360, LLC

426

86757	**Rickettsia**		
	⊞ 0.00 ⚷ 0.00 **FUD** XXX		Ⓠ ▣
	AMA: 2005,Jul,11-12; 2005,Aug,7-8		
86759	**rotavirus**		
	⊞ 0.00 ⚷ 0.00 **FUD** XXX		Ⓠ ▣
	AMA: 2005,Jul,11-12; 2005,Aug,7-8		
86762	**rubella**		
	⊞ 0.00 ⚷ 0.00 **FUD** XXX		Ⓠ ▣
	AMA: 2005,Jul,11-12; 2005,Aug,7-8		
86765	**rubeola**		
	⊞ 0.00 ⚷ 0.00 **FUD** XXX		Ⓠ ▣
	AMA: 2005,Jul,11-12; 2005,Aug,7-8		
86768	**Salmonella**		
	⊞ 0.00 ⚷ 0.00 **FUD** XXX		Ⓠ ▣
	AMA: 2005,Jul,11-12; 2005,Aug,7-8		
86771	**Shigella**		
	⊞ 0.00 ⚷ 0.00 **FUD** XXX		Ⓠ ▣
	AMA: 2005,Jul,11-12; 2005,Aug,7-8		
86774	**tetanus**		
	⊞ 0.00 ⚷ 0.00 **FUD** XXX		Ⓠ ▣
	AMA: 2005,Jul,11-12; 2005,Aug,7-8		
86777	**Toxoplasma**		
	⊞ 0.00 ⚷ 0.00 **FUD** XXX		Ⓠ ▣
	AMA: 2005,Jul,11-12; 2005,Aug,7-8		
86778	**Toxoplasma, IgM**		
	⊞ 0.00 ⚷ 0.00 **FUD** XXX		Ⓠ ▣
	AMA: 2005,Jul,11-12; 2005,Aug,7-8		
86780	**Treponema pallidum**		
	⊞ 0.00 ⚷ 0.00 **FUD** XXX		✖ Ⓐ ▣

EXCLUDES Nontreponemal antibody analysis syphilis testing (86592-86593)

86784	**Trichinella**		
	⊞ 0.00 ⚷ 0.00 **FUD** XXX		Ⓠ ▣
	AMA: 2005,Jul,11-12; 2005,Aug,7-8		
86787	**varicella-zoster**		
	⊞ 0.00 ⚷ 0.00 **FUD** XXX		Ⓠ ▣
	AMA: 2005,Jul,11-12; 2005,Aug,7-8		
86788	**West Nile virus, IgM**		
	⊞ 0.00 ⚷ 0.00 **FUD** XXX		Ⓠ ▣
86789	**West Nile virus**		
	⊞ 0.00 ⚷ 0.00 **FUD** XXX		Ⓠ ▣
86790	**virus, not elsewhere specified**		
	⊞ 0.00 ⚷ 0.00 **FUD** XXX		Ⓠ ▣
	AMA: 2005,Jul,11-12; 2005,Aug,7-8		
86793	**Yersinia**		
	⊞ 0.00 ⚷ 0.00 **FUD** XXX		Ⓠ ▣
	AMA: 2005,Jul,11-12; 2005,Aug,7-8		
86794	**Zika virus, IgM**		
	⊞ 0.00 ⚷ 0.00 **FUD** XXX		Ⓠ ▣
86800	**Thyroglobulin antibody**		

EXCLUDES Thyroglobulin (84432)

	⊞ 0.00 ⚷ 0.00 **FUD** XXX		Ⓠ ▣
	AMA: 2005,Jul,11-12; 2005,Aug,7-8		
86803	**Hepatitis C antibody;**		
	⊞ 0.00 ⚷ 0.00 **FUD** XXX		✖ Ⓠ ▣
	AMA: 2005,Jul,11-12; 2005,Aug,7-8		
86804	**confirmatory test (eg, immunoblot)**		
	⊞ 0.00 ⚷ 0.00 **FUD** XXX		Ⓠ ▣
	AMA: 2018,Jan,8; 2017,Jan,8; 2016,Jan,13; 2015,Jan,16; 2014,Jan,11		

86805-86808 Pre-Transplant Antibody Cross Matching

86805	**Lymphocytotoxicity assay, visual crossmatch; with titration**		
	⊞ 0.00 ⚷ 0.00 **FUD** XXX		Ⓠ ▣
	AMA: 2018,Jan,8; 2017,Jan,8; 2016,Jan,13; 2015,Jan,16; 2014,Jan,11		
86806	**without titration**		
	⊞ 0.00 ⚷ 0.00 **FUD** XXX		Ⓠ ▣
	AMA: 2005,Aug,7-8; 2005,Jul,11-12		
86807	**Serum screening for cytotoxic percent reactive antibody (PRA); standard method**		
	⊞ 0.00 ⚷ 0.00 **FUD** XXX		Ⓠ ▣
	AMA: 2018,Jan,8; 2017,Jan,8; 2016,Jan,13; 2015,Jan,16; 2014,Jan,11		
86808	**quick method**		
	⊞ 0.00 ⚷ 0.00 **FUD** XXX		Ⓠ ▣
	AMA: 2018,Jan,8; 2017,Jan,8; 2016,Jan,13; 2015,Jan,16; 2014,Jan,11		

86812-86826 Histocompatibility Testing

CMS: 100-03,110.23 Stem Cell Transplantation; 100-03,190.1 Histocompatibility Testing; 100-04,3,90.3 Stem Cell Transplantation; 100-04,3,90.3.1 Allogeneic Stem Cell Transplantation; 100-04,3,90.3.3 Billing for Allogeneic Stem Cell Transplants; 100-04,32,90 Billing for Stem Cell Transplantation; 100-04,4,231.11 Billing for Allogeneic Stem Cell Transplants

EXCLUDES HLA typing by molecular pathology techniques (81370-81383)

86812	**HLA typing; A, B, or C (eg, A10, B7, B27), single antigen**		
	⊞ 0.00 ⚷ 0.00 **FUD** XXX		Ⓠ ▣
	AMA: 2018,Jan,8; 2017,Jan,8; 2016,Jan,13; 2015,Jan,16; 2014,Jan,11		
86813	**A, B, or C, multiple antigens**		
	⊞ 0.00 ⚷ 0.00 **FUD** XXX		Ⓠ ▣
	AMA: 2018,Jan,8; 2017,Jan,8; 2016,Jan,13; 2015,Jan,16; 2014,Jan,11		
86816	**DR/DQ, single antigen**		
	⊞ 0.00 ⚷ 0.00 **FUD** XXX		Ⓠ ▣
	AMA: 2018,Jan,8; 2017,Jan,8; 2016,Jan,13; 2015,Jan,16; 2014,Jan,11		
86817	**DR/DQ, multiple antigens**		
	⊞ 0.00 ⚷ 0.00 **FUD** XXX		Ⓠ ▣
	AMA: 2018,Jan,8; 2017,Jan,8; 2016,Jan,13; 2015,Jan,16; 2014,Jan,11		
86821	**lymphocyte culture, mixed (MLC)**		
	⊞ 0.00 ⚷ 0.00 **FUD** XXX		Ⓠ ▣
	AMA: 2018,Jan,8; 2017,Jan,8; 2016,Jan,13; 2015,Jan,16; 2014,Jan,11		
86825	**Human leukocyte antigen (HLA) crossmatch, non-cytotoxic (eg, using flow cytometry); first serum sample or dilution**		
	⊞ 0.00 ⚷ 0.00 **FUD** XXX		Ⓠ ▣

INCLUDES Autologous HLA crossmatch
EXCLUDES B cells (86355)
Flow cytometry (88184-88189)
Lymphocytotoxicity visual crossmatch (86805-86806)
T cells (86359)

+ 86826	**each additional serum sample or sample dilution (List separately in addition to primary procedure)**		
	⊞ 0.00 ⚷ 0.00 **FUD** XXX		Ⓠ ▣

INCLUDES Autologous HLA crossmatch
EXCLUDES B cells (86355)
Flow cytometry (88184-88189)
Lymphocytotoxicity visual crossmatch (86805-86806)
T cells (86359)
Code first (86825)

86828-86849 HLA Antibodies

86828 Antibody to human leukocyte antigens (HLA), solid phase assays (eg, microspheres or beads, ELISA, flow cytometry); qualitative assessment of the presence or absence of antibody(ies) to HLA Class I and Class II HLA antigens

🔧 0.00   ⚕ 0.00   **FUD** XXX   [Q] [▢]

Code also solid phase testing of untreated and treated specimens of either class of HLA after treatment (86828-86833)

86829 qualitative assessment of the presence or absence of antibody(ies) to HLA Class I or Class II HLA antigens

🔧 0.00   ⚕ 0.00   **FUD** XXX   [Q] [▢]

Code also solid phase testing of untreated and treated specimens of either class of HLA after treatment (86828-86833)

86830 antibody identification by qualitative panel using complete HLA phenotypes, HLA Class I

🔧 0.00   ⚕ 0.00   **FUD** XXX   [Q] [▢]

Code also solid phase testing of untreated and treated specimens of either class of HLA after treatment (86828-86833)

86831 antibody identification by qualitative panel using complete HLA phenotypes, HLA Class II

🔧 0.00   ⚕ 0.00   **FUD** XXX   [Q] [▢]

Code also solid phase testing of untreated and treated specimens of either class of HLA after treatment (86828-86833)

86832 high definition qualitative panel for identification of antibody specificities (eg, individual antigen per bead methodology), HLA Class I

🔧 0.00   ⚕ 0.00   **FUD** XXX   [Q] [▢]

Code also solid phase testing of untreated and treated specimens of either class of HLA after treatment (86828-86833)

86833 high definition qualitative panel for identification of antibody specificities (eg, individual antigen per bead methodology), HLA Class II

🔧 0.00   ⚕ 0.00   **FUD** XXX   [Q] [▢]

Code also solid phase testing of untreated and treated specimens of either class of HLA after treatment (86828-86833)

86834 semi-quantitative panel (eg, titer), HLA Class I

🔧 0.00   ⚕ 0.00   **FUD** XXX   [Q] [▢]

86835 semi-quantitative panel (eg, titer), HLA Class II

🔧 0.00   ⚕ 0.00   **FUD** XXX   [Q] [▢]

86849 Unlisted immunology procedure

🔧 0.00   ⚕ 0.00   **FUD** XXX   [N] [▢]

AMA: 2018,Jan,8; 2017,Jan,8; 2016,Jan,13; 2015,Jan,16; 2014,Jan,11

86850-86999 Transfusion Services

EXCLUDES   *Apheresis (36511-36512)*
Therapeutic phlebotomy (99195)

86850 Antibody screen, RBC, each serum technique

🔧 0.00   ⚕ 0.00   **FUD** XXX   [01] [▢]

AMA: 2018,Jan,8; 2017,Jan,8; 2016,Jan,13; 2015,Jan,16; 2014,Jan,11

86860 Antibody elution (RBC), each elution

🔧 0.00   ⚕ 0.00   **FUD** XXX   [01] [▢]

AMA: 2005,Jul,11-12; 2005,Aug,7-8

86870 Antibody identification, RBC antibodies, each panel for each serum technique

🔧 0.00   ⚕ 0.00   **FUD** XXX   [02] [▢]

AMA: 2018,Jan,8; 2017,Jan,8; 2016,Jan,13; 2015,Jan,16; 2014,Jan,11

86880 Antihuman globulin test (Coombs test); direct, each antiserum

🔧 0.00   ⚕ 0.00   **FUD** XXX   [01] [▢]

AMA: 2005,Aug,7-8; 2005,Jul,11-12

86885 indirect, qualitative, each reagent red cell

🔧 0.00   ⚕ 0.00   **FUD** XXX   [01] [▢]

AMA: 2018,Jan,8; 2017,Jan,8; 2016,Jan,13; 2015,Jan,16; 2014,Jan,11

86886 indirect, each antibody titer

EXCLUDES   *Indirect antihuman globulin (Coombs) test for RBC antibody identification using reagent red cell panels (86870)*
Indirect antihuman globulin (Coombs) test for RBC antibody screening (86850)

🔧 0.00   ⚕ 0.00   **FUD** XXX   [01] [▢]

AMA: 2018,Jan,8; 2017,Jan,8; 2016,Jan,13; 2015,Jan,16; 2014,Jan,11

86890 Autologous blood or component, collection processing and storage; predeposited

🔧 0.00   ⚕ 0.00   **FUD** XXX   [01] [▢]

AMA: 2018,Jan,8; 2017,Jan,8; 2016,Jan,13; 2015,Jan,16; 2014,Jan,11

86891 intra- or postoperative salvage

🔧 0.00   ⚕ 0.00   **FUD** XXX   [01] [▢]

AMA: 2005,Aug,7-8; 2005,Jul,11-12

86900 Blood typing, serologic; ABO

🔧 0.00   ⚕ 0.00   **FUD** XXX   [01] [▢]

AMA: 2005,Jul,11-12; 2005,Aug,7-8

86901 Rh (D)

🔧 0.00   ⚕ 0.00   **FUD** XXX   [01] [▢]

AMA: 2018,Jan,8; 2017,Jan,8; 2016,Jan,13; 2015,Jan,16; 2014,Jan,11

86902 antigen testing of donor blood using reagent serum, each antigen test

Code also one time for each antigen for each unit of blood when multiple units are tested for the same antigen

🔧 0.00   ⚕ 0.00   **FUD** XXX   [01] [▢]

AMA: 2010,Dec,7-10

86904 antigen screening for compatible unit using patient serum, per unit screened

🔧 0.00   ⚕ 0.00   **FUD** XXX   [01] [▢]

AMA: 2005,Aug,7-8; 2005,Jul,11-12

86905 RBC antigens, other than ABO or Rh (D), each

🔧 0.00   ⚕ 0.00   **FUD** XXX   [01] [▢]

AMA: 2005,Jul,11-12; 2005,Aug,7-8

86906 Rh phenotyping, complete

EXCLUDES   *Use of molecular pathology procedures for human erythrocyte antigen typing (81403)*

🔧 0.00   ⚕ 0.00   **FUD** XXX   [01] [▢]

AMA: 2005,Jul,11-12; 2005,Aug,7-8

86910 Blood typing, for paternity testing, per individual; ABO, Rh and MN

🔧 0.00   ⚕ 0.00   **FUD** XXX   [E] [▢]

AMA: 2005,Jul,11-12; 2005,Aug,7-8

86911 each additional antigen system

🔧 0.00   ⚕ 0.00   **FUD** XXX   [E] [▢]

AMA: 2005,Jul,11-12; 2005,Aug,7-8

86920 Compatibility test each unit; immediate spin technique

🔧 0.00   ⚕ 0.00   **FUD** XXX   [01] [▢]

AMA: 2018,Jan,8; 2017,Jan,8; 2016,Jan,13; 2015,Jan,16; 2014,Jan,11

86921 incubation technique

🔧 0.00   ⚕ 0.00   **FUD** XXX   [01] [▢]

AMA: 2018,Jan,8; 2017,Jan,8; 2016,Jan,13; 2015,Jan,16; 2014,Jan,11

86922 antiglobulin technique

🔧 0.00   ⚕ 0.00   **FUD** XXX   [01] [▢]

AMA: 2018,Jan,8; 2017,Jan,8; 2016,Jan,13; 2015,Jan,16; 2014,Jan,11

86923 electronic

EXCLUDES   *Other compatibility test techniques (86920-86922)*

🔧 0.00   ⚕ 0.00   **FUD** XXX   [01] [▢]

AMA: 2018,Jan,8; 2017,Jan,8; 2016,Jan,13; 2015,Jan,16; 2014,Jan,11

26/TC PC/TC Only	**A2-Z3** ASC Payment	**50** Bilateral	♂ Male Only	♀ Female Only	🔧 Facility RVU
FUD Follow-up Days	**CMS:** IOM	**AMA:** CPT Asst	**A-Y** OPPSI	**80/80** Surg Assist Allowed / w/Doc	⚕ Non-Facility RVU

Lab Crosswalk   CCI   CLIA   Radiology Crosswalk

CPT © 2019 American Medical Association. All Rights Reserved.

428   © 2019 Optum360, LLC

86927 Fresh frozen plasma, thawing, each unit
🔲 0.00 🔲 0.00 **FUD** XXX ⬜⬜
AMA: 2005,Aug,7-8; 2005,Jul,11-12

86930 Frozen blood, each unit; freezing (includes preparation)
🔲 0.00 🔲 0.00 **FUD** XXX ⬜⬜
AMA: 2018,Jan,8; 2017,Jan,8; 2016,Jan,13; 2015,Jan,16; 2014,Jan,11

86931 thawing
🔲 0.00 🔲 0.00 **FUD** XXX ⬜⬜
AMA: 2018,Jan,8; 2017,Jan,8; 2016,Jan,13; 2015,Jan,16; 2014,Jan,11

86932 freezing (includes preparation) and thawing
🔲 0.00 🔲 0.00 **FUD** XXX ⬜⬜
AMA: 2018,Jan,8; 2017,Jan,8; 2016,Jan,13; 2015,Jan,16; 2014,Jan,11

86940 Hemolysins and agglutinins; auto, screen, each
🔲 0.00 🔲 0.00 **FUD** XXX ⬜⬜
AMA: 2005,Aug,7-8; 2005,Jul,11-12

86941 incubated
🔲 0.00 🔲 0.00 **FUD** XXX ⬜⬜
AMA: 2005,Jul,11-12; 2005,Aug,7-8

86945 Irradiation of blood product, each unit
🔲 0.00 🔲 0.00 **FUD** XXX ⬜⬜
AMA: 2018,Jan,8; 2017,Jan,8; 2016,Jan,13; 2015,Jan,16; 2014,Jan,11

86950 Leukocyte transfusion
EXCLUDES Infusion allogeneic lymphocytes (38242)
Leukapheresis (36511)
🔲 0.00 🔲 0.00 **FUD** XXX ⬜⬜
AMA: 2018,Jan,8; 2017,Jan,8; 2016,Jan,13; 2015,Jan,16

86960 Volume reduction of blood or blood product (eg, red blood cells or platelets), each unit
🔲 0.00 🔲 0.00 **FUD** XXX ⬜⬜
AMA: 2018,Jan,8; 2017,Jan,8; 2016,Jan,13; 2015,Jan,16; 2014,Jan,11

86965 Pooling of platelets or other blood products
EXCLUDES Autologous WBC injection (0481T)
Injection of platelet rich plasma (0232T)
🔲 0.00 🔲 0.00 **FUD** XXX ⬜⬜
AMA: 2018,Jan,8; 2017,Jan,8; 2016,Jan,13; 2015,Jan,16; 2014,Jan,11

86970 Pretreatment of RBCs for use in RBC antibody detection, identification, and/or compatibility testing; incubation with chemical agents or drugs, each
🔲 0.00 🔲 0.00 **FUD** XXX ⬜⬜
AMA: 2005,Jul,11-12; 2005,Aug,7-8

86971 incubation with enzymes, each
🔲 0.00 🔲 0.00 **FUD** XXX ⬜⬜
AMA: 2005,Jul,11-12; 2005,Aug,7-8

86972 by density gradient separation
🔲 0.00 🔲 0.00 **FUD** XXX ⬜⬜
AMA: 2005,Jul,11-12; 2005,Aug,7-8

86975 Pretreatment of serum for use in RBC antibody identification; incubation with drugs, each
🔲 0.00 🔲 0.00 **FUD** XXX ⬜⬜
AMA: 2005,Jul,11-12; 2005,Aug,7-8

86976 by dilution
🔲 0.00 🔲 0.00 **FUD** XXX ⬜⬜
AMA: 2005,Jul,11-12; 2005,Aug,7-8

86977 incubation with inhibitors, each
🔲 0.00 🔲 0.00 **FUD** XXX ⬜⬜
AMA: 2005,Jul,11-12; 2005,Aug,7-8

86978 by differential red cell absorption using patient RBCs or RBCs of known phenotype, each absorption
🔲 0.00 🔲 0.00 **FUD** XXX ⬜⬜
AMA: 2005,Jul,11-12; 2005,Aug,7-8

86985 Splitting of blood or blood products, each unit
🔲 0.00 🔲 0.00 **FUD** XXX ⬜⬜
AMA: 2018,Jan,8; 2017,Jan,8; 2016,Jan,13; 2015,Jan,16; 2014,Jan,11

86999 Unlisted transfusion medicine procedure
🔲 0.00 🔲 0.00 **FUD** XXX ⬜⬜
AMA: 2018,Jan,8; 2017,Jan,8; 2016,Jan,13; 2015,Jan,16; 2014,Jan,11

87003-87118 Identification of Microorganisms

INCLUDES Bacteriology, mycology, parasitology, and virology
EXCLUDES Additional tests using molecular probes, chromatography, nucleic acid resequencing, or immunologic techniques (87140-87158)
Code also modifier 59 for multiple specimens or sites
Code also modifier 91 for repeat procedures performed on the same day

87003 Animal inoculation, small animal, with observation and dissection
🔲 0.00 🔲 0.00 **FUD** XXX ⬜⬜
AMA: 2005,Aug,7-8; 2005,Jul,11-12

87015 Concentration (any type), for infectious agents
EXCLUDES Direct smear for ova and parasites (87177)
🔲 0.00 🔲 0.00 **FUD** XXX ⬜⬜
AMA: 2005,Aug,7-8; 2005,Jul,11-12

87040 Culture, bacterial; blood, aerobic, with isolation and presumptive identification of isolates (includes anaerobic culture, if appropriate)
🔲 0.00 🔲 0.00 **FUD** XXX ⬜⬜
AMA: 2018,Jan,8; 2017,Jan,8; 2016,Jan,13; 2015,Jan,16; 2014,Jan,11

87045 stool, aerobic, with isolation and preliminary examination (eg, KIA, LIA), Salmonella and Shigella species
🔲 0.00 🔲 0.00 **FUD** XXX ⬜⬜
AMA: 2005,Aug,7-8; 2005,Jul,11-12

87046 stool, aerobic, additional pathogens, isolation and presumptive identification of isolates, each plate
🔲 0.00 🔲 0.00 **FUD** XXX ⬜⬜
AMA: 2018,Jan,8; 2017,Jan,8; 2016,Jan,13; 2015,Jan,16; 2014,Jan,11

87070 any other source except urine, blood or stool, aerobic, with isolation and presumptive identification of isolates
EXCLUDES Urine (87088)
🔲 0.00 🔲 0.00 **FUD** XXX ⬜⬜
AMA: 2018,Jan,8; 2017,Jan,8; 2016,Jan,13; 2015,Jan,16; 2014,Jan,11

87071 quantitative, aerobic with isolation and presumptive identification of isolates, any source except urine, blood or stool
EXCLUDES Urine (87088)
🔲 0.00 🔲 0.00 **FUD** XXX ⬜⬜
AMA: 2018,Jan,8; 2017,Jan,8; 2016,Jan,13; 2015,Jan,16; 2014,Jan,11

87073 quantitative, anaerobic with isolation and presumptive identification of isolates, any source except urine, blood or stool
EXCLUDES Definitive identification of isolates (87076, 87077)
Typing of isolates (87140-87158)
🔲 0.00 🔲 0.00 **FUD** XXX ⬜⬜
AMA: 2018,Jan,8; 2017,Jan,8; 2016,Jan,13; 2015,Jan,16; 2014,Jan,11

87075 any source, except blood, anaerobic with isolation and presumptive identification of isolates
🔲 0.00 🔲 0.00 **FUD** XXX ⬜⬜
AMA: 2005,Aug,7-8; 2005,Jul,11-12

87076 anaerobic isolate, additional methods required for definitive identification, each isolate
🔲 0.00 🔲 0.00 **FUD** XXX ⬜⬜
AMA: 2018,Jan,8; 2017,Jan,8; 2016,Jan,13; 2015,Jan,16; 2014,Jan,11

Pathology and Laboratory

87077 — 87169

87077   aerobic isolate, additional methods required for definitive identification, each isolate
🚑 0.00   🔬 0.00   **FUD** XXX   ⊠ 🔲 🔲
AMA: 2018,Jan,8; 2017,Jan,8; 2016,Jan,13; 2015,Jan,16; 2014,Jan,11

87081   Culture, presumptive, pathogenic organisms, screening only;
🚑 0.00   🔬 0.00   **FUD** XXX   🔲 🔲
AMA: 2018,Jan,8; 2017,Jan,8; 2016,Jan,13; 2015,Jan,16; 2014,Jan,11

87084   with colony estimation from density chart
🚑 0.00   🔬 0.00   **FUD** XXX   🔲 🔲
AMA: 2005,Aug,7-8; 2005,Jul,11-12

87086   Culture, bacterial; quantitative colony count, urine
🚑 0.00   🔬 0.00   **FUD** XXX   🔲 🔲
AMA: 2018,Jan,8; 2017,Jan,8; 2016,Jan,13; 2015,Jan,16; 2014,Jan,11

87088   with isolation and presumptive identification of each isolate, urine
🚑 0.00   🔬 0.00   **FUD** XXX   🔲 🔲
AMA: 2018,Jan,8; 2017,Jan,8; 2016,Jan,13; 2015,Jan,16; 2014,Jan,11

87101   Culture, fungi (mold or yeast) isolation, with presumptive identification of isolates; skin, hair, or nail
🚑 0.00   🔬 0.00   **FUD** XXX   🔲 🔲
AMA: 2018,Jan,8; 2017,Jan,8; 2016,Jan,13; 2015,Jan,16; 2014,Jan,11

87102   other source (except blood)
🚑 0.00   🔬 0.00   **FUD** XXX   🔲 🔲
AMA: 2005,Aug,7-8; 2005,Jul,11-12

87103   blood
🚑 0.00   🔬 0.00   **FUD** XXX   🔲 🔲
AMA: 2005,Aug,7-8; 2005,Jul,11-12

87106   Culture, fungi, definitive identification, each organism; yeast
🚑 0.00   🔬 0.00   **FUD** XXX   🔲 🔲
AMA: 2005,Aug,7-8; 2005,Jul,11-12

87107   mold
🚑 0.00   🔬 0.00   **FUD** XXX   🔲 🔲
AMA: 2005,Aug,7-8; 2005,Jul,11-12

87109   Culture, mycoplasma, any source
🚑 0.00   🔬 0.00   **FUD** XXX   🔲 🔲
AMA: 2005,Aug,7-8; 2005,Jul,11-12

87110   Culture, chlamydia, any source
EXCLUDES   Immunofluorescence staining of shell vials (87140)
🚑 0.00   🔬 0.00   **FUD** XXX   🄰 🔲
AMA: 2005,Aug,7-8; 2005,Jul,11-12

87116   Culture, tubercle or other acid-fast bacilli (eg, TB, AFB, mycobacteria) any source, with isolation and presumptive identification of isolates
EXCLUDES   Concentration (87015)
🚑 0.00   🔬 0.00   **FUD** XXX   🔲 🔲
AMA: 2005,Aug,7-8; 2005,Jul,11-12

87118   Culture, mycobacterial, definitive identification, each isolate
🚑 0.00   🔬 0.00   **FUD** XXX   🔲 🔲
AMA: 2005,Aug,7-8; 2005,Jul,11-12

87140-87158 Additional Culture Typing Techniques

INCLUDES   Bacteriology, mycology, parasitology, and virology
EXCLUDES   Use of molecular procedure codes as a substitute for codes in this range (81105-81183 [81173, 81174, 81200, 81201, 81202, 81203, 81204], 81400-81408, [81479])
Code also definitive identification
Code also modifier 59 for multiple specimens or sites
Code also modifier 91 for repeat procedures performed on the same day

87140   Culture, typing; immunofluorescent method, each antiserum
🚑 0.00   🔬 0.00   **FUD** XXX   🔲 🔲
AMA: 2018,Jan,8; 2017,Jan,8; 2016,Jan,13; 2015,Jan,16; 2014,Jan,11

87143   gas liquid chromatography (GLC) or high pressure liquid chromatography (HPLC) method
🚑 0.00   🔬 0.00   **FUD** XXX   🔲 🔲
AMA: 2005,Aug,7-8; 2005,Jul,11-12

87147   immunologic method, other than immunofluorescence (eg, agglutination grouping), per antiserum
🚑 0.00   🔬 0.00   **FUD** XXX   🔲 🔲
AMA: 2018,Jan,8; 2017,Jan,8; 2016,Jan,13; 2015,Jan,16; 2014,Jan,11

87149   identification by nucleic acid (DNA or RNA) probe, direct probe technique, per culture or isolate, each organism probed
🚑 0.00   🔬 0.00   **FUD** XXX   🔲 🔲
AMA: 2018,Jan,8; 2017,Jan,8; 2016,Jan,13; 2015,Jan,16; 2014,Jan,11

87150   identification by nucleic acid (DNA or RNA) probe, amplified probe technique, per culture or isolate, each organism probed
🚑 0.00   🔬 0.00   **FUD** XXX   🔲 🔲
AMA: 2018,Jan,8; 2017,Jan,8; 2016,Jan,13; 2015,Jan,16; 2014,Jan,11

87152   identification by pulse field gel typing
🚑 0.00   🔬 0.00   **FUD** XXX   🔲 🔲
AMA: 2018,Jan,8; 2017,Jan,8; 2016,Jan,13; 2015,Jan,16; 2014,Jan,11

87153   identification by nucleic acid sequencing method, each isolate (eg, sequencing of the 16S rRNA gene)
🚑 0.00   🔬 0.00   **FUD** XXX   🔲 🔲
AMA: 2018,Jan,8; 2017,Jan,8; 2016,Jan,13; 2015,Jan,16

87158   other methods
🚑 0.00   🔬 0.00   **FUD** XXX   🔲 🔲
AMA: 2018,Jan,8; 2017,Jan,8; 2016,Jan,13; 2015,Jan,16; 2014,Jan,11

87164-87255 Identification of Organism from Primary Source and Sensitivity Studies

INCLUDES   Bacteriology, mycology, parasitology, and virology
EXCLUDES   Additional tests using molecular probes, chromatography, or immunologic techniques (87140-87158)
Code also modifier 59 for multiple specimens or sites
Code also modifier 91 for repeat procedures performed on the same day

87164   Dark field examination, any source (eg, penile, vaginal, oral, skin); includes specimen collection
🚑 0.00   🔬 0.00   **FUD** XXX   🔲 80 🔲
AMA: 2005,Jul,11-12; 2005,Aug,7-8

87166   without collection
🚑 0.00   🔬 0.00   **FUD** XXX   🔲 🔲
AMA: 2005,Aug,7-8; 2005,Jul,11-12

87168   Macroscopic examination; arthropod
🚑 0.00   🔬 0.00   **FUD** XXX   🔲 🔲
AMA: 2005,Aug,7-8; 2005,Jul,11-12

87169   parasite
🚑 0.00   🔬 0.00   **FUD** XXX   🔲 🔲
AMA: 2005,Aug,7-8; 2005,Jul,11-12

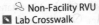

26/TC PC/TC Only   **A2-Z3** ASC Payment   **50** Bilateral   ♂ Male Only   ♀ Female Only   🚑 Facility RVU   🔬 Non-Facility RVU   🔲 CCI   ⊠ CLIA
FUD Follow-up Days   **CMS:** IOM   **AMA:** CPT Asst   **A-Y** OPPSI   **80/80** Surg Assist Allowed / w/Doc   🔲 Lab Crosswalk   🔲 Radiology Crosswalk

430   CPT © 2019 American Medical Association. All Rights Reserved.   © 2019 Optum360, LLC

87172 Pinworm exam (eg, cellophane tape prep)
⚕ 0.00 ⚲ 0.00 **FUD** XXX
AMA: 2005,Aug,7-8; 2005,Jul,11-12

87176 Homogenization, tissue, for culture
⚕ 0.00 ⚲ 0.00 **FUD** XXX
AMA: 2005,Aug,7-8; 2005,Jul,11-12

87177 Ova and parasites, direct smears, concentration and identification
> EXCLUDES Coccidia or microsporidia exam (87207)
> Complex special stain (trichrome, iron hematoxylin) (87209)
> Concentration for infectious agents (87015)
> Direct smears from primary source (87207)
> Nucleic acid probes in cytologic material (88365)

⚕ 0.00 ⚲ 0.00 **FUD** XXX
AMA: 2018,Jan,8; 2017,Jan,8; 2016,Jan,13; 2015,Jan,16; 2014,Jan,11

87181 Susceptibility studies, antimicrobial agent; agar dilution method, per agent (eg, antibiotic gradient strip)
⚕ 0.00 ⚲ 0.00 **FUD** XXX
AMA: 2018,Jan,8; 2017,Jan,8; 2016,Jan,13; 2015,Jan,16; 2014,Jan,11

87184 disk method, per plate (12 or fewer agents)
⚕ 0.00 ⚲ 0.00 **FUD** XXX
AMA: 2018,Jan,8; 2017,Jan,8; 2016,Jan,13; 2015,Jan,16; 2014,Jan,11

87185 enzyme detection (eg, beta lactamase), per enzyme
⚕ 0.00 ⚲ 0.00 **FUD** XXX
AMA: 2018,Jan,8; 2017,Jan,8; 2016,Jan,13; 2015,Jan,16; 2014,Jan,11

87186 microdilution or agar dilution (minimum inhibitory concentration [MIC] or breakpoint), each multi-antimicrobial, per plate
⚕ 0.00 ⚲ 0.00 **FUD** XXX
AMA: 2018,Jan,8; 2017,Jan,8; 2016,Jan,13; 2015,Jan,16; 2014,Jan,11

+ 87187 microdilution or agar dilution, minimum lethal concentration (MLC), each plate (List separately in addition to code for primary procedure)
Code first (87186, 87188)
⚕ 0.00 ⚲ 0.00 **FUD** XXX
AMA: 2018,Jan,8; 2017,Jan,8; 2016,Jan,13; 2015,Jan,16; 2014,Jan,11

87188 macrobroth dilution method, each agent
⚕ 0.00 ⚲ 0.00 **FUD** XXX
AMA: 2018,Jan,8; 2017,Jan,8; 2016,Jan,13; 2015,Jan,16; 2014,Jan,11

87190 mycobacteria, proportion method, each agent
> EXCLUDES Other mycobacterial susceptibility studies (87181, 87184, 87186, 87188)

⚕ 0.00 ⚲ 0.00 **FUD** XXX
AMA: 2005,Aug,7-8; 2005,Jul,11-12

87197 Serum bactericidal titer (Schlichter test)
⚕ 0.00 ⚲ 0.00 **FUD** XXX
AMA: 2005,Aug,7-8; 2005,Jul,11-12

87205 Smear, primary source with interpretation; Gram or Giemsa stain for bacteria, fungi, or cell types
⚕ 0.00 ⚲ 0.00 **FUD** XXX
AMA: 2018,Jan,8; 2017,Jan,8; 2016,Jan,13; 2015,Jan,16; 2014,Jan,11

87206 fluorescent and/or acid fast stain for bacteria, fungi, parasites, viruses or cell types
⚕ 0.00 ⚲ 0.00 **FUD** XXX
AMA: 2005,Aug,7-8; 2005,Jul,11-12

87207 special stain for inclusion bodies or parasites (eg, malaria, coccidia, microsporidia, trypanosomes, herpes viruses)
> EXCLUDES Direct smears with concentration and identification (87177)
> Fat, fibers, meat, nasal eosinophils, starch (89049-89240)
> Thick smear preparation (87015)

⚕ 0.00 ⚲ 0.00 **FUD** XXX
AMA: 2018,Jan,8; 2017,Jan,8; 2016,Jan,13; 2015,Jan,16; 2014,Jan,11

87209 complex special stain (eg, trichrome, iron hemotoxylin) for ova and parasites
⚕ 0.00 ⚲ 0.00 **FUD** XXX
AMA: 2018,Jan,8; 2017,Jan,8; 2016,Jan,13; 2015,Jan,16; 2014,Jan,11

87210 wet mount for infectious agents (eg, saline, India ink, KOH preps)
> EXCLUDES KOH evaluation of skin, hair, or nails (87220)

⚕ 0.00 ⚲ 0.00 **FUD** XXX
AMA: 2018,Jan,8; 2017,Jan,8; 2016,May,13

87220 Tissue examination by KOH slide of samples from skin, hair, or nails for fungi or ectoparasite ova or mites (eg, scabies)
⚕ 0.00 ⚲ 0.00 **FUD** XXX
AMA: 2005,Aug,7-8; 2005,Jul,11-12

87230 Toxin or antitoxin assay, tissue culture (eg, Clostridium difficile toxin)
⚕ 0.00 ⚲ 0.00 **FUD** XXX
AMA: 2005,Aug,7-8; 2005,Jul,11-12

87250 Virus isolation; inoculation of embryonated eggs, or small animal, includes observation and dissection
⚕ 0.00 ⚲ 0.00 **FUD** XXX
AMA: 2005,Aug,7-8; 2005,Jul,11-12

87252 tissue culture inoculation, observation, and presumptive identification by cytopathic effect
⚕ 0.00 ⚲ 0.00 **FUD** XXX
AMA: 2005,Aug,7-8; 2005,Jul,11-12

87253 tissue culture, additional studies or definitive identification (eg, hemabsorption, neutralization, immunofluorescence stain), each isolate
> EXCLUDES Electron microscopy (88348)
> Inclusion bodies in:
> Fluids (88106)
> Smears (87207-87210)
> Tissue sections (88304-88309)

⚕ 0.00 ⚲ 0.00 **FUD** XXX
AMA: 2005,Aug,7-8; 2005,Jul,11-12

87254 centrifuge enhanced (shell vial) technique, includes identification with immunofluorescence stain, each virus
Code also (87252)
⚕ 0.00 ⚲ 0.00 **FUD** XXX
AMA: 2018,Jan,8; 2017,Jan,8; 2016,Jan,13; 2015,Jan,16; 2014,Jan,11

87255 including identification by non-immunologic method, other than by cytopathic effect (eg, virus specific enzymatic activity)
⚕ 0.00 ⚲ 0.00 **FUD** XXX
AMA: 2018,Jan,8; 2017,Jan,8; 2016,Jan,13; 2015,Jan,16; 2014,Jan,11

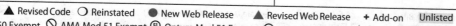

87260-87300 Fluorescence Microscopy by Organism

INCLUDES Primary source only

EXCLUDES Comparable tests on culture material (87140-87158)
Identification of antibodies (86602-86804)
Nonspecific agent detection (87299, 87449-87450, 87797-87799, 87899)

Code also modifier 59 for different species or strains reported by the same code

87260 Infectious agent antigen detection by immunofluorescent technique; adenovirus

🚗 0.00   ⚕ 0.00   **FUD** XXX   🅀 ▣

AMA: 2005,Jul,11-12; 2005,Aug,7-8

87265 Bordetella pertussis/parapertussis

🚗 0.00   ⚕ 0.00   **FUD** XXX   🅀 ▣

AMA: 2005,Jul,11-12; 2005,Aug,7-8

87267 Enterovirus, direct fluorescent antibody (DFA)

🚗 0.00   ⚕ 0.00   **FUD** XXX   🅀 ▣

AMA: 2018,Jan,8; 2017,Jan,8; 2016,Jan,13; 2015,Jan,16;
2014,Jan,11

87269 giardia

🚗 0.00   ⚕ 0.00   **FUD** XXX   🅀 ▣

AMA: 2005,Jul,11-12; 2005,Aug,7-8

87270 Chlamydia trachomatis

🚗 0.00   ⚕ 0.00   **FUD** XXX   🅰 ▣

AMA: 2005,Jul,11-12; 2005,Aug,7-8

87271 Cytomegalovirus, direct fluorescent antibody (DFA)

🚗 0.00   ⚕ 0.00   **FUD** XXX   🅀 ▣

AMA: 2018,Jan,8; 2017,Jan,8; 2016,Jan,13; 2015,Jan,16;
2014,Jan,11

87272 cryptosporidium

🚗 0.00   ⚕ 0.00   **FUD** XXX   🅀 ▣

AMA: 2005,Jul,11-12; 2005,Aug,7-8

87273 Herpes simplex virus type 2

🚗 0.00   ⚕ 0.00   **FUD** XXX   🅀 ▣

AMA: 2005,Jul,11-12; 2005,Aug,7-8

87274 Herpes simplex virus type 1

🚗 0.00   ⚕ 0.00   **FUD** XXX   🅀 ▣

AMA: 2005,Jul,11-12; 2005,Aug,7-8

87275 influenza B virus

🚗 0.00   ⚕ 0.00   **FUD** XXX   🅀 ▣

AMA: 2018,Jan,8; 2017,Jan,8; 2016,Jan,13; 2015,Jan,16;
2014,Jan,11

87276 influenza A virus

🚗 0.00   ⚕ 0.00   **FUD** XXX   🅀 ▣

AMA: 2018,Jan,8; 2017,Jan,8; 2016,Jan,13; 2015,Jan,16;
2014,Jan,11

87278 Legionella pneumophila

🚗 0.00   ⚕ 0.00   **FUD** XXX   🅀 ▣

AMA: 2005,Jul,11-12; 2005,Aug,7-8

87279 Parainfluenza virus, each type

🚗 0.00   ⚕ 0.00   **FUD** XXX   🅀 ▣

AMA: 2005,Jul,11-12; 2005,Aug,7-8

87280 respiratory syncytial virus

🚗 0.00   ⚕ 0.00   **FUD** XXX   🅀 ▣

AMA: 2005,Jul,11-12; 2005,Aug,7-8

87281 Pneumocystis carinii

🚗 0.00   ⚕ 0.00   **FUD** XXX   🅀 ▣

AMA: 2005,Jul,11-12; 2005,Aug,7-8

87283 Rubeola

🚗 0.00   ⚕ 0.00   **FUD** XXX   🅀 ▣

AMA: 2005,Jul,11-12; 2005,Aug,7-8

87285 Treponema pallidum

🚗 0.00   ⚕ 0.00   **FUD** XXX   🅀 ▣

AMA: 2005,Jul,11-12; 2005,Aug,7-8

87290 Varicella zoster virus

🚗 0.00   ⚕ 0.00   **FUD** XXX   🅀 ▣

AMA: 2005,Jul,11-12; 2005,Aug,7-8

87299 not otherwise specified, each organism

🚗 0.00   ⚕ 0.00   **FUD** XXX   🅀 ▣

AMA: 2018,Jan,8; 2017,Jan,8; 2016,Jan,13; 2015,Jan,16;
2014,Jan,11

87300 Infectious agent antigen detection by immunofluorescent technique, polyvalent for multiple organisms, each polyvalent antiserum

EXCLUDES Physician evaluation of infectious disease agents by immunofluorescence (88346)

🚗 0.00   ⚕ 0.00   **FUD** XXX   🅀 ▣

AMA: 2005,Jul,11-12; 2005,Aug,7-8

87301-87451 Enzyme Immunoassay Technique by Organism

INCLUDES Primary source only

EXCLUDES Comparable tests on culture material (87140-87158)
Identification of antibodies (86602-86804)
Nonspecific agent detection (87449-87450, 87797-87799, 87899)

Code also modifier 59 for different species or strains reported by the same code

87301 Infectious agent antigen detection by immunoassay technique, (eg, enzyme immunoassay [EIA], enzyme-linked immunosorbent assay [ELISA], immunochemiluminometric assay [IMCA]) qualitative or semiquantitative, multiple-step method; adenovirus enteric types 40/41

🚗 0.00   ⚕ 0.00   **FUD** XXX   🅀 ▣

AMA: 2018,Jan,8; 2017,Jan,8; 2016,Jan,13; 2015,Jan,16;
2014,Jan,11

87305 Aspergillus

🚗 0.00   ⚕ 0.00   **FUD** XXX   🅀 ▣

87320 Chlamydia trachomatis

🚗 0.00   ⚕ 0.00   **FUD** XXX   🅰 ▣

AMA: 2005,Jul,11-12; 2005,Aug,7-8

87324 Clostridium difficile toxin(s)

🚗 0.00   ⚕ 0.00   **FUD** XXX   🅀 ▣

AMA: 2005,Jul,11-12; 2005,Aug,7-8

87327 Cryptococcus neoformans

EXCLUDES Cryptococcus latex agglutination (86403)

🚗 0.00   ⚕ 0.00   **FUD** XXX   🅀 ▣

AMA: 2005,Jul,11-12; 2005,Aug,7-8

87328 cryptosporidium

🚗 0.00   ⚕ 0.00   **FUD** XXX   🅀 ▣

AMA: 2005,Jul,11-12; 2005,Aug,7-8

87329 giardia

🚗 0.00   ⚕ 0.00   **FUD** XXX   🅀 ▣

AMA: 2005,Jul,11-12; 2005,Aug,7-8

87332 cytomegalovirus

🚗 0.00   ⚕ 0.00   **FUD** XXX   🅀 ▣

AMA: 2005,Jul,11-12; 2005,Aug,7-8

87335 Escherichia coli 0157

EXCLUDES Giardia antigen (87329)

🚗 0.00   ⚕ 0.00   **FUD** XXX   🅀 ▣

AMA: 2005,Jul,11-12; 2005,Aug,7-8

87336 Entamoeba histolytica dispar group

🚗 0.00   ⚕ 0.00   **FUD** XXX   🅀 ▣

AMA: 2005,Jul,11-12; 2005,Aug,7-8

87337 Entamoeba histolytica group

🚗 0.00   ⚕ 0.00   **FUD** XXX   🅀 ▣

AMA: 2005,Jul,11-12; 2005,Aug,7-8

87338 Helicobacter pylori, stool

🚗 0.00   ⚕ 0.00   **FUD** XXX   ☒ 🅀 ▣

AMA: 2018,Jan,8; 2017,Jan,8; 2016,Jan,13; 2015,Jan,16;
2014,Jan,11

87339 **Helicobacter pylori**

EXCLUDES *H. pylori:*
Breath and blood by mass spectrometry (83013-83014)
Liquid scintillation counter (78267-78268)
Stool (87338)

🔧 0.00   ✂ 0.00   **FUD** XXX   Ⓠ ▣

AMA: 2005,Jul,11-12; 2005,Aug,7-8

87340 **hepatitis B surface antigen (HBsAg)**

🔧 0.00   ✂ 0.00   **FUD** XXX   Ⓠ ▣

AMA: 2018,Jan,8; 2017,Jan,8; 2016,Jan,13; 2015,Jan,16; 2014,Jan,11

87341 **hepatitis B surface antigen (HBsAg) neutralization**

🔧 0.00   ✂ 0.00   **FUD** XXX   Ⓐ ▣

AMA: 2005,Jul,11-12; 2005,Aug,7-8

87350 **hepatitis Be antigen (HBeAg)**

🔧 0.00   ✂ 0.00   **FUD** XXX   Ⓠ ▣

AMA: 2005,Jul,11-12; 2005,Aug,7-8

87380 **hepatitis, delta agent**

🔧 0.00   ✂ 0.00   **FUD** XXX   Ⓠ ▣

AMA: 2005,Jul,11-12; 2005,Aug,7-8

87385 **Histoplasma capsulatum**

🔧 0.00   ✂ 0.00   **FUD** XXX   Ⓠ ▣

AMA: 2005,Jul,11-12; 2005,Aug,7-8

87389 **HIV-1 antigen(s), with HIV-1 and HIV-2 antibodies, single result**

🔧 0.00   ✂ 0.00   **FUD** XXX   ☒ Ⓠ ▣

Code also modifier 92 for test performed using a kit or transportable instrument that is all or in part consists of a single-use, disposable analytical chamber

87390 **HIV-1**

🔧 0.00   ✂ 0.00   **FUD** XXX   Ⓠ ▣

AMA: 2005,Jul,11-12; 2005,Aug,7-8

87391 **HIV-2**

🔧 0.00   ✂ 0.00   **FUD** XXX   Ⓠ ▣

AMA: 2005,Jul,11-12; 2005,Aug,7-8

87400 **Influenza, A or B, each**

🔧 0.00   ✂ 0.00   **FUD** XXX   Ⓠ ▣

AMA: 2018,Jan,8; 2017,Jan,8; 2016,Jan,13; 2015,Jan,16; 2014,Jan,11

87420 **respiratory syncytial virus**

🔧 0.00   ✂ 0.00   **FUD** XXX   Ⓠ ▣

AMA: 2005,Jul,11-12; 2005,Aug,7-8

87425 **rotavirus**

🔧 0.00   ✂ 0.00   **FUD** XXX   Ⓠ ▣

AMA: 2005,Jul,11-12; 2005,Aug,7-8

87427 **Shiga-like toxin**

🔧 0.00   ✂ 0.00   **FUD** XXX   Ⓠ ▣

AMA: 2005,Jul,11-12; 2005,Aug,7-8

87430 **Streptococcus, group A**

🔧 0.00   ✂ 0.00   **FUD** XXX   Ⓠ ▣

AMA: 2018,Jan,8; 2017,Jan,8; 2016,Jan,13; 2015,Jan,16

87449 **Infectious agent antigen detection by immunoassay technique, (eg, enzyme immunoassay [EIA], enzyme-linked immunosorbent assay [ELISA], immunochemiluminometric assay [IMCA]), qualitative or semiquantitative; multiple-step method, not otherwise specified, each organism**

🔧 0.00   ✂ 0.00   **FUD** XXX   ☒ Ⓠ ▣

AMA: 2018,Jan,8; 2017,Jan,8; 2016,Jan,13; 2015,Jan,16; 2014,Jan,11

87450 **single step method, not otherwise specified, each organism**

🔧 0.00   ✂ 0.00   **FUD** XXX   Ⓠ ▣

AMA: 2005,Jul,11-12; 2005,Aug,7-8

87451 **multiple step method, polyvalent for multiple organisms, each polyvalent antiserum**

🔧 0.00   ✂ 0.00   **FUD** XXX   Ⓠ ▣

AMA: 2005,Jul,11-12; 2005,Aug,7-8

87471-87801 [87623, 87624, 87625] Detection Infectious Agent by Probe Techniques

INCLUDES Primary source only
EXCLUDES *Comparable tests on culture material (87140-87158)*
Identification of antibodies (86602-86804)
Nonspecific agent detection (87299, 87449-87450, 87797-87799, 87899)
Use of molecular procedure codes as a substitute for codes in this range (81161-81408 [81105, 81106, 81107, 81108, 81109, 81110, 81111, 81112, 81120, 81121, 81161, 81162, 81230, 81231, 81238, 81269, 81283, 81287, 81288, 81334])

Code also modifier 59 for different species or strains reported by the same code

87471 **Infectious agent detection by nucleic acid (DNA or RNA); Bartonella henselae and Bartonella quintana, amplified probe technique**

🔧 0.00   ✂ 0.00   **FUD** XXX   Ⓠ ▣

AMA: 2018,Jan,8; 2017,Jan,8; 2016,Jan,13; 2015,Jan,16

87472 **Bartonella henselae and Bartonella quintana, quantification**

🔧 0.00   ✂ 0.00   **FUD** XXX   Ⓠ ▣

AMA: 2018,Jan,8; 2017,Jan,8; 2016,Jan,13; 2015,Jan,16

87475 **Borrelia burgdorferi, direct probe technique**

🔧 0.00   ✂ 0.00   **FUD** XXX   Ⓠ ▣

AMA: 2018,Jan,8; 2017,Jan,8; 2016,Jan,13; 2015,Jan,16

87476 **Borrelia burgdorferi, amplified probe technique**

🔧 0.00   ✂ 0.00   **FUD** XXX   Ⓠ ▣

AMA: 2018,Jan,8; 2017,Jan,8; 2016,Jan,13; 2015,Jan,16

87480 **Candida species, direct probe technique**

🔧 0.00   ✂ 0.00   **FUD** XXX   Ⓠ ▣

AMA: 2018,Jan,8; 2017,Jan,8; 2016,Jan,13; 2015,Jan,16

87481 **Candida species, amplified probe technique**

🔧 0.00   ✂ 0.00   **FUD** XXX   Ⓠ ▣

AMA: 2018,Jan,8; 2017,Jan,8; 2016,Jan,13; 2015,Jan,16

87482 **Candida species, quantification**

🔧 0.00   ✂ 0.00   **FUD** XXX   Ⓠ ▣

AMA: 2018,Jan,8; 2017,Jan,8; 2016,Jan,13; 2015,Jan,16

87483 **central nervous system pathogen (eg, Neisseria meningitidis, Streptococcus pneumoniae, Listeria, Haemophilus influenzae, E. coli, Streptococcus agalactiae, enterovirus, human parechovirus, herpes simplex virus type 1 and 2, human herpesvirus 6, cytomegalovirus, varicella zoster virus, Cryptococcus), includes multiplex reverse transcription, when performed, and multiplex amplified probe technique, multiple types or subtypes, 12-25 targets**

🔧 0.00   ✂ 0.00   **FUD** XXX   Ⓠ ▣

87485 **Chlamydia pneumoniae, direct probe technique**

🔧 0.00   ✂ 0.00   **FUD** XXX   Ⓠ ▣

AMA: 2018,Jan,8; 2017,Jan,8; 2016,Jan,13; 2015,Jan,16

87486 **Chlamydia pneumoniae, amplified probe technique**

🔧 0.00   ✂ 0.00   **FUD** XXX   Ⓠ ▣

AMA: 2018,Jan,8; 2017,Jan,8; 2016,Jan,13; 2015,Jan,16

87487 **Chlamydia pneumoniae, quantification**

🔧 0.00   ✂ 0.00   **FUD** XXX   Ⓠ ▣

AMA: 2018,Jan,8; 2017,Jan,8; 2016,Jan,13; 2015,Jan,16

87490 **Chlamydia trachomatis, direct probe technique**

🔧 0.00   ✂ 0.00   **FUD** XXX   Ⓐ ▣

AMA: 2018,Jan,8; 2017,Jan,8; 2016,Jan,13; 2015,Jan,16

87491 **Chlamydia trachomatis, amplified probe technique**

🔧 0.00   ✂ 0.00   **FUD** XXX   Ⓐ ▣

AMA: 2018,Jan,8; 2017,Jan,8; 2016,Jan,13; 2015,Jan,16

87492 **Chlamydia trachomatis, quantification**

🔧 0.00   ✂ 0.00   **FUD** XXX   Ⓠ ▣

AMA: 2018,Jan,8; 2017,Jan,8; 2016,Jan,13; 2015,Jan,16

● New Code   ▲ Revised Code   ○ Reinstated   ● New Web Release   ▲ Revised Web Release   + Add-on   Unlisted   Not Covered   # Resequenced
⑤⓪ Optum Mod 50 Exempt   ⊘ AMA Mod 51 Exempt   � Optum Mod 51 Exempt   ㊿ Mod 63 Exempt   ⁄ Non-FDA Drug   ★ Telemedicine   Ⓜ Maternity   Ⓐ Age Edit

87493 Clostridium difficile, toxin gene(s), amplified probe technique
🚑 0.00 ⚕ 0.00 **FUD** XXX 🔲🔲
AMA: 2018,Jan,8; 2017,Jan,8; 2016,Jan,13; 2015,Jan,16; 2014,Jan,11

87495 cytomegalovirus, direct probe technique
🚑 0.00 ⚕ 0.00 **FUD** XXX 🔲🔲
AMA: 2018,Jan,8; 2017,Jan,8; 2016,Jan,13; 2015,Jan,16

87496 cytomegalovirus, amplified probe technique
🚑 0.00 ⚕ 0.00 **FUD** XXX 🔲🔲
AMA: 2018,Jan,8; 2017,Jan,8; 2016,Jan,13; 2015,Jan,16

87497 cytomegalovirus, quantification
🚑 0.00 ⚕ 0.00 **FUD** XXX 🔲🔲
AMA: 2018,Jan,8; 2017,Jan,8; 2016,Jan,13; 2015,Jan,16

87498 enterovirus, amplified probe technique, includes reverse transcription when performed
🚑 0.00 ⚕ 0.00 **FUD** XXX 🔲🔲
AMA: 2018,Jan,8; 2017,Jan,8; 2016,Jan,13; 2015,Jan,16

87500 vancomycin resistance (eg, enterococcus species van A, van B), amplified probe technique
🚑 0.00 ⚕ 0.00 **FUD** XXX 🔲🔲
AMA: 2018,Jan,8; 2017,Jan,8; 2016,Jan,13; 2015,Jan,16; 2014,Jan,11

87501 influenza virus, includes reverse transcription, when performed, and amplified probe technique, each type or subtype
🚑 0.00 ⚕ 0.00 **FUD** XXX 🔲🔲
AMA: 2018,Jan,8; 2017,Jan,8; 2016,Jan,13; 2015,Jan,16

87502 influenza virus, for multiple types or sub-types, includes multiplex reverse transcription, when performed, and multiplex amplified probe technique, first 2 types or sub-types
🚑 0.00 ⚕ 0.00 **FUD** XXX ❌🔲🔲
AMA: 2018,Jan,8; 2017,Jan,8; 2016,Jan,13; 2015,Jan,16

+ **87503** influenza virus, for multiple types or sub-types, includes multiplex reverse transcription, when performed, and multiplex amplified probe technique, each additional influenza virus type or sub-type beyond 2 (List separately in addition to code for primary procedure)
Code first (87502)
🚑 0.00 ⚕ 0.00 **FUD** XXX 🔲🔲
AMA: 2018,Jan,8; 2017,Jan,8; 2016,Jan,13; 2015,Jan,16

87505 gastrointestinal pathogen (eg, Clostridium difficile, E. coli, Salmonella, Shigella, norovirus, Giardia), includes multiplex reverse transcription, when performed, and multiplex amplified probe technique, multiple types or subtypes, 3-5 targets
🚑 0.00 ⚕ 0.00 **FUD** XXX 🔲🔲

87506 gastrointestinal pathogen (eg, Clostridium difficile, E. coli, Salmonella, Shigella, norovirus, Giardia), includes multiplex reverse transcription, when performed, and multiplex amplified probe technique, multiple types or subtypes, 6-11 targets
🚑 0.00 ⚕ 0.00 **FUD** XXX 🔲🔲

87507 gastrointestinal pathogen (eg, Clostridium difficile, E. coli, Salmonella, Shigella, norovirus, Giardia), includes multiplex reverse transcription, when performed, and multiplex amplified probe technique, multiple types or subtypes, 12-25 targets
🚑 0.00 ⚕ 0.00 **FUD** XXX 🔲🔲

87510 Gardnerella vaginalis, direct probe technique
🚑 0.00 ⚕ 0.00 **FUD** XXX 🔲🔲
AMA: 2018,Jan,8; 2017,Jan,8; 2016,Jan,13; 2015,Jan,16

87511 Gardnerella vaginalis, amplified probe technique
🚑 0.00 ⚕ 0.00 **FUD** XXX 🔲🔲
AMA: 2018,Jan,8; 2017,Jan,8; 2016,Jan,13; 2015,Jan,16

87512 Gardnerella vaginalis, quantification
🚑 0.00 ⚕ 0.00 **FUD** XXX 🔲🔲
AMA: 2018,Jan,8; 2017,Jan,8; 2016,Jan,13; 2015,Jan,16

87516 hepatitis B virus, amplified probe technique
🚑 0.00 ⚕ 0.00 **FUD** XXX 🔲🔲
AMA: 2018,Jan,8; 2017,Jan,8; 2016,Jan,13; 2015,Jan,16

87517 hepatitis B virus, quantification
🚑 0.00 ⚕ 0.00 **FUD** XXX 🔲🔲
AMA: 2018,Jan,8; 2017,Jan,8; 2016,Jan,13; 2015,Jan,16

87520 hepatitis C, direct probe technique
🚑 0.00 ⚕ 0.00 **FUD** XXX 🔲🔲
AMA: 2018,Jan,8; 2017,Jan,8; 2016,Jan,13; 2015,Jan,16

87521 hepatitis C, amplified probe technique, includes reverse transcription when performed
🚑 0.00 ⚕ 0.00 **FUD** XXX 🔲🔲
AMA: 2018,Jan,8; 2017,Jan,8; 2016,Jan,13; 2015,Jan,16

87522 hepatitis C, quantification, includes reverse transcription when performed
🚑 0.00 ⚕ 0.00 **FUD** XXX 🔲🔲
AMA: 2018,Jan,8; 2017,Jan,8; 2016,Jan,13; 2015,Jan,16

87525 hepatitis G, direct probe technique
🚑 0.00 ⚕ 0.00 **FUD** XXX 🔲🔲
AMA: 2018,Jan,8; 2017,Jan,8; 2016,Jan,13; 2015,Jan,16

87526 hepatitis G, amplified probe technique
🚑 0.00 ⚕ 0.00 **FUD** XXX 🔲🔲
AMA: 2018,Jan,8; 2017,Jan,8; 2016,Jan,13; 2015,Jan,16

87527 hepatitis G, quantification
🚑 0.00 ⚕ 0.00 **FUD** XXX 🔲🔲
AMA: 2018,Jan,8; 2017,Jan,8; 2016,Jan,13; 2015,Jan,16

87528 Herpes simplex virus, direct probe technique
🚑 0.00 ⚕ 0.00 **FUD** XXX 🔲🔲
AMA: 2018,Jan,8; 2017,Jan,8; 2016,Jan,13; 2015,Jan,16

87529 Herpes simplex virus, amplified probe technique
🚑 0.00 ⚕ 0.00 **FUD** XXX 🔲🔲
AMA: 2018,Jan,8; 2017,Jan,8; 2016,Jan,13; 2015,Jan,16

87530 Herpes simplex virus, quantification
🚑 0.00 ⚕ 0.00 **FUD** XXX 🔲🔲
AMA: 2018,Jan,8; 2017,Jan,8; 2016,Jan,13; 2015,Jan,16

87531 Herpes virus-6, direct probe technique
🚑 0.00 ⚕ 0.00 **FUD** XXX 🔲🔲
AMA: 2018,Jan,8; 2017,Jan,8; 2016,Jan,13; 2015,Jan,16

87532 Herpes virus-6, amplified probe technique
🚑 0.00 ⚕ 0.00 **FUD** XXX 🔲🔲
AMA: 2018,Jan,8; 2017,Jan,8; 2016,Jan,13; 2015,Jan,16

87533 Herpes virus-6, quantification
🚑 0.00 ⚕ 0.00 **FUD** XXX 🔲🔲
AMA: 2018,Jan,8; 2017,Jan,8; 2016,Jan,13; 2015,Jan,16

87534 HIV-1, direct probe technique
🚑 0.00 ⚕ 0.00 **FUD** XXX 🔲🔲
AMA: 2018,Jan,8; 2017,Jan,8; 2016,Jan,13; 2015,Jan,16

87535 HIV-1, amplified probe technique, includes reverse transcription when performed
🚑 0.00 ⚕ 0.00 **FUD** XXX 🔲🔲
AMA: 2018,Jan,8; 2017,Jan,8; 2016,Jan,13; 2015,Jan,16; 2014,Jan,11

87536 HIV-1, quantification, includes reverse transcription when performed
🚑 0.00 ⚕ 0.00 **FUD** XXX 🔲🔲
AMA: 2018,Jan,8; 2017,Jan,8; 2016,Jan,13; 2015,Jan,16; 2014,Jan,11

87537 HIV-2, direct probe technique
🚑 0.00 ⚕ 0.00 **FUD** XXX 🔲🔲
AMA: 2018,Jan,8; 2017,Jan,8; 2016,Jan,13; 2015,Jan,16

87538 HIV-2, amplified probe technique, includes reverse transcription when performed
🗂 0.00   🔬 0.00   **FUD** XXX   [Q] [▯]
AMA: 2018,Jan,8; 2017,Jan,8; 2016,Jan,13; 2015,Jan,16

87539 HIV-2, quantification, includes reverse transcription when performed
🗂 0.00   🔬 0.00   **FUD** XXX   [Q] [▯]
AMA: 2018,Jan,8; 2017,Jan,8; 2016,Jan,13; 2015,Jan,16

\# **87623** Human Papillomavirus (HPV), low-risk types (eg, 6, 11, 42, 43, 44)
🗂 0.00   🔬 0.00   **FUD** XXX   [Q] [▯]

\# **87624** Human Papillomavirus (HPV), high-risk types (eg, 16, 18, 31, 33, 35, 39, 45, 51, 52, 56, 58, 59, 68)
INCLUDES   Low- and high-risk types in one assay
🗂 0.00   🔬 0.00   **FUD** XXX   [Q] [▯]
AMA: 2018,Jan,8; 2017,Jan,8; 2016,Jan,13; 2015,Oct,9

\# **87625** Human Papillomavirus (HPV), types 16 and 18 only, includes type 45, if performed
EXCLUDES   HPV detection (genotyping) (0500T)
🗂 0.00   🔬 0.00   **FUD** XXX   [Q] [▯]
AMA: 2018,Jan,8; 2017,Jan,8; 2016,Jan,13; 2015,Oct,9; 2015,Jun,10

87540 Legionella pneumophila, direct probe technique
🗂 0.00   🔬 0.00   **FUD** XXX   [Q] [▯]
AMA: 2018,Jan,8; 2017,Jan,8; 2016,Jan,13; 2015,Jan,16

87541 Legionella pneumophila, amplified probe technique
🗂 0.00   🔬 0.00   **FUD** XXX   [Q] [▯]
AMA: 2018,Jan,8; 2017,Jan,8; 2016,Jan,13; 2015,Jan,16

87542 Legionella pneumophila, quantification
🗂 0.00   🔬 0.00   **FUD** XXX   [▯]
AMA: 2018,Jan,8; 2017,Jan,8; 2016,Jan,13; 2015,Jan,16

87550 Mycobacteria species, direct probe technique
🗂 0.00   🔬 0.00   **FUD** XXX   [Q] [▯]
AMA: 2018,Jan,8; 2017,Jan,8; 2016,Jan,13; 2015,Jan,16

87551 Mycobacteria species, amplified probe technique
🗂 0.00   🔬 0.00   **FUD** XXX   [Q] [▯]
AMA: 2018,Jan,8; 2017,Jan,8; 2016,Jan,13; 2015,Jan,16

87552 Mycobacteria species, quantification
🗂 0.00   🔬 0.00   **FUD** XXX   [Q] [▯]
AMA: 2018,Jan,8; 2017,Jan,8; 2016,Jan,13; 2015,Jan,16

87555 Mycobacteria tuberculosis, direct probe technique
🗂 0.00   🔬 0.00   **FUD** XXX   [Q] [▯]
AMA: 2018,Jan,8; 2017,Jan,8; 2016,Jan,13; 2015,Jan,16

87556 Mycobacteria tuberculosis, amplified probe technique
🗂 0.00   🔬 0.00   **FUD** XXX   [Q] [▯]
AMA: 2018,Jan,8; 2017,Jan,8; 2016,Jan,13; 2015,Jan,16

87557 Mycobacteria tuberculosis, quantification
🗂 0.00   🔬 0.00   **FUD** XXX   [Q] [▯]
AMA: 2018,Jan,8; 2017,Jan,8; 2016,Jan,13; 2015,Jan,16

87560 Mycobacteria avium-intracellulare, direct probe technique
🗂 0.00   🔬 0.00   **FUD** XXX   [Q] [▯]
AMA: 2018,Jan,8; 2017,Jan,8; 2016,Jan,13; 2015,Jan,16

87561 Mycobacteria avium-intracellulare, amplified probe technique
🗂 0.00   🔬 0.00   **FUD** XXX   [Q] [▯]
AMA: 2018,Jan,8; 2017,Jan,8; 2016,Jan,13; 2015,Jan,16

87562 Mycobacteria avium-intracellulare, quantification
🗂 0.00   🔬 0.00   **FUD** XXX   [Q] [▯]
AMA: 2018,Jan,8; 2017,Jan,8; 2016,Jan,13; 2015,Jan,16

● **87563** Mycoplasma genitalium, amplified probe technique

87580 Mycoplasma pneumoniae, direct probe technique
🗂 0.00   🔬 0.00   **FUD** XXX   [Q] [▯]
AMA: 2018,Jan,8; 2017,Jan,8; 2016,Jan,13; 2015,Jan,16

87581 Mycoplasma pneumoniae, amplified probe technique
🗂 0.00   🔬 0.00   **FUD** XXX   [Q] [▯]
AMA: 2018,Jan,8; 2017,Jan,8; 2016,Jan,13; 2015,Jan,16

87582 Mycoplasma pneumoniae, quantification
🗂 0.00   🔬 0.00   **FUD** XXX   [Q] [▯]
AMA: 2018,Jan,8; 2017,Jan,8; 2016,Jan,13; 2015,Jan,16

87590 Neisseria gonorrhoeae, direct probe technique
🗂 0.00   🔬 0.00   **FUD** XXX   [A] [▯]
AMA: 2018,Jan,8; 2017,Jan,8; 2016,Jan,13; 2015,Jan,16

87591 Neisseria gonorrhoeae, amplified probe technique
🗂 0.00   🔬 0.00   **FUD** XXX   [A] [▯]
AMA: 2018,Jan,8; 2017,Jan,8; 2016,Jan,13; 2015,Jan,16

87592 Neisseria gonorrhoeae, quantification
🗂 0.00   🔬 0.00   **FUD** XXX   [Q] [▯]
AMA: 2018,Jan,8; 2017,Jan,8; 2016,Jan,13; 2015,Jan,16

87623 Resequenced code. See code following 87539.

87624 Resequenced code. See code following 87539.

87625 Resequenced code. See code before 87540.

87631 respiratory virus (eg, adenovirus, influenza virus, coronavirus, metapneumovirus, parainfluenza virus, respiratory syncytial virus, rhinovirus), includes multiplex reverse transcription, when performed, and multiplex amplified probe technique, multiple types or subtypes, 3-5 targets
INCLUDES   Detection of multiple respiratory viruses with one test
EXCLUDES   Assays for typing or subtyping influenza viruses only (87501-87503)
Single test for detection of multiple infectious organisms (87800-87801)
🗂 0.00   🔬 0.00   **FUD** XXX   [✕] [Q] [▯]
AMA: 2018,Jan,8; 2017,Jan,8; 2016,Jan,13; 2015,Jan,16

87632 respiratory virus (eg, adenovirus, influenza virus, coronavirus, metapneumovirus, parainfluenza virus, respiratory syncytial virus, rhinovirus), includes multiplex reverse transcription, when performed, and multiplex amplified probe technique, multiple types or subtypes, 6-11 targets
INCLUDES   Detection of multiple respiratory viruses with one test
EXCLUDES   Assays for typing or subtyping influenza viruses only (87501-87503)
Single test to detect multiple infectious organisms (87800-87801)
🗂 0.00   🔬 0.00   **FUD** XXX   [Q] [▯]
AMA: 2018,Jan,8; 2017,Jan,8; 2016,Jan,13; 2015,Jan,16

87633 respiratory virus (eg, adenovirus, influenza virus, coronavirus, metapneumovirus, parainfluenza virus, respiratory syncytial virus, rhinovirus), includes multiplex reverse transcription, when performed, and multiplex amplified probe technique, multiple types or subtypes, 12-25 targets
INCLUDES   Detection of multiple respiratory viruses with one test
EXCLUDES   Assays for typing or subtyping influenza viruses only (87501-87503)
Single test to detect multiple infectious organisms (87800-87801)
🗂 0.00   🔬 0.00   **FUD** XXX   [✕] [Q] [▯]
AMA: 2018,Jan,8; 2017,Jan,8; 2016,Jan,13; 2015,Jan,16

87634 respiratory syncytial virus, amplified probe technique
🗂 0.00   🔬 0.00   **FUD** XXX   [✕] [Q] [▯]
EXCLUDES   Assays for RSV with other respiratory viruses (87631-87633)

87640 Staphylococcus aureus, amplified probe technique
🗂 0.00   🔬 0.00   **FUD** XXX   [Q] [▯]
AMA: 2018,Jan,8; 2017,Jan,8; 2016,Jan,13; 2015,Jan,16; 2014,Jan,11

87641 Staphylococcus aureus, methicillin resistant, amplified probe technique

> EXCLUDES Assays that detect methicillin resistance and identify Staphylococcus aureus using a single nucleic acid sequence (87641)

🔧 0.00 ⚕ 0.00 **FUD** XXX 🔲🔲

AMA: 2018,Jan,8; 2017,Jan,8; 2016,Jan,13; 2015,Jan,16; 2014,Jan,11

87650 Streptococcus, group A, direct probe technique

🔧 0.00 ⚕ 0.00 **FUD** XXX 🔲🔲

AMA: 2018,Jan,8; 2017,Jan,8; 2016,Jan,13; 2015,Jan,16

87651 Streptococcus, group A, amplified probe technique

🔧 0.00 ⚕ 0.00 **FUD** XXX ❎🔲🔲

AMA: 2018,Jan,8; 2017,Jan,8; 2016,Jan,13; 2015,Jan,16

87652 Streptococcus, group A, quantification

🔧 0.00 ⚕ 0.00 **FUD** XXX 🔲🔲

AMA: 2018,Jan,8; 2017,Jan,8; 2016,Jan,13; 2015,Jan,16

87653 Streptococcus, group B, amplified probe technique

🔧 0.00 ⚕ 0.00 **FUD** XXX 🔲🔲

AMA: 2018,Jan,8; 2017,Jan,8; 2016,Jan,13; 2015,Jan,16; 2014,Jan,11

87660 Trichomonas vaginalis, direct probe technique

🔧 0.00 ⚕ 0.00 **FUD** XXX 🔲🔲

AMA: 2018,Jan,8; 2017,Jan,8; 2016,Jan,13; 2015,Jan,16

87661 Trichomonas vaginalis, amplified probe technique

🔧 0.00 ⚕ 0.00 **FUD** XXX 🔲🔲

87662 Zika virus, amplified probe technique

🔧 0.00 ⚕ 0.00 **FUD** XXX 🔲🔲

87797 Infectious agent detection by nucleic acid (DNA or RNA), not otherwise specified; direct probe technique, each organism

🔧 0.00 ⚕ 0.00 **FUD** XXX 🔲🔲

AMA: 2018,Jan,8; 2017,Jan,8; 2016,Aug,9; 2016,Jan,13; 2015,Jan,16; 2014,Jan,11

87798 amplified probe technique, each organism

🔧 0.00 ⚕ 0.00 **FUD** XXX 🔲🔲

AMA: 2018,Jan,8; 2017,Jan,8; 2016,Jan,13; 2015,Jan,16; 2014,Jan,11

87799 quantification, each organism

🔧 0.00 ⚕ 0.00 **FUD** XXX 🔲🔲

AMA: 2018,Jan,8; 2017,Jan,8; 2016,Jan,13; 2015,Jan,16

87800 Infectious agent detection by nucleic acid (DNA or RNA), multiple organisms; direct probe(s) technique

> INCLUDES Single test to detect multiple infectious organisms
> EXCLUDES Detection of specific infectious agents not otherwise specified (87797-87799)
> Each specific organism nucleic acid detection from a primary source (87471-87660 [87623, 87624, 87625])

🔧 0.00 ⚕ 0.00 **FUD** XXX 🔲🔲

AMA: 2018,Jan,8; 2017,Jan,8; 2016,Aug,9; 2016,Jan,13; 2015,Jan,16

87801 amplified probe(s) technique

> INCLUDES Single test to detect multiple infectious organisms
> EXCLUDES Detection of multiple respiratory viruses with one test (87631-87633)
> Detection of specific infectious agents not otherwise specified (87797-87799)
> Each specific organism nucleic acid detection from a primary source (87471-87660 [87623, 87624, 87625])

🔧 0.00 ⚕ 0.00 **FUD** XXX 🔲🔲

AMA: 2018,Jan,8; 2017,Jan,8; 2016,Jan,13; 2015,Jan,16; 2014,Jan,11

87802-87899 [87806] Detection Infectious Agent by Immunoassay with Direct Optical Observation

87802 Infectious agent antigen detection by immunoassay with direct optical observation; Streptococcus, group B

🔧 0.00 ⚕ 0.00 **FUD** XXX 🔲🔲

AMA: 2005,Aug,7-8; 2005,Jul,11-12

87803 Clostridium difficile toxin A

🔧 0.00 ⚕ 0.00 **FUD** XXX 🔲🔲

AMA: 2005,Aug,7-8; 2005,Jul,11-12

\# **87806** HIV-1 antigen(s), with HIV-1 and HIV-2 antibodies

🔧 0.00 ⚕ 0.00 **FUD** XXX ❎🔲🔲

87804 Influenza

🔧 0.00 ⚕ 0.00 **FUD** XXX ❎🔲🔲

AMA: 2018,Jan,8; 2017,Jan,8; 2016,Jan,13; 2015,Jan,16; 2014,Jan,11

87806 Resequenced code. See code following 87803.

87807 respiratory syncytial virus

🔧 0.00 ⚕ 0.00 **FUD** XXX ❎🔲🔲

AMA: 2005,Jul,11-12; 2005,Aug,7-8

87808 Trichomonas vaginalis

🔧 0.00 ⚕ 0.00 **FUD** XXX ❎🔲🔲

87809 adenovirus

🔧 0.00 ⚕ 0.00 **FUD** XXX ❎🔲🔲

AMA: 2018,Jan,8; 2017,Jan,8; 2016,Jan,13; 2015,Jan,16; 2014,Jan,11

87810 Chlamydia trachomatis

🔧 0.00 ⚕ 0.00 **FUD** XXX 🅰🔲

AMA: 2018,Jan,8; 2017,Jan,8; 2016,Jan,13; 2015,Jan,16; 2014,Jan,11

87850 Neisseria gonorrhoeae

🔧 0.00 ⚕ 0.00 **FUD** XXX 🅰🔲

AMA: 2018,Jan,8; 2017,Jan,8; 2016,Jan,13; 2015,Jan,16; 2014,Jan,11

87880 Streptococcus, group A

🔧 0.00 ⚕ 0.00 **FUD** XXX ❎🔲🔲

AMA: 2018,Jan,8; 2017,Jan,8; 2016,Jan,13; 2015,Jan,16; 2014,Jan,11

87899 not otherwise specified

🔧 0.00 ⚕ 0.00 **FUD** XXX ❎🔲🔲

AMA: 2018,Jan,8; 2017,Jan,8; 2016,Jan,13; 2015,Jan,16; 2014,Jan,11

87900-87999 [87906, 87910, 87912] Drug Sensitivity Genotype/Phenotype

87900 Infectious agent drug susceptibility phenotype prediction using regularly updated genotypic bioinformatics

🔧 0.00 ⚕ 0.00 **FUD** XXX 🔲🔲

AMA: 2018,Jan,8; 2017,Jan,8; 2016,Jan,13; 2015,Dec,18; 2015,Jan,16; 2014,Jan,11

\# **87910** Infectious agent genotype analysis by nucleic acid (DNA or RNA); cytomegalovirus

> EXCLUDES HPV detection (genotyping) (0500T)
> HIV-1 infectious agent phenotype prediction (87900)

🔧 0.00 ⚕ 0.00 **FUD** XXX 🔲🔲

AMA: 2018,Jan,8; 2017,Jan,8; 2016,Jan,13; 2015,Jan,16

87901 HIV-1, reverse transcriptase and protease regions

> EXCLUDES Infectious agent drug susceptibility phenotype prediction for HIV-1 (87900)

🔧 0.00 ⚕ 0.00 **FUD** XXX 🔲🔲

AMA: 2018,Jan,8; 2017,Jan,8; 2016,Jan,13; 2015,Jan,16; 2014,Jan,11

\# **87906** HIV-1, other region (eg, integrase, fusion)

> EXCLUDES HIV-1 infectious agent phenotype prediction (87900)

🔧 0.00 ⚕ 0.00 **FUD** XXX 🔲🔲

AMA: 2018,Jan,8; 2017,Jan,8; 2016,Jan,13; 2015,Jan,16

#	87912	**Hepatitis B virus**		Q ▫

🚑 0.00   ⚕ 0.00   **FUD** XXX

AMA: 2018,Jan,8; 2017,Jan,8; 2016,Jan,13; 2015,Jan,16

87902 **Hepatitis C virus** Q ▫

🚑 0.00   ⚕ 0.00   **FUD** XXX

AMA: 2018,Jan,8; 2017,Jan,8; 2016,Jan,13; 2015,Dec,18; 2015,Nov,10; 2015,Jan,16; 2014,Jan,11

87903 **Infectious agent phenotype analysis by nucleic acid (DNA or RNA) with drug resistance tissue culture analysis, HIV 1; first through 10 drugs tested** Q ▫

🚑 0.00   ⚕ 0.00   **FUD** XXX

AMA: 2018,Jan,8; 2017,Jan,8; 2016,Jan,13; 2015,Jan,16; 2014,Jan,11

+ **87904** **each additional drug tested (List separately in addition to code for primary procedure)** Q ▫

Code first (87903)

🚑 0.00   ⚕ 0.00   **FUD** XXX

AMA: 2018,Jan,8; 2017,Jan,8; 2016,Jan,13; 2015,Jan,16; 2014,Jan,11

87905 **Infectious agent enzymatic activity other than virus (eg, sialidase activity in vaginal fluid)** ✕ Q ▫

🚑 0.00   ⚕ 0.00   **FUD** XXX

EXCLUDES   *Isolation of a virus identified by a nonimmunologic method, and by noncytopathic effect (87255)*

87906 Resequenced code. See code following 87901.

87910 Resequenced code. See code following 87900.

87912 Resequenced code. See code before 87902.

87999 **Unlisted microbiology procedure** N ▫

🚑 0.00   ⚕ 0.00   **FUD** XXX

AMA: 2018,Jan,8; 2017,Jan,8; 2016,Jan,13; 2015,Jan,16; 2014,Jan,11

88000-88099 Autopsy Services

CMS: 100-02,15,80.1 Payment for Clinical Laboratory Services

INCLUDES   Services for physicians only

88000 **Necropsy (autopsy), gross examination only; without CNS** E ▫

🚑 0.00   ⚕ 0.00   **FUD** XXX

AMA: 2018,Jan,8; 2017,Jan,8; 2016,Jan,13; 2015,Jan,16; 2014,Jan,11

88005 **with brain** E ▫

🚑 0.00   ⚕ 0.00   **FUD** XXX

AMA: 2005,Jul,11-12; 2005,Aug,7-8

88007 **with brain and spinal cord** E ▫

🚑 0.00   ⚕ 0.00   **FUD** XXX

AMA: 2005,Jul,11-12; 2005,Aug,7-8

88012 **infant with brain** A

🚑 0.00   ⚕ 0.00   **FUD** XXX   E ▫

AMA: 2005,Jul,11-12; 2005,Aug,7-8

88014 **stillborn or newborn with brain** A

🚑 0.00   ⚕ 0.00   **FUD** XXX   E ▫

AMA: 2005,Jul,11-12; 2005,Aug,7-8

88016 **macerated stillborn** A

🚑 0.00   ⚕ 0.00   **FUD** XXX   E ▫

AMA: 2005,Jul,11-12; 2005,Aug,7-8

88020 **Necropsy (autopsy), gross and microscopic; without CNS** E ▫

🚑 0.00   ⚕ 0.00   **FUD** XXX

AMA: 2005,Jul,11-12; 2005,Aug,7-8

88025 **with brain** E ▫

🚑 0.00   ⚕ 0.00   **FUD** XXX

AMA: 2005,Jul,11-12; 2005,Aug,7-8

88027 **with brain and spinal cord** E ▫

🚑 0.00   ⚕ 0.00   **FUD** XXX

AMA: 2005,Jul,11-12; 2005,Aug,7-8

88028 **infant with brain** A

🚑 0.00   ⚕ 0.00   **FUD** XXX   E ▫

AMA: 2005,Jul,11-12; 2005,Aug,7-8

88029 **stillborn or newborn with brain** A

🚑 0.00   ⚕ 0.00   **FUD** XXX   E ▫

AMA: 2005,Jul,11-12; 2005,Aug,7-8

88036 **Necropsy (autopsy), limited, gross and/or microscopic; regional** E ▫

🚑 0.00   ⚕ 0.00   **FUD** XXX

AMA: 2005,Jul,11-12; 2005,Aug,7-8

88037 **single organ** E ▫

🚑 0.00   ⚕ 0.00   **FUD** XXX

AMA: 2005,Jul,11-12; 2005,Aug,7-8

88040 **Necropsy (autopsy); forensic examination** E ▫

🚑 0.00   ⚕ 0.00   **FUD** XXX

AMA: 2005,Jul,11-12; 2005,Aug,7-8

88045 **coroner's call** E ▫

🚑 0.00   ⚕ 0.00   **FUD** XXX

AMA: 2005,Jul,11-12; 2005,Aug,7-8

88099 **Unlisted necropsy (autopsy) procedure** E ▫

🚑 0.00   ⚕ 0.00   **FUD** XXX

AMA: 2018,Jan,8; 2017,Jan,8; 2016,Jan,13; 2015,Jan,16; 2014,Jan,11

88104-88140 Cytopathology: Other Than Cervical/Vaginal

88104 **Cytopathology, fluids, washings or brushings, except cervical or vaginal; smears with interpretation** 01 80 ▫

🚑 1.98   ⚕ 1.98   **FUD** XXX

AMA: 2018,Jan,8; 2017,Jan,8; 2016,Jan,13; 2015,Jan,16; 2014,Jan,11

88106 **simple filter method with interpretation** 01 80 ▫

EXCLUDES   *Cytopathology smears with interpretation (88104)*
Selective cellular enhancement (nongynecological) including filter transfer techniques (88112)

🚑 1.81   ⚕ 1.81   **FUD** XXX

AMA: 2018,Jan,8; 2017,Jan,8; 2016,Jan,13; 2015,Jan,16; 2014,Jan,11

88108 **Cytopathology, concentration technique, smears and interpretation (eg, Saccomanno technique)** 01 80 ▫

EXCLUDES   *Cervical or vaginal smears (88150-88155)*
Gastric intubation with lavage (43754-43755)

⚡ (74340)

🚑 1.71   ⚕ 1.71   **FUD** XXX

AMA: 2018,Jan,8; 2017,Jan,8; 2016,Jan,13; 2015,Jan,16; 2014,Jan,11

88112 **Cytopathology, selective cellular enhancement technique with interpretation (eg, liquid based slide preparation method), except cervical or vaginal** 01 80 ▫

EXCLUDES   *Cytopathology cellular enhancement technique (88108)*

🚑 1.90   ⚕ 1.90   **FUD** XXX

AMA: 2005,Aug,7-8; 2005,Jul,11-12

88120 **Cytopathology, in situ hybridization (eg, FISH), urinary tract specimen with morphometric analysis, 3-5 molecular probes, each specimen; manual** 02 80 ▫

EXCLUDES   *More than five probes (88399)*
Morphometric in situ hybridization on specimens other than urinary tract (88367-88368 [88373, 88374])

🚑 16.8   ⚕ 16.8   **FUD** XXX

AMA: 2010,Dec,7-10

88121 **using computer-assisted technology** 01 80 ▫

EXCLUDES   *More than five probes (88399)*
Morphometric in situ hybridization on specimens other than urinary tract (88367-88368 [88373, 88374])

🚑 13.5   ⚕ 13.5   **FUD** XXX

AMA: 2010,Dec,7-10

88125 **Cytopathology, forensic (eg, sperm)** 01 80 ▫

🚑 0.75   ⚕ 0.75   **FUD** XXX

AMA: 2005,Aug,7-8; 2005,Jul,11-12

88130 **Sex chromatin identification; Barr bodies** Q ▫

🚑 0.00   ⚕ 0.00   **FUD** XXX

AMA: 2005,Aug,7-8; 2005,Jul,11-12

Pathology and Laboratory

88140 — 88173

88140   peripheral blood smear, polymorphonuclear
         drumsticks
         EXCLUDES *Guard stain (88313)*
         🚗 0.00   ⚖ 0.00   **FUD** XXX   [Q][⌐]
         AMA: 2018,Jan,8; 2017,Jan,8; 2016,Jan,13; 2015,Jan,16;
         2014,Jan,11

88141-88155 Pap Smears
CMS: 100-03,210.2 Screening Pap Smears/Pelvic Examinations for Early Cancer Detection
  EXCLUDES *Non-Bethesda method (88150-88153)*

88141   **Cytopathology, cervical or vaginal (any reporting system),**
         requiring interpretation by physician ♀
         Code also (88142-88153, 88164-88167, 88174-88175)
         🚗 0.90   ⚖ 0.90   **FUD** XXX   [N][80][26][⌐]
         AMA: 2018,Jan,8; 2017,Jan,8; 2016,Jan,13; 2015,Jan,16;
         2014,Jan,11

88142   **Cytopathology, cervical or vaginal (any reporting system),**
         collected in preservative fluid, automated thin layer
         preparation; manual screening under physician
         supervision ♀
         INCLUDES Bethesda or non-Bethesda method
         🚗 0.00   ⚖ 0.00   **FUD** XXX   [Q][⌐]
         AMA: 2018,Jan,8; 2017,Jan,8; 2016,Jan,13; 2015,Jan,16;
         2014,Jan,11

88143   **with manual screening and rescreening under physician**
         supervision ♀
         INCLUDES Bethesda or non-Bethesda method
         EXCLUDES *Automated screening of automated thin layer*
                   preparation (88174-88175)
         🚗 0.00   ⚖ 0.00   **FUD** XXX   [Q][⌐]
         AMA: 2018,Jan,8; 2017,Jan,8; 2016,Jan,13; 2015,Jan,16;
         2014,Jan,11

88147   **Cytopathology smears, cervical or vaginal; screening by**
         automated system under physician supervision ♀
         🚗 0.00   ⚖ 0.00   **FUD** XXX   [Q][⌐]
         AMA: 2018,Jan,8; 2017,Jan,8; 2016,Jan,13; 2015,Jan,16;
         2014,Jan,11

88148   **screening by automated system with manual rescreening**
         under physician supervision ♀
         🚗 0.00   ⚖ 0.00   **FUD** XXX   [Q][⌐]
         AMA: 2018,Jan,8; 2017,Jan,8; 2016,Jan,13; 2015,Jan,16;
         2014,Jan,11

88150   **Cytopathology, slides, cervical or vaginal; manual screening**
         under physician supervision ♀
         EXCLUDES *Bethesda method Pap smears (88164-88167)*
         🚗 0.00   ⚖ 0.00   **FUD** XXX   [Q][⌐]
         AMA: 2018,Jan,8; 2017,Jan,8; 2016,Jan,13; 2015,Jan,16;
         2014,Jan,11

88152   **with manual screening and computer-assisted rescreening**
         under physician supervision ♀
         EXCLUDES *Bethesda method Pap smears (88164-88167)*
         🚗 0.00   ⚖ 0.00   **FUD** XXX   [Q][⌐]
         AMA: 2018,Jan,8; 2017,Jan,8; 2016,Jan,13; 2015,Jan,16;
         2014,Jan,11

88153   **with manual screening and rescreening under physician**
         supervision ♀
         EXCLUDES *Bethesda method Pap smears (88164-88167)*
         🚗 0.00   ⚖ 0.00   **FUD** XXX   [Q][⌐]
         AMA: 2018,Jan,8; 2017,Jan,8; 2016,Jan,13; 2015,Jan,16;
         2014,Jan,11

+ 88155 **Cytopathology, slides, cervical or vaginal, definitive hormonal**
         evaluation (eg, maturation index, karyopyknotic index,
         estrogenic index) (List separately in addition to code[s] for
         other technical and interpretation services) ♀
         Code first (88142-88153, 88164-88167, 88174-88175)
         🚗 0.00   ⚖ 0.00   **FUD** XXX   [Q][⌐]
         AMA: 2018,Jan,8; 2017,Jan,8; 2016,Jan,13; 2015,Jan,16;
         2014,Jan,11

88160-88162 Cytopathology Smears (Other Than Pap)

88160   **Cytopathology, smears, any other source; screening and**
         interpretation
         🚗 2.01   ⚖ 2.01   **FUD** XXX   [01][80][⌐]
         AMA: 2006,Dec,10-12; 2005,Jul,11-12

88161   **preparation, screening and interpretation**
         🚗 1.87   ⚖ 1.87   **FUD** XXX   [01][80][⌐]
         AMA: 2018,Jan,8; 2017,Jan,8; 2016,Jan,13; 2015,Jan,16;
         2014,Jan,11

88162   **extended study involving over 5 slides and/or multiple**
         stains
         EXCLUDES *Aerosol collection of sputum (89220)*
                   Special stains (88312-88314)
         🚗 2.70   ⚖ 2.70   **FUD** XXX   [01][80][⌐]
         AMA: 2005,Aug,7-8; 2005,Jul,11-12

88164-88167 Pap Smears: Bethesda System
CMS: 100-03,210.2 Screening Pap Smears/Pelvic Examinations for Early Cancer Detection
  EXCLUDES *Non-Bethesda method (88150-88153)*

88164   **Cytopathology, slides, cervical or vaginal (the Bethesda**
         System); manual screening under physician supervision ♀
         🚗 0.00   ⚖ 0.00   **FUD** XXX   [Q][⌐]
         AMA: 2018,Jan,8; 2017,Jan,8; 2016,Jan,13; 2015,Jan,16;
         2014,Jan,11

88165   **with manual screening and rescreening under physician**
         supervision ♀
         🚗 0.00   ⚖ 0.00   **FUD** XXX   [Q][⌐]
         AMA: 2018,Jan,8; 2017,Jan,8; 2016,Jan,13; 2015,Jan,16;
         2014,Jan,11

88166   **with manual screening and computer-assisted rescreening**
         under physician supervision ♀
         🚗 0.00   ⚖ 0.00   **FUD** XXX   [Q][⌐]
         AMA: 2018,Jan,8; 2017,Jan,8; 2016,Jan,13; 2015,Jan,16;
         2014,Jan,11

88167   **with manual screening and computer-assisted rescreening**
         using cell selection and review under physician
         supervision ♀
         EXCLUDES *Fine needle aspiration ([10004, 10005, 10006, 10007,*
                   10008, 10009, 10010, 10011, 10012])
         🚗 0.00   ⚖ 0.00   **FUD** XXX   [Q][⌐]
         AMA: 2018,Jan,8; 2017,Jan,8; 2016,Jan,13; 2015,Jan,16;
         2014,Jan,11

88172-88177 [88177] Cytopathology of Needle Biopsy
  EXCLUDES *Fine needle aspiration (10021, [10004, 10005, 10006, 10007, 10008, 10009,*
            10010, 10011, 10012])

88172   **Cytopathology, evaluation of fine needle aspirate; immediate**
         cytohistologic study to determine adequacy for diagnosis,
         first evaluation episode, each site
         INCLUDES The submission of a complete set of cytologic material
                   for evaluation regardless of the number of
                   needle passes performed or slides prepared from
                   each site
         EXCLUDES *Cytologic examination during intraoperative pathology*
                   consultation (88333-88334)
         🚗 1.60   ⚖ 1.60   **FUD** XXX   [01][80][⌐]
         AMA: 2019,Feb,8; 2019,Apr,4; 2018,Jan,8; 2017,Jan,8;
         2016,Jan,13; 2016,Jan,11; 2015,Jan,16; 2014,Jan,11

88173   **interpretation and report**
         INCLUDES The interpretation and report from each anatomical
                   site no matter how many passes or evaluation
                   episodes are performed during the aspiration
         EXCLUDES *Cytologic examination during intraoperative pathology*
                   consultation (88333-88334)
         🚗 4.32   ⚖ 4.32   **FUD** XXX   [01][80][⌐]
         AMA: 2019,Feb,8; 2019,Apr,4; 2018,Jan,8; 2017,Jan,8;
         2016,Jan,13; 2015,Jan,16; 2014,Jan,11

+ # **88177** **immediate cytohistologic study to determine adequacy for diagnosis, each separate additional evaluation episode, same site (List separately in addition to code for primary procedure)**

Code also each additional immediate repeat evaluation episode(s) required from the same site (e.g., previous sample is inadequate)

Code first (88172)

0.84   0.84   **FUD** ZZZ   N 80 ▣

AMA: 2019,Apr,4; 2018,Jan,8; 2017,Jan,8; 2016,Jan,11

88174-88177 Pap Smears: Automated Screening

EXCLUDES *Non-Bethesda method (88150-88153)*

88174 **Cytopathology, cervical or vaginal (any reporting system), collected in preservative fluid, automated thin layer preparation; screening by automated system, under physician supervision** ♀

INCLUDES Bethesda or non-Bethesda method

0.00   0.00   **FUD** XXX   Q ▣

AMA: 2018,Jan,8; 2017,Jan,8; 2016,Jan,13; 2015,Jan,16; 2014,Jan,11

88175 **with screening by automated system and manual rescreening or review, under physician supervision** ♀

INCLUDES Bethesda or non-Bethesda method

EXCLUDES *Manual screening (88142-88143)*

0.00   0.00   **FUD** XXX   Q ▣

AMA: 2018,Jan,8; 2017,Jan,8; 2016,Jan,13; 2015,Jan,16; 2014,Jan,11

88177 Resequenced code. See code following 88173.

88182-88199 Cytopathology Using the Fluorescence-Activated Cell Sorter

88182 **Flow cytometry, cell cycle or DNA analysis**

EXCLUDES *DNA ploidy analysis by morphometric technique (88358)*

3.79   3.79   **FUD** XXX   Q2 80 ▣

AMA: 2018,Jan,8; 2017,Jan,8; 2016,Jan,13; 2015,Jan,16

88184 **Flow cytometry, cell surface, cytoplasmic, or nuclear marker, technical component only; first marker**

1.88   1.88   **FUD** XXX   Q2 80 TC ▣

AMA: 2018,Jan,8; 2017,Jan,8; 2016,Jan,13; 2015,Jan,16; 2014,Jan,11

+ **88185** **each additional marker (List separately in addition to code for first marker)**

Code first (88184)

0.69   0.69   **FUD** ZZZ   N 80 TC ▣

AMA: 2018,Jan,8; 2017,Jan,8; 2016,Jan,13; 2015,Jan,16; 2014,Jan,11

88187 **Flow cytometry, interpretation; 2 to 8 markers**

EXCLUDES *Antibody assessment by flow cytometry (83516-83520, 86000-86849 [86152, 86153])*
Cell enumeration by immunologic selection and identification ([86152, 86153])
Interpretation (86355-86357, 86359-86361, 86367)

1.08   1.08   **FUD** XXX   B 80 26 ▣

AMA: 2018,Jan,8; 2017,Jan,8; 2016,Jan,13; 2015,Jan,16; 2014,Jan,11

88188 **9 to 15 markers**

EXCLUDES *Antibody assessment by flow cytometry (83516-83520, 86000-86849 [86152, 86153])*
Cell enumeration by immunologic selection and identification ([86152, 86153])
Interpretation (86355-86357, 86359-86361, 86367)

1.83   1.83   **FUD** XXX   B 80 26 ▣

AMA: 2018,Jan,8; 2017,Jan,8; 2016,Jan,13; 2015,Jan,16; 2014,Jan,11

88189 **16 or more markers**

EXCLUDES *Antibody assessment by flow cytometry (83516-83520, 86000-86849 [86152, 86153])*
Cell enumeration using immunologic selection and identification in fluid sample ([86152, 86153])
Interpretation (86355-86357, 86359-86361, 86367)

2.45   2.45   **FUD** XXX   B 80 26 ▣

AMA: 2018,Jan,8; 2017,Jan,8; 2016,Jan,13; 2015,Jan,16; 2014,Jan,11

88199 **Unlisted cytopathology procedure**

EXCLUDES *Electron microscopy (88348)*

0.00   0.00   **FUD** XXX   Q1 80 ▣

AMA: 2018,Jan,8; 2017,Jan,8; 2016,Jan,13; 2015,Jan,16; 2014,Jan,11

88230-88299 Cytogenic Studies

CMS: 100-03,190.3 Cytogenic Studies

EXCLUDES *Acetylcholinesterase (82013)*
Alpha-fetoprotein (amniotic fluid or serum) (82105-82106)
Microdissection (88380)
Molecular pathology codes (81105-81383 [81105, 81106, 81107, 81108, 81109, 81110, 81111, 81112, 81120, 81121, 81161, 81162, 81163, 81164, 81165, 81166, 81167, 81173, 81174, 81184, 81185, 81186, 81187, 81188, 81189, 81190, 81200, 81201, 81202, 81203, 81204, 81205, 81206, 81207, 81208, 81209, 81210, 81219, 81227, 81230, 81231, 81233, 81234, 81238, 81239, 81245, 81246, 81250, 81257, 81258, 81259, 81261, 81262, 81263, 81264, 81265, 81266, 81267, 81268, 81269, 81271, 81274, 81283, 81284, 81285, 81286, 81287, 81288, 81289, 81291, 81292, 81293, 81294, 81295, 81301, 81302, 81303, 81304, 81306, 81312, 81320, 81324, 81325, 81326, 81332, 81334, 81336, 81337, 81343, 81344, 81345, 81361, 81362, 81363, 81364], 81400-81408, [81479], 81410-81471 [81448], 81500-81512, 81599)

88230 **Tissue culture for non-neoplastic disorders; lymphocyte**

0.00   0.00   **FUD** XXX   Q ▣

AMA: 2018,Jan,8; 2017,Jan,8; 2016,Jan,13; 2015,Jan,16; 2014,Jan,11

88233 **skin or other solid tissue biopsy**

0.00   0.00   **FUD** XXX   Q ▣

AMA: 2018,Jan,8; 2017,Jan,8; 2016,Jan,13; 2015,Jan,16; 2014,Jan,11

88235 **amniotic fluid or chorionic villus cells** M

0.00   0.00   **FUD** XXX   Q ▣

AMA: 2018,Jan,8; 2017,Jan,8; 2016,Jan,13; 2015,Jan,16; 2014,Jan,11

88237 **Tissue culture for neoplastic disorders; bone marrow, blood cells**

0.00   0.00   **FUD** XXX   Q ▣

AMA: 2018,Jan,8; 2017,Jan,8; 2016,Jan,13; 2015,Jan,16; 2014,Jan,11

88239 **solid tumor**

0.00   0.00   **FUD** XXX   Q ▣

AMA: 2018,Jan,8; 2017,Jan,8; 2016,Jan,13; 2015,Jan,16; 2014,Jan,11

88240 **Cryopreservation, freezing and storage of cells, each cell line**

EXCLUDES *Therapeutic cryopreservation and storage (38207)*

0.00   0.00   **FUD** XXX   Q ▣

AMA: 2018,Jan,8; 2017,Jan,8; 2016,Jan,13; 2015,Jan,16; 2014,Jan,11

88241 **Thawing and expansion of frozen cells, each aliquot**

EXCLUDES *Therapeutic thawing of prior harvest (38208)*

0.00   0.00   **FUD** XXX   Q ▣

AMA: 2018,Jan,8; 2017,Jan,8; 2016,Jan,13; 2015,Jan,16; 2014,Jan,11

88245 **Chromosome analysis for breakage syndromes; baseline Sister Chromatid Exchange (SCE), 20-25 cells**

0.00   0.00   **FUD** XXX   Q ▣

AMA: 2018,Jan,8; 2017,Jan,8; 2016,Jan,13; 2015,Jan,16; 2014,Jan,11

88248 baseline breakage, score 50-100 cells, count 20 cells, 2 karyotypes (eg, for ataxia telangiectasia, Fanconi anemia, fragile X)
   0.00   0.00   **FUD** XXX
   AMA: 2018,Jan,8; 2017,Jan,8; 2016,Jan,13; 2015,Jan,16; 2014,Jan,11

88249 score 100 cells, clastogen stress (eg, diepoxybutane, mitomycin C, ionizing radiation, UV radiation)
   0.00   0.00   **FUD** XXX
   AMA: 2018,Jan,8; 2017,Jan,8; 2016,Jan,13; 2015,Jan,16; 2014,Jan,11

88261 Chromosome analysis; count 5 cells, 1 karyotype, with banding
   0.00   0.00   **FUD** XXX
   AMA: 2018,Jan,8; 2017,Jan,8; 2016,Jan,13; 2015,Jan,16; 2014,Jan,11

88262 count 15-20 cells, 2 karyotypes, with banding
   0.00   0.00   **FUD** XXX
   AMA: 2019,Aug,10; 2018,Jan,8; 2017,Jan,8; 2016,Jan,13; 2015,Jan,16; 2014,Jan,11

88263 count 45 cells for mosaicism, 2 karyotypes, with banding
   0.00   0.00   **FUD** XXX
   AMA: 2018,Jan,8; 2017,Jan,8; 2016,Jan,13; 2015,Jan,16; 2014,Jan,11

88264 analyze 20-25 cells
   0.00   0.00   **FUD** XXX
   AMA: 2019,Aug,10; 2018,Jan,8; 2017,Jan,8; 2016,Jan,13; 2015,Jan,16; 2014,Jan,11

88267 Chromosome analysis, amniotic fluid or chorionic villus, count 15 cells, 1 karyotype, with banding
   0.00   0.00   **FUD** XXX
   AMA: 2018,Jan,8; 2017,Jan,8; 2016,Jan,13; 2015,Jan,16; 2014,Jan,11

88269 Chromosome analysis, in situ for amniotic fluid cells, count cells from 6-12 colonies, 1 karyotype, with banding
   0.00   0.00   **FUD** XXX
   AMA: 2018,Jan,8; 2017,Jan,8; 2016,Jan,13; 2015,Jan,16; 2014,Jan,11

88271 Molecular cytogenetics; DNA probe, each (eg, FISH)
   EXCLUDES   Cytogenomic microarray analysis (81228-81229, 81405-81406, [81479])
      Fetal chromosome analysis using maternal blood (81420-81422)
   0.00   0.00   **FUD** XXX
   AMA: 2018,Jan,8; 2017,Apr,3; 2017,Jan,8; 2016,Jan,13; 2015,Jan,16; 2014,Jan,11

88272 chromosomal in situ hybridization, analyze 3-5 cells (eg, for derivatives and markers)
   0.00   0.00   **FUD** XXX
   AMA: 2018,Jan,8; 2017,Jan,8; 2016,Jan,13; 2015,Jan,16; 2014,Jan,11

88273 chromosomal in situ hybridization, analyze 10-30 cells (eg, for microdeletions)
   0.00   0.00   **FUD** XXX
   AMA: 2018,Jan,8; 2017,Jan,8; 2016,Jan,13; 2015,Jan,16; 2014,Jan,11

88274 interphase in situ hybridization, analyze 25-99 cells
   0.00   0.00   **FUD** XXX
   AMA: 2018,Jan,8; 2017,Jan,8; 2016,Jan,13; 2015,Jan,16; 2014,Jan,11

88275 interphase in situ hybridization, analyze 100-300 cells
   0.00   0.00   **FUD** XXX
   AMA: 2018,Jan,8; 2017,Jan,8; 2016,Jan,13; 2015,Jan,16; 2014,Jan,11

88280 Chromosome analysis; additional karyotypes, each study
   0.00   0.00   **FUD** XXX
   AMA: 2018,Jan,8; 2017,Jan,8; 2016,Jan,13; 2015,Jan,16; 2014,Jan,11

88283 additional specialized banding technique (eg, NOR, C-banding)
   0.00   0.00   **FUD** XXX
   AMA: 2018,Jan,8; 2017,Jan,8; 2016,Jan,13; 2015,Jan,16; 2014,Jan,11

88285 additional cells counted, each study
   0.00   0.00   **FUD** XXX
   AMA: 2018,Jan,8; 2017,Jan,8; 2016,Jan,13; 2015,Jan,16; 2014,Jan,11

88289 additional high resolution study
   0.00   0.00   **FUD** XXX
   AMA: 2018,Jan,8; 2017,Jan,8; 2016,Jan,13; 2015,Jan,16; 2014,Jan,11

88291 Cytogenetics and molecular cytogenetics, interpretation and report
   0.94   0.94   **FUD** XXX
   AMA: 2018,Jan,8; 2017,Jan,8; 2016,Jan,13; 2015,Jan,16; 2014,Jan,11

88299 Unlisted cytogenetic study
   0.00   0.00   **FUD** XXX
   AMA: 2018,Jan,8; 2017,Jan,8; 2016,Jan,13; 2015,Jan,16; 2014,Jan,11

88300 Evaluation of Surgical Specimen: Gross Anatomy

CMS: 100-02,15,80.1 Payment for Clinical Laboratory Services
   INCLUDES   Attainment, examination, and reporting
      Unit of service is the specimen
   EXCLUDES   Additional procedures (88311-88365 [88341, 88350], 88399)
      Microscopic exam (88302-88309)

88300 Level I - Surgical pathology, gross examination only
   0.45   0.45   **FUD** XXX
   AMA: 2018,Jan,8; 2017,Jan,8; 2016,Jan,13; 2015,Jan,16; 2014,Jan,11

88302-88309 Evaluation of Surgical Specimens: Gross and Microscopic Anatomy

CMS: 100-02,15,80.1 Payment for Clinical Laboratory Services
   INCLUDES   Attainment, examination, and reporting
      Unit of service is the specimen
   EXCLUDES   Additional procedures (88311-88365 [88341, 88350], 88399)
      Mohs surgery (17311-17315)

88302 Level II - Surgical pathology, gross and microscopic examination
   INCLUDES   Confirming identification and absence of disease:
      Appendix, incidental
      Fallopian tube, sterilization
      Fingers or toes traumatic amputation
      Foreskin, newborn
      Hernia sac, any site
      Hydrocele sac
      Nerve
      Skin, plastic repair
      Sympathetic ganglion
      Testis, castration
      Vaginal mucosa, incidental
      Vas deferens, sterilization
   0.87   0.87   **FUD** XXX
   AMA: 2018,Jan,8; 2017,Jan,8; 2016,Jan,13; 2015,Jan,16; 2014,Feb,10; 2014,Jan,11

88304 Level III - Surgical pathology, gross and microscopic examination

INCLUDES
Abortion, induced
Abscess
Anal tag
Aneurysm-atrial/ventricular
Appendix, other than incidental
Bartholin's gland cyst
Bone fragment(s), other than pathologic fracture
Bursa/ synovial cyst
Carpal tunnel tissue
Cartilage, shavings
Cholesteatoma
Colon, colostomy stoma
Conjunctiva-biopsy/pterygium
Cornea
Diverticulum-esophagus/small intestine
Dupuytren's contracture tissue
Femoral head, other than fracture
Fissure/fistula
Foreskin, other than newborn
Gallbladder
Ganglion cyst
Hematoma
Hemorrhoids
Hydatid of Morgagni
Intervertebral disc
Joint, loose body
Meniscus
Mucocele, salivary
Neuroma-Morton's/traumatic
Pilonidal cyst/sinus
Polyps, inflammatory-nasal/sinusoidal
Skin-cyst/tag/debridement
Soft tissue, debridement
Soft tissue, lipoma
Spermatocele
Tendon/tendon sheath
Testicular appendage
Thrombus or embolus
Tonsil and/or adenoids
Varicocele
Vas deferens, other than sterilization
Vein, varicosity

1.14 1.14 **FUD** XXX

AMA: 2018,Jan,8; 2017,Jan,8; 2016,Jan,13; 2015,Jan,16; 2014,Feb,10; 2014,Jan,11

88305 Level IV - Surgical pathology, gross and microscopic examination

INCLUDES
Abortion, spontaneous/missed
Artery, biopsy
Bone exostosis
Bone marrow, biopsy
Brain/meninges, other than for tumor resection
Breast biopsy without microscopic assessment of surgical margin
Breast reduction mammoplasty
Bronchus, biopsy
Cell block, any source
Cervix, biopsy
Colon, biopsy
Duodenum, biopsy
Endocervix, curettings/biopsy
Endometrium, curettings/biopsy
Esophagus, biopsy
Extremity, amputation, traumatic
Fallopian tube, biopsy
Fallopian tube, ectopic pregnancy
Femoral head, fracture
Finger/toes, amputation, nontraumatic
Gingiva/oral mucosa, biopsy
Heart valve
Joint resection
Kidney biopsy

Larynx biopsy
Leiomyoma(s), uterine myomectomy-without uterus
Lip, biopsy/wedge resection
Lung, transbronchial biopsy
Lymph node, biopsy
Muscle, biopsy
Nasal mucosa, biopsy
Nasopharynx/oropharynx, biopsy
Nerve biopsy
Odontogenic/dental cyst
Omentum, biopsy
Ovary, biopsy/wedge resection
Ovary with or without tube, nonneoplastic
Parathyroid gland
Peritoneum, biopsy
Pituitary tumor
Placenta, other than third trimester
Pleura/pericardium-biopsy/tissue
Polyp:
  Cervical/endometrial
  Colorectal
  Stomach/small intestine
Prostate:
  Needle biopsy
  TUR
Salivary gland, biopsy
Sinus, paranasal biopsy
Skin, other than cyst/tag/debridement/plastic repair
Small intestine, biopsy
Soft tissue, other than tumor/mas/lipoma/debridement
Spleen
Stomach biopsy
Synovium
Testis, other than tumor/biopsy, castration
Thyroglossal duct/brachial cleft cyst
Tongue, biopsy
Tonsil, biopsy
Trachea biopsy
Ureter, biopsy
Urethra, biopsy
Urinary bladder, biopsy
Uterus, with or without tubes and ovaries, for prolapse
Vagina biopsy
Vulva/labial biopsy

1.95 1.95 **FUD** XXX

AMA: 2018,May,3; 2018,Jan,8; 2017,Jan,8; 2016,Jan,13; 2015,Jan,16; 2014,Feb,10; 2014,Jan,11

88307 **Level V - Surgical pathology, gross and microscopic examination**

INCLUDES Adrenal resection
Bone, biopsy/curettings
Bone fragment(s), pathologic fractures
Brain, biopsy
Brain meninges, tumor resection
Breast, excision of lesion, requiring microscopic evaluation of surgical margins
Breast, mastectomy-partial/simple
Cervix, conization
Colon, segmental resection, other than for tumor
Extremity, amputation, nontraumatic
Eye, enucleation
Kidney, partial/total nephrectomy
Larynx, partial/total resection
Liver
   Biopsy, needle/wedge
   Partial resection
Lung, wedge biopsy
Lymph nodes, regional resection
Mediastinum, mass
Myocardium, biopsy
Odontogenic tumor
Ovary with or without tube, neoplastic
Pancreas, biopsy
Placenta, third trimester
Prostate, except radical resection
Salivary gland
Sentinel lymph node
Small intestine, resection, other than for tumor
Soft tissue mass (except lipoma)-biopsy/simple excision
Stomach-subtotal/total resection, other than for tumor
Testis, biopsy
Thymus, tumor
Thyroid, total/lobe
Ureter, resection
Urinary bladder, TUR
Uterus, with or without tubes and ovaries, other than neoplastic/prolapse

📣 7.59   ⚖ 7.59   **FUD** XXX   02 80 ▭

AMA: 2018,Jan,8; 2017,Jan,8; 2016,Jan,13; 2015,Jan,16; 2014,Feb,10; 2014,Jan,11

88309 **Level VI - Surgical pathology, gross and microscopic examination**

INCLUDES Bone resection
Breast, mastectomy-with regional lymph nodes
Colon:
   Segmental resection for tumor
   Total resection
Esophagus, partial/total resection
Extremity, disarticulation
Fetus, with dissection
Larynx, partial/total resection-with regional lymph nodes
Lung-total/lobe/segment resection
Pancreas, total/subtotal resection
Prostate, radical resection
Small intestine, resection for tumor
Soft tissue tumor, extensive resection
Stomach, subtotal/total resection for tumor
Testis, tumor
Tongue/tonsil, resection for tumor
Urinary bladder, partial/total resection
Uterus, with or without tubes and ovaries, neoplastic
Vulva, total/subtotal resection

EXCLUDES *Evaluation of fine needle aspirate (88172-88173)*
Fine needle aspiration (10021, [10004, 10005, 10006, 10007, 10008, 10009, 10010, 10011, 10012])

📣 11.5   ⚖ 11.5   **FUD** XXX   02 80 ▭

AMA: 2018,Jan,8; 2017,Jan,8; 2016,Jan,13; 2015,Jan,16; 2014,Feb,10; 2014,Jan,11

88311-88399 [88341, 88350, 88364, 88373, 88374, 88377] Additional Surgical Pathology Services

CMS: 100-02,15,80.1 Payment for Clinical Laboratory Services

+ 88311 **Decalcification procedure (List separately in addition to code for surgical pathology examination)**

Code first surgical pathology exam (88302-88309)

📣 0.61   ⚖ 0.61   **FUD** XXX   N 80 ▭

AMA: 2018,Jan,8; 2017,Jan,8; 2016,Jan,13; 2015,Jan,16; 2014,Jan,11

88312 **Special stain including interpretation and report; Group I for microorganisms (eg, acid fast, methenamine silver)**

INCLUDES Reporting one unit for each special stain performed on a surgical pathology block, cytologic sample, or hematologic smear

📣 2.83   ⚖ 2.83   **FUD** XXX   01 80 ▭

AMA: 2018,Jan,8; 2017,Jan,8; 2016,Jan,13; 2015,Jan,16; 2014,Jan,11

88313 **Group II, all other (eg, iron, trichrome), except stain for microorganisms, stains for enzyme constituents, or immunocytochemistry and immunohistochemistry**

INCLUDES Reporting one unit for each special stain performed on a surgical pathology block, cytologic sample, or hematologic smear

EXCLUDES *Immunocytochemistry and immunohistochemistry (88342)*

📣 2.05   ⚖ 2.05   **FUD** XXX   01 80 ▭

AMA: 2018,Jan,8; 2017,Jan,8; 2016,Jan,13; 2015,Jan,16; 2014,Jan,11

+ 88314 **histochemical stain on frozen tissue block (List separately in addition to code for primary procedure)**

INCLUDES Reporting one unit for each special stain on each frozen surgical pathology block

EXCLUDES *Routine frozen section stain during Mohs surgery (17311-17315)*
Special stain performed on frozen tissue section specimen to identify enzyme constituents (88319)

Code also modifier 59 for nonroutine histochemical stain on frozen section during Mohs surgery

Code first (17311-17315, 88302-88309, 88331-88332)

📣 2.60   ⚖ 2.60   **FUD** XXX   N 80 ▭

AMA: 2018,Jan,8; 2017,Jan,8; 2016,Jan,13; 2015,Jan,16; 2014,Jan,11

88319 **Group III, for enzyme constituents**

INCLUDES Reporting one unit for each special stain on each frozen surgical pathology block

EXCLUDES *Detection of enzyme constituents by immunohistochemical or immunocytochemical methodology (88342)*

📣 2.74   ⚖ 2.74   **FUD** XXX   02 80 ▭

AMA: 2018,Jan,8; 2017,Jan,8; 2016,Jan,13; 2015,Jan,16; 2014,Jan,11

88321 **Consultation and report on referred slides prepared elsewhere**

📣 2.42   ⚖ 2.85   **FUD** XXX   01 80 ▭

AMA: 2018,Jan,8; 2017,Jan,8; 2016,Jan,13; 2015,Jan,16; 2014,Jan,11

88323 **Consultation and report on referred material requiring preparation of slides**

📣 3.28   ⚖ 3.28   **FUD** XXX   01 80 ▭

AMA: 2018,Jan,8; 2017,Jan,8; 2016,Jan,13; 2015,Jan,16; 2014,Jan,11

88325 **Consultation, comprehensive, with review of records and specimens, with report on referred material**

📣 4.29   ⚖ 5.12   **FUD** XXX   01 80 ▭

AMA: 2018,Jan,8; 2017,Jan,8; 2016,Jan,13; 2015,Jan,16; 2014,Jan,11

88329 **Pathology consultation during surgery;**

📣 1.04   ⚖ 1.47   **FUD** XXX   01 80 ▭

AMA: 2018,Jan,8; 2017,Jan,8; 2016,Jan,13; 2015,Jan,16; 2014,Feb,10; 2014,Jan,11

26/TC PC/TC Only   A2-Z3 ASC Payment   50 Bilateral   ♂ Male Only   ♀ Female Only   📣 Facility RVU   ⚖ Non-Facility RVU   ▭ CCI   ✖ CLIA
FUD Follow-up Days   CMS: IOM   AMA: CPT Asst   A-Y OPPSI   80/80 Surg Assist Allowed / w/Doc   ▧ Lab Crosswalk   ▨ Radiology Crosswalk

442   CPT © 2019 American Medical Association. All Rights Reserved.   © 2019 Optum360, LLC

88331 **first tissue block, with frozen section(s), single specimen**

Code also cytologic evaluation performed at same time (88334)

🔧 2.75   ⚖ 2.75   **FUD** XXX   01 80 ▣

AMA: 2018,Jan,8; 2017,Jan,8; 2016,Jan,13; 2015,Jan,16; 2014,Feb,10; 2014,Jan,11

+ 88332 **each additional tissue block with frozen section(s) (List separately in addition to code for primary procedure)**

Code first (88331)

🔧 1.51   ⚖ 1.51   **FUD** XXX   N 80 ▣

AMA: 2018,Jan,8; 2017,Jan,8; 2016,Jan,13; 2015,Jan,16; 2014,Feb,10; 2014,Jan,11

88333 **cytologic examination (eg, touch prep, squash prep), initial site**

EXCLUDES   *Intraprocedural cytologic evaluation of fine needle aspirate (88172)*
Nonintraoperative cytologic examination (88160-88162)

🔧 2.53   ⚖ 2.53   **FUD** XXX   02 80 ▣

AMA: 2018,Jan,8; 2017,Jan,8; 2016,Jan,13; 2015,Jan,16; 2014,Feb,10; 2014,Jan,11

+ 88334 **cytologic examination (eg, touch prep, squash prep), each additional site (List separately in addition to code for primary procedure)**

EXCLUDES   *Intraprocedural cytologic evaluation of fine needle aspirate (88172)*
Nonintraoperative cytologic examination (88160-88162)
Percutaneous needle biopsy requiring intraprocedural cytologic examination (88333)

Code first (88331, 88333)

🔧 1.58   ⚖ 1.58   **FUD** ZZZ   N 80 ▣

AMA: 2018,Jan,8; 2017,Jan,8; 2016,Jan,13; 2015,Jan,16; 2014,Feb,10; 2014,Jan,11

88341 **Resequenced code. See code following 88342.**

88342 **Immunohistochemistry or immunocytochemistry, per specimen; initial single antibody stain procedure**

EXCLUDES   *Morphometric analysis, tumor immunohistochemistry, on same antibody (88360-88361)*
Multiplex antibody stain (88344)
Use of code more than one time for each specific antibody

🔧 3.01   ⚖ 3.01   **FUD** XXX   02 80 ▣

AMA: 2018,Jan,8; 2017,Jan,8; 2016,Jan,13; 2015,Jun,10; 2015,Jan,16; 2014,Jun,14; 2014,Jan,11

+ # 88341 **each additional single antibody stain procedure (List separately in addition to code for primary procedure)**

EXCLUDES   *Morphometric analysis (88360-88361)*
Multiplex antibody stain (88344)
Use of code more than one time for each specific antibody

Code first (88342)

🔧 2.62   ⚖ 2.62   **FUD** ZZZ   N 80 ▣

AMA: 2018,Jan,8; 2017,Jan,8; 2016,Jan,13; 2015,Jun,10

88344 **each multiplex antibody stain procedure**

INCLUDES   Staining with multiple antibodies on the same slide
EXCLUDES   *Morphometric analysis, tumor immunohistochemistry, on same antibody (88360-88361)*
Use of code more than one time for each specific antibody

🔧 4.84   ⚖ 4.84   **FUD** XXX   01 80 ▣

AMA: 2018,Jan,8; 2017,Jan,8; 2016,Jan,13; 2015,Jun,10

88346 **Immunofluorescence, per specimen; initial single antibody stain procedure**

EXCLUDES   *Fluorescent in situ hybridization studies (88364-88369 [88364, 88373, 88374, 88377])*
Multiple immunofluorescence analysis (88399)

🔧 3.11   ⚖ 3.11   **FUD** XXX   02 80 ▣

AMA: 2018,Jan,8; 2017,Jan,8; 2016,Jan,13; 2015,Jan,16; 2014,Jan,11

+ # 88350 **each additional single antibody stain procedure (List separately in addition to code for primary procedure)**

🔧 2.18   ⚖ 2.18   **FUD** ZZZ   N 80 ▣

EXCLUDES   *Fluorescent in situ hybridization studies (88364-88369 [88364, 88373, 88374, 88377])*
Multiple immunofluorescence analysis (88399)

Code first (88346)

88348 **Electron microscopy, diagnostic**

🔧 10.1   ⚖ 10.1   **FUD** XXX   02 80 ▣

AMA: 2011,Dec,14-18; 2005,Jul,11-12

88350 **Resequenced code. See code following 88346.**

88355 **Morphometric analysis; skeletal muscle**

🔧 3.75   ⚖ 3.75   **FUD** XXX   01 80 ▣

AMA: 2018,Jan,8; 2017,Jan,8; 2016,Jan,13; 2015,Jan,16; 2014,Jan,11

88356 **nerve**

🔧 6.34   ⚖ 6.34   **FUD** XXX   01 80 ▣

AMA: 2018,Jan,8; 2017,Jan,8; 2016,Jan,13; 2015,Jan,16; 2014,Jun,14; 2014,Jan,11

88358 **tumor (eg, DNA ploidy)**

EXCLUDES   *Special stain, Group II (88313)*

🔧 3.61   ⚖ 3.61   **FUD** XXX   02 80 ▣

AMA: 2018,Jan,8; 2017,Jan,8; 2016,Jan,13; 2015,Jan,16; 2014,Jan,11

88360 **Morphometric analysis, tumor immunohistochemistry (eg, Her-2/neu, estrogen receptor/progesterone receptor), quantitative or semiquantitative, per specimen, each single antibody stain procedure; manual**

EXCLUDES   *Additional stain procedures unless each test is for different antibody (88341, 88342, 88344)*
Morphometric analysis using in situ hybridization techniques (88367-88368 [88373, 88374])

🔧 3.60   ⚖ 3.60   **FUD** XXX   02 80 ▣

AMA: 2018,Jan,8; 2017,Jan,8; 2016,Jan,13; 2015,Jun,10; 2015,Jan,16; 2014,Jun,14; 2014,Jan,11

88361 **using computer-assisted technology**

EXCLUDES   *Additional stain procedures unless each test is for different antibody (88341, 88342, 88344)*
Morphometric analysis using in situ hybridization techniques (88367-88368 [88373, 88374])

🔧 3.72   ⚖ 3.72   **FUD** XXX   02 80 ▣

AMA: 2018,Jan,8; 2017,Jan,8; 2016,Jan,13; 2015,Jun,10; 2015,Jan,16; 2014,Jun,14; 2014,Jan,11

88362 **Nerve teasing preparations**

🔧 5.92   ⚖ 5.92   **FUD** XXX   02 80 ▣

AMA: 2018,Jan,8; 2017,Jan,8; 2016,Jan,13; 2015,Jan,16; 2014,Jan,11

88363 **Examination and selection of retrieved archival (ie, previously diagnosed) tissue(s) for molecular analysis (eg, KRAS mutational analysis)**

INCLUDES   Archival retrieval only

🔧 0.57   ⚖ 0.67   **FUD** XXX   01 80 ▣

AMA: 2018,Jan,8; 2017,Jan,8; 2016,Jan,13; 2015,Jan,16; 2014,Jan,11

88364 **Resequenced code. See code following 88365.**

88365 **In situ hybridization (eg, FISH), per specimen; initial single probe stain procedure**

EXCLUDES   *Morphometric analysis probe stain procedures with same probe (88367, [88374], 88368, [88377])*

🔧 4.99   ⚖ 4.99   **FUD** XXX   01 80 ▣

AMA: 2018,Nov,11; 2018,Jan,8; 2017,Jan,8; 2016,Jan,13; 2015,Jan,16; 2014,Jan,11

+ # 88364 **each additional single probe stain procedure (List separately in addition to code for primary procedure)**

🔧 3.74   ⚖ 3.74   **FUD** ZZZ   N 80 ▣

Code first (88365)

88366   **each multiplex probe stain procedure**
🔹 7.44   ⚬ 7.44   **FUD** XXX   [Q1] [80] 🖵

> *EXCLUDES*   *Morphometric analysis probe stain procedures (88367, [88374], 88368, [88377])*

88367   **Morphometric analysis, in situ hybridization (quantitative or semi-quantitative), using computer-assisted technology, per specimen; initial single probe stain procedure**

> *EXCLUDES*   *In situ hybridization probe stain procedures for same probe (88365, 88366, 88368, [88377])*
> *Morphometric in situ hybridization evaluation of urinary tract cytologic specimens (88120-88121)*

🔹 3.08   ⚬ 3.08   **FUD** XXX   [Q2] [80] 🖵

AMA: 2018,Jan,8; 2017,Jan,8; 2016,Jan,13; 2015,Jan,16; 2014,Jan,11

+ #   **88373**   **each additional single probe stain procedure (List separately in addition to code for primary procedure)**
🔹 2.11   ⚬ 2.11   **FUD** ZZZ   [N] [80] 🖵
Code first (88367)

**88374**   **each multiplex probe stain procedure**
🔹 9.18   ⚬ 9.18   **FUD** XXX   [Q1] [80] 🖵

> *EXCLUDES*   *In situ hybridization probe stain procedures for same probe (88365, 88366, 88368, [88377])*

88368   **Morphometric analysis, in situ hybridization (quantitative or semi-quantitative), manual, per specimen; initial single probe stain procedure**

> *EXCLUDES*   *In situ hybridization probe stain procedures for same probe (88365, 88366-88367, [88374])*
> *Morphometric in situ hybridization evaluation of urinary tract cytologic specimens (88120-88121)*

🔹 3.59   ⚬ 3.59   **FUD** XXX   [Q2] [80] 🖵

AMA: 2018,Jan,8; 2017,Jan,8; 2016,Jan,13; 2015,Jan,16; 2014,Jan,11

+   **88369**   **each additional single probe stain procedure (List separately in addition to code for primary procedure)**
🔹 3.14   ⚬ 3.14   **FUD** ZZZ   [N] [80] 🖵
Code first (88368)

**88377**   **each multiplex probe stain procedure**
🔹 10.9   ⚬ 10.9   **FUD** XXX   [Q1] [80] 🖵

> *EXCLUDES*   *In situ hybridization probe stain procedures for same probe (88365, 88366-88367, [88374])*
> *Morphometric in situ hybridization evaluation, urinary tract cytologic specimens (88120-88121)*

88371   **Protein analysis of tissue by Western Blot, with interpretation and report;**
🔹 0.00   ⚬ 0.00   **FUD** XXX   [N] [80] 🖵

AMA: 2018,Jan,8; 2017,Jan,8; 2016,Jan,13; 2015,Dec,18; 2015,Jan,16; 2014,Jan,11

88372   **immunological probe for band identification, each**
🔹 0.00   ⚬ 0.00   **FUD** XXX   [N] [80] 🖵

AMA: 2018,Jan,8; 2017,Jan,8; 2016,Jan,13; 2015,Jan,16; 2014,Jan,11

88373   **Resequenced code. See code following 88367.**

88374   **Resequenced code. See code following 88367.**

88375   **Optical endomicroscopic image(s), interpretation and report, real-time or referred, each endoscopic session**

> *EXCLUDES*   *Endoscopic procedures that include optical endomicroscopy (43206, 43252, 0397T)*

🔹 1.42   ⚬ 1.42   **FUD** XXX   [B] [80] [26] 🖵

AMA: 2018,Jan,8; 2017,Jan,8; 2016,Jan,13; 2015,Jan,16

88377   **Resequenced code. See code following 88369.**

88380   **Microdissection (ie, sample preparation of microscopically identified target); laser capture**

> *EXCLUDES*   *Microdissection, manual procedure (88381)*

🔹 3.78   ⚬ 3.78   **FUD** XXX   [N] [80] 🖵

AMA: 2018,Aug,3; 2018,Jan,8; 2017,Jan,8; 2016,Jan,13; 2015,Jan,16; 2014,Jan,11

88381   **manual**

> *EXCLUDES*   *Microdissection, laser capture procedure (88380)*

🔹 4.34   ⚬ 4.34   **FUD** XXX   [N] [80] 🖵

AMA: 2018,Aug,3; 2018,Jan,8; 2017,Jan,8; 2016,Jan,13; 2015,Jan,16; 2014,Jan,11

88387   **Macroscopic examination, dissection, and preparation of tissue for non-microscopic analytical studies (eg, nucleic acid-based molecular studies); each tissue preparation (eg, a single lymph node)**

> *EXCLUDES*   *Pathology consultation during surgery (88329-88334, 88388)*
> *Tissue preparation for microbiologic cultures or flow cytometric studies*

🔹 1.00   ⚬ 1.00   **FUD** XXX   [N] [80] 🖵

AMA: 2018,Jan,8; 2017,Jan,8; 2016,Jan,13; 2015,Jan,16; 2014,Jan,11

+   **88388**   **in conjunction with a touch imprint, intraoperative consultation, or frozen section, each tissue preparation (eg, a single lymph node) (List separately in addition to code for primary procedure)**

> *EXCLUDES*   *Tissue preparation for microbiologic cultures or flow cytometric studies*

Code first (88329-88334)
🔹 1.00   ⚬ 1.00   **FUD** XXX   [N] [80] 🖵

AMA: 2018,Jan,8; 2017,Jan,8; 2016,Jan,13; 2015,Jan,16; 2014,Jan,11

88399   **Unlisted surgical pathology procedure**
🔹 0.00   ⚬ 0.00   **FUD** XXX   [Q1] 🖵

AMA: 2018,Jan,8; 2017,Jan,8; 2016,Jan,13; 2015,Jan,16; 2014,Jun,14; 2014,Jan,11

88720-88749 Transcutaneous Procedures

> *EXCLUDES*   *Transcutaneous oxyhemoglobin measurement (0493T)*
> *Wavelength fluorescent spectroscopy of advanced glycation end products (skin) (88749)*

88720   **Bilirubin, total, transcutaneous**

> *EXCLUDES*   *Transdermal oxygen saturation testing (94760-94762)*

🔹 0.00   ⚬ 0.00   **FUD** XXX   [Q] 🖵

AMA: 2018,Jan,8; 2017,Jan,8; 2016,Jan,13; 2015,Jan,16; 2014,Jan,11

88738   **Hemoglobin (Hgb), quantitative, transcutaneous**

> *EXCLUDES*   *In vitro hemoglobin measurement (85018)*

🔹 0.00   ⚬ 0.00   **FUD** XXX   [Q] 🖵

AMA: 2018,Jan,8; 2017,Jan,8; 2016,Jan,13; 2015,Jan,16; 2014,Jan,11

88740   **Hemoglobin, quantitative, transcutaneous, per day; carboxyhemoglobin**

> *EXCLUDES*   *In vitro carboxyhemoglobin measurement (82375)*

🔹 0.00   ⚬ 0.00   **FUD** XXX   [Q] 🖵

AMA: 2018,Jan,8; 2017,Jan,8; 2016,Jan,13; 2015,Jan,16; 2014,Jan,11

88741   **methemoglobin**

> *EXCLUDES*   *In vitro quantitative methemoglobin measurement (83050)*

🔹 0.00   ⚬ 0.00   **FUD** XXX   [Q] 🖵

AMA: 2018,Jan,8; 2017,Jan,8; 2016,Jan,13; 2015,Jan,16; 2014,Jan,11

88749   **Unlisted in vivo (eg, transcutaneous) laboratory service**

> *INCLUDES*   *All in vivo measurements not specifically listed*

🔹 0.00   ⚬ 0.00   **FUD** XXX   [Q] 🖵

AMA: 2010,Dec,7-10

89049-89240 Other Pathology Services

89049   **Caffeine halothane contracture test (CHCT) for malignant hyperthermia susceptibility, including interpretation and report**
🔹 1.77   ⚬ 7.06   **FUD** XXX   [Q1] [80] 🖵

AMA: 2018,Jan,8; 2017,Jan,8; 2016,Jan,13; 2015,Jan,16; 2014,Jan,11

26/[TC] PC/TC Only   [A2-Z3] ASC Payment   [50] Bilateral   ♂ Male Only   ♀ Female Only   🔹 Facility RVU   ⚬ Non-Facility RVU   🖵 CCI   ✖ CLIA
FUD Follow-up Days   **CMS:** IOM   **AMA:** CPT Asst   [A-Y] OPPSI   80/[80] Surg Assist Allowed / w/Doc   🖵 Lab Crosswalk   Radiology Crosswalk

444   CPT © 2019 American Medical Association. All Rights Reserved.   © 2019 Optum360, LLC

89050 Cell count, miscellaneous body fluids (eg, cerebrospinal fluid, joint fluid), except blood;
0.00 0.00 **FUD** XXX
AMA: 2018,Jan,8; 2017,Jan,8; 2016,Jan,13; 2015,Jan,16; 2014,Jan,11

89051 with differential count
0.00 0.00 **FUD** XXX
AMA: 2018,Jan,8; 2017,Jan,8; 2016,Jan,13; 2015,Jan,16; 2014,Jan,11

89055 Leukocyte assessment, fecal, qualitative or semiquantitative
0.00 0.00 **FUD** XXX
AMA: 2018,Jan,8; 2017,Jan,8; 2016,Jan,13; 2015,Jan,16; 2014,Jan,11

89060 Crystal identification by light microscopy with or without polarizing lens analysis, tissue or any body fluid (except urine)
EXCLUDES Crystal identification on paraffin embedded tissue
0.00 0.00 **FUD** XXX
AMA: 2018,Jan,8; 2017,Jan,8; 2016,Jan,13; 2015,Jan,16; 2014,Jan,11

89125 Fat stain, feces, urine, or respiratory secretions
0.00 0.00 **FUD** XXX
AMA: 2018,Jan,8; 2017,Jan,8; 2016,Jan,13; 2015,Jan,16; 2014,Jan,11

89160 Meat fibers, feces
0.00 0.00 **FUD** XXX
AMA: 2018,Jan,8; 2017,Jan,8; 2016,Jan,13; 2015,Jan,16; 2014,Jan,11

89190 Nasal smear for eosinophils
EXCLUDES Occult blood feces (82270)
Paternity tests (86910)
0.00 0.00 **FUD** XXX
AMA: 2018,Jan,8; 2017,Jan,8; 2016,Jan,13; 2015,Jan,16; 2014,Jan,11

89220 Sputum, obtaining specimen, aerosol induced technique (separate procedure)
0.46 0.46 **FUD** XXX
AMA: 2018,Jan,8; 2017,Jan,8; 2016,Jan,13; 2015,Jan,16; 2014,Jan,11

89230 Sweat collection by iontophoresis
0.08 0.08 **FUD** XXX
AMA: 2018,Jan,8; 2017,Jan,8; 2016,Jan,13; 2015,Jan,16; 2014,Jan,11

89240 Unlisted miscellaneous pathology test
0.00 0.00 **FUD** XXX
AMA: 2018,Jan,8; 2017,Jan,8; 2016,Jan,13; 2015,Jan,16; 2014,Jan,11

89250-89398 Infertility Treatment Services
CMS: 100-02,1,100 Treatment for Infertility

89250 Culture of oocyte(s)/embryo(s), less than 4 days;
0.00 0.00 **FUD** XXX
AMA: 2018,Jan,8; 2017,Jan,8; 2016,Jan,13; 2015,Jan,16; 2014,Jan,11

89251 with co-culture of oocyte(s)/embryos
EXCLUDES Extended culture of oocyte(s)/embryo(s) (89272)
0.00 0.00 **FUD** XXX
AMA: 2018,Jan,8; 2017,Jan,8; 2016,Jan,13; 2015,Jan,16; 2014,Jan,11

89253 Assisted embryo hatching, microtechniques (any method)
0.00 0.00 **FUD** XXX
AMA: 2018,Jan,8; 2017,Jan,8; 2016,Jan,13; 2015,Jan,16; 2014,Jan,11

89254 Oocyte identification from follicular fluid
0.00 0.00 **FUD** XXX
AMA: 2018,Jan,8; 2017,Jan,8; 2016,Jan,13; 2015,Jan,16; 2014,Jan,11

89255 Preparation of embryo for transfer (any method)
0.00 0.00 **FUD** XXX
AMA: 2018,Jan,8; 2017,Jan,8; 2016,Jan,13; 2015,Jan,16; 2014,Jan,11

89257 Sperm identification from aspiration (other than seminal fluid)
EXCLUDES Semen analysis (89300-89320)
Sperm identification from testis tissue (89264)
0.00 0.00 **FUD** XXX
AMA: 2018,Jan,8; 2017,Jan,8; 2016,Jan,13; 2015,Jan,16; 2014,Jan,11

89258 Cryopreservation; embryo(s)
0.00 0.00 **FUD** XXX
AMA: 2018,Jan,8; 2017,Jan,8; 2016,Jan,13; 2015,Jan,16; 2014,Jan,11

89259 sperm
EXCLUDES Cryopreservation of testicular reproductive tissue (89335)
0.00 0.00 **FUD** XXX
AMA: 2018,Jan,8; 2017,Jan,8; 2016,Jan,13; 2015,Jan,16; 2014,Jan,11

89260 Sperm isolation; simple prep (eg, sperm wash and swim-up) for insemination or diagnosis with semen analysis
0.00 0.00 **FUD** XXX
AMA: 2018,Jan,8; 2017,Jan,8; 2016,Jan,13; 2015,Jan,16; 2014,Jan,11

89261 complex prep (eg, Percoll gradient, albumin gradient) for insemination or diagnosis with semen analysis
EXCLUDES Semen analysis without sperm wash or swim-up (89320)
0.00 0.00 **FUD** XXX
AMA: 2018,Jan,8; 2017,Jan,8; 2016,Jan,13; 2015,Jan,16; 2014,Jan,11

89264 Sperm identification from testis tissue, fresh or cryopreserved
EXCLUDES Biopsy of testis (54500, 54505)
Semen analysis (89300-89320)
Sperm identification from aspiration (89257)
0.00 0.00 **FUD** XXX
AMA: 2018,Jan,8; 2017,Jan,8; 2016,Jan,13; 2015,Jan,16; 2014,Jan,11

89268 Insemination of oocytes
0.00 0.00 **FUD** XXX
AMA: 2018,Jan,8; 2017,Jan,8; 2016,Jan,13; 2015,Jan,16; 2014,Jan,11

89272 Extended culture of oocyte(s)/embryo(s), 4-7 days
0.00 0.00 **FUD** XXX
AMA: 2018,Jan,8; 2017,Jan,8; 2016,Jan,13; 2015,Jan,16; 2014,Jan,11

89280 Assisted oocyte fertilization, microtechnique; less than or equal to 10 oocytes
0.00 0.00 **FUD** XXX
AMA: 2018,Jan,8; 2017,Jan,8; 2016,Jan,13; 2015,Jan,16; 2014,Jan,11

89281 greater than 10 oocytes
0.00 0.00 **FUD** XXX
AMA: 2018,Jan,8; 2017,Jan,8; 2016,Jan,13; 2015,Jan,16; 2014,Jan,11

89290 Biopsy, oocyte polar body or embryo blastomere, microtechnique (for pre-implantation genetic diagnosis); less than or equal to 5 embryos
0.00 0.00 **FUD** XXX
AMA: 2018,Jan,8; 2017,Jan,8; 2016,Jan,13; 2015,Jan,16; 2014,Jan,11

89291 greater than 5 embryos
0.00 0.00 **FUD** XXX
AMA: 2018,Jan,8; 2017,Jan,8; 2016,Jan,13; 2015,Jan,16; 2014,Jan,11

Pathology and Laboratory *(side tab)*

89300 — 0006U *(side tab)*

89300   **Semen analysis; presence and/or motility of sperm including Huhner test (post coital)** ♀
     🖾 0.00   ⚕ 0.00   **FUD** XXX   [X] [Q] [▭]
     AMA: 2018,Jan,8; 2017,Jan,8; 2016,Jan,13; 2015,Jan,16; 2014,Jan,11

89310   **motility and count (not including Huhner test)** ♂
     🖾 0.00   ⚕ 0.00   **FUD** XXX   [Q] [▭]
     AMA: 2018,Jan,8; 2017,Jan,8; 2016,Jan,13; 2015,Jan,16; 2014,Jan,11

89320   **volume, count, motility, and differential** ♂
     [EXCLUDES]   *Skin testing (86485-86580, 95012-95199)*
     🖾 0.00   ⚕ 0.00   **FUD** XXX   [Q] [▭]
     AMA: 2018,Jan,8; 2017,Jan,8; 2016,Jan,13; 2015,Jan,16; 2014,Jan,11

89321   **sperm presence and motility of sperm, if performed** ♂
     [EXCLUDES]   *Hyaluronan binding assay (HBA) (89398)*
     🖾 0.00   ⚕ 0.00   **FUD** XXX   [X] [Q] [▭]
     AMA: 2018,Jan,8; 2017,Jan,8; 2016,Jan,13; 2015,Jan,16; 2014,Jan,11

89322   **volume, count, motility, and differential using strict morphologic criteria (eg, Kruger)** ♂
     🖾 0.00   ⚕ 0.00   **FUD** XXX   [Q] [▭]
     AMA: 2018,Jan,8; 2017,Jan,8; 2016,Jan,13; 2015,Jan,16; 2014,Jan,11

89325   **Sperm antibodies** ♂
     [EXCLUDES]   *Medicolegal identification of sperm (88125)*
     🖾 0.00   ⚕ 0.00   **FUD** XXX   [Q] [▭]
     AMA: 2018,Jan,8; 2017,Jan,8; 2016,Jan,13; 2015,Jan,16; 2014,Jan,11

89329   **Sperm evaluation; hamster penetration test** ♂
     🖾 0.00   ⚕ 0.00   **FUD** XXX   [Q] [▭]
     AMA: 2018,Jan,8; 2017,Jan,8; 2016,Jan,13; 2015,Jan,16; 2014,Jan,11

89330   **cervical mucus penetration test, with or without spinnbarkeit test** ♂
     🖾 0.00   ⚕ 0.00   **FUD** XXX   [Q] [▭]
     AMA: 2018,Jan,8; 2017,Jan,8; 2016,Jan,13; 2015,Jan,16; 2014,Jan,11

89331   **Sperm evaluation, for retrograde ejaculation, urine (sperm concentration, motility, and morphology, as indicated)** ♂
     [EXCLUDES]   *Detection of sperm in urine (81015)*
     Code also semen analysis on concurrent sperm specimen (89300-89322)
     🖾 0.00   ⚕ 0.00   **FUD** XXX   [Q] [▭]
     AMA: 2018,Jan,8; 2017,Jan,8; 2016,Jan,13; 2015,Jan,16; 2014,Jan,11

89335   **Cryopreservation, reproductive tissue, testicular**
     [EXCLUDES]   *Cryopreservation of:*
           Embryo(s) (89258)
           Mature oocytes (89337)
           Ovarian tissue, oocytes (0058T)
           Sperm (89259)
     🖾 0.00   ⚕ 0.00   **FUD** XXX   [01] [▭]
     AMA: 2018,Jan,8; 2017,Jan,8; 2016,Jan,13; 2015,Jan,16; 2014,Jan,11

89337   **Cryopreservation, mature oocyte(s)** ♀
     [EXCLUDES]   *Cryopreservation of immature oocyte[s] (89398)*
     🖾 0.00   ⚕ 0.00   **FUD** XXX   [01] [▭]
     AMA: 2018,Jan,8; 2017,Jan,8; 2016,Jan,13; 2015,Jan,16

89342   **Storage (per year); embryo(s)**
     🖾 0.00   ⚕ 0.00   **FUD** XXX   [01] [▭]
     AMA: 2018,Jan,8; 2017,Jan,8; 2016,Jan,13; 2015,Jan,16; 2014,Jan,11

89343   **sperm/semen**
     🖾 0.00   ⚕ 0.00   **FUD** XXX   [01] [▭]
     AMA: 2018,Jan,8; 2017,Jan,8; 2016,Jan,13; 2015,Jan,16; 2014,Jan,11

89344   **reproductive tissue, testicular/ovarian**
     🖾 0.00   ⚕ 0.00   **FUD** XXX   [01] [▭]
     AMA: 2018,Jan,8; 2017,Jan,8; 2016,Jan,13; 2015,Jan,16; 2014,Jan,11

89346   **oocyte(s)**
     🖾 0.00   ⚕ 0.00   **FUD** XXX   [02] [▭]
     AMA: 2018,Jan,8; 2017,Jan,8; 2016,Jan,13; 2015,Jan,16; 2014,Jan,11

89352   **Thawing of cryopreserved; embryo(s)**
     🖾 0.00   ⚕ 0.00   **FUD** XXX   [01] [▭]
     AMA: 2018,Jan,8; 2017,Jan,8; 2016,Jan,13; 2015,Jan,16; 2014,Jan,11

89353   **sperm/semen, each aliquot**
     🖾 0.00   ⚕ 0.00   **FUD** XXX   [01] [▭]
     AMA: 2018,Jan,8; 2017,Jan,8; 2016,Jan,13; 2015,Jan,16; 2014,Jan,11

89354   **reproductive tissue, testicular/ovarian**
     🖾 0.00   ⚕ 0.00   **FUD** XXX   [01] [▭]
     AMA: 2018,Jan,8; 2017,Jan,8; 2016,Jan,13; 2015,Jan,16; 2014,Jan,11

89356   **oocytes, each aliquot**
     🖾 0.00   ⚕ 0.00   **FUD** XXX   [01] [▭]
     AMA: 2018,Jan,8; 2017,Jan,8; 2016,Jan,13; 2015,Jan,16; 2014,Jan,11

89398   **Unlisted reproductive medicine laboratory procedure**
     🖾 0.00   ⚕ 0.00   **FUD** XXX   [01] [▭]
     [INCLUDES]   Hyaluronan binding assay (HBA)

0001U-0162U Proprietary Laboratory Analysis (PLA)

[INCLUDES]   All necessary investigative services
            PLA codes take priority over other CPT codes
[EXCLUDES]   *Additional procedures necessary before cell lysis (88380-88381)*

0001U   **Red blood cell antigen typing, DNA, human erythrocyte antigen gene analysis of 35 antigens from 11 blood groups, utilizing whole blood, common RBC alleles reported**
     [INCLUDES]   PreciseType® HEA Test, Immucor, Inc
     🖾 0.00   ⚕ 0.00   **FUD** 000   [A] [▭]
     AMA: 2019,Jun,11

0002U   **Oncology (colorectal), quantitative assessment of three urine metabolites (ascorbic acid, succinic acid and carnitine) by liquid chromatography with tandem mass spectrometry (LC-MS/MS) using multiple reaction monitoring acquisition, algorithm reported as likelihood of adenomatous polyps**
     [INCLUDES]   PolypDX™, Atlantic Diagnostic Laboratories, LLC, Metabolomic Technologies Inc
     🖾 0.00   ⚕ 0.00   **FUD** 000   [Q] [▭]
     AMA: 2018,Aug,3

0003U   **Oncology (ovarian) biochemical assays of five proteins (apolipoprotein A-1, CA 125 II, follicle stimulating hormone, human epididymis protein 4, transferrin), utilizing serum, algorithm reported as a likelihood score**
     🖾 0.00   ⚕ 0.00   **FUD** 000   [Q] [▭]
     [INCLUDES]   Overa (OVA1 Next Generation), Aspira Labs, Inc, Vermillion, Inc

0005U   **Oncology (prostate) gene expression profile by real-time RT-PCR of 3 genes (ERG, PCA3, and SPDEF), urine, algorithm reported as risk score**
     🖾 0.00   ⚕ 0.00   **FUD** 000   [Q] [▭]
     [INCLUDES]   ExosomeDx® Prostate (IntelliScore), Exosome Diagnostics, Inc, Exosome Diagnostics, Inc

0006U   **Detection of interacting medications, substances, supplements and foods, 120 or more analytes, definitive chromatography with mass spectrometry, urine, description and severity of each interaction identified, per date of service**
     🖾 0.00   ⚕ 0.00   **FUD** 000   [Q] [▭]
     [INCLUDES]   Drug-substance Identification and Interaction, Aegis Sciences Corporation

---

0007U Drug test(s), presumptive, with definitive confirmation of positive results, any number of drug classes, urine, includes specimen verification including DNA authentication in comparison to buccal DNA, per date of service

INCLUDES ToxProtect, Genotox Laboratories Ltd

🦠 0.00 🔪 0.00 **FUD** 000 Q ▣

AMA: 2018,Jan,6

▲ **0008U** Helicobacter pylori detection and antibiotic resistance, DNA, 16S and 23S rRNA, gyrA, pbp1, rdxA and rpoB, next-generation sequencing, formalin-fixed paraffin-embedded or fresh tissue or fecal sample, predictive, reported as positive or negative for resistance to clarithromycin, fluoroquinolones, metronidazole, amoxicillin, tetracycline, and rifabutin

🦠 0.00 🔪 0.00 **FUD** 000 A ▣

INCLUDES AmHPR® H. pylori Antibiotic Resistance Panel, American Molecular Laboratories, Inc

0009U Oncology (breast cancer), ERBB2 (HER2) copy number by FISH, tumor cells from formalin fixed paraffin embedded tissue isolated using image-based dielectrophoresis (DEP) sorting, reported as ERBB2 gene amplified or non-amplified

🦠 0.00 🔪 0.00 **FUD** 000 Q ▣

INCLUDES DEPArray™ HER2, PacificDx

0010U Infectious disease (bacterial), strain typing by whole genome sequencing, phylogenetic-based report of strain relatedness, per submitted isolate

🦠 0.00 🔪 0.00 **FUD** 000 A ▣

INCLUDES Bacterial Typing by Whole Genome Sequencing, Mayo Clinic

0011U Prescription drug monitoring, evaluation of drugs present by LC-MS/MS, using oral fluid, reported as a comparison to an estimated steady-state range, per date of service including all drug compounds and metabolites

🦠 0.00 🔪 0.00 **FUD** 000 Q ▣

INCLUDES Cordant CORE™, Cordant Health Solutions

0012U Germline disorders, gene rearrangement detection by whole genome next-generation sequencing, DNA, whole blood, report of specific gene rearrangement(s)

🦠 0.00 🔪 0.00 **FUD** 000 A ▣

INCLUDES MatePair Targeted Rearrangements, Congenital, Mayo Clinic

0013U Oncology (solid organ neoplasia), gene rearrangement detection by whole genome next-generation sequencing, DNA, fresh or frozen tissue or cells, report of specific gene rearrangement(s)

🦠 0.00 🔪 0.00 **FUD** 000 A ▣

INCLUDES MatePair Targeted Rearrangements, Oncology, Mayo Clinic

0014U Hematology (hematolymphoid neoplasia), gene rearrangement detection by whole genome next-generation sequencing, DNA, whole blood or bone marrow, report of specific gene rearrangement(s)

🦠 0.00 🔪 0.00 **FUD** 000 A ▣

INCLUDES MatePair Targeted Rearrangements, Hematologic, Mayo Clinic

0016U Oncology (hematolymphoid neoplasia), RNA, BCR/ABL1 major and minor breakpoint fusion transcripts, quantitative PCR amplification, blood or bone marrow, report of fusion not detected or detected with quantitation

🦠 0.00 🔪 0.00 **FUD** 000 A ▣

INCLUDES BCR-ABL1 major and minor breakpoint fusion transcripts, University of Iowa, Department of Pathology, Asuragen

0017U Oncology (hematolymphoid neoplasia), JAK2 mutation, DNA, PCR amplification of exons 12-14 and sequence analysis, blood or bone marrow, report of JAK2 mutation not detected or detected

🦠 0.00 🔪 0.00 **FUD** 000 A ▣

INCLUDES JAK2 Mutation, University of Iowa, Department of Pathology

0018U Oncology (thyroid), microRNA profiling by RT-PCR of 10 microRNA sequences, utilizing fine needle aspirate, algorithm reported as a positive or negative result for moderate to high risk of malignancy

🦠 0.00 🔪 0.00 **FUD** 000 A ▣

INCLUDES ThyraMIR™, Interpace Diagnostics

0019U Oncology, RNA, gene expression by whole transcriptome sequencing, formalin-fixed paraffin embedded tissue or fresh frozen tissue, predictive algorithm reported as potential targets for therapeutic agents

🦠 0.00 🔪 0.00 **FUD** 000 A ▣

INCLUDES OncoTarget/OncoTreat, Columbia University Department of Pathology and Cell Biology, Darwin Health

0021U Oncology (prostate), detection of 8 autoantibodies (ARF 6, NKX3-1, 5'-UTR-BMI1, CEP 164, 3'-UTR-Ropporin, Desmocollin, AURKAIP-1, CSNK2A2), multiplexed immunoassay and flow cytometry serum, algorithm reported as risk score

🦠 0.00 🔪 0.00 **FUD** 000 Q ▣

INCLUDES Apifiny®, Armune BioScience, Inc

0022U Targeted genomic sequence analysis panel, non-small cell lung neoplasia, DNA and RNA analysis, 23 genes, interrogation for sequence variants and rearrangements, reported as presence/absence of variants and associated therapy(ies) to consider

🦠 0.00 🔪 0.00 **FUD** 000 A ▣

INCLUDES Oncomine™ Dx Target Test, Thermo Fisher Scientific

0023U Oncology (acute myelogenous leukemia), DNA, genotyping of internal tandem duplication, p.D835, p.I836, using mononuclear cells, reported as detection or non-detection of FLT3 mutation and indication for or against the use of midostaurin

🦠 0.00 🔪 0.00 **FUD** 000 A ▣

INCLUDES LeukoStrat® CDx FLT3 Mutation Assay, LabPMM LLC, an Invivoscribe Technologies, Inc Company, Invivoscribe Technologies, Inc

0024U Glycosylated acute phase proteins (GlycA), nuclear magnetic resonance spectroscopy, quantitative

🦠 0.00 🔪 0.00 **FUD** 000 Q ▣

INCLUDES GlycA, Laboratory Corporation of America, Laboratory Corporation of America

0025U Tenofovir, by liquid chromatography with tandem mass spectrometry (LC-MS/MS), urine, quantitative

🦠 0.00 🔪 0.00 **FUD** 000 Q ▣

INCLUDES UrSure Tenofovir Quantification Test, Synergy Medical Laboratories, UrSure Inc

0026U Oncology (thyroid), DNA and mRNA of 112 genes, next-generation sequencing, fine needle aspirate of thyroid nodule, algorithmic analysis reported as a categorical result ("Positive, high probability of malignancy" or "Negative, low probability of malignancy")

🦠 0.00 🔪 0.00 **FUD** 000 A ▣

INCLUDES Thyroseq Genomic Classifier, CBLPath, Inc, University of Pittsburgh Medical Center

0027U JAK2 (Janus kinase 2) (eg, myeloproliferative disorder) gene analysis, targeted sequence analysis exons 12-15

🦠 0.00 🔪 0.00 **FUD** 000 A ▣

INCLUDES JAK2 Exons 12 to 15 Sequencing, Mayo Clinic, Mayo Clinic

---

● New Code ▲ Revised Code ○ Reinstated ● New Web Release ▲ Revised Web Release + Add-on Unlisted Not Covered # Resequenced
㊿ Optum Mod 50 Exempt Ⓢ AMA Mod 51 Exempt ⑤① Optum Mod 51 Exempt ㊿ Mod 63 Exempt ⊮ Non-FDA Drug ★ Telemedicine Ⓜ Maternity Ⓐ Age Edit

CPT © 2019 American Medical Association. All Rights Reserved.

0029U Drug metabolism (adverse drug reactions and drug response), targeted sequence analysis (ie, *CYP1A2, CYP2C19, CYP2C9, CYP2D6, CYP3A4, CYP3A5, CYP4F2, SLCO1B1, VKORC1* and rs12777823)

　　🔬 0.00　　🔎 0.00　　**FUD** 000　　　　　　Ⓐ ▣

　　INCLUDES　　Focused Pharmacogenomics Panel, Mayo Clinic, Mayo Clinic

0030U Drug metabolism (warfarin drug response), targeted sequence analysis (ie, *CYP2C9, CYP4F2, VKORC1,* rs12777823)

　　🔬 0.00　　🔎 0.00　　**FUD** 000　　　　　　Ⓐ ▣

　　INCLUDES　　Warfarin Response Genotype, Mayo Clinic, Mayo Clinic

0031U *CYP1A2 (cytochrome P450 family 1, subfamily A, member 2)*(eg, drug metabolism) gene analysis, common variants (ie, *1F, *1K, *6, *7)

　　🔬 0.00　　🔎 0.00　　**FUD** 000　　　　　　Ⓐ ▣

　　INCLUDES　　Cytochrome P450 1A2 Genotype, Mayo Clinic, Mayo Clinic

0032U *COMT (catechol-O-methyltransferase)(drug metabolism)* gene analysis, c.472G>A (rs4680) variant

　　🔬 0.00　　🔎 0.00　　**FUD** 000　　　　　　Ⓐ ▣

　　INCLUDES　　Catechol-O-Methyltransferase (*COMT*) Genotype, Mayo Clinic, Mayo Clinic

0033U *HTR2A (5-hydroxytryptamine receptor 2A), HTR2C (5-hydroxytryptamine receptor 2C)* (eg, citalopram metabolism) gene analysis, common variants (ie, *HTR2A* rs7997012 [c.614-2211T>C], *HTR2C* rs3813929 [c.-759C>T] and rs1414334 [c.551-3008C>G])

　　🔬 0.00　　🔎 0.00　　**FUD** 000　　　　　　Ⓐ ▣

　　INCLUDES　　Serotonin Receptor Genotype (*HTR2A* and *HTR2C*), Mayo Clinic, Mayo Clinic

0034U *TPMT (thiopurine S-methyltransferase), NUDT15 (nudix hydroxylase 15)(eg, thiopurine metabolism),* gene analysis, common variants (ie, *TPMT* *2, *3A, *3B, *3C, *4, *5, *6, *8, *12; NUDT15* *3, *4, *5)

　　🔬 0.00　　🔎 0.00　　**FUD** 000　　　　　　Ⓐ ▣

　　INCLUDES　　Thiopurine Methyltransferase (*TPMT*) and Nudix Hydrolase (*NUDT15*) Genotyping, Mayo Clinic, Mayo Clinic

0035U Neurology (prion disease), cerebrospinal fluid, detection of prion protein by quaking-induced conformational conversion, qualitative

　　🔬 0.00　　🔎 0.00　　**FUD** 000　　　　　　▣

　　INCLUDES　　Real-time quaking-induced conversion for prion detection (RT-QuIC), National Prion Disease Pathology Surveillance Center

0036U Exome (ie, somatic mutations), paired formalin-fixed paraffin-embedded tumor tissue and normal specimen, sequence analyses

　　🔬 0.00　　🔎 0.00　　**FUD** 000　　　　　　▣

　　INCLUDES　　EXaCT-1 Whole Exome Testing, Lab of Oncology-Molecular Detection, Weill Cornell Medicine- Clinical Genomics Laboratory

0037U Targeted genomic sequence analysis, solid organ neoplasm, DNA analysis of 324 genes, interrogation for sequence variants, gene copy number amplifications, gene rearrangements, microsatellite instability and tumor mutational burden

　　🔬 0.00　　🔎 0.00　　**FUD** 000　　　　　　▣

　　INCLUDES　　FoundationOne CDx™ (F1CDx), Foundation Medicine, Inc, Foundation Medicine, Inc

0038U Vitamin D, 25 hydroxy D2 and D3, by LC-MS/MS, serum microsample, quantitative

　　🔬 0.00　　🔎 0.00　　**FUD** 000　　　　　　▣

　　INCLUDES　　Sensieva™ Droplet 25OH Vitamin D2/D3 Microvolume LC/MS Assay, InSource Diagnostics, InSource Diagnostics

0039U Deoxyribonucleic acid (DNA) antibody, double stranded, high avidity

　　🔬 0.00　　🔎 0.00　　**FUD** 000　　　　　　▣

　　INCLUDES　　Anti-dsDNA, High Salt/Avidity, University of Washington, Department of Laboratory Medicine, Bio-Rad

0040U *BCR/ABL1 (t(9;22))* (eg, chronic myelogenous leukemia) translocation analysis, major breakpoint, quantitative

　　🔬 0.00　　🔎 0.00　　**FUD** 000　　　　　　▣

　　INCLUDES　　MRDx BCR-ABL Test, MolecularMD, MolecularMD

0041U Borrelia burgdorferi, antibody detection of 5 recombinant protein groups, by immunoblot, IgM

　　🔬 0.00　　🔎 0.00　　**FUD** 000　　　　　　▣

　　INCLUDES　　Lyme ImmunoBlot IgM, IGeneX Inc, ID-FISH Technology Inc. (ASR) (Lyme ImmunoBlot IgM Strips Only)

0042U Borrelia burgdorferi, antibody detection of 12 recombinant protein groups, by immunoblot, IgG

　　🔬 0.00　　🔎 0.00　　**FUD** 000　　　　　　▣

　　INCLUDES　　Lyme ImmunoBlot IgG, IGeneX Inc, ID-FISH Technology Inc (ASR) (Lyme ImmunoBlot IgG Strips Only)

0043U Tick-borne relapsing fever Borrelia group, antibody detection to 4 recombinant protein groups, by immunoblot, IgM

　　🔬 0.00　　🔎 0.00　　**FUD** 000　　　　　　▣

　　INCLUDES　　Tick-Borne Relapsing Fever (TBRF) Borrelia ImmunoBlots IgM Test, IGeneX Inc, ID-FISH Technology Inc (Provides TBRF ImmunoBlot IgM Strips)

0044U Tick-borne relapsing fever Borrelia group, antibody detection to 4 recombinant protein groups, by immunoblot, IgG

　　🔬 0.00　　🔎 0.00　　**FUD** 000　　　　　　▣

　　INCLUDES　　Tick-Borne Relapsing Fever (TBRF) Borrelia ImmunoBlots IgG Test, IGeneX Inc., ID-FISH Technology Inc (Provides TBRF ImmunoBlot IgG Strips)

0045U Oncology (breast ductal carcinoma in situ), mRNA, gene expression profiling by real-time RT-PCR of 12 genes (7 content and 5 housekeeping), utilizing formalin-fixed paraffin-embedded tissue, algorithm reported as recurrence score

　　🔬 0.00　　🔎 0.00　　**FUD** 000　　　　　　▣

　　INCLUDES　　The Oncotype DX® Breast DCIS Score™ Test, Genomic Health, Inc, Genomic Health, Inc

0046U *FLT3 (fms-related tyrosine kinase 3)* (eg, acute myeloid leukemia) internal tandem duplication (ITD) variants, quantitative

　　🔬 0.00　　🔎 0.00　　**FUD** 000　　　　　　▣

　　INCLUDES　　FLT3 ITD MRD by NGS, LabPMM LLC, an Invivoscribe Technologies, Inc Company

0047U Oncology (prostate), mRNA, gene expression profiling by real-time RT-PCR of 17 genes (12 content and 5 housekeeping), utilizing formalin-fixed paraffin-embedded tissue, algorithm reported as a risk score

　　🔬 0.00　　🔎 0.00　　**FUD** 000　　　　　　▣

　　INCLUDES　　Oncotype DX Genomic Prostate Score, Genomic Health, Inc, Genomic Health, Inc

0048U Oncology (solid organ neoplasia), DNA, targeted sequencing of protein-coding exons of 468 cancer-associated genes, including interrogation for somatic mutations and microsatellite instability, matched with normal specimens, utilizing formalin-fixed paraffin-embedded tumor tissue, report of clinically significant mutation(s)

　　🔬 0.00　　🔎 0.00　　**FUD** 000　　　　　　▣

　　INCLUDES　　MSK-IMPACT (Integrated Mutation Profiling of Actionable Cancer Targets), Memorial Sloan Kettering Cancer Center

---

0049U NPM1 (nucleophosmin) (eg, acute myeloid leukemia) gene analysis, quantitative

   🚗 0.00   🔪 0.00   **FUD** 000   ▱

INCLUDES   *NPM1* MRD by NGS, LabPMM LLC, an Invivoscribe Technologies, Inc Company

0050U Targeted genomic sequence analysis panel, acute myelogenous leukemia, DNA analysis, 194 genes, interrogation for sequence variants, copy number variants or rearrangements

   🚗 0.00   🔪 0.00   **FUD** 000   ▱

INCLUDES   MyAML NGS Panel, LabPMM LLC, an Invivoscribe Technologies, Inc Company

0051U Prescription drug monitoring, evaluation of drugs present by LC-MS/MS, urine, 31 drug panel, reported as quantitative results, detected or not detected, per date of service

   🚗 0.00   🔪 0.00   **FUD** 000   ▱

INCLUDES   UCompliDx, Elite Medical Laboratory Solutions, LLC, Elite Medical Laboratory Solutions, LLC (LDT)

0052U Lipoprotein, blood, high resolution fractionation and quantitation of lipoproteins, including all five major lipoprotein classes and subclasses of HDL, LDL, and VLDL by vertical auto profile ultracentrifugation

   🚗 0.00   🔪 0.00   **FUD** 000   ▱

INCLUDES   VAP Cholesterol Test, VAP Diagnostics Laboratory, Inc, VAP Diagnostics Laboratory, Inc

0053U Oncology (prostate cancer), FISH analysis of 4 genes (*ASAP1, HDAC9, CHD1* and *PTEN*, needle biopsy specimen, algorithm reported as probability of higher tumor grade

   🚗 0.00   🔪 0.00   **FUD** 000   ▱

INCLUDES   Prostate Cancer Risk Panel, Mayo Clinic, Laboratory Developed Test

0054U Prescription drug monitoring, 14 or more classes of drugs and substances, definitive tandem mass spectrometry with chromatography, capillary blood, quantitative report with therapeutic and toxic ranges, including steady-state range for the prescribed dose when detected, per date of service

   🚗 0.00   🔪 0.00   **FUD** 000   ▱

INCLUDES   AssuranceRx Micro Serum, Firstox Laboratories, LLC, Firstox Laboratories, LLC

0055U Cardiology (heart transplant), cell-free DNA, PCR assay of 96 DNA target sequences (94 single nucleotide polymorphism targets and two control targets), plasma

   🚗 0.00   🔪 0.00   **FUD** 000   ▱

INCLUDES   myTAIHEART, TAI Diagnostics, Inc, TAI Diagnostics, Inc

0056U Hematology (acute myelogenous leukemia), DNA, whole genome next-generation sequencing to detect gene rearrangement(s), blood or bone marrow, report of specific gene rearrangement(s)

   🚗 0.00   🔪 0.00   **FUD** 000   ▱

INCLUDES   MatePair Acute Myeloid Leukemia Panel, Mayo Clinic, Laboratory Developed Test

~~0057U~~ ~~Oncology (solid organ neoplasia), mRNA, gene expression profiling by massively parallel sequencing for analysis of 51 genes, utilizing formalin-fixed paraffin-embedded tissue, algorithm reported as a normalized percentile rank~~

0058U Oncology (Merkel cell carcinoma), detection of antibodies to the Merkel cell polyoma virus oncoprotein (small T antigen), serum, quantitative

   🚗 0.00   🔪 0.00   **FUD** 000   ▱

INCLUDES   Merkel SmT Oncoprotein Antibody Titer, University of Washington, Department of Laboratory Medicine

0059U Oncology (Merkel cell carcinoma), detection of antibodies to the Merkel cell polyoma virus capsid protein (VP1), serum, reported as positive or negative

   🚗 0.00   🔪 0.00   **FUD** 000   ▱

INCLUDES   Merkel Virus VP1 Capsid Antibody, University of Washington, Department of Laboratory Medicine

0060U Twin zygosity, genomic targeted sequence analysis of chromosome 2, using circulating cell-free fetal DNA in maternal blood

   🚗 0.00   🔪 0.00   **FUD** 000   ▱

INCLUDES   Twins Zygosity PLA, Natera, Inc, Natera, Inc

0061U Transcutaneous measurement of five biomarkers (tissue oxygenation [StO2], oxyhemoglobin [ctHbO2], deoxyhemoglobin [ctHbR], papillary and reticular dermal hemoglobin concentrations [ctHb1 and ctHb2]), using spatial frequency domain imaging (SFDI) and multi-spectral analysis

   🚗 0.00   🔪 0.00   **FUD** 000   ▱

INCLUDES   Transcutaneous multispectral measurement of tissue oxygenation and hemoglobin using spatial frequency domain imaging (SFDI), Modulated Imaging, Inc, Modulated Imaging, Inc

● **0062U** Autoimmune (systemic lupus erythematosus), IgG and IgM analysis of 80 biomarkers, utilizing serum, algorithm reported with a risk score

   🚗 0.00   🔪 0.00   **FUD** 000   ▱

INCLUDES   SLE-key® Rule Out, Veracis Inc, Veracis Inc

● **0063U** Neurology (autism), 32 amines by LC-MS/MS, using plasma, algorithm reported as metabolic signature associated with autism spectrum disorder

   🚗 0.00   🔪 0.00   **FUD** 000   ▱

INCLUDES   NPDX ASD ADM Panel I, Stemina Biomarker Discovery, Inc, Stemina Biomarker Discovery, Inc d/b/a NeuroPointDX

● **0064U** Antibody, Treponema pallidum, total and rapid plasma reagin (RPR), immunoassay, qualitative

   🚗 0.00   🔪 0.00   **FUD** 000   ▱

INCLUDES   BioPlex 2200 Syphilis Total & RPR Assay, Bio-Rad Laboratories, Bio-Rad Laboratories

● **0065U** Syphilis test, non-treponemal antibody, immunoassay, qualitative (RPR)

   🚗 0.00   🔪 0.00   **FUD** 000   ▱

INCLUDES   BioPlex 2200 RPR Assay, Bio-Rad Laboratories, Bio-Rad Laboratories

● **0066U** Placental alpha-micro globulin-1 (PAMG-1), immunoassay with direct optical observation, cervico-vaginal fluid, each specimen

   🚗 0.00   🔪 0.00   **FUD** 000   ▱

INCLUDES   PartoSure™ Test, Parsagen Diagnostics, Inc, Parsagen Diagnostics, Inc, a QIAGEN Company

● **0067U** Oncology (breast), immunohistochemistry, protein expression profiling of 4 biomarkers (matrix metalloproteinase-1 [MMP-1], carcinoembryonic antigen-related cell adhesion molecule 6 [CEACAM6], hyaluronoglucosaminidase [HYAL1], highly expressed in cancer protein [HEC1]), formalin-fixed paraffin-embedded precancerous breast tissue, algorithm reported as carcinoma risk score

   🚗 0.00   🔪 0.00   **FUD** 000   ▱

INCLUDES   BBDRisk Dx™, Silbiotech, Inc, Silbiotech, Inc

● **0068U** Candida species panel (*C. albicans, C. glabrata, C. parapsilosis, C. kruseii, C tropicalis, and C. auris*), amplified probe technique with qualitative report of the presence or absence of each species

   🚗 0.00   🔪 0.00   **FUD** 000   ▱

INCLUDES   MYCODART Dual Amplification Real Time PCR Panel for 6 Candida species, RealTime Laboratories, Inc, RealTime Laboratories, Inc

0069U Oncology (colorectal), microRNA, RT-PCR expression profiling of miR-31-3p, formalin-fixed paraffin-embedded tissue, algorithm reported as an expression score

💷 0.00   ⚖ 0.00   **FUD** 000

INCLUDES miR-31now™, GoPath Laboratories, GoPath Laboratories

0070U *CYP2D6 (cytochrome P450, family 2, subfamily D, polypeptide 6) (eg, drug metabolism) gene analysis, common and select rare variants (ie, *2, *3, *4, *4N, *5, *6, *7, *8, *9, *10, *11, *12, *13, *14A, *14B, *15, *17, *29, *35, *36, *41, *57, *61, *63, *68, *83, *xN)*

💷 0.00   ⚖ 0.00   **FUD** 000

INCLUDES CYP2D6 Common Variants and Copy Number, Mayo Clinic, Laboratory Developed Test

+ 0071U *CYP2D6 (cytochrome P450, family 2, subfamily D, polypeptide 6) (eg, drug metabolism) gene analysis, full gene sequence* (List separately in addition to code for primary procedure)

💷 0.00   ⚖ 0.00   **FUD** 000

INCLUDES CYP2D6 Full Gene Sequencing, Mayo Clinic, Laboratory Developed Test

Code first (0070U)

+ 0072U *CYP2D6 (cytochrome P450, family 2, subfamily D, polypeptide 6) (eg, drug metabolism) gene analysis, targeted sequence analysis (ie, CYP2D6-2D7 hybrid gene)* (List separately in addition to code for primary procedure)

💷 0.00   ⚖ 0.00   **FUD** 000

INCLUDES CYP2D6-2D7 Hybrid Gene Targeted Sequence Analysis, Mayo Clinic, Laboratory Developed Test

Code first (0070U)

+ 0073U *CYP2D6 (cytochrome P450, family 2, subfamily D, polypeptide 6) (eg, drug metabolism) gene analysis, targeted sequence analysis (ie, CYP2D7-2D6 hybrid gene)* (List separately in addition to code for primary procedure)

💷 0.00   ⚖ 0.00   **FUD** 000

INCLUDES CYP2D7-2D6 Hybrid Gene Targeted Sequence Analysis, Mayo Clinic, Laboratory Developed Test

Code first (0070U)

+ 0074U *CYP2D6 (cytochrome P450, family 2, subfamily D, polypeptide 6) (eg, drug metabolism) gene analysis, targeted sequence analysis (ie, non-duplicated gene when duplication/multiplication is trans)* (List separately in addition to code for primary procedure)

💷 0.00   ⚖ 0.00   **FUD** 000

INCLUDES CYP2D7-2D6 trans-duplication/multiplication non-duplicated gene targeted sequence analysis, Mayo Clinic, Laboratory Developed Test

Code first (0070U)

+ 0075U *CYP2D6 (cytochrome P450, family 2, subfamily D, polypeptide 6) (eg, drug metabolism) gene analysis, targeted sequence analysis (ie, 5' gene duplication/multiplication)* (List separately in addition to code for primary procedure)

💷 0.00   ⚖ 0.00   **FUD** 000

INCLUDES CYP2D6 5' gene duplication/multiplication targeted sequence analysis, Mayo Clinic, Laboratory Developed Test

Code first (0070U)

+ 0076U *CYP2D6 (cytochrome P450, family 2, subfamily D, polypeptide 6) (eg, drug metabolism) gene analysis, targeted sequence analysis (ie, 3' gene duplication/ multiplication)* (List separately in addition to code for primary procedure)

💷 0.00   ⚖ 0.00   **FUD** 000

INCLUDES CYP2D6 3' gene duplication/multiplication targeted sequence analysis, Mayo Clinic, Laboratory Developed Test

Code first (0070U)

0077U Immunoglobulin paraprotein (M-protein), qualitative, immunoprecipitation and mass spectrometry, blood or urine, including isotype

💷 0.00   ⚖ 0.00   **FUD** 000

INCLUDES M-Protein Detection and Isotyping by MALDI-TOF Mass Spectrometry, Mayo Clinic, Laboratory Developed Test

0078U Pain management (opioid-use disorder) genotyping panel, 16 common variants (ie, *ABCB1, COMT, DAT1, DBH, DOR, DRD1, DRD2, DRD4, GABA, GAL, HTR2A, HTTLPR, MTHFR, MUOR, OPRK1, OPRM1*), buccal swab or other germline tissue sample, algorithm reported as positive or negative risk of opioid-use disorder

💷 0.00   ⚖ 0.00   **FUD** 000

INCLUDES INFINITI® Neural Response Panel, PersonalizeDx Labs, AutoGenomics Inc

0079U Comparative DNA analysis using multiple selected single-nucleotide polymorphisms (SNPs), urine and buccal DNA, for specimen identity verification

💷 0.00   ⚖ 0.00   **FUD** 000

INCLUDES ToxLok™, InSource Diagnostics, InSource Diagnostics

0080U Oncology (lung), mass spectrometric analysis of galectin-3-binding protein and scavenger receptor cysteine-rich type 1 protein M130, with five clinical risk factors (age, smoking status, nodule diameter, nodule-spiculation status and nodule location), utilizing plasma, algorithm reported as a categorical probability of malignancy

💷 0.00   ⚖ 0.00   **FUD** 000

INCLUDES BDX-XL2, Biodesix®, Inc, Biodesix®, Inc, Biodesix®, Inc

0081U ~~Oncology (uveal melanoma), mRNA, gene-expression profiling by real-time RT-PCR of 15 genes (12 content and 3 housekeeping genes), utilizing fine needle aspirate or formalin-fixed paraffin-embedded tissue, algorithm reported as risk of metastasis~~

To report, see (81552)

0082U Drug test(s), definitive, 90 or more drugs or substances, definitive chromatography with mass spectrometry, and presumptive, any number of drug classes, by instrument chemistry analyzer (utilizing immunoassay), urine, report of presence or absence of each drug, drug metabolite or substance with description and severity of significant interactions per date of service

💷 0.00   ⚖ 0.00   **FUD** 000

INCLUDES NextGen Precision™ Testing, Precision Diagnostics, Precision Diagnostics LBN Precision Toxicology, LLC

0083U Oncology, response to chemotherapy drugs using motility contrast tomography, fresh or frozen tissue, reported as likelihood of sensitivity or resistance to drugs or drug combinations

💷 0.00   ⚖ 0.00   **FUD** 000

INCLUDES Onco4D™, Animated Dynamics, Inc, Animated Dynamics, Inc

0084U Red blood cell antigen typing, DNA, genotyping of 10 blood groups with phenotype prediction of 37 red blood cell antigens

INCLUDES BLOODchip®, ID CORE XT™, Grifols Diagnostic Solutions Inc

0085U ~~Cytolethal distending toxin B (CdtB) and vinculin IgG antibodies by immunoassay (ie, ELISA)~~

0086U Infectious disease (bacterial and fungal), organism identification, blood culture, using rRNA FISH, 6 or more organism targets, reported as positive or negative with phenotypic minimum inhibitory concentration (MIC)-based antimicrobial susceptibility

INCLUDES Accelerate PhenoTest™ BC kit, Accelerate Diagnostics, Inc

● **0087U** Cardiology (heart transplant), mRNA gene expression profiling by microarray of 1283 genes, transplant biopsy tissue, allograft rejection and injury algorithm reported as a probability score

> INCLUDES Molecular Microscope® MMDx—Heart, Kashi Clinical Laboratories

● **0088U** Transplantation medicine (kidney allograft rejection), microarray gene expression profiling of 1494 genes, utilizing transplant biopsy tissue, algorithm reported as a probability score for rejection

> INCLUDES Molecular Microscope® MMDx—Kidney, Kashi Clinical Laboratories

● **0089U** Oncology (melanoma), gene expression profiling by RTqPCR, *PRAME* and *LINC00518*, superficial collection using adhesive patch(es)

> INCLUDES Pigmented Lesion Assay (PLA), DermTech

● **0090U** Oncology (cutaneous melanoma), mRNA gene expression profiling by RT-PCR of 23 genes (14 content and 9 housekeeping), utilizing formalin-fixed paraffin-embedded tissue, algorithm reported as a categorical result (ie, benign, indeterminate, malignant)

> INCLUDES myPath® Melanoma, Myriad Genetic Laboratories

● **0091U** Oncology (colorectal) screening, cell enumeration of circulating tumor cells, utilizing whole blood, algorithm, for the presence of adenoma or cancer, reported as a positive or negative result

> INCLUDES FirstSight^CRC, CellMax Life

● **0092U** Oncology (lung), three protein biomarkers, immunoassay using magnetic nanosensor technology, plasma, algorithm reported as risk score for likelihood of malignancy

> INCLUDES REVEAL Lung Nodule Characterization, MagArray, Inc

● **0093U** Prescription drug monitoring, evaluation of 65 common drugs by LC-MS/MS, urine, each drug reported detected or not detected

> INCLUDES ComplyRX, Claro Labs

● **0094U** Genome (eg, unexplained constitutional or heritable disorder or syndrome), rapid sequence analysis

> INCLUDES RCIGM Rapid Whole Genome Sequencing, Rady Children's Institute for Genomic Medicine (RCIGM)

● **0095U** Inflammation (eosinophilic esophagitis), ELISA analysis of eotaxin-3 *(CCL26 [C-C motif chemokine ligand 26])* and major basic protein *(PRG2 [proteoglycan 2, pro eosinophil major basic protein])*, specimen obtained by swallowed nylon string, algorithm reported as predictive probability index for active eosinophilic esophagitis

> INCLUDES Esophageal String Test™ (EST), Cambridge Biomedical, Inc

● **0096U** Human papillomavirus (HPV), high-risk types (ie, 16, 18, 31, 33, 35, 39, 45, 51, 52, 56, 58, 59, 66, 68), male urine

> INCLUDES HPV, High-Risk, Male Urine, Molecular Testing Labs

● **0097U** Gastrointestinal pathogen, multiplex reverse transcription and multiplex amplified probe technique, multiple types or subtypes, 22 targets (Campylobacter [C. jejuni/C. coli/C. upsaliensis], Clostridium difficile [C. difficile] toxin A/B, Plesiomonas shigelloides, Salmonella, Vibrio [V. parahaemolyticus/V. vulnificus/V. cholerae], including specific identification of Vibrio cholerae, Yersinia enterocolitica, Enteroaggregative Escherichia coli [EAEC], Enteropathogenic Escherichia coli [EPEC], Enterotoxigenic Escherichia coli [ETEC] lt/st, Shiga-like toxin-producing Escherichia coli [STEC] stx1/stx2 [including specific identification of the E. coli O157 serogroup within STEC], Shigella/Enteroinvasive Escherichia coli [EIEC], Cryptosporidium, Cyclospora cayetanensis, Entamoeba histolytica, Giardia lamblia [also known as G. intestinalis and G. duodenalis], adenovirus F 40/41, astrovirus, norovirus GI/GII, rotavirus A, sapovirus [Genogroups I, II, IV, and V])

> INCLUDES BioFire® FilmArray® Gastrointestinal (GI) Panel, BioFire® Diagnostics

● **0098U** Respiratory pathogen, multiplex reverse transcription and multiplex amplified probe technique, multiple types or subtypes, 14 targets (adenovirus, coronavirus, human metapneumovirus, influenza A, influenza A subtype H1, influenza A subtype H3, influenza A subtype H1-2009, influenza B, parainfluenza virus, human rhinovirus/enterovirus, respiratory syncytial virus, Bordetella pertussis, Chlamydophila pneumoniae, Mycoplasma pneumoniae)

> INCLUDES BioFire® FilmArray® Respiratory Panel (RP) EZ, BioFire® Diagnostics

● **0099U** Respiratory pathogen, multiplex reverse transcription and multiplex amplified probe technique, multiple types or subtypes, 20 targets (adenovirus, coronavirus 229E, coronavirus HKU1, coronavirus, coronavirus OC43, human metapneumovirus, influenza A, influenza A subtype, influenza A subtype H3, influenza A subtype H1-2009, influenza, parainfluenza virus, parainfluenza virus 2, parainfluenza virus 3, parainfluenza virus 4, human rhinovirus/enterovirus, respiratory syncytial virus, Bordetella pertussis, Chlamydophila pneumonia, Mycoplasma pneumoniae)

> INCLUDES BioFire® FilmArray® Respiratory Panel (RP), BioFire® Diagnostics

● **0100U** Respiratory pathogen, multiplex reverse transcription and multiplex amplified probe technique, multiple types or subtypes, 21 targets (adenovirus, coronavirus 229E, coronavirus HKU1, coronavirus NL63, coronavirus OC43, human metapneumovirus, human rhinovirus/enterovirus, influenza A, including subtypes H1, H1-2009, and H3, influenza B, parainfluenza virus 1, parainfluenza virus 2, parainfluenza virus 3, parainfluenza virus 4, respiratory syncytial virus, Bordetella parapertussis [IS1001], Bordetella pertussis [ptxP], Chlamydia pneumoniae, Mycoplasma pneumoniae)

> INCLUDES BioFire® FilmArray® Respiratory Panel 2 (RP2), BioFire® Diagnostics

● **0101U** Hereditary colon cancer disorders (eg, Lynch syndrome, *PTEN* hamartoma syndrome, Cowden syndrome, familial adenomatosis polyposis), genomic sequence analysis panel utilizing a combination of NGS, Sanger, MLPA, and array CGH, with MRNA analytics to resolve variants of unknown significance when indicated (15 genes [sequencing and deletion/duplication], *EPCAM* and *GREM1* [deletion/duplication only])

> INCLUDES ColoNext®, Ambry Genetics®, Ambry Genetics®

● 0102U **Hereditary breast cancer-related disorders (eg, hereditary breast cancer, hereditary ovarian cancer, hereditary endometrial cancer), genomic sequence analysis panel utilizing a combination of NGS, Sanger, MLPA, and array CGH, with MRNA analytics to resolve variants of unknown significance when indicated (17 genes [sequencing and deletion/duplication])**

INCLUDES BreastNext®, Ambry Genetics®, Ambry Genetics®

● 0103U **Hereditary ovarian cancer (eg, hereditary ovarian cancer, hereditary endometrial cancer), genomic sequence analysis panel utilizing a combination of NGS, Sanger, MLPA, and array CGH, with MRNA analytics to resolve variants of unknown significance when indicated (24 genes [sequencing and deletion/duplication], EPCAM [deletion/duplication only])**

INCLUDES OvaNext®, Ambry Genetics®, Ambry Genetics®

● 0104U ~~Hereditary pan cancer (eg, hereditary breast and ovarian cancer, hereditary endometrial cancer, hereditary colorectal cancer), genomic sequence analysis panel utilizing a combination of NGS, Sanger, MLPA, and array CGH, with MRNA analytics to resolve variants of unknown significance when indicated (32 genes [sequencing and deletion/duplication], EPCAM and GREM1 [deletion/duplication only])~~

● 0105U **Nephrology (chronic kidney disease), multiplex electrochemiluminescent immunoassay (ECLIA) of tumor necrosis factor receptor 1A, receptor superfamily 2 (TNFR1, TNFR2), and kidney injury molecule-1 (KIM-1) combined with longitudinal clinical data, including APOL1 genotype if available, and plasma (isolated fresh or frozen), algorithm reported as probability score for rapid kidney function decline (RKFD)**

INCLUDES KidneyIntelXT™, RenalytixAI, RenalytixAI

● 0106U **Gastric emptying, serial collection of 7 timed breath specimens, non-radioisotope carbon-13 (^{13}C) spirulina substrate, analysis of each specimen by gas isotope ratio mass spectrometry, reported as rate of $^{13}CO_2$ excretion**

INCLUDES 13C-Spirulina Gastric Emptying Breath Test (GEBT), Cairn Diagnostics d/b/a Advanced Breath Diagnostics, LLC, Cairn Diagnostics d/b/a Advanced Breath Diagnostics, LLC

● 0107U **Clostridium difficile toxin(s) antigen detection by immunoassay technique, stool, qualitative, multiple-step method**

INCLUDES Singulex Clarity C.diff toxins A/B assay, Singulex

● 0108U **Gastroenterology (Barrett's esophagus), whole slide-digital imaging, including morphometric analysis, computer-assisted quantitative immunolabeling of 9 protein biomarkers (p16, AMACR, p53, CD68, COX-2, CD45RO, HIF1a, HER-2, K20) and morphology, formalin-fixed paraffin-embedded tissue, algorithm reported as risk of progression to high-grade dysplasia or cancer**

INCLUDES TissueCypher® Barrett's Esophagus Assay, Cernostics, Cernostics

● 0109U **Infectious disease (Aspergillus species), real-time PCR for detection of DNA from 4 species (A. fumigatus, A. terreus, A. niger, and A. flavus), blood, lavage fluid, or tissue, qualitative reporting of presence or absence of each species**

INCLUDES MYCODART Dual Amplification Real Time PCR Panel for 4 Aspergillus species, RealTime Laboratories, Inc/MycoDART, Inc

● 0110U **Prescription drug monitoring, one or more oral oncology drug(s) and substances, definitive tandem mass spectrometry with chromatography, serum or plasma from capillary blood or venous blood, quantitative report with steady-state range for the prescribed drug(s) when detected**

INCLUDES Oral OncolyticAssuranceRX, Firstox Laboratories, LLC, Firstox Laboratories, LLC

● 0111U **Oncology (colon cancer), targeted KRAS (codons 12, 13, and 61) and NRAS (codons 12, 13, and 61) gene analysis utilizing formalin-fixed paraffin-embedded tissue**

INCLUDES Praxis(™) Extended RAS Panel, Illumina, Illumina

● 0112U **Infectious agent detection and identification, targeted sequence analysis (16S and 18S rRNA genes) with drug-resistance gene**

INCLUDES MicroGenDX qPCR & NGS For Infection, MicroGenDX, MicroGenDX

● 0113U **Oncology (prostate), measurement of PCA3 and TMPRSS2-ERG in urine and PSA in serum following prostatic massage, by RNA amplification and fluorescence-based detection, algorithm reported as risk score**

INCLUDES MiPS (Mi-Prostate Score), MLabs, MLabs

● 0114U **Gastroenterology (Barrett's esophagus), VIM and CCNA1 methylation analysis, esophageal cells, algorithm reported as likelihood for Barrett's esophagus**

INCLUDES EsoGuard™, Lucid Diagnostics, Lucid Diagnostics

● 0115U **Respiratory infectious agent detection by nucleic acid (DNA and RNA), 18 viral types and subtypes and 2 bacterial targets, amplified probe technique, including multiplex reverse transcription for RNA targets, each analyte reported as detected or not detected**

INCLUDES ePlex Respiratory Pathogen (RP) Panel, GenMark Diagnostics, Inc, GenMark Diagnostics, Inc

● 0116U **Prescription drug monitoring, enzyme immunoassay of 35 or more drugs confirmed with LC-MS/MS, oral fluid, algorithm results reported as a patient-compliance measurement with risk of drug to drug interactions for prescribed medications**

INCLUDES Snapshot Oral Fluid Compliance, Ethos Laboratories

● 0117U **Pain management, analysis of 11 endogenous analytes (methylmalonic acid, xanthurenic acid, homocysteine, pyroglutamic acid, vanilmandelate, 5-hydroxyindoleacetic acid, hydroxymethylglutarate, ethylmalonate, 3-hydroxypropyl mercapturic acid (3-HPMA), quinolinic acid, kynurenic acid), LC-MS/MS, urine, algorithm reported as a pain-index score with likelihood of atypical biochemical function associated with pain**

INCLUDES Foundation PI⊠, Ethos Laboratories

● 0118U **Transplantation medicine, quantification of donor-derived cell-free DNA using whole genome next-generation sequencing, plasma, reported as percentage of donor-derived cell-free DNA in the total cell-free DNA**

INCLUDES Viracor TRAC™ dd-cfDNA, Viracor Eurofins, Viracor Eurofins

● 0119U **Cardiology, ceramides by liquid chromatography-tandem mass spectrometry, plasma, quantitative report with risk score for major cardiovascular events**

INCLUDES MI-HEART Ceramides, Plasma, Mayo Clinic, Laboratory Developed Test

● 0120U **Oncology (B-cell lymphoma classification), mRNA, gene expression profiling by fluorescent probe hybridization of 58 genes (45 content and 13 housekeeping genes), formalin-fixed paraffin-embedded tissue, algorithm reported as likelihood for primary mediastinal B-cell lymphoma (PMBCL) and diffuse large B-cell lymphoma (DLBCL) with cell of origin subtyping in the latter**

INCLUDES Lymph3Cx Lymphoma Molecular Subtyping Assay, Mayo Clinic, Laboratory Developed Test

● 0121U **Sickle cell disease, microfluidic flow adhesion (VCAM-1), whole blood**

INCLUDES Flow Adhesion of Whole Blood on VCAM-1 (FAB-V), Functional Fluidics, Functional Fluidics

26/16 PC/TC Only | A2-A3 ASC Payment | 50 Bilateral | ♂ Male Only | ♀ Female Only | 📊 Facility RVU | 📈 Non-Facility RVU | 🔲 CCI | ✖ CLIA

FUD Follow-up Days | CMS: IOM | AMA: CPT Asst | A-Y OPPSI | 80/80 Surg Assist Allowed / w/Doc | 📈 Lab Crosswalk | 📊 Radiology Crosswalk

452

CPT © 2019 American Medical Association. All Rights Reserved.

© 2019 Optum360, LLC

● 0122U Sickle cell disease, microfluidic flow adhesion (P-Selectin), whole blood

INCLUDES Flow Adhesion of Whole Blood to P-SELECTIN (WB-PSEL), Functional Fluidics, Functional Fluidics

● 0123U Mechanical fragility, RBC, shear stress and spectral analysis profiling

INCLUDES Mechanical Fragility, RBC by shear stress profiling and spectral analysis, Functional Fluidics, Functional Fluidics

● 0124U Fetal congenital abnormalities, biochemical assays of 3 analytes (free beta-hCG, PAPP-A, AFP), time-resolved fluorescence immunoassay, maternal dried-blood spot, algorithm reported as risk scores for fetal trisomies 13/18 and 21

INCLUDES First Trimester Screen | FßⓍ, Eurofins NTD, LLC, Eurofins NTD, LLC

● 0125U Fetal congenital abnormalities and perinatal complications, biochemical assays of 5 analytes (free beta-hCG, PAPP-A, AFP, placental growth factor, and inhibin-A), time-resolved fluorescence immunoassay, maternal serum, algorithm reported as risk scores for fetal trisomies 13/18, 21, and preeclampsia

INCLUDES Maternal Fetal Screen | T1Ⓧ, Eurofins NTD, LLC, Eurofins NTD, LLC

● 0126U Fetal congenital abnormalities and perinatal complications, biochemical assays of 5 analytes (free beta-hCG, PAPP-A, AFP, placental growth factor, and inhibin-A), time-resolved fluorescence immunoassay, includes qualitative assessment of Y chromosome in cell-free fetal DNA, maternal serum and plasma, predictive algorithm reported as a risk scores for fetal trisomies 13/18, 21, and preeclampsia

INCLUDES Maternal Fetal Screen | T1 + Y Chromosome Ⓧ, Eurofins NTD, LLC, Eurofins NTD, LLC

● 0127U Obstetrics (preeclampsia), biochemical assays of 3 analytes (PAPP-A, AFP, and placental growth factor), time-resolved fluorescence immunoassay, maternal serum, predictive algorithm reported as a risk score for preeclampsia

INCLUDES Preeclampsia Screen | T1Ⓧ, Eurofins NTD, LLC, Eurofins NTD, LLC

● 0128U Obstetrics (preeclampsia), biochemical assays of 3 analytes (PAPP-A, AFP, and placental growth factor), time-resolved fluorescence immunoassay, includes qualitative assessment of Y chromosome in cell-free fetal DNA, maternal serum and plasma, predictive algorithm reported as a risk score for preeclampsia

INCLUDES Preeclampsia Screen | T1 + Y ChromosomeⓍ, Eurofins NTD, LLC, Eurofins NTD, LLC

● 0129U Hereditary breast cancer-related disorders (eg, hereditary breast cancer, hereditary ovarian cancer, hereditary endometrial cancer), genomic sequence analysis and deletion/duplication analysis panel (ATM, BRCA1, BRCA2, CDH1, CHEK2, PALB2, PTEN, and TP53)

INCLUDES BRCAplus, Ambry Genetics

● + 0130U Hereditary colon cancer disorders (eg, Lynch syndrome, PTEN hamartoma syndrome, Cowden syndrome, familial adenomatosis polyposis), targeted mRNA sequence analysis panel (APC, CDH1, CHEK2, MLH1, MSH2, MSH6, MUTYH, PMS2, PTEN, and TP53) (List separately in addition to code for primary procedure)

🖼 0.00   ⚖ 0.00   FUD 000

INCLUDES +RNAinsight™ for ColoNext®, Ambry Genetics Code first (81435, 0101U)

● + 0131U Hereditary breast cancer-related disorders (eg, hereditary breast cancer, hereditary ovarian cancer, hereditary endometrial cancer), targeted mRNA sequence analysis panel (13 genes) (List separately in addition to code for primary procedure)

🖼 0.00   ⚖ 0.00   FUD 000

INCLUDES +RNAinsight™ for BreastNext®, Ambry Genetics Code first ([81162], 81432, 0102U)

● + 0132U Hereditary ovarian cancer-related disorders (eg, hereditary breast cancer, hereditary ovarian cancer, hereditary endometrial cancer), targeted mRNA sequence analysis panel (17 genes) (List separately in addition to code for primary procedure)

🖼 0.00   ⚖ 0.00   FUD 000

INCLUDES +RNAinsight™ for OvaNext®, Ambry Genetics Code first ([81162], 81432, 0103U)

● + 0133U Hereditary prostate cancer-related disorders, targeted mRNA sequence analysis panel (11 genes) (List separately in addition to code for primary procedure)

🖼 0.00   ⚖ 0.00   FUD 000

INCLUDES +RNAinsight™ for ProstateNext®, Ambry Genetics Code first ([81162])

● + 0134U Hereditary pan cancer (eg, hereditary breast and ovarian cancer, hereditary endometrial cancer, hereditary colorectal cancer), targeted mRNA sequence analysis panel (18 genes) (List separately in addition to code for primary procedure)

🖼 0.00   ⚖ 0.00   FUD 000

INCLUDES +RNAinsight™ for CancerNext®, Ambry Genetics Code first ([81162], 81432, 81435)

● + 0135U Hereditary gynecological cancer (eg, hereditary breast and ovarian cancer, hereditary endometrial cancer, hereditary colorectal cancer), targeted mRNA sequence analysis panel (12 genes) (List separately in addition to code for primary procedure)

🖼 0.00   ⚖ 0.00   FUD 000

INCLUDES +RNAinsight™ for GYNPlus®, Ambry Genetics Code first ([81162])

● + 0136U ATM (ataxia telangiectasia mutated) (eg, ataxia telangiectasia) mRNA sequence analysis (List separately in addition to code for primary procedure)

🖼 0.00   ⚖ 0.00   FUD 000

INCLUDES +RNAinsight™ for ATM, Ambry Genetics Code first (81408)

● + 0137U PALB2 (partner and localizer of BRCA2) (eg, breast and pancreatic cancer) mRNA sequence analysis (List separately in addition to code for ...

🖼 0.00   ⚖ 0.00   FUD 000

INCLUDES +RNAinsight™ for PALB2, Ambry Genetics Code first (81406)

● + 0138U BRCA1 (BRCA1, DNA repair associated), BRCA2 (BRCA2, DNA repair associated) (eg, hereditary breast and ovarian cancer) mRNA sequence analysis (List separately in addition to code for primary procedure)

🖼 0.00   ⚖ 0.00   FUD 000

INCLUDES +RNAinsight™ for BRCA1/2, Ambry Genetics Code first ([81162])

● 0139U Neurology (autism spectrum disorder [ASD]), quantitative measurements of 6 central carbon metabolites (ie, α-ketoglutarate, alanine, lactate, phenylalanine, pyruvate, and succinate), LC-MS/MS, plasma, algorithmic analysis with result reported as negative or positive (with metabolic subtypes of ASD)

NPDX ASD Energy Metabolism, Stemina Biomarker Discovery, Inc, Stemina Biomarker Discovery, Inc.

● New Code   ▲ Revised Code   ○ Reinstated   ● New Web Release   ▲ Revised Web Release   + Add-on   Unlisted   Not Covered   # Resequenced
㊿ Optum Mod 50 Exempt   Ⓢ AMA Mod 51 Exempt   �51 Optum Mod 51 Exempt   �63 Mod 63 Exempt   ⚕ Non-FDA Drug   ★ Telemedicine   Ⓜ Maternity   Ⓐ Age Edit

● **0140U** Infectious disease (fungi), fungal pathogen identification, DNA (15 fungal targets), blood culture, amplified probe technique, each target reported as detected or not detected

INCLUDES ePlex® BCID Fungal Pathogens Panel, GenMark Diagnostics, Inc, GenMark Diagnostics, Inc

● **0141U** Infectious disease (bacteria and fungi), gram-positive organism identification and drug resistance element detection, DNA (20 gram-positive bacterial targets, 4 resistance genes, 1 pan gram-negative bacterial target, 1 pan Candida target), blood culture, amplified probe technique, each target reported as detected or not detected

INCLUDES ePlex® BCID Gram-Positive Panel, GenMark Diagnostics, Inc, GenMark Diagnostics, Inc

● **0142U** Infectious disease (bacteria and fungi), gram-negative bacterial identification and drug resistance element detection, DNA (21 gram-negative bacterial targets, 6 resistance genes, 1 pan gram-positive bacterial target, 1 pan Candida target), amplified probe technique, each target reported as detected or not detected

INCLUDES ePlex® BCID Gram-Negative Panel, GenMark Diagnostics, Inc, GenMark Diagnostics, Inc

● **0143U** Drug assay, definitive, 120 or more drugs or metabolites, urine, quantitative liquid chromatography with tandem mass spectrometry (LC-MS/MS) using multiple reaction monitoring (MRM), with drug or metabolite description, comments including sample validation, per date of service

INCLUDES CareViewRx, Newstar Medical Laboratories, LLC, Newstar Medical Laboratories, LLC

EXCLUDES PsychViewRx Plus analysis by Newstar Medical Laboratories, LLC. To report, see (0150U)

● **0144U** Drug assay, definitive, 160 or more drugs or metabolites, urine, quantitative liquid chromatography with tandem mass spectrometry (LC-MS/MS) using multiple reaction monitoring (MRM), with drug or metabolite description, comments including sample validation, per date of service

EXCLUDES CareViewRx Plus, Newstar Medical Laboratories, LLC, Newstar Medical Laboratories, LLC

● **0145U** Drug assay, definitive, 65 or more drugs or metabolites, urine, quantitative liquid chromatography with tandem mass spectrometry (LC-MS/MS) using multiple reaction monitoring (MRM), with drug or metabolite description, comments including sample validation, per date of service

EXCLUDES PainViewRx, Newstar Medical Laboratories, LLC, Newstar Medical Laboratories, LLC

● **0146U** Drug assay, definitive, 80 or more drugs or metabolites, urine, by quantitative liquid chromatography with tandem mass spectrometry (LC-MS/MS) using multiple reaction monitoring (MRM), with drug or metabolite description, comments including sample validation, per date of service

INCLUDES PainViewRx Plus, Newstar Medical Laboratories, LLC, Newstar Medical Laboratories, LLC

● **0147U** Drug assay, definitive, 85 or more drugs or metabolites, urine, quantitative liquid chromatography with tandem mass spectrometry (LC-MS/MS) using multiple reaction monitoring (MRM), with drug or metabolite description, comments including sample validation, per date of service

INCLUDES RiskViewRx, Newstar Medical Laboratories, LLC, Newstar Medical Laboratories, LLC

● **0148U** Drug assay, definitive, 100 or more drugs or metabolites, urine, quantitative liquid chromatography with tandem mass spectrometry (LC-MS/MS) using multiple reaction monitoring (MRM), with drug or metabolite description, comments including sample validation, per date of service

INCLUDES RiskViewRx Plus, Newstar Medical Laboratories, LLC, Newstar Medical Laboratories, LLC

● **0149U** Drug assay, definitive, 60 or more drugs or metabolites, urine, quantitative liquid chromatography with tandem mass spectrometry (LC-MS/MS) using multiple reaction monitoring (MRM), with drug or metabolite description, comments including sample validation, per date of service

INCLUDES PsychViewRx, Newstar Medical Laboratories, LLC, Newstar Medical Laboratories, LLC

● **0150U** Drug assay, definitive, 120 or more drugs or metabolites, urine, quantitative liquid chromatography with tandem mass spectrometry (LC-MS/MS) using multiple reaction monitoring (MRM), with drug or metabolite description, comments including sample validation, per date of service

INCLUDES PsychViewRx Plus, Newstar Medical Laboratories, LLC, Newstar Medical Laboratories, LLC

EXCLUDES CareViewRx analysis by Newstar Medical Laboratories, LLC. To report, see (0143U)

● **0151U** Infectious disease (bacterial or viral respiratory tract infection), pathogen specific nucleic acid (DNA or RNA), 33 targets, real-time semi-quantitative PCR, bronchoalveolar lavage, sputum, or endotracheal aspirate, detection of 33 organismal and antibiotic resistance genes with limited semi-quantitative results

INCLUDES BioFire® FilmArray® Pneumonia Panel, BioFire® Diagnostics, BioFire® Diagnostics

● **0152U** Infectious disease (bacteria, fungi, parasites, and DNA viruses), DNA, PCR and next-generation sequencing, plasma, detection of >1,000 potential microbial organisms for significant positive pathogens

INCLUDES Karius® Test, Karius Inc, Karius Inc

● **0153U** Oncology (breast), mRNA, gene expression profiling by next-generation sequencing of 101 genes, utilizing formalin-fixed paraffin-embedded tissue, algorithm reported as a triple negative breast cancer clinical subtype(s) with information on immune cell involvement

INCLUDES Insight TNBCtype™, Insight Molecular Labs

● **0154U** *FGFR3 (fibroblast growth factor receptor 3)* gene analysis (ie, p.R248C [c.742C>T], p.S249C [c.746C>G], p.G370C [c.1108G>T], p.Y373C [c.1118A>G], FGFR3-TACC3v1, and FGFR3-TACC3v3)

INCLUDES therascreen® *FGFR* RGQ RT-PCR Kit, QIAGEN, QIAGEN GmbH

● **0155U** *PIK3CA (phosphatidylinositol-4,5-bisphosphate 3-kinase, catalytic subunit alpha)* (eg, breast cancer) gene analysis (ie, p.C420R, p.E542K, p.E545A, p.E545D [g.1635G>T only], p.E545G, p.E545K, p.Q546E, p.Q546R, p.H1047L, p.H1047R, p.H1047Y)

INCLUDES therascreen *PIK3CA* RGQ PCR Kit, QIAGEN, QIAGEN GmbH

● **0156U** Copy number (eg, intellectual disability, dysmorphology), sequence analysis

INCLUDES SMASH™, New York Genome Center, Marvel Genomics™

● + **0157U** *APC (APC regulator of WNT signaling pathway)* (eg, familial adenomatosis polyposis [FAP]) mRNA sequence analysis (List separately in addition to code for primary procedure)

🖪 0.00   ⚕ 0.00   **FUD** 000

INCLUDES CustomNext + RNA: *APC*, Ambry Genetics®, Ambry Genetics®

● + **0158U** *MLH1 (mutL homolog 1)* (eg, hereditary non-polyposis colorectal cancer, Lynch syndrome) mRNA sequence analysis (List separately in addition to code for primary procedure)

🖪 0.00   ⚕ 0.00   **FUD** 000

INCLUDES CustomNext + RNA: *MLH1*, Ambry Genetics®, Ambry Genetics®

26/TC PC/TC Only   A2-Z3 ASC Payment   50 Bilateral   ♂ Male Only   ♀ Female Only   🖪 Facility RVU   ⚕ Non-Facility RVU   ▢ CCI   ✖ CLIA
FUD Follow-up Days   CMS: IOM   AMA: CPT Asst   A-Y OPPSI   80/80 Surg Assist Allowed / w/Doc   ▢ Lab Crosswalk   Radiology Crosswalk

454   CPT © 2019 American Medical Association. All Rights Reserved.   © 2019 Optum360, LLC

● + **0159U** *MSH2 (mutS homolog 2) (eg, hereditary colon cancer, Lynch syndrome) mRNA sequence analysis (List separately in addition to code for primary procedure)*

� 0.00　🔧 0.00　**FUD** 000

INCLUDES　CustomNext + RNA: *MSH2,* Ambry Genetics®, Ambry Genetics®

● + **0160U** *MSH6 (mutS homolog 6) (eg, hereditary colon cancer, Lynch syndrome) mRNA sequence analysis (List separately in addition to code for primary procedure)*

🚗 0.00　🔧 0.00　**FUD** 000

INCLUDES　CustomNext + RNA: *MSH6,* Ambry Genetics®, Ambry Genetics®

● + **0161U** *PMS2 (PMS1 homolog 2, mismatch repair system component) (eg, hereditary non-polyposis colorectal cancer, Lynch syndrome) mRNA sequence analysis (List separately in addition to code for primary procedure)*

🚗 0.00　🔧 0.00　**FUD** 000

INCLUDES　CustomNext + RNA: *PMS2,* Ambry Genetics®, Ambry Genetics®

● + **0162U** **Hereditary colon cancer (Lynch syndrome), targeted mRNA sequence analysis panel** *(MLH1, MSH2, MSH6, PMS2)* **(List separately in addition to code for primary procedure)**

🚗 0.00　🔧 0.00　**FUD** 000

INCLUDES　CustomNext + RNA: Lynch *(MLH1, MSH2, MSH6, PMS2),* Ambry Genetics®, Ambry Genetics®

90281-90399 Immunoglobulin Products

INCLUDES Immune globulin product only
    Anti-infectives
    Antitoxins
    Isoantibodies
    Monoclonal antibodies
Code also (96365-96372, 96374-96375)

90281   **Immune globulin (Ig), human, for intramuscular use**

INCLUDES Gamastan

🔲 0.00   🔲 0.00   **FUD** XXX   ⑤ Ⓔ 🔲

AMA: 2018,Jan,8; 2017,Jan,8; 2016,Jan,13; 2015,Jan,16; 2014,Jan,11

90283   **Immune globulin (IgIV), human, for intravenous use**

🔲 0.00   🔲 0.00   **FUD** XXX   ⑤ Ⓔ 🔲

AMA: 2018,Jan,8; 2017,Jan,8; 2016,Jan,13; 2015,Jan,16; 2014,Jan,11

90284   **Immune globulin (SCIg), human, for use in subcutaneous infusions, 100 mg, each**

🔲 0.00   🔲 0.00   **FUD** XXX   ⑤ Ⓔ 🔲

AMA: 2018,Jan,8; 2017,Jan,8; 2016,Jan,13; 2015,Jan,16

90287   **Botulinum antitoxin, equine, any route**

🔲 0.00   🔲 0.00   **FUD** XXX   ⑤ Ⓔ 🔲

AMA: 2018,Jan,8; 2017,Jan,8; 2016,Jan,13; 2015,Jan,16; 2014,Jan,11

90288   **Botulism immune globulin, human, for intravenous use**

🔲 0.00   🔲 0.00   **FUD** XXX   ⑤ Ⓔ 🔲

AMA: 2018,Jan,8; 2017,Jan,8; 2016,Jan,13; 2015,Jan,16; 2014,Jan,11

90291   **Cytomegalovirus immune globulin (CMV-IgIV), human, for intravenous use**

INCLUDES Cytogram

🔲 0.00   🔲 0.00   **FUD** XXX   ⑤ Ⓔ 🔲

AMA: 2018,Jan,8; 2017,Jan,8; 2016,Jan,13; 2015,Jan,16; 2014,Jan,11

90296   **Diphtheria antitoxin, equine, any route**

🔲 0.00   🔲 0.00   **FUD** XXX   ⑤ Ⓔ 🔲

AMA: 2018,Jan,8; 2017,Jan,8; 2016,Jan,13; 2015,Jan,16; 2014,Jan,11

90371   **Hepatitis B immune globulin (HBIg), human, for intramuscular use**

INCLUDES HBIG

🔲 0.00   🔲 0.00   **FUD** XXX   ⑤ Ⓚ K2 🔲

AMA: 2018,Jan,8; 2017,Jan,8; 2016,Jan,13; 2015,Jan,16; 2014,Jan,11

90375   **Rabies immune globulin (RIg), human, for intramuscular and/or subcutaneous use**

INCLUDES HyperRAB

🔲 0.00   🔲 0.00   **FUD** XXX   ⑤ Ⓚ K2 🔲

AMA: 2018,Jan,8; 2017,Jan,8; 2016,Jan,13; 2015,Jan,16

90376   **Rabies immune globulin, heat-treated (RIg-HT), human, for intramuscular and/or subcutaneous use**

🔲 0.00   🔲 0.00   **FUD** XXX   ⑤ Ⓚ K2 🔲

AMA: 2018,Jan,8; 2017,Jan,8; 2016,Jan,13; 2015,Jan,16

90378   **Respiratory syncytial virus, monoclonal antibody, recombinant, for intramuscular use, 50 mg, each**

INCLUDES Synagis

🔲 0.00   🔲 0.00   **FUD** XXX   ⑤ Ⓚ K2 🔲

AMA: 2018,Jan,8; 2017,Jan,8; 2016,Jan,13; 2015,Jan,16; 2014,Jan,11

90384   **Rho(D) immune globulin (RhIg), human, full-dose, for intramuscular use**

🔲 0.00   🔲 0.00   **FUD** XXX   ⑤ Ⓔ 🔲

AMA: 2018,Jan,8; 2017,Jan,8; 2016,Jan,13; 2015,Jan,16; 2014,Jan,11

90385   **Rho(D) immune globulin (RhIg), human, mini-dose, for intramuscular use**

🔲 0.00   🔲 0.00   **FUD** XXX   ⑤ Ⓔ 🔲

AMA: 2018,Jan,8; 2017,Jan,8; 2016,Jan,13; 2015,Jan,16; 2014,Jan,11

90386   **Rho(D) immune globulin (RhIgIV), human, for intravenous use**

🔲 0.00   🔲 0.00   **FUD** XXX   ⑤ Ⓔ 🔲

AMA: 2018,Jan,8; 2017,Jan,8; 2016,Jan,13; 2015,Jan,16; 2014,Jan,11

90389   **Tetanus immune globulin (TIg), human, for intramuscular use**

INCLUDES HyperTET S/D (Tetanus Immune Globulin)

🔲 0.00   🔲 0.00   **FUD** XXX   ⑤ Ⓔ 🔲

AMA: 2018,Jan,8; 2017,Jan,8; 2016,Jan,13; 2015,Jan,16; 2014,Jan,11

90393   **Vaccinia immune globulin, human, for intramuscular use**

🔲 0.00   🔲 0.00   **FUD** XXX   ⑤ Ⓔ 🔲

AMA: 2018,Jan,8; 2017,Jan,8; 2016,Jan,13; 2015,Jan,16; 2014,Jan,11

90396   **Varicella-zoster immune globulin, human, for intramuscular use**

INCLUDES VariZIG

🔲 0.00   🔲 0.00   **FUD** XXX   ⑤ Ⓚ K2 🔲

AMA: 2018,Jan,8; 2017,Jan,8; 2016,Jan,13; 2015,Jan,16; 2014,Jan,11

90399   **Unlisted immune globulin**

🔲 0.00   🔲 0.00   **FUD** XXX   ⑤ Ⓔ 🔲

AMA: 2018,Jan,8; 2017,Jan,8; 2016,Jan,13; 2015,Jan,16; 2014,Jan,11

90460-90461 Injections Provided with Counseling

INCLUDES All components of influenza vaccine, report X 1 only
Combination vaccines which comprise multiple vaccine components
Components (all antigens) in vaccines to prevent disease due to specific organisms
Counseling by physician or other qualified health care professional
Multi-valent antigens or multiple antigen serotypes against single organisms are considered one component
Patient/family face-to-face counseling by doctor or qualified health care professional for patients 18 years of age and younger

EXCLUDES *Administration of influenza and pneumococcal vaccine for Medicare patients (G0008-G0009)*
Allergy testing (95004-95028)
Bacterial/viral/fungal skin tests (86485-86580)
Diagnostic or therapeutic injections (96365-96372, 96374-96375)
Vaccines provided without face-to-face counseling from a physician or qualified health care professional or to patients over the age of 18 (90471-90474)

Code also significant, separately identifiable E&M service when appropriate
Code also toxoid/vaccine (90476-90749 [90620, 90621, 90625, 90630, 90644, 90672, 90673, 90674, 90750, 90756])

90460   **Immunization administration through 18 years of age via any route of administration, with counseling by physician or other qualified health care professional; first or only component of each vaccine or toxoid administered**   Ⓐ

Code also each additional component in a vaccine (e.g., A 5-year-old receives DtaP-IPV IM administration, and MMR/Varicella vaccines SQ administration. Report initial component X 2, and additional components X 6)

🔲 0.47   🔲 0.47   **FUD** XXX   Ⓑ 80 🔲

AMA: 2018,Nov,7; 2018,Jan,8; 2017,Jan,8; 2016,Oct,6; 2016,Jan,13; 2015,May,6; 2015,Apr,9; 2015,Apr,10; 2015,Jan,16; 2014,Mar,10; 2014,Jan,11

+ 90461   each additional vaccine or toxoid component administered
           (List separately in addition to code for primary
           procedure)   Ⓐ
           Code also each additional component in a vaccine (e.g., A
           5-year-old receives DtaP-IPV IM administration, and
           MMR/Varicella vaccines SQ administration. Report initial
           component X 2, and additional components X 6)
           Code first the initial component in each vaccine provided (90460)
           🏥 0.36   🔬 0.36   FUD ZZZ   Ⓑ 80 ▣

           AMA: 2018,Nov,7; 2018,Jan,8; 2017,Jan,8; 2016,Oct,6;
           2016,Jan,13; 2015,May,6; 2015,Apr,10; 2015,Jan,16; 2014,Mar,10;
           2014,Jan,11

90471-90474 Injections and Other Routes of Administration Without Physician Counseling

CMS: 100-04,18,10.4 CWF Edits for Influenza Virus and Pneumococcal Vaccinations

EXCLUDES Administration of influenza and pneumococcal vaccine for Medicare patients
          (G0008-G0009)
          Administration of vaccine with counseling (90460-90461)
          Allergy testing (95004-95028)
          Bacterial/viral/fungal skin tests (86485-86580)
          Diagnostic or therapeutic injections (96365-96371, 96374)
          Patient/family face-to-face counseling
Code also significant separately identifiable E&M service when appropriate
Code also toxoid/vaccine (90476-90749 [90620, 90621, 90625, 90630, 90644, 90672,
90673, 90674, 90750, 90756])

  90471   Immunization administration (includes percutaneous,
           intradermal, subcutaneous, or intramuscular injections); 1
           vaccine (single or combination vaccine/toxoid)
           EXCLUDES Intranasal/oral administration (90473)
           🏥 0.47   🔬 0.47   FUD XXX   01 80 ▣

           AMA: 2019,Jun,11; 2018,Nov,7; 2018,Jan,8; 2017,Jan,8;
           2016,Oct,6; 2016,Jan,13; 2015,May,6; 2015,Apr,9; 2015,Apr,10;
           2015,Jan,16; 2014,Mar,10; 2014,Jan,11

+ 90472   each additional vaccine (single or combination
           vaccine/toxoid) (List separately in addition to code for
           primary procedure)
           EXCLUDES BCG vaccine, intravesical administration (51720, 90586)
                     Immune globulin administration (96365-96371, 96374)
                     Immune globulin product (90281-90399)
           Code first initial vaccine (90460, 90471, 90473)
           🏥 0.36   🔬 0.36   FUD ZZZ   N 80 ▣

           AMA: 2018,Nov,7; 2018,Jan,8; 2017,Jan,8; 2016,Oct,6;
           2016,Jan,13; 2015,May,6; 2015,Apr,10; 2015,Apr,9; 2015,Jan,16;
           2014,Mar,10; 2014,Jan,11

  90473   Immunization administration by intranasal or oral route; 1
           vaccine (single or combination vaccine/toxoid)
           EXCLUDES Administration by injection (90471)
           🏥 0.47   🔬 0.47   FUD XXX   01 80 ▣

           AMA: 2018,Nov,7; 2018,Jan,8; 2017,Jan,8; 2016,Jan,13;
           2015,May,6; 2015,Jan,16; 2014,Mar,10; 2014,Jan,11

+ 90474   each additional vaccine (single or combination
           vaccine/toxoid) (List separately in addition to code for
           primary procedure)
           Code first initial vaccine (90460, 90471, 90473)
           🏥 0.36   🔬 0.36   FUD ZZZ   N 80 ▣

           AMA: 2018,Nov,7; 2018,Jan,8; 2017,Jan,8; 2016,Jan,13;
           2015,May,6; 2015,Apr,9; 2015,Jan,16; 2014,Mar,10; 2014,Jan,11

90476-90756 [90619, 90620, 90621, 90625, 90630, 90644, 90672, 90673, 90674, 90694, 90750, 90756] Vaccination Products

INCLUDES   Patient's age for coding purposes, not for product license
           Vaccine product only
EXCLUDES   Coding of each component of a combination vaccine individually
           Immune globulins and administration (90281-90399, 96365-96375)
Code also administration of vaccine (90460-90474)
Code also significant separately identifiable E&M service when appropriate

  90476   Adenovirus vaccine, type 4, live, for oral use
           INCLUDES Adeno-4
           🏥 0.00   🔬 0.00   FUD XXX   SI N N1 ▣

           AMA: 2018,Jan,8; 2017,Jan,8; 2016,Jan,13; 2015,May,6;
           2015,Jan,16; 2014,Jan,11

  90477   Adenovirus vaccine, type 7, live, for oral use
           INCLUDES Adeno-7
           🏥 0.00   🔬 0.00   FUD XXX   SI M ▣

           AMA: 2018,Jan,8; 2017,Jan,8; 2016,Jan,13; 2015,May,6;
           2015,Jan,16; 2014,Jan,11

  90581   Anthrax vaccine, for subcutaneous or intramuscular use
           INCLUDES BioThrax
           🏥 0.00   🔬 0.00   FUD XXX   SI E ▣

           AMA: 2018,Jan,8; 2017,Jan,8; 2016,Jan,13; 2015,May,6;
           2015,Jan,16; 2014,Jan,11

  90585   Bacillus Calmette-Guerin vaccine (BCG) for tuberculosis, live,
           for percutaneous use
           INCLUDES Mycobax
           🏥 0.00   🔬 0.00   FUD XXX   SI M ▣

           AMA: 2018,Jan,8; 2017,Jan,8; 2016,Jan,13; 2015,May,6;
           2015,Jan,16; 2014,Jan,11

  90586   Bacillus Calmette-Guerin vaccine (BCG) for bladder cancer,
           live, for intravesical use
           INCLUDES TheraCys
                     TICE BCG
           🏥 0.00   🔬 0.00   FUD XXX   SI B ▣

           AMA: 2018,Jan,8; 2017,Jan,8; 2016,Jan,13; 2015,May,6;
           2015,Jan,16; 2014,Jan,11

  90587   Dengue vaccine, quadrivalent, live, 3 dose schedule, for
           subcutaneous use
           🏥 0.00   🔬 0.00   FUD XXX   ✐ SI E ▣

           AMA: 2018,Nov,7; 2018,Jan,8

  90619   Resequenced code. See code following 90734.

  90620   Resequenced code. See code following 90734.

  90621   Resequenced code. See code following 90734.

  90625   Resequenced code. See code following 90723.

  90630   Resequenced code. See code following 90654.

  90632   Hepatitis A vaccine (HepA), adult dosage, for intramuscular
           use   Ⓐ
           INCLUDES Havrix
                     Vaqta
           🏥 0.00   🔬 0.00   FUD XXX   SI N N1 ▣

           AMA: 2018,Jan,8; 2017,Jan,8; 2016,Jan,13; 2015,May,6;
           2015,Jan,16; 2014,Jan,11

  90633   Hepatitis A vaccine (HepA), pediatric/adolescent dosage-2
           dose schedule, for intramuscular use   Ⓐ
           INCLUDES Havrix
                     Vaqta
           🏥 0.00   🔬 0.00   FUD XXX   SI N N1 ▣

           AMA: 2018,Jan,8; 2017,Jan,8; 2016,Jan,13; 2015,May,6;
           2015,Jan,16; 2014,Jan,11

  90634   Hepatitis A vaccine (HepA), pediatric/adolescent dosage-3
           dose schedule, for intramuscular use   Ⓐ
           INCLUDES Havrix
           🏥 0.00   🔬 0.00   FUD XXX   SI N K2 ▣

           AMA: 2018,Jan,8; 2017,Jan,8; 2016,Jan,13; 2015,May,6;
           2015,Jan,16; 2014,Jan,11

  90636   Hepatitis A and hepatitis B vaccine (HepA-HepB), adult
           dosage, for intramuscular use   Ⓐ
           INCLUDES Twinrix
           🏥 0.00   🔬 0.00   FUD XXX   SI N N1 ▣

           AMA: 2018,Jan,8; 2017,Jan,8; 2016,Jan,13; 2015,May,6;
           2015,Jan,16; 2014,Jan,11

  90644   Resequenced code. See code following 90732.

  90647   Haemophilus influenzae type b vaccine (Hib), PRP-OMP
           conjugate, 3 dose schedule, for intramuscular use
           INCLUDES PedvaxHIB
           🏥 0.00   🔬 0.00   FUD XXX   SI N N1 ▣

           AMA: 2018,Jan,8; 2017,Jan,8; 2016,Jan,13; 2015,May,6;
           2015,Jan,16; 2014,Jan,11

90648 Haemophilus influenzae type b vaccine (Hib), PRP-T conjugate, 4 dose schedule, for intramuscular use

INCLUDES ActHIB
Hiberix
OmniHIB

🚫 0.00   ⚕ 0.00   **FUD** XXX   (S) N NI 📄

AMA: 2018,Jan,8; 2017,Jan,8; 2016,Jan,13; 2015,May,6; 2015,Jan,16; 2014,Jan,11

90649 Human Papillomavirus vaccine, types 6, 11, 16, 18, quadrivalent (4vHPV), 3 dose schedule, for intramuscular use

INCLUDES Gardasil

🚫 0.00   ⚕ 0.00   **FUD** XXX   (S) M 📄

AMA: 2018,Jan,8; 2017,Jan,8; 2016,Jan,13; 2015,May,6; 2015,Jan,16; 2014,Jan,11

90650 Human Papillomavirus vaccine, types 16, 18, bivalent (2vHPV), 3 dose schedule, for intramuscular use

INCLUDES Cervarix

🚫 0.00   ⚕ 0.00   **FUD** XXX   (S) M 📄

AMA: 2018,Jan,8; 2017,Jan,8; 2016,Jan,13; 2015,May,6; 2015,Jan,16; 2014,Jan,11

90651 Human Papillomavirus vaccine types 6, 11, 16, 18, 31, 33, 45, 52, 58, nonavalent (9vHPV), 2 or 3 dose schedule, for intramuscular use

INCLUDES GARDASIL 9

🚫 0.00   ⚕ 0.00   **FUD** XXX   (S) M 📄

AMA: 2018,Nov,7; 2018,Jan,8; 2017,Jan,8; 2016,Jan,13; 2015,May,6; 2015,Jan,16

90653 Influenza vaccine, inactivated (IIV), subunit, adjuvanted, for intramuscular use

INCLUDES Fluad

🚫 0.00   ⚕ 0.00   **FUD** XXX   (S) L LI 📄

AMA: 2019,Jun,11; 2018,Jan,8; 2017,Jan,8; 2016,Oct,6; 2016,Jan,13; 2015,May,6; 2015,Jan,16; 2014,Jan,11

90654 Influenza virus vaccine, trivalent (IIV3), split virus, preservative-free, for intradermal use

INCLUDES Fluzone intradermal

🚫 0.00   ⚕ 0.00   **FUD** XXX   (S) L LI 📄

AMA: 2018,Jan,8; 2017,Jan,8; 2016,Jan,13; 2015,May,6; 2015,Apr,9; 2015,Jan,16; 2014,Jan,11

\# **90630** Influenza virus vaccine, quadrivalent (IIV4), split virus, preservative free, for intradermal use

INCLUDES Fluzone Intradermal Quadrivalent

🚫 0.00   ⚕ 0.00   **FUD** XXX   (S) L LI 📄

AMA: 2018,Jan,8; 2017,Jan,8; 2016,Jan,13; 2015,May,6; 2015,Jan,16

90655 Influenza virus vaccine, trivalent (IIV3), split virus, preservative free, 0.25 mL dosage, for intramuscular use   A

INCLUDES Afluria
Fluzone, no preservative, pediatric dose

🚫 0.00   ⚕ 0.00   **FUD** XXX   (S) L LI 📄

AMA: 2018,Jan,8; 2017,Jan,8; 2016,Oct,6; 2016,May,9; 2016,Jan,13; 2015,May,6; 2015,Jan,16; 2014,Jan,11

90656 Influenza virus vaccine, trivalent (IIV3), split virus, preservative free, 0.5 mL dosage, for intramuscular use   A

INCLUDES Afluria

🚫 0.00   ⚕ 0.00   **FUD** XXX   (S) L LI 📄

AMA: 2018,Jan,8; 2017,Jan,8; 2016,Oct,6; 2016,May,9; 2016,Jan,13; 2015,May,6; 2015,Jan,16; 2014,Jan,11

90657 Influenza virus vaccine, trivalent (IIV3), split virus, 0.25 mL dosage, for intramuscular use   A

INCLUDES Afluria
Flulaval
Fluvirin
Fluzone (5 ml vial [0.25ml dose])

🚫 0.00   ⚕ 0.00   **FUD** XXX   (S) L LI 📄

AMA: 2018,Jan,8; 2017,Jan,8; 2016,Oct,6; 2016,May,9; 2016,Jan,13; 2015,May,6; 2015,Jan,16; 2014,Jan,11

90658 Influenza virus vaccine, trivalent (IIV3), split virus, 0.5 mL dosage, for intramuscular use   A

INCLUDES Afluria
Flulaval
Fluvirin
Fluzone

🚫 0.00   ⚕ 0.00   **FUD** XXX   (S) E 📄

AMA: 2018,Jan,8; 2017,Jan,8; 2016,Oct,6; 2016,May,9; 2016,Jan,13; 2015,May,6; 2015,Jan,16; 2014,Jan,11

90660 Influenza virus vaccine, trivalent, live (LAIV3), for intranasal use

INCLUDES FluMist

🚫 0.00   ⚕ 0.00   **FUD** XXX   (S) L LI 📄

AMA: 2018,Jan,8; 2017,Jan,8; 2016,Jan,13; 2015,May,6; 2015,Jan,16; 2014,Jan,11

\# **90672** Influenza virus vaccine, quadrivalent, live (LAIV4), for intranasal use

INCLUDES FluMist Quadrivalent

🚫 0.00   ⚕ 0.00   **FUD** XXX   (S) L LI 📄

AMA: 2018,Jan,8; 2017,Jan,8; 2016,Jan,13; 2015,May,6; 2015,Jan,16; 2014,Jan,11

90661 Influenza virus vaccine (ccIIV3), derived from cell cultures, subunit, preservative and antibiotic free, for intramuscular use

INCLUDES Flucelvax

🚫 0.00   ⚕ 0.00   **FUD** XXX   (S) L LI 📄

AMA: 2018,Jan,8; 2017,Jan,8; 2016,Oct,6; 2016,Jan,13; 2015,May,6; 2015,Jan,16; 2014,Jan,11

\# **90674** Influenza virus vaccine, quadrivalent (ccIIV4), derived from cell cultures, subunit, preservative and antibiotic free, 0.5 mL dosage, for intramuscular use

INCLUDES Flucelvax Quadrivalent

🚫 0.00   ⚕ 0.00   **FUD** XXX   (S) L LI 📄

AMA: 2018,Jan,8; 2017,Jan,8; 2016,Oct,6

\# **90756** Influenza virus vaccine, quadrivalent (ccIIV4), derived from cell cultures, subunit, antibiotic free, 0.5mL dosage, for intramuscular use

INCLUDES Flucelvax Quadrivalent

🚫 0.00   ⚕ 0.00   **FUD** XXX   (S) L LI 📄

AMA: 2018,Nov,7

\# **90673** Influenza virus vaccine, trivalent (RIV3), derived from recombinant DNA, hemagglutinin (HA) protein only, preservative and antibiotic free, for intramuscular use

🚫 0.00   ⚕ 0.00   **FUD** XXX   (S) L LI 📄

AMA: 2018,Jan,8; 2017,Jan,8; 2016,Jan,13; 2015,May,6; 2015,Jan,16; 2014,Mar,10; 2014,Jan,11

90662 Influenza virus vaccine (IIV), split virus, preservative free, enhanced immunogenicity via increased antigen content, for intramuscular use

INCLUDES Fluzone high-dose

🚫 0.00   ⚕ 0.00   **FUD** XXX   (S) L LI 📄

AMA: 2018,Jan,8; 2017,Jan,8; 2016,Jan,13; 2015,May,6; 2015,Jan,16; 2014,Jan,11

90664 Influenza virus vaccine, live (LAIV), pandemic formulation, for intranasal use

🚫 0.00   ⚕ 0.00   **FUD** XXX   (S) E 📄

AMA: 2018,Jan,8; 2017,Jan,8; 2016,Jan,13; 2015,May,6; 2015,Jan,16; 2014,Jan,11

● New Code   ▲ Revised Code   ○ Reinstated   ● New Web Release   ▲ Revised Web Release   + Add-on   Unlisted   Not Covered   \# Resequenced
(50) Optum Mod 50 Exempt   (⚕) AMA Mod 51 Exempt   (S) Optum Mod 51 Exempt   (63) Mod 63 Exempt   ✗ Non-FDA Drug   ★ Telemedicine   M Maternity   A Age Edit

90666 — 90697

90666 Influenza virus vaccine (IIV), pandemic formulation, split virus, preservative free, for intramuscular use
🖥 0.00 ⚕ 0.00 **FUD** XXX ✎ Ⓢ Ⓔ ▱
AMA: 2018,Jan,8; 2017,Jan,8; 2016,Jan,13; 2015,May,6; 2015,Jan,16; 2014,Jan,11

90667 Influenza virus vaccine (IIV), pandemic formulation, split virus, adjuvanted, for intramuscular use
🖥 0.00 ⚕ 0.00 **FUD** XXX ✎ Ⓢ Ⓔ ▱
AMA: 2018,Jan,8; 2017,Jan,8; 2016,Jan,13; 2015,May,6; 2015,Jan,16; 2014,Jan,11

90668 Influenza virus vaccine (IIV), pandemic formulation, split virus, for intramuscular use
🖥 0.00 ⚕ 0.00 **FUD** XXX ✎ Ⓢ Ⓔ ▱
AMA: 2018,Jan,8; 2017,Jan,8; 2016,Jan,13; 2015,May,6; 2015,Jan,16; 2014,Jan,11

90670 Pneumococcal conjugate vaccine, 13 valent (PCV13), for intramuscular use
INCLUDES Prevnar 13
🖥 0.00 ⚕ 0.00 **FUD** XXX Ⓢ Ⓛ Ⓛ1 ▱
AMA: 2018,Jan,8; 2017,Jan,8; 2016,Jan,13; 2015,May,6; 2015,Jan,16; 2014,Jan,11

90672 Resequenced code. See code following 90660.

90673 Resequenced code. See code before 90662.

90674 Resequenced code. See code following 90661.

90675 Rabies vaccine, for intramuscular use
INCLUDES Imovax
RabAvert
🖥 0.00 ⚕ 0.00 **FUD** XXX Ⓢ Ⓚ Ⓚ2 ▱
AMA: 2018,Jan,8; 2017,Jan,8; 2016,Jan,13; 2015,May,6; 2015,Jan,16; 2014,Jan,11

90676 Rabies vaccine, for intradermal use
🖥 0.00 ⚕ 0.00 **FUD** XXX Ⓢ Ⓚ Ⓚ2 ▱
AMA: 2018,Jan,8; 2017,Jan,8; 2016,Jan,13; 2015,May,6; 2015,Jan,16; 2014,Jan,11

90680 Rotavirus vaccine, pentavalent (RV5), 3 dose schedule, live, for oral use
INCLUDES RotaTeq
🖥 0.00 ⚕ 0.00 **FUD** XXX Ⓢ Ⓝ Ⓝ1 ▱
AMA: 2018,Jan,8; 2017,Jan,8; 2016,Jan,13; 2015,May,6; 2015,Jan,16; 2014,Jan,11

90681 Rotavirus vaccine, human, attenuated (RV1), 2 dose schedule, live, for oral use
INCLUDES Rotarix
🖥 0.00 ⚕ 0.00 **FUD** XXX Ⓢ Ⓜ ▱
AMA: 2018,Jan,8; 2017,Jan,8; 2016,Jan,13; 2015,May,6; 2015,Jan,16; 2014,Jan,11

90682 Influenza virus vaccine, quadrivalent (RIV4), derived from recombinant DNA, hemagglutinin (HA) protein only, preservative and antibiotic free, for intramuscular use
INCLUDES Flublok Quadrivalent
🖥 0.00 ⚕ 0.00 **FUD** XXX Ⓢ Ⓛ Ⓛ1 ▱
AMA: 2018,Nov,7; 2018,Jan,8; 2017,Jan,8

90685 Influenza virus vaccine, quadrivalent (IIV4), split virus, preservative free, 0.25 mL, for intramuscular use Ⓐ
INCLUDES Afluria Quadrivalent
Fluzone Quadrivalent
🖥 0.00 ⚕ 0.00 **FUD** XXX Ⓢ Ⓛ Ⓛ1 ▱
AMA: 2018,Jan,8; 2017,Jan,8; 2016,Oct,6; 2016,May,9; 2016,Jan,13; 2015,May,6; 2015,Jan,16; 2014,Mar,10; 2014,Jan,11

90686 Influenza virus vaccine, quadrivalent (IIV4), split virus, preservative free, 0.5 mL dosage, for intramuscular use Ⓐ
INCLUDES Afluria Quadrivalent
Fluarix Quadrivalent
FluLaval Quadrivalent
Fluzone Quadrivalent
🖥 0.00 ⚕ 0.00 **FUD** XXX Ⓢ Ⓛ Ⓛ1 ▱
AMA: 2018,Jan,8; 2017,Jan,8; 2016,Oct,6; 2016,May,9; 2016,Jan,13; 2015,May,6; 2015,Jan,16; 2014,Mar,10; 2014,Jan,11

90687 Influenza virus vaccine, quadrivalent (IIV4), split virus, 0.25 mL dosage, for intramuscular use Ⓐ
INCLUDES Afluria Quadrivalent
Fluzone Quadrivalent
🖥 0.00 ⚕ 0.00 **FUD** XXX Ⓢ Ⓛ Ⓛ1 ▱
AMA: 2018,Jan,8; 2017,Jan,8; 2016,Oct,6; 2016,May,9; 2016,Jan,13; 2015,May,6; 2015,Jan,16; 2014,Mar,10; 2014,Jan,11

90688 Influenza virus vaccine, quadrivalent (IIV4), split virus, 0.5 mL dosage, for intramuscular use Ⓐ
INCLUDES Afluria Quadrivalent
Flulaval Quadrivalent
Fluzone Quadrivalent
🖥 0.00 ⚕ 0.00 **FUD** XXX Ⓢ Ⓛ Ⓛ1 ▱
AMA: 2018,Jan,8; 2017,Jan,8; 2016,Oct,6; 2016,May,9; 2016,Jan,13; 2015,May,6; 2015,Jan,16; 2014,Mar,10; 2014,Jan,11

90689 Influenza virus vaccine quadrivalent (IIV4), inactivated, adjuvanted, preservative free, 0.25 mL dosage, for intramuscular use
🖥 0.00 ⚕ 0.00 **FUD** XXX ✎ Ⓢ Ⓛ1 ▱
AMA: 2019,Jul,10; 2018,Nov,7

● # **90694** Influenza virus vaccine, quadrivalent (aIIV4), inactivated, adjuvanted, preservative free, 0.5 mL dosage, for intramuscular use
🖥 0.00 ⚕ 0.00 **FUD** 000 ✎

90690 Typhoid vaccine, live, oral
INCLUDES Vivotif
🖥 0.00 ⚕ 0.00 **FUD** XXX Ⓢ Ⓝ Ⓝ1 ▱
AMA: 2018,Jan,8; 2017,Jan,8; 2016,Jan,13; 2015,May,6; 2015,Jan,16; 2014,Jan,11

90691 Typhoid vaccine, Vi capsular polysaccharide (ViCPs), for intramuscular use
INCLUDES Typhim Vi
🖥 0.00 ⚕ 0.00 **FUD** XXX Ⓢ Ⓝ Ⓝ1 ▱
AMA: 2018,Jan,8; 2017,Jan,8; 2016,Jan,13; 2015,May,6; 2015,Jan,16; 2014,Jan,11

90694 Resequenced code. See code following 90689.

90696 Diphtheria, tetanus toxoids, acellular pertussis vaccine and inactivated poliovirus vaccine (DTaP-IPV), when administered to children 4 through 6 years of age, for intramuscular use Ⓐ
INCLUDES KINRIX
Quadracel
🖥 0.00 ⚕ 0.00 **FUD** XXX Ⓢ Ⓝ Ⓝ1 ▱
AMA: 2018,Jan,8; 2017,Jan,8; 2016,Jan,13; 2015,May,6; 2015,Jan,16; 2014,Jan,11

90697 Diphtheria, tetanus toxoids, acellular pertussis vaccine, inactivated poliovirus vaccine, Haemophilus influenzae type b PRP-OMP conjugate vaccine, and hepatitis B vaccine (DTaP-IPV-Hib-HepB), for intramuscular use
🖥 0.00 ⚕ 0.00 **FUD** XXX ✎ Ⓢ Ⓜ ▱
AMA: 2018,Jan,8; 2017,Jan,8; 2016,Jan,13; 2015,May,6; 2015,Jan,16

26/TC PC/TC Only   A2-Z3 ASC Payment   50 Bilateral   ♂ Male Only   ♀ Female Only   🖥 Facility RVU   ⚕ Non-Facility RVU   ▱ CCI   ✖ CLIA
FUD Follow-up Days   CMS: IOM   AMA: CPT Asst   A-Y OPPSI   80/80 Surg Assist Allowed / w/Doc   ◤ Lab Crosswalk   ⊞ Radiology Crosswalk

460   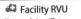 CPT © 2019 American Medical Association. All Rights Reserved.   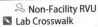 © 2019 Optum360, LLC

90698 Diphtheria, tetanus toxoids, acellular pertussis vaccine, Haemophilus influenzae type b, and inactivated poliovirus vaccine, (DTaP-IPV/Hib), for intramuscular use

INCLUDES Pentacel

🚲 0.00 ⚕ 0.00 **FUD** XXX ⑤ Ⓝ Ⓝ1 🖼

AMA: 2018,Jan,8; 2017,Jan,8; 2016,Jan,13; 2015,May,6; 2015,Jan,16; 2014,Jan,11

90700 Diphtheria, tetanus toxoids, and acellular pertussis vaccine (DTaP), when administered to individuals younger than 7 years, for intramuscular use Ⓐ

INCLUDES Daptacel
Infanrix

🚲 0.00 ⚕ 0.00 **FUD** XXX ⑤ Ⓝ 🖼

AMA: 2018,Jan,8; 2017,Jan,8; 2016,Jan,13; 2015,May,6; 2015,Jan,16; 2014,Jan,11

90702 Diphtheria and tetanus toxoids adsorbed (DT) when administered to individuals younger than 7 years, for intramuscular use Ⓐ

INCLUDES Diphtheria and Tetanus Toxoids Adsorbed USP (For Pediatric Use)

🚲 0.00 ⚕ 0.00 **FUD** XXX ⑤ Ⓝ 🖼

AMA: 2018,Jan,8; 2017,Jan,8; 2016,Jan,13; 2015,May,6; 2015,Jan,16; 2014,Jan,11

90707 Measles, mumps and rubella virus vaccine (MMR), live, for subcutaneous use

INCLUDES M-M-R II

🚲 0.00 ⚕ 0.00 **FUD** XXX ⑤ Ⓝ 🖼

AMA: 2018,Jan,8; 2017,Jan,8; 2016,Jan,13; 2015,May,6; 2015,Jan,16; 2014,Jan,11

90710 Measles, mumps, rubella, and varicella vaccine (MMRV), live, for subcutaneous use

INCLUDES ProQuad

🚲 0.00 ⚕ 0.00 **FUD** XXX ⑤ Ⓝ 🖼

AMA: 2018,Jan,8; 2017,Jan,8; 2016,Jan,13; 2015,May,6; 2015,Jan,16; 2014,Jan,11

90713 Poliovirus vaccine, inactivated (IPV), for subcutaneous or intramuscular use

INCLUDES IPOL

🚲 0.00 ⚕ 0.00 **FUD** XXX ⑤ Ⓝ 🖼

AMA: 2018,Jan,8; 2017,Jan,8; 2016,Jan,13; 2015,May,6; 2015,Jan,16; 2014,Jan,11

90714 Tetanus and diphtheria toxoids adsorbed (Td), preservative free, when administered to individuals 7 years or older, for intramuscular use Ⓐ

INCLUDES Tenivac
Tetanus-diphtheria toxoids absorbed

🚲 0.00 ⚕ 0.00 **FUD** XXX ⑤ Ⓝ 🖼

AMA: 2018,Jan,8; 2017,Jan,8; 2016,Jan,13; 2015,May,6; 2015,Jan,16; 2014,Jan,11

90715 Tetanus, diphtheria toxoids and acellular pertussis vaccine (Tdap), when administered to individuals 7 years or older, for intramuscular use Ⓐ

INCLUDES Adacel
Boostrix

🚲 0.00 ⚕ 0.00 **FUD** XXX ⑤ Ⓝ 🖼

AMA: 2018,Jan,8; 2017,Jan,8; 2016,Jan,13; 2015,May,6; 2015,Jan,16; 2014,Jan,11

90716 Varicella virus vaccine (VAR), live, for subcutaneous use

INCLUDES Varivax

🚲 0.00 ⚕ 0.00 **FUD** XXX ⑤ Ⓜ 🖼

AMA: 2018,Jan,8; 2017,Jan,8; 2016,Jan,13; 2015,May,6; 2015,Mar,3; 2015,Jan,16; 2014,Jan,11

90717 Yellow fever vaccine, live, for subcutaneous use

INCLUDES YF-VAX

🚲 0.00 ⚕ 0.00 **FUD** XXX ⑤ Ⓝ Ⓝ1 🖼

AMA: 2018,Jan,8; 2017,Jan,8; 2016,Jan,13; 2015,May,6; 2015,Jan,16; 2014,Jan,11

90723 Diphtheria, tetanus toxoids, acellular pertussis vaccine, hepatitis B, and inactivated poliovirus vaccine (DTaP-HepB-IPV), for intramuscular use

INCLUDES PEDIARIX

🚲 0.00 ⚕ 0.00 **FUD** XXX ⑤ Ⓜ 🖼

AMA: 2018,Jan,8; 2017,Jan,8; 2016,Jan,13; 2015,May,6; 2015,Jan,16; 2014,Jan,11

\# **90625** Cholera vaccine, live, adult dosage, 1 dose schedule, for oral use Ⓐ

🚲 0.00 ⚕ 0.00 **FUD** XXX ⑤ Ⓔ 🖼

AMA: 2018,Jan,8; 2017,Jan,8; 2016,Oct,6; 2016,Jan,13

90732 Pneumococcal polysaccharide vaccine, 23-valent (PPSV23), adult or immunosuppressed patient dosage, when administered to individuals 2 years or older, for subcutaneous or intramuscular use Ⓐ

INCLUDES Pneumovax 23

🚲 0.00 ⚕ 0.00 **FUD** XXX ⑤ Ⓛ Ⓛ1 🖼

AMA: 2018,Jan,8; 2017,Jan,8; 2016,Jan,13; 2015,May,6; 2015,Jan,16; 2014,Jan,11

\# **90644** Meningococcal conjugate vaccine, serogroups C & Y and Haemophilus influenzae type b vaccine (Hib-MenCY), 4 dose schedule, when administered to children 6 weeks-18 months of age, for intramuscular use Ⓐ

INCLUDES MenHibrix

🚲 0.00 ⚕ 0.00 **FUD** XXX ⑤ Ⓜ 🖼

AMA: 2018,Jan,8; 2017,Jan,8; 2016,Jan,13; 2015,May,6; 2015,Jan,16; 2014,Jan,11

90733 Meningococcal polysaccharide vaccine, serogroups A, C, Y, W-135, quadrivalent (MPSV4), for subcutaneous use

INCLUDES Menomune-A/C/Y/W-135

🚲 0.00 ⚕ 0.00 **FUD** XXX ⑤ Ⓜ 🖼

AMA: 2018,Jan,8; 2017,Jan,8; 2016,Jan,13; 2015,May,6; 2015,Jan,16; 2014,Jan,11

▲ **90734** Meningococcal conjugate vaccine, serogroups A, C, W, Y, quadrivalent, diphtheria toxoid carrier (MenACWY-D) or CRM197 carrier (MenACWY-CRM), for intramuscular use

INCLUDES Menactra
Menveo

🚲 0.00 ⚕ 0.00 **FUD** XXX ⑤ Ⓜ 🖼

AMA: 2018,Jan,8; 2017,Jan,8; 2016,Oct,6; 2016,Jan,13; 2015,May,6; 2015,Jan,16; 2014,Jan,11

● \# **90619** Meningococcal conjugate vaccine, serogroups A, C, W, Y, quadrivalent, tetanus toxoid carrier (MenACWY-TT), for intramuscular use

🚲 0.00 ⚕ 0.00 **FUD** XXX ✗

\# **90620** Meningococcal recombinant protein and outer membrane vesicle vaccine, serogroup B (MenB-4C), 2 dose schedule, for intramuscular use

INCLUDES Bexsero

🚲 0.00 ⚕ 0.00 **FUD** XXX ⑤ Ⓜ 🖼

AMA: 2018,Nov,7; 2018,Jan,8; 2017,Jan,8; 2016,Jan,13; 2015,May,6; 2015,Jan,16

\# **90621** Meningococcal recombinant lipoprotein vaccine, serogroup B (MenB-FHbp), 2 or 3 dose schedule, for intramuscular use

INCLUDES Trumenba

🚲 0.00 ⚕ 0.00 **FUD** XXX ⑤ Ⓜ 🖼

AMA: 2018,Nov,7; 2018,Jan,8; 2017,Jan,8; 2016,Jan,13; 2015,May,6; 2015,Jan,16

90736 Zoster (shingles) vaccine (HZV), live, for subcutaneous injection

INCLUDES Zostavax

🚲 0.00 ⚕ 0.00 **FUD** XXX ⑤ Ⓜ 🖼

AMA: 2018,Nov,7; 2018,Jan,8; 2017,Jan,8; 2016,Jan,13; 2015,May,6; 2015,Jan,16; 2014,Jan,11

● New Code   ▲ Revised Code   ○ Reinstated   ● New Web Release   ▲ Revised Web Release   + Add-on   Unlisted   Not Covered   \# Resequenced
㊿ Optum Mod 50 Exempt   Ⓢ AMA Mod 51 Exempt   ⑤ Optum Mod 51 Exempt   ⓺⓷ Mod 63 Exempt   ✗ Non-FDA Drug   ★ Telemedicine   Ⓜ Maternity   Ⓐ Age Edit

Medicine

 # 90750 Zoster (shingles) vaccine (HZV), recombinant, subunit, adjuvanted, for intramuscular use
📋 0.00   🔧 0.00   **FUD** XXX   ⑤ Ⓜ ▢
AMA: 2018,Nov,7

90738 Japanese encephalitis virus vaccine, inactivated, for intramuscular use
INCLUDES Ixiaro
📋 0.00   🔧 0.00   **FUD** XXX   ⑤ Ⓜ ▢
AMA: 2018,Jan,8; 2017,Jan,8; 2016,Jan,13; 2015,May,6; 2015,Jan,16; 2014,Jan,11

90739 Hepatitis B vaccine (HepB), adult dosage, 2 dose schedule, for intramuscular use
📋 0.00   🔧 0.00   **FUD** XXX   ⑤ Ⓔ ▢
AMA: 2018,Nov,7; 2018,Jan,8; 2017,Jan,8; 2016,Jan,13; 2015,May,6; 2015,Jan,16; 2014,Jan,11

90740 Hepatitis B vaccine (HepB), dialysis or immunosuppressed patient dosage, 3 dose schedule, for intramuscular use
INCLUDES Recombivax HB
📋 0.00   🔧 0.00   **FUD** XXX   ⑤ Ⓕ F4 ▢
AMA: 2018,Jan,8; 2017,Jan,8; 2016,Jan,13; 2015,May,6; 2015,Jan,16; 2014,Jan,11

90743 Hepatitis B vaccine (HepB), adolescent, 2 dose schedule, for intramuscular use   Ⓐ
INCLUDES Energix-B
          Recombivax HB
📋 0.00   🔧 0.00   **FUD** XXX   ⑤ Ⓕ F4 ▢
AMA: 2018,Jan,8; 2017,Jan,8; 2016,Jan,13; 2015,May,6; 2015,Jan,16; 2014,Jan,11

90744 Hepatitis B vaccine (HepB), pediatric/adolescent dosage, 3 dose schedule, for intramuscular use   Ⓐ
INCLUDES Energix-B
          Flucelvax Quadrivalent
          Recombivax HB
📋 0.00   🔧 0.00   **FUD** XXX   ⑤ Ⓕ F4 ▢
AMA: 2018,Jan,8; 2017,Jan,8; 2016,Jan,13; 2015,May,6; 2015,Jan,16; 2014,Jan,11

90746 Hepatitis B vaccine (HepB), adult dosage, 3 dose schedule, for intramuscular use
INCLUDES Energix-B
          Recombivax HB
📋 0.00   🔧 0.00   **FUD** XXX   ⑤ Ⓕ F4 ▢
AMA: 2018,Jan,8; 2017,Jan,8; 2016,Jan,13; 2015,May,6; 2015,Jan,16; 2014,Jan,11

90747 Hepatitis B vaccine (HepB), dialysis or immunosuppressed patient dosage, 4 dose schedule, for intramuscular use
INCLUDES Energix-B
          RECOMBIVAX dialysis
📋 0.00   🔧 0.00   **FUD** XXX   ⑤ Ⓕ F4 ▢
AMA: 2018,Jan,8; 2017,Jan,8; 2016,Jan,13; 2015,May,6; 2015,Jan,16; 2014,Jan,11

90748 Hepatitis B and Haemophilus influenzae type b vaccine (Hib-HepB), for intramuscular use
INCLUDES COMVAX
📋 0.00   🔧 0.00   **FUD** XXX   ⑤ Ⓔ ▢
AMA: 2018,Jan,8; 2017,Jan,8; 2016,Jan,13; 2015,May,6; 2015,Jan,16; 2014,Jan,11

90749 Unlisted vaccine/toxoid
📋 0.00   🔧 0.00   **FUD** XXX   ⑤ Ⓝ N1 ▢
AMA: 2018,Jan,8; 2017,Jan,8; 2016,Jan,13; 2015,May,6; 2015,Jan,16; 2014,Jan,11

90750 Resequenced code. See code following 90736.

90756 Resequenced code. See code following 90661.

90785 Complex Interactive Encounter

CMS: 100-02,15,160 Clinical Psychologist Services; 100-02,15,170 Clinical Social Worker (CSW) Services; 100-03,10.3 Inpatient Pain Rehabilitation Programs; 100-03,10.4 Outpatient Hospital Pain Rehabilitation Programs; 100-03,130.1 Inpatient Stays for Alcoholism Treatment; 100-04,12,100 Teaching Physician Services; 100-04,4,260.1 Special Partial Hospitalization Billing Requirements forHospitals, Community Mental Health Centers, and Critical Access Hospitals; 100-04,4,260.1.1 Bill Review for Partial Hospitalization Services Provided in Community Mental Health Centers (CMHC)

INCLUDES At least one of the following activities:
Discussion of a sentinel event demanding third-party involvement (eg, abuse or neglect reported to a state agency)
Interference by the behavior or emotional state of caregiver to understand and assist in the plan of treatment
Managing discordant communication complicating care among participating members (eg, arguing, reactivity)
Use of nonverbal communication methods (eg, toys, other devices, or translator) to eliminate communication barriers
Complicated issues of communication affecting provision of the psychiatric service
Involved communication with:
Emotionally charged or dissonant family members
Patients wanting others present during the visit (e.g., family member, translator)
Patients with impaired or undeveloped verbal skills
Patients with third parties responsible for their care (eg, parents, guardians)
Third-party involvement (eg, schools, probation and parole officers, child protective agencies)
EXCLUDES *Adaptive behavior assessment/treatment ([97151, 97152, 97153, 97154, 97155, 97156, 97157, 97158], 0362T, 0373T)*
Crisis psychotherapy (90839-90840)

+ 90785 Interactive complexity (List separately in addition to the code for primary procedure)
Code first, when performed (99201-99255 [99224, 99225, 99226], 99304-99337, 99341-99350, 90791-90792, 90832-90834, 90836-90838, 90853)
📋 0.39   🔧 0.42   **FUD** ZZZ   Ⓝ ▢
AMA: 2018,Nov,3; 2018,Jul,12; 2018,Apr,9; 2018,Jan,8; 2017,Jan,8; 2016,Dec,11; 2016,Jan,13; 2015,Jan,16

90791-90792 Psychiatric Evaluations

CMS: 100-02,15,170 Clinical Social Worker (CSW) Services; 100-03,10.3 Inpatient Pain Rehabilitation Programs; 100-03,130.1 Inpatient Stays for Alcoholism Treatment; 100-03,130.2 Outpatient Hospital Services for Alcoholism; 100-04,12,100 Teaching Physician Services; 100-04,12,190.3 List of Telehealth Services; 100-04,12,190.6 Payment Methodology for Physician/Practitioner at the Distant Site ; 100-04,12,190.6.1 Submission of Telehealth Claims for Distant Site Practitioners; 100-04,12,190.7 Contractor Editing of Telehealth Claims; 100-04,4,260.1 Special Partial Hospitalization Billing Requirements forHospitals, Community Mental Health Centers, and Critical Access Hospitals; 100-04,4,260.1.1 Bill Review for Partial Hospitalization Services Provided in Community Mental Health Centers (CMHC)

INCLUDES Diagnostic assessment or reassessment without psychotherapy services
EXCLUDES *Adaptive behavior assessment/treatment ([97151, 97152, 97153, 97154, 97155, 97156, 97157, 97158], 0362T, 0373T)*
Crisis psychotherapy (90839-90840)
E&M services (99201-99337 [99224, 99225, 99226], 99341-99350, 99366-99368, 99401-99443 [99415, 99416, 99421, 99422, 99423], [97151], [97152], [97153], [97154], [97155], [97156], [97157], [97158], 0362T, 0373T)
Code also interactive complexity services when applicable (90785)

90791 Psychiatric diagnostic evaluation
📋 3.54   🔧 3.89   **FUD** XXX   ★ 03 ▢
AMA: 2018,Nov,3; 2018,Jul,12; 2018,Apr,9; 2018,Jan,8; 2017,Nov,3; 2017,Jan,8; 2016,Jan,13; 2015,Jan,16; 2014,Jun,3; 2014,Jan,11

90792 Psychiatric diagnostic evaluation with medical services
📋 4.01   🔧 4.37   **FUD** XXX   ★ 03 ▢
AMA: 2018,Nov,3; 2018,Jul,12; 2018,Apr,9; 2018,Jan,8; 2017,Nov,3; 2017,Jan,8; 2016,Jan,13; 2015,Jan,16; 2014,Jun,3; 2014,Jan,11

90832-90838 Psychotherapy Services

CMS: 100-02,15,160 Clinical Psychologist Services; 100-02,15,170 Clinical Social Worker (CSW) Services; 100-03,130.1 Inpatient Stays for Alcoholism Treatment; 100-03,130.2 Outpatient Hospital Services for Alcoholism; 100-03,130.3 Chemical Aversion Therapy for Treatment of Alcoholism; 100-04,12,100 Teaching Physician Services; 100-04,12,160 Independent Psychologist Services; 100-04,12,170 Clinical Psychologist Services; 100-04,12,190.3 List of Telehealth Services; 100-04,12,190.6 Payment Methodology for Physician/Practitioner at the Distant Site ; 100-04,12,190.6.1 Submission of Telehealth Claims for Distant Site Practitioners; 100-04,12,190.7 Contractor Editing of Telehealth Claims

INCLUDES Face-to-face time with patient (family, other informers may also be present)
Pharmacologic management in time allocated to psychotherapy service codes
Psychotherapy only (90832, 90834, 90837)
Psychotherapy with separately identifiable medical E&M services includes add-on codes (90833, 90836, 90838)
Service times of no less than 16 minutes
Services provided in all settings
Therapeutic communication to:
  Ameliorate the patient's mental and behavioral symptoms
  Modify behavior
  Support and encourage personality growth and development
Treatment for:
  Behavior disturbances
  Mental illness

EXCLUDES *Adaptive behavior assessment/treatment ([97151, 97152, 97153, 97154, 97155, 97156, 97157, 97158], 0362T, 0373T)*
Crisis psychotherapy (90839-90840)
Family psychotherapy (90846-90847)

Code also interactive complexity services with the time the provider spends performing the service reflected in the time for the appropriate psychotherapy code (90785)

90832 **Psychotherapy, 30 minutes with patient**

🛏 1.76 ⚕ 1.90 **FUD** XXX ★ 03 ▢

AMA: 2018,Nov,3; 2018,Jul,12; 2018,Jan,8; 2017,Nov,3; 2017,Sep,11; 2017,Jan,8; 2016,Dec,11; 2016,Jan,13; 2015,Oct,9; 2015,Jan,16; 2014,Aug,5; 2014,Feb,3

+ 90833 **Psychotherapy, 30 minutes with patient when performed with an evaluation and management service (List separately in addition to the code for primary procedure)**

Code first (99201-99255 [99224, 99225, 99226], 99304-99337, 99341-99350)

🛏 1.84 ⚕ 1.97 **FUD** ZZZ ★ N ▢

AMA: 2018,Nov,3; 2018,Jul,12; 2018,Jan,8; 2017,Nov,3; 2017,Jan,8; 2016,Dec,11; 2016,Jan,13; 2015,Oct,9; 2015,Jan,16; 2014,Aug,5; 2014,Feb,3

90834 **Psychotherapy, 45 minutes with patient**

🛏 2.35 ⚕ 2.53 **FUD** XXX ★ 03 ▢

AMA: 2018,Nov,3; 2018,Jul,12; 2018,Jan,8; 2017,Nov,3; 2017,Jan,8; 2016,Dec,11; 2016,Jan,13; 2015,Oct,9; 2015,Jan,16; 2014,Jun,3; 2014,Feb,3

+ 90836 **Psychotherapy, 45 minutes with patient when performed with an evaluation and management service (List separately in addition to the code for primary procedure)**

Code first (99201-99255 [99224, 99225, 99226], 99304-99337, 99341-99350)

🛏 2.33 ⚕ 2.49 **FUD** ZZZ ★ N ▢

AMA: 2018,Nov,3; 2018,Jul,12; 2018,Jan,8; 2017,Nov,3; 2017,Jan,8; 2016,Dec,11; 2016,Jan,13; 2015,Oct,9; 2015,Jan,16; 2014,Feb,3

90837 **Psychotherapy, 60 minutes with patient**

Code also prolonged service for psychotherapy performed without E&M service face-to-face with the patient lasting 90 minutes or longer (99354-99357)

🛏 3.53 ⚕ 3.80 **FUD** XXX ★ 03 ▢

AMA: 2018,Nov,3; 2018,Jul,12; 2018,Jan,8; 2017,Nov,3; 2017,Jan,8; 2016,Dec,11; 2016,Jan,13; 2015,Oct,3; 2015,Oct,9; 2015,Jan,16; 2014,Apr,6; 2014,Feb,3

+ 90838 **Psychotherapy, 60 minutes with patient when performed with an evaluation and management service (List separately in addition to the code for primary procedure)**

Code first (99201-99255 [99224, 99225, 99226], 99304-99337, 99341-99350)

🛏 3.08 ⚕ 3.29 **FUD** ZZZ ★ N ▢

AMA: 2018,Nov,3; 2018,Jul,12; 2018,Jan,8; 2017,Nov,3; 2017,Jan,8; 2016,Dec,11; 2016,Jan,13; 2015,Oct,9; 2015,Jan,16; 2014,Apr,6; 2014,Feb,3

90839-90840 Services for Patients in Crisis

CMS: 100-02,15,170 Clinical Social Worker (CSW) Services; 100-03,130.1 Inpatient Stays for Alcoholism Treatment; 100-03,130.3 Chemical Aversion Therapy for Treatment of Alcoholism; 100-04,12,100 Teaching Physician Services; 100-04,12,160 Independent Psychologist Services; 100-04,12,160.1 Payment of Independent Psychologist Services; 100-04,12,170 Clinical Psychologist Services

INCLUDES 30 minutes or more of face-to-face time with the patient (for all or part of the service) and/or family providing crisis psychotherapy
All time spent exclusively with patient (for all or part of the service) and/or family, even if time is not continuous
Emergent care to a patient in severe distress (eg, life threatening or complex)
Institute interventions to minimize psychological trauma
Measures to ease the crisis and reestablish safety
Psychotherapy

EXCLUDES *Adaptive behavior assessment/treatment ([97151, 97152, 97153, 97154, 97155, 97156, 97157, 97158], 0362T, 0373T)*
Other psychiatric services (90785-90899)

90839 **Psychotherapy for crisis; first 60 minutes**

INCLUDES First 30-74 minutes of crisis psychotherapy per day

EXCLUDES *Use of code more than one time per day, even when service is not continuous on that date.*

🛏 3.69 ⚕ 3.96 **FUD** XXX 03 80 ▢

AMA: 2018,Nov,3; 2018,Jul,12; 2018,Jan,8; 2017,Nov,3; 2017,Jan,8; 2016,Jan,13; 2015,Oct,9; 2015,Jan,16; 2014,Aug,5

+ 90840 **each additional 30 minutes (List separately in addition to code for primary service)**

INCLUDES Up to 30 minutes of time beyond the initial 74 minutes

Code first (90839)

🛏 1.76 ⚕ 1.90 **FUD** ZZZ N 80 ▢

AMA: 2018,Nov,3; 2018,Jul,12; 2018,Jan,8; 2017,Nov,3; 2017,Jan,8; 2016,Jan,13; 2015,Oct,9; 2015,Jan,16; 2014,Aug,5

90845-90863 Additional Psychotherapy Services

CMS: 100-02,15,170 Clinical Social Worker (CSW) Services; 100-03,10.3 Inpatient Pain Rehabilitation Programs; 100-03,10.4 Outpatient Hospital Pain Rehabilitation Programs

EXCLUDES *Adaptive behavior assessment/treatment ([97151, 97152, 97153, 97154, 97155, 97156, 97157, 97158], 0362T, 0373T)*
Analysis/programming of neurostimulators for vagus nerve stimulation therapy (95970, 95976-95977)
Crisis psychotherapy (90839-90840)

90845 **Psychoanalysis**

🛏 2.52 ⚕ 2.70 **FUD** XXX ★ 03 80 ▢

AMA: 2018,Nov,3; 2018,Jul,12; 2018,Jan,8; 2017,Jan,8; 2016,Jan,13; 2015,Oct,9; 2015,Jan,16; 2014,Jan,11

90846 **Family psychotherapy (without the patient present), 50 minutes**

EXCLUDES *Service times of less than 26 minutes*

🛏 2.85 ⚕ 3.06 **FUD** XXX ★ 03 80 ▢

AMA: 2018,Nov,3; 2018,Jul,12; 2018,Jan,8; 2017,Nov,3; 2017,Mar,10; 2017,Jan,8; 2016,Dec,11; 2016,Jan,13; 2015,Oct,9; 2015,Jan,16; 2014,Jan,11

90847 **Family psychotherapy (conjoint psychotherapy) (with patient present), 50 minutes**

EXCLUDES *Service times of less than 26 minutes*
Service times of more than 80 minutes, see prolonged services (99354-99357)

🛏 2.96 ⚕ 3.18 **FUD** XXX ★ 03 80 ▢

AMA: 2018,Nov,3; 2018,Jul,12; 2018,Jan,8; 2017,Nov,3; 2017,Jan,8; 2016,Dec,11; 2016,Jan,13; 2015,Oct,9; 2015,Jan,16; 2014,Jan,11

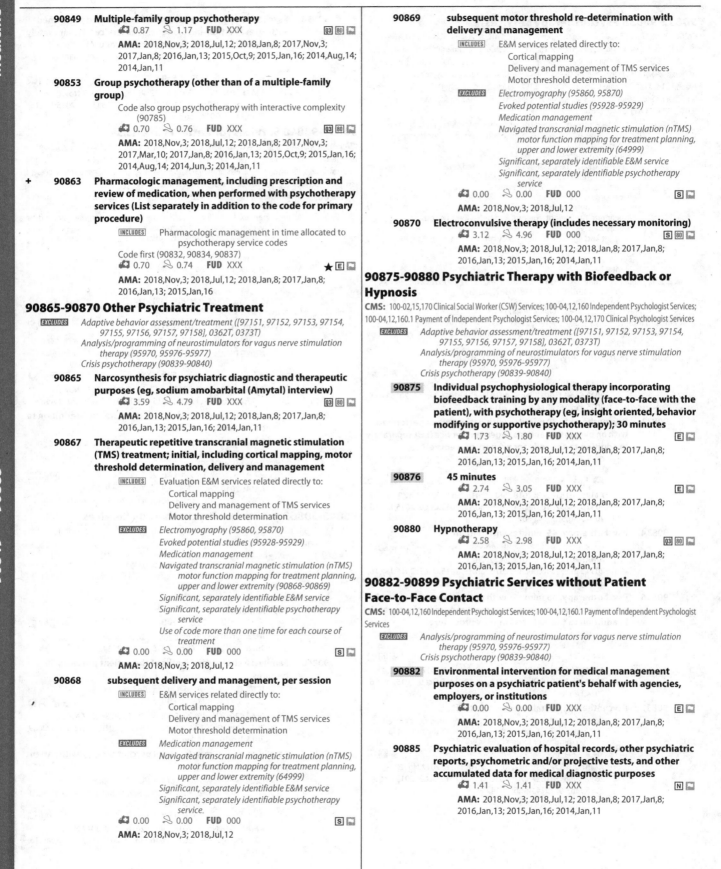

90849   **Multiple-family group psychotherapy**
          💪 0.87   🖐 1.17   **FUD** XXX   Q3 80 ▣
          AMA: 2018,Nov,3; 2018,Jul,12; 2018,Jan,8; 2017,Nov,3;
          2017,Jan,8; 2016,Jan,13; 2015,Oct,9; 2015,Jan,16; 2014,Aug,14;
          2014,Jan,11

90853   **Group psychotherapy (other than of a multiple-family
          group)**
              Code also group psychotherapy with interactive complexity
                 (90785)
          💪 0.70   🖐 0.76   **FUD** XXX   Q3 80 ▣
          AMA: 2018,Nov,3; 2018,Jul,12; 2018,Jan,8; 2017,Nov,3;
          2017,Mar,10; 2017,Jan,8; 2016,Jan,13; 2015,Oct,9; 2015,Jan,16;
          2014,Aug,14; 2014,Jun,3; 2014,Jan,11

+ 90863   **Pharmacologic management, including prescription and
          review of medication, when performed with psychotherapy
          services (List separately in addition to the code for primary
          procedure)**
          INCLUDES   Pharmacologic management in time allocated to
                     psychotherapy service codes
              Code first (90832, 90834, 90837)
          💪 0.70   🖐 0.74   **FUD** XXX   ★ E ▣
          AMA: 2018,Nov,3; 2018,Jul,12; 2018,Jan,8; 2017,Jan,8;
          2016,Jan,13; 2015,Jan,16

90865-90870 Other Psychiatric Treatment

EXCLUDES   *Adaptive behavior assessment/treatment ([97151, 97152, 97153, 97154,
           97155, 97156, 97157, 97158], 0362T, 0373T)*
           *Analysis/programming of neurostimulators for vagus nerve stimulation
           therapy (95970, 95976-95977)*
           Crisis psychotherapy (90839-90840)

90865   **Narcosynthesis for psychiatric diagnostic and therapeutic
          purposes (eg, sodium amobarbital (Amytal) interview)**
          💪 3.59   🖐 4.79   **FUD** XXX   Q3 80 ▣
          AMA: 2018,Nov,3; 2018,Jul,12; 2018,Jan,8; 2017,Jan,8;
          2016,Jan,13; 2015,Jan,16; 2014,Jan,11

90867   **Therapeutic repetitive transcranial magnetic stimulation
          (TMS) treatment; initial, including cortical mapping, motor
          threshold determination, delivery and management**
          INCLUDES   Evaluation E&M services related directly to:
                     Cortical mapping
                     Delivery and management of TMS services
                     Motor threshold determination
          EXCLUDES   *Electromyography (95860, 95870)*
                     Evoked potential studies (95928-95929)
                     Medication management
                     *Navigated transcranial magnetic stimulation (nTMS)
                        motor function mapping for treatment planning,
                        upper and lower extremity (90868-90869)*
                     Significant, separately identifiable E&M service
                     *Significant, separately identifiable psychotherapy
                        service*
                     *Use of code more than one time for each course of
                        treatment*
          💪 0.00   🖐 0.00   **FUD** 000   S ▣
          AMA: 2018,Nov,3; 2018,Jul,12

90868   **subsequent delivery and management, per session**
          INCLUDES   E&M services related directly to:
                     Cortical mapping
                     Delivery and management of TMS services
                     Motor threshold determination
          EXCLUDES   *Medication management*
                     *Navigated transcranial magnetic stimulation (nTMS)
                        motor function mapping for treatment planning,
                        upper and lower extremity (64999)*
                     Significant, separately identifiable E&M service
                     *Significant, separately identifiable psychotherapy
                        service.*
          💪 0.00   🖐 0.00   **FUD** 000   S ▣
          AMA: 2018,Nov,3; 2018,Jul,12

90869   **subsequent motor threshold re-determination with
          delivery and management**
          INCLUDES   E&M services related directly to:
                     Cortical mapping
                     Delivery and management of TMS services
                     Motor threshold determination
          EXCLUDES   *Electromyography (95860, 95870)*
                     Evoked potential studies (95928-95929)
                     Medication management
                     *Navigated transcranial magnetic stimulation (nTMS)
                        motor function mapping for treatment planning,
                        upper and lower extremity (64999)*
                     Significant, separately identifiable E&M service
                     *Significant, separately identifiable psychotherapy
                        service*
          💪 0.00   🖐 0.00   **FUD** 000   S ▣
          AMA: 2018,Nov,3; 2018,Jul,12

90870   **Electroconvulsive therapy (includes necessary monitoring)**
          💪 3.12   🖐 4.96   **FUD** 000   S 80 ▣
          AMA: 2018,Nov,3; 2018,Jul,12; 2018,Jan,8; 2017,Jan,8;
          2016,Jan,13; 2015,Jan,16; 2014,Jan,11

90875-90880 Psychiatric Therapy with Biofeedback or Hypnosis

CMS: 100-02,15,170 Clinical Social Worker (CSW) Services; 100-04,12,160 Independent Psychologist Services;
100-04,12,160.1 Payment of Independent Psychologist Services; 100-04,12,170 Clinical Psychologist Services
EXCLUDES   *Adaptive behavior assessment/treatment ([97151, 97152, 97153, 97154,
           97155, 97156, 97157, 97158], 0362T, 0373T)*
           *Analysis/programming of neurostimulators for vagus nerve stimulation
           therapy (95970, 95976-95977)*
           Crisis psychotherapy (90839-90840)

90875   **Individual psychophysiological therapy incorporating
          biofeedback training by any modality (face-to-face with the
          patient), with psychotherapy (eg, insight oriented, behavior
          modifying or supportive psychotherapy); 30 minutes**
          💪 1.73   🖐 1.80   **FUD** XXX   E ▣
          AMA: 2018,Nov,3; 2018,Jul,12; 2018,Jan,8; 2017,Jan,8;
          2016,Jan,13; 2015,Jan,16; 2014,Jan,11

90876   **45 minutes**
          💪 2.74   🖐 3.05   **FUD** XXX   E ▣
          AMA: 2018,Nov,3; 2018,Jul,12; 2018,Jan,8; 2017,Jan,8;
          2016,Jan,13; 2015,Jan,16; 2014,Jan,11

90880   **Hypnotherapy**
          💪 2.58   🖐 2.98   **FUD** XXX   Q3 80 ▣
          AMA: 2018,Nov,3; 2018,Jul,12; 2018,Jan,8; 2017,Jan,8;
          2016,Jan,13; 2015,Jan,16; 2014,Jan,11

90882-90899 Psychiatric Services without Patient Face-to-Face Contact

CMS: 100-04,12,160 Independent Psychologist Services; 100-04,12,160.1 Payment of Independent Psychologist
Services
EXCLUDES   *Analysis/programming of neurostimulators for vagus nerve stimulation
           therapy (95970, 95976-95977)*
           Crisis psychotherapy (90839-90840)

90882   **Environmental intervention for medical management
          purposes on a psychiatric patient's behalf with agencies,
          employers, or institutions**
          💪 0.00   🖐 0.00   **FUD** XXX   E ▣
          AMA: 2018,Nov,3; 2018,Jul,12; 2018,Jan,8; 2017,Jan,8;
          2016,Jan,13; 2015,Jan,16; 2014,Jan,11

90885   **Psychiatric evaluation of hospital records, other psychiatric
          reports, psychometric and/or projective tests, and other
          accumulated data for medical diagnostic purposes**
          💪 1.41   🖐 1.41   **FUD** XXX   N ▣
          AMA: 2018,Nov,3; 2018,Jul,12; 2018,Jan,8; 2017,Jan,8;
          2016,Jan,13; 2015,Jan,16; 2014,Jan,11

Medicine   90849 — 90885

90887 Interpretation or explanation of results of psychiatric, other medical examinations and procedures, or other accumulated data to family or other responsible persons, or advising them how to assist patient

> EXCLUDES *Adaptive behavior assessment/treatment ([97151, 97152, 97153, 97154, 97155, 97156, 97157, 97158], 0362T, 0373T)*
>
> 🚑 2.14 ⚕ 2.48 **FUD** XXX
>
> [N] 🔲
>
> **AMA:** 2018,Nov,3; 2018,Jul,12; 2018,Jan,8; 2017,Jan,8; 2016,Jan,13; 2015,Jan,16; 2014,Jan,11

90889 Preparation of report of patient's psychiatric status, history, treatment, or progress (other than for legal or consultative purposes) for other individuals, agencies, or insurance carriers

> 🚑 0.00 ⚕ 0.00 **FUD** XXX
>
> [N] 🔲
>
> **AMA:** 2018,Nov,3; 2018,Jul,12; 2018,Jan,8; 2017,Jan,8; 2016,Jan,13; 2015,Jan,16; 2014,Jan,11

90899 Unlisted psychiatric service or procedure

> 🚑 0.00 ⚕ 0.00 **FUD** XXX
>
> [Q3] [80] 🔲
>
> **AMA:** 2018,Nov,3; 2018,Jul,12; 2018,Jan,8; 2017,Jan,8; 2016,Jan,13; 2015,Jan,16; 2014,Jan,11

90901-90913 Biofeedback Therapy

> EXCLUDES *Psychophysiological therapy utilizing biofeedback training (90875-90876)*

90901 Biofeedback training by any modality

> 🚑 0.57 ⚕ 1.13 **FUD** 000
>
> [A] [80] 🔲
>
> **AMA:** 2018,Jan,8; 2017,Jan,8; 2016,Jan,13; 2015,Jan,16; 2014,Jan,11

90911 ~~Biofeedback training, perineal muscles, anorectal or urethral sphincter, including EMG and/or manometry~~

> To report, see (90912-90913)

● **90912** Biofeedback training, perineal muscles, anorectal or urethral sphincter, including EMG and/or manometry, when performed; initial 15 minutes of one-on-one physician or other qualified health care professional contact with the patient

> EXCLUDES *Incontinence treatment using pulsed magnetic neuromodulation (53899)*
> *Testing of rectal sensation, tone, and compliance (91120)*

● + **90913** each additional 15 minutes of one-on-one physician or other qualified health care professional contact with the patient (List separately in addition to code for primary procedure)

> 🚑 0.00 ⚕ 0.00 **FUD** 000
>
> EXCLUDES *Incontinence treatment using pulsed magnetic neuromodulation (53899)*
> *Testing of rectal sensation, tone, and compliance (91120)*
>
> Code first (90912)

90935-90940 Hemodialysis Services: Inpatient ESRD and Outpatient Non-ESRD

CMS: 100-02,11,20 Renal Dialysis Items and Services ; 100-04,3,100.6 Inpatient Renal Services

> EXCLUDES *Attendance by physician or other qualified health care provider for a prolonged period of time (99354-99360 [99415, 99416])*
> *Blood specimen collection from partial/complete implantable venous access device (36591)*
> *Declotting of cannula (36831, 36833, 36860-36861)*
> *Hemodialysis home visit by non-physician health care professional (99512)*
> *Therapeutic apheresis procedures (36511-36516)*
> *Thrombolytic agent declotting of implanted vascular access device/catheter (36593)*

Code also significant separately identifiable E&M service not related to dialysis procedure or renal failure with modifier 25 (99201-99215, 99217-99223 [99224, 99225, 99226], 99231-99239, 99241-99245, 99281-99285, 99291-99292, 99304-99318, 99324-99337, 99341-99350, 99466-99467, 99468-99476, 99477-99480)

90935 Hemodialysis procedure with single evaluation by a physician or other qualified health care professional

> INCLUDES All E&M services related to the patient's renal disease rendered on a day dialysis is performed
> Inpatient ESRD and non-ESRD procedures
> Only one evaluation of the patient related to hemodialysis procedure
> Outpatient non-ESRD dialysis
>
> 🚑 2.07 ⚕ 2.07 **FUD** 000
>
> [S] [80] 🔲
>
> **AMA:** 2018,Jan,8; 2017,Jan,8; 2016,Jan,13; 2015,Jan,16; 2014,Jan,11

90937 Hemodialysis procedure requiring repeated evaluation(s) with or without substantial revision of dialysis prescription

> INCLUDES All E&M services related to the patient's renal disease rendered on a day dialysis is performed
> Inpatient ESRD and non-ESRD procedures
> Outpatient non-ESRD dialysis
> Re-evaluation of the patient during hemodialysis procedure
>
> 🚑 2.95 ⚕ 2.95 **FUD** 000
>
> [B] [80] 🔲
>
> **AMA:** 2018,Jan,8; 2017,Jan,8; 2016,Jan,13; 2015,Jan,16; 2014,Jan,11

90940 Hemodialysis access flow study to determine blood flow in grafts and arteriovenous fistulae by an indicator method

> EXCLUDES *Hemodialysis access duplex scan (93990)*
>
> 🚑 0.00 ⚕ 0.00 **FUD** XXX
>
> [N] 🔲
>
> **AMA:** 2018,Jan,8; 2017,Jan,8; 2016,Jan,13; 2015,Jan,16; 2014,Jan,11

90945-90947 Dialysis Techniques Other Than Hemodialysis

CMS: 100-04,12,40.3 Global Surgery Review; 100-04,3,100.6 Inpatient Renal Services

> INCLUDES All E&M services related to the patient's renal disease rendered on the day dialysis is performed
> Procedures other than hemodialysis:
> Continuous renal replacement therapies
> Hemofiltration
> Peritoneal dialysis
>
> EXCLUDES *Attendance by physician or other qualified health care provider for a prolonged period of time (99354-99360 [99415, 99416])*
> *Hemodialysis*
> *Tunneled intraperitoneal catheter insertion*
> *Open (49421)*
> *Percutaneous (49418)*

Code also significant, separately identifiable E&M service not related to dialysis procedure or renal failure with modifier 25 (99201-99215, 99217-99223 [99224, 99225, 99226], 99231-99239, 99241-99245, 99281-99285, 99291-99292, 99304-99318, 99324-99337, 99341-99350, 99466-99480 [99485, 99486])

90945 Dialysis procedure other than hemodialysis (eg, peritoneal dialysis, hemofiltration, or other continuous renal replacement therapies), with single evaluation by a physician or other qualified health care professional

> INCLUDES Only one evaluation of the patient related to the procedure
>
> EXCLUDES *Peritoneal dialysis home infusion (99601, 99602)*
>
> 🚑 2.42 ⚕ 2.42 **FUD** 000
>
> [V] [80] 🔲
>
> **AMA:** 2018,Jan,8; 2017,Jan,8; 2016,Jan,13; 2015,Jan,16; 2014,Jan,11

90947 Dialysis procedure other than hemodialysis (eg, peritoneal dialysis, hemofiltration, or other continuous renal replacement therapies) requiring repeated evaluations by a physician or other qualified health care professional, with or without substantial revision of dialysis prescription

EXCLUDES Re-evaluation during a procedure

🔧 3.51   ⚕ 3.51   **FUD** 000   B 80 ▢

AMA: 2018,Jan,8; 2017,Jan,8; 2016,Jan,13; 2015,Jan,16; 2014,Jan,11

90951-90962 End-stage Renal Disease Monthly Outpatient Services

CMS: 100-02,11,20 Renal Dialysis Items and Services ; 100-04,12,190.3 List of Telehealth Services; 100-04,12,190.3.4 ESRD-Related Services as a Telehealth Service; 100-04,8,140.1 ESRD-Related Services Under the Monthly Capitation Payment

INCLUDES Establishing dialyzing cycle
Management of dialysis visits
Outpatient E&M of dialysis visits
Patient management during dialysis for a month
Telephone calls

EXCLUDES ESRD/non-ESRD dialysis services performed in an inpatient setting (90935-90937, 90945-90947)
Non-ESRD dialysis services performed in an outpatient setting (90935-90937, 90945-90947)
Non-ESRD related E&M services that cannot be performed during the dialysis session
Services provided during the time transitional care management services are being provided (99495-99496)
Services provided in the same month with chronic care management (99487-99489)

90951 End-stage renal disease (ESRD) related services monthly, for patients younger than 2 years of age to include monitoring for the adequacy of nutrition, assessment of growth and development, and counseling of parents; with 4 or more face-to-face visits by a physician or other qualified health care professional per month   A

🔧 26.6   ⚕ 26.6   **FUD** XXX   ★ M 80 ▢

AMA: 2018,Feb,11; 2018,Jan,8; 2017,Jan,8; 2016,Jan,13; 2015,Jan,16; 2014,Oct,3; 2014,Jan,11

90952 with 2-3 face-to-face visits by a physician or other qualified health care professional per month   A

🔧 0.00   ⚕ 0.00   **FUD** XXX   ★ M 80 ▢

AMA: 2018,Feb,11; 2018,Jan,8; 2017,Jan,8; 2016,Jan,13; 2015,Jan,16; 2014,Oct,3; 2014,Jan,11

90953 with 1 face-to-face visit by a physician or other qualified health care professional per month   A

🔧 0.00   ⚕ 0.00   **FUD** XXX   M 80 ▢

AMA: 2018,Feb,11; 2018,Jan,8; 2017,Jan,8; 2016,Jan,13; 2015,Jan,16; 2014,Oct,3; 2014,Jan,11

90954 End-stage renal disease (ESRD) related services monthly, for patients 2-11 years of age to include monitoring for the adequacy of nutrition, assessment of growth and development, and counseling of parents; with 4 or more face-to-face visits by a physician or other qualified health care professional per month   A

🔧 22.9   ⚕ 22.9   **FUD** XXX   ★ M 80 ▢

AMA: 2018,Feb,11; 2018,Jan,8; 2017,Jan,8; 2016,Jan,13; 2015,Jan,16; 2014,Oct,3; 2014,Jan,11

90955 with 2-3 face-to-face visits by a physician or other qualified health care professional per month   A

🔧 12.9   ⚕ 12.9   **FUD** XXX   ★ M 80 ▢

AMA: 2018,Feb,11; 2018,Jan,8; 2017,Jan,8; 2016,Jan,13; 2015,Jan,16; 2014,Oct,3; 2014,Jan,11

90956 with 1 face-to-face visit by a physician or other qualified health care professional per month   A

🔧 9.00   ⚕ 9.00   **FUD** XXX   M 80 ▢

AMA: 2018,Feb,11; 2018,Jan,8; 2017,Jan,8; 2016,Jan,13; 2015,Jan,16; 2014,Oct,3; 2014,Jan,11

90957 End-stage renal disease (ESRD) related services monthly, for patients 12-19 years of age to include monitoring for the adequacy of nutrition, assessment of growth and development, and counseling of parents; with 4 or more face-to-face visits by a physician or other qualified health care professional per month   A

🔧 18.1   ⚕ 18.1   **FUD** XXX   ★ M 80 ▢

AMA: 2018,Feb,11; 2018,Jan,8; 2017,Jan,8; 2016,Jan,13; 2015,Jan,16; 2014,Oct,3; 2014,Jan,11

90958 with 2-3 face-to-face visits by a physician or other qualified health care professional per month   A

🔧 12.3   ⚕ 12.3   **FUD** XXX   ★ M 80 ▢

AMA: 2018,Feb,11; 2018,Jan,8; 2017,Jan,8; 2016,Jan,13; 2015,Jan,16; 2014,Oct,3; 2014,Jan,11

90959 with 1 face-to-face visit by a physician or other qualified health care professional per month   A

🔧 8.40   ⚕ 8.40   **FUD** XXX   M 80 ▢

AMA: 2018,Feb,11; 2018,Jan,8; 2017,Jan,8; 2016,Jan,13; 2015,Jan,16; 2014,Oct,3; 2014,Jan,11

90960 End-stage renal disease (ESRD) related services monthly, for patients 20 years of age and older; with 4 or more face-to-face visits by a physician or other qualified health care professional per month   A

🔧 8.02   ⚕ 8.02   **FUD** XXX   ★ M 80 ▢

AMA: 2018,Feb,11; 2018,Jan,8; 2017,Jan,8; 2016,Jan,13; 2015,Jan,16; 2014,Oct,3; 2014,Jan,11

90961 with 2-3 face-to-face visits by a physician or other qualified health care professional per month   A

🔧 6.74   ⚕ 6.74   **FUD** XXX   ★ M 80 ▢

AMA: 2018,Feb,11; 2018,Jan,8; 2017,Jan,8; 2016,Jan,13; 2015,Jan,16; 2014,Oct,3; 2014,Jan,11

90962 with 1 face-to-face visit by a physician or other qualified health care professional per month   A

🔧 5.21   ⚕ 5.21   **FUD** XXX   M 80 ▢

AMA: 2018,Feb,11; 2018,Jan,8; 2017,Jan,8; 2016,Jan,13; 2015,Jan,16; 2014,Oct,3; 2014,Jan,11

90963-90966 End-stage Renal Disease Monthly Home Dialysis Services

CMS: 100-02,11,20 Renal Dialysis Items and Services; 100-04,12,190.3.4 ESRD-Related Services as a Telehealth Service; 100-04,8,140.1 ESRD-Related Services Under the Monthly Capitation Payment; 100-04,8,140.1.1 Payment for Managing Patients on Home Dialysis

INCLUDES ESRD services for home dialysis patients
Services provided for a full month

EXCLUDES Services provided during the time transitional care management services are being provided (99495-99496)
Services provided in the same month with chronic care management (99487-99489)

90963 End-stage renal disease (ESRD) related services for home dialysis per full month, for patients younger than 2 years of age to include monitoring for the adequacy of nutrition, assessment of growth and development, and counseling of parents   A

🔧 15.4   ⚕ 15.4   **FUD** XXX   M 80 ▢

AMA: 2018,Feb,11; 2018,Jan,8; 2017,Jan,8; 2016,Jan,13; 2015,Jan,16; 2014,Oct,3; 2014,Jan,11

90964 End-stage renal disease (ESRD) related services for home dialysis per full month, for patients 2-11 years of age to include monitoring for the adequacy of nutrition, assessment of growth and development, and counseling of parents   A

🔧 13.4   ⚕ 13.4   **FUD** XXX   M 80 ▢

AMA: 2018,Feb,11; 2018,Jan,8; 2017,Jan,8; 2016,Jan,13; 2015,Jan,16; 2014,Oct,3; 2014,Jan,11

90965 End-stage renal disease (ESRD) related services for home dialysis per full month, for patients 12-19 years of age to include monitoring for the adequacy of nutrition, assessment of growth and development, and counseling of parents [A]

🔲 12.8 ⚖ 12.8 FUD XXX [M][80][⬜]

AMA: 2018,Feb,11; 2018,Jan,8; 2017,Jan,8; 2016,Jan,13; 2015,Jan,16; 2014,Oct,3; 2014,Jan,11

90966 End-stage renal disease (ESRD) related services for home dialysis per full month, for patients 20 years of age and older [A]

🔲 6.72 ⚖ 6.72 FUD XXX [M][80][⬜]

AMA: 2018,Feb,11; 2018,Jan,8; 2017,Jan,8; 2016,Jan,13; 2015,Jan,16; 2014,Oct,3; 2014,Jan,11

90967-90970 End-stage Renal Disease Services: Partial Month

CMS: 100-02,11,20 Renal Dialysis Items and Services

INCLUDES ESRD services for less than a full month, such as:
A patient who is transient, dies, recovers, or undergoes kidney transplant
Outpatient ESRD-related services initiated prior to completion of assessment
Patient spending part of the month as a hospital inpatient
Services reported on a daily basis, less the days of hospitalization

EXCLUDES Services provided during the time transitional care management services are being provided (99495-99496)
Services provided in the same month with chronic care management (99487-99489)

90967 End-stage renal disease (ESRD) related services for dialysis less than a full month of service, per day; for patients younger than 2 years of age [A]

🔲 0.51 ⚖ 0.51 FUD XXX [M][80][⬜]

AMA: 2018,Feb,11; 2018,Jan,8; 2017,Jan,8; 2016,Jan,13; 2015,Jan,16; 2014,Oct,3; 2014,Jan,11

90968 for patients 2-11 years of age [A]

🔲 0.45 ⚖ 0.45 FUD XXX [M][80][⬜]

AMA: 2018,Feb,11; 2018,Jan,8; 2017,Jan,8; 2016,Jan,13; 2015,Jan,16; 2014,Oct,3; 2014,Jan,11

90969 for patients 12-19 years of age [A]

🔲 0.43 ⚖ 0.43 FUD XXX [M][80][⬜]

AMA: 2018,Feb,11; 2018,Jan,8; 2017,Jan,8; 2016,Jan,13; 2015,Jan,16; 2014,Oct,3; 2014,Jan,11

90970 for patients 20 years of age and older [A]

🔲 0.22 ⚖ 0.22 FUD XXX [M][80][⬜]

AMA: 2018,Feb,11; 2018,Jan,8; 2017,Jan,8; 2016,Jan,13; 2015,Jan,16; 2014,Oct,3; 2014,Jan,11

90989-90993 Dialysis Training Services

CMS: 100-04,3,100.6 Inpatient Renal Services

90989 Dialysis training, patient, including helper where applicable, any mode, completed course

🔲 0.00 ⚖ 0.00 FUD XXX [B][⬜]

AMA: 2018,Feb,11; 2018,Jan,8; 2017,Jan,8; 2016,Jan,13; 2015,Jan,16; 2014,Jan,11

90993 Dialysis training, patient, including helper where applicable, any mode, course not completed, per training session

🔲 0.00 ⚖ 0.00 FUD XXX [B][⬜]

AMA: 2018,Feb,11; 2018,Jan,8; 2017,Jan,8; 2016,Jan,13; 2015,Jan,16; 2014,Jan,11

90997-90999 Hemoperfusion and Unlisted Dialysis Procedures

CMS: 100-04,3,100.6 Inpatient Renal Services

90997 Hemoperfusion (eg, with activated charcoal or resin)

🔲 2.53 ⚖ 2.53 FUD 000 [B][80][⬜]

AMA: 2018,Feb,11

90999 Unlisted dialysis procedure, inpatient or outpatient

🔲 0.00 ⚖ 0.00 FUD XXX [B][80][⬜]

AMA: 2018,Feb,11

91010-91022 Esophageal Manometry

91010 Esophageal motility (manometric study of the esophagus and/or gastroesophageal junction) study with interpretation and report;

EXCLUDES Esophageal motility studies with high-resolution esophageal pressure topography (91299)
Code also for esophageal motility studies with stimulant or perfusion (91013)

🔲 5.38 ⚖ 5.38 FUD 000 [S][80][⬜]

AMA: 2018,Feb,11

+ **91013** with stimulation or perfusion (eg, stimulant, acid or alkali perfusion) (List separately in addition to code for primary procedure)

EXCLUDES Esophageal motility studies with high-resolution esophageal pressure topography (91299)
Use of code more than one time for each session
Code first (91010)

🔲 0.73 ⚖ 0.73 FUD ZZZ [N][80][⬜]

AMA: 2018,Feb,11

91020 Gastric motility (manometric) studies

EXCLUDES Gastrointestinal imaging by wireless capsule (91112)

🔲 7.01 ⚖ 7.01 FUD 000 [S][80][⬜]

AMA: 2018,Feb,11; 2018,Jan,8; 2017,Jan,8; 2016,Jan,13; 2015,Jan,16

Gastric pertains to the stomach; peptic is a term for ulcers caused by digestive juices in the stomach, duodenum or jejunum; duodenal ulcers are more common in young people, gastric in the elderly

Labels: Liver, Stomach, Colon, Small intestine, Esophagus, Mucosal and muscle layers, Fundus, Rugae (folds lining the stomach), Duodenum, Pyloric sphincter, Inner stomach (area where gastric ulcers occur)

91022 Duodenal motility (manometric) study

EXCLUDES Fluoroscopy (76000)
Gastric motility study (91020)
Gastrointestinal imaging by wireless capsule (91112)

🔲 4.79 ⚖ 4.79 FUD 000 [S][80][⬜]

AMA: 2018,Feb,11; 2018,Jan,8; 2017,Jan,8; 2016,Jan,13; 2015,Jan,16

91030-91040 Esophageal Reflux Tests

EXCLUDES Duodenal intubation/aspiration (43756-43757)
Esophagoscopy (43180-43233 [43211, 43212, 43213, 43214])
Insertion of:
Esophageal tamponade tube (43460)
Insertion long gastrointestinal tube (44500)
Radiologic services, gastrointestinal (74210-74363)
Upper gastrointestinal endoscopy (43235-43259 [43233, 43266, 43270])

91030 Esophagus, acid perfusion (Bernstein) test for esophagitis

🔲 3.91 ⚖ 3.91 FUD 000 [S][80][⬜]

AMA: 2018,Feb,11

91034 Esophagus, gastroesophageal reflux test; with nasal catheter pH electrode(s) placement, recording, analysis and interpretation

🔲 5.39 ⚖ 5.39 FUD 000 [S][80][⬜]

AMA: 2018,Feb,11; 2018,Jan,8; 2017,Jan,8; 2016,Jan,13; 2015,Jan,16; 2014,Feb,11; 2014,Jan,11

● New Code ▲ Revised Code ○ Reinstated ● New Web Release ▲ Revised Web Release + Add-on Unlisted Not Covered # Resequenced
⑤⓪ Optum Mod 50 Exempt ⊘ AMA Mod 51 Exempt ⑤① Optum Mod 51 Exempt ⑥③ Mod 63 Exempt ✗ Non-FDA Drug ★ Telemedicine [M] Maternity [A] Age Edit

91035   with mucosal attached telemetry pH electrode placement, recording, analysis and interpretation

INCLUDES   Endoscopy only to place device

📁 13.6   ⚖ 13.6   **FUD** 000   [S] [72] [80] 🖵

AMA: 2018,Feb,11; 2018,Jan,8; 2017,Jan,8; 2016,Jan,13; 2015,Jan,16; 2014,Feb,11; 2014,Jan,11

91037   Esophageal function test, gastroesophageal reflux test with nasal catheter intraluminal impedance electrode(s) placement, recording, analysis and interpretation;

📁 4.66   ⚖ 4.66   **FUD** 000   [S] [80] 🖵

AMA: 2018,Feb,11

91038   prolonged (greater than 1 hour, up to 24 hours)

📁 12.5   ⚖ 12.5   **FUD** 000   [S] [80] 🖵

AMA: 2018,Feb,11; 2018,Jan,8; 2017,Jan,8; 2016,Jan,13; 2015,Jan,16; 2014,Feb,11

91040   Esophageal balloon distension study, diagnostic, with provocation when performed

EXCLUDES   Use of code more than one time for each session

📁 13.5   ⚖ 13.5   **FUD** 000   [S] [80] 🖵

AMA: 2018,Feb,11; 2018,Jan,8; 2017,Jan,6

91065 Breath Analysis

CMS: 100-03,100.5 Diagnostic Breath Analysis

EXCLUDES   H. pylori breath test analysis, radioactive (C-14) or nonradioactive (C-13) (78268, 83013)

Code also each challenge administered

91065   Breath hydrogen or methane test (eg, for detection of lactase deficiency, fructose intolerance, bacterial overgrowth, or oro-cecal gastrointestinal transit)

📁 2.13   ⚖ 2.13   **FUD** 000   [S] [80] 🖵

AMA: 2018,Feb,11; 2018,Jan,8; 2017,Jan,8; 2016,Jan,13; 2015,Jan,16; 2014,Jan,11

91110-91299 Additional Gastrointestinal Diagnostic/Therapeutic Procedures

EXCLUDES   Abdominal paracentesis (49082-49084)
Abdominal paracentesis with medication administration (96440, 96446)
Anoscopy (46600-46615)
Colonoscopy (45378-45393 [45388, 45390, 45398])
Duodenal intubation/aspiration (43756-43757)
Esophagoscopy (43180-43233 [43211, 43212, 43213, 43214])
Proctosigmoidoscopy (45300-45327)
Radiologic services, gastrointestinal (74210-74363)
Sigmoidoscopy (45330-45350 [45346])
Small intestine/stomal endoscopy (44360-44408 [44381, 44401])
Upper gastrointestinal endoscopy (43235-43259 [43233, 43266, 43270])

91110   Gastrointestinal tract imaging, intraluminal (eg, capsule endoscopy), esophagus through ileum, with interpretation and report

EXCLUDES   Imaging of colon (0355T)
Imaging of esophagus through ileum (91111)
Code also modifier 52 if ileum is not visualized

📁 24.9   ⚖ 24.9   **FUD** XXX   [T] [80] 🖵

AMA: 2018,Feb,11; 2018,Jan,8; 2017,Jan,8; 2016,Jan,13; 2015,Jan,16; 2014,Jan,11

91111   Gastrointestinal tract imaging, intraluminal (eg, capsule endoscopy), esophagus with interpretation and report

EXCLUDES   Imaging of colon (0355T)
Imaging of esophagus through ileum (91111)
Use of wireless capsule to measure transit times or pressure in gastrointestinal tract (91112)

📁 22.8   ⚖ 22.8   **FUD** XXX   [T] [80] 🖵

AMA: 2018,Feb,11; 2018,Jan,8; 2017,Jan,8; 2016,Jan,13; 2015,Jan,16

91112   Gastrointestinal transit and pressure measurement, stomach through colon, wireless capsule, with interpretation and report

EXCLUDES   Colon motility study (91117)
Duodenal motility study (91022)
Gastric motility studies (91020)
pH of body fluid (83986)

📁 35.8   ⚖ 35.8   **FUD** XXX   [T] [80] 🖵

AMA: 2018,Feb,11; 2018,Jan,8; 2017,Jan,8; 2016,Jan,13; 2015,Jan,16

91117   Colon motility (manometric) study, minimum 6 hours continuous recording (including provocation tests, eg, meal, intracolonic balloon distension, pharmacologic agents, if performed), with interpretation and report

EXCLUDES   Anal manometry (91122)
Rectal sensation, tone and compliance testing (91120)
Use of code more than one time regardless of the number of provocations
Use of wireless capsule to measure transit times or pressure in gastrointestinal tract (91112)

📁 3.96   ⚖ 3.96   **FUD** 000   [T] [80] 🖵

AMA: 2018,Feb,11; 2018,Jan,8; 2017,Jan,8; 2016,Jan,13; 2015,Jan,16

91120   Rectal sensation, tone, and compliance test (ie, response to graded balloon distention)

EXCLUDES   Anorectal manometry (91122)
Biofeedback training (90912, 90913)
Colon motility study (91117)

📁 12.9   ⚖ 12.9   **FUD** XXX   [S] [80] 🖵

AMA: 2018,Feb,11; 2018,Jan,8; 2017,Jan,8; 2016,Jan,13; 2015,Jan,16; 2014,Jan,11

91122   Anorectal manometry

EXCLUDES   Colon motility study (91117)

📁 6.85   ⚖ 6.85   **FUD** 000   [T] [80] 🖵

AMA: 2018,Feb,11

91132   Electrogastrography, diagnostic, transcutaneous;

📁 6.80   ⚖ 6.80   **FUD** XXX   [S] [80] 🖵

AMA: 2018,Feb,11

91133   with provocative testing

📁 7.44   ⚖ 7.44   **FUD** XXX   [Q1] [80] 🖵

AMA: 2018,Feb,11

91200   Liver elastography, mechanically induced shear wave (eg, vibration), without imaging, with interpretation and report

EXCLUDES   Ultrasound elastography parenchyma (76981-76983)

📁 1.10   ⚖ 1.10   **FUD** XXX   [Q1] [80] 🖵

AMA: 2019,Aug,3; 2018,Feb,11; 2018,Jan,8; 2017,Oct,9; 2014,Dec,13

91299   Unlisted diagnostic gastroenterology procedure

📁 0.00   ⚖ 0.00   **FUD** XXX   [S] [80] 🖵

AMA: 2018,Feb,11; 2018,Jan,8; 2017,Jan,8; 2016,Jan,13; 2015,Jan,16; 2014,Jan,11

26/TC PC/TC Only	A2-Z3 ASC Payment	50 Bilateral	♂ Male Only	♀ Female Only	📁 Facility RVU	⚖ Non-Facility RVU	🖵 CCI	✖ CLIA
FUD Follow-up Days	CMS: IOM	AMA: CPT Asst	A-Y OPPSI	80/80 Surg Assist Allowed / w/Doc		🔲 Lab Crosswalk	🔲 Radiology Crosswalk	

468   CPT © 2019 American Medical Association. All Rights Reserved.   © 2019 Optum360, LLC

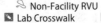

92002-92014 Ophthalmic Medical Services

CMS: 100-02,15,30.4 Optometrist's Services

INCLUDES Routine ophthalmoscopy
Services provided to established patients who have received professional services from the physician or other qualified health care provider or another physician or other qualified health care professional within the same group practice of the exact same specialty and subspecialty within the past three years
Services provided to new patients who have received no professional services from the physician or other qualified health care provider or another physician or other qualified health care professional within the same group practice of the exact same specialty and subspecialty within the past three years

EXCLUDES Retinal polarization scan (0469T)
Surgical procedures on the eye/ocular adnexa (65091-68899 [67810])
Visual screening tests (99173-99174 [99177])

92002   **Ophthalmological services: medical examination and evaluation with initiation of diagnostic and treatment program; intermediate, new patient**

INCLUDES Evaluation of new/existing condition complicated by new diagnostic or management problem
Integrated services where medical decision making cannot be separated from examination methods
Other diagnostic procedures
  Biomicroscopy
  Mydriasis
  Ophthalmoscopy
  Tonometry
Problems not related to primary diagnosis
The following for intermediate services:
  External ocular/adnexal examination
  General medical observation
  History

1.36   2.37   **FUD** XXX   V 80

AMA: 2018,Feb,11; 2018,Feb,3; 2018,Jan,8; 2017,Sep,14; 2017,Jan,8; 2016,Jan,13; 2015,Jan,16; 2014,Jan,11

92004   **comprehensive, new patient, 1 or more visits**

INCLUDES General evaluation of complete visual system
Integrated services where medical decision making cannot be separated from examination methods
Single service that need not be performed at one session
The following for comprehensive services:
  Basic sensorimotor examination
  Biomicroscopy
  Dilation (cycloplegia)
  External examinations
  General medical observation
  Gross visual fields
  History
  Initiation of diagnostic/treatment programs
  Mydriasis
  Ophthalmoscopic examinations
  Other diagnostic procedures
  Prescription of medication
  Special diagnostic/treatment services
  Tonometry

2.81   4.26   **FUD** XXX   V 80

AMA: 2018,Feb,11; 2018,Feb,3; 2018,Jan,8; 2017,Sep,14; 2017,Jan,8; 2016,Nov,9; 2016,Jan,13; 2015,Jan,16; 2014,Jan,11

92012   **Ophthalmological services: medical examination and evaluation, with initiation or continuation of diagnostic and treatment program; intermediate, established patient**

INCLUDES Evaluation of new/existing condition complicated by new diagnostic or management problem
Integrated services where medical decision making cannot be separated from examination methods
Problems not related to primary diagnosis
The following for intermediate services:
  External ocular/adnexal examination
  General medical observation
  History
  Other diagnostic procedures:
    Biomicroscopy
    Mydriasis
    Ophthalmoscopy
    Tonometry

1.49   2.49   **FUD** XXX   V 80

AMA: 2018,Feb,11; 2018,Feb,3; 2018,Jan,8; 2017,Sep,14; 2017,Jan,8; 2016,Jan,13; 2015,Jan,16; 2014,Jan,11

92014   **comprehensive, established patient, 1 or more visits**

INCLUDES General evaluation of complete visual system
Integrated services where medical decision making cannot be separated from examination methods
Single service that need not be performed at one session
The following for comprehensive services:
  Basic sensorimotor examination
  Biomicroscopy
  Dilation (cycloplegia)
  External examinations
  General medical observation
  Gross visual fields
  History
  Initiation of diagnostic/treatment programs
  Mydriasis
  Ophthalmoscopic examinations
  Other diagnostic procedures
  Prescription of medication
  Special diagnostic/treatment services
  Tonometry

2.25   3.57   **FUD** XXX   V 80

AMA: 2018,Feb,11; 2018,Feb,3; 2018,Jan,8; 2017,Sep,14; 2017,Jan,8; 2016,Nov,9; 2016,Jan,13; 2015,Jan,16; 2014,Jan,11

92015-92145 Ophthalmic Special Services

INCLUDES Routine ophthalmoscopy
Surgical procedures on the eye/ocular adnexa (65091-68899 [67810])
Code also E&M services, when performed
Code also general ophthalmological services, when performed (92002-92014)

92015   **Determination of refractive state**

INCLUDES Lens prescription
  Absorptive factor
  Axis
  Impact resistance
  Lens power
  Prism
  Specification of lens type:
    Bifocal
    Monofocal

EXCLUDES Ocular screening, instrument based (99173-99174 [99177])

0.55   0.56   **FUD** XXX   E

AMA: 2018,Feb,11; 2018,Jan,8; 2017,Jan,8; 2016,Mar,10; 2016,Jan,13; 2015,Jan,16; 2014,Jan,11

92018   **Ophthalmological examination and evaluation, under general anesthesia, with or without manipulation of globe for passive range of motion or other manipulation to facilitate diagnostic examination; complete**

4.13   4.13   **FUD** XXX   J 80

AMA: 2018,Feb,11; 2018,Jan,8; 2017,Jan,8; 2016,Jan,13; 2015,Jan,16; 2014,Jan,11

92019 limited
📇 2.05 ⚕ 2.05 **FUD** XXX   J 80 ▭
AMA: 2018,Feb,11; 2018,Jan,8; 2017,Jan,8; 2016,Jan,13; 2015,Jan,16; 2014,Jan,11

92020 Gonioscopy (separate procedure)
EXCLUDES *Gonioscopy under general anesthesia (92018)*
📇 0.60 ⚕ 0.78 **FUD** XXX   Q1 80 ▭
AMA: 2018,Feb,11; 2018,Jan,8; 2017,Jan,8; 2016,Jan,13; 2015,Jan,16; 2014,Jan,11

92025 Computerized corneal topography, unilateral or bilateral, with interpretation and report
EXCLUDES *Corneal transplant procedures (65710-65771)*
Manual keratoscopy
📇 1.07 ⚕ 1.07 **FUD** XXX   Q1 80 ▭
AMA: 2018,Feb,11; 2018,Jan,8; 2017,Jan,8; 2016,Jan,13; 2015,Jan,16; 2014,Jan,11

92060 Sensorimotor examination with multiple measurements of ocular deviation (eg, restrictive or paretic muscle with diplopia) with interpretation and report (separate procedure)
📇 1.82 ⚕ 1.82 **FUD** XXX   Q1 80 ▭
AMA: 2018,Feb,11; 2018,Jan,8; 2017,Jan,8; 2016,Jan,13; 2015,Jan,16; 2014,Jan,11

92065 Orthoptic and/or pleoptic training, with continuing medical direction and evaluation
📇 1.51 ⚕ 1.51 **FUD** XXX   Q1 80 ▭
AMA: 2018,Feb,11; 2018,Jan,8; 2017,Jan,8; 2016,Jan,13; 2015,Jan,16; 2014,Jan,11

92071 Fitting of contact lens for treatment of ocular surface disease
EXCLUDES *Contact lens service for keratoconus (92072)*
Code also supply of lens with appropriate supply code or (99070)
📇 0.95 ⚕ 1.07 **FUD** XXX   N 80 50 ▭
AMA: 2018,Feb,11

92072 Fitting of contact lens for management of keratoconus, initial fitting
EXCLUDES *Contact lens service for disease of ocular surface (92071)*
Subsequent fittings (99211-99215, 92012-92014)
Code also supply of lens with appropriate supply code or (99070)
📇 2.84 ⚕ 3.72 **FUD** XXX   N 80 ▭
AMA: 2018,Feb,11; 2018,Jan,8; 2017,Sep,14; 2017,Jan,8; 2016,Jan,13; 2015,Jan,16; 2014,Jan,11

92081 Visual field examination, unilateral or bilateral, with interpretation and report; limited examination (eg, tangent screen, Autoplot, arc perimeter, or single stimulus level automated test, such as Octopus 3 or 7 equivalent)
INCLUDES Gross visual testing/confrontation testing
📇 0.96 ⚕ 0.96 **FUD** XXX   Q1 80 ▭
AMA: 2018,Feb,11; 2018,Jan,8; 2017,Jan,8; 2016,Jan,13; 2015,Jan,16; 2014,Jan,11

92082 intermediate examination (eg, at least 2 isopters on Goldmann perimeter, or semiquantitative, automated suprathreshold screening program, Humphrey suprathreshold automatic diagnostic test, Octopus program 33)
INCLUDES Gross visual testing/confrontation testing
📇 1.35 ⚕ 1.35 **FUD** XXX   Q1 80 ▭
AMA: 2018,Feb,11; 2018,Jan,8; 2017,Jan,8; 2016,Jan,13; 2015,Jan,16; 2014,Jan,11

92083 extended examination (eg, Goldmann visual fields with at least 3 isopters plotted and static determination within the central 30°, or quantitative, automated threshold perimetry, Octopus program G-1, 32 or 42, Humphrey visual field analyzer full threshold programs 30-2, 24-2, or 30/60-2)
INCLUDES Gross visual field testing/confrontation testing
EXCLUDES *Assessment of visual field by transmission of data by patient to a surveillance center (0378T-0379T)*
📇 1.81 ⚕ 1.81 **FUD** XXX   Q1 80 ▭
AMA: 2018,Feb,11; 2018,Jan,8; 2017,Jan,8; 2016,Jan,13; 2015,Jan,16; 2014,Jan,11

92100 Serial tonometry (separate procedure) with multiple measurements of intraocular pressure over an extended time period with interpretation and report, same day (eg, diurnal curve or medical treatment of acute elevation of intraocular pressure)
EXCLUDES *Intraocular pressure monitoring for 24 hours or more (0329T)*
Ocular blood flow measurements (0198T)
Single-episode tonometry (99201-99215, 92002-92004)
📇 0.96 ⚕ 2.32 **FUD** XXX   N 80 ▭
AMA: 2018,Feb,11; 2018,Jan,8; 2017,Jan,8; 2016,Jan,13; 2015,Jan,16; 2014,May,5; 2014,Jan,11

92132 Scanning computerized ophthalmic diagnostic imaging, anterior segment, with interpretation and report, unilateral or bilateral
EXCLUDES *Imaging of anterior segment with specular microscopy and endothelial cell analysis (92286)*
Scanning computerized ophthalmic diagnostic imaging of optic nerve and retina (92133-92134)
Tear film imaging (0330T)
📇 0.89 ⚕ 0.89 **FUD** XXX   Q1 80 ▭
AMA: 2018,Feb,11; 2018,Jan,8; 2017,Jan,8; 2016,Jan,13; 2015,Jan,16; 2014,May,5; 2014,Jan,11

92133 Scanning computerized ophthalmic diagnostic imaging, posterior segment, with interpretation and report, unilateral or bilateral; optic nerve
EXCLUDES *Remote imaging for retinal disease (92227-92228)*
Scanning computerized ophthalmic imaging of retina at same visit (92134)
📇 1.05 ⚕ 1.05 **FUD** XXX   Q1 80 ▭
AMA: 2018,Feb,11; 2018,Jan,8; 2017,Jan,8; 2016,Jan,13; 2015,Jan,16; 2014,Nov,10; 2014,Jan,11

92134 retina
EXCLUDES *Remote imaging for retinal disease (92227-92228)*
Scanning computerized ophthalmic imaging of optic nerve at same visit (92133)
📇 1.16 ⚕ 1.16 **FUD** XXX   Q1 80 ▭
AMA: 2018,Feb,11; 2018,Jan,8; 2017,Jan,8; 2016,Jan,13; 2015,Jan,16; 2014,Nov,10; 2014,Jan,11

92136 Ophthalmic biometry by partial coherence interferometry with intraocular lens power calculation
EXCLUDES *Tear film imaging (0330T)*
📇 1.98 ⚕ 1.98 **FUD** XXX   Q1 80 ▭
AMA: 2018,Feb,11; 2018,Jan,8; 2017,Jan,8; 2016,Jan,13; 2015,Jan,16; 2014,May,5; 2014,Jan,11

92145 Corneal hysteresis determination, by air impulse stimulation, unilateral or bilateral, with interpretation and report
📇 0.49 ⚕ 0.49 **FUD** XXX   Q1 80 ▭
AMA: 2018,Feb,11

92201-92287 Other Ophthalmology Services
EXCLUDES *Prescription, fitting, and/or medical supervision of ocular prosthesis adaptation by physician (99201-99215, 99241-99245, 92002-92014)*

● **92201** Ophthalmoscopy, extended; with retinal drawing and scleral depression of peripheral retinal disease (eg, for retinal tear, retinal detachment, retinal tumor) with interpretation and report, unilateral or bilateral
EXCLUDES *Fundus photography with interpretation and report (92250)*

26/TC PC/TC Only   N2-Z3 ASC Payment   50 Bilateral   ♂ Male Only   ♀ Female Only   📇 Facility RVU   ⚕ Non-Facility RVU   ▭ CCI   ✖ CLIA
FUD Follow-up Days   **CMS:** IOM   **AMA:** CPT Asst   A-Y OPPSI   80/80 Surg Assist Allowed / w/Doc   ▣ Lab Crosswalk   ▣ Radiology Crosswalk

470   CPT © 2019 American Medical Association. All Rights Reserved.   © 2019 Optum360, LLC

● **92202** with drawing of optic nerve or macula (eg, for glaucoma, macular pathology, tumor) with interpretation and report, unilateral or bilateral

> EXCLUDES *Fundus photography with interpretation and report (92250)*

~~**92225** Ophthalmoscopy, extended, with retinal drawing (eg, for retinal detachment, melanoma), with interpretation and report; initial~~

> To report, see (92201-92202)

~~**92226** subsequent~~

> To report, see (92201-92202)

92227 Remote imaging for detection of retinal disease (eg, retinopathy in a patient with diabetes) with analysis and report under physician supervision, unilateral or bilateral

> EXCLUDES *When services provided with E&M services as part of a single organ system or (92002-92014, 92133-92134, 92228, 92250)*

📷 0.40 🔁 0.40 **FUD** XXX ★ Q1 80 TC 💻

AMA: 2019,Aug,10; 2018,Feb,11; 2018,Jan,8; 2017,Jan,8; 2016,Jul,8; 2016,Jan,13; 2015,Jan,16; 2014,Jan,11

92228 Remote imaging for monitoring and management of active retinal disease (eg, diabetic retinopathy) with physician review, interpretation and report, unilateral or bilateral

> EXCLUDES *When services provided with E&M services as part of a single organ system or (92002-92014, 92133-92134, 92227, 92250)*

📷 0.97 🔁 0.97 **FUD** XXX ★ Q1 80 💻

AMA: 2018,Feb,11; 2018,Jan,8; 2017,Jan,8; 2016,Jan,13; 2015,Jan,16; 2014,Jan,11

92230 Fluorescein angioscopy with interpretation and report

📷 0.95 🔁 1.83 **FUD** XXX Q1 80 💻

AMA: 2018,Feb,11; 2018,Jan,8; 2017,Jan,8; 2016,Jan,13; 2015,Jan,16; 2014,Jan,11

92235 Fluorescein angiography (includes multiframe imaging) with interpretation and report, unilateral or bilateral

> EXCLUDES *Fluorescein and indocyanine-green angiography (92242)*

📷 2.59 🔁 2.59 **FUD** XXX S 80 💻

AMA: 2018,Feb,11; 2018,Jan,8; 2017,Jun,8; 2017,Jan,8; 2016,Jan,13; 2015,Jan,16; 2014,Jan,11

92240 Indocyanine-green angiography (includes multiframe imaging) with interpretation and report, unilateral or bilateral

> EXCLUDES *Fluorescein and indocyanine-green angiography (92242)*

📷 5.83 🔁 5.83 **FUD** XXX S 80 💻

AMA: 2018,Feb,11; 2018,Jan,8; 2017,Jun,8; 2017,Jan,8; 2016,Jan,13; 2015,Jan,16; 2014,Jan,11

92242 Fluorescein angiography and indocyanine-green angiography (includes multiframe imaging) performed at the same patient encounter with interpretation and report, unilateral or bilateral

📷 6.48 🔁 6.48 **FUD** XXX S 80 💻

AMA: 2018,Feb,11; 2018,Jan,8; 2017,Jun,8

92250 Fundus photography with interpretation and report

📷 1.43 🔁 1.43 **FUD** XXX Q1 80 💻

AMA: 2018,Feb,11; 2018,Jan,8; 2017,Jan,8; 2016,Jul,8; 2016,Jan,13; 2015,May,9; 2015,Jan,16; 2014,Dec,16; 2014,Dec,16; 2014,Nov,10; 2014,Jan,11

92260 Ophthalmodynamometry

📷 0.31 🔁 0.55 **FUD** XXX Q1 80 💻

AMA: 2018,Feb,11; 2018,Jan,8; 2017,Jan,8; 2016,Jan,13; 2015,Jan,16; 2014,Jan,11

92265 Needle oculoelectromyography, 1 or more extraocular muscles, 1 or both eyes, with interpretation and report

📷 2.48 🔁 2.48 **FUD** XXX Q1 80 💻

AMA: 2018,Feb,11; 2018,Jan,8; 2017,Jan,8; 2016,Jan,13; 2015,Jan,16; 2014,Jan,11

92270 Electro-oculography with interpretation and report

> EXCLUDES *Recording saccadic eye movement (92700)*
> *Vestibular function testing (92537-92538, 92540-92542, 92544-92549)*

📷 2.70 🔁 2.70 **FUD** XXX Q1 80 💻

AMA: 2018,Feb,11; 2018,Jan,8; 2017,Jan,8; 2016,Jan,13; 2015,Sep,7; 2015,Jan,16; 2014,Jan,11

92273 Electroretinography (ERG), with interpretation and report; full field (ie, ffERG, flash ERG, Ganzfeld ERG)

📷 3.78 🔁 3.78 **FUD** XXX 80 💻

AMA: 2019,Jan,12

92274 multifocal (mfERG)

📷 2.56 🔁 2.56 **FUD** XXX 80 💻

AMA: 2019,Jan,12

92283 Color vision examination, extended, eg, anomaloscope or equivalent

📷 1.52 🔁 1.52 **FUD** XXX Q1 80 💻

AMA: 2018,Feb,11; 2018,Jan,8; 2017,Jan,8; 2016,Jan,13; 2015,Jan,16; 2014,Jan,11

92284 Dark adaptation examination with interpretation and report

📷 1.74 🔁 1.74 **FUD** XXX Q1 80 💻

AMA: 2018,Feb,11; 2018,Jan,8; 2017,Jan,8; 2016,Jan,13; 2015,Jan,16; 2014,Jan,11

92285 External ocular photography with interpretation and report for documentation of medical progress (eg, close-up photography, slit lamp photography, goniophotography, stereo-photography)

📷 0.61 🔁 0.61 **FUD** XXX Q1 80 💻

AMA: 2018,Feb,11; 2018,Jan,8; 2017,Jan,8; 2016,Jan,13; 2015,Jan,16; 2014,May,5; 2014,Jan,11

92286 Anterior segment imaging with interpretation and report; with specular microscopy and endothelial cell analysis

📷 1.10 🔁 1.10 **FUD** XXX Q1 80 💻

AMA: 2018,Feb,11; 2018,Jan,8; 2017,Jan,8; 2016,Jan,13; 2015,Jan,16; 2014,Jan,11

92287 with fluorescein angiography

📷 4.13 🔁 4.13 **FUD** XXX Q1 80 💻

AMA: 2018,Feb,11; 2018,Jan,8; 2017,Jan,8; 2016,Jan,13; 2015,Jan,16; 2014,Jan,11

92310-92326 Services Related to Contact Lenses

CMS: 100-02,15,30.4 Optometrist's Services

> INCLUDES Incidental revision of lens during training period
> Patient training/instruction
> Specification of optical/physical characteristics:
> Curvature
> Flexibility
> Gas-permeability
> Power
> Size

> EXCLUDES *Extended wear lenses follow up (92012-92014)*
> *General ophthalmological services*
> *Therapeutic/surgical use of contact lens (68340, 92071-92072)*

92310 Prescription of optical and physical characteristics of and fitting of contact lens, with medical supervision of adaptation; corneal lens, both eyes, except for aphakia

📷 1.69 🔁 2.80 **FUD** XXX E 💻

AMA: 2018,Feb,11; 2018,Jan,8; 2017,Jan,8; 2016,Jan,13; 2015,Jan,16; 2014,Jan,11

92311 corneal lens for aphakia, 1 eye

📷 1.57 🔁 2.94 **FUD** XXX Q1 80 💻

AMA: 2018,Feb,11; 2018,Jan,8; 2017,Jan,8; 2016,Jan,13; 2015,Jan,16; 2014,Jan,11

92312 corneal lens for aphakia, both eyes

📷 1.81 🔁 3.40 **FUD** XXX Q1 80 💻

AMA: 2018,Feb,11; 2018,Jan,8; 2017,Jan,8; 2016,Jan,13; 2015,Jan,16; 2014,Jan,11

Medicine

92313 — 92516

92313 corneoscleral lens

1.31 2.78 FUD XXX 01 80

AMA: 2018,Feb,11; 2018,Jan,8; 2017,Jan,8; 2016,Jan,13; 2015,Jan,16; 2014,Jan,11

92314 Prescription of optical and physical characteristics of contact lens, with medical supervision of adaptation and direction of fitting by independent technician; corneal lens, both eyes except for aphakia

1.00 2.36 FUD XXX E

AMA: 2018,Feb,11; 2018,Jan,8; 2017,Jan,8; 2016,Jan,13; 2015,Jan,16; 2014,Jan,11

92315 corneal lens for aphakia, 1 eye

0.62 2.19 FUD XXX 01 80

AMA: 2018,Feb,11; 2018,Jan,8; 2017,Jan,8; 2016,Jan,13; 2015,Jan,16; 2014,Jan,11

92316 corneal lens for aphakia, both eyes

0.93 2.72 FUD XXX 01 80

AMA: 2018,Feb,11; 2018,Jan,8; 2017,Jan,8; 2016,Jan,13; 2015,Jan,16; 2014,Jan,11

92317 corneoscleral lens

0.62 2.29 FUD XXX 01 80

AMA: 2018,Feb,11; 2018,Jan,8; 2017,Jan,8; 2016,Jan,13; 2015,Jan,16; 2014,Jan,11

92325 Modification of contact lens (separate procedure), with medical supervision of adaptation

1.24 1.24 FUD XXX 01 80

AMA: 2018,Feb,11; 2018,Jan,8; 2017,Jan,8; 2016,Jan,13; 2015,Jan,16; 2014,Jan,11

92326 Replacement of contact lens

1.05 1.05 FUD XXX 01 80

AMA: 2018,Feb,11; 2018,Jan,8; 2017,Jan,8; 2016,Jan,13; 2015,Jan,16; 2014,Jan,11

92340-92499 Services Related to Eyeglasses

CMS: 100-02,15,30.4 Optometrist's Services

INCLUDES Anatomical facial characteristics measurement
Final adjustment of spectacles to visual axes/anatomical topography
Written laboratory specifications
EXCLUDES Supply of materials

92340 Fitting of spectacles, except for aphakia; monofocal

0.53 0.99 FUD XXX E

AMA: 2018,Feb,11; 2018,Jan,8; 2017,Jan,8; 2016,Jan,13; 2015,Jan,16; 2014,Jan,11

92341 bifocal

0.68 1.14 FUD XXX E

AMA: 2018,Feb,11; 2018,Jan,8; 2017,Jan,8; 2016,Jan,13; 2015,Jan,16; 2014,Jan,11

92342 multifocal, other than bifocal

0.77 1.23 FUD XXX E

AMA: 2018,Feb,11; 2018,Jan,8; 2017,Jan,8; 2016,Jan,13; 2015,Jan,16; 2014,Jan,11

92352 Fitting of spectacle prosthesis for aphakia; monofocal

0.53 1.17 FUD XXX 01

AMA: 2018,Feb,11; 2018,Jan,8; 2017,Jan,8; 2016,Jan,13; 2015,Jan,16; 2014,Jan,11

92353 multifocal

0.72 1.36 FUD XXX 01

AMA: 2018,Feb,11; 2018,Jan,8; 2017,Jan,8; 2016,Jan,13; 2015,Jan,16; 2014,Jan,11

92354 Fitting of spectacle mounted low vision aid; single element system

0.38 0.38 FUD XXX 01

AMA: 2018,Feb,11; 2018,Jan,8; 2017,Jan,8; 2016,Jan,13; 2015,Jan,16; 2014,Jan,11

92355 telescopic or other compound lens system

0.59 0.59 FUD XXX 01

AMA: 2018,Feb,11; 2018,Jan,8; 2017,Jan,8; 2016,Jan,13; 2015,Jan,16; 2014,Jan,11

92358 Prosthesis service for aphakia, temporary (disposable or loan, including materials)

0.32 0.32 FUD XXX 01

AMA: 2018,Feb,11; 2018,Jan,8; 2017,Jan,8; 2016,Jan,13; 2015,Jan,16; 2014,Jan,11

92370 Repair and refitting spectacles; except for aphakia

0.46 0.88 FUD XXX E

AMA: 2018,Feb,11; 2018,Jan,8; 2017,Jan,8; 2016,Jan,13; 2015,Jan,16; 2014,Jan,11

92371 spectacle prosthesis for aphakia

0.33 0.33 FUD XXX 01

AMA: 2018,Feb,11; 2018,Jan,8; 2017,Jan,8; 2016,Jan,13; 2015,Jan,16; 2014,Jan,11

92499 Unlisted ophthalmological service or procedure

0.00 0.00 FUD XXX 01 80

AMA: 2019,Jan,12; 2018,Jul,3; 2018,Feb,11; 2018,Jan,8; 2017,Jan,8; 2016,Jan,13; 2015,Jan,16; 2014,Jan,11

92502-92526 Special Procedures of the Ears/Nose/Throat

INCLUDES Anterior rhinoscopy, tuning fork testing, otoscopy, or removal non-impacted cerumen
Diagnostic/treatment services not generally included in an E&M service
EXCLUDES Laryngoscopy with stroboscopy (31579)

92502 Otolaryngologic examination under general anesthesia

2.73 2.73 FUD 000 T 80

AMA: 2018,Feb,11; 2018,Jan,8; 2017,Jan,8; 2016,Sep,6

92504 Binocular microscopy (separate diagnostic procedure)

0.27 0.83 FUD XXX N 80

AMA: 2018,Feb,11; 2018,Jan,8; 2017,Jan,8; 2016,Sep,6; 2016,Jan,13; 2015,Jan,16; 2014,Jan,11

92507 Treatment of speech, language, voice, communication, and/or auditory processing disorder; individual

EXCLUDES Adaptive behavior treatment ([97153], [97155])
Auditory rehabilitation:
Postlingual hearing loss (92633)
Prelingual hearing loss (92630)
Programming of cochlear implant (92601-92604)

2.23 2.23 FUD XXX A 80

AMA: 2018,Dec,7; 2018,Dec,7; 2018,Nov,3; 2018,Feb,11; 2018,Jan,8; 2017,Jan,8; 2016,Sep,6; 2016,Jan,13; 2015,Jan,16; 2014,Jan,11

92508 group, 2 or more individuals

EXCLUDES Adaptive behavior treatment ([97154], [97158])
Auditory rehabilitation:
Postlingual hearing loss (92633)
Prelingual hearing loss (92630)
Programming of cochlear implant (92601-92604)

0.67 0.67 FUD XXX A 80

AMA: 2018,Nov,3; 2018,Feb,11; 2018,Jan,8; 2017,Jan,8; 2016,Sep,6; 2016,Jan,13; 2015,Jan,16; 2014,Jun,3; 2014,Jan,11

92511 Nasopharyngoscopy with endoscope (separate procedure)

EXCLUDES Diagnostic flexible laryngoscopy (31575)
Transnasal esophagoscopy (43197-43198)

1.08 3.15 FUD 000 T 80

AMA: 2018,Feb,11; 2018,Jan,8; 2017,Jul,7; 2017,Jan,8; 2016,Dec,13; 2016,Sep,6

92512 Nasal function studies (eg, rhinomanometry)

0.80 1.68 FUD XXX S 80

AMA: 2018,Feb,11; 2018,Jan,8; 2017,Jan,8; 2016,Sep,6

92516 Facial nerve function studies (eg, electroneuronography)

0.65 1.94 FUD XXX S 80

AMA: 2018,Feb,11; 2018,Jan,8; 2017,Jan,8; 2016,Sep,6

26/TC PC/TC Only   A2-Z3 ASC Payment   50 Bilateral   ♂ Male Only   ♀ Female Only   Facility RVU   Non-Facility RVU   CCI   CLIA
FUD Follow-up Days   CMS: IOM   AMA: CPT Asst   A-Y OPPSI   80/80 Surg Assist Allowed / w/Doc   Lab Crosswalk   Radiology Crosswalk

92520 **Laryngeal function studies (ie, aerodynamic testing and acoustic testing)**

> EXCLUDES *Other laryngeal function testing (92700)*
> *Swallowing/laryngeal sensory testing with flexible fiberoptic endoscope (92611-92617)*
> Code also modifier 52 for single test

🚑 1.15   𝔈 2.23   **FUD** XXX   [01] [80] ▣

AMA: 2018,Feb,11; 2018,Jan,8; 2017,Jan,8; 2016,Sep,6; 2016,Jan,13; 2015,Jan,16; 2014,Jan,11

92521 **Evaluation of speech fluency (eg, stuttering, cluttering)**

> INCLUDES Ability to execute motor movements needed for speech
> Comprehension of written and verbal expression
> Determination of patient's ability to create and communicate expressive thought
> Evaluation of the ability to produce speech sound

🚑 3.21   𝔈 3.21   **FUD** XXX   [A] [80] ▣

AMA: 2018,Feb,11; 2018,Jan,8; 2017,Jan,8; 2016,Sep,6; 2016,Jan,13; 2015,Jan,16; 2014,Jun,3

92522 **Evaluation of speech sound production (eg, articulation, phonological process, apraxia, dysarthria);**

> INCLUDES Ability to execute motor movements needed for speech
> Comprehension of written and verbal expression
> Determination of patient's ability to create and communicate expressive thought
> Evaluation of the ability to produce speech sound

🚑 2.60   𝔈 2.60   **FUD** XXX   [A] [80] ▣

AMA: 2018,Feb,11; 2018,Jan,8; 2017,Jan,8; 2016,Sep,6; 2016,Jan,13; 2015,Jan,16; 2014,Jun,3

92523 **with evaluation of language comprehension and expression (eg, receptive and expressive language)**

> INCLUDES Ability to execute motor movements needed for speech
> Comprehension of written and verbal expression
> Determination of patient's ability to create and communicate expressive thought
> Evaluation of the ability to produce speech sound

🚑 5.54   𝔈 5.54   **FUD** XXX   [A] [80] ▣

AMA: 2018,Feb,11; 2018,Jan,8; 2017,Jan,8; 2016,Sep,6; 2016,Jan,13; 2015,Jan,16; 2014,Jun,3

92524 **Behavioral and qualitative analysis of voice and resonance**

> INCLUDES Ability to execute motor movements needed for speech
> Comprehension of written and verbal expression
> Determination of patient's ability to create and communicate expressive thought
> Evaluation of the ability to produce speech sound

🚑 2.51   𝔈 2.51   **FUD** XXX   [A] [80] ▣

AMA: 2018,Feb,11; 2018,Jan,8; 2017,Jan,8; 2016,Sep,6; 2016,Jan,13; 2015,Jan,16; 2014,Jun,3

92526 **Treatment of swallowing dysfunction and/or oral function for feeding**

🚑 2.44   𝔈 2.44   **FUD** XXX   [A] [80] ▣

AMA: 2018,Feb,11; 2018,Jan,8; 2017,Jan,8; 2016,Sep,6

92531-92549 Vestibular Function Tests

92531 **Spontaneous nystagmus, including gaze**

> EXCLUDES *When performed with E&M services (99201-99215, 99218-99223 [99224, 99225, 99226], 99231-99236, 99241-99245, 99304-99318, 99324-99337)*

🚑 0.00   𝔈 0.00   **FUD** XXX   [N] ▣

AMA: 2018,Feb,11

92532 **Positional nystagmus test**

> EXCLUDES *When performed with E&M services (99201-99215, 99218-99223 [99224, 99225, 99226], 99231-99236, 99241-99245, 99304-99318, 99324-99337)*

🚑 0.00   𝔈 0.00   **FUD** XXX   [N] ▣

AMA: 2018,Feb,11

92533 **Caloric vestibular test, each irrigation (binaural, bithermal stimulation constitutes 4 tests)**

> INCLUDES Barany caloric test

🚑 0.00   𝔈 0.00   **FUD** XXX   [N] ▣

AMA: 2018,Feb,11; 2018,Jan,8; 2017,Jan,8; 2016,Jan,13; 2015,Jan,16; 2014,Jan,11

92534 **Optokinetic nystagmus test**

🚑 0.00   𝔈 0.00   **FUD** XXX   [N] ▣

AMA: 2018,Feb,11

92537 **Caloric vestibular test with recording, bilateral; bithermal (ie, one warm and one cool irrigation in each ear for a total of four irrigations)**

> EXCLUDES *Electro-oculography (92270)*
> *Monothermal caloric vestibular test (92538)*
> Code also modifier 52 when only three irrigations are performed

🚑 1.16   𝔈 1.16   **FUD** XXX   [S] [80] ▣

AMA: 2018,Feb,11; 2015,Sep,7

92538 **monothermal (ie, one irrigation in each ear for a total of two irrigations)**

> EXCLUDES *Electro-oculography (92270)*
> *Monothermal caloric vestibular test (92538)*
> Code also modifier 52 if only one irrigation is performed

🚑 0.60   𝔈 0.60   **FUD** XXX   [S] [80] ▣

AMA: 2018,Feb,11; 2015,Sep,7

92540 **Basic vestibular evaluation, includes spontaneous nystagmus test with eccentric gaze fixation nystagmus, with recording, positional nystagmus test, minimum of 4 positions, with recording, optokinetic nystagmus test, bidirectional foveal and peripheral stimulation, with recording, and oscillating tracking test, with recording**

> EXCLUDES *Vestibular function tests (92270, 92541-92542, 92544-92545)*

🚑 2.95   𝔈 2.95   **FUD** XXX   [S] [80] ▣

AMA: 2018,Feb,11; 2018,Jan,8; 2017,Jan,8; 2016,Jan,13; 2015,Sep,7

92541 **Spontaneous nystagmus test, including gaze and fixation nystagmus, with recording**

> EXCLUDES *Vestibular function tests (92270, 92540, 92542, 92544-92545)*

🚑 0.71   𝔈 0.71   **FUD** XXX   [01] [80] ▣

AMA: 2019,Jan,12; 2018,Feb,11; 2018,Jan,8; 2017,Jan,8; 2016,Jan,13; 2015,Sep,7; 2015,Jan,16; 2014,Jan,11

92542 **Positional nystagmus test, minimum of 4 positions, with recording**

> EXCLUDES *Vestibular function tests (92270, 92540-92541, 92544-92545)*

🚑 0.82   𝔈 0.82   **FUD** XXX   [01] [80] ▣

AMA: 2018,Feb,11; 2018,Jan,8; 2017,Jan,8; 2016,Jan,13; 2015,Sep,7; 2015,Jan,16; 2014,Jan,11

92544 **Optokinetic nystagmus test, bidirectional, foveal or peripheral stimulation, with recording**

> EXCLUDES *Vestibular function tests (92270, 92540-92542, 92545)*

🚑 0.49   𝔈 0.49   **FUD** XXX   [S] [80] ▣

AMA: 2018,Feb,11; 2018,Jan,8; 2017,Jan,8; 2016,Jan,13; 2015,Sep,7; 2015,Jan,16; 2014,Jan,11

92545 **Oscillating tracking test, with recording**

> EXCLUDES *Vestibular function tests (92270, 92540-92542, 92544)*

🚑 0.46   𝔈 0.46   **FUD** XXX   [S] [80] ▣

AMA: 2018,Feb,11; 2018,Jan,8; 2017,Jan,8; 2016,Jan,13; 2015,Sep,7; 2015,Jan,16; 2014,Jan,11

92546 **Sinusoidal vertical axis rotational testing**

> EXCLUDES *Electro-oculography (92270)*

🚑 2.95   𝔈 2.95   **FUD** XXX   [S] [80] ▣

AMA: 2018,Feb,11; 2018,Jan,8; 2017,Jan,8; 2016,Jan,13; 2015,Sep,7; 2015,Jan,16; 2014,Jan,11

+ **92547** **Use of vertical electrodes (List separately in addition to code for primary procedure)**

EXCLUDES Electro-oculography (92700)

Code first (92540-92546)

🚑 0.21 ⚖ 0.21 **FUD** ZZZ [N] [80] [TC] [▫]

AMA: 2018,Feb,11; 2018,Jan,8; 2017,Jan,8; 2016,Jan,13; 2015,Sep,7; 2015,Jan,16; 2014,Jan,11

▲ **92548** **Computerized dynamic posturography sensory organization test (CDP-SOT), 6 conditions (ie, eyes open, eyes closed, visual sway, platform sway, eyes closed platform sway, platform and visual sway), including interpretation and report;**

EXCLUDES Electro-oculography (92270)

🚑 2.72 ⚖ 2.72 **FUD** XXX [01] [80] [▫]

AMA: 2018,Feb,11; 2018,Jan,8; 2017,Jan,8; 2016,Jan,13; 2015,Sep,7; 2015,Jan,16; 2014,Jan,11

● **92549** **with motor control test (MCT) and adaptation test (ADT)**

EXCLUDES Electro-oculography (92270)

92550-92597 [92558] Hearing and Speech Tests

INCLUDES Diagnostic/treatment services not generally included in a comprehensive otorhinolaryngologic evaluation or office visit
Testing of both ears
Tuning fork and whisper tests
Use of calibrated electronic equipment, recording of results, and a report with interpretation

EXCLUDES Evaluation of speech/language/hearing problems using observation/assessment of performance (92521-92524)

Code also modifier 52 for unilateral testing

92550 **Tympanometry and reflex threshold measurements**

INCLUDES Tympanometry, acoustic reflex testing individual codes (92567-92568)

🚑 0.62 ⚖ 0.62 **FUD** XXX [01] [80] [▫]

AMA: 2018,Feb,11; 2018,Jan,8; 2017,Jan,8; 2016,Jan,13; 2015,Jan,16; 2014,Aug,3

92551 **Screening test, pure tone, air only**

🚑 0.33 ⚖ 0.33 **FUD** XXX [E] [▫]

AMA: 2018,Feb,11; 2018,Jan,8; 2017,Jan,8; 2016,Jan,13; 2015,Jan,16; 2014,Aug,3

92552 **Pure tone audiometry (threshold); air only**

EXCLUDES Automated test (0208T)

🚑 0.89 ⚖ 0.89 **FUD** XXX [01] [80] [TC] [▫]

AMA: 2018,Feb,11; 2018,Jan,8; 2017,Jan,8; 2016,Jan,13; 2015,Jan,16; 2014,Aug,3

92553 **air and bone**

EXCLUDES Automated test (0209T)

🚑 1.08 ⚖ 1.08 **FUD** XXX [01] [80] [TC] [▫]

AMA: 2018,Feb,11; 2018,Jan,8; 2017,Jan,8; 2016,Jan,13; 2015,Jan,16; 2014,Aug,3; 2014,Jan,11

92555 **Speech audiometry threshold;**

EXCLUDES Automated test (0210T)

🚑 0.68 ⚖ 0.68 **FUD** XXX [01] [80] [TC] [▫]

AMA: 2018,Feb,11; 2018,Jan,8; 2017,Jan,8; 2016,Jan,13; 2015,Jan,16; 2014,Aug,3

92556 **with speech recognition**

EXCLUDES Automated test (0211T)

🚑 1.07 ⚖ 1.07 **FUD** XXX [01] [80] [TC] [▫]

AMA: 2018,Feb,11; 2018,Jan,8; 2017,Jan,8; 2016,Jan,13; 2015,Jan,16; 2014,Aug,3; 2014,Jan,11

92557 **Comprehensive audiometry threshold evaluation and speech recognition (92553 and 92556 combined)**

EXCLUDES Automated test (0208T-0212T)
Evaluation/selection of hearing aid (92590-92595)

🚑 0.93 ⚖ 1.08 **FUD** XXX [01] [80] [▫]

AMA: 2018,Feb,11; 2018,Jan,8; 2017,Jan,8; 2016,Jan,13; 2015,Jan,16; 2014,Aug,3; 2014,Jan,11

92558 **Resequenced code. See code following 92586.**

92559 **Audiometric testing of groups**

INCLUDES For group testing, indicate tests performed

🚑 0.00 ⚖ 0.00 **FUD** XXX [E] [▫]

AMA: 2018,Feb,11; 2018,Jan,8; 2017,Jan,8; 2016,Jan,13; 2015,Jan,16; 2014,Aug,3

92560 **Bekesy audiometry; screening**

🚑 0.00 ⚖ 0.00 **FUD** XXX [E] [▫]

AMA: 2018,Feb,11; 2018,Jan,8; 2017,Jan,8; 2016,Jan,13; 2015,Jan,16; 2014,Aug,3

92561 **diagnostic**

🚑 1.10 ⚖ 1.10 **FUD** XXX [01] [80] [TC] [▫]

AMA: 2018,Feb,11; 2018,Jan,8; 2017,Jan,8; 2016,Jan,13; 2015,Jan,16; 2014,Aug,3

92562 **Loudness balance test, alternate binaural or monaural**

INCLUDES ABLB test

🚑 1.28 ⚖ 1.28 **FUD** XXX [01] [80] [TC] [▫]

AMA: 2018,Feb,11; 2018,Jan,8; 2017,Jan,8; 2016,Jan,13; 2015,Jan,16; 2014,Aug,3

92563 **Tone decay test**

🚑 0.87 ⚖ 0.87 **FUD** XXX [01] [80] [TC] [▫]

AMA: 2018,Feb,11; 2018,Jan,8; 2017,Jan,8; 2016,Jan,13; 2015,Jan,16; 2014,Aug,3

92564 **Short increment sensitivity index (SISI)**

🚑 0.71 ⚖ 0.71 **FUD** XXX [01] [80] [TC] [▫]

AMA: 2018,Feb,11; 2018,Jan,8; 2017,Jan,8; 2016,Jan,13; 2015,Jan,16; 2014,Aug,3; 2014,Jan,11

92565 **Stenger test, pure tone**

🚑 0.43 ⚖ 0.43 **FUD** XXX [01] [80] [TC] [▫]

AMA: 2018,Feb,11; 2018,Jan,8; 2017,Jan,8; 2016,Jan,13; 2015,Jan,16; 2014,Aug,3

92567 **Tympanometry (impedance testing)**

🚑 0.31 ⚖ 0.43 **FUD** XXX [01] [80] [▫]

AMA: 2018,Feb,11; 2018,Jan,8; 2017,Jan,8; 2016,Jan,13; 2015,Jan,16; 2014,Aug,3; 2014,Jan,11

92568 **Acoustic reflex testing, threshold**

🚑 0.44 ⚖ 0.45 **FUD** XXX [01] [80] [▫]

AMA: 2018,Feb,11; 2018,Jan,8; 2017,Jan,8; 2016,Jan,13; 2015,Jan,16; 2014,Aug,3; 2014,Jan,11

92570 **Acoustic immittance testing, includes tympanometry (impedance testing), acoustic reflex threshold testing, and acoustic reflex decay testing**

INCLUDES Tympanometry, acoustic reflex testing individual codes (92567-92568)

🚑 0.85 ⚖ 0.92 **FUD** XXX [01] [80] [▫]

AMA: 2018,Feb,11; 2018,Jan,8; 2017,Jan,8; 2016,Jan,13; 2015,Jan,16; 2014,Aug,3

92571 **Filtered speech test**

🚑 0.76 ⚖ 0.76 **FUD** XXX [01] [80] [TC] [▫]

AMA: 2018,Feb,11; 2018,Jan,8; 2017,Jan,8; 2016,Jan,13; 2015,Jan,16; 2014,Aug,3; 2014,Jan,11

92572 **Staggered spondaic word test**

🚑 1.21 ⚖ 1.21 **FUD** XXX [01] [80] [TC] [▫]

AMA: 2018,Feb,11; 2018,Jan,8; 2017,Jan,8; 2016,Jan,13; 2015,Jan,16; 2014,Aug,3; 2014,Jan,11

92575 **Sensorineural acuity level test**

🚑 1.79 ⚖ 1.79 **FUD** XXX [01] [80] [TC] [▫]

AMA: 2018,Feb,11; 2018,Jan,8; 2017,Jan,8; 2016,Jan,13; 2015,Jan,16; 2014,Aug,3

92576 **Synthetic sentence identification test**

🚑 1.03 ⚖ 1.03 **FUD** XXX [01] [80] [TC] [▫]

AMA: 2018,Feb,11; 2018,Jan,8; 2017,Jan,8; 2016,Jan,13; 2015,Jan,16; 2014,Aug,3; 2014,Jan,11

92577 **Stenger test, speech**

🚑 0.39 ⚖ 0.39 **FUD** XXX [01] [80] [TC] [▫]

AMA: 2018,Feb,11; 2018,Jan,8; 2017,Jan,8; 2016,Jan,13; 2015,Jan,16; 2014,Aug,3

92579 Visual reinforcement audiometry (VRA)

🚗 1.09   ⚖ 1.31   **FUD** XXX   `01` `80` 🖥

AMA: 2018,Feb,11; 2018,Jan,8; 2017,Jan,8; 2016,Jan,13; 2015,Jan,16; 2014,Aug,3

92582 Conditioning play audiometry

🚗 2.06   ⚖ 2.06   **FUD** XXX   `01` `80` `TC` 🖥

AMA: 2018,Feb,11; 2018,Jan,8; 2017,Jan,8; 2016,Jan,13; 2015,Jan,16; 2014,Aug,3

92583 Select picture audiometry

🚗 1.35   ⚖ 1.35   **FUD** XXX   `01` `80` `TC` 🖥

AMA: 2018,Feb,11; 2018,Jan,8; 2017,Jan,8; 2016,Jan,13; 2015,Jan,16; 2014,Aug,3

92584 Electrocochleography

🚗 2.09   ⚖ 2.09   **FUD** XXX   `S` `80` `TC` 🖥

AMA: 2018,Feb,11; 2018,Jan,8; 2017,Jan,8; 2016,Jan,13; 2015,Jan,16; 2014,Aug,3; 2014,Jan,11

92585 Auditory evoked potentials for evoked response audiometry and/or testing of the central nervous system; comprehensive

🚗 3.81   ⚖ 3.81   **FUD** XXX   `S` `80` 🖥

AMA: 2018,Feb,11; 2018,Jan,8; 2017,Jan,8; 2016,Jan,13; 2015,Jan,16; 2014,Aug,3

92586 limited

🚗 2.61   ⚖ 2.61   **FUD** XXX   `S` `80` `TC` 🖥

AMA: 2018,Feb,11; 2018,Jan,8; 2017,Jan,8; 2016,Jan,13; 2015,Jan,16; 2014,Aug,3

92558 Evoked otoacoustic emissions, screening (qualitative measurement of distortion product or transient evoked otoacoustic emissions), automated analysis

🚗 0.25   ⚖ 0.28   **FUD** XXX   `E` 🖥

AMA: 2018,Feb,11; 2018,Jan,8; 2017,Jan,8; 2016,Jan,13; 2015,Jan,16; 2014,Aug,3

92587 Distortion product evoked otoacoustic emissions; limited evaluation (to confirm the presence or absence of hearing disorder, 3-6 frequencies) or transient evoked otoacoustic emissions, with interpretation and report

🚗 0.62   ⚖ 0.62   **FUD** XXX   `S` `80` 🖥

AMA: 2018,Feb,11; 2018,Jan,8; 2017,Jan,8; 2016,Jan,13; 2015,Jan,16; 2014,Aug,3; 2014,Jan,11

92588 comprehensive diagnostic evaluation (quantitative analysis of outer hair cell function by cochlear mapping, minimum of 12 frequencies), with interpretation and report

EXCLUDES   *Evaluation of central auditory function (92620-92621)*

🚗 0.94   ⚖ 0.94   **FUD** XXX   `S` `80` 🖥

AMA: 2018,Feb,11; 2018,Jan,8; 2017,Jan,8; 2016,Jan,13; 2015,Jan,16; 2014,Aug,3

92590 Hearing aid examination and selection; monaural

🚗 0.00   ⚖ 0.00   **FUD** XXX   `E` 🖥

AMA: 2018,Feb,11; 2018,Jan,8; 2017,Jan,8; 2016,Jan,13; 2015,Jan,16; 2014,Aug,3; 2014,Jul,4

92591 binaural

🚗 0.00   ⚖ 0.00   **FUD** XXX   `E` 🖥

AMA: 2018,Feb,11; 2018,Jan,8; 2017,Jan,8; 2016,Jan,13; 2015,Jan,16; 2014,Aug,3

92592 Hearing aid check; monaural

🚗 0.00   ⚖ 0.00   **FUD** XXX   `E` 🖥

AMA: 2018,Feb,11; 2018,Jan,8; 2017,Jan,8; 2016,Jan,13; 2015,Jan,16; 2014,Aug,3

92593 binaural

🚗 0.00   ⚖ 0.00   **FUD** XXX   `E` 🖥

AMA: 2018,Feb,11; 2018,Jan,8; 2017,Jan,8; 2016,Jan,13; 2015,Jan,16; 2014,Aug,3

92594 Electroacoustic evaluation for hearing aid; monaural

🚗 0.00   ⚖ 0.00   **FUD** XXX   `E` 🖥

AMA: 2018,Feb,11; 2018,Jan,8; 2017,Jan,8; 2016,Jan,13; 2015,Jan,16; 2014,Aug,3

92595 binaural

🚗 0.00   ⚖ 0.00   **FUD** XXX   `E` 🖥

AMA: 2018,Feb,11; 2018,Jan,8; 2017,Jan,8; 2016,Jan,13; 2015,Jan,16; 2014,Aug,3

92596 Ear protector attenuation measurements

🚗 1.89   ⚖ 1.89   **FUD** XXX   `01` `80` `TC` 🖥

AMA: 2018,Feb,11; 2018,Jan,8; 2017,Jan,8; 2016,Jan,13; 2015,Jan,16; 2014,Aug,3

92597 Resequenced code. See code following 92604.

92601-92609 [92597, 92618] Services Related to Hearing and Speech Devices

INCLUDES   Diagnostic/treatment services not generally included in a comprehensive otorhinolaryngologic evaluation or office visit

92601 Diagnostic analysis of cochlear implant, patient younger than 7 years of age; with programming   `A`

INCLUDES   Connection to cochlear implant
   Postoperative analysis/fitting of previously placed external devices
   Stimulator programming

EXCLUDES   *Cochlear implant placement (69930)*

🚗 3.57   ⚖ 4.68   **FUD** XXX   `S` `80` 🖥

AMA: 2018,Feb,11; 2018,Jan,8; 2017,Jan,8; 2016,Sep,6; 2016,Jan,13; 2015,Jan,16; 2014,Jul,4; 2014,Jan,11

92602 subsequent reprogramming   `A`

INCLUDES   Internal stimulator re-programming
   Subsequent sessions for external transmitter measurements/adjustment

EXCLUDES   *Analysis with programming (92601)*
   Aural rehabilitation services after a cochlear implant (92626-92627, 92630-92633)
   Cochlear implant placement (69930)

🚗 2.02   ⚖ 2.92   **FUD** XXX   `S` `80` 🖥

AMA: 2018,Feb,11; 2018,Jan,8; 2017,Jan,8; 2016,Sep,6; 2016,Jan,13; 2015,Jan,16; 2014,Jul,4; 2014,Jan,11

92603 Diagnostic analysis of cochlear implant, age 7 years or older; with programming   `A`

INCLUDES   Connection to cochlear implant
   Post-operative analysis/fitting of previously placed external devices
   Stimulator programming

EXCLUDES   *Cochlear implant placement (69930)*

🚗 3.47   ⚖ 4.37   **FUD** XXX   `S` `80` 🖥

AMA: 2018,Feb,11; 2018,Jan,8; 2017,Jan,8; 2016,Sep,6; 2016,Jan,13; 2015,Jan,16; 2014,Jul,4; 2014,Jan,11

92604 subsequent reprogramming   `A`

INCLUDES   Internal stimulator re-programming
   Subsequent sessions for external transmitter measurements/adjustment

EXCLUDES   *Analysis with programming (92603)*
   Cochlear implant placement (69930)

🚗 1.94   ⚖ 2.60   **FUD** XXX   `S` `80` 🖥

AMA: 2018,Feb,11; 2018,Jan,8; 2017,Jan,8; 2016,Sep,6; 2016,Jan,13; 2015,Jan,16; 2014,Jul,4; 2014,Jan,11

92597 Evaluation for use and/or fitting of voice prosthetic device to supplement oral speech

EXCLUDES   *Augmentative or alternative communication device services (92605, [92618], 92607-92608)*

🚗 2.06   ⚖ 2.06   **FUD** XXX   `A` `80` 🖥

AMA: 2018,Feb,11; 2018,Jan,8; 2017,Jan,8; 2016,Jan,13; 2015,Jan,16; 2014,Jan,11

92605 Evaluation for prescription of non-speech-generating augmentative and alternative communication device, face-to-face with the patient; first hour

EXCLUDES   *Prosthetic voice device fitting or use evaluation (92597)*

🚗 2.53   ⚖ 2.65   **FUD** XXX   `A` 🖥

AMA: 2018,Feb,11; 2018,Jan,8; 2017,Jan,8; 2016,Jan,13; 2015,Jan,16; 2014,Jan,11

Medicine

92618 — 92626

+ # **92618** **each additional 30 minutes (List separately in addition to code for primary procedure)**
Code first (92605)
🔧 0.94   ⚷ 0.96   **FUD** ZZZ   Ⓐ ▭
AMA: 2018,Feb,11

92606 **Therapeutic service(s) for the use of non-speech-generating device, including programming and modification**
🔧 2.02   ⚷ 2.35   **FUD** XXX   Ⓐ ▭
AMA: 2018,Feb,11; 2018,Jan,8; 2017,Jan,8; 2016,Jan,13; 2015,Jan,16; 2014,Jan,11

92607 **Evaluation for prescription for speech-generating augmentative and alternative communication device, face-to-face with the patient; first hour**
EXCLUDES *Evaluation for prescription of non-speech generating device (92605)*
Evaluation for use/fitting of voice prosthetic (92597)
🔧 3.69   ⚷ 3.69   **FUD** XXX   Ⓐ 80 ▭
AMA: 2018,Feb,11; 2018,Jan,8; 2017,Jan,8; 2016,Jan,13; 2015,Jan,16; 2014,Jan,11

+ **92608** **each additional 30 minutes (List separately in addition to code for primary procedure)**
Code first initial hour (92607)
🔧 1.47   ⚷ 1.47   **FUD** ZZZ   Ⓐ 80 ▭
AMA: 2018,Feb,11; 2018,Jan,8; 2017,Jan,8; 2016,Jan,13; 2015,Jan,16; 2014,Jan,11

92609 **Therapeutic services for the use of speech-generating device, including programming and modification**
EXCLUDES *Therapeutic services for use of non-speech generating device (92606)*
🔧 3.08   ⚷ 3.08   **FUD** XXX   Ⓐ 80 ▭
AMA: 2018,Feb,11; 2018,Jan,8; 2017,Jan,8; 2016,Jan,13; 2015,Jan,16; 2014,Jan,11

92610-92618 Swallowing Evaluations

92610 **Evaluation of oral and pharyngeal swallowing function**
EXCLUDES *Evaluation with flexible endoscope (92612-92617)*
Motion fluoroscopic evaluation of swallowing function (92611)
🔧 2.06   ⚷ 2.45   **FUD** XXX   Ⓐ 80 ▭
AMA: 2018,Feb,11; 2018,Jan,8; 2017,Apr,8; 2017,Jan,8; 2016,Jan,13; 2015,Jan,16; 2014,Jan,11

92611 **Motion fluoroscopic evaluation of swallowing function by cine or video recording**
EXCLUDES *Diagnostic flexible laryngoscopy (31575)*
Evaluation of oral/pharyngeal swallowing function (92610)
🔁 (74230)
🔧 2.55   ⚷ 2.55   **FUD** XXX   Ⓐ 80 ▭
AMA: 2018,Feb,11; 2018,Jan,8; 2017,Apr,8; 2017,Jan,8; 2016,Sep,6; 2016,Jan,13; 2015,Jan,16; 2014,Jul,5; 2014,Jan,11

92612 **Flexible endoscopic evaluation of swallowing by cine or video recording;**
EXCLUDES *Diagnostic flexible fiberoptic laryngoscopy (31575)*
Flexible endoscopic examination/testing without cine or video recording (92700)
🔧 1.94   ⚷ 5.42   **FUD** XXX   Ⓐ 80 ▭
AMA: 2018,Feb,11; 2018,Jan,8; 2017,Jul,7; 2017,Apr,8; 2017,Jan,8; 2016,Dec,13; 2016,Sep,6; 2016,Jan,13; 2015,Jan,16; 2014,Jan,11

92613 **interpretation and report only**
EXCLUDES *Diagnostic flexible laryngoscopy (31575)*
Oral/pharyngeal swallowing function examination (92610)
Swallowing function motion fluoroscopic examination (92611)
🔧 1.07   ⚷ 1.07   **FUD** XXX   Ⓑ 80 ▭
AMA: 2018,Feb,11; 2018,Jan,8; 2017,Jul,7; 2017,Apr,8; 2017,Jan,8; 2016,Dec,13; 2016,Sep,6; 2016,Jan,13; 2015,Jan,16; 2014,Jan,11

92614 **Flexible endoscopic evaluation, laryngeal sensory testing by cine or video recording;**
EXCLUDES *Diagnostic flexible laryngoscopy (31575)*
Flexible endoscopic examination/testing without cine or video recording (92700)
🔧 1.90   ⚷ 4.03   **FUD** XXX   Ⓐ 80 ▭
AMA: 2018,Feb,11; 2018,Jan,8; 2017,Jul,7; 2017,Apr,8; 2017,Jan,8; 2016,Dec,13; 2016,Sep,6; 2016,Jan,13; 2015,Jan,16; 2014,Jan,11

92615 **interpretation and report only**
EXCLUDES *Diagnostic flexible laryngoscopy (31575)*
🔧 0.94   ⚷ 0.94   **FUD** XXX   Ⓔ 80 ▭
AMA: 2018,Feb,11; 2018,Jan,8; 2017,Jul,7; 2017,Apr,8; 2017,Jan,8; 2016,Dec,13; 2016,Sep,6; 2016,Jan,13; 2015,Jan,16; 2014,Jan,11

92616 **Flexible endoscopic evaluation of swallowing and laryngeal sensory testing by cine or video recording;**
EXCLUDES *Diagnostic flexible fiberoptic laryngoscopy (31575)*
Flexible endoscopic examination/testing without cine or video recording (92700)
🔧 2.84   ⚷ 5.85   **FUD** XXX   Ⓐ 80 ▭
AMA: 2018,Feb,11; 2018,Jan,8; 2017,Jul,7; 2017,Apr,8; 2017,Jan,8; 2016,Dec,13; 2016,Sep,6; 2016,Jan,13; 2015,Jan,16; 2014,Jan,11

92617 **interpretation and report only**
EXCLUDES *Diagnostic flexible laryngoscopy (31575)*
🔧 1.18   ⚷ 1.18   **FUD** XXX   Ⓔ 80 ▭
AMA: 2018,Feb,11; 2018,Jan,8; 2017,Jul,7; 2017,Apr,8; 2017,Jan,8; 2016,Dec,13; 2016,Sep,6; 2016,Jan,13; 2015,Jan,16; 2014,Jan,11

92618 **Resequenced code. See code following 92605.**

92620-92700 Diagnostic Hearing Evaluations and Rehabilitation

INCLUDES Diagnostic/treatment services not generally included in a comprehensive otorhinolaryngologic evaluation or office visit

92620 **Evaluation of central auditory function, with report; initial 60 minutes**
EXCLUDES *Voice analysis (92521-92524)*
🔧 2.32   ⚷ 2.67   **FUD** XXX   Ⓠ1 80 ▭
AMA: 2018,Feb,11; 2018,Jan,8; 2017,Jan,8; 2016,Jan,13; 2015,Jan,16; 2014,Aug,3

+ **92621** **each additional 15 minutes (List separately in addition to code for primary procedure)**
EXCLUDES *Voice analysis (92521-92524)*
Code first (92620)
🔧 0.54   ⚷ 0.64   **FUD** ZZZ   Ⓝ 80 ▭
AMA: 2018,Feb,11; 2018,Jan,8; 2017,Jan,8; 2016,Jan,13; 2015,Jan,16; 2014,Aug,3

92625 **Assessment of tinnitus (includes pitch, loudness matching, and masking)**
EXCLUDES *Loudness test (92562)*
Code also modifier 52 for unilateral procedure
🔧 1.78   ⚷ 1.99   **FUD** XXX   Ⓠ1 80 ▭
AMA: 2018,Feb,11; 2018,Jan,8; 2017,Jan,8; 2016,Jan,13; 2015,Jan,16; 2014,Aug,3

▲ **92626** **Evaluation of auditory function for surgically implanted device(s) candidacy or postoperative status of a surgically implanted device(s); first hour**
INCLUDES Assessment to determine patient's proficiency in the use of remaining hearing to identify speech
Face-to-face time spent with the patient or family
EXCLUDES *Hearing aid evaluation, fitting, follow-up, or selection (92590-92591, 92592-92593, 92594-92595)*
🔧 2.16   ⚷ 2.55   **FUD** XXX   Ⓠ1 80 ▭
AMA: 2018,Feb,11; 2018,Jan,8; 2017,Jan,8; 2016,Sep,6; 2016,Jan,13; 2015,Jan,16; 2014,Jul,4; 2014,May,10; 2014,Jan,11

26/TC PC/TC Only   A2-Z3 ASC Payment   50 Bilateral   ♂ Male Only   ♀ Female Only   🔧 Facility RVU   ⚷ Non-Facility RVU   ▭ CCI   ✖ CLIA
FUD Follow-up Days   CMS: IOM   **AMA:** CPT Asst   A-Y OPPSI   80/80 Surg Assist Allowed / w/Doc   Lab Crosswalk   Radiology Crosswalk

476

▲ + **92627** each additional 15 minutes (List separately in addition to code for primary procedure)

    INCLUDES Assessment to determine patient's proficiency in the use of remaining hearing to identify speech
    Face-to-face time spent with the patient or family

    EXCLUDES Hearing aid evaluation, fitting, follow-up, or selection (92590-92591, 92592-92593, 92594-92595)

    Code first initial hour (92626)

    0.51   0.64 **FUD** ZZZ   N 80

    AMA: 2018,Feb,11; 2018,Jan,8; 2017,Jan,8; 2016,Sep,6; 2016,Jan,13; 2015,Jan,16; 2014,Jul,4; 2014,Jan,11

92630 Auditory rehabilitation; prelingual hearing loss

    0.00   0.00 **FUD** XXX   E

    AMA: 2018,Feb,11; 2018,Jan,8; 2017,Jan,8; 2016,Sep,6; 2016,Jan,13; 2015,Jan,16; 2014,Jan,11

92633 postlingual hearing loss

    0.00   0.00 **FUD** XXX   E

    AMA: 2018,Feb,11; 2018,Jan,8; 2017,Jan,8; 2016,Sep,6; 2016,Jan,13; 2015,Jan,16; 2014,Jan,11

92640 Diagnostic analysis with programming of auditory brainstem implant, per hour

    EXCLUDES Nonprogramming services (cardiac monitoring)

    2.73   3.25 **FUD** XXX   S 80

    AMA: 2018,Feb,11

92700 Unlisted otorhinolaryngological service or procedure

    INCLUDES Lombard test

    0.00   0.00 **FUD** XXX   Q1 80

    AMA: 2018,Feb,11; 2018,Jan,8; 2017,Apr,8; 2017,Jan,8; 2016,Sep,6; 2016,Jan,13; 2015,Sep,7; 2015,Sep,12; 2015,Jan,16; 2014,May,10; 2014,Jan,11

92920-92953 Emergency Cardiac Procedures

92920 Resequenced code. See code following 92998.

92921 Resequenced code. See code following 92998.

92924 Resequenced code. See code following 92998.

92925 Resequenced code. See code following 92998.

92928 Resequenced code. See code following 92998.

92929 Resequenced code. See code following 92998.

92933 Resequenced code. See code following 92998.

92934 Resequenced code. See code following 92998.

92937 Resequenced code. See code following 92998.

92938 Resequenced code. See code following 92998.

92941 Resequenced code. See code following 92998.

92943 Resequenced code. See code following 92998.

92944 Resequenced code. See code following 92998.

92950 Cardiopulmonary resuscitation (eg, in cardiac arrest)

    INCLUDES Cardiac defibrillation

    EXCLUDES Critical care services (99291-99292)

    5.35   8.92 **FUD** 000   S 80

    AMA: 2018,Feb,11; 2018,Jan,8; 2017,Jan,8; 2016,Jan,13; 2015,Jan,16; 2014,Jan,11

92953 Temporary transcutaneous pacing

    EXCLUDES Direction of ambulance/rescue personnel by physician or other qualified health care professional (99288)

    0.03   0.03 **FUD** 000   03 80

    AMA: 2019,Aug,8; 2018,Feb,11; 2018,Jan,8; 2017,Jan,8; 2016,Jan,13; 2015,Jan,16; 2014,May,4; 2014,Jan,11

92960-92961 Cardioversion

92960 Cardioversion, elective, electrical conversion of arrhythmia; external

    3.13   4.51 **FUD** 000   S 80

    AMA: 2018,Feb,11; 2018,Jan,8; 2017,Jan,8; 2016,Jan,13; 2015,Jan,16; 2014,Jan,11

92961 internal (separate procedure)

    EXCLUDES Device evaluation for implantable defibrillator/multi-lead pacemaker system (93282-93284, 93287, 93289, 93295-93296)
    Electrophysiological studies (93618-93624, 93631, 93640-93642)
    Intracardiac ablation (93650-93657, 93662)

    7.23   7.23 **FUD** 000   S

    AMA: 2018,Feb,11; 2018,Jan,8; 2017,Jan,8; 2016,Jan,13; 2015,Feb,3; 2015,Jan,16; 2014,Jan,11

92970-92979 Circulatory Assist: External/Internal

    EXCLUDES Atrial septostomy, balloon (92992)
    Catheter placement for use in circulatory assist devices (intra-aortic balloon pump) (33970)

92970 Cardioassist-method of circulatory assist; internal

    5.52   5.52 **FUD** 000   C 80

    AMA: 2018,Feb,11

92971 external

    2.91   2.91 **FUD** 000   C 80

    AMA: 2018,Feb,11

92973 Resequenced code. See code following 92998.

92974 Resequenced code. See code following 92998.

92975 Resequenced code. See code following 92998.

92977 Resequenced code. See code following 92998.

92978 Resequenced code. See code following 92998.

92979 Resequenced code. See code following 92998.

92986-92993 Percutaneous Procedures of Heart Valves and Septum

92986 Percutaneous balloon valvuloplasty; aortic valve

    38.3   38.3 **FUD** 090   J 80

    AMA: 2018,Feb,11; 2018,Jan,8; 2017,Jan,8; 2016,Jan,13; 2015,Feb,3; 2015,Jan,16; 2014,Jan,11

92987 mitral valve

    39.5   39.5 **FUD** 090   J 80

    AMA: 2018,Feb,11; 2018,Jan,8; 2017,Jan,8; 2016,Jan,13; 2015,Feb,3

92990 pulmonary valve

    31.6   31.6 **FUD** 090   J 80

    AMA: 2018,Feb,11; 2018,Jan,8; 2017,Jan,8; 2016,Jan,13; 2015,Jul,10; 2015,Feb,3

92992 Atrial septectomy or septostomy; transvenous method, balloon (eg, Rashkind type) (includes cardiac catheterization)

    0.00   0.00 **FUD** 090   C 80

    AMA: 2018,Feb,11; 2018,Jan,8; 2017,Jan,8; 2016,Jul,3; 2016,Jan,13; 2015,Jan,16; 2014,Jan,11

92993 blade method (Park septostomy) (includes cardiac catheterization)

    0.00   0.00 **FUD** 090   C 80

    AMA: 2018,Feb,11; 2018,Jan,8; 2017,Jan,8; 2016,Jul,3; 2016,Jan,13; 2015,Jan,16; 2014,Jan,11

92997-92998 Percutaneous Angioplasty: Pulmonary Artery

92997 Percutaneous transluminal pulmonary artery balloon angioplasty; single vessel

    19.0   19.0 **FUD** 000   J 80

    AMA: 2018,Feb,11; 2018,Jan,8; 2017,Jul,3; 2017,Jan,8; 2016,Mar,5; 2016,Jan,13; 2015,Feb,3

+ **92998** each additional vessel (List separately in addition to code for primary procedure)

    Code first single vessel (92997)

    9.44   9.44 **FUD** ZZZ   N 80

    AMA: 2018,Feb,11; 2018,Jan,8; 2017,Jul,3; 2017,Jan,8; 2016,Mar,5; 2016,Jan,13; 2015,Feb,3

92920-92944 [92920, 92921, 92924, 92925, 92928, 92929, 92933, 92934, 92937, 92938, 92941, 92943, 92944]

Intravascular Coronary Procedures

Additional procedures performed in a third branch of a major coronary artery

INCLUDES Accessing the vessel

All procedures performed in all segments of branches of coronary arteries
  Branches of left anterior descending (diagonals), left circumflex (marginals), and right (posterior descending, posterolaterals)
  Distal, proximal, and mid segments

All procedures performed in all segments of major coronary arteries through the native vessels:
  Distal, proximal, and mid segments
  Left main, left anterior descending, left circumflex, right, and ramus intermedius arteries

All procedures performed in major coronary arteries or recognized coronary artery branches through a coronary artery bypass graft
  A sequential bypass graft with more than a single distal anastomosis as one graft
  Branching bypass grafts (eg, "Y" grafts) include a coronary vessel for the primary graft, with each branch off the primary graft making up an additional coronary vessel
  Each coronary artery bypass graft denotes a single coronary vessel

Embolic protection devices when used

Arteriotomy closure through the access sheath

Atherectomy (eg, directional, laser, rotational)

Balloon angioplasty (eg, cryoplasty, cutting balloon, wired balloons)

Cardiac catheterization and related procedures when included in the coronary revascularization service (93454-93461, 93563-93564)

Imaging once procedure is complete

Percutaneous coronary interventions (PCI) for disease of coronary vessels, native and bypass grafts

Procedures in branches of the left main and ramus intermedius coronary arteries as they are unrecognized for purposes of individual code assignment

Radiological supervision and interpretation of intervention(s)

Reporting the most comprehensive treatment in a given vessel according to a hierarchy of intensity for the base and add-on codes:
  Add-on codes: 92944 = 92938 > 92934 > 92925 > 92929 > 92921
  Base codes (report only one): 92943 = 92941 = 92933 > 92924 > 92937 = 92928 > 92920

Revascularization achieved with a single procedure when a single lesion continues from one target vessel (major artery, branch, or bypass graft) to ...

Selective vessel catheterization

Stenting (eg, balloon expandable, bare metal, covered, drug eluting, self-expanding)

Traversing of the lesion

EXCLUDES *Application of intravascular radioelements (77770-77772)*
Insertion of device for coronary intravascular brachytherapy (92974)
Reduction of septum (eg, alcohol ablation) (93799)

Code also add-on codes for procedures performed during the same session in additional recognized branches of the target vessel

Code also diagnostic angiography at the time of the interventional procedure when:
  A previous study is available, but documentation states the patient's condition has changed since the previous study or visualization of the anatomy/pathology is inadequate, or a change occurs during the procedure warranting additional evaluation of an area outside the current target area
  No previous catheter-based coronary angiography study is available, and a full diagnostic study is performed, with the decision to perform the intervention based on that study, or

Code also diagnostic angiography performed at a session separate from the interventional procedure

Code also individual base codes for treatment of a segment of a major native coronary artery and another segment of the same artery that requires treatment through a bypass graft when performed at the same time

Code also procedures for both vessels for a bifurcation lesion

Code also procedures performed in second branch of a major coronary artery

Code also treatment of arterial segment requiring access through a bypass graft

---

92920 Percutaneous transluminal coronary angioplasty; single major coronary artery or branch

🔧 15.4   🔪 15.4   **FUD** 000   [J] [80] 🔲

AMA: 2018,Feb,11; 2018,Jan,8; 2017,Jul,3; 2017,Jan,8; 2016,Jan,13; 2015,Jan,16; 2014,Dec,6

Catheter is advanced to affected portion of coronary artery

A stent is placed

Aorta

Left coronary artery

Plaque

Right coronary artery

Inflated balloon

A balloon may be inflated or other intravascular therapy may accompany the procedure

+ # **92921**   **each additional branch of a major coronary artery (List separately in addition to code for primary procedure)**

Code first (92920, 92924, 92928, 92933, 92937, 92941, 92943)

🔧 0.00   🔪 0.00   **FUD** ZZZ   [N] 🔲

AMA: 2018,Feb,11; 2018,Jan,8; 2017,Jul,3; 2017,Jan,8; 2016,Jan,13; 2015,Jan,16; 2014,Dec,6; 2014,Sep,13

**92924**   **Percutaneous transluminal coronary atherectomy, with coronary angioplasty when performed; single major coronary artery or branch**

🔧 18.4   🔪 18.4   **FUD** 000   [J] [80] 🔲

AMA: 2018,Feb,11; 2018,Jan,8; 2017,Jul,3; 2017,Jan,8; 2016,Jan,13; 2015,Jan,16; 2014,Dec,6

+ # **92925**   **each additional branch of a major coronary artery (List separately in addition to code for primary procedure)**

Code first (92924, 92928, 92933, 92937, 92941, 92943)

🔧 0.00   🔪 0.00   **FUD** ZZZ   [N] 🔲

AMA: 2018,Feb,11; 2018,Jan,8; 2017,Jul,3; 2017,Jan,8; 2016,Jan,13; 2015,Jan,16; 2014,Dec,6; 2014,Sep,13

**92928**   **Percutaneous transcatheter placement of intracoronary stent(s), with coronary angioplasty when performed; single major coronary artery or branch**

🔧 17.2   🔪 17.2   **FUD** 000   [J] [80] 🔲

AMA: 2018,Feb,11; 2018,Jan,8; 2017,Jul,3; 2017,Feb,14; 2017,Jan,8; 2017,Jan,6; 2016,Jan,13; 2015,Jan,16; 2014,Dec,6; 2014,Sep,13; 2014,Mar,13; 2014,Jan,3

+ # **92929**   **each additional branch of a major coronary artery (List separately in addition to code for primary procedure)**

Code first (92928, 92933, 92937, 92941, 92943)

🔧 0.00   🔪 0.00   **FUD** ZZZ   [N] 🔲

AMA: 2018,Feb,11; 2018,Jan,8; 2017,Jul,3; 2017,Jan,8; 2017,Jan,6; 2016,Jan,13; 2015,Jan,16; 2014,Dec,6; 2014,Sep,13

| 26/TC PC/TC Only | A2-Z3 ASC Payment | 50 Bilateral | ♂ Male Only | ♀ Female Only | 🔧 Facility RVU | 🔪 Non-Facility RVU | 🔲 CCI | ❌ CLIA |
| **FUD** Follow-up Days | **CMS:** IOM | **AMA:** CPT Asst | A-Y OPPSI | 80/80 Surg Assist Allowed / w/Doc | | 🔲 Lab Crosswalk | 🔲 Radiology Crosswalk | |

478   CPT © 2019 American Medical Association. All Rights Reserved.   © 2019 Optum360, LLC

93227   review and interpretation by a physician or other qualified health care professional

🚑 0.75   ⚖ 0.75   **FUD** XXX

M 80 26 🖵

AMA: 2018,Mar,5; 2018,Feb,11; 2018,Jan,8; 2017,Jan,8; 2016,Jan,13; 2015,Jan,16; 2014,Jan,11

93228-93229 Remote Cardiovascular Telemetry

INCLUDES Cardiac monitoring using in-person as well as remote technology for the assessment of electrocardiographic data
Mobile telemetry monitors with the capacity to:
  Detect arrhythmias
  Real-time data analysis for the evaluation quality of the signal
  Records ECG rhythm on a continuous basis using external electrodes on the patient
  Transmit a tracing at any time
  Transmit data to an attended surveillance center where a technician is available to respond to device or rhythm alerts and contact the physician or qualified health care professional if needed

EXCLUDES Use of code more than one time in a 30-day period

93228   External mobile cardiovascular telemetry with electrocardiographic recording, concurrent computerized real time data analysis and greater than 24 hours of accessible ECG data storage (retrievable with query) with ECG triggered and patient selected events transmitted to a remote attended surveillance center for up to 30 days; review and interpretation with report by a physician or other qualified health care professional

EXCLUDES *Cardiovascular monitors that do not perform automatic ECG triggered transmissions to an attended surveillance center (93224-93227, 93268-93272)*

🚑 0.74   ⚖ 0.74   **FUD** XXX

★ M 80 26 🖵

AMA: 2018,Feb,11; 2018,Jan,8; 2017,Jan,8; 2016,Jan,13; 2015,Jan,16; 2014,Jan,11

93229   technical support for connection and patient instructions for use, attended surveillance, analysis and transmission of daily and emergent data reports as prescribed by a physician or other qualified health care professional

🚑 19.9   ⚖ 19.9   **FUD** XXX

★ S 80 TC 🖵

AMA: 2018,Feb,11; 2018,Jan,8; 2017,Jan,8; 2016,Jan,13; 2015,Jan,16; 2014,Jan,11

93260-93272 Event Monitors

INCLUDES ECG rhythm derived elements, which differ from physiologic data and include rhythm of the heart, rate, ST analysis, heart rate variability, T-wave alternans, among others
Event monitors that:
  Record parts of ECGs in response to patient activation or an automatic detection algorithm (or both)
  Require attended surveillance
  Transmit data upon request (although not immediately when activated)

EXCLUDES *Monitoring of cardiovascular devices (93279-93289 [93260], 93291-93296, 93298)*

93260   Resequenced code. See code following 93284.

93261   Resequenced code. See code following 93289.

93264   Resequenced code. See code before 93279.

93268   External patient and, when performed, auto activated electrocardiographic rhythm derived event recording with symptom-related memory loop with remote download capability up to 30 days, 24-hour attended monitoring; includes transmission, review and interpretation by a physician or other qualified health care professional

EXCLUDES *Implantable patient activated cardiac event recorders (93285, 93291, 93298)*
        Subcutaneous cardiac rhythm monitor (33285)

🚑 5.70   ⚖ 5.70   **FUD** XXX

★ M 80 🖵

AMA: 2018,Feb,11; 2018,Jan,8; 2017,Jan,8; 2016,Jan,13; 2015,Jan,16; 2014,Jan,11

93270   recording (includes connection, recording, and disconnection)

🚑 0.26   ⚖ 0.26   **FUD** XXX

★ Q1 80 TC 🖵

AMA: 2018,Feb,11; 2018,Jan,8; 2017,Jan,8; 2016,Jan,13; 2015,Jan,16; 2014,Jan,11

93271   transmission and analysis

🚑 4.72   ⚖ 4.72   **FUD** XXX

★ S 80 TC 🖵

AMA: 2018,Feb,11; 2018,Jan,8; 2017,Jan,8; 2016,Jan,13; 2015,Jan,16; 2014,Jan,11

93272   review and interpretation by a physician or other qualified health care professional

EXCLUDES *Implantable patient activated cardiac event recorders (93285, 93291, 93298)*
        Subcutaneous cardiac rhythm monitor (33285)

🚑 0.72   ⚖ 0.72   **FUD** XXX

★ M 80 26 🖵

AMA: 2018,Mar,5; 2018,Feb,11; 2018,Jan,8; 2017,Jan,8; 2016,Jan,13; 2015,Jan,16; 2014,Jan,11

93278 Signal-averaged Electrocardiography

EXCLUDES *Echocardiography (93303-93355)*
Code also modifier 26 for the interpretation and report only

93278   Signal-averaged electrocardiography (SAECG), with or without ECG

🚑 0.87   ⚖ 0.87   **FUD** XXX

Q1 80 🖵

AMA: 2018,Feb,11; 2018,Jan,8; 2017,Jan,8; 2016,Jan,13; 2015,Jan,16; 2014,Jan,11

93264 [93264] Wireless Pulmonary Artery Pressure Sensor Monitoring

INCLUDES Collection of data from an internal sensor in pulmonary artery
Downloads, interpretation, analysis, and report that must occur at least one time per week
Transmission and storage of data

EXCLUDES *Use of code if monitoring is for less than a 30-day period*
        Use of code more than one time in 30 days

\# **93264**   Remote monitoring of a wireless pulmonary artery pressure sensor for up to 30 days, including at least weekly downloads of pulmonary artery pressure recordings, interpretation(s), trend analysis, and report(s) by a physician or other qualified health care professional

🚑 1.02   ⚖ 1.44   **FUD** XXX

80 🖵

AMA: 2019,Jun,3

93279-93299 [93260, 93261] Monitoring of Cardiovascular Devices

INCLUDES   Implantable cardiovascular monitor (ICM) interrogation:
    Analysis of at least one recorded physiologic cardiovascular data element from either internal or external sensors
    Programmed parameters
  Implantable defibrillator interrogation:
    Battery
    Capture and sensing functions
    Leads
    Presence or absence of therapy for ventricular tachyarrhythmias
    Programmed parameters
    Underlying heart rhythm
  Implantable loop recorder (ILR) interrogation:
    Heart rate and rhythm during recorded episodes from both patient-initiated and device detected events
    Programmed parameters
  In-person interrogation/device evaluation (93288)
  In-person peri-procedural device evaluation/programming of device system parameters (93286)
  Interrogation evaluation of device
  Pacemaker interrogation:
    Battery
    Capture and sensing functions
    Heart rhythm
    Leads
    Programmed parameters
  Time period established by the initiation of remote monitoring or the 91st day of implantable defibrillator or pacemaker monitoring or the 31st day of ILR monitoring and extending for the succeeding 30- or 90-day period

EXCLUDES   *Wearable device monitoring (93224-93272)*

93279 **Programming device evaluation (in person) with iterative adjustment of the implantable device to test the function of the device and select optimal permanent programmed values with analysis, review and report by a physician or other qualified health care professional; single lead pacemaker system or leadless pacemaker system in one cardiac chamber**

EXCLUDES   *External ECG event recording up to 30 days (93268-93272)*
Peri-procedural and interrogation device evaluation (93286, 93288)
Rhythm strips (93040-93042)

🚑 1.56   Non-Fac 1.56   **FUD** XXX   [01] [80] 🖥

AMA: 2019,Mar,6; 2018,Feb,11; 2018,Jan,8; 2017,Jan,8; 2016,Aug,5; 2016,May,5; 2016,Jan,13; 2015,Jan,16; 2014,Nov,5; 2014,Jul,3; 2014,Jan,11

93280 **dual lead pacemaker system**

EXCLUDES   *External ECG event recording up to 30 days (93268-93272)*
Peri-procedural and interrogation device evaluation (93286, 93288)
Rhythm strips (93040-93042)

🚑 1.83   Non-Fac 1.83   **FUD** XXX   [01] [80] 🖥

AMA: 2018,Feb,11; 2018,Jan,8; 2017,Jan,8; 2016,Aug,5; 2016,May,5; 2016,Jan,13; 2015,Jan,16; 2014,Nov,5; 2014,Jul,3; 2014,Jan,11

93281 **multiple lead pacemaker system**

EXCLUDES   *External ECG event recording up to 30 days (93268-93272)*
Peri-procedural and interrogation device evaluation (93286, 93288)
Rhythm strips (93040-93042)

🚑 1.97   Non-Fac 1.97   **FUD** XXX   [01] [80] 🖥

AMA: 2018,Feb,11; 2018,Jan,8; 2017,Jan,8; 2016,Aug,5; 2016,May,5; 2016,Jan,13; 2015,Jan,16; 2014,Nov,5; 2014,Jul,3; 2014,Jan,11

93282 **single lead transvenous implantable defibrillator system**

EXCLUDES   *Device evaluation subcutaneous lead defibrillator system (93260)*
External ECG event recording up to 30 days (93268-93272)
Peri-procedural and interrogation device evaluation (93287, 93289)
Rhythm strips (93040-93042)
Wearable cardio-defibrillator system services (93745)

🚑 1.90   Non-Fac 1.90   **FUD** XXX   [01] [80] 🖥

AMA: 2018,Feb,11; 2018,Jan,8; 2017,Jan,8; 2016,Aug,5; 2016,Jan,13; 2015,Jan,16; 2014,Nov,5; 2014,Jul,3; 2014,Jan,11

93283 **dual lead transvenous implantable defibrillator system**

EXCLUDES   *External ECG event recording up to 30 days (93268-93272)*
Peri-procedural and interrogation device evaluation (93287, 93289)
Rhythm strips (93040-93042)

🚑 2.39   Non-Fac 2.39   **FUD** XXX   [01] [80]

AMA: 2018,Feb,11; 2018,Jan,8; 2017,Jan,8; 2016,Aug,5; 2016,Jan,13; 2015,Jan,16; 2014,Nov,5; 2014,Jul,3; 2014,Jan,11

93284 **multiple lead transvenous implantable defibrillator system**

EXCLUDES   *External ECG event recording up to 30 days (93268-93272)*
Peri-procedural and interrogation device evaluation (93287, 93289)
Rhythm strips (93040-93042)

🚑 2.59   Non-Fac 2.59   **FUD** XXX   [01] [80] 🖥

AMA: 2018,Feb,11; 2018,Jan,8; 2017,Jan,8; 2016,Aug,5; 2016,Jan,13; 2015,Jan,16; 2014,Nov,5; 2014,Jul,3; 2014,Jan,11

\# **93260** **implantable subcutaneous lead defibrillator system**

EXCLUDES   *Device evaluation (93261, 93282, 93287)*
External ECG event recording up to 30 days (93268-93272)
Insertion/removal/replacement implantable defibrillator (33240, 33241, [33262], [33270, 33271, 33272, 33273])
Rhythm strips (93040-93042)

🚑 1.93   Non-Fac 1.93   **FUD** XXX   [01] [80] 🖥

AMA: 2018,Feb,11; 2018,Jan,8; 2017,Jan,8; 2016,Aug,5; 2016,Jan,13; 2015,Jan,16; 2014,Nov,5

93285 **subcutaneous cardiac rhythm monitor system**

EXCLUDES   *Device evaluation (93279-93284, 93291)*
External ECG event recording up to 30 days (93268-93272)
Insertion subcutaneous cardiac rhythm monitor (33285)
Rhythm strips (93040-93042)

🚑 1.37   Non-Fac 1.37   **FUD** XXX   [01] [80] 🖥

AMA: 2019,Apr,3; 2018,Feb,11; 2018,Jan,8; 2017,Jan,8; 2016,Aug,5; 2016,Jan,13; 2015,Jan,16; 2014,Nov,5; 2014,Jul,3; 2014,Jan,11

26/TC PC/TC Only   **A2-Z3** ASC Payment   **50** Bilateral   ♂ Male Only   ♀ Female Only   🚑 Facility RVU   Non-Facility RVU   🖥 CCI   🗙 CLIA
FUD Follow-up Days   **CMS:** IOM   **AMA:** CPT Asst   **A-Y** OPPSI   **80/80** Surg Assist Allowed / w/Doc   Lab Crosswalk   Radiology Crosswalk

482   CPT © 2019 American Medical Association. All Rights Reserved.   © 2019 Optum360, LLC

93286 Peri-procedural device evaluation (in person) and programming of device system parameters before or after a surgery, procedure, or test with analysis, review and report by a physician or other qualified health care professional; single, dual, or multiple lead pacemaker system, or leadless pacemaker system

INCLUDES One evaluation and programming (if performed once before and once after, report as two units)

EXCLUDES Device evaluation (93279-93281, 93288)
External ECG event recording up to 30 days (93268-93272)
Rhythm strips (93040-93042)
Services related to cardiac contractility modulation systems (0408T-0411T, 0414T-0415T)
Subcutaneous implantable defibrillator peri-procedural device evaluation and programming (93260, 93261)

🚗 0.99   ⚕ 0.99   **FUD** XXX   N 80 ▢

AMA: 2019,Mar,6; 2018,Feb,11; 2018,Jan,8; 2017,Jan,8; 2016,Aug,5; 2016,May,5; 2016,Jan,13; 2015,Jan,16; 2014,Nov,5; 2014,Jul,3; 2014,Jan,11

93287 single, dual, or multiple lead implantable defibrillator system

INCLUDES One evaluation and programming (if performed once before and once after, report as two units)

EXCLUDES Device evaluation (93282-93284, 93289)
External ECG event recording up to 30 days (93268-93272)
Rhythm strips (93040-93042)
Services related to cardiac contractility modulation systems (0408T-0411T, 0414T-0415T)
Subcutaneous implantable defibrillator peri-procedural device evaluation and programming (93260, 93261)

🚗 1.22   ⚕ 1.22   **FUD** XXX   N 80 ▢

AMA: 2018,Feb,11; 2018,Jan,8; 2017,Jan,8; 2016,Aug,5; 2016,May,5; 2016,Jan,13; 2015,Jan,16; 2014,Nov,5; 2014,Jul,3; 2014,Jan,11

93288 Interrogation device evaluation (in person) with analysis, review and report by a physician or other qualified health care professional, includes connection, recording and disconnection per patient encounter; single, dual, or multiple lead pacemaker system, or leadless pacemaker system

EXCLUDES Device evaluation (93279-93281, 93286, 93294-93295)
External ECG event recording up to 30 days (93268-93272)
Rhythm strips (93040-93042)

🚗 1.25   ⚕ 1.25   **FUD** XXX   Q1 80 ▢

AMA: 2019,Mar,6; 2018,Feb,11; 2018,Jan,8; 2017,Jan,8; 2016,Aug,5; 2016,May,5; 2016,Jan,13; 2015,Jan,16; 2014,Nov,5; 2014,Jul,3; 2014,Jan,11

93289 single, dual, or multiple lead transvenous implantable defibrillator system, including analysis of heart rhythm derived data elements

EXCLUDES Monitoring physiologic cardiovascular data elements derived from an implantable defibrillator (93290)

EXCLUDES Device evaluation (93261, 93282-93284, 93287, 93295-93296)
External ECG event recording up to 30 days (93268-93272)
Rhythm strips (93040-93042)

🚗 1.70   ⚕ 1.70   **FUD** XXX   Q1 80 ▢

AMA: 2018,Feb,11; 2018,Jan,8; 2017,Jan,8; 2016,Aug,5; 2016,May,5; 2016,Jan,13; 2015,Jan,16; 2014,Nov,5; 2014,Jul,3; 2014,Jan,11

93261 implantable subcutaneous lead defibrillator system

EXCLUDES Device evaluation (93260, 93287, 93289)
External ECG event recording up to 30 days (93268-93272)
Insertion/removal/replacement implantable defibrillator (33240, 33241, [33262], [33270, 33271, 33272, 33273])
Rhythm strips (93040-93042)

🚗 1.77   ⚕ 1.77   **FUD** XXX   Q1 80 ▢

AMA: 2018,Feb,11; 2018,Jan,8; 2017,Jan,8; 2016,Aug,5; 2016,Jan,13; 2015,Jan,16; 2014,Nov,5

93290 implantable cardiovascular physiologic monitor system, including analysis of 1 or more recorded physiologic cardiovascular data elements from all internal and external sensors

EXCLUDES Device evaluation (93297)
Heart rhythm derived data (93289)

🚗 1.19   ⚕ 1.19   **FUD** XXX   Q1 80 ▢

AMA: 2018,Feb,11; 2018,Jan,8; 2017,Jan,8; 2016,Aug,5; 2016,Jan,13; 2015,Jan,16; 2014,Nov,5; 2014,Jul,3; 2014,Jan,11

93291 subcutaneous cardiac rhythm monitor system, including heart rhythm derived data analysis

EXCLUDES Device evaluation (93288-93290 [93261], 93298)
External ECG event recording up to 30 days (93268-93272)
Insertion subcutaneous cardiac rhythm monitor (33285)
Rhythm strips (93040-93042)

🚗 1.07   ⚕ 1.07   **FUD** XXX   Q1 80 ▢

AMA: 2019,Apr,3; 2018,Feb,11; 2018,Jan,8; 2017,Jan,8; 2016,Aug,5; 2016,Jan,13; 2015,Jan,16; 2014,Nov,5; 2014,Jul,3; 2014,Jan,11

93292 wearable defibrillator system

EXCLUDES External ECG event recording up to 30 days (93268-93272)
Rhythm strips (93040-93042)
Wearable cardioverter-defibrillator system (93745)

🚗 1.14   ⚕ 1.14   **FUD** XXX   Q1 80 ▢

AMA: 2018,Feb,11; 2018,Jan,8; 2017,Jan,8; 2016,Aug,5; 2016,Jan,13; 2015,Jan,16; 2014,Nov,5; 2014,Jul,3; 2014,Jan,11

93293 Transtelephonic rhythm strip pacemaker evaluation(s) single, dual, or multiple lead pacemaker system, includes recording with and without magnet application with analysis, review and report(s) by a physician or other qualified health care professional, up to 90 days

EXCLUDES Device evaluation (93294)
External ECG event recording up to 30 days (93268-93272)
Rhythm strips (93040-93042)
Use of code more than one time in a 90-day period
Use of code when monitoring period is less than 30 days

🚗 1.48   ⚕ 1.48   **FUD** XXX   Q1 80 ▢

AMA: 2018,Feb,11; 2018,Jan,8; 2017,Jan,8; 2016,Aug,5; 2016,Jan,13; 2015,Jan,16; 2014,Nov,5; 2014,Jul,3; 2014,Jan,11

93294 Interrogation device evaluation(s) (remote), up to 90 days; single, dual, or multiple lead pacemaker system, or leadless pacemaker system with interim analysis, review(s) and report(s) by a physician or other qualified health care professional

EXCLUDES Device evaluation (93288, 93293)
External ECG event recording up to 30 days (93268-93272)
Rhythm strips (93040-93042)
Use of code more than one time in a 90-day period
Use of code when monitoring period is less than 30 days

🚗 0.87   ⚕ 0.87   **FUD** XXX   M 80 26 ▢

AMA: 2019,Mar,6; 2018,Feb,11; 2018,Jan,8; 2017,Jan,8; 2016,Aug,5; 2016,Jan,13; 2015,Jan,16; 2014,Nov,5; 2014,Jul,3; 2014,Jan,11

93295 **single, dual, or multiple lead implantable defibrillator system with interim analysis, review(s) and report(s) by a physician or other qualified health care professional**

EXCLUDES Device evaluation (93289)
External ECG event recording up to 30 days (93268-93272)
Remote interrogation device evaluation implantable cardioverter-defibrillator with substernal lead (0578T, 0579T)
Remote monitoring of physiological cardiovascular data (93297)
Rhythm strips (93040-93042)
Use of code more than one time in a 90-day period
Use of code when monitoring period is less than 30 days

📁 1.26 ⚕ 1.26 **FUD** XXX M 80 26 🖦

AMA: 2018,Feb,11; 2018,Jan,8; 2017,Jan,8; 2016,Aug,5; 2016,Jan,13; 2015,Jan,16; 2014,Nov,5; 2014,Jul,3; 2014,Jan,11

93296 **single, dual, or multiple lead pacemaker system, leadless pacemaker system, or implantable defibrillator system, remote data acquisition(s), receipt of transmissions and technician review, technical support and distribution of results**

EXCLUDES Device evaluation (93288-93289)
External ECG event recording up to 30 days (93268-93272)
Remote interrogation device evaluation implantable cardioverter-defibrillator with substernal lead (0578T, 0579T)
Rhythm strips (93040-93042)
Use of code more than one time in a 90-day period
Use of code when monitoring period is less than 30 days

📁 0.72 ⚕ 0.72 **FUD** XXX 01 80 TC 🖦

AMA: 2019,Mar,6; 2019,Jan,6; 2018,Feb,11; 2018,Jan,8; 2017,Jan,8; 2016,Aug,5; 2016,Jan,13; 2015,Jan,16; 2014,Nov,5; 2014,Jul,3; 2014,Jan,11

93297 **Interrogation device evaluation(s), (remote) up to 30 days; implantable cardiovascular physiologic monitor system, including analysis of 1 or more recorded physiologic cardiovascular data elements from all internal and external sensors, analysis, review(s) and report(s) by a physician or other qualified health care professional**

EXCLUDES Collection and interpretation of physiologic data digitally stored and/or transmitted ([99091])
Device evaluation (93290, 93298)
Heart rhythm derived data (93295)
Remote monitoring of a wireless pulmonary artery pressure sensor (93264)
Remote monitoring of physiologic parameter(s) with daily recording(s) or programmed alert(s) ([99454])
Use of code more than one time in a 30-day period
Use of code when monitoring period is less than 10 days

📁 0.75 ⚕ 0.75 **FUD** XXX M 80 26 🖦

AMA: 2018,Feb,11; 2018,Jan,8; 2017,Jan,8; 2016,Aug,5; 2016,Jan,13; 2015,Jan,16; 2014,Nov,5; 2014,Jul,3; 2014,Jan,11

93298 **subcutaneous cardiac rhythm monitor system, including analysis of recorded heart rhythm data, analysis, review(s) and report(s) by a physician or other qualified health care professional**

EXCLUDES Collection and interpretation of physiologic data digitally stored and/or transmitted ([99091])
Device evaluation (93291, 93297)
External ECG event recording up to 30 days (93268-93272)
Implantation of patient-activated cardiac event recorder (33285)
Remote monitoring of physiologic parameter(s) with daily recording(s) or programmed alert(s) ([99454])
Rhythm strips (93040-93042)
Use of code more than one time in a 30-day period
Use of code when monitoring period is less than 10 days

📁 0.75 ⚕ 0.75 **FUD** XXX M 80 26 🖦

AMA: 2019,Apr,3; 2018,Feb,11; 2018,Jan,8; 2017,Jan,8; 2016,Aug,5; 2016,Jan,13; 2015,Jan,16; 2014,Nov,5; 2014,Jul,3; 2014,Jan,11

93299 ~~implantable cardiovascular physiologic monitor system or subcutaneous cardiac rhythm monitor system, remote data acquisition(s), receipt of transmissions and technician review, technical support and distribution of results~~

To report, see (93297-93298)

93303-93356 [93356] Echocardiography

INCLUDES Interpretation and report
Obtaining ultrasonic signals from heart/great arteries
Report of study which includes:
Description of recognized abnormalities
Documentation of all clinically relevant findings which includes obtained quantitative measurements
Interpretation of all information obtained
Two-dimensional image/doppler ultrasonic signal documentation
Ultrasound exam of:
Adjacent great vessels
Cardiac chambers/valves
Pericardium

EXCLUDES Contrast agents and/or drugs used for pharmacological stress
Echocardiography, fetal (76825-76828)
Ultrasound with thorough examination of the organ(s) or anatomic region/documentation of the image/final written report

93303 **Transthoracic echocardiography for congenital cardiac anomalies; complete**

📁 6.65 ⚕ 6.65 **FUD** XXX S 80 🖦

AMA: 2018,Feb,11; 2018,Jan,8; 2017,Jan,8; 2016,Jan,13; 2015,May,10; 2015,Jan,16; 2014,Jan,11

93304 **follow-up or limited study**

📁 4.53 ⚕ 4.53 **FUD** XXX S 80 🖦

AMA: 2018,Feb,11; 2018,Jan,8; 2017,Jan,8; 2016,Jan,13; 2015,May,10; 2015,Jan,16; 2014,Jan,11

93306 **Echocardiography, transthoracic, real-time with image documentation (2D), includes M-mode recording, when performed, complete, with spectral Doppler echocardiography, and with color flow Doppler echocardiography**

INCLUDES Doppler and color flow
Two-dimensional and M-mode

EXCLUDES Transthoracic without spectral and color doppler (93307)

📁 5.84 ⚕ 5.84 **FUD** XXX S 80 🖦

AMA: 2018,Dec,10; 2018,Dec,10; 2018,Feb,11; 2018,Jan,8; 2017,Jan,8; 2016,Apr,8; 2016,Jan,13; 2015,May,10; 2015,Jan,16

93307 **Echocardiography, transthoracic, real-time with image documentation (2D), includes M-mode recording, when performed, complete, without spectral or color Doppler echocardiography**

INCLUDES Additional structures that may be viewed such as pulmonary vein or artery, pulmonic valve, inferior vena cava
Obtaining/recording appropriate measurements
Two-dimensional/selected M-mode exam of:
Adjacent portions of the aorta
Aortic/mitral/tricuspid valves
Left/right atria
Left/right ventricles
Pericardium
Using multiple views as required to obtain a complete functional/anatomic evaluation

EXCLUDES Doppler echocardiography (93320-93321, 93325)

📁 3.97 ⚕ 3.97 **FUD** XXX S 80 🖦

AMA: 2018,Feb,11; 2018,Jan,8; 2017,Jan,8; 2016,Apr,8; 2016,Jan,13; 2015,May,10; 2015,Jan,16; 2014,Jan,11

93308 **Echocardiography, transthoracic, real-time with image documentation (2D), includes M-mode recording, when performed, follow-up or limited study**

INCLUDES An exam that does not evaluate/document the attempt to evaluate all the structures that comprise the complete echocardiographic exam

📁 2.78 ⚕ 2.78 **FUD** XXX S 80 🖦

AMA: 2018,Dec,10; 2018,Dec,10; 2018,Feb,11; 2018,Jan,8; 2017,Jan,8; 2016,Apr,8; 2016,Jan,13; 2015,May,10; 2015,Jan,16; 2014,Jan,11

93312 **Echocardiography, transesophageal, real-time with image documentation (2D) (with or without M-mode recording); including probe placement, image acquisition, interpretation and report**

EXCLUDES *Transesophageal echocardiography (93355)*

📋 6.97   ⚖ 6.97   **FUD** XXX   S 80 ▢

AMA: 2018,Feb,11; 2018,Jan,8; 2017,Jan,8; 2016,Jan,13; 2015,Jan,16; 2014,Jul,8; 2014,Jan,11

93313 **placement of transesophageal probe only**

EXCLUDES *Excludes procedure if performed by same person performing transesophageal echocardiography (93355)*

📋 0.33   ⚖ 0.33   **FUD** XXX   S 80 ▢

AMA: 2018,Feb,11; 2018,Jan,8; 2017,Jan,8; 2016,Jan,13; 2015,Jan,16; 2014,Jul,8; 2014,Jan,11

93314 **image acquisition, interpretation and report only**

EXCLUDES *Transesophageal echocardiography (93355)*

📋 6.73   ⚖ 6.73   **FUD** XXX   N 80 ▢

AMA: 2018,Feb,11; 2018,Jan,8; 2017,Jan,8; 2016,Jan,13; 2015,Jan,16; 2014,Jul,8; 2014,Jan,11

93315 **Transesophageal echocardiography for congenital cardiac anomalies; including probe placement, image acquisition, interpretation and report**

EXCLUDES *Transesophageal echocardiography (93355)*

📋 0.00   ⚖ 0.00   **FUD** XXX   S 80 ▢

AMA: 2018,Feb,11; 2018,Jan,8; 2017,Jan,8; 2016,Jan,13; 2015,Jan,16; 2014,Jul,8; 2014,Jan,11

93316 **placement of transesophageal probe only**

EXCLUDES *Transesophageal echocardiography (93355)*

📋 0.79   ⚖ 0.79   **FUD** XXX   S 80 ▢

AMA: 2018,Feb,11; 2018,Jan,8; 2017,Jan,8; 2016,Jan,13; 2015,Jan,16; 2014,Jan,11

93317 **image acquisition, interpretation and report only**

EXCLUDES *Transesophageal echocardiography (93355)*

📋 0.00   ⚖ 0.00   **FUD** XXX   N 80 ▢

AMA: 2018,Feb,11; 2018,Jan,8; 2017,Jan,8; 2016,Jan,13; 2015,Jan,16; 2014,Jan,11

93318 **Echocardiography, transesophageal (TEE) for monitoring purposes, including probe placement, real time 2-dimensional image acquisition and interpretation leading to ongoing (continuous) assessment of (dynamically changing) cardiac pumping function and to therapeutic measures on an immediate time basis**

EXCLUDES *Transesophageal echocardiography (93355)*

📋 0.00   ⚖ 0.00   **FUD** XXX   S 80 ▢

AMA: 2018,Feb,11; 2018,Jan,8; 2017,Jan,8; 2016,Jan,13; 2015,Jan,16; 2014,Jan,11

+ 93320 **Doppler echocardiography, pulsed wave and/or continuous wave with spectral display (List separately in addition to codes for echocardiographic imaging); complete**

EXCLUDES *Transesophageal echocardiography (93355)*

Code first (93303-93304, 93312, 93314-93315, 93317, 93350-93351)

📋 1.51   ⚖ 1.51   **FUD** ZZZ   N 80 ▢

AMA: 2018,Feb,11; 2018,Jan,8; 2017,Jan,8; 2016,Jan,13; 2015,Jan,16; 2014,Jan,11

+ 93321 **follow-up or limited study (List separately in addition to codes for echocardiographic imaging)**

EXCLUDES *Transesophageal echocardiography (93355)*

Code first (93303-93304, 93308, 93312, 93314-93315, 93317, 93350-93351)

📋 0.76   ⚖ 0.76   **FUD** ZZZ   N 80 ▢

AMA: 2018,Feb,11; 2018,Jan,8; 2017,Jan,8; 2016,Jan,13; 2015,Jan,16; 2014,Jan,11

+ 93325 **Doppler echocardiography color flow velocity mapping (List separately in addition to codes for echocardiography)**

EXCLUDES *Transesophageal echocardiography (93355)*

Code first (76825-76828, 93303-93304, 93308, 93312, 93314-93315, 93317, 93350-93351)

📋 0.71   ⚖ 0.71   **FUD** ZZZ   N 80 ▢

AMA: 2018,Feb,11; 2018,Jan,8; 2017,Jan,8; 2016,Jul,8; 2016,Jan,13; 2015,Jan,16; 2014,Jan,11

93350 **Echocardiography, transthoracic, real-time with image documentation (2D), includes M-mode recording, when performed, during rest and cardiovascular stress test using treadmill, bicycle exercise and/or pharmacologically induced stress, with interpretation and report;**

EXCLUDES *Cardiovascular stress test, complete procedure (93015)*

Code also exercise stress testing (93016-93018)

📋 5.31   ⚖ 5.31   **FUD** XXX   S 80 ▢

AMA: 2018,Feb,11; 2018,Jan,8; 2017,Jan,8; 2016,Apr,8; 2016,Jan,13; 2015,Jan,16; 2014,Jul,8; 2014,Jan,11

93351 **including performance of continuous electrocardiographic monitoring, with supervision by a physician or other qualified health care professional**

INCLUDES *Stress echocardiogram performed with a complete cardiovascular stress test*

EXCLUDES *Cardiovascular stress test (93015-93018)*

Echocardiography (93350)

Professional only components of complete stress test and stress echocardiogram performed in a facility by same physician, report with modifier 26

Use of code for professional component (modifier 26 appended) with (93016, 93018, 93350)

Code also components of cardiovascular stress test when professional services not performed by same physician performing stress echocardiogram (93016-93018)

📋 6.57   ⚖ 6.57   **FUD** XXX   S ▢

AMA: 2018,Feb,11; 2018,Jan,8; 2017,Jan,8; 2016,Apr,8; 2016,Jan,13; 2015,Jan,16; 2014,Jul,8; 2014,Jan,11

● + # 93356 **Myocardial strain imaging using speckle tracking-derived assessment of myocardial mechanics (List separately in addition to codes for echocardiography imaging)**

📋 0.00   ⚖ 0.00   **FUD** 000

EXCLUDES *Use of code more than one time for each session*

Code first (93303-93304, 93306, 93307, 93308, 93350-93351)

+ 93352 **Use of echocardiographic contrast agent during stress echocardiography (List separately in addition to code for primary procedure)**

EXCLUDES *Use of code more than one time for each stress echocardiogram*

Code first (93350, 93351)

📋 0.95   ⚖ 0.95   **FUD** ZZZ   M 80 ▢

AMA: 2018,Feb,11; 2018,Jan,8; 2017,Jan,8; 2016,Jan,13; 2015,Jan,16; 2014,Jan,11

93355 **Echocardiography, transesophageal (TEE) for guidance of a transcatheter intracardiac or great vessel(s) structural intervention(s) (eg, TAVR, transcatheter pulmonary valve replacement, mitral valve repair, paravalvular regurgitation repair, left atrial appendage occlusion/closure, ventricular septal defect closure) (peri-and intra-procedural), real-time image acquisition and documentation, guidance with quantitative measurements, probe manipulation, interpretation, and report, including diagnostic transesophageal echocardiography and, when performed, administration of ultrasound contrast, Doppler, color flow, and 3D**

EXCLUDES *3D rendering (76376-76377)*

Doppler echocardiography (93320-93321, 93325)

Transesophageal echocardiography (93312-93318)

Transesophageal probe positioning by different provider (93313)

📋 6.57   ⚖ 6.57   **FUD** XXX   N 80 ▢

AMA: 2018,Feb,11

93356 **Resequenced code. See code following 93351.**

93451-93505 Heart Catheterization

INCLUDES Access site imaging and placement of closure device
Catheter insertion and positioning
Contrast injection (except as listed below)
Imaging and insertion of closure device
Radiology supervision and interpretation
Roadmapping angiography

EXCLUDES *Congenital cardiac cath procedures (93530-93533)*

Code also separately identifiable:
  Aortography (93567)
  Noncardiac angiography (see radiology and vascular codes)
  Pulmonary angiography (93568)
  Right ventricular or atrial injection (93566)

93451   Right heart catheterization including measurement(s) of oxygen saturation and cardiac output, when performed

INCLUDES Cardiac output review
Insertion catheter into 1+ right cardiac chambers or areas
Obtaining samples for blood gas

EXCLUDES *Catheterization procedures that include right side of heart (93453, 93456-93457, 93460-93461)*
Implantation wireless pulmonary artery pressure sensor (33289)
Indicator dilution studies (93561-93562)
Percutaneous repair congenital interatrial defect (93580)
Swan-Ganz catheter insertion (93503)
Valve repair or annulus reconstruction (33418, 0345T, 0483T, 0484T, 0544T, 0545T)

Code also administration of medication or exercise to repeat assessment of hemodynamic measurement (93463-93464)

🔧 22.1   ⚕ 22.1   **FUD** 000   ⊘ J 62 80 ▭

AMA: 2019,Jun,3; 2019,Mar,6; 2018,Dec,10; 2018,Dec,10; 2018,Feb,11; 2018,Jan,8; 2017,Dec,13; 2017,Jul,3; 2017,Jan,8; 2016,Mar,5; 2016,Jan,13; 2015,Sep,3; 2015,Jan,16; 2014,Jul,3; 2014,Jan,11

Superior vena cava
Aorta
Pulmonary artery
Catheter
Right atrium
Right ventricle
Catheter

93452   Left heart catheterization including intraprocedural injection(s) for left ventriculography, imaging supervision and interpretation, when performed

INCLUDES Insertion of catheter into left cardiac chambers

EXCLUDES *Catheterization procedures that include injections for left ventriculography (93453, 93458-93461)*
Injection procedures (93561-93565)
Percutaneous repair congenital interatrial defect (93580)
Services related to cardiac contractility modulation systems (0408T-0411T, 0414T-0415T)
Swan-Ganz catheter insertion (93503)
Valve repair or annulus reconstruction (33418, 0345T, 0483T, 0484T, 0544T, 0545T)

Code also administration of medication or exercise to repeat assessment of hemodynamic measurement (93463-93464)

Code also transapical or transseptal puncture (93462)

🔧 24.6   ⚕ 24.6   **FUD** 000   J 62 80 ▭

AMA: 2018,Feb,11; 2018,Jan,8; 2017,Jul,3; 2017,Jan,8; 2016,Jan,13; 2015,Jan,16; 2014,Jul,3; 2014,Jan,11

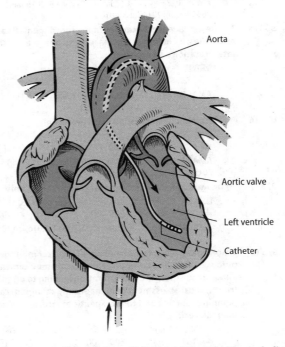

Aorta
Aortic valve
Left ventricle
Catheter

93453   Combined right and left heart catheterization including intraprocedural injection(s) for left ventriculography, imaging supervision and interpretation, when performed

INCLUDES Cardiac output review
Insertion catheter into 1+ right cardiac chambers or areas
Insertion of catheter into left cardiac chambers
Obtaining samples for blood gas

EXCLUDES *Catheterization procedures (93451-93452, 93456-93461)*
Injection procedures (93561-93565)
Percutaneous repair congenital interatrial defect (93580)
Services related to cardiac contractility modulation systems (0408T-0411T, 0414T-0415T)
Swan-Ganz catheter insertion (93503)
Valve repair or annulus reconstruction (33418, 0345T, 0483T, 0484T, 0544T, 0545T)

Code also administration of medication or exercise to repeat assessment of hemodynamic measurement (93463-93464)

Code also transapical or transseptal puncture (93462)

🔧 31.9   ⚕ 31.9   **FUD** 000   J 62 80 ▭

AMA: 2019,Jun,3; 2019,Mar,6; 2018,Feb,11; 2018,Jan,8; 2017,Jul,3; 2017,Jan,8; 2016,Mar,5; 2016,Jan,13; 2015,Sep,3; 2015,Jan,16; 2014,Jul,3; 2014,Jan,11

26/TC PC/TC Only   A2-Z3 ASC Payment   50 Bilateral   ♂ Male Only   ♀ Female Only   🔧 Facility RVU   ⚕ Non-Facility RVU   ▭ CCI   ✖ CLIA
FUD Follow-up Days   **CMS:** IOM   **AMA:** CPT Asst   A-Y OPPSI   80/80 Surg Assist Allowed / w/Doc   ▭ Lab Crosswalk   Radiology Crosswalk

486   CPT © 2019 American Medical Association. All Rights Reserved.   © 2019 Optum360, LLC

93454 Catheter placement in coronary artery(s) for coronary angiography, including intraprocedural injection(s) for coronary angiography, imaging supervision and interpretation;

> *EXCLUDES* *Injection procedures (93561-93565)*
> *Swan-Ganz catheter insertion (93503)*
> *Valve repair or annulus reconstruction (33418, 0345T, 0483T, 0484T, 0544T, 0545T)*

24.8   24.8   **FUD** 000   J G2 80

AMA: 2018,Feb,11; 2018,Jan,8; 2017,Feb,14; 2017,Jan,8; 2016,Mar,5; 2016,Jan,13; 2015,Jan,16; 2014,Dec,6; 2014,Jul,3; 2014,Jan,11

93455 with catheter placement(s) in bypass graft(s) (internal mammary, free arterial, venous grafts) including intraprocedural injection(s) for bypass graft angiography

> *EXCLUDES* *Injection procedures (93561-93565)*
> *Percutaneous repair congenital interatrial defect (93580)*
> *Swan-Ganz catheter insertion (93503)*
> *Valve repair or annulus reconstruction (33418, 0345T, 0483T, 0484T, 0544T, 0545T)*

28.6   28.6   **FUD** 000   J G2 80

AMA: 2018,Feb,11; 2018,Jan,8; 2017,Jan,8; 2016,Mar,5; 2016,Jan,13; 2015,Jan,16; 2014,Dec,6; 2014,Jul,3; 2014,Jan,11

93456 with right heart catheterization

> *INCLUDES* Cardiac output review
> Insertion catheter into 1+ right cardiac chambers or areas
> Obtaining samples for blood gas
> *EXCLUDES* *Injection procedures (93561-93565)*
> *Percutaneous repair congenital interatrial defect (93580)*
> *Swan-Ganz catheter insertion (93503)*
> *Valve repair or annulus reconstruction (33418, 0345T, 0483T, 0484T, 0544T, 0545T)*

Code also administration of medication or exercise to repeat assessment of hemodynamic measurement (93463-93464)

31.4   31.4   **FUD** 000   ⊘ J G2 80

AMA: 2019,Jun,3; 2019,Mar,6; 2018,Feb,11; 2018,Jan,8; 2017,Jul,3; 2017,Jan,8; 2016,Mar,5; 2016,Jan,13; 2015,Sep,3; 2015,Jan,16; 2014,Dec,6; 2014,Jul,3; 2014,Jan,11

93457 with catheter placement(s) in bypass graft(s) (internal mammary, free arterial, venous grafts) including intraprocedural injection(s) for bypass graft angiography and right heart catheterization

> *INCLUDES* Cardiac output review
> Insertion catheter into 1+ right cardiac chambers or areas
> Obtaining samples for blood gas
> *EXCLUDES* *Injection procedures (93561-93565)*
> *Percutaneous repair congenital interatrial defect (93580)*
> *Swan-Ganz catheter insertion (93503)*
> *Valve repair or annulus reconstruction (33418, 0345T, 0483T, 0484T, 0544T, 0545T)*

Code also administration of medication or exercise to repeat assessment of hemodynamic measurement (93463-93464)

35.1   35.1   **FUD** 000   J G2 80

AMA: 2019,Jun,3; 2019,Mar,6; 2018,Feb,11; 2018,Jan,8; 2017,Jan,8; 2016,Mar,5; 2016,Jan,13; 2015,Sep,3; 2015,Jan,16; 2014,Dec,6; 2014,Jul,3; 2014,Jan,11

93458 with left heart catheterization including intraprocedural injection(s) for left ventriculography, when performed

> *INCLUDES* Insertion of catheter into left cardiac chambers
> *EXCLUDES* *Injection procedures (93561-93565)*
> *Percutaneous repair congenital interatrial defect (93580)*
> *Services related to cardiac contractility modulation systems (0408T-0411T, 0414T-0415T)*
> *Swan-Ganz catheter insertion (93503)*
> *Valve repair or annulus reconstruction (33418, 0345T, 0483T, 0484T, 0544T, 0545T)*

Code also administration of medication or exercise to repeat assessment of hemodynamic measurement (93463-93464)
Code also transapical or transseptal puncture (93462)

29.5   29.5   **FUD** 000   J G2 80

AMA: 2018,Feb,11; 2018,Jan,8; 2017,Jul,3; 2017,Jan,8; 2016,Mar,5; 2016,Jan,13; 2015,Sep,3; 2015,Jan,16; 2014,Dec,6; 2014,Jul,3; 2014,Jan,11

93459 with left heart catheterization including intraprocedural injection(s) for left ventriculography, when performed, catheter placement(s) in bypass graft(s) (internal mammary, free arterial, venous grafts) with bypass graft angiography

> *INCLUDES* Insertion of catheter into left cardiac chambers
> *EXCLUDES* *Injection procedures (93561-93565)*
> *Percutaneous repair congenital interatrial defect (93580)*
> *Services related to cardiac contractility modulation systems (0408T-0411T, 0414T-0415T)*
> *Swan-Ganz catheter insertion (93503)*
> *Valve repair or annulus reconstruction (33418, 0345T, 0483T, 0484T, 0544T, 0545T)*

Code also administration of medication or exercise to repeat assessment of hemodynamic measurement (93463-93464)
Code also transapical or transseptal puncture (93462)

32.4   32.4   **FUD** 000   J G2 80

AMA: 2018,Feb,11; 2018,Jan,8; 2017,Jul,3; 2017,Jan,8; 2016,Mar,5; 2016,Jan,13; 2015,Sep,3; 2015,Jan,16; 2014,Dec,6; 2014,Jul,3; 2014,Jan,11

93460 with right and left heart catheterization including intraprocedural injection(s) for left ventriculography, when performed

> *INCLUDES* Cardiac output review
> Insertion catheter into 1+ right cardiac chambers or areas
> Insertion of catheter into left cardiac chambers
> Obtaining samples for blood gas
> *EXCLUDES* *Injection procedures (93561-93565)*
> *Percutaneous repair congenital interatrial defect (93580)*
> *Services related to cardiac contractility modulation systems (0408T-0411T, 0414T-0415T)*
> *Swan-Ganz catheter insertion (93503)*
> *Valve repair or annulus reconstruction (33418, 0345T, 0483T, 0484T, 0544T, 0545T)*

Code also administration of medication or exercise to repeat assessment of hemodynamic measurement (93463-93464)
Code also transapical or transseptal puncture (93462)

35.4   35.4   **FUD** 000   J G2 80

AMA: 2019,Jun,3; 2019,Mar,6; 2018,Feb,11; 2018,Jan,8; 2017,Jul,3; 2017,Jan,8; 2016,Mar,5; 2016,Jan,13; 2015,Sep,3; 2015,Jan,16; 2014,Dec,6; 2014,Jul,3; 2014,Jan,11

93461　**with right and left heart catheterization including intraprocedural injection(s) for left ventriculography, when performed, catheter placement(s) in bypass graft(s) (internal mammary, free arterial, venous grafts) with bypass graft angiography**

INCLUDES　Cardiac output review
　　　　　Insertion catheter into 1+ right cardiac chambers or areas
　　　　　Insertion of catheter into left cardiac chambers
　　　　　Obtaining samples for blood gas

EXCLUDES　*Injection procedures (93561-93565)*
　　　　　Percutaneous repair congenital interatrial defect (93580)
　　　　　Services related to cardiac contractility modulation systems (0408T-0411T, 0414T-0415T)
　　　　　Swan-Ganz catheter insertion (93503)
　　　　　Valve repair or annulus reconstruction (33418, 0345T, 0483T, 0484T, 0544T, 0545T)

Code also administration of medication or exercise to repeat assessment of hemodynamic measurement (93463-93464)
Code also transapical or transseptal puncture (93462)

🖩 40.0　⚕ 40.0　**FUD** 000　　　J G2 80 🖵

AMA: 2019,Jun,3; 2019,Mar,6; 2018,Feb,11; 2018,Jan,8; 2017,Jul,3; 2017,Jan,8; 2016,Mar,5; 2016,Jan,13; 2015,Sep,3; 2015,Jan,16; 2014,Dec,6; 2014,Jul,3; 2014,Jan,11

+ 93462　**Left heart catheterization by transseptal puncture through intact septum or by transapical puncture (List separately in addition to code for primary procedure)**

INCLUDES　Insertion of catheter into left cardiac chambers

EXCLUDES　*Comprehensive electrophysiologic evaluation (93656)*
　　　　　Transseptal approach for percutaneous closure paravalvular leak (93590)
　　　　　Valve repair or annulus reconstruction unless performed with transapical puncture (0345T, 0544T)

Code also percutaneous closure paravalvular leak when a transapical puncture is performed (93590-93591)
Code first (33477, 93452-93453, 93458-93461, 93582, 93653-93654)

🖩 6.11　⚕ 6.11　**FUD** ZZZ　　　N N1 80 🖵

AMA: 2018,Feb,11; 2018,Jan,8; 2017,Sep,3; 2017,Jul,3; 2017,Jan,8; 2016,Jan,13; 2015,Sep,3; 2015,Jan,16; 2014,Jul,3; 2014,Jan,11

+ 93463　**Pharmacologic agent administration (eg, inhaled nitric oxide, intravenous infusion of nitroprusside, dobutamine, milrinone, or other agent) including assessing hemodynamic measurements before, during, after and repeat pharmacologic agent administration, when performed (List separately in addition to code for primary procedure)**

EXCLUDES　*Coronary interventional procedures (92920-92944, 92975, 92977)*
　　　　　Use of code more than one time per catheterization

Code first (33477, 93451-93453, 93456-93461, 93530-93533, 93580-93581)

🖩 2.82　⚕ 2.82　**FUD** ZZZ　　　N 80 🖵

AMA: 2018,Feb,11; 2018,Jan,8; 2017,Jan,8; 2016,Jan,13; 2015,Jan,16; 2014,Dec,6; 2014,Jul,3; 2014,Jan,11

+ 93464　**Physiologic exercise study (eg, bicycle or arm ergometry) including assessing hemodynamic measurements before and after (List separately in addition to code for primary procedure)**

EXCLUDES　*Administration of pharmacologic agent (93463)*
　　　　　Bundle of His recording (93600)
　　　　　Use of code more than one time per catheterization

Code first (33477, 93451-93453, 93456-93461, 93530-93533)

🖩 7.04　⚕ 7.04　**FUD** ZZZ　　　N 80 🖵

AMA: 2018,Feb,11; 2018,Jan,8; 2017,Jan,8; 2016,Jan,13; 2015,Jan,16; 2014,Jul,3; 2014,Jan,11

93503　**Insertion and placement of flow directed catheter (eg, Swan-Ganz) for monitoring purposes**

EXCLUDES　*Diagnostic cardiac catheterization (93451-93461, 93530-93533)*
　　　　　Subsequent monitoring (99356-99357)

🖩 2.55　⚕ 2.55　**FUD** 000　　　⊘ T 80 🖵

AMA: 2018,Feb,11; 2018,Jan,8; 2017,Jan,8; 2016,Jan,13; 2015,Jan,16; 2014,Jan,11

93505　**Endomyocardial biopsy**

EXCLUDES　*Intravascular brachytherapy radionuclide insertion (77770-77772)*
　　　　　Transcatheter insertion of brachytherapy delivery device (92974)

🖩 19.9　⚕ 19.9　**FUD** 000　　　T 80 🖵

AMA: 2018,Feb,11; 2018,Jan,8; 2017,Dec,13; 2017,Jan,8; 2016,Jan,13; 2015,Jan,16; 2014,Jan,11

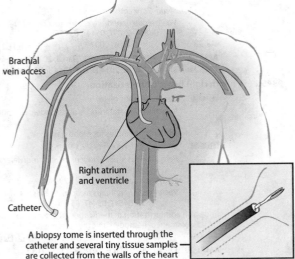

Fluoroscopic guidance may be via brachial, femoral, subclavian, or jugular vein

Brachial vein access

Right atrium and ventricle

Catheter

A biopsy tome is inserted through the catheter and several tiny tissue samples are collected from the walls of the heart

93530-93533 Congenital Heart Defect Catheterization

INCLUDES　Access site imaging and placement of closure device
　　　　　Cardiac output review
　　　　　Insertion catheter into 1+ right cardiac chambers or areas
　　　　　Obtaining samples for blood gas
　　　　　Radiology supervision and interpretation
　　　　　Roadmapping angiography

EXCLUDES　*Cardiac cath on noncongenital heart (93451-93453, 93456-93461)*
　　　　　Percutaneous repair congenital interatrial defect (93580)
　　　　　Swan-Ganz catheter insertion (93503)

Code also (93563-93568)

93530　**Right heart catheterization, for congenital cardiac anomalies**

🖩 0.00　⚕ 0.00　**FUD** 000　　　J 80 🖵

AMA: 2019,Jun,3; 2019,Mar,6; 2018,Feb,11; 2018,Jan,8; 2017,Jul,3; 2017,Jan,8; 2016,Mar,5; 2016,Jan,13; 2015,Sep,3; 2015,Jan,16; 2014,Jul,3; 2014,Jan,11

93531　**Combined right heart catheterization and retrograde left heart catheterization, for congenital cardiac anomalies**

🖩 0.00　⚕ 0.00　**FUD** 000　　　J 80 🖵

AMA: 2019,Jun,3; 2019,Mar,6; 2018,Feb,11; 2018,Jan,8; 2017,Jul,3; 2017,Jan,8; 2016,Mar,5; 2016,Jan,13; 2015,Sep,3; 2015,Jan,16; 2014,Jul,3; 2014,Jan,11

93532 Combined right heart catheterization and transseptal left heart catheterization through intact septum with or without retrograde left heart catheterization, for congenital cardiac anomalies

🚑 0.00 ⚕ 0.00 **FUD** 000 [J] [80] 🖵

AMA: 2019,Jun,3; 2019,Mar,6; 2018,Feb,11; 2018,Jan,8; 2017,Jul,3; 2017,Jan,8; 2016,Mar,5; 2016,Jan,13; 2015,Sep,3; 2015,Jan,16; 2014,Jul,3; 2014,Jan,11

93533 Combined right heart catheterization and transseptal left heart catheterization through existing septal opening, with or without retrograde left heart catheterization, for congenital cardiac anomalies

🚑 0.00 ⚕ 0.00 **FUD** 000 [J] [80] 🖵

AMA: 2019,Jun,3; 2019,Mar,6; 2018,Feb,11; 2018,Jan,8; 2017,Jul,3; 2017,Jan,8; 2016,Mar,5; 2016,Jan,13; 2015,Sep,3; 2015,Jan,16; 2014,Jul,3; 2014,Jan,11

93561-93568 Injection Procedures

INCLUDES Catheter repositioning
Radiology supervision and interpretation
Using automatic power injector

93561 Indicator dilution studies such as dye or thermodilution, including arterial and/or venous catheterization; with cardiac output measurement (separate procedure)

EXCLUDES Cardiac output, radioisotope method (78472-78473, 78481)
Catheterization procedures (93451-93462)
Percutaneous closure patent ductus arteriosus (93582)

🚑 0.00 ⚕ 0.00 **FUD** ZZZ [N] [80] 🖵

AMA: 2019,Aug,8; 2018,Feb,11; 2018,Jan,8; 2017,Jan,8; 2016,Jan,13; 2015,Jan,16; 2014,Jul,3; 2014,Jan,11

93562 subsequent measurement of cardiac output

EXCLUDES Cardiac output, radioisotope method (78472-78473, 78481)
Catheterization procedures (93451-93462)
Percutaneous closure patent ductus arteriosus (93582)

🚑 0.00 ⚕ 0.00 **FUD** ZZZ [N] [80] 🖵

AMA: 2019,Aug,8; 2018,Feb,11; 2018,Jan,8; 2017,Jan,8; 2016,Jan,13; 2015,Jan,16; 2014,Jul,3; 2014,May,4; 2014,Jan,11

+ **93563** Injection procedure during cardiac catheterization including imaging supervision, interpretation, and report; for selective coronary angiography during congenital heart catheterization (List separately in addition to code for primary procedure)

EXCLUDES Catheterization procedures (93452-93461)
Valve repair or annulus reconstruction (33418, 0345T, 0483T, 0484T, 0544T, 0545T)
Code first (93530-93533)

🚑 1.69 ⚕ 1.69 **FUD** ZZZ [N] [80] 🖵

AMA: 2018,Feb,11; 2018,Jan,8; 2017,Jan,8; 2016,Mar,5; 2016,Jan,13; 2015,Jan,16; 2014,Dec,6; 2014,Jan,11

+ **93564** for selective opacification of aortocoronary venous or arterial bypass graft(s) (eg, aortocoronary saphenous vein, free radial artery, or free mammary artery graft) to one or more coronary arteries and in situ arterial conduits (eg, internal mammary), whether native or used for bypass to one or more coronary arteries during congenital heart catheterization, when performed (List separately in addition to code for primary procedure)

Percutaneous repair congenital interatrial defect (93580)
Valve repair or annulus reconstruction (33418, 0345T, 0483T, 0484T, 0544T, 0545T)
Code first (93530-93533)
EXCLUDES Catheterization procedures (93452-93461)

🚑 1.79 ⚕ 1.79 **FUD** ZZZ [N] [80] 🖵

AMA: 2018,Feb,11; 2018,Jan,8; 2017,Jan,8; 2016,Mar,5; 2016,Jan,13; 2015,Jan,16; 2014,Dec,6; 2014,Jan,11

+ **93565** for selective left ventricular or left atrial angiography (List separately in addition to code for primary procedure)

EXCLUDES Catheterization procedures (93452-93461)
Percutaneous repair congenital interatrial defect (93580)
Code first (93530-93533)

🚑 1.31 ⚕ 1.31 **FUD** ZZZ [N] [80] 🖵

AMA: 2018,Feb,11; 2018,Jan,8; 2017,Jan,8; 2016,Jan,13; 2015,Jan,16; 2014,Jan,11

+ **93566** for selective right ventricular or right atrial angiography (List separately in addition to code for primary procedure)

EXCLUDES Annulus reconstruction (0545T)
Percutaneous repair congenital interatrial defect (93580)
Use for right ventriculography when performed during insertion leadless pacemaker ([33274])
Code first (93451, 93453, 93456-93457, 93460-93461, 93530-93533)

🚑 1.35 ⚕ 4.38 **FUD** ZZZ [N] [N1] [80] 🖵

AMA: 2019,Mar,6; 2018,Feb,11; 2018,Jan,8; 2017,Jan,8; 2016,Aug,5; 2016,May,5; 2016,Mar,5; 2016,Jan,13; 2015,May,3; 2015,Jan,16; 2014,Jan,11

+ **93567** for supravalvular aortography (List separately in addition to code for primary procedure)

EXCLUDES Abdominal aortography or non-supravalvular thoracic aortography at same time as cardiac catheterization (36221, 75600-75630)
Code first (93451-93461, 93530-93533)

🚑 1.53 ⚕ 3.71 **FUD** ZZZ [N] [N1] [80] 🖵

AMA: 2018,Feb,11; 2018,Jan,8; 2017,Jan,8; 2016,Mar,5; 2016,Jan,13; 2015,Jan,16; 2014,Jan,11

+ **93568** for pulmonary angiography (List separately in addition to code for primary procedure)

Code first (93451, 93453, 93456-93457, 93460-93461, 93530-93533)

🚑 1.38 ⚕ 3.97 **FUD** ZZZ [N] [N1] [80] 🖵

AMA: 2019,Jun,3; 2019,Apr,10; 2018,Feb,11; 2018,Jan,8; 2017,Jan,8; 2016,Mar,5; 2016,Jan,13; 2015,Jan,16; 2014,Jan,11

93571-93572 Coronary Artery Doppler Studies

INCLUDES Doppler transducer manipulations/repositioning within the vessel examined, during coronary angiography/therapeutic intervention (angioplasty)
EXCLUDES Intraprocedural coronary fractional flow reserve (FFR) ([0523T])

+ **93571** Intravascular Doppler velocity and/or pressure derived coronary flow reserve measurement (coronary vessel or graft) during coronary angiography including pharmacologically induced stress; initial vessel (List separately in addition to code for primary procedure)

Code first (92920, 92924, 92928, 92933, 92937, 92941, 92943, 92975, 93454-93461, 93563-93564)

🚑 0.00 ⚕ 0.00 **FUD** ZZZ [N] [N1] [80] 🖵

AMA: 2018,Feb,11; 2018,Jan,8; 2017,Jan,8; 2016,Jan,13; 2015,Dec,18; 2015,May,10; 2015,Jan,16; 2014,Dec,6; 2014,Jan,11

+ **93572** each additional vessel (List separately in addition to code for primary procedure)

Code first initial vessel (93571)

🚑 0.00 ⚕ 0.00 **FUD** ZZZ [N] [N1] [80] 🖵

AMA: 2018,Feb,11; 2018,Jan,8; 2017,Jan,8; 2016,Jan,13; 2015,Dec,18; 2015,May,10; 2015,Jan,16; 2014,Dec,6; 2014,Jan,11

93580-93583 Percutaneous Repair of Congenital Heart Defects

93580 **Percutaneous transcatheter closure of congenital interatrial communication (ie, Fontan fenestration, atrial septal defect) with implant**

> **INCLUDES** Injection of contrast for right heart atrial/ventricular angiograms (93564-93566)
> Right heart catheterization (93451, 93453, 93456-93457, 93460-93461, 93530-93533)
>
> **EXCLUDES** *Bypass graft angiography (93455)*
> *Injection of contrast for left heart atrial/ventricular angiograms (93458-93459)*
> *Left heart catheterization (93452, 93458-93459)*
> Code also echocardiography, when performed (93303-93317, 93662)

  📋 28.4   ⚕ 28.4   **FUD** 000   J 80 ▢

AMA: 2018,Feb,11; 2018,Jan,8; 2017,Jan,8; 2016,Jan,13; 2015,Jan,16; 2014,Jan,11

93581 **Percutaneous transcatheter closure of a congenital ventricular septal defect with implant**

> **INCLUDES** Injection of contrast for right heart atrial/ventricular angiograms (93564-93566)
> Right heart catheterization (93451, 93453, 93456-93457, 93460-93461, 93530-93533)
>
> **EXCLUDES** *Bypass graft angiography (93455)*
> *Injection of contrast for left heart atrial/ventricular angiograms (93458-93459)*
> *Left heart catheterization (93452, 93458-93459)*
> Code also echocardiography, when performed (93303-93317, 93662)

  📋 38.7   ⚕ 38.7   **FUD** 000   J 80 ▢

AMA: 2018,Feb,11; 2018,Jan,8; 2017,Jan,8; 2016,Jan,13; 2015,Jan,16; 2014,Jan,11

93582 **Percutaneous transcatheter closure of patent ductus arteriosus**

> **INCLUDES** Aorta catheter placement (36200)
> Aortography (75600-75605, 93567)
> Heart catheterization (93451-93461, 93530-93533)
>
> **EXCLUDES** *Catheterization pulmonary artery (36013-36014)*
> *Intracardiac echocardiographic services (93662)*
> *Left heart catheterization performed via transapical puncture or transseptal puncture through intact septum (93462)*
> *Ligation repair (33820, 33822, 33824)*
> *Other cardiac angiographic procedures (93563-93566, 93568)*
> *Other echocardiographic services by different provider (93315-93317)*

  📋 19.4   ⚕ 19.4   **FUD** 000   J 80 ▢

AMA: 2019,Apr,10; 2018,Feb,11; 2018,Jan,8; 2017,Jan,8; 2016,Jan,13; 2015,Jan,16; 2014,Jul,3

93583 **Percutaneous transcatheter septal reduction therapy (eg, alcohol septal ablation) including temporary pacemaker insertion when performed**

> **INCLUDES** Alcohol injection (93463)
> Coronary angiography during the procedure to roadmap, guide the intervention, measure the vessel, and complete the angiography (93454-93461, 93531-93533, 93563, 93563, 93565)
> Left heart catheterization (93452-93453, 93458-93461, 93531-93533)
> Temporary pacemaker insertion (33210)
>
> **EXCLUDES** *Intracardiac echocardiographic services when performed (93662)*
> *Myectomy (surgical ventriculomyotomy) to treat idiopathic hypertrophic subaortic stenosis (33416)*
> *Other echocardiographic services rendered by different provider (93312-93317)*
> Code also diagnostic cardiac catheterization procedures if the patient's condition (clinical indication) has changed since the intervention or prior study, there is no available prior catheter-based diagnostic study of the treatment zone, or the prior study is not adequate (93451, 93454-93457, 93530, 93563-93564, 93566-93568)

  📋 21.6   ⚕ 21.6   **FUD** 000   C 80 ▢

AMA: 2018,Feb,11

93590-93592 Percutaneous Repair Paravalvular Leak

> **INCLUDES** Access with insertion and positioning of device
> Angiography
> Fluoroscopy (76000)
> Imaging guidance
> Left heart catheterization (93452-93453, 93459-93461, 93531-93533)
> Code also diagnostic right heart catheterization and angiography performed:
> If a previous study is available but documentation states the patient's condition has changed since the previous study; visualization is insufficient; or a change necessitates reevaluation; append modifier 59
> When there is no previous study and a complete diagnostic study is performed; append modifier 59

93590 **Percutaneous transcatheter closure of paravalvular leak; initial occlusion device, mitral valve**

> **INCLUDES** Transseptal puncture (93462)
> Code also for transapical puncture (93462)

  📋 31.2   ⚕ 31.2   **FUD** 000   J 80 ▢

AMA: 2018,Feb,11; 2018,Jan,8; 2017,Sep,3

93591 **initial occlusion device, aortic valve**

> **EXCLUDES** *Transapical or transseptal puncture (93462)*

  📋 25.7   ⚕ 25.7   **FUD** 000   J 80 ▢

AMA: 2018,Feb,11; 2018,Jan,8; 2017,Sep,3

+ 93592 **each additional occlusion device (List separately in addition to code for primary procedure)**

> Code first (93590-93591)

  📋 11.3   ⚕ 11.3   **FUD** ZZZ   N 80 ▢

AMA: 2018,Feb,11; 2018,Jan,8; 2017,Sep,3

93600-93603 Recording of Intracardiac Electrograms

> **INCLUDES** Unusual situations where there may be recording/pacing/attempt at arrhythmia induction from only one side of the heart
>
> **EXCLUDES** *Comprehensive electrophysiological studies (93619-93620, 93653-93654, 93656)*

93600 **Bundle of His recording**

  📋 0.00   ⚕ 0.00   **FUD** 000   ⊘ J 80 ▢

AMA: 2018,Feb,11; 2018,Jan,8; 2017,Jan,8; 2016,Jan,13; 2015,Jan,16; 2014,Apr,3; 2014,Jan,11

93602 **Intra-atrial recording**

  📋 0.00   ⚕ 0.00   **FUD** 000   ⊘ J 80 ▢

AMA: 2018,Feb,11; 2018,Jan,8; 2017,Jan,8; 2016,Jan,13; 2015,Jan,16; 2014,Apr,3; 2014,Jan,11

93603 **Right ventricular recording**

  📋 0.00   ⚕ 0.00   **FUD** 000   ⊘ J 80 ▢

AMA: 2018,Feb,11; 2018,Jan,8; 2017,Jan,8; 2016,Jan,13; 2015,Jan,16; 2014,Apr,3; 2014,Jan,11

26/TC PC/TC Only   A2-Z3 ASC Payment   50 Bilateral   ♂ Male Only   ♀ Female Only   📋 Facility RVU   ⚕ Non-Facility RVU   ▢ CCI   CLIA
FUD Follow-up Days   CMS: IOM   AMA: CPT Asst   A-Y OPPSI   80/80 Surg Assist Allowed / w/Doc   Lab Crosswalk   Radiology Crosswalk

490   CPT © 2019 American Medical Association. All Rights Reserved.   © 2019 Optum360, LLC

93609-93613 Intracardiac Mapping and Pacing

+   93609   Intraventricular and/or intra-atrial mapping of tachycardia site(s) with catheter manipulation to record from multiple sites to identify origin of tachycardia (List separately in addition to code for primary procedure)

> EXCLUDES   *Intracardiac 3D mapping (93613)*
> *Intracardiac ablation with 3D mapping (93654)*
> Code first (93620, 93653, 93656)
>
> 🔲 0.00   🔲 0.00   **FUD** ZZZ   Ⓝ 80 ▣
>
> **AMA:** 2018,Feb,11; 2018,Jan,8; 2017,Jan,8; 2016,Jan,13; 2015,Jan,16; 2014,Apr,3; 2014,Jan,11

Sinoatrial node

Atrio-ventricular node

Common bundle (His)

Tachycardia is rapid heartbeat

93610   Intra-atrial pacing

> INCLUDES   Unusual situations where there may be recording/pacing/attempt at arrhythmia induction from only one side of the heart
> EXCLUDES   *Comprehensive electrophysiological studies (93619-93620)*
> *Intracardiac ablation (93653-93654, 93656)*
>
> 🔲 0.00   🔲 0.00   **FUD** 000   Ⓢ Ⓙ 80 ▣
>
> **AMA:** 2018,Feb,11; 2018,Jan,8; 2017,Jan,8; 2016,Jan,13; 2015,Jan,16; 2014,Apr,3; 2014,Jan,11

93612   Intraventricular pacing

> INCLUDES   Unusual situations where there may be recording/pacing/attempt at arrhythmia induction from only one side of the heart
> EXCLUDES   *Comprehensive electrophysiological studies (93619-93622)*
> *Intracardiac ablation (93653-93654, 93656)*
>
> 🔲 0.00   🔲 0.00   **FUD** 000   Ⓢ Ⓙ 80 ▣
>
> **AMA:** 2018,Feb,11; 2018,Jan,8; 2017,Jan,8; 2016,Jan,13; 2015,Jan,16; 2014,Apr,3; 2014,Jan,11

+   93613   Intracardiac electrophysiologic 3-dimensional mapping (List separately in addition to code for primary procedure)

> EXCLUDES   *Intracardiac ablation with 3D mapping (93654)*
> *Mapping of tachycardia site (93609)*
> Code first (93620, 93653, 93656)
>
> 🔲 8.63   🔲 8.63   **FUD** ZZZ   Ⓝ 80 ▣
>
> **AMA:** 2018,Feb,11; 2018,Jan,8; 2017,Jan,8; 2016,Jan,13; 2015,Jan,16; 2014,Apr,3; 2014,Jan,11

93615-93616 Recording and Pacing via Esophagus

93615   Esophageal recording of atrial electrogram with or without ventricular electrogram(s);

> 🔲 0.00   🔲 0.00   **FUD** 000   Ⓢ Ⓙ 80 ▣
>
> **AMA:** 2018,Feb,11; 2018,Jan,8; 2017,Jan,8; 2016,Jan,13; 2015,Jan,16; 2014,Jan,11

93616   with pacing

> 🔲 0.00   🔲 0.00   **FUD** 000   Ⓢ Ⓙ 80 ▣
>
> **AMA:** 2018,Feb,11; 2018,Jan,8; 2017,Jan,8; 2016,Jan,13; 2015,Jan,16; 2014,Jan,11

93618 Pacing to Produce an Arrhythmia

CMS: 100-03,20.12 Diagnostic Endocardial Electrical Stimulation (Pacing)

> INCLUDES   Unusual situations where there may be recording/pacing/attempt at arrhythmia induction from only one side of the heart
> EXCLUDES   *Comprehensive electrophysiological studies (93619-93622)*
> *Intracardiac ablation (93653-93654, 93656)*
> *Intracardiac phonocardiogram (93799)*

93618   Induction of arrhythmia by electrical pacing

> 🔲 0.00   🔲 0.00   **FUD** 000   Ⓢ Ⓙ 80 ▣
>
> **AMA:** 2018,Feb,11; 2018,Jan,8; 2017,Jan,8; 2016,Jan,13; 2015,Jan,16; 2014,Apr,3; 2014,Jan,11

93619-93623 Comprehensive Electrophysiological Studies

CMS: 100-03,20.12 Diagnostic Endocardial Electrical Stimulation (Pacing)

93619   Comprehensive electrophysiologic evaluation with right atrial pacing and recording, right ventricular pacing and recording, His bundle recording, including insertion and repositioning of multiple electrode catheters, without induction or attempted induction of arrhythmia

> INCLUDES   Evaluation of sinus node/atrioventricular node/His-Purkinje conduction system without arrhythmia induction
> EXCLUDES   *Comprehensive electrophysiological studies (93620-93622)*
> *Intracardiac ablation (93653-93657)*
> *Intracardiac pacing (93610, 93612, 93618)*
> *Recording of intracardiac electrograms (93600-93603)*
>
> 🔲 0.00   🔲 0.00   **FUD** 000   Ⓙ 80 ▣
>
> **AMA:** 2018,Feb,11; 2018,Jan,8; 2017,Jan,8; 2016,Jan,13; 2015,Jan,16; 2014,Apr,3; 2014,Jan,11

93620   Comprehensive electrophysiologic evaluation including insertion and repositioning of multiple electrode catheters with induction or attempted induction of arrhythmia; with right atrial pacing and recording, right ventricular pacing and recording, His bundle recording

> INCLUDES   Recording/pacing/attempted arrhythmia induction from one or more site(s) in the heart
> EXCLUDES   *Comprehensive electrophysiological study without induction/attempted induction arrhythmia (93619)*
> *Intracardiac ablation (93653-93657)*
> *Intracardiac pacing (93610, 93612, 93618)*
> *Recording of intracardiac electrograms (93600-93603)*
>
> 🔲 0.00   🔲 0.00   **FUD** 000   Ⓙ 80 ▣
>
> **AMA:** 2018,Feb,11; 2018,Jan,8; 2017,Jan,8; 2016,Jan,13; 2015,Jan,16; 2014,Apr,3; 2014,Jan,11

+   93621   with left atrial pacing and recording from coronary sinus or left atrium (List separately in addition to code for primary procedure)

> INCLUDES   Recording/pacing/attempted arrhythmia induction from one or more site(s) in the heart
> EXCLUDES   *Intracardiac ablation (93656)*
> Code first (93620, 93653-93654)
>
> 🔲 0.00   🔲 0.00   **FUD** ZZZ   Ⓝ 80 ▣
>
> **AMA:** 2018,Feb,11; 2018,Jan,8; 2017,Jan,8; 2016,Jan,13; 2015,Jan,16; 2014,Apr,3; 2014,Jan,11

93609 — 93621

+ 93622 with left ventricular pacing and recording (List separately in addition to code for primary procedure)

> *EXCLUDES*   *Intracardiac ablation (93654)*
> Code first (93620, 93653, 93656)
> 🖪 0.00   ⚕ 0.00   **FUD** ZZZ   N 80 🖿
>
> **AMA:** 2018,Feb,11; 2018,Jan,8; 2017,Jan,8; 2016,Jan,13; 2015,Jan,16; 2014,Apr,3; 2014,Jan,11

+ 93623 Programmed stimulation and pacing after intravenous drug infusion (List separately in addition to code for primary procedure)

> *INCLUDES*   Recording/pacing/attempted arrhythmia induction from one or more site(s) in the heart
> *EXCLUDES*   *Use of code more than one time per day*
> Code first comprehensive electrophysiologic evaluation (93610, 93612, 93619-93620, 93653-93654, 93656)
> 🖪 0.00   ⚕ 0.00   **FUD** ZZZ   N 80 🖿
>
> **AMA:** 2018,Feb,11; 2018,Jan,8; 2017,Jan,8; 2016,Jan,13; 2015,Jan,16; 2014,Apr,3; 2014,Jan,11

93624-93631 Followup and Intraoperative Electrophysiologic Studies

CMS: 100-03,20.12 Diagnostic Endocardial Electrical Stimulation (Pacing)

93624 Electrophysiologic follow-up study with pacing and recording to test effectiveness of therapy, including induction or attempted induction of arrhythmia

> *INCLUDES*   Recording/pacing/attempted arrhythmia induction from one or more site(s) in the heart
> 🖪 0.00   ⚕ 0.00   **FUD** 000   J 80 🖿
>
> **AMA:** 2018,Feb,11; 2018,Jan,8; 2017,Jan,8; 2016,Jan,13; 2015,Jan,16; 2014,Jan,11

93631 Intra-operative epicardial and endocardial pacing and mapping to localize the site of tachycardia or zone of slow conduction for surgical correction

> *EXCLUDES*   *Operative ablation of an arrhythmogenic focus or pathway by a separate provider (33250-33261)*
> 🖪 0.00   ⚕ 0.00   **FUD** 000   N 80 🖿
>
> **AMA:** 2018,Feb,11; 2018,Jan,8; 2017,Jan,8; 2016,Jan,13; 2015,Jan,16; 2014,Jan,11

93640-93644 Electrophysiologic Studies of Cardioverter-Defibrillators

> *INCLUDES*   Recording/pacing/attempted arrhythmia induction from one or more site(s) in the heart

93640 Electrophysiologic evaluation of single or dual chamber pacing cardioverter-defibrillator leads including defibrillation threshold evaluation (induction of arrhythmia, evaluation of sensing and pacing for arrhythmia termination) at time of initial implantation or replacement;

> 🖪 0.00   ⚕ 0.00   **FUD** 000   N 80 🖿
>
> **AMA:** 2018,Feb,11; 2018,Jan,8; 2017,Jan,8; 2016,Jan,13; 2015,Jan,16; 2014,Jan,11

93641 with testing of single or dual chamber pacing cardioverter-defibrillator pulse generator

> *EXCLUDES*   *Single/dual chamber pacing cardioverter-defibrillators reprogramming/electronic analysis, subsequent/periodic (93282-93283, 93289, 93292, 93295, 93642)*
> 🖪 0.00   ⚕ 0.00   **FUD** 000   N 80 🖿
>
> **AMA:** 2018,Feb,11; 2018,Jan,8; 2017,Jan,8; 2016,Jan,13; 2015,Jan,16; 2014,Apr,3; 2014,Jan,11

93642 Electrophysiologic evaluation of single or dual chamber transvenous pacing cardioverter-defibrillator (includes defibrillation threshold evaluation, induction of arrhythmia, evaluation of sensing and pacing for arrhythmia termination, and programming or reprogramming of sensing or therapeutic parameters)

> 🖪 9.78   ⚕ 9.78   **FUD** 000   J 80 🖿
>
> **AMA:** 2018,Feb,11; 2018,Jan,8; 2017,Jan,8; 2016,Jan,13; 2015,Jan,16; 2014,Apr,3; 2014,Jan,11

93644 Electrophysiologic evaluation of subcutaneous implantable defibrillator (includes defibrillation threshold evaluation, induction of arrhythmia, evaluation of sensing for arrhythmia termination, and programming or reprogramming of sensing or therapeutic parameters)

> *EXCLUDES*   *Electrophysiological evaluation subcutaneous implantable defibrillator system with substernal electrode (0577T)*
> *Insertion/replacement subcutaneous implantable defibrillator ([33270])*
> *Subcutaneous cardioverter-defibrillator electrophysiologic evaluation, subsequent/periodic (93260-93261)*
> 🖪 5.65   ⚕ 5.65   **FUD** 000   N 80 🖿
>
> **AMA:** 2018,Feb,11

93650-93657 Intracardiac Ablation

> *INCLUDES*   Ablation services include selective delivery of cryo-energy or radiofrequency to targeted tissue
> Electrophysiologic studies performed in the same session with ablation

93650 Intracardiac catheter ablation of atrioventricular node function, atrioventricular conduction for creation of complete heart block, with or without temporary pacemaker placement

> 🖪 17.2   ⚕ 17.2   **FUD** 000   J 80 🖿
>
> **AMA:** 2018,Feb,11; 2018,Jan,8; 2017,Jan,8; 2016,Jan,13; 2015,Jan,16; 2014,Jan,11

93653 Comprehensive electrophysiologic evaluation including insertion and repositioning of multiple electrode catheters with induction or attempted induction of an arrhythmia with right atrial pacing and recording, right ventricular pacing and recording (when necessary), and His bundle recording (when necessary) with intracardiac catheter ablation of arrhythmogenic focus; with treatment of supraventricular tachycardia by ablation of fast or slow atrioventricular pathway, accessory atrioventricular connection, cavo-tricuspid isthmus or other single atrial focus or source of atrial re-entry

> *EXCLUDES*   *Comprehensive electrophysiological studies (93619-93620)*
> *Electrophysiologic evaluation pacing cardioverter defibrillator (93642)*
> *Intracardiac ablation with transseptal catheterization (93656)*
> *Intracardiac ablation with treatment ventricular arrhythmia (93654)*
> *Intracardiac pacing (93610, 93612, 93618)*
> *Recording of intracardiac electrograms (93600-93603)*
> 🖪 24.3   ⚕ 24.3   **FUD** 000   J 80 🖿
>
> **AMA:** 2018,Feb,11; 2018,Jan,8; 2017,Jan,8; 2016,Jan,13; 2015,Jan,16; 2014,Apr,3

93654 with treatment of ventricular tachycardia or focus of ventricular ectopy including intracardiac electrophysiologic 3D mapping, when performed, and left ventricular pacing and recording, when performed

> *EXCLUDES*   *Comprehensive electrophysiological studies (93619-93620, 93622)*
> *Device evaluation (93279-93284, 93286-93289)*
> *Electrophysiologic evaluation pacing cardioverter defibrillator (93642)*
> *Intracardiac ablation with transseptal catheterization (93656)*
> *Intracardiac ablation with treatment supraventricular tachycardia (93653)*
> *Intracardiac pacing (93609-93613, 93618)*
> *Recording of intracardiac electrograms (93600-93603)*
> 🖪 32.6   ⚕ 32.6   **FUD** 000   J 80 🖿
>
> **AMA:** 2018,Feb,11; 2018,Jan,8; 2017,Jan,8; 2016,Jan,13; 2015,Jan,16; 2014,Apr,3

| 26/TC PC/TC Only | A2-Z3 ASC Payment | 50 Bilateral | ♂ Male Only | ♀ Female Only | 🖪 Facility RVU | ⚕ Non-Facility RVU | CCI | CLIA |
| FUD Follow-up Days | CMS: IOM | AMA: CPT Asst | A-Y OPPSI | 80/80 Surg Assist Allowed / w/Doc | | Lab Crosswalk | Radiology Crosswalk |

492   CPT © 2019 American Medical Association. All Rights Reserved.   © 2019 Optum360, LLC

+ **93655** Intracardiac catheter ablation of a discrete mechanism of arrhythmia which is distinct from the primary ablated mechanism, including repeat diagnostic maneuvers, to treat a spontaneous or induced arrhythmia (List separately in addition to code for primary procedure)

> Code first (93653-93654, 93656)
> 🔲 12.4   ⚬ 12.4   **FUD** ZZZ   N 80 ▢
> **AMA:** 2018,Feb,11; 2018,Jan,8; 2017,Jan,8; 2016,Jan,13; 2015,Jan,16; 2014,Apr,3

93656 Comprehensive electrophysiologic evaluation including transseptal catheterizations, insertion and repositioning of multiple electrode catheters with induction or attempted induction of an arrhythmia including left or right atrial pacing/recording when necessary, right ventricular pacing/recording when necessary, and His bundle recording when necessary with intracardiac catheter ablation of atrial fibrillation by pulmonary vein isolation

> INCLUDES His bundle recording when indicated
> Left atrial pacing/recording
> Right ventricular pacing/recording
> EXCLUDES Comprehensive electrophysiological studies (93619-93621)
> Device evaluation (93279-93284, 93286-93289)
> Electrophysiologic evaluation with treatment ventricular tachycardia (93654)
> Intracardiac ablation with treatment supraventricular tachycardia (93653)
> Intracardiac pacing (93610, 93612, 93618)
> Left heart catheterization by transseptal puncture (93462)
> Recording of intracardiac electrograms (93600-93603)
> 🔲 32.7   ⚬ 32.7   **FUD** 000   J 80 ▢
> **AMA:** 2019,Sep,10; 2018,Feb,11; 2018,Jan,8; 2017,Jan,8; 2016,Jan,13; 2015,Jan,16; 2014,Apr,3

+ **93657** Additional linear or focal intracardiac catheter ablation of the left or right atrium for treatment of atrial fibrillation remaining after completion of pulmonary vein isolation (List separately in addition to code for primary procedure)

> Code first (93656)
> 🔲 12.3   ⚬ 12.3   **FUD** ZZZ   N 80 ▢
> **AMA:** 2019,Sep,10; 2018,Feb,11; 2018,Jan,8; 2017,Jan,8; 2016,Jan,13; 2015,Jan,16; 2014,Apr,3

93660-93662 Other Tests for Cardiac Function

93660 Evaluation of cardiovascular function with tilt table evaluation, with continuous ECG monitoring and intermittent blood pressure monitoring, with or without pharmacological intervention

> EXCLUDES Autonomic nervous system function testing (95921, 95924, [95943])
> 🔲 4.51   ⚬ 4.51   **FUD** 000   S 80 ▢
> **AMA:** 2018,Feb,11; 2018,Jan,8; 2017,Jan,8; 2016,Jan,13; 2015,Jan,16; 2014,Jan,11

+ **93662** Intracardiac echocardiography during therapeutic/diagnostic intervention, including imaging supervision and interpretation (List separately in addition to code for primary procedure)

> EXCLUDES Internal cardioversion (92961)
> Transcatheter tricuspid valve repair with prosthesis, percutaneous approach (0569T-0570T)
> Code first (as appropriate) (92987, 93453, 93460-93462, 93532, 93580-93581, 93620-93622, 93653-93654, 93656)
> 🔲 0.00   ⚬ 0.00   **FUD** ZZZ   N 80 ▢
> **AMA:** 2018,Feb,11; 2018,Jan,8; 2017,Jan,8; 2016,Jan,13; 2015,Jan,16; 2014,Jan,11

93668 Rehabilitation Services: Peripheral Arterial Disease

CMS: 100-03,1,20.35 Supervised Exercise Therapy (SET) for Symptomatic Peripheral Artery Disease (PAD)(Effective May 25, 2017; 100-04,32,390 Supervised exercise therapy (SET) Symptomatic Peripheral Artery Disease; 100-04,32,390.1 General Billing Requirements for Supervised exercise therapy (SET) for PAD; 100-04,32,390.2 Coding Requirements for SET for PAD; 100-04,32,390.3 Special Billing Requirements for Professional Claims; 100-04,32,390.4 Special Billing Requirements for Institutional Claims; 100-04,32,390.5 Common Working File (CWF) Requirements; 100-04,32,390.6 Applicable Medicare Summary Notice (MSN), Remittance Advice Remark Codes (RARCs), and Claim Adjustment Reason Code (CARC) Messaging

> INCLUDES Monitoring:
> Other cardiovascular limitations for adjustment of workload
> Patient's claudication threshold
> Motorized treadmill or track
> Sessions lasting 45-60 minutes
> Supervision by exercise physiologist/nurse
> Code also appropriate E&M service, when performed

93668 Peripheral arterial disease (PAD) rehabilitation, per session

> 🔲 0.50   ⚬ 0.50   **FUD** XXX   S 80 TC ▢
> **AMA:** 2018,Feb,11

93701-93702 Thoracic Electrical Bioimpedance

> EXCLUDES Bioelectrical impedance analysis whole body (0358T)
> Indirect measurement of left ventricular filling pressure by computerized calibration of the arterial waveform response to Valsalva (93799)

93701 Bioimpedance-derived physiologic cardiovascular analysis

> 🔲 0.71   ⚬ 0.71   **FUD** XXX   Q1 80 TC ▢
> **AMA:** 2018,Feb,11; 2018,Jan,8; 2017,Jan,8; 2016,Jan,13; 2015,Jan,16; 2014,Jan,11

93702 Bioimpedance spectroscopy (BIS), extracellular fluid analysis for lymphedema assessment(s)

> 🔲 3.57   ⚬ 3.57   **FUD** XXX   S 80 TC ▢
> **AMA:** 2018,Feb,11

93724 Electronic Analysis of Pacemaker Function

93724 Electronic analysis of antitachycardia pacemaker system (includes electrocardiographic recording, programming of device, induction and termination of tachycardia via implanted pacemaker, and interpretation of recordings)

> 🔲 7.89   ⚬ 7.89   **FUD** 000   S 80 ▢
> **AMA:** 2018,Feb,11; 2018,Jan,8; 2017,Jan,8; 2016,Jan,13; 2015,Jan,16; 2014,Jan,11

93740 Temperature Gradient Assessment

93740 Temperature gradient studies

> 🔲 0.23   ⚬ 0.23   **FUD** XXX   Q1 ▢
> **AMA:** 2018,Feb,11

93745 Wearable Cardioverter-Defibrillator System Services

> EXCLUDES Device evaluation (93282, 93292)

93745 Initial set-up and programming by a physician or other qualified health care professional of wearable cardioverter-defibrillator includes initial programming of system, establishing baseline electronic ECG, transmission of data to data repository, patient instruction in wearing system and patient reporting of problems or events

> 🔲 0.00   ⚬ 0.00   **FUD** XXX   S 80 ▢
> **AMA:** 2018,Feb,11

93750 Ventricular Assist Device (VAD) Interrogation

CMS: 100-03,20.9 Artificial Hearts and Related Devices; 100-03,20.9.1 Ventricular Assist Devices; 100-04,32,320.1 Artificial Hearts Prior to May 1, 2008; 100-04,32,320.2 Coding for Artificial Hearts After May 1, 2008; 100-04,32,320.3 Ventricular Assist Devices; 100-04,32,320.3.1 Post-cardiotomy; 100-04,32,320.3.2 Bridge- to -Transplantation

EXCLUDES Insertion of ventricular assist device (33975-33976, 33979)
Removal/replacement ventricular assist device (33981-33983)

93750 Interrogation of ventricular assist device (VAD), in person, with physician or other qualified health care professional analysis of device parameters (eg, drivelines, alarms, power surges), review of device function (eg, flow and volume status, septum status, recovery), with programming, if performed, and report

1.32 1.58 **FUD** XXX S 80

AMA: 2018,Dec,10; 2018,Dec,10; 2018,Feb,11; 2018,Jan,8; 2017,Jan,8; 2016,Jan,13; 2015,Jan,16; 2014,Jan,11

93770 Peripheral Venous Blood Pressure Assessment

CMS: 100-03,20.19 Ambulatory Blood Pressure Monitoring (20.19)

EXCLUDES Cannulization, central venous (36500, 36555-36556)

93770 Determination of venous pressure

0.23 0.23 **FUD** XXX N

AMA: 2018,Feb,11

93784-93790 Ambulatory Blood Pressure Monitoring

CMS: 100-03,20.19 Ambulatory Blood Pressure Monitoring (20.19); 100-04,32,10.1 Ambulatory Blood Pressure Monitoring Billing Requirements

EXCLUDES Self-measured blood pressure monitoring ([99473, 99474])

▲ **93784** Ambulatory blood pressure monitoring, utilizing report-generating software, automated, worn continuously for 24 hours or longer; including recording, scanning analysis, interpretation and report

1.51 1.51 **FUD** XXX B 80

AMA: 2018,Feb,11

▲ **93786** recording only

0.83 0.83 **FUD** XXX Q1 80 TC

AMA: 2018,Feb,11

▲ **93788** scanning analysis with report

0.15 0.15 **FUD** XXX Q1 80 TC

AMA: 2018,Feb,11

▲ **93790** review with interpretation and report

0.53 0.53 **FUD** XXX M 80 26

AMA: 2018,Feb,11

93792-93793 INR Monitoring

CMS: 100-03,190.11 Home PT/INR Monitoring for Anticoagulation Management; 100-04,32,60.4.1 Anticoagulation Management: Covered Diagnosis Codes

EXCLUDES Chronic care management ([99490], 99487, 99489)
Online digital evaluation and management services by a physician or other qualified health care professional ([99421, 99422, 99423])
Telephone assessment and management service by nonphysician healthcare professional (98966-98968)
Telephone evaluation and management service by physician or other qualified healthcare professional (99441-99443)
Transitional care management (99495-99496)

93792 Patient/caregiver training for initiation of home international normalized ratio (INR) monitoring under the direction of a physician or other qualified health care professional, face-to-face, including use and care of the INR monitor, obtaining blood sample, instructions for reporting home INR test results, and documentation of patient's/caregiver's ability to perform testing and report results

Code also INR home monitoring equipment with appropriate supply code or (99070)
Code also significantly identifiable E&M service on same date of service using modifier 25

1.48 1.48 **FUD** XXX B 80 TC

AMA: 2018,Mar,7; 2018,Feb,11

93793 Anticoagulant management for a patient taking warfarin, must include review and interpretation of a new home, office, or lab international normalized ratio (INR) test result, patient instructions, dosage adjustment (as needed), and scheduling of additional test(s), when performed

EXCLUDES E&M services on same date of service (99201-99215, 99241-99245)
Use of code more than one time per day

0.34 0.34 **FUD** XXX B 80 26

AMA: 2018,Mar,7; 2018,Feb,11; 2018,Jan,8; 2017,Nov,10

93797-93799 Cardiac Rehabilitation

CMS: 100-02,15,232 Cardiac Rehabilitation (CR) and Intensive Cardiac Rehabilitation (ICR) Services Furnished On or After January 1, 2010; 100-04,32,140.2 Cardiac Rehabilitation On or After January 1, 2010; 100-04,32,140.2.1 Coding Cardiac Rehabilitation Services On or After January 1, 2010; 100-04,32,140.2.2.2 Institutional Claims for CR and ICR Services; 100-04,32,140.2.2.4 CR Services Exceeding 36 Sessions; 100-04,32,140.3 Intensive Cardiac Rehabilitation Program Services Furnished On or After January 1, 2010; 100-08,15,4.2.8 Cardiac Rehabilitation (CR) and Intensive Cardiac Rehabilitation (ICR)

93797 Physician or other qualified health care professional services for outpatient cardiac rehabilitation; without continuous ECG monitoring (per session)

0.25 0.46 **FUD** 000 S 80

AMA: 2018,Feb,11

93798 with continuous ECG monitoring (per session)

0.40 0.72 **FUD** 000 S 80

AMA: 2018,Feb,11

93799 Unlisted cardiovascular service or procedure

0.00 0.00 **FUD** XXX S 80

AMA: 2018,Dec,10; 2018,Dec,10; 2018,Sep,10; 2018,Aug,10; 2018,Feb,11; 2018,Jan,8; 2017,Jan,8; 2016,May,5; 2016,Jan,13; 2015,Jan,16; 2014,Jan,11

93880-93895 Noninvasive Tests Extracranial/Intracranial Arteries

INCLUDES Patient care required to perform/supervise studies and interpret results
EXCLUDES Hand-held dopplers that do not provide a hard copy or vascular flow bidirectional analysis (See E&M codes)

93880 Duplex scan of extracranial arteries; complete bilateral study

EXCLUDES Common carotid intima-media thickness (IMT) studies (93895, 0126T)

5.70 5.70 **FUD** XXX S 80

AMA: 2018,Feb,11; 2018,Jan,8; 2017,Jan,8; 2016,Jan,13; 2015,Jan,16; 2014,Jan,11

93882 unilateral or limited study

EXCLUDES Common carotid intima-media thickness (IMT) studies (93895, 0126T)

3.64 3.64 **FUD** XXX S 80

AMA: 2018,Feb,11; 2018,Jan,8; 2017,Jan,8; 2016,Jan,13; 2015,Jan,16; 2014,Jan,11

93886 Transcranial Doppler study of the intracranial arteries; complete study

INCLUDES Complete transcranial doppler (TCD) study
Ultrasound evaluation of right/left anterior circulation territories and posterior circulation territory

7.67 7.67 **FUD** XXX S 80

AMA: 2018,Feb,11; 2018,Jan,8; 2017,Jan,8; 2016,Jan,13; 2015,Jan,16; 2014,Jan,11

93888 limited study

INCLUDES Limited TCD study
Ultrasound examination of two or fewer of these territories (right/left anterior circulation, posterior circulation)

4.47 4.47 **FUD** XXX S 80

AMA: 2018,Feb,11; 2018,Jan,8; 2017,Jan,8; 2016,Jan,13; 2015,Jan,16; 2014,Jan,11

93890 vasoreactivity study

EXCLUDES Limited TCD study (93888)

7.82 7.82 **FUD** XXX Q1 80

AMA: 2018,Feb,11; 2018,Jan,8; 2017,Jan,8; 2016,Jan,13; 2015,Jan,16; 2014,Jan,11

93892   emboli detection without intravenous microbubble injection

EXCLUDES   *Limited TCD study (93888)*

🚑 8.81   ⚕ 8.81   **FUD** XXX   Q1 80 💻

AMA: 2018,Feb,11; 2018,Jan,8; 2017,Jan,8; 2016,Jan,13; 2015,Jan,16; 2014,Jan,11

93893   emboli detection with intravenous microbubble injection

EXCLUDES   *Limited TCD study (93888)*

🚑 9.81   ⚕ 9.81   **FUD** XXX   Q1 80 💻

AMA: 2018,Feb,11; 2018,Jan,8; 2017,Jan,8; 2016,Jan,13; 2015,Jan,16; 2014,Jan,11

93895   Quantitative carotid intima media thickness and carotid atheroma evaluation, bilateral

EXCLUDES   *Common carotid intima-media thickness (IMT) study (0126T)*

Complete and limited duplex studies (93880, 93882)

🚑 0.00   ⚕ 0.00   **FUD** XXX   E 80 💻

AMA: 2018,Feb,11

93922-93971 Noninvasive Vascular Studies: Extremities

CMS: 100-04,8,180 Noninvasive Studies for ESRD Patients

INCLUDES   Patient care required to perform/supervise studies and interpret results

EXCLUDES   *Hand-held dopplers that do not provide a hard copy or provided vascular flow bidirectional analysis (see E&M codes)*

93922   Limited bilateral noninvasive physiologic studies of upper or lower extremity arteries, (eg, for lower extremity: ankle/brachial indices at distal posterior tibial and anterior tibial/dorsalis pedis arteries plus bidirectional, Doppler waveform recording and analysis at 1-2 levels, or ankle/brachial indices at distal posterior tibial and anterior tibial/dorsalis pedis arteries plus volume plethysmography at 1-2 levels, or ankle/brachial indices at distal posterior tibial and anterior tibial/dorsalis pedis arteries with, transcutaneous oxygen tension measurement at 1-2 levels)

INCLUDES   Evaluation of:

Doppler analysis of bidirectional blood flow

Nonimaging physiologic recordings of pressure

Oxygen tension measurements and/or plethysmography

Lower extremity (potential levels include high thigh, low thigh, calf, ankle, metatarsal and toes) limited study includes either:

Ankle/brachial indices at distal posterior tibial and anterior tibial/dorsalis pedis arteries plus bidirectional Doppler waveform recording and analysis as 1-2 levels; OR

Ankle/brachial indices at distal posterior tibial and anterior tibial/dorsalis pedis arteries plus volume plethysmography at 1-2 levels; OR

Ankle/brachial indices at distal posterior tibial and anterior tibial/dorsalis pedis arteries with transcutaneous oxygen tension measurements at 1-2 levels

Unilateral provocative functional measurement

Unilateral study of 3 or move levels

Upper extremity (potential levels include arm, forearm, wrist, and digits) limited study includes:

Doppler-determined systolic pressures and bidirectional waveform recording with analysis at 1-2 levels; OR

Doppler-determined systolic pressures and transcutaneous oxygen tension measurements at 1-2 levels; OR

Doppler-determined systolic pressures and volume plethysmography at 1-2 levels

EXCLUDES   *Transcutaneous oxyhemoglobin measurement (0493T)*

Use of code more than one time for the lower extremity(s)

Use of code more than one time for the upper extremity(s)

Code also modifier 52 for unilateral study of 1-2 levels

Code also twice with modifier 59 for upper and lower extremity study

🚑 2.44   ⚕ 2.44   **FUD** XXX   Q1 80 💻

AMA: 2018,Feb,11; 2018,Jan,8; 2017,Jan,8; 2016,Jan,13; 2015,Jan,16; 2014,Jan,9; 2014,Jan,11

● New Code   ▲ Revised Code   ○ Reinstated   ● New Web Release   ▲ Revised Web Release   + Add-on   Unlisted   Not Covered   # Resequenced
50 Optum Mod 50 Exempt   ⊘ AMA Mod 51 Exempt   51 Optum Mod 51 Exempt   63 Mod 63 Exempt   ✓ Non-FDA Drug   ★ Telemedicine   M Maternity   A Age Edit

© 2019 Optum360, LLC   CPT © 2019 American Medical Association. All Rights Reserved.   495

93923 **Complete bilateral noninvasive physiologic studies of upper or lower extremity arteries, 3 or more levels (eg, for lower extremity: ankle/brachial indices at distal posterior tibial and anterior tibial/dorsalis pedis arteries plus segmental blood pressure measurements with bidirectional Doppler waveform recording and analysis, at 3 or more levels, or ankle/brachial indices at distal posterior tibial and anterior tibial/dorsalis pedis arteries plus segmental volume plethysmography at 3 or more levels, or ankle/brachial indices at distal posterior tibial and anterior tibial/dorsalis pedis arteries plus segmental transcutaneous oxygen tension measurements at 3 or more levels), or single level study with provocative functional maneuvers (eg, measurements with postural provocative tests, or measurements with reactive hyperemia)**

INCLUDES Evaluation of:
Doppler analysis of bidirectional blood flow
Nonimaging physiologic recordings of pressures
Oxygen tension measurements
Lower extremity:
Ankle/brachial indices at distal posterior tibial and anterior tibial/dorsalis pedis arteries plus bidirectional Doppler waveform recording and analysis at 3 or more levels; OR
Ankle/brachial indices at distal posterior tibial and anterior tibial/dorsalis pedis arteries with transcutaneous oxygen tension measurements at 3 or more levels; OR
Ankle/brachial indices at distal posterior tibial and anterior tibial/dorsalis pedis arteries plus volume plethysmography at 3 or more levels; OR
Provocative functional maneuvers and measurement at a single level
Upper extremity complete study:
Doppler-determined systolic pressures and bidirectional waveform recording with analysis at 3 or more levels; OR
Doppler-determined systolic pressures and transcutaneous oxygen tension measurements at 3 or more levels; OR
Doppler-determined systolic pressures and volume plethysmography at 3 or more levels; OR
Provocative functional maneuvers and measurement at a single level

EXCLUDES Unilateral study at 3 or more levels (93922)
Use of code more than one time for the lower extremity(s)
Use of code more than one time for the upper extremity(s)
Code also twice with modifier 59 for upper and lower extremity study
3.78 ☌ 3.78 **FUD** XXX S 80 ▭

AMA: 2018,Feb,11; 2018,Jan,8; 2017,Jan,8; 2016,Jan,13; 2015,Jan,16; 2014,Jan,11; 2014,Jan,9

93924 **Noninvasive physiologic studies of lower extremity arteries, at rest and following treadmill stress testing, (ie, bidirectional Doppler waveform or volume plethysmography recording and analysis at rest with ankle/brachial indices immediately after and at timed intervals following performance of a standardized protocol on a motorized treadmill plus recording of time of onset of claudication or other symptoms, maximal walking time, and time to recovery) complete bilateral study**

INCLUDES Evaluation of:
Doppler analysis of bidirectional blood flow
Non-imaging physiologic recordings of pressures
Oxygen tension measurements
Plethysmography
EXCLUDES Noninvasive vascular studies of extremities (93922-93923)
Other types of exercise
4.67 ☌ 4.67 **FUD** XXX S 80 ▭

AMA: 2018,Feb,11; 2018,Jan,8; 2017,Jan,8; 2016,Jan,13; 2015,Jan,16; 2014,Jan,9; 2014,Jan,11

93925 **Duplex scan of lower extremity arteries or arterial bypass grafts; complete bilateral study**

EXCLUDES Preoperative arterial inflow and venous outflow duplex scan for creation of hemodialysis access, same extremities (93985)
7.25 ☌ 7.25 **FUD** XXX S 80 ▭

AMA: 2018,Feb,11; 2018,Jan,8; 2017,Jan,8; 2016,Sep,9; 2016,Jan,13; 2015,Jan,16; 2014,Jan,11

93926 **unilateral or limited study**

EXCLUDES Preoperative arterial inflow and venous outflow duplex scan for creation of hemodialysis access, same extremity (93986)
4.26 ☌ 4.26 **FUD** XXX S 80 ▭

AMA: 2018,Feb,11; 2018,Jan,8; 2017,Jan,8; 2016,Sep,9; 2016,Jan,13; 2015,Jan,16; 2014,Jan,11

93930 **Duplex scan of upper extremity arteries or arterial bypass grafts; complete bilateral study**

EXCLUDES Preoperative arterial inflow and venous outflow duplex scan for creation of hemodialysis access, same extremity(ies) (93985-93986)
5.82 ☌ 5.82 **FUD** XXX S 80 ▭

AMA: 2018,Feb,11; 2018,Jan,8; 2017,Jan,8; 2016,Sep,9; 2016,Jan,13; 2015,Jan,16; 2014,Jan,11

93931 **unilateral or limited study**

EXCLUDES Preoperative arterial inflow and venous outflow duplex scan for creation of hemodialysis access, same extremity (93985-93986)
3.63 ☌ 3.63 **FUD** XXX S 80 ▭

AMA: 2018,Feb,11; 2018,Jan,8; 2017,Jan,8; 2016,Sep,9; 2016,Jan,13; 2015,Jan,16; 2014,Jan,11

93970 **Duplex scan of extremity veins including responses to compression and other maneuvers; complete bilateral study**

EXCLUDES Endovenous ablation (36475-36476, 36478-36479)
Preoperative arterial inflow and venous outflow duplex scan for creation of hemodialysis access, same extremity(ies) (93985-93986)
5.52 ☌ 5.52 **FUD** XXX S 80 ▭

AMA: 2018,Mar,3; 2018,Feb,11; 2018,Jan,8; 2017,Jan,8; 2016,Nov,3; 2016,Sep,9; 2016,Jan,13; 2015,Jan,16; 2014,Oct,6; 2014,Jan,11

93971 **unilateral or limited study**

EXCLUDES Endovenous ablation (36475-36476, 36478-36479)
Preoperative arterial inflow and venous outflow duplex scan for creation of hemodialysis access, same extremity (93985-93986)
3.42 ☌ 3.42 **FUD** XXX S 80 ▭

AMA: 2018,Mar,3; 2018,Feb,11; 2018,Jan,8; 2017,Jan,8; 2016,Nov,3; 2016,Sep,9; 2016,Jan,13; 2015,Aug,8; 2015,Jan,16; 2014,Oct,6; 2014,Jan,11

93975-93981 Noninvasive Vascular Studies: Abdomen/Chest/Pelvis

93975 **Duplex scan of arterial inflow and venous outflow of abdominal, pelvic, scrotal contents and/or retroperitoneal organs; complete study**
7.88 ☌ 7.88 **FUD** XXX S 80 ▭

AMA: 2018,Feb,11; 2018,Jan,8; 2017,Jan,8; 2016,Aug,9; 2016,Jan,13; 2015,Mar,9; 2015,Jan,16; 2014,Jun,14; 2014,Jan,11

93976 **limited study**
4.64 ☌ 4.64 **FUD** XXX S 80 ▭

AMA: 2018,Feb,11; 2018,Jan,8; 2017,Jan,8; 2016,Aug,9; 2016,Jan,13; 2015,Mar,9; 2015,Jan,16; 2014,Jan,11

93978 **Duplex scan of aorta, inferior vena cava, iliac vasculature, or bypass grafts; complete study**

EXCLUDES Ultrasound screening for abdominal aortic aneurysm (76706)
5.34 ☌ 5.34 **FUD** XXX S 80 ▭

AMA: 2018,Feb,11; 2018,Jan,8; 2017,Jan,8; 2016,Jan,13; 2015,Jan,16; 2014,Jan,11

93979 unilateral or limited study

> EXCLUDES Ultrasound screening for abdominal aortic aneurysm (76706)

🖩 3.40   🔍 3.40   **FUD** XXX   [01] [80] 🖵

AMA: 2018,Feb,11; 2018,Jan,8; 2017,Jan,8; 2016,Jan,13; 2015,Jan,16; 2014,Jun,14; 2014,Jan,11

93980 Duplex scan of arterial inflow and venous outflow of penile vessels; complete study

🖩 3.53   🔍 3.53   **FUD** XXX   [S] [80] 🖵

AMA: 2018,Feb,11; 2018,Jan,8; 2017,Jan,8; 2016,Jan,13; 2015,Jan,16; 2014,Jan,11

93981 follow-up or limited study

🖩 2.15   🔍 2.15   **FUD** XXX   [S] [80] 🖵

AMA: 2018,Feb,11; 2018,Jan,8; 2017,Jan,8; 2016,Jan,13; 2015,Jan,16; 2014,Jan,11

93985-93998 Noninvasive Vascular Studies: Hemodialysis Access

● **93985** Duplex scan of arterial inflow and venous outflow for preoperative vessel assessment prior to creation of hemodialysis access; complete bilateral study

> EXCLUDES Duplex scan of body of hemodialysis access, arterial inflow and venous outflow, same extremity(ies) (93990)
> Duplex scan of extremity arteries only, same extremity(ies) (93925, 93930)
> Duplex scan of extremity veins only, same extremity(ies) (93970)
> Physiologic arterial evaluation of extremities (93922-93924)

● **93986** complete unilateral study

> EXCLUDES Duplex scan of body of hemodialysis access, arterial inflow and venous outflow, same extremity (93990)
> Duplex scan of extremity arteries only, same extremity (93926, 93931)
> Duplex scan of extremity veins only, same extremity (93971)
> Physiologic arterial evaluation of extremities (93922-93924)

93990 Duplex scan of hemodialysis access (including arterial inflow, body of access and venous outflow)

> EXCLUDES Hemodialysis access flow measurement by indicator method (90940)

🖩 4.42   🔍 4.42   **FUD** XXX   [01] [80] 🖵

AMA: 2018,Feb,11; 2018,Jan,8; 2017,Jan,8; 2016,Jan,13; 2015,Jan,16; 2014,Jan,11

93998 Unlisted noninvasive vascular diagnostic study

🖩 0.00   🔍 0.00   **FUD** XXX   [01] [80] 🖵

AMA: 2018,Feb,11; 2018,Jan,8; 2017,Jan,8; 2016,Jan,13; 2015,Jan,16; 2014,Jan,9

94002-94005 Ventilator Management Services

94002 Ventilation assist and management, initiation of pressure or volume preset ventilators for assisted or controlled breathing; hospital inpatient/observation, initial day

> EXCLUDES E&M services

🖩 2.64   🔍 2.64   **FUD** XXX   [03] [80] 🖵

AMA: 2019,Aug,8; 2018,Feb,11; 2018,Jan,8; 2017,Jan,8; 2016,Jan,13; 2015,Jan,16; 2014,Oct,8; 2014,May,4; 2014,Jan,11

94003 hospital inpatient/observation, each subsequent day

> EXCLUDES E&M services

🖩 1.89   🔍 1.89   **FUD** XXX   [03] [80] 🖵

AMA: 2019,Aug,8; 2018,Feb,11; 2018,Jan,8; 2017,Jan,8; 2016,Jan,13; 2015,Jan,16; 2014,Oct,8; 2014,May,4; 2014,Jan,11

94004 nursing facility, per day

> EXCLUDES E&M services

🖩 1.40   🔍 1.40   **FUD** XXX   [B] [80] 🖵

AMA: 2019,Aug,8; 2018,Feb,11; 2018,Jan,8; 2017,Jan,8; 2016,Jan,13; 2015,Jan,16; 2014,Oct,8; 2014,Jan,11

94005 Home ventilator management care plan oversight of a patient (patient not present) in home, domiciliary or rest home (eg, assisted living) requiring review of status, review of laboratories and other studies and revision of orders and respiratory care plan (as appropriate), within a calendar month, 30 minutes or more

> Code also when a different provider reports care plan oversight in the same 30 days (99339-99340, 99374-99378)

🖩 2.61   🔍 2.61   **FUD** XXX   [M] 🖵

AMA: 2018,Feb,11; 2018,Jan,8; 2017,Jan,8; 2016,Jan,13; 2015,Jan,16; 2014,Oct,8; 2014,Jan,11

94010-94799 Respiratory Services: Diagnostic and Therapeutic

> INCLUDES Laboratory procedure(s)
> Test results interpretation
> EXCLUDES Separately identifiable E&M service

94010 Spirometry, including graphic record, total and timed vital capacity, expiratory flow rate measurement(s), with or without maximal voluntary ventilation

> INCLUDES Measurement of expiratory airflow and volumes
> EXCLUDES Diffusing capacity (94729)
> Other respiratory function services (94150, 94200, 94375, 94728)

🖩 1.00   🔍 1.00   **FUD** XXX   [01] [80] 🖵

AMA: 2019,May,10; 2019,Mar,10; 2019,Apr,10; 2018,Feb,11; 2018,Jan,8; 2017,Jan,8; 2016,Jan,13; 2015,Sep,9; 2015,Jan,16; 2014,Mar,11; 2014,Jan,11

94011 Measurement of spirometric forced expiratory flows in an infant or child through 2 years of age

🖩 2.48   🔍 2.48   **FUD** XXX   [01] [80] 🖵

AMA: 2019,Mar,10; 2018,Feb,11; 2018,Jan,8; 2017,Jan,8; 2016,Jan,13; 2015,Jan,16; 2014,Jan,11

94012 Measurement of spirometric forced expiratory flows, before and after bronchodilator, in an infant or child through 2 years of age

🖩 4.02   🔍 4.02   **FUD** XXX   [01] [80] 🖵

AMA: 2019,Mar,10; 2018,Feb,11; 2018,Jan,8; 2017,Jan,8; 2016,Jan,13; 2015,Jan,16; 2014,Jan,11

94013 Measurement of lung volumes (ie, functional residual capacity [FRC], forced vital capacity [FVC], and expiratory reserve volume [ERV]) in an infant or child through 2 years of age

🖩 0.55   🔍 0.55   **FUD** XXX   [S] [80] 🖵

AMA: 2019,Mar,10; 2018,Feb,11; 2018,Jan,8; 2017,Jan,8; 2016,Jan,13; 2015,Jan,16; 2014,Jan,11

94014 Patient-initiated spirometric recording per 30-day period of time; includes reinforced education, transmission of spirometric tracing, data capture, analysis of transmitted data, periodic recalibration and review and interpretation by a physician or other qualified health care professional

🖩 1.58   🔍 1.58   **FUD** XXX   [01] [80] 🖵

AMA: 2019,Mar,10; 2018,Feb,11; 2018,Jan,8; 2017,Jan,8; 2016,Jan,13; 2015,Jan,16; 2014,Jan,11

94015 recording (includes hook-up, reinforced education, data transmission, data capture, trend analysis, and periodic recalibration)

🖩 0.86   🔍 0.86   **FUD** XXX   [01] [80] [TC] 🖵

AMA: 2019,Mar,10; 2018,Feb,11; 2018,Jan,8; 2017,Jan,8; 2016,Jan,13; 2015,Jan,16; 2014,Jan,11

94016 review and interpretation only by a physician or other qualified health care professional

🖩 0.72   🔍 0.72   **FUD** XXX   [A] [80] [26] 🖵

AMA: 2019,Mar,10; 2018,Feb,11; 2018,Jan,8; 2017,Jan,8; 2016,Jan,13; 2015,Jan,16; 2014,Jan,11

94060 **Bronchodilation responsiveness, spirometry as in 94010, pre- and post-bronchodilator administration**

INCLUDES Spirometry performed prior to and after a bronchodilator has been administered

EXCLUDES *Bronchospasm prolonged exercise test with pre- and post-spirometry (94617)*
Diffusing capacity (94729)
Other respiratory function services (94150, 94200, 94375, 94640, 94728)

Code also bronchodilator supply with appropriate supply code or (99070)

⚕ 1.68   ⚖ 1.68   **FUD** XXX   [S] [80] 🖵

AMA: 2019,Mar,10; 2019,Apr,10; 2018,Feb,11; 2018,Jan,8; 2017,Jan,8; 2016,Jan,13; 2015,Sep,9; 2015,Jan,16; 2014,Mar,11; 2014,Jan,11

94070 **Bronchospasm provocation evaluation, multiple spirometric determinations as in 94010, with administered agents (eg, antigen[s], cold air, methacholine)**

EXCLUDES *Diffusing capacity (94729)*
Inhalation treatment (diagnostic or therapeutic) (94640)

Code also antigen(s) administration with appropriate supply code or (99070)

⚕ 1.69   ⚖ 1.69   **FUD** XXX   [S] [80] 🖵

AMA: 2019,Mar,10; 2018,Feb,11; 2018,Jan,8; 2017,Jan,8; 2016,Jan,13; 2015,Sep,9; 2015,Jan,16; 2014,Jan,11

94150 **Vital capacity, total (separate procedure)**

EXCLUDES *Other respiratory function services (94010, 94060, 94728)*
Thoracic gas volumes (94726-94727)

⚕ 0.72   ⚖ 0.72   **FUD** XXX   [01] 🖵

AMA: 2019,Mar,10; 2018,Sep,14; 2018,Feb,11; 2018,Jan,8; 2017,Jan,8; 2016,Jan,13; 2015,Jan,16; 2014,Mar,11; 2014,Jan,11

94200 **Maximum breathing capacity, maximal voluntary ventilation**

EXCLUDES *Other respiratory function services (94010, 94060)*

⚕ 0.78   ⚖ 0.78   **FUD** XXX   [01] [80] 🖵

AMA: 2019,Mar,10; 2018,Feb,11; 2018,Jan,8; 2017,Jan,8; 2016,Jan,13; 2015,Jan,16; 2014,Mar,11; 2014,Jan,11

94250 **Expired gas collection, quantitative, single procedure (separate procedure)**

EXCLUDES *Complex pulmonary stress test (94621)*

⚕ 0.78   ⚖ 0.78   **FUD** XXX   [01] [80] 🖵

AMA: 2019,Mar,10; 2018,Feb,11; 2018,Jan,8; 2017,Oct,3; 2017,Jan,8; 2016,Jan,13; 2015,Dec,16; 2015,Jan,16; 2014,Jan,11

94375 **Respiratory flow volume loop**

INCLUDES Identification of obstruction patterns in central or peripheral airways (inspiratory and/or expiratory)

EXCLUDES *Diffusing capacity (94729)*
Other respiratory function services (94010, 94060, 94728)

⚕ 1.12   ⚖ 1.12   **FUD** XXX   [01] [80] 🖵

AMA: 2019,Mar,10; 2018,Feb,11; 2018,Jan,8; 2017,Jan,8; 2016,Jan,13; 2015,Jan,16; 2014,Mar,11; 2014,Jan,11

94400 **Breathing response to CO2 (CO2 response curve)**

EXCLUDES *Inhalation treatment (diagnostic or therapeutic) (94640)*

⚕ 1.61   ⚖ 1.61   **FUD** XXX   [01] [80] 🖵

AMA: 2019,Mar,10; 2018,Feb,11; 2018,Jan,8; 2017,Jan,8; 2016,Jan,13; 2015,Sep,9; 2015,Jan,16; 2014,Mar,11; 2014,Jan,11

94450 **Breathing response to hypoxia (hypoxia response curve)**

EXCLUDES *HAST - high altitude simulation test (94452, 94453)*

⚕ 2.06   ⚖ 2.06   **FUD** XXX   [01] [80] 🖵

AMA: 2019,Mar,10; 2018,Feb,11; 2018,Jan,8; 2017,Jan,8; 2016,Jan,13; 2015,Jan,16; 2014,Jan,11

94452 **High altitude simulation test (HAST), with interpretation and report by a physician or other qualified health care professional;**

EXCLUDES *HAST test with supplemental oxygen titration (94453)*
Noninvasive pulse oximetry (94760-94761)
Obtaining arterial blood gases (36600)

⚕ 1.55   ⚖ 1.55   **FUD** XXX   [01] [80] 🖵

AMA: 2019,Mar,10; 2018,Feb,11; 2018,Jan,8; 2017,Jan,8; 2016,Jan,13; 2015,Jan,16; 2014,Jan,11

94453 **with supplemental oxygen titration**

EXCLUDES *HAST test without supplemental oxygen titration (94452)*
Noninvasive pulse oximetry (94760-94761)
Obtaining arterial blood gases (36600)

⚕ 2.14   ⚖ 2.14   **FUD** XXX   [01] [80] 🖵

AMA: 2019,Mar,10; 2018,Feb,11; 2018,Jan,8; 2017,Jan,8; 2016,Jan,13; 2015,Jan,16; 2014,Jan,11

94610 **Intrapulmonary surfactant administration by a physician or other qualified health care professional through endotracheal tube**

INCLUDES Reporting once per dosing episode

EXCLUDES *Intubation, endotracheal (31500)*
Neonatal critical care (99468-99472)

⚕ 1.59   ⚖ 1.59   **FUD** XXX   ⊘ [01] [80] 🖵

AMA: 2019,Mar,10; 2018,Feb,11; 2018,Jan,8; 2017,Jan,8; 2016,Jan,13; 2015,Jan,16; 2014,Jan,11

94617 **Exercise test for bronchospasm, including pre- and post-spirometry, electrocardiographic recording(s), and pulse oximetry**

EXCLUDES *Cardiovascular stress test (93015-93018)*
ECG monitoring (93000-93010, 93040-93042)
Pulse oximetry (94760-94761)

⚕ 2.66   ⚖ 2.66   **FUD** XXX   [01] [80] 🖵

AMA: 2019,May,10; 2019,Mar,10; 2018,Feb,11; 2018,Jan,8; 2017,Oct,3

94618 **Pulmonary stress testing (eg, 6-minute walk test), including measurement of heart rate, oximetry, and oxygen titration, when performed**

EXCLUDES *Pulse oximetry (94760-94761)*

⚕ 0.96   ⚖ 0.96   **FUD** XXX   [01] [80] 🖵

AMA: 2019,May,10; 2019,Mar,10; 2018,Feb,11; 2018,Jan,8; 2017,Oct,3

94621 **Cardiopulmonary exercise testing, including measurements of minute ventilation, CO2 production, O2 uptake, and electrocardiographic recordings**

EXCLUDES *Cardiovascular stress test (93015-93018)*
ECG monitoring (93000-93010, 93040-93042)
Expired gas collection (94250)
Oxygen uptake expired gas analysis (94680-94690)
Pulse oximetry (94760-94761)

⚕ 4.54   ⚖ 4.54   **FUD** XXX   [S] [80] 🖵

AMA: 2019,May,10; 2019,Mar,10; 2018,Feb,11; 2018,Jan,8; 2017,Oct,3; 2017,Jan,8; 2016,Jan,13; 2015,Jan,16; 2014,Jan,11

94640 **Pressurized or nonpressurized inhalation treatment for acute airway obstruction for therapeutic purposes and/or for diagnostic purposes such as sputum induction with an aerosol generator, nebulizer, metered dose inhaler or intermittent positive pressure breathing (IPPB) device**

EXCLUDES *1 hour or more of continuous inhalation treatment (94644, 94645)*
Other respiratory function services (94060, 94070, 94400)

Code also modifier 76 when more than 1 inhalation treatment is performed on the same date

⚕ 0.51   ⚖ 0.51   **FUD** XXX   [01] [80] 🖵

AMA: 2019,Mar,10; 2018,Feb,11; 2018,Jan,8; 2017,Jan,8; 2016,Jan,13; 2015,Sep,9; 2015,Jan,16; 2014,Mar,11; 2014,Jan,11

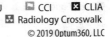

94642 **Aerosol inhalation of pentamidine for pneumocystis carinii pneumonia treatment or prophylaxis**

🔲 0.00 🔲 0.00 **FUD** XXX Q1 80 🖃

AMA: 2019,Mar,10; 2018,Feb,11; 2018,Jan,8; 2017,Jan,8; 2016,Jan,13; 2015,Jan,16; 2014,Jan,11

94644 **Continuous inhalation treatment with aerosol medication for acute airway obstruction; first hour**

EXCLUDES Services that are less than 1 hour (94640)

🔲 1.40 🔲 1.40 **FUD** XXX Q1 80 🖃

AMA: 2019,Mar,10; 2018,Feb,11; 2018,Jan,8; 2017,Jan,8; 2016,Jan,13; 2015,Sep,9; 2015,Jan,16; 2014,Mar,11; 2014,Jan,11

+ 94645 **each additional hour (List separately in addition to code for primary procedure)**

Code first initial hour (94644)

🔲 0.47 🔲 0.47 **FUD** XXX N 80 🖃

AMA: 2019,Mar,10; 2018,Feb,11; 2018,Jan,8; 2017,Jan,8; 2016,Jan,13; 2015,Sep,9; 2015,Jan,16; 2014,Mar,11; 2014,Jan,11

94660 **Continuous positive airway pressure ventilation (CPAP), initiation and management**

🔲 1.09 🔲 1.81 **FUD** XXX Q1 80 🖃

AMA: 2019,Aug,8; 2019,Mar,10; 2018,Feb,11; 2018,Jan,8; 2017,Jan,8; 2016,Jan,13; 2015,Jan,16; 2014,Oct,8; 2014,May,4; 2014,Jan,11

94662 **Continuous negative pressure ventilation (CNP), initiation and management**

🔲 1.03 🔲 1.03 **FUD** XXX Q3 80 🖃

AMA: 2019,Aug,8; 2019,Mar,10; 2018,Feb,11; 2018,Jan,8; 2017,Jan,8; 2016,Jan,13; 2015,Jan,16; 2014,May,4; 2014,Jan,11

94664 **Demonstration and/or evaluation of patient utilization of an aerosol generator, nebulizer, metered dose inhaler or IPPB device**

INCLUDES Reporting only one time per day of service

🔲 0.48 🔲 0.48 **FUD** XXX Q1 80 🖃

AMA: 2019,Mar,10; 2018,Feb,11; 2018,Jan,8; 2017,Jan,8; 2016,Jan,13; 2015,Jan,16; 2014,Jan,11

94667 **Manipulation chest wall, such as cupping, percussing, and vibration to facilitate lung function; initial demonstration and/or evaluation**

🔲 0.71 🔲 0.71 **FUD** XXX Q1 80 🖃

AMA: 2019,Mar,10; 2018,Feb,11; 2018,Jan,8; 2017,Jan,8; 2016,Jan,13; 2015,Sep,9; 2015,Jan,16; 2014,Mar,11; 2014,Jan,11

94668 **subsequent**

🔲 0.92 🔲 0.92 **FUD** XXX Q1 80 🖃

AMA: 2019,Mar,10; 2018,Feb,11; 2018,Jan,8; 2017,Jan,8; 2016,Jan,13; 2015,Sep,9; 2015,Jan,16; 2014,Mar,11; 2014,Jan,11

94669 **Mechanical chest wall oscillation to facilitate lung function, per session**

INCLUDES Application of an external wrap or vest to provide mechanical oscillation

🔲 0.90 🔲 0.90 **FUD** XXX Q1 80 🖃

AMA: 2019,Mar,10; 2018,Feb,11; 2018,Jan,8; 2017,Jan,8; 2016,Jan,13; 2015,Jan,16; 2014,Jan,11

94680 **Oxygen uptake, expired gas analysis; rest and exercise, direct, simple**

EXCLUDES Cardiopulmonary stress testing (94621)

🔲 1.57 🔲 1.57 **FUD** XXX Q1 80 🖃

AMA: 2019,Mar,10; 2018,Feb,11; 2018,Jan,8; 2017,Oct,3; 2017,Jan,8; 2016,Jan,13; 2015,Jan,16; 2014,Jan,11

94681 **including CO2 output, percentage oxygen extracted**

EXCLUDES Cardiopulmonary stress testing (94621)

🔲 1.55 🔲 1.55 **FUD** XXX Q1 80 🖃

AMA: 2019,Mar,10; 2018,Feb,11; 2018,Jan,8; 2017,Oct,3; 2017,Jan,8; 2016,Jan,13; 2015,Jan,16; 2014,Jan,11

94690 **rest, indirect (separate procedure)**

EXCLUDES Arterial puncture (36600)
Cardiopulmonary stress testing (94621)

🔲 1.49 🔲 1.49 **FUD** XXX Q1 80 🖃

AMA: 2019,Mar,10; 2018,Feb,11; 2018,Jan,8; 2017,Oct,3; 2017,Jan,8; 2016,Jan,13; 2015,Jan,16; 2014,Jan,11

94726 **Plethysmography for determination of lung volumes and, when performed, airway resistance**

INCLUDES Airway resistance
Determination of:
Functional residual capacity
Residual volume
Total lung capacity

EXCLUDES Airway resistance (94728)
Bronchial provocation (94070)
Diffusing capacity (94729)
Gas dilution or washout (94727)
Spirometry (94010, 94060)

🔲 1.52 🔲 1.52 **FUD** XXX Q1 80 🖃

AMA: 2019,Mar,10; 2018,Feb,11; 2018,Jan,8; 2017,Jan,8; 2016,Jan,13; 2015,Jan,16; 2014,Jan,11

94727 **Gas dilution or washout for determination of lung volumes and, when performed, distribution of ventilation and closing volumes**

INCLUDES Closing volume
Distribution of ventilation
Lung volume measurement

EXCLUDES Bronchial provocation (94070)
Diffusing capacity (94729)
Plethysmography for lung volume/airway resistance (94726)
Spirometry (94010, 94060)

🔲 1.23 🔲 1.23 **FUD** XXX Q1 80 🖃

AMA: 2019,Mar,10; 2018,Feb,11; 2018,Jan,8; 2017,Jan,8; 2016,Jan,13; 2015,Jan,16; 2014,Jan,11

▲ 94728 **Airway resistance by oscillometry**

EXCLUDES Diffusing capacity (94729)
Gas dilution techniques
Other respiratory function services (94010, 94060, 94070, 94375, 94726)

🔲 1.15 🔲 1.15 **FUD** XXX Q1 80 🖃

AMA: 2019,Mar,10; 2018,Feb,11; 2018,Jan,8; 2017,Jan,8; 2016,Jan,13; 2015,Jan,16; 2014,Mar,11; 2014,Jan,11

+ 94729 **Diffusing capacity (eg, carbon monoxide, membrane) (List separately in addition to code for primary procedure)**

Code first (94010, 94060, 94070, 94375, 94726-94728)

🔲 1.56 🔲 1.56 **FUD** ZZZ N 80 🖃

AMA: 2019,Mar,10; 2018,Feb,11; 2018,Jan,8; 2017,Jan,8; 2016,Jan,13; 2015,Jan,16; 2014,Jan,11

94750 **Pulmonary compliance study (eg, plethysmography, volume and pressure measurements)**

🔲 2.40 🔲 2.40 **FUD** XXX Q1 80 🖃

AMA: 2019,Mar,10; 2018,Feb,11; 2018,Jan,8; 2017,Jan,8; 2016,Jan,13; 2015,Jan,16; 2014,Jan,11

94760 **Noninvasive ear or pulse oximetry for oxygen saturation; single determination**

EXCLUDES Blood gases (82803-82810)
Cardiopulmonary stress testing (94621)
Exercise test for bronchospasm (94617)
Pulmonary stress testing (94618)

🔲 0.07 🔲 0.07 **FUD** XXX N 80 TC 🖃

AMA: 2019,Aug,8; 2019,Mar,10; 2019,Jan,6; 2018,Feb,11; 2018,Jan,8; 2017,Oct,3; 2017,Jan,8; 2016,Jan,13; 2015,Jan,16; 2014,May,4; 2014,Jan,11

● New Code ▲ Revised Code ○ Reinstated ● New Web Release ▲ Revised Web Release + Add-on Unlisted Not Covered # Resequenced

50 Optum Mod 50 Exempt ⊘ AMA Mod 51 Exempt 51 Optum Mod 51 Exempt 63 Mod 63 Exempt ✔ Non-FDA Drug ★ Telemedicine M Maternity A Age Edit

© 2019 Optum360, LLC CPT © 2019 American Medical Association. All Rights Reserved.

499

94761 multiple determinations (eg, during exercise)

EXCLUDES Cardiopulmonary stress testing (94621)
Exercise test for bronchospasm (94617)
Pulmonary stress testing (94618)

💷 0.12 ⚗ 0.12 **FUD** XXX [N] [80] [TC] 🖿

AMA: 2019,Aug,8; 2019,Mar,10; 2018,Feb,11; 2018,Jan,8; 2017,Oct,3; 2017,Jan,8; 2016,Jan,13; 2015,Jan,16; 2014,May,4; 2014,Jan,11

94762 by continuous overnight monitoring (separate procedure)

💷 0.71 ⚗ 0.71 **FUD** XXX [Q3] [80] [TC] 🖿

AMA: 2019,Aug,8; 2019,Mar,10; 2018,Feb,11; 2018,Jan,8; 2017,Jan,8; 2016,Jan,13; 2015,Jan,16; 2014,May,4; 2014,Jan,11

94770 Carbon dioxide, expired gas determination by infrared analyzer

EXCLUDES Arterial catheterization/cannulation (36620)
Arterial puncture (36600)
Bronchoscopy (31622-31654 [31651])
Flow directed catheter placement (93503)
Needle biopsy of the lung (32405)
Orotracheal/nasotracheal intubation (31500)
Placement of central venous catheter (36555-36556)
Therapeutic phlebotomy (99195)
Thoracentesis (32554-32555)
Venipuncture (36410)

💷 0.21 ⚗ 0.21 **FUD** XXX [S] [80] 🖿

AMA: 2019,Mar,10; 2018,Feb,11; 2018,Jan,8; 2017,Jan,8; 2016,Jan,13; 2015,Jan,16; 2014,Mar,11; 2014,Jan,11

94772 Circadian respiratory pattern recording (pediatric pneumogram), 12-24 hour continuous recording, infant [A]

EXCLUDES Electromyograms/EEG/ECG/respiration recordings

💷 0.00 ⚗ 0.00 **FUD** XXX [S] [80] 🖿

AMA: 2019,Mar,10; 2018,Feb,11; 2018,Jan,8; 2017,Jan,8; 2016,Jan,13; 2015,Jan,16; 2014,Jan,11

94774 Pediatric home apnea monitoring event recording including respiratory rate, pattern and heart rate per 30-day period of time; includes monitor attachment, download of data, review, interpretation, and preparation of a report by a physician or other qualified health care professional [A]

INCLUDES Oxygen saturation monitoring
EXCLUDES Event monitors (93268-93272)
Holter monitor (93224-93227)
Pediatric home apnea services (94775-94777)
Remote cardiovascular telemetry (93228-93229)
Sleep testing (95805-95811 [95800, 95801])

💷 0.00 ⚗ 0.00 **FUD** YYY [B] [80] 🖿

AMA: 2019,Mar,10; 2018,Feb,11; 2018,Jan,8; 2017,Jan,8; 2016,Jan,13; 2015,Jan,16; 2014,Jan,11

94775 monitor attachment only (includes hook-up, initiation of recording and disconnection) [A]

INCLUDES Oxygen saturation monitoring
EXCLUDES Event monitors (93268-93272)
Holter monitor (93224-93227)
Remote cardiovascular telemetry (93228-93229)
Sleep testing (95805-95811 [95800, 95801])

💷 0.00 ⚗ 0.00 **FUD** YYY [S] [80] [TC] 🖿

AMA: 2019,Mar,10; 2018,Feb,11; 2018,Jan,8; 2017,Jan,8; 2016,Jan,13; 2015,Jan,16; 2014,Jan,11

94776 monitoring, download of information, receipt of transmission(s) and analyses by computer only [A]

INCLUDES Oxygen saturation monitoring
EXCLUDES Event monitors (93268-93272)
Holter monitor (93224-93227)
Remote cardiovascular telemetry (93228-93229)
Sleep testing (95805-95811 [95800, 95801])

💷 0.00 ⚗ 0.00 **FUD** YYY [S] [80] [TC] 🖿

AMA: 2019,Mar,10; 2018,Feb,11; 2018,Jan,8; 2017,Jan,8; 2016,Jan,13; 2015,Jan,16; 2014,Jan,11

94777 review, interpretation and preparation of report only by a physician or other qualified health care professional [A]

INCLUDES Oxygen saturation monitoring
EXCLUDES Event monitors (93268-93272)
Holter monitor (93224-93227)
Remote cardiovascular telemetry (93228-93229)
Sleep testing (95805-95811 [95800, 95801])

💷 0.00 ⚗ 0.00 **FUD** YYY [B] [80] [26] 🖿

AMA: 2019,Mar,10; 2018,Feb,11; 2018,Jan,8; 2017,Jan,8; 2016,Jan,13; 2015,Jan,16; 2014,Jan,11

94780 Car seat/bed testing for airway integrity, for infants through 12 months of age, with continual clinical staff observation and continuous recording of pulse oximetry, heart rate and respiratory rate, with interpretation and report; 60 minutes [A]

EXCLUDES Pediatric and neonatal critical care services (99468-99476, 99477-99480)
Pulse oximetry (94760-94761)
Rhythm strips (93040-93042)
Use of code for less than 60 minutes of service

💷 0.68 ⚗ 1.45 **FUD** XXX [Q1] 🖿

AMA: 2019,Mar,10; 2018,Feb,11; 2018,Jan,8; 2017,Jan,8; 2016,Jan,13; 2015,May,10; 2015,Jan,16; 2014,Jan,11

\+ **94781** each additional full 30 minutes (List separately in addition to code for primary procedure) [A]

Code first (94780)

💷 0.24 ⚗ 0.57 **FUD** ZZZ [N] 🖿

AMA: 2019,Mar,10; 2018,Feb,11; 2018,Jan,8; 2017,Jan,8; 2016,Jan,13; 2015,May,10; 2015,Jan,16; 2014,Jan,11

94799 Unlisted pulmonary service or procedure

💷 0.00 ⚗ 0.00 **FUD** XXX [Q1] [80] 🖿

AMA: 2019,Mar,10; 2018,Sep,14; 2018,Feb,11; 2018,Jan,8; 2017,Jan,8; 2016,Jan,13; 2015,Dec,16; 2015,May,10; 2015,Jan,16; 2014,Jan,11

95004-95071 Allergy Tests

EXCLUDES Drugs administered for intractable/severe allergic reaction (eg, antihistamines, epinephrine, steroids) (96372)
E&M services when reporting test interpretation/report
Laboratory tests for allergies (86000-86999 [86152, 86153])
Code also medical conferences regarding use of equipment (eg, air filters, humidifiers, dehumidifiers), climate therapy, physical, occupational, and recreation therapy using appropriate E&M codes
Code also significant, separately identifiable E&M services using modifier 25, when performed (99201-99215, 99217-99223 [99224, 99225, 99226], 99231-99233, 99241-99255, 99281-99285, 99304-99318, 99324-99337, 99341-99350, 99381-99429)

95004 Percutaneous tests (scratch, puncture, prick) with allergenic extracts, immediate type reaction, including test interpretation and report, specify number of tests

💷 0.12 ⚗ 0.12 **FUD** XXX [Q1] [80] 🖿

AMA: 2018,Feb,11; 2018,Jan,8; 2017,Jan,8; 2016,Jan,13; 2015,Jan,16; 2014,Jan,11

95012 Nitric oxide expired gas determination

💷 0.57 ⚗ 0.57 **FUD** XXX [Q1] [80] 🖿

AMA: 2018,Feb,11; 2018,Jan,8; 2017,Jan,8; 2016,Jan,13; 2015,Jan,16; 2014,Mar,11; 2014,Jan,11

95017 Allergy testing, any combination of percutaneous (scratch, puncture, prick) and intracutaneous (intradermal), sequential and incremental, with venoms, immediate type reaction, including test interpretation and report, specify number of tests

💷 0.11 ⚗ 0.23 **FUD** XXX [Q1] [80] 🖿

AMA: 2018,Feb,11; 2018,Jan,8; 2017,Jan,8; 2016,Jan,13; 2015,Jul,9; 2015,Jan,16

95018 Allergy testing, any combination of percutaneous (scratch, puncture, prick) and intracutaneous (intradermal), sequential and incremental, with drugs or biologicals, immediate type reaction, including test interpretation and report, specify number of tests
0.21 0.61 **FUD** XXX Q1 80 ▢
AMA: 2018,Feb,11; 2018,Jan,8; 2017,Jan,8; 2016,Jan,13; 2015,Jul,9; 2015,Jan,16

95024 Intracutaneous (intradermal) tests with allergenic extracts, immediate type reaction, including test interpretation and report, specify number of tests
0.03 0.23 **FUD** XXX Q1 80 ▢
AMA: 2018,Feb,11; 2018,Jan,8; 2017,Jan,8; 2016,Jan,13; 2015,Jan,16; 2014,Jan,11

95027 Intracutaneous (intradermal) tests, sequential and incremental, with allergenic extracts for airborne allergens, immediate type reaction, including test interpretation and report, specify number of tests
0.13 0.13 **FUD** XXX Q1 80 ▢
AMA: 2018,Feb,11; 2018,Jan,8; 2017,Jan,8; 2016,Jan,13; 2015,Jan,16; 2014,Jan,11

95028 Intracutaneous (intradermal) tests with allergenic extracts, delayed type reaction, including reading, specify number of tests
0.37 0.37 **FUD** XXX Q1 80 TC ▢
AMA: 2018,Feb,11; 2018,Jan,8; 2017,Jan,8; 2016,Jan,13; 2015,Jan,16; 2014,Jan,11

95044 Patch or application test(s) (specify number of tests)
0.16 0.16 **FUD** XXX Q1 80 ▢
AMA: 2018,Feb,11; 2018,Jan,8; 2017,Jan,8; 2016,Jan,13; 2015,Jan,16; 2014,Jan,11

95052 Photo patch test(s) (specify number of tests)
0.19 0.19 **FUD** XXX Q1 80 ▢
AMA: 2018,Feb,11; 2018,Jan,8; 2017,Jan,8; 2016,Jan,13; 2015,Jan,16; 2014,Jan,11

95056 Photo tests
1.31 1.31 **FUD** XXX Q1 80 ▢
AMA: 2018,Feb,11; 2018,Jan,8; 2017,Jan,8; 2016,Jan,13; 2015,Jan,16; 2014,Jan,11

95060 Ophthalmic mucous membrane tests
0.99 0.99 **FUD** XXX Q1 80 TC ▢
AMA: 2018,Feb,11; 2018,Jan,8; 2017,Jan,8; 2016,Jan,13; 2015,Jan,16; 2014,Jan,11

95065 Direct nasal mucous membrane test
0.74 0.74 **FUD** XXX Q1 80 TC ▢
AMA: 2018,Feb,11; 2018,Jan,8; 2017,Jan,8; 2016,Jan,13; 2015,Jan,16; 2014,Jan,11

95070 Inhalation bronchial challenge testing (not including necessary pulmonary function tests); with histamine, methacholine, or similar compounds
EXCLUDES Pulmonary function tests (94060, 94070)
0.90 0.90 **FUD** XXX S 80 TC ▢
AMA: 2018,Feb,11; 2018,Jan,8; 2017,Jan,8; 2016,Jan,13; 2015,Jan,16; 2014,Jan,11

95071 with antigens or gases, specify
EXCLUDES Pulmonary function tests (94060, 94070)
1.05 1.05 **FUD** XXX Q1 80 TC ▢
AMA: 2018,Feb,11; 2018,Jan,8; 2017,Jan,8; 2016,Jan,13; 2015,Jan,16; 2014,Jan,11

95076-95079 Challenge Ingestion Testing
CMS: 100-03,110.12 Challenge Ingestion Food Testing
INCLUDES Assessment and monitoring for allergic reactions (eg, blood pressure, peak flow meter)
Testing time until the test ends or to the point an E&M service is needed
EXCLUDES Use of code to report testing time less than 61 minutes, such as a positive challenge resulting in ending the test (use E&M codes as appropriate)
Code also interventions when appropriate (eg, injection of epinephrine or steroid)

95076 Ingestion challenge test (sequential and incremental ingestion of test items, eg, food, drug or other substance); initial 120 minutes of testing
INCLUDES First 120 minutes of testing time (not face-to-face time with physician)
2.15 3.43 **FUD** XXX S 80 ▢
AMA: 2018,Feb,11; 2018,Jan,8; 2017,Jan,8; 2016,Jan,13; 2015,Jan,16

+ **95079** each additional 60 minutes of testing (List separately in addition to code for primary procedure)
INCLUDES Includes each 60 minutes of additional testing time (not face-to-face time with physician)
Code first (95076)
1.97 2.42 **FUD** ZZZ N 80 ▢
AMA: 2018,Feb,11; 2018,Jan,8; 2017,Jan,8; 2016,Jan,13; 2015,Jan,16

95115-95199 Allergy Immunotherapy
CMS: 100-03,110.9 Antigens Prepared for Sublingual Administration
INCLUDES Allergen immunotherapy professional services
EXCLUDES Bacterial/viral/fungal extracts skin testing (86485-86580, 95028)
Special reports for allergy patients (99080)
The following procedures for testing: (See Pathology/Immunology section or code:) (95199)
Leukocyte histamine release (LHR)
Lymphocytic transformation test (LTT)
Mast cell degranulation test (MCDT)
Migration inhibitory factor test (MIF)
Nitroblue tetrazolium dye test (NTD)
Radioallergosorbent testing (RAST)
Rat mast cell technique (RMCT)
Transfer factor test (TFT)
Code also significant separately identifiable E&M services, when performed

95115 Professional services for allergen immunotherapy not including provision of allergenic extracts; single injection
0.26 0.26 **FUD** XXX Q1 80 ▢
AMA: 2019,Jun,14; 2018,Feb,11; 2018,Jan,8; 2017,Jan,8; 2016,Jan,13; 2015,Jan,16; 2014,Jan,11

95117 2 or more injections
0.30 0.30 **FUD** XXX Q1 80 ▢
AMA: 2019,Jun,14; 2018,Feb,11; 2018,Jan,8; 2017,Jan,8; 2016,Jan,13; 2015,Jan,16; 2014,Jan,11

95120 Professional services for allergen immunotherapy in the office or institution of the prescribing physician or other qualified health care professional, including provision of allergenic extract; single injection
0.00 0.00 **FUD** XXX E ▢
AMA: 2018,Feb,11; 2018,Jan,8; 2017,Jan,8; 2016,Jan,13; 2015,Jan,16; 2014,Jan,11

95125 2 or more injections
0.00 0.00 **FUD** XXX E ▢
AMA: 2018,Feb,11; 2018,Jan,8; 2017,Jan,8; 2016,Jan,13; 2015,Jan,16; 2014,Jan,11

95130 single stinging insect venom
0.00 0.00 **FUD** XXX E ▢
AMA: 2018,Feb,11; 2018,Jan,8; 2017,Jan,8; 2016,Jan,13; 2015,Jan,16; 2014,Jan,11

95131 2 stinging insect venoms
0.00 0.00 **FUD** XXX E ▢
AMA: 2018,Feb,11; 2018,Jan,8; 2017,Jan,8; 2016,Jan,13; 2015,Jan,16; 2014,Jan,11

Medicine

95132
95251

95132 **3 stinging insect venoms**
🚑 0.00 ⚕ 0.00 **FUD** XXX   E 🖵
AMA: 2018,Feb,11; 2018,Jan,8; 2017,Jan,8; 2016,Jan,13; 2015,Jan,16; 2014,Jan,11

95133 **4 stinging insect venoms**
🚑 0.00 ⚕ 0.00 **FUD** XXX   E 🖵
AMA: 2018,Feb,11; 2018,Jan,8; 2017,Jan,8; 2016,Jan,13; 2015,Jan,16; 2014,Jan,11

95134 **5 stinging insect venoms**
🚑 0.00 ⚕ 0.00 **FUD** XXX   E 🖵
AMA: 2018,Feb,11; 2018,Jan,8; 2017,Jan,8; 2016,Jan,13; 2015,Jan,16; 2014,Jan,11

95144 **Professional services for the supervision of preparation and provision of antigens for allergen immunotherapy, single dose vial(s) (specify number of vials)**
INCLUDES Single dose vial/single dose of antigen administered in one injection
🚑 0.09 ⚕ 0.41 **FUD** XXX   Q1 80 🖵
AMA: 2018,Feb,11; 2018,Jan,8; 2017,Jan,8; 2016,Jan,13; 2015,Jan,16; 2014,Jan,11

95145 **Professional services for the supervision of preparation and provision of antigens for allergen immunotherapy (specify number of doses); single stinging insect venom**
🚑 0.09 ⚕ 0.81 **FUD** XXX   Q1 80 🖵
AMA: 2018,Feb,11; 2018,Jan,8; 2017,Jan,8; 2016,Jan,13; 2015,Jan,16; 2014,Jan,11

95146 **2 single stinging insect venoms**
🚑 0.09 ⚕ 1.50 **FUD** XXX   Q1 80 🖵
AMA: 2018,Feb,11; 2018,Jan,8; 2017,Jan,8; 2016,Jan,13; 2015,Jan,16; 2014,Jan,11

95147 **3 single stinging insect venoms**
🚑 0.09 ⚕ 1.55 **FUD** XXX   Q1 80 🖵
AMA: 2018,Feb,11; 2018,Jan,8; 2017,Jan,8; 2016,Jan,13; 2015,Jan,16; 2014,Jan,11

95148 **4 single stinging insect venoms**
🚑 0.09 ⚕ 2.23 **FUD** XXX   Q1 80 🖵
AMA: 2018,Feb,11; 2018,Jan,8; 2017,Jan,8; 2016,Jan,13; 2015,Jan,16; 2014,Jan,11

95149 **5 single stinging insect venoms**
🚑 0.09 ⚕ 2.97 **FUD** XXX   Q1 80 🖵
AMA: 2018,Feb,11; 2018,Jan,8; 2017,Jan,8; 2016,Jan,13; 2015,Jan,16; 2014,Jan,11

95165 **Professional services for the supervision of preparation and provision of antigens for allergen immunotherapy; single or multiple antigens (specify number of doses)**
🚑 0.09 ⚕ 0.40 **FUD** XXX   Q1 80 🖵
AMA: 2018,Feb,11; 2018,Jan,8; 2017,Jan,8; 2016,Jan,13; 2015,Jan,16; 2014,Jan,11

95170 **whole body extract of biting insect or other arthropod (specify number of doses)**
INCLUDES A dose which is the amount of antigen(s) administered in a single injection from a multiple dose vial
🚑 0.09 ⚕ 0.30 **FUD** XXX   Q1 80 🖵
AMA: 2018,Feb,11; 2018,Jan,8; 2017,Jan,8; 2016,Jan,13; 2015,Jan,16; 2014,Jan,11

95180 **Rapid desensitization procedure, each hour (eg, insulin, penicillin, equine serum)**
🚑 2.96 ⚕ 3.92 **FUD** XXX   Q1 80 🖵
AMA: 2019,Jun,14; 2018,Feb,11; 2018,Jan,8; 2017,Jan,8; 2016,Jan,13; 2015,Jan,16; 2014,Jan,11

95199 **Unlisted allergy/clinical immunologic service or procedure**
🚑 0.00 ⚕ 0.00 **FUD** XXX   Q1 80 🖵
AMA: 2018,Feb,11; 2018,Jan,8; 2017,Jan,8; 2016,Jan,13; 2015,Jan,16; 2014,Jan,11

95249-95251 [95249] Glucose Monitoring By Subcutaneous Device

EXCLUDES *Physiologic data collection/interpretation (99091)*
Code also when data receiver owned by patient for placement of sensor, hook-up, monitor calibration, training, and printout (95999)

95249 **Resequenced code. See code following 95250.**

95250 **Ambulatory continuous glucose monitoring of interstitial tissue fluid via a subcutaneous sensor for a minimum of 72 hours; physician or other qualified health care professional (office) provided equipment, sensor placement, hook-up, calibration of monitor, patient training, removal of sensor, and printout of recording**
EXCLUDES *Subcutaneous pocket with insertion interstitial glucose monitor (0446T)*
Use of code more than one time per month
🚑 4.26 ⚕ 4.26 **FUD** XXX   V 80 TC 🖵
AMA: 2019,Jan,6; 2018,Jun,6; 2018,Mar,5; 2018,Feb,11; 2018,Jan,8; 2017,Jan,8; 2016,Jan,13; 2015,Jan,16; 2014,Jan,11

\# **95249** **patient-provided equipment, sensor placement, hook-up, calibration of monitor, patient training, and printout of recording**
INCLUDES Performing complete collection of initial data in the provider's office
EXCLUDES *Subcutaneous pocket with insertion interstitial glucose monitor (0446T)*
Use of code more than one time during the period the patient owns the data receiver
🚑 1.56 ⚕ 1.56 **FUD** XXX   S 80 TC 🖵
AMA: 2018,Jun,6; 2018,Feb,11

95251 **analysis, interpretation and report**
EXCLUDES *Use of code more than one time per month*
🚑 1.01 ⚕ 1.01 **FUD** XXX   B 80 26 🖵
AMA: 2018,Jun,6; 2018,Mar,5; 2018,Feb,11; 2018,Jan,8; 2017,Jan,8; 2016,Jan,13; 2015,Jan,16; 2014,Jan,11

95700-95783 Sleep Studies

INCLUDES Assessment of sleep disorders in adults and children
Continuous and simultaneous monitoring and recording of physiological sleep parameters of 6 hours or more
Evaluation of patient's response to therapies
Physician:
   Interpretation
   Recording
   Report
Recording sessions may be:
   Attended studies that include the presence of a technologist or qualified health care professional to respond to the needs of the patient or technical issues at the bedside
   Remote without the presence of a technologist or a qualified health professional
   Unattended without the presence of a technologist or qualified health care professional
Testing parameters include:
   Actigraphy: Use of a noninvasive portable device to record gross motor movements to approximate periods of sleep and wakefulness
   Electrooculogram (EOG): Records electrical activity associated with eye movements
   Maintenance of wakefulness test (MWT): An attended study used to determine the patient's ability to stay awake
   Multiple sleep latency test (MSLT): Attended study to determine the tendency of the patient to fall asleep
   Peripheral arterial tonometry (PAT): Pulsatile volume changes in a digit are measured to determine activity in the sympathetic nervous system for respiratory analysis
   Polysomnography: An attended continuous, simultaneous recording of physiological parameters of sleep for at least 6 hours in a sleep laboratory setting that also includes four or more of the following:
      1. Airflow-oral and/or nasal
      2. Bilateral anterior tibialis EMG
      3. Electrocardiogram (ECG)
      4. Oxyhemoglobin saturation, SpO2
      5. Respiratory effort
   Positive airway pressure (PAP): Noninvasive devices used to treat sleep-related disorders
   Respiratory airflow (ventilation): Assessment of air movement during inhalation and exhalation as measured by nasal pressure sensors and thermistor
   Respiratory analysis: Assessment of components of respiration obtained by other methods such as airflow or peripheral arterial tone
   Respiratory effort: Use of the diaphragm and/or intercostal muscle for airflow is measured using transducers to estimate thoracic and abdominal motion
   Respiratory movement: Measures the movement of the chest and abdomen during respiration
   Sleep latency: Pertains to the time it takes to get to sleep
   Sleep staging: Determination of the separate levels of sleep according to physiological measurements
   Total sleep time: Determined by the use of actigraphy and other methods
   Use of portable and in-laboratory technology
EXCLUDES E&M services

95700	Resequenced code. See code following 95967.
95705	Resequenced code. See code following 95967.
95706	Resequenced code. See code following 95967.
95707	Resequenced code. See code following 95967.
95708	Resequenced code. See code following 95967.
95709	Resequenced code. See code following 95967.
95710	Resequenced code. See code following 95967.
95711	Resequenced code. See code following 95967.
95712	Resequenced code. See code following 95967.
95713	Resequenced code. See code following 95967.
95714	Resequenced code. See code following 95967.
95715	Resequenced code. See code following 95967.
95716	Resequenced code. See code following 95967.
95717	Resequenced code. See code following 95967.
95718	Resequenced code. See code following 95967.

95719	Resequenced code. See code following 95967.
95720	Resequenced code. See code following 95967.
95721	Resequenced code. See code following 95967.
95722	Resequenced code. See code following 95967.
95723	Resequenced code. See code following 95967.
95724	Resequenced code. See code following 95967.
95725	Resequenced code. See code following 95967.
95726	Resequenced code. See code following 95967.
95782	Resequenced code. See code following 95811.
95783	Resequenced code. See code following 95811.
95800	Resequenced code. See code following 95806.
95801	Resequenced code. See code following 95806.

95803 **Actigraphy testing, recording, analysis, interpretation, and report (minimum of 72 hours to 14 consecutive days of recording)**

EXCLUDES Sleep studies (95806-95811 [95800, 95801])
Use of code more than one time in a 14-day period
4.06   4.06   FUD XXX   [01] [80]
AMA: 2018,Feb,11; 2018,Jan,8; 2017,Jan,8; 2016,Jan,13; 2015,Jan,16; 2014,Jan,11

95805 **Multiple sleep latency or maintenance of wakefulness testing, recording, analysis and interpretation of physiological measurements of sleep during multiple trials to assess sleepiness**

INCLUDES Physiological sleep parameters as measured by:
   Frontal, central, and occipital EEG leads (3 leads)
   Left and right EOG
   Submental EMG lead
EXCLUDES Polysomnography (95808-95811)
Sleep study, not attended (95806)
Code also modifier 52 when less than four nap opportunities are recorded
11.8   11.8   FUD XXX   [S] [80]
AMA: 2018,Feb,11; 2018,Jan,8; 2017,Jan,8; 2016,Jan,13; 2015,Jan,16; 2014,Jan,11

95806 **Sleep study, unattended, simultaneous recording of, heart rate, oxygen saturation, respiratory airflow, and respiratory effort (eg, thoracoabdominal movement)**

EXCLUDES Arterial waveform analysis (93050)
Event monitors (93268-93272)
Holter monitor (93224-93227)
Remote cardiovascular telemetry (93228-93229)
Rhythm strips (93041-93042)
Unattended sleep study with measurement of a minimum heart rate, oxygen saturation, and respiratory analysis (95801)
Unattended sleep study with measurement of heart rate, oxygen saturation, respiratory analysis, and sleep time (95800)
Code also modifier 52 for fewer than 6 hours of recording
3.90   3.90   FUD XXX   [S] [80]
AMA: 2018,Feb,11; 2018,Jan,8; 2017,Jan,8; 2016,Jan,13; 2015,Jan,16; 2014,Jan,11

\# **95800** **Sleep study, unattended, simultaneous recording; heart rate, oxygen saturation, respiratory analysis (eg, by airflow or peripheral arterial tone), and sleep time**

4.79   4.79   FUD XXX   [S] [80]
AMA: 2018,Feb,11; 2018,Jan,8; 2017,Jan,8; 2016,Jan,13; 2015,Jan,16; 2014,Jan,11

\# **95801** **minimum of heart rate, oxygen saturation, and respiratory analysis (eg, by airflow or peripheral arterial tone)**

2.57   2.57   FUD XXX   [01] [80]
AMA: 2018,Feb,11; 2018,Jan,8; 2017,Jan,8; 2016,Jan,13; 2015,Jan,16; 2014,Jan,11

95807

95807 **Sleep study, simultaneous recording of ventilation, respiratory effort, ECG or heart rate, and oxygen saturation, attended by a technologist**

> EXCLUDES *Polysomnography (95808-95811)*
> *Sleep study, not attended (95806)*
> Code also modifier 52 for fewer than 6 hours of recording
> 🔲 12.1 ⚲ 12.1 **FUD** XXX S 80 🔲
>
> **AMA:** 2018,Feb,11; 2018,Jan,8; 2017,Jan,8; 2016,Jan,13; 2015,Jan,16; 2014,Jan,11

95808 **Polysomnography; any age, sleep staging with 1-3 additional parameters of sleep, attended by a technologist**

> EXCLUDES *Sleep study, not attended (95806)*
> 🔲 18.9 ⚲ 18.9 **FUD** XXX S 80 🔲
>
> **AMA:** 2018,Feb,11; 2018,Jan,8; 2017,Jan,8; 2016,Jan,13; 2015,Jan,16; 2014,Jan,11

95810 **age 6 years or older, sleep staging with 4 or more additional parameters of sleep, attended by a technologist** A

> EXCLUDES *Sleep study, not attended (95806)*
> Code also modifier 52 for fewer than 6 hours of recording
> 🔲 17.3 ⚲ 17.3 **FUD** XXX S 80 🔲
>
> **AMA:** 2018,Feb,11; 2018,Jan,8; 2017,Jan,8; 2016,Jan,13; 2015,Jan,16; 2014,Jan,11

95811 **age 6 years or older, sleep staging with 4 or more additional parameters of sleep, with initiation of continuous positive airway pressure therapy or bilevel ventilation, attended by a technologist** A

> EXCLUDES *Sleep study, not attended (95806)*
> Code also modifier 52 for fewer than 6 hours of recording
> 🔲 18.1 ⚲ 18.1 **FUD** XXX S 80 🔲
>
> **AMA:** 2018,Feb,11; 2018,Jan,8; 2017,Jan,8; 2016,Jan,13; 2015,Jan,16; 2014,Oct,8; 2014,Jan,11

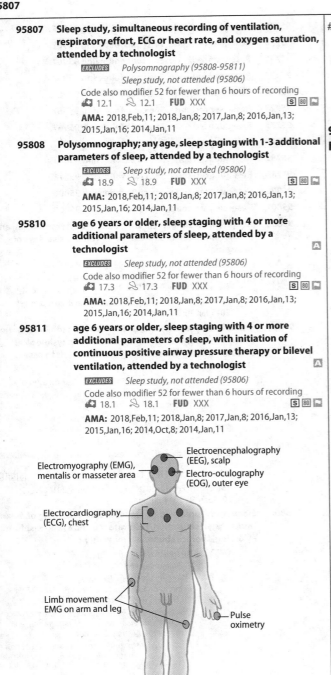

Electroencephalography (EEG), scalp
Electromyography (EMG), mentalis or masseter area
Electro-oculography (EOG), outer eye
Electrocardiography (ECG), chest
Limb movement EMG on arm and leg
Pulse oximetry

Core areas of monitoring for polysomnography

\# 95782 **younger than 6 years, sleep staging with 4 or more additional parameters of sleep, attended by a technologist** A

> 🔲 25.6 ⚲ 25.6 **FUD** XXX S 80 🔲
>
> **AMA:** 2018,Feb,11; 2018,Jan,8; 2017,Jan,8; 2016,Jan,13; 2015,Jan,16; 2014,Jan,11

\# 95783 **younger than 6 years, sleep staging with 4 or more additional parameters of sleep, with initiation of continuous positive airway pressure therapy or bi-level ventilation, attended by a technologist** A

> Code also modifier 52 for fewer than 7 hours of recording
> 🔲 27.3 ⚲ 27.3 **FUD** XXX S 80 🔲
>
> **AMA:** 2018,Feb,11; 2018,Jan,8; 2017,Jan,8; 2016,Jan,13; 2015,Jan,16; 2014,Oct,8; 2014,Jan,11

95812-95830 Evaluation of Brain Activity by Electroencephalogram

> INCLUDES Only time when time is being recorded and data are being collected and does not include set-up and take-down
> EXCLUDES E&M services

95812 **Electroencephalogram (EEG) extended monitoring; 41-60 minutes**

> INCLUDES Hyperventilation
> Photic stimulation
> Physician interpretation
> Recording of 41-60 minutes
> Report
>
> EXCLUDES *EEG digital analysis (95957)*
> *EEG during nonintracranial surgery (95955)*
> *Long-term EEG (two hours or more) ([95700, 95705, 95706, 95707, 95708, 95709, 95710, 95711, 95712, 95713, 95714, 95715, 95716, 95717, 95718, 95719, 95720, 95721, 95722, 95723, 95724, 95725, 95726])*
> *Wada test (95958)*
> Code also modifier 26 for physician interpretation only
> 🔲 9.19 ⚲ 9.19 **FUD** XXX S 80 🔲
>
> **AMA:** 2018,Dec,3; 2018,Dec,3; 2018,Feb,11; 2018,Jan,8; 2017,Jan,8; 2016,Jan,13; 2015,Jan,16; 2014,Jan,11

▲ 95813 **61-119 minutes**

> INCLUDES Hyperventilation
> Photic stimulation
> Physician interpretation
> Recording of 61 minutes or more
> Report
>
> EXCLUDES *EEG digital analysis (95957)*
> *EEG during nonintracranial surgery (95955)*
> *Long-term EEG (two hours or more) ([95700, 95705, 95706, 95707, 95708, 95709, 95710, 95711, 95712, 95713, 95714, 95715, 95716, 95717, 95718, 95719, 95720, 95721, 95722, 95723, 95724, 95725, 95726])*
> *Wada test (95958)*
> Code also modifier 26 for physician interpretation only
> 🔲 11.4 ⚲ 11.4 **FUD** XXX S 80 🔲
>
> **AMA:** 2018,Dec,3; 2018,Dec,3; 2018,Feb,11; 2018,Jan,8; 2017,Jan,8; 2016,Jan,13; 2015,Jan,16; 2014,Jan,11

95816 **Electroencephalogram (EEG); including recording awake and drowsy**

> INCLUDES Photic stimulation
> Physician interpretation
> Recording of 20-40 minutes
> Report
>
> EXCLUDES *EEG digital analysis (95957)*
> *EEG during nonintracranial surgery (95955)*
> *Long-term EEG (two hours or more) ([95700, 95705, 95706, 95707, 95708, 95709, 95710, 95711, 95712, 95713, 95714, 95715, 95716, 95717, 95718, 95719, 95720, 95721, 95722, 95723, 95724, 95725, 95726])*
> *Wada test (95958)*
> Code also modifier 26 for physician interpretation only
> 🔲 10.2 ⚲ 10.2 **FUD** XXX S 80 🔲
>
> **AMA:** 2018,Dec,3; 2018,Dec,3; 2018,Feb,11; 2018,Jan,8; 2017,Jan,8; 2016,Jan,13; 2015,Dec,16; 2015,Jan,16; 2014,Jan,11

Medicine

95819 including recording awake and asleep

INCLUDES
Hyperventilation
Photic stimulation
Physician interpretation
Recording of 20-40 minutes
Report

EXCLUDES
EEG digital analysis (95957)
EEG during nonintracranial surgery (95955)
Long-term EEG (two hours or more) ([95700, 95705, 95706, 95707, 95708, 95709, 95710, 95711, 95712, 95713, 95714, 95715, 95716, 95717, 95718, 95719, 95720, 95721, 95722, 95723, 95724, 95725, 95726])
Wada test (95958)

Code also modifier 26 for interpretation only
🔲 12.0 🔲 12.0 FUD XXX [S] [80] 🔲

AMA: 2018,Dec,3; 2018,Dec,3; 2018,Feb,11; 2018,Jan,8; 2017,Jan,8; 2016,Jan,13; 2015,Dec,16; 2015,Jan,16; 2014,Jan,11

95822 recording in coma or sleep only

INCLUDES
Hyperventilation
Photic stimulation
Physician interpretation
Recording of 20-40 minutes
Report

EXCLUDES
EEG digital analysis (95957)
EEG during nonintracranial surgery (95955)
Long-term EEG (two hours or more) ([95700, 95705, 95706, 95707, 95708, 95709, 95710, 95711, 95712, 95713, 95714, 95715, 95716, 95717, 95718, 95719, 95720, 95721, 95722, 95723, 95724, 95725, 95726])
Wada test (95958)

Code also modifier 26 for interpretation only
🔲 10.9 🔲 10.9 FUD XXX [S] [80] 🔲

AMA: 2018,Dec,3; 2018,Dec,3; 2018,Feb,11; 2018,Jan,8; 2017,Jan,8; 2016,Jan,13; 2015,Jan,16; 2014,Dec,18; 2014,Jan,11

95824 cerebral death evaluation only

INCLUDES
Physician interpretation
Recording
Report

EXCLUDES
EEG digital analysis (95957)
EEG during nonintracranial surgery (95955)
Long-term EEG (two hours or more) ([95700, 95705, 95706, 95707, 95708, 95709, 95710, 95711, 95712, 95713, 95714, 95715, 95716, 95717, 95718, 95719, 95720, 95721, 95722, 95723, 95724, 95725, 95726])
Wada test (95958)

Code also modifier 26 for physician interpretation only
🔲 0.00 🔲 0.00 FUD XXX [S] [80] 🔲

AMA: 2018,Feb,11

95827 all night recording

To report, see ([97505-95707], [95711], [95713], [95717-95718])

95829 Resequenced code. See code following 95830.

95830 Insertion by physician or other qualified health care professional of sphenoidal electrodes for electroencephalographic (EEG) recording
🔲 2.64 🔲 10.9 FUD XXX [B] [80] 🔲

AMA: 2018,Feb,11

[95829, 95836] Evaluation of Brain Activity by Electrocorticography

\# 95829 Electrocorticogram at surgery (separate procedure)

INCLUDES
EEG recording from electrodes placed in or on the brain
Interpretation and review during the surgical procedure

Code also modifier 26 for interpretation only
🔲 53.6 🔲 53.6 FUD XXX [N] [80] 🔲

AMA: 2018,Dec,3; 2018,Dec,3; 2018,Feb,11

\# 95836 Electrocorticogram from an implanted brain neurostimulator pulse generator/transmitter, including recording, with interpretation and written report, up to 30 days

INCLUDES
Intracranial recordings for up to 30 days (unattended) with storage for review at a later time

EXCLUDES
Programming of neurostimulator during the 30-day period ([95983, 95984])
Use of code more than one time for the documented 30-day period

🔲 3.14 🔲 3.14 FUD XXX [80] 🔲

AMA: 2018,Dec,3; 2018,Dec,3

95831-95857 Evaluation of Muscles and Range of Motion

CMS: 100-02,15,230.4 Services By a Physical/Occupational Therapist in Private Practice

EXCLUDES E&M services

95831 ~~Muscle testing, manual (separate procedure) with report; extremity (excluding hand) or trunk~~

To report, see ([97161], [97162], [97163], [97164], [97165], [97166], [97167], [97168], [97169], [97170], [97171], [97172])

95832 ~~hand, with or without comparison with normal side~~

To report, see ([97161], [97162], [97163], [97164], [97165], [97166], [97167], [97168], [97169], [97170], [97171], [97172])

95833 ~~total evaluation of body, excluding hands~~

To report, see ([97161], [97162], [97163], [97164], [97165], [97166], [97167], [97168], [97169], [97170], [97171], [97172])

95834 ~~total evaluation of body, including hands~~

To report, see ([97161], [97162], [97163], [97164], [97165], [97166], [97167], [97168], [97169], [97170], [97171], [97172])

95836 Resequenced code. See code following 95830.

95851 Range of motion measurements and report (separate procedure); each extremity (excluding hand) or each trunk section (spine)
🔲 0.22 🔲 0.59 FUD XXX [A] [80] 🔲

AMA: 2018,Feb,11; 2018,Jan,8; 2017,Jan,8; 2016,Dec,16; 2016,Jan,13; 2015,Jan,16; 2014,Jan,11

95852 hand, with or without comparison with normal side
🔲 0.17 🔲 0.53 FUD XXX [A] [80] 🔲

AMA: 2018,Feb,11; 2018,Jan,8; 2017,Jan,8; 2016,Jan,13; 2015,Jan,16; 2014,Jan,11

95857 Cholinesterase inhibitor challenge test for myasthenia gravis
🔲 0.85 🔲 1.54 FUD XXX [S] [80] 🔲

AMA: 2018,Feb,11; 2018,Jan,8; 2017,Jan,8; 2016,Jan,13; 2015,Jan,16; 2014,Jan,11

95860-95887 [95885, 95886, 95887] Evaluation of Nerve and Muscle Function: EMGs with/without Nerve Conduction Studies

INCLUDES
Physician interpretation
Recording
Report

EXCLUDES E&M services

95860 Needle electromyography; 1 extremity with or without related paraspinal areas

INCLUDES
Testing of five or more muscles per extremity

EXCLUDES
Dynamic electromyography during motion analysis studies (96002-96003)
Guidance for chemodenervation (95873-95874)

Code also modifier 26 for interpretation only
🔲 3.43 🔲 3.43 FUD XXX [Q1] [80] 🔲

AMA: 2018,Feb,11; 2018,Jan,8; 2017,Jan,8; 2016,Jan,13; 2015,Mar,6; 2015,Jan,16; 2014,Jan,11

95861 **2 extremities with or without related paraspinal areas**

INCLUDES Testing of five or more muscles per extremity

EXCLUDES *Dynamic electromyography during motion analysis studies (96002-96003)*
Guidance for chemodenervation (95873-95874)

Code also modifier 26 for interpretation only

4.90 4.90 **FUD** XXX Q1 80

AMA: 2018,Feb,11; 2018,Jan,8; 2017,Jan,8; 2016,Jan,13; 2015,Mar,6; 2015,Jan,16; 2014,Jan,11

95863 **3 extremities with or without related paraspinal areas**

INCLUDES Testing of five or more muscles per extremity

EXCLUDES *Dynamic electromyography during motion analysis studies (96002-96003)*
Guidance for chemodenervation (95873-95874)

Code also modifier 26 for interpretation only

6.15 6.15 **FUD** XXX S 80

AMA: 2018,Feb,11; 2018,Jan,8; 2017,Jan,8; 2016,Jan,13; 2015,Mar,6; 2015,Jan,16; 2014,Jan,11

95864 **4 extremities with or without related paraspinal areas**

INCLUDES Testing of five or more muscles per extremity

EXCLUDES *Dynamic electromyography during motion analysis studies (96002-96003)*
Guidance for chemodenervation (95873-95874)

Code also modifier 26 for interpretation only

7.07 7.07 **FUD** XXX S 80

AMA: 2018,Feb,11; 2018,Jan,8; 2017,Jan,8; 2016,Jan,13; 2015,Mar,6; 2015,Jan,16; 2014,Jan,11

95865 **larynx**

EXCLUDES *Dynamic electromyography during motion analysis studies (96002-96003)*
Guidance for chemodenervation (95873-95874)

Code also modifier 26 for interpretation only
Code also modifier 52 for unilateral procedure

4.25 4.25 **FUD** XXX Q1 80

AMA: 2018,Feb,11; 2018,Jan,8; 2017,Jan,8; 2016,Jan,13; 2015,Mar,6; 2015,Jan,16; 2014,Jan,6; 2014,Jan,11

95866 **hemidiaphragm**

EXCLUDES *Dynamic electromyography during motion analysis studies (96002-96003)*
Guidance for chemodenervation (95873-95874)

Code also modifier 26 for interpretation only

3.90 3.90 **FUD** XXX Q1 80

AMA: 2018,Feb,11; 2018,Jan,8; 2017,Jan,8; 2016,Jan,13; 2015,Mar,6; 2015,Jan,16; 2014,Jan,11

95867 **cranial nerve supplied muscle(s), unilateral**

EXCLUDES *Guidance for chemodenervation (95873-95874)*

Code also modifier 26 for interpretation only

3.00 3.00 **FUD** XXX S 80

AMA: 2018,Feb,11; 2018,Jan,8; 2017,Jan,8; 2016,Jan,13; 2015,Mar,6; 2015,Jan,16; 2014,Jan,11

95868 **cranial nerve supplied muscles, bilateral**

EXCLUDES *Guidance for chemodenervation (95873-95874)*

3.93 3.93 **FUD** XXX S 80

AMA: 2018,Feb,11; 2018,Jan,8; 2017,Jan,8; 2016,Jan,13; 2015,Mar,6; 2015,Jan,16; 2014,Jan,11

95869 **thoracic paraspinal muscles (excluding T1 or T12)**

EXCLUDES *Dynamic electromyography during motion analysis studies (96002-96003)*
Guidance for chemodenervation (95873-95874)

2.67 2.67 **FUD** XXX Q1 80

AMA: 2018,Feb,11; 2018,Jan,8; 2017,Jan,8; 2016,Jan,13; 2015,Mar,6; 2015,Jan,16; 2014,Jan,11

95870 **limited study of muscles in 1 extremity or non-limb (axial) muscles (unilateral or bilateral), other than thoracic paraspinal, cranial nerve supplied muscles, or sphincters**

INCLUDES Adson test
Testing of four or less muscles per extremity

EXCLUDES *Anal/urethral sphincter/detrusor/urethra/perineum musculature (51785-51792)*
Complete study of extremities (95860-95864)
Dynamic electromyography during motion analysis studies (96002-96003)
Eye muscles (92265)
Guidance for chemodenervation (95873-95874)

2.58 2.58 **FUD** XXX Q1 80

AMA: 2018,Feb,11; 2018,Jan,8; 2017,Jan,8; 2016,Jan,13; 2015,Mar,6; 2015,Jan,16; 2014,Jan,11

95872 **Needle electromyography using single fiber electrode, with quantitative measurement of jitter, blocking and/or fiber density, any/all sites of each muscle studied**

EXCLUDES *Dynamic electromyography during motion analysis studies (96002-96003)*

5.64 5.64 **FUD** XXX S 80

AMA: 2018,Feb,11; 2018,Jan,8; 2017,Jan,8; 2016,Jan,13; 2015,Mar,6; 2015,Jan,16; 2014,Jan,11

+ # **95885** **Needle electromyography, each extremity, with related paraspinal areas, when performed, done with nerve conduction, amplitude and latency/velocity study; limited (List separately in addition to code for primary procedure)**

1.73 1.73 **FUD** ZZZ N 80

AMA: 2018,Feb,11; 2018,Jan,8; 2017,Jul,10; 2017,Jan,8; 2016,Jan,13; 2015,Mar,6; 2015,Jan,16; 2014,Jan,11

+ # **95886** **complete, five or more muscles studied, innervated by three or more nerves or four or more spinal levels (List separately in addition to code for primary procedure)**

2.68 2.68 **FUD** ZZZ N 80

AMA: 2018,Feb,11; 2018,Jan,8; 2017,Jul,10; 2017,Jan,8; 2016,Jan,13; 2015,Mar,6; 2015,Jan,16; 2014,Jan,11

+ # **95887** **Needle electromyography, non-extremity (cranial nerve supplied or axial) muscle(s) done with nerve conduction, amplitude and latency/velocity study (List separately in addition to code for primary procedure)**

2.33 2.33 **FUD** ZZZ N 80

AMA: 2018,Feb,11; 2018,Jan,8; 2017,Jul,10; 2017,Jan,8; 2016,Jan,13; 2015,Mar,6; 2015,Jan,16; 2014,Jan,11; 2014,Jan,8

Trigeminal nerve branches in infratemporal fossa

Mandibular branch V3

Inferior alveolar nerve

Lingual nerve

Mental nerve

Cranial nerves: trigeminal branches of lower face and select facial nerves

Needle EMG is performed to determine conduction, amplitude, and latency/velocity

26/TC **PC/TC Only** A2-Z3 **ASC Payment** 50 **Bilateral** ♂ **Male Only** ♀ **Female Only** **Facility RVU** **Non-Facility RVU** **CCI** **CLIA**
FUD Follow-up Days **CMS: IOM** **AMA: CPT Asst** A-Y **OPPSI** 80/80 **Surg Assist Allowed / w/Doc** **Lab Crosswalk** **Radiology Crosswalk**

95861 — 95887

506

CPT © 2019 American Medical Association. All Rights Reserved. © 2019 Optum360, LLC

+ 95873 **Electrical stimulation for guidance in conjunction with chemodenervation (List separately in addition to code for primary procedure)**

> EXCLUDES *Chemodenervation larynx (64617)*
> *Injection of anesthetic or steroid, sacroiliac joint (64451)*
> *Needle electromyography (95860-95870)*
> *Needle electromyography guidance for chemodenervation (95874)*
> *Radiofrequency ablation, sacroiliac joint ([64625])*
> *Use of more than one guidance code for each code for chemodenervation*
>
> Code first chemodenervation (64612, 64615-64616, 64642-64647)

🚑 2.13 ⚕ 2.13 **FUD** ZZZ N 80 ▭

AMA: 2019,Apr,9; 2018,Feb,11; 2018,Jan,8; 2017,Jan,8; 2016,Jan,13; 2015,Mar,6; 2015,Jan,16; 2014,Jan,6; 2014,Jan,11

+ 95874 **Needle electromyography for guidance in conjunction with chemodenervation (List separately in addition to code for primary procedure)**

> EXCLUDES *Chemodenervation larynx (64617)*
> *Injection of anesthetic or steroid, sacroiliac joint (64451)*
> *Needle electromyography (95860-95870)*
> *Needle electromyography guidance for chemodenervation (95873)*
> *Radiofrequency ablation, sacroiliac joint ([64625])*
> *Use of more than one guidance code for each code for chemodenervation*
>
> Code first chemodenervation (64612, 64615-64616, 64642-64647)

🚑 2.18 ⚕ 2.18 **FUD** ZZZ N 80 ▭

AMA: 2019,Apr,9; 2018,Feb,11; 2018,Jan,8; 2017,Jan,8; 2016,Jan,13; 2015,Mar,6; 2015,Jan,16; 2014,Oct,14; 2014,Jan,6; 2014,Jan,11

95875 **Ischemic limb exercise test with serial specimen(s) acquisition for muscle(s) metabolite(s)**

🚑 3.75 ⚕ 3.75 **FUD** XXX S 80 ▭

AMA: 2018,Feb,11; 2018,Jan,8; 2017,Jan,8; 2016,Jan,13; 2015,Mar,6; 2015,Jan,16; 2014,Jan,11

95885 Resequenced code. See code following 95872.

95886 Resequenced code. See code following 95872.

95887 Resequenced code. See code before 95873.

95905-95913 Evaluation of Nerve Function: Nerve Conduction Studies

> INCLUDES Conduction studies of motor and sensory nerves
> Reports from on-site examiner including the work product of the interpretation of results using established methodologies, calculations, comparisons to normal studies, and interpretation by physician or other qualified health care professional
> Single conduction study comprising a sensory and motor conduction test with/without F or H wave testing, and all orthodromic and antidromic impulses
> Total number of tests performed indicate which code is appropriate
>
> EXCLUDES *Use of code for more than one study when multiple sites on the same nerve are tested*
>
> Code also electromyography performed with nerve conduction studies, as appropriate ([95885, 95886, 95887])

95905 **Motor and/or sensory nerve conduction, using preconfigured electrode array(s), amplitude and latency/velocity study, each limb, includes F-wave study when performed, with interpretation and report**

> INCLUDES Study with preconfigured electrodes that are customized to a specific body location
>
> EXCLUDES *Needle electromyography ([95885, 95886])*
> *Nerve conduction studies (95907-95913)*
> *Use of this code more than one time for each limb studied*

🚑 1.80 ⚕ 1.80 **FUD** XXX ⊘ 01 80 ▭

AMA: 2018,Feb,11; 2018,Jan,8; 2017,Jan,8; 2016,Jan,13; 2015,Jan,16; 2014,Jan,11

95907 **Nerve conduction studies; 1-2 studies**

🚑 2.72 ⚕ 2.72 **FUD** XXX S 80 ▭

AMA: 2018,Aug,10; 2018,Feb,11; 2018,Jan,8; 2017,Dec,14; 2017,Jan,8; 2016,Jan,13; 2015,Jan,16; 2014,Jan,11

95908 **3-4 studies**

🚑 3.52 ⚕ 3.52 **FUD** XXX S 80 ▭

AMA: 2018,Aug,10; 2018,Feb,11; 2018,Jan,8; 2017,Jan,8; 2016,Jan,13; 2015,Mar,6; 2015,Jan,16; 2014,Jan,11

95909 **5-6 studies**

🚑 4.20 ⚕ 4.20 **FUD** XXX S 80 ▭

AMA: 2018,Aug,10; 2018,Feb,11; 2018,Jan,8; 2017,Jan,8; 2016,Jan,13; 2015,Jan,16; 2014,Jan,11

95910 **7-8 studies**

🚑 5.51 ⚕ 5.51 **FUD** XXX S 80 ▭

AMA: 2018,Aug,10; 2018,Feb,11; 2018,Jan,8; 2017,Jan,8; 2016,Jan,13; 2015,Jan,16; 2014,Jan,11

95911 **9-10 studies**

🚑 6.62 ⚕ 6.62 **FUD** XXX S 80 ▭

AMA: 2018,Aug,10; 2018,Feb,11; 2018,Jan,8; 2017,Jan,8; 2016,Jan,13; 2015,Jan,16; 2014,Jan,11

95912 **11-12 studies**

🚑 7.44 ⚕ 7.44 **FUD** XXX S 80 ▭

AMA: 2018,Aug,10; 2018,Feb,11; 2018,Jan,8; 2017,Jan,8; 2016,Jan,13; 2015,Jan,16; 2014,Jan,11

95913 **13 or more studies**

🚑 8.59 ⚕ 8.59 **FUD** XXX S 80 ▭

AMA: 2018,Aug,10; 2018,Feb,11; 2018,Jan,8; 2017,Jan,8; 2016,Jan,13; 2015,Jan,16; 2014,Jan,11

95940-95941 [95940, 95941] Intraoperative Neurophysiological Monitoring

> INCLUDES Monitoring, testing, and data evaluation during surgical procedures by a monitoring professional dedicated only to performing the necessary testing and monitoring
> Monitoring services provided by the anesthesiologist or surgeon separately
>
> EXCLUDES *Baseline neurophysiologic monitoring*
> *EEG during nonintracranial surgery (95955)*
> *Electrocorticography (95829)*
> *Intraoperative cortical and subcortical mapping (95961-95962)*
> *Neurostimulator programming/analysis (95971-95972, 95976-95977, [95983, 95984])*
> *Time required for set-up, recording, interpretation, and removal of electrodes*
>
> Code also baseline studies (eg, EMGs, NCVs), no more than one time per operative session
> Code also services provided after midnight using the date when monitoring started and the total monitoring time
> Code also standby time prior to procedure (99360)
> Code first (92585, 95822, 95860-95870, 95907-95913, 95925-95937 [95938, 95939])

+ # 95940 **Continuous intraoperative neurophysiology monitoring in the operating room, one on one monitoring requiring personal attendance, each 15 minutes (List separately in addition to code for primary procedure)**

> INCLUDES 15 minute increments of monitoring service
> A total of all monitoring time for procedures overlapping midnight
> Based on time spent monitoring, regardless of number of tests or parameters monitored
> Continuous intraoperative neurophysiologic monitoring by a dedicated monitoring professional in the operating room providing one-on-one patient care
> Monitoring time may begin prior to the incision
> Monitoring time that is distinct from baseline neurophysiologic study/s time or other services (eg, mapping)
>
> EXCLUDES *Time spent in executing or interpreting the baseline neurophysiologic study or studies*
>
> Code also monitoring from outside of the operative room, when applicable ([95941])

🚑 0.93 ⚕ 0.93 **FUD** XXX N 80 ▭

AMA: 2018,Feb,11; 2018,Jan,8; 2017,Aug,8; 2017,Jan,8; 2016,Jan,13; 2015,Jan,16; 2014,Apr,5; 2014,Apr,10

+ # **95941** **Continuous intraoperative neurophysiology monitoring, from outside the operating room (remote or nearby) or for monitoring of more than one case while in the operating room, per hour (List separately in addition to code for primary procedure)**

INCLUDES Based on time spent monitoring, regardless of number of tests or parameters monitored

Monitoring time that is distinct from baseline neurophysiologic study/s time or other services (eg, mapping)

One hour increments of monitoring service

🔲 0.00   ⚕ 0.00   **FUD** XXX   N ▣

AMA: 2018,Feb,11; 2018,Jan,8; 2017,Aug,8; 2017,Jan,8; 2016,Jan,13; 2015,Jan,16; 2014,Dec,18; 2014,Apr,10; 2014,Apr,5; 2014,Jan,11

95921-95943 [95943] Evaluation of Autonomic Nervous System

INCLUDES Physician interpretation

Recording

Report

Testing for autonomic dysfunction including site and autonomic subsystems

95921 **Testing of autonomic nervous system function; cardiovagal innervation (parasympathetic function), including 2 or more of the following: heart rate response to deep breathing with recorded R-R interval, Valsalva ratio, and 30:15 ratio**

INCLUDES Display on a monitor

Minimum of two of the following elements are performed:

Cardiovascular function as indicated by a 30:15 ration (R/R interval at beat 30)/(R-R interval at beat 15)

Heart rate response to deep breathing obtained by visual quantitative analysis of recordings with patient taking 5-6 breaths per minute

Valsalva ratio (at least 2) obtained by dividing the highest heart rate by the lowest

Monitoring of heart rate by electrocardiography of rate obtained from time between two successive R waves (R-R interval)

Storage of data for waveform analysis

Testing most usually in prone position

Tilt table testing, when performed

EXCLUDES *Autonomic nervous system testing with sympathetic adrenergic function testing (95922, 95924)*

Simultaneous measures of parasympathetic and sympathetic function ([95943])

🔲 2.36   ⚕ 2.36   **FUD** XXX   S 80 ▣

AMA: 2018,Feb,11; 2018,Jan,8; 2017,Jan,8; 2016,Jan,13; 2015,Jan,16; 2014,Jan,11

95922 **vasomotor adrenergic innervation (sympathetic adrenergic function), including beat-to-beat blood pressure and R-R interval changes during Valsalva maneuver and at least 5 minutes of passive tilt**

EXCLUDES *Autonomic nervous system testing with parasympathetic function (95921, 95924)*

Simultaneous measures of parasympathetic and sympathetic function ([95943])

🔲 2.70   ⚕ 2.70   **FUD** XXX   Q1 80 ▣

AMA: 2018,Feb,11; 2018,Jan,8; 2017,Jan,8; 2016,Jan,13; 2015,Jan,16; 2014,Jan,11

95923 **sudomotor, including 1 or more of the following: quantitative sudomotor axon reflex test (QSART), silastic sweat imprint, thermoregulatory sweat test, and changes in sympathetic skin potential**

🔲 3.64   ⚕ 3.64   **FUD** XXX   Q1 80 ▣

AMA: 2018,Feb,11; 2018,Jan,8; 2017,Jan,8; 2016,Jan,13; 2015,Jan,16; 2014,Jan,11

95924 **combined parasympathetic and sympathetic adrenergic function testing with at least 5 minutes of passive tilt**

INCLUDES Tilt table testing of adrenergic and parasympathetic function

EXCLUDES *Autonomic nervous system testing with parasympathetic function (95921-95922)*

Simultaneous measures of parasympathetic and sympathetic function ([95943])

🔲 4.25   ⚕ 4.25   **FUD** XXX   S 80 ▣

AMA: 2018,Feb,11; 2018,Jan,8; 2017,Jan,8; 2016,Jan,13; 2015,Jan,16

95943 **Simultaneous, independent, quantitative measures of both parasympathetic function and sympathetic function, based on time-frequency analysis of heart rate variability concurrent with time-frequency analysis of continuous respiratory activity, with mean heart rate and blood pressure measures, during rest, paced (deep) breathing, Valsalva maneuvers, and head-up postural change**

EXCLUDES *Autonomic nervous system testing (95921-95922, 95924)*

Rhythm ECG (93040)

🔲 0.00   ⚕ 0.00   **FUD** XXX   S 80 ▣

AMA: 2018,Feb,11; 2018,Jan,8; 2017,Jan,8; 2016,Jan,13; 2015,Jan,16

95925-95943 [95938, 95939] Neurotransmission Studies

95925 **Short-latency somatosensory evoked potential study, stimulation of any/all peripheral nerves or skin sites, recording from the central nervous system; in upper limbs**

EXCLUDES *Auditory evoked potentials (92585)*

Evoked potential study in both upper and lower limbs ([95938])

Evoked potential study in lower limbs (95926)

🔲 3.73   ⚕ 3.73   **FUD** XXX   S 80 ▣

AMA: 2018,Feb,11; 2018,Jan,8; 2017,Jan,8; 2016,Jan,13; 2015,Jan,16; 2014,Jan,11

95926 **in lower limbs**

EXCLUDES *Auditory evoked potentials (92585)*

Evoked potential study in both upper and lower limbs ([95938])

Evoked potential study in upper limbs (95925)

🔲 3.61   ⚕ 3.61   **FUD** XXX   S 80 ▣

AMA: 2018,Feb,11; 2018,Jan,8; 2017,Jan,8; 2016,Jan,13; 2015,Jan,16; 2014,Jan,11

95938 **in upper and lower limbs**

🔲 9.79   ⚕ 9.79   **FUD** XXX   S 80 ▣

AMA: 2018,Feb,11; 2018,Jan,8; 2017,Jan,8; 2016,Jan,13; 2015,Jan,16; 2014,Jan,11

95927 **in the trunk or head**

EXCLUDES *Auditory evoked potentials (92585)*

Code also modifier 52 for unilateral test

🔲 3.74   ⚕ 3.74   **FUD** XXX   S 80 ▣

AMA: 2018,Feb,11; 2018,Jan,8; 2017,Jan,8; 2016,Jan,13; 2015,Jan,16; 2014,Jan,11

95928 **Central motor evoked potential study (transcranial motor stimulation); upper limbs**

EXCLUDES *Central motor evoked potential study lower limbs (95929)*

🔲 6.20   ⚕ 6.20   **FUD** XXX   S 80 ▣

AMA: 2018,Feb,11; 2018,Jan,8; 2017,Jan,8; 2016,Jan,13; 2015,Jan,16

95929 **lower limbs**

EXCLUDES *Central motor evoked potential study upper limbs (95928)*

🔲 6.35   ⚕ 6.35   **FUD** XXX   S 80 ▣

AMA: 2018,Feb,11; 2018,Jan,8; 2017,Jan,8; 2016,Jan,13; 2015,Jan,16; 2014,Dec,6

26/TC PC/TC Only   A2-Z3 ASC Payment   50 Bilateral   ♂ Male Only   ♀ Female Only   🔲 Facility RVU   ⚕ Non-Facility RVU   ▣ CCI   ☒ CLIA

FUD Follow-up Days   **CMS:** IOM   **AMA:** CPT Asst   A-Y OPPSI   80/80 Surg Assist Allowed / w/Doc   ▣ Lab Crosswalk   ▣ Radiology Crosswalk

**95939** **in upper and lower limbs**

> EXCLUDES Central motor evoked potential study of either lower or upper limbs (95928-95929)

📷 14.5 ⚖ 14.5 **FUD** XXX 〔S〕〔80〕▱

AMA: 2018,Feb,11; 2018,Jan,8; 2017,Jan,8; 2016,Jan,13; 2015,Jan,16; 2014,Jan,11

95930 **Visual evoked potential (VEP) checkerboard or flash testing, central nervous system except glaucoma, with interpretation and report**

> EXCLUDES Visual acuity screening using automated visual evoked potential devices (0333T)
> Visual evoked glaucoma testing ([0464T])

📷 1.94 ⚖ 1.94 **FUD** XXX 〔S〕〔80〕▱

AMA: 2018,Feb,11; 2018,Feb,3; 2018,Jan,8; 2017,Jan,8; 2016,Jan,13; 2015,Jan,16; 2014,Aug,8

95933 **Orbicularis oculi (blink) reflex, by electrodiagnostic testing**

📷 2.30 ⚖ 2.30 **FUD** XXX 〔01〕〔80〕▱

AMA: 2018,Feb,11; 2018,Jan,8; 2017,Jul,10; 2017,Jan,8; 2016,Jan,13; 2015,Jan,16

95937 **Neuromuscular junction testing (repetitive stimulation, paired stimuli), each nerve, any 1 method**

📷 2.48 ⚖ 2.48 **FUD** XXX 〔S〕〔80〕▱

AMA: 2018,Feb,11; 2018,Jan,8; 2017,Jan,8; 2016,Feb,13; 2016,Jan,13; 2015,Jan,16; 2014,Jan,11

Nerve

Muscle

Nerve fascicles

Model of normal neuromuscular junction

Acetylcholine reaction

A selected neuromusular junction is repeatedly stimulated. The test is useful to demonstrate reduced muscle action potential from fatigue

95938 Resequenced code. See code following 95926.

95939 Resequenced code. See code following 95929.

95940 Resequenced code. See code following 95913.

95941 Resequenced code. See code following 95913.

95943 Resequenced code. See code following 95924.

95950-95962 Electroencephalography For Seizure Monitoring/Intraoperative Use

> EXCLUDES E&M services

95950 ~~Monitoring for identification and lateralization of cerebral seizure focus, electroencephalographic (eg, 8 channel EEG) recording and interpretation, each 24 hours~~

> To report, see ([95700-95726])

95951 ~~Monitoring for localization of cerebral seizure focus by cable or radio, 16 or more channel telemetry, combined electroencephalographic (EEG) and video recording and interpretation (eg, for presurgical localization), each 24 hours~~

> To report, see ([95700-95726])

95953 ~~Monitoring for localization of cerebral seizure focus by computerized portable 16 or more channel EEG, electroencephalographic (EEG) recording and interpretation, each 24 hours, unattended~~

> To report, see ([95700-95726])

95954 **Pharmacological or physical activation requiring physician or other qualified health care professional attendance during EEG recording of activation phase (eg, thiopental activation test)**

📷 11.3 ⚖ 11.3 **FUD** XXX 〔S〕〔80〕▱

AMA: 2018,Feb,11; 2018,Jan,8; 2017,Jan,8; 2016,Jan,13; 2015,Jan,16; 2014,Jan,11

95955 **Electroencephalogram (EEG) during nonintracranial surgery (eg, carotid surgery)**

📷 5.95 ⚖ 5.95 **FUD** XXX 〔N〕〔80〕▱

AMA: 2018,Feb,11; 2018,Jan,8; 2017,Jan,8; 2016,Jan,13; 2015,Jan,16; 2014,Dec,18

95956 ~~Monitoring for localization of cerebral seizure focus by cable or radio, 16 or more channel telemetry, electroencephalographic (EEG) recording and interpretation, each 24 hours, attended by a technologist or nurse~~

> To report, see ([95700-95726])

95957 **Digital analysis of electroencephalogram (EEG) (eg, for epileptic spike analysis)**

> EXCLUDES Use of automated spike and seizure detection/trending software, when performed ([95700, 95705, 95706, 95707, 95708, 95709, 95710, 95711, 95712, 95713, 95714, 95715, 95716, 95717, 95718, 95719, 95720, 95721, 95722, 95723, 95724, 95725, 95726])

📷 7.62 ⚖ 7.62 **FUD** XXX 〔N〕〔80〕▱

AMA: 2018,Dec,3; 2018,Dec,3; 2018,Feb,11; 2018,Jan,8; 2017,Jan,8; 2016,Jan,13; 2015,Jan,16; 2014,Jan,11

95958 **Wada activation test for hemispheric function, including electroencephalographic (EEG) monitoring**

📷 16.3 ⚖ 16.3 **FUD** XXX 〔S〕〔80〕▱

AMA: 2018,Feb,11

95961 **Functional cortical and subcortical mapping by stimulation and/or recording of electrodes on brain surface, or of depth electrodes, to provoke seizures or identify vital brain structures; initial hour of attendance by a physician or other qualified health care professional**

> INCLUDES One hour of attendance by physician or other qualified health care professional

Code also each additional hour of attendance by physician or other qualified health care professional, when appropriate (95962)

Code also long-term EEG (two hours or more), when performed ([95700, 95705, 95706, 95707, 95708, 95709, 95710, 95711, 95712, 95713, 95714, 95715, 95716, 95717, 95718, 95719, 95720, 95721, 95722, 95723, 95724, 95725, 95726])

Code also modifier 52 for 30 minutes or less of attendance by physician or other qualified health care professional

📷 8.69 ⚖ 8.69 **FUD** XXX 〔S〕〔80〕▱

AMA: 2018,Dec,3; 2018,Dec,3; 2018,Feb,11; 2018,Jan,8; 2017,Jan,8; 2016,Jan,13; 2015,Jan,16; 2014,Jan,11

+ 95962 **each additional hour of attendance by a physician or other qualified health care professional (List separately in addition to code for primary procedure)**

> INCLUDES One hour of attendance by physician or other qualified health care professional

Code also long-term EEG (two hours or more), when performed ([95700, 95705, 95706, 95707, 95708, 95709, 95710, 95711, 95712, 95713, 95714, 95715, 95716, 95717, 95718, 95719, 95720, 95721, 95722, 95723, 95724, 95725, 95726])

Code first initial hour (95961)

📷 7.46 ⚖ 7.46 **FUD** ZZZ 〔N〕〔80〕▱

AMA: 2018,Feb,11; 2018,Jan,8; 2017,Jan,8; 2016,Jan,13; 2015,Jan,16; 2014,Jan,11

95965-95967 Magnetoencephalography

INCLUDES Physician interpretation
Recording
Report

EXCLUDES CT provided along with magnetoencephalography (70450-70470, 70496)
Electroencephalography provided along with magnetoencephalography
(95812-95824)
E&M services
MRI provided along with magnetoencephalography (70551-70553)
Somatosensory evoked potentials/auditory evoked potentials/visual evoked
potentials provided along with magnetic evoked field responses (92585,
95925, 95926, 95930)

95965 **Magnetoencephalography (MEG), recording and analysis; for spontaneous brain magnetic activity (eg, epileptic cerebral cortex localization)**

🔲 0.00   ⌇ 0.00   **FUD** XXX   Ⓢ 80 🔲

AMA: 2018,Feb,11

95966 **for evoked magnetic fields, single modality (eg, sensory, motor, language, or visual cortex localization)**

🔲 0.00   ⌇ 0.00   **FUD** XXX   Ⓢ 80 🔲

AMA: 2018,Feb,11

+ **95967** **for evoked magnetic fields, each additional modality (eg, sensory, motor, language, or visual cortex localization) (List separately in addition to code for primary procedure)**

Code first single modality (95966)

🔲 0.00   ⌇ 0.00   **FUD** ZZZ   Ⓝ 80 🔲

AMA: 2018,Feb,11

95700-95726 [95700, 95705, 95706, 95707, 95708, 95709, 95710, 95711, 95712, 95713, 95714, 95715, 95716, 95717, 95718, 95719, 95720, 95721, 95722, 95723, 95724, 95725, 95726] Electronencephalogram (EEG)

INCLUDES Determination of:
Eligibility for epilepsy surgery
Location and type of seizures
Differentiation of seizures from other conditions
Monitoring of:
Seizure treatment
Status epilepticus
Use of automated spike and seizure detection/trending software, when
performed

EXCLUDES Diagnostic EEG recording time less than two hours
Routine EEG (95812-95813, 95816, 95819, 95822)
Code also cortical or subcortical mapping, when performed (95961-95962)

● # **95700** **Electroencephalogram (EEG) continuous recording, with video when performed, setup, patient education, and takedown when performed, administered in person by EEG technologist, minimum of 8 channels**

🔲 0.00   ⌇ 0.00   **FUD** 000

INCLUDES Technical component

EXCLUDES EEG performed using patient-placed electrodes,
performed by non-EEG technologist, or remote
supervision by an EEG technologist (95999)
Use of code more than one time for each session

● # **95705** **Electroencephalogram (EEG), without video, review of data, technical description by EEG technologist, 2-12 hours; unmonitored**

🔲 0.00   ⌇ 0.00   **FUD** 000

INCLUDES Technical component

EXCLUDES Use of code more than one time to capture complete
long-term EEG session or final 2-12 hour segment
past 26 hours

● # **95706** **with intermittent monitoring and maintenance**

🔲 0.00   ⌇ 0.00   **FUD** 000

INCLUDES Technical component

EXCLUDES Use of code more than one time to capture complete
long-term EEG session or final 2-12 hour segment
past 26 hours

● # **95707** **with continuous, real-time monitoring and maintenance**

🔲 0.00   ⌇ 0.00   **FUD** 000

INCLUDES Technical component

EXCLUDES Use of code more than one time to capture complete
long-term EEG session or final 2-12 hour segment
past 26 hours

● # **95708** **Electroencephalogram (EEG), without video, review of data, technical description by EEG technologist, each increment of 12-26 hours; unmonitored**

🔲 0.00   ⌇ 0.00   **FUD** 000

INCLUDES Technical component

● # **95709** **with intermittent monitoring and maintenance**

🔲 0.00   ⌇ 0.00   **FUD** 000

INCLUDES Technical component

● # **95710** **with continuous, real-time monitoring and maintenance**

🔲 0.00   ⌇ 0.00   **FUD** 000

INCLUDES Technical component

● # **95711** **Electroencephalogram with video (VEEG), review of data, technical description by EEG technologist, 2-12 hours; unmonitored**

🔲 0.00   ⌇ 0.00   **FUD** 000

INCLUDES Technical component

EXCLUDES Use of code more than one time to capture complete
long-term EEG session or final 2-12 hour segment
past 26 hours

● # **95712** **with intermittent monitoring and maintenance**

🔲 0.00   ⌇ 0.00   **FUD** 000

INCLUDES Technical component

EXCLUDES Use of code more than one time to capture complete
long-term EEG session or final 2-12 hour segment
past 26 hours

● # **95713** **with continuous, real-time monitoring and maintenance**

🔲 0.00   ⌇ 0.00   **FUD** 000

INCLUDES Technical component

EXCLUDES Use of code more than one time to capture complete
long-term EEG session or final 2-12 hour segment
past 26 hours

● # **95714** **Electroencephalogram with video (VEEG), review of data, technical description by EEG technologist, each increment of 12-26 hours; unmonitored**

🔲 0.00   ⌇ 0.00   **FUD** 000

INCLUDES Technical component

● # **95715** **with intermittent monitoring and maintenance**

🔲 0.00   ⌇ 0.00   **FUD** 000

INCLUDES Technical component

● # **95716** **with continuous, real-time monitoring and maintenance**

🔲 0.00   ⌇ 0.00   **FUD** 000

INCLUDES Technical component

● # **95717** **Electroencephalogram (EEG), continuous recording, physician or other qualified health care professional review of recorded events, analysis of spike and seizure detection, interpretation and report, 2-12 hours of EEG recording; without video**

🔲 0.00   ⌇ 0.00   **FUD** 000

INCLUDES Professional component

EXCLUDES Professional interpretation for recordings greater than
36 hours and for which the entire professional
report is generated retroactively ([95721, 95722,
95723, 95724, 95725, 95726])
Use of code more than one time to capture complete
long-term EEG session or final 2-12 hour segment
past 24 hours

 # 95718   **with video (VEEG)**

🚑 0.00   ✂ 0.00   **FUD** 000

INCLUDES   Professional component

EXCLUDES   *Professional interpretation for recordings greater than 36 hours and for which the entire professional report is generated retroactively ([95721, 95722, 95723, 95724, 95725, 95726])*

Use of code more than one time to capture complete long-term EEG session or final 2-12 hour segment past 24 hours

 # 95719   **Electroencephalogram (EEG), continuous recording, physician or other qualified health care professional review of recorded events, analysis of spike and seizure detection, each increment of greater than 12 hours, up to 26 hours of EEG recording, interpretation and report after each 24-hour period; without video**

🚑 0.00   ✂ 0.00   **FUD** 000

INCLUDES   Professional component

Single report or multiple reports during the 26-hour reporting period

EXCLUDES   *Professional interpretation for recordings greater than 36 hours and for which the entire professional report is generated retroactively ([95721, 95722, 95723, 95724, 95725, 95726])*

Use of code more than one time to capture of 12 to 26 hours

EEG, 2-12 hours for studies longer than 26 hours ([95717, 95718])

Repeat use of code for multiple day studies after each 24-hour period during extended EEG recording time ([95719, 95720])

 # 95720   **with video (VEEG)**

🚑 0.00   ✂ 0.00   **FUD** 000

INCLUDES   Professional component

Single report or multiple reports during the 26-hour reporting period

EXCLUDES   *Professional interpretation for recordings greater than 36 hours and for which the entire professional report is generated retroactively ([95721, 95722, 95723, 95724, 95725, 95726])*

Use of code more than one time to capture of 12 to 26 hours

EEG, 2-12 hours for studies longer than 26 hours ([95717, 95718])

Repeat use of code for multiple day studies after each 24-hour period during extended EEG recording time ([95719, 95720])

 # 95721   **Electroencephalogram (EEG), continuous recording, physician or other qualified health care professional review of recorded events, analysis of spike and seizure detection, interpretation, and summary report, complete study; greater than 36 hours, up to 60 hours of EEG recording, without video**

🚑 0.00   ✂ 0.00   **FUD** 000

INCLUDES   Professional interpretation for recordings greater than 36 hours and for which the entire professional report is generated retroactively

EXCLUDES   *EEG, continuous recording, less than 36 hours ([95717, 95718, 95719, 95720])*

 # 95722   **greater than 36 hours, up to 60 hours of EEG recording, with video (VEEG)**

🚑 0.00   ✂ 0.00   **FUD** 000

INCLUDES   Professional interpretation for recordings greater than 36 hours and for which the entire professional report is generated retroactively

EXCLUDES   *EEG, continuous recording, less than 36 hours ([95717, 95718, 95719, 95720])*

 # 95723   **greater than 60 hours, up to 84 hours of EEG recording, without video**

🚑 0.00   ✂ 0.00   **FUD** 000

INCLUDES   Professional interpretation for recordings greater than 36 hours and for which the entire professional report is generated retroactively

EXCLUDES   *EEG, continuous recording, less than 36 hours ([95717, 95718, 95719, 95720])*

 # 95724   **greater than 60 hours, up to 84 hours of EEG recording, with video (VEEG)**

🚑 0.00   ✂ 0.00   **FUD** 000

INCLUDES   Professional interpretation for recordings greater than 36 hours and for which the entire professional report is generated retroactively

EXCLUDES   *EEG, continuous recording, less than 36 hours ([95717, 95718, 95719, 95720])*

 # 95725   **greater than 84 hours of EEG recording, without video**

INCLUDES   Professional interpretation for recordings greater than 36 hours and for which the entire professional report is generated retroactively

EXCLUDES   *EEG, continuous recording, less than 36 hours ([95717, 95718, 95719, 95720])*

🚑 0.00   ✂ 0.00   **FUD** 000

AMA: 2011,Jan,11; 2009,Jan,11-31

 # 95726   **greater than 84 hours of EEG recording, with video (VEEG)**

🚑 0.00   ✂ 0.00   **FUD** 000

INCLUDES   Professional interpretation for recordings greater than 36 hours and for which the entire professional report is generated retroactively

EXCLUDES   *EEG, continuous recording, less than 36 hours ([95717, 95718, 95719, 95720])*

95970-95984 [95983, 95984] Evaluation of Implanted Neurostimulator with/without Programming

INCLUDES   Documentation of settings and electrode impedances of system parameters before programming

Insertion of electrode array(s) into target area (permanent or trial)

Multiple adjustments to parameters necessary during a programming session

Neurostimulators distinguished by area of nervous system stimulated:

Brain: Deep brain stimulation or cortical stimulation (surface of brain)

Cranial nerves: Includes the 12 pairs of cranial nerves, branches, divisions, intracranial and extracranial segments

Spinal cord and peripheral nerves: Nerves originating in spinal cord and nerves and ganglia outside spinal cord

Parameters (vary by system) include:

Amplitude
Burst
Cycling on/off
Detection algorithms
Dose lockout
Frequency
Pulse width
Responsive neurostimulation

EXCLUDES   *Implantation/replacement neurostimulator electrodes (43647, 43881, 61850-61870, 63650-63655, 64553-64581)*

Neurostimulation system, posterior tibial nerve (0587T-0590T)

Neurostimulator pulse generator/receiver:

Insertion (61885-61886, 63685, 64568, 64590)

Revision/removal (61888, 63688, 64569, 64595)

Revision/removal neurostimulator electrodes (43648, 43882, 61880, 63661-63664, 64569-64570, 64585)

95970   **Electronic analysis of implanted neurostimulator pulse generator/transmitter (eg, contact group[s], interleaving, amplitude, pulse width, frequency [Hz], on/off cycling, burst, magnet mode, dose lockout, patient selectable parameters, responsive neurostimulation, detection algorithms, closed loop parameters, and passive parameters) by physician or other qualified health care professional; with brain, cranial nerve, spinal cord, peripheral nerve, or sacral nerve, neurostimulator pulse generator/transmitter, without programming**

INCLUDES   Analysis of implanted neurostimulator without programming

EXCLUDES   *Programming with analysis (95971-95972, 95976-95977, [95983, 95984])*

🚑 0.53   ✂ 0.54   **FUD** XXX   Q1 80 ⬛

AMA: 2019,Feb,6; 2018,Oct,8; 2018,Feb,11; 2018,Jan,8; 2017,Jan,8; 2016,Jul,7; 2016,Jan,13; 2015,Jan,16; 2014,Jan,11

95971 with simple spinal cord or peripheral nerve (eg, sacral nerve) neurostimulator pulse generator/transmitter programming by physician or other qualified health care professional

EXCLUDES *Programming of neurostimulator for complex spinal cord or peripheral nerve (95972)*

⚙ 1.17 ⚕ 1.44 **FUD** XXX Ⓢ 80 ▱

AMA: 2019,Feb,6; 2018,Oct,8; 2018,Feb,11; 2018,Jan,8; 2017,Jan,8; 2016,Jul,7; 2016,Jan,13; 2015,Jan,16; 2014,Jan,11

95972 with complex spinal cord or peripheral nerve (eg, sacral nerve) neurostimulator pulse generator/transmitter programming by physician or other qualified health care professional

⚙ 1.19 ⚕ 1.62 **FUD** XXX Ⓢ 80 ▱

AMA: 2019,Feb,6; 2018,Oct,8; 2018,Feb,11; 2018,Jan,8; 2017,Jan,8; 2016,Jul,7; 2016,Jan,13; 2015,Jan,16; 2014,Aug,5; 2014,Jan,11

95976 with simple cranial nerve neurostimulator pulse generator/transmitter programming by physician or other qualified health care professional

EXCLUDES *Programming of neurostimulator for complex cranial nerve (95977)*

⚙ 1.14 ⚕ 1.16 **FUD** XXX 80 ▱

AMA: 2019,Feb,6

95977 with complex cranial nerve neurostimulator pulse generator/transmitter programming by physician or other qualified health care professional

⚙ 1.52 ⚕ 1.54 **FUD** XXX 80 ▱

AMA: 2019,Feb,6

 # 95983 with brain neurostimulator pulse generator/transmitter programming, first 15 minutes face-to-face time with physician or other qualified health care professional

⚙ 1.44 ⚕ 1.46 **FUD** XXX 80 ▱

AMA: 2019,Feb,6; 2018,Dec,3; 2018,Dec,3

+ # 95984 with brain neurostimulator pulse generator/transmitter programming, each additional 15 minutes face-to-face time with physician or other qualified health care professional (List separately in addition to code for primary procedure)

Code first ([95983])

⚙ 1.26 ⚕ 1.27 **FUD** ZZZ 80 ▱

AMA: 2019,Feb,6; 2018,Dec,3; 2018,Dec,3

95980 Electronic analysis of implanted neurostimulator pulse generator system (eg, rate, pulse amplitude and duration, configuration of wave form, battery status, electrode selectability, output modulation, cycling, impedance and patient measurements) gastric neurostimulator pulse generator/transmitter; intraoperative, with programming

INCLUDES *Gastric neurostimulator of lesser curvature*

EXCLUDES *Analysis, with programming when performed, of vagus nerve trunk stimulator for morbid obesity (0312T, 0317T)*

⚙ 1.32 ⚕ 1.32 **FUD** XXX Ⓝ 80 ▱

AMA: 2018,Feb,11; 2018,Jan,8; 2017,Jan,8; 2016,Jul,7; 2016,Jan,13; 2015,Jan,16; 2014,Jan,11

95981 subsequent, without reprogramming

EXCLUDES *Analysis, with programming when performed, of vagus nerve trunk stimulator for morbid obesity (0312T, 0317T)*

⚙ 0.51 ⚕ 0.97 **FUD** XXX 01 80 ▱

AMA: 2018,Feb,11; 2018,Jan,8; 2017,Jan,8; 2016,Jul,7; 2016,Jan,13; 2015,Jan,16; 2014,Jan,11

95982 subsequent, with reprogramming

EXCLUDES *Analysis, with programming when performed, of vagus nerve trunk stimulator for morbid obesity (0312T, 0317T)*

⚙ 1.04 ⚕ 1.55 **FUD** XXX 01 80 ▱

AMA: 2018,Feb,11; 2018,Jan,8; 2017,Jan,8; 2016,Jul,7; 2016,Jan,13; 2015,Jan,16; 2014,Jan,11

95983 Resequenced code. See code following 95977.

95984 Resequenced code. See code following 95977.

95990-95991 Refill/Upkeep of Implanted Drug Delivery Pump to Central Nervous System

EXCLUDES *Analysis/reprogramming of implanted pump for infusion (62367-62370) E&M services*

95990 Refilling and maintenance of implantable pump or reservoir for drug delivery, spinal (intrathecal, epidural) or brain (intraventricular), includes electronic analysis of pump, when performed;

⚙ 2.62 ⚕ 2.62 **FUD** XXX Ⓢ 80 ▱

AMA: 2018,Feb,11; 2018,Jan,8; 2017,Jan,8; 2016,Jan,13; 2015,Jan,16; 2014,Jan,11

95991 requiring skill of a physician or other qualified health care professional

⚙ 1.14 ⚕ 3.30 **FUD** XXX Ⓣ 80 ▱

AMA: 2018,Feb,11; 2018,Jan,8; 2017,Jan,8; 2016,Jan,13; 2015,Jan,16; 2014,Jan,11

95992-95999 Other and Unlisted Neurological Procedures

95992 Canalith repositioning procedure(s) (eg, Epley maneuver, Semont maneuver), per day

EXCLUDES *Nystagmus testing (92531-92532)*

⚙ 1.07 ⚕ 1.25 **FUD** XXX ⊘ Ⓐ 80 ▱

AMA: 2018,Feb,11; 2018,Jan,8; 2017,Jan,8; 2016,Jan,13; 2015,Jan,16; 2014,Jan,11

95999 Unlisted neurological or neuromuscular diagnostic procedure

⚙ 0.00 ⚕ 0.00 **FUD** XXX 01 80 ▱

AMA: 2018,Aug,10; 2018,Feb,11; 2018,Jan,8; 2017,Jan,8; 2016,Jan,13; 2015,Aug,8; 2015,Jan,16; 2014,Jan,11

96000-96004 Motion Analysis Studies

CMS: 100-02,15,230.4 Services By a Physical/Occupational Therapist in Private Practice

INCLUDES *Services provided as part of major therapeutic/diagnostic decision making*
Services provided in a dedicated motion analysis department capable of:
3-D kinetics/dynamic electromyography
Computerized 3-D kinematics
Videotaping from the front/back/both sides

EXCLUDES *E&M services*
Gait training (97116)
Needle electromyography (95860-95872 [95885, 95886, 95887])

96000 Comprehensive computer-based motion analysis by video-taping and 3D kinematics;

⚙ 2.72 ⚕ 2.72 **FUD** XXX Ⓢ 80 ▱

AMA: 2018,Feb,11; 2018,Jan,8; 2017,Jan,8; 2016,Jan,13; 2015,Jan,16; 2014,Jan,11

96001 with dynamic plantar pressure measurements during walking

⚙ 3.65 ⚕ 3.65 **FUD** XXX Ⓢ 80 ▱

AMA: 2018,Feb,11; 2018,Jan,8; 2017,Jan,8; 2016,Jan,13; 2015,Jan,16; 2014,Jan,11

96002 Dynamic surface electromyography, during walking or other functional activities, 1-12 muscles

⚙ 0.63 ⚕ 0.63 **FUD** XXX Ⓢ 80 ▱

AMA: 2018,Feb,11; 2018,Jan,8; 2017,Jan,8; 2016,Jan,13; 2015,Aug,8; 2015,Jan,16; 2014,Jan,11

96003 Dynamic fine wire electromyography, during walking or other functional activities, 1 muscle

⚙ 0.49 ⚕ 0.49 **FUD** XXX 01 80 ▱

AMA: 2018,Feb,11; 2018,Jan,8; 2017,Jan,8; 2016,Jan,13; 2015,Jan,16; 2014,Jan,11

26/TC PC/TC Only   A2-Z3 ASC Payment   50 Bilateral   ♂ Male Only   ♀ Female Only   ⚙ Facility RVU   ⚕ Non-Facility RVU   ▱ CCI   ✖ CLIA
FUD Follow-up Days   **CMS:** IOM   **AMA:** CPT Asst   A-Y OPPSI   80/80 Surg Assist Allowed / w/Doc   Lab Crosswalk   Radiology Crosswalk

Medicine

97152

96004 Review and interpretation by physician or other qualified health care professional of comprehensive computer-based motion analysis, dynamic plantar pressure measurements, dynamic surface electromyography during walking or other functional activities, and dynamic fine wire electromyography, with written report

🔔 3.27 👤 3.27 **FUD** XXX ☐ B 80 26 ☐

AMA: 2018,Feb,11; 2018,Jan,8; 2017,Jan,8; 2016,Jan,13; 2015,Aug,8; 2015,Jan,16; 2014,Jan,11

96020 Neurofunctional Brain Testing

INCLUDES Selection/administration of testing of:
  Cognition
  Determination of validity of neurofunctional testing relative to separately interpreted functional magnetic resonance images
  Functional neuroimaging
  Language
  Memory
  Monitoring performance of testing
  Movement
  Other neurological functions
  Sensation

EXCLUDES *Clinical depression treatment by repetitive transcranial magnetic stimulation (90867-90868)*
  Developmental test administration (96112-96113)
  E&M services on the same date
  MRI of the brain (70554-70555)
  Neurobehavioral status examination (96116, 96121)
  Neuropsychological testing (96132-96133)
  Psychological testing (96130-96131)

96020 Neurofunctional testing selection and administration during noninvasive imaging functional brain mapping, with test administered entirely by a physician or other qualified health care professional (ie, psychologist), with review of test results and report

🔔 0.00 👤 0.00 **FUD** XXX ☐ N 80 ☐

AMA: 2018,Feb,11; 2018,Jan,8; 2017,Jan,8; 2016,Jan,13; 2015,Jan,16; 2014,Jan,11

96040 Genetic Counseling Services

INCLUDES Analysis for genetic risk assessment
  Counseling of patient/family
  Counseling services
  Face-to-face interviews
  Obtaining structured family genetic history
  Pedigree construction
  Review of medical data/family information
  Services provided by trained genetic counselor
  Services provided during one or more sessions
  Thirty minutes of face-to-face time and is reported one time for each 16-30 minutes of the service

EXCLUDES *Education/genetic counseling by a physician or other qualified health care provider to a group (99078)*
  Education/genetic counseling by a physician or other qualified health care provider to an individual; use appropriate E&M code
  Education regarding genetic risks by a nonphysician to a group (98961, 98962)
  Genetic counseling and/or risk factor reduction intervention from a physician or other qualified health care provider provided to patients without symptoms/diagnosis (99401-99412)
  Use of code when 15 minutes or less of face-to-face time is provided

96040 Medical genetics and genetic counseling services, each 30 minutes face-to-face with patient/family

🔔 1.30 👤 1.30 **FUD** XXX ★ B ☐

AMA: 2018,Feb,11; 2018,Jan,8; 2017,Jan,8; 2016,Jan,13; 2015,Jan,16; 2014,Jan,11

97151-97158 [97151, 97152, 97153, 97154, 97155, 97156, 97157, 97158] Adaptive Behavior Assessments and Treatments

INCLUDES Adaptive behavior deficits (e.g., impairment in social, communication, self care skills)
  Assessment and treatment that focuses on:
    Maladaptive behaviors (e.g., repetitive movements, risk of harm to self, others, property)
    Secondary functional impairment due to consequences of deficient adaptive and maladaptive behaviors (e.g. communication, play, leisure, social interactions)
  Treatment determined based on goals and targets identified in assessments

\# **97151** Behavior identification assessment, administered by a physician or other qualified health care professional, each 15 minutes of the physician's or other qualified health care professional's time face-to-face with patient and/or guardian(s)/caregiver(s) administering assessments and discussing findings and recommendations, and non-face-to-face analyzing past data, scoring/interpreting the assessment, and preparing the report/treatment plan

EXCLUDES *Health and behavior assessment and intervention (96156, 96158-96159, [96164, 96165], [96167, 96168], [96170, 96171])*
  Medical team conference (99366-99368)
  Neurobehavioral status examination (96116, 96121)
  Neuropsychological testing (96132-96133, 96136-96139, 96146)
  Psychiatric diagnostic evaluation (90791-90792)
  Speech evaluations (92521-92524)

Code also more than one time on same or different days until assessment is complete
Code also supporting assessment depending on time patient spends face-to-face with one or more technicians (counting only the time spent by one of the technicians) ([97152], 0362T)

🔔 0.00 👤 0.00 **FUD** XXX ☐ 80 ☐

AMA: 2018,Nov,3

\# **97152** Behavior identification-supporting assessment, administered by one technician under the direction of a physician or other qualified health care professional, face-to-face with the patient, each 15 minutes

EXCLUDES *Health and behavior assessment and intervention (96156, 96158-96159, [96164, 96165], [96167, 96168], [96170, 96171])*
  Medical team conference (99366-99368)
  Neurobehavioral status examination (96116, 96121)
  Neuropsychological testing (96132-96133, 96136-96139, 96146)
  Psychiatric diagnostic evaluation (90791-90792)
  Speech evaluations (92521-92524)

Code also more than one time on same or different days until assessment is complete
Code also supporting assessment depending on time patient spends face-to-face with one or more technicians (counting only the time spent by one of the technicians) ([97151], 0362T)

🔔 0.00 👤 0.00 **FUD** XXX ☐ 80 ☐

AMA: 2018,Nov,3

97153 — 97158

Medicine

97153 Adaptive behavior treatment by protocol, administered by technician under the direction of a physician or other qualified health care professional, face-to-face with one patient, each 15 minutes

INCLUDES Face-to-face service with one patient only
Provided by technician under physician/other qualified healthcare professional direction

EXCLUDES Aphasia and cognitive performance testing (96105, [96125])
Behavioral/developmental screening/testing (96110-96113 [96127])
Health and behavior assessment and intervention (96156, 96158-96159, [96164, 96165], [96167, 96168], [96170, 96171])
Health risk assessment (96160-96161)
Neurobehavioral status examination (96116, 96121)
Psychiatric services (90785-90899)
Testing administration with scoring (96136-96139, 96146)
Testing evaluation (96130-96133)
Therapeutic procedure(s), individual patient (97129)
Treatment speech disorders (individual) (92507)

🚑 0.00   ⚕ 0.00   **FUD** XXX   80 ▱

AMA: 2018,Nov,3

97154 Group adaptive behavior treatment by protocol, administered by technician under the direction of a physician or other qualified health care professional, face-to-face with two or more patients, each 15 minutes

INCLUDES Face-to-face service with one patient only
Provided by technician under physician/other qualified healthcare professional direction

EXCLUDES Aphasia and cognitive performance testing (96105, [96125])
Behavioral/developmental screening/testing (96110-96113, [96127])
Health and behavior assessment and intervention (96156, 96158-96159, [96164, 96165], [96167, 96168], [96170, 96171])
Neurobehavioral status examination (96116, 96121)
Psychiatric services (90785-90899)
Testing administration with scoring (96136-96139, 96146)
Testing evaluation (96130-96133)
Therapeutic procedure(s) group of two or more patients (97150)
Treatment speech disorders (group) (92508)

🚑 0.00   ⚕ 0.00   **FUD** XXX   80 ▱

AMA: 2018,Nov,3

97155 Adaptive behavior treatment with protocol modification, administered by physician or other qualified health care professional, which may include simultaneous direction of technician, face-to-face with one patient, each 15 minutes

INCLUDES Face-to-face service with one patient only
Provided by technician under physician/other qualified healthcare professional direction

EXCLUDES Aphasia and cognitive performance testing (96105, [96125])
Behavioral/developmental screening/testing (96110-96113, [96127])
Health and behavior assessment and intervention (96156, 96158-96159, [96164, 96165], [96167, 96168], [96170, 96171])
Neurobehavioral status examination (96116, 96121)
Psychiatric services (90785-90899)
Testing administration with scoring (96136-96139, 96146)
Testing evaluation (96130-96133)
Therapeutic procedure(s), individual patient (97129)
Treatment speech disorders (individual) (92507)

🚑 0.00   ⚕ 0.00   **FUD** XXX   80 ▱

AMA: 2018,Nov,3

97156 Family adaptive behavior treatment guidance, administered by physician or other qualified health care professional (with or without the patient present), face-to-face with guardian(s)/caregiver(s), each 15 minutes

INCLUDES Provided by physician/other qualified healthcare professional
Without patient presence

EXCLUDES Aphasia and cognitive performance testing (96105, [96125])
Behavioral/developmental screening/testing (96110-96113 [96127])
Health and behavior assessment and intervention (96156, 96158-96159, [96164, 96165], [96167, 96168], [96170, 96171])
Neurobehavioral status examination (96116, 96121)
Psychiatric services (90785-90899)
Testing administration with scoring (96136-96139, 96146)
Testing evaluation (96130-96133)

🚑 0.00   ⚕ 0.00   **FUD** XXX   80 ▱

AMA: 2018,Nov,3

97157 Multiple-family group adaptive behavior treatment guidance, administered by physician or other qualified health care professional (without the patient present), face-to-face with multiple sets of guardians/caregivers, each 15 minutes

INCLUDES Provided by physician/other qualified healthcare professional
Without patient presence

EXCLUDES Aphasia and cognitive performance testing (96105, [96125])
Behavioral/developmental screening/testing (96110-96113 [96127])
Groups of more than 8 families
Health and behavior assessment and intervention (96156, 96158-96159, [96164, 96165], [96167, 96168], [96170, 96171])
Neurobehavioral status examination (96116, 96121)
Psychiatric services (90785-90899)
Testing administration with scoring (96136-96139, 96146)
Testing evaluation (96130-96133)

🚑 0.00   ⚕ 0.00   **FUD** XXX   80 ▱

AMA: 2018,Nov,3

97158 Group adaptive behavior treatment with protocol modification, administered by physician or other qualified health care professional, face-to-face with multiple patients, each 15 minutes

INCLUDES Face-to-face service with one patient only
Provided by technician under physician/other qualified healthcare professional direction

EXCLUDES Aphasia and cognitive performance testing (96105, [96125])
Behavioral/developmental screening/testing (96110-96113 [96127])
Groups of more than 8 patients
Health and behavior assessment and intervention (96156, 96158-96159, [96164, 96165], [96167, 96168], [96170, 96171])
Neurobehavioral status examination (96116, 96121)
Psychiatric services (90785-90899)
Testing administration with scoring (96136-96139, 96146)
Testing evaluation (96130-96133)
Therapeutic procedure(s) group of two or more patients (97150)
Treatment speech disorders (group) (92508)

🚑 0.00   ⚕ 0.00   **FUD** XXX   80 ▱

AMA: 2018,Nov,3

26/TC PC/TC Only   A2-Z3 ASC Payment   50 Bilateral   ♂ Male Only   ♀ Female Only   🚑 Facility RVU   ⚕ Non-Facility RVU   ▱ CCI   ✖ CLIA
FUD Follow-up Days   CMS: IOM   AMA: CPT Asst   A-Y OPPSI   80/80 Surg Assist Allowed / w/Doc   ▨ Lab Crosswalk   ▧ Radiology Crosswalk

514   CPT © 2019 American Medical Association. All Rights Reserved.   © 2019 Optum360, LLC

96105-96146 [96125, 96127] Testing Services

INCLUDES   Interpretation and report when performed by qualified healthcare professional
Results when automatically generated

EXCLUDES   Adaptive behavior assessments and treatments ([97151, 97152, 97153, 97154, 97155, 97156, 97157, 97158], 0362T, 0373T)
Cognitive skills development (97129, 97533)

96105   Assessment of aphasia (includes assessment of expressive and receptive speech and language function, language comprehension, speech production ability, reading, spelling, writing, eg, by Boston Diagnostic Aphasia Examination) with interpretation and report, per hour

EXCLUDES   Use of code for less than 31 minutes of time

2.96   2.96   **FUD** XXX   [A] [80] [▢]

AMA: 2018,Nov,3; 2018,Oct,5; 2018,Feb,11; 2018,Jan,8; 2017,Jan,8; 2016,Jan,13; 2015,Aug,5; 2015,Jan,16; 2014,Jan,11

\# **96125**   Standardized cognitive performance testing (eg, Ross Information Processing Assessment) per hour of a qualified health care professional's time, both face-to-face time administering tests to the patient and time interpreting these test results and preparing the report

EXCLUDES   Neuropsychological testing (96132-96139, 96146)

3.12   3.12   **FUD** XXX   [A] [80] [▢]

AMA: 2018,Nov,3; 2018,Oct,5; 2018,Feb,11; 2018,Jan,8; 2017,Jan,8; 2016,Jan,13; 2015,Aug,5; 2015,Jan,16; 2014,Jan,11

96110   Developmental screening (eg, developmental milestone survey, speech and language delay screen), with scoring and documentation, per standardized instrument

EXCLUDES   Emotional/behavioral assessment ([96127])

0.28   0.28   **FUD** XXX   [E] [▢]

AMA: 2018,Nov,3; 2018,Feb,11; 2018,Jan,8; 2017,Feb,14; 2017,Jan,8; 2016,Jan,13; 2015,Aug,5; 2015,Jan,16; 2014,Jun,3; 2014,Jan,11

96112   Developmental test administration (including assessment of fine and/or gross motor, language, cognitive level, social, memory and/or executive functions by standardized developmental instruments when performed), by physician or other qualified health care professional, with interpretation and report; first hour

EXCLUDES   Use of code for less than 31 minutes of time

3.61   3.83   **FUD** XXX   [80] [▢]

AMA: 2018,Nov,3

+ **96113**   each additional 30 minutes (List separately in addition to code for primary procedure)

EXCLUDES   Use of code for less than 16 minutes of time

1.65   1.71   **FUD** ZZZ   [80] [▢]

AMA: 2018,Nov,3

\# **96127**   Brief emotional/behavioral assessment (eg, depression inventory, attention-deficit/hyperactivity disorder [ADHD] scale), with scoring and documentation, per standardized instrument

0.15   0.15   **FUD** XXX   [Q1] [80] [TC] [▢]

AMA: 2018,Nov,3; 2018,Oct,5; 2018,Apr,9; 2018,Feb,11; 2018,Jan,8; 2017,Feb,14; 2017,Jan,8; 2016,Jan,13; 2015,Aug,5

96116   Neurobehavioral status exam (clinical assessment of thinking, reasoning and judgment, [eg, acquired knowledge, attention, language, memory, planning and problem solving, and visual spatial abilities]), by physician or other qualified health care professional, both face-to-face time with the patient and time interpreting test results and preparing the report; first hour

EXCLUDES   Neuropsychological testing (96132-96139, 96146)
Use of code for less than 31 minutes of time

2.41   2.70   **FUD** XXX   [★] [Q3] [80] [▢]

AMA: 2018,Nov,3; 2018,Oct,5; 2018,Feb,11; 2018,Jan,8; 2017,Jan,8; 2016,Jan,13; 2015,Aug,5; 2015,Jan,16; 2014,Jun,3; 2014,Jan,11

+ **96121**   each additional hour (List separately in addition to code for primary procedure)

EXCLUDES   Use of code for less than 31 minutes of time
Code first (96116)

2.21   2.32   **FUD** ZZZ   [80] [▢]

AMA: 2018,Nov,3

96125   Resequenced code. See code following 96105.

96127   Resequenced code. See code following 96113.

96130   Psychological testing evaluation services by physician or other qualified health care professional, including integration of patient data, interpretation of standardized test results and clinical data, clinical decision making, treatment planning and report, and interactive feedback to the patient, family member(s) or caregiver(s), when performed; first hour

EXCLUDES   Use of code for less than 31 minutes of time

3.10   3.30   **FUD** XXX   [80] [▢]

AMA: 2019,Sep,10; 2018,Nov,3

+ **96131**   each additional hour (List separately in addition to code for primary procedure)

EXCLUDES   Use of code for less than 31 minutes of time

2.36   2.51   **FUD** ZZZ   [80] [▢]

AMA: 2019,Sep,10; 2018,Nov,3

96132   Neuropsychological testing evaluation services by physician or other qualified health care professional, including integration of patient data, interpretation of standardized test results and clinical data, clinical decision making, treatment planning and report, and interactive feedback to the patient, family member(s) or caregiver(s), when performed; first hour

EXCLUDES   Use of code for less than 31 minutes of time

3.04   3.71   **FUD** XXX   [80] [▢]

AMA: 2019,Sep,10; 2018,Nov,3

+ **96133**   each additional hour (List separately in addition to code for primary procedure)

EXCLUDES   Use of code for less than 31 minutes of time

2.33   2.83   **FUD** ZZZ   [80] [▢]

AMA: 2019,Sep,10; 2018,Nov,3

96136   Psychological or neuropsychological test administration and scoring by physician or other qualified health care professional, two or more tests, any method; first 30 minutes

EXCLUDES   Use of code for less than 16 minutes of time
Code also testing evaluation on same or different days (96130-96133)

0.70   1.33   **FUD** XXX   [80] [▢]

AMA: 2019,Sep,10; 2018,Nov,3

+ **96137**   each additional 30 minutes (List separately in addition to code for primary procedure)

EXCLUDES   Use of code for less than 16 minutes of time
Code also testing evaluation on same or different days (96130-96133)

0.55   1.23   **FUD** ZZZ   [80] [▢]

AMA: 2019,Sep,10; 2018,Nov,3

96138   Psychological or neuropsychological test administration and scoring by technician, two or more tests, any method; first 30 minutes

EXCLUDES   Use of code for less than 16 minutes of time
Code also testing evaluation on same or different days (96130-96133)

1.08   1.08   **FUD** XXX   [80] [▢]

AMA: 2018,Nov,3

+ **96139**   each additional 30 minutes (List separately in addition to code for primary procedure)

EXCLUDES   Use of code for less than 16 minutes of time
Code also testing evaluation on same or different days (96130-96133)

1.08   1.08   **FUD** ZZZ   [80] [▢]

AMA: 2018,Nov,3

● New Code   ▲ Revised Code   ○ Reinstated   ● New Web Release   ▲ Revised Web Release   + Add-on   Unlisted   Not Covered   # Resequenced
50 Optum Mod 50 Exempt   ⊘ AMA Mod 51 Exempt   51 Optum Mod 51 Exempt   63 Mod 63 Exempt   ⁄ Non-FDA Drug   ★ Telemedicine   Ⓜ Maternity   A Age Edit

CPT © 2019 American Medical Association. All Rights Reserved.

Medicine

96146   **Psychological or neuropsychological test administration, with single automated, standardized instrument via electronic platform, with automated result only**

> EXCLUDES   *Testing provided by physician, other qualified healthcare professional, or technician ([96127], 96136-96139)*
>
> 🔹 0.06   🔸 0.06   **FUD** XXX   80 ▫
>
> **AMA:** 2018,Nov,3

96150-96171 [96164, 96165, 96167, 96168, 96170, 96171] Biopsychosocial Assessment/Intervention

INCLUDES   Services for patients that have primary physical illnesses/diagnoses/symptoms who may benefit from assessments/interventions that focus on the biopsychosocial factors related to the patient's health status

Services used to identify the following factors which are important to the prevention/treatment/management of physical health problems:
- Behavioral
- Cognitive
- Emotional
- Psychological
- Social

EXCLUDES   *Adaptive behavior services ([97151, 97152, 97153, 97154, 97155, 97156, 97157, 97158], 0362T, 0373T)*
E&M services on the same date
Health and behavior assessment and intervention (96156, 96158-96159)
Preventive medicine counseling services (99401-99412)

96150   ~~Health and behavior assessment (eg, health-focused clinical interview, behavioral observations, psychophysiological monitoring, health-oriented questionnaires), each 15 minutes face-to-face with the patient; initial assessment~~

> To report, see (96156, 96158-96159)

96151   ~~re-assessment~~

> To report, see (96156, 96158-96159)

96152   ~~Health and behavior intervention, each 15 minutes, face-to-face; individual~~

> To report, see (96156, 96158-96159)

96153   ~~group (2 or more patients)~~

> To report, see ([96164-96165])

96154   ~~family (with the patient present)~~

> To report, see ([96167-96168])

96155   ~~family (without the patient present)~~

> To report, see ([96170-96171])

●   **96156**   **Health behavior assessment, or re-assessment (ie, health-focused clinical interview, behavioral observations, clinical decision making)**

> EXCLUDES   *Psychotherapy services (90785-90899)*

●   **96158**   **Health behavior intervention, individual, face-to-face; initial 30 minutes**

> EXCLUDES   *Psychotherapy services (90785-90899)*

● +   **96159**   **each additional 15 minutes (List separately in addition to code for primary service)**

> 🔹 0.00   🔸 0.00   **FUD** 000
>
> EXCLUDES   *Psychotherapy services (90785-90899)*
> Code first (96158)

● #   **96164**   **Health behavior intervention, group (2 or more patients), face-to-face; initial 30 minutes**

> 🔹 0.00   🔸 0.00   **FUD** 000
>
> EXCLUDES   *Psychotherapy services (90785-90899)*

● + #   **96165**   **each additional 15 minutes (List separately in addition to code for primary service)**

> 🔹 0.00   🔸 0.00   **FUD** 000
>
> EXCLUDES   *Psychotherapy services (90785-90899)*
> Code first ([96164])

● #   **96167**   **Health behavior intervention, family (with the patient present), face-to-face; initial 30 minutes**

> 🔹 0.00   🔸 0.00   **FUD** 000
>
> EXCLUDES   *Psychotherapy services (90785-90899)*

● + #   **96168**   **each additional 15 minutes (List separately in addition to code for primary service)**

> 🔹 0.00   🔸 0.00   **FUD** 000
>
> EXCLUDES   *Psychotherapy services (90785-90899)*
> Code first ([96167])

● #   **96170**   **Health behavior intervention, family (without the patient present), face-to-face; initial 30 minutes**

> 🔹 0.00   🔸 0.00   **FUD** 000
>
> EXCLUDES   *Psychotherapy services (90785-90899)*

● + #   **96171**   **each additional 15 minutes (List separately in addition to code for primary service)**

> 🔹 0.00   🔸 0.00   **FUD** 000
>
> EXCLUDES   *Psychotherapy services (90785-90899)*
> Code first ([96170])

96160-96171 Health Risk Assessments

96160   **Administration of patient-focused health risk assessment instrument (eg, health hazard appraisal) with scoring and documentation, per standardized instrument**

> 🔹 0.11   🔸 0.11   **FUD** ZZZ   S ▫
>
> **AMA:** 2018,Feb,11; 2018,Jan,8; 2017,Feb,14; 2017,Jan,8; 2016,Nov,5

96161   **Administration of caregiver-focused health risk assessment instrument (eg, depression inventory) for the benefit of the patient, with scoring and documentation, per standardized instrument**

> 🔹 0.11   🔸 0.11   **FUD** ZZZ   S ▫
>
> **AMA:** 2018,Feb,11; 2018,Jan,8; 2017,Feb,14; 2017,Jan,8; 2016,Nov,5

96164   Resequenced code. See code following 96159.

96165   Resequenced code. See code following 96159.

96167   Resequenced code. See code following 96159.

96168   Resequenced code. See code following 96159.

96170   Resequenced code. See code following 96159.

96171   Resequenced code. See code following 96159.

96360-96361 Intravenous Fluid Infusion for Hydration (Nonchemotherapy)

CMS: 100-04,4,230.2 OPPS Drug Administration

INCLUDES Administration of prepackaged fluids and electrolytes
Coding hierarchy rules for facility reporting only:
Chemotherapy services are primary to diagnostic, prophylactic, and therapeutic services
Diagnostic, prophylactic, and therapeutic services are primary to hydration services
Infusions are primary to pushes
Pushes are primary to injections
Constant observance/attendance of person administering the drug or substance
Infusion of 15 minutes or less
Direct supervision by physician or other qualified health care provider:
Direction of personnel
Minimal supervision for:
Consent
Safety oversight
Supervision of personnel
Report the initial code for the primary reason for the visit regardless of the order in which the infusions or injections are given
The following if done to facilitate the injection/infusion:
Flush at the end of infusion
Indwelling IV, subcutaneous catheter/port access
Local anesthesia
Start of IV
Supplies/tubing/syringes
Treatment plan verification

EXCLUDES *Catheter/port declotting (36593)*
Drugs/other substances
Minimal infusion to keep the vein open or during other therapeutic infusions
Services provided by physicians or other qualified health care providers in facility settings
Significant separately identifiable E&M service if performed
Use of a code for a second initial service on the same date for accessing a multi-lumen catheter, restarting an IV, or when two IV lines are needed to meet an infusion rate
Use of code for infusion for hydration that is 31 minutes or less

96360 **Intravenous infusion, hydration; initial, 31 minutes to 1 hour**

EXCLUDES *Use of code if service is performed as a concurrent infusion*

1.07 1.07 **FUD** XXX S 80

AMA: 2019,Jun,5; 2018,Feb,11; 2018,Jan,8; 2017,Jan,8; 2016,Jan,13; 2015,Jan,16; 2014,May,10; 2014,Jan,11

+ 96361 **each additional hour (List separately in addition to code for primary procedure)**

INCLUDES Hydration infusion of more than 30 minutes beyond 1 hour
Hydration provided as a secondary or subsequent service after a different initial service via the same IV access site

Code first (96360)
0.38 0.38 **FUD** ZZZ S 80

AMA: 2019,Jun,5; 2018,Feb,11; 2018,Jan,8; 2017,Jan,8; 2016,Jan,13; 2015,Jan,16; 2014,May,10; 2014,Jan,11

96365-96371 Infusions: Diagnostic/Preventive/Therapeutic

CMS: 100-04,4,230.2 OPPS Drug Administration

INCLUDES Administration of fluid
Administration of substances/drugs
An infusion of 16 minutes or more
Coding hierarchy rules for facility reporting:
Chemotherapy services are primary to diagnostic, prophylactic, and therapeutic services
Diagnostic, prophylactic, and therapeutic services are primary to hydration services
Infusions are primary to pushes
Pushes are primary to injections
Constant presence of health care professional administering the substance/drug
Direct supervision of physician or other qualified health care provider:
Consent
Direction of personnel
Patient assessment
Safety oversight
Supervision of personnel
The following if done to facilitate the injection/infusion:
Flush at the end of infusion
Indwelling IV, subcutaneous catheter/port access
Local anesthesia
Start of IV
Supplies/tubing/syringes
Training to assess patient and monitor vital signs
Training to prepare/dose/dispose
Treatment plan verification

EXCLUDES *Catheter/port declotting (36593)*
Services provided by physicians or other qualified health care providers in facility settings
Significant separately identifiable E&M service, when performed
Use of a code for a second initial service on the same date for accessing a multi-lumen catheter, restarting an IV, or when two IV lines are needed to meet an infusion rate
Use of code with other procedures for which IV push or infusion is an integral part of the procedure

Code also drugs/materials

96365 **Intravenous infusion, for therapy, prophylaxis, or diagnosis (specify substance or drug); initial, up to 1 hour**

Code also second initial service with modifier 59 when patient's condition or drug protocol mandates the use of two IV lines
2.02 2.02 **FUD** XXX S 80

AMA: 2018,Dec,8; 2018,Dec,8; 2018,Sep,14; 2018,May,10; 2018,Feb,11; 2018,Jan,8; 2017,Jan,8; 2016,Jan,13; 2015,Jan,16; 2014,Jan,11

+ 96366 **each additional hour (List separately in addition to code for primary procedure)**

INCLUDES Additional hours of sequential infusion
Infusion intervals of more than 30 minutes beyond one hour
Second and subsequent infusions of the same drug or substance

Code also additional infusion, when appropriate (96367)
Code first (96365)
0.61 0.61 **FUD** ZZZ S 80

AMA: 2018,Sep,14; 2018,Feb,11; 2018,Jan,8; 2017,Jan,8; 2016,Jan,13; 2015,Jan,16; 2014,Jan,11

+ 96367 **additional sequential infusion of a new drug/substance, up to 1 hour (List separately in addition to code for primary procedure)**

INCLUDES A secondary or subsequent service with a new drug or substance after a different initial service via the same IV access

EXCLUDES *Use of code more than one time per sequential infusion of the same mix*

Code first (96365, 96374, 96409, 96413)
0.88 0.88 **FUD** ZZZ S 80

AMA: 2018,Feb,11; 2018,Jan,8; 2017,Jan,8; 2016,Jan,13; 2015,Jan,16; 2014,Jan,11

+ 96368 concurrent infusion (List separately in addition to code for primary procedure)

　　EXCLUDES *Use of code more than one time per date of service*

　　Code first (96365, 96366, 96413, 96415, 96416)

　　📋 0.59　　🔧 0.59　　**FUD** ZZZ　　　　N 80 ▭

　　AMA: 2018,Feb,11; 2018,Jan,8; 2017,Jan,8; 2016,Jan,13; 2015,Jan,16; 2014,Jan,11

96369 Subcutaneous infusion for therapy or prophylaxis (specify substance or drug); initial, up to 1 hour, including pump set-up and establishment of subcutaneous infusion site(s)

　　EXCLUDES *Infusions of 15 minutes or less (96372)*

　　　　　　Use of code more than one time per encounter

　　📋 4.69　　🔧 4.69　　**FUD** XXX　　　　S 80 ▭

　　AMA: 2018,Feb,11; 2018,Jan,8; 2017,Jan,8; 2016,Jan,13; 2015,Jan,16; 2014,Jan,11

+ 96370 each additional hour (List separately in addition to code for primary procedure)

　　INCLUDES Infusions of more than 30 minutes beyond one hour

　　Code first (96369)

　　📋 0.44　　🔧 0.44　　**FUD** ZZZ　　　　S 80 ▭

　　AMA: 2018,Feb,11; 2018,Jan,8; 2017,Jan,8; 2016,Jan,13; 2015,Jan,16; 2014,Jan,11

+ 96371 additional pump set-up with establishment of new subcutaneous infusion site(s) (List separately in addition to code for primary procedure)

　　EXCLUDES *Use of code more than one time per encounter*

　　Code first (96369)

　　📋 1.84　　🔧 1.84　　**FUD** ZZZ　　　　01 80 ▭

　　AMA: 2018,Feb,11; 2018,Jan,8; 2017,Jan,8; 2016,Jan,13; 2015,Jan,16; 2014,Jan,11

96372-96379 Injections: Diagnostic/Preventive/Therapeutic

CMS: 100-04,4,230.2 OPPS Drug Administration

　INCLUDES Administration of fluid
　　Administration of substances/drugs
　　Coding hierarchy rules for facility reporting:
　　　Chemotherapy services are primary to diagnostic, prophylactic, and therapeutic services
　　　Infusions are primary to pushes
　　　Pushes are primary to injections
　　Constant presence of health care professional administering the substance/drug
　　Direct supervision by physician or other qualified health care provider:
　　　Consent
　　　Direction of personnel
　　　Patient assessment
　　　Safety oversight
　　　Supervision of personnel
　　Infusion of 15 minutes or less
　　The following if done to facilitate the injection/infusion:
　　　Flush at the end of infusion
　　　Indwelling IV, subcutaneous catheter/port access
　　　Local anesthesia
　　　Start of IV
　　　Supplies/tubing/syringes
　　Training to assess patient and monitor vital signs
　　Training to prepare/dose/dispose
　　Treatment plan verification

　EXCLUDES *Catheter/port declotting (36593)*
　　Services provided by physicians or other qualified health care providers in facility settings
　　Significant separately identifiable E&M service, when performed
　　Use of a code for a second initial service on the same date for accessing a multi-lumen catheter, restarting an IV, or when two IV lines are needed to meet an infusion rate
　　Use of code with other procedures for which IV push or infusion is an integral part of the procedure

Code also drugs/materials

96372 Therapeutic, prophylactic, or diagnostic injection (specify substance or drug); subcutaneous or intramuscular

　　INCLUDES Direct supervision by physician or other qualified health care provider when reported by the physician/other qualified health care provider. When reported by a hospital, physician/other qualified health care provider need not be present.
　　　Hormonal therapy injections (non-antineoplastic) (96372)

　　EXCLUDES *Administration of vaccines/toxoids (90460-90474)*
　　　Allergen immunotherapy injections (95115-95117)
　　　Antineoplastic hormonal injections (96402)
　　　Antineoplastic nonhormonal injections (96401)
　　　Injections administered without direct supervision by physician or other qualified health care provider (99211)

　　📋 0.47　　🔧 0.47　　**FUD** XXX　　　　01 80 ▭

　　AMA: 2018,Dec,10; 2018,Dec,10; 2018,Feb,11; 2018,Jan,8; 2017,Jan,8; 2016,Oct,9; 2016,Jan,13; 2015,Jan,16; 2014,Jan,11; 2014,Jan,9

96373 intra-arterial

　　📋 0.53　　🔧 0.53　　**FUD** XXX　　　　S 80 ▭

　　AMA: 2018,Feb,11; 2018,Jan,8; 2017,Jan,8; 2016,Jan,13; 2015,Jan,16; 2014,Jan,11

96374 intravenous push, single or initial substance/drug

　　Code also second initial service with modifier 59 when patient's condition or drug protocol mandates the use of two IV lines

　　📋 1.10　　🔧 1.10　　**FUD** XXX　　　　S 80 ▭

　　AMA: 2019,Sep,5; 2019,Jun,9; 2018,Feb,11; 2018,Jan,8; 2017,Jan,8; 2016,Jan,13; 2015,Nov,3; 2015,Jan,16; 2014,Jan,11

+ **96375** **each additional sequential intravenous push of a new substance/drug (List separately in addition to code for primary procedure)**

INCLUDES IV push of a new substance/drug provided as a secondary or subsequent service after a different initial service via same IV access site

Code first (96365, 96374, 96409, 96413)

⚐ 0.47 ⚐ 0.47 **FUD** ZZZ   S 80 ▭

AMA: 2019,Sep,5; 2018,Feb,11; 2018,Jan,8; 2017,Jan,8; 2016,Jan,13; 2015,Nov,3; 2015,Jan,16; 2014,Jan,11

+ **96376** **each additional sequential intravenous push of the same substance/drug provided in a facility (List separately in addition to code for primary procedure)**

INCLUDES Facilities only

EXCLUDES IV push performed within 30 minutes of a reported push of the same substance or drug
Services performed by any nonfacilty provider

Code first (96365, 96374, 96409, 96413)

⚐ 0.00 ⚐ 0.00 **FUD** ZZZ   N ▭

AMA: 2018,Dec,8; 2018,Dec,8; 2018,Feb,11; 2018,Jan,8; 2017,Jan,8; 2016,Jan,13; 2015,Jan,16; 2014,Nov,14; 2014,Jan,11

96377 **Application of on-body injector (includes cannula insertion) for timed subcutaneous injection**

⚐ 0.57 ⚐ 0.57 **FUD** XXX   Q1 80 ▭

AMA: 2018,Feb,11; 2018,Jan,8; 2017,Jan,8; 2016,Oct,9

96379 **Unlisted therapeutic, prophylactic, or diagnostic intravenous or intra-arterial injection or infusion**

⚐ 0.00 ⚐ 0.00 **FUD** XXX   Q1 80 ▭

AMA: 2018,Feb,11; 2018,Jan,8; 2017,Jan,8; 2016,Jan,13; 2015,Jan,16; 2014,Jan,11

96401-96411 Chemotherapy and Other Complex Drugs, Biologicals: Injection and IV Push

CMS: 100-03,110.2 Certain Drugs Distributed by the National Cancer Institute; 100-03,110.6 Scalp Hypothermia During Chemotherapy, to Prevent Hair Loss; 100-04,4,230.2 OPPS Drug Administration

INCLUDES Highly complex services that require direct supervision for:
Consent
Patient assessment
Safety oversight
Supervision
More intense work and monitoring of clinical staff by physician or other qualified health care provider due to greater risk of severe patient reactions
Parenteral administration of:
Anti-neoplastic agents for noncancer diagnoses
Monoclonal antibody agents
Nonradionuclide antineoplastic drugs
Other biologic response modifiers

EXCLUDES Use of a code for a second initial service on the same date for accessing a multi-lumen catheter, restarting an IV, or when two IV lines are needed to meet an infusion rate

96401 **Chemotherapy administration, subcutaneous or intramuscular; non-hormonal anti-neoplastic**

EXCLUDES Services performed by physicians or other qualified health care providers in facility settings

⚐ 2.24 ⚐ 2.24 **FUD** XXX   Q1 80 ▭

AMA: 2018,Feb,11; 2018,Jan,8; 2017,Jan,8; 2016,Jan,13; 2015,Jan,16; 2014,Jan,11

96402 **hormonal anti-neoplastic**

EXCLUDES Services performed by physicians or other qualified health care providers in facility settings

⚐ 0.87 ⚐ 0.87 **FUD** XXX   Q1 80 ▭

AMA: 2018,Feb,11; 2018,Jan,8; 2017,Jan,8; 2016,Jan,13; 2015,Jan,16; 2014,Jan,11

96405 **Chemotherapy administration; intralesional, up to and including 7 lesions**

⚐ 0.84 ⚐ 2.31 **FUD** 000   Q1 ▭

AMA: 2018,Feb,11; 2018,Jan,8; 2017,Jan,8; 2016,Jan,13; 2015,Jan,16; 2014,Jan,11

96406 **intralesional, more than 7 lesions**

⚐ 1.31 ⚐ 3.46 **FUD** 000   S ▭

AMA: 2018,Feb,11; 2018,Jan,8; 2017,Jan,8; 2016,Jan,13; 2015,Jan,16; 2014,Jan,11

96409 **intravenous, push technique, single or initial substance/drug**

INCLUDES Push technique includes:
Administration of injection directly into vessel or access line by health care professional; or
Infusion less than or equal to 15 minutes

EXCLUDES Insertion of arterial and venous cannula(s) for extracorporeal circulation (36823)
Services performed by physicians or other qualified health care providers in facility settings

Code also second initial service with modifier 59 when patient's condition or drug protocol mandates the use of two IV lines

⚐ 3.05 ⚐ 3.05 **FUD** XXX   S 80 ▭

AMA: 2018,Feb,11; 2018,Jan,8; 2017,Jan,8; 2016,Jan,13; 2015,Jan,16; 2014,Jan,11

+ **96411** **intravenous, push technique, each additional substance/drug (List separately in addition to code for primary procedure)**

INCLUDES Push technique includes:
Administration of injection directly into vessel or access line by health care professional; or
Infusion less than or equal to 15 minutes

EXCLUDES Insertion of arterial and venous cannula(s) for extracorporeal circulation (36823)
Services performed by physicians or other qualified health care providers in facility settings

Code first initial substance/drug (96409, 96413)

⚐ 1.65 ⚐ 1.65 **FUD** ZZZ   S 80 ▭

AMA: 2018,Feb,11; 2018,Jan,8; 2017,Jan,8; 2016,Jan,13; 2015,Jan,16; 2014,Jan,11

96413-96417 Chemotherapy and Complex Drugs, Biologicals: Intravenous Infusion

CMS: 100-03,110.2 Certain Drugs Distributed by the National Cancer Institute; 100-03,110.6 Scalp Hypothermia During Chemotherapy, to Prevent Hair Loss; 100-04,4,230.2 OPPS Drug Administration

INCLUDES   Highly complex services that require direct supervision for:
    Consent
    Patient assessment
    Safety oversight
    Supervision
    More intense work and monitoring of clinical staff by physician or other qualified health care provider due to greater risk of severe patient reactions
    Parenteral administration of:
    Anti-neoplastic agents for noncancer diagnoses
    Monoclonal antibody agents
    Nonradionuclide antineoplastic drugs
    Other biologic response modifiers
    The following in the administration:
    Access to IV/catheter/port
    Drug preparation
    Flushing at the completion of the infusion
    Hydration fluid
    Routine tubing/syringe/supplies
    Starting the IV
    Use of local anesthesia

EXCLUDES   *Administration of nonchemotherapy agents such as antibiotics/steroids/analgesics*
Declotting of catheter/port (36593)
Home infusion (99601-99602)
Insertion of arterial and venous cannula(s) for extracorporeal circulation (36823)
Services provided by physicians or other qualified health care providers in facility settings
Use of a code for a second initial service on the same date for accessing a multi-lumen catheter, restarting an IV, or when two IV lines are needed to meet an infusion rate

Code also drug or substance
Code also significant separately identifiable E&M service, when performed

96413 **Chemotherapy administration, intravenous infusion technique; up to 1 hour, single or initial substance/drug**

    INCLUDES   Push technique includes:
    Administration of injection directly into vessel or access line by health care professional; or
    Infusion less than or equal to 15 minutes

    EXCLUDES   *Hydration administered as secondary or subsequent service via same IV access site (96361)*
Therapeutic/prophylactic/diagnostic drug infusion/injection through the same intravenous access (96366, 96367, 96375)
Code also second initial service with modifier 59 when patient's condition or drug protocol mandates the use of two IV lines

    🚑 3.97   ⚕ 3.97   **FUD** XXX   S 80 ▣

    AMA: 2018,Feb,11; 2018,Jan,8; 2017,Jan,8; 2016,Jan,13; 2015,Jan,16; 2014,Jan,11

+ **96415** **each additional hour (List separately in addition to code for primary procedure)**

    INCLUDES   Infusion intervals of more than 30 minutes past 1-hour increments
Code first initial hour (96413)

    🚑 0.86   ⚕ 0.86   **FUD** ZZZ   S 80 ▣

    AMA: 2018,Feb,11; 2018,Jan,8; 2017,Jan,8; 2016,Jan,13; 2015,Jan,16; 2014,Jan,11

96416 **initiation of prolonged chemotherapy infusion (more than 8 hours), requiring use of a portable or implantable pump**

    EXCLUDES   *Portable or implantable infusion pump/reservoir refilling/maintenance for drug delivery (96521-96523)*

    🚑 3.98   ⚕ 3.98   **FUD** XXX   S 80 ▣

    AMA: 2018,Feb,11; 2018,Jan,8; 2017,Jan,8; 2016,Jan,13; 2015,Jan,16; 2014,Jan,11

+ **96417** **each additional sequential infusion (different substance/drug), up to 1 hour (List separately in addition to code for primary procedure)**

    INCLUDES   Push technique includes:
    Administration of injection directly into vessel or access line by health care professional; or
    Infusion less than or equal to 15 minutes

    EXCLUDES   *Additional hour(s) of sequential infusion (96415)*
Use of code more than one time per sequential infusion
Code first initial substance/drug (96413)

    🚑 1.92   ⚕ 1.92   **FUD** ZZZ   S 80 ▣

    AMA: 2018,Feb,11; 2018,Jan,8; 2017,Jan,8; 2016,Jan,13; 2015,Jan,16; 2014,Jan,11

96420-96425 Chemotherapy and Complex Drugs, Biologicals: Intra-arterial

CMS: 100-03,110.2 Certain Drugs Distributed by the National Cancer Institute; 100-03,110.6 Scalp Hypothermia During Chemotherapy, to Prevent Hair Loss; 100-04,4,230.2 OPPS Drug Administration

INCLUDES   Highly complex services that require direct supervision for:
    Consent
    Patient assessment
    Safety oversight
    Supervision
    More intense work and monitoring of clinical staff by physician or other qualified health care provider due to greater risk of severe patient reactions
    Parenteral administration of:
    Anti-neoplastic agents for noncancer diagnoses
    Monoclonal antibody agents
    Non-radionuclide antineoplastic drugs
    Other biologic response modifiers
    The following in the administration:
    Access to IV/catheter/port
    Drug preparation
    Flushing at the completion of the infusion
    Hydration fluid
    Routine tubing/syringe/supplies
    Starting the IV
    Use of local anesthesia

EXCLUDES   *Administration of non-chemotherapy agents such as antibiotics/steroids/analgesics*
Declotting of catheter/port (36593)
Home infusion (99601-99602)
Services provided by physicians or other qualified health care providers in facility settings
Use of a code for a second initial service on the same date for accessing a multi-lumen catheter, restarting an IV, or when two IV lines are needed

Code also drug or substance
Code also significant separately identifiable E&M service, when performed

96420 **Chemotherapy administration, intra-arterial; push technique**

    INCLUDES   Push technique includes:
    Administration of injection directly into vessel or access line by health care professional; or
    Infusion less than or equal to 15 minutes
    Regional chemotherapy perfusion

    EXCLUDES   *Insertion of arterial and venous cannula(s) for extracorporeal circulation (36823)*
Placement of intra-arterial catheter

    🚑 2.95   ⚕ 2.95   **FUD** XXX   S 80 ▣

    AMA: 2018,Feb,11; 2018,Jan,8; 2017,Jan,8; 2016,Mar,3; 2016,Jan,13; 2015,Nov,3; 2015,Jan,16; 2014,Jan,11

96422 **infusion technique, up to 1 hour**

    INCLUDES   Push technique includes:
    Administration of injection directly into vessel or access line by health care professional; or
    Infusion less than or equal to 15 minutes
    Regional chemotherapy perfusion

    EXCLUDES   *Insertion of arterial and venous cannula(s) for extracorporeal circulation (36823)*
Placement of intra-arterial catheter

    🚑 4.85   ⚕ 4.85   **FUD** XXX   S 80 ▣

    AMA: 2018,Feb,11; 2018,Jan,8; 2017,Jan,8; 2016,Mar,3; 2016,Jan,13; 2015,Nov,3; 2015,Jan,16; 2014,Jan,11

+ **96423** infusion technique, each additional hour (List separately in addition to code for primary procedure)

INCLUDES Infusion intervals of more than 30 minutes past 1-hour increments
Regional chemotherapy perfusion

EXCLUDES Insertion of arterial and venous cannula(s) for extracorpororeal circulation (36823)
Placement of intra-arterial catheter

Code first initial hour (96422)
2.24 2.24 **FUD** ZZZ [S] [80] [▭]

AMA: 2018,Feb,11; 2018,Jan,8; 2017,Jan,8; 2016,Mar,3; 2016,Jan,13; 2015,Nov,3; 2015,Jan,16; 2014,Jan,11

96425 infusion technique, initiation of prolonged infusion (more than 8 hours), requiring the use of a portable or implantable pump

INCLUDES Regional chemotherapy perfusion

EXCLUDES Insertion of arterial and venous cannula(s) for extracorpororeal circulation (36823)
Placement of intra-arterial catheter
Portable or implantable infusion pump/reservoir refilling/maintenance for drug delivery (96521-96523)

5.14 5.14 **FUD** XXX [S] [80] [▭]

AMA: 2018,Feb,11; 2018,Jan,8; 2017,Jan,8; 2016,Mar,3; 2016,Jan,13; 2015,Nov,3; 2015,Jan,16; 2014,Jan,11

96440-96450 Chemotherapy Administration: Intrathecal/Peritoneal Cavity/Pleural Cavity

CMS: 100-03,110.2 Certain Drugs Distributed by the National Cancer Institute; 100-04,4,230.2 OPPS Drug Administration

96440 Chemotherapy administration into pleural cavity, requiring and including thoracentesis
3.57 23.6 **FUD** 000 [S] [80] [▭]

AMA: 2018,Feb,11; 2018,Jan,8; 2017,Jan,8; 2016,Jan,13; 2015,Jan,16; 2014,Jan,11

96446 Chemotherapy administration into the peritoneal cavity via indwelling port or catheter
0.79 5.78 **FUD** XXX [S] [80] [▭]

AMA: 2018,Feb,11; 2018,Jan,8; 2017,Jan,8; 2016,Jan,13; 2015,Jan,16; 2014,Jan,11

96450 Chemotherapy administration, into CNS (eg, intrathecal), requiring and including spinal puncture

EXCLUDES Chemotherapy administration, intravesical/bladder (51720)
Fluoroscopy (77003)
Insertion of catheter/reservoir:
Intraventricular (61210, 61215)
Subarachnoid (62350-62351, 62360-62362)

2.27 5.13 **FUD** 000 [S] [80] [▭]

AMA: 2018,Feb,11; 2018,Jan,8; 2017,Jan,8; 2016,Jan,13; 2015,Jan,16; 2014,Jan,11

96521-96523 Refill/Upkeep of Drug Delivery Device

CMS: 100-04,4,230.2 OPPS Drug Administration

INCLUDES Highly complex services that require direct supervision for:
Consent
Patient assessment
Safety oversight
Supervision
Parenteral administration of:
Anti-neoplastic agents for noncancer diagnoses
Monoclonal antibody agents
Non-radionuclide antineoplastic drugs
Other biologic response modifiers
The following in the administration:
Access to IV/catheter/port
Drug preparation
Flushing at the completion of the infusion
Hydration fluid
Routine tubing/syringe/supplies
Starting the IV
Use of local anesthesia
Therapeutic drugs other than chemotherapy

EXCLUDES Administration of non-chemotherapy agents such as antibiotics/steroids/analgesics
Blood specimen collection from completely implantable venous access device (36591)
Declotting of catheter/port (36593)
Home infusion (99601-99602)
Services provided by physicians or other qualified health care providers in facility settings

Code also drug or substance
Code also significant separately identifiable E&M service, when performed

96521 Refilling and maintenance of portable pump
4.13 4.13 **FUD** XXX [S] [80] [▭]

AMA: 2018,Feb,11; 2018,Jan,8; 2017,Jan,8; 2016,Jan,13; 2015,Jan,16; 2014,Jan,11

96522 Refilling and maintenance of implantable pump or reservoir for drug delivery, systemic (eg, intravenous, intra-arterial)

EXCLUDES Implantable infusion pump refilling/maintenance for spinal/brain drug delivery (95990-95991)

3.39 3.39 **FUD** XXX [S] [80] [▭]

AMA: 2018,Feb,11; 2018,Jan,8; 2017,Jan,8; 2016,Jan,13; 2015,Jan,16; 2014,Jan,11

96523 Irrigation of implanted venous access device for drug delivery systems

EXCLUDES Direct supervision by physician or other qualified health care provider in facility settings
Use of code with any other services on the same date of service

0.77 0.77 **FUD** XXX [Q1] [80] [▭]

AMA: 2018,Feb,11; 2018,Jan,8; 2017,Jan,8; 2016,Jan,13; 2015,Jan,16; 2014,Jan,11

Medicine (sidebar)

96542 — 96904 (sidebar)

96542-96549 Chemotherapy Injection Into Brain

CMS: 100-04,4,230.2 OPPS Drug Administration

INCLUDES Highly complex services that require direct supervision for:
Consent
Patient assessment
Safety oversight
Supervision
Parenteral administration of:
Anti-neoplastic agents for noncancer diagnoses
Monoclonal antibody agents
Non-radionuclide antineoplastic drugs
Other biologic response modifiers
The following in the administration:
Access to IV/catheter/port
Drug preparation
Flushing at the completion of the infusion
Hydration fluid
Routine tubing/syringe/supplies
Starting the IV
Use of local anesthesia

EXCLUDES *Administration of non-chemotherapy agents such as antibiotics/steroids/analgesics*
Blood specimen collection from completely implantable venous access device (36591)
Declotting of catheter/port (36593)
Home infusion (99601-99602)

Code also drug or substance
Code also significant separately identifiable E&M service, when performed

96542 **Chemotherapy injection, subarachnoid or intraventricular via subcutaneous reservoir, single or multiple agents**

EXCLUDES *Oral radioactive isotope therapy (79005)*

1.19 3.77 **FUD** XXX   S 80

AMA: 2018,Feb,11; 2018,Jan,8; 2017,Jan,8; 2016,Jan,13; 2015,Jan,16; 2014,Jan,11

96549 **Unlisted chemotherapy procedure**

0.00 0.00 **FUD** XXX   Q1 80

AMA: 2018,Feb,11; 2018,Jan,8; 2017,Jan,8; 2016,Jan,13; 2015,Jan,16; 2014,Jan,11

96567-96574 Destruction of Lesions: Photodynamic Therapy

EXCLUDES *Ocular photodynamic therapy (67221)*

96567 **Photodynamic therapy by external application of light to destroy premalignant lesions of the skin and adjacent mucosa with application and illumination/activation of photosensitive drug(s), per day**

INCLUDES Services provided without direct participation by physician or other qualified healthcare professional

3.50 3.50 **FUD** XXX   Q1 80

AMA: 2018,Jul,14; 2018,Feb,10; 2018,Feb,11; 2018,Jan,8; 2017,Jan,8; 2016,Jan,13; 2015,Jan,16; 2014,Jan,11

+ **96570** **Photodynamic therapy by endoscopic application of light to ablate abnormal tissue via activation of photosensitive drug(s); first 30 minutes (List separately in addition to code for endoscopy or bronchoscopy procedures of lung and gastrointestinal tract)**

Code also for 38-52 minutes (96571)
Code also modifier 52 when services with report are less than 23 minutes
Code first (31641, 43229)

1.48 1.48 **FUD** ZZZ   N

AMA: 2018,Feb,11; 2018,Jan,8; 2017,Jan,8; 2016,Jan,13; 2015,Jan,16; 2014,Jan,11

+ **96571** **each additional 15 minutes (List separately in addition to code for endoscopy or bronchoscopy procedures of lung and gastrointestinal tract)**

EXCLUDES *23-37 minutes of service (96570)*
Code first (96570)
Code first when appropriate (31641, 43229)

0.83 0.83 **FUD** ZZZ   N

AMA: 2018,Feb,11; 2018,Jan,8; 2017,Jan,8; 2016,Jan,13; 2015,Jan,16; 2014,Jan,11

96573 **Photodynamic therapy by external application of light to destroy premalignant lesions of the skin and adjacent mucosa with application and illumination/activation of photosensitizing drug(s) provided by a physician or other qualified health care professional, per day**

INCLUDES Application of photosensitizer to lesions at an anatomical site
Debridement, when performed
Use of light to activate photosensitizer for destruction of premalignant lesions

EXCLUDES *Debridement lesion with photodynamic therapy provided by physician or other qualified healthcare professional (96574)*
Photodynamic therapy by external application of light to same anatomical site (96567)
Services provided to same area on same date of services as photodynamic therapy:
Biopsy (11102-11107)
Debridement (11000-11001, 11004-11005)
Excision of lesion (11400-11471)
Shaving of lesion (11300-11313)

5.70 5.70 **FUD** 000   Q1 80

AMA: 2018,Jul,14; 2018,Feb,11; 2018,Feb,10

96574 **Debridement of premalignant hyperkeratotic lesion(s) (ie, targeted curettage, abrasion) followed with photodynamic therapy by external application of light to destroy premalignant lesions of the skin and adjacent mucosa with application and illumination/activation of photosensitizing drug(s) provided by a physician or other qualified health care professional, per day**

INCLUDES Application of photosensitizer to lesions at an anatomical site
Debridement, when performed
Use of light to activate photosensitizer for destruction of premalignant lesions

EXCLUDES *Photodynamic therapy by external application of light for destruction of premalignant lesions (96573)*
Photodynamic therapy by external application of light to same anatomical site (96567)
Services provided to same area on same date of services as photodynamic therapy:
Biopsy (11102-11107)
Debridement (11000-11001, 11004-11005)
Excision of lesion (11400-11471)
Shaving of lesion (11300-11313)

7.25 7.25 **FUD** 000   Q1 80

AMA: 2018,Feb,10; 2018,Feb,11

96900-96999 Diagnostic/Therapeutic Skin Procedures

EXCLUDES *E&M services*
Injection, intralesional (11900-11901)

96900 **Actinotherapy (ultraviolet light)**

EXCLUDES *Rhinophototherapy (30999)*
(88160-88161)

0.61 0.61 **FUD** XXX   Q1 80

AMA: 2018,Feb,11; 2018,Jan,8; 2017,Jan,8; 2016,Nov,9; 2016,Sep,3; 2016,Jan,13; 2015,Jan,16; 2014,Jan,11

96902 **Microscopic examination of hairs plucked or clipped by the examiner (excluding hair collected by the patient) to determine telogen and anagen counts, or structural hair shaft abnormality**

(88160-88161)

0.59 0.62 **FUD** XXX   N

AMA: 2018,Feb,11

96904 **Whole body integumentary photography, for monitoring of high risk patients with dysplastic nevus syndrome or a history of dysplastic nevi, or patients with a personal or familial history of melanoma**

(88160-88161)

1.82 1.82 **FUD** XXX   N 80

AMA: 2018,Feb,11

26/TC PC/TC Only   A2-Z3 ASC Payment   50 Bilateral   ♂ Male Only   ♀ Female Only   Facility RVU   Non-Facility RVU   CCI   CLIA
FUD Follow-up Days   **CMS:** IOM   **AMA:** CPT Asst   A-Y OPPSI   80/80 Surg Assist Allowed / w/Doc   Lab Crosswalk   Radiology Crosswalk

96910 Photochemotherapy; tar and ultraviolet B (Goeckerman treatment) or petrolatum and ultraviolet B
🔲 (88160-88161)
🚑 3.24 ⚕ 3.24 **FUD** XXX
Q1 80 🔲
AMA: 2018,Feb,11; 2018,Jan,8; 2017,Jan,8; 2016,Sep,3; 2016,Jan,13; 2015,Jan,16; 2014,Jan,11

96912 psoralens and ultraviolet A (PUVA)
🔲 (88160-88161)
🚑 2.75 ⚕ 2.75 **FUD** XXX
Q1 80 🔲
AMA: 2018,Feb,11; 2018,Jan,8; 2017,Jan,8; 2016,Sep,3; 2016,Jan,13; 2015,Jan,16; 2014,Jan,11

96913 Photochemotherapy (Goeckerman and/or PUVA) for severe photoresponsive dermatoses requiring at least 4-8 hours of care under direct supervision of the physician (includes application of medication and dressings)
🔲 (88160-88161)
🚑 3.91 ⚕ 3.91 **FUD** XXX
T 80 🔲
AMA: 2018,Feb,11; 2018,Jan,8; 2017,Jan,8; 2016,Sep,3

96920 Laser treatment for inflammatory skin disease (psoriasis); total area less than 250 sq cm
EXCLUDES Destruction by laser of:
Benign lesions (17110-17111)
Cutaneous vascular proliferative lesions (17106-17108)
Malignant lesions (17260-17286)
Premalignant lesions (17000-17004)
🔲 (88160-88161)
🚑 1.90 ⚕ 4.64 **FUD** 000
Q1 🔲
AMA: 2018,Feb,11; 2018,Jan,8; 2017,Jan,8; 2016,Sep,3; 2016,Jan,13; 2015,Jan,16; 2014,Jan,11

96921 250 sq cm to 500 sq cm
EXCLUDES Destruction by laser of:
Benign lesions (17110-17111)
Cutaneous vascular proliferative lesions (17106-17108)
Malignant lesions (17260-17286)
Premalignant lesions (17000-17004)
🔲 (88160-88161)
🚑 2.14 ⚕ 5.09 **FUD** 000
Q1 🔲
AMA: 2018,Feb,11; 2018,Jan,8; 2017,Jan,8; 2016,Sep,3; 2016,Jan,13; 2015,Jan,16; 2014,Jan,11

96922 over 500 sq cm
EXCLUDES Destruction by laser of:
Benign lesions (17110-17111)
Cutaneous vascular proliferative lesions (17106-17108)
Malignant lesions (17260-17286)
Premalignant lesions (17000-17004)
🔲 (88160-88161)
🚑 3.43 ⚕ 6.91 **FUD** 000
Q1 🔲
AMA: 2018,Feb,11; 2018,Jan,8; 2017,Jan,8; 2016,Sep,3; 2016,Jan,13; 2015,Jan,16; 2014,Jan,11

96931 Reflectance confocal microscopy (RCM) for cellular and sub-cellular imaging of skin; image acquisition and interpretation and report, first lesion
EXCLUDES Optical coherence tomography for skin imaging (0470T-0471T)
Reflectance confocal microscopy examination without generated mosaic images (96999)
🚑 4.83 ⚕ 4.83 **FUD** XXX
M 80 🔲
AMA: 2018,Feb,11; 2018,Jan,8; 2017,Sep,9

96932 image acquisition only, first lesion
EXCLUDES Optical coherence tomography for skin imaging (0470T-0471T)
Reflectance confocal microscopy examination without generated mosaic images (96999)
🚑 3.51 ⚕ 3.51 **FUD** XXX
Q1 80 TC 🔲
AMA: 2018,Feb,11; 2018,Jan,8; 2017,Sep,9

96933 interpretation and report only, first lesion
EXCLUDES Optical coherence tomography for skin imaging (0470T-0471T)
Reflectance confocal microscopy examination without generated mosaic images (96999)
🚑 1.32 ⚕ 1.32 **FUD** XXX
B 80 26 🔲
AMA: 2018,Feb,11; 2018,Jan,8; 2017,Sep,9

+ **96934** image acquisition and interpretation and report, each additional lesion (List separately in addition to code for primary procedure)
EXCLUDES Optical coherence tomography for skin imaging (0470T-0471T)
Reflectance confocal microscopy examination without generated mosaic images (96999)
Code first (96931)
🚑 2.74 ⚕ 2.74 **FUD** ZZZ
N 80 🔲
AMA: 2018,Feb,11; 2018,Jan,8; 2017,Sep,9

+ **96935** image acquisition only, each additional lesion (List separately in addition to code for primary procedure)
EXCLUDES Optical coherence tomography for skin imaging (0470T-0471T)
Reflectance confocal microscopy examination without generated mosaic images (96999)
Code first (96932)
🚑 1.26 ⚕ 1.26 **FUD** ZZZ
N 80 TC 🔲
AMA: 2018,Feb,11; 2018,Jan,8; 2017,Sep,9

+ **96936** interpretation and report only, each additional lesion (List separately in addition to code for primary procedure)
EXCLUDES Optical coherence tomography for skin imaging (0470T-0471T)
Reflectance confocal microscopy examination without generated mosaic images (96999)
Code first (96933)
🚑 1.26 ⚕ 1.26 **FUD** ZZZ
N 80 26 🔲
AMA: 2018,Feb,11; 2018,Jan,8; 2017,Sep,9

96999 Unlisted special dermatological service or procedure
🚑 0.00 ⚕ 0.00 **FUD** XXX
Q1 80 🔲
AMA: 2018,Feb,11; 2018,Jan,8; 2017,Sep,9; 2017,Jan,8; 2016,Sep,3; 2016,Jan,13; 2015,Jan,16; 2014,Jan,11

97161-97164 [97161, 97162, 97163, 97164] Assessment: Physical Therapy

CMS: 100-02,15,220 Coverage of Outpatient Rehabilitation Therapy Services; 100-02,15,220.4 Functional Reporting; 100-02,15,230 Practice of Physical Therapy, Occupational Therapy, and Speech-Language Pathology; 100-02,15,230.1 Practice of Physical Therapy; 100-02,15,230.4 Services By a Physical/Occupational Therapist in Private Practice; 100-04,5,10.3.2 Therapy Cap Exceptions; 100-04,5,10.3.3 Use of the KX Modifier; 100-04,5,10.6 Functional Reporting; 100-04,5,20.2 Reporting Units of Service

INCLUDES Creation of care plan
Evaluation of body systems as defined in the 1997 E&M documentation guidelines:
Cardiovascular system: Vital signs, edema of extremities
Integumentary system: Inspection for abnormalities of skin
Mental status: Orientation, judgment, thought processes
Musculoskeletal system: Evaluation of gait and station, range of motion, muscle strength, height and weight
Neuromuscular evaluation: Balance, abnormal movements

EXCLUDES Biofeedback traning via EMG (90901)
Joint range of motion (95851-95852)
Transcutaneous nerve stimulation (TENS) (97014, 97032)

\# **97161** Physical therapy evaluation: low complexity, requiring these components: A history with no personal factors and/or comorbidities that impact the plan of care; An examination of body system(s) using standardized tests and measures addressing 1-2 elements from any of the following: body structures and functions, activity limitations, and/or participation restrictions; A clinical presentation with stable and/or uncomplicated characteristics; and Clinical decision making of low complexity using standardized patient assessment instrument and/or measurable assessment of functional outcome. Typically, 20 minutes are spent face-to-face with the patient and/or family.

2.38   2.38   **FUD** XXX   A 80

AMA: 2018,May,5; 2018,Feb,11; 2018,Jan,8; 2017,Aug,3; 2017,Jun,6; 2017,Jan,8

\# **97162** Physical therapy evaluation: moderate complexity, requiring these components: A history of present problem with 1-2 personal factors and/or comorbidities that impact the plan of care; An examination of body systems using standardized tests and measures in addressing a total of 3 or more elements from any of the following: body structures and functions, activity limitations, and/or participation restrictions; An evolving clinical presentation with changing characteristics; and Clinical decision making of moderate complexity using standardized patient assessment instrument and/or measurable assessment of functional outcome. Typically, 30 minutes are spent face-to-face with the patient and/or family.

2.38   2.38   **FUD** XXX   A 80

AMA: 2018,May,5; 2018,Feb,11; 2018,Jan,8; 2017,Aug,3; 2017,Jun,6; 2017,Jan,8

\# **97163** Physical therapy evaluation: high complexity, requiring these components: A history of present problem with 3 or more personal factors and/or comorbidities that impact the plan of care; An examination of body systems using standardized tests and measures addressing a total of 4 or more elements from any of the following: body structures and functions, activity limitations, and/or participation restrictions; A clinical presentation with unstable and unpredictable characteristics; and Clinical decision making of high complexity using standardized patient assessment instrument and/or measurable assessment of functional outcome. Typically, 45 minutes are spent face-to-face with the patient and/or family.

2.38   2.38   **FUD** XXX   A 80

AMA: 2018,May,5; 2018,Feb,11; 2018,Jan,8; 2017,Aug,3; 2017,Jun,6; 2017,Jan,8

\# **97164** Re-evaluation of physical therapy established plan of care, requiring these components: An examination including a review of history and use of standardized tests and measures is required; and Revised plan of care using a standardized patient assessment instrument and/or measurable assessment of functional outcome Typically, 20 minutes are spent face-to-face with the patient and/or family.

1.61   1.61   **FUD** XXX   A 80

AMA: 2018,May,5; 2018,Feb,11; 2018,Jan,8; 2017,Aug,3; 2017,Jun,6; 2017,Jan,8

97165-97168 [97165, 97166, 97167, 97168] Assessment: Occupational Therapy

CMS: 100-02,15,220 Coverage of Outpatient Rehabilitation Therapy Services; 100-02,15,220.4 Functional Reporting; 100-02,15,230 Practice of Physical Therapy, Occupational Therapy, and Speech-Language Pathology; 100-02,15,230.1 Practice of Physical Therapy; 100-02,15,230.2 Practice of Occupational Therapy; 100-02,15,230.4 Services By a Physical/Occupational Therapist in Private Practice; 100-04,5,10.3.2 Exceptions Process; 100-04,5,10.3.3 Use of the KX Modifier; 100-04,5,10.6 Functional Reporting; 100-04,5,20.2 Reporting Units of Service

INCLUDES Creation of care plan
Evaluations as appropriate
Medical history
Occupational status
Past history of therapy

\# **97165** Occupational therapy evaluation, low complexity, requiring these components: An occupational profile and medical and therapy history, which includes a brief history including review of medical and/or therapy records relating to the presenting problem; An assessment(s) that identifies 1-3 performance deficits (ie, relating to physical, cognitive, or psychosocial skills) that result in activity limitations and/or participation restrictions; and Clinical decision making of low complexity, which includes an analysis of the occupational profile, analysis of data from problem-focused assessment(s), and consideration of a limited number of treatment options. Patient presents with no comorbidities that affect occupational performance. Modification of tasks or assistance (eg, physical or verbal) with assessment(s) is not necessary to enable completion of evaluation component. Typically, 30 minutes are spent face-to-face with the patient and/or family.

2.57   2.57   **FUD** XXX   A 80

AMA: 2018,May,5; 2018,Feb,11; 2018,Jan,8; 2017,Jun,6; 2017,Feb,3; 2017,Jan,8

\# **97166** Occupational therapy evaluation, moderate complexity, requiring these components: An occupational profile and medical and therapy history, which includes an expanded review of medical and/or therapy records and additional review of physical, cognitive, or psychosocial history related to current functional performance; An assessment(s) that identifies 3-5 performance deficits (ie, relating to physical, cognitive, or psychosocial skills) that result in activity limitations and/or participation restrictions; and Clinical decision making of moderate analytic complexity, which includes an analysis of the occupational profile, analysis of data from detailed assessment(s), and consideration of several treatment options. Patient may present with comorbidities that affect occupational performance. Minimal to moderate modification of tasks or assistance (eg, physical or verbal) with assessment(s) is necessary to enable patient to complete evaluation component. Typically, 45 minutes are spent face-to-face with the patient and/or family.

2.57   2.57   **FUD** XXX   A 80

AMA: 2018,May,5; 2018,Feb,11; 2018,Jan,8; 2017,Jun,6; 2017,Feb,3; 2017,Jan,8

26/TC PC/TC Only   A2-Z3 ASC Payment   50 Bilateral   ♂ Male Only   ♀ Female Only   Facility RVU   Non-Facility RVU   CCI   CLIA
FUD Follow-up Days   CMS: IOM   AMA: CPT Asst   A-Y OPPSI   80/80 Surg Assist Allowed / w/Doc   Lab Crosswalk   Radiology Crosswalk

524   CPT © 2019 American Medical Association. All Rights Reserved.   © 2019 Optum360, LLC

97167

97167 Occupational therapy evaluation, high complexity, requiring these components: An occupational profile and medical and therapy history, which includes review of medical and/or therapy records and extensive additional review of physical, cognitive, or psychosocial history related to current functional performance; An assessment(s) that identifies 5 or more performance deficits (ie, relating to physical, cognitive, or psychosocial skills) that result in activity limitations and/or participation restrictions; and Clinical decision making of high analytic complexity, which includes an analysis of the patient profile, analysis of data from comprehensive assessment(s), and consideration of multiple treatment options. Patient presents with comorbidities that affect occupational performance. Significant modification of tasks or assistance (eg, physical or verbal) with assessment(s) is necessary to enable patient to complete evaluation component. Typically, 60 minutes are spent face-to-face with the patient and/or family.

🚑 2.58 ⚕ 2.58 **FUD** XXX Ⓐ 80 ▱

AMA: 2018,May,5; 2018,Feb,11; 2018,Jan,8; 2017,Jun,6; 2017,Feb,3; 2017,Jan,8

97168 Re-evaluation of occupational therapy established plan of care, requiring these components: An assessment of changes in patient functional or medical status with revised plan of care; An update to the initial occupational profile to reflect changes in condition or environment that affect future interventions and/or goals; and A revised plan of care. A formal reevaluation is performed when there is a documented change in functional status or a significant change to the plan of care is required. Typically, 30 minutes are spent face-to-face with the patient and/or family.

🚑 1.75 ⚕ 1.75 **FUD** XXX Ⓐ 80 ▱

AMA: 2018,May,5; 2018,Feb,11; 2018,Jan,8; 2017,Jun,6; 2017,Feb,3; 2017,Jan,8

97169-97172 [97169, 97170, 97171, 97172] Assessment: Athletic Training

CMS: 100-02,15,220 Coverage of Outpatient Rehabilitation Therapy Services; 100-02,15,230 Practice of Physical Therapy, Occupational Therapy, and Speech-Language Pathology; 100-02,15,230.1 Practice of Physical Therapy

INCLUDES Creation of care plan
Evaluation of body systems as defined in the 1997 E&M documentation guidelines:
Cardiovascular system: Vital signs, edema of extremities
Integumentary system: Inspection for abnormalities of skin
Musculoskeletal system: Evaluation of gait and station, range of motion, muscle strength, height and weight
Neuromuscular evaluation: Balance, abnormal movements

97169 Athletic training evaluation, low complexity, requiring these components: A history and physical activity profile with no comorbidities that affect physical activity; An examination of affected body area and other symptomatic or related systems addressing 1-2 elements from any of the following: body structures, physical activity, and/or participation deficiencies; and Clinical decision making of low complexity using standardized patient assessment instrument and/or measurable assessment of functional outcome. Typically, 15 minutes are spent face-to-face with the patient and/or family.

🚑 0.00 ⚕ 0.00 **FUD** XXX Ⓔ ▱

AMA: 2018,May,5; 2018,Feb,11; 2018,Jan,8; 2017,Jun,6; 2017,Jan,8

97170 Athletic training evaluation, moderate complexity, requiring these components: A medical history and physical activity profile with 1-2 comorbidities that affect physical activity; An examination of affected body area and other symptomatic or related systems addressing a total of 3 or more elements from any of the following: body structures, physical activity, and/or participation deficiencies; and Clinical decision making of moderate complexity using standardized patient assessment instrument and/or measurable assessment of functional outcome. Typically, 30 minutes are spent face-to-face with the patient and/or family.

🚑 0.00 ⚕ 0.00 **FUD** XXX Ⓔ ▱

AMA: 2018,May,5; 2018,Feb,11; 2018,Jan,8; 2017,Jun,6; 2017,Jan,8

97171 Athletic training evaluation, high complexity, requiring these components: A medical history and physical activity profile, with 3 or more comorbidities that affect physical activity; A comprehensive examination of body systems using standardized tests and measures addressing a total of 4 or more elements from any of the following: body structures, physical activity, and/or participation deficiencies; Clinical presentation with unstable and unpredictable characteristics; and Clinical decision making of high complexity using standardized patient assessment instrument and/or measurable assessment of functional outcome. Typically, 45 minutes are spent face-to-face with the patient and/or family.

🚑 0.00 ⚕ 0.00 **FUD** XXX Ⓔ ▱

AMA: 2018,May,5; 2018,Feb,11; 2018,Jan,8; 2017,Jun,6; 2017,Jan,8

97172 Re-evaluation of athletic training established plan of care requiring these components: An assessment of patient's current functional status when there is a documented change; and A revised plan of care using a standardized patient assessment instrument and/or measurable assessment of functional outcome with an update in management options, goals, and interventions. Typically, 20 minutes are spent face-to-face with the patient and/or family.

🚑 0.00 ⚕ 0.00 **FUD** XXX Ⓔ ▱

AMA: 2018,May,5; 2018,Feb,11; 2018,Jan,8; 2017,Jun,6; 2017,Jan,8

97010-97028 Physical Therapy Treatment Modalities: Supervised

CMS: 100-02,15,220 Coverage of Outpatient Rehabilitation Therapy Services; 100-02,15,220.4 Functional Reporting; 100-02,15,230 Practice of Physical Therapy, Occupational Therapy, and Speech-Language Pathology; 100-02,15,230.1 Practice of Physical Therapy; 100-02,15,230.2 Practice of Occupational Therapy; 100-02,15,230.4 Services By a Physical/Occupational Therapist in Private Practice; 100-03,10.3 Inpatient Pain Rehabilitation Programs; 100-03,10.4 Outpatient Hospital Pain Rehabilitation Programs; 100-03,160.17 Payment for L-Dopa /Associated Inpatient Hospital Services; 100-04,5,10 Part B Outpatient Rehabilitation and Comprehensive Outpatient Rehabilitation Facility (CORF) Services - General; 100-04,5,10.2 Financial Limitation for Outpatient Rehabilitation Services; 100-04,5,10.3.2 Therapy Cap Exceptions; 100-04,5,10.3.3 Use of the KX Modifier; 100-04,5,20.2 Reporting Units of Service

INCLUDES Adding incremental intervals of treatment time for the same visit to calculate the total service time

EXCLUDES *Direct patient contact by the provider*
Electromyography (95860-95872 [95885, 95886, 95887])
EMG biofeedback training (90901)
Muscle and range of motion tests ([97161, 97162, 97163, 97164, 97165, 97166, 97167, 97168, 97169, 97170, 97171, 97172])
Nerve conduction studies (95905-95913)

97010 Application of a modality to 1 or more areas; hot or cold packs

🚑 0.18 ⚕ 0.18 **FUD** XXX Ⓢ Ⓐ ▱

AMA: 2018,May,5; 2018,Feb,11; 2018,Jan,8; 2017,Jan,8; 2016,Jun,8; 2016,Jan,13; 2015,Jan,16; 2014,Jan,11

97012 traction, mechanical

🚑 0.42 ⚕ 0.42 **FUD** XXX Ⓢ Ⓐ 80 ▱

AMA: 2018,May,5; 2018,Feb,11; 2018,Jan,8; 2017,Jan,8; 2016,Jun,8; 2016,Jan,13; 2015,Jan,16; 2014,Jan,11

97014 — 97124

97014 **electrical stimulation (unattended)**
EXCLUDES *Acupuncture with electrical stimulation (97813, 97814)*
0.42 0.42 **FUD** XXX Ⓢ Ⓔ ▭
AMA: 2019,Jul,10; 2018,Oct,11; 2018,Oct,8; 2018,May,5; 2018,Feb,11; 2018,Jan,8; 2017,Jan,8; 2016,Jan,13; 2015,Jan,16; 2014,Jan,11

97016 **vasopneumatic devices**
0.36 0.36 **FUD** XXX Ⓢ Ⓐ 80 ▭
AMA: 2018,May,5; 2018,Feb,11; 2018,Jan,8; 2017,Jan,8; 2016,Jan,13; 2015,Jan,16; 2014,Jan,11

97018 **paraffin bath**
0.20 0.20 **FUD** XXX Ⓢ Ⓐ 80 ▭
AMA: 2018,May,5; 2018,Feb,11; 2018,Jan,8; 2017,Jan,8; 2016,Jan,13; 2015,Jan,16; 2014,Jan,11

97022 **whirlpool**
0.51 0.51 **FUD** XXX Ⓢ Ⓐ 80 ▭
AMA: 2018,May,5; 2018,Feb,11; 2018,Jan,8; 2017,Jan,8; 2016,Jan,13; 2015,Jan,16; 2014,Jan,11

97024 **diathermy (eg, microwave)**
0.20 0.20 **FUD** XXX Ⓢ Ⓐ 80 ▭
AMA: 2018,May,5; 2018,Feb,11; 2018,Jan,8; 2017,Jan,8; 2016,Jan,13; 2015,Jan,16; 2014,Jan,11

97026 **infrared**
0.18 0.18 **FUD** XXX Ⓢ Ⓐ 80 ▭
AMA: 2018,May,5; 2018,Feb,11; 2018,Jan,8; 2017,Jan,8; 2016,Jan,13; 2015,Jan,16; 2014,Jan,11

97028 **ultraviolet**
0.23 0.23 **FUD** XXX Ⓢ Ⓐ 80 ▭
AMA: 2018,May,5; 2018,Feb,11; 2018,Jan,8; 2017,Jan,8; 2016,Jan,13; 2015,Jan,16; 2014,Jan,11

97032-97039 Physical Therapy Treatment Modalities: Constant Attendance

CMS: 100-02,15,220 Coverage of Outpatient Rehabilitation Therapy Services; 100-02,15,220.4 Functional Reporting; 100-02,15,230 Practice of Physical Therapy, Occupational Therapy, and Speech-Language Pathology; 100-02,15,230.1 Practice of Physical Therapy; 100-02,15,230.2 Practice of Occupational Therapy; 100-02,15,230.4 Services By a Physical/Occupational Therapist in Private Practice; 100-03,10.3 Inpatient Pain Rehabilitation Programs; 100-03,10.4 Outpatient Hospital Pain Rehabilitation Programs; 100-03,160.17 Payment for L-Dopa /Associated Inpatient Hospital Services; 100-04,5,10 Part B Outpatient Rehabilitation and Comprehensive Outpatient Rehabilitation Facility (CORF) Services - General; 100-04,5,10.3.2 Exceptions Process; 100-04,5,10.3.3 Use of the KX Modifier; 100-04,5,20.2 Reporting Units of Service

INCLUDES Adding incremental intervals of treatment time for the same visit to calculate the total service time
Direct patient contact by the provider
EXCLUDES *Electromyography (95860-95872 [95885, 95886, 95887])*
EMG biofeedback training (90901)
Muscle and range of motion tests ([97161, 97162, 97163, 97164, 97165, 97166, 97167, 97168, 97169, 97170, 97171, 97172])
Nerve conduction studies (95905-95913)

97032 **Application of a modality to 1 or more areas; electrical stimulation (manual), each 15 minutes**
EXCLUDES *Transcutaneous electrical modulation pain reprocessing (TEMPR) (scrambler therapy) (0278T)*
0.42 0.42 **FUD** XXX Ⓐ 80 ▭
AMA: 2019,Jul,10; 2018,Oct,11; 2018,Oct,8; 2018,May,5; 2018,Feb,11; 2018,Jan,8; 2017,Jan,8; 2016,Jan,13; 2015,Jan,16; 2014,Jan,11

97033 **iontophoresis, each 15 minutes**
0.59 0.59 **FUD** XXX Ⓢ Ⓐ 80 ▭
AMA: 2018,May,5; 2018,Feb,11; 2018,Jan,8; 2017,Jan,8; 2016,Jan,13; 2015,Jan,16; 2014,Jan,11

97034 **contrast baths, each 15 minutes**
0.43 0.43 **FUD** XXX Ⓢ Ⓐ 80 ▭
AMA: 2018,May,5; 2018,Feb,11; 2018,Jan,8; 2017,Jan,8; 2016,Jan,13; 2015,Jan,16; 2014,Jan,11

97035 **ultrasound, each 15 minutes**
0.39 0.39 **FUD** XXX Ⓢ Ⓐ 80 ▭
AMA: 2018,May,5; 2018,Feb,11; 2018,Jan,8; 2017,Jan,8; 2016,Jan,13; 2015,Jan,16; 2014,Jan,11

97036 **Hubbard tank, each 15 minutes**
0.99 0.99 **FUD** XXX Ⓢ Ⓐ 80 ▭
AMA: 2018,May,5; 2018,Feb,11; 2018,Jan,8; 2017,Jan,8; 2016,Jan,13; 2015,Jan,16; 2014,Jan,11

97039 **Unlisted modality (specify type and time if constant attendance)**
0.00 0.00 **FUD** XXX Ⓐ 80 ▭
AMA: 2018,May,5; 2018,Feb,11; 2018,Jan,8; 2017,Jan,8; 2016,Nov,9; 2016,Jun,8; 2016,Jan,13; 2015,Jan,16; 2014,Jan,11

97110-97546 Other Therapeutic Techniques With Direct Patient Contact

CMS: 100-02,15,220 Coverage of Outpatient Rehabilitation Therapy Services; 100-02,15,230 Practice of Physical Therapy, Occupational Therapy, and Speech-Language Pathology; 100-02,15,230.1 Practice of Physical Therapy; 100-02,15,230.2 Practice of Occupational Therapy; 100-02,15,230.4 Services By a Physical/Occupational Therapist in Private Practice; 100-03,10.3 Inpatient Pain Rehabilitation Programs; 100-03,10.4 Outpatient Hospital Pain Rehabilitation Programs; 100-04,5,10 Part B Outpatient Rehabilitation and Comprehensive Outpatient Rehabilitation Facility (CORF) Services - General; 100-04,5,10.2 Financial Limitation for Outpatient Rehabilitation Services; 100-04,5,20.2 Reporting Units of Service

INCLUDES Application of clinical skills/services to improve function
Direct patient contact by the provider
EXCLUDES *Electromyography (95860-95872 [95885, 95886, 95887])*
EMG biofeedback training (90901)
Muscle and range of motion tests ([97161, 97162, 97163, 97164, 97165, 97166, 97167, 97168, 97169, 97170, 97171, 97172])
Nerve conduction studies (95905-95913)

97110 **Therapeutic procedure, 1 or more areas, each 15 minutes; therapeutic exercises to develop strength and endurance, range of motion and flexibility**
0.87 0.87 **FUD** XXX Ⓢ Ⓐ 80 ▭
AMA: 2019,Jun,14; 2018,Dec,7; 2018,Dec,7; 2018,May,5; 2018,Feb,11; 2018,Jan,8; 2017,Dec,14; 2017,Jan,8; 2016,Jun,8; 2016,Jan,13; 2015,Jan,16; 2014,Aug,5; 2014,Mar,13; 2014,Jan,11

97112 **neuromuscular reeducation of movement, balance, coordination, kinesthetic sense, posture, and/or proprioception for sitting and/or standing activities**
0.99 0.99 **FUD** XXX Ⓢ Ⓐ 80 ▭
AMA: 2018,May,5; 2018,Feb,11; 2018,Jan,8; 2017,Jan,8; 2016,Jan,13; 2015,Jan,16; 2014,Mar,13; 2014,Jan,11

97113 **aquatic therapy with therapeutic exercises**
1.10 1.10 **FUD** XXX Ⓢ Ⓐ 80 ▭
AMA: 2018,May,5; 2018,Feb,11; 2018,Jan,8; 2017,Jan,8; 2016,Jan,13; 2015,Jan,16; 2014,Mar,13; 2014,Jan,11

97116 **gait training (includes stair climbing)**
EXCLUDES *Comprehensive gait/motion analysis (96000-96003)*
0.86 0.86 **FUD** XXX Ⓢ Ⓐ 80 ▭
AMA: 2018,May,5; 2018,Feb,11; 2018,Jan,8; 2017,Jan,8; 2016,Jan,13; 2015,Jan,16; 2014,Mar,13; 2014,Jan,11

97124 **massage, including effleurage, petrissage and/or tapotement (stroking, compression, percussion)**
EXCLUDES *Myofascial release (97140)*
0.81 0.81 **FUD** XXX Ⓢ Ⓐ 80 ▭
AMA: 2019,Jun,14; 2018,May,5; 2018,Feb,11; 2018,Jan,8; 2017,Jan,8; 2016,Jun,8; 2016,Jan,13; 2015,Jan,16; 2014,Mar,13; 2014,Jan,11

97127 ~~Therapeutic interventions that focus on cognitive function (eg, attention, memory, reasoning, executive function, problem solving, and/or pragmatic functioning) and compensatory strategies to manage the performance of an activity (eg, managing time or schedules, initiating, organizing and sequencing tasks), direct (one-on-one) patient contact~~
To report, see (97129)

● **97129** **Therapeutic interventions that focus on cognitive function (eg, attention, memory, reasoning, executive function, problem solving, and/or pragmatic functioning) and compensatory strategies to manage the performance of an activity (eg, managing time or schedules, initiating, organizing, and sequencing tasks), direct (one-on-one) patient contact; initial 15 minutes**
🚑 0.00 ⚕ 0.00 **FUD** 000 ⑤⑴
EXCLUDES Adaptive behavior treatment ([97153], [97155])
Use of code more than one time per-day

● + **97130** **each additional 15 minutes (List separately in addition to code for primary procedure)**
🚑 0.00 ⚕ 0.00 **FUD** 000 ⑤⑴
EXCLUDES Adaptive behavior treatment ([97153], [97155])
Code first (97129)

97139 **Unlisted therapeutic procedure (specify)**
🚑 0.00 ⚕ 0.00 **FUD** XXX A 80
AMA: 2018,May,5; 2018,Feb,11; 2018,Jan,8; 2017,Jan,8; 2016,Jan,13; 2015,Jan,16; 2014,Mar,13; 2014,Jan,11

97140 **Manual therapy techniques (eg, mobilization/manipulation, manual lymphatic drainage, manual traction), 1 or more regions, each 15 minutes**
EXCLUDES Insertion of needle without injection ([20560, 20561])
🚑 0.79 ⚕ 0.79 **FUD** XXX ⑤⑴ A 80
AMA: 2019,Jun,14; 2018,May,5; 2018,Feb,11; 2018,Jan,8; 2017,Jan,8; 2016,Nov,9; 2016,Sep,9; 2016,Aug,3; 2016,Jan,13; 2015,Mar,9; 2015,Jan,16; 2014,Mar,13; 2014,Jan,11

97150 **Therapeutic procedure(s), group (2 or more individuals)**
INCLUDES Constant attendance by the physician/therapist
Reporting this procedure for each member of group
EXCLUDES Adaptive behavior services ([97154], [97158])
Osteopathic manipulative treatment (98925-98929)
🚑 0.52 ⚕ 0.52 **FUD** XXX ⑤⑴ A 80
AMA: 2018,Nov,3; 2018,May,5; 2018,Feb,11; 2018,Jan,8; 2017,Jan,8; 2016,Jan,13; 2015,Jan,16; 2014,Mar,13; 2014,Jan,11

97151 Resequenced code. See code following 96040.
97152 Resequenced code. See code following 96040.
97153 Resequenced code. See code following 96040.
97154 Resequenced code. See code following 96040.
97155 Resequenced code. See code following 96040.
97156 Resequenced code. See code following 96040.
97157 Resequenced code. See code following 96040.
97158 Resequenced code. See code following 96040.
97161 Resequenced code. See code before 97010.
97162 Resequenced code. See code before 97010.
97163 Resequenced code. See code before 97010.
97164 Resequenced code. See code before 97010.
97165 Resequenced code. See code before 97010.
97166 Resequenced code. See code before 97010.
97167 Resequenced code. See code before 97010.
97168 Resequenced code. See code before 97010.
97169 Resequenced code. See code before 97010.
97170 Resequenced code. See code before 97010.
97171 Resequenced code. See code before 97010.
97172 Resequenced code. See code before 97010.

97530 **Therapeutic activities, direct (one-on-one) patient contact (use of dynamic activities to improve functional performance), each 15 minutes**
🚑 1.13 ⚕ 1.13 **FUD** XXX ⑤⑴ A 80
AMA: 2018,Dec,7; 2018,Dec,7; 2018,May,5; 2018,Feb,11; 2018,Jan,8; 2017,Jan,8; 2016,Jan,13; 2015,Jan,16; 2014,Mar,13; 2014,Jan,11

97533 **Sensory integrative techniques to enhance sensory processing and promote adaptive responses to environmental demands, direct (one-on-one) patient contact, each 15 minutes**
🚑 1.21 ⚕ 1.21 **FUD** XXX ⑤⑴ A 80
AMA: 2018,May,5; 2018,Feb,11; 2018,Jan,8; 2017,Jan,8; 2016,Jan,13; 2015,Jan,16; 2014,Mar,13; 2014,Jan,11

97535 **Self-care/home management training (eg, activities of daily living (ADL) and compensatory training, meal preparation, safety procedures, and instructions in use of assistive technology devices/adaptive equipment) direct one-on-one contact, each 15 minutes**
🚑 0.97 ⚕ 0.97 **FUD** XXX ⑤⑴ A 80
AMA: 2018,May,5; 2018,Feb,11; 2018,Jan,8; 2017,Jan,8; 2016,Aug,3; 2016,Jan,13; 2015,Jun,10; 2015,Mar,9; 2015,Jan,16; 2014,Mar,13; 2014,Jan,11

97537 **Community/work reintegration training (eg, shopping, transportation, money management, avocational activities and/or work environment/modification analysis, work task analysis, use of assistive technology device/adaptive equipment), direct one-on-one contact, each 15 minutes**
EXCLUDES Wheelchair management/propulsion training (97542)
🚑 0.93 ⚕ 0.93 **FUD** XXX ⑤⑴ A 80
AMA: 2018,May,5; 2018,Feb,11; 2018,Jan,8; 2017,Jan,8; 2016,Jan,13; 2015,Jan,16; 2014,Mar,13; 2014,Jan,11

97542 **Wheelchair management (eg, assessment, fitting, training), each 15 minutes**
🚑 0.94 ⚕ 0.94 **FUD** XXX ⑤⑴ A 80
AMA: 2018,May,5; 2018,Feb,11; 2018,Jan,8; 2017,Jan,8; 2016,Jan,13; 2015,Jun,10; 2015,Jan,16; 2014,Mar,13; 2014,Jan,11

97545 **Work hardening/conditioning; initial 2 hours**
🚑 0.00 ⚕ 0.00 **FUD** XXX ⑤⑴ A 80
AMA: 2018,May,5; 2018,Feb,11; 2018,Jan,8; 2017,Jan,8; 2016,Jan,13; 2015,Jan,16; 2014,Mar,13; 2014,Jan,11

+ **97546** **each additional hour (List separately in addition to code for primary procedure)**
Code first initial 2 hours (97545)
🚑 0.00 ⚕ 0.00 **FUD** ZZZ ⑤⑴ A 80
AMA: 2018,May,5; 2018,Feb,11; 2018,Jan,8; 2017,Jan,8; 2016,Jan,13; 2015,Jan,16; 2014,Mar,13; 2014,Jan,11

97597-97610 Treatment of Wounds

CMS: 100-02,15,220.4 Functional Reporting; 100-02,15,230.4 Services By a Physical/Occupational Therapist in Private Practice; 100-03,270.3 Blood-derived Products for Chronic Nonhealing Wounds; 100-04,4,200.9 Billing for "Sometimes Therapy" Services that May be Paid as Non-Therapy Services; 100-04,5,10 Part B Outpatient Rehabilitation and Comprehensive Outpatient Rehabilitation Facility (CORF) Services - General; 100-04,5,10.3.2 Exceptions Process; 100-04,5,10.3.3 Use of the KX Modifier

INCLUDES Direct patient contact
Removing devitalized/necrotic tissue and promoting healing

EXCLUDES *Burn wound debridement (16020-16030)*

97597 Debridement (eg, high pressure waterjet with/without suction, sharp selective debridement with scissors, scalpel and forceps), open wound, (eg, fibrin, devitalized epidermis and/or dermis, exudate, debris, biofilm), including topical application(s), wound assessment, use of a whirlpool, when performed and instruction(s) for ongoing care, per session, total wound(s) surface area; first 20 sq cm or less

INCLUDES Chemical cauterization (17250)

🔁 0.68   🔀 2.52   **FUD** 000   SI T 80 ▣

AMA: 2018,May,5; 2018,Feb,11; 2018,Jan,8; 2017,Jan,8; 2016,Oct,3; 2016,Aug,9; 2016,Jan,13; 2015,Jan,16; 2014,Jun,11; 2014,Jan,11

Wound may be washed, addressed with scissors, and/or tweezers and scalpel

+ 97598 each additional 20 sq cm, or part thereof (List separately in addition to code for primary procedure)

INCLUDES Chemical cauterization (17250)
Code first (97597)

🔁 0.32   🔀 0.79   **FUD** ZZZ   SI N 80 ▣

AMA: 2018,May,5; 2018,Feb,11; 2018,Jan,8; 2017,Jan,8; 2016,Oct,3; 2016,Aug,9; 2016,Jan,13; 2015,Jan,16; 2014,Jun,11; 2014,Jan,11

97602 Removal of devitalized tissue from wound(s), non-selective debridement, without anesthesia (eg, wet-to-moist dressings, enzymatic, abrasion, larval therapy), including topical application(s), wound assessment, and instruction(s) for ongoing care, per session

INCLUDES Chemical cauterization (17250)

🔁 0.00   🔀 0.00   **FUD** XXX   SI Q1 ▣

AMA: 2018,May,5; 2018,Feb,11; 2018,Jan,8; 2017,Jan,8; 2016,Oct,3; 2016,Jan,13; 2015,Jan,16; 2014,Jun,11; 2014,Jan,11

97605 Negative pressure wound therapy (eg, vacuum assisted drainage collection), utilizing durable medical equipment (DME), including topical application(s), wound assessment, and instruction(s) for ongoing care, per session; total wound(s) surface area less than or equal to 50 square centimeters

EXCLUDES *Negative pressure wound therapy using disposable medical equipment (97607-97608)*

🔁 0.74   🔀 1.24   **FUD** XXX   SI Q1 80 ▣

AMA: 2018,May,5; 2018,Feb,11; 2018,Jan,8; 2017,Jan,8; 2016,Feb,13; 2016,Jan,13; 2015,Jan,16; 2014,Nov,8; 2014,Jan,11

97606 total wound(s) surface area greater than 50 square centimeters

EXCLUDES *Negative pressure wound therapy using disposable medical equipment (97607-97608)*

🔁 0.80   🔀 1.46   **FUD** XXX   SI Q1 80 ▣

AMA: 2018,May,5; 2018,Feb,11; 2018,Jan,8; 2017,Jan,8; 2016,Feb,13; 2016,Jan,13; 2015,Jan,16; 2014,Nov,8; 2014,Jan,11

97607 Negative pressure wound therapy, (eg, vacuum assisted drainage collection), utilizing disposable, non-durable medical equipment including provision of exudate management collection system, topical application(s), wound assessment, and instructions for ongoing care, per session; total wound(s) surface area less than or equal to 50 square centimeters

EXCLUDES *Negative pressure wound therapy using durable medical equipment (97605-97606)*

🔁 0.00   🔀 0.00   **FUD** XXX   SI T 80 ▣

AMA: 2018,May,5; 2018,Feb,11; 2018,Jan,8; 2017,Jan,8; 2016,Jan,13; 2015,Jan,16; 2014,Nov,8

97608 total wound(s) surface area greater than 50 square centimeters

EXCLUDES *Negative pressure wound therapy using durable medical equipment (97605-97606)*

🔁 0.00   🔀 0.00   **FUD** XXX   SI T 80 ▣

AMA: 2018,May,5; 2018,Feb,11; 2018,Jan,8; 2017,Jan,8; 2016,Jan,13; 2015,Jan,16; 2014,Nov,8

97610 Low frequency, non-contact, non-thermal ultrasound, including topical application(s), when performed, wound assessment, and instruction(s) for ongoing care, per day

🔁 0.48   🔀 6.39   **FUD** XXX   SI Q1 80 ▣

AMA: 2018,May,5; 2018,Feb,11; 2018,Jan,8; 2017,Jan,8; 2016,Jan,13; 2015,Jan,16; 2014,Jun,11

97750-97799 Assessments and Training

CMS: 100-02,15,220 Coverage of Outpatient Rehabilitation Therapy Services; 100-02,15,220.4 Functional Reporting; 100-02,15,230 Practice of Physical Therapy, Occupational Therapy, and Speech-Language Pathology; 100-02,15,230.1 Practice of Physical Therapy; 100-02,15,230.2 Practice of Occupational Therapy; 100-02,15,230.4 Services By a Physical/Occupational Therapist in Private Practice; 100-04,5,10 Part B Outpatient Rehabilitation and Comprehensive Outpatient Rehabilitation Facility (CORF) Services - General; 100-04,5,10.3.2 Therapy Cap Exceptions; 100-04,5,10.3.3 Use of the KX Modifier

97750 Physical performance test or measurement (eg, musculoskeletal, functional capacity), with written report, each 15 minutes

INCLUDES Direct patient contact
EXCLUDES *Electromyography (95860-95872, [95885, 95886, 95887])*
Joint range of motion (95851-95852)
Nerve velocity determination (95905, 95907-95913)

🔁 0.99   🔀 0.99   **FUD** XXX   SI A 80 ▣

AMA: 2018,May,5; 2018,Feb,11; 2018,Jan,8; 2017,Jan,8; 2016,Jan,13; 2015,Jan,16; 2014,Jan,11

26/TC PC/TC Only   A2-Z3 ASC Payment   50 Bilateral   ♂ Male Only   ♀ Female Only   🔁 Facility RVU   🔀 Non-Facility RVU   ▣ CCI   ✖ CLIA
FUD Follow-up Days   CMS: IOM   AMA: CPT Asst   A-Y OPPSI   80/80 Surg Assist Allowed / w/Doc   Lab Crosswalk   Radiology Crosswalk

CPT © 2019 American Medical Association. All Rights Reserved.
© 2019 Optum360, LLC

528

97755 Assistive technology assessment (eg, to restore, augment or compensate for existing function, optimize functional tasks and/or maximize environmental accessibility), direct one-on-one contact, with written report, each 15 minutes

> INCLUDES Direct patient contact
> EXCLUDES Augmentative/alternative communication device (92605, 92607)
> Electromyography (95860-95872, [95885, 95886, 95887])
> Joint range of motion (95851-95852)
> Nerve velocity determination (95905, 95907-95913)
>
> 📷 1.08 ✂ 1.08 **FUD** XXX   �51 Ⓐ 80 💻
>
> **AMA:** 2018,May,5; 2018,Feb,11

97760 Orthotic(s) management and training (including assessment and fitting when not otherwise reported), upper extremity(ies), lower extremity(ies) and/or trunk, initial orthotic(s) encounter, each 15 minutes

> EXCLUDES Gait training, if performed on the same extremity (97116)
>
> 📷 1.35 ✂ 1.35 **FUD** XXX   �51 Ⓐ 80 💻
>
> **AMA:** 2018,May,5; 2018,Feb,11; 2018,Jan,8; 2017,Jan,8; 2016,Jan,13; 2015,Jan,16; 2014,Jan,11

97761 Prosthetic(s) training, upper and/or lower extremity(ies), initial prosthetic(s) encounter, each 15 minutes

> 📷 1.16 ✂ 1.16 **FUD** XXX   �51 Ⓐ 80 💻
>
> **AMA:** 2018,May,5; 2018,Feb,11; 2018,Jan,8; 2017,Jan,8; 2016,Jan,13; 2015,Jan,16; 2014,Jan,11

97763 Orthotic(s)/prosthetic(s) management and/or training, upper extremity(ies), lower extremity(ies), and/or trunk, subsequent orthotic(s)/prosthetic(s) encounter, each 15 minutes

> EXCLUDES Initial encounter for orthotics and prosthetics management and training (97760-97761)
>
> 📷 1.43 ✂ 1.43 **FUD** XXX   �51 Ⓐ 80 💻
>
> **AMA:** 2018,May,5; 2018,Feb,11

97799 Unlisted physical medicine/rehabilitation service or procedure

> 📷 0.00 ✂ 0.00 **FUD** XXX   Ⓐ 80 💻
>
> **AMA:** 2018,May,5; 2018,Feb,11; 2018,Jan,8; 2017,Jan,8; 2016,Nov,9; 2016,Jan,13; 2015,Jan,16; 2014,Jan,11

97802-97804 Medical Nutrition Therapy Services

CMS: 100-02,13,220 Preventive Health Services; 100-03,180.1 Medical Nutrition Therapy; 100-04,12,190.3 List of Telehealth Services; 100-04,12,190.6 Payment Methodology for Physician/Practitioner at the Distant Site ; 100-04,12,190.6.1 Submission of Telehealth Claims for Distant Site Practitioners; 100-04,12,190.7 Contractor Editing of Telehealth Claims; 100-04,4,300 Medical Nutrition Therapy Services; 100-04,4,300.6 CWF Edits for MNT/DSMT

> EXCLUDES Medical nutrition therapy assessment/intervention provided by physician or other qualified health care provider; use appropriate E&M codes

97802 Medical nutrition therapy; initial assessment and intervention, individual, face-to-face with the patient, each 15 minutes

> 📷 0.96 ✂ 1.05 **FUD** XXX   ★ Ⓐ 80 💻
>
> **AMA:** 2018,Feb,11; 2018,Jan,8; 2017,Jan,8; 2016,Jan,13; 2015,Jan,16; 2014,Jan,11

97803 re-assessment and intervention, individual, face-to-face with the patient, each 15 minutes

> 📷 0.82 ✂ 0.91 **FUD** XXX   ★ Ⓐ 80 💻
>
> **AMA:** 2018,Feb,11; 2018,Jan,8; 2017,Jan,8; 2016,Jan,13; 2015,Jan,16; 2014,Jan,11

97804 group (2 or more individual(s)), each 30 minutes

> 📷 0.45 ✂ 0.48 **FUD** XXX   ★ Ⓐ 80 💻
>
> **AMA:** 2018,Feb,11; 2018,Jan,8; 2017,Jan,8; 2016,Jan,13; 2015,Jan,16; 2014,Jan,11

97810-97814 Acupuncture

CMS: 100-03,10.3 Inpatient Pain Rehabilitation Programs; 100-03,10.4 Outpatient Hospital Pain Rehabilitation Programs; 100-03,30.3 Acupuncture; 100-03,30.3.1 Acupuncture for Fibromyalgia; 100-03,30.3.2 Acupuncture for Osteoarthritis

> INCLUDES 15 minute increments of face-to-face contact with the patient
> Reporting only one code for each 15 minute increment
> EXCLUDES Insertion of needle without injection ([20560, 20561])
> Code also significant separately identifiable E&M service using modifier 25, when performed

97810 Acupuncture, 1 or more needles; without electrical stimulation, initial 15 minutes of personal one-on-one contact with the patient

> EXCLUDES Treatment with electrical stimulation (97813-97814)
>
> 📷 0.87 ✂ 1.03 **FUD** XXX   E 💻
>
> **AMA:** 2018,Feb,11; 2018,Jan,8; 2017,Jan,8; 2016,Jan,13; 2015,Jan,16; 2014,Jan,11

+ 97811 without electrical stimulation, each additional 15 minutes of personal one-on-one contact with the patient, with re-insertion of needle(s) (List separately in addition to code for primary procedure)

> EXCLUDES Treatment with electrical stimulation (97813-97814)
> Code first initial 15 minutes (97810)
>
> 📷 0.72 ✂ 0.78 **FUD** ZZZ   E 💻
>
> **AMA:** 2018,Feb,11; 2018,Jan,8; 2017,Jan,8; 2016,Jan,13; 2015,Jan,16; 2014,Jan,11

97813 with electrical stimulation, initial 15 minutes of personal one-on-one contact with the patient

> EXCLUDES Treatment without electrical stimulation (97813-97814)
>
> 📷 0.94 ✂ 1.13 **FUD** XXX   E 💻
>
> **AMA:** 2018,Feb,11; 2018,Jan,8; 2017,Jan,8; 2016,Jan,13; 2015,Jan,16; 2014,Jan,11

+ 97814 with electrical stimulation, each additional 15 minutes of personal one-on-one contact with the patient, with re-insertion of needle(s) (List separately in addition to code for primary procedure)

> EXCLUDES Treatment without electrical stimulation (97813-97814)
> Code first initial 15 minutes (97813)
>
> 📷 0.79 ✂ 0.91 **FUD** ZZZ   E 💻
>
> **AMA:** 2018,Feb,11; 2018,Jan,8; 2017,Jan,8; 2016,Jan,13; 2015,Jan,16; 2014,Jan,11

98925-98929 Osteopathic Manipulation

CMS: 100-03,150.1 Manipulation

> INCLUDES Physician applied manual treatment done to eliminate/alleviate somatic dysfunction and related disorders using a variety of techniques
> The following body regions:
> Abdomen/visceral region
> Cervical region
> Head region
> Lower extremities
> Lumbar region
> Pelvic region
> Rib cage region
> Sacral region
> Thoracic region
> Upper extremities
> Code also significant separately identifiable E&M service using modifier 25, when performed

98925 Osteopathic manipulative treatment (OMT); 1-2 body regions involved

> 📷 0.68 ✂ 0.89 **FUD** 000   🔾1 80 💻
>
> **AMA:** 2018,Aug,9; 2018,Feb,11; 2018,Jan,8; 2017,Dec,14; 2017,Jan,8; 2016,Jan,13; 2015,Jan,16; 2014,Jan,11

98926 3-4 body regions involved

> 📷 1.02 ✂ 1.28 **FUD** 000   🔾1 80 💻
>
> **AMA:** 2018,Aug,9; 2018,Feb,11; 2018,Jan,8; 2017,Jan,8; 2016,Jan,13; 2015,Jan,16; 2014,Jan,11

98927 5-6 body regions involved

> 📷 1.35 ✂ 1.68 **FUD** 000   🔾1 80 💻
>
> **AMA:** 2018,Aug,9; 2018,Feb,11; 2018,Jan,8; 2017,Jan,8; 2016,Jan,13; 2015,Jan,16; 2014,Jan,11

98928 7-8 body regions involved
🔶 1.69 ⚕ 2.04 **FUD** 000 `01` `80` ▭
AMA: 2018,Aug,9; 2018,Feb,11; 2018,Jan,8; 2017,Jan,8; 2016,Jan,13; 2015,Jan,16; 2014,Jan,11

98929 9-10 body regions involved
🔶 2.05 ⚕ 2.44 **FUD** 000 `01` `80` ▭
AMA: 2018,Aug,9; 2018,Feb,11; 2018,Jan,8; 2017,Jan,8; 2016,Jan,13; 2015,Jan,16; 2014,Jan,11

98940-98943 Chiropractic Manipulation

CMS: 100-01,5,70.6 Chiropractors; 100-02,15,240 Chiropractic Services - General; 100-02,15,240.1.3 Necessity for Treatment; 100-02,15,30.5 Chiropractor's Services; 100-03,150.1 Manipulation

INCLUDES Form of manual treatment performed to influence joint/neurophysical function
The following five extraspinal regions:
Abdomen
Head, including temporomandibular joint, excluding atlanto-occipital region
Lower extremities
Rib cage, not including costotransverse/costovertebral joints
Upper extremities
The following five spinal regions:
Cervical region (atlanto-occipital joint)
Lumbar region
Pelvic region (sacro-iliac joint)
Sacral region
Thoracic region (costovertebral/costotransverse joints)
Code also significant separately identifiable E&M service using modifier 25 when performed

98940 Chiropractic manipulative treatment (CMT); spinal, 1-2 regions
🔶 0.64 ⚕ 0.80 **FUD** 000 `01` `80` ▭
AMA: 2018,Nov,11; 2018,Feb,11; 2018,Jan,8; 2017,Jan,8; 2016,Jan,13; 2015,Jan,16; 2014,Jan,11

98941 spinal, 3-4 regions
🔶 0.98 ⚕ 1.16 **FUD** 000 `01` `80` ▭
AMA: 2018,Nov,11; 2018,Feb,11; 2018,Jan,8; 2017,Jan,8; 2016,Jan,13; 2015,Jan,16; 2014,Jan,11

98942 spinal, 5 regions
🔶 1.33 ⚕ 1.50 **FUD** 000 `01` `80` ▭
AMA: 2018,Nov,11; 2018,Feb,11; 2018,Jan,8; 2017,Jan,8; 2016,Jan,13; 2015,Jan,16; 2014,Jan,11

98943 extraspinal, 1 or more regions
🔶 0.67 ⚕ 0.77 **FUD** XXX `E` ▭
AMA: 2018,Nov,11; 2018,Feb,11; 2018,Jan,8; 2017,Jan,8; 2016,Jan,13; 2015,Jan,16; 2014,Jan,11

98960-98962 Self-Management Training

INCLUDES Education/training services:
Prescribed by a physician or other qualified health care professional
Provided by a qualified nonphysician health care provider
Standardized curriculum that may be modified as necessary for:
Clinical needs
Cultural norms
Health literacy
Teaching the patient how to manage the illness/delay the comorbidity(s)

EXCLUDES *Genetic counseling education services (96040, 98961-98962)*
Health and behavior assessment and intervention (96156, 96158-96159, [96164, 96165], [96167, 96168], [96170, 96171])
Medical nutrition therapy (97802-97804)
The following services:
Counseling/education to a group (99078)
Collection/interpretation of physiologic data ([99091])
Complex chronic care management (99487, 99489)
Counseling/risk factor reduction without symptoms/established disease (99401-99412)
Physician supervision in home, domiciliary, or rest home (99339, 99340, 99374-99375, 99379-99380)
Services provided with cumulative time of less than 5 minutes
Services provided in which time would be reported with other services
Supervision of hospice patient (99377-99378)
Transitional care management (99495, 99496)

98960 Education and training for patient self-management by a qualified, nonphysician health care professional using a standardized curriculum, face-to-face with the patient (could include caregiver/family) each 30 minutes; individual patient
🔶 0.77 ⚕ 0.77 **FUD** XXX ★ `E` ▭
AMA: 2018,Aug,6; 2018,Feb,11; 2018,Jan,8; 2017,Jan,8; 2016,Jan,13; 2015,Jan,16; 2014,Oct,3; 2014,Jan,11

98961 2-4 patients
INCLUDES Group education regarding genetic risks
🔶 0.38 ⚕ 0.38 **FUD** XXX ★ `E` ▭
AMA: 2018,Aug,6; 2018,Feb,11; 2018,Jan,8; 2017,Jan,8; 2016,Jan,13; 2015,Jan,16; 2014,Oct,3; 2014,Jan,11

98962 5-8 patients
INCLUDES Group education regarding genetic risks
🔶 0.28 ⚕ 0.28 **FUD** XXX ★ `E` ▭
AMA: 2018,Aug,6; 2018,Feb,11; 2018,Jan,8; 2017,Jan,8; 2016,Jan,13; 2015,Jan,16; 2014,Oct,3; 2014,Jan,11

98966-98968 Nonphysician Telephone Services

INCLUDES Assessment and management services provided by telephone by a qualified health care professional
Episode of care initiated by an established patient or his/her guardian

EXCLUDES *Call initiated by the qualified health care professional*
Calls during the postoperative period of a procedure
Decision to see the patient at the next available urgent care appointment
Decision to see the patient within 24 hours of the call
Monitoring of INR (93792-93793)
Patient management services during same time frame as (99487-99489, 99495-99496)
Telephone services provided by a physician (99441-99443)
Telephone services that are considered a part of a previous or subsequent service
Use of codes if same codes billed within the past seven days

98966 Telephone assessment and management service provided by a qualified nonphysician health care professional to an established patient, parent, or guardian not originating from a related assessment and management service provided within the previous 7 days nor leading to an assessment and management service or procedure within the next 24 hours or soonest available appointment; 5-10 minutes of medical discussion
🔶 0.36 ⚕ 0.39 **FUD** XXX `E` ▭
AMA: 2018,Mar,7; 2018,Feb,11; 2018,Jan,8; 2017,Jan,8; 2016,Jan,13; 2015,Jan,16; 2014,Oct,3; 2014,Jan,11

98967 11-20 minutes of medical discussion
🔶 0.72 ⚕ 0.76 **FUD** XXX `E` ▭
AMA: 2018,Mar,7; 2018,Feb,11; 2018,Jan,8; 2017,Jan,8; 2016,Jan,13; 2015,Jan,16; 2014,Oct,3; 2014,Jan,11

| 26/TC PC/TC Only | A2-Z3 ASC Payment | 50 Bilateral | ♂ Male Only | ♀ Female Only | 🔶 Facility RVU | ⚕ Non-Facility RVU | ▭ CCI | ✖ CLIA |
| FUD Follow-up Days | CMS: IOM | AMA: CPT Asst | A-Y OPPSI | 80/80 Surg Assist Allowed / w/Doc | ⬛ Lab Crosswalk | ⬛ Radiology Crosswalk |

530   CPT © 2019 American Medical Association. All Rights Reserved.   © 2019 Optum360, LLC

98968 **21-30 minutes of medical discussion**
🔷 1.08   🔶 1.12   **FUD** XXX   E ▣

AMA: 2018,Mar,7; 2018,Feb,11; 2018,Jan,8; 2017,Jan,8; 2016,Jan,13; 2015,Jan,16; 2014,Oct,3; 2014,Jan,11

98969-98972 Nonphysician Online Service

Timely reply to the patient as well as:
Ordering laboratory services
Permanent record of the service; either hard copy or electronic
Providing a prescription
Related telephone calls

EXCLUDES *Monitoring of INR (93792-93793)*
Online digital assessment and management service provided by a qualified health care professional ([99421, 99422, 99423])
Online evaluation service:
Provided during the postoperative period of a procedure
Provided more than once in a seven day period
Related to a service provided in the previous seven days
Provided with cumulative time of less than 5 minutes
Where time would be reported as part of another service
Patient management services during same time frame as:
Collection/interpretation of physiologic data ([99091])
Complex chronic care management (99487-99489)
Physician supervision in home, domiciliary, or rest home (99339-99340, 99374-99375, 99379-99380)
Supervision of hospice patient (99377-99378)
Transitional care management (99495-99496)

98969 ~~Online assessment and management service provided by a qualified nonphysician health care professional to an established patient or guardian, not originating from a related assessment and management service provided within the previous 7 days, using the Internet or similar electronic communications network~~

To report, see (98970-98972)

● **98970** **Qualified nonphysician health care professional online digital evaluation and management service, for an established patient, for up to 7 days, cumulative time during the 7 days; 5-10 minutes**

● **98971** **11-20 minutes**

● **98972** **21 or more minutes**

99000-99091 Supplemental Services and Supplies

INCLUDES Supplemental reporting for services adjunct to the basic service provided

99000 **Handling and/or conveyance of specimen for transfer from the office to a laboratory**
🔷 0.00   🔶 0.00   **FUD** XXX   E ▣

AMA: 2018,Dec,10; 2018,Dec,10; 2018,Feb,11; 2018,Jan,8; 2017,Jan,8; 2016,Jan,13; 2015,Jan,16; 2014,Jan,11

99001 **Handling and/or conveyance of specimen for transfer from the patient in other than an office to a laboratory (distance may be indicated)**
🔷 0.00   🔶 0.00   **FUD** XXX   E ▣

AMA: 2018,Dec,10; 2018,Dec,10; 2018,Feb,11; 2018,Jan,8; 2017,Jan,8; 2016,Jan,13; 2015,Jan,16; 2014,Jan,11

99002 **Handling, conveyance, and/or any other service in connection with the implementation of an order involving devices (eg, designing, fitting, packaging, handling, delivery or mailing) when devices such as orthotics, protectives, prosthetics are fabricated by an outside laboratory or shop but which items have been designed, and are to be fitted and adjusted by the attending physician or other qualified health care professional**

EXCLUDES *Venous blood routine collection (36415)*
🔷 0.00   🔶 0.00   **FUD** XXX   B ▣

AMA: 2018,Dec,10; 2018,Dec,10; 2018,Feb,11; 2018,Jan,8; 2017,Jan,8; 2016,Jan,13; 2015,Jan,16; 2014,Jan,11

99024 **Postoperative follow-up visit, normally included in the surgical package, to indicate that an evaluation and management service was performed during a postoperative period for a reason(s) related to the original procedure**
🔷 0.00   🔶 0.00   **FUD** XXX   B ▣

AMA: 2018,Dec,10; 2018,Dec,10; 2018,Feb,11; 2018,Jan,8; 2017,Jul,9; 2017,Jan,3; 2017,Jan,8; 2016,Jan,13; 2015,Mar,3; 2015,Jan,16; 2014,Jan,11

99026 **Hospital mandated on call service; in-hospital, each hour**
EXCLUDES *Physician stand-by services with prolonged physician attendance (99360)*
Time spent providing procedures or services that may be separately reported
🔷 0.00   🔶 0.00   **FUD** XXX   E ▣

AMA: 2018,Dec,10; 2018,Dec,10; 2018,Feb,11; 2018,Jan,8; 2017,Jan,8; 2016,Jan,13; 2015,Jan,16; 2014,Jan,11

99027 **out-of-hospital, each hour**
EXCLUDES *Physician stand-by services with prolonged physician attendance (99360)*
Time spent providing procedures or services that may be separately reported
🔷 0.00   🔶 0.00   **FUD** XXX   E ▣

AMA: 2018,Dec,10; 2018,Dec,10; 2018,Feb,11; 2018,Jan,8; 2017,Jan,8; 2016,Jan,13; 2015,Jan,16; 2014,Jan,11

99050 **Services provided in the office at times other than regularly scheduled office hours, or days when the office is normally closed (eg, holidays, Saturday or Sunday), in addition to basic service**

Code also more than one adjunct code per encounter when appropriate
Code first basic service provided
🔷 0.00   🔶 0.00   **FUD** XXX   ⑤① B ▣

AMA: 2018,Dec,10; 2018,Dec,10; 2018,Feb,11; 2018,Jan,8; 2017,Jan,8; 2016,Jan,13; 2015,Jan,16; 2014,Jan,11

99051 **Service(s) provided in the office during regularly scheduled evening, weekend, or holiday office hours, in addition to basic service**

Code also more than one adjunct code per encounter when appropriate
Code first basic service provided
🔷 0.00   🔶 0.00   **FUD** XXX   ⑤① B ▣

AMA: 2018,Dec,10; 2018,Dec,10; 2018,Feb,11; 2018,Jan,8; 2017,Jan,8; 2016,Jan,13; 2015,Jan,16; 2014,Jan,11

99053 **Service(s) provided between 10:00 PM and 8:00 AM at 24-hour facility, in addition to basic service**

Code also more than one adjunct code per encounter when appropriate
Code first basic service provided
🔷 0.00   🔶 0.00   **FUD** XXX   ⑤① B ▣

AMA: 2018,Dec,10; 2018,Dec,10; 2018,Feb,11; 2018,Jan,8; 2017,Jan,8; 2016,Jan,13; 2015,Jan,16; 2014,Jan,11

99056 **Service(s) typically provided in the office, provided out of the office at request of patient, in addition to basic service**

Code also more than one adjunct code per encounter when appropriate
Code first basic service provided
🔷 0.00   🔶 0.00   **FUD** XXX   ⑤① B ▣

AMA: 2018,Dec,10; 2018,Dec,10; 2018,Feb,11; 2018,Jan,8; 2017,Jan,8; 2016,Jan,13; 2015,Jan,16; 2014,Jan,11

99058 **Service(s) provided on an emergency basis in the office, which disrupts other scheduled office services, in addition to basic service**

Code also more than one adjunct code per encounter when appropriate
Code first basic service provided
🔷 0.00   🔶 0.00   **FUD** XXX   ⑤① B ▣

AMA: 2018,Dec,10; 2018,Dec,10; 2018,Feb,11; 2018,Jan,8; 2017,Jan,8; 2016,Jan,13; 2015,Jan,16; 2014,Jan,11

Medicine

99060 Service(s) provided on an emergency basis, out of the office, which disrupts other scheduled office services, in addition to basic service

> Code also more than one adjunct code per encounter when appropriate
> Code first basic service provided
> 🚑 0.00 ⚬ 0.00 **FUD** XXX Ⓢ Ⓑ 🖃
> **AMA:** 2018,Dec,10; 2018,Dec,10; 2018,Feb,11; 2018,Jan,8; 2017,Jan,8; 2016,Jan,13; 2015,Jan,16; 2014,Jan,11

99070 Supplies and materials (except spectacles), provided by the physician or other qualified health care professional over and above those usually included with the office visit or other services rendered (list drugs, trays, supplies, or materials provided)

> EXCLUDES Spectacles supply
> 🚑 0.00 ⚬ 0.00 **FUD** XXX Ⓑ 🖃
> **AMA:** 2019,Apr,10; 2019,Feb,10; 2018,Dec,10; 2018,Dec,10; 2018,Jun,11; 2018,Mar,7; 2018,Jan,8; 2018,Jan,3; 2017,Sep,14; 2017,Jan,6; 2017,Jan,8; 2016,Jan,13; 2015,Jan,16; 2014,Mar,11; 2014,Jan,11

99071 Educational supplies, such as books, tapes, and pamphlets, for the patient's education at cost to physician or other qualified health care professional

> 🚑 0.00 ⚬ 0.00 **FUD** XXX Ⓑ 🖃
> **AMA:** 2018,Dec,10; 2018,Dec,10; 2018,Jan,8; 2017,Jan,8; 2016,Jan,13; 2015,Jan,16; 2014,Oct,3; 2014,Jan,11

99075 Medical testimony

> 🚑 0.00 ⚬ 0.00 **FUD** XXX Ⓔ 🖃
> **AMA:** 2018,Dec,10; 2018,Dec,10; 2018,Jan,8; 2017,Jan,8; 2016,Jan,13; 2015,Jan,16; 2014,Jan,11

99078 Physician or other qualified health care professional qualified by education, training, licensure/regulation (when applicable) educational services rendered to patients in a group setting (eg, prenatal, obesity, or diabetic instructions)

> 🚑 0.00 ⚬ 0.00 **FUD** XXX Ⓝ 🖃
> **AMA:** 2018,Dec,10; 2018,Dec,10; 2018,Jan,8; 2017,Jan,8; 2016,Jan,13; 2015,Jan,16; 2014,Oct,3; 2014,Jan,11

99080 Special reports such as insurance forms, more than the information conveyed in the usual medical communications or standard reporting form

> EXCLUDES Completion of workmen's compensation forms (99455-99456)
> 🚑 0.00 ⚬ 0.00 **FUD** XXX Ⓑ 🖃
> **AMA:** 2018,Dec,10; 2018,Dec,10; 2018,Jan,8; 2017,Jan,8; 2016,Jan,13; 2015,Jan,16; 2014,Oct,3; 2014,Jan,11

99082 Unusual travel (eg, transportation and escort of patient)

> 🚑 0.00 ⚬ 0.00 **FUD** XXX Ⓑ 80 🖃
> **AMA:** 2018,Dec,10; 2018,Dec,10; 2018,Jan,8; 2017,Jan,8; 2016,Jan,13; 2015,Jan,16; 2014,Jan,11

99091 Resequenced code. See code following resequenced code 99454.

99100-99140 Modifying Factors for Anesthesia Services

CMS: 100-04,12,140.3 Payment for Qualified Nonphysician Anesthetists; 100-04,12,140.3.3 Billing Modifiers; 100-04,12,140.3.4 General Billing Instructions; 100-04,12,140.4.1 Anesthesiologist/Qualified Nonphysican Anesthetist; 100-04,12,140.4.2 Anesthetist and Anesthesiologist in a Single Procedure; 100-04,12,140.4.4 Conversion Factors for Anesthesia Services; 100-04,4,250.3.2 Anesthesia in a Hospital Outpatient Setting

> Code first primary anesthesia procedure

+ **99100** Anesthesia for patient of extreme age, younger than 1 year and older than 70 (List separately in addition to code for primary anesthesia procedure) Ⓐ

> EXCLUDES Anesthesia services for infants one year old or less at the time of surgery (00326, 00561, 00834, 00836)
> 🚑 0.00 ⚬ 0.00 **FUD** ZZZ Ⓑ 🖃
> **AMA:** 2018,Jan,8; 2017,Dec,8; 2017,Jan,8; 2016,Jan,13; 2015,Jan,16; 2014,Jan,11

+ **99116** Anesthesia complicated by utilization of total body hypothermia (List separately in addition to code for primary anesthesia procedure)

> EXCLUDES Anesthesia for procedures on heart/pericardial sac/great vessels of chest with pump oxygenator (00561)
> 🚑 0.00 ⚬ 0.00 **FUD** ZZZ 🖃
> **AMA:** 2018,Jan,8; 2017,Dec,8; 2017,Jan,8; 2016,Jan,13; 2015,Jan,16; 2014,Jan,11

+ **99135** Anesthesia complicated by utilization of controlled hypotension (List separately in addition to code for primary anesthesia procedure)

> EXCLUDES Anesthesia for procedures on heart/pericardial sac/great vessels of chest with pump oxygenator (00561)
> 🚑 0.00 ⚬ 0.00 **FUD** ZZZ Ⓑ 🖃
> **AMA:** 2018,Jan,8; 2017,Dec,8; 2017,Jan,8; 2016,Jan,13; 2015,Jan,16; 2014,Jan,11

+ **99140** Anesthesia complicated by emergency conditions (specify) (List separately in addition to code for primary anesthesia procedure)

> INCLUDES Conditions where postponement of treatment could be dangerous to life or health
> 🚑 0.00 ⚬ 0.00 **FUD** ZZZ Ⓑ 🖃
> **AMA:** 2018,Jan,8; 2017,Dec,8; 2017,Jan,8; 2016,Jan,13; 2015,Jan,16; 2014,Jan,11

99151-99157 Moderate Sedation Services

> INCLUDES Intraservice work that begins with administration of the sedation drugs and ends when the procedure is over
> Monitoring of:
> Patient response to the drugs
> Vital signs
> Ordering and providing the drug to the patient (first and subsequent)
> Pre- and postservice procedures

99151 Moderate sedation services provided by the same physician or other qualified health care professional performing the diagnostic or therapeutic service that the sedation supports, requiring the presence of an independent trained observer to assist in the monitoring of the patient's level of consciousness and physiological status; initial 15 minutes of intraservice time, patient younger than 5 years of age

> INCLUDES First 15 minutes of intraservice time for patients under age 5
> Services provided to patients by same provider of the service for which moderate sedation is necessary with monitoring by a trained observer
> 🚑 0.70 ⚬ 2.20 **FUD** XXX ⊘ Ⓝ 🖃
> **AMA:** 2019,Feb,10; 2018,Jan,8; 2017,Sep,11; 2017,Jun,3; 2017,Jan,3

99152 initial 15 minutes of intraservice time, patient age 5 years or older

> INCLUDES First 15 minutes of intraservice time for patients age 5 and over
> Services provided to patients by same provider of the service for which moderate sedation is necessary with monitoring by a trained observer
> 🚑 0.36 ⚬ 1.46 **FUD** XXX ⊘ Ⓝ 🖃
> **AMA:** 2019,May,10; 2019,Feb,10; 2018,Jan,8; 2017,Sep,11; 2017,Jun,3; 2017,Jan,3

+ **99153** each additional 15 minutes intraservice time (List separately in addition to code for primary service)

> INCLUDES Services provided to patients by same provider of the service for which moderate sedation is necessary with monitoring by a trained observer (99155-99157)
> EXCLUDES Services provided to patients by a physician/other qualified health care professional other than the provider rendering the service
> Code first (99151-99152)
> 🚑 0.31 ⚬ 0.31 **FUD** ZZZ Ⓝ 🇹🇨
> **AMA:** 2019,May,10; 2019,Feb,10; 2018,Jan,8; 2017,Sep,11; 2017,Jun,3; 2017,Jan,3

26/TC PC/TC Only A2-Z3 ASC Payment 50 Bilateral ♂ Male Only ♀ Female Only 🚑 Facility RVU ⚬ Non-Facility RVU 🖃 CCI 🗙 CLIA
FUD Follow-up Days **CMS:** IOM **AMA:** CPT Asst A-Y OPPSI 80/80 Surg Assist Allowed / w/Doc Lab Crosswalk Radiology Crosswalk

CPT © 2019 American Medical Association. All Rights Reserved.

532

© 2019 Optum360, LLC

99155 Moderate sedation services provided by a physician or other qualified health care professional other than the physician or other qualified health care professional performing the diagnostic or therapeutic service that the sedation supports; initial 15 minutes of intraservice time, patient younger than 5 years of age

INCLUDES First 15 minutes of intraservice time for patients under age 5

Services provided to patients by a physician/other qualified health care professional other than the provider rendering the service for which moderate sedation is necessary

🔲 2.74 ⚕ 2.74 **FUD** XXX 🅽 🔲

AMA: 2019,Feb,10; 2018,Jan,8; 2017,Sep,11; 2017,Jun,3; 2017,Jan,3

99156 initial 15 minutes of intraservice time, patient age 5 years or older

INCLUDES First 15 minutes of intraservice time for patients age 5 and over

Services provided to patients by a physician/other qualified health care professional other than the provider rendering the service for which moderate sedation is necessary

🔲 2.15 ⚕ 2.15 **FUD** XXX 🅽 🔲

AMA: 2019,Feb,10; 2018,Jan,8; 2017,Sep,11; 2017,Jun,3; 2017,Jan,3

+ **99157** each additional 15 minutes intraservice time (List separately in addition to code for primary service)

INCLUDES Each subsequent 15 minutes of services

Services provided to patients by a physician/other qualified health care professional other than the provider rendering the service for which moderate sedation is necessary (99151-99152)

EXCLUDES Services provided to patients by same provider of-the service for which moderate sedation is necessary with monitoring by a trained observer (99151-99152)

Code first (99155-99156)

🔲 1.64 ⚕ 1.64 **FUD** ZZZ 🅽 🔲

AMA: 2019,Feb,10; 2018,Jan,8; 2017,Sep,11; 2017,Jun,3; 2017,Jan,3

99170 Specialized Examination of Child

EXCLUDES Moderate sedation (99151-99157)

99170 Anogenital examination, magnified, in childhood for suspected trauma, including image recording when performed 🅰

🔲 2.47 ⚕ 4.48 **FUD** 000 🆃 🔲

AMA: 2018,Jan,8; 2017,Jan,8; 2016,Jan,13; 2015,Jan,16; 2014,Sep,7; 2014,Jan,11

99172-99173 Visual Acuity Screening Tests

INCLUDES Graduated visual acuity stimuli that allow a quantitative determination/estimation of visual acuity

EXCLUDES General ophthalmological or E&M services

99172 Visual function screening, automated or semi-automated bilateral quantitative determination of visual acuity, ocular alignment, color vision by pseudoisochromatic plates, and field of vision (may include all or some screening of the determination[s] for contrast sensitivity, vision under glare)

EXCLUDES Screening for visual acuity, amblyogenic factors, retinal polarization scan (99173, 99174 [99177], 0469T)

🔲 0.00 ⚕ 0.00 **FUD** XXX 🅴 🔲

AMA: 2018,Jan,8; 2017,Jan,8; 2016,Jan,13; 2015,Jan,16; 2014,Jan,11

99173 Screening test of visual acuity, quantitative, bilateral

EXCLUDES Screening for visual function, amblyogenic factors (99172, 99174, [99177])

🔲 0.08 ⚕ 0.08 **FUD** XXX 🅴 🔲

AMA: 2018,Jan,8; 2017,Jan,8; 2016,Jan,13; 2015,Jan,16; 2014,Jan,11

99174-99177 [99177] Screening For Amblyogenic Factors

EXCLUDES General ophthalmological services (92002-92014)
Screening for visual acuity (99172-99173, [99177])

99174 Instrument-based ocular screening (eg, photoscreening, automated-refraction), bilateral; with remote analysis and report

EXCLUDES Ocular screening on-site analysis ([99177])

🔲 0.16 ⚕ 0.16 **FUD** XXX 🅴 🔲

AMA: 2018,Feb,3; 2018,Jan,8; 2017,Jan,8; 2016,Mar,10; 2016,Jan,13; 2015,Jan,16; 2014,Jan,11

\# **99177** with on-site analysis

EXCLUDES Remote ocular screening (99174)
Retinal polarization scan (0469T)

🔲 0.13 ⚕ 0.13 **FUD** XXX 🅴 🔲

AMA: 2018,Feb,3; 2018,Jan,8; 2017,Jan,8; 2016,Mar,10

99175-99177 Drug Administration to Induce Vomiting

EXCLUDES Diagnostic gastric lavage (43754-43755)
Diagnostic gastric intubation (43754-43755)

99175 Ipecac or similar administration for individual emesis and continued observation until stomach adequately emptied of poison

🔲 0.73 ⚕ 0.73 **FUD** XXX 🅽 80 🔲

AMA: 1997,Nov,1

99177 **Resequenced code. See code following 99174.**

99183-99184 Hyperbaric Oxygen Therapy

CMS: 100-03,20.29 Hyperbaric Oxygen Therapy; 100-04,32,30.1 HBO Therapy for Lower Extremity Diabetic Wounds

EXCLUDES E&M services, when performed
Other procedures such as wound debridement, when performed

99183 Physician or other qualified health care professional attendance and supervision of hyperbaric oxygen therapy, per session

🔲 3.12 ⚕ 3.12 **FUD** XXX 🅱 80 26 🔲

AMA: 2018,Jan,8; 2017,Jan,8; 2016,Jan,13; 2015,Jan,16; 2014,Jan,11

99184 Initiation of selective head or total body hypothermia in the critically ill neonate, includes appropriate patient selection by review of clinical, imaging and laboratory data, confirmation of esophageal temperature probe location, evaluation of amplitude EEG, supervision of controlled hypothermia, and assessment of patient tolerance of cooling 🅰

EXCLUDES Use of code more than one time per hospitalization

🔲 6.33 ⚕ 6.33 **FUD** XXX 🅲 80 🔲

AMA: 2018,Jan,8; 2017,Jan,8; 2016,Jan,13; 2015,Oct,8

99188 Topical Fluoride Application

99188 Application of topical fluoride varnish by a physician or other qualified health care professional

🔲 0.29 ⚕ 0.35 **FUD** XXX 🅴 80 🔲

99190-99192 Assemble and Manage Pump with Oxygenator/Heat Exchange

99190 Assembly and operation of pump with oxygenator or heat exchanger (with or without ECG and/or pressure monitoring); each hour

🔲 0.00 ⚕ 0.00 **FUD** XXX 🅲 🔲

AMA: 1997,Nov,1

99191 45 minutes

🔲 0.00 ⚕ 0.00 **FUD** XXX 🅲 🔲

AMA: 1997,Nov,1

99192 30 minutes

🔲 0.00 ⚕ 0.00 **FUD** XXX 🅲 🔲

AMA: 1997,Nov,1

Medicine

99195—99607

99195-99199 Therapeutic Phlebotomy and Unlisted Procedures

99195   Phlebotomy, therapeutic (separate procedure)
🔲 2.86   🔲 2.86   **FUD** XXX   01 80 🔲

AMA: 2018,Jan,8; 2017,Jan,8; 2016,Jan,13; 2015,Jan,16; 2014,Jan,11

99199   Unlisted special service, procedure or report
🔲 0.00   🔲 0.00   **FUD** XXX   B 80 🔲

AMA: 2018,Jan,8; 2017,Jan,8; 2016,Jan,13; 2015,Jan,16; 2014,Jan,11

99500-99602 Home Visit By Non-Physician Professionals

INCLUDES Services performed by non-physician providers
Services provided in patient's:
     Assisted living apartment
     Custodial care facility
     Group home
     Non-traditional private home
     Residence
     School
EXCLUDES Home visits performed by physicians (99341-99350)
     Other services/procedures provided by physicians to patients at home
Code also home visit E&M codes if health care provider is authorized to use (99341-99350)
Code also significant separately identifiable E&M service, when performed

99500   Home visit for prenatal monitoring and assessment to include fetal heart rate, non-stress test, uterine monitoring, and gestational diabetes monitoring   M ♀
🔲 0.00   🔲 0.00   **FUD** XXX   E 🔲

AMA: 2018,Jan,8; 2017,Jan,8; 2016,Jan,13; 2015,Jan,16; 2014,Jan,11

99501   Home visit for postnatal assessment and follow-up care   M ♀
🔲 0.00   🔲 0.00   **FUD** XXX   E 🔲

AMA: 2018,Jan,8; 2017,Jan,8; 2016,Jan,13; 2015,Jan,16; 2014,Jan,11

99502   Home visit for newborn care and assessment   A
🔲 0.00   🔲 0.00   **FUD** XXX   E 🔲

AMA: 2018,Jan,8; 2017,Jan,8; 2016,Jan,13; 2015,Jan,16; 2014,Jan,11

99503   Home visit for respiratory therapy care (eg, bronchodilator, oxygen therapy, respiratory assessment, apnea evaluation)
🔲 0.00   🔲 0.00   **FUD** XXX   E 🔲

AMA: 2018,Jan,8; 2017,Jan,8; 2016,Jan,13; 2015,Jan,16; 2014,Jan,11

99504   Home visit for mechanical ventilation care
🔲 0.00   🔲 0.00   **FUD** XXX   E 🔲

AMA: 2018,Jan,8; 2017,Jan,8; 2016,Jan,13; 2015,Jan,16; 2014,Jan,11

99505   Home visit for stoma care and maintenance including colostomy and cystostomy
🔲 0.00   🔲 0.00   **FUD** XXX   E 🔲

AMA: 2018,Jan,8; 2017,Jan,8; 2016,Jan,13; 2015,Jan,16; 2014,Jan,11

99506   Home visit for intramuscular injections
🔲 0.00   🔲 0.00   **FUD** XXX   E 🔲

AMA: 2018,Jan,8; 2017,Jan,8; 2016,Jan,13; 2015,Jan,16; 2014,Jan,11

99507   Home visit for care and maintenance of catheter(s) (eg, urinary, drainage, and enteral)
🔲 0.00   🔲 0.00   **FUD** XXX   E 🔲

AMA: 2018,Jan,8; 2017,Jan,8; 2016,Jan,13; 2015,Jan,16; 2014,Jan,11

99509   Home visit for assistance with activities of daily living and personal care
EXCLUDES Medical nutrition therapy/assessment home services (97802-97804)
     Self-care/home management training (97535)
     Speech therapy home services (92507-92508)
🔲 0.00   🔲 0.00   **FUD** XXX   E 🔲

AMA: 2018,Jan,8; 2017,Jan,8; 2016,Jan,13; 2015,Jan,16; 2014,Jan,11

99510   Home visit for individual, family, or marriage counseling
🔲 0.00   🔲 0.00   **FUD** XXX   E 🔲

AMA: 2018,Jan,8; 2017,Jan,8; 2016,Jan,13; 2015,Jan,16; 2014,Jan,11

99511   Home visit for fecal impaction management and enema administration
🔲 0.00   🔲 0.00   **FUD** XXX   E 🔲

AMA: 2018,Jan,8; 2017,Jan,8; 2016,Jan,13; 2015,Jan,16; 2014,Jan,11

99512   Home visit for hemodialysis
EXCLUDES Peritoneal dialysis home infusion (99601-99602)
🔲 0.00   🔲 0.00   **FUD** XXX   E 🔲

AMA: 2018,Jan,8; 2017,Jan,8; 2016,Jan,13; 2015,Jan,16; 2014,Jan,11

99600   Unlisted home visit service or procedure
🔲 0.00   🔲 0.00   **FUD** XXX   E 🔲

AMA: 2018,Jan,8; 2017,Jan,8; 2016,Jan,13; 2015,Jan,16; 2014,Jan,11

99601   Home infusion/specialty drug administration, per visit (up to 2 hours);
🔲 0.00   🔲 0.00   **FUD** XXX   E 🔲

AMA: 2005,Nov,1-9; 2003,Oct,7

+ 99602   each additional hour (List separately in addition to code for primary procedure)
Code first (99601)
🔲 0.00   🔲 0.00   **FUD** XXX   E 🔲

AMA: 2005,Nov,1-9; 2003,Oct,7

99605-99607 Medication Management By Pharmacist

INCLUDES Direct (face-to-face) assessment and intervention by a pharmacist for the purpose of:
     Managing medication complications and/or interactions
     Maximizing the patient's response to drug therapy
Documenting the following required elements:
     Advice given regarding improvement of treatment compliance and outcomes
     Profile of medications (prescription and nonprescription)
     Review of applicable patient history
EXCLUDES Routine tasks associated with dispensing and related activities (e.g., providing product information)

99605   Medication therapy management service(s) provided by a pharmacist, individual, face-to-face with patient, with assessment and intervention if provided; initial 15 minutes, new patient
🔲 0.00   🔲 0.00   **FUD** XXX   E 🔲

AMA: 2018,Apr,9; 2018,Jan,8; 2017,Jan,8; 2016,Jan,13; 2015,Jan,16; 2014,Oct,3; 2014,Jan,11

99606   initial 15 minutes, established patient
🔲 0.00   🔲 0.00   **FUD** XXX   E 🔲

AMA: 2018,Apr,9; 2018,Jan,8; 2017,Jan,8; 2016,Jan,13; 2015,Jan,16; 2014,Oct,3; 2014,Jan,11

+ 99607   each additional 15 minutes (List separately in addition to code for primary service)
Code first (99605, 99606)
🔲 0.00   🔲 0.00   **FUD** XXX   E 🔲

AMA: 2018,Apr,9; 2018,Jan,8; 2017,Jan,8; 2016,Jan,13; 2015,Jan,16; 2014,Oct,3; 2014,Jan,11

Evaluation and Management (E/M) Services Guidelines

Information unique to this section is defined or identified below.

For additional information about evaluation and management services, see Appendix C: Evaluation and Management Extended Guidelines. This appendix includes comprehensive explanations and instructions for the correct selection of an E&M service code based on federal documentation standards.

Classification of Evaluation and Management (E/M) Services

The E/M section is divided into broad categories such as office visits, hospital visits, and consultations. Most of the categories are further divided into two or more subcategories of E/M services. For example, there are two subcategories of office visits (new patient and established patient) and there are two subcategories of hospital visits (initial and subsequent). The subcategories of E/M services are further classified into levels of E/M services that are identified by specific codes. This classification is important because the nature of work varies by type of service, place of service, and the patient's status.

The basic format of the levels of E/M services is the same for most categories. First, a unique code number is listed. Second, the place and/or type of service is specified, eg, office consultation. Third, the content of the service is defined, eg, comprehensive history and comprehensive examination. (See "Levels of E/M Services," for details on the content of E/M services.) Fourth, the nature of the presenting problem(s) usually associated with a given level is described. Fifth, the time typically required to provide the service is specified. (A detailed discussion of time is provided separately.)

Definitions of Commonly Used Terms

Certain key words and phrases are used throughout the E/M section. The following definitions are intended to reduce the potential for differing interpretations and to increase the consistency of reporting by physicians in differing specialties. E/M services may also be reported by other qualified health care professionals who are authorized to perform such services within the scope of their practice.

New and Established Patient

Solely for the purposes of distinguishing between new and established patients, professional services are those face-to-face services rendered by physicians and other qualified health care professionals who may report E/M services with a specific CPT® code or codes. A new patient is one who has not received any professional services from the physician/qualified health care professional or another physician/qualified health care professional of the exact same specialty and subspecialty who belongs to the same group practice, within the past three years.

An established patient is one who has received professional services from the physician/qualified health care professional or another physician/qualified health care professional of the exact same specialty and subspecialty who belongs to the same group practice, within the past three years. See the decision tree at right.

When a physician/qualified health care professional is on call or covering for another physician/qualified health care professional, the patient's encounter is classified as it would have been by the physician/qualified health care professional who is not available. When advanced practice nurses and physician assistants are working with physicians, they are considered as working in the exact same specialty and exact same subspecialties as the physician.

No distinction is made between new and established patients in the emergency department. E/M services in the emergency department category may be reported for any new or established patient who presents for treatment in the emergency department.

The decision tree in the next column is provided to aid in determining whether to report the E/M service provided as a new or an established patient encounter.

Chief Complaint

A chief complaint is a concise statement describing the symptom, problem, condition, diagnosis, or other factor that is the reason for the encounter, usually stated in the patient's words.

Concurrent Care and Transfer of Care

Concurrent care is the provision of similar services (e.g., hospital visits) to the same patient by more than one physician or other qualified health care professional on the same day. When concurrent care is provided, no special reporting is required. Transfer of care is the process whereby a physician or other qualified health care professional who is managing some or all of a patient's problems relinquishes this responsibility to another physician or other qualified health care professional who explicitly agrees to accept this responsibility and who, from the initial encounter, is not providing consultative services. The physician or other qualified health care professional transferring care is then no longer providing care for these problems though he or she may continue providing care for other conditions when appropriate. Consultation codes should not be reported by the physician or other qualified health care professional who has agreed to accept transfer of care before an initial evaluation, but they are appropriate to report if the decision to accept transfer of care cannot be made until after the initial consultation evaluation, regardless of site of service.

Decision Tree for New vs Established Patients

Counseling

Counseling is a discussion with a patient and/or family concerning one or more of the following areas:

- Diagnostic results, impressions, and/or recommended diagnostic studies
- Prognosis
- Risks and benefits of management (treatment) options
- Instructions for management (treatment) and/or follow-up
- Importance of compliance with chosen management (treatment) options
- Risk factor reduction
- Patient and family education
  (For psychotherapy, see 90832–90834, 90836–90840)

Evaluation and Management (E/M) Services Guidelines

Family History

A review of medical events in the patient's family that includes significant information about:

- The health status or cause of death of parents, siblings, and children

- Specific diseases related to problems identified in the Chief Complaint or History of the Present Illness, and/or System Review

- Diseases of family members that may be hereditary or place the patient at risk

History of Present Illness

A chronological description of the development of the patient's present illness from the first sign and/or symptom to the present. This includes a description of location, quality, severity, timing, context, modifying factors, and associated signs and symptoms significantly related to the presenting problem(s).

Levels of E/M Services

Within each category or subcategory of E/M service, there are three to five levels of E/M services available for reporting purposes. Levels of E/M services are not interchangeable among the different categories or subcategories of service. For example, the first level of E/M services in the subcategory of office visit, new patient, does not have the same definition as the first level of E/M services in the subcategory of office visit, established patient.

The levels of E/M services include examinations, evaluations, treatments, conferences with or concerning patients, preventive pediatric and adult health supervision, and similar medical services, such as the determination of the need and/or location for appropriate care. Medical screening includes the history, examination, and medical decision-making required to determine the need and/or location for appropriate care and treatment of the patient (eg, office and other outpatient setting, emergency department, nursing facility). The levels of E/M services encompass the wide variations in skill, effort, time, responsibility, and medical knowledge required for the prevention or diagnosis and treatment of illness or injury and the promotion of optimal health. Each level of E/M services may be used by all physicians or other qualified health care professionals.

The descriptors for the levels of E/M services recognize seven components, six of which are used in defining the levels of E/M services. These components are:

- History
- Examination
- Medical decision making
- Counseling
- Coordination of care
- Nature of presenting problem
- Time

The first three of these components (history, examination, and medical decision making) are considered the key components in selecting a level of E/M services. (See "Determine the Extent of History Obtained.")

The next three components (counseling, coordination of care, and the nature of the presenting problem) are considered contributory factors in the majority of encounters. Although the first two of these contributory factors are important E/M services, it is not required that these services be provided at every patient encounter.

Coordination of care with other physicians, other qualified health care professionals, or agencies without a patient encounter on that day is reported using the case management codes.

The final component, time, is discussed in detail below.

Any specifically identifiable procedure (ie, identified with a specific CPT code) performed on or subsequent to the date of initial or subsequent E/M services should be reported separately.

The actual performance and/or interpretation of diagnostic tests/studies ordered during a patient encounter are not included in the levels of E/M services. Physician performance of diagnostic tests/studies for which specific CPT codes are available may be reported separately, in addition to the appropriate E/M code. The physician's interpretation of the results of diagnostic tests/studies (ie, professional component) with preparation of a separate distinctly identifiable signed written report may also be reported separately, using the appropriate CPT code with modifier 26 appended.

The physician or other health care professional may need to indicate that on the day a procedure or service identified by a CPT code was performed, the patient's condition required a significant separately identifiable E/M service above and beyond other services provided or beyond the usual preservice and postservice care associated with the procedure that was performed. The E/M service may be caused or prompted by the symptoms or condition for which the procedure and/or service was provided. This circumstance may be reported by adding modifier 25 to the appropriate level of E/M service. As such, different diagnoses are not required for reporting of the procedure and the E/M services on the same date.

Nature of Presenting Problem

A presenting problem is a disease, condition, illness, injury, symptom, sign, finding, complaint, or other reason for encounter, with or without a diagnosis being established at the time of the encounter. The E/M codes recognize five types of presenting problems that are defined as follows:

Minimal: A problem that may not require the presence of the physician or other qualified health care professional, but service is provided under the physician's or other qualified health care professional's supervision.

Self-limited or minor: A problem that runs a definite and prescribed course, is transient in nature, and is not likely to permanently alter health status OR has a good prognosis with management/compliance.

Low severity: A problem where the risk of morbidity without treatment is low; there is little to no risk of mortality without treatment; full recovery without functional impairment is expected.

Moderate severity: A problem where the risk of morbidity without treatment is moderate; there is moderate risk of mortality without treatment; uncertain prognosis OR increased probability of prolonged functional impairment.

High severity: A problem where the risk of morbidity without treatment is high to extreme; there is a moderate to high risk of mortality without treatment OR high probability of severe, prolonged functional impairment.

Past History

A review of the patient's past experiences with illnesses, injuries, and treatments that includes significant information about:

- Prior major illnesses and injuries
- Prior operations
- Prior hospitalizations
- Current medications
- Allergies (eg, drug, food)
- Age appropriate immunization status
- Age appropriate feeding/dietary status

Social History

An age appropriate review of past and current activities that includes significant information about:

- Marital status and/or living arrangements
- Current employment
- Occupational history
- Military history
- Use of drugs, alcohol, and tobacco
- Level of education
- Sexual history
- Other relevant social factors

System Review (Review of Systems)

An inventory of body systems obtained through a series of questions seeking to identify signs and/or symptoms that the patient may be experiencing or has experienced. For the purposes of the CPT codebook the following elements of a system review have been identified:

- Constitutional symptoms (fever, weight loss, etc)
- Eyes
- Ears, nose, mouth, throat
- Cardiovascular
- Respiratory
- Gastrointestinal
- Genitourinary
- Musculoskeletal
- Integumentary (skin and/or breast)
- Neurological
- Psychiatric
- Endocrine
- Hematologic/lymphatic
- Allergic/immunologic

The review of systems helps define the problem, clarify the differential diagnosis, identify needed testing, or serves as baseline data on other systems that might be affected by any possible management options.

Time

The inclusion of time in the definitions of levels of E/M services has been implicit in prior editions of the CPT codebook. The inclusion of time as an explicit factor beginning in *CPT 1992* is done to assist in selecting the most appropriate level of E/M services. It should be recognized that the specific times expressed in the visit code descriptors are averages and, therefore, represent a range of times that may be higher or lower depending on actual clinical circumstances.

Time is not a descriptive component for the emergency department levels of E/M services because emergency department services are typically provided on a variable intensity basis, often involving multiple encounters with several patients over an extended period of time. Therefore, it is often difficult to provide accurate estimates of the time spent face-to-face with the patient.

Studies to establish levels of E/M services employed surveys of practicing physicians to obtain data on the amount of time and work associated with typical E/M services. Since "work" is not easily quantifiable, the codes must rely on other objective, verifiable measures that correlate with physicians' estimates of their "work." It has been demonstrated that estimations of intraservice time, both within and across specialties, is a variable that is predictive of the "work" of E/M services. This same research has shown there is a strong relationship between intraservice time and total time for E/M services. Intraservice time, rather than total time, was chosen for inclusion with the codes because of its relative ease of measurement and because of its direct correlation with measurements of the total amount of time and work associated with typical E/M services.

Intraservice times are defined as face-to-face time for office and other outpatient visits and as unit/floor time for hospital and other inpatient visits. This distinction is necessary because most of the work of typical office visits takes place during the face-to-face time with the patient, while most of the work of typical hospital visits takes place during the time spent on the patient's floor or unit. When prolonged time occurs in either the office or the inpatient areas, the appropriate add-on code should be reported.

Face-to-face time (office and other outpatient visits and office consultations): For coding purposes, face-to-face time for these services is defined as only that time spent face-to-face with the patient and/or family. This includes the time spent performing such tasks as obtaining a history, performing an examination, and counseling the patient.

Time is also spent doing work before or after the face-to-face time with the patient, performing such tasks as reviewing records and tests, arranging for further services, and communicating further with other professionals and the patient through written reports and telephone contact.

This non-face-to-face time for office services—also called pre- and postencounter time—is not included in the time component described in the E/M codes. However, the pre- and post-non-face-to-face work associated with an encounter was included in calculating the total work of typical services in physician surveys.

Thus, the face-to-face time associated with the services described by any E/M code is a valid proxy for the total work done before, during, and after the visit.

Unit/floor time (hospital observation services, inpatient hospital care, initial inpatient hospital consultations, nursing facility): For reporting purposes, intraservice time for these services is defined as unit/floor time, which includes the time present on the patient's hospital unit and at the bedside rendering services for that patient. This includes the time to establish and/or review the patient's chart, examine the patient, write notes, and communicate with other professionals and the patient's family.

In the hospital, pre- and post-time includes time spent off the patient's floor performing such tasks as reviewing pathology and radiology findings in another part of the hospital.

This pre- and postvisit time is not included in the time component described in these codes. However, the pre- and postwork performed during the time spent off the floor or unit was included in calculating the total work of typical services in physician surveys.

Thus, the unit/floor time associated with the services described by any code is a valid proxy for the total work done before, during, and after the visit.

Unlisted Service

An E/M service may be provided that is not listed in this section of the CPT codebook. When reporting such a service, the appropriate unlisted code may be used to indicate the service, identifying it by "Special Report," as discussed in the following paragraph. The "Unlisted Services" and accompanying codes for the E/M section are as follows:

99429	**Unlisted preventive medicine service**
99499	**Unlisted evaluation and management service**

Special Report

An unlisted service or one that is unusual, variable, or new may require a special report demonstrating the medical appropriateness of the service. Pertinent information should include an adequate definition or description of the nature, extent, and need for the procedure and the time, effort, and equipment necessary to provide the service. Additional items that may be included are complexity of symptoms, final diagnosis, pertinent physical findings, diagnostic and therapeutic procedures, concurrent problems, and follow-up care.

Instructions for Selecting a Level of E/M Service

Review the Reporting Instructions for the Selected Category or Subcategory

Most of the categories and many of the subcategories of service have special guidelines or instructions unique to that category or subcategory. Where these are indicated, eg, "Inpatient Hospital Care," special instructions will be presented preceding the levels of E/M services.

Review the Level of E/M Service Descriptors and Examples in the Selected Category or Subcategory

The descriptors for the levels of E/M services recognize seven components, six of which are used in defining the levels of E/M services. These components are:

- History
- Examination
- Medical decision making

- Counseling
- Coordination of care
- Nature of presenting problem
- Time

The first three of these components (ie, history, examination, and medical decision making) should be considered the key components in selecting the level of E/M services. An exception to this rule is in the case of visits that consist predominantly of counseling or coordination of care.

The nature of the presenting problem and time are provided in some levels to assist the physician in determining the appropriate level of E/M service.

Determine the Extent of History Obtained
The extent of the history is dependent upon clinical judgment and on the nature of the presenting problem(s). The levels of E/M services recognize four types of history that are defined as follows:

Problem focused: Chief complaint; brief history of present illness or problem.

Expanded problem focused: Chief complaint; brief history of present illness; problem pertinent system review.

Detailed: Chief complaint; extended history of present illness; problem pertinent system review extended to include a review of a limited number of additional systems; pertinent past, family, and/or social history directly related to the patient's problems.

Comprehensive: Chief complaint; extended history of present illness; review of systems that is directly related to the problem(s) identified in the history of the present illness plus a review of all additional body systems; complete past, family, and social history.

The comprehensive history obtained as part of the preventive medicine E/M service is not problem-oriented and does not involve a chief complaint or present illness. It does, however, include a comprehensive system review and comprehensive or interval past, family, and social history as well as a comprehensive assessment/history of pertinent risk factors.

Determine the Extent of Examination Performed
The extent of the examination performed is dependent on clinical judgment and on the nature of the presenting problem(s). The levels of E/M services recognize four types of examination that are defined as follows:

Problem focused: A limited examination of the affected body area or organ system.

Expanded problem focused: A limited examination of the affected body area or organ system and other symptomatic or related organ system(s).

Detailed: An extended examination of the affected body area(s) and other symptomatic or related organ system(s).

Comprehensive: A general multisystem examination or a complete examination of a single organ system. Note: The comprehensive examination performed as part of the preventive medicine E/M service is multisystem, but its extent is based on age and risk factors identified.

For the purposes of these CPT definitions, the following body areas are recognized:

- Head, including the face
- Neck
- Chest, including breasts and axilla
- Abdomen
- Genitalia, groin, buttocks
- Back
- Each extremity

For the purposes of these CPT definitions, the following organ systems are recognized:

- Eyes
- Ears, nose, mouth, and throat
- Cardiovascular
- Respiratory
- Gastrointestinal
- Genitourinary
- Musculoskeletal
- Skin
- Neurologic
- Psychiatric
- Hematologic/lymphatic/immunologic

Determine the Complexity of Medical Decision Making
Medical decision making refers to the complexity of establishing a diagnosis and/or selecting a management option as measured by:

- The number of possible diagnoses and/or the number of management options that must be considered
- The amount and/or complexity of medical records, diagnostic tests, and/or other information that must be obtained, reviewed, and analyzed
- The risk of significant complications, morbidity, and/or mortality, as well as comorbidities associated with the patient's presenting problem(s), the diagnostic procedure(s), and/or the possible management options

Four types of medical decision making are recognized: straightforward, low complexity, moderate complexity, and high complexity. To qualify for a given type of decision making, two of the three elements in Table 1 must be met or exceeded.

Comorbidities and underlying diseases, in and of themselves, are not considered in selecting a level of E/M services unless their presence significantly increases the complexity of the medical decision making.

Select the Appropriate Level of E/M Services Based on the Following
For the following categories/subcategories, all of the key components, ie, history, examination, and medical decision making, must meet or exceed the stated requirements to qualify for a particular level of E/M service: office, new patient; hospital observation services; initial hospital care; office consultations; initial inpatient consultations; emergency department services; initial nursing facility care; domiciliary care, new patient; and home, new patient.

For the following categories/subcategories, two of the three key components (ie, history, examination, and medical decision making) must meet or exceed the stated requirements to qualify for a particular level of E/M services: office, established patient; subsequent hospital care; subsequent nursing facility care; domiciliary care, established patient; and home, established patient.

When counseling and/or coordination of care dominates (more than 50 percent) the encounter with the patient and/or family (face-to-face time in the office or other outpatient setting or floor/unit time in the hospital or nursing facility), then time shall be considered the key or controlling factor to qualify for a particular level of E/M services. This includes time spent with parties who have assumed responsibility for the care of the patient or decision making whether or not they are family members (e.g., foster parents, person acting in loco parentis, legal guardian). The extent of counseling and/or coordination of care must be documented in the medical record.

CONSULTATION CODES AND MEDICARE REIMBURSEMENT

The Centers for Medicare and Medicaid Services (CMS) no longer provides benefits for CPT consultation codes. CMS has, however, redistributed the value of the consultation codes across the other E/M codes for services which are covered by Medicare. CMS has retained codes 99241 - 99251 in the Medicare Physician Fee Schedule for those private payers that use this data for reimbursement. Note that private payers may choose to follow CMS or CPT guidelines, and the use of consultation codes should be verified with individual payers.

Table 1

Complexity of Medical Decision Making

Number of Diagnoses or Management Options	Amount and/or Complexity of Data to Be Reviewed	Risk of Complications and/or Morbidity or Mortality	Type of Decision Making
minimal	minimal or none	minimal	straightforward
limited	limited	low	low complexity
multiple	moderate	moderate	moderate complexity
extensive	extensive	high	high complexity

Evaluation and Management

99201 — 99211

99201-99215 Outpatient and Other Visits

CMS: 100-04,11,40.1.3 Independent Attending Physician Services; 100-04,12,190.3 List of Telehealth Services; 100-04,12,190.6 Payment Methodology for Physician/Practitioner at the Distant Site ; 100-04,12,190.6.1 Submission of Telehealth Claims for Distant Site Practitioners; 100-04,12,190.7 Contractor Editing of Telehealth Claims; 100-04,12,230 Primary Care Incentive Payment Program; 100-04,12,230.1 Definition of Primary Care Practitioners and Services; 100-04,12,230.2 Coordination with Other Payments; 100-04,12,230.3 Claims Processing and Payment; 100-04,12,30.6.10 Consultation Services; 100-04,12,30.6.15.1 Prolonged Services With Direct Face-to-Face Patient Contact; 100-04,12,30.6.4 Services Furnished Incident to Physician's Service; 100-04,12,30.6.7 Payment for Office or Other Outpatient E&M Visits; 100-04,12,40.3 Global Surgery Review; 100-04,18,80.2 Contractor Billing Requirements; 100-04,32,12.1 Counseling to Prevent Tobacco Use HCPCS and Diagnosis Coding; 100-04,32,130.1 Billing and Payment of External counterpulsation (ECP)

INCLUDES Established patients: received prior professional services from the physician or qualified health care professional or another physician or qualified health care professional in the practice of the exact same specialty and subspecialty in the previous three years (99211-99215)
New patients: have not received professional services from the physician or qualified health care professional or any other physician or qualified health care professional in the same practice in the exact same specialty and subspecialty in the previous three years (99201-99205)
Office visits
Outpatient services (including services prior to a formal admission to a facility)

EXCLUDES Services provided in:
Emergency department (99281-99285)
Hospital observation (99217-99220 [99224, 99225, 99226])
Hospital observation or inpatient with same day admission and discharge (99234-99236)

99201 Office or other outpatient visit for the evaluation and management of a new patient, which requires these 3 key components: A problem focused history; A problem focused examination; Straightforward medical decision making. Counseling and/or coordination of care with other physicians, other qualified health care professionals, or agencies are provided consistent with the nature of the problem(s) and the patient's and/or family's needs. Usually, the presenting problem(s) are self limited or minor. Typically, 10 minutes are spent face-to-face with the patient and/or family.
🔑 0.76   🔑 1.29   **FUD** XXX   ★ B 80 ▭
AMA: 2019,Feb,3; 2019,Jan,3; 2018,Sep,14; 2018,Apr,10; 2018,Apr,9; 2018,Mar,7; 2018,Jan,8; 2017,Aug,3; 2017,Jun,6; 2017,Jan,8; 2016,Dec,11; 2016,Sep,6; 2016,Mar,10; 2016,Jan,7; 2016,Jan,13; 2015,Dec,3; 2015,Oct,3; 2015,Jan,16; 2015,Jan,12; 2014,Nov,14; 2014,Oct,3; 2014,Oct,8; 2014,Aug,3; 2014,Jan,11

99202 Office or other outpatient visit for the evaluation and management of a new patient, which requires these 3 key components: An expanded problem focused history; An expanded problem focused examination; Straightforward medical decision making. Counseling and/or coordination of care with other physicians, other qualified health care professionals, or agencies are provided consistent with the nature of the problem(s) and the patient's and/or family's needs. Usually, the presenting problem(s) are of low to moderate severity. Typically, 20 minutes are spent face-to-face with the patient and/or family.
🔑 1.43   🔑 2.15   **FUD** XXX   ★ B 80 ▭
AMA: 2019,Feb,3; 2019,Jan,3; 2018,Sep,14; 2018,Apr,10; 2018,Apr,9; 2018,Mar,7; 2018,Jan,8; 2017,Aug,3; 2017,Jun,6; 2017,Jan,8; 2016,Dec,11; 2016,Sep,6; 2016,Mar,10; 2016,Jan,7; 2016,Jan,13; 2015,Dec,3; 2015,Oct,3; 2015,Jan,16; 2015,Jan,12; 2014,Nov,14; 2014,Oct,3; 2014,Oct,8; 2014,Aug,3; 2014,Jan,11

99203 Office or other outpatient visit for the evaluation and management of a new patient, which requires these 3 key components: A detailed history; A detailed examination; Medical decision making of low complexity. Counseling and/or coordination of care with other physicians, other qualified health care professionals, or agencies are provided consistent with the nature of the problem(s) and the patient's and/or family's needs. Usually, the presenting problem(s) are of moderate severity. Typically, 30 minutes are spent face-to-face with the patient and/or family.
🔑 2.15   🔑 3.05   **FUD** XXX   ★ B 80 ▭
AMA: 2019,Feb,3; 2019,Jan,3; 2018,Sep,14; 2018,Apr,9; 2018,Apr,10; 2018,Mar,7; 2018,Jan,8; 2017,Aug,3; 2017,Jun,6; 2017,Jan,8; 2016,Dec,11; 2016,Sep,6; 2016,Mar,10; 2016,Jan,7; 2016,Jan,13; 2015,Dec,3; 2015,Oct,3; 2015,Jan,12; 2015,Jan,16; 2014,Nov,14; 2014,Oct,3; 2014,Oct,8; 2014,Aug,3; 2014,Jan,11

99204 Office or other outpatient visit for the evaluation and management of a new patient, which requires these 3 key components: A comprehensive history; A comprehensive examination; Medical decision making of moderate complexity. Counseling and/or coordination of care with other physicians, other qualified health care professionals, or agencies are provided consistent with the nature of the problem(s) and the patient's and/or family's needs. Usually, the presenting problem(s) are of moderate to high severity. Typically, 45 minutes are spent face-to-face with the patient and/or family.
🔑 3.64   🔑 4.63   **FUD** XXX   ★ B 80 ▭
AMA: 2019,Feb,3; 2019,Jan,3; 2018,Sep,14; 2018,Apr,9; 2018,Apr,10; 2018,Mar,7; 2018,Jan,8; 2017,Aug,3; 2017,Jun,6; 2017,Jan,8; 2016,Dec,11; 2016,Sep,6; 2016,Mar,10; 2016,Jan,7; 2016,Jan,13; 2015,Dec,3; 2015,Oct,3; 2015,Jan,12; 2015,Jan,16; 2014,Nov,14; 2014,Oct,3; 2014,Oct,8; 2014,Aug,3; 2014,Jan,11

99205 Office or other outpatient visit for the evaluation and management of a new patient, which requires these 3 key components: A comprehensive history; A comprehensive examination; Medical decision making of high complexity. Counseling and/or coordination of care with other physicians, other qualified health care professionals, or agencies are provided consistent with the nature of the problem(s) and the patient's and/or family's needs. Usually, the presenting problem(s) are of moderate to high severity. Typically, 60 minutes are spent face-to-face with the patient and/or family.
🔑 4.75   🔑 5.82   **FUD** XXX   ★ B 80 ▭
AMA: 2019,Feb,3; 2019,Jan,3; 2018,Sep,14; 2018,Apr,9; 2018,Apr,10; 2018,Mar,7; 2018,Jan,8; 2017,Aug,3; 2017,Jun,6; 2017,Jan,8; 2016,Dec,11; 2016,Sep,6; 2016,Mar,10; 2016,Jan,7; 2016,Jan,13; 2015,Dec,3; 2015,Oct,3; 2015,Jan,12; 2015,Jan,16; 2014,Nov,14; 2014,Oct,3; 2014,Oct,8; 2014,Aug,3; 2014,Jan,11

99211 Office or other outpatient visit for the evaluation and management of an established patient, that may not require the presence of a physician or other qualified health care professional. Usually, the presenting problem(s) are minimal. Typically, 5 minutes are spent performing or supervising these services.
🔑 0.26   🔑 0.64   **FUD** XXX   B 80 ▭
AMA: 2019,Feb,3; 2019,Jan,3; 2018,Sep,14; 2018,Apr,10; 2018,Apr,9; 2018,Mar,7; 2018,Jan,8; 2017,Aug,3; 2017,Jun,6; 2017,Mar,10; 2017,Jan,8; 2016,Dec,11; 2016,Sep,6; 2016,Mar,10; 2016,Jan,7; 2016,Jan,13; 2015,Dec,3; 2015,Oct,3; 2015,Jan,12; 2015,Jan,16; 2014,Nov,14; 2014,Oct,3; 2014,Oct,8; 2014,Aug,3; 2014,Mar,13; 2014,Jan,11

99212   Office or other outpatient visit for the evaluation and management of an established patient, which requires at least 2 of these 3 key components: A problem focused history; A problem focused examination; Straightforward medical decision making. Counseling and/or coordination of care with other physicians, other qualified health care professionals, or agencies are provided consistent with the nature of the problem(s) and the patient's and/or family's needs. Usually, the presenting problem(s) are self limited or minor. Typically, 10 minutes are spent face-to-face with the patient and/or family.

🔲 0.72   ⚕ 1.27   **FUD** XXX   ★ B 80 🖳

AMA: 2019,Feb,3; 2019,Jan,3; 2018,Sep,14; 2018,Apr,9; 2018,Apr,10; 2018,Mar,7; 2018,Jan,8; 2017,Oct,5; 2017,Aug,3; 2017,Jun,6; 2017,Jan,8; 2016,Dec,11; 2016,Sep,6; 2016,Mar,10; 2016,Jan,7; 2016,Jan,13; 2015,Dec,3; 2015,Oct,3; 2015,Jan,12; 2015,Jan,16; 2014,Nov,14; 2014,Oct,3; 2014,Oct,8; 2014,Aug,3; 2014,Jan,11

99213   Office or other outpatient visit for the evaluation and management of an established patient, which requires at least 2 of these 3 key components: An expanded problem focused history; An expanded problem focused examination; Medical decision making of low complexity. Counseling and coordination of care with other physicians, other qualified health care professionals, or agencies are provided consistent with the nature of the problem(s) and the patient's and/or family's needs. Usually, the presenting problem(s) are of low to moderate severity. Typically, 15 minutes are spent face-to-face with the patient and/or family.

🔲 1.44   ⚕ 2.09   **FUD** XXX   ★ B 80 🖳

AMA: 2019,Feb,3; 2019,Jan,3; 2018,Sep,14; 2018,Apr,9; 2018,Apr,10; 2018,Mar,7; 2018,Jan,8; 2017,Aug,3; 2017,Jun,6; 2017,Jan,8; 2016,Dec,11; 2016,Sep,6; 2016,Mar,10; 2016,Jan,7; 2016,Jan,13; 2015,Dec,3; 2015,Oct,3; 2015,Jan,12; 2015,Jan,16; 2014,Nov,14; 2014,Oct,8; 2014,Oct,3; 2014,Aug,3; 2014,Jan,11

99214   Office or other outpatient visit for the evaluation and management of an established patient, which requires at least 2 of these 3 key components: A detailed history; A detailed examination; Medical decision making of moderate complexity. Counseling and/or coordination of care with other physicians, other qualified health care professionals, or agencies are provided consistent with the nature of the problem(s) and the patient's and/or family's needs. Usually, the presenting problem(s) are of moderate to high severity. Typically, 25 minutes are spent face-to-face with the patient and/or family.

🔲 2.22   ⚕ 3.06   **FUD** XXX   ★ B 80 🖳

AMA: 2019,Feb,3; 2019,Jan,3; 2018,Sep,14; 2018,Apr,9; 2018,Apr,10; 2018,Mar,7; 2018,Jan,8; 2017,Aug,3; 2017,Jun,6; 2017,Jan,8; 2016,Dec,11; 2016,Sep,6; 2016,Mar,10; 2016,Jan,13; 2016,Jan,7; 2015,Dec,3; 2015,Oct,3; 2015,Jan,12; 2015,Jan,16; 2014,Nov,14; 2014,Oct,3; 2014,Aug,3; 2014,Jan,11

99215   Office or other outpatient visit for the evaluation and management of an established patient, which requires at least 2 of these 3 key components: A comprehensive history; A comprehensive examination; Medical decision making of high complexity. Counseling and/or coordination of care with other physicians, other qualified health care professionals, or agencies are provided consistent with the nature of the problem(s) and the patient's and/or family's needs. Usually, the presenting problem(s) are of moderate to high severity. Typically, 40 minutes are spent face-to-face with the patient and/or family.

🔲 3.13   ⚕ 4.10   **FUD** XXX   ★ B 80 🖳

AMA: 2019,Feb,3; 2019,Jan,3; 2018,Sep,14; 2018,Apr,9; 2018,Apr,10; 2018,Mar,7; 2018,Jan,8; 2017,Aug,3; 2017,Jun,6; 2017,Jan,8; 2016,Dec,11; 2016,Sep,6; 2016,Mar,10; 2016,Jan,7; 2016,Jan,13; 2015,Dec,3; 2015,Oct,3; 2015,Jan,12; 2015,Jan,16; 2014,Nov,14; 2014,Oct,3; 2014,Aug,3; 2014,Jan,11

99217-99220 Facility Observation Visits: Initial and Discharge

CMS: 100-04,11,40.1.3 Independent Attending Physician Services; 100-04,12,30.6.4 Services Furnished Incident to Physician's Service; 100-04,12,30.6.8 Payment for Hospital Observation Services; 100-04,12,40.3 Global Surgery Review; 100-04,32,130.1 Billing and Payment of External counterpulsation (ECP)

INCLUDES   Services provided on the same date in other settings or departments associated with the observation status admission (99201-99215, 99281-99285, 99304-99318, 99324-99337, 99341-99350, 99381-99429)

Services provided to new and established patients admitted to a hospital specifically for observation (not required to be a designated area of the hospital)

EXCLUDES   *Services provided by physicians or another qualified health care professional other than the admitting physician ([99224, 99225, 99226], 99241-99245)*

Services provided to a patient admitted and discharged from observation status on the same date (99234-99236)

Services provided to a patient admitted to the hospital following observation status (99221-99223)

Services provided to a patient discharged from inpatient care (99238-99239)

99217   Observation care discharge day management (This code is to be utilized to report all services provided to a patient on discharge from outpatient hospital "observation status" if the discharge is on other than the initial date of "observation status." To report services to a patient designated as "observation status" or "inpatient status" and discharged on the same date, use the codes for Observation or Inpatient Care Services [including Admission and Discharge Services, 99234-99236 as appropriate.])

INCLUDES   Discussing the observation admission with the patient

Final patient evaluation:

Discharge instructions

Sign off on discharge medical records

🔲 2.06   ⚕ 2.06   **FUD** XXX   B 80 🖳

AMA: 2019,Jul,10; 2018,Jan,8; 2017,Aug,3; 2017,Jun,6; 2017,Jan,8; 2016,Dec,11; 2016,Jan,13; 2016,Jan,7; 2015,Dec,3; 2015,Jan,16; 2014,Nov,14; 2014,Oct,8; 2014,Jan,11

99218   Initial observation care, per day, for the evaluation and management of a patient which requires these 3 key components: A detailed or comprehensive history; A detailed or comprehensive examination; and Medical decision making that is straightforward or of low complexity. Counseling and/or coordination of care with other physicians, other qualified health care professionals, or agencies are provided consistent with the nature of the problem(s) and the patient's and/or family's needs. Usually, the problem(s) requiring admission to outpatient hospital "observation status" are of low severity. Typically, 30 minutes are spent at the bedside and on the patient's hospital floor or unit.

🔲 2.81   ⚕ 2.81   **FUD** XXX   B 80 🖳

AMA: 2019,Jul,10; 2018,Dec,8; 2018,Dec,8; 2018,Jan,8; 2017,Aug,3; 2017,Jun,6; 2017,Jan,8; 2016,Dec,11; 2016,Jan,7; 2016,Jan,13; 2015,Dec,3; 2015,Jul,3; 2015,Mar,3; 2015,Jan,16; 2014,Nov,14; 2014,Oct,8; 2014,Jan,11

99219   Initial observation care, per day, for the evaluation and management of a patient, which requires these 3 key components: A comprehensive history; A comprehensive examination; and Medical decision making of moderate complexity. Counseling and/or coordination of care with other physicians, other qualified health care professionals, or agencies are provided consistent with the nature of the problem(s) and the patient's and/or family's needs. Usually, the problem(s) requiring admission to outpatient hospital "observation status" are of moderate severity. Typically, 50 minutes are spent at the bedside and on the patient's hospital floor or unit.

🔲 3.83   ⚕ 3.83   **FUD** XXX   B 80 🖳

AMA: 2019,Jul,10; 2018,Dec,8; 2018,Dec,8; 2018,Jan,8; 2017,Aug,3; 2017,Jun,6; 2017,Jan,8; 2016,Dec,11; 2016,Jan,7; 2016,Jan,13; 2015,Dec,3; 2015,Jul,3; 2015,Jan,16; 2014,Nov,14; 2014,Oct,8; 2014,Jan,11

● New Code   ▲ Revised Code   ○ Reinstated   ● New Web Release   ▲ Revised Web Release   + Add-on   Unlisted   Not Covered   # Resequenced

㊿ Optum Mod 50 Exempt   Ⓢ AMA Mod 51 Exempt   � Optum Mod 51 Exempt   ㊿ Mod 63 Exempt   ✗ Non-FDA Drug   ★ Telemedicine   Ⓜ Maternity   Ⓐ Age Edit

© 2019 Optum360, LLC   CPT © 2019 American Medical Association. All Rights Reserved.   **541**

Evaluation and Management

99220 — 99222

99220 Initial observation care, per day, for the evaluation and management of a patient, which requires these 3 key components: A comprehensive history; A comprehensive examination; and Medical decision making of high complexity. Counseling and/or coordination of care with other physicians, other qualified health care professionals, or agencies are provided consistent with the nature of the problem(s) and the patient's and/or family's needs. Usually, the problem(s) requiring admission to outpatient hospital "observation status" are of high severity. Typically, 70 minutes are spent at the bedside and on the patient's hospital floor or unit.

🔧 5.23   ⚖ 5.23   **FUD** XXX   [B] [80] 🖥

AMA: 2019,Jul,10; 2018,Dec,8; 2018,Dec,8; 2018,Jan,8; 2017,Aug,3; 2017,Jun,6; 2017,Jan,8; 2016,Dec,11; 2016,Jan,7; 2016,Jan,13; 2015,Dec,3; 2015,Jul,3; 2015,Jan,16; 2014,Nov,14; 2014,Oct,8; 2014,Jan,11

99224-99226 [99224, 99225, 99226] Facility Observation Visits: Subsequent

CMS: 100-04,11,40.1.3 Independent Attending Physician Services; 100-04,12,30.6.4 Services Furnished Incident to Physician's Service; 100-04,12,30.6.8 Payment for Hospital Observation Services; 100-04,12,30.6.9.1 Initial Hospital Care and Observation or Inpatient Care Services

INCLUDES Changes in patient's status (e.g., physical condition, history; response to medical management)
Medical record review
Review of diagnostic test results
Services provided on the same date in other settings or departments associated with the observation status admission (99201-99215, 99281-99285, 99304-99318, 99324-99337, 99341-99350, 99381-99429)

EXCLUDES *Observation admission and discharge on the same day (99234-99236)*

\# 99224 Subsequent observation care, per day, for the evaluation and management of a patient, which requires at least 2 of these 3 key components: Problem focused interval history; Problem focused examination; Medical decision making that is straightforward or of low complexity. Counseling and/or coordination of care with other physicians, other qualified health care professionals, or agencies are provided consistent with the nature of the problem(s) and the patient's and/or family's needs. Usually, the patient is stable, recovering, or improving. Typically, 15 minutes are spent at the bedside and on the patient's hospital floor or unit.

🔧 1.12   ⚖ 1.12   **FUD** XXX   [B] [80] 🖥

AMA: 2019,Jul,10; 2018,Jan,8; 2017,Aug,3; 2017,Jun,6; 2017,Jan,8; 2016,Dec,11; 2016,Jan,7; 2016,Jan,13; 2015,Dec,3; 2015,Jan,16; 2014,Nov,14; 2014,Oct,8; 2014,Jan,11

\# 99225 Subsequent observation care, per day, for the evaluation and management of a patient, which requires at least 2 of these 3 key components: An expanded problem focused interval history; An expanded problem focused examination; Medical decision making of moderate complexity. Counseling and/or coordination of care with other physicians, other qualified health care professionals, or agencies are provided consistent with the nature of the problem(s) and the patient's and/or family's needs. Usually, the patient is responding inadequately to therapy or has developed a minor complication. Typically, 25 minutes are spent at the bedside and on the patient's hospital floor or unit.

🔧 2.06   ⚖ 2.06   **FUD** XXX   [B] [80] 🖥

AMA: 2019,Jul,10; 2018,Jan,8; 2017,Aug,3; 2017,Jun,6; 2017,Jan,8; 2016,Dec,11; 2016,Jan,7; 2016,Jan,13; 2015,Dec,3; 2015,Jan,16; 2014,Nov,14; 2014,Oct,8; 2014,Jan,11

\# 99226 Subsequent observation care, per day, for the evaluation and management of a patient, which requires at least 2 of these 3 key components: A detailed interval history; A detailed examination; Medical decision making of high complexity. Counseling and/or coordination of care with other physicians, other qualified health care professionals, or agencies are provided consistent with the nature of the problem(s) and the patient's and/or family's needs. Usually, the patient is unstable or has developed a significant complication or a significant new problem. Typically, 35 minutes are spent at the bedside and on the patient's hospital floor or unit.

🔧 2.95   ⚖ 2.95   **FUD** XXX   [B] [80] 🖥

AMA: 2019,Jul,10; 2018,Jan,8; 2017,Aug,3; 2017,Jun,6; 2017,Jan,8; 2016,Dec,11; 2016,Jan,7; 2016,Jan,13; 2015,Dec,3; 2015,Jan,16; 2014,Nov,14; 2014,Oct,8; 2014,Jan,11

99221-99233 Inpatient Hospital Visits: Initial and Subsequent

CMS: 100-04,11,40.1.3 Independent Attending Physician Services; 100-04,12,30.6.10 Consultation Services; 100-04,12,30.6.15.1 Prolonged Services With Direct Face-to-Face Patient Contact; 100-04,12,30.6.4 Services Furnished Incident to Physician's Service; 100-04,12,30.6.9 Hospital Visit and Critical Care on Same Day

INCLUDES Initial physician services provided to the patient in the hospital or "partial" hospital settings (99221-99223)
Services provided on the date of admission in other settings or departments associated with an observation status admission (99201-99215, 99281-99285, 99304-99318, 99324-99337, 99341-99350, 99381-99397)
Services provided to a new or established patient

EXCLUDES *Inpatient admission and discharge on the same date (99234-99236)*
Inpatient E&M services provided by other than the admitting physician

99221 Initial hospital care, per day, for the evaluation and management of a patient, which requires these 3 key components: A detailed or comprehensive history; A detailed or comprehensive examination; and Medical decision making that is straightforward or of low complexity. Counseling and/or coordination of care with other physicians, other qualified health care professionals, or agencies are provided consistent with the nature of the problem(s) and the patient's and/or family's needs. Usually, the problem(s) requiring admission are of low severity. Typically, 30 minutes are spent at the bedside and on the patient's hospital floor or unit.

🔧 2.86   ⚖ 2.86   **FUD** XXX   [B] [80] 🖥

AMA: 2018,Dec,8; 2018,Dec,8; 2018,Jan,8; 2017,Aug,3; 2017,Jun,6; 2017,Jan,8; 2016,Dec,11; 2016,Mar,10; 2016,Jan,13; 2016,Jan,7; 2015,Dec,3; 2015,Dec,18; 2015,Jul,3; 2015,Jan,16; 2014,Nov,14; 2014,Oct,8; 2014,Jan,11

99222 Initial hospital care, per day, for the evaluation and management of a patient, which requires these 3 key components: A comprehensive history; A comprehensive examination; and Medical decision making of moderate complexity. Counseling and/or coordination of care with other physicians, other qualified health care professionals, or agencies are provided consistent with the nature of the problem(s) and the patient's and/or family's needs. Usually, the problem(s) requiring admission are of moderate severity. Typically, 50 minutes are spent at the bedside and on the patient's hospital floor or unit.

🔧 3.86   ⚖ 3.86   **FUD** XXX   [B] [80] 🖥

AMA: 2018,Dec,8; 2018,Dec,8; 2018,Jan,8; 2017,Aug,3; 2017,Jun,6; 2017,Jan,8; 2016,Dec,11; 2016,Mar,10; 2016,Jan,7; 2016,Jan,13; 2015,Dec,3; 2015,Dec,18; 2015,Jul,3; 2015,Mar,3; 2015,Jan,16; 2014,Nov,14; 2014,Oct,8; 2014,Jan,11

99223 Initial hospital care, per day, for the evaluation and management of a patient, which requires these 3 key components: A comprehensive history; A comprehensive examination; and Medical decision making of high complexity. Counseling and/or coordination of care with other physicians, other qualified health care professionals, or agencies are provided consistent with the nature of the problem(s) and the patient's and/or family's needs. Usually, the problem(s) requiring admission are of high severity. Typically, 70 minutes are spent at the bedside and on the patient's hospital floor or unit.

🖐 5.70   🔧 5.70   **FUD** XXX   Ⓑ 80 ▭

AMA: 2018,Dec,8; 2018,Dec,8; 2018,Jan,8; 2017,Aug,3; 2017,Jun,6; 2017,Jan,8; 2016,Dec,11; 2016,Mar,10; 2016,Jan,7; 2016,Jan,13; 2015,Dec,3; 2015,Dec,18; 2015,Jul,3; 2015,Jan,16; 2014,Nov,14; 2014,Oct,8; 2014,Jan,11

99224 Resequenced code. See code following 99220.

99225 Resequenced code. See code following 99220.

99226 Resequenced code. See code following 99220.

99231 Subsequent hospital care, per day, for the evaluation and management of a patient, which requires at least 2 of these 3 key components: A problem focused interval history; A problem focused examination; Medical decision making that is straightforward or of low complexity. Counseling and/or coordination of care with other physicians, other qualified health care professionals, or agencies are provided consistent with the nature of the problem(s) and the patient's and/or family's needs. Usually, the patient is stable, recovering or improving. Typically, 15 minutes are spent at the bedside and on the patient's hospital floor or unit.

🖐 1.11   🔧 1.11   **FUD** XXX   ★ Ⓑ 80 ▭

AMA: 2018,Dec,8; 2018,Dec,8; 2018,Jan,8; 2017,Aug,3; 2017,Jun,6; 2017,Jan,8; 2016,Dec,11; 2016,Jan,13; 2016,Jan,7; 2015,Dec,3; 2015,Jul,3; 2015,Jan,16; 2014,Nov,14; 2014,Oct,8; 2014,May,4; 2014,Jan,11

99232 Subsequent hospital care, per day, for the evaluation and management of a patient, which requires at least 2 of these 3 key components: An expanded problem focused interval history; An expanded problem focused examination; Medical decision making of moderate complexity. Counseling and/or coordination of care with other physicians, other qualified health care professionals, or agencies are provided consistent with the nature of the problem(s) and the patient's and/or family's needs. Usually, the patient is responding inadequately to therapy or has developed a minor complication. Typically, 25 minutes are spent at the bedside and on the patient's hospital floor or unit.

🖐 2.05   🔧 2.05   **FUD** XXX   ★ Ⓑ 80 ▭

AMA: 2018,Dec,8; 2018,Dec,8; 2018,Jan,8; 2017,Aug,3; 2017,Jun,6; 2017,Jan,8; 2016,Dec,11; 2016,Oct,8; 2016,Jan,7; 2016,Jan,13; 2015,Dec,3; 2015,Jul,3; 2015,Jan,16; 2014,Nov,14; 2014,Oct,8; 2014,Jan,11

99233 Subsequent hospital care, per day, for the evaluation and management of a patient, which requires at least 2 of these 3 key components: A detailed interval history; A detailed examination; Medical decision making of high complexity. Counseling and/or coordination of care with other physicians, other qualified health care professionals, or agencies are provided consistent with the nature of the problem(s) and the patient's and/or family's needs. Usually, the patient is unstable or has developed a significant complication or a significant new problem. Typically, 35 minutes are spent at the bedside and on the patient's hospital floor or unit.

🖐 2.93   🔧 2.93   **FUD** XXX   ★ Ⓑ 80 ▭

AMA: 2018,Dec,8; 2018,Dec,8; 2018,Jan,8; 2017,Aug,3; 2017,Jun,6; 2017,Jan,8; 2016,Dec,11; 2016,Oct,8; 2016,Jan,13; 2016,Jan,7; 2015,Dec,3; 2015,Jul,3; 2015,Jan,16; 2014,Nov,14; 2014,Oct,8; 2014,May,4; 2014,Jan,11

99234-99236 Observation/Inpatient Visits: Admitted/Discharged on Same Date

CMS: 100-04,11,40.1.3 Independent Attending Physician Services; 100-04,12,30.6.4 Services Furnished Incident to Physician's Service; 100-04,12,30.6.8 Payment for Hospital Observation Services; 100-04,12,30.6.9 Payment for Inpatient Hospital Visits - General; 100-04,12,30.6.9.1 Initial Hospital Care and Observation or Inpatient Care Services; 100-04,12,30.6.9.2 Subsequent Hospital Visit and Discharge Management; 100-04,12,40.3 Global Surgery Review

INCLUDES   Admission and discharge services on the same date in an observation or inpatient setting
All services provided by admitting physician or other qualified health care professional on same date of service, even when initiated in another setting (e.g., emergency department, nursing facility, office)

EXCLUDES   *Services provided to patients admitted to observation and discharged on a different date (99217-99220, [99224, 99225, 99226])*

99234 Observation or inpatient hospital care, for the evaluation and management of a patient including admission and discharge on the same date, which requires these 3 key components: A detailed or comprehensive history; A detailed or comprehensive examination; and Medical decision making that is straightforward or of low complexity. Counseling and/or coordination of care with other physicians, other qualified health care professionals, or agencies are provided consistent with the nature of the problem(s) and the patient's and/or family's needs. Usually the presenting problem(s) requiring admission are of low severity. Typically, 40 minutes are spent at the bedside and on the patient's hospital floor or unit.

🖐 3.75   🔧 3.75   **FUD** XXX   Ⓑ 80 ▭

AMA: 2018,Dec,8; 2018,Dec,8; 2018,Apr,10; 2018,Jan,8; 2017,Aug,3; 2017,Jun,6; 2017,Jan,8; 2016,Dec,11; 2016,Jan,13; 2015,Jul,3; 2015,Jan,16; 2014,Oct,8; 2014,Jan,11

99235 Observation or inpatient hospital care, for the evaluation and management of a patient including admission and discharge on the same date, which requires these 3 key components: A comprehensive history; A comprehensive examination; and Medical decision making of moderate complexity. Counseling and/or coordination of care with other physicians, other qualified health care professionals, or agencies are provided consistent with the nature of the problem(s) and the patient's and/or family's needs. Usually the presenting problem(s) requiring admission are of moderate severity. Typically, 50 minutes are spent at the bedside and on the patient's hospital floor or unit.

🖐 4.77   🔧 4.77   **FUD** XXX   Ⓑ 80 ▭

AMA: 2018,Dec,8; 2018,Dec,8; 2018,Apr,10; 2018,Jan,8; 2017,Aug,3; 2017,Jun,6; 2017,Jan,8; 2016,Dec,11; 2016,Jan,13; 2015,Jul,3; 2015,Jan,16; 2014,Oct,8; 2014,Jan,11

99236 Observation or inpatient hospital care, for the evaluation and management of a patient including admission and discharge on the same date, which requires these 3 key components: A comprehensive history; A comprehensive examination; and Medical decision making of high complexity. Counseling and/or coordination of care with other physicians, other qualified health care professionals, or agencies are provided consistent with the nature of the problem(s) and the patient's and/or family's needs. Usually the presenting problem(s) requiring admission are of high severity. Typically, 55 minutes are spent at the bedside and on the patient's hospital floor or unit.

🖐 6.13   🔧 6.13   **FUD** XXX   Ⓑ 80 ▭

AMA: 2018,Dec,8; 2018,Dec,8; 2018,Apr,10; 2018,Jan,8; 2017,Aug,3; 2017,Jun,6; 2017,Jan,8; 2016,Dec,11; 2016,Jan,13; 2015,Jul,3; 2015,Jan,16; 2014,Oct,8; 2014,Jan,11

Evaluation and Management

99238 — 99242

99238-99239 Inpatient Hospital Discharge Services

CMS: 100-04,11,40.1.3 Independent Attending Physician Services; 100-04,12,30.6.4 Services Furnished Incident to Physician's Service; 100-04,12,30.6.9 Swing Bed Visits; 100-04,12,30.6.9.1 Initial Hospital Care and Observation or Inpatient Care Services; 100-04,12,30.6.9.2 Subsequent Hospital Visit and Discharge Management; 100-04,12,40.3 Global Surgery Review

INCLUDES All services on discharge day when discharge and admission are not the same day
Discharge instructions
Final patient evaluation
Final preparation of the patient's medical records
Provision of prescriptions/referrals, as needed
Review of the inpatient admission

EXCLUDES *Admission/discharge on same date (99234-99236)*
Discharge from observation (99217)
Discharge from nursing facility (99315-99316)
Healthy newborn evaluated and discharged on same date (99463)
Services provided by other than attending physician or other qualified health care professional on date of discharge (99231-99233)

99238 **Hospital discharge day management; 30 minutes or less**
 🖩 2.06 ⚕ 2.06 **FUD** XXX Ⓑ 80 ▭
AMA: 2018,Dec,8; 2018,Dec,8; 2018,Jan,8; 2017,Aug,3; 2017,Jun,6; 2017,Jan,8; 2016,Dec,11; 2016,Jan,13; 2015,Jan,16; 2014,Oct,8; 2014,Jan,11

99239 **more than 30 minutes**
 🖩 3.02 ⚕ 3.02 **FUD** XXX Ⓑ 80 ▭
AMA: 2018,Dec,8; 2018,Dec,8; 2018,Jan,8; 2017,Aug,3; 2017,Jun,6; 2017,Jan,8; 2016,Dec,11; 2015,Jan,16; 2014,Oct,8; 2014,Jan,11

99241-99245 Consultations: Office and Outpatient

CMS: 100-04,11,40.1.3 Independent Attending Physician Services; 100-04,12,190.6 Payment Methodology for Physician/Practitioner at the Distant Site ; 100-04,12,190.6.1 Submission of Telehealth Claims for Distant Site Practitioners; 100-04,12,190.7 Contractor Editing of Telehealth Claims; 100-04,12,30.6.10 Consultation Services; 100-04,12,30.6.15.1 Prolonged Services With Direct Face-to-Face Patient Contact; 100-04,12,30.6.4 Services Furnished Incident to Physician's Service; 100-04,12,30.6.9.1 Initial Hospital Care and Observation or Inpatient Care Services; 100-04,12,40.3 Global Surgery Review; 100-04,32,130.1 Billing and Payment of External counterpulsation (ECP); 100-04,4,160 Clinic and Emergency Visits Under OPPS

INCLUDES A third-party mandated consultation; append modifier 32
All outpatient consultations provided in the office, outpatient or other ambulatory facility, domiciliary/rest home, emergency department, patient's home, and hospital observation
Documentation of a request for a consultation from an appropriate source
Documentation of the need for consultation in the patient's medical record
One consultation per consultant
Provision by a physician or qualified nonphysician practitioner whose advice, opinion, recommendation, suggestion, direction, or counsel, etc., is requested for evaluating/treating a patient since that individual's expertise in a specific medical area is beyond the scope of knowledge of the requesting physician
Provision of a written report of findings/recommendations to the consultant to the referring physician

EXCLUDES *Another appropriately requested and documented consultation pertaining to the same/new problem; repeat use of consultation codes*
Any distinctly recognizable procedure/service provided on or following the consultation
Assumption of care (all or partial); report subsequent codes as appropriate for the place of service (99211-99215, 99334-99337, 99347-99350)
Consultation prompted by the patient/family; report codes for office, domiciliary/rest home, or home visits instead (99201-99215, 99324-99337, 99341-99350)
Services provided to Medicare patients; E&M code as appropriate for the place of service or HCPCS code (99201-99215, 99221-99223, 99231-99233, G0406-G0408, G0425-G0427)

99241 **Office consultation for a new or established patient, which requires these 3 key components: A problem focused history; A problem focused examination; and Straightforward medical decision making. Counseling and/or coordination of care with other physicians, other qualified health care professionals, or agencies are provided consistent with the nature of the problem(s) and the patient's and/or family's needs. Usually, the presenting problem(s) are self limited or minor. Typically, 15 minutes are spent face-to-face with the patient and/or family.**
 🖩 0.92 ⚕ 1.34 **FUD** XXX ★ Ⓔ ▭
AMA: 2018,Apr,9; 2018,Apr,10; 2018,Mar,7; 2018,Jan,8; 2017,Aug,3; 2017,Jun,6; 2017,Jan,8; 2016,Dec,11; 2016,Sep,6; 2016,Jan,13; 2016,Jan,7; 2015,Jan,12; 2015,Jan,16; 2014,Nov,14; 2014,Oct,8; 2014,Sep,13; 2014,Aug,3; 2014,Jan,11

99242 **Office consultation for a new or established patient, which requires these 3 key components: An expanded problem focused history; An expanded problem focused examination; and Straightforward medical decision making. Counseling and/or coordination of care with other physicians, other qualified health care professionals, or agencies are provided consistent with the nature of the problem(s) and the patient's and/or family's needs. Usually, the presenting problem(s) are of low severity. Typically, 30 minutes are spent face-to-face with the patient and/or family.**
 🖩 1.93 ⚕ 2.52 **FUD** XXX ★ Ⓔ ▭
AMA: 2018,Apr,10; 2018,Apr,9; 2018,Mar,7; 2018,Jan,8; 2017,Aug,3; 2017,Jun,6; 2017,Jun,8; 2017,Jan,8; 2016,Dec,11; 2016,Sep,6; 2016,Jan,7; 2016,Jan,13; 2015,Jan,12; 2015,Jan,16; 2014,Nov,14; 2014,Oct,8; 2014,Sep,13; 2014,Aug,3; 2014,Jan,11

99243 Office consultation for a new or established patient, which requires these 3 key components: A detailed history; A detailed examination; and Medical decision making of low complexity. Counseling and/or coordination of care with other physicians, other qualified health care professionals, or agencies are provided consistent with the nature of the problem(s) and the patient's and/or family's needs. Usually, the presenting problem(s) are of moderate severity. Typically, 40 minutes are spent face-to-face with the patient and/or family.

🚑 2.70   ⚖ 3.45   **FUD** XXX   ★ E 🖵

AMA: 2018,Apr,10; 2018,Apr,9; 2018,Mar,7; 2018,Jan,8; 2017,Aug,3; 2017,Jun,6; 2017,Jan,8; 2016,Dec,11; 2016,Sep,6; 2016,Jan,7; 2016,Jan,13; 2015,Jan,16; 2015,Jan,12; 2014,Nov,14; 2014,Oct,8; 2014,Sep,13; 2014,Aug,3; 2014,Jan,11

99244 Office consultation for a new or established patient, which requires these 3 key components: A comprehensive history; A comprehensive examination; and Medical decision making of moderate complexity. Counseling and/or coordination of care with other physicians, other qualified health care professionals, or agencies are provided consistent with the nature of the problem(s) and the patient's and/or family's needs. Usually, the presenting problem(s) are of moderate to high severity. Typically, 60 minutes are spent face-to-face with the patient and/or family.

🚑 4.34   ⚖ 5.16   **FUD** XXX   ★ E 🖵

AMA: 2018,Apr,10; 2018,Apr,9; 2018,Mar,7; 2018,Jan,8; 2017,Aug,3; 2017,Jun,6; 2017,Jan,8; 2016,Dec,11; 2016,Sep,6; 2016,Jan,7; 2016,Jan,13; 2015,Jan,16; 2015,Jan,12; 2014,Nov,14; 2014,Oct,8; 2014,Sep,13; 2014,Aug,3; 2014,Jan,11

99245 Office consultation for a new or established patient, which requires these 3 key components: A comprehensive history; A comprehensive examination; and Medical decision making of high complexity. Counseling and/or coordination of care with other physicians, other qualified health care professionals, or agencies are provided consistent with the nature of the problem(s) and the patient's and/or family's needs. Usually, the presenting problem(s) are of moderate to high severity. Typically, 80 minutes are spent face-to-face with the patient and/or family.

🚑 5.37   ⚖ 6.29   **FUD** XXX   ★ E 🖵

AMA: 2018,Apr,10; 2018,Apr,9; 2018,Mar,7; 2018,Jan,8; 2017,Aug,3; 2017,Jun,6; 2017,Jan,8; 2016,Dec,11; 2016,Sep,6; 2016,Jan,7; 2016,Jan,13; 2015,Jan,16; 2015,Jan,12; 2014,Nov,14; 2014,Oct,8; 2014,Sep,13; 2014,Aug,3; 2014,Jan,11

99251-99255 Consultations: Inpatient

CMS: 100-04,11,40.1.3 Independent Attending Physician Services; 100-04,12,190.6 Payment Methodology for Physician/Practitioner at the Distant Site ; 100-04,12,190.6.1 Submission of Telehealth Claims for Distant Site Practitioners; 100-04,12,190.7 Contractor Editing of Telehealth Claims; 100-04,12,30.6.10 Consultation Services; 100-04,12,30.6.15.1 Prolonged Services With Direct Face-to-Face Patient Contact; 100-04,12,30.6.4 Services Furnished Incident to Physician's Service; 100-04,12,30.6.9.1 Initial Hospital Care and Observation or Inpatient Care Services; 100-04,12,40.3 Global Surgery Review

INCLUDES A third-party mandated consultation; append modifier 32
All inpatient consultations include services provided in the hospital inpatient or partial hospital settings and nursing facilities
Consultation services provided outpatient for the same inpatient hospitalization (99241-99245)
Documentation of a request for a consultation from an appropriate source
Documentation of the need for consultation in the patient's medical record
One consultation by consultant per admission
Provision by a physician or qualified nonphysician practitioner whose advice, opinion, recommendation, suggestion, direction, or counsel, etc. is requested for evaluating/treating a patient since that individual's expertise in a specific medical area is beyond the scope of knowledge of the requesting physician
Provision of a written report of findings/recommendations from the consultant to the referring physician

EXCLUDES *Another appropriately requested and documented consultation pertaining to the same/new problem: repeat use of consultation codes*
Any distinctly recognizable procedure/service provided on or following the consultation
Assumption of care (all or partial): report subsequent codes as appropriate for the place of service (99231-99233, 99307-99310)
Consultation prompted by the patient/family: report codes for office, domiciliary/rest home, or home visits instead (99201-99215, 99324-99337, 99341-99350)
Services provided to Medicare patients; E&M code as appropriate for the place of service or HCPCS code (99201-99215, 99221-99223, 99231-99233, G0406-G0408, G0425-G0427)

99251 Inpatient consultation for a new or established patient, which requires these 3 key components: A problem focused history; A problem focused examination; and Straightforward medical decision making. Counseling and/or coordination of care with other physicians, other qualified health care professionals, or agencies are provided consistent with the nature of the problem(s) and the patient's and/or family's needs. Usually, the presenting problem(s) are self limited or minor. Typically, 20 minutes are spent at the bedside and on the patient's hospital floor or unit.

🚑 1.38   ⚖ 1.38   **FUD** XXX   ★ E 🖵

AMA: 2018,Jan,8; 2017,Aug,3; 2017,Jun,6; 2017,Jan,8; 2016,Dec,11; 2016,Jan,7; 2016,Jan,13; 2015,Jan,16; 2014,Nov,14; 2014,Oct,8; 2014,Jan,11

99252 Inpatient consultation for a new or established patient, which requires these 3 key components: An expanded problem focused history; An expanded problem focused examination; and Straightforward medical decision making. Counseling and/or coordination of care with other physicians, other qualified health care professionals, or agencies are provided consistent with the nature of the problem(s) and the patient's and/or family's needs. Usually, the presenting problem(s) are of low severity. Typically, 40 minutes are spent at the bedside and on the patient's hospital floor or unit.

🚑 2.11   ⚖ 2.11   **FUD** XXX   ★ E 🖵

AMA: 2018,Jan,8; 2017,Aug,3; 2017,Jun,6; 2017,Jan,8; 2016,Dec,11; 2016,Jan,7; 2016,Jan,13; 2015,Jan,16; 2014,Nov,14; 2014,Oct,8; 2014,Jan,11

99253 Inpatient consultation for a new or established patient, which requires these 3 key components: A detailed history; A detailed examination; and Medical decision making of low complexity. Counseling and/or coordination of care with other physicians, other qualified health care professionals, or agencies are provided consistent with the nature of the problem(s) and the patient's and/or family's needs. Usually, the presenting problem(s) are of moderate severity. Typically, 55 minutes are spent at the bedside and on the patient's hospital floor or unit.

 3.25 3.25 **FUD** XXX ★ E 🖵

AMA: 2018,Jan,8; 2017,Aug,3; 2017,Jun,6; 2017,Jan,8; 2016,Dec,11; 2016,Jan,7; 2016,Jan,13; 2015,Jan,16; 2014,Nov,14; 2014,Oct,8; 2014,Jan,11

99254 Inpatient consultation for a new or established patient, which requires these 3 key components: A comprehensive history; A comprehensive examination; and Medical decision making of moderate complexity. Counseling and/or coordination of care with other physicians, other qualified health care professionals, or agencies are provided consistent with the nature of the problem(s) and the patient's and/or family's needs. Usually, the presenting problem(s) are of moderate to high severity. Typically, 80 minutes are spent at the bedside and on the patient's hospital floor or unit.

 4.72 4.72 **FUD** XXX ★ E 🖵

AMA: 2018,Jan,8; 2017,Aug,3; 2017,Jun,6; 2017,Jan,8; 2016,Dec,11; 2016,Jan,7; 2016,Jan,13; 2015,Jan,16; 2014,Nov,14; 2014,Oct,8; 2014,Jan,11

99255 Inpatient consultation for a new or established patient, which requires these 3 key components: A comprehensive history; A comprehensive examination; and Medical decision making of high complexity. Counseling and/or coordination of care with other physicians, other qualified health care professionals, or agencies are provided consistent with the nature of the problem(s) and the patient's and/or family's needs. Usually, the presenting problem(s) are of moderate to high severity. Typically, 110 minutes are spent at the bedside and on the patient's hospital floor or unit.

 5.68 5.68 **FUD** XXX ★ E 🖵

AMA: 2018,Jan,8; 2017,Aug,3; 2017,Jun,6; 2017,Jan,8; 2016,Dec,11; 2016,Jan,7; 2016,Jan,13; 2015,Jan,16; 2014,Nov,14; 2014,Oct,8; 2014,Jan,11

99281-99288 Emergency Department Visits

CMS: 100-04,11,40.1.3 Independent Attending Physician Services; 100-04,12,30.6.11 Emergency Department Visits; 100-04,4,160 Clinic and Emergency Visits Under OPPS

INCLUDES Any amount of time spent with the patient, which usually involves a series of encounters while the patient is in the emergency department
Care provided to new and established patients

EXCLUDES *Critical care services (99291-99292)*
Observation services (99217-99220, 99234-99236)

99281 Emergency department visit for the evaluation and management of a patient, which requires these 3 key components: A problem focused history; A problem focused examination; and Straightforward medical decision making. Counseling and/or coordination of care with other physicians, other qualified health care professionals, or agencies are provided consistent with the nature of the problem(s) and the patient's and/or family's needs. Usually, the presenting problem(s) are self limited or minor.

 0.60 0.60 **FUD** XXX J 80 🖵

AMA: 2019,Jul,10; 2018,Jan,8; 2017,Aug,3; 2017,Jun,6; 2017,Jan,8; 2016,Jan,7; 2016,Jan,13; 2015,Jan,16; 2015,Jan,12; 2014,Nov,14; 2014,Oct,8; 2014,Jan,11

99282 Emergency department visit for the evaluation and management of a patient, which requires these 3 key components: An expanded problem focused history; An expanded problem focused examination; and Medical decision making of low complexity. Counseling and/or coordination of care with other physicians, other qualified health care professionals, or agencies are provided consistent with the nature of the problem(s) and the patient's and/or family's needs. Usually, the presenting problem(s) are of low to moderate severity.

 1.17 1.17 **FUD** XXX J 80 🖵

AMA: 2019,Jul,10; 2018,Jan,8; 2017,Aug,3; 2017,Jun,6; 2017,Jan,8; 2016,Jan,7; 2016,Jan,13; 2015,Jan,16; 2015,Jan,12; 2014,Nov,14; 2014,Oct,8; 2014,Jan,11

99283 Emergency department visit for the evaluation and management of a patient, which requires these 3 key components: An expanded problem focused history; An expanded problem focused examination; and Medical decision making of moderate complexity. Counseling and/or coordination of care with other physicians, other qualified health care professionals, or agencies are provided consistent with the nature of the problem(s) and the patient's and/or family's needs. Usually, the presenting problem(s) are of moderate severity.

 1.75 1.75 **FUD** XXX J 80 🖵

AMA: 2019,Jul,10; 2018,Jan,8; 2017,Aug,3; 2017,Jun,6; 2017,Jan,8; 2016,Jan,13; 2016,Jan,7; 2015,Jan,16; 2015,Jan,12; 2014,Nov,14; 2014,Oct,8; 2014,Jan,11

99284 Emergency department visit for the evaluation and management of a patient, which requires these 3 key components: A detailed history; A detailed examination; and Medical decision making of moderate complexity. Counseling and/or coordination of care with other physicians, other qualified health care professionals, or agencies are provided consistent with the nature of the problem(s) and the patient's and/or family's needs. Usually, the presenting problem(s) are of high severity, and require urgent evaluation by the physician, or other qualified health care professionals but do not pose an immediate significant threat to life or physiologic function.

 3.32 3.32 **FUD** XXX J 80 🖵

AMA: 2019,Jul,10; 2018,Jan,8; 2017,Aug,3; 2017,Jun,6; 2017,Jan,8; 2016,Jan,7; 2016,Jan,13; 2015,Jan,16; 2015,Jan,12; 2014,Nov,14; 2014,Oct,8; 2014,Jan,11

99285 Emergency department visit for the evaluation and management of a patient, which requires these 3 key components within the constraints imposed by the urgency of the patient's clinical condition and/or mental status: A comprehensive history; A comprehensive examination; and Medical decision making of high complexity. Counseling and/or coordination of care with other physicians, other qualified health care professionals, or agencies are provided consistent with the nature of the problem(s) and the patient's and/or family's needs. Usually, the presenting problem(s) are of high severity and pose an immediate significant threat to life or physiologic function.

 4.89 4.89 **FUD** XXX J 80 🖵

AMA: 2019,Jul,10; 2018,Jan,8; 2017,Aug,3; 2017,Jun,6; 2017,Jan,8; 2016,Jan,7; 2016,Jan,13; 2015,Jan,16; 2015,Jan,12; 2014,Nov,14; 2014,Oct,8; 2014,Jan,11

99288 Physician or other qualified health care professional direction of emergency medical systems (EMS) emergency care, advanced life support

INCLUDES Management provided by an emergency/intensive care based physician or other qualified health care professional via voice contact to ambulance/rescue staff for services such as heart monitoring and drug administration

🔷 0.00 ⚕ 0.00 **FUD** XXX [B] 🖵

AMA: 2018,Jan,8; 2017,Aug,3; 2017,Jun,6; 2017,Jan,8; 2016,Jan,13; 2015,Jan,16; 2014,Oct,8; 2014,Jan,11

99291-99292 Critical Care Visits: Patients 72 Months of Age and Older

CMS: 100-04,11,40.1.3 Independent Attending Physician Services; 100-04,12,30.6.4 Services Furnished Incident to Physician's Service; 100-04,12,30.6.9 Swing Bed Visits; 100-04,12,40.3 Global Surgery Review; 100-04,4,160 Clinic and Emergency Visits Under OPPS; 100-04,4,160.1 Critical Care Services

INCLUDES 30 minutes or more of direct care provided by the physician or other qualified health care professional to a critically ill or injured patient, regardless of the location

All activities performed outside of the unit or off the floor

All time spent exclusively with patient/family/caregivers on the nursing unit or elsewhere

Outpatient critical care provided to neonates and pediatric patients up through 71 months of age

Physician or other qualified health care professional presence during interfacility transfer for critically ill/injured patients over 24 months of age

Professional services for interpretation of:
Blood gases
Chest films (71045-71046)
Measurement of cardiac output (93561-93562)
Other computer stored information
Pulse oximetry (94760-94762)
Professional services for:
Gastric intubation (43752-43753)
Transcutaneous pacing, temporary (92953)
Venous access, arterial puncture (36000, 36410, 36415, 36591, 36600)
Ventilation assistance and management, includes CPAP, CNP (94002-94004, 94660, 94662)

EXCLUDES All services that are less than 30 minutes; report appropriate E&M code

Inpatient critical care services provided to child 2 through 5 years of age (99475-99476)

Inpatient critical care services provided to infants 29 days through 24 months of age (99471-99472)

Inpatient critical care services provided to neonates that are age 28 days or less (99468-99469)

Other procedures not listed as included performed by the physician or other qualified health care professional rendering critical care

Patients who are not critically ill but in the critical care department (report appropriate E&M code)

Physician or other qualified health care professional presence during interfacility transfer for critically ill/injured patients under 24 months of age (99466-99467)

Supervisory services of control physician during interfacility transfer for critically ill/injured patients under 24 months of age ([99485, 99486])

99291 Critical care, evaluation and management of the critically ill or critically injured patient; first 30-74 minutes

🔷 6.28 ⚕ 7.82 **FUD** XXX [J] 80 🖵

AMA: 2019,Aug,8; 2019,Jul,10; 2018,Dec,8; 2018,Dec,8; 2018,Jun,9; 2018,Jan,8; 2017,Aug,3; 2017,Jun,6; 2017,Jan,8; 2016,Oct,8; 2016,Aug,9; 2016,May,3; 2016,Jan,13; 2015,Jul,3; 2015,Feb,10; 2015,Jan,16; 2014,Oct,8; 2014,Oct,14; 2014,Aug,5; 2014,May,4; 2014,Jan,11

+ **99292** each additional 30 minutes (List separately in addition to code for primary service)

Code first (99291)

🔷 3.15 ⚕ 3.46 **FUD** ZZZ [N] 80 🖵

AMA: 2019,Aug,8; 2019,Jul,10; 2018,Dec,8; 2018,Dec,8; 2018,Jun,9; 2018,Jan,8; 2017,Aug,3; 2017,Jun,6; 2017,Jan,8; 2016,Aug,9; 2016,May,3; 2016,Jan,13; 2015,Jul,3; 2015,Feb,10; 2015,Jan,16; 2014,Oct,8; 2014,Oct,14; 2014,Aug,5; 2014,May,4; 2014,Jan,11

99304-99310 Nursing Facility Visits

CMS: 100-04,11,40.1.3 Independent Attending Physician Services; 100-04,12,230 Primary Care Incentive Payment Program; 100-04,12,230.1 Definition of Primary Care Practitioners and Services; 100-04,12,230.2 Coordination with Other Payments; 100-04,12,230.3 Claims Processing and Payment; 100-04,12,30.6.10 Consultation Services; 100-04,12,30.6.13 Nursing Facility Visits; 100-04,12,30.6.15.1 Prolonged Services With Direct Face-to-Face Patient Contact; 100-04,12,30.6.4 Services Furnished Incident to Physician's Service; 100-04,12,30.6.9 Swing Bed Visits

INCLUDES All E&M services provided by the admitting physician on the date of nursing facility admission in other locations (e.g., office, emergency department)

Initial care, subsequent care, discharge, and yearly assessments

Initial services include patient assessment and physician participation in developing a plan of care (99304-99306)

Services provided in a psychiatric residential treatment center

Services provided to new and established patients in a nursing facility (skilled, intermediate, and long-term care facilities)

Subsequent services include physician review of medical records, reassessment, and review of test results (99307-99310)

EXCLUDES Care plan oversight services (99379-99380)

Code also hospital discharge services on the same date of admission or readmission to the nursing home (99217, 99234-99236, 99238-99239)

99304 Initial nursing facility care, per day, for the evaluation and management of a patient, which requires these 3 key components: A detailed or comprehensive history; A detailed or comprehensive examination; and Medical decision making that is straightforward or of low complexity. Counseling and/or coordination of care with other physicians, other qualified health care professionals, or agencies are provided consistent with the nature of the problem(s) and the patient's and/or family's needs. Usually, the problem(s) requiring admission are of low severity. Typically, 25 minutes are spent at the bedside and on the patient's facility floor or unit.

🔷 2.54 ⚕ 2.54 **FUD** XXX [B] 80 🖵

AMA: 2018,Jan,8; 2017,Aug,3; 2017,Jun,6; 2017,Jan,8; 2016,Dec,11; 2016,Jan,13; 2016,Jan,7; 2015,Jan,16; 2014,Nov,14; 2014,Oct,8; 2014,Jan,11

99305 Initial nursing facility care, per day, for the evaluation and management of a patient, which requires these 3 key components: A comprehensive history; A comprehensive examination; and Medical decision making of moderate complexity. Counseling and/or coordination of care with other physicians, other qualified health care professionals, or agencies are provided consistent with the nature of the problem(s) and the patient's and/or family's needs. Usually, the problem(s) requiring admission are of moderate severity. Typically, 35 minutes are spent at the bedside and on the patient's facility floor or unit.

🔷 3.67 ⚕ 3.67 **FUD** XXX [B] 80 🖵

AMA: 2018,Jan,8; 2017,Aug,3; 2017,Jun,6; 2017,Jan,8; 2016,Dec,11; 2016,Jan,13; 2016,Jan,7; 2015,Jan,16; 2014,Nov,14; 2014,Oct,8; 2014,Jan,11

99306 Initial nursing facility care, per day, for the evaluation and management of a patient, which requires these 3 key components: A comprehensive history; A comprehensive examination; and Medical decision making of high complexity. Counseling and/or coordination of care with other physicians, other qualified health care professionals, or agencies are provided consistent with the nature of the problem(s) and the patient's and/or family's needs. Usually, the problem(s) requiring admission are of high severity. Typically, 45 minutes are spent at the bedside and on the patient's facility floor or unit.

🔷 4.70 ⚕ 4.70 **FUD** XXX [B] 80 🖵

AMA: 2018,Jan,8; 2017,Aug,3; 2017,Jun,6; 2017,Jan,8; 2016,Dec,11; 2016,Jan,13; 2016,Jan,7; 2015,Jan,16; 2014,Nov,14; 2014,Oct,8; 2014,Jan,11

99307 Subsequent nursing facility care, per day, for the evaluation and management of a patient, which requires at least 2 of these 3 key components: A problem focused interval history; A problem focused examination; Straightforward medical decision making. Counseling and/or coordination of care with other physicians, other qualified health care professionals, or agencies are provided consistent with the nature of the problem(s) and the patient's and/or family's needs. Usually, the patient is stable, recovering, or improving. Typically, 10 minutes are spent at the bedside and on the patient's facility floor or unit.

    🔲 1.24　🔲 1.24　**FUD** XXX　　　　★ B 80 ▭

    AMA: 2018,Jan,8; 2017,Aug,3; 2017,Jun,6; 2017,Jan,8; 2016,Dec,11; 2016,Jan,13; 2016,Jan,7; 2015,Jan,16; 2014,Nov,14; 2014,Oct,8; 2014,Jan,11

99308 Subsequent nursing facility care, per day, for the evaluation and management of a patient, which requires at least 2 of these 3 key components: An expanded problem focused interval history; An expanded problem focused examination; Medical decision making of low complexity. Counseling and/or coordination of care with other physicians, other qualified health care professionals, or agencies are provided consistent with the nature of the problem(s) and the patient's and/or family's needs. Usually, the patient is responding inadequately to therapy or has developed a minor complication. Typically, 15 minutes are spent at the bedside and on the patient's facility floor or unit.

    🔲 1.94　🔲 1.94　**FUD** XXX　　　　★ B 80 ▭

    AMA: 2018,Jan,8; 2017,Aug,3; 2017,Jun,6; 2017,Jan,8; 2016,Dec,11; 2016,Jan,13; 2016,Jan,7; 2015,Jan,16; 2014,Nov,14; 2014,Oct,8; 2014,Jan,11

99309 Subsequent nursing facility care, per day, for the evaluation and management of a patient, which requires at least 2 of these 3 key components: A detailed interval history; A detailed examination; Medical decision making of moderate complexity. Counseling and/or coordination of care with other physicians, other qualified health care professionals, or agencies are provided consistent with the nature of the problem(s) and the patient's and/or family's needs. Usually, the patient has developed a significant complication or a significant new problem. Typically, 25 minutes are spent at the bedside and on the patient's facility floor or unit.

    🔲 2.58　🔲 2.58　**FUD** XXX　　　　★ B 80 ▭

    AMA: 2018,Jan,8; 2017,Aug,3; 2017,Jun,6; 2017,Jan,8; 2016,Dec,11; 2016,Jan,13; 2016,Jan,7; 2015,Jan,16; 2014,Nov,14; 2014,Oct,8; 2014,Jan,11

99310 Subsequent nursing facility care, per day, for the evaluation and management of a patient, which requires at least 2 of these 3 key components: A comprehensive interval history; A comprehensive examination; Medical decision making of high complexity. Counseling and/or coordination of care with other physicians, other qualified health care professionals, or agencies are provided consistent with the nature of the problem(s) and the patient's and/or family's needs. The patient may be unstable or may have developed a significant new problem requiring immediate physician attention. Typically, 35 minutes are spent at the bedside and on the patient's facility floor or unit.

    🔲 3.82　🔲 3.82　**FUD** XXX　　　　★ B 80 ▭

    AMA: 2018,Jan,8; 2017,Aug,3; 2017,Jun,6; 2017,Jan,8; 2016,Dec,11; 2016,Jan,13; 2016,Jan,7; 2015,Jan,16; 2014,Nov,14; 2014,Oct,8; 2014,Jan,11

99315-99316 Nursing Home Discharge

CMS: 100-04,11,40.1.3 Independent Attending Physician Services; 100-04,12,230 Primary Care Incentive Payment Program; 100-04,12,230.1 Definition of Primary Care Practitioners and Services; 100-04,12,230.2 Coordination with Other Payments; 100-04,12,230.3 Claims Processing and Payment; 100-04,12,30.6.13 Nursing Facility Visits; 100-04,12,30.6.4 Services Furnished Incident to Physician's Service; 100-04,12,40.3 Global Surgery Review

  INCLUDES　Discharge services include all time spent by the physician or other qualified health care professional for:
    Completion of discharge records
    Discharge instructions for patient and caregivers
    Discussion regarding the stay in the facility
    Final patient examination
    Provide prescriptions and referrals as appropriate

99315 Nursing facility discharge day management; 30 minutes or less

    🔲 2.07　🔲 2.07　**FUD** XXX　　　　B 80 ▭

    AMA: 2018,Jan,8; 2017,Aug,3; 2017,Jun,6; 2017,Jan,8; 2016,Dec,11; 2016,Jan,13; 2016,Jan,7; 2015,Jan,16; 2014,Nov,14; 2014,Oct,8; 2014,Jan,11

99316 more than 30 minutes

    🔲 2.98　🔲 2.98　**FUD** XXX　　　　B 80 ▭

    AMA: 2018,Jan,8; 2017,Aug,3; 2017,Jun,6; 2017,Jan,8; 2016,Dec,11; 2016,Jan,13; 2016,Jan,7; 2015,Jan,16; 2014,Nov,14; 2014,Oct,8; 2014,Jan,11

99318 Annual Nursing Home Assessment

CMS: 100-04,11,40.1.3 Independent Attending Physician Services; 100-04,12,230 Primary Care Incentive Payment Program; 100-04,12,230.1 Definition of Primary Care Practitioners and Services; 100-04,12,230.2 Coordination with Other Payments; 100-04,12,230.3 Claims Processing and Payment; 100-04,12,30.6.13 Nursing Facility Visits; 100-04,12,30.6.15.1 Prolonged Services With Direct Face-to-Face Patient Contact; 100-04,12,30.6.4 Services Furnished Incident to Physician's Service; 100-04,12,30.6.9 Swing Bed Visits

  INCLUDES　Includes nursing facility visits on same date of service as (99304-99316)

99318 Evaluation and management of a patient involving an annual nursing facility assessment, which requires these 3 key components: A detailed interval history; A comprehensive examination; and Medical decision making that is of low to moderate complexity. Counseling and/or coordination of care with other physicians, other qualified health care professionals, or agencies are provided consistent with the nature of the problem(s) and the patient's and/or family's needs. Usually, the patient is stable, recovering, or improving. Typically, 30 minutes are spent at the bedside and on the patient's facility floor or unit.

    🔲 2.70　🔲 2.70　**FUD** XXX　　　　B 80 ▭

    AMA: 2018,Jan,8; 2017,Aug,3; 2017,Jun,6; 2017,Jan,8; 2016,Dec,11; 2016,Jan,7; 2016,Jan,13; 2015,Jan,16; 2014,Nov,14; 2014,Oct,8; 2014,Jan,11

99324-99337 Domiciliary Care, Rest Home, Assisted Living Visits

CMS: 100-04,12,230 Primary Care Incentive Payment Program; 100-04,12,230.1 Definition of Primary Care Practitioners and Services; 100-04,12,230.2 Coordination with Other Payments; 100-04,12,230.3 Claims Processing and Payment; 100-04,12,30.6.14 Domiciliary Care, Rest Home, Assisted Living Visits; 100-04,12,30.6.15.1 Prolonged Services With Direct Face-to-Face Patient Contact; 100-04,12,30.6.4 Services Furnished Incident to Physician's Service

INCLUDES E&M services for patients residing in assisted living, domiciliary care, and rest homes where medical care is not included
Services provided to new patients or established patients (99324-99328, 99334-99337)

EXCLUDES *Care plan oversight services provided to a patient in a rest home under the care of a home health agency (99374-99375)*
Care plan oversight services provided to a patient under the care of a hospice agency (99377-99378)

99324 Domiciliary or rest home visit for the evaluation and management of a new patient, which requires these 3 key components: A problem focused history; A problem focused examination; and Straightforward medical decision making. Counseling and/or coordination of care with other physicians, other qualified health care professionals, or agencies are provided consistent with the nature of the problem(s) and the patient's and/or family's needs. Usually, the presenting problem(s) are of low severity. Typically, 20 minutes are spent with the patient and/or family or caregiver.
1.56 ⚖ 1.56 **FUD** XXX   B 80 ▭
AMA: 2018,Apr,9; 2018,Jan,8; 2017,Aug,3; 2017,Jun,6; 2017,Jan,8; 2016,Dec,11; 2016,Jan,13; 2016,Jan,7; 2015,Jan,16; 2014,Nov,14; 2014,Oct,8; 2014,Oct,3; 2014,Jan,11

99325 Domiciliary or rest home visit for the evaluation and management of a new patient, which requires these 3 key components: An expanded problem focused history; An expanded problem focused examination; and Medical decision making of low complexity. Counseling and/or coordination of care with other physicians, other qualified health care professionals, or agencies are provided consistent with the nature of the problem(s) and the patient's and/or family's needs. Usually, the presenting problem(s) are of moderate severity. Typically, 30 minutes are spent with the patient and/or family or caregiver.
2.26 ⚖ 2.26 **FUD** XXX   B 80 ▭
AMA: 2018,Apr,9; 2018,Jan,8; 2017,Aug,3; 2017,Jun,6; 2017,Jan,8; 2016,Dec,11; 2016,Jan,13; 2016,Jan,7; 2015,Jan,16; 2014,Nov,14; 2014,Oct,8; 2014,Oct,3; 2014,Jan,11

99326 Domiciliary or rest home visit for the evaluation and management of a new patient, which requires these 3 key components: A detailed history; A detailed examination; and Medical decision making of moderate complexity. Counseling and/or coordination of care with other physicians, other qualified health care professionals, or agencies are provided consistent with the nature of the problem(s) and the patient's and/or family's needs. Usually, the presenting problem(s) are of moderate to high severity. Typically, 45 minutes are spent with the patient and/or family or caregiver.
3.92 ⚖ 3.92 **FUD** XXX   B 80 ▭
AMA: 2018,Apr,9; 2018,Jan,8; 2017,Aug,3; 2017,Jun,6; 2017,Jan,8; 2016,Dec,11; 2016,Jan,13; 2016,Jan,7; 2015,Jan,16; 2014,Nov,14; 2014,Oct,8; 2014,Oct,3; 2014,Jan,11

99327 Domiciliary or rest home visit for the evaluation and management of a new patient, which requires these 3 key components: A comprehensive history; A comprehensive examination; and Medical decision making of moderate complexity. Counseling and/or coordination of care with other physicians, other qualified health care professionals, or agencies are provided consistent with the nature of the problem(s) and the patient's and/or family's needs. Usually, the presenting problem(s) are of high severity. Typically, 60 minutes are spent with the patient and/or family or caregiver.
5.26 ⚖ 5.26 **FUD** XXX   B 80 ▭
AMA: 2018,Apr,9; 2018,Jan,8; 2017,Aug,3; 2017,Jun,6; 2017,Jan,8; 2016,Dec,11; 2016,Jan,13; 2016,Jan,7; 2015,Jan,16; 2014,Nov,14; 2014,Oct,8; 2014,Oct,3; 2014,Jan,11

99328 Domiciliary or rest home visit for the evaluation and management of a new patient, which requires these 3 key components: A comprehensive history; A comprehensive examination; and Medical decision making of high complexity. Counseling and/or coordination of care with other physicians, other qualified health care professionals, or agencies are provided consistent with the nature of the problem(s) and the patient's and/or family's needs. Usually, the patient is unstable or has developed a significant new problem requiring immediate physician attention. Typically, 75 minutes are spent with the patient and/or family or caregiver.
6.19 ⚖ 6.19 **FUD** XXX   B 80 ▭
AMA: 2018,Apr,9; 2018,Jan,8; 2017,Aug,3; 2017,Jun,6; 2017,Jan,8; 2016,Dec,11; 2016,Jan,13; 2016,Jan,7; 2015,Jan,16; 2014,Nov,14; 2014,Oct,8; 2014,Oct,3; 2014,Jan,11

99334 Domiciliary or rest home visit for the evaluation and management of an established patient, which requires at least 2 of these 3 key components: A problem focused interval history; A problem focused examination; Straightforward medical decision making. Counseling and/or coordination of care with other physicians, other qualified health care professionals, or agencies are provided consistent with the nature of the problem(s) and the patient's and/or family's needs. Usually, the presenting problem(s) are self-limited or minor. Typically, 15 minutes are spent with the patient and/or family or caregiver.
1.70 ⚖ 1.70 **FUD** XXX   B 80 ▭
AMA: 2018,Apr,9; 2018,Jan,8; 2017,Aug,3; 2017,Jun,6; 2017,Jan,8; 2016,Dec,11; 2016,Jan,13; 2016,Jan,7; 2015,Jan,16; 2014,Nov,14; 2014,Oct,8; 2014,Oct,3; 2014,Jan,11

99335 Domiciliary or rest home visit for the evaluation and management of an established patient, which requires at least 2 of these 3 key components: An expanded problem focused interval history; An expanded problem focused examination; Medical decision making of low complexity. Counseling and/or coordination of care with other physicians, other qualified health care professionals, or agencies are provided consistent with the nature of the problem(s) and the patient's and/or family's needs. Usually, the presenting problem(s) are of low to moderate severity. Typically, 25 minutes are spent with the patient and/or family or caregiver.
2.68 ⚖ 2.68 **FUD** XXX   B 80 ▭
AMA: 2018,Apr,9; 2018,Jan,8; 2017,Aug,3; 2017,Jun,6; 2017,Jan,8; 2016,Dec,11; 2016,Jan,13; 2016,Jan,7; 2015,Jan,16; 2014,Nov,14; 2014,Oct,8; 2014,Oct,3; 2014,Jan,11

Evaluation and Management

99336 — 99343

99336 Domiciliary or rest home visit for the evaluation and management of an established patient, which requires at least 2 of these 3 key components: A detailed interval history; A detailed examination; Medical decision making of moderate complexity. Counseling and/or coordination of care with other physicians, other qualified health care professionals, or agencies are provided consistent with the nature of the problem(s) and the patient's and/or family's needs. Usually, the presenting problem(s) are of moderate to high severity. Typically, 40 minutes are spent with the patient and/or family or caregiver.

  📖 3.82   ⚕ 3.82   **FUD** XXX   B 80 ▭

  AMA: 2018,Apr,9; 2018,Jan,8; 2017,Aug,3; 2017,Jun,6; 2017,Jan,8; 2016,Dec,11; 2016,Jan,13; 2016,Jan,7; 2015,Jan,16; 2014,Nov,14; 2014,Oct,8; 2014,Oct,3; 2014,Jan,11

99337 Domiciliary or rest home visit for the evaluation and management of an established patient, which requires at least 2 of these 3 key components: A comprehensive interval history; A comprehensive examination; Medical decision making of moderate to high complexity. Counseling and/or coordination of care with other physicians, other qualified health care professionals, or agencies are provided consistent with the nature of the problem(s) and the patient's and/or family's needs. Usually, the presenting problem(s) are of moderate to high severity. The patient may be unstable or may have developed a significant new problem requiring immediate physician attention. Typically, 60 minutes are spent with the patient and/or family or caregiver.

  📖 5.47   ⚕ 5.47   **FUD** XXX   B 80 ▭

  AMA: 2018,Apr,9; 2018,Jan,8; 2017,Aug,3; 2017,Jun,6; 2017,Jan,8; 2016,Dec,11; 2016,Jan,13; 2016,Jan,7; 2015,Jan,16; 2014,Nov,14; 2014,Oct,8; 2014,Oct,3; 2014,Jan,11

99339-99340 Care Plan Oversight: Rest Home, Domiciliary Care, Assisted Living, and Home

CMS: 100-04,12,180 Payment of Care Plan Oversight (CPO); 100-04,12,180.1 Billing for Care Plan Oversight (CPO); 100-04,12,230 Primary Care Incentive Payment Program; 100-04,12,230.1 Definition of Primary Care Practitioners and Services; 100-04,12,230.2 Coordination with Other Payments; 100-04,12,230.3 Claims Processing and Payment; 100-04,12,30.6.14 Domiciliary Care, Rest Home, Assisted Living Visits; 100-04,12,30.6.4 Services Furnished Incident to Physician's Service

  INCLUDES Care plan oversight for patients residing in assisted living, domiciliary care, private residences, and rest homes
            Patient management services during same time frame as ([99421, 99422, 99423], 99441-99443, 98966-98969)

  EXCLUDES *Care plan oversight services furnished under a home health agency, nursing facility, or hospice (99374-99380)*

99339 Individual physician supervision of a patient (patient not present) in home, domiciliary or rest home (eg, assisted living facility) requiring complex and multidisciplinary care modalities involving regular physician development and/or revision of care plans, review of subsequent reports of patient status, review of related laboratory and other studies, communication (including telephone calls) for purposes of assessment or care decisions with health care professional(s), family member(s), surrogate decision maker(s) (eg, legal guardian) and/or key caregiver(s) involved in patient's care, integration of new information into the medical treatment plan and/or adjustment of medical therapy, within a calendar month; 15-29 minutes

  📖 2.17   ⚕ 2.17   **FUD** XXX   B ▭

  AMA: 2019,Jan,6; 2018,Oct,9; 2018,Jan,8; 2017,Aug,3; 2017,Jun,6; 2017,Jan,8; 2016,Jan,13; 2015,Jan,16; 2014,Oct,3; 2014,Oct,8; 2014,Jan,11

99340 30 minutes or more

  📖 3.05   ⚕ 3.05   **FUD** XXX   B ▭

  AMA: 2019,Jan,6; 2018,Oct,9; 2018,Jan,8; 2017,Aug,3; 2017,Jun,6; 2017,Jan,8; 2016,Jan,13; 2015,Jan,16; 2014,Oct,3; 2014,Oct,8; 2014,Jan,11

99341-99350 Home Visits

CMS: 100-04,11,40.1.3 Independent Attending Physician Services; 100-04,12,230 Primary Care Incentive Payment Program; 100-04,12,230.1 Definition of Primary Care Practitioners and Services; 100-04,12,230.2 Coordination with Other Payments; 100-04,12,230.3 Claims Processing and Payment; 100-04,12,30.6.14 Domiciliary Care, Rest Home, Assisted Living Visits; 100-04,12,30.6.14.1 Home Visits; 100-04,12,30.6.15.1 Prolonged Services With Direct Face-to-Face Patient Contact; 100-04,12,30.6.4 Services Furnished Incident to Physician's Service; 100-04,12,40.3 Global Surgery Review; 100-04,30.6.14.1 Home Services (Codes 99341 - 99350)

  INCLUDES Services for a new patient or an established patient (99341-99345, 99347-99350)
            Services provided to a patient in a private home (e.g., private residence, temporary or short-term housing such as campground, cruise ship, hostel or hotel)

  EXCLUDES *Services provided to patients under home health agency or hospice care (99374-99378)*

99341 Home visit for the evaluation and management of a new patient, which requires these 3 key components: A problem focused history; A problem focused examination; and Straightforward medical decision making. Counseling and/or coordination of care with other physicians, other qualified health care professionals, or agencies are provided consistent with the nature of the problem(s) and the patient's and/or family's needs. Usually, the presenting problem(s) are of low severity. Typically, 20 minutes are spent face-to-face with the patient and/or family.

  📖 1.56   ⚕ 1.56   **FUD** XXX   B 80 ▭

  AMA: 2018,Apr,9; 2018,Jan,8; 2017,Aug,3; 2017,Jun,6; 2017,Jan,8; 2016,Dec,11; 2016,Jan,13; 2016,Jan,7; 2015,Jan,16; 2014,Nov,14; 2014,Oct,8; 2014,Oct,3; 2014,Jan,11

99342 Home visit for the evaluation and management of a new patient, which requires these 3 key components: An expanded problem focused history; An expanded problem focused examination; and Medical decision making of low complexity. Counseling and/or coordination of care with other physicians, other qualified health care professionals, or agencies are provided consistent with the nature of the problem(s) and the patient's and/or family's needs. Usually, the presenting problem(s) are of moderate severity. Typically, 30 minutes are spent face-to-face with the patient and/or family.

  📖 2.25   ⚕ 2.25   **FUD** XXX   B 80 ▭

  AMA: 2018,Apr,9; 2018,Jan,8; 2017,Aug,3; 2017,Jun,6; 2017,Jan,8; 2016,Dec,11; 2016,Jan,13; 2016,Jan,7; 2015,Jan,16; 2014,Nov,14; 2014,Oct,8; 2014,Oct,3; 2014,Jan,11

99343 Home visit for the evaluation and management of a new patient, which requires these 3 key components: A detailed history; A detailed examination; and Medical decision making of moderate complexity. Counseling and/or coordination of care with other physicians, other qualified health care professionals, or agencies are provided consistent with the nature of the problem(s) and the patient's and/or family's needs. Usually, the presenting problem(s) are of moderate to high severity. Typically, 45 minutes are spent face-to-face with the patient and/or family.

  📖 3.67   ⚕ 3.67   **FUD** XXX   B 80 ▭

  AMA: 2018,Apr,9; 2018,Jan,8; 2017,Aug,3; 2017,Jun,6; 2017,Jan,8; 2016,Dec,11; 2016,Jan,13; 2016,Jan,7; 2015,Jan,16; 2014,Nov,14; 2014,Oct,8; 2014,Oct,3; 2014,Jan,11

99344 Home visit for the evaluation and management of a new patient, which requires these 3 key components: A comprehensive history; A comprehensive examination; and Medical decision making of moderate complexity. Counseling and/or coordination of care with other physicians, other qualified health care professionals, or agencies are provided consistent with the nature of the problem(s) and the patient's and/or family's needs. Usually, the presenting problem(s) are of high severity. Typically, 60 minutes are spent face-to-face with the patient and/or family.

🚑 5.14   ⚗ 5.14   **FUD** XXX   [B] [80] [💻]

AMA: 2018,Apr,9; 2018,Jan,8; 2017,Aug,3; 2017,Jun,6; 2017,Jan,8; 2016,Dec,11; 2016,Jan,7; 2016,Jan,13; 2015,Jan,16; 2014,Nov,14; 2014,Oct,8; 2014,Oct,3; 2014,Jan,11

99345 Home visit for the evaluation and management of a new patient, which requires these 3 key components: A comprehensive history; A comprehensive examination; and Medical decision making of high complexity. Counseling and/or coordination of care with other physicians, other qualified health care professionals, or agencies are provided consistent with the nature of the problem(s) and the patient's and/or family's needs. Usually, the patient is unstable or has developed a significant new problem requiring immediate physician attention. Typically, 75 minutes are spent face-to-face with the patient and/or family.

🚑 6.25   ⚗ 6.25   **FUD** XXX   [B] [80] [💻]

AMA: 2018,Apr,9; 2018,Jan,8; 2017,Aug,3; 2017,Jun,6; 2017,Jan,8; 2016,Dec,11; 2016,Jan,7; 2016,Jan,13; 2015,Jan,16; 2014,Nov,14; 2014,Oct,8; 2014,Oct,3; 2014,Jan,11

99347 Home visit for the evaluation and management of an established patient, which requires at least 2 of these 3 key components: A problem focused interval history; A problem focused examination; Straightforward medical decision making. Counseling and/or coordination of care with other physicians, other qualified health care professionals, or agencies are provided consistent with the nature of the problem(s) and the patient's and/or family's needs. Usually, the presenting problem(s) are self limited or minor. Typically, 15 minutes are spent face-to-face with the patient and/or family.

🚑 1.56   ⚗ 1.56   **FUD** XXX   [B] [80] [💻]

AMA: 2018,Apr,9; 2018,Jan,8; 2017,Aug,3; 2017,Jun,6; 2017,Jan,8; 2016,Dec,11; 2016,Jan,7; 2016,Jan,13; 2015,Jan,16; 2014,Nov,14; 2014,Oct,8; 2014,Oct,3; 2014,Jan,11

99348 Home visit for the evaluation and management of an established patient, which requires at least 2 of these 3 key components: An expanded problem focused interval history; An expanded problem focused examination; Medical decision making of low complexity. Counseling and/or coordination of care with other physicians, other qualified health care professionals, or agencies are provided consistent with the nature of the problem(s) and the patient's and/or family's needs. Usually, the presenting problem(s) are of low to moderate severity. Typically, 25 minutes are spent face-to-face with the patient and/or family.

🚑 2.37   ⚗ 2.37   **FUD** XXX   [B] [80] [💻]

AMA: 2018,Apr,9; 2018,Jan,8; 2017,Aug,3; 2017,Jun,6; 2017,Jan,8; 2016,Dec,11; 2016,Jan,7; 2016,Jan,13; 2015,Jan,16; 2014,Nov,14; 2014,Oct,8; 2014,Oct,3; 2014,Jan,11

99349 Home visit for the evaluation and management of an established patient, which requires at least 2 of these 3 key components: A detailed interval history; A detailed examination; Medical decision making of moderate complexity. Counseling and/or coordination of care with other physicians, other qualified health care professionals, or agencies are provided consistent with the nature of the problem(s) and the patient's and/or family's needs. Usually, the presenting problem(s) are moderate to high severity. Typically, 40 minutes are spent face-to-face with the patient and/or family.

🚑 3.64   ⚗ 3.64   **FUD** XXX   [B] [80] [💻]

AMA: 2018,Apr,9; 2018,Jan,8; 2017,Aug,3; 2017,Jun,6; 2017,Jan,8; 2016,Dec,11; 2016,Jan,7; 2016,Jan,13; 2015,Jan,16; 2014,Nov,14; 2014,Oct,8; 2014,Oct,3; 2014,Jan,11

99350 Home visit for the evaluation and management of an established patient, which requires at least 2 of these 3 key components: A comprehensive interval history; A comprehensive examination; Medical decision making of moderate to high complexity. Counseling and/or coordination of care with other physicians, other qualified health care professionals, or agencies are provided consistent with the nature of the problem(s) and the patient's and/or family's needs. Usually, the presenting problem(s) are of moderate to high severity. The patient may be unstable or may have developed a significant new problem requiring immediate physician attention. Typically, 60 minutes are spent face-to-face with the patient and/or family.

🚑 5.05   ⚗ 5.05   **FUD** XXX   [B] [80] [💻]

AMA: 2018,Apr,9; 2018,Jan,8; 2017,Aug,3; 2017,Jun,6; 2017,Jan,8; 2016,Dec,11; 2016,Jan,7; 2016,Jan,13; 2015,Jan,16; 2014,Nov,14; 2014,Oct,8; 2014,Oct,3; 2014,Jan,11

99354-99357 Prolonged Services Direct Contact

CMS: 100-04,11,40.1.3 Independent Attending Physician Services; 100-04,12,30.6.15.1 Prolonged Services With Direct Face-to-Face Patient Contact; 100-04,12,30.6.4 Services Furnished Incident to Physician's Service

INCLUDES Personal contact with the patient by the physician or other qualified health professional
Services extending beyond the customary service provided in the inpatient or outpatient setting
Time spent providing additional indirect contact services on the floor or unit of the hospital or nursing facility during the same session as the direct contact
Time spent providing prolonged services on a date of service, even when the time is not continuous

EXCLUDES Services less than 30 minutes, less than 15 minutes after the first hour, or after the final 30 minutes
Services provided independent of the date of personal contact with the patient (99358-99359)

Code first E&M service code, as appropriate

+ 99354 Prolonged evaluation and management or psychotherapy service(s) (beyond the typical service time of the primary procedure) in the office or other outpatient setting requiring direct patient contact beyond the usual service; first hour (List separately in addition to code for office or other outpatient Evaluation and Management or psychotherapy service)

EXCLUDES Prolonged service provided by clinical staff under supervision ([99415, 99416])
Use of code more than one time per date of service

Code first (99201-99215, 99241-99245, 99324-99337, 99341-99350, 90837, 90847)

🚑 3.44   ⚗ 3.67   **FUD** ZZZ   [★] [N] [80] [💻]

AMA: 2019,Jun,7; 2018,Jan,8; 2017,Jan,8; 2016,Dec,11; 2016,Jan,13; 2015,Oct,9; 2015,Oct,3; 2015,Jan,16; 2014,Oct,8; 2014,Jun,14; 2014,Apr,6; 2014,Jan,11

+   99355   **each additional 30 minutes (List separately in addition to code for prolonged service)**

> EXCLUDES   *Prolonged service provided by clinical staff under supervision ([99415, 99416])*
> Code first (99354)
> 🚑 2.60   ⚕ 2.80   **FUD** ZZZ   ★ N 80 ▣

AMA: 2019,Jun,7; 2018,Jan,8; 2017,Jan,8; 2016,Dec,11; 2016,Jan,13; 2015,Oct,9; 2015,Oct,3; 2015,Jan,16; 2014,Oct,8; 2014,Jun,14; 2014,Apr,6; 2014,Jan,11

+   99356   **Prolonged service in the inpatient or observation setting, requiring unit/floor time beyond the usual service; first hour (List separately in addition to code for inpatient Evaluation and Management service)**

> EXCLUDES   *Use of code more than one time per date of service*
> Code first (99218-99223 [99224, 99225, 99226], 99231-99236, 99251-99255, 99304-99310, 90837, 90847)
> 🚑 2.60   ⚕ 2.60   **FUD** ZZZ   C 80 ▣

AMA: 2019,Jun,7; 2018,Jan,8; 2017,Jan,8; 2016,Dec,11; 2016,Jan,13; 2015,Oct,9; 2015,Oct,3; 2015,Jan,16; 2014,Oct,8; 2014,Jun,14; 2014,Apr,6; 2014,Jan,11

+   99357   **each additional 30 minutes (List separately in addition to code for prolonged service)**

> Code first (99356)
> 🚑 2.61   ⚕ 2.61   **FUD** ZZZ   C 80 ▣

AMA: 2019,Jun,7; 2018,Jan,8; 2017,Jan,8; 2016,Dec,11; 2016,Jan,13; 2015,Oct,9; 2015,Oct,3; 2015,Jan,16; 2014,Oct,8; 2014,Jun,14; 2014,Apr,6; 2014,Jan,11

99358-99359 Prolonged Services Indirect Contact

CMS: 100-04,11,40.1.3 Independent Attending Physician Services; 100-04,12,30.6.15.2 Prolonged Services Without Face to Face Service; 100-04,12,30.6.4 Services Furnished Incident to Physician's Service

> INCLUDES   Services extending beyond the customary service
> Time spent providing indirect contact services by the physician or other qualified health care professional in relation to patient management where face-to-face services have or will occur on a different date
> Time spent providing prolonged services performed on a date of service (which may be other than the date of the primary service) that are not continuous

> EXCLUDES   *Any additional unit or floor time in the hospital or nursing facility during the same evaluation and management session*
> *Behavioral health integration care management services (99484)*
> *Care plan oversight (99339-99340, 99374-99380)*
> *Chronic care management services provided during the same month ([99490], [99491])*
> *INR monitoring services (93792-93793)*
> *Online medical services ([99421, 99422, 99423])*
> *Patient management services during same time frame as (99487-99489, 99495-99496)*
> *Psychiatric collaborative care management services during the same month (99492-99494)*
> *Services less than 30 minutes, less than 15 minutes after the first hour, or after the final 30 minutes*
> *Time spent in medical team conference (99366-99368)*
> *Use of code more than one time per date of service*
> Code also E&M or other services provided

99358   **Prolonged evaluation and management service before and/or after direct patient care; first hour**

> EXCLUDES   *Use of code more than one time per date of service*
> 🚑 3.15   ⚕ 3.15   **FUD** XXX   N 80 ▣

AMA: 2019,Jun,7; 2019,Jan,13; 2018,Oct,9; 2018,Jan,8; 2017,Jan,8; 2016,Jan,13; 2015,Jan,16; 2014,Oct,8; 2014,Oct,3; 2014,Jan,11

+   99359   **each additional 30 minutes (List separately in addition to code for prolonged service)**

> Code first (99358)
> 🚑 1.52   ⚕ 1.52   **FUD** ZZZ   N 80 ▣

AMA: 2019,Jun,7; 2019,Jan,13; 2018,Oct,9; 2018,Jan,8; 2017,Jan,8; 2016,Jan,13; 2015,Jan,16; 2014,Oct,8; 2014,Oct,3; 2014,Jan,11

99415-99416 [99415, 99416] Prolonged Clinical Staff Services Under Supervision

CMS: 100-04,11,40.1.3 Independent Attending Physician Services

> INCLUDES   Time spent by clinical staff providing prolonged face-to-face services extending beyond the customary service under the supervision of a physician or other qualified health professional
> Time spent by clinical staff providing prolonged services on a date of service, even when the time is not continuous

> EXCLUDES   *Prolonged service provided by physician or other qualified health care professional (99354-99357)*
> *Services less than 45 minutes*
> *Services provided to more than two patients at the same time*
> Code also E&M or other services provided

+ #   99415   **Prolonged clinical staff service (the service beyond the typical service time) during an evaluation and management service in the office or outpatient setting, direct patient contact with physician supervision; first hour (List separately in addition to code for outpatient Evaluation and Management service)**

> EXCLUDES   *Use of code more than one time per date of service*
> Code first (99201-99215)
> 🚑 0.28   ⚕ 0.28   **FUD** ZZZ   N 80 TC ▣

AMA: 2018,Jan,8; 2017,Jan,8; 2016,Mar,8; 2016,Feb,13; 2016,Jan,13; 2015,Oct,3

+ #   99416   **each additional 30 minutes (List separately in addition to code for prolonged service)**

> EXCLUDES   *Services less than 30 minutes, less than 15 minutes after the first hour, or after the final 30 minutes*
> Code first ([99415])
> 🚑 0.12   ⚕ 0.12   **FUD** ZZZ   N 80 TC ▣

AMA: 2018,Jan,8; 2017,Jan,8; 2016,Mar,8; 2016,Feb,13; 2016,Jan,13; 2015,Oct,3

99360 Standby Services

CMS: 100-04,11,40.1.3 Independent Attending Physician Services; 100-04,12,30.6.15.3 Standby Services; 100-04,12,30.6.4 Services Furnished Incident to Physician's Service

> INCLUDES   Services requested by physician or qualified health care professional that involve no direct patient contact
> Total standby time for the day

> EXCLUDES   *Delivery attendance (99464)*
> *Less than 30 minutes of standby time*
> *On-call services mandated by the hospital (99026-99027)*
> Code also as appropriate (99460, 99465)

99360   **Standby service, requiring prolonged attendance, each 30 minutes (eg, operative standby, standby for frozen section, for cesarean/high risk delivery, for monitoring EEG)**

> 🚑 1.73   ⚕ 1.73   **FUD** XXX   B ▣

AMA: 2018,Jan,8; 2017,Jan,8; 2016,Jan,13; 2015,Jan,16; 2014,Oct,8; 2014,Apr,5; 2014,Jan,11

26/TC PC/TC Only   A2-Z3 ASC Payment   50 Bilateral   ♂ Male Only   ♀ Female Only   🚑 Facility RVU   ⚕ Non-Facility RVU   ▣ CCI   ✖ CLIA
FUD Follow-up Days   CMS: IOM   AMA: CPT Asst   A-Y OPPSI   80/80 Surg Assist Allowed / w/Doc   ✖ Lab Crosswalk   ✖ Radiology Crosswalk

552   CPT © 2019 American Medical Association. All Rights Reserved.   © 2019 Optum360, LLC

99366-99368 Interdisciplinary Conferences

CMS: 100-04,11,40.1.3 Independent Attending Physician Services

INCLUDES Documentation of participation, contribution, and recommendations of the conference
Face-to-face participation by minimum of three qualified people from different specialties or disciplines
Only participants who have performed face-to-face evaluations or direct treatment to the patient within the previous 60 days
Start of the review of an individual patient and ends at conclusion of review

EXCLUDES *Conferences of less than 30 minutes (not reportable)*
More than one individual from the same specialty at the same encounter
Patient management services during same time frame as (99487-99489, 99495-99496)
Time spent record keeping or writing a report

99366 **Medical team conference with interdisciplinary team of health care professionals, face-to-face with patient and/or family, 30 minutes or more, participation by nonphysician qualified health care professional**

INCLUDES Team conferences of 30 minutes or more
EXCLUDES *Team conferences by a physician with patient or family present, see appropriate evaluation and management service code*

🚑 1.19 ⚗ 1.21 **FUD** XXX N ▭

AMA: 2018,Apr,9; 2018,Jan,8; 2017,Jan,8; 2016,Jan,13; 2015,Jan,16; 2014,Oct,8; 2014,Oct,3; 2014,Jun,3; 2014,Jan,11

99367 **Medical team conference with interdisciplinary team of health care professionals, patient and/or family not present, 30 minutes or more; participation by physician**

INCLUDES Team conferences of 30 minutes or more
🚑 1.60 ⚗ 1.60 **FUD** XXX N ▭

AMA: 2018,Apr,9; 2018,Jan,8; 2017,Jan,8; 2016,Jan,13; 2015,Jan,16; 2014,Oct,8; 2014,Jun,3; 2014,Jan,11

99368 **participation by nonphysician qualified health care professional**

INCLUDES Team conferences of 30 minutes or more
🚑 1.04 ⚗ 1.04 **FUD** XXX N ▭

AMA: 2018,Apr,9; 2018,Jan,8; 2017,Jan,8; 2016,Jan,13; 2015,Jan,16; 2014,Oct,8; 2014,Oct,3; 2014,Jun,3; 2014,Jan,11

99374-99380 Care Plan Oversight: Patient Under Care of HHA, Hospice, or Nursing Facility

CMS: 100-04,11,40.1.3 Independent Attending Physician Services; 100-04,12,180 Payment of Care Plan Oversight (CPO); 100-04,12,180.1 Billing for Care Plan Oversight (CPO); 100-04,12,30.6.4 Services Furnished Incident to Physician's Service

INCLUDES Analysis of reports, diagnostic tests, treatment plans
Discussions with other health care providers, outside of the practice, involved in the patient's care
Establishment of and revisions to care plans within a 30-day period
Payment to one physician per month for covered care plan oversight services (must be the same one who signed the plan of care)

EXCLUDES *Care plan oversight services provided in a hospice agency (99377-99378)*
Care plan oversight services provided in assisted living, domiciliary care, or private residence, not under care of a home health agency or hospice (99339-99340)
Patient management services during same time frame as ([99421, 99422, 99423], 99441-99443, 98966-98968)
Routine postoperative care provided during a global surgery period
Time discussing treatment with patient and/or caregivers

Code also office/outpatient visits, hospital, home, nursing facility, domiciliary, or non-face-to-face services

99374 **Supervision of a patient under care of home health agency (patient not present) in home, domiciliary or equivalent environment (eg, Alzheimer's facility) requiring complex and multidisciplinary care modalities involving regular development and/or revision of care plans by that individual, review of subsequent reports of patient status, review of related laboratory and other studies, communication (including telephone calls) for purposes of assessment or care decisions with health care professional(s), family member(s), surrogate decision maker(s) (eg, legal guardian) and/or key caregiver(s) involved in patient's care, integration of new information into the medical treatment plan and/or adjustment of medical therapy, within a calendar month; 15-29 minutes**

🚑 1.60 ⚗ 1.96 **FUD** XXX B ▭

AMA: 2019,Jan,6; 2018,Jan,8; 2017,Jan,8; 2016,Jan,13; 2015,Jan,16; 2014,Oct,8; 2014,Oct,3; 2014,Jan,11

99375 **30 minutes or more**

🚑 2.50 ⚗ 2.94 **FUD** XXX E ▭

AMA: 2019,Jan,6; 2018,Jan,8; 2017,Jan,8; 2016,Jan,13; 2015,Jan,16; 2014,Oct,8; 2014,Oct,3; 2014,Jan,11

99377 **Supervision of a hospice patient (patient not present) requiring complex and multidisciplinary care modalities involving regular development and/or revision of care plans by that individual, review of subsequent reports of patient status, review of related laboratory and other studies, communication (including telephone calls) for purposes of assessment or care decisions with health care professional(s), family member(s), surrogate decision maker(s) (eg, legal guardian) and/or key caregiver(s) involved in patient's care, integration of new information into the medical treatment plan and/or adjustment of medical therapy, within a calendar month; 15-29 minutes**

🚑 1.60 ⚗ 1.96 **FUD** XXX B ▭

AMA: 2019,Jan,6; 2018,Jan,8; 2017,Jan,8; 2016,Jan,13; 2015,Jan,16; 2014,Oct,8; 2014,Oct,3; 2014,Jan,11

99378 **30 minutes or more**

🚑 2.50 ⚗ 2.94 **FUD** XXX E ▭

AMA: 2019,Jan,6; 2018,Jan,8; 2017,Jan,8; 2016,Jan,13; 2015,Jan,16; 2014,Oct,8; 2014,Oct,3; 2014,Jan,11

99379 Supervision of a nursing facility patient (patient not present) requiring complex and multidisciplinary care modalities involving regular development and/or revision of care plans by that individual, review of subsequent reports of patient status, review of related laboratory and other studies, communication (including telephone calls) for purposes of assessment or care decisions with health care professional(s), family member(s), surrogate decision maker(s) (eg, legal guardian) and/or key caregiver(s) involved in patient's care, integration of new information into the medical treatment plan and/or adjustment of medical therapy, within a calendar month; 15-29 minutes

     1.60   1.96   **FUD** XXX   B

     AMA: 2019,Jan,6; 2018,Jan,8; 2017,Jan,8; 2016,Jan,13; 2015,Jan,16; 2014,Oct,8; 2014,Oct,3; 2014,Jan,11

99380 30 minutes or more

     2.50   2.94   **FUD** XXX   B

     AMA: 2019,Jan,6; 2018,Jan,8; 2017,Jan,8; 2016,Jan,13; 2015,Jan,16; 2014,Oct,8; 2014,Oct,3; 2014,Jan,11

99381-99397 Preventive Medicine Visits

CMS: 100-04,11,40.1.3 Independent Attending Physician Services; 100-04,12,30.6.2 Medically Necessary and Preventive Medicine Service on Same Date; 100-04,12,30.6.4 Services Furnished Incident to Physician's Service

INCLUDES Care of a small problem or preexisting condition that requires no extra work
New patients or established patients (99381-99387, 99391-99397)
Regular preventive care (e.g., well-child exams) for all age groups

EXCLUDES *Behavioral change interventions (99406-99409)*
Counseling/risk factor reduction interventions not provided with a preventive medical examination (99401-99412)
Diagnostic tests and other procedures
Code also immunization counseling, administration, and product (90460-90461, 90471-90474, 90476-90749 [90620, 90621, 90625, 90630, 90644, 90672, 90673, 90674, 90750, 90756])
Code also significant, separately identifiable E&M service on the same date for substantial problems requiring additional work using modifier 25 and (99201-99215)

99381 Initial comprehensive preventive medicine evaluation and management of an individual including an age and gender appropriate history, examination, counseling/anticipatory guidance/risk factor reduction interventions, and the ordering of laboratory/diagnostic procedures, new patient; infant (age younger than 1 year)   A

     2.17   3.13   **FUD** XXX   E

     AMA: 2018,Jan,8; 2017,Jan,8; 2016,Mar,8; 2016,Jan,13; 2015,Jan,16; 2014,Oct,8; 2014,Jan,11

99382 early childhood (age 1 through 4 years)   A

     2.32   3.28   **FUD** XXX   E

     AMA: 2018,Jan,8; 2017,Jan,8; 2016,Mar,8; 2016,Jan,13; 2015,Jan,16; 2014,Oct,8; 2014,Jan,11

99383 late childhood (age 5 through 11 years)   A

     2.46   3.41   **FUD** XXX   E

     AMA: 2018,Jan,8; 2017,Jan,8; 2016,Mar,8; 2016,Jan,13; 2015,Jan,16; 2014,Oct,8; 2014,Jan,11

99384 adolescent (age 12 through 17 years)   A

     2.88   3.85   **FUD** XXX   E

     AMA: 2018,Jan,8; 2017,Jan,8; 2016,Mar,8; 2016,Jan,13; 2015,Jan,12; 2015,Jan,16; 2014,Oct,8; 2014,Jan,11

99385 18-39 years   A

     2.76   3.72   **FUD** XXX   E

     AMA: 2018,Jan,8; 2017,Jan,8; 2016,Mar,8; 2016,Jan,13; 2015,Jan,12; 2015,Jan,16; 2014,Oct,8; 2014,Jan,11

99386 40-64 years   A

     3.36   4.32   **FUD** XXX   E

     AMA: 2018,Jan,8; 2017,Jan,8; 2016,Mar,8; 2016,Jan,13; 2015,Jan,12; 2015,Jan,16; 2014,Oct,8; 2014,Jan,11

99387 65 years and older   A

     3.61   4.68   **FUD** XXX   E

     AMA: 2018,Jan,8; 2017,Jan,8; 2016,Mar,8; 2016,Jan,13; 2015,Jan,16; 2014,Oct,8; 2014,Jan,11

99391 Periodic comprehensive preventive medicine reevaluation and management of an individual including an age and gender appropriate history, examination, counseling/anticipatory guidance/risk factor reduction interventions, and the ordering of laboratory/diagnostic procedures, established patient; infant (age younger than 1 year)   A

     1.98   2.82   **FUD** XXX   E

     AMA: 2018,Jan,8; 2017,Jan,8; 2016,Mar,8; 2016,Jan,13; 2015,Jan,16; 2014,Oct,8; 2014,Jan,11

99392 early childhood (age 1 through 4 years)   A

     2.17   3.01   **FUD** XXX   E

     AMA: 2018,Jan,8; 2017,Jan,8; 2016,Mar,8; 2016,Jan,13; 2015,Jan,16; 2014,Oct,8; 2014,Jan,11

99393 late childhood (age 5 through 11 years)   A

     2.17   3.00   **FUD** XXX   E

     AMA: 2018,Jan,8; 2017,Jan,8; 2016,Mar,8; 2016,Jan,13; 2015,Jan,16; 2014,Oct,8; 2014,Jan,11

99394 adolescent (age 12 through 17 years)   A

     2.46   3.29   **FUD** XXX   E

     AMA: 2018,Jan,8; 2017,Jan,8; 2016,Mar,8; 2016,Jan,13; 2015,Jan,12; 2015,Jan,16; 2014,Oct,8; 2014,Jan,11

99395 18-39 years   A

     2.53   3.36   **FUD** XXX   E

     AMA: 2018,Jan,8; 2017,Jan,8; 2016,Mar,8; 2016,Jan,13; 2015,Jan,16; 2015,Jan,12; 2014,Oct,8; 2014,Jan,11

99396 40-64 years   A

     2.74   3.58   **FUD** XXX   E

     AMA: 2018,Jan,8; 2017,Sep,11; 2017,Jan,8; 2016,Mar,8; 2016,Jan,13; 2015,Jan,12; 2015,Jan,16; 2014,Oct,8; 2014,Jan,11

99397 65 years and older   A

     2.88   3.85   **FUD** XXX   E

     AMA: 2018,Jan,8; 2017,Jan,8; 2016,Mar,8; 2016,Jan,13; 2015,Jan,16; 2014,Oct,8; 2014,Jan,11

99401-99423 Counseling Services: Risk Factor and Behavioral Change Modification

INCLUDES Face-to-face services for new and established patients based on time increments of 15 to 60 minutes
Health and behavioral services provided on the same day (96156-96159 [96164, 96165, 96167, 96168, 96170, 96171])
Issues such as a healthy diet, exercise, alcohol and drug abuse
Services provided by a physician or other qualified healthcare professional for the purpose of promoting health and reducing illness and injury

EXCLUDES *Counseling and risk factor reduction interventions included in preventive medicine services (99381-99397)*
Counseling services provided to patient groups with existing symptoms or illness (99078)
Code also significant, separately identifiable E&M services when performed and append modifier 25 to that service

99401 Preventive medicine counseling and/or risk factor reduction intervention(s) provided to an individual (separate procedure); approximately 15 minutes

     0.70   1.10   **FUD** XXX   E

     AMA: 2018,Jan,8; 2017,Jan,8; 2016,Mar,8; 2016,Jan,13; 2015,Jan,16; 2014,Oct,8; 2014,Aug,5; 2014,Jan,11

99402 approximately 30 minutes

     1.42   1.81   **FUD** XXX   E

     AMA: 2018,Jan,8; 2017,Jan,8; 2016,Mar,8; 2016,Jan,13; 2015,Jan,16; 2014,Oct,8; 2014,Aug,5; 2014,Jan,11

99403 approximately 45 minutes

     2.12   2.51   **FUD** XXX   E

     AMA: 2018,Jan,8; 2017,Jan,8; 2016,Mar,8; 2016,Jan,13; 2015,Jan,16; 2014,Oct,8; 2014,Aug,5; 2014,Jan,11

99404 approximately 60 minutes

     2.81   3.21   **FUD** XXX   E

     AMA: 2018,Jan,8; 2017,Jan,8; 2016,Mar,8; 2016,Jan,13; 2015,Jan,16; 2014,Oct,8; 2014,Aug,5; 2014,Jan,11

26/TC PC/TC Only   A2-Z3 ASC Payment   50 Bilateral   ♂ Male Only   ♀ Female Only   Facility RVU   Non-Facility RVU   CCI   CLIA
FUD Follow-up Days   **CMS:** IOM   **AMA:** CPT Asst   A-Y OPPSI   80/80 Surg Assist Allowed / w/Doc   Lab Crosswalk   Radiology Crosswalk

554   CPT © 2019 American Medical Association. All Rights Reserved.   © 2019 Optum360, LLC

99406 Smoking and tobacco use cessation counseling visit; intermediate, greater than 3 minutes up to 10 minutes

　0.35 　0.42 **FUD** XXX ★ S 80 ▭

AMA: 2018,Jan,8; 2017,Nov,3; 2017,Jan,8; 2016,Mar,8; 2016,Jan,13; 2015,Jan,16; 2014,Oct,8; 2014,Jan,11

99407 intensive, greater than 10 minutes

INCLUDES Time duration of (99406)

　0.73 　0.80 **FUD** XXX ★ S 80 ▭

AMA: 2018,Jan,8; 2017,Nov,3; 2017,Jan,8; 2016,Mar,8; 2016,Jan,13; 2015,Jan,16; 2014,Oct,8; 2014,Jan,11

99408 Alcohol and/or substance (other than tobacco) abuse structured screening (eg, AUDIT, DAST), and brief intervention (SBI) services; 15 to 30 minutes

INCLUDES Health risk assessment (96160-96161)
Only initial screening and brief intervention
Services of 15 minutes or more

　0.94 　1.01 **FUD** XXX ★ E ▭

AMA: 2018,Jan,8; 2017,Nov,3; 2017,Jan,8; 2016,Nov,5; 2016,Mar,8; 2016,Jan,13; 2015,Jan,16; 2014,Oct,8; 2014,Jan,11

99409 greater than 30 minutes

INCLUDES Health risk assessment (96160-96161)
Only initial screening and brief intervention
Time duration of (99408)

　1.88 　1.95 **FUD** XXX ★ E ▭

AMA: 2018,Jan,8; 2017,Nov,3; 2017,Jan,8; 2016,Nov,5; 2016,Mar,8; 2016,Jan,13; 2015,Jan,16; 2014,Oct,8; 2014,Jan,11

99411 Preventive medicine counseling and/or risk factor reduction intervention(s) provided to individuals in a group setting (separate procedure); approximately 30 minutes

　0.22 　0.55 **FUD** XXX E ▭

AMA: 2018,Jan,8; 2017,Jan,8; 2016,Mar,8; 2016,Jan,13; 2015,Jan,16; 2014,Oct,8; 2014,Jan,11

99412 approximately 60 minutes

　0.36 　0.69 **FUD** XXX E ▭

AMA: 2018,Jan,8; 2017,Jan,8; 2016,Mar,8; 2016,Jan,13; 2015,Jan,16; 2014,Oct,8; 2014,Jan,11

99415 Resequenced code. See code following 99359.

99416 Resequenced code. See code following 99359.

99421 Resequenced code. See code following 99443.

99422 Resequenced code. See code following 99443.

99423 Resequenced code. See code following 99443.

99429 Other Preventive Medicine

99429 Unlisted preventive medicine service

　0.00 　0.00 **FUD** XXX E ▭

AMA: 2018,Jan,8; 2017,Jan,8; 2016,Mar,8; 2016,Jan,13; 2015,Jan,16; 2014,Oct,8; 2014,Jan,11

99441-99443 Telephone Calls for Patient Management

CMS: 100-04,11,40.1.3 Independent Attending Physician Services

INCLUDES Episodes of care initiated by an established patient or the patient or guardian of an established patient
Non-face-to-face E&M services provided by a physician or other health care provider qualified to report E&M services
Related E&M services provided within:
Postoperative period of a completed procedure
Seven days prior to the service

EXCLUDES Patient management services during same time frame as (99339-99340, 99374-99380, 99487-99489, 99495-99496, 93792-93793)
Services provided by a qualified nonphysician health care professional unable to report E&M codes (98966-98968)
Use of codes more than one time for telephone and online services when reported within a seven day period of time by the same provider

99441 Telephone evaluation and management service by a physician or other qualified health care professional who may report evaluation and management services provided to an established patient, parent, or guardian not originating from a related E/M service provided within the previous 7 days nor leading to an E/M service or procedure within the next 24 hours or soonest available appointment; 5-10 minutes of medical discussion

　0.36 　0.39 **FUD** XXX E ▭

AMA: 2019,Mar,8; 2018,Mar,7; 2018,Jan,8; 2017,Jan,8; 2016,Jan,13; 2015,Jan,16; 2014,Oct,3; 2014,Oct,8; 2014,Jan,11

99442 11-20 minutes of medical discussion

　0.72 　0.76 **FUD** XXX E ▭

AMA: 2019,Mar,8; 2018,Mar,7; 2018,Jan,8; 2017,Jan,8; 2016,Jan,13; 2015,Jan,16; 2014,Oct,3; 2014,Oct,8; 2014,Jan,11

99443 21-30 minutes of medical discussion

　1.08 　1.12 **FUD** XXX E ▭

AMA: 2019,Mar,8; 2018,Mar,7; 2018,Jan,8; 2017,Jan,8; 2016,Jan,13; 2015,Jan,16; 2014,Oct,3; 2014,Oct,8; 2014,Jan,11

99421-99423 [99421, 99422, 99423] Digital Evaluation and Management Services

CMS: 100-04,11,40.1.3 Independent Attending Physician Services

INCLUDES Cumulative service time within a 7 day time frame needed to evaluate, assess, and manage the patient:
Ordering of tests
Prescription generation
Separate digital inquiry for new and unrelated problem
Subsequent communication that is digitally supported (i.e., email, online, telephone)
Digital service initiated by an established patient

EXCLUDES Clinical staff time
Digital evaluation by a qualified nonphysician health care professional (98970-98972)
Digital evaluation peformed with separately reportable E&M services during same time frame for new or established patient:
Inquiries related to previously completed procedure and within the postoperative period
INR monitoring (93792-93793)
Office consultation (99241-99245)
Office or other outpatient visit (99201-99205, 99212-99215)
Patient management services (99339-99340, 99374-99380, [99091], 99487-99489, 99495-99496)
Digital service less than 5 minutes
Use of code more than one time in 7 days

● # **99421** Online digital evaluation and management service, for an established patient, for up to 7 days, cumulative time during the 7 days; 5-10 minutes

　0.00 　0.00 **FUD** 000

● # **99422** 11-20 minutes

　0.00 　0.00 **FUD** 000

● # **99423** 21 or more minutes

　0.00 　0.00 **FUD** 000

99444 Online Patient Management Services

99444 ~~Online evaluation and management service provided by a physician or other qualified health care professional who may report evaluation and management services provided to an established patient or guardian, not originating from a related E/M service provided within the previous 7 days, using the Internet or similar electronic communications network~~

To report, see (99421-99423)

99446-99452 [99451, 99452] Online and Telephone Consultative Services

INCLUDES   Multiple telephone and/or internet contact needed to complete the consultation (e.g., test result(s) follow-up)
New or established patient with new problem or exacerbation of existing problem and not seen within the last 14 days
Review of pertinent lab, imaging and/or pathology studies, medical records, medications

EXCLUDES   Any service less than 5 minutes
Communication with family with or without the patient present ([99421, 99422, 99423], 99441-99443, 98966-98967)
Transfer of care only

99446   Interprofessional telephone/Internet/electronic health record assessment and management service provided by a consultative physician, including a verbal and written report to the patient's treating/requesting physician or other qualified health care professional; 5-10 minutes of medical consultative discussion and review

INCLUDES   Verbal and written reports from the consultant to the requesting provider

EXCLUDES   Prolonged services without direct patient contact (99358-99359)
Use of code more than one time in 7 days

🚑 0.51   ⚕ 0.51   **FUD** XXX   E 80 ▢

AMA: 2019,Jun,7; 2019,Jan,3; 2018,Jan,8; 2017,Jan,8; 2016,Jan,13; 2015,Jan,16; 2014,Oct,8; 2014,Jun,14

99447   11-20 minutes of medical consultative discussion and review

INCLUDES   Verbal and written reports from the consultant to the requesting provider

EXCLUDES   Prolonged services without direct patient contact (99358-99359)
Use of code more than one time in 7 days

🚑 1.01   ⚕ 1.01   **FUD** XXX   E 80 ▢

AMA: 2019,Jun,7; 2019,Jan,3; 2018,Jan,8; 2017,Jan,8; 2016,Jan,13; 2015,Jan,16; 2014,Oct,8; 2014,Jun,14

99448   21-30 minutes of medical consultative discussion and review

INCLUDES   Verbal and written reports from the consultant to the requesting provider

EXCLUDES   Prolonged services without direct patient contact (99358-99359)
Use of code more than one time in 7 days

🚑 1.52   ⚕ 1.52   **FUD** XXX   E 80 ▢

AMA: 2019,Jun,7; 2019,Jan,3; 2018,Jan,8; 2017,Jan,8; 2016,Jan,13; 2015,Jan,16; 2014,Oct,8; 2014,Jun,14

99449   31 minutes or more of medical consultative discussion and review

INCLUDES   Verbal and written reports from the consultant to the requesting provider

EXCLUDES   Prolonged services without direct patient contact (99358-99359)
Use of code more than one time in 7 days

🚑 2.02   ⚕ 2.02   **FUD** XXX   E 80 ▢

AMA: 2019,Jun,7; 2019,Jan,3; 2018,Jan,8; 2017,Jan,8; 2016,Jan,13; 2015,Jan,16; 2014,Oct,8; 2014,Jun,14

\# **99451**   Interprofessional telephone/Internet/electronic health record assessment and management service provided by a consultative physician, including a written report to the patient's treating/requesting physician or other qualified health care professional, 5 minutes or more of medical consultative time

INCLUDES   Verbal and written reports from the consultant to the requesting provider

EXCLUDES   Prolonged services without direct patient contact (99358-99359)
Use of code more than one time in 7 days

🚑 1.04   ⚕ 1.04   **FUD** XXX   80 ▢

AMA: 2019,Jun,7; 2019,Jan,3

\# **99452**   Interprofessional telephone/Internet/electronic health record referral service(s) provided by a treating/requesting physician or other qualified health care professional, 30 minutes

INCLUDES   Time preparing for referral of 16 to 30 minutes

EXCLUDES   Requesting physician's time 30 minutes over the typical E&M service, patient not on site (99358-99359)
Requesting physician's time 30 minutes over the typical E&M service, patient on site (99354-99357)
Use of code more than one time every 14 days

🚑 1.04   ⚕ 1.04   **FUD** XXX   80 ▢

AMA: 2019,Jun,7; 2019,Jan,3

99453-99474 [99091, 99453, 99454, 99473, 99474] Remote Monitoring/Collection Biological Data

\# **99453**   Remote monitoring of physiologic parameter(s) (eg, weight, blood pressure, pulse oximetry, respiratory flow rate), initial; set-up and patient education on use of equipment

INCLUDES   30 day period of physiologic monitoring of parameters such as weight, blood pressure, pulse oximetry
Services ordered by physician or other qualified healthcare professional
Services provided for each episode of care (starts when monitoring begins and ends when treatment goals achieved)
Set-up and instructions for use
Use of device approved by the FDA

EXCLUDES   Use for monitoring of less than 16 days
Use of codes when services are included in other monitoring services (e.g., 93296, 94760, 95250)

🚑 0.54   ⚕ 0.54   **FUD** XXX   80 ▢

AMA: 2019,Mar,10; 2019,Jan,3; 2019,Jan,6

\# **99454**   device(s) supply with daily recording(s) or programmed alert(s) transmission, each 30 days

INCLUDES   30 day period of physiologic monitoring of parameters such as weight, blood pressure, pulse oximetry
Service ordered by physician or other qualified healthcare professional
Supply of device
Use of device approved by the FDA

EXCLUDES   Remote monitoring treatment management
Self-measured blood pressure monitoring ([99473, 99474])
Use for monitoring of less than 16 days
Use of codes when services are included in other monitoring services (e.g., 93296, 94760, 95250)

🚑 1.78   ⚕ 1.78   **FUD** XXX   80 ▢

AMA: 2019,Mar,10; 2019,Jan,3; 2019,Jan,6

26/TC PC/TC Only   A2-Z3 ASC Payment   50 Bilateral   ♂ Male Only   ♀ Female Only   🚑 Facility RVU   ⚕ Non-Facility RVU   ▢ CCI   ✖ CLIA
FUD Follow-up Days   CMS: IOM   AMA: CPT Asst   A-Y OPPSI   80/80 Surg Assist Allowed / w/Doc   ▢ Lab Crosswalk   ▢ Radiology Crosswalk

CPT © 2019 American Medical Association. All Rights Reserved.

556   © 2019 Optum360, LLC

Evaluation and Management

 # 99091 Collection and interpretation of physiologic data (eg, ECG, blood pressure, glucose monitoring) digitally stored and/or transmitted by the patient and/or caregiver to the physician or other qualified health care professional, qualified by education, training, licensure/regulation (when applicable) requiring a minimum of 30 minutes of time, each 30 days

INCLUDES E&M services provided on the same date of service

EXCLUDES *Care plan oversight services within 30 days (99339-99340, 99374-99375, 99378-99380)*
Remote physiologic monitoring treatment management within 30 days ([99457])
Use of code more than one time in 30 days
Use of codes when services are included in other monitoring services such as (93227, 93272, 95250)

1.62 1.62 **FUD** XXX N 80 ⌨

AMA: 2019,Jun,3; 2019,Jan,6; 2018,Dec,10; 2018,Dec,10; 2018,Jun,6; 2018,Mar,5; 2018,Feb,7; 2018,Jan,8; 2017,Jan,8; 2016,Jan,13; 2015,Jan,16; 2014,Oct,3; 2014,Jan,11

● # 99473 Self-measured blood pressure using a device validated for clinical accuracy; patient education/training and device calibration

0.00 0.00 **FUD** 000

EXCLUDES *Use of codes when services are included in the same calendar month as:*
Ambulatory blood pressure monitoring (93784-93790)
Chronic care management service ([99490, 99491], 99487-99489)
Remote physiologic monitoring, collection and interpretation ([99453, 99454], [99091], [99457])
Use of code more than once per device

● # 99474 separate self-measurements of two readings one minute apart, twice daily over a 30-day period (minimum of 12 readings), collection of data reported by the patient and/or caregiver to the physician or other qualified health care professional, with report of average systolic and diastolic pressures and subsequent communication of a treatment plan to the patient

0.00 0.00 **FUD** 000

EXCLUDES *Use of codes when services are included in the same calendar month as:*
Ambulatory blood pressure monitoring (93784-93790)
Chronic care management services ([99490, 99491], 99487-99489)
Remote physiologic monitoring, collection and interpretation services ([99453, 99454], [99091], [99457])
Use of code more than once per calendar month

99457-99458 [99457, 99458] Remote Monitoring Management

CMS: 100-04,11,40.1.3 Independent Attending Physician Services

INCLUDES Interactive live communication with patient for at least 20 minutes per month
Results of remote monitoring used for patient management
Service ordered by physician or other qualified healthcare professional
Time managing care when more specific service codes are not available
Use of code each 30 days no matter the number of parameters monitored
Use of device approved by the FDA

EXCLUDES *Use of code for services lasting less than 20 mintues*
Use of code on same date of service as E&M services (99201-99215, 99221-99223, 99231-99233, 99251-99255, 99324-99328, 99334-99337, 99341-99350)

▲ # 99457 Remote physiologic monitoring treatment management services, clinical staff/physician/other qualified health care professional time in a calendar month requiring interactive communication with the patient/caregiver during the month; first 20 minutes

EXCLUDES *Collection and interpretation of physiologic data ([99091])*

0.90 1.43 **FUD** XXX 80 ⌨

AMA: 2019,Jun,3; 2019,Jan,3; 2019,Jan,6

● + # 99458 each additional 20 minutes (List separately in addition to code for primary procedure)

0.00 0.00 **FUD** 000

EXCLUDES *Use of code if 20 minutes of additional treatment time is not obtained ([99457])*

Code first ([99457])

99450-99458 Life/Disability Insurance Eligibility Visits

INCLUDES Assessment services for insurance eligibility and work-related disability without medical management of the patient's illness/injury
Services provided to new/established patients at any site of service

EXCLUDES *Any additional E&M services or procedures performed on the same date of service: report with appropriate code*

99450 Basic life and/or disability examination that includes: Measurement of height, weight, and blood pressure; Completion of a medical history following a life insurance pro forma; Collection of blood sample and/or urinalysis complying with "chain of custody" protocols; and Completion of necessary documentation/certificates.

0.00 0.00 **FUD** XXX E ⌨

AMA: 2019,Jun,7; 2018,Jan,8; 2017,Jan,8; 2016,Jan,13; 2015,Jan,16; 2014,Oct,8; 2014,Jan,11

99451 Resequenced code. See code following 99449.

99452 Resequenced code. See code following 99449.

99453 Resequenced code. See code following 99449.

99454 Resequenced code. See code following 99449.

99455 Work related or medical disability examination by the treating physician that includes: Completion of a medical history commensurate with the patient's condition; Performance of an examination commensurate with the patient's condition; Formulation of a diagnosis, assessment of capabilities and stability, and calculation of impairment; Development of future medical treatment plan; and Completion of necessary documentation/certificates and report.

INCLUDES Special reports (99080)

0.00 0.00 **FUD** XXX B 80 ⌨

AMA: 2018,Jan,8; 2017,Jan,8; 2016,Jan,13; 2015,Jan,16; 2014,Oct,8; 2014,Jan,11

99456 Work related or medical disability examination by other than the treating physician that includes: Completion of a medical history commensurate with the patient's condition; Performance of an examination commensurate with the patient's condition; Formulation of a diagnosis, assessment of capabilities and stability, and calculation of impairment; Development of future medical treatment plan; and Completion of necessary documentation/certificates and report.

INCLUDES Special reports (99080)

0.00 0.00 **FUD** XXX B 80 ⌨

AMA: 2018,Jan,8; 2017,Jan,8; 2016,Jan,13; 2015,Jan,16; 2014,Oct,8; 2014,Jan,11

99457 Resequenced code. See code before resequenced code 99474.

99458 Resequenced code. See code before 99450.

99460-99463 Evaluation and Management Services for Age 28 Days or Less

CMS: 100-04,12,30.6.4 Services Furnished Incident to Physician's Service

INCLUDES
Family consultation
Healthy newborn history and physical
Medical record documentation
Ordering of diagnostic test and treatments
Services provided to healthy newborns age 28 days or less

EXCLUDES
Neonatal intensive and critical care services (99466-99469 [99485, 99486], 99477-99480)
Newborn follow up services in an office or outpatient setting (99201-99215, 99381, 99391)
Newborn hospital discharge services if provided on a date subsequent to the admission date (99238-99239)
Nonroutine neonatal inpatient evaluation and management services (99221-99233)

Code also attendance at delivery (99464)
Code also circumcision (54150)
Code also emergency resuscitation services (99465)

99460 Initial hospital or birthing center care, per day, for evaluation and management of normal newborn infant   A

    2.71   2.71   **FUD** XXX   V 80

AMA: 2018,Jan,8; 2017,Jan,8; 2016,Jan,13; 2015,Jan,16; 2014,Oct,8; 2014,Jan,11

99461 Initial care, per day, for evaluation and management of normal newborn infant seen in other than hospital or birthing center   A

    1.78   2.58   **FUD** XXX   M 80

AMA: 2018,Jan,8; 2017,Jan,8; 2016,Jan,13; 2015,Jan,16; 2014,Oct,8; 2014,Jan,11

99462 Subsequent hospital care, per day, for evaluation and management of normal newborn   A

    1.19   1.19   **FUD** XXX   C 80

AMA: 2018,Jan,8; 2017,Jan,8; 2016,Jan,13; 2015,Jan,16; 2014,Oct,8; 2014,Jan,11

99463 Initial hospital or birthing center care, per day, for evaluation and management of normal newborn infant admitted and discharged on the same date   A

    3.13   3.13   **FUD** XXX   V 80

AMA: 2018,Jan,8; 2017,Jan,8; 2016,Jan,13; 2015,Jan,16; 2014,Oct,8; 2014,Jan,11

99464-99465 Newborn Delivery Attendance/Resuscitation

CMS: 100-04,12,30.6.4 Services Furnished Incident to Physician's Service

99464 Attendance at delivery (when requested by the delivering physician or other qualified health care professional) and initial stabilization of newborn   A

EXCLUDES   *Resuscitation at delivery (99465)*

    2.12   2.12   **FUD** XXX   N 80

AMA: 2018,Jan,8; 2017,Jan,8; 2016,Jan,13; 2015,Jan,16; 2014,Oct,8; 2014,Jan,11

99465 Delivery/birthing room resuscitation, provision of positive pressure ventilation and/or chest compressions in the presence of acute inadequate ventilation and/or cardiac output   A

EXCLUDES   *Attendance at delivery (99464)*

Code also any necessary procedures performed as part of the resuscitation

    4.13   4.13   **FUD** XXX   S 80

AMA: 2018,Jan,8; 2017,Jan,8; 2016,Jan,13; 2015,Jan,16; 2014,Oct,8; 2014,Jan,11

99466-99467 Critical Care Transport Age 24 Months or Younger

CMS: 100-04,12,30.6.4 Services Furnished Incident to Physician's Service

INCLUDES
Face-to-face care starting when the physician assumes responsibility of the patient at the referring facility until the receiving facility accepts the patient
Physician presence during interfacility transfer of critically ill/injured patient 24 months of age or less
Services provided by the physician during transport:
    Blood gases
    Chest x-rays (71045-71046)
    Data stored in computers (e.g., ECGs, blood pressures, hematologic data)
    Gastric intubation (43752-43753)
    Interpretation of cardiac output measurements (93562)
    Pulse oximetry (94760-94762)
    Routine monitoring:
      Heart rate
      Respiratory rate
    Temporary transcutaneous pacing (92953)
    Vascular access procedures (36000, 36400, 36405-36406, 36415, 36591, 36600)
    Ventilatory management (94002-94003, 94660, 94662)

EXCLUDES
Neonatal hypothermia (99184)
Patient critical care transport services with personal contact with patient of less than 30 minutes
Physician directed emergency care via two-way voice communication with transporting staff (99288, [99485, 99486])
Services less than 30 minutes in duration (see E&M codes)
Services of the physician directing transport (control physician) ([99485, 99486])

Code also any services not designated as included in the critical care transport service

99466 Critical care face-to-face services, during an interfacility transport of critically ill or critically injured pediatric patient, 24 months of age or younger; first 30-74 minutes of hands-on care during transport

    6.75   6.75   **FUD** XXX   N 80

AMA: 2018,Jun,9; 2018,Jan,8; 2017,Jan,8; 2016,Jan,13; 2015,Jan,16; 2014,Oct,8; 2014,Jan,11

+ 99467 each additional 30 minutes (List separately in addition to code for primary service)   A

Code first (99466)

    3.37   3.37   **FUD** ZZZ   N 80

AMA: 2018,Jun,9; 2018,Jan,8; 2017,Jan,8; 2016,Jan,13; 2015,Jan,16; 2014,Oct,8; 2014,Jan,11

99485-99486 [99485, 99486] Critical Care Transport Supervision Age 24 Months or Younger

INCLUDES
Advice for treatment to the transport team from the control physician
Non face-to-face care starts with first contact by the control physician with the transport team and ends when patient responsibility is assumed by the receiving facility

EXCLUDES
Emergency systems physician direction for pediatric patient older than 24 months (99288)
Services provided by transport team
Services less than 15 minutes
Services performed by control physician for the same time period
Services performed by same physician providing critical care transport (99466-99467)

 # 99485 Supervision by a control physician of interfacility transport care of the critically ill or critically injured pediatric patient, 24 months of age or younger, includes two-way communication with transport team before transport, at the referring facility and during the transport, including data interpretation and report; first 30 minutes   A

    2.17   2.17   **FUD** XXX   B

AMA: 2018,Jun,9; 2018,Jan,8; 2017,Jan,8; 2016,Jan,13; 2015,Jan,16; 2014,Oct,8

+ # 99486 each additional 30 minutes (List separately in addition to code for primary procedure)   A

Code first ([99485])

    1.88   1.88   **FUD** XXX   B

AMA: 2018,Jun,9; 2018,Jan,8; 2017,Jan,8; 2016,Jan,13; 2015,Jan,16; 2014,Oct,8

26/TC PC/TC Only   A2-Z3 ASC Payment   50 Bilateral   ♂ Male Only   ♀ Female Only   Facility RVU   Non-Facility RVU   CCI   CLIA
FUD Follow-up Days   CMS: IOM   AMA: CPT Asst   A-Y OPPSI   80/80 Surg Assist Allowed / w/Doc   Lab Crosswalk   Radiology Crosswalk

558   CPT © 2019 American Medical Association. All Rights Reserved.   © 2019 Optum360, LLC

99468-99476 Critical Care Age 5 Years or Younger

CMS: 100-04,12,30.6.4 Services Furnished Incident to Physician's Service

INCLUDES All services included in codes 99291-99292 as well as the following which may be reported by facilities only:
Administration of blood/blood components (36430, 36440)
Administration of intravenous fluids (96360-96361)
Administration of surfactant (94610)
Bladder aspiration, suprapubic (51100)
Bladder catheterization (51701, 51702)
Car seat evaluation (94780-94781)
Catheterization umbilical artery (36660)
Catheterization umbilical vein (36510)
Central venous catheter, centrally inserted (36555)
Endotracheal intubation (31500)
Lumbar puncture (62270)
Oral or nasogastric tube placement (43752)
Pulmonary function testing, performed at the bedside (94375)
Pulse or ear oximetry (94760-94762)
Vascular access, arteries (36140, 36620)
Vascular access, venous (36400-36406, 36420, 36600)
Ventilatory management (94002-94004, 94660)
Initial and subsequent care provided to a critically ill infant or child
Other hospital care or intensive care services by same group or individual done on same day that patient was transferred to initial neonatal/pediatric critical care
Readmission to critical unit on same day or during the same stay (subsequent care)

EXCLUDES *Critical care services for patients 6 years of age or older (99291-99292)*
Critical care services provided by a second physician or physician of a different specialty (99291-99292)
Interfacility transport services by same or different individual of same or different specialty or group on same date of service (99466-99467, [99485, 99486])
Neonatal hypothermia (99184)
Services performed by individual in another group receiving a patient transferred to a lower level of care (99231-99233, 99478-99480)
Services performed by individual transferring a patient to a lower level of care (99231-99233, 99291-99292)
Services performed by same or different individual in same group on same day (99291-99292)
Services performed by transferring individual prior to transfer of patient to an individual in a different group (99221-99233, 99291-99292, 99460-99462, 99477-99480)

Code also normal newborn care if done on same day by same group or individual that provides critical care. Report modifier 25 with initial critical care code (99460-99462)

99468 Initial inpatient neonatal critical care, per day, for the evaluation and management of a critically ill neonate, 28 days of age or younger Ⓐ

🕐 26.0 ⚕ 26.0 **FUD** XXX C 80 🔲

AMA: 2018,Dec,8; 2018,Dec,8; 2018,Jun,9; 2018,Jan,8; 2017,Jan,8; 2016,May,3; 2016,Jan,13; 2015,Oct,8; 2015,Jul,3; 2015,Feb,10; 2015,Jan,16; 2014,Oct,8; 2014,May,4; 2014,Jan,11

99469 Subsequent inpatient neonatal critical care, per day, for the evaluation and management of a critically ill neonate, 28 days of age or younger Ⓐ

🕐 11.2 ⚕ 11.2 **FUD** XXX C 80 🔲

AMA: 2018,Dec,8; 2018,Dec,8; 2018,Jun,9; 2018,Jan,8; 2017,Jan,8; 2016,May,3; 2016,Jan,13; 2015,Oct,8; 2015,Jul,3; 2015,Feb,10; 2015,Jan,16; 2014,Oct,8; 2014,May,4; 2014,Jan,11

99471 Initial inpatient pediatric critical care, per day, for the evaluation and management of a critically ill infant or young child, 29 days through 24 months of age Ⓐ

🕐 22.5 ⚕ 22.5 **FUD** XXX C 80 🔲

AMA: 2018,Dec,8; 2018,Dec,8; 2018,Jun,9; 2018,Jan,8; 2017,Jan,8; 2016,May,3; 2016,Jan,13; 2015,Jul,3; 2015,Feb,10; 2015,Jan,16; 2014,Oct,8; 2014,Jan,11

99472 Subsequent inpatient pediatric critical care, per day, for the evaluation and management of a critically ill infant or young child, 29 days through 24 months of age Ⓐ

🕐 11.5 ⚕ 11.5 **FUD** XXX C 80 🔲

AMA: 2018,Dec,8; 2018,Dec,8; 2018,Jun,9; 2018,Jan,8; 2017,Jan,8; 2016,May,3; 2016,Jan,13; 2015,Jul,3; 2015,Feb,10; 2015,Jan,16; 2014,Oct,8; 2014,Jan,11

99473 Resequenced code. See code before 99450.

99474 Resequenced code. See code before 99450.

99475 Initial inpatient pediatric critical care, per day, for the evaluation and management of a critically ill infant or young child, 2 through 5 years of age Ⓐ

🕐 15.8 ⚕ 15.8 **FUD** XXX C 80 🔲

AMA: 2018,Dec,8; 2018,Dec,8; 2018,Jun,9; 2018,Jan,8; 2017,Jan,8; 2016,May,3; 2016,Jan,13; 2015,Jul,3; 2015,Feb,10; 2015,Jan,16; 2014,Oct,8; 2014,Jan,11

99476 Subsequent inpatient pediatric critical care, per day, for the evaluation and management of a critically ill infant or young child, 2 through 5 years of age Ⓐ

🕐 9.86 ⚕ 9.86 **FUD** XXX C 80 🔲

AMA: 2018,Dec,8; 2018,Dec,8; 2018,Jun,9; 2018,Jan,8; 2017,Jan,8; 2016,May,3; 2016,Jan,13; 2015,Jul,3; 2015,Feb,10; 2015,Jan,16; 2014,Oct,8; 2014,Jan,11

99477-99480 Initial Inpatient Neonatal Intensive Care and Other Services

CMS: 100-04,12,30.6.4 Services Furnished Incident to Physician's Service

INCLUDES All services included in codes 99291-99292 as well as the following that may be reported by facilities only:
Adjustments to enteral and/or parenteral nutrition
Airway and ventilator management (31500, 94002-94004, 94375, 94610, 94660)
Bladder catheterization (51701-51702)
Blood transfusion (36430, 36440)
Car seat evaluation (94780-94781)
Constant and/or frequent monitoring of vital signs
Continuous observation by the healthcare team
Heat maintenance
Intensive cardiac or respiratory monitoring
Oral or nasogastric tube insertion (43752)
Oxygen saturation (94760-94762)
Spinal puncture (62270)
Suprapubic catheterization (51100)
Vascular access procedures (36000, 36140, 36400, 36405-36406, 36420, 36510, 36555, 36600, 36620, 36660)

EXCLUDES *Critical care services for patient transferred after initial or subsequent intensive care is provided (99291-99292)*
Initial day intensive care provided by transferring individual same day neonate/infant transferred to a lower level of care (99477)
Inpatient neonatal/pediatric critical care services received on same day (99468-99476)
Necessary resuscitation services done as part of delivery care prior to admission
Neonatal hypothermia (99184)
Services provided by receiving individual when patient is transferred for critical care (99468-99476)
Services for receiving provider when patient improves after the initial day and is transferred to a lower level of care (99231-99233, 99478-99480)
Subsequent care of a sick neonate, under 28 days of age, more than 5000 grams, not requiring critical or intensive care services (99231-99233)

Code also care provided by receiving individual when patient is transferred to an individual in different group (99231-99233, 99462)
Code also initial neonatal intensive care service when physician or other qualified health care professional is present for delivery and/or neonate requires resuscitation (99464-99465); append modifier 25 to (99477)

99477 Initial hospital care, per day, for the evaluation and management of the neonate, 28 days of age or younger, who requires intensive observation, frequent interventions, and other intensive care services Ⓐ

EXCLUDES *Initiation of care of a critically ill neonate (99468)*
Initiation of inpatient care of a normal newborn (99460)

🕐 9.85 ⚕ 9.85 **FUD** XXX C 80 🔲

AMA: 2018,Dec,8; 2018,Dec,8; 2018,Jan,8; 2017,Jan,8; 2016,Jan,13; 2015,Jul,3; 2015,Jan,16; 2014,Oct,8; 2014,Jan,11

99478 Subsequent intensive care, per day, for the evaluation and management of the recovering very low birth weight infant (present body weight less than 1500 grams) Ⓐ

🕐 3.87 ⚕ 3.87 **FUD** XXX C 80 🔲

AMA: 2018,Dec,8; 2018,Dec,8; 2018,Jun,11; 2018,Jan,8; 2017,Jan,8; 2016,Jan,13; 2015,Jul,3; 2015,Jan,16; 2014,Oct,8; 2014,Jan,11

Evaluation and Management (sidebar)

99479 — 99491 (sidebar)

99479 Subsequent intensive care, per day, for the evaluation and management of the recovering low birth weight infant (present body weight of 1500-2500 grams) Ⓐ

3.52 3.52 **FUD** XXX Ⓒ 80 ▭

AMA: 2018,Dec,8; 2018,Dec,8; 2018,Jun,11; 2018,Jan,8; 2017,Jan,8; 2016,Jan,13; 2015,Jul,3; 2015,Jan,16; 2014,Oct,8; 2014,Jan,11

99480 Subsequent intensive care, per day, for the evaluation and management of the recovering infant (present body weight of 2501-5000 grams) Ⓐ

3.37 3.37 **FUD** XXX Ⓒ 80 ▭

AMA: 2018,Dec,8; 2018,Dec,8; 2018,Jun,11; 2018,Jan,8; 2017,Jan,8; 2016,Jan,13; 2015,Jul,3; 2015,Jan,16; 2014,Oct,8; 2014,Jan,11

99483-99486 Cognitive Impairment Services

INCLUDES Evaluation and care plans for new or existing patients with symptoms of cognitive impairment
Assessment and care plan services during the same time frame as:
E&M services (99201-99215, 99241-99245, 99324-99337, 99341-99350, 99366-99368, 99497-99498)
Medication management (99605-99607)
Need for services evaluation (e.g., legal, financial, meals, personal care)
Patient and caregiver focused risk assessment (96160-96161)
Psychiatric and psychological services (90785, 90791-90792, [96127])
Psychological or neuropsychological tests (96146)
Consideration of other conditions that may cause cognitive impairment (e.g., infection, hydrocephalus, stroke, medications)

EXCLUDES Use of code more than one time per 180 day period

99483 Assessment of and care planning for a patient with cognitive impairment, requiring an independent historian, in the office or other outpatient, home or domiciliary or rest home, with all of the following required elements: Cognition-focused evaluation including a pertinent history and examination; Medical decision making of moderate or high complexity; Functional assessment (eg, basic and instrumental activities of daily living), including decision-making capacity; Use of standardized instruments for staging of dementia (eg, functional assessment staging test [FAST], clinical dementia rating [CDR]); Medication reconciliation and review for high-risk medications; Evaluation for neuropsychiatric and behavioral symptoms, including depression, including use of standardized screening instrument(s); Evaluation of safety (eg, home), including motor vehicle operation; Identification of caregiver(s), caregiver knowledge, caregiver needs, social supports, and the willingness of caregiver to take on caregiving tasks; Development, updating or revision, or review of an Advance Care Plan; Creation of a written care plan, including initial plans to address any neuropsychiatric symptoms, neuro-cognitive symptoms, functional limitations, and referral to community resources as needed (eg, rehabilitation services, adult day programs, support groups) shared with the patient and/or caregiver with initial education and support. Typically, 50 minutes are spent face-to-face with the patient and/or family or caregiver.

5.09 7.32 **FUD** XXX Ⓢ 80 ▭

AMA: 2018,Jul,12; 2018,Apr,9; 2018,Jan,8

99484 Resequenced code. See code following 99498.

99485 Resequenced code. See code following 99467.

99486 Resequenced code. See code following 99467.

99490-99491 [99490, 99491] Coordination of Services for Chronic Care

CMS: 100-04,11,40.1.3 Independent Attending Physician Services

INCLUDES Case management services provided to patients that:
Have two or more conditions anticipated to endure more than 12 months or until the patient's death
Require at least 20 minutes of staff time monthly
Risk is high that conditions will result in decompensation, deterioration, or death
Patient management services during same time frame as (99339-99340, 99487-99489)

EXCLUDES Psychiatric collaborative care management (99484, 99492-99494)
Use of code with ESRD services during the same month (90951-90970)

\# **99490** Chronic care management services, at least 20 minutes of clinical staff time directed by a physician or other qualified health care professional, per calendar month, with the following required elements: multiple (two or more) chronic conditions expected to last at least 12 months, or until the death of the patient; chronic conditions place the patient at significant risk of death, acute exacerbation/decompensation, or functional decline; comprehensive care plan established, implemented, revised, or monitored.

INCLUDES Patient management services during same time frame as (99358-99359, 99366-99368, 99374-99380, [99421, 99422, 99423], 99441-99443, [99091], 99495-99496, 93792-93793, 98960-98962, 99071, 99078, 99080, 99605-99607)

EXCLUDES Chronic care management provided personally by physician or other qualified health care professional ([99491])

0.90 1.17 **FUD** XXX Ⓢ 80 ▭

AMA: 2019,Jan,6; 2018,Oct,9; 2018,Jul,12; 2018,Apr,9; 2018,Mar,5; 2018,Mar,7; 2018,Feb,7; 2018,Jan,8; 2017,Jan,8; 2016,Jan,13; 2015,Feb,3; 2015,Jan,16; 2014,Oct,3

\# **99491** Chronic care management services, provided personally by a physician or other qualified health care professional, at least 30 minutes of physician or other qualified health care professional time, per calendar month, with the following required elements: multiple (two or more) chronic conditions expected to last at least 12 months, or until the death of the patient; chronic conditions place the patient at significant risk of death, acute exacerbation/decompensation, or functional decline; comprehensive care plan established, implemented, revised, or monitored

2.33 2.33 **FUD** XXX 80 ▭

EXCLUDES Chronic care management provided by medically directed clinical staff only ([99490])

26/TC PC/TC Only   A2-Z3 ASC Payment   50 Bilateral   ♂ Male Only   ♀ Female Only   🔾 Facility RVU   Non-Facility RVU   CCI   CLIA
FUD Follow-up Days   **CMS:** IOM   **AMA:** CPT Asst   A-Y OPPSI   80/80 Surg Assist Allowed / w/Doc   Lab Crosswalk   Radiology Crosswalk

560   CPT © 2019 American Medical Association. All Rights Reserved.   © 2019 Optum360, LLC

99487-99491 [99490, 99491] Coordination of Complex Services for Chronic Care

INCLUDES
All clinical non-face-to-face time with patient, family, and caregivers

Only services given by physician or other qualified health caregiver who has the role of care coordination for the patient for the month

Patient management services during same time frame as (99339-99340, 99358-99359, 99374-99380, 99441-99443, [99091], 99495-99496, 90951-90970, 93792-93793, 98960-98962, 98966-98968, 99071, 99078, 99080, 99605-99607)

Services provided to patients in a rest home, domiciliary, assisted living facility, or at home that include:

Caregiver education to family or patient, addressing independent living and self-management

Communication with patient and all caregivers and professionals regarding care

Determining which community and health resources would benefit the patient

Developing and maintaining a care plan

Facilitation of services and care

Health outcomes data and registry documentation

Providing communication with home health and other patient utilized services

Support for treatment and medication adherence

Services that address activities of daily living, psychosocial, and medical needs

EXCLUDES
E&M services by same/different individual during time frame of care management services

Psychiatric collaborative care management (99484, 99492-99494)

99487 **Complex chronic care management services, with the following required elements: multiple (two or more) chronic conditions expected to last at least 12 months, or until the death of the patient, chronic conditions place the patient at significant risk of death, acute exacerbation/decompensation, or functional decline, establishment or substantial revision of a comprehensive care plan, moderate or high complexity medical decision making; 60 minutes of clinical staff time directed by a physician or other qualified health care professional, per calendar month**

INCLUDES
Clinical services, 60 to 74 minutes, during a calendar month

🚑 1.47   ⚕ 2.58   **FUD** XXX   Ⓢ 80 ▢

AMA: 2019,Jan,6; 2018,Oct,9; 2018,Jul,12; 2018,Apr,9; 2018,Mar,5; 2018,Mar,7; 2018,Feb,7; 2018,Jan,8; 2017,Apr,9; 2017,Jan,8; 2016,Jan,13; 2015,Jan,16; 2014,Oct,8; 2014,Oct,3; 2014,Jun,3; 2014,Feb,3; 2014,Jan,11

+ **99489** **each additional 30 minutes of clinical staff time directed by a physician or other qualified health care professional, per calendar month (List separately in addition to code for primary procedure)**

EXCLUDES
Clinical services less than 30 minutes beyond the initial 60 minutes of care, per calendar month

Code first (99487)

🚑 0.74   ⚕ 1.29   **FUD** ZZZ   Ⓝ 80 ▢

AMA: 2019,Jan,6; 2018,Oct,9; 2018,Jul,12; 2018,Apr,9; 2018,Mar,5; 2018,Mar,7; 2018,Feb,7; 2018,Jan,8; 2017,Apr,9; 2017,Jan,8; 2016,Jan,13; 2015,Jan,16; 2014,Oct,8; 2014,Oct,3; 2014,Jun,3; 2014,Jan,11

99490 **Resequenced code. See code before 99487.**

99491 **Resequenced code. See code before 99487.**

99492-99494 Psychiatric Collaborative Care

INCLUDES
Services provided during a calendar month by a physician or other qualified healthcare profession for patients with a psychiatric diagnosis

Assessment of behavioral health status

Creation of and updating a care plan

Treatment provided during an episode of care during which goals may be met, not achieved, or there is a lack of services during a period of six months

EXCLUDES
Additional services provided by a behavioral health care manager during the same calendar month period (do not count as time for 99492-99494):

Psychiatric evaluation (90791-90792)

Psychotherapy (99406-99407, 99408-99409, 90832-90834, 90836-90838, 90839-90840, 90846-90847, 90849, 90853)

Services provided by a psychiatric consultant (do not count as time for 99492-99494): (E&M services) and psychiatric evaluation (90791-90792)

99492 **Initial psychiatric collaborative care management, first 70 minutes in the first calendar month of behavioral health care manager activities, in consultation with a psychiatric consultant, and directed by the treating physician or other qualified health care professional, with the following required elements: outreach to and engagement in treatment of a patient directed by the treating physician or other qualified health care professional; initial assessment of the patient, including administration of validated rating scales, with the development of an individualized treatment plan; review by the psychiatric consultant with modifications of the plan if recommended; entering patient in a registry and tracking patient follow-up and progress using the registry, with appropriate documentation, and participation in weekly caseload consultation with the psychiatric consultant; and provision of brief interventions using evidence-based techniques such as behavioral activation, motivational interviewing, and other focused treatment strategies.**

EXCLUDES
Services of less than 36 minutes

Subsequent collaborative care managment in same calendar month (99493)

🚑 2.51   ⚕ 4.50   **FUD** XXX   Ⓢ 80 ▢

AMA: 2019,Jan,6; 2018,Jul,12; 2018,Mar,5; 2018,Feb,7; 2018,Jan,8; 2017,Nov,3

99493 **Subsequent psychiatric collaborative care management, first 60 minutes in a subsequent month of behavioral health care manager activities, in consultation with a psychiatric consultant, and directed by the treating physician or other qualified health care professional, with the following required elements: tracking patient follow-up and progress using the registry, with appropriate documentation; participation in weekly caseload consultation with the psychiatric consultant; ongoing collaboration with and coordination of the patient's mental health care with the treating physician or other qualified health care professional and any other treating mental health providers; additional review of progress and recommendations for changes in treatment, as indicated, including medications, based on recommendations provided by the psychiatric consultant; provision of brief interventions using evidence-based techniques such as behavioral activation, motivational interviewing, and other focused treatment strategies; monitoring of patient outcomes using validated rating scales; and relapse prevention planning with patients as they achieve remission of symptoms and/or other treatment goals and are prepared for discharge from active treatment.**

EXCLUDES
Initial collaborative care managment in same calendar month (99492)

🚑 2.27   ⚕ 3.59   **FUD** XXX   Ⓢ 80 ▢

AMA: 2019,Jan,6; 2018,Jul,12; 2018,Mar,5; 2018,Feb,7; 2018,Jan,8; 2017,Nov,3

● New Code ▲ Revised Code ○ Reinstated ● New Web Release ▲ Revised Web Release + Add-on Unlisted Not Covered # Resequenced
⑨⓪ Optum Mod 50 Exempt Ⓢ AMA Mod 51 Exempt ⑤① Optum Mod 51 Exempt ⑥③ Mod 63 Exempt ⊮ Non-FDA Drug ★ Telemedicine Ⓜ Maternity Ⓐ Age Edit

561

Evaluation and Management

99494 — 99499

+   99494   Initial or subsequent psychiatric collaborative care management, each additional 30 minutes in a calendar month of behavioral health care manager activities, in consultation with a psychiatric consultant, and directed by the treating physician or other qualified health care professional (List separately in addition to code for primary procedure)

INCLUDES   Coordination of care with emergency department staff

Code first (99492, 99493)

🔧 1.22   ⚕ 1.86   **FUD** ZZZ   N 80 ▭

AMA: 2019,Jan,6; 2018,Jul,12; 2018,Mar,5; 2018,Feb,7; 2018,Jan,8; 2017,Nov,3

99495-99496 Management of Transitional Care Services

CMS: 100-02,13,230.1 Transitional Care Management Services; 100-04,11,40.1.3 Independent Attending Physician Services; 100-04,12,190.3 List of Telehealth Services

INCLUDES   First interaction (face-to-face, by telephone, or electronic) with patient or his/her caregiver and must be done within 2 working days of discharge
Initial face-to-face; must be done within code time frame and include medication management
New or established patient with moderate to high complexity medical decision making needs during care transitions
Patient management services during same time frame as (99339-99340, 99358-99359, 99366-99368, 99374-99380, 99441-99443, [99091], 99487-99489, 90951-90970, 93792-93793, 98960-98962, 98966-98968, 99071, 99078, 99080, 99605-99607)
Services from discharge day up to 29 days post discharge
Subsequent discharge within 30 days
Without face-to-face patient care given by physician or other qualified health care professional includes:
    Arrangement of follow-up and referrals with community resources and providers
    Contacting qualified health care professionals for specific problems of patient
    Discharge information review
    Need for follow-up care review based on tests and treatments
    Patient, family, and caregiver education
Without face-to-face patient care given by staff under the guidance of physician or other qualified health care professional includes:
    Caregiver education to family or patient, addressing independent living and self-management
    Communication with patient and all caregivers and professionals regarding care
    Determining which community and health resources would benefit the patient
    Providing communication with home health and other patient utilized services
    Support for treatment and medication adherence
    The facilitation of services and care

EXCLUDES   E&M services after the first face-to-face visit

99495   Transitional Care Management Services with the following required elements: Communication (direct contact, telephone, electronic) with the patient and/or caregiver within 2 business days of discharge Medical decision making of at least moderate complexity during the service period Face-to-face visit, within 14 calendar days of discharge

🔧 3.11   ⚕ 4.62   **FUD** XXX   ★ V 80 ▭

AMA: 2019,Jan,6; 2018,Jul,12; 2018,Apr,9; 2018,Mar,5; 2018,Mar,7; 2018,Feb,7; 2018,Jan,8; 2017,Jan,8; 2016,Jan,13; 2015,Jan,16; 2014,Oct,3; 2014,Oct,8; 2014,Mar,13; 2014,Jan,11

99496   Transitional Care Management Services with the following required elements: Communication (direct contact, telephone, electronic) with the patient and/or caregiver within 2 business days of discharge Medical decision making of high complexity during the service period Face-to-face visit, within 7 calendar days of discharge

🔧 4.51   ⚕ 6.52   **FUD** XXX   ★ V 80 ▭

AMA: 2019,Jan,6; 2018,Jul,12; 2018,Apr,9; 2018,Mar,5; 2018,Mar,7; 2018,Feb,7; 2018,Jan,8; 2017,Jan,8; 2016,Jan,13; 2015,Jan,16; 2014,Oct,3; 2014,Oct,8; 2014,Mar,13; 2014,Jan,11

99497-99498 Advance Directive Guidance

CMS: 100-02,15,280.5.1 Advance Care Planning with an Annual Wellness Visit; 100-04,11,40.1.3 Independent Attending Physician Services; 100-04,18,140.8 Advance Care Planning with an Annual Wellness Visit (AWV); 100-04,4,200.11 Advance Care Planning as an Optional Element of an Annual Wellness Visit

EXCLUDES   Critical care services (99291-99292, 99468-99469, 99471-99472, 99475-99476, 99477-99480)
Services for cognitive care (99483)
Treatment/management for an active problem (see appropriate E&M service)

99497   Advance care planning including the explanation and discussion of advance directives such as standard forms (with completion of such forms, when performed), by the physician or other qualified health care professional; first 30 minutes, face-to-face with the patient, family member(s), and/or surrogate

🔧 2.23   ⚕ 2.40   **FUD** XXX   Q1 80 ▭

AMA: 2018,Apr,9; 2018,Jan,8; 2017,Jan,8; 2016,Feb,7; 2016,Jan,13; 2015,Jan,16; 2014,Dec,11

+   99498   each additional 30 minutes (List separately in addition to code for primary procedure)

Code first (99497)

🔧 2.10   ⚕ 2.11   **FUD** ZZZ   N 80 ▭

AMA: 2018,Apr,9; 2018,Jan,8; 2017,Jan,8; 2016,Feb,7; 2016,Jan,13; 2015,Jan,16; 2014,Dec,11

99484 [99484] Behavioral Health Integration Care

CMS: 100-02,13,230.2 Chronic Care Management and General Behavioral Health Integration Services

INCLUDES   Care management services requiring 20 minutes or more per calendar month
Coordination of care with emergency department staff
Face to face services when necessary
Provided as an outpatient service
Provision of services by clinical staff and reported by supervising physician or other qualified healthcare professional
Provision of services to patients with whom there is an ongoing relationship
Treatment plan and specific service components

EXCLUDES   Other services for which the time or activities associated with that service aren't used to meet requirements for 99484:
Chronic care management ([99490], 99487-99489)
Psychiatric collaborative care in same calendar month (99492-99494)
Psychotherapy services (90785-90899)

 #   99484   Care management services for behavioral health conditions, at least 20 minutes of clinical staff time, directed by a physician or other qualified health care professional, per calendar month, with the following required elements: initial assessment or follow-up monitoring, including the use of applicable validated rating scales; behavioral health care planning in relation to behavioral/psychiatric health problems, including revision for patients who are not progressing or whose status changes; facilitating and coordinating treatment such as psychotherapy, pharmacotherapy, counseling and/or psychiatric consultation; and continuity of care with a designated member of the care team.

🔧 0.91   ⚕ 1.35   **FUD** XXX   S 80 ▭

AMA: 2019,Jan,6; 2018,Jul,12; 2018,Mar,5; 2018,Feb,7; 2018,Jan,8

99499 Unlisted Evaluation and Management Services

CMS: 100-04,12,30.6.10 Consultation Services; 100-04,12,30.6.4 Services Furnished Incident to Physician's Service; 100-04,12,30.6.9.1 Initial Hospital Care and Observation or Inpatient Care Services

99499   Unlisted evaluation and management service

🔧 0.00   ⚕ 0.00   **FUD** XXX   B 80 ▭

AMA: 2019,Aug,8; 2018,Jan,8; 2017,Jan,8; 2016,Jan,13; 2015,Jan,16; 2014,Oct,8; 2014,Jan,11

26/TC PC/TC Only   A2-Z3 ASC Payment   50 Bilateral   ♂ Male Only   ♀ Female Only   🔧 Facility RVU   ⚕ Non-Facility RVU   ▭ CCI   CLIA
FUD Follow-up Days   CMS: IOM   AMA: CPT Asst   A-Y OPPSI   80/80 Surg Assist Allowed / w/Doc   Lab Crosswalk   Radiology Crosswalk

562   CPT © 2019 American Medical Association. All Rights Reserved.   © 2019 Optum360, LLC

0001F-0015F Quality Measures with Multiple Components

INCLUDES   Several measures grouped within a single code descriptor to make possible reporting for clinical conditions when all of the components have been met

0001F   **Heart failure assessed (includes assessment of all the following components) (CAD): Blood pressure measured (2000F) Level of activity assessed (1003F) Clinical symptoms of volume overload (excess) assessed (1004F) Weight, recorded (2001F) Clinical signs of volume overload (excess) assessed (2002F)**

INCLUDES   Blood pressure measured (2000F)
Clinical signs of volume overload (excess) assessed (2002F)
Clinical symptoms of volume overload (excess) assessed (1004F)
Level of activity assessed (1003F)
Weight recorded (2001F)

📋 0.00   ⚖ 0.00   **FUD** XXX   E

AMA: 2018,Jan,8; 2017,Jan,8; 2016,Jan,13; 2015,Jan,16; 2014,Jan,11

0005F   **Osteoarthritis assessed (OA) Includes assessment of all the following components: Osteoarthritis symptoms and functional status assessed (1006F) Use of anti-inflammatory or over-the-counter (OTC) analgesic medications assessed (1007F) Initial examination of the involved joint(s) (includes visual inspection, palpation, range of motion) (2004F)**

INCLUDES   Initial examination of the involved joint(s) (includes visual inspection/palpation/range of motion) (2004F)
Osteoarthritis symptoms and functional status assessed (1006F)
Use of anti-inflammatory or over-the-counter (OTC) analgesic medications assessed (1007F)

📋 0.00   ⚖ 0.00   **FUD** XXX   E

AMA: 2005,Oct,1-5

0012F   **Community-acquired bacterial pneumonia assessment (includes all of the following components) (CAP): Co-morbid conditions assessed (1026F) Vital signs recorded (2010F) Mental status assessed (2014F) Hydration status assessed (2018F)**

📋 0.00   ⚖ 0.00   **FUD** XXX   E

INCLUDES   Co-morbid conditions assessed (1026F)
Hydration status assessed (2018F)
Mental status assessed (2014F)
Vital signs recorded (2010F)

0014F   **Comprehensive preoperative assessment performed for cataract surgery with intraocular lens (IOL) placement (includes assessment of all of the following components) (EC): Dilated fundus evaluation performed within 12 months prior to cataract surgery (2020F) Pre-surgical (cataract) axial length, corneal power measurement and method of intraocular lens power calculation documented (must be performed within 12 months prior to surgery) (3073F) Preoperative assessment of functional or medical indication(s) for surgery prior to the cataract surgery with intraocular lens placement (must be performed within 12 months prior to cataract surgery) (3325F)**

INCLUDES   Evaluation of dilated fundus done within 12 months prior to surgery (2020F)
Preoperative assessment of functional or medical indications done within 12 months prior to surgery (3325F)
Presurgical measurement of axial length, corneal power, and IOL power calculation performed within 12 months prior to surgery (3073F)

📋 0.00   ⚖ 0.00   **FUD** XXX   E

AMA: 2008,Mar,8-12

0015F   **Melanoma follow up completed (includes assessment of all of the following components) (ML): History obtained regarding new or changing moles (1050F) Complete physical skin exam performed (2029F) Patient counseled to perform a monthly self skin examination (5005F)**

INCLUDES   Complete physical skin exam (2029F)
Counseling to perform monthly skin self-examination (5005F)
History obtained of new or changing moles (1050F)

📋 0.00   ⚖ 0.00   **FUD** XXX   E

AMA: 2008,Mar,8-12

0500F-0584F Care Provided According to Prevailing Guidelines

INCLUDES   Measures of utilization or patient care provided for certain clinical purposes

0500F   **Initial prenatal care visit (report at first prenatal encounter with health care professional providing obstetrical care. Report also date of visit and, in a separate field, the date of the last menstrual period [LMP]) (Prenatal)**   M ♀

📋 0.00   ⚖ 0.00   **FUD** XXX   E

AMA: 2018,Jan,8; 2017,Jan,8; 2016,Jan,13; 2015,Jan,16; 2014,Jan,11

0501F   **Prenatal flow sheet documented in medical record by first prenatal visit (documentation includes at minimum blood pressure, weight, urine protein, uterine size, fetal heart tones, and estimated date of delivery). Report also: date of visit and, in a separate field, the date of the last menstrual period [LMP] (Note: If reporting 0501F Prenatal flow sheet, it is not necessary to report 0500F Initial prenatal care visit) (Prenatal)**   M ♀

📋 0.00   ⚖ 0.00   **FUD** XXX   E

AMA: 2004,Nov,1

0502F   **Subsequent prenatal care visit (Prenatal) [Excludes: patients who are seen for a condition unrelated to pregnancy or prenatal care (eg, an upper respiratory infection; patients seen for consultation only, not for continuing care)]**   M ♀

EXCLUDES   Patients seen for an unrelated pregnancy/prenatal care condition (e.g., upper respiratory infection; patients seen for consultation only, not for continuing care)

📋 0.00   ⚖ 0.00   **FUD** XXX   E

AMA: 2004,Nov,1

0503F   **Postpartum care visit (Prenatal)**   M ♀

📋 0.00   ⚖ 0.00   **FUD** XXX   E

AMA: 2004,Nov,1

0505F   **Hemodialysis plan of care documented (ESRD, P-ESRD)**

📋 0.00   ⚖ 0.00   **FUD** XXX   E

AMA: 2008,Mar,8-12

0507F   **Peritoneal dialysis plan of care documented (ESRD)**

📋 0.00   ⚖ 0.00   **FUD** XXX   E

AMA: 2008,Mar,8-12

0509F   **Urinary incontinence plan of care documented (GER)**

📋 0.00   ⚖ 0.00   **FUD** XXX   M

0513F   **Elevated blood pressure plan of care documented (CKD)**

📋 0.00   ⚖ 0.00   **FUD** XXX   M

AMA: 2008,Mar,8-12

0514F   **Plan of care for elevated hemoglobin level documented for patient receiving Erythropoiesis-Stimulating Agent therapy (ESA) (CKD)**

📋 0.00   ⚖ 0.00   **FUD** XXX   E

AMA: 2008,Mar,8-12

0516F   **Anemia plan of care documented (ESRD)**

📋 0.00   ⚖ 0.00   **FUD** XXX   E

AMA: 2008,Mar,8-12

0517F   **Glaucoma plan of care documented (EC)**

📋 0.00   ⚖ 0.00   **FUD** XXX   M

AMA: 2008,Mar,8-12

0518F Falls plan of care documented (GER)
🔲 0.00   ⅋ 0.00   **FUD** XXX   [M]
AMA: 2008,Mar,8-12

0519F Planned chemotherapy regimen, including at a minimum: drug(s) prescribed, dose, and duration, documented prior to initiation of a new treatment regimen (ONC)
🔲 0.00   ⅋ 0.00   **FUD** XXX   [E]
AMA: 2008,Mar,8-12

0520F Radiation dose limits to normal tissues established prior to the initiation of a course of 3D conformal radiation for a minimum of 2 tissue/organ (ONC)
🔲 0.00   ⅋ 0.00   **FUD** XXX   [M]
AMA: 2008,Mar,8-12

0521F Plan of care to address pain documented (COA) (ONC)
🔲 0.00   ⅋ 0.00   **FUD** XXX   [M]
AMA: 2008,Mar,8-12

0525F Initial visit for episode (BkP)
🔲 0.00   ⅋ 0.00   **FUD** XXX   [E]
AMA: 2008,Mar,8-12

0526F Subsequent visit for episode (BkP)
🔲 0.00   ⅋ 0.00   **FUD** XXX   [M]
AMA: 2008,Mar,8-12

0528F Recommended follow-up interval for repeat colonoscopy of at least 10 years documented in colonoscopy report (End/Polyp)
🔲 0.00   ⅋ 0.00   **FUD** XXX   [M]

0529F Interval of 3 or more years since patient's last colonoscopy, documented (End/Polyp)
🔲 0.00   ⅋ 0.00   **FUD** XXX   [M]

0535F Dyspnea management plan of care, documented (Pall Cr)
🔲 0.00   ⅋ 0.00   **FUD** XXX   [E]

0540F Glucorticoid Management Plan Documented (RA)
🔲 0.00   ⅋ 0.00   **FUD** XXX   [M]

0545F Plan for follow-up care for major depressive disorder, documented (MDD ADOL)
🔲 0.00   ⅋ 0.00   **FUD** XXX   [E]

0550F Cytopathology report on routine nongynecologic specimen finalized within two working days of accession date (PATH)
🔲 0.00   ⅋ 0.00   **FUD** XXX   [E]

0551F Cytopathology report on nongynecologic specimen with documentation that the specimen was non-routine (PATH)
🔲 0.00   ⅋ 0.00   **FUD** XXX   [E]

0555F Symptom management plan of care documented (HF)
🔲 0.00   ⅋ 0.00   **FUD** XXX   [E]

0556F Plan of care to achieve lipid control documented (CAD)
🔲 0.00   ⅋ 0.00   **FUD** XXX   [E]

0557F Plan of care to manage anginal symptoms documented (CAD)
🔲 0.00   ⅋ 0.00   **FUD** XXX   [E]

0575F HIV RNA control plan of care, documented (HIV)
🔲 0.00   ⅋ 0.00   **FUD** XXX   [E]

0580F Multidisciplinary care plan developed or updated (ALS)
🔲 0.00   ⅋ 0.00   **FUD** XXX   [E]

0581F Patient transferred directly from anesthetizing location to critical care unit (Peri2)
🔲 0.00   ⅋ 0.00   **FUD** XXX   [M]

0582F Patient not transferred directly from anesthetizing location to critical care unit (Peri2)
🔲 0.00   ⅋ 0.00   **FUD** XXX   [E]

0583F Transfer of care checklist used (Peri2)
🔲 0.00   ⅋ 0.00   **FUD** XXX   [M]

0584F Transfer of care checklist not used (Peri2)
🔲 0.00   ⅋ 0.00   **FUD** XXX   [E]

1000F-1505F Elements of History/Review of Systems

INCLUDES   Measures for specific aspects of patient history or review of systems

1000F Tobacco use assessed (CAD, CAP, COPD, PV) (DM)
🔲 0.00   ⅋ 0.00   **FUD** XXX   [E]
AMA: 2018,Jan,8; 2017,Jan,8; 2016,Jan,13; 2015,Jan,16; 2014,Jan,11

1002F Anginal symptoms and level of activity assessed (NMA-No Measure Associated)
🔲 0.00   ⅋ 0.00   **FUD** XXX   [E]
AMA: 2004,Nov,1

1003F Level of activity assessed (NMA-No Measure Associated)
🔲 0.00   ⅋ 0.00   **FUD** XXX   [E]
AMA: 2006,Dec,10-12

1004F Clinical symptoms of volume overload (excess) assessed (NMA-No Measure Associated)
🔲 0.00   ⅋ 0.00   **FUD** XXX   [E]
AMA: 2006,Dec,10-12

1005F Asthma symptoms evaluated (includes documentation of numeric frequency of symptoms or patient completion of an asthma assessment tool/survey/questionnaire) (NMA-No Measure Associated)
🔲 0.00   ⅋ 0.00   **FUD** XXX   [E]

1006F Osteoarthritis symptoms and functional status assessed (may include the use of a standardized scale or the completion of an assessment questionnaire, such as the SF-36, AAOS Hip & Knee Questionnaire) (OA) [Instructions: Report when osteoarthritis is addressed during the patient encounter]
🔲 0.00   ⅋ 0.00   **FUD** XXX   [M]

INCLUDES   Osteoarthritis when it is addressed during the patient encounter

1007F Use of anti-inflammatory or analgesic over-the-counter (OTC) medications for symptom relief assessed (OA)
🔲 0.00   ⅋ 0.00   **FUD** XXX   [E]

1008F Gastrointestinal and renal risk factors assessed for patients on prescribed or OTC non-steroidal anti-inflammatory drug (NSAID) (OA)
🔲 0.00   ⅋ 0.00   **FUD** XXX   [E]

1010F Severity of angina assessed by level of activity (CAD)
🔲 0.00   ⅋ 0.00   **FUD** XXX   [E]

1011F Angina present (CAD)
🔲 0.00   ⅋ 0.00   **FUD** XXX   [E]

1012F Angina absent (CAD)
🔲 0.00   ⅋ 0.00   **FUD** XXX   [E]

1015F Chronic obstructive pulmonary disease (COPD) symptoms assessed (Includes assessment of at least 1 of the following: dyspnea, cough/sputum, wheezing), or respiratory symptom assessment tool completed (COPD)
🔲 0.00   ⅋ 0.00   **FUD** XXX   [E]

1018F Dyspnea assessed, not present (COPD)
🔲 0.00   ⅋ 0.00   **FUD** XXX   [E]

1019F Dyspnea assessed, present (COPD)
🔲 0.00   ⅋ 0.00   **FUD** XXX   [E]

1022F Pneumococcus immunization status assessed (CAP, COPD)
🔲 0.00   ⅋ 0.00   **FUD** XXX   [E]
AMA: 2010,Jul,3-5; 2008,Mar,8-12

1026F Co-morbid conditions assessed (eg, includes assessment for presence or absence of: malignancy, liver disease, congestive heart failure, cerebrovascular disease, renal disease, chronic obstructive pulmonary disease, asthma, diabetes, other co-morbid conditions) (CAP)
🔲 0.00   ⅋ 0.00   **FUD** XXX   [E]

1030F Influenza immunization status assessed (CAP)
🔲 0.00   ⅋ 0.00   **FUD** XXX   [E]
AMA: 2008,Mar,8-12

1031F Smoking status and exposure to second hand smoke in the home assessed (Asthma)
🚑 0.00   ⚕ 0.00   **FUD** XXX   E

1032F Current tobacco smoker or currently exposed to secondhand smoke (Asthma)
🚑 0.00   ⚕ 0.00   **FUD** XXX   E

1033F Current tobacco non-smoker and not currently exposed to secondhand smoke (Asthma)
🚑 0.00   ⚕ 0.00   **FUD** XXX   E

1034F Current tobacco smoker (CAD, CAP, COPD, PV) (DM)
🚑 0.00   ⚕ 0.00   **FUD** XXX   E
AMA: 2008,Mar,8-12

1035F Current smokeless tobacco user (eg, chew, snuff) (PV)
🚑 0.00   ⚕ 0.00   **FUD** XXX   E
AMA: 2008,Mar,8-12

1036F Current tobacco non-user (CAD, CAP, COPD, PV) (DM) (IBD)
🚑 0.00   ⚕ 0.00   **FUD** XXX   M
AMA: 2008,Mar,8-12

1038F Persistent asthma (mild, moderate or severe) (Asthma)
🚑 0.00   ⚕ 0.00   **FUD** XXX   M
AMA: 2018,Jan,8; 2017,Jan,8; 2016,Jan,13; 2015,Jan,16; 2014,Jan,11

1039F Intermittent asthma (Asthma)
🚑 0.00   ⚕ 0.00   **FUD** XXX   M
AMA: 2018,Jan,8; 2017,Jan,8; 2016,Jan,13; 2015,Jan,16; 2014,Jan,11

1040F DSM-5 criteria for major depressive disorder documented at the initial evaluation (MDD, MDD ADOL)
🚑 0.00   ⚕ 0.00   **FUD** XXX   E
AMA: 2008,Mar,8-12

1050F History obtained regarding new or changing moles (ML)
🚑 0.00   ⚕ 0.00   **FUD** XXX   E
AMA: 2008,Mar,8-12

1052F Type, anatomic location, and activity all assessed (IBD)
🚑 0.00   ⚕ 0.00   **FUD** XXX   E

1055F Visual functional status assessed (EC)
🚑 0.00   ⚕ 0.00   **FUD** XXX   E

1060F Documentation of permanent or persistent or paroxysmal atrial fibrillation (STR)
🚑 0.00   ⚕ 0.00   **FUD** XXX   E

1061F Documentation of absence of permanent and persistent and paroxysmal atrial fibrillation (STR)
🚑 0.00   ⚕ 0.00   **FUD** XXX   E

1065F Ischemic stroke symptom onset of less than 3 hours prior to arrival (STR)
🚑 0.00   ⚕ 0.00   **FUD** XXX   E

1066F Ischemic stroke symptom onset greater than or equal to 3 hours prior to arrival (STR)
🚑 0.00   ⚕ 0.00   **FUD** XXX   E

1070F Alarm symptoms (involuntary weight loss, dysphagia, or gastrointestinal bleeding) assessed; none present (GERD)
🚑 0.00   ⚕ 0.00   **FUD** XXX   E

1071F 1 or more present (GERD)
🚑 0.00   ⚕ 0.00   **FUD** XXX   E

1090F Presence or absence of urinary incontinence assessed (GER)
🚑 0.00   ⚕ 0.00   **FUD** XXX   M

1091F Urinary incontinence characterized (eg, frequency, volume, timing, type of symptoms, how bothersome) (GER)
🚑 0.00   ⚕ 0.00   **FUD** XXX   E

1100F Patient screened for future fall risk; documentation of 2 or more falls in the past year or any fall with injury in the past year (GER)
🚑 0.00   ⚕ 0.00   **FUD** XXX   M
AMA: 2008,Mar,8-12

1101F documentation of no falls in the past year or only 1 fall without injury in the past year (GER)
🚑 0.00   ⚕ 0.00   **FUD** XXX   M
AMA: 2008,Mar,8-12

1110F Patient discharged from an inpatient facility (eg, hospital, skilled nursing facility, or rehabilitation facility) within the last 60 days (GER)
🚑 0.00   ⚕ 0.00   **FUD** XXX   E

1111F Discharge medications reconciled with the current medication list in outpatient medical record (COA) (GER)
🚑 0.00   ⚕ 0.00   **FUD** XXX   M

1116F Auricular or periauricular pain assessed (AOE)
🚑 0.00   ⚕ 0.00   **FUD** XXX   E
AMA: 2008,Mar,8-12

1118F GERD symptoms assessed after 12 months of therapy (GERD)
🚑 0.00   ⚕ 0.00   **FUD** XXX   E
AMA: 2008,Mar,8-12

1119F Initial evaluation for condition (HEP C)(EPI, DSP)
🚑 0.00   ⚕ 0.00   **FUD** XXX   E
AMA: 2008,Mar,8-12

1121F Subsequent evaluation for condition (HEP C)(EPI)
🚑 0.00   ⚕ 0.00   **FUD** XXX   E
AMA: 2008,Mar,8-12

1123F Advance Care Planning discussed and documented advance care plan or surrogate decision maker documented in the medical record (DEM) (GER, Pall Cr)
🚑 0.00   ⚕ 0.00   **FUD** XXX   M
AMA: 2008,Mar,8-12

1124F Advance Care Planning discussed and documented in the medical record, patient did not wish or was not able to name a surrogate decision maker or provide an advance care plan (DEM) (GER, Pall Cr)
🚑 0.00   ⚕ 0.00   **FUD** XXX   M
AMA: 2008,Mar,8-12

1125F Pain severity quantified; pain present (COA) (ONC)
🚑 0.00   ⚕ 0.00   **FUD** XXX   M
AMA: 2008,Mar,8-12

1126F no pain present (COA) (ONC)
🚑 0.00   ⚕ 0.00   **FUD** XXX   M
AMA: 2008,Mar,8-12

1127F New episode for condition (NMA-No Measure Associated)
🚑 0.00   ⚕ 0.00   **FUD** XXX   E
AMA: 2008,Mar,8-12

1128F Subsequent episode for condition (NMA-No Measure Associated)
🚑 0.00   ⚕ 0.00   **FUD** XXX   E
AMA: 2008,Mar,8-12

1130F Back pain and function assessed, including all of the following: Pain assessment and functional status and patient history, including notation of presence or absence of "red flags" (warning signs) and assessment of prior treatment and response, and employment status (BkP)
🚑 0.00   ⚕ 0.00   **FUD** XXX   E
AMA: 2008,Mar,8-12

1134F Episode of back pain lasting 6 weeks or less (BkP)
🚑 0.00   ⚕ 0.00   **FUD** XXX   E
AMA: 2008,Mar,8-12

1135F Episode of back pain lasting longer than 6 weeks (BkP)
🖪 0.00   ⚕ 0.00   **FUD** XXX   E
AMA: 2008,Mar,8-12

1136F Episode of back pain lasting 12 weeks or less (BkP)
🖪 0.00   ⚕ 0.00   **FUD** XXX   E
AMA: 2008,Mar,8-12

1137F Episode of back pain lasting longer than 12 weeks (BkP)
🖪 0.00   ⚕ 0.00   **FUD** XXX   E
AMA: 2008,Mar,8-12

1150F Documentation that a patient has a substantial risk of death within 1 year (Pall Cr)
🖪 0.00   ⚕ 0.00   **FUD** XXX   E

1151F Documentation that a patient does not have a substantial risk of death within one year (Pall Cr)
🖪 0.00   ⚕ 0.00   **FUD** XXX   E

1152F Documentation of advanced disease diagnosis, goals of care prioritize comfort (Pall Cr)
🖪 0.00   ⚕ 0.00   **FUD** XXX   E

1153F Documentation of advanced disease diagnosis, goals of care do not prioritize comfort (Pall Cr)
🖪 0.00   ⚕ 0.00   **FUD** XXX   E

1157F Advance care plan or similar legal document present in the medical record (COA)
🖪 0.00   ⚕ 0.00   **FUD** XXX   E

1158F Advance care planning discussion documented in the medical record (COA)
🖪 0.00   ⚕ 0.00   **FUD** XXX   M

1159F Medication list documented in medical record (COA)
🖪 0.00   ⚕ 0.00   **FUD** XXX   E

1160F Review of all medications by a prescribing practitioner or clinical pharmacist (such as, prescriptions, OTCs, herbal therapies and supplements) documented in the medical record (COA)
🖪 0.00   ⚕ 0.00   **FUD** XXX   E

1170F Functional status assessed (COA) (RA)
🖪 0.00   ⚕ 0.00   **FUD** XXX   M

1175F Functional status for dementia assessed and results reviewed (DEM)
🖪 0.00   ⚕ 0.00   **FUD** XXX   E

1180F All specified thromboembolic risk factors assessed (AFIB)
🖪 0.00   ⚕ 0.00   **FUD** XXX   E

1181F Neuropsychiatric symptoms assessed and results reviewed (DEM)
🖪 0.00   ⚕ 0.00   **FUD** XXX   E

1182F Neuropsychiatric symptoms, one or more present (DEM)
🖪 0.00   ⚕ 0.00   **FUD** XXX   E

1183F Neuropsychiatric symptoms, absent (DEM)
🖪 0.00   ⚕ 0.00   **FUD** XXX   E

1200F Seizure type(s) and current seizure frequency(ies) documented (EPI)
🖪 0.00   ⚕ 0.00   **FUD** XXX   E

1205F Etiology of epilepsy or epilepsy syndrome(s) reviewed and documented (EPI)
🖪 0.00   ⚕ 0.00   **FUD** XXX   E

1220F Patient screened for depression (SUD)
🖪 0.00   ⚕ 0.00   **FUD** XXX   E

1400F Parkinson's disease diagnosis reviewed (Prkns)
🖪 0.00   ⚕ 0.00   **FUD** XXX   E

1450F Symptoms improved or remained consistent with treatment goals since last assessment (HF)
🖪 0.00   ⚕ 0.00   **FUD** XXX   E

1451F Symptoms demonstrated clinically important deterioration since last assessment (HF)
🖪 0.00   ⚕ 0.00   **FUD** XXX   E

1460F Qualifying cardiac event/diagnosis in previous 12 months (CAD)
🖪 0.00   ⚕ 0.00   **FUD** XXX   M

1461F No qualifying cardiac event/diagnosis in previous 12 months (CAD)
🖪 0.00   ⚕ 0.00   **FUD** XXX   M

1490F Dementia severity classified, mild (DEM)
🖪 0.00   ⚕ 0.00   **FUD** XXX   E

1491F Dementia severity classified, moderate (DEM)
🖪 0.00   ⚕ 0.00   **FUD** XXX   E

1493F Dementia severity classified, severe (DEM)
🖪 0.00   ⚕ 0.00   **FUD** XXX   E

1494F Cognition assessed and reviewed (DEM)
🖪 0.00   ⚕ 0.00   **FUD** XXX   E

1500F Symptoms and signs of distal symmetric polyneuropathy reviewed and documented (DSP)
🖪 0.00   ⚕ 0.00   **FUD** XXX   E

1501F Not initial evaluation for condition (DSP)
🖪 0.00   ⚕ 0.00   **FUD** XXX   E

1502F Patient queried about pain and pain interference with function using a valid and reliable instrument (DSP)
🖪 0.00   ⚕ 0.00   **FUD** XXX   E

1503F Patient queried about symptoms of respiratory insufficiency (ALS)
🖪 0.00   ⚕ 0.00   **FUD** XXX   E

1504F Patient has respiratory insufficiency (ALS)
🖪 0.00   ⚕ 0.00   **FUD** XXX   E

1505F Patient does not have respiratory insufficiency (ALS)
🖪 0.00   ⚕ 0.00   **FUD** XXX   E

2000F-2060F [2033F] Elements of Examination

[INCLUDES]   Components of clinical assessment or physical exam

2000F Blood pressure measured (CKD)(DM)
🖪 0.00   ⚕ 0.00   **FUD** XXX   M
AMA: 2018,Jan,8; 2017,Jan,8; 2016,Jan,13; 2015,Jan,16; 2014,Jan,11

2001F Weight recorded (PAG)
🖪 0.00   ⚕ 0.00   **FUD** XXX   E
AMA: 2006,Dec,10-12

2002F Clinical signs of volume overload (excess) assessed (NMA-No Measure Associated)
🖪 0.00   ⚕ 0.00   **FUD** XXX   E
AMA: 2006,Dec,10-12

2004F Initial examination of the involved joint(s) (includes visual inspection, palpation, range of motion) (OA) [Instructions: Report only for initial osteoarthritis visit or for visits for new joint involvement]
[INCLUDES]   Visits for initial osteoarthritis examination or new joint involvement
🖪 0.00   ⚕ 0.00   **FUD** XXX   E
AMA: 2004,Feb,3; 2003,Aug,1

2010F Vital signs (temperature, pulse, respiratory rate, and blood pressure) documented and reviewed (CAP) (EM)
🖪 0.00   ⚕ 0.00   **FUD** XXX   E

2014F Mental status assessed (CAP) (EM)
🖪 0.00   ⚕ 0.00   **FUD** XXX   E

2015F Asthma impairment assessed (Asthma)
🖪 0.00   ⚕ 0.00   **FUD** XXX   E

2016F Asthma risk assessed (Asthma)
🖪 0.00   ⚕ 0.00   **FUD** XXX   E

2018F Hydration status assessed (normal/mildly dehydrated/severely dehydrated) (CAP)
🗐 0.00 ✑ 0.00 **FUD** XXX
E

2019F Dilated macular exam performed, including documentation of the presence or absence of macular thickening or hemorrhage and the level of macular degeneration severity (EC)
🗐 0.00 ✑ 0.00 **FUD** XXX
E

2020F Dilated fundus evaluation performed within 12 months prior to cataract surgery (EC)
🗐 0.00 ✑ 0.00 **FUD** XXX
E
AMA: 2008,Mar,8-12

2021F Dilated macular or fundus exam performed, including documentation of the presence or absence of macular edema and level of severity of retinopathy (EC)
🗐 0.00 ✑ 0.00 **FUD** XXX
E

▲ 2022F Dilated retinal eye exam with interpretation by an ophthalmologist or optometrist documented and reviewed; with evidence of retinopathy (DM)
🗐 0.00 ✑ 0.00 **FUD** XXX
M
AMA: 2008,Mar,8-12

2023F without evidence of retinopathy (DM)
🗐 0.00 ✑ 0.00 **FUD** 000

▲ 2024F 7 standard field stereoscopic retinal photos with interpretation by an ophthalmologist or optometrist documented and reviewed; with evidence of retinopathy (DM)
🗐 0.00 ✑ 0.00 **FUD** XXX
M
AMA: 2008,Mar,8-12

2025F without evidence of retinopathy (DM)
🗐 0.00 ✑ 0.00 **FUD** 000

▲ 2026F Eye imaging validated to match diagnosis from 7 standard field stereoscopic retinal photos results documented and reviewed; with evidence of retinopathy (DM)
🗐 0.00 ✑ 0.00 **FUD** XXX
M
AMA: 2008,Mar,8-12

● # 2033F without evidence of retinopathy (DM)
🗐 0.00 ✑ 0.00 **FUD** 000

2027F Optic nerve head evaluation performed (EC)
🗐 0.00 ✑ 0.00 **FUD** XXX
M

2028F Foot examination performed (includes examination through visual inspection, sensory exam with monofilament, and pulse exam - report when any of the 3 components are completed) (DM)
🗐 0.00 ✑ 0.00 **FUD** XXX
E

2029F Complete physical skin exam performed (ML)
🗐 0.00 ✑ 0.00 **FUD** XXX
E
AMA: 2008,Mar,8-12

2030F Hydration status documented, normally hydrated (PAG)
🗐 0.00 ✑ 0.00 **FUD** XXX
E

2031F Hydration status documented, dehydrated (PAG)
🗐 0.00 ✑ 0.00 **FUD** XXX
E

2033F Resequenced code. See code following 2026F.

2035F Tympanic membrane mobility assessed with pneumatic otoscopy or tympanometry (OME)
🗐 0.00 ✑ 0.00 **FUD** XXX
E
AMA: 2008,Mar,8-12

2040F Physical examination on the date of the initial visit for low back pain performed, in accordance with specifications (BkP)
🗐 0.00 ✑ 0.00 **FUD** XXX
E
AMA: 2008,Mar,8-12

2044F Documentation of mental health assessment prior to intervention (back surgery or epidural steroid injection) or for back pain episode lasting longer than 6 weeks (BkP)
🗐 0.00 ✑ 0.00 **FUD** XXX
E
AMA: 2008,Mar,8-12

2050F Wound characteristics including size and nature of wound base tissue and amount of drainage prior to debridement documented (CWC)
🗐 0.00 ✑ 0.00 **FUD** XXX
E

2060F Patient interviewed directly on or before date of diagnosis of major depressive disorder (MDD ADOL)
🗐 0.00 ✑ 0.00 **FUD** XXX
E

3006F-3776F [3051F, 3052F] Findings from Diagnostic or Screening Tests

INCLUDES Results and medical decision making with regards to ordered tests:
Clinical laboratory tests
Other examination procedures
Radiological examinations

3006F Chest X-ray results documented and reviewed (CAP)
🗐 0.00 ✑ 0.00 **FUD** XXX
E
AMA: 2018,Jan,8; 2017,Jan,8; 2016,Jan,13; 2015,Jan,16; 2014,Jan,11

3008F Body Mass Index (BMI), documented (PV)
🗐 0.00 ✑ 0.00 **FUD** XXX
E

3011F Lipid panel results documented and reviewed (must include total cholesterol, HDL-C, triglycerides and calculated LDL-C) (CAD)
🗐 0.00 ✑ 0.00 **FUD** XXX
E

3014F Screening mammography results documented and reviewed (PV)
🗐 0.00 ✑ 0.00 **FUD** XXX
E
AMA: 2008,Mar,8-12

3015F Cervical cancer screening results documented and reviewed (PV)
🗐 0.00 ✑ 0.00 **FUD** XXX
♀
E

3016F Patient screened for unhealthy alcohol use using a systematic screening method (PV) (DSP)
🗐 0.00 ✑ 0.00 **FUD** XXX
E

3017F Colorectal cancer screening results documented and reviewed (PV)
🗐 0.00 ✑ 0.00 **FUD** XXX
M
AMA: 2008,Mar,8-12

3018F Pre-procedure risk assessment and depth of insertion and quality of the bowel prep and complete description of polyp(s) found, including location of each polyp, size, number and gross morphology and recommendations for follow-up in final colonoscopy report documented (End/Polyp)
🗐 0.00 ✑ 0.00 **FUD** XXX
E

3019F Left ventricular ejection fraction (LVEF) assessment planned post discharge (HF)
🗐 0.00 ✑ 0.00 **FUD** XXX
E

3020F Left ventricular function (LVF) assessment (eg, echocardiography, nuclear test, or ventriculography) documented in the medical record (Includes quantitative or qualitative assessment results) (NMA-No Measure Associated)
🗐 0.00 ✑ 0.00 **FUD** XXX
E
AMA: 2006,Dec,10-12

3021F Left ventricular ejection fraction (LVEF) less than 40% or documentation of moderately or severely depressed left ventricular systolic function (CAD, HF)
🗐 0.00 ✑ 0.00 **FUD** XXX
M

3022F Left ventricular ejection fraction (LVEF) greater than or equal to 40% or documentation as normal or mildly depressed left ventricular systolic function (CAD, HF)
🏥 0.00 🔲 0.00 **FUD** XXX ⓜ

3023F Spirometry results documented and reviewed (COPD)
🏥 0.00 🔲 0.00 **FUD** XXX ⓜ

3025F Spirometry test results demonstrate FEV1/FVC less than 70% with COPD symptoms (eg, dyspnea, cough/sputum, wheezing) (CAP, COPD)
🏥 0.00 🔲 0.00 **FUD** XXX Ⓔ

3027F Spirometry test results demonstrate FEV1/FVC greater than or equal to 70% or patient does not have COPD symptoms (COPD)
🏥 0.00 🔲 0.00 **FUD** XXX Ⓔ

3028F Oxygen saturation results documented and reviewed (includes assessment through pulse oximetry or arterial blood gas measurement) (CAP, COPD) (EM)
🏥 0.00 🔲 0.00 **FUD** XXX Ⓔ

3035F Oxygen saturation less than or equal to 88% or a PaO2 less than or equal to 55 mm Hg (COPD)
🏥 0.00 🔲 0.00 **FUD** XXX Ⓔ

3037F Oxygen saturation greater than 88% or PaO2 greater than 55 mm Hg (COPD)
🏥 0.00 🔲 0.00 **FUD** XXX Ⓔ

3038F Pulmonary function test performed within 12 months prior to surgery (Lung/Esop Cx)
🏥 0.00 🔲 0.00 **FUD** XXX Ⓔ

3040F Functional expiratory volume (FEV1) less than 40% of predicted value (COPD)
🏥 0.00 🔲 0.00 **FUD** XXX Ⓔ

3042F Functional expiratory volume (FEV1) greater than or equal to 40% of predicted value (COPD)
🏥 0.00 🔲 0.00 **FUD** XXX Ⓔ

3044F Most recent hemoglobin A1c (HbA1c) level less than 7.0% (DM)
🏥 0.00 🔲 0.00 **FUD** XXX ⓜ

● # **3051F** Most recent hemoglobin A1c (HbA1c) level greater than or equal to 7.0% and less than 8.0% (DM)
🏥 0.00 🔲 0.00 **FUD** 000

3045F Most recent hemoglobin A1c (HbA1c) level 7.0-9.0% (DM)
To report, see ([3051F], [3052F])

● # **3052F** Most recent hemoglobin A1c (HbA1c) level greater than or equal to 8.0% and less than or equal to 9.0% (DM)
🏥 0.00 🔲 0.00 **FUD** 000

▲ **3046F** Most recent hemoglobin A1c level greater than 9.0% (DM)
🏥 0.00 🔲 0.00 **FUD** XXX ⓜ
EXCLUDES Levels of hemoglobin A1c less than or equal to 9.0% (3044F, [3051F], [3052F])

3048F Most recent LDL-C less than 100 mg/dL (CAD) (DM)
🏥 0.00 🔲 0.00 **FUD** XXX Ⓔ

3049F Most recent LDL-C 100-129 mg/dL (CAD) (DM)
🏥 0.00 🔲 0.00 **FUD** XXX Ⓔ

3050F Most recent LDL-C greater than or equal to 130 mg/dL (CAD) (DM)
🏥 0.00 🔲 0.00 **FUD** XXX Ⓔ

3051F Resequenced code. See code following 3044F.

3052F Resequenced code. See code before 3046F.

3055F Left ventricular ejection fraction (LVEF) less than or equal to 35% (HF)
🏥 0.00 🔲 0.00 **FUD** XXX Ⓔ

3056F Left ventricular ejection fraction (LVEF) greater than 35% or no LVEF result available (HF)
🏥 0.00 🔲 0.00 **FUD** XXX Ⓔ

3060F Positive microalbuminuria test result documented and reviewed (DM)
🏥 0.00 🔲 0.00 **FUD** XXX ⓜ

3061F Negative microalbuminuria test result documented and reviewed (DM)
🏥 0.00 🔲 0.00 **FUD** XXX ⓜ

3062F Positive macroalbuminuria test result documented and reviewed (DM)
🏥 0.00 🔲 0.00 **FUD** XXX ⓜ

3066F Documentation of treatment for nephropathy (eg, patient receiving dialysis, patient being treated for ESRD, CRF, ARF, or renal insufficiency, any visit to a nephrologist) (DM)
🏥 0.00 🔲 0.00 **FUD** XXX ⓜ

3072F Low risk for retinopathy (no evidence of retinopathy in the prior year) (DM)
🏥 0.00 🔲 0.00 **FUD** XXX ⓜ
AMA: 2008,Mar,8-12

3073F Pre-surgical (cataract) axial length, corneal power measurement and method of intraocular lens power calculation documented within 12 months prior to surgery (EC)
🏥 0.00 🔲 0.00 **FUD** XXX Ⓔ
AMA: 2008,Mar,8-12

3074F Most recent systolic blood pressure less than 130 mm Hg (DM), (HTN, CKD, CAD)
🏥 0.00 🔲 0.00 **FUD** XXX Ⓔ
AMA: 2008,Mar,8-12

3075F Most recent systolic blood pressure 130-139 mm Hg (DM) (HTN, CKD, CAD)
🏥 0.00 🔲 0.00 **FUD** XXX Ⓔ
AMA: 2008,Mar,8-12

3077F Most recent systolic blood pressure greater than or equal to 140 mm Hg (HTN, CKD, CAD) (DM)
🏥 0.00 🔲 0.00 **FUD** XXX Ⓔ
AMA: 2008,Mar,8-12

3078F Most recent diastolic blood pressure less than 80 mm Hg (HTN, CKD, CAD) (DM)
🏥 0.00 🔲 0.00 **FUD** XXX Ⓔ
AMA: 2008,Mar,8-12

3079F Most recent diastolic blood pressure 80-89 mm Hg (HTN, CKD, CAD) (DM)
🏥 0.00 🔲 0.00 **FUD** XXX Ⓔ
AMA: 2008,Mar,8-12

3080F Most recent diastolic blood pressure greater than or equal to 90 mm Hg (HTN, CKD, CAD) (DM)
🏥 0.00 🔲 0.00 **FUD** XXX Ⓔ
AMA: 2008,Mar,8-12

3082F Kt/V less than 1.2 (Clearance of urea [Kt]/volume [V]) (ESRD, P-ESRD)
🏥 0.00 🔲 0.00 **FUD** XXX Ⓔ
AMA: 2008,Mar,8-12

3083F Kt/V equal to or greater than 1.2 and less than 1.7 (Clearance of urea [Kt]/volume [V]) (ESRD, P-ESRD)
🏥 0.00 🔲 0.00 **FUD** XXX Ⓔ
AMA: 2008,Mar,8-12

3084F Kt/V greater than or equal to 1.7 (Clearance of urea [Kt]/volume [V]) (ESRD, P-ESRD)
🏥 0.00 🔲 0.00 **FUD** XXX Ⓔ
AMA: 2008,Mar,8-12

3085F Suicide risk assessed (MDD, MDD ADOL)
🏥 0.00 🔲 0.00 **FUD** XXX Ⓔ

3088F Major depressive disorder, mild (MDD)
🏥 0.00 🔲 0.00 **FUD** XXX Ⓔ

3089F Major depressive disorder, moderate (MDD)
🏥 0.00 🔲 0.00 **FUD** XXX Ⓔ

3090F Major depressive disorder, severe without psychotic features (MDD)
🔲 0.00 🔾 0.00 **FUD** XXX
[E]

3091F Major depressive disorder, severe with psychotic features (MDD)
🔲 0.00 🔾 0.00 **FUD** XXX
[E]

3092F Major depressive disorder, in remission (MDD)
🔲 0.00 🔾 0.00 **FUD** XXX
[E]

3093F Documentation of new diagnosis of initial or recurrent episode of major depressive disorder (MDD)
🔲 0.00 🔾 0.00 **FUD** XXX
[E]
AMA: 2008,Mar,8-12

3095F Central dual-energy X-ray absorptiometry (DXA) results documented (OP)(IBD)
🔲 0.00 🔾 0.00 **FUD** XXX
[M]

3096F Central dual-energy X-ray absorptiometry (DXA) ordered (OP)(IBD)
🔲 0.00 🔾 0.00 **FUD** XXX
[E]

3100F Carotid imaging study report (includes direct or indirect reference to measurements of distal internal carotid diameter as the denominator for stenosis measurement) (STR, RAD)
🔲 0.00 🔾 0.00 **FUD** XXX
[M]
AMA: 2008,Mar,8-12

3110F Documentation in final CT or MRI report of presence or absence of hemorrhage and mass lesion and acute infarction (STR)
🔲 0.00 🔾 0.00 **FUD** XXX
[E]

3111F CT or MRI of the brain performed in the hospital within 24 hours of arrival or performed in an outpatient imaging center, to confirm initial diagnosis of stroke, TIA or intracranial hemorrhage (STR)
🔲 0.00 🔾 0.00 **FUD** XXX
[E]

3112F CT or MRI of the brain performed greater than 24 hours after arrival to the hospital or performed in an outpatient imaging center for purpose other than confirmation of initial diagnosis of stroke, TIA, or intracranial hemorrhage (STR)
🔲 0.00 🔾 0.00 **FUD** XXX
[E]

3115F Quantitative results of an evaluation of current level of activity and clinical symptoms (HF)
🔲 0.00 🔾 0.00 **FUD** XXX
[E]

3117F Heart failure disease specific structured assessment tool completed (HF)
🔲 0.00 🔾 0.00 **FUD** XXX
[E]

3118F New York Heart Association (NYHA) Class documented (HF)
🔲 0.00 🔾 0.00 **FUD** XXX
[E]

3119F No evaluation of level of activity or clinical symptoms (HF)
🔲 0.00 🔾 0.00 **FUD** XXX
[E]

3120F 12-Lead ECG Performed (EM)
🔲 0.00 🔾 0.00 **FUD** XXX
[E]

3126F Esophageal biopsy report with a statement about dysplasia (present, absent, or indefinite, and if present, contains appropriate grading) (PATH)
🔲 0.00 🔾 0.00 **FUD** XXX
[M]

3130F Upper gastrointestinal endoscopy performed (GERD)
🔲 0.00 🔾 0.00 **FUD** XXX
[E]

3132F Documentation of referral for upper gastrointestinal endoscopy (GERD)
🔲 0.00 🔾 0.00 **FUD** XXX
[E]

3140F Upper gastrointestinal endoscopy report indicates suspicion of Barrett's esophagus (GERD)
🔲 0.00 🔾 0.00 **FUD** XXX
[E]

3141F Upper gastrointestinal endoscopy report indicates no suspicion of Barrett's esophagus (GERD)
🔲 0.00 🔾 0.00 **FUD** XXX
[E]

3142F Barium swallow test ordered (GERD)
🔲 0.00 🔾 0.00 **FUD** XXX
[E]
INCLUDES Documentation of barium swallow test

3150F Forceps esophageal biopsy performed (GERD)
🔲 0.00 🔾 0.00 **FUD** XXX
[E]

3155F Cytogenetic testing performed on bone marrow at time of diagnosis or prior to initiating treatment (HEM)
🔲 0.00 🔾 0.00 **FUD** XXX
[M]

3160F Documentation of iron stores prior to initiating erythropoietin therapy (HEM)
🔲 0.00 🔾 0.00 **FUD** XXX
[M]
AMA: 2008,Mar,8-12

3170F Flow cytometry studies performed at time of diagnosis or prior to initiating treatment (HEM)
🔲 0.00 🔾 0.00 **FUD** XXX
[M]
AMA: 2008,Mar,8-12

3200F Barium swallow test not ordered (GERD)
🔲 0.00 🔾 0.00 **FUD** XXX
[E]

3210F Group A Strep Test Performed (PHAR)
🔲 0.00 🔾 0.00 **FUD** XXX
[M]
AMA: 2008,Mar,8-12

3215F Patient has documented immunity to Hepatitis A (HEP-C)
🔲 0.00 🔾 0.00 **FUD** XXX
[E]
AMA: 2008,Mar,8-12

3216F Patient has documented immunity to Hepatitis B (HEP-C)(IBD)
🔲 0.00 🔾 0.00 **FUD** XXX
[E]
AMA: 2008,Mar,8-12

3218F RNA testing for Hepatitis C documented as performed within 6 months prior to initiation of antiviral treatment for Hepatitis C (HEP-C)
🔲 0.00 🔾 0.00 **FUD** XXX
[E]
AMA: 2008,Mar,8-12

3220F Hepatitis C quantitative RNA testing documented as performed at 12 weeks from initiation of antiviral treatment (HEP-C)
🔲 0.00 🔾 0.00 **FUD** XXX
[E]
AMA: 2008,Mar,8-12

3230F Documentation that hearing test was performed within 6 months prior to tympanostomy tube insertion (OME)
🔲 0.00 🔾 0.00 **FUD** XXX
[E]
AMA: 2008,Mar,8-12

3250F Specimen site other than anatomic location of primary tumor (PATH)
🔲 0.00 🔾 0.00 **FUD** XXX
[M]

3260F pT category (primary tumor), pN category (regional lymph nodes), and histologic grade documented in pathology report (PATH)
🔲 0.00 🔾 0.00 **FUD** XXX
[M]
AMA: 2008,Mar,8-12

3265F Ribonucleic acid (RNA) testing for Hepatitis C viremia ordered or results documented (HEP C)
🔲 0.00 🔾 0.00 **FUD** XXX
[E]
AMA: 2008,Mar,8-12

3266F Hepatitis C genotype testing documented as performed prior to initiation of antiviral treatment for Hepatitis C (HEP C)
🔲 0.00 🔾 0.00 **FUD** XXX
[E]
AMA: 2008,Mar,8-12

3267F Pathology report includes pT category, pN category, Gleason score, and statement about margin status (PATH)
🔲 0.00 🔾 0.00 **FUD** XXX
[M]

3268F Prostate-specific antigen (PSA), and primary tumor (T) stage, and Gleason score documented prior to initiation of treatment (PRCA)

    🖫 0.00   ☌ 0.00   **FUD** XXX   E

    AMA: 2008,Mar,8-12

3269F Bone scan performed prior to initiation of treatment or at any time since diagnosis of prostate cancer (PRCA)

    🖫 0.00   ☌ 0.00   **FUD** XXX   M

    AMA: 2008,Mar,8-12

3270F Bone scan not performed prior to initiation of treatment nor at any time since diagnosis of prostate cancer (PRCA)

    🖫 0.00   ☌ 0.00   **FUD** XXX   M

    AMA: 2008,Mar,8-12

3271F Low risk of recurrence, prostate cancer (PRCA)

    🖫 0.00   ☌ 0.00   **FUD** XXX   E

    AMA: 2008,Mar,8-12

3272F Intermediate risk of recurrence, prostate cancer (PRCA)

    🖫 0.00   ☌ 0.00   **FUD** XXX   E

    AMA: 2008,Mar,8-12

3273F High risk of recurrence, prostate cancer (PRCA)

    🖫 0.00   ☌ 0.00   **FUD** XXX   E

    AMA: 2008,Mar,8-12

3274F Prostate cancer risk of recurrence not determined or neither low, intermediate nor high (PRCA)

    🖫 0.00   ☌ 0.00   **FUD** XXX   E

    AMA: 2008,Mar,8-12

3278F Serum levels of calcium, phosphorus, intact Parathyroid Hormone (PTH) and lipid profile ordered (CKD)

    🖫 0.00   ☌ 0.00   **FUD** XXX   E

    AMA: 2008,Mar,8-12

3279F Hemoglobin level greater than or equal to 13 g/dL (CKD, ESRD)

    🖫 0.00   ☌ 0.00   **FUD** XXX   E

    AMA: 2008,Mar,8-12

3280F Hemoglobin level 11 g/dL to 12.9 g/dL (CKD, ESRD)

    🖫 0.00   ☌ 0.00   **FUD** XXX   E

    AMA: 2008,Mar,8-12

3281F Hemoglobin level less than 11 g/dL (CKD, ESRD)

    🖫 0.00   ☌ 0.00   **FUD** XXX   E

    AMA: 2008,Mar,8-12

3284F Intraocular pressure (IOP) reduced by a value of greater than or equal to 15% from the pre-intervention level (EC)

    🖫 0.00   ☌ 0.00   **FUD** XXX   M

    AMA: 2008,Mar,8-12

3285F Intraocular pressure (IOP) reduced by a value less than 15% from the pre-intervention level (EC)

    🖫 0.00   ☌ 0.00   **FUD** XXX   M

    AMA: 2008,Mar,8-12

3288F Falls risk assessment documented (GER)

    🖫 0.00   ☌ 0.00   **FUD** XXX   M

3290F Patient is D (Rh) negative and unsensitized (Pre-Cr)

    🖫 0.00   ☌ 0.00   **FUD** XXX   E

    AMA: 2008,Mar,8-12

3291F Patient is D (Rh) positive or sensitized (Pre-Cr)

    🖫 0.00   ☌ 0.00   **FUD** XXX   E

    AMA: 2008,Mar,8-12

3292F HIV testing ordered or documented and reviewed during the first or second prenatal visit (Pre-Cr)

    🖫 0.00   ☌ 0.00   **FUD** XXX   E

3293F ABO and Rh blood typing documented as performed (Pre-Cr)

    🖫 0.00   ☌ 0.00   **FUD** XXX   E

3294F Group B Streptococcus (GBS) screening documented as performed during week 35-37 gestation (Pre-Cr)

    🖫 0.00   ☌ 0.00   **FUD** XXX   E

3300F American Joint Committee on Cancer (AJCC) stage documented and reviewed (ONC)

    🖫 0.00   ☌ 0.00   **FUD** XXX   M

    AMA: 2008,Mar,8-12

3301F Cancer stage documented in medical record as metastatic and reviewed (ONC)

    EXCLUDES   *Cancer staging measures (3321F-3390F)*

    🖫 0.00   ☌ 0.00   **FUD** XXX   M

    AMA: 2008,Mar,8-12

3315F Estrogen receptor (ER) or progesterone receptor (PR) positive breast cancer (ONC)

    🖫 0.00   ☌ 0.00   **FUD** XXX   E

    AMA: 2008,Mar,8-12

3316F Estrogen receptor (ER) and progesterone receptor (PR) negative breast cancer (ONC)

    🖫 0.00   ☌ 0.00   **FUD** XXX   E

    AMA: 2008,Mar,8-12

3317F Pathology report confirming malignancy documented in the medical record and reviewed prior to the initiation of chemotherapy (ONC)

    🖫 0.00   ☌ 0.00   **FUD** XXX   E

    AMA: 2008,Mar,8-12

3318F Pathology report confirming malignancy documented in the medical record and reviewed prior to the initiation of radiation therapy (ONC)

    🖫 0.00   ☌ 0.00   **FUD** XXX   E

    AMA: 2008,Mar,8-12

3319F 1 of the following diagnostic imaging studies ordered: chest x-ray, CT, Ultrasound, MRI, PET, or nuclear medicine scans (ML)

    🖫 0.00   ☌ 0.00   **FUD** XXX   M

    AMA: 2008,Mar,8-12

3320F None of the following diagnostic imaging studies ordered: chest X-ray, CT, Ultrasound, MRI, PET, or nuclear medicine scans (ML)

    🖫 0.00   ☌ 0.00   **FUD** XXX   M

    AMA: 2008,Mar,8-12

3321F AJCC Cancer Stage 0 or IA Melanoma, documented (ML)

    🖫 0.00   ☌ 0.00   **FUD** XXX   M

3322F Melanoma greater than AJCC Stage 0 or IA (ML)

    🖫 0.00   ☌ 0.00   **FUD** XXX   M

3323F Clinical tumor, node and metastases (TNM) staging documented and reviewed prior to surgery (Lung/Esop Cx)

    🖫 0.00   ☌ 0.00   **FUD** XXX   E

3324F MRI or CT scan ordered, reviewed or requested (EPI)

    🖫 0.00   ☌ 0.00   **FUD** XXX   E

3325F Preoperative assessment of functional or medical indication(s) for surgery prior to the cataract surgery with intraocular lens placement (must be performed within 12 months prior to cataract surgery) (EC)

    🖫 0.00   ☌ 0.00   **FUD** XXX   E

    AMA: 2008,Mar,8-12

3328F Performance status documented and reviewed within 2 weeks prior to surgery (Lung/Esop Cx)

    🖫 0.00   ☌ 0.00   **FUD** XXX   E

3330F Imaging study ordered (BkP)

    🖫 0.00   ☌ 0.00   **FUD** XXX   E

    AMA: 2008,Mar,8-12

3331F Imaging study not ordered (BkP)

    🖫 0.00   ☌ 0.00   **FUD** XXX   E

    AMA: 2008,Mar,8-12

3340F   Mammogram assessment category of "incomplete: need additional imaging evaluation" documented (RAD)
    🔲 0.00   🔲 0.00   **FUD** XXX   Ⓜ
    AMA: 2008,Mar,8-12

3341F   Mammogram assessment category of "negative," documented (RAD)
    🔲 0.00   🔲 0.00   **FUD** XXX   Ⓜ
    AMA: 2008,Mar,8-12

3342F   Mammogram assessment category of "benign," documented (RAD)
    🔲 0.00   🔲 0.00   **FUD** XXX   Ⓜ
    AMA: 2008,Mar,8-12

3343F   Mammogram assessment category of "probably benign," documented (RAD)
    🔲 0.00   🔲 0.00   **FUD** XXX   Ⓜ
    AMA: 2008,Mar,8-12

3344F   Mammogram assessment category of "suspicious," documented (RAD)
    🔲 0.00   🔲 0.00   **FUD** XXX   Ⓜ
    AMA: 2008,Mar,8-12

3345F   Mammogram assessment category of "highly suggestive of malignancy," documented (RAD)
    🔲 0.00   🔲 0.00   **FUD** XXX   Ⓜ
    AMA: 2008,Mar,8-12

3350F   Mammogram assessment category of "known biopsy proven malignancy," documented (RAD)
    🔲 0.00   🔲 0.00   **FUD** XXX   Ⓜ
    AMA: 2008,Mar,8-12

3351F   Negative screen for depressive symptoms as categorized by using a standardized depression screening/assessment tool (MDD)
    🔲 0.00   🔲 0.00   **FUD** XXX   Ⓔ

3352F   No significant depressive symptoms as categorized by using a standardized depression assessment tool (MDD)
    🔲 0.00   🔲 0.00   **FUD** XXX   Ⓔ

3353F   Mild to moderate depressive symptoms as categorized by using a standardized depression screening/assessment tool (MDD)
    🔲 0.00   🔲 0.00   **FUD** XXX   Ⓔ

3354F   Clinically significant depressive symptoms as categorized by using a standardized depression screening/assessment tool (MDD)
    🔲 0.00   🔲 0.00   **FUD** XXX   Ⓔ

3370F   AJCC Breast Cancer Stage 0 documented (ONC)
    🔲 0.00   🔲 0.00   **FUD** XXX   Ⓔ

3372F   AJCC Breast Cancer Stage I: T1mic, T1a or T1b (tumor size ≤ 1 cm) documented (ONC)
    🔲 0.00   🔲 0.00   **FUD** XXX   Ⓔ

3374F   AJCC Breast Cancer Stage I: T1c (tumor size > 1 cm to 2 cm) documented (ONC)
    🔲 0.00   🔲 0.00   **FUD** XXX   Ⓔ

3376F   AJCC Breast Cancer Stage II documented (ONC)
    🔲 0.00   🔲 0.00   **FUD** XXX   Ⓔ

3378F   AJCC Breast Cancer Stage III documented (ONC)
    🔲 0.00   🔲 0.00   **FUD** XXX   Ⓔ

3380F   AJCC Breast Cancer Stage IV documented (ONC)
    🔲 0.00   🔲 0.00   **FUD** XXX   Ⓔ

3382F   AJCC colon cancer, Stage 0 documented (ONC)
    🔲 0.00   🔲 0.00   **FUD** XXX   Ⓔ

3384F   AJCC colon cancer, Stage I documented (ONC)
    🔲 0.00   🔲 0.00   **FUD** XXX   Ⓔ

3386F   AJCC colon cancer, Stage II documented (ONC)
    🔲 0.00   🔲 0.00   **FUD** XXX   Ⓔ

3388F   AJCC colon cancer, Stage III documented (ONC)
    🔲 0.00   🔲 0.00   **FUD** XXX   Ⓔ

3390F   AJCC colon cancer, Stage IV documented (ONC)
    🔲 0.00   🔲 0.00   **FUD** XXX   Ⓔ

3394F   Quantitative HER2 immunohistochemistry (IHC) evaluation of breast cancer consistent with the scoring system defined in the ASCO/CAP guidelines (PATH)
    🔲 0.00   🔲 0.00   **FUD** XXX   Ⓜ

3395F   Quantitative non-HER2 immunohistochemistry (IHC) evaluation of breast cancer (eg, testing for estrogen or progesterone receptors [ER/PR]) performed (PATH)
    🔲 0.00   🔲 0.00   **FUD** XXX   Ⓜ

3450F   Dyspnea screened, no dyspnea or mild dyspnea (Pall Cr)
    🔲 0.00   🔲 0.00   **FUD** XXX   Ⓔ

3451F   Dyspnea screened, moderate or severe dyspnea (Pall Cr)
    🔲 0.00   🔲 0.00   **FUD** XXX   Ⓔ

3452F   Dyspnea not screened (Pall Cr)
    🔲 0.00   🔲 0.00   **FUD** XXX   Ⓔ

3455F   TB screening performed and results interpreted within six months prior to initiation of first-time biologic disease modifying anti-rheumatic drug therapy for RA (RA)
    🔲 0.00   🔲 0.00   **FUD** XXX   Ⓜ

3470F   Rheumatoid arthritis (RA) disease activity, low (RA)
    🔲 0.00   🔲 0.00   **FUD** XXX   Ⓜ

3471F   Rheumatoid arthritis (RA) disease activity, moderate (RA)
    🔲 0.00   🔲 0.00   **FUD** XXX   Ⓜ

3472F   Rheumatoid arthritis (RA) disease activity, high (RA)
    🔲 0.00   🔲 0.00   **FUD** XXX   Ⓜ

3475F   Disease prognosis for rheumatoid arthritis assessed, poor prognosis documented (RA)
    🔲 0.00   🔲 0.00   **FUD** XXX   Ⓜ

3476F   Disease prognosis for rheumatoid arthritis assessed, good prognosis documented (RA)
    🔲 0.00   🔲 0.00   **FUD** XXX   Ⓜ

3490F   History of AIDS-defining condition (HIV)
    🔲 0.00   🔲 0.00   **FUD** XXX   Ⓔ

3491F   HIV indeterminate (infants of undetermined HIV status born of HIV-infected mothers) (HIV)
    🔲 0.00   🔲 0.00   **FUD** XXX   Ⓔ

3492F   History of nadir CD4+ cell count <350 cells/mm3 (HIV)
    🔲 0.00   🔲 0.00   **FUD** XXX   Ⓔ

3493F   No history of nadir CD4+ cell count <350 cells/mm3 and no history of AIDS-defining condition (HIV)
    🔲 0.00   🔲 0.00   **FUD** XXX   Ⓔ

3494F   CD4+ cell count <200 cells/mm3 (HIV)
    🔲 0.00   🔲 0.00   **FUD** XXX   Ⓔ

3495F   CD4+ cell count 200 - 499 cells/mm3 (HIV)
    🔲 0.00   🔲 0.00   **FUD** XXX   Ⓔ

3496F   CD4+ cell count ≥ 500 cells/mm3 (HIV)
    🔲 0.00   🔲 0.00   **FUD** XXX   Ⓔ

3497F   CD4+ cell percentage <15% (HIV)
    🔲 0.00   🔲 0.00   **FUD** XXX   Ⓔ

3498F   CD4+ cell percentage ≥ 15% (HIV)
    🔲 0.00   🔲 0.00   **FUD** XXX   Ⓔ

3500F   CD4+ cell count or CD4+ cell percentage documented as performed (HIV)
    🔲 0.00   🔲 0.00   **FUD** XXX   Ⓔ

3502F   HIV RNA viral load below limits of quantification (HIV)
    🔲 0.00   🔲 0.00   **FUD** XXX   Ⓔ

3503F   HIV RNA viral load not below limits of quantification (HIV)
    🔲 0.00   🔲 0.00   **FUD** XXX   Ⓔ

● New Code ▲ Revised Code ○ Reinstated ● New Web Release ▲ Revised Web Release + Add-on Unlisted Not Covered # Resequenced
㊿ Optum Mod 50 Exempt Ⓝ AMA Mod 51 Exempt �51 Optum Mod 51 Exempt �63 Mod 63 Exempt ✗ Non-FDA Drug ★ Telemedicine Ⓜ Maternity Ⓐ Age Edit

    CPT © 2019 American Medical Association. All Rights Reserved.

3510F Documentation that tuberculosis (TB) screening test performed and results interpreted (HIV) (IBD)
🖭 0.00   ⚖ 0.00   **FUD** XXX   E

3511F Chlamydia and gonorrhea screenings documented as performed (HIV)
🖭 0.00   ⚖ 0.00   **FUD** XXX   E

3512F Syphilis screening documented as performed (HIV)
🖭 0.00   ⚖ 0.00   **FUD** XXX   E

3513F Hepatitis B screening documented as performed (HIV)
🖭 0.00   ⚖ 0.00   **FUD** XXX   E

3514F Hepatitis C screening documented as performed (HIV)
🖭 0.00   ⚖ 0.00   **FUD** XXX   E

3515F Patient has documented immunity to Hepatitis C (HIV)
🖭 0.00   ⚖ 0.00   **FUD** XXX   E

3517F Hepatitis B Virus (HBV) status assessed and results interpreted within one year prior to receiving a first course of anti-TNF (tumor necrosis factor) therapy (IBD)
🖭 0.00   ⚖ 0.00   **FUD** XXX   E

3520F Clostridium difficile testing performed (IBD)
🖭 0.00   ⚖ 0.00   **FUD** XXX   E

3550F Low risk for thromboembolism (AFIB)
🖭 0.00   ⚖ 0.00   **FUD** XXX   E

3551F Intermediate risk for thromboembolism (AFIB)
🖭 0.00   ⚖ 0.00   **FUD** XXX   E

3552F High risk for thromboembolism (AFIB)
🖭 0.00   ⚖ 0.00   **FUD** XXX   E

3555F Patient had International Normalized Ratio (INR) measurement performed (AFIB)
🖭 0.00   ⚖ 0.00   **FUD** XXX   E
AMA: 2010,Jul,3-5

3570F Final report for bone scintigraphy study includes correlation with existing relevant imaging studies (eg, X-ray, MRI, CT) corresponding to the same anatomical region in question (NUC_MED)
🖭 0.00   ⚖ 0.00   **FUD** XXX   M

3572F Patient considered to be potentially at risk for fracture in a weight-bearing site (NUC_MED)
🖭 0.00   ⚖ 0.00   **FUD** XXX   E

3573F Patient not considered to be potentially at risk for fracture in a weight-bearing site (NUC_MED)
🖭 0.00   ⚖ 0.00   **FUD** XXX   E

3650F Electroencephalogram (EEG) ordered, reviewed or requested (EPI)
🖭 0.00   ⚖ 0.00   **FUD** XXX   E

3700F Psychiatric disorders or disturbances assessed (Prkns)
🖭 0.00   ⚖ 0.00   **FUD** XXX   E

3720F Cognitive impairment or dysfunction assessed (Prkns)
🖭 0.00   ⚖ 0.00   **FUD** XXX   M

3725F Screening for depression performed (DEM)
🖭 0.00   ⚖ 0.00   **FUD** XXX   M

3750F Patient not receiving dose of corticosteroids greater than or equal to 10mg/day for 60 or greater consecutive days (IBD)
🖭 0.00   ⚖ 0.00   **FUD** XXX   E

3751F Electrodiagnostic studies for distal symmetric polyneuropathy conducted (or requested), documented, and reviewed within 6 months of initial evaluation for condition (DSP)
🖭 0.00   ⚖ 0.00   **FUD** XXX   E

3752F Electrodiagnostic studies for distal symmetric polyneuropathy not conducted (or requested), documented, or reviewed within 6 months of initial evaluation for condition (DSP)
🖭 0.00   ⚖ 0.00   **FUD** XXX   E

3753F Patient has clear clinical symptoms and signs that are highly suggestive of neuropathy AND cannot be attributed to another condition, AND has an obvious cause for the neuropathy (DSP)
🖭 0.00   ⚖ 0.00   **FUD** XXX   E

3754F Screening tests for diabetes mellitus reviewed, requested, or ordered (DSP)
🖭 0.00   ⚖ 0.00   **FUD** XXX   E

3755F Cognitive and behavioral impairment screening performed (ALS)
🖭 0.00   ⚖ 0.00   **FUD** XXX   E

3756F Patient has pseudobulbar affect, sialorrhea, or ALS-related symptoms (ALS)
🖭 0.00   ⚖ 0.00   **FUD** XXX   E

3757F Patient does not have pseudobulbar affect, sialorrhea, or ALS-related symptoms (ALS)
🖭 0.00   ⚖ 0.00   **FUD** XXX   E

3758F Patient referred for pulmonary function testing or peak cough expiratory flow (ALS)
🖭 0.00   ⚖ 0.00   **FUD** XXX   E

3759F Patient screened for dysphagia, weight loss, and impaired nutrition, and results documented (ALS)
🖭 0.00   ⚖ 0.00   **FUD** XXX   E

3760F Patient exhibits dysphagia, weight loss, or impaired nutrition (ALS)
🖭 0.00   ⚖ 0.00   **FUD** XXX   E

3761F Patient does not exhibit dysphagia, weight loss, or impaired nutrition (ALS)
🖭 0.00   ⚖ 0.00   **FUD** XXX   E

3762F Patient is dysarthric (ALS)
🖭 0.00   ⚖ 0.00   **FUD** XXX   E

3763F Patient is not dysarthric (ALS)
🖭 0.00   ⚖ 0.00   **FUD** XXX   E

3775F Adenoma(s) or other neoplasm detected during screening colonoscopy (SCADR)
🖭 0.00   ⚖ 0.00   **FUD** XXX   E

3776F Adenoma(s) or other neoplasm not detected during screening colonoscopy (SCADR)
🖭 0.00   ⚖ 0.00   **FUD** XXX   E

4000F-4563F Therapies Provided (Includes Preventive Services)

INCLUDES Behavioral/pharmacologic/procedural therapies
Preventive services including patient education/counseling

4000F Tobacco use cessation intervention, counseling (COPD, CAP, CAD, Asthma) (DM) (PV)
🖭 0.00   ⚖ 0.00   **FUD** XXX   E
AMA: 2018,Jan,8; 2017,Jan,8; 2016,Jan,13; 2015,Jan,16; 2014,Jan,11

4001F Tobacco use cessation intervention, pharmacologic therapy (COPD, CAD, CAP, PV, Asthma) (DM) (PV)
🖭 0.00   ⚖ 0.00   **FUD** XXX   E
AMA: 2008,Mar,8-12; 2004,Nov,1

4003F Patient education, written/oral, appropriate for patients with heart failure, performed (NMA-No Measure Associated)
🖭 0.00   ⚖ 0.00   **FUD** XXX   E
AMA: 2004,Nov,1

4004F Patient screened for tobacco use and received tobacco cessation intervention (counseling, pharmacotherapy, or both), if identified as a tobacco user (PV, CAD)
🖭 0.00   ⚖ 0.00   **FUD** XXX   M

4005F Pharmacologic therapy (other than minerals/vitamins) for osteoporosis prescribed (OP) (IBD)
🖭 0.00   ⚖ 0.00   **FUD** XXX   E

4008F Beta-blocker therapy prescribed or currently being taken (CAD,HF)

🚗 0.00 ⚕ 0.00 **FUD** XXX

Ⓜ

4010F Angiotensin Converting Enzyme (ACE) Inhibitor or Angiotensin Receptor Blocker (ARB) therapy prescribed or currently being taken (CAD, CKD, HF) (DM)

🚗 0.00 ⚕ 0.00 **FUD** XXX

Ⓜ

4011F Oral antiplatelet therapy prescribed (CAD)

🚗 0.00 ⚕ 0.00 **FUD** XXX

Ⓔ

AMA: 2004,Nov,1

4012F Warfarin therapy prescribed (NMA-No Measure Associated)

🚗 0.00 ⚕ 0.00 **FUD** XXX

Ⓔ

4013F Statin therapy prescribed or currently being taken (CAD)

🚗 0.00 ⚕ 0.00 **FUD** XXX

Ⓔ

4014F Written discharge instructions provided to heart failure patients discharged home (Instructions include all of the following components: activity level, diet, discharge medications, follow-up appointment, weight monitoring, what to do if symptoms worsen) (NMA-No Measure Associated)

🚗 0.00 ⚕ 0.00 **FUD** XXX

Ⓔ

4015F Persistent asthma, preferred long term control medication or an acceptable alternative treatment, prescribed (NMA-No Measure Associated)

🚗 0.00 ⚕ 0.00 **FUD** XXX

Ⓔ

EXCLUDES Use of code with modifier 1P
Code also modifier 2P for patient reasons for not prescribing

4016F Anti-inflammatory/analgesic agent prescribed (OA) (Use for prescribed or continued medication[s], including over-the-counter medication[s])

🚗 0.00 ⚕ 0.00 **FUD** XXX

Ⓔ

INCLUDES Over-the-counter medication(s)
Prescribed/continued medication(s)

4017F Gastrointestinal prophylaxis for NSAID use prescribed (OA)

🚗 0.00 ⚕ 0.00 **FUD** XXX

Ⓔ

4018F Therapeutic exercise for the involved joint(s) instructed or physical or occupational therapy prescribed (OA)

🚗 0.00 ⚕ 0.00 **FUD** XXX

Ⓔ

4019F Documentation of receipt of counseling on exercise and either both calcium and vitamin D use or counseling regarding both calcium and vitamin D use (OP)

🚗 0.00 ⚕ 0.00 **FUD** XXX

Ⓔ

4025F Inhaled bronchodilator prescribed (COPD)

🚗 0.00 ⚕ 0.00 **FUD** XXX

Ⓔ

4030F Long-term oxygen therapy prescribed (more than 15 hours per day) (COPD)

🚗 0.00 ⚕ 0.00 **FUD** XXX

Ⓔ

4033F Pulmonary rehabilitation exercise training recommended (COPD)

🚗 0.00 ⚕ 0.00 **FUD** XXX

Ⓔ

Code also dyspnea assessed, present (1019F)

4035F Influenza immunization recommended (COPD) (IBD)

🚗 0.00 ⚕ 0.00 **FUD** XXX

Ⓔ

AMA: 2008,Mar,8-12

4037F Influenza immunization ordered or administered (COPD, PV, CKD, ESRD)(IBD)

🚗 0.00 ⚕ 0.00 **FUD** XXX

Ⓔ

AMA: 2008,Mar,8-12

4040F Pneumococcal vaccine administered or previously received (COPD) (PV), (IBD)

🚗 0.00 ⚕ 0.00 **FUD** XXX

Ⓜ

AMA: 2008,Mar,8-12

4041F Documentation of order for cefazolin OR cefuroxime for antimicrobial prophylaxis (PERI 2)

🚗 0.00 ⚕ 0.00 **FUD** XXX

Ⓔ

4042F Documentation that prophylactic antibiotics were neither given within 4 hours prior to surgical incision nor given intraoperatively (PERI 2)

🚗 0.00 ⚕ 0.00 **FUD** XXX

Ⓔ

4043F Documentation that an order was given to discontinue prophylactic antibiotics within 48 hours of surgical end time, cardiac procedures (PERI 2)

🚗 0.00 ⚕ 0.00 **FUD** XXX

Ⓔ

4044F Documentation that an order was given for venous thromboembolism (VTE) prophylaxis to be given within 24 hours prior to incision time or 24 hours after surgery end time (PERI 2)

🚗 0.00 ⚕ 0.00 **FUD** XXX

Ⓜ

4045F Appropriate empiric antibiotic prescribed (CAP), (EM)

🚗 0.00 ⚕ 0.00 **FUD** XXX

Ⓔ

4046F Documentation that prophylactic antibiotics were given within 4 hours prior to surgical incision or given intraoperatively (PERI 2)

🚗 0.00 ⚕ 0.00 **FUD** XXX

Ⓔ

4047F Documentation of order for prophylactic parenteral antibiotics to be given within 1 hour (if fluoroquinolone or vancomycin, 2 hours) prior to surgical incision (or start of procedure when no incision is required) (PERI 2)

🚗 0.00 ⚕ 0.00 **FUD** XXX

Ⓔ

4048F Documentation that administration of prophylactic parenteral antibiotic was initiated within 1 hour (if fluoroquinolone or vancomycin, 2 hours) prior to surgical incision (or start of procedure when no incision is required) as ordered (PERI 2)

🚗 0.00 ⚕ 0.00 **FUD** XXX

Ⓔ

4049F Documentation that order was given to discontinue prophylactic antibiotics within 24 hours of surgical end time, non-cardiac procedure (PERI 2)

🚗 0.00 ⚕ 0.00 **FUD** XXX

Ⓔ

4050F Hypertension plan of care documented as appropriate (NMA-No Measure Associated)

🚗 0.00 ⚕ 0.00 **FUD** XXX

Ⓔ

4051F Referred for an arteriovenous (AV) fistula (ESRD, CKD)

🚗 0.00 ⚕ 0.00 **FUD** XXX

Ⓔ

AMA: 2008,Mar,8-12

4052F Hemodialysis via functioning arteriovenous (AV) fistula (ESRD)

🚗 0.00 ⚕ 0.00 **FUD** XXX

Ⓔ

AMA: 2008,Mar,8-12

4053F Hemodialysis via functioning arteriovenous (AV) graft (ESRD)

🚗 0.00 ⚕ 0.00 **FUD** XXX

Ⓔ

AMA: 2008,Mar,8-12

4054F Hemodialysis via catheter (ESRD)

🚗 0.00 ⚕ 0.00 **FUD** XXX

Ⓔ

AMA: 2008,Mar,8-12

4055F Patient receiving peritoneal dialysis (ESRD)

🚗 0.00 ⚕ 0.00 **FUD** XXX

Ⓔ

AMA: 2008,Mar,8-12

4056F Appropriate oral rehydration solution recommended (PAG)

🚗 0.00 ⚕ 0.00 **FUD** XXX

Ⓔ

4058F Pediatric gastroenteritis education provided to caregiver (PAG)

🚗 0.00 ⚕ 0.00 **FUD** XXX

Ⓔ

● New Code ▲ Revised Code ○ Reinstated ● New Web Release ▲ Revised Web Release + Add-on Unlisted Not Covered # Resequenced
⑤⓪ Optum Mod 50 Exempt Ⓢ AMA Mod 51 Exempt ⑤⓵ Optum Mod 51 Exempt ⑥③ Mod 63 Exempt ✐ Non-FDA Drug ★ Telemedicine Ⓜ Maternity Ⓐ Age Edit

CPT © 2019 American Medical Association. All Rights Reserved.

4060F Psychotherapy services provided (MDD, MDD ADOL)
0.00   0.00   **FUD** XXX   E

4062F Patient referral for psychotherapy documented (MDD, MDD ADOL)
0.00   0.00   **FUD** XXX   E

4063F Antidepressant pharmacotherapy considered and not prescribed (MDD ADOL)
0.00   0.00   **FUD** XXX   E

4064F Antidepressant pharmacotherapy prescribed (MDD, MDD ADOL)
0.00   0.00   **FUD** XXX   E

4065F Antipsychotic pharmacotherapy prescribed (MDD)
0.00   0.00   **FUD** XXX   E

4066F Electroconvulsive therapy (ECT) provided (MDD)
0.00   0.00   **FUD** XXX   E

4067F Patient referral for electroconvulsive therapy (ECT) documented (MDD)
0.00   0.00   **FUD** XXX   E

4069F Venous thromboembolism (VTE) prophylaxis received (IBD)
0.00   0.00   **FUD** XXX   E

4070F Deep vein thrombosis (DVT) prophylaxis received by end of hospital day 2 (STR)
0.00   0.00   **FUD** XXX   E

4073F Oral antiplatelet therapy prescribed at discharge (STR)
0.00   0.00   **FUD** XXX   E

4075F Anticoagulant therapy prescribed at discharge (STR)
0.00   0.00   **FUD** XXX   E

4077F Documentation that tissue plasminogen activator (t-PA) administration was considered (STR)
0.00   0.00   **FUD** XXX   E

4079F Documentation that rehabilitation services were considered (STR)
0.00   0.00   **FUD** XXX   E

4084F Aspirin received within 24 hours before emergency department arrival or during emergency department stay (EM)
0.00   0.00   **FUD** XXX   E

4086F Aspirin or clopidogrel prescribed or currently being taken (CAD)
0.00   0.00   **FUD** XXX   M

4090F Patient receiving erythropoietin therapy (HEM)
0.00   0.00   **FUD** XXX   M
AMA: 2008,Mar,8-12

4095F Patient not receiving erythropoietin therapy (HEM)
0.00   0.00   **FUD** XXX   E
AMA: 2008,Mar,8-12

4100F Bisphosphonate therapy, intravenous, ordered or received (HEM)
0.00   0.00   **FUD** XXX   M
AMA: 2008,Mar,8-12

4110F Internal mammary artery graft performed for primary, isolated coronary artery bypass graft procedure (CABG)
0.00   0.00   **FUD** XXX   M

4115F Beta blocker administered within 24 hours prior to surgical incision (CABG)
0.00   0.00   **FUD** XXX   M

4120F Antibiotic prescribed or dispensed (URI, PHAR), (A-BRONCH)
0.00   0.00   **FUD** XXX   M
AMA: 2008,Mar,8-12

4124F Antibiotic neither prescribed nor dispensed (URI, PHAR), (A-BRONCH)
0.00   0.00   **FUD** XXX   M
AMA: 2008,Mar,8-12

4130F Topical preparations (including OTC) prescribed for acute otitis externa (AOE)
0.00   0.00   **FUD** XXX   M
AMA: 2010,Jan,6-7; 2008,Mar,8-12

4131F Systemic antimicrobial therapy prescribed (AOE)
0.00   0.00   **FUD** XXX   M
AMA: 2008,Mar,8-12

4132F Systemic antimicrobial therapy not prescribed (AOE)
0.00   0.00   **FUD** XXX   M
AMA: 2008,Mar,8-12

4133F Antihistamines or decongestants prescribed or recommended (OME)
0.00   0.00   **FUD** XXX   E
AMA: 2008,Mar,8-12

4134F Antihistamines or decongestants neither prescribed nor recommended (OME)
0.00   0.00   **FUD** XXX   E
AMA: 2008,Mar,8-12

4135F Systemic corticosteroids prescribed (OME)
0.00   0.00   **FUD** XXX   E
AMA: 2008,Mar,8-12

4136F Systemic corticosteroids not prescribed (OME)
0.00   0.00   **FUD** XXX   E
AMA: 2008,Mar,8-12

4140F Inhaled corticosteroids prescribed (Asthma)
0.00   0.00   **FUD** XXX   E

4142F Corticosteroid sparing therapy prescribed (IBD)
0.00   0.00   **FUD** XXX   E

4144F Alternative long-term control medication prescribed (Asthma)
0.00   0.00   **FUD** XXX   E

4145F Two or more anti-hypertensive agents prescribed or currently being taken (CAD, HTN)
0.00   0.00   **FUD** XXX   E

4148F Hepatitis A vaccine injection administered or previously received (HEP-C)
0.00   0.00   **FUD** XXX   E

4149F Hepatitis B vaccine injection administered or previously received (HEP-C, HIV) (IBD)
0.00   0.00   **FUD** XXX   E

4150F Patient receiving antiviral treatment for Hepatitis C (HEP-C)
0.00   0.00   **FUD** XXX   E
AMA: 2008,Mar,8-12

4151F Patient did not start or is not receiving antiviral treatment for Hepatitis C during the measurement period (HEP-C)
0.00   0.00   **FUD** XXX   E
AMA: 2008,Mar,8-12

4153F Combination peginterferon and ribavirin therapy prescribed (HEP-C)
0.00   0.00   **FUD** XXX   E
AMA: 2008,Mar,8-12

4155F Hepatitis A vaccine series previously received (HEP-C)
0.00   0.00   **FUD** XXX   E
AMA: 2008,Mar,8-12

4157F Hepatitis B vaccine series previously received (HEP-C)
0.00   0.00   **FUD** XXX   E
AMA: 2008,Mar,8-12

26/10 PC/TC Only   A2-Z3 ASC Payment   50 Bilateral   ♂ Male Only   ♀ Female Only   Facility RVU   Non-Facility RVU   CCI   CLIA
FUD Follow-up Days   **CMS:** IOM   **AMA:** CPT Asst   A-Y OPPSI   80/80 Surg Assist Allowed / w/Doc   Lab Crosswalk   Radiology Crosswalk

CPT © 2019 American Medical Association. All Rights Reserved.
© 2019 Optum360, LLC

574

4158F Patient counseled about risks of alcohol use (HEP-C)
🚗 0.00　🔌 0.00　**FUD** XXX　　　E
AMA: 2008,Mar,8-12

4159F Counseling regarding contraception received prior to initiation of antiviral treatment (HEP-C)
🚗 0.00　🔌 0.00　**FUD** XXX　　　E
AMA: 2008,Mar,8-12

4163F Patient counseling at a minimum on all of the following treatment options for clinically localized prostate cancer: active surveillance, and interstitial prostate brachytherapy, and external beam radiotherapy, and radical prostatectomy, provided prior to initiation of treatment (PRCA)
🚗 0.00　🔌 0.00　**FUD** XXX　　　E
AMA: 2008,Mar,8-12

4164F Adjuvant (ie, in combination with external beam radiotherapy to the prostate for prostate cancer) hormonal therapy (gonadotropin-releasing hormone [GnRH] agonist or antagonist) prescribed/administered (PRCA)
🚗 0.00　🔌 0.00　**FUD** XXX　　　E
AMA: 2008,Mar,8-12

4165F 3-dimensional conformal radiotherapy (3D-CRT) or intensity modulated radiation therapy (IMRT) received (PRCA)
🚗 0.00　🔌 0.00　**FUD** XXX　　　E
AMA: 2008,Mar,8-12

4167F Head of bed elevation (30-45 degrees) on first ventilator day ordered (CRIT)
🚗 0.00　🔌 0.00　**FUD** XXX　　　E
AMA: 2008,Mar,8-12

4168F Patient receiving care in the intensive care unit (ICU) and receiving mechanical ventilation, 24 hours or less (CRIT)
🚗 0.00　🔌 0.00　**FUD** XXX　　　E
AMA: 2008,Mar,8-12

4169F Patient either not receiving care in the intensive care unit (ICU) OR not receiving mechanical ventilation OR receiving mechanical ventilation greater than 24 hours (CRIT)
🚗 0.00　🔌 0.00　**FUD** XXX　　　E
AMA: 2008,Mar,8-12

4171F Patient receiving erythropoiesis-stimulating agents (ESA) therapy (CKD)
🚗 0.00　🔌 0.00　**FUD** XXX　　　E
AMA: 2008,Mar,8-12

4172F Patient not receiving erythropoiesis-stimulating agents (ESA) therapy (CKD)
🚗 0.00　🔌 0.00　**FUD** XXX　　　E
AMA: 2008,Mar,8-12

4174F Counseling about the potential impact of glaucoma on visual functioning and quality of life, and importance of treatment adherence provided to patient and/or caregiver(s) (EC)
🚗 0.00　🔌 0.00　**FUD** XXX　　　E
AMA: 2008,Mar,8-12

4175F Best-corrected visual acuity of 20/40 or better (distance or near) achieved within the 90 days following cataract surgery (EC)
🚗 0.00　🔌 0.00　**FUD** XXX　　　M
AMA: 2008,Mar,8-12

4176F Counseling about value of protection from UV light and lack of proven efficacy of nutritional supplements in prevention or progression of cataract development provided to patient and/or caregiver(s) (NMA-No Measure Associated)
🚗 0.00　🔌 0.00　**FUD** XXX　　　E

4177F Counseling about the benefits and/or risks of the Age-Related Eye Disease Study (AREDS) formulation for preventing progression of age-related macular degeneration (AMD) provided to patient and/or caregiver(s) (EC)
🚗 0.00　🔌 0.00　**FUD** XXX　　　M
AMA: 2008,Mar,8-12

4178F Anti-D immune globulin received between 26 and 30 weeks gestation (Pre-Cr)　　　M
🚗 0.00　🔌 0.00　**FUD** XXX　　　E
AMA: 2008,Mar,8-12

4179F Tamoxifen or aromatase inhibitor (AI) prescribed (ONC)
🚗 0.00　🔌 0.00　**FUD** XXX　　　E
AMA: 2008,Mar,8-12

4180F Adjuvant chemotherapy referred, prescribed, or previously received for Stage III colon cancer (ONC)
🚗 0.00　🔌 0.00　**FUD** XXX　　　E
AMA: 2008,Mar,8-12

4181F Conformal radiation therapy received (NMA-No Measure Associated)
🚗 0.00　🔌 0.00　**FUD** XXX　　　E

4182F Conformal radiation therapy not received (NMA-No Measure Associated)
🚗 0.00　🔌 0.00　**FUD** XXX　　　E

4185F Continuous (12-months) therapy with proton pump inhibitor (PPI) or histamine H2 receptor antagonist (H2RA) received (GERD)
🚗 0.00　🔌 0.00　**FUD** XXX　　　E

4186F No continuous (12-months) therapy with either proton pump inhibitor (PPI) or histamine H2 receptor antagonist (H2RA) received (GERD)
🚗 0.00　🔌 0.00　**FUD** XXX　　　E

4187F Disease modifying anti-rheumatic drug therapy prescribed or dispensed (RA)
🚗 0.00　🔌 0.00　**FUD** XXX　　　E

4188F Appropriate angiotensin converting enzyme (ACE)/angiotensin receptor blockers (ARB) therapeutic monitoring test ordered or performed (AM)
🚗 0.00　🔌 0.00　**FUD** XXX　　　E

4189F Appropriate digoxin therapeutic monitoring test ordered or performed (AM)
🚗 0.00　🔌 0.00　**FUD** XXX　　　E
AMA: 2008,Mar,8-12

4190F Appropriate diuretic therapeutic monitoring test ordered or performed (AM)
🚗 0.00　🔌 0.00　**FUD** XXX　　　E
AMA: 2008,Mar,8-12

4191F Appropriate anticonvulsant therapeutic monitoring test ordered or performed (AM)
🚗 0.00　🔌 0.00　**FUD** XXX　　　E
AMA: 2008,Mar,8-12

4192F Patient not receiving glucocorticoid therapy (RA)
🚗 0.00　🔌 0.00　**FUD** XXX　　　M

4193F Patient receiving <10 mg daily prednisone (or equivalent), or RA activity is worsening, or glucocorticoid use is for less than 6 months (RA)
🚗 0.00　🔌 0.00　**FUD** XXX　　　M

4194F Patient receiving ≥10 mg daily prednisone (or equivalent) for longer than 6 months, and improvement or no change in disease activity (RA)
🚗 0.00　🔌 0.00　**FUD** XXX　　　M

4195F Patient receiving first-time biologic disease modifying anti-rheumatic drug therapy for rheumatoid arthritis (RA)
🚗 0.00　🔌 0.00　**FUD** XXX　　　M

4196F Patient not receiving first-time biologic disease modifying anti-rheumatic drug therapy for rheumatoid arthritis (RA)
🚗 0.00　🔌 0.00　**FUD** XXX　　　M

4200F External beam radiotherapy as primary therapy to prostate with or without nodal irradiation (PRCA)
    🚑 0.00   ⚖ 0.00   **FUD** XXX   E
    AMA: 2008,Mar,8-12

4201F External beam radiotherapy with or without nodal irradiation as adjuvant or salvage therapy for prostate cancer patient (PRCA)
    🚑 0.00   ⚖ 0.00   **FUD** XXX   E
    AMA: 2008,Mar,8-12

4210F Angiotensin converting enzyme (ACE) or angiotensin receptor blockers (ARB) medication therapy for 6 months or more (MM)
    🚑 0.00   ⚖ 0.00   **FUD** XXX   E
    AMA: 2008,Mar,8-12

4220F Digoxin medication therapy for 6 months or more (MM)
    🚑 0.00   ⚖ 0.00   **FUD** XXX   E
    AMA: 2008,Mar,8-12

4221F Diuretic medication therapy for 6 months or more (MM)
    🚑 0.00   ⚖ 0.00   **FUD** XXX   E
    AMA: 2008,Mar,8-12

4230F Anticonvulsant medication therapy for 6 months or more (MM)
    🚑 0.00   ⚖ 0.00   **FUD** XXX   E
    AMA: 2008,Mar,8-12

4240F Instruction in therapeutic exercise with follow-up provided to patients during episode of back pain lasting longer than 12 weeks (BkP)
    🚑 0.00   ⚖ 0.00   **FUD** XXX   E
    AMA: 2008,Mar,8-12

4242F Counseling for supervised exercise program provided to patients during episode of back pain lasting longer than 12 weeks (BkP)
    🚑 0.00   ⚖ 0.00   **FUD** XXX   E
    AMA: 2008,Mar,8-12

4245F Patient counseled during the initial visit to maintain or resume normal activities (BkP)
    🚑 0.00   ⚖ 0.00   **FUD** XXX   E
    AMA: 2008,Mar,8-12

4248F Patient counseled during the initial visit for an episode of back pain against bed rest lasting 4 days or longer (BkP)
    🚑 0.00   ⚖ 0.00   **FUD** XXX   E
    AMA: 2008,Mar,8-12

4250F Active warming used intraoperatively for the purpose of maintaining normothermia, or at least 1 body temperature equal to or greater than 36 degrees Centigrade (or 96.8 degrees Fahrenheit) recorded within the 30 minutes immediately before or the 15 minutes immediately after anesthesia end time (CRIT)
    🚑 0.00   ⚖ 0.00   **FUD** XXX   E
    AMA: 2008,Mar,8-12

4255F Duration of general or neuraxial anesthesia 60 minutes or longer, as documented in the anesthesia record (CRIT) (Peri2)
    🚑 0.00   ⚖ 0.00   **FUD** XXX   M

4256F Duration of general or neuraxial anesthesia less than 60 minutes, as documented in the anesthesia record (CRIT) (Peri2)
    🚑 0.00   ⚖ 0.00   **FUD** XXX   E

4260F Wound surface culture technique used (CWC)
    🚑 0.00   ⚖ 0.00   **FUD** XXX   E

4261F Technique other than surface culture of the wound exudate used (eg, Levine/deep swab technique, semi-quantitative or quantitative swab technique) or wound surface culture technique not used (CWC)
    🚑 0.00   ⚖ 0.00   **FUD** XXX   E

4265F Use of wet to dry dressings prescribed or recommended (CWC)
    🚑 0.00   ⚖ 0.00   **FUD** XXX   E

4266F Use of wet to dry dressings neither prescribed nor recommended (CWC)
    🚑 0.00   ⚖ 0.00   **FUD** XXX   E

4267F Compression therapy prescribed (CWC)
    🚑 0.00   ⚖ 0.00   **FUD** XXX   E

4268F Patient education regarding the need for long term compression therapy including interval replacement of compression stockings received (CWC)
    🚑 0.00   ⚖ 0.00   **FUD** XXX   E

4269F Appropriate method of offloading (pressure relief) prescribed (CWC)
    🚑 0.00   ⚖ 0.00   **FUD** XXX   E

4270F Patient receiving potent antiretroviral therapy for 6 months or longer (HIV)
    🚑 0.00   ⚖ 0.00   **FUD** XXX   E

4271F Patient receiving potent antiretroviral therapy for less than 6 months or not receiving potent antiretroviral therapy (HIV)
    🚑 0.00   ⚖ 0.00   **FUD** XXX   E

4274F Influenza immunization administered or previously received (HIV) (P-ESRD)
    🚑 0.00   ⚖ 0.00   **FUD** XXX   E

4276F Potent antiretroviral therapy prescribed (HIV)
    🚑 0.00   ⚖ 0.00   **FUD** XXX   E

4279F Pneumocystis jiroveci pneumonia prophylaxis prescribed (HIV)
    🚑 0.00   ⚖ 0.00   **FUD** XXX   E

4280F Pneumocystis jiroveci pneumonia prophylaxis prescribed within 3 months of low CD4+ cell count or percentage (HIV)
    🚑 0.00   ⚖ 0.00   **FUD** XXX   E

4290F Patient screened for injection drug use (HIV)
    🚑 0.00   ⚖ 0.00   **FUD** XXX   E

4293F Patient screened for high-risk sexual behavior (HIV)
    🚑 0.00   ⚖ 0.00   **FUD** XXX   E

4300F Patient receiving warfarin therapy for nonvalvular atrial fibrillation or atrial flutter (AFIB)
    🚑 0.00   ⚖ 0.00   **FUD** XXX   E

4301F Patient not receiving warfarin therapy for nonvalvular atrial fibrillation or atrial flutter (AFIB)
    🚑 0.00   ⚖ 0.00   **FUD** XXX   E

4305F Patient education regarding appropriate foot care and daily inspection of the feet received (CWC)
    🚑 0.00   ⚖ 0.00   **FUD** XXX   E

4306F Patient counseled regarding psychosocial and pharmacologic treatment options for opioid addiction (SUD)
    🚑 0.00   ⚖ 0.00   **FUD** XXX   E

4320F Patient counseled regarding psychosocial and pharmacologic treatment options for alcohol dependence (SUD)
    🚑 0.00   ⚖ 0.00   **FUD** XXX   E

4322F Caregiver provided with education and referred to additional resources for support (DEM)
    🚑 0.00   ⚖ 0.00   **FUD** XXX   M

4324F Patient (or caregiver) queried about Parkinson's disease medication related motor complications (Prkns)
    🚑 0.00   ⚖ 0.00   **FUD** XXX   E

4325F Medical and surgical treatment options reviewed with patient (or caregiver) (Prkns)
    🚑 0.00   ⚖ 0.00   **FUD** XXX   M

4326F Patient (or caregiver) queried about symptoms of autonomic dysfunction (Prkns)
🚑 0.00   ⚕ 0.00   **FUD** XXX   E

4328F Patient (or caregiver) queried about sleep disturbances (Prkns)
🚑 0.00   ⚕ 0.00   **FUD** XXX   E

4330F Counseling about epilepsy specific safety issues provided to patient (or caregiver(s)) (EPI)
🚑 0.00   ⚕ 0.00   **FUD** XXX   E

4340F Counseling for women of childbearing potential with epilepsy (EPI)
🚑 0.00   ⚕ 0.00   **FUD** XXX   M

4350F Counseling provided on symptom management, end of life decisions, and palliation (DEM)
🚑 0.00   ⚕ 0.00   **FUD** XXX   E

4400F Rehabilitative therapy options discussed with patient (or caregiver) (Prkns)
🚑 0.00   ⚕ 0.00   **FUD** XXX   M

4450F Self-care education provided to patient (HF)
🚑 0.00   ⚕ 0.00   **FUD** XXX   E

4470F Implantable cardioverter-defibrillator (ICD) counseling provided (HF)
🚑 0.00   ⚕ 0.00   **FUD** XXX   E

4480F Patient receiving ACE inhibitor/ARB therapy and beta-blocker therapy for 3 months or longer (HF)
🚑 0.00   ⚕ 0.00   **FUD** XXX   E

4481F Patient receiving ACE inhibitor/ARB therapy and beta-blocker therapy for less than 3 months or patient not receiving ACE inhibitor/ARB therapy and beta-blocker therapy (HF)
🚑 0.00   ⚕ 0.00   **FUD** XXX   E

4500F Referred to an outpatient cardiac rehabilitation program (CAD)
🚑 0.00   ⚕ 0.00   **FUD** XXX   M

4510F Previous cardiac rehabilitation for qualifying cardiac event completed (CAD)
🚑 0.00   ⚕ 0.00   **FUD** XXX   M

4525F Neuropsychiatric intervention ordered (DEM)
🚑 0.00   ⚕ 0.00   **FUD** XXX   E

4526F Neuropsychiatric intervention received (DEM)
🚑 0.00   ⚕ 0.00   **FUD** XXX   E

4540F Disease modifying pharmacotherapy discussed (ALS)
🚑 0.00   ⚕ 0.00   **FUD** XXX   E

4541F Patient offered treatment for pseudobulbar affect, sialorrhea, or ALS-related symptoms (ALS)
🚑 0.00   ⚕ 0.00   **FUD** XXX   E

4550F Options for noninvasive respiratory support discussed with patient (ALS)
🚑 0.00   ⚕ 0.00   **FUD** XXX   E

4551F Nutritional support offered (ALS)
🚑 0.00   ⚕ 0.00   **FUD** XXX   E

4552F Patient offered referral to a speech language pathologist (ALS)
🚑 0.00   ⚕ 0.00   **FUD** XXX   E

4553F Patient offered assistance in planning for end of life issues (ALS)
🚑 0.00   ⚕ 0.00   **FUD** XXX   E

4554F Patient received inhalational anesthetic agent (Peri2)
🚑 0.00   ⚕ 0.00   **FUD** XXX   M

4555F Patient did not receive inhalational anesthetic agent (Peri2)
🚑 0.00   ⚕ 0.00   **FUD** XXX   E

4556F Patient exhibits 3 or more risk factors for post-operative nausea and vomiting (Peri2)
🚑 0.00   ⚕ 0.00   **FUD** XXX   M

4557F Patient does not exhibit 3 or more risk factors for post-operative nausea and vomiting (Peri2)
🚑 0.00   ⚕ 0.00   **FUD** XXX   E

4558F Patient received at least 2 prophylactic pharmacologic anti-emetic agents of different classes preoperatively and intraoperatively (Peri2)
🚑 0.00   ⚕ 0.00   **FUD** XXX   E

4559F At least 1 body temperature measurement equal to or greater than 35.5 degrees Celsius (or 95.9 degrees Fahrenheit) recorded within the 30 minutes immediately before or the 15 minutes immediately after anesthesia end time (Peri2)
🚑 0.00   ⚕ 0.00   **FUD** XXX   E

4560F Anesthesia technique did not involve general or neuraxial anesthesia (Peri2)
🚑 0.00   ⚕ 0.00   **FUD** XXX   E

4561F Patient has a coronary artery stent (Peri2)
🚑 0.00   ⚕ 0.00   **FUD** XXX   E

4562F Patient does not have a coronary artery stent (Peri2)
🚑 0.00   ⚕ 0.00   **FUD** XXX   E

4563F Patient received aspirin within 24 hours prior to anesthesia start time (Peri2)
🚑 0.00   ⚕ 0.00   **FUD** XXX   E

5005F-5250F Results Conveyed and Documented

INCLUDES   Patient's:
Functional status
Morbidity/mortality
Satisfaction/experience with care
Review/communication of test results to patients

5005F Patient counseled on self-examination for new or changing moles (ML)
🚑 0.00   ⚕ 0.00   **FUD** XXX   E
AMA: 2008,Mar,8-12

5010F Findings of dilated macular or fundus exam communicated to the physician or other qualified health care professional managing the diabetes care (EC)
🚑 0.00   ⚕ 0.00   **FUD** XXX   M

5015F Documentation of communication that a fracture occurred and that the patient was or should be tested or treated for osteoporosis (OP)
🚑 0.00   ⚕ 0.00   **FUD** XXX   M

5020F Treatment summary report communicated to physician(s) or other qualified health care professional(s) managing continuing care and to the patient within 1 month of completing treatment (ONC)
🚑 0.00   ⚕ 0.00   **FUD** XXX   E
AMA: 2008,Mar,8-12

5050F Treatment plan communicated to provider(s) managing continuing care within 1 month of diagnosis (ML)
🚑 0.00   ⚕ 0.00   **FUD** XXX   M
AMA: 2008,Mar,8-12

5060F Findings from diagnostic mammogram communicated to practice managing patient's on-going care within 3 business days of exam interpretation (RAD)
🚑 0.00   ⚕ 0.00   **FUD** XXX   E
AMA: 2008,Mar,8-12

5062F Findings from diagnostic mammogram communicated to the patient within 5 days of exam interpretation (RAD)
🚑 0.00   ⚕ 0.00   **FUD** XXX   E
AMA: 2008,Mar,8-12

5100F — 9007F
Category II Codes

5100F Potential risk for fracture communicated to the referring physician or other qualified health care professional within 24 hours of completion of the imaging study (NUC_MED)
📁 0.00   ⚕ 0.00   **FUD** XXX   E

5200F Consideration of referral for a neurological evaluation of appropriateness for surgical therapy for intractable epilepsy within the past 3 years (EPI)
📁 0.00   ⚕ 0.00   **FUD** XXX   E

5250F Asthma discharge plan provided to patient (Asthma)
📁 0.00   ⚕ 0.00   **FUD** XXX   E

6005F-6150F Elements Related to Patient Safety Processes

INCLUDES   Patient safety practices

6005F Rationale (eg, severity of illness and safety) for level of care (eg, home, hospital) documented (CAP)
📁 0.00   ⚕ 0.00   **FUD** XXX   E
AMA: 2018,Jan,8; 2017,Jan,8; 2016,Jan,13; 2015,Jan,16; 2014,Jan,11

6010F Dysphagia screening conducted prior to order for or receipt of any foods, fluids, or medication by mouth (STR)
📁 0.00   ⚕ 0.00   **FUD** XXX   E

6015F Patient receiving or eligible to receive foods, fluids, or medication by mouth (STR)
📁 0.00   ⚕ 0.00   **FUD** XXX   E

6020F NPO (nothing by mouth) ordered (STR)
📁 0.00   ⚕ 0.00   **FUD** XXX   E

6030F All elements of maximal sterile barrier technique, hand hygiene, skin preparation and, if ultrasound is used, sterile ultrasound techniques followed (CRIT)
📁 0.00   ⚕ 0.00   **FUD** XXX   M
AMA: 2008,Mar,8-12

6040F Use of appropriate radiation dose reduction devices OR manual techniques for appropriate moderation of exposure, documented (RAD)
📁 0.00   ⚕ 0.00   **FUD** XXX   E

6045F Radiation exposure or exposure time in final report for procedure using fluoroscopy, documented (RAD)
📁 0.00   ⚕ 0.00   **FUD** XXX   E
AMA: 2008,Mar,8-12

6070F Patient queried and counseled about anti-epileptic drug (AED) side effects (EPI)
📁 0.00   ⚕ 0.00   **FUD** XXX   E

6080F Patient (or caregiver) queried about falls (Prkns, DSP)
📁 0.00   ⚕ 0.00   **FUD** XXX   E

6090F Patient (or caregiver) counseled about safety issues appropriate to patient's stage of disease (Prkns)
📁 0.00   ⚕ 0.00   **FUD** XXX   E

6100F Timeout to verify correct patient, correct site, and correct procedure, documented (PATH)
📁 0.00   ⚕ 0.00   **FUD** XXX   E

6101F Safety counseling for dementia provided (DEM)
📁 0.00   ⚕ 0.00   **FUD** XXX   E

6102F Safety counseling for dementia ordered (DEM)
📁 0.00   ⚕ 0.00   **FUD** XXX   E

6110F Counseling provided regarding risks of driving and the alternatives to driving (DEM)
📁 0.00   ⚕ 0.00   **FUD** XXX   E

6150F Patient not receiving a first course of anti-TNF (tumor necrosis factor) therapy (IBD)
📁 0.00   ⚕ 0.00   **FUD** XXX   E

7010F-7025F Recall/Reminder System in Place

INCLUDES   Capabilities of the provider
Measures that address the setting or system of care provided

7010F Patient information entered into a recall system that includes: target date for the next exam specified and a process to follow up with patients regarding missed or unscheduled appointments (ML)
📁 0.00   ⚕ 0.00   **FUD** XXX   M
AMA: 2008,Mar,8-12

7020F Mammogram assessment category (eg, Mammography Quality Standards Act [MQSA], Breast Imaging Reporting and Data System [BI-RADS], or FDA approved equivalent categories) entered into an internal database to allow for analysis of abnormal interpretation (recall) rate (RAD)
📁 0.00   ⚕ 0.00   **FUD** XXX   E
AMA: 2008,Mar,8-12

7025F Patient information entered into a reminder system with a target due date for the next mammogram (RAD)
📁 0.00   ⚕ 0.00   **FUD** XXX   M
AMA: 2008,Mar,8-12

9001F-9007F No Measure Associated

INCLUDES   Aspects of care not associated with measures at the current time

9001F Aortic aneurysm less than 5.0 cm maximum diameter on centerline formatted CT or minor diameter on axial formatted CT (NMA-No Measure Associated)
📁 0.00   ⚕ 0.00   **FUD** XXX   E

9002F Aortic aneurysm 5.0 - 5.4 cm maximum diameter on centerline formatted CT or minor diameter on axial formatted CT (NMA-No Measure Associated)
📁 0.00   ⚕ 0.00   **FUD** XXX   E

9003F Aortic aneurysm 5.5 - 5.9 cm maximum diameter on centerline formatted CT or minor diameter on axial formatted CT (NMA-No Measure Associated)
📁 0.00   ⚕ 0.00   **FUD** XXX   M

9004F Aortic aneurysm 6.0 cm or greater maximum diameter on centerline formatted CT or minor diameter on axial formatted CT (NMA-No Measure Associated)
📁 0.00   ⚕ 0.00   **FUD** XXX   M

9005F Asymptomatic carotid stenosis: No history of any transient ischemic attack or stroke in any carotid or vertebrobasilar territory (NMA-No Measure Associated)
📁 0.00   ⚕ 0.00   **FUD** XXX   E

9006F Symptomatic carotid stenosis: Ipsilateral carotid territory TIA or stroke less than 120 days prior to procedure (NMA-No Measure Associated)
📁 0.00   ⚕ 0.00   **FUD** XXX   M

9007F Other carotid stenosis: Ipsilateral TIA or stroke 120 days or greater prior to procedure or any prior contralateral carotid territory or vertebrobasilar TIA or stroke (NMA-No Measure Associated)
📁 0.00   ⚕ 0.00   **FUD** XXX   M

0042T

0042T Cerebral perfusion analysis using computed tomography with contrast administration, including post-processing of parametric maps with determination of cerebral blood flow, cerebral blood volume, and mean transit time

0.00 0.00 **FUD** XXX N 80

AMA: 2003,Nov,5

0054T-0055T

+ **0054T** Computer-assisted musculoskeletal surgical navigational orthopedic procedure, with image-guidance based on fluoroscopic images (List separately in addition to code for primary procedure)

Code first primary procedure

0.00 0.00 **FUD** XXX N 80

AMA: 2018,Jan,8; 2017,Jan,8; 2016,Jan,13; 2015,Jan,16; 2014,Jan,11

+ **0055T** Computer-assisted musculoskeletal surgical navigational orthopedic procedure, with image-guidance based on CT/MRI images (List separately in addition to code for primary procedure)

INCLUDES Performance of both CT and MRI in same session (1 unit)

Code first primary procedure

0.00 0.00 **FUD** XXX N 80

AMA: 2018,Jan,8; 2017,Jan,8; 2016,Jan,13; 2015,Jan,16; 2014,Jan,11

0058T

EXCLUDES Cryopreservation of:
Embryos (89258)
Oocyte(s), immature (89398)
Oocyte(s), mature (89337)
Sperm (89259)
Testicular reproductive tissue (89335)

0058T Cryopreservation; reproductive tissue, ovarian

0.00 0.00 **FUD** XXX Q1 80

AMA: 2004,Apr,1; 2004,Jun,7

0071T-0072T

EXCLUDES Insertion bladder catheter (51702)
MRI guidance for parenchymal tissue ablation (77022)

0071T Focused ultrasound ablation of uterine leiomyomata, including MR guidance; total leiomyomata volume less than 200 cc of tissue ♀

0.00 0.00 **FUD** XXX J 80

AMA: 2005,Mar,1-6; 2005,Dec,3-6

0072T total leiomyomata volume greater or equal to 200 cc of tissue ♀

0.00 0.00 **FUD** XXX J 80

AMA: 2005,Mar,1-6; 2005,Dec,3-6

0075T-0076T

INCLUDES All diagnostic services for stenting
Ipsilateral extracranial vertebral selective catheterization when confirming the need for stenting

EXCLUDES Selective catheterization and imaging when stenting is not required (report only selective catheterization codes)

0075T Transcatheter placement of extracranial vertebral artery stent(s), including radiologic supervision and interpretation, open or percutaneous; initial vessel

0.00 0.00 **FUD** XXX C 80

AMA: 2018,Jan,8; 2017,Jan,8; 2016,Jan,13; 2015,Jan,16; 2014,Mar,8

+ **0076T** each additional vessel (List separately in addition to code for primary procedure)

Code first (0075T)

0.00 0.00 **FUD** XXX C 80

AMA: 2018,Jan,8; 2017,Jan,8; 2016,Jan,13; 2015,Jan,16; 2014,Mar,8

0085T

0085T Breath test for heart transplant rejection

0.00 0.00 **FUD** XXX E

AMA: 2005,May,7-12

0095T-0098T

INCLUDES Fluoroscopy

+ **0095T** Removal of total disc arthroplasty (artificial disc), anterior approach, each additional interspace, cervical (List separately in addition to code for primary procedure)

EXCLUDES Lumbar disc (0164T)
Revision of total disc arthroplasty, cervical (22861)
Revision of total disc arthroplasty, lumbar (22862)

Code first (22864)

0.00 0.00 **FUD** XXX C 80

AMA: 2006,Feb,1-6; 2005,Jun,6-8

+ **0098T** Revision including replacement of total disc arthroplasty (artificial disc), anterior approach, each additional interspace, cervical (List separately in addition to code for primary procedure)

EXCLUDES Application of intervertebral biomechanical device(s) at the same level (22853-22854, [22859])
Removal of total disc arthroplasty (0095T)
Spinal cord decompression (63001-63048)

Code first (22861)

0.00 0.00 **FUD** XXX C 80

AMA: 2006,Feb,1-6; 2005,Jun,6-8

0100T

0100T Placement of a subconjunctival retinal prosthesis receiver and pulse generator, and implantation of intra-ocular retinal electrode array, with vitrectomy

EXCLUDES Evaluation and initial programming of implantable retinal electrode array device (0472T)

0.00 0.00 **FUD** XXX T J8 80

AMA: 2018,Feb,3; 2018,Jan,8; 2017,Jan,8; 2016,Jan,13; 2015,Jan,16; 2014,Jan,11

0101T-0513T [0512T, 0513T]

0101T Extracorporeal shock wave involving musculoskeletal system, not otherwise specified, high energy

EXCLUDES Extracorporeal shock wave therapy of the integumentary system not otherwise specified ([0512T, 0513T])

0.00 0.00 **FUD** XXX J G2 80

AMA: 2018,Dec,5; 2018,Dec,5; 2018,Jan,8; 2017,Jan,8; 2016,Jan,13; 2015,Jan,16; 2014,Jan,11

0102T Extracorporeal shock wave, high energy, performed by a physician, requiring anesthesia other than local, involving lateral humeral epicondyle

0.00 0.00 **FUD** XXX J G2 80

AMA: 2019,Jun,11; 2018,Dec,5; 2018,Dec,5; 2018,Jan,8; 2017,Jan,8; 2016,Jan,13; 2015,Jan,16; 2014,Jan,11

0512T Extracorporeal shock wave for integumentary wound healing, high energy, including topical application and dressing care; initial wound

0.00 0.00 **FUD** YYY R2 80

AMA: 2018,Dec,5; 2018,Dec,5

+ # **0513T** each additional wound (List separately in addition to code for primary procedure)

Code first ([0512T])

0.00 0.00 **FUD** ZZZ N1 80

AMA: 2018,Dec,5; 2018,Dec,5

0106T-0110T

0106T Quantitative sensory testing (QST), testing and interpretation per extremity; using touch pressure stimuli to assess large diameter sensation

0.00 0.00 **FUD** XXX Q1 80

AMA: 2018,Jan,8; 2017,Jan,8; 2016,Jan,13; 2015,Jan,16; 2014,Jan,11

0107T using vibration stimuli to assess large diameter fiber sensation
🔢 0.00 ⚕ 0.00 **FUD** XXX [01] [80] [▭]
AMA: 2018,Jan,8; 2017,Jan,8; 2016,Jan,13; 2015,Jan,16; 2014,Jan,11

0108T using cooling stimuli to assess small nerve fiber sensation and hyperalgesia
🔢 0.00 ⚕ 0.00 **FUD** XXX [01] [80] [▭]
AMA: 2018,Jan,8; 2017,Jan,8; 2016,Jan,13; 2015,Jan,16; 2014,Jan,11

0109T using heat-pain stimuli to assess small nerve fiber sensation and hyperalgesia
🔢 0.00 ⚕ 0.00 **FUD** XXX [01] [80] [▭]
AMA: 2018,Jan,8; 2017,Jan,8; 2016,Jan,13; 2015,Jan,16; 2014,Jan,11

0110T using other stimuli to assess sensation
🔢 0.00 ⚕ 0.00 **FUD** XXX [01] [80] [▭]
AMA: 2018,Jan,8; 2017,Jan,8; 2016,Jan,13; 2015,Jan,16; 2014,Jan,11

0111T-0126T

0111T Long-chain (C20-22) omega-3 fatty acids in red blood cell (RBC) membranes
EXCLUDES Very long chain fatty acids (82726)
🔢 0.00 ⚕ 0.00 **FUD** XXX [A] [▭]
AMA: 2018,Jan,8; 2017,Jan,8; 2016,Jan,13; 2015,Jan,16; 2014,Jan,11

0126T Common carotid intima-media thickness (IMT) study for evaluation of atherosclerotic burden or coronary heart disease risk factor assessment
EXCLUDES Duplex scan extracranial arteries (93880-93882)
Evaluation carotid intima media and atheroma (93895)
🔢 0.00 ⚕ 0.00 **FUD** XXX [01] [80] [▭]
AMA: 2018,Jan,8; 2017,Jan,8; 2016,Jan,13; 2015,Jan,16; 2014,Jan,11

0163T-0165T

CMS: 100-03,150.10 Lumbar Artificial Disc Replacement (LADR)
INCLUDES Fluoroscopy
EXCLUDES Application of intervertebral biomechanical device(s) at the same level (22853-22854, [22859])
Cervical disc procedures (22856)
Decompression (63001-63048)
Exploration retroperitoneal area at same level (49010)

+ 0163T Total disc arthroplasty (artificial disc), anterior approach, including discectomy to prepare interspace (other than for decompression), each additional interspace, lumbar (List separately in addition to code for primary procedure)
Code first (22857)
🔢 0.00 ⚕ 0.00 **FUD** YYY [C] [80] [▭]
AMA: 2018,Jan,8; 2017,Jan,8; 2016,Jan,13; 2015,Jan,16; 2014,Jan,11

+ 0164T Removal of total disc arthroplasty, (artificial disc), anterior approach, each additional interspace, lumbar (List separately in addition to code for primary procedure)
Code first (22865)
🔢 0.00 ⚕ 0.00 **FUD** YYY [C] [80] [▭]
AMA: 2018,Jan,8; 2017,Jan,8; 2016,Jan,13; 2015,Jan,16; 2014,Jan,11

+ 0165T Revision including replacement of total disc arthroplasty (artificial disc), anterior approach, each additional interspace, lumbar (List separately in addition to code for primary procedure)
Code first (22862)
🔢 0.00 ⚕ 0.00 **FUD** YYY [C] [80] [▭]
AMA: 2018,Jan,8; 2017,Jan,8; 2016,Jan,13; 2015,Jan,16; 2014,Jan,11

0174T-0175T

+ 0174T Computer-aided detection (CAD) (computer algorithm analysis of digital image data for lesion detection) with further physician review for interpretation and report, with or without digitization of film radiographic images, chest radiograph(s), performed concurrent with primary interpretation (List separately in addition to code for primary procedure)
Code first (71045-71048)
🔢 0.00 ⚕ 0.00 **FUD** XXX [N] [80] [▭]
AMA: 2018,Apr,7

0175T Computer-aided detection (CAD) (computer algorithm analysis of digital image data for lesion detection) with further physician review for interpretation and report, with or without digitization of film radiographic images, chest radiograph(s), performed remote from primary interpretation
INCLUDES Chest x-rays (71045-71048)
🔢 0.00 ⚕ 0.00 **FUD** XXX [N] [80] [▭]
AMA: 2018,Apr,7

0184T

0184T Excision of rectal tumor, transanal endoscopic microsurgical approach (ie, TEMS), including muscularis propria (ie, full thickness)
INCLUDES Operating microscope (66990)
Proctosigmoidoscopy (45300, 45308-45309, 45315, 45317, 45320)
EXCLUDES Nonendoscopic excision of rectal tumor (45160, 45171-45172)
🔢 0.00 ⚕ 0.00 **FUD** XXX [J] [80] [▭]
AMA: 2018,Feb,11; 2018,Jan,8; 2017,Jan,8; 2016,Feb,12; 2016,Jan,13; 2015,Jan,16; 2014,Jan,11

0191T-0253T [0253T, 0376T]

0191T Insertion of anterior segment aqueous drainage device, without extraocular reservoir, internal approach, into the trabecular meshwork; initial insertion
🔢 0.00 ⚕ 0.00 **FUD** XXX [J] [J8] [80] [▭]
AMA: 2018,Jul,3; 2018,Feb,3; 2018,Jan,8; 2017,Jan,8; 2016,Jan,13; 2015,Jan,16; 2014,Jan,11

+ # 0376T each additional device insertion (List separately in addition to code for primary procedure)
Code first (0191T)
🔢 0.00 ⚕ 0.00 **FUD** XXX [N] [N1] [80] [▭]
AMA: 2018,Jul,3; 2018,Feb,3

0253T Insertion of anterior segment aqueous drainage device, without extraocular reservoir, internal approach, into the suprachoroidal space
EXCLUDES Insertion aqueous drainage device, external approach (66183)
🔢 0.00 ⚕ 0.00 **FUD** YYY [J] [G2] [80] [▭]
AMA: 2018,Jul,3

0198T

0198T Measurement of ocular blood flow by repetitive intraocular pressure sampling, with interpretation and report
🔢 0.00 ⚕ 0.00 **FUD** XXX [01] [80] [▭]
AMA: 2018,Jan,8; 2017,Jan,8; 2016,Jan,13; 2015,Jan,16; 2014,Jan,11

0200T-0201T

INCLUDES Deep bone biopsy (20225)

0200T Percutaneous sacral augmentation (sacroplasty), unilateral injection(s), including the use of a balloon or mechanical device, when used, 1 or more needles, includes imaging guidance and bone biopsy, when performed
🔢 0.00 ⚕ 0.00 **FUD** XXX [J] [G2] [80] [50] [▭]
AMA: 2018,Jan,8; 2017,Jan,8; 2016,Jan,13; 2015,Dec,18; 2015,Apr,8; 2015,Jan,8

0201T Percutaneous sacral augmentation (sacroplasty), bilateral injections, including the use of a balloon or mechanical device, when used, 2 or more needles, includes imaging guidance and bone biopsy, when performed

    0.00   0.00   **FUD** XXX   J G2 80

    AMA: 2018,Jan,8; 2017,Jan,8; 2016,Jan,13; 2015,Dec,18; 2015,Apr,8; 2015,Jan,8

0202T-0563T [0563T]

0202T Posterior vertebral joint(s) arthroplasty (eg, facet joint[s] replacement), including facetectomy, laminectomy, foraminotomy, and vertebral column fixation, injection of bone cement, when performed, including fluoroscopy, single level, lumbar spine

    0.00   0.00   **FUD** XXX   C 80

    INCLUDES Instrumentation (22840, 22853-22854, [22859])
    Laminectomy (63005, 63012, 63017, 63047)
    Laminotomy (63030, 63042)
    Lumbar arthroplasty (22857)
    Percutaneous lumbar vertebral augmentation (22514)
    Percutaneous vertebroplasty (22511)
    Spinal cord decompression (63056)

0205T ~~Intravascular catheter-based coronary vessel or graft spectroscopy (eg, infrared) during diagnostic evaluation and/or therapeutic intervention including imaging supervision, interpretation, and report, each vessel (List separately in addition to code for primary procedure)~~

0206T ~~Computerized database analysis of multiple cycles of digitized cardiac electrical data from two or more ECG leads, including transmission to a remote center, application of multiple nonlinear mathematical transformations, with coronary artery obstruction severity assessment~~

0207T Evacuation of meibomian glands, automated, using heat and intermittent pressure, unilateral

    EXCLUDES Evacuation using:
    Heat through wearable device ([0563T])
    Manual expression only, report appropriate E&M code

    0.00   0.00   **FUD** XXX   01 80

    AMA: 2018,Jan,8; 2017,Jan,8; 2016,Jan,13; 2015,Jan,16; 2014,May,5

● # **0563T** Evacuation of meibomian glands, using heat delivered through wearable, open-eye eyelid treatment devices and manual gland expression, bilateral

    0.00   0.00   **FUD** 000

    EXCLUDES Evacuation using:
    Heat and intermittent pressure (0207T)
    Manual expression only, report appropriate E&M code

0208T-0212T

EXCLUDES Manual audiometric testing by a qualified health care professional, using audiometers (92551-92557)

0208T Pure tone audiometry (threshold), automated; air only

    0.00   0.00   **FUD** XXX   01 80 TC

    AMA: 2018,Jan,8; 2017,Jan,8; 2016,Jan,13; 2015,Jan,16; 2014,Aug,3

0209T air and bone

    0.00   0.00   **FUD** XXX   01 80 TC

    AMA: 2018,Jan,8; 2017,Jan,8; 2016,Jan,13; 2015,Jan,16; 2014,Aug,3; 2014,Jan,11

0210T Speech audiometry threshold, automated;

    0.00   0.00   **FUD** XXX   01 80 TC

    AMA: 2014,Aug,3

0211T with speech recognition

    0.00   0.00   **FUD** XXX   01 80 TC

    AMA: 2018,Jan,8; 2017,Jan,8; 2016,Jan,13; 2015,Jan,16; 2014,Aug,3; 2014,Jan,11

0212T Comprehensive audiometry threshold evaluation and speech recognition (0209T, 0211T combined), automated

    0.00   0.00   **FUD** XXX   01 80 TC

    AMA: 2018,Jan,8; 2017,Jan,8; 2016,Jan,13; 2015,Jan,16; 2014,Aug,3; 2014,Jan,11

0213T-0215T

0213T Injection(s), diagnostic or therapeutic agent, paravertebral facet (zygapophyseal) joint (or nerves innervating that joint) with ultrasound guidance, cervical or thoracic; single level

    0.00   0.00   **FUD** XXX   T R2 80 50

    AMA: 2018,Jan,8; 2017,Jan,8; 2016,Jan,13; 2015,Jan,16; 2014,Jan,11

+ **0214T** second level (List separately in addition to code for primary procedure)

    EXCLUDES Reporting with modifier 50. Report once for each side when performed bilaterally
    Code first (0213T)

    0.00   0.00   **FUD** ZZZ   50 N N1 80

    AMA: 2018,Jan,8; 2017,Jan,8; 2016,Jan,13; 2015,Jan,16; 2014,Jan,11

+ **0215T** third and any additional level(s) (List separately in addition to code for primary procedure)

    EXCLUDES Reporting with modifier 50. Report once for each side when performed bilaterally
    Use of code more than one time per date of service
    Code first (0213T-0214T)

    0.00   0.00   **FUD** ZZZ   50 N N1 80

    AMA: 2018,Jan,8; 2017,Jan,8; 2016,Jan,13; 2015,Jan,16; 2014,Jan,11

0216T-0218T

EXCLUDES Injection with CT or fluoroscopic guidance (64490-64495)

0216T Injection(s), diagnostic or therapeutic agent, paravertebral facet (zygapophyseal) joint (or nerves innervating that joint) with ultrasound guidance, lumbar or sacral; single level

    0.00   0.00   **FUD** XXX   T R2 80 50

    AMA: 2018,Jan,8; 2017,Jan,8; 2016,Jan,13; 2015,Jan,16; 2014,Jan,11

+ **0217T** second level (List separately in addition to code for primary procedure)

    EXCLUDES Reporting with modifier 50. Report once for each side when performed bilaterally
    Code first (0216T)

    0.00   0.00   **FUD** ZZZ   50 N N1 80

    AMA: 2018,Jan,8; 2017,Jan,8; 2016,Jan,13; 2015,Jan,16; 2014,Jan,11

+ **0218T** third and any additional level(s) (List separately in addition to code for primary procedure)

    EXCLUDES Reporting with modifier 50. Report once for each side when performed bilaterally
    Use of code more than one time per date of service
    Code first (0216T-0217T)

    0.00   0.00   **FUD** ZZZ   50 N N1 80

    AMA: 2018,Jan,8; 2017,Jan,8; 2016,Jan,13; 2015,Jan,16; 2014,Jan,11

0219T-0222T

INCLUDES Allografts at same level (20930-20931)
    Application of intervertebral biomechanical device(s) at the same level (22853-22854, [22859])
    Arthrodesis at same level (22600-22614)
    Instrumentation at same level (22840)
    Radiologic services

0219T Placement of a posterior intrafacet implant(s), unilateral or bilateral, including imaging and placement of bone graft(s) or synthetic device(s), single level; cervical

    0.00   0.00   **FUD** XXX   C 80

    AMA: 2018,Jan,8; 2017,Jan,8; 2016,Jan,13; 2015,Jan,16; 2014,Jan,11

0220T

	0220T	**thoracic**

    📱 0.00   ✂ 0.00   **FUD** XXX   [C] [80] 🖳

    AMA: 2018,Jan,8; 2017,Jan,8; 2016,Jan,13; 2015,Jan,16; 2014,Jan,11

  0221T **lumbar**

    📱 0.00   ✂ 0.00   **FUD** XXX   [J] [80] 🖳

    AMA: 2018,Jan,8; 2017,Jan,8; 2016,Jan,13; 2015,Jan,16; 2014,Jan,11

\+ 0222T **each additional vertebral segment (List separately in addition to code for primary procedure)**

    Code first (0219T-0221T)

    📱 0.00   ✂ 0.00   **FUD** ZZZ   [N] [80] 🖳

    AMA: 2018,Jan,8; 2017,Jan,8; 2016,Jan,13; 2015,Jan,16; 2014,Jan,11

0228T-0231T

INCLUDES   Ultrasound guidance (76942, 76998-76999)

EXCLUDES   *Injection performed with CT of fluoroscopic guidance (64479-64484)*

  0228T **Injection(s), anesthetic agent and/or steroid, transforaminal epidural, with ultrasound guidance, cervical or thoracic; single level**

    📱 0.00   ✂ 0.00   **FUD** XXX   [T] [G2] [50] 🖳

    AMA: 2018,Jan,8; 2017,Jan,8; 2016,Jan,13; 2015,Jan,16; 2014,Jan,11

\+ 0229T **each additional level (List separately in addition to code for primary procedure)**

    Code first (0228T)

    📱 0.00   ✂ 0.00   **FUD** XXX   [N] [N1] [50] 🖳

    AMA: 2018,Jan,8; 2017,Jan,8; 2016,Jan,13; 2015,Jan,16; 2014,Jan,11

  0230T **Injection(s), anesthetic agent and/or steroid, transforaminal epidural, with ultrasound guidance, lumbar or sacral; single level**

    📱 0.00   ✂ 0.00   **FUD** XXX   [T] [G2] [50] 🖳

    AMA: 2018,Jan,8; 2017,Jan,8; 2016,Jan,13; 2015,Jan,16; 2014,Jan,11

\+ 0231T **each additional level (List separately in addition to code for primary procedure)**

    Code first (0230T)

    📱 0.00   ✂ 0.00   **FUD** XXX   [N] [N1] [50] 🖳

    AMA: 2018,Jan,8; 2017,Jan,8; 2016,Jan,13; 2015,Jan,16; 2014,Jan,11

0232T

INCLUDES   Arthrocentesis (20600-20611)
    Blood collection (36415, 36592)
    Fat and other soft tissue grafts ([15769], 15771-15774)
    Imaging guidance (76942, 77002, 77012, 77021)
    Injections (20550-20551)
    Platelet/blood product pooling (86965)

EXCLUDES   *Aspiration of bone marrow for grafting, biopsy, harvesting for transplant (38220-38221, 38230)*
    Injections white cell concentrate (0481T)

  0232T **Injection(s), platelet rich plasma, any site, including image guidance, harvesting and preparation when performed**

    📱 0.00   ✂ 0.00   **FUD** XXX   [Q1] [N1] 🖳

    AMA: 2019,Apr,10; 2018,May,3; 2018,Jan,8; 2017,Jan,8; 2016,Jan,13; 2015,Jan,16; 2014,Jan,11

0234T-0238T

INCLUDES   Atherectomy by any technique in arteries above the inguinal ligaments
    Radiology supervision and interpretation

EXCLUDES   *Accessing and catheterization of the vessel*
    Atherectomy performed below the inguinal ligaments (37225, 37227, 37229, 37231, 37233, 37235)
    Closure of the arteriotomy by any technique
    Negotiating the lesion
    Other interventions to the same or different vessels
    Protection from embolism

  0234T **Transluminal peripheral atherectomy, open or percutaneous, including radiological supervision and interpretation; renal artery**

    📱 0.00   ✂ 0.00   **FUD** YYY   [J] [80] 🖳

    AMA: 2018,Jan,8; 2017,Jan,8; 2016,Jan,13; 2015,Jan,16; 2014,Jan,11

  0235T **visceral artery (except renal), each vessel**

    📱 0.00   ✂ 0.00   **FUD** YYY   [C] [80] 🖳

    AMA: 2018,Jan,8; 2017,Jan,8; 2016,Jan,13; 2015,Jan,16; 2014,Jan,11

  0236T **abdominal aorta**

    📱 0.00   ✂ 0.00   **FUD** YYY   [J] [80] 🖳

    AMA: 2018,Jan,8; 2017,Jan,8; 2016,Jan,13; 2015,Jan,16; 2014,Jan,11

  0237T **brachiocephalic trunk and branches, each vessel**

    📱 0.00   ✂ 0.00   **FUD** YYY   [J] [80] 🖳

    AMA: 2018,Jan,8; 2017,Jan,8; 2016,Jan,13; 2015,Jan,16; 2014,Jan,11

  0238T **iliac artery, each vessel**

    📱 0.00   ✂ 0.00   **FUD** YYY   [J] [G2] [80] 🖳

    AMA: 2018,Jan,8; 2017,Jan,8; 2016,Jan,13; 2015,Jan,16; 2014,Jan,11

0249T-0254T [0253T]

  ~~0249T~~ ~~**Ligation, hemorrhoidal vascular bundle(s), including ultrasound guidance**~~

    To report, see (46948)

  0253T **Resequenced code. See code before 0198T.**

  ~~0254T~~ ~~**Endovascular repair of iliac artery bifurcation (eg, aneurysm, pseudoaneurysm, arteriovenous malformation, trauma, dissection) using bifurcated endograft from the common iliac artery into both the external and internal iliac artery, including all selective and/or nonselective catheterization(s) required for device placement and all associated radiological supervision and interpretation, unilateral**~~

    To report, see ([34717-34718])

0263T-0265T

EXCLUDES   *Bone marrow and stem cell services (38204-38242 [38243])*

  0263T **Intramuscular autologous bone marrow cell therapy, with preparation of harvested cells, multiple injections, one leg, including ultrasound guidance, if performed; complete procedure including unilateral or bilateral bone marrow harvest**

    📱 0.00   ✂ 0.00   **FUD** XXX   [S] [G2] [80] 🖳

    INCLUDES Duplex scan (93925-93926)
                Ultrasound guidance (76942)

  0264T **complete procedure excluding bone marrow harvest**

    📱 0.00   ✂ 0.00   **FUD** XXX   [S] [G2] [80] 🖳

    INCLUDES Bone marrow harvest only (0265T)
                Duplex scan (93925-93926)
                Ultrasound guidance (76942)

  0265T **unilateral or bilateral bone marrow harvest only for intramuscular autologous bone marrow cell therapy**

    📱 0.00   ✂ 0.00   **FUD** XXX   [S] [G2] [80] 🖳

    EXCLUDES *Complete procedure (0263T-0264T)*

26/TC PC/TC Only	A2-Z3 ASC Payment	50 Bilateral	♂ Male Only	♀ Female Only	📱 Facility RVU	✂ Non-Facility RVU	🖳 CCI	☒ CLIA
FUD Follow-up Days	CMS: IOM	AMA: CPT Asst	A-Y OPPSI		80/80 Surg Assist Allowed / w/Doc		☒ Lab Crosswalk	☒ Radiology Crosswalk

582   CPT © 2019 American Medical Association. All Rights Reserved.   © 2019 Optum360, LLC

0266T-0273T

0266T Implantation or replacement of carotid sinus baroreflex activation device; total system (includes generator placement, unilateral or bilateral lead placement, intra-operative interrogation, programming, and repositioning, when performed)

🏥 0.00   ⚕ 0.00   **FUD** YYY   C 80 ▣

INCLUDES   Components of complete procedure (0267T-0268T)

0267T lead only, unilateral (includes intra-operative interrogation, programming, and repositioning, when performed)

🏥 0.00   ⚕ 0.00   **FUD** YYY   T 80 ▣

EXCLUDES   Complete procedure (0266T)
Device interrogation (0272T-0273T)
Removal/revision device or components (0269T-0271T)

0268T pulse generator only (includes intra-operative interrogation, programming, and repositioning, when performed)

🏥 0.00   ⚕ 0.00   **FUD** YYY   J 80 ▣

EXCLUDES   Complete procedure (0266T)
Device interrogation (0272T-0273T)
Removal/revision device or components (0269T-0271T)

0269T Revision or removal of carotid sinus baroreflex activation device; total system (includes generator placement, unilateral or bilateral lead placement, intra-operative interrogation, programming, and repositioning, when performed)

🏥 0.00   ⚕ 0.00   **FUD** XXX   02 G2 80 ▣

EXCLUDES   Device interrogation (0272T-0273T)
Implantation/replacement device and/or components (0266T-0268T)
Removal/revision device or components (0270T-0271T)

0270T lead only, unilateral (includes intra-operative interrogation, programming, and repositioning, when performed)

🏥 0.00   ⚕ 0.00   **FUD** XXX   02 G2 80 ▣

EXCLUDES   Device interrogation (0272T-0273T)
Implantation/replacement device and/or components (0266T-0269T)
Removal/revision device or components (0271T)

0271T pulse generator only (includes intra-operative interrogation, programming, and repositioning, when performed)

🏥 0.00   ⚕ 0.00   **FUD** XXX   02 G2 80 ▣

EXCLUDES   Device interrogation (0272T-0273T)
Implantation/replacement device and/or components (0266T-0268T)
Removal/revision device or components (0271T-0273T)

0272T Interrogation device evaluation (in person), carotid sinus baroreflex activation system, including telemetric iterative communication with the implantable device to monitor device diagnostics and programmed therapy values, with interpretation and report (eg, battery status, lead impedance, pulse amplitude, pulse width, therapy frequency, pathway mode, burst mode, therapy start/stop times each day);

🏥 0.00   ⚕ 0.00   **FUD** XXX   S 80 ▣

EXCLUDES   Device interrogation (0273T)
Implantation/replacement device and/or components (0266T-0268T)
Removal/revision device or components (0269T-0271T)

0273T with programming

🏥 0.00   ⚕ 0.00   **FUD** XXX   S 80 ▣

EXCLUDES   Device interrogation (0272T)
Implantation/replacement device and/or components (0266T-0268T)
Removal/revision device or components (0269T-0271T)

0274T-0275T

EXCLUDES   Laminotomy/hemilaminectomy by open and endoscopically assisted approach (63020-63035)
Percutaneous decompression of nucleus pulposus of intervertebral disc by needle-based technique (62287)

0274T Percutaneous laminotomy/laminectomy (interlaminar approach) for decompression of neural elements, (with or without ligamentous resection, discectomy, facetectomy and/or foraminotomy), any method, under indirect image guidance (eg, fluoroscopic, CT), single or multiple levels, unilateral or bilateral; cervical or thoracic

🏥 0.00   ⚕ 0.00   **FUD** YYY   J G2 80 ▣

AMA: 2018,Jan,8; 2017,Feb,12; 2017,Jan,8; 2016,Jan,13; 2015,Jan,16; 2014,Jan,11

0275T lumbar

🏥 0.00   ⚕ 0.00   **FUD** YYY   J G2 80 ▣

AMA: 2018,Jan,8; 2017,Feb,12; 2017,Jan,8; 2016,Jan,13; 2015,Jan,16; 2014,Jan,11

0278T

0278T Transcutaneous electrical modulation pain reprocessing (eg, scrambler therapy), each treatment session (includes placement of electrodes)

🏥 0.00   ⚕ 0.00   **FUD** XXX   01 N1 80 ▣

0290T

+ **0290T** Corneal incisions in the recipient cornea created using a laser, in preparation for penetrating or lamellar keratoplasty (List separately in addition to code for primary procedure)

Code first (65710, 65730, 65750, 65755)

🏥 0.00   ⚕ 0.00   **FUD** ZZZ   N N1 80 ▣

AMA: 2018,Jan,8; 2017,Jan,8; 2016,Jan,13; 2015,Jan,16; 2014,Jan,11

0295T-0298T

EXCLUDES   External echocardiograph monitoring up to 48 hours (93224-93227)
External electrocardiographic monitoring (93260-93272)
Mobile cardiovascular telemetry with echocardiograph recording (93228-93229)

0295T External electrocardiographic recording for more than 48 hours up to 21 days by continuous rhythm recording and storage; includes recording, scanning analysis with report, review and interpretation

🏥 0.00   ⚕ 0.00   **FUD** XXX   M 80 ▣

AMA: 2018,Jan,8; 2017,Jan,8; 2016,Jan,13; 2015,Jan,16; 2014,Jan,11

0296T recording (includes connection and initial recording)

🏥 0.00   ⚕ 0.00   **FUD** XXX   01 80 ▣

AMA: 2018,Jan,8; 2017,Jan,8; 2016,Jan,13; 2015,Jan,16; 2014,Jan,11

0297T scanning analysis with report

🏥 0.00   ⚕ 0.00   **FUD** XXX   01 80 ▣

AMA: 2018,Jan,8; 2017,Jan,8; 2016,Jan,13; 2015,Jan,16; 2014,Jan,11

0298T review and interpretation

🏥 0.00   ⚕ 0.00   **FUD** XXX   M 80 ▣

AMA: 2018,Jan,8; 2017,Jan,8; 2016,Jan,13; 2015,Jan,16; 2014,Jan,11

0308T

0308T Insertion of ocular telescope prosthesis including removal of crystalline lens or intraocular lens prosthesis

INCLUDES   Injection procedures (66020, 66030)
Iridectomy when performed (66600-66635, 66761)
Operating microscope (69990)
Repositioning of intraocular lens (66825)

EXCLUDES   Cataract extraction (66982-66986)

🏥 0.00   ⚕ 0.00   **FUD** YYY   J J8 50 ▣

AMA: 2018,Jan,8; 2017,Jan,8; 2016,Jan,13; 2015,Jan,16; 2014,Jan,11

0312T-0317T

EXCLUDES *Analysis and/or programming (or reprogramming) of vagus nerve stimulator (95970, 95976-95977)*
Implantation, replacement, removal, and/or revision of vagus nerve neurostimulator (electrode array and/or pulse generator) for stimulation of vagus nerve other than at the esophagogastric junction (64568-64570)

0312T **Vagus nerve blocking therapy (morbid obesity); laparoscopic implantation of neurostimulator electrode array, anterior and posterior vagal trunks adjacent to esophagogastric junction (EGJ), with implantation of pulse generator, includes programming**

0.00   0.00   **FUD** XXX   J 80

AMA: 2018,Jan,8; 2017,Jan,8; 2016,Jan,13; 2015,Jan,16

0313T **laparoscopic revision or replacement of vagal trunk neurostimulator electrode array, including connection to existing pulse generator**

0.00   0.00   **FUD** XXX   T 02

AMA: 2018,Jan,8; 2017,Jan,8; 2016,Jan,13; 2015,Jan,16

0314T **laparoscopic removal of vagal trunk neurostimulator electrode array and pulse generator**

0.00   0.00   **FUD** XXX   02 02 80

AMA: 2018,Jan,8; 2017,Jan,8; 2016,Jan,13; 2015,Jan,16

0315T **removal of pulse generator**

EXCLUDES *Removal with replacement pulse generator (0316T)*

0.00   0.00   **FUD** XXX   02 02 80

AMA: 2018,Jan,8; 2017,Jan,8; 2016,Jan,13; 2015,Jan,16

0316T **replacement of pulse generator**

EXCLUDES *Removal without replacement pulse generator (0315T)*

0.00   0.00   **FUD** XXX   J J8 80

AMA: 2018,Jan,8; 2017,Jan,8; 2016,Jan,13; 2015,Jan,16

0317T **neurostimulator pulse generator electronic analysis, includes reprogramming when performed**

EXCLUDES *Analysis and/or programming (or reprogramming) of vagus nerve stimulator (95970, 95976-95977)*

0.00   0.00   **FUD** XXX   01 80

AMA: 2018,Jan,8; 2017,Jan,8; 2016,Jan,13; 2015,Jan,16

0329T-0330T

0329T **Monitoring of intraocular pressure for 24 hours or longer, unilateral or bilateral, with interpretation and report**

0.00   0.00   **FUD** YYY   E

AMA: 2018,Jan,8; 2017,Jan,8; 2016,Jan,13; 2015,Jan,16; 2014,May,5

0330T **Tear film imaging, unilateral or bilateral, with interpretation and report**

0.00   0.00   **FUD** YYY   01 N1

AMA: 2018,Jan,8; 2017,Jan,8; 2016,Jan,13; 2015,Jan,16; 2014,May,5

0331T-0332T

EXCLUDES *Myocardial infarction avid imaging (78466, 78468, 78469)*

0331T **Myocardial sympathetic innervation imaging, planar qualitative and quantitative assessment;**

0.00   0.00   **FUD** YYY   S Z2

AMA: 2018,Jan,8; 2017,Jan,8; 2016,Jan,13; 2015,Jan,16; 2014,Jun,14

0332T **with tomographic SPECT**

0.00   0.00   **FUD** YYY   S Z2

AMA: 2018,Jan,8; 2017,Jan,8; 2016,Jan,13; 2015,Jan,16; 2014,Jun,14

0333T-0464T [0464T]

0333T **Visual evoked potential, screening of visual acuity, automated, with report**

EXCLUDES *Visual evoked potential testing for glaucoma ([0464T])*

0.00   0.00   **FUD** YYY   E

AMA: 2018,Feb,3; 2018,Jan,8; 2017,Jan,8; 2016,Jan,13; 2015,Jan,16; 2014,Aug,8

\# **0464T** **Visual evoked potential, testing for glaucoma, with interpretation and report**

EXCLUDES *Visual evoked potential for visual acuity (0333T)*

0.00   0.00   **FUD** YYY   S

AMA: 2018,Feb,3

0335T-0511T [0510T, 0511T]

0335T **Insertion of sinus tarsi implant**

0.00   0.00   **FUD** YYY   J J8

EXCLUDES *Arthroscopic subtalar arthrodesis (29907)*
Open talotarsal joint dislocation repair (28585)
Subtalar arthodesis (28725)

\# **0510T** **Removal of sinus tarsi implant**

0.00   0.00   **FUD** YYY   02 50

\# **0511T** **Removal and reinsertion of sinus tarsi implant**

0.00   0.00   **FUD** YYY   J8 50

0338T-0339T

INCLUDES Selective catheter placement renal arteries (36251-36254)

0338T **Transcatheter renal sympathetic denervation, percutaneous approach including arterial puncture, selective catheter placement(s) renal artery(ies), fluoroscopy, contrast injection(s), intraprocedural roadmapping and radiological supervision and interpretation, including pressure gradient measurements, flush aortogram and diagnostic renal angiography when performed; unilateral**

0.00   0.00   **FUD** YYY   J 02

0339T **bilateral**

0.00   0.00   **FUD** YYY   J 02

0341T-0342T

~~0341T~~ ~~Quantitative pupillometry with interpretation and report, unilateral or bilateral~~

0342T **Therapeutic apheresis with selective HDL delipidation and plasma reinfusion**

0.00   0.00   **FUD** YYY   S 02

0345T-0347T

0345T **Transcatheter mitral valve repair percutaneous approach via the coronary sinus**

INCLUDES Coronary angiography (93563-93564)

EXCLUDES *Diagnostic cardiac catheterization procedures integral to valve procedure (93451-93461, 93530-93533, 93563-93564)*
Repair of mitral valve including transseptal puncture (33418-33419)
Transcatheter implantation/replacement mitral valve (TMVI) (0483T-0484T)
Transcatheter mitral valve annulus reconstruction (0544T)

0.00   0.00   **FUD** YYY   C

AMA: 2018,Jan,8; 2017,Jan,8; 2016,Jan,13; 2015,Sep,3

0347T **Placement of interstitial device(s) in bone for radiostereometric analysis (RSA)**

0.00   0.00   **FUD** YYY   01 N1

AMA: 2018,Jan,8; 2017,Jan,8; 2016,Jan,13; 2015,Jun,8

0348T-0350T

0348T **Radiologic examination, radiostereometric analysis (RSA); spine, (includes cervical, thoracic and lumbosacral, when performed)**

0.00   0.00   **FUD** YYY   01 N1

AMA: 2018,Jan,8; 2017,Jan,8; 2016,Jan,13; 2015,Jun,8

0349T **upper extremity(ies), (includes shoulder, elbow, and wrist, when performed)**

0.00   0.00   **FUD** YYY   01 N1

AMA: 2018,Jan,8; 2017,Jan,8; 2016,Jan,13; 2015,Jun,8

26/TC PC/TC Only   A2-Z3 ASC Payment   50 Bilateral   ♂ Male Only   ♀ Female Only   Facility RVU   Non-Facility RVU   CCI   CLIA
FUD Follow-up Days   CMS: IOM   AMA: CPT Asst   A-Y OPPSI   80/80 Surg Assist Allowed / w/Doc   Lab Crosswalk   Radiology Crosswalk

584

CPT © 2019 American Medical Association. All Rights Reserved.

© 2019 Optum360, LLC

0350T lower extremity(ies), (includes hip, proximal femur, knee, and ankle, when performed)

🚑 0.00   ⚕ 0.00   **FUD** YYY   [Q1] [N1] ▣

AMA: 2018,Jan,8; 2017,Jan,8; 2016,Jan,13; 2015,Jun,8

0351T-0354T

0351T Optical coherence tomography of breast or axillary lymph node, excised tissue, each specimen; real-time intraoperative

[INCLUDES]   Interpretation and report (0352T)

🚑 0.00   ⚕ 0.00   **FUD** YYY   [N] [N1] ▣

AMA: 2018,Jan,8; 2017,Jan,8; 2016,Jan,13; 2015,Apr,6

0352T interpretation and report, real-time or referred

[INCLUDES]   Interpretation and report (0351T)

🚑 0.00   ⚕ 0.00   **FUD** YYY   [B] ▣

AMA: 2018,Jan,8; 2017,Jan,8; 2016,Jan,13; 2015,Apr,6

0353T Optical coherence tomography of breast, surgical cavity; real-time intraoperative

[INCLUDES]   Interpretation and report (0354T)

[EXCLUDES]   *Use of code more than one time per session*

🚑 0.00   ⚕ 0.00   **FUD** YYY   [N] [N1] ▣

AMA: 2018,Jan,8; 2017,Jan,8; 2016,Jan,13; 2015,Apr,6

0354T interpretation and report, real time or referred

🚑 0.00   ⚕ 0.00   **FUD** YYY   [B] ▣

AMA: 2018,Jan,8; 2017,Jan,8; 2016,Jan,13; 2015,Apr,6

0355T-0358T

0355T Gastrointestinal tract imaging, intraluminal (eg, capsule endoscopy), colon, with interpretation and report

🚑 0.00   ⚕ 0.00   **FUD** YYY   [J] ▣

[INCLUDES]   Distal ileum imaging when performed

[EXCLUDES]   *Capsule endoscopy esophagus only (91111)*
         Capsule endoscopy esophagus through ileum (91110)

0356T Insertion of drug-eluting implant (including punctal dilation and implant removal when performed) into lacrimal canaliculus, each

[EXCLUDES]   *Drug-eluting ocular insert (0444T-0445T)*

🚑 0.00   ⚕ 0.00   **FUD** YYY   [Q1] [N1] ▣

AMA: 2018,Jan,8; 2017,Aug,7

~~**0357T** immature oocyte(s)~~

0358T Bioelectrical impedance analysis whole body composition assessment, with interpretation and report

🚑 0.00   ⚕ 0.00   **FUD** YYY   [Q1] ▣

0362T-0373T

[INCLUDES]   Only the time of one technician when more than one is in attendance
         Provided by physician/other qualified healthcare professional while on-site (immediately available during procedure), but does not need to be face-to-face
         Provided in environment appropriate for patient
         Provided to patients with destructive behaviors

[EXCLUDES]   *Adaptive behavior services ([97153, 97154, 97155, 97156, 97157, 97158])*
         Aphasia assessment (96105)
         Behavioral/developmental screening/testing (96110-96113, [96127])
         Behavior/health assessment (96156-96159 [96164, 96165, 96167, 96168, 96170, 96171])
         Cognitive testing ([96125])
         Neurobehavioral testing (96116-96121)
         Psychiatric evaluations/psychotherapy/interactive complexity (90785-90899)
         Psychological/neuropsychological evaluation/testing (96130-96146)

0362T Behavior identification supporting assessment, each 15 minutes of technicians' time face-to-face with a patient, requiring the following components: administration by the physician or other qualified health care professional who is on site; with the assistance of two or more technicians; for a patient who exhibits destructive behavior; completion in an environment that is customized to the patient's behavior.

[INCLUDES]   Comprises:
         Functional analysis and behavioral assessment
         Procedures and instruments to assess functional impairment and levels of behavior
         Structured observation with data collection not including direct patient involvement

[EXCLUDES]   *Conferences by medical team (99366-99368)*
         Occupational therapy evaluation ([97165, 97166, 97167, 97168])
         Speech evaluation (92521-92524)

Code also when performed on different days until completion of behavioral and supporting assessments are complete

🚑 0.00   ⚕ 0.00   **FUD** YYY   [S] ▣

AMA: 2018,Nov,3; 2018,Jan,8; 2017,Jan,8; 2016,Jan,13; 2015,Jan,16; 2014,Jun,3

0373T Adaptive behavior treatment with protocol modification, each 15 minutes of technicians' time face-to-face with a patient, requiring the following components: administration by the physician or other qualified health care professional who is on site; with the assistance of two or more technicians; for a patient who exhibits destructive behavior; completion in an environment that is customized to the patient's behavior.

🚑 0.00   ⚕ 0.00   **FUD** YYY   [S] ▣

AMA: 2018,Nov,3; 2018,Jan,8; 2017,Jan,8; 2016,Jan,13; 2015,Jan,16; 2014,Jun,3

0375T

~~**0375T** Total disc arthroplasty (artificial disc), anterior approach, including discectomy with end plate preparation (includes osteophytectomy for nerve root or spinal cord decompression and microdissection), cervical, three or more levels~~

0376T-0377T [0376T]

0376T **Resequenced code. See code following 0191T.**

~~**0377T** Anoscopy with directed submucosal injection of bulking agent for fecal incontinence~~

0378T-0380T

0378T Visual field assessment, with concurrent real time data analysis and accessible data storage with patient initiated data transmitted to a remote surveillance center for up to 30 days; review and interpretation with report by a physician or other qualified health care professional

🚑 0.00   ⚕ 0.00   **FUD** XXX   [B] [80] ▣

AMA: 2018,Jan,8; 2017,Jan,8; 2016,Jan,13; 2015,Jan,10

● New Code   ▲ Revised Code   ○ Reinstated   ● New Web Release   ▲ Revised Web Release   + Add-on   Unlisted   Not Covered   # Resequenced
🔟 Optum Mod 50 Exempt   ⊘ AMA Mod 51 Exempt   🔟 Optum Mod 51 Exempt   63 Mod 63 Exempt   ⚡ Non-FDA Drug   ★ Telemedicine   [M] Maternity   [A] Age Edit

0379T technical support and patient instructions, surveillance, analysis and transmission of daily and emergent data reports as prescribed by a physician or other qualified health care professional

🔲 0.00   ✂ 0.00   **FUD** XXX   [Q1] [N1] [80] [▭]

AMA: 2018,Jan,8; 2017,Jan,8; 2016,Jan,13; 2015,Jan,10

~~0380T~~ ~~Computer-aided animation and analysis of time series retinal images for the monitoring of disease progression, unilateral or bilateral, with interpretation and report~~

0381T-0386T

0381T External heart rate and 3-axis accelerometer data recording up to 14 days to assess changes in heart rate and to monitor motion analysis for the purposes of diagnosing nocturnal epilepsy seizure events; includes report, scanning analysis with report, review and interpretation by a physician or other qualified health care professional

🔲 0.00   ✂ 0.00   **FUD** XXX   [M] [80] [▭]

EXCLUDES   *External heart rate and data recording for 15 days or more (0383T-0386T)*

0382T review and interpretation only

🔲 0.00   ✂ 0.00   **FUD** XXX   [M] [80] [▭]

EXCLUDES   *External heart rate and data recording for 15 days or more (0383T-0386T)*

0383T External heart rate and 3-axis accelerometer data recording from 15 to 30 days to assess changes in heart rate and to monitor motion analysis for the purposes of diagnosing nocturnal epilepsy seizure events; includes report, scanning analysis with report, review and interpretation by a physician or other qualified health care professional

🔲 0.00   ✂ 0.00   **FUD** XXX   [M] [80] [▭]

EXCLUDES   *External heart rate and data recording for 14 days or less (0381T-0382T)*
External heart rate and data recording for 30 days or more (0385T-0386T)

0384T review and interpretation only

🔲 0.00   ✂ 0.00   **FUD** XXX   [M] [80] [▭]

EXCLUDES   *External heart rate and data recording for 14 days or less (0381T-0382T)*
External heart rate and data recording for 30 days or more (0385T-0386T)

0385T External heart rate and 3-axis accelerometer data recording more than 30 days to assess changes in heart rate and to monitor motion analysis for the purposes of diagnosing nocturnal epilepsy seizure events; includes report, scanning analysis with report, review and interpretation by a physician or other qualified health care professional

🔲 0.00   ✂ 0.00   **FUD** XXX   [M] [80] [▭]

EXCLUDES   *External heart rate and data recording for 30 days or less (0381T-0384T)*

0386T review and interpretation only

🔲 0.00   ✂ 0.00   **FUD** XXX   [M] [80] [▭]

EXCLUDES   *External heart rate and data recording for 30 days or less (0381T-0384T)*

0394T-0395T

EXCLUDES   *Radiation oncology procedures (77261-77263, 77300, 77306-77307, 77316-77318, 77332-77334, 77336, 77427-77499, 77761-77772, 77778, 77789)*

0394T High dose rate electronic brachytherapy, skin surface application, per fraction, includes basic dosimetry, when performed

🔲 0.00   ✂ 0.00   **FUD** XXX   [S] [Z2] [80] [▭]

EXCLUDES   *Superficial non-brachytherapy radiation (77401)*

0395T High dose rate electronic brachytherapy, interstitial or intracavitary treatment, per fraction, includes basic dosimetry, when performed

🔲 0.00   ✂ 0.00   **FUD** XXX   [S] [Z2] [80] [▭]

EXCLUDES   *High dose rate skin surface application (0394T)*

0396T-0399T

+ 0396T Intra-operative use of kinetic balance sensor for implant stability during knee replacement arthroplasty (List separately in addition to code for primary procedure)

🔲 0.00   ✂ 0.00   **FUD** XXX   [N] [N1] [80] [▭]

Code first (27445-27447, 27486-27488)

+ 0397T Endoscopic retrograde cholangiopancreatography (ERCP), with optical endomicroscopy (List separately in addition to code for primary procedure)

🔲 0.00   ✂ 0.00   **FUD** XXX   [N] [N1] [80] [▭]

INCLUDES   Optical endomicroscopic image(s) (88375)

EXCLUDES   *Use of code more than one time per operative session*
Code first (43260-43265, [43274], [43275], [43276], [43277], [43278])

0398T Magnetic resonance image guided high intensity focused ultrasound (MRgFUS), stereotactic ablation lesion, intracranial for movement disorder including stereotactic navigation and frame placement when performed

🔲 0.00   ✂ 0.00   **FUD** XXX   [S] [80] [▭]

INCLUDES   Application stereotactic headframe (61800)
Stereotactic computer-assisted navigation (61781)

~~0399T~~ ~~Myocardial strain imaging (quantitative assessment of myocardial mechanics using image-based analysis of local myocardial dynamics) (List separately in addition to code for primary procedure)~~

To report, see (93356)

0400T-0401T

0400T Multi-spectral digital skin lesion analysis of clinically atypical cutaneous pigmented lesions for detection of melanomas and high risk melanocytic atypia; one to five lesions

🔲 0.00   ✂ 0.00   **FUD** XXX   [N] [N1] [80] [▭]

0401T six or more lesions

🔲 0.00   ✂ 0.00   **FUD** XXX   [N] [N1] [80] [▭]

INCLUDES   Treatment of one to five lesions (0400T)

0402T

▲ 0402T Collagen cross-linking of cornea, including removal of the corneal epithelium and intraoperative pachymetry, when performed (Report medication separately)

INCLUDES   Corneal epithelium removal (65435)
Corneal pachymetry (76514)
Operating microscope (69990)

🔲 0.00   ✂ 0.00   **FUD** XXX   [J] [R2] [80] [▭]

AMA: 2018,Jun,11; 2018,Jan,8; 2017,Jan,8; 2016,Feb,12

0403T-0488T [0488T]

INCLUDES   Intensive behavioral counseling by trained lifestyle coach
Standardized course with an emphasis on weight, exercise, stress management, and nutrition

0403T Preventive behavior change, intensive program of prevention of diabetes using a standardized diabetes prevention program curriculum, provided to individuals in a group setting, minimum 60 minutes, per day

EXCLUDES   *Online/electronic diabetes prevention program ([0488T])*
Self-management training and education by nonphysician health care professional (98960-98962)

🔲 0.00   ✂ 0.00   **FUD** XXX   [E] [80] [▭]

AMA: 2018,Aug,6; 2015,Aug,4

---

[26]/[10] PC/TC Only   [A2]-[Z3] ASC Payment   [50] Bilateral   ♂ Male Only   ♀ Female Only   🔲 Facility RVU   ✂ Non-Facility RVU   [▭] CCI   [✖] CLIA
FUD Follow-up Days   **CMS:** IOM   **AMA:** CPT Asst   [A]-[Y] OPPSI   [80]/[80] Surg Assist Allowed / w/Doc   [▭] Lab Crosswalk   [▭] Radiology Crosswalk

586   CPT © 2019 American Medical Association. All Rights Reserved.   © 2019 Optum360, LLC

0488T
Preventive behavior change, online/electronic structured intensive program for prevention of diabetes using a standardized diabetes prevention program curriculum, provided to an individual, per 30 days

INCLUDES In person elements when appropriate
EXCLUDES *Group diabetes prevention program (0403T)*
Self-management training and education by nonphysician health care professional (98960-98962)

0.00   0.00   FUD XXX   E

AMA: 2018,Aug,6

0404T-0405T

0404T Transcervical uterine fibroid(s) ablation with ultrasound guidance, radiofrequency ♀
0.00   0.00   FUD XXX   J 80

0405T Oversight of the care of an extracorporeal liver assist system patient requiring review of status, review of laboratories and other studies, and revision of orders and liver assist care plan (as appropriate), within a calendar month, 30 minutes or more of non-face-to-face time
0.00   0.00   FUD XXX   B 80

0408T-0418T

0408T Insertion or replacement of permanent cardiac contractility modulation system, including contractility evaluation when performed, and programming of sensing and therapeutic parameters; pulse generator with transvenous electrodes
0.00   0.00   FUD XXX   J J8 80

INCLUDES Device evaluation (93286-93287, 0415T, 0417T-0418T)
Insertion or replacement of entire system
EXCLUDES *Cardiac catheterization (93452-93453, 93456-93461)*
Code also removal of each electrode when pulse generator and electrodes are removed and replaced (0410T-0411T)

0409T pulse generator only
0.00   0.00   FUD XXX   J J8 80

INCLUDES Device evaluation (93286-93287, 0415T, 0417T-0418T)
EXCLUDES *Cardiac catheterization (93452-93453, 93456-93461)*

0410T atrial electrode only
0.00   0.00   FUD XXX   J J8 80

INCLUDES Device evaluation (93286-93287, 0415T, 0417T-0418T)
Each atrial electrode inserted or replaced
EXCLUDES *Cardiac catheterization (93452-93453, 93456-93461)*

0411T ventricular electrode only
0.00   0.00   FUD XXX   J J8 80

INCLUDES Device evaluation (93286-93287, 0415T, 0417T-0418T)
Each ventricular electrode inserted or replaced
EXCLUDES *Cardiac catheterization (93452-93453, 93456-93461)*
Insertion or replacement of complete CCM system (0408T)

0412T Removal of permanent cardiac contractility modulation system; pulse generator only
0.00   0.00   FUD XXX   Q2 G2 80

EXCLUDES *Device evaluation (0417T-0418T)*
Insertion or replacement of complete CCM system (0408T)

0413T transvenous electrode (atrial or ventricular)
0.00   0.00   FUD XXX   Q2 G2 80

INCLUDES Each electrode removed
EXCLUDES *Device evaluation (0417T-0418T)*
Insertion or replacement of complete CCM system (0408T)
Code also removal and replacement of electrode(s), as appropriate (0410T-0411T)
Code also removal of pulse generator when leads also removed (0412T)

0414T Removal and replacement of permanent cardiac contractility modulation system pulse generator only
0.00   0.00   FUD XXX   J J8 80

INCLUDES Device evaluation (93286-93287, 0417T-0418T)
EXCLUDES *Cardiac catheterization (93452-93453, 93456-93461)*
Code also replacement of pulse generator when leads also removed and replaced (0408T, 0412T-0413T)

0415T Repositioning of previously implanted cardiac contractility modulation transvenous electrode, (atrial or ventricular lead)
0.00   0.00   FUD XXX   T G2 80

INCLUDES Device evaluation (93286-93287, 0417T-0418T)
EXCLUDES *Cardiac catheterization (93452-93453, 93456-93461)*
Insertion or replacement of entire system or components (0408T-0411T)

0416T Relocation of skin pocket for implanted cardiac contractility modulation pulse generator
0.00   0.00   FUD XXX   T G2 80

0417T Programming device evaluation (in person) with iterative adjustment of the implantable device to test the function of the device and select optimal permanent programmed values with analysis, including review and report, implantable cardiac contractility modulation system
0.00   0.00   FUD XXX   Q1 80

EXCLUDES *Insertion/replacement/removal/repositioning of device or components (0408T-0415T, 0418T)*

0418T Interrogation device evaluation (in person) with analysis, review and report, includes connection, recording and disconnection per patient encounter, implantable cardiac contractility modulation system
0.00   0.00   FUD XXX   Q1 80

EXCLUDES *Insertion/replacement/removal/repositioning of device or components (0408T-0415T, 0417T)*

0419T-0420T

EXCLUDES *Neurofibroma excision (64792)*
Use of code more than one time per session

0419T Destruction of neurofibroma, extensive (cutaneous, dermal extending into subcutaneous); face, head and neck, greater than 50 neurofibromas
0.00   0.00   FUD XXX   T R2 80

AMA: 2018,Jan,8; 2017,Jan,8; 2016,Apr,3

0420T trunk and extremities, extensive, greater than 100 neurofibromas
0.00   0.00   FUD XXX   T R2 80

AMA: 2018,Jan,8; 2017,Jan,8; 2016,Apr,3

0421T-0423T

0421T Transurethral waterjet ablation of prostate, including control of post-operative bleeding, including ultrasound guidance, complete (vasectomy, meatotomy, cystourethroscopy, urethral calibration and/or dilation, and internal urethrotomy are included when performed) ♂
0.00   0.00   FUD XXX   J G2 80

EXCLUDES *Transrectal ultrasound (76872)*
Transurethral prostate resection (52500, 52630)

0422T Tactile breast imaging by computer-aided tactile sensors, unilateral or bilateral
0.00   0.00   FUD XXX   Q1 Z2 80

0423T Secretory type II phospholipase A2 (sPLA2-IIA)
0.00   0.00   FUD XXX   A

EXCLUDES *Lipoprotein-associated phospholipase A2 [LpPLA2] (83698)*

0424T-0436T

INCLUDES Phrenic nerve stimulation system includes:
Pulse generator
Sensing lead (placed in azygos vein)
Stimulation lead (placed into right brachiocephalic vein or left periocardiophrenic vein)

0424T **Insertion or replacement of neurostimulator system for treatment of central sleep apnea; complete system (transvenous placement of right or left stimulation lead, sensing lead, implantable pulse generator)**

🖧 0.00   ⚕ 0.00   **FUD** XXX   J J8 80 ▱

INCLUDES Device evaluation (0434T-0436T)
Insertion or replacement system components (0425T-0427T)
Repositioning of leads (0432T-0433T)
Code also when pulse generator and all leads are removed and replaced (0428T-0430T)

0425T **sensing lead only**

🖧 0.00   ⚕ 0.00   **FUD** XXX   J G2 80 ▱

EXCLUDES Device evaluation (0434T-0436T)
Insertion/replacement complete system (0424T)
Repositioning of leads (0432T-0433T)

0426T **stimulation lead only**

🖧 0.00   ⚕ 0.00   **FUD** XXX   J G2 80 ▱

EXCLUDES Device evaluation (0434T-0436T)
Insertion/replacement complete system (0424T)
Repositioning of leads (0432T-0433T)

0427T **pulse generator only**

🖧 0.00   ⚕ 0.00   **FUD** XXX   J G2 80 ▱

EXCLUDES Device evaluation (0434T-0436T)
Insertion/replacement complete system (0424T)
Repositioning of leads (0432T-0433T)

0428T **Removal of neurostimulator system for treatment of central sleep apnea; pulse generator only**

🖧 0.00   ⚕ 0.00   **FUD** XXX   Q2 G2 80 ▱

EXCLUDES Device evaluation (0434T-0436T)
Removal with replacement of pulse generator and all leads (0424T, 0429T-0430T)
Repositioning of leads (0432T-0433T)
Code also when a lead is removed (0429T-0430T)

0429T **sensing lead only**

🖧 0.00   ⚕ 0.00   **FUD** XXX   Q2 G2 80 ▱

INCLUDES Removal of one sensing lead
EXCLUDES Device evaluation (0434T-0436T)

0430T **stimulation lead only**

INCLUDES Removal of one stimulation lead
EXCLUDES Device evaluation (0434T-0436T)

🖧 0.00   ⚕ 0.00   **FUD** XXX   Q2 G2 80 ▱

AMA: 2015,Aug,4

0431T **Removal and replacement of neurostimulator system for treatment of central sleep apnea, pulse generator only**

🖧 0.00   ⚕ 0.00   **FUD** XXX   J G2 80 ▱

EXCLUDES Device evaluation (0434T-0436T)
Removal with replacement of generator and all three leads (0424T, 0428T-0430T)

0432T **Repositioning of neurostimulator system for treatment of central sleep apnea; stimulation lead only**

🖧 0.00   ⚕ 0.00   **FUD** XXX   T G2 80 ▱

EXCLUDES Device evaluation (0434T-0436T)
Insertion/replacement complete system or components (0424T-0427T)

0433T **sensing lead only**

🖧 0.00   ⚕ 0.00   **FUD** XXX   T G2 80 ▱

EXCLUDES Device evaluation (0434T-0436T)
Insertion/replacement complete system or components (0424T-0427T)

0434T **Interrogation device evaluation implanted neurostimulator pulse generator system for central sleep apnea**

🖧 0.00   ⚕ 0.00   **FUD** XXX   S G2 80 ▱

EXCLUDES Insertion/replacement complete system or components (0424T-0427T)
Removal of system or components (0428T-0431T)
Repositioning leads (0432T-0433T)

0435T **Programming device evaluation of implanted neurostimulator pulse generator system for central sleep apnea; single session**

🖧 0.00   ⚕ 0.00   **FUD** XXX   S 80 ▱

EXCLUDES Device evaluation (0436T)
Insertion/replacement complete system or components (0424T-0427T)
Removal of system or components (0428T-0431T)
Repositioning leads (0432T-0433T)

0436T **during sleep study**

🖧 0.00   ⚕ 0.00   **FUD** XXX   S 80 ▱

EXCLUDES Device evaluation (0435T)
Insertion/replacement complete system or components (0424T-0427T)
Removal of system or components (0428T-0431T)
Repositioning leads (0432T-0433T)
Use of code more than one time for each sleep study

0437T-0439T

+ **0437T** **Implantation of non-biologic or synthetic implant (eg, polypropylene) for fascial reinforcement of the abdominal wall (List separately in addition to code for primary procedure)**

🖧 0.00   ⚕ 0.00   **FUD** ZZZ   N N1 80 ▱

EXCLUDES Implantation mesh, other material for repair incisional or ventral hernia (49560-49561, 49565-49566, 49568)
Insertion mesh, other material for closure of wound caused by necrotizing soft tissue infection (11004-11006, 49568)

+ **0439T** **Myocardial contrast perfusion echocardiography, at rest or with stress, for assessment of myocardial ischemia or viability (List separately in addition to code for primary procedure)**

Code first (93306-93308, 93350-93351)
🖧 0.00   ⚕ 0.00   **FUD** ZZZ   N N1 80 ▱

AMA: 2018,Jan,8; 2017,Jan,8; 2016,Apr,8

0440T-0442T

0440T **Ablation, percutaneous, cryoablation, includes imaging guidance; upper extremity distal/peripheral nerve**

🖧 0.00   ⚕ 0.00   **FUD** YYY   J G2 80 ▱

AMA: 2019,Apr,9; 2018,Jan,8

0441T **lower extremity distal/peripheral nerve**

🖧 0.00   ⚕ 0.00   **FUD** YYY   J G2 80 ▱

AMA: 2019,Apr,9; 2018,Jan,8

0442T **nerve plexus or other truncal nerve (eg, brachial plexus, pudendal nerve)**

🖧 0.00   ⚕ 0.00   **FUD** YYY   J G2 80 ▱

AMA: 2019,Apr,9; 2018,Jan,8

0443T

+ **0443T** **Real-time spectral analysis of prostate tissue by fluorescence spectroscopy, including imaging guidance (List separately in addition to code for primary procedure)** ♂

🖧 0.00   ⚕ 0.00   **FUD** ZZZ   N N1 80 ▱

EXCLUDES Use of code more than one time for each session
Code also (55700)

CPT © 2019 American Medical Association. All Rights Reserved.   © 2019 Optum360, LLC

0444T-0445T

EXCLUDES   *Insertion/removal drug-eluting stent into canaliculus (0356T)*

0444T   **Initial placement of a drug-eluting ocular insert under one or more eyelids, including fitting, training, and insertion, unilateral or bilateral**

 0.00   0.00   **FUD** YYY   N N1 80

AMA: 2018,Jan,8; 2017,Aug,7

0445T   **Subsequent placement of a drug-eluting ocular insert under one or more eyelids, including re-training, and removal of existing insert, unilateral or bilateral**

 0.00   0.00   **FUD** YYY   N N1 80

AMA: 2018,Jan,8; 2017,Aug,7

0446T-0448T

EXCLUDES   *Placement non-implantable interstitial glucose sensor without pocket (95250)*

0446T   **Creation of subcutaneous pocket with insertion of implantable interstitial glucose sensor, including system activation and patient training**

EXCLUDES   *Interpretation/report of ambulatory glucose monitoring of interstitial tissue (95251)*
Removal interstitial glucose sensor (0447T-0448T)

 0.00   0.00   **FUD** YYY   T G2

AMA: 2018,Jun,6

0447T   **Removal of implantable interstitial glucose sensor from subcutaneous pocket via incision**

 0.00   0.00   **FUD** YYY   02 G2

0448T   **Removal of implantable interstitial glucose sensor with creation of subcutaneous pocket at different anatomic site and insertion of new implantable sensor, including system activation**

 0.00   0.00   **FUD** YYY   T G2

EXCLUDES   *Initial insertion of sensor (0446T)*
Removal of sensor (0447T)

0449T-0450T

EXCLUDES   *Removal by internal approach of aqueous drainage device without extraocular reservoir in subconjunctival space (92499)*

0449T   **Insertion of aqueous drainage device, without extraocular reservoir, internal approach, into the subconjunctival space; initial device**

 0.00   0.00   **FUD** YYY   J J8

AMA: 2018,Sep,3; 2018,Jul,3

\+   **0450T**   **each additional device (List separately in addition to code for primary procedure)**

Code first (0449T)

 0.00   0.00   **FUD** YYY   N N1

AMA: 2018,Jul,3

0451T-0463T

INCLUDES   Access procedures (36000-36010)
Catheterization of vessel (36200-36228)
Diagnostic angiography (75600-75774)
Imaging guidance (76000, 76936-76937, 77001-77002, 77011-77012, 77021)
Injection procedures (93561-93572)
Radiological supervision and interpretation

EXCLUDES   *Cardiac catheterization (93451-93533)*

0451T   **Insertion or replacement of a permanently implantable aortic counterpulsation ventricular assist system, endovascular approach, and programming of sensing and therapeutic parameters; complete system (counterpulsation device, vascular graft, implantable vascular hemostatic seal, mechano-electrical skin interface and subcutaneous electrodes)**

EXCLUDES   *Aortic counterpulsation ventricular assist system procedures (0452T-0458T)*
Insertion intra-aortic balloon assist device (33967, 33970, 33973)
Insertion/replacement extracorporeal ventricular assist device (33975-33976, 33981)
Insertion/replacement intracorporeal ventricular assist device (33979, 33982-33983)
Insertion ventricular assist device (33990-33991)

 0.00   0.00   **FUD** YYY   C

AMA: 2017,Dec,3

0452T   **aortic counterpulsation device and vascular hemostatic seal**

EXCLUDES   *Insertion intra-aortic balloon assist device (33973)*
Insertion intracorporeal ventricular assist device (33979, 33982-33983)
Insertion/replacement counterpulsation ventricular assist system procedures (0451T)
Insertion ventricular assist device (33990-33991)
Removal counterpulsation ventricular assist system (0455T-0456T)

 0.00   0.00   **FUD** YYY   C

AMA: 2017,Dec,3

0453T   **mechano-electrical skin interface**

 0.00   0.00   **FUD** YYY   J

EXCLUDES   *Insertion intra-aortic balloon assist device (33973)*
Insertion intracorporeal ventricular assist device (33979, 33982-33983)
Insertion/replacement counterpulsation ventricular assist system procedures (0451T)
Insertion ventricular assist device (33990-33991)
Removal counterpulsation ventricular assist system (0455T, 0457T)

0454T   **subcutaneous electrode**

 0.00   0.00   **FUD** YYY   J

INCLUDES   Each electrode inserted or replaced

EXCLUDES   *Insertion intra-aortic balloon assist device (33973, 33982-33983)*
Insertion/replacement counterpulsation ventricular assist system (0451T)
Insertion/replacement intracorporeal ventricular assist device (33979, 33982-33983)
Insertion ventricular assist device (33990-33991)
Removal device or component (0455T, 0458T)

0455T   **Removal of permanently implantable aortic counterpulsation ventricular assist system; complete system (aortic counterpulsation device, vascular hemostatic seal, mechano-electrical skin interface and electrodes)**

> EXCLUDES   *Insertion/replacement system or component (0451T-0454T)*
> *Removal:*
>   *Extracorporeal ventricular assist device (33977-33978)*
>   *Intra-aortic balloon assist device (33968, 33971, 33974)*
>   *Intracorporeal ventricular assist device (33980)*
>   *Percutaneous ventricular assist device (33992)*
>   *System or component (0456T-0458T)*

🔲 0.00   ⚕ 0.00   **FUD** YYY   C ▭

AMA: 2017,Dec,3

0456T   **aortic counterpulsation device and vascular hemostatic seal**

> EXCLUDES   *Insertion/replacement system or component (0451T-0452T)*
> *Removal:*
>   *Aortic counterpulsation ventricular assist system (0455T)*
>   *Intra-aortic balloon assist device (33974)*
>   *Intracorporeal ventricular assist device (33980)*
>   *Percutaneous ventricular assist device (33992)*

🔲 0.00   ⚕ 0.00   **FUD** YYY   C ▭

AMA: 2017,Dec,3

0457T   **mechano-electrical skin interface**

🔲 0.00   ⚕ 0.00   **FUD** YYY   02 ▭

> EXCLUDES   *Insertion/replacement system or component (0451T, 0453T)*
> *Removal:*
>   *Aortic counterpulsation ventricular assist system (0455T)*
>   *Intra-aortic balloon assist device (33974)*
>   *Intracorporeal ventricular assist device (33980)*
>   *Percutaneous ventricular assist device (33992)*

0458T   **subcutaneous electrode**

🔲 0.00   ⚕ 0.00   **FUD** YYY   02 ▭

> INCLUDES   Each electrode removed
> EXCLUDES   *Insertion/replacement system or component (0451T, 0454T)*
> *Removal:*
>   *Aortic counterpulsation ventricular assist system (0455T)*
>   *Intra-aortic balloon assist device (33974)*
>   *Intracorporeal ventricular assist device (33980)*
>   *Percutaneous ventricular assist device (33992)*

0459T   **Relocation of skin pocket with replacement of implanted aortic counterpulsation ventricular assist device, mechano-electrical skin interface and electrodes**

🔲 0.00   ⚕ 0.00   **FUD** YYY   C ▭

> EXCLUDES   *Repositioning percutaneous ventricular assist device (33993)*

0460T   **Repositioning of previously implanted aortic counterpulsation ventricular assist device; subcutaneous electrode**

🔲 0.00   ⚕ 0.00   **FUD** YYY   T ▭

> INCLUDES   Reporting for repositioning of each electrode
> EXCLUDES   *Insertion/replacement system or component (0451T, 0454T)*
> *Repositioning of percutaneous ventricular assist device (33993)*

0461T   **aortic counterpulsation device**

🔲 0.00   ⚕ 0.00   **FUD** YYY   C ▭

> EXCLUDES   *Repositioning percutaneous ventricular assist device (33993)*

0462T   **Programming device evaluation (in person) with iterative adjustment of the implantable mechano-electrical skin interface and/or external driver to test the function of the device and select optimal permanent programmed values with analysis, including review and report, implantable aortic counterpulsation ventricular assist system, per day**

🔲 0.00   ⚕ 0.00   **FUD** YYY   S ▭

> EXCLUDES   *Device evaluation (0463T)*
> *Insertion/replacement system or component (0451T-0454T)*
> *Relocation of pocket (0459T)*
> *Removal system or component (0455T-0458T)*
> *Repositioning device (0460T-0461T)*

0463T   **Interrogation device evaluation (in person) with analysis, review and report, includes connection, recording and disconnection per patient encounter, implantable aortic counterpulsation ventricular assist system, per day**

🔲 0.00   ⚕ 0.00   **FUD** YYY   S ▭

> EXCLUDES   *Device evaluation (0462T)*
> *Insertion/replacement system or component (0451T-0454T)*
> *Relocation of pocket (0459T)*
> *Removal system or component (0455T-0458T)*
> *Repositioning device (0460T-0461T)*

0464T [0464T]

0464T   **Resequenced code. See code following 0333T.**

0465T-0469T

> EXCLUDES   *Replacement/revision cranial nerve neurostimulator electrode array (64569)*

0465T   **Suprachoroidal injection of a pharmacologic agent (does not include supply of medication)**

> EXCLUDES   *Intravitreal implantation or injection (67025-67028)*

🔲 0.00   ⚕ 0.00   **FUD** YYY   T R2 ▭

AMA: 2018,Feb,3

+ 0466T   **Insertion of chest wall respiratory sensor electrode or electrode array, including connection to pulse generator (List separately in addition to code for primary procedure)**

> EXCLUDES   *Revision/removal chest wall respiratory sensor electrode or array (0467T-0468T)*
> Code first (64568)

🔲 0.00   ⚕ 0.00   **FUD** YYY   N N1 ▭

AMA: 2018,Mar,9; 2018,Jan,8; 2017,Jan,8; 2016,Nov,6

0467T   **Revision or replacement of chest wall respiratory sensor electrode or electrode array, including connection to existing pulse generator**

> EXCLUDES   *Insertion/removal chest wall respiratory sensor electrode or array (0466T, 0468T)*
> *Replacement/revision cranial nerve neurostimulator electrode array (64569)*

🔲 0.00   ⚕ 0.00   **FUD** YYY   02 N1 ▭

AMA: 2018,Mar,9; 2018,Jan,8; 2017,Jan,8; 2016,Nov,6

0468T   **Removal of chest wall respiratory sensor electrode or electrode array**

> EXCLUDES   *Insertion/removal chest wall respiratory sensor electrode or array (0466T-0467T)*
> *Removal cranial neurostimulator electrode array (64570)*

🔲 0.00   ⚕ 0.00   **FUD** YYY   02 N1 ▭

AMA: 2018,Mar,9; 2018,Jan,8; 2017,Jan,8; 2016,Nov,6

0469T   **Retinal polarization scan, ocular screening with on-site automated results, bilateral**

> INCLUDES   Ophthalmic medical services (92002-92014)
> EXCLUDES   *Ocular screening (99174, [99177])*

🔲 0.00   ⚕ 0.00   **FUD** XXX   E ▭

AMA: 2018,Feb,3

26/TC PC/TC Only   A2-Z3 ASC Payment   50 Bilateral   ♂ Male Only   ♀ Female Only   🔲 Facility RVU   ⚕ Non-Facility RVU   ▭ CCI   ✖ CLIA

FUD Follow-up Days   **CMS:** IOM   **AMA:** CPT Asst   A-Y OPPSI   80/80 Surg Assist Allowed / w/Doc   ▪ Lab Crosswalk   ▪ Radiology Crosswalk

590   CPT © 2019 American Medical Association. All Rights Reserved.   © 2019 Optum360, LLC

0470T-0471T

EXCLUDES *Optical coherence tomography of coronary vessel or graft (92978-92979)*
Reflectance confocal microscopy (RCM) for cellular and subcellular skin imaging (96931-96936)

0470T **Optical coherence tomography (OCT) for microstructural and morphological imaging of skin, image acquisition, interpretation, and report; first lesion**

🔲 0.00 🔲 0.00 **FUD** XXX `M` `▢`

+ 0471T **each additional lesion (List separately in addition to code for primary procedure)**

🔲 0.00 🔲 0.00 **FUD** XXX `N` `N1` `▢`

Code first (0470T)

0472T-0474T

0472T **Device evaluation, interrogation, and initial programming of intraocular retinal electrode array (eg, retinal prosthesis), in person, with iterative adjustment of the implantable device to test functionality, select optimal permanent programmed values with analysis, including visual training, with review and report by a qualified health care professional**

🔲 0.00 🔲 0.00 **FUD** XXX `01` `▢`

AMA: 2018,Feb,3

0473T **Device evaluation and interrogation of intraocular retinal electrode array (eg, retinal prosthesis), in person, including reprogramming and visual training, when performed, with review and report by a qualified health care professional**

INCLUDES Reprogramming of device (0473T)
EXCLUDES *Placement of intra-ocular retinal electrode display (0100T)*

🔲 0.00 🔲 0.00 **FUD** XXX `01` `▢`

AMA: 2018,Feb,3

0474T **Insertion of anterior segment aqueous drainage device, with creation of intraocular reservoir, internal approach, into the supraciliary space**

🔲 0.00 🔲 0.00 **FUD** XXX `J` `▢`

AMA: 2018,Dec,8; 2018,Dec,8; 2018,Jul,3; 2018,Feb,3

0475T-0478T

0475T **Recording of fetal magnetic cardiac signal using at least 3 channels; patient recording and storage, data scanning with signal extraction, technical analysis and result, as well as supervision, review, and interpretation of report by a physician or other qualified health care professional**

🔲 0.00 🔲 0.00 **FUD** XXX `M` `▢`

0476T **patient recording, data scanning, with raw electronic signal transfer of data and storage**

🔲 0.00 🔲 0.00 **FUD** XXX `01` `▢`

0477T **signal extraction, technical analysis, and result**

🔲 0.00 🔲 0.00 **FUD** XXX `01` `▢`

0478T **review, interpretation, report by physician or other qualified health care professional**

🔲 0.00 🔲 0.00 **FUD** XXX `M` `▢`

0479T-0480T

EXCLUDES *Ablative laser treatment for additional square cm for open wound (0492T)*
Cicatricial lesion excision (11400-11446)
Use of code more than one time per day

0479T **Fractional ablative laser fenestration of burn and traumatic scars for functional improvement; first 100 cm2 or part thereof, or 1% of body surface area of infants and children**

🔲 0.00 🔲 0.00 **FUD** 000 `T` `62` `▢`

AMA: 2018,Jan,8; 2017,Dec,13

+ 0480T **each additional 100 cm2, or each additional 1% of body surface area of infants and children, or part thereof (List separately in addition to code for primary procedure)**

Code first (0479T)

🔲 0.00 🔲 0.00 **FUD** ZZZ `N` `N1` `▢`

AMA: 2018,Jan,8; 2017,Dec,13

0481T-0482T

0481T **Injection(s), autologous white blood cell concentrate (autologous protein solution), any site, including image guidance, harvesting and preparation, when performed**

🔲 0.00 🔲 0.00 **FUD** 000 `01` `▢`

EXCLUDES *Blood collection (36415, 36592)*
Bone marrow procedures (38220-38222, 38230)
Imaging guidance (76942, 77002, 77012, 77021)
Injection of platelet rich plasma (0232T)
Injections to tendon, ligament, or fascia (20550-20551)
Joint aspiration or injection (20600-20611)
Other tissue grafts ([15769], 15771-15774)
Pooling of platelets (86965)

~~**0482T** **Absolute quantitation of myocardial blood flow, positron emission tomography (PET), rest and stress (List separately in addition to code for primary procedure)**~~

0483T-0484T

INCLUDES Access and closure
Angiography
Balloon valvuloplasty
Contrast injections
Fluoroscopy
Radiological supervision and interpretation
Valve deployment and repositioning
Ventriculography

EXCLUDES *Diagnostic heart catheterization (93451-93453, 93456-93461, 93530-93533)*
Transcatheter mitral valve annulus reconstruction (0544T)
Transcatheter mitral valve repair through coronary sinus (0345T)
Transcatheter mitral valve repair with transseptal puncture, when performed (33418-33419)
Transcatheter tricuspid valve annulus reconstruction (0545T)
Code also cardiopulmonary bypass when provided (33367-33369)
Code also diagnostic cardiac catheterization procedures if there is no previous study available and append modifier 59 when:
The condition of the patient has changed
The previous study is inadequate

0483T **Transcatheter mitral valve implantation/replacement (TMVI) with prosthetic valve; percutaneous approach, including transseptal puncture, when performed**

🔲 0.00 🔲 0.00 **FUD** 000 `C` `80` `▢`

0484T **transthoracic exposure (eg, thoracotomy, transapical)**

🔲 0.00 🔲 0.00 **FUD** 000 `C` `80` `▢`

0485T-0486T

0485T **Optical coherence tomography (OCT) of middle ear, with interpretation and report; unilateral**

🔲 0.00 🔲 0.00 **FUD** XXX `01` `50` `▢`

0486T **bilateral**

🔲 0.00 🔲 0.00 **FUD** XXX `01` `▢`

0487T-0488T [0488T]

0487T **Biomechanical mapping, transvaginal, with report**

🔲 0.00 🔲 0.00 **FUD** XXX `01` `N1` `▢`

0488T **Resequenced code. See code following 0403T.**

0489T-0490T

EXCLUDES *Joint injection/aspiration (20600, 20604)*
Liposuction procedures (15876-15879)
Tissue grafts ([15769], 15771-15774)
Code also for complete procedure report both codes (0489T-0490T)

0489T **Autologous adipose-derived regenerative cell therapy for scleroderma in the hands; adipose tissue harvesting, isolation and preparation of harvested cells including incubation with cell dissociation enzymes, removal of non-viable cells and debris, determination of concentration and dilution of regenerative cells**

🔲 0.00 🔲 0.00 **FUD** 000 `E` `▢`

AMA: 2018,Sep,12

0490T **multiple injections in one or both hands**

EXCLUDES *Single injections*

🔲 0.00 🔲 0.00 **FUD** 000 `E` `▢`

AMA: 2018,Sep,12

0491T-0493T

0491T   Ablative laser treatment, non-contact, full field and fractional ablation, open wound, per day, total treatment surface area; first 20 sq cm or less

   📷 0.00   ✂ 0.00   **FUD** 000   T 62 ▭

+ 0492T   each additional 20 sq cm, or part thereof (List separately in addition to code for primary procedure)

   📷 0.00   ✂ 0.00   **FUD** ZZZ   N N1 ▭

   EXCLUDES   *Laser fenestration for scars (0479T-0480T)*
     Code first (0491T)

0493T   Near-infrared spectroscopy studies of lower extremity wounds (eg, for oxyhemoglobin measurement)

   📷 0.00   ✂ 0.00   **FUD** XXX   N N1 ▭

0494T-0496T

0494T   Surgical preparation and cannulation of marginal (extended) cadaver donor lung(s) to ex vivo organ perfusion system, including decannulation, separation from the perfusion system, and cold preservation of the allograft prior to implantation, when performed

   📷 0.00   ✂ 0.00   **FUD** XXX   C 80 ▭

0495T   Initiation and monitoring marginal (extended) cadaver donor lung(s) organ perfusion system by physician or qualified health care professional, including physiological and laboratory assessment (eg, pulmonary artery flow, pulmonary artery pressure, left atrial pressure, pulmonary vascular resistance, mean/peak and plateau airway pressure, dynamic compliance and perfusate gas analysis), including bronchoscopy and X ray when performed; first two hours in sterile field

   📷 0.00   ✂ 0.00   **FUD** XXX   C ▭

+ 0496T   each additional hour (List separately in addition to code for primary procedure)

   📷 0.00   ✂ 0.00   **FUD** ZZZ   C ▭

     Code first (0495T)

0497T-0498T

   EXCLUDES   *ECG event monitoring (93268, 93271-93272)*
     ECG rhythm strips (93040-93042)
     External ECG monitoring for more than 48 hours and less than 21 days (0295T-0298T)
     Remote telemetry (93228-93229)

0497T   External patient-activated, physician- or other qualified health care professional-prescribed, electrocardiographic rhythm derived event recorder without 24 hour attended monitoring; in-office connection

   📷 0.00   ✂ 0.00   **FUD** XXX   01 TC ▭

0498T   review and interpretation by a physician or other qualified health care professional per 30 days with at least one patient-generated triggered event

   📷 0.00   ✂ 0.00   **FUD** XXX   M 26 ▭

0499T-0500T

0499T   Cystourethroscopy, with mechanical dilation and urethral therapeutic drug delivery for urethral stricture or stenosis, including fluoroscopy, when performed

   📷 0.00   ✂ 0.00   **FUD** 000   E ▭

   EXCLUDES   *Cystourethroscopy for stricture (52281, 52283)*

0500T   Infectious agent detection by nucleic acid (DNA or RNA), human papillomavirus (HPV) for five or more separately reported high-risk HPV types (eg, 16, 18, 31, 33, 35, 39, 45, 51, 52, 56, 58, 59, 68) (ie, genotyping)

   📷 0.00   ✂ 0.00   **FUD** XXX   A ▭

   EXCLUDES   *Less than five high-risk HPV types ([87624, 87625])*

0501T-0523T [0523T]

   EXCLUDES   *Use of code more than one time for each CT angiogram*

0501T   Noninvasive estimated coronary fractional flow reserve (FFR) derived from coronary computed tomography angiography data using computation fluid dynamics physiologic simulation software analysis of functional data to assess the severity of coronary artery disease; data preparation and transmission, analysis of fluid dynamics and simulated maximal coronary hyperemia, generation of estimated FFR model, with anatomical data review in comparison with estimated FFR model to reconcile discordant data, interpretation and report

   INCLUDES   All components of complete test (0501T-0504T)
   📷 0.00   ✂ 0.00   **FUD** XXX   M ▭
   AMA: 2018,Sep,10

0502T   data preparation and transmission

   📷 0.00   ✂ 0.00   **FUD** XXX   N N1 TC ▭
   AMA: 2018,Sep,10

0503T   analysis of fluid dynamics and simulated maximal coronary hyperemia, and generation of estimated FFR model

   📷 0.00   ✂ 0.00   **FUD** XXX   S N1 TC ▭
   AMA: 2018,Sep,10

0504T   anatomical data review in comparison with estimated FFR model to reconcile discordant data, interpretation and report

   📷 0.00   ✂ 0.00   **FUD** XXX   M 26 ▭
   AMA: 2018,Sep,10

+ # 0523T   Intraprocedural coronary fractional flow reserve (FFR) with 3D functional mapping of color-coded FFR values for the coronary tree, derived from coronary angiogram data, for real-time review and interpretation of possible atherosclerotic stenosis(es) intervention (List separately in addition to code for primary procedure)

   📷 0.00   ✂ 0.00   **FUD** ZZZ   N1 80 ▭

   EXCLUDES   *3-D rendering with interpretation (76376-76377)*
     Coronary artery doppler studies (93571-93572)
     Noninvasive estimated coronary fractional flow reserve (FFR) (0501T-0504T)
     Procedure reported more than one time for each session
     Code first (93454-93461)

0505T-0514T [0510T, 0511T, 0512T, 0513T]

0505T   Endovascular femoral-popliteal arterial revascularization, with transcatheter placement of intravascular stent graft(s) and closure by any method, including percutaneous or open vascular access, ultrasound guidance for vascular access when performed, all catheterization(s) and intraprocedural roadmapping and imaging guidance necessary to complete the intervention, all associated radiological supervision and interpretation, when performed, with crossing of the occlusive lesion in an extraluminal fashion

   📷 0.00   ✂ 0.00   **FUD** YYY   80 ▭

   INCLUDES   All procedures performed on the same side:
     Catheterization (arterial and venous)
     Diagnostic imaging for arteriography
     Radiologic supervision and interpretation
     Ultrasound guidance (76937)

   EXCLUDES   *Balloon angioplasty of arteries other than dialysis circuit ([37248, 37249])*
     Revascularization femoral or popliteal artery (37224-37227)
     Venous stenting (37238-37239)

0506T   Macular pigment optical density measurement by heterochromatic flicker photometry, unilateral or bilateral, with interpretation and report

   📷 0.00   ✂ 0.00   **FUD** XXX   80 ▭

   AMA: 2018,Dec,6; 2018,Dec,6

26/TC PC/TC Only   A2-Z3 ASC Payment   50 Bilateral   ♂ Male Only   ♀ Female Only   📷 Facility RVU   ✂ Non-Facility RVU   ▭ CCI   ✗ CLIA
FUD Follow-up Days   CMS: IOM   AMA: CPT Asst   A-Y OPPSI   80/80 Surg Assist Allowed / w/Doc   🔲 Lab Crosswalk   🔲 Radiology Crosswalk

592   CPT © 2019 American Medical Association. All Rights Reserved.   © 2019 Optum360, LLC

0507T Near-infrared dual imaging (ie, simultaneous reflective and trans-illuminated light) of meibomian glands, unilateral or bilateral, with interpretation and report

⚙ 0.00   ⚒ 0.00   **FUD** XXX   80 ▣

EXCLUDES   *External ocular photography (92285)*
Tear film imaging (0330T)

0508T Pulse-echo ultrasound bone density measurement resulting in indicator of axial bone mineral density, tibia

⚙ 0.00   ⚒ 0.00   **FUD** XXX   72 80 ▣

0509T Electroretinography (ERG) with interpretation and report, pattern (PERG)

EXCLUDES   *Full field ERG (92273)*
Multifocal ERG (92274)

⚙ 2.24   ⚒ 2.24   **FUD** XXX   80 ▣

AMA: 2019,Jan,12

0510T Resequenced code. See code following 0335T.

0511T Resequenced code. See code following 0335T.

0512T Resequenced code. See code following 0102T.

0513T Resequenced code. See code following 0102T.

+ **0514T** Intraoperative visual axis identification using patient fixation (List separately in addition to code for primary procedure)

Code first (66982, 66984)

⚙ 0.00   ⚒ 0.00   **FUD** ZZZ   N1 ▣

AMA: 2018,Dec,6; 2018,Dec,6

0515T-0523T [0523T]

INCLUDES   Complete system with two components
Pulse generator comprised of battery and transmitter
Wireless endocardial left ventricular electrode

0515T Insertion of wireless cardiac stimulator for left ventricular pacing, including device interrogation and programming, and imaging supervision and interpretation, when performed; complete system (includes electrode and generator [transmitter and battery])

⚙ 0.00   ⚒ 0.00   **FUD** YYY   ▣

INCLUDES   Catheterization (93452-93453, 93458-93461, 93531-93533)
Creation of pockets
Electrode insertion
Imaging guidance (76000, 76998, 93303-93355)
Insertion complete wireless cardiac stimulator system
Interrogation of device (0521T)
Programming of device (0522T)
Pulse generator (battery and transmitter) (0517T)
Revision and repositioning

EXCLUDES   *Insertion of electrode as a separate procedure (0516T)*
Removal/replacement device or components (0518T-0520T)

0516T electrode only

⚙ 0.00   ⚒ 0.00   **FUD** YYY   ▣

INCLUDES   Catheterization (93452-93453, 93458-93461, 93531-93533)
Imaging guidance (76000, 76998, 93303-93355)
Interrogation of device (0521T)
Programming of device (0522T)

EXCLUDES   *Removal/replacement device or components (0518T-0520T)*

0517T pulse generator component(s) (battery and/or transmitter) only

⚙ 0.00   ⚒ 0.00   **FUD** YYY   ▣

INCLUDES   Catheterization (93452-93453, 93458-93461, 93531-93533)
Imaging guidance (76000, 76998, 93303-93355)
Interrogation of device (0521T)
Programming of device (0522T)

EXCLUDES   *Removal/replacement device or components (0518T-0520T)*

0518T Removal of only pulse generator component(s) (battery and/or transmitter) of wireless cardiac stimulator for left ventricular pacing

⚙ 0.00   ⚒ 0.00   **FUD** YYY   ▣

INCLUDES   Catheterization (93452-93453, 93458-93461, 93531-93533)
Imaging guidance (76000, 76998, 93303-93355)
Interrogation of device (0521T)
Programming of device (0522T)
Pulse generator (battery and transmitter) (0517T)

EXCLUDES   *Complete procedure (0515T)*
Insertion electrode only (0516T)
Removal/replacement device or components (0519T-0520T)

0519T Removal and replacement of wireless cardiac stimulator for left ventricular pacing; pulse generator component(s) (battery and/or transmitter)

⚙ 0.00   ⚒ 0.00   **FUD** YYY   ▣

INCLUDES   Catheterization (93452-93453, 93458-93461, 93531-93533)
Imaging guidance (76000, 76998, 93303-93355)
Interrogation of device (0521T)
Programming of device (0522T)
Pulse generator (battery and transmitter) (0517T)

EXCLUDES   *Complete procedure (0515T)*
Insertion electrode only (0516T)
Removal/replacement device or components (0518T)

0520T pulse generator component(s) (battery and/or transmitter), including placement of a new electrode

⚙ 0.00   ⚒ 0.00   **FUD** YYY   ▣

INCLUDES   Catheterization (93452-93453, 93458-93461, 93531-93533)
Imaging guidance (76000, 76998, 93303-93355)
Interrogation of device (0521T)
Programming of device (0522T)
Pulse generator (battery and transmitter) (0517T)

EXCLUDES   *Complete procedure (0515T)*
Insertion electrode only (0516T)
Removal only of device or components (0518T)

0521T Interrogation device evaluation (in person) with analysis, review and report, includes connection, recording, and disconnection per patient encounter, wireless cardiac stimulator for left ventricular pacing

⚙ 0.00   ⚒ 0.00   **FUD** XXX   ▣

INCLUDES   Programming of device (0522T)
Pulse generator (battery and transmitter) (0517T)

EXCLUDES   *Complete procedure (0515T)*
Insertion electrode only (0516T)
Removal/replacement device or components (0518T-0520T)

0522T Programming device evaluation (in person) with iterative adjustment of the implantable device to test the function of the device and select optimal permanent programmed values with analysis, including review and report, wireless cardiac stimulator for left ventricular pacing

⚙ 0.00   ⚒ 0.00   **FUD** XXX   ▣

INCLUDES   Interrogation of device (0521T)
Pulse generator (battery and transmitter) (0517T)

EXCLUDES   *Complete procedure (0515T)*
Insertion electrode only (0516T)
Interrogation of device (0521T)
Removal/replacement device or components (0518T-0520T)

0523T Resequenced code. See code following 0504T.

Category III Codes

0524T

0524T Endovenous catheter directed chemical ablation with balloon isolation of incompetent extremity vein, open or percutaneous, including all vascular access, catheter manipulation, diagnostic imaging, imaging guidance and monitoring
🕮 0.00   ⚕ 0.00   **FUD** YYY   [G2] [50] [▣]

0525T-0532T

0525T Insertion or replacement of intracardiac ischemia monitoring system, including testing of the lead and monitor, initial system programming, and imaging supervision and interpretation; complete system (electrode and implantable monitor)
🕮 0.00   ⚕ 0.00   **FUD** YYY   [J8] [▣]

INCLUDES Electrocardiography (93000, 93005, 93010)
Interrogation of device (0529T)
Programming of device (0528T)

EXCLUDES Removal of intracardiac ischemia monitor or components (0530T-0532T)

0526T electrode only
🕮 0.00   ⚕ 0.00   **FUD** YYY   [J8] [▣]

INCLUDES Electrocardiography (93000, 93005, 93010)
Interrogation of device (0529T)
Programming of device (0528T)

EXCLUDES Removal of intracardiac ischemia monitor or components (0530T-0532T)

0527T implantable monitor only
🕮 0.00   ⚕ 0.00   **FUD** YYY   [G2] [▣]

INCLUDES Electrocardiography (93000, 93005, 93010)
Interrogation of device (0529T)
Programming of device (0528T)

EXCLUDES Removal of intracardiac ischemia monitor or components (0530T-0532T)

0528T Programming device evaluation (in person) of intracardiac ischemia monitoring system with iterative adjustment of programmed values, with analysis, review, and report
🕮 0.00   ⚕ 0.00   **FUD** XXX   [▣]

INCLUDES Electrocardiography (93000, 93005, 93010)

EXCLUDES Insertion/replacement intracardiac ischemia monitor or components (0525T-0527T)
Interrogation of device (0529T)
Removal of intracardiac ischemia monitor or components (0530T-0532T)

0529T Interrogation device evaluation (in person) of intracardiac ischemia monitoring system with analysis, review, and report
🕮 0.00   ⚕ 0.00   **FUD** XXX   [▣]

INCLUDES Electrocardiography (93000, 93005, 93010)

EXCLUDES Insertion/replacement electrode only (0526T)
Insertion/replacement intracardiac ischemia monitor or comoponents (0525T-0527T)
Programming of device (0528T)
Removal of intracardiac ischemia monitor or components (0530T-0532T)

0530T Removal of intracardiac ischemia monitoring system, including all imaging supervision and interpretation; complete system (electrode and implantable monitor)
🕮 0.00   ⚕ 0.00   **FUD** YYY   [G2] [▣]

EXCLUDES Interrogation of device (0529T)
Programming of device (0528T)

0531T electrode only
🕮 0.00   ⚕ 0.00   **FUD** YYY   [G2] [▣]

EXCLUDES Interrogation of device (0529T)
Programming of device (0528T)

0532T implantable monitor only
🕮 0.00   ⚕ 0.00   **FUD** YYY   [G2] [▣]

EXCLUDES Interrogation of device (0529T)
Programming of device (0528T)

0533T-0536T

0533T Continuous recording of movement disorder symptoms, including bradykinesia, dyskinesia, and tremor for 6 days up to 10 days; includes set-up, patient training, configuration of monitor, data upload, analysis and initial report configuration, download review, interpretation and report
🕮 0.00   ⚕ 0.00   **FUD** XXX   [▣]

0534T set-up, patient training, configuration of monitor
🕮 0.00   ⚕ 0.00   **FUD** XXX   [▣]

0535T data upload, analysis and initial report configuration
🕮 0.00   ⚕ 0.00   **FUD** XXX   [▣]

0536T download review, interpretation and report
🕮 0.00   ⚕ 0.00   **FUD** XXX   [▣]

0537T-0540T

INCLUDES Administration of genetically modified cells for the treatment of serious diseases (e.g., cancer)
Evaluation prior to, during, and after CAR-T cell administration
Infusion of fluids and supportive medications provided with administration
Management of clinical staff
Management of untoward events (e.g, nausea)
Physician certification of processing of cells
Physician presence during cell administration
Code also care provided that is not directly related to CAR-T cell administration (e.g., other medical problems) may be reported separately using appropriate E&M code and modifier 25

0537T Chimeric antigen receptor T-cell (CAR-T) therapy; harvesting of blood-derived T lymphocytes for development of genetically modified autologous CAR-T cells, per day

EXCLUDES Use more than one time per day despite number of times cells are collected

🕮 0.00   ⚕ 0.00   **FUD** XXX   [▣]

AMA: 2019,Jun,5

0538T preparation of blood-derived T lymphocytes for transportation (eg, cryopreservation, storage)
🕮 0.00   ⚕ 0.00   **FUD** XXX   [▣]

AMA: 2019,Jun,5

0539T receipt and preparation of CAR-T cells for administration
🕮 0.00   ⚕ 0.00   **FUD** XXX   [▣]

AMA: 2019,Jun,5

0540T CAR-T cell administration, autologous

EXCLUDES Use more than one time per day despite number of units administered

🕮 0.00   ⚕ 0.00   **FUD** YYY   [▣]

AMA: 2019,Jun,5

0541T-0542T

0541T Myocardial imaging by magnetocardiography (MCG) for detection of cardiac ischemia, by signal acquisition using minimum 36 channel grid, generation of magnetic-field time-series images, quantitative analysis of magnetic dipoles, machine learning-derived clinical scoring, and automated report generation, single study;
🕮 0.00   ⚕ 0.00   **FUD** XXX   [TC] [▣]

0542T interpretation and report
🕮 0.00   ⚕ 0.00   **FUD** XXX   [26] [▣]

0543T

EXCLUDES Transesophageal echocardiography (93355)

● **0543T** Transapical mitral valve repair, including transthoracic echocardiography, when performed, with placement of artificial chordae tendineae
🕮 0.00   ⚕ 0.00   **FUD** YYY   [80]

0544T-0545T

INCLUDES Adjustment/deployment of reconstruction device
Catheterization
Insertion temporary pacemaker
Vascular access and closure

EXCLUDES Fluoroscopic guidance (76000)
Percutaneous mitral valve repair
Transcatheter implantation/replacement mitral valve

Code also diagnostic angiography or catheterizIation and append modifier 59, when:
Prior study available but inadequate or the patient's condition has changed
Prior study not available and full diagnostic study performed

Code also when performed:
Balloon pump insertion (33967, 33970, 33973)
Central bypass (33369)
Peripheral bypass (33367-33368)
Ventricular assist device (33990-33993)

● **0544T** **Transcatheter mitral valve annulus reconstruction, with implantation of adjustable annulus reconstruction device, percutaneous approach including transseptal puncture**

    🔲 0.00   ⚕ 0.00   **FUD** YYY   80

      EXCLUDES Transcatheter implantation/replacement mitral valve (0483T)
                Transcatheter mitral valve repair (33418-33419)
                Transcatheter mitral valve repair via coronary sinus (0345T)

● **0545T** **Transcatheter tricuspid valve annulus reconstruction with implantation of adjustable annulus reconstruction device, percutaneous approach**

    🔲 0.00   ⚕ 0.00   **FUD** YYY   80

      EXCLUDES Repositioning/plication of tricuspid valve (33468)

0546T

EXCLUDES Use of code for re-excision of site
Use of code more than one time per partial mastectomy site

● **0546T** **Radiofrequency spectroscopy, real time, intraoperative margin assessment, at the time of partial mastectomy, with report**

    🔲 0.00   ⚕ 0.00   **FUD** YYY   80

0547T

● **0547T** **Bone-material quality testing by microindentation(s) of the tibia(s), with results reported as a score**

    🔲 0.00   ⚕ 0.00   **FUD** XXX   80

0548T-0551T

● **0548T** **Transperineal periurethral balloon continence device; bilateral placement, including cystoscopy and fluoroscopy**

    🔲 0.00   ⚕ 0.00   **FUD** YYY   J8 80

● **0549T** **unilateral placement, including cystoscopy and fluoroscopy**

    🔲 0.00   ⚕ 0.00   **FUD** YYY   J8 80

● **0550T** **removal, each balloon**

    🔲 0.00   ⚕ 0.00   **FUD** YYY   G2 80

● **0551T** **adjustment of balloon(s) fluid volume**

    🔲 0.00   ⚕ 0.00   **FUD** YYY   R2 80

      EXCLUDES Insertion or removal periurethral balloon continence device (0548T-0550T)

0552T

● **0552T** **Low-level laser therapy, dynamic photonic and dynamic thermokinetic energies, provided by a physician or other qualified health care professional**

    🔲 0.00   ⚕ 0.00   **FUD** YYY   80

0553T

EXCLUDES Angiography of extremity (75710)
Endovascular revascularization (37220-37221, 37224, 37226, 37238)
Injection for venography (36005)
Insertion catheter/needle, upper or lower extremity artery (36140)
Selective catheter placement (36011-36012, 36245-36246)
Transluminal balloon angioplasty ([37248])
Venography (75820)

● **0553T** **Percutaneous transcatheter placement of iliac arteriovenous anastomosis implant, inclusive of all radiological supervision and interpretation, intraprocedural roadmapping, and imaging guidance necessary to complete the intervention**

    🔲 0.00   ⚕ 0.00   **FUD** YYY   80

0554T-0557T

● **0554T** **Bone strength and fracture risk using finite element analysis of functional data, and bone-mineral density, utilizing data from a computed tomography scan; retrieval and transmission of the scan data, assessment of bone strength and fracture risk and bone mineral density, interpretation and report**

    🔲 0.00   ⚕ 0.00   **FUD** XXX   80

      INCLUDES Assessment, interpretation and report, and retrieval and transmission of data (0555T-0557T)

● **0555T** **retrieval and transmission of the scan data**

    🔲 0.00   ⚕ 0.00   **FUD** XXX   80

● **0556T** **assessment of bone strength and fracture risk and bone mineral density**

    🔲 0.00   ⚕ 0.00   **FUD** XXX   80

● **0557T** **interpretation and report**

    🔲 0.00   ⚕ 0.00   **FUD** XXX   80

0558T

EXCLUDES Computed tomography:
    abdominal aorta (75635)
    abdomen/pelvis (72191-72194, 74150-74178)
    chest/thorax (71250-71270, 71275)
    colonography (74261-74263)
    heart (75571-75574)
    spine (72125-72133)
    whole body (78816)

● **0558T** **Computed tomography scan taken for the purpose of biomechanical computed tomography analysis**

    🔲 0.00   ⚕ 0.00   **FUD** XXX   Z2 80

0559T-0562T

EXCLUDES 3D rendering (76376-76377)

● **0559T** **Anatomic model 3D-printed from image data set(s); first individually prepared and processed component of an anatomic structure**

    🔲 0.00   ⚕ 0.00   **FUD** XXX   80

      INCLUDES 3D printed anatomical model production

● + **0560T** **each additional individually prepared and processed component of an anatomic structure (List separately in addition to code for primary procedure)**

    🔲 0.00   ⚕ 0.00   **FUD** ZZZ   80

      INCLUDES 3D printed anatomical model production
      Code first (0559T)

● **0561T** **Anatomic guide 3D-printed and designed from image data set(s); first anatomic guide**

    🔲 0.00   ⚕ 0.00   **FUD** XXX   80

      INCLUDES 3D printed cutting or drilling guides for use during surgery

● + **0562T** **each additional anatomic guide (List separately in addition to code for primary procedure)**

    🔲 0.00   ⚕ 0.00   **FUD** ZZZ   80

      INCLUDES 3D printed cutting or drilling guides for use during surgery
      Code first (0561T)

0563T-0564T [0563T]

0563T   **Resequenced code. See code before numeric code 0208T.**

● New Code   ▲ Revised Code   ○ Reinstated   ● New Web Release   ▲ Revised Web Release   + Add-on   Unlisted   Not Covered   # Resequenced
50 Optum Mod 50 Exempt   ⊘ AMA Mod 51 Exempt   51 Optum Mod 51 Exempt   63 Mod 63 Exempt   ✗ Non-FDA Drug   ★ Telemedicine   M Maternity   A Age Edit

- **0564T** Oncology, chemotherapeutic drug cytotoxicity assay of cancer stem cells (CSCs), from cultured CSCs and primary tumor cells, categorical drug response reported based on percent of cytotoxicity observed, a minimum of 14 drugs or drug combinations

0565T-0566T

- **0565T** Autologous cellular implant derived from adipose tissue for the treatment of osteoarthritis of the knees; tissue harvesting and cellular implant creation

  > _EXCLUDES_ Other tissue grafts ([15769], 15771-15774)

- **0566T** injection of cellular implant into knee joint including ultrasound guidance, unilateral

  > _INCLUDES_ Guidance for needle placement:
  > Fluoroscopy (77002)
  > Ultrasound (76942)
  > _EXCLUDES_ Arthrocentesis, with or without imaging guidance (20610-20611)

0567T-0568T

- **0567T** Permanent fallopian tube occlusion with degradable biopolymer implant, transcervical approach, including transvaginal ultrasound

  > _INCLUDES_ Transvaginal ultrasound (76830)
  > _EXCLUDES_ Catheter insertion and introduction of saline/contrast for sonohysterography or hysterosalpingography (58340)
  > Hysterosalpingography (74740)
  > Nonobstetric pelvic ultrasound (76856-76857)
  > Surgical hysteroscopy with bilateral occlusion of fallopian tube (58565)
  > Transcervical catheterization of fallopian tube (74742)

- **0568T** Introduction of mixture of saline and air for sonosalpingography to confirm occlusion of fallopian tubes, transcervical approach, including transvaginal ultrasound and pelvic ultrasound

  > _INCLUDES_ Transvaginal ultrasound (76830)
  > _EXCLUDES_ Catheter insertion and introduction of saline/contrast for sonohysterography or hysterosalpingography (58340)
  > Hysterosalpingography (74740)
  > Nonobstetric pelvic ultrasound (76856-76857)
  > Sonohysterography (SIS) (76831)
  > Surgical hysteroscopy with bilateral occlusion of fallopian tube (58565)
  > Transcervical catheterization of fallopian tube (74742)

0569T-0570T

> _INCLUDES_ Adjustment/deployment of prosthetic device
> Catheterization
> Fluoroscopic guidance (76000)
> Intracardiac echocardiography (93662)
> Vascular access and closure
> _EXCLUDES_ Open tricuspid valve procedures (33460, 33463-33465, 33468)

Code also diagnostic angiography or catheteriziation and append modifier 59, when:
Prior study available but inadequate or the patient's condition has changed
Prior study not available and full diagnostic study performed
Code also when performed:
Balloon pump insertion (33967, 33970, 33973)
Central bypass (33369)
Peripheral bypass (33367-33368)
Ventricular assist device (33990-33993)
TEE, when done by different operator (93355)

- **0569T** Transcatheter tricuspid valve repair, percutaneous approach; initial prosthesis

  > _EXCLUDES_ Use of code more than once per session

- **+ 0570T** each additional prosthesis during same session (List separately in addition to code for primary procedure)

  🔷 0.00   ⚖ 0.00   **FUD** 000

  Code first (0569T)

0571T-0580T

> _EXCLUDES_ Defibrillator or pacemaker device evaluations (93279-93284, 93285-93289, 93290-93298)
> Implantable defibrillator procedures (33215-33220, 33223-33226, 33240-33249 [33230, 33231, 33262, 33263, 33264])
> Pacemaker procedures (33202-33220 [33221], 33222-33226, 33233-33238 [33227, 33228, 33229])
> Subcutaneous implantable defibrillator system procedures:
> Electrophysiological evaluation (93644)
> Insertion of electrode ([33271])
> Insertion/replacement entire system ([33270])
> Interrogation ([93261])
> Programming ([93260])
> Removal of electrode ([33272])
> Repositioning of electrode ([33273])
> Transcatheter permanent leadless pacemaker procedures:
> Insertion or replacement ([33274])

- **0571T** Insertion or replacement of implantable cardioverter-defibrillator system with substernal electrode(s), including all imaging guidance and electrophysiological evaluation (includes defibrillation threshold evaluation, induction of arrhythmia, evaluation of sensing for arrhythmia termination, and programming or reprogramming of sensing or therapeutic parameters), when performed

  > _INCLUDES_ Imaging guidance
  > Programming, interrogation, and electrophysiological evaluations (0575T-0577T)
  > _EXCLUDES_ Substernal electrode insertion only (0572T)

  Code also removal of implantable cardioverter-defibrillator generator and substernal electrode(s), when total system is replaced:
  Electrode(s) (0573T)
  Generator (0580T)

- **0572T** Insertion of substernal implantable defibrillator electrode

  > _INCLUDES_ Imaging guidance
  > Programming, interrogation, and electrophysiological evaluations (0575T-0577T)
  > _EXCLUDES_ Insertion of generator and electrode (0571T)

- **0573T** Removal of substernal implantable defibrillator electrode

  > _INCLUDES_ Imaging guidance
  > _EXCLUDES_ Programming, interrogation, and electrophysiological evaluations (0575T-0577T)

  Code also removal of implantable cardioverter-defibrillator generator and insertion of new generator/electrode, when total system is replaced:
  Insertion of new system (0571T)
  Removal of generator (0580T)

- **0574T** Repositioning of previously implanted substernal implantable defibrillator-pacing electrode

  > _INCLUDES_ Imaging guidance
  > _EXCLUDES_ Programming, interrogation, and electrophysiological evaluations (0575T-0577T)

- **0575T** Programming device evaluation (in person) of implantable cardioverter-defibrillator system with substernal electrode, with iterative adjustment of the implantable device to test the function of the device and select optimal permanent programmed values with analysis, review and report by a physician or other qualified health care professional

  > _EXCLUDES_ Interrogation of device (0576T)
  > Programming at time of:
  > Electrode insertion (0572T)
  > Electrode removal (0573T)
  > Electrode repositioning (0574T)
  > Generator removal (0580T)
  > Insertion/replacement entire system (0571T)

26/TC PC/TC Only   A2-Z3 ASC Payment   50 Bilateral   ♂ Male Only   ♀ Female Only   🔷 Facility RVU   ⚖ Non-Facility RVU   CCI   CLIA
FUD Follow-up Days   CMS: IOM   AMA: CPT Asst   A-Y OPPSI   80/80 Surg Assist Allowed / w/Doc   Lab Crosswalk   Radiology Crosswalk

CPT © 2019 American Medical Association. All Rights Reserved.   © 2019 Optum360, LLC

596

● 0576T **Interrogation device evaluation (in person) of implantable cardioverter-defibrillator system with substernal electrode, with analysis, review and report by a physician or other qualified health care professional, includes connection, recording and disconnection per patient encounter**

EXCLUDES *Interrogation at time of:*
Electrode insertion (0572T)
Electrode removal (0573T)
Electrode repositioning (0574T)
Insertion/replacement entire system (0571T)
Programming of device (0575T)

● 0577T **Electrophysiological evaluation of implantable cardioverter-defibrillator system with substernal electrode (includes defibrillation threshold evaluation, induction of arrhythmia, evaluation of sensing for arrhythmia termination, and programming or reprogramming of sensing or therapeutic parameters)**

EXCLUDES *Electrophysiological evaluation at time of:*
Electrode insertion (0572T)
Electrode removal (0573T)
Electrode repositioning (0574T)
Generator removal (0580T)
Insertion/replacement entire system (0571T)

● 0578T **Interrogation device evaluation(s) (remote), up to 90 days, substernal lead implantable cardioverter-defibrillator system with interim analysis, review(s) and report(s) by a physician or other qualified health care professional**

EXCLUDES *In person device interrogation (0576T)*
Use of code more than once per 90 days

● 0579T **Interrogation device evaluation(s) (remote), up to 90 days, substernal lead implantable cardioverter-defibrillator system, remote data acquisition(s), receipt of transmissions and technician review, technical support and distribution of results**

EXCLUDES *In person device interrogation (0576T)*
Use of code more than once per 90 days

● 0580T **Removal of substernal implantable defibrillator pulse generator only**

EXCLUDES *Programming, interrogation, and electrophysiological evaluations (0575T-0577T)*
Code also removal of substernal electrode and insertion of new generator/electrode, when total system is replaced:
Insertion of new system (0571T)
Removal of electrode (0573T)

0581T-0582T

● 0581T **Ablation, malignant breast tumor(s), percutaneous, cryotherapy, including imaging guidance when performed, unilateral**

INCLUDES Ultrasound for:
Breast imaging (76641-76642)
Monitoring of tissue ablation (76940)
Needle placement (76942)

EXCLUDES *Cryoablation for breast fibroadenoma(s) (19105)*
Use of code more than once per treated breast

● 0582T **Transurethral ablation of malignant prostate tissue by high-energy water vapor thermotherapy, including intraoperative imaging and needle guidance**

INCLUDES 3D rendering (76376-76377)
Cystourethroscopy (52000)
Imaging guidance for:
Needle placement (76942, 77021)
Tissue ablation monitoring (76940, 77022)
MRI of pelvis (72195-72197)
Transrectal ultrasound (76872)

EXCLUDES *Destruction by radiofrequency-generated water vapor thermotherapy for benign prostatic hypertrophy (BPH) (53854)*

0583T

● 0583T **Tympanostomy (requiring insertion of ventilating tube), using an automated tube delivery system, iontophoresis local anesthesia**

INCLUDES Binocular microscopy (92504)
Iontophoresis (97033)
Operating microscope (69990)

EXCLUDES *Myringotomy (69420-69421)*
Removal of impacted cerumen (69209-69210)
Tympanostomy without the use of automated delivery system (69433, 69436)

0584T-0586T

● 0584T **Islet cell transplant, includes portal vein catheterization and infusion, including all imaging, including guidance, and radiological supervision and interpretation, when performed; percutaneous**

● 0585T **laparoscopic**

● 0586T **open**

0587T-0590T

● 0587T **Percutaneous implantation or replacement of integrated single device neurostimulation system including electrode array and receiver or pulse generator, including analysis, programming, and imaging guidance when performed, posterior tibial nerve**

INCLUDES Electronic analysis (95970-95972, 0589T-0590T)

EXCLUDES *Insertion of other neurostimulator devices (64555, 64566, 64575, 64590)*
Revision or removal of integrated neurostimulation system (0588T)

● 0588T **Revision or removal of integrated single device neurostimulation system including electrode array and receiver or pulse generator, including analysis, programming, and imaging guidance when performed, posterior tibial nerve**

INCLUDES Electronic analysis (95970-95972, 0589T-0590T)

EXCLUDES *Initial insertion or replacement of integrated neurostimulation system (0587T)*
Insertion of other neurostimulator devices (64555, 64566, 64575, 64590)

● 0589T **Electronic analysis with simple programming of implanted integrated neurostimulation system (eg, electrode array and receiver), including contact group(s), amplitude, pulse width, frequency (Hz), on/off cycling, burst, dose lockout, patient-selectable parameters, responsive neurostimulation, detection algorithms, closed-loop parameters, and passive parameters, when performed by physician or other qualified health care professional, posterior tibial nerve, 1-3 parameters**

EXCLUDES *Electronic analysis of other implanted neurostimulators (95970-95977, [95983, 95984])*
Electronic analysis with complex programming (0590T)
Use of code at time of insertion, replacement, revision, or removal of integrated neurostimulation system (0587T-0588T)
Use of code at time of insertion, replacement, revision, or removal of other neurostimulator device (generator and/or electrode) (43647-43648, 43881-43882, 61850-61888, 63650, 63655, 63661-63688, 64553-64595)

● **0590T** **Electronic analysis with complex programming of implanted integrated neurostimulation system (eg, electrode array and receiver), including contact group(s), amplitude, pulse width, frequency (Hz), on/off cycling, burst, dose lockout, patient-selectable parameters, responsive neurostimulation, detection algorithms, closed-loop parameters, and passive parameters, when performed by physician or other qualified health care professional, posterior tibial nerve, 4 or more parameters**

> EXCLUDES *Electronic analysis of other implanted neurostimulators (95970-95977, [95983, 95984])*
> *Electronic analysis with simple programming (0589T)*
> *Use of code at time of insertion, replacement, revision, or removal of integrated neurostimulation system (0587T-0588T)*
> *Use of code at time of insertion, replacement, revision, or removal of other neurostimulator device (generator and/or electrode) (43647-43648, 43881-43882, 61850-61888, 63650, 63655, 63661-63688, 64553-64595)*

0591T-0593T

> INCLUDES Nonphysician health care professional coach trained to assist patients in obtaining improved health and well-being goals through the use of:
> Accountability
> Active learning processes
> *Self discovery*

● **0591T** **Health and well-being coaching face-to-face; individual, initial assessment**

> EXCLUDES *Health and well-being coaching, follow-up session (0592T)*
> *Health and well-being coaching, group session (0593T)*

● **0592T** **individual, follow-up session, at least 30 minutes**

> EXCLUDES *Diabetic preventative behavior change program ([0488T])*
> *Education/training for self-management (98960)*
> *Health and well-being coaching, group session (0593T)*
> *Health and well-being coaching, initial session (0591T)*
> *Health behavior assessment/intervention (96156-96159)*
> *Medical nutrition therapy (97802-97804)*

● **0593T** **group (2 or more individuals), at least 30 minutes**

> EXCLUDES *Diabetic preventative behavior change program (0403T)*
> *Education/training for self-management (98961-98962)*
> *Group therapy procedure (97150)*
> *Health and well-being coaching, individual (0591T-0592T)*
> *Health behavior assessment/intervention ([96164, 96165])*

Appendix A — Modifiers

CPT Modifiers

A modifier is a two-position alpha or numeric code appended to a CPT® code to clarify the services being billed. Modifiers provide a means by which a service can be altered without changing the procedure code. They add more information, such as the anatomical site, to the code. In addition, they help to eliminate the appearance of duplicate billing and unbundling. Modifiers are used to increase accuracy in reimbursement, coding consistency, editing, and to capture payment data.

22   **Increased Procedural Services:** When the work required to provide a service is substantially greater than typically required, it may be identified by adding modifier 22 to the usual procedure code. Documentation must support the substantial additional work and the reason for the additional work (ie, increased intensity, time, technical difficulty of procedure, severity of patient's condition, physical and mental effort required).
Note: This modifier should not be appended to an E/M service.

23   **Unusual Anesthesia:** Occasionally, a procedure, which usually requires either no anesthesia or local anesthesia, because of unusual circumstances must be done under general anesthesia. This circumstance may be reported by adding modifier 23 to the procedure code of the basic service.

24   **Unrelated Evaluation and Management Service by the Same Physician or Other Qualified Health Care Professional During a Postoperative Period:** The physician or other qualified health care professional may need to indicate that an evaluation and management service was performed during a postoperative period for a reason(s) unrelated to the original procedure. This circumstance may be reported by adding modifier 24 to the appropriate level of E/M service.

25   **Significant, Separately Identifiable Evaluation and Management Service by the Same Physician or Other Qualified Health Care Professional on the Same Day of the Procedure or Other Service:** It may be necessary to indicate that on the day a procedure or service identified by a CPT code was performed, the patient's condition required a significant, separately identifiable E/M service above and beyond the other service provided or beyond the usual preoperative and postoperative care associated with the procedure that was performed. A significant, separately identifiable E/M service is defined or substantiated by documentation that satisfies the relevant criteria for the respective E/M service to be reported (see Evaluation and Management Services Guidelines for instructions on determining level of E/M service). The E/M service may be prompted by the symptom or condition for which the procedure and/or service was provided. As such, different diagnoses are not required for reporting of the E/M services on the same date. This circumstance may be reported by adding modifier 25 to the appropriate level of E/M service.
Note: This modifier is not used to report an E/M service that resulted in a decision to perform surgery. See modifier 57. For significant, separately identifiable non-E/M services, see modifier 59.

26   **Professional Component:** Certain procedures are a combination of a physician or other qualified health care professional component and a technical component. When the physician or other qualified health care professional component is reported separately, the service may be identified by adding modifier 26 to the usual procedure number.

32   **Mandated Services:** Services related to mandated consultation and/or related services (eg, third party payer, governmental, legislative or regulatory requirement) may be identified by adding modifier 32 to the basic procedure.

33   **Preventive Services:** When the primary purpose of the service is the delivery of an evidence based service in accordance with a US Preventive Services Task Force A or B rating in effect and other preventive services identified in preventive services mandates (legislative or regulatory), the service may be identified by adding 33 to the procedure. For separately reported services specifically identified as preventive, the modifier should not be used.

47   **Anesthesia by Surgeon:** Regional or general anesthesia provided by the surgeon may be reported by adding modifier 47 to the basic service. (This does not include local anesthesia.)
Note: Modifier 47 would not be used as a modifier for the anesthesia procedures.

50   **Bilateral Procedure:** Unless otherwise identified in the listings, bilateral procedures that are performed at the same session should be identified by adding modifier 50 to the appropriate 5 digit code.
Note: This modifier should not be appended to designated "add-on" codes (see Appendix F).

51   **Multiple Procedures:** When multiple procedures, other than E/M services, Physical Medicine and Rehabilitation services or provision of supplies (eg, vaccines), are performed at the same session by the same individual, the primary procedure or service may be reported as listed. The additional procedure(s) or service(s) may be identified by appending modifier 51 to the additional procedure or service code(s).
Note: This modifier should not be appended to designated "add-on" codes (see Appendix F).

52   **Reduced Services:** Under certain circumstances a service or procedure is partially reduced or eliminated at the discretion of the physician or other qualified health care professional. Under these circumstances the service provided can be identified by its usual procedure number and the addition of modifier 52, signifying that the service is reduced. This provides a means of reporting reduced services without disturbing the identification of the basic service.
Note: For hospital outpatient reporting of a previously scheduled procedure/service that is partially reduced or cancelled as a result of extenuating circumstances or those that threaten the well-being of the patient prior to or after administration of anesthesia, see modifiers 73 and 74 (see modifiers approved for ASC hospital outpatient use).

53   **Discontinued Procedure:** Under certain circumstances, the physician or other qualified health care professional may elect to terminate a surgical or diagnostic procedure. Due to extenuating circumstances or those that threaten the well being of the patient, it may be necessary to indicate that a surgical or diagnostic procedure was started but discontinued. This circumstance may be reported by adding modifier 53 to the code reported by the physician for the discontinued procedure.
Note: This modifier is not used to report the elective cancellation of a procedure prior to the patient's anesthesia induction and/or surgical preparation in the operating suite. For outpatient hospital/ambulatory surgery center (ASC) reporting of a previously scheduled procedure/service that is partially reduced or cancelled as a result of extenuating circumstances or those that threaten the well being of the patient prior to or after administration of anesthesia, see modifiers 73 and 74 (see modifiers approved for ASC hospital outpatient use).

54   **Surgical Care Only:** When 1 physician or other qualified health care professional performs a surgical procedure and another provides preoperative and/or postoperative management, surgical services may be identified by adding modifier 54 to the usual procedure number.

55   **Postoperative Management Only:** When 1 physician or other qualified health care professional performed the postoperative management and another performed the surgical procedure, the postoperative component may be identified by adding modifier 55 to the usual procedure number.

56   **Preoperative Management Only:** When 1 physician or other qualified health care professional performed the preoperative care and evaluation and another performed the surgical procedure, the preoperative component may be identified by adding modifier 56 to the usual procedure number.

57   **Decision for Surgery:** An evaluation and management service that resulted in the initial decision to perform the surgery may be identified by adding modifier 57 to the appropriate level of E/M service.

58   Staged or Related Procedure or Service by the Same Physician or Other Qualified Health Care Professional During the Postoperative Period: It may be necessary to indicate that the performance of a procedure or service during the postoperative period was (a) planned or anticipated (staged); (b) more extensive than the original procedure; or (c) for therapy following a surgical procedure. This circumstance may be reported by adding modifier 58 to the staged or related procedure.
Note: For treatment of a problem that requires a return to the operating/procedure room (eg, unanticipated clinical condition), see modifier 78.

59   Distinct Procedural Service: Under certain circumstances, it may be necessary to indicate that a procedure or service was distinct or independent from other non-E/M services performed on the same day. Modifier 59 is used to identify procedures/services, other than E/M services, that are not normally reported together but are appropriate under the circumstances. Documentation must support a different session, different procedure or surgery, different site or organ system, separate incision/excision, separate lesion, or separate injury (or area of injury in extensive injuries) not ordinarily encountered or performed on the same day by the same individual. However, when another already established modifier is appropriate it should be used rather than modifier 59. Only if no more descriptive modifier is available, and the use of modifier 59 best explains the circumstances, should modifier 59 be used.
Note: Modifier 59 should not be appended to an E/M service. To report a separate and distinct E/M service with a non-E/M service performed on the same date, see modifier 25.

62   Two Surgeons: When 2 surgeons work together as primary surgeons performing distinct part(s) of a procedure, each surgeon should report his/her distinct operative work by adding modifier 62 to the procedure code and any associated add-on code(s) for that procedure as long as both surgeons continue to work together as primary surgeons. Each surgeon should report the co-surgery once using the same procedure code. If additional procedure(s) (including add-on procedure[s]) are performed during the same surgical session, separate code(s) may also be reported with modifier 62 added.
Note: If a co-surgeon acts as an assistant in the performance of additional procedure(s), other than those reported with the modifier 62, during the same surgical session, those services may be reported using separate procedure code(s) with modifier 80 or modifier 82 added, as appropriate.

63   Procedure Performed on Infants less than 4 kg: Procedures performed on neonates and infants up to a present body weight of 4 kg may involve significantly increased complexity and physician or other qualified health care professional work commonly associated with these patients. This circumstance may be reported by adding modifier 63 to the procedure number.
Note: Unless otherwise designated, this modifier may only be appended to procedures/services listed in the 20100-69990 code series and 92920, 92928, 92953, 92960, 92986, 92987, 92990, 92997, 92998, 93312, 93313, 93314, 93315, 93316, 93317, 93318, 93452, 93505, 93530, 93531, 93532, 93533, 93561, 93562, 93563, 93564, 93568, 93580, 93582, 93590, 93591, 93592, 93615, 93616 from the Medicine/Cardiovascular section.

Modifier 63 should not be appended to any CPT codes listed in the Evaluation and Management Services, Anesthesia, Radiology, Pathology/Laboratory, or Medicine sections (other than those identified above from the Medicine/Cardiovascular section).

66   Surgical Team: Under some circumstances, highly complex procedures (requiring the concomitant services of several physicians or other qualified health care professionals, often of different specialties, plus other highly skilled, specially trained personnel, various types of complex equipment) are carried out under the "surgical team" concept. Such circumstances may be identified by each participating individual with the addition of modifier 66 to the basic procedure number used for reporting services.

76   Repeat Procedure or Service by Same Physician or Other Qualified Health Care Professional: It may be necessary to indicate that a procedure or service was repeated by the same physician or other qualified health care professional subsequent to the original procedure or service. This circumstance may be reported by adding modifier 76 to the repeated procedure or service.
Note: This modifier should not be appended to an E/M service.

77   Repeat Procedure by Another Physician or Other Qualified Health Care Professional: It may be necessary to indicate that a basic procedure or service was repeated by another physician or other qualified health care professional subsequent to the original procedure or service. This circumstance may be reported by adding modifier 77 to the repeated procedure or service.
Note: This modifier should not be appended to an E/M service.

78   Unplanned Return to the Operating/Procedure Room by the Same Physician or Other Qualified Health Care Professional Following Initial Procedure for a Related Procedure During the Postoperative Period: It may be necessary to indicate that another procedure was performed during the postoperative period of the initial procedure (unplanned procedure following initial procedure). When this procedure is related to the first, and requires the use of an operating/procedure room, it may be reported by adding modifier 78 to the related procedure. (For repeat procedures, see modifier 76.)

79   Unrelated Procedure or Service by the Same Physician or Other Qualified Health Care Professional During the Postoperative Period: The individual may need to indicate that the performance of a procedure or service during the postoperative period was unrelated to the original procedure. This circumstance may be reported by using modifier 79. (For repeat procedures on the same day, see modifier 76.)

80   Assistant Surgeon: Surgical assistant services may be identified by adding modifier 80 to the usual procedure number(s).

81   Minimum Assistant Surgeon: Minimum surgical assistant services are identified by adding modifier 81 to the usual procedure number.

82   Assistant Surgeon (when qualified resident surgeon not available): The unavailability of a qualified resident surgeon is a prerequisite for use of modifier 82 appended to the usual procedure code number(s).

90   Reference (Outside) Laboratory: When laboratory procedures are performed by a party other than the treating or reporting physician or other qualified health care professional, the procedure may be identified by adding modifier 90 to the usual procedure number.

91   Repeat Clinical Diagnostic Laboratory Test: In the course of treatment of the patient, it may be necessary to repeat the same laboratory test on the same day to obtain subsequent (multiple) test results. Under these circumstances, the laboratory test performed can be identified by its usual procedure number and the addition of modifier 91.
Note: This modifier may not be used when tests are rerun to confirm initial results; due to testing problems with specimens or equipment; or for any other reason when a normal, one-time, reportable result is all that is required. This modifier may not be used when other code(s) describe a series of test results (eg, glucose tolerance tests, evocative/suppression testing). This modifier may only be used for laboratory test(s) performed more than once on the same day on the same patient.

92   Alternative Laboratory Platform Testing: When laboratory testing is being performed using a kit or transportable instrument that wholly or in part consists of a single use, disposable analytical chamber, the service may be identified by adding modifier 92 to the usual laboratory procedure code (HIV testing 86701-86703, and 87389). The test does not require permanent dedicated space, hence by its design may be hand carried or transported to the vicinity of the patient for immediate testing at that site, although location of the testing is not in itself determinative of the use of this modifier.

95 **Synchronous Telemedicine Service Rendered Via a Real-Time Interactive Audio and Video Telecommunications System:** Synchronous telemedicine service is defined as a **real-time** interaction between a physician or other qualified health care professional and a patient who is located at a distant site from the physician or other qualified health care professional. The totality of the communication of information exchanged between the physician or other qualified health care professional and patient during the course of the synchronous telemedicine service must be of an amount and nature that would be sufficient to meet the key components and/or requirements of the same service when rendered via a face-to-face interaction. Modifier 95 may only be appended to the services listed in Appendix F. Appendix F is the list of CPT codes for services that are typically performed face-to-face, but may be rendered via real-time (synchronous) interactive audio and video telecommunications system.

96 **Habilitative Services:** When a service or procedure that may be either habilitative or rehabilitative in nature is provided for habilitative purposes, the physician or other qualified health care professional may add modifier 96 to the service or procedure code to indicate that the service or procedure provided was a habilitative service. Habilitative services help an individual learn skills and functioning for daily living that the individual has not yet developed, and then keep and/or improve those learned skills. Habilitative services also help an individual keep, learn, or improve skills and functioning for daily living.

97 **Rehabilitative Services:** When a service or procedure that may be either habilitative or rehabilitative in nature is provided for rehabilitative purposes, the physician or other qualified health care professional may add modifier 97 to the service or procedure code to indicate that the service or procedure provided was a rehabilitative service. Rehabilitative services help an individual keep, get back, or improve skills and functioning for daily living that have been lost or impaired because the individual was sick, hurt, or disabled.

99 **Multiple Modifiers:** Under certain circumstances 2 or more modifiers may be necessary to completely delineate a service. In such situations modifier 99 should be added to the basic procedure, and other applicable modifiers may be listed as part of the description of the service.

Anesthesia Physical Status Modifiers

All anesthesia services are reported by use of the five-digit anesthesia procedure code with the appropriate physical status modifier appended.

Under certain circumstances, when other modifier(s) are appropriate, they should be reported in addition to the physical status modifier.

P1 A normal healthy patient

P2 A patient with mild systemic disease

P3 A patient with severe systemic disease

P4 A patient with severe systemic disease that is a constant threat to life

P5 A moribund patient who is not expected to survive without the operation

P6 A declared brain-dead patient whose organs are being removed for donor purposes

Modifiers Approved for Ambulatory Surgery Center (ASC) Hospital Outpatient Use

CPT Level I Modifiers

25 **Significant, Separately Identifiable Evaluation and Management Service by the Same Physician or Other Qualified Health Care Professional on the Same Day of the Procedure or Other Service:** It may be necessary to indicate that on the day a procedure or service identified by a CPT code was performed, the patient's condition required a significant, separately identifiable E/M service above and beyond the other service provided or beyond the usual preoperative and postoperative care associated with the procedure that was performed. A significant, separately identifiable E/M service is defined or substantiated by documentation that satisfies the relevant criteria for the respective E/M service to be reported (see Evaluation and Management Services Guidelines for instructions on determining level of E/M service). The E/M service may be prompted by the symptom or condition for which the procedure and/or service was provided. As such, different diagnoses are not required for reporting of the E/M services on the same date. This circumstance may be reported by adding modifier 25 to the appropriate level of E/M service.
Note: This modifier is not used to report an E/M service that resulted in a decision to perform surgery. See modifier 57. For significant, separately identifiable non-E/M services, see modifier 59.

27 **Multiple Outpatient Hospital E/M Encounters on the Same Date:** For hospital outpatient reporting purposes, utilization of hospital resources related to separate and distinct E/M encounters performed in multiple outpatient hospital settings on the same date may be reported by adding modifier 27 to each appropriate level outpatient and/or emergency department E/M code(s). This modifier provides a means of reporting circumstances involving evaluation and management services provided by a physician(s) in more than one (multiple) outpatient hospital setting(s) (eg, hospital emergency department, clinic).
Note: This modifier is not to be used for physician reporting of multiple E/M services performed by the same physician on the same date. For physician reporting of all outpatient evaluation and management services provided by the same physician on the same date and performed in multiple outpatient settings (eg, hospital emergency department, clinic), see Evaluation and Management, Emergency Department, or Preventive Medicine Services codes.

33 **Preventive Services:** When the primary purpose of the service is the delivery of an evidence based service in accordance with a US Preventive Services Task Force A or B rating in effect and other preventive services identified in preventive services mandates (legislative or regulatory), the service may be identified by adding 33 to the procedure. For separately reported services specifically identified as preventive, the modifier should not be used.

50 **Bilateral Procedure:** Unless otherwise identified in the listings, bilateral procedures that are performed at the same session should be identified by adding modifier 50 to the appropriate 5 digit code.
Note: This modifier should not be appended to designated "add-on" codes (see appendix F).

52 **Reduced Services:** Under certain circumstances a service or procedure is partially reduced or eliminated at the discretion of the physician or other qualified health care professional. Under these circumstances the service provided can be identified by its usual procedure number and the addition of modifier 52, signifying that the service is reduced. This provides a means of reporting reduced services without disturbing the identification of the basic service.
Note: For hospital outpatient reporting of a previously scheduled procedure/service that is partially reduced or cancelled as a result of extenuating circumstances or those that threaten the well-being of the patient prior to or after administration of anesthesia, see modifiers 73 and 74 (see modifiers approved for ASC hospital outpatient use).

58 **Staged or Related Procedure or Service by the Same Physician or Other Qualified Health Care Professional During the Postoperative Period:** It may be necessary to indicate that the performance of a procedure or service during the postoperative period was (a) planned or anticipated (staged); (b) more extensive than the original procedure; or (c) for therapy following a surgical procedure. This circumstance may be reported by adding modifier 58 to the staged or related procedure.
Note: For treatment of a problem that requires a return to the operating or procedure room (eg, unanticipated clinical condition), see modifier 78.

59 **Distinct Procedural Service:** Under certain circumstances, it may be necessary to indicate that a procedure or service was distinct or independent from other non-E/M services performed on the same day. Modifier 59 is used to identify procedures/services, other than E/M services, that are not normally reported together but are appropriate under the circumstances. Documentation must support a different session, different procedure or surgery, different site or organ system, separate incision/excision, separate lesion, or separate injury (or area of injury in extensive injuries) not ordinarily encountered or performed on the same day by the same individual. However, when another already established modifier is appropriate it should be used rather than modifier 59. Only if no more descriptive modifier is available, and the use of modifier 59 best explains the circumstances, should modifier 59 be used. **Note:** Modifier 59 should not be appended to an E/M service. To report a separate and distinct E/M service with a non-E/M service performed on the same date, see modifier 25.

73 **Discontinued Out-Patient Hospital/Ambulatory Surgery Center (ASC) Procedure Prior to the Administration of Anesthesia:** Due to extenuating circumstances or those that threaten the well being of the patient, the physician may cancel a surgical or diagnostic procedure subsequent to the patient's surgical preparation (including sedation when provided, and being taken to the room where the procedure is to be performed), but prior to the administration of anesthesia (local, regional block(s) or general). Under these circumstances, the intended service that is prepared for but cancelled can be reported by its usual procedure number and the addition of modifier 73.
Note: The elective cancellation of a service prior to the administration of anesthesia and/or surgical preparation of the patient should not be reported. For physician reporting of a discontinued procedure, see modifier 53.

74 **Discontinued Out-Patient Hospital/Ambulatory Surgery Center (ASC) Procedure After Administration of Anesthesia:** Due to extenuating circumstances or those that threaten the well being of the patient, the physician may terminate a surgical or diagnostic procedure after the administration of anesthesia (local, regional block(s), general) or after the procedure was started (incision made, intubation started, scope inserted, etc.). Under these circumstances, the procedure started but terminated can be reported by its usual procedure number and the addition of modifier 74.
Note: The elective cancellation of a service prior to the administration of anesthesia and/or surgical preparation of the patient should not be reported. For physician reporting of a discontinued procedure, see modifier 53.

76 **Repeat Procedure or Service by Same Physician or Other Qualified Health Care Professional:** It may be necessary to indicate that a procedure or service was repeated by the same physician or other qualified health care professional subsequent to the original procedure or service. This circumstance may be reported by adding modifier 76 to the repeated procedure or service.
Note: This modifier should not be appended to an E/M service.

77 **Repeat Procedure by Another Physician or Other Qualified Health Care Professional:** It may be necessary to indicate that a basic procedure or service was repeated by another physician or other qualified health care professional subsequent to the original procedure or service. This circumstance may be reported by adding modifier 77 to the repeated procedure or service.
Note: This modifier should not be appended to an E/M service.

78 **Unplanned Return to the Operating/Procedure Room by the Same Physician or Other Qualified Health Care Professional Following Initial Procedure for a Related Procedure During the Postoperative Period:** It may be necessary to indicate that another procedure was performed during the postoperative period of the initial procedure (unplanned procedure following initial procedure). When this procedure is related to the first, and requires the use of an operating/procedure room, it may be reported by adding modifier 78 to the related procedure. (For repeat procedures, see modifier 76.)

79 **Unrelated Procedure or Service by the Same Physician During the Postoperative Period:** The individual may need to indicate that the performance of a procedure or service during the postoperative period was unrelated to the original procedure. This circumstance may be reported by using modifier 79. (For repeat procedures on the same day, see modifier 76.)

91 **Repeat Clinical Diagnostic Laboratory Test:** In the course of treatment of the patient, it may be necessary to repeat the same laboratory test on the same day to obtain subsequent (multiple) test results. Under these circumstances, the laboratory test performed can be identified by its usual procedure number and the addition of modifier 91.
Note: This modifier may not be used when tests are rerun to confirm initial results; due to testing problems with specimens or equipment; or for any other reason when a normal, one-time, reportable result is all that is required. This modifier may not be used when other code(s) describe a series of test results (eg, glucose tolerance tests, evocative/suppression testing). This modifier may only be used for laboratory test(s) performed more than once on the same day on the same patient.

Level II (HCPCS/National) Modifiers

The HCPCS Level II modifiers included here are those most commonly used when coding procedures. See your 2020 HCPCS Level II book for a complete listing.

Anatomical Modifiers

E1	Upper left, eyelid
E2	Lower left, eyelid
E3	Upper right, eyelid
E4	Lower right, eyelid
F1	Left hand, second digit
F2	Left hand, third digit
F3	Left hand, fourth digit
F4	Left hand, fifth digit
F5	Right hand, thumb
F6	Right hand, second digit
F7	Right hand, third digit
F8	Right hand, fourth digit
F9	Right hand, fifth digit
FA	Left hand, thumb
LT	Left side (used to identify procedures performed on the left side of the body)
RT	Right side (used to identify procedures performed on the right side of the body)
T1	Left foot, second digit
T2	Left foot, third digit
T3	Left foot, fourth digit
T4	Left foot, fifth digit
T5	Right foot, great toe
T6	Right foot, second digit
T7	Right foot, third digit
T8	Right foot, fourth digit
T9	Right foot, fifth digit
TA	Left foot, great toe

Anesthesia Modifiers

AA	Anesthesia services performed personally by anesthesiologist
AD	Medical supervision by a physician: more than four concurrent anesthesia procedures
G8	Monitored anesthesia care (MAC) for deep complex, complicated, or markedly invasive surgical procedure
G9	Monitored anesthesia care for patient who has history of severe cardiopulmonary condition
QK	Medical direction of two, three, or four concurrent anesthesia procedures involving qualified individuals
QS	Monitored anesthesiology care service
QX	CRNA service: with medical direction by a physician
QY	Medical direction of one certified registered nurse anesthetist (CRNA) by an anesthesiologist
QZ	CRNA service: without medical direction by a physician

Coronary Artery Modifiers

LC Left circumflex coronary artery

LD Left anterior descending coronary artery

LM Left main coronary artery

RC Right coronary artery

RI Ramus intermedius coronary artery

Other Modifiers

CT Computed tomography services furnished using equipment that does not meet each of the attributes of the national electrical manufacturers association (NEMA) XR-29-2013 standard

EA Erythropoetic stimulating agent (ESA) administered to treat anemia due to anticancer chemotherapy

EB Erythropoetic stimulating agent (ESA) administered to treat anemia due to anticancer radiotherapy

EC Erythropoetic stimulating agent (ESA) administered to treat anemia not due to anticancer radiotherapy or anticancer chemotherapy

FP Service provided as part of family planning program

FX X-ray taken using film

G7 Pregnancy resulted from rape or incest or pregnancy certified by physician as life threatening

GA Waiver of liability statement issued as required by payer policy, individual case

GG Performance and payment of a screening mammogram and diagnostic mammogram on the same patient, same day

GH Diagnostic mammogram converted from screening mammogram on same day

GQ Via asynchronous telecommunications system

GT Via interactive audio and video telecommunication systems

GU Waiver of liability statement issued as required by payer policy, routine notice

GX Notice of liability issued, voluntary under payer policy

GY Item or service statutorily excluded, does not meet the definition of any Medicare benefit or, for non-Medicare insurers, is not a contract benefit

GZ Item or service expected to be denied as not reasonable and necessary

PI Positron emission tomography (PET) or PET/computed tomography (CT) to inform the initial treatment strategy of tumors that are biopsy proven or strongly suspected of being cancerous based on other diagnostic testing

PS Positron emission tomography (PET) or PET/computed tomography (CT) to inform the subsequent treatment strategy of cancerous tumors when the beneficiary's treating physician determines that the PET study is needed to inform subsequent antitumor strategy

PT Colorectal cancer screening test; converted to diagnostic test or other procedure

Q7 One Class A finding

Q8 Two Class B findings

Q9 One Class B and two Class C findings

QC Single channel monitoring

QM Ambulance service provided under arrangement by a provider of services

QN Ambulance service furnished directly by a provider of services

QW CLIA waived test

TC Technical component; under certain circumstances, a charge may be made for the technical component alone; under those circumstances the technical component charge is identified by adding modifier TC to the usual procedure number; technical component charges are institutional charges and not billed separately by physicians; however, portable x-ray suppliers only bill for technical component and should utilize modifier TC; the charge data from portable x-ray suppliers will then be used to build customary and prevailing profiles

* XE Separate encounter, a service that is distinct because it occurred during a separate encounter

* XP Separate practitioner, a service that is distinct because it was performed by a different practitioner

* XS Separate structure, a service that is distinct because it was performed on a separate organ/structure

* XU Unusual nonoverlapping service, the use of a service that is distinct because it does not overlap usual components of the main service

* CMS instituted additional HCPCS modifiers to define explicit subsets of modifier 59 Distinct Procedural Service.

Category II Modifiers

1P Performance Measure Exclusion Modifier due to Medical Reasons

Reasons include:

- Not indicated (absence of organ/limb, already received/performed, other)
- Contraindicated (patient allergic history, potential adverse drug interaction, other)
- Other medical reasons

2P Performance Measure Exclusion Modifier due to Patient Reasons

Reasons include:

- Patient declined
- Economic, social, or religious reasons
- Other patient reasons

3P Performance Measure Exclusion Modifier due to System Reasons

Reasons include:

- Resources to perform the services not available
- Insurance coverage/payor-related limitations
- Other reasons attributable to health care delivery system

Modifier 8P is intended to be used as a "reporting modifier" to allow the reporting of circumstances when an action described in a measure's numerator is not performed and the reason is not otherwise specified.

8P Performance measure reporting modifier-action not performed, reason not otherwise specified

Appendix B — New, Revised, and Deleted Codes

New Codes

0563T Evacuation of meibomian glands, using heat delivered through wearable, open-eye eyelid treatment devices and manual gland expression, bilateral

0564T Oncology, chemotherapeutic drug cytotoxicity assay of cancer stem cells (CSCs), from cultured CSCs and primary tumor cells, categorical drug response reported based on percent of cytotoxicity observed, a minimum of 14 drugs or drug combinations

0565T Autologous cellular implant derived from adipose tissue for the treatment of osteoarthritis of the knees; tissue harvesting and cellular implant creation

0566T Autologous cellular implant derived from adipose tissue for the treatment of osteoarthritis of the knees; injection of cellular implant into knee joint including ultrasound guidance, unilateral

0567T Permanent fallopian tube occlusion with degradable biopolymer implant, transcervical approach, including transvaginal ultrasound

0568T Introduction of mixture of saline and air for sonosalpingography to confirm occlusion of fallopian tubes, transcervical approach, including transvaginal ultrasound and pelvic ultrasound

0569T Transcatheter tricuspid valve repair, percutaneous approach; initial prosthesis

0570T Transcatheter tricuspid valve repair, percutaneous approach; each additional prosthesis during same session (List separately in addition to code for primary procedure)

0571T Insertion or replacement of implantable cardioverter-defibrillator system with substernal electrode(s), including all imaging guidance and electrophysiological evaluation (includes defibrillation threshold evaluation, induction of arrhythmia, evaluation of sensing for arrhythmia termination, and programming or reprogramming of sensing or therapeutic parameters), when performed

0572T Insertion of substernal implantable defibrillator electrode

0573T Removal of substernal implantable defibrillator electrode

0574T Repositioning of previously implanted substernal implantable defibrillator-pacing electrode

0575T Programming device evaluation (in person) of implantable cardioverter-defibrillator system with substernal electrode, with iterative adjustment of the implantable device to test the function of the device and select optimal permanent programmed values with analysis, review and report by a physician or other qualified health care professional

0576T Interrogation device evaluation (in person) of implantable cardioverter-defibrillator system with substernal electrode, with analysis, review and report by a physician or other qualified health care professional, includes connection, recording and disconnection per patient encounter

0577T Electrophysiological evaluation of implantable cardioverter-defibrillator system with substernal electrode (includes defibrillation threshold evaluation, induction of arrhythmia, evaluation of sensing for arrhythmia termination, and programming or reprogramming of sensing or therapeutic parameters)

0578T Interrogation device evaluation(s) (remote), up to 90 days, substernal lead implantable cardioverter-defibrillator system with interim analysis, review(s) and report(s) by a physician or other qualified health care professional

0579T Interrogation device evaluation(s) (remote), up to 90 days, substernal lead implantable cardioverter-defibrillator system, remote data acquisition(s), receipt of transmissions and technician review, technical support and distribution of results

0580T Removal of substernal implantable defibrillator pulse generator only

0581T Ablation, malignant breast tumor(s), percutaneous, cryotherapy, including imaging guidance when performed, unilateral

0582T Transurethral ablation of malignant prostate tissue by high-energy water vapor thermotherapy, including intraoperative imaging and needle guidance

0583T Tympanostomy (requiring insertion of ventilating tube), using an automated tube delivery system, iontophoresis local anesthesia

0584T Islet cell transplant, includes portal vein catheterization and infusion, including all imaging, including guidance, and radiological supervision and interpretation, when performed; percutaneous

0585T Islet cell transplant, includes portal vein catheterization and infusion, including all imaging, including guidance, and radiological supervision and interpretation, when performed; laparoscopic

0586T Islet cell transplant, includes portal vein catheterization and infusion, including all imaging, including guidance, and radiological supervision and interpretation, when performed; open

0587T Percutaneous implantation or replacement of integrated single device neurostimulation system including electrode array and receiver or pulse generator, including analysis, programming, and imaging guidance when performed, posterior tibial nerve

0588T Revision or removal of integrated single device neurostimulation system including electrode array and receiver or pulse generator, including analysis, programming, and imaging guidance when performed, posterior tibial nerve

0589T Electronic analysis with simple programming of implanted integrated neurostimulation system (eg, electrode array and receiver), including contact group(s), amplitude, pulse width, frequency (Hz), on/off cycling, burst, dose lockout, patient-selectable parameters, responsive neurostimulation, detection algorithms, closed-loop parameters, and passive parameters, when performed by physician or other qualified health care professional, posterior tibial nerve, 1-3 parameters

0590T Electronic analysis with complex programming of implanted integrated neurostimulation system (eg, electrode array and receiver), including contact group(s), amplitude, pulse width, frequency (Hz), on/off cycling, burst, dose lockout, patient-selectable parameters, responsive neurostimulation, detection algorithms, closed-loop parameters, and passive parameters, when performed by physician or other qualified health care professional, posterior tibial nerve, 4 or more parameters

0591T Health and well-being coaching face-to-face; individual, initial assessment

0592T Health and well-being coaching face-to-face; individual, follow-up session, at least 30 minutes

0593T Health and well-being coaching face-to-face; group (2 or more individuals), at least 30 minutes

15769 Grafting of autologous soft tissue, other, harvested by direct excision (eg, fat, dermis, fascia)

15771 Grafting of autologous fat harvested by liposuction technique to trunk, breasts, scalp, arms, and/or legs; 50 cc or less injectate

15772 Grafting of autologous fat harvested by liposuction technique to trunk, breasts, scalp, arms, and/or legs; each additional 50 cc injectate, or part thereof (List separately in addition to code for primary procedure)

15773 Grafting of autologous fat harvested by liposuction technique to face, eyelids, mouth, neck, ears, orbits, genitalia, hands, and/or feet; 25 cc or less injectate

15774 Grafting of autologous fat harvested by liposuction technique to face, eyelids, mouth, neck, ears, orbits, genitalia, hands, and/or feet; each additional 25 cc injectate, or part thereof (List separately in addition to code for primary procedure)

20560 Needle insertion(s) without injection(s); 1 or 2 muscle(s)

20561 Needle insertion(s) without injection(s); 3 or more muscles

20700 Manual preparation and insertion of drug-delivery device(s), deep (eg, subfascial) (List separately in addition to code for primary procedure)

20701 Removal of drug-delivery device(s), deep (eg, subfascial) (List separately in addition to code for primary procedure)

20702 Manual preparation and insertion of drug-delivery device(s), intramedullary (List separately in addition to code for primary procedure)

20703 Removal of drug-delivery device(s), intramedullary (List separately in addition to code for primary procedure)

20704 Manual preparation and insertion of drug-delivery device(s), intra-articular (List separately in addition to code for primary procedure)

20705 Removal of drug-delivery device(s), intra-articular (List separately in addition to code for primary procedure)

21601 Excision of chest wall tumor including rib(s)

21602 Excision of chest wall tumor involving rib(s), with plastic reconstruction; without mediastinal lymphadenectomy

21603 Excision of chest wall tumor involving rib(s), with plastic reconstruction; with mediastinal lymphadenectomy

33016 Pericardiocentesis, including imaging guidance, when performed

33017 Pericardial drainage with insertion of indwelling catheter, percutaneous, including fluoroscopy and/or ultrasound guidance, when performed; 6 years and older without congenital cardiac anomaly

33018 Pericardial drainage with insertion of indwelling catheter, percutaneous, including fluoroscopy and/or ultrasound guidance, when performed; birth through 5 years of age or any age with congenital cardiac anomaly

33019 Pericardial drainage with insertion of indwelling catheter, percutaneous, including CT guidance

33858 Ascending aorta graft, with cardiopulmonary bypass, includes valve suspension, when performed; for aortic dissection

33859 Ascending aorta graft, with cardiopulmonary bypass, includes valve suspension, when performed; for aortic disease other than dissection (eg, aneurysm)

33871 Transverse aortic arch graft, with cardiopulmonary bypass, with profound hypothermia, total circulatory arrest and isolated cerebral perfusion with reimplantation of arch vessel(s) (eg, island pedicle or individual arch vessel reimplantation)

34717 Endovascular repair of iliac artery at the time of aorto-iliac artery endograft placement by deployment of an iliac branched endograft including pre-procedure sizing and device selection, all ipsilateral selective iliac artery catheterization(s), all associated radiological supervision and interpretation, and all endograft extension(s) proximally to the aortic bifurcation and distally in the internal iliac, external iliac, and common femoral artery(ies), and treatment zone angioplasty/stenting, when performed, for rupture or other than rupture (eg, for aneurysm, pseudoaneurysm, dissection, arteriovenous malformation, penetrating ulcer, traumatic disruption), unilateral (List separately in addition to code for primary procedure)

34718 Endovascular repair of iliac artery, not associated with placement of an aorto-iliac artery endograft at the same session, by deployment of an iliac branched endograft, including pre-procedure sizing and device selection, all ipsilateral selective iliac artery catheterization(s), all associated radiological supervision and interpretation, and all endograft extension(s) proximally to the aortic bifurcation and distally in the internal iliac, external iliac, and common femoral artery(ies), and treatment zone angioplasty/stenting, when performed, for other than rupture (eg, for aneurysm, pseudoaneurysm, dissection, arteriovenous malformation, penetrating ulcer), unilateral

35702 Exploration not followed by surgical repair, artery; upper extremity (eg, axillary, brachial, radial, ulnar)

35703 Exploration not followed by surgical repair, artery; lower extremity (eg, common femoral, deep femoral, superficial femoral, popliteal, tibial, peroneal)

46948 Hemorrhoidectomy, internal, by transanal hemorrhoidal dearterialization, 2 or more hemorrhoid columns/groups, including ultrasound guidance, with mucopexy, when performed

49013 Preperitoneal pelvic packing for hemorrhage associated with pelvic trauma, including local exploration

49014 Re-exploration of pelvic wound with removal of preperitoneal pelvic packing, including repacking, when performed

62328 Spinal puncture, lumbar, diagnostic; with fluoroscopic or CT guidance

62329 Spinal puncture, therapeutic, for drainage of cerebrospinal fluid (by needle or catheter); with fluoroscopic or CT guidance

64451 Injection(s), anesthetic agent(s) and/or steroid; nerves innervating the sacroiliac joint, with image guidance (ie, fluoroscopy or computed tomography)

64454 Injection(s), anesthetic agent(s) and/or steroid; genicular nerve branches, including imaging guidance, when performed

64624 Destruction by neurolytic agent, genicular nerve branches including imaging guidance, when performed

64625 Radiofrequency ablation, nerves innervating the sacroiliac joint, with image guidance (ie, fluoroscopy or computed tomography)

66987 Extracapsular cataract removal with insertion of intraocular lens prosthesis (1-stage procedure), manual or mechanical technique (eg, irrigation and aspiration or phacoemulsification), complex, requiring devices or techniques not generally used in routine cataract surgery (eg, iris expansion device, suture support for intraocular lens, or primary posterior capsulorrhexis) or performed on patients in the amblyogenic developmental stage; with endoscopic cyclophotocoagulation

66988 Extracapsular cataract removal with insertion of intraocular lens prosthesis (1 stage procedure), manual or mechanical technique (eg, irrigation and aspiration or phacoemulsification); with endoscopic cyclophotocoagulation

74221 Radiologic examination, esophagus, including scout chest radiograph(s) and delayed image(s), when performed; double-contrast (eg, high-density barium and effervescent agent) study

74248 Radiologic small intestine follow-through study, including multiple serial images (List separately in addition to code for primary procedure for upper GI radiologic examination)

78429 Myocardial imaging, positron emission tomography (PET), metabolic evaluation study (including ventricular wall motion[s] and/or ejection fraction[s], when performed), single study; with concurrently acquired computed tomography transmission scan

78430 Myocardial imaging, positron emission tomography (PET), perfusion study (including ventricular wall motion[s] and/or ejection fraction[s], when performed); single study, at rest or stress (exercise or pharmacologic), with concurrently acquired computed tomography transmission scan

78431 Myocardial imaging, positron emission tomography (PET), perfusion study (including ventricular wall motion[s] and/or ejection fraction[s], when performed); multiple studies at rest and stress (exercise or pharmacologic), with concurrently acquired computed tomography transmission scan

78432 Myocardial imaging, positron emission tomography (PET), combined perfusion with metabolic evaluation study (including ventricular wall motion[s] and/or ejection fraction[s], when performed), dual radiotracer (eg, myocardial viability);

78433 Myocardial imaging, positron emission tomography (PET), combined perfusion with metabolic evaluation study (including ventricular wall motion[s] and/or ejection fraction[s], when performed), dual radiotracer (eg, myocardial viability); with concurrently acquired computed tomography transmission scan

78434 Absolute quantitation of myocardial blood flow (AQMBF), positron emission tomography (PET), rest and pharmacologic stress (List separately in addition to code for primary procedure)

78830 Radiopharmaceutical localization of tumor, inflammatory process or distribution of radiopharmaceutical agent(s) (includes vascular flow and blood pool imaging, when performed); tomographic (SPECT) with concurrently acquired computed tomography (CT) transmission scan for anatomical review, localization and determination/detection of pathology, single area (eg, head, neck, chest, pelvis), single day imaging

78831 Radiopharmaceutical localization of tumor, inflammatory process or distribution of radiopharmaceutical agent(s) (includes vascular flow and blood pool imaging, when performed); tomographic (SPECT), minimum 2 areas (eg, pelvis and knees, abdomen and pelvis), single day imaging, or single area imaging over 2 or more days

78832 Radiopharmaceutical localization of tumor, inflammatory process or distribution of radiopharmaceutical agent(s) (includes vascular flow and blood pool imaging, when performed); tomographic (SPECT) with concurrently acquired computed tomography (CT) transmission scan for anatomical review, localization and determination/detection of pathology, minimum 2 areas (eg, pelvis and knees, abdomen and pelvis), single day imaging, or single area imaging over 2 or more days

78835 Radiopharmaceutical quantification measurement(s) single area (List separately in addition to code for primary procedure)

80145 Adalimumab

80187 Posaconazole

80230 Infliximab

80235 Lacosamide

80280 Vedolizumab

80285 Voriconazole

81277 Cytogenomic neoplasia (genome-wide) microarray analysis, interrogation of genomic regions for copy number and loss-of-heterozygosity variants for chromosomal abnormalities

81307 PALB2 (partner and localizer of BRCA2) (eg, breast and pancreatic cancer) gene analysis; full gene sequence

81308 PALB2 (partner and localizer of BRCA2) (eg, breast and pancreatic cancer) gene analysis; known familial variant

81309 PIK3CA (phosphatidylinositol-4, 5-biphosphate 3-kinase, catalytic subunit alpha) (eg, colorectal and breast cancer) gene analysis, targeted sequence analysis (eg, exons 7, 9, 20)

81522 Oncology (breast), mRNA, gene expression profiling by RT-PCR of 12 genes (8 content and 4 housekeeping), utilizing formalin-fixed paraffin-embedded tissue, algorithm reported as recurrence risk score

81542 Oncology (prostate), mRNA, microarray gene expression profiling of 22 content genes, utilizing formalin-fixed paraffin-embedded tissue, algorithm reported as metastasis risk score

81552 Oncology (uveal melanoma), mRNA, gene expression profiling by real-time RT-PCR of 15 genes (12 content and 3 housekeeping), utilizing fine needle aspirate or formalin-fixed paraffin-embedded tissue, algorithm reported as risk of metastasis

87563 Infectious agent detection by nucleic acid (DNA or RNA); Mycoplasma genitalium, amplified probe technique

90694 Influenza virus vaccine, quadrivalent (aIIV4), inactivated, adjuvanted, preservative free, 0.5 mL dosage, for intramuscular use

90912 Biofeedback training, perineal muscles, anorectal or urethral sphincter, including EMG and/or manometry, when performed; initial 15 minutes of one-on-one physician or other qualified health care professional contact with the patient

90913 Biofeedback training, perineal muscles, anorectal or urethral sphincter, including EMG and/or manometry, when performed; each additional 15 minutes of one-on-one physician or other qualified health care professional contact with the patient (List separately in addition to code for primary procedure)

92201 Ophthalmoscopy, extended; with retinal drawing and scleral depression of peripheral retinal disease (eg, for retinal tear, retinal detachment, retinal tumor) with interpretation and report, unilateral or bilateral

92202 Ophthalmoscopy, extended; with drawing of optic nerve or macula (eg, for glaucoma, macular pathology, tumor) with interpretation and report, unilateral or bilateral

92549 Computerized dynamic posturography sensory organization test (CDP-SOT), 6 conditions (ie, eyes open, eyes closed, visual sway, platform sway, eyes closed platform sway, platform and visual sway), including interpretation and report; with motor control test (MCT) and adaptation test (ADT)

93356 Myocardial strain imaging using speckle tracking-derived assessment of myocardial mechanics (List separately in addition to codes for echocardiography imaging)

93985 Duplex scan of arterial inflow and venous outflow for preoperative vessel assessment prior to creation of hemodialysis access; complete bilateral study

93986 Duplex scan of arterial inflow and venous outflow for preoperative vessel assessment prior to creation of hemodialysis access; complete unilateral study

95700 Electroencephalogram (EEG) continuous recording, with video when performed, setup, patient education, and takedown when performed, administered in person by EEG technologist, minimum of 8 channels

95705 Electroencephalogram (EEG), without video, review of data, technical description by EEG technologist, 2-12 hours; unmonitored

95706 Electroencephalogram (EEG), without video, review of data, technical description by EEG technologist, 2-12 hours; with intermittent monitoring and maintenance

95707 Electroencephalogram (EEG), without video, review of data, technical description by EEG technologist, 2-12 hours; with continuous, real-time monitoring and maintenance

95708 Electroencephalogram (EEG), without video, review of data, technical description by EEG technologist, each increment of 12-26 hours; unmonitored

95709 Electroencephalogram (EEG), without video, review of data, technical description by EEG technologist, each increment of 12-26 hours; with intermittent monitoring and maintenance

95710 Electroencephalogram (EEG), without video, review of data, technical description by EEG technologist, each increment of 12-26 hours; with continuous, real-time monitoring and maintenance

95711 Electroencephalogram with video (VEEG), review of data, technical description by EEG technologist, 2-12 hours; unmonitored

95712 Electroencephalogram with video (VEEG), review of data, technical description by EEG technologist, 2-12 hours; with intermittent monitoring and maintenance

95713 Electroencephalogram with video (VEEG), review of data, technical description by EEG technologist, 2-12 hours; with continuous, real-time monitoring and maintenance

95714 Electroencephalogram with video (VEEG), review of data, technical description by EEG technologist, each increment of 12-26 hours; unmonitored

95715 Electroencephalogram with video (VEEG), review of data, technical description by EEG technologist, each increment of 12-26 hours; with intermittent monitoring and maintenance

95716 Electroencephalogram with video (VEEG), review of data, technical description by EEG technologist, each increment of 12-26 hours; with continuous, real-time monitoring and maintenance

95717 Electroencephalogram (EEG), continuous recording, physician or other qualified health care professional review of recorded events, analysis of spike and seizure detection, interpretation and report, 2-12 hours of EEG recording; without video

95718 Electroencephalogram (EEG), continuous recording, physician or other qualified health care professional review of recorded events, analysis of spike and seizure detection, interpretation and report, 2-12 hours of EEG recording; with video (VEEG)

95719 Electroencephalogram (EEG), continuous recording, physician or other qualified health care professional review of recorded events, analysis of spike and seizure detection, each increment of greater than 12 hours, up to 26 hours of EEG recording, interpretation and report after each 24-hour period; without video

95720 Electroencephalogram (EEG), continuous recording, physician or other qualified health care professional review of recorded events, analysis of spike and seizure detection, each increment of greater than 12 hours, up to 26 hours of EEG recording, interpretation and report after each 24-hour period; with video (VEEG)

95721 Electroencephalogram (EEG), continuous recording, physician or other qualified health care professional review of recorded events, analysis of spike and seizure detection, interpretation, and summary report, complete study; greater than 36 hours, up to 60 hours of EEG recording, without video

95722 Electroencephalogram (EEG), continuous recording, physician or other qualified health care professional review of recorded events, analysis of spike and seizure detection, interpretation, and summary report, complete study; greater than 36 hours, up to 60 hours of EEG recording, with video (VEEG)

95723 Electroencephalogram (EEG), continuous recording, physician or other qualified health care professional review of recorded events, analysis of spike and seizure detection, interpretation, and summary report, complete study; greater than 60 hours, up to 84 hours of EEG recording, without video

95724 Electroencephalogram (EEG), continuous recording, physician or other qualified health care professional review of recorded events, analysis of spike and seizure detection, interpretation, and summary report, complete study; greater than 60 hours, up to 84 hours of EEG recording, with video (VEEG)

95725 Electroencephalogram (EEG), continuous recording, physician or other qualified health care professional review of recorded events, analysis of spike and seizure detection, interpretation, and summary report, complete study; greater than 84 hours of EEG recording, without video

95726 Electroencephalogram (EEG), continuous recording, physician or other qualified health care professional review of recorded events, analysis of spike and seizure detection, interpretation, and summary report, complete study; greater than 84 hours of EEG recording, with video (VEEG)

96156 Health behavior assessment, or re-assessment (ie, health-focused clinical interview, behavioral observations, clinical decision making)

96158 Health behavior intervention, individual, face-to-face; initial 30 minutes

96159 Health behavior intervention, individual, face-to-face; each additional 15 minutes (List separately in addition to code for primary service)

96164 Health behavior intervention, group (2 or more patients), face-to-face; initial 30 minutes

96165 Health behavior intervention, group (2 or more patients), face-to-face; each additional 15 minutes (List separately in addition to code for primary service)

96167 Health behavior intervention, family (with the patient present), face-to-face; initial 30 minutes

96168 Health behavior intervention, family (with the patient present), face-to-face; each additional 15 minutes (List separately in addition to code for primary service)

96170 Health behavior intervention, family (without the patient present), face-to-face; initial 30 minutes

96171 Health behavior intervention, family (without the patient present), face-to-face; each additional 15 minutes (List separately in addition to code for primary service)

97129 Therapeutic interventions that focus on cognitive function (eg, attention, memory, reasoning, executive function, problem solving, and/or pragmatic functioning) and compensatory strategies to manage the performance of an activity (eg, managing time or schedules, initiating, organizing, and sequencing tasks), direct (one-on-one) patient contact; initial 15 minutes

97130 Therapeutic interventions that focus on cognitive function (eg, attention, memory, reasoning, executive function, problem solving, and/or pragmatic functioning) and compensatory strategies to manage the performance of an activity (eg, managing time or schedules, initiating, organizing, and sequencing tasks), direct (one-on-one) patient contact; each additional 15 minutes (List separately in addition to code for primary procedure)

98970 Qualified nonphysician health care professional online digital evaluation and management service, for an established patient, for up to 7 days, cumulative time during the 7 days; 5-10 minutes

98971 Qualified nonphysician health care professional online digital evaluation and management service, for an established patient, for up to 7 days, cumulative time during the 7 days; 11-20 minutes

98972 Qualified nonphysician health care professional online digital evaluation and management service, for an established patient, for up to 7 days, cumulative time during the 7 days; 21 or more minutes

99421 Online digital evaluation and management service, for an established patient, for up to 7 days, cumulative time during the 7 days; 5-10 minutes

99422 Online digital evaluation and management service, for an established patient, for up to 7 days, cumulative time during the 7 days; 11-20 minutes

99423 Online digital evaluation and management service, for an established patient, for up to 7 days, cumulative time during the 7 days; 21 or more minutes

99458 Remote physiologic monitoring treatment management services, clinical staff/physician/other qualified health care professional time in a calendar month requiring interactive communication with the patient/caregiver during the month; each additional 20 minutes (List separately in addition to code for primary procedure)

99473 Self-measured blood pressure using a device validated for clinical accuracy; patient education/training and device calibration

99474 Self-measured blood pressure using a device validated for clinical accuracy; separate self-measurements of two readings one minute apart, twice daily over a 30-day period (minimum of 12 readings), collection of data reported by the patient and/or caregiver to the physician or other qualified health care professional, with report of average systolic and diastolic pressures and subsequent communication of a treatment plan to the patient

Revised Codes

31233 Nasal/sinus endoscopy, diagnostic ~~with maxillary sinusoscopy (via inferior meatus or canine fossa puncture)~~; with maxillary sinusoscopy (via inferior meatus or canine fossa puncture)

31235 with sphenoid sinusoscopy (via puncture of sphenoidal face or cannulation of ostium)

31292 Nasal/sinus endoscopy, surgical, with orbital decompression; ~~with~~ medial or inferior ~~orbital wall decompression~~

31293 ~~with~~ medial ~~orbital wall~~ and inferior ~~orbital wall decompression~~

31294 Nasal/sinus endoscopy, surgical, with optic nerve decompression; ~~with optic nerve decompression~~

31295 Nasal/sinus endoscopy, surgical, with dilation (eg, balloon dilation); ~~with dilation of~~ maxillary sinus ostium ~~(eg, balloon dilation)~~, transnasal or via canine fossa

31296 ~~with dilation of~~ frontal sinus ostium ~~(eg, balloon dilation)~~

31297 ~~with dilation of~~ sphenoid sinus ostium ~~(eg, balloon dilation)~~

31298 ~~with dilation of~~ frontal and sphenoid sinus ostia ~~(eg, balloon dilation)~~

33275 Transcatheter removal of permanent leadless pacemaker, right ventricular, including imaging guidance (eg, fluoroscopy, venous ultrasound, ventriculography, femoral venography), when performed

35701 Exploration ~~(not followed by surgical repair,)~~, ~~with or without lysis of artery;~~ neck (eg, carotid ~~artery, subclavian~~)

46945 Hemorrhoidectomy, internal, by ligation other than rubber band; single hemorrhoid column/group, without imaging guidance

46946 2 or more hemorrhoid columns/groups, without imaging guidance

54640 Orchiopexy, inguinal ~~approach, with or without hernia repair~~ scrotal approach

62270 Spinal puncture, lumbar, diagnostic;

62272 Spinal puncture, therapeutic, for drainage of cerebrospinal fluid (by needle or catheter);

64400 Injection(s), anesthetic agent(s) and/or steroid; trigeminal nerve, ~~any division or branch~~each branch (ie, ophthalmic, maxillary, mandibular)

64405   greater occipital nerve

64408   vagus nerve

64415   brachial plexus~~, single~~

64416   brachial plexus, continuous infusion by catheter (including catheter placement)

64417   axillary nerve

64418   suprascapular nerve

64420   intercostal nerve, single level

64421   intercostal nerve, ~~multiple, regional block~~ each additional level (List separately in addition to code for primary procedure)

64425   ilioinguinal, iliohypogastric nerves

64430   pudendal nerve

64435   paracervical (uterine) nerve

64445   sciatic nerve~~, single~~

64446   sciatic nerve, continuous infusion by catheter (including catheter placement)

64447   femoral nerve~~, single~~

64448   femoral nerve, continuous infusion by catheter (including catheter placement)

64449   lumbar plexus, posterior approach, continuous infusion by catheter (including catheter placement)

64450   other peripheral nerve or branch

66711 Ciliary body destruction; cyclophotocoagulation, endoscopic, without concomitant removal of crystalline lens

66982 Extracapsular cataract removal with insertion of intraocular lens prosthesis (1-stage procedure), manual or mechanical technique (eg, irrigation and aspiration or phacoemulsification), complex, requiring devices or techniques not generally used in routine cataract surgery (eg, iris expansion device, suture support for intraocular lens, or primary posterior capsulorrhexis) or performed on patients in the amblyogenic developmental stage; without endoscopic cyclophotocoagulation

66984 Extracapsular cataract removal with insertion of intraocular lens prosthesis (1 stage procedure), manual or mechanical technique (eg, irrigation and aspiration or phacoemulsification); without endoscopic cyclophotocoagulation

74022 Radiologic examination, ~~abdomen;~~ complete acute abdomen series, including 2 or more views of the abdomen (eg, supine, erect, ~~and/or~~ decubitus ~~views~~), and a single view chest

74210 Radiologic examination, pharynx and/or cervical esophagus, including scout neck radiograph(s) and delayed image(s), when performed, contrast (eg, barium) study~~; pharynx and/or cervical esophagus~~

74220 Radiologic examination, esophagus, including scout chest radiograph(s) and delayed image(s), when performed; ~~esophagus~~single-contrast (eg, barium) study

74230 ~~Swallowing~~Radiologic examination, swallowing function, with cineradiography/videoradiography, including scout neck radiograph(s) and delayed image(s), when performed, contrast (eg, barium) study

74240 Radiologic examination, upper gastrointestinal tract, including scout abdominal radiograph(s) and delayed image(s), ~~upper~~ when performed; ~~with or without delayed images~~single-contrast (eg, ~~without KUB~~ barium) study

74246   with or without delayed images double-contrast (eg, high-density barium and effervescent agent) study, including glucagon, ~~without KUB~~ when administered

74250 Radiologic examination, small intestine, ~~includes~~including multiple serial images and scout abdominal radiograph(s), when performed; single-contrast (eg, barium) study

74251   double-contrast (eg, high-density barium and air via enteroclysis tube) study, including glucagon, when administered

74270 Radiologic examination, colon, including scout abdominal radiograph(s) and delayed image(s), when performed; single-contrast (eg, barium) ~~enema, with or without KUB~~study

74280   air double-contrast ~~with specific~~(eg, high density barium and air) study, ~~with or without glucagon~~including glucagon, when administered

78459 Myocardial imaging, positron emission tomography (PET), metabolic evaluation study (including ventricular wall motion[s] and/or ejection fraction[s], when performed), single study;

78491 Myocardial imaging, positron emission tomography (PET), perfusion study (including ventricular wall motion[s] and/or ejection fraction[s], when performed); single study, at rest or stress (exercise or pharmacologic)

78492   multiple studies at rest and~~/or~~ stress (exercise or pharmacologic)

78800 Radiopharmaceutical localization of tumor, inflammatory process or distribution of radiopharmaceutical agent(s) (includes vascular flow and blood pool imaging, when performed); ~~limited~~planar, single area (eg, head, neck, chest, pelvis), single day imaging

78801   multiple planar, 2 or more areas (eg, abdomen and pelvis, head and chest), 1 or more days imaging or single area imaging over 2 or more days

78802   planar, whole body, single day imaging

78803   tomographic (SPECT), single area (eg, head, neck, chest, pelvis), single day imaging

78804   planar, whole body, requiring 2 or more days imaging

81350 UGT1A1 (UDP glucuronosyltransferase 1 family, polypeptide A1) (eg, ~~irinotecan~~ drug metabolism, hereditary unconjugated hyperbilirubinemia [Gilbert syndrome]), gene analysis, common variants (eg, *28, *36, *37)

81404 Molecular pathology procedure, Level 5 (eg, analysis of 2-5 exons by DNA sequence analysis, mutation scanning or duplication/deletion variants of 6-10 exons, or characterization of a dynamic mutation disorder/triplet repeat by Southern blot analysis) ~~PIK3CA (phosphatidylinositol-4,5-bisphosphate 3-kinase, catalytic subunit alpha) (eg, colorectal cancer), targeted sequence analysis (eg, exons 9 and 20)~~ UGT1A1 (UDP glucuronosyltransferase 1 family, polypeptide A1) (eg, hereditary unconjugated hyperbilirubinemia [Crigler-Najjar syndrome]) full gene sequence

81406 Molecular pathology procedure, Level 7 (eg, analysis of 11-25 exons by DNA sequence analysis, mutation scanning or duplication/deletion variants of 26-50 exons, ~~cytogenomic array analysis for neoplasia) Cytogenomic microarray analysis, neoplasia (eg, interrogation of copy number, and loss-of-heterozygosity via single nucleotide polymorphism [SNP]-based comparative genomic hybridization [CGH] microarray analysis)~~ PALB2 (partner and localizer of BRCA2) (eg, breast and pancreatic cancer), full gene sequence

81407 Molecular pathology procedure, Level 8 (eg, analysis of 26-50 exons by DNA sequence analysis, mutation scanning or duplication/deletion variants of >50 exons, sequence analysis of multiple genes on one platform) APOB (apolipoprotein B) (eg, familial hypercholesterolemia type B) full gene sequence

90734 Meningococcal conjugate vaccine, serogroups A, C, W, Y ~~and W-135, quadrivalent (MCV4,~~ quadrivalent, diphtheria toxoid carrier (MenACWY-D) or ~~MenACWY~~CRM197 carrier (MenACWY-CRM), for intramuscular use

92548 Computerized dynamic posturography sensory organization test (CDP-SOT), 6 conditions (ie, eyes open, eyes closed, visual sway, platform sway, eyes closed platform sway, platform and visual sway), including interpretation and report;

92626 Evaluation of auditory ~~rehabilitation~~function for surgically implanted device(s) candidacy or postoperative status of a surgically implanted device(s); first hour

92627   each additional 15 minutes (List separately in addition to code for primary procedure)

93784 Ambulatory blood pressure monitoring, utilizing ~~a system such as magnetic tape and/or computer disk,~~report-generating software, automated, worn continuously for 24 hours or longer; including recording, scanning analysis, interpretation and report

93786   recording only

93788   scanning analysis with report

93790   review with interpretation and report

94728   Airway resistance by ~~impulse~~ oscillometry

95813   Electroencephalogram (EEG) extended monitoring; ~~greater than 1 hour~~ 61-119 minutes

99457   Remote physiologic monitoring treatment management services, ~~20 minutes or more of~~ clinical staff/physician/other qualified health care professional time in a calendar month requiring interactive communication with the patient/caregiver during the month; first 20 minutes

0008U   Helicobacter pylori detection and antibiotic resistance, DNA, 16S and 23S rRNA, gyrA, pbp1, rdxA and rpoB, next generation sequencing, formalin-fixed paraffin-embedded or fresh tissue or fecal sample, predictive, reported as positive or negative for resistance to clarithromycin, fluoroquinolones, metronidazole, amoxicillin, tetracycline, and rifabutin

0402T   Collagen cross-linking of cornea ~~(~~, including removal of the corneal epithelium and intraoperative pachymetry, when performed (Report medication separately)

2022F   Dilated retinal eye exam with interpretation by an ophthalmologist or optometrist documented and reviewed; with evidence of retinopathy (DM)[2,4]

2024F   7 standard field stereoscopic retinal photos with interpretation by an ophthalmologist or optometrist documented and reviewed; with evidence of retinopathy (DM)[2,4]

2026F   Eye imaging validated to match diagnosis from 7 standard field stereoscopic retinal photos results documented and reviewed; with evidence of retinopathy (DM)[2,4]

Deleted Codes

0009M	0081U	0104U	0205T	0206T	0249T	0254T
0341T	0357T	0375T	0377T	0380T	0399T	0482T
19260	19271	19272	19304	20926	33010	33011
33015	33860	33870	35721	35741	35761	43401
64402	64410	64413	74241	74245	74247	74249
74260	76930	78205	78206	78320	78607	78647
78710	78805	78806	78807	90911	92225	92226
93299	95827	95831	95832	95833	95834	95950
95951	95953	95956	96150	96151	96152	96153
96154	96155	97127	98969	99444		

Resequenced Icon Added

15769	20560	20561	46948	62328	62329	64624
64625	66987	66988	78429	78430	78431	78432
78433	78434	78804	78830	78831	78832	78835
80230	80235	80280	80285	81277	81307	81308
81309	81433	81522	90619	90694	93356	95700
95705	95706	95707	95708	95709	95710	95711
95712	95713	95714	95715	95716	95717	95718
95719	95720	95721	95722	95723	95724	95725
95726	96164	96165	96167	96168	96170	96171
2033F	3051F	3052F	99421	99422	99423	99458
99473	99474					

Web Release New and Revised Codes

Codes indicated as "Web Release" codes indicate CPT codes that are in *Current Procedural Coding Expert* for the current year, but will not be in the AMA CPT book until the following year. This can also include those codes designated by the AMA as new or revised for 2020 but that actually appeared in the 2019 Optum360 book. These codes will have the appropriate new or revised icon appended to match the CPT code book, however. See the complete list that follows:

New codes, deleted codes, and revisions to codes in the 2020 *Current Procedural Coding Expert* that will not appear in the CPT code book until 2021

These codes are indicated with the following icons: ● ▲ These icons will be green in the body of the book.

New Codes

0139U   Neurology (autism spectrum disorder [ASD]), quantitative measurements of 6 central carbon metabolites (ie, α-ketoglutarate, alanine, lactate, phenylalanine, pyruvate, and succinate), LC-MS/MS, plasma, algorithmic analysis with result reported as negative or positive (with metabolic subtypes of ASD)

0140U   Infectious disease (fungi), fungal pathogen identification, DNA (15 fungal targets), blood culture, amplified probe technique, each target reported as detected or not detected

0141U   Infectious disease (bacteria and fungi), gram-positive organism identification and drug resistance element detection, DNA (20 gram-positive bacterial targets, 4 resistance genes, 1 pan gram-negative bacterial target, 1 pan Candida target), blood culture, amplified probe technique, each target reported as detected or not detected

0142U   Infectious disease (bacteria and fungi), gram-negative bacterial identification and drug resistance element detection, DNA (21 gram-negative bacterial targets, 6 resistance genes, 1 pan gram-positive bacterial target, 1 pan Candida target), amplified probe technique, each target reported as detected or not detected

0143U   Drug assay, definitive, 120 or more drugs or metabolites, urine, quantitative liquid chromatography with tandem mass spectrometry (LC-MS/MS) using multiple reaction monitoring (MRM), with drug or metabolite description, comments including sample validation, per date of service

0144U   Drug assay, definitive, 160 or more drugs or metabolites, urine, quantitative liquid chromatography with tandem mass spectrometry (LC-MS/MS) using multiple reaction monitoring (MRM), with drug or metabolite description, comments including sample validation, per date of service

0145U   Drug assay, definitive, 65 or more drugs or metabolites, urine, quantitative liquid chromatography with tandem mass spectrometry (LC-MS/MS) using multiple reaction monitoring (MRM), with drug or metabolite description, comments including sample validation, per date of service

0146U   Drug assay, definitive, 80 or more drugs or metabolites, urine, by quantitative liquid chromatography with tandem mass spectrometry (LC-MS/MS) using multiple reaction monitoring (MRM), with drug or metabolite description, comments including sample validation, per date of service

0147U   Drug assay, definitive, 85 or more drugs or metabolites, urine, quantitative liquid chromatography with tandem mass spectrometry (LC-MS/MS) using multiple reaction monitoring (MRM), with drug or metabolite description, comments including sample validation, per date of service

0148U   Drug assay, definitive, 100 or more drugs or metabolites, urine, quantitative liquid chromatography with tandem mass spectrometry (LC-MS/MS) using multiple reaction monitoring (MRM), with drug or metabolite description, comments including sample validation, per date of service

0149U   Drug assay, definitive, 60 or more drugs or metabolites, urine, quantitative liquid chromatography with tandem mass spectrometry (LC-MS/MS) using multiple reaction monitoring (MRM), with drug or metabolite description, comments including sample validation, per date of service

0150U   Drug assay, definitive, 120 or more drugs or metabolites, urine, quantitative liquid chromatography with tandem mass spectrometry (LC-MS/MS) using multiple reaction monitoring (MRM), with drug or metabolite description, comments including sample validation, per date of service

0151U   Infectious disease (bacterial or viral respiratory tract infection), pathogen specific nucleic acid (DNA or RNA), 33 targets, real-time semi-quantitative PCR, bronchoalveolar lavage, sputum, or endotracheal aspirate, detection of 33 organismal and antibiotic resistance genes with limited semi-quantitative results

0152U Infectious disease (bacteria, fungi, parasites, and DNA viruses), DNA, PCR and next-generation sequencing, plasma, detection of >1,000 potential microbial organisms for significant positive pathogens

0153U Oncology (breast), mRNA, gene expression profiling by next-generation sequencing of 101 genes, utilizing formalin-fixed paraffin-embedded tissue, algorithm reported as a triple negative breast cancer clinical subtype(s) with information on immune cell involvement

0154U *FGFR3 (fibroblast growth factor receptor 3)* gene analysis (ie, p.R248C [c.742C>T], p.S249C [c.746C>G], p.G370C [c.1108G>T], p.Y373C [c.1118A>G], FGFR3-TACC3v1, and FGFR3-TACC3v3)

0155U *PIK3CA (phosphatidylinositol-4,5-bisphosphate 3-kinase, catalytic subunit alpha)* (eg, breast cancer) gene analysis (ie, p.C420R, p.E542K, p.E545A, p.E545D [g.1635G>T only], p.E545G, p.E545K, p.Q546E, p.Q546R, p.H1047L, p.H1047R, p.H1047Y)

0156U Copy number (eg, intellectual disability, dysmorphology), sequence analysis

0157U *APC (APC regulator of WNT signaling pathway)* (eg, familial adenomatosis polyposis [FAP]) mRNA sequence analysis (List separately in addition to code for primary procedure)

0158U *MLH1 (mutL homolog 1)* (eg, hereditary non-polyposis colorectal cancer, Lynch syndrome) mRNA sequence analysis (List separately in addition to code for primary procedure)

0159U *MSH2 (mutS homolog 2)* (eg, hereditary colon cancer, Lynch syndrome) mRNA sequence analysis (List separately in addition to code for primary procedure)

0160U *MSH6 (mutS homolog 6)* (eg, hereditary colon cancer, Lynch syndrome) mRNA sequence analysis (List separately in addition to code for primary procedure)

0161U *PMS2 (PMS1 homolog 2, mismatch repair system component)* (eg, hereditary non-polyposis colorectal cancer, Lynch syndrome) mRNA sequence analysis (List separately in addition to code for primary procedure)

0162U Hereditary colon cancer (Lynch syndrome), targeted mRNA sequence analysis panel *(MLH1, MSH2, MSH6, PMS2)* (List separately in addition to code for primary procedure)

Deleted Codes

0011M Oncology, prostate cancer, mRNA expression assay of 12 genes (10 content and 2 housekeeping), RT-PCR test utilizing blood plasma and urine, algorithms to predict high-grade prostate cancer risk

0012M Oncology (urothelial), mRNA, gene expression profiling by real-time quantitative PCR of five genes (*MDK, HOXA13, CDC2 [CDK1], IGFBP5,* and *CXCR2*), utilizing urine, algorithm reported as a risk score for having urothelial carcinoma

0013M Oncology (urothelial), mRNA, gene expression profiling by real-time quantitative PCR of five genes (*MDK, HOXA13, CDC2 [CDK1], IGFBP5,* and *CXCR2*), utilizing urine, algorithm reported as a risk score for having recurrent urothelial carcinoma

81518 Oncology (breast), mRNA, gene expression profiling by real-time RT-PCR of 11 genes (7 content and 4 housekeeping), utilizing formalin-fixed paraffin-embedded tissue, algorithms reported as percentage risk for metastatic recurrence and likelihood of benefit from extended endocrine therapy

0062U Autoimmune (systemic lupus erythematosus), IgG and IgM analysis of 80 biomarkers, utilizing serum, algorithm reported with a risk score

0063U Neurology (autism), 32 amines by LC-MS/MS, using plasma, algorithm reported as metabolic signature associated with autism spectrum disorder

0064U Antibody, Treponema pallidum, total and rapid plasma reagin (RPR), immunoassay, qualitative

0065U Syphilis test, non-treponemal antibody, immunoassay, qualitative (RPR)

0066U Placental alpha-micro globulin-1 (PAMG-1), immunoassay with direct optical observation, cervico-vaginal fluid, each specimen

0067U Oncology (breast), immunohistochemistry, protein expression profiling of 4 biomarkers (matrix metalloproteinase-1 [MMP-1], carcinoembryonic antigen-related cell adhesion molecule 6 [CEACAM6], hyaluronoglucosaminidase [HYAL1], highly expressed in cancer protein [HEC1]), formalin-fixed paraffin-embedded precancerous breast tissue, algorithm reported as carcinoma risk score

0068U Candida species panel (*C. albicans, C. glabrata, C. parapsilosis, C. kruseii, C tropicalis, and C. auris*), amplified probe technique with qualitative report of the presence or absence of each species

0069U Oncology (colorectal), microRNA, RT-PCR expression profiling of miR-31-3p, formalin-fixed paraffin-embedded tissue, algorithm reported as an expression score

0070U *CYP2D6 (cytochrome P450, family 2, subfamily D, polypeptide 6)* (eg, drug metabolism) gene analysis, common and select rare variants (ie, *2, *3, *4, *4N, *5, *6, *7, *8, *9, *10, *11, *12, *13, *14A, *14B, *15, *17, *29, *35, *36, *41, *57, *61, *63, *68, *83, *xN)

0071U *CYP2D6 (cytochrome P450, family 2, subfamily D, polypeptide 6)* (eg, drug metabolism) gene analysis, full gene sequence (List separately in addition to code for primary procedure)

0072U *CYP2D6 (cytochrome P450, family 2, subfamily D, polypeptide 6)* (eg, drug metabolism) gene analysis, targeted sequence analysis (ie, CYP2D6-2D7 hybrid gene) (List separately in addition to code for primary procedure)

0073U *CYP2D6 (cytochrome P450, family 2, subfamily D, polypeptide 6)* (eg, drug metabolism) gene analysis, targeted sequence analysis (ie, CYP2D7-2D6 hybrid gene) (List separately in addition to code for primary procedure)

0074U *CYP2D6 (cytochrome P450, family 2, subfamily D, polypeptide 6)* (eg, drug metabolism) gene analysis, targeted sequence analysis (ie, non-duplicated gene when duplication/multiplication is trans) (List separately in addition to code for primary procedure)

0075U *CYP2D6 (cytochrome P450, family 2, subfamily D, polypeptide 6)* (eg, drug metabolism) gene analysis, targeted sequence analysis (ie, 5' gene duplication/multiplication) (List separately in addition to code for primary procedure)

0076U *CYP2D6 (cytochrome P450, family 2, subfamily D, polypeptide 6)* (eg, drug metabolism) gene analysis, targeted sequence analysis (ie, 3' gene duplication/ multiplication) (List separately in addition to code for primary procedure)

0077U Immunoglobulin paraprotein (M-protein), qualitative, immunoprecipitation and mass spectrometry, blood or urine, including isotype

0078U Pain management (opioid-use disorder) genotyping panel, 16 common variants (ie, *ABCB1, COMT, DAT1, DBH, DOR, DRD1, DRD2, DRD4, GABA, GAL, HTR2A, HTTLPR, MTHFR, MUOR, OPRK1, OPRM1*), buccal swab or other germline tissue sample, algorithm reported as positive or negative risk of opioid-use disorder

0079U Comparative DNA analysis using multiple selected single-nucleotide polymorphisms (SNPs), urine and buccal DNA, for specimen identity verification

This appendix provides an overview of evaluation and management (E/M) services, tables that identify the documentation elements associated with each code, and the federal documentation guidelines with emphasis on the 1997 exam guidelines. This set of guidelines represents the most complete discussion of the elements of the currently accepted versions. The 1997 version identifies both general multi-system physical examinations and single-system examinations, but providers may also use the original 1995 version of the E/M guidelines; both are currently supported by the Centers for Medicare and Medicaid Services (CMS) for audit purposes.

The levels of E/M services define the wide variations in skill, effort, and time and are required for preventing and/or diagnosing and treating illness or injury, and promoting optimal health. These codes are intended to represent physician work, and because much of this work involves the amount of training, experience, expertise, and knowledge that a provider may employ when treating a given patient, the true indications of the level of this work may be difficult to recognize without some explanation.

Providers

The AMA advises coders that while a particular service or procedure may be assigned to a specific section, the service or procedure itself is not limited to use only by that specialty group (see paragraphs 2 and 3 under "Instructions for Use of the CPT® Codebook" on page xii of the AMA CPT Book). Additionally, the procedures and services listed throughout the book are for use by any qualified physician or other qualified health care professional or entity (e.g., hospitals, laboratories, or home health agencies).

The use of the phrase "physician or other qualified health care professional" (OQHCP) was adopted to identify a health care provider other than a physician. This type of provider is further described in CPT as an individual "qualified by education, training, licensure/regulation (when applicable), and facility privileging (when applicable)." State licensure guidelines determine the scope of practice and an OQHCP must practice within these guidelines, even if more restrictive than the CPT guidelines. The OQHCP may report services independently or under incident-to guidelines. The professionals within this definition are separate from "clinical staff" and are able to practice independently. CPT defines clinical staff as "a person who works under the supervision of a physician or OQHCP and who is allowed, by law, regulation, and facility policy to perform or assist in the performance of a specified professional service, but who does not individually report that professional service." Keep in mind that there may be other policies or guidance that can affect who may report a specific service.

Types of E/M Services

When approaching E/M, the first choice that a provider must make is what type of code to use. The following tables outline the E/M codes for different levels of care for:

- Office or other outpatient services—new patient
- Office or other outpatient services—established patient
- Hospital observation services—initial care, subsequent, and discharge
- Hospital inpatient services—initial care, subsequent, and discharge
- Observation or inpatient care (including admission and discharge services)
- Consultations—office or other outpatient
- Consultations—inpatient
- Emergency department services
- Critical care
- Nursing facility—initial services
- Nursing facility—subsequent services
- Nursing facility—discharge and annual assessment
- Domiciliary, rest home, or custodial care—new patient
- Domiciliary, rest home, or custodial care—established patient
- Home services—new patient

- Home services—established patient
- Newborn care services
- Neonatal and pediatric interfacility transport
- Neonatal and pediatric critical care—inpatient
- Neonate and infant intensive care services—initial and continuing

The specifics of the code components that determine code selection are listed in the table and discussed in the next section. Before a level of service is decided upon, the correct type of service is identified.

A new patient is a patient who has not received any face-to-face professional services from the physician or OQHCP within the past three years. An established patient is a patient who has received face-to-face professional services from the physician or OQHCP within the past three years. In the case of group practices, if a physician or OQHCP of the exact same specialty or subspecialty has seen the patient within three years, the patient is considered established.

If a physician or OQHCP is on call or covering for another physician or OQHCP, the patient's encounter is classified as it would have been by the physician or OQHCP who is not available. Thus, a locum tenens physician or OQHCP who sees a patient on behalf of the patient's attending physician or OQHCP may not bill a new patient code unless the attending physician or OQHCP has not seen the patient for any problem within three years.

Office or other outpatient services are E/M services provided in the physician or OQHCP office, the outpatient area, or other ambulatory facility. Until the patient is admitted to a health care facility, he/she is considered to be an outpatient. Hospital observation services are E/M services provided to patients who are designated or admitted as "observation status" in a hospital.

Codes 99218-99220 are used to indicate initial observation care. These codes include the initiation of the observation status, supervision of patient care including writing orders, and the performance of periodic reassessments. These codes are used only by the provider "admitting" the patient for observation.

Codes 99234-99236 are used to indicate evaluation and management services to a patient who is admitted to and discharged from observation status or hospital inpatient on the same day. If the patient is admitted as an inpatient from observation on the same day, use the appropriate level of Initial Hospital Care (99221-99223).

Code 99217 indicates discharge from observation status. It includes the final physical examination of the patient, instructions, and preparation of the discharge records. It should not be used when admission and discharge are on the same date of service. As mentioned above, report codes 99234-99236 to appropriately describe same day observation services.

If a patient is in observation longer than one day, subsequent observation care codes 99224-99226 should be reported. If the patient is discharged on the second day, observation discharge code 99217 should be reported. If the patient status is changed to inpatient on a subsequent date, the appropriate inpatient code, 99221-99233, should be reported.

Initial hospital care is defined as E/M services provided during the first hospital inpatient encounter with the patient by the admitting provider. (If a physician other than the admitting physician performs the initial inpatient encounter, refer to consultations or subsequent hospital care in the CPT book.) Subsequent hospital care includes all follow-up encounters with the patient by all physicians or OQHCP. As there may only be one admitting physician, HCPCS Level II modifier AI Principal physician of record, should be appended to the initial hospital care code by the attending physician or OQHCP.

A consultation is the provision of a physician or OQHCP's opinion or advice about a patient for a specific problem at the request of another physician or other appropriate source. CPT also states that a consultation may be performed when a physician or OQHCP is determining whether to accept the transfer of patient care at the request of another physician or appropriate source. An office or other outpatient consultation is a consultation provided in the consultant's office, in the emergency department, or in an outpatient or other ambulatory facility including hospital observation services, home services, domiciliary, rest home, or custodial care. An inpatient consultation is a consultation provided in the hospital or partial hospital nursing facility setting. Report only one inpatient consultation by a consultant for each admission to the hospital or nursing facility.

If a consultant participates in the patient's management after the opinion or advice is provided, use codes for subsequent hospital or observation care or for office or other outpatient services (established patient), as appropriate.

Under CMS guidelines, the inpatient and office/outpatient consultation codes contained in the CPT manual are not covered services.

All outpatient consultation services will be reported for Medicare using the appropriate new or established evaluation and management (E/M) codes. Inpatient consultation services for the initial encounter should be reported by the physician providing the service using initial hospital care codes 99221–99223, and subsequent inpatient care codes 99231–99233.

Codes 99487, 99489, 99490, and 99491 are used to report evaluation and management services for chronic care management. These codes

represent management and support services provided by clinical staff, under the direction of a physician or OQHCP, to patients residing at home or in a domiciliary, rest home, or assisted living facility. The qualified provider oversees the management and/or coordination of services for all medical conditions, psychosocial needs, and activities of daily living. These codes are reported only once per calendar month and have specific time-based thresholds.

Codes 99497-99498 are used to report the discussion and explanation of advanced directives by a physician or OQHCP. These codes represent a face-to-face service between the provider and a patient, family member, or surrogate. These codes are time-based codes and, since no active management of the problem(s) is undertaken during this time, may be reported on the same day as another E/M service.

Certain codes that CPT considers appropriate telehealth services are identified with the ★ icon and reported with modifier 95 Synchronous telemedicine service rendered via a real-time interactive audio and video telecommunications system. Medicare recognizes certain CPT and HCPCS Level II G codes as telehealth services reported with modifier GT. Check with individual payers for telehealth modifier guidance.

Office or Other Outpatient Services—New Patient

CMS PROPOSED CHANGES FOR E&M SERVICES, CODES 99201–99215

The Centers for Medicare and Medicaid Services (CMS) has announced the following changes that are scheduled to become effective January 1, 2021:

- Separate payment will be assigned for each level of office/outpatient E&M services codes, as revised by the CPT Editorial Panel effective January 1, 2021, and resurveyed by the AMA RUC, with minor refinement. This would include deletion of CPT code 99201 (Level 1 new patient office/outpatient E&M visit) and adoption of the revised CPT code descriptors for CPT codes 99202–99215.
- The use of history and/or physical exam to select among code levels will be eliminated.
- Either time or medical decision making can be used to decide the level of office/outpatient E&M visit (using the revised CPT interpretive guidelines for medical decision making), with the exception of 99211 and emergency department levels.
- Time is face-to-face and will include non-face-to-face time before and after the encounter.
- CMS will adopt updated E&M guidelines.
- CPT descriptions will be revised.
- A new CPT add-on code will be created for level 5 to capture prolonged/extended visits of at least 15 additional minutes.

E/M Code	History[1]	Exam[1]	Medical Decision Making[1]	Problem Severity	Coordination of Care; Counseling	Time Spent Face-to-Face (avg.)
99201	Problem-focused	Problem-focused	Straight-forward	Minor or self-limited	Consistent with problem(s) and patient's needs	10 min.
99202	Expanded problem-focused	Expanded problem-focused	Straight-forward	Low to moderate	Consistent with problem(s) and patient's needs	20 min.
99203	Detailed	Detailed	Low complexity	Moderate	Consistent with problem(s) and patient's needs	30 min.
99204	Comprehensive	Comprehensive	Moderate complexity	Moderate to high	Consistent with problem(s) and patient's needs	45 min.
99205	Comprehensive	Comprehensive	High complexity	Moderate to high	Consistent with problem(s) and patient's needs	60 min.

1 Key component. For new patients, all three components (history, exam, and medical decision making) are crucial for selecting the correct code.

Office or Other Outpatient Services—Established Patient[1]

E/M Code	History[2]	Exam[2]	Medical Decision Making[2]	Problem Severity	Coordination of Care; Counseling	Time Spent Face-to-Face (avg.)
99211	—	—	Physician supervision, but presence not required	Minimal	Consistent with problem(s) and patient's needs	5 min.
99212	Problem-focused	Problem-focused	Straight-forward	Minor or self-limited	Consistent with problem(s) and patient's needs	10 min.
99213	Expanded problem-focused	Expanded problem-focused	Low complexity	Low to moderate	Consistent with problem(s) and patient's needs	15 min.
99214	Detailed	Detailed	Moderate complexity	Moderate to high	Consistent with problem(s) and patient's needs	25 min.
99215	Comprehensive	Comprehensive	High complexity	Moderate to high	Consistent with problem(s) and patient's needs	40 min.

1 Includes follow-up, periodic reevaluation, and evaluation and management of new problems.

2 Key component. For established patients, at least two of the three components (history, exam, and medical decision making) are needed to select the correct code.

Hospital Observation Services

E/M Code	History[1]	Exam[1]	Medical Decision Making[1]	Problem Severity	Coordination of Care; Counseling	Time Spent Bedside and on Unit/Floor (avg.)
99217	Observation care discharge day management					
99218	Detailed or comprehensive	Detailed or comprehensive	Straight-forward or low complexity	Low	Consistent with problem(s) and patient's needs	30 min.
99219	Comprehensive	Comprehensive	Moderate complexity	Moderate	Consistent with problem(s) and patient's needs	50 min.
99220	Comprehensive	Comprehensive	High complexity	High	Consistent with problem(s) and patient's needs	70 min.

1 Key component. All three components (history, exam, and medical decision making) are crucial for selecting the correct code.

Subsequent Hospital Observation Services[1]

E/M Code[2]	History[3]	Exam[3]	Medical Decision Making[3]	Problem Severity	Coordination of Care; Counseling	Time Spent Bedside and on Unit/Floor (avg.)
99224	Problem-focused interval	Problem-focused	Straight-forward or low complexity	Stable, recovering, or improving	Consistent with problem(s) and patient's needs	15 min.
99225	Expanded problem-focused interval	Expanded problem-focused	Moderate complexity	Inadequate response to treatment; minor complications	Consistent with problem(s) and patient's needs	25 min.
99226	Detailed interval	Detailed	High complexity	Unstable; significant new problem or significant complication	Consistent with problem(s) and patient's needs	35 min.

1 All subsequent levels of service include reviewing the medical record, diagnostic studies, and changes in the patient's status, such as history, physical condition, and response to treatment since the last assessment.

2 These codes are resequenced in CPT and are printed following codes 99217-99220.

3 Key component. For subsequent care, at least two of the three components (history, exam, and medical decision making) are needed to select the correct code.

Hospital Inpatient Services—Initial Care[1]

E/M Code	History[2]	Exam[2]	Medical Decision Making[2]	Problem Severity	Coordination of Care; Counseling	Time Spent Bedside and on Unit/Floor (avg.)
99221	Detailed or comprehensive	Detailed or comprehensive	Straight-forward or low complexity	Low	Consistent with problem(s) and patient's needs	30 min.
99222	Comprehensive	Comprehensive	Moderate complexity	Moderate	Consistent with problem(s) and patient's needs	50 min.
99223	Comprehensive	Comprehensive	High complexity	High	Consistent with problem(s) and patient's needs	70 min.

1 The admitting physician should append modifier AI, Principal physician of record, for Medicare patients

2 Key component. For initial care, all three components (history, exam, and medical decision making) are crucial for selecting the correct code.

Hospital Inpatient Services—Subsequent Care[1]

E/M Code	History[2]	Exam[2]	Medical Decision Making[2]	Problem Severity	Coordination of Care; Counseling	Time Spent Bedside and on Unit/Floor (avg.)
99231	Problem-focused interval	Problem-focused	Straight-forward or low complexity	Stable, recovering or Improving	Consistent with problem(s) and patient's needs	15 min.
99232	Expanded problem-focused interval	Expanded problem-focused	Moderate complexity	Inadequate response to treatment; minor complications	Consistent with problem(s) and patient's needs	25 min.
99233	Detailed interval	Detailed	High complexity	Unstable; significant new problem or significant complication	Consistent with problem(s) and patient's needs	35 min.
99238	Hospital discharge day management					30 min. or less
99239	Hospital discharge day management					> 30 min.

1 All subsequent levels of service include reviewing the medical record, diagnostic studies, and changes in the patient's status, such as history, physical condition, and response to treatment since the last assessment.

2 Key component. For subsequent care, at least two of the three components (history, exam, and medical decision making) are needed to select the correct code.

Observation or Inpatient Care Services (Including Admission and Discharge Services)

E/M Code	History[1]	Exam[1]	Medical Decision Making[1]	Problem Severity	Coordination of Care; Counseling	Time
99234	Detailed or comprehensive	Detailed or comprehensive	Straight-forward or low complexity	Low	Consistent with problem(s) and patient's needs	40 min.
99235	Comprehensive	Comprehensive	Moderate	Moderate	Consistent with problem(s) and patient's needs	50 min.
99236	Comprehensive	Comprehensive	High	High	Consistent with problem(s) and patient's needs	55 min.

1 Key component. All three components (history, exam, and medical decision making) are crucial for selecting the correct code.

Consultations—Office or Other Outpatient

E/M Code	History[1]	Exam[1]	Medical Decision Making[1]	Problem Severity	Coordination of Care; Counseling	Time Spent Face-to-Face (avg.)
99241	Problem-focused	Problem-focused	Straight-forward	Minor or self-limited	Consistent with problem(s) and patient's needs	15 min.
99242	Expanded problem-focused	Expanded problem-focused	Straight-forward	Low	Consistent with problem(s) and patient's needs	30 min.
99243	Detailed	Detailed	Low complexity	Moderate	Consistent with problem(s) and patient's needs	40 min.
99244	Comprehensive	Comprehensive	Moderate complexity	Moderate to high	Consistent with problem(s) and patient's needs	60 min.
99245	Comprehensive	Comprehensive	High complexity	Moderate to high	Consistent with problem(s) and patient's needs	80 min.

1 Key component. For office or other outpatient consultations, all three components (history, exam, and medical decision making) are crucial for selecting the correct code.

Consultations—Inpatient[1]

E/M Code	History[2]	Exam[2]	Medical Decision Making[2]	Problem Severity	Coordination of Care; Counseling	Time Spent Bedside and on Unit/Floor (avg.)
99251	Problem-focused	Problem-focused	Straight-forward	Minor or self-limited	Consistent with problem(s) and patient's needs	20 min.
99252	Expanded problem-focused	Expanded problem-focused	Straight-forward	Low	Consistent with problem(s) and patient's needs	40 min.
99253	Detailed	Detailed	Low complexity	Moderate	Consistent with problem(s) and patient's needs	55 min.
99254	Comprehensive	Comprehensive	Moderate complexity	Moderate to high	Consistent with problem(s) and patient's needs	80 min.
99255	Comprehensive	Comprehensive	High complexity	Moderate to high	Consistent with problem(s) and patient's needs	110 min.

1 These codes are used for hospital inpatients, residents of nursing facilities or patients in a partial hospital setting.
2 Key component. For initial inpatient consultations, all three components (history, exam, and medical decision making) are crucial for selecting the correct code.

Emergency Department Services, New or Established Patient

E/M Code	History[1]	Exam[1]	Medical Decision Making[1]	Problem Severity[3]	Coordination of Care; Counseling	Time Spent[2] Face-to-Face (avg.)
99281	Problem-focused	Problem-focused	Straight-forward	Minor or self-limited	Consistent with problem(s) and patient's needs	N/A
99282	Expanded problem-focused	Expanded problem-focused	Low complexity	Low to moderate	Consistent with problem(s) and patient's needs	N/A
99283	Expanded problem-focused	Expanded problem-focused	Moderate complexity	Moderate	Consistent with problem(s) and patient's needs	N/A
99284	Detailed	Detailed	Moderate complexity	High; requires urgent evaluation	Consistent with problem(s) and patient's needs	N/A
99285	Comprehensive	Comprehensive	High complexity	High; poses immediate/significant threat to life or physiologic function	Consistent with problem(s) and patient's needs	N/A
99288[4]			High complexity			N/A

1 Key component. For emergency department services, all three components (history, exam, and medical decision making) are crucial for selecting the correct code and must be adequately documented in the medical record to substantiate the level of service reported.

2 Typical times have not been established for this category of services.

3 NOTE: The severity of the patient's problem, while taken into consideration when evaluating and treating the patient, does not automatically determine the level of E/M service unless the medical record documentation reflects the severity of the patient's illness, injury, or condition in the details of the history, physical examination, and medical decision making process. Federal auditors will "downcode" the level of E/M service despite the nature of the patient's problem when the documentation does not support the E/M code reported.

4 Code 99288 is used to report two-way communication with emergency medical services personnel in the field.

Critical Care

E/M Code	Patient Status	Physician Attendance	Time[1]
99291	Critically ill or critically injured	Constant	First 30–74 minutes
99292	Critically ill or critically injured	Constant	Each additional 30 minutes beyond the first 74 minutes

1 Per the guidelines for time in *CPT 2016 page xv*, "A unit of time is attained when the mid-point is passed. For example, an hour is attained when 31 minutes have elapsed (more than midway between zero and 60 minutes)."

Nursing Facility Services—Initial Nursing Facility Care[1]

E/M Code	History[1]	Exam[1]	Medical Decision Making[1]	Problem Severity	Coordination of Care; Counseling
99304	Detailed or comprehensive	Detailed or comprehensive	Straight-forward or low complexity	Low	25 min.
99305	Comprehensive	Comprehensive	Moderate complexity	Moderate	35 min.
99306	Comprehensive	Comprehensive	High complexity	High	45 min.

1 These services must be performed by the physician. See CPT Corrections Document – CPT 2013 page 3 or guidelines CPT 2016 page 26.

2 Key component. For new patients, all three components (history, exam, and medical decision making) are crucial for selecting the correct code.

Nursing Facility Services—Subsequent Nursing Facility Care

E/M Code	History[1]	Exam[1]	Medical Decision Making[2]	Problem Severity	Coordination of Care; Counseling
99307	Problem-focused interval	Problem-focused	Straight-forward	Stable, recovering or improving	10 min.
99308	Expanded problem-focused interval	Expanded problem-focused	Low complexity	Responding inadequately or has developed a minor complication	15 min.
99309	Detailed interval	Detailed	Moderate complexity	Significant complication or a significant new problem	25 min.
99310	Comprehensive interval	Comprehensive	High complexity	Developed a significant new problem requiring immediate attention	35 min.

1 Key component. For established patients, at least two of the three components (history, exam, and medical decision making) are needed for selecting the correct code.

Nursing Facility Discharge and Annual Assessment

E/M Code	History[1]	Exam[1]	Medical Decision Making[1]	Problem Severity	Time Spent Bedside and on Unit/Floor (avg.)
99315	Nursing facility discharge day management				30 min. or less
99316	Nursing facility discharge day management				more than 30 min.
99318	Detailed interval	Comprehensive	Low to moderate complexity	Stable, recovering or improving	30 min.

1 Key component. For annual nursing facility assessment, all three components (history, exam, and medical decision making) are crucial for selecting the correct code.

Domiciliary, Rest Home (e.g., Boarding Home) or Custodial Care Services—New Patient

E/M Code	History[1]	Exam[1]	Medical Decision Making[1]	Problem Severity	Coordination of Care; Counseling	Time Spent Face-to-Face (avg.)
99324	Problem-focused	Problem-focused	Straight-forward	Low	Consistent with problem(s) and patient's needs	20 min.
99325	Expanded problem-focused	Expanded problem-focused	Low complexity	Moderate	Consistent with problem(s) and patient's needs	30 min.
99326	Detailed	Detailed	Moderate complexity	Moderate to high	Consistent with problem(s) and patient's needs	45 min.
99327	Comprehensive	Comprehensive	Moderate complexity	High	Consistent with problem(s) and patient's needs	60 min.
99328	Comprehensive	Comprehensive	High complexity	Unstable or developed a new problem requiring immediate physician attention	Consistent with problem(s) and patient's needs	75 min.

1 Key component. For new patients, all three components (history, exam, and medical decision making) are crucial for selecting the correct code and must be adequately documented in the medical record to substantiate the level of service reported.

Domiciliary, Rest Home (e.g., Boarding Home) or Custodial Care Services— Established Patient

E/M Code	History[1]	Exam[1]	Medical Decision Making[1]	Problem Severity	Coordination of Care; Counseling	Time Spent Face-to-Face (avg.)
99334	Problem-focused interval	Problem-focused	Straight-forward	Minor or self-limited	Consistent with problem(s) and patient's needs	15 min.
99335	Expanded problem-focused interval	Expanded problem-focused	Low complexity	Low to moderate	Consistent with problem(s) and patient's needs	25 min.
99336	Detailed interval	Detailed	Moderate complexity	Moderate to high	Consistent with problem(s) and patient's needs	40 min.
99337	Comprehensive interval	Comprehensive	Moderate to high complexity	Moderate to high	Consistent with problem(s) and patient's needs	60 min.

1 Key component. For established patients, at least two of the three components (history, exam, and medical decision making) are needed for selecting the correct code.

Domiciliary, Rest Home (e.g., Assisted Living Facility), or Home Care Plan Oversight Services

E/M Code	Intent of Service	Presence of Patient	Time
99339	Individual physician supervision of a patient (patient not present) in home, domiciliary or rest home (e.g., assisted living facility) requiring complex and multidisciplinary care modalities involving regular physician development and/or revision of care plans, review of subsequent reports of patient status, review of related laboratory and other studies, communication (including telephone calls) for purposes of assessment or care decisions with health care professional(s), family member(s), surrogate decision maker(s) (e.g., legal guardian) and/or key caregiver(s) involved in patient's care, integration of new information into the medical treatment plan and/or adjustment of medical therapy, within a calendar month	Patient not present	15–29 min.
99340	Same as 99339	Patient not present	30 min. or more

Home Services—New Patient

E/M Code	History[1]	Exam[1]	Medical Decision Making[1]	Problem Severity	Coordination of Care; Counseling	Time Spent Face-to-Face (avg.)
99341	Problem-focused	Problem-focused	Straight-forward complexity	Low	Consistent with problem(s) and patient's needs	20 min.
99342	Expanded problem-focused	Expanded problem-focused	Low complexity	Moderate	Consistent with problem(s) and patient's needs	30 min.
99343	Detailed	Detailed	Moderate complexity	Moderate to high	Consistent with problem(s) and patient's needs	45 min.
99344	Comprehensive	Comprehensive	Moderate complexity	High	Consistent with problem(s) and patient's needs	60 min.
99345	Comprehensive	Comprehensive	High complexity	Usually the patient has developed a significant new problem requiring immediate physician attention	Consistent with problem(s) and patient's needs	75 min.

1 Key component. For new patients, all three components (history, exam, and medical decision making) are crucial for selecting the correct code and must be adequately documented in the medical record to substantiate the level of service reported.

Home Services—Established Patient

E/M Code	History[1]	Exam[1]	Medical Decision Making[1]	Problem Severity	Coordination of Care; Counseling	Time Spent Face-to-Face (avg.)
99347	Problem-focused interval	Problem-focused	Straight-forward	Minor or self-limited	Consistent with problem(s) and patient's needs	15 min.
99348	Expanded problem-focused interval	Expanded problem-focused	Low complexity	Low to moderate	Consistent with problem(s) and patient's needs	25 min.
99349	Detailed interval	Detailed	Moderate complexity	Moderate to high	Consistent with problem(s) and patient's needs	40 min.
99350	Comprehensive interval	Comprehensive	Moderate to high complexity	Moderate to high Usually the patient has developed a significant new problem requiring immediate physician attention	Consistent with problem(s) and patient's needs	60 min.

1 Key component. For established patients, at least two of the three components (history, exam, and medical decision making) are needed for selecting the correct code.

Newborn Care Services

E/M Code	Patient Status	Type of Visit
99460	Normal newborn	Inpatient initial inpatient hospital or birthing center per day
99461	Normal newborn	Inpatient initial treatment not in hospital or birthing center per day
99462	Normal newborn	Inpatient subsequent per day
99463	Normal newborn	Inpatient initial inpatient and discharge in hospital or birthing center per day
99464	Unstable newborn	Attendance at delivery
99465	High-risk newborn at delivery	Resuscitation, ventilation, and cardiac treatment

Neonatal and Pediatric Interfacility Transportation

E/M Code	Patient Status	Type of Visit
99466	Critically ill or injured infant or young child, to 24 months	Face-to-face transportation from one facility to another, initial 30-74 minutes
99467	Critically ill or injured infant or young child, to 24 months	Face-to-face transportation from one facility to another, each additional 30 minutes
99485[1]	Critically ill or injured infant or young child, to 24 months	Supervision of patient transport from one facility to another, initial 30 minutes
99486[1]	Critically ill or injured infant or young child, to 24 months	Supervision of patient transport from one facility to another, each additional 30 minutes

1 These codes are resequenced in CPT and are printed following codes 99466-99467.

Inpatient Neonatal and Pediatric Critical Care

E/M Code	Patient Status	Type of Visit
99468[1]	Critically ill neonate, aged 28 days or less	Inpatient initial per day
99469[2]	Critically ill neonate, aged 28 days or less	Inpatient subsequent per day
99471	Critically ill infant or young child, aged 29 days to 24 months	Inpatient initial per day
99472	Critically ill infant or young child, aged 29 days to 24 months	Inpatient subsequent per day
99475	Critically ill infant or young child, 2 to 5 years[3]	Inpatient initial per day
99476	Critically ill infant or young child, 2 to 5 years	Inpatient subsequent per day

1 Codes 99468, 99471, and 99475 may be reported only once per admission.
2 Codes 99469, 99472, and 99476 may be reported only once per day and by only one provider.
3 See 99291-99292 for patients 6 years of age and older.

Neonate and Infant Initial and Continuing Intensive Care Services

E/M Code	Patient Status	Type of Visit
99477	Neonate, aged 28 days or less	Inpatient initial per day
99478	Infant with present body weight of less than 1500 grams, no longer critically ill	Inpatient subsequent per day
99479	Infant with present body weight of 1500-2500 grams, no longer critically ill	Inpatient subsequent per day
99480	Infant with present body weight of 2501-5000 grams, no longer critically ill	Inpatient subsequent per day

Levels of E/M Services

Confusion may be experienced when first approaching E/M due to the way that each description of a code component or element seems to have another layer of description beneath. The three key components—history, exam, and decision making—are each comprised of elements that combine to create varying levels of that component.

For example, an expanded problem-focused history includes the chief complaint, a brief history of the present illness, and a system review focusing on the patient's problems. The level of exam is not made up of different elements but rather distinguished by the extent of exam across body areas or organ systems.

The single largest source of confusion are the "labels" or names applied to the varying degrees of history, exam, and decision-making. Terms such as expanded problem-focused, detailed, and comprehensive are somewhat meaningless unless they are defined. The lack of definition in CPT guidelines relative to these terms is precisely what caused the first set of federal guidelines to be developed in 1995 and again in 1997.

Documentation Guidelines for Evaluation and Management Services

Both versions of the federal guidelines go well beyond CPT guidelines in defining specific code requirements. The current version of the CPT guidelines does not explain the number of history of present illness (HPI) elements or the specific number of organ systems or body areas to be examined as they are in the federal guidelines. Adherence to some version of the guidelines is required when billing E/M to federal payers, but at this time, the CPT guidelines do not incorporate this level of detail into the code definitions. Although that could be interpreted to mean that non-governmental payers have a lesser documentation standard, it is best to adopt one set of the federal versions for all payer types for both consistency and ease of use.

The 1997 guidelines supply a great amount of detail relative to history and exam and will give the provider clear direction to follow when documenting elements. With that stated, the 1995 guidelines are equally valid and place a lesser documentation burden on the provider in regards to the physical exam.

The 1995 guidelines ask only for a notation of "normal" on systems with normal findings. The only narrative required is for abnormal findings. The 1997 version calls for much greater detail, or an "elemental" or "bullet-point" approach to organ systems, although a notation of normal is sufficient when addressing the elements within a system. The 1997 version works well in a template or electronic health record (EHR) format for recording E/M services.

The 1997 version did produce the single system specialty exam guidelines. When reviewing the complete guidelines listed below, note the differences between exam requirements in the 1995 and 1997 versions.

A Comparison of 1995 and 1997 Exam Guidelines

There are four types of exams indicated in the levels of E/M codes. Although the descriptors or labels are the same under 1995 and 1997 guidelines, the degree of detail required is different. The remaining content on this topic references the 1997 general multi-system specialty examination, at the end of this chapter.

The levels under each set of guidelines are:

1995 Exam Guidelines:

Problem focused:	One body area or system
Expanded problem focused:	Two to seven body areas or organ systems
Detailed:	Two to seven body areas or organ systems
Comprehensive:	Eight or more organ systems or a complete single-system examination

1997 Exam Guidelines:

Problem-focused:	Perform and document examination of one to five bullet point elements in one or more organ systems/body areas from the general multi-system examination
OR	
	Perform or document examination of one to five bullet point elements from one of the 10 single-organ-system examinations, shaded or unshaded boxes
Expanded problem-focused:	Perform and document examination of at least six bullet point elements in one or more organ systems from the general multi-system examination
OR	
	Perform and document examination of at least six bullet point elements from one of the 10 single-organ-system examinations, shaded or unshaded boxes
Detailed:	Perform and document examination of at least six organ systems or body areas, including at least two bullet point elements for each organ system or body area from the general multi-system examination
OR	
	Perform and document examination of at least 12 bullet point elements in two or more organ systems or body areas from the general multisystem examination
OR	
	Perform and document examination of at least 12 bullet elements from one of the single-organ-system examinations, shaded or unshaded boxes
Comprehensive:	Perform and document examination of at least nine organ systems or body areas, with all bullet elements for each organ system or body area (unless specific instructions are expected to limit examination content with at least two bullet elements for each organ system or body area) from the general multi-system examination

OR

Perform and document examination of all bullet point elements from one of the 10 single-organ system examinations with documentation of every element in shaded boxes and at least one element in each unshaded box from the single-organ-system examination.

The Documentation Guidelines

The following guidelines were developed jointly by the American Medical Association (AMA) and the Centers for Medicare and Medicaid Services (CMS). Their mutual goal was to provide physicians and claims reviewers with advice about preparing or reviewing documentation for Evaluation and Management (E/M) services.

I. Introduction

What is Documentation and Why Is It Important?

Medical record documentation is required to record pertinent facts, findings, and observations about an individual's health history, including past and present illnesses, examinations, tests, treatments, and outcomes. The medical record chronologically documents the care of the patient and is an important element contributing to high quality care. The medical record facilitates:

- The ability of the physician and other health care professionals to evaluate and plan the patient's immediate treatment and to monitor his/her health care over time
- Communication and continuity of care among physicians and other health care professionals involved in the patient's care
- Accurate and timely claims review and payment
- Appropriate utilization review and quality of care evaluations
- Collection of data that may be useful for research and education

An appropriately documented medical record can reduce many of the problems associated with claims processing and may serve as a legal document to verify the care provided, if necessary.

What Do Payers Want and Why?

Because payers have a contractual obligation to enrollees, they may require reasonable documentation that services are consistent with the insurance coverage provided. They may request information to validate:

- The site of service
- The medical necessity and appropriateness of the diagnostic and/or therapeutic services provided
- Services provided have been accurately reported

II. General Principles of Medical Record Documentation

The principles of documentation listed below are applicable to all types of medical and surgical services in all settings. For Evaluation and Management (E/M) services, the nature and amount of physician work and documentation varies by type of service, place of service, and the patient's status. The general principles listed below may be modified to account for these variable circumstances in providing E/M services.

- The medical record should be complete and legible
- The documentation of each patient encounter should include:
  - A reason for the encounter and relevant history, physical examination findings, and prior diagnostic test results
  - Assessment, clinical impression, or diagnosis
  - Plan for care
  - Date and legible identity of the practitioner
- If not documented, the rationale for ordering diagnostic and other ancillary services should be easily inferred
- Past and present diagnoses should be accessible to the treating and/or consulting physician
- Appropriate health risk factors should be identified
- The patient's progress, response to, and changes in treatment and revision of diagnosis should be documented
- The CPT and ICD-9-CM codes reported on the health insurance claim form or billing statement should be supported by the documentation in the medical record

III. Documentation of E/M Services 1995 and 1997

The following information provides definitions and documentation guidelines for the three key components of E/M services and for visits that consist predominately of counseling or coordination of care. The three key components—history, examination, and medical decision making—appear in the descriptors for office and other outpatient services, hospital observation services, hospital inpatient services, consultations, emergency department services, nursing facility services, domiciliary care services, and home services. While some of the text of the CPT guidelines has been repeated in this document, the reader should refer to CMS or CPT for the complete descriptors for E/M services and instructions for selecting a level of service. Documentation guidelines are identified by the symbol DG.

The descriptors for the levels of E/M services recognize seven components that are used in defining the levels of E/M services. These components are:

- History
- Examination
- Medical decision making
- Counseling
- Coordination of care
- Nature of presenting problem
- Time

The first three of these components (i.e., history, examination, and medical decision making) are the key components in selecting the level of E/M services. In the case of visits that consist predominately of counseling or coordination of care, time is the key or controlling factor to qualify for a particular level of E/M service.

Because the level of E/M service is dependent on two or three key components, performance and documentation of one component (e.g., examination) at the highest level does not necessarily mean that the encounter in its entirety qualifies for the highest level of E/M service.

These Documentation Guidelines for E/M services reflect the needs of the typical adult population. For certain groups of patients, the recorded information may vary slightly from that described here. Specifically, the medical records of infants, children, adolescents, and pregnant women may have additional or modified information, as appropriate, recorded in each history and examination area.

As an example, newborn records may include under history of the present illness (HPI) the details of the mother's pregnancy and the infant's status at birth; social history will focus on family structure; and family history will focus on congenital anomalies and hereditary disorders in the family. In addition, the content of a pediatric examination will vary with the age and development of the child. Although not specifically defined in these documentation guidelines, these patient group variations on history and examination are appropriate.

A. Documentation of History

The levels of E/M services are based on four types of history (Problem Focused, Expanded Problem Focused, Detailed, and Comprehensive). Each type of history includes some or all of the following elements:

- Chief complaint (CC)
- History of present illness (HPI)
- Review of systems (ROS)
- Past, family, and/or social history (PFSH)

The extent of history of present illness, review of systems, and past, family, and/or social history that is obtained and documented is dependent upon clinical judgment and the nature of the presenting problem.

The chart below shows the progression of the elements required for each type of history. To qualify for a given type of history all three elements in the table must be met. (A chief complaint is indicated at all levels.)

- DG: The CC, ROS, and PFSH may be listed as separate elements of history or they may be included in the description of the history of present illness

- DG: A ROS and/or a PFSH obtained during an earlier encounter does not need to be re-recorded if there is evidence that the physician reviewed and updated the previous information. This may occur when a physician updates his/her own record or in an institutional setting or group practice where many physicians use a common record. The review and update may be documented by:

  – Describing any new ROS and/or PFSH information or noting there has been no change in the information

  – Noting the date and location of the earlier ROS and/or PFSH

- DG: The ROS and/or PFSH may be recorded by ancillary staff or on a form completed by the patient. To document that the physician reviewed the information, there must be a notation supplementing or confirming the information recorded by others

- DG: If the physician is unable to obtain a history from the patient or other source, the record should describe the patient's condition or other circumstance that precludes obtaining a history

Definitions and specific documentation guidelines for each of the elements of history are listed below.

Chief Complaint (CC)

The CC is a concise statement describing the symptom, problem, condition, diagnosis, physician recommended return, or other factor that is the reason for the encounter, usually stated in the patient's words.

- DG: The medical record should clearly reflect the chief complaint

History of Present Illness (HPI)

The HPI is a chronological description of the development of the patient's present illness from the first sign and/or symptom or from the previous encounter to the present. It includes the following elements:

- Location
- Quality
- Severity
- Duration
- Timing
- Context
- Modifying factors
- Associated signs and symptoms

Brief and extended HPIs are distinguished by the amount of detail needed to accurately characterize the clinical problem.

A brief HPI consists of one to three elements of the HPI.

- DG: The medical record should describe one to three elements of the present illness (HPI)

An extended HPI consists of at least four elements of the HPI or the status of at least three chronic or inactive conditions.

- DG: The medical record should describe at least four elements of the present illness (HPI) or the status of at least three chronic or inactive conditions

Beginning with services performed on or after September 10, 2013, CMS has stated that physicians and OQHCP will be able to use the 1997 guidelines for an extended history of present illness (HPI) in combination with other elements from the 1995 documentation guidelines to document a particular level of evaluation and management service.

History of Present Illness	Review of systems (ROS)	PFSH	Type of History
Brief	N/A	N/A	Problem-focused
Brief	Problem Pertinent	N/A	Expanded Problem-Focused
Extended	Extended	Pertinent	Detailed
Extended	Complete	Complete	Comprehensive

Review of Systems (ROS)

A ROS is an inventory of body systems obtained through a series of questions seeking to identify signs and/or symptoms that the patient may be experiencing or has experienced. For purposes of ROS, the following systems are recognized:

- Constitutional symptoms (e.g., fever, weight loss)
- Eyes
- Ears, nose, mouth, throat
- Cardiovascular
- Respiratory
- Gastrointestinal
- Genitourinary
- Musculoskeletal
- Integumentary (skin and/or breast)
- Neurological
- Psychiatric
- Endocrine
- Hematologic/lymphatic
- Allergic/immunologic

A problem pertinent ROS inquires about the system directly related to the problem identified in the HPI.

- DG: The patient's positive responses and pertinent negatives for the system related to the problem should be documented

An extended ROS inquires about the system directly related to the problem identified in the HPI and a limited number of additional systems.

- DG: The patient's positive responses and pertinent negatives for two to nine systems should be documented

A complete ROS inquires about the system directly related to the problem identified in the HPI plus all additional body systems.

- DG: At least 10 organ systems must be reviewed. Those systems with positive or pertinent negative responses must be individually documented. For the remaining systems, a notation indicating all other systems are negative is permissible. In the absence of such a notation, at least 10 systems must be individually documented

Past, Family, and/or Social History (PFSH)

The PFSH consists of a review of three areas:

- Past history (the patient's past experiences with illnesses, operations, injuries, and treatment)
- Family history (a review of medical events in the patient's family, including diseases that may be hereditary or place the patient at risk)
- Social history (an age appropriate review of past and current activities)

For certain categories of E/M services that include only an interval history, it is not necessary to record information about the PFSH. Those categories are subsequent hospital care, follow-up inpatient consultations, and subsequent nursing facility care.

A pertinent PFSH is a review of the history area directly related to the problem identified in the HPI.

- DG: At least one specific item from any of the three history areas must be documented for a pertinent PFSH

A complete PFSH is a review of two or all three of the PFSH history areas, depending on the category of the E/M service. A review of all three history areas is required for services that by their nature include a comprehensive assessment or reassessment of the patient. A review of two of the three history areas is sufficient for other services.

- DG: A least one specific item from two of the three history areas must be documented for a complete PFSH for the following categories of E/M services: office or other outpatient services, established patient; emergency department; domiciliary care, established patient; and home care, established patient

- DG: At least one specific item from each of the three history areas must be documented for a complete PFSH for the following categories of E/M services: office or other outpatient services, new patient; hospital observation services; hospital inpatient services, initial care; consultations; comprehensive nursing facility assessments; domiciliary care, new patient; and home care, new patient

B. Documentation of Examination 1997 Guidelines

The levels of E/M services are based on four types of examination:

- Problem Focused: A limited examination of the affected body area or organ system
- Expanded Problem Focused: A limited examination of the affected body area or organ system and any other symptomatic or related body area or organ system
- Detailed: An extended examination of the affected body area or organ system and any other symptomatic or related body area or organ system
- Comprehensive: A general multi-system examination or complete examination of a single organ system and other symptomatic or related body area or organ system

These types of examinations have been defined for general multi-system and the following single organ systems:

- Cardiovascular
- Ears, nose, mouth, and throat
- Eyes
- Genitourinary (Female)
- Genitourinary (Male)
- Hematologic/lymphatic/immunologic
- Musculoskeletal
- Neurological
- Psychiatric
- Respiratory
- Skin

Any physician regardless of specialty may perform a general multi-system examination or any of the single organ system examinations. The type (general multi-system or single organ system) and content of examination are selected by the examining physician and are based upon clinical judgment, the patient's history, and the nature of the presenting problem.

The content and documentation requirements for each type and level of examination are summarized below and described in detail in a table found later on in this document. In the table, organ systems and body areas recognized by CPT for purposes of describing examinations are shown in the left column. The content, or individual elements, of the examination pertaining to that body area or organ system are identified by bullets (•) in the right column.

Parenthetical examples "(e.g., ...)," have been used for clarification and to provide guidance regarding documentation. Documentation for each element must satisfy any numeric requirements (such as "Measurement of any three of the following seven...") included in the description of the element. Elements with multiple components but with no specific numeric requirement (such as "Examination of liver and spleen") require documentation of at least one component. It is possible for a given examination to be expanded beyond what is defined here. When that occurs, findings related to the additional systems and/or areas should be documented.

- DG: Specific abnormal and relevant negative findings from the examination of the affected or symptomatic body area or organ system should be documented. A notation of "abnormal" without elaboration is insufficient

- DG: Abnormal or unexpected findings from the examination of any asymptomatic body area or organ system should be described

- DG: A brief statement or notation indicating "negative" or "normal" is sufficient to document normal findings related to an unaffected areas or asymptomatic organ system

General Multi-System Examinations

General multi-system examinations are described in detail later in this document. To qualify for a given level of multi-system examination, the following content and documentation requirements should be met:

- Problem Focused Examination: It should include performance and documentation of one to five elements identified by a bullet (•) in one or more organ systems or body areas
- Expanded Problem Focused Examination: It should include performance and documentation of at least six elements identified by a bullet (•) in one or more organ systems or body areas
- Detailed Examination: It should include at least six organ systems or body areas. For each system/area selected, performance and documentation of at least two elements identified by a bullet (•) is expected. Alternatively, a detailed examination may include

performance and documentation of at least 12 elements identified by a bullet (•) in two or more organ systems or body areas
- Comprehensive Examination: It should include at least nine organ systems or body areas. For each system/area selected, all elements of the examination identified by a bullet (•) should be performed, unless specific directions limit the content of the examination. For each area/system, documentation of at least two elements identified by a bullet (•) is expected

Single Organ System Examinations

The single organ system examinations recognized by CMS include eyes; ears, nose, mouth, and throat; cardiovascular; respiratory; genitourinary (male and female); musculoskeletal; neurologic; hematologic, lymphatic, and immunologic; skin; and psychiatric. Note that for each specific single organ examination type, the performance and documentation of the stated number of elements, identified by a bullet (•) should be included, whether in a box with a shaded or unshaded border. The following content and documentation requirements must be met to qualify for a given level:

- Problem Focused Examination: one to five elements
- Expanded Problem Focused Examination: at least six elements
- Detailed Examination: at least 12 elements (other than eye and psychiatric examinations)
- Comprehensive Examination: all elements (Documentation of every element in a box with a shaded border and at least one element in a box with an unshaded border is expected)

Content and Documentation Requirements

General Multisystem Examination 1997

System/Body Area	Elements of Examination
Constitutional	• Measurement of any three of the following seven vital signs: 1) sitting or standing blood pressure, 2) supine blood pressure, 3) pulse rate and regularity, 4) respiration, 5) temperature, 6) height, 7) weight (May be measured and recorded by ancillary staff). • General appearance of patient (e.g., development, nutrition, body habitus, deformities attention to grooming)
Eyes	• Inspection of conjunctivae and lids • Examination of pupils and irises (e.g., reaction to light and accommodation, size and symmetry) • Ophthalmoscopic examination of optic discs (e.g., size, C/D ratio, appearance) and posterior segments (e.g., vessel changes, exudates, hemorrhages)
Ears, nose, mouth, and throat	• External inspection of ears and nose (e.g., overall appearance, scars, lesions, masses) • Otoscopic examination of external auditory canals and tympanic membranes • Assessment of hearing (e.g., whispered voice, finger rub, tuning fork) • Inspection of nasal mucosa, septum and turbinates • Inspection of lips, teeth and gums • Examination of oropharynx: oral mucosa, salivary glands, hard and soft palates, tongue, tonsils and posterior pharynx
Neck	• Examination of neck (e.g., masses, overall appearance, symmetry, tracheal position, crepitus) • Examination of thyroid (e.g., enlargement, tenderness, mass)
Respiratory	• Assessment of respiratory effort (e.g., intercostal retractions, use of accessory muscles, diaphragmatic movement) • Percussion of chest (e.g., dullness, flatness, hyperresonance) • Palpation of chest (e.g., tactile fremitus) • Auscultation of lungs (e.g., breath sounds, adventitious sounds, rubs)

Cardiovascular	• Palpation of heart (e.g., location, size, thrills)
	• Auscultation of heart with notation of abnormal sounds and murmurs
	• Examination of:
	  — carotid arteries (e.g., pulse amplitude, bruits)
	  — abdominal aorta (e.g., size, bruits)
	  — femoral arteries (e.g., pulse amplitude, bruits)
	  — pedal pulses (e.g., pulse amplitude)
	  — extremities for edema and/or varicosities

Chest (Breasts)	• Inspection of breasts (e.g., symmetry, nipple discharge) • Palpation of breasts and axillae (e.g., masses or lumps, tenderness)
Gastrointestinal (Abdomen)	• Examination of abdomen with notation of presence of masses or tenderness • Examination of liver and spleen • Examination for presence or absence of hernia • Examination (when indicated) of anus, perineum and rectum, including sphincter tone, presence of hemorrhoids, rectal masses • Obtain stool sample for occult blood test when indicated

System/Body Area	Elements of Examination

Genitourinary	**Male:**
	• Examination of the scrotal contents (e.g., hydrocele, spermatocele, tenderness of cord, testicular mass)
	• Examination of the penis
	• Digital rectal examination of prostate gland (e.g., size, symmetry, nodularity tenderness)
	Female:
	• Pelvic examination (with or without specimen collection for smears and cultures), including:
	  — examination of external genitalia (e.g., general appearance, hair distribution, lesions) and vagina (e.g., general appearance, estrogen effect, discharge, lesions, pelvic support, cystocele, rectocele)
	  — examination of urethra (e.g., masses, tenderness, scarring)
	  — examination of bladder (e.g., fullness, masses, tenderness)
	• Cervix (e.g., general appearance, lesions, discharge)
	• Uterus (e.g., size, contour, position, mobility, tenderness, consistency, descent or support)
	• Adnexa/parametria (e.g., masses, tenderness)

Lymphatic	Palpation of lymph nodes in **two or more** areas: • Neck • Groin • Axillae • Other
Musculoskeletal	• Examination of gait and station *(if circled, add to total at bottom of column to the left) • Inspection and/or palpation of digits and nails (e.g., clubbing, cyanosis, inflammatory conditions, petechiae, ischemia, infections, nodes) *(if circled, add to total at bottom of column to the left) Examination of joints, bones and muscles of **one or more of the following six** areas: 1) head and neck; 2) spine, ribs, and pelvis; 3) right upper extremity; 4) left upper extremity; 5) right lower extremity; and 6) left lower extremity. The examination of a given area includes: • Inspection and/or palpation with notation of presence of any misalignment, asymmetry, crepitation, defects, tenderness, masses, effusions • Assessment of range of motion with notation of any pain, crepitation or contracture • Assessment of stability with notation of any dislocation (luxation), subluxation, or laxity • Assessment of muscle strength and tone (e.g., flaccid, cog wheel, spastic) with notation of any atrophy or abnormal movements
Skin	• Inspection of skin and subcutaneous tissue (e.g., rashes, lesions, ulcers) • Palpation of skin and subcutaneous tissue (e.g., induration, subcutaneous nodules, tightening)
Neurologic	• Test cranial nerves with notation of any deficits • Examination of deep tendon reflexes with notation of pathological reflexes (e.g., Babinski) • Examination of sensation (e.g., by touch, pin, vibration, proprioception)

Psychiatric	• Description of patient's judgment and insight
	• Brief assessment of mental status including:
	  — Orientation to time, place and person
	  — Recent and remote memory
	  — Mood and affect (e.g., depression, anxiety, agitation)

Content and Documentation Requirements

Level of exam	Perform and document
Problem focused	**One to five** elements identified by a bullet
Expanded problem focused	**At least six** elements identified by a bullet
Detailed	**At least 12** elements identified by a bullet, whether in a box with a shaded or unshaded border
Comprehensive	Performance of **all** elements identified by a bullet; whether in a box or with a shaded or unshaded box. Documentation of every element in each with a shaded border and at least one element in a box with un shaded border is expected

Number of Diagnoses or Management Options	Amount and/or Complexity of Data to be Reviewed	Risk of Complications and/or Morbidity or Mortality	Type of Decision Making
Minimal	Minimal or None	Minimal	Straightforward
Limited	Limited	Low	Low Complexity
Multiple	Moderate	Moderate	Moderate Complexity
Extensive	Extensive	High	High Complexity

C. Documentation of the Complexity of Medical Decision Making 1995 and 1997

The levels of E/M services recognize four types of medical decision-making (straightforward, low complexity, moderate complexity, and high complexity). Medical decision-making refers to the complexity of establishing a diagnosis and/or selecting a management option as measured by:

- The number of possible diagnoses and/or the number of management options that must be considered
- The amount and/or complexity of medical records, diagnostic tests, and/or other information that must be obtained, reviewed, and analyzed
- The risk of significant complications, morbidity, and/or mortality, as well as comorbidities, associated with the patient's presenting problem, the diagnostic procedure, and/or the possible management options

The following chart shows the progression of the elements required for each level of medical decision-making. To qualify for a given type of decision-making, two of the three elements in the table must be either met or exceeded.

Each of the elements of medical decision-making is described below.

Number of Diagnoses or Management Options

The number of possible diagnoses and/or the number of management options that must be considered is based on the number and types of problems addressed during the encounter, the complexity of establishing a diagnosis, and the management decisions that are made by the physician.

Generally, decision making with respect to a diagnosed problem is easier than that for an identified but undiagnosed problem. The number and type of diagnostic tests employed may be an indicator of the number of possible diagnoses. Problems that are improving or resolving are less complex than those that are worsening or failing to change as expected. The need to seek advice from others is another indicator of complexity of diagnostic or management problems.

- DG: For each encounter, an assessment, clinical impression, or diagnosis should be documented. It may be explicitly stated or implied in documented decisions regarding management plans and/or further evaluation

  - For a presenting problem with an established diagnosis, the record should reflect whether the problem is: a) improved, well controlled, resolving, or resolved; or b) inadequately controlled, worsening, or failing to change as expected

  - For a presenting problem without an established diagnosis, the assessment or clinical impression may be stated in the form of a differential diagnosis or as a "possible," "probable," or "rule-out" (R/O) diagnosis

- DG: The initiation of, or changes in, treatment should be documented. Treatment includes a wide range of management options including patient instructions, nursing instructions, therapies, and medications

- DG: If referrals are made, consultations requested, or advice sought, the record should indicate to whom or where the referral or consultation is made or from whom the advice is requested

Amount and/or Complexity of Data to be Reviewed

The amount and complexity of data to be reviewed is based on the types of diagnostic testing ordered or reviewed. A decision to obtain and review old medical records and/or obtain history from sources other than the patient increases the amount and complexity of data to be reviewed.

Discussion of contradictory or unexpected test results with the physician who performed or interpreted the test is an indication of the complexity of data being reviewed. On occasion, the physician who ordered a test may personally review the image, tracing, or specimen to supplement information from the physician who prepared the test report or interpretation; this is another indication of the complexity of data being reviewed.

- DG: If a diagnostic service (test or procedure) is ordered, planned, scheduled, or performed at the time of the E/M encounter, the type of service (e.g., lab or x-ray) should be documented

- DG: The review of lab, radiology, and/or other diagnostic tests should be documented. A simple notation such as WBC elevated" or "chest x-ray unremarkable" is acceptable. Alternatively, the review may be documented by initialing and dating the report containing the test results

- DG: A decision to obtain old records or a decision to obtain additional history from the family, caretaker, or other source to supplement that obtained from the patient should be documented

- DG: Relevant findings from the review of old records and/or the receipt of additional history from the family, caretaker, or other source to supplement that obtained from the patient should be documented. If there is no relevant information beyond that already obtained, that fact should be documented. A notation of "old records reviewed" or "additional history obtained from family" without elaboration is insufficient

- DG: The results of discussion of laboratory, radiology, or other diagnostic tests with the physician who performed or interpreted the study should be documented

- DG: The direct visualization and independent interpretation of an image, tracing, or specimen previously or subsequently interpreted by another physician should be documented

Risk of Significant Complications, Morbidity, and/or Mortality

The risk of significant complications, morbidity, and/or mortality is based on the risks associated with the presenting problem, the diagnostic procedure, and the possible management options.

- DG: Comorbidities/underlying disease or other factors that increase the complexity of medical decision making by increasing the risk of complications, morbidity, and/or mortality should be documented

- DG: If a surgical or invasive diagnostic procedure is ordered, planned, or scheduled at the time of the E/M encounter, the type of procedure (e.g., laparoscopy) should be documented

- DG: If a surgical or invasive diagnostic procedure is performed at the time of the E/M encounter, the specific procedure should be documented

- DG: The referral for or decision to perform a surgical or invasive diagnostic procedure on an urgent basis should be documented or implied

The following Table of Risk may be used to help determine whether the risk of significant complications, morbidity, and/or mortality is minimal, low, moderate, or high. Because the determination of risk is complex and not readily quantifiable, the table includes common clinical examples rather than absolute measures of risk. The assessment of risk of the presenting problem is based on the risk related to the disease process anticipated between the present encounter and the next one. The assessment of risk of selecting diagnostic procedures and management options is based on the risk during and immediately following any procedures or treatment. The highest level of risk in any one category (presenting problem, diagnostic procedure, or management options) determines the overall risk.

Table of Risk

Level of Risk	Presenting Problem(s)	Diagnostic Procedure(s) Ordered	Management Options Selected
Minimal	One self-limited or minor problem (e.g., cold, insect bite, tinea corporis)	Laboratory test requiring venipuncture Chest x-rays EKG/EEG Urinalysis Ultrasound (e.g., echocardiography) KOH prep	Rest Gargles Elastic bandages Superficial dressings
Low	Two or more self-limited or minor problems One stable chronic illness (e.g., well controlled hypertension, non-insulin dependent diabetes, cataract, BPH) Acute, uncomplicated illness or injury (e.g., cystitis, allergic rhinitis, simple sprain)	Physiologic tests not under stress (e.g., pulmonary function tests) Non-cardiovascular imaging studies with contrast (e.g., barium enema) Superficial needle biopsies Clinical laboratory tests requiring arterial puncture Skin biopsies	Over-the-counter drugs Minor surgery with no identified risk factors Physical therapy Occupational therapy IV fluids without additives
Moderate	One or more chronic illnesses with mild exacerbation, progression or side effects of treatment Two or more stable chronic illnesses Undiagnosed new problem with uncertain prognosis (e.g., lump in breast) Acute illness with systemic symptoms (e.g., pyelonephritis, pneumonitis, colitis) Acute complicated injury (e.g., head injury with brief loss of consciousness)	Physiologic tests not under stress (e.g., cardiac stress test, fetal contraction stress test) Diagnostic endoscopies with no identified risk factors Deep needle or incisional biopsy Cardiovascular imaging studies with contrast and no identified risk factors (e.g., arteriogram, cardiac catheterization) Obtain fluid from body cavity (e.g., lumbar puncture, thoracentesis, culdocentesis)	Minor surgery with identified risk factors Effective major surgery (open, percutaneous or endoscopic) with no identified risk factors Prescription drug management Therapeutic nuclear medicine IV fluids with additives Closed treatment of fracture or dislocation without manipulation
High	One or more chronic illnesses with severe exacerbation, progression or side effects of treatment Acute/chronic illnesses that may pose a threat to life or bodily function (e.g., multiple trauma, acute MI, pulmonary embolus, severe respiratory distress, progressive severe rheumatoid arthritis, psychiatric illness with potential threat to self or others, peritonitis, acute renal failure An abrupt change in neurologic status (e.g., seizure, TIA, weakness or sensory loss)	Cardiovascular imaging studies with contrast with identified risk factors Cardiac electrophysiological tests Diagnostic endoscopies with identified risk factors Discography	Elective major surgery (open, percutaneous or endoscopic) with identified risk factors Emergency major surgery (open, percutaneous or endoscopic) Parenteral controlled substances Drug therapy requiring intensive monitoring for toxicity Decision not to resuscitate or to de-escalate care because of poor prognosis

D. Documentation of an Encounter Dominated by Counseling or Coordination of Care

In the case where counseling and/or coordination of care dominates (more than 50 percent) the physician/patient and/or family encounter (face-to-face time in the office or other outpatient setting or floor-unit time in the hospital or nursing facility), time is considered the key or controlling factor to qualify for a particular level of E/M service.

- DG: If the physician elects to report the level of service based on counseling and/or coordination of care, the total length of time of the encounter (face-to-face or floor time, as appropriate) should be documented and the record should describe the counseling and/or activities to coordinate care

Appendix D — Crosswalk of Deleted Codes

The deleted code crosswalk is meant to be used as a reference tool to find active codes that could be used in place of the deleted code. This will not always be an exact match. Please review the code descriptions and guidelines before selecting a code.

Code	Cross reference
19260	To report, see 21601
19271	To report, see 21602
19272	To report, see 21603
33010	To report, see 33016-33019
33011	To report, see 33016-33019
33015	To report, see 33017-33019
33860	To report, see 33858-33859
33870	To report, see 33871
64402	To report, see 64999
64410	To report, see 64999
64413	To report, see 64999
74241	To report, see 74240
74245	To report, see 74240, 74248
74247	To report, see 74246
74249	To report, see 74246, 74248
74260	To report, see 74251
76930	To report, see 33016-33018
78205	To report, see 78803
78206	To report, see 78803

Code	Cross reference
78320	To report, see 78803
78607	To report, see 78803
78647	To report, see 78803
78710	To report, see 78803
78805	To report, see 78300, 78305-78306, 78315, 78800-78803, 78830-78332
78806	To report, see 78300, 78305-78306, 78315, 78800-78803, 78830-78332
78807	To report, see 78300, 78305-78306, 78315, 78800-78803, 78830-78332
90911	To report, see 90912-90913
92225	To report, see 92201-92202
92226	To report, see 92201-92202
93299	To report, see 93297-93298
95827	To report, see 95705-95707, 95711-95713, 95717-95718
95831	To report, see [97161-97172]
95832	To report, see [97161-97172]
95833	To report, see [97161-97172]
95834	To report, see [97161-97172]
95950	To report, see [95700-95726]

Code	Cross reference
95951	To report, see [95700-95726]
95953	To report, see [95700-95726]
95956	To report, see [95700-95726]
96150	To report, see 96156, 96158-96159
96151	To report, see 96156, 96158-96159
96152	To report, see 96156, 96158-96159
96153	To report, see [96164-96165]
96154	To report, see [96167-96168]
96155	To report, see [96170-9617]
97127	To report, see 97129
98969	To report, see 98970-98972
99444	To report, see [99421-99423]
3045F	To report, see 3051F, 3052F
0249T	To report, see 46948
0254T	To report, see 34717-34718
0399T	To report, see 93356
0081U	To report, see 81552

Appendix E — Resequenced Codes

Code	Reference
10004	See code following 10021.
10005	See code following 10021.
10006	See code following 10021.
10007	See code following 10021.
10008	See code following 10021.
10009	See code following 10021.
10010	See code following 10021.
10011	See code following 10021.
10012	See code following 10021.
11045	See code following 11042.
11046	See code following 11043.
15769	See code following 15770.
20560	See code following 20553.
20561	See code before 20555.
21552	See code following 21555.
21554	See code following 21556.
22858	See code following 22856.
22859	See code following 22854.
23071	See code following 23075.
23073	See code following 23076.
24071	See code following 24075.
24073	See code following 24076.
25071	See code following 25075.
25073	See code following 25076.
26111	See code following 26115.
26113	See code following 26116.
27043	See code following 27047.
27045	See code following 27048.
27059	See code following 27049.
27329	See code following 27360.
27337	See code following 27327.
27339	See code before 27330.
27632	See code following 27618.
27634	See code following 27619.
28039	See code following 28043.
28041	See code following 28045.
28295	See code following 28296.
29914	See code following 29863.
29915	See code following 29863.
29916	See code before 29866.
31253	See code following 31255.
31257	See code following 31255.
31259	See code following 31255.
31551	See code following 31580.
31552	See code following 31580.
31553	See code following 31580.
31554	See code following 31580.
31572	See code following 31578.
31573	See code following 31578.
31574	See code following 31578.

Code	Reference
31651	See code following 31647.
32994	See code following 32998.
33221	See code following 33213.
33227	See code following 33233.
33228	See code following 33233.
33229	See code before 33234.
33230	See code following 33240.
33231	See code before 33241.
33262	See code following 33241.
33263	See code following 33241.
33264	See code before 33243.
33270	See code following 33249.
33271	See code following 33249.
33272	See code following 33249.
33273	See code following 33249.
33274	See code following 33249.
33275	See code following 33249.
33440	See code following 33410.
33962	See code following 33959.
33963	See code following 33959.
33964	See code following 33959.
33965	See code following 33959.
33966	See code following 33959.
33969	See code following 33959.
33984	See code following 33959.
33985	See code following 33959.
33986	See code following 33959.
33987	See code following 33959.
33988	See code following 33959.
33989	See code following 33959.
34717	See code following 34708.
34718	See code following 34709.
34812	See code following 34713.
34820	See code following 34714.
34833	See code following 34714.
34834	See code following 34714.
36465	See code following 36471.
36466	See code following 36471.
36482	See code following 36479.
36483	See code following 36479.
36572	See code following 36569.
36573	See code following 36569.
37246	See code following 37235.
37247	See code following 37235.
37248	See code following 37235.
37249	See code following 37235.
38243	See code following 38241.
43210	See code following 43259.
43211	See code following 43217.
43212	See code following 43217.
43213	See code following 43220.

Code	Reference
43214	See code following 43220.
43233	See code following 43249.
43266	See code following 43255.
43270	See code following 43257.
43274	See code following numeric code 43270.
43275	See code following numeric code 43270.
43276	See code following numeric code 43270.
43277	See code following numeric code 43270.
43278	See code following numeric code 43270.
44381	See code following 44382.
44401	See code following 44392.
45346	See code following 45338.
45388	See code following 45382.
45390	See code following 45392.
45398	See code following 45393.
45399	See code before 45990.
46220	See code before 46230.
46320	See code following 46230.
46945	See code following 46221.
46946	See code following resequenced code 46945.
46947	See code following 46761.
46948	See code before resequenced code 46220.
50430	See code following 50396.
50431	See code following 50396.
50432	See code following 50396.
50433	See code following 50396.
50434	See code following 50396.
50435	See code following 50396.
50436	See code following 50391.
50437	See code following 50391.
51797	See code following 51729.
52356	See code following 52353.
58674	See code before 58541.
62328	See code following 62270.
62329	See code following 62272.
64461	See code following 64484.
64462	See code following 64484.
64463	See code following 64484.
64624	See code following 64610.
64625	See code before 64611.
64633	See code following 64620.
64634	See code following 64620.
64635	See code following 64620.
64636	See code before 64630.
66987	See code following 66982.
66988	See code following 66984.

Code	Reference
67810	See code following 67715.
77085	See code following 77081.
77086	See code before 77084.
77295	See code before 77300.
77385	See code following 77417.
77386	See code following 77417.
77387	See code following 77417.
77424	See code following 77417.
77425	See code following 77417.
78429	See code following 78459.
78430	See code following 78491.
78431	See code following 78492.
78432	See code following 78492.
78433	See code following 78492.
78434	See code following 78492.
78804	See code following 78802.
78830	See code following numeric code 78804.
78831	See code following numeric code 78804.
78832	See code following numeric code 78804.
78835	See code following numeric code 78804.
80081	See code following 80055.
80164	See code following 80201.
80165	See code following 80201.
80171	See code following 80169.
80230	See code following 80173.
80235	See code before 80175.
80280	See code following 80202.
80285	See code before 80203.
80305	See code before 80145.
80306	See code before 80145.
80307	See code before 80145.
80320	See code before 80145.
80321	See code before 80145.
80322	See code before 80145.
80323	See code before 80145.
80324	See code before 80145.
80325	See code before 80145.
80326	See code before 80145.
80327	See code before 80145.
80328	See code before 80145.
80329	See code before 80145.
80330	See code before 80145.
80331	See code before 80145.
80332	See code before 80145.
80333	See code before 80145.
80334	See code before 80145.
80335	See code before 80145.
80336	See code before 80145.
80337	See code before 80145.
80338	See code before 80145.
80339	See code before 80145.

Code	Reference
80340	See code before 80145.
80341	See code before 80145.
80342	See code before 80145.
80343	See code before 80145.
80344	See code before 80145.
80345	See code before 80145.
80346	See code before 80145.
80347	See code before 80145.
80348	See code before 80145.
80349	See code before 80145.
80350	See code before 80145.
80351	See code before 80145.
80352	See code before 80145.
80353	See code before 80145.
80354	See code before 80145.
80355	See code before 80145.
80356	See code before 80145.
80357	See code before 80145.
80358	See code before 80145.
80359	See code before 80145.
80360	See code before 80145.
80361	See code before 80145.
80362	See code before 80145.
80363	See code before 80145.
80364	See code before 80145.
80365	See code before 80145.
80366	See code before 80145.
80367	See code before 80145.
80368	See code before 80145.
80369	See code before 80145.
80370	See code before 80145.
80371	See code before 80145.
80372	See code before 80145.
80373	See code before 80145.
80374	See code before 80145.
80375	See code before 80145.
80376	See code before 80145.
80377	See code before 80145.
81105	See code before 81260.
81106	See code before 81260.
81107	See code before 81260.
81108	See code before 81260.
81109	See code before 81260.
81110	See code before 81260.
81111	See code before 81260.
81112	See code before 81260.
81120	See code before 81260.
81121	See code before 81260.
81161	See code following numeric code 81231.
81162	See code following resequenced code 81210.
81163	See code following resequenced code 81210.

Code	Reference
81164	See code following resequenced code 81210.
81165	See code following 81212.
81166	See code following 81212.
81167	See code following 81216.
81173	See code following resequenced code 81204.
81174	See code following resequenced code 81204.
81184	See code following resequenced code 81233.
81185	See code following resequenced code 81233.
81186	See code following resequenced code 81233.
81187	See code following resequenced code 81268.
81188	See code following resequenced code 81266.
81189	See code following resequenced code 81266.
81190	See code following resequenced code 81266.
81200	See code before 81175.
81201	See code following numeric code 81174.
81202	See code following numeric code 81174.
81203	See code following numeric code 81174.
81204	See code following numeric code 81174.
81205	See code following numeric code 81210.
81206	See code following numeric code 81210.
81207	See code following numeric code 81210.
81208	See code following numeric code 81210.
81209	See code following numeric code 81210.
81210	See code following numeric code 81210.
81219	See code before 81218.
81227	See code before 81225.
81230	See code following numeric code 81227.
81231	See code following numeric code 81227.
81233	See code following 81217.
81234	See code following numeric code 81231.
81238	See code following 81241.
81239	See code before 81232.
81245	See code following 81242.
81246	See code following 81242.
81250	See code before 81247.
81257	See code following 81254.
81258	See code following 81254.

Code	Reference
81259	See code following 81254.
81261	See code before 81260.
81262	See code before 81260.
81263	See code before 81260.
81264	See code before 81260.
81265	See code following resequenced code 81187.
81266	See code following resequenced code 81187.
81267	See code following 81224.
81268	See code following 81224.
81269	See code following resequenced code 81259.
81271	See code following numeric code 81259.
81274	See code following resequenced code 81271.
81277	See code following 81229.
81283	See code following resequenced code 81121.
81284	See code following numeric code 81246.
81285	See code following numeric code 81246.
81286	See code following numeric code 81246.
81287	See code following resequenced code 81304.
81288	See code following resequenced code 81292.
81289	See code following numeric code 81246.
81291	See code before 81305.
81292	See code before numeric code 81291.
81293	See code before numeric code 81291.
81294	See code before numeric code 81291.
81295	See code before numeric code 81291.
81301	See code following resequenced code 81287.
81302	See code following 81290.
81303	See code following 81290.
81304	See code following 81290.
81306	See code following resequenced code 81312.
81307	See code before 81313.
81308	See code before 81313.
81309	See code following 81314.
81312	See code following numeric code 81312.
81320	See code before 81315.
81324	See code following 81316.
81325	See code following 81316.
81326	See code following 81316.
81332	See code following 81327.
81334	See code following numeric code 81326.
81336	See code following 81329.
81337	See code following 81329.

Code	Reference
81343	See code following numeric code 81320.
81344	See code following numeric code 81332.
81345	See code following numeric code 81332.
81361	See code following 81254.
81362	See code following 81254.
81363	See code following 81254.
81364	See code following 81254.
81443	See code following 81422.
81448	See code following 81438.
81479	See code following 81408.
81522	See code following 81518.
82042	See code following 82045.
82652	See code following 82306.
83992	See code following resequenced code 80365.
86152	See code folowing 86147.
86153	See code before 86148.
87623	See code following 87539.
87624	See code following 87539.
87625	See code before 87540.
87806	See code following 87803.
87906	See code following 87901.
87910	See code following 87900.
87912	See code before 87902.
88177	See code following 88173.
88341	See code following 88342.
88350	See code following 88346.
88364	See code following 88365.
88373	See code following 88367.
88374	See code following 88367.
88377	See code following 88369.
90619	See code following 90734.
90620	See code following 90734.
90621	See code following 90734.
90625	See code following 90723.
90630	See code following 90654.
90644	See code following 90732.
90672	See code following 90660.
90673	See code before 90662.
90674	See code following 90661.
90694	See code following 90689.
90750	See code following 90736.
90756	See code following 90661.
92558	See code following 92586.
92597	See code following 92604.
92618	See code following 92605.
92920	See code following 92998.
92921	See code following 92998.
92924	See code following 92998.
92925	See code following 92998.
92928	See code following 92998.
92929	See code following 92998.

Code	Reference
92933	See code following 92998.
92934	See code following 92998.
92937	See code following 92998.
92938	See code following 92998.
92941	See code following 92998.
92943	See code following 92998.
92944	See code following 92998.
92973	See code following 92998.
92974	See code following 92998.
92975	See code following 92998.
92977	See code following 92998.
92978	See code following 92998.
92979	See code following 92998.
93260	See code following 93284.
93261	See code following 93289.
93264	See code before 93279.
93356	See code following 93351.
95249	See code following 95250.
95700	See code following 95967.
95705	See code following 95967.
95706	See code following 95967.
95707	See code following 95967.
95708	See code following 95967.
95709	See code following 95967.
95710	See code following 95967.
95711	See code following 95967.
95712	See code following 95967.
95713	See code following 95967.
95714	See code following 95967.
95715	See code following 95967.
95716	See code following 95967.
95717	See code following 95967.
95718	See code following 95967.
95719	See code following 95967.
95720	See code following 95967.
95721	See code following 95967.
95722	See code following 95967.
95723	See code following 95967.
95724	See code following 95967.
95725	See code following 95967.
95726	See code following 95967.
95782	See code following 95811.
95783	See code following 95811.
95800	See code following 95806.
95801	See code following 95806.
95829	See code following 95830.
95836	See code following 95830.
95885	See code following 95872.
95886	See code following 95872.
95887	See code before 95873.
95938	See code following 95926.
95939	See code following 95929.
95940	See code following 95913.
95941	See code following 95913.

Code	Reference
95943	See code following 95924.
95983	See code following 95977.
95984	See code following 95977.
96125	See code following 96105.
96127	See code following 96113.
96164	See code following 96159.
96165	See code following 96159.
96167	See code following 96159.
96168	See code following 96159.
96170	See code following 96159.
96171	See code following 96159.
97151	See code following 96040.
97152	See code following 96040.
97153	See code following 96040.
97154	See code following 96040.
97155	See code following 96040.
97156	See code following 96040.
97157	See code following 96040.
97158	See code following 96040.
97161	See code before 97010.
97162	See code before 97010.
97163	See code before 97010.
97164	See code before 97010.

Code	Reference
97165	See code before 97010.
97166	See code before 97010.
97167	See code before 97010.
97168	See code before 97010.
97169	See code before 97010.
97170	See code before 97010.
97171	See code before 97010.
97172	See code before 97010.
99091	See code following resequenced code 99454.
99177	See code following 99174.
99224	See code following 99220.
99225	See code following 99220.
99226	See code following 99220.
99415	See code following 99359.
99416	See code following 99359.
99421	See code following 99443.
99422	See code following 99443.
99423	See code following 99443.
99451	See code following 99449.
99452	See code following 99449.
99453	See code following 99449.
99454	See code following 99449.

Code	Reference
99457	See code before 99450.
99458	See code before 99450.
99473	See code before 99450.
99474	See code before 99450.
99484	See code following 99498.
99485	See code following 99467.
99486	See code following 99467.
99490	See code before 99487.
99491	See code before 99487.
2033F	See code following 2026F.
3051F	See code following 3044F.
3052F	See code before 3046F.
0253T	See code before 0198T.
0376T	See code following 0191T.
0464T	See code following 0333T.
0488T	See code following 0403T.
0510T	See code following 0335T.
0511T	See code following 0335T.
0512T	See code following 0102T.
0513T	See code following 0102T.
0523T	See code following 0504T.
0563T	See code following 0207T.

Appendix F — Add-on Codes, Optum Modifier 50 Exempt, Modifier 51 Exempt, Optum Modifier 51 Exempt, Modifier 63 Exempt, and Modifier 95 Telemedicine Services

Codes specified as add-on, exempt from modifiers 50, 51 and 63, and modifier 95 (telemedicine services) are listed. The lists are designed to be read left to right rather than vertically.

Add-on Codes

0054T	0055T	0071U	0072U	0073U	0074U	0075U
0076T	0076U	0095T	0098T	0130U	0131U	0132U
0133U	0134U	0135U	0136U	0137U	0138U	0157U
0158U	0159T	0159U	0160U	0161U	0162U	0163T
0164T	0165T	0174T	0189T	0190T	01953	01968
01969	0196T	0205T	0214T	0215T	0217T	0218T
0222T	0229T	0231T	0290T	0346T	0361T	0363T
0365T	0367T	0369T	0374T	0376T	0396T	0397T
0399T	0437T	0439T	0443T	0450T	0466T	0471T
0480T	0482T	0492T	0496T	0513T	0514T	0523T
0560T	0562T	0570T	10004	10006	10008	10010
10012	10036	11001	11008	11045	11046	11047
11101	11103	11105	11107	11201	11732	11922
13102	13122	13133	13153	14302	15003	15005
15101	15111	15116	15121	15131	15136	15151
15152	15156	15157	15201	15221	15241	15261
15272	15274	15276	15278	15772	15774	15777
15787	15847	16036	17003	17312	17314	17315
19001	19082	19084	19086	19126	19282	19284
19286	19288	19294	19297	20700	20701	20702
20703	20704	20705	20930	20931	20932	20933
20934	20936	20937	20938	20939	20985	22103
22116	22208	22216	22226	22328	22512	22515
22527	22534	22552	22585	22614	22632	22634
22840	22841	22842	22843	22844	22845	22846
22847	22848	22853	22854	22858	22859	22868
22870	26125	26861	26863	27358	27692	29826
31627	31632	31633	31637	31649	31651	31654
32501	32506	32507	32667	32668	32674	33141
33225	33257	33258	33259	33367	33368	33369
33419	33508	33517	33518	33519	33521	33522
33523	33530	33572	33768	33866	33884	33924
33929	33987	34709	34711	34713	34714	34715
34716	34717	34808	34812	34813	34820	34833
34834	35306	35390	35400	35500	35572	35600
35681	35682	35683	35685	35686	35697	35700
36218	36227	36228	36248	36474	36476	36479
36483	36907	36908	36909	37185	37186	37222
37223	37232	37233	37234	37235	37237	37239
37247	37249	37252	37253	38102	38746	38747
38900	43273	43283	43338	43635	44015	44121
44128	44139	44203	44213	44701	44955	47001
47542	47543	47544	47550	48400	49326	49327
49412	49435	49568	49905	50706	50705	50706
51797	52442	56606	57267	58110	58611	59525
60512	61316	61517	61610	61611	61612	61641
61642	61651	61781	61782	61783	61797	61799
61800	61864	61868	62148	62160	63035	63043
63044	63048	63057	63066	63076	63078	63082
63086	63088	63091	63103	63295	63308	63621
64421	64462	64480	64484	64491	64492	64494
64495	64634	64636	64643	64645	64727	64778
64783	64787	64832	64837	64859	64872	64874
64876	64901	64902	64913	65757	66990	67225
67331	67331	67332	67334	67335	67340	69990
74248	74301	74713	75565	75774	76125	76802
76810	76812	76814	76937	76979	76983	77001
77002	77003	77063	77293	78020	78434	78496
78730	78835	81266	81416	81426	81536	82952
86826	87187	87503	87904	88155	88177	88185
88311	88314	88332	88334	88341	88350	88364
88369	88373	88388	90461	90472	90474	90785
90833	90836	90838	90840	90863	90913	91013
92547	92608	92618	92621	92627	92921	92925
92929	92934	92938	92944	92973	92974	92978
92979	92998	93320	93321	93325	93352	93356
93462	93463	93464	93563	93564	93565	93566
93567	93568	93571	93572	93592	93609	93613
93621	93622	93623	93655	93657	93662	94645
94729	94781	95079	95873	95874	95885	95886
95887	95940	95941	95962	95967	95975	95979
95984	96113	96121	96131	96133	96137	96139
96159	96165	96168	96171	96361	96366	96367
96368	96370	96371	96375	96376	96411	96415
96417	96423	96570	96571	96934	96935	96936
97130	97546	97598	97811	97814	99100	99116
99135	99140	99153	99157	99292	99354	99355
99356	99357	99359	99415	99416	99458	99467
99486	99489	99494	99498	99602	99607	

Optum Modifier 50 Exempt Codes

0214T	0215T	0217T	0218T	15777	20939	34713
34714	34715	34716	34717	34812	34820	34833
34834	35572	36227	36228	49568	63035	63043
63044	64421	64462	64480	64484	64491	64492
64494	64495	64634	64636			

AMA Modifier 51 Exempt Codes

20697	20974	20975	44500	61107	93600	93602
93603	93610	93612	93615	93616	93618	94610
95905	99151	99152				

Optum Modifier 51 Exempt Codes

90281	90283	90284	90287	90288	90291	90296
90371	90375	90376	90378	90384	90385	90386
90389	90393	90396	90399	90476	90477	90581
90585	90586	90587	90620	90621	90625	90630
90632	90633	90634	90636	90644	90647	90648
90649	90650	90651	90653	90654	90655	90656
90657	90658	90660	90661	90662	90664	90666
90667	90668	90670	90672	90673	90674	90675
90676	90680	90681	90682	90685	90686	90687
90688	90689	90690	90691	90696	90697	90698
90700	90702	90707	90710	90713	90714	90715
90716	90717	90723	90732	90733	90734	90736
90738	90739	90740	90743	90744	90746	90747
90748	90749	90750	90756	97010	97012	97014
97016	97018	97022	97024	97026	97028	97032
97033	97034	97035	97036	97110	97112	97113
97116	97124	97129	97130	97140	97150	97530
97533	97535	97537	97542	97545	97546	97597
97598	97602	97605	97606	97607	97608	97610
97750	97755	97760	97761	97763	99050	99051
99053	99056	99058	99060			

Modifier 63 Exempt Codes

30540	30545	31520	33470	33502	33503	33505
33506	33610	33611	33619	33647	33670	33690
33694	33730	33732	33735	33736	33750	33755
33762	33778	33786	33922	33946	33947	33948
33949	36415	36420	36450	36456	36460	36510
36660	39503	43313	43314	43520	43831	44055
44126	44127	44128	46070	46705	46715	46716
46730	46735	46740	46742	46744	47700	47701

49215	49491	49492	49495	49496	49600	49605
49606	49610	49611	53025	54000	54150	54160
63700	63702	63704	63706	65820		

Telemedicine Services Codes

The codes on the following list may be used to report telemedicine services when modifier 95 Synchronous Telemedicine Service Rendered via a Real-Time Interactive Audio and Visual Telecommunications System, is appended.

90791	90792	90832	90833	90834	90836	90837
90838	90845	90846	90847	90863	90951	90952
90954	90955	90957	90958	90960	90961	92227
92228	93228	93229	93268	93270	93271	93272
96040	96116	97802	97803	97804	98960	98961
98962	99201	99202	99203	99204	99205	99212
99213	99214	99215	99231	99232	99233	*99241
*99242	*99243	*99244	*99245	*99251	*99252	*99253
*99254	*99255	99307	99308	99309	99310	99354
99355	99406	99407	99408	99409	99495	99496

* Consultations are noncovered by Medicare

Appendix G — Medicare Internet-only Manuals (IOMs)

The Centers for Medicare and Medicaid Services restructured its paper-based manual system as a web-based system on October 1, 2003. Called the online CMS manual system, it combines all of the various program instructions into internet-only manuals (IOMs), which are used by all CMS programs and contractors. In many instances, the references from the online manuals in appendix G contain a mention of the old paper manuals from which the current information was obtained when the manuals were converted. This information is shown in the header of the text, in the following format, when applicable, as A3-3101, HO-210, and B3-2049. Complete versions of all of the manuals can be found at https://www.cms.gov/Regulations-and-Guidance/Guidance/Manuals/Internet-Only-Manuals-IOMs.html.

Effective with implementation of the IOMs, the former method of publishing program memoranda (PMs) to communicate program instructions was replaced by the following four templates:

- One-time notification
- Manual revisions
- Business requirements
- Confidential requirements

The web-based system has been organized by functional area (e.g., eligibility, entitlement, claims processing, benefit policy, program integrity) in an effort to eliminate redundancy within the manuals, simplify updating, and make CMS program instructions available more quickly. The web-based system contains the functional areas included below:

Pub. 100	Introduction
Pub. 100-01	Medicare General Information, Eligibility, and Entitlement Manual
Pub. 100-02	Medicare Benefit Policy Manual
Pub. 100-03	Medicare National Coverage Determinations (NCD) Manual
Pub. 100-04	Medicare Claims Processing Manual
Pub. 100-05	Medicare Secondary Payer Manual
Pub. 100-06	Medicare Financial Management Manual
Pub. 100-07	State Operations Manual
Pub. 100-08	Medicare Program Integrity Manual
Pub. 100-09	Medicare Contractor Beneficiary and Provider Communications Manual
Pub. 100-10	Quality Improvement Organization Manual
Pub. 100-11	Programs of All-Inclusive Care for the Elderly (PACE) Manual
Pub. 100-12	State Medicaid Manual (under development)
Pub. 100-13	Medicaid State Children's Health Insurance Program (under development)
Pub. 100-14	Medicare ESRD Network Organizations Manual
Pub. 100-15	Medicaid Integrity Program (MIP)
Pub. 100-16	Medicare Managed Care Manual
Pub. 100-17	CMS/Business Partners Systems Security Manual
Pub. 100-18	Medicare Prescription Drug Benefit Manual
Pub. 100-19	Demonstrations
Pub. 100-20	One-Time Notification
Pub. 100-21	Recurring Update Notification
Pub. 100-22	Medicare Quality Reporting Incentive Programs Manual
Pub. 100-24	State Buy-In Manual
Pub. 100-25	Information Security Acceptable Risk Safeguards Manual

A brief description of the Medicare manuals primarily used for *CPC Expert* follows:

The ***National Coverage Determinations Manual*** (NCD), is organized according to categories such as diagnostic services, supplies, and medical procedures. The table of contents lists each category and subject within that category. Revision transmittals identify any new or background material, recap the changes, and provide an effective date for the change.

When complete, the manual will contain two chapters. Chapter 1 currently includes a description of CMS's national coverage determinations. When available, chapter 2 will contain a list of HCPCS codes related to each coverage determination. The manual is organized in accordance with CPT category sequences.

The ***Medicare Benefit Policy Manual*** contains Medicare general coverage instructions that are not national coverage determinations. As a general rule, in the past these instructions have been found in chapter II of the ***Medicare Carriers Manual,*** the ***Medicare Intermediary Manual***, other provider manuals, and program memoranda.

The ***Medicare Claims Processing Manual*** contains instructions for processing claims for contractors and providers.

The ***Medicare Program Integrity Manual*** communicates the priorities and standards for the Medicare integrity programs.

Medicare IOM references

100-01, 3, 20.5

Blood Deductibles (Part A and Part B)
(Rev. 1, 09-11-02)

Program payment may not be made for the first 3 pints of whole blood or equivalent units of packed red cells received under Part A and Part B combined in a calendar year. However, blood processing (e.g., administration, storage) is not subject to the deductible.

The blood deductibles are in addition to any other applicable deductible and coinsurance amounts for which the patient is responsible.

The deductible applies only to the first 3 pints of blood furnished in a calendar year, even if more than one provider furnished blood.

100-01, 5, 70.6

Chiropractors
(Rev. 1, 09-11-02)

A. General

A licensed chiropractor who meets uniform minimum standards (see subsection C) is a physician for specified services. Coverage extends only to treatment by means of manual manipulation of the spine to correct a subluxation demonstrated by X-ray, provided such treatment is legal in the State where performed. All other services furnished or ordered by chiropractors are not covered. An X-ray obtained by a chiropractor for his or her own diagnostic purposes before commencing treatment may suffice for claims documentation purposes. This means that if a chiropractor orders, takes, or interprets an X-ray to demonstrate a subluxation of the spine, the X-ray can be used for claims processing purposes. However, there is no coverage or payment for these services or for any other diagnostic or therapeutic service ordered or furnished by the chiropractor. In addition, in performing manual manipulation of the spine, some chiropractors use manual devices that are hand-held with the thrust of the force of the device being controlled manually. While such manual manipulation may be covered, there is no separate payment permitted for use of this device.

B. Licensure and Authorization to Practice

A chiropractor must be licensed or legally authorized to furnish chiropractic services by the State or jurisdiction in which the services are furnished.

C. Uniform Minimum Standards

I. Prior to July 1, 1974, Chiropractors licensed or authorized to practice prior to July 1, 1974, and those individuals who commenced their studies in a chiropractic college before that date must meet all of the following minimum standards to render payable services under the program:

  a. Preliminary education equal to the requirements for graduation from an accredited high school or other secondary school;

b. Graduation from a college of chiropractic approved by the State's chiropractic examiners that included the completion of a course of study covering a period of not less than 3 school years of 6 months each year in actual continuous attendance covering adequate course of study in the subjects of anatomy, physiology, symptomatology and diagnosis, hygiene and sanitation, chemistry, histology, pathology, and principles and practice of chiropractic, including clinical instruction in vertebral palpation, nerve tracing and adjusting; and

c. Passage of an examination prescribed by the State's chiropractic examiners covering the subjects listed in subsection b.

2. After June 30, 1974 - Individuals commencing their studies in a chiropractic college after June 30, 1974, must meet all of the following additional requirements:

a. Satisfactory completion of 2 years of pre-chiropractic study at the college level;

b. Satisfactory completion of a 4-year course of 8 months each year (instead of a 3-year course of 6 months each year) at a college or school of chiropractic that includes not less than 4,000 hours in the scientific and chiropractic courses specified in subsection1.b, plus courses in the use and effect of X-ray and chiropractic analysis; and

c. The practitioner must be over 21 years of age.

100-02, 1, 90
Termination of Pregnancy
(Rev. 1, 10-01-03) B3-4276.1,.2

Effective for services furnished on or after October 1, 1998, Medicare will cover abortions procedures in the following situations:

1. If the pregnancy is the result of an act or rape or incest; or

2. In the case where a woman suffers from a physical disorder, physical injury, or physical illness, including a life-endangering physical condition caused by the pregnancy itself that would, as certified by a physician, place the woman in danger of death unless an abortion is performed.

NOTE: The "G7" modifier must be used with the following CPT codes in order for these services to be covered when the pregnancy resulted from rape or incest, or the pregnancy is certified by a physician as life threatening to the mother:

59840, 59841, 59850, 59851, 59852, 59855, 59856, 59857, 59866

100-02, 1, 100
Treatment for Infertility
(Rev. 1, 10-01-03) A3-3101.13

Effective for services rendered on or after January 15, 1980, reasonable and necessary services associated with treatment for infertility are covered under Medicare. Like pregnancy (see Sec. 80 above), infertility is a condition sufficiently at variance with the usual state of health to make it appropriate for a person who normally would be expected to be fertile to seek medical consultation and treatment. Contractors should coordinate with QIOs to see that utilization guidelines are established for this treatment if inappropriate utilization or abuse is suspected.

100-02, 11, 20
Renal Dialysis Items and Services
(Rev.199, Issued: 11-14-14-Effective: 01-01-15, Implementation: 01-05-15)

Medicare provides payment under the ESRD PPS for all renal dialysis services for outpatient maintenance dialysis when they are furnished to Medicare ESRD patients for the treatment of ESRD by a Medicare certified ESRD facility or a special purpose dialysis facility. Renal dialysis services are the items and services included under the composite rate and the ESRD-related items and services that were separately paid as of December 31, 2010 that were used for the treatment of ESRD.

Renal dialysis services are furnished in various settings including hospital outpatient ESRD facilities, independent ESRD facilities, or in the patient's home. Renal dialysis items and services furnished at ESRD facilities differ according to the types of patients being treated, the types of equipment and supplies used, the preferences of the treating physician, and the capability and makeup of the staff. Although not all facilities provide an identical range of services, the most common elements of dialysis treatment include:

- Laboratory Tests;
- Drugs and Biologicals;
- Equipment and supplies - dialysis machine use and maintenance;
- Personnel services;
- Administrative services;
- Overhead costs;
- Monitoring access and related declotting or referring the patient, and
- Direct nursing services include registered nurses, licensed practical nurses, technicians, social workers, and dietitians.

100-02, 11, 20.2
Laboratory Services
(Rev. 224, Issued: 06-03-16, Effective: 01-01-16, Implementation: 09-06-16)

All laboratory services furnished to individuals for the treatment of ESRD are included in the ESRD PPS as Part B services and are not paid separately as of January 1, 2011. The laboratory services include but are not limited to:

- Laboratory tests included under the composite rate as of December 31, 2010 (discussed below); and
- Former separately billable Part B laboratory tests that were billed by ESRD facilities and independent laboratories for ESRD patients.

Composite rate laboratory tests are listed in §20.2.E of this chapter. More information regarding composite rate laboratory tests can be found in Pub. 100-4, Medicare Claims Processing Manual, chapter 8, §50.1, §60.1, and §80. As discussed below, composite rate laboratory services should not be reported on claims.

The distinction of what is considered to be a renal dialysis laboratory test is a clinical decision determined by the ESRD patient's ordering practitioner. If a laboratory test is ordered for the treatment of ESRD, then the laboratory test is not paid separately.

Payment for all renal dialysis laboratory tests furnished under the ESRD PPS is made directly to the ESRD facility responsible for the patient's care. The ESRD facility must furnish the laboratory tests directly or under arrangement and report renal dialysis laboratory tests on the ESRD facility claim (with the exception of composite rate laboratory services).

An ESRD facility must report renal dialysis laboratory services on its claims in order for the laboratory tests to be included in the outlier payment calculation. Renal dialysis laboratory services that were or would have been paid separately under Medicare Part B prior to January 1, 2011, are priced for the outlier payment calculation using the Clinical Laboratory Fee Schedule. Further information regarding the outlier policy can be found in §60.D of this chapter.

Certain laboratory services will be subject to Part B consolidated billing requirements and will no longer be separately payable when provided to ESRD beneficiaries by providers other than the renal dialysis facility. The list below includes the renal dialysis laboratory tests that are routinely performed for the treatment of ESRD. Payment for the laboratory tests identified on this list is included in the ESRD PPS. The laboratory tests listed in the table are used to enforce consolidated billing edits to ensure that payment is not made for renal dialysis laboratory tests outside of the ESRD PPS. The list of renal dialysis laboratory tests is not an all-inclusive list. If any laboratory test is ordered for the treatment of ESRD, then the laboratory test is considered to be included in the ESRD PPS and is the responsibility of the ESRD facility. Additional renal dialysis laboratory tests may be added through administrative issuances in the future.

LABS SUBJECT TO ESRD CONSOLIDATED BILLING

CPT/ HCPCS	Short Description
80047	Basic Metabolic Panel (Calcium, ionized)
80048	Basic Metabolic Panel (Calcium, total)
80051	Electrolyte Panel
80053	Comprehensive Metabolic Panel
80061	Lipid Panel
80069	Renal Function Panel
80076	Hepatic Function Panel
82040	Assay of serum albumin
82108	Assay of aluminum
82306	Vitamin d, 25 hydroxy
82310	Assay of calcium
82330	Assay of calcium, Ionized
82374	Assay, blood carbon dioxide
82379	Assay of carnitine
82435	Assay of blood chloride
82565	Assay of creatinine
82570	Assay of urine creatinine
82575	Creatinine clearance test
82607	Vitamin B-12
82652	Vit d 1, 25-dihydroxy
82668	Assay of erythropoietin
82728	Assay of ferritin
82746	Blood folic acid serum
83540	Assay of iron
83550	Iron binding test
83735	Assay of magnesium
83970	Assay of parathormone
84075	Assay alkaline phosphatase
84100	Assay of phosphorus
84132	Assay of serum potassium

CPT/ HCPCS	Short Description
84134	Assay of prealbumin
84155	Assay of protein, serum
84157	Assay of protein by other source
84295	Assay of serum sodium
84466	Assay of transferrin
84520	Assay of urea nitrogen
84540	Assay of urine/urea-n
84545	Urea-N clearance test
85014	Hematocrit
85018	Hemoglobin
85025	Complete (cbc), automated (HgB, Hct, RBC, WBC, and Platelet count) and automated differential WBC count.
85027	Complete (cbc), automated (HgB, Hct, RBC, WBC, and Platelet count)
85041	Automated rbc count
85044	Manual reticulocyte count
85045	Automated reticulocyte count
85046	Reticyte/hgb concentrate
85048	Automated leukocyte count
86704	Hep b core antibody, total
86705	Hep b core antibody, igm
86706	Hep b surface antibody
87040	Blood culture for bacteria
87070	Culture, bacteria, other
87071	Culture bacteri aerobic othr
87073	Culture bacteria anaerobic
87075	Cultr bacteria, except blood
87076	Culture anaerobe ident, each
87077	Culture aerobic identify
87081	Culture screen only
87340	Hepatitis b surface ag, eia
G0306	CBC/diff WBC w/o platelet
G0307	CBC without platelet

A. Automated Multi-Channel Chemistry (AMCC) Tests

During the ESRD PPS transition period (see §70 of this chapter) ESRD facilities are required to report the renal dialysis AMCC tests with the appropriate modifiers (CD, CE, or CF) on their claims for purposes of applying the 50/50 rule under the composite rate portion of the blended payment. Refer to §70.B of this chapter for additional information regarding the composite rate portion of the blended payment during the transition.

The 50/50 rule is necessary for those ESRD facilities that chose to go through the transition period. If the 50/50 rule allows for separate payment, then the laboratory tests are priced using the clinical laboratory fee schedule. Information regarding the 50/50 rule can be found in §20.2.E of this chapter and in Pub. 100-4, Medicare Claims Processing Manual, chapter 16, §40.6.

NOTE: An ESRD facility billing a renal dialysis AMCC test must use the CF modifier when the AMCC is not in the composite rate but is a renal dialysis service. AMCC tests that are furnished to individuals for reasons other than for the treatment of ESRD should be billed with the AY modifier to Medicare directly by the entity furnishing the service with the AY modifier.

B. Laboratory Services Furnished for Reasons Other Than for the Treatment of ESRD

1. Independent Laboratory

A patient's physician or practitioner may order a laboratory test that is included on the list of items and services subject to consolidated billing edits for reasons other than for the treatment of ESRD. When this occurs, the patient's physician or practitioner should notify the independent laboratory or the ESRD facility (with the appropriate clinical laboratory certification in accordance with the Clinical Laboratory Improvement Act) that furnished the laboratory service that the test is not a renal dialysis service and that entity may bill Medicare separately using the AY modifier. The AY modifier serves as an attestation that the item or service is medically necessary for the patient but is not being used for the treatment of ESRD.

2. Hospital-Based Laboratory

Hospital outpatient clinical laboratories furnishing renal dialysis laboratory tests to ESRD patients for reasons other than for the treatment of ESRD may submit a claim for separate payment using the AY modifier. The AY modifier serves as an attestation that the item or service is medically necessary for the patient but is not being used for the treatment of ESRD.

C. Laboratory Services Performed in Emergency Rooms or Emergency Departments

In an emergency room or emergency department, the ordering physician or practitioner may not know at the time the laboratory test is being ordered, if it is being ordered as a renal dialysis service. Consequently, emergency rooms or emergency departments are not required to append an AY modifier to these laboratory tests when submitting claims with dates of service on or after January 1, 2012.

When a renal dialysis laboratory service is furnished to an ESRD patient in an emergency room or emergency department on a different date of service, hospitals can append an ET modifier to the laboratory tests furnished to ESRD patients to indicate that the laboratory test was furnished in conjunction with the emergency visit. Appending the ET modifier indicates that the laboratory service being furnished on a day other than the emergency visit is related to the emergency visit and at the time the ordering physician was unable to determine if the test was ordered for reasons of treating the patient's ESRD.

Allowing laboratory testing to bypass consolidated billing edits in the emergency room or department does not mean that ESRD facilities should send patients to other settings for routine laboratory testing for the purpose of not assuming financial responsibility of renal dialysis items and services. For additional information regarding laboratory services furnished in a variety of settings, see Pub. 100-4, Medicare Claims Processing Manual, chapter 16, §30.3 and §40.6.

D. Hepatitis B Laboratory Services for Transient Patients

Laboratory testing for hepatitis B is a renal dialysis service. Effective January 1, 2011, hepatitis B testing is included in the ESRD PPS and therefore cannot be billed separately to Medicare.

The Conditions for Coverage for ESRD facilities require routine hepatitis B testing (42 CFR §494.30(a)(1)). The ESRD facility is responsible for the payment of the laboratory test, regardless of frequency. If an ESRD patient wishes to travel, the patient's home ESRD facility should have systems in place for communicating hepatitis B test results to the destination ESRD facility.

E. Laboratory Services Included Under Composite Rate

Prior to the implementation of the ESRD PPS, the costs of certain ESRD laboratory services furnished for outpatient maintenance dialysis by either the ESRD facility's staff or an independent laboratory, were included in the composite rate calculations. Therefore, payment for all of these laboratory tests was included in the ESRD facility's composite rate and the tests could not have been billed separately to the Medicare program.

All laboratory services that were included under the composite rate are included under the ESRD PPS unless otherwise specified. Payments for these laboratory tests are included in the ESRD PPS and are not paid separately under the composite rate portion of the blended payment and are not eligible for outlier payments. Therefore, composite rate laboratory services should not be reported on the claim. Laboratory tests included in the composite payment rate are identified below.

1. Routinely Covered Tests Paid Under Composite Rate

The tests listed below are usually performed for dialysis patients and were routinely covered at the frequency specified in the absence of indications to the contrary, (i.e., no documentation of medical necessity was required other than knowledge of the patient's status as an ESRD beneficiary). When any of these tests were performed at a frequency greater than that specified, the additional tests were separately billable and were covered only if they were medically justified by accompanying documentation. A diagnosis of ESRD alone was not sufficient medical evidence to warrant coverage of the additional tests. The nature of the illness or injury (diagnosis, complaint, or symptom) requiring the performance of the test(s) must have been present, along with ICD diagnosis coding, on the claim for payment.

a. Hemodialysis, IPD, CCPD, and Hemofiltration

- Per Treatment - All hematocrit, hemoglobin, and clotting time tests furnished incident to dialysis treatments;

- Weekly - Prothrombin time for patients on anticoagulant therapy and Serum Creatinine;

- Weekly or Thirteen Per Quarter - BUN;

- Monthly - Serum Calcium, Serum Potassium, Serum Chloride, CBC, Serum Bicarbonate, Serum Phosphorous, Total Protein, Serum Albumin, Alkaline Phosphatase, aspartate amino transferase (AST) (SGOT) and LDH; and

- Automated Multi-Channel Chemistry (AMCC) - If an automated battery of tests, such as the SMA-12, is performed and contains most of the tests listed in one of the weekly or monthly categories, it is not necessary to separately identify any tests in the battery that are not listed. Further information concerning automated tests and the "50 percent rule" can be found below and in Pub. 100-4, Medicare Claims Processing Manual, chapter 16, §40.6.1.

b. CAPD

- Monthly – BUN, Creatinine, Sodium, Potassium, CO2, Calcium, Magnesium, Phosphate, Total Protein, Albumin, Alkaline Phosphatase, LDH, AST, SGOT, HCT, Hbg, and Dialysate Protein.

Under the ESRD PPS, frequency requirements do not apply for the purpose of payment. However, laboratory tests should be ordered as necessary and should not be restricted because of financial reasons.

2. Separately Billable Tests Under the Composite Rate

The following list identifies certain separately billable laboratory tests that were covered routinely and without documentation of medical necessity other than knowledge of the patient's status as an ESRD beneficiary, when furnished at specified frequencies. If they were performed at a frequency greater than that specified, they were covered only if accompanied by medical documentation. A diagnosis of ESRD alone was not sufficient documentation. The medical necessity of the test(s), the nature of the illness or injury (diagnosis, complaint or symptom) requiring the performance of the test(s) must have been furnished on claims using the ICD diagnosis coding system.

— Separately Billable Tests for Hemodialysis, IPD, CCPD, and Hemofiltration

Serum Aluminum - one every 3 months

Serum Ferritin - one every 3 months

— Separately Billable Tests for CAPD

WBC, RBC, and Platelet count – One every 3 months

Residual renal function and 24 hour urine volume – One every 6 months

Under the ESRD PPS frequency requirements do not apply for the purpose of payment. However, laboratory tests should be ordered as necessary and should not be restricted because of financial reasons.

3. **Automated Multi-Channel Chemistry (AMCC) Tests Under the Composite Rate**

Clinical diagnostic laboratory tests that comprise the AMCC (listed in Appendix A and B) could be considered to be composite rate and non-composite rate laboratory services. Composite rate payment was paid by the A/B MAC (A). To determine if separate payment was allowed for non-composite rate tests for a particular date of service, 50 percent or more of the covered tests must be non-composite rate tests. This policy also applies to the composite rate portion of the blended payment during the transition. Beginning January 1, 2014, the 50 percent rule will no longer apply and no separate payment will be made under the composite rate portion of the blended payment.

Medicare applied the following to AMCC tests for ESRD beneficiaries:

— Payment was the lowest rate for services performed by the same provider, for the same beneficiary, for the same date of service.

— The A/B MAC identified, for a particular date of service, the AMCC tests ordered that were included in the composite rate and those that were not included. The composite rate tests were defined for Hemodialysis, IPD, CCPD, and Hemofiltration (see Appendix A) and for CAPD (see Appendix B).

— If 50 percent or more of the covered tests were included under the composite rate payment, then all submitted tests were included within the composite payment. In this case, no separate payment in addition to the composite rate was made for any of the separately billable tests.

— If less than 50 percent of the covered tests were composite rate tests, all AMCC tests submitted for that Date of Service (DOS) were separately payable.

— A non-composite rate test was defined as any test separately payable outside of the composite rate or beyond the normal frequency covered under the composite rate that was reasonable and necessary.

Three pricing modifiers identify the different payment situations for ESRD AMCC tests. The physician who ordered the tests was responsible for identifying the appropriate modifier when ordering the tests.

— CD - AMCC test had been ordered by an ESRD facility or Medicare capitation payment (MCP) physician that was part of the composite rate and was not separately billable

— CE - AMCC test had been ordered by an ESRD facility or MCP physician that was a composite rate test but was beyond the normal frequency covered under the rate and was separately reimbursable based on medical necessity

— CF - AMCC test had been ordered by an ESRD facility or MCP physician that was not part of the composite rate and was separately billable

The ESRD clinical diagnostic laboratory tests identified with modifiers "CD", "CE" or "CF" may not have been billed as organ or disease panels. Effective October 1, 2003, all ESRD clinical diagnostic laboratory tests must be billed individually. See Pub. 100-4, Medicare Claims Processing Manual, chapter 16, §40.6.1, for additional billing and payment instructions as well as examples of the 50/50 rule.

For ESRD dialysis patients, CPT code 82330 Calcium; ionized shall be included in the calculation for the 50/50 rule (Pub. 100-4, Medicare Claims Processing Manual, chapter 16, §40.6.1). When CPT code 82330 is billed as a substitute for CPT code 82310, Calcium; total, it shall be billed with modifier CD or CE. When CPT code 82330 is billed in addition to CPT 82310, it shall be billed with CF modifier.

100-02, 12, 30.1

(Rev.255, Issued: 01-25-19, Effective: 01- 01- 19, Implementation: 02-26-19)

Rules for Payment of CORF Services

The payment basis for CORF services is 80 percent of the lesser of: (1) the actual charge for the service or (2) the physician fee schedule amount for the service when the physician fee schedule establishes a payment amount for such service. Payment for CORF services under the physician fee schedule is made for physical therapy, occupational therapy, speech-language pathology and respiratory therapy services, as well as the nursing and social and/or psychological services, which are a part of, or directly relate to, the rehabilitation plan of treatment.

Payment for covered durable medical equipment, orthotic and prosthetic (DMEPOS) devices and supplies provided by a CORF is based upon: the lesser of 80 percent of actual charges or the payment amount established under the DMEPOS fee schedule;

or, the single payment amount established under the DMEPOS competitive bidding program, provided that payment for such an item is not included in the payment amount for other CORF services.

If there is no fee schedule amount for a covered CORF item or service, payment should be based on the lesser of 80 percent of the actual charge for the service provided or an amount determined by the local Medicare contractor.

The following conditions apply to CORF physical therapy, occupational therapy, and speech-language pathology services;

• Claims must contain the required functional reporting. (Reference: Sections 42 CFR 410.105.) Refer to Pub. 100-04, Medicare Claims Processing Manual, chapter 5, section 10.6. NOTE: Functional reporting and documentation requirements are no longer applicable for claims for dates of service on and after January 1, 2019. For more information, refer to subsection F in section 30 above.

• The functional reporting on claims must be consistent with the functional limitations identified as part of the patient's therapy plan of care and expressed as part of the patient's therapy goals; effective for claims with dates of service on and after January, 1, 2013. (Reference: 42 CFR 410.105.) See Pub. 100-04, Medicare Claims Processing Manual, chapter 5, section 10.6. NOTE: Functional reporting and documentation requirements are no longer applicable for claims for dates of service on and after January 1, 2019. For more information, refer to subsection F in section 30 above.

• The National Provider Identifier (NPI) of the certifying physician identified for a CORF physical therapy, occupational therapy, and speech-language pathology plan of treatment must be included on the therapy claim. This requirement is effective for claims with dates of service on or after October 1, 2012. (See Pub. 100-04, Medicare Claims Processing Manual, chapter 5, section 10.3.)

Payment for CORF social and/or psychological services is made under the physician fee schedule only for HCPCS code G0409, as appropriate, and only when billed using revenue codes 0560, 0569, 0910, 0911, 0914 and 0919.

Payment for CORF respiratory therapy services is made under the physician fee schedule when provided by a respiratory therapist as defined at 42CFR485.70(j) and, only to the extent that these services support or are an adjunct to the rehabilitation plan of treatment, when billed using revenue codes 0410, 0412 and 0419. Separate payment is not made for diagnostic tests or for services related to physiologic monitoring services which are bundled into other respiratory therapy services appropriately performed by a respiratory therapist, such as HCPCS codes G0237, G0238 and G0239.

Payment for CORF nursing services is made under the physician fee schedule only when provided by a registered nurse as defined at 42CFR485.70(h) for nursing services only to the extent that these services support or are an adjunct to the rehabilitation plan of treatment. In addition, payment for CORF nursing services is made only when provided by a registered nurse. HCPCS code G0128 is used to bill for these services and only with revenue codes 0550 and 0559.

For specific payment requirements for CORF items and services see Pub. 100-04, Medicare Claims Processing Manual, Chapter 5, Part B Outpatient Rehabilitation and CORF/OPT Services.

100-02, 13, 220

Preventive Health Services

(Rev. 230, Issued: 12-09-16, Effective: 03-09-17, Implementation: 03-09-17)

RHCs and FQHCs are paid for the professional component of allowable preventive services when all of the program requirements are met and frequency limits (where applicable) have not been exceeded. The beneficiary copayment and deductible (where applicable) is waived by the Affordable Care Act for the IPPE and AWV, and for Medicare-covered preventive services recommended by the USPSTF with a grade or A or B.

100-02, 13, 220.1

Preventive Health Services in RHCs

(Rev. 230, Issued: 12-09-16, Effective: 03-09-17, Implementation: 03-09-17)

Influenza (G0008) and Pneumococcal Vaccines (G0009)

Influenza and pneumococcal vaccines and their administration are paid at 100 percent of reasonable cost through the cost report. No visit is billed, and these costs should not be included on the claim. The beneficiary coinsurance and deductible are waived.

Hepatitis B Vaccine (G0010)

Hepatitis B vaccine and its administration is included in the RHC visit and is not separately billable. The cost of the vaccine and its administration can be included in the line item for the otherwise qualifying visit. A visit cannot be billed if vaccine administration is the only service the RHC provides. The beneficiary coinsurance and deductible are waived.

Initial Preventive Physical Exam (G0402)

The IPPE is a face-to-face one-time exam that must occur within the first 12 months following the beneficiary's enrollment. The IPPE can be billed as a stand-alone visit if it is the only medical service provided on that day with an RHC practitioner. If an IPPE visit is furnished on the same day as another billable visit, two visits may be billed. The beneficiary coinsurance and deductible are waived.

Annual Wellness Visit (G0438 and G0439)

The AWV is a personalized face-to-face prevention visit for beneficiaries who are not within the first 12 months of their first Part B coverage period and have not received an IPPE or AWV within the past 12 months. The AWV can be billed as a stand-alone visit if it is the only medical service provided on that day with an RHC practitioner. If the AWV is furnished on the same day as another medical visit, it is not a separately billable visit. The beneficiary coinsurance and deductible are waived.

Diabetes Self-Management Training (G0108) and Medical Nutrition Therapy (97802 and 97803)

Diabetes self-management training or medical nutrition therapy provided by a registered dietician or nutritional professional at an RHC may be considered incident to a visit with an RHC practitioner provided all applicable conditions are met. DSMT and MNT are not billable visits in an RHC, although the cost may be allowable on the cost report. RHCs cannot bill a visit for services furnished by registered dieticians or nutritional professionals. However, RHCs are permitted to become certified providers of DSMT services and report the cost of such services on their cost report for inclusion in the computation of their AIR. The beneficiary coinsurance and deductible apply.

Screening Pelvic and Clinical Breast Examination (G0101)

Screening pelvic and clinical breast examination can be billed as a stand-alone visit if it is the only medical service provided on that day with an RHC practitioner. If it is furnished on the same day as another medical visit, it is not a separately billable visit. The beneficiary coinsurance and deductible are waived.

Screening Papanicolaou Smear (Q0091)

Screening Papanicolaou smear can be billed as a stand-alone visit if it is the only medical service provided on that day with an RHC practitioner. If it is furnished on the same day as another medical visit, it is not a separately billable visit. The beneficiary coinsurance and deductible are waived.

Prostate Cancer Screening (G0102)

Prostate cancer screening can be billed as a stand-alone visit if it is the only medical service provided on that day with an RHC practitioner. If it is furnished on the same day as another medical visit, it is not a separately billable visit. The beneficiary coinsurance and deductible apply.

Glaucoma Screening (G0117 and G0118)

Glaucoma screening for high risk patients can be billed as a stand-alone visit if it is the only medical service provided on that day with an RHC practitioner. If it is furnished on the same day as another medical visit, it is not a separately billable visit. The beneficiary coinsurance and deductible apply.

Lung Cancer Screening Using Low Dose Computed Tomography (LDCT) (G0296)

LDCT can be billed as a stand-alone visit if it is the only medical service provided on that day with an RHC practitioner. If it is furnished on the same day as another medical visit, it is not a separately billable visit. The beneficiary coinsurance and deductible are waived.

NOTE: Hepatitis C Screening (GO472) is a technical service only and therefore it is not paid as part of the RHC visit.

100-02, 13, 220.3

Preventive Health Services in FQHCs

(Rev. 230, Issued: 12-09-16, Effective: 03-09-17, Implementation: 03-09-17)

FQHCs must provide preventive health services on site or by arrangement with another provider. These services must be furnished by or under the direct supervision of a physician, NP, PA, CNM, CP, or CSW. Section 330(b)(1)(A)(i)(III) of the Public Health Service (PHS) Act required preventive health services can be found at http://bphc.hrsa.gov/policiesregulations/legislation/index.html, and include:

- prenatal and perinatal services;
- appropriate cancer screening;
- well-child services;
- immunizations against vaccine-preventable diseases;
- screenings for elevated blood lead levels, communicable diseases, and cholesterol;
- pediatric eye, ear, and dental screenings to determine the need for vision and hearing correction and dental care;
- voluntary family planning services; and
- preventive dental services.

NOTE: The cost of providing these services may be included in the FQHC cost report but they do not necessarily qualify as FQHC billable visits or for the waiver of the beneficiary coinsurance.

Influenza (G0008) and Pneumococcal Vaccines (G0009)

Influenza and pneumococcal vaccines and their administration are paid at 100 percent of reasonable cost through the cost report. The cost is included in the cost report and no visit is billed. FQHCs must include these charges on the claim if furnished as part of an encounter. The beneficiary coinsurance is waived.

Hepatitis B Vaccine (G0010)

Hepatitis B vaccine and its administration is included in the FQHC visit and is not separately billable. The cost of the vaccine and its administration can be included in the line item for the otherwise qualifying visit. A visit cannot be billed if vaccine administration is the only service the FQHC provides. The beneficiary coinsurance is waived.

Initial Preventive Physical Exam (G0402)

The IPPE is a one-time exam that must occur within the first 12 months following the beneficiary's enrollment. The IPPE can be billed as a stand-alone visit if it is the only medical service provided on that day with a FQHC practitioner. If an IPPE visit is furnished on the same day as another billable visit, FQHCs may not bill for a separate visit. These FQHCs will have an adjustment of 1.3416 to their PPS rate. The beneficiary coinsurance is waived.

Annual Wellness Visit (G0438 and G0439)

The AWV is a personalized prevention plan for beneficiaries who are not within the first 12 months of their first Part B coverage period and have not received an IPPE or AWV within the past 12 months. The AWV can be billed as a stand-alone visit if it is the only medical service provided on that day with a FQHC practitioner. If the AWV is furnished on the same day as another medical visit, it is not a separately billable visit. FQHCs that are authorized to bill under the FQHC PPS will have an adjustment of 1.3416 to their PPS rate. The beneficiary coinsurance is waived.

Diabetes Self-Management Training (G0108) and Medical Nutrition Therapy (97802 and 97803)

DSMT and MNT furnished by certified DSMT and MNT providers are billable visits in FQHCs when they are provided in a one-on-one, face-to-face encounter and all program requirements are met. Other diabetes counseling or medical nutrition services provided by a registered dietician at the FQHC may be considered incident to a visit with a FQHC provider. The beneficiary coinsurance is waived for MNT services and is applicable for DSMT.

DSMT must be furnished by a certified DSMT practitioner, and MNT must be furnished by a registered dietitian or nutrition professional. Program requirements for DSMT services are set forth in 42 CFR 410 Subpart H for DSMT and in Part 410, Subpart G for MNT services, and additional guidance can be found at Pub. 100-02, chapter 15, section 300.

Screening Pelvic and Clinical Breast Examination (G0101)

Screening pelvic and clinical breast examination can be billed as a stand-alone visit if it is the only medical service provided on that day with a FQHC practitioner. If it is furnished on the same day as another medical visit, it is not a separately billable visit. The beneficiary coinsurance is waived.

Screening Papanicolaou Smear (Q0091)

Screening Papanicolaou smear can be billed as a stand-alone visit if it is the only medical service provided on that day with a FQHC practitioner. If it is furnished on the same day as another medical visit, it is not a separately billable visit. The beneficiary coinsurance is waived.

Prostate Cancer Screening (G0102)

Prostate cancer screening can be billed as a stand-alone visit if it is the only medical service provided on that day with a FQHC practitioner. If it is furnished on the same day as another medical visit, it is not a separately billable visit. The beneficiary coinsurance applies.

Glaucoma Screening (G0117 and G0118)

Glaucoma screening for high risk patients can be billed as a stand-alone visit if it is the only medical service provided on that day with a FQHC practitioner. If it is furnished on the same day as another medical visit, it is not a separately billable visit. The beneficiary coinsurance applies.

Lung Cancer Screening Using Low Dose Computed Tomography (LDCT) (G0296)

LDCT can be billed as a stand-alone visit if it is the only medical service provided on that day with a FQHC practitioner. If it is furnished on the same day as another medical visit, it is not a separately billable visit. The beneficiary coinsurance is waived.

NOTE: Hepatitis C Screening (GO472) is a technical service only and therefore not paid as part of the FQHC visit.

100-02, 13, 230

Care Management Services

(Rev. 239, Issued: 01-09-18, Effective: 1-22-18, Implementation: 1-22-18)

Care management services are RHC and FQHC services. Except for TCM services, care management services are paid separately from the RHC AIR or FQHC PPS payment methodology.

100-02, 13, 230.1

Transitional Care Management Services

(Rev. 239, Issued: 01-09-18, Effective: 1-22-18, Implementation: 1-22-18)

Effective January 1, 2013, RHCs and FQHCs are paid for TCM services furnished by an RHC or FQHC practitioner when all TCM requirements are met. TCM services must be furnished within 30 days of the date of the patient's discharge from a hospital (including outpatient observation or partial hospitalization), SNF, or community mental health center.

Communication (direct contact, telephone, or electronic) with the patient or caregiver must commence within 2 business days of discharge, and a face-to-face visit must occur within 14 days of discharge for moderate complexity decision making (CPT code 99495), or within 7 days of discharge for high complexity decision making (CPT code 99496). The TCM visit is billed on the day that the TCM visit takes place, and only one TCM visit may be paid per beneficiary for services furnished during that 30 day post-discharge period. The TCM visit is subject to applicable copayments and deductibles.

TCM services can be billed as a stand-alone visit if it is the only medical service provided on that day with an RHC or FQHC practitioner and it meets the TCM billing requirements. If it is furnished on the same day as another visit, only one visit can be billed. Beginning on January 1, 2017, services furnished by auxiliary personnel incident to a TCM visit may be furnished under general supervision.

100-02, 13, 230.2

General Care Management Services – Chronic Care Management and General Behavioral Health Integration Services

(Rev. 239, Issued: 01-09-18, Effective: 1-22-18, Implementation: 1-22-18)

Chronic Care Management (CCM)

Effective January 1, 2016, RHCs and FQHCs are paid for CCM services when a minimum of 20 minutes of qualifying CCM services during a calendar month is furnished to patients with multiple chronic conditions that are expected to last at least 12 months or until the death of the patient, and that place the patient at significant risk of death, acute exacerbation/decompensation, or functional decline. For CCM services furnished between January 1, 2016, and December 31, 2017, payment is based on the PFS national average non-facility payment rate when CPT code 99490 is billed alone or with other payable services on an RHC or FQHC claim.

CCM Service Requirements

- Structured recording of patient health information using Certified EHR Technology including demographics, problems, medications, and medication allergies that inform the care plan, care coordination, and ongoing clinical care;

- 24/7 access to physicians or other qualified health care professionals or clinical staff including providing patients/caregivers with a means to make contact with health care professionals in the practice to address urgent needs regardless of the time of day or day of week, and continuity of care with a designated member of the care team with whom the patient is able to schedule successive routine appointments;

- Comprehensive care management including systematic assessment of the patient's medical, functional, and psychosocial needs; system-based approaches to ensure timely receipt of all recommended preventive care services; medication reconciliation with review of adherence and potential interactions; and oversight of patient self-management of medications;

- Comprehensive care plan including the creation, revision, and/or monitoring of an electronic care plan based on a physical, mental, cognitive, psychosocial, functional, and environmental (re)assessment and an inventory of resources and supports; a comprehensive care plan for all health issues with particular focus on the chronic conditions being managed;

- Care plan information made available electronically (including fax) in a timely manner within and outside the RHC or FQHC as appropriate and a copy of the plan of care given to the patient and/or caregiver;

- Management of care transitions between and among health care providers and settings, including referrals to other clinicians; follow-up after an emergency department visit; and follow-up after discharges from hospitals, skilled nursing facilities, or other health care facilities; timely creation and exchange/transmit continuity of care document(s) with other practitioners and providers;

- Coordination with home- and community-based clinical service providers, and documentation of communication to and from home- and community-based providers regarding the patient's psychosocial needs and functional deficits in the patient's medical record; and

- Enhanced opportunities for the patient and any caregiver to communicate with the practitioner regarding the patient's care through not only telephone access, but also through the use of secure messaging, Internet, or other asynchronous non-face-to-face consultation methods.

General Behavioral Health Integration (BHI)

General BHI is a team-based, collaborative approach to care that focuses on integrative treatment of patients with primary care and mental or behavioral health conditions. Patients are eligible to receive BHI services if they have one or more new or pre-existing behavioral health or psychiatric conditions being treated by the RHC or FQHC primary care practitioner, including substance use disorders, that, in the clinical judgment of the RHC or FQHC primary care practitioner, warrants BHI services.

General BHI Service Requirements

- An initial assessment and ongoing monitoring using validated clinical rating scales;

- Behavioral health care planning in relation to behavioral/psychiatric health problems, including revision for patients who are not progressing or whose status changes;

- Facilitating and coordinating treatment such as psychotherapy, pharmacotherapy, counseling and/or psychiatric consultation; and

- Continuity of care with a designated member of the care team.

Care Management Payment

Effective January 1, 2018, RHCs and FQHCs are paid for CCM or general BHI services when general care management G code, G0511, is on an RHC or FQHC claim, either alone or with other payable services, for CCM or BHI services furnished on or after January 1, 2018.

A separately billable initiating visit with an RHC or FQHC primary care practitioner (physician, NP, PA, or CNM) is required before care management services can be furnished. This visit can be an E/M, AWV, or IPPE visit, and must occur no more than one-year prior to commencing care management services.

Documentation that the beneficiary has consented to receive CCM or BHI services must be in the beneficiary's medical record before CCM or BHI services are furnished. This should include that the beneficiary has

- Given permission to consult with relevant specialists as needed;

- Been informed that there may be cost-sharing (e.g. deductible and coinsurance in RHCs, and coinsurance in FQHCs) for both in-person and non-face-to-face services that are provided

- Been informed that only one practitioner/facility can furnish and be paid for these services during a calendar month; and

- Been informed that they can stop care management services at any time, effective at the end of the calendar month.

Payment for G0511 is set at the average of the national non-facility PFS payment rate for CPT codes 99490 (30 minutes or more of CCM services), 99487 (60 minutes or more of complex CCM services), and 99484 (20 minutes or more of general behavioral health integration services). This rate is updated annually based on the PFS amounts.

RHCs and FQHCs can bill G0511 when the requirements for either CPT codes 99490, 99487, or 99484 are met. G0511 can be billed alone or in addition to other services furnished during an RHC or FQHC visit. Coinsurance and deductibles are applied as applicable to RHC claims, and coinsurance is applied as applicable to FQHC claims. General Care Management services furnished by auxiliary personnel may be provided under general supervision and the face-to-face requirements are waived.

RHCs and FQHCs may not bill for care management services for a patient if another practitioner or facility has already billed for care management services for the same beneficiary during the same time period. RHCs and FQHCs may not bill for care management and TCM services, or another program that provides additional payment for care management services (outside of the RHC AIR or FQHC PPS payment), for the same beneficiary during the same time period.

100-02, 13, 230.3

Psychiatric Collaborative Care Model (CoCM) Services

(Rev. 239, Issued: 01-09-18, Effective: 1-22-18, Implementation: 1-22-18)

Effective January 1, 2018, RHCs and FQHCs are paid for psychiatric CoCM services when psychiatric CoCM G code, G0512, is on an RHC or FQHC claim, either alone or with other payable services. At least 70 minutes in the first calendar month, and at least 60 minutes in subsequent calendar months, of psychiatric CoCM services must have been furnished in order to bill for this service.

Psychiatric CoCM is a specific model of care provided by a primary care team consisting of a primary care provider and a health care manager who work in collaboration with a psychiatric consultant to integrate primary health care services with care management support for patients receiving behavioral health treatment. It includes regular psychiatric inter-specialty consultation with the primary care team, particularly regarding patients whose conditions are not improving. Patients with mental health, behavioral health, or psychiatric conditions, including substance use disorders, who are being treated by an RHC or FQHC practitioner may be eligible for psychiatric CoCM services, as determined by the RHC or FQHC practitioner.

The psychiatric CoCM team must include the RHC or FQHC practitioner, a behavioral health care manager, and a psychiatric consultant. The primary care team regularly reviews the beneficiary's treatment plan and status with the psychiatric consultant and maintains or adjusts treatment, including referral to behavioral health specialty care, as needed.

RHC or FQHC Practitioner Requirements

The RHC or FQHC practitioner is a primary care physician, NP, PA, or CNM who:

- Directs the behavioral health care manager and any other clinical staff;

- Oversees the beneficiary's care, including prescribing medications, providing treatments for medical conditions, and making referrals to specialty care when needed; and

- Remains involved through ongoing oversight, management, collaboration and reassessment.

Behavioral Health Care Manager Requirements

The behavioral health care manager is a designated individual with formal education or specialized training in behavioral health, including social work, nursing, or psychology, and has a minimum of a bachelor's degree in a behavioral health field (such as in clinical social work or psychology), or is a clinician with behavioral health training, including RNs and LPNs. The behavioral health care manager furnishes both face-to-face and non-face-to-face services under the general supervision of the RHC or FQHC practitioner and may be employed by or working under contract to the RHC or FQHC. The behavioral health care manager:

- Provides assessment and care management services, including the administration of validated rating scales;

- Provides behavioral health care planning in relation to behavioral/psychiatric health problems, including revision for patients who are not progressing or whose status changes;

- Provides brief psychosocial interventions;

- Maintains ongoing collaboration with the RHC or FQHC practitioner;

- Maintains a registry that tracks patient follow-up and progress;

- Acts in consultation with the psychiatric consultant;

- Is available to provide services face-to-face with the beneficiary; and

- Has a continuous relationship with the patient and a collaborative, integrated relationship with the rest of the care team.

Psychiatric Consultant Requirements

The psychiatric consultant is a medical professional trained in psychiatry and qualified to prescribe the full range of medications. The psychiatric consultant is not required to be on site or to have direct contact with the patient and does not prescribe medications or furnish treatment to the beneficiary directly. The psychiatric consultant:

- Participates in regular reviews of the clinical status of patients receiving psychiatric CoCM services;

- Advises the RHC or FQHC practitioner regarding diagnosis and options for resolving issues with beneficiary adherence and tolerance of behavioral health treatment; making adjustments to behavioral health treatment for beneficiaries who are not progressing; managing any negative interactions between beneficiaries' behavioral health and medical treatments; and

- Facilitates referral for direct provision of psychiatric care when clinically indicated.

A separately billable initiating visit with an RHC or FQHC primary care practitioner (physician, NP, PA, or CNM) is required before psychiatric CoCM services can be furnished. This visit can be an E/M, AWV, or IPPE visit, and must occur no more than one-year prior to commencing psychiatric CoCM services.

Documentation that the beneficiary has consented to receive psychiatric CoCM services must be in the beneficiary's medical record before CCM or BHI services are furnished. This should include that the beneficiary has

- Given permission to consult with relevant specialists as needed;

- Been informed that there may be cost-sharing (e.g. deductible and coinsurance in RHCs, and coinsurance in FQHCs) for both in-person and non-face-to-face services that are provided;

- Been informed that only one practitioner/facility can furnish and be paid for these services during a calendar month; and

- Been informed that they can stop care management services at any time, effective at the end of the calendar month.

RHCs and FQHCs can bill G0512 when the requirements for either initial or subsequent psychiatric CoCM services are met. G0512 can be billed alone or in addition to other services furnished during an RHC or FQHC visit. To prevent duplication of payment, this code can only be billed once per month per beneficiary, and cannot be billed if other care management services are billed for the same time period.

Payment for G0512 is set at the average of the national non-facility PFS payment rate for CPT code 99492 (70 minutes or more of initial psychiatric CoCM services) and CPT code 99493 (60 minutes or more of subsequent psychiatric CoCM services). This rate is updated annually based on the PFS amounts. Coinsurance is applied as applicable to FQHC claims, and coinsurance and deductibles are applied as applicable to RHC claims. Psychiatric CoCM services furnished by auxiliary personnel may be provided under general supervision and the face-to-face requirements are waived.

100-02, 15, 20.1

Physician Expense for Surgery, Childbirth, and Treatment for Infertility

(Rev. 1, 10-01-03) B3-2005.I

A. Surgery and Childbirth

Skilled medical management is covered throughout the events of pregnancy, beginning with diagnosis, continuing through delivery and ending after the necessary postnatal care. Similarly, in the event of termination of pregnancy, regardless of whether terminated spontaneously or for therapeutic reasons (i.e., where the life of the mother would be endangered if the fetus were brought to term), the need for skilled medical management and/or medical services is equally important as in those cases carried to full term. After the infant is delivered and is a separate individual, items and services furnished to the infant are not covered on the basis of the mother's eligibility.

Most surgeons and obstetricians bill patients an all-inclusive package charge intended to cover all services associated with the surgical procedure or delivery of the child. All expenses for surgical and obstetrical care, including preoperative/prenatal examinations and tests and post-operative/postnatal services, are considered incurred on the date of surgery or delivery, as appropriate. This policy applies whether the physician bills on a package charge basis, or itemizes the bill separately for these items.

Occasionally, a physician's bill may include charges for additional services not directly related to the surgical procedure or the delivery. Such charges are considered incurred on the date the additional services are furnished.

The above policy applies only where the charges are imposed by one physician or by a clinic on behalf of a group of physicians. Where more than one physician imposes charges for surgical or obstetrical services, all preoperative/prenatal and post-operative/postnatal services performed by the physician who performed the surgery or delivery are considered incurred on the date of the surgery or delivery. Expenses for services rendered by other physicians are considered incurred on the date they were performed.

B. Treatment for Infertility

Reasonable and necessary services associated with treatment for infertility are covered under Medicare. Infertility is a condition sufficiently at variance with the usual state of health to make it appropriate for a person who normally is expected to be fertile to seek medical consultation and treatment.

100-02, 15, 30.4

Optometrist's Services

(Rev. 1, 10-01-03) B3-2020.25

Effective April 1, 1987, a doctor of optometry is considered a physician with respect to all services the optometrist is authorized to perform under State law or regulation. To be covered under Medicare, the services must be medically reasonable and necessary for the diagnosis or treatment of illness or injury, and must meet all applicable coverage requirements. See the Medicare Benefit Policy Manual, Chapter 16, "General Exclusions from Coverage," for exclusions from coverage that apply to vision care services, and the Medicare Claims Processing Manual, Chapter 12, "Physician/Practitioner Billing," for information dealing with payment for items and services furnished by optometrists.

A. FDA Monitored Studies of Intraocular Lenses

Special coverage rules apply to situations in which an ophthalmologist is involved in a Food and Drug Administration (FDA) monitored study of the safety and efficacy of an investigational Intraocular Lens (IOL). The investigation process for IOLs is unique in that there is a core period and an adjunct period. The core study is a traditional, well-controlled clinical investigation with full record keeping and reporting requirements. The adjunct study is essentially an extended distribution phase for lenses in which only limited safety data are compiled. Depending on the lens being evaluated, the adjunct study may be an extension of the core study or may be the only type of investigation to which the lens may be subject.

All eye care services related to the investigation of the IOL must be provided by the investigator (i.e., the implanting ophthalmologist) or another practitioner (including a doctor of optometry) who provides services at the direction or under the supervision of the investigator and who has an agreement with the investigator that information on the patient is given to the investigator so that he or she may report on the patient to the IOL manufacturer. Eye care services furnished by anyone other than the investigator (or a practitioner who assists the investigator, as described in the preceding paragraph) are not covered during the period the IOL is being investigated, unless the services are not related to the investigation.

B. Concurrent Care

Where more than one practitioner furnishes concurrent care, services furnished to a beneficiary by both an ophthalmologist and another physician (including an optometrist) may be recognized for payment if it is determined that each practitioner's services were reasonable and necessary. (See Sec.30.E.)

100-02, 15, 30.5

Chiropractor's Services

(Rev. 23, Issued: 10-08-04, Effective: 10-01-04, Implementation: 10-04-04) B3-2020.26

A chiropractor must be licensed or legally authorized to furnish chiropractic services by the State or jurisdiction in which the services are furnished. In addition, a licensed chiropractor must meet the following uniform minimum standards to be considered a physician for Medicare coverage. Coverage extends only to treatment by means of manual manipulation of the spine to correct a subluxation provided such treatment is legal in the State where performed. All other services furnished or ordered by chiropractors are not covered. If a chiropractor orders, takes, or interprets an x-ray or other diagnostic procedure to demonstrate a subluxation of the spine, the x-ray can be used for documentation. However, there is no coverage or payment for these services or for any other diagnostic or therapeutic service ordered or furnished by the chiropractor. For detailed information on using x-rays to determine subluxation, see Sec.240.1.2. In addition, in performing manual manipulation of the spine, some chiropractors use manual devices that are hand-held with the thrust of the force of the device being controlled manually. While such manual manipulation may be covered, there is no separate payment permitted for use of this device.

A. Uniform Minimum Standards

Prior to July 1, 1974

Chiropractors licensed or authorized to practice prior to July 1, 1974, and those individuals who commenced their studies in a chiropractic college before that date must meet all of the following three minimum standards to render payable services under the program:

- Preliminary education equal to the requirements for graduation from an accredited high school or other secondary school;

- Graduation from a college of chiropractic approved by the State's chiropractic examiners that included the completion of a course of study covering a period of not less than 3 school years of 6 months each year in actual continuous attendance covering adequate course of study in the subjects of anatomy, physiology, symptomatology and diagnosis, hygiene and sanitation, chemistry, histology, pathology, and principles and practice of chiropractic, including clinical instruction in vertebral palpation, nerve tracing, and adjusting; and

- Passage of an examination prescribed by the State's chiropractic examiners covering the subjects listed above.

After June 30, 1974

Individuals commencing their studies in a chiropractic college after June 30, 1974, must meet all of the above three standards and all of the following additional requirements:

- Satisfactory completion of 2 years of pre-chiropractic study at the college level;

- Satisfactory completion of a 4-year course of 8 months each year (instead of a 3-year course of 6 months each year) at a college or school of chiropractic that includes not less than 4,000 hours in the scientific and chiropractic courses specified in the second bullet under "Prior to July 1, 1974" above, plus courses in the use and effect of x-ray and chiropractic analysis; and

- The practitioner must be over 21 years of age.

B. Maintenance Therapy

Under the Medicare program, Chiropractic maintenance therapy is not considered to be medically reasonable or necessary, and is therefore not payable. Maintenance therapy is defined as a treatment plan that seeks to prevent disease, promote health, and prolong and enhance the quality of life; or therapy that is performed to maintain or prevent deterioration of a chronic condition. When further clinical improvement cannot reasonably be expected from continuous ongoing care, and the chiropractic treatment becomes supportive rather than corrective in nature, the treatment is then considered maintenance therapy. For information on how to indicate on a claim a treatment is or is not maintenance, see Sec.240.1.3.

100-02, 15, 50.4.4.2

Immunizations

(Rev. 202, Issued: 12-31-14, Effective: 09-19-14, Imp: 02-02-15)

Vaccinations or inoculations are excluded as immunizations unless they are directly related to the treatment of an injury or direct exposure to a disease or condition, such as anti-rabies treatment, tetanus antitoxin or booster vaccine, botulin antitoxin, antivenin sera, or immune globulin. In the absence of injury or direct exposure, preventive immunization (vaccination or inoculation) against such diseases as smallpox, polio, diphtheria, etc., is not covered. However, pneumococcal, hepatitis B, and influenza virus vaccines are exceptions to this rule. (See items A, B, and C below.) In cases where a vaccination or inoculation is excluded from coverage, related charges are also not covered.

A. Pneumococcal Pneumonia Vaccinations

1. Background and History of Coverage:

   Section 1861(s)(10)(A) of the Social Security Act and regulations at 42 CFR 410.57 authorize Medicare coverage under Part B for pneumococcal vaccine and its administration.

   For services furnished on or after May 1, 1981 through September 18, 2014, the Medicare Part B program covered pneumococcal pneumonia vaccine and its administration when furnished in compliance with any applicable State law by any provider of services or any entity or individual with a supplier number. Coverage included an initial vaccine administered only to persons at high risk of serious pneumococcal disease (including all people 65 and older; immunocompetent adults at increased risk of pneumococcal disease or its complications because of chronic illness; and individuals with compromised immune systems), with revaccination administered only to persons at highest risk of serious pneumococcal infection and those likely to have a rapid decline in pneumococcal antibody levels, provided that at least 5 years had passed since the previous dose of pneumococcal vaccine.

   Those administering the vaccine did not require the patient to present an immunization record prior to administering the pneumococcal vaccine, nor were they compelled to review the patient's complete medical record if it was not available, relying on the patient's verbal history to determine prior vaccination status.

   Effective July 1, 2000, Medicare no longer required for coverage purposes that a doctor of medicine or osteopathy order the vaccine. Therefore, a beneficiary could receive the vaccine upon request without a physician's order and without physician supervision.

2. Coverage Requirements:

   Effective for claims with dates of service on and after September 19, 2014, an initial pneumococcal vaccine may be administered to all Medicare beneficiaries who have never received a pneumococcal vaccination under Medicare Part B. A different, second pneumococcal vaccine may be administered 1 year after the first vaccine was administered (i.e., 11 full months have passed following the month in which the last pneumococcal vaccine was administered).

   Those administering the vaccine should not require the patient to present an immunization record prior to administering the pneumococcal vaccine, nor should they feel compelled to review the patient's complete medical record if it is

not available. Instead, provided that the patient is competent, it is acceptable to rely on the patient's verbal history to determine prior vaccination status.

Medicare does not require for coverage purposes that a doctor of medicine or osteopathy order the vaccine. Therefore, the beneficiary may receive the vaccine upon request without a physician's order and without physician supervision.

B. Hepatitis B Vaccine

Effective for services furnished on or after September 1, 1984, P.L. 98-369 provides coverage under Part B for hepatitis B vaccine and its administration, furnished to a Medicare beneficiary who is at high or intermediate risk of contracting hepatitis B. High-risk groups currently identified include (see exception below):

- ESRD patients;

- Hemophiliacs who receive Factor VIII or IX concentrates;

- Clients of institutions for the mentally retarded;

- Persons who live in the same household as a Hepatitis B Virus (HBV) carrier;

- Homosexual men;

- Illicit injectable drug abusers; and

- Persons diagnosed with diabetes mellitus.

Intermediate risk groups currently identified include:

- Staff in institutions for the mentally retarded; and

- Workers in health care professions who have frequent contact with blood or blood-derived body fluids during routine work.

EXCEPTION: Persons in both of the above-listed groups in paragraph B, would not be considered at high or intermediate risk of contracting hepatitis B, however, if there were laboratory evidence positive for antibodies to hepatitis B. (ESRD patients are routinely tested for hepatitis B antibodies as part of their continuing monitoring and therapy.)

For Medicare program purposes, the vaccine may be administered upon the order of a doctor of medicine or osteopathy, by a doctor of medicine or osteopathy, or by home health agencies, skilled nursing facilities, ESRD facilities, hospital outpatient departments, and persons recognized under the incident to physicians' services provision of law.

A charge separate from the ESRD composite rate will be recognized and paid for administration of the vaccine to ESRD patients.

C. Influenza Virus Vaccine

Effective for services furnished on or after May 1, 1993, the Medicare Part B program covers influenza virus vaccine and its administration when furnished in compliance with any applicable State law by any provider of services or any entity or individual with a supplier number. Typically, these vaccines are administered once a flu season. Medicare does not require, for coverage purposes, that a doctor of medicine or osteopathy order the vaccine. Therefore, the beneficiary may receive the vaccine upon request without a physician's order and without physician supervision.

100-02, 15, 80.1

Clinical Laboratory Services

(Rev. 80; Issued: 11-11-08; Effective: 01-01-03; Implementation: 11-19-07)

Section 1833 and 1861 of the Act provides for payment of clinical laboratory services under Medicare Part B. Clinical laboratory services involve the biological, microbiological, serological, chemical, immunohematological, hematological, biophysical, cytological, pathological, or other examination of materials derived from the human body for the diagnosis, prevention, or treatment of a disease or assessment of a medical condition. Laboratory services must meet all applicable requirements of the Clinical Laboratory Improvement Amendments of 1988 (CLIA), as set forth at 42 CFR part 493. Section 1862(a)(1)(A) of the Act provides that Medicare payment may not be made for services that are not reasonable and necessary. Clinical laboratory services must be ordered and used promptly by the physician who is treating the beneficiary as described in 42 CFR 410.32(a), or by a qualified nonphysician practitioner, as described in 42 CFR 410.32(a)(3).

See section 80.6 of this manual for related physician ordering instructions.

See the Medicare Claims Processing Manual Chapter 16 for related claims processing instructions.

100-02, 15, 80.2

Psychological Tests and Neuropsychological Tests

(Rev. 85, Issued: 02-29-08, Effective: 01-01-06, Implementation: 12-28-06)

Medicare Part B coverage of psychological tests and neuropsychological tests is authorized under section 1861(s)(3) of the Social Security Act. Payment for psychological and neuropsychological tests is authorized under section 1842(b)(2)(A) of the Social Security Act. The payment amounts for the new psychological and neuropsychological tests (CPT codes 96102, 96103, 96119 and 96120) that are effective January 1, 2006, and are billed for tests administered by a technician or a computer reflect a site of service payment differential for the facility and non-facility settings.

Additionally, there is no authorization for payment for diagnostic tests when performed on an "incident to" basis.

Under the diagnostic tests provision, all diagnostic tests are assigned a certain level of supervision. Generally, regulations governing the diagnostic tests provision require that only physicians can provide the assigned level of supervision for diagnostic tests.

However, there is a regulatory exception to the supervision requirement for diagnostic psychological and neuropsychological tests in terms of who can provide the supervision.

That is, regulations allow a clinical psychologist (CP) or a physician to perform the general supervision assigned to diagnostic psychological and neuropsychological tests.

In addition, nonphysician practitioners such as nurse practitioners (NPs), clinical nurse specialists (CNSs) and physician assistants (PAs) who personally perform diagnostic psychological and neuropsychological tests are excluded from having to perform these tests under the general supervision of a physician or a CP. Rather, NPs and CNSs must perform such tests under the requirements of their respective benefit instead of the requirements for diagnostic psychological and neuropsychological tests. Accordingly, NPs and CNSs must perform tests in collaboration (as defined under Medicare law at section 1861(aa)(6) of the Act) with a physician. PAs perform tests under the general supervision of a physician as required for services furnished under the PA benefit.

Furthermore, physical therapists (PTs), occupational therapists (OTs) and speech language pathologists (SLPs) are authorized to bill three test codes as "sometimes therapy" codes. Specifically, CPT codes 96105, 96110 and 96111 may be performed by these therapists. However, when PTs, OTs and SLPs perform these three tests, they must be performed under the general supervision of a physician or a CP.

Who May Bill for Diagnostic Psychological and Neuropsychological Tests CPs - see qualifications under chapter 15, section 160 of the Benefits Policy Manual, Pub. 100-2.

- NPs -to the extent authorized under State scope of practice. See qualifications under chapter 15, section 200 of the Benefits Policy Manual, Pub. 100-2.

- CNSs -to the extent authorized under State scope of practice. See qualifications under chapter 15, section 210 of the Benefits Policy Manual, Pub. 100-2.

- PAs - to the extent authorized under State scope of practice. See qualifications under chapter 15, section 190 of the Benefits Policy Manual, Pub. 100-2.

- Independently Practicing Psychologists (IPPs) PTs, OTs and SLPs - see qualifications under chapter 15, sections 220-230.6 of the Benefits Policy Manual, Pub. 100-2.

Psychological and neuropsychological tests performed by a psychologist (who is not a CP) practicing independently of an institution, agency, or physician's office are covered when a physician orders such tests. An IPP is any psychologist who is licensed or certified to practice psychology in the State or jurisdiction where furnishing services or, if the jurisdiction does not issue licenses, if provided by any practicing psychologist. (It is CMS' understanding that all States, the District of Columbia, and Puerto Rico license psychologists, but that some trust territories do not. Examples of psychologists, other than CPs, whose psychological and neuropsychological tests are covered under the diagnostic tests provision include, but are not limited to, educational psychologists and counseling psychologists.)

The carrier must secure from the appropriate State agency a current listing of psychologists holding the required credentials to determine whether the tests of a particular IPP are covered under Part B in States that have statutory licensure or certification. In States or territories that lack statutory licensing or certification, the carrier checks individual qualifications before provider numbers are issued. Possible reference sources are the national directory of membership of the American Psychological Association, which provides data about the educational background of individuals and indicates which members are board-certified, the records and directories of the State or territorial psychological association, and the National Register of Health Service Providers. If qualification is dependent on a doctoral degree from a currently accredited program, the carrier verifies the date of accreditation of the school involved, since such accreditation is not retroactive. If the listed reference sources do not provide enough information (e.g., the psychologist is not a member of one of these sources), the carrier contacts the psychologist personally for the required information. Generally, carriers maintain a continuing list of psychologists whose qualifications have been verified.

NOTE: When diagnostic psychological tests are performed by a psychologist who is not practicing independently, but is on the staff of an institution, agency, or clinic, that entity bills for the psychological tests.

The carrier considers psychologists as practicing independently when:

- They render services on their own responsibility, free of the administrative and professional control of an employer such as a physician, institution or agency;

- The persons they treat are their own patients; and

- They have the right to bill directly, collect and retain the fee for their services.

A psychologist practicing in an office located in an institution may be considered an independently practicing psychologist when both of the following conditions exist:

- The office is confined to a separately-identified part of the facility which is used solely as the psychologist's office and cannot be construed as extending throughout the entire institution; and

- The psychologist conducts a private practice, i.e., services are rendered to patients from outside the institution as well as to institutional patients.

Payment for Diagnostic Psychological and Neuropsychological Tests

Expenses for diagnostic psychological and neuropsychological tests are not subject to the outpatient mental health treatment limitation, that is, the payment limitation on treatment services for mental, psychoneurotic and personality disorders as authorized under Section 1833(c) of the Act. The payment amount for the new psychological and neuropsychological tests (CPT codes 96102, 96103, 96119 and 96120) that are billed for tests performed by a technician or a computer reflect a site of service payment differential for the facility and non-facility settings. CPs, NPs, CNSs and PAs are required by law to accept assigned payment for psychological and neuropsychological tests. However, while IPPs are not required by law to accept assigned payment for these tests, they must report the name and address of the physician who ordered the test on the claim form when billing for tests.

CPT Codes for Diagnostic Psychological and Neuropsychological Tests

The range of CPT codes used to report psychological and neuropsychological tests is 96101-96120. CPT codes 96101, 96102, 96103, 96105, 96110, and 96111 are appropriate for use when billing for psychological tests. CPT codes 96116, 96118, 96119 and 96120 are appropriate for use when billing for neuropsychological tests.

All of the tests under this CPT code range 96101-96120 are indicated as active codes under the physician fee schedule database and are covered if medically necessary.

Payment and Billing Guidelines for Psychological and Neuropsychological Tests

The technician and computer CPT codes for psychological and neuropsychological tests include practice expense, malpractice expense and professional work relative value units.

Accordingly, CPT psychological test code 96101 should not be paid when billed for the same tests or services performed under psychological test codes 96102 or 96103. CPT neuropsychological test code 96118 should not be paid when billed for the same tests or services performed under neuropsychological test codes 96119 or 96120. However, CPT codes 96101 and 96118 can be paid separately on the rare occasion when billed on the same date of service for different and separate tests from 96102, 96103, 96119 and 96120.

Under the physician fee schedule, there is no payment for services performed by students or trainees. Accordingly, Medicare does not pay for services represented by CPT codes 96102 and 96119 when performed by a student or a trainee. However, the presence of a student or a trainee while the test is being administered does not prevent a physician, CP, IPP, NP, CNS or PA from performing and being paid for the psychological test under 96102 or the neuropsychological test under 96119.

100-02, 15, 80.5.5

Frequency Standards

(Rev.70, Issued: 05-11-07, Effective: 01-01-07, Implementation: 07-02-07)

Medicare pays for a screening BMM once every 2 years (at least 23 months have passed since the month the last covered BMM was performed).

When medically necessary, Medicare may pay for more frequent BMMs. Examples include, but are not limited to, the following medical circumstances:

- Monitoring beneficiaries on long-term glucocorticoid (steroid) therapy of more than 3 months.

- Confirming baseline BMMs to permit monitoring of beneficiaries in the future.

100-02, 15, 150.1

Treatment of Temporomandibular Joint (TMJ) Syndrome

(Rev. 1, 10-01-03)

There are a wide variety of conditions that can be characterized as TMJ, and an equally wide variety of methods for treating these conditions. Many of the procedures fall within the Medicare program's statutory exclusion that prohibits payment for items and services that have not been demonstrated to be reasonable and necessary for the diagnosis and treatment of illness or injury (§1862(a)(1) of the Act). Other services and appliances used to treat TMJ fall within the Medicare program's statutory exclusion at 1862(a)(12), which prohibits payment "for services in connection with the care, treatment, filling, removal, or replacement of teeth or structures directly supporting teeth...." For these reasons, a diagnosis of TMJ on a claim is insufficient. The actual condition or symptom must be determined.

100-02, 15, 160

Clinical Psychologist Services

(Rev. 51, Issued: 06-23-06, Effective: 01-01-05, Implementation: 09-21-06)

A. Clinical Psychologist (CP) Defined

To qualify as a clinical psychologist (CP), a practitioner must meet the following requirements: Hold a doctoral degree in psychology; Be licensed or certified, on the basis of the doctoral degree in psychology, by the State in which he or she practices, at the independent practice level of psychology to furnish diagnostic, assessment, preventive, and therapeutic services directly to individuals.

B. Qualified Clinical Psychologist Services Defined

Effective July 1, 1990, the diagnostic and therapeutic services of CPs and services and supplies furnished incident to such services are covered as the services furnished by a physician or as incident to physician's services are covered. However, the CP must be legally authorized to perform the services under applicable licensure laws of the State in which they are furnished.

C. Types of Clinical Psychologist Services

That May Be Covered Diagnostic and therapeutic services that the CP is legally authorized to perform in accordance with State law and/or regulation. Carriers pay all qualified CPs based on the physician fee schedule for the diagnostic and therapeutic services. (Psychological tests by practitioners who do not meet the requirements for a CP may be covered under the provisions for diagnostic tests as described in Sec. 80.2.

Services and supplies furnished incident to a CP's services are covered if the requirements that apply to services incident to a physician's services, as described in Sec.60 are met. These services must be:

- Mental health services that are commonly furnished in CPs' offices;

- An integral, although incidental, part of professional services performed by the CP;

- Performed under the direct personal supervision of the CP; i.e., the CP must be physically present and immediately available;

- Furnished without charge or included in the CP's bill; and

- Performed by an employee of the CP (or an employee of the legal entity that employs the supervising CP) under the common law control test of the Act, as set forth in 20 CFR 404.1007 and Sec.RS 2101.020 of the Retirement and Survivors Insurance part of the Social Security Program Operations Manual System.

- Diagnostic psychological testing services when furnished under the general supervision of a CP.

Carriers are required to familiarize themselves with appropriate State laws and/or regulations governing a CP's scope of practice.

D. Noncovered Services

The services of CPs are not covered if the service is otherwise excluded from Medicare coverage even though a clinical psychologist is authorized by State law to perform them.

For example, Sec.1862(a)(1)(A) of the Act excludes from coverage services that are not "reasonable and necessary for the diagnosis or treatment of an illness or injury or to improve the functioning of a malformed body member." Therefore, even though the services are authorized by State law, the services of a CP that are determined to be not reasonable and necessary are not covered. Additionally, any therapeutic services that are billed by CPs under CPT psychotherapy codes that include medical evaluation and management services are not covered.

E. Requirement for Consultation

When applying for a Medicare provider number, a CP must submit to the carrier a signed Medicare provider/supplier enrollment form that indicates an agreement to the effect that, contingent upon the patient's consent, the CP will attempt to consult with the patient's attending or primary care physician in accordance with accepted professional ethical norms, taking into consideration patient confidentiality.

If the patient assents to the consultation, the CP must attempt to consult with the patient's physician within a reasonable time after receiving the consent. If the CP's attempts to consult directly with the physician are not successful, the CP must notify the physician within a reasonable time that he or she is furnishing services to the patient. Additionally, the CP must document, in the patient's medical record, the date the patient consented or declined consent to consultations, the date of consultation, or, if attempts to consult did not succeed, that date and manner of notification to the physician.

The only exception to the consultation requirement for CPs is in cases where the patient's primary care or attending physician refers the patient to the CP. Also, neither a CP nor a primary care nor attending physician may bill Medicare or the patient for this required consultation.

F. Outpatient Mental Health Services Limitation

All covered therapeutic services furnished by qualified CPs are subject to the outpatient mental health services limitation in Pub 100-1, Medicare General Information, Eligibility, and Entitlement Manual, Chapter 3, "Deductibles, Coinsurance Amounts, and Payment Limitations," Sec.30, (i.e., only 62 1/2 percent of expenses for these services are considered incurred expenses for Medicare purposes). The limitation does not apply to diagnostic services.

G. Assignment Requirement Assignment iSec. required.

100-02, 15, 170

Clinical Social Worker (CSW) Services

(Rev. 1, 10-01-03) B3-2152

See the Medicare Claims Processing Manual Chapter 12, Physician/Nonphysician Practitioners, §150, "Clinical Social Worker Services," for payment requirements.

A. Clinical Social Worker Defined

Section 1861(hh) of the Act defines a "clinical social worker" as an individual who:

- Possesses a master's or doctor's degree in social work;

- Has performed at least two years of supervised clinical social work; and

- Is licensed or certified as a clinical social worker by the State in which the services are performed; or

- In the case of an individual in a State that does not provide for licensure or certification, has completed at least 2 years or 3,000 hours of post master's degree supervised clinical social work practice under the supervision of a master's level social worker in an appropriate setting such as a hospital, SNF, or clinic.

B. Clinical Social Worker Services Defined

Section 1861(hh)(2) of the Act defines "clinical social worker services" as those services that the CSW is legally authorized to perform under State law (or the State regulatory mechanism provided by State law) of the State in which such services are performed for the diagnosis and treatment of mental illnesses. Services furnished to an inpatient of a hospital or an inpatient of a SNF that the SNF is required to provide as a requirement for participation are not included. The services that are covered are those that are otherwise covered if furnished by a physician or as incident to a physician's professional service.

C. Covered Services

Coverage is limited to the services a CSW is legally authorized to perform in accordance with State law (or State regulatory mechanism established by State law). The services of a CSW may be covered under Part B if they are:

- The type of services that are otherwise covered if furnished by a physician, or as incident to a physician's service. (See §30 for a description of physicians' services and §70 of Pub 100-1, the Medicare General Information, Eligibility, and Entitlement Manual, Chapter 5, for the definition of a physician.);

- Performed by a person who meets the definition of a CSW (See subsection A.); and

- Not otherwise excluded from coverage. Carriers should become familiar with the State law or regulatory mechanism governing a CSW's scope of practice in their service area.

D. Noncovered Services

Services of a CSW are not covered when furnished to inpatients of a hospital or to inpatients of a SNF if the services furnished in the SNF are those that the SNF is required to furnish as a condition of participation in Medicare. In addition, CSW services are not covered if they are otherwise excluded from Medicare coverage even though a CSW is authorized by State law to perform them. For example, the Medicare law excludes from coverage services that are not "reasonable and necessary for the diagnosis or treatment of an illness or injury or to improve the functioning of a malformed body member."

E. Outpatient Mental Health Services Limitation

All covered therapeutic services furnished by qualified CSWs are subject to the outpatient psychiatric services limitation in Pub 100-1, Medicare General Information, Eligibility, and Entitlement Manual, Chapter 3, "Deductibles, Coinsurance Amounts, and Payment Limitations," §30, (i.e., only 62 1/2 percent of expenses for these services are considered incurred expenses for Medicare purposes). The limitation does not apply to diagnostic services.

F. Assignment Requirement

Assignment is required.

100-02, 15, 180

Nurse-Midwife (CNM) Services

(Rev. 1, 10-01-03) B3-2154

A. General

Effective on or after July 1, 1988, the services provided by a certified nurse-midwife or incident to the certified nurse-midwife's services are covered. Payment is made under assignment only. See the Medicare Claims Processing Manual, Chapter 12, "Physician and Nonphysician Practitioners," §130, for payment methodology for nurse midwife services.

B. Certified Nurse-Midwife Defined

A certified nurse-midwife is a registered nurse who has successfully completed a program of study and clinical experience in nurse-midwifery, meeting guidelines prescribed by the Secretary, or who has been certified by an organization recognized by the Secretary. The Secretary has recognized certification by the American College of Nurse-Midwives and State qualifying requirements in those States that specify a program of education and clinical experience for nurse-midwives for these purposes. A nurse-midwife must:

- Be currently licensed to practice in the State as a registered professional nurse; and

- Meet one of the following requirements:

  1. Be legally authorized under State law or regulations to practice as a nurse-midwife and have completed a program of study and clinical experience for nurse-midwives, as specified by the State; or

  2. If the State does not specify a program of study and clinical experience that nurse-midwives must complete to practice in that State, the nurse-midwife must:

     a. Be currently certified as a nurse-midwife by the American College of Nurse-Midwives;

     b. Have satisfactorily completed a formal education program (of at least one academic year) that, upon completion, qualifies the nurse to take the certification examination offered by the American College of Nurse-Midwives; or

c. Have successfully completed a formal education program for preparing registered nurses to furnish gynecological and obstetrical care to women during pregnancy, delivery, and the postpartum period, and care to normal newborns, and have practiced as a nurse-midwife for a total of 12 months during any 18-month period from August 8, 1976, to July 16, 1982.

C. Covered Services

1. General - Effective January 1, 1988, through December 31, 1993, the coverage of nurse-midwife services was restricted to the maternity cycle. The maternity cycle is a period that includes pregnancy, labor, and the immediate postpartum period.

   Beginning with services furnished on or after January 1, 1994, coverage is no longer limited to the maternity cycle. Coverage is available for services furnished by a nurse-midwife that he or she is legally authorized to perform in the State in which the services are furnished and that would otherwise be covered if furnished by a physician, including obstetrical and gynecological services.

2. Incident To- Services and supplies furnished incident to a nurse midwife's service are covered if they would have been covered when furnished incident to the services of a doctor of medicine or osteopathy, as described in §60.

D. Noncovered Services

The services of nurse-midwives are not covered if they are otherwise excluded from Medicare coverage even though a nurse-midwife is authorized by State law to perform them. For example, the Medicare program excludes from coverage routine physical checkups and services that are not reasonable and necessary for the diagnosis or treatment of an illness or injury or to improve the functioning of a malformed body member. Coverage of service to the newborn continues only to the point that the newborn is or would normally be treated medically as a separate individual. Items and services furnished the newborn from that point are not covered on the basis of the mother's eligibility.

E. Relationship With Physician

Most States have licensure and other requirements applicable to nurse-midwives. For example, some require that the nurse-midwife have an arrangement with a physician for the referral of the patient in the event a problem develops that requires medical attention. Others may require that the nurse-midwife function under the general supervision of a physician. Although these and similar State requirements must be met in order for the nurse-midwife to provide Medicare covered care, they have no effect on the nurse-midwife's right to personally bill for and receive direct Medicare payment. That is, billing does not have to flow through a physician or facility. See §60.2 for coverage of services performed by nurse-midwives incident to the service of physicians.

F. Place of Service

There is no restriction on place of service. Therefore, nurse-midwife services are covered if provided in the nurse-midwife's office, in the patient's home, or in a hospital or other facility, such as a clinic or birthing center owned or operated by a nurse-midwife.

G. Assignment Requirement

Assignment is required.

100-02, 15, 220

Coverage of Outpatient Rehabilitation Therapy Services (Physical Therapy, Occupational Therapy, and Speech-Language Pathology Services) Under Medical Insurance

(Rev. 194, Issued: 09-03-14, Effective: Upon Implementation of ICD-10)

A comprehensive knowledge of the policies that apply to therapy services cannot be obtained through manuals alone. The most definitive policies are Local Coverage Determinations found at the Medicare Coverage Database www.cms.hhs.gov/mcd. A list of Medicare contractors is found at the CMS Web site. Specific questions about all Medicare policies should be addressed to the contractors through the contact information supplied on their Web sites. General Medicare questions may be addressed to the Medicare regional offices http://www.cms.hhs.gov/RegionalOffices/.

A. Definitions

The following defines terms used in this section and §230:

ACTIVE PARTICIPATION of the clinician in treatment means that the clinician personally furnishes in its entirety at least 1 billable service on at least 1 day of treatment.

ASSESSMENT is separate from evaluation, and is included in services or procedures, (it is not separately payable). The term assessment as used in Medicare manuals related to therapy services is distinguished from language in Current Procedural Terminology (CPT) codes that specify assessment, e.g., 97755, Assistive Technology Assessment, which may be payable). Assessments shall be provided only by clinicians, because assessment requires professional skill to gather data by observation and patient inquiry and may include limited objective testing and measurement to make clinical judgments regarding the patient's condition(s). Assessment determines, e.g., changes in the patient's status since the last visit/treatment day and whether the planned procedure or service should be modified. Based on these assessment data, the professional may make judgments about progress toward goals and/or determine that a more complete evaluation or re-evaluation (see definitions below) is indicated. Routine weekly assessments of expected progression in accordance with the plan are not payable as re-evaluations.

CERTIFICATION is the physician's/nonphysician practitioner's (NPP) approval of the plan of care. Certification requires a dated signature on the plan of care or some other document that indicates approval of the plan of care.

The CLINICIAN is a term used in this manual and in Pub 100-4, chapter 5, section 10 or section 20, to refer to only a physician, nonphysician practitioner or a therapist (but not to an assistant, aide or any other personnel) providing a service within their scope of practice and consistent with state and local law. Clinicians make clinical judgments and are responsible for all services they are permitted to supervise. Services that require the skills of a therapist, may be appropriately furnished by clinicians, that is, by or under the supervision of qualified physicians/NPPs when their scope of practice, state and local laws allow it and their personal professional training is judged by Medicare contractors as sufficient to provide to the beneficiary skills equivalent to a therapist for that service.

COMPLEXITIES are complicating factors that may influence treatment, e.g., they may influence the type, frequency, intensity and/or duration of treatment. Complexities may be represented by diagnoses (ICD codes), by patient factors such as age, severity, acuity, multiple conditions, and motivation, or by the patient's social circumstances such as the support of a significant other or the availability of transportation to therapy.

A DATE may be in any form (written, stamped or electronic). The date may be added to the record in any manner and at any time, as long as the dates are accurate. If they are different, refer to both the date a service was performed and the date the entry to the record was made. For example, if a physician certifies a plan and fails to date it, staff may add "Received Date" in writing or with a stamp. The received date is valid for certification/re-certification purposes. Also, if the physician faxes the referral, certification, or re-certification and forgets to date it, the date that prints out on the fax is valid. If services provided on one date are documented on another date, both dates should be documented.

The EPISODE of Outpatient Therapy – For the purposes of therapy policy, an outpatient therapy episode is defined as the period of time, in calendar days, from the first day the patient is under the care of the clinician (e.g., for evaluation or treatment) for the current condition(s) being treated by one therapy discipline (PT, or OT, or SLP) until the last date of service for that discipline in that setting.

During the episode, the beneficiary may be treated for more than one condition; including conditions with an onset after the episode has begun. For example, a beneficiary receiving PT for a hip fracture who, after the initial treatment session, develops low back pain would also be treated under a PT plan of care for rehabilitation of low back pain. That plan may be modified from the initial plan, or it may be a separate plan specific to the low back pain, but treatment for both conditions concurrently would be considered the same episode of PT treatment. If that same patient developed a swallowing problem during intubation for the hip surgery, the first day of treatment by the SLP would be a new episode of SLP care.

EVALUATION is a separately payable comprehensive service provided by a clinician, as defined above, that requires professional skills to make clinical judgments about conditions for which services are indicated based on objective measurements and subjective evaluations of patient performance and functional abilities. Evaluation is warranted e.g., for a new diagnosis or when a condition is treated in a new setting. These evaluative judgments are essential to development of the plan of care, including goals and the selection of interventions.

FUNCTIONAL REPORTING, which is required on claims for all outpatient therapy services pursuant to 42CFR410.59, 410.60, and 410.62, uses nonpayable G-codes and related modifiers to convey information about the patient's functional status at specified points during therapy. (See Pub 100-4, chapter 5, section 10.6)

RE-EVALUATION provides additional objective information not included in other documentation. Re-evaluation is separately payable and is periodically indicated during an episode of care when the professional assessment of a clinician indicates a significant improvement, or decline, or change in the patient's condition or functional status that was not anticipated in the plan of care. Although some state regulations and state practice acts require re-evaluation at specific times, for Medicare payment, reevaluations must also meet Medicare coverage guidelines. The decision to provide a reevaluation shall be made by a clinician.

INTERVAL of certified treatment (certification interval) consists of 90 calendar days or less, based on an individual's needs. A physician/NPP may certify a plan of care for an interval length that is less than 90 days. There may be more than one certification interval in an episode of care. The certification interval is not the same as a Progress Report period.

MAINTENANCE PROGRAM (MP) means a program established by a therapist that consists of activities and/or mechanisms that will assist a beneficiary in maximizing or maintaining the progress he or she has made during therapy or to prevent or slow further deterioration due to a disease or illness.

NONPHYSICIAN PRACTITIONERS (NPP) means physician assistants, clinical nurse specialists, and nurse practitioners, who may, if state and local laws permit it, and when appropriate rules are followed, provide, certify or supervise therapy services.

PHYSICIAN with respect to outpatient rehabilitation therapy services means a doctor of medicine, osteopathy (including an osteopathic practitioner), podiatric medicine, or optometry (for low vision rehabilitation only). Chiropractors and doctors of dental surgery or dental medicine are not considered physicians for therapy services and may neither refer patients for rehabilitation therapy services nor establish therapy plans of care.

PATIENT, client, resident, and beneficiary are terms used interchangeably to indicate enrolled recipients of Medicare covered services.

PROVIDERS of services are defined in §1861(u) of the Act, 42CFR400.202 and 42CFR485 Subpart H as participating hospitals, critical access hospitals (CAH), skilled nursing facilities (SNF), comprehensive outpatient rehabilitation facilities (CORF), home health agencies (HHA), hospices, participating clinics, rehabilitation agencies or outpatient rehabilitation facilities (ORF). Providers are also defined as public health agencies with agreements only to furnish outpatient therapy services, or community mental health centers with agreements only to furnish partial hospitalization services. To qualify as providers of services, these providers must meet certain conditions enumerated in the law and enter into an agreement with the Secretary in which they agree not to charge any beneficiary for covered services for which the program will pay and to refund any erroneous collections made. Note that the word PROVIDER in sections 220 and 230 is not used to mean a person who provides a service, but is used as in the statute to mean a facility or agency such as rehabilitation agency or home health agency.

QUALIFIED PROFESSIONAL means a physical therapist, occupational therapist, speech-language pathologist, physician, nurse practitioner, clinical nurse specialist, or physician's assistant, who is licensed or certified by the state to furnish therapy services, and who also may appropriately furnish therapy services under Medicare policies. Qualified professional may also include a physical therapist assistant (PTA) or an occupational therapy assistant (OTA), who is working within the state scope of practice in the state in which the services are furnished. Assistants are limited in the services they may furnish (see section 230.1 and 230.2) and may not supervise other therapy caregivers.

QUALIFIED PERSONNEL means staff (auxiliary personnel) who have been educated and trained as therapists and qualify to furnish therapy services only under direct supervision incident to a physician or NPP. See §230.5 of this chapter. Qualified personnel may or may not be licensed as therapists but meet all of the requirements for therapists with the exception of licensure.

SIGNATURE means a legible identifier of any type acceptable according to policies in Pub. 100-08, Medicare Program Integrity Manual, chapter 3, §3.3.2.4 concerning signatures.

SUPERVISION LEVELS for outpatient rehabilitation therapy services are the same as those for diagnostic tests defined in 42CFR410.32. Depending on the setting, the levels include personal supervision (in the room), direct supervision (in the office suite), and general supervision (physician/NPP is available but not necessarily on the premises).

SUPPLIERS of therapy services include individual practitioners such as physicians, NPPs, physical therapists and occupational therapists who have Medicare provider numbers. Regulatory references on physical therapists in private practice (PTPPs) and occupational therapists in private practice (OTPPs) are at 42CFR410.60 (C)(1), 485.701-729, and 486.150-163.

THERAPIST refers only to qualified physical therapists, occupational therapists and speech-language pathologists, as defined in §230. Qualifications that define therapists are in §§230.1, 230.2, and 230.3. Skills of a therapist are defined by the scope of practice for therapists in the state.

THERAPY (or outpatient rehabilitation services) includes only outpatient physical therapy (PT), occupational therapy (OT) and speech-language pathology (SLP) services paid using the Medicare Physician Fee Schedule or the same services when provided in hospitals that are exempt from the hospital Outpatient Prospective Payment System and paid on a reasonable cost basis, including critical access hospitals.

Therapy services referred to in this chapter are those skilled services furnished according to the standards and conditions in CMS manuals, (e.g., in this chapter and in Pub. 100-4, Medicare Claims Processing Manual, chapter 5), within their scope of practice by qualified professionals or qualified personnel, as defined in this section, represented by procedures found in the American Medical Association's "Current Procedural Terminology (CPT)." A list of CPT (HCPCS) codes is provided in Pub. 100-4, chapter 5, §20, and in Local Coverage Determinations developed by contractors.

TREATMENT DAY means a single calendar day on which treatment, evaluation and/or reevaluation is provided. There could be multiple visits, treatment sessions/encounters on a treatment day.

VISITS OR TREATMENT SESSIONS begin at the time the patient enters the treatment area (of a building, office, or clinic) and continue until all services (e.g., activities, procedures, services) have been completed for that session and the patient leaves that area to participate in a non-therapy activity. It is likely that not all minutes in the visits/treatment sessions are billable (e.g., rest periods). There may be two treatment sessions in a day, for example, in the morning and afternoon. When there are two visits/ treatment sessions in a day, plans of care indicate treatment amount of twice a day.

B. References

Paper Manuals. The following manuals, now outdated, were resources for the Internet Only Manuals:

- Part A Medicare Intermediary Manual, (Pub. 13)
- Part B Medicare Carrier Manual, (Pub. 14)
- Hospital Manual, (Pub. 10)
- Outpatient Physical Therapy/CORF Manual, (Pub. 9)

Regulation and Statute. The information in this section is based in part on the following current references:

- 42CFR refers to Title 42, Code of Federal Regulation (CFR).
- The Act refers to the Social Security Act.

Internet Only Manuals. Current Policies that concern providers and suppliers of therapy services are located in many places throughout CMS Manuals. Sites that may be of interest include:

- Pub.100-1 GENERAL INFORMATION, ELIGIBILITY, AND ENTITLEMENT
  — Chapter 1- General Overview
    – 10.1 - Hospital Insurance (Part A) for Inpatient Hospital, Hospice, Home Health and SNF Services - A Brief Description
    – 10.2 - Home Health Services
    – 10.3 - Supplementary Medical Insurance (Part B) - A Brief Description
    – 20.2 - Discrimination Prohibited
- Pub. 100-2, MEDICARE BENEFIT POLICY MANUAL
  — Ch 6 - Hospital Services Covered Under Part B
    – 10 - Medical and Other Health Services Furnished to Inpatients of Participating Hospitals
    – 20 - Outpatient Hospital Services
    – 20.2 - Outpatient Defined
    – 20.4.1 - Diagnostic Services Defined
    – 70 - Outpatient Hospital Psychiatric Services
  — Ch 8 - Coverage of Extended Care (SNF) Services Under Hospital Insurance
    – 30.4. - Direct Skilled Rehabilitation Services to Patients
    – 40 - Physician Certification and Recertification for Extended Care Services
    – 50.3 - Physical Therapy, Speech-Language Pathology, and Occupational Therapy Furnished by the Skilled Nursing Facility or by Others Under Arrangements with the Facility and Under Its Supervision
    – 70.3 - Inpatient Physical Therapy, Occupational Therapy, and Speech Pathology Services
  — Ch 12 - Comprehensive Outpatient Rehabilitation Facility (CORF) Coverage
    – 10 - Comprehensive Outpatient Rehabilitation Facility (CORF) Services Provided by Medicare
    – 20 - Required and Optional CORF Services
    – 20.1 - Required Services
    – 20.2 - Optional CORF Services
    – 30 - Rules for Provision of Services
    – 30.1 - Rules for Payment of CORF Services
    – 40 - Specific CORF Services
    – 40.1 - Physicians' Services
    – 40.2 - Physical Therapy Services
    – 40.3 - Occupational Therapy Services
    – 40.4 – Speech Language Pathology Services
- Pub. 100-3 MEDICARE NATIONAL COVERAGE DETERMINATIONS MANUAL
  — Part 1
    – 20.10 - Cardiac Rehabilitation Programs
    – 30.1 - Biofeedback Therapy
    – 30.1.1 - Biofeedback Therapy for the Treatment of Urinary Incontinence
    – 50.1 – Speech Generating Devices
    – 50.2 - Electronic Speech Aids
    – 50.4 - Tracheostomy Speaking Valve
  — Part 2
    – 150.2 - Osteogenic Stimulator
    – 160.7 - Electrical Nerve Stimulators
    – 160.12 - Neuromuscular Electrical Stimulation (NMES)
    – 160.13 - Supplies Used in the Delivery of Transcutaneous Electrical Nerve Stimulation (TENS) and Neuromuscular Electrical Stimulation (NMES)
    – 160.17 - L-Dopa

- Part 3
  - 170.1 - Institutional and Home Care Patient Education Programs
  - 170.2 - Melodic Intonation Therapy
  - 170.3 - Speech Pathology Services for the Treatment of Dysphagia
  - 180 – Nutrition
- Part 4
  - 230.8 - Non-implantable Pelvic Flood Electrical Stimulator
  - 240.7 - Postural Drainage Procedures and Pulmonary Exercises
  - 270.1 -Electrical Stimulation (ES) and Electromagnetic Therapy for the Treatment of Wounds
  - 270.4 - Treatment of Decubitus Ulcers
  - 280.3 - Mobility Assisted Equipment (MAE)
  - 280.4 - Seat Lift
  - 280.13 - Transcutaneous Electrical Nerve Stimulators (TENS)
  - 290.1 - Home Health Visits to A Blind Diabetic
- Pub. 100-08 PROGRAM INTEGRITY MANUAL
  - Chapter 3 - Verifying Potential Errors and Taking Corrective Actions
    - 3.4.1.1 - Linking LCD and NCD ID Numbers to Edits
  - Chapter 13 - Local Coverage Determinations
    - 13.5.1 - Reasonable and Necessary Provisions in LCDs

Specific policies may differ by setting. Other policies concerning therapy services are found in other manuals. When a therapy service policy is specific to a setting, it takes precedence over these general outpatient policies. For special rules on:

- CORFs - See chapter 12 of this manual and also Pub. 100-4, chapter 5;
- SNF - See chapter 8 of this manual and also Pub. 100-4, chapter 6, for SNF claims/billing;
- HHA - See chapter 7 of this manual, and Pub. 100-4, chapter 10;
- GROUP THERAPY AND STUDENTS - See Pub. 100-2, chapter 15, §230;
- ARRANGEMENTS - Pub. 100-1, chapter 5, §10.3;
- COVERAGE is described in the Medicare Program Integrity Manual, Pub. 100-08, chapter 13, §13.5.1; and .
- THERAPY CAPS - See Pub. 100-4, chapter 5, §10.2, for a complete description of this financial limitation.

C. General

Therapy services are a covered benefit in §§1861(g), 1861(p), and 1861(ll) of the Act. Therapy services may also be provided incident to the services of a physician/NPP under §§1861(s)(2) and 1862(a)(20) of the Act.

Covered therapy services are furnished by providers, by others under arrangements with and under the supervision of providers, or furnished by suppliers (e.g., physicians, NPP, enrolled therapists), who meet the requirements in Medicare manuals for therapy services.

Where a prospective payment system (PPS) applies, therapy services are paid when services conform to the requirements of that PPS. Reimbursement for therapy provided to Part A inpatients of hospitals or residents of SNFs in covered stays is included in the respective PPS rates.

Payment for therapy provided by an HHA under a plan of treatment is included in the home health PPS rate. Therapy may be billed by an HHA on bill type 34x if there are no home health services billed under a home health plan of care at the same time (e.g., the patient is not homebound), and there is a valid therapy plan of treatment.

In addition to the requirements described in this chapter, the services must be furnished in accordance with health and safety requirements set forth in regulations at 42CFR484, and 42CFR485.

When therapy services may be furnished appropriately in a community pool by a clinician in a physical therapist or occupational therapist private practice, physician office, outpatient hospital, or outpatient SNF, the practice/office or provider shall rent or lease the pool, or a specific portion of the pool. The use of that part of the pool during specified times shall be restricted to the patients of that practice or provider. The written agreement to rent or lease the pool shall be available for review on request. When part of the pool is rented or leased, the agreement shall describe the part of the pool that is used exclusively by the patients of that practice/office or provider and the times that exclusive use applies. Other providers, including rehabilitation agencies (previously referred to as OPTs and ORFs) and CORFs, are subject to the requirements outlined in the respective State Operations Manual regarding rented or leased community pools.

100-02, 15, 220.4

(Rev.255, Issued: 01-25-19, Effective: 01- 01- 19, Implementation: 02-26-19)

Functional Reporting

NOTE: In the calendar year (CY) 2019 Physician Fee Schedule (PFS) final rule, CMS-1693-F, after consideration of stakeholder comments for burden reduction, a review of all of the requirements under section 3005(g) of Middle Class Tax Relief and Jobs Creation Act of 2012 (MCTRJCA), and in light of the statutory amendments to section 1833(g) of the Act, via section 50202 of Bipartisan Budget Act of 2018 to

repeal the therapy caps, CMS concluded that continued collection of functional reporting data through the same or reduced format would not yield additional information to inform future analyses or to serve as a basis for reforms to the payment system for therapy services. To reduce the burden of reporting for providers of therapy services, the CY 2019 PFS final rule ended the requirements of reporting the functional limitation nonpayable HCPCS G-codes and severity modifiers on claims for therapy services and the associated documentation requirements in medical records, effective for dates of service on and after January 1, 2019. The rule also revised regulation text at 42 CFR 410.59, 410.60, 410.61, 410.62, 410.105, accordingly.

The instructions below apply only to dates of service when the functional reporting requirements were effective, January 1, 2013 through December 31, 2018.

A. Selecting the G-codes to Use in Functional Reporting.

There are 42 functional G-codes, 14 sets of three codes each, for that can be used in identifying the functional limitation being reported. Six of the G-code sets are generally for PT and OT functional limitations and eight sets of G-codes are for SLP functional limitations. (For a list of these codes and descriptors, see Pub. 100-04, Medicare Claims Processing Manual, chapter 5, section 10.6 F.)

Only one functional limitation shall be reported at a time. Consequently, the clinician must select the G-code set for the functional limitation that most closely relates to the primary functional limitation being treated or the one that is the primary reason for treatment. When the beneficiary has more than one functional limitation, the clinician may need to make a determination as to which functional limitation is primary. In these cases, the clinician may choose the functional limitation that is:

The instructions below apply only to dates of service when the functional reporting requirements were effective, January 1, 2013 through December 31, 2018.

A. Selecting the G-codes to Use in Functional Reporting.

There are 42 functional G-codes, 14 sets of three codes each, for that can be used in identifying the functional limitation being reported. Six of the G-code sets are generally for PT and OT functional limitations and eight sets of G-codes are for SLP functional limitations. (For a list of these codes and descriptors, see Pub. 100-04, Medicare Claims Processing Manual, chapter 5, section 10.6 F.)

Only one functional limitation shall be reported at a time. Consequently, the clinician must select the G-code set for the functional limitation that most closely relates to the primary functional limitation being treated or the one that is the primary reason for treatment. When the beneficiary has more than one functional limitation, the clinician may need to make a determination as to which functional limitation is primary. In these cases, the clinician may choose the functional limitation that is:

- Most clinically relevant to a successful outcome for the beneficiary;
- The one that would yield the quickest and/or greatest functional progress; or
- The one that is the greatest priority for the beneficiary.

In all cases, this primary functional limitation should reflect the predominant limitation that the furnished therapy services are intended to address.

For services typically reported as PT or OT, the clinician reports one of the "Other PT/OT" functional G-codes sets to report when one of the four PT/OT categorical code sets does not describe the beneficiary's functional limitation, as follows:

- a beneficiary's functional limitation that is not defined by one of the four categories;
- a beneficiary whose therapy services are not intended to treat a functional limitation; or
- a beneficiary's functional limitation where an overall, composite, or other score from a functional assessment tool is used and does not clearly represent a functional limitation defined by one of the above four categorical PT/OT code sets.

In addition, the subsequent "Other PT/OT" G-code set is only reported after the primary "Other PT/OT" G-code set has been reported for the beneficiary during the same episode of care.

For services typically reported as SLP services, the clinician uses the "Other SLP" functional G-code to report when the functional limitation being treated is not represented by one of the seven categorical SLP functional measures. In addition, the "Other SLP" G-code set is used to report where an overall, composite, or other score from an assessment tool that does not clearly represent a functional limitation defined by one of the seven categorical SLP measures.

B. Selecting the severity modifiers to use in functional reporting/documenting.

Each G-code requires one of the following severity modifiers. When the clinician reports any of the following a modifier is used to convey the severity of the functional limitation: current status, the goal status and the discharge status.

Modifier	Impairment Limitation Restriction
CH	0 percent impaired, limited or restricted
CI	At least 1 percent but less than 20 percent impaired, limited or restricted
CJ	At least 20 percent but less than 40 percent impaired, limited or restricted
CK	At least 40 percent but less than 60 percent impaired, limited or restricted
CL	At least 60 percent but less than 80 percent impaired, limited or restricted
CM	At least 80 percent but less than 100 percent impaired, limited or restricted
CN	100 percent impaired, limited or restricted

The severity modifier reflects the beneficiary's percentage of functional impairment as determined by the clinician furnishing the therapy services for each functional status: current, goal, or discharge. In selecting the severity modifier, the clinician:

- Uses the severity modifier that reflects the score from a functional assessment tool or other performance measurement instrument, as appropriate.

- Uses his/her clinical judgment to combine the results of multiple measurement tools used during the evaluative process to inform clinical decision making to determine a functional limitation percentage.

- Uses his/her clinical judgment in the assignment of the appropriate modifier.

- Uses the CH modifier to reflect a zero percent impairment when the therapy services being furnished are not intended to treat (or address) a functional limitation.

In some cases the modifier will be the same for current status and goal status. For example: where improvement is expected but it is not expected to be enough to move to another modifier, such as from 10 percent to 15 percent, the same severity modifier would be used in reporting the current and goal status. Also, when the clinician does not expect improvement, such as for individuals receiving maintenance therapy, the modifier used for projected goal status will be the same as the one for current status. In these cases, the discharge status may also include the same modifier.

Therapists must document in the medical record how they made the modifier selection so that the same process can be followed at succeeding assessment intervals.

C. Documentation of G-code and Severity Modifier Selection.

Documentation of the nonpayable G-codes and severity modifiers regarding functional limitations reported on claims must be included in the patient's medical record of therapy services for each required reporting. (See Pub. 100-04, Medicare Claims Processing Manual, chapter 5, section 10.6 for details about the functional reporting requirements on claims for therapy services, including PT, OT, and SLP services furnished in CORFs.)

Documentation of functional reporting in the medical record of therapy services must be completed by the clinician furnishing the therapy services:

- The qualified therapist furnishing the therapy services

- The physician/NPP personally furnishing the therapy services

- The qualified therapist furnishing services incident to the physician/NPP

- The physician/NPP for incident to services furnished by qualified personnel, who are not qualified therapists.

The qualified therapist furnishing the PT, OT, or SLP services in a CORF

A. Selecting the G-codes to Use in Functional Reporting.

There are 42 functional G-codes, 14 sets of three codes each, for that can be used in identifying the functional limitation being reported. Six of the G-code sets are generally for PT and OT functional limitations and eight sets of G-codes are for SLP functional limitations. (For a list of these codes and descriptors, see Pub. 100-04, Medicare Claims Processing Manual, chapter 5, section 10.6 F.)

Only one functional limitation shall be reported at a time. Consequently, the clinician must select the G-code set for the functional limitation that most closely relates to the primary functional limitation being treated or the one that is the primary reason for treatment. When the beneficiary has more than one functional limitation, the clinician may need to make a determination as to which functional limitation is primary. In these cases, the clinician may choose the functional limitation that is:

- Most clinically relevant to a successful outcome for the beneficiary;

- The one that would yield the quickest and/or greatest functional progress; or

- The one that is the greatest priority for the beneficiary.

In all cases, this primary functional limitation should reflect the predominant limitation that the furnished therapy services are intended to address.

For services typically reported as PT or OT, the clinician reports one of the "Other PT/OT" functional G-codes sets to report when one of the four PT/OT categorical code sets does not describe the beneficiary's functional limitation, as follows:

- a beneficiary's functional limitation that is not defined by one of the four categories;

- a beneficiary whose therapy services are not intended to treat a functional limitation; or

- a beneficiary's functional limitation where an overall, composite, or other score from a functional assessment tool is used and does not clearly represent a functional limitation defined by one of the above four categorical PT/OT code sets.

In addition, the subsequent "Other PT/OT" G-code set is only reported after the primary "Other PT/OT" G-code set has been reported for the beneficiary during the same episode of care.

For services typically reported as SLP services, the clinician uses the "Other SLP" functional G-code to report when the functional limitation being treated is not represented by one of the seven categorical SLP functional measures. In addition, the "Other SLP" G-code set is used to report where an overall, composite, or other score from an assessment tool that does not clearly represent a functional limitation defined by one of the seven categorical SLP measures.

B. Selecting the severity modifiers to use in functional reporting/documenting.

Each G-code requires one of the following severity modifiers. When the clinician reports any of the following a modifier is used to convey the severity of the functional limitation: current status, the goal status and the discharge status.

Modifier	Impairment Limitation Restriction
CH	0 percent impaired, limited or restricted
CI	At least 1 percent but less than 20 percent impaired, limited or restricted
CJ	At least 20 percent but less than 40 percent impaired, limited or restricted
CK	At least 40 percent but less than 60 percent impaired, limited or restricted
CL	At least 60 percent but less than 80 percent impaired, limited or restricted
CM	At least 80 percent but less than 100 percent impaired, limited or restricted
CN	100 percent impaired, limited or restricted

The severity modifier reflects the beneficiary's percentage of functional impairment as determined by the clinician furnishing the therapy services for each functional status: current, goal, or discharge. In selecting the severity modifier, the clinician:

- Uses the severity modifier that reflects the score from a functional assessment tool or other performance measurement instrument, as appropriate.

- Uses his/her clinical judgment to combine the results of multiple measurement tools used during the evaluative process to inform clinical decision making to determine a functional limitation percentage.

- Uses his/her clinical judgment in the assignment of the appropriate modifier.

- Uses the CH modifier to reflect a zero percent impairment when the therapy services being furnished are not intended to treat (or address) a functional limitation.

In some cases the modifier will be the same for current status and goal status. For example: where improvement is expected but it is not expected to be enough to move to another modifier, such as from 10 percent to 15 percent, the same severity modifier would be used in reporting the current and goal status. Also, when the clinician does not expect improvement, such as for individuals receiving maintenance therapy, the modifier used for projected goal status will be the same as the one for current status. In these cases, the discharge status may also include the same modifier.

Therapists must document in the medical record how they made the modifier selection so that the same process can be followed at succeeding assessment intervals.

C. Documentation of G-code and Severity Modifier Selection.

Documentation of the nonpayable G-codes and severity modifiers regarding functional limitations reported on claims must be included in the patient's medical record of therapy services for each required reporting. (See Pub. 100-04, Medicare Claims Processing Manual, chapter 5, section 10.6 for details about the functional reporting requirements on claims for therapy services, including PT, OT, and SLP services furnished in CORFs.)

Documentation of functional reporting in the medical record of therapy services must be completed by the clinician furnishing the therapy services:

- The qualified therapist furnishing the therapy services

- The physician/NPP personally furnishing the therapy services

- The qualified therapist furnishing services incident to the physician/NPP

- The physician/NPP for incident to services furnished by qualified personnel, who are not qualified therapists.

The qualified therapist furnishing the PT, OT, or SLP services in a CORF

100-02, 15, 230

Practice of Physical Therapy, Occupational Therapy, and Speech-Language Pathology

(Rev. 63, Issued: 12-29-06, Effective: 01-01-07, Implementation: on or before 01-29-07)

A. Group Therapy Services.

Contractors pay for outpatient physical therapy services (which includes outpatient speech-language pathology services) and outpatient occupational therapy services provided simultaneously to two or more individuals by a practitioner as group therapy services (97150). The individuals can be, but need not be performing the same activity. The physician or therapist involved in group therapy services must be in constant attendance, but one-on-one patient contact is not required.

B. Therapy Students
1. General

Only the services of the therapist can be billed and paid under Medicare Part B. The services performed by a student are not reimbursed even if provided under "line of sight" supervision of the therapist; however, the presence of the student "in the room" does not make the service unbillable. Pay for the direct (one-to-one) patient contact services of the physician or therapist provided to Medicare Part B patients. Group therapy services performed by a therapist or physician may be billed when a student is also present "in the room".

EXAMPLES:

Therapists may bill and be paid for the provision of services in the following scenarios:

— The qualified practitioner is present and in the room for the entire session. The student participates in the delivery of services when the qualified practitioner is directing the service, making the skilled judgment, and is responsible for the assessment and treatment.

— The qualified practitioner is present in the room guiding the student in service delivery when the therapy student and the therapy assistant student are participating in the provision of services, and the practitioner is not engaged in treating another patient or doing other tasks at the same time.

— The qualified practitioner is responsible for the services and as such, signs all documentation. (A student may, of course, also sign but it is not necessary since the Part B payment is for the clinician's service, not for the student's services).

2. Therapy Assistants as Clinical Instructors

Physical therapist assistants and occupational therapy assistants are not precluded from serving as clinical instructors for therapy students, while providing services within their scope of work and performed under the direction and supervision of a licensed physical or occupational therapist to a Medicare beneficiary.

3. Services Provided Under Part A and Part B

The payment methodologies for Part A and B therapy services rendered by a student are different. Under the MPFS (Medicare Part B), Medicare pays for services provided by physicians and practitioners that are specifically authorized by statute. Students do not meet the definition of practitioners under Medicare Part B. Under SNF PPS, payments are based upon the case mix or Resource Utilization Group (RUG) category that describes the patient. In the rehabilitation groups, the number of therapy minutes delivered to the patient determines the RUG category. Payment levels for each category are based upon the costs of caring for patients in each group rather than providing specific payment for each therapy service as is done in Medicare Part B.

100-02, 15, 230.1

Practice of Physical Therapy

(Rev. 88, Issued: 05-07-08, Effective: 01-01-08, Implementation: 06-09-08)

A. General

Physical therapy services are those services provided within the scope of practice of physical therapists and necessary for the diagnosis and treatment of impairments, functional limitations, disabilities or changes in physical function and health status. (See Pub. 100-3, the Medicare National Coverage Determinations Manual, for specific conditions or services.) For descriptions of aquatic therapy in a community center pool see section 220C of this chapter.

B. Qualified Physical Therapist Defined
Reference: 42CFR484.4

The new personnel qualifications for physical therapists were discussed in the 2008 Physician Fee Schedule. See the Federal Register of November 27, 2007, for the full text. See also the correction notice for this rule, published in the Federal Register on January 15, 2008.

The regulation provides that a qualified physical therapist (PT) is a person who is licensed, if applicable, as a PT by the state in which he or she is practicing unless licensure does not apply, has graduated from an accredited PT education program and passed a national examination approved by the state in which PT services are provided.

The phrase, "by the state in which practicing" includes any authorization to practice provided by the same state in which the service is provided, including temporary licensure, regardless of the location of the entity billing the services. The curriculum accreditation is provided by the Commission on Accreditation in Physical Therapy Education (CAPTE) or, for those who graduated before CAPTE, curriculum approval was provided by the American Physical Therapy Association (APTA). For internationally educated PTs, curricula are approved by a credentials evaluation organization either approved by the APTA or identified in 8 CFR 212.15(e) as it relates to PTs. For example, in 2007, 8 CFR 212.15(e) approved the credentials evaluation provided by the Federation of State Boards of Physical Therapy (FSBPT) and the Foreign Credentialing Commission on Physical Therapy (FCCPT). The requirements above apply to all PTs effective January 1, 2010, if they have not met any of the following requirements prior to January 1, 2010.

Physical therapists whose current license was obtained on or prior to December 31, 2009, qualify to provide PT services to Medicare beneficiaries if they:

- graduated from a CAPTE approved program in PT on or before December 31, 2009 (examination is not required); or,

- graduated on or before December 31, 2009, from a PT program outside the U.S. that is determined to be substantially equivalent to a U.S. program by a credentials evaluating organization approved by either the APTA or identified in 8 CFR 212.15(e) and also passed an examination for PTs approved by the state in which practicing.

Or, PTs whose current license was obtained before January 1, 2008, may meet the requirements in place on that date (i.e., graduation from a curriculum approved by either the APTA, the Committee on Allied Health Education and Accreditation of the American Medical Association, or both).

Or, PTs meet the requirements who are currently licensed and were licensed or qualified as a PT on or before December 31, 1977, and had 2 years appropriate experience as a PT, and passed a proficiency examination conducted, approved, or sponsored by the U.S. Public Health Service.

Or, PTs meet the requirements if they are currently licensed and before January 1, 1966, they were:

— admitted to membership by the APTA; or

— admitted to registration by the American Registry of Physical Therapists; or

— graduated from a 4-year PT curriculum approved by a State Department of Education; or

— licensed or registered and prior to January 1, 1970, they had 15 years of fulltime experience in PT under the order and direction of attending and referring doctors of medicine or osteopathy.

Or, PTs meet requirements if they are currently licensed and they were trained outside the U.S. before January 1, 2008, and after 1928 graduated from a PT curriculum approved in the country in which the curriculum was located, if that country had an organization that was a member of the World Confederation for Physical Therapy, and that PT qualified as a member of the organization.

For outpatient PT services that are provided incident to the services of physicians/NPPs, the requirement for PT licensure does not apply; all other personnel qualifications do apply. The qualified personnel providing PT services incident to the services of a physician/NPP must be trained in an accredited PT curriculum. For example, a person who, on or before December 31, 2009, graduated from a PT curriculum accredited by CAPTE, but who has not passed the national examination or obtained a license, could provide Medicare outpatient PT therapy services incident to the services of a physician/NPP if the physician assumes responsibility for the services according to the incident to policies. On or after January 1, 2010, although licensure does not apply, both education and examination requirements that are effective January 1, 2010, apply to qualified personnel who provide PT services incident to the services of a physician/NPP.

C. Services of Physical Therapy Support Personnel
Reference: 42CFR 484.4

Personnel Qualifications. The new personnel qualifications for physical therapist assistants (PTA) were discussed in the 2008 Physician Fee Schedule. See the Federal Register of November 27, 2007, for the full text. See also the correction notice for this rule, published in the Federal Register on January 15, 2008.

The regulation provides that a qualified PTA is a person who is licensed as a PTA unless licensure does not apply, is registered or certified, if applicable, as a PTA by the state in which practicing, and graduated from an approved curriculum for PTAs, and passed a national examination for PTAs. The phrase, "by the state in which practicing" includes any authorization to practice provided by the same state in which the service is provided, including temporary licensure, regardless of the location or the entity billing for the services. Approval for the curriculum is provided by CAPTE or, if internationally or military trained PTAs apply, approval will be through a credentialing body for the curriculum for PTAs identified by either the American Physical Therapy Association or identified in 8 CFR 212.15(e). A national examination for PTAs is, for example the one furnished by the Federation of State Boards of Physical Therapy. These requirements above apply to all PTAs effective January 1, 2010, if they have not met any of the following requirements prior to January 1, 2010.

Those PTAs also qualify who, on or before December 31, 2009, are licensed, registered or certified as a PTA and met one of the two following requirements:

1. Is licensed or otherwise regulated in the state in which practicing; or

2. In states that have no licensure or other regulations, or where licensure does not apply, PTAs have:

— graduated on or before December 31, 2009, from a 2-year college-level program approved by the APTA or CAPTE; and

— effective January 1, 2010, those PTAs must have both graduated from a CAPTE approved curriculum and passed a national examination for PTAs; or

— PTAs may also qualify if they are licensed, registered or certified as a PTA, if applicable and meet requirements in effect before January 1, 2008, that is,

- they have graduated before January 1, 2008, from a 2 year college level program approved by the APTA; or

- on or before December 31, 1977, they were licensed or qualified as a PTA and passed a proficiency examination conducted, approved, or sponsored by the U.S. Public Health Service.

Services. The services of PTAs used when providing covered therapy benefits are included as part of the covered service. These services are billed by the supervising physical therapist. PTAs may not provide evaluation services, make clinical judgments or decisions or take responsibility for the service. They act at the direction and under the supervision of the treating physical therapist and in accordance with state laws.

A physical therapist must supervise PTAs. The level and frequency of supervision differs by setting (and by state or local law). General supervision is required for PTAs in all settings except private practice (which requires direct supervision) unless state practice requirements are more stringent, in which case state or local requirements must be followed. See specific settings for details. For example, in clinics, rehabilitation services, either on or off the organization's premises, those services are supervised by a qualified physical therapist who makes an onsite supervisory visit at least once every 30 days or more frequently if required by state or local laws or regulation.

The services of a PTA shall not be billed as services incident to a physician/NPP's service, because they do not meet the qualifications of a therapist.

The cost of supplies (e.g., theraband, hand putty, electrodes) used in furnishing covered therapy care is included in the payment for the HCPCS codes billed by the physical therapist, and are, therefore, not separately billable. Separate coverage and billing provisions apply to items that meet the definition of brace in Sec.130.

Services provided by aides, even if under the supervision of a therapist, are not therapy services and are not covered by Medicare. Although an aide may help the therapist by providing unskilled services, those services that are unskilled are not covered by Medicare and shall be denied as not reasonable and necessary if they are billed as therapy services.

D. Application of Medicare Guidelines to PT Services
This subsection will be used in the future to illustrate the application of the above guidelines to some of the physical therapy modalities and procedures utilized in the treatment of patients.

100-02, 15, 230.2
Practice of Occupational Therapy
(Rev. 88, Issued: 05-07-08, Effective: 01-01-08, Implementation: 06-09-08)

A. General
Occupational therapy services are those services provided within the scope of practice of occupational therapists and necessary for the diagnosis and treatment of impairments, functional disabilities or changes in physical function and health status. (See Pub. 100- 03, the Medicare National Coverage Determinations Manual, for specific conditions or services.)

Occupational therapy is medically prescribed treatment concerned with improving or restoring functions which have been impaired by illness or injury or, where function has been permanently lost or reduced by illness or injury, to improve the individual's ability to perform those tasks required for independent functioning. Such therapy may involve:

- The evaluation, and reevaluation as required, of a patient's level of function by administering diagnostic and prognostic tests;

- The selection and teaching of task-oriented therapeutic activities designed to restore physical function; e.g., use of woodworking activities on an inclined table to restore shoulder, elbow, and wrist range of motion lost as a result of burns;

- The planning, implementing, and supervising of individualized therapeutic activity programs as part of an overall "active treatment" program for a patient with a diagnosed psychiatric illness; e.g., the use of sewing activities which require following a pattern to reduce confusion and restore reality orientation in a schizophrenic patient;

- The planning and implementing of therapeutic tasks and activities to restore sensoryintegrative function; e.g., providing motor and tactile activities to increase sensory input and improve response for a stroke patient with functional loss resulting in a distorted body image;

- The teaching of compensatory technique to improve the level of independence in the activities of daily living, for example:

  — Teaching a patient who has lost the use of an arm how to pare potatoes and chop vegetables with one hand;

  — Teaching an upper extremity amputee how to functionally utilize a prosthesis;

  — Teaching a stroke patient new techniques to enable the patient to perform feeding, dressing, and other activities as independently as possible; or

  — Teaching a patient with a hip fracture/hip replacement techniques of standing tolerance and balance to enable the patient to perform such functional activities as dressing and homemaking tasks.

The designing, fabricating, and fitting of orthotics and self-help devices; e.g., making a hand splint for a patient with rheumatoid arthritis to maintain the hand in a functional position or constructing a device which would enable an individual to hold a utensil and feed independently; or Vocational and prevocational assessment and training, subject to the limitations specified in item B below.

Only a qualified occupational therapist has the knowledge, training, and experience required to evaluate and, as necessary, reevaluate a patient's level of function, determine whether an occupational therapy program could reasonably be expected to improve, restore, or compensate for lost function and, where appropriate, recommend to the physician/NPP a plan of treatment.

B. Qualified Occupational Therapist Defined
Reference: 42CFR484.4 The new personnel qualifications for occupational therapists (OT) were discussed in the 2008 Physician Fee Schedule. See the Federal Register of November 27, 2007, for the full text. See also the correction notice for this rule, published in the Federal Register on January 15, 2008.

The regulation provides that a qualified OT is an individual who is licensed, if licensure applies, or otherwise regulated, if applicable, as an OT by the state in which practicing, and graduated from an accredited education program for OTs, and is eligible to take or has passed the examination for OTs administered by the National

Board for Certification in Occupational Therapy, Inc. (NBCOT). The phrase, "by the state in which practicing" includes any authorization to practice provided by the same state in which the service is provided, including temporary licensure, regardless of the location of the entity billing the services. The education program for U.S. trained OTs is accredited by the Accreditation Council for Occupational Therapy Education (ACOTE). The requirements above apply to all OTs effective January 1, 2010, if they have not met any of the following requirements prior to January 1, 2010.

The OTs may also qualify if on or before December 31, 2009:

- they are licensed or otherwise regulated as an OT in the state in which practicing (regardless of the qualifications they met to obtain that licensure or regulation); or

- when licensure or other regulation does not apply, OTs have graduated from an OT education program accredited by ACOTE and are eligible to take, or have successfully completed the NBCOT examination for OTs.

Also, those OTs who met the Medicare requirements for OTs that were in 42CFR484.4 prior to January 1, 2008, qualify to provide OT services for Medicare beneficiaries if:

- on or before January 1, 2008, they graduated an OT program approved jointly by the American Medical Association and the AOTA, or

- they are eligible for the National Registration Examination of AOTA or the National Board for Certification in OT.

Also, they qualify who on or before December 31, 1977, had 2 years of appropriate experience as an occupational therapist, and had achieved a satisfactory grade on a proficiency examination conducted, approved, or sponsored by the U.S. Public Health Service.

Those educated outside the U.S. may meet the same qualifications for domestic trained OTs. For example, they qualify if they were licensed or otherwise regulated by the state in which practicing on or before December 31, 2009. Or they are qualified if they:

- graduated from an OT education program accredited as substantially equivalent to a U.S. OT education program by ACOTE, the World Federation of Occupational Therapists, or a credentialing body approved by AOTA; and

- passed the NBCOT examination for OT; and

- Effective January 1, 2010, are licensed or otherwise regulated, if applicable as an OT by the state in which practicing.

For outpatient OT services that are provided incident to the services of physicians/NPPs, the requirement for OT licensure does not apply; all other personnel qualifications do apply. The qualified personnel providing OT services incident to the services of a physician/NPP must be trained in an accredited OT curriculum. For example, a person who, on or before December 31, 2009, graduated from an OT curriculum accredited by ACOTE and is eligible to take or has successfully completed the entry-level certification examination for OTs developed and administered by NBCOT, could provide Medicare outpatient OT services incident to the services of a physician/NPP if the physician assumes responsibility for the services according to the incident to policies. On or after January 1, 2010, although licensure does not apply, both education and examination requirements that are effective January 1, 2010, apply to qualified personnel who provide OT services incident to the services of a physician/NPP.

C. Services of Occupational Therapy Support Personnel
Reference: 42CFR 484.4

The new personnel qualifications for occupational therapy assistants were discussed in the 2008 Physician Fee Schedule. See the Federal Register of November 27, 2007, for the full text. See also the correction notice for this rule, published in the Federal Register on January 15, 2008.

The regulation provides that an occupational therapy assistant is a person who is licensed, unless licensure does not apply, or otherwise regulated, if applicable, as an OTA by the state in which practicing, and graduated from an OTA education program accredited by ACOTE and is eligible to take or has successfully completed the NBCOT examination for OTAs. The phrase, "by the state in which practicing" includes any authorization to practice provided by the same state in which the service is provided, including temporary licensure, regardless of the location of the entity billing the services.

If the requirements above are not met, an OTA may qualify if, on or before December 31, 2009, the OTA is licensed or otherwise regulated as an OTA, if applicable, by the state in which practicing, or meets any qualifications defined by the state in which practicing.

Or, where licensure or other state regulation does not apply, OTAs may qualify if they have, on or before December 31, 2009:

- completed certification requirements to practice as an OTA established by a credentialing organization approved by AOTA; and

- after January 1, 2010, they have also completed an education program accredited by ACOTE and passed the NBCOT examination for OTAs.

OTAs who qualified under the policies in effect prior to January 1, 2008, continue to qualify to provide OT directed and supervised OTA services to Medicare beneficiaries.

Therefore, OTAs qualify who after December 31, 1977, and on or before December 31, 2007:

- completed certification requirements to practice as an OTA established by a credentialing organization approved by AOTA; or

- completed the requirements to practice as an OTA applicable in the state in which practicing.

Those OTAs who were educated outside the U.S. may meet the same requirements as domestically trained OTAs. Or, if educated outside the U.S. on or after January 1, 2008, they must have graduated from an OTA program accredited as substantially equivalent to OTA entry level education in the U.S. by ACOTE, its successor organization, or the World Federation of Occupational Therapists or a credentialing body approved by AOTA. In addition, they must have passed an exam for OTAs administered by NBCOT.

Services. The services of OTAs used when providing covered therapy benefits are included as part of the covered service. These services are billed by the supervising occupational therapist. OTAs may not provide evaluation services, make clinical judgments or decisions or take responsibility for the service. They act at the direction and under the supervision of the treating occupational therapist and in accordance with state laws.

An occupational therapist must supervise OTAs. The level and frequency of supervision differs by setting (and by state or local law). General supervision is required for OTAs in all settings except private practice (which requires direct supervision) unless state practice requirements are more stringent, in which case state or local requirements must be followed. See specific settings for details. For example, in clinics, rehabilitation agencies, and public health agencies, 42CFR485.713 indicates that when an OTA provides services, either on or off the organization's premises, those services are supervised by a qualified occupational therapist who makes an onsite supervisory visit at least once every 30 days or more frequently if required by state or local laws or regulation.

The services of an OTA shall not be billed as services incident to a physician/NPP's service, because they do not meet the qualifications of a therapist.

The cost of supplies (e.g., looms, ceramic tiles, or leather) used in furnishing covered therapy care is included in the payment for the HCPCS codes billed by the occupational therapist and are, therefore, not separately billable. Separate coverage and billing provisions apply to items that meet the definition of brace in Sec.130 of this manual.

Services provided by aides, even if under the supervision of a therapist, are not therapy services in the outpatient setting and are not covered by Medicare. Although an aide may help the therapist by providing unskilled services, those services that are unskilled are not covered by Medicare and shall be denied as not reasonable and necessary if they are billed as therapy services.

D. Application of Medicare Guidelines to Occupational Therapy Services

Occupational therapy may be required for a patient with a specific diagnosed psychiatric illness. If such services are required, they are covered assuming the coverage criteria are met. However, where an individual's motivational needs are not related to a specific diagnosed psychiatric illness, the meeting of such needs does not usually require an individualized therapeutic program. Such needs can be met through general activity programs or the efforts of other professional personnel involved in the care of the patient. Patient motivation is an appropriate and inherent function of all health disciplines, which is interwoven with other functions performed by such personnel for the patient. Accordingly, since the special skills of an occupational therapist are not required, an occupational therapy program for individuals who do not have a specific diagnosed psychiatric illness is not to be considered reasonable and necessary for the treatment of an illness or injury. Services furnished under such a program are not covered.

Occupational therapy may include vocational and prevocational assessment and training. When services provided by an occupational therapist are related solely to specific employment opportunities, work skills, or work settings, they are not reasonable or necessary for the diagnosis or treatment of an illness or injury and are not covered. However, carriers and intermediaries exercise care in applying this exclusion, because the assessment of level of function and the teaching of compensatory techniques to improve the level of function, especially in activities of daily living, are services which occupational therapists provide for both vocational and nonvocational purposes. For example, an assessment of sitting and standing tolerance might be nonvocational for a mother of young children or a retired individual living alone, but could also be a vocational test for a sales clerk. Training an amputee in the use of prosthesis for telephoning is necessary for everyday activities as well as for employment purposes. Major changes in life style may be mandatory for an individual with a substantial disability. The techniques of adjustment cannot be considered exclusively vocational or nonvocational.

100-02, 15, 230.4

Services Furnished by a Therapist in Private Practice
(Rev. 179, Issued: 01-14-14, Effective: 01-07-14, Implementation: 01-07-14)

A. General

See section 220 of this chapter for definitions. Therapist refers only to a qualified physical therapist, occupational therapist or speech-language pathologist. TPP refers to therapists in private practice (qualified physical therapists, occupational therapists and speech-language pathologists).

In order to qualify to bill Medicare directly as a therapist, each individual must be enrolled as a private practitioner and employed in one of the following practice types: an unincorporated solo practice, unincorporated partnership, unincorporated group practice, physician/NPP group or groups that are not professional corporations, if allowed by state and local law. Physician/NPP group practices may employ TPP if state and local law permits this employee relationship.

For purposes of this provision, a physician/NPP group practice is defined as one or more physicians/NPPs enrolled with Medicare who may bill as one entity. For further details on issues concerning enrollment, see the provider enrollment Web site at www.cms.hhs.gov/MedicareProviderSupEnroll and Pub. 100-08, Medicare Program Integrity Manual, chapter15, section 15.4.4.9.

Private practice also includes therapists who are practicing therapy as employees of another supplier, of a professional corporation or other incorporated therapy practice. Private practice does not include individuals when they are working as employees of an institutional provider.

Services should be furnished in the therapist's or group's office or in the patient's home. The office is defined as the location(s) where the practice is operated, in the state(s) where the therapist (and practice, if applicable) is legally authorized to furnish services, during the hours that the therapist engages in the practice at that location. If services are furnished in a private practice office space, that space shall be owned, leased, or rented by the practice and used for the exclusive purpose of operating the practice. For descriptions of aquatic therapy in a community center pool see section 220C of this chapter.

Therapists in private practice must be approved as meeting certain requirements, but do not execute a formal provider agreement with the Secretary.

If therapists who have their own Medicare National Provider Identifier (NPI) are employed by therapist groups, physician/NPP groups, or groups that are not professional organizations, the requirement that therapy space be owned, leased, or rented may be satisfied by the group that employs the therapist. Each therapist employed by a group should enroll as a TPP.

When therapists with a Medicare NPI provide services in the physician's/NPP's office in which they are employed, and bill using their NPI for each therapy service, then the direct supervision requirement for enrolled staff apply.

When the therapist who has a Medicare NPI is employed in a physician's/NPP's office the services are ordinarily billed as services of the therapist, with the therapist identified on the claim as the supplier of services. However, services of the therapist who has a Medicare NPI may also be billed by the physician/NPP as services incident to the physician's/NPP's service. (See §230.5 for rules related to therapy services incident to a physician.) In that case, the physician/NPP is the supplier of service, the NPI of the supervising physician/NPP is reported on the claim with the service and all the rules for both therapy services and incident to services (§230.5) must be followed.

B. Private Practice Defined

Reference: Federal Register November, 1998, pages 58863-58869; 42CFR 410.38(b), 42CFR410.59, 42CFR410.60, 42CFR410.62

The contractor considers a therapist to be in private practice if the therapist maintains office space at his or her own expense and furnishes services only in that space or the patient's home. Or, a therapist is employed by another supplier and furnishes services in facilities provided at the expense of that supplier.

The therapist need not be in full-time private practice but must be engaged in private practice on a regular basis; i.e., the therapist is recognized as a private practitioner and for that purpose has access to the necessary equipment to provide an adequate program of therapy.

The therapy services must be provided either by or under the direct supervision of the TPP. Each TPP should be enrolled as a Medicare provider. If a therapist is not enrolled, the services of that therapist must be directly supervised by an enrolled therapist. Direct supervision requires that the supervising private practice therapist be present in the office suite at the time the service is performed. These direct supervision requirements apply only in the private practice setting and only for therapists and their assistants. In other outpatient settings, supervision rules differ. The services of support personnel must be included in the therapist's bill. The supporting personnel, including other therapists, must be W-2 or 1099 employees of the TPP or other qualified employer.

Coverage of outpatient therapy under Part B includes the services of a qualified TPP when furnished in the therapist's office or the beneficiary's home. For this purpose, "home" includes an institution that is used as a home, but not a hospital, CAH or SNF, (Federal Register Nov. 2, 1998, pg 58869).

C. Assignment

Reference: Nov. 2, 1998 Federal Register, pg. 58863

See also Pub. 100-4 chapter 1, §30.2.

When physicians, NPPs, or TPPs obtain provider numbers, they have the option of accepting assignment (participating) or not accepting assignment (nonparticipating). In contrast, providers, such as outpatient hospitals, SNFs, rehabilitation agencies, and CORFs, do not have the option. For these providers, assignment is mandatory.

If physicians/NPPs, or TPPs accept assignment (are participating), they must accept the Medicare Physician Fee Schedule amount as payment. Medicare pays 80% and the patient is responsible for 20%. In contrast, if they do not accept assignment, Medicare will only pay 95% of the fee schedule amount. However, when these services are not furnished on an assignment-related basis, the limiting charge applies. (See §1848(g)(2)(c) of the Act.)

NOTE: Services furnished by a therapist in the therapist's office under arrangements with hospitals in rural communities and public health agencies (or services provided in the beneficiary's home under arrangements with a provider of outpatient physical or occupational therapy services) are not covered under this provision. See section 230.6.

100-02, 15, 232

Cardiac Rehabilitation (CR) and Intensive Cardiac Rehabilitation (ICR) Services Furnished On or After January 1, 2010

(Rev. 256, Issued: 02-01-19, Effective: 02-09-18, Implementation: 03-19-19)

Cardiac rehabilitation (CR) services mean a physician-supervised program that furnishes physician prescribed exercise, cardiac risk factor modification, including education, counseling, and behavioral intervention; psychosocial assessment, outcomes assessment, and other items/services as determined by the Secretary under certain conditions. Intensive cardiac rehabilitation (ICR) services mean a physician-supervised program that furnishes the same items/services under the same conditions as a CR program but must also demonstrate, as shown in peer-reviewed published research, that it improves patients' cardiovascular disease through specific outcome measurements described in 42 CFR 410.49(c). Effective January 1, 2010, Medicare Part B pays for CR/ICR programs and related items/services if specific criteria is met by the Medicare beneficiary, the CR/ICR program itself, the setting in which is it administered, and the physician administering the program, as outlined below:

CR/ICR Program Beneficiary Requirements:

Medicare covers CR/ICR program services for beneficiaries who have experienced one or more of the following:

- Acute myocardial infarction within the preceding 12 months;
- Coronary artery bypass surgery;
- Current stable angina pectoris;
- Heart valve repair or replacement;
- Percutaneous transluminal coronary angioplasty (PTCA) or coronary stenting;
- Heart or heart-lung transplant.

For cardiac rehabilitation only: Stable, chronic heart failure defined as patients with left ventricular ejection fraction of 35% or less and New York Heart Association (NYHA) class II to IV symptoms despite being on optimal heart failure therapy for at least 6 weeks. (Effective February 18, 2014.)

Effective February 9, 2018, section 51004 of the Bipartisan Budget Act (BBA) of 2018, Pub. L. No. 115-123 (2018), amended section 1861(eee)(4)(B) of the Social Security Act to expand coverage in an intensive cardiac rehabilitation program to additional conditions:

- Stable, chronic heart failure defined as patients with left ventricular ejection fraction of 35% or less and New York Heart Association (NYHA) class II to IV symptoms despite being on optimal heart failure therapy for at least 6 weeks; or
- Any additional condition for which the Secretary has determined that a cardiac rehabilitation program shall be covered, unless the Secretary determines, using the same process used to determine that the condition is covered for a cardiac rehabilitation program, that such coverage is not supported by the clinical evidence.

NOTE: CMS plans to amend our intensive cardiac rehabilitation regulations specified at 42 CFR 410.49 to reflect this expanded coverage. CMS anticipates that the changes will be included in the 2020 Medicare Physician Fee Schedule notice of proposed rulemaking. However, because the expanded coverage under the statutory change was effective on enactment, expanded coverage for these conditions will be made effective for services furnished on or after February 9, 2018.

CR/ICR Program Component Requirements:

- Physician-prescribed exercise. This physical activity includes aerobic exercise combined with other types of exercise (i.e., strengthening, stretching) as determined to be appropriate for individual patients by a physician each day CR/ICR items/services are furnished.
- Cardiac risk factor modification. This includes education, counseling, and behavioral intervention, tailored to the patients' individual needs.
- Psychosocial assessment. This assessment means an evaluation of an individual's mental and emotional functioning as it relates to the individual's rehabilitation. It should include: (1) an assessment of those aspects of the individual's family and home situation that affects the individual's rehabilitation treatment, and, (2) a psychosocial evaluation of the individual's response to, and rate of progress under, the treatment plan.
- Outcomes assessment. These should include: (i) minimally, assessments from the commencement and conclusion of CR/ICR, based on patient-centered outcomes which must be measured by the physician immediately at the beginning and end of the program, and, (ii) objective clinical measures of the effectiveness of the CR/ICR program for the individual patient, including exercise performance and self-reported measures of exertion and behavior.
- Individualized treatment plan. This plan should be written and tailored to each individual patient and include (i) a description of the individual's diagnosis; (ii) the type, amount, frequency, and duration of the CR/ICR items/services furnished; and (iii) the goals set for the individual under the plan. The individualized treatment plan must be established, reviewed, and signed by a physician every 30 days.

As specified at 42 CFR 410.49(f)(1), CR sessions are limited to a maximum of 2 1-hour sessions per day for up to 36 sessions over up to 36 weeks with the option for an additional 36 sessions over an extended period of time if approved by the contractor under section 1862(a)(1)(A) of the Act. ICR sessions are limited to 72 1-hour sessions (as defined in section 1848(b)(5) of the Act), up to 6 sessions per day, over a period of up to 18 weeks.

CR/ICR Program Setting Requirements:

CR/ICR services must be furnished in a physician's office or a hospital outpatient setting (for ICR, the hospital outpatient setting must provide ICR using an approved ICR program). All settings must have a physician immediately available and accessible for medical consultations and emergencies at all times when items/services are being furnished under the program. This provision is satisfied if the physician meets the requirements for direct supervision of physician office services as specified at 42 CFR 410.26, and for hospital outpatient services as specified at 42 CFR 410.27.

ICR Program Approval Requirements:

All prospective ICR programs must be approved through the national coverage determination (NCD) process. To be approved as an ICR program, it must demonstrate through peer-reviewed, published research that it has accomplished one or more of the following for its patients: (i) positively affected the progression of coronary heart disease, (ii) reduced the need for coronary bypass surgery, or, (iii) reduced the need for percutaneous coronary interventions.

An ICR program must also demonstrate through peer-reviewed, published research that it accomplished a statistically significant reduction in five or more of the following measures for patients from their levels before CR services to after CR services: (i) low density lipoprotein, (ii) triglycerides, (iii) body mass index, (iv) systolic blood pressure, (v) diastolic blood pressure, and (vi) the need for cholesterol, blood pressure, and diabetes medications.

A list of approved ICR programs, identified through the NCD process, will be posted to the CMS Web site and listed in the Federal Register.

Once an ICR program is approved through the NCD process, all prospective ICR sites wishing to furnish ICR items/services via an approved ICR program may enroll with their local contractor to become an ICR program supplier using the designated forms as specified at 42 CFR 424.510, and report specialty code 31 to be identified as an enrolled ICR supplier. For purposes of appealing an adverse determination concerning site approval, an ICR site is considered a supplier (or prospective supplier) as defined in 42 CFR 498.2.

CR/ICR Program Physician Requirements:

Physicians responsible for CR/ICR programs are identified as medical directors who oversee or supervise the CR/ICR program at a particular site. The medical director, in consultation with staff, is involved in directing the progress of individuals in the program. The medical director, as well as physicians acting as the supervising physician, must possess all of the following: (1) expertise in the management of individuals with cardiac pathophysiology, (2) cardiopulmonary training in basic life support or advanced cardiac life support, and (3) licensed to practice medicine in the state in which the CR/ICR program is offered. Direct physician supervision may be provided by a supervising physician or the medical director.

(See Pub. 100-3, Medicare National Coverage Determinations Manual, Chapter 1, Part 1, section 20.10.1, Pub. 100-4, Medicare Claims Processing Manual, Chapter 32, section 140, Pub. 100-08, Medicare Program Integrity Manual, Chapter 15, section 15.4.2.8, for specific claims processing, coding, and billing requirements for CR/ICR program services.)

100-02, 15, 240

Chiropractic Services - General

(Rev. 1, 10-01-03) B3-2250, B3-4118

The term "physician" under Part B includes a chiropractor who meets the specified qualifying requirements set forth in Sec.30.5 but only for treatment by means of manual manipulation of the spine to correct a subluxation.

Effective for claims with dates of services on or after January 1, 2000, an x-ray is not required to demonstrate the subluxation.

Implementation of the chiropractic benefit requires an appreciation of the differences between chiropractic theory and experience and traditional medicine due to fundamental differences regarding etiology and theories of the pathogenesis of disease. Judgments about the reasonableness of chiropractic treatment must be based on the application of chiropractic principles. So that Medicare beneficiaries receive equitable adjudication of claims based on such principles and are not deprived of the benefits intended by the law, carriers may use chiropractic consultation in carrier review of Medicare chiropractic claims.

Payment is based on the physician fee schedule and made to the beneficiary or, on assignment, to the chiropractor.

A. Verification of Chiropractor's Qualifications

Carriers must establish a reference file of chiropractors eligible for payment as physicians under the criteria in Sec.30.1. They pay only chiropractors on file. Information needed to establish such files is furnished by the CMS RO.

The RO is notified by the appropriate State agency which chiropractors are licensed and whether each meets the national uniform standards.

100-02, 15, 240.1.3

Necessity for Treatment

(Rev. 23, Issued: 10-08-04, Effective: 10-01-04, Implementation: 10-04-04)

The patient must have a significant health problem in the form of a neuromusculoskeletal condition necessitating treatment, and the manipulative services rendered must have a direct therapeutic relationship to the patient's condition and provide reasonable expectation of recovery or improvement of function. The patient must have a subluxation of the spine as demonstrated by x-ray or physical exam, as described above.

Most spinal joint problems fall into the following categories:

- Acute subluxation-A patient's condition is considered acute when the patient is being treated for a new injury, identified by x-ray or physical exam as specified above. The result of chiropractic manipulation is expected to be an improvement in, or arrest of progression, of the patient's condition.

- Chronic subluxation-A patient's condition is considered chronic when it is not expected to significantly improve or be resolved with further treatment (as is the case with an acute condition), but where the continued therapy can be expected to result in some functional improvement. Once the clinical status has remained stable for a given condition, without expectation of additional objective clinical improvements, further manipulative treatment is considered maintenance therapy and is not covered.

For Medicare purposes, a chiropractor must place an AT modifier on a claim when providing active/corrective treatment to treat acute or chronic subluxation. However the presence of the AT modifier may not in all instances indicate that the service is reasonable and necessary. As always, contractors may deny if appropriate after medical review.

A. Maintenance Therapy

Maintenance therapy includes services that seek to prevent disease, promote health and prolong and enhance the quality of life, or maintain or prevent deterioration of a chronic condition. When further clinical improvement cannot reasonably be expected from continuous ongoing care, and the chiropractic treatment becomes supportive rather than corrective in nature, the treatment is then considered maintenance therapy. The AT modifier must not be placed on the claim when maintenance therapy has been provided. Claims without the AT modifier will be considered as maintenance therapy and denied. Chiropractors who give or receive from beneficaries an ABN shall follow the instructions in Pub. 100-4, Medicare Claims Processing Manual, chapter 23, section 20.9.1.1 and include a GA (or in rare instances a GZ) modifier on the claim.

B. Contraindications

Dynamic thrust is the therapeutic force or maneuver delivered by the physician during manipulation in the anatomic region of involvement. A relative contraindication is a condition that adds significant risk of injury to the patient from dynamic thrust, but does not rule out the use of dynamic thrust. The doctor should discuss this risk with the patient and record this in the chart. The following are relative contraindications to dynamic thrust:

- Articular hyper mobility and circumstances where the stability of the joint is uncertain;

- Severe demineralization of bone;

- Benign bone tumors (spine);

- Bleeding disorders and anticoagulant therapy; and

- Radiculopathy with progressive neurological signs.

- Dynamic thrust is absolutely contraindicated near the site of demonstrated subluxation and proposed manipulation in the following:

- Acute arthropathies characterized by acute inflammation and ligamentous laxity and anatomic subluxation or dislocation; including acute rheumatoid arthritis and ankylosing spondylitis;

- Acute fractures and dislocations or healed fractures and dislocations with signs of instability;

- An unstable os odontoideum;

- Malignancies that involve the vertebral column;

- Infection of bones or joints of the vertebral column;

- Signs and symptoms of myelopathy or cauda equina syndrome;

- For cervical spinal manipulations, vertebrobasilar insufficiency syndrome; and

- A significant major artery aneurysm near the proposed manipulation.

100-02, 15, 280.5.1

Advance Care Planning (ACP) Furnished as an Optional Element with an Annual Wellness Visit (AWV) Upon Agreement with the Patient

(Rev. 216 Issued: 12-22-15, Effective: 01-01-16, Implementation: 01-04-16)

Beginning in CY 2016, CMS will treat an AWV and voluntary ACP that are furnished on the same day and by the same provider as a preventive service. Voluntary ACP services, upon agreement with the patient, will be an optional element of the AWV. (See section 1861(hhh)(2)(G) of the Act.) When ACP services are furnished as a part of

an AWV, according to sections 1833(a)(1) and 1833(b)(10) of the Act, the coinsurance and deductible are waived.

Voluntary advance care planning means the face-to-face service between a physician (or other qualified health care professional) and the patient discussing advance directives, with or without completing relevant legal forms. An advance directive is a document appointing an agent and/or recording the wishes of a patient pertaining to his/her medical treatment at a future time should he/she lack decisional capacity at that time.

See Pub. 100-04, Medicare Claims Processing Manual, chapter 18, section 140.8 for claims processing and billing instructions.

100-02, 15, 290

Foot Care

(Rev. 1, 10-01-03)

A. Treatment of Subluxation of Foot

Subluxations of the foot are defined as partial dislocations or displacements of joint surfaces, tendons ligaments, or muscles of the foot. Surgical or nonsurgical treatments undertaken for the sole purpose of correcting a subluxated structure in the foot as an isolated entity are not covered.

However, medical or surgical treatment of subluxation of the ankle joint (talo-crural joint) is covered. In addition, reasonable and necessary medical or surgical services, diagnosis, or treatment for medical conditions that have resulted from or are associated with partial displacement of structures is covered. For example, if a patient has osteoarthritis that has resulted in a partial displacement of joints in the foot, and the primary treatment is for the osteoarthritis, coverage is provided.

B. Exclusions from Coverage

The following foot care services are generally excluded from coverage under both Part A and Part B. (See Sec. 290.F and Sec. 290.G for instructions on applying foot care exclusions.)

1. Treatment of Flat Foot

   The term "flat foot" is defined as a condition in which one or more arches of the foot have flattened out. Services or devices directed toward the care or correction of such conditions, including the prescription of supportive devices, are not covered.

2. Routine Foot Care

   Except as provided above, routine foot care is excluded from coverage. Services that normally are considered routine and not covered by Medicare include the following:

   — The cutting or removal of corns and calluses;

   — The trimming, cutting, clipping, or debriding of nails; and

   — Other hygienic and preventive maintenance care, such as cleaning and soaking the feet, the use of skin creams to maintain skin tone of either ambulatory or bedfast patients, and any other service performed in the absence of localized illness, injury, or symptoms involving the foot.

3. Supportive Devices for Feet Orthopedic shoes and other supportive devices for the feet generally are not covered.

   However, this exclusion does not apply to such a shoe if it is an integral part of a leg brace, and its expense is included as part of the cost of the brace. Also, this exclusion does not apply to therapeutic shoes furnished to diabetics.

C. Exceptions to Routine Foot Care Exclusion

1. Necessary and Integral Part of Otherwise Covered Services

   In certain circumstances, services ordinarily considered to be routine may be covered if they are performed as a necessary and integral part of otherwise covered services, such as diagnosis and treatment of ulcers, wounds, or infections.

2. Treatment of Warts on Foot

   The treatment of warts (including plantar warts) on the foot is covered to the same extent as services provided for the treatment of warts located elsewhere on the body.

3. Presence of Systemic Condition

   The presence of a systemic condition such as metabolic, neurologic, or peripheral vascular disease may require scrupulous foot care by a professional that in the absence of such condition(s) would be considered routine (and, therefore, excluded from coverage). Accordingly, foot care that would otherwise be considered routine may be covered when systemic condition(s) result in severe circulatory embarrassment or areas of diminished sensation in the individual's legs or feet. (See subsection A.)

   In these instances, certain foot care procedures that otherwise are considered routine (e.g., cutting or removing corns and calluses, or trimming, cutting, clipping, or debriding nails) may pose a hazard when performed by a nonprofessional person on patients with such systemic conditions. (See Sec.290.G for procedural instructions.)

4. Mycotic Nails

   In the absence of a systemic condition, treatment of mycotic nails may be covered.

The treatment of mycotic nails for an ambulatory patient is covered only when the physician attending the patient's mycotic condition documents that (1) there is clinical evidence of mycosis of the toenail, and (2) the patient has marked limitation of ambulation, pain, or secondary infection resulting from the thickening and dystrophy of the infected toenail plate.

The treatment of mycotic nails for a nonambulatory patient is covered only when the physician attending the patient's mycotic condition documents that (1) there is clinical evidence of mycosis of the toenail, and (2) the patient suffers from pain or secondary infection resulting from the thickening and dystrophy of the infected toenail plate.

For the purpose of these requirements, documentation means any written information that is required by the carrier in order for services to be covered. Thus, the information submitted with claims must be substantiated by information found in the patient's medical record. Any information, including that contained in a form letter, used for documentation purposes is subject to carrier verification in order to ensure that the information adequately justifies coverage of the treatment of mycotic nails.

D. Systemic Conditions That Might Justify Coverage
Although not intended as a comprehensive list, the following metabolic, neurologic, and peripheral vascular diseases (with synonyms in parentheses) most commonly represent the underlying conditions that might justify coverage for routine foot care.

Diabetes mellitus *

Arteriosclerosis obliterans (A.S.O., arteriosclerosis of the extremities, occlusive peripheral arteriosclerosis)

Buerger's disease (thromboangiitis obliterans)

Chronic thrombophlebitis *

Peripheral neuropathies involving the feet -

— Associated with malnutrition and vitamin deficiency *
  – Malnutrition (general, pellagra)
  – Alcoholism
  – Malabsorption (celiac disease, tropical sprue)
  – Pernicious anemia Associated with carcinoma *
— Associated with diabetes mellitus *
— Associated with drugs and toxins *
— Associated with multiple sclerosis *
— Associated with uremia (chronic renal disease) *
— Associated with traumatic injury
— Associated with leprosy or neurosyphilis
— Associated with hereditary disorders
  – Hereditary sensory radicular neuropathy
  – Angiokeratoma corporis diffusum (Fabry's)
  – Amyloid neuropathy

When the patient's condition is one of those designated by an asterisk (*), routine procedures are covered only if the patient is under the active care of a doctor of medicine or osteopathy who documents the condition.

E. Supportive Devices for Feet Orthopedic shoes and other supportive devices for the feet generally are not covered.
However, this exclusion does not apply to such a shoe if it is an integral part of a leg brace, and its expense is included as part of the cost of the brace. Also, this exclusion does not apply to therapeutic shoes furnished to diabetics.

F. Presumption of Coverage
In evaluating whether the routine services can be reimbursed, a presumption of coverage may be made where the evidence available discloses certain physical and/or clinical findings consistent with the diagnosis and indicative of severe peripheral involvement.

For purposes of applying this presumption the following findings are pertinent:

Class A Findings
Nontraumatic amputation of foot or integral skeletal portion thereof.

Class B Findings
Absent posterior tibial pulse;

Advanced trophic changes as: hair growth (decrease or absence) nail changes (thickening) pigmentary changes (discoloration) skin texture (thin, shiny) skin color (rubor or redness) (Three required); and

Absent dorsalis pedis pulse.

Class C Findings
Claudication;

Temperature changes (e.g., cold feet);

Edema;

Paresthesias (abnormal spontaneous sensations in the feet); and

Burning.

The presumption of coverage may be applied when the physician rendering the routine foot care has identified:

1. A Class A finding;
2. Two of the Class B findings; or
3. One Class B and two Class C findings.

Cases evidencing findings falling short of these alternatives may involve podiatric treatment that may constitute covered care and should be reviewed by the intermediary's medical staff and developed as necessary.

For purposes of applying the coverage presumption where the routine services have been rendered by a podiatrist, the contractor may deem the active care requirement met if the claim or other evidence available discloses that the patient has seen an M.D. or D.O. for treatment and/or evaluation of the complicating disease process during the 6-month period prior to the rendition of the routine-type services. The intermediary may also accept the podiatrist's statement that the diagnosing and treating M.D. or D.O. also concurs with the podiatrist's findings as to the severity of the peripheral involvement indicated.

Services ordinarily considered routine might also be covered if they are performed as a necessary and integral part of otherwise covered services, such as diagnosis and treatment of diabetic ulcers, wounds, and infections.

G. Application of Foot Care Exclusions to Physician's Services
The exclusion of foot care is determined by the nature of the service. Thus, payment for an excluded service should be denied whether performed by a podiatrist, osteopath, or a doctor of medicine, and without regard to the difficulty or complexity of the procedure.

When an itemized bill shows both covered services and noncovered services not integrally related to the covered service, the portion of charges attributable to the noncovered services should be denied. (For example, if an itemized bill shows surgery for an ingrown toenail and also removal of calluses not necessary for the performance of toe surgery, any additional charge attributable to removal of the calluses should be denied.) In reviewing claims involving foot care, the carrier should be alert to the following exceptional situations:

1. Payment may be made for incidental noncovered services performed as a necessary and integral part of, and secondary to, a covered procedure. For example, if trimming of toenails is required for application of a cast to a fractured foot, the carrier need not allocate and deny a portion of the charge for the trimming of the nails. However, a separately itemized charge for such excluded service should be disallowed. When the primary procedure is covered the administration of anesthesia necessary for the performance of such procedure is also covered.

2. Payment may be made for initial diagnostic services performed in connection with a specific symptom or complaint if it seems likely that its treatment would be covered even though the resulting diagnosis may be one requiring only noncovered care.

The name of the M.D. or D.O. who diagnosed the complicating condition must be submitted with the claim. In those cases, where active care is required, the approximate date the beneficiary was last seen by such physician must also be indicated.

NOTE: Section 939 of P.L. 96-499 removed "warts" from the routine foot care exclusion effective July 1, 1981.

Relatively few claims for routine-type care are anticipated considering the severity of conditions contemplated as the basis for this exception. Claims for this type of foot care should not be paid in the absence of convincing evidence that nonprofessional performance of the service would have been hazardous for the beneficiary because of an underlying systemic disease. The mere statement of a diagnosis such as those mentioned in Sec.D above does not of itself indicate the severity of the condition. Where development is indicated to verify diagnosis and/or severity the carrier should follow existing claims processing practices, which may include review of carrier's history and medical consultation as well as physician contacts.

The rules in Sec.290.F concerning presumption of coverage also apply.

Codes and policies for routine foot care and supportive devices for the feet are not exclusively for the use of podiatrists. These codes must be used to report foot care services regardless of the specialty of the physician who furnishes the services. Carriers must instruct physicians to use the most appropriate code available when billing for routine foot care.

100-02, 16, 10

General Exclusions From Coverage
(Rev. 1, 10-01-03) A3-3150, HO-260, HHA-232, B3-2300

No payment can be made under either the hospital insurance or supplementary medicalinsurance program for certain items and services, when the following conditions exist:

- Not reasonable and necessary (§20);
- No legal obligation to pay for or provide (§40);
- Paid for by a governmental entity (§50);
- Not provided within United States (§60);
- Resulting from war (§70);

- Personal comfort (§80);
- Routine services and appliances (§90);
- Custodial care (§110);
- Cosmetic surgery (§120);
- Charges by immediate relatives or members of household (§130);
- Dental services (§140);
- Paid or expected to be paid under workers' compensation (§150);
- Nonphysician services provided to a hospital inpatient that were not provided directly or arranged for by the hospital (§170);
- Services Related to and Required as a Result of Services Which are not Covered Under Medicare (§180);
- Excluded foot care services and supportive devices for feet (§30); or
- Excluded investigational devices (See Chapter 14, §30).

100-02, 16, 100

Hearing Aids and Auditory Implants

(Rev. 39; Issued: 11-10-05; Effective: 11-10-05; Implementation: 12-12-05)

Section 1862(a)(7) of the Social Security Act states that no payment may be made under part A or part B for any expenses incurred for items or services "where such expenses are for . . . hearing aids or examinations therefore. . . ." This policy is further reiterated at 42 CFR 411.15(d) which specifically states that "hearing aids or examination for the purpose of prescribing, fitting, or changing hearing aids" are excluded from coverage.

Hearing aids are amplifying devices that compensate for impaired hearing. Hearing aids include air conduction devices that provide acoustic energy to the cochlea via stimulation of the tympanic membrane with amplified sound. They also include bone conduction devices that provide mechanical energy to the cochlea via stimulation of the scalp with amplified mechanical vibration or by direct contact with the tympanic membrane or middle ear ossicles.

Certain devices that produce perception of sound by replacing the function of the middle ear, cochlea or auditory nerve are payable by Medicare as prosthetic devices. These devices are indicated only when hearing aids are medically inappropriate or cannot be utilized due to congenital malformations, chronic disease, severe sensorineural hearing loss or surgery. The following are prosthetic devices:

- Cochlear implants and auditory brainstem implants, i.e., devices that replace the function of cochlear structures or auditory nerve and provide electrical energy to auditory nerve fibers and other neural tissue via implanted electrode arrays.
- Osseointegrated implants, i.e., devices implanted in the skull that replace the function of the middle ear and provide mechanical energy to the cochlea via a mechanical transducer.

Medicare contractors deny payment for an item or service that is associated with any hearing aid as defined above. See Sec.180 for policy for the medically necessary treatment of complications of implantable hearing aids, such as medically necessary removals of implantable hearing aids due to infection.

100-02, 16, 120

Cosmetic Surgery

(Rev. 1, 10-01-03) A3-3160, HO-260.11, B3-2329

Cosmetic surgery or expenses incurred in connection with such surgery is not covered. Cosmetic surgery includes any surgical procedure directed at improving appearance, except when required for the prompt (i.e., as soon as medically feasible) repair of accidental injury or for the improvement of the functioning of a malformed body member. For example, this exclusion does not apply to surgery in connection with treatment of severe burns or repair of the face following a serious automobile accident, or to surgery for therapeutic purposes which coincidentally also serves some cosmetic purpose.

100-02, 16, 180

Services Related to and Required as a Result of Services Which Are Not Covered Under Medicare

(Rev. 1, 10-03-03) B3-2300.1, A3-3101.14, HO-210.12

Medical and hospital services are sometimes required to treat a condition that arises as a result of services that are not covered because they are determined to be not reasonable and necessary or because they are excluded from coverage for other reasons. Services "related to" noncovered services (e.g., cosmetic surgery, noncovered organ transplants, noncovered artificial organ implants, etc.), including services related to follow-up care and complications of noncovered services which require treatment during a hospital stay in which the noncovered service was performed, are not covered services under Medicare. Services "not related to" noncovered services are covered under Medicare. Following are examples of services "related to" and "not related to" noncovered services while the beneficiary is an inpatient:

- A beneficiary was hospitalized for a noncovered service and broke a leg while in the hospital. Services related to care of the broken leg during this stay is a clear example of "not related to" services and are covered under Medicare.

- A beneficiary was admitted to the hospital for covered services, but during the course of hospitalization became a candidate for a noncovered transplant or implant and actually received the transplant or implant during that hospital stay. When the original admission was entirely unrelated to the diagnosis that led to a recommendation for a noncovered transplant or implant, the services related to the admitting condition would be covered.

- A beneficiary was admitted to the hospital for covered services related to a condition which ultimately led to identification of a need for transplant and receipt of a transplant during the same hospital stay. If, on the basis of the nature of the services and a comparison of the date they are received with the date on which the beneficiary is identified as a transplant candidate, the services could reasonably be attributed to preparation for the noncovered transplant, the services would be "related to" noncovered services and would also be noncovered.

Following is an example of services received subsequent to a noncovered inpatient stay:

- After a beneficiary has been discharged from the hospital stay in which the beneficiary received noncovered services, medical and hospital services required to treat a condition or complication that arises as a result of the prior noncovered services may be covered when they are reasonable and necessary in all other respects. Thus, coverage could be provided for subsequent inpatient stays or outpatient treatment ordinarily covered by Medicare, even if the need for treatment arose because of a previous noncovered procedure. Some examples of services that may be found to be covered under this policy are the reversal of intestinal bypass surgery for obesity, repair of complications from transsexual surgery or from cosmetic surgery, removal of a noncovered bladder stimulator, or treatment of any infection at the surgical site of a noncovered transplant that occurred following discharge from the hospital.

However, any subsequent services that could be expected to have been incorporated into a global fee are considered to have been paid in the global fee, and may not be paid again. Thus, where a patient undergoes cosmetic surgery and the treatment regimen calls for a series of postoperative visits to the surgeon for evaluating the patient's progress, these visits are not paid.

100-03, 10.2

NCD for Transcutaneous Electrical Nerve Stimulation (TENS) for Acute Post-Operative Pain (10.2)

(Rev. 173, Issued: 9-4-14, Effective: With Implementation I-10)

Indications and Limitations of Coverage

The use of Transcutaneous Electrical Nerve Stimulation (TENS) for the relief of acute post-operative pain is covered under Medicare. TENS may be covered whether used as an adjunct to the use of drugs, or as an alternative to drugs, in the treatment of acute pain resulting from surgery.

TENS devices, whether durable or disposable, may be used in furnishing this service. When used for the purpose of treating acute post-operative pain, TENS devices are considered supplies. As such they may be hospital supplies furnished inpatients covered under Part A, or supplies incident to a physician's service when furnished in connection with surgery done on an outpatient basis, and covered under Part B.

It is expected that TENS, when used for acute post-operative pain, will be necessary for relatively short periods of time, usually 30 days or less. In cases when TENS is used for longer periods, Medicare Administrative Contractors should attempt to ascertain whether TENS is no longer being used for acute pain but rather for chronic pain, in which case the TENS device may be covered as durable medical equipment as described in §160.27.

Cross-references: Medicare Benefit Policy Manual, Chapter 1, "Inpatient Hospital Services," §40; Medicare Benefit Policy Manual, Chapter 2, "Hospital Services Covered Under Part B," §§20, 20.4, and 80; Medicare Benefit Policy Manual, Chapter 15, "Covered Medical and other Health Services, §110."

100-03, 10.3

NCD for Inpatient Hospital Pain Rehabilitation Programs (10.3)

(Rev. 1, 10-03-03)

Since pain rehabilitation programs of a lesser scope than that described above would raise a question as to whether the program could be provided in a less intensive setting than on an inpatient hospital basis, carefully evaluate such programs to determine whether the program does, in fact, necessitate a hospital level of care. Some pain rehabilitation programs may utilize services and devices which are excluded from coverage, e.g., acupuncture (see 35-8), biofeedback (see 35-27), dorsal column stimulator (see 65-8), and family counseling services (see 35-I4). In determining whether the scope of a pain program does necessitate inpatient hospital care, evaluate only those services and devices which are covered. Although diagnostic tests may be an appropriate part of pain rehabilitation programs, such tests would be covered in an individual case only where they can be reasonably related to a patient's illness, complaint, symptom, or injury and where they do not represent an unnecessary duplication of tests previously performed.

An inpatient program of 4 weeks' duration is generally required to modify pain behavior. After this period it would be expected that any additional rehabilitation services which might be required could be effectively provided on an outpatient basis under an outpatient pain rehabilitation program (see 10.4 of the NCD Manual) or other outpatient program. The first 7-10 days of such an inpatient program constitute, in effect, an evaluation period. If a patient is unable to adjust to the program within this period, it is generally concluded that it is unlikely that the program will be effective and the patient is discharged from the program. On occasions a program longer than 4 weeks may be required in a particular case. In such a case there should be documentation to substantiate that inpatient care beyond a 4-week period was reasonable and necessary. Similarly, where it appears that a patient participating in a program is being granted frequent outside passes, a question would exist as to whether an inpatient program is reasonable and necessary for the treatment of the patient's condition.

An inpatient hospital stay for the purpose of participating in a pain rehabilitation program would be covered as reasonable and necessary to the treatment of a patient's condition where the pain is attributable to a physical cause, the usual methods of treatment have not been successful in alleviating it, and a significant loss of ability to function independently has resulted from the pain. Chronic pain patients often have psychological problems which accompany or stem from the physical pain and it is appropriate to include psychological treatment in the multidisciplinary approach. However, patients whose pain symptoms result from a mental condition, rather than from any physical cause, generally cannot be successfully treated in a pain rehabilitation program.

100-03, 10.4

NCD for Outpatient Hospital Pain Rehabilitation Programs (10.4)

(Rev. 173, Issued: 9-4-14, Effective: With Implementation I-10)

Coverage of services furnished under outpatient hospital pain rehabilitation programs, including services furnished in group settings under individualized plans of treatment, is available if the patient's pain is attributable to a physical cause, the usual methods of treatment have not been successful in alleviating it, and a significant loss of ability by the patient to function independently has resulted from the pain. If a patient meets these conditions and the program provides services of the types discussed in §10.3, the services provided under the program may be covered. Non-covered services (e.g., vocational counseling, meals for outpatients, or acupuncture) continue to be excluded from coverage, and A/B Medicare Administrative Contractors would not be precluded from finding, in the case of particular patients, that the pain rehabilitation program is not reasonable and necessary under §1862(a)(1) of the Social Security Act for the treatment of their conditions.

100-03, 10.5

NCD for Autogenous Epidural Blood Graft (10.5)

(Rev. 1, 10-03-03)

Autogenous epidural blood grafts are considered a safe and effective remedy for severe headaches that may occur after performance of spinal anesthesia, spinal taps or myelograms, and are covered.

100-03, 10.6

NCD for Anesthesia in Cardiac Pacemaker Surgery (10.6)

(Rev. 173, Issued: 9-4-14, Effective: With Implementation I-10)

The use of general or monitored anesthesia during transvenous cardiac pacemaker surgery may be reasonable and necessary and therefore covered under Medicare only if adequate documentation of medical necessity is provided on a case-by-case basis. The Medicare Administrative Contractor obtains advice from its medical consultants or from appropriate specialty physicians or groups in its locality regarding the adequacy of documentation before deciding whether a particular claim should be covered.

A second type of pacemaker surgery that is sometimes performed involves the use of the thoracic method of implantation which requires open surgery. Where the thoracic method is employed, general anesthesia is always used and should not require special medical documentation.

100-03, 20.2

NCD for Extracranial-Intracranial (EC-IC) Arterial Bypass Surgery (20.2)

(Rev. 1, 10-03-03)

Extracranial-Intracranial (EC-IC) arterial bypass surgery is not a covered procedure when it is performed as a treatment for ischemic cerebrovascular disease of the carotid or middle cerebral arteries which includes the treatment or prevention of strokes. The premise that this procedure which bypasses narrowed arterial segments, improves the blood supply to the brain and reduces the risk of having a stroke has not been demonstrated to be any more effective than no surgical intervention. Accordingly, EC-IC arterial bypass surgery is not considered reasonable and necessary within the meaning of §1862(a)(1) of the Act when it is performed as a treatment for ischemic cerebrovascular disease of the carotid or middle cerebral arteries.

100-03, 20.8.4

Leadless Pacemakers

(Rev. 201, Issued: 07-28-17, Effective: 01-18-18, Implementation: 08-29-17- for MAC local edits; January 2, 2018 - for MCS shared edits)

A. General

The leadless pacemaker eliminates the need for a device pocket and insertion of a pacing lead which are integral elements of traditional pacing systems. The removal of these elements eliminate an important source of complications associated with traditional pacing systems while providing similar benefits. Leadless pacemakers are delivered via catheter to the heart, and function similarly to other transvenous single-chamber ventricular pacemakers.

B. Nationally Covered Indications

Effective January 18, 2017, the Centers for Medicare & Medicaid Services (CMS) covers leadless pacemakers through Coverage with Evidence Development (CED). CMS covers leadless pacemakers when procedures are performed in Food and Drug Administration (FDA) approved studies. CMS also covers, in prospective longitudinal studies, leadless pacemakers that are used in accordance with the FDA approved label for devices that have either:

- an associated ongoing FDA approved post-approval study; or
- completed an FDA post-approval study.

Each study must be approved by CMS and as a fully-described, written part of its protocol, must address the following research questions:

- What are the peri-procedural and post-procedural complications of leadless pacemakers?
- What are the long term outcomes of leadless pacemakers?
- What are the effects of patient characteristics (age, gender, comorbidities) on the use and health effects of leadless pacemakers?

CMS will review studies to determine if they meet the 13 criteria listed below. If CMS determines that they meet these criteria, the study will be posted on CMS' CED website (https://www.cms.gov/Medicare/Coverage/Coverage-with-Evidence-Development/index.html).

a. The principal purpose of the study is to test whether the item or service meaningfully improves health outcomes of affected beneficiaries who are represented by the enrolled subjects.

b. The rationale for the study is well supported by available scientific and medical evidence.

c. The study results are not anticipated to unjustifiably duplicate existing knowledge.

d. The study design is methodologically appropriate and the anticipated number of enrolled subjects is sufficient to answer the research question(s) being asked in the National Coverage Determination.

e. The study is sponsored by an organization or individual capable of completing it successfully.

f. The research study is in compliance with all applicable Federal regulations concerning the protection of human subjects found in the Code of Federal Regulations (CFR) at 45 CFR Part 46. If a study is regulated by the Food and Drug Administration (FDA), it is also in compliance with 21 CFR Parts 50 and 56. In addition, to further enhance the protection of human subjects in studies conducted under CED, the study must provide and obtain meaningful informed consent from patients regarding the risks associated with the study items and/or services, and the use and eventual disposition of the collected data.

g. All aspects of the study are conducted according to appropriate standards of scientific integrity.

h. The study has a written protocol that clearly demonstrates adherence to the standards listed here as Medicare requirements.

i. The study is not designed to exclusively test toxicity or disease pathophysiology in healthy individuals. Such studies may meet this requirement only if the disease or condition being studied is life threatening as defined in 21 CFR §312.81(a) and the patient has no other viable treatment options.

j. The clinical research studies and registries are registered on the www.ClinicalTrials.gov website by the principal sponsor/investigator prior to the enrollment of the first study subject. Registries are also registered in the Agency for Healthcare Research and Quality (AHRQ) Registry of Patient Registries (RoPR).

k. The research study protocol specifies the method and timing of public release of all prespecified outcomes to be measured including release of outcomes if outcomes are negative or study is terminated early. The results must be made public within 12 months of the study's primary completion date, which is the date the final subject had final data collection for the primary endpoint, even if the trial does not achieve its primary aim. The results must include number started/completed, summary results for primary and secondary outcome measures, statistical analyses, and adverse events. Final results must be reported in a publicly accessibly manner; either in a peer-reviewed scientific journal (in print or on-line), in an on-line publicly accessible registry dedicated to the dissemination of clinical trial information such as ClinicalTrials.gov, or in journals willing to publish in abbreviated format (e.g., for studies with negative or incomplete results).

l. The study protocol must explicitly discuss beneficiary subpopulations affected by the item or service under investigation, particularly traditionally underrepresented groups in clinical studies, how the inclusion and exclusion criteria effect enrollment of these populations, and a plan for the retention and reporting of said populations in the trial. If the inclusion and exclusion criteria are expected to have a negative effect on the recruitment or retention of underrepresented populations, the protocol must discuss why these criteria are necessary.

m. The study protocol explicitly discusses how the results are or are not expected to be generalizable to affected beneficiary subpopulations. Separate discussions in the protocol may be necessary for populations eligible for Medicare due to age, disability or Medicaid eligibility.

Consistent with section 1142 of the Act, the Agency for Healthcare Research and Quality (AHRQ) supports clinical research studies that CMS determines meet the above-listed standards and address the above-listed research questions.

All clinical research study protocols must be reviewed and approved by CMS. The principal investigator must submit the complete study protocol, identify the relevant CMS research question(s) that will be addressed and cite the location of the detailed analysis plan for those questions in the protocol, plus provide a statement addressing how the study satisfies each of the standards of scientific integrity (a. through m. listed above), as well as the investigator's contact information, to the address below. The information will be reviewed, and approved studies will be identified on the CMS website.

Director, Coverage and Analysis Group
Re: Leadless Pacemakers CED
Centers for Medicare & Medicaid Services (CMS)
7500 Security Blvd., Mail Stop S3-02-01
Baltimore, MD 21244-1850

Email address for protocol submissions: clinicalstudynotification@cms.hhs.gov

Email subject line: "CED [NCD topic (i.e. Leadless Pacemakers)] [name of sponsor/primary investigator]"

C. Nationally Non-Covered Indications
Leadless pacemakers are non-covered when furnished outside of a CMS approved CED study.

D. Other
NA

100-03, 20.9

Artificial Hearts and Related Devices (Various Effective Dates Below)
(Rev.172, Issued: 08-29-14, Effective:10-30-13, Implementation: 09- 30-14)

A. General
An artificial heart is a biventricular replacement device which requires removal of a substantial part of the native heart, including both ventricles. Removal of this device is not compatible with life, unless the patient has a heart transplant.

B. Nationally Covered Indications
1. Bridge-to-transplant (BTT) (effective for services performed on or after May 1, 2008)

   An artificial heart for bridge-to-transplantation (BTT) is covered when performed under coverage with evidence development (CED) when a clinical study meets all of the criteria listed below. The clinical study must address at least one of the following questions:

   — Were there unique circumstances such as expertise available in a particular facility or an unusual combination of conditions in particular patients that affected their outcomes?

   — What will be the average time to device failure when the device is made available to larger numbers of patients?

   — Do results adequately give a reasonable indication of the full range of outcomes (both positive and negative) that might be expected from more widespread use?

   The clinical study must meet all of the criteria stated in Section D of this policy. The above information should be mailed to: Director, Coverage and Analysis Group, Centers for Medicare & Medicaid Services (CMS), Re: Artificial Heart, Mailstop S3-02-01, 7500 Security Blvd, Baltimore, MD 21244-1850.

   Clinical studies that are determined by CMS to meet the above requirements will be listed on the CMS Web site at: http://www.cms.gov/Medicare/Coverage/Coverage-with-Evidence-Development/Artificial-Hearts.html.

2. Destination therapy (DT) (effective for services performed on or after May 1, 2008)

   An artificial heart for destination therapy (DT) is covered when performed under CED when a clinical study meets all of the criteria listed below. The clinical study must address at least one of the following questions:

   — Were there unique circumstances such as expertise available in a particular facility or an unusual combination of conditions in particular patients that affected their outcomes?

   — What will be the average time to device failure when the device is made available to larger numbers of patients?

   — Do results adequately give a reasonable indication of the full range of outcomes (both positive and negative) that might be expected from more widespread use?

The clinical study must meet all of the criteria stated in Section D of this policy. The above information should be mailed to: Director, Coverage and Analysis Group, Centers for Medicare & Medicaid Services, Re: Artificial Heart, Mailstop S3-02-01, 7500 Security Blvd, Baltimore, MD 21244-1850.

Clinical studies that are determined by CMS to meet the above requirements will be listed on the CMS Web site at: http://www.cms.gov/Medicare/Coverage/Coverage-with-Evidence-Development/Artificial-Hearts.html.

C. Nationally Non-Covered Indications
All other indications for the use of artificial hearts not otherwise listed remain non-covered, except in the context of Category B investigational device exemption clinical trials (42 CFR 405) or as a routine cost in clinical trials defined under section 310.1 of the National Coverage Determinations (NCD) Manual.

D. Other
Clinical study criteria:

· The study must be reviewed and approved by the Food and Drug Administration (FDA).

· The principal purpose of the research study is to test whether a particular intervention potentially improves the participants' health outcomes.

· The research study is well supported by available scientific and medical information, or it is intended to clarify or establish the health outcomes of interventions already in common clinical use.

· The research study does not unjustifiably duplicate existing studies.

· The research study design is appropriate to answer the research question being asked in the study.

· The research study is sponsored by an organization or individual capable of executing the proposed study successfully.

· The research study is in compliance with all applicable Federal regulations concerning the protection of human subjects found at 45 CFR Part 46. If a study is FDA-regulated it also must be in compliance with 21 CFR Parts 50 and 56.

· All aspects of the research study are conducted according to appropriate standards of scientific integrity (see http://www.icmje.org).

· The research study has a written protocol that clearly addresses, or incorporates by reference, the standards listed here as Medicare requirements for CED.

· The clinical research study is not designed to exclusively test toxicity or disease pathophysiology in healthy individuals. Trials of all medical technologies measuring therapeutic outcomes as one of the objectives meet this standard only if the disease or condition being studied is life threatening as defined in 21 CFR §312.81(a) and the patient has no other viable treatment options.

· The clinical research study is registered on the www.ClinicalTrials.gov Web site by the principal sponsor/investigator as demonstrated by having a Clinicaltrials.gov Identifier.

· The research study protocol specifies the method and timing of public release of all pre-specified outcomes to be measured including release of outcomes if outcomes are negative or study is terminated early. The results must be made public within 24 months of the end of data collection. If a report is planned to be published in a peer-reviewed journal, then that initial release may be an abstract that meets the requirements of the International Committee of Medical Journal Editors (ICMJE) (http://www.icmje.org). However a full report of the outcomes must be made public no later than three (3) years after the end of data collection.

· The research study protocol must explicitly discuss subpopulations affected by the treatment under investigation, particularly traditionally under-represented groups in clinical studies, how the inclusion and exclusion criteria effect enrollment of these populations, and a plan for the retention and reporting of said populations in the trial. If the inclusion and exclusion criteria are expected to have a negative effect on the recruitment or retention of under-represented populations, the protocol must discuss why these criteria are necessary.

· The research study protocol explicitly discusses how the results are or are not expected to be generalizable to the Medicare population to infer whether Medicare patients may benefit from the intervention. Separate discussions in the protocol may be necessary for populations eligible for Medicare due to age, disability, or Medicaid eligibility.

Consistent with section 1142 of the Social Security Act (the Act), the Agency for Healthcare Research and Quality (AHRQ) supports clinical research studies that CMS determines meet the above-listed standards and address the above-listed research questions.

The principal investigator of an artificial heart clinical study seeking Medicare payment should submit the following documentation to CMS and should expect to be notified when the CMS review is complete:

· Complete study protocol (must be dated or identified with a version number);

· Protocol summary;

· Statement that the submitted protocol version has been agreed upon by the FDA;

- Statement that the above study standards are met;
- Statement that the study addresses at least one of the above questions related to artificial hearts;
- Complete contact information (phone number, email address, and mailing address); and,
- Clinicaltrials.gov Identifier.

100-03, 20.9.1

Ventricular Assist Devices (Various Effective Dates Below)

(Rev.172, Issued: 08-29-14, Effective: 10-30-13, Implementation: 09- 30-14)

A. General

A ventricular assist device (VAD) is surgically attached to one or both intact ventricles and is used to assist or augment the ability of a damaged or weakened native heart to pump blood. Improvement in the performance of the native heart may allow the device to be removed.

B. Nationally Covered Indications

1. Post-cardiotomy (effective for services performed on or after October 18, 1993) Post-cardiotomy is the period following open-heart surgery. VADs used for support of blood circulation post-cardiotomy are covered only if they have received approval from the Food and Drug Administration (FDA) for that purpose, and the VADs are used according to the FDA-approved labeling instructions.

2. Bridge-to-Transplant (effective for services performed on or after January 22, 1996)

   The VADs used for bridge to transplant are covered only if they have received approval from the FDA for that purpose, and the VADs are used according to FDA-approved labeling instructions. All of the following criteria must be fulfilled in order for Medicare coverage to be provided for a VAD used as a bridge to transplant:

   — The patient is approved for heart transplantation by a Medicare-approved heart transplant center and is active on the Organ Procurement and Transplantation Network (OPTN) heart transplant waitlist.

   — The implanting site, if different than the Medicare-approved transplant center, must receive written permission from the Medicare-approved transplant center under which the patient is listed prior to implantation of the VAD.

3. Destination Therapy (DT) (effective for services performed on or after October 1, 2003)

   Destination therapy (DT) is for patients that require mechanical cardiac support. The VADs used for DT are covered only if they have received approval from the FDA for that purpose.

   Patient Selection (effective November 9, 2010):

   The VADs are covered for patients who have chronic end-stage heart failure (New York Heart Association Class IV end-stage left ventricular failure) who are not candidates for heart transplantation at the time of VAD implant, and meet the following conditions:Have failed to respond to optimal medical management (including beta-blockers and ACE inhibitors if tolerated) for 45 of the last 60 days, or have been balloon pump-dependent for 7 days, or IV inotrope-dependent for 14 days; and,

   — Have a left ventricular ejection fraction (LVEF) <25%; and,

   — Have demonstrated functional limitation with a peak oxygen consumption of =14 ml/kg/min unless balloon pump- or inotrope-dependent or physically unable to perform the test. Facility Criteria (effective October 30, 2013):

   Facilities currently credentialed by the Joint Commission for placement of VADs as DT may continue as Medicare-approved facilities until October 30, 2014. At the conclusion of this transition period, these facilities must be in compliance with the following criteria as determined by a credentialing organization. As of the effective date, new facilities must meet the following criteria as a condition of coverage of this procedure as DT under section 1862(a)(1)(A) of the Social Security Act (the Act):

   Beneficiaries receiving VADs for DT must be managed by an explicitly identified cohesive, multidisciplinary team of medical professionals with the appropriate qualifications, training, and experience. The team embodies collaboration and dedication across medical specialties to offer optimal patient-centered care. Collectively, the team must ensure that patients and caregivers have the knowledge and support necessary to participate in shared decision making and to provide appropriate informed consent. The team members must be based at the facility and must include individuals with experience working with patients before and after placement of a VAD.

   The team must include, at a minimum:

   — At least one physician with cardiothoracic surgery privileges and individual experience implanting at least 10 durable, intracorporeal, left VADs as BTT or DT over the course of the previous 36 months with activity in the last year.

   — At least one cardiologist trained in advanced heart failure with clinical competence in medical and device-based management including VADs,

and clinical competence in the management of patients before and after heart transplant.

   — A VAD program coordinator.

   — A social worker.

   — A palliative care specialist. Facilities must be credentialed by an organization approved by the Centers for Medicare & Medicaid Services.

C. Nationally Non-Covered Indications

All other indications for the use of VADs not otherwise listed remain non-covered, except in the context of Category B investigational device exemption clinical trials (42 CFR 405) or as a routine cost in clinical trials defined under section 310.1 of the National Coverage Determinations (NCD) Manual.

D. Other

This policy does not address coverage of VADs for right ventricular support, biventricular support, use in beneficiaries under the age of 18, use in beneficiaries with complex congenital heart disease, or use in beneficiaries with acute heart failure without a history of chronic heart failure. Coverage under section 1862(a)(1)(A) of the Act for VADs in these situations will be made by local Medicare Administrative Contractors within their respective jurisdictions.

100-03, 20.12

NCD for Diagnostic Endocardial Electrical Stimulation (Pacing) (20.12)

(Rev. 1, 10-03-03)

Diagnostic endocardial electrical stimulation (EES), also called programmed electrical stimulation of the heart, is covered under Medicare when used for patients with severe cardiac arrhythmias.

100-03, 20.19

NCD for Ambulatory Blood Pressure Monitoring (20.19)

(Rev. 1, 10-03-03)

ABPM must be performed for at least 24 hours to meet coverage criteria.

ABPM is only covered for those patients with suspected white coat hypertension. Suspected white coat hypertension is defined as

1) office blood pressure > 140/90 mm Hg on at least three separate clinic/office visits with two separate measurements made at each visit;

2) at least two documented blood pressure measurements taken outside the office which are < 140/90 mm Hg; and

3) no evidence of end-organ damage.

The information obtained by ABPM is necessary in order to determine the appropriate management of the patient. ABPM is not covered for any other uses. In the rare circumstance that ABPM needs to be performed more than once in a patient, the qualifying criteria described above must be met for each subsequent ABPM test.

For those patients that undergo ABPM and have an ambulatory blood pressure of < 135/85 with no evidence of end-organ damage, it is likely that their cardiovascular risk is similar to that of normotensives. They should be followed over time. Patients for which ABPM demonstrates a blood pressure of > 135/85 may be at increased cardiovascular risk, and a physician may wish to consider antihypertensive therapy.

100-03, 20.26

NCD for Partial Ventriculectomy (20.26)

(Rev. 1, 10-03-03)

Since the mortality rate is high and there are no published scientific articles or clinical studies regarding partial ventriculectomy, this procedure cannot be considered reasonable and necessary within the meaning of Sec.1862(a)(1) of the Act. Therefore, partial ventriculectomy is not covered by Medicare.

100-03, 20.28

NCD for Therapeutic Embolization (20.28)

(Rev. 1, 10-03-03)

Therapeutic embolization is covered when done for hemorrhage, and for other conditions amenable to treatment by the procedure, when reasonable and necessary for the individual patient. Renal embolization for the treatment of renal adenocarcinoma continues to be covered, effective December 15, 1978, as one type of therapeutic embolization, to:

- Reduce tumor vascularity preoperatively;
- Reduce tumor bulk in inoperable cases; or
- Palliate specific symptoms.

100-03, 20.29

NCD for Hyperbaric Oxygen Therapy (20.29)

(Rev.203, Issued:11-17-17, Effective: 04- 03-17, Implementation: 12-18-17)

A. Covered Conditions

Program reimbursement for HBO therapy will be limited to that which is administered in a chamber (including the one man unit) and is limited to the following conditions:

1. Acute carbon monoxide intoxication,

2. Decompression illness,

3. Gas embolism,

4. Gas gangrene,

5. Acute traumatic peripheral ischemia. HBO therapy is a valuable adjunctive treatment to be used in combination with accepted standard therapeutic measures when loss of function, limb, or life is threatened.

6. Crush injuries and suturing of severed limbs. As in the previous conditions, HBO therapy would be an adjunctive treatment when loss of function, limb, or life is threatened.

7. Progressive necrotizing infections (necrotizing fasciitis),

8. Acute peripheral arterial insufficiency,

9. Preparation and preservation of compromised skin grafts (not for primary management of wounds),

10. Chronic refractory osteomyelitis, unresponsive to conventional medical and surgical management,

11. Osteoradionecrosis as an adjunct to conventional treatment,

12. Soft tissue radionecrosis as an adjunct to conventional treatment,

13. Cyanide poisoning,

14. Actinomycosis, only as an adjunct to conventional therapy when the disease process is refractory to antibiotics and surgical treatment,

14. Diabetic wounds of the lower extremities in patients who meet the following three criteria:

    a. Patient has type I or type II diabetes and has a lower extremity wound that is due to diabetes;

    b. Patient has a wound classified as Wagner grade III or higher; and

    c. Patient has failed an adequate course of standard wound therapy.

The use of HBO therapy is covered as adjunctive therapy only after there are no measurable signs of healing for at least 30 -days of treatment with standard wound therapy and must be used in addition to standard wound care. Standard wound care in patients with diabetic wounds includes: assessment of a patient's vascular status and correction of any vascular problems in the affected limb if possible, optimization of nutritional status, optimization of glucose control, debridement by any means to remove devitalized tissue, maintenance of a clean, moist bed of granulation tissue with appropriate moist dressings, appropriate off-loading, and necessary treatment to resolve any infection that might be present. Failure to respond to standard wound care occurs when there are no measurable signs of healing for at least 30 consecutive days. Wounds must be evaluated at least every 30 days during administration of HBO therapy. Continued treatment with HBO therapy is not covered if measurable signs of healing have not been demonstrated within any 30-day period of treatment.

B. Noncovered Conditions

All other indications not specified under Sec.270.4(A) are not covered under the Medicare program. No program payment may be made for any conditions other than those listed in Sec. 270.4(A).

No program payment may be made for HBO in the treatment of the following conditions:

1. Cutaneous, decubitus, and stasis ulcers.

2. Chronic peripheral vascular insufficiency.

3. Anaerobic septicemia and infection other than clostridial.

4. Skin burns (thermal).

5. Senility.

6. Myocardial infarction.

7. Cardiogenic shock.

8. Sickle cell anemia.

9. Acute thermal and chemical pulmonary damage, i.e., smoke inhalation with pulmonary insufficiency.

10. Acute or chronic cerebral vascular insufficiency.

11. Hepatic necrosis.

12. Aerobic septicemia.

13. Nonvascular causes of chronic brain syndrome (Pick's disease, Alzheimer's disease, Korsakoff's disease).

14. Tetanus.

15. Systemic aerobic infection.

16. Organ transplantation.

17. Organ storage.

18. Pulmonary emphysema.

19. Exceptional blood loss anemia.

20. Multiple Sclerosis.

21. Arthritic Diseases.

22. Acute cerebral edema.

C. Topical Application of Oxygen

This method of administering oxygen does not meet the definition of HBO therapy as stated above. Also, its clinical efficacy has not been established. Therefore, no Medicare reimbursement may be made for the topical application of oxygen.

100-03, 20.30

Microvolt T-Wave Alternans (MTWA)

(Rev. 182, Issued: 05-22-15, Effective: 01-13- 15, Implementation: 06-23-15)

A. General

Microvolt T-wave Alternans (MTWA) testing is a non-invasive diagnostic test that detects minute electrical activity in a portion of the electrocardiogram (ECG) known as the T-wave. MTWA testing has a role in the stratification of patients who may be at risk for sudden cardiac death (SCD) from ventricular arrhythmias.

Within patient groups that may be considered candidates for implantable cardioverter defibrillator (ICD) therapy, a negative MTWA test may be useful in identifying low-risk patients who are unlikely to benefit from, and who may experience worse outcomes from, ICD placement.

Spectral analysis (SA) is a sensitive mathematical method of measuring and comparing time and the ECG signals. It requires specialized propriety electrodes to calculate minute T-wave voltage changes. Software then analyzes these microvolt changes and produces a report to be interpreted by a physician. The Modified Moving Average (MMA) method uses a temporal domain in which T-wave alternans are assessed as a continuous variable along the complete ECG. The MMA method of MTWA testing is performed using standard ambulatory ECG equipment.

B. Nationally Covered Indications

Effective for dates of service on and after March 21, 2006, MTWA diagnostic testing is covered for the evaluation of patients at risk for SCD, only when the SA method is used.

C. Nationally Non-Covered Indications

N/A

D. Other

Effective for dates of service on and after January 21, 2015, Medicare Administrative Contractors (MACs) acting within their respective jurisdictions may determine coverage of MTWA diagnostic testing for the evaluation of patients at risk for SCD using all other methods.

(This NCD last reviewed January 2015.)

100-03, 20.32

Transcatheter Aortic Valve Replacement (TAVR)

(Rev. 147, Issued: 09-24-12, Effective: 05-01-12, Implementation: 01-07-13)

A. General

Transcatheter aortic valve replacement (TAVR - also known as TAVI or transcatheter aortic valve implantation) is used in the treatment of aortic stenosis. A bioprosthetic valve is inserted percutaneously using a catheter and implanted in the orifice of the aortic valve.

B. Nationally Covered Indications

The Centers for Medicare & Medicaid Services (CMS) covers transcatheter aortic valve replacement (TAVR) under Coverage with Evidence Development (CED) with the following conditions:

A. TAVR is covered for the treatment of symptomatic aortic valve stenosis when furnished according to a Food and Drug Administration (FDA)-approved indication and when all of the following conditions are met:

   1. The procedure is furnished with a complete aortic valve and implantation system that has received FDA premarket approval (PMA) for that system's FDA approved indication.

   2. Two cardiac surgeons have independently examined the patient face-to-face and evaluated the patient's suitability for open aortic valve replacement (AVR) surgery; and both surgeons have documented the rationale for their clinical judgment and the rationale is available to the heart team.

   3. The patient (preoperatively and postoperatively) is under the care of a heart team: a cohesive, multi-disciplinary, team of medical professionals. The heart team concept embodies collaboration and dedication across medical specialties to offer optimal patient-centered care.

   TAVR must be furnished in a hospital with the appropriate infrastructure that includes but is not limited to:

   a. On-site heart valve surgery program,

   b. Cardiac catheterization lab or hybrid operating room/catheterization lab equipped with a fixed radiographic imaging system with flat-panel fluoroscopy, offering quality imaging,

   c. Non-invasive imaging such as echocardiography, vascular ultrasound, computed tomography (CT) and magnetic resonance (MR),

d. Sufficient space, in a sterile environment, to accommodate necessary equipment for cases with and without complications,

e. Post-procedure intensive care facility with personnel experienced in managing patients who have undergone open-heart valve procedures,

f. Appropriate volume requirements per the applicable qualifications below.

There are two sets of qualifications; the first set outlined below is for hospital programs and heart teams without previous TAVR experience and the second set is for those with TAVR experience.

Qualifications to begin a TAVR program for hospitals without TAVR experience:

The hospital program must have the following:

a. ≥ 50 total AVRs in the previous year prior to TAVR, including = 10 high-risk patients, and;

b. ≥ 2 physicians with cardiac surgery privileges, and;

c. ≥ 1000 catheterizations per year, including = 400 percutaneous coronary interventions (PCIs) per year.

Qualifications to begin a TAVR program for heart teams without TAVR experience:

The heart team must include:

a. Cardiovascular surgeon with:

   i. ≥ 100 career AVRs including 10 high-risk patients; or,

   ii. ≥ 25 AVRs in one year; or,

   iii. ≥ 50 AVRs in 2 years; and which include at least 20 AVRs in the last year prior to TAVR initiation; and,

b. Interventional cardiologist with:

   i. Professional experience with 100 structural heart disease procedures lifetime; or,

   ii. 30 left-sided structural procedures per year of which 60% should be balloon aortic valvuloplasty (BAV). Atrial septal defect and patent foramen ovale closure are not considered left-sided procedures; and,

c. Additional members of the heart team such as echocardiographers, imaging specialists, heart failure specialists, cardiac anesthesiologists, intensivists, nurses, and social workers; and,

d. Device-specific training as required by the manufacturer.

Qualifications for hospital programs with TAVR experience:

The hospital program must maintain the following:

a. ≥ 20 AVRs per year or = 40 AVRs every 2 years; and,

b. ≥ 2 physicians with cardiac surgery privileges; and,

c. ≥ 1000 catheterizations per year, including = 400 percutaneous coronary interventions (PCIs) per year.

Qualifications for heart teams with TAVR experience:

The heart team must include:

a. cardiovascular surgeon and an interventional cardiologist whose combined experience maintains the following:

   i. ≥ 20 TAVR procedures in the prior year, or,

   ii. ≥ 40 TAVR procedures in the prior 2 years; and,

b. Additional members of the heart team such as echocardiographers, imaging specialists, heart failure specialists, cardiac anesthesiologists, intensivists, nurses, and social workers.

4. The heart team's interventional cardiologist(s) and cardiac surgeon(s) must jointly participate in the intra-operative technical aspects of TAVR.

5. The heart team and hospital are participating in a prospective, national, audited registry that: 1) consecutively enrolls TAVR patients; 2) accepts all manufactured devices; 3) follows the patient for at least one year; and, 4) complies with relevant regulations relating to protecting human research subjects, including 45 CFR Part 46 and 21 CFR Parts 50 & 56. The following outcomes must be tracked by the registry; and the registry must be designed to permit identification and analysis of patient, practitioner and facility level variables that predict each of these outcomes:

   i. Stroke;

   ii. All cause mortality;

   iii. Transient Ischemic Attacks (TIAs);

   iv. Major vascular events;

   v. Acute kidney injury;

   vi. Repeat aortic valve procedures;

   vii. Quality of Life (QoL).

The registry should collect all data necessary and have a written executable analysis plan in place to address the following questions (to appropriately

address some questions, Medicare claims or other outside data may be necessary):

– When performed outside a controlled clinical study, how do outcomes and adverse events compare to the pivotal clinical studies?

– How do outcomes and adverse events in subpopulations compare to patients in the pivotal clinical studies?

– What is the long term (≥ 5 year) durability of the device?

– What are the long term (≥ 5 year) outcomes and adverse events?

– How do the demographics of registry patients compare to the pivotal studies?

Consistent with section 1142 of the Act, the Agency for Healthcare Research and Quality (AHRQ) supports clinical research studies that CMS determines meet the above-listed standards and address the above-listed research questions.

B. TAVR is covered for uses that are not expressly listed as an FDA-approved indication when performed within a clinical study that fulfills all of the following.

1. The heart team's interventional cardiologist(s) and cardiac surgeon(s) must jointly participate in the intra-operative technical aspects of TAVR.

2. As a fully-described, written part of its protocol, the clinical research study must critically evaluate not only each patient's quality of life pre- and post-TAVR (minimum of 1 year), but must also address at least one of the following questions: § What is the incidence of stroke?

– What is the rate of all cause mortality?

– What is the incidence of transient ischemic attacks (TIAs)?

– What is the incidence of major vascular events?

– What is the incidence of acute kidney injury?

– What is the incidence of repeat aortic valve procedures?

3. The clinical study must adhere to the following standards of scientific integrity and relevance to the Medicare population:

a. The principal purpose of the research study is to test whether a particular intervention potentially improves the participants' health outcomes.

b. The research study is well supported by available scientific and medical information or it is intended to clarify or establish the health outcomes of interventions already in common clinical use.

c. The research study does not unjustifiably duplicate existing studies.

d. The research study design is appropriate to answer the research question being asked in the study.

e. The research study is sponsored by an organization or individual capable of executing the proposed study successfully.

f. The research study is in compliance with all applicable Federal regulations concerning the protection of human subjects found in the Code of Federal Regulations (CFR) at 45 CFR Part 46. If a study is regulated by the Food and Drug Administration (FDA), it also must be in compliance with 21 CFR Parts 50 and 56. In particular, the informed consent includes a straightforward explanation of the reported increased risks of stroke and vascular complications that have been published for TAVR.

g. All aspects of the research study are conducted according to appropriate standards of scientific integrity (see http://www.icmje.org).

h. The research study has a written protocol that clearly addresses, or incorporates by reference, the standards listed as Medicare coverage requirements.

i. The clinical research study is not designed to exclusively test toxicity or disease pathophysiology in healthy individuals. Trials of all medical technologies measuring therapeutic outcomes as one of the objectives meet this standard only if the disease or condition being studied is life threatening as defined in 21 CFR §312.81(a) and the patient has no other viable treatment options.

j. The clinical research study is registered on the www.ClinicalTrials.gov website by the principal sponsor/investigator prior to the enrollment of the first study subject.

k. The research study protocol specifies the method and timing of public release of all pre-specified outcomes to be measured including release of outcomes if outcomes are negative or study is terminated early. The results must be made public within 24 months of the end of data collection. If a report is planned to be published in a peer reviewed journal, then that initial release may be an abstract that meets the requirements of the International Committee of Medical Journal Editors (http://www.icmje.org). However a full report of the outcomes must be made public no later than three (3) years after the end of data collection.

l. The research study protocol must explicitly discuss subpopulations affected by the treatment under investigation, particularly traditionally underrepresented groups in clinical studies, how the inclusion and exclusion criteria affect enrollment of these populations, and a plan for the retention and reporting of said populations on the trial. If the inclusion and exclusion criteria are expected to have a negative effect on

m. The research study protocol explicitly discusses how the results are or are not expected to be generalizable to the Medicare population to infer whether Medicare patients may benefit from the intervention. Separate discussions in the protocol may be necessary for populations eligible for Medicare due to age, disability or Medicaid eligibility. Consistent with section 1142 of the Act, AHRQ supports clinical research studies that CMS determines meet the above-listed standards and address the above-listed research questions.

4. The principal investigator must submit the complete study protocol, identify the relevant CMS research question(s) that will be addressed, and cite the location of the detailed analysis plan for those questions in the protocol, plus provide a statement addressing how the study satisfies each of the standards of scientific integrity (a. through m. listed above), as well as the investigator's contact information, to the address below. The information will be reviewed, and approved studies will be identified on the CMS Website.

> Director, Coverage and Analysis Group
> Re: TAVR CED
> Centers for Medicare & Medicaid Services (CMS)
> 7500 Security Blvd., Mail Stop S3-02-01
> Baltimore, MD 21244-1850

C. Nationally Non-Covered Indications

TAVR is not covered for patients in whom existing co-morbidities would preclude the expected benefit from correction of the aortic stenosis.

D.

NA

(This NCD last reviewed May 2012.)

100-03, 20.34

Percutaneous Left Atrial Appendage Closure (LAAC)

(Rev. 192, Issued: 05-06-16, Effective: 02-08-16, Implementation: 10-03-16)

A. General

Patients with atrial fibrillation (AF), an irregular heartbeat, are at an increased risk of stroke. The left atrial appendage (LAA) is a tubular structure that opens into the left atrium and has been shown to be one potential source for blood clots that can cause strokes. While thinning the blood with anticoagulant medications has been proven to prevent strokes, percutaneous LAA closure (LAAC) has been studied as a non-pharmacologic alternative for patients with AF.

B. Nationally Covered Indications

The Centers for Medicare & Medicaid Services (CMS) covers percutaneous LAAC for non-valvular atrial fibrillation (NVAF) through Coverage with Evidence Development (CED) with the following conditions:

a. LAAC devices are covered when the device has received Food and Drug Administration (FDA) Premarket Approval (PMA) for that device's FDA-approved indication and meet all of the conditions specified below:

The patient must have:

- A CHADS2 score ≥ 2 (Congestive heart failure, Hypertension, Age >75, Diabetes, Stroke/transient ischemia attack/thromboembolism) or CHA2DS2-VASc score ≥ 3 (Congestive heart failure, Hypertension, Age ≥ 65, Diabetes, Stroke/transient ischemia attack/thromboembolism, Vascular disease, Sex category)

- A formal shared decision making interaction with an independent non-interventional physician using an evidence-based decision tool on oral anticoagulation in patients with NVAF prior to LAAC. Additionally, the shared decision making interaction must be documented in the medical record.

- A suitability for short-term warfarin but deemed unable to take long-term oral anticoagulation following the conclusion of shared decision making, as LAAC is only covered as a second line therapy to oral anticoagulants. The patient (preoperatively and postoperatively) is under the care of a cohesive, multidisciplinary team (MDT) of medical professionals. The procedure must be furnished in a hospital with an established structural heart disease (SHD) and/or electrophysiology (EP) program.

The procedure must be performed by an interventional cardiologist(s), electrophysiologist(s), or cardiovascular surgeon (s) that meet the following criteria:

- Has received training prescribed by the manufacturer on the safe and effective use of the device prior to performing LAAC; and,

- Has performed ≥ 25 interventional cardiac procedures that involve transseptal puncture through an intact septum; and,

- Continues to perform ≥ 25 interventional cardiac procedures that involve transseptal puncture through an intact septum, of which at least 12 are LAAC, over a 2-year period.

The patient is enrolled in, and the MDT and hospital must participate in, a prospective, national, audited registry that: 1) consecutively enrolls LAAC patients, and, 2) tracks the following annual outcomes for each patient for a period of at least 4 years from the time of the LAAC:

- Operator-specific complications

- Device-specific complications including device thrombosis
- Stroke, adjudicated, by type
- Transient Ischemic Attack (TIA)
- Systemic embolism
- Death
- Major bleeding, by site and severity

The registry must be designed to permit identification and analysis of patient, practitioner, and facility level factors that predict patient risk for these outcomes. The registry must collect all data necessary to conduct analyses adjusted for relevant confounders, and have a written executable analysis plan in place to address the following questions:

- How do the outcomes listed above compare to outcomes in the pivotal clinical trials in the short term (≤12 months) and in the long term (≥ 4 years)?
- What is the long term (≥ 4 year) durability of the device?
- What are the short term (≤12 months) and the long term (≥4 years) device-specific complications including device thromboses?

To appropriately address some of these questions, Medicare claims or other outside data may be necessary.

Registries must be reviewed and approved by CMS. Potential registry sponsors must submit all registry documentation to CMS for approval, including the written executable analysis plan and auditing plan. CMS will review the qualifications of candidate registries to ensure that the approved registry follows standard data collection practices, and collects data necessary to evaluate the patient outcomes specified above. The registry's national clinical trial number must be recorded on the claim.

Consistent with section 1142 of the Social Security Act (the Act), the Agency for Healthcare Research and Quality (AHRQ) supports clinical research studies that CMS determines address the above-listed research questions and the a-m criteria listed in Section c. of this decision.

All approved registries will be posted on the CED website located at: https://www.cms.gov/Medicare/Coverage/Coverage-with-Evidence-Development/index.html.

b. LAAC is covered for NVAF patients not included in Section a. of this decision when performed within an FDA-approved randomized controlled trial (RCT) if such trials meet the criteria established below:

As a fully-described written part of its protocol, the RCT must critically answer, in comparison to optimal medical therapy, the following questions:

- As a primary endpoint, what is the true incidence of ischemic stroke and systemic embolism?
- As a secondary endpoint, what is cardiovascular mortality and all-cause mortality?

FDA-approved RCTs must be reviewed and approved by CMS. Consistent with section 1142 of the Act, AHRQ supports clinical research studies that CMS determines address the above-listed research questions and the a-m criteria listed in Section c. of this decision.

The principal investigator must submit the complete study protocol, identify the relevant CMS research question(s) that will be addressed, and cite the location of the detailed analysis plan for those questions in the protocol, plus provide a statement addressing how the study satisfies each of the standards of scientific integrity a. through m. listed in section c. of this decision, as well as the investigator's contact information, to the address below.

Director, Coverage and Analysis Group Re: LAAC CED Centers for Medicare & Medicaid Services 7500 Security Blvd., Mail Stop S3-02-01 Baltimore, MD 21244-1850

c. All clinical studies, RCTs and registries submitted for review must adhere to the following standards of scientific integrity and relevance to the Medicare population:

a. The principal purpose of the study is to test whether the item or service meaningfully improves health outcomes of affected beneficiaries who are represented by the enrolled subjects.

b. The rationale for the study is well supported by available scientific and medical evidence.

c. The study results are not anticipated to unjustifiably duplicate existing knowledge.

d. The study design is methodologically appropriate and the anticipated number of enrolled subjects is sufficient to answer the research question(s) being asked in the National Coverage Determination.

e. The study is sponsored by an organization or individual capable of completing it successfully.

f. The research study is in compliance with all applicable Federal regulations concerning the protection of human subjects found in the Code of Federal Regulations (CFR) at 45 CFR Part 46. If a study is regulated by the FDA, it is also in compliance with 21 CFR Parts 50 and 56. In addition, to further enhance the protection of human subjects in studies conducted under CED, the study must provide and obtain meaningful informed consent from patients regarding the risks associated with the study items and/or services, and the use and eventual disposition of the collected data.

g. All aspects of the study are conducted according to appropriate standards of scientific integrity.

h. The study has a written protocol that clearly demonstrates adherence to the standards listed here as Medicare requirements.

i. The study is not designed to exclusively test toxicity or disease pathophysiology in healthy individuals. Such studies may meet this requirement only if the disease or condition being studied is life threatening as defined in 21 CFR §312.81(a) and the patient has no other viable treatment options.

j. The clinical research studies and registries are registered on the www.ClinicalTrials.gov website by the principal sponsor/investigator prior to the enrollment of the first study subject. Registries are also registered in the AHRQ Registry of Patient Registries (RoPR).

k. The research study protocol specifies the method and timing of public release of all prespecified outcomes to be measured including release of outcomes if outcomes are negative or study is terminated early. The results must be made public within 12 months of the study's primary completion date, which is the date the final subject had final data collection for the primary endpoint, even if the trial does not achieve its primary aim. The results must include number started/completed, summary results for primary and secondary outcome measures, statistical analyses, and adverse events. Final results must be reported in a publicly accessibly manner; either in a peer-reviewed scientific journal (in print or on-line), in an on-line publicly accessible registry dedicated to the dissemination of clinical trial information such as ClinicalTrials.gov, or in journals willing to publish in abbreviated format (e.g., for studies with negative or incomplete results).

l. The study protocol must explicitly discuss beneficiary subpopulations affected by the item or service under investigation, particularly traditionally underrepresented groups in clinical studies, how the inclusion and exclusion criteria effect enrollment of these populations, and a plan for the retention and reporting of said populations in the trial. If the inclusion and exclusion criteria are expected to have a negative effect on the recruitment or retention of underrepresented populations, the protocol must discuss why these criteria are necessary.

m. The study protocol explicitly discusses how the results are or are not expected to be generalizable to affected beneficiary subpopulations. Separate discussions in the protocol may be necessary for populations eligible for Medicare due to age, disability, or Medicaid eligibility.

C. Nationally Non-Covered Indications
LAAC is non-covered for the treatment of NVAF when not furnished under CED according to the above-noted criteria.

(This NCD last reviewed February 2016.)

100-03, 20.35

Supervised Exercise Therapy (SET) for Symptomatic Peripheral Artery Disease (PAD)
(Rev. 207, Issued: 05-11-18, Effective: 05-25-17, Implementation: 07-02-18)

A. General
Research has shown supervised exercise therapy (SET) to be an effective, minimally invasive method to alleviate the most common symptom associated with peripheral artery disease (PAD) – intermittent claudication (IC). SET has been shown to be significantly more effective than unsupervised exercise, and could prevent the progression of PAD and lower the risk of cardiovascular events that are prevalent in these patients. SET has also been shown to perform at least as well as more invasive revascularization treatments that are covered by Medicare.

B. Nationally Covered Indications
Effective for services performed on or after May 25, 2017, the Centers for Medicare & Medicaid Services has determined that the evidence is sufficient to cover SET for beneficiaries with IC for the treatment of symptomatic PAD. Up to 36 sessions over a 12-week period are covered if all of the following components of a SET program are met. The SET program must:

- consist of sessions lasting 30-60 minutes comprising a therapeutic exercise-training program for PAD in patients with claudication;

- be conducted in a physician's office;

- be delivered by qualified auxiliary personnel necessary to ensure benefits exceed harms, and who are trained in exercise therapy for PAD; and

- be under the direct supervision of a physician (as defined in 1861(r)(1)), physician assistant, or nurse practitioner/clinical nurse specialist (as identified in 1861(aa)(5)) who must be trained in both basic and advanced life support techniques.

Beneficiaries must have a face-to-face visit with the physician responsible for PAD treatment to obtain the referral for SET. At this visit, the beneficiary must receive information regarding cardiovascular disease and PAD risk factor reduction, which could include education, counseling, behavioral interventions, and outcome assessments.

C. Nationally Non-Covered Indications
SET is non-covered for beneficiaries with absolute contraindications to exercise as determined by their primary physician.

D. Other
Medicare Administrative Contractors (MACs) have the discretion to cover SET beyond the nationally covered 36 sessions over a 12-week period. MACs may cover an additional 36 sessions over an extended period of time. A second referral is required for these additional sessions.

(This NCD last reviewed May 2017.)

100-03, 20.4

Implantable Cardioverter Defibrillators (ICDs)
(Rev.213, Issued: 02-15-19)

A. General
An ICD is an electronic device designed to diagnose and treat life-threatening ventricular tachyarrhythmias.

B. Nationally Covered Indications
Effective for services performed on or after February 15, 2018, CMS has determined that the evidence is sufficient to conclude that the use of ICDs, (also referred to as defibrillators) is reasonable and necessary:

1. Patients with a personal history of sustained Ventricular Tachyarrhythmia (VT) or cardiac arrest due to Ventricular Fibrillation (VF). Patients must have demonstrated: • An episode of sustained VT, either spontaneous or induced by an Electrophysiology (EP) study, not associated with an acute Myocardial Infarction (MI) and not due to a transient or reversible cause; or

   - An episode of cardiac arrest due to VF, not due to a transient or reversible cause.

2. Patients with a prior MI and a measured Left Ventricular Ejection Fraction (LVEF) ≤ 0.30. Patients must not have: • New York Heart Association (NYHA) classification IV heart failure; or,

   - Had a Coronary Artery Bypass Graft (CABG), or Percutaneous Coronary Intervention (PCI) with angioplasty and/or stenting, within the past three (3) months; or,

   - Had an MI within the past 40 days; or,

   - Clinical symptoms and findings that would make them a candidate for coronary revascularization.

   For these patients identified in B2, a formal shared decision making encounter must occur between the patient and a physician (as defined in Section 1861(r)(1) of the Social Security Act (the Act))or qualified non-physician practitioner (meaning a physician assistant, nurse practitioner, or clinical nurse specialist as defined in §1861(aa)(5) of the Act) using an evidence-based decision tool on ICDs prior to initial ICD implantation. The shared decision making encounter may occur at a separate visit.

3. Patients who have severe, ischemic, dilated cardiomyopathy but no personal history of sustained VT or cardiac arrest due to VF, and have NYHA Class II or III heart failure, LVEF < 35%. Additionally, patients must not have: • Had a CABG, or PCI with angioplasty and/or stenting, within the past three (3) months; or,

   - Had an MI within the past 40 days; or,

   - Clinical symptoms and findings that would make them a candidate for coronary revascularization.

   For these patients identified in B3, a formal shared decision making encounter must occur between the patient and a physician (as defined in Section 1861(r)(1) of the Actor qualified non-physician practitioner (meaning a physician assistant, nurse practitioner, or clinical nurse specialist as defined in §1861(aa)(5) of the Act) using an evidence-based decision tool on ICDs prior to initial ICD implantation. The shared decision making encounter may occur at a separate visit.

4. Patients who have severe, non-ischemic, dilated cardiomyopathy but no personal history of cardiac arrest or sustained VT, NYHA Class II or III heart failure, LVEF < 35%, been on optimal medical therapy for at least three (3) months. Additionally, patients must not have: • Had a CABG or PCI with angioplasty and/or stenting, within the past three (3) months; or,

   - Had an MI within the past 40 days; or,

   - Clinical symptoms and findings that would make them a candidate for coronary revascularization.

   For these patients identified in B4, a formal shared decision making encounter must occur between the patient and a physician (as defined in Section 1861(r)(1) of the Act) or qualified non-physician practitioner (meaning a physician assistant, nurse practitioner, or clinical nurse specialist as defined in §1861(aa)(5) of the Act) using an evidence-based decision tool on ICDs prior to initial ICD implantation. The shared decision making encounter may occur at a separate visit.

5. Patients with documented, familial or genetic disorders with a high risk of life-threatening tachyarrhythmias (sustained VT or VF, to include, but not limited to, long QT syndrome or hypertrophic cardiomyopathy.

   For these patients identified in B5, a formal shared decision making encounter must occur between the patient and a physician (as defined in Section 1861(r)(1) of the Act) or qualified non-physician practitioner (meaning a physician assistant, nurse practitioner, or clinical nurse specialist as defined in §1861(aa)(5) of the Act) using an evidence-based decision tool on ICDs prior to initial ICD implantation. The shared decision making encounter may occur at a separate visit.

6. Patients with an existing ICD may receive an ICD replacement if it is required due to the end of battery life, Elective Replacement Indicator (ERI), or device/lead malfunction.

For each of the six (6) covered indications above, the following additional criteria must also be met:

1. Patients must be clinically stable (e.g., not in shock, from any etiology);

2. LVEF must be measured by echocardiography, radionuclide (nuclear medicine) imaging, cardiac Magnetic Resonance Imaging (MRI), or catheter angiography;

3. Patients must not have:

   – Significant, irreversible brain damage; or,

   – Any disease, other than cardiac disease (e.g., cancer, renal failure, liver failure) associated with a likelihood of survival less than one (1) year; or,

   – Supraventricular tachycardia such as atrial fibrillation with a poorly controlled ventricular rate.

Exceptions to waiting periods for patients that have had a CABG, or PCI with angioplasty and/or stenting, within the past three (3) months, or had an MI within the past 40 days:

Cardiac Pacemakers: Patients who meet all CMS coverage requirements for cardiac pacemakers, and who meet the criteria in this national coverage determination for an ICD, may receive the combined devices in one procedure, at the time the pacemaker is clinically indicated;

Replacement of ICDs: Patients with an existing ICD may receive an ICD replacement if it is required due to the end of battery life, ERI, or device/lead malfunction.

C. Nationally Non-Covered Indications
N/A

D. Other
For patients that are candidates for heart transplantation on the United Network for Organ Sharing (UNOS) transplant list awaiting a donor heart, coverage of ICDs, as with cardiac resynchronization therapy, as a bridge-to-transplant to prolong survival until a donor becomes available, is determined by the local Medicare Administrative Contractors (MACs).

All other indications for ICDs not currently covered in accordance with this decision may be covered under Category B Investigational Device Exemption (IDE) trials (42 CFR 405.201).

(This NCD last reviewed February 2018.)

100-03, 30.3

NCD for Acupuncture (30.3)
(Rev. 1, 10-03-03)

Although acupuncture has been used for thousands of years in China and for decades in parts of Europe, it is a new agent of unknown use and efficacy in the United States. Even in those areas of the world where it has been widely used, its mechanism is not known. Three units of the National Institutes of Health, the National Institute of General Medical Sciences, National Institute of Neurological Diseases and Stroke, and Fogarty International Center have been designed to assess and identify specific opportunities and needs for research attending the use of acupuncture for surgical anesthesia and relief of chronic pain. Until the pending scientific assessment of the technique has been completed and its efficacy has been established, Medicare reimbursement for acupuncture, as an anesthetic or as an analgesic or for other therapeutic purposes, may not be made. Accordingly, acupuncture is not considered reasonable and necessary within the meaning of §1862(a)(1) of the Act.

100-03, 30.3.1

NCD for Acupuncture for Fibromyalgia (30.3.1)
(Rev. 11, 04-16-04)

General
Although acupuncture has been used for thousands of years in China and for decades in parts of Europe, it is still a relatively new agent of unknown use and efficacy in the United States. Even in those areas of the world where it has been widely used, its mechanism is not known. Three units of the National Institutes of Health, the National Institute of General Medical Sciences, National Institute of Neurological Diseases and Stroke, and Fogarty International Center were designated to assess and identify specific opportunities and needs for research attending the use of acupuncture for surgical anesthesia and relief of chronic pain. Following thorough review, and pending completion of the scientific assessment and efficacy of the technique, CMS initially issued a national noncoverage determination for acupuncture in May 1980.

Nationally Covered Indications
Not applicable.

Nationally Noncovered Indications
After careful reconsideration of its initial noncoverage determination for acupuncture, CMS concludes that there is no convincing evidence for the use of acupuncture for pain relief in patients with fibromyalgia. Study design flaws presently prohibit assessing acupuncture's utility for improving health outcomes. Accordingly, CMS determines that acupuncture is not considered reasonable and necessary for the treatment of fibromyalgia within the meaning of §1862(a)(1) of the Social Security Act, and the national noncoverage determination for acupuncture continues.

(This NCD last reviewed April 2004.)

100-03, 30.3.2

NCD for Acupuncture for Osteoarthritis (30.3.2)
(Rev. 11, 04-16-04)

General
Although acupuncture has been used for thousands of years in China and for decades in parts of Europe, it is still a relatively new agent of unknown use and efficacy in the United States. Even in those areas of the world where it has been widely used, its mechanism is not known. Three units of the National Institutes of Health, the National Institute of General Medical Sciences, National Institute of Neurological Diseases and Stroke, and Fogarty International Center were designated to assess and identify specific opportunities and needs for research attending the use of acupuncture for surgical anesthesia and relief of chronic pain. Following thorough review, and pending completion of the scientific assessment and efficacy of the technique, CMS initially issued a national noncoverage determination for acupuncture in May 1980.

Nationally Covered Indications
Not applicable.

Nationally Noncovered Indications
After careful reconsideration of its initial noncoverage determination for acupuncture, CMS concludes that there is no convincing evidence for the use of acupuncture for pain relief in patients with osteoarthritis. Study design flaws presently prohibit assessing acupuncture's utility for improving health outcomes. Accordingly, CMS determines that acupuncture is not considered reasonable and necessary for the treatment of osteoarthritis within the meaning of §1862(a)(1) of the Social Security Act, and the national noncoverage determination for acupuncture continues.

(This NCD last reviewed April 2004.)

100-03, 80.7

NCD for Refractive Keratoplasty (80.7)
(Rev. 1, 10-03-03)

The correction of common refractive errors by eyeglasses, contact lenses or other prosthetic devices is specifically excluded from coverage. The use of radial keratotomy and/or keratoplasty for the purpose of refractive error compensation is considered a substitute or alternative to eye glasses or contact lenses, which are specifically excluded by Sec.1862(a)(7) of the Act (except in certain cases in connection with cataract surgery). In addition, many in the medical community consider such procedures cosmetic surgery, which is excluded by section Sec.1862(a)(10) of the Act. Therefore, radial keratotomy and keratoplasty to treat refractive defects are not covered.

Keratoplasty that treats specific lesions of the cornea, such as phototherapeutic keratectomy that removes scar tissue from the visual field, deals with an abnormality of the eye and is not cosmetic surgery. Such cases may be covered under Sec.1862(a)(1)(A) of the Act.

The use of lasers to treat ophthalmic disease constitutes opthalmalogic surgery. Coverage is restricted to practitioners who have completed an approved training program in ophthalmologic surgery.

100-03, 80.10

NCD for Phaco-Emulsification procedure - cataract extraction (80.10)
(Rev. 1, 10-03-03)

In view of recommendations of authoritative sources in the field of ophthalmology, the subject technique is viewed as an accepted procedure for removal of cataracts. Accordingly, program reimbursement may be made for necessary services furnished in connection with cataract extraction utilizing the phaco-emulsification procedure.

100-03, 80.12

NCD for Intraocular Lenses (IOLs) (80.12)
(Rev. 1, 10-03-03)

Intraocular lens implantation services, as well as the lens itself, may be covered if reasonable and necessary for the individual. Implantation services may include hospital, surgical, and other medical services, including pre-implantation ultrasound (A-scan) eye measurement of one or both eyes.

100-03, 90.2

Next Generation Sequencing (NGS) for Patients with Advanced Cancer

(Rev.215, Issued: 04-10-19)

A. General

Clinical laboratory diagnostic tests can include tests that, for example, predict the risk associated with one or more genetic variations. In addition, in vitro companion diagnostic laboratory tests provide a report of test results of genetic variations and are essential for the safe and effective use of a corresponding therapeutic product. Next Generation Sequencing (NGS) is one technique that can measure one or more genetic variations as a laboratory diagnostic test, such as when used as a companion in vitro diagnostic test.

Patients with cancer can have recurrent, relapsed, refractory, metastatic, and/or advanced stages III or IV of cancer. Clinical studies show that genetic variations in a patient's cancer can, in concert with clinical factors, predict how each individual responds to specific treatments.

In application, a report of results of a diagnostic laboratory test using NGS (i.e., information on the cancer's genetic variations) can contribute to predicting a patient's response to a given drug: good, bad, or none at all. Applications of NGS to predict a patient's response to treatment occurs ideally prior to initiation of such treatment.

B. Nationally Covered Indications

Effective for services performed on or after March 16, 2018, the Centers for Medicare & Medicaid Services (CMS) has determined that Next Generation Sequencing (NGS) as a diagnostic laboratory test is reasonable and necessary and covered nationally, when performed in a Clinical Laboratory Improvement Amendments (CLIA)-certified laboratory, when ordered by a treating physician, and when all of the following requirements are met:

1. Patient has:
   - either recurrent, relapsed, refractory, metastatic, or advanced stage III or IV cancer; and,
   - either not been previously tested using the same NGS test for the same primary diagnosis of cancer, or repeat testing using the same NGS test only when a new primary cancer diagnosis is made by the treating physician; and,
   - decided to seek further cancer treatment (e.g., therapeutic chemotherapy).

2. The diagnostic laboratory test using NGS must have:
   - Food & Drug Administration (FDA) approval or clearance as a companion in vitro diagnostic; and,
   - an FDA-approved or -cleared indication for use in that patient's cancer; and,
   - results provided to the treating physician for management of the patient using a report template to specify treatment options.

C. Nationally Non-Covered

Effective for services performed on or after March 16, 2018, NGS as a diagnostic laboratory test for patients with cancer are non-covered if the cancer patient does not meet the criteria noted in section B.1. above.

D. Other

1. Effective for services performed on or after March 16, 2018, Medicare Administrative Contractors (MACs) may determine coverage of other NGS as a diagnostic laboratory test for patients with cancer only when the test is performed in a CLIA-certified laboratory, ordered by a treating physician, and the patient has:
   - either recurrent, relapsed, refractory, metastatic, or advanced stages III or IV cancer; and,
   - either not been previously tested using the same NGS test for the same primary diagnosis of cancer or repeat testing using the same NGS test was performed only when a new primary cancer diagnosis is made by the treating physician; and,
   - decided to seek further cancer treatment (e.g., therapeutic chemotherapy).

(This NCD last reviewed March 2018.)

ICD-10-CM	ICD-10-CM Code Descriptor 0037U: Effective Date: 04/01/2018
C00.0	Malignant neoplasm of external upper lip
C00.1	Malignant neoplasm of external lower lip
	Note that claims for F1CDx test 03/16/2018-03/31/2018 will be recognized with NOC/NOS code 81455 coverable under this policy.
C00.2	Malignant neoplasm of external lip, unspecified
C00.3	Malignant neoplasm of upper lip, inner aspect
C00.4	Malignant neoplasm of lower lip, inner aspect
C00.5	Malignant neoplasm of lip, unspecified, inner aspect
C00.6	Malignant neoplasm of commissure of lip, unspecified
C00.8	Malignant neoplasm of overlapping sites of lip
C00.9	Malignant neoplasm of lip, unspecified
C01	Malignant neoplasm of base of tongue
C02.0	Malignant neoplasm of dorsal surface of tongue

ICD-10-CM	ICD-10-CM Code Descriptor 0037U: Effective Date: 04/01/2018
C02.1	Malignant neoplasm of border of tongue
C02.2	Malignant neoplasm of ventral surface of tongue
C02.3	Malignant neoplasm of anterior two-thirds of tongue, part unspecified
C02.4	Malignant neoplasm of lingual tonsil
C02.8	Malignant neoplasm of overlapping sites of tongue
C02.9	Malignant neoplasm of tongue, unspecified
C03.0	Malignant neoplasm of upper gum
C03.1	Malignant neoplasm of lower gum
C03.9	Malignant neoplasm of gum, unspecified
C04.0	Malignant neoplasm of anterior floor of mouth
C04.1	Malignant neoplasm of lateral floor of mouth
C04.8	Malignant neoplasm of overlapping sites of floor of mouth
C04.9	Malignant neoplasm of floor of mouth, unspecified
C05.0	Malignant neoplasm of hard palate
C05.1	Malignant neoplasm of soft palate
C05.2	Malignant neoplasm of uvula
C05.8	Malignant neoplasm of overlapping sites of palate
C05.9	Malignant neoplasm of palate, unspecified
C06.0	Malignant neoplasm of cheek mucosa
C06.1	Malignant neoplasm of vestibule of mouth
C06.2	Malignant neoplasm of retromolar area
C06.80	Malignant neoplasm of overlapping sites of unspecified parts of mouth
C06.89	Malignant neoplasm of overlapping sites of other parts of mouth
C06.9	Malignant neoplasm of mouth, unspecified
C07	Malignant neoplasm of parotid gland
C08.0	Malignant neoplasm of submandibular gland
C08.1	Malignant neoplasm of sublingual gland
C08.9	Malignant neoplasm of major salivary gland, unspecified
C09.0	Malignant neoplasm of tonsillar fossa
C09.1	Malignant neoplasm of tonsillar pillar (anterior) (posterior)
C09.8	Malignant neoplasm of overlapping sites of tonsil
C09.9	Malignant neoplasm of tonsil, unspecified
C10.0	Malignant neoplasm of vallecula
C10.1	Malignant neoplasm of anterior surface of epiglottis
C10.2	Malignant neoplasm of lateral wall of oropharynx
C10.3	Malignant neoplasm of posterior wall of oropharynx
C10.4	Malignant neoplasm of branchial cleft
C10.8	Malignant neoplasm of overlapping sites of oropharynx
C10.9	Malignant neoplasm of oropharynx, unspecified
C11.0	Malignant neoplasm of superior wall of nasopharynx
C11.1	Malignant neoplasm of posterior wall of nasopharynx
C11.2	Malignant neoplasm of lateral wall of nasopharynx
C11.3	Malignant neoplasm of anterior wall of nasopharynx
C11.8	Malignant neoplasm of overlapping sites of nasopharynx
C11.9	Malignant neoplasm of nasopharynx, unspecified
C12	Malignant neoplasm of pyriform sinus
C13.0	Malignant neoplasm of postcricoid region
C13.1	Malignant neoplasm of aryepiglottic fold, hypopharyngeal aspect
C13.2	Malignant neoplasm of posterior wall of hypopharynx
C13.8	Malignant neoplasm of overlapping sites of hypopharynx
C13.9	Malignant neoplasm of hypopharynx, unspecified
C14.0	Malignant neoplasm of pharynx, unspecified
C14.2	Malignant neoplasm of Waldeyer's ring
C14.8	Malignant neoplasm of overlapping sites of lip, oral cavity and pharynx
C15.3	Malignant neoplasm of upper third of esophagus
C15.4	Malignant neoplasm of middle third of esophagus
C15.5	Malignant neoplasm of lower third of esophagus
C15.8	Malignant neoplasm of overlapping sites of esophagus
C15.9	Malignant neoplasm of esophagus, unspecified
C16.0	Malignant neoplasm of cardia
C16.1	Malignant neoplasm of fundus of stomach
C16.2	Malignant neoplasm of body of stomach
C16.3	Malignant neoplasm of pyloric antrum

ICD-10-CM	ICD-10-CM Code Descriptor 0037U: Effective Date: 04/01/2018
C16.4	Malignant neoplasm of pylorus
C16.5	Malignant neoplasm of lesser curvature of stomach, unspecified
C16.6	Malignant neoplasm of greater curvature of stomach, unspecified
C16.8	Malignant neoplasm of overlapping sites of stomach
C16.9	Malignant neoplasm of stomach, unspecified
C17.0	Malignant neoplasm of duodenum
C17.1	Malignant neoplasm of jejunum
C17.2	Malignant neoplasm of ileum
C17.3	Meckel's diverticulum, malignant
C17.8	Malignant neoplasm of overlapping sites of small intestine
C17.9	Malignant neoplasm of small intestine, unspecified
C18.0	Malignant neoplasm of cecum
C18.1	Malignant neoplasm of appendix
C18.2	Malignant neoplasm of ascending colon
C18.3	Malignant neoplasm of hepatic flexure
C18.4	Malignant neoplasm of transverse colon
C18.5	Malignant neoplasm of splenic flexure
C18.6	Malignant neoplasm of descending colon
C18.7	Malignant neoplasm of sigmoid colon
C18.8	Malignant neoplasm of overlapping sites of colon
C18.9	Malignant neoplasm of colon, unspecified
C19	Malignant neoplasm of rectosigmoid junction
C20	Malignant neoplasm of rectum
C21.0	Malignant neoplasm of anus, unspecified
C21.1	Malignant neoplasm of anal canal
C21.2	Malignant neoplasm of cloacogenic zone
C21.8	Malignant neoplasm of overlapping sites of rectum, anus and anal canal
C22.0	Liver cell carcinoma
C22.1	Intrahepatic bile duct carcinoma
C22.2	Hepatoblastoma
C22.3	Angiosarcoma of liver
C22.4	Other sarcomas of liver
C22.7	Other specified carcinomas of liver
C22.8	Malignant neoplasm of liver, primary, unspecified as to type
C22.9	Malignant neoplasm of liver, not specified as primary or secondary
C23	Malignant neoplasm of gallbladder
C24.0	Malignant neoplasm of extrahepatic bile duct
C24.1	Malignant neoplasm of ampulla of Vater
C24.8	Malignant neoplasm of overlapping sites of biliary tract
C24.9	Malignant neoplasm of biliary tract, unspecified
C25.0	Malignant neoplasm of head of pancreas
C25.1	Malignant neoplasm of body of pancreas
C25.2	Malignant neoplasm of tail of pancreas
C25.3	Malignant neoplasm of pancreatic duct
C25.4	Malignant neoplasm of endocrine pancreas
C25.7	Malignant neoplasm of other parts of pancreas
C25.8	Malignant neoplasm of overlapping sites of pancreas
C25.9	Malignant neoplasm of pancreas, unspecified
C26.0	Malignant neoplasm of intestinal tract, part unspecified
C26.1	Malignant neoplasm of spleen
C26.9	Malignant neoplasm of ill-defined sites within the digestive system
C30.0	Malignant neoplasm of nasal cavity
C30.1	Malignant neoplasm of middle ear
C31.0	Malignant neoplasm of maxillary sinus
C31.1	Malignant neoplasm of ethmoidal sinus
C31.2	Malignant neoplasm of frontal sinus
C31.3	Malignant neoplasm of sphenoid sinus
C31.8	Malignant neoplasm of overlapping sites of accessory sinuses
C31.9	Malignant neoplasm of accessory sinus, unspecified
C32.0	Malignant neoplasm of glottis
C32.1	Malignant neoplasm of supraglottis
C32.2	Malignant neoplasm of subglottis
C32.3	Malignant neoplasm of laryngeal cartilage

ICD-10-CM	ICD-10-CM Code Descriptor 0037U: Effective Date: 04/01/2018
C32.8	Malignant neoplasm of overlapping sites of larynx
C32.9	Malignant neoplasm of larynx, unspecified
C33	Malignant neoplasm of trachea
C34.00	Malignant neoplasm of unspecified main bronchus
C34.01	Malignant neoplasm of right main bronchus
C34.02	Malignant neoplasm of left main bronchus
C34.10	Malignant neoplasm of upper lobe, unspecified bronchus or lung
C34.11	Malignant neoplasm of upper lobe, right bronchus or lung
C34.12	Malignant neoplasm of upper lobe, left bronchus or lung
C34.2	Malignant neoplasm of middle lobe, bronchus or lung
C34.30	Malignant neoplasm of lower lobe, unspecified bronchus or lung
C34.31	Malignant neoplasm of lower lobe, right bronchus or lung
C34.32	Malignant neoplasm of lower lobe, left bronchus or lung
C34.80	Malignant neoplasm of overlapping sites of unspecified bronchus and lung
C34.81	Malignant neoplasm of overlapping sites of right bronchus and lung
C34.82	Malignant neoplasm of overlapping sites of left bronchus and lung
C34.90	Malignant neoplasm of unspecified part of unspecified bronchus or lung
C34.91	Malignant neoplasm of unspecified part of right bronchus or lung
C34.92	Malignant neoplasm of unspecified part of left bronchus or lung
C37	Malignant neoplasm of thymus
C38.0	Malignant neoplasm of heart
C38.1	Malignant neoplasm of anterior mediastinum
C38.2	Malignant neoplasm of posterior mediastinum
C38.3	Malignant neoplasm of mediastinum, part unspecified
C38.4	Malignant neoplasm of pleura
C38.8	Malignant neoplasm of overlapping sites of heart, mediastinum and pleura
C39.0	Malignant neoplasm of upper respiratory tract, part unspecified
C39.9	Malignant neoplasm of lower respiratory tract, part unspecified
C40.00	Malignant neoplasm of scapula and long bones of unspecified upper limb
C40.01	Malignant neoplasm of scapula and long bones of right upper limb
C40.02	Malignant neoplasm of scapula and long bones of left upper limb
C40.10	Malignant neoplasm of short bones of unspecified upper limb
C40.11	Malignant neoplasm of short bones of right upper limb
C40.12	Malignant neoplasm of short bones of left upper limb
C40.20	Malignant neoplasm of long bones of unspecified lower limb
C40.21	Malignant neoplasm of long bones of right lower limb
C40.22	Malignant neoplasm of long bones of left lower limb
C40.30	Malignant neoplasm of short bones of unspecified lower limb
C40.31	Malignant neoplasm of short bones of right lower limb
C40.32	Malignant neoplasm of short bones of left lower limb
C40.80	Malignant neoplasm of overlapping sites of bone and articular cartilage of unspecified limb
C40.81	Malignant neoplasm of overlapping sites of bone and articular cartilage of right limb
C40.82	Malignant neoplasm of overlapping sites of bone and articular cartilage of left limb
C40.90	Malignant neoplasm of unspecified bones and articular cartilage of unspecified limb
C40.91	Malignant neoplasm of unspecified bones and articular cartilage of right limb
C40.92	Malignant neoplasm of unspecified bones and articular cartilage of left limb
C41.0	Malignant neoplasm of bones of skull and face
C41.1	Malignant neoplasm of mandible
C41.2	Malignant neoplasm of vertebral column
C41.3	Malignant neoplasm of ribs, sternum and clavicle
C41.4	Malignant neoplasm of pelvic bones, sacrum and coccyx
C41.9	Malignant neoplasm of bone and articular cartilage, unspecified
C43.0	Malignant melanoma of lip
C43.10	Malignant melanoma of unspecified eyelid, including canthus
C43.11	Malignant melanoma of right eyelid, including canthus Expired 9/30/2018

ICD-10-CM	ICD-10-CM Code Descriptor 0037U: Effective Date: 04/01/2018
C43.111	Malignant melanoma of right upper eyelid, including canthus Effective 10/1/2018
C43.112	Malignant melanoma of right lower eyelid, including canthus Effective 10/1/2018
C43.12	Malignant melanoma of left eyelid, including canthus Expired 9/30/2018
C43.121	Malignant melanoma of left upper eyelid, including canthus Effective 10/1/2018
C43.122	Malignant melanoma of left lower eyelid, including canthus Effective 10/1/2018
C43.20	Malignant melanoma of unspecified ear and external auricular canal
C43.21	Malignant melanoma of right ear and external auricular canal
C43.22	Malignant melanoma of left ear and external auricular canal
C43.30	Malignant melanoma of unspecified part of face
C43.31	Malignant melanoma of nose
C43.39	Malignant melanoma of other parts of face
C43.4	Malignant melanoma of scalp and neck
C43.51	Malignant melanoma of anal skin
C43.52	Malignant melanoma of skin of breast
C43.59	Malignant melanoma of other part of trunk
C43.60	Malignant melanoma of unspecified upper limb, including shoulder
C43.61	Malignant melanoma of right upper limb, including shoulder
C43.62	Malignant melanoma of left upper limb, including shoulder
C43.70	Malignant melanoma of unspecified lower limb, including hip
C43.71	Malignant melanoma of right lower limb, including hip
C43.72	Malignant melanoma of left lower limb, including hip
C43.8	Malignant melanoma of overlapping sites of skin
C43.9	Malignant melanoma of skin, unspecified
C44.00	Unspecified malignant neoplasm of skin of lip
C44.01	Basal cell carcinoma of skin of lip
C44.02	Squamous cell carcinoma of skin of lip
C44.09	Other specified malignant neoplasm of skin of lip
C44.101	Unspecified malignant neoplasm of skin of unspecified eyelid, including canthus
C44.102	Unspecified malignant neoplasm of skin of right eyelid, including canthus Expired 9/30/2018
C44.1021	Unspecified malignant neoplasm of skin of right upper eyelid, including canthus Effective 10/1/2018
C44.1022	Unspecified malignant neoplasm of skin of right lower eyelid, including canthus Effective 10/1/2018
C44.109	Unspecified malignant neoplasm of skin of left eyelid, including canthus Expired 9/30/2018
C44.1091	Unspecified malignant neoplasm of skin of left upper eyelid, including canthus Effective 10/1/2018
C44.1092	Unspecified malignant neoplasm of skin of left lower eyelid, including canthus Effective 10/1/2018
C44.111	Basal cell carcinoma of skin of unspecified eyelid, including canthus
C44.112	Basal cell carcinoma of skin of right eyelid, including canthus Expired 9/30/2018
C44.1121	Basal cell carcinoma of skin of right upper eyelid, including canthus Effective 10/1/2018
C44.1122	Basal cell carcinoma of skin of right lower eyelid, including canthus Effective 10/1/2018
C44.119	Basal cell carcinoma of skin of left eyelid, including canthus Expired 9/30/2018
C44.1191	Basal cell carcinoma of skin of left upper eyelid, including canthus Effective 10/1/2018
C44.1192	Basal cell carcinoma of skin of left lower eyelid, including canthus Effective 10/1/2018

ICD-10-CM	ICD-10-CM Code Descriptor 0037U: Effective Date: 04/01/2018
C44.121	Squamous cell carcinoma of skin of unspecified eyelid, including canthus
C44.122	Squamous cell carcinoma of skin of right eyelid, including canthus Expired 9/30/2018
C44.1221	Squamous cell carcinoma of skin of right upper eyelid, including canthus Effective 10/1/2018
C44.1222	Squamous cell carcinoma of skin of right lower eyelid, including canthus Effective 10/1/2018
C44.129	Squamous cell carcinoma of skin of left eyelid, including canthus Expired 9/30/2018
C44.1291	Squamous cell carcinoma of skin of left upper eyelid, including canthus Effective 10/1/2018
C44.1292	Squamous cell carcinoma of skin of left lower eyelid, including canthus Effective 10/1/2018
C44.191	Other specified malignant neoplasm of skin of unspecified eyelid, including canthus
C44.192	Other specified malignant neoplasm of skin of right eyelid, including canthus Expired 9/30/2018
C44.1921	Other specified malignant neoplasm of skin of right upper eyelid, including canthus Effective 10/1/2018
C44.1922	Other specified malignant neoplasm of skin of right lower eyelid, including canthus Effective 10/1/2018
C44.199	Other specified malignant neoplasm of skin of left eyelid, including canthus Expired 9/30/2018
C44.1991	Other specified malignant neoplasm of skin of left upper eyelid, including canthus Effective 10/1/2018
C44.1992	Other specified malignant neoplasm of skin of left lower eyelid, including canthus Effective 10/1/2018
C44.201	Unspecified malignant neoplasm of skin of unspecified ear and external auricular canal
C44.202	Unspecified malignant neoplasm of skin of right ear and external auricular canal
C44.209	Unspecified malignant neoplasm of skin of left ear and external auricular canal
C44.211	Basal cell carcinoma of skin of unspecified ear and external auricular canal
C44.212	Basal cell carcinoma of skin of right ear and external auricular canal
C44.219	Basal cell carcinoma of skin of left ear and external auricular canal
C44.221	Squamous cell carcinoma of skin of unspecified ear and external auricular canal
C44.222	Squamous cell carcinoma of skin of right ear and external auricular canal
C44.229	Squamous cell carcinoma of skin of left ear and external auricular canal
C44.291	Other specified malignant neoplasm of skin of unspecified ear and external auricular canal
C44.292	Other specified malignant neoplasm of skin of right ear and external auricular canal
C44.299	Other specified malignant neoplasm of skin of left ear and external auricular canal
C44.300	Unspecified malignant neoplasm of skin of unspecified part of face
C44.301	Unspecified malignant neoplasm of skin of nose
C44.309	Unspecified malignant neoplasm of skin of other parts of face
C44.310	Basal cell carcinoma of skin of unspecified parts of face
C44.311	Basal cell carcinoma of skin of nose
C44.319	Basal cell carcinoma of skin of other parts of face
C44.320	Squamous cell carcinoma of skin of unspecified parts of face
C44.321	Squamous cell carcinoma of skin of nose
C44.329	Squamous cell carcinoma of skin of other parts of face

ICD-10-CM	ICD-10-CM Code Descriptor 0037U: Effective Date: 04/01/2018
C44.390	Other specified malignant neoplasm of skin of unspecified parts of face
C44.391	Other specified malignant neoplasm of skin of nose
C44.399	Other specified malignant neoplasm of skin of other parts of face
C44.40	Unspecified malignant neoplasm of skin of scalp and neck
C44.41	Basal cell carcinoma of skin of scalp and neck
C44.42	Squamous cell carcinoma of skin of scalp and neck
C44.49	Other specified malignant neoplasm of skin of scalp and neck
C44.500	Unspecified malignant neoplasm of anal skin
C44.501	Unspecified malignant neoplasm of skin of breast
C44.509	Unspecified malignant neoplasm of skin of other part of trunk
C44.510	Basal cell carcinoma of anal skin
C44.511	Basal cell carcinoma of skin of breast
C44.519	Basal cell carcinoma of skin of other part of trunk
C44.520	Squamous cell carcinoma of anal skin
C44.521	Squamous cell carcinoma of skin of breast
C44.529	Squamous cell carcinoma of skin of other part of trunk
C44.590	Other specified malignant neoplasm of anal skin
C44.591	Other specified malignant neoplasm of skin of breast
C44.599	Other specified malignant neoplasm of skin of other part of trunk
C44.601	Unspecified malignant neoplasm of skin of unspecified upper limb, including shoulder
C44.602	Unspecified malignant neoplasm of skin of right upper limb, including shoulder
C44.609	Unspecified malignant neoplasm of skin of left upper limb, including shoulder
C44.611	Basal cell carcinoma of skin of unspecified upper limb, including shoulder
C44.612	Basal cell carcinoma of skin of right upper limb, including shoulder
C44.619	Basal cell carcinoma of skin of left upper limb, including shoulder
C44.621	Squamous cell carcinoma of skin of unspecified upper limb, including shoulder
C44.622	Squamous cell carcinoma of skin of right upper limb, including shoulder
C44.629	Squamous cell carcinoma of skin of left upper limb, including shoulder
C44.691	Other specified malignant neoplasm of skin of unspecified upper limb, including shoulder
C44.692	Other specified malignant neoplasm of skin of right upper limb, including shoulder
C44.699	Other specified malignant neoplasm of skin of left upper limb, including shoulder
C44.701	Unspecified malignant neoplasm of skin of unspecified lower limb, including hip
C44.702	Unspecified malignant neoplasm of skin of right lower limb, including hip
C44.709	Unspecified malignant neoplasm of skin of left lower limb, including hip
C44.711	Basal cell carcinoma of skin of unspecified lower limb, including hip
C44.712	Basal cell carcinoma of skin of right lower limb, including hip
C44.719	Basal cell carcinoma of skin of left lower limb, including hip
C44.721	Squamous cell carcinoma of skin of unspecified lower limb, including hip
C44.722	Squamous cell carcinoma of skin of right lower limb, including hip
C44.729	Squamous cell carcinoma of skin of left lower limb, including hip
C44.791	Other specified malignant neoplasm of skin of unspecified lower limb, including hip
C44.792	Other specified malignant neoplasm of skin of right lower limb, including hip
C44.799	Other specified malignant neoplasm of skin of left lower limb, including hip
C44.80	Unspecified malignant neoplasm of overlapping sites of skin
C44.81	Basal cell carcinoma of overlapping sites of skin
C44.82	Squamous cell carcinoma of overlapping sites of skin
C44.89	Other specified malignant neoplasm of overlapping sites of skin
C44.90	Unspecified malignant neoplasm of skin, unspecified
C44.91	Basal cell carcinoma of skin, unspecified
C44.92	Squamous cell carcinoma of skin, unspecified
C44.99	Other specified malignant neoplasm of skin, unspecified

ICD-10-CM	ICD-10-CM Code Descriptor 0037U: Effective Date: 04/01/2018
C45.0	Mesothelioma of pleura
C45.1	Mesothelioma of peritoneum
C45.2	Mesothelioma of pericardium
C45.7	Mesothelioma of other sites
C45.9	Mesothelioma, unspecified
C47.0	Malignant neoplasm of peripheral nerves of head, face and neck
C47.10	Malignant neoplasm of peripheral nerves of unspecified upper limb, including shoulder
C47.11	Malignant neoplasm of peripheral nerves of right upper limb, including shoulder
C47.12	Malignant neoplasm of peripheral nerves of left upper limb, including shoulder
C47.20	Malignant neoplasm of peripheral nerves of unspecified lower limb, including hip
C47.21	Malignant neoplasm of peripheral nerves of right lower limb, including hip
C47.22	Malignant neoplasm of peripheral nerves of left lower limb, including hip
C47.3	Malignant neoplasm of peripheral nerves of thorax
C47.4	Malignant neoplasm of peripheral nerves of abdomen
C47.5	Malignant neoplasm of peripheral nerves of pelvis
C47.6	Malignant neoplasm of peripheral nerves of trunk, unspecified
C47.8	Malignant neoplasm of overlapping sites of peripheral nerves and autonomic nervous system
C47.9	Malignant neoplasm of peripheral nerves and autonomic nervous system, unspecified
C48.0	Malignant neoplasm of retroperitoneum
C48.1	Malignant neoplasm of specified parts of peritoneum
C48.2	Malignant neoplasm of peritoneum, unspecified
C48.8	Malignant neoplasm of overlapping sites of retroperitoneum and peritoneum
C49.0	Malignant neoplasm of connective and soft tissue of head, face and neck
C49.10	Malignant neoplasm of connective and soft tissue of unspecified upper limb, including shoulder
C49.11	Malignant neoplasm of connective and soft tissue of right upper limb, including shoulder
C49.12	Malignant neoplasm of connective and soft tissue of left upper limb, including shoulder
C49.20	Malignant neoplasm of connective and soft tissue of unspecified lower limb, including hip
C49.21	Malignant neoplasm of connective and soft tissue of right lower limb, including hip
C49.22	Malignant neoplasm of connective and soft tissue of left lower limb, including hip
C49.3	Malignant neoplasm of connective and soft tissue of thorax
C49.4	Malignant neoplasm of connective and soft tissue of abdomen
C49.5	Malignant neoplasm of connective and soft tissue of pelvis
C49.6	Malignant neoplasm of connective and soft tissue of trunk, unspecified
C49.8	Malignant neoplasm of overlapping sites of connective and soft tissue
C49.9	Malignant neoplasm of connective and soft tissue, unspecified
C49.A0	Gastrointestinal stromal tumor, unspecified site
C49.A1	Gastrointestinal stromal tumor of esophagus
C49.A2	Gastrointestinal stromal tumor of stomach
C49.A3	Gastrointestinal stromal tumor of small intestine
C49.A4	Gastrointestinal stromal tumor of large intestine
C49.A5	Gastrointestinal stromal tumor of rectum
C49.A9	Gastrointestinal stromal tumor of other sites
C4A.0	Merkel cell carcinoma of lip
C4A.10	Merkel cell carcinoma of unspecified eyelid, including canthus
C4A.11	Merkel cell carcinoma of right eyelid, including canthus Expired 9/30/2018
C4A.111	Merkel cell carcinoma of right upper eyelid, including canthus Effective 10/1/2018
C4A.112	Merkel cell carcinoma of right lower eyelid, including canthus Effective 10/1/2018

ICD-10-CM	ICD-10-CM Code Descriptor 0037U: Effective Date: 04/01/2018
C4A.12	Merkel cell carcinoma of left eyelid, including canthus Expired 9/30/2018
C4A.121	Merkel cell carcinoma of left upper eyelid, including canthus Effective 10/1/2018
C4A.122	Merkel cell carcinoma of left lower eyelid, including canthus Effective 10/1/2018
C4A.20	Merkel cell carcinoma of unspecified ear and external auricular canal
C4A.21	Merkel cell carcinoma of right ear and external auricular canal
C4A.22	Merkel cell carcinoma of left ear and external auricular canal
C4A.30	Merkel cell carcinoma of unspecified part of face
C4A.31	Merkel cell carcinoma of nose
C4A.39	Merkel cell carcinoma of other parts of face
C4A.4	Merkel cell carcinoma of scalp and neck
C4A.51	Merkel cell carcinoma of anal skin
C4A.52	Merkel cell carcinoma of skin of breast
C4A.59	Merkel cell carcinoma of other part of trunk
C4A.60	Merkel cell carcinoma of unspecified upper limb, including shoulder
C4A.61	Merkel cell carcinoma of right upper limb, including shoulder
C4A.62	Merkel cell carcinoma of left upper limb, including shoulder
C4A.70	Merkel cell carcinoma of unspecified lower limb, including hip
C4A.71	Merkel cell carcinoma of right lower limb, including hip
C4A.72	Merkel cell carcinoma of left lower limb, including hip
C4A.8	Merkel cell carcinoma of overlapping sites
C4A.9	Merkel cell carcinoma, unspecified
C50.011	Malignant neoplasm of nipple and areola, right female breast
C50.012	Malignant neoplasm of nipple and areola, left female breast
C50.019	Malignant neoplasm of nipple and areola, unspecified female breast
C50.021	Malignant neoplasm of nipple and areola, right male breast
C50.022	Malignant neoplasm of nipple and areola, left male breast
C50.029	Malignant neoplasm of nipple and areola, unspecified male breast
C50.111	Malignant neoplasm of central portion of right female breast
C50.112	Malignant neoplasm of central portion of left female breast
C50.119	Malignant neoplasm of central portion of unspecified female breast
C50.121	Malignant neoplasm of central portion of right male breast
C50.122	Malignant neoplasm of central portion of left male breast
C50.129	Malignant neoplasm of central portion of unspecified male breast
C50.211	Malignant neoplasm of upper-inner quadrant of right female breast
C50.212	Malignant neoplasm of upper-inner quadrant of left female breast
C50.219	Malignant neoplasm of upper-inner quadrant of unspecified female breast
C50.221	Malignant neoplasm of upper-inner quadrant of right male breast
C50.222	Malignant neoplasm of upper-inner quadrant of left male breast
C50.229	Malignant neoplasm of upper-inner quadrant of unspecified male breast
C50.311	Malignant neoplasm of lower-inner quadrant of right female breast
C50.312	Malignant neoplasm of lower-inner quadrant of left female breast
C50.319	Malignant neoplasm of lower-inner quadrant of unspecified female breast
C50.321	Malignant neoplasm of lower-inner quadrant of right male breast
C50.322	Malignant neoplasm of lower-inner quadrant of left male breast
C50.329	Malignant neoplasm of lower-inner quadrant of unspecified male breast
C50.411	Malignant neoplasm of upper-outer quadrant of right female breast
C50.412	Malignant neoplasm of upper-outer quadrant of left female breast
C50.419	Malignant neoplasm of upper-outer quadrant of unspecified female breast
C50.421	Malignant neoplasm of upper-outer quadrant of right male breast
C50.422	Malignant neoplasm of upper-outer quadrant of left male breast
C50.429	Malignant neoplasm of upper-outer quadrant of unspecified male breast
C50.511	Malignant neoplasm of lower-outer quadrant of right female breast
C50.512	Malignant neoplasm of lower-outer quadrant of left female breast
C50.519	Malignant neoplasm of lower-outer quadrant of unspecified female breast
C50.521	Malignant neoplasm of lower-outer quadrant of right male breast

ICD-10-CM	ICD-10-CM Code Descriptor 0037U: Effective Date: 04/01/2018
C50.522	Malignant neoplasm of lower-outer quadrant of left male breast
C50.529	Malignant neoplasm of lower-outer quadrant of unspecified male breast
C50.611	Malignant neoplasm of axillary tail of right female breast
C50.612	Malignant neoplasm of axillary tail of left female breast
C50.619	Malignant neoplasm of axillary tail of unspecified female breast
C50.621	Malignant neoplasm of axillary tail of right male breast
C50.622	Malignant neoplasm of axillary tail of left male breast
C50.629	Malignant neoplasm of axillary tail of unspecified male breast
C50.811	Malignant neoplasm of overlapping sites of right female breast
C50.812	Malignant neoplasm of overlapping sites of left female breast
C50.819	Malignant neoplasm of overlapping sites of unspecified female breast
C50.821	Malignant neoplasm of overlapping sites of right male breast
C50.822	Malignant neoplasm of overlapping sites of left male breast
C50.829	Malignant neoplasm of overlapping sites of unspecified male breast
C50.911	Malignant neoplasm of unspecified site of right female breast
C50.912	Malignant neoplasm of unspecified site of left female breast
C50.919	Malignant neoplasm of unspecified site of unspecified female breast
C50.921	Malignant neoplasm of unspecified site of right male breast
C50.922	Malignant neoplasm of unspecified site of left male breast
C50.929	Malignant neoplasm of unspecified site of unspecified male breast
C51.0	Malignant neoplasm of labium majus
C51.1	Malignant neoplasm of labium minus
C51.2	Malignant neoplasm of clitoris
C51.8	Malignant neoplasm of overlapping sites of vulva
C51.9	Malignant neoplasm of vulva, unspecified
C52	Malignant neoplasm of vagina
C53.0	Malignant neoplasm of endocervix
C53.1	Malignant neoplasm of exocervix
C53.8	Malignant neoplasm of overlapping sites of cervix uteri
C53.9	Malignant neoplasm of cervix uteri, unspecified
C54.0	Malignant neoplasm of isthmus uteri
C54.1	Malignant neoplasm of endometrium
C54.2	Malignant neoplasm of myometrium
C54.3	Malignant neoplasm of fundus uteri
C54.8	Malignant neoplasm of overlapping sites of corpus uteri
C54.9	Malignant neoplasm of corpus uteri, unspecified
C55	Malignant neoplasm of uterus, part unspecified
C56.1	Malignant neoplasm of right ovary
C56.2	Malignant neoplasm of left ovary
C56.9	Malignant neoplasm of unspecified ovary
C57.00	Malignant neoplasm of unspecified fallopian tube
C57.01	Malignant neoplasm of right fallopian tube
C57.02	Malignant neoplasm of left fallopian tube
C57.10	Malignant neoplasm of unspecified broad ligament
C57.11	Malignant neoplasm of right broad ligament
C57.12	Malignant neoplasm of left broad ligament
C57.20	Malignant neoplasm of unspecified round ligament
C57.21	Malignant neoplasm of right round ligament
C57.22	Malignant neoplasm of left round ligament
C57.3	Malignant neoplasm of parametrium
C57.4	Malignant neoplasm of uterine adnexa, unspecified
C57.7	Malignant neoplasm of other specified female genital organs
C57.8	Malignant neoplasm of overlapping sites of female genital organs
C57.9	Malignant neoplasm of female genital organ, unspecified
C58	Malignant neoplasm of placenta
C60.0	Malignant neoplasm of prepuce
C60.1	Malignant neoplasm of glans penis
C60.2	Malignant neoplasm of body of penis
C60.8	Malignant neoplasm of overlapping sites of penis
C60.9	Malignant neoplasm of penis, unspecified
C61	Malignant neoplasm of prostate
C62.00	Malignant neoplasm of unspecified undescended testis
C62.01	Malignant neoplasm of undescended right testis

ICD-10-CM	ICD-10-CM Code Descriptor 0037U: Effective Date: 04/01/2018
C62.02	Malignant neoplasm of undescended left testis
C62.10	Malignant neoplasm of unspecified descended testis
C62.11	Malignant neoplasm of descended right testis
C62.12	Malignant neoplasm of descended left testis
C62.90	Malignant neoplasm of unspecified testis, unspecified whether descended or undescended
C62.91	Malignant neoplasm of right testis, unspecified whether descended or undescended
C62.92	Malignant neoplasm of left testis, unspecified whether descended or undescended
C63.00	Malignant neoplasm of unspecified epididymis
C63.01	Malignant neoplasm of right epididymis
C63.02	Malignant neoplasm of left epididymis
C63.10	Malignant neoplasm of unspecified spermatic cord
C63.11	Malignant neoplasm of right spermatic cord
C63.12	Malignant neoplasm of left spermatic cord
C63.2	Malignant neoplasm of scrotum
C63.7	Malignant neoplasm of other specified male genital organs
C63.8	Malignant neoplasm of overlapping sites of male genital organs
C63.9	Malignant neoplasm of male genital organ, unspecified
C64.1	Malignant neoplasm of right kidney, except renal pelvis
C64.2	Malignant neoplasm of left kidney, except renal pelvis
C64.9	Malignant neoplasm of unspecified kidney, except renal pelvis
C65.1	Malignant neoplasm of right renal pelvis
C65.2	Malignant neoplasm of left renal pelvis
C65.9	Malignant neoplasm of unspecified renal pelvis
C66.1	Malignant neoplasm of right ureter
C66.2	Malignant neoplasm of left ureter
C66.9	Malignant neoplasm of unspecified ureter
C67.0	Malignant neoplasm of trigone of bladder
C67.1	Malignant neoplasm of dome of bladder
C67.2	Malignant neoplasm of lateral wall of bladder
C67.3	Malignant neoplasm of anterior wall of bladder
C67.4	Malignant neoplasm of posterior wall of bladder
C67.5	Malignant neoplasm of bladder neck
C67.6	Malignant neoplasm of ureteric orifice
C67.7	Malignant neoplasm of urachus
C67.8	Malignant neoplasm of overlapping sites of bladder
C67.9	Malignant neoplasm of bladder, unspecified
C68.0	Malignant neoplasm of urethra
C68.1	Malignant neoplasm of paraurethral glands
C68.8	Malignant neoplasm of overlapping sites of urinary organs
C68.9	Malignant neoplasm of urinary organ, unspecified
C69.00	Malignant neoplasm of unspecified conjunctiva
C69.01	Malignant neoplasm of right conjunctiva
C69.02	Malignant neoplasm of left conjunctiva
C69.10	Malignant neoplasm of unspecified cornea
C69.11	Malignant neoplasm of right cornea
C69.12	Malignant neoplasm of left cornea
C69.20	Malignant neoplasm of unspecified retina
C69.21	Malignant neoplasm of right retina
C69.22	Malignant neoplasm of left retina
C69.30	Malignant neoplasm of unspecified choroid
C69.31	Malignant neoplasm of right choroid
C69.32	Malignant neoplasm of left choroid
C69.40	Malignant neoplasm of unspecified ciliary body
C69.41	Malignant neoplasm of right ciliary body
C69.42	Malignant neoplasm of left ciliary body
C69.50	Malignant neoplasm of unspecified lacrimal gland and duct
C69.51	Malignant neoplasm of right lacrimal gland and duct
C69.52	Malignant neoplasm of left lacrimal gland and duct
C69.60	Malignant neoplasm of unspecified orbit
C69.61	Malignant neoplasm of right orbit
C69.62	Malignant neoplasm of left orbit

ICD-10-CM	ICD-10-CM Code Descriptor 0037U: Effective Date: 04/01/2018
C69.80	Malignant neoplasm of overlapping sites of unspecified eye and adnexa
C69.81	Malignant neoplasm of overlapping sites of right eye and adnexa
C69.82	Malignant neoplasm of overlapping sites of left eye and adnexa
C69.90	Malignant neoplasm of unspecified site of unspecified eye
C69.91	Malignant neoplasm of unspecified site of right eye
C69.92	Malignant neoplasm of unspecified site of left eye
C70.0	Malignant neoplasm of cerebral meninges
C70.1	Malignant neoplasm of spinal meninges
C70.9	Malignant neoplasm of meninges, unspecified
C71.0	Malignant neoplasm of cerebrum, except lobes and ventricles
C71.1	Malignant neoplasm of frontal lobe
C71.2	Malignant neoplasm of temporal lobe
C71.3	Malignant neoplasm of parietal lobe
C71.4	Malignant neoplasm of occipital lobe
C71.5	Malignant neoplasm of cerebral ventricle
C71.6	Malignant neoplasm of cerebellum
C71.7	Malignant neoplasm of brain stem
C71.8	Malignant neoplasm of overlapping sites of brain
C71.9	Malignant neoplasm of brain, unspecified
C72.0	Malignant neoplasm of spinal cord
C72.1	Malignant neoplasm of cauda equina
C72.20	Malignant neoplasm of unspecified olfactory nerve
C72.21	Malignant neoplasm of right olfactory nerve
C72.22	Malignant neoplasm of left olfactory nerve
C72.30	Malignant neoplasm of unspecified optic nerve
C72.31	Malignant neoplasm of right optic nerve
C72.32	Malignant neoplasm of left optic nerve
C72.40	Malignant neoplasm of unspecified acoustic nerve
C72.41	Malignant neoplasm of right acoustic nerve
C72.42	Malignant neoplasm of left acoustic nerve
C72.50	Malignant neoplasm of unspecified cranial nerve
C72.59	Malignant neoplasm of other cranial nerves
C72.9	Malignant neoplasm of central nervous system, unspecified
C73	Malignant neoplasm of thyroid gland
C74.00	Malignant neoplasm of cortex of unspecified adrenal gland
C74.01	Malignant neoplasm of cortex of right adrenal gland
C74.02	Malignant neoplasm of cortex of left adrenal gland
C74.10	Malignant neoplasm of medulla of unspecified adrenal gland
C74.11	Malignant neoplasm of medulla of right adrenal gland
C74.12	Malignant neoplasm of medulla of left adrenal gland
C74.90	Malignant neoplasm of unspecified part of unspecified adrenal gland
C74.91	Malignant neoplasm of unspecified part of right adrenal gland
C74.92	Malignant neoplasm of unspecified part of left adrenal gland
C75.0	Malignant neoplasm of parathyroid gland
C75.1	Malignant neoplasm of pituitary gland
C75.2	Malignant neoplasm of craniopharyngeal duct
C75.3	Malignant neoplasm of pineal gland
C75.4	Malignant neoplasm of carotid body
C75.5	Malignant neoplasm of aortic body and other paraganglia
C75.8	Malignant neoplasm with pluriglandular involvement, unspecified
C75.9	Malignant neoplasm of endocrine gland, unspecified
C76.0	Malignant neoplasm of head, face and neck
C76.1	Malignant neoplasm of thorax
C76.2	Malignant neoplasm of abdomen
C76.3	Malignant neoplasm of pelvis
C76.40	Malignant neoplasm of unspecified upper limb
C76.41	Malignant neoplasm of right upper limb
C76.42	Malignant neoplasm of left upper limb
C76.50	Malignant neoplasm of unspecified lower limb
C76.51	Malignant neoplasm of right lower limb
C76.52	Malignant neoplasm of left lower limb
C76.8	Malignant neoplasm of other specified ill-defined sites
C7A.00	Malignant carcinoid tumor of unspecified site

ICD-10-CM	ICD-10-CM Code Descriptor 0037U: Effective Date: 04/01/2018
C7A.010	Malignant carcinoid tumor of the duodenum
C7A.011	Malignant carcinoid tumor of the jejunum
C7A.012	Malignant carcinoid tumor of the ileum
C7A.019	Malignant carcinoid tumor of the small intestine, unspecified portion
C7A.020	Malignant carcinoid tumor of the appendix
C7A.021	Malignant carcinoid tumor of the cecum
C7A.022	Malignant carcinoid tumor of the ascending colon
C7A.023	Malignant carcinoid tumor of the transverse colon
C7A.024	Malignant carcinoid tumor of the descending colon
C7A.025	Malignant carcinoid tumor of the sigmoid colon
C7A.026	Malignant carcinoid tumor of the rectum
C7A.029	Malignant carcinoid tumor of the large intestine, unspecified portion
C7A.090	Malignant carcinoid tumor of the bronchus and lung
C7A.091	Malignant carcinoid tumor of the thymus
C7A.092	Malignant carcinoid tumor of the stomach
C7A.093	Malignant carcinoid tumor of the kidney
C7A.094	Malignant carcinoid tumor of the foregut, unspecified
C7A.095	Malignant carcinoid tumor of the midgut, unspecified
C7A.096	Malignant carcinoid tumor of the hindgut, unspecified
C7A.098	Malignant carcinoid tumors of other sites
C7A.1	Malignant poorly differentiated neuroendocrine tumors
C7A.8	Other malignant neuroendocrine tumors
C80.0	Disseminated malignant neoplasm, unspecified
C80.1	Malignant (primary) neoplasm, unspecified
C80.2	Malignant neoplasm associated with transplanted organ

ICD-10-CM	ICD-10-CM Code Descriptor 0022U: Effective Date: 03/16/2018
C33	Malignant neoplasm of trachea
C34.00	Malignant neoplasm of unspecified main bronchus
C34.01	Malignant neoplasm of right main bronchus
C34.02	Malignant neoplasm of left main bronchus
C34.10	Malignant neoplasm of upper lobe, unspecified bronchus or lung
C34.11	Malignant neoplasm of upper lobe, right bronchus or lung
C34.12	Malignant neoplasm of upper lobe, left bronchus or lung
C34.2	Malignant neoplasm of middle lobe, bronchus or lung
C34.30	Malignant neoplasm of lower lobe, unspecified bronchus or lung
C34.31	Malignant neoplasm of lower lobe, right bronchus or lung
C34.32	Malignant neoplasm of lower lobe, left bronchus or lung
C34.80	Malignant neoplasm of overlapping sites of unspecified bronchus and lung
C34.81	Malignant neoplasm of overlapping sites of right bronchus and lung
C34.82	Malignant neoplasm of overlapping sites of left bronchus and lung
C34.90	Malignant neoplasm of unspecified part of unspecified bronchus or lung
C34.91	Malignant neoplasm of unspecified part of right bronchus or lung
C34.92	Malignant neoplasm of unspecified part of left bronchus or lung

100-03, 100.1

100.1 - Bariatric Surgery for Treatment of Co-Morbid Conditions Related to Morbid Obesity

(Rev.158, Issued: 12-23-13, Effective: 09-24-13, Implementation: 12-17-13)

Please note, sections 40.5, 100.8, 100.11, and 100.14 have been removed from the National Coverage Determination (NCD) Manual and incorporated into NCD 100.1.

A. General

Obesity may be caused by medical conditions such as hypothyroidism, Cushing's disease, and hypothalamic lesions, or can aggravate a number of cardiac and respiratory diseases as well as diabetes and hypertension. Non-surgical services in connection with the treatment of obesity are covered when such services are an integral and necessary part of a course of treatment for one of these medical conditions.

In addition, supplemented fasting is a type of very low calorie weight reduction regimen used to achieve rapid weight loss. The reduced calorie intake is supplemented by a mixture of protein, carbohydrates, vitamins, and minerals. Serious questions exist about the safety of prolonged adherence for 2 months or more to a very low calorie weight reduction regimen as a general treatment for obesity,

because of instances of cardiopathology and sudden death, as well as possible loss of body protein.

Bariatric surgery procedures are performed to treat comorbid conditions associated with morbid obesity. Two types of surgical procedures are employed. Malabsorptive procedures divert food from the stomach to a lower part of the digestive tract where the normal mixing of digestive fluids and absorption of nutrients cannot occur. Restrictive procedures restrict the size of the stomach and decrease intake. Surgery can combine both types of procedures.

The following are descriptions of bariatric surgery procedures:

1. Roux-en-Y Gastric Bypass (RYGBP)

   The RYGBP achieves weight loss by gastric restriction and malabsorption. Reduction of the stomach to a small gastric pouch (30 cc) results in feelings of satiety following even small meals. This small pouch is connected to a segment of the jejunum, bypassing the duodenum and very proximal small intestine, thereby reducing absorption. RYGBP procedures can be open or laparoscopic.

2. Biliopancreatic Diversion with Duodenal Switch (BPD/DS) or Gastric Reduction Duodenal Switch (BPD/GRDS)

   The BPD achieves weight loss by gastric restriction and malabsorption. The stomach is partially resected, but the remaining capacity is generous compared to that achieved with RYGBP. As such, patients eat relatively normal-sized meals and do not need to restrict intake radically, since the most proximal areas of the small intestine (i.e., the duodenum and jejunum) are bypassed, and substantial malabsorption occurs. The partial BPD/DS or BPD/GRDS is a variant of the BPD procedure. It involves resection of the greater curvature of the stomach, preservation of the pyloric sphincter, and transection of the duodenum above the ampulla of Vater with a duodeno-ileal anastomosis and a lower ileo-ileal anastomosis. BPD/DS or BPD/GRDS procedures can be open or laparoscopic.

3. Adjustable Gastric Banding (AGB)

   The AGB achieves weight loss by gastric restriction only. A band creating a gastric pouch with a capacity of approximately 15 to 30 cc's encircles the uppermost portion of the stomach. The band is an inflatable doughnut-shaped balloon, the diameter of which can be adjusted in the clinic by adding or removing saline via a port that is positioned beneath the skin. The bands are adjustable, allowing the size of the gastric outlet to be modified as needed, depending on the rate of a patient's weight loss. AGB procedures are laparoscopic only.

4. Sleeve Gastrectomy

   Sleeve gastrectomy is a 70%-80% greater curvature gastrectomy (sleeve resection of the stomach) with continuity of the gastric lesser curve being maintained while simultaneously reducing stomach volume. In the past, sleeve gastrectomy was the first step in a two-stage procedure when performing RYGBP, but more recently has been offered as a stand-alone surgery. Sleeve gastrectomy procedures can be open or laparoscopic.

5. Vertical Gastric Banding (VGB)

   The VGB achieves weight loss by gastric restriction only. The upper part of the stomach is stapled, creating a narrow gastric inlet or pouch that remains connected with the remainder of the stomach. In addition, a non-adjustable band is placed around this new inlet in an attempt to prevent future enlargement of the stoma (opening). As a result, patients experience a sense of fullness after eating small meals. Weight loss from this procedure results entirely from eating less. VGB procedures are essentially no longer performed.

B. Nationally Covered Indications

Effective for services performed on and after February 21, 2006, Open and laparoscopic Roux-en-Y gastric bypass (RYGBP), open and laparoscopic Biliopancreatic Diversion with Duodenal Switch (BPD/DS) or Gastric Reduction Duodenal Switch (BPD/GRDS), and laparoscopic adjustable gastric banding (LAGB) are covered for Medicare beneficiaries who have a body-mass index = 35, have at least one co-morbidity related to obesity, and have been previously unsuccessful with medical treatment for obesity.

Effective for dates of service on and after February 21, 2006, these procedures are only covered when performed at facilities that are: (1) certified by the American College of Surgeons as a Level 1 Bariatric Surgery Center (program standards and requirements in effect on February 15, 2006); or (2) certified by the American Society for Bariatric Surgery as a Bariatric Surgery Center of Excellence (program standards and requirements in effect on February 15, 2006). Effective for dates of service on and after September 24, 2013, facilities are no longer required to be certified.

Effective for services performed on and after February 12, 2009, the Centers for Medicare & Medicaid Services (CMS) determines that Type 2 diabetes mellitus is a co-morbidity for purposes of this NCD.

A list of approved facilities and their approval dates are listed and maintained on the CMS Coverage Web site at http://www.cms.gov/Medicare/Medicare-General-Information/MedicareApprovedFacilitie/Bariatric-Surgery.html, and published in the Federal Register for services provided up to and including date of service September 23, 2013.

C. Nationally Non-Covered Indications

Treatments for obesity alone remain non-covered.

Supplemented fasting is not covered under the Medicare program as a general treatment for obesity (see section D. below for discretionary local coverage).

The following bariatric surgery procedures are non-covered for all Medicare beneficiaries:

- Open adjustable gastric banding;
- Open sleeve gastrectomy;
- Laparoscopic sleeve gastrectomy (prior to June 27, 2012);
- Open and laparoscopic vertical banded gastroplasty;
- Intestinal bypass surgery; and,
- Gastric balloon for treatment of obesity.

D. Other

Effective for services performed on and after June 27, 2012, Medicare Administrative Contractors (MACs) acting within their respective jurisdictions may determine coverage of stand-alone laparoscopic sleeve gastrectomy (LSG) for the treatment of co-morbid conditions related to obesity in Medicare beneficiaries only when all of the following conditions a.-c. are satisfied.

a. The beneficiary has a body-mass index (BMI) = 35 kg/m2,

b. The beneficiary has at least one co-morbidity related to obesity, and,

c. The beneficiary has been previously unsuccessful with medical treatment for obesity.

The determination of coverage for any bariatric surgery procedures that are not specifically identified in an NCD as covered or non-covered, for Medicare beneficiaries who have a body-mass index = 35, have at least one co-morbidity related to obesity, and have been previously unsuccessful with medical treatment for obesity, is left to the local MACs.

Where weight loss is necessary before surgery in order to ameliorate the complications posed by obesity when it coexists with pathological conditions such as cardiac and respiratory diseases, diabetes, or hypertension (and other more conservative techniques to achieve this end are not regarded as appropriate), supplemented fasting with adequate monitoring of the patient is eligible for coverage on a case-by-case basis or pursuant to a local coverage determination. The risks associated with the achievement of rapid weight loss must be carefully balanced against the risk posed by the condition requiring surgical treatment.

100-03, 100.5

NCD for Diagnostic Breath Analyses (100.5)

(Rev. 1, 10-03-03)

The Following Breath Test is Covered:

- Lactose breath hydrogen to detect lactose malabsorption.

The Following Breath Tests are Excluded from Coverage;

- Lactulose breath hydrogen for diagnosing small bowel bacterial overgrowth and measuring small bowel transit time.
- CO_2 for diagnosing bile acid malabsorption.
- CO_2 for diagnosing fat malabsorption.

100-03, 100.13

NCD for Laparoscopic Cholecystectomy (100.13)

(Rev. 173, Issued: 09-04-14, Effective: Upon Implementation: of ICD-10)

Laparoscopic cholecystectomy is a covered surgical procedure in which a diseased gall bladder is removed through the use of instruments introduced via cannulae, with vision of the operative field maintained by use of a high-resolution television camera-monitor system (video laparoscope). For inpatient claims, use ICD-9-CM code 51.23, Laparoscopic cholecystectomy. For all other claims, use CPT codes 49310 for laparoscopy, surgical; cholecystectomy (any method), and 49311 for laparoscopy, surgical: cholecystectomy with cholangiography.

100-03, 110.1

NCD for Hyperthermia for Treatment of Cancer (110.1)

(Rev. 1, 10-03-03)

Local hyperthermia is covered under Medicare when used in connection with radiation therapy for the treatment of primary or metastatic cutaneous or subcutaneous superficial malignancies. It is not covered when used alone or in connection with chemotherapy.

100-03, 110.2

NCD for Certain Drugs Distributed by the National Cancer Institute (110.2)

(Rev. 173, Issued: 09-04-14, Effective: Upon Implementation: of ICD-10)

Under its Cancer Therapy Evaluation, the Division of Cancer Treatment of the National Cancer Institute (NCI), in cooperation with the Food and Drug Administration, approves and distributes certain drugs for use in treating terminally ill cancer patients. One group of these drugs, designated as Group C drugs, unlike other drugs distributed by the NCI, is not limited to use in clinical trials for the purpose of testing their efficacy. Drugs are classified as Group C drugs only if there is sufficient evidence demonstrating their efficacy within a tumor type and that they can be safely administered.

A physician is eligible to receive Group C drugs from the Divison of Cancer Treatment only if the following requirements are met:

- A physician must be registered with the NCI as an investigator by having completed an FD-Form 1573;
- A written request for the drug, indicating the disease to be treated, must be submitted to the NCI;
- The use of the drug must be limited to indications outlined in the NCI's guidelines; and
- All adverse reactions must be reported to the Investigational Drug Branch of the Division of Cancer Treatment.

In view of these NCI controls on distribution and use of Group C drugs, A/B Medicare Adminstrative Contractors (MACs) may assume, in the absence of evidence to the contrary, that a Group C drug and the related hospital stay are covered if all other applicable coverage requirements are satisfied.

If there is reason to question coverage in a particular case, the matter should be resolved with the assistance of the Quality Improvement Organization (QIO), or if there is none, the assistance of the MAC's medical consultants.

Information regarding those drugs which are classified as Group C drugs may be obtained from:

Chief, Investigational Drug Branch
Cancer Therapy Evaluation Program
Executive Plaza North, Suite 7134
National Cancer Institute
Rockville, Maryland 20852-7426

100-03, 110.4

Extracorporeal Photopheresis

(Rev.143, Issued: 05-18-12, Effective: 04-30-12, Implementation: 10-01-12)

A. General

Extracorporeal photopheresis is a medical procedure in which a patient's white blood cells are exposed first to a drug called 8-methoxypsoralen (8-MOP) and then to ultraviolet A (UVA) light. The procedure starts with the removal of the patient's blood, which is centrifuged to isolate the white blood cells. The drug is typically administered directly to the white blood cells after they have been removed from the patient (referred to as ex vivo administration) but the drug can alternatively be administered directly to the patient before the white blood cells are withdrawn. After UVA light exposure, the treated white blood cells are then re-infused into the patient.

B. Nationally Covered Indications

The Centers for Medicare & Medicaid Services (CMS) has determined that extracorporeal photopheresis is reasonable and necessary under §1862(a)(1)(A) of the Social Security Act (the Act) under the following circumstances:

1. Effective April 8, 1988, Medicare provides coverage for:

   Palliative treatment of skin manifestations of cutaneous T-cell lymphoma that has not responded to other therapy.

2. Effective December 19, 2006, Medicare also provides coverage for:

   Patients with acute cardiac allograft rejection whose disease is refractory to standard immunosuppressive drug treatment; and,

   Patients with chronic graft versus host disease whose disease is refractory to standard immunosuppressive drug treatment.

3. Effective April 30, 2012, Medicare also provides coverage for:

   Extracorporeal photopheresis for the treatment of bronchiolitis obliterans syndrome (BOS) following lung allograft transplantation only when extracorporeal photopheresis is provided under a clinical research study that meets the following conditions:

   The clinical research study meets the requirements specified below to assess the effect of extracorporeal photopheresis for the treatment of BOS following lung allograft transplantation. The clinical study must address one or more aspects of the following question:

   Prospectively, do Medicare beneficiaries who have received lung allografts, developed BOS refractory to standard immunosuppressive therapy, and received extracorporeal photopheresis , experience improved patient-centered health outcomes as indicated by:

   a. improved forced expiratory volume in one second (FEV1);

   b. improved survival after transplant; and/or,

   c. improved quality of life?

   The required clinical study must adhere to the following standards of scientific integrity and relevance to the Medicare population:

   a. The principal purpose of the research study is to test whether extracorporeal photopheresis potentially improves the participants' health outcomes.

   b. The research study is well supported by available scientific and medical information or it is intended to clarify or establish the health outcomes of interventions already in common clinical use.

   c. The research study does not unjustifiably duplicate existing studies.

d. The research study design is appropriate to answer the research question being asked in the study.

e. The research study is sponsored by an organization or individual capable of successfully executing the proposed study.

f. The research study is in compliance with all applicable Federal regulations concerning the protection of human subjects found at 45 CFR Part 46. If a study is regulated by the Food and Drug Administration (FDA), it must also be in compliance with 21 CFR parts 50 and 56.

g. All aspects of the research study are conducted according to appropriate standards of scientific integrity (see http://www.icmje.org).

h. The research study has a written protocol that clearly addresses, or incorporates by reference, the standards listed here as Medicare requirements for coverage with evidence development.

i. The clinical research study is not designed to exclusively test toxicity or disease pathophysiology in healthy individuals. Trials of all medical technologies measuring therapeutic outcomes as one of the objectives meet this standard only if the disease or condition being studied is life threatening as defined in 21 CFR § 312.81(a) and the patient has no other viable treatment options.

j. The clinical research study is registered on the ClinicalTrials.gov website by the principal sponsor/investigator prior to the enrollment of the first study subject.

k. The research study protocol specifies the method and timing of public release of all prespecified outcomes to be measured including release of outcomes if outcomes are negative or study is terminated early. The results must be made public within 24 months of the end of data collection. If a report is planned to be published in a peer-reviewed journal, then that initial release may be an abstract that meets the requirements of the International Committee of Medical Journal Editors (http://www.icmje.org).

l. The research study protocol must explicitly discuss subpopulations affected by the treatment under investigation, particularly traditionally underrepresented groups in clinical studies, how the inclusion and exclusion criteria effect enrollment of these populations, and a plan for the retention and reporting of said populations on the trial. If the inclusion and exclusion criteria are expected to have a negative effect on the recruitment or retention of underrepresented populations, the protocol must discuss why these criteria are necessary.

m. The research study protocol explicitly discusses how the results are or are not expected to be generalizable to the Medicare population to infer whether Medicare patients may benefit from the intervention. Separate discussions in the protocol may be necessary for populations eligible for Medicare due to age, disability or Medicaid eligibility.

Consistent with section 1142 of the Act, the Agency for Healthcare Research and Quality supports clinical research studies that CMS determines meet the above-listed standards and address the above-listed research questions.

Any clinical study under which there is coverage of extracorporeal photopheresis for this indication pursuant to this national coverage determination (NCD) must be approved by April 30, 2014. If there are no approved clinical studies on this date, this NCD will expire and coverage of extracorporeal photopheresis for BOS will revert to the coverage policy in effect prior to the issuance of the final decision memorandum for this NCD.

C. Nationally Non-Covered Indications

All other indications for extracorporeal photopheresis not otherwise indicated above as covered remain non-covered.

D. Other

Claims processing instructions can be found in chapter 32, section 190 of the Medicare Claims Processing Manual.

(This NCD last reviewed April 2012.)

100-03, 110.6

NCD for Scalp Hypothermia During Chemotherapy, to Prevent Hair Loss (110.6)

(Rev. 1, 10-03-03)

While ice-filled bags or bandages or other devices used for scalp hypothermia during chemotherapy may be covered as supplies of the kind commonly furnished without a separate charge, no separate charge for them would be recognized.

100-03, 110.7

NCD for Blood Transfusions (110.7)

(Rev. 1, 10-03-03)

Blood transfusions are used to restore blood volume after hemorrhage, to improve the oxygen carrying capacity of blood in severe anemia, and to combat shock in acute hemolytic anemia.

A. Definitions

1. Homologous Blood Transfusion

Homologous blood transfusion is the infusion of blood or blood components that have been collected from the general public.

2. Autologous Blood Transfusion

An autologous blood transfusion is the precollection and subsequent infusion of a patient's own blood.

3. Donor Directed Blood Transfusion

A donor directed blood transfusion is the infusion of blood or blood components that have been precollected from a specific individual(s) other than the patient and subsequently infused into the specific patient for whom the blood is designated. For example, patient B's brother predeposits his blood for use by patient B during upcoming surgery.

4. Perioperative Blood Salvage

Perioperative blood salvage is the collection and reinfusion of blood lost during and immediately after surgery.

B. Policy Governing Transfusions

For Medicare coverage purposes, it is important to distinguish between a transfusion itself and preoperative blood services; e.g., collection, processing, storage. Medically necessary transfusion of blood, regardless of the type, may generally be a covered service under both Part A and Part B of Medicare. Coverage does not make a distinction between the transfusion of homologous, autologous, or donor-directed blood. With respect to the coverage of the services associated with the preoperative collection, processing, and storage of autologous and donor-directed blood, the following policies apply.

1. Hospital Part A and B Coverage and Payment

Under Sec.1862(a)(14) of the Act, non-physician services furnished to hospital patients are covered and paid for as hospital services. As provided in Sec.1886 of the Act, under the prospective [payment system (PPS), the diagnosis related group (DRG) payment to the hospital includes all covered blood and blood processing expenses, whether or not the blood is eventually used.

Under its provider agreement, a hospital is required to furnish or arrange for all covered services furnished to hospital patients. medicare payment is made to the hospital, under PPS or cost reimbursement, for covered inpatient services, and it is intended to reflect payment for all costs of furnishing those services.

2. Nonhospital Part B Coverage

Under Part B, to be eligible for separate coverage, a service must fit the definition of one of the services authorized by Sec.1832 of the Act. These services are defined in 42 CFR 410.10 and do not include a separate category for a supplier's services associated with blood donation services, either autologous or donor-directed. That is, the collection, processing, and storage of blood for later transfusion into the beneficiary is not recognized as a separate service under Part B. Therefore, there is no avenue through which a blood supplier can receive direct payment under Part B for blood donation services.

C. Perioperative Blood Salvage

When the perioperative blood salvage process is used in surgery on a hospital patient, payment made to the hospital (under PPS or through cost reimbursement) for the procedure in which that process is used is intended to encompass payment for all costs relating to that process.

100-03, 110.8

NCD for Blood Platelet Transfusions (110.8)

(Rev. 1, 10-03-03)

Blood platelet transplants are safe and effective for the correction of thrombocytopenia and other blood defects. It is covered under Medicare when treatment is reasonable and necessary for the individual patient.

100-03, 110.9

NCD for Antigens Prepared for Sublingual Administration (110.9)

(Rev. 1, 10-03-03)

For antigens provided to patients on or after November 17, 1996, Medicare does not cover such antigens if they are to be administered sublingually, i.e., by placing drops under the patient's tongue. This kind of allergy therapy has not been proven to be safe and effective. Antigens are covered only if they are administered by injection.

100-03, 110.12

NCD for Challenge Ingestion Food Testing (110.12)

(Rev. 1, 10-03-03)

This procedure is covered when it is used on an outpatient basis if it is reasonable and necessary for the individual patient.

Challenge ingestion food testing has not been proven to be effective in the diagnosis of rheumatoid arthritis, depression, or respiratory disorders. Accordingly, its use in the diagnosis of these conditions is not reasonable and necessary within the meaning of section 1862(a)(1) of the Medicare law, and no program payment is made for this procedure when it is so used.

100-03, 110.14

NCD for Apheresis (Therapeutic Pheresis) (110.14)

(Rev. 1, 10-03-03)

A. General

Apheresis (also known as pheresis or therapeutic pheresis) is a medical procedure utilizing specialized equipment to remove selected blood constituents (plasma, leukocytes, plataelets, or cells) from whole blood. The remainder is retransfused into the person from whom the blood was taken.

For purposes of Medicare coverage, apheresis is defined as an autologous procedure, i.e., blood is taken from the patient, processed, and returned to the patient as part of a continuous procedure (as distinguished from the procedure in which a patient donates blood preoperatively and is transfused with the donated blood at a later date).

B. Indications

Apheresis is covered for the following indications:

- Plasma exchange for acquired myasthenia gravis;
- Leukapheresis in the treatment of leukemekia
- Plasmapheresis in the treatment of primary macroglobulinemia (Waldenstrom);
- Treatment of hyperglobulinemias, including (but not limited to) multiple myelomas, cryoglobulinemia and hyperviscosity syndromes;
- Plasmapheresis or plasma exchange as a last resort treatment of thromobotic thrombocytopenic purpura (TTP);
- Plasmapheresis or plasma exchange in the last resort treatment of life threatening rheumatoid vasculitis;
- Plasma perfusion of charcoal filters for treatment of pruritis of cholestatic liver disease;
- Plasma exchange in the treatment of Goodpasture's Syndrome;
- Plasma exchange in the treatment of glomerulonephritis associated with antiglomerular basement membrane antibodies and advancing renal failure or pulmonary hemorrhage;
- Treatment of chronic relapsing polyneuropathy for patients with severe or life threatening symptoms who have failed to respond to conventional therapy;
- Treatment of life threatening scleroderma and polymyositis when the patient is unresponsive to conventional therapy;
- Treatment of Guillain-Barre Syndrome; and
- Treatment of last resort for life threatening systemic lupus erythematosus (SLE) when conventional therapy has failed to prevent clinical deterioration.

C. Settings

Apheresis is covered only when performed in a hospital setting (either inpatient or outpatient). or in a nonhospital setting. e.g. physician directed clinic when the following conditions are met:

- A physician (or a number of physicians) is present to perform medical services and to respond to medical emergencies at all times during patient care hours;
- Each patient is under the care of a physician; and
- All nonphysician services are furnished under the direct, personal supervision of a physician.

100-03, 110.16

NCD for Nonselective (Random) Transfusions and Living Related Donor Specific Transfusions (DST) in Kidney Transplantation (110.16)

(Rev. 1, 10-03-03)

These pretransplant transfusions are covered under Medicare without a specific limitation on the number of transfusions, subject to the normal Medicare blood deductible provisions. Where blood is given directly to the transplant patient; e.g., in the case of donor specific transfusions, the blood is considered replaced for purposes of the blood deductible provisions.

100-03, 110.23

Stem Cell Transplantation (Formerly 110.8.1) (Various Effective Dates Below)

(Rev. 193, Issued; 07-01-16, Effective: 01-27-16, Implementation: 10-03-16)

A. General

Stem cell transplantation is a process in which stem cells are harvested from either a patient's (autologous) or donor's (allogeneic) bone marrow or peripheral blood for intravenous infusion. Autologous stem cell transplantation (AuSCT) is a technique for restoring stem cells using the patient's own previously stored cells. AuSCT must be used to effect hematopoietic reconstitution following severely myelotoxic doses of chemotherapy (HDCT) and/or radiotherapy used to treat various malignancies. Allogeneic hematopoietic stem cell transplantation (HSCT) is a procedure in which a portion of a healthy donor's stem cell or bone marrow is obtained and prepared for intravenous infusion. Allogeneic HSCT may be used to restore function in recipients having an inherited or acquired deficiency or defect. Hematopoietic stem cells are

multi-potent stem cells that give rise to all the blood cell types; these stem cells form blood and immune cells. A hematopoietic stem cell is a cell isolated from blood or bone marrow that can renew itself, differentiate to a variety of specialized cells, can mobilize out of the bone marrow into circulating blood, and can undergo programmed cell death, called apoptosis - a process by which cells that are unneeded or detrimental will self-destruct.

The Centers for Medicare & Medicaid Services (CMS) is clarifying that bone marrow and peripheral blood stem cell transplantation is a process which includes mobilization, harvesting, and transplant of bone marrow or peripheral blood stem cells and the administration of high dose chemotherapy or radiotherapy prior to the actual transplant. When bone marrow or peripheral blood stem cell transplantation is covered, all necessary steps are included in coverage. When bone marrow or peripheral blood stem cell transplantation is non-covered, none of the steps are covered.

B. Nationally Covered Indications

I. Allogeneic Hematopoietic Stem Cell Transplantation (HSCT)

   a) Effective for services performed on or after August 1, 1978, for the treatment of leukemia, leukemia in remission, or aplastic anemia when it is reasonable and necessary,

   b) Effective for services performed on or after June 3, 1985, for the treatment of severe combined immunodeficiency disease (SCID) and for the treatment of Wiskott-Aldrich syndrome.

   c) Effective for services performed on or after August 4, 2010, for the treatment of Myelodysplastic Syndromes (MDS) pursuant to Coverage with Evidence Development (CED) in the context of a Medicare-approved, prospective clinical study.

MDS refers to a group of diverse blood disorders in which the bone marrow does not produce enough healthy, functioning blood cells. These disorders are varied with regard to clinical characteristics, cytologic and pathologic features, and cytogenetics. The abnormal production of blood cells in the bone marrow leads to low blood cell counts, referred to as cytopenias, which are a hallmark feature of MDS along with a dysplastic and hypercellular-appearing bone marrow

Medicare payment for these beneficiaries will be restricted to patients enrolled in an approved clinical study. In accordance with the Stem Cell Therapeutic and Research Act of 2005 (US Public Law 109-129) a standard dataset is collected for all allogeneic transplant patients in the United States by the Center for International Blood and Marrow Transplant Research. The elements in this dataset, comprised of two mandatory forms plus one additional form, encompass the information we require for a study under CED.

A prospective clinical study seeking Medicare payment for treating a beneficiary with allogeneic HSCT for MDS pursuant to CED must meet one or more aspects of the following questions:

1. Prospectively, compared to Medicare beneficiaries with MDS who do not receive HSCT, do Medicare beneficiaries with MDS who receive HSCT have improved outcomes as indicated by:

   – Relapse-free mortality,
   – progression free survival,
   – relapse, and
   – overall survival?

2. Prospectively, in Medicare beneficiaries with MDS who receive HSCT, how do International Prognostic Scoring System (IPSS) scores, patient age, cytopenias, and comorbidities predict the following outcomes:

   – Relapse-free mortality,
   – progression free survival,
   – relapse, and
   – overall survival?

3. Prospectively, in Medicare beneficiaries with MDS who receive HSCT, what treatment facility characteristics predict meaningful clinical improvement in the following outcomes:

   – Relapse-free mortality,
   – progression free survival,
   – relapse, and
   – overall survival?

In addition, the clinical study must adhere to the following standards of scientific integrity and relevance to the Medicare population:

a. The principal purpose of the research study is to test whether a particular intervention potentially improves the participants' health outcomes.

b. The research study is well supported by available scientific and medical information or it is intended to clarify or establish the health outcomes of interventions already in common clinical use.

c. The research study does not unjustifiably duplicate existing studies.

d. The research study design is appropriate to answer the research question being asked in the study.

e. The research study is sponsored by an organization or individual capable of executing the proposed study successfully.

f. The research study is in compliance with all applicable Federal regulations concerning the protection of human subjects found at 45 CFR Part 46. If a study is regulated by the Food and Drug Administration (FDA), it must be in compliance with 21 CFR parts 50 and 56.

g. All aspects of the research study are conducted according to appropriate standards of scientific integrity (see http://www.icmje.org).

h. The research study has a written protocol that clearly addresses, or incorporates by reference, the standards listed here as Medicare requirements for CED coverage.

i. The clinical research study is not designed to exclusively test toxicity or disease pathophysiology in healthy individuals. Trials of all medical technologies measuring therapeutic outcomes as one of the objectives meet this standard only if the disease or condition being studied is life threatening as defined in 21 CFR §312.81(a) and the patient has no other viable treatment options.

j. The clinical research study is registered on the ClinicalTrials.gov Web site by the principal sponsor/investigator prior to the enrollment of the first study subject.

k. The research study protocol specifies the method and timing of public release of all pre-specified outcomes to be measured including release of outcomes if outcomes are negative or study is terminated early. The results must be made public within 24 months of the end of data collection. If a report is planned to be published in a peer-reviewed journal, then that initial release may be an abstract that meets the requirements of the International Committee of Medical Journal Editors (http://www.icmje.org). However a full report of the outcomes must be made public no later than 3 years after the end of data collection.

l. The research study protocol must explicitly discuss subpopulations affected by the treatment under investigation, particularly traditionally underrepresented groups in clinical studies, how the inclusion and exclusion criteria effect enrollment of these populations, and a plan for the retention and reporting of said populations on the trial. If the inclusion and exclusion criteria are expected to have a negative effect on the recruitment or retention of underrepresented populations, the protocol must discuss why these criteria are necessary.

m. The research study protocol explicitly discusses how the results are or are not expected to be generalizable to the Medicare population to infer whether Medicare patients may benefit from the intervention. Separate discussions in the protocol may be necessary for populations eligible for Medicare due to age, disability or Medicaid eligibility.

Consistent with section 1142 of the Social Security Act, the Agency for Health Research and Quality (AHRQ) supports clinical research studies that CMS determines meet the above-listed standards and address the above-listed research questions.

The clinical research study should also have the following features:

- It should be a prospective, longitudinal study with clinical information from the period before HSCT and short- and long-term follow-up information.
- Outcomes should be measured and compared among pre-specified subgroups within the cohort.
- The study should be powered to make inferences in subgroup analyses.
- Risk stratification methods should be used to control for selection bias. Data elements to be used in risk stratification models should include:

Patient selection:

- Patient Age at diagnosis of MDS and at transplantation
- Date of onset of MDS
- Disease classification (specific MDS subtype at diagnosis prior to preparative/conditioning regimen using World Health Organization (WHO) classifications). Include presence/absence of refractory cytopenias
- Comorbid conditions
- IPSS score (and WHO-adapted Prognostic Scoring System (WPSS) score, if applicable) at diagnosis and prior to transplantation
- Score immediately prior to transplantation and one year post-transplantation
- Disease assessment at diagnosis at start of preparative regimen and last assessment prior to preparative regimen Subtype of MDS (refractory anemia with or without blasts, degree of blasts, etc.)
- Type of preparative/conditioning regimen administered (myeloabalative, non-myeloablative, reduced–intensity conditioning)
- Donor type
- Cell Source

Facilities must submit the required transplant essential data to the Stem Cell Therapeutics Outcomes Database.

d) Effective for claims with dates of service on or after January 27, 2016, allogeneic HSCT for multiple myeloma is covered by Medicare only for beneficiaries with Durie-Salmon Stage II or III multiple myeloma, or International Staging System (ISS) Stage II or Stage III multiple myeloma, and participating in an approved prospective clinical study that meets the criteria below. There must be appropriate statistical techniques to control for selection bias and confounding by age, duration of diagnosis, disease classification, International Myeloma Working Group (IMWG) classification, ISS stage, comorbid conditions, type of preparative/conditioning regimen, graft vs. host disease (GVHD) prophylaxis, donor type and cell source.

A prospective clinical study seeking Medicare coverage for allogeneic HSCT for multiple myeloma pursuant to CED must address the following question:

Compared to patients who do not receive allogeneic HSCT, do Medicare beneficiaries with multiple myeloma who receive allogeneic HSCT have improved outcomes as indicated by:

- Graft vs. host disease (acute and chronic);
- Other transplant-related adverse events;
- Overall survival; and
- (optional) Quality of life?

All CMS-approved clinical studies and registries must adhere to the below listed standards of scientific integrity and relevance to the Medicare population as listed in section g.

e) Effective for claims with dates of service on or after January 27, 2016, allogeneic HSCT for myelofibrosis (MF) is covered by Medicare only for beneficiaries with Dynamic International Prognostic Scoring System (DIPSSplus) intermediate-2 or High primary or secondary MF and participating in an approved prospective clinical study. All Medicare approved studies must use appropriate statistical techniques in the analysis to control for selection bias and potential confounding by age, duration of diagnosis, disease classification, DIPSSplus score, comorbid conditions, type of preparative/conditioning regimen, graft vs. host disease (GVHD) prophylaxis, donor type and cell source.

A prospective clinical study seeking Medicare coverage for allogeneic HSCT for myelofibrosis pursuant to Coverage with Evidence Development (CED) must address the following question:

Compared to patients who do not receive allogeneic HSCT, do Medicare beneficiaries with MF who receive allogeneic HSCT transplantation have improved outcomes as indicated by:

- Graft vs. host disease (acute and chronic);
- Other transplant-related adverse events;
- Overall survival; and
- (optional) Quality of life?

All CMS-approved clinical studies and registries must adhere to the below listed standards of scientific integrity and relevance to the Medicare population as listed in section g.

f) Effective for claims with dates of service on or after January 27, 2016, allogeneic HSCT for sickle cell disease (SCD) is covered by Medicare only for beneficiaries with severe, symptomatic SCD who participate in an approved prospective clinical study.

A prospective clinical study seeking Medicare coverage for allogeneic HSCT for sickle cell disease pursuant to Coverage with Evidence Development (CED) must address the following question:

Compared to patients who do not receive allogeneic HSCT, do Medicare beneficiaries with SCD who receive allogeneic HSCT have improved outcomes as indicated by:

- Graft vs. host disease (acute and chronic),
- Other transplant-related adverse events;
- Overall survival; and
- (optional) Quality of life?

All CMS-approved clinical studies and registries must adhere to the below listed standards of scientific integrity and relevance to the Medicare population listed in section g:

g) All CMS-approved clinical studies and registries in sections d, e and f must adhere to the below listed standards of scientific integrity and relevance to the Medicare population:

a. The principal purpose of the study is to test whether the item or service meaningfully improves health outcomes of affected beneficiaries who are represented by the enrolled subjects.

b. The rationale for the study is well supported by available scientific and medical evidence.

c. The study results are not anticipated to unjustifiably duplicate existing knowledge.

d. The study design is methodologically appropriate and the anticipated number of enrolled subjects is sufficient to answer the research question(s) being asked in the National Coverage Determination.

e. The study is sponsored by an organization or individual capable of completing it successfully.

f. The research study is in compliance with all applicable Federal regulations concerning the protection of human subjects found in the Code of Federal Regulations (CFR) at 45 CFR Part 46. If a study is regulated by the Food and Drug Administration (FDA), it is also in compliance with 21 CFR Parts 50 and 56. In addition, to further enhance the protection of human subjects in studies conducted under CED, the study must provide and obtain meaningful informed consent from patients regarding the risks associated with the study items and/or services, and the use and eventual disposition of the collected data.

g. All aspects of the study are conducted according to appropriate standards of scientific integrity.

h. The study has a written protocol that clearly demonstrates adherence to the standards listed here as Medicare requirements.

i. The study is not designed to exclusively test toxicity or disease pathophysiology in healthy individuals. Such studies may meet this requirement only if the disease or condition being studied is life threatening as defined in 21 CFR §312.81(a) and the patient has no other viable treatment options.

j. The clinical research studies and registries are registered on the www.ClinicalTrials.gov website by the principal sponsor/investigator prior to the enrollment of the first study subject. Registries are also registered in the Agency for Healthcare Quality (AHRQ) Registry of Patient Registries (RoPR).

k. The research study protocol specifies the method and timing of public release of all prespecified outcomes to be measured including release of outcomes if outcomes are negative or study is terminated early. The results must be made public within 12 months of the study's primary completion date, which is the date the final subject had final data collection for the primary endpoint, even if the trial does not achieve its primary aim. The results must include number started/completed, summary results for primary and secondary outcome measures, statistical analyses, and adverse events. Final results must be reported in a publicly accessibly manner; either in a peer-reviewed scientific journal (in print or on-line), in an on-line publicly accessible registry dedicated to the dissemination of clinical trial information such as ClinicalTrials.gov, or in journals willing to publish in abbreviated format (e.g., for studies with negative or incomplete results).

l. The study protocol must explicitly discuss beneficiary subpopulations affected by the item or service under investigation, particularly traditionally underrepresented groups in clinical studies, how the inclusion and exclusion criteria effect enrollment of these populations, and a plan for the retention and reporting of said populations in the trial. If the inclusion and exclusion criteria are expected to have a negative effect on the recruitment or retention of underrepresented populations, the protocol must discuss why these criteria are necessary.

m. The study protocol explicitly discusses how the results are or are not expected to be generalizable to affected beneficiary subpopulations. Separate discussions in the protocol may be necessary for populations eligible for Medicare due to age, disability or Medicaid eligibility.

Consistent with section 1142 of the Act, the Agency for Healthcare Research and Quality (AHRQ) supports clinical research studies that CMS determines meet the above-listed standards and address the above-listed research questions.

II. Autologous Stem Cell Transplantation (AuSCT)

a) Effective for services performed on or after April 28, 1989, AuSCT is considered reasonable and necessary under §1862(a)(1)(A) of the Act for the following conditions and is covered under Medicare for patients with:

1. Acute leukemia in remission who have a high probability of relapse and who have no human leucocyte antigens (HLA)-matched;

2. Resistant non-Hodgkin's lymphomas or those presenting with poor prognostic features following an initial response;

3. Recurrent or refractory neuroblastoma; or,

4. Advanced Hodgkin's disease who have failed conventional therapy and have no HLA-matched donor.

b) Effective October 1, 2000, single AuSCT is only covered for Durie-Salmon Stage II or III patients that fit the following requirements:

– Newly diagnosed or responsive multiple myeloma. This includes those patients with previously untreated disease, those with at least a partial response to prior chemotherapy (defined as a 50% decrease either in measurable paraprotein [serum and/or urine] or in bone marrow infiltration, sustained for at least 1 month), and those in responsive relapse; and

– Adequate cardiac, renal, pulmonary, and hepatic function.

c) Effective for services performed on or after March 15, 2005, when recognized clinical risk factors are employed to select patients for transplantation, high

dose melphalan (HDM) together with AuSCT is reasonable and necessary for Medicare beneficiaries of any age group with primary amyloid light chain (AL) amyloidosis who meet the following criteria:

– Amyloid deposition in 2 or fewer organs; and,

– Cardiac left ventricular ejection fraction (EF) greater than 45%.

C. Nationally Non-Covered Indications

I. Allogeneic Hematopoietic Stem Cell Transplantation (HSCT)

Effective for claims with dates of service on or after May 24, 1996, through January 26, 2016, allogeneic HSCT is not covered as treatment for multiple myeloma.

II. Autologous Stem Cell Transplantation (AuSCT)

Insufficient data exist to establish definite conclusions regarding the efficacy of AuSCT for the following conditions:

a) Acute leukemia not in remission;

b) Chronic granulocytic leukemia;

c) Solid tumors (other than neuroblastoma);

d) Up to October 1, 2000, multiple myeloma;

e) Tandem transplantation (multiple rounds of AuSCT) for patients with multiple myeloma;

f) Effective October 1, 2000, non primary AL amyloidosis; and,

g) Effective October 1, 2000, through March 14, 2005, primary AL amyloidosis for Medicare beneficiaries age 64 or older.

In these cases, AuSCT is not considered reasonable and necessary within the meaning of §l862(a)(1)(A) of the Act and is not covered under Medicare.

D. Other

All other indications for stem cell transplantation not otherwise noted above as covered or non-covered remain at local Medicare Administrative Contractor discretion.

(This NCD last reviewed January 2016.)

100-03, 130.1
NCD for Inpatient Hospital Stays for Treatment of Alcoholism (130.1)
(Rev. 1, 10-03-03)

A. Inpatient Hospital Stay for Alcohol Detoxification

Many hospitals provide detoxification services during the more acute stages of alcoholism or alcohol withdrawal. When the high probability or occurrence of medical complications (e.g., delirium, confusion, trauma, or unconsciousness) during detoxification for acute alcoholism or alcohol withdrawal necessitates the constant availability of physicians and/or complex medical equipment found only in the hospital setting, inpatient hospital care during this period is considered reasonable and necessary and is therefore covered under the program. Generally, detoxification can be accomplished within two to three days with an occasional need for up to five days where the patient's condition dictates. This limit (five days) may be extended in an individual case where there is a need for a longer period for detoxification for a particular patient.

In such cases, however, there should be documentation by a physician which substantiates that a longer period of detoxification was reasonable and necessary. When the detoxification needs of an individual no longer require an inpatient hospital setting, coverage should be denied on the basis that inpatient hospital care is not reasonable and necessary as required by §1862(a)(l) of the Social Security Act (the Act). Following detoxification a patient may be transferred to an inpatient rehabilitation unit or discharged to a residential treatment program or outpatient treatment setting.

B. Inpatient Hospital Stay for Alcohol Rehabilitation

Hospitals may also provide structured inpatient alcohol rehabilitation programs to the chronic alcoholic. These programs are composed primarily of coordinated educational and psychotherapeutic services provided on a group basis. Depending on the subject matter, a series of lectures, discussions, films, and group therapy sessions are led by either physicians, psychologists, or alcoholism counselors from the hospital or various outside organizations. In addition, individual psychotherapy and family counseling (see §70.1) may be provided in selected cases. These programs are conducted under the supervision and direction of a physician. Patients may directly enter an inpatient hospital rehabilitation program after having undergone detoxification in the same hospital or in another hospital or may enter an inpatient hospital rehabilitation program without prior hospitalization for detoxification.

Alcohol rehabilitation can be provided in a variety of settings other than the hospital setting. In order for an inpatient hospital stay for alcohol rehabilitation to be covered under Medicare it must be medically necessary for the care to be provided in the inpatient hospital setting rather than in a less costly facility or on an outpatient basis. Inpatient hospital care for receipt of an alcohol rehabilitation program would generally be medically necessary where either (l) there is documentation by the physician that recent alcohol rehabilitation services in a less intensive setting or on an outpatient basis have proven unsuccessful and, as a consequence, the patient requires the supervision and intensity of services which can only be found in the controlled environment of the hospital, or (2) only the hospital environment can assure the medical management or control of the patient's concomitant conditions during the course of alcohol rehabilitation. (However, a patient's concomitant condition may make the use of certain alcohol treatment modalities medically inappropriate.)

In addition, the "active treatment" criteria (see the Medicare Benefit Policy Manual, Chapter 2, "Inpatient Psychiatric Hospital Services," §20) should be applied to psychiatric care in the general hospital as well as to psychiatric care in a psychiatric hospital. Since alcoholism is classifiable as a psychiatric condition the "active treatment" criteria must also be met in order for alcohol rehabilitation services to be covered under Medicare. (Thus, it is the combined need for "active treatment" and for covered care which can only be provided in the inpatient hospital setting, rather than the fact that rehabilitation immediately follows a period of detoxification which provides the basis for coverage of inpatient hospital alcohol rehabilitation programs.)

Generally 16-19 days of rehabilitation services are sufficient to bring a patient to a point where care could be continued in other than an inpatient hospital setting. An inpatient hospital stay for alcohol rehabilitation may be extended beyond this limit in an individual case where a longer period of alcohol rehabilitation is medically necessary. In such cases, however, there should be documentation by a physician which substantiates the need for such care. Where the rehabilitation needs of an individual no longer require an inpatient hospital setting, coverage should be denied on the basis that inpatient hospital care is not reasonable and necessary as required by §1862 (a)(I) of the Act.

Subsequent admissions to the inpatient hospital setting for alcohol rehabilitation follow-up, reinforcement, or "recap" treatments are considered to be readmissions (rather than an extension of the original stay) and must meet the requirements of this section for coverage under Medicare. Prior admissions to the inpatient hospital setting - either in the same hospital or in a different hospital - may be an indication that the "active treatment" requirements are not met (i.e., there is no reasonable expectation of improvement) and the stay should not be covered. Accordingly, there should be documentation to establish that "readmission" to the hospital setting for alcohol rehabilitation services can reasonably be expected to result in improvement of the patient's condition. For example, the documentation should indicate what changes in the patient's medical condition, social or emotional status, or treatment plan make improvement likely, or why the patient's initial hospital treatment was not sufficient.

C. Combined Alcohol Detoxification/Rehabilitation Programs

Medicare Administrative Contractors (MACs) should apply the guidelines in A. and B. above to both phases of a combined inpatient hospital alcohol detoxification/rehabilitation program. Not all patients who require the inpatient hospital setting for detoxification also need the inpatient hospital setting for rehabilitation. (See §130.1 for coverage of outpatient hospital alcohol rehabilitation services.) Where the inpatient hospital setting is medically necessary for both alcohol detoxification and rehabilitation, generally a 3-week period is reasonable and necessary to bring the patient to the point where care can be continued in other than an inpatient hospital setting.

Decisions regarding reasonableness and necessity of treatment, the need for an inpatient hospital level of care, and length of treatment should be made by A/B MAC (A) based on accepted medical practice with the advice of their medical consultant. (In hospitals under PSRO review, PSRO determinations of medical necessity of services and appropriateness of the level of care at which services are provided are binding on A/B MAC (A) for purposes of adjudicating claims for payment.)

100-03, 130.2

NCD for Outpatient Hospital Services for Treatment of Alcoholism (130.2)

(Rev. 1, 10-03-03)

Coverage is available for both diagnostic and therapeutic services furnished for the treatment of alcoholism by the hospital to outpatients subject to the same rules applicable to outpatient hospital services in general. While there is no coverage for day hospitalization programs, per se, individual services which meet the requirements in the Medicare Benefit Policy Manual, Chapter 6, Sec.20 may be covered. (Meals, transportation and recreational and social activities do not fall within the scope of covered outpatient hospital services under Medicare.)

All services must be reasonable and necessary for diagnosis or treatment of the patient's condition (see the Medicare Benefit Policy Manual, chapter 16 Sec.20). Thus, educational services and family counseling would only be covered where they are directly related to treatment of the patient's condition. The frequency of treatment and period of time over which it occurs must also be reasonable and necessary.

100-03, 130.3

NCD for Chemical Aversion Therapy for Treatment of Alcoholism (130.3)

(Rev. 173, Issued: 09-04-14, Effective: Upon Implementation: of ICD-10, Implementation: Upon Implementation of ICD-10)

Chemical aversion therapy is a behavior modification technique that is used in the treatment of alcoholism. Chemical aversion therapy facilitates alcohol abstinence through the development of conditioned aversions to the taste, smell, and sight of alcohol beverages. This is accomplished by repeatedly pairing alcohol with unpleasant symptoms (e.g., nausea) which have been induced by one of several

chemical agents. While a number of drugs have been employed in chemical aversion therapy, the three most commonly used are emetine, apomorphine, and lithium. None of the drugs being used, however, have yet been approved by the Food and Drug Administration specifically for use in chemical aversion therapy for alcoholism. Accordingly, when these drugs are being employed in conjunction with this therapy, patients undergoing this treatment need to be kept under medical observation.

Available evidence indicates that chemical aversion therapy may be an effective component of certain alcoholism treatment programs, particularly as part of multi-modality treatment programs which include other behavioral techniques and therapies, such as psychotherapy. Based on this evidence, the Centers for Medicare & Medicaid Services' medical consultants have recommended that chemical aversion therapy be covered under Medicare. However, since chemical aversion therapy is a demanding therapy which may not be appropriate for all Medicare beneficiaries needing treatment for alcoholism, a physician should certify to the appropriateness of chemical aversion therapy in the individual case. Therefore, if chemical aversion therapy for treatment of alcoholism is determined to be reasonable and necessary for an individual patient, it is covered under Medicare.

When it is medically necessary for a patient to receive chemical aversion therapy as a hospital inpatient, coverage for care in that setting is available. (See §130.1 regarding coverage of multi-modality treatment programs.) Follow-up treatments for chemical aversion therapy can generally be provided on an outpatient basis. Thus, where a patient is admitted as an inpatient for receipt of chemical aversion therapy, there must be documentation by the physician of the need in the individual case for the inpatient hospital admission.

Decisions regarding reasonableness and necessity of treatment and the need for an inpatient hospital level of care should be made by the A/B MAC (A) based on accepted medical practice with the advice of their medical consultant. (In hospitals under Quality Improvement Organization (QIO) review, QIO determinations of medical necessity of services and appropriateness of the level of care at which services are provided are binding on the A/B MAC (A) for purposes of adjudicating claims for payment.)

100-03, 140.1

NCD for Abortion (140.1)

(Rev. 48, Issued: 03-17-06; Effective/Implementation Dates: 06-19-06)

Abortions are not covered Medicare procedures except:

1. If the pregnancy is the result of an act of rape or incest; or

2. In the case where a woman suffers from a physical disorder, physical injury, or physical illness, including a life-endangering physical condition caused by or arising from the pregnancy itself, that would, as certified by a physician, place the woman in danger of death unless an abortion is performed.

100-03, 140.2

NCD for Breast Reconstruction Following Mastectomy (140.2)

(Rev. 1, 10-03-03)

CIM 35-47

Reconstruction of the affected and the contralateral unaffected breast following a medically necessary mastectomy is considered a relatively safe and effective noncosmetic procedure. Accordingly, program payment may be made for breast reconstruction surgery following removal of a breast for any medical reason.

Program payment may not be made for breast reconstruction for cosmetic reasons. (Cosmetic surgery is excluded from coverage under Sec.I862(a)(I0) of the Social Security Act.)

100-03, 140.5

NCD for Laser Procedures (140.5)

(Rev. 173, Issued: 09-04-14, Effective: Upon Implementation: of ICD-10)

Medicare recognizes the use of lasers for many medical indications. Procedures performed with lasers are sometimes used in place of more conventional techniques. In the absence of a specific noncoverage instruction, and where a laser has been approved for marketing by the Food and Drug Administration, Medicare Administrative Contractor discretion may be used to determine whether a procedure performed with a laser is reasonable and necessary and, therefore, covered.

The determination of coverage for a procedure performed using a laser is made on the basis that the use of lasers to alter, revise, or destroy tissue is a surgical procedure. Therefore, coverage of laser procedures is restricted to practitioners with training in the surgical management of the disease or condition being treated.

100-03, 150.1

NCD for Manipulation (150.1)

(Rev. 1, 10-03-03)

CIM 35-2

A. Manipulation of the Rib Cage

Manual manipulation of the rib cage contributes to the treatment of respiratory conditions such as bronchitis, emphysema, and asthma as part of a regimen that includes other elements of therapy, and is covered only under such circumstances.

B. Manipulation of the Head

Manipulation of the occipitocervical or temporomandibular regions of the head when indicated for conditions affecting those portions of the head and neck is a covered service.

100-03, 150.2

NCD for Osteogenic Stimulators (150.2)

(Rev. 41, Issued: 06-24-05, Effective: 04-27-05, Implementation: 08-01-05)

Electrical Osteogenic Stimulators

A. General

Electrical stimulation to augment bone repair can be attained either invasively or non-invasively. Invasive devices provide electrical stimulation directly at the fracture site either through percutaneously placed cathodes or by implantation of a coiled cathode wire into the fracture site. The power pack for the latter device is implanted into soft tissue near the fracture site and subcutaneously connected to the cathode, creating a self-contained system with no external components. The power supply for the former device is externally placed and the leads connected to the inserted cathodes. With the non-invasive device, opposing pads, wired to an external power supply, are placed over the cast. An electromagnetic field is created between the pads at the fracture site.

B. Nationally Covered Indications

1. Noninvasive Stimulator.

   The noninvasive stimulator device is covered only for the following indications:

   — Nonunion of long bone fractures;

   — Failed fusion, where a minimum of nine months has elapsed since the last surgery;

   — Congenital pseudarthroses; and

   — Effective July 1, 1996, as an adjunct to spinal fusion surgery for patients at high risk of pseudarthrosis due to previously failed spinal fusion at the same site or for those undergoing multiple level fusion. A multiple level fusion involves 3 or more vertebrae (e.g., L3-L5, L4-S1, etc).

   — Effective September 15, 1980, nonunion of long bone fractures is considered to exist only after 6 or more months have elapsed without healing of the fracture.

   — Effective April 1, 2000, nonunion of long bone fractures is considered to exist only when serial radiographs have confirmed that fracture healing has ceased for 3 or more months prior to starting treatment with the electrical osteogenic stimulator. Serial radiographs must include a minimum of 2 sets of radiographs, each including multiple views of the fracture site, separated by a minimum of 90 days.

2. Invasive (Implantable) Stimulator.

   The invasive stimulator device is covered only for the following indications:

   — Nonunion of long bone fractures

   — Effective July 1, 1996, as an adjunct to spinal fusion surgery for patients at high risk of pseudarthrosis due to previously failed spinal fusion at the same site or for those undergoing multiple level fusion. A multiple level fusion involves 3 or more vertebrae (e.g., L3-5, L4-S1, etc.).

   — Effective September 15, 1980, nonunion of long bone fractures is considered to exist only after 6 or more months have elapsed without healing of the fracture.

   — Effective April 1, 2000, non union of long bone fractures is considered to exist only when serial radiographs have confirmed that fracture healing has ceased for 3 or more months prior to starting treatment with the electrical osteogenic stimulator. Serial radiographs must include a minimum of 2 sets of radiographs, each including multiple views of the fracture site, separated by a minimum of 90 days.

   — Effective for services performed on or after January 1, 2001, ultrasonic osteogenic stimulators are covered as medically reasonable and necessary for the treatment of non-union fractures. In demonstrating nonunion of fractures, we would expect:

     – A minimum of two sets of radiographs obtained prior to starting treatment with the osteogenic stimulator, separated by a minimum of 90 days. Each radiograph must include multiple views of the fracture site accompanied with a written interpretation by a physician stating that there has been no clinically significant evidence of fracture healing between the two sets of radiographs.

     – Indications that the patient failed at least one surgical intervention for the treatment of the fracture.

   — Effective April 27, 2005, upon the recommendation of the ultrasound stimulation for nonunion fracture healing, CMS determins that the evidence is adequate to condlude that noninvasive ultrasound stimulation for the treatment of nonunion bone fractures prior to surfical intervention is reasonable and necessary. In demonstrating non-union fracturs, CMS expects:

     – A minimum of 2 sets of radiographs, obtained prior to starting treating with the osteogenic stimulator, separated by a minimum of 90 days. Each radiograph set must include multiple views of the fracture site accompanied with a written interpretation by a physician stating that there has been no clinically significant evidence of fracture healing between the 2 sets of radiographs.

C. Nationally Non-Covered Indications

Nonunion fractures of the skull, vertebrae and those that are tumor-related are excluded from coverage.

Ultrasonic osteogenic stimulators may not be used concurrently with other non-invasive osteogenic devices.

Ultrasonic osteogenic stimulators for fresh fracturs and delayed unions remain non-covered.

(This NCD last reviewed June 2005)

100-03, 150.7

NCD for Prolotherapy, Joint Sclerotherapy, and Ligamentous Injections with Sclerosing Agents (150.7)

(Rev. 1, 10-03-03)

CIM 35-13

Not Covered

The medical effectiveness of the above therapies has not been verified by scientifically controlled studies. Accordingly, reimbursement for these modalities should be denied on the ground that they are not reasonable and necessary as required by Sec.1862(a)(1) of the Act.

100-03, 150.10

NCD for Lumbar Artificial Disc Replacement (LADR) (150.10)

(Rev. 173, Issued: 09-04-14, Effective: Upon Implementation: of ICD–10)

A. General

The lumbar artificial disc replacement (LADR) is a surgical procedure on the lumbar spine that involves complete removal of the damaged or diseased lumbar intervertebral disc and implantation of an artificial disc. The procedure may be done as an alternative to lumbar spinal fusion and is intended to reduce pain, increase movement at the site of surgery and restore intervertebral disc height. The Food and Drug Administration has approved the use of LADR for spine arthroplasty in skeletally mature patients with degenerative or discogenic disc disease at one level for L3 to S1.

B. Nationally Covered Indications

N/A

C. Nationally Non-Covered Indications

Effective for services performed from May 16, 2006 through August 13, 2007, the Centers for Medicare and Medicaid Services (CMS) has found that LADR with the ChariteTM lumbar artificial disc is not reasonable and necessary for the Medicare population over 60 years of age; therefore, LADR with the ChariteTM lumbar artificial disc is non-covered for Medicare beneficiaries over 60 years of age.

Effective for services performed on or after August 14, 2007, CMS has found that LADR is not reasonable and necessary for the Medicare population over 60 years of age; therefore, LADR is non-covered for Medicare beneficiaries over 60 years of age.

D. Other

For Medicare beneficiaries 60 years of age and younger, there is no national coverage determination for LADR, leaving such determinations to continue to be made by the local Medicare Administrative Contractors.

For dates of service May 16, 2006 through August 13, 2007, Medicare coverage under the investigational device exemption (IDE) for LADR with a disc other than the ChariteTM lumbar disc in eligible clinical trials is not impacted.

100-03, 160.8

NCD for Electroencephalographic (EEG) Monitoring During Surgical Procedures Involving the Cerebral Vasculature (160.8)

(Rev. 48, Issued: 03-17-06; Effective/Implementation Dates: 06-19-06)

CIM 35-57

Electroencephalographic (EEG) monitoring is a safe and reliable technique for the assessment of gross cerebral blood flow during general anesthesia and is covered under Medicare. Very characteristic changes in the EEG occur when cerebral perfusion is inadequate for cerebral function. EEG monitoring as an indirect measure of cerebral perfusion requires the expertise of an electroencephalographer, a neurologist trained in EEG, or an advanced EEG technician for its proper interpretation.

The EEG monitoring may be covered routinely in carotid endarterectomies and in other neurological procedures where cerebral perfusion could be reduced. Such other procedures might include aneurysm surgery where hypotensive anesthesia is used or other cerebral vascular procedures where cerebral blood flow may be interrupted.

100-03, 160.17

NCD for L-DOPA (160.17)

(Rev. 1, 10-03-03)

A. Part A Payment for L-Dopa and Associated Inpatient Hospital Services

A hospital stay and related ancillary services for the administration of L-Dopa are covered if medically required for this purpose. Whether a drug represents an allowable inpatient hospital cost during such stay depends on whether it meets the definition of a drug in Sec.1861(t) of the Act; i.e., on its inclusion in the compendia named in the Act or approval by the hospital's pharmacy and drug therapeutics (P&DT) or equivalent committee. (Levodopa (L-Dopa) has been favorably evaluated for the treatment of Parkinsonism by A.M.A. Drug Evaluations, First Edition 1971, the replacement compendia for "New Drugs.")

Inpatient hospital services are frequently not required in many cases when L-Dopa therapy is initiated. Therefore, determine the medical need for inpatient hospital services on the basis of medical facts in the individual case. It is not necessary to hospitalize the typical, well-functioning, ambulatory Parkinsonian patient who has no concurrent disease at the start of L-Dopa treatment. It is reasonable to provide inpatient hospital services for Parkinsonian patients with concurrent diseases, particularly of the cardiovascular, gastrointestinal, and neuropsychiatric systems. Although many patients require hospitalization for a period of under 2 weeks, a 4-week period of inpatient care is not unreasonable.

Laboratory tests in connection with the administration of L-Dopa - The tests medically warranted in connection with the achievement of optimal dosage and the control of the side effects of L-Dopa include a complete blood count, liver function tests such as SGOT, SGPT, and/or alkaline phosphatase, BUN or creatinine and urinalysis, blood sugar, and electrocardiogram.

Whether or not the patient is hospitalized, laboratory tests in certain cases are reasonable at weekly intervals although some physicians prefer to perform the tests much less frequently.

Physical therapy furnished in connection with administration of L-Dopa - Where, following administration of the drug, the patient experiences a reduction of rigidity which permits the reestablishment of a restorative goal for him/her, physical therapy services required to enable him/her to achieve this goal are payable provided they require the skills of a qualified physical therapist and are furnished by or under the supervision of such a therapist. However, once the individual's restoration potential has been achieved, the services required to maintain him/her at this level do not generally require the skills of a qualified physical therapist. In such situations, the role of the therapist is to evaluate the patient's needs in consultation with his/her physician and design a program of exercise appropriate to the capacity and tolerance of the patient and treatment objectives of the physician, leaving to others the actual carrying out of the program. While the evaluative services rendered by a qualified physical therapist are payable as physical therapy, services furnished by others in connection with the carrying out of the maintenance program established by the therapist are not.

B. Part A Reimbursement for L-Dopa Therapy in SNFs

Initiation of L-Dopa therapy can be appropriately carried out in the SNF setting, applying the same guidelines used for initiation of L-Dopa therapy in the hospital, including the types of patients who should be covered for inpatient services, the role of physical therapy, and the use of laboratory tests. (See subsection A.) Where inpatient care is required and L-Dopa therapy is initiated in the SNF, limit the stay to a maximum of 4 weeks; but in many cases the need may be no longer than 1 or 2 weeks, depending upon the patient's condition. However, where L-Dopa therapy is begun in the hospital and the patient is transferred to an SNF for continuation of the therapy, a combined length of stay in hospital and SNF of no longer than 4 weeks is reasonable (i.e., 1 week hospital stay followed by 3 weeks SNF stay; or 2 weeks hospital stay followed by 2 weeks SNF stay; etc.). Medical need must be demonstrated in cases where the combined length of stay in hospital and SNF is longer than 4 weeks. The choice of hospital or SNF, and the decision regarding the relative length of time spent in each, should be left to the medical judgment of the treating physician.

C. L-Dopa Coverage Under Part B

Part B reimbursement may not be made for the drug L-Dopa since it is a self-administrable drug. However, physician services rendered in connection with its administration and control of its side effects are covered if determined to be reasonable and necessary. Initiation of L-Dopa therapy on an outpatient basis is possible in most cases. Visit frequency ranging from every week to every 2 or 3 months is acceptable. However, after half a year of therapy, visits more frequent than every month would usually not be reasonable.

100-03, 180.1

NCD for Medical Nutrition Therapy (180.1)

(Rev. 1, 10-03-03)

Effective October 1, 2002, basic coverage of MNT for the first year a beneficiary receives MNT with either a diagnosis of renal disease or diabetes as defined at 42 CFR Sec.410.130 is 3 hours. Also effective October 1, 2002, basic coverage in subsequent years for renal disease or diabetes is 2 hours. The dietitian/nutritionist may choose how many units are performed per day as long as all of the other requirements in this NCD and 42 CFR Secs.410.130-410.134 are met. Pursuant to the exception at 42 CFR Sec.410.132(b)(5), additional hours are considered to be medically necessary and covered if the treating physician determines that there is a change in medical condition, diagnosis, or treatment regimen that requires a change in MNT and orders additional hours during that episode of care.

Effective October 1, 2002, if the treating physician determines that receipt of both MNT and DSMT is medically necessary in the same episode of care, Medicare will cover both DSMT and MNT initial and subsequent years without decreasing either benefit as long as DSMT and MNT are not provided on the same date of service. The dietitian/nutritionist may choose how many units are performed per day as long as all of the other requirements in the NCD and 42 CFR Secs.410.130-410.134 are met. Pursuant to the exception at 42 CFR 410.132(b)(5), additional hours are considered to be medically necessary and covered if the treating physician determines that there is a change in medical condition, diagnosis, or treatment regimen that requires a change in MNT and orders additional hours during that episode of care.

100-03, 190.1

NCD for Histocompatibility Testing (190.1)

(Rev. 1, 10-03-03)

This testing is safe and effective when it is performed on patients:

- In preparation for a kidney transplant;
- In preparation for bone marrow transplantation;
- In preparation for blood platelet transfusions (particularly where multiple infusions are involved); or
- Who are suspected of having ankylosing spondylitis.

This testing is covered under Medicare when used for any of the indications listed in A, B, and C and if it is reasonable and necessary for the patient.

It is covered for ankylosing spondylitis in cases where other methods of diagnosis would not be appropriate or have yielded inconclusive results. Request documentation supporting the medical necessity of the test from the physician in all cases where ankylosing spondylitis is indicated as the reason for the test.

100-03, 190.3

NCD for Cytogenetic Studies (190.3)

(Rev. 1, 10-03-03)

Medicare covers these tests when they are reasonable and necessary for the diagnosis or treatment of the following conditions:

- Genetic disorders (e.g., mongolism) in a fetus (See Medicare Benefit Policy Manual, Chapter 15, "Covered medical and Other health Services," Sec. 20.1)
- Failure of sexual development;
- Chronic myelogenous leukemia;
- Acute leukemias lymphoid (FAB L1-L3), myeloid (FAB M0-M7), and unclassified; or
- Mylodysplasia

100-03, 190.8

NCD for Lymphocyte Mitogen Response Assays (190.8)

(Rev. 1, 10-03-03)

It is a covered test under Medicare when it is medically necessary to assess lymphocytic function in diagnosed immunodeficiency diseases and to monitor immunotherapy.

It is not covered when it is used to monitor the treatment of cancer, because its use for that purpose is experimental.

100-03, 190.9

NCD for Serologic Testing for Acquired Immunodeficiency Syndrome (AIDS) (190.9)

(Rev. 1, 10-03-03)

These tests may be covered when performed to help determine a diagnosis for symptomatic patients. They are not covered when furnished as part of a screening program for asymptomatic persons.

Note: Two enzyme-linked immunosorbent assay (ELISA) tests that were conducted on the same specimen must both be positive before Medicare will cover the Western blot test.

100-03, 190.11

NCD for Home Prothrombin Time International Normalized Ratio (INR) Monitoring for Anticoagulation Management (190.11)

(Rev. 90, Issued: 07-25-08, Effective: 03-19-08, Implementation: 08-25-08)

A. General

Use of the International Normalized Ratio (INR) or prothrombin time (PT) - standard measurement for reporting the blood's clotting time) - allows physicians to determine the level of anticoagulation in a patient independent of the laboratory reagents used. The INR is the ratio of the patient's PT (extrinsic or tissue-factor dependent coagulation pathway) compared to the mean PT for a group of normal individuals. Maintaining patients within his/her prescribed therapeutic range minimizes adverse events associated with inadequate or excessive anticoagulation such as serious bleeding or thromboembolic events. Patient self-testing and self-management through the use of a home INR monitor may be used to improve the time in therapeutic rate (TTR) for select groups of patients. Increased TTR leads to improved clinical outcomes and reductions in thromboembolic and hemorrhagic events.

Warfarin (also prescribed under other trade names, e.g., Coumadin(R)) is a self-administered, oral anticoagulant (blood thinner) medication that affects the vitamin K- dependent clotting factors II, VII, IX and X. It is widely used for various medical conditions, and has a narrow therapeutic index, meaning it is a drug with less than a 2-fold difference between median lethal dose and median effective dose. For this reason, since October 4, 2006, it falls under the category of a Food and Drug dministration (FDA) "black-box" drug whose dosage must be closely monitored to avoid serious complications. A PT/INR monitoring system is a portable testing device that includes a finger-stick and an FDA-cleared meter that measures the time it takes for a person's blood plasma to clot.

B. Nationally Covered Indications

For services furnished on or after March 19, 2008, Medicare will cover the use of home PT/INR monitoring for chronic, oral anticoagulation management for patients with mechanical heart valves, chronic atrial fibrillation, or venous thromboembolism (inclusive of deep venous thrombosis and pulmonary embolism) on warfarin. The monitor and the home testing must be prescribed by a treating physician as provided at 42 CFR 410.32(a), and all of the following requirements must be met:

1. The patient must have been anticoagulated for at least 3 months prior to use of the home INR device; and,

2. The patient must undergo a face-to-face educational program on anticoagulation anagement and must have demonstrated the correct use of the device prior to its use in the home; and,

3. The patient continues to correctly use the device in the context of the management of the anticoagulation therapy following the initiation of home monitoring; and,

4. Self-testing with the device should not occur more frequently than once a week.

C. Nationally Non-Covered Indications

N/A

D. Other

1. All other indications for home PT/INR monitoring not indicated as nationally covered above remain at local Medicare contractor discretion.

2. This national coverage determination (NCD) is distinct from, and makes no changes to, the PT clinical laboratory NCD at section 190.17 of Publication 100-3 of the NCD Manual.

100-03, 190.14

NCD for Human Immunodeficiency Virus (HIV) Testing (Diagnosis) (190.14)

(Rev. 113, Issued: 02-19-10, Effective: 12-08-09, Implementation; 07-06-10)

Indications and Limitations of Coverage

Indications

Diagnostic testing to establish HIV infection may be indicated when there is a strong clinical suspicion supported by one or more of the following clinical findings:

- The patient has a documented, otherwise unexplained, AIDS-defining or AIDS-associated opportunistic infection.

- The patient has another documented sexually transmitted disease which identifies significant risk of exposure to HIV and the potential for an early or subclinical infection.

- The patient has documented acute or chronic hepatitis B or C infection that identifies a significant risk of exposure to HIV and the potential for an early or subclinical infection.

- The patient has a documented AIDS-defining or AIDS-associated neoplasm.

- The patient has a documented AIDS-associated neurologic disorder or otherwise unexplained dementia.

- The patient has another documented AIDS-defining clinical condition, or a history of other severe, recurrent, or persistent conditions which suggest an underlying immune deficiency (for example, cutaneous or mucosal disorders).

- The patient has otherwise unexplained generalized signs and symptoms suggestive of a chronic process with an underlying immune deficiency (for example, fever, weight loss, malaise, fatigue, chronic diarrhea, failure to thrive, chronic cough, hemoptysis, shortness of breath, or lymphadenopathy).

- The patient has otherwise unexplained laboratory evidence of a chronic disease process with an underlying immune deficiency (for example, anemia, leukopenia, pancytopenia, lymphopenia, or low CD4+ lymphocyte count).

- The patient has signs and symptoms of acute retroviral syndrome with fever, malaise, lymphadenopathy, and skin rash.

- The patient has documented exposure to blood or body fluids known to be capable of transmitting HIV (for example, needlesticks and other significant blood exposures) and antiviral therapy is initiated or anticipated to be initiated.

- The patient is undergoing treatment for rape. (HIV testing is a part of the rape treatment protocol.)

Limitations

HIV antibody testing in the United States is usually performed using HIV-1 or HIV-½ combination tests. HIV-2 testing is indicated if clinical circumstances suggest HIV-2 is likely (that is, compatible clinical findings and HIV-1 test negative). HIV-2 testing may also be indicated in areas of the country where there is greater prevalence of HIV-2 infections.

The Western Blot test should be performed only after documentation that the initial EIA tests are repeatedly positive or equivocal on a single sample.

- The HIV antigen tests currently have no defined diagnostic usage.

- Direct viral RNA detection may be performed in those situations where serologic testing does not establish a diagnosis but strong clinical suspicion persists (for example, acute retroviral syndrome, nonspecific serologic evidence of HIV, or perinatal HIV infection).

- If initial serologic tests confirm an HIV infection, repeat testing is not indicated.

- If initial serologic tests are HIV EIA negative and there is no indication for confirmation of infection by viral RNA detection, the interval prior to retesting is 3-6 months.

- Testing for evidence of HIV infection using serologic methods may be medically appropriate in situations where there is a risk of exposure to HIV. However, in the absence of a documented AIDS defining or HIV- associated disease, an HIV associated sign or symptom, or documented exposure to a known HIV-infected source, the testing is considered by Medicare to be screening and thus is not covered by Medicare (for example, history of multiple blood component transfusions, exposure to blood or body fluids not resulting in consideration of therapy, history of transplant, history of illicit drug use, multiple sexual partners, same-sex encounters, prostitution, or contact with prostitutes).

- The CPT Editorial Panel has issued a number of codes for infectious agent detection by direct antigen or nucleic acid probe techniques that have not yet been developed or are only being used on an investigational basis. Laboratory providers are advised to remain current on FDA-approval status for these tests.

100-03, 190.15

NCD for Blood Counts (190.15)

(Rev. 17, Issued: 07-02-04) (Effective/Implementation: Not Applicable)

Indications

Indications for a CBC or hemogram include red cell, platelet, and white cell disorders. Examples of these indications are enumerated individually below.

1. Indications for a CBC generally include the evaluation of bone marrow dysfunction as a result of neoplasms, therapeutic agents, exposure to toxic substances, or pregnancy. The CBC is also useful in assessing peripheral destruction of blood cells, suspected bone marrow failure or bone marrow infiltrate, suspected myeloproliferative, myelodysplastic, or lymphoproliferative processes, and immune disorders.

2. Indications for hemogram or CBC related to red cell (RBC) parameters of the hemogram include signs, symptoms, test results, illness, or disease that can be associated with anemia or other red blood cell disorder (e.g., pallor, weakness, fatigue, weight loss, bleeding, acute injury associated with blood loss or suspected blood loss, abnormal menstrual bleeding, hematuria, hematemesis, hematochezia, positive fecal occult blood test, malnutrition, vitamin deficiency, malabsorption, neuropathy, known malignancy, presence of acute or chronic disease that may have associated anemia, coagulation or hemostatic disorders, postural dizziness, syncope, abdominal pain, change in bowel habits, chronic marrow hypoplasia or decreased RBC production, tachycardia, systolic heart murmur, congestive heart failure, dyspnea, angina, nailbed deformities, growth retardation, jaundice, hepatomegaly, splenomegaly, lymphadenopathy, ulcers on the lower extremities).

3. Indications for hemogram or CBC related to red cell (RBC) parameters of the hemogram include signs, symptoms, test results, illness, or disease that can be associated with polycythemia (for example, fever, chills, ruddy skin, conjunctival redness, cough, wheezing, cyanosis, clubbing of the fingers, orthopnea, heart murmur, headache, vague cognitive changes including memory changes, sleep apnea, weakness, pruritus, dizziness, excessive sweating, visual symptoms, weight loss, massive obesity, gastrointestinal bleeding, paresthesias, dyspnea, joint symptoms, epigastric distress, pain and erythema of the fingers or toes, venous or arterial thrombosis, thromboembolism, myocardial infarction, stroke, transient ischemic attacks, congenital heart disease, chronic obstructive pulmonary disease, increased erythropoietin production associated with neoplastic, renal or hepatic disorders, androgen or diuretic use, splenomegaly, hepatomegaly, diastolic hypertension.)

4. Specific indications for CBC with differential count related to the WBC include signs, symptoms, test results, illness, or disease associated with leukemia, infections or inflammatory processes, suspected bone marrow failure or bone marrow infiltrate, suspected myeloproliferative, myelodysplastic or lymphoproliferative disorder, use of drugs that may cause leukopenia, and immune disorders (e.g., fever, chills, sweats, shock, fatigue, malaise, tachycardia, tachypnea, heart murmur, seizures, alterations of consciousness, meningismus, pain such as headache, abdominal pain, arthralgia, odynophagia, or dysuria, redness or swelling of skin, soft tissue bone, or joint, ulcers of the skin or mucous

membranes, gangrene, mucous membrane discharge, bleeding, thrombosis, respiratory failure, pulmonary infiltrate, jaundice, diarrhea, vomiting, hepatomegaly, splenomegaly, lymphadenopathy, opportunistic infection such as oral candidiasis.)

5. Specific indications for CBC related to the platelet count include signs, symptoms, test results, illness, or disease associated with increased or decreased platelet production and destruction, or platelet dysfunction (e.g., gastrointestinal bleeding, genitourinary tract bleeding, bilateral epistaxis, thrombosis, ecchymosis, purpura, jaundice, petechiae, fever, heparin therapy, suspected DIC, shock, pre-eclampsia, neonate with maternal ITP, massive transfusion, recent platelet transfusion, cardiopulmonary bypass, hemolytic uremic syndrome, renal diseases, lymphadenopathy, hepatomegaly, splenomegaly, hypersplenism, neurologic abnormalities, viral or other infection, myeloproliferative, myelodysplastic, or lymphoproliferative disorder, thrombosis, exposure to toxic agents, excessive alcohol ingestion, autoimmune disorders (SLE, RA and other).

6. Indications for hemogram or CBC related to red cell (RBC) parameters of the hemogram include, in addition to those already listed, thalassemia, suspected hemoglobinopathy, lead poisoning, arsenic poisoning, and spherocytosis.

7. Specific indications for CBC with differential count related to the WBC include, in addition to those already listed, storage diseases; mucopolysaccharidoses, and use of drugs that cause leukocytosis such as G-CSF or GM-CSF.

8. Specific indications for CBC related to platelet count include, in addition to those already listed, May-Hegglin syndrome and Wiskott-Aldrich syndrome.

Limitations

1. Testing of patients who are asymptomatic, or who do not have a condition that could be expected to result in a hematological abnormality, is screening and is not a covered service.

2. In some circumstances it may be appropriate to perform only a hemoglobin or hematocrit to assess the oxygen carrying capacity of the blood. When the ordering provider requests only a hemoglobin or hematocrit, the remaining components of the CBC are not covered.

3. When a blood count is performed for an end-stage renal disease (ESRD) patient, and is billed outside the ESRD rate, documentation of the medical necessity for the blood count must be submitted with the claim.

4. In some patients presenting with certain signs, symptoms or diseases, a single CBC may be appropriate. Repeat testing may not be indicated unless abnormal results are found, or unless there is a change in clinical condition. If repeat testing is performed, a more descriptive diagnosis code (e.g., anemia) should be reported to support medical necessity. However, repeat testing may be indicated where results are normal in patients with conditions where there is a continued risk for the development of hematologic abnormality.

100-03, 190.18

Serum Iron Studies

(Rev. 17, Issued: 07-02-04) (Effective/Implementation: Not Applicable)

Indications:

1. Ferritin (82728), iron (83540) and either iron binding capacity (83550) or transferrin (84466) are useful in the differential diagnosis of iron deficiency, anemia, and for iron overload conditions.

   a. The following presentations are examples that may support the use of these studies for evaluating iron deficiency:

   – Certain abnormal blood count values (i.e., decreased mean corpuscular volume (MCV), decreased hemoglobin/hematocrit when the MCV is low or normal, or increased red cell distribution width (RDW) and low or normal MCV);

   – Abnormal appetite (pica);

   – Acute or chronic gastrointestinal blood loss;

   – Hematuria;

   – Menorrhagia;

   – Malabsorption;

   – Status post-gastrectomy;

   – Status post-gastrojejunostomy;

   – Malnutrition;

   – Preoperative autologous blood collection(s);

   – Malignant, chronic inflammatory and infectious conditions associated with anemia which may present in a similar manner to iron deficiency anemia;

   – Following a significant surgical procedure where blood loss had occurred and had not been repaired with adequate iron replacement.

   b. The following presentations are examples that may support the use of these studies for evaluating iron overload:

   – Chronic Hepatitis;

   – Diabetes;

   – Hyperpigmentation of skin;

– Arthropathy;

– Cirrhosis;

– Hypogonadism;

– Hypopituitarism;

– Impaired porphyrin metabolism;

– Heart failure;

– Multiple transfusions;

– Sideroblastic anemia;

– Thalassemia major;

– Cardiomyopathy, cardiac dysrhythmias and conduction disturbances.

2. Follow-up testing may be appropriate to monitor response to therapy, e.g., oral or parenteral iron, ascorbic acid, and erythropoietin.

3. Iron studies may be appropriate in patients after treatment for other nutritional deficiency anemias, such as folate and vitamin B12, because iron deficiency may not be revealed until such a nutritional deficiency is treated.

4. Serum ferritin may be appropriate for monitoring iron status in patients with chronic renal disease with or without dialysis.

5. Serum iron may also be indicated for evaluation of toxic effects of iron and other metals (e.g., nickel, cadmium, aluminum, lead) whether due to accidental, intentional exposure or metabolic causes.

Limitations:

1. Iron studies should be used to diagnose and manage iron deficiency or iron overload states. These tests are not to be used solely to assess acute phase reactants where disease management will be unchanged. For example, infections and malignancies are associated with elevations in acute phase reactants such as ferritin, and decreases in serum iron concentration, but iron studies would only be medically necessary if results of iron studies might alter the management of the primary diagnosis or might warrant direct treatment of an iron disorder or condition.

2. If a normal serum ferritin level is documented, repeat testing would not ordinarily be medically necessary unless there is a change in the patient's condition, and ferritin assessment is needed for the ongoing management of the patient. For example, a patient presents with new onset insulin-dependent diabetes mellitus and has a serum ferritin level performed for the suspicion of hemochromatosis. If the ferritin level is normal, the repeat ferritin for diabetes mellitus would not be medically necessary.

3. When an End Stage Renal Disease (ESRD) patient is tested for ferritin, testing more frequently than every three months (the frequency authorized by 3167.3, Fiscal Intermediary manual) requires documentation of medical necessity [e.g., other than "Chronic Renal Failure" (ICD-9-CM 585) or "Renal Failure, Unspecified" (ICD-9-CM 586)].

4. It is ordinarily not necessary to measure both transferrin and TIBC at the same time because TIBC is an indirect measure of transferrin. When transferrin is ordered as part of the nutritional assessment for evaluating malnutrition, it is not necessary to order other iron studies unless iron deficiency or iron overload is suspected as well.

5. It is not ordinarily necessary to measure both iron/TIBC (or transferrin) and ferritin in initial patient testing. If clinically indicated after evaluation of the initial iron studies, it may be appropriate to perform additional iron studies either on the initial specimen or on a subsequently obtained specimen. After a diagnosis of iron deficiency or iron overload is established, either iron/TIBC (or transferrin) or ferritin may be medically necessary for monitoring, but not both.

6. It would not ordinarily be considered medically necessary to do a ferritin as a preoperative test except in the presence of anemia or recent autologous blood collections prior to the surgery.

100-03, 190.19

Collagen Crosslinks, Any Method

(Rev. 17, Issued: 07-02-04) (Effective/Implementation: Not Applicable)

Indications:

Generally speaking, collagen crosslink testing is useful mostly in "fast losers" of bone. The age when these bone markers can help direct therapy is often pre-Medicare. By the time a fast loser of bone reaches age 65, she will most likely have been stabilized by appropriate therapy or have lost so much bone mass that further testing is useless. Coverage for bone marker assays may be established, however, for younger Medicare beneficiaries and for those men and women who might become fast losers because of some other therapy such as glucocorticoids. Safeguards should be incorporated to prevent excessive use of tests in patients for whom they have no clinical relevance.

Collagen crosslinks testing is used to:

• Identify individuals with elevated bone resorption, who have osteoporosis in whom response to treatment is being monitored;

• Predict response (as assessed by bone mass measurements) to FDA approved antiresorptive therapy in postmenopausal women; and

• Assess response to treatment of patients with osteoporosis, Paget's disease of the bone, or risk for osteoporosis where treatment may include FDA approved antiresorptive agents, anti-estrogens or selective estrogen receptor moderators.

Limitations:

Because of significant specimen to specimen collagen crosslink physiologic variability (15-20%), current recommendations for appropriate utilization include: one or two base-line assays from specified urine collections on separate days; followed by a repeat assay about three months after starting anti-resorptive therapy; followed by a repeat assay in 12 months after the three-month assay; and thereafter not more than annually, unless there is a change in therapy in which circumstance an additional test may be indicated three months after the initiation of new therapy.

Some collagen crosslink assays may not be appropriate for use in some disorders, according to FDA labeling restrictions.

Note: Scroll down for links to the quarterly Covered Code Lists (including narrative).

100-03, 190.20

NCD for Blood Glucose Testing (190.20)

(Rev. 28, Issued: 02-11-05, Effective: 01-01-05, Implementation: 03-11-05)

Indications:

Blood glucose values are often necessary for the management of patients with diabetes mellitus, where hyperglycemia and hypoglycemia are often present. They are also critical in the determination of control of blood glucose levels in the patient with impaired fasting glucose (FPG 110-125 mg/dL), the patient with insulin resistance syndrome and/or carbohydrate intolerance (excessive rise in glucose following ingestion of glucose or glucose sources of food), in the patient with a hypoglycemia disorder such as nesidioblastosis or insulinoma, and in patients with a catabolic or malnutrition state. In addition to those conditions already listed, glucose testing may be medically necessary in patients with tuberculosis, unexplained chronic or recurrent infections, alcoholism, coronary artery disease (especially in women), or unexplained skin conditions (including pruritus, local skin infections, ulceration and gangrene without an established cause).

Many medical conditions may be a consequence of a sustained elevated or depressed glucose level. These include comas, seizures or epilepsy, confusion, abnormal hunger, abnormal weight loss or gain, and loss of sensation. Evaluation of glucose may also be indicated in patients on medications known to affect carbohydrate metabolism.

Effective January 1, 2005, the Medicare law expanded coverage to diabetic screening services. Some forms of blood glucode testing covered under this national coverage determination may be covered for screening purposes subject to specified frequencies. See 42 CFR 410.18 and section 90, chapter 18 of the Claims Processing Manual, for a full description of this screening benefit.

Limitations:

Frequent home blood glucose testing by diabetic patients should be encouraged. In stable, non-hospitalized patients who are unable or unwilling to do home monitoring, it may be reasonable and necessary to measure quantitative blood glucose up to four times annually.

Depending upon the age of the patient, type of diabetes, degree of control, complications of diabetes, and other co-morbid conditions, more frequent testing than four times annually may be reasonable and necessary.

In some patients presenting with nonspecific signs, symptoms, or diseases not normally associated with disturbances in glucose metabolism, a single blood glucose test may be medically necessary. Repeat testing may not be indicated unless abnormal results are found or unless there is a change in clinical condition. If repeat testing is performed, a specific diagnosis code (e.g., diabetes) should be reported to support medical necessity. However, repeat testing may be indicated where results are normal in patients with conditions where there is a confirmed continuing risk of glucose metabolism abnormality (e.g., monitoring glucocorticoid therapy).

100-03, 190.22

NCD for Thyroid Testing (190.22)

(Rev. 17, Issued: 07-02-04) (Effective/Implementation: Not Applicable)

Indications

Thyroid function tests are used to define hyper function, euthyroidism, or hypofunction of thyroid disease. Thyroid testing may be reasonable and necessary to:

- Distinguish between primary and secondary hypothyroidism;
- Confirm or rule out primary hypothyroidism;
- Monitor thyroid hormone levels (for example, patients with goiter, thyroid nodules, or thyroid cancer);
- Monitor drug therapy in patients with primary hypothyroidism;
- Confirm or rule out primary hyperthyroidism; and
- Monitor therapy in patients with hyperthyroidism.

Thyroid function testing may be medically necessary in patients with disease or neoplasm of the thyroid and other endocrine glands. Thyroid function testing may also be medically necessary in patients with metabolic disorders; malnutrition; hyperlipidemia; certain types of anemia; psychosis and non-psychotic personality disorders; unexplained depression; ophthalmologic disorders; various cardiac arrhythmias; disorders of menstruation; skin conditions; myalgias; and a wide array of signs and symptoms, including alterations in consciousness; malaise; hypothermia; symptoms of the nervous and musculoskeletal system; skin and integumentary system; nutrition and metabolism; cardiovascular; and gastrointestinal system.

It may be medically necessary to do follow-up thyroid testing in patients with a personal history of malignant neoplasm of the endocrine system and in patients on long-term thyroid drug therapy.

Limitations

Testing may be covered up to two times a year in clinically stable patients; more frequent testing may be reasonable and necessary for patients whose thyroid therapy has been altered or in whom symptoms or signs of hyperthyroidism or hypothyroidism are noted.

100-03, 190.23

NCD for Lipid Testing (190.23)

(Rev. 28, Issued: 02-11-05, Effective: 01-01-05, Implementation: 03-11-05)

Indications and Limitations of Coverage

Indications

The medical community recognizes lipid testing as appropriate for evaluating atherosclerotic cardiovascular disease. Conditions in which lipid testing may be indicated include:

- Assessment of patients with atherosclerotic cardiovascular disease.
- Evaluation of primary dyslipidemia.
- Any form of atherosclerotic disease, or any disease leading to the formation of atherosclerotic disease.
- Diagnostic evaluation of diseases associated with altered lipid metabolism, such as: nephrotic syndrome, pancreatitis, hepatic disease, and hypo and hyperthyroidism.
- Secondary dyslipidemia, including diabetes mellitus, disorders of gastrointestinal absorption, chronic renal failure.
- Signs or symptoms of dyslipidemias, such as skin lesions.
- As follow-up to the initial screen for coronary heart disease (total cholesterol + HDL cholesterol) when total cholesterol is determined to be high (>240 mg/dL), or borderline-high (200-240 mg/dL) plus two or more coronary heart disease risk factors, or an HDL cholesterol, <35 mg/dl.

To monitor the progress of patients on anti-lipid dietary management and pharmacologic therapy for the treatment of elevated blood lipid disorders, total cholesterol, HDL cholesterol and LDL cholesterol may be used. Triglycerides may be obtained if this lipid fraction is also elevated or if the patient is put on drugs (for example, thiazide diuretics, beta blockers, estrogens, glucocorticoids, and tamoxifen) which may raise the triglyceride level.

When monitoring long term anti-lipid dietary or pharmacologic therapy and when following patients with borderline high total or LDL cholesterol levels, it may be reasonable to perform the lipid panel annually. A lipid panel at a yearly interval will usually be adequate while measurement of the serum total cholesterol or a measured LDL should suffice for interim visits if the patient does not have hypertriglyceridemia.

Any one component of the panel or a measured LDL may be reasonable and necessary up to six times the first year for monitoring dietary or pharmacologic therapy. More frequent total cholesterol HDL cholesterol, LDL cholesterol and triglyceride testing may be indicated for marked elevations or for changes to anti-lipid therapy due to inadequate initial patient response to dietary or pharmacologic therapy. The LDL cholesterol or total cholesterol may be measured three times yearly after treatment goals have been achieved.

Electrophoretic or other quantitation of lipoproteins may be indicated if the patient has a primary disorder of lipid metabolism.

Effective January 1, 2005, the Medicare law expanded coverage to cardiovascular screening services. Several of the procedures included in this NCD may be covered for screening purposes subject to specified frequencies. See 42 CFR 410.17 and section 100, chapter 18, of the Claims Processing Manual, for a full description of this benefit.

Limitations

Lipid panel and hepatic panel testing may be used for patients with severe psoriasis which has not responded to conventional therapy and for which the retinoid etretinate has been prescribed and who have developed hyperlipidemia or hepatic toxicity. Specific examples include erythrodermia and generalized pustular type and psoriasis associated with arthritis.

Routine screening and prophylactic testing for lipid disorder are not covered by Medicare. While lipid screening may be medically appropriate, Medicare by statute does not pay for it. Lipid testing in asymptomatic individuals is considered to be screening regardless of the presence of other risk factors such as family history, tobacco use, etc.

Once a diagnosis is established, one or several specific tests are usually adequate for monitoring the course of the disease. Less specific diagnoses (for example, other chest pain) alone do not support medical necessity of these tests.

When monitoring long term anti-lipid dietary or pharmacologic therapy and when following patients with borderline high total or LDL cholesterol levels, it is reasonable to perform the lipid panel annually. A lipid panel at a yearly interval will usually be adequate while measurement of the serum total cholesterol or a measured LDL should suffice for interim visits if the patient does not have hypertriglyceridemia.

Any one component of the panel or a measured LDL may be medically necessary up to six times the first year for monitoring dietary or pharmacologic therapy. More frequent total cholesterol HDL cholesterol, LDL cholesterol and triglyceride testing may be indicated for marked elevations or for changes to anti-lipid therapy due to inadequate initial patient response to dietary or pharmacologic therapy. The LDL cholesterol or total cholesterol may be measured three times yearly after treatment goals have been achieved.

If no dietary or pharmacological therapy is advised, monitoring is not necessary.

When evaluating non-specific chronic abnormalities of the liver (for example, elevations of transaminase, alkaline phosphatase, abnormal imaging studies, etc.), a lipid panel would generally not be indicated more than twice per year.

100-03, 190.26

NCD for Carcinoembryonic Antigen (CEA)

(Rev. 17, Issued: 07-02-04)

Carcinoembryonic antigen (CEA) is a protein polysaccharide found in some carcinomas. It is effective as a biochemical marker for monitoring the response of certain malignancies to therapy.

Indications

CEA may be medically necessary for follow-up of patients with colorectal carcinoma. It would however only be medically necessary at treatment decision-making points. In some clinical situations (e.g. adenocarcinoma of the lung, small cell carcinoma of the lung, and some gastrointestinal carcinomas) when a more specific marker is not expressed by the tumor, CEA may be a medically necessary alternative marker for monitoring. Preoperative CEA may also be helpful in determining the post-operative adequacy of surgical resection and subsequent medical management. In general, a single tumor marker will suffice in following patients with colorectal carcinoma or other malignancies that express such tumor markers.

In following patients who have had treatment for colorectal carcinoma, ASCO guideline suggests that if resection of liver metastasis would be indicated, it is recommended that post-operative CEA testing be performed every two to three months in patients with initial stage II or stage III disease for at least two years after diagnosis.

For patients with metastatic solid tumors which express CEA, CEA may be measured at the start of the treatment and with subsequent treatment cycles to assess the tumor's response to therapy.

Limitations:

Serum CEA determinations are generally not indicated more frequently than once per chemotherapy treatment cycle for patients with metastatic solid tumors which express CEA or every two months post-surgical treatment for patients who have had colorectal carcinoma. However, it may be proper to order the test more frequently in certain situations, for example, when there has been a significant change from prior CEA level or a significant change in patient status which could reflect disease progression or recurrence.

Testing with a diagnosis of an in situ carcinoma is not reasonably done more frequently than once, unless the result is abnormal, in which case the test may be repeated once.

100-03, 190.31

NCD for Prostate Specific Antigen (PSA) (190.31)

(Rev. 17, Issued: 07-02-04) (Effective/Implementation: Not Applicable)

Indications:

PSA is of proven value in differentiating benign from malignant disease in men with lower urinary tract signs and symptoms (e.g., hematuria, slow urine stream, hesitancy, urgency, frequency, nocturia and incontinence) as well as with patients with palpably abnormal prostate glands on physician exam, and in patients with other laboratory or imaging studies that suggest the possibility of a malignant prostate disorder. PSA is also a marker used to follow the progress of prostate cancer once a diagnosis has been established, such as in detecting metastatic or persistent disease in patients who may require additional treatment. PSA testing may also be useful in the differential diagnosis of men presenting with as yet undiagnosed disseminated metastatic disease.

Limitations:

Generally, for patients with lower urinary tract signs or symptoms, the test is performed only once per year unless there is a change in the patient's medical condition.

Testing with a diagnosis of in situ carcinoma is not reasonably done more frequently than once, unless the result is abnormal, in which case the test may be repeated once.

100-03, 210.1

NCD for Prostate Cancer Screening Tests (210.1)

(Rev. 48, Issued: 03-17-06; Effective/Implementation Dates: 06-19-06)

Indications and Limitations of Coverage

CIM 50-55

Covered

A. General

Section 4103 of the Balanced Budget Act of 1997 provides for coverage of certain prostate cancer screening tests subject to certain coverage, frequency, and payment

limitations. Medicare will cover prostate cancer screening tests/procedures for the early detection of prostate cancer. Coverage of prostate cancer screening tests includes the following procedures furnished to an individual for the early detection of prostate cancer:

- Screening digital rectal examination; and
- Screening prostate specific antigen blood test

B. Screening Digital Rectal Examinations

Screening digital rectal examinations are covered at a frequency of once every 12 months for men who have attained age 50 (at least 11 months have passed following the month in which the last Medicare-covered screening digital rectal examination was performed). Screening digital rectal examination means a clinical examination of an individual's prostate for nodules or other abnormalities of the prostate. This screening must be performed by a doctor of medicine or osteopathy (as defined in §1861(r)(1) of the Act), or by a physician assistant, nurse practitioner, clinical nurse specialist, or certified nurse midwife (as defined in §1861(aa) and §1861(gg) of the Act) who is authorized under State law to perform the examination, fully knowledgeable about the beneficiary's medical condition, and would be responsible for using the results of any examination performed in the overall management of the beneficiary's specific medical problem.

C. Screening Prostate Specific Antigen Tests

Screening prostate specific antigen tests are covered at a frequency of once every 12 months for men who have attained age 50 (at least 11 months have passed following the month in which the last Medicare-covered screening prostate specific antigen test was performed). Screening prostate specific antigen tests (PSA) means a test to detect the marker for adenocarcinoma of prostate. PSA is a reliable immunocytochemical marker for primary and metastatic adenocarcinoma of prostate. This screening must be ordered by the beneficiary's physician or by the beneficiary's physician assistant, nurse practitioner, clinical nurse specialist, or certified nurse midwife (the term "attending physician"; is defined in §1861(r)(1) of the Act to mean a doctor of medicine or osteopathy and the terms ";physician assistant, nurse practitioner, clinical nurse specialist, or certified nurse midwife"; are defined in §1861(aa) and §1861(gg) of the Act) who is fully knowledgeable about the beneficiary's medical condition, and who would be responsible for using the results of any examination (test) performed in the overall management of the beneficiary's specific medical problem.

100-03, 210.2

NCD for Screening Pap Smears and Pelvic Examinations for Early Detection of Cervical or Vaginal Cancer (210.2)

(Rev. 173, Issued: 09-04-14, Effective: Upon Implementation: of ICD–10)

Screening Pap Smear

A screening pap smear and related medically necessary services provided to a woman for the early detection of cervical cancer (including collection of the sample of cells and a physician's interpretation of the test results) and pelvic examination (including clinical breast examination) are covered under Medicare Part B when ordered by a physician (or authorized practitioner) under one of the following conditions:

- She has not had such a test during the preceding two years or is a woman of childbearing age (§1861(nn) of the Social Security Act (the Act).
- There is evidence (on the basis of her medical history or other findings) that she is at high risk of developing cervical cancer and her physician (or authorized practitioner) recommends that she have the test performed more frequently than every two years.

High risk factors for cervical and vaginal cancer are:

- Early onset of sexual activity (under 16 years of age)
- Multiple sexual partners (five or more in a lifetime)
- History of sexually transmitted disease (including HIV infection)
- Fewer than three negative or any pap smears within the previous seven years; and
- DES (diethylstilbestrol) - exposed daughters of women who took DES during pregnancy.

NOTE: Claims for pap smears must indicate the beneficiary's low or high risk status by including the appropriate diagnosis code on the line item (Item 24E of the Form CMS-1500).

Definitions

A woman as described in §1861(nn) of the Act is a woman who is of childbearing age and has had a pap smear test during any of the preceding 3 years that indicated the presence of cervical or vaginal cancer or other abnormality, or is at high risk of developing cervical or vaginal cancer.

A woman of childbearing age is one who is premenopausal and has been determined by a physician or other qualified practitioner to be of childbearing age, based upon the medical history or other findings.

Other qualified practitioner, as defined in 42 CFR 410.56(a) includes a certified nurse midwife (as defined in §1861(gg) of the Act), or a physician assistant, nurse practitioner, or clinical nurse specialist (as defined in §1861(aa) of the Act) who is authorized under State law to perform the examination.

Screening Pelvic Examination

Section 4102 of the Balanced Budget Act of 1997 provides for coverage of screening pelvic examinations (including a clinical breast examination) for all female beneficiaries, subject to certain frequency and other limitations. A screening pelvic examination (including a clinical breast examination) should include at least seven of the following eleven elements:

- Inspection and palpation of breasts for masses or lumps, tenderness, symmetry, or nipple discharge.
- Digital rectal examination including sphincter tone, presence of hemorrhoids, and rectal masses. Pelvic examination (with or without specimen collection for smears and cultures) including:
- External genitalia (for example, general appearance, hair distribution, or lesions).
- Urethral meatus (for example, size, location, lesions, or prolapse).
- Urethra (for example, masses, tenderness, or scarring).
- Bladder (for example, fullness, masses, or tenderness).
- Vagina (for example, general appearance, estrogen effect, discharge lesions, pelvic support, cystocele, or rectocele).
- Cervix (for example, general appearance, lesions, or discharge).
- Uterus (for example, size, contour, position, mobility, tenderness, consistency, descent, or support).
- Adnexa/parametria (for example, masses, tenderness, organomegaly, or nodularity).
- Anus and perineum.

This description is from Documentation Guidelines for Evaluation and Management Services, published in May 1997 and was developed by the Centers for Medicare & Medicaid Services and the American Medical Association.

100-03, 210.2.1

Screening for Cervical Cancer with Human Papillomavirus (HPV) Testing (Effective July 9, 2015)

(Rev. 189, Issued: 02-05-16, Effective: 07-05-16; Implementation: 03-07-16 - for non-shared MAC edits; 07-05-16 - CWF analysis and design; 10-03-16 - CWF Coding, Testing and Implementation, MCS, and FISS Implementation; 01-03-17 - Requirement BR9434.04.8.2)

A. General

Medicare covers a screening pelvic examination and Pap test for all female beneficiaries at 12 or 24 month intervals, based on specific risk factors. See 42 C.F.R. §410.56; Medicare National Coverage Determinations Manual, §210.2.1 Current Medicare coverage does not include the HPV testing. Pursuant to §1861(ddd) of the Social Security Act, the Secretary may add coverage of "additional preventive services" if certain statutory requirements are met.

B. Nationally Covered Indications

Effective for services performed on or after July 9, 2015, CMS has determined that the evidence is sufficient to add Human Papillomavirus (HPV) testing once every five years as an additional preventive service benefit under the Medicare program for asymptomatic beneficiaries aged 30 to 65 years in conjunction with the Pap smear test. CMS will cover screening for cervical cancer with the appropriate U.S. Food and Drug Administration (FDA) approved/cleared laboratory tests, used consistent with FDA approved labeling and in compliance with the Clinical Laboratory Improvement Act (CLIA) regulations.

C. Nationally Non-Covered Indications

Unless specifically covered in this NCD, any other NCD, by statute or regulation, preventive services are non-covered by Medicare.

D. Other

(This NCD last reviewed July 2015.)

100-03, 210.4.1

Counseling to Prevent Tobacco Use (Effective August 25, 2010)

(Rev.202, Issued: 08-25-17, Effective: 09-26-17, Implementation: 09- 26-17)

A. General

Tobacco use remains the leading cause of preventable morbidity and mortality in the U.S. and is a major contributor to the nation's increasing medical costs. Despite the growing list of adverse health effects associated with smoking, more than 45 million U.S. adults continue to smoke and approximately 1,200 die prematurely each day from tobacco-related diseases. Annual smoking-attributable expenditures can be measured both in direct medical costs ($96 billion) and in lost productivity ($97 billion), but the results of national surveys have raised concerns that recent declines in smoking prevalence among U.S. adults may have come to an end. According to the U.S. Department of Health and Human Services (DHHS) Public Health Service (PHS) Clinical Practice Guideline on Treating Tobacco Use and Dependence (2008), 4.5 million adults over 65 years of age smoke cigarettes. Even smokers over age 65, however, can benefit greatly from abstinence, and older smokers who quit can reduce their risk of death from coronary heart disease, chronic obstructive lung disease and lung cancer, as well as decrease their risk of osteoporosis.

B. Nationally Covered Indications

Effective for claims with dates of service on or after August 25, 2010, CMS will cover tobacco cessation counseling for outpatient and hospitalized Medicare beneficiaries

1. Who use tobacco, regardless of whether they have signs or symptoms of tobacco-related disease;
2. Who are competent and alert at the time that counseling is provided; and,
3. Whose counseling is furnished by a qualified physician or other Medicare-recognized practitioner.

Intermediate and intensive smoking cessation counseling services will be covered under Medicare Part B when the above conditions of coverage are met, subject to frequency and other limitations. That is, similar to existing tobacco cessation counseling for symptomatic individuals, CMS will allow 2 individual tobacco cessation counseling attempts per 12-month period. Each attempt may include a maximum of 4 intermediate OR intensive sessions, with a total benefit covering up to 8 sessions per 12-month period per Medicare beneficiary who uses tobacco. The practitioner and patient have the flexibility to choose between intermediate (more than 3 minutes but less than 10 minutes), or intensive (more than 10 minutes) cessation counseling sessions for each attempt.

C. Nationally Non-Covered Indications

Inpatient hospital stays with the principal diagnosis of tobacco use disorder are not reasonable and necessary for the effective delivery of tobacco cessation counseling services. Therefore, we will not cover tobacco cessation services if tobacco cessation is the primary reason for the patient's hospital stay.

D. Other

Section 4104 of the Affordable Care Act provided for a waiver of the Medicare coinsurance and Part B deductible requirements for this service effective on or after January 1, 2011. Until that time, this service will continue to be subject to the standard Medicare coinsurance and Part B deductible requirements.

100-03, 220.2

(Rev. 173, Issued: 09-04-14, Effective: Upon Implementation: of ICD-10, Implementation: Upon Implementation of ICD-10)

A. General

1. Method of Operation

   Magnetic Resonance Imaging (MRI), formerly called nuclear magnetic resonance (NMR), is a non-invasive method of graphically representing the distribution of water and other hydrogen-rich molecules in the human body. In contrast to conventional radiographs or computed tomography (CT) scans, in which the image is produced by x-ray beam attenuation by an object, MRI is capable of producing images by several techniques. In fact, various combinations of MRI image production methods may be employed to emphasize particular characteristics of the tissue or body part being examined. The basic elements by which MRI produces an image are the density of hydrogen nuclei in the object being examined, their motion, and the relaxation times, and the period of time required for the nuclei to return to their original states in the main, static magnetic field after being subjected to a brief additional magnetic field. These relaxation times reflect the physical-chemical properties of tissue and the molecular environment of its hydrogen nuclei. Only hydrogen atoms are present in human tissues in sufficient concentration for current use in clinical MRI.

   Magnetic Resonance Angiography (MRA) is a non-invasive diagnostic test that is an application of MRI. By analyzing the amount of energy released from tissues exposed to a strong magnetic field, MRA provides images of normal and diseased blood vessels, as well as visualization and quantification of blood flow through these vessels.

2. General Clinical Utility

   Overall, MRI is a useful diagnostic imaging modality that is capable of demonstrating a wide variety of soft-tissue lesions with contrast resolution equal or superior to CT scanning in various parts of the body.

   Among the advantages of MRI are the absence of ionizing radiation and the ability to achieve high levels of tissue contrast resolution without injected iodinated radiological contrast agents. Recent advances in technology have resulted in development and Food and Drug Administration (FDA) approval of new paramagnetic contrast agents for MRI which allow even better visualization in some instances. Multi-slice imaging and the ability to image in multiple planes, especially sagittal and coronal, have provided flexibility not easily available with other modalities. Because cortical (outer layer) bone and metallic prostheses do not cause distortion of MR images, it has been possible to visualize certain lesions and body regions with greater certainty than has been possible with CT. The use of MRI on certain soft tissue structures for the purpose of detecting disruptive, neoplastic, degenerative, or inflammatory lesions has now become established in medical practice.

   Phase contrast (PC) and time-of-flight (TOF) are some of the available MRA techniques at the time these instructions are being issued. PC measures the difference between the phases of proton spins in tissue and blood and measures both the venous and arterial blood flow at any point in the cardiac cycle. TOF measures the difference between the amount of magnetization of tissue and blood and provides information on the structure of blood vessels, thus indirectly indicating blood flow. Two-dimensional (2D) and three-dimensional (3D) images can be obtained using each method.

Contrast-enhanced MRA (CE-MRA) involves blood flow imaging after the patient receives an intravenous injection of a contrast agent. Gadolinium, a non-ionic element, is the foundation of all contrast agents currently in use. Gadolinium affects the way in which tissues respond to magnetization, resulting in better visualization of structures when compared to un-enhanced studies. Unlike ionic (i.e., iodine-based) contrast agents used in conventional contrast angiography (CA), allergic reactions to gadolinium are extremely rare. Additionally, gadolinium does not cause the kidney failure occasionally seen with ionic contrast agents. Digital subtraction angiography (DSA) is a computer-augmented form of CA that obtains digital blood flow images as contrast agent courses through a blood vessel. The computer "subtracts" bone and other tissue from the image, thereby improving visualization of blood vessels. Physicians elect to use a specific MRA or CA technique based upon clinical information from each patient.

B. Nationally Covered MRI and MRA Indications

1. MRI

   Although several uses of MRI are still considered investigational and some uses are clearly contraindicated (see subsection C), MRI is considered medically efficacious for a number of uses. Use the following descriptions as general guidelines or examples of what may be considered covered rather than as a restrictive list of specific covered indications. Coverage is limited to MRI units that have received FDA premarket approval, and such units must be operated within the parameters specified by the approval. In addition, the services must be reasonable and necessary for the diagnosis or treatment of the specific patient involved.

   a. Effective November 22, 1985, MRI is useful in examining the head, central nervous system, and spine. Multiple sclerosis can be diagnosed with MRI and the contents of the posterior fossa are visible. The inherent tissue contrast resolution of MRI makes it an appropriate standard diagnostic modality for general neuroradiology.

   b. Effective November 22, 1985, MRI can assist in the differential diagnosis of mediastinal and retroperitoneal masses, including abnormalities of the large vessels such as aneurysms and dissection. When a clinical need exists to visualize the parenchyma of solid organs to detect anatomic disruption or neoplasia, this can be accomplished in the liver, urogenital system, adrenals, and pelvic organs without the use of radiological contrast materials. When MRI is considered reasonable and necessary, the use of paramagnetic contrast materials may be covered as part of the study. MRI may also be used to detect and stage pelvic and retroperitoneal neoplasms and to evaluate disorders of cancellous bone and soft tissues. It may also be used in the detection of pericardial thickening. Primary and secondary bone neoplasm and aseptic necrosis can be detected at an early stage and monitored with MRI. Patients with metallic prostheses, especially of the hip, can be imaged in order to detect the early stages of infection of the bone to which the prosthesis is attached.

   c. Effective March 22, 1994, MRI may also be covered to diagnose disc disease without regard to whether radiological imaging has been tried first to diagnose the problem.

   d. Effective March 4, 1991, MRI with gating devices and surface coils, and gating devices that eliminate distorted images caused by cardiac and respiratory movement cycles are now considered state of the art techniques and may be covered. Surface and other specialty coils may also be covered, as they are used routinely·for high resolution imaging where small limited regions of the body are studied. They produce high signal-to-noise ratios resulting in images of enhanced anatomic detail.

2. MRA (MRI for Blood Flow)

   Currently covered indications include using MRA for specific conditions to evaluate flow in internal carotid vessels of the head and neck, peripheral arteries of lower extremities, abdomen and pelvis, and the chest. Coverage is limited to MRA units that have received FDA premarket approval, and such units must be operated within the parameters specified by the approval. In addition, the services must be reasonable and necessary for the diagnosis or treatment of the specific patient involved.

   a. Head and Neck

   Effective April 15, 2003, studies have proven that MRA is effective for evaluating flow in internal carotid vessels of the head and neck. However, not all potential applications of MRA have been shown to be reasonable and necessary. All of the following criteria must apply in order for Medicare to provide coverage for MRA of the head and neck:

   – MRA is used to evaluate the carotid arteries, the circle of Willis, the anterior, middle or posterior cerebral arteries, the vertebral or basilar arteries or the venous sinuses;

   – MRA is performed on patients with conditions of the head and neck for which surgery is anticipated and may be found to be appropriate based on the MRA. These conditions include, but are not limited to, tumor, aneurysms, vascular malformations, vascular occlusion or thrombosis.

   Within this broad category of disorders, medical necessity is the underlying determinant of the need for an MRA in specific diseases. The medical records should clearly justify and demonstrate the existence of medical necessity; and

   – MRA and CA are not expected to be performed on the same patient for diagnostic purposes prior to the application of anticipated therapy. Only

one of these tests will be covered routinely unless the physician can demonstrate the medical need to perform both tests.

   b. Peripheral Arteries of Lower Extremities

   Effective April 15, 2003, studies have proven that MRA of peripheral arteries is useful in determining the presence and extent of peripheral vascular disease in lower extremities. This procedure is non-invasive and has been shown to find occult vessels in some patients for which those vessels were not apparent when CA was performed. Medicare will cover either MRA or CA to evaluate peripheral arteries of the lower extremities. However, both MRA and CA may be useful in some cases, such as:

   – A patient has had CA and this test was unable to identify a viable run-off vessel for bypass. When exploratory surgery is not believed to be a reasonable medical course of action for this patient, MRA may be performed to identify the viable runoff vessel; or

   – A patient has had MRA, but the results are inconclusive.

   c. Abdomen and Pelvis

   i. Pre-operative Evaluation of Patients Undergoing Elective Abdominal Aortic Aneurysm (AAA) Repair

   Effective July 1, 1999, MRA is covered for pre-operative evaluation of patients undergoing elective AAA repair if the scientific evidence reveals MRA is considered comparable to CA in determining the extent of AAA, as well as in evaluating aortoiliac occlusion disease and renal artery pathology that may be necessary in the surgical planning of AAA repair. These studies also reveal that MRA could provide a net benefit to the patient. If preoperative CA is avoided, then patients are not exposed to the risks associated with invasive procedures, contrast media, end-organ damage, or arterial injury.

   ii. Imaging the Renal Arteries and the Aortoiliac Arteries in the Absence of AAA or Aortic Dissection

   Effective July 1, 2003, MRA coverage is expanded to include imaging the renal arteries and the aortoiliac arteries in the absence of AAA or aortic dissection. MRA should be obtained in those circumstances in which using MRA is expected to avoid obtaining CA, when physician history, physical examination, and standard assessment tools provide insufficient information for patient management, and obtaining an MRA has a high probability of positively affecting patient management. However, CA may be ordered after obtaining the results of an MRA in those rare instances where medical necessity is demonstrated.

   d. Chest

   i. Diagnosis of Pulmonary Embolism

   Current scientific data has shown that diagnostic pulmonary MRAs are improving due to recent developments such as faster imaging capabilities and gadolinium-enhancement. However, these advances in MRA are not significant enough to warrant replacement of pulmonary angiography in the diagnosis of pulmonary embolism for patients who have no contraindication to receiving intravenous iodinated contrast material. Patients who are allergic to iodinated contrast material face a high risk of developing complications if they undergo pulmonary angiography or computed tomography angiography. Therefore, Medicare will cover MRA of the chest for diagnosing a suspected pulmonary embolism when it is contraindicated for the patient to receive intravascular iodinated contrast material.

   ii. Evaluation of Thoracic Aortic Dissection and Aneurysm

   Studies have shown that MRA of the chest has a high level of diagnostic accuracy for pre-operative and post-operative evaluation of aortic dissection of aneurysm. Depending on the clinical presentation, MRA may be used as an alternative to other non-invasive imaging technologies, such as transesophageal echocardiography and CT. Generally, Medicare will provide coverage only for MRA or for CA when used as a diagnostic test. However, if both MRA and CA of the chest are used, the physician must demonstrate the medical need for performing these tests.

   While the intent of this policy is to provide reimbursement for either RA or CA, the Centers for Medicare & Medicaid Services (CMS) is also allowing flexibility for physicians to make appropriate decisions concerning the use of these tests based on the needs of individual patients. CMS anticipates, however, low utilization of the combined use of MRA and CA. As a result, CMS encourages the Medicare Administrative Contractors (MACs) to monitor the use of these tests and, where indicated, require evidence of the need to perform both MRA and CA.

C. Contraindications and Nationally Non-Covered Indications

1. Contraindications

   The MRI is not covered when the following patient-specific contraindications are present:

   MRI is not covered for patients with cardiac pacemakers or with metallic clips on vascular aneurysms unless the Medicare beneficiary meets the provisions of the following exceptions:

   Effective July 7, 2011, the contraindications will not apply to pacemakers when used according to the FDA-approved labeling in an MRI environment, or

Effective February 24, 2011, CMS believes that the evidence is promising although not yet convincing that MRI will improve patient health outcomes if certain safeguards are in place to ensure that the exposure of the device to an MRI environment adversely affects neither the interpretation of the MRI result nor the proper functioning of the implanted device itself. We believe that specific precautions (as listed below) could maximize benefits of MRI exposure for beneficiaries enrolled in clinical trials designed to assess the utility and safety of MRI exposure. Therefore, CMS determines that MRI will be covered by Medicare when provided in a clinical study under section 1862(a)(1)(E) (consistent with section 1142 of the Social Security Act (the Act)) through the Coverage with Study Participation (CSP) form of Coverage with Evidence Development (CED) if the study meets the criteria in each of the three paragraphs below:

The approved prospective clinical study of MRI must, with appropriate methodology, address one or more aspects of the following questions:

1. Do results of MRI in implanted permanent pacemaker (PM)/implantable cardioverter defibrillator (ICD) beneficiaries with implanted cardiac devices affect physician decision making related to:

    a. Clinical management strategy (e.g., in oncology, toward palliative or curative care)?

    b. Planning of treatment interventions?; or

    c. Prevention of unneeded diagnostic studies or interventions, or preventable exposures?

2. Do results of MRI in PM/ICD beneficiaries with implanted cardiac devices affect patient outcomes related to:

    a. Survival?

    b. Quality of life?; or

    c. Adverse events during and after MR scanning?

In addition, the prospective clinical study of MRI must include safety criteria for all participants. Such required safety measures for such studies, as further explained in guidance documents from professional societies must include, but are not limited to:

1. MRI should be done on a case-by-case and site-by-site basis.

2. MRI scan sequences, field intensity, and field(s) of exposure should be selected to minimize risk to the patient while gaining needed diagnostic information for diagnosis or for managing therapy.

3. MRI scanning should be done only if the site is staffed with individuals with the appropriate radiology and cardiology knowledge and expertise on hand.

4. Implanted device patients who are candidates for recruitment for an MRI clinical study should be advised that life-threatening arrhythmias might occur during MRI and serious device malfunction might occur, requiring replacement of the device.

5. Radiology and cardiology personnel and a fully stocked crash cart should be readily available throughout the procedure in case a significant arrhythmia develops during the examination that does not terminate with the cessation of the MRI study. The cardiologist should be familiar with the patient's arrhythmia history and the implanted device. A programmer that can be used to adjust the device as necessary should be readily available.

6. All such patients should be actively monitored for cardiac and respiratory function throughout the examination. At a minimum, ECG and pulse oximetry should be used. Visual and verbal contact with the patient must be maintained throughout the MRI scan. The patient should be instructed to alert the MRI staff on hand to any unusual sensations, pains, or to any problems.

7. At the conclusion of the examination, the cardiologist should examine the device to confirm that the function is consistent with its pre-examination state.

8. Follow-up should include a check of the patient's device at a time remote (1-6 weeks) after the scan to confirm appropriate function.

9. If the implanted device manufacturer has indicated additional safety precautions appropriate for safe MRI performance, these must be included in the study protocol.

The clinical study must adhere to the following standards of scientific integrity and relevance to the Medicare population:

a. The principal purpose of the research study is to test whether a particular intervention potentially improves the participants' health outcomes.

b. The research study is well supported by available scientific and medical information or it is intended to clarify or establish the health outcomes of interventions already in common clinical use.

c. The research study does not unjustifiably duplicate existing studies.

d. The research study design is appropriate to answer the research question being asked in the study.

e. The research study is sponsored by an organization or individual capable of executing the proposed study successfully.

f. The research study is in compliance with all applicable Federal regulations concerning the protection of human subjects found at 45 CFR Part 46. If a study is regulated by the FDA, it must be in compliance with 21 CFR Parts 50 and 56.

g. All aspects of the research study are conducted according to appropriate standards of scientific integrity (see http://www.icmje.org).

h. The research study has a written protocol that clearly addresses, or incorporates by reference, the standards listed here as Medicare requirements for CED coverage.

i. The clinical research study is not designed to exclusively test toxicity or disease pathophysiology in healthy individuals. Trials of all medical technologies measuring therapeutic outcomes as one of the objectives meet this standard only if the disease or condition being studied is life threatening as defined in 21 CFR §312.81(a) and the patient has no other viable treatment options.

j. The clinical research study is registered on the www.ClinicalTrials.gov website by the principal sponsor/investigator prior to the enrollment of the first study subject.

k. The research study protocol specifies the method and timing of public release of all pre-specified outcomes to be measured, including release of outcomes if outcomes are negative or study is terminated early. The results must be made public within 24 months of the end of data collection. If a report is planned to be published in a peer reviewed journal, then that initial release may be an abstract that meets the requirements of the International Committee of Medical Journal Editors (http://www.icmje.org). However, a full report of the outcomes must be made public no later than three (3) years after the end of data collection.

l. The research study protocol must explicitly discuss subpopulations affected by the treatment under investigation, particularly traditionally underrepresented groups in clinical studies, how the inclusion and exclusion criteria effect enrollment of these populations, and a plan for the retention and reporting of said populations in the trial. If the inclusion and exclusion criteria are expected to have a negative effect on the recruitment or retention of underrepresented populations, the protocol must discuss why these criteria are necessary.

m. The research study protocol explicitly discusses how the results are or are not expected to be generalizable to the Medicare population to infer whether Medicare patients may benefit from the intervention. Separate discussions in the protocol may be necessary for populations eligible for Medicare due to age, disability, or Medicaid eligibility.

Consistent with section 1142 of the Act, the Agency for Healthcare Research and Quality supports clinical research studies that CMS determines meet the above-listed standards and address the above-listed research questions.

- MRI during a viable pregnancy is also contraindicated at this time.

- The danger inherent in bringing ferromagnetic materials within range of MRI units generally constrains the use of MRI on acutely ill patients requiring life support systems and monitoring devices that employ ferromagnetic materials.

- In addition, the long imaging time and the enclosed position of the patient may result in claustrophobia, making patients who have a history of claustrophobia unsuitable candidates for MRI procedures.

2. Nationally Non-Covered Indications

CMS has determined that MRI of cortical bone and calcifications, and procedures involving spatial resolution of bone and calcifications, are not considered reasonable and necessary indications within the meaning of section 1862(a)(1)(A) of the Act, and are therefore non-covered.

D. Other

Effective June 3, 2010, all other uses of MRI or MRA for which CMS has not specifically indicated coverage or non-coverage continue to be eligible for coverage through individual MAC discretion.

100-03, 220.6.9

NCD for PET (FDG) for Refractory Seizures (220.6.9)

(Rev. 120; Issued: 05-06-10; Effective Date: 04-03-09; Implementation Date: 10-30-09)

Beginning July 1, 2001, Medicare covers FDG PET for pre-surgical evaluation for the purpose of localization of a focus of refractory seizure activity.

Limitations: Covered only for pre-surgical evaluation.

Documentation that these conditions are met should be maintained by the referring physician in the beneficiary's medical record, as is normal business practice.

(This NCD last reviewed June 2001.)

100-03, 220.6.17

NCD for Positron Emission Tomography (FDG) for Oncologic Conditions (220.6.17)

(Rev. 173, Issued: 09-04-14, Effective: Upon Implementation: of ICD–10)

A. General

FDG (2-[F18] fluoro-2-deoxy-D-glucose) Positron Emission Tomography (PET) is a minimally-invasive diagnostic imaging procedure used to evaluate glucose metabolism in normal tissue as well as in diseased tissues in conditions such as cancer, ischemic heart disease, and some neurologic disorders. FDG is an injected radionuclide (or radiopharmaceutical) that emits sub-atomic particles, known as positrons, as it decays. FDG PET uses a positron camera (tomograph) to measure the decay of FDG. The rate of FDG decay provides biochemical information on glucose metabolism in the tissue being studied. As malignancies can cause abnormalities of metabolism and blood flow, FDG PET evaluation may indicate the probable presence or absence of a malignancy based upon observed differences in biologic activity compared to adjacent tissues.

The Centers for Medicare and Medicaid Services (CMS) was asked by the National Oncologic PET Registry (NOPR) to reconsider section 220.6 of the National Coverage Determinations (NCD) Manual to end the prospective data collection requirements under Coverage with Evidence Development (CED) across all oncologic indications of FDG PET imaging. The CMS received public input indicating that the current coverage framework of prospective data collection under CED be ended for all oncologic uses of FDG PET imaging.

1. Framework

   Effective for claims with dates of service on and after June 11, 2013, CMS is adopting a coverage framework that ends the prospective data collection requirements by NOPR under CED for all oncologic uses of FDG PET imaging. CMS is making this change for all NCDs that address coverage of FDG PET for oncologic uses addressed in this decision. This decision does not change coverage for any use of PET imaging using radiopharmaceuticals NaF-18 (fluorine-18 labeled sodium fluoride), ammonia N-13, or rubidium-82 (Rb-82).

2. Initial Anti-Tumor Treatment Strategy

   CMS continues to believe that the evidence is adequate to determine that the results of FDG PET imaging are useful in determining the appropriate initial anti-tumor treatment strategy for beneficiaries with suspected cancer and improve health outcomes and thus are reasonable and necessary under §1862(a)(1)(A) of the Social Security Act (the Act).

   Therefore, CMS continues to nationally cover one FDG PET study for beneficiaries who have cancers that are biopsy proven or strongly suspected based on other diagnostic testing when the beneficiary's treating physician determines that the FDG PET study is needed to determine the location and/or extent of the tumor for the following therapeutic purposes related to the initial anti-tumor treatment strategy:

   — To determine whether or not the beneficiary is an appropriate candidate for an invasive diagnostic or therapeutic procedure; or

   — To determine the optimal anatomic location for an invasive procedure; or

   — To determine the anatomic extent of tumor when the recommended antitumor treatment reasonably depends on the extent of the tumor.

   See the table at the end of this section for a synopsis of all nationally covered and noncovered oncologic uses of FDG PET imaging.

   #### B.1. Initial Anti-Tumor Treatment Strategy Nationally Covered Indications

   a. CMS continues to nationally cover FDG PET imaging for the initial anti-tumor treatment strategy for male and female breast cancer only when used in staging distant metastasis.

   b. CMS continues to nationally cover FDG PET to determine initial anti-tumor treatment strategy for melanoma other than for the evaluation of regional lymph nodes.

   c. CMS continues to nationally cover FDG PET imaging for the detection of pre-treatment metastasis (i.e., staging) in newly diagnosed cervical cancers following conventional imaging.

   #### C.1. Initial Anti-Tumor Treatment Strategy Nationally Non-Covered Indications

   a. CMS continues to nationally non-cover initial anti-tumor treatment strategy in Medicare beneficiaries who have adenocarcinoma of the prostate.

   b. CMS continues to nationally non-cover FDG PET imaging for diagnosis of breast cancer and initial staging of axillary nodes.

   c. CMS continues to nationally non-cover FDG PET imaging for initial anti-tumor treatment strategy for the evaluation of regional lymph nodes in melanoma.

   d. CMS continues to nationally non-cover FDG PET imaging for the diagnosis of cervical cancer related to initial anti-tumor treatment strategy.

3. Subsequent Anti-Tumor Treatment Strategy

   #### B.2. Subsequent Anti-Tumor Treatment Strategy Nationally Covered Indications

   Three FDG PET scans are nationally covered when used to guide subsequent management of anti-tumor treatment strategy after completion of initial anti-cancer therapy. Coverage of more than three FDG PET scans to guide subsequent management of anti-tumor treatment strategy after completion of initial anti-cancer therapy shall be determined by the local Medicare Administrative Contractors.

4. Synopsis of Coverage of FDG PET for Oncologic Conditions

   Effective for claims with dates of service on and after June 11, 2013, the chart below summarizes national FDG PET coverage for oncologic conditions:

FDG PET for Cancers Tumor Type	Initial Treatment Strategy (formerly "diagnosis" & "staging")	Subsequent Treatment Strategy (formerly "restaging" & "monitoring response to treatment")
Colorectal	Cover	Cover
Esophagus	Cover	Cover
Head & Neck (not Thyroid, CNS)	Cover	Cover
Lymphoma	Cover	Cover
Non-Small Cell Lung	Cover	Cover
Ovary	Cover	Cover
Brain	Cover	Cover
Cervix	Cover w/exception*	Cover
Small Cell Lung	Cover	Cover
Soft Tissue Sarcoma	Cover	Cover
Pancreas	Cover	Cover
Testes	Cover	Cover
Prostate	Non-cover	Cover
Thyroid	Cover	Cover
Breast (male and female)	Cover w/exception*	Cover
Melanoma	Cover w/exception*	Cover
All Other Solid Tumors	Cover	Cover
Myeloma	Cover	Cover
All other cancers not listed	Cover	Cover

* Cervix: Nationally non-covered for the initial diagnosis of cervical cancer related to initial anti-tumor treatment strategy. All other indications for initial anti-tumor treatment strategy for cervical cancer are nationally covered.

* Breast: Nationally non-covered for initial diagnosis and/or staging of axillary lymph nodes. Nationally covered for initial staging of metastatic disease. All other indications for initial anti-tumor treatment strategy for breast cancer are nationally covered.

* Melanoma: Nationally non-covered for initial staging of regional lymph nodes. All other indications for initial anti-tumor treatment strategy for melanoma are nationally covered.

D. Other

N/A

100-03, 220.6.19

Positron Emission Tomography NaF-18 (NaF-18 PET) to Identify Bone Metastasis of Cancer (Effective February 26, 2010)

(Rev.119, Issued: 03-26-10, Effective: 02-26-10, Implementation: 07-06-10)

A. General

Positron Emission Tomography (PET) is a non-invasive, diagnostic imaging procedure that assesses the level of metabolic activity and perfusion in various organ systems of the body. A positron camera (tomograph) is used to produce cross-sectional tomographic images, which are obtained from positron-emitting radioactive tracer substances (radiopharmaceuticals) such as F-18 sodium fluoride. NaF-18 PET has been recognized as an excellent technique for imaging areas of altered osteogenic activity in bone. The clinical value of detecting and assessing the initial extent of metastatic cancer in bone is attested by a number of professional guidelines for oncology. Imaging to detect bone metastases is also recommended when a patient, following completion of initial treatment, is symptomatic with bone pain suspicious for metastases from a known primary tumor.

B. Nationally Covered Indications

Effective February 26, 2010, the Centers for Medicare & Medicaid Services (CMS) will cover NaF-18 PET imaging when the beneficiary's treating physician determines that the NaF-18 PET study is needed to inform the initial antitumor treatment strategy or to guide subsequent antitumor treatment strategy after the completion of initial treatment, and when the beneficiary is enrolled in, and the NaF-18 PET provider is participating in, the following type of prospective clinical study:

   A NaF-18 PET clinical study that is designed to collect additional information at the time of the scan to assist in initial antitumor treatment planning or to guide subsequent treatment strategy by the identification, location and quantification of bone metastases in beneficiaries in whom bone metastases are strongly suspected based on clinical symptoms or the results of other diagnostic studies. Qualifying clinical studies must ensure that specific hypotheses are addressed; appropriate data elements are collected; hospitals and providers are qualified to provide the PET scan and interpret the results; participating hospitals and providers accurately report data on all enrolled patients not included in other qualifying trials through adequate auditing mechanisms; and all patient confidentiality, privacy, and other Federal laws must be followed.

The clinical studies for which Medicare will provide coverage must answer one or more of the following questions:

Prospectively, in Medicare beneficiaries whose treating physician determines that the NaF-18 PET study results are needed to inform the initial antitumor treatment strategy or to guide subsequent antitumor treatment strategy after the completion of initial treatment, does the addition of NaF-18 PET imaging lead to:

- A change in patient management to more appropriate palliative care; or
- A change in patient management to more appropriate curative care; or
- Improved quality of life; or Improved survival?

The study must adhere to the following standards of scientific integrity and relevance to the Medicare population:

a. The principal purpose of the research study is to test whether a particular intervention potentially improves the participants' health outcomes.

b. The research study is well-supported by available scientific and medical information or it is intended to clarify or establish the health outcomes of interventions already in common clinical use.

c. The research study does not unjustifiably duplicate existing studies.

d. The research study design is appropriate to answer the research question being asked in the study.

e. The research study is sponsored by an organization or individual capable of executing the proposed study successfully.

f. The research study is in compliance with all applicable Federal regulations concerning the protection of human subjects found in the Code of Federal Regulations (CFR) at 45 CFR Part 46. If a study is regulated by the Food and Drug Administration (FDA), it also must be in compliance with 21 CFR Parts 50 and 56.

g. All aspects of the research study are conducted according to the appropriate standards of scientific integrity.

h. The research study has a written protocol that clearly addresses, or incorporates by reference, the Medicare standards.

i. The clinical research study is not designed to exclusively test toxicity or disease pathophysiology in healthy individuals. Trials of all medical technologies measuring therapeutic outcomes as one of the objectives meet this standard only if the disease or condition being studied is life-threatening as defined in 21 CFR Sec.312.81(a) and the patient has no other viable treatment options.

j. The clinical research study is registered on the www.ClinicalTrials.gov Web site by the principal sponsor/investigator prior to the enrollment of the first study subject.

k. The research study protocol specifies the method and timing of public release of all pre-specified outcomes to be measured including release of outcomes if outcomes are negative or study is terminated early. The results must be made public within 24 months of the end of data collection. If a report is planned to be published in a peer-reviewed journal, then that initial release may be an abstract that meets the requirements of the International Committee of Medical Journal Editors. However, a full report of the outcomes must be made public no later than three (3) years after the end of data collection.

l. The research study protocol must explicitly discuss subpopulations affected by the treatment under investigation, particularly traditionally underrepresented groups in clinical studies, how the inclusion and exclusion criteria affect enrollment of these populations, and a plan for the retention and reporting of said populations on the trial. If the inclusion and exclusion criteria are expected to have a negative effect on the recruitment or retention of underrepresented populations, the protocol must discuss why these criteria are necessary.

m. The research study protocol explicitly discusses how the results are or are not expected to be generalizable to the Medicare population to infer whether Medicare patients may benefit from the intervention. Separate discussions in the protocol may be necessary for populations eligible for Medicare due to age, disability or Medicaid eligibility.

Consistent with section 1142 of the Social Security Act (the Act), the Agency for Healthcare Research and Quality (AHRQ) supports clinical research studies that the Centers for Medicare and Medicaid Services (CMS) determines meet the above-listed standards and address the above-listed research questions.

C. Nationally Non-Covered Indications

Effective February 26, 2010, CMS determines that the evidence is not sufficient to determine that the results of NaF-18 PET imaging to identify bone metastases improve health outcomes of beneficiaries with cancer and is not reasonable and necessary under Sec.1862(a)(1)(A) of the Act unless it is to inform initial antitumor treatment strategy or to guide subsequent antitumor treatment strategy after completion of initial treatment, and then only under CED. All other uses and clinical indications of NaF-18 PET are nationally non-covered.

D. Other

The only radiopharmaceutical diagnostic imaging agents covered by Medicare for PET cancer imaging are 2-[F-18] Fluoro-D-Glucose (FDG) and NaF-18 (sodium fluoride-18). All other PET radiopharmaceutical diagnostic imaging agents are non-covered for this indication.

(This NCD was last reviewed in February 2010.)

100-03, 220.13

NCD for Percutaneous Image-Guided Breast Biopsy (220.13)

(Rev. 173, Issued: 09-04-14, Effective: Upon Implementation: of ICD–10)

Percutaneous image-guided breast biopsy is a method of obtaining a breast biopsy through a percutaneous incision by employing image guidance systems. Image guidance systems may be either ultrasound or stereotactic.

The Breast Imaging Reporting and Data System (or BIRADS system) employed by the American College of Radiology provides a standardized lexicon with which radiologists may report their interpretation of a mammogram. The BIRADS grading of mammograms is as follows: Grade I-Negative, Grade II-Benign finding, Grade III-Probably benign, Grade IV-Suspicious abnormality, and Grade V-Highly suggestive of malignant neoplasm.

A. Non-Palpable Breast Lesions

Effective January 1, 2003, Medicare covers percutaneous image-guided breast biopsy using stereotactic or ultrasound imaging for a radiographic abnormality that is non-palpable and is graded as a BIRADS III, IV, or V.

B. Palpable Breast Lesions

Effective January 1, 2003, Medicare covers percutaneous image guided breast biopsy using stereotactic or ultrasound imaging for palpable lesions that are difficult to biopsy using palpation alone. Medicare Administrative Contractors have the discretion to decide what types of palpable lesions are difficult to biopsy using palpation.

100-03, 230.1

NCD for Treatment of Kidney Stones (230.1)

(Rev. 1, 10-03-03)

In addition to the traditional surgical/endoscopic techniques for the treatment of kidney stones, the following lithotripsy techniques are also covered for services rendered on or after March 15, 1985.

Extracorporeal Shock Wave Lithotripsy.--Extracorporeal Shock Wave Lithotripsy (ESWL) is a non-invasive method of treating kidney stones using a device called a lithotriptor. The lithotriptor uses shock waves generated outside of the body to break up upper urinary tract stones. It focuses the shock waves specifically on stones under X-ray visualization, pulverizing them by repeated shocks. ESWL is covered under Medicare for use in the treatment of upper urinary tract kidney stones.

Percutaneous Lithotripsy.--Percutaneous lithotripsy (or nephrolithotomy) is an invasive method of treating kidney stones by using ultrasound, electrohydraulic or mechanical lithotripsy. A probe is inserted through an incision in the skin directly over the kidney and applied to the stone. A form of lithotripsy is then used to fragment the stone. Mechanical or electrohydraulic lithotripsy may be used as an alternative or adjunct to ultrasonic lithotripsy. Percutaneous lithotripsy of kidney stones by ultrasound or by the related techniques of electrohydraulic or mechanical lithotripsy is covered under Medicare.

The following is covered for services rendered on or after January 16, 1988.

Transurethral Ureteroscopic Lithotripsy.--Transurethral ureteroscopic lithotripsy is a method of fragmenting and removing ureteral and renal stones through a cystoscope. The cystoscope is inserted through the urethra into the bladder. Catheters are passed through the scope into the opening where the ureters enter the bladder. Instruments passed through this opening into the ureters are used to manipulate and ultimately disintegrate stones, using either mechanical crushing, transcystoscopic electrohydraulic shock waves, ultrasound or laser. Transurethral ureteroscopic lithotripsy for the treatment of urinary tract stones of the kidney or ureter is covered under Medicare.

100-03, 230.3

NCD for Sterilization (230.3)

(Rev. 173, Issued: 09-04-14, Effective: Upon Implementation: of ICD-10, Implementation: Upon Implementation of ICD-10)

A. Nationally Covered Conditions

Payment may be made only where sterilization is a necessary part of the treatment of an illness or injury, e.g., removal of a uterus because of a tumor, removal of diseased ovaries.

Sterilization of a mentally challenged beneficiary is covered if it is a necessary part of the treatment of an illness or injury (bilateral oophorectomy or bilateral orchidectomy in a case of cancer of the prostate). The Medicare Administrative Contractor denies claims when the pathological evidence of the necessity to perform any such procedures to treat an illness or injury is absent; and

Monitor such surgeries closely and obtain the information needed to determine whether in fact the surgery was performed as a means of treating an illness or injury or only to achieve sterilization.

B. Nationally Non-Covered Conditions

- Elective hysterectomy, tubal ligation, and vasectomy, if the primary indication for these procedures is sterilization;

- A sterilization that is performed because a physician believes another pregnancy would endanger the overall general health of the woman is not considered to be reasonable and necessary for the diagnosis or treatment of illness or injury within the meaning of §1862(a)(1) of the Social Security Act. The same conclusion would apply where the sterilization is performed only as a measure to prevent the possible development of, or effect on, a mental condition should the individual become pregnant; and sterilization of a mentally retarded person where the purpose is to prevent conception, rather than the treatment of an illness or injury.

100-03, 230.4

NCD for Diagnosis and Treatment of Impotence (230.4)

(Rev. 1, 10-03-03)

Program payment may be made for diagnosis and treatment of sexual impotence. Impotence is a failure of a body part for which the diagnosis, and frequently the treatment, require medical expertise. Depending on the cause of the condition, treatment may be surgical; e.g., implantation of a penile prosthesis, or nonsurgical; e.g., medical or psychotherapeutic treatment. Since causes and, therefore, appropriate treatment vary, if abuse is suspected it may be necessary to request documentation of appropriateness in individual cases. If treatment is furnished to patients (other than hospital inpatients) in connection with a mental condition, apply the psychiatric service limitation described in the Medicare General Information, Eligibility, and Entitlement Manual, Chapter 3.

100-03, 230.10

NCD for Incontinence Control Devices (230.10)

(Rev. 1, 10-03-03)

A - Mechanical/Hydraulic Incontinence Control Devices

Mechanical/hydraulic incontinence control devices are accepted as safe and effective in the management of urinary incontinence in patients with permanent anatomic and neurologic dysfunctions of the bladder. This class of devices achieves control of urination by compression of the urethra. The materials used and the success rate may vary somewhat from device to device. Such a device is covered when its use is reasonable and necessary for the individual patient.

B - Collagen Implant

A collagen implant, which is injected into the submucosal tissues of the urethra and/or the bladder neck and into tissues adjacent to the urethra, is a prosthetic device used in the treatment of stress urinary incontinence resulting from intrinsic sphincter deficiency (ISD). ISD is a cause of stress urinary incontinence in which the urethral sphincter is unable to contract and generate sufficient resistance in the bladder, especially during stress maneuvers.

Prior to collagen implant therapy, a skin test for collagen sensitivity must be administered and evaluated over a 4 week period.

In male patients, the evaluation must include a complete history and physical examination and a simple cystometrogram to determine that the bladder fills and stores properly. The patient then is asked to stand upright with a full bladder and to cough or otherwise exert abdominal pressure on his bladder. If the patient leaks, the diagnosis of ISD is established.

In female patients, the evaluation must include a complete history and physical examination (including a pelvic exam) and a simple cystometrogram to rule out abnormalities of bladder compliance and abnormalities of urethral support. Following that determination, an abdominal leak point pressure (ALLP) test is performed. Leak point pressure, stated in cm H2O, is defined as the intra-abdominal pressure at which leakage occurs from the bladder (around a catheter) when the bladder has been filled with a minimum of 150 cc fluid. If the patient has an ALLP of less than 100 cm H₂O, the diagnosis of ISD is established.

To use a collagen implant, physicians must have urology training in the use of a cystoscope and must complete a collagen implant training program.

Coverage of a collagen implant, and the procedure to inject it, is limited to the following types of patients with stress urinary incontinence due to ISD:

- Male or female patients with congenital sphincter weakness secondary to conditions such as myelomeningocele or epispadias;
- Male or female patients with acquired sphincter weakness secondary to spinal cord lesions;
- Male patients following trauma, including prostatectomy and/or radiation; and
- Female patients without urethral hypermobility and with abdominal leak point pressures of 100 cm H2O or less.

Patients whose incontinence does not improve with 5 injection procedures (5 separate treatment sessions) are considered treatment failures, and no further treatment of urinary incontinence by collagen implant is covered. Patients who have a reoccurrence of incontinence following successful treatment with collagen implants in the past (e.g., 6-12 months previously) may benefit from additional treatment sessions. Coverage of additional sessions may be allowed but must be supported by medical justification.

100-03, 260.1

Adult Liver Transplantation

(Rev.146, Issued: 08-03-12, Effective: 06-21-12, Implementation; 09-04-12)

A. General

Liver transplantation, which is in situ replacement of a patient's liver with a donor liver, in certain circumstances, may be an accepted treatment for patients with end-stage liver disease due to a variety of causes. The procedure is used in selected patients as a treatment for malignancies, including primary liver tumors and certain metastatic tumors, which are typically rare but lethal with very limited treatment options. It has also been used in the treatment of patients with extrahepatic perihilar malignancies. Examples of malignancies include extrahepatic unresectable cholangiocarcinoma (CCA), liver metastases due to a neuroendocrine tumor (NET), and, hemangioendothelioma (HAE). Despite potential short- and long-term complications, transplantation may offer the only chance of cure for selected patients while providing meaningful palliation for some others.

B. Nationally Covered Indications

Effective July 15, 1996, adult liver transplantation when performed on beneficiaries with end- stage liver disease other than hepatitis B or malignancies is covered under Medicare when performed in a facility which is approved by the Centers for Medicare & Medicaid Services (CMS) as meeting institutional coverage criteria.

Effective December 10, 1999, adult liver transplantation when performed on beneficiaries with end-stage liver disease other than malignancies is covered under Medicare when performed in a facility which is approved by CMS as meeting institutional coverage criteria.

Effective September 1, 2001, Medicare covers adult liver transplantation for hepatocellular carcinoma when the following conditions are met:

- The patient is not a candidate for subtotal liver resection;
- The patient's tumor(s) is less than or equal to 5 cm in diameter;
- There is no macrovascular involvement;
- There is no identifiable extrahepatic spread of tumor to surrounding lymph nodes, lungs, abdominal organs or bone; and,
- The transplant is furnished in a facility that is approved by CMS as meeting institutional coverage criteria for liver transplants (see 65 FR 15006).

Effective June 21, 2012, Medicare Adminstrative Contractors acting within their respective jurisdictions may determine coverage of adult liver transplantation for the following malignancies: (1) extrahepatic unresectable cholangiocarcinoma (CCA); (2) liver metastases due to a neuroendocrine tumor (NET); and, (3) hemangioendothelioma (HAE).

1. Follow-Up Care
   Follow-up care or re-transplantation required as a result of a covered liver transplant is covered, provided such services are otherwise reasonable and necessary. Follow-up care is also covered for patients who have been discharged from a hospital after receiving non-covered liver transplant. Coverage for follow-up care is for items and services that are reasonable and necessary as determined by Medicare guidelines.
2. Immunosuppressive Drugs
   See the Medicare Benefit Policy Manual, Chapter 15, "Covered Medical and Other Health Services," §50.5.1 and the Medicare Claims Processing Manual, Chapter 17, "Drugs and Biologicals," §80.3.

C. Nationally Non-Covered Indications

Adult liver transplantation for other malignancies remains excluded from coverage.

D. Other

Coverage of adult liver transplantation is effective as of the date of the facility's approval, but for applications received before July 13, 1991, can be effective as early as March 8, 1990. (See 56 FR 15006 dated April 12, 1991.)

(This NCD last reviewed June 2012.)

100-03, 260.2

NCD for Pediatric Liver Transplantation (260.2)

(Rev. 1, 10-03-03)

Liver transplantation is covered for children (under age 18) with extrahepatic biliary atresia or any other form of end stage liver disease, except that coverage is not provided for children with a malignancy extending beyond the margins of the liver or those with persistent viremia.

Liver transplantation is covered for Medicare beneficiaries when performed in a pediatric hospital that performs pediatric liver transplants if the hospital submits an application which CMS approves documenting that:

- The hospital's pediatric liver transplant program is operated jointly by the hospital and another facility that has been found by CMS to meet the institutional coverage criteria in the "Federal Register" notice of April 12, 1991;
- The unified program shares the same transplant surgeons and quality assurance program (including oversight committee, patient protocol, and patient selection criteria); and
- The hospital is able to provide the specialized facilities, services, and personnel that are required by pediatric liver transplant patients.

100-03, 260.3

NCD for Pancreas Transplants (260.3)

(Rev. 56, Issued: 05-19-06, Effective: 04-26-06, Implementation: 07-03-06)

A. General

Pancreas transplantation is performed to induce an insulin-independent, euglycemic state in diabetic patients. The procedure is generally limited to those patients with severe secondary complications of diabetes, including kidney failure. However, pancreas transplantation is sometimes performed on patients with labile diabetes and hypoglycemic unawareness.

B. Nationally Covered Indications

Effective for services performed on or after July 1, 1999, whole organ pancreas transplantation is nationally covered by Medicare when performed simultaneous with or after a kidney transplant. If the pancreas transplant occurs after the kidney transplant, immunosuppressive therapy begins with the date of discharge from the inpatient stay for the pancreas transplant.

Effective for services performed on or after April 26, 2006, pancreas transplants alone (PA) are reasonable and necessary for Medicare beneficiaries in the following limited circumstances:

1. PA will be limited to those facilities that are Medicare-approved for kidney transplantation. (Approved centers can be found at http://www.cms.hhs.gov/ESRDGeneralInformation/02_Data.asp#TopOfPage

2. Patients must have a diagnosis of type I diabetes:

    — Patient with diabetes must be beta cell autoantibody positive; or

    — Patient must demonstrate insulinopenia defined as a fasting C-peptide level that is less than or equal to 110% of the lower limit of normal of the laboratory's measurement method. Fasting C-peptide levels will only be considered valid with a concurrently obtained fasting glucose <225 mg/dL;

3. Patients must have a history of medically-uncontrollable labile (brittle) insulin-dependent diabetes mellitus with documented recurrent, severe, acutely life-threatening metabolic complications that require hospitalization. Aforementioned complications include frequent hypoglycemia unawareness or recurring severe ketoacidosis, or recurring severe hypoglycemic attacks;

4. Patients must have been optimally and intensively managed by an endocrinologist for at least 12 months with the most medically-recognized advanced insulin formulations and delivery systems;

5. Patients must have the emotional and mental capacity to understand the significant risks associated with surgery and to effectively manage the lifelong need for immunosuppression; and,

6. Patients must otherwise be a suitable candidate for transplantation.

C. Nationally Non-Covered Indications

The following procedure is not considered reasonable and necessary within the meaning of section 1862(a)(1)(A) of the Social Security Act:

1. Transplantation of partial pancreatic tissue or islet cells (except in the context of a clinical trial (see section 260.3.1 of the National Coverage Determinations Manual).

D. Other

Not applicable.

(This NCD last reviewed April 2006.)

100-03, 260.5

NCD for Intestinal and Multi-Visceral Transplantation (260.5)

(Rev. 58, Issued: 05-26-06; Effective: 05-11-06; Implementation: 06-26-06)

A. General

Medicare covers intestinal and multi-visceral transplantation for the purpose of restoring intestinal function in patients with irreversible intestinal failure. Intestinal failure is defined as the loss of absorptive capacity of the small bowel secondary to severe primary gastrointestinal disease or surgically induced short bowel syndrome. It may be associated with both mortality and profound morbidity. Multi-visceral transplantation includes organs in the digestive system (stomach, duodenum, pancreas, liver and intestine).

The evidence supports the fact that aged patients generally do not survive as well as younger patients receiving intestinal transplantation. Nonetheless, some older patients who are free from other contraindications have received the procedure and are progressing well, as evidenced by the United Network for Organ Sharing (UNOS) data. Thus, it is not appropriate to include specific exclusions from coverage, such as an age limitation, in the national coverage policy.

B. Nationally Covered Indications

Effective for services performed on or after April 1, 2001, this procedure is covered only when performed for patients who have failed total parenteral nutrition (TPN) and only when performed in centers that meet approval criteria.

1. Failed TPN

    The TPN delivers nutrients intravenously, avoiding the need for absorption through the small bowel. TPN failure includes the following:

    — Impending or overt liver failure due to TPN induced liver injury. The clinical manifestations include elevated serum bilirubin and/or liver enzymes,

splenomegaly, thrombocytopenia, gastroesophageal varices, coagulopathy, stomal bleeding or hepatic fibrosis/cirrhosis.

— Thrombosis of the major central venous channels; jugular, subclavian, and femoral veins. Thrombosis of two or more of these vessels is considered a life threatening complication and failure of TPN therapy. The sequelae of central venous thrombosis are lack of access for TPN infusion, fatal sepsis due to infected thrombi, pulmonary embolism, Superior Vena Cava syndrome, or chronic venous insufficiency.

— Frequent line infection and sepsis. The development of two or more episodes of systemic sepsis secondary to line infection per year that requires hospitalization indicates failure of TPN therapy. A single episode of line related fungemia, septic shock and/or Acute Respiratory Distress Syndrome are considered indicators of TPN failure.

— Frequent episodes of severe dehydration despite intravenous fluid supplement in addition to TPN. Under certain medical conditions such as secretory diarrhea and non-constructable gastrointestinal tract, the loss of the gastrointestinal and pancreatobiliary secretions exceeds the maximum intravenous infusion rates that can be tolerated by the cardiopulmonary system. Frequent episodes of dehydration are deleterious to all body organs particularly kidneys and the central nervous system with the development of multiple kidney stones, renal failure, and permanent brain damage.

2. Approved Transplant Facilities

    Intestinal transplantation is covered by Medicare if performed in an approved facility. The criteria for approval of centers will be based on a volume of 10 intestinal transplants per year with a 1-year actuarial survival of 65 percent using the Kaplan-Meier technique.

C. Nationally Non-covered Indications

All other indications remain non-covered.

D. Other

NA.

(This NCD last reviewed May 2006.)

100-03, 260.9

NCD for Heart Transplants (260.9)

(Rev. 95; Issued: 09-10-08; Effective Date: 05-01-08; Implementation Date: 12-01-08)

A. General

Cardiac transplantation is covered under Medicare when performed in a facility which is approved by Medicare as meeting institutional coverage criteria. (See CMS Ruling 87-1.)

B. Exceptions

In certain limited cases, exceptions to the criteria may be warranted if there is justification and if the facility ensures our objectives of safety and efficacy. Under no circumstances will exceptions be made for facilities whose transplant programs have been in existence for less than two years, and applications from consortia will not be approved.

Although consortium arrangements will not be approved for payment of Medicare heart transplants, consideration will be given to applications from heart transplant facilities that consist of more than one hospital where all of the following conditions exist:

*   The hospitals are under the common control or have a formal affiliation arrangement with each other under the auspices of an organization such as a university or a legally-constituted medical research institute; and

*   The hospitals share resources by routinely using the same personnel or services in their transplant programs. The sharing of resources must be supported by the submission of operative notes or other information that documents the routine use of the same personnel and services in all of the individual hospitals. At a minimum, shared resources means:

*   The individual members of the transplant team, consisting of the cardiac transplant surgeons, cardiologists and pathologists, must practice in all the hospitals and it can be documented that they otherwise function as members of the transplant team;

*   The same organ procurement organization, immunology, and tissue-typing services must be used by all the hospitals;

*   The hospitals submit, in the manner required (Kaplan-Meier method) their individual and pooled experience and survival data; and

*   The hospitals otherwise meet the remaining Medicare criteria for heart transplant facilities; that is, the criteria regarding patient selection, patient management, program commitment, etc.

C. Pediatric Hospitals

Cardiac transplantation is covered for Medicare beneficiaries when performed in a pediatric hospital that performs pediatric heart transplants if the hospital submits an application which CMS approves as documenting that:

*   The hospital's pediatric heart transplant program is operated jointly by the hospital and another facility that has been found by CMS to meet the institutional coverage criteria in CMS Ruling 87-1;

- The unified program shares the same transplant surgeons and quality assurance program (including oversight committee, patient protocol, and patient selection criteria); and
- The hospital is able to provide the specialized facilities, services, and personnel that are required by pediatric heart transplant patients.

D. Follow-Up Care

Follow-up care required as a result of a covered heart transplant is covered, provided such services are otherwise reasonable and necessary. Follow-up care is also covered for patients who have been discharged from a hospital after receiving a noncovered heart transplant. Coverage for follow-up care would be for items and services that are reasonable and necessary, as determined by Medicare guidelines. (See the Medicare Benefit Policy Manual, Chapter 16, "General Exclusions from Coverage," Sec.180.)

E. Immunosuppressive Drugs

See the Medicare Claims Processing Manual, Chapter 17, "Drugs and Biologicals," Sec.80.3.1, and Chapter 8, "Outpatient ESRD Hospital, Independent Facility, and Physician/Supplier Claims," Sec.120.1.

F. Artificial Hearts

Medicare does not cover the use of artificial hearts as a permanent replacement for a human heart or as a temporary life-support system until a human heart becomes available for transplant (often referred to as a "bridge to transplant"). Medicare does cover a ventricular assist device (VAD) when used in conjunction with specific criteria listed in Sec.20.9 of the NCD Manual.

100-03, 270.3

NCD for Blood-Derived Products for Chronic Non-Healing Wounds (270.3)

(Rev. 154, Issued: 06-10-13, Effective: 08-02-12, Implementation: 07-01-13)

A. General

Wound healing is a dynamic, interactive process that involves multiple cells and proteins. There are three progressive stages of normal wound healing, and the typical wound healing duration is about 4 weeks. While cutaneous wounds are a disruption of the normal, anatomic structure and function of the skin, subcutaneous wounds involve tissue below the skin's surface. Wounds are categorized as either acute, in where the normal wound healing stages are not yet completed but it is presumed they will be, resulting in orderly and timely wound repair, or chronic, in where a wound has failed to progress through the normal wound healing stages and repair itself within a sufficient time period.

Platelet-rich plasma (PRP) is produced in an autologous or homologous manner. Autologous PRP is comprised of blood from the patient who will ultimately receive the PRP. Alternatively, homologous PRP is derived from blood from multiple donors.

Blood is donated by the patient and centrifuged to produce an autologous gel for treatment of chronic, non-healing cutaneous wounds that persists for 30 days or longer and fail to properly complete the healing process. Autologous blood derived products for chronic, non-healing wounds includes both: (1) platelet derived growth factor (PDGF) products (such as Procuren), and (2) PRP (such as AutoloGel).

The PRP is different from previous products in that it contains whole cells including white cells, red cells, plasma, platelets, fibrinogen, stem cells, macrophages, and fibroblasts.

The PRP is used by physicians in clinical settings in treating chronic, non-healing wounds, open, cutaneous wounds, soft tissue, and bone. Alternatively, PDGF does not contain cells and was previously marketed as a product to be used by patients at home.

B. Nationally Covered Indications

Effective August 2, 2012, upon reconsideration, The Centers for Medicare and Medicaid Services (CMS) has determined that platelet-rich plasma (PRP) – an autologous blood-derived product, will be covered only for the treatment of chronic non-healing diabetic, venous and/or pressure wounds and only when the following conditions are met:

The patient is enrolled in a clinical trial that addresses the following questions using validated and reliable methods of evaluation. Clinical study applications for coverage pursuant to this National coverage Determination (NCD) must be received by August 2, 2014.

The clinical research study must meet the requirements specified below to assess the effect of PRP for the treatment of chronic non-healing diabetic, venous and/or pressure wounds. The clinical study must address:

Prospectively, do Medicare beneficiaries that have chronic non-healing diabetic, venous and/or pressure wounds who receive well-defined optimal usual care along with PRP therapy, experience clinically significant health outcomes compared to patients who receive well-defined optimal usual care for chronic non-healing diabetic, venous and/or pressure wounds as indicated by addressing at least one of the following:

a. Complete wound healing?

b. Ability to return to previous function and resumption of normal activities?

c. Reduction of wound size or healing trajectory which results in the patient's ability to return to previous function and resumption of normal activities?

The required clinical trial of PRP must adhere to the following standards of scientific integrity and relevance to the Medicare population:

a. The principal purpose of the CLINICAL STUDY is to test whether PRP improves the participants' health outcomes.

b. The CLINICAL STUDY is well supported by available scientific and medical information or it is intended to clarify or establish the health outcomes of interventions already in common clinical use.

c. The CLINICAL STUDY does not unjustifiably duplicate existing studies.

d. The CLINICAL STUDY design is appropriate to answer the research question being asked in the study.

e. The CLINICAL STUDY is sponsored by an organization or individual capable of executing the proposed study successfully.

f. The CLINICAL STUDY is in compliance with all applicable Federal regulations concerning the protection of human subjects found at 45 CFR Part 46.

g. All aspects of the CLINICAL STUDY are conducted according to appropriate standards of scientific integrity set by the International Committee of Medical Journal Editors (http://www.icmje.org).

h. The CLINICAL STUDY has a written protocol that clearly addresses, or incorporates by reference, the standards listed here as Medicare requirements for coverage with evidence development (CED).

i. The CLINICAL STUDY is not designed to exclusively test toxicity or disease pathophysiology in healthy individuals. Trials of all medical technologies measuring therapeutic outcomes as one of the objectives meet this standard only if the disease or condition being studied is life threatening as defined in 21 CFR §312.81(a) and the patient has no other viable treatment options.

j. The CLINICAL STUDY is registered on the ClinicalTrials.gov website by the principal sponsor/investigator prior to the enrollment of the first study subject.

k. The CLINICAL STUDY protocol specifies the method and timing of public release of all pre-specified outcomes to be measured including release of outcomes if outcomes are negative or study is terminated early. The results must be made public within 24 months of the end of data collection. If a report is planned to be published in a peer reviewed journal, then that initial release may be an abstract that meets the requirements of the International Committee of Medical Journal Editors (http://www.icmje.org). However a full report of the outcomes must be made public no later than three (3) years after the end of data collection.

l. The CLINICAL STUDY protocol must explicitly discuss subpopulations affected by the treatment under investigation, particularly traditionally underrepresented groups in clinical studies, how the inclusion and exclusion criteria effect enrollment of these populations, and a plan for the retention and reporting of said populations on the trial. If the inclusion and exclusion criteria are expected to have a negative effect on the recruitment or retention of underrepresented populations, the protocol must discuss why these criteria are necessary.

m. The CLINICAL STUDY protocol explicitly discusses how the results are or are not expected to be generalizable to the Medicare population to infer whether Medicare patients may benefit from the intervention. Separate discussions in the protocol may be necessary for populations eligible for Medicare due to age, disability or Medicaid eligibility. Consistent with §1142 of the Social Security Act (the Act), the Agency for Healthcare Research and Quality (AHRQ) supports clinical research studies that CMS determines meet the above-listed standards and address the above-listed research questions.

Any clinical study undertaken pursuant to this NCD must be approved no later than August 2, 2014. If there are no approved clinical studies on or before August 2, 2014, this CED will expire. Any clinical study approved will adhere to the timeframe designated in the approved clinical study protocol.

C. Nationally Non-Covered Indications

1. Effective December 28, 1992, the Centers for Medicare & Medicaid Services (CMS) issued a national non-coverage determination for platelet-derived wound-healing formulas intended to treat patients with chronic, non-healing wounds. This decision was based on a lack of sufficient published data to determine safety and efficacy, and a public health service technology assessment.

100-04, 3, 90.1

Kidney Transplant - General

(Rev.1341, Issued: 09-21-07, Effective: 06-28-07, Implementation: 10-22-07)

A3-3612, HO-E414

A major treatment for patients with ESRD is kidney transplantation. This involves removing a kidney, usually from a living relative of the patient or from an unrelated person who has died, and surgically placing the kidney into the patient. After the beneficiary receives a kidney transplant, Medicare pays the transplant hospital for the transplant and appropriate standard acquisition charges. Special provisions apply to payment. For the list of approved Medicare certified transplant facilities, refer to the following Web site:

http://www.cms.hhs.gov/CertificationandComplianc/20_Transplant.asp#TopOfPage

A transplant hospital may acquire cadaver kidneys by:

- Excising kidneys from cadavers in its own hospital; and

- Arrangements with a freestanding organ procurement organization (OPO) that provides cadaver kidneys to any transplant hospital or by a hospital based OPO.

A transplant hospital that is also a certified organ procurement organization may acquire cadaver kidneys by:

- Having its organ procurement team excise kidneys from cadavers in other hospitals;

- Arrangements with participating community hospitals, whether they excise kidneys on a regular or irregular basis; and

- Arrangements with an organ procurement organization that services the transplant hospital as a member of a network.

When the transplant hospital also excises the cadaver kidney, the cost of the procedure is included in its kidney acquisition costs and is considered in arriving at its standard cadaver kidney acquisition charge. When the transplant hospital excises a kidney to provide another hospital, it may use its standard cadaver kidney acquisition charge or its standard detailed departmental charges to bill that hospital.

When the excising hospital is not a transplant hospital, it bills its customary charges for services used in excising the cadaver kidney to the transplant hospital or organ procurement agency.

If the transplanting hospital's organ procurement team excises the cadaver kidney at another hospital, the cost of operating such a team is included in the transplanting hospital's kidney acquisition costs, along with the reasonable charges billed by the other hospital of its services.

100-04, 3, 90.1.1

The Standard Kidney Acquisition Charge

(Rev. 3030, Issued: 08-22-14, Effective: Upon Implementation of ICD-10)

There are two basic standard charges that must be developed by transplant hospitals from costs expected to be incurred in the acquisition of kidneys:

- The standard charge for acquiring a live donor kidney; and

- The standard charge for acquiring a cadaver kidney.

The standard charge is not a charge representing the acquisition cost of a specific kidney; rather, it is a charge that reflects the average cost associated with each type of kidney acquisition.

When the transplant hospital bills the program for the transplant, it shows its standard kidney acquisition charge on revenue code 081X. Kidney acquisition charges are not considered for the IPPS outlier calculation.

Acquisition services are billed from the excising hospital to the transplant hospital. A billing form is not submitted from the excising hospital to the FI. The transplant hospital keeps an itemized statement that identifies the services furnished, the charges, the person receiving the service (donor/recipient), and whether this is a potential transplant donor or recipient. These charges are reflected in the transplant hospital's kidney acquisition costcenter and are used in determining the hospital's standard charge for acquiring a live donor's kidney or a cadaver's kidney. The standard charge is not a charge representing the acquisition cost of a specific kidney. Rather, it is a charge that reflects the average cost associated with each type of kidney acquisition. Also, it is an all-inclusive charge for all services required in acquisition of a kidney, i.e., tissue typing, post-operative evaluation.

A. Billing For Blood And Tissue Typing of the Transplant Recipient Whether or Not Medicare Entitlement Is Established

Tissue typing and pre-transplant evaluation can be reflected only through the kidney acquisition charge of the hospital where the transplant will take place. The transplant hospital includes in its kidney acquisition cost center the reasonable charges it pays to the independent laboratory or other hospital which typed the potential transplant recipient, either before or after his entitlement. It also includes reasonable charges paid for physician tissue typing services, applicable to live donors and recipients (during the preentitlement period and after entitlement, but prior to hospital admission for transplantation).

B. Billing for Blood and Tissue Typing and Other Pre-Transplant Evaluation of Live Donors

The entitlement date of the beneficiary who will receive the transplant is not a consideration in reimbursing for the services to donors, since no bill is submitted directly to Medicare. All charges for services to donors prior to admission into the hospital for excision are "billed" indirectly to Medicare through the live donor acquisition charge of transplanting hospitals.

C. Billing Donor And Recipient Pre-Transplant Services (Performed by Transplant Hospitals or Other Providers) to the Kidney Acquisition Cost Center

The transplant hospital prepares an itemized statement of the services rendered for submittal to its cost accounting department. Regular Medicare billing forms are not necessary for this purpose, since no bills are submitted to the A/B MAC (A) at this point.

The itemized statement should contain information that identifies the person receiving the service (donor/recipient), the health care insurance number, the service rendered and the charge for the service, as well as a statement as to whether this is a potential transplant donor or recipient. If it is a potential donor, the provider must identify the prospective recipient.

EXAMPLE:

Mary Jones
Health care insurance number
200 Adams St.
Anywhere, MS

Transplant donor evaluation services for recipient:

John Jones
Health care insurance number
200 Adams St.
Anywhere, MS

Services performed in a hospital other than the potential transplant hospital or by an independent laboratory are billed by that facility to the potential transplant hospital. This holds true regardless of where in the United States the service is performed. For example, if the donor services are performed in a Florida hospital and the transplant is to take place in a California hospital, the Florida hospital bills the California hospital (as described in above). The Florida hospital is paid by the California hospital, which recoups the monies through the kidney acquisition cost center.

D. Billing for Cadaveric Donor Services

Normally, various tests are performed to determine the type and suitability of a cadaver kidney. Such tests may be performed by the excising hospital (which may also be a transplant hospital) or an independent laboratory. When the excising-only hospital performs the tests, it includes the related charges on its bill to the transplant hospital or to the organ procurement agency. When the tests are performed by the transplant hospital, it uses the related costs in establishing the standard charge for acquiring the cadaver kidney. The transplant hospital includes the costs and charges in the appropriate departments for final cost settlement purposes. When the tests are performed by an independent laboratory for the excising-only hospital or the transplant hospital, the laboratory bills the hospital that engages its services or the organ procurement agency. The excising-only hospital includes such charges in its charges to the transplant hospital, which then includes the charges in developing its standard charge for acquiring the cadaver kidney. It is the transplant hospitals' responsibility to assure that the independent laboratory does not bill both hospitals. The cost of these services cannot be billed directly to the program, since such tests and other procedures performed on a cadaver are not identifiable to a specific patient.

E. Billing For Physicians' Services Prior to Transplantation

Physicians' services applicable to kidney excisions involving live donors and recipients (during the pre-entitlement period and after entitlement, but prior to entrance into the hospital for transplantation) as well as all physicians' services applicable to cadavers are considered Part A hospital services (kidney acquisition costs).

F. Billing for Physicians' Services After Transplantation

All physicians' services rendered to the living donor and all physicians' services rendered to the transplant recipient are billed to the Medicare program in the same manner as all Medicare Part B services are billed. All donor physicians' services must be billed to the account of the recipient (i.e., the recipient's Medicare number).

G. Billing For Physicians' Renal Transplantation Services

To ensure proper payment when submitting a Part B bill for the renal surgeon's services to the recipient, the appropriate HCPCS codes must be submitted, including HCPCS codes for concurrent surgery, as applicable.

The bill must include all living donor physicians' services, e.g., Revenue Center code 081X.

100-04, 3, 90.1.2

Billing for Kidney Transplant and Acquisition Services

(Rev. 3030, Issued: 8/22/14, Eff. ASC X12: January 1, 2012, I-10: w/Imp I -10, ASC X12: 9/23/2014)

Applicable standard kidney acquisition charges are identified separately by revenue code 0811 (Living Donor Kidney Acquisition) or 0812 (Cadaver Donor Kidney Acquisition). Where interim bills are submitted, the standard acquisition charge appears on the billing form for the period during which the transplant took place. This charge is in addition to the hospital's charges for services rendered directly to the Medicare recipient.

The contractor deducts kidney acquisition charges for PPS hospitals for processing through Pricer. These costs, incurred by approved kidney transplant hospitals, are not included in the kidney transplant prospective payment. They are paid on a reasonable cost basis. Interim payment is paid as a "pass through" item. (See the Provider Reimbursement Manual, Part 1, §2802 B.8.) The contractor includes kidney acquisition charges under the appropriate revenue code in CWF.

Bill Review Procedures

The Medicare Code Editor (MCE) creates a Limited Coverage edit for kidney transplant procedure codes. Where these procedure codes are identified by MCE, the contractor checks the provider number to determine if the provider is an approved transplant center, and checks the effective approval date. The contractor shall also determine if the facility is certified for adults and/or pediatric transplants dependent upon the patient's age. If payment is appropriate (i.e., the center is approved and the service is on or after the approval date) it overrides the limited coverage edit.

100-04, 3, 90.2

Heart Transplants

(Rev. 3030, Issued: 8/22/14, Eff. ASC X12: January 1, 2012, I-10: w/Imp I -10, ASC X12: 9/23/2014)

Cardiac transplantation is covered under Medicare when performed in a facility which is approved by Medicare as meeting institutional coverage criteria. On April 6, 1987, CMS Ruling 87-1, "Criteria for Medicare Coverage of Heart Transplants" was published in the "Federal Register." For Medicare coverage purposes, heart transplants are medically reasonable and necessary when performed in facilities that meet these criteria. If a hospital wishes to bill Medicare for heart transplants, it must submit an application and documentation, showing its ongoing compliance with each criterion.

If a contractor has any questions concerning the effective or approval dates of its hospitals, it should contact its RO.

For a complete list of approved transplant centers, visit:

http://www.cms.hhs.gov/CertificationandComplianc/20_Transplant.asp#TopOfPage

A. Effective Dates

The effective date of coverage for heart transplants performed at facilities applying after July 6, 1987, is the date the facility receives approval as a heart transplant facility. Coverage is effective for discharges October 17, 1986 for facilities that would have qualified and that applied by July 6, 1987. All transplant hospitals will be recertified under the final rule, Federal Register / Vol. 72, No. 61 / Friday, March 30, 2007, / Rules and Regulations.

The CMS informs each hospital of its effective date in an approval letter.

B. Drugs

Medicare Part B covers immunosuppressive drugs following a covered transplant in an approved facility.

C. Noncovered Transplants

Medicare will not cover transplants or re-transplants in facilities that have not been approved as meeting the facility criteria. If a beneficiary is admitted for and receives a heart transplant from a hospital that is not approved, physicians' services, and inpatient services associated with the transplantation procedure are not covered.

If a beneficiary received a heart transplant from a hospital while it was not an approved facility and later requires services as a result of the noncovered transplant, the services are covered when they are reasonable and necessary in all other respects.

D. Charges for Heart Acquisition Services

The excising hospital bills the OPO, who in turn bills the transplant (implant) hospital for applicable services. It should not submit a bill to its contractor. The transplant hospital must keep an itemized statement that identifies the services rendered, the charges, the person receiving the service (donor/recipient), and whether this person is a potential transplant donor or recipient. These charges are reflected in the transplant hospital's heart acquisition cost center and are used in determining its standard charge for acquiring a donor's heart. The standard charge is not a charge representing the acquisition cost of a specific heart; rather, it reflects the average cost associated with each type of heart acquisition. Also, it is an all inclusive charge for all services required in acquisition of a heart, i.e., tissue typing, post-operative evaluation, etc.

E. Bill Review Procedures

The contractor takes the following actions to process heart transplant bills. It may accomplish them manually or modify its MCE and Grouper interface programs to handle the processing.

1. MCE Interface

   The MCE creates a Limited Coverage edit for heart transplant procedure codes. Where these procedure codes are identified by MCE, the contractor checks the provider number to determine if the provider is an approved transplant center, and checks the effective approval date. The contractor shall also determine if the facility is certified for adults and/or pediatric transplants dependent upon the patient's age. If payment is appropriate (i.e., the center is approved and the service is on or after the approval date) it overrides the limited coverage edit.

2. Handling Heart Transplant Billings From Nonapproved Hospitals

   Where a heart transplant and covered services are provided by a nonapproved hospital, the bill data processed through Grouper and Pricer must exclude transplant procedure codes and related charges.

100-04, 3, 90.3

Stem Cell Transplantation

(Rev. 3556, Issued: 07-01-16; Effective: 1-27-16; Implementation: 10-3-16)

A. General

Stem cell transplantation is a process in which stem cells are harvested from either a patient's (autologous) or donor's (allogeneic) bone marrow or peripheral blood for intravenous infusion. Autologous stem cell transplantation (AuSCT) is a technique for restoring stem cells using the patient's own previously stored cells. AuSCT must be used to effect hematopoietic reconstitution following severely myelotoxic doses of chemotherapy (HDCT) and/or radiotherapy used to treat various malignances. Allogeneic hematopoietic stem cell transplantation (HSCT) is a procedure in which a

portion of a healthy donor's stem cell or bone marrow is obtained and prepared for intravenous infusion. Allogeneic HSCT may be used to restore function in recipients having an inherited or acquired deficiency or defect. Hematopoietic stem cells are multi-potent stem cells that give rise to all the blood cell types; these stem cells form blood and immune cells. A hematopoietic stem cell is a cell isolated from blood or bone marrow that can renew itself, differentiate to a variety of specialized cells, can mobilize out of the bone marrow into circulating blood, and can undergo programmed cell death, called apoptosis - a process by which cells that are unneeded or detrimental will self-destruct.

The Centers for Medicare & Medicaid Services (CMS) is clarifying that bone marrow and peripheral blood stem cell transplantation is a process which includes mobilization, harvesting, and transplant of bone marrow or peripheral blood stem cells and the administration of high dose chemotherapy or radiotherapy prior to the actual transplant. When bone marrow or peripheral blood stem cell transplantation is covered, all necessary steps are included in coverage. When bone marrow or peripheral blood stem cell transplantation is non-covered, none of the steps are covered.

Allogeneic and autologous stem cell transplants are covered under Medicare for specific diagnoses. Effective October 1, 1990, these cases were assigned to MS-DRG 009, Bone Marrow Transplant.

The A/B MAC (A)'s Medicare Code Editor (MCE) will edit stem cell transplant procedure codes against diagnosis codes to determine which cases meet specified coverage criteria. Cases with a diagnosis code for a covered condition will pass (as covered) the MCE noncovered procedure edit. When a stem cell transplant case is selected for review based on the random selection of beneficiaries, the QIO will review the case on a post-payment basis to assure proper coverage decisions.

Bone marrow transplant codes that are reported with an ICD-9-CM that is "not otherwise specified" are returned to the hospital for a more specific procedure code. ICD-10-PCS codes are more precise and clearly identify autologous and nonautologous stem cells.

The A/B MAC (A) may choose to review if data analysis deems it a priority.

B. Nationally Covered Indications

I. Allogeneic Hematopoietic Stem Cell Transplantation (HSCT)

   a. General

     Allogeneic stem cell transplantation (ICD-9-CM Procedure Codes 41.02, 41.03, 41.05, and 41.08,; ICD-10-PCS codes 30230G1, 30230Y1, 30233G1, 30233Y1, 30240G1, 30240Y1, 30243G1, 30243Y1, 30250G1, 30250Y1, 30253G1, 30253Y1, 30260G1, 30260Y1, 30263G1, and 30263Y1) is a procedure in which a portion of a healthy donor's stem cells are obtained and prepared for intravenous infusion to restore normal hematopoietic function in recipients having an inherited or acquired hematopoietic deficiency or defect. See Pub. 100-03, National Coverage Determinations (NCD) Manual, chapter 1, section 110.23, for further information about this policy, and Pub. 100-04, CPM, chapter 32, section 90, for information on coding.

     Expenses incurred by a donor are a covered benefit to the recipient/beneficiary but, except for physician services, are not paid separately. Services to the donor include physician services, hospital care in connection with screening the stem cell, and ordinary follow-up care.

   b. Covered Conditions

     i. Effective for services performed on or after August 1, 1978: For the treatment of leukemia, leukemia in remission, or aplastic anemia when it is reasonable and necessary;

     ii. Effective for services performed on or after June 3, 1985: For the treatment of severe combined immunodeficiency disease (SCID), and for the treatment of Wiskott-Aldrich syndrome;

     iii. Effective for services performed on or after August 4, 2010: For the treatment of Myelodysplastic Syndromes (MDS) pursuant to Coverage with Evidence Development (CED) in the context of a Medicare-approved, prospective clinical study.

     iv. Effective for claims with dates of service on or after January 27, 2016:

1. Allogeneic HSCT for multiple myeloma is covered by Medicare only for beneficiaries with Durie-Salmon Stage II or III multiple myeloma, or International Staging System (ISS) Stage II or Stage III multiple myeloma, and participating in an approved prospective clinical study.

2. Allogeneic HSCT for myelofibrosis (MF) is covered by Medicare only for beneficiaries with Dynamic International Prognostic Scoring System (DIPSSplus) intermediate-2 or High primary or secondary MF and participating in an approved prospective clinical study.

3. Allogeneic HSCT for sickle cell disease (SCD) is covered by Medicare only for beneficiaries with severe, symptomatic SCD who participate in an approved prospective clinical study.

II. Autologous Stem Cell Transplantation (AuSCT)

   a. General

     Autologous stem cell transplantation (ICD-9-CM Procedure Codes 41.01, 41.04, 41.07, and 41.09; ICD-10-PCS codes 30230AZ, 30230G0, 30230Y0, 30233G0, 30233Y0, 30240G0, 30240Y0, 30243G0, 30243Y0, 30250G0, 30250Y0, 30253G0, 30253Y0, 30260G0, 30260Y0, 30263G0, and 30263Y0) is a technique for restoring stem cells using the patient's own previously stored cells. AuSCT must be used to effect hematopoietic reconstitution following severely myelotoxic doses of chemotherapy (high dose chemotherapy (HDCT)) and/or radiotherapy used to treat various malignancies. Refer to Pub. 100-03, NCD Manual, chapter 1, section 110.23, for further information about this policy, and Pub. 100-04, CPM, chapter 32, section 90, for information on coding.

  b. Covered Conditions

    1. Effective for services performed on or after April 28, 1989: Acute leukemia in remission who have a high probability of relapse and who have no human leucocyte antigens (HLA)-matched; Resistant non-Hodgkin's lymphomas or those presenting with poor prognostic features following an initial response; Recurrent or refractory neuroblastoma; or, Advanced Hodgkin's disease who have failed conventional therapy and have no HLA-matched donor.

    2. Effective for services performed on or after October 1, 2000: Single AuSCT is only covered for Durie-Salmon Stage II or III patients that fit the following requirements:

      • Newly diagnosed or responsive multiple myeloma. This includes those patients with previously untreated disease, those with at least a partial response to prior chemotherapy (defined as a 50% decrease either in measurable paraprotein [serum and/or urine] or in bone marrow infiltration, sustained for at least 1 month), and those in responsive relapse; and

      • Adequate cardiac, renal, pulmonary, and hepatic function.

    3. Effective for services performed on or after March 15, 2005: When recognized clinical risk factors are employed to select patients for transplantation, high dose melphalan (HDM) together with AuSCT is reasonable and necessary for Medicare beneficiaries of any age group with primary amyloid light chain (AL) amyloidosis who meet the following criteria:

      • Amyloid deposition in 2 or fewer organs; and,

      • Cardiac left ventricular ejection fraction (EF) greater than 45%.

C. Nationally Non-Covered Indications

I. Allogeneic Hematopoietic Stem Cell Transplantation (HSCT)

Effective for claims with dates of service on or after May 24, 1996, through January 26, 2016, allogeneic HSCT is not covered as treatment for multiple myeloma. Refer to Pub. 100-03, NCD Manual, chapter 1, section 110.23, for further information about this policy, and Pub. 100-04, CPM, chapter 32, section 90, for information on coding.

II. Autologous Stem Cell Transplantation (AuSCT)

Insufficient data exist to establish definite conclusions regarding the efficacy of AuSCT for the following conditions:

  a) Acute leukemia not in remission;

  b) Chronic granulocytic leukemia;

  c) Solid tumors (other than neuroblastoma); Up to October 1, 2000, multiple myeloma;

  e) Tandem transplantation (multiple rounds of AuSCT) for patients with multiple myeloma;

  f) Effective October 1, 2000, non primary AL amyloidosis; and,

  g) Effective October 1, 2000, through March 14, 2005, primary AL amyloidosis for Medicare beneficiaries age 64 or older. In these cases, AuSCT is not considered reasonable and necessary within the meaning of §I862(a)(1)(A) of the Act and is not covered under Medicare. Refer to Pub. 100-03, NCD Manual, chapter 1, section 110.23, for further information about this policy, and Pub. 100-04, CPM, chapter 32, section 90, for information on coding.

D. Other

All other indications for stem cell transplantation not otherwise noted above as covered or non-covered remain at local Medicare Administrative Contractor discretion.

100-04, 3, 90.3.1
Billing for Stem Cell Transplantation
(Rev. 3571, Issued: 07-29-16; Effective: 01-01-17; Implementation; 01-03-17)

A. Billing for Allogeneic Stem Cell Transplants

1. Definition of Acquisition Charges for Allogeneic Stem Cell Transplants

Acquisition charges for allogeneic stem cell transplants include, but are not limited to, charges for the costs of the following services:

• National Marrow Donor Program fees, if applicable, for stem cells from an unrelated donor;

• Tissue typing of donor and recipient;

• Donor evaluation;

• Physician pre-admission/pre-procedure donor evaluation services;

• Costs associated with harvesting procedure (e.g., general routine and special care services, procedure/operating room and other ancillary services, apheresis services, etc.);

• Post-operative/post-procedure evaluation of donor; and

• Preparation and processing of stem cells.

Payment for these acquisition services is included in the MS-DRG payment for the allogeneic stem cell transplant when the transplant occurs in the inpatient setting, and in the OPPS APC payment for the allogeneic stem cell transplant when the transplant occurs in the outpatient setting. The Medicare contractor does not make separate payment for these acquisition services, because hospitals may bill and receive payment only for services provided to the Medicare beneficiary who is the recipient of the stem cell transplant and whose illness is being treated with the stem cell transplant. Unlike the acquisition costs of solid organs for transplant (e.g., hearts and kidneys), which are paid on a reasonable cost basis, acquisition costs for allogeneic stem cells are included in prospective payment.

Acquisition charges for stem cell transplants apply only to allogeneic transplants, for which stem cells are obtained from a donor (other than the recipient himself or herself). Acquisition charges do not apply to autologous transplants (transplanted stem cells are obtained from the recipient himself or herself), because autologous transplants involve services provided to the beneficiary only (and not to a donor), for which the hospital may bill and receive payment (see Pub. 100-04, chapter 4, §231.10 and paragraph B of this section for information regarding billing for autologous stem cell transplants).

2. Billing for Acquisition Services

The hospital bills and shows acquisition charges for allogeneic stem cell transplants based on the status of the patient (i.e., inpatient or outpatient) when the transplant is furnished. See Pub. 100-04, chapter 4, §231.11 for instructions regarding billing for acquisition services for allogeneic stem cell transplants that are performed in the outpatient setting.

When the allogeneic stem cell transplant occurs in the inpatient setting, the hospital identifies stem cell acquisition charges for allogeneic bone marrow/stem cell transplants separately by using revenue code 0815 (Stem Cell Acquisition). Revenue code 0815 charges should include all services required to acquire stem cells from a donor, as defined above.

On the recipient's transplant bill, the hospital reports the acquisition charges, cost report days, and utilization days for the donor's hospital stay (if applicable) and/or charges for other encounters in which the stem cells were obtained from the donor. The donor is covered for medically necessary inpatient hospital days of care or outpatient care provided in connection with the allogeneic stem cell transplant under Part A. Expenses incurred for complications are paid only if they are directly and immediately attributable to the stem cell donation procedure. The hospital reports the acquisition charges on the billing form for the recipient, as described in the first paragraph of this section. It does not charge the donor's days of care against the recipient's utilization record. For cost reporting purposes, it includes the covered donor days and charges as Medicare days and charges.

The transplant hospital keeps an itemized statement that identifies the services furnished, the charges, the person receiving the service (donor/recipient), and whether this is a potential transplant donor or recipient. These charges will be reflected in the transplant hospital's stem cell/bone marrow acquisition cost center. For allogeneic stem cell acquisition services in cases that do not result in transplant, due to death of the intended recipient or other causes, hospitals include the costs associated with the acquisition services on the Medicare cost report.

The hospital shows charges for the transplant itself in revenue center code 0362 or another appropriate cost center. Selection of the cost center is up to the hospital.

B. Billing for Autologous Stem Cell Transplants

The hospital bills and shows all charges for autologous stem cell harvesting, processing, and transplant procedures based on the status of the patient (i.e., inpatient or outpatient) when the services are furnished. It shows charges for the actual transplant, in revenue center code 0362 or another appropriate cost center. ICD-9-CM or ICD-10-PCS codes are used to identify inpatient procedures.

The HCPCS codes describing autologous stem cell harvesting procedures may be billed and are separately payable under the OPPS when provided in the hospital outpatient setting of care. Autologous harvesting procedures are distinct from the acquisition services described in Pub. 100-04, chapter 4, §231.11 and section A. above for allogeneic stem cell transplants, which include services provided when stem cells are obtained from a donor and not from the patient undergoing the stem cell transplant. The HCPCS codes describing autologous stem cell processing procedures also may be billed and are separately payable under the OPPS when provided to hospital outpatients.

Payment for autologous stem cell harvesting procedures performed in the hospital inpatient setting of care, with transplant also occurring in the inpatient setting of care, is included in the MS-DRG payment for the autologous stem cell transplant.

100-04, 3, 90.3.2

Autologous Stem Cell Transplantation (AuSCT)

(Rev. 3030, Issued: 8/22/14, Eff. ASC X12: January 1, 2012, I-10: w/Imp I -10, ASC X12: 9/23/2014)

Autologous Stem Cell Transplantation (AuSCT)

A. General

Autologous stem cell transplantation (AuSCT) (ICD-9-CM procedure code 41.01, 41.04, 41.07, and 41.09 and CPT-4 code 38241) is a technique for restoring stem cells using the patient's own previously stored cells. AuSCT must be used to effect hematopoietic reconstitution following severely myelotoxic doses of chemotherapy (high dose chemotherapy (HDCT)) and/or radiotherapy used to treat various malignancies.

If ICD-9-CM is applicable, use the following Procedure Codes and Descriptions

ICD-9-CM Code	Description
41.01	Autologous bone marrow transplant without purging
41.04	Autologous hematopoietic stem cell transplant without purging
41.07	Autologous hematopoietic stem cell transplant with purging
41.09	Autologous bone marrow transplant with purging

If ICD-10-PCS is applicable, use the following Procedure Codes and Descriptions

ICD-10-PCS Code	Description
30230AZ	Transfusion of Embryonic Stem Cells into Peripheral Vein, Open Approach
30230G0	Transfusion of Autologous Bone Marrow into Peripheral Vein, Open Approach
30230Y0	Transfusion of Autologous Hematopoietic Stem Cells into Peripheral Vein, Open Approach
30233G0	Transfusion of Autologous Bone Marrow into Peripheral Vein, Percutaneous Approach
30233Y0	Transfusion of Autologous Hematopoietic Stem Cells into Peripheral Vein, Percutaneous Approach
30240G0	Transfusion of Autologous Bone Marrow into Central Vein, Open Approach
30240Y0	Transfusion of Autologous Bone Marrow into Central Vein, Open Approach
30243G0	Transfusion of Autologous Bone Marrow into Central Vein, Percutaneous Approach
30243Y0	Transfusion of Autologous Hematopoietic Stem Cells into Central Vein, Percutaneous Approach
30250G0	Transfusion of Autologous Bone Marrow into Peripheral Artery, Open Approach
30250Y0	Transfusion of Autologous Hematopoietic Stem Cells into Peripheral Artery, Open Approach
30253G0	Transfusion of Autologous Bone Marrow into Peripheral Artery, Percutaneous Approach
30253Y0	Transfusion of Autologous Hematopoietic Stem Cells into Peripheral Artery, Percutaneous Approach
30260G0	Transfusion of Autologous Bone Marrow into Central Artery, Open Approach
30260Y0	Transfusion of Autologous Hematopoietic Stem Cells into Central Artery, Open Approach
30263G0	Transfusion of Autologous Bone Marrow into Central Artery, Percutaneous Approach
30263Y0	Transfusion of Autologous Hematopoietic Stem Cells into Central Artery, Percutaneous Approach

B. Covered Conditions

1. Effective for services performed on or after April 28, 1989:

For acute leukemia in remission for patients who have a high probability of relapse and who have no human leucocyte antigens (HLA)-matched the following diagnosis codes are reported:

If ICD-9-CM is applicable, use the following Diagnosis Codes and Descriptions

Diagnosis Code	Description
204.01	Lymphoid leukemia, acute, in remission
205.01	Myeloid leukemia, acute, in remission
206.01	Monocytic leukemia, acute, in remission
207.01	Acute erythremia and erythroleukemia, in remission
208.01	Leukemia of unspecified cell type, acute, in remission

If ICD-10-CM is applicable, use the following Diagnosis Codes and Descriptions

Diagnosis Code	Description
C91.01	Acute lymphoblastic leukemia, in remission
C92.01	Acute myeloblastic leukemia, in remission
C92.41	Acute promyelocytic leukemia, in remission
C92.51	Acute myelomonocytic leukemia, in remission
C92.61	Acute myeloid leukemia with 11q23-abnormality in remission
C92.A1	Acute myeloid leukemia with multilineage dysplasia, in remission
C93.01	Acute monoblastic/monocytic leukemia, in remission
C94.01	Acute erythroid leukemia, in remission
C94.21	Acute megakaryoblastic leukemia, in remission
C94.41	Acute parmyelosis with myelofibrosis, in remission
C95.01	Acute leukemia of unspecified cell type, in remission

For resistant non-Hodgkin's lymphomas (or those presenting with poor prognostic features following an initial response the following diagnosis codes are reported:

If ICD-9-CM is applicable, use the following code ranges:

200.00 - 200.08,

200.10 - 00.18,

200.20 - 200.28,

200.80 - 200.88,

202.00 - 202.08,

202.80 - 202.88, and

202.90 - 202.98.

If ICD-10-CM is applicable use the following code ranges:

C82.00 - C85.29,

C85.80 - C86.6,

C96.4, and

C96.Z - C96.9.

For recurrent or refractory neuroblastoma (see ICD-9-CM Neoplasm by site, malignant for the appropriate diagnosis code)

If ICD-10-CM is applicable the following ranges are reported:

C00 - C96, and

D00 - D09 Resistant non-Hodgkin's lymphomas

For advanced Hodgkin's disease patients who have failed conventional therapy and have no HLA-matched donor the following diagnosis codes are reported:

If ICD-9-CM is applicable, 201.00-201.98.

If ICD-10-CM is applicable, C81.00 – C81.99.

2. Effective for services performed on or after October 1, 2000:

Durie-Salmon Stage II or III that fit the following requirement are covered: Newly diagnosed or responsive multiple myeloma (if ICD-9-CM is applicable, diagnosis codes 203.00 and 238.6, and, if ICD-10-CM is applicable, diagnosis codes C90.00 and D47.Z9). This includes those patients with previously untreated disease, those with at least a partial response to prior chemotherapy (defined as a 50% decrease either in measurable paraprotein [serum and/or urine] or in bone marrow infiltration, sustained for at least 1 month), and those in responsive relapse, and adequate cardiac, renal, pulmonary, and hepatic function.

3. Effective for Services On or After March 15, 2005

Effective for services performed on or after March 15, 2005 when recognized clinical risk factors are employed to select patients for transplantation, high-dose melphalan (HDM), together with AuSCT, in treating Medicare beneficiaries of any age group with primary amyloid light-chain (AL) amyloidosis who meet the following criteria:

Amyloid deposition in 2 or fewer organs; and,

Cardiac left ventricular ejection fraction (EF) of 45% or greater.

C. Noncovered Conditions

Insufficient data exist to establish definite conclusions regarding the efficacy of autologous stem cell transplantation for the following conditions:

- Acute leukemia not in remission:
  — If ICD-9-CM is applicable, diagnosis codes 204.00, 205.00, 206.00, 207.00 and 208.00 are noncovered;
  — If ICD-10-CM is applicable, diagnosis codes C91.00, C92.00, C92.40, C92.50, C92.60, C92.A0, C93.00, C94.00, and C95.00 are noncovered.
- Chronic granulocytic leukemia:
  — If ICD-9-CM is applicable, diagnosis codes 205.10 and 205.11;
  — If ICD-10-CM is applicable, diagnosis codes C92.10 and C92.11.
- Solid tumors (other than neuroblastoma):
  — If ICD-9-CM is applicable, diagnosis codes 140.0-199.1;

- If ICD-10-CM is applicable, diagnosis codes C00.0 - C80.2 and D00.0 - D09.9. Multiple myeloma (ICD-9-CM codes 203.00 and 238.6), through September 30, 2000.

- Tandem transplantation (multiple rounds of autologous stem cell transplantation) for patients with multiple myeloma

  - If ICD-9-CM is applicable, diagnosis codes 203.00 and 238.6 and,

  - If ICD-10-CM is applicable, diagnosis codes C90.00 and D47.Z9)

- Non-primary (AL) amyloidosis,

  - If ICD-9-CM is applicable, diagnosis code 277.3. Effective October 1, 2000; ICD-9-CM code 277.3 was expanded to codes 277.30, 277.31, and 277.39 effective October 1, 2006.

  - If ICD-10-CM is applicable, diagnosis codes are E85.0 – E85.9. or

- Primary (AL) amyloidosis

  - If ICD-9-CM is applicable, diagnosis codes 277.30, 277.31, and 277.39 and for Medicare beneficiaries age 64 or older, effective October 1, 2000, through March 14, 2005.

  - If ICD-10-CM is applicable, diagnosis codes are E85.0 – E85.9.

NOTE: Coverage for conditions other than these specifically designated as covered or non-covered is left to the discretion of the A/B MAC (A).

100-04, 3, 90.3.3

Billing for Stem Cell Transplantation

(Rev. 3030, Issued: 8/22/14, Eff. ASC X12: January 1, 2012, I-10: w/Imp I -10, ASC X12: 9/23/2014)

A. Billing for Allogeneic Stem Cell Transplants

1. Definition of Acquisition Charges for Allogeneic Stem Cell Transplants

   Acquisition charges for allogeneic stem cell transplants include, but are not limited to, charges for the costs of the following services:

   - National Marrow Donor Program fees, if applicable, for stem cells from an unrelated donor;

   - Tissue typing of donor and recipient;

   - Donor evaluation;

   - Physician pre-admission/pre-procedure donor evaluation services;

   - Costs associated with harvesting procedure (e.g., general routine and special care services, procedure/operating room and other ancillary services, apheresis services, etc.);

   - Post-operative/post-procedure evaluation of donor; and

   - Preparation and processing of stem cells.

   Payment for these acquisition services is included in the MS-DRG payment for the allogeneic stem cell transplant when the transplant occurs in the inpatient setting, and in the OPPS APC payment for the allogeneic stem cell transplant when the transplant occurs in the outpatient setting. The Medicare contractor does not make separate payment for these acquisition services, because hospitals may bill and receive payment only for services provided to the Medicare beneficiary who is the recipient of the stem cell transplant and whose illness is being treated with the stem cell transplant. Unlike the acquisition costs of solid organs for transplant (e.g., hearts and kidneys), which are paid on a reasonable cost basis, acquisition costs for allogeneic stem cells are included in prospective payment.

   Acquisition charges for stem cell transplants apply only to allogeneic transplants, for which stem cells are obtained from a donor (other than the recipient himself or herself). Acquisition charges do not apply to autologous transplants (transplanted stem cells are obtained from the recipient himself or herself), because autologous transplants involve services provided to the beneficiary only (and not to a donor), for which the hospital may bill and receive payment (see Pub. 100-4, chapter 4, §231.10 and paragraph B of this section for information regarding billing for autologous stem cell transplants).

2. Billing for Acquisition Services

   The hospital bills and shows acquisition charges for allogeneic stem cell transplants based on the status of the patient (i.e., inpatient or outpatient) when the transplant is furnished. See Pub. 100-4, chapter 4, §231.11 for instructions regarding billing for acquisition services for allogeneic stem cell transplants that are performed in the outpatient setting.

   When the allogeneic stem cell transplant occurs in the inpatient setting, the hospital identifies stem cell acquisition charges for allogeneic bone marrow/stem cell transplants separately in FL 42 of Form CMS-1450 (or electronic equivalent) by using revenue code 0819 (Other Organ Acquisition). Revenue code 0819 charges should include all services required to acquire stem cells from a donor, as defined above.

   On the recipient's transplant bill, the hospital reports the acquisition charges, cost report days, and utilization days for the donor's hospital stay (if applicable) and/or charges for other encounters in which the stem cells were obtained from the donor. The donor is covered for medically necessary inpatient hospital days of care or outpatient care provided in connection with the allogeneic stem cell transplant under Part A. Expenses incurred for complications are paid only if they are directly and immediately attributable to the stem cell donation procedure. The hospital reports the acquisition charges on the billing form for the recipient, as described in the first paragraph of this section. It does not charge the donor's days of care against the recipient's utilization record. For cost reporting purposes, it includes the covered donor days and charges as Medicare days and charges.

The transplant hospital keeps an itemized statement that identifies the services furnished, the charges, the person receiving the service (donor/recipient), and whether this is a potential transplant donor or recipient. These charges will be reflected in the transplant hospital's stem cell/bone marrow acquisition cost center. For allogeneic stem cell acquisition services in cases that do not result in transplant, due to death of the intended recipient or other causes, hospitals include the costs associated with the acquisition services on the Medicare cost report.

The hospital shows charges for the transplant itself in revenue center code 0362 or another appropriate cost center. Selection of the cost center is up to the hospital.

B. Billing for Autologous Stem Cell Transplants

The hospital bills and shows all charges for autologous stem cell harvesting, processing, and transplant procedures based on the status of the patient (i.e., inpatient or outpatient) when the services are furnished. It shows charges for the actual transplant, described by the appropriate ICD-9-CM procedure or CPT codes, in revenue center code 0362 or another appropriate cost center. ICD-9-CM or ICD-10-PCS codes are used to identify inpatient procedures.

The CPT codes describing autologous stem cell harvesting procedures may be billed and are separately payable under the OPPS when provided in the hospital outpatient setting of care. Autologous harvesting procedures are distinct from the acquisition services described in Pub. 100-4, chapter 4, §231.11 and section A. above for allogeneic stem cell transplants, which include services provided when stem cells are obtained from a donor and not from the patient undergoing the stem cell transplant. The CPT codes describing autologous stem cell processing procedures also may be billed and are separately payable under the OPPS when provided to hospital outpatients.

Payment for autologous stem cell harvesting procedures performed in the hospital inpatient setting of care, with transplant also occurring in the inpatient setting of care, is included in the MS-DRG payment for the autologous stem cell transplant.

100-04, 3, 90.4

Liver Transplants

(Rev. 2513, Issued: 08-03-12, Effective: 06-21-12, Implementation: 09-04-12)

A. Background

For Medicare coverage purposes, liver transplants are considered medically reasonable and necessary for specified conditions when performed in facilities that meet specific criteria. Coverage guidelines may be found in Publication 100-3, Section 260.1.

Effective for claims with dates of service June 21, 2012 and later, contractors may, at their discretion cover adult liver transplantation for patients with extrahepatic unresectable cholangiocarcinoma (CCA), (2) liver metastases due to a neuroendocrine tumor (NET) or (3) hemangioendothelimo (HAE) when furnished in an approved Liver Transplant Center (below). All other nationally non-covered malignancies continue to remain nationally non-covered.

To review the current list of approved Liver Transplant Centers, see http://www.cms.hhs.gov/CertificationandCompliance/20_Transplant.asp#TopOfPage

100-04, 3, 90.4.1

Standard Liver Acquisition Charge

(Rev. 1, 10-01-03) A3-3615.1, A3-3615.3

Each transplant facility must develop a standard charge for acquiring a cadaver liver from costs it expects to incur in the acquisition of livers.

This standard charge is not a charge that represents the acquisition cost of a specific liver. Rather, it is a charge that reflects the average cost associated with a liver acquisition.

Services associated with liver acquisition are billed from the organ procurement organization or, in some cases, the excising hospital to the transplant hospital. The excising hospital does not submit a billing form to the FI. The transplant hospital keeps an itemized statement that identifies the services furnished, the charges, the person receiving the service (donor/recipient), and the potential transplant donor. These charges are reflected in the transplant hospital's liver acquisition cost center and are used in determining the hospital's standard charge for acquiring a cadaver's liver. The standard charge is not a charge representing the acquisition cost of a specific liver. Rather, it is a charge that reflects the average cost associated with liver acquisition. Also, it is an all inclusive charge for all services required in acquisition of a liver, e.g., tissue typing, transportation of organ, and surgeons' retrieval fees.

100-04, 3, 90.4.2

Billing for Liver Transplant and Acquisition Services

(Rev. 3030, Issued: 8/22/14, Eff. ASC X12: January 1, 2012, I-10: w/Imp I -10, ASC X12: 9/23/2014)

The inpatient claim is completed in accordance with instructions in chapter 25 for the beneficiary who receives a covered liver transplant. Applicable standard liver acquisition charges are identified separately in FL 42 by revenue code 0817 (Donor-Liver). Where interim bills are submitted, the standard acquisition charge appears on the billing form for the period during which the transplant took place. This charge is in addition to the hospital's charge for services furnished directly to the Medicare recipient.

The contractor deducts liver acquisition charges for IPPS hospitals prior to processing through Pricer. Costs of liver acquisition incurred by approved liver transplant facilities are not included in prospective payment DRG 480 (Liver Transplant). They are paid on a reasonable cost basis. This item is a "pass-through" cost for which interim payments are made. (See the Provider Reimbursement Manual, Part 1, §2802 B.8.) The contractor includes liver acquisition charges under revenue code 0817 in the HUIP record that it sends to CWF and the QIO.

A. Bill Review Procedures

The contractor takes the following actions to process liver transplant bills.

1. Operative Report

   The contractor requires the operative report with all claims for liver transplants, or sends a development request to the hospital for each liver transplant with a diagnosis code for a covered condition.

2. MCE Interface

   The MCE contains a limited coverage edit for liver transplant procedures using ICD-9-CM code 50.59 if ICD-9 is applicable, and, if ICD-10 is applicable, using ICD-10-PCS codes 0FY00Z0, 0FY00Z1, and 0FY00Z2.

   Where a liver transplant procedure code is identified by the MCE, the contractor shall check the provider number and effective date to determine if the provider is an approved liver transplant facility at the time of the transplant, and the contractor shall also determine if the facility is certified for adults and/or pediatric transplants dependent upon the patient's age. If yes, the claim is suspended for review of the operative report to determine whether the beneficiary has at least one of the covered conditions when the diagnosis code is for a covered condition. If payment is appropriate (i.e., the facility is approved, the service is furnished on or after the approval date, and the beneficiary has a covered condition), the contractor sends the claim to Grouper and Pricer.

   If none of the diagnoses codes are for a covered condition, or if the provider is not an approved liver transplant facility, the contractor denies the claim.

   NOTE: Some noncovered conditions are included in the covered diagnostic codes. (The diagnostic codes are broader than the covered conditions. Do not pay for noncovered conditions.

3. Grouper

   If the bill shows a discharge date before March 8, 1990, the liver transplant procedure is not covered. If the discharge date is March 8, 1990 or later, the contractor processes the bill through Grouper and Pricer. If the discharge date is after March 7, 1990, and before October 1, 1990, Grouper assigned CMS DRG 191 or 192. The contractor sent the bill to Pricer with review code 08. Pricer would then overlay CMS DRG 191 or 192 with CMS DRG 480 and the weights and thresholds for CMS DRG 480 to price the bill. If the discharge date is after September 30, 1990, Grouper assigns CMS DRG 480 and Pricer is able to price without using review code 08. If the discharge date is after September 30, 2007, Grouper assigns MS-DRG 005 or 006 (Liver transplant with MCC or Intestinal Transplant or Liver transplant without MCC, respectively) and Pricer is able to price without using review code 08.

4. Liver Transplant Billing From Non-approved Hospitals

   Where a liver transplant and covered services are provided by a non-approved hospital, the bill data processed through Grouper and Pricer must exclude transplant procedure codes and related charges.

   When CMS approves a hospital to furnish liver transplant services, it informs the hospital of the effective date in the approval letter. The contractor will receive a copy of the letter.

100-04, 3, 90.5

Pancreas Transplants Kidney Transplants

(Rev. 3481, Issued: 03-18-16. Effective: 06-20-16, Implementation: 06-20-16)

A. Background

Effective July 1, 1999, Medicare covered pancreas transplantation when performed simultaneously with or following a kidney transplant if ICD-9 is applicable, ICD-9-CM procedure code 55.69. If ICD-10 is applicable, the following ICD-10-PCS codes will be used:

0TY00Z0, 0TY00Z1, 0TY00Z2, 0TY10Z0. 0TY10Z1, and 0TY10Z2.

Pancreas transplantation is performed to induce an insulin independent, euglycemic state in diabetic patients. The procedure is generally limited to those patients with severe secondary complications of diabetes including kidney failure. However, pancreas transplantation is sometimes performed on patients with labile diabetes and hypoglycemic unawareness.

Medicare has had a policy of not covering pancreas transplantation. The Office of Health Technology Assessment performed an assessment on pancreas-kidney transplantation in 1994. They found reasonable graft survival outcomes for patients receiving either simultaneous pancreas-kidney (SPK) transplantation or pancreas after kidney (PAK) transplantation. For a list of facilities approved to perform SPK or PAK, refer to the following Web site: https://www.cms.gov/Medicare/Provider-Enrollment-and-Certification/CertificationandComplianc/downloads/ApprovedTransplantPrograms.pdf

B. Billing for Pancreas Transplants

There are no special provisions related to managed care participants. Managed care plans are required to provide all Medicare covered services. Medicare does not restrict which hospitals or physicians may perform pancreas transplantation.

The transplant procedure and revenue code 0360 for the operating room are paid under these codes. Procedures must be reported using the current ICD-9-CM procedure codes for pancreas and kidney transplants. Providers must place at least one of the following transplant procedure codes on the claim:

If ICD-9 Is Applicable

52.80 Transplant of pancreas

52.82 Homotransplant of pancreas

The Medicare Code Editor (MCE) has been updated to include 52.80 and 52.82 as limited coverage procedures. The contractor must determine if the facility is approved for the transplant and certified for either pediatric or adult transplants dependent upon the age of the patient.

Effective October 1, 2000, ICD-9-CM code 52.83 was moved in the MCE to non-covered. The contractor must override any deny edit on claims that came in with 52.82 prior to October 1, 2000 and adjust, as 52.82 is the correct code.

If the discharge date is July 1, 1999, or later: the contractor processes the bill through Grouper and Pricer.

If ICD-10 is applicable, the following procedure codes (ICD-10-PCS) are:

0FYG0Z0 Transplantation of Pancreas, Allogeneic, Open Approach

0FYG0Z1 Transplantation of Pancreas, Syngeneic, Open Approach

Pancreas transplantation is reasonable and necessary for the following diagnosis codes. However, since this is not an all-inclusive list, the contractor is permitted to determine if any additional diagnosis codes will be covered for this procedure.

If ICD-9-CM is applicable, Diabetes Diagnosis Codes and Descriptions

ICD-9-CM Code	Description
250.00	Diabetes mellitus without mention of complication, type II (non-insulin dependent) (NIDDM) (adult onset) or unspecified type, not stated as uncontrolled.
250.01	Diabetes mellitus without mention of complication, type I (insulin dependent) (IDDM) (juvenile), not stated as uncontrolled.
250.02	Diabetes mellitus without mention of complication, type II (non-insulin dependent) (NIDDM) (adult onset) or unspecified type, uncontrolled.
250.03	Diabetes mellitus without mention of complication, type I (insulin dependent) (IDDM) (juvenile), uncontrolled.
250.1X	Diabetes with ketoacidosis
250.2X	Diabetes with hyperosmolarity
250.3X	Diabetes with coma
250.4X	Diabetes with renal manifestations
250.5X	Diabetes with ophthalmic manifestations
250.6X	Diabetes with neurological manifestations
250.7X	Diabetes with peripheral circulatory disorders
250.8X	Diabetes with other specified manifestations
250.9X	Diabetes with unspecified complication

NOTE: X=0-3

If ICD-10-CM is applicable, the diagnosis codes are: E10.10 - E10.9

Hypertensive Renal Diagnosis Codes and Descriptions if ICD-9-CM is applicable :

ICD-9-CM Code	Description
403.01	Malignant hypertensive renal disease, with renal failure
403.11	Benign hypertensive renal disease, with renal failure
403.91	Unspecified hypertensive renal disease, with renal failure
404.02	Malignant hypertensive heart and renal disease, with renal failure
404.03	Malignant hypertensive heart and renal disease, with congestive heart failure or renal failure
404.12	Benign hypertensive heart and renal disease, with renal failure

ICD-9-CM Code	Description
404.13	Benign hypertensive heart and renal disease, with congestive heart failure or renal failure
404.92	Unspecified hypertensive heart and renal disease, with renal failure
404.93	Unspecified hypertensive heart and renal disease, with congestive heart failure or renal failure
585.1–585.6, 585.9	Chronic Renal Failure Code

If ICD-10-CM is applicable, diagnosis codes and descriptions are:

ICD-10-CM code	Description
I12.0	Hypertensive chronic kidney disease with stage 5 chronic kidney disease or end stage renal disease
I13.11	Hypertensive heart and chronic kidney disease without heart failure, with stage 5 chronic kidney disease, or end stage renal disease
I13.2	Hypertensive heart and chronic kidney disease with heart failure and with stage 5 chronic kidney disease, or end stage renal disease
N18.1	Chronic kidney disease, stage 1
N18.2	Chronic kidney disease, stage 2 (mild)
N18.3	Chronic kidney disease, stage 3 (moderate)
N18.4	Chronic kidney disease, stage 4 (severe)
N18.5	Chronic kidney disease, stage 5
N18.6	End stage renal disease
N18.9	Chronic kidney disease, unspecified

NOTE: If a patient had a kidney transplant that was successful, the patient no longer has chronic kidney failure, therefore it would be inappropriate for the provider to bill ICD-9-CM codes 585.1 - 585.6, 585.9 or, if ICD-10-CM is applicable, the diagnosis codes N18.1 - N18.9 on such a patient. In these cases one of the following codes should be present on the claim or in the beneficiary's history.

The provider uses the following ICD-9-CM status codes only when a kidney transplant was performed before the pancreas transplant and ICD-9 is applicable:

ICD-9-CM code	Description
V42.0	Organ or tissue replaced by transplant kidney
V43.89	Organ tissue replaced by other means, kidney or pancreas

If ICD-10-CM is applicable, the following ICD-10-CM status codes will be used:

ICD-10-CM code	Description
Z48.22	Encounter for aftercare following kidney transplant
Z94.0	Kidney transplant status

NOTE: If a kidney and pancreas transplants are performed simultaneously, the claim should contain a diabetes diagnosis code and a renal failure code or one of the hypertensive renal failure diagnosis codes. The claim should also contain two transplant procedure codes. If the claim is for a pancreas transplant only, the claim should contain a diabetes diagnosis code and a status code to indicate a previous kidney transplant. If the status code is not on the claim for the pancreas transplant, the contractor will search the beneficiary's claim history for a status code indicating a prior kidney transplant.

C. Drugs
If the pancreas transplant occurs after the kidney transplant, immunosuppressive therapy will begin with the date of discharge from the inpatient stay for the pancreas transplant.

D. Charges for Pancreas Acquisition Services
A separate organ acquisition cost center has been established for pancreas transplantation. The Medicare cost report will include a separate line to account for pancreas transplantation costs. The 42 CFR 412.2(e)(4) was changed to include pancreas in the list of organ acquisition costs that are paid on a reasonable cost basis.

Acquisition costs for pancreas transplantation as well as kidney transplants will occur in Revenue Center 081X. The contractor overrides any claims that suspend due to repetition of revenue code 081X on the same claim if the patient had a simultaneous kidney/pancreas transplant. It pays for acquisition costs for both kidney and pancreas organs if transplants are performed simultaneously. It will not pay for more than two organ acquisitions on the same claim.

E. Medicare Summary Notices (MSN) and Remittance Advice Messages
If the provider submits a claim for simultaneous pancreas kidney transplantation or pancreas transplantation following a kidney transplant, and omits one of the appropriate diagnosis/procedure codes, the contractor shall reject the claim.

The following reflects the remittance advice messages and associated codes that will appear when rejecting/denying claims under this policy. This CARC/RARC combination is compliant with CAQH CORE Business Scenario 3.

Group Code: CO

CARC: B15

RARC: N/A

MSN: 16.32

If no evidence of a prior kidney transplant is presented, then the contractor shall deny the claim.

The following reflects the remittance advice messages and associated codes that will appear when rejecting/denying claims under this policy. This CARC/RARC combination is compliant with CAQH CORE Business Scenario 3.

Group Code: CO

CARC: 50

RARC: MA126

MSN: 15.4

100-04, 3, 90.5.1
Pancreas Transplants Alone (PA)
Rev.3481, Issued: 03-18-16. Effective: 06-20-16, Implementation: 06-20-16

A. General

Pancreas transplantation is performed to induce an insulin-independent, euglycemic state in diabetic patients. The procedure is generally limited to those patients with severe secondary complications of diabetes, including kidney failure. However, pancreas transplantation is sometimes performed on patients with labile diabetes and hypoglycemic unawareness. Medicare has had a long-standing policy of not covering pancreas transplantation, as the safety and effectiveness of the procedure had not been demonstrated. The Office of Health Technology Assessment performed an assessment of pancreas-kidney transplantation in 1994. It found reasonable graft survival outcomes for patients receiving either simultaneous pancreas-kidney transplantation or pancreas-after-kidney transplantation.

B. Nationally Covered Indications

CMS determines that whole organ pancreas transplantation will be nationally covered by Medicare when performed simultaneous with or after a kidney transplant. If the pancreas transplant occurs after the kidney transplant, immunosuppressive therapy will begin with the date of discharge from the inpatient stay for the pancreas transplant.

C. Billing and Claims Processing

Contractors shall pay for Pancreas Transplantation Alone (PA) effective for services on or after April 26, 2006 when performed in those facilities that are Medicare-approved for kidney transplantation. Approved facilities are located at the following address: https://www.cms.gov/Medicare/Provider-Enrollment-and-Certification/CertificationandComplianc/downloads/ApprovedTransplantPrograms.pdf

Contractors who receive claims for PA services that were performed in an unapproved facility, should reject such claims. The following reflects the remittance advice messages and associated codes that will appear when rejecting/denying claims under this policy. This CARC/RARC combination is compliant with CAQH CORE Business Scenario 3.

Group Code: CO

CARC: 58

RARC: N/A

MSN: 16.2.

Payment will be made for a PA service performed in an approved facility, and which meets the coverage guidelines mentioned above for beneficiaries with type I diabetes.

All-Inclusive List of Covered Diagnosis Codes for PA if ICD-9-CM is applicable (NOTE: "X" = 1 and 3 only)

ICD-9-CM code	Description
250.0X	Diabetes mellitus without mention of complication, type I (insulin dependent) (IDDM) (juvenile), not stated as uncontrolled.
250.1X	Diabetes with ketoacidosis
250.2X	Diabetes with hyperosmolarity
250.3X	Diabetes with coma
250.4X	Diabetes with renal manifestations
250.5X	Diabetes with ophthalmic manifestations
250.6X	Diabetes with neurological manifestations
250.7X	Diabetes with peripheral circulatory disorders
250.8X	Diabetes with other specified manifestations
250.9X	Diabetes with unspecified complication

If ICD-10-CM is applicable, the provider uses the following range of ICD-10-CM codes:
E10.10 – E10.9.

Procedure Codes

If ICD-9 CM is applicable

52.80 - Transplant of pancreas

52.82 - Homotransplant of pancreas

If ICD-10 is applicable, the provider uses the following ICD-10-PCS codes:

ØFYGØZØ Transplantation of Pancreas, Allogeneic, Open Approach

ØFYGØZ1 Transplantation of Pancreas, Syngeneic, Open Approach

Contractors who receive claims for PA that are not billed using the covered diagnosis/procedure codes listed above shall reject such claims. The MCE edits to ensure that the transplant is covered based on the diagnosis. The MCE also considers ICD-9-CM codes 52.80 and 52.82 and ICD-10-PCS codes ØFYGØZØ and ØFYGØZ1 as limited coverage dependent upon whether the facility is approved to perform the transplant and is certified for the age of the patient.

The following reflects the remittance advice messages and associated codes that will appear when rejecting/denying claims under this policy. This CARC/RARC combination is compliant with CAQH CORE Business Scenario 3.

Group Code: CO

CARC: 50

RARC: N/A

MSN: 15.4

Contractors shall hold the provider liable for denied\rejected claims unless the hospital issues a Hospital Issued Notice of Non-coverage (HINN) or a physician issues an Advanced Beneficiary Notice (ABN) for Part-B for physician services.

D. Charges for Pancreas Alone Acquisition Services

A separate organ acquisition cost center has been established for pancreas transplantation. The Medicare cost report will include a separate line to account for pancreas transplantation costs. The 42 CFR 412.2(e)(4) was changed to include PA in the list of organ acquisition costs that are paid on a reasonable cost basis.

Acquisition costs for PA transplantation are billed in Revenue Code 081X. The contractor removes acquisition charges prior to sending the claims to Pricer so such charges are not included in the outlier calculation.

100-04, 3, 90.6

Intestinal and Multi-Visceral Transplants

(Rev. 3481, Issued: 03-18-16. Effective: 06-20-16, Implementation: 06-20-16)

A. Background

Effective for services on or after April 1, 2001, Medicare covers intestinal and multi-visceral transplantation for the purpose of restoring intestinal function in patients with irreversible intestinal failure. Intestinal failure is defined as the loss of absorptive capacity of the small bowel secondary to severe primary gastrointestinal disease or surgically induced short bowel syndrome. Intestinal failure prevents oral nutrition and may be associated with both mortality and profound morbidity. Multi-Visceral transplantation includes organs in the digestive system (stomach, duodenum, liver, and intestine). See §260.5 of the National Coverage Determinations Manual for further information.

B. Approved Transplant Facilities

Medicare will cover intestinal transplantation if performed in an approved facility. The approved facilities are located at: https://www.cms.gov/Medicare/Provider-Enrollment-and-Certification/Certificationa ndComplianc/downloads/ApprovedTransplantPrograms.pdf

C. Billing

If ICD-9-CM is applicable, ICD-9-CM procedure code 46.97 is effective for discharges on or after April 1, 2001. If ICD-10 is applicable, the ICD-10-PCS procedure codes are ØDY80ZØ, ØDY80Z1, ØDY80Z2, ØDYE0ZØ, ØDYE0Z1, and ØDYE0Z2. The Medicare Code Editor (MCE) lists these codes as limited coverage procedures. The contractor shall override the MCE when this procedure code is listed and the coverage criteria are met in an approved transplant facility, and also determine if the facility is certified for adults and/or pediatric transplants dependent upon the patient's age.

For these procedures where the provider is approved as transplant facility and certified for the adult and/or pediatric population, and the service is performed on or after the transplant approval date, the contractor must suspend the claim for clerical review of the operative report to determine whether the beneficiary has at least one of the covered conditions listed when the diagnosis code is for a covered condition.

This review is not part of the contractor's medical review workload. Instead, the contractor should complete this review as part of its claims processing workload.

If ICD-9-CM is applicable, charges for ICD-9-CM procedure code 46.97, and, if ICD-10 is applicable, the ICD-10-PCS procedure codes ØDY80ZØ, ØDY80Z1, ØDY80Z2, ØDYE0ZØ, ØDYE0Z1, or ØDYE0Z2 should be billed under revenue code 0360, Operating Room Services.

For discharge dates on or after October 1, 2001, acquisition charges are billed under revenue code 081X, Organ Acquisition. For discharge dates between April 1, 2001, and September 30, 2001, hospitals were to report the acquisition charges on the claim, but there was no interim pass-through payment made for these costs.

Bill the procedure used to obtain the donor's organ on the same claim, using appropriate ICD procedure codes.

The 11X bill type should be used when billing for intestinal transplants.

Immunosuppressive therapy for intestinal transplantation is covered and should be billed consistent with other organ transplants under the current rules.

If ICD-9-CM is applicable, there is no specific ICD-9-CM diagnosis code for intestinal failure. Diagnosis codes exist to capture the causes of intestinal failure. Some examples of intestinal failure include but are not limited to the following conditions and their associated ICD-9-CM codes:

- Volvulus 560.2,
- Volvulus gastroschisis 756.79, other [congenital] anomalies of abdominal wall,
- Volvulus gastroschisis 569.89, other specified disorders of intestine,
- Necrotizing enterocolitis 777.5, necrotizing enterocolitis in fetus or newborn,
- Necrotizing enterocolitis 014.8, other tuberculosis of intestines, peritoneum, and mesenteric,
- Necrotizing enterocolitis and splanchnic vascular thrombosis 557.0, acute vascular insufficiency of intestine,
- Inflammatory bowel disease 569.9, unspecified disorder of intestine,
- Radiation enteritis 777.5, necrotizing enterocolitis in fetus or newborn, and
- Radiation enteritis 558.1.

If ICD-10-CM is applicable, some diagnosis codes that may be used for intestinal failure are:

- Volvulus K56.2,
- Enteroptosis K63.4,
- Other specified diseases of intestine K63.89,
- Other specified diseases of the digestive system K92.89,
- Postsurgical malabsorption, not elsewhere classified K91.2,
- Other congenital malformations of abdominal wall Q79.59,
- Necrotizing enterocolitis in newborn, unspecified P77.9,
- Stage 1 necrotizing enterocolitis in newborn P77.1,
- Stage 2 necrotizing enterocolitis in newborn P77.2, and
- Stage 3 necrotizing enterocolitis in newborn P77.3

D. Acquisition Costs

A separate organ acquisition cost center was established for acquisition costs incurred on or after October 1, 2001. The Medicare Cost Report will include a separate line to account for these transplantation costs.

For intestinal and multi-visceral transplants performed between April 1, 2001, and October 1, 2001, the DRG payment was payment in full for all hospital services related to this procedure.

E. Medicare Summary Notices (MSN), Remittance Advice Messages, and Notice of Utilization Notices (NOU)

If an intestinal transplant is billed by an unapproved facility after April 1, 2001, the contractor shall deny the claim.

The following reflects the remittance advice messages and associated codes that will appear when rejecting/denying claims under this policy. This CARC/RARC combination is compliant with CAQH CORE Business Scenario 3.

Group Code: CO

CARC: 171

RARC: N/A

MSN: 21.6 or 21.18 or 16.2

100-04, 3, 100.1

Billing for Abortion Services

(Rev. 3481, Issued: 03-18-16. Effective: 06-20-16, Implementation: 06-20-16)

Effective October 1, 1998, abortions are not covered under the Medicare program except for instances where the pregnancy is a result of an act of rape or incest; or the woman suffers from a physical disorder, physical injury, or physical illness, including a life endangering physical condition caused by the pregnancy itself that would, as certified by a physician, place the woman in danger of death unless an abortion is performed.

A. "G" Modifier

The "G7" modifier is defined as "the pregnancy resulted from rape or incest, or pregnancy certified by physician as life threatening."

Beginning July 1, 1999, providers should bill for abortion services using the new Modifier G7. This modifier can be used on claims with dates of services October 1, 1998, and after. CWF will be able to recognize the modifier beginning July 1, 1999.

B. A/B MAC (A) Billing Instructions
1. Hospital Inpatient Billing

Hospitals use bill type 11X. Medicare will pay only when one of the following condition codes is reported:

Condition Code	Description
AA	Abortion Performed due to Rape
AB	Abortion Performed due to Incest
AD	Abortion Performed due to life endangering physical condition

With one of the following:

If ICD-9-CM Is Applicable:

- an appropriate ICD principal diagnosis code that will group to DRG 770 (Abortion W D&C, Aspiration Curettage Or Hysterotomy) or

- an appropriate ICD principal diagnosis code and one of the following ICD-9-CM operating room procedure that will group to DRG 779 (Abortion W/O D&C):69.01, 69.02, 69.51, 74.91.

If ICD-10-CM is applicable, one of the following ICD-10-PCS codes are used:

ICD-10-PCS code	Description
10A07ZZ	Abortion of Products of Conception, Via Natural or Artificial Opening
10A08ZZ	Abortion of Products of Conception, Via Natural or Artificial Opening Endoscopic
10D17ZZ	Extraction of Products of Conception, Retained, Via Natural or Artificial Opening
10D18ZZ	Extraction of Products of Conception, Retained, Via Natural or Artificial Opening Endoscopic
10A07ZZ	Abortion of Products of Conception, Via Natural or Artificial Opening
10A08ZZ	Abortion of Products of Conception, Via Natural or Artificial Opening Endoscopic
10A00ZZ	Abortion of Products of Conception, Open Approach
10A03ZZ	Abortion of Products of Conception, Percutaneous Approach
10A04ZZ	Abortion of Products of Conception, Percutaneous Endoscopic Approach

Providers must use ICD-9-CM codes 69.01 and 69.02 if ICD-9-CM is applicable, or, if ICD-10-CM is applicable, the related 1CD-10-PCS codes to describe exactly the procedure or service performed.

The A/B MAC (A) must manually review claims with the above ICD-9-CM/ICD-10-PCS procedure codes to verify that all of the above conditions are met.

2. Outpatient Billing

Hospitals will use bill type 13X and 85X. Medicare will pay only if one of the following CPT codes is used with the "G7" modifier.

59840	59851	59856	59841	59852
59857	59850	59855	59866	

C. Common Working File (CWF) Edits

For hospital outpatient claims, CWF will bypass its edits for a managed care beneficiary who is having an abortion outside their plan and the claim is submitted with the "G7" modifier and one of the above CPT codes.

For hospital inpatient claims, CWF will bypass its edits for a managed care beneficiary who is having an abortion outside their plan and the claim is submitted with one of the above inpatient procedure codes.

D. Medicare Summary Notices (MSN)/Explanation of Your Medicare Benefits Remittance Advice Message

If a claim is submitted with one of the above CPT procedure codes but no "G7" modifier, the claim is denied.

The following reflects the remittance advice messages and associated codes that will appear when rejecting/denying claims under this policy. This CARC/RARC combination is compliant with CAQH CORE Business Scenario 3.

Group Code: CO

CARC: 272

RARC: N/A

MSN: 21.21

100-04, 3, 100.6

Inpatient Renal Services

(Rev. 1, 10-01-03) HO-E400

Section 405.103l of Subpart J of Regulation 5 stipulates that only approved hospitals may bill for ESRD services. Hence, to allow hospitals to bill and be reimbursed for inpatient dialysis services furnished under arrangements, both facilities participating in the arrangement must meet the conditions of 405.2120 and 405.2160 of Subpart U of Regulation 5. In order for renal dialysis facilities to have a written arrangement with

each other to provide inpatient dialysis care both facilities must meet the minimum utilization rate requirement, i.e., two dialysis stations with a performance capacity of at least four dialysis treatments per week.

Dialysis may be billed by an SNF as a service if: (a) it is provided by a hospital with which the facility has a transfer agreement in effect, and that hospital is approved to provide staff-assisted dialysis for the Medicare program; or (b) it is furnished directly by an SNF meeting all nonhospital maintenance dialysis facility requirements, including minimum utilization requirements. (See 1861(h)(6), 1861(h)(7), title XVIII.)

100-04, 4, 20.6.12

Use of HCPCS Modifier – CT

(Rev. 3425, Issued: 12-18-15, Effective: 01-01-16, Implementation: 01-04-16)

Effective January 1, 2016, the definition of modifier – CT is "Computed tomography services furnished using equipment that does not meet each of the attributes of the National Electrical Manufacturers Association (NEMA) XR-29-2013 standard." This modifier is required to be reported on claims for computed tomography (CT) scans described by applicable HCPCS codes that are furnished on non-NEMA Standard XR-29-2013-compliant equipment. The applicable CT services are identified by HCPCS codes 70450 through 70498; 71250 through 71275; 72125 through 72133; 72191 through 72194; 73200 through 73206; 73700 through 73706; 74150 through 74178; 74261 through 74263; and 75571 through 75574 (and any succeeding codes).

This modifier should not be reported with codes that describe CT scans not listed above.

100-04, 4, 160

Clinic and Emergency Visits

(Rev. 1445, Issued: 02-08-08; Effective: 01-01-08; Implementation: 03-10-08)

CMS has acknowledged from the beginning of the OPPS that CMS believes that CPT Evaluation and Management (E/M) codes were designed to reflect the activities of physicians and do not describe well the range and mix of services provided by hospitals during visits of clinic and emergency department patients. While awaiting the development of a national set of facility-specific codes and guidelines, providers should continue to apply their current internal guidelines to the existing CPT codes. Each hospital's internal guidelines should follow the intent of the CPT code descriptors, in that the guidelines should be designed to reasonably relate the intensity of hospital resources to the different levels of effort represented by the codes. Hospitals should ensure that their guidelines accurately reflect resource distinctions between the five levels of codes.

Effective January 1, 2007, CMS is distinguishing between two types of emergency departments: Type A emergency departments and Type B emergency departments.

A Type A emergency department is defined as an emergency department that is available 24 hours a day, 7 days a week and is either licensed by the State in which it is located under applicable State law as an emergency room or emergency department or it is held out to the public (by name, posted signs, advertising, or other means) as a place that provides care for emergency medical conditions on an urgent basis without requiring a previously scheduled appointment.

A Type B emergency department is defined as an emergency department that meets the definition of a "dedicated emergency department" as defined in 42 CFR 489.24 under the EMTALA regulations. It must meet at least one of the following requirements: (1) It is licensed by the State in which it is located under applicable State law as an emergency room or emergency department; (2) It is held out to the public (by name, posted signs, advertising, or other means) as a place that provides care for emergency medical conditions on an urgent basis without requiring a previously scheduled appointment; or (3) During the calendar year immediately preceding the calendar year in which a determination under 42 CFR 489.24 is being made, based on a representative sample of patient visits that occurred during that calendar year, it provides at least one-third of all of its outpatient visits for the treatment of emergency medical conditions on an urgent basis without requiring a previously scheduled appointment.

Hospitals must bill for visits provided in Type A emergency departments using CPT emergency department E/M codes. Hospitals must bill for visits provided in Type B emergency departments using the G-codes that describe visits provided in Type B emergency departments.

Hospitals that will be billing the new Type B ED visit codes may need to update their internal guidelines to report these codes.

Emergency department and clinic visits are paid in some cases separately and in other cases as part of a composite APC payment. See section 10.2.1 of this chapter for further details.

100-04, 4, 200.1

Billing for Corneal Tissue

(Rev. 3425, Issued: 12-18-15, Effective: 01-01-16, Implementation: 01-04-16)

Corneal tissue will be paid on a cost basis, not under OPPS, only when it is used in a corneal transplant procedure described by one of the following CPT codes: 65710, 65730, 65750, 65755, 65756, 65765, 65767, and any successor code or new code describing a new type of corneal transplant procedure that uses eye banked corneal tissue. In all other procedures cornea tissue is packaged. To receive cost based reimbursement hospitals must bill charges for corneal tissue using HCPCS code V2785.

100-04, 4, 200.3.1

Billing Instructions for IMRT Planning and Delivery

(Rev. 3685, Issued: 12-22-16, Effective: 01-01-17, Implementation: 01-03-17)

Payment for the services identified by CPT codes 77014, 77280, 77285, 77290, 77295, 77306 through 77321, 77331, and 77370 are included in the APC payment for CPT code 77301 (IMRT planning). These codes should not be reported in addition to CPT code 77301 when provided prior to or as part of the development of the IMRT plan. In addition, CPT codes 77280-77290 (simulation-aided field settings) should not be reported for verification of the treatment field during a course of IMRT.

100-04, 4, 200.3.2

Billing for Multi-Source Photon (Cobalt 60-Based) Stereotactic Radiosurgery (SRS) Planning and Delivery

(Rev. 3685, Issued: 12-22-16, Effective: 01-01-17, Implementation: 01-03-17)

Effective for services furnished on or after January 1, 2014, hospitals must report SRS planning and delivery services using only the CPT codes that accurately describe the service furnished. For the delivery services, hospitals must report CPT code 77371, 77372, or 77373.

CPT Code	Long Descriptor
77371	Radiation treatment delivery, stereotactic radiosurgery (srs), complete course of treatment of cranial lesion(s) consisting of 1 session; multi- source cobalt 60 based
77372	Radiation treatment delivery, stereotactic radiosurgery (srs), complete course of treatment of cranial lesion(s) consisting of 1 session; linear accelerator based
77373	Stereotactic body radiation therapy, treatment delivery, per fraction to 1 or more lesions, including image guidance, entire course not to exceed 5 fractions

As instructed in the CY 2014 OPPS/ASC final rule, CPT code 77371 is to be used only for single session cranial SRS cases performed with a Cobalt-60 device, and CPT code 77372 is to be used only for single session cranial SRS cases performed with a linac-based device. The term "cranial" means that the pathological lesion(s) that are the target of the radiation is located in the patient's cranium or head. The term "single session" means that the entire intracranial lesion(s) that comprise the patient's diagnosis are treated in their entirety during a single treatment session on a single day. CPT code 77372 is never to be used for the first fraction or any other fraction of a fractionated SRS treatment. CPT code 77372 is to be used only for single session cranial linac-based SRS treatment. Fractionated SRS treatment is any SRS delivery service requiring more thana single session of SRS treatment for a cranial lesion, up to a total of no more than five fractions, and one to five sessions (but no more than five) for non-cranial lesions. CPT code 77373 is to be used for any fraction (including the first fraction) in any series of fractionated treatments, regardless of the anatomical location of the lesion or lesions being radiated. Fractionated cranial SRS is any cranial SRS that exceeds one treatment session and fractionated non-cranial SRS is any non-cranial SRS, regardless of the number of fractions but never more than five. Therefore, CPT code 77373 is the exclusive code (and the use of no other SRS treatment delivery code is permitted) for any and all fractionated SRS treatment services delivered anywhere in the body, including, but not limited to, the cranium or head. 77372 is not to be used for the first fraction of a fractionated cranial SRS treatment series and must only be used in cranial SRS when there is a single treatment session to treat the patient's entire condition.

In addition, for the planning services, hospitals must report the specific CPT code that accurately describes the service provided. The planning services may include but are not limited to CPT code 77290, 77295, 77300, 77334, or 77370.

CPT Code	Long Descriptor
77290	Therapeutic radiology simulation-aided field setting; complex
77295	Therapeutic radiology simulation-aided field setting; 3-dimensional
77300	Basic radiation dosimetry calculation, central axis depth dose calculation, tdf, nsd, gap calculation, off axis factor, tissue inhomogeneity factors, calculation of non-ionizing radiation surface and depth dose, as required during course of treatment, only when prescribed by the treating physician
77334	Treatment devices, design and construction; complex (irregular blocks, special shields, compensators, wedges, molds or casts)
77370	Special medical radiation physics consultation

Effective for cranial single session stereotactic radiosurgery procedures (CPT code 77371 or 77372) furnished on or after January 1, 2016 until December 31, 2017, costs for certain adjunctive services (e.g., planning and preparation) are not factored into the APC payment rate for APC 5627 (Level 7 Radiation Therapy). Rather, the ten planning and preparation codes listed in table below, will be paid according to their assigned status indicator when furnished 30 days prior or 30 days post SRS treatment delivery.

In addition, hospitals must report modifier "CP" (Adjunctive service related to a procedure assigned to a comprehensive ambulatory payment classification [C-APC] procedure) on TOB 13X claims for any other services (excluding the ten codes in table below) that are adjunctive or related to SRS treatment but billed on a different claim and within either 30 days prior or 30 days after the date of service for either CPT code 77371 (Radiation treatment delivery, stereotactic radiosurgery, complete course of treatment cranial lesion(s) consisting of 1 session; multi-source Cobalt 60-based) or CPT code 77372 (Linear accelerator based). The "CP" modifier need not be reported with the ten planning and preparation CPT codes table below. Adjunctive/related services include but are not necessarily limited to imaging, clinical treatment planning/preparation, and consultations. Any service related to the SRS delivery should have the CP modifier appended. We would not expect the "CP" modifier to be reported with services such as chemotherapy administration as this is considered to be a distinct service that is not directly adjunctive, integral, or dependent on delivery of SRS treatment.

Excluded Planning and Preparation CPT Codes

CPT Code	CY 2017 Short Descriptor	CY 2017 Opps Status Indicator
70551	Mri brain stem w/o dye	Q3
70552	Mri brain stem w/dye	Q3
70553	Mri brain stem w/o & w/dye	Q3
77011	Ct scan for localization	N
77014	Ct scan for therapy guide	N
77280	Set radiation therapy field	S
77285	Set radiation therapy field	S
77290	Set radiation therapy field	S
77295	3-d radiotherapy plan	S
77336	Radiation physics consult	S

100-04, 4, 200.11

Billing Advance Care Planning (ACP) as an Optional Element of an Annual Wellness Visit (AWV)

(Rev. 3739, Issued: 03-17-17, Effective: 01-01-16, Implementation: 06-19-17)

Effective January 1, 2016 payment for the service described by CPT code 99497 (Advance care planning including the explanation and discussion of advance directives such as standard forms (with completion of such forms, when performed), by the physician or other qualified health care professional; first 30 minutes, face-to-face with the patient, family member(s), and/or surrogate) is conditionally packaged under the OPPS and is consequently assigned to a conditionally packaged payment status indicator of "Q1." When this service is furnished with another service paid under the OPPS, payment is packaged; when it is the only service furnished, payment is made separately. CPT code 99498 (Advance care planning including the explanation and discussion of advance directives such as standard forms (with completion of such forms, when performed), by the physician or other qualified health care professional; each additional 30 minutes (List separately in addition to code for primary procedure)) is an add-on code and therefore payment for the service described by this code is unconditionally packaged (assigned status indicator "N") in the OPPS in accordance with 42 CFR 419.2(b)(18).

In addition, for services furnished on or after January 1, 2016, Advance Care Planning (ACP) is treated as a preventive service when furnished with an AWV. The Medicare coinsurance and Part B deductible are waived for ACP when furnished as an optional element of an AWV.

The codes for the optional ACP services furnished as part of an AWV are 99497 (Advance care planning including the explanation and discussion of advance directives such as standard forms (with completion of such forms, when performed), by the physician or other qualified health professional; first 30 minutes, face-to-face with the patient, family member(s) and/or surrogate;) and an add-on code 99498 (each additional 30 minutes (List separately in addition to code for primary procedure)). When ACP services are provided as a part of an AWV, practitioners would report CPT code 99497 (and add-on CPT code 99498 when applicable) for the ACP services in addition to either of the AWV codes (G0438 or G0439).

The deductible and coinsurance for ACP will only be waived when billed on the same day and on the same claim as an AWV (code G0438 or G0439), and must also be furnished by the same provider. Waiver of the deductible and coinsurance for ACP is limited to once per year. Payment for an AWV is limited to once per year. If the AWV billed with ACP is denied for exceeding the once per year limit, the deductible and coinsurance will be applied to the ACP.

Also see Pub. 100-02, Medicare Benefit Policy Manual, chapter 15, section 280.5.1 for more information.

100-04, 4, 231.10

Billing for Autologous Stem Cell Transplants

(Rev.3556, Issued: 07-01-2016; Effective: 1-27-16; Implementation: 10-3-16)

The hospital bills and shows all charges for autologous stem cell harvesting, processing, and transplant procedures based on the status of the patient (i.e., inpatient or outpatient) when the services are furnished. It shows charges for the actual transplant, described by the appropriate ICD procedure or CPT codes in

Revenue Center 0362 (Operating Room Services; Organ Transplant, Other than Kidney) or another appropriate cost center.

The CPT codes describing autologous stem cell harvesting procedures may be billed and are separately payable under the Outpatient Prospective Payment System (OPPS) when provided in the hospital outpatient setting of care. Autologous harvesting procedures are distinct from the acquisition services described in Pub. 100-04, Chapter 3, §90.3.1 and §231.11 of this chapter for allogeneic stem cell transplants, which include services provided when stem cells are obtained from a donor and not from the patient undergoing the stem cell transplant.

The CPT codes describing autologous stem cell processing procedures also may be billed and are separately payable under the OPPS when provided to hospital outpatients.

100-04, 4, 231.11

Billing for Allogeneic Stem Cell Transplants
(Rev. 3571, Issued: 07-29-16, Effective: 01-01-17, Implementation: 01-03-17)

1. Definition of Acquisition Charges for Allogeneic Stem Cell Transplants
Acquisition charges for allogeneic stem cell transplants include, but are not limited to, charges for the costs of the following services:

- National Marrow Donor Program fees, if applicable, for stem cells from an unrelated donor;
- Tissue typing of donor and recipient;
- Donor evaluation;
- Physician pre-procedure donor evaluation services;
- Costs associated with harvesting procedure (e.g., general routine and special care services, procedure/operating room and other ancillary services, apheresis services, etc.);
- Post-operative/post-procedure evaluation of donor; and
- Preparation and processing of stem cells.

Payment for these acquisition services is included in the OPPS C-APC payment for the allogeneic stem cell transplant when the transplant occurs in the hospital outpatient setting, and in the MS-DRG payment for the allogeneic stem cell transplant when the transplant occurs in the inpatient setting. The Medicare contractor does not make separate payment for these acquisition services, because hospitals may bill and receive payment only for services provided to the Medicare beneficiary who is the recipient of the stem cell transplant and whose illness is being treated with the stem cell transplant. Unlike the acquisition costs of solid organs for transplant (e.g., hearts and kidneys), which are paid on a reasonable cost basis, acquisition costs for allogeneic stem cells are included in prospective payment. Recurring update notifications describing changes to and billing instructions for various payment policies implemented in the OPPS are issued annually.

Acquisition charges for stem cell transplants apply only to allogeneic transplants, for which stem cells are obtained from a donor (other than the recipient himself or herself). Acquisition charges do not apply to autologous transplants (transplanted stem cells are obtained from the recipient himself or herself), because autologous transplants involve services provided to the beneficiary only (and not to a donor), for which the hospital may bill and receive payment (see Pub. 100-04, chapter 3, §90.3.1 and §231.10 of this chapter for information regarding billing for autologous stem cell transplants).

2. Billing for Acquisition Services
The hospital bills and shows acquisition charges for allogeneic stem cell transplants based on the status of the patient (i.e., inpatient or outpatient) when the transplant is furnished. See Pub. 100-04, chapter 3, §90.3.1 for instructions regarding billing for acquisition services for allogeneic stem cell transplants that are performed in the inpatient setting.

Effective January 1, 2017, when the allogeneic stem cell transplant occurs in the outpatient setting, the hospital identifies stem cell acquisition charges for allogeneic bone marrow/stem cell transplants separately in FL 42 of Form CMS-1450 (or electronic equivalent) by using revenue code 0815 (Other Organ Acquisition). Revenue code 0815 charges should include all services required to acquire stem cells from a donor, as defined above, and should be reported on the same date of service as the transplant procedure in order to be appropriately packaged for payment purposes.

The transplant hospital keeps an itemized statement that identifies the services furnished, the charges, the person receiving the service (donor/recipient), and whether this is a potential transplant donor or recipient. These charges will be reflected in the transplant hospital's stem cell/bone marrow acquisition cost center. For allogeneic stem cell acquisition services in cases that do not result in transplant, due to death of the intended recipient or other causes, hospitals include the costs associated with the acquisition services on the Medicare cost report.

In the case of an allogeneic transplant in the hospital outpatient setting, the hospital reports the transplant itself with the appropriate CPT code, and a charge under revenue center code 0362 or another appropriate cost center. Selection of the cost center is up to the hospital.

100-04, 4, 250.16

Multiple Procedure Payment Reduction (MPPR) on Certain Diagnostic Imaging Procedures Rendered by Physicians
(Rev. 3578, Issued: 08-05 Effective: 01-01-17, Implementation: 01-03-17)

Diagnostic imaging procedures rendered by a physician that has reassigned their billing rights to a Method II CAH are payable by Medicare when the procedures are eligible and billed on type of bill 85x with revenue code (RC) 096x, 097x and/or 098x.

The MPPR on diagnostic imaging applies when multiple services are furnished by the same physician to the same patient in the same session on the same day. Full payment is made for each service with the highest payment under the MPFS. Effective for dates of services on or after January 1, 2012, payment is made at 75 percent for each subsequent service; and effective for dates of services on or after January 1, 2017, payment is made at 95 percent for each subsequent service.

100-04, 4, 250.18

Incomplete Colonoscopies (Codes 44388, 45378, G0105 and G0121)
(Rev. 4153, Issued: 10-26-18, Effective: 04-01-19, Implementation: 04-01-19)

An incomplete colonoscopy, e.g., the inability to advance the colonoscope to the cecum or colon-small intestine anastomosis due to unforeseen circumstances, is billed and paid using colonoscopy through stoma code 44388, colonoscopy code 45378, and screening colonoscopy codes G0105 and G0121 with modifier "-53." (Code 44388 is valid with modifier 53 beginning January 1, 2016.) The Medicare physician fee schedule database has specific values for codes 44388-53, 45378-53, G0105-53 and G0121-53. An incomplete colonoscopy performed prior to January 1, 2016, is paid at the same rate as a sigmoidoscopy. Beginning January 1, 2016, Medicare will pay for the interrupted colonoscopy at a rate that is calculated using one-half the value of the inputs for the codes.

As such, instruct CAHs that elect Method II payment to use modifier "-53" to identify an incomplete screening colonoscopy (physician professional service(s) billed in revenue code 096X, 097X, and/or 098X).

CAH Method II shall be consistent with the guidelines outlined in PUB. 100-04, chapter 12, section 30.1 and chapter 18, section 60.2.

100-04, 4, 260.1

Special Partial Hospitalization Billing Requirements forHospitals, Community Mental Health Centers, and Critical Access Hospitals
(Rev. 4204, Issued: 01-17-19, Effective: 01-01-19, Implementation: 01-07-19)

Medicare Part B coverage is available for hospital outpatient partial hospitalization services.

A. Billing Requirement
Section 1861 (http://www.socialsecurity.gov/OP_Home/ssact/title18/1800.htm) of the Act defines the services under the partial hospitalization benefit in a hospital.

Section 1866(e)(2) of the Act (http://www.socialsecurity.gov/OP_Home/ssact/title18/1800.htm)recognizes CMHCs as "providers of services" but only for furnishing partial hospitalization services. See §261.1.1 of this chapter for CMHC partial hospitalization bill review directions.

Hospitals and CAHs report condition code 41 in FLs 18-28 (or electronic equivalent) to indicate the claim is for partial hospitalization services. They must also report a revenue code and the charge for each individual covered service furnished. In addition, hospital outpatient departments are required to report HCPCS codes. CAHs are not required to report HCPCS code for this benefit.

Under component billing, hospitals are required to report a revenue code and the charge for each individual covered service furnished under a partial hospitalization program. In addition, hospital outpatient departments are required to report HCPCS codes. Component billing assures that only those partial hospitalization services covered under §1861(ff) of the Act are paid by the Medicare program.

Effective January 1, 2017, non-excepted off-campus provider-based departments of a hospital are required to report a "PN" modifier on each claim line for non-excepted items and services. The use of modifier "PN" will trigger a payment rate under the Medicare Physician Fee Schedule. We expect the PN modifier to be reported with each non-excepted item and service including those for which payment will not be adjusted, such as separately payable drugs, clinical laboratory tests, and therapy services.

Excepted off-campus provider-based departments of a hospital must continue to report existing modifier "PO" (Services, procedures and/or surgeries provided at off-campus provider-based outpatient departments) for all excepted items and services furnished. Use of the off-campus PBD modifier became mandatory beginning January 1, 2016.

All hospitals are required to report condition code 41 in FLs 18-28 to indicate the claim is for partial hospitalization services. Hospitals use bill type 13X and CAHs use bill type 85X. The following special procedures apply.

Bills must contain an acceptable revenue code. They are as follows:

Revenue Code	Description
0250	Drugs and Biologicals
043X	Occupational Therapy
0900	Behavioral Health Treatment/Services
0904	Activity Therapy
0910	Psychiatric/Psychological Services (Dates of Service prior to October 16, 2003)
0914	Individual Therapy
0915	Group Therapy
0916	Family Therapy
0918	Behavioral Health/Testing
0942	Education/Training

Psychiatric diagnostic evaluation (no medical services) completed by a non-physician.

*****The definition of code 90792 is as follows:

Psychiatric diagnostic evaluation (with medical services) completed by a physician.

Codes G0129 and G0176 are used only for partial hospitalization programs.

Code G0177 may be used in both partial hospitalization program and outpatient mental health settings.

Revenue code 250 does not require HCPCS coding. However, Medicare does not cover drugs that can be self-administered.

Edit to assure that HCPCS are present when the above revenue codes are billed and that they are valid HCPCS codes. Do not edit for the matching of revenue code to HCPCS.

B. Professional Services
The professional services listed below when provided in all hospital outpatient departments are separately covered and paid as the professional services of physicians and other practitioners. These professional services are unbundled and these practitioners (other than physician assistants (PA) bill the Medicare A/B MAC (B) directly for the professional services furnished to hospital outpatient partial hospitalization patients. The hospital can also serve as a billing agent for these professionals by billing the A/B MAC (B) on their behalf under their billing number for their professional services. The professional services of a PA can be billed to the A/B MAC (B) only by the PAs employer. The employer of a PA may be such entities or individuals as a physician, medical group, professional corporation, hospital, SNF, or nursing facility. For example, if a physician is the employer of the PA and the PA renders services in the hospital, the physician and not the hospital would be responsible for billing the A/B MAC (B) on Form CMS-1500 for the services of the PA. The following direct professional services are unbundled and not paid as partial hospitalization services.

- Physician services that meet the criteria of 42 CFR 415.102, for payment on a fee schedule basis;
- Physician assistant (PA) services as defined in §1861(s)(2)(K)(i) of the Act;
- Nurse practitioner and clinical nurse specialist services, as defined in §1861(s)(2)(K)(ii) of the Act; and
- Clinical psychologist services as defined in §1861(ii) of the Act.

The services of other practitioners (including clinical social workers and occupational therapists), are bundled when furnished to hospital patients, including partial hospitalization patients. The hospital must bill the contractor for such nonphysician practitioner services as partial hospitalization services. Make payment for the services to the hospital.

C. Outpatient Mental Health Treatment Limitation
The outpatient mental health treatment limitation may apply to services to treat mental, psychoneurotic, and

personality disorders when furnished by physicians, clinical psychologists, NPs, CNSs, and PAs to partial hospitalization patients. However, the outpatient mental health treatment limitation does not apply to such mental health treatment services billed to the A/B MAC (A) by a CMHC or hospital outpatient department as partial hospitalization services.

D. Reporting of Service Units
Hospitals report the number of times the service or procedure, as defined by the HCPCS code, was performed. CAHs report the number of times the revenue code visit was performed.

NOTE: Service units are not required to be reported for drugs and biologicals (Revenue Code 250).

E. Line Item Date of Service Reporting
Hospitals other than CAHs are required to report line item dates of service per revenue code line for partial hospitalization claims. This means each service (revenue code) provided must be repeated on a separate line item along with the specific date the service was provided for every occurrence. Line item dates of service are reported in FL 45 "Service Date" (MMDDYY). See §260.5 for a detailed explanation.

F. Payment
Starting in CY 2017 and subsequent years, the payment structure for partial hospitalization services provided in hospital outpatient departments and CMHCs has been reduced from four APCs (two for CMHCs and two for hospital-based PHPs) to a single APC by provider type. Effective January 2, 2017, we are replacing existing CMHC APCs 5851 (Level 1 Partial Hospitalization (3 services)) and 5852 (Level 2 Partial Hospitalization (4 or more services)) with a new CMHC APC 5853 (Partial Hospitalization (3 or More Services Per Day)), and replacing existing hospital-based PHP APCs 5861 (Level 1 Partial Hospitalization (3 services)) and 5862 (Level 2 Partial Hospitalization (4 or more services)) with a new hospital-based PHP APC 5863 (Partial Hospitalization (3 or More Services Per Day)). The following chart displays the CMHC and hospital-based PHPAPCs:

Hospital-Based and Community Mental Health Center PHP APCs CY 2017 APC	Group Title
5853	Partial Hospitalization (3 or more services per day) for CMHCs
5863	Partial Hospitalization (3 or more services per day) for hospital-based PHPs

Apply Part B deductible, if any, and coinsurance.

G. Data for CWF and PS&R
Include revenue codes, HCPCS/CPT codes, units, and covered charges in the financial data section (fields 65a - 65j), as appropriate. Report the billed charges in field 65h, "Charges," of the CWF record.

Include in the financial data portion of the PS&R UNIBILL, revenue codes, HCPCS/CPT codes, units, and charges, as appropriate.

Future updates will be issued in a Recurring Update Notification.

100-04, 4, 260.1.1

Bill Review for Partial Hospitalization Services Provided in Community Mental Health Centers (CMHC)
(Rev. 4204, Issued: 01-17-19, Effective: 01-01-19, Implementation: 01-07-19)

A. General
Medicare Part B coverage for partial hospitalization services provided by CMHCs is available effective for services provided on or after October 1, 1991.

B. Special Requirements
Section 1866(e)(2) (http://www.socialsecurity.gov/OP_Home/ssact/title18/1800.htm) of the Act recognizes CMHCs as "providers of services" but only for furnishing partial hospitalization services. Applicable provider ranges are 1400-1499, 4600-4799, and 4900-4999.

C. Billing Requirements
The CMHCs bill for partial hospitalization services under bill type 76X. The A/B MACs (A) follow bill review instructions in chapter 25 of this manual, except for those listed below.

The acceptable revenue codes are as follows:

Revenue Code	Description
0250	Drugs and Biologicals
043X	Occupational Therapy
0900	Behavioral Health Treatments/Services
0904	Activity Therapy
0910	Psychiatric/Psychological Services (Dates of Service prior to October 16, 2003)
0914	Individual Therapy
0915	Group Therapy
0916	Family Therapy
0918	Behavioral Health/Testing
0942	Education/Training

The A/B MAC(s) (A) edit to assure that HCPCS are present when the above revenue codes are billed and that they are valid HCPCS codes. They do not edit for the matching of revenue codes to HCPCS.

Definitions each of the asterisked HCPCS codes follows:

*The definition of code G0129 is as follows:

Occupational therapy services requiring the skills of a qualified occupational therapist, furnished as a component of a partial hospitalization treatment program, per session (45 minutes or more).

**The definition of code G0176 is as follows:

Activity therapy, such as music, dance, art or play therapies not for recreation, related to the care and treatment of patient's disabling mental health problems, per session (45 minutes or more).

***The definition of code G0177 is as follows:

Training and educational services related to the care and treatment of patient's disabling mental health problems, per session (45 minutes or more).

****The definition of code 90791 is as follows:

Psychiatric diagnostic evaluation (no medical services) completed by a non-physician.

*****The definition of code 90792 is as follows:

Psychiatric diagnostic evaluation (with medical services) completed by a physician.

Codes G0129 and G0176 are used only for partial hospitalization programs.

Code G0177 may be used in both partial hospitalization program and outpatient mental health settings.

Revenue code 0250 does not require HCPCS coding. However, drugs that can be self-administered are not covered by Medicare.

HCPCS includes CPT-4 codes. See the ASC X12 837 institutional claim guide for how to report HCPCS electronically. CMHCs report HCPCS codes on Form CMS-1450 in FL44, "HCPCS/Rates." HCPCS code reporting is effective for claims with dates of service on or after April 1, 2000.

The A/B MACs (A) are to advise their CMHCs of these requirements. CMHCs should complete the remaining items on the claim in accordance with the ASC X12 837 Institutional Claim implementation guide and the Form CMS-1450 instructions in Chapter 25 of this manual.

The professional services listed below are separately covered and are paid as the professional services of physicians and other practitioners. These professional services are unbundled and these practitioners (other than physician assistants (PAs)) bill the A/B MAC (B) directly for the professional services furnished to CMHC partial hospitalization patients. The ASC X12 837 professional claim format or the paper form 1500 is used. The CMHC can also serve as a billing agent for these professionals by billing the A/B MAC (B) on their behalf for their professional services. The professional services of a PA can be billed to the A/B MAC (B) only by the PAs employer. The employer of a PA may be such entities or individuals as a physician, medical group, professional corporation, hospital, SNF, or nursing facility. For example, if a physician is the employer of the PA and the PA renders services in the CMHC, the physician and not the CMHC would be responsible for billing the A/B MAC (B) for the services of the PA.

The following professional services are unbundled and not paid as partial hospitalization services:

- Physician services that meet the criteria of 42 CFR 415.102, for payment on a fee schedule basis;

- PA services, as defined in §1861(s)(2)(K)(i) (http://www.socialsecurity.gov/OP_Home/ssact/title18/1800.htm) of the Act;

- Nurse practitioner and clinical nurse specialist services, as defined in §1861(s)(2)(K)(ii) (http://www.socialsecurity.gov/OP_Home/ssact/title18/1800.htm) of the Act; and,

- Clinical psychologist services, as defined in §1861(ii) (http://www.socialsecurity.gov/OP_Home/ssact/title18/1800.htm) of the Act.

The services of other practitioners (including clinical social workers and occupational therapists) are bundled when furnished to CMHC patients. The CMHC must bill the A/B MAC (A) for such nonphysician practitioner services as partial hospitalization services. The A/B MAC (A) makes payment for the services to the CMHC.

D. Outpatient Mental Health Treatment Limitation

The outpatient mental health treatment limitation may apply to services to treat mental, psychoneurotic, and personality disorders when furnished by physicians, clinical psychologists, NPs, CNSs, and PAs to partial hospitalization patients. However, the outpatient mental health treatment limitation does not apply to such mental health treatment services billed to the A/B MAC (A) as partial hospitalization services.

E. Reporting of Service Units

Visits should no longer be reported as units. Instead, CMHCs report in the field, "Service Units," the number of times the service or procedure, as defined by the HCPCS code, was performed when billing for partial hospitalization services identified by revenue code in subsection C.

EXAMPLE: A beneficiary received psychological testing performed by a physician for a total of 3 hours during one day (HCPCS code 96130, first hour; HCPCS code 96131 for 2 additional hours). The CMHC reports revenue code 0918, HCPCS code 96130, and 1 unit; and a second line on the claim showing revenue code 918, HCPCS code 96131, and 2 units.

When reporting service units for HCPCS codes where the definition of the procedure does not include any reference to time (either minutes, hours or days), CMHCs should not bill for sessions of less than 45 minutes.

The CMHC need not report service units for drugs and biologicals (Revenue Code 0250)

NOTE: Information regarding the Form CMS-1450 form locators that correspond with these fields is found in Chapter 25 of this manual. See the ASC X12 837 Institutional Claim implementation guide for related guidelines for the electronic claim.

F. Line Item Date of Service Reporting

Dates of service per revenue code line for partial hospitalization claims that span two or more dates. This means each service (revenue code) provided must be repeated on a separate line item along with the specific date the service was provided for every

occurrence. Line item dates of service are reported in "Service Date". See examples below of reporting line item dates of service. These examples are for group therapy services provided twice during a billing period.

For claims, report as follows:

Revenue Code	HCPCS	Dates of Service	Units	Total Charges
0915	G0176	20090505	1	$80
0915	G0176	20090529	2	$160

NOTE: Information regarding the Form CMS-1450 form locators that correspond with these fields is found in Chapter 25 of this manual. See the ASC X12 837 Institutional Claim Implementation Guide for related guidelines for the electronic claim.

The A/B MACs (A) return to provider claims that span two or more dates if a line item date of service is not entered for each HCPCS code reported or if the line item dates of service reported are outside of the statement covers period. Line item date of service reporting is effective for claims with dates of service on or after June 5, 2000.

G. Payment

Section 1833(a)(2)(B) (http://www.socialsecurity.gov/OP_Home/ssact/title18/1800.htm) of the Act provides the statutory authority governing payment for partial hospitalization services provided by a CMHC. A/B MAC(s) (A) made payment on a reasonable cost basis until OPPS was implemented. The Part B deductible and coinsurance applied.

Payment principles applicable to partial hospitalization services furnished in CMHCs are contained in §2400 of the Medicare Provider Reimbursement Manual.

The A/B MACs (A) make payment on a per diem basis under the hospital outpatient prospective payment system for partial hospitalization services. CMHCs must continue to maintain documentation to support medical necessity of each service provided, including the beginning and ending time.

Effective January 1, 2011, there were four separate APC payment rates for PHP: two for CMHCs (for Level I and Level II services based on only CMHC data) and two for hospital-based PHPs (for Level I and Level II services based on only hospital-based PHP data).

The two CMHC APCS for providing partial hospitalization services were: APC 5851 (Level 1 Partial Hospitalization (3 services)) and APC 5852 (Level 2 Partial Hospitalization (4 or more services)). Effective January 1, 2017, we are combining APCs 5851 and 5852 into one new APC 5853 (Partial Hospitalization (3 or more services) for CMHCs).

Community Mental Health Center PHP APC APC	Group Title
5853	Partial Hospitalization (3 or more services per day) for CMHCs

NOTE: Occupational therapy services provided to partial hospitalization patients are not subject to the prospective payment system for outpatient rehabilitation services, and therefore the financial limitation required under §4541 of the Balanced Budget Act (BBA) does not apply.

H. Medical Review

The A/B MACs (A) follow medical review guidelines in Pub. 100-08, Medicare Program Integrity Manual.

I. Coordination with CWF

See chapter 27 of this manual. All edits for bill type 74X apply, except provider number ranges 4600-4799 are acceptable only for services provided on or after October 1, 1991.

100-04, 4, 290.5.3

Billing and Payment for Observation Services Furnished Beginning January 1, 2016

(Rev. 3425, Issued: 12-18-15, Effective: 01-01-16, Implementation: 01-04-16)

Observation services are reported using HCPCS code G0378 (Hospital observation service, per hour). Beginning January 1, 2008, HCPCS code G0378 for hourly observation services is assigned status indicator N, signifying that its payment is always packaged. No separate payment is made for observation services reported with HCPCS code G0378, and APC 0339 is deleted as of January 1, 2008. In most circumstances, observation services are supportive and ancillary to the other services provided to a patient. Beginning January 1, 2016, in certain circumstances when observation services are billed in conjunction with a clinic visit, Type A emergency department visit (Level 1 through 5), Type B emergency department visit (Level 1 through 5), critical care services, or a direct referral as an integral part of a patient's extended encounter of care, comprehensive payment may be made for all services on the claim including, the entire extended care encounter through comprehensive APC 8011 (Comprehensive Observation Services) when certain criteria are met. For information about comprehensive APCs, see §10.2.3 (Comprehensive APCs) of this chapter.

There is no limitation on diagnosis for payment of APC 8011; however, comprehensive APC payment will not be made when observation services are reported in association with a surgical procedure (T status procedure) or the hours of observation care reported are less than 8. The I/OCE evaluates every claim received to determine if payment through a comprehensive APC is appropriate. If payment through a comprehensive APC is inappropriate, the I/OCE, in conjunction with the Pricer, determines the appropriate status indicator, APC, and payment for every code on a claim.

All of the following requirements must be met in order for a hospital to receive a comprehensive APC payment through the Comprehensive Observation Services APC (APC 8011):

1. Observation Time

    a. Observation time must be documented in the medical record.

    b. Hospital billing for observation services begins at the clock time documented in the patient's medical record, which coincides with the time that observation services are initiated in accordance with a physician's order for observation services.

    c. A beneficiary's time receiving observation services (and hospital billing) ends when all clinical or medical interventions have been completed, including follow-up care furnished by hospital staff and physicians that may take place after a physician has ordered the patient be released or admitted as an inpatient.

    d. The number of units reported with HCPCS code G0378 must equal or exceed 8 hours.

2. Additional Hospital Services

    a. The claim for observation services must include one of the following services in addition to the reported observation services. The additional services listed below must have a line item date of service on the same day or the day before the date reported for observation:

        • A Type A or B emergency department visit (CPT codes 99281 through 99285 or HCPCS codes G0380 through G0384); or

        • A clinic visit (HCPCS code G0463); or

        • Critical care (CPT code 99291); or

        • Direct referral for observation care reported with HCPCS code G0379 (APC 5013) must be reported on the same date of service as the date reported for observation services.

    b. No procedure with a T status indicator or a J1 status indicator can be reported on the claim.

3. Physician Evaluation

    a. The beneficiary must be in the care of a physician during the period of observation, as documented in the medical record by outpatient registration, discharge, and other appropriate progress notes that are timed, written, and signed by the physician.

    b. The medical record must include documentation that the physician explicitly assessed patient risk to determine that the beneficiary would benefit from observation care.

Criteria 1 and 3 related to observation care beginning and ending time and physician evaluation apply regardless of whether the hospital believes that the criteria will be met for payment of the extended encounter through the Comprehensive Observation Services APC (APC 8011).

Only visits, critical care and observation services that are billed on a 13X bill type may be considered for a comprehensive APC payment through the Comprehensive Observation Services APC (APC 8011).

Non-repetitive services provided on the same day as either direct referral for observation care or observation services must be reported on the same claim because the OCE claim-by-claim logic cannot function properly unless all services related to the episode of observation care, including hospital clinic visits, emergency department visits, critical care services, and T status procedures, are reported on the same claim. Additional guidance can be found in chapter 1, section 50.2.2 of this manual.

If a claim for services provided during an extended assessment and management encounter including observation care does not meet all of the requirements listed above, then the usual APC logic will apply to separately payable items and services on the claim; the special logic for direct admission will apply, and payment for the observation care will be packaged into payments for other separately payable services provided to the beneficiary in the same encounter.

100-04, 5, 10

Part B Outpatient Rehabilitation and Comprehensive Outpatient Rehabilitation Facility (CORF) Services - General

(Rev. 3454, Issued: 02-04-16, Effective: 07-01-16, Implementation: 07-05-16)

Language in this section is defined or described in Pub. 100-02, chapter 15, sections 220 and 230.

Section §1834(k)(5) to the Social Security Act (the Act), requires that all claims for outpatient rehabilitation services and comprehensive outpatient rehabilitation facility (CORF) services, be reported using a uniform coding system. The CMS chose HCPCS (Healthcare Common Procedure Coding System) as the coding system to be used for the reporting of these services. This coding requirement is effective for all claims for outpatient rehabilitation services and CORF services submitted on or after April 1, 1998.

The Act also requires payment under a prospective payment system for outpatient rehabilitation services including CORF services. Effective for claims with dates of service on or after January 1, 1999, the Medicare Physician Fee Schedule (MPFS) became the method of payment for outpatient therapy services furnished by:

    • Comprehensive outpatient rehabilitation facilities (CORFs);

    • Outpatient physical therapy providers (OPTs), also known as rehabilitation agencies;

    • Hospitals (to outpatients and inpatients who are not in a covered Part A stay);

    • Skilled nursing facilities (SNFs) (to residents not in a covered Part A stay and to nonresidents who receive outpatient rehabilitation services from the SNF); and

    • Home health agencies (HHAs) (to individuals who are not homebound or otherwise are not receiving services under a home health plan of care (POC)).

NOTE: No provider or supplier other than the SNF will be paid for therapy services during the time the beneficiary is in a covered SNF Part A stay. For information regarding SNF consolidated billing see chapter 6, section 10 of this manual.

Similarly, under the HH prospective payment system, HHAs are responsible to provide, either directly or under arrangements, all outpatient rehabilitation therapy services to beneficiaries receiving services under a home health POC. No other provider or supplier will be paid for these services during the time the beneficiary is in a covered Part A stay. For information regarding HH consolidated billing see chapter 10, section 20 of this manual.

Section 143 of the Medicare Improvements for Patients and Provider's Act of 2008 (MIPPA) authorizes the Centers for Medicare & Medicaid Services (CMS) to enroll speech-language pathologists (SLP) as suppliers of Medicare services and for SLPs to begin billing Medicare for outpatient speech-language pathology services furnished in private practice beginning July 1, 2009. Enrollment will allow SLPs in private practice to bill Medicare and receive direct payment for their services. Previously, the Medicare program could only pay SLP services if an institution, physician or nonphysician practitioner billed them.

In Chapter 23, as part of the CY 2009 Medicare Physician Fee Schedule Database, the descriptor for PC/TC indicator "7", as applied to certain HCPCS/CPT codes, is described as specific to the services of privately practicing therapists. Payment may not be made if the service is provided to either a hospital outpatient or a hospital inpatient by a physical therapist, occupational therapist, or speech-language pathologist in private practice.

The MPFS is used as a method of payment for outpatient rehabilitation services furnished under arrangement with any of these providers.

In addition, the MPFS is used as the payment system for CORF services identified by the HCPCS codes in §20. Assignment is mandatory.

Services that are paid subject to the MPFS are adjusted based on the applicable payment locality. Rehabilitation agencies and CORFs with service locations in different payment localities shall follow the instructions for multiple service locations in chapter 1, section 170.1.1.

The Medicare allowed charge for the services is the lower of the actual charge or the MPFS amount. The Medicare payment for the services is 80 percent of the allowed charge after the Part B deductible is met. Coinsurance is made at 20 percent of the lower of the actual charge or the MPFS amount. The general coinsurance rule (20 percent of the actual charges) does not apply when making payment under the MPFS. This is a final payment.

The MPFS does not apply to outpatient rehabilitation services furnished by critical access hospitals (CAHs) or hospitals in Maryland. CAHs are to be paid on a reasonable cost basis. Maryland hospitals are paid under the Maryland All-Payer Model.

Contractors process outpatient rehabilitation claims from hospitals, including CAHs, SNFs, HHAs, CORFs, outpatient rehabilitation agencies, and outpatient physical therapy providers for which they have received a tie in notice from the Regional Office (RO). These provider types submit their claims to the contractors using the ASC X12 837 institutional claim format or the CMS-1450 paper form when permissible. Contractors also process claims from physicians, certain nonphysician practitioners (NPPs), therapists in private practices (TPPs), (which are limited to physical and occupational therapists, and speech-language pathologists in private practices), and physician-directed clinics that bill for services furnished incident to a physician's service (see Pub. 100-02, Medicare Benefit Policy Manual, chapter 15, for a definition of "incident to"). These provider types submit their claims to the contractor using the ASC X 12 837 professional claim format or the CMS-1500 paper form when permissible.

There are different fee rates for nonfacility and facility services. Chapter 23 describes the differences in these two rates. (See fields 28 and 29 of the record therein described). Facility rates apply to professional services performed in a facility other than the professional's office. Nonfacility rates apply when the service is performed in the professional's office. The nonfacility rate (that is paid when the provider performs the services in its own facility) accommodates overhead and indirect expenses the provider incurs by operating its own facility. Thus it is somewhat higher than the facility rate.

Contractors pay the nonfacility rate on institutional claims for services performed in the provider's facility. Contractors may pay professional claims using the facility or nonfacility rate depending upon where the service is performed (place of service on the claim), and the provider specialty.

Contractors pay the codes in §20 under the MPFS on professional claims regardless of whether they may be considered rehabilitation services. However, contractors must use this list for institutional claims to determine whether to pay under outpatient rehabilitation rules or whether payment rules for other types of service may apply, e.g., OPPS for hospitals, reasonable costs for CAHs.

Note that because a service is considered an outpatient rehabilitation service does not automatically imply payment for that service. Additional criteria, including coverage, plan of care and physician certification must also be met. These criteria are described in Pub. 100-02, Medicare Benefit Policy Manual, chapters 1 and 15.

Payment for rehabilitation services provided to Part A inpatients of hospitals or SNFs is included in the respective PPS rate. Also, for SNFs (but not hospitals), if the beneficiary has Part B, but not Part A coverage (e.g., Part A benefits are exhausted), the SNF must bill for any rehabilitation service.

Payment for rehabilitation therapy services provided by home health agencies under a home health plan of care is included in the home health PPS rate. HHAs may submit bill type 34X and be paid under the MPFS if there are no home health services billed under a home health plan of care at the same time, and there is a valid rehabilitation POC (e.g., the patient is not homebound).

An institutional employer (other than a SNF) of the TPPs, or physician performing outpatient services, (e.g., hospital, CORF, etc.), or a clinic billing on behalf of the physician or therapist may bill the contractor on a professional claim.

The MPFS is the basis of payment for outpatient rehabilitation services furnished by TPPs, physicians, and certain nonphysician practitioners or for diagnostic tests provided incident to the services of such physicians or nonphysician practitioners. (See Pub. 100-02, Medicare Benefit Policy Manual, Chapter 15, for a definition of "incident to, therapist, therapy and related instructions.") Such services are billed to the contractor on the professional claim format. Assignment is mandatory.

The following table identifies the provider and supplier types, and identifies which claim format they may use to submit claims for outpatient therapy services to the contractor.

"Provider/Supplier Service" Type	Format	Bill Type	Comment
Inpatient SNF Part A	Institutional	21X	Included in PPS
Inpatient hospital Part B	Institutional	12X	Hospital may obtain services under arrangements and bill, or rendering provider may bill.
Inpatient SNF Part B (audiology tests are not included)	Institutional	22X	SNF must provide and bill, or obtain under arrangements and bill.
Outpatient hospital	Institutional	13X	Hospital may provide and bill or obtain under arrangements and bill.
Outpatient SNF	Institutional	23X	SNF must provide and bill or obtain under arrangements and bill.
HHA billing for services not rendered under a Part A or Part B home health plan of care, but rendered under a therapy plan of care.	Institutional	34X	Service not under home health plan of care.
Outpatient physical therapy providers (OPTs), also known as rehabilitation agencies	Institutional	74X	Paid MPFS for outpatient rehabilitation services.
Comprehensive Outpatient Rehabilitation Facility (CORF)	Institutional	75X	Paid MPFS for outpatient rehabilitation services and all other services except drugs. Drugs are paid 95% of the AWP.
Physician, NPPs, TPPs, (therapy services in hospital or SNF)	Professional	See Chapter 26 for place of service coding.	Payment may not be made for therapy services to Part A inpatients of hospitals or SNFs, or for Part B SNF residents. **NOTE:** Payment may be made to physicians and NPPs for their professional services defined as "sometimes therapy" (not part of a therapy plan) in certain situations; for example, when furnished to a beneficiary registered as an outpatient of a hospital.

"Provider/Supplier Service" Type	Format	Bill Type	Comment
Physician/NPP/TPPs office, or patient's home	Professional	See Chapter 26 for place of service coding.	Paid via MPFS.
Critical Access Hospital - inpatient Part B	Institutional	12X	Rehabilitation services are paid at cost.
Critical Access Hospital – outpatient Part B	Institutional	85X	Rehabilitation services are paid at cost.

For a list of the outpatient rehabilitation HCPCS codes see §20.

If a contractor receives an institutional claim for one of these HCPCS codes with dates of service on or after July 1, 2003, that does not appear on the supplemental file it currently uses to pay the therapy claims, it contacts its professional claims area to obtain the non-facility price in order to pay the claim.

NOTE: The list of codes in §20 contains commonly utilized codes for outpatient rehabilitation services. Contractors may consider other codes on institutional claims for payment under the MPFS as outpatient rehabilitation services to the extent that such codes are determined to be medically reasonable and necessary and could be performed within the scope of practice of the therapist providing the service.

100-04, 5, 10.2

The Financial Limitation Legislation

(Rev. 2073, Issued:10-22-10, Effective: 01-01-11, Implementation: 01-03-11)

A. Legislation on Limitations

The dollar amount of the limitations (caps) on outpatient therapy services is established by statute. The updated amount of the caps is released annually via Recurring Update Notifications and posted on the CMS Website www.cms.gov/TherapyServices, on contractor Websites, and on each beneficiary's Medicare Summary Notice. Medicare contractors shall publish the financial limitation amount in educational articles. It is also available at 1-800-Medicare.

Section 4541(a)(2) of the Balanced Budget Act (BBA) (P.L. 105-33) of 1997, which added §1834(k)(5) to the Act, required payment under a prospective payment system (PPS) for outpatient rehabilitation services (except those furnished by or under arrangements with a hospital). Outpatient rehabilitation services include the following services:

- Physical therapy

- Speech-language pathology; and

- Occupational therapy.

Section 4541(c) of the BBA required application of financial limitations to all outpatient rehabilitation services (except those furnished by or under arrangements with a hospital).

In 1999, an annual per beneficiary limit of $1,500 was applied, including all outpatient physical therapy services and speech-language pathology services. A separate limit applied to all occupational therapy services. The limits were based on incurred expenses and included applicable deductible and coinsurance. The BBA provided that the limits be indexed by the Medicare Economic Index (MEI) each year beginning in 2002.

Since the limitations apply to outpatient services, they do not apply to skilled nursing facility (SNF) residents in a covered Part A stay, including patients occupying swing beds. Rehabilitation services are included within the global Part A per diem payment that the SNF receives under the prospective payment system (PPS) for the covered stay. Also, limitations do not apply to any therapy services covered under prospective payment systems for home health or inpatient hospitals, including critical access hospitals.

The limitation is based on therapy services the Medicare beneficiary receives, not the type of practitioner who provides the service. Physical therapists, speech-language pathologists, and occupational therapists, as well as physicians and certain nonphysician practitioners, could render a therapy service.

B. Moratoria and Exceptions for Therapy Claims

Since the creation of therapy caps, Congress has enacted several moratoria. The Deficit Reduction Act of 2005 directed CMS to develop exceptions to therapy caps for calendar year 2006 and the exceptions have been extended periodically. The cap exception for therapy services billed by outpatient hospitals was part of the original legislation and applies as long as caps are in effect. Exceptions to caps based on the medical necessity of the service are in effect only when Congress legislates the exceptions.

C. Repeal of Original Legislation and Replacement with Thresholds to Ensure Appropriate Therapy.

Section 50202 of the Bipartisan Budget Act of 2018 repeals application of the Medicare outpatient therapy caps but retains the former cap amounts as a threshold of incurred expenses above which claims must include a modifier as a confirmation that services are medically necessary as justified by appropriate documentation in the medical record. This is termed the KX modifier threshold.

Along with this KX modifier threshold, the new law retains the targeted medical review process but at a lower threshold amount of $3,000. For more information about the medical review (MR) threshold see the below section 10.3.4.

100-04, 5, 10.3.2

Exceptions Process

(Rev. 3670, Issued: 12-01-16, Effective: 01-01-17, Implementation: 01-03-17)

An exception may be made when the patient's condition is justified by documentation indicating that the beneficiary requires continued skilled therapy, i.e., therapy beyond the amount payable under the therapy cap, to achieve their prior functional status or maximum expected functional status within a reasonable amount of time.

No special documentation is submitted to the contractor for exceptions. The clinician is responsible for consulting guidance in the Medicare manuals and in the professional literature to determine if the beneficiary may qualify for the exception because documentation justifies medically necessary services above the caps. The clinician's opinion is not binding on the Medicare contractor who makes the final determination concerning whether the claim is payable.

Documentation justifying the services shall be submitted in response to any Additional Documentation Request (ADR) for claims that are selected for medical review. Follow the documentation requirements in Pub. 100-02, chapter 15, section 220.3. If medical records are requested for review, clinicians may include, at their discretion, a summary that specifically addresses the justification for therapy cap exception.

In making a decision about whether to utilize the exception, clinicians shall consider, for example, whether services are appropriate to--

The patient's condition, including the diagnosis, complexities, and severity;

The services provided, including their type, frequency, and duration;

The interaction of current active conditions and complexities that directly and significantly influence the treatment such that it causes services to exceed caps.

In addition, the following should be considered before using the exception process:

1. Exceptions for Evaluation Services

Evaluation. The CMS will accept therapy evaluations from caps after the therapy caps are reached when evaluation is necessary, e.g., to determine if the current status of the beneficiary requires therapy services. For example, the following CPT codes for evaluation procedures may be appropriate:

> 92521, 92522, 92523, 92524, 92597, 92607, 92608, 92610, 92611, 92612, 92614, 92616, 96105, 96125. 97161, 97162, 97163, 97164, 97165, 97166, 97167, and 97168.

These codes will continue to be reported as outpatient therapy procedures as listed in the Annual Therapy Update for the current year at: http://www.cms.gov/TherapyServices/05_Annual_Therapy_Update.asp#TopOfPage.

They are not diagnostic tests. Definitions of evaluations and documentation are found in Pub. 100-02, chapter 15, sections 220 and 230.

Other Services. There are a number of sources that suggest the amount of certain services that may be typical, either per service, per episode, per condition, or per discipline. For example, see the CSC - Therapy Cap Report, 3/21/2008, and CSC – Therapy Edits Tables 4/14/2008 at www.cms.hhs.gov/TherapyServices (Studies and Reports), or more recent utilization reports. Professional literature and guidelines from professional associations also provide a basis on which to estimate whether the type, frequency, and intensity of services are appropriate to an individual. Clinicians and contractors should utilize available evidence related to the patient's condition to justify provision of medically necessary services to individual beneficiaries, especially when they exceed caps. Contractors shall not limit medically necessary services that are justified by scientific research applicable to the beneficiary. Neither contractors nor clinicians shall utilize professional literature and scientific reports to justify payment for continued services after an individual's goals have been met earlier than is typical. Conversely, professional literature and scientific reports shall not be used as justification to deny payment to patients whose needs are greater than is typical or when the patient's condition is not represented by the literature.

2. Exceptions for Medically Necessary Services

Clinicians may utilize the process for exception for any diagnosis or condition for which they can justify services exceeding the cap. Regardless of the diagnosis or condition, the patient must also meet other requirements for coverage.

Bill the most relevant diagnosis. As always, when billing for therapy services, the diagnosis code that best relates to the reason for the treatment shall be on the claim, unless there is a compelling reason to report another diagnosis code. For example, when a patient with diabetes is being treated with therapy for gait training due to amputation, the preferred diagnosis is abnormality of gait (which characterizes the treatment). Where it is possible in accordance with State and local laws and the contractors' local coverage determinations, avoid using vague or general diagnoses. When a claim includes several types of services, or where the physician/NPP must supply the diagnosis, it may not be possible to use the most relevant therapy diagnosis code in the primary position. In that case, the relevant diagnosis code should, if possible, be on the claim in another position.

Codes representing the medical condition that caused the treatment are used when there is no code representing the treatment. Complicating conditions are preferably used in non-primary positions on the claim and are billed in the primary position only in the rare circumstance that there is no more relevant code.

The condition or complexity that caused treatment to exceed caps must be related to the therapy goals and must either be the condition that is being treated or a complexity that directly **and significantly impacts the rate of recovery of the condition being treated** such that it is appropriate to exceed the caps. Documentation for an exception should indicate how the complexity (or combination of complexities) directly and significantly affects treatment for a therapy condition.

If the contractor has determined that certain codes do not characterize patients who require medically necessary services, providers/suppliers may not use those codes, but must utilize a billable diagnosis code allowed by their contractor to describe the patient's condition. Contractors shall not apply therapy caps to services based on the patient's condition, but only on the medical necessity of the service for the condition. If a service would be payable before the cap is reached and is still medically necessary after the cap is reached, that service is excepted.

Contact your contractor for interpretation if you are not sure that a service is applicable for exception.

It is very important to recognize that most conditions would not ordinarily result in services exceeding the cap. Use the KX modifier only in cases where the condition of the individual patient is such that services are APPROPRIATELY provided in an episode that exceeds the cap. Routine use of the KX modifier for all patients with these conditions will likely show up on data analysis as aberrant and invite inquiry. Be sure that documentation is sufficiently detailed to support the use of the modifier.

In justifying exceptions for therapy caps, clinicians and contractors should not only consider the medical diagnoses and medical complications that might directly and significantly influence the amount of treatment required. Other variables (such as the availability of a caregiver at home) that affect appropriate treatment shall also be considered. Factors that influence the need for treatment should be supportable by published research, clinical guidelines from professional sources, and/or clinical or common sense. See Pub. 100-02, chapter 15, section 220.3 for information related to documentation of the evaluation, and section 220.2 on medical necessity for some factors that complicate treatment.

NOTE: The patient's lack of access to outpatient hospital therapy services alone, when outpatient hospital therapy services are excluded from the limitation, does not justify excepted services. Residents of skilled nursing facilities prevented by consolidated billing from accessing hospital services, debilitated patients for whom transportation to the hospital is a physical hardship, or lack of therapy services at hospitals in the beneficiary's county may or may not qualify as justification for continued services above the caps. The patient's condition and complexities might justify extended services, but their location does not. For dates of service on or after October 1, 2012, therapy services furnished in an outpatient hospital are not excluded from the limitation.

100-04, 5, 10.6

Functional Reporting

(Rev. 3670, Issued: 12-01-16, Effective: 01-01-17, Implementation: 01-03-17)

A. General

Section 3005(g) of the Middle Class Tax Relief and Jobs Creation Act (MCTRJCA) amended Section 1833(g) of the Act to require a claims-based data collection system for outpatient therapy services, including physical therapy (PT), occupational therapy (OT) and speech-language pathology (SLP) services. 42 CFR 410.59, 410.60, 410.61, 410.62 and 410.105 implement this requirement. The system will collect data on beneficiary function during the course of therapy services in order to better understand beneficiary conditions, outcomes, and expenditures.

Beneficiary unction information is reported using 42 nonpayable functional G-codes and seven severity/complexity modifiers on claims for PT, OT, and SLP services. Functional reporting on one functional limitation at a time is required periodically throughout an entire PT, OT, or SLP therapy episode of care.

The nonpayable G-codes and severity modifiers provide information about the beneficiary's functional status at the outset of the therapy episode of care, including projected goal status, at specified points during treatment, and at the time of discharge. These G-codes, along with the associated modifiers, are required at specified intervals on all claims for outpatient therapy services – not just those over the cap.

B. Application of New Coding Requirements

This functional data reporting and collection system is effective for therapy services with dates of service on and after January 1, 2013. A testing period will be in effect from January 1, 2013, until July 1, 2013, to allow providers and practitioners to use the new coding requirements to assure that systems work. Claims for therapy services furnished on and after July 1, 2013, that do not contain the required functional G-code/modifier information will be returned or rejected, as applicable.

C. Services Affected

These requirements apply to all claims for services furnished under the Medicare Part B outpatient therapy benefit and the PT, OT, and SLP services furnished under the CORF benefit. They also apply to the therapy services furnished personally by and incident to the service of a physician or a nonphysician practitioner (NPP), including a nurse practitioner (NP), a certified nurse specialist (CNS), or a physician assistant (PA), as applicable.

D. Providers and Practitioners Affected.

The functional reporting requirements apply to the therapy services furnished by the following providers: hospitals, CAHs, SNFs, CORFs, rehabilitation agencies, and HHAs (when the beneficiary is not under a home health plan of care). It applies to the following practitioners: physical therapists, occupational therapists, and speech-language pathologists in private practice (TPPs), physicians, and NPPs as noted above. The term "clinician" is applied to these practitioners throughout this manual section. (See definition section of Pub. 100-02, chapter 15, section 220.)

E. Function-related G-codes

There are 42 functional G-codes, 14 sets of three codes each. Six of the G-code sets are generally for PT and OT functional limitations and eight sets of G-codes are for SLP functional limitations.

The following G-codes are for functional limitations typically seen in beneficiaries receiving PT or OT services. The first four of these sets describe categories of functional limitations and the final two sets describe "other" functional limitations, which are to be used for functional limitations not described by one of the four categories.

NONPAYABLE G-CODES FOR FUNCTIONAL LIMITATIONS

	Long Descriptor	Short Descriptor
Mobility G-code Set		
G8978	Mobility: walking & moving around functional limitation, current status, at therapy episode outset and at reporting intervals	Mobility current status
G8979	Mobility: walking & moving around functional limitation, projected goal status, at therapy episode outset, at reporting intervals, and at discharge or to end reporting	Mobility goal status
G8980	Mobility: walking & moving around functional limitation, discharge status, at discharge from therapy or to end reporting	Mobility D/C status
Changing & Maintaining Body Position G-code Set		
G8981	Changing & maintaining body position functional limitation, current status, at therapy episode outset and at reporting intervals	Body pos current status
G8982	Changing & maintaining body position functional limitation, projected goal status, at therapy episode outset, at reporting intervals, and at discharge or to end reporting	Body pos goal status
G8983	Changing & maintaining body position functional limitation, discharge status, at discharge from therapy or to end reporting	Body pos D/C status
Carrying, Moving & Handling Objects G-code Set		
G8984	Carrying, moving & handling objects functional limitation, current status, at therapy episode outset and at reporting intervals	Carry current status
G8985	Carrying, moving & handling objects functional limitation, projected goal status, at therapy episode outset, at reporting intervals, and at discharge or to end reporting	Carry goal status
G8986	Carrying, moving & handling objects functional limitation, discharge status, at discharge from therapy or to end reporting	Carry D/C status
Self Care G-code Set		
G8987	Self care functional limitation, current status, at therapy episode outset and at reporting intervals	Self care current status
G8988	Self care functional limitation, projected goal status, at therapy episode outset, at reporting intervals, and at discharge or to end reporting	Self care goal status
G8989	Self care functional limitation, discharge status, at discharge from therapy or to end reporting	Self care D/C status

- The following "other PT/OT" functional G-codes are used to report:
- a beneficiary's functional limitation that is not defined by one of the above four categories;
- a beneficiary whose therapy services are not intended to treat a functional limitation;
- or a beneficiary's functional limitation when an overall, composite or other score from a functional assessment too is used and it does not clearly represent a functional limitation defined by one of the above four code sets.

	Long Descriptor	Short Descriptor
Other PT/OT Primary G-code Set		
G8990	Other physical or occupational therapy primary functional limitation, current status, at therapy episode outset and at reporting intervals	Other PT/OT current status

	Long Descriptor	Short Descriptor
G8991	Other physical or occupational therapy primary functional limitation, projected goal status, at therapy episode outset, at reporting intervals, and at discharge or to end reporting	Other PT/OT goal status
G8992	Other physical or occupational therapy primary functional limitation, discharge status, at discharge from therapy or to end reporting	Other PT/OT D/C status
Other PT/OT Subsequent G-code Set		
G8993	Other physical or occupational therapy subsequent functional limitation, current status, at therapy episode outset and at reporting intervals	Sub PT/OT current status
G8994	Other physical or occupational therapy subsequent functional limitation, projected goal status, at therapy episode outset, at reporting intervals, and at discharge or to end reporting	Sub PT/OT goal status
G8995	Other physical or occupational subsequent functional limitation, discharge from therapy or end reporting.	Sub PT/OT D/C status

The following G-codes are for functional limitations typically seen in beneficiaries receiving SLP services. Seven are for specific functional communication measures, which are modeled after the National Outcomes Measurement System (NOMS), and one is for any "other" measure not described by one of the other seven.

	Long Descriptor	Short Descriptor
Swallowing G-code Set		
G8996	Swallowing functional limitation, current status, at therapy episode outset and at reporting intervals	Swallow current status
G8997	Swallowing functional limitation, projected goal status, at therapy episode outset, at reporting intervals, and at discharge or to end reporting	Swallow goal status
G8998	Swallowing functional limitation, discharge status, at discharge from therapy or to end reporting	Swallow D/C status
Motor Speech G-code Set (Note: These codes are not sequentially numbered)		
G8999	Motor speech functional limitation, current status, at therapy episode outset and at reporting intervals	Motor speech current status
G9186	Motor speech functional limitation, projected goal status at therapy episode outset, at reporting intervals, and at discharge or to end reporting	Motor speech goal status
G9158	Motor speech functional limitation, discharge status, at discharge from therapy or to end reporting	Motor speech D/C status
Spoken Language Comprehension G-code Set		
G9159	Spoken language comprehension functional limitation, current status, at therapy episode outset and at reporting intervals	Lang comp current status
G9160	Spoken language comprehension functional limitation, projected goal status, at therapy episode outset, at reporting intervals, and at discharge or to end reporting	Lang comp goal status
G9161	Spoken language comprehension functional limitation, discharge status, at discharge from therapy or to end reporting	Lang comp D/C status
Spoken Language Expressive G-code Set		
G9162	Spoken language expression functional limitation, current status, at therapy episode outset and at reporting intervals	Lang express current status
G9163	Spoken language expression functional limitation, projected goal status, at therapy episode outset, at reporting intervals, and at discharge or to end reporting	Lang press goal status
G9164	Spoken language expression functional limitation, discharge status, at discharge from therapy or to end reporting	Lang express D/C status
Attention G-code Set		
G9165	Attention functional limitation, current status, at therapy episode outset and at reporting intervals	Atten current status
G9166	Attention functional limitation, projected goal status, at therapy episode outset, at reporting intervals, and at discharge or to end reporting	Atten goal status

	Long Descriptor	Short Descriptor
G9167	Attention functional limitation, discharge status, at discharge from therapy or to end reporting	Atten D/C status

Memory G-code Set

	Long Descriptor	Short Descriptor
G9168	Memory functional limitation, current status, at therapy episode outset and at reporting intervals	Memory current status
G9169	Memory functional limitation, projected goal status, at therapy episode outset, at reporting intervals, and at discharge or to end reporting	Memory goal status
G9170	Memory functional limitation, discharge status, at discharge from therapy or to end reporting	Memory D/C status

Voice G-code Set

	Long Descriptor	Short Descriptor
G9171	Voice functional limitation, current status, at therapy episode outset and at reporting intervals	Voice current status
G9172	Voice functional limitation, projected goal status, at therapy episode outset, at reporting intervals, and at discharge or to end reporting	Voice goal status
G9173	Voice functional limitation, discharge status, at discharge from therapy or to end reporting	Voice D/C status

The following "other SLP" G-code set is used to report:

- on one of the other eight NOMS-defined functional measures not described by the above code sets; or
- to report an overall, composite or other score from assessment tool that does not clearly represent one of the above seven categorical SLP functional measures.

	Long Descriptor	Short Descriptor
Other Speech Language Pathology G-code Set		
G9174	Other speech language pathology functional limitation, current status, at therapy episode outset and at reporting intervals	Speech lang current status
G9175	Other speech language pathology functional limitation, projected goal status, at therapy episode outset, at reporting intervals, and at discharge or to end reporting	Speech lang goal status
G9176	Other speech language pathology functional limitation, discharge status, at discharge from therapy or to end reporting	Speech lang D/C status

F. Severity/Complexity Modifiers

For each nonpayable functional G-code, one of the modifiers listed below must be used to report the severity/complexity for that functional limitation.

Modifier	Impairment Limitation Restriction
CH	0 percent impaired, limited or restricted
CI	At least 1 percent but less than 20 percent impaired, limited or restricted
CJ	At least 20 percent but less than 40 percent impaired, limited or restricted
CK	At least 40 percent but less than 60 percent impaired, limited or restricted
CL	At least 60 percent but less than 80 percent impaired, limited or restricted
CM	At least 80 percent but less than 100 percent impaired, limited or restricted
CN	100 percent impaired, limited or restricted

The severity modifiers reflect the beneficiary's percentage of functional impairment as determined by the clinician furnishing the therapy services.

G. Required Reporting of Functional G-codes and Severity Modifiers

The functional G-codes and severity modifiers listed above are used in the required reporting on therapy claims at certain specified points during therapy episodes of care. Claims containing these functional G-codes must also contain another billable and separately payable (non-bundled) service. Only one functional limitation shall be reported at a given time for each related therapy plan of care (POC).

Functional reporting using the G-codes and corresponding severity modifiers is required reporting on specified therapy claims. Specifically, they are required on claims:

- At the outset of a therapy episode of care (i.e., on the claim for the date of service (DOS) of the initial therapy service);
- At least once every 10 treatment days, which corresponds with the progress reporting period;
- When an evaluative procedure, including a re-evaluative one, (HCPCS/CPT codes 92521, 92522, 92523, 92524, 92597, 92607, 92608, 92610, 92611, 92612, 92614,

92616, 96105, 96125, 97161, 97162, 97163, 97164, 97165, 97166, 97167, 97168) is furnished and billed;

- At the time of discharge from the therapy episode of care–(i.e., on the date services related to the discharge [progress] report are furnished); and
- At the time reporting of a particular functional limitation is ended in cases where the need for further therapy is necessary.
- At the time reporting is begun for a new or different functional limitation within the same episode of care (i.e., after the reporting of the prior functional limitation is ended)

Functional reporting is required on claims throughout the entire episode of care. When the beneficiary has reached his or her goal or progress has been maximized on the initially selected functional limitation, but the need for treatment continues, reporting is required for a second functional limitation using another set of G-codes. In these situations two or more functional limitations will be reported for a beneficiary during the therapy episode of care. Thus, reporting on more than one functional limitation may be required for some beneficiaries but not simultaneously.

When the beneficiary stops coming to therapy prior to discharge, the clinician should report the functional information on the last claim. If the clinician is unaware that the beneficiary is not returning for therapy until after the last claim is submitted, the clinician cannot report the discharge status.

When functional reporting is required on a claim for therapy services, two G-codes will generally be required.

Two exceptions exist:

1. Therapy services under more than one therapy POC. Claims may contain more than two nonpayable functional G-codes when in cases where a beneficiary receives therapy services under multiple POCs (PT, OT, and/or SLP) from the same therapy provider.
2. One-Time Therapy Visit. When a beneficiary is seen and future therapy services are either not medically indicated or are going to be furnished by another provider, the clinician reports on the claim for the DOS of the visit, all three G-codes in the appropriate code set (current status, goal status and discharge status), along with corresponding severity modifiers. Each reported functional G-code must also contain the following line of service information:

- Functional severity modifier
- Therapy modifier indicating the related discipline/POC -- GP, GO or GN -- for PT, OT, and SLP services, respectively
- Date of the related therapy service
- Nominal charge, e.g., a penny, for institutional claims submitted to the FIs and A/MACs. For professional claims, a zero charge is acceptable for the service line. If provider billing software requires an amount for professional claims, a nominal charge, e.g., a penny, may be included. Note: The KX modifier is not required on the claim line for nonpayable G-codes, but would be required with the procedure code for medically necessary therapy services furnished once the beneficiary's annual cap has been reached.

The following example demonstrates how the G-codes and modifiers are used. In this example, the clinician determines that the beneficiary's mobility restriction is the most clinically relevant functional limitation and selects the Mobility G-code set (G8978 – G8980) to represent the beneficiary's functional limitation. The clinician also determines the severity/complexity of the beneficiary's functional limitation and selects the appropriate modifier. In this example, the clinician determines that the beneficiary has a 75 percent mobility restriction for which the CL modifier is applicable. The clinician expects that at the end of therapy the beneficiaries will have only a 15 percent mobility restriction for which the CI modifier is applicable. When the beneficiary attains the mobility goal, therapy continues to be medically necessary to addresss a functional limitation for which there is no categorical G-code. The clinician reports this using (G8990 – G8992).

At the outset of therapy. On the DOS for which the initial evaluative procedure is furnished or the initial treatment day of a therapy POC, the claim for the service will also include two G-codes as shown below.

- G8978-CL to report the functional limitation (Mobility with current mobility limitation of "at least 60 percent but less than 80 percent impaired, limited or restricted")
- G8979-CI to report the projected goal for a mobility restriction of "at least 1 percent but less than 20 percent impaired, limited or restricted."

At the end of each progress reporting period. On the claim for the DOS when the services related to the progress report (which must be done at least once each 10 treatment days) are furnished, the clinician will report the same two G-codes but the modifier for the current status may be different.

- G8978 with the appropriate modifier are reported to show the beneficiary's current status as of this DOS. So if thebeneficiary has made no progress, this claim will include G8978-CL. If the beneficiary made progress and now has a mobility restriction of 65 percent CL will still be the appropriate modifier for 65 percent, and G8978-CL would be reported in this case. If the beneficiary now has a mobility restriction of 45 percent, G8978-CK would be reported.
- G8979-CI would be reported to show the projected goal. This severity modifier would not change unless the clinician adjusts the beneficiary's goal. This step is repeated as necessary and clinically appropriate, adjusting the current status modifier used as the beneficiary progresses through therapy.

- At the time the beneficiary is discharged from the therapy episode. The final claim for therapy episode will include two G-codes.
- G8979-CI would be reported to show the projected goal. G8980-CI would be reported if the beneficiary attained the 15 percent mobility goal. Alternatively, if the beneficiary's mobility restriction only reached 25 percent; G8980-CJ would be reported. To end reporting of one functional limitation. As noted above, functional reporting is required to continue throughout the entire episode of care. Accordingly, when further therapy is medically necessary after the beneficiary attains the goal for the first reported functional limitation, the clinician would end reporting of the first functional limitation by using the same G-codes and modifiers that would be used at the time of discharge. Using the mobility example, to end reporting of the mobility functional limitation, G8979-CI and G8980-CI would be reported on the same DOS that coincides with end of that progress reporting period.

To begin reporting of a second functional limitation. At the time reporting is begun for a new and different functional limitation, within the same episode of care (i.e., after the reporting of the prior functional limitation is ended). Reporting on the second functional limitation, however, is not begun until the DOS of the next treatment day -- which is day one of the new progress reporting period. When the next functional limitation to be reported is NOT defined by one of the other three PT/OT categorical codes, the G-code set (G8990 - G8992) for the "other PT/OT primary" functional limitation is used, rather than the G-code set for the "other PT/OT subsequent" because it is the first reported "other PT/OT" functional limitation. This reporting begins on the DOS of the first treatment day following the mobility "discharge" reporting, which is counted as the initial service for the "other PT/OT primary" functional limitation and the first treatment day of the new progress reporting period. In this case, G8990 and G8991, along with the corresponding modifiers, are reported on the claim for therapy services.

The table below illustrates when reporting is required using this example and what G-codes would be used.

Example of Required Reporting

Key: Reporting Period (RP)	Begin RP #1 for Mobility at Episode Outset	End RP#1for Mobility at Progress Report	Mobility RP #2 Begins Next Treatment Day	End RP#2 for Mobility at Progress Report	Mobility RP #3 Begins Next Treatment Day	D/C or End Reporting for \Mobility	Begin RP #1 for Other PT/OT Primary
Mobility: Walking & Moving Around							
G8978 – Current Status	X	X		X			
G 8979– Goal Status	X	X		X		X	
G8980 – Discharge Status						X	
Other PT/OT Primary							
G8990 – Current Status							X
G8991 – Goal Status							X
G8992 – Discharge Status							
No Functional Reporting Req'd			X		X		

H. Required Tracking and Documentation of Functional G-codes and Severity Modifiers

The clinician who furnishes the services must not only report the functional information on the therapy claim, but, he/she must track and document the G-codes and severity modifiers used for this reporting in the beneficiary's medical record of therapy services.

For details related to the documentation requirements, refer to Pub. 100-02, Medicare Benefit Policy Manual, chapter 15, section 220.4, - MCTRJCA-required Functional Reporting. For coverage rules related to MCTRJCA and therapy goals, refer to Pub. 100-02: a) for outpatient therapy services, see chapter 15, section 220.1.2 B and b) for instructions specific to PT, OT, and SLP services in the CORF, see chapter 12, section 10.

100-04, 5, 20.2

Reporting of Service Units With HCPCS

(Rev. 3670, Issued: 12-01-16, Effective: 01-01-17, Implementation: 01-03-17)

A. General

Effective with claims submitted on or after April 1, 1998, providers billing on the ASC X12 837 institutional claim format or Form CMS-1450 were required to report the number of units for outpatient rehabilitation services based on the procedure or service, e.g., based on the HCPCS code reported instead of the revenue code. This was already in effect for billing on the Form CMS-1500, and CORFs were required to report their full range of CORF services on the institutional claim. These unit-reporting requirements continue with the standards required for electronically submitting health care claims under the Health Insurance Portability and Accountability Act of 1996 (HIPAA) - the currently adopted version of the ASC X12 837 transaction standards and implementation guides. The Administrative Simplification Compliance

Act mandates that claims be sent to Medicare electronically unless certain exceptions are met.

B. Timed and Untimed Codes

When reporting service units for HCPCS codes where the procedure is not defined by a specific timeframe ("untimed" HCPCS), the provider enters "1" in the field labeled units. For timed codes, units are reported based on the number of times the procedure is performed, as described in the HCPCS code definition.

EXAMPLE: A beneficiary received a speech-language pathology evaluation represented by HCPCS "untimed" code 92521. Regardless of the number of minutes spent providing this service only one unit of service is appropriately billed on the same day.

Several CPT codes used for therapy modalities, procedures, and tests and measurements specify that the direct (one on one) time spent in patient contact is 15 minutes. Providers report these "timed" procedure codes for services delivered on any single calendar day using CPT codes and the appropriate number of 15 minute units of service.

EXAMPLE: A beneficiary received a total of 60 minutes of occupational therapy, e.g., HCPCS "timed" code 97530 which is defined in 15 minute units, on a given date of service. The provider would then report 4 units of 97530.

C. Counting Minutes for Timed Codes in 15 Minute Units

When only one service is provided in a day, providers should not bill for services performed for less than 8 minutes. For any single timed CPT code in the same day measured in 15 minute units, providers bill a single 15-minute unit for treatment greater than or equal to 8 minutes through and including 22 minutes. If the duration of a single modality or procedure in a day is greater than or equal to 23 minutes, through and including 37 minutes, then 2 units should be billed. Time intervals for 1 through 8 units are as follows:

Units Number of Minutes

1 unit: ≥ 8 minutes through 22 minutes

2 units:≥ 23 minutes through 37 minutes

3 units:≥ 38 minutes through 52 minutes

4 units:≥ 53 minutes through 67 minutes

5 units:≥ 68 minutes through 82 minutes

6 units:≥ 83 minutes through 97 minutes

7 units:≥ 98 minutes through 112 minutes

8 units:≥ 113 minutes through 127 minutes

The pattern remains the same for treatment times in excess of 2 hours.

If a service represented by a 15 minute timed code is performed in a single day for at least 15 minutes, that service shall be billed for at least one unit. If the service is performed for at least 30 minutes, that service shall be billed for at least two units, etc. It is not appropriate to count all minutes of treatment in a day toward the units for one code if other services were performed for more than 15 minutes. See examples 2 and 3 below.

When more than one service represented by 15 minute timed codes is performed in a single day, the total number of minutes of service (as noted on the chart above) determines the number of timed units billed. See example 1 below.

If any 15 minute timed service that is performed for 7 minutes or less than 7 minutes on the same day as another 15 minute timed service that was also performed for 7 minutes or less and the total time of the two is 8 minutes or greater than 8 minutes, then bill one unit for the service performed for the most minutes. This is correct because the total time is greater than the minimum time for one unit. The same logic is applied when three or more different services are provided for 7 minutes or less than 7 minutes. See example 5 below.

The expectation (based on the work values for these codes) is that a provider's direct patient contact time for each unit will average 15 minutes in length. If a provider has a consistent practice of billing less than 15 minutes for a unit, these situations should be highlighted for review.

If more than one 15 minute timed CPT code is billed during a single calendar day, then the total number of timed units that can be billed is constrained by the total treatment minutes for that day. See all examples below.

Pub. 100-02, Medicare Benefit Policy Manual, Chapter 15, Section 220.3B, Documentation Requirements for Therapy Services, indicates that the amount of time for each specific intervention/modality provided to the patient is not required to be documented in the Treatment Note. However, the total number of timed minutes must be documented. These examples indicate how to count the appropriate number of units for the total therapy minutes provided.

Example 1 –

24 minutes of neuromuscular reeducation, code 97112,

23 minutes of therapeutic exercise, code 97110,

Total timed code treatment time was 47 minutes.

See the chart above. The 47 minutes falls within the range for 3 units = 38 to 52 minutes.

Appropriate billing for 47 minutes is only 3 timed units. Each of the codes is performed for more than 15 minutes, so each shall be billed for at least 1 unit. The correct coding is 2 units of code 97112 and one unit of code 97110, assigning more timed units to the service that took the most time.

Example 2 –

20 minutes of neuromuscular reeducation (97112)

20 minutes therapeutic exercise (97110),

40 Total timed code minutes.

Appropriate billing for 40 minutes is 3 units. Each service was done at least 15 minutes and should be billed for at least one unit, but the total allows 3 units. Since the time for each service is the same, choose either code for 2 units and bill the other for 1 unit. Do not bill 3 units for either one of the codes.

Example 3 –

33 minutes of therapeutic exercise (97110),

7 minutes of manual therapy (97140),

40 Total timed minutes

Appropriate billing for 40 minutes is for 3 units. Bill 2 units of 97110 and 1 unit of 97140. Count the first 30 minutes of 97110 as two full units. Compare the remaining time for 97110 (33-30 = 3 minutes) to the time spent on 97140 (7 minutes) and bill the larger, which is 97140.

Example 4 –

18 minutes of therapeutic exercise (97110),

13 minutes of manual therapy (97140),

10 minutes of gait training (97116),

8 minutes of ultrasound (97035),

49 Total timed minutes

Appropriate billing is for 3 units. Bill the procedures you spent the most time providing. Bill 1 unit each of 97110, 97116, and 97140. You are unable to bill for the ultrasound because the total time of timed units that can be billed is constrained by the total timed code treatment minutes (i.e., you may not bill 4 units for less than 53 minutes regardless of how many services were performed). You would still document the ultrasound in the treatment notes.

Example 5 –

7 minutes of neuromuscular reeducation (97112)

7 minutes therapeutic exercise (97110)

7 minutes manual therapy (97140)

21 Total timed minutes

Appropriate billing is for one unit. The qualified professional (See definition in Pub. 100-02, chapter 15, section 220) shall select one appropriate CPT code (97112, 97110, 97140) to bill since each unit was performed for the same amount of time and only one unit is allowed.

NOTE: The above schedule of times is intended to provide assistance in rounding time into 15-minute increments. It does not imply that any minute until the eighth should be excluded from the total count. The total minutes of active treatment counted for all 15 minute timed codes includes all direct treatment time for the timed codes. Total treatment minutes - including minutes spent providing services represented by untimed codes - are also documented. For documentation in the medical record of the services provided see Pub. 100-02, chapter 15, section 220.3.

D. Specific Limits for HCPCS

The Deficit Reduction Act of 2005, section 5107 requires the implementation of clinically appropriate code edits to eliminate improper payments for outpatient therapy services. The following codes may be billed, when covered, only at or below the number of units indicated on the chart per treatment day. When higher amounts of units are billed than those indicated in the table below, the units on the claim line that exceed the limit shall be denied as medically unnecessary (according to 1862(a)(1)(A)). Denied claims may be appealed and an ABN is appropriate to notify the beneficiary of liability.

This chart does not include all of the codes identified as therapy codes; refer to section 20 of this chapter for further detail on these and other therapy codes. For example, therapy codes called "always therapy" must always be accompanied by therapy modifiers identifying the type of therapy plan of care under which the service is provided.

Use the chart in the following manner:

The codes that are allowed one unit for "Allowed Units" in the chart below may be billed no more than once per provider, per discipline, per date of service, per patient.

The codes allowed 0 units in the column for "Allowed Units", may not be billed under a plan of care indicated by the discipline in that column. Some codes may be billed by one discipline (e.g., PT) and not by others (e.g., OT or SLP).

When physicians/NPPs bill "always therapy" codes they must follow the policies of the type of therapy they are providing e.g., utilize a plan of care, bill with the appropriate therapy modifier (GP, GO, GN), bill the allowed units on the chart below for PT, OT or SLP depending on the plan. A physician/NPP shall not bill an "always therapy" code unless the service is provided under a therapy plan of care. Therefore, NA stands for "Not Applicable" in the chart below.

When a "sometimes therapy" code is billed by a physician/NPP, but as a medical service, and not under a therapy plan of care, the therapy modifier shall not be used, but the number of units billed must not exceed the number of units indicated in the chart below per patient, per provider/supplier, per day.

NOTE: As of April 1, 2017, the chart below uses the CPT Consumer Friendly Code Descriptions which are intended only to assist the reader in identifying the service related to the CPT/HCPCS code. The reader is reminded that these descriptions cannot be used in place of the CPT long descriptions which officially define each of the services. The table below no longer contains a column noting whether a code is "timed" or "untimed" as this notation is not relevant to the number of units allowed per code on claims for the listed therapy services. We note that the official long descriptors for the CPT codes can be found in the latest CPT code book.

CPT/ HCPCS Code	CPT Consumer Friendly Code Descriptions and Claim Line Outlier/Edit Details	PT Allowed Units	OT Allowed Units	SLP Allowed Units	Physician /NPP Not Under Therapy POC
92521	Evaluation of speech fluency	0	0	1	NA
92522	Evaluation of speech sound production	0	0	1	NA
92523	Evaluation of speech sound production with evaluation of language comprehension and expression	0	0	1	NA
92524	Behavioral and qualitative analysis of voice and resonance	0	0	1	NA
92597	Evaluation for use and/or fitting of voice prosthetic device to supplement oral speech	0	0	1	NA
92607	Evaluation of patient with prescription of speech-generating and alternative communication device	0	0	1	NA
92611	Fluoroscopic and video recorded motion evaluation of swallowing function	0	1	1	1
92612	Evaluation and recording of swallowing using an endoscope Evaluation and recording of swallowing using an endoscope	0	1	1	1
92614	Evaluation and recording of voice box sensory function using an endoscope	0	1	1	1
92616	Evaluation and recording of swallowing and voice box sensory function using an endoscope	0	1	1	1
95833	Manual muscle testing of whole body	1	1	0	1
95834	Manual muscle testing of whole body including hands	1	1	0	1
96110	Developmental screening	1	1	1	1
96111	Developmental testing	1	1	1	1
97161	Evaluation of physical therapy, typically 20 minutes	1	0	0	NA
97162	Evaluation of physical therapy, typically 30 minutes	1	0	0	NA
97163	Evaluation of physical therapy, typically 45 minutes	1	0	0	NA
97164	Re-evaluation of physical therapy, typically 20 minutes	1	0	0	NA
97165	Evaluation of occupational therapy, typically 30 minutes	0	1	0	NA
97166	Evaluation of occupational therapy, typically 45 minutes	0	1	0	NA
97167	Evaluation of occupational therapy, typically 60 minutes	0	1	0	NA
97168	Re-evaluation of occupational therapy established plan of care, typically 30 minutes	0	1	0	NA

100-04, 8, 60.4.2

Facility Billing Requirements for ESAs

(Rev.4105, Issued: 08- 03-18, Effective: 01-01-19, Implementation: 01-07-19)

Hematocrit and Hemoglobin Levels

Renal dialysis facilities are required to report hematocrit or hemoglobin levels for their Medicare patients receiving erythropoietin products. Hematocrit levels are reported in value code 49 and reflect the most recent reading taken before the start of the billing period. Hemoglobin readings before the start of the billing period are reported in value code 48.

To report a hemoglobin or hematocrit reading for a new patient on or after January 1, 2006, the provider should report the reading that prompted the treatment of epoetin alfa. The provider may use results documented on form CMS 2728 or the patient's medical records from a transferring facility.

Effective January 1, 2012, ESRD facilities are required to report hematocrit or hemoglobin levels on all ESRD claims. Reporting the value 99.99 is not permitted when billing for an ESA.

The revenue codes for reporting Epoetin Alfa are 0634 and 0635. All other ESAs are reported using revenue code 0636. The HCPCS code for the ESA must be included:

HCPCS	HCPCS Description	Dates of Service
Q4055	Injection, Epoetin Alfa, 1,000 units (for ESRD on Dialysis)	1/1/2004 through 12/31/2005
J0886	Injection, Epoetin Alfa, 1,000 units (for ESRD on Dialysis)	1/1/2006 through 12/31/2006
Q4081	Injection, Epoetin alfa, 100	1/1/2007 through 7/1/2015
Q5105	Injection, epoetin alfa, biosimilar, (Retacrit) (For ESRD on Dialysis), 100 units	7/1/2018 to present

Each administration of an ESA is reported on a separate line item with the units reported used as a multiplier by the dosage description in the HCPCS to arrive at the dosage per administration.

Route of Administration Modifiers

Patients with end stage renal disease (ESRD) receiving administrations of erythropoiesis stimulating agents (ESA) for the treatment of anemia may receive intravenous administration or subcutaneous administrations of the ESA. Effective for claims with dates of services on or after January 1, 2012, all facilities billing for injections of ESA for ESRD beneficiaries must include the modifier JA on the claim to indicate an intravenous administration or modifier JB to indicate a subcutaneous administration. ESRD claims containing ESA administrations that are submitted without the route of administration modifiers will be returned to the provider for correction. Renal dialysis facilities claim including charges for administrations of the ESA by both methods must report separate lines to identify the number of administration provided using each method.

Effective July 1, 2013, providers must identify when a drug is administered via the dialysate by appending the modifier JE (administered via dialysate).

ESA Monitoring Policy Modifiers

Append modifiers ED, EE and GS as applicable, see instructions in section 60.4.1.

Maximum Allowable Administrations

The maximum number of administrations of EPO for a billing cycle is 13 times in 30 days and 14 times in 31 days.

The maximum number of administrations of Aranesp for a billing cycle is 5 times in 30/31days.

The maximum number of administrations of Peginesatide is 1 time in 30/31days.

100-04, 8, 140.1

Payment for ESRD-Related Services Under the Monthly Capitation Payment (Center Based Patients)

(Rev. 2269, Issued: 08-05-11, Effective: 01-01-11, Implementation: 11-07-11)

Physicians and practitioners managing center based patients on dialysis are paid a monthly rate for most outpatient dialysis-related physician services furnished to a Medicare ESRD beneficiary. The payment amount varies based on the number of visits provided within each month and the age of the ESRD beneficiary. Under this methodology, separate codes are billed for providing one visit per month, two to three visits per month and four or more visits per month. The lowest payment amount applies when a physician provides one visit per month; a higher payment is provided for two to three visits per month. To receive the highest payment amount, a physician or practitioner would have to provide at least four ESRD-related visits per month. The MCP is reported once per month for services performed in an outpatient setting that are related to the patients' ESRD.

The physician or practitioner who provides the complete assessment, establishes the patient's plan of care, and provides the ongoing management is the physician or practitioner who submits the bill for the monthly service.

a. Month defined.

For purposes of billing for physician and practitioner ESRD related services, the term 'month' means a calendar month. The first month the beneficiary begins dialysis treatments is the date the dialysis treatments begin through the end of the calendar month. Thereafter, the term 'month' refers to a calendar month.

b. Determination of the age of beneficiary.

The beneficiary's age at the end of the month is the age of the patient for determining the appropriate age related ESRD-related services code.

c. Qualifying Visits Under the MCP

- General policy.

Visits must be furnished face-to-face by a physician, clinical nurse specialist, nurse practitioner, or physician's assistant.

- Visits furnished by another physician or practitioner (who is not the MCP physician or practitioner).

The MCP physician or practitioner may use other physicians or qualified nonphysician practitioners to provide some of the visits during the month. The MCP physician or practitioner does not have to be present when these other physicians or practitioners provide visits. In this instance, the rules are consistent with the requirements for hospital split/shared evaluation and management visits. The non-MCP physician or practitioner must be a partner, an employee of the same group practice, or an employee of the MCP physician or practitioner. For example, the physician or practitioner furnishing visits under the MCP may be either a W-2 employee or 1099 independent contractor.

When another physician is used to furnish some of the visits during the month, the physician who provides the complete assessment, establishes the patient's plan of care, and provides the ongoing management should bill for the MCP service.

If the nonphysician practitioner is the practitioner who performs the complete assessment and establishes the plan of care, then the MCP service should be billed under the PIN of the clinical nurse specialist, nurse practitioner, or physician assistant.

- Residents, interns and fellows.

Patient visits by residents, interns and fellows enrolled in an approved Medicare graduate medical education (GME) program may be counted towards the MCP visits if the teaching MCP physician is present during the visit.

- Patients designated/admitted as hospital observation status.

ESRD-related visits furnished to patients in hospital observation status that occur on or after January 1, 2005, should be counted for purposes of billing the MCP codes. Visits furnished to patients in hospital observation status are included when submitting MCP claims for ESRD-related services.

- ESRD-related visits furnished to beneficiaries residing in a SNF.

ESRD-related visits furnished to beneficiaries residing in a SNF should be counted for purposes of billing the MCP codes.

- SNF residents admitted as an inpatient.

Inpatient visits are not counted for purposes of the MCP service. If the beneficiary residing in a SNF is admitted to the hospital as an inpatient, the appropriate inpatient visit code should be billed.

- ESRD Related Visits as a Telehealth Service

ESRD-related services with 2 or 3 visits per month and ESRD-related services with 4 or more visits per month may be furnished as a telehealth service. However, at least one visit per month is required in person to examine the vascular access site. A clinical examination of the vascular access site must be furnished face-to-face (not as a telehealth service) by a physician, nurse practitioner or physician's assistant. For more information on how ESRD-related visits may be furnished as a Medicare telehealth service and for general Medicare telehealth policy see Pub. 100-2, Medicare Benefit Policy manual, chapter 15, section 270. For claims processing instructions see Pub. 100-4, Medicare Claims Processing manual chapter 12, section 190.

100-04, 8, 140.1.1

Payment for Managing Patients on Home Dialysis

(Rev. 2269, Issued: 08-05-11, Effective: 01-01-11, Implementation: 11-07-11)

Physicians and practitioners managing ESRD patients who dialyze at home are paid a single monthly rate based on the age of the beneficiary. The MCP physician (or practitioner) must furnish at least one face-to-face patient visit per month for the home dialysis MCP service. Documentation by the MCP physician (or practitioner) should support at least one face-to-face encounter per month with the home dialysis patient. Medicare contractors may waive the requirement for a monthly face-to-face visit for the home dialysis MCP service on a case by case basis, for example, when the nephrologist's notes indicate that the physician actively and adequately managed the care of the home dialysis patient throughout the month. The management of home dialysis patients who remain a home dialysis patient the entire month should be coded using the ESRD-related services for home dialysis patients HCPCS codes.

When another physician is used to furnish some of the visits during the month, the physician who provides the complete assessment, establishes the patient's plan of care, and provides the ongoing management should bill for the MCP service.

If the nonphysician practitioner is the practitioner who performs the complete assessment and establishes the plan of care, then the MCP service should be billed under the PIN of the clinical nurse specialist, nurse practitioner, or physician assistant.

Residents, interns and fellows. Patient visits by residents, interns and fellows enrolled in an approved Medicare graduate medical education (GME) program may be counted towards the MCP visits if the teaching MCP physician is present during the visit.

    a. Month defined.

For purposes of billing for physician and practitioner ESRD related services, the term 'month' means a calendar month. The first month the beneficiary begins dialysis treatments is the date the dialysis treatments begin through the end of the calendar month. Thereafter, the term 'month' refers to a calendar month.

    b. Qualifying Visits under the MCP

- General policy.

Visits must be furnished face-to-face by a physician, clinical nurse specialist, nurse practitioner, or physician's assistant.

- Visits furnished by another physician or practitioner (who is not the MCP physician or practitioner).

The MCP physician or practitioner may use other physicians or qualified nonphysician practitioners to provide the visit(s) during the month. The MCP physician or practitioner does not have to be present when these other physicians or practitioners provide visit(s). The non-MCP physician or practitioner must be a partner, an employee of the same group practice, or an employee of the MCP physician or practitioner. For example, the physician or practitioner furnishing visits under the MCP may be either a W-2 employee or 1099 independent contractor.

When another physician is used to furnish some of the visits during the month, the physician who provides the complete assessment, establishes the patient's plan of care, and provides the ongoing management should bill for the MCP service.

If the nonphysician practitioner is the practitioner who performs the complete assessment and establishes the plan of care, then the MCP service should be billed under the PIN of the clinical nurse specialist, nurse practitioner, or physician assistant.

- Residents, interns and fellows.

Patient visits by residents, interns and fellows enrolled in an approved Medicare graduate medical education (GME) program may be counted towards the MCP visits if the teaching MCP physician is present during the visit.

100-04, 8, 180
Noninvasive Studies for ESRD Patients - Facility and Physician Services
(Rev. 3650, Issued: 11-10-16, Effective: 02-10-17, Implementation: 02-10-17)

For Medicare coverage of noninvasive vascular studies, see the Medicare Benefit Policy Manual, Chapter 11.

For dialysis to take place there must be a means of access so that the exchange of waste products may occur. As part of the dialysis treatment, ESRD facilities are responsible for monitoring access, and when occlusions occur, either declot the access or refer the patient for appropriate treatment. Procedures associated with monitoring access involve taking venous pressure, aspirating thrombus, observing elevated recirculation time, reduced urea reduction ratios, or collapsed shunt, etc. All such procedures are covered under the composite rate.

ESRD facilities may not monitor access through noninvasive vascular studies such as duplex and Doppler flow scans and bill separately for these procedures. Noninvasive vascular studies are not covered as a separately billable service if used to monitor a patient's vascular access site.

Medicare pays for the technical component of the procedure in the composite payment rate.

Where there are signs and symptoms of vascular access problems, Doppler flow studies may be used as a means to obtain diagnostic information to permit medical intervention to address the problem. Doppler flow studies may be considered medically necessary in the presence of signs or symptoms of possible failure of the ESRD patient's vascular access site, and when the results are used in determining the clinical course of the treatment for the patient.

The only Current Procedural Terminology (CPT) billing code for noninvasive vascular testing of a hemodialysis access site is 93990. A/B MACs (B) must deny separate billing of the technical component of this code if it is performed on any patient for whom the ESRD composite rate for dialysis is being paid, unless there is appropriate medical indication of the need for a Doppler flow study.

When a dialysis patient exhibits signs and symptoms of compromise to the vascular access site, Doppler flow studies may provide diagnostic information that will determine the appropriate medical intervention. Medicare considers a Doppler flow study medically necessary when the beneficiary's dialysis access site manifests signs or symptoms associated with vascular compromise, and when the results of this test are necessary to determine the clinical course of treatment.

Examples supporting the medical necessity for Doppler flow studies include:

    a. Elevated dynamic venous pressure >200mm HG when measured during dialysis with the blood pump set on a 200cc/min.,

    b. Access recirculation of 12 percent or greater,

    c. An otherwise unexplained urea reduction ration <60 oercebtm abd

    d. An access with a palpable "water hammer" pulse on examination, (which implies venous outflow obstruction).

Unless the documentation is provided supporting the necessity of more than one study, Medicare will limit payment to either a Doppler flow study or an arteriogram (fistulogram, venogram), but not both.

An example of when both studies may be clinically necessary is when a Doppler flow study demonstrates reduced flow (blood flow rate less than 800cc/min or a decreased flow of 25 percent or greater from previous study) and the physician requires an arteriogram to further define the extent of the problem. The patient's medical record(s) must provide documentation supporting the need for more than one imaging study.

This policy is applicable to claims from ESRD facilities and all other sources, such as independent diagnostic testing facilities, and hospital outpatient departments.

A/B MACs (B) shall develop LMRP for Doppler flow studies if this service meets the criteria listed in the Medicare Program Integrity Manual, Chapter 1. This provides guidance to contractors on the scope, purpose, and meaning of LMRP.

The professional component of the procedure is included in the monthly capitation payment (MCP) (See §140 above.) The professional component should be denied for code 93990 if billed by the MCP physician. Medically necessary services that are included or bundled into the MCP (e.g., test interpretations) are separately payable when furnished by physicians other than the MCP physician.

The contractor shall use the following remittance advice messages and associated codes when rejecting/denying claims under this policy. This CARC/RARC combination is compliant with CAQH CORE Business Scenario Four.

    Group Code: CO
    CARC: 24
    RARC: N/A
    MSN:16.32

Billing for monitoring of hemodialysis access using CPT codes for noninvasive vascular studies other than 93990 is considered a misrepresentation of the service actually provided and contractors will consider this action for fraud investigation. They will conduct data analysis on a periodic basis for noninvasive diagnostic studies of the extremities (including CPT codes 93922, 93923, 93924, 93925, 93926, 93930, 93931, 93965, 93970, 93971). Contractors should handle aberrant findings under normal program safeguard processes by taking whatever corrective action is deemed necessary.

100-04, 11, 40.1.3
Independent Attending Physician Services
(Rev. 4280, Issued: 04-19-2019, Effective: 07-21-19, Implementation: 07-21-19)

When hospice coverage is elected, the beneficiary waives all rights to Medicare Part B payments for professional services that are related to the treatment and management of his/her terminal illness during any period his/her hospice benefit election is in force, except for professional services of an independent attending physician, who is not an employee of the designated hospice nor receives compensation from the hospice for those services. For purposes of administering the hospice benefit provisions, an "attending physician" means an individual who:

- Is a doctor of medicine or osteopathy or

- A nurse practitioner (for professional services related to the terminal illness that are furnished on or after December 8, 2003); and

- Is identified by the individual, at the time he/she elects hospice coverage, as having the most significant role in the determination and delivery of their medical care.

Hospices should reiterate with patients that they must not see independent physicians for care related to their terminal illness other than their independent attending physician unless the hospice arranges it.

Even though a beneficiary elects hospice coverage, he/she may designate and use an independent attending physician, who is not employed by nor receives compensation from the hospice for professional services furnished, in addition to the services of hospice-employed physicians. The professional services of an independent attending physician, who may be a nurse practitioner as defined in Chapter 9, that are reasonable and necessary for the treatment and management of a hospice patient's terminal illness are not considered Medicare Part A hospice services.

Where the service is related to the hospice patient's terminal illness but was furnished by someone other than the designated "attending physician" [or a physician substituting for the attending physician]) the physician or other provider must look to the hospice for payment.

Professional services related to the hospice patient's terminal condition that were furnished by an independent attending physician, who may be a nurse practitioner, are billed to the Medicare contractor through Medicare Part B. When the independent attending physician furnishes a terminal illness related service that includes both a professional and technical component (e.g., x-rays), he/she bills the professional component of such services to the Medicare contractor on a professional claim and looks to the hospice for payment for the technical component. Likewise, the independent attending physician, who may be a nurse practitioner, would look to the hospice for payment for terminal illness related services furnished that have no professional component (e.g., clinical lab tests). The remainder of this section explains this in greater detail.

When a Medicare beneficiary elects hospice coverage he/she may designate an attending physician, who may be a nurse practitioner, not employed by the hospice, in addition to receiving care from hospice-employed physicians. The professional services of a non-hospice affiliated attending physician for the treatment and management of a hospice patient's terminal illness are not considered Medicare Part A "hospice services." These independent attending physician services are billed through Medicare Part B to the Medicare contractor, provided they were not furnished under a payment arrangement with the hospice. The independent attending physician codes services with the GV modifier "Attending physician not employed or paid under agreement by the patient's hospice provider" when billing his/her professional services furnished for the treatment and management of a hospice patient's terminal condition. The Medicare contractor makes payment to the independent attending physician or beneficiary, as appropriate, based on the payment and deductible rules applicable to each covered service.

Payments for the services of an independent attending physician are not counted in determining whether the hospice cap amount has been exceeded because Part B services provided by an independent attending physician are not part of the hospice's care.

Services provided by an independent attending physician who may be a nurse practitioner must be coordinated with any direct care services provided by hospice physicians.

Only the direct professional services of an independent attending physician, who may be a nurse practitioner, to a patient may be billed; the costs for services such as lab or x-rays are not to be included in the bill.

If another physician covers for a hospice patient's designated attending physician, the services of the substituting physician are billed by the designated attending physician under the reciprocal or locum tenens billing instructions. In such instances, the attending physician bills using the GV modifier in conjunction with either the Q5 or Q6 modifier.

When services related to a hospice patient's terminal condition are furnished under a payment arrangement with the hospice by the designated attending physician who may be a nurse practitioner (i.e., by a non-independent physician/nurse practitioner), the physician must look to the hospice for payment. In this situation the physicians' services are Part A hospice services and are billed by the hospice to its Medicare contractor.

Medicare contractors must process and pay for covered, medically necessary Part B services that physicians furnish to patients after their hospice benefits are revoked even if the patient remains under the care of the hospice. Such services are billed without the GV or GW modifiers. Make payment based on applicable Medicare payment and deductible rules for each covered service even if the beneficiary continues to be treated by the hospice after hospice benefits are revoked.

The CWF response contains the periods of hospice entitlement. This information is a permanent part of the notice and is furnished on all CWF replies and automatic notices. Medicare contractor use the CWF reply for validating dates of hospice coverage and to research, examine and adjudicate services coded with the GV or GW modifiers.

100-04, 12, 20.4.7

Services That Do Not Meet the National Electrical Manufacturers Association (NEMA) Standard XR-29-2013
(Rev. 3820, Issued: 11-21-17, Effective: 01-01-18, Implementation; 01-02-18)

Several provisions provide for a payment reduction to the technical component (and the technical component of the global fee) for X-rays and imaging services under certain circumstances. Please see Chapter 13, Section 20.2 of this publication for more information.

100-04, 12, 30.1

Digestive System
(Rev. 3368, Issued: 10-09-15, Effective: 01-01-16, Implementation: 01-01-16)

A. Upper Gastrointestinal Endoscopy Including Endoscopic Ultrasound (EUS) (Code 43259)

If the person performing the original diagnostic endoscopy has access to the EUS and the clinical situation requires an EUS, the EUS may be done at the same time. The procedure, diagnostic and EUS, is reported under the same code, CPT 43259. This code conforms to CPT guidelines for the indented codes. The service represented by the indented code, in this case code 43259 for EUS, includes the service represented by the unintended code preceding the list of indented codes. Therefore, when a diagnostic examination of the upper gastrointestinal tract "including esophagus, stomach, and either the duodenum or jejunum as appropriate," includes the use of endoscopic ultrasonography, the service is reported by a single code, namely 43259.

Interpretation, whether by a radiologist or endoscopist, is reported under CPT code 76975-26. These codes may both be reported on the same day.

B. Incomplete Colonoscopies (Codes 44388, 45378, G0105 and G0121)

An incomplete colonoscopy, e.g., the inability to advance the colonoscope to the cecum or colon-small intestine anastomosis due to unforeseen circumstances, is billed and paid using colonoscopy through stoma code 44388, colonoscopy code 45378, and screening colonoscopy codes G0105 and G0121 with modifier "-53." (Code 44388 is valid with modifier 53 beginning January 1, 2016.) The Medicare physician fee schedule database has specific values for codes 44388-53, 45378-53, G0105-53 and G0121-53. An incomplete colonoscopy performed prior to January 1, 2016, is paid at the same rate as a sigmoidoscopy. Beginning January 1, 2016, Medicare will pay for the interrupted colonoscopy at a rate that is calculated using one-half the value of the inputs for the codes.

100-04, 12, 30.6.2

Billing for Medically Necessary Visit on Same Occasion as Preventive Medicine Service
(Rev. 1, 10-01-03)

See Chapter 18 for payment for covered preventive services.

When a physician furnishes a Medicare beneficiary a covered visit at the same place and on the same occasion as a noncovered preventive medicine service (CPT codes 99381- 99397), consider the covered visit to be provided in lieu of a part of the preventive medicine service of equal value to the visit. A preventive medicine service (CPT codes 99381-99397) is a noncovered service. The physician may charge the beneficiary, as a charge for the noncovered remainder of the service, the amount by which the physician's current established charge for the preventive medicine service exceeds his/her current established charge for the covered visit. Pay for the covered visit based on the lesser of the fee schedule amount or the physician's actual charge for the visit. The physician is not required to give the beneficiary written advance notice of noncoverage of the part of the visit that constitutes a routine preventive visit. However, the physician is responsible for notifying the patient in advance of his/her liability for the charges for services that are not medically necessary to treat the illness or injury.

There could be covered and noncovered procedures performed during this encounter (e.g., screening x-ray, EKG, lab tests.). These are considered individually. Those procedures which are for screening for asymptomatic conditions are considered noncovered and, therefore, no payment is made. Those procedures ordered to diagnose or monitor a symptom, medical condition, or treatment are evaluated for medical necessity and, if covered, are paid.

100-04, 12, 30.6.4

Evaluation and Management (E/M) Services Furnished Incident to Physician's Service by Nonphysician Practitioners
(Rev. 1, 10-01-03)

When evaluation and management services are furnished incident to a physician's service by a nonphysician practitioner, the physician may bill the CPT code that describes the evaluation and management service furnished.

When evaluation and management services are furnished incident to a physician's service by a nonphysician employee of the physician, not as part of a physician service, the physician bills code 99211 for the service.

A physician is not precluded from billing under the "incident to" provision for services provided by employees whose services cannot be paid for directly under the Medicare program. Employees of the physician may provide services incident to the physician's service, but the physician alone is permitted to bill Medicare.

Services provided by employees as "incident to" are covered when they meet all the requirements for incident to and are medically necessary for the individual needs of the patient.

100-04, 12, 30.6.7

Payment for Office or Other Outpatient Evaluation and Management (E/M) Visits
(Rev. 3315, Issued: 08-06-15, Effective: 01-01-16, Implementation: 01-04-16)

A. Definition of New Patient for Selection of E/M Visit Code

Interpret the phrase "new patient" to mean a patient who has not received any professional services, i.e., E/M service or other face-to-face service (e.g., surgical procedure) from the physician or physician group practice (same physician specialty) within the previous 3 years. For example, if a professional component of a previous procedure is billed in a 3 year time period, e.g., a lab interpretation is billed and no E/M service or other face-to-face service with the patient is performed, then this patient remains a new patient for the initial visit. An interpretation of a diagnostic test, reading an x-ray or EKG etc., in the absence of an E/M service or other face-to-face service with the patient does not affect the designation of a new patient.

B. Office/Outpatient E/M Visits Provided on Same Day for Unrelated Problems

As for all other E/M services except where specifically noted, the Medicare Administrative Contractors (MACs) may not pay two E/M office visits billed by a physician (or physician of the same specialty from the same group practice) for the same beneficiary on the same day unless the physician documents that the visits were for unrelated problems in the office, off campus-outpatient hospital, or on campus-outpatient hospital setting which could not be provided during the same encounter (e.g., office visit for blood pressure medication evaluation, followed five hours later by a visit for evaluation of leg pain following an accident).

C. Office/Outpatient or Emergency Department E/M Visit on Day of Admission to Nursing Facility
MACs may not pay a physician for an emergency department visit or an office visit and a comprehensive nursing facility assessment on the same day. Bundle E/M visits on the same date provided in sites other than the nursing facility into the initial nursing facility care code when performed on the same date as the nursing facility admission by the same physician.

D. Drug Administration Services and E/M Visits Billed on Same Day of Service
MACs must advise physicians that CPT code 99211 cannot be paid if it is billed with a drug administration service such as a chemotherapy or nonchemotherapy drug infusion code (effective January 1, 2004). This drug administration policy was expanded in the Physician Fee Schedule Final Rule, November 15, 2004, to also include a therapeutic or diagnostic injection code (effective January 1, 2005). Therefore, when a medically necessary, significant and separately identifiable E/M service (which meets a higher complexity level than CPT code 99211) is performed, in addition to one of these drug administration services, the appropriate E/M CPT code should be reported with modifier -25. Documentation should support the level of E/M service billed. For an E/M service provided on the same day, a different diagnosis is not required.

100-04, 12, 30.6.8

Payment for Hospital Observation Services and Observation or Inpatient Care Services (Including Admission and Discharge Services)
(Rev. 2282, Issued: 08-26-11, Effective: 01-01-11, Implementation: 11-28-11)

A. Who May Bill Observation Care Codes
Observation care is a well-defined set of specific, clinically appropriate services, which include ongoing short term treatment, assessment, and reassessment, that are furnished while a decision is being made regarding whether patients will require further treatment as hospital inpatients or if they are able to be discharged from the hospital. Observation services are commonly ordered for patients who present to the emergency department and who then require a significant period of treatment or monitoring in order to make a decision concerning their admission or discharge.

In only rare and exceptional cases do reasonable and necessary outpatient observation services span more than 48 hours. In the majority of cases, the decision whether to discharge a patient from the hospital following resolution of the reason for the observation care or to admit the patient as an inpatient can be made in less than 48 hours, usually in less than 24 hours.

Contractors pay for initial observation care billed by only the physician who ordered hospital outpatient observation services and was responsible for the patient during his/her observation care. A physician who does not have inpatient admitting privileges but who is authorized to furnish hospital outpatient observation services may bill these codes.

For a physician to bill observation care codes, there must be a medical observation record for the patient which contains dated and timed physician's orders regarding the observation services the patient is to receive, nursing notes, and progress notes prepared by the physician while the patient received observation services. This record must be in addition to any record prepared as a result of an emergency department or outpatient clinic encounter.

Payment for an initial observation care code is for all the care rendered by the ordering physician on the date the patient's observation services began. All other physicians who furnish consultations or additional evaluations or services while the patient is receiving hospital outpatient observation services must bill the appropriate outpatient service codes.

For example, if an internist orders observation services and asks another physician to additionally evaluate the patient, only the internist may bill the initial and subsequent observation care codes. The other physician who evaluates the patient must bill the new or established office or other outpatient visit codes as appropriate.

For information regarding hospital billing of observation services, see Chapter 4, §290.

B. Physician Billing for Observation Care Following Initiation of Observation Services
Similar to initial observation codes, payment for a subsequent observation care code is for all the care rendered by the treating physician on the day(s) other than the initial or discharge date. All other physicians who furnish consultations or additional evaluations or services while the patient is receiving hospital outpatient observation services must bill the appropriate outpatient service codes.

When a patient receives observation care for less than 8 hours on the same calendar date, the Initial Observation Care, from CPT code range 99218 – 99220, shall be reported by the physician. The Observation Care Discharge Service, CPT code 99217, shall not be reported for this scenario.

When a patient is admitted for observation care and then is discharged on a different calendar date, the physician shall report Initial Observation Care, from CPT code range 99218 – 99220, and CPT observation care discharge CPT code 99217. On the rare occasion when a patient remains in observation care for 3 days, the physician shall report an initial observation care code (99218-99220) for the first day of observation care, a subsequent observation care code (99224-99226) for the second

day of observation care, and an observation care discharge CPT code 99217 for the observation care on the discharge date. When observation care continues beyond 3 days, the physician shall report a subsequent observation care code (99224-99226) for each day between the first day of observation care and the discharge date.

When a patient receives observation care for a minimum of 8 hours, but less than 24 hours, and is discharged on the same calendar date, Observation or Inpatient Care Services (Including Admission and Discharge Services) from CPT code range 99234 – 99236 shall be reported. The observation discharge, CPT code 99217, cannot also be reported for this scenario.

C. Documentation Requirements for Billing Observation or Inpatient Care Services (Including Admission and Discharge Services)
The physician shall satisfy the E/M documentation guidelines for furnishing observation care or inpatient hospital care. In addition to meeting the documentation requirements for history, examination, and medical decision making, documentation in the medical record shall include:

- Documentation stating the stay for observation care or inpatient hospital care involves 8 hours, but less than 24 hours;
- Documentation identifying the billing physician was present and personally performed the services; and
- Documentation identifying the order for observation services, progress notes, and discharge notes were written by the billing physician.

In the rare circumstance when a patient receives observation services for more than 2 calendar dates, the physician shall bill observation services furnished on day(s) other than the initial or discharge date using subsequent observation care codes. The physician may not use the subsequent hospital care codes since the patient is not an inpatient of the hospital.

D. Admission to Inpatient Status Following Observation Care
If the same physician who ordered hospital outpatient observation services also admits the patient to inpatient status before the end of the date on which the patient began receiving hospital outpatient observation services, pay only an initial hospital visit for the evaluation and management services provided on that date. Medicare payment for the initial hospital visit includes all services provided to the patient on the date of admission by that physician, regardless of the site of service. The physician may not bill an initial or subsequent observation care code for services on the date that he or she admits the patient to inpatient status. If the patient is admitted to inpatient status from hospital outpatient observation care subsequent to the date of initiation of observation services, the physician must bill an initial hospital visit for the services provided on that date. The physician may not bill the hospital observation discharge management code (code 99217) or an outpatient/office visit for the care provided while the patient received hospital outpatient observation services on the date of admission to inpatient status.

E. Hospital Observation Services During Global Surgical Period
The global surgical fee includes payment for hospital observation (codes 99217, 99218, 99219, 99220, 99224, 99225, 99226, 99234, 99235, and 99236) services unless the criteria for use of CPT modifiers "-24," "-25," or "-57" are met. Contractors must pay for these services in addition to the global surgical fee only if both of the following requirements are met:

- The hospital observation service meets the criteria needed to justify billing it with CPT modifiers "-24," "-25," or "-57" (decision for major surgery); and
- The hospital observation service furnished by the surgeon meets all of the criteria for the hospital observation code billed.

Examples of the decision for surgery during a hospital observation period are:

- An emergency department physician orders hospital outpatient observation services for a patient with a head injury. A neurosurgeon is called in to evaluate the need for surgery while the patient is receiving observation services and decides that the patient requires surgery. The surgeon would bill a new or established office or other outpatient visit code as appropriate with the "-57" modifier to indicate that the decision for surgery was made during the evaluation. The surgeon must bill the office or other outpatient visit code because the patient receiving hospital outpatient observation services is not an inpatient of the hospital. Only the physician who ordered hospital outpatient observation services may bill for observation care.
- A neurosurgeon orders hospital outpatient observation services for a patient with a head injury. During the observation period, the surgeon makes the decision for surgery. The surgeon would bill the appropriate level of hospital observation code with the "-57" modifier to indicate that the decision for surgery was made while the surgeon was providing hospital observation care.

Examples of hospital observation services during the postoperative period of a surgery are:

- A surgeon orders hospital outpatient observation services for a patient with abdominal pain from a kidney stone on the 80th day following a TURP (performed by that surgeon). The surgeon decides that the patient does not require surgery. The surgeon would bill the observation code with CPT modifier "-24" and documentation to support that the observation services are unrelated to the surgery.
- A surgeon orders hospital outpatient observation services for a patient with abdominal pain on the 80th day following a TURP (performed by that surgeon). While the patient is receiving hospital outpatient observation services, the surgeon decides that the patient requires kidney surgery. The surgeon would bill the observation code with HCPCS modifier "-57" to indicate that the decision for

surgery was made while the patient was receiving hospital outpatient observation services. The subsequent surgical procedure would be reported with modifier "-79."

- A surgeon orders hospital outpatient observation services for a patient with abdominal pain on the 20th day following a resection of the colon (performed by that surgeon). The surgeon determines that the patient requires no further colon surgery and discharges the patient. The surgeon may not bill for the observation services furnished during the global period because they were related to the previous surgery.

An example of a billable hospital observation service on the same day as a procedure is when a physician repairs a laceration of the scalp in the emergency department for a patient with a head injury and then subsequently orders hospital outpatient observation services for that patient. The physician would bill the observation code with a CPT modifier 25 and the procedure code.

100-04, 12, 30.6.9

Payment for Inpatient Hospital Visits - General
(Rev. 2282, Issued: 08-26-11, Effective: 01-01-11, Implementation: 11-28-11)

A. Hospital Visit and Critical Care on Same Day
When a hospital inpatient or office/outpatient evaluation and management service (E/M) are furnished on a calendar date at which time the patient does not require critical care and the patient subsequently requires critical care both the critical Care Services (CPT codes 99291 and 99292) and the previous E/M service may be paid on the same date of service. Hospital emergency department services are not paid for the same date as critical care services when provided by the same physician to the same patient.

During critical care management of a patient those services that do not meet the level of critical care shall be reported using an inpatient hospital care service with CPT Subsequent Hospital Care using a code from CPT code range 99231 – 99233.

Both Initial Hospital Care (CPT codes 99221 – 99223) and Subsequent Hospital Care codes are "per diem" services and may be reported only once per day by the same physician or physicians of the same specialty from the same group practice.

Physicians and qualified nonphysician practitioners (NPPs) are advised to retain documentation for discretionary contractor review should claims be questioned for both hospital care and critical care claims. The retained documentation shall support claims for critical care when the same physician or physicians of the same specialty in a group practice report critical care services for the same patient on the same calendar date as other E/M services.

B. Two Hospital Visits Same Day
Contractors pay a physician for only one hospital visit per day for the same patient, whether the problems seen during the encounters are related or not. The inpatient hospital visit descriptors contain the phrase "per day" which means that the code and the payment established for the code represent all services provided on that date. The physician should select a code that reflects all services provided during the date of the service.

C. Hospital Visits Same Day But by Different Physicians
In a hospital inpatient situation involving one physician covering for another, if physician A sees the patient in the morning and physician B, who is covering for A, sees the same patient in the evening, contractors do not pay physician B for the second visit. The hospital visit descriptors include the phrase "per day" meaning care for the day.

If the physicians are each responsible for a different aspect of the patient's care, pay both visits if the physicians are in different specialties and the visits are billed with different diagnoses. There are circumstances where concurrent care may be billed by physicians of the same specialty.

D. Visits to Patients in Swing Beds
If the inpatient care is being billed by the hospital as inpatient hospital care, the hospital care codes apply. If the inpatient care is being billed by the hospital as nursing facility care, then the nursing facility codes apply.

100-04, 12, 30.6.9.1

Payment for Initial Hospital Care Services and Observation or Inpatient Care Services (Including Admission and Discharge Services)
(Rev. 2282, Issued: 08-26-11, Effective: 01-01-11, Implementation: 11-28-11)

A. Initial Hospital Care From Emergency Room
Contractors pay for an initial hospital care service if a physician sees a patient in the emergency room and decides to admit the person to the hospital. They do not pay for both E/M services. Also, they do not pay for an emergency department visit by the same physician on the same date of service. When the patient is admitted to the hospital via another site of service (e.g., hospital emergency department, physician's office, nursing facility), all services provided by the physician in conjunction with that admission are considered part of the initial hospital care when performed on the same date as the admission.

B. Initial Hospital Care on Day Following Visit
Contractors pay both visits if a patient is seen in the office on one date and admitted to the hospital on the next date, even if fewer than 24 hours has elapsed between the visit and the admission.

C. Initial Hospital Care and Discharge on Same Day
When the patient is admitted to inpatient hospital care for less than 8 hours on the same date, then Initial Hospital Care, from CPT code range 99221 – 99223, shall be reported by the physician. The Hospital Discharge Day Management service, CPT codes 99238 or 99239, shall not be reported for this scenario.

When a patient is admitted to inpatient initial hospital care and then discharged on a different calendar date, the physician shall report an Initial Hospital Care from CPT code range 99221 – 99223 and a Hospital Discharge Day Management service, CPT code 99238 or 99239.

When a patient has been admitted to inpatient hospital care for a minimum of 8 hours but less than 24 hours and discharged on the same calendar date, Observation or Inpatient Hospital Care Services (Including Admission and Discharge Services), from CPT code range 99234 – 99236, shall be reported.

D. Documentation Requirements for Billing Observation or Inpatient Care Services (Including Admission and Discharge Services)
The physician shall satisfy the E/M documentation guidelines for admission to and discharge from inpatient observation or hospital care. In addition to meeting the documentation requirements for history, examination and medical decision making documentation in the medical record shall include:

- Documentation stating the stay for hospital treatment or observation care status involves 8 hours but less than 24 hours;
- Documentation identifying the billing physician was present and personally performed the services; and
- Documentation identifying the admission and discharge notes were written by the billing physician.

E. Physician Services Involving Transfer From One Hospital to Another; Transfer Within Facility to Prospective Payment System (PPS) Exempt Unit of Hospital; Transfer From One Facility to Another Separate Entity Under Same Ownership and/or Part of Same Complex; or Transfer From One Department to Another Within Single Facility
Physicians may bill both the hospital discharge management code and an initial hospital care code when the discharge and admission do not occur on the same day if the transfer is between:

- Different hospitals;
- Different facilities under common ownership which do not have merged records; or
- Between the acute care hospital and a PPS exempt unit within the same hospital when there are no merged records.

In all other transfer circumstances, the physician should bill only the appropriate level of subsequent hospital care for the date of transfer.

F. Initial Hospital Care Service History and Physical That Is Less Than Comprehensive
When a physician performs a visit that meets the definition of a Level 5 office visit several days prior to an admission and on the day of admission performs less than a comprehensive history and physical, he or she should report the office visit that reflects the services furnished and also report the lowest level initial hospital care code (i.e., code 99221) for the initial hospital admission. Contractors pay the office visit as billed and the Level 1 initial hospital care code.

Physicians who provide an initial visit to a patient during inpatient hospital care that meets the minimum key component work and/or medical necessity requirements shall report an initial hospital care code (99221-99223). The principal physician of record shall append modifier "-AI" (Principal Physician of Record) to the claim for the initial hospital care code. This modifier will identify the physician who oversees the patient's care from all other physicians who may be furnishing specialty care.

Physicians may bill initial hospital care service codes (99221-99223), for services that were reported with CPT consultation codes (99241 – 99255) prior to January 1, 2010, when the furnished service and documentation meet the minimum key component work and/or medical necessity requirements. Physicians must meet all the requirements of the initial hospital care codes, including "a detailed or comprehensive history" and "a detailed or comprehensive examination" to report CPT code 99221, which are greater than the requirements for consultation codes 99251 and 99252.

Subsequent hospital care CPT codes 99231 and 99232, respectively, require "a problem focused interval history" and "an expanded problem focused interval history." An E/M service that could be described by CPT consultation code 99251 or 99252 could potentially meet the component work and medical necessity requirements to report 99231 or 99232. Physicians may report a subsequent hospital care CPT code for services that were reported as CPT consultation codes (99241 – 99255) prior to January 1, 2010, where the medical record appropriately demonstrates that the work and medical necessity requirements are met for reporting a subsequent hospital care code (under the level selected), even though the reported code is for the provider's first E/M service to the inpatient during the hospital stay.

Reporting CPT code 99499 (Unlisted evaluation and management service) should be limited to cases where there is no other specific E/M code payable by Medicare that describes that service.

Reporting CPT code 99499 requires submission of medical records and contractor manual medical review of the service prior to payment. Contractors shall expect reporting under these circumstances to be unusual.

G. Initial Hospital Care Visits by Two Different M.D.s or D.O.s When They Are Involved in Same Admission

In the inpatient hospital setting all physicians (and qualified nonphysician practitioners where permitted) who perform an initial evaluation may bill the initial hospital care codes (99221 – 99223) or nursing facility care codes (99304 – 99306). Contractors consider only one M.D. or D.O. to be the principal physician of record (sometimes referred to as the admitting physician.) The principal physician of record is identified in Medicare as the physician who oversees the patient's care from other physicians who may be furnishing specialty care. Only the principal physician of record shall append modifier "-AI" (Principal Physician of Record) in addition to the E/M code. Follow-up visits in the facility setting shall be billed as subsequent hospital care visits and subsequent nursing facility care visits.

100-04, 12, 30.6.9.2

Subsequent Hospital Visit and Hospital Discharge Day Management (Codes 99231–99239)
(Rev. 1460, Issued: 02-22-08, Effective: 04-01-08, Implementation: 04-07-08)

A. Subsequent Hospital Visits During the Global Surgery Period
(Refer to Secs.40-40.4 on global surgery) The Medicare physician fee schedule payment amount for surgical procedures includes all services (e.g., evaluation and management visits) that are part of the global surgery payment; therefore, contractors shall not pay more than that amount when a bill is fragmented for staged procedures.

B. Hospital Discharge Day Management Service Hospital Discharge Day
Management Services, CPT code 99238 or 99239 is a face-to-face evaluation and management (E/M) service between the attending physician and the patient. The E/M discharge day management visit shall be reported for the date of the actual visit by the physician or qualified nonphysician practitioner even if the patient is discharged from the facility on a different calendar date. Only one hospital discharge day management service is payable per patient per hospital stay.

Only the attending physician of record reports the discharge day management service. Physicians or qualified nonphysician practitioners, other than the attending physician, who have been managing concurrent health care problems not primarily managed by the attending physician, and who are not acting on behalf of the attending physician, shall use Subsequent Hospital Care (CPT code range 99231 - 99233) for a final visit.

Medicare pays for the paperwork of patient discharge day management through the pre- and post- service work of an E/M service.

C. Subsequent Hospital Visit and Discharge Management on Same Day
Pay only the hospital discharge management code on the day of discharge (unless it is also the day of admission, in which case, refer to Sec.30.6.9.1 C for the policy on Observation or Inpatient Care Services (Including Admission and Discharge Services CPT Codes 99234 - 99236). Contractors do not pay both a subsequent hospital visit in addition to hospital discharge day management service on the same day by the same physician. Instruct physicians that they may not bill for both a hospital visit and hospital discharge management for the same date of service.

D. Hospital Discharge Management (CPT Codes 99238 and 99239) and Nursing Facility Admission Code When Patient Is Discharged From Hospital and Admitted to Nursing Facility on Same Day
Contractors pay the hospital discharge code (codes 99238 or 99239) in addition to a nursing facility admission code when they are billed by the same physician with the same date of service.

If a surgeon is admitting the patient to the nursing facility due to a condition that is not as a result of the surgery during the postoperative period of a service with the global surgical period, he/she bills for the nursing facility admission and care with a modifier "-24" and provides documentation that the service is unrelated to the surgery (e.g., return of an elderly patient to the nursing facility in which he/she has resided for five years following discharge from the hospital for cholecystectomy).

Contractors do not pay for a nursing facility admission by a surgeon in the postoperative period of a procedure with a global surgical period if the patient's admission to the nursing facility is to receive post operative care related to the surgery (e.g., admission to a nursing facility to receive physical therapy following a hip replacement). Payment for the nursing facility admission and subsequent nursing facility services are included in the global fee and cannot be paid separately.

E. Hospital Discharge Management and Death Pronouncement
Only the physician who personally performs the pronouncement of death shall bill for the face-to-face Hospital Discharge Day Management Service, CPT code 99238 or 99239. The date of the pronouncement shall reflect the calendar date of service on the day it was performed even if the paperwork is delayed to a subsequent date.

100-04, 12, 30.6.10

Consultation Services
(Rev. 2282, Issued: 08-26-11, Effective: 01-01-11, Implementation: 11-28-11)

Consultation Services versus Other Evaluation and Management (E/M) Visits

Effective January 1, 2010, the consultation codes are no longer recognized for Medicare Part B payment. Physicians shall code patient evaluation and management visits with E/M codes that represent where the visit occurs and that identify the complexity of the visit performed.

In the inpatient hospital setting and the nursing facility setting, physicians (and qualified nonphysician practitioners where permitted) may bill the most appropriate initial hospital care code (99221-99223), subsequent hospital care code (99231 and 99232), initial nursing facility care code (99304-99306), or subsequent nursing facility care code (99307-99310) that reflects the services the physician or practitioner furnished. Subsequent hospital care codes could potentially meet the component work and medical necessity requirements to be reported for an E/M service that could be described by CPT consultation code 99251 or 99252. Contractors shall not find fault in cases where the medical record appropriately demonstrates that the work and medical necessity requirements are met for reporting a subsequent hospital care code (under the level selected), even though the reported code is for the provider's first E/M service to the inpatient during the hospital stay. Unlisted evaluation and management service (code 99499) shall only be reported for consultation services when an E/M service that could be described by codes 99251 or 99252 is furnished, and there is no other specific E/M code payable by Medicare that describes that service. Reporting code 99499 requires submission of medical records and contractor manual medical review of the service prior to payment. CMS expects reporting under these circumstances to be unusual. T he principal physician of record is identified in Medicare as the physician who oversees the patient's care from other physicians who may be furnishing specialty care. The principal physician of record shall append modifier "-AI" (Principal Physician of Record), in addition to the E/M code. Follow-up visits in the facility setting shall be billed as subsequent hospital care visits and subsequent nursing facility care visits.

In the CAH setting, those CAHs that use method II shall bill the appropriate new or established visit code for those physician and non-physician practitioners who have reassigned their billing rights, depending on the relationship status between the physician and patient.

In the office or other outpatient setting where an evaluation is performed, physicians and qualified nonphysician practitioners shall use the CPT codes (99201 – 99215) depending on the complexity of the visit and whether the patient is a new or established patient to that physician. All physicians and qualified nonphysician practitioners shall follow the E/M documentation guidelines for all E/M services. These rules are applicable for Medicare secondary payer claims as well as for claims in which Medicare is the primary payer.

100-04, 12, 30.6.11

Emergency Department Visits (Codes 99281–99288)
(Rev. 1875, Issued: 12-14-09, Effective: 01-01-10, Implementation: 01-04-10)

A. Use of Emergency Department Codes by Physicians Not Assigned to Emergency Department
Any physician seeing a patient registered in the emergency department may use emergency department visit codes (for services matching the code description). It is not required that the physician be assigned to the emergency department.

B. Use of Emergency Department Codes In Office
Emergency department coding is not appropriate if the site of service is an office or outpatient setting or any sight of service other than an emergency department. The emergency department codes should only be used if the patient is seen in the emergency department and the services described by the HCPCS code definition are provided. The emergency department is defined as an organized hospital-based facility for the provision of unscheduled or episodic services to patients who present for immediate medical attention.

C. Use of Emergency Department Codes to Bill Nonemergency Services
Services in the emergency department may not be emergencies. However the codes (99281 - 99288) are payable if the described services are provided.

However, if the physician asks the patient to meet him or her in the emergency department as an alternative to the physician's office and the patient is not registered as a patient in the emergency department, the physician should bill the appropriate office/outpatient visit codes. Normally a lower level emergency department code would be reported for a nonemergency condition.

D. Emergency Department or Office/Outpatient Visits on Same Day As Nursing Facility Admission
Emergency department visit provided on the same day as a comprehensive nursing facility assessment are not paid. Payment for evaluation and management services on the same date provided in sites other than the nursing facility are included in the payment for initial nursing facility care when performed on the same date as the nursing facility admission.

E. Physician Billing for Emergency Department Services Provided to Patient by Both Patient's Personal Physician and Emergency Department Physician
If a physician advises his/her own patient to go to an emergency department (ED) of a hospital for care and the physician subsequently is asked by the ED physician to come to the hospital to evaluate the patient and to advise the ED physician as to

whether the patient should be admitted to the hospital or be sent home, the physicians should bill as follows:

If the patient is admitted to the hospital by the patient's personal physician, then the patient's regular physician should bill only the appropriate level of the initial hospital care (codes 99221 - 99223) because all evaluation and management services provided by that physician in conjunction with that admission are considered part of the initial hospital care when performed on the same date as the admission. The ED physician who saw the patient in the emergency department should bill the appropriate level of the ED codes.

If the ED physician, based on the advice of the patient's personal physician who came to the emergency department to see the patient, sends the patient home, then the ED physician should bill the appropriate level of emergency department service. The patient's personal physician should also bill the level of emergency department code that describes the service he or she provided in the emergency department. If the patient's personal physician does not come to the hospital to see the patient, but only advises the emergency department physician by telephone, then the patient's personal physician may not bill.

F. Emergency Department Physician Requests Another Physician to See the Patient in Emergency Department or Office/Outpatient Setting

If the emergency department physician requests that another physician evaluate a given patient, the other physician should bill an emergency department visit code. If the patient is admitted to the hospital by the second physician performing the evaluation, he or she should bill an initial hospital care code and not an emergency department visit code.

100-04, 12, 30.6.13

Nursing Facility Services

(Rev. 2282, Issued: 08-26-11, Effective: 01-01-11, Implementation: 11-28-11)

A. Visits to Perform the Initial Comprehensive Assessment and Annual Assessments

The distinction made between the delegation of physician visits and tasks in a skilled nursing facility (SNF) and in a nursing facility (NF) is based on the Medicare Statute. Section 1819 (b) (6) (A) of the Social Security Act (the Act) governs SNFs while section 1919 (b) (6) (A) of the Act governs NFs. For further information refer to Medlearn Matters article number SE0418 at www.cms.hhs.gov/medlearn/matters.

The federally mandated visits in a SNF and NF must be performed by the physician except as otherwise permitted (42 CFR 483.40 (c) (4) and (f)). The principal physician of record must append the modifier "-AI", (Principal Physician of Record), to the initial nursing facility care code. This modifier will identify the physician who oversees the patient's care from other physicians who may be furnishing specialty care. All other physicians or qualified NPPs who perform an initial evaluation in the NF or SNF may bill the initial nursing facility care code. The initial federally mandated visit is defined in S&C-04-08 (see www.cms.hhs.gov/medlearn/matters) as the initial comprehensive visit during which the physician completes a thorough assessment, develops a plan of care, and writes or verifies admitting orders for the nursing facility resident. For Survey and Certification requirements, a visit must occur no later than 30 days after admission.

Further, per the Long Term Care regulations at 42 CFR 483.40 (c) (4) and (e) (2), in a SNF the physician may not delegate a task that the physician must personally perform. Therefore, as stated in S&C-04-08 the physician may not delegate the initial federally mandated comprehensive visit in a SNF.

The only exception, as to who performs the initial visit, relates to the NF setting. In the NF setting, a qualified NPP (i.e., a nurse practitioner (NP), physician assistant (PA), or a clinical nurse specialist (CNS)), who is not employed by the facility, may perform the initial visit when the State law permits. The evaluation and management (E/M) visit shall be within the State scope of practice and licensure requirements where the E/M visit is performed and the requirements for physician collaboration and physician supervision shall be met.

Under Medicare Part B payment policy, other medically necessary E/M visits may be performed and reported prior to and after the initial visit, if the medical needs of the patient require an E/M visit. A qualified NPP may perform medically necessary E/M visits prior to and after the initial visit if all the requirements for collaboration, general physician supervision, licensure, and billing are met.

The CPT Nursing Facility Services codes shall be used with place of service (POS) 31 (SNF) if the patient is in a Part A SNF stay. They shall be used with POS 32 (nursing facility) if the patient does not have Part A SNF benefits or if the patient is in a NF or in a non-covered SNF stay (e.g., there was no preceding 3-day hospital stay). The CPT Nursing Facility code definition also includes POS 54 (Intermediate Care Facility/Mentally Retarded) and POS 56 (Psychiatric Residential Treatment Center). For further guidance on POS codes and associated CPT codes refer to §30.6.14.

Effective January 1, 2006, the Initial Nursing Facility Care codes 99301– 99303 are deleted.

Beginning January 1, 2006, the new CPT codes, Initial Nursing Facility Care, per day, (99304 – 99306) shall be used to report the initial federally mandated visit. Only a physician may report these codes for an initial federally mandated visit performed in a SNF or NF (with the exception of the qualified NPP in the NF setting who is not employed by the facility and when State law permits, as explained above).

A readmission to a SNF or NF shall have the same payment policy requirements as an initial admission in both the SNF and NF settings.

A physician who is employed by the SNF/NF may perform the E/M visits and bill independently to Medicare Part B for payment. An NPP who is employed by the SNF or NF may perform and bill Medicare Part B directly for those services where it is permitted as discussed above. The employer of the PA shall always report the visits performed by the PA. A physician, NP or CNS has the option to bill Medicare directly or to reassign payment for his/her professional service to the facility.

As with all E/M visits for Medicare Part B payment policy, the E/M documentation guidelines apply.

Medically Necessary Visits

Qualified NPPs may perform medically necessary E/M visits prior to and after the physician's initial federally mandated visit in both the SNF and NF. Medically necessary E/M visits for the diagnosis or treatment of an illness or injury or to improve the functioning of a malformed body member are payable under the physician fee schedule under Medicare Part B. A physician or NPP may bill the most appropriate initial nursing facility care code (CPT codes 99304-99306) or subsequent nursing facility care code (CPT codes 99307-99310), even if the E/M service is provided prior to the initial federally mandated visit.

SNF Setting--Place of Service Code 31

Following the initial federally mandated visit by the physician, the physician may delegate alternate federally mandated physician visits to a qualified NPP who meets collaboration and physician supervision requirements and is licensed as such by the State and performing within the scope of practice in that State.

NF Setting--Place of Service Code 32

Per the regulations at 42 CFR 483.40 (f), a qualified NPP, who meets the collaboration and physician supervision requirements, the State scope of practice and licensure requirements, and who is not employed by the NF, may at the option of the State, perform the initial federally mandated visit in a NF, and may perform any other federally mandated physician visit in a NF in addition to performing other medically necessary E/M visits.

Questions pertaining to writing orders or certification and recertification issues in the SNF and NF settings shall be addressed to the appropriate State Survey and Certification Agency departments for clarification.

B. Visits to Comply With Federal Regulations (42 CFR 483.40 (c) (1)) in the SNF and NF

Payment is made under the physician fee schedule by Medicare Part B for federally mandated visits. Following the initial federally mandated visit by the physician or qualified NPP where permitted, payment shall be made for federally mandated visits that monitor and evaluate residents at least once every 30 days for the first 90 days after admission and at least once every 60 days thereafter.

Effective January 1, 2006, the Subsequent Nursing Facility Care, per day, codes 99311– 99313 are deleted.

Beginning January 1, 2006, the new CPT codes, Subsequent Nursing Facility Care, per day, (99307 – 99310) shall be used to report federally mandated physician E/M visits and medically necessary E/M visits.

Carriers shall not pay for more than one E/M visit performed by the physician or qualified NPP for the same patient on the same date of service. The Nursing Facility Services codes represent a "per day" service.

The federally mandated E/M visit may serve also as a medically necessary E/M visit if the situation arises (i.e., the patient has health problems that need attention on the day the scheduled mandated physician E/M visit occurs). The physician/qualified NPP shall bill only one E/M visit.

Beginning January 1, 2006, the new CPT code, Other Nursing Facility Service (99318), may be used to report an annual nursing facility assessment visit on the required schedule of visits on an annual basis. For Medicare Part B payment policy, an annual nursing facility assessment visit code may substitute as meeting one of the federally mandated physician visits if the code requirements for CPT code 99318 are fully met and in lieu of reporting a Subsequent Nursing Facility Care, per day, service (codes 99307 – 99310). It shall not be performed in addition to the required number of federally mandated physician visits. The new CPT annual assessment code does not represent a new benefit service for Medicare Part B physician services.

Qualified NPPs, whether employed or not by the SNF, may perform alternating federally mandated physician visits, at the option of the physician, after the initial federally mandated visit by the physician in a SNF.

Qualified NPPs in the NF setting, who are not employed by the NF and who are working in collaboration with a physician, may perform federally mandated physician visits, at the option of the State.

Medicare Part B payment policy does not pay for additional E/M visits that may be required by State law for a facility admission or for other additional visits to satisfy facility or other administrative purposes. E/M visits, prior to and after the initial federally mandated physician visit, that are reasonable and medically necessary to meet the medical needs of the individual patient (unrelated to any State requirement or administrative purpose) are payable under Medicare Part B.

C. Visits by Qualified Nonphysician Practitioners

All E/M visits shall be within the State scope of practice and licensure requirements where the visit is performed and all the requirements for physician collaboration and physician supervision shall be met when performed and reported by qualified NPPs. General physician supervision and employer billing requirements shall be met for PA services in addition to the PA meeting the State scope of practice and licensure requirements where the E/M visit is performed.

Medically Necessary Visits

Qualified NPPs may perform medically necessary E/M visits prior to and after the physician's initial visit in both the SNF and NF. Medically necessary E/M visits for the diagnosis or treatment of an illness or injury or to improve the functioning of a malformed body member are payable under the physician fee schedule under Medicare Part B. A physician or NPP may bill the most appropriate initial nursing facility care code (CPT codes 99304-99306) or subsequent nursing facility care code (CPT codes 99307-99310), even if the E/M service is provided prior to the initial federally mandated visit.

SNF Setting--Place of Service Code 31

Following the initial federally mandated visit by the physician, the physician may delegate alternate federally mandated physician visits to a qualified NPP who meets collaboration and physician supervision requirements and is licensed as such by the State and performing within the scope of practice in that State.

NF Setting--Place of Service Code 32

Per the regulations at 42 CFR 483.40 (f), a qualified NPP, who meets the collaboration and physician supervision requirements, the State scope of practice and licensure requirements, and who is not employed by the NF, may at the option of the State, perform the initial federally mandated visit in a NF, and may perform any other federally mandated physician visit in a NF in addition to performing other medically necessary E/M visits.

Questions pertaining to writing orders or certification and recertification issues in the SNF and NF settings shall be addressed to the appropriate State Survey and Certification Agency departments for clarification.

D. Medically Complex Care

Payment is made for E/M visits to patients in a SNF who are receiving services for medically complex care upon discharge from an acute care facility when the visits are reasonable and medically necessary and documented in the medical record. Physicians and qualified NPPs shall report initial nursing facility care codes for their first visit with the patient. The principal physician of record must append the modifier "-AI" (Principal Physician of Record), to the initial nursing facility care code when billed to identify the physician who oversees the patient's care from other physicians who may be furnishing specialty care. Follow-up visits shall be billed as subsequent nursing facility care visits.

E. Incident to Services

Where a physician establishes an office in a SNF/NF, the "incident to" services and requirements are confined to this discrete part of the facility designated as his/her office. "Incident to" E/M visits, provided in a facility setting, are not payable under the Physician Fee Schedule for Medicare Part B. Thus, visits performed outside the designated "office" area in the SNF/NF would be subject to the coverage and payment rules applicable to the SNF/NF setting and shall not be reported using the CPT codes for office or other outpatient visits or use place of service code 11.

F. Use of the Prolonged Services Codes and Other Time-Related Services

Beginning January 1, 2008, typical/average time units for E/M visits in the SNF/NF settings are reestablished. Medically necessary prolonged services for E/M visits (codes 99356 and 99357) in a SNF or NF may be billed with the Nursing Facility Services in the code ranges (99304 – 99306, 99307 – 99310 and 99318).

Counseling and Coordination of Care Visits

With the reestablishment of typical/average time units, medically necessary E/M visits for counseling and coordination of care, for Nursing Facility Services in the code ranges (99304 – 99306, 99307 – 99310 and 99318) that are time-based services, may be billed with the appropriate prolonged services codes (99356 and 99357).

G. Multiple Visits

The complexity level of an E/M visit and the CPT code billed must be a covered and medically necessary visit for each patient (refer to §§1862 (a)(1)(A) of the Act). Claims for an unreasonable number of daily E/M visits by the same physician to multiple patients at a facility within a 24-hour period may result in medical review to determine medical necessity for the visits. The E/M visit (Nursing Facility Services) represents a "per day" service per patient as defined by the CPT code. The medical record must be personally documented by the physician or qualified NPP who performed the E/M visit and the documentation shall support the specific level of E/M visit to each individual patient.

H. Split/Shared E/M Visit

A split/shared E/M visit cannot be reported in the SNF/NF setting. A split/shared E/M visit is defined by Medicare Part B payment policy as a medically necessary encounter with a patient where the physician and a qualified NPP each personally perform a substantive portion of an E/M visit face-to-face with the same patient on the same date of service. A substantive portion of an E/M visit involves all or some portion of the history, exam or medical decision making key components of an E/M service. The physician and the qualified NPP must be in the same group practice or be employed by the same employer. The split/shared E/M visit applies only to selected E/M visits and settings (i.e., hospital inpatient, hospital outpatient, hospital observation, emergency department, office and non facility clinic visits, and prolonged visits associated with these E/M visit codes). The split/shared E/M policy does not apply to critical care services or procedures.

I. SNF/NF Discharge Day Management Service

Medicare Part B payment policy requires a face-to-face visit with the patient provided by the physician or the qualified NPP to meet the SNF/NF discharge day management service as defined by the CPT code. The E/M discharge day management visit shall be reported for the date of the actual visit by the physician or qualified NPP even if the patient is discharged from the facility on a different calendar date. The CPT codes 99315 – 99316 shall be reported for this visit. The Discharge Day Management Service may be reported using CPT code 99315 or 99316, depending on the code requirement, for a patient who has expired, but only if the physician or qualified NPP personally performed the death pronouncement.

100-04, 12, 30.6.14

Home Care and Domiciliary Care Visits (Codes 99324–99350)

(Rev. 775, Issued: 12-02-05, Effective: 01-01-06, Implementation: 01-03-06)

Physician Visits to Patients Residing in Various Places of Service

The American Medical Association's Current Procedural Terminology (CPT) 2006 new patient codes 99324 - 99328 and established patient codes 99334 - 99337(new codes beginning January 2006), for Domiciliary, Rest Home (e.g., Boarding Home), or Custodial Care Services, are used to report evaluation and management (E/M) services to residents residing in a facility which provides room, board, and other personal assistance services, generally on a long-term basis. These CPT codes are used to report E/M services in facilities assigned places of service (POS) codes 13 (Assisted Living Facility), 14 (Group Home), 33 (Custodial Care Facility) and 55 (Residential Substance Abuse Facility). Assisted living facilities may also be known as adult living facilities.

Physicians and qualified nonphysician practitioners (NPPs) furnishing E/M services to residents in a living arrangement described by one of the POS listed above must use the level of service code in the CPT code range 99324 - 99337 to report the service they provide. The CPT codes 99321 - 99333 for Domiciliary, Rest Home (e.g., Boarding Home), or Custodial Care Services are deleted beginning January, 2006.

Beginning in 2006, reasonable and medically necessary, face-to-face, prolonged services, represented by CPT codes 99354 - 99355, may be reported with the appropriate companion E/M codes when a physician or qualified NPP, provides a prolonged service involving direct (face-to-face) patient contact that is beyond the usual E/M visit service for a Domiciliary, Rest Home (e.g., Boarding Home) or Custodial Care Service. All the requirements for prolonged services at Sec.30.6.15.1 must be met.

The CPT codes 99341 through 99350, Home Services codes, are used to report E/M services furnished to a patient residing in his or her own private residence (e.g., private home, apartment, town home) and not residing in any type of congregate/shared facility living arrangement including assisted living facilities and group homes. The Home Services codes apply only to the specific 2-digit POS 12 (Home). Home Services codes may not be used for billing E/M services provided in settings other than in the private residence of an individual as described above.

Beginning in 2006, E/M services provided to patients residing in a Skilled Nursing Facility (SNF) or a Nursing Facility (NF) must be reported using the appropriate CPT level of service code within the range identified for Initial Nursing Facility Care (new CPT codes 99304 - 99306) and Subsequent Nursing Facility Care (new CPT codes 99307 - 99310). Use the CPT code, Other Nursing Facility Services (new CPT code 99318), for an annual nursing facility assessment. Use CPT codes 99315 - 99316 for SNF/NF discharge services. The CPT codes 99301 - 99303 and 99311 - 99313 are deleted beginning January, 2006. The Home Services codes should not be used for these places of service.

The CPT SNF/NF code definition includes intermediate care facilities (ICFs) and long term care facilities (LTCFs). These codes are limited to the specific 2-digit POS 31 (SNF), 32 (Nursing Facility), 54 (Intermediate Care Facility/Mentally Retarded) and 56 (Psychiatric Residential Treatment Center).

The CPT nursing facility codes should be used with POS 31 (SNF) if the patient is in a Part A SNF stay and POS 32 (nursing facility) if the patient does not have Part A SNF benefits. There is no longer a different payment amount for a Part A or Part B benefit period in these POS settings.

100-04, 12, 30.6.14.1

Home Care and Domiciliary Care Visits (Codes 99324–99350)

(Rev. 775, Issued: 12-02-05, Effective: 01-01-06, Implementation: 01-03-06)

Physician Visits to Patients Residing in Various Places of Service

The American Medical Association's Current Procedural Terminology (CPT) 2006 new patient codes 99324 - 99328 and established patient codes 99334 - 99337(new codes beginning January 2006), for Domiciliary, Rest Home (e.g., Boarding Home), or Custodial Care Services, are used to report evaluation and management (E/M) services to residents residing in a facility which provides room, board, and other personal assistance services, generally on a long-term basis. These CPT codes are used to report E/M services in facilities assigned places of service (POS) codes 13 (Assisted Living Facility), 14 (Group Home), 33 (Custodial Care Facility) and 55 (Residential Substance Abuse Facility). Assisted living facilities may also be known as adult living facilities.

Physicians and qualified nonphysician practitioners (NPPs) furnishing E/M services to residents in a living arrangement described by one of the POS listed above must use the level of service code in the CPT code range 99324 - 99337 to report the service they provide. The CPT codes 99321 - 99333 for Domiciliary, Rest Home (e.g., Boarding Home), or Custodial Care Services are deleted beginning January, 2006.

Beginning in 2006, reasonable and medically necessary, face-to-face, prolonged services, represented by CPT codes 99354 - 99355, may be reported with the appropriate companion E/M codes when a physician or qualified NPP, provides a prolonged service involving direct (face-to-face) patient contact that is beyond the usual E/M visit service for a Domiciliary, Rest Home (e.g., Boarding Home) or Custodial Care Service. All the requirements for prolonged services at §30.6.15.1 must be met.

The CPT codes 99341 through 99350, Home Services codes, are used to report E/M services furnished to a patient residing in his or her own private residence (e.g., private home, apartment, town home) and not residing in any type of congregate/shared facility living arrangement including assisted living facilities and group homes. The Home Services codes apply only to the specific 2-digit POS 12 (Home). Home Services codes may not be used for billing E/M services provided in settings other than in the private residence of an individual as described above.

Beginning in 2006, E/M services provided to patients residing in a Skilled Nursing Facility (SNF) or a Nursing Facility (NF) must be reported using the appropriate CPT level of service code within the range identified for Initial Nursing Facility Care (new CPT codes 99304 - 99306) and Subsequent Nursing Facility Care (new CPT codes 99307 - 99310). Use the CPT code, Other Nursing Facility Services (new CPT code 99318), for an annual nursing facility assessment. Use CPT codes 99315 - 99316 for SNF/NF discharge services. The CPT codes 99301 - 99303 and 99311 - 99313 are deleted beginning January, 2006. The Home Services codes should not be used for these places of service.

The CPT SNF/NF code definition includes intermediate care facilities (ICFs) and long term care facilities (LTCFs). These codes are limited to the specific 2-digit POS 31 (SNF), 32 (Nursing Facility), 54 (Intermediate Care Facility/Mentally Retarded) and 56 (Psychiatric Residential Treatment Center).

The CPT nursing facility codes should be used with POS 31 (SNF) if the patient is in a Part A SNF stay and POS 32 (nursing facility) if the patient does not have Part A SNF benefits. There is no longer a different payment amount for a Part A or Part B benefit period in these POS settings.

100-04, 12, 30.6.15.1

Prolonged Services With Direct Face-to-Face Patient Contact Service (ZZZ codes)

(Rev. 2282, Issued: 08-26-11, Effective: 01-01-11, Implementation: 11-28-11)

A. Definition

Prolonged physician services (CPT code 99354) in the office or other outpatient setting with direct face-to-face patient contact which require 1 hour beyond the usual service are payable when billed on the same day by the same physician or qualified nonphysician practitioner (NPP) as the companion evaluation and management codes. The time for usual service refers to the typical/average time units associated with the companion evaluation and management service as noted in the CPT code. Each additional 30 minutes of direct face-to-face patient contact following the first hour of prolonged services may be reported by CPT code 99355.

Prolonged physician services (code 99356) in the inpatient setting, with direct face-to-face patient contact which require 1 hour beyond the usual service are payable when they are billed on the same day by the same physician or qualified NPP as the companion evaluation and management codes. Each additional 30 minutes of direct face-to-face patient contact following the first hour of prolonged services may be reported by CPT code 99357.

Prolonged service of less than 30 minutes total duration on a given date is not separately reported because the work involved is included in the total work of the evaluation and management codes.

Code 99355 or 99357 may be used to report each additional 30 minutes beyond the first hour of prolonged services, based on the place of service. These codes may be used to report the final 15 – 30 minutes of prolonged service on a given date, if not otherwise billed. Prolonged service of less than 15 minutes beyond the first hour or less than 15 minutes beyond the final 30 minutes is not reported separately.

B. Required Companion Codes

- The companion evaluation and management codes for 99354 are the Office or Other Outpatient visit codes (99201 - 99205, 99212 – 99215), the Domiciliary, Rest Home, or Custodial Care Services codes (99324 – 99328, 99334 – 99337), the Home Services codes (99341 - 99345, 99347 – 99350);

- The companion codes for 99355 are 99354 and one of the evaluation and management codes required for 99354 to be used;

- The companion evaluation and management codes for 99356 are the Initial Hospital Care codes and Subsequent Hospital Care codes (99221 - 99223, 99231 – 99233); Nursing Facility Services codes (99304 -99318); or

- The companion codes for 99357 are 99356 and one of the evaluation and management codes required for 99356 to be used.

Prolonged services codes 99354 – 99357 are not paid unless they are accompanied by the companion codes as indicated.

C. Requirement for Physician Presence

Physicians may count only the duration of direct face-to-face contact between the physician and the patient (whether the service was continuous or not) beyond the typical/average time of the visit code billed to determine whether prolonged services can be billed and to determine the prolonged services codes that are allowable. In the case of prolonged office services, time spent by office staff with the patient, or time the patient remains unaccompanied in the office cannot be billed. In the case of prolonged hospital services, time spent reviewing charts or discussion of a patient with house medical staff and not with direct face-to-face contact with the patient, or

waiting for test results, for changes in the patient's condition, for end of a therapy, or for use of facilities cannot be billed as prolonged services.

D. Documentation

Documentation is not required to accompany the bill for prolonged services unless the physician has been selected for medical review. Documentation is required in the medical record about the duration and content of the medically necessary evaluation and management service and prolonged services billed. The medical record must be appropriately and sufficiently documented by the physician or qualified NPP to show that the physician or qualified NPP personally furnished the direct face-to-face time with the patient specified in the CPT code definitions. The start and end times of the visit shall be documented in the medical record along with the date of service.

E. Use of the Codes

Prolonged services codes can be billed only if the total duration of the physician or qualified NPP direct face-to-face service (including the visit) equals or exceeds the threshold time for the evaluation and management service the physician or qualified NPP provided (typical/average time associated with the CPT E/M code plus 30 minutes). If the total duration of direct face-to-face time does not equal or exceed the threshold time for the level of evaluation and management service the physician or qualified NPP provided, the physician or qualified NPP may not bill for prolonged services.

F. Threshold Times for Codes 99354 and 99355 (Office or Other Outpatient Setting)

If the total direct face-to-face time equals or exceeds the threshold time for code 99354, but is less than the threshold time for code 99355, the physician should bill the evaluation and management visit code and code 99354. No more than one unit of 99354 is acceptable. If the total direct face-to-face time equals or exceeds the threshold time for code 99355 by no more than 29 minutes, the physician should bill the visit code 99354 and one unit of code 99355. One additional unit of code 99355 is billed for each additional increment of 30 minutes extended duration. Contractors use the following threshold times to determine if the prolonged services codes 99354 and/or 99355 can be billed with the office or other outpatient settings including domiciliary, rest home, or custodial care services and home services codes.

Threshold Time for Prolonged Visit Codes 99354 and/or 99355 Billed with Office/Outpatient Code

Code	Typical Time for Code	Threshold Time to Bill Code 99354	Threshold Time to Bill Codes 99354 and 99355
99201	10	40	85
99202	20	50	95
99203	30	60	105
99204	45	75	120
99205	60	90	135
99212	10	40	85
99213	15	45	90
99214	25	55	100
99215	40	70	115
99324	20	50	95
99325	30	60	105
99326	45	75	120
99327	60	90	135
99328	75	105	150
99334	15	45	90
99335	25	55	100
99336	40	70	115
99337	60	90	135
99341	20	50	95
99342	30	60	105
99343	45	75	120
99344	60	90	135
99345	75	105	150
99347	15	45	90
99348	25	55	100
99349	40	70	115
99350	60	90	135

G. Threshold Times for Codes 99356 and 99357

(Inpatient Setting) If the total direct face-to-face time equals or exceeds the threshold time for code 99356, but is less than the threshold time for code 99357, the physician should bill the visit and code 99356. Contractors do not accept more than one unit of code 99356. If the total direct face-to-face time equals or exceeds the threshold time for code 99356 by no more than 29 minutes, the physician bills the visit code 99356 and one unit of code 99357. One additional unit of code 99357 is billed for each additional increment of 30 minutes extended duration. Contractors use the following threshold times to determine if the prolonged services codes 99356 and/or 99357 can be billed with the inpatient setting codes.

Threshold Time for Prolonged Visit Codes 99356 and/or 99357 Billed with Inpatient Setting Codes Code

Code	Typical Time for Code	Threshold Time to Bill Code 99356	Threshold Time to Bill Codes 99356 and 99357
99221	30	60	105
99222	50	80	125
99223	70	100	145
99231	15	45	90
99232	25	55	100
99233	35	65	110
99304	25	55	100
99305	35	65	110
99306	45	75	120
99307	10	40	85
99308	15	45	90
99309	25	55	100
99310	35	65	110
99318	30	60	10

Add 30 minutes to the threshold time for billing codes 99356 and 99357 to get the threshold time for billing code 99356 and two units of 99357.

H. Prolonged Services Associated With Evaluation and Management Services Based on Counseling and/or Coordination of Care (Time-Based)

When an evaluation and management service is dominated by counseling and/or coordination of care (the counseling and/or coordination of care represents more than 50% of the total time with the patient) in a face-to-face encounter between the physician or qualified NPP and the patient in the office/clinic or the floor time (in the scenario of an inpatient service), then the evaluation and management code is selected based on the typical/average time associated with the code levels. The time approximation must meet or exceed the specific CPT code billed (determined by the typical/average time associated with the evaluation and management code) and should not be "rounded" to the next higher level.

In those evaluation and management services in which the code level is selected based on time, prolonged services may only be reported with the highest code level in that family of codes as the companion code.

I. Examples of Billable Prolonged Services

EXAMPLE 1

A physician performed a visit that met the definition of an office visit code 99213 and the total duration of the direct face-to-face services (including the visit) was 65 minutes. The physician bills code 99213 and one unit of code 99354.

EXAMPLE 2

A physician performed a visit that met the definition of a domiciliary, rest home care visit code 99327 and the total duration of the direct face-to-face contact (including the visit) was 140 minutes. The physician bills codes 99327, 99354, and one unit of code 99355.

EXAMPLE 3

A physician performed an office visit to an established patient that was predominantly counseling, spending 75 minutes (direct face-to-face) with the patient. The physician should report CPT code 99215 and one unit of code 99354.

J. Examples of Nonbillable Prolonged Services

EXAMPLE 1

A physician performed a visit that met the definition of visit code 99212 and the total duration of the direct face-to-face contact (including the visit) was 35 minutes. The physician cannot bill prolonged services because the total duration of direct face-to-face service did not meet the threshold time for billing prolonged services.

EXAMPLE 2

A physician performed a visit that met the definition of code 99213 and, while the patient was in the office receiving treatment for 4 hours, the total duration of the direct face-to-face service of the physician was 40 minutes. The physician cannot bill prolonged services because the total duration of direct face-to-face service did not meet the threshold time for billing prolonged services.

EXAMPLE 3

A physician provided a subsequent office visit that was predominantly counseling, spending 60 minutes (face-to-face) with the patient. The physician cannot code 99214, which has a typical time of 25 minutes, and one unit of code 99354. The physician must bill the highest level code in the code family (99215 which has 40 minutes typical/average time units associated with it). The additional time spent beyond this code is 20 minutes and does not meet the threshold time for billing prolonged services.

100-04, 12, 30.6.15.2

Prolonged Services Without Direct Face-to-Face Patient Contact Service (Codes 99358 - 99359)

(Rev. 3678, Issued: 12-16-16, Effective: 01-01-17, Implementation: 01-03-17)

Until CY 2017, CPT codes 99358 and 99359 were not separately payable and were bundled (included for payment) under the related face-to-face E/M service code. Practitioners were not permitted to bill the patient for services described by CPT codes 99358 and 99359 since they are Medicare covered services and payment was included in the payment for other billable services.

Beginning in CY 2017, CPT codes 99358 and 99359 are separately payable under the physician fee schedule. The CPT prefatory language and reporting rules for these codes apply for Medicare billing. For example, CPT codes 99358 and 99359 cannot be reported during the same service period as complex chronic care management (CCM) services or transitional care management services. They are not reported for time spent in non-face-to-face care described by more specific codes having no upper time limit in the CPT code set. We have posted a file that notes the times assumed to be typical for purposes of PFS rate-setting. That file is available on our website under downloads for our annual regulation at http://www.cms.gov/Medicare/Medicare-Fee-for-Service-Payment/PhysicianFeeSched/PFS-Federal-Regulation-Notices.html. We note that while these typical times are not required to bill the displayed codes, we would expect that only time spent in excess of these times would be reported under CPT codes 99358 and 99359. We note that CPT codes 99358 and 99359 can only be used to report extended qualifying time of the billing physician or other practitioner (not clinical staff). Prolonged services cannot be reported in association with a companion E/M code that also qualifies as the initiating visit for CCM services. Practitioners should instead report the add-on code for CCM initiation, if applicable.

100-04, 12, 30.6.15.3

Physician Standby Service (Code 99360)

(Rev. 1, 10-01-03)

Standby services are not payable to physicians. Physicians may not bill Medicare or beneficiaries for standby services. Payment for standby services is included in the Part A payment to the facility. Such services are a part of hospital costs to provide quality care. If hospitals pay physicians for standby services, such services are part of hospital costs to provide quality care.

100-04, 12, 30.6.17

Physician Management Associated with Superficial Radiation Treatment

(Rev. 4339, Issued: 07-25-19, Effective: 01-01-19, Implementation: 08-27-19)

Evaluation and management codes for levels I through III (99211, 99212, and 99213) may be billed with modifier 25 when performed for the purpose of reporting physician work associated with radiation therapy planning, radiation treatment device construction, and radiation treatment management when performed on the same date of service as superficial radiation treatment delivery. See chapter 13, section 70.2, of this manual for information regarding services bundled into treatment management codes.

100-04, 12, 40.3

Claims Review for Global Surgeries

(Rev. 2997, Issued: 07-25-14, Effective: Upon implementation of ICD-10; 01-01- 2012 - ASC X12, Implementation: 08-25-2014 - ASC X12; Upon Implementation of ICD-10)

A. Relationship to Correct Coding Initiative (CCI)

The CCI policy and computer edits allow A/B MACs (B) to detect instances of fragmented billing for certain intra-operative services and other services furnished on the same day as the surgery that are considered to be components of the surgical procedure and, therefore, included in the global surgical fee. When both correct coding and global surgery edits apply to the same claim, A/B MACs (B) first apply the correct coding edits, then, apply the global surgery edits to the correctly coded services.

B. Prepayment Edits to Detect Separate Billing of Services Included in the Global Package

In addition to the correct coding edits, A/B MACs (B) must be capable of detecting certain other services included in the payment for a major or minor surgery or for an endoscopy. On a prepayment basis, A/B MACs (B) identify the services that meet the following conditions:

- Preoperative services that are submitted on the same claim or on a subsequent claim as a surgical procedure; or

- Same day or postoperative services that are submitted on the same claim or on a subsequent claim as a surgical procedure or endoscopy;

   and -

- Services that were furnished within the prescribed global period of the surgical procedure;

- Services that are billed without modifier "-78," "-79," "-24," "25," or "-57" or are billed with modifier "-24" but without the required documentation; and

- Services that are billed with the same provider or group number as the surgical procedure or endoscopy. Also, edit for any visits billed separately during the postoperative period without modifier "-24" by a physician who billed for the postoperative care only with modifier "-55."

A/B MACs (B) use the following evaluation and management codes in establishing edits for visits included in the global package. CPT codes 99241, 99242, 99243, 99244, 99245, 99251, 99252, 99253, 99254, 99255, 99271, 99272, 99273, 99274, and 99275 have been transferred from the excluded category and are now included in the global surgery edits.

Evaluation and Management Codes for A/B MAC (B) Edits

92012	92014	99211	99212	99213	99214	99215
99217	99218	99219	99220	99221	99222	99223
99231	99232	99233	99234	99235	99236	99238
99239	99241	99242	99243	99244	99245	99251
99252	99253	99254	99255	99261	99262	99263
99271	99272	99273	99274	99275	99291	99292
99301	99302	99303	99311	99312	99313	99315
99316	99331	99332	99333	99347	99348	99349
99350	99374	99375	99377	99378		

NOTE: In order for codes 99291 or 99292 to be paid for services furnished during the preoperative or postoperative period, modifier "-25" or "-24," respectively, must be used to indicate that the critical care was unrelated to the specific anatomic injury or general surgical procedure performed.

If a surgeon is admitting a patient to a nursing facility for a condition not related to the global surgical procedure, the physician should bill for the nursing facility admission and care with a "-24" modifier and appropriate documentation. If a surgeon is admitting a patient to a nursing facility and the patient's admission to that facility relates to the global surgical procedure, the nursing facility admission and any services related to the global surgical procedure are included in the global surgery fee.

C. Exclusions from Prepayment Edits
A/B MACs (B) exclude the following services from the prepayment audit process and allow separate payment if all usual requirements are met:

- Services listed in §40.1.B; and
- Services billed with the modifier "-25," "-57," "-58," "-78," or "-79."

Exceptions

See §§40.2.A.8, 40.2.A.9, and 40.4.A for instances where prepayment review is required for modifier "-25." In addition, prepayment review is necessary for CPT codes 90935, 90937, 90945, and 90947 when a visit and modifier "-25" are billed with these services.

Exclude the following codes from the prepayment edits required in §40.3.B.

92002	92004	99201	99202	99203	99204	99205
99281	99282	99283	99284	99285	99321	99322
99323	99341	99342	99343	99344	99345	

100-04, 12, 40.7

Claims for Bilateral Surgeries
(Rev. 1, 10-01-03) B3-4827, B3-15040

A. General
Bilateral surgeries are procedures performed on both sides of the body during the same operative session or on the same day.

The terminology for some procedure codes includes the terms "bilateral" (e.g., code 27395; Lengthening of the hamstring tendon; multiple, bilateral.) or "unilateral or bilateral" (e.g., code 52290; cystourethroscopy; with ureteral meatotomy, unilateral or bilateral). The payment adjustment rules for bilateral surgeries do not apply to procedures identified by CPT as "bilateral" or "unilateral or bilateral" since the fee schedule reflects any additional work required for bilateral surgeries.

Field 22 of the MFSDB indicates whether the payment adjustment rules apply to a surgical procedure.

B. Billing Instructions for Bilateral Surgeries
If a procedure is not identified by its terminology as a bilateral procedure (or unilateral or bilateral), physicians must report the procedure with modifier "-50." They report such procedures as a single line item. (NOTE: This differs from the CPT coding guidelines which indicate that bilateral procedures should be billed as two line items.)

If a procedure is identified by the terminology as bilateral (or unilateral or bilateral), as in codes 27395 and 52290, physicians do not report the procedure with modifier "-50."

C. Claims Processing System Requirements
Carriers must be able to:

1. Identify bilateral surgeries by the presence on the claim form or electronic submission of the "-50" modifier or of the same code on separate lines reported once with modifier "-LT" and once with modifier "-RT";

2. Access Field 34 or 35 of the MFSDB to determine the Medicare payment amount;

3. Access Field 22 of the MFSDB:

   — If Field 22 contains an indicator of "0," "2," or "3," the payment adjustment rules for bilateral surgeries do not apply. Base payment on the lower of the billed amount or 100 percent of the fee schedule amount (Field 34 or 35) unless other payment adjustment rules apply.

   NOTE: Some codes which have a bilateral indicator of "0" in the MFSDB may be performed more than once on a given day. These are services that would never be considered bilateral and thus should not be billed with modifier "-50." Where such a code is billed on multiple line items or with more than 1 in the units field and carriers have determined that the code may be reported more than once, bypass the "0" bilateral indicator and refer to the multiple surgery field for pricing;

   — If Field 22 contains an indicator of "1," the standard adjustment rules apply. Base payment on the lower of the billed amount or 150 percent of the fee schedule amount (Field 34 or 35). (Multiply the payment amount in Field 34 or 35 for the surgery by 150 percent and round to the nearest cent.)

4. Apply the requirements 40 - 40.4 on global surgeries to bilateral surgeries; and

5. Retain the "-50" modifier in history for any bilateral surgeries paid at the adjusted amount.

   (NOTE: The "-50" modifier is not retained for surgeries which are bilateral by definition such as code 27395.)

100-04, 12, 40.8

Claims for Co-Surgeons and Team Surgeons
(Rev. 3721, Issued: 02-24-17, Effective: 05-25-17, Implementation: 05-25-17)

A. General
Under some circumstances, the individual skills of two or more surgeons are required to perform surgery on the same patient during the same operative session. This may be required because of the complex nature of the procedure(s) and/or the patient's condition.

In these cases, the additional physicians are not acting as assistants-at-surgery.

B. Billing Instructions
The following billing procedures apply when billing for a surgical procedure or procedures that required the use of two surgeons or a team of surgeons:

- If two surgeons (each in a different specialty) are required to perform a specific procedure, each surgeon bills for the procedure with a modifier "-62. " Co-surgery also refers to surgical procedures involving two surgeons performing the parts of the procedure simultaneously, i.e., heart transplant or bilateral knee replacements. Documentation of the medical necessity for two surgeons is required for certain services identified in the MFSDB. (See 40.8.C.5.);

- If a team of surgeons (more than 2 surgeons of different specialties) is required to perform a specific procedure, each surgeon bills for the procedure with a modifier "-66." Field 25 of the MFSDB identifies certain services submitted with a "-66" modifier which must be sufficiently documented to establish that a team was medically necessary. All claims for team surgeons must contain sufficient information to allow pricing "by report."

- If surgeons of different specialties are each performing a different procedure (with specific CPT codes), neither co-surgery nor multiple surgery rules apply (even if the procedures are performed through the same incision). If one of the surgeons performs multiple procedures, the multiple procedure rules apply to that surgeon's services. (See 40.6 for multiple surgery payment rules.)

For co-surgeons (modifier 62), the fee schedule amount applicable to the payment for each co-surgeon is 62.5 percent of the global surgery fee schedule amount. Team surgery (modifier 66) is paid for on a "By Report" basis.

C. Claims Processing System Requirements
Carriers must be able to:

1. Identify a surgical procedure performed by two surgeons or a team of surgeons by the presence on the claim form or electronic submission of the "-62" or "-66" modifier;

2. Access Field 34 or 35 of the MFSDB to determine the fee schedule payment amount for the surgery;

3. Access Field 24 or 25, as appropriate, of the MFSDB. These fields provide guidance on whether two or team surgeons are generally required for the surgical procedure;

4. If the surgery is billed with a "-62" or "-66" modifier and Field 24 or 25 contains an indicator of "0," payment adjustment rules for two or team surgeons do not apply:

   — Carriers pay the first bill submitted, and base payment on the lower of the billed amount or 100 percent of the fee schedule amount (Field 34 or 35) unless other payment adjustment rules apply;

   — Carriers deny bills received subsequently from other physicians and use the appropriate MSN message in 40.8.D. As these are medical necessity denials, the instructions in the Program Integrity Manual regarding denial of unassigned claims for medical necessity are applied;

5. If the surgery is billed with a "-62" modifier and Field 24 contains an indicator of "1," suspend the claim for manual review of any documentation submitted with the claim. If the documentation supports the need for co-surgeons, base payment for each physician on the lower of the billed amount or 62.5 percent of the fee schedule amount (Field 34 or 35);

6. If the surgery is billed with a "-62" modifier and Field 24 contains an indicator of "2," payment rules for two surgeons apply. Carriers base payment for each physician on the lower of the billed amount or 62.5 percent of the fee schedule amount (Field 34 or 35);

7. If the surgery is billed with a "-66" modifier and Field 25 contains an indicator of "1," carriers suspend the claim for manual review. If carriers determine that team surgeons were medically necessary, each physician is paid on a "by report" basis;

8. If the surgery is billed with a "-66" modifier and Field 25 contains an indicator of "2," carriers pay "by report";

NOTE: A Medicare fee may have been established for some surgical procedures that are billed with the "-66" modifier. In these cases, all physicians on the team must agree on the percentage of the Medicare payment amount each is to receive.

If carriers receive a bill with a "-66" modifier after carriers have paid one surgeon the full Medicare payment amount (on a bill without the modifier), deny the subsequent claim.

9. Apply the rules global surgical packages to each of the physicians participating in a co- or team surgery; and

10. Retain the "-62" and "-66" modifiers in history for any co- or team surgeries.

D. Beneficiary Liability on Denied Claims for Assistant, Co- surgeon and Team Surgeons

When the procedure is subject to the statutory restriction against payment for assistants-at-surgery, such payment shall be denied.

The following reflects the remittance advice messages and associated codes that will appear when rejecting/denying claims under this policy. This CARC/RARC combination is compliant with CAQH CORE Business Scenario 3.

    Group Code: CO
    CARC: 54
    RARC: N/A
    MSN: 15.11

Carriers include the following statement in the MSN:

"You cannot be charged for this service." (Unnumbered add-on message.)

If Field 23 of the MFSDB contains an indicator of "0" or "1" (assistant-at-surgery may not be paid) for procedures CMS has determined that an assistant surgeon is not generally medically necessary.

The following reflects the remittance advice messages and associated codes that will appear when rejecting/denying claims under this policy. This CARC/RARC combination is compliant with CAQH CORE Business Scenario 3.

    Group Code: CO
    CARC: 54
    RARC: N/A
    MSN: 15.12

For those procedures with an indicator of "0," the limitation on liability provisions described in Chapter 30 apply to assigned claims. Therefore, carriers include the appropriate limitation of liability language from Chapter 21. For unassigned claims, apply the rules in the Program Integrity Manual concerning denial for medical necessity.

Where payment may not be made for a co- or team surgeon, deny the claim

The following reflects the remittance advice messages and associated codes that will appear when rejecting/denying claims under this policy. This CARC/RARC combination is compliant with CAQH CORE Business Scenario 3.

    Group Code: CO
    CARC: 54
    RARC: N/A
    MSN: 15.13

Where payment may not be made for a two surgeons, deny the claim.

The following reflects the remittance advice messages and associated codes that will appear when rejecting/denying claims under this policy. This CARC/RARC combination is compliant with CAQH CORE Business Scenario 3.

    Group Code: CO
    CARC: 54
    RARC: N/A
    MSN: 15.12

Also see limitation of liability remittance notice Remittance Advice Remark Code Alert M27 and use when appropriate.

100-04, 12, 50
Payment for Anesthesiology Services
(Rev. 3747; Issued: 04-14-17; Effective: 01-01-17; Implementation: 05-15-17)

A. General Payment Rule
The fee schedule amount for physician anesthesia services furnished is, with the exceptions noted, based on allowable base and time units multiplied by an anesthesia conversion factor specific to that locality. The base unit for each anesthesia procedure is communicated to the A/B MACs by means of the HCPCS file released annually. CMS releases the conversion factor annually. The base units and conversion factor are available on the CMS website at: https://www.cms.gov/Center/Provider-Type/Anesthesiologists-Center.html.

B. Payment at Personally Performed Rate
The A/B MAC must determine the fee schedule payment, recognizing the base unit for the anesthesia code and one time unit per 15 minutes of anesthesia time if:

- The physician personally performed the entire anesthesia service alone;

- The physician is involved with one anesthesia case with a resident, the physician is a teaching physician as defined in §100;

- The physician is involved in the training of physician residents in a single anesthesia case, two concurrent anesthesia cases involving residents or a single anesthesia case involving a resident that is concurrent to another case that meets the requirements for payment at the medically directed rate. The physician meets the teaching physician criteria in §100.1.4;

- The physician is continuously involved in a single case involving a student nurse anesthetist;

- If the physician is involved with a single case with a qualified nonphysician anesthetist (a certified registered nurse anesthetist (CRNA) or an anesthesiologist's assistant), A/B MACs may pay the physician service and the qualified nonphysician anesthetist service in accordance with the requirements for payment at the medically directed rate;

Or

- The physician and the CRNA (or anesthesiologist's assistant) are involved in one anesthesia case and the services of each are found to be medically necessary. Documentation must be submitted by both the CRNA and the physician to support payment of the full fee for each of the two providers. The physician reports the AA modifier and the CRNA reports the QZ modifier.

C. Payment at the Medically Directed Rate
The A/B MAC determines payment at the medically directed rate for the physician on the basis of 50 percent of the allowance for the service performed by the physician alone. Payment will be made at the medically directed rate if the physician medically directs qualified individuals (all of whom could be CRNAs, anesthesiologists' assistants, interns, residents, or combinations of these individuals) in two, three, or four concurrent cases and the physician performs the followingactivities.

- Performs a pre-anesthetic examination and evaluation;

- Prescribes the anesthesia plan;

- Personally participates in the most demanding procedures in the anesthesia plan, including, if applicable, induction and emergence;

- Ensures that any procedures in the anesthesia plan that he or she does not perform are performed by a qualified individual;

- Monitors the course of anesthesia administration at frequent intervals;

- Remains physically present and available for immediate diagnosis and treatment of emergencies; and

- Provides indicated post-anesthesia care.

The physician must document in the medical record that he or she performed the pre-anesthetic examination and evaluation. Physicians must also document that they provided indicated post-anesthesia care, were present during some portion of the anesthesia monitoring, and were present during the most demanding procedures in the anesthesia plan, including induction and emergence, where indicated.

NOTE: Concurrency refers to to the maximum number of procedures that the physician is medically directing within the context of a single procedure andwhether these other procedures overlap each other. Concurrency is not dependent on each of the cases involving a Medicare patient. For example, if an anesthesiologist medically directs three concurrent procedures, two of which involve non-Medicare patients and the remaining a Medicare patient, this represents three concurrent cases.

The requirements for payment at the medically directed rate also apply to cases involving student nurse anesthetists if the physician medically directs two concurrent cases, with each of the two cases involving a student nurse anesthetist, or the physician directs one case involving a student nurse anesthetist and another involving a qualified individual (for example: CRNA, anesthesiologist's assistant, intern or resident).

The requirements for payment at the medically directed rate do not apply to a single resident case that is concurrent to another anesthesia case paid at the medically directed rate or to two concurrent anesthesia cases involving residents.

If anesthesiologists are in a group practice, one physician member may provide the pre- anesthesia examination and evaluation while another fulfills the other criteria. Similarly, one physician member of the group may provide post-anesthesia care while another member of the group furnishes the other component parts of the anesthesia service. However, the medical record must indicate that the services were furnished by physicians and identify the physicians who furnished them.

A physician who is concurrently furnishing services that meet the requirements for payment at the medically directed rate cannot ordinarily be involved in furnishing additional services to other patients. However, addressing an emergency of short duration in the immediate area, administering an epidural or caudal anesthetic to ease labor pain, periodic (rather than continuous) monitoring of an obstetrical patient, receiving patients entering the operating suite for the next surgery, checking or discharging patients in the recovery room, or handling scheduling matters, do not substantially diminish the scope of control exercised by the physician and do not constitute a separate service for the purpose of determining whether the requirements for payment at the medically directed rate are met.

However, if the physician leaves the immediate area of the operating suite for other than short durations or devotes extensive time to an emergency case or is otherwise not available to respond to the immediate needs of the surgical patients, the physician's services to the surgical patients would not meet the requirements for payment at the medically directed rate. A/B MACs may not make payment under the feeschedule.

D. Payment at Medically Supervised Rate
The A/B MAC may allow only three base units per procedure when the anesthesiologist is involved in furnishing more than four procedures concurrently or is performing other services while directing the concurrent procedures. An additional time unit may be recognized if the physician can document he or she was present atinduction.

E. Billing and Payment for Multiple Anesthesia Procedures
Physicians bill for the anesthesia services associated with multiple bilateral surgeries by reporting the anesthesia procedure with the highest base unit value with the multiple procedure modifier -51. They report the total time for all procedures in the line item with the highest base unit value.

If the same anesthesia CPT code applies to two or more of the surgical procedures, billers enter the anesthesia code with the -51 modifier and the number of surgeries to which the modified CPT code applies.

Payment can be made under the fee schedule for anesthesia services associated with multiple surgical procedures or multiple bilateral procedures. Payment is determined based on the base unit of the anesthesia procedure with the highest base unit value and time units based on the actual anesthesia time of the multiple procedures. See §§40.6-40.7 for billing and claims processing instructions for multiple and bilateral surgeries.

F. Payment for Medical and Surgical Services Furnished in Addition to Anesthesia Procedure
Payment may be made under the fee schedule for specific medical and surgical services furnished by the anesthesiologist as long as these services are reasonable and medically necessary or provided that other rebundling provisions (see §30 and Chapter 23) do not preclude separate payment. These services may be furnished in conjunction with the anesthesia procedure to the patient or may be furnished as single services, e.g., during the day of or the day before the anesthesia service. These services include the insertion of a Swan Ganz catheter, the insertion of central venous pressure lines, emergency intubation, and critical care visits.

G. Anesthesia Time and Calculation of Anesthesia TimeUnits
Anesthesia time is defined as the period during which an anesthesia practitioner is present with the patient. It starts when the anesthesia practitioner begins to prepare the patient for anesthesia services in the operating room or an equivalent area and ends when the anesthesia practitioner is no longer furnishing anesthesia services to the patient, that is, when the patient may be placed safely under postoperative care. Anesthesia time is a continuous time period from the start of anesthesia to the end of an anesthesia service. In counting anesthesia time for services furnished, the anesthesia practitioner can add blocks of time around an interruption in anesthesia time as long as the anesthesia practitioner is furnishing continuous anesthesia care within the time periods around the interruption.

Actual anesthesia time in minutes is reported on the claim. For anesthesia services furnished, the A/B MAC computes time units by dividing reported anesthesia time by 15 minutes. Round the time unit to one decimal place. The A/B MAC does not recognize time units for CPT code 01996 (daily hospital management of epidural or subarachnoid continuous drug administration).

For purposes of this section, anesthesia practitioner means:

- a physician who performs the anesthesia service alone,
- a CRNA who is furnishing services that do not meet the requirements for payment at the medically directed rate,
- a qualified nonphysician anesthetist who is furnishing services that meet the requirements for payment at the medically directed rate.

The physician who medically directs the qualified nonphysician anesthetist would ordinarily report the same time as the qualified nonphysician anesthetist reports for the service.

H. Monitored Anesthesia Care
Monitored anesthesia care involves the intra-operative monitoring by a physician or qualified individual under the medical direction of a physician or of the patient's vital physiological signs in anticipation of the need for administration of general anesthesia or of the development of adverse physiological patient reaction to the surgical procedure. It also includes the performance of a pre-anesthetic examination and evaluation, prescription of the anesthesia care required, administration of any

necessary oral or parenteral medications (e.g., atropine, demerol, valium) and provision of indicated postoperative anesthesia care.

The A/B MAC pays for reasonable and medically necessary monitored anesthesia care services on the same basis as other anesthesia services. If the physician personally performs the monitored anesthesia care case, payment is made under the fee schedule using the payment rules for payment at the personally performed rate. If the physician medically directs four or fewer concurrent cases and monitored anesthesia care represents one or more of these concurrentcases, payment is made under the fee schedule using the payment rules for payment at the medically directed rate. Anesthesiologists use the QS modifier to report monitored anesthesia care cases, in addition to reporting the actual anesthesia time and one of the payment modifiers on the claim.

I. Anesthesia Claims Modifiers
Physicians report the appropriate modifier to denote whether the service meets the requirements for payment at the personally performed rate, medically directed rate, or medically supervised rate.

AA Anesthesia Services performed personally by the anesthesiologist

AD Medical Supervision by a physician; more than 4 concurrent anesthesia procedures

G8 Monitored anesthesia care (MAC) for deep complex, complicated, or markedly invasive surgical procedures

G9 Monitored anesthesia care for patient who has a history of severe cardio-pulmonary condition

QK Medical direction of two, three or four concurrent anesthesia procedures involving qualified individuals

QS Monitored anesthesia care service

NOTE: The QS modifier can be used by a physician or a qualified nonphysician anesthetist and is for informational purposes. Providers must report actual anesthesia time and one of the payment modifiers on the claim.

QY Medical direction of one qualified nonphysician anesthetist by an anesthesiologist

GC These services have been performed by a resident under the direction of a teaching physician.

NOTE: The GC modifier is reported by the teaching physician to indicate he/she rendered the service in compliance with the teaching physician requirements in §100 of this chapter. One of the payment modifiers must be used in conjunction with the GC modifier.

The A/B MAC must determine payment for anesthesia in accordance with these instructions. They must be able to determine the uniform base unit that is assigned to the anesthesia code and apply the appropriate reduction where the anesthesia procedure meets the requirements for payment at the medically directed rate. They must also be able to determine the number of anesthesia time units from actual anesthesia time reported on the claim. The A/B MAC must multiply allowable units by the anesthesia-specific conversion factor used to determine fee schedule payment for the payment area.

J. Moderate Sedation Services Furnished in Conjunction with and in Support of Procedural Services
Anesthesia services range in complexity. The continuum of anesthesia services, from least intense to most intense in complexity is as follows: local or topical anesthesia, moderate (conscious) sedation, regional anesthesia and general anesthesia. Moderate sedation is a drug induced depression of consciousness during which the patient responds purposefully to verbal commands, either alone or accompanied by light tactile stimulation. Moderate sedation does not include minimal sedation, deep sedation or monitored anesthesia care.

Practitioners will report the appropriate CPT and/or HCPCS code that describes the moderate sedation services furnished during a patient encounter, which are furnished in conjunction with and in support of a procedural service, consistent with CPT guidance.

Refer to §50 and §140 of this chapter for information regarding reporting of anesthesia services furnished in conjunction with and in support of procedural services.

K. Anesthesia for Diagnostic or Therapeutic Nerve Blocks and Services Lower in Intensity than Moderate Sedation
If the anesthesiologist or CRNA provides anesthesia for diagnostic or therapeutic nerve blocks or injections and a different provider performs the block or injection, then the anesthesiologist or CRNA may report the anesthesia service using the appropriate CPT code consistent with CPT guidance. The service must meet the criteria for monitored anesthesia care as described in this section. If the anesthesiologist or CRNA provides both the anesthesia service and the block or injection, then the anesthesiologist or CRNA may report the anesthesia service and the injection or block. However, the anesthesia service must meet the requirements for moderate sedation and if a lower level complexity anesthesia service is provided, then the moderate sedation code should not be reported.

If the physician performing the medical or surgical procedure also provides a level of anesthesia lower in intensity than moderate sedation, such as a local or topical anesthesia, then the moderate sedation code should not be reported and no separate payment should be allowed by the A/B MAC.

100-04, 12, 100

Teaching Physician Services
(Rev. 811, Issued: 01-13-06, Effective: 01-01-06, Implementation: 02-13-06)

Definitions
For purposes of this section, the following definitions apply.

Resident -An individual who participates in an approved graduate medical education (GME) program or a physician who is not in an approved GME program but who is authorized to practice only in a hospital setting. The term includes interns and fellows in GME programs recognized as approved for purposes of direct GME payments made by the FI. Receiving a staff or faculty appointment or participating in a fellowship does not by itself alter the status of "resident". Additionally, this status remains unaffected regardless if a hospital includes the physician in its full time equivalency count of residents.

Student- An individual who participates in an accredited educational program (e.g., a medical school) that is not an approved GME program. A student is never considered to be an intern or a resident. Medicare does not pay for any service furnished by a student. See 100.1.1B for a discussion concerning E/M service documentation performed by students.

Teaching Physician -A physician (other than another resident) who involves residents in the care of his or her patients.

Direct Medical and Surgical Services -Services to individual beneficiaries that are either personally furnished by a physician or furnished by a resident under the supervision of a physician in a teaching hospital making the reasonable cost election for physician services furnished in teaching hospitals. All payments for such services are made by the FI for the hospital.

Teaching Hospital -A hospital engaged in an approved GME residency program in medicine, osteopathy, dentistry, or podiatry.

Teaching Setting -Any provider, hospital-based provider, or nonprovider setting in which Medicare payment for the services of residents is made by the FI under the direct graduate medical education payment methodology or freestanding SNF or HHA in which such payments are made on a reasonable cost basis.

Critical or Key Portion- That part (or parts) of a service that the teaching physician determines is (are) a critical or key portion(s). For purposes of this section, these terms are interchangeable.

Documentation- Notes recorded in the patient's medical records by a resident, and/or teaching physician or others as outlined in the specific situations below regarding the service furnished. Documentation may be dictated and typed or hand-written, or computer-generated and typed or handwritten. Documentation must be dated and include a legible signature or identity. Pursuant to 42 CFR 415.172 (b), documentation must identify, at a minimum, the service furnished, the participation of the teaching physician in providing the service, and whether the teaching physician was physically present. In the context of an electronic medical record, the term 'macro' means a command in a computer or dictation application that automatically generates predetermined text that is not edited by the user.

When using an electronic medical record, it is acceptable for the teaching physician to use a macro as the required personal documentation if the teaching physician adds it personally in a secured (password protected) system. In addition to the teaching physician's macro, either the resident or the teaching physician must provide customized information that is sufficient to support a medical necessity determination. The note in the electronic medical record must sufficiently describe the specific services furnished to the specific patient on the specific date. It is insufficient documentation if both the resident and the teaching physician use macros only.

Physically Present- The teaching physician is located in the same room (or partitioned or curtained area, if the room is subdivided to accommodate multiple patients) as the patient and/or performs a face-to-face service.

100-04, 12, 100.1.1

Evaluation and Management (E/M) Services
(Rev. 4283, Issued: 04- 26-19, Effective: 01-01-19, 07-29-19)

A. General Documentation Requirements
Evaluation and Management (E/M) Services -- For a given encounter, the selection of the appropriate level of E/M service should be determined according to the code definitions in the American Medical Association's Current Procedural Terminology (CPT) book and any applicable documentation guidelines.

For purposes of payment, E/M services billed by teaching physicians require that the medical records must demonstrate:

- That the teaching physician performed the service or was physically present during the key or critical portions of the service when performed by the resident; and

- The participation of the teaching physician in the management of the patient.

The presence of the teaching physician during E/M services may be demonstrated by the notes in the medical records made by physicians, residents, or nurses.

B. E/M Service Documentation Provided By Students
Any contribution and participation of students to the performance of a billable service (other than the review of systems and/or past family/social history which are not separately billable, but are taken as part of an E/M service) must be performed in the physical presence of a teaching physician or physical presence of a resident in a service meeting the requirements set forth in this section for teaching physician billing.

Students may document services in the medical record. However, the teaching physician must verify in the medical record all student documentation or findings, including history, physical exam and/or medical decision making. The teaching physician must personally perform (or re-perform) the physical exam and medical decision making activities of the E/M service being billed, but may verify any student documentation of them in the medical record, rather than re-documenting this work.

C. Exception for E/M Services Furnished in Certain Primary CareCenters
Teaching physicians providing E/M services with a GME program granted a primary care exception may bill Medicare for lower and mid-level E/M services provided by residents. For the E/M codes listed below, teaching physicians may submit claims for services furnished by residents in the absence of a teaching physician:

New Patient	Established Patient
99201	99211
99202	99212
99203	99213

Effective January 1, 2005, the following code is included under the primary care exception: HCPCS code G0402 (Initial preventive physical examination; face-to-face visit services limited to new beneficiary during the first 12 months of Medicare enrollment).

Effective January 1, 2011, the following codes are included under the primary care exception: HCPCS codes G0438 (Annual wellness visit, including personal preventive plan service, first visit) and G0439 (Annual wellness visit, including personal preventive plan service, subsequent visit).

If a service other than those listed above needs to be furnished, then the general teaching physician policy set forth in §100.1 applies. For this exception to apply, a center must attest in writing that all the following conditions are met for a particular residency program. Prior approval is not necessary, but centers exercising the primary care exception must maintain records demonstrating that they qualify for the exception.

The services must be furnished in a center located in the outpatient department of a hospital or another ambulatory care entity in which the time spent by residents in patient care activities is included in determining direct GME payments to a teaching hospital by the hospital's A/B MAC (A). This requirement is not met when the resident is assigned to a physician's office away from the center or makes home visits. In the case of a nonhospital entity, verify with the A/B MAC (A) that the entity meets the requirements of a written agreement between the hospital and the entity set forth at 42 CFR 413.78(e)(3)(ii).

Under this exception, residents providing the billable patient care service without the physical presence of a teaching physician must have completed at least 6 months of a GME approved residency program. Centers must maintain information under the provisions at 42 CFR 413.79(a)(6).

Teaching physicians submitting claims under this exception may not supervise more than four residents at any given time and must direct the care from such proximity as to constitute immediate availability. Teaching physicians may include residents with less than 6 months in a GME approved residency program in the mix of four residents under the teaching physician's supervision. However, the teaching physician must be physically present for the critical or key portions of services furnished by the residents with less than 6 months in a GME approved residency program. That is, the primary care exception does not apply in the case of residents with less than 6 months in a GME approved residency program.

Teaching physicians submitting claims under this exception must:

- Not have other responsibilities (including the supervision of other personnel) at the time the service was provided by the residents;

- Have the primary medical responsibility for patients cared for by the residents;

- Ensure that the care provided was reasonable and necessary;

- Review the care provided by the residents during or immediately after each visit. This must include a review of the patient's medical history, the resident's findings on physical examination, the patient's diagnosis, and treatment plan (i.e., record of tests and therapies); and

Patients under this exception should consider the center to be their primary location for health care services. The residents must be expected to generally provide care to the same group of established patients during their residency training. The types of services furnished by residents under this exception include:

- Acute care for undifferentiated problems or chronic care for ongoing conditions including chronic mental illness;

- Coordination of care furnished by other physicians and providers; and,

- Comprehensive care not limited by organ system or diagnosis.

Residency programs most likely qualifying for this exception include family practice, general internal medicine, geriatric medicine, pediatrics, and obstetrics/gynecology.

Certain GME programs in psychiatry may qualify in special situations such as when the program furnishes

comprehensive care for chronically mentally ill patients. These would be centers in which the range of services the residents are trained to furnish, and actually do furnish, include comprehensive medical care as well as psychiatric care. For example, antibiotics are being prescribed as well as psychotropic drugs.

The patient medical record must document the extent of the teaching physician's participation in the review and direction of the services furnished to each beneficiary. The extent of the teaching physician's participation may be demonstrated by the notes in the medical records made by physicians, residents, or nurses.

100-04, 12, 140.1

Qualified Nonphysician Anesthetists
(Rev. 3747; Issued: 04-14-17; Effective: 01-01-17; Implementation: 05-15-17)

For payment purposes, the term "qualified nonphysician anesthetist" is used to refer to both certified registered nurse anesthetists (CRNAs) and anesthesiologists' assistants unless otherwise separately discussed.

An anesthesiologist's assistant means a person who:

- Works under the direction of an anesthesiologist;
- Is in compliance with all applicable requirements of State law, including any licensure requirements the state imposes on nonphysician anesthetists; and
- Is a graduate of a medical school based anesthesiologist assistant educational program that –
  — Is accredited by the Committee on Allied Health Education and Accreditation;

And

  — Includes approximately two years of specialized basic science and clinical education in anesthesia at a level that builds on a premedical undergraduate science background.

A CRNA is a registered nurse who:

- is licensed as a registered professional nurse by the State in which the nurse practices;
- Meets any licensure requirements the State imposes with respect to nonphysician anesthetists;
- Has graduated from a nurse anesthesia educational program that meets the standards of the Council on Accreditation of Nurse Anesthesia Programs; and
- Meets the following criteria:
  — Has passed a certification examination of the Council on Certification of Nurse Anesthetists or the Council on Recertification of Nurse Anesthetists;

Or

  — Is a graduate of a nurse anesthesia educational program that meets the standards of the Council of Accreditation of Nurse Anesthesia Educational Programs, and within 24 months of graduation, has passed a certification examination of the Council on Certification of Nurse Anesthetists or the Council on Recertification of Nurse Anesthetists.

100-04, 12, 140.2

Entity or Individual to Whom Fee Schedule is Payable for Qualified Nonphysician Anesthetists
(Rev. 3747; Issued: 04-14-17; Effective: 01-01-17; Implementation: 05-15-17)

Payment for the services of a qualified nonphysician anesthetist may be made directly to the qualified nonphysician anesthetist who furnished the anesthesia services or to a hospital, physician, group practice, or ASC with which the qualified nonphysician anesthetist has an employment or contractual relationship.

100-04, 12, 140.3

Anesthesia Fee Schedule Payment for Qualified Nonphysician Anesthetists
(Rev. 3747; Issued: 04-14-17; Effective: 01-01-17; Implementation: 05-15-17)

Payment for the services furnished by qualified nonphysician anesthetists are subject to the usual Part B coinsurance and deductible, and are made only on an assignment basis. The assignment agreed to by the qualified nonphysician anesthetist is binding upon any other person or entity claiming payment for the service. Except for deductible and coinsurance amounts, any person who knowingly and willfully presents or causes to be presented to a Medicare beneficiary a bill or request for payment for services of a qualified nonphysician anesthetist for which payment may be made on an assignment-related basis is subject to civil monetary penalties.

The fee schedule for anesthesia services furnished by qualified nonphysician anesthetists is the least of 80 percent of:

- The actual charge;
- The applicable locality anesthesia conversion factor multiplied by the sum of allowable base and time units.

100-04, 12, 140.3.1

Conversion Factors Used for Qualified Nonphysician Anesthetists
(Rev. 3747; Issued: 04-14-17; Effective: 01-01-17; Implementation: 05-15-17)

The conversion factors applicable to anesthesia services are increased by the update factor used to update physicians' services under the physician fee schedule. They are generally published in November of the year preceding the year in which they apply.

100-04, 12, 140.3.2

Anesthesia Time and Calculation of Anesthesia TimeUnits
(Rev. 3747; Issued: 04-14-17; Effective: 01-01-17; Implementation: 05-15-17)

Anesthesia time means the time during which a qualified nonphysician anesthetist is present with the patient. It starts when the qualified nonphysician anesthetist begins to prepare the patient for anesthesia services in the operating room or an equivalent area and ends when the qualified nonphysician anesthetist is no longer furnishing anesthesia services to the patient, that is, when the patient may be placed safely under postoperative care. Anesthesia time is a continuous time period from the start of anesthesia to the end of an anesthesia service. In counting anesthesia time, the qualified nonphysician anesthetist can add blocks of time around an interruption in anesthesia time as long as the qualified nonphysician anesthetist is furnishing continuous anesthesia care within the time periods around the interruption.

100-04, 12, 140.3.3

Billing Modifiers
(Rev. 3747; Issued: 04-14-17; Effective: 01-01-17; Implementation: 05-15-17)

The following modifiers are used by qualified nonphysician anesthetists when billing for anesthesia services:

- QX – Qualified nonphysician anesthetist service: With medical direction by a physician.
- QZ – CRNA service: Without medical direction by a physician.
- QS – Monitored anesthesia care services
  — NOTE: The QS modifier can be used by a physician or a qualified nonphysician anesthetist and is for informational purposes. Providers must report actual anesthesia time and one of the payment modifiers on the claim.

100-04, 12, 140.3.4

General Billing Instructions
(Rev. 3747; Issued: 04-14-17; Effective: 01-01-17; Implementation: 05-15-17)

Claims for reimbursement for qualified nonphysician anesthetist services should be completed in accordance with existing billing instructions for anesthesiologists with the following additions.

- If an employer-physician furnishes concurrent medical direction for a procedure involving CRNAs and the medical direction service is unassigned, the physician should bill on an assigned basis on a separate claim for the qualified nonphysician anesthetist service. If the physician is participating or takes assignment, both services should be billed on one claim but as separate line items.
- All claims forms must have the provider billing number of the qualified nonphysician anesthetist and/or the employer of the qualified nonphysician anesthetist performing the service in either block 24.H of the Form CMS-1500 and/or block 31 as applicable. Verify that the billing number is valid before making payment.

Payments should be calculated in accordance with Medicare payment rules in §140.3. The A/B MAC must institute all necessary payment edits to assure that duplicate payments are not made to physicians for qualified nonphysician anesthetist services or to a qualified nonphysician anesthetist directly for bills submitted on their behalf by qualified billers.

A CRNA is identified on the provider file by specialty code 43. An anesthesiologist's assistant is identified on the provider file by specialty code 32.

100-04, 12, 140.4.1

An Anesthesiologist and Qualified Nonphysician Anesthetist Work Together
(Rev. 3747; Issued: 04-14-17; Effective: 01-01-17; Implementation: 05-15-17)

A/B MACs will distribute educational releases and use other established means to ensure that anesthesiologists understand the requirements for medical direction of qualified nonphysician anesthetists.

A/B MACs will perform reviews of payments for anesthesiology services to identify situations in which an excessive number of concurrent anesthesiology services may have been performed. They will use peer practice and their experience in developing review criteria. They will also periodically review a sample of claims for medical direction of four or fewer concurrent anesthesia procedures. During this process physicians may be requested to submit documentation of the names of procedures performed and the names of the anesthetists medically directed.

Physicians who cannot supply the necessary documentation for the sample claims must submit documentation with all subsequent claims before payment will be made.

100-04, 12, 140.4.2

Qualified Nonphysician Anesthetist and an Anesthesiologist in a Single Anesthesia Procedure

(Rev. 3747; Issued: 04-14-17; Effective: 01-01-17; Implementation: 05-15-17)

Where a single anesthesia procedure involves both a physician medical direction service and the service of the medically directed qualified nonphysician anesthetist, the payment amount for the service of each is 50 percent of the allowance otherwise recognized had the service been furnished by the anesthesiologist alone. For the single medically directed service, the physician will use the QY modifier and the qualified nonphysician anesthetist will use the QX modifier.

In unusual circumstances when it is medically necessary for both the CRNA and the anesthesiologist to be completely and fully involved during a procedure, full payment for the services of each provider is allowed. The physician would report using the AA modifier and the CRNA would report using the QZ modifier. Documentation must be submitted by each provider to support payment of the full fee.

100-04, 12, 140.4.3

Payment for Medical or Surgical Services Furnished by CRNAs

(Rev. 3747; Issued: 04-14-17; Effective: 01-01-17; Implementation: 05-15-17)

Payment shall be made for reasonable and necessary medical or surgical services furnished by CRNAs if they are legally authorized to perform these services in the state in which services are furnished. Payment is determined under the physician fee schedule on the basis of the national physician fee schedule conversion factor, the geographic adjustment factor, and the resource-based relative value units for the medical or surgical service.

100-04, 12, 140.5

Payment for Anesthesia Services Furnished by a Teaching CRNA

(Rev. 3747; Issued: 04-14-17; Effective: 01-01-17; Implementation: 05-15-17)

Payment can be made under Part B to a teaching CRNA who supervises a single case involving a student nurse anesthetist where the CRNA is continuously present. The CRNA reports the service using the QZ modifier. No payment is made under Part B for the service provided by a student nurse anesthetist.

The A/B MAC may allow payment, as follows, if a teaching CRNA is involved in cases with two student nurse anesthetists:

- Recognize the full base units (assigned to the anesthesia code) where the teaching CRNA is present with the student nurse anesthetist throughout pre and post anesthesia care; and
- Recognize the actual time the teaching CRNA is personally present with the student nurse anesthetist. Anesthesia time may be discontinuous. For example, a teaching CRNA is involved in two concurrent cases with student nurse anesthetists. Case 1 runs from 9:00 a.m. to 11:00 a.m. and case 2 runs from 9:45a.m. to 11:30 a.m. The teaching CRNA is present in case 1 from 9:00 a.m. to 9:30 a.m. and from 10:15 a.m. to 10:30 a.m. From 9:45 a.m. to 10:14 a.m. and from 10:31 a.m. to 11:30 a.m., the CRNA is present in case 2. The CRNA may report 45 minutes of anesthesia time for case 1 (i.e., 3 time units) and 88 minutes (i.e., 5.9 units) of anesthesia time for case 2.

The teaching CRNA must document his/her involvement in cases with student nurse anesthetists. The documentation must be sufficient to support the payment of the fee and available for review upon request.

The teaching CRNA (not under the medical direction of a physician), can be paid for his or her involvement in each of two concurrent cases with student nurse anesthetists; allow payment at the regular fee schedule rate. The teaching CRNA reports the anesthesia service using the QZmodifier.

To bill the anesthesia base units, the teaching CRNA must be present with the student nurse anesthetist during pre and post anesthesia care for each of the two cases. To bill anesthesia time for each case, the teaching CRNA must continue to devote his or her time to the two concurrent cases and not be involved in other activities. The teaching CRNA can decide how to allocate his or her time to optimize patient care in the two cases based on the complexity of the anesthesia cases, the experience and skills of the student nurse anesthetists, and the patients' health status and other factors. The teaching CRNA must document his or her involvement in the cases with the student nurse anesthetists.

100-04, 12, 160

Independent Psychologist Services

(Rev. 1, 10-01-03) B3-2150, B3-2070.2

See the Medicare Benefit Policy Manual, Chapter 15, for coverage requirements.

There are a number of types of psychologists. Educational psychologists engage in identifying and treating education-related issues. In contrast, counseling psychologists provide services that include a broader realm including phobias, familial issues, etc.

Psychometrists are psychologists who have been trained to administer and interpret tests.

However, clinical psychologists are defined as a provider of diagnostic and therapeutic services. Because of the differences in services provided, services provided by psychologists who do not provide clinical services are subject to different billing guidelines. One service often provided by nonclinical psychologist is diagnostic testing.

NOTE: Diagnostic psychological testing services performed by persons who meet these requirements are covered as other diagnostic tests. When, however, the psychologist is not practicing independently, but is on the staff of an institution, agency, or clinic, that entity bills for the diagnostic services.

Expenses for such testing are not subject to the payment limitation on treatment for mental, psychoneurotic, and personality disorders. Independent psychologists are not required by law to accept assignment when performing psychological tests. However, regardless of whether the psychologist accepts assignment, he or she must report on the claim form the name and address of the physician who ordered the test.

100-04, 12, 160.1

Payment

(Rev. 1, 10-01-03)

Diagnostic testing services are not subject to the outpatient mental health limitation. Refer to §210, below, for a discussion of the outpatient mental health limitation. The diagnostic testing services performed by a psychologist (who is not a clinical psychologist) practicing independently of an institution, agency, or physician's office are covered as other diagnostic tests if a physician orders such testing. Medicare covers this type of testing as an outpatient service if furnished by any psychologist who is licensed or certified to practice psychology in the State or jurisdiction where he or she is furnishing services or, if the jurisdiction does not issue licenses, if provided by any practicing psychologist. (It is CMS' understanding that all States, the District of Columbia, and Puerto Ricolicense psychologists, but that some trust territories do not. Examples of psychologists, other than clinical psychologists, whose services are covered under this provision include, but are not limited to, educational psychologists and counseling psychologists.)

To determine whether the diagnostic psychological testing services of a particular independent psychologist are covered under Part B in States which have statutory licensure or certification, carriers must secure from the appropriate State agency a current listing of psychologists holding the required credentials. In States or territories which lack statutory licensing and certification, carriers must check individual qualifications as claims are submitted. Possible reference sources are the national directory of membership of the American Psychological Association, which provides data about the educational background of individuals and indicates which members are board-certified, and records and directories of the State or territorial psychological association. If qualification is dependent on a doctoral degree from a currently accredited program, carriers must verify the date of accreditation of the school involved, since such accreditation is not retroactive. If the reference sources listed above do not provide enough information (e.g., the psychologist is not a member of the association), carriers must contact the psychologist personally for the required information. Carriers may wish to maintain a continuing list of psychologists whose qualifications have been verified.

Medicare excludes expenses for diagnostic testing from the payment limitation on treatment for mental/psychoneurotic/personality disorders.

Carriers must identify the independent psychologist's choice whether or not to accept assignment when performing psychological tests.

Carriers must accept an independent psychologist claim only if the psychologist reports the name/UPIN of the physician who ordered a test.

Carriers pay nonparticipating independent psychologists at 95 percent of the physician fee schedule allowed amount.

Carriers pay participating independent psychologists at 100 percent of the physician fee schedule allowed amount. Independent psychologists are identified on the provider file by specialty code 62 and provider type 35.

100-04, 12, 170

Clinical Psychologist Services

(Rev. 1, 10-01-03)

B3-2150 See Medicare Benefit Policy Manual, Chapter 15, for general coverage requirements.

Direct payment may be made under Part B for professional services. However, services furnished incident to the professional services of CPs to hospital patients remain bundled.

Therefore, payment must continue to be made to the hospital (by the FI) for such "incident to" services.

100-04, 12, 180

Care Plan Oversight Services

(Rev. 999, Issued: 07-14-06; Effective: 01-01-05; Implementation: 10-02-06)

The Medicare Benefit Policy Manual, Chapter 15, contains requirements for coverage for medical and other health services including those of physicians and non-physician practitioners.

Care plan oversight (CPO) is the physician supervision of a patient receiving complex and/or multidisciplinary care as part of Medicare-covered services provided by a participating home health agency or Medicare approved hospice.

CPO services require complex or multidisciplinary care modalities involving:

- Regular physician development and/or revision of care plans;
- Review of subsequent reports of patient status;
- Review of related laboratory and other studies;
- Communication with other health professionals not employed in the same practice who are involved in the patient's care;
- Integration of new information into the medical treatment plan; and/or
- Adjustment of medical therapy.

The CPO services require recurrent physician supervision of a patient involving 30 or more minutes of the physician's time per month. Services not countable toward the 30 minutes threshold that must be provided in order to bill for CPO include, but are not limited to:

- Time associated with discussions with the patient, his or her family or friends to adjust medication or treatment;
- Time spent by staff getting or filing charts;
- Travel time; and/or Physician's time spent telephoning prescriptions into the pharmacist unless the telephone conversation involves discussions of pharmaceutical therapies.

Implicit in the concept of CPO is the expectation that the physician has coordinated an aspect of the patient's care with the home health agency or hospice during the month for which CPO services were billed. The physician who bills for CPO must be the same physician who signs the plan of care.

Nurse practitioners, physician assistants, and clinical nurse specialists, practicing within the scope of State law, may bill for care plan oversight. These non-physician practitioners must have been providing ongoing care for the beneficiary through evaluation and management services. These non-physician practitioners may not bill for CPO if they have been involved only with the delivery of the Medicare-covered home health or hospice service.

A. Home Health CPO

Non-physician practitioners can perform CPO only if the physician signing the plan of care provides regular ongoing care under the same plan of care as does the NPP billing for CPO and either:

- The physician and NPP are part of the same group practice; or
- If the NPP is a nurse practitioner or clinical nurse specialist, the physician signing the plan of care also has a collaborative agreement with the NPP; or
- If the NPP is a physician assistant, the physician signing the plan of care is also the physician who provides general supervision of physician assistant services for the practice.

Billing may be made for care plan oversight services furnished by an NPP when:

- The NPP providing the care plan oversight has seen and examined the patient;
- The NPP providing care plan oversight is not functioning as a consultant whose participation is limited to a single medical condition rather than multidisciplinary coordination of care; and
- The NPP providing care plan oversight integrates his or her care with that of the physician who signed the plan of care.

NPPs may not certify the beneficiary for home health care.

B. Hospice CPO

The attending physician or nurse practitioner (who has been designated as the attending physician) may bill for hospice CPO when they are acting as an "attending physician".

An "attending physician" is one who has been identified by the individual, at the time he/she elects hospice coverage, as having the most significant role in the determination and delivery of their medical care. They are not employed nor paid by the hospice. The care plan oversight services are billed using Form CMS-1500 or electronic equivalent.

For additional information on hospice CPO, see Chapter 11, 40.1.3.1 of this manual.

100-04, 12, 180.1

Care Plan Oversight Billing Requirements
(Rev. 999, Issued: 07-14-06; Effective: 01-01-05; Implementation: 10-02-06)

A. Codes for Which Separate Payment May Be Made

Effective January 1, 1995, separate payment may be made for CPO oversight services for 30 minutes or more if the requirements specified in the Medicare Benefits Policy Manual, Chapter 15 are met.

Providers billing for CPO must submit the claim with no other services billed on that claim and may bill only after the end of the month in which the CPO services were rendered. CPO services may not be billed across calendar months and should be submitted (and paid) only for one unit of service.

Physicians may bill and be paid separately for CPO services only if all the criteria in the Medicare Benefit Policy Manual, Chapter 15 are met.

B. Physician Certification and Recertification of Home Health Plans of Care

Effective 2001, two new HCPCS codes for the certification and recertification and development of plans of care for Medicare-covered home health services were created.

See the Medicare General Information, Eligibility, and Entitlement Manual, Pub. 100-1, Chapter 4, "Physician Certification and Recertification of Services," 10-60, and the Medicare Benefit Policy Manual, Pub. 100-2, Chapter 7, "Home Health Services", 30.

The home health agency certification code can be billed only when the patient has not received Medicare-covered home health services for at least 60 days. The home health agency recertification code is used after a patient has received services for at least 60 days (or one certification period) when the physician signs the certification after the initial certification period. The home health agency recertification code will be reported only once every 60 days, except in the rare situation when the patient starts a new episode before 60 days elapses and requires a new plan of care to start a new episode.

C. Provider Number of Home Health Agency (HHA) or Hospice

For claims for CPO submitted on or after January 1, 1997, physicians must enter on the Medicare claim form the 6-character Medicare provider number of the HHA or hospice providing Medicare-covered services to the beneficiary for the period during which CPO services was furnished and for which the physician signed the plan of care. Physicians are responsible for obtaining the HHA or hospice Medicare provider numbers.

Additionally, physicians should provide their UPIN to the HHA or hospice furnishing services to their patient.

NOTE: There is currently no place on the HIPAA standard ASC X12N 837 professional format to specifically include the HHA or hospice provider number required for a care plan oversight claim. For this reason, the requirement to include the HHA or hospice provider number on a care plan oversight claim is temporarily waived until a new version of this electronic standard format is adopted under HIPAA and includes a place to provide the HHA and hospice provider numbers for care plan oversight claims.

100-04, 12, 190.3

List of Medicare Telehealth Services
(Rev. 3476, Issued: 03-11-16, Effective: 01-01-15, Effective: 04-11-16)

The use of a telecommunications system may substitute for an in-person encounter for professional consultations, office visits, office psychiatry services, and a limited number of other physician fee schedule (PFS) services. The various services and corresponding current procedure terminology (CPT) or Healthcare Common Procedure Coding System (HCPCS) codes are listed on the CMS website at www.cms.gov/Medicare/Medicare-General-Information/Telehealth/.

NOTE: Beginning January 1, 2010, CMS eliminated the use of all consultation codes, except for inpatient telehealth consultation G-codes. CMS no longer recognizes office/outpatient or inpatient consultation CPT codes for payment of office/outpatient or inpatient visits. Instead, physicians and practitioners are instructed to bill a new or established patient office/outpatient visit CPT code or appropriate hospital or nursing facility care code, as appropriate to the particular patient, for all office/outpatient or inpatient visits.

100-04, 12, 190.3.4

Payment for ESRD-Related Services as a Telehealth Service
(Rev. 3476, Issued: 03-11-16, Effective: 01-01-15, Effective: 04-11-16)

The ESRD-related services included in the monthly capitation payment (MCP) with 2 or 3 visits per month and ESRD-related services with 4 or more visits per month may be paid as Medicare telehealth services. However, at least 1 visit must be furnished face-to-face "hands on" to examine the vascular access site by a physician, clinical nurse specialist, nurse practitioner, or physician assistant. An interactive audio and video telecommunications system may be used for providing additional visits required under the 2-to-3 visit MCP and the 4-or-more visit MCP. The medical record must indicate that at least one of the visits was furnished face-to-face "hands on" by a physician, clinical nurse specialist, nurse practitioner, or physician assistant.

The MCP physician, for example, the physician or practitioner who is responsible for the complete monthly assessment of the patient and establishes the patient's plan of care, may use other physicians and practitioners to furnish ESRD-related visits through an interactive audio and video telecommunications system. The non-MCP physician or practitioner must have a relationship with the billing physician or practitioner such as a partner, employees of the same group practice or an employee of the MCP physician, for example, the non MCP physician or practitioner is either a W-2 employee or 1099 independent contractor. However, the physician or practitioner who is responsible for the complete monthly assessment and establishes the ESRD beneficiary's plan of care should bill for the MCP in any given month.

Clinical Criteria

The visit, including a clinical examination of the vascular access site, must be conducted face-to-face "hands on" by a physician, clinical nurse specialist, nurse practitioner or physician's assistant. For additional visits, the physician or practitioner at the distant site is required, at a minimum, to use an interactive audio and video telecommunications system that allows the physician or practitioner to provide medical management services for a maintenance dialysis beneficiary. For example, an

ESRD-related visit conducted via telecommunications system must permit the physician or practitioner at the distant site to perform an assessment of whether the dialysis is working effectively and whether the patient is tolerating the procedure well (physiologically and psychologically). During this assessment, the physician or practitioner at the distant site must be able to determine whether alteration in any aspect of the beneficiary's prescription is indicated, due to such changes as the estimate of the patient's dry weight.

100-04, 12, 190.3.5

Payment for Subsequent Hospital Care Services and Subsequent Nursing Facility Care Services as Telehealth Services

(Rev. 3476, Issued: 03-11-16, Effective: 01-01-15, Effective: 04-11-16)

Subsequent hospital care services are limited to one telehealth visit every 3 days. The frequency limit of the benefit is not intended to apply to consulting physicians or practitioners, who should continue to report initial or follow-up inpatient telehealth consultations using the applicable HCPCS G-codes.

Similarly, subsequent nursing facility care services are limited to one telehealth visit every 30 days. Furthermore, subsequent nursing facility care services reported for a Federally-mandated periodic visit under 42 CFR 483.40(c) may not be furnished through telehealth. The frequency limit of the benefit is not intended to apply to consulting physicians or practitioners, who should continue to report initial or follow-up inpatient telehealth consultations using the applicable HCPCS G-codes.

Inpatient telehealth consultations are furnished to beneficiaries in hospitals or skilled nursing facilities via telehealth at the request of the physician of record, the attending physician, or another appropriate source. The physician or practitioner who furnishes the initial inpatient consultation via telehealth cannot be the physician or practitioner of record or the attending physician or practitioner, and the initial inpatient telehealth consultation would be distinct from the care provided by the physician or practitioner of record or the attending physician or practitioner. Counseling and coordination of care with other providers or agencies is included as well, consistent with the nature of the problem(s) and the patient's needs. Initial and follow-up inpatient telehealth consultations are subject to the criteria for inpatient telehealth consultation services, as described in section 190.3 of this chapter.

100-04, 12, 190.3.6

Payment for Diabetes Self-Management Training (DSMT) as a Telehealth Service

(Rev. 3476, Issued: 03-11-16, Effective: 01-01-15, Effective: 04-11-16)

Individual and group DSMT services may be paid as a Medicare telehealth service; however, at least 1 hour of the 10 hour benefit in the year following the initial DSMT service must be furnished in-person to allow for effective injection training. The injection training may be furnished through either individual or group DSMT services. By reporting the –GT or –GQ modifier with HCPCS code G0108 (Diabetes outpatient self-management training services, individual, per 30 minutes) or G0109 (Diabetes outpatient self-management training services, group session (2 or more), per 30 minutes), the distant site practitioner certifies that the beneficiary has received or will receive 1 hour of in-person DSMT services for purposes of injection training during the year following the initial DSMT service.

As specified in 42 CFR 410.141(e) and stated in Pub. 100-02, Medicare Benefit Policy Manual, chapter 15, section 300.2, individual DSMT services may be furnished by a physician, individual, or entity that furnishes other services for which direct Medicare payment may be made and that submits necessary documentation to, and is accredited by, an accreditation organization approved by CMS. However, consistent with the statutory requirements of section 1834(m)(1) of the Act, as provided in 42 CFR 410.78(b)(1) and (b)(2) and stated in section 190.6 of this chapter, Medicare telehealth services, including individual DSMT services furnished as a telehealth service, could only be furnished by a licensed PA, NP, CNS, CNM, clinical psychologist, clinical social worker, or registered dietitian or nutrition professional.

100-04, 12, 190.5

Originating Site Facility Fee Payment Methodology

(Rev. 3476, Issued: 03-11-16, Effective: 01-01-15, Effective: 04-11-16)

1. Originating site defined

The term originating site means the location of an eligible Medicare beneficiary at the time the service being furnished via a telecommunications system occurs. For asynchronous, store and forward telecommunications technologies, an originating site is only a Federal telemedicine demonstration program conducted in Alaska or Hawaii.

2. Facility fee for originating site

The originating site facility fee is a separately billable Part B payment. The contractor pays it outside of other payment methodologies. This fee is subject to post payment verification.

For telehealth services furnished from October 1, 2001, through December 31, 2002, the originating site facility fee was the lesser of $20 or the actual charge. For services furnished on or after January 1 of each subsequent year, the originating site facility fee is updated by the Medicare Economic Index. The updated fee is included in the Medicare Physician Fee Schedule (MPFS) Final Rule, which is published by November 1 prior to the start of the calendar year for which it is effective. The updated fee for

each calendar year is also issued annually in a Recurring Update Notification instruction for January of each year.

3. Payment amount:

The originating site facility fee is a separately billable Part B payment. The payment amount to the originating site is the lesser of 80 percent of the actual charge or 80 percent of the originating site facility fee, except CAHs. The beneficiary is responsible for any unmet deductible amount and Medicare coinsurance.

The originating site facility fee payment methodology for each type of facility is clarified below.

Hospital outpatient department. When the originating site is a hospital outpatient department, payment for the originating site facility fee must be made as described above and not under the OPPS. Payment is not based on the OPPS payment methodology.

Hospital inpatient. For hospital inpatients, payment for the originating site facility fee must be made outside the diagnostic related group (DRG) payment, since this is a Part B benefit, similar to other services paid separately from the DRG payment, (e.g., hemophilia blood clotting factor).

Critical access hospitals. When the originating site is a critical access hospital, make payment separately from the cost-based reimbursement methodology. For CAH's, the payment amount is 80 percent of the originating site facility fee.

Federally qualified health centers (FQHCs) and rural health clinics (RHCs). The originating site facility fee for telehealth services is not an FQHC or RHC service. When an FQHC or RHC serves as the originating site, the originating site facility fee must be paid separately from the center or clinic all-inclusive rate.

Physicians' and practitioners' offices. When the originating site is a physician's or practitioner's office, the payment amount, in accordance with the law, is the lesser of 80 percent of the actual charge or 80 percent of the originating site facility fee, regardless of geographic location. The A/B MAC (B) shall not apply the geographic practice cost index (GPCI) to the originating site facility fee. This fee is statutorily set and is not subject to the geographic payment adjustments authorized under the MPFS.

Hospital-based or critical access-hospital based renal dialysis center (or their satellites). When a hospital-based or critical access hospital-based renal dialysis center (or their satellites) serves as the originating site, the originating site facility fee is covered in addition to any composite rate or MCP amount.

Skilled nursing facility (SNF). The originating site facility fee is outside the SNF prospective payment system bundle and, as such, is not subject to SNF consolidated billing. The originating site facility fee is a separately billable Part B payment.

Community Mental Health Center (CMHC). The originating site facility fee is not a partial hospitalization service. The originating site facility fee does not count towards the number of services used to determine payment for partial hospitalization services. The originating site facility fee is not bundled in the per diem payment for partial hospitalization. The originating site facility fee is a separately billable Part B payment.

To receive the originating facility site fee, the provider submits claims with HCPCS code "Q3014, telehealth originating site facility fee"; short description "telehealth facility fee." The type of service for the telehealth originating site facility fee is "9, other items and services." For A/B MAC (B) processed claims, the "office" place of service (code 11) is the only payable setting for code Q3014. There is no participation payment differential for code Q3014. Deductible and coinsurance rules apply to Q3014. By submitting Q3014 HCPCS code, the originating site authenticates they are located in either a rural HPSA or non-MSA county.

This benefit may be billed on bill types 12X, 13X, 22X, 23X, 71X, 72X, 73X, 76X, and 85X. Unless otherwise applicable, report the originating site facility fee under revenue code 078X and include HCPCS code "Q3014, telehealth originating site facility fee."

Hospitals and critical access hospitals bill their A/B/MAC (A) for the originating site facility fee. Telehealth bills originating in inpatient hospitals must be submitted on a 12X TOB using the date of discharge as the line item date of service.

Independent and provider-based RHCs and FQHCs bill the appropriate A/B/MAC (A) using the RHC or FQHC bill type and billing number. HCPCS code Q3014 is the only non-RHC/FQHC service that is billed using the clinic/center bill type and provider number. All RHCs and FQHCs must use revenue code 078X when billing for the originating site facility fee. For all other non-RHC/FQHC services, provider based RHCs and FQHCs must bill using the base provider's bill type and billing number. Independent RHCs and FQHCs must bill the A/B MAC (B) for all other non-RHC/FQHC services. If an RHC/FQHC visit occurs on the same day as a telehealth service, the RHC/FQHC serving as an originating site must bill for HCPCS code Q3014 telehealth originating site facility fee on a separate revenue line from the RHC/FQHC visit using revenue code 078X.

Hospital-based or CAH-based renal dialysis centers (including satellites) bill their A/B/MAC (A) for the originating site facility fee. Telehealth bills originating in renal dialysis centers must be submitted on a 72X TOB. All hospital-based or CAH-based renal dialysis centers (including satellites) must use revenue code 078X when billing for the originating site facility fee. The renal dialysis center serving as an originating site must bill for HCPCS code Q3014, telehealth originating site facility fee, on a separate revenue line from any other services provided to the beneficiary.

Skilled nursing facilities (SNFs) bill their A/B/MAC (A) for the originating site facility fee. Telehealth bills originating in SNFs must be submitted on TOB 22X or 23X. For SNF inpatients in a covered Part A stay, the originating site facility fee must be submitted on a 22X TOB. All SNFs must use revenue code 078X when billing for the originating site facility fee. The SNF serving as an originating site must bill for HCPCS code Q3014, telehealth originating site facility fee, on a separate revenue line from any other services provided to the beneficiary.

Community mental health centers (CMHCs) bill their A/B/MAC (A) for the originating site facility fee. Telehealth bills originating in CMHCs must be submitted on a 76X TOB. All CMHCs must use revenue code 078X when billing for the originating site facility fee. The CMHC serving as an originating site must bill for HCPCS code Q3014, telehealth originating site facility fee, on a separate revenue line from any other services provided to the beneficiary. Note that Q3014 does not count towards the number of services used to determine per diem payments for partial hospitalization services.

The beneficiary is responsible for any unmet deductible amount and Medicare coinsurance.

100-04, 12, 190.6

Payment Methodology for Physician/Practitioner at the Distant Site

(Rev. 3586, Issued: 08-12-16, Effective: 01-01-17, Effective: 01-03-17)

1. Distant Site Defined

The term "distant site" means the site where the physician or practitioner, providing the professional service, is located at the time the service is provided via a telecommunications system.

2. Payment Amount (professional fee)

The payment amount for the professional service provided via a telecommunications system by the physician or practitioner at the distant site is equal to the current fee schedule amount for the service provided at the facility rate. Payment for an office visit, consultation, individual psychotherapy or pharmacologic management via a telecommunications system should be made at the same facility amount as when these services are furnished without the use of a telecommunications system. For Medicare payment to occur, the service must be within a practitioner's scope of practice under State law. The beneficiary is responsible for any unmet deductible amount and applicable coinsurance.

3. Medicare Practitioners Who May Receive Payment at the Distant Site (i.e., at a site other than where beneficiary is)

As a condition of Medicare Part B payment for telehealth services, the physician or practitioner at the distant site must be licensed to provide the service under state law. When the physician or practitioner at the distant site is licensed under state law to provide a covered telehealth service (i.e., professional consultation, office and other outpatient visits, individual psychotherapy, and pharmacologic management) then he or she may bill for and receive payment for this service when delivered via a telecommunications system.

If the physician or practitioner at the distant site is located in a CAH that has elected Method II, and the physician or practitioner has reassigned his/her benefits to the CAH, the CAH bills its regular A/B/MAC (A) for the professional services provided at the distant site via a telecommunications system, in any of the revenue codes 096x, 097x or 098x. All requirements for billing distant site telehealth services apply.

4. Medicare Practitioners Who May Bill for Covered Telehealth Services are Listed Below (subject to State law)

- Physician
- Nurse practitioner
- Physician assistant
- Nurse-midwife
- Clinical nurse specialist
- Clinical psychologist*
- Clinical social worker*
- Registered dietitian or nutrition professional
- Certified registered nurse anesthetist

*Clinical psychologists and clinical social workers cannot bill for psychotherapy services that include medical evaluation and management services under Medicare. These practitioners may not bill or receive payment for the following CPT codes: 90805, 90807, and 90809.

100-04, 12, 190.6.1

Submission of Telehealth Claims for Distant Site Practitioners

(Rev. 3586, Issued: 08-12-16, Effective: 01-01-17, Implementation: 01-03-17)

Claims for telehealth services are submitted to the contractors that process claims for the performing physician/practitioner's service area. Physicians/practitioners submit the appropriate HCPCS procedure code for covered professional telehealth services with place of service code 02 (Telehealth) along with the "GT" modifier ("via interactive audio and video telecommunications system"). By coding and billing the "GT" modifier with a covered telehealth procedure code, the distant site physician/practitioner certifies that the beneficiary was present at an eligible originating site when the telehealth service was furnished. By coding and billing the "GT" modifier with a covered ESRD-related service telehealth code, the distant site physician/practitioner certifies that 1 visit per month was furnished face-to-face

"hands on" to examine the vascular access site. Refer to section 190.3.4 of this chapter for the conditions of telehealth payment for ESRD-related services.

In situations where a CAH has elected payment Method II for CAH outpatients, and the practitioner has reassigned his/her benefits to the CAH, A/B/MACs (A) should make payment for telehealth services provided by the physician or practitioner at 80 percent of the MPFS facility amount for the distant site service. In all other cases, except for MNT services as discussed in Section 190.7- A/B MAC (B) Editing of Telehealth Claims, telehealth services provided by the physician or practitioner at the distant site are billed to the A/B/MAC (B).

Physicians and practitioners at the distant site bill their A/B/MAC (B) for covered telehealth services, for example, "99245 GT." Physicians' and practitioners' offices serving as a telehealth originating site bill their A/B/MAC (B) for the originating site facility fee.

100-04, 12, 190.7

A/B MAC (B) Editing of Telehealth Claims

(Rev. 3721, Issued: 02-24-17, Effective: 05-25-17, Implementation: 05-25-17)

Medicare telehealth services (as listed in section 190.3) are billed with either the "GT" or "GQ" modifier. The contractor shall approve covered telehealth services if the physician or practitioner is licensed under State law to provide the service. Contractors must familiarize themselves with licensure provisions of States for which they process claims and disallow telehealth services furnished by physicians or practitioners who are not authorized to furnish the applicable telehealth service under State law. For example, if a nurse practitioner is not licensed to provide individual psychotherapy under State law, he or she would not be permitted to receive payment for individual psychotherapy under Medicare. The contractor shall install edits to ensure that only properly licensed physicians and practitioners are paid for covered telehealth services.

If a contractor receives claims for professional telehealth services coded with the "GQ" modifier (representing "via asynchronous telecommunications system"), it shall approve/pay for these services only if the physician or practitioner is affiliated with a Federal telemedicine demonstration conducted in Alaska or Hawaii. The contractor may require the physician or practitioner at the distant site to document his or her participation in a Federal telemedicine demonstration program conducted in Alaska or Hawaii prior to paying for telehealth services provided via asynchronous, store and forward technologies.

Contractors shall deny telehealth services if the physician or practitioner is not eligible to bill for them.

The following reflects the remittance advice messages and associated codes that will appear when rejecting/denying claims under this policy. This CARC/RARC combination is compliant with CAQH CORE Business Scenario 3.

> Group Code: CO
> CARC: 185
> RARC: N/A
> MSN: 21.18

If a service is billed with one of the telehealth modifiers and the procedure code is not designated as a covered telehealth service, the contractor denies the service.

The following reflects the remittance advice messages and associated codes that will appear when rejecting/denying claims under this policy. This CARC/RARC combination is compliant with CAQH CORE Business Scenario 3.

> Group Code: CO
> CARC: 96
> RARC: N776
> MSN: 9.4

The only claims from institutional facilities that FIs shall pay for telehealth services at the distant site, except for MNT services, are for physician or practitioner services when the distant site is located in a CAH that has elected Method II, and the physician or practitioner has reassigned his/her benefits to the CAH. The CAH bills its regular FI for the professional services provided at the distant site via a telecommunications system, in any of the revenue codes 096x, 097x or 098x. All requirements for billing distant site telehealth services apply.

Claims from hospitals or CAHs for MNT services are submitted to the hospital's or CAH's regular FI. Payment is based on the non-facility amount on the Medicare Physician Fee Schedule for the particular HCPCS codes.

100-04, 12, 230

Primary Care Incentive Payment Program (PCIP)

(Rev. 2161, Issued: 02-25-11, Effective: 01-01-11- Analysis/04-04-11-Design, Implementation: 01-01-11)

Section 5501(a) of the Affordable Care Act revises Section 1833 of the Social Security Act (the Act) by adding a new paragraph, (x), "Incentive Payments for Primary Care Services." Section 1833(x) of the Act states that in the case of primary care services furnished on or after January 1, 2011, and before January 1, 2016, there shall be a 10 percent incentive payment for such services under Part B when furnished by a primary care practitioner.

Information regarding Primary Care Incentive Payment Program (PCIP) payments made to critical access hospitals (CAHs) paid under the optional method can be found in Pub. 100-4, Chapter 4, §250.12 of this manual.

100-04, 12, 230.1

Definition of Primary Care Practitioners and Primary Care Services

(Rev. 2161, Issued: 02-25-11, Effective: 01-01-11- Analysis/04-04-11-Design, Implementation: 01-01-11)

Primary care practitioners are defined as:

1. A physician who has a primary specialty designation of family medicine, internal medicine, geriatric medicine, or pediatric medicine for whom primary care services accounted for at least 60 percent of the allowed charges under Part B for the practitioner in a prior period as determined appropriate by the Secretary; or

2. A nurse practitioner, clinical nurse specialist, or physician assistant for whom primary care services accounted for at least 60 percent of the allowed charges under Part B for the practitioner in a prior period as determined appropriate by the Secretary.

Primary care services are defined as HCPCS Codes:

1. 99201 through 99215 for new and established patient office or outpatient evaluation and management (E/M) visits;

2. 99304 through 99340 for initial, subsequent, discharge, and other nursing facility E/M services; new and established patient domiciliary, rest home or custodial care E/M services; and domiciliary, rest home or home care plan oversight services; and

3. 99341 through 99350 for new and established patient home E/M visits.

Practitioner Identification

Eligible practitioners will be identified on claims by the National Provider Identifier (NPI) number of the rendering practitioner. If the claim is submitted by a practitioner's group practice, the rendering practitioner's NPI must be included on the line-item for the primary care service and reflect an eligible HCPCS as identified. In order to be eligible for the PCIP, physician assistants, clinical nurse specialists, and nurse practitioners must be billing for their services under their own NPI and not furnishing services incident to physicians' services. Regardless of the specialty area in which they may be practicing, the specific nonphysician practitioners are eligible for the PCIP based on their profession and historical percentage of allowed charges as primary care services that equals or exceeds the 60 percent threshold.

Beginning in calendar year (CY) 2011, primary care practitioners will be identified based on their primary specialty of enrollment in Medicare and percentage of allowed charges for primary care services that equals or exceeds the 60 percent threshold from Medicare claims data 2 years prior to the bonus payment year.

Eligible practitioners for PCIP payments in a given calendar year (CY) will be listed by eligible NPI in the Primary Care Incentive Payment Program Eligibility File, available after January 31, of the payment year on their Medicare contractor's website. Practitioners should contact their contractor with any questions regarding their eligibility for the PCIP.

100-04, 12, 230.2

Coordination with Other Payments

(Rev. 2161, Issued: 02-25-11, Effective: 01-01-11- Analysis/04-04-11-Design, Implementation: 01-01-11)

Section 5501(a)(3) of the Affordable Care Act provides payment under the PCIP as an additional payment amount for specified primary care services without regard to any additional payment for the service under Section 1833(m) of the Act. Therefore, an eligible primary care physician furnishing a primary care service in a health professional shortage area (HPSA) may receive both a HPSA physician bonus payment (as described in the Medicare Claims Processing Manual, Pub. 100-4, Chapter 12, §90.4) under the HPSA physician bonus program and a PCIP incentive payment under the new program beginning in CY 2011.

100-04, 12, 230.3

Claims Processing and Payment

(Rev. 2161, Issued: 02-25-11, Effective: 01-01-11- Analysis/04-04-11-Design, Implementation: 01-01-11)

A. General Overview

Incentive payments will be made on a quarterly basis and shall be equal to 10 percent of the amount paid for such services under the Medicare Physician Fee Schedule (PFS) for those services furnished during the bonus payment year. For information on PCIP payments to CAHs paid under the optional method, see the Medicare Claims Processing Manual, Pub. 100-4, Chapter 4, §250.12.

On an annual basis Medicare contractors shall receive a Primary Care Incentive Payment Program Eligibility File that they shall post to their website. The file will list the NPIs of all practitioners who are eligible to receive PCIP payments for the upcoming CY.

B. Method of Payment

- Calculate and pay qualifying primary care practitioners an additional 10 percent incentive payment;

- Calculate the payment based on the amount actually paid for the services, not the Medicare approved amounts;

- Combine the PCIP incentive payments, when appropriate, with other incentive payments, including the HPSA physician bonus payment, and the HPSA Surgical Incentive Payment Program (HSIP) payment;

- Provide a special remittance form that is forwarded with the incentive payment so that physicians and practitioners can identify which type of incentive payment (HPSA physician and/or PCIP) was paid for which services.

- Practitioners should contact their contractor with any questions regarding PCIP payments.

C. Changes for Contractor Systems

The Medicare Carrier System, (MCS), Common Working File (CWF) and the National Claims History (NCH) shall be modified to accept a new PCIP indicator on the claim line. Once the type of incentive payment has been identified by the shared systems, the shared system shall modify their systems to set the indicator on the claim line as follows:

1 = HPSA;

2 = PSA;

3 = HPSA and PSA;

4 = HSIP;

5 = HPSA and HSIP;

6 = PCIP;

7 = HPSA and PCIP; and

Space = Not Applicable.

The contractor shared system shall send the HIGLAS 810 invoice for incentive payment invoices, including the new PCIP payment. The contractor shall also combine the provider's HPSA physician bonus, physician scarcity (PSA) bonus (if it should become available at a later date), HSIP payment and/or PCIP payment invoice per provider. The contractor shall receive the HIGLAS 835 payment file from HIGLAS showing a single incentive payment per provider.

100-04, 13, 30.1.3.1

A/B MAC (A) Payment for Low Osmolar Contrast Material (LOCM) (Radiology)

(Rev. 3227, Issued: 04-02-15, Effective--multiple effective dates)

The LOCM is paid on a reasonable cost basis when rendered by a SNF to its Part B patients (in addition to payment for the radiology procedure) when it is used in one of the situations listed below.

The following HCPCS are used when billing for LOCM.

HCPCS Code	Description (January 1. 1994, and later)
A4644	Supply of low osmolar contrast material (100-199 mgs of iodine);
A4645	Supply of low osmolar contrast material (200-299 mgs of iodine); or
A4646	Supply of low osmolar contrast material (300-399 mgs of iodine).

When billing for LOCM, SNFs use revenue code 0636. If the SNF charge for the radiology procedure includes a charge for contrast material, the SNF must adjust the charge for the radiology procedure to exclude any amount for the contrast material.

NOTE: LOCM is never billed with revenue code 0255 or as part of the radiology procedure.

The A/B MAC (A) will edit for the intrathecal procedure codes and the following codes to determine if payment for LOCM is to be made. If an intrathecal procedure code is not present, or one of the ICD codes is not present to indicate that a required medical condition is met, the A/B MAC (A) will deny payment for LOCM. In these instances, LOCM is not covered and should not be billed to Medicare.

When LOCM Is Separately Billable and Related Coding Requirements

- In all intrathecal injections. HCPCS codes that indicate intrathecal injections are:

  70010, 70015, 72240, 72255, 72265, 72270, 72285, 72295

  One of these must be included on the claim; or

- In intravenous and intra-arterial injections only when certain medical conditions are present in an outpatient. The SNF must verify the existence of at least one of the following medical conditions, and report the applicable diagnosis code(s) either as a principal diagnosis code or other diagnosis codes on the claim:

  — A history of previous adverse reaction to contrast material. The applicable ICD-9-CM codes are V14.8 and V14.9. The applicable ICD-10-CM codes are Z88.8 and Z88.9. The conditions which should not be considered adverse reactions are a sensation of heat, flushing, or a single episode of nausea or vomiting. If the adverse reaction occurs on that visit with the induction of contrast material, codes describing hives, urticaria, etc. should also be present, as well as a code describing the external cause of injury and poisoning, ICD-9-CM code E947.8. The applicable ICD-10 CM codes are: T50.8X5A Adverse effect of diagnostic agents, initial encounter, T50.8X5S Adverse effect of diagnostic agents, sequela , T50.995A Adverse effect of other drugs, medicaments and biological substances, initial encounter, or

T50.995S Adverse effect of other drugs, medicaments and biological substances, sequela;

— A history or condition of asthma or allergy. The applicable ICD-9-CM codes are V07.1, V14.0 through V14.9, V15.0, 493.00, 493.01, 493.10, 493.11, 493.20, 493.21, 493.90, 493.91, 495.0, 495.1, 495.2, 495.3, 495.4, 495.5, 495.6, 495.7, 495.8, 495.9, 995.0, 995.1, 995.2, and 995.3. The applicable ICD-10-CM codes are in the table below:

ICD-10-CM Codes

J44.0	J44.9	J45.20	J45.22	J45.30	J45.32	J45.40
J45.42	J45.50	J45.52	J45.902	J45.909	J45.998	J67.0
J67.1	JJ67.2	J67.3	J67.4	J67.5	J67.6	J67.7
J67.8	J67.9	J96.00	J96.01	J96.02	J96.90	J96.91
J96.92	T36.0X5A	T36.1X5A	T36.2X5A	T36.3X5A	T36.4X5A	T36.5X5A
T36.6X5A	T36.7X5A	T36.8X5A	T36.95XA	T37.0X5A	T37.1X5A	T37.2X5A
T37.3X5A	T37.8X5A	T37.95XA	T38.0X5A	T38.1X5A	T38.2X5A	T38.3X5A
T38.4X5A	T38.6X5A	T38.7X5A	T38.805A	T38.815A	T38.895A	T38.905A
T38.995A	T39.015A	T39.095A	T39.1X5A	T39.2X5A	T39.2X5A	T39.315A
T39.395A	T39.4X5A	T39.8X5A	T39.95XA	T40.0X5A	T40.1X5A	T40.2X5A
T40.3X5A	T40.4X5A	T40.5X5A	T40.605A	T40.695A	T40.7X5A	T40.8X5A
T40.905A	T40.995A	T41.0X5A	T41.1X5A	T41.205A	T41.295A	T41.3X5A
T41.4X5A	T41.X5A	T41.5X5A	T42.0X5A	T42.1X5A	T42.2X5A	T42.3X5A
T42.4X5A	T42.5X5A	T42.6X5A	427.5XA	428.X5A	T43.015A	T43.025A
T43.1X5A	T43.205A	T43.215A	T43.225A	T43.295A	T43.3X5A	T43.4X5A
T43.505A	T43.595A	T43.605A	T43.615A	T43.625A	T43.635A	T43.695A
T43.8X5A	T43.95XA	T44.0X5A	T44.1X5A	T44.2X5A	T44.3X5A	T44.6X5A
T44.7X5A	T44.8X5A	T44.905A	T44.995A	T45.0X5A	T45.1X5A	T45.2X5A
T45.3X5A	T45.4X5A	T45.515A	T45.525A	T45.605A	T45.615A	T45.625A
T45.695A	T45.7X5A	T45.8X5A	T45.95XA	T46.0X5A	T46.1X5A	T46.2X5A
T46.3X5A	T46.4X5A	T46.5X5A	T46.6X5A	T46.7X5A	T46.8X5A	T46.905A
T46.995A	T47.0X5A	T47.1X5A	T47.2X5A	T47.3X5A	T47.4X5A	T47.5X5A
T47.6X5A	T47.7X5A	T47.8X5A	T47.95XA	T48.0X5A	T48.1X5A	T48.205A
T48.295A	T48.3X5A	T48.4X5A	T48.5X5A	T48.6X5A	T48.905A	T48.995A
T49.0X5A	T49.1X5A	T49.2X5A	T49.3X5A	T49.4X5A	T49.5X5A	T49.6X5A
T49.6X5A	T47.X5A9	T49.8X5A	T49.95XA	T50.0X5A	T50.1X5A	T50.2X5A
T50.3X5A	T50.4X5A	T50.5X5A	T50.6X5A	T50.7X5A	T50.8X5A	T50.905a
T50.Z95A	T50.A15A	T50.A25A	T50.A95A	T50.B15A	T50.B95A	T50.Z15A
T50.Z95A	T78.2XXA	T78.3XXA	T78.40XA	T78.41XA	T88.52XA	T88.59XA
T88.6XXA	Z51.89	Z88.0	Z88.1	Z88.2	Z88.3	Z88.4
Z88.5	Z88.6	Z88.7	Z88.8	Z88.9	Z91.010	

— Significant cardiac dysfunction including recent or imminent cardiac decompensation, severe arrhythmia, unstable angina pectoris, recent myocardial infarction, and pulmonary hypertension. The applicable ICD-9-CM codes are:

ICD-9-CM

402.00	402.01	402.10	402.11	402.90	402.91	404.00
404.01	404.02	404.03	404.10	404.11	404.12	404.13
404.90	404.91	404.92	404.93	410.00	410.01	410.02
410.10	410.11	410.12	410.20	410.21	410.22	410.30
410.31	410.32	410.40	410.41	410.42	410.50	410.51
410.52	410.60	410.61	410.62	410.70	410.71	410.72
410.80	410.81	410.82	410.90	410.91	410.92	411.1
415.0	416.0	416.1	416.8	416.9	420.0	420.90
420.91	420.99	424.90	424.91	424.99	427.0	427.1
427.2	427.31	427.32	427.41	427.42	427.5	427.60
427.61	427.69	427.81	427.89	427.9	428.0	428.1
428.9	429.0	429.1	429.2	429.3	429.4	429.5
429.6	429.71	429.79	429.81	429.82	429.89	429.9
785.50	785.51	785.59				

— The applicable ICD-10-CM codes are in the table below:

ICD-10-CM Codes

A18.84	I11.0	I11.9	I13.0	I13.10	I13.11	I13.2
I20.0	I21.01	I21.02	I21.09	I21.11	I21.19	I21.21
I21.29	I21.3	I21.4	I22.1	I22.2	I22.8	I23.0
I23.1	I23.2	I23.3	I23.4	I23.5	I23.6	I23.7
I23.8	I25.10	I25.110	I25.700	I25.710	I25.720	I25.730

I25.750	I25.760	I25.790	I26.01	I26.02	I26.09	I27.0
I27.1	I27.2	I27.81	I27.89	I27.9	I30.0	I30.1
I30.8	I30.9	I32	I38	I39	I46.2	I46.8
I46.9	I47.0	I471	I472	I47.9	I48.0	I48.1
I48.1	I48.2	I48.3	I48.4	I48.91	I48.92	I49.01
I49.02	I49.1	I49.2	I49.3	I49.40	I49.49	I49.5
I49.8	I49.9	I50.1	I50.20	I50.21	I50.22	I50.23
I50.30	I50.31	I50.32	I50.33	I50.40	I50.41	I50.42
I50.43	I50.9	I51	I51.0	I51.1	I51.2	I51.3
I51.4	I51.5	I51.7	I51.89	I51.9	I52	I97.0
I97.110	I97.111	I97.120	I97.121	I97.130	I97.131	I97.190
I97.191	M32.11	M32.12	R00.1	R57.0	R57.8	R57.9

— Generalized severe debilitation. The applicable ICD-9-CM codes are: 203.00, 203.01, all codes for diabetes mellitus, 518.81, 585, 586, 799.3, 799.4, and V46.1. The applicable ICD-10-CM codes are: J96.850, J96.00 through J96.02, J96.90 through J96.91, N18.1 through N19, R53.81, R64, and Z99.11 through Z99.12. Or

— Sickle Cell disease. The applicable ICD-9-CM codes are 282.4, 282.60, 282.61, 282.62, 282.63, and 282.69. The applicable ICD-10-CM codes are D56.0 through D56.3, D56.5 through D56.9, D57.00 through D57.1, D57.20, D57.411 through D57.419, and D57.811 through D57.819.

100-04, 13, 40

Magnetic Resonance Imaging (MRI) Procedures

(Rev. 4147, Issued: 10-19-18, Effective: 04- 10-18, Implementation: 12-10-18)

The Centers for Medicare & Medicaid Services (CMS) finds that the non-coverage of magnetic resonance imaging (MRI) for blood flow determination is no longer supported by the available evidence. CMS is removing the phrase "blood flow measurement" and local Medicare contractors will have the discretion to cover (or not cover).

Consult Publication (Pub.) 100-03, National Coverage Determinations (NCD) Manual, chapter 1, section 220.2, for specific coverage and non-coverage indications associated with MRI and MRA (Magnetic Resonance Angiography).

A/B MACs (B) do not make additional payments for three or more MRI sequences. The relative value units (RVUs) reflect payment levels for two sequences.

The technical component (TC) RVUs for MRI procedures that specify "with contrast" include payment for paramagnetic contrast media. A/B MACs (B) do not make separate payment under code A4647.

A diagnostic technique has been developed under which an MRI of the brain or spine is first performed without contrast material, then another MRI is performed with a standard (0.1mmol/kg) dose of contrast material and, based on the need to achieve a better image, a third MRI is performed with an additional double dosage (0.2mmol/kg) of contrast material. When the high-dose contrast technique is utilized, A/B MACs (B):

- Do not pay separately for the contrast material used in the second MRI procedure;

- Pay for the contrast material given for the third MRI procedure through supply code Q9952, the replacement code for A4643, when billed with Current Procedural Terminology (CPT) codes 70553, 72156, 72157, and 72158;

- Do not pay for the third MRI procedure. For example, in the case of an MRI of the brain, if CPT code 70553 (without contrast material, followed by with contrast material(s) and further sequences) is billed, make no payment for CPT code 70551 (without contrast material(s)), the additional procedure given for the purpose of administering the double dosage, furnished during the same session. Medicare does not pay for the third procedure (as distinguished from the contrast material) because the CPT definition of code 70553 includes all further sequences; and

- Do not apply the payment criteria for low osmolar contrast media in §30.1.2 to billings for code Q9952, the replacement code for A4643. Effective January 1; 2008, Q9952 is replaced with A9579.

With the implementation for calendar year 2007 of a bottom-up methodology, which utilizes the direct inputs to determine the practice expense (PE) relative value units (RVUs), the cost of the contrast media is not included in the PE RVUs. Therefore, a separate payment for the contrast media used in various imaging procedures is paid. In addition to the CPT code representing the imaging procedure, separately bill the appropriate HCPCS "Q" code (Q9945 – Q9954; Q9958-Q9964) for the contrast medium utilized in performing the service. Effective January 1, 2008, HCPCS code ranges changed to Q9950-Q9954, Q9958-Q9967.

For claims with dates of service on or after February 24, 2011, through April 9, 2018, Medicare will allow for coverage of MRI for beneficiaries with implanted pacemakers (PMs) or cardioverter defibrillators

(ICDs) for use in an MRI environment in a Medicare-approved clinical study as described in section 220.C.1 of the NCD Manual.

For claims with dates of service on or after July 7, 2011, through April 9, 2018, Medicare will allow for coverage of MRI for beneficiaries with implanted PMs when the PMs are used according to the Food and Drug Administration (FDA)-approved labeling for use in an MRI environment as described in section 220.2.C.1 of the NCD Manual.

For claims with dates of service on or after April 10, 2018, Medicare will allow for coverage for MRIs for beneficiaries with implanted PMs, ICDs, cardiac resynchronization therapy pacemakers (CRT-Ps), or cardiac resynchronization therapy defibrillators (CRT-Ds), both on and off FDA label, for use in an MRI environment as described in section 220.2.B.3 of the NCD Manual. The data collection requirement under coverage with evidence development ceases April 9, 2018.

100-04, 13, 40.1.1

Magnetic Resonance Angiography (MRA) Coverage Summary

(Rev. 2171, Issued: 03-04-11, Effective: 02-24-11, Implementation: 04-04-11)

Section 1861(s)(2)(C) of the Social Security Act provides for coverage of diagnostic testing. Coverage of magnetic resonance angiography (MRA) of the head and neck, and MRA of the peripheral vessels of the lower extremities is limited as described in Publication (Pub.) 100-3, the Medicare National Coverage Determinations (NCD) Manual. This instruction has been revised as of July 1, 2003, based on a determination that coverage is reasonable and necessary in additional circumstances. Under that instruction, MRA is generally covered only to the extent that it is used as a substitute for contrast angiography, except to the extent that there are documented circumstances consistent with that instruction that demonstrates the medical necessity of both tests. Prior to June 3, 2010, there was no coverage of MRA outside of the indications and circumstances described in that instruction.

Effective for claims with dates of service on or after June 3, 2010, contractors have the discretion to cover or not cover all indications of MRA (and magnetic resonance imaging (MRI)) that are not specifically nationally covered or nationally non-covered as stated in section 220.2 of the NCD Manual.

Because the status codes for HCPCS codes 71555, 71555-TC, 71555-26, 74185, 74185-TC, and 74185-26 were changed in the Medicare Physician Fee Schedule Database from 'N' to 'R' on April 1, 1998, any MRA claims with those HCPCS codes with dates of service between April 1, 1998, and June 30, 1999, are to be processed according to the contractor's discretionary authority to determine payment in the absence of national policy.

Effective for claims with dates of service on or after February 24, 2011, Medicare will provide coverage for MRIs for beneficiaries with implanted cardiac pacemakers or implantable cardioverter defibrillators if the beneficiary is enrolled in an approved clinical study under the Coverage with Study Participation form of Coverage with Evidence Development that meets specific criteria per Pub. 100-3, the NCD Manual, chapter 1, section 220.2.C.1

100-04, 13, 40.1.2

HCPCS Coding Requirements

(Rev. 1472, Issued: 03-06-08, Effective: 05-23-07, Implementation: 04-07-08)

Providers must report HCPCS codes when submitting claims for MRA of the chest, abdomen, head, neck or peripheral vessels of lower extremities. The following HCPCS codes should be used to report these services:

MRA of head	70544, 70544-26, 70544-TC
MRA of head	70545, 70545-26, 70545-TC
MRA of head	70546, 70546-26, 70546-TC
MRA of neck	70547, 70547-26, 70547-TC
MRA of neck	70548, 70548-26, 70548-TC
MRA of neck	70549, 70549-26, 70549-TC
MRA of chest	71555, 71555-26, 71555-TC
MRA of pelvis	72198, 72198-26, 72198-TC
MRA of abdomen (dates of service on or after July 1, 2003) – see below.	74185, 74185-26, 74185-TC
MRA of peripheral vessels of lower extremities	73725, 73725-26, 73725-TC

100-04, 13, 60

Positron Emission Tomography (PET) Scans - General Information

(Rev. 1833; Issued: 10-16-09; Effective Date: 04-03-09; Implementation Date: 10-30-09)

Positron emission tomography (PET) is a noninvasive imaging procedure that assesses perfusion and the level of metabolic activity in various organ systems of the human body. A positron camera (tomograph) is used to produce cross-sectional tomographic images which are obtained by detecting radioactivity from a radioactive tracer substance radiopharmaceutical) that emits a radioactive tracer substance (radiopharmaceutical FDG) such as 2 -[F-18] flouro-D-glucose FDG, that is administered intravenously to the patient.

The Medicare National Coverage Determinations (NCD) Manual, Chapter 1, Sec.220.6, contains additional coverage instructions to indicate the conditions under which a PET scan is performed.

A. Definitions

For all uses of PET, excluding Rubidium 82 for perfusion of the heart, myocardial viability and refractory seizures, the following definitions apply:

- **Diagnosis:** PET is covered only in clinical situations in which the PET results may assist in avoiding an invasive diagnostic procedure, or in which the PET results may assist in determining the optimal anatomical location to perform an invasive diagnostic procedure. In general, for most solid tumors, a tissue diagnosis is made prior to the performance of PET scanning. PET scans following a tissue diagnosis are generally performed for the purpose of staging, rather than diagnosis. Therefore, the use of PET in the diagnosis of lymphoma, esophageal and colorectal cancers, as well as in melanoma, should be rare. PET is not covered for other diagnostic uses, and is not covered for screening (testing of patients without specific signs and symptoms of disease).

- **Staging:** PET is covered in clinical situations in which (1) (a) the stage of the cancer remains in doubt after completion of a standard diagnostic workup, including conventional imaging (computed tomography, magnetic resonance imaging, or ultrasound) or, (b) the use of PET would also be considered reasonable and necessary if it could potentially replace one or more conventional imaging studies when it is expected that conventional study information is insufficient for the clinical management of the patient and, (2) clinical management of the patient would differ depending on the stage of the cancer identified.

  NOTE: Effective for services on or after April 3, 2009, the terms "diagnosis" and "staging" will be replaced with "Initial Treatment Strategy." For further information on this new term, refer to Pub. 100-3, NCD Manual, section 220.6.17.

- **Restaging:** PET will be covered for restaging: (1) after the completion of treatment for the purpose of detecting residual disease, (2) for detecting suspected recurrence, or metastasis, (3) to determine the extent of a known recurrence, or (4) if it could potentially replace one or more conventional imaging studies when it is expected that conventional study information is to determine the extent of a known recurrence, or if study information is insufficient for the clinical management of the patient. Restaging applies to testing after a course of treatment is completed and is covered subject to the conditions above.

- **Monitoring:** Use of PET to monitor tumor response to treatment during the planned course of therapy (i.e., when a change in therapy is anticipated).

  NOTE: Effective for services on or after April 3, 2009, the terms "restaging" and "monitoring" will be replaced with "Subsequent Treatment Strategy." For further information on this new term, refer to Pub. 100-3, NCD Manual, section 220.6.17.

B. Limitations

For staging and restaging: PET is covered in either/or both of the following circumstances:

- The stage of the cancer remains in doubt after completion of a standard diagnostic workup, including conventional imaging (computed tomography, magnetic resonance imaging, or ultrasound); and/or

- The clinical management of the patient would differ depending on the stage of the cancer identified. PET will be covered for restaging after the completion of treatment for the purpose of detecting residual disease, for detecting suspected recurrence, or to determine the extent of a known recurrence. Use of PET would also be considered reasonable and necessary if it could potentially replace one or more conventional imaging studies when it is expected that conventional study information is insufficient for the clinical management of the patient.

The PET is not covered for other diagnostic uses, and is not covered for screening (testing of patients without specific symptoms). Use of PET to monitor tumor response during the planned course of therapy (i.e. when no change in therapy is being contemplated) is not covered.

100-04, 13, 60.2

Use of Gamma Cameras and Full Ring and Partial Ring PET Scanners for PET Scans

(Rev. 527, Issued: 04-15-05, Effective: 01-28-05, Implementation: 04-18-05)

See the Medicare NCD Manual, Section 220.6, concerning 2-[F-18] Fluoro-D-Glucose (FDG) PET scanners and details about coverage.

On July 1, 2001, HCPCS codes G0210 - G0230 were added to allow billing for all currently covered indications for FDG PET. Although the codes do not indicate the type of PET scanner, these codes were used until January 1, 2002, by providers to bill for services in a manner consistent with the coverage policy.

Effective January 1, 2002, HCPCS codes G0210 - G0230 were updated with new descriptors to properly reflect the type of PET scanner used. In addition, four new HCPCS codes became effective for dates of service on and after January 1, 2002, (G0231, G0232, G0233, G0234) for covered conditions that may be billed if a gamma camera is used for the PET scan. For services performed from January 1, 2002, through January 27, 2005, providers should bill using the revised HCPCS codes G0210 - G0234.

Beginning January 28, 2005 providers should bill using the appropriate CPT code.

100-04, 13, 60.3

PET Scan Qualifying Conditions and HCPCS Code Chart

(Rev. 527, Issued: 04-15-05, Effective: 01-28-05, Implementation: 04-18-05)

Below is a summary of all covered PET scan conditions, with effective dates.

NOTE: The G codes below except those a # can be used to bill for PET Scan services through January 27, 2005. Effective for dates of service on or after January 28, 2005, providers must bill for PET Scan services using the appropriate CPT codes. See section 60.3.1. The G codes with a # can continue to be used for billing after January 28, 2005 and these remain non-covered by Medicare. (NOTE: PET Scanners must be FDA-approved.)

Conditions	Coverage Effective Date	****HCPCS/CPT
*Myocardial perfusion imaging (following previous PET G0030-G0047) single study, rest or stress (exercise and/or pharmacologic)	3/14/95	G0030
*Myocardial perfusion imaging (following previous PET G0030-G0047) multiple studies, rest or stress (exercise and/or pharmacologic)	3/14/95	G0031
*Myocardial perfusion imaging (following rest SPECT, 78464); single study, rest or stress (exercise and/or pharmacologic)	3/14/95	G0032
*Myocardial perfusion imaging (following rest SPECT 78464); multiple studies, rest or stress (exercise and/or pharmacologic)	3/14/95	G0033
*Myocardial perfusion (following stress SPECT 78465); single study, rest or stress (exercise and/or pharmacologic)	3/14/95	G0034
*Myocardial Perfusion Imaging (following stress SPECT 78465); multiple studies, rest or stress (exercise and/or pharmacologic)	3/14/95	G0035
*Myocardial Perfusion Imaging (following coronary angiography 93510-93529); single study, rest or stress (exercise and/or pharmacologic)	3/14/95	G0036
*Myocardial Perfusion Imaging, (following coronary angiography), 93510-93529); multiple studies, rest or stress (exercise and/or pharmacologic)	3/14/95	G0037
*Myocardial Perfusion Imaging (following stress planar myocardial perfusion, 78460); single study, rest or stress (exercise and/or pharmacologic)	3/14/95	G0038
*Myocardial Perfusion Imaging (following stress planar myocardial perfusion, 78460); multiple studies, rest or stress (exercise and/or pharmacologic)	3/14/95	G0039
*Myocardial Perfusion Imaging (following stress echocardiogram 93350); single study, rest or stress (exercise and/or pharmacologic)	3/14/95	G0040
*Myocardial Perfusion Imaging (following stress echocardiogram, 93350); multiple studies, rest or stress (exercise and/or pharmacologic)	3/14/95	G0041
*Myocardial Perfusion Imaging (following stress nuclear ventriculogram 78481 or 78483); single study, rest or stress (exercise and/or pharmacologic)	3/14/95	G0042
*Myocardial Perfusion Imaging (following stress nuclear ventriculogram 78481 or 78483); multiple studies, rest or stress (exercise and/or pharmacologic)	3/14/95	G0043
*Myocardial Perfusion Imaging (following stress ECG, 93000); single study, rest or stress (exercise and/or pharmacologic)	3/14/95	G0044
*Myocardial perfusion (following stress ECG, 93000), multiple studies; rest or stress (exercise and/or pharmacologic)	3/14/95	G0045
*Myocardial perfusion (following stress ECG, 93015), single study; rest or stress (exercise and/or pharmacologic)	3/14/95	G0046
*Myocardial perfusion (following stress ECG, 93015); multiple studies, rest or stress (exercise and/or pharmacologic)	3/14/95	G0047
PET imaging regional or whole body; single pulmonary nodule	1/1/98	G0125
Lung cancer, non-small cell (PET imaging whole body) Diagnosis, Initial Staging, Restaging	7/1/01	G0210 G0211 G0212

Conditions	Coverage Effective Date	****HCPCS/CPT
Colorectal cancer (PET imaging whole body) Diagnosis, Initial Staging, Restaging	7/1/01	G0213 G0214 G0215
Melanoma (PET imaging whole body) Diagnosis, Initial Staging, Restaging	7/1/01	G0216 G0217 G0218
Melanoma for non-covered indications	7/1/01	#G0219
Lymphoma (PET imaging whole body) Diagnosis, Initial Staging, Restaging	7/1/01	G0220 G0221 G0222
Head and neck cancer; excluding thyroid and CNS cancers (PET imaging whole body or regional) Diagnosis, Initial Staging, Restaging	7/1/01	G0223 G0224 G0225
Esophageal cancer (PET imaging whole body) Diagnosis, Initial Staging, Restaging	7/1/01	G0226 G0227 G0228
Metabolic brain imaging for pre-surgical evaluation of refractory seizures	7/1/01	G0229
Metabolic assessment for myocardial viability following inconclusive SPECT study	7/1/01	G0230
Recurrence of colorectal or colorectal metastatic cancer (PET whole body, gamma cameras only)	1/1/02	G0231
Staging and characterization of lymphoma (PET whole body, gamma cameras only)	1/1/02	G0232
Recurrence of melanoma or melanoma metastatic cancer (PET whole body, gamma cameras only)	1/1/02	G0233
Regional or whole body, for solitary pulmonary nodule following CT, or for initial staging of nonsmall cell lung cancer (gamma cameras only)	1/1/02	G0234
Non-Covered Service PET imaging, any site not otherwise specified	1/28/05	#G0235
Non-Covered Service Initial diagnosis of breast cancer and/or surgical planning for breast cancer (e.g., initial staging of axillary lymph nodes), not covered (full- and partialring PET scanners only)	10/1/02	#G0252
Breast cancer, staging/restaging of local regional recurrence or distant metastases, i.e., staging/restaging after or prior to course of treatment (full- and partial-ring PET scanners only)	10/1/02	G0253
Breast cancer, evaluation of responses to treatment, performed during course of treatment (full- and partial-ring PET scanners only)	10/1/02	G0254
Myocardial imaging, positron emission tomography (PET), metabolic evaluation)	10/1/02	78459
Restaging or previously treated thyroid cancer of follicular cell origin following negative I-131 whole body scan (full- and partial-ring PET scanner only)	10/1/03	G0296
Tracer Rubidium**82 (Supply of Radiopharmaceutical Diagnostic Imaging Agent) (This is only billed through Outpatient Perspective Payment System, OPPS.) (Carriers must use HCPCS Code A4641).	10/1/03	Q3000
Supply of Radiopharmaceutical Diagnostic Imaging Agent, Ammonia N-13	01/1/04	A9526
PET imaging, brain imaging for the differential diagnosis of Alzheimer's disease with aberrant features vs. fronto-temporal dementia	09/15/04	Appropriate CPT Code from section 60.3.1
PET Cervical Cancer Staging as adjunct to conventional imaging, other staging, diagnosis, restaging, monitoring	1/28/05	Appropriate CPT Code from section 60.3.1

*   NOTE: Carriers must report A4641 for the tracer Rubidium 82 when used with PET scan codes G0030 through G0047 for services performed on or before January 27, 2005

**   NOTE: Not FDG PET

*** NOTE: For dates of service October 1, 2003, through December 31, 2003, use temporary code Q4078 for billing this radiopharmaceutical.

100-04, 13, 60.3.1

Appropriate CPT Codes Effective for PET Scans for Services Performed on or After January 28, 2005

(Rev. 1301, Issued: 07-20-07, Effective: 01-28-05 CPT Code 78609/01-01-08 HCPCS Code A4641, Implementation: 01-07-08)

NOTE: All PET scan services require the use of a radiopharmaceutical diagnostic imaging agent (tracer). The applicable tracer code should be billed when billing for a PET scan service. See section 60.3.2 below for applicable tracer codes.

CPT Code	Description
78459	Myocardial imaging, positron emission tomography (PET), metabolic evaluation
78491	Myocardial imaging, positron emission tomography (PET), perfusion, single study at rest or stress
78492	Myocardial imaging, positron emission tomography (PET), perfusion, multiple studies at rest and/or stress
78608	Brain imaging, positron emission tomography (PET); metabolic evaluation
78811	Tumor imaging, positron emission tomography (PET); limited area (eg, chest, head/neck)
78812	Tumor imaging, positron emission tomography (PET); skull base to mid-thigh
78813	Tumor imaging, positron emission tomography (PET); whole body
78814	Tumor imaging, positron emission tomography (PET) with concurrently acquired computed tomography (CT) for attenuation correction and anatomical localization; limited area (eg, chest, head/neck)
78815	Tumor imaging, positron emission tomography (PET) with concurrently acquired computed tomography (CT) for attenuation correction and anatomical localization; skull base to mid-thigh
78816	Tumor imaging, positron emission tomography (PET) with concurrently acquired computed tomography (CT) for attenuation correction and anatomical localization; whole body

100-04, 13, 60.3.2

Tracer Codes Required for Positron Emission Tomography (PET) Scans

(Rev.3911, Issued: 11-09-17, Effective: 01-01-18, Implementation: 12-11-17)

An applicable tracer/radiopharmaceutical code, along with an applicable Current Procedural Technology (CPT) code, is necessary for claims processing of any Positron Emission Tomography (PET) scan services. While there are a number of PET tracers already billable for a diverse number of medical indications, there have been, and may be in the future, additional PET indications that might require a new PET tracer. Under those circumstances, the process to request/approve/implement a new code could be time-intensive. To help alleviate inordinate spans of time between when a national coverage determination is made, or when the Food and Drug Administration (FDA) approves a particular radiopharmaceutical for an oncologic indication already approved by the Centers for Medicare & Medicaid Services (CMS), and when it can be fully implemented via valid claims processing, CMS has created two new PET radiopharmaceutical unclassified tracer codes that can be used temporarily. This time period would be pending the creation/approval/implementation of permanent CPT codes that would later specifically define their function by CMS in official instructions.

Effective with dates of service on or after January 1, 2018, the following Healthcare Common Procedure Coding System (HCPCS) codes shall be used ONLY AS NECESSARY FOR AN INTERIM PERIOD OF TIME under the circumstances explained here. Specifically, there are two circumstances that would warrant use of the below codes: (1) After FDA approval of a PET oncologic indication, or, (2) after CMS approves coverage of a new PET indication, and ONLY if either of those situations requires the use of a dedicated PET radiopharmaceutical/tracer that is currently non-existent. Once permanent replacement codes are officially implemented by CMS, use of the temporary code for that particular indication will simultaneously be discontinued.

NOTE: The following two codes were effective as of January 1, 2017, with the January 2017 quarterly HCPCS update.

A9597 - Positron emission tomography radiopharmaceutical, diagnostic, for tumor identification, not otherwise classified

A9598 - Positron emission tomography radiopharmaceutical, diagnostic, for non-tumor identification, not otherwise classified

Effective for claims with dates of service on and after January 1, 2018, when PET tracer code A9597 or A9598 are present on a claim, that claim must also include:

- an appropriate PET HCPCS code, either 78459, 78491, 78492, 78608, 78811, 78812, 78813, 78814, 78815, or 78816,
- if tumor-related, either the -PI or -PS modifier as appropriate,
- if clinical trial, registry, or study-related outside of NCD220.6.17, PET for Solid Tumors, clinical trial modifier –Q0,
- if clinical trial, registry, or study-related, all claims require the 8-digit clinical trial number,

- if Part A OP and clinical trial, registry, or study-related outside of NCD220.6.17, PET for Solid Tumors, also include condition code 30 and ICD-10 diagnosis Z00.6.

Effective for claims with dates of service on and after January 1, 2018, A/Medicare Administrative Contractors (MACs) shall line-item deny, and B/MACs shall line-item reject, PET claims for A9597 or A9598 that don't include the elements noted above as appropriate.

Contractors shall use the following messaging when line-item denying (Part A) or line-item rejecting (Part B) PET claims containing HCPCS A9597 or A9598:

Remittance Advice Remark Codes (RARC) N386

Claim Adjustment Reason Code (CARC) 50, 96, and/or 119.

Group Code CO (Contractual Obligation) assigning financial liability to the provider (if a claim is received with a GZ modifier indicating no signed ABN is on file).

(The above new verbiage will supersede any existing verbiage in chapter 13, section 60.3.2.)

100-04, 13, 60.12

Coverage for PET Scans for Dementia and Neurodegenerative Diseases

(Rev. 3650, Issued: 11-10-16, Effective: 02-10-17, Implementation: 02-10-17)

Effective for dates of service on or after September 15, 2004, Medicare will cover FDG PET scans for a differential diagnosis of fronto-temporal dementia (FTD) and Alzheimer's disease OR; its use in a CMS-approved practical clinical trial focused on the utility of FDG-PET in the diagnosis or treatment of dementing neurodegenerative diseases. Refer to Pub. 100-03, NCD Manual, section 220.6.13, for complete coverage conditions and clinical trial requirements and section 60.15 of this manual for claims processing information.

A. A/B MAC (A and B) Billing Requirements for PET Scan Claims for FDG-PET for the Differential Diagnosis of Fronto-temporal Dementia and Alzheimer's Disease:

CPT Code for PET Scans for Dementia and Neurodegenerative Diseases

Contractors shall advise providers to use the appropriate CPT code from section 60.3.1 for dementia and neurodegenerative diseases for services performed on or after January 28, 2005.

Diagnosis Codes for PET Scans for Dementia and Neurodegenerative Diseases

The contractor shall ensure one of the following appropriate diagnosis codes is present on claims for PET Scans for AD:

- If ICD-9-CM is applicable, ICD-9 codes are: 290.0, 290.10 - 290.13, 290.20 - 290, 21, 290.3, 331.0, 331.11, 331.19, 331.2, 331.9, 780.93
- If ICD-10-CM is applicable, ICD-10 codes are: F03.90, F03.90 plus F05, G30.9, G31.01, G31.9, R41.2 or R41.3

Medicare contractors shall deny claims when submitted with an appropriate CPT code from section 60.3.1 and with a diagnosis code other than the range of codes listed above.

Medicare contractors shall instruct providers to issue an Advanced Beneficiary Notice to beneficiaries advising them of potential financial liability prior to delivering the service if one of the appropriate diagnosis codes will not be present on the claim.

The contractor shall use the following remittance advice messages and associated codes when rejecting/denying claims under this policy. This CARC/RARC combination is compliant with CAQH CORE Business Scenario Three.

Group Code: PR (if claim is received with a GA modifier) otherwise CO

CARC: 11

RARC: N/A

MSN: 16.48

Provider Documentation Required with the PET Scan Claim

Medicare contractors shall inform providers to ensure the conditions mentioned in the NCD Manual, section 220.6.13, have been met. The information must also be maintained in the beneficiary's medical record:

- Date of onset of symptoms;
  - Diagnosis of clinical syndrome (normal aging, mild cognitive impairment or MCI: mild, moderate, or severe dementia);
  - Mini mental status exam (MMSE) or similar test score;
  - Presumptive cause (possible, probably, uncertain AD);
  - Any neuropsychological testing performed;
  - Results of any structural imaging (MRI, CT) performed;
  - Relevant laboratory tests (B12, thyroid hormone); and,
  - Number and name of prescribed medications.

B. Billing Requirements for Beta Amyloid Positron Emission Tomography (PET) in Dementia and Neurodegenerative Disease:

Effective for claims with dates of service on and after September 27, 2013, Medicare will only allow coverage with evidence development (CED) for Positron Emission Tomography (PET) beta amyloid (also referred to as amyloid-beta (Aβ)) imaging (HCPCS A9586)or (HCPCS A9599) (one PET Aβ scan per patient).

NOTE: Please note that effective January 1, 2014 the following code A9599 will be updated in the IOCE and HCPCS update. This code will be contractor priced.

Medicare Summary Notices, Remittance Advice Remark Codes, and Claim Adjustment Reason Codes

Effective for dates of service on or after September 27, 2013, contractors shall return as unprocessable/return to provider claims for PET Aβ imaging, through CED during a clinical trial, not containing the following:

- Condition code 30, (A/B MAC (A) only)
- Modifier Q0 and/or modifier Q1 as appropriate
- ICD-9 dx code V70.7/ICD-10 dx code Z00.6 (on either the primary/secondary position)
- A PET HCPCS code (78811 or 78814)
- At least, one Dx code from the table below

ICD-9 Codes	Corresponding ICD-10 Codes
290.0 Senile dementia, uncomplicated	F03.90 Unspecified dementia without behavioral disturbance
290.10 Presenile dementia, uncomplicated	F03.90 Unspecified dementia without behavioral disturbance
290.11 Presenile dementia with delirium	F03.90 Unspecified dementia without behavioral disturbance
290.12 Presenile dementia with delusional features	F03.90 Unspecified dementia without behavioral disturbance
290.13 Presenile dementia with depressive features	F03.90 Unspecified dementia without behavioral disturbance
290.20 Senile dementia with delusional features	F03.90 Unspecified dementia without behavioral disturbance
290.21 Senile dementia with depressive features	F03.90 Unspecified dementia without behavioral disturbance
290.3 Senile dementia with delirium	F03.90 Unspecified dementia without behavioral disturbance
290.40 Vascular dementia, uncomplicated	F01.50 Vascular dementia without behavioral disturbance
290.41 Vascular dementia with delirium	F01.51 Vascular dementia with behavioral disturbance
290.42 Vascular dementia with delusions	F01.51 Vascular dementia with behavioral disturbance
290.43 Vascular dementia with depressed mood	F01.51 Vascular dementia with behavioral disturbance
294.10 Dementia in conditions classified elsewhere without behavioral disturbance	F02.80 Dementia in other diseases classified elsewhere without behavioral disturbance
294.11 Dementia in conditions classified elsewhere with behavioral disturbance	F02.81 Dementia in other diseases classified elsewhere with behavioral disturbance
294.20 Dementia, unspecified, without behavioral disturbance	F03.90 Unspecified dementia without behavioral disturbance
294.21 Dementia, unspecified, with behavioral disturbance	F03.91 Unspecified dementia with behavioral disturbance
331.11 Pick's Disease	G31.01 Pick's disease
331.19 Other Frontotemporal dementia	G31.09 Other frontotemporal dementia
331.6 Corticobasal degeneration	G31.85 Corticobasal degeneration
331.82 Dementia with Lewy Bodies	G31.83 Dementia with Lewy bodies
331.83 Mild cognitive impairment, so stated	G31.84 Mild cognitive impairment, so stated
ICD-9 Codes	Corresponding ICD-10 Codes
780.93 Memory Loss	R41.1 Anterograde amnesia
	R41.2 Retrograde amnesia
	R41.3 Other amnesia (Amnesia NOS, Memory loss NOS)
V70.7 Examination for normal comparison or control in clinical	Z00.6 Encounter for examination for normal comparison and control in clinical research program

and

- Aβ HCPCS code A9586 or A9599

The contractor shall use the following remittance advice messages and associated codes when returning claims under this policy. This CARC/RARC combination is compliant with CAQH CORE Business Scenario Two.

  Group Code: CO
  CARC: 4
  RARC: N517, N519
  MSN: N/A

Contractors shall line-item deny claims for PET Aβ, HCPCS code A9586 or A9599, where a previous PET Aβ, HCPCS code A9586 or A9599 is paid in history.

The contractor shall use the following remittance advice messages and associated codes when rejecting/denying claims under this policy. This CARC/RARC combination is compliant with CAQH CORE Business Scenario Three.

Group Code: PR (if claim is received with a GA modifier) otherwise CO

  CARC: 149
  RARC: N587
  MSN: 20.12

100-04, 13, 60.13

Billing Requirements for PET Scans for Specific Indications of Cervical Cancer for Services Performed on or After January 28, 2005

(Rev. 1888; Issued: 01-06-10, Effective date: 11-10-09; Implementation Date: 01-04-10)

Contractors shall accept claims for these services with the appropriate CPT code listed in section 60.3.1. Refer to Pub. 100-3, section 220.6.17, for complete coverage guidelines for this new PET oncology indication. The implementation date for these CPT codes will be April 18, 2005. Also see section 60.17, of this chapter for further claims processing instructions for cervical cancer indications.

100-04, 13, 60.15

Billing Requirements for CMS - Approved Clinical Trials and Coverage With Evidence Development Claims for PET Scans for Neurodegenerative Diseases, Previously Specified Cancer Indications, and All Other Cancer Indications Not Previously Specified

(Rev. 3227, Issued: 04-02-15, Multiple effective dates)

A/B MACs (A and B)

Effective for services on or after January 28, 2005, contractors shall accept and pay for claims for Positron Emission Tomography (PET) scans for lung cancer, esophageal cancer, colorectal cancer, lymphoma, melanoma, head & neck cancer, breast cancer, thyroid cancer, soft tissue sarcoma, brain cancer, ovarian cancer, pancreatic cancer, small cell lung cancer, and testicular cancer, as well as for neurodegenerative diseases and all other cancer indications not previously mentioned in this chapter, if these scans were performed as part of a Centers for Medicare & Medicaid (CMS)-approved clinical trial. (See Pub. 100-3, National Coverage Determinations (NCD) Manual, sections 220.6.13 and 220.6.17.)

Contractors shall also be aware that PET scans for all cancers not previously specified at Pub. 100-3, NCD Manual, section 220.6.17, remain nationally non-covered unless performed in conjunction with a CMS-approved clinical trial.

Effective for dates of service on or after June 11, 2013, Medicare has ended the coverage with evidence development (CED) requirement for FDG (2-[F18] fluoro-2-deoxy-D-glucose) PET and PET/computed tomography (CT) and PET/magnetic resonance imaging (MRI) for all oncologic indications contained in section 220.6.17 of the NCD Manual. Modifier -Q0 (Investigational clinical service provided in a clinical research study that is in an approved clinical research study) or -Q1 (routine clinical service provided in a clinical research study that is in an approved clinical research study) is no longer mandatory for these services when performed on or after June 11, 2013.

A/B MACs (B) Only

A/B MACs (B) shall pay claims for PET scans for beneficiaries participating in a CMS-approved clinical trial submitted with an appropriate current procedural terminology (CPT) code from section 60.3.1 of this chapter and modifier Q0/Q1 for services performed on or after January 1, 2008, through June 10, 2013. (NOTE: Modifier QR (Item or service provided in a Medicare specified study) and QA (FDA investigational device exemption) were replaced by modifier Q0 effective January 1, 2008.) Modifier QV (item or service provided as routine care in a Medicare qualifying clinical trial) was replaced by modifier Q1 effective January 1, 2008.) Beginning with services performed on or after June 11, 2013, modifier Q0/Q1 is no longer required for PET FDG services.

A/B MACs (A) Only

In order to pay claims for PET scans on behalf of beneficiaries participating in a CMS-approved clinical trial, A/B MACs (A) require providers to submit claims with, if ICD-9-CM is applicable, ICD-9 code V70.7; if ICD-10-CM is applicable, ICD-10 code Z00.6 in the primary/secondary diagnosis position using the ASC X12 837 institutional claim format or on Form CMS-1450, with the appropriate principal diagnosis code and an appropriate CPT code from section 60.3.1. Effective for PET scan claims for dates of service on or after January 28, 2005, through December 31, 2007, A/B MACs (A) shall accept claims with the QR, QV, or QA modifier on other than inpatient claims. Effective for services on or after January 1, 2008, through June 10, 2013, modifier Q0 replaced the QR and QA modifier, modifier Q1 replaced the QV modifier. Modifier Q0/Q1 is no longer required for services performed on or after June 11, 2013.

100-04, 13, 60.16

Billing and Coverage Changes for PET Scans Effective for Services on or After April 3, 2009

(Rev. 3650, Issued: 11-10-16, Effective: 02-10-17, Implementation: 02-10-17)

A. Summary of Changes

Effective for services on or after April 3, 2009, Medicare will not cover the use of FDG PET imaging to determine initial treatment strategy in patients with adenocarcinoma of the prostate.

Medicare will also not cover FDG PET imaging for subsequent treatment strategy for tumor types other than breast, cervical, colorectal, esophagus, head and neck (non-CNS/thyroid), lymphoma, melanoma, myeloma, non-small cell lung, and ovarian, unless the FDG PET is provided under the coverage with evidence development (CED) paradigm (billed with modifier -Q0/-Q1, see section 60.15 of this chapter).

Medicare will cover FDG PET imaging for initial treatment strategy for myeloma.

Effective for services performed on or after June 11, 2013, Medicare has ended the CED requirement for FDG PET and PET/CT and PET/MRI for all oncologic indications contained in section 220.6.17 of the NCD Manual. Effective for services on or after June 11, 2013, the Q0/Q1 modifier is no longer required.

Beginning with services performed on or after June 11, 2013, contractors shall pay for up to three (3) FDG PET scans when used to guide subsequent management of anti-tumor treatment strategy (modifier PS) after completion of initial anti-cancer therapy (modifier PI) for the exact same cancer diagnosis.

Coverage of any additional FDG PET scans (that is, beyond 3) used to guide subsequent management of anti-tumor treatment strategy after completion of initial anti-tumor therapy for the same cancer diagnosis will be determined by the A/B MACs (A or B). Claims will include the KX modifier indicating the coverage criteria is met for coverage of four or more FDG PET scans for subsequent treatment strategy for the same cancer diagnosis under this NCD.

A different cancer diagnosis whether submitted with a PI or a PS modifier will begin the count of one initial and three subsequent FDG PET scans not requiring the KX modifier and four or more FDG PET scans for subsequent treatment strategy for the same cancer diagnosis requiring the KX modifier.

NOTE: The presence or absence of an initial treatment strategy claim in a beneficiary's record does not impact the frequency criteria for subsequent treatment strategy claims for the same cancer diagnosis.

NOTE: Providers please refer to the following link for a list of appropriate diagnosis codes, http://cms.gov/medicare/coverage/determinationprocess/downloads/petforsolidtumorsoncologicdxcodesattachment_NCD220_6_17.pdf

For further information regarding the changes in coverage, refer to Pub.100-03, NCD Manual, section 220.6.17.

B. Modifiers for PET Scans

Effective for claims with dates of service on or after April 3, 2009, the following modifiers have been created for use to inform for the initial treatment strategy of biopsy-proven or strongly suspected tumors or subsequent treatment strategy of cancerous tumors:

PI Positron Emission Tomography (PET) or PET/Computed Tomography (CT) to inform the initial treatment strategy of tumors that are biopsy proven or strongly suspected of being cancerous based on other diagnostic testing.

Short descriptor: PET tumor init tx strat

PS Positron Emission Tomography (PET) or PET/Computed Tomography (CT) to inform the subsequent treatment strategy of cancerous tumors when the beneficiary's treatment physician determines that the PET study is needed to inform subsequent anti-tumor strategy.

Short descriptor: PS - PET tumor subsq tx strategy

C. Billing for A/B MACs (A and B)

Effective for claims with dates of service on or after April 3, 2009, contractors shall accept FDG PET claims billed to inform initial treatment strategy with the following CPT codes AND modifier PI: 78608, 78811, 78812, 78813, 78814, 78815, 78816.

Effective for claims with dates of service on or after April 3, 2009, contractors shall accept FDG PET claims with modifier PS for the subsequent treatment strategy for solid tumors using a CPT code above AND a cancer diagnosis code.

Contractors shall also accept FDG PET claims billed to inform initial treatment strategy or subsequent treatment strategy when performed under CED with one of the PET or PET/CT CPT codes above AND modifier PI OR modifier PS AND a cancer diagnosis code AND modifier Q0/Q1. Effective for services performed on or after June 11, 2013, the CED requirement has ended and modifier Q0/Q1, along with condition code 30 (institutional claims only), or ICD-9 code V70.7, (both institutional and practitioner claims) are no longer required.

D. Medicare Summary Notices, Remittance Advice Remark Codes, and Claim Adjustment Reason Codes

Effective for dates of service on or after April 3, 2009, contractors shall return as unprocessable/return to provider claims that do not include the PI modifier with one of the PET/PET/CT CPT codes listed in subsection C. above when billing for the initial treatment strategy for solid tumors in accordance with Pub.100-03, NCD Manual, section 220.6.17.

In addition, contractors shall return as unprocessable/return to provider claims that do not include the PS modifier with one of the CPT codes listed in subsection C. above when billing for the subsequent treatment strategy for solid tumors in accordance with Pub.100-03, NCD Manual, section 220.6.17.

The contractor shall use the following remittance advice messages and associated codes when returning claims under this policy. This CARC/RARC combination is compliant with CAQH CORE Business Scenario Two.

Group Code: CO
CARC: 4
RARC: MA130
MSN: N/A

Effective for claims with dates of service on or after April 3, 2009, through June 10, 2013, contractors shall return as unprocessable/return to provider FDG PET claims billed to inform initial treatment strategy or subsequent treatment strategy when performed under CED without one of the PET/PET/CT CPT codes listed in subsection C. above AND modifier PI OR modifier PS AND a cancer diagnosis code AND modifier Q0/Q1.

The contractor shall use the following remittance advice messages and associated codes when returning claims under this policy. This CARC/RARC combination is compliant with CAQH CORE Business Scenario Two.

Group Code: CO
CARC: 4
RARC: MA130
MSN: N/A

Effective April 3, 2009, contractors shall deny claims with ICD-9/ICD-10 diagnosis code 185/C61 for FDG PET imaging for the initial treatment strategy of patients with adenocarcinoma of the prostate.

For dates of service prior to June 11, 2013, contractors shall also deny claims for FDG PET imaging for subsequent treatment strategy for tumor types other than breast, cervical, colorectal, esophagus, head and neck (non-CNS/thyroid), lymphoma, melanoma, myeloma, non-small cell lung, and ovarian, unless the FDG PET is provided under CED (submitted with the Q0/Q1 modifier) and use the following messages:

The contractor shall use the following remittance advice messages and associated codes when rejecting/denying claims under this policy. This CARC/RARC combination is compliant with CAQH CORE Business Scenario Three.

Group Code: PR (if claim is received with a GA modifier) otherwise CO
CARC: 50
RARC: N/A
MSN: 15.4

Effective for dates of service on or after June 11, 2013, contractors shall use the following messages when denying claims in excess of three for PET FDG scans for subsequent treatment strategy when the KX modifier is not included, identified by CPT codes 78608, 78811, 78812, 78813, 78814, 78815, or 78816, modifier PS, HCPCS A9552, and the same cancer diagnosis code.

The contractor shall use the following remittance advice messages and associated codes when rejecting/denying claims under this policy. This CARC/RARC combination is compliant with CAQH CORE Business Scenario Three.

Group Code: PR (if claim is received with a GA modifier) otherwise CO
CARC: 96
RARC: N435
MSN: 23.17

100-04, 13, 60.17

Billing and Coverage Changes for PET Scans for Cervical Cancer Effective for Services on or After November 10, 2009

(Rev. 3650, Issued: 11-10-16, Effective: 02-10-17, Implementation: 02-10-17)

A. Billing Changes for A/B MACs (A and B)

Effective for claims with dates of service on or after November 10, 2009, contractors shall accept FDG PET oncologic claims billed to inform initial treatment strategy; specifically for staging in beneficiaries who have biopsy-proven cervical cancer when the beneficiary's treating physician determines the FDG PET study is needed to determine the location and/or extent of the tumor as specified in Pub. 100-03, section 220.6.17.

EXCEPTION: CMS continues to non-cover FDG PET for initial diagnosis of cervical cancer related to initial treatment strategy.

NOTE: Effective for claims with dates of service on and after November 10, 2009, the –Q0 modifier is no longer necessary for FDG PET for cervical cancer.

B. Medicare Summary Notices, Remittance Advice Remark Codes, and Claim Adjustment Reason Codes

Additionally, contractors shall return as unprocessable /return to provider for FDG PET for cervical cancer for initial treatment strategy billed without the following: one of the PET/PET/ CT CPT codes listed in 60.16 C above AND modifier PI AND a cervical cancer diagnosis code.

The contractor shall use the following remittance advice messages and associated codes when returning claims under this policy. This CARC/RARC combination is compliant with CAQH CORE Business Scenario Two.

Group Code: CO
CARC: 4
RARC: MA130
MSN: N/A

100-04, 13, 60.18

Billing and Coverage Changes for PET (NaF-18) Scans to Identify Bone Metastasis of Cancer Effective for Claims With Dates of Services on or After February 26, 2010

(Rev. 3650, Issued: 11-10-16, Effective: 02-10-17, Implementation: 02-10-17)

A. Billing Changes for A/B MACs (A and B)

Effective for claims with dates of service on and after February 26, 2010, contractors shall pay for NaF-18 PET oncologic claims to inform of initial treatment strategy (PI) or subsequent treatment strategy (PS) for suspected or biopsy proven bone metastasis ONLY in the context of a clinical study and as specified in Pub. 100-03, section 220.6. All other claims for NaF-18 PET oncology claims remain non-covered.

B. Medicare Summary Notices, Remittance Advice Remark Codes, and Claim Adjustment Reason Codes

Effective for claims with dates of service on or after February 26, 2010, contractors shall return as unprocessable NaF-18 PET oncologic claims billed with modifier TC or globally (for A/B MACs (A) modifier TC or globally does not apply) and HCPCS A9580 to inform the initial treatment strategy or subsequent treatment strategy for bone metastasis that do not include ALL of the following:

- PI or PS modifier AND
- PET or PET/CT CPT code (78811, 78812, 78813, 78814, 78815, 78816) AND
- Cancer diagnosis code AND
- Q0 modifier - Investigational clinical service provided in a clinical research study, are present on the claim.

NOTE: For institutional claims, continue to include ICD-9 diagnosis code V70.7 or ICD-10 diagnosis code Z00.6 and condition code 30 to denote a clinical study.

The contractor shall use the following remittance advice messages and associated codes when returning claims under this policy. This CARC/RARC combination is compliant with CAQH CORE Business Scenario Two.

Group Code: CO
CARC: 4
RARC: MA130
MSN: N/A

Effective for claims with dates of service on or after February 26, 2010, contractors shall accept PET oncologic claims billed with modifier 26 and modifier KX to inform the initial treatment strategy or subsequent treatment strategy for bone metastasis that include the following:

- PI or PS modifier AND
- PET or PET/CT CPT code (78811, 78812, 78813, 78814, 78815, 78816) AND
- Cancer diagnosis code AND
- Q0 modifier - Investigational clinical service provided in a clinical research study, are present on the claim.

NOTE: If modifier KX is present on the professional component service, Contractors shall process the service as PET NaF-18 rather than PET with FDG.

Contractors shall also return as unprocessable NaF-18 PET oncologic professional component claims (i.e., claims billed with modifiers 26 and KX) to inform the initial treatment strategy or subsequent treatment strategy for bone metastasis billed with HCPCS A9580.

The contractor shall use the following remittance advice messages and associated codes when returning claims under this policy. This CARC/RARC combination is compliant with CAQH CORE Business Scenario Two.

Group Code: CO
CARC: 4
RARC: MA130
MSN: N/A

Claim Adjustment Reason Code 97 – The benefit for this service is included in the payment/allowance for another service/procedure that has already been adjudicated.

NOTE: Refer to the 835 Healthcare Policy identification Segment (loop 2110 Service Payment Information REF), if present.

100-04, 13, 70.2

Services Bundled Into Treatment Management Codes

(Rev.4267, Issued: 03-27-19, Effective: 01-01-19, Implementation: 03-25-19)

A/B MACs (B) do not make separate payment for services rendered by the radiation oncologists or in conjunction with radiation therapy.

11920 Tattooing, intradermal introduction of insoluble opaque pigments to correct color defects of skin; 6.0 sq. cm or less

11921 6.11 to 20.0 sq. cm

11922 Each additional 20.0 sq. cm

16000 Initial treatment, first-degree burn, when no more than local treatment is required

16010 Dressings and/or debridement, initial or subsequent; under anesthesia, small

16015 Under anesthesia, medium or large, or with major debridement

16020 Without anesthesia, office or hospital, small

16025 Without anesthesia, medium (e.g., whole face or whole extremity)

16030 Without anesthesia, large (e.g., more than one extremity)

36425 Venipuncture, cut down age 1 or over

53670 Catheterization, urethra; simple

53675 Complicated (may include difficult removal of balloon catheter)

99211 Office or other outpatient visit, established patient; Level I*

99212 Level II*

99213 Level III*

99214 Level IV

99215 Level V

99238 Hospital discharge day management

99281 Emergency department visit, new or established patient; Level I

99282 Level II

99283 Level III

99284 Level IV

99285 Level V

90780 IV Infusion therapy, administered by physician or under direct supervision of physician; up to one hour

90781 Each additional hour, up to 8 hours

90847 Family medical psychotherapy (conjoint psychotherapy) by a physician, with continuing medical diagnostic evaluation, and drug management when indicated

99050 Services requested after office hours in addition to basic service

99052 Services requested between 10:00 PM and 8:00 AM in addition to basic service

99054 Services requested on Sundays and holidays in addition to basic service

99058 Office services provided on an emergency basis

99071 Educational supplies, such as books, tapes, and pamphlets, provided by the physician for the patient's education at cost to physician

99090 Analysis of information data stored in computers (e.g., ECG, blood pressures, hematologic data)

99185 Hypothermia; regional

99371 Telephone call by a physician to patient or for consultation or medical management or for coordinating medical management with other health care professionals; simple or brief (e.g., to report on tests and/or laboratory results, to clarify or alter previous instructions, to integrate new information from other health professionals into the medical treatment plan, or to adjust therapy)

99372 Intermediate (e.g., to provide advice to an established patient on a new problem, to initiate therapy that can be handled by telephone, to discuss test results in detail, to coordinate medical management of a new problem in an established patient, to discuss and evaluate new information and details, or to initiate a new plan of care)

99373 Complex or lengthy (e.g., lengthy counseling session with anxious or distraught patient, detailed or prolonged discussion with family members regarding seriously ill patient, lengthy communication necessary to coordinate complex services or several different health professionals working on different aspects of the total patient care plan)

- Anesthesia (whatever code billed)
- Care of Infected Skin (whatever code billed)
- Checking of Treatment Charts
- Verification of Dosage, As Needed (whatever code billed)
- Continued Patient Evaluation, Examination, Written Progress Notes, As Needed (whatever code billed)
- Final Physical Examination (whatever code billed)
- Medical Prescription Writing (whatever code billed
- Nutritional Counseling (whatever code billed)
- Pain Management (whatever code billed)
- Review & Revision of Treatment Plan (whatever code billed)
- Routine Medical Management of Unrelated Problem (whatever code billed)
- Special Care of Ostomy (whatever code billed)
- Written Reports, Progress Note (whatever code billed)

- Follow-up Examination and Care for 90 Days After Last Treatment (whatever code billed)

*NOTE: May be billed with Radiation Treatment Delivery, superficial and/or ortho voltage, for the purpose of reporting physician services consisting of radiation therapy planning (including, but not limited to clinical treatment planning, isodose planning, physics consultation), radiation treatment device construction, and radiation treatment management when performed on the same date of service as treatment delivery. Billing with modifier 25 may be necessary if National Correct Coding Initiative (NCCI) edits apply.

100-04, 13, 70.4

Clinical Brachytherapy (CPT Codes 77750 - 77799)

(Rev. 1, 10-01-03)

A/B MACs (B) must apply the bundled services policy to procedures in this family of codes other than CPT code 77776. For procedures furnished in settings in which TC payments are made, A/B MACs (B) must pay separately for the expendable source associated with these procedures under CPT code 79900 except in the case of remote after-loading high intensity brachytherapy procedures (CPT codes 77781-77784). In the four codes cited, the expendable source is included in the RVUs for the TC of the procedures.

100-04, 13, 70.5

Radiation Physics Services (CPT Codes 77300 - 77399)

(Rev. 1, 10-01-03)

A/B MACs (B) pay for the PC and TC of CPT codes 77300-77334 and 77399 on the same basis as they pay for radiologic services generally. For professional component billings in all settings, A/B MACs (B) presume that the radiologist participated in the provision of the service, e.g., reviewed/validated the physicist's calculation. CPT codes 77336 and 77370 are technical services only codes that are payable by A/B MACs (B) in settings in which only technical component is are payable.

100-04, 13, 80.1

Physician Presence

(Rev. 1, 10-01-03)

Radiologic supervision and interpretation (S&I) codes are used to describe the personal supervision of the performance of the radiologic portion of a procedure by one or more physicians and the interpretation of the findings. In order to bill for the supervision aspect of the procedure, the physician must be present during its performance. This kind of personal supervision of the performance of the procedure is a service to an individual beneficiary and differs from the type of general supervision of the radiologic procedures performed in a hospital for which FIs pay the costs as physician services to the hospital. The interpretation of the procedure may be performed later by another physician. In situations in which a cardiologist, for example, bills for the supervision (the "S") of the S&I code, and a radiologist bills for the interpretation (the "I") of the code, both physicians should use a "-52" modifier indicating a reduced service, e.g., only one of supervision and/or interpretation. Payment for the fragmented S&I code is no more than if a single physician furnished both aspects of the procedure.

100-04, 13, 80.2

Multiple Procedure Reduction

(Rev. 1, 10-01-03)

A/B MACs (B) make no multiple procedure reductions in the S&I or primary non-radiologic codes in these types of procedures, or in any procedure codes for which the descriptor and RVUs reflect a multiple service reduction. For additional procedure codes that do not reflect such a reduction, A/B MACs (B) apply the multiple procedure reductions.

100-04, 13, 140.1

Payment Methodology and HCPCS Coding

(Rev.4150, Issued: 10-26-2018, Effective: 04-01-19, Implementation: 04-01-19)

A/B MACs (B) pay for BMM procedures based on the Medicare physician fee schedule. Claims from physicians, other practitioners, or suppliers where assignment was not taken are subject to the Medicare limiting charge.

The A/B MACs (A) pay for BMM procedures under the current payment methodologies for radiology services according to the type of provider.

Do not pay BMM procedure claims for dual photon absorptiometry, CPT procedure code 78351.

Deductible and coinsurance do not apply.

Any of the following CPT procedure codes may be used when billing for BMMs through December 31, 2006. All of these codes are bone densitometry measurements except code 76977, which is bone sonometry measurements. CPT procedure codes are applicable to billing A/B MACs (A and B).

76070 76071 76075 76076 76078 76977 78350 G0130

Effective for dates of services on and after January 1, 2007, the following changes apply to BMM:

New 2007 CPT bone mass procedure codes have been assigned for BMM. The following codes will replace current codes, however the CPT descriptors for the services remain the same:

77078 replaces 76070

77079 replaces 76071

77080 replaces 76075

77081 replaces 76076

77083 replaces 76078

Effective for dates of service on and after January 1, 2015, contractors shall pay for bone mass procedure code 77085 (Dual-energy X-ray absorptiometry (DXA), bone density study, 1 or more sites, axial skeleton, (e.g., hips, pelvis, spine), including vertebral fracture assessment.)

Certain BMM tests are covered when used to screen patients for osteoporosis subject to the frequency standards described in chapter 15, section 80.5.5 of the Medicare Benefit Policy Manual.

Contractors will pay claims for screening tests when coded as follows:

Contains CPT procedure code 77078, 77079, 77080, 77081, 77083, 76977 or G0130, and

Contains a valid diagnosis code indicating the reason for the test is postmenopausal female, vertebral fracture, hyperparathyroidism, or steroid therapy. Contractors are to maintain local lists of valid codes for the benefit's screening categories.

Contractors will deny claims for screening tests when coded as follows:

Contains CPT procedure code 77078, 77079, 77081, 77083, 76977 or G0130, but

Does not contain a valid diagnosis code from the local lists of valid diagnosis codes maintained by the contractor for the benefit's screening categories indicating the reason for the test is postmenopausal female, vertebral fracture, hyperparathyroidism, or steroid therapy.

Dual-energy x-ray absorptiometry (axial) tests are covered when used to monitor FDA-approved osteoporosis drug therapy subject to the 2-year frequency standards described in chapter 15, section 80.5.5 of the Medicare Benefit Policy Manual.

Contractors will pay claims for monitoring tests when coded as follows:

Contains CPT procedure code 77080 or 77085, and

Contains 733.00, 733.01, 733.02, 733.03, 733.09, 733.90, or 255.0 as the ICD-9-CM diagnosis code or M81.0, M81.8, M81.6 or M94.9 as the ICD-10-CM diagnosis code.

Contractors will deny claims for monitoring tests when coded as follows:

Contains CPT procedure code 77078, 77079, 77081, 77083, 76977 or G0130, and

Contains 733.00, 733.01, 733.02, 733.03, 733.09, 733.90, or 255.0 as the ICD-9-CM diagnosis code, but

Does not contain a valid ICD-9-CM diagnosis code from the local lists of valid ICD-9-CM diagnosis codes maintained by the contractor for the benefit's screening categories indicating the reason for the test is postmenopausal female, vertebral fracture, hyperparathyroidism, or steroid therapy.

Does not contain a valid ICD-10-CM diagnosis code from the local lists of valid ICD-10-CM diagnosis codes maintained by the contractor for the benefit's screening categories indicating the reason for the test is postmenopausal female, vertebral fracture, hyperparathyroidism, or steroid therapy.

Single photon absorptiometry tests are not covered. Contractors will deny CPT procedure code 78350.

The A/B MACs (A) are billed using the ASC X12 837 institutional claim format or hardcopy Form CMS-1450. The appropriate bill types are: 12X, 13X, 22X, 23X, 34X, 71X (Provider-based and independent), 72X, 77X (Provider-based and freestanding), 83X, and 85X. Effective April 1, 2006, type of bill 14X is for non-patient laboratory specimens and is no longer applicable for bone mass measurements. Information regarding the claim form locators that correspond to the HCPCS/CPT code or Type of Bill are found in chapter 25.

Providers must report HCPCS codes for bone mass measurements under revenue code 320 with number of units and line item dates of service per revenue code line for each bone mass measurement reported.

A/B MACs (B) are billed for bone mass measurement procedures using the ASC X12 837 professional claim format or hardcopy Form CMS-1500.

100-04, 15, 20.4

Ambulance InflationFactor (AIF)

(Rev. 4172, Issued: 11-30-18, Effective: 01-01-19, Implementation: 01-07-19)

Section 1834(l)(3)(B) of the Social Security Act (the Act) provides the basis for an update to the payment limits for ambulance services that is equal to the percentage increase in the consumer price index for all urban consumers (CPI-U) for the 12-month period ending with June of the previous year. Section 3401 of the Affordable Care Act amended Section 1834(l)(3) of the Act to apply a productivity adjustment to this update equal to the 10-year moving average of changes in economy-wide private nonfarm business multi- factor productivity beginning January 1, 2011. The resulting update percentage is referred to as the Ambulance Inflation Factor (AIF). These updated percentages are issued via Recurring Update Notifications.

Part B coinsurance and deductible requirements apply to payments under the ambulance fee schedule. Following is a chart tracking the history of the AIF:

CY	AIF
2003	1.1
2004	2.1
2005	3.3
2006	2.5
2007	4.3
2008	2.7
2009	5.0
2010	0.0
2011	-0.1
2012	2.4
2013	0.8
2014	1.0
2015	1.5
2016	-0.4
2017	0.7
2018	1.1
2019	2.3

100-04, 16, 40.6.1

Automated Multi-Channel Chemistry (AMCC) Tests for ESRD Beneficiaries

(Rev. 3116, Issued: 11-06-14, Effective: 04-01-15, Implementation: 04-06-15)

Instructions for Services Provided on and After January 1, 2011

Section 153b of the MIPPA requires that all ESRD-related laboratory tests must be reported by the ESRD facility whether provided directly or under arrangements with an independent laboratory. When laboratory services are billed by providers other than the ESRD facility and the laboratory test furnished is designated as a laboratory test that is included in the ESRD PPS (ESRD-related), the claim will be rejected or denied. In the event that an ESRD-related laboratory test was furnished to an ESRD beneficiary for reasons other than for the treatment of ESRD, the provider may submit a claim for separate payment using modifier AY. The AY modifier serves as an attestation that the item or service is medically necessary for the dialysis patient but is not being used for the treatment of ESRD. The items and services subject to consolidated billing located on the CMS website includes the list of ESRD-related laboratory tests that are routinely performed for the treatment of ESRD.

For services provided on or after January 1, 2011, the 50/50 rule no longer applies to independent laboratory claims for AMCC tests furnished to ESRD beneficiaries. The 50/50 rule modifiers (CD, CE, and CF) are no longer required for independent laboratories effective for dates of service on and after January 1, 2011. However, for services provided between January 1, 2011 and March 31, 2015, the 50/50 rule modifiers are still required for use by ESRD facilities that are receiving the transitional blended payment amount (the transition ends in CY 2014). For services provided on or after April 1, 2015, the 50/50 rule modifiers are no longer required for use by ESRD facilities.

Effective for dates of service on and after January 1, 2012, contractors shall allow organ disease panel codes (i.e., HCPCS codes 80047, 80048, 80051, 80053, 80061, 80069, and 80076) to be billed by independent laboratories for AMCC panel tests furnished to ESRD eligible beneficiaries if:

- The beneficiary is not receiving dialysis treatment for any reason (e.g., post-transplant beneficiaries), or
- The test is not related to the treatment of ESRD, in which case the supplier would append modifier "AY".

Contractors shall make payment for organ disease panels according to the Clinical Laboratory Fee Schedule and shall apply the normal ESRD PPS editing rules for independent laboratory claims. The aforementioned organ disease panel codes were added to the list of bundled ESRD PPS laboratory tests in January 2012.

Effective for dates of service on and after April 1, 2015, contractors shall allow organ disease panel codes (i.e., HCPCS codes 80047, 80048, 80051, 80053, 80061, 80069, and 80076) to be billed by ESRD facilities for AMCC panel tests furnished to ESRD eligible beneficiaries if:

- These codes best describe the laboratory services provided to the beneficiary, which are paid under the ESRD PPS, or

- The test is not related to the treatment of ESRD, in which case the ESRD facility would append modifier "AY" and the service may be paid separately from the ESRD PPS.

Instructions for Services Provided Prior to January 1, 2011

For claims with dates of service prior to January 1, 2011, Medicare will apply the following rules to Automated Multi-Channel Chemistry (AMCC) tests for ESRD beneficiaries:

- Payment is at the lowest rate for tests performed by the same provider, for the same beneficiary, for the same date of service.
- The facility/laboratory must identify, for a particular date of service, the AMCC tests ordered that are included in the composite rate and those that are not included. See Publication 100-02, Chapter 11, Section 30.2.2 for the chart detailing the composite rate tests for Hemodialysis, Intermittent Peritoneal Dialysis (IPD), Continuous Cycling Peritoneal Dialysis (CCPD), and Hemofiltration as well as a second chart detailing the composite rate tests for Continuous Ambulatory Peritoneal Dialysis (CAPD).
- If 50 percent or more of the covered tests are included under the composite rate payment, then all submitted tests are included within the composite payment. In this case, no separate payment in addition to the composite rate is made for any of the separately billable tests.
- If less than 50 percent of the covered tests are composite rate tests, all AMCC tests submitted for that Date of Service (DOS) for that beneficiary are separately payable.
- A noncomposite rate test is defined as any test separately payable outside of the composite rate or beyond the normal frequency covered under the composite rate that is reasonable and necessary.
- For carrier processed claims, all chemistries ordered for beneficiaries with chronic dialysis for ESRD must be billed individually and must be rejected when billed as a panel.

(See §100.6UH for details regarding pricing modifiers.)

Implementation of this Policy:

ESRD facilities when ordering an ESRD-related AMCC must specify for each test within the AMCC whether the test:

a. Is part of the composite rate and not separately payable;

b. Is a composite rate test but is, on the date of the order, beyond the frequency covered under the composite rate and thus separately payable; or

c. Is not part of the ESRD composite rate and thus separately payable.

Laboratories must:

a. Identify which tests, if any, are not included within the ESRD facility composite rate payment

b. Identify which tests ordered for chronic dialysis for ESRD as follows:

1) Modifier CD: AMCC Test has been ordered by an ESRD facility or MCP physician that is part of the composite rate and is not separately billable.

2) Modifier CE: AMCC Test has been ordered by an ESRD facility or MCP physician that is a composite rate test but is beyond the normal frequency covered under the rate and is separately reimbursable based on medical necessity.

3) Modifier CF: AMCC Test has been ordered by an ESRD facility or MCP physician that is not part of the composite rate and is separately billable.

c. Bill all tests ordered for a chronic dialysis ESRD beneficiary individually and not as a panel.

The shared system must calculate the number of AMCC tests provided for any given date of service. Sum all AMCC tests with a CD modifier and divide the sum of all tests with a CD, CE, and CF modifier for the same beneficiary and provider for any given date of service.

If the result of the calculation for a date of service is 50 percent or greater, do not pay for the tests.

If the result of the calculation for a date of service is less than 50 percent, pay for all of the tests.

For FI processed claims, all tests for a date of service must be billed on the monthly ESRD bill. Providers that submit claims to a FI must send in an adjustment if they identify additional tests that have not been billed.

Carrier standard systems shall adjust the previous claim when the incoming claim for a date of service is compared to a claim on history and the action is adjust payment. Carrier standard systems shall spread the payment amount over each line item on both claims (the claim on history and the incoming claim).

The organ and disease oriented panels (80048, 80051, 80053, and 80076) are subject to the 50 percent rule. However, clinical diagnostic laboratories shall not bill these services as panels, they must be billed individually. Laboratory tests that are not covered under the composite rate and that are furnished to CAPD end stage renal disease (ESRD) patients dialyzing at home are billed in the same way as any other test furnished home patients.

FI Business Requirements for ESRD Reimbursement of AMCC Tests:

Requirement #	Requirements	Responsibility
1.1	The FI shared system must RTP a claim for AMCC tests when a claim for that date of service has already been submitted.	Shared system
1.2	Based upon the presence of the CD, CE and CF payment modifiers, identify the AMCC tests ordered that are included and not included in the composite rate payment.	Shared System
1.3	Based upon the determination of requirement 1.2, if 50 percent or more of the covered tests are included under the composite rate, no separate payment is made.	Shared System
1.4	Based upon the determination of requirement 1.2, if less than 50 percent are covered tests included under the composite rate, all AMCC tests for that date of service are payable.	Shared System
1.5	Effective for claims with dates of service on or after January 1, 2006, include any line items with a modifier 91 used in conjunction with the "CD," "CE," or "CF" modifier in the calculation of the 50/50 rule.	Shared System
1.6	FIs must return any claims for additional tests for any date of service within the billing period when the provider has already submitted a claim. Instruct the provider to adjust the first claim.	FI or Shared System
1.7	After the calculation of the 50/50 rule, services used to determine the payment amount may never exceed 22. Effective for claims with dates of service on or after January 1, 2006, accept all valid line items submitted for the date of service and pay a maximum of the ATP 22 rate.	Shared System

Carrier Business Requirements for ESRD Reimbursement of AMCC Tests:

Requirement #	Requirements	Responsibility
1	The standard systems shall calculate payment at the lowest rate for these automated tests even if reported on separate claims for services performed by the same provider, for the same beneficiary, for the same date of service.	Standard Systems
2	Standard Systems shall identify the AMCC tests ordered that are included and are not included in the composite rate payment based upon the presence of the "CD," "CE" and "CF" modifiers.	Standard Systems
3	Based upon the determination of requirement 2 if 50 percent or more of the covered services are included under the composite rate payment, Standard Systems shall indicate that no separate payment is provided for the services submitted for that date of service.	Standard Systems
4	Based upon the determination of requirement 2 if less than 50 percent are covered services included under the composite rate, Standard Systems shall indicate that all AMCC tests for that date of service are payable under the 50/50 rule.	Standard Systems
5	Effective for claims with dates of service on or after January 1, 2006, include any line items with a modifier 91 used in conjunction with the "CD," "CE," or "CF" modifier in the calculation of the 50/50 rule.	Standard Systems
6	Standard Systems shall adjust the previous claim when the incoming claim is compared to the claim on history and the action is to deny the previous claim. Spread the payment amount over each line item on both claims (the adjusted claim and the incoming claim).	Standard Systems
7	Standard Systems shall spread the adjustment across the incoming claim unless the adjusted amount would exceed the submitted amount of the services on the claim.	Standard System
8	After the calculation of the 50/50 rule, services used to determine the payment amount may never exceed 22. Accept all valid line items for the date of service and pay a maximum of the ATP 22 rate.	Standard Systems

Examples of the Application of the 50/50 Rule

The following examples are to illustrate how claims should be paid. The percentages in the action section represent the number of composite rate tests over the total tests. If this percentage is 50 percent or greater, no payment should be made for the claim.

Example 1:
Provider Name: Jones Hospital
DOS 2/1/02

Claim/Services
82040 Mod CD
82310 Mod CD
82374 Mod CD
82435 Mod CD
82947 Mod CF
84295 Mod CF
82040 Mod CD (Returned as duplicate)
84075 Mod CE
82310 Mod CE
84155 Mod CE

ACTION: 9 services total, 2 non-composite rate tests, 3 composite rate tests beyond the frequency, 4 composite rate tests; 4/9 = 44.4%<50% pay at ATP 09

Example 2:
Provider Name: Bon Secours Renal Facility
DOS 2/15/02

Claim/Services
82040 Mod CE and Mod 91
84450 Mod CE
82310 Mod CE
82247 Mod CF
82465 No modifier present
82565 Mod CE
84550 Mod CF
82040 Mod CD
84075 Mod CE
82435 Mod CE
82550 Mod CF
82947 Mod CF
82977 Mod CF

ACTION: 12 services total, 5 non-composite rate tests, 6 composite rate tests beyond the frequency, 1 composite rate test; 1/12 = 8.3%<50% pay at ATP 12

Example 3:
Provider Name: Sinai Hospital Renal Facility
DOS 4/02/02

Claim/Services
82565 Mod CD
83615 Mod CD
82247 Mod CF
82248 Mod CF
82040 Mod CD
84450 Mod CD
82565 Mod CE
84550 Mod CF
82248 Mod CF (Duplicate

ACTION: 8 services total, 3 non-composite rate tests, 4 composite rate tests, 1 composite rate test beyond the frequency; 4/8 = 50%, therefore no payment is made

Example 4:
Provider Name: Dr. Andrew Ross
DOS 6/01/02

Claim/Services
84460 Mod CF
82247 Mod CF
82248 Mod CF
82040 Mod CD
84075 Mod CD
84450 Mod CD

ACTION: 6 services total, 3 non-composite rate tests and 3 composite rate tests; 3/6 = 50%, therefore no payment

Example 5: (Carrier Processing Example Only)
Payment for first claim, second creates a no payment for either claim
Provider Name: Dr. Andrew Ross
DOS 6/01/06

Claim/Services
84460 Mod CF
82247 Mod CF
82248 Mod CF

ACTION: 3 services total, 3 non-composite rate tests, 0 composite rate tests beyond the frequency, and 0 composite rate tests, 0/3 = 0%, therefore ATP 03

Provider Name: Dr. Andrew Ross
DOS 6/01/06
Claim/Services   82040 Mod CD
                            84075 Mod CD
                            84450 Mod CD

ACTION: An additional 3 services are billed, 0 non-composite rate tests, 8 composite rate test beyond the frequency, 3 composite rate tests. For both claims there are 6 services total, 3 non-composite rate tests and 3 composite rate tests; 3/6 = 50% U>U 50%, therefore no payment. An overpayment should be recovered for the ATP 03 payment.

100-04, 16, 60.2

Travel Allowance

(Rev. 4199, Issued: 01-11-19, Effective: 01-01-19, Implementation: 02-12-19)

In addition to a specimen collection fee allowed under §60.1, Medicare, under Part B, covers a specimen collection fee and travel allowance for a laboratory technician to draw a specimen from either a nursing home patient or homebound patient under §1833(h)(3) of the Act and payment is made based on the clinical laboratory fee schedule. The travel allowance is intended to cover the estimated travel costs of collecting a specimen and to reflect the technician's salary and travel costs.

The additional allowance can be made only where a specimen collection fee is also payable, i.e., no travel allowance is made where the technician merely performs a messenger service to pick up a specimen drawn by a physician or nursing home personnel. The travel allowance may not be paid to a physician unless the trip to the home, or to the nursing home was solely for the purpose of drawing a specimen. Otherwise travel costs are considered to be associated with the other purposes of the trip.

The travel allowance is not distributed by CMS. Instead, the carrier must calculate the travel allowance for each claim using the following rules for the particular Code. The following HCPCS codes are used for travel allowances:

Per Mile Travel Allowance (P9603)

- The minimum "per mile travel allowance" is $1.03. The per mile travel allowance is to be used in situations where the average trip to patients' homes is longer than 20 miles round trip, and is to be pro-rated in situations where specimens are drawn or picked up from non-Medicare patients in the same trip. - one way, in connection with medically necessary laboratory specimen collection drawn from homebound or nursing home bound patient; prorated miles actually traveled (carrier allowance on per mile basis); or

- The per mile allowance was computed using the Federal mileage rate plus an additional 45 cents a mile to cover the technician's time and travel costs. Contractors have the option of establishing a higher per mile rate in excess of the minimum ($1.03 a mile in CY 2019) if local conditions warrant it. The minimum mileage rate will be reviewed and updated in conjunction with the clinical lab fee schedule as needed. At no time will the laboratory be allowed to bill for more miles than are reasonable or for miles not actually traveled by the laboratory technician.

Example 1: In CY 2019, a laboratory technician travels 60 miles round trip from a lab in a city to a remote rural location, and back to the lab to draw a single Medicare patient's blood. The total reimbursement would be $61.80 (60 miles x $1.03 a mile), plus the specimen collection fee.

Example 2: In CY 2019, a laboratory technician travels 40 miles from the lab to a Medicare patient's home to draw blood, and then travels an additional 10 miles to a non-Medicare patient's home and then travels 30 miles to return to the lab. The total miles traveled would be 80 miles. The claim submitted would be for one half of the miles traveled or $41.20 (40 x $1.03), plus the specimen collection fee.

Flat Rate (P9604)

The CMS will pay a minimum of $10.30 (based on CY 2019) one way flat rate travel allowance. The flat rate travel allowance is to be used in areas where average trips are less than 20 miles round trip. The flat rate travel fee is to be pro-rated for more than one blood drawn at the same address, and for stops at the homes of Medicare and non-Medicare patients. The laboratory does the pro-ration when the claim is submitted based on the number of patients seen on that trip. The specimen collection fee will be paid for each patient encounter.

This rate is based on an assumption that a trip is an average of 15 minutes and up to 10 miles one way. It uses the Federal mileage rate and a laboratory technician's time of $17.66 an hour, including overhead. Contractors have the option of establishing a flat rate in excess of the minimum of $10.00, if local conditions warrant it. The minimum national flat rate will be reviewed and updated in conjunction with the clinical laboratory fee schedule, as necessitated by adjustments in the Federal travel allowance and salaries.

The claimant identifies round trip travel by use of the LR modifier

Example 3: A laboratory technician travels from the laboratory to a single Medicare patient's home and returns to the laboratory without making any other stops. The flat rate would be calculated as follows: 2 x $10.30 for a total trip reimbursement of $20.60, plus the specimen collection fee.

Example 4: A laboratory technician travels from the laboratory to the homes of five patients to draw blood, four of the patients are Medicare patients and one is not. An additional flat rate would be charged to cover the 5 stops and the return trip to the lab (6 x $10.30 = $61.80). Each of the claims submitted would be for $12.36 ($61.80/5

= $12.36). Since one of the patients is non-Medicare, four claims would be submitted for $12.36 each, plus the specimen collection fee for each.

Example 5: A laboratory technician travels from a laboratory to a nursing home and draws blood from 5 patients and returns to the laboratory. Four of the patients are on Medicare and one is not. The $10.30 flat rate is multiplied by two to cover the return trip to the laboratory (2 x $10.30 = $20.60) and then divided by five (1/5 of $20.60 = $4.12). Since one of the patients is non-Medicare, four claims would be submitted for $4.12 each, plus the specimen collection fee.

If a carrier determines that it results in equitable payment, the carrier may extend the former payment allowances for additional travel (such as to a distant rural nursing home) to all circumstances where travel is required. This might be appropriate, for example, if the carrier's former payment allowance was on a per mile basis. Otherwise, it should establish an appropriate allowance and inform the suppliers in its service area. If a carrier decides to establish a new allowance, one method is to consider developing a travel allowance consisting of:

- The current Federal mileage allowance for operating personal automobiles, plus a personnel allowance per mile to cover personnel costs based upon an estimate of average hourly wages and average driving speed.

Carriers must prorate travel allowance amounts claimed by suppliers by the number of patients (including Medicare and non-Medicare patients) from whom specimens were drawn on a given trip.

The carrier may determine that payment in addition to the routine travel allowance determined under this section is appropriate if:

- The patient from whom the specimen must be collected is in a nursing home or is homebound; and

- The clinical laboratory tests are needed on an emergency basis outside the general business hours of the laboratory making the collection.

- Subsequent updated travel allowance amounts will be issued by CMS via Recurring Update Notification (RUN) on an annual basis.

100-04, 16, 70.8

Certificate of Waiver

(Rev. 1652, Issued: 12-19-08, Effective: 01-01-09, Implementation: 01-05-09)

Effective September 1, 1992, all laboratory testing sites (except as provided in 42 CFR 493.3(b)) must have either a CLIA certificate of waiver, certificate for provider-performed microscopy procedures, certificate of registration, certificate of compliance, or certificate of accreditation to legally perform clinical laboratory testing on specimens from individuals in the United States.

The Food and Drug Administration approves CLIA waived tests on a flow basis. The CMS identifies CLIA waived tests by providing an updated list of waived tests to the Medicare contractors on a quarterly basis via a Recurring Update Notification. To be recognized as a waived test, some CLIA waived tests have unique HCPCS procedure codes and some must have a QW modifier included with the HCPCS code.

For a list of specific HCPCS codes subject to CLIA see

http://www.cms.hhs.gov/CLIA/downloads/waivetbl.pdf

100-04, 16, 90.2

Organ or Disease Oriented Panels

(Rev. 4299; Issued: 05-03-19; Effective: 01-01-19; Implementation: 10-07-19)

Prior to January 1, 2018, organ or disease panels must be paid at the lower of the billed charge, the fee amount for the panel, or the sum of the fee amounts for all components. When panels contain one or more automated tests, the A/B MAC (A) or (B) determines the correct price for the panel by comparing the price for the automated profile laboratory tests with the sum of the fee amounts for individual tests. Payment for the total panel may not exceed the sum total of the fee amounts for individual covered tests. All Medicare coverage rules apply.

The Medicare shared systems must calculate the correct payment amount. The CMS furnishes fee prices for each code but the A/B MAC (A) or (B) system must compare individual codes billed with codes and prices for related individual tests. (With each HCPCS update, HCPCS codes are reviewed and the system is updated). Once the codes are identified, A/B MACs (A) and (B) publish panel codes to providers.

The only acceptable Medicare definition for the component tests included in the CPT codes for organ or disease oriented panels is the American Medical Association (AMA) definition of component tests. The CMS will not pay for the panel code unless all of the tests in the definition are performed. If the laboratory has a custom panel that includes other tests, in addition to those in the defined CPT or HCPCS panels, the additional tests, whether on the list of automated tests or not, are billed separately in addition to the CPT or HCPCS panel code.

NOTE: If a laboratory chooses, it can bill each of the component tests of these panels individually, but payment will be based upon the above rules.

Effective for claims with dates of service on or after January 1, 2019, laboratories shall bill the HCPCS panel test code and not unbundle the individual components if all components of the HCPCS panel are performed. Claims will be returned as unprocessable/rejected if the HCPCS panel test code is not billed. Providers and suppliers are required to submit all AMCC laboratory test HCPCS for the same beneficiary, performed on the same date of service on the same claim. This billing policy applies when:

a). Submitting a complete organ disease panel; or

b). Submitting individual component tests of an organ disease panel when all components of the panel were not performed.

TABLE OF CHEMISTRY PANELS

Chemistry	CPT	Hepatic Function Panel 80076	Basic Metabolic Panel (Calcium, ionized) 80047	Basic Metabolic Panel (Calcium, total) 80048	Comprehensive Metabolic Panel 80053	Renal Function Panel 80069	Lipid[1] Panel 80061	Electrolyte Panel 80051
Albumin	82040	X			X	X		
Alkaline phosphatase	84075	X			X			
ALT (SGPT)	84460	X			X			
AST (SGOT)	84450	X			X			
Bilirubin, total	82247	X			X			
Bilirubin, direct	82248	X						
Calcium	82310			X	X	X		
Calcium ionized	82330		X					
Chloride	82435		X	X	X	X		X
Cholesterol	82465						X	
CK, CPK	82550							
CO2 (bicarbonate)	82374		X	X	X	X		X
Creatinine	82565		X	X	X	X		
GGT	82977							
Glucose	82947		X	X	X	X		
LDH	83615							
Phosphorus	84100					X		
Potassium	84132		X	X	X	X		X
Protein	84155	X			X			
Sodium	84295		X	X	X	X		X
Triglycerides	84478						X	
Urea nitrogen (BUN)	84520		X	X	X	X		
Uric Acid	84550							

1   CPT code 83718 is billed with Organ/Disease Panel 80061 but is not included in the AMCC bundling.

100-04, 18, 1.2

Table of Preventive and Screening Services

(Rev. 4150, Issued: 10-26-2018, Effective: 04-01-19, Implementation: 04-01-19)

Service	CPT/ HCPCS	Long Descriptor	USPSTF Rating	Coins./ Deductible
Initial Preventive Physical Examination, IPPE	G0402	Initial preventive physical examination; face to face visits, services limited to new beneficiary during the first 12 months of Medicare enrollment	*Not Rated	WAIVED
	G0403	Electrocardiogram, routine ECG with 12 leads; performed as a screening for the initial preventive physical examination with interpretation and report		Not Waived
	G0404	Electrocardiogram, routine ECG with 12 leads; tracing only, without interpretation and report, performed as a screening for the initial preventive physical examination		Not Waived
	G0405	Electrocardiogram, routine ECG with 12 leads; interpretation and report only, performed as a screening for the initial preventive physical examination		Not Waived

Service	CPT/ HCPCS	Long Descriptor	USPSTF Rating	Coins./ Deductible
Ultrasound Screening for Abdominal Aortic Aneurysm (AAA) furnished prior to January 1, 2017	G0389	Ultrasound, B-scan and/or real time with image documentation; for abdominal aortic aneurysm (AAA) ultrasound screening	B	WAIVED
Ultrasound Screening for Abdominal Aortic Aneurysm (AAA) services furnished on or after January 1, 2017	76706	Ultrasound, abdominal aorta, real time with image documentation, screening study for abdominal aortic aneurysm (AAA)		WAIVED
Cardio-vascular Disease Screening	80061	Lipid panel	A	WAIVED
	82465	Cholesterol, serum or whole blood, total		WAIVED
	83718	Lipoprotein, direct measurement; high density cholesterol (hdl cholesterol)		WAIVED
	84478	Triglycerides		WAIVED
Diabetes Screening Tests	82947	Glucose; quantitative, blood (except reagent strip)	B	WAIVED
	82950	Glucose; post glucose dose (includes glucose)		WAIVED
	82951	Glucose; tolerance test (gtt), three specimens (includes glucose)	*Not Rated	WAIVED
Diabetes Self-Management Training Services (DSMT)	G0108	Diabetes outpatient self-management training services, individual, per 30 minutes	*Not Rated	Not Waived
	G0109	Diabetes outpatient self-management training services, group session (2 or more), per 30 minutes		Not Waived
Medical Nutrition Therapy (MNT) Services	97802	Medical nutrition therapy; initial assessment and intervention, individual, face-to-face with the patient, each 15 minutes	B	WAIVED
	97803	Medical nutrition therapy; re-assessment and intervention, individual, face-to-face with the patient, each 15 minutes		WAIVED
	97804	Medical nutrition therapy; group (2 or more individual(s)), each 30 minutes		WAIVED
	G0270	Medical nutrition therapy; reassessment and subsequent intervention(s) following second referral in same year for change in diagnosis, medical condition or treatment regimen (including additional hours needed for renal disease), individual, face to face with the patient, each 15 minutes	B	WAIVED
	G0271	Medical nutrition therapy, reassessment and subsequent intervention(s) following second referral in same year for change in diagnosis, medical condition, or treatment regimen (including additional hours needed for renal disease), group (2 or more individuals), each 30 minutes		WAIVED

Service	CPT/HCPCS	Long Descriptor	USPSTF Rating	Coins./Deductible
Screening Pap Test	G0123	Screening cytopathology, cervical or vaginal (any reporting system), collected in preservative fluid, automated thin layer preparation, screening by cytotechnologist under physician supervision	A	WAIVED
	G0124	Screening cytopathology, cervical or vaginal (any reporting system), collected in preservative fluid, automated thin layer preparation, requiring interpretation by physician		WAIVED
	G0141	Screening cytopathology smears, cervical or vaginal, performed by automated system, with manual rescreening, requiring interpretation by physician	A	WAIVED
	G0143	Screening cytopathology, cervical or vaginal (any reporting system), collected in preservative fluid, automated thin layer preparation, with manual screening and rescreening by cytotechnologist under physician supervision	A	WAIVED
	G0144	Screening cytopathology, cervical or vaginal (any reporting system), collected in preservative fluid, automated thin layer preparation, with screening by automated system, under physician supervision	A	WAIVED
	G0145	Screening cytopathology, cervical or vaginal (any reporting system), collected in preservative fluid, automated thin layer preparation, with screening by automated system and manual rescreening under physician supervision	A	WAIVED
	G0147	Screening cytopathology smears, cervical or vaginal, performed by automated system under physician supervision	A	WAIVED
	G0148	Screening cytopathology smears, cervical or vaginal, performed by automated system with manual rescreening	A	WAIVED
	P3000	Screening papanicolaou smear, cervical or vaginal, up to three smears, by technician under physician supervision		WAIVED
	P3001	Screening papanicolaou smear, cervical or vaginal, up to three smears, requiring interpretation by physician		WAIVED
	Q0091	Screening papanicolaou smear; obtaining, preparing and conveyance of cervical or vaginal smear to laboratory		WAIVED
Screening Pelvic Exam	G0101	Cervical or vaginal cancer screening; pelvic and clinical breast examination	A	WAIVED
Screening Mammography	77052	Computer-aided detection (computer algorithm analysis of digital image data for lesion detection) with further physician review for interpretation, with or without digitization of film radiographic images; screening mammography (list separately in addition to code for primary procedure)	B	WAIVED
	77057	Screening mammography, bilateral (2-view film study of each breast)	B	WAIVED
	77063	Screening digital breast tomosynthesis, bilateral		WAIVED

Service	CPT/HCPCS	Long Descriptor	USPSTF Rating	Coins./Deductible
Screening Mammography (continued)	77067	Screening mammography, bilateral (2-view study of each breast), including computer-aided detection (CAD) when performed	B	WAIVED
Bone Mass Measurement	G0130	Single energy x-ray absorptiometry (sexa) bone density study, one or more sites; appendicular skeleton (peripheral) (e.g., radius, wrist, heel)		WAIVED
	77078	Computed tomography, bone mineral density study, 1 or more sites; axial skeleton (e.g., hips, pelvis, spine)	B	WAIVED
	77079	Computed tomography, bone mineral density study, 1 or more sites; appendicular skeleton (peripheral) (e.g., radius, wrist, heel)		WAIVED
	77080	Dual-energy x-ray absorptiometry (dxa), bone density study, 1 or more sites; axial skeleton (e.g., hips, pelvis, spine)		WAIVED
	77081	Dual-energy x-ray absorptiometry (dxa), bone density study, 1 or more sites; appendicular skeleton (peripheral) (e.g., radius, wrist, heel)		WAIVED
	77083	Radiographic absorptiometry (e.g., photo densitometry, radiogrammetry), 1 or more sites		WAIVED
	77085	Dual-energy X-ray absorptiometry (DXA), bone density study, 1 or more sites, axial skeleton, (e.g., hips, pelvis, spine), including vertebral fracture assessment.		WAIVED
	76977	Ultrasound bone density measurement and interpretation, peripheral site(s), any method		WAIVED

NOTE: Anesthesia services furnished in conjunction with and in support of a screening colonoscopy are reported with CPT code 00812 and coinsurance and deductible are waived. When a screening colonoscopy becomes a diagnostic colonoscopy, anesthesia services are reported with CPT code 00811 and with the PT modifier; only the deductible is waived.

Coinsurance and deductible are waived for moderate sedation services (reported with G0500 or 99153) when furnished in conjunction with and in support of a screening colonoscopy service and when reported with modifier 33. When a screening colonoscopy becomes a diagnostic colonoscopy, moderate sedation services (G0500 or 99153) are reported with only the PT modifier; only the deductible is waived.

Service	CPT/HCPCS	Long Descriptor	USPSTF Rating	Coins./Deductible
Colorectal Cancer Screening	G0104	Colorectal cancer screening; flexible sigmoidoscopy	A	WAIVED
	G0105	Colorectal cancer screening; colonoscopy on individual at high risk		WAIVED
	G0106	Colorectal cancer screenng; alternative to G0104, screening sigmoidoscopy, barium enema	*Not Rated	Coins. Applies & Ded. is waived
	G0120	Colorectal cancer screening; alternative to G0105, screening colonoscopy, barium enema.i		Coins. Applies & Ded. is waived
	G0121	Colorectal cancer screening; colonoscopy on individual not meeting criteria for high risk		WAIVED
	82270	Blood, occult, by peroxidase activity (e.g., guaiac), qualitative; feces, consecutive	A	WAIVED
	G0328	Colorectal cancer screening; fecal occult blood test, immunoassay, 1-3 simultaneous		WAIVED
Prostate Cancer Screening	G0102	Prostate cancer screening; digital rectal examination	D	Not Waived
	G0103	Prostate cancer screening; prostate specific antigen test (PSA)		WAIVED

Service	CPT/HCPCS	Long Descriptor	USPSTF Rating	Coins./Deductible
Glaucoma Screening	G0117	Glaucoma screening for high risk patients furnished by an optometrist or ophthalmologist	I	Not Waived
	G0118	Glaucoma screening for high risk patient furnished under the direct supervision of an optometrist or ophthalmologist		Not Waived
Influenza Virus Vaccine	90630	Influenza virus vaccine, quadrivalent (IIV4), split virus, preservative free, for intradermal use	B	WAIVED
	90653	Influenza virus vaccine, inactivated, subunit, adjuvanted, for intramuscular use		WAIVED
	90654	Influenza virus vaccine, split virus, preservative free, for intradermal use, for adults ages 18-64		WAIVED
	90655	Influenza virus vaccine, split virus, preservative free, when administered to children 6-35 months of age, for intramuscular use		WAIVED
	90656	Influenza virus vaccine, split virus, preservative free, when administered to individuals 3 years and older, for intramuscular use		WAIVED
	90657	Influenza virus vaccine, split virus, when administered to children 6-35 months of age, for intramuscular use		WAIVED
	90658	Influenza virus vaccine, trivalent (IIV3), split virus, 0.5 mL dosage, for intramuscular use		WAIVED
	90660	Influenza virus vaccine, live, for intranasal use		WAIVED
	90661	Influenza virus vaccine, derived from cell cultures, subunit, preservative and antibiotic free, for intramuscular use		WAIVED
	90662	Influenza virus vaccine, split virus, preservative free, enhanced immunogenicity via increased antigen content, for intramuscular use		WAIVED
	90672	Influenza virus vaccine, live, quadrivalent, for intranasal use		WAIVED
	90673	Influenza virus vaccine, trivalent, derived from recombinant DNA (RIV3), hemagglutinin (HA) protein only, preservative and antibiotic free, for intramuscular use		WAIVED
	90674	Influenza virus vaccine, quadrivalent (ccIIV4), derived from cell cultures, subunit, preservative and antibiotic free, 0.5 mL dosage, for intramuscular use		WAIVED
	90682	Influenza virus vaccine, quadrivalent (RIV4), derived from recombinant DNA, hemagglutinin (HA) protein only, preservative and antibiotic free, for intramuscular use		WAIVED
	90685	Influenza virus vaccine, quadrivalent, split virus, preservative free, when administered to children 6-35 months of age, for intramuscular use		WAIVED

Service	CPT/HCPCS	Long Descriptor	USPSTF Rating	Coins./Deductible
Influenza Virus Vaccine (continued)	90686	Influenza virus vaccine, quadrivalent, split virus, preservative free, when administered to individuals 3 years of age and older, for intramuscular use		WAIVED
	90687	Influenza virus vaccine, quadrivalent, split virus, when administered to children 6-35 months of age, for intramuscular use		WAIVED
	90688	Influenza virus vaccine, quadrivalent, split virus, when administered to individuals 3 years of age and older, for intramuscular use		WAIVED
	90689	Influenza virus vaccine, quadrivalent (IIV4), inactivated, adjuvanted, preservative free, 0.25 mL dosage, for INtramuscular use		WAIVED
	90756	Influenza virus vaccine, quadrivalent (ccIIV4), derived from cell cultures, subunit, antibiotic free, 0.5mL dosage, for intramuscular use		WAIVED
	G0008	Administration of influenza virus vaccine		WAIVED
Pneumococcal Vaccine	90669	Pneumococcal conjugate vaccine, polyvalent, when administered to children younger than 5 years, for intramuscular use	B	WAIVED
	90670	Pneumococcal conjugate vaccine, 13 valent, for intramuscular use		WAIVED
	90732	Pneumococcal polysaccharide vaccine, 23-valent, adult or immunosuppressed patient dosage, when administered to individuals 2 years or older, for subcutaneous or intramuscular use		WAIVED
	G0009	Administration of pneumococcal vaccine		WAIVED
Hepatitis B Vaccine	90739	Hepatitis B vaccine, adult dosage (2 dose schedule), for intramuscular use	A	WAIVED
	90740	Hepatitis B vaccine, dialysis or immunosuppressed patient dosage (3 dose schedule), for intramuscular use		WAIVED
	90743	Hepatitis B vaccine, adolescent (2 dose schedule), for intramuscular use		WAIVED
	90744	Hepatitis B vaccine, pediatric/adolescent dosage (3 dose schedule), for intramuscular use		WAIVED
	90746	Hepatitis B vaccine, adult dosage, for intramuscular use		WAIVED
	90747	Hepatitis B vaccine, dialysis or immunosuppressed patient dosage (4 dose schedule), for intramuscular use		WAIVED
	G0010	Administration of Hepatitis B vaccine	A	WAIVED
Hepatitis C Virus Screening	G0472	Screening for Hepatitis C antibody	B	WAIVED

Service	CPT/HCPCS	Long Descriptor	USPSTF Rating	Coins./Deductible
HIV Screening	G0432	Infectious agent antigen detection by enzyme immunoassay (EIA) technique, qualitative or semi-qualitative, multiple-step method, HIV-1 or HIV-2, screening	A	WAIVED
	G0433	Infectious agent antigen detection by enzyme-linked immunosorbent assay (ELISA) technique, antibody, HIV-1 or HIV-2, screening		WAIVED
	G0435	Infectious agent antigen detection by rapid antibody test of oral mucosa transudate, HIV-1 or HIV-2, screening		WAIVED
Smoking Cessation for services furnished prior to October 1, 2016	G0436	Smoking and tobacco cessation counseling visit for the asymptomatic patient; intermediate, greater than 3 minutes, up to 10 minutes	A	WAIVED
	G0437	Smoking and tobacco cessation counseling visit for the asymptomatic patient intensive, greater than 10 minutes		WAIVED
Smoking Cessation for services furnished on or after October 1, 2016	99406	Smoking and tobacco cessation counseling visit for the asymptomatic patient; intermediate, greater than 3 minutes, up to 10 minutes	A	WAIVED
	99407	Smoking and tobacco cessation counseling visit for the asymptomatic patient intensive, greater than 10 minutes		WAIVED
Annual Wellness Visit	G0438	Annual wellness visit, including PPPS, first visit	*Not Rated	WAIVED
	G0439	Annual wellness visit, including PPPS, subsequent visit		WAIVED
Intensive Behavioral Therapy for Obesity	G0447	Face-to-Face Behavioral Counseling for Obesity, 15 minutes	B	WAIVED
	G0473	Face-to-face behavioral counseling for obesity, group (2-10), 30 minute(s)		WAIVED
Lung Cancer Screening	G0296	Counseling visit to discuss need for lung cancer screening (LDCT) using low dose CT scan (service is for eligibility determination and shared decision making)	B	WAIVED
	G0297	Low dose CT scan (LDCT) for lung cancer screening		

100-04, 18, 10.2.1

Healthcare Common Procedure Coding System (HCPCS) and Diagnosis Codes

(Rev. 4100, Issued: 08-03-18; Effective: 01-01-19; Implementation: 01-07-19)

Vaccines and their administration are reported using separate codes. The following codes are for reporting the vaccines only.

HCPCS	Definition
90630	Influenza virus vaccine, quadrivalent (IIV4), split virus, preservative free, for intradermal use
90653	Influenza virus vaccine, inactivated, subunit, adjuvanted, for intramuscular use
90654	Influenza virus vaccine, split virus, preservative-free, for intradermal use, for adults ages 18 – 64;
90655	Influenza virus vaccine, split virus, preservative free, for children 6-35 months of age, for intramuscular use;
90656	Influenza virus vaccine, split virus, preservative free, for use in individuals 3 years and above, for intramuscular use;
90657	Influenza virus vaccine, split virus, for children 6-35 months of age, for intramuscular use;
90658	Influenza virus vaccine, trivalent (IIV3), split virus, 0.5 mL dosage, for intramuscular use
90660	Influenza virus vaccine, live, for intranasal use;
90661	Influenza virus vaccine, derived from cell cultures, subunit, preservative and antibiotic free, for intramuscular use
90662	Influenza virus vaccine, split virus, preservative free, enhanced immunogenicity via increased antigen content, for intramuscular use

HCPCS	Definition
90669	Pneumococcal conjugate vaccine, polyvalent, for children under 5 years, for intramuscular use
90670	Pneumococcal conjugate vaccine, 13 valent, for intramuscular use
90672	Influenza virus vaccine, live, quadrivalent, for intranasal use
90673	Influenza virus vaccine, trivalent, derived from recombinant DNA (RIV3), hemagglutinin (HA) protein only, preservative and antibiotic free, for intramuscular use
90674	Influenza virus vaccine, quadrivalent (ccIIV4), derived from cell cultures, subunit, preservative and antibiotic free, 0.5 mL dosage, for intramuscular use
90682	Influenza virus vaccine, quadrivalent (RIV4), derived from recombinant DNA, hemagglutinin (HA) protein only, preservative and antibiotic free, for intramuscular use
90685	Influenza virus vaccine, quadrivalent, split virus, preservative free, when administered to children 6-35 months of age, for intramuscular use
90686	Influenza virus vaccine, quadrivalent, split virus, preservative free, when administered to individuals 3 years of age and older, for intramuscular use
90687	Influenza virus vaccine, quadrivalent, split virus, when administered to children 6-35 months of age, for intramuscular use
90688	Influenza virus vaccine, quadrivalent, split virus, when administered to individuals 3 years of age and older, for intramuscular use
90689	Influenza virus vaccine, quadrivalent (IIV4), inactivated, adjuvanted, preservative free, 0.25mL dosage, for intramuscular use
90732	Pneumococcal polysaccharide vaccine, 23-valent, adult or immunosuppressed patient dosage, for use in individuals 2 years or older, for subcutaneous or intramuscular use;
90739	Hepatitis B vaccine, adult dosage (2 dose schedule), for intramuscular use
90740	Hepatitis B vaccine, dialysis or immunosuppressed patient dosage (3 dose schedule), for intramuscular use;
90743	Hepatitis B vaccine, adolescent (2 dose schedule), for intramuscular use;
90744	Hepatitis B vaccine, pediatric/adolescent dosage (3 dose schedule), for intramuscular use;
90746	Hepatitis B vaccine, adult dosage, for intramuscular use; and
90747	Hepatitis B vaccine, dialysis or immunosuppressed patient dosage (4 dose schedule), for intramuscular use.
90756	Influenza virus vaccine, quadrivalent (ccIIV4), derived from cell cultures, subunit, antibiotic free, 0.5mL dosage, for intramuscular use

The following codes are for reporting administration of the vaccines only. The administration of the vaccines is billed using:

HCPCS	Definition
G0008	Administration of influenza virus vaccine;
G0009	Administration of pneumococcal vaccine; and
*G0010	Administration of hepatitis B vaccine.
*90471	Immunization administration. (For OPPS hospitals billing for the hepatitis B vaccine administration)
*90472	Each additional vaccine. (For OPPS hospitals billing for the hepatitis B vaccine administration)

* NOTE: For claims with dates of service prior to January 1, 2006, OPPS and non-OPPS hospitals report G0010 for hepatitis B vaccine administration. For claims with dates of service January 1, 2006 until December 31, 2010, OPPS hospitals report 90471 or 90472 for hepatitis B vaccine administration as appropriate in place of G0010. Beginning January 1, 2011, providers should report G0010 for billing under the OPPS rather than 90471 or 90472 to ensure correct waiver of coinsurance and deductible for the administration of hepatitis B vaccine.

One of the following diagnosis codes must be reported as appropriate. If the sole purpose for the visit is to receive a vaccine or if a vaccine is the only service billed on a claim, the applicable following diagnosis code may be used.

ICD-9-CM Diagnosis Code	Description
V03.82	Pneumococcus
V04.81**	Influenza
V06.6***	Pneumococcus and Influenza
V05.3	Hepatitis B

**Effective for influenza virus claims with dates of service October 1, 2003 and later.

***Effective October 1, 2006, providers may report ICD-9-CM diagnosis code V06.6 on claims for pneumococcus and/or influenza virus vaccines when the purpose of the visit was to receive both vaccines.

NOTE: ICD-10-CM diagnosis code Z23 may be used for an encounter for immunizations effective October 1, 2015, when ICD-10 was implemented.

If a diagnosis code for pneumococcus, hepatitis B, or influenza virus vaccination is not reported on a claim, contractors may not enter the diagnosis on the claim. Contractors must follow current resolution processes for claims with missing diagnosis codes.

If the diagnosis code and the narrative description are correct, but the HCPCS code is incorrect, the A/B MAC (A or B) may correct the HCPCS code and pay the claim. For example, if the reported diagnosis code is V04.81 and the narrative description (if annotated on the claim) says "flu shot" but the HCPCS code is incorrect, contractors may change the HCPCS code and pay for the flu vaccine. Effective October 1, 2006, A/B MACs (B) should follow the instructions in Pub. 100-04, Chapter 1, Section 80.3.2.1.1 (A/B MAC (B) Data Element Requirements) for claims submitted without a HCPCS code.

Claims for hepatitis B vaccinations must report the I.D. Number of the referring physician. In addition, if a doctor of medicine or osteopathy does not order the influenza virus vaccine, the A/B MACs (A) claims require:

- UPIN code SLF000 to be reported on claims submitted prior to May 23, 2008, when Medicare began accepting NPIs, only
- The provider's own NPI to be reported in the NPI field for the attending physician on claims submitted on or after May 23, 2008, when NPI requirements were implemented.

100-04, 18, 10.2.2.1

Payment for Pneumococcal Pneumonia Virus, Influenza Virus, and Hepatitis B Virus Vaccines and Their Administration on Institutional Claims

(Rev. 3754, Issued: 04-21-17; Effective: 07-01-17; Implementation: 07-03-17)

Payment for Vaccines

Payment for these vaccines is as follows:

Facility	Type of Bill	Payment
Hospitals, other than Indian Health Service (IHS) Hospitals and Critical Access Hospitals (CAHs)	012x, 013x	Reasonable cost
IHS Hospitals	012x, 013x, 083x	95% of AWP
IHS CAHs	085x	95% of AWP
CAHs Method I and Method II	085x	Reasonable cost
Skilled Nursing Facilities	022x, 023x	Reasonable cost
Home Health Agencies	034x	Reasonable cost
Hospice	081x, 082x	95% of the AWP
Comprehensive Outpatient Rehabilitation Facilities	075x	95% of the AWP
Independent Renal Dialysis Facilities	072x	95% of the AWP
Hospital-based Renal Dialysis Facilities	072x	Reasonable cost

Payment for Vaccine Administration

Payment for the administration of Influenza Virus and PPV vaccines is as follows:

Facility	Type of Bill	Payment
Hospitals, other than IHS Hospitals and CAHs	012x, 013x	Outpatient Prospective Payment System (OPPS) for hospitals subject to OPPS Reasonable cost for hospitals not subject to OPPS
IHS Hospitals	012x, 013x, 083x	MPFS as indicated in guidelines below.
IHS CAHs	085x	MPFS as indicated in guidelines below.
CAHs Method I and II	085x	Reasonable cost
Skilled Nursing Facilities	022x, 023x	MPFS
Home Health Agencies	034x	OPPS
Hospices	081x, 082x	MPFS
Comprehensive Outpatient Rehabilitation Facilities	075x	MPFS
Independent RDFs	072x	MPFS
Hospital-based RDFs	072x	Reasonable cost

Payment for the administration of Hepatitis B vaccine is as follows:

Facility	Type of Bill	Payment
Hospitals other than IHS hospitals and CAHs	012x, 013x	Outpatient Prospective Payment System (OPPS) for hospitals subject to OPPS Reasonable cost for hospitals not subject to OPPS
IHS Hospitals	012x, 013x, 083x	MPFS
CAHs	085x	Reasonable cost
Method I and II		
IHS CAHs	085x	MPFS
Skilled Nursing Facilities	022x, 023x	MPFS
Home Health Agencies	034x	OPPS
Hospices	081x, 082x	MPFS
Comprehensive Outpatient Rehabilitation Facilities	075x	MPFS
Independent RDFs	072x	MPFS
Hospital-based RDFs	072x	Reasonable cost

100-04, 18, 10.4.1

CWF Edits on A/B MAC (A) Claims

(Rev. 4100, Issued: 08-03-18; Effective: 01-01-19; Implementation: 01-07-19)

In order to prevent duplicate payment by the same A/B MAC (A), CWF edits by line item on the A/B MAC (A) number, the beneficiary Health Insurance Claim (HIC) number, and the date of service, the influenza virus procedure codes 90630, 90653, 90654, 90655, 90656, 90657, 90658, 90660, 90661, 90662, 90672, 90673, 90674, 90682, 90685, 90686, 90687, 90688, 90689, or 90756 and the pneumococcal procedure codes 90669, 90670, or 90732, and the administration codes G0008 or G0009.

If CWF receives a claim with either HCPCS codes 90630, 90653, 90654, 90655, 90656, 90657, 90658, 90660, 90661, 90662, 90672, 90673, 90674, 90682, 90685, 90686, 90687, 90688, 90689, or 90756 and it already has on record a claim with the same HIC number, same A/B MAC (A) number, same date of service, and any one of those HCPCS codes, the second claim submitted to CWF rejects.

If CWF receives a claim with HCPCS codes 90669, 90670, or 90732 and it already has on record a claim with the same HIC number, same A/B MAC (A) number, same date of service, and the same HCPCS code, the second claim submitted to CWF rejects when all four items match.

If CWF receives a claim with HCPCS administration codes G0008 or G0009 and it already has on record a claim with the same HIC number, same A/B MAC (A) number, same date of service, and same procedure code, CWF rejects the second claim submitted when all four items match.

CWF returns to the A/B MAC (A) a reject code "7262" for this edit. A/B MACs (A) must deny the second claim and use the same messages they currently use for the denial of duplicate claims.

100-04, 18, 10.4.2

CWF Edits on A/B MAC (B) Claims

(Rev. 4100, Issued: 08-03-18; Effective: 01-01-19; Implementation: 01-07-19)

In order to prevent duplicate payment by the same A/B MAC (B), CWF will edit by line item on the A/B MAC (B) number, the HIC number, the date of service, the influenza virus procedure codes 90630, 90653, 90654, 90655, 90656, 90657, 90658, 90660, 90661, 90662, 90672, 90673, 90674, 90682, 90685, 90686, 90687, 90688, 90689, or 90756; the pneumococcal procedure codes 90669, 90670, or 90732; and the administration code G0008 or G0009.

If CWF receives a claim with either HCPCS codes 90630, 90653, 90654, 90655, 90656, 90657, 90658, 90660, 90661, 90662, 90672, 90673, 90674, 90682, 90685, 90686, 90687, 90688, 90689, or 90756 and it already has on record a claim with the same HIC number, same A/B MAC (B) number, same date of service, and any one of those HCPCS codes, the second claim submitted to CWF will reject.

If CWF receives a claim with HCPCS codes 90669, 90670, or 90732 and it already has on record a claim with the same HIC number, same A/B MAC (B) number, same date of service, and the same HCPCS code, the second claim submitted to CWF will reject when all four items match.

If CWF receives a claim with HCPCS administration codes G0008 or G0009 and it already has on record a claim with the same HIC number, same A/B MAC (B) number, same date of service, and same procedure code, CWF will reject the second claim submitted.

CWF will return to the A/B MAC (B) a specific reject code for this edit. A/B MACs (B) must deny the second claim and use the same messages they currently use for the denial of duplicate claims.

In order to prevent duplicate payment by the centralized billing contractor and local A/B MAC (B), CWF will edit by line item for A/B MAC (B) number, same HIC number, same date of service, the influenza virus procedure codes 90630, 90653, 90654, 90655, 90656, 90657, 90658, 90660, 90661, 90662, 90672, 90673, 90674, 90682,

90685, 90686, 90687, 90688, 90689, or 90756; the pneumococcal procedure codes 90669, 90670, or 90732; and the administration code G0008 or G0009.

If CWF receives a claim with either HCPCS codes 90630, 90653, 90654, 90655, 90656, 90657, 90658, 90660, 90661, 90662, 90672, 90673, 90674, 90682, 90685, 90686, 90687, 90688, 90689, or 90756 and it already has on record a claim with a different A/B MAC (B) number, but same HIC number, same date of service, and any one of those same HCPCS codes, the second claim submitted to CWF will reject.

If CWF receives a claim with HCPCS codes 90669, 90670, or 90732 and it already has on record a claim with the same HIC number, different A/B MAC (B) number, same date of service, and the same HCPCS code, the second claim submitted to CWF will reject.

If CWF receives a claim with HCPCS administration codes G0008 or G0009 and it already has on record a claim with a different A/B MAC (B) number, but the same HIC number, same date of service, and same procedure code, CWF will reject the second claim submitted.

CWF will return a specific reject code for this edit. A/B MACs (B) must deny the second claim. For the second edit, the reject code should automatically trigger the following Medicare Summary Notice (MSN) and Remittance Advice (RA) messages.

MSN: 7.2 – "This is a duplicate of a claim processed by another contractor. You should receive a Medicare Summary Notice from them."

Claim Adjustment Reason Code 18 – Exact duplicate claim/service

100-04, 18, 10.4.3

CWF Crossover Edits A/B MAC (B) Claims
(Rev. 4100, Issued: 08-03-18; Effective: 01-01-19; Implementation: 01-07-19)

When CWF receives a claim from the A/B MAC (B), it will review Part B outpatient claims history to verify that a duplicate claim has not already been posted.

CWF will edit on the beneficiary HIC number; the date of service; the influenza virus procedure codes 90630, 90653, 90654, 90655, 90656, 90657, 90658, 90660, 90661, 90662, 90672, 90673, 90674, 90682, 90685, 90686, 90687, 90688, 90689, or 90756; the pneumococcal procedure codes 90669, 90670, or 90732; and the administration code G0008 or G0009.

CWF will return a specific reject code for this edit. A/B MACs (B) must deny the second claim and use the same messages they currently use for the denial of duplicate claims.

100-04, 18, 20.2

HCPCS and Diagnosis Codes for Mammography Services
(Rev. 3844, Issued: 08-18-17, Effective: 01-01-18, Implementation: 01-02-18)
The following HCPCS codes are used to bill for mammography services.

HCPCS Code	Definition
77065* (G0206*)	Diagnostic mammography, including computer-aided detection (CAD) when performed; unilateral
77066* (G0204*)	Diagnostic mammography, including computer-aided detection (CAD) when performed; bilateral
77067* (G0202*)	Screening mammography, bilateral (2-view study of each breast), including computer-aided detection (CAD) when performed
77063**	Screening Breast Tomosynthesis; bilateral (list separately in addition to code for primary procedure).
G0279**	Diagnostic digital breast tomosynthesis, unilateral or bilateral (List separately in addition to code for primary procedure)

*   NOTE: For claims with dates of service January 1, 2017 through December 31, 2017 providers report HCPCS codes G0202, G0204, and G0206. For claims with dates of service on or after January 1, 2018 providers report CPT codes 77067, 77066, and 77065 respectively.

**   NOTE: HCPCS codes 77063 and G0279 are effective for claims with dates of service on or after January 1, 2015.

New Modifier "-GG": Performance and payment of a screening mammography and diagnostic mammography on same patient same day - This is billed with the Diagnostic Mammography code to show the test changed from a screening test to a diagnostic test. A/B MACs (A) and (B) will pay both the screening and diagnostic mammography tests. This modifier is for tracking purposes only. This applies to claims with dates of service on or after January 1, 2002.

A. Diagnosis for Services On or After January 1, 1998
The BBA of 1997 eliminated payment based on high-risk indicators. However, to ensure proper coding, one of the following diagnosis codes should be reported on screening mammography claims as appropriate:

ICD-9-CM

V76.11 - "Special screening for malignant neoplasm, screening mammogram for high- risk patients" or;

V76.12 - "Special screening for malignant neoplasm, other screening mammography."

ICD-10-CM

Z12.31 - Encounter for screening mammogram for malignant neoplasm of breast.

Beginning October 1, 2003, A/B MACs (B) are not permitted to plug the code for a screening mammography when the screening mammography claim has no diagnosis code. Screening mammography claims with no diagnosis code must be returned as unprocessable for assigned claims. For unassigned claims, deny the claim.

In general, providers report diagnosis codes in accordance with the instructions in the appropriate ASC X12 837 claim technical report 3 (institutional or professional) and the paper claim form instructions found in chapters 25 (institutional) and 26 (professional).

In addition, for institutional claims, providers report diagnosis code V76.11 or V76.12 (ICD-9-CM) or Z12.31 (if ICD-10-CM is applicable) in "Principal Diagnosis Code" if the screening mammography is the only service reported on the claim. If the claim contains other services in addition to the screening mammography, these diagnostic codes V76.11 or V76.12 (ICD-9-CM) or Z12.31 (ICD-10-CM) are reported, as appropriate, in "Other Diagnostic Codes." NOTE: Information regarding the form locator number that corresponds to the principal and other diagnosis codes is found in chapter 25.

A/B MACs (B) receive this diagnosis in field 21 and field 24E with the appropriate pointer code of Form CMS-1500 or in Loop 2300 of ASC- X12 837 professional claim format.

Diagnosis codes for a diagnostic mammography will vary according to diagnosis.

100-04, 18, 20.2.2

Claim Adjustment Reason Codes (CARCs), Remittance Advice Remark Codes (RARCs), Group Codes, and Medicare Summary Notice (MSN) Messages
(Rev. 3844, Issued: 08-18-17, Effective: 01-01-18, Implementation: 01-02-18)

When denying claim lines for HCPCS code 77063 that are not submitted with the diagnosis code V76.11 or V76.12, the contractor shall use the following remittance advice messages and associated codes when rejecting/denying claims under this policy. This CARC/RARC combination is compliant with CAQH CORE Business Scenario Three.

CARC: 167 RARC: N386

MSN: 14.9

Group Code PR (Patient Responsibility) assigning financial responsibility to the beneficiary (if a claim is received with a GA modifier indicating a signed ABN is on file).

Group Code CO (Contractual Obligation) assigning financial liability to the provider (if a claim is received with a GZ modifier indicating no signed ABN is on file).

When denying claim lines for HCPCS code G0279 that are not submitted with HCPCS 77066 or 77065.

100-04, 18, 20.4.1

Rural Health Clinics and Federally Qualified Health Centers
(Rev. 4225, Issues: 02-01-19, Effective: 07-01-19, Implementation: 07-01-19)

A. Provider-Based RHC & FQHC - Technical Component
The technical component of a screening or diagnostic mammography is outside the scope of the RHC/FQHC benefit. In a provider-based RHC or FQHC, the technical component is billed by the base provider to the A/B MAC (A) under bill type 12X, 13X, 22X, 23X or 85X as appropriate using the base provider's outpatient provider number (not the RHC/FQHC provider number). The revenue code for a screening mammography is 0403, and the HCPCS code is 77067*, (G0202)*). The revenue code for a diagnostic mammography is 0401, and the HCPCS codes are 77065* (G0206*), 77066* (G0204*). Payment is based on the payment method for the base provider.

** G0236 is a deleted code after December 31, 2003. Use 76082* for claims with dates of service January 1, 2004 through December 31, 2006, and code 77051 for claims with dates of service January 1, 2007 and later.

*   For claims with dates of service January 1, 2017 through December 31, 2017, report CPT codes G0206, G0204, and G0202. For claims with dates of service January 1, 2018 and later, report CPT codes 77065, 77066, and 77067 respectively.

B. Independent RHCs and Freestanding FQHCs - Technical Component
The technical component of a screening or diagnostic mammography is outside the scope of the RHC/FQHC benefit. The practitioner that renders the technical service bills their A/B MACs (B) using Form CMS-1500. Payment is based on the MPFS national non- facility rate.

C. Provider-Based RHC & FQHC, Independent RHCs and Freestanding FQHCs - Professional Component
The professional component of a screening or diagnostic mammography is within the scope of the RHC/FQHC benefit and is billed under the RHC AIR or the FQHC PPS payment methodology with revenue code 052X. A/B MACs (A) should assure payment is not made for revenue code 0403 (screening mammography) or 0401 (diagnostic mammography). No payment is made on the line item reporting revenue code 0403.

For claims with dates of service on or after April 1, 2005, RHCs and FQHCs bill the A/B MAC (A) under bill type 71X or 77X for the professional component of a diagnostic mammography. No payment is made for the professional component of a diagnostic mammography unless there is a qualifying visit on the same day. The services should be billed with the appropriate revenue code. HCPCS coding is required for the diagnostic mammography.

100-04, 18, 20.6

Instructions When an Interpretation Results in Additional Films

(Rev. 3844, Issued: 08-18-17, Effective: 01-01-18, Implementation: 01-02-18)

A radiologist who interprets a screening mammography is allowed to order and interpret additional films based on the results of the screening mammogram while a beneficiary is still at the facility for the screening exam. When a radiologist's interpretation results in additional films, Medicare will pay for both the screening and diagnostic mammogram.

A/B MACs (B) Claims

For A/B MACs (B) claims, providers submitting a claim for a screening mammography and a diagnostic mammography for the same patient on the same day, attach modifier "- GG" to the diagnostic mammography. A modifier "-GG" is appended to the claim for the diagnostic mammogram for tracking and data collection purposes. Medicare will reimburse both the screening mammography and the diagnostic mammography.

A/B MAC (A) Claims

A/B MACs (A) require the diagnostic claim be prepared reflecting the diagnostic revenue code (0401) along with HCPCS code 77065*(G0206*), 77066*(G0204*), or G0279 and modifier "-GG" "Performance and payment of a screening mammogram and diagnostic mammogram on the same patient, same day." Reporting of this modifier is needed for data collection purposes. Regular billing instructions remain in place for a screening mammography that does not fit this situation.

Both A/B MACs (A) and (B) systems must accept the GH and GG modifiers where appropriate.

For claims with dates of service prior to January 1, 2017 thru December 31, 2017, providers report CPT codes G0206 and G0204. For claims with dates of service January 1, 2018 and later, providers report CPT codes 77065 and 77066 respectively.

100-04, 18, 60

Colorectal Cancer Screening

(Rev. 3436, Issued: 12-30-15, Effective: 10-09-14, Implementation: 09-08-15 for non-shared MAC edits; 01-04-16 - For all shared system changes.)

See the Medicare Benefit Policy Manual, Chapter 15, and the Medicare National Coverage Determinations (NCD) Manual, Chapter 1, Section 210.3 for Medicare Part B coverage requirements and effective dates of colorectal cancer screening services.

Effective for services furnished on or after January 1, 1998, payment may be made for colorectal cancer screening for the early detection of cancer. For screening colonoscopy services (one of the types of services included in this benefit) prior to July 2001, coverage was limited to high-risk individuals. For services July 1, 2001, and later screening colonoscopies are covered for individuals not at high risk.

The following services are considered colorectal cancer screening services:

- Fecal-occult blood test (FOBT),1-3 simultaneous determinations (guaiac-based);
- Flexible sigmoidoscopy;
- Colonoscopy; and,
- Barium enema

Effective for services on or after January 1, 2004, payment may be made for the following colorectal cancer screening service as an alternative for the guaiac-based FOBT, 1-3 simultaneous determinations:

- Fecal-occult blood test, immunoassay, 1-3 simultaneous determinations

Effective for claims with dates of service on or after October 9, 2014, payment may be made for colorectal cancer screening using the Cologuard™ multitarget stool DNA (sDNA) test:

G0464 (Colorectal cancer screening; stool-based DNA and fecal occult hemoglobin (e.g., KRAS, NDRG4 and BMP3).

Note: HCPCS code G0464 expired on December 31, 2015 and has been replaced in the 2016 Clinical Laboratory Fee Schedule with CPT code 81528, Oncology (colorectal) screening, quantitative real-time target and signal amplification of 10 DNA markers (KRAS mutations, promoter methylation of NDRG4 and BMP3) and fecal hemoglobin, utilizing stool, algorithm reported as a positive or negative result.

100-04, 18, 80.2

A/B Medicare Administrative Contractor (MAC) (B) Billing Requirements

(Rev. 3329, Issued: 08-14-15, Effective: 01-01-12, Implementation: 09-14-15)

Effective for dates of service on and after January 1, 2005, through December 31, 2008, contractors shall recognize the HCPCS codes G0344, G0366, G0367, and G0368

shown above in §80.1 for an IPPE. The type of service (TOS) for each of these codes is as follows:

G0344: TOS = 1

G0366: TOS = 5

G0367: TOS = 5

G0368: TOS = 5

Contractors shall pay physicians or qualified nonphysician practitioners for only one IPPE performed not later than 6 months after the date the individual's first coverage begins under Medicare Part B, but only if that coverage period begins on or after January 1, 2005.

Effective for dates of service on and after January 1, 2009, contractors shall recognize the HCPCS codes G0402, G0403, G0404, and G0405 shown above in §80.1 for an IPPE. The TOS for each of these codes is as follows:

G0402: TOS = 1

G0403: TOS = 5

G0404: TOS = 5

G0405: TOS = 5

Under the MIPPA of 2008, contractors shall pay physicians or qualified nonphysician practitioners for only one IPPE performed not later than 12 months after the date the individual's first coverage begins under Medicare Part B only if that coverage period begins on or after January 1, 2009.

Contractors shall allow payment for a medically necessary Evaluation and Management (E/M) service at the same visit as the IPPE when it is clinically appropriate. Physicians and qualified nonphysician practitioners shall use CPT codes 99201-99215 to report an E/M with CPT modifier 25 to indicate that the E/M is a significant, separately identifiable service from the IPPE code reported (G0344 or G0402, whichever applies based on the date the IPPE is performed). Refer to chapter 12, § 30.6.1.1, of this manual for the physician/practitioner billing correct coding and payment policy regarding E/M services.

If the EKG performed as a component of the IPPE is not performed by the primary physician or qualified NPP during the IPPE visit, another physician or entity may perform and/or interpret the EKG. The referring physician or qualified NPP needs to make sure that the performing physician or entity bills the appropriate G code for the screening EKG, and not a CPT code in the 93000 series. **Both the IPPE and the EKG should be billed in order for the beneficiary to receive the complete IPPE service.** Effective for dates of service on and after January 1, 2009, the screening EKG is optional and is no longer a mandated service of an IPPE if performed as a result of a referral from an IPPE.

Should the same physician or NPP need to perform an additional medically necessary EKG in the 93000 series on the same day as the IPPE, report the appropriate EKG CPT code(s) with modifier 59, indicating that the EKG is a distinct procedural service.

Physicians or qualified nonphysician practitioners shall bill the contractor the appropriate HCPCS codes for IPPE on the Form CMS-1500 claim or an approved electronic format. The HCPCS codes for an IPPE and screening EKG are paid under the Medicare Physician Fee Schedule (MPFS).

See §1.3 of this chapter for waiver of cost sharing requirements of coinsurance, copayment and deductible for furnished preventive services available in Medicare.

100-04, 18, 140.8

Advance Care Planning (ACP) as an Optional Element of an Annual Wellness Visit (AWV)

(Rev. 3428 Issued: 12-22-15, Effective: 01-01-16, Implementation: 01-04-16)

For services furnished on or after January 1, 2016, Advance Care Planning (ACP) is treated as a preventive service when furnished with an AWV. The Medicare coinsurance and Part B deductible are waived for ACP when furnished as an optional element of an AWV.

The codes for the optional ACP services furnished as part of an AWV are 99497 (Advance care planning including the explanation and discussion of advance directives such as standard forms (with completion of such forms, when performed), by the physician or other qualified health professional; first 30 minutes, face-to-face with the patient, family member(s) and/or surrogate;) and an add-on code 99498 (each additional 30 minutes (List separately in addition to code for primary procedure)). When ACP services are provided as a part of an AWV, practitioners would report CPT code 99497 (and add-on CPT code 99498 when applicable) for the ACP services in addition to either of the AWV codes (G0438 or G0439).

The deductible and coinsurance for ACP will only be waived when billed with modifier 33 on the same day and on the same claim as an AWV (code G0438 or G0439), and must also be furnished by the same provider. Waiver of the deductible and coinsurance for ACP is limited to once per year. Payment for an AWV is limited to once per year. If the AWV billed with ACP is denied for exceeding the once per year limit, the deductible and coinsurance will be applied to the ACP.

Also see Pub. 100-02, *Medicare Benefit Policy Manual*, chapter 15, section 280.5.1 for more information.

100-04, 23, 30.2

MPFSDB Record Layout

(Rev. 4298, Issued: 05-03-19, Effective: 01-01-19, Implementation 10-07-19)

The CMS MPFSDB includes the total fee schedule amount, related component parts, and payment policy indicators. The record layout is provided in the Addendum below.

Addendum - MPFSDB File Record Layout and Field Descriptions

(Rev. 4298, Issued: 05-03-19, Effective: 01-01-19, Implementation 10-07-19)

The CMS MPFSDB includes the total fee schedule amount, related component parts, and payment policy indicators. The record layout is provided below. Beginning with the 2019 MPFSDB, and thereafter, the MPFSDB File Record Layout will no longer be revised annually in this section for the sole purpose of changing the calendar year, but will only be revised when there is a change to a field. Previous MPFSDB file layouts (for 2018 and prior) can be found on the CMS web site on the Physician Fee Schedule web page at: https://www.cms.gov/Medicare/Medicare-Fee-for-Service-Payment/PhysicianFeeSched/index.html.

MPFSDB File Layout

HEADER RECORD

FIELD #	DATA ELEMENT NAME	LOCATION	PIC
1	Header ID	1-4	x(4) Value "Head"
2	Header Number	5	x(1)
3	Data Set Name	6-50	x(45)
4	Record Length	51-53	x(3)
5	Filler	54-54	x(1)
6	Block size	55-58	x(4)
7	Filler	59-59	x(1)
8	Number of Records Number does not include this header record.		
		60-69	9(10)
9	Date Created	70-77	x(8) YYYYMMDD
10	Blanks	78-345	x(268)

DATA RECORD

FIELD # & ITEM	LENGTH & PIC
1 File Year This field displays the effective year of the file.	4 Pic x(4)
2 A/B MAC (B) Number This field represents the 5-digit number assigned to the A/B MAC (B).	5 Pic x(5)
3 Locality This 2-digit code identifies the pricing locality used.	2 Pic x(2)
4 HCPCS Code This field represents the procedure code. Each A/B MAC (B) Current Procedural Terminology (CPT) code (other than codes for Multianalyte Assays with Algorithmic Analyses (MAAA) and Proprietary Laboratory Analyses (PLA)) and alpha-numeric HCPCS codes other than B, C, E, K and L codes will be included. The standard sort for this field is blanks, alpha, and numeric in ascending order. Note: MAAA and PLA are alpha-numeric CPT codes.	5 Pic x(5)

FIELD # & ITEM	LENGTH & PIC
5 Modifier For diagnostic tests, a blank in this field denotes the global service and the following modifiers identify the components: 26 = Professional component TC = Technical component For services other than those with a professional and/or technical component, a blank will appear in this field with one exception: the presence of CPT modifier -53 which indicates that separate Relative Value Units (RVUs) and a fee schedule amount have been established for procedures which the physician terminated before completion. This modifier is used only with colonoscopy through stoma code 44388, colonoscopy code 45378 and screening colonoscopy codes G0105 and G0121. Any other codes billed with modifier -53 are subject to medical review and priced by individual consideration. Modifier-53 = Discontinued Procedure - Under certain circumstances, the physician may elect to terminate a surgical or diagnostic procedure. Due to extenuating circumstances, or those that threaten the well being of the patient, it may be necessary to indicate that a surgical or diagnostic procedure was started but discontinued.	2 Pic x(2)
6 Descriptor This field will include a brief description of each procedure code.	50 Pic x(50)
7 Code Status This 1 position field provides the status of each code under the full fee schedule. Each status code is explained in §30.2.2.	1 Pic x(1)
8 Conversion Factor This field displays the multiplier which transforms relative values into payment amounts. The file will contain the conversion factor for the File Year which will reflect all adjustments.	8 Pic 9(4)v9999
9 Update Factor This update factor has been included in the conversion factor in Field 8.	6 Pic 9(2)v9999
10 Work Relative Value Unit This field displays the unit value for the physician work RVU.	9 Pic 9(7)v99
11 Filler	9 Pic 9(7)v99
12 Malpractice Relative Value Unit This field displays the unit value for the malpractice expense RVU.	9 Pic 9(7)v99
13 Work Geographic Practice Cost Indices (GPCIs) This field displays a work geographic adjustment factor used in computing the fee schedule amount.	5 Pic 99v999
14 Practice Expense GPCI This field displays a practice expense geographic adjustment factor used in computing the fee schedule amount.	5 Pic 99v999
15 Malpractice GPCI This field displays a malpractice expense geographic adjustment factor used in computing the fee schedule amount.	5 Pic 99v999

FIELD # & ITEM	LENGTH & PIC
16	3 Pic x(3)

Global Surgery

This field provides the postoperative time frames that apply to payment for each surgical procedure or another indicator that describes the applicability of the global concept to the service.

000 = Endoscopic or minor procedure with related preoperative and postoperative relative values on the day of the procedure only included in the fee schedule payment amount; evaluation and management services on the day of the procedure generally not payable.

010 = Minor procedure with preoperative relative values on the day of the procedure and postoperative relative values during a 10-day postoperative period included in the fee schedule amount; evaluation and management services on the day of the procedure and during this 10-day postoperative period generally not payable.

090 = Major surgery with a 1-day preoperative period and 90-day postoperative period included in the fee schedule payment amount.

MMM = Maternity codes; usual global period does not apply.

XXX = Global concept does not apply.

YYY = A/B MAC (B) determines whether global concept applies and establishes postoperative period, if appropriate, at time of pricing.

ZZZ = Code related to another service and is always included in the global period of the other service. (Note: Physician work is associated with intra-service time and in some instances the post service time.)

FIELD # & ITEM	LENGTH & PIC
17	6 Pic 9v9(5)

Preoperative Percentage (Modifier 56)

This field contains the percentage (shown in decimal format) for the preoperative portion of the global package. For example, 10 percent will be shown as 010000. The total of fields 17, 18, and 19 will usually equal one. Any variance is slight and results from rounding.

FIELD # & ITEM	LENGTH & PIC
18	6 Pic 9v9(5)

Intraoperative Percentage (Modifier 54)

This field contains the percentage (shown in decimal format) for the intraoperative portion of the global package including postoperative work in the hospital. For example, 63 percent will be shown as 063000. The total of fields 17, 18, and 19 will usually equal one. Any variance is slight and results from rounding.

FIELD # & ITEM	LENGTH & PIC
19	6 Pic 9v9(5)

Postoperative Percentage (Modifier 55)

This field contains the percentage (shown in decimal format) for the postoperative portion of the global package that is provided in the office after discharge from the hospital. For example, 17 percent will be shown as 017000. The total of fields 17, 18, and 19 will usually equal one. Any variance is slight and results from rounding.

FIELD # & ITEM	LENGTH & PIC
20	

Professional Component (PC)/Technical Component (TC) Indicator

0 = Physician service codes: This indicator identifies codes that describe physician services. Examples include visits, consultations, and surgical procedures. The concept of PC/TC does not apply since physician services cannot be split into professional and technical components. Modifiers 26 & TC cannot be used with these codes. The total Relative Value Units (RVUs) include values for physician work, practice expense and malpractice expense. There are some codes with no work RVUs.

1 = Diagnostic tests or radiology services: This indicator identifies codes that describe diagnostic tests, e.g., pulmonary function tests, or therapeutic radiology procedures, e.g., radiation therapy. These codes generally have both a professional and technical component. Modifiers 26 and TC can be used with these codes.

The total RVUs for codes reported with a 26 modifier include values for physician work, practice expense, and malpractice expense.

The total RVUs for codes reported with a TC modifier include values for practice expense and malpractice expense only. The total RVUs for codes reported without a modifier equals the sum of RVUs for both the professional and technical component.

2 = Professional component only codes: This indicator identifies stand alone codes that describe the physician work portion of selected diagnostic tests for which there is an associated code that

describes the technical component of the diagnostic test only and another associated code that describes the global test.

An example of a professional component only code is 93010, Electrocardiogram; interpretation and report. Modifiers 26 and TC cannot be used with these codes. The total RVUs for professional component only codes include values for physician work, practice expense, and malpractice expense.

3 = Technical component only codes: This indicator identifies stand alone codes that describe the technical component (i.e., staff and equipment costs) of selected diagnostic tests for which there is an associated code that describes the professional component of the diagnostic tests only.

An example of a technical component code is 93005, Electrocardiogram, tracing only, without interpretation and report. It also identifies codes that are covered only as diagnostic tests and therefore do not have a related professional code. Modifiers 26 and TC cannot be used with these codes.

The total RVUs for technical component only codes include values for practice expense and malpractice expense only.

4 = Global test only codes: This indicator identifies stand alone codes for which there are associated codes that describe: a) the professional component of the test only and b) the technical component of the test only. Modifiers 26 and TC cannot be used with these codes. The total RVUs for global procedure only codes include values for physician work, practice expense, and malpractice expense. The total RVUs for global procedure only codes equals the sum of the total RVUs for the professional and technical components only codes combined.

5 = Incident to codes: This indicator identifies codes that describe services covered incident to a physicians service when they are provided by auxiliary personnel employed by the physician and working under his or her direct supervision.

Payment may not be made by A/B MACs (B) for these services when they are provided to hospital inpatients or patients in a hospital outpatient department. Modifiers 26 and TC cannot be used with these codes.

6 = Laboratory physician interpretation codes: This indicator identifies clinical laboratory codes for which separate payment for interpretations by laboratory physicians may be made. Actual performance of the tests is paid for under the lab fee schedule. Modifier TC cannot be used with these codes. The total RVUs for laboratory physician interpretation codes include values for physician work, practice expense and malpractice expense.

7 = Private practice therapist's service: Payment may not be made if the service is provided to either a hospital outpatient or a hospital inpatient by a physical therapist, occupational therapist, or speech-language pathologist in private practice.

8 = Physician interpretation codes: This indicator identifies the professional component of clinical laboratory codes for which separate payment may be made only if the physician interprets an abnormal smear for hospital inpatient. This applies only to code

85060. No TC billing is recognized because payment for the underlying clinical laboratory test is made to the hospital, generally through the PPS rate.

No payment is recognized for code 85060 furnished to hospital outpatients or non-hospital patients. The physician interpretation is paid through the clinical laboratory fee schedule payment for the clinical laboratory test.

9 = Concept of a professional/technical component does not apply.

FIELD # & ITEM	LENGTH & PIC
21	

Multiple Procedure (Modifier 51)

Indicator indicates which payment adjustment rule for multiple procedures applies to the service.

0 = No payment adjustment rules for multiple procedures apply. If procedure is reported on the same day as another procedure, base payment on the lower of: (a) the actual charge or (b) the fee schedule amount for the procedure.

1 = Standard payment adjustment rules in effect before January 1, 1996, for multiple procedures apply. In the 1996 MPFSDB, this indicator only applies to codes with procedure status of "D." If a procedure is reported on the same day as another procedure with an indicator of 1,2, or 3, rank the procedures by fee schedule amount and apply the appropriate reduction to this code (100 percent, 50 percent, 25 percent, 25 percent, 25 percent, and by report). Base payment on the lower of: (a) the actual charge or (b) the fee schedule amount reduced by the appropriate percentage.

2 = Standard payment adjustment rules for multiple procedures apply. If procedure is reported on the same day as another procedure with an indicator of 1, 2, or 3, rank the procedures by fee schedule amount and apply the appropriate reduction to this code (100 percent, 50 percent, 50 percent, 50 percent, 50 percent, and by report). Base payment on the lower of: (a) the actual charge or (b) the fee schedule amount reduced by the appropriate percentage.

3 = Special rules for multiple endoscopic procedures apply if procedure is billed with another endoscopy in the same family (i.e., another endoscopy that has the same base procedure). The base procedure for each code with this indicator is identified in field 31G.

Apply the multiple endoscopy rules to a family before ranking the family with other procedures performed on the same day (for example, if multiple endoscopies in the same family are reported on the same day as endoscopies in another family or on the same day as a non-endoscopic procedure).

If an endoscopic procedure is reported with only its base procedure, do not pay separately for the base procedure. Payment for the base procedure is included in the payment for the other endoscopy.

4 = Subject to 25% reduction of the TC diagnostic imaging (effective for services January 1, 2006 through June 30, 2010). Subject to 50% reduction of the TC diagnostic imaging (effective for services July 1, 2010 and after). Subject to 25% reduction of the PC of diagnostic imaging (effective for services January 1, 2012 through December 31, 2016). Subject to 5% reduction of the PC of diagnostic imaging (effective for services January 1, 2017 and after).

5 = Subject to 20% reduction of the practice expense component for certain therapy services furnished in office and other non-institutional settings, and 25% reduction of the practice expense component for certain therapy services furnished in institutional settings (effective for services January 1, 2011 and after). Subject to 50% reduction of the practice expense component for certain therapy services furnished in both institutional and non-institutional settings (effective for services April 1, 2013 and after).

6 = Subject to 25% reduction of the TC diagnostic cardiovascular services (effective for services January 1, 2013 and after).

7 = Subject to 20% reduction of the TC diagnostic ophthalmology services (effective for services January 1, 2013 and after).

9 = Concept does not apply.

FIELD # & ITEM	LENGTH & PIC
22	1 Pic (x)1

Bilateral Surgery Indicator (Modifier 50)

This field provides an indicator for services subject to a payment adjustment.

0 = 150 percent payment adjustment for bilateral procedures does not apply. If procedure is reported with modifier -50 or with modifiers RT and LT, base payment for the two sides on the lower of: (a) the total actual charge for both sides or (b) 100 percent of the fee schedule amount for a single code. Example: The fee schedule amount for code XXXXX is $125. The physician reports code XXXXX-LT with an actual charge of $100 and XXXXX-RT with an actual charge of $100.

Payment would be based on the fee schedule amount ($125) since it is lower than the total actual charges for the left and right sides ($200).

The bilateral adjustment is inappropriate for codes in this category because of (a) physiology or anatomy or (b) because the code descriptor specifically states that it is a unilateral procedure and there is an existing code for the bilateral procedure.

1 = 150 percent payment adjustment for bilateral procedures applies. If code is billed with the bilateral modifier or is reported twice on the same day by any other means (e.g., with RT and LT modifiers or with a 2 in the units field), base payment for these codes when reported as bilateral procedures on the lower of: (a) the total actual charge for both sides or (b) 150 percent of the fee schedule amount for a single code.

If code is reported as a bilateral procedure and is reported with other procedure codes on the same day, apply the bilateral adjustment before applying any applicable multiple procedure rules.

2 = 150 percent payment adjustment for bilateral procedure does not apply. RVUs are already based on the procedure being performed as a bilateral procedure. If procedure is reported with modifier -50 or is reported twice on the same day by any other means (e.g., with RT and LT modifiers with a 2 in the units field), base payment for both sides on the lower of (a) the total actual charges by the physician for both sides or (b) 100 percent of the fee schedule amount for a single

1 Pic (x)1 code.

Example: The fee schedule amount for code YYYYY is $125. The physician reports code YYYYY-LT with an actual charge of $100 and YYYYY-RT with an actual charge of $100. Payment would be based on the fee schedule amount ($125) since it is lower than the total actual charges for the left and right sides ($200).

The RVUs are based on a bilateral procedure because: (a) the code descriptor specifically states that the procedure is bilateral; (b) the code descriptor states that the procedure may be performed either unilaterally or bilaterally; or (c) the procedure is usually performed as a bilateral procedure.

3 = The usual payment adjustment for bilateral procedures does not apply. If procedure is reported with modifier -50 or is reported for both sides on the same day by any other means (e.g., with RT and LT modifiers or with a 2 in the units field), base payment for each side or organ or site of a paired organ on the lower of: (a) the actual charge for each side or (b) 100% of the fee schedule amount for each side. If procedure is reported as a bilateral procedure and with other procedure codes on the same day, determine the fee schedule amount for a bilateral procedure before applying any applicable multiple procedure rules.

Services in this category are generally radiology procedures or other diagnostic tests which are not subject to the special payment rules for other bilateral procedures.

9 = Concept does not apply.

FIELD # & ITEM	LENGTH & PIC
23	1 Pic (x)1
Assistant at Surgery	

This field provides an indicator for services where an assistant at surgery is never paid for per IOM.

0 = Payment restriction for assistants at surgery applies to this procedure unless supporting documentation is submitted to establish medical necessity.

1 = Statutory payment restriction for assistants at surgery applies to this procedure. Assistant at surgery may not be paid.

2 = Payment restriction for assistants at surgery does not apply to this procedure. Assistant at surgery may be paid.

9 = Concept does not apply. 24

Co-Surgeons (Modifier 62)

This field provides an indicator for services for which two surgeons, each in a different specialty, may be paid.

0 = Co-surgeons not permitted for this procedure.

1 = Co-surgeons could be paid; supporting documentation required to establish medical necessity of two surgeons for the procedure.

2 = Co-surgeons permitted; no documentation required if two specialty requirements are met.

9 = Concept does not apply.

FIELD # & ITEM	LENGTH & PIC
25	1 Pic (x)1

9 Pic 9(7)v99

Team Surgeons (Modifier 66)

This field provides an indicator for services for which team surgeons may be paid.

0 = Team surgeons not permitted for this procedure.

1 = Team surgeons could be paid; supporting documentation required to establish medical necessity of a team; pay by report.

2 = Team surgeons permitted; pay by report.

9 = Concept does not apply.

FIELD # & ITEM	LENGTH & PIC
26	1 Pic (x)1
Filler	
27	1 Pic (x)1
Site of Service Differential	

For 1999 and beyond, the site of service differential no longer applies. The following definitions will apply for all years after 1998:

0 = Facility pricing does not apply.

1 = Facility pricing applies.

9 = Concept does not apply. 28

Non-Facility Fee Schedule Amount

This field shows the fee schedule amount for the non-facility setting. This amount equals Field 34.

Note: Field 33 D indicates if an additional adjustment should be applied to this formula.

Non-Facility Pricing Amount for the File Year

[(Work RVU * Work GPCI) +

(Non-Facility PE RVU * PE GPCI) +

(MP RVU * MP GPCI)] * Conversion Factor

FIELD # & ITEM	LENGTH & PIC
29	9 Pic 9(7)v99
Facility Fee Schedule Amount	

This field shows the fee schedule amount for the facility setting. This amount equals Field 35.

Note: Field 33D indicates if an additional adjustment should be applied to this formula.

Facility Pricing Amount for the File Year

[(Work RVU * Work GPCI) +

(Facility PE RVU * PE GPCI) +

(MP RVU * MP GPCI)] * Conversion Factor

Place of service codes to be used to identify facilities.

02 – Telehealth-Medicare pays telehealth services at the facility rate.

19 – Off Campus-Outpatient Hospital

21 - Inpatient Hospital

22 – On Campus-Outpatient Hospital

23 - Emergency Room - Hospital

FIELD # & ITEM	LENGTH & PIC
24 - Ambulatory Surgical Center – In a Medicare approved ASC, for an approved procedure on the ASC list, Medicare pays the lower facility fee to physicians. Beginning with dates of service January 1, 2008, in a Medicare approved ASC, for procedures NOT on the ASC list of approved procedures, contractors will also pay the lower facility fee to physicians.	

26 - Military Treatment Facility

31 - Skilled Nursing Facility

34 - Hospice

41 - Ambulance - Land

42 - Ambulance Air or Water

51 - Inpatient Psychiatric Facility

52 - Psychiatric Facility Partial Hospitalization

53 - Community Mental Health Center

56 - Psychiatric Residential Treatment Facility

61 - Comprehensive Inpatient Rehabilitation Facility

FIELD # & ITEM	LENGTH & PIC
29A	1 Pic x
Anti-markup Test Indicator	

This field providers an indicator for Anti-markup Test HCPCS codes:

'1' = Anti-markup Test HCPCS.

'9' = Concept does not apply.

FIELD # & ITEM	LENGTH & PIC
30	8 Pic x(8)
Record Effective Date	

This field identifies the effective date for the MPFSDB record for each HCPCS. The field is in YYYYMMDD format.

NOTE: This is not the date the HCPCS code was created. It is the date the code was updated or added to the MPFSDB file for the current file year. This field is set to January 1 for all codes during the annual update process.

FIELD # & ITEM	LENGTH & PIC
31	28 Pic x(28)
Filler	
31EE	9Pic(7)v99
Reduced therapy fee schedule amount	
31DD	1Pic x(2)
Filler	
31CC	1Pic x(1)
Imaging Cap Indicator	

A value of "1" means subject to OPPS payment cap determination.

A value of "9" means not subject to OPPS payment cap determination.

FIELD # & ITEM	LENGTH & PIC
31BB	9Pic(7)v99
Non-Facility Imaging Payment Amount	
31AA	9Pic(7)v99
Facility Imaging Payment Amount	

FIELD # & ITEM	LENGTH & PIC
31A	2 Pic x(2)
Physician Supervision of Diagnostic Procedures	
This field is for use in post payment review.	
01 = Procedure must be performed under the general supervision of a physician.	
02 = Procedure must be performed under the direct supervision of a physician.	
03 = Procedure must be performed under the personal supervision of a physician.	
(Diagnostic imaging procedures performed by a Registered Radiologist Assistant (RRA) who is certified and registered by The American Registry of Radiologic Technologists (ARRT) or a Radiology Practitioner Assistant (RPA) who is certified by the Certification Board for Radiology Practitioner Assistants (CBRPA), and is authorized to furnish the procedure under state law, may be performed under direct supervision.)	
04 = Physician supervision policy does not apply when procedure is furnished by a qualified, independent psychologist or a clinical psychologist; otherwise must be performed under the general supervision of a physician.	
05 = Not subject to supervision when furnished personally by a qualified audiologist, physician or non physician practitioner. Direct supervision by a physician is required for those parts of the test that may be furnished by a qualified technician when appropriate to the circumstances of the test.	
06 = Procedure must be personally performed by a physician or a physical therapist (PT) who is certified by the American Board of Physical Therapy Specialties (ABPTS) as a qualified electrophysiological clinical specialist and is permitted to provide the procedure under State law. Procedure may also be performed by a PT with ABPTS certification without physician supervision.	
21 = Procedure may be performed by a technician with certification under general supervision of a physician; otherwise must be performed under direct supervision of a physician. Procedure may also be performed by a PT with ABPTS certification without physician supervision.	
22 = May be performed by a technician with on-line real-time contact with physician.	
66 = May be personally performed by a physician or by a physical therapist with ABPTS certification and certification in this specific procedure.	
6A = Supervision standards for level 66 apply; in addition, the PT with ABPTS certification may personally supervise another PT, but only the PT with ABPTS certification may bill.	
77 = Procedure must be performed by a PT with ABPTS certification (TC & PC) or by a PT without certification under direct supervision of a physician (TC & PC), or by a technician with certification under general supervision of a physician (TC only; PC always physician).	1 Pic x(1)
7A = Supervision standards for level 77 apply; in addition, the PT with ABPTS certification may personally supervise another PT, but only the PT with ABPTS certification may bill.	
09 = Concept does not apply.	
31B	
This field has been deleted to allow for the expansion of field 31A.	
31C	9 Pic(7)v99
Facility Setting Practice Expense Relative Value Units	
31D	9 Pic(7)v99
Non-Facility Setting Practice Expense Relative Value Units	
31E	9 Pic(7)v99
Filler	
31F	
Filler	
Reserved for future use.	1 Pic x(1)
31G	5 Pic x(5)
Endoscopic Base Codes	
This field identifies an endoscopic base code for each code with a multiple surgery indicator of 3.	
32A	9 Pic 9(7)v99
1996 Transition/Fee Schedule Amount	
This field is no longer applicable since transitioning ended in 1996. This field will contain a zero.	

FIELD # & ITEM	LENGTH & PIC
32B	1 Pic x(1)
1996 Transition/Fee Schedule	
This field is no longer applicable since transitioning ended in 1996. This field will contain spaces.	
32C	9 Pic 9(7)v99
1996 Transition/Fee Schedule Amount When Site or Service Differential Applies	
This field is no longer applicable since transitioning ended in 1996. This field will contain a zero. 33A	
Units Payment Rule Indicator	
Reserved for future use.	
9 = Concept does not apply.	
33B	1 Pic x(1)
Mapping Indicator	
This field is no longer applicable since transitioning ended in 1996.	
	3 Pic x (3)
This field will contain spaces.	
33C	2 Pic x(2)
Anti-markup Locality—Informational Use—Locality used for reporting utilization of anti-markup services.	
NOT FOR A/B MAC (B) USE: These Medicare Advantage encounter pricing localities are for Shared System Maintainer purposes only. The locality values were developed to facilitate centralized processing of encounter data by the Medicare Advantage organizations.	
33D	1 Pic x(1)
Calculation Flag	
This field is informational only; the SSMs do not need to add this field. The intent is to assist A/B MACs (B) to understand how the fee schedule amount in fields 28 and 29 are calculated. The MMA mandates an additional adjustment to selected HCPCS codes. A value of "1" indicates an additional fee schedule adjustment of 1.32 in 2004 and 1.03 in 2005. A value of "0" indicates no additional adjustment needed. A value of "2" indicates an additional fee schedule adjustment of 1.05 effective 7/1/2008.	
33 E	2 Pic x(2)
Diagnostic Imaging Family Indicator	
For services effective January 1, 2011, and after, family indicators 01 - 11 will not be populated.	
01 = Family 1 Ultrasound (Chest/Abdomen/Pelvis – Non Obstetrical	
02 = Family 2 CT and CTA (Chest/Thorax/Abd/Pelvis)	
03 = Family 3 CT and CTA (Head/Brain/Orbit/Maxillofacial/Neck)	
04 = Family 4 MRI and MRA (Chest/Abd/Pelvis)	
05 = Family 5 MRI and MRA (Head/Brain/Neck)	
06 = Family 6 MRI and MRA (spine)	
07 = Family 7 CT (spine)	
08 = Family 8 MRI and MRA (lower extremities)	
09 = Family 9 CT and CTA (lower extremities)	
10 = Family 10 Mr and MRI (upper extremities and joints)	
11 = Family 11 CT and CTA (upper extremities)	
88 = Subject to the reduction of the TC diagnostic imaging (effective for services January 1, 2011, and after). Subject to the reduction of the PC diagnostic imaging (effective for services January 1, 2012 and after).	
99 = Concept Does Not Apply	
33F	1 Pic x (1)
Performance Payment Indicator	
(For future use) 33G	
National Level Future Expansion	
34	9 Pic 9(7)v99
Non-Facility Fee Schedule Amount	
This field replicates field 28.	
35	9 Pic 9(7)v99
Facility Fee Schedule Amount	
This field replicates field 29.	
36	1 Pic x(1)
Filler	

FIELD # & ITEM	LENGTH & PIC
37	7 Pic x(7)
Future Local Level Expansion**	
The Updated 1992 Transition Amount was previously stored in this field. A/B MACs (B) can continue to maintain the updated transition amount in this field.	
38A	7 Pic x(7)
Future Local Level Expansion**	
The adjusted historical payment basis (AHPB) was previously stored in this field. A/B MACs (B) can continue to maintain the AHPB in this field.	
38 B	8 Pix x(8)
Filler	
This field was originally established for 15 spaces. Since AHPB data will only use 7 of the 15 spaces, A/B MACs (B) have 8 remaining spaces for their purposes.	
** These fields will be appended by each A/B MAC (B) at the local level.	

100-04, 32, 10.1

Ambulatory Blood Pressure Monitoring (ABPM) Billing Requirements

(Rev. 2998, Issued: 07-25-14, Effective: Upon implementation of ICD-10; 01-01-12 - ASC X12, Implementation: 08-25-2014 - ASC X12; Upon Implementation of ICD-10)

A. Coding Applicable to A/B MACs (A and B)

Effective April 1, 2002, a National Coverage Decision was made to allow for Medicare coverage of ABPM for those beneficiaries with suspected "white coat hypertension" (WCH). ABPM involves the use of a non-invasive device, which is used to measure blood pressure in 24-hour cycles. These 24-hour measurements are stored in the device and are later interpreted by a physician. Suspected "WCH" is defined as: (1) Clinic/office blood pressure >140/90 mm Hg on at least three separate clinic/office visits with two separate measurements made at each visit; (2) At least two documented separate blood pressure measurements taken outside the clinic/office which are < 140/90 mm Hg; and (3) No evidence of end-organ damage. ABPM is not covered for any other uses. Coverage policy can be found in Medicare National Coverage Determinations Manual, Chapter 1, Part 1, §20.19. (http://www.cms.hhs.gov/manuals/103_cov_determ/ncd103index.asp).

The ABPM must be performed for at least 24 hours to meet coverage criteria. Payment is not allowed for institutionalized beneficiaries, such as those receiving Medicare covered skilled nursing in a facility. In the rare circumstance that ABPM needs to be performed more than once for a beneficiary, the qualifying criteria described above must be met for each subsequent ABPM test.

Effective dates for applicable Common Procedure Coding System (HCPCS) codes for ABPM for suspected WCH and their covered effective dates are as follows:

HCPCS	Definition	Effective Date
93784	ABPM, utilizing a system such as magnetic tape and/or computer disk, for 24 hours or longer; including recording, scanning analysis, interpretation and report.	04/01/2002
93786	ABPM, utilizing a system such as magnetic tape and/or computer disk, for 24 hours or longer; recording only.	04/01/2002
93788	ABPM, utilizing a system such as magnetic tape and/or computer disk, for 24 hours or longer; scanning analysis with report.	01/01/2004
93790	ABPM, utilizing a system such as magnetic tape and/or computer disk, for 24 hours or longer; physician review with interpretation and report.	04/01/2002

In addition, one of the following diagnosis codes must be present:

	Diagnosis Code	Description
If ICD-9-CM is applicable	796.2	Elevated blood pressure reading without diagnosis of hypertension.
If ICD-10-CM is applicable	R03.0	Elevated blood pressure reading without diagnosis of hypertension

B. A/B MAC (A) Billing Instructions

The applicable types of bills acceptable when billing for ABPM services are 13X, 23X, 71X, 73X, 75X, and 85X. Chapter 25 of this manual provides general billing instructions that must be followed for bills submitted to A/B MACs (A). The A/B MACs (A) pay for hospital outpatient ABPM services billed on a 13X type of bill with HCPCS 93786 and/or 93788 as follows: (1) Outpatient Prospective Payment System (OPPS) hospitals pay based on the Ambulatory Payment Classification (APC); (2) non-OPPS hospitals (Indian Health Services Hospitals, Hospitals that provide Part B services only, and hospitals located in American Samoa, Guam, Saipan and the Virgin Islands) pay based on reasonable cost, except for Maryland Hospitals which are paid based on

a percentage of cost. Effective 4/1/06, type of bill 14X is for non-patient laboratory specimens and is no longer applicable for ABPM.

The A/B MACs (A) pay for comprehensive outpatient rehabilitation facility (CORF) ABPM services billed on a 75x type of bill with HCPCS code 93786 and/or 93788 based on the Medicare Physician Fee Schedule (MPFS) amount for that HCPCS code.

The A/B MACs (A) pay for ABPM services for critical access hospitals (CAHs) billed on a 85x type of bill as follows: (1) for CAHs that elected the Standard Method and billed HCPCS code 93786 and/or 93788, pay based on reasonable cost for that HCPCS code; and (2) for CAHs that elected the Optional Method and billed any combination of HCPCS codes 93786, 93788 and 93790 pay based on reasonable cost for HCPCS 93786 and 93788 and pay 115% of the MPFS amount for HCPCS 93790.

The A/B MACs (A) pay for ABPM services for skilled nursing facility (SNF) outpatients billed on a 23x type of bill with HCPCS code 93786 and/or 93788, based on the MPFS.

The A/B MACs (A) accept independent and provider-based rural health clinic (RHC) bills for visits under the all-inclusive rate when the RHC bills on a 71x type of bill with revenue code 052x for providing the professional component of ABPM services. The A/B MACs (A) should not make a separate payment to a RHC for the professional component of ABPM services in addition to the all-inclusive rate. RHCs are not required to use ABPM HCPCS codes for professional services covered under the all-inclusive rate.

The A/B MACs (A) accept free-standing and provider-based federally qualified health center (FQHC) bills for visits under the all-inclusive rate when the FQHC bills on a 73x type of bill with revenue code 052x for providing the professional component of ABPM services.

The A/B MACs (A) should not make a separate payment to a FQHC for the professional component of ABPM services in addition to the all-inclusive rate. FQHCs are not required to use ABPM HCPCS codes for professional services covered under the all-inclusive rate.

The A/B MACs (A) pay provider-based RHCs/FQHCs for the technical component of ABPM services when billed under the base provider's number using the above requirements for that particular base provider type, i.e., a OPPS hospital based RHC would be paid for the ABPM technical component services under the OPPS using the APC for code 93786 and/or 93788 when billed on a 13x type of bill.

Independent and free-standing RHC/FQHC practitioners are only paid for providing the technical component of ABPM services when billed to the A/B MAC (B) following the MAC's instructions.

C. A/B MAC (B) Claims

A/B MACs (B) pay for ABPM billed with ICD-9-CM diagnosis code 796.2 (if ICD-9 is applicable) or, if ICD-10 is applicable, ICD-10-CM diagnosis code R03.0 and HCPCS codes 93784 or for any combination of 93786, 93788 and 93790, based on the MPFS for the specific HCPCS code billed.

D. Coinsurance and Deductible

The A/B MACs (A and B) shall apply coinsurance and deductible to payments for ABPM services except for services billed to the A/B MAC (A) by FQHCs. For FQHCs only co-insurance applies.

100-04, 32, 12

Counseling to Prevent Tobacco Use

(Rev.3848, Issued: 08-25-17, Effective: 09-26-17, Implementation: 09-26-17)

Background: Effective for services furnished on or after March 22, 2005, a National Coverage Determination (NCD) provided for coverage of smoking and tobacco-use cessation counseling services located at Medicare National Coverage Determinations Manual, Publication 100-03 section 210.4. CMS established a related policy entitled Counseling to Prevent Tobaccos Use at NCD Manual 210.4.1 effective August 25, 2010. However, effective September 30, 2016, the conditions of Medicare Part A and Medicare Part B coverage for smoking and tobacco-use cessation counseling services (210.4) were deleted. The remaining NCD entitled Counseling to Prevent Tobacco Use (210.4.1), remains in effect, along with HCPCS codes 99406 and 99407, specifically payable for counseling to prevent tobacco use effective October 1, 2016.

100-04, 32, 12.1

Counseling to Prevent Tobacco Use HCPCS and Diagnosis Coding

(Rev. 4237, Issued: 02-08-19, Effective: 03-12-19, Implementation: 03-12-19)

The following HCPCS codes should be reported when billing for counseling to prevent tobacco use services:

99406 Smoking and tobacco-use cessation counseling visit; intermediate, greater than 3 minutes up to 10 minutes

99407 Smoking and tobacco-use cessation counseling visit; intensive, greater than 10 minutes

Note the above codes were effective for dates of service on or after January 1, 2008, and specifically effective for counseling to prevent tobacco use claims on or after October 1, 2016.

Contractors shall allow payment for a medically necessary E/M service on the same day as the counseling to prevent tobacco use service when it is clinically appropriate. Physicians and qualified non-physician practitioners shall use an appropriate HCPCS code, such as HCPCS 99201– 99215, to report an E/M service with modifier 25 to indicate that the E/M service is a separately identifiable service from 99406 or 99407.

Contractors shall only pay for 8 counseling to prevent tobacco use sessions in a 12-month period. The beneficiary may receive another 8 sessions during a second or subsequent year after 11 full months have passed since the first Medicare covered counseling session was performed. To start the count for the second or subsequent 12-month period, begin with the month after the month in which the first Medicare covered counseling session was performed and count until 11 full months have elapsed.

Claims for counseling to prevent tobacco use services shall be submitted with an appropriate diagnosis code.

NOTE: This decision does not modify existing coverage for minimal cessation counseling (defined as 3 minutes or less in duration) which is already considered to be covered as part of each Evaluation and Management (E/M) visit and is not separately billable.

Claims for counseling to prevent tobacco use services shall be submitted with an applicable diagnosis code:

ICD-9-CM (prior to October 1, 2015)

V15.82, personal history of tobacco use, or

305.1, non-dependent tobacco use disorder

989.84, toxic effect of tobacco

ICD-10-CM (effective October 1, 2015)

F17.210, nicotine dependence, cigarettes, uncomplicated,

F17.211, nicotine dependence, cigarettes, in remission,

F17.213 Nicotine dependence, cigarettes, with withdrawal

F17.218 Nicotine dependence, cigarettes, with other nicotine-induced disorders

F17.219 Nicotine dependence, cigarettes, with unspecified nicotine-induced disorders

F17.220, nicotine dependence, chewing tobacco, uncomplicated,

F17.221, nicotine dependence, chewing tobacco, in remission,

F17.223 Nicotine dependence, chewing tobacco, with withdrawal

F17.228 Nicotine dependence, chewing tobacco, with other nicotine-induced disorders

F17.229 Nicotine dependence, chewing tobacco, with unspecified nicotine-induced disorders

F17.290, nicotine dependence, other tobacco product, uncomplicated,

F17.291, nicotine dependence, other tobacco product, in remission, or

F17.293 Nicotine dependence, other tobacco product, with withdrawal

F17.298 Nicotine dependence, other tobacco product, with other nicotine-induced disorders

F17.299 Nicotine dependence, other tobacco product, with unspecified nicotine-induced disorders

Z87.891, personal history of nicotine dependence, unspecified, uncomplicated.

T65.211A, Toxic effect of chewing tobacco, accidental (unintentional), initial encounter

T65.212A, Toxic effect of chewing tobacco, intentional self-harm, initial encounter

T65.213A, Toxic effect of chewing tobacco, assault, initial encounter

T65.214A, Toxic effect of chewing tobacco, undetermined, initial encounter

T65.221A, Toxic effect of tobacco cigarettes, accidental (unintentional), initial encounter

T65.222A, Toxic effect of tobacco cigarettes, intentional self-harm, initial encounter

T65.223A, Toxic effect of tobacco cigarettes, assault, initial encounter

T65.224A, Toxic effect of tobacco cigarettes, undetermined, initial encounter

T65.291A, Toxic effect of other tobacco and nicotine, accidental (unintentional), initial encounter

T65.292A, Toxic effect of other tobacco and nicotine, intentional self-harm, initial encounter

T65.293A, Toxic effect of other tobacco and nicotine, assault, initial encounter

T65.294A, Toxic effect of other tobacco and nicotine, undetermined, initial encounter

100-04, 32, 30.1

Billing Requirements for HBO Therapy for the Treatment of Diabetic Wounds of the Lower Extremities

(Rev. 2998, Issued: 07-25-14, Effective: Upon implementation of ICD-10; 01-01-12 - ASC X12, Implementation: 08-25-2014 - ASC X12; Upon Implementation of ICD-10)

Hyperbaric Oxygen Therapy is a modality in which the entire body is exposed to oxygen under increased atmospheric pressure. Effective April 1, 2003, a National Coverage Decision expanded the use of HBO therapy to include coverage for the treatment of diabetic wounds of the lower extremities. For specific coverage criteria

for HBO Therapy, refer to the National Coverage Determinations Manual, Chapter 1, section 20.29.

NOTE: Topical application of oxygen does not meet the definition of HBO therapy as stated above. Also, its clinical efficacy has not been established. Therefore, no Medicare reimbursement may be made for the topical application of oxygen.

I. Billing Requirements for A/B MACs (A)

Claims for HBO therapy should be submitted using the ASC X12 837 institutional claim format or, in rare cases, on Form CMS-1450.

a. Applicable Bill Types

The applicable hospital bill types are 11X, 13X and 85X.

b. Procedural Coding

99183– Physician attendance and supervision of hyperbaric oxygen therapy, per session.

C1300 – Hyperbaric oxygen under pressure, full body chamber, per 30-minute interval.

NOTE: Code C1300 is not available for use other than in a hospital outpatient department. In skilled nursing facilities (SNFs), HBO therapy is part of the SNF PPS payment for beneficiaries in covered Part A stays.

For hospital inpatients and critical access hospitals (CAHs) not electing Method I, HBO therapy is reported under revenue code 940 without any HCPCS code. For inpatient services, if ICD-9-is applicable, show ICD-9-CM procedure code 93.59. If ICD-10 is applicable, show ICD-10-PCS code 5A05121.

For CAHs electing Method I, HBO therapy is reported under revenue code 940 along with HCPCS code 99183.

c. Payment Requirements for A/B MACs (A)

Payment is as follows:

A/B MAC (A) payment is allowed for HBO therapy for diabetic wounds of the lower extremities when performed as a physician service in a hospital outpatient setting and for inpatients. Payment is allowed for claims with valid diagnosis codes as shown above with dates of service on or after April 1, 2003. Those claims with invalid codes should be denied as not medically necessary.

For hospitals, payment will be based upon the Ambulatory Payment Classification (APC) or the inpatient Diagnosis Related Group (DRG). Deductible and coinsurance apply.

Payment to Critical Access Hospitals (electing Method I) is made under cost reimbursement. For Critical Access Hospitals electing Method II, the technical component is paid under cost reimbursement and the professional component is paid under the Physician Fee Schedule.

II. A/B MAC (B) Billing Requirements

Claims for this service should be submitted using the ASC X12 837 professional claim format or Form CMS-1500.

The following HCPCS code applies:

99183 – Physician attendance and supervision of hyperbaric oxygen therapy, per session.

a. Payment Requirements for A/B MACs (B)

Payment and pricing information will occur through updates to the Medicare Physician Fee Schedule Database (MPFSDB). Pay for this service on the basis of the MPFSDB. Deductible and coinsurance apply. Claims from physicians or other practitioners where assignment was not taken, are subject to the Medicare limiting charge.

III. Medicare Summary Notices (MSNs)

Use the following MSN Messages where appropriate:

In situations where the claim is being denied on the basis that the condition does not meet our coverage requirements, use one of the following MSN Messages:

"Medicare does not pay for this item or service for this condition." (MSN Message 16.48)

The Spanish version of the MSN message should read:

"Medicare no paga por este articulo o servicio para esta afeccion."

In situations where, based on the above utilization policy, medical review of the claim results in a determination that the service is not medically necessary, use the following MSN message:

"The information provided does not support the need for this service or item." (MSN Message 15.4)

The Spanish version of the MSN message should read:

"La informacion proporcionada no confirma la necesidad para este servicio o articulo."

IV. Remittance Advice Notices

Use appropriate existing remittance advice remark codes and claim adjustment reason codes at the line level to express the specific reason if you deny payment for HBO therapy for the treatment of diabetic wounds of lower extremities.

100-04, 32, 60.4.1

Allowable Covered Diagnosis Codes

(Rev. 2998, Issued: 07-25-14, Effective: Upon implementation of ICD-10; 01-01-12 -
ASC X12, Implementation: 08-25-2014 - ASC X12; Upon Implementation of ICD-10)

For services furnished on or after July 1, 2002, the applicable ICD-9-CM diagnosis code for this benefit is V43.3, organ or tissue replaced by other means; heart valve.

For services furnished on or after March 19, 2008, the applicable ICD-9-CM diagnosis codes for this benefit are:

- V43.3 (organ or tissue replaced by other means; heart valve),
- 289.81 (primary hypercoagulable state),
- 451.0-451.9 (includes 451.11, 451.19, 451.2, 451.80-451.84, 451.89) (phlebitis & thrombophlebitis),
- 453.0-453.3 (other venous embolism & thrombosis),
- 453.40-453.49 (includes 453.40-453.42, 453.8-453.9) (venous embolism and thrombosis of the deep vessels of the lower extremity, and other specified veins/unspecified sites)
- 415.11-415.12, 415.19 (pulmonary embolism & infarction) or,
- 427.31 (atrial fibrillation (established) (paroxysmal)).

For services furnished on or after the implementation of ICD-10 the applicable ICD-10-CM diagnosis codes for this benefit are:

Heart Valve Replacement
- Z95.2 - Presence of prosthetic heart valve

Primary Hypercoagulable State

ICD-10-CM	Code Description
D68.51	Activated protein C resistance
D68.52	Prothrombin gene mutation
D68.59	Other primary thrombophilia
D68.61	Antiphospholipid syndrome
D68.62	Lupus anticoagulant syndrome

Phlebitis & Thrombophlebitis

ICD-10-CM	Code Description
I80.00	Phlebitis and thrombophlebitis of superficial vessels of unspecified lower extremity
I80.01	Phlebitis and thrombophlebitis of superficial vessels of right lower extremity
I80.02	Phlebitis and thrombophlebitis of superficial vessels of left lower extremity
I80.03	Phlebitis and thrombophlebitis of superficial vessels of lower extremities, bilateral
I80.10	Phlebitis and thrombophlebitis of unspecified femoral vein
I80.11	Phlebitis and thrombophlebitis of right femoral vein
I80.12	Phlebitis and thrombophlebitis of left femoral vein
I80.13	Phlebitis and thrombophlebitis of femoral vein, bilateral
I80.201	Phlebitis and thrombophlebitis of unspecified deep vessels of right lower extremity
I80.202	Phlebitis and thrombophlebitis of unspecified deep vessels of left lower extremity
I80.203	Phlebitis and thrombophlebitis of unspecified deep vessels of lower extremities, bilateral
I80.209	Phlebitis and thrombophlebitis of unspecified deep vessels of unspecified lower extremity
I80.221	Phlebitis and thrombophlebitis of right popliteal vein
I80.222	Phlebitis and thrombophlebitis of left popliteal vein
I80.223	Phlebitis and thrombophlebitis of popliteal vein, bilateral
I80.229	Phlebitis and thrombophlebitis of unspecified popliteal vein
I80.231	Phlebitis and thrombophlebitis of right tibial vein
I80.232	Phlebitis and thrombophlebitis of left tibial vein
I80.233	Phlebitis and thrombophlebitis of tibial vein, bilateral
I80.239	Phlebitis and thrombophlebitis of unspecified tibial vein
I80.291	Phlebitis and thrombophlebitis of other deep vessels of right lower extremity
I80.292	Phlebitis and thrombophlebitis of other deep vessels of left lower extremity
I80.293	Phlebitis and thrombophlebitis of other deep vessels of lower extremity, bilateral
I80.299	Phlebitis and thrombophlebitis of other deep vessels of unspecified lower extremity
I80.3	Phlebitis and thrombophlebitis of lower extremities, unspecified

ICD-10-CM	Code Description
I80.211	Phlebitis and thrombophlebitis of right iliac vein
I80.212	Phlebitis and thrombophlebitis of left iliac vein
I80.213	Phlebitis and thrombophlebitis of iliac vein, bilateral
I80.219	Phlebitis and thrombophlebitis of unspecified iliac vein
I80.8	Phlebitis and thrombophlebitis of other sites
I80.9	Phlebitis and thrombophlebitis of unspecified site

Other Venous Embolism & Thrombosis

ICD-10-CM	Code Description
I82.0	Budd- Chiari syndrome
I82.1	Thrombophlebitis migrans
I82.211	Chronic embolism and thrombosis of superior vena cava
I82.220	Acute embolism and thrombosis of inferior vena cava
I82.221	Chronic embolism and thrombosis of inferior vena cava
I82.291	Chronic embolism and thrombosis of other thoracic veins
I82.3	Embolism and thrombosis of renal vein

Venous Embolism and thrombosis of the deep vessels of the lower extremity, and other specified veins/unspecified sites

ICD-10-CM	Code Description
I82.401	Acute embolism and thrombosis of unspecified deep veins of right lower extremity
I82.402	Acute embolism and thrombosis of unspecified deep veins of left lower extremity
I82.403	Acute embolism and thrombosis of unspecified deep veins of lower extremity, bilateral
I82.409	Acute embolism and thrombosis of unspecified deep veins of unspecified lower extremity
I82.411	Acute embolism and thrombosis of right femoral vein
I82.412	Acute embolism and thrombosis of left femoral vein
I82.413	Acute embolism and thrombosis of femoral vein, bilateral
I82.419	Acute embolism and thrombosis of unspecified femoral vein
I82.421	Acute embolism and thrombosis of right iliac vein
I82.422	Acute embolism and thrombosis of left iliac vein
I82.423	Acute embolism and thrombosis of iliac vein, bilateral
I82.429	Acute embolism and thrombosis of unspecified iliac vein
I82.431	Acute embolism and thrombosis of right popliteal vein
I82.432	Acute embolism and thrombosis of left popliteal vein
I82.433	Acute embolism and thrombosis of popliteal vein, bilateral
I82.439	Acute embolism and thrombosis of unspecified popliteal vein
I82.4Y1	Acute embolism and thrombosis of unspecified deep veins of right proximal lower extremity
I82.4Y2	Acute embolism and thrombosis of unspecified deep veins of left proximal lower extremity
I82.4Y3	Acute embolism and thrombosis of unspecified deep veins of proximal lower extremity, bilateral
I82.4Y9	Acute embolism and thrombosis of unspecified deep veins of unspecified proximal lower extremity
I82.441	Acute embolism and thrombosis of right tibial vein
I82.442	Acute embolism and thrombosis of left tibial vein
I82.443	Acute embolism and thrombosis of tibial vein, bilateral
I82.449	Acute embolism and thrombosis of unspecified tibial vein
I82.491	Acute embolism and thrombosis of other specified deep vein of right lower extremity
I82.492	Acute embolism and thrombosis of other specified deep vein of left lower extremity
I82.493	Acute embolism and thrombosis of other specified deep vein of lower extremity, bilateral
I82.499	Acute embolism and thrombosis of other specified deep vein of unspecified lower extremity
I82.4Z1	Acute embolism and thrombosis of unspecified deep veins of right distal lower extremity
I82.4Z2	Acute embolism and thrombosis of unspecified deep veins of left distal lower extremity
I82.4Z3	Acute embolism and thrombosis of unspecified deep veins of distal lower extremity, bilateral
I82.4Z9	Acute embolism and thrombosis of unspecified deep veins of unspecified distal lower extremity
I82.501	Chronic embolism and thrombosis of unspecified deep veins of right lower extremity

ICD-10-CM	Code Description
I82.502	Chronic embolism and thrombosis of unspecified deep veins of left lower extremity
I82.503	Chronic embolism and thrombosis of unspecified deep veins of lower extremity, bilateral
I82.509	Chronic embolism and thrombosis of unspecified deep veins of unspecified lower extremity
I82.591	Chronic embolism and thrombosis of other specified deep vein of right lower extremity
I82.592	Chronic embolism and thrombosis of other specified deep vein of left lower extremity
I82.593	Chronic embolism and thrombosis of other specified deep vein of lower extremity, bilateral
I82.599	Chronic embolism and thrombosis of other specified deep vein of unspecified lower extremity
I82.511	Chronic embolism and thrombosis of right femoral vein
I82.512	Chronic embolism and thrombosis of left femoral vein
I82.513	Chronic embolism and thrombosis of femoral vein, bilateral
I82.519	Chronic embolism and thrombosis of unspecified femoral vein
I82.521	Chronic embolism and thrombosis of right iliac vein
I82.522	Chronic embolism and thrombosis of left iliac vein
I82.523	Chronic embolism and thrombosis of iliac vein, bilateral
I82.529	Chronic embolism and thrombosis of unspecified iliac vein
I82.531	Chronic embolism and thrombosis of right popliteal vein
I82.532	Chronic embolism and thrombosis of left popliteal vein
I82.533	Chronic embolism and thrombosis of popliteal vein, bilateral
I82.539	Chronic embolism and thrombosis of unspecified popliteal vein
I82.5Y1	Chronic embolism and thrombosis of unspecified deep veins of right proximal lower extremity
I82.5Y2	Chronic embolism and thrombosis of unspecified deep veins of left proximal lower extremity
I82.5Y3	Chronic embolism and thrombosis of unspecified deep veins of proximal lower extremity, bilateral
I82.5Y9	Chronic embolism and thrombosis of unspecified deep veins of unspecified proximal lower extremity
I82.541	Chronic embolism and thrombosis of right tibial vein
I82.542	Chronic embolism and thrombosis of left tibial vein
I82.543	Chronic embolism and thrombosis of tibial vein, bilateral
I82.549	Chronic embolism and thrombosis of unspecified tibial vein
I82.5Z1	Chronic embolism and thrombosis of unspecified deep veins of right distal lower extremity
I82.5Z2	Chronic embolism and thrombosis of unspecified deep veins of left distal lower extremity
I82.5Z3	Chronic embolism and thrombosis of unspecified deep veins of distal lower extremity, bilateral
I82.5Z9	Chronic embolism and thrombosis of unspecified deep veins of unspecified distal lower extremity
I82.611	Acute embolism and thrombosis of superficial veins of right upper extremity
I82.612	Acute embolism and thrombosis of superficial veins of left upper extremity
I82.613	Acute embolism and thrombosis of superficial veins of upper extremity, bilateral
I82.619	Acute embolism and thrombosis of superficial veins of unspecified upper extremity
I82.621	Acute embolism and thrombosis of deep veins of right upper extremity
I82.622	Acute embolism and thrombosis of deep veins of left upper extremity
I82.623	Acute embolism and thrombosis of deep veins of upper extremity, bilateral
I82.629	Acute embolism and thrombosis of deep veins of unspecified upper extremity
I82.601	Acute embolism and thrombosis of unspecified veins of right upper extremity
I82.602	Acute embolism and thrombosis of unspecified veins of left upper extremity
I82.603	Acute embolism and thrombosis of unspecified veins of upper extremity, bilateral
I82.609	Acute embolism and thrombosis of unspecified veins of unspecified upper extremity
I82.A11	Acute embolism and thrombosis of right axillary vein
I82.A12	Acute embolism and thrombosis of left axillary vein

ICD-10-CM	Code Description
I82.A13	Acute embolism and thrombosis of axillary vein, bilateral
I82.A19	Acute embolism and thrombosis of unspecified axillary vein
I82.A21	Chronic embolism and thrombosis of right axillary vein
I82.A22	Chronic embolism and thrombosis of left axillary vein
I82.A23	Chronic embolism and thrombosis of axillary vein, bilateral
I82.A29	Chronic embolism and thrombosis of unspecified axillary vein
I82.B11	Acute embolism and thrombosis of right subclavian vein
I82.B12	Acute embolism and thrombosis of left subclavian vein
I82.B13	Acute embolism and thrombosis of subclavian vein, bilateral
I82.B19	Acute embolism and thrombosis of unspecified subclavian vein
I82.B21	Chronic embolism and thrombosis of right subclavian vein
I82.B22	Chronic embolism and thrombosis of left subclavian vein
I82.B23	Chronic embolism and thrombosis of subclavian vein, bilateral
I82.B29	Chronic embolism and thrombosis of unspecified subclavian vein
I82.C11	Acute embolism and thrombosis of right internal jugular vein
I82.C12	Acute embolism and thrombosis of left internal jugular vein
I82.C13	Acute embolism and thrombosis of internal jugular vein, bilateral
I82.C19	Acute embolism and thrombosis of unspecified internal jugular vein
I82.C21	Chronic embolism and thrombosis of right internal jugular vein
I82.C22	Chronic embolism and thrombosis of left internal jugular vein
I82.C23	Chronic embolism and thrombosis of internal jugular vein, bilateral
I82.C29	Chronic embolism and thrombosis of unspecified internal jugular vein
I82.210	Acute embolism and thrombosis of superior vena cava
I82.290	Acute embolism and thrombosis of other thoracic veins
I82.701	Chronic embolism and thrombosis of unspecified veins of right upper extremity
I82.702	Chronic embolism and thrombosis of unspecified veins of left upper extremity
I82.703	Chronic embolism and thrombosis of unspecified veins of upper extremity, bilateral
I82.709	Chronic embolism and thrombosis of unspecified veins of unspecified upper extremity
I82.711	Chronic embolism and thrombosis of superficial veins of right upper extremity
I82.712	Chronic embolism and thrombosis of superficial veins of left upper extremity
I82.713	Chronic embolism and thrombosis of superficial veins of upper extremity, bilateral
I82.719	Chronic embolism and thrombosis of superficial veins of unspecified upper extremity
I82.721	Chronic embolism and thrombosis of deep veins of right upper extremity
I82.722	Chronic embolism and thrombosis of deep veins of left upper extremity
I82.723	Chronic embolism and thrombosis of deep veins of upper extremity, bilateral
I82.729	Chronic embolism and thrombosis of deep veins of unspecified upper extremity
I82.811	Embolism and thrombosis of superficial veins of right lower extremities
I82.812	Embolism and thrombosis of superficial veins of left lower extremities
I82.813	Embolism and thrombosis of superficial veins of lower extremities, bilateral
I82.819	Embolism and thrombosis of superficial veins of unspecified lower extremities
I82.890	Acute embolism and thrombosis of other specified veins
I82.891	Chronic embolism and thrombosis of other specified veins
I82.90	Acute embolism and thrombosis of unspecified vein
I82.91	Chronic embolism and thrombosis of unspecified vein

Pulmonary Embolism & Infarction

ICD-10-CM	Code Description
I26.90	Septic pulmonary embolism without acute cor pulmonale
I26.99	Other pulmonary embolism without acute cor pulmonale
I26.01	Septic pulmonary embolism with acute cor pulmonale
I26.90	Septic pulmonary embolism without acute cor pulmonale
I26.09	Other pulmonary embolism with acute cor pulmonale
I26.99	Other pulmonary embolism without acute cor pulmonale

Atrial Fibrillation

ICD-10-CM	Code Description
I48.0	Paroxysmal atrial fibrillation
I48.2	Chronic atrial fibrillation
I48	-91 Unspecified atrial fibrillation Other
I23.6	Thrombosis of atrium, auricular appendage, and ventricle as current complications following acute myocardial infarction
I27.82	Chronic pulmonary embolism
I67.6	Nonpyogenic thrombosis of intracranial venous system
O22.50	Cerebral venous thrombosis in pregnancy, unspecified trimester
O22.51	Cerebral venous thrombosis in pregnancy, first trimester
O22.52	Cerebral venous thrombosis in pregnancy, second trimester
O22.53	Cerebral venous thrombosis in pregnancy, third trimester
O87.3	Cerebral venous thrombosis in the puerperium
Z79.01	Long term (current) use of anticoagulants

Coverage policy can be found in Pub. 100-3, Medicare National Coverage Determinations Manual, Chapter 1, section 190.11 PT/INR. (http://www.cms.hhs.gov/manuals/103_cov_determ/ncd103index.asp

100-04, 32, 60.5.2

Applicable Diagnosis Codes for A/B Macs

(Rev. 2998, Issued: 07-25-14, Effective: Upon implementation of ICD-10; 01-01-12 - ASC X12, Implementation: 08-25-2014 - ASC X12; Upon Implementation of ICD-10)

For services furnished on or after July 1, 2002, the applicable ICD-9-CM diagnosis code for this benefit is V43.3, organ or tissue replaced by other means; heart valve.

For services furnished on or after March 19, 2008, the applicable ICD-9-CM diagnosis codes for this benefit are:

- V43.3 (organ or tissue replaced by other means; heart valve),
- 289.81 (primary hypercoagulable state),
- 451.0-451.9 (includes 451.11, 451.19, 451.2, 451.80-451.84, 451.89) (phlebitis & thrombophlebitis),
- 453.0-453.3 (other venous embolism & thrombosis),
- 453.40-453.49 (includes 453.40-453.42, 453.8-453.9) (venous embolism and thrombosis of the deep vessels of the lower extremity, and other specified veins/unspecified sites)
- 415.11-415.12, 415.19 (pulmonary embolism & infarction) or,
- 427.31 (atrial fibrillation (established) (paroxysmal)).

For services furnished on or after implementation of ICD-10 the applicable ICD-10-CM diagnosis codes for this benefit are:

Heart Valve Replacement
- Z95.2 - Presence of prosthetic heart valve

Primary Hypercoagulable State

ICD-10-CM	Code Description
D68.51	Activated protein C resistance
D68.52	Prothrombin gene mutation
D68.59	Other primary thrombophilia
D68.61	Antiphospholipid syndrome
D68.62	Lupus anticoagulant syndrome

Phlebitis & Thrombophlebitis

ICD-10-CM	Code Description
I80.00	Phlebitis and thrombophlebitis of superficial vessels of unspecified lower extremity
I80.01	Phlebitis and thrombophlebitis of superficial vessels of right lower extremity
I80.02	Phlebitis and thrombophlebitis of superficial vessels of left lower extremity
I80.03	Phlebitis and thrombophlebitis of superficial vessels of lower extremities, bilateral
I80.10	Phlebitis and thrombophlebitis of unspecified femoral vein
I80.11	Phlebitis and thrombophlebitis of right femoral vein
I80.12	Phlebitis and thrombophlebitis of left femoral vein
I80.13	Phlebitis and thrombophlebitis of femoral vein, bilateral
I80.201	Phlebitis and thrombophlebitis of unspecified deep vessels of right lower extremity
I80.202	Phlebitis and thrombophlebitis of unspecified deep vessels of left lower extremity
I80.203	Phlebitis and thrombophlebitis of unspecified deep vessels of lower extremities, bilateral

ICD-10-CM	Code Description
I80.209	Phlebitis and thrombophlebitis of unspecified deep vessels of unspecified lower extremity
I80.221	Phlebitis and thrombophlebitis of right popliteal vein
I80.222	Phlebitis and thrombophlebitis of left popliteal vein
I80.223	Phlebitis and thrombophlebitis of popliteal vein, bilateral
I80.229	Phlebitis and thrombophlebitis of unspecified popliteal vein
I80.231	Phlebitis and thrombophlebitis of right tibial vein
I80.232	Phlebitis and thrombophlebitis of left tibial vein
I80.233	Phlebitis and thrombophlebitis of tibial vein, bilateral
I80.239	Phlebitis and thrombophlebitis of unspecified tibial vein
I80.291	Phlebitis and thrombophlebitis of other deep vessels of right lower extremity
I80.292	Phlebitis and thrombophlebitis of other deep vessels of left lower extremity
I80.293	Phlebitis and thrombophlebitis of other deep vessels of lower extremity, bilateral
I80.299	Phlebitis and thrombophlebitis of other deep vessels of unspecified lower extremity
I80.3	Phlebitis and thrombophlebitis of lower extremities, unspecified
I80.211	Phlebitis and thrombophlebitis of right iliac vein
I80.212	Phlebitis and thrombophlebitis of left iliac vein
I80.213	Phlebitis and thrombophlebitis of iliac vein, bilateral
I80.219	Phlebitis and thrombophlebitis of unspecified iliac vein
I80.8	Phlebitis and thrombophlebitis of other sites
I80.9	Phlebitis and thrombophlebitis of unspecified site

Other Venous Embolism & Thrombosis

ICD-10-CM	Code Description
I82.0	Budd- Chiari syndrome
I82.1	Thrombophlebitis migrans
I82.211	Chronic embolism and thrombosis of superior vena cava
I82220	Acute embolism and thrombosis of inferior vena cava
I82.221	Chronic embolism and thrombosis of inferior vena cava
I82.291	Chronic embolism and thrombosis of other thoracic veins
I82.3	Embolism and thrombosis of renal vein

Venous Embolism and thrombosis of the deep vessels of the lower extremity, and other specified veins/unspecified sites

ICD-10-CM	Code Description
I82.401	Acute embolism and thrombosis of unspecified deep veins of right lower extremity
I82.402	Acute embolism and thrombosis of unspecified deep veins of left lower extremity
I82.403	Acute embolism and thrombosis of unspecified deep veins of lower extremity, bilateral
I82. 409	Acute embolism and thrombosis of unspecified deep veins of unspecified lower extremity
I82.411	Acute embolism and thrombosis of right femoral vein
I82.412	Acute embolism and thrombosis of left femoral vein
I82.413	Acute embolism and thrombosis of femoral vein, bilateral
I82.419	Acute embolism and thrombosis of unspecified femoral vein
I82.421	Acute embolism and thrombosis of right iliac vein
I82.422	Acute embolism and thrombosis of left iliac vein
I82.423	Acute embolism and thrombosis of iliac vein, bilateral
I82.429	Acute embolism and thrombosis of unspecified iliac vein
I82.431	Acute embolism and thrombosis of right popliteal vein
I82.432	Acute embolism and thrombosis of left popliteal vein
I82.433	Acute embolism and thrombosis of popliteal vein, bilateral
I82.439	Acute embolism and thrombosis of unspecified popliteal vein
I82.4Y1	Acute embolism and thrombosis of unspecified deep veins of right proximal lower extremity
I82.4Y2	Acute embolism and thrombosis of unspecified deep veins of left proximal lower extremity
I82.4Y3	Acute embolism and thrombosis of unspecified deep veins of proximal lower extremity, bilateral
I82.4Y9	Acute embolism and thrombosis of unspecified deep veins of unspecified proximal lower extremity
I82.441	Acute embolism and thrombosis of right tibial vein
I82.442	Acute embolism and thrombosis of left tibial vein

ICD-10-CM	Code Description
I82.443	Acute embolism and thrombosis of tibial vein, bilateral
I82.449	Acute embolism and thrombosis of unspecified tibial vein
I82.491	Acute embolism and thrombosis of other specified deep vein of right lower extremity
I82.492	Acute embolism and thrombosis of other specified deep vein of left lower extremity
I82.493	Acute embolism and thrombosis of other specified deep vein of lower extremity, bilateral
I82.499	Acute embolism and thrombosis of other specified deep vein of unspecified lower extremity
I82.4Z1	Acute embolism and thrombosis of unspecified deep veins of right distal lower extremity
I82.4Z2	Acute embolism and thrombosis of unspecified deep veins of left distal lower extremity
I82.4Z3	Acute embolism and thrombosis of unspecified deep veins of distal lower extremity, bilateral
I82.4Z9	Acute embolism and thrombosis of unspecified deep veins of unspecified distal lower extremity
I82.501	Chronic embolism and thrombosis of unspecified deep veins of right lower extremity
I82.502	Chronic embolism and thrombosis of unspecified deep veins of left lower extremity
I82.503	Chronic embolism and thrombosis of unspecified deep veins of lower extremity, bilateral
I82.509	Chronic embolism and thrombosis of unspecified deep veins of unspecified lower extremity
I82.591	Chronic embolism and thrombosis of other specified deep vein of right lower extremity
I82.592	Chronic embolism and thrombosis of other specified deep vein of left lower extremity
I82.593	Chronic embolism and thrombosis of other specified deep vein of lower extremity, bilateral
I82.599	Chronic embolism and thrombosis of other specified deep vein of unspecified lower extremity
I82.511	Chronic embolism and thrombosis of right femoral vein
I82.512	Chronic embolism and thrombosis of left femoral vein
I82.513	Chronic embolism and thrombosis of femoral vein, bilateral
I82.519	Chronic embolism and thrombosis of unspecified femoral vein
I82.521	Chronic embolism and thrombosis of right iliac vein
I82.522	Chronic embolism and thrombosis of left iliac vein
I82.523	Chronic embolism and thrombosis of iliac vein, bilateral
I82.529	Chronic embolism and thrombosis of unspecified iliac vein
I82.531	Chronic embolism and thrombosis of right popliteal vein
I82.532	Chronic embolism and thrombosis of left popliteal vein
I82.533	Chronic embolism and thrombosis of popliteal vein, bilateral
I82.539	Chronic embolism and thrombosis of unspecified popliteal vein
I82.5Y1	Chronic embolism and thrombosis of unspecified deep veins of right proximal lower extremity
I82.5Y2	Chronic embolism and thrombosis of unspecified deep veins of left proximal lower extremity
I82.5Y3	Chronic embolism and thrombosis of unspecified deep veins of proximal lower extremity, bilateral
I82.5Y9	Chronic embolism and thrombosis of unspecified deep veins of unspecified proximal lower extremity
I82.541	Chronic embolism and thrombosis of right tibial vein
I82.42	Chronic embolism and thrombosis of left tibial vein
I82.543	Chronic embolism and thrombosis of tibial vein, bilateral
I82.549	Chronic embolism and thrombosis of unspecified tibial vein
I82.5Z1	Chronic embolism and thrombosis of unspecified deep veins of right distal lower extremity
I82.5Z2	Chronic embolism and thrombosis of unspecified deep veins of left distal lower extremity
I82.5Z3	Chronic embolism and thrombosis of unspecified deep veins of distal lower extremity, bilateral
I82.5Z9	Chronic embolism and thrombosis of unspecified deep veins of unspecified distal lower extremity
I82.611	Acute embolism and thrombosis of superficial veins of right upper extremity
I82.612	Acute embolism and thrombosis of superficial veins of left upper extremity

ICD-10-CM	Code Description
I82.613	Acute embolism and thrombosis of superficial veins of upper extremity, bilateral
I82.619	Acute embolism and thrombosis of superficial veins of unspecified upper extremity
I82.621	Acute embolism and thrombosis of deep veins of right upper extremity
I82.622	Acute embolism and thrombosis of deep veins of left upper extremity
I82.623	Acute embolism and thrombosis of deep veins of upper extremity, bilateral
I82.629	Acute embolism and thrombosis of deep veins of unspecified upper extremity
I82.601	Acute embolism and thrombosis of unspecified veins of right upper extremity
I82.602	Acute embolism and thrombosis of unspecified veins of left upper extremity
I82.603	Acute embolism and thrombosis of unspecified veins of upper extremity, bilateral
I82.609	Acute embolism and thrombosis of unspecified veins of unspecified upper extremity
I82.A11	Acute embolism and thrombosis of right axillary vein
I82.A12	Acute embolism and thrombosis of left axillary vein
I82.A13	Acute embolism and thrombosis of axillary vein, bilateral
I82.A19	Acute embolism and thrombosis of unspecified axillary vein
I82.A21	Chronic embolism and thrombosis of right axillary vein
I82.A22	Chronic embolism and thrombosis of left axillary vein
I82.A23	Chronic embolism and thrombosis of axillary vein, bilateral
I82.A29	Chronic embolism and thrombosis of unspecified axillary vein
I82.B11	Acute embolism and thrombosis of right subclavian vein
I82.B12	Acute embolism and thrombosis of left subclavian vein
I82.B13	Acute embolism and thrombosis of subclavian vein, bilateral
I82.B19	Acute embolism and thrombosis of unspecified subclavian vein
I82.B21	Chronic embolism and thrombosis of right subclavian vein
I82.B22	Chronic embolism and thrombosis of left subclavian vein
I82.B23	Chronic embolism and thrombosis of subclavian vein, bilateral
I82.B29	Chronic embolism and thrombosis of unspecified subclavian vein
I82.C11	Acute embolism and thrombosis of right internal jugular vein
I82.C12	Acute embolism and thrombosis of left internal jugular vein
I82.C13	Acute embolism and thrombosis of internal jugular vein, bilateral
I82.C19	Acute embolism and thrombosis of unspecified internal jugular vein
I82.C21	Chronic embolism and thrombosis of right internal jugular vein
I82.C22	Chronic embolism and thrombosis of left internal jugular vein
I82.C23	Chronic embolism and thrombosis of internal jugular vein, bilateral
I82.C29	Chronic embolism and thrombosis of unspecified internal jugular vein
I82.210	Acute embolism and thrombosis of superior vena cava
I82.290	Acute embolism and thrombosis of other thoracic veins
I82.701	Chronic embolism and thrombosis of unspecified veins of right upper extremity
I82.702	Chronic embolism and thrombosis of unspecified veins of left upper extremity
I82.703	Chronic embolism and thrombosis of unspecified veins of upper extremity, bilateral
I82.709	Chronic embolism and thrombosis of unspecified veins of unspecified upper extremity
I82.711	Chronic embolism and thrombosis of superficial veins of right upper extremity
I82.712	Chronic embolism and thrombosis of superficial veins of left upper extremity
I82.713	Chronic embolism and thrombosis of superficial veins of upper extremity, bilateral
I82.719	Chronic embolism and thrombosis of superficial veins of unspecified upper extremity
I82.721	Chronic embolism and thrombosis of deep veins of right upper extremity
I82.722	Chronic embolism and thrombosis of deep veins of left upper extremity
I82.723	Chronic embolism and thrombosis of deep veins of upper extremity, bilateral
I82.729	Chronic embolism and thrombosis of deep veins of unspecified upper extremity

ICD-10-CM	Code Description
I82.811	Embolism and thrombosis of superficial veins of right lower extremities
I82.812	Embolism and thrombosis of superficial veins of left lower extremities
I82.813	Embolism and thrombosis of superficial veins of lower extremities, bilateral
I82.819	Embolism and thrombosis of superficial veins of unspecified lower extremities
I82.890	Acute embolism and thrombosis of other specified veins
I82.891	Chronic embolism and thrombosis of other specified veins
I82.90	Acute embolism and thrombosis of unspecified vein
I82.91	Chronic embolism and thrombosis of unspecified vein

Pulmonary Embolism & Infarction

ICD-10-CM	Code Description
I26.01	Septic pulmonary embolism with acute cor pulmonale
I26.90	Septic pulmonary embolism without acute cor pulmonale
I26.09	Other pulmonary embolism with acute cor pulmonale
I26.99	Other pulmonary embolism without acute cor pulmonale

Atrial Fibrillation

ICD-10-CM	Code Description
I48.0	Paroxysmal atrial fibrillation
I48.2	Chronic atrial fibrillation
I48.	-91 Unspecified atrial fibrillation Other
I23.6	Thrombosis of atrium, auricular appendage, and ventricle as current complications following acute myocardial infarction
I27.82	Chronic pulmonary embolism
I67.6	Nonpyogenic thrombosis of intracranial venous system
O22.50	Cerebral venous thrombosis in pregnancy, unspecified trimester
O22.51	Cerebral venous thrombosis in pregnancy, first trimester
O22.52	Cerebral venous thrombosis in pregnancy, second trimester
O22.53	Cerebral venous thrombosis in pregnancy, third trimester
O87.3	Cerebral venous thrombosis in the puerperium
Z79.01	Long term (current) use of anticoagulants
Z86.718	Personal history of other venous thrombosis and embolism
Z95.4	Presence of other heart

Coverage policy can be found in Pub. 100-3, Medicare National Coverage Determinations Manual, Chapter 1, section 190.11 PT/INR. (http://www.cms.hhs.gov/manuals/103_cov_determ/ncd103index.asp

100-04, 32, 80.8

CWF Utilization Edits

(Rev. 1742, Issued: 05-22-09, Effective: 06-08-09, Implementation: 06-08-09)

Edit 1

Should CWF receive a claim from an FI for G0245 or G0246 and a second claim from a contractor for either G0245 or G0246 (or vice versa) and they are different dates of service and less than 6 months apart, the second claim will reject. CWF will edit to allow G0245 or G0246 to be paid no more than every 6 months for a particular beneficiary, regardless of who furnished the service. If G0245 has been paid, regardless of whether it was posted as a facility or professional claim, it must be 6 months before G0245 can be paid again or G0246 can be paid. If G0246 has been paid, regardless of whether it was posted as a facility or professional claim, it must be 6 months before G0246 can be paid again or G0245 can be paid. CWF will not impose limits on how many times each code can be paid for a beneficiary as long as there has been 6 months between each service.

The CWF will return a specific reject code for this edit to the contractors and FIs that will be identified in the CWF documentation. Based on the CWF reject code, the contractors and FIs must deny the claims and return the following messages:

MSN 18.4 -- This service is being denied because it has not been ___ months since your last examination of this kind (NOTE: Insert 6 as the appropriate number of months.)

RA claim adjustment reason code 96 - Non-covered charges, along with remark code M86 - Service denied because payment already made for same/similar procedure within set time frame.

Edit 2

The CWF will edit to allow G0247 to pay only if either G0245 or G0246 has been submitted and accepted as payable on the same date of service. CWF will return a specific reject code for this edit to the contractors and FIs that will be identified in the CWF documentation. Based on this reject code, contractors and FIs will deny the claims and return the following messages:

MSN 21.21 - This service was denied because Medicare only covers this service under certain circumstances.

RA claim adjustment reason code 107 - The related or qualifying claim/service was not identified on this claim.

Edit 3

Once a beneficiary's condition has progressed to the point where routine foot care becomes a covered service, payment will no longer be made for LOPS evaluation and management services. Those services would be considered to be included in the regular exams and treatments afforded to the beneficiary on a routine basis. The physician or provider must then just bill the routine foot care codes, per Pub 100-2, Chapter 15, Sec. 290.

The CWF will edit to reject LOPS codes G0245, G0246, and/or G0247 when on the beneficiary's record it shows that one of the following routine foot care codes were billed and paid within the prior 6 months: 11055, 11056, 11057, 11719, 11720, and/or 11721.

The CWF will return a specific reject code for this edit to the contractors and FIs that will be identified in the CWF documentation. Based on the CWF reject code, the contractors and FIs must deny the claims and return the following messages:

MSN 21.21 - This service was denied because Medicare only covers this service under certain circumstances.

The RA claim adjustment reason code 96 - Non-covered charges, along with remark code M86 - Service denied because payment already made for same/similar procedure within set time frame.

100-04, 32, 90

Stem Cell Transplantation

(Rev. 3556, Issued: 07-01-2016; Effective: 1-27-16; Implementation: 10-3-16)

A. General

Stem cell transplantation is a process in which stem cells are harvested from either a patient's (autologous) or donor's (allogeneic) bone marrow or peripheral blood for intravenous infusion.

Allogeneic and autologous stem cell transplants are covered under Medicare for specific diagnoses. See Pub. 100-03, National Coverage Determinations Manual, section 110.23, for a complete description of covered and noncovered conditions. For Part A hospital inpatient claims processing instructions, refer to Pub. 100-04, Chapter 3, section 90. The following sections contain claims processing instructions for all other claims.

B. Nationally Covered Indications

I.   Allogeneic Hematopoietic Stem Cell Transplantation (HSCT)

HCPCS Code 38240

ICD-9-CM Procedure Codes 41.02, 41.03, 41.05, and 41.08

ICD-10-PCS Procedure Codes 30230G1, 30230Y1, 30233G1, 30233Y1, 30240G1, 30240Y1, 30243G1, 30243Y1, 30250G1, 30250Y1, 30253G1, 30253Y1, 30260G1, 30260Y1, 30263G1, and 30263Y1

a.   Effective for services performed on or after August 1, 1978:

i.   For the treatment of leukemia, leukemia in remission (ICD-9-CM codes 204.00 through 208.91; see table below for ICD-10-CM codes)

ICD-10	Description
C91.01	Acute lymphoblastic leukemia, in remission
C91.11	Chronic lymphocytic leukemia of B-cell type in remission
C91.31	Prolymphocytic leukemia of B-cell type, in remission
C91.51	Adult T-cell lymphoma/leukemia (HTLV-1-associated), in remission
C91.61	Prolymphocytic leukemia of T-cell type, in remission
C91.91	Lymphoid leukemia, unspecified, in remission
C91.A1	Mature B-cell leukemia Burkitt-type, in remission
C91.Z1	Other lymphoid leukemia, in remission
C92.01	Acute myeloblastic leukemia, in remission
C92.11	Chronic myeloid leukemia, BCR/ABL-positive, in remission
C92.21	Atypical chronic myeloid leukemia, BCR/ABL-negative, in remission
C92.31	Myeloid sarcoma, in remission
C92.41	Acute promyelocytic leukemia, in remission
C92.51	Acute myelomonocytic leukemia, in remission
C92.61	Acute myeloid leukemia with 11q23-abnormality in remission
C92.91	Myeloid leukemia, unspecified in remission
C92.A1	Acute myeloid leukemia with multilineage dysplasia, in remission
C92.Z1	Other myeloid leukemia, in remission
C93.01	Acute monoblastic/monocytic leukemia, in remission
C93.11	Chronic myelomonocytic leukemia, in remission
C93.31	Juvenile myelomonocytic leukemia, in remission
C93.91	Monocytic leukemia, unspecified in remission

ICD-10	Description
C93.Z1	Other monocytic leukemia, in remission
C94.01	Acute erythroid leukemia, in remission
C94.21	Acute megakaryoblastic leukemia, in remission
C94.31	Mast cell leukemia, in remission
C94.81	Other specified leukemias, in remission
C95.01	Acute leukemia of unspecified cell type, in remission
C95.11	Chronic leukemia of unspecified cell type, in remission
C95.91	Leukemia, unspecified, in remission
D45	Polycythemia vera

ii. For the treatment of aplastic anemia (ICD-9-CM codes 284.0 through 284.9; see table below for ICD-10-CM codes)

ICD-10	Description
D60.0	Chronic acquired pure red cell aplasia
D60.1	Transient acquired pure red cell aplasia
D60.8	Other acquired pure red cell aplasias
D60.9	Acquired pure red cell aplasia, unspecified
D61.01	Constitutional (pure) red blood cell aplasia
D61.09	Other constitutional aplastic anemia
D61.1	Drug-induced aplastic anemia
D61.2	Aplastic anemia due to other external agents
D61.3	Idiopathic aplastic anemia
D61.810	Antineoplastic chemotherapy induced pancytopenia
D61.811	Other drug-induced pancytopenia
D61.818	Other pancytopenia
D61.82	Myelophthisis
D61.89	Other specified aplastic anemias and other bone marrow failure syndromes
D61.9	Aplastic anemia, unspecified

b. Effective for services performed on or after June 3, 1985:

   i. For the treatment of severe combined immunodeficiency disease (SCID) (ICD-9-CM code 279.2; ICD-10-CM codes D81.0, D81.1, D81.2, D81.6, D81.7, D81.89, and D81.9). ii. For the treatment of Wiskott-Aldrich syndrome (ICD-9-CM code 279.12; ICD-10-CM code D82.0)

c. Effective for services performed on or after August 4, 2010: For the treatment of Myelodysplastic Syndromes (MDS) (ICD-9-CM codes 238.72, 238.73, 238.74, 238.75 and ICD-10-CM codes D46.A, D46.B, D46.C, D46.0, D46.1, D46.20, D46.21, D46.22, D46.4, D46.9, D46.Z) pursuant to Coverage with Evidence Development (CED) in the context of a Medicare-approved, prospective clinical study. Refer to Pub. 100-03, NCD Manual, chapter 1, section 110.23, for further information about this policy. See section F below for billing instructions.

d. Effective for services performed on or after January 27, 2016:

   i. Allogeneic HSCT for multiple myeloma (ICD-10-CM codes C90.00, C90.01, and C90.02) is covered by Medicare only for beneficiaries with Durie-Salmon Stage II or III multiple myeloma, or International Staging System (ISS) Stage II or Stage III multiple myeloma, and participating in an approved prospective clinical study. Refer to Pub. 100-03, NCD Manual, chapter 1, section 110.23, for further information about this policy. See section F below for billing instructions.

   ii. Allogeneic HSCT for myelofibrosis (MF) (ICD-10-CM codes C94.40, C94.41, C94.42, D47.4, and D75.81) is covered by Medicare only for beneficiaries with Dynamic International Prognostic Scoring System (DIPSSplus) intermediate-2 or High primary or secondary MF and participating in an approved prospective clinical study. Refer to Pub. 100-03, NCD Manual, chapter 1, section 110.23, for further information about this policy. See section F below for billing instructions.

   iii. Allogeneic HSCT for sickle cell disease (SCD) (ICD-10-CM codes D57.00, D57.01, D57.02, D57.1, D57.20, D57.211, D57.212, D57.219, D57.40, D57.411, D57.412, D57.419, D57.80, D57.811, D57.812, and D57.819) is covered by Medicare only for beneficiaries with severe, symptomatic SCD who participate in an approved prospective clinical study. Refer to Pub. 100-03, NCD Manual, chapter 1, section 110.23, for further information about this policy. See section F below for billing instructions.

II. Autologous Stem Cell Transplantation (AuSCT)

HCPCS Code 38241

ICD-9-CM Procedure Codes 41.01, 41.04, 41.07, and 41.09;

ICD-10-PCS Procedure Codes 30230AZ, 30230G0, 30230Y0, 30233G0, 30233Y0, 30240G0, 30240Y0, 30243G0, 30243Y0, 30250G0, 30250Y0, 30253G0, 30253Y0, 30260G0, 30260Y0, 30263G0, and 30263Y0

a. Effective for services performed on or after April 28, 1989: Acute leukemia in remission who have a high probability of relapse and who have no human leucocyte antigens (HLA)-matched (ICD-9-CM codes 204.01, 205.01, 206.01, 207.01, 208.01; ICD-10-CM diagnosis codes C91.01, C92.01, C92,41, C92.51, C92.61, C92.A1, C93.01, C94.01, C94.21, C94.41, C95.01); Resistant non-Hodgkin's lymphomas or those presenting with poor prognostic features following an initial response (ICD-9-CM codes 200.00 - 200.08, 200.10-200.18, 200.20-200.28, 200.80-200.88, 202.00-202.08, 202.80-202.88 or 202.90-202.98; ICD-10-CM diagnosis codes C82.00-C85.29, C85.80-C86.6, C96.4, and C96.Z-C96.9); Recurrent or refractory neuroblastoma (see ICD-9-CM codes Neoplasm by site, malignant for the appropriate diagnosis code; if ICD-10-CM is applicable the following ranges are reported: C00 - C96, and D00 - D09 Resistant non-Hodgkin's lymphomas); or, Advanced Hodgkin's disease who have failed conventional therapy and have no HLA-matched donor (ICD-9-CM codes 201.00 - 201.98; ICD-10-CM code C81.00 - C81.99).

b. Effective for services performed on or after October 1, 2000: Single AuSCT is only covered for Durie-Salmon Stage II or III multiple myeloma patients (ICD-9-CM codes 203.00 or 238.6; ICD-10-CM codes C90.00, C90.01, C90.02 and D47.Z9) that fit the following requirements:

   • Newly diagnosed or responsive multiple myeloma. This includes those patients with previously untreated disease, those with at least a partial response to prior chemotherapy (defined as a 50% decrease either in measurable paraprotein [serum and/or urine] or in bone marrow infiltration, sustained for at least 1 month), and those in responsive relapse; and • Adequate cardiac, renal, pulmonary, and hepatic function.

c. Effective for services performed on or after March 15, 2005: When recognized clinical risk factors are employed to select patients for transplantation, high dose melphalan (HDM) together with AuSCT is reasonable and necessary for Medicare beneficiaries of any age group with primary amyloid light chain (AL) amyloidosis (ICD-9-CM code 277.3 or 277.39) who meet the following criteria:

   • Amyloid deposition in 2 or fewer organs; and,

   • Cardiac left ventricular ejection fraction (EF) greater than 45%.

ICD-9-CM code	Description	ICD-10-CM code	Description
277.30	Amyloidosis, unspecified	E85.9	Amyloidosis, unspecified
277.39	Other amyloidosis	E85.8	Other amyloidosis
		E85.4	Organ-limited amyloidosis

As the ICD-9-CM codes 277.3, and 277.39 for amyloidosis do not differentiate between primary and non-primary, A/B MACs (B) should perform prepay reviews on all claims with a diagnosis of ICD-9-CM code 277.3 to determine whether payment is appropriate.

If ICD-10-CM is applicable, as the applicable ICD-10 CM codes E85.4, E85.8, and E85.9 for amyloidosis do not differentiate between primary and non-primary, A/B MACs (B) should perform prepay reviews on all claims with a diagnosis of ICD-10-CM code E85.4, E85.8, and E85.9 to determine whether payment is appropriate.

C. Nationally Non-Covered Indications

I. Allogeneic Hematopoietic Stem Cell Transplantation (HSCT)

Effective for claims with dates of service on or after May 24, 1996, through January 27, 2016, allogeneic HSCT is not covered as treatment for multiple myeloma (if ICD-9-CM is applicable, ICD-9-CM code 203.00 and 203.01; or if ICD-10-CM is applicable, ICD-10-CMcodes C90.00, C90.01, C90.02 and D47.Z9).

II. Autologous Stem Cell Transplantation (AuSCT)

AuSCT is not considered reasonable and necessary within the meaning of §l862(a)(1)(A) of the Act and is not covered under Medicare for the following conditions:

a) Acute leukemia not in remission (if ICD-9-CM is applicable, ICD-9-CM codes 204.00, 205.00, 206.00, 207.00 and 208.00; or if ICD-10-CM is applicable, ICD-10-CM codes C91.00, C92.00, C93.00, C94.00, andC95.00)

b) Chronic granulocytic leukemia (if ICD-9-CM is applicable, ICD-9-CM codes 205.10 and 205.11; or if ICD-10-CM is applicable, ICD-10-CM codes C92.10 andC92.11);

c) Solid tumors (other than neuroblastoma) (if ICD-9-CM is applicable, ICD-9-CM codes 140.0 through 199.1; or if ICD-10-CM is applicable, ICD-10-CM codesC00.0 – C80.2 and D00.0 – D09.9);

d) Up to October 1, 2000, multiple myeloma (if ICD-9-CM is applicable, ICD-9-CM code 203.00 and 203.01; or if ICD-10-CM is applicable, ICD-10-CM codes C90.00, C90.01, C90.02 and D47.Z9);

e) Tandem transplantation (multiple rounds of AuSCT) for patients with multiple myeloma (if ICD-9-CM is applicable, ICD-9-CM code 203.00 and 203.01; or if ICD-10-CM is applicable, ICD-10-CM codes C90.00, C90.01, C90.02 and D47.Z9);

f) Effective October 1, 2000, non-primary AL amyloidosis (see table below for applicable ICD codes); and,

g) Effective October 1, 2000, through March 14, 2005, primary AL amyloidosis for Medicare beneficiaries age 64 or older (see table below for applicable ICD codes).

ICD-9-CM codes	Description	ICD-10-CM codes	Description
277.30	Amyloidosis, unspecified	E85.9	Amyloidosis, unspecified
277.31	Familial Mediterranean fever	E85.0	Non-neuropathic heredofamilial amyloidosis
277.39	Other amyloidosis	E85.8	Other amyloidosis
		E85.1	Neuropathic heredofamilial amyloidosis
		E85.2	Heredofamilial amyloidosis, unspecified
		E85.3	Secondary systemic amyloidosis
		E85.4	Organ-limited amyloidosis

As the ICD-9-CM code 277.3 and 277.39 for amyloidosis do not differentiate between primary and non-primary, A/B MACs (B) should perform prepay reviews on all claims with a diagnosis of ICD-9-CM code 277.3 and 277.39 to determine whether payment is appropriate.

If ICD-10-CM is applicable, as the applicable ICD-10 CM codes E85.4, E85.8, and E85.9 for amyloidosis do not differentiate between primary and non-primary, A/B MACs (B) should perform prepay reviews on all claims with a diagnosis of ICD-10-CM code E85.4, E85.8, and E85.9 to determine whether payment is appropriate.

D. Other

All other indications for stem cell transplantation not otherwise noted above as covered or non-covered remain at local Medicare Administrative Contractor discretion.

E. Suggested MSN and RA Messages

The contractor shall use an appropriate MSN and RA message such as the following:

MSN - 15.4, The information provided does not support the need for this service or item;

RA - 150, Payment adjusted because the payer deems the information submitted does not support this level of service.

F. Clinical Trials for Allogeneic Hematopoietic Stem Cell Transplantation (HSCT) for Myelodysplastic Syndrome (MDS), Multiple Myeloma, Myelofibrosis (MF), and for Sickle Cell Disease (SCD)

I. Background

Effective for services performed on or after August 4, 2010, contractors shall pay for claims for allogeneic HSCT for the treatment of Myelodysplastic Syndromes (MDS) pursuant to Coverage with Evidence Development (CED) in the context of a Medicare-approved, prospective clinical study.

Effective for services performed on or after January 27, 2016, contractors shall pay for claims for allogeneic HSCT for the treatment of multiple myeloma, myelofibrosis (MF), and for sickle cell disease (SCD) pursuant to CED, in the context of a Medicare-approved, prospective clinical study.

Refer to Pub.100-03, National Coverage Determinations Manual, Chapter 1, section 110.23, for more information about this policy, and Pub. 100-04, Medicare Claims Processing Manual, Chapter 3, section 90.3, for information on inpatient billing of this CED.

II. Adjudication Requirements Payable Conditions. For claims with dates of service on and after August 4, 2010, contractors shall pay for claims for allogeneic HSCT for MDS when the service was provided pursuant to a Medicare-approved clinical study under CED; these services are paid only in the inpatient setting (Type of Bill (TOB) 11X), as outpatient Part B (TOB 13X), and in Method II critical access hospitals (TOB 85X).

Contractors shall require the following coding in order to pay for these claims:

- Existing Medicare-approved clinical trial coding conventions, as required in Pub. 100-04, Medicare Claims Processing Manual, Chapter 32, section 69, and inpatient billing requirements regarding acquisition of stem cells in Pub. 100-04, Medicare Claims Processing Manual, Chapter 3, section 90.3.1.

- If ICD-9-CM is applicable, for Inpatient Hospital Claims: ICD-9-CM procedure codes 41.02, 41.03, 41.05, and 41.08 or,

- If ICD-10-CM is applicable, ICD-10-PCS, procedure codes 30230G1, 30230Y1, 30233G1, 30233Y1, 30240G1, 30240Y1, 30243G1, 30243Y1, 30250G1,30250Y1, 30253G1, 30253Y1, 30260G1, 30260Y1, and 30263Y1

- If Outpatient Hospital or Professional Claims: HCPCS procedure code 38240

- If ICD-9-CM is applicable, ICD-9-CM diagnosis codes 238.72, 238.73, 238.74, 238.75 or,

- If ICD-10-CM is applicable, ICD-10-CM codes D46.A, D46.B, D46.C, D46.0, D46.1, D46.20, D46.21, D46.22, D46.4, D46.9, D46.Z,

- Professional claims only: place of service codes 19, 21, or 22.

Payable Conditions. For claims with dates of service on and after January 27, 2016, contractors shall pay for claims for allogeneic HSCT for multiple myeloma, myelofibrosis (MF), and for sickle cell disease (SCD) when the service was provided pursuant to a Medicare-approved clinical study under CED; these services are paid only in the inpatient setting (Type of Bill (TOB) 11X), as outpatient Part B (TOB 13X), and in Method II critical access hospitals (TOB 85X).

Contractors shall require the following coding in order to pay for these claims:

- Existing Medicare-approved clinical trial coding conventions, as required in Pub. 100-04, Medicare Claims Processing Manual, Chapter 32, section 69, and inpatient billing requirements regarding acquisition of stem cells in Pub. 100-04, Medicare Claims Processing Manual, Chapter 3, section 90.3.1.

- ICD-10-PCS codes 30230G1, 30230Y1, 30233G1, 30233Y1, 30240G1, 30240Y1, 30243G1, 30243Y1, 30250G1, 30250Y1, 30253G1, 30253Y1, 30260G1, 30260Y1, 30263G1, and 30263Y1

- If Outpatient Hospital or Professional Claims: HCPCS procedure code 38240

- ICD-10-CM diagnosis codes C90.00, C90.01, C90.02, C94.40, C94.41, C94.42, D47.4, D75.81, D57.00, D57.01, D57.02, D57.1, D57.20, D57.211, D57.212, D57.219, D57.40, D57.411, D57.412, D57.419, D57.80, D57.811, D57.812, and D57.819

- Professional claims only: place of service codes 19, 21, or 22.

Denials. Contractors shall deny claims failing to meet any of the above criteria. In addition, contractors shall apply the following requirements:

- Providers shall issue a hospital issued notice of non-coverage (HINN) or advance beneficiary notice (ABN) to the beneficiary if the services performed are not provided in accordance with CED.

- Contractors shall deny claims that do not meet the criteria for coverage with the following messages:

CARC 50 - These are non-covered services because this is not deemed a 'medical necessity' by the payer.

NOTE: Refer to the 835 Healthcare Policy Identification Segment (loop 2110 Service Payment Information REF), if present.

RARC N386 - This decision was based on a National Coverage Determination (NCD). An NCD provides a coverage determination as to whether a particular item or service is covered. A copy of this policy is available at http:www.cms.hhs.gov/mcd/search.asp. If you do not have web access, you may contact the contractor to request a copy of the NCD.

Group Code – Patient Responsibility (PR) if HINN/ABN issued, otherwise Contractual Obligation (CO)

MSN 16.77 – This service/item was not covered because it was not provided as part of a qualifying trial/study. (Este servicio/artículo no fue cubierto porque no estaba incluido como parte de un ensayo clínico/estudio calificado.)

MSN 15.20 – The following policies [NCD 110.23] were used when we made this decision. (Las siguientes políticas [NCD 110.23] fueron utilizadas cuando se tomó esta decisión.)

100-04, 32, 90.2

HCPCS and Diagnosis Coding
(Rev. 2998, Issued: 07-25-14, Effective: Upon implementation of ICD-10; 01-01-12 - ASC X12, Implementation: 08-25-2014 - ASC X12; Upon Implementation of ICD-10)

Allogeneic Stem Cell Transplantation
- Effective for services performed on or after August 1, 1978:

  — For the treatment of leukemia or leukemia in remission, providers shall use ICD-9-CM codes 204.00 through 208.91 and HCPCS code 38240.

  — For the treatment of aplastic anemia, providers shall use ICD-9-CM codes 284.0 through 284.9 and HCPCS code 38240.

- Effective for services performed on or after June 3, 1985:

  — For the treatment of severe combined immunodeficiency disease, providers shall use ICD-9-CM code 279.2 and HCPCS code 38240.

  — For the treatment of Wiskott-Aldrich syndrome, providers shall use ICD-9-CM code 279.12 and HCPCS code 38240.

- Effective for services performed on or after May 24, 1996:

  — Allogeneic stem cell transplantation, HCPCS code 38240 is not covered as treatment for the diagnosis of multiple myeloma ICD-9-CM codes 203.00 or 203.01.

Autologous Stem Cell Transplantation.--Is covered under the following circumstances effective for services performed on or after April 28, 1989:

- For the treatment of patients with acute leukemia in remission who have a high probability of relapse and who have no human leucocyte antigens (HLA) matched, providers shall use ICD-9-CM code 204.01 lymphoid; ICD-9-CM code 205.01 myeloid; ICD-9-CM code 206.01 monocytic; or ICD-9-CM code 207.01 acute erythremia and erythroleukemia; or ICD-9-CM code 208.01 unspecified cell type and HCPCS code 38241.

- For the treatment of resistant non-Hodgkin's lymphomas for those patients presenting with poor prognostic features following an initial response, providers shall use ICD-9-CM codes 200.00 - 200.08, 200.10-200.18, 200.20-200.28,

200.80-200.88, 202.00-202.08, 202.80-202.88 or 202.90-202.98 and HCPCS code 38241.

- For the treatment of recurrent or refractory neuroblastoma, providers shall use ICD-9-CM codes Neoplasm by site, malignant, the appropriate HCPCS code and HCPCS code 38241.

- For the treatment of advanced Hodgkin's disease for patients who have failed conventional therapy and have no HLA-matched donor, providers shall use ICD-9-CM codes 201.00 - 201.98 and HCPCS code 38241.

Autologous Stem Cell Transplantation.--Is covered under the following circumstances effective for services furnished on or after October 1, 2000:

- For the treatment of multiple myeloma (only for beneficiaries who are less than age 78, have Durie-Salmon stage II or III newly diagnosed or responsive multiple myeloma, and have adequate cardiac, renal, pulmonary and hepatic functioning), providers shall use ICD-9-CM code 203.00 or 238.6 and HCPCS code 38241.

- For the treatment of recurrent or refractory neuroblastoma, providers shall use appropriate code (see ICD-9-CM neoplasm by site, malignant) and HCPCS code 38241.

- Effective for services performed on or after March 15, 2005, when recognized clinical risk factors are employed to select patients for transplantation, high-dose melphalan (HDM) together with autologous stem cell transplantation (HDM/AuSCT) is reasonable and necessary for Medicare beneficiaries of any age group for the treatment of primary amyloid light chain (AL) amyloidosis, ICD-9-CM code 277.3 who meet the following criteria:

- Amyloid deposition in 2 or fewer organs; and,

- Cardiac left ventricular ejection fraction (EF) greater than 45%.

100-04, 32, 90.2.1

HCPCS and Diagnosis Coding for Stem Cell Transplantation - ICD-10-CM Applicable

(Rev. 2998, Issued: 07-25-14, Effective: Upon implementation of ICD-10; 01-01-12 - ASC X12, Implementation: 08-25-2014 - ASC X12; Upon Implementation of ICD-10)

ICD-10 is applicable to services on and after the implementation of ICD-.

For services provided use the appropriate code from the ICD-10 CM codes in the table below. See §90.2 for a list of covered conditions.

ICD-10	Description
C91.01	Acute lymphoblastic leukemia, in remission
C91.11	Chronic lymphocytic leukemia of B-cell type in remission
C91.31	Prolymphocytic leukemia of B-cell type, in remission
C91.51	Adult T-cell lymphoma/leukemia (HTLV-1-associated), in remission
C91.61	Prolymphocytic leukemia of T-cell type, in remission
C91.91	Lymphoid leukemia, unspecified, in remission
C91.A1	Mature B-cell leukemia Burkitt-type, in remission
C91.Z1	Other lymphoid leukemia, in remission
C92.01	Acute myeloblastic leukemia, in remission
C92.11	Chronic myeloid leukemia, BCR/ABL-positive, in remission
C92.21	Atypical chronic myeloid leukemia, BCR/ABL-negative, in remission
C92.31	Myeloid sarcoma, in remission
C92.41	Acute promyelocytic leukemia, in remission
C92.51	Acute myelomonocytic leukemia, in remission
C92.61	Acute myeloid leukemia with 11q23-abnormality in remission
C92.91	Myeloid leukemia, unspecified in remission
C92.A1	Acute myeloid leukemia with multilineage dysplasia, in remission
C92.Z1	Other myeloid leukemia, in remission
C93.01	Acute monoblastic/monocytic leukemia, in remission
C93.11	Chronic myelomonocytic leukemia, in remission
C93.31	Juvenile myelomonocytic leukemia, in remission
C93.91	Monocytic leukemia, unspecified in remission
C93.91	Monocytic leukemia, unspecified in remission
C93.Z1	Other monocytic leukemia, in remission
C94.01	Acute erythroid leukemia, in remission
C94.21	Acute megakaryoblastic leukemia, in remission
C94.31	Mast cell leukemia, in remission
C94.81	Other specified leukemias, in remission
C95.01	Acute leukemia of unspecified cell type, in remission
C95.11	Chronic leukemia of unspecified cell type, in remission
C95.91	Leukemia, unspecified, in remission
D45	Polycythemia vera
D61.01	Constitutional (pure) red blood cell aplasia
D61.09	Other constitutional aplastic anemia

ICD-10	Description
D82.0	Wiskott-Aldrich syndrome
D81.0	Severe combined immunodeficiency [SCID] with reticular dysgenesis
D81.1	Severe combined immunodeficiency [SCID] with low T- and B-cell numbers
D81.2	Severe combined immunodeficiency [SCID] with low or normal B-cell numbers
D81.6	Major histocompatibility complex class I deficiency
D81.7	Major histocompatibility complex class II deficiency
D81.89	Other combined immunodeficiencies
D81.9	Combined immunodeficiency, unspecified
D81.2	Severe combined immunodeficiency [SCID] with low or normal B-cell numbers
D81.6	Major histocompatibility complex class I deficiency
D60.0	Chronic acquired pure red cell aplasia
D60.1	Transient acquired pure red cell aplasia
D60.8	Other acquired pure red cell aplasias
D60.9	Acquired pure red cell aplasia, unspecified
D61.01	Constitutional (pure) red blood cell aplasia
D61.09	Other constitutional aplastic anemia
D61.1	Drug-induced aplastic anemia
D61.2	Aplastic anemia due to other external agents
D61.3	Idiopathic aplastic anemia
D61.810	Antineoplastic chemotherapy induced pancytopenia
D61.811	Other drug-induced pancytopenia
D61.818	Other pancytopenia
D61.82	Myelophthisis
D61.89	Other specified aplastic anemias and other bone marrow failure syndromes
D61.9	Aplastic anemia, unspecified

- If ICD-10-CM is applicable, the following ranges of ICD-10-CM codes are also covered for AuSCT: Resistant non-Hodgkin's lymphomas, ICD-10-CM diagnosis codes C82.00-C85.29, C85.80-C86.6, C96.4, and C96.Z-C96.9.

- Tandem transplantation (multiple rounds of autologous stem cell transplantation) for patients with multiple myeloma, ICD-10-CM codes C90.00 and D47.Z9

NOTE: The following conditions are not covered:

- Acute leukemia not in remission

- Chronic granulocytic leukemia

- Solid tumors (other than neuroblastoma)

- Multiple myeloma

- For Medicare beneficiaries age 64 or older, all forms of amyloidosis, primary and non-primary

- Non-primary amyloidosis

Also coverage for conditions other than those specifically designated as covered in §90.2 or specifically designated as non-covered in this section or in §90.3 will be at the discretion of the individual contractor.

100-04, 32, 90.3

Non-Covered Conditions

(Rev. 2998, Issued: 07-25-14, Effective: Upon implementation of ICD-10; 01-01-12 - ASC X12, Implementation: 08-25-2014 - ASC X12; Upon Implementation of ICD-10)

Autologous stem cell transplantation is not covered for the following conditions:

- Acute leukemia not in remission (If ICD-9-CM is applicable, ICD-9-CM codes 204.00, 205.00, 206.00, 207.00 and 208.00) or (If ICD-10-CM is applicable, ICD-10-CM codes C91.00, C92.00, C93.00, C94.00, and C95.00)

- Chronic granulocytic leukemia (ICD-9-CM codes 205.10 and 205.11 if ICD-9-CM is applicable) or (if ICD-10-CM is applicable, ICD-10-CM codes C92.10 and C92.11);

- Solid tumors (other than neuroblastoma) (ICD-9-CM codes 140.0 through 199.1 if ICD-9-CM is applicable or if ICD-10-CM is applicable, ICD-10-CM codes C00.0 – C80.2 and D00.0 – D09.9.)

- Effective for services rendered on or after May 24, 1996 through September 30, 2000, multiple myeloma (ICD-9-CM code 203.00 and 203.01 if ICD-9-CM is applicable or if ICD-10-CM is applicable, ICD-10-CM codes C90.00 and D47.Z9);

- Effective for services on or after October 1, 2000, through March 14, 2005, for Medicare beneficiaries age 64 or older, all forms of amyloidosis, primary and non-primary

- Effective for services on or after 10/01/00, for all Medicare beneficiaries, non-primary amyloidosis

ICD-9-CM	Description	ICD-10-CM	Description
277.30	Amyloidosis, unspecified	E85.9	Amyloidosis, unspecified
277.31	Familial Mediterranean fever	E85.0	Non-neuropathic heredofamilial amyloidosis
277.39	Other amyloidosis	E85.1	Neuropathic heredofamilial amyloidosis
277.39	Other amyloidosis	E85.2	Heredofamilial amyloidosis, unspecified
277.39	Other amyloidosis	E85.3	Secondary systemic amyloidosis
277.39	Other amyloidosis	E85.4	Organ-limited amyloidosis
277.39	Other amyloidosis	E85.8	Other amyloidosis

NOTE: Coverage for conditions other than those specifically designated as covered in 90.2 or 90.2.1 or specifically designated as non-covered in this section will be at the discretion of the individual A/B MAC (B).

100-04, 32, 90.4

Edits

(Rev. 2998, Issued: 07-25-14, Effective: Upon implementation of ICD-10; 01-01-12 - ASC X12, Implementation: 08-25-2014 - ASC X12; Upon Implementation of ICD-10)

NOTE: Coverage for conditions other than those specifically designated as covered in 80.2 or specifically designated as non-covered in this section will be at the discretion of the individual A/B MAC (B).

Appropriate diagnosis to procedure code edits should be implemented for the non-covered conditions and services in 90.2 90.2.1, and 90.3 as applicable.

As the ICD-9-CM code 277.3 for amyloidosis does not differentiate between primary and non-primary, A/B MACs (B) should perform prepay reviews on all claims with a diagnosis of ICD-9-CM code 277.3 and a HCPCS procedure code of 38241 to determine whether payment is appropriate.

If ICD-10-CM is applicable, the applicable ICD-10 CM codes are: E85.0, E85.1, E85.2, E85.3, E85.4, E85.8, and E85.9.

100-04, 32, 90.6

Clinical Trials for Allogeneic Hematopoietic Stem Cell Transplantation (HSCT) for Myelodysplastic Syndrome (MDS)

(Rev. 2998, Issued: 07-25-14, Effective: Upon implementation of ICD-10; 01-01-12 - ASC X12, Implementation: 08-25-2014 - ASC X12; Upon Implementation of ICD-10)

A. Background
Myelodysplastic Syndrome (MDS) refers to a group of diverse blood disorders in which the bone marrow does not produce enough healthy, functioning blood cells. These disorders are varied with regard to clinical characteristics, cytologic and pathologic features, and cytogenetics.

On August 4, 2010, the Centers for Medicare & Medicaid Services (CMS) issued a national coverage determination (NCD) stating that CMS believes that the evidence does not demonstrate that the use of allogeneic hematopoietic stem cell transplantation (HSCT) improves health outcomes in Medicare beneficiaries with MDS. Therefore, allogeneic HSCT for MDS is not reasonable and necessary under §1862(a)(1)(A) of the Social Security Act (the Act). However, allogeneic HSCT for MDS is reasonable and necessary under §1862(a)(1)(E) of the Act and therefore covered by Medicare ONLY if provided pursuant to a Medicare-approved clinical study under Coverage with Evidence Development (CED). Refer to Pub.100-3, NCD Manual, Chapter 1, section 110.8.1, for more information about this policy, and Pub. 100-4, MCP Manual, Chapter 3, section 90.3.1, for information on CED.

B. Adjudication Requirements
Payable Conditions. For claims with dates of service on and after August 4, 2010, contractors shall pay for claims for HSCT for MDS when the service was provided pursuant to a Medicare-approved clinical study under CED; these services are paid only in the inpatient setting (Type of Bill (TOB) 11X), as outpatient Part B (TOB 13X), and in Method II critical access hospitals (TOB 85X). Contractors shall require the following coding in order to pay for these claims:

- Existing Medicare-approved clinical trial coding conventions, as required in Pub. 100-4, MCP Manual, Chapter 32, section 69, and inpatient billing requirements regarding acquisition of stem cells in Pub. 100-4, MCP Manual, Chapter 3, section 90.3.3.
- If ICD-9-CM is applicable, for Inpatient Hospital Claims: ICD-9-CM procedure codes 41.02, 41.03, 41.05, and 41.08 or,
- If ICD-10-CM is applicable, ICD-10-PCS, procedure codes 30230G1, 30230Y1, 3023G1, 30233Y1, 30240G1, 30240Y1, 30243G1, 30243Y1, 30250G1,30250Y1, 30253G1, 30253Y1, 30260G1, 30260Y1, 30263G1, and 30263Y1
- If Outpatient Hospital or Professional Claims: HCPCS procedure code 38240
- If ICD-9-CM is applicable, ICD-9-CM diagnosis code 238.75 or If ICD-10-CM is applicable, ICD-10-CM diagnosis codes D46.9, D46.Z, or Z00.6 Professional claims only: place of service codes 21 or 22.

Denials. Contractors shall deny claims failing to meet any of the above criteria. In addition, contractors shall apply the following requirements:

- Providers shall issue a hospital issued notice of non-coverage (HINN) or advance beneficiary notice (ABN) to the beneficiary if the services performed are not provided in accordance with CED.
- Contractors shall deny claims that do not meet the criteria for coverage with the following messages:

CARC 50 - These are non-covered services because this is not deemed a 'medical necessity' by the payer.

NOTE: Refer to the 835 Healthcare Policy Identification Segment (loop 2110 Service Payment Information REF), if present.

RARC N386 - This decision was based on a National Coverage Determination (NCD). An NCD provides a coverage determination as to whether a particular item or service is covered. A copy of this policy is available at http://www.cms.hhs.gov/mcd/search.asp. If you do not have web access, you may contact the contractor to request a copy of the NCD.

Group Code – Patient Responsibility (PR) if HINN/ABN issued, otherwise Contractual Obligation (CO)

MSN 16.77 – This service/item was not covered because it was not provided as part of a qualifying trial/study. (Este servicio/artículo no fue cubierto porque no estaba incluido como parte de un ensayo clínico/estudio calificado.)

100-04, 32, 120.2

Coding and General Billing Requirements

(Rev. 1430; Issued: 02-01-08; Effective: 01-01-08; Implementation: 03-03-08)

Physicians and hospitals must report one of the following Current Procedural Terminology (CPT) codes on the claim:

66982 Extracapsular cataract removal with insertion of intraocular lens prosthesis (one stage procedure), manual or mechanical technique (e.g., irrigation and aspiration or phacoemulsification), complex requiring devices or techniques not generally used in routine cataract surgery (e.g., iris expansion device, suture support for intraocular lens, or primary posterior capsulorrhexis) or performed on patients in the amblyogenic development stage.

66983 Intracapsular cataract with insertion of intraocular lens prosthesis (one stage procedure)

66984 Extracapsular cataract removal with insertion of intraocular lens prosthesis (one stage procedure), manual or mechanical technique (e.g., irrigation and aspiration or phacoemulsification)

66985 Insertion of intraocular lens prosthesis (secondary implant), not associated with concurrent cataract extraction

66986 Exchange of intraocular lens

In addition, physicians inserting a P-C IOL or A-C IOL in an office setting may bill code V2632 (posterior chamber intraocular lens) for the IOL. Medicare will make payment for the lens based on reasonable cost for a conventional IOL. Place of Service (POS) = 11.

Effective for dates of service on and after January 1, 2006, physician, hospitals and ASCs may also bill the non-covered charges related to the P-C function of the IOL using HCPCS code V2788. Effective for dates of service on and after January 22, 2007 through January 1, 2008, non-covered charges related to A-C function of the IOL can be billed using HCPCS code V2788. The type of service indicator for the non-covered billed charges is Q. (The type of service is applied by the Medicare carrier and not the provider). Effective for A-C IOL insertion services on or after January 1, 2008, physicians, hospitals and ASCs should use V2787 rather than V2788 to report any additional charges that accrue.

When denying the non-payable charges submitted with V2787 or V2788, contractors shall use an appropriate Medical Summary Notice (MSN) such as 16.10 (Medicare does not pay for this item or service) and an appropriate claim adjustment reason code such as 96 (non-covered charges) for claims submitted with the non-payable charges.

Hospitals and physicians may use the proper CPT code(s) to bill Medicare for evaluation and management services usually associated with services following cataract extraction surgery, if appropriate.

A - Applicable Bill Types
The hospital applicable bill types are 12X, 13X, 83X and 85X.

B - Other Special Requirements for Hospitals
Hospitals shall continue to pay CAHs method 2 claims under current payment methodologies for conditional IOLs.

100-04, 32, 130.1

Billing and Payment Requirements

(Rev. 898, Issued: 03-31-06; Effective/Implementation Dates: 03-31-06)

Effective for dates of service on or after January 1, 2000, use HCPCS code G0166 (External counterpulsation, per session) to report ECP services. The codes for external cardiac assist (92971), ECG rhythm strip and report (93040 or 93041), pulse oximetry (94760 or 94761) and plethysmography (93922 or 93923) or other monitoring tests for examining the effects of this treatment are not clinically necessary with this service and should not be paid on the same day, unless they occur in a clinical setting not connected with the delivery of the ECP. Daily evaluation and management service, e.g., 99201-99205, 99211-99215, 99217-99220, 99241-99245, cannot be billed with the ECP treatments. Any evaluation and management service must be justified with adequate documentation of the medical necessity of the visit. Deductible and coinsurance apply.

100-04, 32, 140.2

Cardiac Rehabilitation Program Services Furnished On or After January 1, 2010

(Rev. 3058, Issued: 08-29-14, Effective: 02-18-14, Implementation: 08-18-14)

As specified at 42 CFR 410.49, Medicare covers cardiac rehabilitation items and services for patients who have experienced one or more of the following:

- An acute myocardial infarction within the preceding 12 months; or
- A coronary artery bypass surgery; or
- Current stable angina pectoris; or
- Heart valve repair or replacement; or
- Percutaneous transluminal coronary angioplasty (PTCA) or coronary stenting; or
- A heart or heart-lung transplant or;
- Stable, chronic heart failure defined as patients with left ventricular ejection fraction of 35% or less and New York Heart Association (NYHA) class II to IV symptoms despite being on optimal heart failure therapy for at least 6 weeks (effective February 18, 2014).

Cardiac rehabilitation programs must include the following components:

- Physician-prescribed exercise each day cardiac rehabilitation items and services are furnished;
- Cardiac risk factor modification, including education, counseling, and behavioral intervention at least once during the program, tailored to patients' individual needs;
- Psychosocial assessment;
- Outcomes assessment; and
- An individualized treatment plan detailing how components are utilized for each patient.

Cardiac rehabilitation items and services must be furnished in a physician's office or a hospital outpatient setting. All settings must have a physician immediately available and accessible for medical consultations and emergencies at all times items and services are being furnished under the program. This provision is satisfied if the physician meets the requirements for the direct supervision of physician's office services as specified at 42 CFR 410.26 and for hospital outpatient therapeutic services as specified at 42 CFR 410.27.

As specified at 42 CFR 410.49(f)(1), cardiac rehabilitation program sessions are limited to a maximum of 2 1-hour sessions per day for up to 36 sessions over up to 36 weeks, with the option for an additional 36 sessions over an extended period of time if approved by the Medicare contractor.

100-04, 32, 140.2.1

Coding Requirements for Cardiac Rehabilitation Services Furnished On or After January 1, 2010

(Rev. 1882, Issued: 12-21-09; Effective Date: 01-01-10; Implementation Date: 01-04-10)

The following are the applicable CPT codes for cardiac rehabilitation services: 93797 - Physician services for outpatient cardiac rehabilitation; without continuous ECG monitoring (per session) and 93798 - Physician services for outpatient cardiac rehabilitation; with continuous ECG monitoring (per session) Effective for dates of service on or after January 1, 2010, hospitals and practitioners may report a maximum of 2 1-hour sessions per day. In order to report one session of cardiac rehabilitation services in a day, the duration of treatment must be at least 31 minutes. Two sessions of cardiac rehabilitation services may only be reported in the same day if the duration of treatment is at least 91 minutes. In other words, the first session would account for 60 minutes and the second session would account for at least 31 minutes if two sessions are reported. If several shorter periods of cardiac rehabilitation services are furnished on a given day, the minutes of service during those periods must be added together for reporting in 1-hour session increments.

Example: If the patient receives 20 minutes of cardiac rehabilitation services in the day, no cardiac rehabilitation session may be reported because less than 31 minutes of services were furnished.

Example: If a patient receives 20 minutes of cardiac rehabilitation services in the morning and 35 minutes of cardiac rehabilitation services in the afternoon of a single day, the hospital or practitioner would report 1 session of cardiac rehabilitation services under 1 unit of the appropriate CPT code for the total duration of 55 minutes of cardiac rehabilitation services on that day.

Example: If the patient receives 70 minutes of cardiac rehabilitation services in the morning and 25 minutes of cardiac rehabilitation services in the afternoon of a single day, the hospital or practitioner would report two sessions of cardiac rehabilitation

services under the appropriate CPT code(s) because the total duration of cardiac rehabilitation services on that day of 95 minutes exceeds 90 minutes.

Example: If the patient receives 70 minutes of cardiac rehabilitation services in the morning and 85 minutes of cardiac rehabilitation services in the afternoon of a single day, the hospital or practitioner would report two sessions of cardiac rehabilitation services under the appropriate CPT code(s) for the total duration of cardiac rehabilitation services of 155 minutes. A maximum of two sessions per day may be reported, regardless of the total duration of cardiac rehabilitation services.

100-04, 32, 140.2.2.2

Requirements for CR and ICR Services on Institutional Claims

(Rev. 3084, Issued: 10-03-14, Effective: 05-06-14, Implementation: 11-04-14)

Effective for claims with dates of service on and after January 1, 2010, contractors shall pay for CR and ICR services when submitted on Types of Bill (TOBs) 13X and 85X only. All other TOBs shall be denied.

The following messages shall be used when contractors deny CR and ICR claims for TOBs 13X and 85X:

Claim Adjustment Reason Code (CARC) 171 – Payment is denied when performed/billed by this type of provider in this type of facility.

Remittance Advice Remark Code (RARC) N428 - Service/procedure not covered when performed in this place of service.

Medicare Summary Notice (MSN) 21.25 - This service was denied because Medicare only covers this service in certain settings.

Group Code PR (Patient Responsibility) – Where a claim is received with the GA modifier indicating that a signed ABN is on file.

Group Code CO (Contractor Responsibility) – Where a claim is received with the GZ modifier indicating that no signed ABN is on file.

100-04, 32, 140.2.2.4

Edits for CR Services Exceeding 36 Sessions

(Rev. 3058, Issued: 08-29-14, Effective: 02-18-14, Implementation: 08-18-14)

Effective for claims with dates of service on or after January 1, 2010, contractors shall deny all claims with HCPCS 93797 and 93798 (both professional and institutional claims) that exceed 36 CR sessions when a KX modifier is not included on the claim line.

The following messages shall be used when contractors deny CR claims that exceed 36 sessions, when a KX modifier is not included on the claim line:

Claim Adjustment Reason Code (CARC) 119 – Benefit maximum for this period or occurrence has been reached.

RARC N435 - Exceeds number/frequency approved/allowed within time period without support documentation.

MSN 23.17- Medicare won't cover these services because they are not considered medically necessary.

Spanish Version - Medicare no cubrirá estos servicios porque no son considerados necesarios por razones médicas.

Group Code PR (Patient Responsibility) – Where a claim is received with the GA modifier indicating that a signed ABN is on file.

Group Code CO (Contractor Responsibility) – Where a claim is received with the GZ modifier indicating that no signed ABN is on file.

Contractors shall not research and adjust CR claims paid for more than 36 sessions processed prior to the implementation of CWF edits. However, contractors may adjust claims brought to their attention.

100-04, 32, 140.3

Intensive Cardiac Rehabilitation Program Services Furnished On or After January 1, 2010

(Rev. 4222, Issued: 02-01-19, Effective: 02-09-18, Implementation: 03-19-19)

As specified at 42 CFR 410.49, Medicare covers intensive cardiac rehabilitation items and services for patients who have experienced one or more of the following:

- An acute myocardial infarction within the preceding 12 months;
- A coronary artery bypass surgery;
- Current stable angina pectoris;
- Heart valve repair or replacement;
- Percutaneous transluminal coronary angioplasty or coronary stenting;
- A heart or heart-lung transplant.

Effective February 9, 2018, section 51004 of the Bipartisan Budget Act (BBA) of 2018, Pub. L. No. 115-123 (2018), amended section 1861(eee)(4)(B) of the Social Security Act to expand coverage in an intensive cardiac rehabilitation program to additional conditions:

- Stable, chronic heart failure defined as patients with left ventricular ejection fraction of 35% or less and New York Heart Association (NYHA) class II to IV symptoms despite being on optimal heart failure therapy for at least 6 weeks; or

- Any additional condition for which the Secretary has determined that a cardiac rehabilitation program shall be covered, unless the Secretary determines, using the same process used to determine that the condition is covered for a cardiac rehabilitation program, that such coverage is not supported by the clinical evidence.

NOTE: CMS plans to amend our intensive cardiac rehabilitation regulations specified at 42 CFR 410.49 to reflect this expanded coverage. CMS anticipates that the changes will be included in the 2020 Medicare Physician Fee Schedule notice of proposed rulemaking. However, because the expanded coverage under the statutory change was effective on enactment, expanded coverage for these conditions will be made effective for services furnished on or after February 9, 2018.

Intensive cardiac rehabilitation programs must include the following components:

- Physician-prescribed exercise each day cardiac rehabilitation items and services are furnished;

- Cardiac risk factor modification, including education, counseling, and behavioral intervention at least once during the program, tailored to patients' individual needs;

- Psychosocial assessment;

- Outcomes assessment; and,

- An individualized treatment plan detailing how components are utilized for each patient.

Intensive cardiac rehabilitation programs must be approved by Medicare. In order to be approved, a program must demonstrate through peer-reviewed published research that it has accomplished one or more of the following for its patients:

- Positively affected the progression of coronary heart disease;

- Reduced the need for coronary bypass surgery; and,

- Reduced the need for percutaneous coronary interventions.

An intensive cardiac rehabilitation program must also demonstrate through peer-reviewed published research that it accomplished a statistically significant reduction in five or more of the following measures for patients from their levels before cardiac rehabilitation services to after cardiac rehabilitation services:

- Low density lipoprotein;

- Triglycerides;

- Body mass index;

- Systolic blood pressure;

- Diastolic blood pressure; and,

- The need for cholesterol, blood pressure, and diabetes medications.

Intensive cardiac rehabilitation items and services must be furnished in a physician's office or a hospital outpatient setting. All settings must have a physician immediately available and accessible for medical consultations and emergencies at all times items and services are being furnished under the program. This provision is satisfied if the physician meets the requirements for direct supervision of physician office services as specified at 42 CFR 410.26 and for hospital outpatient therapeutic services as specified at 42 CFR 410.27. As specified at 42 CFR 410.49(f)(2), ICR program sessions are limited to 72 1-hour sessions, up to 6 sessions per day, over a period of up to 18 weeks.

100-04, 32, 150.1

Bariatric Surgery for Treatment of Co-Morbid Conditions Related to Morbid Obesity

(Rev. 2841, Issued: 12-23-13, Effective: 09-24-13, Implementation: 12-17-13)

Effective for services on or after February 21, 2006, Medicare has determined that the following bariatric surgery procedures are reasonable and necessary under certain conditions for the treatment of morbid obesity. The patient must have a body-mass index (BMI) =35, have at least one co-morbidity related to obesity, and have been previously unsuccessful with medical treatment for obesity. This medical information must be documented in the patient's medical record. In addition, the procedure must be performed at an approved facility. A list of approved facilities may be found at http://www.cms.gov/Medicare/Medicare-General-Information/MedicareApprovedFacilitie/Bariatric-Surgery.html

Effective for services performed on and after February 12, 2009, Medicare has determined that Type 2 diabetes mellitus is a co-morbidity for purposes of processing bariatric surgery claims.

Effective for dates of service on and after September 24, 2013, the Centers for Medicare & Medicaid Services (CMS) has removed the certified facility requirements for Bariatric Surgery for Treatment of Co-Morbid Conditions Related to Morbid Obesity.

Please note the additional national coverage determinations related to bariatric surgery will be consolidated and subsumed into Publication 100-3, Chapter 1, section 100.1. These include sections 40.5, 100.8, 100.11 and 100.14.

- Open Roux-en-Y gastric bypass (RYGBP)

- Laparoscopic Roux-en-Y gastric bypass (RYGBP)

- Laparoscopic adjustable gastric banding (LAGB)

- Open biliopancreatic diversion with duodenal switch (BPD/DS) or gastric reduction duodenal switch (BPD/GRDS)

- Laparoscopic biliopancreatic diversion with duodenal switch (BPD/DS) or gastric reduction duodenal switch (BPD/GRDS)

- Laparoscopic sleeve gastrectomy (LSG) (Effective June 27, 2012, covered at Medicare Administrative Contractor (MAC) discretion.

100-04, 32, 150.2

HCPCS Procedure Codes for Bariatric Surgery

(Rev. 2641, Issued: 01-29-13, Effective: 06-27-12, Implementation: 02-28-13)

A. Covered HCPCS Procedure Codes

For services on or after February 21, 2006, the following HCPCS procedure codes are covered for bariatric surgery:

43770 Laparoscopy, surgical, gastric restrictive procedure; placement of adjustable gastric band (gastric band and subcutaneous port components).

43644 Laparoscopy, surgical, gastric restrictive procedure; with gastric bypass and Roux-en-Y gastroenterostomy (roux limb 150 cm or less).

43645 Laparoscopy with gastric bypass and small intestine reconstruction to limit absorption. (Do not report 43645 in conjunction with 49320, 43847.)

43845 Gastric restrictive procedure with partial gastrectomy, pylorus-preserving duodenoileostomy and ileoieostomy (50 to 100 cm common channel) to limit absorption (biliopancreatic diversion with duodenal switch).

43846 Gastric restrictive procedure, with gastric bypass for morbid obesity; with short limb (150 cm or less Roux-en-Y gastroenterostomy. (For greater than 150 cm, use 43847.) (For laparoscopic procedure, use 43644.)

43847 With small intestine reconstruction to limit absorption.

43775 Laparoscopy, surgical, gastric restrictive procedure; longitudinal gastrectomy (i.e., sleeve gastrectomy) (Effective June 27, 2012, covered at contractor's discretion.)

B. Noncovered HCPCS Procedure Codes

For services on or after February 21, 2006, the following HCPCS procedure codes are non-covered for bariatric surgery:

43842 Gastric restrictive procedure, without gastric bypass, for morbid obesity; vertical banded gastroplasty.

NOC code 43999 used to bill for:

Laparoscopic vertical banded gastroplasty

Open sleeve gastrectomy

Laparoscopic sleeve gastrectomy (for contractor non-covered instances)

Open adjustable gastric banding

100-04, 32, 150.5

ICD Diagnosis Codes for BMI Greater Than or Equal to 35

(Rev. 2841, Issued: 12-23-13, Effective: 09-24-13, Implementation: 12-17-13)

The following ICD-9 diagnosis codes identify BMI >=35 :

V85.35 - Body Mass Index 35.0-35.9, adult

V85.36 - Body Mass Index 36.0-36.9, adult

V85.37 - Body Mass Index 37.0-37.9, adult

V85.38 - Body Mass Index 38.0-38.9, adult

V85.39 - Body Mass Index 39.0-39.9, adult

V85.41 - Body Mass Index 40.0-44.9, adult

V85.42 - Body Mass Index 45.0-49.9, adult

V85.43 - Body Mass Index 50.0-59.9, adult

V85.44 - Body Mass Index 60.0-69.9, adult

V85.45 - Body Mass Index 70.0 and over, adult

The following ICD-10 diagnosis codes identify BMI >=35:

Z6835 - Body Mass Index 35.0-35.9, adult

Z6836 - Body Mass Index 36.0-36.9, adult.

Z6837 - Body Mass Index 37.0-37.9, adult

Z6838 - Body Mass Index 38.0-38.9, adult

Z6839 - Body Mass Index 39.0-39.9, adult

Z6841 - Body Mass Index 40.0-44.9, adult

Z6842 - Body Mass Index 45.0-49.9, adult

Z6843 - Body Mass Index 50.0-59.9, adult

Z6844 - Body Mass Index 60.0-69.9, adult

Z6845 - Body Mass Index 70.0 and over, adult

100-04, 32, 150.6

Claims Guidance for Payment

(Rev. 2841, Issued: 12-23-13, Effective: 09-24-13, Implementation: 12-17-13)

Covered Bariatric Surgery Procedures for Treatment of Co-Morbid Conditions Related to Morbid Obesity

Contractors shall process covered bariatric surgery claims as follows:

1. Identify bariatric surgery claims.

    Contractors identify inpatient bariatric surgery claims by the presence of ICD-9/ICD-10 diagnosis code 278.01/E66.01as the primary diagnosis (for morbid obesity) and one of the covered ICD-9/ICD-10 procedure codes listed in §150.3.

    Contractors identify practitioner bariatric surgery claims by the presence of ICD-9/ICD-10 diagnosis code 278.01/E66.01 as the primary diagnosis (for morbid obesity) and one of the covered HCPCS procedure codes listed in §150.2.

2. Perform facility certification validation for all bariatric surgery claims on a pre-pay basis up to and including date of service September 23, 2013.

    A list of approved facilities are found at the link noted in section 150.1, section A, above.

3. Review bariatric surgery claims data and determine whether a pre- or post-pay sample of bariatric surgery claims need further review to assure that the beneficiary has a BMI =35 (V85.35-V85.45/Z68.35-Z68.45) (see ICD-10 equivalents above in section 150.5), and at least one co-morbidity related to obesity

    The A/B MAC medical director may define the appropriate method for addressing the obesity-related co-morbid requirement.

    Effective for dates of service on and after September 24, 2013, CMS has removed the certified facility requirements for Bariatric Surgery for Treatment of Co-Morbid Conditions Related to Morbid Obesity.

NOTE: If ICD-9/ICD-10 diagnosis code 278.01/E66.01 is present, but a covered procedure code (listed in §150.2 or §150.3) is/are not present, the claim is not for bariatric surgery and should be processed under normal procedures.

100-04, 32, 161

Intracranial Percutaneous Transluminal Angioplasty (PTA) With Stenting

(Rev. 2998, Issued: 07-25-14, Effective: Upon implementation of ICD-10; 01-01-12 - ASC X12, Implementation: 08-25-2014 - ASC X12; Upon Implementation of ICD-10)

A. Background

In the past, PTA to treat obstructive lesions of the cerebral arteries was non-covered by Medicare because the safety and efficacy of the procedure had not been established. This national coverage determination (NCD) meant that the procedure was also non-covered for beneficiaries participating in Food and Drug Administration (FDA)-approved investigational device exemption (IDE) clinical trials.

B. Policy

On February 9, 2006, a request for reconsideration of this NCD initiated a national coverage analysis. CMS reviewed the evidence and determined that intracranial PTA with stenting is reasonable and necessary under §1862(a)(1)(A) of the Social Security Act for the treatment of cerebral vessels (as specified in The National Coverage Determinations Manual, Chapter 1, part 1, section 20.7) only when furnished in accordance with FDA-approved protocols governing Category B IDE clinical trials. All other indications for intracranial PTA with stenting remain non-covered.

C. Billing

Providers of covered intracranial PTA with stenting shall use Category B IDE billing requirements, as listed above in section 68.4. In addition to these requirements, providers must bill the appropriate procedure and diagnosis codes for the date of service to receive payment. That is, under Part A, providers must bill intracranial PTA using ICD-9-CM procedure codes 00.62 and 00.65, if ICD-9-CM is applicable, or, if ICD-10-PCS is applicable, ICD-10-PCS procedure codes 037G34Z, 037G3DZ, 037G3ZZ, 037G44Z, 037G4DZ, 037G4ZZ, 03CG3ZZ, 057L3DZ, 057L4DZ and 05CL3ZZ. ICD-9-CM diagnosis code 437.0 or ICD-10-CM diagnosis code 167.2applies, depending on the date of service.

Under Part B, providers must bill HCPCS procedure code 37799. If ICD-9-CM is applicable ICD-9-CM diagnosis code 437.0 or if ICD-10-CM is applicable,ICD-10-CM diagnosis code 167.2 applies.

NOTE: ICD- codes are subject to modification. Providers must always ensure they are using the latest and most appropriate codes.

100-04, 32, 190

Billing Requirements for Extracorporeal Photopheresis

(Rev. 3050, Issued: 08-22-14, Effective: 09-23-14, ICD-10: Upon Implementation of ICD-10, Implementation: 09-23-14, ICD-10: Upon Implementation of ICD-10)

Effective for dates of services on and after December 19, 2006, Medicare has expanded coverage for extracorporeal photopheresis for patients with acute cardiac

allograft rejection whose disease is refractory to standard immunosuppresive drug treatment and patients with chronic graft versus host disease whose disease is refractory to standard immunosuppresive drug treatment. (See Pub. 100-3, chapter 1, section 110.4, for complete coverage guidelines).

Effective for claims with dates of service on or after April 30, 2012, CMS has expanded coverage for extracorporeal photopheresis for the treatment of BOS following lung allograft transplantation only when extracorporeal photopheresis is provided under a clinical research study that meets specific requirements to assess the effect of extracorporeal photopheresis for the treatment of BOS following lung allograft transplantation. Further coverage criteria is outlined in Publication 100-3, Section 110.4 of the NCD.

100-04, 32, 190.2

Healthcare Common Procedural Coding System (HCPCS), Applicable Diagnosis Codes and Procedure Code

(Rev. 3050, Issued: 08-22-14, Effective: 09-23-14, ICD-10: Upon Implementation of ICD-10, Implementation: 09-23-14, ICD-10: Upon Implementation of ICD-10)

The following HCPCS procedure code is used for billing extracorporeal photopheresis:

*   36522 - Photopheresis, extracorporeal

The following are the applicable ICD-9-CM diagnosis codes for the new expanded coverage:

*   996.83 - Complications of transplanted heart, or,
*   996.85 - Complications of transplanted bone marrow, or,
*   996.88 - Complications of transplanted organ, stem cell

Effective for services for BOS following lung allograft transplantation the following is a list of applicable ICD-9-CM diagnosis codes:

*   996.84 - Complications of transplanted lung
*   491.9 - Unspecified chronic bronchitis
*   491.20 – Obstructive chronic bronchitis without exacerbation
*   491.21 – Obstructive chronic bronchitis with (acute) exacerbation
*   496 – Chronic airway obstruction, not elsewhere classified

The following is the applicable ICD-9-CM procedure code for the new expanded coverage:

*   99.88 - Therapeutic photopheresis

NOTE: Contractors shall edit for an appropriate oncological and autoimmune disorder diagnosis for payment of extracorporeal photopheresis according to the NCD.

Effective for claims with dates of service on or after April 30, 2012, in addition to HCPCS 36522, the following ICD-9-CM codes are applicable for extracorporeal photopheresis for the treatment of BOS following lung allograft transplantation only when extracorporeal photopheresis is provided under a clinical research study as outlined in Section 190 above:

A reference listing of ICD-9 CM and ICD-10-CM coding and descriptions is listed V70.7 below:

ICD9	Long Description	ICD10	ICD10 Description
491.20	Obstructive chronic	J44.9	Chronic obstructive bronchitis without exacerbation pulmonary disease, unspecified
491.21	Obstructive chronic bronchitis with (acute) exacerbation	J44.1	Chronic obstructive pulmonary disease with (acute) exacerbation
491.9	Unspecified chronic bronchitis	J42	Unspecified chronic bronchitis
496	Chronic airway obstruction, not elsewhere classified	J44.9	Chronic obstructive pulmonary disease, unspecified
996.84	Complications of transplanted lung	T86.810	Lung transplant rejection
996.84	Complications of transplanted lung	T86.811	Lung transplant failure
996.84	Complications of transplanted lung	T86.812	Lung transplant infection (not recommended for extracorporeal photopheresis coverage)
996.84	Complications of transplanted lung	T86.818	Other complications of lung transplant
996.84	Complications of transplanted lung	T86.819	Unspecified complication of lung transplant
996.88	Complications of Transplanted organ, Stem cell	T86.5	Complications of Stem Cell Transplant
V70.7	Examination of participant in clinical trial	Z00.6	Encounter for examination for normal comparison and control in clinical research program (needed for CED)

Contractors must also report modifier Q0 - (investigational clinical service provided in a clinical research study that is in an approved research study) or Q1 (routine clinical service provided in a clinical research study that is in an approved clinical research study) as appropriate on these claims. Contractors must use diagnosis code V70.7/Z00.6 and condition code 30 (A/B MAC (A) only), along with value code D4 and the 8-digit clinical identifier number (A/MACs only) for these claims.

100-04, 32, 190.3

Medicare Summary Notices (MSNs), Remittance Advice Remark Codes (RAs) and Claim Adjustment Reason Code

(Rev. 3050, Issued: 08-22-14, Effective: 09-23-14, ICD-10: Upon Implementation of ICD-10, Implementat)

Contractors shall continue to use the appropriate existing messages that they have in place when denying claims submitted that do not meet the Medicare coverage criteria for extracorporeal photopheresis.

Medicare coverage for extracorporeal photopheresis is restricted to the inpatient or outpatient hospital settings specifically for BOS, and not for the other covered diagnosis (including chronic graft versus host disease) which remain covered in the hospital inpatient, hospital outpatient, and non-facility (physician-directed clinic or office settings) settings.

Contractors shall deny claims for extracorporeal photopheresis for BOS when the service is not rendered to an inpatient or outpatient of a hospital, including critical access hospitals using the following codes:

- Claim Adjustment Reason Code (CARC) 96 – Non-covered charge(s). At least one Remark Code must be provided (may be comprised of either the NCPDP Reject Reason [sic] Code, or Remittance Advice Remark Code that is not an ALERT.) NOTE: Refer to the 835 Healthcare Policy Identification Segment (loop 2110 Service Payment Information REF), if present.

- CARC 171 – Payment is denied when performed/billed by this type of provider in this type of facility. NOTE: Refer to the 835 Healthcare Policy Identification Segment (loop 2110 Service Payment Information REF), if present.

- Medicare Summary Notice 16.2 - This service cannot be paid when provided in this location/facility." Spanish translation: "Este servicio no se puede pagar cuando es suministrado en esta sitio/facilidad. (Include either MSN 36.1 or 36.2 dependent on liability.)

- Remittance Advice Remark Code (RARC) N428 – Not covered when performed in this place of service. (A/MACs only) Group Code CO (Contractual Obligations) or PR (Patient Responsibility) dependent on liability.

Contractors shall return to provider/ return as unprocessable claims for BOS containing HCPCS procedure code 36522 along with one of the following ICD-9-CM diagnosis codes: 996.84, 491.9, 491.20, 491.21, and 496 but is missing diagnosis code V70.7 (as primary/secondary diagnosis, institutional only), condition code 30 (institutional claims only), clinical trial modifier Q0/Q1, and value code D4 with an 8-digit clinical trial identifier number (A/MACs only). Use the following messages:

- CARC 4 – The procedure code is inconsistent with the modifier used or a required modifier is missing. NOTE: Refer to the 835 Healthcare Policy Identification Segment (loop 2110 Service Payment Information REF), if present.

- RARC N517 – Resubmit a new claim with the requested information.

100-04, 32, 220.1

220.1 - General

(Rev. 1646, Issued: 12-09-08, Effective: 09-29-08, Implementation: 01-05-09)

Effective for services on or after September 29, 2008, the Center for Medicare & Medicaid Services (CMS) made the decision that Thermal Intradiscal Procedures (TIPS) are not reasonable and necessary for the treatment of low back pain. Therefore, TIPs are non-covered. Refer to Pub.100-3, Medicare National Coverage Determination (NCD) Manual Chapter 1, Part 2, Section 150.11, for further information on the NCD.

100-04, 32, 290.1.1

Coding Requirements for TAVR Services Furnished on or After January 1, 2013

(Rev. 2827. Issued: 11-29-13, Effective: 01-01-14, Implementation: 01-06-14)

Beginning January 1, 2013, the following are the applicable Current Procedural Terminology (CPT) codes for TAVR:

33361 Transcatheter aortic valve replacement (TAVR/TAVI) with prosthetic valve; percutaneous femoral artery approach

33362 Transcatheter aortic valve replacement (TAVR/TAVI) with prosthetic valve; open femoral approach

33363 Transcatheter aortic valve replacement (TAVR/TAVI) with prosthetic valve; open axillary artery approach

33364 Transcatheter aortic valve replacement (TAVR/TAVI) with prosthetic valve; open iliac artery approach

3336 Transcatheter aortic valve replacement (TAVR/TAVI) with prosthetic valve; transaortic approach (e.g., median sternotomy, mediastinotomy)

0318T Transcatheter aortic valve replacement (TAVR/TAVI) with prosthetic valve; transapical approach (e.g., left thoracotomy)

Beginning January 1, 2014, temporary CPT code 0318T above is retired. TAVR claims with dates of service on and after January 1, 2014 shall instead use permanent CPT code:

33366 Transcatheter aortic valve replacement (TAVR/TAVI) with prosthetic valve; transapical exposure (e.g., left thoracotomy)

100-04, 32, 290.2

Claims Processing Requirements for TAVR Services on Professional Claims

(Rev. 2827. Issued: 11-29-13, Effective: 01-01-14, Implementation: 01-06-14)

Place of Service (POS) Professional Claims

Effective for claims with dates of service on and after May 1, 2012, place of service (POS) code 21 shall be used for TAVR services. All other POS codes shall be denied.

The following messages shall be used when Medicare contractors deny TAVR claims for POS:

Claim Adjustment Reason Code (CARC) 58: "Treatment was deemed by the payer to have been rendered in an inappropriate or invalid place of service. NOTE: Refer to the 835 Healthcare Policy Identification Segment (loop 2110 Service Payment Information REF), if present."

Remittance advice remark code (RARC) N428: "Not covered when performed in this place of service."

Medicare Summary Notice (MSN) 21.25: "This service was denied because Medicare only covers this service in certain settings."

Spanish Version: "El servicio fue denegado porque Medicare solamente lo cubre en ciertas situaciones."

Professional Claims Modifier -62

For TAVR claims processed on or after July 1, 2013, contractors shall pay claim lines with 0256T, 0257T, 0258T, 0259T, 33361, 33362, 33363, 33364, 33365 & 0318T only when billed with modifier -62. Claim lines billed without modifier -62 shall be returned as unprocessable.

Beginning January 1, 2014, temporary CPT code 0318T above is retired. TAVR claims with dates of service on and after January 1, 2014 shall instead use permanent CPT code 33366.

The following messages shall be used when Medicare contractors return TAVR claims billed without modifier -62 as unprocessable:

CARC 4: "The procedure code is inconsistent with the modifier used or a required modifier is missing. Note: Refer to the 835 Healthcare Policy Identification Segment (loop 2110 Service Payment Information REF), if present."

RARC N29: "Missing documentation/orders/notes/summary/report/chart."

RARC MA130: "Your claim contains incomplete and/or invalid information, and no appeal rights are afforded because the claim is unprocessable. Please submit a new claim with the complete/correct information."

Professional Claims Modifier -Q0

For claims processed on or after July 1, 2013, contractors shall pay TAVR claim lines for 0256T, 0257T, 0258T, 0259T, 33361, 33362, 33363, 33364, 33365 & 0318T when billed with modifier -Q0. Claim lines billed without modifier -Q0 shall be returned as unprocessable.

Beginning January 1, 2014, temporary CPT code 0318T above is retired. TAVR claims with dates of service on and after January 1, 2014 shall instead use permanent CPT code 33366.

The following messages shall be used when Medicare contractors return TAVR claims billed without modifier -Q0 as unprocessable:

CARC 4: "The procedure code is inconsistent with the modifier used or a required modifier is missing. Note: Refer to the 835 Healthcare Policy Identification Segment (loop 2110 Service Payment Information REF), if present."

RARC N29: "Missing documentation/orders/notes/summary/report/chart."

RARC MA130: "Your claim contains incomplete and/or invalid information, and no appeal rights are afforded because the claim is unprocessable. Please submit a new claim with the complete/correct information."

For claims processed on or after July 1, 2013, contractors shall pay TAVR claim lines for 0256T, 0257T, 0258T, 0259T, 33361, 33362, 33363, 33364, 33365 & 0318T when billed with diagnosis code V70.7 (ICD-10=Z00.6). Claim lines billed without diagnosis code V70.7 (ICD-10=Z00.6) shall be returned as unprocessable.

Beginning January 1, 2014, temporary CPT code 0318T above is retired. TAVR claims with dates of service on and after January 1, 2014 shall instead use permanent CPT code 33366.

The following messages shall be used when Medicare contractors return TAVR claims billed without diagnosis code V70.7 (ICD-10=Z00.6) as unprocessable:

CARC 16: "Claim/service lacks information which is needed for adjudication. At least one Remark Code must be provided (may be comprised of either the NCPDP Reject Reason Code, or Remittance Advice Remark Code that is not an ALERT)."

RARC M76: "Missing/incomplete/invalid diagnosis or condition"

RARC MA130: "Your claim contains incomplete and/or invalid information, and no appeal rights are afforded because the claim is unprocessable. Please submit a new claim with the complete/correct information."

Professional Claims 8-digit ClinicalTrials.gov Identifier Number

For claims processed on or after July 1, 2013, contractors shall pay TAVR claim lines for 0256T, 0257T, 0258T, 0259T, 33361, 33362, 33363, 33364, 33365 & 0318T when billed with the numeric, 8-digit clinicaltrials.gov identifier number preceded by the two alpha characters "CT" when placed in Field 19 of paper Form CMS-1500, or when entered without the "CT" prefix in the electronic 837P in Loop 2300REF02(REF01=P4). Claim lines billed without an 8-digit clinicaltrials.gov identifier number shall be returned as unprocessable.

Beginning January 1, 2014, temporary CPT code 0318T above is retired. TAVR claims with dates of service on and after January 1, 2014 shall instead use permanent CPT code 33366.

The following messages shall be used when Medicare contractors return TAVR claims billed without an 8-digit clinicaltrials.gov identifier number as unprocessable:

CARC 16: "Claim/service lacks information which is needed for adjudication. At least one Remark Code must be provided (may be comprised of either NCPDP Reject Reason Code, or Remittance Advice Remark Code that is not an ALERT)."

RARC MA50: "Missing/incomplete/invalid Investigational Device Exemption number for FDA-approved clinical trial services."

RARC MA130: "Your claim contains incomplete and/or invalid information, and no appeal rights are afforded because the claim is unprocessable. Please submit a new claim with the complete/correct information."

NOTE: Clinicaltrials.gov identifier numbers for TAVR are listed on our website:

(http://www.cms.gov/Medicare/Coverage/Coverage-with-Evidence-Development/Transcatheter-Aortic-Valve-Replacement-TAVR-.html)

100-04, 32, 290.3

Claims Processing Requirements for TAVR Services on Inpatient Hospital Claims

(Rev.2827. Issued: 11-29-13, Effective: 01-01-14, Implementation: 01-06-14)

Inpatient hospitals shall bill for TAVR on an 11X TOB effective for discharges on or after May 1, 2012. Refer to Section 69 of this chapter for further guidance on billing under CED.

Inpatient hospital discharges for TAVR shall be covered when billed with:

- V70.7 and Condition Code 30.
- An 8-digit clinicaltrials.gov identifier number listed on the CMS website (effective July 1, 2013)

Inpatient hospital discharges for TAVR shall be rejected when billed without:

- V70.7 and Condition Code 30.
- An 8-digit clinicaltrials.gov identifier number listed on the CMS website (effective July 1, 2013)

Claims billed by hospitals not participating in the trial/registry shall be rejected with the following messages:

CARC: 50 -These are non-covered services because this is not deemed a "medical necessity" by the payer.

RARC N386 - This decision was based on a National Coverage Determination (NCD). An NCD provides a coverage determination as to whether a particular item or service is covered. A copy of this policy is available at http://www.cms.hhs.gov/mcd/search.asp. If you do not have web access, you may contact the contractor to request a copy of the NCD.

Group Code –Contractual Obligation (CO)

MSN 16.77 – This service/item was not covered because it was not provided as part of a qualifying trial/study. (Este servicio/artículo no fue cubierto porque no estaba incluido como parte de un ensayo clínico/estudio calificado.)

100-04, 32, 290.4

Claims Processing Requirements for TAVR Services for Medicare Advantage (MA) Plan Participants

(Rev. 3943; Issued: 12-22-17; Effective: 04- 01-15; Implementation: 04-02-18)

MA plans are responsible for payment of TAVR services for MA plan participants. Medicare coverage for TAVR is not included under section 310.1 of the NCD Manual (Routine Costs in Clinical Trials).

100-04, 32, 320.1

Coding Requirements for Artificial Hearts Furnished Before May 1, 2008

(Rev. 3054, Issued: 08-29-14, Effective: 10-30- 13, Implementation: 09-30-14)

Effective for discharges before May 1, 2008, Medicare does not cover the use of artificial hearts, either as a permanent replacement for a human heart or as a temporary life-support system until a human heart becomes available for transplant (often referred to a "bridge to transplant").

100-04, 32, 320.2

Coding Requirements for Artificial Hearts Furnished On or After May 1, 2008

(Rev. 3054, Issued: 08-29-14, Effective: 10-30- 13, Implementation: 09-30-14)

Effective for discharges on or after May 1, 2008, the use of artificial hearts will be covered by Medicare under Coverage with Evidence Development (CED) when beneficiaries are enrolled in a clinical study that meets all of the criteria listed in IOM Pub. 100-3, Medicare NCD Manual, section 20.9.

Claims Coding

For claims with dates of service on or after May 1, 2008, artificial hearts in the context of an approved clinical study for a Category A IDE, refer to section 69 in this manual for more detail on CED billing. Appropriate ICD-10 diagnosis and procedure codes are included below:

ICD-10 Diagnosis Code	Definition	Discharges Effective
I09.81	Rheumatic heart failure	On or After ICD-10 Implementation
I11.0	Hypertensive heart disease with heart failure	
I13.0	Hypertensive heart and chronic kidney disease with heart failure and stage 1 through stage 4 chronic kidney disease, or unspecified chronic kidney disease	
I13.2	Hypertensive heart and chronic kidney disease with heart failure and with stage 5 chronic kidney disease, or end stage renal disease	
I20.0	Unstable angina	
I21.01	ST elevation (STEMI) myocardial infarction involving left main coronary artery	
I21.02	ST elevation (STEMI) myocardial infarction involving left anterior descending coronary artery	
I21.09	ST elevation (STEMI) myocardial infarction involving other coronary artery of anterior wall	
I21.11	ST elevation (STEMI) myocardial infarction involving right coronary artery	
I21.19	ST elevation (STEMI) myocardial infarction involving other coronary artery of inferior wall	
I21.21	ST elevation (STEMI) myocardial infarction involving left circumflex coronary artery	
I21.29	ST elevation (STEMI) myocardial infarction involving other sites	
I21.3	ST elevation (STEMI) myocardial infarction of unspecified site	
I21.4	Non-ST elevation (NSTEMI) myocardial infarction	
I22.0	Subsequent ST elevation (STEMI) myocardial infarction of anterior wall	
I22.1	Subsequent ST elevation (STEMI) myocardial infarction of inferior wall	
I22.2	Subsequent non-ST elevation (NSTEMI) myocardial infarction	
I22.8	Subsequent ST elevation (STEMI) myocardial infarction of other sites	
I22.9	Subsequent ST elevation (STEMI) myocardial infarction of unspecified site	
I24.0	Acute coronary thrombosis not resulting in myocardial infarction	
I24.1	Dressler's syndrome	
I24.8	Other forms of acute ischemic heart disease	
I24.9	Acute ischemic heart disease, unspecified	
I25.10	Atherosclerotic heart disease of native coronary artery without angina pectoris	
I25.110	Atherosclerotic heart disease of native coronary artery with unstable angina pectoris	
I25.111	Atherosclerotic heart disease of native coronary artery with angina pectoris with documented spasm	
I25.118	Atherosclerotic heart disease of native coronary artery with other forms of angina pectoris	
I25.119	Atherosclerotic heart disease of native coronary artery with unspecified angina pectoris	
I25.5	Ischemic cardiomyopathy	
I25.6	Silent myocardial ischemia	

ICD-10 Diagnosis Code	Definition	Discharges Effective
I25.700	Atherosclerosis of coronary artery bypass graft(s), unspecified, with unstable angina pectoris	On or After ICD-10 Implementation
I25.701	Atherosclerosis of coronary artery bypass graft(s), unspecified, with angina pectoris with documented spasm	
I25.708	Atherosclerosis of coronary artery bypass graft(s), unspecified, with other forms of angina pectoris	
I25.709	Atherosclerosis of coronary artery bypass graft(s), unspecified, with unspecified angina pectoris	
I25.710	Atherosclerosis of autologous vein coronary artery bypass graft(s) with unstable angina pectoris	
I25.711	Atherosclerosis of autologous vein coronary artery bypass graft(s) with angina pectoris with documented spasm	
I25.718	Atherosclerosis of autologous vein coronary artery bypass graft(s) with other forms of angina pectoris	
I25.719	Atherosclerosis of autologous vein coronary artery bypass graft(s) with unspecified angina pectoris	
I25.720	Atherosclerosis of autologous artery coronary artery bypass graft(s) with unstable angina pectoris	
I25.721	Atherosclerosis of autologous artery coronary artery bypass graft(s) with angina pectoris with documented spasm	
I25.728	Atherosclerosis of autologous artery coronary artery bypass graft(s) with other forms of angina pectoris	
I25.729	Atherosclerosis of autologous artery coronary artery bypass graft(s) with unspecified angina pectoris	
I25.730	Atherosclerosis of nonautologous biological coronary artery bypass graft(s) with unstable angina pectoris	
I25.731	Atherosclerosis of nonautologous biological coronary artery bypass graft(s) with angina pectoris with documented spasm	
I25.738	Atherosclerosis of nonautologous biological coronary artery bypass graft(s) with other forms of angina pectoris	
I25.739	Atherosclerosis of nonautologous biological coronary artery bypass graft(s) with unspecified angina pectoris	
I25.750	Atherosclerosis of native coronary artery of transplanted heart with unstable angina	
I25.751	Atherosclerosis of native coronary artery of transplanted heart with angina pectoris with documented spasm	
I25.758	Atherosclerosis of native coronary artery of transplanted heart with other forms of angina pectoris	
I25.759	Atherosclerosis of native coronary artery of transplanted heart with unspecified angina pectoris	
I25.760	Atherosclerosis of bypass graft of coronary artery of transplanted heart with unstable angina	
I25.761	Atherosclerosis of bypass graft of coronary artery of transplanted heart with angina pectoris with documented spasm	
I25.768	Atherosclerosis of bypass graft of coronary artery of transplanted heart with other forms of angina pectoris	
I25.769	Atherosclerosis of bypass graft of coronary artery of transplanted heart with unspecified angina pectoris	
I25.790	Atherosclerosis of other coronary artery bypass graft(s) with unstable angina pectoris	
I25.791	Atherosclerosis of other coronary artery bypass graft(s) with angina pectoris with documented spasm	

ICD-10 Diagnosis Code	Definition	Discharges Effective
I25.798	Atherosclerosis of other coronary artery bypass graft(s) with other forms of angina pectoris	On or After ICD-10 Implementation
I25.799	Atherosclerosis of other coronary artery bypass graft(s) with unspecified angina pectoris	
I25.810	Atherosclerosis of coronary artery bypass graft(s) without angina pectoris	
I25.811	Atherosclerosis of native coronary artery of transplanted heart without angina pectoris	
I25.812	Atherosclerosis of bypass graft of coronary artery of transplanted heart without angina pectoris	
I25.89	Other forms of chronic ischemic heart disease	
I25.9	Chronic ischemic heart disease, unspecified	
I34.0	Nonrheumatic mitral (valve) insufficiency	
I34.1	Nonrheumatic mitral (valve) prolapse	
I34.2	Nonrheumatic mitral (valve) stenosis	
I34.8	Other nonrheumatic mitral valve disorders	
I34.9	Nonrheumatic mitral valve disorder, unspecified	
I35.0	Nonrheumatic aortic (valve) stenosis	
I35.1	Nonrheumatic aortic (valve) insufficiency	
I35.2	Nonrheumatic aortic (valve) stenosis with insufficiency	
I35.8	Other nonrheumatic aortic valve disorders	
I35.9	Nonrheumatic aortic valve disorder, unspecified	
I36.0	Nonrheumatic tricuspid (valve) stenosis	
I36.1	Nonrheumatic tricuspid (valve) insufficiency	
I36.2	Nonrheumatic tricuspid (valve) stenosis with insufficiency	
I36.8	Other nonrheumatic tricuspid valve disorders	
I36.9	Nonrheumatic tricuspid valve disorder, unspecified	
I37.0	Nonrheumatic pulmonary valve stenosis	
I37.1	Nonrheumatic pulmonary valve insufficiency	
I37.2	Nonrheumatic pulmonary valve stenosis with insufficiency	
I37.8	Other nonrheumatic pulmonary valve disorders	
I37.9	Nonrheumatic pulmonary valve disorder, unspecified	
I38	Endocarditis, valve unspecified	
I39	Endocarditis and heart valve disorders in diseases classified elsewhere	
I42.0	Dilated cardiomyopathy	
I42.2	Other hypertrophic cardiomyopathy	
I42.3	Endomyocardial (eosinophilic) disease	
I42.4	Endocardial fibroelastosis	
I42.5	Other restrictive cardiomyopathy	
I42.6	Alcoholic cardiomyopathy	
I42.7	Cardiomyopathy due to drug and external agent	
I42.8	Other cardiomyopathies	
I42.9	Cardiomyopathy, unspecified	
I43	Cardiomyopathy in diseases classified elsewhere	
I46.2	Cardiac arrest due to underlying cardiac condition	
I46.8	Cardiac arrest due to other underlying condition	
I46.9	Cardiac arrest, cause unspecified	
I47.0	Re-entry ventricular arrhythmia	
I47.1	Supraventricular tachycardia	
I47.2	Ventricular tachycardia	
I47.9	Paroxysmal tachycardia, unspecified	
I48.0	Atrial fibrillation	
I48.1	Atrial flutter	
I49.01	Ventricular fibrillation	
I49.02	Ventricular flutter	
I49.1	Atrial premature depolarization	

ICD-10 Diagnosis Code	Definition	Discharges Effective
I49.2	Junctional premature depolarization	On or After ICD-10 Implementation
I49.3	Ventricular premature depolarization	
I49.40	Unspecified premature depolarization	
I49.49	Other premature depolarization	
I49.5	Sick sinus syndrome	
I49.8	Other specified cardiac arrhythmias	
I49.9	Cardiac arrhythmia, unspecified	
I50.1	Left ventricular failure	
I50.20	Unspecified systolic (congestive) heart failure	
I50.21	Acute systolic (congestive) heart failure	
I50.22	Chronic systolic (congestive) heart failure	
I50.23	Acute on chronic systolic (congestive) heart failure	
I50.30	Unspecified diastolic (congestive) heart failure	
I50.31	Acute diastolic (congestive) heart failure	
I50.32	Chronic diastolic (congestive) heart failure	
I50.33	Acute on chronic diastolic (congestive) heart failure	
I50.40	Unspecified combined systolic (congestive) and diastolic (congestive) heart failure	
I50.41	Acute combined systolic (congestive) and diastolic (congestive) heart failure	
I50.42	Chronic combined systolic (congestive) and diastolic (congestive) heart failure	
I50.43	Acute on chronic combined systolic (congestive) and diastolic (congestive) heart failure	
I50.9	Heart failure, unspecified	
I51.4	Myocarditis, unspecified	
I51.9	Heart disease, unspecified	
I52	Other heart disorders in diseases classified elsewhere	
I97.0	Postcardiotomy syndrome	
I97.110	Postprocedural cardiac insufficiency following cardiac surgery	
I97.111	Postprocedural cardiac insufficiency following other surgery	
I97.120	Postprocedural cardiac arrest following cardiac surgery	
I97.121	Postprocedural cardiac arrest following other surgery	
I97.130	Postprocedural heart failure following cardiac surgery	
I97.131	Postprocedural heart failure following other surgery	
I97.190	Other postprocedural cardiac functional disturbances following cardiac surgery	
I97.191	Other postprocedural cardiac functional disturbances following other surgery	
I97.710	Intraoperative cardiac arrest during cardiac surgery	
I97.711	Intraoperative cardiac arrest during other surgery	
I97.790	Other intraoperative cardiac functional disturbances during cardiac surgery	
I97.791	Other intraoperative cardiac functional disturbances during other surgery	
I97.88	Other intraoperative complications of the circulatory system, not elsewhere classified	
I97.89	Other postprocedural complications and disorders of the circulatory system, not elsewhere classified	
M32.11	Endocarditis in systemic lupus erythematosus	
O90.89	Other complications of the puerperium, not elsewhere classified	
Q20.0	Common arterial trunk	
Q20.1	Double outlet right ventricle	
Q20.2	Double outlet left ventricle	
Q20.3	Discordant ventriculoarterial connection	
Q20.4	Double inlet ventricle	

ICD-10 Diagnosis Code	Definition	Discharges Effective
Q20.5	Discordant atrioventricular connection	On or After ICD-10 Implementation
Q20.6	Isomerism of atrial appendages	
Q20.8	Other congenital malformations of cardiac chambers and connections	
Q20.9	Congenital malformation of cardiac chambers and connections, unspecified	
Q21.0	Ventricular septal defect	
Q21.1	Atrial septal defect	
Q21.2	Atrioventricular septal defect	
Q21.3	Tetralogy of Fallot	
Q21.4	Aortopulmonary septal defect	
Q21.8	Other congenital malformations of cardiac septa	
Q21.9	Congenital malformation of cardiac septum, unspecified	
Q22.0	Pulmonary valve atresia	
Q22.1	Congenital pulmonary valve stenosis	
Q22.2	Congenital pulmonary valve insufficiency	
Q22.3	Other congenital malformations of pulmonary valve	
Q22.4	Congenital tricuspid stenosis	
Q22.5	Ebstein's anomaly	
Q22.6	Hypoplastic right heart syndrome	
Q22.8	Other congenital malformations of tricuspid valve	
Q22.9	Congenital malformation of tricuspid valve, unspecified	
Q23.0	Congenital stenosis of aortic valve	
Q23.1	Congenital insufficiency of aortic valve	
Q23.2	Congenital mitral stenosis	
Q23.3	Congenital mitral insufficiency	
Q23.4	Hypoplastic left heart syndrome	
Q23.8	Other congenital malformations of aortic and mitral valves	
Q23.9	Congenital malformation of aortic and mitral valves, unspecified	
Q24.0	Dextrocardia	
Q24.1	Levocardia	
Q24.2	Cor triatriatum	
Q24.3	Pulmonary infundibular stenosis	
Q24.4	Congenital subaortic stenosis	
Q24.5	Malformation of coronary vessels	
Q24.6	Congenital heart block	
Q24.8	Other specified congenital malformations of heart	
Q24.9	Congenital malformation of heart, unspecified	
R00.1	Bradycardia, unspecified	
R57.0	Cardiogenic shock	
T82.221A	Breakdown (mechanical) of biological heart valve graft, initial encounter	
T82.222A	Displacement of biological heart valve graft, initial encounter	
T82.223A	Leakage of biological heart valve graft, initial encounter	
T82.228A	Other mechanical complication of biological heart valve graft, initial encounter	
T82.512A	Breakdown (mechanical) of artificial heart, initial encounter	
T82.514A	Breakdown (mechanical) of infusion catheter, initial encounter	
T82.518A	Breakdown (mechanical) of other cardiac and vascular devices and implants, initial encounter	
T82.519A	Breakdown (mechanical) of unspecified cardiac and vascular devices and implants, initial encounter	
T82.522A	Displacement of artificial heart, initial encounter	
T82.524A	Displacement of infusion catheter, initial encounter	

ICD-10 Diagnosis Code	Definition	Discharges Effective
T82.528A	Displacement of other cardiac and vascular devices and implants, initial encounter	On or After ICD-10 Implementation
T82.529A	Displacement of unspecified cardiac and vascular devices and implants, initial encounter	On or After ICD-10 Implementation
T82.532A	Leakage of artificial heart, initial encounter	
T82.534A	Leakage of infusion catheter, initial encounter	
T82.538A	Leakage of other cardiac and vascular devices and implants, initial encounter	
T82.539A	Leakage of unspecified cardiac and vascular devices and implants, initial encounter	
T82.592A	Other mechanical complication of artificial heart, initial encounter	
T82.594A	Other mechanical complication of infusion catheter, initial encounter	
T82.598A	Other mechanical complication of other cardiac and vascular devices and implants, initial encounter	
T82.599A	Other mechanical complication of unspecified cardiac and vascular devices and implants, initial encounter	
T86.20	Unspecified complication of heart transplant	
T86.21	Heart transplant rejection	
T86.22	Heart transplant failure	
T86.23	Heart transplant infection	
T86.290	Cardiac allograft vasculopathy	
T86.298	Other complications of heart transplant	
T86.30	Unspecified complication of heart-lung transplant	
T86.31	Heart-lung transplant rejection	
T86.32	Heart-lung transplant failure	
T86.33	Heart-lung transplant infection	
T86.39	Other complications of heart-lung transplant	
Z48.21	Encounter for aftercare following heart transplant	
Z48.280	Encounter for aftercare following heart-lung transplant	
Z94.1	Heart transplant status	
Z94.3	Heart and lungs transplant status	
Z95.9	Presence of cardiac and vascular implant and graft, unspecified	
Q24.0	Dextrocardia	
Q24.1	Levocardia	
Q24.2	Cor triatriatum	
Q24.3	Pulmonary infundibular stenosis	
Q24.4	Congenital subaortic stenosis	
Q24.5	Malformation of coronary vessels	
Q24.6	Congenital heart block	
Q24.8	Other specified congenital malformations of heart	
Q24.9	Congenital malformation of heart, unspecified	
R00.1	Bradycardia, unspecified	
R57.0	Cardiogenic shock	
T82.221A	Breakdown (mechanical) of biological heart valve graft, initial encounter	
T82.222A	Displacement of biological heart valve graft, initial encounter	
T82.223A	Leakage of biological heart valve graft, initial encounter	
T82.228A	Other mechanical complication of biological heart valve graft, initial encounter	
T82.512A	Breakdown (mechanical) of artificial heart, initial encounter	
T82.514A	Breakdown (mechanical) of infusion catheter, initial encounter	
T82.518A	Breakdown (mechanical) of other cardiac and vascular devices and implants, initial encounter	
T82.519A	Breakdown (mechanical) of unspecified cardiac and vascular devices and implants, initial encounter	

ICD-10 Diagnosis Code	Definition	Discharges Effective
T82.522A	Displacement of artificial heart, initial encounter	On or After ICD-10 Implementation
T82.524A	Displacement of infusion catheter, initial encounter	
T82.528A	Displacement of other cardiac and vascular devices and implants, initial encounter	
T82.529A	Displacement of unspecified cardiac and vascular devices and implants, initial encounter	
T82.532A	Leakage of artificial heart, initial encounter	
T82.534A	Leakage of infusion catheter, initial encounter	
T82.538A	Leakage of other cardiac and vascular devices and implants, initial encounter	
T82.539A	Leakage of unspecified cardiac and vascular devices and implants, initial encounter	
T82.592A	Other mechanical complication of artificial heart, initial encounter	
T82.594A	Other mechanical complication of infusion catheter, initial encounter	
T82.598A	Other mechanical complication of other cardiac and vascular devices and implants, initial encounter	
T82.599A	Other mechanical complication of unspecified cardiac and vascular devices and implants, initial encounter	
T86.20	Unspecified complication of heart transplant	
T86.21	Heart transplant rejection	
T86.22	Heart transplant failure	
T86.23	Heart transplant infection	
T86.290	Cardiac allograft vasculopathy	
T86.298	Other complications of heart transplant	
T86.30	Unspecified complication of heart-lung transplant	
T86.31	Heart-lung transplant rejection	
T86.32	Heart-lung transplant failure	
T86.33	Heart-lung transplant infection	
T86.39	Other complications of heart-lung transplant	
Z48.21	Encounter for aftercare following heart transplant	
Z48.280	Encounter for aftercare following heart-lung transplant	
Z94.1	Heart transplant status	
Z94.3	Heart and lungs transplant status	
Z95.9	Presence of cardiac and vascular implant and graft, unspecified	
02RK0JZ	Replacement of Right Ventricle with Synthetic Substitute, Open Approach	
02RL0JZ	Revision of Synthetic Substitute in Heart, Open Approach	
02WA0JZ	Revision of Synthetic Substitute in Heart, Open Approach	

NOTE: Total artificial heart is reported with a "cluster" of 2 codes for open replacement with synthetic substitute of the right and left ventricles- 02RK0JZ + 02RL0JZ

100-04, 32, 320.3
Ventricular Assist Devices
(Rev. 3054, Issued: 08-29-14, Effective: 10-30-13, Implementation: 09-30-14)

Medicare may cover a Ventricular Assist Device (VAD). A VAD is used to assist a damaged or weakened heart in pumping blood. VADs are used as a bridge to a heart transplant, for support of blood circulation post-cardiotomy or destination therapy. Refer to the IOM Pub. 100-3, NCD Manual, section 20.9.1 for coverage criteria.

100-04, 32, 320.3.1
Post-cardiotomy
(Rev. 3054, Issued: 08-29-14, Effective: 10-30-13, Implementation: 09-30-14)

Post-cardiotomy is the period following open-heart surgery. VADs used for support of blood circulation post-cardiotomy are covered only if they have received approval from the Food and Drug Administration (FDA) for that purpose, and the VADs are used according to the FDA-approved labeling instructions.

100-04, 32, 320.3.2

Bridge- to -Transplantation (BTT)

(Rev. 3054, Issued: 08-29-14, Effective: 10-30-13, Implementation: 09-30-14)

Coverage for BTT is restricted to patients listed for heart transplantation. The Centers for Medicare & Medicaid Services (CMS) has clearly identified that the patient must be active on the waitlist maintained by the Organ Procurement and Transplantation Network. CMS has also removed the general time requirement that patients receive a transplant as soon as medically reasonable.

100-04, 32, 370

Microvolt T-wave Alternans (MTWA)

(Rev. 3265, Issued: 05-22-15, Effective: 01-13-15, Implementation: 06-23-15)

On March 21, 2006, the Centers for Medicare & Medicaid Services (CMS) began national coverage of microvolt T-wave Alternans (MTWA) diagnostic testing when it was performed using only the spectral analysis (SA) method for the evaluation of patients at risk for sudden cardiac death (SCD) from ventricular arrhythmias and patients who may be candidates for Medicare coverage of the placement of an implantable cardiac defibrillator (ICD).

Effective for claims with dates of service on and after January 13, 2015, Medicare Administrative Contractors (MACs) may determine coverage of MTWA diagnostic testing when it is performed using methods of analysis other than SA for the evaluation of patients at risk for SCD from ventricular arrhythmias. Further information can be found at Publication 100-3, section 20.30, of the National Coverage Determinations Manual.

100-04, 32, 370.1

Coding and Claims Processing for MTWA

(Rev. 3265, Issued: 05-22-15, Effective: 01-13-15, Implementation: 06-23-15)

Effective for claims with dates of service on and after March 21, 2006, MACs shall accept CPT 93025 (MTWA for assessment of ventricular arrhythmias) for MTWA diagnostic testing for the evaluation of patients at risk for SCD with the SA method of analysis only. All other methods of analysis for MTWA are non-covered.

Effective for claims with dates of service on and after January 13, 2015, MACs shall at their discretion determine coverage for CPT 93025 for MTWA diagnostic testing for the evaluation of patients at risk for SCD with methods of analysis other than SA. The –KX modifier shall be used as an attestation by the practitioner and/or provider of the service that documentation is on file verifying the MTWA was performed using a method of analysis other than SA for the evaluation of patients at risk for SCD from ventricular arrhythmias and that all other NCD criteria was met.

NOTE: The –KX modifier is NOT required on MTWA claims for the evaluation of patients at risk for SCD if the SA analysis method is used.

NOTE: This diagnosis code list/translation was approved by CMS/Coverage. It may or may not be a complete list of covered indications/diagnosis codes that are covered but should serve as a finite starting point.

As this policy indicates, individual A/B MACs within their respective jurisdictions have the discretion to make coverage determinations they deem reasonable and necessary under section 1862(a)1)(A) of the Social Security Act. Therefore, A/B MACs may have additional covered diagnosis codes in their individual policies where contractor discretion is appropriate.

ICD-9 Codes

410.11	Acute myocardial infarction of other anterior wall, initial episode of care
410.11	Acute myocardial infarction of other anterior wall, initial episode of care
410.01	Acute myocardial infarction of anterolateral wall, initial episode of care
410.11	Acute myocardial infarction of other anterior wall, initial episode of care
410.31	Acute myocardial infarction of inferoposterior wall, initial episode of care
410.21	Acute myocardial infarction of inferolateral wall, initial episode of care
410.41	Acute myocardial infarction of other inferior wall, initial episode of care
410.81	Acute myocardial infarction of other specified sites, initial episode of care
410.51	Acute myocardial infarction of other lateral wall, initial episode of care
410.61	True posterior wall infarction, initial episode of care
410.81	Acute myocardial infarction of other specified sites, initial episode of care
410.91	Acute myocardial infarction of unspecified site, initial episode of care
410.71	Subendocardial infarction, initial episode of care
410.01	Acute myocardial infarction of anterolateral wall, initial episode of care
410.11	Acute myocardial infarction of other anterior wall, initial episode of care
410.21	Acute myocardial infarction of inferolateral wall, initial episode of care
410.31	Acute myocardial infarction of inferoposterior wall, initial episode of care
410.41	Acute myocardial infarction of other inferior wall, initial episode of care
410.71	Subendocardial infarction, initial episode of care
410.51	Acute myocardial infarction of other lateral wall, initial episode of care
410.61	True posterior wall infarction, initial episode of care

410.81	Acute myocardial infarction of other specified sites, initial episode of care
410.91	Acute myocardial infarction of unspecified site, initial episode of care
411.89	Other acute and subacute forms of ischemic heart disease, other
411.89	Other acute and subacute forms of ischemic heart disease, other
427.1	Paroxysmal ventricular tachycardia
427.1	Paroxysmal ventricular tachycardia
427.41	Ventricular fibrillation
427.42	Ventricular flutter
780.2	Syncope and collapse
V45.89	Other postprocedural status

ICD-10 Codes

I21.01	ST elevation (STEMI) myocardial infarction involving left main coronary artery
I21.02	ST elevation (STEMI) myocardial infarction involving left anterior descending coron
I21.09	ST elevation (STEMI) myocardial infarction involving other coronary artery of anteri
I21.09	ST elevation (STEMI) myocardial infarction involving other coronary artery of anteri
I21.11	ST elevation (STEMI) myocardial infarction involving right coronary artery
I21.19	ST elevation (STEMI) myocardial infarction involving other coronary artery of inferi
I21.19	ST elevation (STEMI) myocardial infarction involving other coronary artery of inferi
I21.21	ST elevation (STEMI) myocardial infarction involving left circumflex coronary artery
I21.29	ST elevation (STEMI) myocardial infarction involving other sites
I21.29	ST elevation (STEMI) myocardial infarction involving other sites
I21.29	ST elevation (STEMI) myocardial infarction involving other sites
I21.3	ST elevation (STEMI) myocardial infarction of unspecified site
I21.4	Non-ST elevation (NSTEMI) myocardial infarction
I22.0	Subsequent ST elevation (STEMI) myocardial infarction of anterior wall
I22.0	Subsequent ST elevation (STEMI) myocardial infarction of anterior wall
I22.1	Subsequent ST elevation (STEMI) myocardial infarction of inferior wall
I22.1	Subsequent ST elevation (STEMI) myocardial infarction of inferior wall
I22.1	Subsequent ST elevation (STEMI) myocardial infarction of inferior wall
I22.2	Subsequent non-ST elevation (NSTEMI) myocardial infarction
I22.8	Subsequent ST elevation (STEMI) myocardial infarction of other sites
I22.8	Subsequent ST elevation (STEMI) myocardial infarction of other sites
I22.8	Subsequent ST elevation (STEMI) myocardial infarction of other sites
I22.9	Subsequent ST elevation (STEMI) myocardial infarction of unspecified site
I24.8	Other forms of acute ischemic heart disease
I24.9	Acute ischemic heart disease, unspecified
I47.0	Re-entry ventricular arrhythmia
I47.2	Ventricular tachycardia
I49.01	Ventricular fibrillation
I49.02	Ventricular flutter
R55	Syncope and collapse
Z98.89	Other specified postprocedural states

100-04, 32, 370.2

Messaging for MTWA

(Rev. 3265, Issued: 05-22-15, Effective: 01-13-15, Implementation: 06-23-15)

Effective for claims with dates of service on and after January 13, 2015, MACs shall deny claims for MTWA CPT 93025 with methods of analysis other than SA without modifier -KX using the following messages:

CARC 4: "The procedure code is inconsistent with the modifier used or a required modifier is missing. Note: Refer to the 835 Healthcare Policy Identification Segment (loop 2110 Service Payment Information REF), if present."

RARC N657 – This should be billed with the appropriate code for these services.

Group Code: CO (Contractual Obligation) assigning financial liability to the provider

MSN 15.20 - The following policies [NCD 20.30] were used when we made this decision

Spanish Equivalent - 15.20 - Las siguientes políticas [NCD 20.30] fueron utilizadas cuando se tomó esta decisión.

100-04, 32, 380

Leadless Pacemakers

(Rev. 3815, Issued: 07-28-17, Effective: 01-18-18, Implementation: 08-29-17 - for MAC local edits; January 2, 2018 - for MCS shared edits)

Effective for dates of service on or after January 18, 2017, contractors shall cover leadless pacemakers through Coverage with Evidence Development (CED) when procedures are performed in CMS-approved CED studies. Please refer to the National Coverage Determinations Manual (Publication 100-03, Section 20.8.4) for more information.

100-04, 32, 380.1

Leadless Pacemaker Coding and Billing Requirements for Professional Claims

(Rev. 3815, Issued: 07-28-17, Effective: 01-18-18, Implementation: 08-29-17 - for MAC local edits; January 2, 2018 - for MCS shared edits)

Effective for dates of service on or after January 18, 2017, contractors shall allow the following procedure codes on claims for leadless pacemakers:

0387T Transcatheter insertion or replacement of permanent leadless pacemaker, ventricular

0389T Programming device evaluation (in person) with iterative adjustment of the implantable device to test the function of the device and select optimal permanent programmed values with analysis, review and report, leadless pacemaker system.

0390T Peri-procedural device evaluation (in person) and programming of device system parameters before or after surgery, procedure or test with analysis, review and report, leadless pacemaker system.

0391T Interrogation device evaluation (in person) with analysis, review and report, includes connection, recording and disconnection per patient encounter, leadless pacemaker system.

Effective for dates of service on or after January 18, 2017, contractors shall allow the following ICD-10 diagnosis codes on claims for leadless pacemakers:

Z00.6 – Encounter for examination for normal comparison and control in clinical research program.

100-04, 32, 380.1.1

Leadless Pacemaker Place of Service Restrictions

(Rev. 3815, Issued: 07-28-17, Effective: 01-18-18, Implementation: 08-29-17 - for MAC local edits; January 2, 2018 - for MCS shared edits)

Effective for dates of service on or after January 18, 2017, contractors shall only pay claims for leadless pacemakers when services are provided in one of the following places of service (POS):

POS 06 – Indian Health Service Provider Based Facility

POS 21 – Inpatient Hospital

POS 22 - On Campus-Outpatient Hospital

POS 26 – Military Treatment Facility

100-04, 32, 380.1.2

Leadless Pacemaker Modifier

(Rev. 3815, Issued: 07-28-17, Effective: 01-18-18, Implementation: 08-29-17 - for MAC local edits; January 2, 2018 - for MCS shared edits)

Effective for claims with dates of service on or after January 18, 2017, modifier Q0 – Investigational clinical service provided in a clinical research study that is an approved clinical research study, must also be included.

100-04, 32, 390

Supervised exercise therapy (SET) Symptomatic Peripheral Artery Disease

(Rev. 4049, Issued: 05- 11-18, Effective: 05-25-17, Implementation: 07-02-18)

Effective for claims with dates of service on or after May 25, 2017, the Centers for Medicare and Medicaid Services (CMS) will cover supervised exercise therapy (SET) for beneficiaries with intermittent claudication (IC) for the treatment of symptomatic peripheral artery disease (PAD). Up to 36 sessions over a 12 week period are covered if all of the following components of a SET program are met:

The SET program must:

- consist of sessions lasting 30-60 minutes comprising a therapeutic exercise-training program for PAD in patients with claudication;

- be conducted in a physician's office;

- be delivered by qualified auxiliary personnel necessary to ensure benefits exceed harms, and who are trained in exercise therapy for PAD; and

- be under the direct supervision of a physician (as defined in 1861(r)(1)) of the Social Security Act (the Act)), physician assistant, or nurse practitioner/clinical

nurse specialist (as identified in 1861(aa)(5)) of (the Act) who must be trained in both basic and advanced life support techniques.

Beneficiaries must have a face-to-face visit with the physician responsible for PAD treatment to obtain the referral for SET. At this visit, the beneficiary must receive information regarding cardiovascular disease and PAD risk factor reduction, which could include education, counseling, behavioral interventions, and outcome assessments.

SET is non-covered for beneficiaries with absolute contraindications to exercise as determined by their primary attending physician.

Please refer to the National Coverage Determinations Manual (Publication 100-03, Section 20.35) for more information.

100-04, 32, 390.1

General Billing Requirements

(Rev. 4049, Issued: 05- 11-18, Effective: 05-25-17, Implementation: 07-02-18)

Effective for claims with date of services on or after May 25, 2017, contractors shall pay claims for SET for beneficiaries with IC for the treatment of symptomatic PAD, with a referral from the physician responsible for PAD treatment.

Medicare Administrative Contractors (MACs) have the discretion to cover SET beyond 36 sessions over 12 weeks and may cover an additional 36 sessions over an extended period of time. Contractors shall accept the inclusion of the KX modifier on the claim line(s) as an attestation by the provider of the services that documentation is on file verifying that further treatment beyond the 36 sessions of SET over a 12 week period meets the requirements of the medical policy.

100-04, 32, 390.2

Coding Requirements for SET for PAD

(Rev. 4229, Issued: 02-01-19, Effective: 05-25-17, Implementation: 03-19-19)

- CPT 93668 Peripheral arterial disease (PAD) rehabilitation, per session
- ICD-10 Codes

  I70.211 Atherosclerosis of native arteries of extremities with intermittent claudication, right leg

  I70.212 Atherosclerosis of native arteries of extremities with intermittent claudication, left leg

  I70.213 Atherosclerosis of native arteries of extremities with intermittent claudication, bilateral legs

  I70.218 Atherosclerosis of native arteries of extremities with intermittent claudication, other extremity

  I70.311 Atherosclerosis of unspecified type of bypass graft(s) of the extremities with intermittent claudication, right leg

  I70.312 Atherosclerosis of unspecified type of bypass graft(s) of the extremities with intermittent claudication, left leg

  I70.313 Atherosclerosis of unspecified type of bypass graft(s) of the extremities with intermittent claudication, bilateral legs

  I70.318 Atherosclerosis of unspecified type of bypass graft(s) of the extremities with intermittent claudication, other extremity

  I70.411 Atherosclerosis of autologous vein bypass graft(s) of the extremities with intermittent claudication, right leg

  I70.412 Atherosclerosis of autologous vein bypass graft(s) of the extremities with intermittent claudication, left leg

  I70.413 Atherosclerosis of autologous vein bypass graft(s) of the extremities with intermittent claudication, bilateral legs

  I70.418 Atherosclerosis of autologous vein bypass graft(s) of the extremities with intermittent claudication, other extremity

  I70.511 Atherosclerosis of nonautologous biological bypass graft(s) of the extremities with intermittent claudication, right leg

  I70.512 Atherosclerosis of nonautologous biological bypass graft(s) of the extremities with intermittent claudication, left leg

  I70.513 Atherosclerosis of nonautologous biological bypass graft(s) of the extremities with intermittent claudication, bilateral legs

  I70.518 Atherosclerosis of nonautologous biological bypass graft(s) of the extremities with intermittent claudication, other extremity

  I70.611 Atherosclerosis of nonbiological bypass graft(s) of the extremities with intermittent claudication, right leg

  I70.612 Atherosclerosis of nonbiological bypass graft(s) of the extremities with intermittent claudication, left leg

  I70.613 Atherosclerosis of nonbiological bypass graft(s) of the extremities with intermittent claudication, bilateral legs

  I70.618 Atherosclerosis of nonbiological bypass graft(s) of the extremities with intermittent claudication, other extremity

  I70.711 Atherosclerosis of other type of bypass graft(s) of the extremities with intermittent claudication, right leg

I70.712 Atherosclerosis of other type of bypass graft(s) of the extremities with intermittent claudication, left leg

I70.713 Atherosclerosis of other type of bypass graft(s) of the extremities with intermittent claudication, bilateral legs

I70.718 Atherosclerosis of other type of bypass graft(s) of the extremities with intermittent claudication, other extremity

100-04, 32, 390.3

Special Billing Requirements for Institutional Claims

(Rev. 4229, Issued: 02-01-19, Effective: 05-25-17, Implementation: 03-19-19)

Professional claim services for SET are only allowed in place of service (POS) 11. All other POS for SET will be denied. See section 390.4 for hospital outpatient center billing requirements.

100-04, 32, 390.4

Common Working File (CWF) Requirements

(Rev. 4049, Issued: 05- 11-18, Effective: 05-25-17, Implementation: 07-02-18)

Contractors shall pay claims for SET services containing CPT code 93668 on Types of Bill (TOBs) 13X under OPPS and 85X based on reasonable cost.

Contractors shall not pay claims for SET services containing CPT 93668 with revenue codes 096X, 097X, or 098X when billed on TOB 85X Method II.

100-04, 32, 390.5

Common Working File (CWF) Requirements

(Rev. 4229, Issued: 02-01-19, Effective: 05-25-17, Implementation: 03-19-19)

CWF shall create a new edit for CPT 93668 to reject claims when a beneficiary has reached 36 SET sessions within 84 days after the date of the first SET session and the -KX modifier is not included on the claim, or to reject any SET session provided after 84 days from the date of the first session and the -KX modifier is not included on the claim.

CWF shall determine the remaining SET sessions.

The CWF determination, to parallel claims processing, shall include all applicable factors including:

- Beneficiary entitlement status
- Beneficiary claims history
- Utilization rules

CWF shall update the determination when any changes occur to the beneficiary master data or claims data that would result in a change to the calculation.

CWF shall display the remaining SET sessions on all CWF provider query screens.

The Multi-Carrier System Desktop Tool (MCSDT) shall display the remaining SET sessions in a format equivalent to the CWF HIMR screen(s).

100-04, 32, 390.6

Applicable Medicare Summary Notice (MSN), Remittance Advice Remark Codes (RARCs), and Claim Adjustment Reason Code (CARC) Messaging

(Rev. 4229, Issued: 02-01-19, Effective: 05-25-17, Implementation: 03-19-19)

- Effective for claims with dates of service on or after May 25, 2017, contractor shall deny claims for SET in Place of Service (POS) other than 11, office using the following messages:

  Medicare Summary Notice (MSN) 15.20: "The following policies National Coverage Determination 20.35 (NCD) were used when we made this decision." Spanish Version: "Las siguientes políticas NCD 20.35 fueron utilizadas cuando se tomó esta decisión."

  Claim Adjustment Reason Code (CARC) 58: "Treatment was deemed by the payer to have been rendered in an inappropriate or invalid place of service. NOTE: Refer to the 835 Healthcare Policy Identification Segment (loop 2110 Service payment Information REF), if present."

  Remittance Advice Remark Code (RARC) N386: "This decision was based on a NCD 20.35. An NCD provides a coverage determination as to whether a particular item or service is covered. A copy of this policy is available at www.cms.gov/mcd/search.asp. If you do not have web access, you may contact the contractor to request a copy of the NCD."

  Contractors shall use Group Code CO (Contractual Obligation) assigning financial liability to the provider, if a claim is received with a GZ modifier indicating no signed Advance Beneficiary Notice (ABN) is on file.

- Contractors shall deny claims for SET when services are provided on other than TOBs 13X and 85X using the following messages:

  MSN 15.20: "The following policies NCD 20.35 were used when we made this decision."

Spanish Version: "Las siguientes políticas NCD 20.35 fueron utilizadas cuando se tomó esta decisión."

(Part A only) MSN 15.19: "Local Coverage Determinations (LCDs) help Medicare decide what is covered. An LCD was used for your claim. You can compare your case to the LCD, and send information from your doctor if you think it could change our decision. Call 1-800-MEDICARE (1-800-633-4227) for a copy of the LCD."

Spanish Version: "Las Determinaciones Locales de Cobertura (LCDs en inglés) le ayudan a decidir a Medicare lo que está cubierto. Un LCD se usó para su reclamación. Usted puede comparar su caso con la determinación y enviar información de su médico si piensa que puede cambiar nuestra decisión. Para obtener una copia del LCD, llame al 1-800-MEDICARE (1800-633-4227)."

CARC 58: "Treatment was deemed by the payer to have been rendered in an inappropriate or invalid place of service. NOTE: Refer to the 835 Healthcare Policy Identification Segment (loop 2110 Service payment Information REF), if present.

RARC N386: This decision was based on a National Coverage Determination (NCD) 20.35. An NCD provides a coverage determination as to whether a particular item or service is covered. A copy of this policy is available at www.cms.gov/mcd/search.asp. If you do not have web access, you may contact the contractor to request a copy of the NCD.

Contractors shall use Group Code CO (Contractual Obligation) assigning financial liability to the provider, if a claim is received with a GZ modifier indicating no signed ABN is on file.

For professional claims only, contractors shall deny line items on claims for SET services performed in POS other than POS 11 and use the following messages:

MSN 15.20: "The following policies NCD 20.35 were used when we made this decision."

Spanish Version: "Las siguientes políticas NCD 20.35 fueron utilizadas cuando se tomó esta decisión." CARC 58: "Treatment was deemed by the payer to have been rendered in an inappropriate or invalid place of service. NOTE: Refer to the 835 Healthcare Policy Identification Segment (loop 2110 Service payment Information REF), if present.

RARC N386: "This decision was based on a National Coverage Determination 20.35 (NCD). An NCD provides a coverage determination as to whether a particular item or service is covered. A copy of this policy is available at www.cms.gov/mcd/search.asp. If you do not have web access, you may contact the contractor to request a copy of the NCD.

Contractors shall use Group Code CO (Contractual Obligation) assigning financial liability to the provider, if a claim is received with a GZ modifier indicating no signed ABN is on file.

- Contractors shall deny/reject claim lines for CPT 93668 without one of the diagnosis codes listed in section 390.2 above and use the following messages:

  MSN 15.20: "The following policies NCD 20.35 were used when we made this decision."

  Spanish Version: "Las siguientes políticas NCD 20.35 fueron utilizadas cuando se tomó esta decisión."

  (Part A only) MSN 15.19: "Local Coverage Determinations (LCDs) help Medicare decide what is covered. An LCD was used for your claim. You can compare your case to the LCD, and send information from your doctor if you think it could change our decision. Call 1-800-MEDICARE (1-800-633-4227) for a copy of the LCD".

  Spanish Version: "Las Determinaciones Locales de Cobertura (LCDs en inglés) le ayudan a decidir a Medicare lo que está cubierto. Un LCD se usó para su reclamación. Usted puede comparar su caso con la determinación y enviar información de su médico si piensa que puede cambiar nuestra decisión. Para obtener una copia del LCD, llame al 1-800-MEDICARE (1800-633-4227)."

  CARC 167: "This (these) diagnosis(es) is (are) not covered. Note: Refer to the 835 Healthcare Policy Identification Segment (loop 2110 Service Payment Information REF), if present."

  RARC N386: "This decision was based on a National Coverage Determination (NCD). An NCD provides a coverage determination as to whether a particular item or service is covered. A copy of this policy is available at

  www.cms.gov/mcd/search.asp. If you do not have web access, you may contact the contractor to request a copy of the NCD."

  Contractors shall use Group Code PR (Patient Responsibility) assigning financial liability to the beneficiary if a claim is received with a GA modifier indicating a signed ABN is on file.

  Contractors shall use Group Code CO (Contractual Obligation) assigning financial liability to the provider, if a claim is received with a GZ modifier indicating no signed ABN is on file.

- Contractors shall reject claims with CPT 93668 which exceed 36 sessions within 84 days from the date of the first session when the -KX modifier is not included on the claim line OR any SET session provided after 84 days from the date of the first session and the -KX modifier is not included on the claim and use the following messages:

CARC 96: "Non-covered charge(s). At least one Remark Code must be provided (may be comprised of either the NCPDP Reject Reason [sic] Code, or Remittance Advice Remark Code that is not an ALERT.) Note: Refer to the 835 Healthcare Policy Identification Segment (loop 2110 Service Payment Information REF), if present."

RARC N640: "Exceeds number/frequency approved/allowed within time period."

Group Code CO (Contractual Obligation) assigning financial liability to the provider (if a claim line-item is received with a GZ modifier indicating no signed ABN is on file and occurrence code 32 is not present).

• Contractors shall deny/reject claim lines with CPT 93668 when 73 sessions have been reached using the following messages:

MSN 15.20: "The following policies NCD 20.35 were used when we made this decision." Spanish Version: "Las siguientes políticas NCD 20.35 fueron utilizadas cuando se tomó esta decisión."

(Part A only) MSN 15.19: "Local Coverage Determinations (LCDs) help Medicare decide what is covered. An LCD was used for your claim. You can compare your case to the LCD, and send information from your doctor if you think it could change our decision. Call 1-800-MEDICARE (1-800-633-4227) for a copy of the LCD".

Spanish Version: "Las Determinaciones Locales de Cobertura (LCDs en inglés) le ayudan a decidir a Medicare lo que está cubierto. Un LCD se usó para su reclamación. Usted puede comparar su caso con la determinación y enviar información de su médico si piensa que puede cambiar nuestra decisión. Para obtener una copia del LCD, llame al 1-800-MEDICARE (1800-633-4227)."

CARC 119: "Benefit maximum for this time period or occurrence has been reached."

RARC N386: "This decision was based on a National Coverage Determination (NCD). An NCD provides a coverage determination as to whether a particular item or service is covered. A copy of this policy is available at www.cms.gov/mcd/search.asp. If you do not have web access, you may contact the contractor to request a copy of the NCD."

Group Code PR (Patient Responsibility) assigning financial responsibility to the beneficiary (if a claim is received with occurrence code 32 with or without a GA modifier or a claim-line is received with a GA modifier indicating a signed ABN is on file)

Group Code CO (Contractual Obligation) assigning financial liability to the provider (if a claim line-item is received with a GZ modifier indicating no signed ABN is on file and occurrence code 32 is not present

• Contractors shall deny claim line-items for SET, CPT 93668, when 73 sessions have been reached with or without the -KX modifier present using the following messages:

MSN 15.20: "The following policies NCD 20.35 were used when we made this decision."

Spanish Version: "Las siguientes políticas NCD 20.35 fueron utilizadas cuando se tomó esta decisión."

(Part A only) MSN 15.19: "Local Coverage Determinations (LCDs) help Medicare decide what is covered. An LCD was used for your claim. You can compare your case to the LCD, and send information from your doctor if you think it could change our decision. Call 1-800-MEDICARE (1-800-633-4227) for a copy of the LCD".

Spanish Version: "Las Determinaciones Locales de Cobertura (LCDs en inglés) le ayudan a decidir a Medicare lo que está cubierto. Un LCD se usó para su reclamación. Usted puede comparar su caso con la determinación y enviar información de su médico si piensa que puede cambiar nuestra decisión. Para obtener una copia del LCD, llame al 1-800- MEDICARE (1800-633-4227)."

CARC 119: "Benefit maximum for this time period or occurrence has been reached."

RARC N386: "This decision was based on a National Coverage Determination (NCD). An NCD provides a coverage determination as to whether a particular item or service is covered. A copy of this policy is available at www.cms.gov/mcd/search.asp. If you do not have web access, you may contact the contractor to request a copy of the NCD."

Group Code PR (Patient Responsibility) assigning financial responsibility to the beneficiary (if a claim is received with occurrence code 32 with or without a GA modifier or a claim-line is received with a GA modifier indicating a signed ABN is on file)

Group Code CO (Contractual Obligation) assigning financial liability to the provider (if a claim line-item is received with a GZ modifier indicating no signed ABN is on file and occurrence code 32 is not present).

100-05, 10.3.2

Exceptions Process

(Rev. 3367 Issued: 10-07-2015, Effective: 01-01-2016, Implementation: 01-04-2016)

An exception may be made when the patient's condition is justified by documentation indicating that the beneficiary requires continued skilled therapy, i.e.,

therapy beyond the amount payable under the therapy cap, to achieve their prior functional status or maximum expected functional status within a reasonable amount of time.

No special documentation is submitted to the contractor for exceptions. The clinician is responsible for consulting guidance in the Medicare manuals and in the professional literature to determine if the beneficiary may qualify for the exception because documentation justifies medically necessary services above the caps. The clinician's opinion is not binding on the Medicare contractor who makes the final determination concerning whether the claim is payable.

Documentation justifying the services shall be submitted in response to any Additional Documentation Request (ADR) for claims that are selected for medical review. Follow the documentation requirements in Pub. 100-02, chapter 15, section 220.3. If medical records are requested for review, clinicians may include, at their discretion, a summary that specifically addresses the justification for therapy cap exception.

In making a decision about whether to utilize the exception, clinicians shall consider, for example, whether services are appropriate to--

The patient's condition, including the diagnosis, complexities, and severity;

The services provided, including their type, frequency, and duration;

The interaction of current active conditions and complexities that directly and significantly influence the treatment such that it causes services to exceed caps.

In addition, the following should be considered before using the exception process:

1. Exceptions for Evaluation Services

Evaluation. The CMS will except therapy evaluations from caps after the therapy caps are reached when evaluation is necessary, e.g., to determine if the current status of the beneficiary requires therapy services. For example, the following CPT codes for evaluation procedures may be appropriate:

92521, 92522, 92523, 92524, 92597, 92607, 92608, 92610, 92611, 92612, 92614, 92616, 96105, 96125, 97001, 97002, 97003, 97004.

These codes will continue to be reported as outpatient therapy procedures as listed in the Annual Therapy Update for the current year at: http://www.cms.gov/TherapyServices/05_Annual_Therapy_Update.asp#TopOfPage.

They are not diagnostic tests. Definitions of evaluations and documentation are found in Pub. 100-02, chapter 15, sections 220 and 230.

Other Services. There are a number of sources that suggest the amount of certain services that may be typical, either per service, per episode, per condition, or per discipline. For example, see the CSC - Therapy Cap Report, 3/21/2008, and CSC – Therapy Edits Tables 4/14/2008 at www.cms.hhs.gov/TherapyServices (Studies and Reports), or more recent utilization reports. Professional literature and guidelines from professional associations also provide a basis on which to estimate whether the type, frequency, and intensity of services are appropriate to an individual. Clinicians and contractors should utilize available evidence related to the patient's condition to justify provision of medically necessary services to individual beneficiaries, especially when they exceed caps. Contractors shall not limit medically necessary services that are justified by scientific research applicable to the beneficiary. Neither contractors nor clinicians shall utilize professional literature and scientific reports to justify payment for continued services after an individual's goals have been met earlier than is typical. Conversely, professional literature and scientific reports shall not be used as justification to deny payment to patients whose needs are greater than is typical or when the patient's condition is not represented by the literature.

2. Exceptions for Medically Necessary Services

Clinicians may utilize the process for exception for any diagnosis or condition for which they can justify services exceeding the cap. Regardless of the diagnosis or condition, the patient must also meet other requirements for coverage.

Bill the most relevant diagnosis. As always, when billing for therapy services, the diagnosis code that best relates to the reason for the treatment shall be on the claim, unless there is a compelling reason to report another diagnosis code. For example, when a patient with diabetes is being treated with therapy for gait training due to amputation, the preferred diagnosis is abnormality of gait (which characterizes the treatment). Where it is possible in accordance with State and local laws and the contractors' local coverage determinations, avoid using vague or general diagnoses. When a claim includes several types of services, or where the physician/NPP must supply the diagnosis, it may not be possible to use the most relevant therapy diagnosis code in the primary position. In that case, the relevant diagnosis code should, if possible, be on the claim in another position.

Codes representing the medical condition that caused the treatment are used when there is no code representing the treatment. Complicating conditions are preferably used in non-primary positions on the claim and are billed in the primary position only in the rare circumstance that there is no more relevant code.

The condition or complexity that caused treatment to exceed caps must be related to the therapy goals and must either be the condition that is being treated or a complexity that directly and significantly impacts the rate of recovery of the condition being treated such that it is appropriate to exceed the caps. Documentation for an exception should indicate how the complexity (or combination of complexities) directly and significantly affects treatment for a therapy condition.

If the contractor has determined that certain codes do not characterize patients who require medically necessary services, providers/suppliers may not use those codes, but must utilize a billable diagnosis code allowed by their contractor to describe the patient's condition. Contractors shall not apply therapy caps to services based on the patient's condition, but only on the medical necessity of the service for the condition. If a service would be payable before the cap is reached and is still medically necessary after the cap is reached, that service is excepted.

Contact your contractor for interpretation if you are not sure that a service is applicable for exception.

It is very important to recognize that most conditions would not ordinarily result in services exceeding the cap. Use the KX modifier only in cases where the condition of the individual patient is such that services are APPROPRIATELY provided in an episode that exceeds the cap. Routine use of the KX modifier for all patients with these conditions will likely show up on data analysis as aberrant and invite inquiry. Be sure that documentation is sufficiently detailed to support the use of the modifier.

In justifying exceptions for therapy caps, clinicians and contractors should not only consider the medical diagnoses and medical complications that might directly and significantly influence the amount of treatment required. Other variables (such as the availability of a caregiver at home) that affect appropriate treatment shall also be considered. Factors that influence the need for treatment should be supportable by published research, clinical guidelines from professional sources, and/or clinical or common sense. See Pub. 100-02, chapter 15, section 220.3 for information related to documentation of the evaluation, and section 220.2 on medical necessity for some factors that complicate treatment.

NOTE: The patient's lack of access to outpatient hospital therapy services alone, when outpatient hospital therapy services are excluded from the limitation, does not justify excepted services. Residents of skilled nursing facilities prevented by consolidated billing from accessing hospital services, debilitated patients for whom transportation to the hospital is a physical hardship, or lack of therapy services at hospitals in the beneficiary's county may or may not qualify as justification for continued services above the caps. The patient's condition and complexities might justify extended services, but their location does not. For dates of service on or after October 1, 2012, therapy services furnished in an outpatient hospital are not excluded from the limitation.

Appendix H — Quality Payment Program

In 2015, Congress passed the Medicare Access and CHIP Reauthorization Act (MACRA), which included sweeping changes for practitioners who provide services reimbursed under the Medicare physician fee schedule (MPFS). The act focused on repealing the faulty Medicare sustainable growth rate, focusing on quality of patient outcomes, and controlling Medicare spending.

A MACRA final rule in October 2016 established the Quality Payment Program (QPP) that was effective January 1, 2017.

The QPP has two tracks:

- The merit-based incentive payment system (MIPS)
- Alternative payment models (APMs)

MIPS uses the existing quality and value reporting systems—Physician Quality Reporting System (PQRS) (which ends January 1, 2019), Medicare meaningful use (MU), and value-based modifier (VBM) programs—to define certain performance categories that determine an overall score. Eligible clinicians (ECs) can obtain a composite performance score (CPS) of up to 100 points from these weighted performance categories. This performance score then defines the payment adjustments in the second calendar year after the year the score is obtained. For instance, the score obtained for the 2017 performance year is linked to payment for Medicare Part B services in 2019.

The performance categories, along with the weights used to determine the overall score, are:

- Quality
- Advancing care information (previously called meaningful use)
- Clinical practice improvement activities (CPIA)
- Resource use

ECs may also choose to participate in APMs. These payment models, created in conjunction with the clinician community, provide additional incentives to those clinicians in the APM who provide high-quality care as cost-efficiently as possible. APMs can be created around specific clinical conditions, a care episode, or a patient population type. An APM can also be described as a new way of paying the healthcare provider for the care rendered to Medicare patients.

Advanced APMs are a subset of APMs; practices participating in an advanced APM can earn even more incentives because the ECs take on risk related to their patients' outcomes. For calendar years 2019 through 2024, clinicians participating in advanced APMs have the potential to earn an additional 5 percent incentive payment; furthermore, they are exempt from having to participate in MIPS as long as they have sufficiently participated in the advanced APM.

Eligible clinicians have three flexible options for submitting data to the MIPS and a fourth option to join advanced APMs. Under the QPP, providers can receive increased payment by providing high-quality care and by controlling costs. ECs who successfully report determined criteria—defined by the pathway chosen—receive a larger payment depending on how successful they are at meeting performance thresholds. Those who do not participate or who do not fulfill the defined requirements receive a negative penalty; failure to participate in a track in 2020 results in 9 percent payment reduction in 2022.

ECs can receive incentives under the QPP. Once the performance threshold is established, ALL ECs who score above that threshold are eligible to receive a positive payment adjustment. Keep in mind that the key requirement is that an EC **submit data** to avoid the negative payment adjustment and receive the incentives. CMS has redesigned the scoring so that clinicians are able to know how well they are doing in the program, as benchmarks are known in advance of participating.

Proposed 2020 Changes

A number of revisions have been proposed for 2020. As noted earlier, in 2020, the maximum negative payment for payment adjustment is negative 9 percent. The positive payment, not including additional positive payments adjustments for exceptional performance is also up to a 9 percent adjustment. CMS is proposing additions, revisions, and deletions to many of the current reporting measures. Other proposals affecting the MIPS program for 2020 include:

- In the MIPS performance category CMS proposes to reduce the Quality performance category weight from 45 percent to 40 percent and to increase the Cost performance category weight from 15 percent to 20 percent. This is in accordance with CMS's effort to equalize weighting between the Quality and Cost performance categories by 2022 as indicated in MACRA.

- The data completeness requirements for 2020 are proposed to increase to 70 percent of the Quality performance category. This is up from 2019, which had a 60 percent requirement.

- New specialty sets would be added for Speech Language Pathology, Audiology, Clinical Social Work, Chiropractic Medicine, Pulmonology, Nutrition/Dietician, and Endocrinology.

- CMS proposes 10 new episode-based measures and revisions to two current measures (Medicare Spending Per Beneficiary Clinician and Total Per Capita Cost measures) to the Cost performance category.

- In the Improvement Activities performance category, CMS recommends modifying the definition of rural areas, removing the accreditation from criteria for patient-centered medical home designation, and increasing the participation threshold for group reporting from a single clinician to 50 percent of the practice clinicians.

Within the advanced alternative payment models (APMs). CMS has proposed MIPS quality reporting options for APM participants. Previously, CMS has tried to streamline APM participation in MIPS; however, the agency feels that allowing MIPS quality measures reported by the APMs would offer flexibility and improve meaningful measurement.

Appendix I — Medically Unlikely Edits (MUEs)

The Centers for Medicare & Medicaid Services (CMS) began to publish many of the edits used in the medically unlikely edits (MUE) program for the first time effective October 2008. What follows below is a list of the published CPT codes that have MUEs assigned to them and the number of units allowed with each code. CMS publishes the updates on a quarterly basis. Not all MUEs will be published, however. MUEs intended to detect and discourage any questionable payments will not be published as the agency feels the efficacy of these edits would be compromised. CMS added another component to the MUEs—the MUE Adjudication Indicator (MAI). The appropriate MAI can be found in parentheses following the MUE in this table and specify the maximum units of service (UOS) for a CPT/HCPCS code for the service. The MAI designates whether the UOS edit is applied to the line or claim.

The three MAIs are defined as follows:

MAI 1 (Line Edit) This MAI will continue to be adjudicated as the line edit on the claim and is auto-adjudicated by the contractor.

MAI 2 (Date of Service Edit, Policy) This MAI is considered to be the "absolute date of service edit" and is based on policy. The total unit of services (UOS) for that CPT code and that date of service (DOS) are combined for this edit. Medicare contractors are required to review all claims for the same patient, same date of service, and same provider.

MAI 3 (Date of Service Edit: Clinical) This MAI is also a date-of-service edit but is based upon clinical standards. The review takes current and previously submitted claims for the same patient, same date of service, and same provider into account. When medical necessity is clearly documented, the edit may be bypassed or the claim resubmitted.

The quarterly updates are published on the CMS website at http://www.cms.gov/NationalCorrectCodInitEd/MUE.html.

Professional

CPT	MUE	CPT	MUE	CPT	MUE	CPT	MUE	CPT	MUE	CPT	MUE	CPT	MUE	CPT	MUE
0001U	1(2)	0040U	1(2)	0076U	1(2)	0216T	1(2)	0316T	1(3)	0399T	1(3)	0446T	1(3)	0490T	1(2)
0002M	1(3)	0041U	1(2)	0077U	2(2)	0217T	1(2)	0317T	1(3)	0400T	1(2)	0447T	1(3)	0491T	1(2)
0002U	1(2)	0042T	1(3)	0078U	1(2)	0218T	1(2)	0329T	1(2)	0401T	1(2)	0448T	1(3)	0492T	4(3)
0003M	1(3)	0042U	1(2)	0079U	0(3)	0219T	1(2)	0330T	1(2)	0402T	2(2)	0449T	1(2)	0493T	1(3)
0003U	1(2)	0043U	1(2)	0080U	1(2)	0220T	1(2)	0331T	1(3)	0403T	1(2)	0450T	1(3)	0494T	1(2)
0004M	1(2)	0044U	1(2)	0081U	1(3)	0221T	1(2)	0332T	1(3)	0404T	1(2)	0451T	1(3)	0495T	1(2)
0005U	1(2)	0045U	1(3)	0082U	1(2)	0222T	1(3)	0333T	1(3)	0405T	1(2)	0452T	1(3)	0496T	4(3)
0006M	1(2)	0046U	1(3)	0083U	1(3)	0228T	1(2)	0335T	2(2)	0408T	1(3)	0453T	1(3)	0497T	1(3)
0006U	1(2)	0047U	1(3)	0085T	0(3)	0229T	2(3)	0338T	1(2)	0409T	1(3)	0454T	3(3)	0498T	1(2)
0007M	1(2)	0048U	1(3)	0095T	1(3)	0230T	1(2)	0339T	1(2)	0410T	1(3)	0455T	1(3)	0499T	1(2)
0007U	1(2)	0049U	1(3)	0098T	2(3)	0231T	2(3)	0341T	1(2)	0411T	1(3)	0456T	1(3)	0500T	1(2)
0008U	1(3)	0050U	1(3)	0100T	1(2)	0232T	1(3)	0342T	1(3)	0412T	1(2)	0457T	1(3)	0501T	1(2)
0009M	1(2)	0051U	1(2)	0101T	1(3)	0234T	2(3)	0345T	1(2)	0413T	1(3)	0458T	3(3)	0502T	1(2)
0009U	2(3)	0052U	1(2)	0102T	2(2)	0235T	2(3)	0347T	1(3)	0414T	1(2)	0459T	1(3)	0503T	1(2)
0010U	2(3)	0053U	1(3)	0106T	4(2)	0236T	1(2)	0348T	1(3)	0415T	1(3)	0460T	3(3)	0504T	1(2)
0011M	1(2)	0054T	1(3)	0107T	4(2)	0237T	2(3)	0349T	1(3)	0416T	1(3)	0461T	1(3)	0505T	1(3)
0011U	1(2)	0054U	1(2)	0108T	4(2)	0238T	2(3)	0350T	1(3)	0417T	1(3)	0462T	1(2)	0506T	1(2)
0012M	1(2)	0055T	1(3)	0109T	4(2)	0249T	1(2)	0351T	5(3)	0418T	1(3)	0463T	1(2)	0507T	1(2)
0012U	1(2)	0055U	1(2)	0110T	4(2)	0253T	1(3)	0352T	5(3)	0419T	1(2)	0464T	1(2)	0508T	1(3)
0013M	1(2)	0056U	1(3)	0111T	1(3)	0254T	2(2)	0353T	2(3)	0420T	1(2)	0465T	1(3)	0509T	1(2)
0013U	1(3)	0057U	1(3)	0126T	1(3)	0263T	1(3)	0354T	2(3)	0421T	1(2)	0466T	1(3)	0510T	1(2)
0014U	1(3)	0058T	1(2)	0163T	1(3)	0264T	1(3)	0355T	1(2)	0422T	1(3)	0467T	1(3)	0511T	1(2)
0016U	1(3)	0058U	1(2)	0164T	4(2)	0265T	1(3)	0356T	4(2)	0423T	1(3)	0468T	1(3)	0512T	1(2)
0017U	1(3)	0059U	1(2)	0165T	4(2)	0266T	1(2)	0357T	1(2)	0424T	1(3)	0469T	1(2)	0513T	2(3)
0018U	1(1)	0060U	1(2)	0174T	1(3)	0267T	1(3)	0358T	1(2)	0425T	1(3)	0470T	1(2)	0514T	2(2)
0019U	1(3)	0061U	1(2)	0175T	1(3)	0268T	1(3)	0362T	8(3)	0426T	1(3)	0471T	2(1)	0515T	1(3)
0021U	1(2)	0062U	1(2)	0184T	1(3)	0269T	1(2)	0373T	24(3)	0427T	1(3)	0472T	1(2)	0516T	1(3)
0022U	2(3)	0063U	1(2)	0191T	2(2)	0270T	1(3)	0375T	1(2)	0428T	1(2)	0473T	1(2)	0517T	1(3)
0023U	1(2)	0064U	2(3)	0198T	2(2)	0271T	1(2)	0376T	2(3)	0429T	1(2)	0474T	2(2)	0518T	1(3)
0024U	1(2)	0065U	2(3)	01996	1(2)	0272T	1(3)	0377T	1(2)	0430T	1(2)	0475T	1(3)	0519T	1(3)
0025U	1(2)	0066U	1(3)	0200T	1(2)	0273T	1(3)	0378T	1(2)	0431T	1(2)	0476T	1(3)	0520T	1(3)
0026U	1(3)	0067U	2(3)	0201T	1(2)	0274T	1(2)	0379T	1(2)	0432T	1(3)	0477T	1(3)	0521T	1(3)
0027U	1(2)	0068U	1(3)	0202T	1(3)	0275T	1(2)	0380T	1(2)	0433T	1(3)	0478T	1(3)	0522T	1(3)
0029U	1(2)	0069U	1(3)	0205T	3(3)	0278T	1(3)	0381T	1(2)	0434T	1(2)	0479T	1(2)	0523T	1(3)
0030U	1(2)	0070U	1(2)	0206T	1(3)	0290T	1(3)	0382T	1(2)	0435T	1(3)	0480T	4(1)	0524T	3(3)
0031U	1(2)	0071T	1(2)	0207T	2(2)	0295T	1(2)	0383T	1(2)	0436T	1(3)	0481T	1(3)	0525T	1(3)
0032U	1(2)	0071U	1(2)	0208T	1(3)	0296T	1(2)	0384T	1(2)	0437T	1(3)	0482T	1(3)	0526T	1(3)
0033U	1(2)	0072T	1(2)	0209T	1(3)	0297T	1(2)	0385T	1(2)	0439T	1(3)	0483T	1(2)	0527T	1(3)
0034U	1(2)	0072U	1(2)	0210T	1(3)	0298T	1(2)	0386T	1(2)	0440T	3(3)	0484T	1(2)	0528T	1(3)
0035U	1(2)	0073U	1(2)	0211T	1(3)	0308T	1(3)	0394T	2(3)	0441T	3(3)	0485T	1(2)	0529T	1(3)
0036U	1(3)	0074U	1(2)	0212T	1(3)	0312T	1(3)	0395T	2(3)	0442T	3(3)	0486T	1(2)	0530T	1(3)
0037U	1(3)	0075T	1(2)	0213T	1(2)	0313T	1(3)	0396T	2(2)	0443T	1(2)	0487T	1(3)	0531T	1(3)
0038U	1(2)	0075U	1(2)	0214T	1(2)	0314T	1(3)	0397T	1(3)	0444T	1(2)	0488T	1(2)	0532T	1(3)
0039U	1(2)	0076U	1(2)	0215T	1(2)	0315T	1(3)	0398T	1(3)	0445T	1(2)	0489T	1(2)	0533T	1(2)

CPT	MUE	CPT	MUE	CPT	MUE	CPT	MUE	CPT	MUE	CPT	MUE	CPT	MUE	CPT	MUE
0534T	1(2)	11308	2(3)	11922	1(3)	14041	3(3)	15758	2(3)	15956	2(3)	19272	1(3)	20552	1(2)
0535T	1(2)	11310	4(3)	11950	1(2)	14060	2(3)	15760	2(3)	15958	2(3)	19281	1(2)	20553	1(2)
0536T	1(2)	11311	4(3)	11951	1(2)	14061	2(3)	15770	2(3)	15999	1(3)	19282	2(3)	20555	1(3)
0537T	1(2)	11312	3(3)	11952	1(2)	14301	2(3)	15775	1(2)	16000	1(2)	19283	1(2)	20600	6(3)
0538T	1(3)	11313	3(3)	11954	1(3)	14302	8(3)	15776	1(2)	16020	1(3)	19284	2(3)	20604	4(3)
0539T	1(3)	11400	3(3)	11960	2(3)	14350	2(3)	15777	1(3)	16025	1(3)	19285	1(2)	20605	2(3)
0540T	1(3)	11401	3(3)	11970	2(3)	15002	1(2)	15780	1(2)	16030	1(3)	19286	2(3)	20606	2(3)
0541T	1(3)	11402	3(3)	11971	2(3)	15003	60(3)	15781	1(3)	16035	1(2)	19287	1(2)	20610	2(3)
0542T	1(3)	11403	2(3)	11976	1(2)	15004	1(2)	15782	1(3)	16036	8(3)	19288	2(3)	20611	2(3)
10004	3(3)	11404	2(3)	11980	1(2)	15005	19(3)	15783	1(3)	17000	1(2)	19294	2(3)	20612	2(3)
10005	1(2)	11406	2(3)	11981	1(3)	15040	1(2)	15786	1(2)	17003	13(2)	19296	1(3)	20615	1(3)
10006	3(3)	11420	3(3)	11982	1(3)	15050	1(3)	15787	2(3)	17004	1(2)	19297	2(3)	20650	4(3)
10007	1(2)	11421	3(3)	11983	1(3)	15100	1(2)	15788	1(2)	17106	1(2)	19298	1(2)	20660	1(2)
10008	3(3)	11422	3(3)	12001	1(2)	15101	40(3)	15789	1(2)	17107	1(2)	19300	1(2)	20661	1(2)
10009	1(2)	11423	2(3)	12002	1(2)	15110	1(2)	15792	1(3)	17108	1(2)	19301	1(2)	20662	1(2)
10010	3(3)	11424	2(3)	12004	1(2)	15111	5(3)	15793	1(3)	17110	1(2)	19302	1(2)	20663	1(2)
10011	1(2)	11426	2(3)	12005	1(2)	15115	1(2)	15819	1(2)	17111	1(2)	19303	1(2)	20664	1(2)
10012	3(3)	11440	4(3)	12006	1(2)	15116	2(3)	15820	1(2)	17250	4(3)	19304	1(2)	20665	1(2)
10021	1(2)	11441	3(3)	12007	1(2)	15120	1(2)	15821	1(2)	17260	7(3)	19305	1(2)	20670	3(3)
10030	2(3)	11442	3(3)	12011	1(2)	15121	8(3)	15822	1(2)	17261	7(3)	19306	1(2)	20680	3(3)
10035	1(2)	11443	2(3)	12013	1(2)	15130	1(2)	15823	1(2)	17262	6(3)	19307	1(2)	20690	2(3)
10036	2(3)	11444	2(3)	12014	1(2)	15131	2(3)	15824	1(2)	17263	3(3)	19316	1(2)	20692	2(3)
10040	1(2)	11446	2(3)	12015	1(2)	15135	1(2)	15825	1(2)	17264	3(3)	19318	1(2)	20693	2(3)
10060	1(2)	11450	1(2)	12016	1(2)	15136	1(3)	15826	1(2)	17266	2(3)	19324	1(2)	20694	2(3)
10061	1(2)	11451	1(2)	12017	1(2)	15150	1(2)	15828	1(2)	17270	6(3)	19325	1(2)	20696	2(3)
10080	1(3)	11462	1(2)	12018	1(2)	15151	1(2)	15829	1(2)	17271	4(3)	19328	1(2)	20697	4(3)
10081	1(3)	11463	1(2)	12020	2(3)	15152	5(3)	15830	1(2)	17272	5(3)	19330	1(2)	20802	1(2)
10120	3(3)	11470	3(2)	12021	3(3)	15155	1(2)	15832	1(2)	17273	4(3)	19340	1(2)	20805	1(2)
10121	2(3)	11471	2(3)	12031	1(2)	15156	1(2)	15833	1(2)	17274	2(3)	19342	1(2)	20808	1(2)
10140	2(3)	11600	2(3)	12032	1(2)	15157	1(3)	15834	1(2)	17276	2(3)	19350	1(2)	20816	3(3)
10160	3(3)	11601	2(3)	12034	1(2)	15200	1(2)	15835	1(3)	17280	6(3)	19355	1(2)	20822	3(3)
10180	2(3)	11602	3(3)	12035	1(2)	15201	7(3)	15836	1(2)	17281	5(3)	19357	1(2)	20824	1(2)
11000	1(2)	11603	2(3)	12036	1(2)	15220	1(2)	15837	2(3)	17282	4(3)	19361	1(2)	20827	1(2)
11001	1(3)	11604	2(3)	12037	1(2)	15221	9(3)	15838	1(2)	17283	4(3)	19364	1(2)	20838	1(2)
11004	1(2)	11606	2(3)	12041	1(2)	15240	1(2)	15839	2(3)	17284	2(3)	19366	1(2)	20900	2(3)
11005	1(2)	11620	2(3)	12042	1(2)	15241	9(3)	15840	1(3)	17286	2(3)	19367	1(2)	20902	2(3)
11006	1(2)	11621	2(3)	12044	1(2)	15260	1(2)	15841	2(3)	17311	4(3)	19368	1(2)	20910	1(3)
11008	1(2)	11622	2(3)	12045	1(2)	15261	6(3)	15842	2(3)	17312	6(3)	19369	1(2)	20912	1(3)
11010	2(3)	11623	2(3)	12046	1(2)	15271	1(2)	15845	2(3)	17313	3(3)	19370	1(2)	20920	1(3)
11011	1(2)	11624	2(3)	12047	1(2)	15272	3(3)	15847	1(2)	17314	4(3)	19371	1(2)	20922	1(3)
11012	2(3)	11626	2(3)	12051	1(2)	15273	1(2)	15850	0(3)	17315	15(3)	19380	1(2)	20924	2(3)
11042	1(2)	11640	2(3)	12052	1(2)	15274	60(3)	15851	1(2)	17340	1(2)	19396	1(2)	20926	2(3)
11043	1(2)	11641	2(3)	12053	1(2)	15275	1(2)	15852	1(3)	17360	1(2)	19499	1(3)	20930	0(3)
11044	1(2)	11642	3(3)	12054	1(2)	15276	3(2)	15860	1(3)	17380	1(3)	20100	2(3)	20931	1(2)
11045	12(3)	11643	2(3)	12055	1(2)	15277	1(2)	15876	1(2)	17999	1(3)	20101	2(3)	20932	1(3)
11046	10(3)	11644	2(3)	12056	1(2)	15278	15(3)	15877	1(2)	19000	2(3)	20102	3(3)	20933	1(3)
11047	10(3)	11646	2(3)	12057	1(2)	15570	2(3)	15878	1(2)	19001	5(3)	20103	3(3)	20934	1(3)
11055	1(2)	11719	1(2)	13100	1(2)	15572	2(3)	15879	1(2)	19020	2(3)	20150	2(3)	20936	0(3)
11056	1(2)	11720	1(2)	13101	1(2)	15574	2(3)	15920	1(3)	19030	1(2)	20200	2(3)	20937	1(2)
11057	1(2)	11721	1(2)	13102	9(3)	15576	2(3)	15922	1(3)	19081	1(2)	20205	3(3)	20938	1(2)
11102	1(2)	11730	1(2)	13120	1(2)	15600	2(3)	15931	1(3)	19082	2(3)	20206	3(3)	20939	1(3)
11103	6(3)	11732	4(3)	13121	1(2)	15610	2(3)	15933	1(3)	19083	1(2)	20220	3(3)	20950	2(3)
11104	1(2)	11740	2(3)	13122	9(3)	15620	2(3)	15934	1(3)	19084	2(3)	20225	2(3)	20955	1(3)
11105	3(3)	11750	6(3)	13131	1(2)	15630	2(3)	15935	1(3)	19085	1(2)	20240	4(3)	20956	1(3)
11106	1(2)	11755	2(3)	13132	1(2)	15650	1(3)	15936	1(3)	19086	2(3)	20245	3(3)	20957	1(3)
11107	2(3)	11760	4(3)	13133	7(3)	15730	1(3)	15937	1(3)	19100	4(3)	20250	1(3)	20962	1(3)
11200	1(2)	11762	2(3)	13151	1(2)	15731	1(3)	15940	2(3)	19101	3(3)	20251	2(3)	20969	2(3)
11201	0(3)	11765	4(3)	13152	1(2)	15733	2(3)	15941	2(3)	19105	2(3)	20500	2(3)	20970	2(3)
11300	5(3)	11770	1(3)	13153	2(3)	15734	4(3)	15944	2(3)	19110	1(3)	20501	1(3)	20972	2(3)
11301	6(3)	11771	1(3)	13160	2(3)	15736	2(3)	15945	2(3)	19112	2(3)	20520	2(3)	20973	1(2)
11302	4(3)	11772	1(3)	14000	2(3)	15738	3(3)	15946	2(3)	19120	1(3)	20525	4(3)	20974	1(3)
11303	3(3)	11900	1(3)	14001	2(3)	15740	2(3)	15950	2(3)	19125	1(2)	20526	1(2)	20975	1(3)
11305	4(3)	11901	1(2)	14020	2(3)	15750	2(3)	15951	2(3)	19126	3(3)	20527	2(3)	20979	1(3)
11306	4(3)	11920	1(2)	14021	2(3)	15756	2(3)	15952	2(3)	19260	2(3)	20550	5(3)	20982	1(2)
11307	3(3)	11921	1(2)	14040	2(3)	15757	2(3)	15953	2(3)	19271	1(3)	20551	5(3)	20983	1(2)

CPT	MUE	CPT	MUE	CPT	MUE	CPT	MUE	CPT	MUE	CPT	MUE	CPT	MUE
20985	2(3)	21175	1(2)	21366	1(2)	21820	1(2)	22614	13(3)	23101	1(3)	23570	1(2)
20999	1(3)	21179	1(2)	21385	1(2)	21825	1(2)	22630	1(2)	23105	1(2)	23575	1(2)
21010	1(2)	21180	1(2)	21386	1(2)	21899	1(3)	22632	4(2)	23106	1(2)	23585	1(2)
21011	4(3)	21181	1(3)	21387	1(2)	21920	2(3)	22633	1(2)	23107	1(2)	23600	1(2)
21012	3(3)	21182	1(2)	21390	1(2)	21925	2(3)	22634	4(2)	23120	1(2)	23605	1(2)
21013	2(3)	21183	1(2)	21395	1(2)	21930	5(3)	22800	1(2)	23125	1(2)	23615	1(2)
21014	2(3)	21184	1(2)	21400	1(2)	21931	3(3)	22802	1(2)	23130	1(2)	23616	1(2)
21015	1(3)	21188	1(2)	21401	1(2)	21932	1(3)	22804	1(2)	23140	1(3)	23620	1(2)
21016	2(3)	21193	1(2)	21406	1(2)	21933	2(3)	22808	1(2)	23145	1(3)	23625	1(2)
21025	2(3)	21194	1(2)	21407	1(2)	21935	1(3)	22810	1(2)	23146	1(3)	23630	1(2)
21026	2(3)	21195	1(2)	21408	1(2)	21936	1(3)	22812	1(2)	23150	1(3)	23650	1(2)
21029	1(3)	21196	1(2)	21421	1(2)	22010	2(3)	22818	1(2)	23155	1(3)	23655	1(2)
21030	1(3)	21198	1(3)	21422	1(2)	22015	2(3)	22819	1(2)	23156	1(3)	23660	1(2)
21031	2(3)	21199	1(2)	21423	1(2)	22100	1(2)	22830	1(2)	23170	1(3)	23665	1(2)
21032	1(3)	21206	1(3)	21431	1(2)	22101	1(2)	22840	1(3)	23172	1(3)	23670	1(2)
21034	1(3)	21208	1(3)	21432	1(2)	22102	1(2)	22841	0(3)	23174	1(3)	23675	1(2)
21040	2(3)	21209	1(3)	21433	1(2)	22103	3(3)	22842	1(3)	23180	1(3)	23680	1(2)
21044	1(3)	21210	2(3)	21435	1(2)	22110	1(2)	22843	1(3)	23182	1(3)	23700	1(2)
21045	1(3)	21215	2(3)	21436	1(2)	22112	1(2)	22844	1(3)	23184	1(3)	23800	1(2)
21046	2(3)	21230	2(3)	21440	2(2)	22114	1(2)	22845	1(3)	23190	1(3)	23802	1(2)
21047	2(3)	21235	2(3)	21445	2(2)	22116	3(3)	22846	1(3)	23195	1(2)	23900	1(2)
21048	2(3)	21240	1(2)	21450	1(2)	22206	1(2)	22847	1(3)	23200	1(3)	23920	1(2)
21049	1(3)	21242	1(2)	21451	1(2)	22207	1(2)	22848	1(2)	23210	1(3)	23921	1(2)
21050	1(2)	21243	1(2)	21452	1(2)	22208	5(3)	22849	1(2)	23220	1(3)	23929	1(3)
21060	1(2)	21244	1(2)	21453	1(2)	22210	1(2)	22850	1(2)	23330	2(3)	23930	2(3)
21070	1(2)	21245	2(3)	21454	1(2)	22212	1(2)	22852	1(2)	23333	1(3)	23931	2(3)
21073	1(2)	21246	2(3)	21461	1(2)	22214	1(2)	22853	4(3)	23334	1(2)	23935	2(3)
21076	1(2)	21247	1(2)	21462	1(2)	22216	6(3)	22854	4(3)	23335	1(2)	24000	1(2)
21077	1(2)	21248	2(3)	21465	1(2)	22220	1(2)	22855	1(2)	23350	1(2)	24006	1(2)
21079	1(2)	21249	2(3)	21470	1(2)	22222	1(2)	22856	1(2)	23395	1(2)	24065	2(3)
21080	1(2)	21255	1(2)	21480	1(2)	22224	1(2)	22857	1(2)	23397	1(3)	24066	2(3)
21081	1(2)	21256	1(2)	21485	1(2)	22226	4(3)	22858	1(2)	23400	1(2)	24071	2(3)
21082	1(2)	21260	1(2)	21490	1(2)	22310	1(2)	22859	4(3)	23405	2(3)	24073	2(3)
21083	1(2)	21261	1(2)	21497	1(2)	22315	1(2)	22861	1(2)	23406	1(2)	24075	5(3)
21084	1(2)	21263	1(2)	21499	1(3)	22318	1(2)	22862	1(2)	23410	1(2)	24076	4(3)
21085	1(3)	21267	1(2)	21501	3(3)	22319	1(2)	22864	1(2)	23412	1(2)	24077	1(3)
21086	1(2)	21268	1(2)	21502	1(3)	22325	1(2)	22865	1(2)	23415	1(2)	24079	1(3)
21087	1(2)	21270	1(2)	21510	1(3)	22326	1(2)	22867	1(2)	23420	1(2)	24100	1(2)
21088	1(2)	21275	1(2)	21550	2(3)	22327	1(2)	22868	1(2)	23430	1(2)	24101	1(2)
21089	1(3)	21280	1(2)	21552	2(3)	22328	6(3)	22869	1(2)	23440	1(2)	24102	1(2)
21100	1(2)	21282	1(2)	21554	2(3)	22505	1(2)	22870	1(2)	23450	1(2)	24105	1(2)
21110	2(3)	21295	1(2)	21555	2(3)	22510	1(2)	22899	1(3)	23455	1(2)	24110	1(3)
21116	1(2)	21296	1(2)	21556	2(3)	22511	1(2)	22900	3(3)	23460	1(2)	24115	1(3)
21120	1(2)	21299	1(3)	21557	1(3)	22512	3(3)	22901	2(3)	23462	1(2)	24116	1(3)
21121	1(2)	21310	1(2)	21558	1(3)	22513	1(2)	22902	4(3)	23465	1(2)	24120	1(3)
21122	1(2)	21315	1(2)	21600	5(3)	22514	1(2)	22903	3(3)	23466	1(2)	24125	1(3)
21123	1(2)	21320	1(2)	21610	1(3)	22515	4(3)	22904	1(3)	23470	1(2)	24126	1(3)
21125	2(2)	21325	1(2)	21615	1(2)	22526	0(3)	22905	1(3)	23472	1(2)	24130	1(2)
21127	2(3)	21330	1(2)	21616	1(2)	22527	0(3)	22999	1(3)	23473	1(2)	24134	1(3)
21137	1(2)	21335	1(2)	21620	1(2)	22532	1(2)	23000	1(2)	23474	1(2)	24136	1(3)
21138	1(2)	21336	1(2)	21627	1(2)	22533	1(2)	23020	1(2)	23480	1(2)	24138	1(3)
21139	1(2)	21337	1(2)	21630	1(2)	22534	3(3)	23030	2(3)	23485	1(2)	24140	1(3)
21141	1(2)	21338	1(2)	21632	1(2)	22548	1(2)	23031	1(3)	23490	1(2)	24145	1(3)
21142	1(2)	21339	1(2)	21685	1(2)	22551	1(2)	23035	1(3)	23491	1(2)	24147	1(2)
21143	1(2)	21340	1(2)	21700	1(2)	22552	5(3)	23040	1(2)	23500	1(2)	24149	1(2)
21145	1(2)	21343	1(2)	21705	1(2)	22554	1(2)	23044	1(3)	23505	1(2)	24150	1(3)
21146	1(2)	21344	1(2)	21720	1(3)	22556	1(2)	23065	2(3)	23515	1(2)	24152	1(3)
21147	1(2)	21345	1(2)	21725	1(3)	22558	1(2)	23066	2(3)	23520	1(2)	24155	1(2)
21150	1(2)	21346	1(2)	21740	1(2)	22585	5(3)	23071	2(3)	23525	1(2)	24160	1(2)
21151	1(2)	21347	1(2)	21742	1(2)	22586	1(2)	23073	2(3)	23530	1(2)	24164	1(2)
21154	1(2)	21348	1(2)	21743	1(2)	22590	1(2)	23075	2(3)	23532	1(2)	24200	3(3)
21155	1(2)	21355	1(2)	21750	1(2)	22595	1(2)	23076	2(3)	23540	1(2)	24201	3(3)
21159	1(2)	21356	1(2)	21811	1(2)	22600	1(2)	23077	1(3)	23545	1(2)	24220	1(2)
21160	1(2)	21360	1(2)	21812	1(2)	22610	1(2)	23078	1(3)	23550	1(2)	24300	1(2)
21172	1(3)	21365	1(2)	21813	1(2)	22612	1(2)	23100	1(2)	23552	1(2)	24301	2(3)

CPT	MUE
24305	4(3)
24310	2(3)
24320	2(3)
24330	1(3)
24331	1(3)
24332	1(2)
24340	1(2)
24341	2(3)
24342	2(3)
24343	1(2)
24344	1(2)
24345	1(2)
24346	1(2)
24357	1(3)
24358	1(3)
24359	2(3)
24360	1(2)
24361	1(2)
24362	1(2)
24363	1(2)
24365	1(2)
24366	1(2)
24370	1(2)
24371	1(2)
24400	1(3)
24410	1(2)
24420	1(2)
24430	1(3)
24435	1(3)
24470	1(2)
24495	1(2)
24498	1(2)
24500	1(2)
24505	1(2)
24515	1(2)
24516	1(2)
24530	1(2)
24535	1(2)
24538	1(2)
24545	1(2)
24546	1(2)
24560	1(3)
24565	1(3)
24566	1(3)
24575	1(3)
24576	1(3)
24577	1(3)
24579	1(3)
24582	1(3)
24586	1(3)
24587	1(2)
24600	1(2)
24605	1(2)
24615	1(2)
24620	1(2)
24635	1(2)
24640	1(2)
24650	1(2)
24655	1(2)
24665	1(2)
24666	1(2)
24670	1(2)
24675	1(2)
24685	1(2)
24800	1(2)

CPT	MUE	CPT	MUE	CPT	MUE	CPT	MUE	CPT	MUE	CPT	MUE	CPT	MUE	CPT	MUE
24802	1(2)	25275	2(3)	25609	1(2)	26135	4(3)	26499	2(3)	26756	2(3)	27096	1(2)	27267	1(2)
24900	1(2)	25280	9(3)	25622	1(2)	26140	2(3)	26500	3(3)	26765	3(3)	27097	1(3)	27268	1(2)
24920	1(2)	25290	10(3)	25624	1(2)	26145	6(3)	26502	2(3)	26770	3(3)	27098	1(2)	27269	1(2)
24925	1(2)	25295	9(3)	25628	1(2)	26160	4(3)	26508	1(2)	26775	2(3)	27100	1(2)	27275	2(2)
24930	1(2)	25300	1(2)	25630	1(3)	26170	4(3)	26510	4(3)	26776	4(3)	27105	1(3)	27279	1(2)
24931	1(2)	25301	1(2)	25635	1(3)	26180	4(3)	26516	1(2)	26785	3(3)	27110	1(2)	27280	1(2)
24935	1(2)	25310	5(3)	25645	1(3)	26185	1(3)	26517	1(2)	26820	1(2)	27111	1(2)	27282	1(2)
24940	1(2)	25312	4(3)	25650	1(2)	26200	2(3)	26518	1(2)	26841	1(2)	27120	1(2)	27284	1(2)
24999	1(3)	25315	1(3)	25651	1(2)	26205	1(3)	26520	4(3)	26842	1(2)	27122	1(2)	27286	1(2)
25000	2(3)	25316	1(3)	25652	1(2)	26210	2(3)	26525	4(3)	26843	2(3)	27125	1(2)	27290	1(2)
25001	1(3)	25320	1(2)	25660	1(2)	26215	2(3)	26530	4(3)	26844	2(3)	27130	1(2)	27295	1(2)
25020	1(2)	25332	1(2)	25670	1(2)	26230	2(3)	26531	4(3)	26850	5(3)	27132	1(2)	27299	1(3)
25023	1(2)	25335	1(2)	25671	1(2)	26235	2(3)	26535	3(3)	26852	2(3)	27134	1(2)	27301	3(3)
25024	1(2)	25337	1(2)	25675	1(2)	26236	2(3)	26536	4(3)	26860	1(2)	27137	1(2)	27303	2(3)
25025	1(2)	25350	1(3)	25676	1(2)	26250	2(3)	26540	4(3)	26861	4(3)	27138	1(2)	27305	1(2)
25028	4(3)	25355	1(3)	25680	1(2)	26260	1(3)	26541	4(3)	26862	1(2)	27140	1(2)	27306	1(2)
25031	2(3)	25360	1(3)	25685	1(2)	26262	1(3)	26542	4(3)	26863	2(3)	27146	1(3)	27307	1(2)
25035	2(3)	25365	1(3)	25690	1(2)	26320	4(3)	26545	4(3)	26910	4(3)	27147	1(3)	27310	1(2)
25040	1(3)	25370	1(2)	25695	1(2)	26340	4(3)	26546	2(3)	26951	8(3)	27151	1(3)	27323	2(3)
25065	2(3)	25375	1(2)	25800	1(2)	26341	2(3)	26548	3(3)	26952	4(3)	27156	1(2)	27324	3(3)
25066	2(3)	25390	1(2)	25805	1(2)	26350	6(3)	26550	1(2)	26989	1(3)	27158	1(2)	27325	1(2)
25071	3(3)	25391	1(2)	25810	1(2)	26352	2(3)	26551	1(2)	26990	2(3)	27161	1(2)	27326	1(2)
25073	2(3)	25392	1(2)	25820	1(2)	26356	4(3)	26553	1(3)	26991	1(3)	27165	1(2)	27327	5(3)
25075	6(3)	25393	1(2)	25825	1(2)	26357	2(3)	26554	1(3)	26992	2(3)	27170	1(2)	27328	3(3)
25076	3(3)	25394	1(3)	25830	1(2)	26358	2(3)	26555	2(3)	27000	1(3)	27175	1(2)	27329	1(3)
25077	1(3)	25400	1(2)	25900	1(2)	26370	3(3)	26556	2(3)	27001	1(3)	27176	1(2)	27330	1(2)
25078	1(3)	25405	1(2)	25905	1(2)	26372	1(3)	26560	2(3)	27003	1(2)	27177	1(2)	27331	1(2)
25085	1(2)	25415	1(2)	25907	1(2)	26373	2(3)	26561	2(3)	27005	1(2)	27178	1(2)	27332	1(2)
25100	1(2)	25420	1(2)	25909	1(2)	26390	2(3)	26562	2(3)	27006	1(2)	27179	1(2)	27333	1(2)
25101	1(2)	25425	1(2)	25915	1(2)	26392	2(3)	26565	2(3)	27025	1(3)	27181	1(2)	27334	1(2)
25105	1(2)	25426	1(2)	25920	1(2)	26410	4(3)	26567	3(3)	27027	1(2)	27185	1(2)	27335	1(2)
25107	1(2)	25430	1(3)	25922	1(2)	26412	3(3)	26568	2(3)	27030	1(2)	27187	1(2)	27337	3(3)
25109	4(3)	25431	1(3)	25924	1(2)	26415	2(3)	26580	1(2)	27033	1(2)	27197	1(2)	27339	4(3)
25110	2(3)	25440	1(2)	25927	1(2)	26416	2(3)	26587	2(3)	27035	1(2)	27198	1(2)	27340	1(2)
25111	1(3)	25441	1(2)	25929	1(2)	26418	4(3)	26590	2(3)	27036	1(2)	27200	1(2)	27345	1(2)
25112	1(3)	25442	1(2)	25931	1(2)	26420	3(3)	26591	4(3)	27040	2(3)	27202	1(2)	27347	1(2)
25115	1(3)	25443	1(2)	25999	1(3)	26426	4(3)	26593	8(3)	27041	3(3)	27215	0(3)	27350	1(2)
25116	1(3)	25444	1(2)	26010	2(3)	26428	2(3)	26596	1(3)	27043	2(3)	27216	0(3)	27355	1(3)
25118	5(3)	25445	1(2)	26011	3(3)	26432	2(3)	26600	2(3)	27045	3(3)	27217	0(3)	27356	1(3)
25119	1(2)	25446	1(2)	26020	4(3)	26433	2(3)	26605	3(3)	27047	2(3)	27218	0(3)	27357	1(3)
25120	1(3)	25447	4(3)	26025	1(2)	26434	2(3)	26607	2(3)	27048	2(3)	27220	1(2)	27358	1(3)
25125	1(3)	25449	1(2)	26030	1(2)	26437	4(3)	26608	4(3)	27049	1(3)	27222	1(2)	27360	2(3)
25126	1(3)	25450	1(2)	26034	2(3)	26440	6(3)	26615	3(3)	27050	1(2)	27226	1(2)	27364	1(3)
25130	1(3)	25455	1(2)	26035	1(3)	26442	5(3)	26641	1(2)	27052	1(2)	27227	1(2)	27365	1(3)
25135	1(3)	25490	1(2)	26037	1(3)	26445	5(3)	26645	1(2)	27054	1(2)	27228	1(2)	27369	1(2)
25136	1(3)	25491	1(2)	26040	1(2)	26449	5(3)	26650	1(2)	27057	1(2)	27230	1(2)	27372	2(3)
25145	1(3)	25492	1(2)	26045	1(2)	26450	6(3)	26665	1(2)	27059	1(3)	27232	1(2)	27380	1(2)
25150	1(3)	25500	1(2)	26055	5(3)	26455	6(3)	26670	2(3)	27060	1(2)	27235	1(2)	27381	1(2)
25151	1(3)	25505	1(2)	26060	5(3)	26460	4(3)	26675	1(3)	27062	1(2)	27236	1(2)	27385	2(3)
25170	1(3)	25515	1(2)	26070	2(3)	26471	4(3)	26676	2(3)	27065	1(3)	27238	1(2)	27386	2(3)
25210	2(3)	25520	1(2)	26075	3(3)	26474	4(3)	26685	3(3)	27066	1(3)	27240	1(2)	27390	1(2)
25215	1(2)	25525	1(2)	26080	3(3)	26476	4(3)	26686	3(3)	27067	1(3)	27244	1(2)	27391	1(2)
25230	1(2)	25526	1(2)	26100	1(3)	26477	2(3)	26700	2(3)	27070	1(3)	27245	1(2)	27392	1(2)
25240	1(2)	25530	1(2)	26105	2(3)	26478	6(3)	26705	3(3)	27071	1(3)	27246	1(2)	27393	1(2)
25246	1(2)	25535	1(2)	26110	2(3)	26479	4(3)	26706	2(3)	27075	1(3)	27248	1(2)	27394	1(2)
25248	3(3)	25545	1(2)	26111	4(3)	26480	4(3)	26715	3(3)	27076	1(2)	27250	1(2)	27395	1(2)
25250	1(2)	25560	1(2)	26113	3(3)	26483	4(3)	26720	4(3)	27077	1(2)	27252	1(2)	27396	1(2)
25251	1(2)	25565	1(2)	26115	4(3)	26485	4(3)	26725	3(3)	27078	1(2)	27253	1(2)	27397	1(2)
25259	1(2)	25574	1(2)	26116	2(3)	26489	4(3)	26727	3(3)	27080	1(2)	27254	1(2)	27400	1(2)
25260	9(3)	25575	1(2)	26117	2(3)	26490	3(3)	26735	4(3)	27086	1(3)	27256	1(2)	27403	1(3)
25263	4(3)	25600	1(2)	26118	1(3)	26492	2(3)	26740	3(3)	27087	1(3)	27257	1(2)	27405	2(2)
25265	4(3)	25605	1(2)	26121	1(2)	26494	1(3)	26742	3(3)	27090	1(2)	27258	1(2)	27407	2(2)
25270	8(3)	25606	1(2)	26123	1(2)	26496	1(3)	26746	3(3)	27091	1(2)	27259	1(2)	27409	1(2)
25272	4(3)	25607	1(2)	26125	4(3)	26497	2(3)	26750	3(3)	27093	1(2)	27265	1(2)	27412	1(2)
25274	4(3)	25608	1(2)	26130	1(3)	26498	1(3)	26755	2(3)	27095	1(2)	27266	1(2)	27415	1(2)

CPT	MUE	CPT	MUE	CPT	MUE	CPT	MUE	CPT	MUE	CPT	MUE	CPT	MUE	CPT	MUE
27416	1(2)	27550	1(2)	27692	4(3)	27880	1(2)	28171	1(3)	28445	1(2)	29058	1(3)	29843	1(2)
27418	1(2)	27552	1(2)	27695	1(2)	27881	1(2)	28173	2(3)	28446	1(2)	29065	1(3)	29844	1(2)
27420	1(2)	27556	1(2)	27696	1(2)	27882	1(2)	28175	2(3)	28450	2(3)	29075	1(3)	29845	1(2)
27422	1(2)	27557	1(2)	27698	2(2)	27884	1(2)	28190	3(3)	28455	3(3)	29085	1(3)	29846	1(2)
27424	1(2)	27558	1(2)	27700	1(2)	27886	1(2)	28192	2(3)	28456	2(3)	29086	2(3)	29847	1(2)
27425	1(2)	27560	1(2)	27702	1(2)	27888	1(2)	28193	2(3)	28465	3(3)	29105	1(2)	29848	1(2)
27427	1(2)	27562	1(2)	27703	1(2)	27889	1(2)	28200	4(3)	28470	2(3)	29125	1(2)	29850	1(2)
27428	1(2)	27566	1(2)	27704	1(2)	27892	1(2)	28202	2(3)	28475	5(3)	29126	1(2)	29851	1(2)
27429	1(2)	27570	1(2)	27705	1(3)	27893	1(2)	28208	4(3)	28476	4(3)	29130	3(3)	29855	1(2)
27430	1(2)	27580	1(2)	27707	1(3)	27894	1(2)	28210	2(3)	28485	5(3)	29131	2(3)	29856	1(2)
27435	1(2)	27590	1(2)	27709	1(3)	27899	1(3)	28220	1(2)	28490	1(2)	29200	1(2)	29860	1(2)
27437	1(2)	27591	1(2)	27712	1(2)	28001	2(3)	28222	1(2)	28495	1(2)	29240	1(2)	29861	1(2)
27438	1(2)	27592	1(2)	27715	1(2)	28002	3(3)	28225	1(2)	28496	1(2)	29260	1(2)	29862	1(2)
27440	1(2)	27594	1(2)	27720	1(2)	28003	2(3)	28226	1(2)	28505	1(2)	29280	2(3)	29863	1(2)
27441	1(2)	27596	1(2)	27722	1(2)	28005	3(3)	28230	1(2)	28510	4(3)	29305	1(3)	29866	1(2)
27442	1(2)	27598	1(2)	27724	1(2)	28008	2(3)	28232	6(3)	28515	4(3)	29325	1(3)	29867	1(2)
27443	1(2)	27599	1(3)	27725	1(2)	28010	4(3)	28234	6(3)	28525	4(3)	29345	1(3)	29868	1(3)
27445	1(2)	27600	1(2)	27726	1(2)	28011	4(3)	28238	1(2)	28530	1(2)	29355	1(3)	29870	1(2)
27446	1(2)	27601	1(2)	27727	1(2)	28020	2(3)	28240	1(2)	28531	1(2)	29358	1(3)	29871	1(2)
27447	1(2)	27602	1(2)	27730	1(2)	28022	3(3)	28250	1(2)	28540	1(3)	29365	1(3)	29873	1(2)
27448	1(3)	27603	2(3)	27732	1(2)	28024	4(3)	28260	1(2)	28545	1(3)	29405	1(3)	29874	1(2)
27450	1(3)	27604	2(3)	27734	1(2)	28035	1(2)	28261	1(3)	28546	1(3)	29425	1(3)	29875	1(2)
27454	1(2)	27605	1(2)	27740	1(2)	28039	2(3)	28262	1(2)	28555	1(3)	29435	1(3)	29876	1(2)
27455	1(3)	27606	1(2)	27742	1(2)	28041	2(3)	28264	1(2)	28570	1(2)	29440	1(2)	29877	1(2)
27457	1(3)	27607	2(3)	27745	1(2)	28043	4(3)	28270	6(3)	28575	1(2)	29445	1(3)	29879	1(2)
27465	1(2)	27610	1(2)	27750	1(2)	28045	4(3)	28272	6(3)	28576	1(2)	29450	1(3)	29880	1(2)
27466	1(2)	27612	1(2)	27752	1(2)	28046	1(3)	28280	1(2)	28585	1(3)	29505	1(2)	29881	1(2)
27468	1(2)	27613	3(3)	27756	1(2)	28047	1(3)	28285	4(3)	28600	2(3)	29515	1(2)	29882	1(2)
27470	1(2)	27614	3(3)	27758	1(2)	28050	2(3)	28286	1(2)	28605	2(3)	29520	1(2)	29883	1(2)
27472	1(2)	27615	1(3)	27759	1(2)	28052	2(3)	28288	4(3)	28606	3(3)	29530	1(2)	29884	1(2)
27475	1(2)	27616	1(3)	27760	1(2)	28054	2(3)	28289	1(2)	28615	5(3)	29540	1(2)	29885	1(2)
27477	1(2)	27618	3(3)	27762	1(2)	28055	1(3)	28291	1(2)	28630	2(3)	29550	1(2)	29886	1(2)
27479	1(2)	27619	2(3)	27766	1(2)	28060	1(2)	28292	1(2)	28635	2(3)	29580	1(2)	29887	1(2)
27485	1(2)	27620	1(2)	27767	1(2)	28062	1(2)	28295	1(2)	28636	4(3)	29581	1(2)	29888	1(2)
27486	1(2)	27625	1(2)	27768	1(2)	28070	2(3)	28296	1(2)	28645	4(3)	29584	1(2)	29889	1(2)
27487	1(2)	27626	1(2)	27769	1(2)	28072	4(3)	28297	1(2)	28660	4(3)	29700	2(3)	29891	1(2)
27488	1(2)	27630	2(3)	27780	1(2)	28080	3(3)	28298	1(2)	28665	3(3)	29705	1(3)	29892	1(2)
27495	1(2)	27632	3(3)	27781	1(2)	28086	2(3)	28299	1(2)	28666	4(3)	29710	1(2)	29893	1(2)
27496	1(2)	27634	2(3)	27784	1(2)	28088	2(3)	28300	1(2)	28675	3(3)	29720	1(2)	29894	1(2)
27497	1(2)	27635	1(3)	27786	1(2)	28090	2(3)	28302	1(2)	28705	1(2)	29730	1(3)	29895	1(2)
27498	1(2)	27637	1(3)	27788	1(2)	28092	2(3)	28304	1(3)	28715	1(2)	29740	1(3)	29897	1(2)
27499	1(2)	27638	1(3)	27792	1(2)	28100	1(3)	28305	1(3)	28725	1(2)	29750	1(3)	29898	1(2)
27500	1(2)	27640	1(3)	27808	1(2)	28102	1(3)	28306	1(2)	28730	1(2)	29799	1(3)	29899	1(2)
27501	1(2)	27641	1(3)	27810	1(2)	28103	1(3)	28307	1(2)	28735	1(2)	29800	1(2)	29900	2(3)
27502	1(2)	27645	1(3)	27814	1(2)	28104	2(3)	28308	4(3)	28737	1(2)	29804	1(2)	29901	2(3)
27503	1(2)	27646	1(3)	27816	1(2)	28106	1(3)	28309	1(2)	28740	1(2)	29805	1(2)	29902	2(3)
27506	1(2)	27647	1(3)	27818	1(2)	28107	1(3)	28310	1(2)	28750	1(2)	29806	1(2)	29904	1(2)
27507	1(2)	27648	1(2)	27822	1(2)	28108	2(3)	28312	4(3)	28755	1(2)	29807	1(2)	29905	1(2)
27508	1(2)	27650	1(2)	27823	1(2)	28110	1(2)	28313	4(3)	28760	1(2)	29819	1(2)	29906	1(2)
27509	1(2)	27652	1(2)	27824	1(2)	28111	1(2)	28315	1(2)	28800	1(2)	29820	1(2)	29907	1(2)
27510	1(2)	27654	1(2)	27825	1(2)	28112	4(3)	28320	1(2)	28805	1(2)	29821	1(2)	29914	1(2)
27511	1(2)	27656	1(3)	27826	1(2)	28113	1(2)	28322	2(3)	28810	5(3)	29822	1(2)	29915	1(2)
27513	1(2)	27658	2(3)	27827	1(2)	28114	1(2)	28340	2(3)	28820	6(3)	29823	1(2)	29916	1(2)
27514	1(2)	27659	2(3)	27828	1(2)	28116	1(2)	28341	2(3)	28825	8(2)	29824	1(2)	29999	1(3)
27516	1(2)	27664	2(3)	27829	1(2)	28118	1(2)	28344	1(2)	28890	1(2)	29825	1(2)	30000	1(3)
27517	1(2)	27665	2(3)	27830	1(2)	28119	1(2)	28345	2(3)	28899	1(3)	29826	1(2)	30020	1(3)
27519	1(2)	27675	1(2)	27831	1(2)	28120	2(3)	28360	1(2)	29000	1(3)	29827	1(2)	30100	2(3)
27520	1(2)	27676	1(2)	27832	1(2)	28122	4(3)	28400	1(2)	29010	1(3)	29828	1(2)	30110	1(2)
27524	1(2)	27680	2(3)	27840	1(2)	28124	4(3)	28405	1(2)	29015	1(3)	29830	1(2)	30115	1(2)
27530	1(2)	27681	1(2)	27842	1(2)	28126	4(3)	28406	1(2)	29035	1(3)	29834	1(2)	30117	2(3)
27532	1(2)	27685	2(3)	27846	1(2)	28130	1(2)	28415	1(2)	29040	1(3)	29835	1(2)	30118	1(3)
27535	1(2)	27686	3(3)	27848	1(2)	28140	3(3)	28420	1(2)	29044	1(3)	29836	1(2)	30120	1(2)
27536	1(2)	27687	1(2)	27860	1(2)	28150	4(3)	28430	1(2)	29046	1(3)	29837	1(2)	30124	2(3)
27538	1(2)	27690	2(3)	27870	1(2)	28153	4(3)	28435	1(2)	29049	1(3)	29838	1(2)	30125	1(3)
27540	1(2)	27691	2(3)	27871	1(3)	28160	5(3)	28436	1(2)	29055	1(3)	29840	1(2)	30130	1(2)

CPT	MUE	CPT	MUE	CPT	MUE	CPT	MUE	CPT	MUE	CPT	MUE	CPT	MUE	CPT	MUE
30140	1(2)	31241	1(2)	31573	1(2)	31780	1(2)	32650	1(2)	33214	1(3)	33365	1(2)	33536	1(2)
30150	1(2)	31253	1(2)	31574	1(2)	31781	1(2)	32651	1(2)	33215	2(3)	33366	1(3)	33542	1(2)
30160	1(2)	31254	1(2)	31575	1(3)	31785	1(3)	32652	1(2)	33216	1(3)	33367	1(2)	33545	1(2)
30200	1(2)	31255	1(2)	31576	1(3)	31786	1(3)	32653	1(3)	33217	1(3)	33368	1(2)	33548	1(2)
30210	1(3)	31256	1(2)	31577	1(3)	31800	1(3)	32654	1(3)	33218	1(3)	33369	1(2)	33572	3(2)
30220	1(2)	31257	1(2)	31578	1(3)	31805	1(3)	32655	1(3)	33220	1(3)	33390	1(2)	33600	1(3)
30300	1(3)	31259	1(2)	31579	1(2)	31820	1(2)	32656	1(2)	33221	1(3)	33391	1(2)	33602	1(3)
30310	1(3)	31267	1(2)	31580	1(2)	31825	1(2)	32658	1(3)	33222	1(3)	33404	1(2)	33606	1(2)
30320	1(3)	31276	1(2)	31584	1(2)	31830	1(2)	32659	1(2)	33223	1(3)	33405	1(2)	33608	1(2)
30400	1(2)	31287	1(2)	31587	1(2)	31899	1(3)	32661	1(3)	33224	1(3)	33406	1(2)	33610	1(2)
30410	1(2)	31288	1(2)	31590	1(2)	32035	1(2)	32662	1(3)	33225	1(3)	33410	1(2)	33611	1(2)
30420	1(2)	31290	1(2)	31591	1(2)	32036	1(3)	32663	1(3)	33226	1(3)	33411	1(2)	33612	1(2)
30430	1(2)	31291	1(2)	31592	1(2)	32096	1(3)	32664	1(2)	33227	1(3)	33412	1(2)	33615	1(2)
30435	1(2)	31292	1(2)	31599	1(3)	32097	1(3)	32665	1(2)	33228	1(3)	33413	1(2)	33617	1(2)
30450	1(2)	31293	1(2)	31600	1(2)	32098	1(2)	32666	1(3)	33229	1(3)	33414	1(2)	33619	1(2)
30460	1(2)	31294	1(2)	31601	1(2)	32100	1(3)	32667	3(3)	33230	1(3)	33415	1(2)	33620	1(2)
30462	1(2)	31295	1(2)	31603	1(2)	32110	1(3)	32668	2(3)	33231	1(3)	33416	1(2)	33621	1(3)
30465	1(2)	31296	1(2)	31605	1(2)	32120	1(3)	32669	2(3)	33233	1(2)	33417	1(2)	33622	1(2)
30520	1(2)	31297	1(2)	31610	1(2)	32124	1(3)	32670	1(2)	33234	1(2)	33418	1(3)	33641	1(2)
30540	1(2)	31298	1(2)	31611	1(2)	32140	1(3)	32671	1(2)	33235	1(2)	33419	1(2)	33645	1(2)
30545	1(2)	31299	1(3)	31612	1(3)	32141	1(3)	32672	1(3)	33236	1(2)	33420	1(2)	33647	1(2)
30560	1(2)	31300	1(2)	31613	1(2)	32150	1(3)	32673	1(2)	33237	1(2)	33422	1(2)	33660	1(2)
30580	2(3)	31360	1(2)	31614	1(2)	32151	1(3)	32674	1(2)	33238	1(2)	33425	1(2)	33665	1(2)
30600	1(3)	31365	1(2)	31615	1(3)	32160	1(3)	32701	1(2)	33240	1(3)	33426	1(2)	33670	1(2)
30620	1(2)	31367	1(2)	31622	1(3)	32200	2(3)	32800	1(3)	33241	1(2)	33427	1(2)	33675	1(2)
30630	1(2)	31368	1(2)	31623	1(3)	32215	1(2)	32810	1(3)	33243	1(2)	33430	1(2)	33676	1(2)
30801	1(2)	31370	1(2)	31624	1(3)	32220	1(2)	32815	1(3)	33244	1(2)	33440	1(2)	33677	1(2)
30802	1(2)	31375	1(2)	31625	1(2)	32225	1(2)	32820	1(2)	33249	1(3)	33460	1(2)	33681	1(2)
30901	1(3)	31380	1(2)	31626	1(2)	32310	1(3)	32850	1(2)	33250	1(2)	33463	1(2)	33684	1(2)
30903	1(3)	31382	1(2)	31627	1(3)	32320	1(3)	32851	1(2)	33251	1(2)	33464	1(2)	33688	1(2)
30905	1(2)	31390	1(2)	31628	1(2)	32400	2(3)	32852	1(2)	33254	1(2)	33465	1(2)	33690	1(2)
30906	1(3)	31395	1(2)	31629	1(2)	32405	2(3)	32853	1(2)	33255	1(2)	33468	1(2)	33692	1(2)
30915	1(3)	31400	1(3)	31630	1(3)	32440	1(2)	32854	1(2)	33256	1(2)	33470	1(2)	33694	1(2)
30920	1(3)	31420	1(2)	31631	1(2)	32442	1(2)	32855	1(2)	33257	1(2)	33471	1(2)	33697	1(2)
30930	1(2)	31500	2(3)	31632	2(3)	32445	1(2)	32856	1(2)	33258	1(2)	33474	1(2)	33702	1(2)
30999	1(3)	31502	1(3)	31633	2(3)	32480	1(2)	32900	1(2)	33259	1(2)	33475	1(2)	33710	1(2)
31000	1(2)	31505	1(3)	31634	1(3)	32482	1(2)	32905	1(2)	33261	1(2)	33476	1(2)	33720	1(2)
31002	1(2)	31510	1(2)	31635	1(2)	32484	2(3)	32906	1(2)	33262	1(3)	33477	1(2)	33722	1(3)
31020	1(2)	31511	1(3)	31636	1(2)	32486	1(3)	32940	1(3)	33263	1(3)	33478	1(2)	33724	1(2)
31030	1(2)	31512	1(3)	31637	2(3)	32488	1(2)	32960	1(2)	33264	1(3)	33496	1(3)	33726	1(2)
31032	1(2)	31513	1(3)	31638	1(3)	32491	1(2)	32994	1(2)	33265	1(2)	33500	1(3)	33730	1(2)
31040	1(2)	31515	1(3)	31640	1(3)	32501	1(3)	32997	1(2)	33266	1(2)	33501	1(3)	33732	1(2)
31050	1(2)	31520	1(3)	31641	1(3)	32503	1(2)	32998	1(2)	33270	1(3)	33502	1(3)	33735	1(2)
31051	1(2)	31525	1(3)	31643	1(2)	32504	1(2)	32999	1(3)	33271	1(3)	33503	1(3)	33736	1(2)
31070	1(2)	31526	1(3)	31645	1(2)	32505	1(2)	33010	1(2)	33272	1(3)	33504	1(3)	33737	1(2)
31075	1(2)	31527	1(2)	31646	2(3)	32506	3(3)	33011	1(3)	33273	1(3)	33505	1(3)	33750	1(3)
31080	1(2)	31528	1(2)	31647	1(2)	32507	2(3)	33015	1(3)	33274	1(3)	33506	1(3)	33755	1(2)
31081	1(2)	31529	1(3)	31648	1(2)	32540	1(3)	33020	1(3)	33275	1(3)	33507	1(3)	33762	1(2)
31084	1(2)	31530	1(3)	31649	2(3)	32550	2(3)	33025	1(2)	33285	1(3)	33508	1(2)	33764	1(3)
31085	1(2)	31531	1(3)	31651	3(3)	32551	2(3)	33030	1(2)	33286	1(3)	33510	1(2)	33766	1(2)
31086	1(2)	31535	1(3)	31652	1(2)	32552	2(2)	33031	1(2)	33289	1(3)	33511	1(2)	33767	1(2)
31087	1(2)	31536	1(3)	31653	1(2)	32553	1(2)	33050	1(2)	33300	1(3)	33512	1(2)	33768	1(2)
31090	1(2)	31540	1(3)	31654	1(3)	32554	2(3)	33120	1(3)	33305	1(3)	33513	1(2)	33770	1(2)
31200	1(2)	31541	1(3)	31660	1(2)	32555	2(3)	33130	1(3)	33310	1(2)	33514	1(2)	33771	1(2)
31201	1(2)	31545	1(2)	31661	1(2)	32556	2(3)	33140	1(2)	33315	1(2)	33516	1(2)	33774	1(2)
31205	1(2)	31546	1(2)	31717	1(3)	32557	2(3)	33141	1(2)	33320	1(3)	33517	1(2)	33775	1(2)
31225	1(2)	31551	1(2)	31720	1(3)	32560	1(3)	33202	1(2)	33321	1(3)	33518	1(2)	33776	1(2)
31230	1(2)	31552	1(2)	31725	1(3)	32561	1(2)	33203	1(2)	33322	1(3)	33519	1(2)	33777	1(2)
31231	1(2)	31553	1(2)	31730	1(3)	32562	1(2)	33206	1(3)	33330	1(3)	33521	1(2)	33778	1(2)
31233	1(2)	31554	1(2)	31750	1(2)	32601	1(3)	33207	1(3)	33335	1(3)	33522	1(2)	33779	1(2)
31235	1(2)	31560	1(2)	31755	1(2)	32604	1(3)	33208	1(3)	33340	1(2)	33523	1(2)	33780	1(2)
31237	1(2)	31561	1(2)	31760	1(2)	32606	1(3)	33210	1(3)	33361	1(2)	33530	1(2)	33781	1(2)
31238	1(3)	31570	1(2)	31766	1(2)	32607	1(3)	33211	1(3)	33362	1(2)	33533	1(2)	33782	1(2)
31239	1(2)	31571	1(2)	31770	2(3)	32608	1(3)	33212	1(3)	33363	1(2)	33534	1(2)	33783	1(2)
31240	1(2)	31572	1(2)	31775	1(3)	32609	1(3)	33213	1(3)	33364	1(2)	33535	1(2)	33786	1(2)

CPT	MUE	CPT	MUE	CPT	MUE	CPT	MUE	CPT	MUE	CPT	MUE	CPT	MUE
33788	1(2)	33968	1(3)	34832	1(2)	35305	1(2)	35642	1(3)	36227	1(3)	36575	2(3)	37195	1(3)
33800	1(2)	33969	1(3)	34833	1(2)	35306	2(3)	35645	1(3)	36228	4(3)	36576	2(3)	37197	2(3)
33802	1(3)	33970	1(3)	34834	1(2)	35311	1(2)	35646	1(3)	36245	6(3)	36578	2(3)	37200	2(3)
33803	1(3)	33971	1(3)	34839	1(2)	35321	1(2)	35647	1(3)	36246	4(3)	36580	2(3)	37211	1(2)
33813	1(2)	33973	1(3)	34841	1(2)	35331	1(2)	35650	1(3)	36247	3(3)	36581	2(3)	37212	1(2)
33814	1(2)	33974	1(3)	34842	1(2)	35341	3(3)	35654	1(3)	36248	6(3)	36582	2(3)	37213	1(2)
33820	1(2)	33975	1(3)	34843	1(2)	35351	1(3)	35656	1(3)	36251	1(3)	36583	2(3)	37214	1(2)
33822	1(2)	33976	1(3)	34844	1(2)	35355	1(3)	35661	1(3)	36252	1(3)	36584	2(3)	37215	1(2)
33824	1(2)	33977	1(3)	34845	1(2)	35361	1(2)	35663	1(3)	36253	1(3)	36585	2(3)	37216	0(3)
33840	1(2)	33978	1(3)	34846	1(2)	35363	1(2)	35665	1(3)	36254	1(3)	36589	2(3)	37217	1(2)
33845	1(2)	33979	1(3)	34847	1(2)	35371	1(2)	35666	2(3)	36260	1(2)	36590	2(3)	37218	1(2)
33851	1(2)	33980	1(3)	34848	1(2)	35372	1(2)	35671	2(3)	36261	1(2)	36591	2(3)	37220	1(2)
33852	1(2)	33981	1(3)	35001	1(2)	35390	1(3)	35681	1(3)	36262	1(2)	36592	1(3)	37221	1(2)
33853	1(2)	33982	1(3)	35002	1(2)	35400	1(3)	35682	1(2)	36299	1(3)	36593	2(3)	37222	2(3)
33860	1(2)	33983	1(3)	35005	1(2)	35500	2(3)	35683	1(2)	36400	1(3)	36595	2(3)	37223	2(2)
33863	1(2)	33984	1(3)	35011	1(2)	35501	1(3)	35685	2(3)	36405	1(3)	36596	2(3)	37224	1(2)
33864	1(2)	33985	1(3)	35013	1(2)	35506	1(3)	35686	1(3)	36406	1(3)	36597	2(3)	37225	1(2)
33866	1(2)	33986	1(3)	35021	1(2)	35508	1(3)	35691	1(3)	36410	3(3)	36598	2(3)	37226	1(2)
33870	1(2)	33987	1(3)	35022	1(2)	35509	1(3)	35693	1(3)	36415	2(3)	36600	4(3)	37227	1(2)
33875	1(2)	33988	1(3)	35045	1(3)	35510	1(3)	35694	1(3)	36416	0(3)	36620	3(3)	37228	1(2)
33877	1(2)	33989	1(3)	35081	1(2)	35511	1(3)	35695	1(3)	36420	2(3)	36625	2(3)	37229	1(2)
33880	1(2)	33990	1(3)	35082	1(2)	35512	1(3)	35697	2(3)	36425	2(3)	36640	1(3)	37230	1(2)
33881	1(2)	33991	1(3)	35091	1(2)	35515	1(3)	35700	2(3)	36430	1(2)	36660	1(3)	37231	1(2)
33883	1(2)	33992	1(2)	35092	1(2)	35516	1(3)	35701	1(2)	36440	1(3)	36680	1(3)	37232	2(3)
33884	2(3)	33993	1(3)	35102	1(2)	35518	1(3)	35721	1(2)	36450	1(3)	36800	1(3)	37233	2(3)
33886	1(2)	33999	1(3)	35103	1(2)	35521	1(3)	35741	1(2)	36455	1(3)	36810	1(3)	37234	2(3)
33889	1(2)	34001	1(3)	35111	1(2)	35522	1(3)	35761	2(3)	36456	1(3)	36815	1(3)	37235	2(3)
33891	1(2)	34051	1(3)	35112	1(2)	35523	1(3)	35800	2(3)	36460	2(3)	36818	1(3)	37236	1(2)
33910	1(3)	34101	1(3)	35121	1(3)	35525	1(3)	35820	2(3)	36465	1(2)	36819	1(3)	37237	2(3)
33915	1(3)	34111	2(3)	35122	1(3)	35526	1(3)	35840	2(3)	36466	1(2)	36820	1(3)	37238	1(2)
33916	1(3)	34151	1(3)	35131	1(2)	35531	1(3)	35860	2(3)	36468	2(3)	36821	2(3)	37239	2(3)
33917	1(2)	34201	1(3)	35132	1(2)	35533	1(3)	35870	1(3)	36470	1(2)	36823	1(3)	37241	2(3)
33920	1(2)	34203	1(2)	35141	1(2)	35535	1(3)	35875	2(3)	36471	1(2)	36825	1(3)	37242	2(3)
33922	1(2)	34401	1(3)	35142	1(2)	35536	1(3)	35876	2(3)	36473	1(3)	36830	2(3)	37243	1(3)
33924	1(2)	34421	1(3)	35151	1(2)	35537	1(3)	35879	2(3)	36474	1(3)	36831	1(3)	37244	2(3)
33925	1(2)	34451	1(3)	35152	1(2)	35538	1(3)	35881	1(3)	36475	1(3)	36832	2(3)	37246	1(2)
33926	1(2)	34471	1(2)	35180	2(3)	35539	1(3)	35883	1(3)	36476	2(3)	36833	1(3)	37247	2(3)
33927	1(3)	34490	1(2)	35182	2(3)	35540	1(3)	35884	1(3)	36478	1(3)	36835	1(3)	37248	1(2)
33928	1(3)	34501	1(2)	35184	2(3)	35556	1(3)	35901	1(3)	36479	2(3)	36838	1(3)	37249	3(3)
33929	1(3)	34502	1(2)	35188	2(3)	35558	1(3)	35903	2(3)	36481	1(3)	36860	2(3)	37252	1(2)
33930	1(2)	34510	2(3)	35189	1(3)	35560	1(3)	35905	1(3)	36482	1(3)	36861	2(3)	37253	5(3)
33933	1(2)	34520	1(3)	35190	2(3)	35563	1(3)	35907	1(3)	36483	2(3)	36901	1(3)	37500	1(3)
33935	1(2)	34530	1(2)	35201	2(3)	35565	1(3)	36000	4(3)	36500	4(3)	36902	1(3)	37501	1(3)
33940	1(2)	34701	1(2)	35206	2(3)	35566	1(3)	36002	2(3)	36510	1(3)	36903	1(3)	37565	1(2)
33944	1(2)	34702	1(2)	35207	3(3)	35570	1(3)	36005	2(3)	36511	1(3)	36904	1(3)	37600	1(3)
33945	1(2)	34703	1(2)	35211	3(3)	35571	1(3)	36010	2(3)	36512	1(3)	36905	1(3)	37605	1(3)
33946	1(2)	34704	1(2)	35216	2(3)	35572	2(3)	36011	4(3)	36513	1(3)	36906	1(3)	37606	1(3)
33947	1(2)	34705	1(2)	35221	3(3)	35583	1(2)	36012	4(3)	36514	1(3)	36907	1(3)	37607	1(3)
33948	1(2)	34706	1(2)	35226	3(3)	35585	2(3)	36013	2(3)	36516	1(3)	36908	1(3)	37609	1(2)
33949	1(2)	34707	1(2)	35231	2(3)	35587	1(3)	36014	2(3)	36522	1(3)	36909	1(3)	37615	2(3)
33951	1(3)	34708	1(2)	35236	2(3)	35600	2(3)	36015	4(3)	36555	2(3)	37140	1(2)	37616	1(3)
33952	1(3)	34709	3(3)	35241	2(3)	35601	1(3)	36100	2(3)	36556	2(3)	37145	1(3)	37617	3(3)
33953	1(3)	34710	1(2)	35246	2(3)	35606	1(3)	36140	3(3)	36557	2(3)	37160	1(3)	37618	2(3)
33954	1(3)	34711	2(3)	35251	2(3)	35612	1(3)	36160	2(3)	36558	2(3)	37180	1(2)	37619	1(2)
33955	1(3)	34712	1(2)	35256	2(3)	35616	1(3)	36200	2(3)	36560	2(3)	37181	1(2)	37650	1(2)
33956	1(3)	34713	1(2)	35261	1(3)	35621	1(3)	36215	6(3)	36561	2(3)	37182	1(2)	37660	1(2)
33957	1(3)	34714	1(2)	35266	2(3)	35623	1(3)	36216	4(3)	36563	1(3)	37183	1(2)	37700	1(2)
33958	1(3)	34715	1(2)	35271	2(3)	35626	3(3)	36217	2(3)	36565	1(3)	37184	1(2)	37718	1(2)
33959	1(3)	34716	1(2)	35276	2(3)	35631	4(3)	36218	6(3)	36566	1(3)	37185	2(3)	37722	1(2)
33962	1(3)	34808	1(3)	35281	2(3)	35632	1(3)	36221	1(3)	36568	2(3)	37186	2(3)	37735	1(2)
33963	1(3)	34812	1(2)	35286	2(3)	35633	1(3)	36222	1(3)	36569	2(3)	37187	1(3)	37760	1(2)
33964	1(3)	34813	1(2)	35301	2(3)	35634	1(3)	36223	1(3)	36570	2(3)	37188	1(3)	37761	1(2)
33965	1(3)	34820	1(2)	35302	1(2)	35636	1(3)	36224	1(3)	36571	2(3)	37191	1(3)	37765	1(2)
33966	1(3)	34830	1(2)	35303	1(2)	35637	1(3)	36225	1(3)	36572	1(3)	37192	1(3)	37766	1(2)
33967	1(3)	34831	1(2)	35304	1(2)	35638	1(3)	36226	1(3)	36573	1(3)	37193	1(3)	37780	1(2)

CPT	MUE	CPT	MUE	CPT	MUE	CPT	MUE	CPT	MUE	CPT	MUE	CPT	MUE	CPT	MUE
37785	1(2)	38780	1(2)	41015	2(3)	42227	1(2)	42960	1(3)	43245	1(2)	43405	1(2)	43850	1(2)
37788	1(2)	38790	1(2)	41016	1(3)	42235	1(2)	42961	1(3)	43246	1(2)	43410	1(3)	43855	1(2)
37790	1(2)	38792	1(3)	41017	2(3)	42260	1(3)	42962	1(3)	43247	1(2)	43415	1(3)	43860	1(2)
37799	1(3)	38794	1(2)	41018	2(3)	42280	1(2)	42970	1(3)	43248	1(3)	43420	1(3)	43865	1(2)
38100	1(2)	38900	1(3)	41019	1(2)	42281	1(2)	42971	1(3)	43249	1(3)	43425	1(3)	43870	1(2)
38101	1(3)	38999	1(3)	41100	2(3)	42299	1(3)	42972	1(3)	43250	1(3)	43450	1(3)	43880	1(3)
38102	1(2)	39000	1(2)	41105	2(3)	42300	2(3)	42999	1(3)	43251	1(2)	43453	1(3)	43881	1(3)
38115	1(3)	39010	1(2)	41108	2(3)	42305	2(3)	43020	1(2)	43252	1(2)	43460	1(3)	43882	1(3)
38120	1(2)	39200	1(2)	41110	2(3)	42310	2(3)	43030	1(2)	43253	1(3)	43496	1(3)	43886	1(2)
38129	1(3)	39220	1(2)	41112	2(3)	42320	2(3)	43045	1(2)	43254	1(3)	43499	1(3)	43887	1(2)
38200	1(3)	39401	1(3)	41113	2(3)	42330	1(3)	43100	1(3)	43255	2(3)	43500	1(2)	43888	1(2)
38204	0(3)	39402	1(3)	41114	2(3)	42335	2(2)	43101	1(3)	43257	1(2)	43501	1(3)	43999	1(3)
38205	1(3)	39499	1(3)	41115	1(2)	42340	1(2)	43107	1(2)	43259	1(2)	43502	1(2)	44005	1(2)
38206	1(3)	39501	1(3)	41116	2(3)	42400	2(3)	43108	1(2)	43260	1(3)	43510	1(2)	44010	1(2)
38207	0(3)	39503	1(2)	41120	1(2)	42405	2(3)	43112	1(2)	43261	1(2)	43520	1(2)	44015	1(2)
38208	0(3)	39540	1(2)	41130	1(2)	42408	1(3)	43113	1(2)	43262	2(2)	43605	1(2)	44020	2(3)
38209	0(3)	39541	1(2)	41135	1(2)	42409	1(3)	43116	1(2)	43263	1(2)	43610	2(3)	44021	1(3)
38210	0(3)	39545	1(2)	41140	1(2)	42410	1(2)	43117	1(2)	43264	1(2)	43611	2(3)	44025	1(3)
38211	0(3)	39560	1(3)	41145	1(2)	42415	1(2)	43118	1(2)	43265	1(2)	43620	1(2)	44050	1(2)
38212	0(3)	39561	1(3)	41150	1(2)	42420	1(2)	43121	1(2)	43266	1(3)	43621	1(2)	44055	1(2)
38213	0(3)	39599	1(3)	41153	1(2)	42425	1(2)	43122	1(2)	43270	1(3)	43622	1(2)	44100	1(2)
38214	0(3)	40490	2(3)	41155	1(2)	42426	1(2)	43123	1(2)	43273	1(2)	43631	1(2)	44110	1(2)
38215	0(3)	40500	2(3)	41250	2(3)	42440	1(2)	43124	1(2)	43274	2(3)	43632	1(2)	44111	1(2)
38220	1(3)	40510	2(3)	41251	2(3)	42450	1(3)	43130	1(3)	43275	1(3)	43633	1(2)	44120	1(2)
38221	1(3)	40520	2(3)	41252	2(3)	42500	2(3)	43135	1(3)	43276	2(3)	43634	1(2)	44121	2(3)
38222	1(2)	40525	2(3)	41510	1(2)	42505	2(3)	43180	1(2)	43277	3(3)	43635	1(2)	44125	1(2)
38230	1(2)	40527	2(3)	41512	1(2)	42507	1(2)	43191	1(3)	43278	1(3)	43640	1(2)	44126	1(2)
38232	1(2)	40530	2(3)	41520	1(3)	42509	1(2)	43192	1(3)	43279	1(2)	43641	1(2)	44127	1(2)
38240	1(3)	40650	2(3)	41530	1(3)	42510	1(2)	43193	1(3)	43280	1(2)	43644	1(2)	44128	2(3)
38241	1(2)	40652	2(3)	41599	1(3)	42550	2(3)	43194	1(3)	43281	1(2)	43645	1(2)	44130	2(3)
38242	1(2)	40654	2(3)	41800	2(3)	42600	1(3)	43195	1(3)	43282	1(2)	43647	1(2)	44132	1(2)
38243	1(3)	40700	1(2)	41805	1(3)	42650	2(3)	43196	1(3)	43283	1(2)	43648	1(2)	44133	1(2)
38300	1(3)	40701	1(2)	41806	1(3)	42660	2(3)	43197	1(3)	43284	1(2)	43651	1(2)	44135	1(2)
38305	1(3)	40702	1(2)	41820	4(2)	42665	2(3)	43198	1(3)	43285	1(2)	43652	1(2)	44136	1(2)
38308	1(3)	40720	1(2)	41821	2(3)	42699	1(3)	43200	1(3)	43286	1(2)	43653	1(2)	44137	1(2)
38380	1(2)	40761	1(2)	41822	1(2)	42700	2(3)	43201	1(2)	43287	1(2)	43659	1(3)	44139	1(2)
38381	1(2)	40799	1(3)	41823	1(2)	42720	1(3)	43202	1(2)	43288	1(2)	43752	2(3)	44140	2(3)
38382	1(2)	40800	2(3)	41825	2(3)	42725	1(3)	43204	1(2)	43289	1(3)	43753	1(3)	44141	1(3)
38500	2(3)	40801	2(3)	41826	2(3)	42800	3(3)	43205	1(2)	43300	1(2)	43754	1(3)	44143	1(2)
38505	2(3)	40804	1(3)	41827	2(3)	42804	1(3)	43206	1(2)	43305	1(2)	43755	1(3)	44144	1(3)
38510	1(2)	40805	2(3)	41828	4(2)	42806	1(3)	43210	1(2)	43310	1(2)	43756	1(2)	44145	1(2)
38520	1(2)	40806	2(2)	41830	2(3)	42808	2(3)	43211	1(3)	43312	1(2)	43757	1(2)	44146	1(2)
38525	1(2)	40808	2(3)	41850	2(3)	42809	1(3)	43212	1(3)	43313	1(2)	43761	2(3)	44147	1(3)
38530	1(2)	40810	2(3)	41870	2(3)	42810	1(3)	43213	1(2)	43314	1(2)	43762	2(3)	44150	1(2)
38531	1(2)	40812	2(3)	41872	4(2)	42815	1(3)	43214	1(3)	43320	1(2)	43763	2(3)	44151	1(2)
38542	1(2)	40814	4(3)	41874	4(2)	42820	1(2)	43215	1(3)	43325	1(2)	43770	1(2)	44155	1(2)
38550	1(3)	40816	2(3)	41899	1(3)	42821	1(2)	43216	1(2)	43327	1(2)	43771	1(2)	44156	1(2)
38555	1(3)	40818	2(3)	42000	1(3)	42825	1(2)	43217	1(2)	43328	1(2)	43772	1(2)	44157	1(2)
38562	1(2)	40819	2(2)	42100	2(3)	42826	1(2)	43220	1(3)	43330	1(2)	43773	1(2)	44158	1(2)
38564	1(2)	40820	2(3)	42104	2(3)	42830	1(2)	43226	1(3)	43331	1(2)	43774	1(2)	44160	1(2)
38570	1(2)	40830	2(3)	42106	2(3)	42831	1(2)	43227	1(3)	43332	1(2)	43775	1(2)	44180	1(2)
38571	1(2)	40831	2(3)	42107	2(3)	42835	1(2)	43229	1(3)	43333	1(2)	43800	1(2)	44186	1(2)
38572	1(2)	40840	1(2)	42120	1(2)	42836	1(2)	43231	1(2)	43334	1(2)	43810	1(2)	44187	1(3)
38573	1(2)	40842	1(2)	42140	1(2)	42842	1(3)	43232	1(2)	43335	1(2)	43820	1(2)	44188	1(3)
38589	1(3)	40843	1(2)	42145	1(2)	42844	1(3)	43233	1(3)	43336	1(2)	43825	1(2)	44202	1(2)
38700	1(2)	40844	1(2)	42160	1(3)	42845	1(3)	43235	1(3)	43337	1(2)	43830	1(2)	44203	2(3)
38720	1(2)	40845	1(3)	42180	1(3)	42860	1(2)	43236	1(2)	43338	1(2)	43831	1(2)	44204	2(3)
38724	1(2)	40899	1(3)	42182	1(3)	42870	1(3)	43237	1(2)	43340	1(2)	43832	1(2)	44205	1(2)
38740	1(2)	41000	1(3)	42200	1(2)	42890	1(2)	43238	1(2)	43341	1(2)	43840	2(3)	44206	1(2)
38745	1(2)	41005	1(3)	42205	1(2)	42892	1(3)	43239	1(2)	43351	1(2)	43842	0(3)	44207	1(2)
38746	1(2)	41006	2(3)	42210	1(2)	42894	1(3)	43240	1(2)	43352	1(2)	43843	1(2)	44208	1(2)
38747	1(2)	41007	2(3)	42215	1(2)	42900	1(3)	43241	1(3)	43360	1(2)	43845	1(2)	44210	1(2)
38760	1(2)	41008	2(3)	42220	1(2)	42950	1(2)	43242	1(2)	43361	1(2)	43846	1(2)	44211	1(2)
38765	1(2)	41009	2(3)	42225	1(2)	42953	1(3)	43243	1(2)	43400	1(2)	43847	1(2)	44212	1(2)
38770	1(2)	41010	1(2)	42226	1(2)	42955	1(2)	43244	1(2)	43401	1(2)	43848	1(2)	44213	1(2)

CPT	MUE	CPT	MUE	CPT	MUE	CPT	MUE	CPT	MUE	CPT	MUE	CPT	MUE	CPT	MUE
44227	1(3)	44721	2(3)	45381	1(2)	46600	1(3)	47350	1(3)	47999	1(3)	49411	1(2)	49659	1(3)
44238	1(3)	44799	1(3)	45382	1(3)	46601	1(3)	47360	1(3)	48000	1(2)	49412	1(2)	49900	1(3)
44300	1(3)	44800	1(3)	45384	1(2)	46604	1(2)	47361	1(2)	48001	1(2)	49418	1(3)	49904	1(3)
44310	2(3)	44820	1(3)	45385	1(2)	46606	1(2)	47362	1(3)	48020	1(3)	49419	1(2)	49905	1(3)
44312	1(2)	44850	1(3)	45386	1(2)	46607	1(2)	47370	1(2)	48100	1(3)	49421	1(2)	49906	1(3)
44314	1(2)	44899	1(3)	45388	1(2)	46608	1(3)	47371	1(2)	48102	1(3)	49422	1(2)	49999	1(3)
44316	1(2)	44900	1(2)	45389	1(3)	46610	1(2)	47379	1(3)	48105	1(2)	49423	2(3)	50010	1(2)
44320	1(2)	44950	1(2)	45390	1(3)	46611	1(2)	47380	1(2)	48120	1(3)	49424	3(3)	50020	1(2)
44322	1(2)	44955	1(2)	45391	1(2)	46612	1(2)	47381	1(2)	48140	1(2)	49425	1(2)	50040	1(2)
44340	1(2)	44960	1(2)	45392	1(2)	46614	1(3)	47382	1(2)	48145	1(2)	49426	1(3)	50045	1(2)
44345	1(2)	44970	1(2)	45393	1(3)	46615	1(2)	47383	1(2)	48146	1(2)	49427	1(3)	50060	1(2)
44346	1(2)	44979	1(3)	45395	1(2)	46700	1(2)	47399	1(3)	48148	1(2)	49428	1(2)	50065	1(2)
44360	1(3)	45000	1(3)	45397	1(2)	46705	1(2)	47400	1(3)	48150	1(2)	49429	1(2)	50070	1(2)
44361	1(2)	45005	1(3)	45398	1(2)	46706	1(3)	47420	1(2)	48152	1(2)	49435	1(2)	50075	1(2)
44363	1(3)	45020	1(3)	45399	1(3)	46707	1(3)	47425	1(2)	48153	1(2)	49436	1(2)	50080	1(2)
44364	1(2)	45100	2(3)	45400	1(2)	46710	1(3)	47460	1(2)	48154	1(2)	49440	1(3)	50081	1(2)
44365	1(2)	45108	1(2)	45402	1(2)	46712	1(3)	47480	1(2)	48155	1(2)	49441	1(3)	50100	1(2)
44366	1(3)	45110	1(2)	45499	1(3)	46715	1(2)	47490	1(2)	48160	0(3)	49442	1(3)	50120	1(2)
44369	1(2)	45111	1(2)	45500	1(2)	46716	1(2)	47531	2(3)	48400	1(3)	49446	1(2)	50125	1(2)
44370	1(2)	45112	1(2)	45505	1(2)	46730	1(2)	47532	1(3)	48500	1(3)	49450	1(3)	50130	1(2)
44372	1(2)	45113	1(2)	45520	1(2)	46735	1(2)	47533	1(3)	48510	1(3)	49451	1(3)	50135	1(2)
44373	1(2)	45114	1(2)	45540	1(2)	46740	1(2)	47534	2(3)	48520	1(3)	49452	1(3)	50200	1(3)
44376	1(3)	45116	1(2)	45541	1(2)	46742	1(2)	47535	1(3)	48540	1(3)	49460	1(3)	50205	1(3)
44377	1(2)	45119	1(2)	45550	1(2)	46744	1(2)	47536	2(3)	48545	1(3)	49465	1(3)	50220	1(2)
44378	1(3)	45120	1(2)	45560	1(2)	46746	1(2)	47537	1(3)	48547	1(2)	49491	1(2)	50225	1(2)
44379	1(2)	45121	1(2)	45562	1(2)	46748	1(2)	47538	2(3)	48548	1(2)	49492	1(2)	50230	1(2)
44380	1(3)	45123	1(2)	45563	1(2)	46750	1(2)	47539	2(3)	48550	1(2)	49495	1(2)	50234	1(2)
44381	1(3)	45126	1(2)	45800	1(3)	46751	1(2)	47540	2(3)	48551	1(2)	49496	1(2)	50236	1(2)
44382	1(2)	45130	1(2)	45805	1(3)	46753	1(2)	47541	1(3)	48552	2(3)	49500	1(2)	50240	1(2)
44384	1(3)	45135	1(2)	45820	1(3)	46754	1(3)	47542	2(3)	48554	1(2)	49501	1(2)	50250	1(3)
44385	1(3)	45136	1(2)	45825	1(3)	46760	1(2)	47543	1(3)	48556	1(2)	49505	1(2)	50280	1(2)
44386	1(2)	45150	1(2)	45900	1(2)	46761	1(2)	47544	1(3)	48999	1(3)	49507	1(2)	50290	1(3)
44388	1(3)	45160	1(3)	45905	1(2)	46900	1(2)	47550	1(3)	49000	1(2)	49520	1(2)	50300	1(2)
44389	1(2)	45171	2(3)	45910	1(2)	46910	1(2)	47552	1(3)	49002	1(3)	49521	1(2)	50320	1(2)
44390	1(3)	45172	2(3)	45915	1(2)	46916	1(2)	47553	1(2)	49010	1(3)	49525	1(2)	50323	1(2)
44391	1(3)	45190	1(3)	45990	1(2)	46917	1(2)	47554	1(3)	49020	2(3)	49540	1(2)	50325	1(2)
44392	1(2)	45300	1(3)	45999	1(3)	46922	1(2)	47555	1(2)	49040	2(3)	49550	1(2)	50327	2(3)
44394	1(2)	45303	1(3)	46020	2(3)	46924	1(2)	47556	1(2)	49060	2(3)	49553	1(2)	50328	1(3)
44401	1(2)	45305	1(2)	46030	1(3)	46930	1(2)	47562	1(2)	49062	1(3)	49555	1(2)	50329	1(3)
44402	1(3)	45307	1(3)	46040	2(3)	46940	1(2)	47563	1(2)	49082	1(3)	49557	1(2)	50340	1(2)
44403	1(3)	45308	1(2)	46045	2(3)	46942	1(3)	47564	1(2)	49083	2(3)	49560	2(3)	50360	1(2)
44404	1(3)	45309	1(2)	46050	2(3)	46945	1(2)	47570	1(2)	49084	1(3)	49561	1(3)	50365	1(2)
44405	1(3)	45315	1(2)	46060	2(3)	46946	1(2)	47579	1(3)	49180	2(3)	49565	2(3)	50370	1(2)
44406	1(3)	45317	1(3)	46070	1(2)	46947	1(2)	47600	1(2)	49185	2(3)	49566	2(3)	50380	1(2)
44407	1(2)	45320	1(2)	46080	1(2)	46999	1(3)	47605	1(2)	49203	1(2)	49568	2(3)	50382	1(3)
44408	1(3)	45321	1(2)	46083	2(3)	47000	3(3)	47610	1(2)	49204	1(2)	49570	1(3)	50384	1(3)
44500	1(3)	45327	1(2)	46200	1(3)	47001	3(3)	47612	1(2)	49205	1(2)	49572	1(3)	50385	1(3)
44602	1(2)	45330	1(3)	46220	1(2)	47010	1(3)	47620	1(2)	49215	1(2)	49580	1(2)	50386	1(3)
44603	1(2)	45331	1(2)	46221	1(2)	47015	1(2)	47700	1(2)	49220	1(2)	49582	1(2)	50387	1(3)
44604	1(2)	45332	1(3)	46230	1(2)	47100	3(3)	47701	1(2)	49250	1(2)	49585	1(2)	50389	1(3)
44605	1(2)	45333	1(2)	46250	1(2)	47120	2(3)	47711	1(2)	49255	1(2)	49587	1(2)	50390	2(3)
44615	3(3)	45334	1(3)	46255	1(2)	47122	1(2)	47712	1(2)	49320	1(3)	49590	1(2)	50391	1(3)
44620	2(3)	45335	1(2)	46257	1(2)	47125	1(2)	47715	1(2)	49321	1(2)	49600	1(2)	50396	1(3)
44625	1(3)	45337	1(2)	46258	1(2)	47130	1(2)	47720	1(2)	49322	1(2)	49605	1(2)	50400	1(2)
44626	1(3)	45338	1(2)	46260	1(2)	47133	1(2)	47721	1(2)	49323	1(2)	49606	1(2)	50405	1(2)
44640	2(3)	45340	1(2)	46261	1(2)	47135	1(2)	47740	1(2)	49324	1(2)	49610	1(2)	50430	2(3)
44650	2(3)	45341	1(2)	46262	1(2)	47140	1(2)	47741	1(2)	49325	1(2)	49611	1(2)	50431	2(3)
44660	1(3)	45342	1(2)	46270	1(3)	47141	1(2)	47760	1(2)	49326	1(2)	49650	1(2)	50432	2(3)
44661	1(3)	45346	1(2)	46275	1(3)	47142	1(2)	47765	1(2)	49327	1(2)	49651	1(2)	50433	2(3)
44680	1(3)	45347	1(3)	46280	1(2)	47143	1(2)	47780	1(2)	49329	1(3)	49652	2(3)	50434	2(3)
44700	1(2)	45349	1(3)	46285	1(3)	47144	1(2)	47785	1(2)	49400	1(3)	49653	2(3)	50435	2(3)
44701	1(2)	45350	1(2)	46288	1(3)	47145	1(2)	47800	1(2)	49402	1(3)	49654	1(3)	50436	1(3)
44705	1(3)	45378	1(3)	46320	2(3)	47146	2(3)	47801	1(3)	49405	2(3)	49655	1(3)	50437	1(3)
44715	1(2)	45379	1(3)	46500	1(2)	47147	1(3)	47802	1(2)	49406	2(3)	49656	1(3)	50500	1(3)
44720	2(3)	45380	1(2)	46505	1(2)	47300	2(3)	47900	1(2)	49407	1(3)	49657	1(3)	50520	1(3)

CPT	MUE	CPT	MUE	CPT	MUE	CPT	MUE	CPT	MUE	CPT	MUE	CPT	MUE	CPT	MUE
50525	1(3)	50845	1(2)	51784	1(3)	52351	1(3)	53605	1(3)	54400	1(2)	55559	1(3)	57105	2(3)
50526	1(3)	50860	1(2)	51785	1(3)	52352	1(2)	53620	1(2)	54401	1(2)	55600	1(2)	57106	1(2)
50540	1(2)	50900	1(3)	51792	1(3)	52353	1(3)	53621	1(3)	54405	1(2)	55605	1(2)	57107	1(2)
50541	1(2)	50920	2(3)	51797	1(3)	52354	1(3)	53660	1(2)	54406	1(2)	55650	1(2)	57109	1(2)
50542	1(2)	50930	2(3)	51798	1(3)	52355	1(3)	53661	1(3)	54408	1(2)	55680	1(3)	57110	1(2)
50543	1(2)	50940	1(2)	51800	1(2)	52356	1(2)	53665	1(3)	54410	1(2)	55700	1(2)	57111	1(2)
50544	1(2)	50945	1(2)	51820	1(2)	52400	1(2)	53850	1(2)	54411	1(2)	55705	1(2)	57112	1(2)
50545	1(2)	50947	1(2)	51840	1(2)	52402	1(2)	53852	1(2)	54415	1(2)	55706	1(2)	57120	1(2)
50546	1(2)	50948	1(2)	51841	1(2)	52441	1(2)	53854	1(2)	54416	1(2)	55720	1(3)	57130	1(2)
50547	1(2)	50949	1(3)	51845	1(2)	52442	6(3)	53855	1(2)	54417	1(2)	55725	1(3)	57135	2(3)
50548	1(2)	50951	1(3)	51860	1(3)	52450	1(2)	53860	1(2)	54420	1(2)	55801	1(2)	57150	1(3)
50549	1(3)	50953	1(3)	51865	1(3)	52500	1(2)	53899	1(3)	54430	1(2)	55810	1(2)	57155	1(3)
50551	1(3)	50955	1(2)	51880	1(2)	52601	1(2)	54000	1(2)	54435	1(2)	55812	1(2)	57156	1(3)
50553	1(3)	50957	1(2)	51900	1(3)	52630	1(2)	54001	1(2)	54437	1(2)	55815	1(2)	57160	1(2)
50555	1(2)	50961	1(2)	51920	1(3)	52640	1(2)	54015	1(3)	54438	1(2)	55821	1(2)	57170	1(2)
50557	1(2)	50970	1(3)	51925	1(2)	52647	1(2)	54050	1(2)	54440	1(2)	55831	1(2)	57180	1(3)
50561	1(2)	50972	1(3)	51940	1(2)	52648	1(2)	54055	1(2)	54450	1(2)	55840	1(2)	57200	1(3)
50562	1(3)	50974	1(2)	51960	1(2)	52649	1(2)	54056	1(2)	54500	1(3)	55842	1(2)	57210	1(2)
50570	1(3)	50976	1(2)	51980	1(2)	52700	1(3)	54057	1(2)	54505	1(3)	55845	1(2)	57220	1(2)
50572	1(3)	50980	1(2)	51990	1(2)	53000	1(2)	54060	1(2)	54512	1(3)	55860	1(2)	57230	1(2)
50574	1(2)	51020	1(2)	51992	1(2)	53010	1(2)	54065	1(2)	54520	1(2)	55862	1(2)	57240	1(2)
50575	1(2)	51030	1(2)	51999	1(3)	53020	1(2)	54100	2(3)	54522	1(2)	55865	1(2)	57250	1(2)
50576	1(2)	51040	1(3)	52000	1(3)	53025	1(2)	54105	2(3)	54530	1(2)	55866	1(2)	57260	1(2)
50580	1(2)	51045	2(3)	52001	1(3)	53040	1(3)	54110	1(2)	54535	1(2)	55870	1(2)	57265	1(2)
50590	1(2)	51050	1(3)	52005	2(3)	53060	1(3)	54111	1(2)	54550	1(2)	55873	1(2)	57267	2(3)
50592	1(2)	51060	1(3)	52007	1(2)	53080	1(3)	54112	1(3)	54560	1(2)	55874	1(2)	57268	1(2)
50593	1(2)	51065	1(3)	52010	1(2)	53085	1(3)	54115	1(3)	54600	1(2)	55875	1(2)	57270	1(2)
50600	1(3)	51080	1(3)	52204	1(2)	53200	1(3)	54120	1(2)	54620	1(2)	55876	1(2)	57280	1(2)
50605	1(3)	51100	1(3)	52214	1(2)	53210	1(2)	54125	1(2)	54640	1(2)	55899	1(3)	57282	1(2)
50606	1(3)	51101	1(3)	52224	1(2)	53215	1(2)	54130	1(2)	54650	1(2)	55920	1(2)	57283	1(2)
50610	1(2)	51102	1(3)	52234	1(2)	53220	1(3)	54135	1(2)	54660	1(2)	55970	1(2)	57284	1(2)
50620	1(2)	51500	1(2)	52235	1(2)	53230	1(3)	54150	1(2)	54670	1(3)	55980	1(2)	57285	1(2)
50630	1(2)	51520	1(2)	52240	1(2)	53235	1(3)	54160	1(2)	54680	1(2)	56405	2(3)	57287	1(2)
50650	1(2)	51525	1(2)	52250	1(2)	53240	1(3)	54161	1(2)	54690	1(2)	56420	1(3)	57288	1(2)
50660	1(3)	51530	1(2)	52260	1(2)	53250	1(3)	54162	1(2)	54692	1(2)	56440	1(3)	57289	1(2)
50684	1(3)	51535	1(2)	52265	1(2)	53260	1(2)	54163	1(2)	54699	1(3)	56441	1(2)	57291	1(2)
50686	2(3)	51550	1(2)	52270	1(2)	53265	1(3)	54164	1(2)	54700	1(3)	56442	1(2)	57292	1(2)
50688	2(3)	51555	1(2)	52275	1(2)	53270	1(2)	54200	1(2)	54800	1(2)	56501	1(2)	57295	1(2)
50690	2(3)	51565	1(2)	52276	1(2)	53275	1(2)	54205	1(2)	54830	1(2)	56515	1(2)	57296	1(2)
50693	2(3)	51570	1(2)	52277	1(2)	53400	1(2)	54220	1(3)	54840	1(2)	56605	1(2)	57300	1(3)
50694	2(3)	51575	1(2)	52281	1(2)	53405	1(2)	54230	1(3)	54860	1(2)	56606	6(3)	57305	1(3)
50695	2(3)	51580	1(2)	52282	1(2)	53410	1(2)	54231	1(3)	54861	1(2)	56620	1(2)	57307	1(3)
50700	1(2)	51585	1(2)	52283	1(2)	53415	1(2)	54235	1(3)	54865	1(3)	56625	1(2)	57308	1(3)
50705	2(3)	51590	1(2)	52285	1(2)	53420	1(2)	54240	1(2)	54900	1(2)	56630	1(2)	57310	1(3)
50706	2(3)	51595	1(2)	52287	1(2)	53425	1(2)	54250	1(2)	54901	1(2)	56631	1(2)	57311	1(3)
50715	1(2)	51596	1(2)	52290	1(2)	53430	1(2)	54300	1(2)	55000	1(3)	56632	1(2)	57320	1(3)
50722	1(2)	51597	1(2)	52300	1(2)	53431	1(2)	54304	1(2)	55040	1(2)	56633	1(2)	57330	1(3)
50725	1(3)	51600	1(3)	52301	1(2)	53440	1(2)	54308	1(2)	55041	1(2)	56634	1(2)	57335	1(2)
50727	1(3)	51605	1(3)	52305	1(2)	53442	1(2)	54312	1(2)	55060	1(2)	56637	1(2)	57400	1(2)
50728	1(3)	51610	1(3)	52310	1(3)	53444	1(3)	54316	1(2)	55100	2(3)	56640	1(2)	57410	1(2)
50740	1(2)	51700	1(3)	52315	2(3)	53445	1(2)	54318	1(2)	55110	1(2)	56700	1(2)	57415	1(3)
50750	1(2)	51701	2(3)	52317	1(3)	53446	1(2)	54322	1(2)	55120	1(3)	56740	1(3)	57420	1(3)
50760	1(2)	51702	2(3)	52318	1(3)	53447	1(2)	54324	1(2)	55150	1(2)	56800	1(2)	57421	1(3)
50770	1(2)	51703	2(3)	52320	1(2)	53448	1(2)	54326	1(2)	55175	1(2)	56805	1(2)	57423	1(2)
50780	1(2)	51705	1(3)	52325	1(3)	53449	1(2)	54328	1(2)	55180	1(2)	56810	1(2)	57425	1(2)
50782	1(2)	51710	1(3)	52327	1(2)	53450	1(2)	54332	1(2)	55200	1(2)	56820	1(2)	57426	1(2)
50783	1(2)	51715	1(2)	52330	1(2)	53460	1(2)	54336	1(2)	55250	1(2)	56821	1(2)	57452	1(3)
50785	1(2)	51720	1(3)	52332	1(2)	53500	1(2)	54340	1(2)	55300	1(2)	57000	1(3)	57454	1(3)
50800	1(2)	51725	1(3)	52334	1(2)	53502	1(3)	54344	1(2)	55400	1(2)	57010	1(3)	57455	1(3)
50810	1(3)	51726	1(3)	52341	1(2)	53505	1(3)	54348	1(2)	55500	1(2)	57020	1(3)	57456	1(3)
50815	1(2)	51727	1(3)	52342	1(2)	53510	1(3)	54352	1(2)	55520	1(2)	57022	1(3)	57460	1(3)
50820	1(2)	51728	1(3)	52343	1(2)	53515	1(3)	54360	1(2)	55530	1(2)	57023	1(3)	57461	1(3)
50825	1(3)	51729	1(3)	52344	1(2)	53520	1(3)	54380	1(2)	55535	1(2)	57061	1(2)	57500	1(3)
50830	1(3)	51736	1(3)	52345	1(2)	53600	1(3)	54385	1(2)	55540	1(2)	57065	1(2)	57505	1(3)
50840	1(2)	51741	1(3)	52346	1(2)	53601	1(3)	54390	1(2)	55550	1(2)	57100	2(3)	57510	1(3)

CPT	MUE	CPT	MUE	CPT	MUE	CPT	MUE	CPT	MUE	CPT	MUE	CPT	MUE	CPT	MUE
57511	1(3)	58554	1(2)	59030	2(3)	60240	1(2)	61512	1(3)	61618	2(3)	62142	2(3)	62380	2(3)
57513	1(3)	58555	1(3)	59050	2(3)	60252	1(2)	61514	2(3)	61619	2(3)	62143	2(3)	63001	1(2)
57520	1(3)	58558	1(3)	59051	2(3)	60254	1(2)	61516	1(3)	61623	2(3)	62145	2(3)	63003	1(2)
57522	1(3)	58559	1(3)	59070	2(3)	60260	1(2)	61517	1(3)	61624	2(3)	62146	2(3)	63005	1(2)
57530	1(3)	58560	1(3)	59072	2(3)	60270	1(2)	61518	1(3)	61626	2(3)	62147	1(3)	63011	1(2)
57531	1(2)	58561	1(3)	59074	2(3)	60271	1(2)	61519	1(3)	61630	1(3)	62148	1(3)	63012	1(2)
57540	1(2)	58562	1(3)	59076	2(3)	60280	1(3)	61520	1(3)	61635	2(3)	62160	1(3)	63015	1(2)
57545	1(3)	58563	1(3)	59100	1(2)	60281	1(3)	61521	1(3)	61640	0(3)	62161	1(3)	63016	1(2)
57550	1(3)	58565	1(2)	59120	1(3)	60300	2(3)	61522	1(3)	61641	0(3)	62162	1(3)	63017	1(2)
57555	1(2)	58570	1(3)	59121	1(3)	60500	1(2)	61524	2(3)	61642	0(3)	62163	1(3)	63020	1(2)
57556	1(2)	58571	1(2)	59130	1(3)	60502	1(3)	61526	1(3)	61645	1(3)	62164	1(3)	63030	1(2)
57558	1(3)	58572	1(3)	59135	1(3)	60505	1(3)	61530	1(3)	61650	1(2)	62165	1(2)	63035	4(3)
57700	1(3)	58573	1(2)	59136	1(3)	60512	1(3)	61531	1(2)	61651	2(2)	62180	1(3)	63040	1(2)
57720	1(3)	58575	1(2)	59140	1(2)	60520	1(2)	61533	2(3)	61680	1(3)	62190	1(3)	63042	1(2)
57800	1(3)	58578	1(3)	59150	1(3)	60521	1(3)	61534	1(3)	61682	1(3)	62192	1(3)	63043	4(3)
58100	1(3)	58579	1(3)	59151	1(3)	60522	1(3)	61535	2(3)	61684	1(3)	62194	1(3)	63044	4(2)
58110	1(3)	58600	1(2)	59160	1(2)	60540	1(2)	61536	1(3)	61686	1(3)	62200	1(2)	63045	1(2)
58120	1(3)	58605	1(2)	59200	1(3)	60545	1(2)	61537	1(3)	61690	1(3)	62201	1(2)	63046	1(2)
58140	1(3)	58611	1(2)	59300	1(2)	60600	1(3)	61538	1(2)	61692	1(3)	62220	1(3)	63047	1(2)
58145	1(3)	58615	1(2)	59320	1(2)	60605	1(3)	61539	1(3)	61697	2(3)	62223	1(3)	63048	5(3)
58146	1(3)	58660	1(2)	59325	1(2)	60650	1(2)	61540	1(3)	61698	1(3)	62225	2(3)	63050	1(2)
58150	1(3)	58661	1(2)	59350	1(2)	60659	1(3)	61541	1(2)	61700	2(3)	62230	2(3)	63051	1(2)
58152	1(2)	58662	1(2)	59400	1(2)	60699	1(3)	61543	1(2)	61702	1(3)	62252	2(3)	63055	1(2)
58180	1(3)	58670	1(2)	59409	2(3)	61000	1(2)	61544	1(3)	61703	1(3)	62256	1(3)	63056	1(2)
58200	1(2)	58671	1(2)	59410	1(2)	61001	1(2)	61545	1(2)	61705	1(3)	62258	1(3)	63057	3(3)
58210	1(2)	58672	1(2)	59412	1(3)	61020	2(3)	61546	1(3)	61708	1(3)	62263	1(2)	63064	1(2)
58240	1(3)	58673	1(2)	59414	1(3)	61026	2(3)	61548	1(2)	61710	1(3)	62264	1(2)	63066	1(3)
58260	1(3)	58674	1(2)	59425	1(2)	61050	1(3)	61550	1(2)	61711	1(3)	62267	2(3)	63075	1(2)
58262	1(3)	58679	1(3)	59426	1(2)	61055	1(3)	61552	1(2)	61720	1(3)	62268	1(3)	63076	3(3)
58263	1(2)	58700	1(2)	59430	1(2)	61070	2(3)	61556	1(3)	61735	1(3)	62269	2(3)	63077	1(2)
58267	1(2)	58720	1(2)	59510	1(2)	61105	1(3)	61557	1(2)	61750	2(3)	62270	2(3)	63078	3(3)
58270	1(2)	58740	1(2)	59514	1(3)	61107	1(3)	61558	1(3)	61751	2(3)	62272	1(3)	63081	1(2)
58275	1(2)	58750	1(2)	59515	1(2)	61108	1(3)	61559	1(3)	61760	1(2)	62273	2(3)	63082	6(2)
58280	1(2)	58752	1(2)	59525	1(2)	61120	1(3)	61563	2(3)	61770	1(2)	62280	1(3)	63085	1(2)
58285	1(3)	58760	1(2)	59610	1(2)	61140	1(3)	61564	1(2)	61781	1(3)	62281	1(3)	63086	2(3)
58290	1(3)	58770	1(2)	59612	2(3)	61150	1(3)	61566	1(3)	61782	1(3)	62282	1(3)	63087	1(2)
58291	1(2)	58800	1(2)	59614	1(2)	61151	1(3)	61567	1(2)	61783	1(3)	62284	1(3)	63088	3(3)
58292	1(2)	58805	1(2)	59618	1(2)	61154	1(3)	61570	1(3)	61790	1(2)	62287	1(3)	63090	1(2)
58293	1(2)	58820	1(2)	59620	1(2)	61156	1(3)	61571	1(3)	61791	1(2)	62290	5(2)	63091	3(3)
58294	1(2)	58822	1(3)	59622	1(2)	61210	1(3)	61575	1(2)	61796	1(2)	62291	4(3)	63101	1(2)
58300	0(3)	58825	1(2)	59812	1(2)	61215	1(3)	61576	1(2)	61797	4(3)	62292	1(2)	63102	1(2)
58301	1(3)	58900	1(2)	59820	1(2)	61250	1(3)	61580	1(2)	61798	1(2)	62294	1(3)	63103	3(3)
58321	1(2)	58920	1(2)	59821	1(2)	61253	1(3)	61581	1(2)	61799	4(3)	62302	1(3)	63170	1(3)
58322	1(2)	58925	1(3)	59830	1(2)	61304	1(3)	61582	1(2)	61800	1(2)	62303	1(3)	63172	1(3)
58323	1(3)	58940	1(2)	59840	1(2)	61305	1(3)	61583	1(2)	61850	1(3)	62304	1(3)	63173	1(3)
58340	1(3)	58943	1(2)	59841	1(2)	61312	2(3)	61584	1(2)	61860	1(3)	62305	1(3)	63180	1(2)
58345	1(3)	58950	1(2)	59850	1(2)	61313	2(3)	61585	1(3)	61863	1(2)	62320	1(3)	63182	1(2)
58346	1(2)	58951	1(2)	59851	1(2)	61314	2(3)	61586	1(3)	61864	1(3)	62321	1(3)	63185	1(2)
58350	1(2)	58952	1(2)	59852	1(2)	61315	1(3)	61590	1(2)	61867	1(2)	62322	1(3)	63190	1(2)
58353	1(3)	58953	1(2)	59855	1(2)	61316	1(3)	61591	1(2)	61868	2(3)	62323	1(3)	63191	1(2)
58356	1(3)	58954	1(2)	59856	1(2)	61320	2(3)	61592	1(2)	61870	1(3)	62324	1(3)	63194	1(2)
58400	1(3)	58956	1(2)	59857	1(2)	61321	1(3)	61595	1(2)	61880	1(2)	62325	1(3)	63195	1(2)
58410	1(2)	58957	1(2)	59866	1(2)	61322	1(3)	61596	1(2)	61885	1(3)	62326	1(3)	63196	1(2)
58520	1(2)	58958	1(2)	59870	1(2)	61323	1(3)	61597	1(2)	61886	1(3)	62327	1(3)	63197	1(2)
58540	1(3)	58960	1(2)	59871	1(2)	61330	1(2)	61598	1(3)	61888	1(3)	62350	1(3)	63198	1(2)
58541	1(3)	58970	1(3)	59897	1(3)	61333	1(2)	61600	1(3)	62000	1(3)	62351	1(3)	63199	1(2)
58542	1(2)	58974	1(3)	59898	1(3)	61340	1(2)	61601	1(3)	62005	1(3)	62355	1(3)	63200	1(2)
58543	1(3)	58976	2(3)	59899	1(3)	61343	1(2)	61605	1(3)	62010	1(3)	62360	1(2)	63250	1(3)
58544	1(2)	58999	1(3)	60000	1(3)	61345	1(3)	61606	1(3)	62100	1(3)	62361	1(2)	63251	1(3)
58545	1(2)	59000	2(3)	60100	3(3)	61450	1(3)	61607	1(3)	62115	1(2)	62362	1(2)	63252	1(3)
58546	1(2)	59001	2(3)	60200	2(3)	61458	1(2)	61608	1(3)	62117	1(2)	62365	1(2)	63265	1(3)
58548	1(2)	59012	2(3)	60210	1(2)	61460	1(2)	61611	1(3)	62120	1(2)	62367	1(3)	63266	1(3)
58550	1(3)	59015	2(3)	60212	1(2)	61500	1(3)	61613	1(3)	62121	1(2)	62368	1(3)	63267	1(3)
58552	1(3)	59020	2(3)	60220	1(3)	61501	1(3)	61615	1(3)	62140	1(3)	62369	1(3)	63268	1(3)
58553	1(3)	59025	2(3)	60225	1(2)	61510	1(3)	61616	1(3)	62141	1(3)	62370	1(3)	63270	1(3)

CPT	MUE	CPT	MUE	CPT	MUE	CPT	MUE	CPT	MUE	CPT	MUE	CPT	MUE	CPT	MUE
63271	1(3)	64447	1(3)	64681	1(2)	64872	1(3)	65756	1(2)	66825	1(2)	67346	1(3)	67999	1(3)
63272	1(3)	64448	1(2)	64702	2(3)	64874	1(3)	65757	1(3)	66830	1(2)	67399	1(3)	68020	1(3)
63273	1(3)	64449	1(2)	64704	4(3)	64876	1(3)	65760	0(3)	66840	1(2)	67400	1(2)	68040	1(2)
63275	1(3)	64450	10(3)	64708	3(3)	64885	1(3)	65765	0(3)	66850	1(2)	67405	1(2)	68100	1(3)
63276	1(3)	64455	1(2)	64712	1(2)	64886	1(3)	65767	0(3)	66852	1(2)	67412	1(2)	68110	1(3)
63277	1(3)	64461	1(2)	64713	1(2)	64890	2(3)	65770	1(2)	66920	1(2)	67413	1(2)	68115	1(3)
63278	1(3)	64462	1(2)	64714	1(2)	64891	2(3)	65771	0(3)	66930	1(2)	67414	1(2)	68130	1(3)
63280	1(3)	64463	1(3)	64716	2(3)	64892	2(3)	65772	1(2)	66940	1(2)	67415	1(3)	68135	1(3)
63281	1(3)	64479	1(2)	64718	1(2)	64893	2(3)	65775	1(2)	66982	1(2)	67420	1(2)	68200	1(3)
63282	1(3)	64480	4(3)	64719	1(2)	64895	2(3)	65778	1(2)	66983	1(2)	67430	1(2)	68320	1(2)
63283	1(3)	64483	1(2)	64721	1(2)	64896	2(3)	65779	1(2)	66984	1(2)	67440	1(2)	68325	1(2)
63285	1(3)	64484	4(3)	64722	4(3)	64897	2(3)	65780	1(2)	66985	1(2)	67445	1(2)	68326	1(2)
63286	1(3)	64486	1(3)	64726	2(3)	64898	2(3)	65781	1(2)	66986	1(2)	67450	1(2)	68328	1(2)
63287	1(3)	64487	1(2)	64727	2(3)	64901	2(3)	65782	1(2)	66990	1(3)	67500	1(3)	68330	1(3)
63290	1(3)	64488	1(3)	64732	1(2)	64902	1(3)	65785	1(2)	66999	1(3)	67505	1(3)	68335	1(3)
63295	1(2)	64489	1(2)	64734	1(2)	64905	1(3)	65800	1(2)	67005	1(2)	67515	1(3)	68340	1(3)
63300	1(2)	64490	1(2)	64736	1(2)	64907	1(3)	65810	1(2)	67010	1(2)	67550	1(3)	68360	1(3)
63301	1(2)	64491	1(2)	64738	1(2)	64910	3(3)	65815	1(3)	67015	1(2)	67560	1(2)	68362	1(3)
63302	1(2)	64492	1(2)	64740	1(2)	64911	2(3)	65820	1(2)	67025	1(2)	67570	1(2)	68371	1(3)
63303	1(2)	64493	1(2)	64742	1(2)	64912	3(3)	65850	1(2)	67027	1(2)	67599	1(3)	68399	1(3)
63304	1(2)	64494	1(2)	64744	1(2)	64913	3(3)	65855	1(2)	67028	1(3)	67700	2(3)	68400	1(2)
63305	1(2)	64495	1(2)	64746	1(2)	64999	1(3)	65860	1(2)	67030	1(2)	67710	1(2)	68420	1(2)
63306	1(2)	64505	1(3)	64755	1(2)	65091	1(2)	65865	1(2)	67031	1(2)	67715	1(3)	68440	2(3)
63307	1(2)	64510	1(3)	64760	1(2)	65093	1(2)	65870	1(2)	67036	1(2)	67800	1(2)	68500	1(2)
63308	3(3)	64517	1(3)	64763	1(2)	65101	1(2)	65875	1(2)	67039	1(2)	67801	1(2)	68505	1(2)
63600	2(3)	64520	1(3)	64766	1(2)	65103	1(2)	65880	1(2)	67040	1(2)	67805	1(2)	68510	1(2)
63610	1(3)	64530	1(3)	64771	2(3)	65105	1(2)	65900	1(3)	67041	1(2)	67808	1(2)	68520	1(2)
63620	1(2)	64553	1(3)	64772	2(3)	65110	1(2)	65920	1(2)	67042	1(2)	67810	2(3)	68525	1(2)
63621	2(2)	64555	2(3)	64774	2(3)	65112	1(2)	65930	1(3)	67043	1(2)	67820	1(2)	68530	1(2)
63650	2(3)	64561	1(3)	64776	1(2)	65114	1(2)	66020	1(3)	67101	1(2)	67825	1(2)	68540	1(2)
63655	1(3)	64566	1(3)	64778	1(3)	65125	1(2)	66030	1(3)	67105	1(2)	67830	1(2)	68550	1(2)
63661	1(2)	64568	1(3)	64782	2(2)	65130	1(2)	66130	1(3)	67107	1(2)	67835	1(2)	68700	1(2)
63662	1(2)	64569	1(3)	64783	2(3)	65135	1(2)	66150	1(2)	67108	1(2)	67840	3(3)	68705	2(3)
63663	1(3)	64570	1(3)	64784	3(3)	65140	1(2)	66155	1(2)	67110	1(2)	67850	3(3)	68720	1(2)
63664	1(3)	64575	2(3)	64786	1(3)	65150	1(2)	66160	1(2)	67113	1(2)	67875	1(2)	68745	1(2)
63685	1(3)	64580	2(3)	64787	4(3)	65155	1(2)	66170	1(2)	67115	1(2)	67880	1(2)	68750	1(2)
63688	1(3)	64581	2(3)	64788	5(3)	65175	1(2)	66172	1(2)	67120	1(2)	67882	1(2)	68760	4(2)
63700	1(3)	64585	2(3)	64790	1(3)	65205	1(3)	66174	1(2)	67121	1(2)	67900	1(2)	68761	4(2)
63702	1(3)	64590	1(3)	64792	2(3)	65210	1(3)	66175	1(2)	67141	1(2)	67901	1(2)	68770	1(3)
63704	1(3)	64595	1(3)	64795	2(3)	65220	1(3)	66179	1(2)	67145	1(2)	67902	1(2)	68801	4(2)
63706	1(3)	64600	2(3)	64802	1(2)	65222	1(3)	66180	1(2)	67208	1(2)	67903	1(2)	68810	1(2)
63707	1(3)	64605	1(2)	64804	1(2)	65235	1(3)	66183	1(3)	67210	1(2)	67904	1(2)	68811	1(2)
63709	1(3)	64610	1(2)	64809	1(2)	65260	1(3)	66184	1(2)	67218	1(2)	67906	1(2)	68815	1(2)
63710	1(3)	64611	1(2)	64818	1(2)	65265	1(3)	66185	1(2)	67220	1(2)	67908	1(2)	68816	1(2)
63740	1(3)	64612	1(2)	64820	4(3)	65270	1(3)	66225	1(2)	67221	1(2)	67909	1(2)	68840	1(2)
63741	1(3)	64615	1(2)	64821	1(2)	65272	1(3)	66250	1(2)	67225	1(2)	67911	2(3)	68850	1(3)
63744	1(3)	64616	1(2)	64822	1(2)	65273	1(3)	66500	1(2)	67227	1(2)	67912	1(2)	68899	1(3)
63746	1(2)	64617	1(2)	64823	1(2)	65275	1(3)	66505	1(2)	67228	1(2)	67914	2(3)	69000	1(3)
64400	4(3)	64620	5(3)	64831	1(2)	65280	1(3)	66600	1(2)	67229	1(2)	67915	2(3)	69005	1(3)
64402	1(3)	64630	1(3)	64832	3(3)	65285	1(3)	66605	1(2)	67250	1(2)	67916	2(3)	69020	1(3)
64405	1(3)	64632	1(2)	64834	1(2)	65286	1(3)	66625	1(2)	67255	1(2)	67917	2(3)	69090	0(3)
64408	1(3)	64633	1(2)	64835	1(2)	65290	1(3)	66630	1(2)	67299	1(3)	67921	2(3)	69100	3(3)
64410	1(3)	64634	4(3)	64836	1(2)	65400	1(3)	66635	1(2)	67311	1(2)	67922	2(3)	69105	1(3)
64413	1(3)	64635	1(2)	64837	2(3)	65410	1(3)	66680	1(2)	67312	1(2)	67923	2(3)	69110	1(2)
64415	1(3)	64636	4(2)	64840	1(2)	65420	1(2)	66682	1(2)	67314	1(2)	67924	2(3)	69120	1(3)
64416	1(2)	64640	5(3)	64856	2(3)	65426	1(2)	66700	1(2)	67316	1(2)	67930	2(3)	69140	1(2)
64417	1(3)	64642	1(2)	64857	2(3)	65430	1(2)	66710	1(2)	67318	1(2)	67935	2(3)	69145	1(3)
64418	1(3)	64643	3(2)	64858	1(2)	65435	1(2)	66711	1(2)	67320	2(3)	67938	2(3)	69150	1(3)
64420	3(3)	64644	1(2)	64859	2(3)	65436	1(2)	66720	1(2)	67331	1(2)	67950	2(2)	69155	1(3)
64421	3(3)	64645	3(2)	64861	1(2)	65450	1(3)	66740	1(2)	67332	1(2)	67961	2(3)	69200	1(2)
64425	1(3)	64646	1(2)	64862	1(2)	65600	1(3)	66761	1(2)	67334	1(2)	67966	2(3)	69205	1(3)
64430	1(3)	64647	1(2)	64864	2(3)	65710	1(2)	66762	1(2)	67335	1(2)	67971	1(2)	69209	1(2)
64435	1(3)	64650	1(2)	64865	1(3)	65730	1(2)	66770	1(3)	67340	2(2)	67973	1(2)	69210	1(2)
64445	1(3)	64653	1(2)	64866	1(3)	65750	1(2)	66820	1(2)	67343	1(2)	67974	1(2)	69220	1(2)
64446	1(2)	64680	1(2)	64868	1(3)	65755	1(2)	66821	1(2)	67345	1(3)	67975	1(2)	69222	1(2)

Current Procedural Coding Expert — Appendix I — Medically Unlikely Edits (MUEs)

CPT	MUE	CPT	MUE	CPT	MUE	CPT	MUE	CPT	MUE	CPT	MUE	CPT	MUE	CPT	MUE
69300	1(2)	69915	1(3)	70551	2(3)	72193	1(3)	73630	3(3)	74430	1(3)	75902	2(3)	76828	2(3)
69310	1(2)	69930	1(2)	70552	2(3)	72194	1(3)	73650	2(3)	74440	1(2)	75956	1(2)	76830	1(3)
69320	1(2)	69949	1(3)	70553	2(3)	72195	1(3)	73660	2(3)	74445	1(2)	75957	1(2)	76831	1(3)
69399	1(3)	69950	1(2)	70554	1(3)	72196	1(3)	73700	2(3)	74450	1(3)	75958	2(3)	76856	1(3)
69420	1(2)	69955	1(2)	70555	1(3)	72197	1(3)	73701	2(3)	74455	1(3)	75959	1(3)	76857	1(3)
69421	1(2)	69960	1(2)	70557	1(3)	72198	1(3)	73702	2(3)	74470	2(2)	75970	1(3)	76870	1(2)
69424	1(2)	69970	1(3)	70558	1(3)	72200	2(3)	73706	2(3)	74485	2(3)	75984	2(3)	76872	1(3)
69433	1(2)	69979	1(3)	70559	1(3)	72202	1(3)	73718	2(3)	74710	1(3)	75989	2(3)	76873	1(2)
69436	1(2)	69990	1(3)	71045	4(3)	72220	1(3)	73719	2(3)	74712	1(3)	76000	3(3)	76881	2(3)
69440	1(2)	70010	1(3)	71046	2(3)	72240	1(2)	73720	2(3)	74713	2(3)	76010	2(3)	76882	2(3)
69450	1(2)	70015	1(3)	71047	1(3)	72255	1(2)	73721	3(3)	74740	1(3)	76080	3(3)	76885	1(2)
69501	1(3)	70030	2(2)	71048	1(3)	72265	1(2)	73722	2(3)	74742	2(2)	76098	3(3)	76886	1(2)
69502	1(2)	70100	2(3)	71100	2(3)	72270	1(2)	73723	2(3)	74775	1(2)	76100	2(3)	76930	1(3)
69505	1(2)	70110	2(3)	71101	2(3)	72275	1(3)	73725	2(3)	75557	1(3)	76101	1(3)	76932	1(2)
69511	1(2)	70120	1(3)	71110	1(3)	72285	4(3)	74018	3(3)	75559	1(3)	76102	1(3)	76936	1(3)
69530	1(2)	70130	1(3)	71111	1(3)	72295	5(3)	74019	2(3)	75561	1(3)	76120	1(3)	76937	2(3)
69535	1(2)	70134	1(3)	71120	1(3)	73000	2(3)	74021	2(3)	75563	1(3)	76125	1(3)	76940	1(3)
69540	1(3)	70140	2(3)	71130	1(3)	73010	2(3)	74022	2(3)	75565	1(3)	76140	0(3)	76941	3(3)
69550	1(3)	70150	1(3)	71250	2(3)	73020	2(3)	74150	1(3)	75571	1(3)	76376	2(3)	76942	1(3)
69552	1(2)	70160	1(3)	71260	2(3)	73030	4(3)	74160	1(3)	75572	1(3)	76377	2(3)	76945	1(3)
69554	1(2)	70170	2(2)	71270	1(3)	73040	2(3)	74170	1(3)	75573	1(3)	76380	2(3)	76946	1(3)
69601	1(2)	70190	1(2)	71275	1(3)	73050	1(3)	74174	1(3)	75574	1(3)	76390	0(3)	76948	1(2)
69602	1(2)	70200	2(3)	71550	1(3)	73060	2(3)	74175	1(3)	75600	1(3)	76391	1(3)	76965	2(3)
69603	1(2)	70210	1(3)	71551	1(3)	73070	2(3)	74176	2(3)	75605	1(3)	76496	1(3)	76970	2(3)
69604	1(2)	70220	1(3)	71552	1(3)	73080	2(3)	74177	2(3)	75625	1(3)	76497	1(3)	76975	1(3)
69605	1(2)	70240	1(2)	71555	1(3)	73085	2(2)	74178	1(3)	75630	1(3)	76498	1(3)	76977	1(2)
69610	1(2)	70250	2(3)	72020	4(3)	73090	2(3)	74181	1(3)	75635	1(3)	76499	1(3)	76978	1(3)
69620	1(2)	70260	1(3)	72040	3(3)	73092	2(3)	74182	1(3)	75705	20(3)	76506	1(2)	76979	3(3)
69631	1(2)	70300	1(3)	72050	1(3)	73100	2(3)	74183	1(3)	75710	2(3)	76510	2(2)	76981	1(3)
69632	1(3)	70310	1(3)	72052	1(3)	73110	3(3)	74185	1(3)	75716	1(3)	76511	2(2)	76982	1(2)
69633	1(2)	70320	1(3)	72070	1(3)	73115	2(2)	74190	1(3)	75726	3(3)	76512	2(2)	76983	3(3)
69635	1(3)	70328	1(3)	72072	1(3)	73120	2(3)	74210	1(3)	75731	1(3)	76513	2(3)	76998	1(3)
69636	1(3)	70330	1(3)	72074	1(3)	73130	3(3)	74220	1(3)	75733	1(3)	76514	1(2)	76999	1(3)
69637	1(3)	70332	2(3)	72080	1(3)	73140	3(3)	74230	1(3)	75736	2(3)	76516	1(2)	77001	2(3)
69641	1(2)	70336	1(3)	72081	1(3)	73200	2(3)	74235	1(3)	75741	1(3)	76519	2(2)	77002	1(3)
69642	1(2)	70350	1(3)	72082	1(3)	73201	2(3)	74240	2(3)	75743	1(3)	76529	2(2)	77003	1(3)
69643	1(2)	70355	1(3)	72083	1(3)	73202	2(3)	74241	1(3)	75746	1(3)	76536	1(3)	77011	1(3)
69644	1(2)	70360	2(3)	72084	1(3)	73206	2(3)	74245	1(3)	75756	2(3)	76604	1(3)	77012	1(3)
69645	1(2)	70370	1(3)	72100	2(3)	73218	2(3)	74246	1(3)	75774	7(3)	76641	2(2)	77013	1(3)
69646	1(2)	70371	1(2)	72110	1(3)	73219	2(3)	74247	1(3)	75801	1(3)	76642	2(2)	77014	2(3)
69650	1(2)	70380	2(3)	72114	1(3)	73220	2(3)	74249	1(3)	75803	1(3)	76700	1(3)	77021	1(3)
69660	1(2)	70390	2(3)	72120	1(3)	73221	2(3)	74250	1(3)	75805	1(2)	76705	2(3)	77022	1(3)
69661	1(2)	70450	3(3)	72125	1(3)	73222	2(3)	74251	1(3)	75807	1(2)	76706	1(2)	77046	1(2)
69662	1(2)	70460	1(3)	72126	1(3)	73223	2(3)	74260	1(2)	75809	1(3)	76770	1(3)	77047	1(2)
69666	1(2)	70470	2(3)	72127	1(3)	73225	2(3)	74261	1(2)	75810	1(3)	76775	2(3)	77048	1(2)
69667	1(2)	70480	1(3)	72128	1(3)	73501	2(3)	74262	1(2)	75820	2(3)	76776	2(3)	77049	1(2)
69670	1(2)	70481	1(3)	72129	1(3)	73502	2(3)	74263	0(3)	75822	1(3)	76800	1(3)	77053	2(2)
69676	1(2)	70482	1(3)	72130	1(3)	73503	2(3)	74270	1(3)	75825	1(3)	76801	1(2)	77054	2(2)
69700	1(3)	70486	1(3)	72131	1(3)	73521	2(3)	74280	1(3)	75827	1(3)	76802	2(3)	77061	1(2)
69710	0(3)	70487	1(3)	72132	1(3)	73522	2(3)	74283	1(3)	75831	1(3)	76805	1(2)	77062	1(2)
69711	1(2)	70488	1(3)	72133	1(3)	73523	2(3)	74290	1(3)	75833	1(3)	76810	1(3)	77063	1(2)
69714	1(2)	70490	1(3)	72141	1(3)	73525	2(2)	74300	1(3)	75840	1(3)	76811	1(2)	77065	1(2)
69715	1(3)	70491	1(3)	72142	1(3)	73551	2(3)	74301	1(3)	75842	1(3)	76812	2(3)	77066	1(2)
69717	1(2)	70492	1(3)	72146	1(3)	73552	2(3)	74328	1(3)	75860	2(3)	76813	1(2)	77067	1(2)
69718	1(2)	70496	2(3)	72147	1(3)	73560	4(3)	74329	1(3)	75870	1(3)	76814	2(3)	77071	1(3)
69720	1(2)	70498	2(3)	72148	1(3)	73562	3(3)	74330	1(3)	75872	1(3)	76815	1(2)	77072	1(2)
69725	1(2)	70540	1(3)	72149	1(3)	73564	4(3)	74340	1(3)	75880	1(3)	76816	2(3)	77073	1(2)
69740	1(2)	70542	1(3)	72156	1(3)	73565	1(3)	74355	1(3)	75885	1(3)	76817	1(3)	77074	1(2)
69745	1(2)	70543	1(3)	72157	1(3)	73580	2(2)	74360	1(3)	75887	1(3)	76818	2(3)	77075	1(2)
69799	1(3)	70544	2(3)	72158	1(3)	73590	3(3)	74363	2(3)	75889	1(3)	76819	2(3)	77076	1(2)
69801	1(3)	70545	1(3)	72159	1(3)	73592	2(3)	74400	1(3)	75891	1(3)	76820	3(3)	77077	1(2)
69805	1(3)	70546	1(3)	72170	2(3)	73600	2(3)	74410	1(3)	75893	2(3)	76821	2(3)	77078	1(2)
69806	1(3)	70547	1(3)	72190	1(3)	73610	3(3)	74415	1(3)	75894	2(3)	76825	2(3)	77080	1(2)
69905	1(2)	70548	1(3)	72191	1(3)	73615	2(2)	74420	2(3)	75898	2(3)	76826	2(3)	77081	1(2)
69910	1(2)	70549	1(3)	72192	1(3)	73620	2(3)	74425	2(3)	75901	1(3)	76827	2(3)	77084	1(2)

© 2019 Optum360, LLC   CPT © 2019 American Medical Association. All Rights Reserved.   795

CPT	MUE	CPT	MUE	CPT	MUE	CPT	MUE	CPT	MUE	CPT	MUE	CPT	MUE	CPT	MUE
77085	1(2)	77772	2(3)	78428	1(3)	78813	1(2)	80321	1(3)	80416	1(3)	81190	1(2)	81267	1(3)
77086	1(2)	77778	1(3)	78445	1(3)	78814	1(2)	80322	1(3)	80417	1(3)	81200	1(2)	81268	4(3)
77261	1(3)	77789	2(3)	78451	1(2)	78815	1(2)	80323	1(3)	80418	1(3)	81201	1(2)	81269	1(2)
77262	1(3)	77790	1(3)	78452	1(2)	78816	1(2)	80324	1(3)	80420	1(2)	81202	1(3)	81270	1(2)
77263	1(3)	77799	1(3)	78453	1(2)	78999	1(3)	80325	1(3)	80422	1(3)	81203	1(3)	81271	1(2)
77280	2(3)	78012	1(3)	78454	1(2)	79005	1(3)	80326	1(3)	80424	1(3)	81204	1(2)	81272	1(3)
77285	1(3)	78013	1(3)	78456	1(3)	79101	1(3)	80327	1(3)	80426	1(3)	81205	1(3)	81273	1(3)
77290	1(3)	78014	1(2)	78457	1(2)	79200	1(3)	80328	1(3)	80428	1(3)	81206	1(3)	81274	1(2)
77293	1(3)	78015	1(3)	78458	1(2)	79300	1(3)	80329	1(3)	80430	1(3)	81207	1(3)	81275	1(3)
77295	1(3)	78016	1(3)	78459	1(3)	79403	1(3)	80330	1(3)	80432	1(3)	81208	1(3)	81276	1(3)
77299	1(3)	78018	1(2)	78466	1(3)	79440	1(3)	80331	1(3)	80434	1(3)	81209	1(3)	81283	1(2)
77300	10(3)	78020	1(3)	78468	1(3)	79445	1(3)	80332	1(3)	80435	1(3)	81210	1(3)	81284	1(2)
77301	1(3)	78070	1(2)	78469	1(3)	79999	1(3)	80333	1(3)	80436	1(3)	81212	1(2)	81285	1(2)
77306	1(3)	78071	1(3)	78472	1(2)	80047	2(3)	80334	1(3)	80438	1(3)	81215	1(2)	81286	1(2)
77307	1(3)	78072	1(3)	78473	1(2)	80048	2(3)	80335	1(3)	80439	1(3)	81216	1(2)	81287	1(3)
77316	1(3)	78075	1(2)	78481	1(2)	80050	0(3)	80336	1(3)	80500	1(3)	81217	1(2)	81288	1(3)
77317	1(3)	78099	1(3)	78483	1(2)	80051	2(3)	80337	1(3)	80502	1(3)	81218	1(3)	81289	1(2)
77318	1(3)	78102	1(2)	78491	1(3)	80053	1(3)	80338	1(3)	81000	2(3)	81219	1(3)	81290	1(3)
77321	1(2)	78103	1(2)	78492	1(2)	80055	1(3)	80339	1(3)	81001	2(3)	81220	1(3)	81291	1(3)
77331	3(3)	78104	1(2)	78494	1(3)	80061	1(3)	80340	1(3)	81002	2(3)	81221	1(3)	81292	1(2)
77332	4(3)	78110	1(2)	78496	1(3)	80069	1(3)	80341	1(3)	81003	2(3)	81222	1(3)	81293	1(3)
77333	2(3)	78111	1(2)	78499	1(3)	80074	1(2)	80342	1(3)	81005	2(3)	81223	1(2)	81294	1(3)
77334	10(3)	78120	1(2)	78579	1(3)	80076	1(3)	80343	1(3)	81007	1(3)	81224	1(3)	81295	1(2)
77336	1(2)	78121	1(2)	78580	1(3)	80081	1(2)	80344	1(3)	81015	2(3)	81225	1(3)	81296	1(3)
77338	1(3)	78122	1(2)	78582	1(3)	80150	2(3)	80345	1(3)	81020	1(3)	81226	1(3)	81297	1(3)
77370	1(3)	78130	1(2)	78597	1(3)	80155	1(3)	80346	1(3)	81025	1(3)	81227	1(3)	81298	1(2)
77371	1(3)	78135	1(3)	78598	1(3)	80156	2(3)	80347	1(3)	81050	2(3)	81228	1(3)	81299	1(3)
77372	1(2)	78140	1(3)	78599	1(3)	80157	2(3)	80348	1(3)	81099	1(3)	81229	1(3)	81300	1(3)
77373	1(3)	78185	1(2)	78600	1(3)	80158	1(3)	80349	1(3)	81105	1(2)	81230	1(2)	81301	1(3)
77385	1(3)	78191	1(2)	78601	1(3)	80159	2(3)	80350	1(3)	81106	1(2)	81231	1(2)	81302	1(3)
77386	1(3)	78195	1(2)	78605	1(3)	80162	2(3)	80351	1(3)	81107	1(2)	81232	1(2)	81303	1(3)
77387	1(3)	78199	1(3)	78606	1(3)	80163	1(3)	80352	1(3)	81108	1(2)	81233	1(3)	81304	1(3)
77399	1(3)	78201	1(3)	78607	1(3)	80164	2(3)	80353	1(3)	81109	1(2)	81234	1(2)	81305	1(3)
77401	1(2)	78202	1(3)	78608	1(3)	80165	1(3)	80354	1(3)	81110	1(2)	81235	1(3)	81306	1(2)
77402	2(3)	78205	1(3)	78609	0(3)	80168	2(3)	80355	1(3)	81111	1(2)	81236	1(3)	81310	1(3)
77407	2(3)	78206	1(3)	78610	1(3)	80169	1(3)	80356	1(3)	81112	1(2)	81237	1(3)	81311	1(3)
77412	2(3)	78215	1(3)	78630	1(3)	80170	2(3)	80357	1(3)	81120	1(3)	81238	1(2)	81312	1(2)
77417	1(2)	78216	1(3)	78635	1(3)	80171	1(3)	80358	1(3)	81121	1(3)	81239	1(2)	81313	1(3)
77423	1(3)	78226	1(3)	78645	1(3)	80173	2(3)	80359	1(3)	81161	1(3)	81240	1(2)	81314	1(3)
77424	1(2)	78227	1(3)	78647	1(3)	80175	1(3)	80360	1(3)	81162	1(2)	81241	1(2)	81315	1(3)
77425	1(3)	78230	1(3)	78650	1(3)	80176	1(3)	80361	1(3)	81163	1(2)	81242	1(3)	81316	1(2)
77427	1(2)	78231	1(3)	78660	1(2)	80177	1(3)	80362	1(3)	81164	1(2)	81243	1(3)	81317	1(3)
77431	1(2)	78232	1(3)	78699	1(3)	80178	2(3)	80363	1(3)	81165	1(2)	81244	1(3)	81318	1(3)
77432	1(2)	78258	1(3)	78700	1(3)	80180	1(3)	80364	1(3)	81166	1(2)	81245	1(3)	81319	1(2)
77435	1(2)	78261	1(2)	78701	1(3)	80183	1(3)	80365	1(3)	81167	1(2)	81246	1(3)	81320	1(3)
77469	1(2)	78262	1(2)	78707	1(2)	80184	2(3)	80366	1(3)	81170	1(2)	81247	1(2)	81321	1(3)
77470	1(2)	78264	1(2)	78708	1(3)	80185	2(3)	80367	1(3)	81171	1(2)	81248	1(2)	81322	1(3)
77499	1(3)	78265	1(2)	78709	1(2)	80186	2(3)	80368	1(3)	81172	1(2)	81249	1(2)	81323	1(3)
77520	1(3)	78266	1(2)	78710	1(3)	80188	2(3)	80369	1(3)	81173	1(2)	81250	1(3)	81324	1(3)
77522	1(3)	78267	1(2)	78725	1(3)	80190	2(3)	80370	1(3)	81174	1(2)	81251	1(3)	81325	1(3)
77523	1(3)	78268	1(2)	78730	1(3)	80192	2(3)	80371	1(3)	81175	1(3)	81252	1(3)	81326	1(3)
77525	1(3)	78278	2(3)	78740	1(2)	80194	2(3)	80372	1(3)	81176	1(3)	81253	1(3)	81327	1(2)
77600	1(3)	78282	1(2)	78761	1(2)	80195	2(3)	80373	1(3)	81177	1(2)	81254	1(3)	81328	1(2)
77605	1(3)	78290	1(3)	78799	1(3)	80197	2(3)	80374	1(3)	81178	1(2)	81255	1(3)	81329	1(2)
77610	1(3)	78291	1(3)	78800	1(2)	80198	2(3)	80375	1(3)	81179	1(2)	81256	1(2)	81330	1(3)
77615	1(3)	78299	1(3)	78801	1(2)	80199	1(3)	80376	1(3)	81180	1(2)	81257	1(2)	81331	1(3)
77620	1(3)	78300	1(2)	78802	1(2)	80200	2(3)	80377	1(3)	81181	1(2)	81258	1(2)	81332	1(3)
77750	1(3)	78305	1(2)	78803	1(2)	80201	2(3)	80400	1(3)	81182	1(2)	81259	1(2)	81333	1(3)
77761	1(3)	78306	1(2)	78804	1(2)	80202	2(3)	80402	1(3)	81183	1(2)	81260	1(3)	81334	1(3)
77762	1(3)	78315	1(2)	78805	1(3)	80203	1(3)	80406	1(3)	81184	1(2)	81261	1(3)	81335	1(2)
77763	1(3)	78320	1(2)	78806	1(2)	80299	3(3)	80408	1(3)	81185	1(2)	81262	1(3)	81336	1(2)
77767	2(3)	78350	0(3)	78807	1(3)	80305	1(2)	80410	1(3)	81186	1(2)	81263	1(3)	81337	1(2)
77768	2(3)	78351	0(3)	78808	1(2)	80306	1(2)	80412	1(3)	81187	1(2)	81264	1(3)	81340	1(3)
77770	2(3)	78399	1(3)	78811	1(2)	80307	1(2)	80414	1(3)	81188	1(2)	81265	1(3)	81341	1(3)
77771	2(3)	78414	1(2)	78812	1(2)	80320	1(3)	80415	1(3)	81189	1(2)	81266	2(3)	81342	1(3)

CPT	MUE	CPT	MUE	CPT	MUE	CPT	MUE	CPT	MUE	CPT	MUE	CPT	MUE	CPT	MUE
81343	1(2)	81470	1(2)	82160	1(3)	82565	2(3)	82960	1(2)	83662	4(3)	84132	2(3)	84443	4(2)
81344	1(2)	81471	1(2)	82163	1(3)	82570	3(3)	82962	2(3)	83663	3(3)	84133	2(3)	84445	1(2)
81345	1(3)	81479	3(3)	82164	1(3)	82575	1(3)	82963	1(3)	83664	3(3)	84134	1(3)	84446	1(2)
81346	1(2)	81490	1(2)	82172	2(3)	82585	1(2)	82965	1(3)	83670	1(3)	84135	1(3)	84449	1(3)
81350	1(3)	81493	1(2)	82175	2(3)	82595	1(3)	82977	1(3)	83690	2(3)	84138	1(3)	84450	1(3)
81355	1(3)	81500	1(2)	82180	1(2)	82600	1(3)	82978	1(3)	83695	1(3)	84140	1(3)	84460	1(3)
81361	1(2)	81503	1(2)	82190	2(3)	82607	1(2)	82979	1(3)	83698	1(3)	84143	2(3)	84466	1(3)
81362	1(2)	81504	1(3)	82232	2(3)	82608	1(2)	82985	1(3)	83700	1(2)	84144	1(3)	84478	1(3)
81363	1(2)	81506	1(2)	82239	1(3)	82610	1(3)	83001	1(3)	83701	1(3)	84145	1(3)	84479	1(3)
81364	1(2)	81507	1(2)	82240	1(3)	82615	1(3)	83002	1(3)	83704	1(3)	84146	3(3)	84480	1(2)
81370	1(2)	81508	1(2)	82247	2(3)	82626	1(3)	83003	5(3)	83718	1(3)	84150	2(3)	84481	1(2)
81371	1(2)	81509	1(2)	82248	2(3)	82627	1(3)	83006	1(2)	83719	1(3)	84152	1(2)	84482	1(2)
81372	1(2)	81510	1(2)	82252	1(3)	82633	1(3)	83009	1(3)	83721	1(3)	84153	1(2)	84484	2(3)
81373	2(2)	81511	1(2)	82261	1(3)	82634	1(3)	83010	1(3)	83722	1(2)	84154	1(2)	84485	1(3)
81374	1(3)	81512	1(2)	82270	1(3)	82638	1(3)	83012	1(2)	83727	1(3)	84155	1(3)	84488	1(3)
81375	1(2)	81518	1(3)	82271	1(3)	82642	1(2)	83013	1(3)	83735	4(3)	84156	1(3)	84490	1(2)
81376	5(3)	81519	1(2)	82272	1(3)	82652	1(2)	83014	1(2)	83775	1(3)	84157	2(3)	84510	1(3)
81377	2(3)	81520	1(3)	82274	1(3)	82656	1(3)	83015	1(2)	83785	1(3)	84160	2(3)	84512	1(3)
81378	1(2)	81521	1(3)	82286	1(3)	82657	2(3)	83018	4(3)	83789	4(3)	84163	1(3)	84520	1(3)
81379	1(2)	81525	1(3)	82300	1(3)	82658	2(3)	83020	2(3)	83825	2(3)	84165	1(2)	84525	1(3)
81380	2(2)	81528	1(3)	82306	1(2)	82664	2(3)	83021	2(3)	83835	2(3)	84166	2(3)	84540	2(3)
81381	3(3)	81535	1(2)	82308	1(3)	82668	1(3)	83026	1(3)	83857	1(3)	84181	3(3)	84545	1(3)
81382	6(3)	81536	11(3)	82310	2(3)	82670	2(3)	83030	1(3)	83861	2(2)	84182	6(3)	84550	1(3)
81383	2(3)	81538	1(2)	82330	2(3)	82671	1(3)	83033	1(3)	83864	1(2)	84202	1(2)	84560	2(3)
81400	2(3)	81539	1(2)	82331	1(3)	82672	1(3)	83036	1(2)	83872	2(3)	84203	1(2)	84577	1(3)
81401	2(3)	81540	1(3)	82340	1(3)	82677	1(3)	83037	1(2)	83873	1(3)	84206	1(2)	84578	1(3)
81402	1(3)	81541	1(2)	82355	2(3)	82679	1(3)	83045	1(3)	83874	2(3)	84207	1(2)	84580	1(3)
81403	4(3)	81545	1(3)	82360	2(3)	82693	2(3)	83050	1(3)	83876	1(3)	84210	1(3)	84583	1(3)
81404	5(3)	81551	1(2)	82365	2(3)	82696	1(3)	83051	1(3)	83880	1(3)	84220	1(3)	84585	1(2)
81405	2(3)	81595	1(2)	82370	2(3)	82705	1(3)	83060	1(3)	83883	4(3)	84228	1(3)	84586	1(2)
81406	2(3)	81596	1(2)	82373	1(3)	82710	1(3)	83065	1(2)	83885	2(3)	84233	1(3)	84588	1(3)
81407	1(3)	81599	1(3)	82374	1(3)	82715	3(3)	83068	1(2)	83915	1(3)	84234	1(3)	84590	1(3)
81408	2(3)	82009	1(3)	82375	1(3)	82725	1(3)	83069	1(3)	83916	2(3)	84235	1(3)	84591	1(3)
81410	1(2)	82010	1(3)	82376	1(3)	82726	1(3)	83070	1(2)	83918	2(3)	84238	3(3)	84597	1(3)
81411	1(2)	82013	1(3)	82378	1(3)	82728	1(3)	83080	2(3)	83919	1(3)	84244	2(3)	84600	2(3)
81412	1(2)	82016	1(3)	82379	1(3)	82731	1(3)	83088	1(3)	83921	2(3)	84252	1(2)	84620	1(2)
81413	1(2)	82017	1(3)	82380	1(3)	82735	1(3)	83090	2(3)	83930	2(3)	84255	2(3)	84630	2(3)
81414	1(2)	82024	4(3)	82382	1(2)	82746	1(2)	83150	1(3)	83935	2(3)	84260	1(3)	84681	1(3)
81415	1(2)	82030	1(3)	82383	1(3)	82747	1(2)	83491	1(3)	83937	1(3)	84270	1(3)	84702	2(3)
81416	2(3)	82040	1(3)	82384	2(3)	82757	1(2)	83497	1(3)	83945	2(3)	84275	1(3)	84703	1(3)
81417	1(3)	82042	2(3)	82387	1(3)	82759	1(3)	83498	2(3)	83950	1(2)	84285	1(3)	84704	1(3)
81420	1(2)	82043	1(3)	82390	1(2)	82760	1(3)	83500	1(3)	83951	1(2)	84295	1(3)	84830	1(2)
81422	1(2)	82044	1(3)	82397	3(3)	82775	1(3)	83505	1(3)	83970	2(3)	84300	2(3)	84999	1(3)
81425	1(2)	82045	1(3)	82415	1(3)	82776	1(2)	83516	4(3)	83986	2(3)	84302	1(3)	85002	1(3)
81426	2(3)	82075	2(3)	82435	1(3)	82777	1(3)	83518	1(3)	83987	1(3)	84305	1(3)	85004	1(3)
81427	1(3)	82085	1(3)	82436	1(3)	82784	6(3)	83519	5(3)	83992	2(3)	84307	1(3)	85007	1(3)
81430	1(2)	82088	2(3)	82438	1(3)	82785	1(3)	83520	8(3)	83993	1(3)	84311	2(3)	85008	1(3)
81431	1(2)	82103	1(3)	82441	1(2)	82787	4(3)	83525	4(3)	84030	1(2)	84315	1(3)	85009	1(3)
81432	1(2)	82104	1(2)	82465	1(3)	82800	1(3)	83527	1(3)	84035	1(2)	84375	1(3)	85013	1(3)
81433	1(2)	82105	1(3)	82480	2(3)	82803	2(3)	83528	1(3)	84060	1(3)	84376	1(3)	85014	2(3)
81434	1(2)	82106	2(3)	82482	1(3)	82805	2(3)	83540	2(3)	84066	1(3)	84377	1(3)	85018	2(3)
81435	1(2)	82107	1(3)	82485	1(3)	82810	2(3)	83550	1(3)	84075	2(3)	84378	2(3)	85025	2(3)
81436	1(2)	82108	1(3)	82495	1(2)	82820	1(3)	83570	1(3)	84078	1(2)	84379	1(3)	85027	2(3)
81437	1(2)	82120	1(3)	82507	1(3)	82930	1(3)	83582	1(3)	84080	1(3)	84392	1(3)	85032	1(3)
81438	1(2)	82127	1(3)	82523	1(3)	82938	1(3)	83586	1(3)	84081	1(3)	84402	1(3)	85041	1(3)
81439	1(2)	82128	2(3)	82525	2(3)	82941	1(3)	83593	1(3)	84085	1(2)	84403	2(3)	85044	1(2)
81440	1(2)	82131	2(3)	82528	1(3)	82943	1(3)	83605	1(3)	84087	1(3)	84410	1(2)	85045	1(2)
81442	1(2)	82135	1(3)	82530	4(3)	82945	4(3)	83615	2(3)	84100	2(3)	84425	1(2)	85046	1(2)
81443	1(2)	82136	2(3)	82533	5(3)	82946	1(2)	83625	1(3)	84105	1(3)	84430	1(3)	85048	2(3)
81445	1(2)	82139	2(3)	82540	1(3)	82947	5(3)	83630	1(3)	84106	1(2)	84431	1(3)	85049	2(3)
81448	1(2)	82140	2(3)	82542	6(3)	82948	2(3)	83631	1(3)	84110	1(3)	84432	1(2)	85055	1(3)
81450	1(2)	82143	2(3)	82550	3(3)	82950	3(3)	83632	1(3)	84112	1(3)	84436	1(2)	85060	1(3)
81455	1(2)	82150	2(3)	82552	3(3)	82951	1(2)	83633	1(3)	84119	1(2)	84437	1(2)	85097	2(3)
81460	1(2)	82154	1(3)	82553	3(3)	82952	3(3)	83655	2(3)	84120	1(3)	84439	1(2)	85130	1(3)
81465	1(2)	82157	1(3)	82554	1(3)	82955	1(2)	83661	3(3)	84126	1(3)	84442	1(2)	85170	1(3)

Appendix I — Medically Unlikely Edits (MUEs)—Professional

CPT	MUE	CPT	MUE	CPT	MUE	CPT	MUE	CPT	MUE	CPT	MUE	CPT	MUE	CPT	MUE
85175	1(3)	85612	1(3)	86331	12(3)	86666	4(3)	86813	1(2)	87081	2(3)	87299	1(3)	87525	1(3)
85210	2(3)	85613	3(3)	86332	1(3)	86668	2(3)	86816	1(2)	87084	1(3)	87300	2(3)	87526	1(3)
85220	2(3)	85635	1(3)	86334	2(2)	86671	3(3)	86817	1(2)	87086	3(3)	87301	1(3)	87527	1(3)
85230	2(3)	85651	1(2)	86335	2(3)	86674	3(3)	86821	1(3)	87088	3(3)	87305	1(3)	87528	1(3)
85240	2(3)	85652	1(2)	86336	1(3)	86677	3(3)	86825	1(3)	87101	2(3)	87320	1(3)	87529	2(3)
85244	1(3)	85660	2(3)	86337	1(2)	86682	2(3)	86826	2(3)	87102	4(3)	87324	2(3)	87530	2(3)
85245	2(3)	85670	2(3)	86340	1(2)	86684	2(3)	86828	1(3)	87103	2(3)	87327	1(3)	87531	1(3)
85246	2(3)	85675	1(3)	86341	1(3)	86687	1(3)	86829	1(3)	87106	3(3)	87328	2(3)	87532	1(3)
85247	2(3)	85705	1(3)	86343	1(3)	86688	1(3)	86830	2(3)	87107	4(3)	87329	2(3)	87533	1(3)
85250	2(3)	85730	4(3)	86344	1(2)	86689	2(3)	86831	2(3)	87109	2(3)	87332	1(3)	87534	1(3)
85260	2(3)	85732	4(3)	86352	1(3)	86692	2(3)	86832	2(3)	87110	2(3)	87335	1(3)	87535	1(3)
85270	2(3)	85810	2(3)	86353	7(3)	86694	2(3)	86833	1(3)	87116	2(3)	87336	1(3)	87536	1(3)
85280	2(3)	85999	1(3)	86355	1(2)	86695	2(3)	86834	1(3)	87118	3(3)	87337	1(3)	87537	1(3)
85290	2(3)	86000	6(3)	86356	7(3)	86696	2(3)	86835	1(3)	87140	3(3)	87338	1(3)	87538	1(3)
85291	1(3)	86001	20(3)	86357	1(2)	86698	3(3)	86849	1(3)	87143	2(3)	87339	1(3)	87539	1(3)
85292	1(3)	86005	2(3)	86359	1(2)	86701	1(3)	86850	3(3)	87149	4(3)	87340	1(2)	87540	1(3)
85293	1(3)	86008	20(3)	86360	1(2)	86702	2(3)	86860	2(3)	87150	12(3)	87341	1(2)	87541	1(3)
85300	2(3)	86021	1(2)	86361	1(2)	86703	1(2)	86870	2(3)	87152	1(3)	87350	1(2)	87542	1(3)
85301	1(3)	86022	1(2)	86367	1(3)	86704	1(2)	86880	4(3)	87153	3(3)	87380	1(2)	87550	1(3)
85302	1(3)	86023	3(3)	86376	2(3)	86705	1(2)	86885	2(3)	87158	1(3)	87385	2(3)	87551	2(3)
85303	2(3)	86038	1(3)	86382	3(3)	86706	2(3)	86886	3(3)	87164	2(3)	87389	1(3)	87552	1(3)
85305	2(3)	86039	1(3)	86384	1(3)	86707	1(3)	86890	1(3)	87166	2(3)	87390	1(3)	87555	1(3)
85306	2(3)	86060	1(3)	86386	1(2)	86708	1(2)	86891	1(3)	87168	2(3)	87391	1(3)	87556	1(3)
85307	2(3)	86063	1(3)	86403	2(3)	86709	1(2)	86900	1(3)	87169	2(3)	87400	2(3)	87557	1(3)
85335	2(3)	86077	1(2)	86406	2(3)	86710	4(3)	86901	1(3)	87172	1(3)	87420	1(3)	87560	1(3)
85337	1(3)	86078	1(3)	86430	2(3)	86711	2(3)	86902	6(3)	87176	2(3)	87425	1(3)	87561	1(3)
85345	1(3)	86079	1(3)	86431	2(3)	86713	3(3)	86904	2(3)	87177	3(3)	87427	2(3)	87562	1(3)
85347	3(3)	86140	1(2)	86480	1(3)	86717	8(3)	86905	8(3)	87181	12(3)	87430	1(3)	87580	1(3)
85348	1(3)	86141	1(3)	86481	1(3)	86720	2(3)	86906	1(2)	87184	8(3)	87449	3(3)	87581	1(3)
85360	1(3)	86146	3(3)	86485	1(2)	86723	2(3)	86910	0(3)	87185	4(3)	87450	2(3)	87582	1(3)
85362	2(3)	86147	4(3)	86486	2(3)	86727	2(3)	86911	0(3)	87186	12(3)	87451	2(3)	87590	1(3)
85366	1(3)	86148	3(3)	86490	1(2)	86732	2(3)	86920	9(3)	87187	3(3)	87471	1(3)	87591	3(3)
85370	1(3)	86152	1(3)	86510	1(2)	86735	2(3)	86921	2(3)	87188	6(3)	87472	1(3)	87592	1(3)
85378	1(3)	86153	1(3)	86580	1(2)	86738	2(3)	86922	5(3)	87190	9(3)	87475	1(3)	87623	1(2)
85379	2(3)	86155	1(3)	86590	1(3)	86741	2(3)	86923	10(3)	87197	1(3)	87476	1(3)	87624	1(3)
85380	1(3)	86156	1(2)	86592	2(3)	86744	2(3)	86927	2(3)	87205	3(3)	87480	1(3)	87625	1(3)
85384	2(3)	86157	1(2)	86593	2(3)	86747	2(3)	86930	0(3)	87206	6(3)	87481	5(3)	87631	1(3)
85385	1(3)	86160	4(3)	86602	3(3)	86750	4(3)	86931	1(3)	87207	3(3)	87482	1(3)	87632	1(3)
85390	3(3)	86161	2(3)	86603	2(3)	86753	3(3)	86932	1(3)	87209	4(3)	87483	1(2)	87633	1(3)
85396	1(2)	86162	1(2)	86609	14(3)	86756	2(3)	86940	1(3)	87210	4(3)	87485	1(3)	87634	1(3)
85397	2(3)	86171	2(3)	86611	4(3)	86757	6(3)	86941	1(3)	87220	3(3)	87486	1(3)	87640	1(3)
85400	1(3)	86200	1(3)	86612	2(3)	86759	2(3)	86945	2(3)	87230	2(3)	87487	1(3)	87641	1(3)
85410	1(3)	86215	1(3)	86615	6(3)	86762	2(3)	86950	1(3)	87250	1(3)	87490	1(3)	87650	1(3)
85415	2(3)	86225	1(3)	86617	2(3)	86765	2(3)	86960	1(3)	87252	2(3)	87491	3(3)	87651	1(3)
85420	2(3)	86226	1(3)	86618	2(3)	86768	5(3)	86965	1(3)	87253	2(3)	87492	1(3)	87652	1(3)
85421	*1(3)	86235	10(3)	86619	2(3)	86771	2(3)	86970	1(3)	87254	7(3)	87493	2(3)	87653	1(3)
85441	1(2)	86255	5(3)	86622	2(3)	86774	2(3)	86971	1(3)	87255	2(3)	87495	1(3)	87660	1(3)
85445	1(2)	86256	9(3)	86625	1(3)	86777	2(3)	86972	1(3)	87260	1(3)	87496	1(3)	87661	1(3)
85460	1(3)	86277	1(3)	86628	3(3)	86778	2(3)	86975	1(3)	87265	1(3)	87497	2(3)	87662	2(3)
85461	1(2)	86280	1(3)	86631	6(3)	86780	2(3)	86976	1(3)	87267	1(3)	87498	1(3)	87797	3(3)
85475	1(3)	86294	1(3)	86632	3(3)	86784	1(3)	86977	1(3)	87269	1(3)	87500	1(3)	87798	13(3)
85520	1(3)	86300	2(3)	86635	4(3)	86787	2(3)	86978	1(3)	87270	1(3)	87501	1(3)	87799	3(3)
85525	2(3)	86301	1(2)	86638	6(3)	86788	2(3)	86985	1(3)	87271	1(3)	87502	1(3)	87800	2(3)
85530	1(3)	86304	1(2)	86641	2(3)	86789	2(3)	86999	1(3)	87272	1(3)	87503	1(3)	87801	3(3)
85536	1(2)	86305	1(2)	86644	2(3)	86790	4(3)	87003	1(3)	87273	1(3)	87505	1(2)	87802	2(3)
85540	1(2)	86308	1(2)	86645	1(3)	86793	2(3)	87015	3(3)	87274	1(3)	87506	1(2)	87803	3(3)
85547	1(2)	86309	1(2)	86648	2(3)	86794	1(3)	87040	2(3)	87275	1(3)	87507	1(2)	87804	3(3)
85549	1(3)	86310	1(2)	86651	2(3)	86800	1(3)	87045	3(3)	87276	1(3)	87510	1(3)	87806	1(2)
85555	1(2)	86316	2(3)	86652	2(3)	86803	1(3)	87046	6(3)	87278	1(3)	87511	1(3)	87807	2(3)
85557	1(2)	86317	6(3)	86653	2(3)	86804	1(2)	87070	3(3)	87279	1(3)	87512	1(3)	87808	1(3)
85576	7(3)	86318	2(3)	86654	2(3)	86805	2(3)	87071	2(3)	87280	1(3)	87516	1(3)	87809	2(3)
85597	1(3)	86320	1(2)	86658	12(3)	86806	2(3)	87073	2(3)	87281	1(3)	87517	1(3)	87810	2(3)
85598	1(3)	86325	2(3)	86663	2(3)	86807	2(3)	87075	6(3)	87283	1(3)	87520	1(3)	87850	1(3)
85610	4(3)	86327	1(3)	86664	2(3)	86808	1(3)	87076	2(3)	87285	1(3)	87521	1(3)	87880	2(3)
85611	2(3)	86329	3(3)	86665	2(3)	86812	1(2)	87077	4(3)	87290	1(3)	87522	1(3)	87899	4(3)

Appendix I — Medically Unlikely Edits (MUEs)—Professional

CPT	MUE	CPT	MUE	CPT	MUE	CPT	MUE	CPT	MUE	CPT	MUE	CPT	MUE	CPT	MUE
87900	1(2)	88235	2(3)	88373	3(3)	90287	0(3)	90687	1(2)	90935	1(3)	92083	1(2)	92538	1(2)
87901	1(2)	88237	4(3)	88374	5(3)	90288	0(3)	90688	1(2)	90937	1(3)	92100	1(2)	92540	1(3)
87902	1(2)	88239	3(3)	88375	1(3)	90291	0(3)	90689	1(2)	90940	1(3)	92132	1(2)	92541	1(3)
87903	1(2)	88240	1(3)	88377	5(3)	90296	1(2)	90690	1(2)	90945	1(3)	92133	1(2)	92542	1(3)
87904	14(3)	88241	3(3)	88380	1(3)	90371	10(3)	90691	1(2)	90947	1(3)	92134	1(2)	92544	1(3)
87905	2(3)	88245	1(2)	88381	1(3)	90375	20(3)	90696	1(2)	90951	1(2)	92136	2(2)	92545	1(3)
87906	2(3)	88248	1(2)	88387	2(3)	90376	20(3)	90697	1(2)	90952	1(2)	92145	1(2)	92546	1(3)
87910	1(3)	88249	1(2)	88388	1(3)	90378	4(3)	90698	1(2)	90953	1(2)	92225	2(2)	92547	1(3)
87912	1(3)	88261	2(3)	88399	1(3)	90384	0(3)	90700	1(2)	90954	1(2)	92226	2(2)	92548	1(3)
87999	1(3)	88262	2(3)	88720	1(3)	90385	1(2)	90702	1(2)	90955	1(2)	92227	1(2)	92550	1(2)
88000	0(3)	88263	1(3)	88738	1(3)	90386	0(3)	90707	1(2)	90956	1(2)	92228	1(2)	92551	0(3)
88005	0(3)	88264	1(3)	88740	1(2)	90389	0(3)	90710	1(2)	90957	1(2)	92230	2(2)	92552	1(2)
88007	0(3)	88267	2(3)	88741	1(2)	90393	1(2)	90713	1(2)	90958	1(2)	92235	1(2)	92553	1(2)
88012	0(3)	88269	2(3)	88749	1(3)	90396	1(2)	90714	1(2)	90959	1(2)	92240	1(2)	92555	1(2)
88014	0(3)	88271	16(3)	89049	1(3)	90399	0(3)	90715	1(2)	90960	1(2)	92242	1(2)	92556	1(2)
88016	0(3)	88272	12(3)	89050	2(3)	90460	9(3)	90716	1(2)	90961	1(2)	92250	1(2)	92557	1(2)
88020	0(3)	88273	3(3)	89051	2(3)	90461	8(3)	90717	1(2)	90962	1(2)	92260	1(2)	92558	0(3)
88025	0(3)	88274	5(3)	89055	2(3)	90471	1(2)	90723	0(3)	90963	1(2)	92265	1(2)	92559	0(3)
88027	0(3)	88275	12(3)	89060	2(3)	90472	8(3)	90732	1(2)	90964	1(2)	92270	1(2)	92560	0(3)
88028	0(3)	88280	1(3)	89125	2(3)	90473	1(2)	90733	1(2)	90965	1(2)	92273	1(2)	92561	1(2)
88029	0(3)	88283	5(3)	89160	1(3)	90474	1(3)	90734	1(2)	90966	1(2)	92274	1(2)	92562	1(2)
88036	0(3)	88285	10(3)	89190	1(3)	90476	1(2)	90736	1(2)	90967	1(2)	92283	1(2)	92563	1(2)
88037	0(3)	88289	1(3)	89220	1(2)	90477	1(2)	90738	1(2)	90968	1(2)	92284	1(2)	92564	1(2)
88040	0(3)	88291	1(3)	89230	1(2)	90581	1(2)	90739	1(2)	90969	1(2)	92285	1(2)	92565	1(2)
88045	0(3)	88299	1(3)	89240	1(3)	90585	1(2)	90740	1(2)	90970	1(2)	92286	1(2)	92567	1(2)
88099	0(3)	88300	4(3)	89250	1(2)	90586	1(2)	90743	1(2)	90989	1(2)	92287	1(2)	92568	1(2)
88104	5(3)	88302	4(3)	89251	1(2)	90587	1(2)	90744	1(2)	90993	1(3)	92310	0(3)	92570	1(2)
88106	5(3)	88304	5(3)	89253	1(3)	90620	1(2)	90746	1(2)	90997	1(3)	92311	1(2)	92571	1(2)
88108	6(3)	88305	16(3)	89254	1(3)	90621	1(2)	90747	1(2)	90999	1(3)	92312	1(2)	92572	1(2)
88112	6(3)	88307	8(3)	89255	1(3)	90625	1(2)	90748	0(3)	91010	1(2)	92313	1(3)	92575	1(2)
88120	2(3)	88309	3(3)	89257	1(3)	90630	1(2)	90749	1(3)	91013	1(3)	92314	0(3)	92576	1(2)
88121	2(3)	88311	4(3)	89258	1(2)	90632	1(2)	90750	1(2)	91020	1(2)	92315	1(2)	92577	1(2)
88125	1(3)	88312	9(3)	89259	1(2)	90633	1(2)	90756	1(2)	91022	1(2)	92316	1(2)	92579	1(2)
88130	1(2)	88313	8(3)	89260	1(2)	90634	1(2)	90785	3(3)	91030	1(2)	92317	1(3)	92582	1(2)
88140	1(2)	88314	6(3)	89261	1(2)	90636	1(2)	90791	1(3)	91034	1(2)	92325	1(3)	92583	1(2)
88141	1(3)	88319	11(3)	89264	1(3)	90644	1(2)	90792	1(3)	91035	1(2)	92326	2(2)	92584	1(2)
88142	1(3)	88321	1(2)	89268	1(2)	90647	1(2)	90832	2(3)	91037	1(2)	92340	0(3)	92585	1(2)
88143	1(3)	88323	1(2)	89272	1(2)	90648	1(2)	90833	2(3)	91038	1(2)	92341	0(3)	92586	1(2)
88147	1(3)	88325	1(2)	89280	1(2)	90649	1(2)	90834	2(3)	91040	1(2)	92342	0(3)	92587	1(2)
88148	1(3)	88329	2(3)	89281	1(2)	90650	1(2)	90836	2(3)	91065	2(2)	92352	0(3)	92588	1(2)
88150	1(3)	88331	11(3)	89290	1(2)	90651	1(2)	90837	2(3)	91110	1(2)	92353	0(3)	92590	0(3)
88152	1(3)	88332	13(3)	89291	1(2)	90653	1(2)	90838	2(3)	91111	1(2)	92354	0(3)	92591	0(3)
88153	1(3)	88333	4(3)	89300	1(2)	90654	1(2)	90839	1(2)	91112	1(3)	92355	0(3)	92592	0(3)
88155	1(3)	88334	5(3)	89310	1(2)	90655	1(2)	90840	3(3)	91117	1(2)	92358	0(3)	92593	0(3)
88160	4(3)	88341	13(3)	89320	1(2)	90656	1(2)	90845	1(2)	91120	1(2)	92370	0(3)	92594	0(3)
88161	4(3)	88342	3(3)	89321	1(2)	90657	1(2)	90846	1(3)	91122	1(2)	92371	0(3)	92595	0(3)
88162	3(3)	88344	6(3)	89322	1(2)	90658	1(2)	90847	1(3)	91132	1(3)	92499	1(3)	92596	1(2)
88164	1(3)	88346	2(3)	89325	1(2)	90660	1(2)	90849	1(3)	91133	1(3)	92502	1(3)	92597	1(3)
88165	1(3)	88348	1(3)	89329	1(2)	90661	1(2)	90853	1(3)	91200	1(2)	92504	1(3)	92601	1(3)
88166	1(3)	88350	8(3)	89330	1(2)	90662	1(2)	90863	1(3)	91299	1(3)	92507	1(3)	92602	1(3)
88167	1(3)	88355	1(3)	89331	1(2)	90664	1(2)	90865	1(3)	92002	1(2)	92508	1(3)	92603	1(3)
88172	5(3)	88356	3(3)	89335	1(3)	90666	1(2)	90867	1(2)	92004	1(2)	92511	1(3)	92604	1(3)
88173	5(3)	88358	2(3)	89337	1(2)	90667	1(2)	90868	1(3)	92012	1(3)	92512	1(2)	92605	0(3)
88174	1(3)	88360	6(3)	89342	1(2)	90668	1(2)	90869	1(3)	92014	1(3)	92516	1(3)	92606	0(3)
88175	1(3)	88361	6(3)	89343	1(2)	90670	1(2)	90870	2(3)	92015	0(3)	92520	1(2)	92607	1(3)
88177	6(3)	88362	1(3)	89344	1(2)	90672	1(2)	90875	0(3)	92018	1(2)	92521	1(2)	92608	4(3)
88182	2(3)	88363	2(3)	89346	1(2)	90673	1(2)	90876	0(3)	92019	1(2)	92522	1(2)	92609	1(3)
88184	2(3)	88364	3(3)	89352	1(2)	90674	1(2)	90880	1(3)	92020	1(2)	92523	1(2)	92610	1(2)
88185	35(3)	88365	4(3)	89353	1(3)	90675	1(2)	90882	0(3)	92025	1(2)	92524	1(2)	92611	1(3)
88187	2(3)	88366	2(3)	89354	1(3)	90676	1(2)	90885	0(3)	92060	1(2)	92526	1(2)	92612	1(3)
88188	2(3)	88367	3(3)	89356	2(3)	90680	1(2)	90887	0(3)	92065	1(2)	92531	0(3)	92613	1(2)
88189	2(3)	88368	3(3)	89398	1(3)	90681	1(2)	90889	0(3)	92071	2(2)	92532	0(3)	92614	1(3)
88199	1(3)	88369	3(3)	90281	0(3)	90682	1(2)	90899	1(3)	92072	1(2)	92533	0(3)	92615	1(2)
88230	2(3)	88371	1(3)	90283	0(3)	90685	1(2)	90901	1(3)	92081	1(2)	92534	0(3)	92616	1(3)
88233	2(3)	88372	1(3)	90284	0(3)	90686	1(2)	90911	1(3)	92082	1(2)	92537	1(2)	92617	1(2)

CPT	MUE	CPT	MUE	CPT	MUE	CPT	MUE	CPT	MUE	CPT	MUE	CPT	MUE	CPT	MUE
92618	1(3)	93270	1(2)	93562	1(3)	93888	1(3)	94760	1(3)	95822	1(3)	95965	1(3)	96401	3(3)
92620	1(2)	93271	1(2)	93563	1(3)	93890	1(3)	94761	1(2)	95824	1(3)	95966	1(3)	96402	2(3)
92621	2(3)	93272	1(2)	93564	1(3)	93892	1(3)	94762	1(2)	95827	1(2)	95967	3(3)	96405	1(2)
92625	1(2)	93278	1(3)	93565	1(3)	93893	1(3)	94770	1(3)	95829	1(3)	95970	1(3)	96406	1(2)
92626	1(2)	93279	1(3)	93566	1(3)	93895	1(3)	94772	1(2)	95830	1(3)	95971	1(3)	96409	1(3)
92627	6(3)	93280	1(3)	93567	1(3)	93922	2(2)	94774	1(2)	95831	5(2)	95972	1(3)	96411	3(3)
92630	0(3)	93281	1(3)	93568	1(3)	93923	2(2)	94775	1(2)	95832	1(3)	95976	1(3)	96413	1(3)
92633	0(3)	93282	1(3)	93571	1(3)	93924	1(2)	94776	1(2)	95833	1(3)	95977	1(3)	96415	8(3)
92640	1(3)	93283	1(3)	93572	2(3)	93925	1(3)	94777	1(2)	95834	1(3)	95980	1(3)	96416	1(3)
92700	1(3)	93284	1(3)	93580	1(3)	93926	1(3)	94780	1(2)	95836	1(2)	95981	1(3)	96417	3(3)
92920	3(3)	93285	1(3)	93581	1(3)	93930	1(3)	94781	2(3)	95851	3(3)	95982	1(3)	96420	1(3)
92921	6(2)	93286	2(3)	93582	1(2)	93931	1(3)	94799	1(3)	95852	1(3)	95983	1(2)	96422	2(3)
92924	2(3)	93287	2(3)	93583	1(2)	93970	1(3)	95004	80(3)	95857	1(2)	95984	11(3)	96423	1(3)
92925	6(2)	93288	1(3)	93590	1(3)	93971	1(3)	95012	1(2)	95860	1(3)	95990	1(3)	96425	1(3)
92928	3(3)	93289	1(3)	93591	1(2)	93975	1(3)	95017	27(3)	95861	1(3)	95991	1(3)	96440	1(3)
92929	6(2)	93290	1(3)	93592	2(3)	93976	1(3)	95018	19(3)	95863	1(3)	95992	1(2)	96446	1(3)
92933	2(3)	93291	1(3)	93600	1(3)	93978	1(3)	95024	40(3)	95864	1(3)	95999	1(3)	96450	1(3)
92934	6(2)	93292	1(3)	93602	1(3)	93979	1(3)	95027	90(3)	95865	1(3)	96000	1(2)	96521	2(3)
92937	2(3)	93293	1(2)	93603	1(3)	93980	1(3)	95028	30(3)	95866	1(3)	96001	1(2)	96522	1(3)
92938	6(3)	93294	1(2)	93609	1(3)	93981	1(3)	95044	80(3)	95867	1(3)	96002	1(3)	96523	1(3)
92941	1(3)	93295	1(2)	93610	1(3)	93990	2(3)	95052	20(3)	95868	1(3)	96003	1(3)	96542	1(3)
92943	2(3)	93296	1(2)	93612	1(3)	93998	1(3)	95056	1(2)	95869	1(3)	96004	1(2)	96549	1(3)
92944	3(3)	93297	1(2)	93613	1(3)	94002	1(2)	95060	1(2)	95870	4(3)	96020	1(2)	96567	1(3)
92950	2(3)	93298	1(2)	93615	1(3)	94003	1(2)	95065	1(3)	95872	4(3)	96040	4(3)	96570	1(2)
92953	2(3)	93299	1(2)	93616	1(3)	94004	1(2)	95070	1(3)	95873	1(2)	96105	3(3)	96571	2(3)
92960	2(3)	93303	1(3)	93618	1(3)	94005	0(3)	95071	1(2)	95874	1(2)	96110	3(3)	96573	1(2)
92961	1(3)	93304	1(3)	93619	1(3)	94010	1(3)	95076	1(2)	95875	2(3)	96112	1(2)	96574	1(2)
92970	1(3)	93306	1(3)	93620	1(3)	94011	1(3)	95079	2(3)	95885	4(2)	96113	6(3)	96900	1(3)
92971	1(3)	93307	1(3)	93621	1(3)	94012	1(3)	95115	1(2)	95886	4(2)	96116	1(2)	96902	0(3)
92973	2(3)	93308	1(3)	93622	1(3)	94013	1(3)	95117	1(2)	95887	1(2)	96121	3(3)	96904	1(2)
92974	1(3)	93312	1(3)	93623	1(3)	94014	1(3)	95120	0(3)	95905	2(3)	96125	2(3)	96910	1(3)
92975	1(3)	93313	1(3)	93624	1(3)	94015	1(2)	95125	0(3)	95907	1(2)	96127	2(3)	96912	1(3)
92977	1(3)	93314	1(3)	93631	1(3)	94016	1(2)	95130	0(3)	95908	1(2)	96130	1(2)	96913	1(3)
92978	1(3)	93315	1(3)	93640	1(3)	94060	1(3)	95131	0(3)	95909	1(2)	96131	7(3)	96920	1(2)
92979	2(3)	93316	1(3)	93641	1(2)	94070	1(2)	95132	0(3)	95910	1(2)	96132	1(2)	96921	1(2)
92986	1(2)	93317	1(3)	93642	1(3)	94150	0(3)	95133	0(3)	95911	1(2)	96133	7(3)	96922	1(2)
92987	1(3)	93318	1(3)	93644	1(3)	94200	1(3)	95134	0(3)	95912	1(2)	96136	1(2)	96931	1(2)
92990	1(2)	93320	1(3)	93650	1(2)	94250	1(3)	95144	30(3)	95913	1(2)	96137	11(3)	96932	1(2)
92992	1(2)	93321	1(3)	93653	1(3)	94375	1(3)	95145	10(3)	95921	1(3)	96138	1(2)	96933	1(2)
92993	1(2)	93325	1(3)	93654	1(3)	94400	1(3)	95146	10(3)	95922	1(3)	96139	11(3)	96934	2(3)
92997	1(2)	93350	1(2)	93655	2(3)	94450	1(3)	95147	10(3)	95923	1(3)	96146	1(2)	96935	2(3)
92998	2(3)	93351	1(2)	93656	1(3)	94452	1(2)	95148	10(3)	95924	1(3)	96150	8(3)	96936	2(3)
93000	3(3)	93352	1(3)	93657	1(3)	94453	1(2)	95149	10(3)	95925	1(3)	96151	6(3)	96999	1(3)
93005	3(3)	93355	1(3)	93660	1(3)	94610	2(3)	95165	30(3)	95926	1(3)	96152	6(3)	97010	0(3)
93010	5(3)	93451	1(3)	93662	1(3)	94617	1(3)	95170	10(3)	95927	1(3)	96153	8(3)	97012	1(3)
93015	1(3)	93452	1(3)	93668	1(3)	94618	1(3)	95180	6(3)	95928	1(3)	96154	8(3)	97014	0(3)
93016	1(3)	93453	1(3)	93701	1(2)	94621	1(3)	95199	1(3)	95929	1(3)	96155	0(3)	97016	1(3)
93017	1(3)	93454	1(3)	93702	1(2)	94640	4(3)	95249	1(2)	95930	1(3)	96160	3(3)	97018	1(3)
93018	1(3)	93455	1(3)	93724	1(3)	94642	1(3)	95250	1(2)	95933	1(3)	96161	1(3)	97022	1(3)
93024	1(3)	93456	1(3)	93740	0(3)	94644	1(2)	95251	1(2)	95937	4(3)	96360	1(3)	97024	1(3)
93025	1(2)	93457	1(3)	93745	1(2)	94645	2(3)	95782	1(2)	95938	1(3)	96361	8(3)	97026	1(3)
93040	3(3)	93458	1(3)	93750	4(3)	94660	1(2)	95783	1(2)	95939	1(3)	96365	1(3)	97028	1(3)
93041	2(3)	93459	1(3)	93770	0(3)	94662	1(2)	95800	1(2)	95940	32(3)	96366	8(3)	97032	4(3)
93042	3(3)	93460	1(3)	93784	1(2)	94664	1(3)	95801	1(2)	95941	0(3)	96367	4(3)	97033	4(3)
93050	1(3)	93461	1(3)	93786	1(2)	94667	1(2)	95803	1(2)	95943	1(3)	96368	1(2)	97034	2(3)
93224	1(2)	93462	1(3)	93788	1(2)	94668	2(3)	95805	1(2)	95950	1(2)	96369	1(2)	97035	2(3)
93225	1(2)	93463	1(3)	93790	1(2)	94669	2(3)	95806	1(2)	95951	1(2)	96370	3(3)	97036	3(3)
93226	1(2)	93464	1(3)	93792	1(2)	94680	1(3)	95807	1(2)	95953	1(2)	96371	1(3)	97039	1(3)
93227	1(2)	93503	2(3)	93793	1(2)	94681	1(3)	95808	1(2)	95954	1(3)	96372	4(3)	97110	6(3)
93228	1(2)	93505	1(2)	93797	2(2)	94690	1(3)	95810	1(2)	95955	1(3)	96373	2(3)	97112	4(3)
93229	1(2)	93530	1(3)	93798	2(2)	94726	1(3)	95811	1(2)	95956	1(2)	96374	1(3)	97113	6(3)
93260	1(2)	93531	1(3)	93799	1(3)	94727	1(3)	95812	1(3)	95957	1(3)	96375	6(3)	97116	4(3)
93261	1(3)	93532	1(3)	93880	1(3)	94728	1(3)	95813	1(3)	95958	1(3)	96376	0(3)	97124	4(3)
93264	1(2)	93533	1(3)	93882	1(3)	94729	1(3)	95816	1(3)	95961	1(2)	96377	1(3)	97127	1(2)
93268	1(2)	93561	1(3)	93886	1(3)	94750	1(3)	95819	1(3)	95962	5(3)	96379	1(3)	97139	1(3)

CPT	MUE	CPT	MUE	CPT	MUE	CPT	MUE	CPT	MUE	CPT	MUE	CPT	MUE	CPT	MUE
97140	6(3)	98969	0(3)	99232	1(3)	99374	0(3)	99479	1(2)	A0428	2(3)	A4285	0(3)	A4388	1(3)
97150	1(3)	99000	0(3)	99233	1(3)	99375	0(3)	99480	1(2)	A0429	2(3)	A4286	0(3)	A4389	2(3)
97151	8(3)	99001	0(3)	99234	1(3)	99377	0(3)	99483	1(2)	A0430	1(3)	A4290	2(3)	A4390	1(3)
97152	8(3)	99002	0(3)	99235	1(3)	99378	0(3)	99484	1(2)	A0431	1(3)	A4300	0(3)	A4391	1(3)
97153	32(3)	99024	1(3)	99236	1(3)	99379	0(3)	99485	1(3)	A0432	1(3)	A4301	1(2)	A4392	2(3)
97154	12(3)	99026	0(3)	99238	1(2)	99380	0(3)	99486	4(1)	A0433	1(3)	A4305	0(3)	A4393	1(3)
97155	24(3)	99027	0(3)	99239	1(2)	99381	0(3)	99487	1(2)	A0434	2(3)	A4306	0(3)	A4394	1(3)
97156	16(3)	99050	0(3)	99241	0(3)	99382	0(3)	99489	10(3)	A0435	999(3)	A4310	0(3)	A4395	3(3)
97157	16(3)	99051	0(3)	99242	0(3)	99383	0(3)	99490	1(2)	A0436	300(3)	A4311	0(3)	A4396	2(3)
97158	16(3)	99053	0(3)	99243	0(3)	99384	0(3)	99491	1(2)	A0888	0(3)	A4312	0(3)	A4397	0(3)
97161	1(2)	99056	0(3)	99244	0(3)	99385	0(3)	99492	1(2)	A0998	0(3)	A4313	0(3)	A4398	0(3)
97162	1(2)	99058	0(3)	99245	0(3)	99386	0(3)	99493	1(2)	A0999	1(3)	A4314	0(3)	A4399	0(3)
97163	1(2)	99060	0(3)	99251	0(3)	99387	0(3)	99494	2(3)	A4206	0(3)	A4315	0(3)	A4400	0(3)
97164	1(2)	99070	0(3)	99252	0(3)	99391	0(3)	99495	1(2)	A4207	0(3)	A4316	0(3)	A4402	0(3)
97165	1(2)	99071	0(3)	99253	0(3)	99392	0(3)	99496	1(2)	A4208	0(3)	A4320	0(3)	A4404	0(3)
97166	1(2)	99075	0(3)	99254	0(3)	99393	0(3)	99497	1(2)	A4209	0(3)	A4321	1(3)	A4405	1(3)
97167	1(2)	99078	0(3)	99255	0(3)	99394	0(3)	99498	3(3)	A4210	0(3)	A4322	0(3)	A4406	1(3)
97168	1(2)	99080	0(3)	99281	1(3)	99395	0(3)	99499	1(3)	A4211	0(3)	A4326	0(3)	A4407	2(3)
97169	0(3)	99082	1(3)	99282	1(3)	99396	0(3)	99500	0(3)	A4212	0(3)	A4327	0(3)	A4408	1(3)
97170	0(3)	99091	1(2)	99283	1(3)	99397	0(3)	99501	0(3)	A4213	0(3)	A4328	0(3)	A4409	1(3)
97171	0(3)	99100	1(3)	99284	1(3)	99401	0(3)	99502	0(3)	A4215	0(3)	A4330	0(3)	A4410	2(3)
97172	0(3)	99116	0(3)	99285	1(3)	99402	0(3)	99503	0(3)	A4216	0(3)	A4331	1(3)	A4411	1(3)
97530	6(3)	99135	0(3)	99288	0(3)	99403	0(3)	99504	0(3)	A4217	0(3)	A4332	2(3)	A4412	1(3)
97533	4(3)	99140	0(3)	99291	1(2)	99404	0(3)	99505	0(3)	A4218	0(3)	A4333	1(3)	A4413	2(3)
97535	8(3)	99151	1(3)	99292	8(3)	99406	1(2)	99506	0(3)	A4220	1(3)	A4334	1(3)	A4414	1(3)
97537	6(3)	99152	2(3)	99304	1(2)	99407	1(2)	99507	0(3)	A4221	0(3)	A4335	0(3)	A4415	1(3)
97542	8(3)	99153	9(3)	99305	1(2)	99408	0(3)	99509	0(3)	A4222	0(3)	A4336	1(3)	A4416	2(3)
97545	1(2)	99155	1(3)	99306	1(2)	99409	0(3)	99510	0(3)	A4223	0(3)	A4337	0(3)	A4417	2(3)
97546	2(3)	99156	1(3)	99307	1(2)	99411	0(3)	99511	0(3)	A4224	0(3)	A4338	0(3)	A4418	2(3)
97597	1(3)	99157	6(3)	99308	1(2)	99412	0(3)	99512	0(3)	A4225	0(3)	A4340	0(3)	A4419	2(3)
97598	8(3)	99170	1(3)	99309	1(2)	99415	1(2)	99600	0(3)	A4230	0(3)	A4344	0(3)	A4420	1(3)
97602	0(3)	99172	0(3)	99310	1(2)	99416	3(3)	99601	0(3)	A4231	0(3)	A4346	0(3)	A4422	7(3)
97605	1(3)	99173	0(3)	99315	1(2)	99429	0(3)	99602	0(3)	A4232	0(3)	A4349	1(3)	A4423	2(3)
97606	1(3)	99174	0(3)	99316	1(2)	99441	0(3)	99605	0(2)	A4233	0(3)	A4351	0(3)	A4424	1(3)
97607	1(3)	99175	1(3)	99318	1(2)	99442	0(3)	99606	0(3)	A4234	0(3)	A4352	0(3)	A4425	1(3)
97608	1(3)	99177	1(2)	99324	1(2)	99443	0(3)	99607	0(3)	A4235	0(3)	A4353	1(3)	A4426	2(3)
97610	1(2)	99183	1(3)	99325	1(2)	99444	0(3)	A0021	0(3)	A4236	0(3)	A4354	0(3)	A4427	1(3)
97750	8(3)	99184	1(2)	99326	1(2)	99446	1(2)	A0080	0(3)	A4244	0(3)	A4355	0(3)	A4428	1(3)
97755	8(3)	99188	1(2)	99327	1(2)	99447	1(2)	A0090	0(3)	A4245	0(3)	A4356	0(3)	A4429	2(3)
97760	6(3)	99190	1(3)	99328	1(2)	99448	1(2)	A0100	0(3)	A4246	0(3)	A4357	0(3)	A4430	1(3)
97761	6(3)	99191	1(3)	99334	1(3)	99449	1(2)	A0110	0(3)	A4247	0(3)	A4358	0(3)	A4431	1(3)
97763	6(3)	99192	1(3)	99335	1(3)	99450	0(3)	A0120	0(3)	A4248	0(3)	A4360	1(3)	A4432	2(3)
97799	1(3)	99195	2(3)	99336	1(3)	99451	1(2)	A0130	0(3)	A4250	0(3)	A4361	0(3)	A4433	1(3)
97802	8(3)	99199	1(3)	99337	1(3)	99452	1(2)	A0140	0(3)	A4252	0(3)	A4362	0(3)	A4434	1(3)
97803	8(3)	99201	1(2)	99339	0(3)	99453	1(2)	A0160	0(3)	A4253	0(3)	A4363	1(3)	A4435	2(3)
97804	6(3)	99202	1(2)	99340	0(3)	99454	1(2)	A0170	0(3)	A4255	0(3)	A4364	0(3)	A4450	0(3)
97810	0(3)	99203	1(2)	99341	1(2)	99455	1(3)	A0180	0(3)	A4256	0(3)	A4366	1(3)	A4452	0(3)
97811	0(3)	99204	1(2)	99342	1(2)	99456	1(3)	A0190	0(3)	A4257	0(3)	A4367	0(3)	A4455	0(3)
97813	0(3)	99205	1(2)	99343	1(2)	99457	1(2)	A0200	0(3)	A4258	0(3)	A4368	1(3)	A4458	0(3)
97814	0(3)	99211	1(3)	99344	1(2)	99460	1(2)	A0210	0(3)	A4259	0(3)	A4369	1(3)	A4459	0(3)
98925	1(2)	99212	2(3)	99345	1(2)	99461	1(2)	A0225	0(3)	A4261	0(3)	A4371	1(3)	A4461	2(3)
98926	1(2)	99213	2(3)	99347	1(3)	99462	1(2)	A0380	0(3)	A4262	0(3)	A4372	0(3)	A4463	0(3)
98927	1(2)	99214	2(3)	99348	1(3)	99463	1(2)	A0382	0(3)	A4263	0(3)	A4373	1(3)	A4465	0(3)
98928	1(2)	99215	1(3)	99349	1(3)	99464	1(2)	A0384	0(3)	A4264	0(3)	A4375	2(3)	A4467	0(3)
98929	1(2)	99217	1(2)	99350	1(3)	99465	1(2)	A0390	0(3)	A4265	0(3)	A4376	2(3)	A4470	0(3)
98940	1(2)	99218	1(2)	99354	1(2)	99466	1(2)	A0392	0(3)	A4266	0(3)	A4377	2(3)	A4480	0(3)
98941	1(2)	99219	1(2)	99355	4(3)	99467	4(3)	A0394	0(3)	A4267	0(3)	A4378	2(3)	A4481	0(3)
98942	1(2)	99220	1(2)	99356	1(2)	99468	1(2)	A0396	0(3)	A4268	0(3)	A4379	2(3)	A4483	0(3)
98943	0(3)	99221	1(3)	99357	4(3)	99469	1(2)	A0398	0(3)	A4269	0(3)	A4380	2(3)	A4490	0(3)
98960	0(3)	99222	1(3)	99358	1(2)	99471	1(2)	A0420	0(3)	A4270	0(3)	A4381	2(3)	A4495	0(3)
98961	0(3)	99223	1(3)	99359	2(3)	99472	1(2)	A0422	0(3)	A4280	0(3)	A4382	2(3)	A4500	0(3)
98962	0(3)	99224	1(2)	99360	1(3)	99475	1(2)	A0424	0(3)	A4281	0(3)	A4383	2(3)	A4510	0(3)
98966	0(3)	99225	1(2)	99366	0(3)	99476	1(2)	A0425	250(1)	A4282	0(3)	A4384	2(3)	A4520	0(3)
98967	0(3)	99226	1(2)	99367	0(3)	99477	1(2)	A0426	2(3)	A4283	0(3)	A4385	2(3)	A4550	0(3)
98968	0(3)	99231	1(3)	99368	0(3)	99478	1(2)	A0427	2(3)	A4284	0(3)	A4387	1(3)	A4553	0(3)

Appendix I — Medically Unlikely Edits (MUEs)—Professional

CPT	MUE	CPT	MUE	CPT	MUE	CPT	MUE	CPT	MUE	CPT	MUE	CPT	MUE	CPT	MUE
A4554	0(3)	A4690	0(3)	A5121	0(3)	A6241	0(3)	A6534	0(3)	A7523	0(3)	A9547	2(3)	B4157	0(3)
A4555	0(3)	A4706	0(3)	A5122	0(3)	A6242	0(3)	A6535	0(3)	A7524	0(3)	A9548	2(3)	B4158	0(3)
A4556	0(3)	A4707	0(3)	A5126	0(3)	A6243	0(3)	A6536	0(3)	A7525	0(3)	A9550	1(3)	B4159	0(3)
A4557	0(3)	A4708	0(3)	A5131	0(3)	A6244	0(3)	A6537	0(3)	A7526	0(3)	A9551	1(3)	B4160	0(3)
A4558	0(3)	A4709	0(3)	A5200	2(3)	A6245	0(3)	A6538	0(3)	A7527	0(3)	A9552	1(3)	B4161	0(3)
A4559	0(3)	A4714	0(3)	A5500	0(3)	A6246	0(3)	A6539	0(3)	A8000	0(3)	A9553	1(3)	B4162	0(3)
A4561	1(3)	A4719	0(3)	A5501	0(3)	A6247	0(3)	A6540	0(3)	A8001	0(3)	A9554	1(3)	B4164	0(3)
A4562	1(3)	A4720	0(3)	A5503	0(3)	A6248	0(3)	A6541	0(3)	A8002	0(3)	A9555	2(3)	B4168	0(3)
A4563	1(2)	A4721	0(3)	A5504	0(3)	A6250	0(3)	A6544	0(3)	A8003	0(3)	A9556	10(3)	B4172	0(3)
A4565	2(3)	A4722	0(3)	A5505	0(3)	A6251	0(3)	A6545	0(3)	A8004	0(3)	A9557	2(3)	B4176	0(3)
A4566	0(3)	A4723	0(3)	A5506	0(3)	A6252	0(3)	A6549	0(3)	A9152	0(3)	A9558	7(3)	B4178	0(3)
A4570	0(3)	A4724	0(3)	A5507	0(3)	A6253	0(3)	A6550	0(3)	A9153	0(3)	A9559	1(3)	B4180	0(3)
A4575	0(3)	A4725	0(3)	A5508	0(3)	A6254	0(3)	A7000	0(3)	A9155	1(3)	A9560	2(3)	B4185	0(3)
A4580	0(3)	A4726	0(3)	A5510	0(3)	A6255	0(3)	A7001	0(3)	A9180	0(3)	A9561	1(3)	B4189	0(3)
A4590	0(3)	A4728	0(3)	A5512	0(3)	A6256	0(3)	A7002	0(3)	A9270	0(3)	A9562	2(3)	B4193	0(3)
A4595	0(3)	A4730	0(3)	A5513	0(3)	A6257	0(3)	A7003	0(3)	A9272	0(3)	A9563	10(3)	B4197	0(3)
A4600	0(3)	A4736	0(3)	A5514	0(3)	A6258	0(3)	A7004	0(3)	A9273	0(3)	A9564	20(3)	B4199	0(3)
A4601	0(3)	A4737	0(3)	A6000	0(3)	A6259	0(3)	A7005	0(3)	A9274	0(3)	A9566	1(3)	B4216	0(3)
A4602	0(3)	A4740	0(3)	A6010	0(3)	A6260	0(3)	A7006	0(3)	A9275	0(3)	A9567	2(3)	B4220	0(3)
A4604	0(3)	A4750	0(3)	A6011	0(3)	A6261	0(3)	A7007	0(3)	A9276	0(3)	A9568	0(3)	B4222	0(3)
A4605	0(3)	A4755	0(3)	A6021	0(3)	A6262	0(3)	A7008	0(3)	A9277	0(3)	A9569	1(3)	B4224	0(3)
A4606	0(3)	A4760	0(3)	A6022	0(3)	A6266	0(3)	A7009	0(3)	A9278	0(3)	A9570	1(3)	B5000	0(3)
A4608	0(3)	A4765	0(3)	A6023	0(3)	A6402	0(3)	A7010	0(3)	A9279	0(3)	A9571	1(3)	B5100	0(3)
A4611	0(3)	A4766	0(3)	A6024	0(3)	A6403	0(3)	A7012	0(3)	A9280	0(3)	A9572	1(3)	B5200	0(3)
A4612	0(3)	A4770	0(3)	A6025	0(3)	A6404	0(3)	A7013	0(3)	A9281	0(3)	A9575	300(3)	B9002	0(3)
A4613	0(3)	A4771	0(3)	A6154	0(3)	A6407	0(3)	A7014	0(3)	A9282	0(3)	A9576	40(3)	B9004	0(3)
A4614	0(3)	A4772	0(3)	A6196	0(3)	A6410	2(3)	A7015	0(3)	A9283	0(3)	A9577	50(3)	B9006	0(3)
A4615	0(3)	A4773	0(3)	A6197	0(3)	A6411	0(3)	A7016	0(3)	A9284	0(3)	A9578	50(3)	B9998	0(3)
A4616	0(3)	A4774	0(3)	A6198	0(3)	A6412	0(3)	A7017	0(3)	A9285	0(3)	A9579	100(3)	B9999	0(3)
A4617	0(3)	A4802	0(3)	A6199	0(3)	A6413	0(3)	A7018	0(3)	A9286	0(3)	A9580	1(3)	C1713	20(3)
A4618	1(3)	A4860	0(3)	A6203	0(3)	A6441	0(3)	A7020	0(3)	A9300	0(3)	A9581	20(3)	C1714	4(3)
A4619	0(3)	A4870	0(3)	A6204	0(3)	A6442	0(3)	A7025	0(3)	A9500	3(3)	A9582	1(3)	C1715	45(3)
A4620	0(3)	A4890	0(3)	A6205	0(3)	A6443	0(3)	A7026	0(3)	A9501	1(3)	A9583	18(3)	C1716	4(3)
A4623	0(3)	A4911	0(3)	A6206	0(3)	A6444	0(3)	A7027	0(3)	A9502	3(3)	A9584	1(3)	C1717	10(3)
A4624	0(3)	A4913	0(3)	A6207	0(3)	A6445	0(3)	A7028	0(3)	A9503	1(3)	A9585	300(3)	C1719	99(3)
A4625	30(3)	A4918	0(3)	A6208	0(3)	A6446	0(3)	A7029	0(3)	A9504	1(3)	A9586	1(3)	C1721	1(3)
A4626	0(3)	A4927	0(3)	A6209	0(3)	A6447	0(3)	A7030	0(3)	A9505	4(3)	A9587	54(3)	C1722	1(3)
A4627	0(3)	A4928	0(3)	A6210	0(3)	A6448	0(3)	A7031	0(3)	A9507	1(3)	A9588	10(3)	C1724	5(3)
A4628	0(3)	A4929	0(3)	A6211	0(3)	A6449	0(3)	A7032	0(3)	A9508	2(3)	A9589	1(3)	C1725	9(3)
A4629	0(3)	A4930	0(3)	A6212	0(3)	A6450	0(3)	A7033	0(3)	A9509	5(3)	A9600	7(3)	C1726	5(3)
A4630	0(3)	A4931	0(3)	A6213	0(3)	A6451	0(3)	A7034	0(3)	A9510	1(3)	A9604	1(3)	C1727	4(3)
A4633	0(3)	A4932	0(3)	A6214	0(3)	A6452	0(3)	A7035	0(3)	A9512	30(3)	A9606	224(3)	C1728	5(3)
A4634	0(3)	A5051	0(3)	A6215	0(3)	A6453	0(3)	A7036	0(3)	A9513	200(3)	A9698	2(3)	C1729	6(3)
A4635	0(3)	A5052	0(3)	A6216	0(3)	A6454	0(3)	A7037	0(3)	A9515	1(3)	A9700	0(3)	C1730	4(3)
A4636	0(3)	A5053	0(3)	A6217	0(3)	A6455	0(3)	A7038	0(3)	A9516	4(3)	A9900	1(3)	C1731	2(3)
A4637	0(3)	A5054	0(3)	A6218	0(3)	A6456	0(3)	A7039	0(3)	A9517	200(3)	A9901	0(3)	C1732	3(3)
A4638	0(3)	A5055	0(3)	A6219	0(3)	A6457	0(3)	A7040	2(3)	A9520	1(3)	A9999	1(3)	C1733	3(3)
A4639	0(3)	A5056	90(3)	A6220	0(3)	A6460	1(1)	A7041	2(3)	A9521	2(3)	B4034	0(3)	C1749	1(3)
A4640	0(3)	A5057	90(3)	A6221	0(3)	A6461	1(1)	A7044	0(3)	A9524	10(3)	B4035	0(3)	C1750	2(3)
A4642	1(3)	A5061	0(3)	A6222	0(3)	A6501	0(3)	A7045	0(3)	A9526	2(3)	B4036	0(3)	C1751	3(3)
A4648	5(3)	A5062	0(3)	A6223	0(3)	A6502	0(3)	A7046	0(3)	A9527	195(3)	B4081	0(3)	C1752	2(3)
A4649	1(3)	A5063	0(3)	A6224	0(3)	A6503	0(3)	A7047	0(3)	A9528	10(3)	B4082	0(3)	C1753	2(3)
A4650	3(3)	A5071	0(3)	A6228	0(3)	A6504	0(3)	A7048	2(3)	A9529	10(3)	B4083	0(3)	C1754	2(3)
A4651	0(3)	A5072	0(3)	A6229	0(3)	A6505	0(3)	A7501	0(3)	A9530	200(3)	B4087	0(3)	C1755	2(3)
A4652	0(3)	A5073	0(3)	A6230	0(3)	A6506	0(3)	A7502	0(3)	A9531	100(3)	B4088	0(3)	C1756	2(3)
A4653	0(3)	A5081	0(3)	A6231	0(3)	A6507	0(3)	A7503	0(3)	A9532	10(3)	B4100	0(3)	C1757	6(3)
A4657	0(3)	A5082	0(3)	A6232	0(3)	A6508	0(3)	A7504	0(3)	A9536	1(3)	B4102	0(3)	C1758	2(3)
A4660	0(3)	A5083	5(3)	A6233	0(3)	A6509	0(3)	A7505	0(3)	A9537	1(3)	B4103	0(3)	C1759	2(3)
A4663	0(3)	A5093	0(3)	A6234	0(3)	A6510	0(3)	A7506	0(3)	A9538	1(3)	B4104	0(3)	C1760	4(3)
A4670	0(3)	A5102	0(3)	A6235	0(3)	A6511	0(3)	A7507	0(3)	A9539	2(3)	B4149	0(3)	C1762	4(3)
A4671	0(3)	A5105	0(3)	A6236	0(3)	A6513	0(3)	A7508	0(3)	A9540	2(3)	B4150	0(3)	C1763	4(3)
A4672	0(3)	A5112	0(3)	A6237	0(3)	A6530	0(3)	A7509	0(3)	A9541	1(3)	B4152	0(3)	C1764	1(3)
A4673	0(3)	A5113	0(3)	A6238	0(3)	A6531	0(3)	A7520	0(3)	A9542	1(3)	B4153	0(3)	C1765	4(3)
A4674	0(3)	A5114	0(3)	A6239	0(3)	A6532	0(3)	A7521	0(3)	A9543	1(3)	B4154	0(3)	C1766	4(3)
A4680	0(3)	A5120	150(3)	A6240	0(3)	A6533	0(3)	A7522	0(3)	A9546	1(3)	B4155	0(3)	C1767	2(3)

CPT	MUE	CPT	MUE	CPT	MUE	CPT	MUE	CPT	MUE	CPT	MUE	CPT	MUE	CPT	MUE
C1768	3(3)	C2618	4(3)	C8936	2(3)	C9753	3(3)	D9946	0(3)	E0217	0(3)	E0430	0(3)	E0635	0(3)
C1769	9(3)	C2619	1(3)	C8937	2(2)	C9754	1(2)	D9950	1(3)	E0218	0(3)	E0431	0(3)	E0636	0(3)
C1770	3(3)	C2620	1(3)	C8957	2(3)	C9755	1(2)	D9951	1(3)	E0221	0(3)	E0433	0(3)	E0637	0(3)
C1771	1(3)	C2621	1(3)	C9035	675(3)	D0150	1(3)	D9952	1(3)	E0225	0(3)	E0434	0(3)	E0638	0(3)
C1772	1(3)	C2622	1(3)	C9036	300(3)	D0240	1(3)	D9961	0(3)	E0231	0(3)	E0435	0(3)	E0639	0(3)
C1773	3(3)	C2623	2(3)	C9037	240(3)	D0250	2(3)	D9990	0(3)	E0232	0(3)	E0439	0(3)	E0640	0(3)
C1776	10(3)	C2624	1(3)	C9038	160(3)	D0270	1(3)	E0100	0(3)	E0235	0(3)	E0440	0(3)	E0641	0(3)
C1777	2(3)	C2625	4(3)	C9039	500(3)	D0272	1(3)	E0105	0(3)	E0236	0(3)	E0441	0(3)	E0642	0(3)
C1778	4(3)	C2626	1(3)	C9040	675(3)	D0274	1(3)	E0110	0(3)	E0239	0(3)	E0442	0(3)	E0650	0(3)
C1779	2(3)	C2627	2(3)	C9041	180(3)	D0277	1(3)	E0111	0(3)	E0240	0(3)	E0443	0(3)	E0651	0(3)
C1780	2(3)	C2628	4(3)	C9043	300(3)	D0412	0(3)	E0112	0(3)	E0241	0(3)	E0444	0(3)	E0652	0(3)
C1781	4(3)	C2629	4(3)	C9044	350(3)	D0416	1(3)	E0113	0(3)	E0242	0(3)	E0445	0(3)	E0655	0(3)
C1782	1(3)	C2630	3(3)	C9045	600(3)	D0431	1(3)	E0114	0(3)	E0243	0(3)	E0446	0(3)	E0656	0(3)
C1783	2(3)	C2631	1(3)	C9046	160(3)	D0460	1(2)	E0116	0(3)	E0244	0(3)	E0447	0(3)	E0657	0(3)
C1784	2(3)	C2634	24(3)	C9113	10(3)	D0484	1(2)	E0117	0(3)	E0245	0(3)	E0455	0(3)	E0660	0(3)
C1785	1(3)	C2635	124(3)	C9132	5500(3)	D0485	1(2)	E0118	0(3)	E0246	0(3)	E0457	0(3)	E0665	0(3)
C1786	1(3)	C2636	690(3)	C9248	25(3)	D0601	1(2)	E0130	0(3)	E0247	0(3)	E0459	0(3)	E0666	0(3)
C1787	2(3)	C2637	0(3)	C9250	1(3)	D0602	1(2)	E0135	0(3)	E0248	0(3)	E0462	0(3)	E0667	0(3)
C1788	2(3)	C2638	150(3)	C9254	400(3)	D0603	1(2)	E0140	0(3)	E0249	0(3)	E0465	0(3)	E0668	0(3)
C1789	2(3)	C2639	150(3)	C9257	5(3)	D1510	2(2)	E0141	0(3)	E0250	0(3)	E0466	0(3)	E0669	0(3)
C1813	1(3)	C2640	150(3)	C9285	2(3)	D1516	1(2)	E0143	0(3)	E0251	0(3)	E0467	0(3)	E0670	0(3)
C1814	2(3)	C2641	150(3)	C9290	266(3)	D1517	1(2)	E0144	0(3)	E0255	0(3)	E0470	0(3)	E0671	0(3)
C1815	1(3)	C2642	120(3)	C9293	700(3)	D1520	2(2)	E0147	0(3)	E0256	0(3)	E0471	0(3)	E0672	0(3)
C1816	2(3)	C2643	120(3)	C9352	3(3)	D1526	1(2)	E0148	0(3)	E0260	0(3)	E0472	0(3)	E0673	0(3)
C1817	1(3)	C2644	500(1)	C9353	4(3)	D1527	1(2)	E0149	0(3)	E0261	0(3)	E0480	0(3)	E0675	0(3)
C1818	2(3)	C2645	4608(3)	C9354	300(3)	D1550	2(3)	E0153	0(3)	E0265	0(3)	E0481	0(3)	E0676	1(3)
C1819	4(3)	C5271	1(2)	C9355	3(3)	D1575	4(2)	E0154	0(3)	E0266	0(3)	E0482	0(3)	E0691	0(3)
C1820	2(3)	C5272	3(2)	C9356	125(3)	D4260	4(2)	E0155	0(3)	E0270	0(3)	E0483	0(3)	E0692	0(3)
C1821	4(3)	C5273	1(2)	C9358	800(3)	D4263	4(2)	E0156	0(3)	E0271	0(3)	E0484	0(3)	E0693	0(3)
C1822	1(3)	C5274	35(3)	C9359	30(3)	D4264	3(3)	E0157	0(3)	E0272	0(3)	E0485	0(3)	E0694	0(3)
C1823	1(3)	C5275	1(2)	C9360	300(3)	D4270	4(3)	E0158	0(3)	E0273	0(3)	E0486	0(3)	E0700	0(3)
C1830	2(3)	C5276	3(2)	C9361	10(3)	D4273	1(2)	E0159	2(3)	E0274	0(3)	E0487	0(3)	E0705	0(3)
C1840	1(3)	C5277	1(2)	C9362	60(3)	D4277	1(2)	E0160	0(3)	E0275	0(3)	E0500	0(3)	E0710	0(3)
C1841	1(2)	C5278	15(3)	C9363	500(3)	D4278	3(3)	E0161	0(3)	E0276	0(3)	E0550	0(3)	E0720	0(3)
C1842	1(2)	C8900	1(3)	C9364	600(3)	D4355	1(2)	E0162	0(3)	E0277	0(3)	E0555	0(3)	E0730	0(3)
C1874	5(3)	C8901	1(3)	C9407	15(3)	D4381	12(3)	E0163	0(3)	E0280	0(3)	E0560	0(3)	E0731	0(3)
C1875	4(3)	C8902	1(3)	C9408	510(3)	D5282	0(3)	E0165	0(3)	E0290	0(3)	E0561	0(3)	E0740	0(3)
C1876	5(3)	C8903	1(3)	C9447	1(3)	D5283	0(3)	E0167	0(3)	E0291	0(3)	E0562	0(3)	E0744	0(3)
C1877	5(3)	C8905	1(3)	C9460	1(3)	D5876	0(3)	E0168	0(3)	E0292	0(3)	E0565	0(3)	E0745	0(3)
C1878	2(3)	C8906	1(3)	C9462	600(3)	D5911	1(3)	E0170	0(3)	E0293	0(3)	E0570	0(3)	E0746	1(3)
C1880	2(3)	C8908	1(3)	C9482	150(3)	D5912	1(2)	E0171	0(3)	E0294	0(3)	E0572	0(3)	E0747	0(3)
C1881	2(3)	C8909	1(3)	C9488	20(3)	D5983	1(3)	E0172	0(3)	E0295	0(3)	E0574	0(3)	E0748	0(3)
C1882	1(3)	C8910	1(3)	C9600	3(3)	D5984	1(3)	E0175	0(3)	E0296	0(3)	E0575	0(3)	E0749	1(3)
C1883	4(3)	C8911	1(3)	C9601	2(3)	D5985	1(3)	E0181	0(3)	E0297	0(3)	E0580	0(3)	E0755	0(3)
C1884	4(3)	C8912	1(3)	C9602	2(3)	D7111	20(3)	E0182	0(3)	E0300	0(3)	E0585	0(3)	E0760	0(3)
C1885	2(3)	C8913	1(3)	C9603	2(3)	D7140	32(2)	E0184	0(3)	E0301	0(3)	E0600	0(3)	E0761	0(3)
C1886	1(3)	C8914	1(3)	C9604	2(3)	D7210	32(2)	E0185	0(3)	E0302	0(3)	E0601	0(3)	E0762	0(3)
C1887	7(3)	C8918	1(3)	C9605	2(3)	D7220	6(3)	E0186	0(3)	E0303	0(3)	E0602	0(3)	E0764	0(3)
C1888	2(3)	C8919	1(3)	C9606	1(3)	D7230	6(3)	E0187	0(3)	E0304	0(3)	E0603	0(3)	E0765	0(3)
C1889	1(3)	C8920	1(3)	C9607	1(2)	D7240	6(3)	E0188	0(3)	E0305	0(3)	E0604	0(3)	E0766	0(3)
C1891	1(3)	C8921	1(3)	C9608	2(3)	D7241	6(3)	E0189	0(3)	E0310	0(3)	E0605	0(3)	E0769	0(3)
C1892	6(3)	C8922	1(3)	C9725	1(3)	D7250	32(2)	E0190	0(3)	E0315	0(3)	E0606	0(3)	E0770	1(3)
C1893	6(3)	C8923	1(3)	C9726	2(3)	D7260	1(3)	E0191	0(3)	E0316	0(3)	E0607	0(3)	E0776	0(3)
C1894	6(3)	C8924	1(3)	C9727	1(2)	D7261	1(3)	E0193	0(3)	E0325	0(3)	E0610	0(3)	E0779	0(3)
C1895	2(3)	C8925	1(3)	C9728	1(2)	D7283	4(3)	E0194	0(3)	E0326	0(3)	E0615	0(3)	E0780	0(3)
C1896	2(3)	C8926	1(3)	C9733	1(3)	D7288	2(3)	E0196	0(3)	E0328	0(3)	E0616	1(2)	E0781	1(2)
C1897	2(3)	C8927	1(3)	C9734	1(3)	D7321	4(2)	E0197	0(3)	E0329	0(3)	E0617	0(3)	E0782	1(2)
C1898	2(3)	C8928	1(2)	C9738	1(3)	D9110	1(3)	E0198	0(3)	E0350	0(3)	E0618	0(3)	E0783	1(2)
C1899	2(3)	C8929	1(3)	C9739	1(2)	D9130	0(3)	E0199	0(3)	E0352	0(3)	E0619	0(3)	E0784	0(3)
C1900	1(3)	C8930	1(2)	C9740	1(2)	D9230	1(3)	E0200	0(3)	E0370	0(3)	E0620	0(3)	E0785	1(2)
C2613	2(3)	C8931	1(3)	C9745	2(2)	D9248	1(3)	E0202	0(3)	E0371	0(3)	E0621	0(3)	E0786	1(2)
C2614	3(3)	C8932	1(3)	C9747	1(2)	D9613	0(3)	E0203	0(3)	E0372	0(3)	E0625	0(3)	E0791	0(3)
C2615	2(3)	C8933	1(3)	C9749	1(2)	D9930	1(2)	E0205	0(3)	E0373	0(3)	E0627	0(3)	E0830	0(3)
C2616	1(3)	C8934	2(3)	C9751	1(3)	D9944	0(3)	E0210	0(3)	E0424	0(3)	E0629	0(3)	E0840	0(3)
C2617	4(3)	C8935	2(3)	C9752	1(2)	D9945	0(3)	E0215	0(3)	E0425	0(3)	E0630	0(3)	E0849	0(3)

CPT	MUE	CPT	MUE	CPT	MUE	CPT	MUE	CPT	MUE	CPT	MUE	CPT	MUE	CPT	MUE
E0850	0(3)	E1011	0(3)	E1250	0(3)	E1818	0(3)	E2341	0(3)	E2615	0(3)	G0166	2(3)	G0383	0(3)
E0855	0(3)	E1012	0(3)	E1260	0(3)	E1820	0(3)	E2342	0(3)	E2616	0(3)	G0168	2(3)	G0384	0(3)
E0856	0(3)	E1014	0(3)	E1270	0(3)	E1821	0(3)	E2343	0(3)	E2617	0(3)	G0175	1(3)	G0390	0(3)
E0860	0(3)	E1015	0(3)	E1280	0(3)	E1825	0(3)	E2351	0(3)	E2619	0(3)	G0177	0(3)	G0396	1(2)
E0870	0(3)	E1016	0(3)	E1285	0(3)	E1830	0(3)	E2358	0(3)	E2620	0(3)	G0179	1(2)	G0397	1(2)
E0880	0(3)	E1017	0(3)	E1290	0(3)	E1831	0(3)	E2359	0(3)	E2621	0(3)	G0180	1(2)	G0398	1(2)
E0890	0(3)	E1018	0(3)	E1295	0(3)	E1840	0(3)	E2360	0(3)	E2622	0(3)	G0181	1(2)	G0399	1(2)
E0900	0(3)	E1020	0(3)	E1296	0(3)	E1841	0(3)	E2361	0(3)	E2623	0(3)	G0182	1(2)	G0400	1(2)
E0910	0(3)	E1028	0(3)	E1297	0(3)	E1902	0(3)	E2362	0(3)	E2624	0(3)	G0186	1(2)	G0402	1(2)
E0911	0(3)	E1029	0(3)	E1298	0(3)	E2000	0(3)	E2363	0(3)	E2625	0(3)	G0219	0(3)	G0403	1(2)
E0912	0(3)	E1030	0(3)	E1300	0(3)	E2100	0(3)	E2364	0(3)	E2626	0(3)	G0235	1(3)	G0404	1(2)
E0920	0(3)	E1031	0(3)	E1310	0(3)	E2101	0(3)	E2365	0(3)	E2627	0(3)	G0237	8(3)	G0405	1(2)
E0930	0(3)	E1035	0(3)	E1352	0(3)	E2120	0(3)	E2366	0(3)	E2628	0(3)	G0238	8(3)	G0406	1(3)
E0935	0(3)	E1036	0(3)	E1353	0(3)	E2201	0(3)	E2367	0(3)	E2629	0(3)	G0239	1(3)	G0407	1(3)
E0936	0(3)	E1037	0(3)	E1354	0(3)	E2202	0(3)	E2368	0(3)	E2630	0(3)	G0245	1(2)	G0408	1(3)
E0940	0(3)	E1038	0(3)	E1355	0(3)	E2203	0(3)	E2369	0(3)	E2631	0(3)	G0246	1(2)	G0410	4(3)
E0941	0(3)	E1039	0(3)	E1356	0(3)	E2204	0(3)	E2370	0(3)	E2632	0(3)	G0247	1(2)	G0411	4(3)
E0942	0(3)	E1050	0(3)	E1357	0(3)	E2205	0(3)	E2371	0(3)	E2633	0(3)	G0248	1(2)	G0412	1(2)
E0944	0(3)	E1060	0(3)	E1358	0(3)	E2206	0(3)	E2372	0(3)	E8000	0(3)	G0249	3(3)	G0413	1(2)
E0945	0(3)	E1070	0(3)	E1372	0(3)	E2207	0(3)	E2373	0(3)	E8001	0(3)	G0250	1(2)	G0414	1(2)
E0946	0(3)	E1083	0(3)	E1390	0(3)	E2208	0(3)	E2374	0(3)	E8002	0(3)	G0252	0(3)	G0415	1(2)
E0947	0(3)	E1084	0(3)	E1391	0(3)	E2209	0(3)	E2375	0(3)	G0008	1(2)	G0255	0(3)	G0416	1(2)
E0948	0(3)	E1085	0(3)	E1392	0(3)	E2210	0(3)	E2376	0(3)	G0009	1(2)	G0257	0(3)	G0420	2(3)
E0950	0(3)	E1086	0(3)	E1399	1(3)	E2211	0(3)	E2377	0(3)	G0010	1(3)	G0259	2(3)	G0421	2(3)
E0951	0(3)	E1087	0(3)	E1405	0(3)	E2212	0(3)	E2378	0(3)	G0027	1(2)	G0260	2(3)	G0422	6(2)
E0952	0(3)	E1088	0(3)	E1406	0(3)	E2213	0(3)	E2381	0(3)	G0068	16(3)	G0268	1(2)	G0423	6(2)
E0953	0(3)	E1089	0(3)	E1500	0(3)	E2214	0(3)	E2382	0(3)	G0069	16(3)	G0269	0(3)	G0424	2(2)
E0954	0(3)	E1090	0(3)	E1510	0(3)	E2215	0(3)	E2383	0(3)	G0070	16(3)	G0270	8(3)	G0425	1(3)
E0955	0(3)	E1092	0(3)	E1520	0(3)	E2216	0(3)	E2384	0(3)	G0071	1(3)	G0271	4(3)	G0426	1(3)
E0956	0(3)	E1093	0(3)	E1530	0(3)	E2217	0(3)	E2385	0(3)	G0076	1(3)	G0276	1(3)	G0427	1(3)
E0957	0(3)	E1100	0(3)	E1540	0(3)	E2218	0(3)	E2386	0(3)	G0077	1(3)	G0277	5(3)	G0428	0(3)
E0958	0(3)	E1110	0(3)	E1550	0(3)	E2219	0(3)	E2387	0(3)	G0078	1(3)	G0278	1(2)	G0429	1(2)
E0959	0(3)	E1130	0(3)	E1560	0(3)	E2220	0(3)	E2388	0(3)	G0079	1(3)	G0279	1(2)	G0432	1(2)
E0960	0(3)	E1140	0(3)	E1570	0(3)	E2221	0(3)	E2389	0(3)	G0080	1(3)	G0281	1(3)	G0433	1(2)
E0961	0(3)	E1150	0(3)	E1575	0(3)	E2222	0(3)	E2390	0(3)	G0081	1(3)	G0282	0(3)	G0435	1(2)
E0966	0(3)	E1160	0(3)	E1580	0(3)	E2224	0(3)	E2391	0(3)	G0082	1(3)	G0283	1(3)	G0438	1(2)
E0967	0(3)	E1161	0(3)	E1590	0(3)	E2225	0(3)	E2392	0(3)	G0083	1(3)	G0288	1(2)	G0439	1(2)
E0968	0(3)	E1170	0(3)	E1592	0(3)	E2226	0(3)	E2394	0(3)	G0084	1(3)	G0289	1(2)	G0442	1(2)
E0969	0(3)	E1171	0(3)	E1594	0(3)	E2227	0(3)	E2395	0(3)	G0085	1(3)	G0293	1(2)	G0443	1(2)
E0970	0(3)	E1172	0(3)	E1600	0(3)	E2228	0(3)	E2396	0(3)	G0086	1(3)	G0294	1(2)	G0444	1(2)
E0971	0(3)	E1180	0(3)	E1610	0(3)	E2230	0(3)	E2397	0(3)	G0087	1(3)	G0295	0(3)	G0445	1(2)
E0973	0(3)	E1190	0(3)	E1615	0(3)	E2231	0(3)	E2402	0(3)	G0101	1(2)	G0296	1(2)	G0446	1(3)
E0974	0(3)	E1195	0(3)	E1620	0(3)	E2291	1(2)	E2500	0(3)	G0102	1(2)	G0297	1(2)	G0448	1(3)
E0978	0(3)	E1200	0(3)	E1625	0(3)	E2292	1(2)	E2502	0(3)	G0103	1(2)	G0302	1(2)	G0451	1(3)
E0980	0(3)	E1220	0(3)	E1630	0(3)	E2293	1(2)	E2504	0(3)	G0104	1(2)	G0303	1(2)	G0452	6(3)
E0981	0(3)	E1221	0(3)	E1632	0(3)	E2294	1(2)	E2506	0(3)	G0105	1(2)	G0304	1(2)	G0453	40(3)
E0982	0(3)	E1222	0(3)	E1634	0(3)	E2295	0(3)	E2508	0(3)	G0106	1(2)	G0305	1(2)	G0454	1(2)
E0983	0(3)	E1223	0(3)	E1635	0(3)	E2300	0(3)	E2510	0(3)	G0108	6(3)	G0306	1(3)	G0455	1(2)
E0984	0(3)	E1224	0(3)	E1636	0(3)	E2301	0(3)	E2511	0(3)	G0109	12(3)	G0307	1(3)	G0458	1(3)
E0985	0(3)	E1225	0(3)	E1637	0(3)	E2310	0(3)	E2512	0(3)	G0117	1(2)	G0328	1(2)	G0459	1(3)
E0986	0(3)	E1226	0(3)	E1639	0(3)	E2311	0(3)	E2599	0(3)	G0118	1(2)	G0329	1(3)	G0460	1(3)
E0988	0(3)	E1227	0(3)	E1699	0(3)	E2312	0(3)	E2601	0(3)	G0120	1(2)	G0333	0(3)	G0463	0(3)
E0990	0(3)	E1228	0(3)	E1700	0(3)	E2313	0(3)	E2602	0(3)	G0121	1(2)	G0337	1(2)	G0466	1(2)
E0992	0(3)	E1229	0(3)	E1701	0(3)	E2321	0(3)	E2603	0(3)	G0122	0(3)	G0339	1(2)	G0467	1(3)
E0994	0(3)	E1230	0(3)	E1702	0(3)	E2322	0(3)	E2604	0(3)	G0123	1(3)	G0340	1(3)	G0468	1(2)
E0995	0(3)	E1231	0(3)	E1800	0(3)	E2323	0(3)	E2605	0(3)	G0124	1(2)	G0341	1(2)	G0469	1(2)
E1002	0(3)	E1232	0(3)	E1801	0(3)	E2324	0(3)	E2606	0(3)	G0127	1(2)	G0342	1(2)	G0470	1(3)
E1003	0(3)	E1233	0(3)	E1802	0(3)	E2325	0(3)	E2607	0(3)	G0128	1(3)	G0343	1(2)	G0471	2(3)
E1004	0(3)	E1234	0(3)	E1805	0(3)	E2326	0(3)	E2608	0(3)	G0130	1(2)	G0365	2(3)	G0472	1(2)
E1005	0(3)	E1235	0(3)	E1806	0(3)	E2327	0(3)	E2609	0(3)	G0141	1(3)	G0372	1(2)	G0473	1(3)
E1006	0(3)	E1236	0(3)	E1810	0(3)	E2328	0(3)	E2610	0(3)	G0143	1(3)	G0378	0(3)	G0475	1(2)
E1007	0(3)	E1237	0(3)	E1811	0(3)	E2329	0(3)	E2611	0(3)	G0144	1(3)	G0379	0(3)	G0476	1(2)
E1008	0(3)	E1238	0(3)	E1812	0(3)	E2330	0(3)	E2612	0(3)	G0145	1(3)	G0380	0(3)	G0480	1(2)
E1009	0(3)	E1239	0(3)	E1815	0(3)	E2331	0(3)	E2613	0(3)	G0147	1(3)	G0381	0(3)	G0481	1(2)
E1010	0(3)	E1240	0(3)	E1816	0(3)	E2340	0(3)	E2614	0(3)	G0148	1(3)	G0382	0(3)	G0482	1(2)

CPT	MUE	CPT	MUE	CPT	MUE	CPT	MUE	CPT	MUE	CPT	MUE	CPT	MUE	CPT	MUE
G0483	1(2)	G9156	1(2)	J0364	6(3)	J0714	4(3)	J1301	60(3)	J1670	1(3)	J2300	4(3)	J2790	1(3)
G0490	1(3)	G9157	1(2)	J0365	0(3)	J0715	0(3)	J1320	0(3)	J1675	0(3)	J2310	4(3)	J2791	15(3)
G0491	1(3)	G9187	1(3)	J0380	1(3)	J0716	4(3)	J1322	150(3)	J1700	0(3)	J2315	380(3)	J2792	450(3)
G0492	1(3)	G9480	1(3)	J0390	0(3)	J0717	400(3)	J1324	108(3)	J1710	0(3)	J2320	4(3)	J2793	320(3)
G0493	1(3)	G9481	1(3)	J0395	0(3)	J0720	15(3)	J1325	1(3)	J1720	10(3)	J2323	300(3)	J2794	100(3)
G0494	1(3)	G9482	1(3)	J0400	39(3)	J0725	10(3)	J1327	1(3)	J1726	28(3)	J2325	0(3)	J2795	200(3)
G0495	1(3)	G9483	1(3)	J0401	400(3)	J0735	50(3)	J1330	1(3)	J1729	25(3)	J2326	120(3)	J2796	150(3)
G0496	1(3)	G9484	1(3)	J0456	4(3)	J0740	2(3)	J1335	2(3)	J1730	0(3)	J2350	600(3)	J2797	333(3)
G0498	1(2)	G9485	1(3)	J0461	200(3)	J0743	16(3)	J1364	2(3)	J1740	3(3)	J2353	60(3)	J2800	3(3)
G0499	1(2)	G9486	1(3)	J0470	2(3)	J0744	6(3)	J1380	4(3)	J1741	8(3)	J2354	60(3)	J2805	3(3)
G0500	1(3)	G9487	1(3)	J0475	8(3)	J0745	2(3)	J1410	4(3)	J1742	2(3)	J2355	2(3)	J2810	5(3)
G0501	0(3)	G9488	1(3)	J0476	2(3)	J0770	5(3)	J1428	450(3)	J1743	66(3)	J2357	90(3)	J2820	15(3)
G0506	1(2)	G9489	1(3)	J0480	1(3)	J0775	180(3)	J1430	10(3)	J1744	30(3)	J2358	405(3)	J2840	160(3)
G0508	1(2)	G9490	1(3)	J0485	1500(3)	J0780	4(3)	J1435	1(3)	J1745	150(3)	J2360	2(3)	J2850	16(3)
G0509	1(2)	G9678	1(2)	J0490	160(3)	J0795	100(3)	J1436	0(3)	J1746	200(3)	J2370	2(3)	J2860	170(3)
G0511	1(2)	G9685	1(3)	J0500	4(3)	J0800	3(3)	J1438	2(3)	J1750	45(3)	J2400	4(3)	J2910	0(3)
G0512	1(2)	G9978	1(3)	J0515	3(3)	J0834	3(3)	J1439	750(3)	J1756	500(3)	J2405	64(3)	J2916	20(3)
G0513	1(2)	G9979	1(3)	J0517	30(3)	J0840	6(3)	J1442	1500(3)	J1786	680(3)	J2407	120(3)	J2920	25(3)
G0514	1(1)	G9980	1(3)	J0520	0(3)	J0841	20(3)	J1443	272(3)	J1790	2(3)	J2410	2(3)	J2930	25(3)
G0515	8(3)	G9981	1(3)	J0558	24(3)	J0850	9(3)	J1444	272(3)	J1800	6(3)	J2425	125(3)	J2941	8(3)
G0516	1(2)	G9982	1(3)	J0561	24(3)	J0875	300(3)	J1447	960(3)	J1810	0(3)	J2426	819(3)	J2950	0(3)
G0517	1(2)	G9983	1(3)	J0565	200(3)	J0878	1500(3)	J1450	4(3)	J1815	8(3)	J2430	3(3)	J2993	2(3)
G0518	1(2)	G9984	1(3)	J0567	300(3)	J0881	500(3)	J1451	1(3)	J1817	0(3)	J2440	4(3)	J2995	0(3)
G0659	1(2)	G9985	1(3)	J0570	4(3)	J0882	300(3)	J1452	0(3)	J1826	1(3)	J2460	0(3)	J2997	8(3)
G2000	1(3)	G9986	1(3)	J0571	0(3)	J0883	1125(3)	J1453	150(3)	J1830	1(3)	J2469	10(3)	J3000	2(3)
G2001	1(3)	G9987	1(3)	J0572	0(3)	J0884	1125(3)	J1454	1(3)	J1833	372(3)	J2501	2(3)	J3010	100(3)
G2002	1(3)	J0120	1(3)	J0573	0(3)	J0885	60(3)	J1455	18(3)	J1835	0(3)	J2502	60(3)	J3030	1(3)
G2003	1(3)	J0129	100(3)	J0574	0(3)	J0887	360(3)	J1457	0(3)	J1840	3(3)	J2503	2(3)	J3060	760(3)
G2004	1(3)	J0130	4(3)	J0575	0(3)	J0888	360(3)	J1458	100(3)	J1850	4(3)	J2504	15(3)	J3070	3(3)
G2005	1(3)	J0131	400(3)	J0583	250(3)	J0890	0(3)	J1459	300(3)	J1885	8(3)	J2505	1(3)	J3090	200(3)
G2006	1(3)	J0132	12(3)	J0584	90(3)	J0894	100(3)	J1555	480(3)	J1890	0(3)	J2507	8(3)	J3095	150(3)
G2007	1(3)	J0133	1200(3)	J0585	600(3)	J0895	12(3)	J1556	300(3)	J1930	120(3)	J2510	4(3)	J3101	50(3)
G2008	1(3)	J0135	8(3)	J0586	300(3)	J0897	120(3)	J1557	300(3)	J1931	377(3)	J2513	1(3)	J3105	2(3)
G2009	1(3)	J0153	180(3)	J0587	300(3)	J0945	4(3)	J1559	300(3)	J1940	6(3)	J2515	1(3)	J3110	2(3)
G2010	1(3)	J0171	20(3)	J0588	600(3)	J1000	1(3)	J1560	1(2)	J1942	1064(3)	J2540	75(3)	J3121	400(3)
G2011	1(2)	J0178	4(3)	J0592	6(3)	J1020	8(3)	J1561	300(3)	J1945	0(3)	J2543	16(3)	J3145	750(3)
G2012	1(3)	J0180	125(3)	J0594	320(3)	J1030	8(3)	J1562	0(3)	J1950	12(3)	J2545	1(3)	J3230	2(3)
G2013	1(3)	J0185	130(3)	J0595	8(3)	J1040	4(3)	J1566	300(3)	J1953	300(3)	J2547	600(3)	J3240	1(3)
G2014	1(3)	J0190	0(3)	J0596	840(3)	J1050	1000(3)	J1568	300(3)	J1955	11(3)	J2550	3(3)	J3243	150(3)
G2015	1(3)	J0200	0(3)	J0597	250(3)	J1071	400(3)	J1569	300(3)	J1956	4(3)	J2560	1(3)	J3245	100(3)
G6001	2(3)	J0202	12(3)	J0598	100(3)	J1094	0(3)	J1570	4(3)	J1960	0(3)	J2562	48(3)	J3246	1(3)
G6002	2(3)	J0205	0(3)	J0599	900(3)	J1095	517(1)	J1571	20(3)	J1980	2(3)	J2590	3(3)	J3250	2(3)
G6003	2(3)	J0207	4(3)	J0600	3(3)	J1100	120(3)	J1572	300(3)	J1990	0(3)	J2597	45(3)	J3260	8(3)
G6004	2(3)	J0210	4(3)	J0606	150(3)	J1110	3(3)	J1573	130(3)	J2001	60(3)	J2650	0(3)	J3262	800(3)
G6005	2(3)	J0215	30(3)	J0610	15(3)	J1120	2(3)	J1575	650(3)	J2010	10(3)	J2670	0(3)	J3265	0(3)
G6006	2(3)	J0220	1(3)	J0620	1(3)	J1130	300(3)	J1580	9(3)	J2020	6(3)	J2675	1(3)	J3280	0(3)
G6007	2(3)	J0221	250(3)	J0630	1(3)	J1160	2(3)	J1595	1(3)	J2060	4(3)	J2680	4(3)	J3285	1(3)
G6008	2(3)	J0256	1600(3)	J0636	100(3)	J1162	1(3)	J1599	300(3)	J2062	10(3)	J2690	4(3)	J3300	160(3)
G6009	2(3)	J0257	1400(3)	J0637	20(3)	J1165	50(3)	J1600	2(3)	J2150	8(3)	J2700	48(3)	J3301	16(3)
G6010	2(3)	J0270	32(3)	J0638	150(3)	J1170	350(3)	J1602	300(3)	J2170	8(3)	J2704	80(3)	J3302	0(3)
G6011	2(3)	J0275	1(3)	J0640	24(3)	J1180	0(3)	J1610	2(3)	J2175	4(3)	J2710	2(3)	J3303	24(3)
G6012	2(3)	J0278	15(3)	J0641	1200(3)	J1190	8(3)	J1620	0(3)	J2180	0(3)	J2720	5(3)	J3304	64(2)
G6013	2(3)	J0280	7(3)	J0670	10(3)	J1200	8(3)	J1626	30(3)	J2182	300(3)	J2724	3500(3)	J3305	0(3)
G6014	2(3)	J0282	5(3)	J0690	12(3)	J1205	4(3)	J1627	100(3)	J2185	30(3)	J2725	0(3)	J3310	0(3)
G6015	2(3)	J0285	5(3)	J0692	12(3)	J1212	1(3)	J1628	100(3)	J2186	600(3)	J2730	2(3)	J3315	6(3)
G6016	2(3)	J0287	50(3)	J0694	8(3)	J1230	3(3)	J1630	5(3)	J2210	1(3)	J2760	2(3)	J3316	6(3)
G6017	2(3)	J0288	0(3)	J0695	60(3)	J1240	6(3)	J1631	9(3)	J2212	240(3)	J2765	10(3)	J3320	0(3)
G9143	1(2)	J0289	50(3)	J0696	16(3)	J1245	6(3)	J1640	672(3)	J2248	150(3)	J2770	6(3)	J3350	0(3)
G9147	0(3)	J0290	24(3)	J0697	4(3)	J1250	2(3)	J1642	100(3)	J2250	22(3)	J2778	10(3)	J3355	1(3)
G9148	1(3)	J0295	12(3)	J0698	10(3)	J1260	2(3)	J1644	40(3)	J2260	4(3)	J2780	16(3)	J3357	90(3)
G9149	1(3)	J0300	8(3)	J0702	18(3)	J1265	20(3)	J1645	10(3)	J2265	400(3)	J2783	60(3)	J3358	520(3)
G9150	1(3)	J0330	10(3)	J0706	1(3)	J1267	150(3)	J1650	30(3)	J2270	9(3)	J2785	4(3)	J3360	6(3)
G9151	1(3)	J0348	200(3)	J0710	0(3)	J1270	8(3)	J1652	20(3)	J2274	250(3)	J2786	500(3)	J3364	0(3)
G9152	1(3)	J0350	0(3)	J0712	120(3)	J1290	30(3)	J1655	0(3)	J2278	1000(3)	J2787	1(3)	J3365	0(3)
G9153	1(3)	J0360	2(3)	J0713	12(3)	J1300	120(3)			J2280	4(3)	J2788	1(3)		

CPT	MUE	CPT	MUE	CPT	MUE	CPT	MUE	CPT	MUE	CPT	MUE	CPT	MUE	CPT	MUE
J3370	12(3)	J7207	7500(1)	J7610	0(3)	J8565	0(3)	J9207	90(3)	K0004	0(3)	K0801	0(3)	L0113	0(3)
J3380	300(3)	J7208	12000(1)	J7611	10(3)	J8597	0(3)	J9208	15(3)	K0005	0(3)	K0802	0(3)	L0120	0(3)
J3385	80(3)	J7209	7500(1)	J7612	10(3)	J8600	0(3)	J9209	55(3)	K0006	0(3)	K0806	0(3)	L0130	0(3)
J3396	150(3)	J7210	22000(1)	J7613	10(3)	J8610	0(3)	J9211	6(3)	K0007	0(3)	K0807	0(3)	L0140	0(3)
J3397	600(3)	J7211	22000(1)	J7614	10(3)	J8650	0(3)	J9212	0(3)	K0008	0(3)	K0808	0(3)	L0150	0(3)
J3398	150(2)	J7296	0(3)	J7615	0(3)	J8655	1(3)	J9213	12(3)	K0009	0(3)	K0812	0(3)	L0160	0(3)
J3400	0(3)	J7297	0(3)	J7620	6(3)	J8670	0(3)	J9214	100(3)	K0010	0(3)	K0813	0(3)	L0170	0(3)
J3410	8(3)	J7298	0(3)	J7622	0(3)	J8700	0(3)	J9215	0(3)	K0011	0(3)	K0814	0(3)	L0172	0(3)
J3411	4(3)	J7300	0(3)	J7624	0(3)	J8705	0(3)	J9216	2(3)	K0012	0(3)	K0815	0(3)	L0174	0(3)
J3415	6(3)	J7301	0(3)	J7626	2(3)	J8999	0(3)	J9217	6(3)	K0013	0(3)	K0816	0(3)	L0180	0(3)
J3420	1(3)	J7303	0(3)	J7627	0(3)	J9000	20(3)	J9218	1(3)	K0014	0(3)	K0820	0(3)	L0190	0(3)
J3430	25(3)	J7304	0(3)	J7628	0(3)	J9015	1(3)	J9219	1(3)	K0015	0(3)	K0821	0(3)	L0200	0(3)
J3465	40(3)	J7306	0(3)	J7629	0(3)	J9017	30(3)	J9225	1(3)	K0017	0(3)	K0822	0(3)	L0220	0(3)
J3470	3(3)	J7307	0(3)	J7631	4(3)	J9019	60(3)	J9226	1(3)	K0018	0(3)	K0823	0(3)	L0450	0(3)
J3471	999(2)	J7308	3(3)	J7632	0(3)	J9020	0(3)	J9228	1100(3)	K0019	0(3)	K0824	0(3)	L0452	0(3)
J3472	2(3)	J7309	1(3)	J7633	0(3)	J9022	168(3)	J9229	27(3)	K0020	0(3)	K0825	0(3)	L0454	0(3)
J3473	450(3)	J7310	0(3)	J7634	0(3)	J9023	140(3)	J9230	5(3)	K0037	0(3)	K0826	0(3)	L0455	0(3)
J3475	20(3)	J7311	1(3)	J7635	0(3)	J9025	300(3)	J9245	9(3)	K0038	0(3)	K0827	0(3)	L0456	0(3)
J3480	40(3)	J7312	14(3)	J7636	0(3)	J9027	100(3)	J9250	25(3)	K0039	0(3)	K0828	0(3)	L0457	0(3)
J3485	160(3)	J7313	38(3)	J7637	0(3)	J9030	50(3)	J9260	20(3)	K0040	0(3)	K0829	0(3)	L0458	0(3)
J3486	4(3)	J7315	2(3)	J7638	0(3)	J9032	300(3)	J9261	80(3)	K0041	0(3)	K0830	0(3)	L0460	0(3)
J3489	5(3)	J7316	3(2)	J7639	3(3)	J9033	300(3)	J9262	700(3)	K0042	0(3)	K0831	0(3)	L0462	0(3)
J3520	0(3)	J7318	120(3)	J7640	0(3)	J9034	360(3)	J9263	700(3)	K0043	0(3)	K0835	0(3)	L0464	0(3)
J3530	0(3)	J7320	50(3)	J7641	0(3)	J9035	170(3)	J9264	600(3)	K0044	0(3)	K0836	0(3)	L0466	0(3)
J3535	0(3)	J7321	2(2)	J7642	0(3)	J9036	360(3)	J9266	2(3)	K0045	0(3)	K0837	0(3)	L0467	0(3)
J3570	0(3)	J7322	48(3)	J7643	0(3)	J9039	210(3)	J9267	750(3)	K0046	0(3)	K0838	0(3)	L0468	0(3)
J7030	5(3)	J7323	2(2)	J7644	3(3)	J9040	4(3)	J9268	1(3)	K0047	0(3)	K0839	0(3)	L0469	0(3)
J7040	6(3)	J7324	2(2)	J7645	0(3)	J9041	35(3)	J9270	0(3)	K0050	0(3)	K0840	0(3)	L0470	0(3)
J7042	6(3)	J7325	96(3)	J7647	0(3)	J9042	200(3)	J9271	300(3)	K0051	0(3)	K0841	0(3)	L0472	0(3)
J7050	10(3)	J7326	2(2)	J7648	0(3)	J9043	60(3)	J9280	12(3)	K0052	0(3)	K0842	0(3)	L0480	0(3)
J7060	10(3)	J7327	2(2)	J7649	0(3)	J9044	35(3)	J9285	200(3)	K0053	0(3)	K0843	0(3)	L0482	0(3)
J7070	4(3)	J7328	336(3)	J7650	0(3)	J9045	22(3)	J9293	8(3)	K0056	0(3)	K0848	0(3)	L0484	0(3)
J7100	2(3)	J7329	50(2)	J7657	0(3)	J9047	160(3)	J9295	800(3)	K0065	0(3)	K0849	0(3)	L0486	0(3)
J7110	2(3)	J7330	1(3)	J7658	0(3)	J9050	6(3)	J9299	480(3)	K0069	0(3)	K0850	0(3)	L0488	0(3)
J7120	4(3)	J7336	1120(3)	J7659	0(3)	J9055	120(3)	J9301	100(3)	K0070	0(3)	K0851	0(3)	L0490	0(3)
J7121	4(3)	J7340	1(3)	J7660	0(3)	J9057	60(3)	J9302	200(3)	K0071	0(3)	K0852	0(3)	L0491	0(3)
J7131	500(3)	J7342	10(3)	J7665	0(3)	J9060	24(3)	J9303	90(3)	K0072	0(3)	K0853	0(3)	L0492	0(3)
J7170	1800(3)	J7345	200(3)	J7667	0(3)	J9065	100(3)	J9305	150(3)	K0073	0(3)	K0854	0(3)	L0621	0(3)
J7175	9000(1)	J7500	0(3)	J7668	0(3)	J9070	55(3)	J9306	840(3)	K0077	0(3)	K0855	0(3)	L0622	0(3)
J7177	10500(3)	J7501	1(3)	J7669	0(3)	J9098	5(3)	J9307	60(3)	K0098	0(3)	K0856	0(3)	L0623	0(3)
J7178	7700(1)	J7502	0(3)	J7670	0(3)	J9100	120(3)	J9308	280(3)	K0105	0(3)	K0857	0(3)	L0624	0(3)
J7179	7500(1)	J7503	0(3)	J7674	100(3)	J9120	5(3)	J9311	160(3)	K0108	0(3)	K0858	0(3)	L0625	0(3)
J7180	6000(1)	J7504	15(3)	J7676	0(3)	J9130	24(3)	J9312	150(3)	K0195	0(3)	K0859	0(3)	L0626	0(3)
J7181	3850(1)	J7505	1(3)	J7677	175(3)	J9145	240(3)	J9315	40(3)	K0455	0(3)	K0860	0(3)	L0627	0(3)
J7182	22000(1)	J7507	0(3)	J7680	0(3)	J9150	12(3)	J9320	4(3)	K0462	0(3)	K0861	0(3)	L0628	0(3)
J7183	7500(1)	J7508	0(3)	J7681	0(3)	J9151	10(3)	J9325	400(3)	K0553	0(3)	K0862	0(3)	L0629	0(3)
J7185	22000(1)	J7509	0(3)	J7682	2(3)	J9153	132(3)	J9328	400(3)	K0554	0(3)	K0863	0(3)	L0630	0(3)
J7186	7500(1)	J7510	0(3)	J7683	0(3)	J9155	240(3)	J9330	50(3)	K0602	0(3)	K0864	0(3)	L0631	0(3)
J7187	7500(1)	J7511	9(3)	J7684	0(3)	J9160	7(3)	J9340	4(3)	K0604	0(3)	K0868	0(3)	L0632	0(3)
J7188	22000(1)	J7512	0(3)	J7685	0(3)	J9165	0(3)	J9351	120(3)	K0605	0(3)	K0869	0(3)	L0633	0(3)
J7189	13000(1)	J7513	0(3)	J7686	1(3)	J9171	240(3)	J9352	40(3)	K0606	0(3)	K0870	0(3)	L0634	0(3)
J7190	22000(1)	J7515	0(3)	J7699	1(3)	J9173	150(3)	J9354	600(3)	K0607	0(3)	K0871	0(3)	L0635	0(3)
J7191	0(3)	J7516	1(3)	J7799	2(3)	J9175	10(3)	J9355	105(3)	K0608	0(3)	K0877	0(3)	L0636	0(3)
J7192	22000(1)	J7517	0(3)	J7999	2(3)	J9176	3000(3)	J9356	60(3)	K0609	0(3)	K0878	0(3)	L0637	0(3)
J7193	4000(1)	J7518	0(3)	J8498	0(3)	J9178	150(3)	J9357	4(3)	K0669	0(3)	K0879	0(3)	L0638	0(3)
J7194	9000(1)	J7520	0(3)	J8499	0(3)	J9179	50(3)	J9360	40(3)	K0672	0(3)	K0880	0(3)	L0639	0(3)
J7195	6000(1)	J7525	2(3)	J8501	0(3)	J9181	100(3)	J9370	4(3)	K0730	0(3)	K0884	0(3)	L0640	0(3)
J7196	175(3)	J7527	0(3)	J8510	0(3)	J9185	2(3)	J9371	5(3)	K0733	0(3)	K0885	0(3)	L0641	0(3)
J7197	6300(1)	J7599	1(3)	J8515	0(3)	J9190	20(3)	J9390	36(3)	K0738	0(3)	K0886	0(3)	L0642	0(3)
J7198	6000(1)	J7604	0(3)	J8520	0(3)	J9200	5(3)	J9395	20(3)	K0740	0(3)	K0890	0(3)	L0643	0(3)
J7200	20000(1)	J7605	2(3)	J8521	0(3)	J9201	20(3)	J9400	500(3)	K0743	0(3)	K0891	0(3)	L0648	0(3)
J7201	9000(1)	J7606	2(3)	J8530	0(3)	J9202	3(3)	J9600	4(3)	K0744	0(3)	K0898	1(2)	L0649	0(3)
J7202	11550(1)	J7607	0(3)	J8540	0(3)	J9203	180(3)	K0001	0(3)	K0745	0(3)	K0899	0(3)	L0650	0(3)
J7203	12000(1)	J7608	3(3)	J8560	0(3)	J9205	215(3)	K0002	0(3)	K0746	0(3)	K0900	0(3)	L0651	0(3)
J7205	9750(1)	J7609	0(3)	J8562	0(3)	J9206	42(3)	K0003	0(3)	K0800	0(3)	L0112	0(3)	L0700	0(3)

CPT	MUE	CPT	MUE	CPT	MUE	CPT	MUE	CPT	MUE	CPT	MUE	CPT	MUE	CPT	MUE
L0710	0(3)	L1830	0(3)	L2188	0(3)	L2795	0(3)	L3350	0(3)	L3912	0(3)	L5010	0(3)	L5645	0(3)
L0810	0(3)	L1831	0(3)	L2190	0(3)	L2800	0(3)	L3360	0(3)	L3913	0(3)	L5020	0(3)	L5646	0(3)
L0820	0(3)	L1832	0(3)	L2192	0(3)	L2810	0(3)	L3370	0(3)	L3915	0(3)	L5050	0(3)	L5647	0(3)
L0830	0(3)	L1833	0(3)	L2200	0(3)	L2820	0(3)	L3380	0(3)	L3916	0(3)	L5060	0(3)	L5648	0(3)
L0859	0(3)	L1834	0(3)	L2210	0(3)	L2830	0(3)	L3390	0(3)	L3917	0(3)	L5100	0(3)	L5649	0(3)
L0861	0(3)	L1836	0(3)	L2220	0(3)	L2840	0(3)	L3400	0(3)	L3918	0(3)	L5105	0(3)	L5650	0(3)
L0970	0(3)	L1840	0(3)	L2230	0(3)	L2850	0(3)	L3410	0(3)	L3919	0(3)	L5150	0(3)	L5651	0(3)
L0972	0(3)	L1843	0(3)	L2232	0(3)	L2861	0(3)	L3420	0(3)	L3921	0(3)	L5160	0(3)	L5652	0(3)
L0974	0(3)	L1844	0(3)	L2240	0(3)	L2999	0(3)	L3430	0(3)	L3923	0(3)	L5200	0(3)	L5653	0(3)
L0976	0(3)	L1845	0(3)	L2250	0(3)	L3000	0(3)	L3440	0(3)	L3924	0(3)	L5210	0(3)	L5654	0(3)
L0978	0(3)	L1846	0(3)	L2260	0(3)	L3001	0(3)	L3450	0(3)	L3925	0(3)	L5220	0(3)	L5655	0(3)
L0980	0(3)	L1847	0(3)	L2265	0(3)	L3002	0(3)	L3455	0(3)	L3927	0(3)	L5230	0(3)	L5656	0(3)
L0982	0(3)	L1848	0(3)	L2270	0(3)	L3003	0(3)	L3460	0(3)	L3929	0(3)	L5250	0(3)	L5658	0(3)
L0984	0(3)	L1850	0(3)	L2275	0(3)	L3010	0(3)	L3465	0(3)	L3930	0(3)	L5270	0(3)	L5661	0(3)
L0999	0(3)	L1851	0(3)	L2280	0(3)	L3020	0(3)	L3470	0(3)	L3931	0(3)	L5280	0(3)	L5665	0(3)
L1000	0(3)	L1852	0(3)	L2300	0(3)	L3030	0(3)	L3480	0(3)	L3933	0(3)	L5301	0(3)	L5666	0(3)
L1001	0(3)	L1860	0(3)	L2310	0(3)	L3031	0(3)	L3485	0(3)	L3935	0(3)	L5312	0(3)	L5668	0(3)
L1005	0(3)	L1900	0(3)	L2320	0(3)	L3040	0(3)	L3500	0(3)	L3956	0(3)	L5321	0(3)	L5670	0(3)
L1010	0(3)	L1902	0(3)	L2330	0(3)	L3050	0(3)	L3510	0(3)	L3960	0(3)	L5331	0(3)	L5671	0(3)
L1020	0(3)	L1904	0(3)	L2335	0(3)	L3060	0(3)	L3520	0(3)	L3961	0(3)	L5341	0(3)	L5672	0(3)
L1025	0(3)	L1906	0(3)	L2340	0(3)	L3070	0(3)	L3530	0(3)	L3962	0(3)	L5400	0(3)	L5673	0(3)
L1030	0(3)	L1907	0(3)	L2350	0(3)	L3080	0(3)	L3540	0(3)	L3967	0(3)	L5410	0(3)	L5676	0(3)
L1040	0(3)	L1910	0(3)	L2360	0(3)	L3090	0(3)	L3550	0(3)	L3971	0(3)	L5420	0(3)	L5677	0(3)
L1050	0(3)	L1920	0(3)	L2370	0(3)	L3100	0(3)	L3560	0(3)	L3973	0(3)	L5430	0(3)	L5678	0(3)
L1060	0(3)	L1930	0(3)	L2375	0(3)	L3140	0(3)	L3570	0(3)	L3975	0(3)	L5450	0(3)	L5679	0(3)
L1070	0(3)	L1932	0(3)	L2380	0(3)	L3150	0(3)	L3580	0(3)	L3976	0(3)	L5460	0(3)	L5680	0(3)
L1080	0(3)	L1940	0(3)	L2385	0(3)	L3160	0(3)	L3590	0(3)	L3977	0(3)	L5500	0(3)	L5681	0(3)
L1085	0(3)	L1945	0(3)	L2387	0(3)	L3170	0(3)	L3595	0(3)	L3978	0(3)	L5505	0(3)	L5682	0(3)
L1090	0(3)	L1950	0(3)	L2390	0(3)	L3201	0(3)	L3600	0(3)	L3980	0(3)	L5510	0(3)	L5683	0(3)
L1100	0(3)	L1951	0(3)	L2395	0(3)	L3202	0(3)	L3610	0(3)	L3981	0(3)	L5520	0(3)	L5684	0(3)
L1110	0(3)	L1960	0(3)	L2397	0(3)	L3203	0(3)	L3620	0(3)	L3982	0(3)	L5530	0(3)	L5685	0(3)
L1120	0(3)	L1970	0(3)	L2405	0(3)	L3204	0(3)	L3630	0(3)	L3984	0(3)	L5535	0(3)	L5686	0(3)
L1200	0(3)	L1971	0(3)	L2415	0(3)	L3206	0(3)	L3640	0(3)	L3995	0(3)	L5540	0(3)	L5688	0(3)
L1210	0(3)	L1980	0(3)	L2425	0(3)	L3207	0(3)	L3649	0(3)	L3999	0(3)	L5560	0(3)	L5690	0(3)
L1220	0(3)	L1990	0(3)	L2430	0(3)	L3208	0(3)	L3650	0(3)	L4000	0(3)	L5570	0(3)	L5692	0(3)
L1230	0(3)	L2000	0(3)	L2492	0(3)	L3209	0(3)	L3660	0(3)	L4002	0(3)	L5580	0(3)	L5694	0(3)
L1240	0(3)	L2005	0(3)	L2500	0(3)	L3211	0(3)	L3670	0(3)	L4010	0(3)	L5585	0(3)	L5695	0(3)
L1250	0(3)	L2010	0(3)	L2510	0(3)	L3212	0(3)	L3671	0(3)	L4020	0(3)	L5590	0(3)	L5696	0(3)
L1260	0(3)	L2020	0(3)	L2520	0(3)	L3213	0(3)	L3674	0(3)	L4030	0(3)	L5595	0(3)	L5697	0(3)
L1270	0(3)	L2030	0(3)	L2525	0(3)	L3214	0(3)	L3675	0(3)	L4040	0(3)	L5600	0(3)	L5698	0(3)
L1280	0(3)	L2034	0(3)	L2526	0(3)	L3215	0(3)	L3677	0(3)	L4045	0(3)	L5610	0(3)	L5699	0(3)
L1290	0(3)	L2035	0(3)	L2530	0(3)	L3216	0(3)	L3678	0(3)	L4050	0(3)	L5611	0(3)	L5700	0(3)
L1300	0(3)	L2036	0(3)	L2540	0(3)	L3217	0(3)	L3702	0(3)	L4055	0(3)	L5613	0(3)	L5701	0(3)
L1310	0(3)	L2037	0(3)	L2550	0(3)	L3219	0(3)	L3710	0(3)	L4060	0(3)	L5614	0(3)	L5702	0(3)
L1499	1(3)	L2038	0(3)	L2570	0(3)	L3221	0(3)	L3720	0(3)	L4070	0(3)	L5616	0(3)	L5703	0(3)
L1600	0(3)	L2040	0(3)	L2580	0(3)	L3222	0(3)	L3730	0(3)	L4080	0(3)	L5617	0(3)	L5704	0(3)
L1610	0(3)	L2050	0(3)	L2600	0(3)	L3224	0(3)	L3740	0(3)	L4090	0(3)	L5618	0(3)	L5705	0(3)
L1620	0(3)	L2060	0(3)	L2610	0(3)	L3225	0(3)	L3760	0(3)	L4100	0(3)	L5620	0(3)	L5706	0(3)
L1630	0(3)	L2070	0(3)	L2620	0(3)	L3230	0(3)	L3761	0(3)	L4110	0(3)	L5622	0(3)	L5707	0(3)
L1640	0(3)	L2080	0(3)	L2622	0(3)	L3250	0(3)	L3762	0(3)	L4130	0(3)	L5624	0(3)	L5710	0(3)
L1650	0(3)	L2090	0(3)	L2624	0(3)	L3251	0(3)	L3763	0(3)	L4205	0(3)	L5626	0(3)	L5711	0(3)
L1652	0(3)	L2106	0(3)	L2627	0(3)	L3252	0(3)	L3764	0(3)	L4210	0(3)	L5628	0(3)	L5712	0(3)
L1660	0(3)	L2108	0(3)	L2628	0(3)	L3253	0(3)	L3765	0(3)	L4350	0(3)	L5629	0(3)	L5714	0(3)
L1680	0(3)	L2112	0(3)	L2630	0(3)	L3254	0(3)	L3766	0(3)	L4360	0(3)	L5630	0(3)	L5716	0(3)
L1685	0(3)	L2114	0(3)	L2640	0(3)	L3255	0(3)	L3806	0(3)	L4361	0(3)	L5631	0(3)	L5718	0(3)
L1686	0(3)	L2116	0(3)	L2650	0(3)	L3257	0(3)	L3807	0(3)	L4370	0(3)	L5632	0(3)	L5722	0(3)
L1690	0(3)	L2126	0(3)	L2660	0(3)	L3260	0(3)	L3808	0(3)	L4386	0(3)	L5634	0(3)	L5724	0(3)
L1700	0(3)	L2128	0(3)	L2670	0(3)	L3265	0(3)	L3809	0(3)	L4387	0(3)	L5636	0(3)	L5726	0(3)
L1710	0(3)	L2132	0(3)	L2680	0(3)	L3300	0(3)	L3891	0(3)	L4392	0(3)	L5637	0(3)	L5728	0(3)
L1720	0(3)	L2134	0(3)	L2750	0(3)	L3310	0(3)	L3900	0(3)	L4394	0(3)	L5638	0(3)	L5780	0(3)
L1730	0(3)	L2136	0(3)	L2755	0(3)	L3320	0(3)	L3901	0(3)	L4396	0(3)	L5639	0(3)	L5781	0(3)
L1755	0(3)	L2180	0(3)	L2760	0(3)	L3330	0(3)	L3904	0(3)	L4397	0(3)	L5640	0(3)	L5782	0(3)
L1810	0(3)	L2182	0(3)	L2768	0(3)	L3332	0(3)	L3905	0(3)	L4398	0(3)	L5642	0(3)	L5785	0(3)
L1812	0(3)	L2184	0(3)	L2780	0(3)	L3334	0(3)	L3906	0(3)	L4631	0(3)	L5643	0(3)	L5790	0(3)
L1820	0(3)	L2186	0(3)	L2785	0(3)	L3340	0(3)	L3908	0(3)	L5000	0(3)	L5644	0(3)	L5795	0(3)

Appendix I — Medically Unlikely Edits (MUEs)—Professional

CPT	MUE	CPT	MUE	CPT	MUE	CPT	MUE	CPT	MUE	CPT	MUE	CPT	MUE	CPT	MUE
L5810	0(3)	L6300	0(3)	L6692	0(3)	L7400	0(3)	L8605	4(3)	P9022	2(3)	Q0477	1(1)	Q4018	2(3)
L5811	0(3)	L6310	0(3)	L6693	0(3)	L7401	0(3)	L8606	5(3)	P9023	2(3)	Q0478	1(3)	Q4021	2(3)
L5812	0(3)	L6320	0(3)	L6694	0(3)	L7402	0(3)	L8607	20(3)	P9031	12(3)	Q0479	1(3)	Q4025	1(3)
L5814	0(3)	L6350	0(3)	L6695	0(3)	L7403	0(3)	L8609	1(3)	P9032	12(3)	Q0480	1(3)	Q4026	1(3)
L5816	0(3)	L6360	0(3)	L6696	0(3)	L7404	0(3)	L8610	1(3)	P9033	12(3)	Q0481	1(2)	Q4027	1(3)
L5818	0(3)	L6370	0(3)	L6697	0(3)	L7405	0(3)	L8612	1(3)	P9034	2(3)	Q0482	1(3)	Q4028	1(3)
L5822	0(3)	L6380	0(3)	L6698	0(3)	L7499	0(3)	L8613	1(3)	P9035	2(3)	Q0483	1(3)	Q4030	2(3)
L5824	0(3)	L6382	0(3)	L6703	0(3)	L7510	4(3)	L8614	1(3)	P9036	2(3)	Q0484	1(3)	Q4037	2(3)
L5826	0(3)	L6384	0(3)	L6704	0(3)	L7600	0(3)	L8615	2(3)	P9037	2(3)	Q0485	1(3)	Q4042	2(3)
L5828	0(3)	L6386	0(3)	L6706	0(3)	L7700	0(3)	L8616	2(3)	P9038	2(3)	Q0486	1(3)	Q4046	2(3)
L5830	0(3)	L6388	0(3)	L6707	0(3)	L7900	0(3)	L8617	2(3)	P9039	2(3)	Q0487	1(3)	Q4050	2(3)
L5840	0(3)	L6400	0(3)	L6708	0(3)	L7902	0(3)	L8618	2(3)	P9040	3(3)	Q0488	1(3)	Q4051	2(3)
L5845	0(3)	L6450	0(3)	L6709	0(3)	L8000	0(3)	L8619	2(3)	P9041	5(3)	Q0489	1(3)	Q4074	3(3)
L5848	0(3)	L6500	0(3)	L6711	0(3)	L8001	0(3)	L8621	360(3)	P9043	5(3)	Q0490	1(3)	Q4081	100(3)
L5850	0(3)	L6550	0(3)	L6712	0(3)	L8002	0(3)	L8622	2(3)	P9044	10(3)	Q0491	1(3)	Q4103	0(3)
L5855	0(3)	L6570	0(3)	L6713	0(3)	L8010	0(3)	L8625	1(3)	P9045	20(3)	Q0492	1(3)	Q5101	1500(3)
L5856	0(3)	L6580	0(3)	L6714	0(3)	L8015	0(3)	L8627	2(2)	P9046	25(3)	Q0493	1(3)	Q5103	150(3)
L5857	0(3)	L6582	0(3)	L6715	0(3)	L8020	0(3)	L8628	2(2)	P9047	20(3)	Q0494	1(3)	Q5104	150(3)
L5858	0(3)	L6584	0(3)	L6721	0(3)	L8030	0(3)	L8629	2(2)	P9048	1(3)	Q0495	1(3)	Q5105	100(3)
L5859	0(3)	L6586	0(3)	L6722	0(3)	L8031	0(3)	L8631	1(3)	P9050	1(3)	Q0496	1(3)	Q5106	60(3)
L5910	0(3)	L6588	0(3)	L6805	0(3)	L8032	0(3)	L8641	4(3)	P9051	2(3)	Q0497	2(3)	Q5107	170(3)
L5920	0(3)	L6590	0(3)	L6810	0(3)	L8035	0(3)	L8642	2(3)	P9052	2(3)	Q0498	1(3)	Q5108	12(3)
L5925	0(3)	L6600	0(3)	L6880	0(3)	L8039	0(3)	L8658	2(3)	P9053	2(3)	Q0499	1(3)	Q5109	150(3)
L5930	0(3)	L6605	0(3)	L6881	0(3)	L8040	0(3)	L8659	2(3)	P9054	2(3)	Q0501	1(3)	Q5110	1500(3)
L5940	0(3)	L6610	0(3)	L6882	0(3)	L8041	0(3)	L8670	2(3)	P9055	2(3)	Q0502	1(3)	Q5111	12(3)
L5950	0(3)	L6611	0(3)	L6883	0(3)	L8042	0(3)	L8679	1(3)	P9056	2(3)	Q0503	3(3)	Q5112	120(3)
L5960	0(3)	L6615	0(3)	L6884	0(3)	L8043	0(3)	L8681	1(3)	P9057	2(3)	Q0504	1(3)	Q5113	120(3)
L5961	0(3)	L6616	0(3)	L6885	0(3)	L8044	0(3)	L8682	2(3)	P9058	2(3)	Q0506	8(3)	Q5114	120(3)
L5962	0(3)	L6620	0(3)	L6890	0(3)	L8045	0(3)	L8683	1(3)	P9059	2(3)	Q0507	1(3)	Q5115	120(3)
L5964	0(3)	L6621	0(3)	L6895	0(3)	L8046	0(3)	L8684	1(3)	P9060	2(3)	Q0508	4(3)	Q9950	5(3)
L5966	0(3)	L6623	0(3)	L6900	0(3)	L8047	0(3)	L8685	1(3)	P9070	2(3)	Q0509	2(3)	Q9951	0(3)
L5968	0(3)	L6624	0(3)	L6905	0(3)	L8048	1(3)	L8686	2(3)	P9071	2(3)	Q0510	0(3)	Q9953	10(3)
L5969	0(3)	L6625	0(3)	L6910	0(3)	L8049	0(3)	L8687	1(3)	P9073	2(3)	Q0511	0(3)	Q9954	18(3)
L5970	0(3)	L6628	0(3)	L6915	0(3)	L8300	0(3)	L8688	1(3)	P9100	2(3)	Q0512	0(3)	Q9955	0(3)
L5971	0(3)	L6629	0(3)	L6920	0(3)	L8310	0(3)	L8689	1(3)	P9603	300(3)	Q0513	0(3)	Q9956	9(3)
L5972	0(3)	L6630	0(3)	L6925	0(3)	L8320	0(3)	L8690	2(2)	P9604	2(3)	Q0514	0(3)	Q9957	3(3)
L5973	0(3)	L6632	0(3)	L6930	0(3)	L8330	0(3)	L8691	1(3)	P9612	1(3)	Q0515	0(3)	Q9958	300(3)
L5974	0(3)	L6635	0(3)	L6935	0(3)	L8400	0(3)	L8692	0(3)	P9615	1(3)	Q1004	2(2)	Q9959	0(3)
L5975	0(3)	L6637	0(3)	L6940	0(3)	L8410	0(3)	L8693	1(3)	Q0035	1(3)	Q1005	2(2)	Q9960	250(3)
L5976	0(3)	L6638	0(3)	L6945	0(3)	L8415	0(3)	L8694	1(3)	Q0081	1(3)	Q2004	1(3)	Q9961	200(3)
L5978	0(3)	L6640	0(3)	L6950	0(3)	L8417	0(3)	L8695	1(3)	Q0083	1(3)	Q2009	100(3)	Q9962	150(3)
L5979	0(3)	L6641	0(3)	L6955	0(3)	L8420	0(3)	L8696	1(3)	Q0084	1(3)	Q2017	12(3)	Q9963	240(3)
L5980	0(3)	L6642	0(3)	L6960	0(3)	L8430	0(3)	L8701	0(3)	Q0085	1(3)	Q2026	45(3)	Q9964	0(3)
L5981	0(3)	L6645	0(3)	L6965	0(3)	L8435	0(3)	L8702	0(3)	Q0091	1(3)	Q2028	1470(3)	Q9966	250(3)
L5982	0(3)	L6646	0(3)	L6970	0(3)	L8440	0(3)	M0075	0(3)	Q0111	2(3)	Q2034	1(2)	Q9967	300(3)
L5984	0(3)	L6647	0(3)	L6975	0(3)	L8460	0(3)	M0076	0(3)	Q0112	3(3)	Q2035	1(2)	Q9969	3(3)
L5985	0(3)	L6648	0(3)	L7007	0(3)	L8465	0(3)	M0100	0(3)	Q0113	1(3)	Q2036	1(2)	Q9982	1(3)
L5986	0(3)	L6650	0(3)	L7008	0(3)	L8470	0(3)	M0300	0(3)	Q0114	1(3)	Q2037	1(2)	Q9983	1(3)
L5987	0(3)	L6655	0(3)	L7009	0(3)	L8480	0(3)	M0301	0(3)	Q0115	1(3)	Q2038	1(2)	Q9991	1(3)
L5988	0(3)	L6660	0(3)	L7040	0(3)	L8485	0(3)	P2028	1(2)	Q0138	510(3)	Q2039	1(2)	Q9992	1(3)
L5990	0(3)	L6665	0(3)	L7045	0(3)	L8499	1(3)	P2029	1(2)	Q0139	510(3)	Q2043	1(2)	R0070	2(3)
L5999	0(3)	L6670	0(3)	L7170	0(3)	L8500	0(3)	P2031	0(3)	Q0144	0(3)	Q2049	14(3)	R0075	2(3)
L6000	0(3)	L6672	0(3)	L7180	0(3)	L8501	0(3)	P2033	1(2)	Q0161	0(3)	Q2050	14(3)	R0076	1(3)
L6010	0(3)	L6675	0(3)	L7181	0(3)	L8505	0(3)	P2038	1(2)	Q0162	0(3)	Q2052	1(3)	V2020	0(3)
L6020	0(3)	L6676	0(3)	L7185	0(3)	L8507	0(3)	P3000	1(3)	Q0163	0(3)	Q3014	1(3)	V2025	0(3)
L6026	0(3)	L6677	0(3)	L7186	0(3)	L8509	1(3)	P3001	1(3)	Q0164	0(3)	Q3027	30(3)	V2100	0(3)
L6050	0(3)	L6680	0(3)	L7190	0(3)	L8510	0(3)	P7001	0(3)	Q0166	0(3)	Q3028	0(3)	V2101	0(3)
L6055	0(3)	L6682	0(3)	L7191	0(3)	L8511	1(3)	P9010	2(3)	Q0167	0(3)	Q3031	1(3)	V2102	0(3)
L6100	0(3)	L6684	0(3)	L7259	0(3)	L8512	1(3)	P9011	2(3)	Q0169	0(3)	Q4001	1(3)	V2103	0(3)
L6110	0(3)	L6686	0(3)	L7360	0(3)	L8513	1(3)	P9012	8(3)	Q0173	0(3)	Q4002	1(3)	V2104	0(3)
L6120	0(3)	L6687	0(3)	L7362	0(3)	L8514	1(3)	P9016	3(3)	Q0174	0(3)	Q4003	2(3)	V2105	0(3)
L6130	0(3)	L6688	0(3)	L7364	0(3)	L8515	1(3)	P9017	2(3)	Q0175	0(3)	Q4004	2(3)	V2106	0(3)
L6200	0(3)	L6689	0(3)	L7366	0(3)	L8600	2(3)	P9019	2(3)	Q0177	0(3)	Q4012	2(3)	V2107	0(3)
L6205	0(3)	L6690	0(3)	L7367	0(3)	L8603	4(3)	P9020	2(3)	Q0180	0(3)	Q4013	2(3)	V2108	0(3)
L6250	0(3)	L6691	0(3)	L7368	0(3)	L8604	3(3)	P9021	3(3)	Q0181	0(3)	Q4014	2(3)	V2109	0(3)

CPT	MUE	CPT	MUE	CPT	MUE	CPT	MUE	CPT	MUE	CPT	MUE	CPT	MUE	CPT	MUE
V2110	0(3)	V2215	0(3)	V2320	0(3)	V2623	0(3)	V2770	0(3)	V5095	0(3)	V5244	0(3)	V5268	0(3)
V2111	0(3)	V2218	0(3)	V2321	0(3)	V2624	0(3)	V2780	0(3)	V5100	0(3)	V5245	0(3)	V5269	0(3)
V2112	0(3)	V2219	0(3)	V2399	0(3)	V2625	0(3)	V2781	0(2)	V5110	0(3)	V5246	0(3)	V5270	0(3)
V2113	0(3)	V2220	0(3)	V2410	0(3)	V2626	0(3)	V2782	0(3)	V5120	0(3)	V5247	0(3)	V5271	0(3)
V2114	0(3)	V2221	0(3)	V2430	0(3)	V2627	0(3)	V2783	0(3)	V5130	0(3)	V5248	0(3)	V5272	0(3)
V2115	0(3)	V2299	0(3)	V2499	2(3)	V2628	0(3)	V2784	0(3)	V5140	0(3)	V5249	0(3)	V5273	0(3)
V2118	0(3)	V2300	0(3)	V2500	0(3)	V2629	0(3)	V2785	2(2)	V5150	0(3)	V5250	0(3)	V5274	0(3)
V2121	0(3)	V2301	0(3)	V2501	0(3)	V2630	2(2)	V2786	0(3)	V5160	0(3)	V5251	0(3)	V5275	0(3)
V2199	2(3)	V2302	0(3)	V2502	0(3)	V2631	2(2)	V2787	0(3)	V5171	0(3)	V5252	0(3)	V5281	0(3)
V2200	0(3)	V2303	0(3)	V2503	0(3)	V2632	2(2)	V2788	0(3)	V5172	0(3)	V5253	0(3)	V5282	0(3)
V2201	0(3)	V2304	0(3)	V2510	0(3)	V2700	0(3)	V2790	1(3)	V5181	0(3)	V5254	0(3)	V5283	0(3)
V2202	0(3)	V2305	0(3)	V2511	0(3)	V2702	0(3)	V2797	0(3)	V5190	0(3)	V5255	0(3)	V5284	0(3)
V2203	0(3)	V2306	0(3)	V2512	0(3)	V2710	0(3)	V5008	0(3)	V5200	0(3)	V5256	0(3)	V5285	0(3)
V2204	0(3)	V2307	0(3)	V2513	0(3)	V2715	0(3)	V5010	0(3)	V5211	0(3)	V5257	0(3)	V5286	0(3)
V2205	0(3)	V2308	0(3)	V2520	2(3)	V2718	0(3)	V5011	0(3)	V5212	0(3)	V5258	0(3)	V5287	0(3)
V2206	0(3)	V2309	0(3)	V2521	2(3)	V2730	0(3)	V5014	0(3)	V5213	0(3)	V5259	0(3)	V5288	0(3)
V2207	0(3)	V2310	0(3)	V2522	2(3)	V2744	0(3)	V5020	0(3)	V5214	0(3)	V5260	0(3)	V5289	0(3)
V2208	0(3)	V2311	0(3)	V2523	2(3)	V2745	0(3)	V5030	0(3)	V5215	0(3)	V5261	0(3)	V5290	0(3)
V2209	0(3)	V2312	0(3)	V2530	0(3)	V2750	0(3)	V5040	0(3)	V5221	0(3)	V5262	0(3)	V5298	0(3)
V2210	0(3)	V2313	0(3)	V2531	0(3)	V2755	0(3)	V5050	0(3)	V5230	0(3)	V5263	0(3)	V5299	1(3)
V2211	0(3)	V2314	0(3)	V2599	2(3)	V2756	0(3)	V5060	0(3)	V5240	0(3)	V5264	0(3)	V5336	0(3)
V2212	0(3)	V2315	0(3)	V2600	0(2)	V2760	0(3)	V5070	0(3)	V5241	0(3)	V5265	0(3)	V5362	0(3)
V2213	0(3)	V2318	0(3)	V2610	0(2)	V2761	0(2)	V5080	0(3)	V5242	0(3)	V5266	0(3)	V5363	0(3)
V2214	0(3)	V2319	0(3)	V2615	0(2)	V2762	0(3)	V5090	0(3)	V5243	0(3)	V5267	0(3)	V5364	0(3)

OPPS

CPT	MUE	CPT	MUE	CPT	MUE	CPT	MUE	CPT	MUE	CPT	MUE	CPT	MUE	CPT	MUE
0001U	1(2)	0057U	1(3)	0212T	1(3)	0350T	1(3)	0437T	1(3)	0502T	1(2)	11000	1(2)	11602	3(3)
0002M	1(3)	0058T	1(2)	0213T	1(2)	0351T	5(3)	0439T	1(3)	0503T	1(2)	11001	1(3)	11603	2(3)
0002U	1(2)	0058U	1(2)	0214T	1(2)	0352T	5(3)	0440T	3(3)	0504T	1(2)	11004	1(2)	11604	2(3)
0003M	1(3)	0059U	1(2)	0215T	1(2)	0353T	2(3)	0441T	3(3)	0505T	1(3)	11005	1(2)	11606	2(3)
0003U	1(2)	0060U	1(2)	0216T	1(2)	0354T	2(3)	0442T	3(3)	0506T	1(2)	11006	1(2)	11620	2(3)
0004M	1(2)	0061U	1(2)	0217T	1(2)	0355T	1(2)	0443T	1(2)	0507T	1(2)	11008	1(2)	11621	2(3)
0005U	1(2)	0062U	1(2)	0218T	1(2)	0356T	4(2)	0444T	1(2)	0508T	1(3)	11010	2(3)	11622	2(3)
0006M	1(2)	0063U	1(2)	0219T	1(2)	0357T	1(2)	0445T	1(2)	0509T	1(2)	11011	2(3)	11623	2(3)
0006U	1(2)	0064U	2(3)	0220T	1(2)	0358T	1(2)	0446T	1(3)	0510T	1(2)	11012	2(3)	11624	2(3)
0007M	1(2)	0065U	2(3)	0221T	1(2)	0362T	8(3)	0447T	1(3)	0511T	1(2)	11042	1(2)	11626	2(3)
0007U	1(2)	0066U	1(3)	0222T	1(3)	0373T	24(3)	0448T	1(3)	0512T	1(2)	11043	1(2)	11640	2(3)
0008U	1(3)	0067U	2(3)	0228T	1(2)	0375T	1(2)	0449T	1(2)	0513T	2(3)	11044	1(2)	11641	2(3)
0009M	1(2)	0068U	1(3)	0229T	2(3)	0376T	2(3)	0450T	1(3)	0514T	2(2)	11045	12(3)	11642	3(3)
0009U	2(3)	0069U	1(3)	0230T	1(2)	0377T	1(2)	0451T	1(3)	0515T	1(3)	11046	4(3)	11643	2(3)
0010U	2(3)	0070U	1(2)	0231T	2(3)	0378T	1(2)	0452T	1(3)	0516T	1(3)	11047	4(3)	11644	2(3)
0011M	1(2)	0071T	1(2)	0232T	1(3)	0379T	1(2)	0453T	1(3)	0517T	1(3)	11055	1(2)	11646	2(3)
0011U	1(2)	0071U	1(2)	0234T	2(3)	0380T	1(2)	0454T	3(3)	0518T	1(3)	11056	1(2)	11719	1(2)
0012M	1(2)	0072T	1(2)	0235T	2(3)	0381T	1(2)	0455T	1(3)	0519T	1(3)	11057	1(2)	11720	1(2)
0012U	1(2)	0072U	1(2)	0236T	1(2)	0382T	1(2)	0456T	1(3)	0520T	1(3)	11102	1(2)	11721	1(2)
0013M	1(2)	0073U	1(2)	0237T	2(3)	0383T	1(2)	0457T	1(3)	0521T	1(3)	11103	6(3)	11730	1(2)
0013U	1(3)	0074U	1(2)	0238T	2(3)	0384T	1(2)	0458T	3(3)	0522T	1(3)	11104	1(2)	11732	4(3)
0014U	1(3)	0075T	1(2)	0249T	1(2)	0385T	1(2)	0459T	1(3)	0523T	1(3)	11105	3(3)	11740	2(3)
0016U	1(3)	0075U	1(2)	0253T	1(3)	0386T	1(2)	0460T	3(3)	0524T	3(3)	11106	1(2)	11750	6(3)
0017U	1(3)	0076T	1(2)	0254T	2(2)	0394T	2(3)	0461T	1(3)	0525T	1(3)	11107	2(3)	11755	2(3)
0018U	1(1)	0076U	1(2)	0263T	1(3)	0395T	2(3)	0462T	1(2)	0526T	1(3)	11200	1(2)	11760	4(3)
0019U	1(3)	0077U	2(2)	0264T	1(3)	0396T	2(2)	0463T	1(2)	0527T	1(3)	11201	0(3)	11762	2(3)
0021U	1(2)	0078U	1(2)	0265T	1(3)	0397T	1(3)	0464T	1(2)	0528T	1(3)	11300	5(3)	11765	4(3)
0022U	2(3)	0079U	0(3)	0266T	1(2)	0398T	1(3)	0465T	1(2)	0529T	1(3)	11301	6(3)	11770	1(3)
0023U	1(2)	0080U	1(2)	0267T	1(3)	0399T	1(3)	0466T	1(3)	0530T	1(3)	11302	4(3)	11771	1(3)
0024U	1(2)	0081U	1(3)	0268T	1(3)	0400T	1(2)	0467T	1(3)	0531T	1(3)	11303	3(3)	11772	1(3)
0025U	1(2)	0082U	1(2)	0269T	1(2)	0401T	1(2)	0468T	1(3)	0532T	1(3)	11305	4(3)	11900	1(2)
0026U	1(3)	0083U	1(3)	0270T	1(3)	0402T	2(2)	0469T	1(2)	0533T	1(2)	11306	4(3)	11901	1(2)
0027U	1(2)	0085T	0(3)	0271T	1(3)	0403T	0(3)	0470T	1(2)	0534T	1(2)	11307	3(3)	11920	1(2)
0029U	1(2)	0095T	1(3)	0272T	1(3)	0404T	1(2)	0471T	2(1)	0535T	1(2)	11308	2(3)	11921	1(2)
0030U	1(2)	0098T	2(3)	0273T	1(3)	0405T	1(2)	0472T	1(2)	0536T	1(2)	11310	4(3)	11922	1(3)
0031U	1(2)	0100T	1(2)	0274T	1(2)	0408T	1(3)	0473T	1(2)	0537T	1(2)	11311	1(3)	11950	1(2)
0032U	1(2)	0101T	1(3)	0275T	1(2)	0409T	1(3)	0474T	2(2)	0538T	1(3)	11312	3(3)	11951	1(2)
0033U	1(2)	0102T	2(2)	0278T	1(3)	0410T	1(3)	0475T	1(3)	0539T	1(3)	11313	3(3)	11952	1(2)
0034U	1(2)	0106T	4(2)	0290T	1(3)	0411T	1(3)	0476T	1(3)	0540T	1(3)	11400	3(3)	11954	1(3)
0035U	1(2)	0107T	4(2)	0295T	1(2)	0412T	1(2)	0477T	1(3)	0541T	1(3)	11401	3(3)	11960	2(3)
0036U	1(3)	0108T	4(2)	0296T	1(2)	0413T	1(3)	0478T	1(3)	0542T	1(3)	11402	3(3)	11970	2(3)
0037U	1(3)	0109T	4(2)	0297T	1(2)	0414T	1(2)	0479T	1(2)	10004	3(3)	11403	2(3)	11971	2(3)
0038U	1(2)	0110T	4(2)	0298T	1(2)	0415T	1(3)	0480T	4(1)	10005	1(2)	11404	2(3)	11976	1(2)
0039U	1(2)	0111T	1(3)	0308T	1(3)	0416T	1(3)	0481T	1(3)	10006	3(3)	11406	2(3)	11980	1(2)
0040U	1(2)	0126T	1(3)	0312T	1(3)	0417T	1(3)	0482T	1(3)	10007	1(2)	11420	3(3)	11981	1(3)
0041U	1(2)	0163T	1(3)	0313T	1(3)	0418T	1(3)	0483T	1(2)	10008	3(3)	11421	3(3)	11982	1(3)
0042T	1(3)	0164T	4(2)	0314T	1(3)	0419T	1(2)	0484T	1(2)	10009	1(2)	11422	3(3)	11983	1(3)
0042U	1(2)	0165T	4(2)	0315T	1(3)	0420T	1(2)	0485T	1(2)	10010	3(3)	11423	2(3)	12001	1(2)
0043U	1(2)	0174T	1(3)	0316T	1(3)	0421T	1(2)	0486T	1(2)	10011	1(2)	11424	2(3)	12002	1(2)
0044U	1(2)	0175T	1(3)	0317T	1(3)	0422T	1(3)	0487T	1(3)	10012	3(3)	11426	2(3)	12004	1(2)
0045U	1(3)	0184T	1(3)	0329T	0(3)	0423T	1(3)	0488T	1(2)	10021	1(2)	11440	4(3)	12005	1(2)
0046U	1(3)	0191T	2(2)	0330T	1(2)	0424T	1(3)	0489T	1(2)	10030	2(3)	11441	3(3)	12006	1(2)
0047U	1(3)	0198T	2(2)	0331T	1(3)	0425T	1(3)	0490T	1(2)	10035	1(2)	11442	3(3)	12007	1(2)
0048U	1(3)	01996	1(2)	0332T	1(3)	0426T	1(3)	0491T	1(2)	10036	3(3)	11443	2(3)	12011	1(2)
0049U	1(3)	0200T	1(2)	0333T	0(3)	0427T	1(3)	0492T	4(3)	10040	1(2)	11444	2(3)	12013	1(2)
0050U	1(3)	0201T	1(2)	0335T	2(2)	0428T	1(2)	0493T	1(3)	10060	1(2)	11446	2(3)	12014	1(2)
0051U	1(2)	0202T	1(3)	0338T	1(2)	0429T	1(2)	0494T	1(2)	10061	1(2)	11450	1(2)	12015	1(2)
0052U	1(3)	0205T	3(3)	0339T	1(2)	0430T	1(2)	0495T	1(2)	10080	1(3)	11451	1(2)	12016	1(2)
0053U	1(3)	0206T	1(3)	0341T	1(2)	0431T	1(2)	0496T	4(3)	10081	1(3)	11462	1(2)	12017	1(2)
0054T	1(3)	0207T	2(2)	0342T	1(3)	0432T	1(3)	0497T	1(3)	10120	3(3)	11463	1(2)	12018	1(2)
0054U	1(2)	0208T	1(3)	0345T	1(2)	0433T	1(3)	0498T	1(2)	10121	2(3)	11470	3(2)	12020	2(3)
0055T	1(3)	0209T	1(3)	0347T	1(3)	0434T	1(3)	0499T	1(2)	10140	2(3)	11471	2(3)	12021	3(3)
0055U	1(2)	0210T	1(3)	0348T	1(3)	0435T	1(3)	0500T	1(3)	10160	3(3)	11600	2(3)	12031	1(2)
0056U	1(3)	0211T	1(3)	0349T	1(3)	0436T	1(3)	0501T	1(2)	10180	2(3)	11601	2(3)	12032	1(2)

CPT	MUE	CPT	MUE	CPT	MUE	CPT	MUE	CPT	MUE	CPT	MUE	CPT	MUE	CPT	MUE
12034	1(2)	15200	1(2)	15835	1(3)	17280	6(3)	19355	1(2)	20822	3(3)	21080	1(2)	21255	1(2)
12035	1(2)	15201	7(3)	15836	1(2)	17281	5(3)	19357	1(2)	20824	1(2)	21081	1(2)	21256	1(2)
12036	1(2)	15220	1(2)	15837	2(3)	17282	4(3)	19361	1(2)	20827	1(2)	21082	1(2)	21260	1(2)
12037	1(2)	15221	9(3)	15838	1(2)	17283	4(3)	19364	1(2)	20838	1(2)	21083	1(2)	21261	1(2)
12041	1(2)	15240	1(2)	15839	2(3)	17284	2(3)	19366	1(2)	20900	2(3)	21084	1(2)	21263	1(2)
12042	1(2)	15241	9(3)	15840	1(3)	17286	2(3)	19367	1(2)	20902	2(3)	21085	1(3)	21267	1(2)
12044	1(2)	15260	1(2)	15841	2(3)	17311	4(3)	19368	1(2)	20910	1(3)	21086	1(2)	21268	1(2)
12045	1(2)	15261	6(3)	15842	2(3)	17312	6(3)	19369	1(2)	20912	1(3)	21087	1(2)	21270	1(2)
12046	1(2)	15271	1(2)	15845	2(3)	17313	3(3)	19370	1(2)	20920	1(3)	21088	1(2)	21275	1(2)
12047	1(2)	15272	3(3)	15847	1(2)	17314	4(3)	19371	1(2)	20922	1(3)	21089	1(3)	21280	1(2)
12051	1(2)	15273	1(2)	15850	1(2)	17315	15(3)	19380	1(2)	20924	2(3)	21100	1(2)	21282	1(2)
12052	1(2)	15274	6(3)	15851	1(2)	17340	1(2)	19396	1(2)	20926	2(3)	21110	2(3)	21295	1(2)
12053	1(2)	15275	1(2)	15852	1(3)	17360	1(2)	19499	1(3)	20930	1(3)	21116	1(2)	21296	1(2)
12054	1(2)	15276	3(2)	15860	1(3)	17380	1(3)	20100	2(3)	20931	1(2)	21120	1(2)	21299	1(3)
12055	1(2)	15277	1(2)	15876	1(2)	17999	1(3)	20101	2(3)	20932	1(3)	21121	1(2)	21310	1(2)
12056	1(2)	15278	3(3)	15877	1(2)	19000	2(3)	20102	3(3)	20933	1(3)	21122	1(2)	21315	1(2)
12057	1(2)	15570	2(3)	15878	1(2)	19001	5(3)	20103	3(3)	20934	1(2)	21123	1(2)	21320	1(2)
13100	1(2)	15572	2(3)	15879	1(2)	19020	2(3)	20150	2(3)	20936	1(3)	21125	2(2)	21325	1(2)
13101	1(2)	15574	2(3)	15920	1(3)	19030	1(2)	20200	2(3)	20937	1(2)	21127	2(3)	21330	1(2)
13102	9(3)	15576	2(3)	15922	1(3)	19081	1(2)	20205	3(3)	20938	1(2)	21137	1(2)	21335	1(2)
13120	1(2)	15600	2(3)	15931	1(3)	19082	2(3)	20206	3(3)	20939	1(3)	21138	1(2)	21336	1(2)
13121	1(2)	15610	2(3)	15933	1(3)	19083	1(2)	20220	3(3)	20950	2(3)	21139	1(2)	21337	1(2)
13122	9(3)	15620	2(3)	15934	1(3)	19084	2(3)	20225	2(3)	20955	1(3)	21141	1(2)	21338	1(2)
13131	1(2)	15630	2(3)	15935	1(3)	19085	1(2)	20240	4(3)	20956	1(3)	21142	1(2)	21339	1(2)
13132	1(2)	15650	1(3)	15936	1(3)	19086	2(3)	20245	3(3)	20957	1(3)	21143	1(2)	21340	1(2)
13133	7(3)	15730	1(3)	15937	1(3)	19100	4(3)	20250	1(3)	20962	1(3)	21145	1(2)	21343	1(2)
13151	1(2)	15731	1(3)	15940	2(3)	19101	3(3)	20251	2(3)	20969	2(3)	21146	1(2)	21344	1(2)
13152	1(2)	15733	2(3)	15941	2(3)	19105	2(3)	20500	2(3)	20970	1(3)	21147	1(2)	21345	1(2)
13153	2(3)	15734	4(3)	15944	2(3)	19110	1(3)	20501	2(3)	20972	2(3)	21150	1(2)	21346	1(2)
13160	2(3)	15736	2(3)	15945	2(3)	19112	2(3)	20520	2(3)	20973	1(2)	21151	1(2)	21347	1(2)
14000	2(3)	15738	3(3)	15946	2(3)	19120	1(2)	20525	4(3)	20974	1(3)	21154	1(2)	21348	1(2)
14001	2(3)	15740	2(3)	15950	2(3)	19125	1(2)	20526	1(2)	20975	1(3)	21155	1(2)	21355	1(2)
14020	2(3)	15750	2(3)	15951	2(3)	19126	3(3)	20527	2(3)	20979	1(3)	21159	1(2)	21356	1(2)
14021	2(3)	15756	2(3)	15952	2(3)	19260	2(3)	20550	5(3)	20982	1(2)	21160	1(2)	21360	1(2)
14040	2(3)	15757	2(3)	15953	2(3)	19271	1(3)	20551	5(3)	20983	1(2)	21172	1(3)	21365	1(2)
14041	3(3)	15758	2(3)	15956	2(3)	19272	1(3)	20552	1(2)	20985	2(3)	21175	1(2)	21366	1(2)
14060	2(3)	15760	2(3)	15958	2(3)	19281	1(2)	20553	1(2)	20999	1(3)	21179	1(2)	21385	1(2)
14061	2(3)	15770	2(3)	15999	1(3)	19282	2(3)	20555	1(3)	21010	1(2)	21180	1(2)	21386	1(2)
14301	2(3)	15775	1(2)	16000	1(2)	19283	1(2)	20600	6(3)	21011	4(3)	21181	1(3)	21387	1(2)
14302	8(3)	15776	1(2)	16020	1(3)	19284	2(3)	20604	4(3)	21012	3(3)	21182	1(2)	21390	1(2)
14350	2(3)	15777	1(3)	16025	1(3)	19285	1(2)	20605	2(3)	21013	2(3)	21183	1(2)	21395	1(2)
15002	1(2)	15780	1(2)	16030	1(3)	19286	2(3)	20606	2(3)	21014	2(3)	21184	1(2)	21400	1(2)
15003	9(3)	15781	1(3)	16035	1(2)	19287	1(2)	20610	2(3)	21015	1(3)	21188	1(2)	21401	1(2)
15004	1(2)	15782	1(3)	16036	2(3)	19288	2(3)	20611	2(3)	21016	2(3)	21193	1(2)	21406	1(2)
15005	2(3)	15783	1(3)	17000	1(2)	19294	2(3)	20612	2(3)	21025	2(3)	21194	1(2)	21407	1(2)
15040	1(2)	15786	1(2)	17003	13(2)	19296	1(3)	20615	1(3)	21026	2(3)	21195	1(2)	21408	1(2)
15050	1(3)	15787	2(3)	17004	1(2)	19297	2(3)	20650	4(3)	21029	1(3)	21196	1(2)	21421	1(2)
15100	1(2)	15788	1(2)	17106	1(2)	19298	1(2)	20660	1(2)	21030	1(3)	21198	1(3)	21422	1(2)
15101	9(3)	15789	1(2)	17107	1(2)	19300	1(2)	20661	1(2)	21031	2(3)	21199	1(2)	21423	1(2)
15110	1(2)	15792	1(3)	17108	1(2)	19301	1(2)	20662	1(2)	21032	1(3)	21206	1(3)	21431	1(2)
15111	2(3)	15793	1(3)	17110	1(2)	19302	1(2)	20663	1(2)	21034	1(3)	21208	1(3)	21432	1(2)
15115	1(2)	15819	1(2)	17111	1(2)	19303	1(2)	20664	1(2)	21040	2(3)	21209	1(3)	21433	1(2)
15116	2(3)	15820	1(2)	17250	4(3)	19304	1(2)	20665	1(2)	21044	1(3)	21210	2(3)	21435	1(2)
15120	1(2)	15821	1(2)	17260	7(3)	19305	1(2)	20670	3(3)	21045	1(3)	21215	2(3)	21436	1(2)
15121	5(3)	15822	1(2)	17261	7(3)	19306	1(2)	20680	3(3)	21046	2(3)	21230	2(3)	21440	2(2)
15130	1(2)	15823	1(2)	17262	6(3)	19307	1(2)	20690	2(3)	21047	2(3)	21235	2(3)	21445	2(2)
15131	2(3)	15824	1(2)	17263	3(3)	19316	1(2)	20692	2(3)	21048	2(3)	21240	1(2)	21450	1(2)
15135	1(2)	15825	1(2)	17264	3(3)	19318	1(2)	20693	2(3)	21049	1(3)	21242	1(2)	21451	1(2)
15136	1(3)	15826	1(2)	17266	2(3)	19324	1(2)	20694	2(3)	21050	1(2)	21243	1(2)	21452	1(2)
15150	1(2)	15828	1(2)	17270	6(3)	19325	1(2)	20696	2(3)	21060	1(2)	21244	1(2)	21453	1(2)
15151	1(2)	15829	1(2)	17271	4(3)	19328	1(2)	20697	4(3)	21070	1(2)	21245	2(2)	21454	1(2)
15152	2(3)	15830	1(2)	17272	5(3)	19330	1(2)	20802	1(2)	21073	1(2)	21246	2(2)	21461	1(2)
15155	1(2)	15832	1(2)	17273	4(3)	19340	1(2)	20805	1(2)	21076	1(2)	21247	1(2)	21462	1(2)
15156	1(2)	15833	1(2)	17274	2(3)	19342	1(2)	20808	1(2)	21077	1(2)	21248	2(3)	21465	1(2)
15157	1(3)	15834	1(2)	17276	2(3)	19350	1(2)	20816	3(3)	21079	1(2)	21249	2(3)	21470	1(2)

Appendix I — Medically Unlikely Edits (MUEs)—OPPS

CPT	MUE	CPT	MUE	CPT	MUE	CPT	MUE	CPT	MUE	CPT	MUE	CPT	MUE	CPT	MUE
21480	1(2)	22224	1(2)	22857	1(2)	23397	1(3)	24066	2(3)	24495	1(2)	25105	1(2)	25426	1(2)
21485	1(2)	22226	4(3)	22858	1(2)	23400	1(2)	24071	2(3)	24498	1(2)	25107	1(2)	25430	1(3)
21490	1(2)	22310	1(2)	22859	4(3)	23405	2(3)	24073	2(3)	24500	1(2)	25109	4(3)	25431	1(3)
21497	1(2)	22315	1(2)	22861	1(2)	23406	1(3)	24075	5(3)	24505	1(2)	25110	2(3)	25440	1(2)
21499	1(3)	22318	1(2)	22862	1(2)	23410	1(2)	24076	4(3)	24515	1(2)	25111	1(3)	25441	1(2)
21501	3(3)	22319	1(2)	22864	1(2)	23412	1(2)	24077	1(3)	24516	1(2)	25112	1(3)	25442	1(2)
21502	1(3)	22325	1(2)	22865	1(2)	23415	1(2)	24079	1(3)	24530	1(2)	25115	1(3)	25443	1(2)
21510	1(3)	22326	1(2)	22867	1(2)	23420	1(2)	24100	1(2)	24535	1(2)	25116	1(3)	25444	1(2)
21550	2(3)	22327	1(2)	22868	1(2)	23430	1(2)	24101	1(2)	24538	1(2)	25118	5(3)	25445	1(2)
21552	2(3)	22328	6(3)	22869	1(2)	23440	1(2)	24102	1(2)	24545	1(2)	25119	1(2)	25446	1(2)
21554	2(3)	22505	1(2)	22870	1(2)	23450	1(2)	24105	1(2)	24546	1(2)	25120	1(3)	25447	4(3)
21555	2(3)	22510	1(2)	22899	1(3)	23455	1(2)	24110	1(3)	24560	1(3)	25125	1(3)	25449	1(2)
21556	2(3)	22511	1(2)	22900	3(3)	23460	1(2)	24115	1(3)	24565	1(3)	25126	1(3)	25450	1(2)
21557	1(3)	22512	3(3)	22901	2(3)	23462	1(2)	24116	1(3)	24566	1(3)	25130	1(3)	25455	1(2)
21558	1(3)	22513	1(2)	22902	4(3)	23465	1(2)	24120	1(3)	24575	1(3)	25135	1(3)	25490	1(2)
21600	5(3)	22514	1(2)	22903	3(3)	23466	1(2)	24125	1(3)	24576	1(3)	25136	1(3)	25491	1(2)
21610	1(3)	22515	4(3)	22904	1(3)	23470	1(2)	24126	1(3)	24577	1(3)	25145	1(3)	25492	1(2)
21615	1(2)	22526	0(3)	22905	1(3)	23472	1(2)	24130	1(2)	24579	1(3)	25150	1(3)	25500	1(2)
21616	1(2)	22527	0(3)	22999	1(3)	23473	1(2)	24134	1(3)	24582	1(3)	25151	1(3)	25505	1(2)
21620	1(2)	22532	1(2)	23000	1(2)	23474	1(2)	24136	1(3)	24586	1(3)	25170	1(3)	25515	1(2)
21627	1(2)	22533	1(2)	23020	1(2)	23480	1(2)	24138	1(3)	24587	1(2)	25210	2(3)	25520	1(2)
21630	1(2)	22534	3(3)	23030	2(3)	23485	1(2)	24140	1(3)	24600	1(2)	25215	1(2)	25525	1(2)
21632	1(2)	22548	1(2)	23031	1(3)	23490	1(2)	24145	1(3)	24605	1(2)	25230	1(2)	25526	1(2)
21685	1(2)	22551	1(2)	23035	1(3)	23491	1(2)	24147	1(3)	24615	1(2)	25240	1(2)	25530	1(2)
21700	1(2)	22552	5(3)	23040	1(2)	23500	1(2)	24149	1(2)	24620	1(2)	25246	1(2)	25535	1(2)
21705	1(2)	22554	1(2)	23044	1(3)	23505	1(2)	24150	1(3)	24635	1(2)	25248	3(3)	25545	1(2)
21720	1(3)	22556	1(2)	23065	2(3)	23515	1(2)	24152	1(3)	24640	1(2)	25250	1(2)	25560	1(2)
21725	1(3)	22558	1(2)	23066	2(3)	23520	1(2)	24155	1(2)	24650	1(2)	25251	1(2)	25565	1(2)
21740	1(2)	22585	5(3)	23071	2(3)	23525	1(2)	24160	1(2)	24655	1(2)	25259	1(2)	25574	1(2)
21742	1(2)	22586	1(2)	23073	2(3)	23530	1(2)	24164	1(2)	24665	1(2)	25260	7(3)	25575	1(2)
21743	1(2)	22590	1(2)	23075	2(3)	23532	1(2)	24200	3(3)	24666	1(2)	25263	4(3)	25600	1(2)
21750	1(2)	22595	1(2)	23076	2(3)	23540	1(2)	24201	3(3)	24670	1(2)	25265	4(3)	25605	1(2)
21811	1(2)	22600	1(2)	23077	1(3)	23545	1(2)	24220	1(2)	24675	1(2)	25270	8(3)	25606	1(2)
21812	1(2)	22610	1(2)	23078	1(3)	23550	1(2)	24300	1(2)	24685	1(2)	25272	4(3)	25607	1(2)
21813	1(2)	22612	1(2)	23100	1(2)	23552	1(2)	24301	2(3)	24800	1(2)	25274	4(3)	25608	1(2)
21820	1(2)	22614	13(3)	23101	1(3)	23570	1(2)	24305	4(3)	24802	1(2)	25275	2(3)	25609	1(2)
21825	1(2)	22630	1(2)	23105	1(2)	23575	1(2)	24310	2(3)	24900	1(2)	25280	9(3)	25622	1(2)
21899	1(3)	22632	4(2)	23106	1(2)	23585	1(2)	24320	2(3)	24920	1(2)	25290	10(3)	25624	1(2)
21920	2(3)	22633	1(2)	23107	1(2)	23600	1(2)	24330	1(3)	24925	1(2)	25295	9(3)	25628	1(2)
21925	2(3)	22634	4(2)	23120	1(2)	23605	1(2)	24331	1(3)	24930	1(2)	25300	1(2)	25630	1(3)
21930	5(3)	22800	1(2)	23125	1(2)	23615	1(2)	24332	1(2)	24931	1(2)	25301	1(2)	25635	1(3)
21931	3(3)	22802	1(2)	23130	1(2)	23616	1(2)	24340	1(2)	24935	1(2)	25310	5(3)	25645	1(3)
21932	2(3)	22804	1(2)	23140	1(3)	23620	1(2)	24341	2(3)	24940	1(2)	25312	4(3)	25650	1(2)
21933	2(3)	22808	1(2)	23145	1(3)	23625	1(2)	24342	2(3)	24999	1(3)	25315	1(3)	25651	1(2)
21935	1(3)	22810	1(2)	23146	1(3)	23630	1(2)	24343	1(2)	25000	2(3)	25316	1(3)	25652	1(2)
21936	1(3)	22812	1(2)	23150	1(3)	23650	1(2)	24344	1(2)	25001	1(3)	25320	1(2)	25660	1(2)
22010	2(3)	22818	1(2)	23155	1(3)	23655	1(2)	24345	1(2)	25020	1(2)	25332	1(2)	25670	1(2)
22015	2(3)	22819	1(2)	23156	1(3)	23660	1(2)	24346	1(2)	25023	1(2)	25335	1(2)	25671	1(2)
22100	1(2)	22830	1(2)	23170	1(3)	23665	1(2)	24357	1(3)	25024	1(2)	25337	1(2)	25675	1(2)
22101	1(2)	22840	1(3)	23172	1(3)	23670	1(2)	24358	1(3)	25025	1(2)	25350	1(3)	25676	1(2)
22102	1(2)	22841	0(3)	23174	1(3)	23675	1(2)	24359	2(3)	25028	4(3)	25355	1(3)	25680	1(2)
22103	3(3)	22842	1(3)	23180	1(3)	23680	1(2)	24360	1(2)	25031	2(3)	25360	1(3)	25685	1(2)
22110	1(2)	22843	1(3)	23182	1(3)	23700	1(2)	24361	1(2)	25035	2(3)	25365	1(3)	25690	1(2)
22112	1(2)	22844	1(3)	23184	1(3)	23800	1(2)	24362	1(2)	25040	1(3)	25370	1(2)	25695	1(2)
22114	1(2)	22845	1(3)	23190	1(3)	23802	1(2)	24363	1(2)	25065	2(3)	25375	1(2)	25800	1(2)
22116	3(3)	22846	1(3)	23195	1(2)	23900	1(2)	24365	1(2)	25066	2(3)	25390	1(2)	25805	1(2)
22206	1(2)	22847	1(3)	23200	1(3)	23920	1(2)	24366	1(2)	25071	3(3)	25391	1(2)	25810	1(2)
22207	1(2)	22848	1(2)	23210	1(3)	23921	1(2)	24370	1(2)	25073	2(3)	25392	1(2)	25820	1(2)
22208	5(3)	22849	1(2)	23220	1(3)	23929	1(3)	24371	1(2)	25075	6(3)	25393	1(2)	25825	1(2)
22210	1(2)	22850	1(2)	23330	2(3)	23930	2(3)	24400	1(3)	25076	3(3)	25394	1(3)	25830	1(2)
22212	1(2)	22852	1(2)	23333	1(3)	23931	2(3)	24410	1(2)	25077	1(3)	25400	1(2)	25900	1(2)
22214	1(2)	22853	4(3)	23334	1(2)	23935	2(3)	24420	1(2)	25078	1(3)	25405	1(2)	25905	1(2)
22216	6(3)	22854	4(3)	23335	1(2)	24000	1(2)	24430	1(3)	25085	1(2)	25415	1(2)	25907	1(2)
22220	1(2)	22855	1(2)	23350	1(2)	24006	1(2)	24435	1(3)	25100	1(2)	25420	1(2)	25909	1(2)
22222	1(2)	22856	1(2)	23395	1(2)	24065	2(3)	24470	1(2)	25101	1(2)	25425	1(2)	25915	1(2)

CPT	MUE	CPT	MUE	CPT	MUE	CPT	MUE	CPT	MUE	CPT	MUE	CPT	MUE	CPT	MUE
25920	1(2)	26410	4(3)	26567	3(3)	27027	1(2)	27185	1(2)	27335	1(2)	27475	1(2)	27616	1(3)
25922	1(2)	26412	3(3)	26568	2(3)	27030	1(2)	27187	1(2)	27337	3(3)	27477	1(2)	27618	3(3)
25924	1(2)	26415	2(3)	26580	1(2)	27033	1(2)	27197	1(2)	27339	4(3)	27479	1(2)	27619	2(3)
25927	1(2)	26416	4(3)	26587	2(3)	27035	1(2)	27198	1(2)	27340	1(2)	27485	1(2)	27620	1(2)
25929	1(2)	26418	4(3)	26590	2(3)	27036	1(2)	27200	1(2)	27345	1(2)	27486	1(2)	27625	1(2)
25931	1(2)	26420	3(3)	26591	4(3)	27040	2(3)	27202	1(2)	27347	1(2)	27487	1(2)	27626	1(2)
25999	1(3)	26426	4(3)	26593	8(3)	27041	3(3)	27215	0(3)	27350	1(2)	27488	1(2)	27630	2(3)
26010	2(3)	26428	2(3)	26596	1(3)	27043	2(3)	27216	0(3)	27355	1(3)	27495	1(2)	27632	3(3)
26011	3(3)	26432	2(3)	26600	2(3)	27045	3(3)	27217	0(3)	27356	1(3)	27496	1(2)	27634	2(3)
26020	4(3)	26433	2(3)	26605	3(3)	27047	2(3)	27218	0(3)	27357	1(3)	27497	1(2)	27635	1(3)
26025	1(2)	26434	2(3)	26607	2(3)	27048	2(3)	27220	1(2)	27358	1(3)	27498	1(2)	27637	1(3)
26030	1(2)	26437	4(3)	26608	4(3)	27049	1(3)	27222	1(2)	27360	2(3)	27499	1(2)	27638	1(3)
26034	2(3)	26440	6(3)	26615	3(3)	27050	1(2)	27226	1(2)	27364	1(3)	27500	1(2)	27640	1(3)
26035	1(3)	26442	5(3)	26641	1(2)	27052	1(2)	27227	1(2)	27365	1(2)	27501	1(2)	27641	1(3)
26037	1(3)	26445	5(3)	26645	1(2)	27054	1(2)	27228	1(2)	27369	1(2)	27502	1(2)	27645	1(3)
26040	1(2)	26449	5(3)	26650	1(2)	27057	1(2)	27230	1(2)	27372	2(3)	27503	1(2)	27646	1(3)
26045	1(2)	26450	6(3)	26665	1(2)	27059	1(3)	27232	1(2)	27380	1(2)	27506	1(2)	27647	1(3)
26055	5(3)	26455	6(3)	26670	2(3)	27060	1(2)	27235	1(2)	27381	1(2)	27507	1(2)	27648	1(2)
26060	5(3)	26460	4(3)	26675	1(3)	27062	1(2)	27236	1(2)	27385	2(3)	27508	1(2)	27650	1(2)
26070	2(3)	26471	4(3)	26676	2(3)	27065	1(3)	27238	1(2)	27386	2(3)	27509	1(2)	27652	1(2)
26075	3(3)	26474	4(3)	26685	3(3)	27066	1(3)	27240	1(2)	27390	1(2)	27510	1(2)	27654	1(2)
26080	3(3)	26476	4(3)	26686	3(3)	27067	1(3)	27244	1(2)	27391	1(2)	27511	1(2)	27656	1(3)
26100	1(3)	26477	2(3)	26700	2(3)	27070	1(3)	27245	1(2)	27392	1(2)	27513	1(2)	27658	2(3)
26105	2(3)	26478	6(3)	26705	3(3)	27071	1(3)	27246	1(2)	27393	1(2)	27514	1(2)	27659	2(3)
26110	2(3)	26479	4(3)	26706	2(3)	27075	1(3)	27248	1(2)	27394	1(2)	27516	1(2)	27664	2(3)
26111	4(3)	26480	4(3)	26715	3(3)	27076	1(2)	27250	1(2)	27395	1(2)	27517	1(2)	27665	2(3)
26113	3(3)	26483	4(3)	26720	4(3)	27077	1(2)	27252	1(2)	27396	1(2)	27519	1(2)	27675	1(2)
26115	4(3)	26485	4(3)	26725	3(3)	27078	1(2)	27253	1(2)	27397	1(2)	27520	1(2)	27676	1(2)
26116	2(3)	26489	2(3)	26727	4(3)	27080	1(2)	27254	1(2)	27400	1(2)	27524	1(2)	27680	2(3)
26117	2(3)	26490	3(3)	26735	4(3)	27086	1(3)	27256	1(2)	27403	1(3)	27530	1(2)	27681	1(2)
26118	1(3)	26492	2(3)	26740	3(3)	27087	1(3)	27257	1(2)	27405	2(2)	27532	1(2)	27685	2(3)
26121	1(2)	26494	1(3)	26742	3(3)	27090	1(2)	27258	1(2)	27407	2(2)	27535	1(2)	27686	3(3)
26123	1(2)	26496	1(3)	26746	3(3)	27091	1(2)	27259	1(2)	27409	1(2)	27536	1(2)	27687	1(2)
26125	4(3)	26497	2(3)	26750	3(3)	27093	1(2)	27265	1(2)	27412	1(2)	27538	1(2)	27690	2(3)
26130	1(3)	26498	1(3)	26755	2(3)	27095	1(2)	27266	1(2)	27415	1(2)	27540	1(2)	27691	2(3)
26135	4(3)	26499	2(3)	26756	2(3)	27096	1(2)	27267	1(2)	27416	1(2)	27550	1(2)	27692	4(3)
26140	2(3)	26500	3(3)	26765	3(3)	27097	1(3)	27268	1(2)	27418	1(2)	27552	1(2)	27695	1(2)
26145	6(3)	26502	2(3)	26770	3(3)	27098	1(2)	27269	1(2)	27420	1(2)	27556	1(2)	27696	1(2)
26160	4(3)	26508	1(2)	26775	2(3)	27100	1(2)	27275	2(2)	27422	1(2)	27557	1(2)	27698	2(2)
26170	4(3)	26510	4(3)	26776	4(3)	27105	1(3)	27279	1(2)	27424	1(2)	27558	1(2)	27700	1(2)
26180	4(3)	26516	1(2)	26785	3(3)	27110	1(2)	27280	1(2)	27425	1(2)	27560	1(2)	27702	1(2)
26185	1(3)	26517	1(2)	26820	1(2)	27111	1(2)	27282	1(2)	27427	1(2)	27562	1(2)	27703	1(2)
26200	2(3)	26518	1(2)	26841	1(2)	27120	1(2)	27284	1(2)	27428	1(2)	27566	1(2)	27704	1(2)
26205	1(3)	26520	4(3)	26842	1(2)	27122	1(2)	27286	1(2)	27429	1(2)	27570	1(2)	27705	1(3)
26210	2(3)	26525	4(3)	26843	2(3)	27125	1(2)	27290	1(2)	27430	1(2)	27580	1(2)	27707	1(3)
26215	2(3)	26530	4(3)	26844	2(3)	27130	1(2)	27295	1(2)	27435	1(2)	27590	1(2)	27709	1(3)
26230	2(3)	26531	4(3)	26850	5(3)	27132	1(2)	27299	1(3)	27437	1(2)	27591	1(2)	27712	1(2)
26235	2(3)	26535	3(3)	26852	2(3)	27134	1(2)	27301	3(3)	27438	1(2)	27592	1(2)	27715	1(2)
26236	2(3)	26536	4(3)	26860	1(2)	27137	1(2)	27303	2(3)	27440	1(2)	27594	1(2)	27720	1(2)
26250	2(3)	26540	4(3)	26861	4(3)	27138	1(2)	27305	1(2)	27441	1(2)	27596	1(2)	27722	1(2)
26260	1(3)	26541	4(3)	26862	1(2)	27140	1(2)	27306	1(2)	27442	1(2)	27598	1(2)	27724	1(2)
26262	1(3)	26542	4(3)	26863	2(3)	27146	1(3)	27307	1(2)	27443	1(2)	27599	1(3)	27725	1(2)
26320	4(3)	26545	4(3)	26910	4(3)	27147	1(2)	27310	1(2)	27445	1(2)	27600	1(2)	27726	1(2)
26340	4(3)	26546	2(3)	26951	8(3)	27151	1(3)	27323	2(3)	27446	1(2)	27601	1(2)	27727	1(2)
26341	2(3)	26548	3(3)	26952	4(3)	27156	1(2)	27324	3(3)	27447	1(2)	27602	1(2)	27730	1(2)
26350	6(3)	26550	1(2)	26989	1(3)	27158	1(2)	27325	1(2)	27448	1(3)	27603	2(3)	27732	1(2)
26352	2(3)	26551	1(2)	26990	2(3)	27161	1(2)	27326	1(2)	27450	1(2)	27604	2(3)	27734	1(2)
26356	4(3)	26553	1(3)	26991	1(3)	27165	1(2)	27327	5(3)	27454	1(2)	27605	1(2)	27740	1(2)
26357	2(3)	26554	1(3)	26992	2(3)	27170	1(2)	27328	3(3)	27455	1(3)	27606	1(2)	27742	1(2)
26358	2(3)	26555	2(3)	27000	1(3)	27175	1(2)	27329	1(3)	27457	1(3)	27607	2(3)	27745	1(2)
26370	3(3)	26556	2(3)	27001	1(3)	27176	1(2)	27330	1(2)	27465	1(2)	27610	1(2)	27750	1(2)
26372	1(3)	26560	2(3)	27003	1(2)	27177	1(2)	27331	1(2)	27466	1(2)	27612	1(2)	27752	1(2)
26373	2(3)	26561	2(3)	27005	1(2)	27178	1(2)	27332	1(2)	27468	1(2)	27613	3(3)	27756	1(2)
26390	2(3)	26562	2(3)	27006	1(2)	27179	1(2)	27333	1(2)	27470	1(2)	27614	3(3)	27758	1(2)
26392	2(3)	26565	2(3)	27025	1(3)	27181	1(2)	27334	1(2)	27472	1(2)	27615	1(3)	27759	1(2)

CPT	MUE	CPT	MUE	CPT	MUE	CPT	MUE	CPT	MUE	CPT	MUE	CPT	MUE
27760	1(2)	28054	2(3)	28289	1(2)	28615	5(3)	29540	1(2)	29885	1(2)	30905	1(2)
27762	1(2)	28055	1(3)	28291	1(2)	28630	2(3)	29550	1(2)	29886	1(2)	30906	1(3)
27766	1(2)	28060	1(2)	28292	1(2)	28635	2(3)	29580	1(2)	29887	1(2)	30915	1(3)
27767	1(2)	28062	1(2)	28295	1(2)	28636	4(3)	29581	1(2)	29888	1(2)	30920	1(3)
27768	1(2)	28070	2(3)	28296	1(2)	28645	4(3)	29584	1(2)	29889	1(2)	30930	1(2)
27769	1(2)	28072	4(3)	28297	1(2)	28660	4(3)	29700	2(3)	29891	1(2)	30999	1(3)
27780	1(2)	28080	3(3)	28298	1(2)	28665	3(3)	29705	1(3)	29892	1(2)	31000	1(2)
27781	1(2)	28086	2(3)	28299	1(2)	28666	4(3)	29710	1(2)	29893	1(2)	31002	1(2)
27784	1(2)	28088	2(3)	28300	1(2)	28675	3(3)	29720	1(2)	29894	1(2)	31020	1(2)
27786	1(2)	28090	2(3)	28302	1(2)	28705	1(2)	29730	1(3)	29895	1(2)	31030	1(2)
27788	1(2)	28092	2(3)	28304	1(3)	28715	1(2)	29740	1(3)	29897	1(2)	31032	1(2)
27792	1(2)	28100	1(3)	28305	1(3)	28725	1(2)	29750	1(3)	29898	1(2)	31040	1(2)
27808	1(2)	28102	1(3)	28306	1(2)	28730	1(2)	29799	1(3)	29899	1(2)	31050	1(2)
27810	1(2)	28103	1(3)	28307	1(2)	28735	1(2)	29800	1(2)	29900	2(3)	31051	1(2)
27814	1(2)	28104	2(3)	28308	4(3)	28737	1(2)	29804	1(2)	29901	2(3)	31070	1(2)
27816	1(2)	28106	1(3)	28309	1(2)	28740	1(2)	29805	1(2)	29902	2(3)	31075	1(2)
27818	1(2)	28107	1(3)	28310	1(2)	28750	1(2)	29806	1(2)	29904	1(2)	31080	1(2)
27822	1(2)	28108	2(3)	28312	4(3)	28755	1(2)	29807	1(2)	29905	1(2)	31081	1(2)
27823	1(2)	28110	1(2)	28313	4(3)	28760	1(2)	29819	1(2)	29906	1(2)	31084	1(2)
27824	1(2)	28111	1(2)	28315	1(2)	28800	1(2)	29820	1(2)	29907	1(2)	31085	1(2)
27825	1(2)	28112	4(3)	28320	1(2)	28805	1(2)	29821	1(2)	29914	1(2)	31086	1(2)
27826	1(2)	28113	1(2)	28322	2(3)	28810	5(3)	29822	1(2)	29915	1(2)	31087	1(2)
27827	1(2)	28114	1(2)	28340	2(3)	28820	6(3)	29823	1(2)	29916	1(2)	31090	1(2)
27828	1(2)	28116	1(2)	28341	2(3)	28825	8(2)	29824	1(2)	29999	1(3)	31200	1(2)
27829	1(2)	28118	1(2)	28344	1(2)	28890	1(2)	29825	1(2)	30000	1(3)	31201	1(2)
27830	1(2)	28119	1(2)	28345	2(3)	28899	1(3)	29826	1(2)	30020	1(3)	31205	1(2)
27831	1(2)	28120	2(3)	28360	1(2)	29000	1(3)	29827	1(2)	30100	2(3)	31225	1(2)
27832	1(2)	28122	4(3)	28400	1(2)	29010	1(3)	29828	1(2)	30110	1(2)	31230	1(2)
27840	1(2)	28124	4(3)	28405	1(2)	29015	1(3)	29830	1(2)	30115	1(2)	31231	1(2)
27842	1(2)	28126	4(3)	28406	1(2)	29035	1(3)	29834	1(2)	30117	2(3)	31233	1(2)
27846	1(2)	28130	1(2)	28415	1(2)	29040	1(3)	29835	1(2)	30118	1(3)	31235	1(2)
27848	1(2)	28140	3(3)	28420	1(2)	29044	1(3)	29836	1(2)	30120	1(2)	31237	1(2)
27860	1(2)	28150	4(3)	28430	1(2)	29046	1(3)	29837	1(2)	30124	2(3)	31238	1(3)
27870	1(2)	28153	4(3)	28435	1(2)	29049	1(3)	29838	1(2)	30125	1(3)	31239	1(2)
27871	1(3)	28160	5(3)	28436	1(2)	29055	1(3)	29840	1(2)	30130	1(2)	31240	1(2)
27880	1(2)	28171	1(3)	28445	1(2)	29058	1(3)	29843	1(2)	30140	1(2)	31241	1(2)
27881	1(2)	28173	2(3)	28446	1(2)	29065	1(3)	29844	1(2)	30150	1(2)	31253	1(2)
27882	1(2)	28175	2(3)	28450	2(3)	29075	1(3)	29845	1(2)	30160	1(2)	31254	1(2)
27884	1(2)	28190	3(3)	28455	3(3)	29085	1(3)	29846	1(2)	30200	1(2)	31255	1(2)
27886	1(2)	28192	2(3)	28456	2(3)	29086	2(3)	29847	1(2)	30210	1(3)	31256	1(2)
27888	1(2)	28193	2(3)	28465	3(3)	29105	1(2)	29848	1(2)	30220	1(2)	31257	1(2)
27889	1(2)	28200	4(3)	28470	2(3)	29125	1(2)	29850	1(2)	30300	1(3)	31259	1(2)
27892	1(2)	28202	2(3)	28475	5(3)	29126	1(2)	29851	1(2)	30310	1(3)	31267	1(2)
27893	1(2)	28208	4(3)	28476	4(3)	29130	3(3)	29855	1(2)	30320	1(3)	31276	1(2)
27894	1(2)	28210	2(3)	28485	5(3)	29131	2(3)	29856	1(2)	30400	1(2)	31287	1(2)
27899	1(3)	28220	1(2)	28490	1(2)	29200	1(2)	29860	1(2)	30410	1(2)	31288	1(2)
28001	2(3)	28222	1(2)	28495	1(2)	29240	1(2)	29861	1(2)	30420	1(2)	31290	1(2)
28002	3(3)	28225	1(2)	28496	1(2)	29260	1(3)	29862	1(2)	30430	1(2)	31291	1(2)
28003	2(3)	28226	1(2)	28505	1(2)	29280	2(3)	29863	1(2)	30435	1(2)	31292	1(2)
28005	3(3)	28230	1(2)	28510	4(3)	29305	1(3)	29866	1(2)	30450	1(2)	31293	1(2)
28008	2(3)	28232	6(3)	28515	4(3)	29325	1(3)	29867	1(2)	30460	1(2)	31294	1(2)
28010	4(3)	28234	6(3)	28525	4(3)	29345	1(3)	29868	1(3)	30462	1(2)	31295	1(2)
28011	4(3)	28238	1(2)	28530	1(2)	29355	1(3)	29870	1(2)	30465	1(2)	31296	1(2)
28020	2(3)	28240	1(2)	28531	1(2)	29358	1(3)	29871	1(2)	30520	1(2)	31297	1(2)
28022	3(3)	28250	1(2)	28540	1(3)	29365	1(3)	29873	1(2)	30540	1(2)	31298	1(2)
28024	4(3)	28260	1(2)	28545	1(3)	29405	1(3)	29874	1(2)	30545	1(2)	31299	1(3)
28035	1(2)	28261	1(3)	28546	1(3)	29425	1(3)	29875	1(2)	30560	1(2)	31300	1(2)
28039	2(3)	28262	1(2)	28555	1(3)	29435	1(3)	29876	1(2)	30580	2(3)	31360	1(2)
28041	2(3)	28264	1(2)	28570	1(2)	29440	1(2)	29877	1(2)	30600	1(3)	31365	1(2)
28043	4(3)	28270	6(3)	28575	1(2)	29445	1(3)	29879	1(2)	30620	1(2)	31367	1(2)
28045	4(3)	28272	6(3)	28576	1(2)	29450	1(3)	29880	1(2)	30630	1(2)	31368	1(2)
28046	1(3)	28280	1(2)	28585	1(3)	29505	1(2)	29881	1(2)	30801	1(2)	31370	1(2)
28047	1(3)	28285	4(3)	28600	2(3)	29515	1(2)	29882	1(2)	30802	1(2)	31375	1(2)
28050	2(3)	28286	1(2)	28605	2(3)	29520	1(2)	29883	1(2)	30901	1(3)	31380	1(2)
28052	2(3)	28288	4(3)	28606	3(3)	29530	1(2)	29884	1(2)	30903	1(3)	31382	1(2)
												31390	1(2)
												31395	1(2)
												31400	1(3)
												31420	1(2)
												31500	2(3)
												31502	1(3)
												31505	1(3)
												31510	1(2)
												31511	1(3)
												31512	1(3)
												31513	1(3)
												31515	1(3)
												31520	1(3)
												31525	1(3)
												31526	1(3)
												31527	1(2)
												31528	1(2)
												31529	1(3)
												31530	1(3)
												31531	1(3)
												31535	1(3)
												31536	1(3)
												31540	1(3)
												31541	1(3)
												31545	1(2)
												31546	1(2)
												31551	1(2)
												31552	1(2)
												31553	1(2)
												31554	1(2)
												31560	1(2)
												31561	1(2)
												31570	1(2)
												31571	1(2)
												31572	1(2)
												31573	1(2)
												31574	1(2)
												31575	1(3)
												31576	1(3)
												31577	1(3)
												31578	1(3)
												31579	1(2)
												31580	1(2)
												31584	1(2)
												31587	1(2)
												31590	1(2)
												31591	1(2)
												31592	1(2)
												31599	1(3)
												31600	1(2)
												31601	1(2)
												31603	1(2)
												31605	1(2)
												31610	1(2)
												31611	1(2)
												31612	1(3)
												31613	1(2)
												31614	1(2)
												31615	1(3)
												31622	1(3)
												31623	1(3)
												31624	1(3)
												31625	1(2)
												31626	1(2)
												31627	1(3)

CPT	MUE	CPT	MUE	CPT	MUE	CPT	MUE	CPT	MUE	CPT	MUE	CPT	MUE	CPT	MUE
31628	1(2)	32400	2(3)	32852	1(2)	33254	1(2)	33465	1(2)	33690	1(2)	33916	1(3)	34151	1(3)
31629	1(2)	32405	2(3)	32853	1(2)	33255	1(2)	33468	1(2)	33692	1(2)	33917	1(2)	34201	1(3)
31630	1(3)	32440	1(2)	32854	1(2)	33256	1(2)	33470	1(2)	33694	1(2)	33920	1(2)	34203	1(2)
31631	1(2)	32442	1(2)	32855	1(2)	33257	1(2)	33471	1(2)	33697	1(2)	33922	1(2)	34401	1(3)
31632	2(3)	32445	1(2)	32856	1(2)	33258	1(2)	33474	1(2)	33702	1(2)	33924	1(2)	34421	1(3)
31633	2(3)	32480	1(2)	32900	1(2)	33259	1(2)	33475	1(2)	33710	1(2)	33925	1(2)	34451	1(3)
31634	1(3)	32482	1(2)	32905	1(2)	33261	1(2)	33476	1(2)	33720	1(2)	33926	1(2)	34471	1(2)
31635	1(3)	32484	2(3)	32906	1(2)	33262	1(3)	33477	1(2)	33722	1(3)	33927	1(3)	34490	1(2)
31636	1(2)	32486	1(3)	32940	1(3)	33263	1(3)	33478	1(2)	33724	1(2)	33928	1(3)	34501	1(2)
31637	2(3)	32488	1(2)	32960	1(2)	33264	1(3)	33496	1(3)	33726	1(2)	33929	1(3)	34502	1(2)
31638	1(3)	32491	1(2)	32994	1(2)	33265	1(2)	33500	1(3)	33730	1(2)	33930	1(2)	34510	2(3)
31640	1(3)	32501	1(3)	32997	1(2)	33266	1(2)	33501	1(3)	33732	1(2)	33933	1(2)	34520	1(3)
31641	1(3)	32503	1(2)	32998	1(2)	33270	1(3)	33502	1(3)	33735	1(2)	33935	1(2)	34530	1(2)
31643	1(2)	32504	1(2)	32999	1(3)	33271	1(2)	33503	1(3)	33736	1(2)	33940	1(2)	34701	1(2)
31645	1(2)	32505	1(2)	33010	1(2)	33272	1(3)	33504	1(3)	33737	1(2)	33944	1(2)	34702	1(2)
31646	2(3)	32506	3(3)	33011	1(3)	33273	1(3)	33505	1(3)	33750	1(3)	33945	1(2)	34703	1(2)
31647	1(2)	32507	2(3)	33015	1(3)	33274	1(3)	33506	1(3)	33755	1(2)	33946	1(2)	34704	1(2)
31648	1(2)	32540	1(3)	33020	1(3)	33275	1(3)	33507	1(3)	33762	1(2)	33947	1(2)	34705	1(2)
31649	2(3)	32550	2(3)	33025	1(2)	33285	1(3)	33508	1(2)	33764	1(3)	33948	1(2)	34706	1(2)
31651	3(3)	32551	2(3)	33030	1(2)	33286	1(3)	33510	1(2)	33766	1(2)	33949	1(2)	34707	1(2)
31652	1(2)	32552	2(2)	33031	1(2)	33289	1(3)	33511	1(2)	33767	1(2)	33951	1(3)	34708	1(2)
31653	1(2)	32553	1(2)	33050	1(2)	33300	1(3)	33512	1(2)	33768	1(2)	33952	1(3)	34709	3(3)
31654	1(3)	32554	2(3)	33120	1(3)	33305	1(3)	33513	1(2)	33770	1(2)	33953	1(2)	34710	1(2)
31660	1(2)	32555	2(3)	33130	1(3)	33310	1(2)	33514	1(2)	33771	1(2)	33954	1(2)	34711	2(3)
31661	1(2)	32556	2(3)	33140	1(2)	33315	1(2)	33516	1(3)	33774	1(2)	33955	1(3)	34712	1(2)
31717	1(3)	32557	2(3)	33141	1(2)	33320	1(3)	33517	1(2)	33775	1(2)	33956	1(3)	34713	1(2)
31720	3(3)	32560	1(3)	33202	1(2)	33321	1(3)	33518	1(2)	33776	1(2)	33957	1(3)	34714	1(2)
31725	1(3)	32561	1(2)	33203	1(2)	33322	1(3)	33519	1(2)	33777	1(2)	33958	1(3)	34715	1(2)
31730	1(3)	32562	1(2)	33206	1(3)	33330	1(3)	33521	1(2)	33778	1(2)	33959	1(3)	34716	1(2)
31750	1(2)	32601	1(3)	33207	1(3)	33335	1(3)	33522	1(2)	33779	1(2)	33962	1(3)	34808	1(3)
31755	1(2)	32604	1(3)	33208	1(3)	33340	1(2)	33523	1(2)	33780	1(2)	33963	1(3)	34812	1(2)
31760	1(2)	32606	1(3)	33210	1(3)	33361	1(2)	33530	1(2)	33781	1(2)	33964	1(3)	34813	1(2)
31766	1(2)	32607	1(3)	33211	1(3)	33362	1(2)	33533	1(2)	33782	1(2)	33965	1(3)	34820	1(2)
31770	2(3)	32608	1(3)	33212	1(3)	33363	1(2)	33534	1(2)	33783	1(2)	33966	1(3)	34830	1(2)
31775	1(3)	32609	1(3)	33213	1(3)	33364	1(2)	33535	1(2)	33786	1(2)	33967	1(3)	34831	1(2)
31780	1(2)	32650	1(2)	33214	1(3)	33365	1(2)	33536	1(2)	33788	1(2)	33968	1(3)	34832	1(2)
31781	1(2)	32651	1(2)	33215	2(3)	33366	1(3)	33542	1(2)	33800	1(2)	33969	1(3)	34833	1(2)
31785	1(3)	32652	1(2)	33216	1(3)	33367	1(2)	33545	1(2)	33802	1(3)	33970	1(3)	34834	1(2)
31786	1(3)	32653	1(3)	33217	1(3)	33368	1(2)	33548	1(2)	33803	1(3)	33971	1(3)	34839	1(2)
31800	1(3)	32654	1(3)	33218	1(3)	33369	1(2)	33572	3(2)	33813	1(2)	33973	1(3)	34841	1(2)
31805	1(3)	32655	1(3)	33220	1(3)	33390	1(2)	33600	1(3)	33814	1(2)	33974	1(3)	34842	1(2)
31820	1(2)	32656	1(2)	33221	1(3)	33391	1(2)	33602	1(3)	33820	1(2)	33975	1(3)	34843	1(2)
31825	1(2)	32658	1(3)	33222	1(3)	33404	1(2)	33606	1(2)	33822	1(2)	33976	1(3)	34844	1(2)
31830	1(2)	32659	1(2)	33223	1(3)	33405	1(2)	33608	1(2)	33824	1(2)	33977	1(3)	34845	1(2)
31899	1(3)	32661	1(3)	33224	1(3)	33406	1(2)	33610	1(2)	33840	1(2)	33978	1(3)	34846	1(2)
32035	1(2)	32662	1(3)	33225	1(3)	33410	1(2)	33611	1(2)	33845	1(2)	33979	1(3)	34847	1(2)
32036	1(3)	32663	1(3)	33226	1(3)	33411	1(2)	33612	1(2)	33851	1(2)	33980	1(3)	34848	1(2)
32096	1(3)	32664	1(2)	33227	1(3)	33412	1(2)	33615	1(2)	33852	1(2)	33981	1(3)	35001	1(2)
32097	1(3)	32665	1(2)	33228	1(3)	33413	1(2)	33617	1(2)	33853	1(2)	33982	1(3)	35002	1(2)
32098	1(2)	32666	1(3)	33229	1(3)	33414	1(2)	33619	1(2)	33860	1(2)	33983	1(3)	35005	1(2)
32100	1(3)	32667	3(3)	33230	1(3)	33415	1(2)	33620	1(2)	33863	1(2)	33984	1(3)	35011	1(2)
32110	1(3)	32668	2(3)	33231	1(3)	33416	1(2)	33621	1(3)	33864	1(2)	33985	1(3)	35013	1(2)
32120	1(3)	32669	2(3)	33233	1(2)	33417	1(2)	33622	1(2)	33866	1(2)	33986	1(3)	35021	1(2)
32124	1(3)	32670	1(2)	33234	1(2)	33418	1(3)	33641	1(2)	33870	1(2)	33987	1(3)	35022	1(2)
32140	1(3)	32671	1(2)	33235	1(2)	33419	1(2)	33645	1(2)	33875	1(2)	33988	1(3)	35045	1(3)
32141	1(3)	32672	1(3)	33236	1(2)	33420	1(2)	33647	1(2)	33877	1(2)	33989	1(3)	35081	1(2)
32150	1(3)	32673	1(2)	33237	1(2)	33422	1(2)	33660	1(2)	33880	1(2)	33990	1(3)	35082	1(2)
32151	1(3)	32674	1(2)	33238	1(2)	33425	1(2)	33665	1(2)	33881	1(2)	33991	1(3)	35091	1(2)
32160	1(3)	32701	1(2)	33240	1(3)	33426	1(2)	33670	1(2)	33883	1(2)	33992	1(2)	35092	1(2)
32200	2(3)	32800	1(3)	33241	1(2)	33427	1(2)	33675	1(2)	33884	2(3)	33993	1(3)	35102	1(2)
32215	1(2)	32810	1(3)	33243	1(2)	33430	1(2)	33676	1(2)	33886	1(2)	33999	1(3)	35103	1(2)
32220	1(2)	32815	1(3)	33244	1(2)	33440	1(2)	33677	1(2)	33889	1(2)	34001	1(3)	35111	1(2)
32225	1(2)	32820	1(2)	33249	1(3)	33460	1(2)	33681	1(2)	33891	1(2)	34051	1(3)	35112	1(2)
32310	1(3)	32850	1(2)	33250	1(2)	33463	1(2)	33684	1(2)	33910	1(3)	34101	1(3)	35121	1(3)
32320	1(3)	32851	1(2)	33251	1(2)	33464	1(2)	33688	1(2)	33915	1(3)	34111	2(3)	35122	1(3)

CPT © 2019 American Medical Association. All Rights Reserved.

CPT	MUE	CPT	MUE	CPT	MUE	CPT	MUE	CPT	MUE	CPT	MUE	CPT	MUE	CPT	MUE
35131	1(2)	35531	1(3)	35860	2(3)	36468	2(3)	36821	2(3)	37239	2(3)	38242	1(2)	40654	2(3)
35132	1(2)	35533	1(3)	35870	1(3)	36470	1(3)	36823	1(3)	37241	2(3)	38243	1(3)	40700	1(2)
35141	1(2)	35535	1(3)	35875	2(3)	36471	1(2)	36825	1(3)	37242	2(3)	38300	1(3)	40701	1(2)
35142	1(2)	35536	1(3)	35876	2(3)	36473	1(3)	36830	2(3)	37243	1(3)	38305	1(3)	40702	1(2)
35151	1(2)	35537	1(3)	35879	2(3)	36474	1(3)	36831	1(3)	37244	2(3)	38308	1(3)	40720	1(2)
35152	1(2)	35538	1(3)	35881	1(3)	36475	1(3)	36832	2(3)	37246	1(2)	38380	1(2)	40761	1(2)
35180	2(3)	35539	1(3)	35883	1(3)	36476	2(3)	36833	1(3)	37247	2(3)	38381	1(2)	40799	1(3)
35182	2(3)	35540	1(3)	35884	1(3)	36478	1(3)	36835	1(3)	37248	1(2)	38382	1(2)	40800	2(3)
35184	2(3)	35556	1(3)	35901	1(3)	36479	2(3)	36838	1(3)	37249	3(3)	38500	2(3)	40801	2(3)
35188	2(3)	35558	1(3)	35903	2(3)	36481	1(3)	36860	2(3)	37252	1(2)	38505	2(3)	40804	1(3)
35189	1(3)	35560	1(3)	35905	1(3)	36482	1(3)	36861	2(3)	37253	5(3)	38510	1(2)	40805	2(3)
35190	2(3)	35563	1(3)	35907	1(3)	36483	2(3)	36901	1(3)	37500	1(3)	38520	1(2)	40806	2(2)
35201	2(3)	35565	1(3)	36000	4(3)	36500	4(3)	36902	1(3)	37501	1(3)	38525	1(2)	40808	2(3)
35206	2(3)	35566	1(3)	36002	2(3)	36510	1(3)	36903	1(3)	37565	1(2)	38530	1(2)	40810	2(3)
35207	3(3)	35570	1(3)	36005	2(3)	36511	1(3)	36904	1(3)	37600	1(3)	38531	1(2)	40812	2(3)
35211	3(3)	35571	1(3)	36010	2(3)	36512	1(3)	36905	1(3)	37605	1(3)	38542	1(2)	40814	4(3)
35216	2(3)	35572	2(3)	36011	4(3)	36513	1(3)	36906	1(3)	37606	1(3)	38550	1(3)	40816	2(3)
35221	3(3)	35583	1(2)	36012	4(3)	36514	1(3)	36907	1(3)	37607	1(3)	38555	1(3)	40818	2(3)
35226	3(3)	35585	2(3)	36013	2(3)	36516	1(3)	36908	1(3)	37609	1(2)	38562	1(2)	40819	2(2)
35231	2(3)	35587	1(3)	36014	2(3)	36522	1(3)	36909	1(3)	37615	2(3)	38564	1(2)	40820	2(3)
35236	2(3)	35600	2(3)	36015	4(3)	36555	2(3)	37140	1(2)	37616	1(3)	38570	1(2)	40830	2(3)
35241	2(3)	35601	1(3)	36100	2(3)	36556	2(3)	37145	1(3)	37617	3(3)	38571	1(2)	40831	2(3)
35246	2(3)	35606	1(3)	36140	3(3)	36557	2(3)	37160	1(3)	37618	2(3)	38572	1(2)	40840	1(2)
35251	2(3)	35612	1(3)	36160	2(3)	36558	2(3)	37180	1(2)	37619	1(2)	38573	1(2)	40842	1(2)
35256	2(3)	35616	1(3)	36200	2(3)	36560	2(3)	37181	1(2)	37650	1(2)	38589	1(3)	40843	1(2)
35261	1(3)	35621	1(3)	36215	2(3)	36561	2(3)	37182	1(2)	37660	1(2)	38700	1(2)	40844	1(2)
35266	2(3)	35623	1(3)	36216	2(3)	36563	1(3)	37183	1(2)	37700	1(2)	38720	1(2)	40845	1(3)
35271	2(3)	35626	3(3)	36217	2(3)	36565	1(3)	37184	1(2)	37718	1(2)	38724	1(2)	40899	1(3)
35276	2(3)	35631	4(3)	36218	2(3)	36566	1(3)	37185	2(3)	37722	1(2)	38740	1(2)	41000	1(3)
35281	2(3)	35632	1(3)	36221	1(3)	36568	2(3)	37186	2(3)	37735	1(2)	38745	1(2)	41005	1(3)
35286	2(3)	35633	1(3)	36222	1(3)	36569	2(3)	37187	1(3)	37760	1(2)	38746	1(2)	41006	2(3)
35301	2(3)	35634	1(3)	36223	1(3)	36570	2(3)	37188	1(3)	37761	1(2)	38747	1(2)	41007	2(3)
35302	1(2)	35636	1(3)	36224	1(3)	36571	2(3)	37191	1(3)	37765	1(2)	38760	1(2)	41008	2(3)
35303	1(2)	35637	1(3)	36225	1(3)	36572	1(3)	37192	1(3)	37766	1(2)	38765	1(2)	41009	2(3)
35304	1(2)	35638	1(3)	36226	1(3)	36573	1(3)	37193	1(3)	37780	1(2)	38770	1(2)	41010	1(2)
35305	1(2)	35642	1(3)	36227	1(3)	36575	2(3)	37195	1(3)	37785	1(2)	38780	1(2)	41015	2(3)
35306	2(3)	35645	1(3)	36228	2(3)	36576	2(3)	37197	2(3)	37788	1(2)	38790	1(2)	41016	1(3)
35311	1(2)	35646	1(3)	36245	3(3)	36578	2(3)	37200	2(3)	37790	1(2)	38792	1(3)	41017	2(3)
35321	1(2)	35647	1(3)	36246	4(3)	36580	2(3)	37211	1(2)	37799	1(3)	38794	1(3)	41018	2(3)
35331	1(2)	35650	1(3)	36247	2(3)	36581	2(3)	37212	1(2)	38100	1(2)	38900	1(3)	41019	1(2)
35341	3(3)	35654	1(3)	36248	2(3)	36582	2(3)	37213	1(2)	38101	1(3)	38999	1(3)	41100	2(3)
35351	1(3)	35656	1(3)	36251	1(3)	36583	2(3)	37214	1(2)	38102	1(2)	39000	1(2)	41105	2(3)
35355	1(2)	35661	1(3)	36252	1(3)	36584	2(3)	37215	1(2)	38115	1(3)	39010	1(2)	41108	2(3)
35361	1(2)	35663	1(3)	36253	1(3)	36585	2(3)	37216	0(3)	38120	1(2)	39200	1(2)	41110	2(3)
35363	1(2)	35665	1(3)	36254	1(3)	36589	2(3)	37217	1(2)	38129	1(3)	39220	1(2)	41112	2(3)
35371	1(2)	35666	2(3)	36260	1(2)	36590	2(3)	37218	1(2)	38200	1(3)	39401	1(3)	41113	2(3)
35372	1(2)	35671	2(3)	36261	1(2)	36591	2(3)	37220	1(2)	38204	1(2)	39402	1(3)	41114	2(3)
35390	1(3)	35681	1(3)	36262	1(2)	36592	1(3)	37221	1(2)	38205	1(3)	39499	1(3)	41115	1(2)
35400	1(3)	35682	1(2)	36299	1(3)	36593	2(3)	37222	2(2)	38206	1(3)	39501	1(3)	41116	2(3)
35500	2(3)	35683	1(2)	36400	1(3)	36595	2(3)	37223	2(2)	38207	1(3)	39503	1(2)	41120	1(2)
35501	1(3)	35685	2(3)	36405	1(3)	36596	2(3)	37224	1(2)	38208	1(3)	39540	1(2)	41130	1(2)
35506	1(3)	35686	1(3)	36406	1(3)	36597	2(3)	37225	1(2)	38209	1(3)	39541	1(2)	41135	1(2)
35508	1(3)	35691	1(3)	36410	3(3)	36598	2(3)	37226	1(2)	38210	1(3)	39545	1(2)	41140	1(2)
35509	1(3)	35693	1(3)	36415	2(3)	36600	4(3)	37227	1(2)	38211	1(3)	39560	1(3)	41145	1(2)
35510	1(3)	35694	1(3)	36416	6(3)	36620	3(3)	37228	1(2)	38212	1(3)	39561	1(3)	41150	1(2)
35511	1(3)	35695	1(3)	36420	2(3)	36625	2(3)	37229	1(2)	38213	1(3)	39599	1(3)	41153	1(2)
35512	1(3)	35697	2(3)	36425	2(3)	36640	1(3)	37230	1(2)	38214	1(3)	40490	2(3)	41155	1(2)
35515	1(3)	35700	2(3)	36430	1(2)	36660	1(3)	37231	1(2)	38215	1(3)	40500	2(3)	41250	2(3)
35516	1(3)	35701	1(2)	36440	1(3)	36680	1(3)	37232	2(3)	38220	1(3)	40510	2(3)	41251	2(3)
35518	1(3)	35721	1(2)	36450	1(3)	36800	1(3)	37233	2(3)	38221	1(3)	40520	2(3)	41252	2(3)
35521	1(3)	35741	1(2)	36455	1(3)	36810	1(3)	37234	2(3)	38222	1(2)	40525	2(3)	41510	1(2)
35522	1(3)	35761	2(3)	36456	1(3)	36815	1(3)	37235	2(3)	38230	1(2)	40527	2(3)	41512	1(2)
35523	1(3)	35800	2(3)	36460	2(3)	36818	1(3)	37236	1(2)	38232	1(2)	40530	2(3)	41520	1(3)
35525	1(3)	35820	2(3)	36465	1(2)	36819	1(3)	37237	2(3)	38240	1(3)	40650	2(3)	41530	1(3)
35526	1(3)	35840	2(3)	36466	1(2)	36820	1(3)	37238	1(2)	38241	1(2)	40652	2(3)	41599	1(3)

CPT	MUE	CPT	MUE	CPT	MUE	CPT	MUE	CPT	MUE	CPT	MUE	CPT	MUE	CPT	MUE
41800	2(3)	42600	1(3)	43195	1(3)	43282	1(2)	43647	1(2)	44132	1(2)	44385	1(3)	45136	1(2)
41805	1(3)	42650	2(3)	43196	1(3)	43283	1(2)	43648	1(2)	44133	1(2)	44386	1(2)	45150	1(2)
41806	1(3)	42660	2(3)	43197	1(3)	43284	1(2)	43651	1(2)	44135	1(2)	44388	1(3)	45160	1(3)
41820	4(2)	42665	2(3)	43198	1(3)	43285	1(2)	43652	1(2)	44136	1(2)	44389	1(2)	45171	2(3)
41821	2(3)	42699	1(3)	43200	1(3)	43286	1(2)	43653	1(2)	44137	1(2)	44390	1(3)	45172	2(3)
41822	1(2)	42700	2(3)	43201	1(2)	43287	1(2)	43659	1(3)	44139	1(2)	44391	1(3)	45190	1(3)
41823	1(2)	42720	1(3)	43202	1(2)	43288	1(2)	43752	2(3)	44140	2(3)	44392	1(2)	45300	1(3)
41825	2(3)	42725	1(3)	43204	1(2)	43289	1(3)	43753	1(3)	44141	1(3)	44394	1(2)	45303	1(3)
41826	2(3)	42800	3(3)	43205	1(2)	43300	1(2)	43754	1(3)	44143	1(2)	44401	1(2)	45305	1(2)
41827	2(3)	42804	1(3)	43206	1(2)	43305	1(2)	43755	1(3)	44144	1(3)	44402	1(3)	45307	1(3)
41828	4(2)	42806	1(3)	43210	1(2)	43310	1(2)	43756	1(2)	44145	1(2)	44403	1(3)	45308	1(2)
41830	2(3)	42808	2(3)	43211	1(3)	43312	1(2)	43757	1(2)	44146	1(2)	44404	1(3)	45309	1(2)
41850	2(3)	42809	1(3)	43212	1(3)	43313	1(2)	43761	2(3)	44147	1(3)	44405	1(3)	45315	1(2)
41870	2(3)	42810	1(3)	43213	1(2)	43314	1(2)	43762	2(3)	44150	1(2)	44406	1(3)	45317	1(3)
41872	4(2)	42815	1(3)	43214	1(3)	43320	1(2)	43763	2(3)	44151	1(2)	44407	1(2)	45320	1(2)
41874	4(2)	42820	1(2)	43215	1(3)	43325	1(2)	43770	1(2)	44155	1(2)	44408	1(3)	45321	1(2)
41899	1(3)	42821	1(2)	43216	1(2)	43327	1(2)	43771	1(2)	44156	1(2)	44500	1(3)	45327	1(2)
42000	1(3)	42825	1(2)	43217	1(2)	43328	1(2)	43772	1(2)	44157	1(2)	44602	1(2)	45330	1(3)
42100	2(3)	42826	1(2)	43220	1(3)	43330	1(2)	43773	1(2)	44158	1(2)	44603	1(2)	45331	1(2)
42104	2(3)	42830	1(2)	43226	1(3)	43331	1(2)	43774	1(2)	44160	1(2)	44604	1(2)	45332	1(2)
42106	2(3)	42831	1(2)	43227	1(3)	43332	1(2)	43775	1(2)	44180	1(2)	44605	1(2)	45333	1(2)
42107	2(3)	42835	1(2)	43229	1(3)	43333	1(2)	43800	1(2)	44186	1(2)	44615	3(3)	45334	1(3)
42120	1(2)	42836	1(2)	43231	1(2)	43334	1(2)	43810	1(2)	44187	1(3)	44620	2(3)	45335	1(2)
42140	1(2)	42842	1(3)	43232	1(2)	43335	1(2)	43820	1(2)	44188	1(3)	44625	1(3)	45337	1(2)
42145	1(2)	42844	1(3)	43233	1(3)	43336	1(2)	43825	1(2)	44202	1(2)	44626	1(3)	45338	1(2)
42160	1(3)	42845	1(3)	43235	1(3)	43337	1(2)	43830	1(2)	44203	2(3)	44640	2(3)	45340	1(2)
42180	1(3)	42860	1(3)	43236	1(2)	43338	1(2)	43831	1(2)	44204	2(3)	44650	2(3)	45341	1(2)
42182	1(3)	42870	1(3)	43237	1(2)	43340	1(2)	43832	1(2)	44205	1(2)	44660	1(3)	45342	1(2)
42200	1(2)	42890	1(2)	43238	1(2)	43341	1(2)	43840	2(3)	44206	1(2)	44661	1(3)	45346	1(2)
42205	1(2)	42892	1(3)	43239	1(2)	43351	1(2)	43842	0(3)	44207	1(2)	44680	1(3)	45347	1(3)
42210	1(2)	42894	1(3)	43240	1(2)	43352	1(2)	43843	1(2)	44208	1(2)	44700	1(2)	45349	1(3)
42215	1(2)	42900	1(3)	43241	1(3)	43360	1(2)	43845	1(2)	44210	1(2)	44701	1(2)	45350	1(2)
42220	1(2)	42950	1(2)	43242	1(2)	43361	1(2)	43846	1(2)	44211	1(2)	44705	1(3)	45378	1(3)
42225	1(2)	42953	1(3)	43243	1(2)	43400	1(2)	43847	1(2)	44212	1(2)	44715	1(2)	45379	1(3)
42226	1(2)	42955	1(2)	43244	1(2)	43401	1(2)	43848	1(2)	44213	1(2)	44720	2(3)	45380	1(2)
42227	1(2)	42960	1(3)	43245	1(2)	43405	1(2)	43850	1(2)	44227	1(3)	44721	2(3)	45381	1(2)
42235	1(2)	42961	1(3)	43246	1(2)	43410	1(3)	43855	1(2)	44238	1(3)	44799	1(3)	45382	1(3)
42260	1(3)	42962	1(3)	43247	1(2)	43415	1(3)	43860	1(2)	44300	1(2)	44800	1(3)	45384	1(2)
42280	1(2)	42970	1(3)	43248	1(3)	43420	1(3)	43865	1(2)	44310	2(3)	44820	1(3)	45385	1(2)
42281	1(2)	42971	1(3)	43249	1(3)	43425	1(3)	43870	1(2)	44312	1(2)	44850	1(3)	45386	1(2)
42299	1(3)	42972	1(3)	43250	1(2)	43450	1(3)	43880	1(3)	44314	1(2)	44899	1(3)	45388	1(2)
42300	2(3)	42999	1(3)	43251	1(2)	43453	1(3)	43881	1(3)	44316	1(2)	44900	1(2)	45389	1(3)
42305	2(3)	43020	1(2)	43252	1(2)	43460	1(3)	43882	1(3)	44320	1(2)	44950	1(2)	45390	1(3)
42310	2(3)	43030	1(2)	43253	1(3)	43496	1(3)	43886	1(2)	44322	1(2)	44955	1(2)	45391	1(2)
42320	2(3)	43045	1(2)	43254	1(3)	43499	1(3)	43887	1(2)	44340	1(2)	44960	1(2)	45392	1(2)
42330	1(3)	43100	1(3)	43255	2(3)	43500	1(2)	43888	1(2)	44345	1(2)	44970	1(2)	45393	1(3)
42335	2(2)	43101	1(3)	43257	1(2)	43501	1(3)	43999	1(3)	44346	1(2)	44979	1(3)	45395	1(2)
42340	1(2)	43107	1(2)	43259	1(2)	43502	1(2)	44005	1(2)	44360	1(3)	45000	1(3)	45397	1(2)
42400	2(3)	43108	1(2)	43260	1(3)	43510	1(2)	44010	1(2)	44361	1(2)	45005	1(3)	45398	1(2)
42405	2(3)	43112	1(2)	43261	1(2)	43520	1(2)	44015	1(2)	44363	1(3)	45020	1(3)	45399	1(3)
42408	1(3)	43113	1(2)	43262	2(2)	43605	1(2)	44020	2(3)	44364	1(2)	45100	2(3)	45400	1(2)
42409	1(3)	43116	1(2)	43263	1(2)	43610	2(3)	44021	1(3)	44365	1(2)	45108	1(2)	45402	1(2)
42410	1(2)	43117	1(2)	43264	1(2)	43611	2(3)	44025	1(3)	44366	1(3)	45110	1(2)	45499	1(3)
42415	1(2)	43118	1(2)	43265	1(2)	43620	1(2)	44050	1(2)	44369	1(2)	45111	1(2)	45500	1(2)
42420	1(2)	43121	1(2)	43266	1(3)	43621	1(2)	44055	1(2)	44370	1(2)	45112	1(2)	45505	1(2)
42425	1(2)	43122	1(2)	43270	1(3)	43622	1(2)	44100	1(2)	44372	1(2)	45113	1(2)	45520	1(2)
42426	1(2)	43123	1(2)	43273	1(2)	43631	1(2)	44110	1(2)	44373	1(2)	45114	1(2)	45540	1(2)
42440	1(2)	43124	1(2)	43274	2(3)	43632	1(2)	44111	1(2)	44376	1(3)	45116	1(2)	45541	1(2)
42450	1(3)	43130	1(3)	43275	1(3)	43633	1(2)	44120	1(2)	44377	1(2)	45119	1(2)	45550	1(2)
42500	2(3)	43135	1(3)	43276	2(3)	43634	1(2)	44121	2(3)	44378	1(3)	45120	1(2)	45560	1(2)
42505	2(3)	43180	1(2)	43277	3(3)	43635	1(2)	44125	1(2)	44379	1(2)	45121	1(2)	45562	1(2)
42507	1(2)	43191	1(3)	43278	1(3)	43640	1(2)	44126	1(2)	44380	1(3)	45123	1(2)	45563	1(2)
42509	1(2)	43192	1(3)	43279	1(2)	43641	1(2)	44127	1(2)	44381	1(3)	45126	1(2)	45800	1(3)
42510	1(2)	43193	1(3)	43280	1(2)	43644	1(2)	44128	2(3)	44382	1(2)	45130	1(2)	45805	1(3)
42550	2(3)	43194	1(3)	43281	1(2)	43645	1(2)	44130	2(3)	44384	1(3)	45135	1(2)	45820	1(3)

CPT	MUE	CPT	MUE	CPT	MUE	CPT	MUE	CPT	MUE	CPT	MUE	CPT	MUE	CPT	MUE
45825	1(3)	46760	1(2)	47543	1(3)	48556	1(2)	49505	1(2)	50280	1(2)	50610	1(2)	51102	1(3)
45900	1(2)	46761	1(2)	47544	1(3)	48999	1(3)	49507	1(2)	50290	1(3)	50620	1(2)	51500	1(2)
45905	1(2)	46900	1(2)	47550	1(3)	49000	1(2)	49520	1(2)	50300	1(2)	50630	1(2)	51520	1(2)
45910	1(2)	46910	1(2)	47552	1(3)	49002	1(3)	49521	1(2)	50320	1(2)	50650	1(2)	51525	1(2)
45915	1(2)	46916	1(2)	47553	1(2)	49010	1(3)	49525	1(2)	50323	1(2)	50660	1(3)	51530	1(2)
45990	1(2)	46917	1(2)	47554	1(3)	49020	2(3)	49540	1(2)	50325	1(2)	50684	1(3)	51535	1(2)
45999	1(3)	46922	1(2)	47555	1(2)	49040	2(3)	49550	1(2)	50327	2(3)	50686	2(3)	51550	1(2)
46020	2(3)	46924	1(2)	47556	1(2)	49060	2(3)	49553	1(2)	50328	1(3)	50688	2(3)	51555	1(2)
46030	1(3)	46930	1(2)	47562	1(2)	49062	1(3)	49555	1(2)	50329	1(3)	50690	2(3)	51565	1(2)
46040	2(3)	46940	1(2)	47563	1(2)	49082	1(3)	49557	1(2)	50340	1(2)	50693	2(3)	51570	1(2)
46045	2(3)	46942	1(3)	47564	1(2)	49083	2(3)	49560	2(3)	50360	1(2)	50694	2(3)	51575	1(2)
46050	2(3)	46945	1(2)	47570	1(2)	49084	1(3)	49561	1(3)	50365	1(2)	50695	2(3)	51580	1(2)
46060	2(3)	46946	1(2)	47579	1(3)	49180	2(3)	49565	2(3)	50370	1(2)	50700	1(2)	51585	1(2)
46070	1(2)	46947	1(2)	47600	1(2)	49185	2(3)	49566	2(3)	50380	1(2)	50705	2(3)	51590	1(2)
46080	1(2)	46999	1(3)	47605	1(2)	49203	1(2)	49568	2(3)	50382	1(3)	50706	2(3)	51595	1(2)
46083	2(3)	47000	3(3)	47610	1(2)	49204	1(2)	49570	1(3)	50384	1(3)	50715	1(2)	51596	1(2)
46200	1(3)	47001	3(3)	47612	1(2)	49205	1(2)	49572	1(3)	50385	1(3)	50722	1(2)	51597	1(2)
46220	1(2)	47010	1(3)	47620	1(2)	49215	1(2)	49580	1(2)	50386	1(3)	50725	1(3)	51600	1(3)
46221	1(2)	47015	1(2)	47700	1(2)	49220	1(2)	49582	1(2)	50387	1(3)	50727	1(3)	51605	1(3)
46230	1(2)	47100	3(3)	47701	1(2)	49250	1(2)	49585	1(2)	50389	1(3)	50728	1(3)	51610	1(3)
46250	1(2)	47120	2(3)	47711	1(2)	49255	1(2)	49587	1(2)	50390	2(3)	50740	1(2)	51700	1(3)
46255	1(2)	47122	1(2)	47712	1(2)	49320	1(3)	49590	1(2)	50391	1(3)	50750	1(2)	51701	2(3)
46257	1(2)	47125	1(2)	47715	1(2)	49321	1(2)	49600	1(2)	50396	1(3)	50760	1(2)	51702	2(3)
46258	1(2)	47130	1(2)	47720	1(2)	49322	1(2)	49605	1(2)	50400	1(2)	50770	1(2)	51703	2(3)
46260	1(2)	47133	1(2)	47721	1(2)	49323	1(2)	49606	1(2)	50405	1(2)	50780	1(2)	51705	2(3)
46261	1(2)	47135	1(2)	47740	1(2)	49324	1(2)	49610	1(2)	50430	2(3)	50782	1(2)	51710	1(3)
46262	1(2)	47140	1(2)	47741	1(2)	49325	1(2)	49611	1(2)	50431	2(3)	50783	1(2)	51715	1(2)
46270	1(3)	47141	1(2)	47760	1(2)	49326	1(2)	49650	1(2)	50432	2(3)	50785	1(2)	51720	1(3)
46275	1(3)	47142	1(2)	47765	1(2)	49327	1(2)	49651	1(2)	50433	2(3)	50800	1(2)	51725	1(3)
46280	1(2)	47143	1(2)	47780	1(2)	49329	1(3)	49652	2(3)	50434	2(3)	50810	1(3)	51726	1(3)
46285	1(3)	47144	1(2)	47785	1(2)	49400	1(3)	49653	2(3)	50435	2(3)	50815	1(2)	51727	1(3)
46288	1(3)	47145	1(2)	47800	1(2)	49402	1(3)	49654	1(3)	50436	1(3)	50820	1(2)	51728	1(3)
46320	2(3)	47146	2(3)	47801	1(3)	49405	2(3)	49655	1(3)	50437	1(3)	50825	1(3)	51729	1(3)
46500	1(2)	47147	1(3)	47802	1(2)	49406	2(3)	49656	1(3)	50500	1(3)	50830	1(3)	51736	1(3)
46505	1(2)	47300	2(3)	47900	1(2)	49407	1(3)	49657	1(3)	50520	1(3)	50840	1(2)	51741	1(3)
46600	1(3)	47350	1(3)	47999	1(3)	49411	1(2)	49659	1(3)	50525	1(3)	50845	1(2)	51784	1(3)
46601	1(3)	47360	1(3)	48000	1(2)	49412	1(2)	49900	1(3)	50526	1(3)	50860	1(2)	51785	1(3)
46604	1(2)	47361	1(3)	48001	1(2)	49418	1(2)	49904	1(3)	50540	1(2)	50900	1(3)	51792	1(3)
46606	1(2)	47362	1(3)	48020	1(3)	49419	1(2)	49905	1(3)	50541	1(2)	50920	2(3)	51797	1(3)
46607	1(2)	47370	1(2)	48100	1(3)	49421	1(2)	49906	1(3)	50542	1(2)	50930	2(3)	51798	1(3)
46608	1(3)	47371	1(3)	48102	1(3)	49422	1(2)	49999	1(3)	50543	1(2)	50940	1(2)	51800	1(2)
46610	1(2)	47379	1(3)	48105	1(2)	49423	2(3)	50010	1(2)	50544	1(2)	50945	1(2)	51820	1(2)
46611	1(2)	47380	1(2)	48120	1(3)	49424	3(3)	50020	1(3)	50545	1(2)	50947	1(2)	51840	1(2)
46612	1(2)	47381	1(2)	48140	1(2)	49425	1(2)	50040	1(2)	50546	1(2)	50948	1(2)	51841	1(2)
46614	1(3)	47382	1(2)	48145	1(2)	49426	1(3)	50045	1(2)	50547	1(2)	50949	1(3)	51845	1(2)
46615	1(2)	47383	1(2)	48146	1(2)	49427	1(3)	50060	1(2)	50548	1(2)	50951	1(3)	51860	1(3)
46700	1(2)	47399	1(3)	48148	1(2)	49428	1(2)	50065	1(2)	50549	1(3)	50953	1(3)	51865	1(3)
46705	1(2)	47400	1(3)	48150	1(2)	49429	1(2)	50070	1(2)	50551	1(3)	50955	1(2)	51880	1(2)
46706	1(3)	47420	1(2)	48152	1(2)	49435	1(2)	50075	1(2)	50553	1(3)	50957	1(2)	51900	1(3)
46707	1(3)	47425	1(2)	48153	1(2)	49436	1(2)	50080	1(2)	50555	1(3)	50961	1(2)	51920	1(3)
46710	1(3)	47460	1(2)	48154	1(2)	49440	1(3)	50081	1(2)	50557	1(3)	50970	1(3)	51925	1(2)
46712	1(3)	47480	1(2)	48155	1(2)	49441	1(3)	50100	1(2)	50561	1(3)	50972	1(3)	51940	1(2)
46715	1(2)	47490	1(2)	48160	0(3)	49442	1(3)	50120	1(2)	50562	1(3)	50974	1(2)	51960	1(2)
46716	1(2)	47531	2(3)	48400	1(3)	49446	1(2)	50125	1(2)	50570	1(3)	50976	1(2)	51980	1(2)
46730	1(2)	47532	1(3)	48500	1(3)	49450	1(3)	50130	1(2)	50572	1(3)	50980	1(2)	51990	1(2)
46735	1(2)	47533	1(3)	48510	1(3)	49451	1(3)	50135	1(2)	50574	1(2)	51020	1(3)	51992	1(2)
46740	1(2)	47534	2(3)	48520	1(3)	49452	1(3)	50200	1(3)	50575	1(2)	51030	1(2)	51999	1(3)
46742	1(2)	47535	1(3)	48540	1(3)	49460	1(3)	50205	1(3)	50576	1(2)	51040	1(3)	52000	1(3)
46744	1(2)	47536	2(3)	48545	1(3)	49465	1(3)	50220	1(2)	50580	1(2)	51045	2(3)	52001	1(3)
46746	1(2)	47537	1(3)	48547	1(2)	49491	1(2)	50225	1(2)	50590	1(2)	51050	1(3)	52005	2(3)
46748	1(2)	47538	2(3)	48548	1(2)	49492	1(2)	50230	1(2)	50592	1(2)	51060	1(3)	52007	1(2)
46750	1(2)	47539	2(3)	48550	1(2)	49495	1(2)	50234	1(2)	50593	1(2)	51065	1(3)	52010	1(2)
46751	1(2)	47540	2(3)	48551	1(2)	49496	1(2)	50236	1(2)	50600	1(3)	51080	1(3)	52204	1(2)
46753	1(2)	47541	1(3)	48552	2(3)	49500	1(2)	50240	1(2)	50605	1(3)	51100	1(3)	52214	1(2)
46754	1(3)	47542	2(3)	48554	1(2)	49501	1(2)	50250	1(3)	50606	1(3)	51101	1(3)	52224	1(2)

CPT	MUE	CPT	MUE	CPT	MUE	CPT	MUE	CPT	MUE	CPT	MUE	CPT	MUE	CPT	MUE
52234	1(2)	53220	1(3)	54135	1(2)	54660	1(2)	55970	1(2)	57284	1(2)	58267	1(2)	58720	1(2)
52235	1(2)	53230	1(3)	54150	1(2)	54670	1(3)	55980	1(2)	57285	1(2)	58270	1(2)	58740	1(2)
52240	1(2)	53235	1(3)	54160	1(2)	54680	1(2)	56405	2(3)	57287	1(2)	58275	1(2)	58750	1(2)
52250	1(2)	53240	1(3)	54161	1(2)	54690	1(2)	56420	1(3)	57288	1(2)	58280	1(2)	58752	1(2)
52260	1(2)	53250	1(3)	54162	1(2)	54692	1(2)	56440	1(3)	57289	1(2)	58285	1(3)	58760	1(2)
52265	1(2)	53260	1(2)	54163	1(2)	54699	1(3)	56441	1(2)	57291	1(2)	58290	1(3)	58770	1(2)
52270	1(2)	53265	1(3)	54164	1(2)	54700	1(3)	56442	1(2)	57292	1(2)	58291	1(2)	58800	1(2)
52275	1(2)	53270	1(2)	54200	1(2)	54800	1(2)	56501	1(2)	57295	1(2)	58292	1(2)	58805	1(2)
52276	1(2)	53275	1(2)	54205	1(2)	54830	1(2)	56515	1(2)	57296	1(2)	58293	1(2)	58820	1(3)
52277	1(2)	53400	1(2)	54220	1(3)	54840	1(2)	56605	1(2)	57300	1(3)	58294	1(2)	58822	1(3)
52281	1(2)	53405	1(2)	54230	1(3)	54860	1(2)	56606	6(3)	57305	1(3)	58300	0(3)	58825	1(2)
52282	1(2)	53410	1(2)	54231	1(2)	54861	1(2)	56620	1(2)	57307	1(3)	58301	1(3)	58900	1(2)
52283	1(2)	53415	1(2)	54235	1(3)	54865	1(3)	56625	1(2)	57308	1(3)	58321	1(2)	58920	1(2)
52285	1(2)	53420	1(2)	54240	1(2)	54900	1(2)	56630	1(2)	57310	1(3)	58322	1(2)	58925	1(3)
52287	1(2)	53425	1(2)	54250	1(2)	54901	1(2)	56631	1(2)	57311	1(3)	58323	1(3)	58940	1(2)
52290	1(2)	53430	1(2)	54300	1(2)	55000	1(3)	56632	1(2)	57320	1(3)	58340	1(3)	58943	1(2)
52300	1(2)	53431	1(2)	54304	1(2)	55040	1(2)	56633	1(2)	57330	1(3)	58345	1(3)	58950	1(2)
52301	1(2)	53440	1(2)	54308	1(2)	55041	1(2)	56634	1(2)	57335	1(2)	58346	1(2)	58951	1(2)
52305	1(2)	53442	1(2)	54312	1(2)	55060	1(2)	56637	1(2)	57400	1(2)	58350	1(2)	58952	1(2)
52310	1(3)	53444	1(3)	54316	1(2)	55100	2(3)	56640	1(2)	57410	1(2)	58353	1(3)	58953	1(2)
52315	2(3)	53445	1(2)	54318	1(2)	55110	1(2)	56700	1(2)	57415	1(3)	58356	1(3)	58954	1(2)
52317	1(3)	53446	1(2)	54322	1(2)	55120	1(3)	56740	1(3)	57420	1(3)	58400	1(2)	58956	1(2)
52318	1(3)	53447	1(2)	54324	1(2)	55150	1(2)	56800	1(2)	57421	1(3)	58410	1(2)	58957	1(2)
52320	1(2)	53448	1(2)	54326	1(2)	55175	1(2)	56805	1(2)	57423	1(2)	58520	1(2)	58958	1(2)
52325	1(3)	53449	1(2)	54328	1(2)	55180	1(2)	56810	1(2)	57425	1(2)	58540	1(3)	58960	1(2)
52327	1(2)	53450	1(2)	54332	1(2)	55200	1(2)	56820	1(2)	57426	1(2)	58541	1(3)	58970	1(3)
52330	1(2)	53460	1(2)	54336	1(2)	55250	1(2)	56821	1(2)	57452	1(3)	58542	1(2)	58974	1(3)
52332	1(2)	53500	1(2)	54340	1(2)	55300	1(2)	57000	1(3)	57454	1(3)	58543	1(3)	58976	2(3)
52334	1(2)	53502	1(3)	54344	1(2)	55400	1(2)	57010	1(3)	57455	1(3)	58544	1(2)	58999	1(3)
52341	1(2)	53505	1(3)	54348	1(2)	55500	1(2)	57020	1(3)	57456	1(3)	58545	1(2)	59000	2(3)
52342	1(2)	53510	1(3)	54352	1(2)	55520	1(2)	57022	1(3)	57460	1(3)	58546	1(2)	59001	2(3)
52343	1(2)	53515	1(2)	54360	1(2)	55530	1(2)	57023	1(3)	57461	1(3)	58548	1(2)	59012	2(3)
52344	1(2)	53520	1(3)	54380	1(2)	55535	1(2)	57061	1(2)	57500	1(3)	58550	1(3)	59015	2(3)
52345	1(2)	53600	1(3)	54385	1(2)	55540	1(2)	57065	1(2)	57505	1(3)	58552	1(3)	59020	2(3)
52346	1(2)	53601	1(3)	54390	1(2)	55550	1(2)	57100	2(3)	57510	1(3)	58553	1(3)	59025	2(3)
52351	1(3)	53605	1(3)	54400	1(2)	55559	1(3)	57105	2(3)	57511	1(3)	58554	1(2)	59030	2(3)
52352	1(2)	53620	1(2)	54401	1(2)	55600	1(3)	57106	1(2)	57513	1(3)	58555	1(3)	59050	2(3)
52353	1(2)	53621	1(3)	54405	1(2)	55605	1(2)	57107	1(2)	57520	1(3)	58558	1(3)	59051	2(3)
52354	1(3)	53660	1(2)	54406	1(2)	55650	1(2)	57109	1(2)	57522	1(3)	58559	1(3)	59070	2(3)
52355	1(3)	53661	1(3)	54408	1(2)	55680	1(3)	57110	1(2)	57530	1(3)	58560	1(3)	59072	2(3)
52356	1(2)	53665	1(3)	54410	1(2)	55700	1(2)	57111	1(2)	57531	1(2)	58561	1(3)	59074	2(3)
52400	1(2)	53850	1(2)	54411	1(2)	55705	1(2)	57112	1(2)	57540	1(2)	58562	1(3)	59076	2(3)
52402	1(2)	53852	1(2)	54415	1(2)	55706	1(2)	57120	1(2)	57545	1(3)	58563	1(3)	59100	1(2)
52441	1(2)	53854	1(2)	54416	1(2)	55720	1(3)	57130	1(2)	57550	1(3)	58565	1(2)	59120	1(3)
52442	6(3)	53855	1(2)	54417	1(2)	55725	1(3)	57135	2(3)	57555	1(2)	58570	1(2)	59121	1(3)
52450	1(2)	53860	1(2)	54420	1(2)	55801	1(2)	57150	1(3)	57556	1(2)	58571	1(2)	59130	1(3)
52500	1(2)	53899	1(3)	54430	1(2)	55810	1(2)	57155	1(3)	57558	1(3)	58572	1(3)	59135	1(3)
52601	1(2)	54000	1(2)	54435	1(2)	55812	1(2)	57156	1(3)	57700	1(3)	58573	1(2)	59136	1(3)
52630	1(2)	54001	1(2)	54437	1(2)	55815	1(2)	57160	1(2)	57720	1(3)	58575	1(2)	59140	1(2)
52640	1(2)	54015	1(3)	54438	1(2)	55821	1(2)	57170	1(2)	57800	1(3)	58578	1(3)	59150	1(3)
52647	1(2)	54050	1(2)	54440	1(2)	55831	1(2)	57180	1(3)	58100	1(3)	58579	1(3)	59151	1(3)
52648	1(2)	54055	1(2)	54450	1(2)	55840	1(2)	57200	1(3)	58110	1(3)	58600	1(2)	59160	1(2)
52649	1(2)	54056	1(2)	54500	1(3)	55842	1(2)	57210	1(3)	58120	1(3)	58605	1(2)	59200	1(3)
52700	1(3)	54057	1(2)	54505	1(3)	55845	1(2)	57220	1(2)	58140	1(3)	58611	1(2)	59300	1(2)
53000	1(2)	54060	1(2)	54512	1(3)	55860	1(2)	57230	1(2)	58145	1(3)	58615	1(2)	59320	1(2)
53010	1(2)	54065	1(2)	54520	1(2)	55862	1(2)	57240	1(2)	58146	1(3)	58660	1(2)	59325	1(2)
53020	1(2)	54100	2(3)	54522	1(2)	55865	1(2)	57250	1(2)	58150	1(3)	58661	1(2)	59350	1(2)
53025	1(2)	54105	2(3)	54530	1(2)	55866	1(2)	57260	1(2)	58152	1(2)	58662	1(2)	59400	1(2)
53040	1(3)	54110	1(2)	54535	1(2)	55870	1(2)	57265	1(2)	58180	1(3)	58670	1(2)	59409	2(3)
53060	1(3)	54111	1(2)	54550	1(2)	55873	1(2)	57267	2(3)	58200	1(2)	58671	1(2)	59410	1(2)
53080	1(3)	54112	1(3)	54560	1(2)	55874	1(2)	57268	1(2)	58210	1(2)	58672	1(2)	59412	1(3)
53085	1(3)	54115	1(3)	54600	1(2)	55875	1(2)	57270	1(2)	58240	1(2)	58673	1(2)	59414	1(3)
53200	1(3)	54120	1(2)	54620	1(2)	55876	1(2)	57280	1(2)	58260	1(3)	58674	1(2)	59425	1(2)
53210	1(2)	54125	1(2)	54640	1(2)	55899	1(3)	57282	1(2)	58262	1(3)	58679	1(3)	59426	1(2)
53215	1(2)	54130	1(2)	54650	1(2)	55920	1(2)	57283	1(2)	58263	1(2)	58700	1(2)	59430	1(2)

CPT	MUE	CPT	MUE	CPT	MUE	CPT	MUE	CPT	MUE	CPT	MUE	CPT	MUE
59510	1(2)	61105	1(3)	61557	1(2)	61750	2(3)	62270	2(3)	63078	3(3)	63655	1(3)	64566	1(3)
59514	1(3)	61107	1(3)	61558	1(3)	61751	2(3)	62272	2(3)	63081	1(2)	63661	1(2)	64568	1(3)
59515	1(2)	61108	1(3)	61559	1(3)	61760	1(2)	62273	2(3)	63082	6(2)	63662	1(2)	64569	1(3)
59525	1(2)	61120	1(3)	61563	2(3)	61770	1(2)	62280	1(3)	63085	1(2)	63663	1(3)	64570	1(3)
59610	1(2)	61140	1(3)	61564	1(2)	61781	1(3)	62281	1(3)	63086	2(3)	63664	1(3)	64575	2(3)
59612	2(3)	61150	1(3)	61566	1(3)	61782	1(3)	62282	1(3)	63087	1(2)	63685	1(3)	64580	2(3)
59614	1(2)	61151	1(3)	61567	1(2)	61783	1(3)	62284	1(3)	63088	3(3)	63688	1(3)	64581	2(3)
59618	1(2)	61154	1(3)	61570	1(3)	61790	1(2)	62287	1(2)	63090	1(2)	63700	1(3)	64585	2(3)
59620	1(2)	61156	1(3)	61571	1(3)	61791	1(2)	62290	5(2)	63091	3(3)	63702	1(3)	64590	1(3)
59622	1(2)	61210	1(3)	61575	1(2)	61796	1(2)	62291	4(3)	63101	1(2)	63704	1(3)	64595	1(3)
59812	1(2)	61215	1(3)	61576	1(2)	61797	4(3)	62292	1(2)	63102	1(2)	63706	1(3)	64600	2(3)
59820	1(2)	61250	1(3)	61580	1(2)	61798	1(2)	62294	1(3)	63103	3(3)	63707	1(3)	64605	1(2)
59821	1(2)	61253	1(3)	61581	1(2)	61799	4(3)	62302	1(3)	63170	1(3)	63709	1(3)	64610	1(2)
59830	1(2)	61304	1(3)	61582	1(2)	61800	1(2)	62303	1(3)	63172	1(3)	63710	1(3)	64611	1(2)
59840	1(2)	61305	1(3)	61583	1(2)	61850	1(3)	62304	1(3)	63173	1(3)	63740	1(3)	64612	1(2)
59841	1(2)	61312	2(3)	61584	1(2)	61860	1(3)	62305	1(3)	63180	1(2)	63741	1(3)	64615	1(2)
59850	1(2)	61313	2(3)	61585	1(2)	61863	1(2)	62320	1(3)	63182	1(2)	63744	1(3)	64616	1(2)
59851	1(2)	61314	2(3)	61586	1(3)	61864	1(3)	62321	1(3)	63185	1(2)	63746	1(2)	64617	1(2)
59852	1(2)	61315	1(2)	61590	1(2)	61867	1(2)	62322	1(3)	63190	1(2)	64400	4(3)	64620	5(3)
59855	1(2)	61316	1(3)	61591	1(2)	61868	2(3)	62323	1(3)	63191	1(2)	64402	1(3)	64630	1(3)
59856	1(2)	61320	2(3)	61592	1(2)	61870	1(3)	62324	1(3)	63194	1(2)	64405	1(3)	64632	1(2)
59857	1(2)	61321	1(3)	61595	1(2)	61880	1(2)	62325	1(3)	63195	1(2)	64408	1(3)	64633	1(2)
59866	1(2)	61322	1(3)	61596	1(2)	61885	1(3)	62326	1(3)	63196	1(2)	64410	1(3)	64634	4(3)
59870	1(2)	61323	1(3)	61597	1(2)	61886	1(3)	62327	1(3)	63197	1(2)	64413	1(3)	64635	1(2)
59871	1(2)	61330	1(2)	61598	1(3)	61888	1(3)	62350	1(3)	63198	1(2)	64415	1(3)	64636	4(2)
59897	1(3)	61333	1(2)	61600	1(3)	62000	1(3)	62351	1(3)	63199	1(2)	64416	1(2)	64640	5(3)
59898	1(3)	61340	1(2)	61601	1(3)	62005	1(3)	62355	1(3)	63200	1(2)	64417	1(3)	64642	1(2)
59899	1(3)	61343	1(2)	61605	1(3)	62010	1(3)	62360	1(3)	63250	1(3)	64418	1(3)	64643	3(2)
60000	1(3)	61345	1(3)	61606	1(3)	62100	1(3)	62361	1(2)	63251	1(3)	64420	3(3)	64644	1(2)
60100	3(3)	61450	1(3)	61607	1(3)	62115	1(2)	62362	1(2)	63252	1(3)	64421	3(3)	64645	3(2)
60200	2(3)	61458	1(2)	61608	1(3)	62117	1(2)	62365	1(2)	63265	1(3)	64425	1(3)	64646	1(2)
60210	1(2)	61460	1(2)	61611	1(3)	62120	1(2)	62367	1(3)	63266	1(3)	64430	1(3)	64647	1(2)
60212	1(2)	61500	1(3)	61613	1(3)	62121	1(2)	62368	1(3)	63267	1(3)	64435	1(3)	64650	1(2)
60220	1(3)	61501	1(3)	61615	1(3)	62140	1(2)	62369	1(3)	63268	1(3)	64445	1(3)	64653	1(2)
60225	1(2)	61510	1(3)	61616	1(3)	62141	1(3)	62370	1(3)	63270	1(3)	64446	1(2)	64680	1(2)
60240	1(2)	61512	1(3)	61618	2(3)	62142	2(3)	62380	2(3)	63271	1(3)	64447	1(3)	64681	1(2)
60252	1(2)	61514	2(3)	61619	2(3)	62143	2(3)	63001	1(2)	63272	1(3)	64448	1(2)	64702	2(3)
60254	1(2)	61516	1(3)	61623	2(3)	62145	1(3)	63003	1(2)	63273	1(3)	64449	1(2)	64704	4(3)
60260	1(2)	61517	1(3)	61624	2(3)	62146	2(3)	63005	1(2)	63275	1(3)	64450	10(3)	64708	3(3)
60270	1(2)	61518	1(3)	61626	2(3)	62147	1(3)	63011	1(2)	63276	1(3)	64455	1(2)	64712	1(2)
60271	1(2)	61519	1(3)	61630	1(3)	62148	1(3)	63012	1(2)	63277	1(3)	64461	1(2)	64713	1(2)
60280	1(3)	61520	1(3)	61635	2(3)	62160	1(3)	63015	1(2)	63278	1(3)	64462	1(2)	64714	1(2)
60281	1(3)	61521	1(3)	61640	0(3)	62161	1(3)	63016	1(2)	63280	1(3)	64463	1(3)	64716	2(3)
60300	2(3)	61522	1(3)	61641	0(3)	62162	1(3)	63017	1(2)	63281	1(3)	64479	1(2)	64718	1(2)
60500	1(2)	61524	2(3)	61642	0(3)	62163	1(3)	63020	1(2)	63282	1(3)	64480	4(3)	64719	1(2)
60502	1(3)	61526	1(3)	61645	1(3)	62164	1(3)	63030	1(2)	63283	1(3)	64483	1(2)	64721	1(2)
60505	1(3)	61530	1(3)	61650	1(2)	62165	1(2)	63035	4(3)	63285	1(3)	64484	4(3)	64722	4(3)
60512	1(3)	61531	1(2)	61651	2(2)	62180	1(3)	63040	1(2)	63286	1(3)	64486	1(3)	64726	2(3)
60520	1(2)	61533	2(3)	61680	1(3)	62190	1(3)	63042	1(2)	63287	1(3)	64487	1(2)	64727	2(3)
60521	1(2)	61534	1(3)	61682	1(3)	62192	1(3)	63043	4(3)	63290	1(3)	64488	1(3)	64732	1(2)
60522	1(2)	61535	2(3)	61684	1(3)	62194	1(3)	63044	4(2)	63295	1(2)	64489	1(2)	64734	1(2)
60540	1(2)	61536	1(3)	61686	1(3)	62200	1(2)	63045	1(2)	63300	1(2)	64490	1(2)	64736	1(2)
60545	1(2)	61537	1(3)	61690	1(3)	62201	1(2)	63046	1(2)	63301	1(2)	64491	1(2)	64738	1(2)
60600	1(3)	61538	1(2)	61692	1(3)	62220	1(3)	63047	1(2)	63302	1(2)	64492	1(2)	64740	1(2)
60605	1(3)	61539	1(3)	61697	2(3)	62223	1(3)	63048	5(3)	63303	1(2)	64493	1(2)	64742	1(2)
60650	1(2)	61540	1(3)	61698	1(3)	62225	2(3)	63050	1(2)	63304	1(2)	64494	1(2)	64744	1(2)
60659	1(3)	61541	1(2)	61700	2(3)	62230	2(3)	63051	1(2)	63305	1(2)	64495	1(2)	64746	1(2)
60699	1(3)	61543	1(2)	61702	1(3)	62252	2(3)	63055	1(2)	63306	1(2)	64505	1(3)	64755	1(2)
61000	1(2)	61544	1(3)	61703	1(3)	62256	1(3)	63056	1(2)	63307	1(2)	64510	1(3)	64760	1(2)
61001	1(2)	61545	1(2)	61705	1(3)	62258	1(3)	63057	3(3)	63308	3(3)	64517	1(3)	64763	1(2)
61020	2(3)	61546	1(2)	61708	1(3)	62263	1(2)	63064	1(2)	63600	2(3)	64520	1(3)	64766	1(2)
61026	2(3)	61548	1(2)	61710	1(3)	62264	1(2)	63066	1(3)	63610	1(3)	64530	1(3)	64771	2(3)
61050	1(3)	61550	1(2)	61711	1(3)	62267	2(3)	63075	1(2)	63620	1(2)	64553	1(3)	64772	2(3)
61055	1(3)	61552	1(2)	61720	1(3)	62268	1(3)	63076	3(3)	63621	2(2)	64555	2(3)	64774	2(3)
61070	2(3)	61556	1(3)	61735	1(3)	62269	2(3)	63077	1(2)	63650	2(3)	64561	1(3)	64776	1(2)

CPT	MUE	CPT	MUE	CPT	MUE	CPT	MUE	CPT	MUE	CPT	MUE	CPT	MUE	CPT	MUE
64778	1(3)	65125	1(2)	66030	1(3)	67105	1(2)	67830	1(2)	68550	1(2)	69633	1(2)	70320	1(3)
64782	2(2)	65130	1(2)	66130	1(3)	67107	1(2)	67835	1(2)	68700	1(2)	69635	1(3)	70328	1(3)
64783	2(3)	65135	1(2)	66150	1(2)	67108	1(2)	67840	3(3)	68705	2(3)	69636	1(3)	70330	1(3)
64784	3(3)	65140	1(2)	66155	1(2)	67110	1(2)	67850	3(3)	68720	1(2)	69637	1(2)	70332	2(3)
64786	1(3)	65150	1(2)	66160	1(2)	67113	1(2)	67875	1(2)	68745	1(2)	69641	1(2)	70336	1(3)
64787	4(3)	65155	1(2)	66170	1(2)	67115	1(2)	67880	1(2)	68750	1(2)	69642	1(2)	70350	1(3)
64788	5(3)	65175	1(2)	66172	1(2)	67120	1(2)	67882	1(2)	68760	4(2)	69643	1(2)	70355	1(3)
64790	1(3)	65205	1(3)	66174	1(2)	67121	1(2)	67900	1(2)	68761	4(2)	69644	1(2)	70360	2(3)
64792	2(3)	65210	1(3)	66175	1(2)	67141	1(2)	67901	1(2)	68770	1(3)	69645	1(2)	70370	1(3)
64795	2(3)	65220	1(3)	66179	1(2)	67145	1(2)	67902	1(2)	68801	4(2)	69646	1(2)	70371	1(2)
64802	1(2)	65222	1(3)	66180	1(2)	67208	1(2)	67903	1(2)	68810	1(2)	69650	1(2)	70380	2(3)
64804	1(2)	65235	1(3)	66183	1(3)	67210	1(2)	67904	1(2)	68811	1(2)	69660	1(2)	70390	2(3)
64809	1(2)	65260	1(3)	66184	1(2)	67218	1(2)	67906	1(2)	68815	1(2)	69661	1(2)	70450	3(3)
64818	1(2)	65265	1(3)	66185	1(2)	67220	1(2)	67908	1(2)	68816	1(2)	69662	1(2)	70460	1(3)
64820	4(3)	65270	1(3)	66225	1(2)	67221	1(2)	67909	1(2)	68840	1(2)	69666	1(2)	70470	2(3)
64821	1(2)	65272	1(3)	66250	1(2)	67225	1(2)	67911	2(3)	68850	1(3)	69667	1(2)	70480	1(3)
64822	1(2)	65273	1(3)	66500	1(2)	67227	1(2)	67912	1(2)	68899	1(3)	69670	1(2)	70481	1(3)
64823	1(2)	65275	1(3)	66505	1(2)	67228	1(2)	67914	2(3)	69000	1(3)	69676	1(2)	70482	1(3)
64831	1(2)	65280	1(3)	66600	1(2)	67229	1(2)	67915	2(3)	69005	1(3)	69700	1(3)	70486	1(3)
64832	3(3)	65285	1(3)	66605	1(2)	67250	1(2)	67916	2(3)	69020	1(3)	69710	0(3)	70487	1(3)
64834	1(2)	65286	1(3)	66625	1(2)	67255	1(2)	67917	2(3)	69090	0(3)	69711	1(2)	70488	1(3)
64835	1(2)	65290	1(3)	66630	1(2)	67299	1(3)	67921	2(3)	69100	3(3)	69714	1(2)	70490	1(3)
64836	1(2)	65400	1(3)	66635	1(2)	67311	1(2)	67922	2(3)	69105	1(3)	69715	1(3)	70491	1(3)
64837	2(3)	65410	1(3)	66680	1(2)	67312	1(2)	67923	2(3)	69110	1(2)	69717	1(2)	70492	1(3)
64840	1(2)	65420	1(2)	66682	1(2)	67314	1(2)	67924	2(3)	69120	1(3)	69718	1(2)	70496	2(3)
64856	2(3)	65426	1(2)	66700	1(2)	67316	1(2)	67930	2(3)	69140	1(2)	69720	1(2)	70498	2(3)
64857	2(3)	65430	1(2)	66710	1(2)	67318	1(2)	67935	2(3)	69145	1(2)	69725	1(2)	70540	1(3)
64858	1(2)	65435	1(2)	66711	1(2)	67320	2(3)	67938	2(3)	69150	1(3)	69740	1(2)	70542	1(3)
64859	2(3)	65436	1(2)	66720	1(2)	67331	1(2)	67950	2(2)	69155	1(3)	69745	1(2)	70543	1(3)
64861	1(2)	65450	1(3)	66740	1(2)	67332	1(2)	67961	2(3)	69200	1(2)	69799	1(3)	70544	2(3)
64862	1(2)	65600	1(2)	66761	1(2)	67334	1(2)	67966	2(3)	69205	1(3)	69801	1(3)	70545	1(3)
64864	2(3)	65710	1(2)	66762	1(2)	67335	1(2)	67971	1(2)	69209	1(2)	69805	1(3)	70546	1(3)
64865	1(3)	65730	1(2)	66770	1(3)	67340	2(2)	67973	1(2)	69210	1(2)	69806	1(3)	70547	1(3)
64866	1(3)	65750	1(2)	66820	1(2)	67343	1(2)	67974	1(2)	69220	1(2)	69905	1(2)	70548	1(3)
64868	1(3)	65755	1(2)	66821	1(2)	67345	1(3)	67975	1(2)	69222	1(2)	69910	1(2)	70549	1(3)
64872	1(3)	65756	1(2)	66825	1(2)	67346	1(3)	67999	1(3)	69300	1(2)	69915	1(3)	70551	2(3)
64874	1(3)	65757	1(3)	66830	1(2)	67399	1(3)	68020	1(3)	69310	1(2)	69930	1(2)	70552	2(3)
64876	1(3)	65760	0(3)	66840	1(2)	67400	1(2)	68040	1(2)	69320	1(2)	69949	1(3)	70553	2(3)
64885	1(2)	65765	0(3)	66850	1(2)	67405	1(2)	68100	1(3)	69399	1(3)	69950	1(2)	70554	1(3)
64886	1(3)	65767	0(3)	66852	1(2)	67412	1(2)	68110	1(3)	69420	1(2)	69955	1(2)	70555	1(3)
64890	2(3)	65770	1(2)	66920	1(2)	67413	1(2)	68115	1(3)	69421	1(2)	69960	1(2)	70557	1(3)
64891	2(3)	65771	0(3)	66930	1(2)	67414	1(2)	68130	1(3)	69424	1(2)	69970	1(3)	70558	1(3)
64892	2(3)	65772	1(2)	66940	1(2)	67415	1(3)	68135	1(3)	69433	1(2)	69979	1(3)	70559	1(3)
64893	2(3)	65775	1(2)	66982	1(2)	67420	1(2)	68200	1(3)	69436	1(2)	69990	1(3)	71045	4(3)
64895	2(3)	65778	1(2)	66983	1(2)	67430	1(2)	68320	1(2)	69440	1(2)	70010	1(3)	71046	3(3)
64896	2(3)	65779	1(2)	66984	1(2)	67440	1(2)	68325	1(2)	69450	1(2)	70015	1(3)	71047	2(3)
64897	2(3)	65780	1(2)	66985	1(2)	67445	1(2)	68326	1(2)	69501	1(3)	70030	2(2)	71048	1(3)
64898	2(3)	65781	1(2)	66986	1(2)	67450	1(2)	68328	1(2)	69502	1(2)	70100	2(3)	71100	2(3)
64901	2(3)	65782	1(2)	66990	1(3)	67500	1(3)	68330	1(3)	69505	1(2)	70110	2(3)	71101	2(3)
64902	1(3)	65785	1(2)	66999	1(3)	67505	1(3)	68335	1(3)	69511	1(2)	70120	1(3)	71110	1(3)
64905	1(3)	65800	1(2)	67005	1(2)	67515	1(3)	68340	1(3)	69530	1(2)	70130	1(3)	71111	1(3)
64907	1(3)	65810	1(2)	67010	1(2)	67550	1(2)	68360	1(3)	69535	1(2)	70134	1(3)	71120	1(3)
64910	3(3)	65815	1(3)	67015	1(2)	67560	1(2)	68362	1(3)	69540	1(3)	70140	2(3)	71130	1(3)
64911	2(3)	65820	1(2)	67025	1(2)	67570	1(2)	68371	1(3)	69550	1(3)	70150	1(3)	71250	2(3)
64912	3(3)	65850	1(2)	67027	1(2)	67599	1(3)	68399	1(3)	69552	1(2)	70160	1(3)	71260	2(3)
64913	3(3)	65855	1(2)	67028	1(3)	67700	2(3)	68400	1(2)	69554	1(2)	70170	2(2)	71270	1(3)
64999	1(3)	65860	1(2)	67030	1(2)	67710	1(2)	68420	1(2)	69601	1(2)	70190	1(2)	71275	1(3)
65091	1(2)	65865	1(2)	67031	1(2)	67715	1(3)	68440	2(3)	69602	1(2)	70200	2(3)	71550	1(3)
65093	1(2)	65870	1(2)	67036	1(2)	67800	1(2)	68500	1(2)	69603	1(2)	70210	1(3)	71551	1(3)
65101	1(2)	65875	1(2)	67039	1(2)	67801	1(2)	68505	1(2)	69604	1(2)	70220	1(3)	71552	1(3)
65103	1(2)	65880	1(2)	67040	1(2)	67805	1(2)	68510	1(2)	69605	1(2)	70240	1(2)	71555	1(3)
65105	1(2)	65900	1(3)	67041	1(2)	67808	1(2)	68520	1(2)	69610	1(2)	70250	2(3)	72020	4(3)
65110	1(2)	65920	1(2)	67042	1(2)	67810	2(3)	68525	1(2)	69620	1(2)	70260	1(3)	72040	3(3)
65112	1(2)	65930	1(3)	67043	1(2)	67820	1(2)	68530	1(2)	69631	1(2)	70300	1(3)	72050	1(3)
65114	1(2)	66020	1(3)	67101	1(2)	67825	1(2)	68540	1(2)	69632	1(3)	70310	1(3)	72052	1(3)

CPT	MUE	CPT	MUE	CPT	MUE	CPT	MUE	CPT	MUE	CPT	MUE	CPT	MUE	CPT	MUE
72070	1(3)	73115	2(2)	74190	1(3)	75726	3(3)	76512	2(2)	76983	3(3)	77386	2(3)	78195	1(2)
72072	1(3)	73120	2(3)	74210	1(3)	75731	1(3)	76513	2(2)	76998	1(3)	77387	2(3)	78199	1(3)
72074	1(3)	73130	3(3)	74220	1(3)	75733	1(3)	76514	1(2)	76999	1(3)	77399	1(3)	78201	1(3)
72080	1(3)	73140	3(3)	74230	1(3)	75736	2(3)	76516	1(2)	77001	2(3)	77401	1(2)	78202	1(3)
72081	1(3)	73200	2(3)	74235	1(3)	75741	1(3)	76519	1(3)	77002	1(3)	77402	2(3)	78205	1(3)
72082	1(3)	73201	2(3)	74240	2(3)	75743	1(3)	76529	2(2)	77003	1(3)	77407	2(3)	78206	1(3)
72083	1(3)	73202	2(3)	74241	1(3)	75746	1(3)	76536	1(3)	77011	1(3)	77412	2(3)	78215	1(3)
72084	1(3)	73206	2(3)	74245	1(3)	75756	2(3)	76604	1(3)	77012	1(3)	77417	1(2)	78216	1(3)
72100	2(3)	73218	2(3)	74246	1(3)	75774	7(3)	76641	2(2)	77013	1(3)	77423	1(3)	78226	1(3)
72110	1(3)	73219	2(3)	74247	1(3)	75801	1(3)	76642	2(2)	77014	2(3)	77424	1(2)	78227	1(3)
72114	1(3)	73220	2(3)	74249	1(3)	75803	1(3)	76700	1(3)	77021	1(3)	77425	1(3)	78230	1(3)
72120	1(3)	73221	2(3)	74250	1(3)	75805	1(2)	76705	2(3)	77022	1(3)	77427	1(2)	78231	1(3)
72125	1(3)	73222	2(3)	74251	1(3)	75807	1(2)	76706	1(2)	77046	1(2)	77431	1(3)	78232	1(3)
72126	1(3)	73223	2(3)	74260	1(2)	75809	1(3)	76770	1(3)	77047	1(2)	77432	1(2)	78258	1(2)
72127	1(3)	73225	2(3)	74261	1(2)	75810	1(3)	76775	2(3)	77048	1(2)	77435	1(2)	78261	1(2)
72128	1(3)	73501	2(3)	74262	1(2)	75820	2(3)	76776	2(3)	77049	1(2)	77469	1(2)	78262	1(2)
72129	1(3)	73502	2(3)	74263	0(3)	75822	1(3)	76800	1(3)	77053	2(2)	77470	1(2)	78264	1(2)
72130	1(3)	73503	2(3)	74270	1(3)	75825	1(3)	76801	1(2)	77054	2(2)	77499	1(3)	78265	1(2)
72131	1(3)	73521	2(3)	74280	1(3)	75827	1(3)	76802	2(3)	77061	1(2)	77520	2(3)	78266	1(2)
72132	1(3)	73522	2(3)	74283	1(3)	75831	1(3)	76805	1(2)	77062	1(2)	77522	2(3)	78267	1(2)
72133	1(3)	73523	2(3)	74290	1(3)	75833	1(3)	76810	2(3)	77063	1(2)	77523	2(3)	78268	1(2)
72141	1(3)	73525	2(2)	74300	1(3)	75840	1(3)	76811	1(2)	77065	1(2)	77525	2(3)	78278	2(3)
72142	1(3)	73551	2(3)	74301	1(3)	75842	1(3)	76812	2(3)	77066	1(2)	77600	1(3)	78282	1(2)
72146	1(3)	73552	2(3)	74328	1(3)	75860	2(3)	76813	1(2)	77067	1(2)	77605	1(3)	78290	1(3)
72147	1(3)	73560	4(3)	74329	1(3)	75870	1(3)	76814	2(3)	77071	1(3)	77610	1(3)	78291	1(3)
72148	1(3)	73562	3(3)	74330	1(3)	75872	1(3)	76815	1(2)	77072	1(2)	77615	1(3)	78299	1(3)
72149	1(3)	73564	4(3)	74340	1(3)	75880	1(3)	76816	2(3)	77073	1(2)	77620	1(3)	78300	1(2)
72156	1(3)	73565	1(3)	74355	1(3)	75885	1(3)	76817	1(3)	77074	1(2)	77750	1(3)	78305	1(2)
72157	1(3)	73580	2(2)	74360	1(3)	75887	1(3)	76818	2(3)	77075	1(2)	77761	1(3)	78306	1(2)
72158	1(3)	73590	3(3)	74363	2(3)	75889	1(3)	76819	2(3)	77076	1(2)	77762	1(3)	78315	1(2)
72159	1(3)	73592	3(3)	74400	1(3)	75891	1(3)	76820	3(3)	77077	1(2)	77763	1(3)	78320	1(2)
72170	2(3)	73600	2(3)	74410	1(3)	75893	2(3)	76821	2(3)	77078	1(2)	77767	2(3)	78350	0(3)
72190	1(3)	73610	3(3)	74415	1(3)	75894	2(3)	76825	2(3)	77080	1(2)	77768	2(3)	78351	0(3)
72191	1(3)	73615	2(2)	74420	2(3)	75898	2(3)	76826	2(3)	77081	1(2)	77770	2(3)	78399	1(3)
72192	1(3)	73620	2(3)	74425	2(3)	75901	1(3)	76827	2(3)	77084	1(2)	77771	2(3)	78414	1(2)
72193	1(3)	73630	3(3)	74430	1(3)	75902	2(3)	76828	2(3)	77085	1(2)	77772	2(3)	78428	1(3)
72194	1(3)	73650	2(3)	74440	1(2)	75956	1(2)	76830	1(3)	77086	1(2)	77778	1(3)	78445	1(3)
72195	1(3)	73660	2(3)	74445	1(2)	75957	1(2)	76831	1(3)	77261	1(3)	77789	2(3)	78451	1(2)
72196	1(3)	73700	2(3)	74450	1(3)	75958	2(3)	76856	1(3)	77262	1(3)	77790	1(3)	78452	1(2)
72197	1(3)	73701	2(3)	74455	1(3)	75959	1(2)	76857	1(3)	77263	1(3)	77799	1(3)	78453	1(2)
72198	1(3)	73702	2(3)	74470	2(2)	75970	1(3)	76870	1(2)	77280	2(3)	78012	1(3)	78454	1(2)
72200	2(3)	73706	2(3)	74485	2(3)	75984	2(3)	76872	1(3)	77285	1(3)	78013	1(3)	78456	1(3)
72202	1(3)	73718	2(3)	74710	1(3)	75989	2(3)	76873	1(2)	77290	1(3)	78014	1(2)	78457	1(2)
72220	1(3)	73719	2(3)	74712	1(3)	76000	3(3)	76881	2(3)	77293	1(3)	78015	1(3)	78458	1(2)
72240	1(2)	73720	2(3)	74713	2(3)	76010	2(3)	76882	2(3)	77295	1(3)	78016	1(3)	78459	1(3)
72255	1(2)	73721	3(3)	74740	1(3)	76080	3(3)	76885	1(2)	77299	1(3)	78018	1(2)	78466	1(3)
72265	1(2)	73722	2(3)	74742	2(2)	76098	3(3)	76886	1(2)	77300	10(3)	78020	1(3)	78468	1(3)
72270	1(2)	73723	2(3)	74775	1(2)	76100	2(3)	76930	1(3)	77301	1(3)	78070	1(2)	78469	1(3)
72275	1(3)	73725	2(3)	75557	1(3)	76101	1(3)	76932	1(2)	77306	1(3)	78071	1(3)	78472	1(2)
72285	4(3)	74018	3(3)	75559	1(3)	76102	1(3)	76936	1(3)	77307	1(3)	78072	1(3)	78473	1(2)
72295	5(3)	74019	2(3)	75561	1(3)	76120	1(3)	76937	2(3)	77316	1(3)	78075	1(2)	78481	1(2)
73000	2(3)	74021	2(3)	75563	1(3)	76125	1(3)	76940	1(3)	77317	1(3)	78099	1(3)	78483	1(2)
73010	2(3)	74022	2(3)	75565	1(3)	76140	0(3)	76941	3(3)	77318	1(3)	78102	1(2)	78491	1(3)
73020	2(3)	74150	1(3)	75571	1(3)	76376	2(3)	76942	1(3)	77321	1(2)	78103	1(2)	78492	1(2)
73030	4(3)	74160	1(3)	75572	1(3)	76377	2(3)	76945	1(3)	77331	3(3)	78104	1(2)	78494	1(3)
73040	2(2)	74170	1(3)	75573	1(3)	76380	2(3)	76946	1(3)	77332	4(3)	78110	1(2)	78496	1(3)
73050	1(3)	74174	1(3)	75574	1(3)	76390	0(3)	76948	1(2)	77333	2(3)	78111	1(2)	78499	1(3)
73060	2(3)	74175	1(3)	75600	1(3)	76391	1(3)	76965	2(3)	77334	10(3)	78120	1(2)	78579	1(3)
73070	2(3)	74176	2(3)	75605	1(3)	76496	1(3)	76970	2(3)	77336	1(2)	78121	1(2)	78580	1(3)
73080	2(3)	74177	2(3)	75625	1(3)	76497	1(3)	76975	1(3)	77338	1(3)	78122	1(2)	78582	1(3)
73085	2(2)	74178	1(3)	75630	1(3)	76498	1(3)	76977	1(2)	77370	1(3)	78130	1(2)	78597	1(3)
73090	2(3)	74181	1(3)	75635	1(3)	76499	1(3)	76978	1(2)	77371	1(2)	78135	1(3)	78598	1(3)
73092	2(3)	74182	1(3)	75705	20(3)	76506	1(2)	76979	3(3)	77372	1(2)	78140	1(3)	78599	1(3)
73100	2(3)	74183	1(3)	75710	2(3)	76510	2(2)	76981	1(3)	77373	1(3)	78185	1(2)	78600	1(3)
73110	3(3)	74185	1(3)	75716	1(3)	76511	2(2)	76982	1(2)	77385	2(3)	78191	1(2)	78601	1(3)

CPT	MUE	CPT	MUE	CPT	MUE	CPT	MUE	CPT	MUE	CPT	MUE	CPT	MUE	CPT	MUE
78605	1(3)	80162	2(3)	80351	1(3)	81107	1(2)	81232	1(2)	81303	1(3)	81406	3(3)	81596	1(2)
78606	1(3)	80163	1(3)	80352	1(3)	81108	1(2)	81233	1(3)	81304	1(3)	81407	1(3)	81599	1(3)
78607	1(3)	80164	2(3)	80353	1(3)	81109	1(2)	81234	1(2)	81305	1(3)	81408	1(3)	82009	3(3)
78608	1(3)	80165	1(3)	80354	1(3)	81110	1(2)	81235	1(3)	81306	1(2)	81410	1(2)	82010	3(3)
78609	0(3)	80168	2(3)	80355	1(3)	81111	1(2)	81236	1(3)	81310	1(3)	81411	1(2)	82013	1(3)
78610	1(3)	80169	2(3)	80356	1(3)	81112	1(2)	81237	1(3)	81311	1(3)	81412	1(2)	82016	1(3)
78630	1(3)	80170	2(3)	80357	1(3)	81120	1(3)	81238	1(2)	81312	1(2)	81413	1(2)	82017	1(3)
78635	1(3)	80171	1(3)	80358	1(3)	81121	1(3)	81239	1(2)	81313	1(3)	81414	1(2)	82024	4(3)
78645	1(3)	80173	2(3)	80359	1(3)	81161	1(3)	81240	1(2)	81314	1(3)	81415	1(2)	82030	1(3)
78647	1(3)	80175	1(3)	80360	1(3)	81162	1(2)	81241	1(2)	81315	1(3)	81416	2(3)	82040	1(3)
78650	1(3)	80176	1(3)	80361	2(3)	81163	1(3)	81242	1(3)	81316	1(2)	81417	1(3)	82042	2(3)
78660	1(2)	80177	1(3)	80362	1(3)	81164	1(2)	81243	1(3)	81317	1(3)	81420	1(2)	82043	1(3)
78699	1(3)	80178	2(3)	80363	1(3)	81165	1(2)	81244	1(3)	81318	1(3)	81422	1(2)	82044	1(3)
78700	1(3)	80180	1(3)	80364	1(3)	81166	1(2)	81245	1(3)	81319	1(2)	81425	1(2)	82045	1(3)
78701	1(3)	80183	1(3)	80365	2(3)	81167	1(2)	81246	1(3)	81320	1(3)	81426	2(3)	82075	2(3)
78707	1(2)	80184	2(3)	80366	1(3)	81170	1(2)	81247	1(2)	81321	1(3)	81427	1(3)	82085	1(3)
78708	1(2)	80185	2(3)	80367	1(3)	81171	1(2)	81248	1(2)	81322	1(3)	81430	1(2)	82088	2(3)
78709	1(2)	80186	2(3)	80368	1(3)	81172	1(2)	81249	1(2)	81323	1(3)	81431	1(2)	82103	1(3)
78710	1(3)	80188	2(3)	80369	1(3)	81173	1(3)	81250	1(3)	81324	1(3)	81432	1(2)	82104	1(2)
78725	1(3)	80190	2(3)	80370	1(3)	81174	1(2)	81251	1(3)	81325	1(3)	81433	1(2)	82105	1(3)
78730	1(2)	80192	2(3)	80371	1(3)	81175	1(3)	81252	1(3)	81326	1(3)	81434	1(2)	82106	2(3)
78740	1(2)	80194	2(3)	80372	1(3)	81176	1(3)	81253	1(3)	81327	1(2)	81435	1(2)	82107	1(3)
78761	1(2)	80195	2(3)	80373	1(3)	81177	1(2)	81254	1(3)	81328	1(2)	81436	1(2)	82108	1(3)
78799	1(3)	80197	2(3)	80374	1(3)	81178	1(2)	81255	1(3)	81329	1(2)	81437	1(2)	82120	1(3)
78800	1(2)	80198	2(3)	80375	1(3)	81179	1(3)	81256	1(2)	81330	1(3)	81438	1(2)	82127	1(3)
78801	1(2)	80199	1(3)	80376	1(3)	81180	1(2)	81257	1(2)	81331	1(3)	81439	1(2)	82128	2(3)
78802	1(2)	80200	2(3)	80377	1(3)	81181	1(2)	81258	1(2)	81332	1(3)	81440	1(2)	82131	2(3)
78803	1(2)	80201	2(3)	80400	1(3)	81182	1(2)	81259	1(2)	81333	1(3)	81442	1(2)	82135	1(3)
78804	1(2)	80202	2(3)	80402	1(3)	81183	1(2)	81260	1(3)	81334	1(3)	81443	1(2)	82136	2(3)
78805	1(3)	80203	1(3)	80406	1(3)	81184	1(2)	81261	1(3)	81335	1(2)	81445	1(2)	82139	2(3)
78806	1(2)	80299	3(3)	80408	1(3)	81185	1(2)	81262	1(3)	81336	1(2)	81448	1(2)	82140	2(3)
78807	1(3)	80305	1(2)	80410	1(3)	81186	1(2)	81263	1(3)	81337	1(2)	81450	1(2)	82143	2(3)
78808	1(2)	80306	1(2)	80412	1(3)	81187	1(2)	81264	1(3)	81340	1(3)	81455	1(2)	82150	4(3)
78811	1(2)	80307	1(2)	80414	1(3)	81188	1(2)	81265	1(3)	81341	1(3)	81460	1(2)	82154	1(3)
78812	1(2)	80320	2(3)	80415	1(3)	81189	1(2)	81266	2(3)	81342	1(3)	81465	1(2)	82157	1(3)
78813	1(2)	80321	1(3)	80416	1(3)	81190	1(2)	81267	1(3)	81343	1(2)	81470	1(2)	82160	1(3)
78814	1(2)	80322	1(3)	80417	1(3)	81200	1(2)	81268	4(3)	81344	1(2)	81471	1(2)	82163	1(3)
78815	1(2)	80323	1(3)	80418	1(3)	81201	1(2)	81269	1(2)	81345	1(3)	81479	3(3)	82164	1(3)
78816	1(2)	80324	1(3)	80420	1(2)	81202	1(3)	81270	1(2)	81346	1(2)	81490	1(2)	82172	2(3)
78999	1(3)	80325	1(3)	80422	1(3)	81203	1(3)	81271	1(2)	81350	1(3)	81493	1(2)	82175	2(3)
79005	1(3)	80326	1(3)	80424	1(3)	81204	1(2)	81272	1(3)	81355	1(3)	81500	1(2)	82180	1(2)
79101	1(3)	80327	1(3)	80426	1(3)	81205	1(3)	81273	1(3)	81361	1(2)	81503	1(2)	82190	1(3)
79200	1(3)	80328	1(3)	80428	1(3)	81206	1(3)	81274	1(2)	81362	1(2)	81504	1(3)	82232	2(3)
79300	1(3)	80329	2(3)	80430	1(3)	81207	1(3)	81275	1(3)	81363	1(2)	81506	1(2)	82239	1(3)
79403	1(3)	80330	1(3)	80432	1(3)	81208	1(3)	81276	1(3)	81364	1(2)	81507	1(2)	82240	1(3)
79440	1(3)	80331	1(3)	80434	1(3)	81209	1(3)	81283	1(2)	81370	1(2)	81508	1(2)	82247	2(3)
79445	1(3)	80332	1(3)	80435	1(3)	81210	1(3)	81284	1(2)	81371	1(2)	81509	1(2)	82248	2(3)
79999	1(3)	80333	1(3)	80436	1(3)	81212	1(2)	81285	1(2)	81372	1(2)	81510	1(2)	82252	1(3)
80047	2(3)	80334	1(3)	80438	1(3)	81215	1(2)	81286	1(2)	81373	2(2)	81511	1(2)	82261	1(3)
80048	2(3)	80335	1(3)	80439	1(3)	81216	1(2)	81287	1(3)	81374	1(3)	81512	1(2)	82270	1(3)
80050	0(3)	80336	1(3)	80500	1(3)	81217	1(2)	81288	1(3)	81375	1(2)	81518	1(3)	82271	3(3)
80051	4(3)	80337	1(3)	80502	1(3)	81218	1(3)	81289	1(2)	81376	5(3)	81519	1(2)	82272	1(3)
80053	1(3)	80338	1(3)	81000	2(3)	81219	1(3)	81290	1(3)	81377	2(3)	81520	1(3)	82274	1(3)
80055	1(3)	80339	2(3)	81001	2(3)	81220	1(3)	81291	1(3)	81378	1(2)	81521	1(3)	82286	1(3)
80061	1(3)	80340	1(3)	81002	2(3)	81221	1(3)	81292	1(2)	81379	1(2)	81525	1(3)	82300	1(3)
80069	1(3)	80341	1(3)	81003	2(3)	81222	1(3)	81293	1(3)	81380	2(2)	81528	1(2)	82306	1(2)
80074	1(2)	80342	1(3)	81005	2(3)	81223	1(2)	81294	1(3)	81381	3(3)	81535	1(2)	82308	1(3)
80076	1(3)	80343	1(3)	81007	1(3)	81224	1(3)	81295	1(2)	81382	6(3)	81536	11(3)	82310	4(3)
80081	1(2)	80344	1(3)	81015	2(3)	81225	1(3)	81296	1(3)	81383	2(3)	81538	1(2)	82330	4(3)
80150	2(3)	80345	2(3)	81020	1(3)	81226	1(3)	81297	1(3)	81400	2(3)	81539	1(2)	82331	1(3)
80155	1(3)	80346	1(3)	81025	1(3)	81227	1(3)	81298	1(2)	81401	3(3)	81540	1(3)	82340	1(3)
80156	2(3)	80347	1(3)	81050	2(3)	81228	1(3)	81299	1(3)	81402	1(3)	81541	1(2)	82355	2(3)
80157	2(3)	80348	1(3)	81099	1(3)	81229	1(3)	81300	1(3)	81403	3(3)	81545	1(3)	82360	2(3)
80158	2(3)	80349	1(3)	81105	1(2)	81230	1(2)	81301	1(3)	81404	3(3)	81551	1(2)	82365	2(3)
80159	2(3)	80350	1(3)	81106	1(2)	81231	1(2)	81302	1(3)	81405	2(3)	81595	1(2)	82370	2(3)

Appendix I — Medically Unlikely Edits (MUEs)—OPPS

CPT	MUE	CPT	MUE	CPT	MUE	CPT	MUE	CPT	MUE	CPT	MUE	CPT	MUE	CPT	MUE
82373	1(3)	82710	1(3)	83070	1(2)	83918	2(3)	84238	3(3)	84597	1(3)	85378	2(3)	86153	1(3)
82374	2(3)	82715	3(3)	83080	2(3)	83919	1(3)	84244	2(3)	84600	2(3)	85379	2(3)	86155	1(3)
82375	4(3)	82725	1(3)	83088	1(3)	83921	2(3)	84252	1(2)	84620	1(2)	85380	2(3)	86156	1(2)
82376	2(3)	82726	1(3)	83090	2(3)	83930	2(3)	84255	2(3)	84630	2(3)	85384	2(3)	86157	1(2)
82378	1(3)	82728	1(3)	83150	1(3)	83935	2(3)	84260	1(3)	84681	1(3)	85385	1(3)	86160	4(3)
82379	1(3)	82731	1(3)	83491	1(3)	83937	1(3)	84270	1(3)	84702	2(3)	85390	3(3)	86161	2(3)
82380	1(3)	82735	1(3)	83497	1(3)	83945	2(3)	84275	1(3)	84703	1(3)	85396	1(2)	86162	1(2)
82382	1(2)	82746	1(2)	83498	2(3)	83950	1(2)	84285	1(3)	84704	1(3)	85397	2(3)	86171	2(3)
82383	1(3)	82747	1(2)	83500	1(3)	83951	1(2)	84295	2(3)	84830	1(2)	85400	1(3)	86200	1(3)
82384	2(3)	82757	1(2)	83505	1(3)	83970	4(3)	84300	2(3)	84999	1(3)	85410	1(3)	86215	1(3)
82387	1(3)	82759	1(3)	83516	5(3)	83986	2(3)	84302	1(3)	85002	1(3)	85415	2(3)	86225	1(3)
82390	1(2)	82760	1(3)	83518	1(3)	83987	1(3)	84305	1(3)	85004	2(3)	85420	2(3)	86226	1(3)
82397	4(3)	82775	1(3)	83519	5(3)	83992	2(3)	84307	1(3)	85007	1(3)	85421	1(3)	86235	10(3)
82415	1(3)	82776	1(2)	83520	8(3)	83993	1(3)	84311	2(3)	85008	1(3)	85441	1(2)	86255	5(3)
82435	2(3)	82777	1(3)	83525	4(3)	84030	1(2)	84315	1(3)	85009	1(3)	85445	1(2)	86256	9(3)
82436	1(3)	82784	6(3)	83527	1(3)	84035	1(2)	84375	1(3)	85013	1(3)	85460	1(3)	86277	1(3)
82438	1(3)	82785	1(3)	83528	1(3)	84060	1(3)	84376	1(3)	85014	4(3)	85461	1(3)	86280	1(3)
82441	1(2)	82787	4(3)	83540	2(3)	84066	1(3)	84377	1(3)	85018	4(3)	85475	1(3)	86294	1(3)
82465	1(3)	82800	2(3)	83550	1(3)	84075	2(3)	84378	2(3)	85025	4(3)	85520	3(3)	86300	2(3)
82480	2(3)	82805	3(3)	83570	1(3)	84078	1(2)	84379	1(3)	85027	4(3)	85525	2(3)	86301	1(2)
82482	1(3)	82810	4(3)	83582	1(3)	84080	1(3)	84392	1(3)	85032	2(3)	85530	1(3)	86304	1(3)
82485	1(3)	82820	1(3)	83586	1(3)	84081	1(3)	84402	1(3)	85041	1(3)	85536	1(2)	86305	1(2)
82495	1(2)	82930	1(3)	83593	1(3)	84085	1(2)	84403	2(3)	85044	1(2)	85540	1(2)	86308	1(2)
82507	1(3)	82938	1(3)	83605	2(3)	84087	1(3)	84410	1(2)	85045	1(2)	85547	1(2)	86309	1(2)
82523	1(3)	82941	1(3)	83615	3(3)	84100	2(3)	84425	1(2)	85046	1(2)	85549	1(3)	86310	1(2)
82525	2(3)	82943	1(3)	83625	1(3)	84105	1(3)	84430	1(3)	85048	2(3)	85555	1(2)	86316	2(3)
82528	1(3)	82945	4(3)	83630	1(3)	84106	1(2)	84431	1(3)	85049	2(3)	85557	1(2)	86317	6(3)
82530	4(3)	82946	1(2)	83631	1(3)	84110	1(3)	84432	1(2)	85055	1(3)	85576	7(3)	86318	2(3)
82533	5(3)	82947	5(3)	83632	1(3)	84112	1(3)	84436	1(2)	85060	1(3)	85597	1(3)	86320	1(2)
82540	1(3)	82950	3(3)	83633	1(3)	84119	1(2)	84437	1(2)	85097	2(3)	85598	1(3)	86325	2(3)
82542	6(3)	82951	1(2)	83655	2(3)	84120	1(3)	84439	1(2)	85130	1(3)	85610	4(3)	86327	1(3)
82550	3(3)	82952	3(3)	83661	3(3)	84126	1(3)	84442	1(2)	85170	1(3)	85611	2(3)	86329	3(3)
82552	3(3)	82955	1(2)	83662	4(3)	84132	3(3)	84443	4(2)	85175	1(3)	85612	1(3)	86331	12(3)
82553	3(3)	82960	1(2)	83663	3(3)	84133	2(3)	84445	1(2)	85210	2(3)	85613	3(3)	86332	1(3)
82554	2(3)	82963	1(3)	83664	3(3)	84134	1(3)	84446	1(2)	85220	2(3)	85635	1(3)	86334	2(2)
82565	2(3)	82965	1(3)	83670	1(3)	84135	1(3)	84449	1(3)	85230	2(3)	85651	1(2)	86335	2(3)
82570	3(3)	82977	1(3)	83690	2(3)	84138	1(3)	84450	1(3)	85240	2(3)	85652	1(2)	86336	1(3)
82575	1(3)	82978	1(3)	83695	1(3)	84140	1(3)	84460	1(3)	85244	1(3)	85660	2(3)	86337	1(2)
82585	1(2)	82979	1(3)	83698	1(3)	84143	2(3)	84466	1(3)	85245	2(3)	85670	2(3)	86340	1(2)
82595	1(3)	82985	1(3)	83700	1(2)	84144	1(3)	84478	1(3)	85246	2(3)	85675	1(3)	86341	1(3)
82600	1(3)	83001	1(3)	83701	1(3)	84145	1(3)	84479	1(3)	85247	2(3)	85705	1(3)	86343	1(3)
82607	1(2)	83002	1(3)	83704	1(3)	84146	3(3)	84480	1(2)	85250	2(3)	85730	4(3)	86344	1(2)
82608	1(2)	83003	5(3)	83718	1(3)	84150	2(3)	84481	1(2)	85260	2(3)	85732	4(3)	86352	1(3)
82610	1(3)	83006	1(2)	83719	1(3)	84152	1(2)	84482	1(2)	85270	2(3)	85810	2(3)	86353	7(3)
82615	1(3)	83009	1(3)	83721	1(3)	84153	1(2)	84484	4(3)	85280	2(3)	85999	1(3)	86355	1(2)
82626	1(3)	83010	1(3)	83722	1(2)	84154	1(2)	84485	1(3)	85290	2(3)	86000	6(3)	86356	7(3)
82627	1(3)	83012	1(2)	83727	1(3)	84155	1(3)	84488	1(3)	85291	1(3)	86001	20(3)	86357	1(2)
82633	1(3)	83013	1(3)	83735	4(3)	84156	1(3)	84490	1(2)	85292	1(3)	86005	6(3)	86359	1(2)
82634	1(3)	83014	1(2)	83775	1(3)	84157	2(3)	84510	1(3)	85293	1(3)	86008	20(3)	86360	1(2)
82638	1(3)	83015	1(2)	83785	1(3)	84160	2(3)	84512	3(3)	85300	2(3)	86021	1(2)	86361	1(2)
82642	1(2)	83018	4(3)	83789	4(3)	84163	1(3)	84520	2(3)	85301	1(3)	86022	1(2)	86367	2(3)
82652	1(2)	83020	2(3)	83825	2(3)	84165	1(2)	84525	1(3)	85302	1(3)	86023	3(3)	86376	2(3)
82656	1(3)	83021	2(3)	83835	2(3)	84166	2(3)	84540	2(3)	85303	2(3)	86038	1(3)	86382	3(3)
82657	2(3)	83026	1(3)	83857	1(3)	84181	3(3)	84545	1(3)	85305	2(3)	86039	1(3)	86384	1(3)
82658	2(3)	83030	1(3)	83861	2(2)	84182	6(3)	84550	1(3)	85306	2(3)	86060	1(3)	86386	1(2)
82664	2(3)	83033	1(3)	83864	1(2)	84202	1(2)	84560	2(3)	85307	2(3)	86063	1(3)	86403	3(3)
82668	1(3)	83036	1(2)	83872	2(3)	84203	1(2)	84577	1(3)	85335	2(3)	86077	1(2)	86406	2(3)
82670	2(3)	83037	1(2)	83873	1(3)	84206	1(2)	84578	1(3)	85337	1(3)	86078	1(3)	86430	2(3)
82671	1(3)	83045	1(3)	83874	4(3)	84207	1(2)	84580	1(3)	85345	1(3)	86079	1(3)	86431	2(3)
82672	1(3)	83050	2(3)	83876	1(3)	84210	1(3)	84583	1(3)	85347	9(3)	86140	1(2)	86480	1(3)
82677	1(3)	83051	1(3)	83880	1(3)	84220	1(3)	84585	1(2)	85348	4(3)	86141	1(2)	86481	1(3)
82679	1(3)	83060	1(3)	83883	4(3)	84228	1(3)	84586	1(2)	85360	1(3)	86146	3(3)	86485	1(2)
82693	2(3)	83065	1(2)	83885	2(3)	84233	1(3)	84588	1(3)	85362	2(3)	86147	4(3)	86486	2(3)
82696	1(3)	83068	1(2)	83915	1(3)	84234	1(3)	84590	1(2)	85366	1(3)	86148	3(3)	86490	1(2)
82705	1(3)	83069	1(3)	83916	2(3)	84235	1(3)	84591	1(3)	85370	1(3)	86152	1(3)	86510	1(2)

CPT	MUE	CPT	MUE	CPT	MUE	CPT	MUE	CPT	MUE	CPT	MUE	CPT	MUE	CPT	MUE
86580	1(2)	86738	2(3)	86930	3(3)	87254	10(3)	87493	2(3)	87653	1(3)	88161	4(3)	88342	3(3)
86590	1(3)	86741	2(3)	86931	4(3)	87255	2(3)	87495	1(3)	87660	1(3)	88162	3(3)	88344	6(3)
86592	2(3)	86744	2(3)	86940	3(3)	87260	1(3)	87496	1(3)	87661	1(3)	88164	1(3)	88346	2(3)
86593	2(3)	86747	2(3)	86941	3(3)	87265	1(3)	87497	2(3)	87662	2(3)	88165	1(3)	88348	1(3)
86602	3(3)	86750	4(3)	86945	5(3)	87267	1(3)	87498	1(3)	87797	3(3)	88166	1(3)	88350	8(3)
86603	2(3)	86753	3(3)	86950	1(3)	87269	1(3)	87500	1(3)	87798	21(3)	88167	1(3)	88355	1(3)
86609	14(3)	86756	2(3)	86960	3(3)	87270	1(3)	87501	1(3)	87799	3(3)	88172	7(3)	88356	3(3)
86611	4(3)	86757	6(3)	86965	4(3)	87271	1(3)	87502	1(3)	87800	2(3)	88173	7(3)	88358	2(3)
86612	2(3)	86759	2(3)	86971	6(3)	87272	1(3)	87503	1(3)	87801	3(3)	88174	1(3)	88360	6(3)
86615	6(3)	86762	2(3)	86972	2(3)	87273	1(3)	87505	1(2)	87802	2(3)	88175	1(3)	88361	6(3)
86617	2(3)	86765	2(3)	86975	2(3)	87274	1(3)	87506	1(2)	87803	3(3)	88177	6(3)	88362	1(3)
86618	2(3)	86768	5(3)	86976	2(3)	87275	1(3)	87507	1(2)	87804	3(3)	88182	2(3)	88363	2(3)
86619	2(3)	86771	2(3)	86977	2(3)	87276	1(3)	87510	1(3)	87806	1(2)	88184	2(3)	88364	3(3)
86622	2(3)	86774	2(3)	86999	1(3)	87278	1(3)	87511	1(3)	87807	2(3)	88185	35(3)	88365	4(3)
86625	1(3)	86777	2(3)	87003	1(3)	87279	1(3)	87512	1(3)	87808	1(3)	88187	2(3)	88366	2(3)
86628	3(3)	86778	2(3)	87015	3(3)	87280	1(3)	87516	1(3)	87809	2(3)	88188	2(3)	88367	3(3)
86631	6(3)	86780	2(3)	87045	3(3)	87281	1(3)	87517	1(3)	87810	2(3)	88189	2(3)	88368	3(3)
86632	3(3)	86784	1(3)	87046	6(3)	87283	1(3)	87520	1(3)	87850	1(3)	88199	1(3)	88369	3(3)
86635	4(3)	86787	2(3)	87071	2(3)	87285	1(3)	87521	1(3)	87880	2(3)	88230	2(3)	88371	1(3)
86638	6(3)	86788	2(3)	87073	2(3)	87290	1(3)	87522	1(3)	87899	6(3)	88233	2(3)	88372	1(3)
86641	2(3)	86789	2(3)	87075	6(3)	87299	1(3)	87525	1(3)	87900	1(2)	88235	2(3)	88373	3(3)
86644	2(3)	86790	4(3)	87076	4(3)	87300	2(3)	87526	1(3)	87901	1(2)	88237	4(3)	88374	5(3)
86645	1(3)	86793	2(3)	87077	6(3)	87301	1(3)	87527	1(3)	87902	1(2)	88239	3(3)	88375	1(3)
86648	2(3)	86794	1(3)	87081	4(3)	87305	1(3)	87528	1(3)	87903	1(2)	88240	3(3)	88377	5(3)
86651	2(3)	86800	1(3)	87084	1(3)	87320	1(3)	87529	2(3)	87904	14(3)	88241	3(3)	88380	1(3)
86652	2(3)	86803	1(3)	87086	3(3)	87324	2(3)	87530	2(3)	87905	2(3)	88245	1(2)	88381	1(3)
86653	2(3)	86804	1(2)	87088	3(3)	87327	1(3)	87531	1(3)	87906	2(3)	88248	1(2)	88387	2(3)
86654	2(3)	86805	12(3)	87101	3(3)	87328	2(3)	87532	1(3)	87910	1(3)	88249	1(2)	88388	1(3)
86658	12(3)	86806	2(3)	87102	4(3)	87329	2(3)	87533	1(3)	87912	1(3)	88261	2(3)	88399	1(3)
86663	2(3)	86807	2(3)	87103	2(3)	87332	1(3)	87534	1(3)	87999	1(3)	88262	2(3)	88720	1(3)
86664	2(3)	86808	1(3)	87106	4(3)	87335	1(3)	87535	1(3)	88000	0(3)	88263	1(3)	88738	1(3)
86665	2(3)	86812	1(2)	87107	4(3)	87336	1(3)	87536	1(3)	88005	0(3)	88264	1(3)	88740	1(2)
86666	4(3)	86813	1(2)	87109	2(3)	87337	1(3)	87537	1(3)	88007	0(3)	88267	2(3)	88741	1(2)
86668	2(3)	86816	1(2)	87110	2(3)	87338	1(3)	87538	1(3)	88012	0(3)	88269	2(3)	88749	1(3)
86671	3(3)	86817	1(2)	87118	3(3)	87339	1(3)	87539	1(3)	88014	0(3)	88271	16(3)	89049	1(3)
86674	3(3)	86821	1(3)	87140	3(3)	87340	1(2)	87540	1(3)	88016	0(3)	88272	12(3)	89050	2(3)
86677	3(3)	86825	1(3)	87143	2(3)	87341	1(2)	87541	1(3)	88020	0(3)	88273	3(3)	89051	2(3)
86682	2(3)	86826	8(3)	87149	11(3)	87350	1(2)	87542	1(3)	88025	0(3)	88274	5(3)	89055	2(3)
86684	2(3)	86828	2(3)	87150	12(3)	87380	1(2)	87550	1(3)	88027	0(3)	88275	12(3)	89060	2(3)
86687	1(3)	86829	2(3)	87152	1(3)	87385	2(3)	87551	2(3)	88028	0(3)	88280	1(3)	89125	2(3)
86688	1(3)	86830	2(3)	87153	3(3)	87389	1(3)	87552	1(3)	88029	0(3)	88283	5(3)	89160	1(3)
86689	2(3)	86831	2(3)	87164	2(3)	87390	1(3)	87555	1(3)	88036	0(3)	88285	10(3)	89190	1(3)
86692	2(3)	86832	2(3)	87166	2(3)	87391	1(3)	87556	1(3)	88037	0(3)	88289	1(3)	89220	2(3)
86694	2(3)	86833	1(3)	87168	2(3)	87400	2(3)	87557	1(3)	88040	0(3)	88291	0(3)	89230	1(2)
86695	2(3)	86834	1(3)	87169	2(3)	87420	1(3)	87560	1(3)	88045	0(3)	88299	1(3)	89240	1(3)
86696	2(3)	86835	1(3)	87172	1(3)	87425	2(3)	87561	1(3)	88099	0(3)	88300	4(3)	89250	1(2)
86698	3(3)	86849	1(3)	87176	3(3)	87427	2(3)	87562	1(3)	88104	5(3)	88302	4(3)	89251	1(2)
86701	1(3)	86850	3(3)	87177	3(3)	87430	1(3)	87580	1(3)	88106	5(3)	88304	5(3)	89253	1(3)
86702	2(3)	86860	2(3)	87181	12(3)	87449	3(3)	87581	1(3)	88108	6(3)	88305	16(3)	89254	1(3)
86703	1(2)	86870	6(3)	87184	8(3)	87450	2(3)	87582	1(3)	88112	6(3)	88307	8(3)	89255	1(3)
86704	1(2)	86880	4(3)	87185	4(3)	87451	2(3)	87590	1(3)	88120	2(3)	88309	3(3)	89257	1(3)
86705	1(2)	86885	3(3)	87186	12(3)	87471	1(3)	87591	3(3)	88121	2(3)	88311	4(3)	89258	1(2)
86706	2(3)	86886	3(3)	87187	3(3)	87472	1(3)	87592	1(3)	88125	1(3)	88312	9(3)	89259	1(2)
86707	1(3)	86890	2(3)	87188	14(3)	87475	1(3)	87623	1(2)	88130	1(2)	88313	8(3)	89260	1(2)
86708	1(2)	86891	2(3)	87190	10(3)	87476	1(3)	87624	1(3)	88140	1(2)	88314	6(3)	89261	1(3)
86709	1(2)	86900	3(3)	87197	1(3)	87480	1(3)	87625	1(3)	88141	1(3)	88319	11(3)	89264	1(3)
86710	4(3)	86901	3(3)	87206	6(3)	87481	6(3)	87631	1(3)	88142	1(3)	88321	1(2)	89268	1(2)
86711	2(3)	86902	40(3)	87207	3(3)	87482	1(3)	87632	1(3)	88143	1(3)	88323	1(2)	89272	1(2)
86713	3(3)	86905	28(3)	87209	4(3)	87483	1(2)	87633	1(3)	88147	1(3)	88325	1(2)	89280	1(2)
86717	8(3)	86906	1(2)	87210	4(3)	87485	1(3)	87634	1(3)	88148	1(3)	88329	2(3)	89281	1(2)
86720	2(3)	86910	0(3)	87220	3(3)	87486	1(3)	87640	1(3)	88150	1(3)	88331	11(3)	89290	1(2)
86723	2(3)	86911	0(3)	87230	2(3)	87487	1(3)	87641	1(3)	88152	1(3)	88332	13(3)	89291	1(2)
86727	2(3)	86920	19(3)	87250	1(3)	87490	1(3)	87650	1(3)	88153	1(3)	88333	4(3)	89300	1(2)
86732	2(3)	86922	10(3)	87252	4(3)	87491	3(3)	87651	1(3)	88155	1(3)	88334	5(3)	89310	1(2)
86735	2(3)	86923	10(3)	87253	3(3)	87492	1(3)	87652	1(3)	88160	4(3)	88341	13(3)	89320	1(2)

CPT	MUE	CPT	MUE	CPT	MUE	CPT	MUE	CPT	MUE	CPT	MUE	CPT	MUE	CPT	MUE
89321	1(2)	90657	1(2)	90846	2(3)	91122	1(2)	92371	1(3)	92595	0(3)	93015	1(3)	93452	1(3)
89322	1(2)	90658	1(2)	90847	2(3)	91132	1(3)	92499	1(3)	92596	1(2)	93016	1(3)	93453	1(3)
89325	1(2)	90660	1(2)	90849	2(3)	91133	1(3)	92502	1(3)	92597	1(3)	93017	1(3)	93454	1(3)
89329	1(2)	90661	1(2)	90853	4(3)	91200	1(3)	92504	1(3)	92601	1(3)	93018	1(3)	93455	1(3)
89330	1(2)	90662	1(2)	90863	1(3)	91299	1(3)	92507	1(3)	92602	1(3)	93024	1(3)	93456	1(3)
89331	1(2)	90664	1(2)	90865	1(3)	92002	1(2)	92508	1(3)	92603	1(3)	93025	1(2)	93457	1(3)
89335	1(3)	90666	1(2)	90867	1(2)	92004	1(2)	92511	1(3)	92604	1(3)	93040	3(3)	93458	1(3)
89337	1(2)	90667	1(2)	90868	1(3)	92012	1(2)	92512	1(2)	92605	1(2)	93041	3(3)	93459	1(3)
89342	1(2)	90668	1(2)	90869	1(3)	92014	1(3)	92516	1(3)	92606	1(2)	93042	3(3)	93460	1(3)
89343	1(2)	90670	1(2)	90870	2(3)	92015	0(3)	92520	1(2)	92607	1(3)	93050	1(3)	93461	1(3)
89344	1(2)	90672	1(2)	90875	0(3)	92018	1(2)	92521	1(2)	92608	4(3)	93224	1(2)	93462	1(3)
89346	1(2)	90673	1(2)	90876	0(3)	92019	1(2)	92522	1(2)	92609	1(3)	93225	1(2)	93463	1(3)
89352	1(2)	90674	1(2)	90880	1(3)	92020	1(2)	92523	1(2)	92610	1(2)	93226	1(2)	93464	1(3)
89353	1(3)	90675	1(2)	90882	0(3)	92025	1(2)	92524	1(2)	92611	1(3)	93227	1(2)	93503	2(3)
89354	1(3)	90676	1(2)	90885	1(3)	92060	1(2)	92526	1(2)	92612	1(3)	93228	1(2)	93505	1(2)
89356	2(3)	90680	1(2)	90887	1(3)	92065	1(2)	92531	1(3)	92613	1(2)	93229	1(2)	93530	1(3)
89398	1(3)	90681	1(2)	90889	1(3)	92071	2(2)	92532	1(3)	92614	1(3)	93260	1(2)	93531	1(3)
90281	0(3)	90682	1(2)	90899	1(3)	92072	1(2)	92533	4(2)	92615	1(2)	93261	1(3)	93532	1(3)
90283	0(3)	90685	1(2)	90901	1(3)	92081	1(2)	92534	1(3)	92616	1(3)	93264	1(2)	93533	1(3)
90284	0(3)	90686	1(2)	90911	1(3)	92082	1(2)	92537	1(2)	92617	1(2)	93268	1(2)	93561	1(3)
90287	0(3)	90687	1(2)	90935	1(3)	92083	1(2)	92538	1(2)	92618	1(3)	93270	1(2)	93562	1(3)
90288	0(3)	90688	1(2)	90937	1(3)	92100	1(2)	92540	1(3)	92620	1(2)	93271	1(2)	93563	1(3)
90291	0(3)	90689	1(2)	90940	1(3)	92132	1(2)	92541	1(3)	92621	4(3)	93272	1(2)	93564	1(3)
90296	1(2)	90690	1(2)	90945	1(3)	92133	1(2)	92542	1(3)	92625	1(2)	93278	1(3)	93565	1(3)
90371	10(3)	90691	1(2)	90947	1(3)	92134	1(2)	92544	1(3)	92626	1(2)	93279	1(3)	93566	1(3)
90375	20(3)	90696	1(2)	90951	1(2)	92136	1(3)	92545	1(3)	92627	6(3)	93280	1(3)	93567	1(3)
90376	20(3)	90697	1(2)	90952	1(2)	92145	1(2)	92546	1(3)	92630	0(3)	93281	1(3)	93568	1(3)
90378	4(3)	90698	1(2)	90953	1(2)	92225	2(2)	92547	1(3)	92633	0(3)	93282	1(3)	93571	1(3)
90384	0(3)	90700	1(2)	90954	1(2)	92226	2(2)	92548	1(3)	92640	1(3)	93283	1(3)	93572	2(3)
90385	0(3)	90702	1(2)	90955	1(2)	92227	1(2)	92550	1(2)	92700	1(3)	93284	1(3)	93580	1(3)
90386	0(3)	90707	1(2)	90956	1(2)	92228	1(2)	92551	0(3)	92920	3(3)	93285	1(3)	93581	1(3)
90389	0(3)	90710	1(2)	90957	1(2)	92230	2(2)	92552	1(2)	92921	6(2)	93286	2(3)	93582	1(2)
90393	1(2)	90713	1(2)	90958	1(2)	92235	1(2)	92553	1(2)	92924	2(3)	93287	2(3)	93583	1(2)
90396	1(2)	90714	1(2)	90959	1(2)	92240	1(2)	92555	1(2)	92925	6(2)	93288	1(3)	93590	1(2)
90399	0(3)	90715	1(2)	90960	1(2)	92242	1(2)	92556	1(2)	92928	3(3)	93289	1(3)	93591	1(2)
90460	9(3)	90716	1(2)	90961	1(2)	92250	1(2)	92557	1(2)	92929	6(2)	93290	1(3)	93592	2(3)
90461	8(3)	90717	1(2)	90962	1(2)	92260	1(2)	92558	0(3)	92933	2(3)	93291	1(3)	93600	1(3)
90471	1(2)	90723	0(3)	90963	1(2)	92265	1(2)	92559	0(3)	92934	6(2)	93292	1(3)	93602	1(3)
90472	8(3)	90732	1(2)	90964	1(2)	92270	1(2)	92560	0(3)	92937	2(3)	93293	1(2)	93603	1(3)
90473	1(2)	90733	1(2)	90965	1(2)	92273	1(2)	92561	1(2)	92938	6(3)	93294	1(2)	93609	1(3)
90474	1(3)	90734	1(2)	90966	1(2)	92274	1(2)	92562	1(2)	92941	1(3)	93295	1(2)	93610	1(3)
90476	1(2)	90736	1(2)	90967	1(2)	92283	1(2)	92563	1(2)	92943	2(3)	93296	1(2)	93612	1(3)
90477	1(2)	90738	1(2)	90968	1(2)	92284	1(2)	92564	1(2)	92944	3(3)	93297	1(2)	93613	1(3)
90581	1(2)	90739	1(2)	90969	1(2)	92285	1(2)	92565	1(2)	92950	2(3)	93298	1(2)	93615	1(3)
90585	1(2)	90740	1(2)	90970	1(2)	92286	1(2)	92567	1(2)	92953	2(3)	93299	1(2)	93616	1(3)
90586	1(2)	90743	1(2)	90989	1(2)	92287	1(2)	92568	1(2)	92960	2(3)	93303	1(3)	93618	1(3)
90587	1(2)	90744	1(2)	90993	1(3)	92310	0(3)	92570	1(2)	92961	1(3)	93304	1(3)	93619	1(3)
90620	1(2)	90746	1(2)	90997	1(3)	92311	1(2)	92571	1(2)	92970	1(3)	93306	1(3)	93620	1(3)
90621	1(2)	90747	1(2)	90999	1(3)	92312	1(2)	92572	1(2)	92971	1(3)	93307	1(3)	93621	1(3)
90625	1(2)	90748	0(3)	91010	1(2)	92313	1(3)	92575	1(2)	92973	2(3)	93308	1(3)	93622	1(3)
90630	1(2)	90749	1(3)	91013	1(3)	92314	0(3)	92576	1(2)	92974	1(3)	93312	1(3)	93623	1(3)
90632	1(2)	90750	1(2)	91020	1(2)	92315	1(2)	92577	1(2)	92975	1(3)	93313	1(3)	93624	1(3)
90633	1(2)	90756	1(2)	91022	1(2)	92316	1(2)	92579	1(2)	92977	1(3)	93314	1(3)	93631	1(3)
90634	1(2)	90785	3(3)	91030	1(2)	92317	1(3)	92582	1(2)	92978	1(3)	93315	1(3)	93640	1(3)
90636	1(2)	90791	1(3)	91034	1(2)	92325	1(3)	92583	1(2)	92979	2(3)	93316	1(3)	93641	1(2)
90644	1(2)	90792	2(3)	91035	1(2)	92326	2(2)	92584	1(2)	92986	1(2)	93317	1(3)	93642	1(3)
90647	1(2)	90832	3(3)	91037	1(2)	92340	0(3)	92585	1(2)	92987	1(2)	93318	1(3)	93644	1(3)
90648	1(2)	90833	3(3)	91038	1(2)	92341	0(3)	92586	1(2)	92990	1(2)	93320	1(3)	93650	1(2)
90649	1(2)	90834	3(3)	91040	1(2)	92342	0(3)	92587	1(2)	92992	1(2)	93321	1(3)	93653	1(3)
90650	1(2)	90836	3(3)	91065	2(2)	92352	1(3)	92588	1(2)	92993	1(2)	93325	1(3)	93654	1(3)
90651	1(2)	90837	3(3)	91110	1(2)	92353	1(3)	92590	0(3)	92997	1(2)	93350	1(2)	93655	2(3)
90653	1(2)	90838	3(3)	91111	1(2)	92354	1(3)	92591	0(3)	92998	2(3)	93351	1(2)	93656	1(3)
90654	1(2)	90839	1(2)	91112	1(3)	92355	1(3)	92592	0(3)	93000	3(3)	93352	1(3)	93657	1(3)
90655	1(2)	90840	4(3)	91117	1(2)	92358	1(3)	92593	0(3)	93005	5(3)	93355	1(3)	93660	1(3)
90656	1(2)	90845	1(2)	91120	1(2)	92370	0(3)	92594	0(3)	93010	5(3)	93451	1(3)	93662	1(3)

CPT	MUE	CPT	MUE	CPT	MUE	CPT	MUE	CPT	MUE	CPT	MUE	CPT	MUE	CPT	MUE
93668	1(3)	94618	1(3)	95180	8(3)	95928	1(3)	96154	8(3)	97014	0(3)	97804	6(3)	99202	1(2)
93701	1(2)	94621	1(3)	95199	1(3)	95929	1(3)	96155	0(3)	97016	1(3)	97810	0(3)	99203	1(2)
93702	1(2)	94640	1(3)	95249	1(2)	95930	1(3)	96160	3(3)	97018	1(3)	97811	0(3)	99204	1(2)
93724	1(3)	94642	1(3)	95250	1(2)	95933	1(3)	96161	1(3)	97022	1(3)	97813	0(3)	99205	1(2)
93740	1(3)	94644	1(2)	95251	1(2)	95937	4(3)	96360	2(3)	97024	1(3)	97814	0(3)	99211	2(3)
93745	1(2)	94645	4(3)	95782	1(2)	95938	1(3)	96361	24(3)	97026	1(3)	98925	1(2)	99212	2(3)
93750	1(3)	94660	1(2)	95783	1(2)	95939	1(3)	96365	2(3)	97028	1(3)	98926	1(2)	99213	2(3)
93770	1(3)	94662	1(2)	95800	1(2)	95940	20(3)	96366	24(3)	97032	4(3)	98927	1(2)	99214	2(3)
93784	1(2)	94664	1(3)	95801	1(2)	95941	8(3)	96367	4(3)	97033	4(3)	98928	1(2)	99215	2(3)
93786	1(2)	94667	1(2)	95803	1(2)	95943	1(3)	96368	1(2)	97034	2(3)	98929	1(2)	99217	1(2)
93788	1(2)	94668	5(3)	95805	1(2)	95950	1(2)	96369	1(2)	97035	2(3)	98940	1(2)	99218	1(2)
93790	1(2)	94669	4(3)	95806	1(2)	95951	1(2)	96370	3(3)	97036	3(3)	98941	1(2)	99219	1(2)
93792	1(2)	94680	1(3)	95807	1(2)	95953	1(2)	96371	1(3)	97039	1(3)	98942	1(2)	99220	1(2)
93793	1(2)	94681	1(3)	95808	1(2)	95954	1(3)	96372	5(3)	97110	8(3)	98943	0(3)	99221	0(3)
93797	2(2)	94690	1(3)	95810	1(3)	95955	1(3)	96373	3(3)	97112	6(3)	98960	0(3)	99222	0(3)
93798	2(2)	94726	1(3)	95811	1(2)	95956	1(2)	96374	1(3)	97113	6(3)	98961	0(3)	99223	0(3)
93799	1(3)	94727	1(3)	95812	1(3)	95957	1(3)	96375	6(3)	97116	4(3)	98962	0(3)	99224	1(2)
93880	1(3)	94728	1(3)	95813	1(3)	95958	1(3)	96376	10(3)	97124	4(3)	98966	0(3)	99225	1(2)
93882	1(3)	94729	1(3)	95816	1(3)	95961	1(2)	96377	1(3)	97127	1(2)	98967	0(3)	99226	1(2)
93886	1(3)	94750	1(3)	95819	1(3)	95962	3(3)	96379	2(3)	97139	1(3)	98968	0(3)	99231	0(3)
93888	1(3)	94760	1(3)	95822	1(3)	95965	1(3)	96401	4(3)	97140	6(3)	98969	0(3)	99232	0(3)
93890	1(3)	94761	1(2)	95824	1(3)	95966	1(3)	96402	2(3)	97150	2(3)	99000	0(3)	99233	0(3)
93892	1(3)	94762	1(2)	95827	1(2)	95967	3(3)	96405	1(2)	97151	8(3)	99001	0(3)	99234	1(3)
93893	1(3)	94770	1(3)	95829	1(3)	95970	1(3)	96406	1(2)	97152	8(3)	99002	1(3)	99235	1(3)
93895	1(3)	94772	1(2)	95830	1(3)	95971	1(3)	96409	1(3)	97153	32(3)	99024	1(3)	99236	1(3)
93922	2(2)	94774	1(2)	95831	5(2)	95972	1(3)	96411	3(3)	97154	12(3)	99026	0(3)	99238	0(3)
93923	2(2)	94775	1(2)	95832	1(3)	95976	1(3)	96413	1(3)	97155	24(3)	99027	0(3)	99239	0(3)
93924	1(2)	94776	1(2)	95833	1(3)	95977	1(3)	96415	8(3)	97156	16(3)	99050	1(3)	99241	0(3)
93925	1(3)	94777	1(2)	95834	1(3)	95980	1(3)	96416	1(3)	97157	16(3)	99051	1(3)	99242	0(3)
93926	1(3)	94780	1(2)	95836	1(2)	95981	1(3)	96417	3(3)	97158	16(3)	99053	1(3)	99243	0(3)
93930	1(3)	94781	2(3)	95851	3(3)	95982	1(3)	96420	2(3)	97161	1(2)	99056	1(3)	99244	0(3)
93931	1(3)	94799	1(3)	95852	1(3)	95983	1(2)	96422	2(3)	97162	1(2)	99058	1(3)	99245	0(3)
93970	1(3)	95004	80(3)	95857	1(2)	95984	11(3)	96423	2(3)	97163	1(2)	99060	1(3)	99251	0(3)
93971	1(3)	95012	2(3)	95860	1(3)	95990	1(3)	96425	1(3)	97164	1(2)	99070	1(3)	99252	0(3)
93975	1(3)	95017	27(3)	95861	1(3)	95991	1(3)	96440	1(3)	97165	1(2)	99071	1(3)	99253	0(3)
93976	1(3)	95018	19(3)	95863	1(3)	95992	1(2)	96446	1(3)	97166	1(2)	99075	0(3)	99254	0(3)
93978	1(3)	95024	40(3)	95864	1(3)	95999	1(3)	96450	1(3)	97167	1(2)	99078	3(3)	99255	0(3)
93979	1(3)	95027	90(3)	95865	1(3)	96000	1(2)	96521	2(3)	97168	1(2)	99080	1(3)	99281	2(3)
93980	1(3)	95028	30(3)	95866	1(3)	96001	1(2)	96522	1(3)	97169	0(3)	99082	1(3)	99282	2(3)
93981	1(3)	95044	80(3)	95867	1(3)	96002	1(3)	96523	2(3)	97170	0(3)	99091	1(2)	99283	2(3)
93990	2(3)	95052	20(3)	95868	1(3)	96003	1(3)	96542	1(3)	97171	0(3)	99100	1(3)	99284	2(3)
93998	1(3)	95056	1(2)	95869	1(3)	96004	1(2)	96549	1(3)	97172	0(3)	99116	1(3)	99285	2(3)
94002	1(2)	95060	1(2)	95870	4(3)	96020	1(2)	96567	1(3)	97530	6(3)	99135	1(3)	99288	1(3)
94003	1(2)	95065	1(3)	95872	4(3)	96040	4(3)	96570	1(2)	97533	4(3)	99140	2(3)	99291	1(2)
94004	1(2)	95070	1(3)	95873	1(2)	96105	3(3)	96571	2(3)	97535	8(3)	99151	1(3)	99292	8(3)
94005	0(3)	95071	1(2)	95874	1(2)	96110	3(3)	96573	1(2)	97537	8(3)	99152	2(3)	99304	1(2)
94010	1(3)	95076	1(2)	95875	2(3)	96112	1(2)	96574	1(2)	97542	8(3)	99153	12(3)	99305	1(2)
94011	1(3)	95079	2(3)	95885	4(2)	96113	6(3)	96900	1(3)	97545	1(2)	99155	1(3)	99306	1(2)
94012	1(3)	95115	1(2)	95886	4(2)	96116	1(2)	96902	1(3)	97546	2(3)	99156	1(3)	99307	1(2)
94013	1(3)	95117	1(2)	95887	1(2)	96121	3(3)	96904	1(2)	97597	1(3)	99157	6(3)	99308	1(2)
94014	1(2)	95120	0(3)	95905	2(3)	96125	2(3)	96910	1(3)	97598	8(3)	99170	1(3)	99309	1(2)
94015	1(2)	95125	0(3)	95907	1(2)	96127	2(3)	96912	1(3)	97602	1(3)	99172	0(3)	99310	1(2)
94016	1(2)	95130	0(3)	95908	1(2)	96130	1(2)	96913	1(3)	97605	1(3)	99173	0(3)	99315	1(2)
94060	1(3)	95131	0(3)	95909	1(2)	96131	7(3)	96920	1(2)	97606	1(3)	99174	0(3)	99316	1(2)
94070	1(2)	95132	0(3)	95910	1(2)	96132	1(2)	96921	1(2)	97607	1(3)	99175	1(3)	99318	1(2)
94150	2(3)	95133	0(3)	95911	1(2)	96133	7(3)	96922	1(2)	97608	1(3)	99177	1(2)	99324	1(2)
94200	1(3)	95134	0(3)	95912	1(2)	96136	1(2)	96931	1(3)	97610	1(2)	99183	1(3)	99325	1(2)
94250	1(3)	95144	30(3)	95913	1(2)	96137	11(3)	96932	1(2)	97750	8(3)	99184	1(2)	99326	1(2)
94375	1(3)	95145	10(3)	95921	1(3)	96138	1(2)	96933	1(2)	97755	8(3)	99188	1(2)	99327	1(2)
94400	1(3)	95146	10(3)	95922	1(3)	96139	11(3)	96934	2(3)	97760	6(3)	99190	1(3)	99328	1(2)
94450	1(3)	95147	10(3)	95923	1(3)	96146	1(2)	96935	2(3)	97761	6(3)	99191	1(3)	99334	1(3)
94452	1(2)	95148	10(3)	95924	1(3)	96150	8(3)	96936	2(3)	97763	6(3)	99192	1(3)	99335	1(3)
94453	1(2)	95149	10(3)	95925	1(3)	96151	6(3)	96999	1(3)	97799	1(3)	99195	2(3)	99336	1(3)
94610	2(3)	95165	30(3)	95926	1(3)	96152	6(3)	97010	1(3)	97802	8(3)	99199	1(3)	99337	1(3)
94617	1(3)	95170	10(3)	95927	1(3)	96153	12(3)	97012	1(3)	97803	8(3)	99201	1(2)	99339	1(2)

CPT	MUE	CPT	MUE	CPT	MUE	CPT	MUE	CPT	MUE	CPT	MUE	CPT	MUE	CPT	MUE
99340	1(2)	99454	1(2)	A0170	0(3)	A4255	0(3)	A4369	1(3)	A4461	2(3)	A4648	3(3)	A5063	1(3)
99341	1(2)	99455	1(3)	A0180	0(3)	A4256	1(3)	A4371	1(3)	A4463	2(3)	A4650	3(3)	A5071	2(3)
99342	1(2)	99456	1(3)	A0190	0(3)	A4257	0(3)	A4372	1(3)	A4465	1(3)	A4651	2(3)	A5072	1(3)
99343	1(2)	99457	1(2)	A0200	0(3)	A4258	0(3)	A4373	1(3)	A4467	0(3)	A4652	2(3)	A5073	1(3)
99344	1(2)	99460	1(2)	A0210	0(3)	A4259	0(3)	A4375	2(3)	A4470	1(3)	A4653	0(3)	A5081	2(3)
99345	1(2)	99461	1(2)	A0225	0(3)	A4261	0(3)	A4376	2(3)	A4480	1(3)	A4657	0(3)	A5082	1(3)
99347	1(3)	99462	1(2)	A0380	0(3)	A4262	4(2)	A4377	2(3)	A4481	2(3)	A4660	0(3)	A5083	5(3)
99348	1(3)	99463	1(2)	A0382	0(3)	A4263	4(2)	A4378	2(3)	A4483	1(3)	A4663	0(3)	A5093	2(3)
99349	1(3)	99464	1(2)	A0384	0(3)	A4264	0(3)	A4379	2(3)	A4490	0(3)	A4670	0(3)	A5102	1(3)
99350	1(3)	99465	1(2)	A0390	0(3)	A4265	1(3)	A4380	2(3)	A4495	0(3)	A4671	0(3)	A5105	1(3)
99354	1(2)	99466	1(2)	A0392	0(3)	A4266	0(3)	A4381	2(3)	A4500	0(3)	A4672	0(3)	A5112	2(3)
99355	4(3)	99467	4(3)	A0394	0(3)	A4267	2(3)	A4382	2(3)	A4510	0(3)	A4673	0(3)	A5113	0(3)
99356	1(2)	99468	1(2)	A0396	0(3)	A4268	0(3)	A4383	2(3)	A4520	0(3)	A4674	0(3)	A5114	0(3)
99357	1(3)	99469	1(2)	A0398	0(3)	A4269	0(3)	A4384	2(3)	A4550	3(3)	A4680	0(3)	A5120	150(3)
99358	1(2)	99471	1(2)	A0420	0(3)	A4270	3(3)	A4385	2(3)	A4553	0(3)	A4690	0(3)	A5121	1(3)
99359	1(3)	99472	1(2)	A0422	0(3)	A4280	1(3)	A4387	1(3)	A4554	0(3)	A4706	0(3)	A5122	1(3)
99360	1(3)	99475	1(2)	A0424	0(3)	A4281	0(3)	A4388	1(3)	A4555	0(3)	A4707	0(3)	A5126	2(3)
99366	2(3)	99476	1(2)	A0425	250(1)	A4282	0(3)	A4389	2(3)	A4556	2(3)	A4708	0(3)	A5131	1(3)
99367	1(3)	99477	1(2)	A0426	2(3)	A4283	0(3)	A4390	1(3)	A4557	2(3)	A4709	0(3)	A5200	2(3)
99368	2(3)	99478	1(2)	A0427	2(3)	A4284	0(3)	A4391	1(3)	A4558	1(3)	A4714	0(3)	A5500	0(3)
99374	1(2)	99479	1(2)	A0428	2(3)	A4285	0(3)	A4392	2(3)	A4559	1(3)	A4719	0(3)	A5501	0(3)
99375	0(3)	99480	1(2)	A0429	2(3)	A4286	0(3)	A4393	1(3)	A4561	1(3)	A4720	0(3)	A5503	0(3)
99377	1(2)	99483	1(2)	A0430	1(3)	A4290	2(3)	A4394	1(3)	A4562	1(3)	A4721	0(3)	A5504	0(3)
99378	0(3)	99484	1(2)	A0431	1(3)	A4300	4(3)	A4395	3(3)	A4563	1(2)	A4722	0(3)	A5505	0(3)
99379	1(2)	99485	1(3)	A0432	1(3)	A4301	1(2)	A4396	2(3)	A4565	2(3)	A4723	0(3)	A5506	0(3)
99380	1(2)	99486	4(1)	A0433	1(3)	A4305	2(3)	A4397	1(3)	A4566	0(3)	A4724	0(3)	A5507	0(3)
99381	0(3)	99487	1(2)	A0434	2(3)	A4306	2(3)	A4398	2(3)	A4570	0(3)	A4725	0(3)	A5508	0(3)
99382	0(3)	99489	4(3)	A0435	999(3)	A4310	2(3)	A4399	1(3)	A4575	0(3)	A4726	0(3)	A5510	0(3)
99383	0(3)	99490	1(2)	A0436	300(3)	A4311	2(3)	A4400	1(3)	A4580	0(3)	A4728	0(3)	A5512	0(3)
99384	0(3)	99491	1(2)	A0888	0(3)	A4312	1(3)	A4402	1(3)	A4590	0(3)	A4730	0(3)	A5513	0(3)
99385	0(3)	99492	1(2)	A0998	0(3)	A4313	1(3)	A4404	1(3)	A4595	2(3)	A4736	0(3)	A5514	0(3)
99386	0(3)	99493	1(2)	A0999	1(3)	A4314	2(3)	A4405	1(3)	A4600	0(3)	A4737	0(3)	A6000	0(3)
99387	0(3)	99494	2(3)	A4206	1(3)	A4315	2(3)	A4406	1(3)	A4601	0(3)	A4740	0(3)	A6010	3(3)
99391	0(3)	99495	1(2)	A4207	1(3)	A4316	1(3)	A4407	2(3)	A4602	1(3)	A4750	0(3)	A6011	20(3)
99392	0(3)	99496	1(2)	A4208	4(3)	A4320	2(3)	A4408	1(3)	A4604	1(3)	A4755	0(3)	A6024	1(3)
99393	0(3)	99497	1(2)	A4209	6(3)	A4321	1(3)	A4409	1(3)	A4605	1(3)	A4760	0(3)	A6025	4(3)
99394	0(3)	99498	3(3)	A4210	0(3)	A4322	2(3)	A4410	2(3)	A4606	1(3)	A4765	0(3)	A6154	1(3)
99395	0(3)	99499	1(3)	A4211	1(3)	A4326	1(3)	A4411	1(3)	A4608	1(3)	A4766	0(3)	A6205	1(3)
99396	0(3)	99500	0(3)	A4212	2(3)	A4327	2(3)	A4412	1(3)	A4611	0(3)	A4770	0(3)	A6221	9(3)
99397	0(3)	99501	0(3)	A4213	5(3)	A4328	1(3)	A4413	2(3)	A4612	0(3)	A4771	0(3)	A6228	2(3)
99401	0(3)	99502	0(3)	A4215	9(3)	A4330	1(3)	A4414	1(3)	A4613	0(3)	A4772	0(3)	A6230	1(3)
99402	0(3)	99503	0(3)	A4216	25(3)	A4331	3(3)	A4415	1(3)	A4614	1(2)	A4773	0(3)	A6236	1(3)
99403	0(3)	99504	0(3)	A4217	4(3)	A4332	2(3)	A4416	2(3)	A4615	2(3)	A4774	0(3)	A6238	3(3)
99404	0(3)	99505	0(3)	A4218	20(3)	A4335	1(3)	A4417	2(3)	A4616	1(3)	A4802	0(3)	A6239	1(3)
99406	1(2)	99506	0(3)	A4220	1(3)	A4336	1(3)	A4418	2(3)	A4617	1(3)	A4860	0(3)	A6240	2(3)
99407	1(2)	99507	0(3)	A4221	1(3)	A4337	2(3)	A4419	2(3)	A4618	1(3)	A4870	0(3)	A6241	1(3)
99408	0(3)	99509	0(3)	A4222	2(3)	A4338	3(3)	A4420	1(3)	A4619	1(3)	A4890	0(3)	A6244	1(3)
99409	0(3)	99510	0(3)	A4223	1(3)	A4340	2(3)	A4423	2(3)	A4620	1(3)	A4911	0(3)	A6246	3(3)
99411	0(3)	99511	0(3)	A4224	1(2)	A4344	2(3)	A4424	1(3)	A4623	10(3)	A4913	0(3)	A6247	2(3)
99412	0(3)	99512	0(3)	A4225	1(3)	A4346	2(3)	A4425	1(3)	A4624	2(3)	A4918	0(3)	A6250	1(3)
99415	1(2)	99600	0(3)	A4230	1(3)	A4351	2(3)	A4426	2(3)	A4625	30(3)	A4927	0(3)	A6256	3(3)
99416	3(3)	99601	0(3)	A4231	1(3)	A4352	2(3)	A4427	1(3)	A4626	1(3)	A4928	0(3)	A6259	3(3)
99429	0(3)	99602	0(3)	A4232	0(3)	A4353	3(3)	A4428	1(3)	A4627	0(3)	A4929	0(3)	A6261	3(3)
99441	0(3)	99605	0(2)	A4233	0(3)	A4354	2(3)	A4429	2(3)	A4628	1(3)	A4930	0(3)	A6262	3(3)
99442	0(3)	99606	0(3)	A4234	0(3)	A4355	2(3)	A4430	1(3)	A4629	1(3)	A4931	0(3)	A6404	2(3)
99443	0(3)	99607	0(3)	A4235	1(3)	A4356	2(3)	A4431	1(3)	A4630	0(3)	A4932	0(3)	A6407	4(3)
99444	0(3)	A0021	0(3)	A4236	0(3)	A4357	2(3)	A4432	2(3)	A4633	0(3)	A5051	1(3)	A6410	2(3)
99446	1(2)	A0080	0(3)	A4244	1(3)	A4360	1(3)	A4433	1(3)	A4634	1(3)	A5052	1(3)	A6411	2(3)
99447	1(2)	A0090	0(3)	A4245	1(3)	A4361	1(3)	A4434	1(3)	A4635	0(3)	A5053	2(3)	A6412	2(3)
99448	1(2)	A0100	0(3)	A4246	1(3)	A4362	2(3)	A4435	2(3)	A4636	0(3)	A5054	1(3)	A6413	0(3)
99449	1(2)	A0110	0(3)	A4247	1(3)	A4363	0(3)	A4450	20(3)	A4637	0(3)	A5055	1(3)	A6441	8(3)
99450	0(3)	A0120	0(3)	A4248	10(3)	A4364	2(3)	A4452	4(3)	A4638	0(3)	A5056	90(3)	A6442	8(3)
99451	1(2)	A0130	0(3)	A4250	0(3)	A4366	1(3)	A4455	1(3)	A4639	0(3)	A5057	90(3)	A6443	8(3)
99452	1(2)	A0140	0(3)	A4252	0(3)	A4367	1(3)	A4458	1(3)	A4640	0(3)	A5061	2(3)	A6444	4(3)
99453	1(2)	A0160	0(3)	A4253	0(3)	A4368	1(3)	A4459	1(3)	A4642	1(3)	A5062	1(3)	A6445	8(3)

CPT	MUE	CPT	MUE	CPT	MUE	CPT	MUE	CPT	MUE	CPT	MUE	CPT	MUE	CPT	MUE
A6446	14(3)	A7029	0(3)	A9504	1(3)	A9586	1(3)	C1721	1(3)	C1874	5(3)	C8900	1(3)	C9407	15(3)
A6447	6(3)	A7030	0(3)	A9505	4(3)	A9587	54(3)	C1722	1(3)	C1875	4(3)	C8901	1(3)	C9408	510(3)
A6448	24(3)	A7031	0(3)	A9507	1(3)	A9588	10(3)	C1724	5(3)	C1876	5(3)	C8902	1(3)	C9447	1(3)
A6449	12(3)	A7032	0(3)	A9508	2(3)	A9589	1(3)	C1725	9(3)	C1877	5(3)	C8903	1(3)	C9460	100(3)
A6450	8(3)	A7033	0(3)	A9509	5(3)	A9600	7(3)	C1726	5(3)	C1878	2(3)	C8905	1(3)	C9462	600(3)
A6451	8(3)	A7034	0(3)	A9510	1(3)	A9604	1(3)	C1727	4(3)	C1880	2(3)	C8906	1(3)	C9482	300(3)
A6452	22(3)	A7035	0(3)	A9512	30(3)	A9606	224(3)	C1728	5(3)	C1881	2(3)	C8908	1(3)	C9488	40(3)
A6453	6(3)	A7036	0(3)	A9513	200(3)	A9698	3(3)	C1729	6(3)	C1882	1(3)	C8909	1(3)	C9600	3(3)
A6454	25(3)	A7037	0(3)	A9515	1(3)	A9700	2(3)	C1730	4(3)	C1883	4(3)	C8910	1(3)	C9601	2(3)
A6455	4(3)	A7038	0(3)	A9516	4(3)	A9900	0(3)	C1731	2(3)	C1884	4(3)	C8911	1(3)	C9602	2(3)
A6456	20(3)	A7039	0(3)	A9517	200(3)	A9901	0(3)	C1732	3(3)	C1885	2(3)	C8912	1(3)	C9603	2(3)
A6457	12(3)	A7040	2(3)	A9520	1(3)	A9999	0(3)	C1733	3(3)	C1886	1(3)	C8913	1(3)	C9604	2(3)
A6460	1(1)	A7041	2(3)	A9521	2(3)	B4034	0(3)	C1749	1(3)	C1887	7(3)	C8914	1(3)	C9605	2(3)
A6461	1(1)	A7044	0(3)	A9524	10(3)	B4035	0(3)	C1750	2(3)	C1888	2(3)	C8918	1(3)	C9606	1(3)
A6501	1(3)	A7045	0(3)	A9526	2(3)	B4036	0(3)	C1751	3(3)	C1889	2(3)	C8919	1(3)	C9607	1(2)
A6502	1(3)	A7046	0(3)	A9527	195(3)	B4081	0(3)	C1752	2(3)	C1891	1(3)	C8920	1(3)	C9608	2(3)
A6503	1(3)	A7047	1(3)	A9528	10(3)	B4082	0(3)	C1753	2(3)	C1892	6(3)	C8921	1(3)	C9725	1(3)
A6504	2(3)	A7048	2(3)	A9529	10(3)	B4083	0(3)	C1754	2(3)	C1893	6(3)	C8922	1(3)	C9726	2(3)
A6505	2(3)	A7501	1(3)	A9530	200(3)	B4087	1(3)	C1755	2(3)	C1894	6(3)	C8923	1(3)	C9727	1(2)
A6506	2(3)	A7502	1(3)	A9531	100(3)	B4088	1(3)	C1756	2(3)	C1895	2(3)	C8924	1(3)	C9728	1(3)
A6507	2(3)	A7503	1(3)	A9532	10(3)	B4100	0(3)	C1757	6(3)	C1896	2(3)	C8925	1(3)	C9733	1(3)
A6508	2(3)	A7504	180(3)	A9536	1(3)	B4102	0(3)	C1758	2(3)	C1897	2(3)	C8926	1(3)	C9734	1(3)
A6509	1(3)	A7505	1(3)	A9537	1(3)	B4103	0(3)	C1759	2(3)	C1898	2(3)	C8927	1(3)	C9738	1(3)
A6510	1(3)	A7506	0(3)	A9538	1(3)	B4104	0(3)	C1760	4(3)	C1899	2(3)	C8928	1(2)	C9739	1(2)
A6511	1(3)	A7507	200(3)	A9539	2(3)	B4149	0(3)	C1762	4(3)	C1900	1(3)	C8929	1(3)	C9740	1(2)
A6513	1(3)	A7508	0(3)	A9540	2(3)	B4150	0(3)	C1763	4(3)	C2613	2(3)	C8930	1(2)	C9745	1(2)
A6530	0(3)	A7509	0(3)	A9541	1(3)	B4152	0(3)	C1764	1(3)	C2614	3(3)	C8931	1(3)	C9747	1(2)
A6531	2(3)	A7520	1(3)	A9542	1(3)	B4153	0(3)	C1765	4(3)	C2615	2(3)	C8932	1(3)	C9749	1(2)
A6532	2(3)	A7521	1(3)	A9543	1(3)	B4154	0(3)	C1766	4(3)	C2616	1(3)	C8933	1(3)	C9751	1(3)
A6533	0(3)	A7522	0(3)	A9546	1(3)	B4155	0(3)	C1767	2(3)	C2617	4(3)	C8934	2(3)	C9752	1(2)
A6534	0(3)	A7523	0(3)	A9547	2(3)	B4157	0(3)	C1768	3(3)	C2618	4(3)	C8935	2(3)	C9753	3(3)
A6535	0(3)	A7524	1(3)	A9548	2(3)	B4158	0(3)	C1769	9(3)	C2619	1(3)	C8936	2(3)	C9754	1(2)
A6536	0(3)	A7525	0(3)	A9550	1(3)	B4159	0(3)	C1770	3(3)	C2620	1(3)	C8937	2(2)	C9755	1(2)
A6537	0(3)	A7526	0(3)	A9551	1(3)	B4160	0(3)	C1771	1(3)	C2621	1(3)	C8957	2(3)	C9898	1(3)
A6538	0(3)	A7527	1(3)	A9552	1(3)	B4161	0(3)	C1772	1(3)	C2622	1(3)	C9035	675(3)	D0150	1(3)
A6539	0(3)	A8000	0(3)	A9553	1(3)	B4162	0(3)	C1773	3(3)	C2623	4(3)	C9036	300(3)	D0240	1(3)
A6540	0(3)	A8001	0(3)	A9554	1(3)	B4164	0(3)	C1776	10(3)	C2624	1(3)	C9037	240(3)	D0250	2(3)
A6541	0(3)	A8002	0(3)	A9555	2(3)	B4168	0(3)	C1777	2(3)	C2625	4(3)	C9038	160(3)	D0270	1(3)
A6544	0(3)	A8003	0(3)	A9556	10(3)	B4172	0(3)	C1778	4(3)	C2626	1(3)	C9039	500(3)	D0272	1(3)
A6545	2(3)	A8004	0(3)	A9557	2(3)	B4176	0(3)	C1779	2(3)	C2627	2(3)	C9040	675(3)	D0274	1(3)
A6549	0(3)	A9152	0(3)	A9558	7(3)	B4178	0(3)	C1780	2(3)	C2628	4(3)	C9041	180(3)	D0277	1(3)
A6550	1(3)	A9153	0(3)	A9559	1(3)	B4180	0(3)	C1781	4(3)	C2629	4(3)	C9043	600(3)	D0412	0(3)
A7000	0(3)	A9155	1(3)	A9560	2(3)	B4185	0(3)	C1782	1(3)	C2630	3(3)	C9044	350(3)	D0416	1(3)
A7001	0(3)	A9180	0(3)	A9561	1(3)	B4189	0(3)	C1783	2(3)	C2631	1(3)	C9045	600(3)	D0431	1(3)
A7002	0(3)	A9270	0(3)	A9562	2(3)	B4193	0(3)	C1784	2(3)	C2634	24(3)	C9046	160(3)	D0460	1(2)
A7003	0(3)	A9272	0(3)	A9563	10(3)	B4197	0(3)	C1785	1(3)	C2635	124(3)	C9113	10(3)	D0484	1(2)
A7004	0(3)	A9273	0(3)	A9564	0(3)	B4199	0(3)	C1786	1(3)	C2636	690(3)	C9132	5500(3)	D0485	1(2)
A7005	0(3)	A9274	0(3)	A9566	1(3)	B4216	0(3)	C1787	2(3)	C2637	0(3)	C9248	25(3)	D0601	0(3)
A7006	0(3)	A9275	0(3)	A9567	2(3)	B4220	0(3)	C1788	2(3)	C2638	150(3)	C9250	5(3)	D0602	0(3)
A7007	0(3)	A9276	0(3)	A9568	0(3)	B4222	0(3)	C1789	2(3)	C2639	150(3)	C9254	400(3)	D0603	0(3)
A7008	0(3)	A9277	0(3)	A9569	1(3)	B4224	0(3)	C1813	1(3)	C2640	150(3)	C9257	8000(3)	D1510	2(2)
A7009	0(3)	A9278	0(3)	A9570	1(3)	B5000	0(3)	C1814	2(3)	C2641	150(3)	C9285	2(3)	D1516	1(2)
A7010	0(3)	A9279	0(3)	A9571	1(3)	B5100	0(3)	C1815	1(3)	C2642	120(3)	C9290	266(3)	D1517	1(2)
A7012	0(3)	A9280	0(3)	A9572	1(3)	B5200	0(3)	C1816	2(3)	C2643	120(3)	C9293	700(3)	D1520	2(2)
A7013	0(3)	A9281	0(3)	A9575	300(3)	B9002	0(3)	C1817	1(3)	C2644	500(1)	C9352	3(3)	D1526	1(2)
A7014	0(3)	A9282	0(3)	A9576	100(3)	B9004	0(3)	C1818	2(3)	C2645	4608(3)	C9353	4(3)	D1527	1(2)
A7015	0(3)	A9283	0(3)	A9577	50(3)	B9006	0(3)	C1819	4(3)	C5271	1(2)	C9354	300(3)	D1550	2(3)
A7016	0(3)	A9284	0(3)	A9578	50(3)	B9998	0(3)	C1820	2(3)	C5272	3(2)	C9355	3(3)	D1575	4(2)
A7017	0(3)	A9285	0(3)	A9579	100(3)	B9999	0(3)	C1821	4(3)	C5273	1(2)	C9356	125(3)	D1999	0(3)
A7018	0(3)	A9286	0(3)	A9580	1(3)	C1713	20(3)	C1822	1(3)	C5274	35(3)	C9358	800(3)	D4260	4(2)
A7020	0(3)	A9300	0(3)	A9581	20(3)	C1714	4(3)	C1823	1(3)	C5275	1(2)	C9359	30(3)	D4263	4(2)
A7025	0(3)	A9500	3(3)	A9582	1(3)	C1715	45(3)	C1830	2(3)	C5276	3(2)	C9360	300(3)	D4264	3(3)
A7026	0(3)	A9501	1(3)	A9583	18(3)	C1716	4(3)	C1840	1(3)	C5277	1(2)	C9361	10(3)	D4270	4(3)
A7027	0(3)	A9502	3(3)	A9584	1(3)	C1717	10(3)	C1841	1(2)	C5278	15(3)	C9362	60(3)	D4273	1(2)
A7028	0(3)	A9503	1(3)	A9585	300(3)	C1719	99(3)	C1842	0(3)			C9363	500(3)	D4277	0(3)
												C9364	600(3)		

CPT	MUE	CPT	MUE	CPT	MUE	CPT	MUE	CPT	MUE	CPT	MUE	CPT	MUE	CPT	MUE
D4278	0(3)	E0159	0(3)	E0274	0(3)	E0487	0(3)	E0705	1(2)	E0958	0(3)	E1110	0(3)	E1550	0(3)
D4355	1(2)	E0160	0(3)	E0275	0(3)	E0500	0(3)	E0710	0(3)	E0959	2(2)	E1130	0(3)	E1560	0(3)
D4381	12(3)	E0161	0(3)	E0276	0(3)	E0550	0(3)	E0720	0(3)	E0960	0(3)	E1140	0(3)	E1570	0(3)
D5282	0(3)	E0162	0(3)	E0277	0(3)	E0555	0(3)	E0730	0(3)	E0961	2(2)	E1150	0(3)	E1575	0(3)
D5283	0(3)	E0163	0(3)	E0280	0(3)	E0560	0(3)	E0731	0(3)	E0966	1(2)	E1160	0(3)	E1580	0(3)
D5876	0(3)	E0165	0(3)	E0290	0(3)	E0561	0(3)	E0740	0(3)	E0967	0(3)	E1161	0(3)	E1590	0(3)
D5911	1(3)	E0167	0(3)	E0291	0(3)	E0562	0(3)	E0744	0(3)	E0968	0(3)	E1170	0(3)	E1592	0(3)
D5912	1(2)	E0168	0(3)	E0292	0(3)	E0565	0(3)	E0745	0(3)	E0969	0(3)	E1171	0(3)	E1594	0(3)
D5951	0(3)	E0170	0(3)	E0293	0(3)	E0570	0(3)	E0746	1(3)	E0970	0(3)	E1172	0(3)	E1600	0(3)
D5983	1(3)	E0171	0(3)	E0294	0(3)	E0572	0(3)	E0747	0(3)	E0971	2(3)	E1180	0(3)	E1610	0(3)
D5984	1(3)	E0172	0(3)	E0295	0(3)	E0574	0(3)	E0748	0(3)	E0973	2(3)	E1190	0(3)	E1615	0(3)
D5985	1(3)	E0175	0(3)	E0296	0(3)	E0575	0(3)	E0749	1(3)	E0974	2(3)	E1195	0(3)	E1620	0(3)
D6052	0(3)	E0181	0(3)	E0297	0(3)	E0580	0(3)	E0755	0(3)	E0978	1(3)	E1200	0(3)	E1625	0(3)
D7111	20(3)	E0182	0(3)	E0300	0(3)	E0585	0(3)	E0760	0(3)	E0980	0(3)	E1220	0(3)	E1630	0(3)
D7140	32(2)	E0184	0(3)	E0301	0(3)	E0600	0(3)	E0761	0(3)	E0981	0(3)	E1221	0(3)	E1632	0(3)
D7210	32(2)	E0185	0(3)	E0302	0(3)	E0601	0(3)	E0762	1(3)	E0982	0(3)	E1222	0(3)	E1634	0(3)
D7220	6(3)	E0186	0(3)	E0303	0(3)	E0602	0(3)	E0764	0(3)	E0983	0(3)	E1223	0(3)	E1635	0(3)
D7230	6(3)	E0187	0(3)	E0304	0(3)	E0603	0(3)	E0765	0(3)	E0984	0(3)	E1224	0(3)	E1636	0(3)
D7240	6(3)	E0188	0(3)	E0305	0(3)	E0604	0(3)	E0766	0(3)	E0985	0(3)	E1225	0(3)	E1637	0(3)
D7241	6(3)	E0189	0(3)	E0310	0(3)	E0605	0(3)	E0769	0(3)	E0986	0(3)	E1226	1(2)	E1639	0(3)
D7250	32(2)	E0190	0(3)	E0315	0(3)	E0606	0(3)	E0770	1(3)	E0988	0(3)	E1227	0(3)	E1699	1(3)
D7260	1(3)	E0191	0(3)	E0316	0(3)	E0607	0(3)	E0776	0(3)	E0990	2(2)	E1228	0(3)	E1700	0(3)
D7261	1(3)	E0193	0(3)	E0325	0(3)	E0610	0(3)	E0779	0(3)	E0992	1(2)	E1229	0(3)	E1701	0(3)
D7283	4(3)	E0194	0(3)	E0326	0(3)	E0615	0(3)	E0780	0(3)	E0994	0(3)	E1230	0(3)	E1702	0(3)
D7288	2(3)	E0196	0(3)	E0328	0(3)	E0616	1(2)	E0781	0(3)	E0995	2(2)	E1231	0(3)	E1800	0(3)
D7321	4(2)	E0197	0(3)	E0329	0(3)	E0617	0(3)	E0782	1(2)	E1002	0(3)	E1232	0(3)	E1801	0(3)
D9110	1(3)	E0198	0(3)	E0350	0(3)	E0618	0(3)	E0783	1(2)	E1003	0(3)	E1233	0(3)	E1802	0(3)
D9130	0(3)	E0199	0(3)	E0352	0(3)	E0619	0(3)	E0784	0(3)	E1004	0(3)	E1234	0(3)	E1805	0(3)
D9230	1(3)	E0200	0(3)	E0370	0(3)	E0620	0(3)	E0785	1(3)	E1005	0(3)	E1235	0(3)	E1806	0(3)
D9248	1(3)	E0202	0(3)	E0371	0(3)	E0621	0(3)	E0786	1(2)	E1006	0(3)	E1236	0(3)	E1810	0(3)
D9613	0(3)	E0203	0(3)	E0372	0(3)	E0625	0(3)	E0791	0(3)	E1007	0(3)	E1237	0(3)	E1811	0(3)
D9930	1(2)	E0205	0(3)	E0373	0(3)	E0627	0(3)	E0830	0(3)	E1008	0(3)	E1238	0(3)	E1812	0(3)
D9944	2(2)	E0210	0(3)	E0424	0(3)	E0629	0(3)	E0840	0(3)	E1009	0(3)	E1239	0(3)	E1815	0(3)
D9945	2(2)	E0215	0(3)	E0425	0(3)	E0630	0(3)	E0849	0(3)	E1010	0(3)	E1240	0(3)	E1816	0(3)
D9946	2(2)	E0217	0(3)	E0430	0(3)	E0635	0(3)	E0850	0(3)	E1011	0(3)	E1250	0(3)	E1818	0(3)
D9950	1(3)	E0218	0(3)	E0431	0(3)	E0636	0(3)	E0855	0(3)	E1012	0(3)	E1260	0(3)	E1820	0(3)
D9951	1(3)	E0221	0(3)	E0433	0(3)	E0637	0(3)	E0856	0(3)	E1014	0(3)	E1270	0(3)	E1821	0(3)
D9952	1(3)	E0225	0(3)	E0434	0(3)	E0638	0(3)	E0860	0(3)	E1015	0(3)	E1280	0(3)	E1825	0(3)
D9961	0(3)	E0231	0(3)	E0435	0(3)	E0639	0(3)	E0870	0(3)	E1016	0(3)	E1285	0(3)	E1830	0(3)
D9990	0(3)	E0232	0(3)	E0439	0(3)	E0640	0(3)	E0880	0(3)	E1017	0(3)	E1290	0(3)	E1831	0(3)
E0100	0(3)	E0235	0(3)	E0440	0(3)	E0641	0(3)	E0890	0(3)	E1018	0(3)	E1295	0(3)	E1840	0(3)
E0105	0(3)	E0236	0(3)	E0441	0(3)	E0642	0(3)	E0900	0(3)	E1020	0(3)	E1296	0(3)	E1841	0(3)
E0110	0(3)	E0239	0(3)	E0442	0(3)	E0650	0(3)	E0910	0(3)	E1028	0(3)	E1297	0(3)	E1902	0(3)
E0111	0(3)	E0240	0(3)	E0443	0(3)	E0651	0(3)	E0911	0(3)	E1029	0(3)	E1298	0(3)	E2000	0(3)
E0112	0(3)	E0241	0(3)	E0444	0(3)	E0652	0(3)	E0912	0(3)	E1030	0(3)	E1300	0(3)	E2100	0(3)
E0113	0(3)	E0242	0(3)	E0445	0(3)	E0655	0(3)	E0920	0(3)	E1031	0(3)	E1310	0(3)	E2101	0(3)
E0114	0(3)	E0243	0(3)	E0446	0(3)	E0656	0(3)	E0930	0(3)	E1035	0(3)	E1352	0(3)	E2120	0(3)
E0116	0(3)	E0244	0(3)	E0447	0(3)	E0657	0(3)	E0935	0(3)	E1036	0(3)	E1353	0(3)	E2201	0(3)
E0117	0(3)	E0245	0(3)	E0455	0(3)	E0660	0(3)	E0936	0(3)	E1037	0(3)	E1354	0(3)	E2202	0(3)
E0118	0(3)	E0246	0(3)	E0457	0(3)	E0665	0(3)	E0940	0(3)	E1038	0(3)	E1355	0(3)	E2203	0(3)
E0130	0(3)	E0247	0(3)	E0459	0(3)	E0666	0(3)	E0941	0(3)	E1039	0(3)	E1356	0(3)	E2204	0(3)
E0135	0(3)	E0248	0(3)	E0462	0(3)	E0667	0(3)	E0942	0(3)	E1050	0(3)	E1357	0(3)	E2205	0(3)
E0140	0(3)	E0249	0(3)	E0465	0(3)	E0668	0(3)	E0944	0(3)	E1060	0(3)	E1358	0(3)	E2206	0(3)
E0141	0(3)	E0250	0(3)	E0466	0(3)	E0669	0(3)	E0945	0(3)	E1070	0(3)	E1372	0(3)	E2207	0(3)
E0143	0(3)	E0251	0(3)	E0467	0(3)	E0670	0(3)	E0946	0(3)	E1083	0(3)	E1390	0(3)	E2208	0(3)
E0144	0(3)	E0255	0(3)	E0470	0(3)	E0671	0(3)	E0947	0(3)	E1084	0(3)	E1391	0(3)	E2209	0(3)
E0147	0(3)	E0256	0(3)	E0471	0(3)	E0672	0(3)	E0948	0(3)	E1085	0(3)	E1392	0(3)	E2210	0(3)
E0148	0(3)	E0260	0(3)	E0472	0(3)	E0673	0(3)	E0950	0(3)	E1086	0(3)	E1399	0(3)	E2211	0(3)
E0149	0(3)	E0261	0(3)	E0480	0(3)	E0675	0(3)	E0951	0(3)	E1087	0(3)	E1405	0(3)	E2212	0(3)
E0153	0(3)	E0265	0(3)	E0481	0(3)	E0676	1(3)	E0952	0(3)	E1088	0(3)	E1406	0(3)	E2213	0(3)
E0154	0(3)	E0266	0(3)	E0482	0(3)	E0691	0(3)	E0953	0(3)	E1089	0(3)	E1500	0(3)	E2214	0(3)
E0155	0(3)	E0270	0(3)	E0483	0(3)	E0692	0(3)	E0954	0(3)	E1090	0(3)	E1510	0(3)	E2215	0(3)
E0156	0(3)	E0271	0(3)	E0484	0(3)	E0693	0(3)	E0955	0(3)	E1092	0(3)	E1520	0(3)	E2216	0(3)
E0157	0(3)	E0272	0(3)	E0485	0(3)	E0694	0(3)	E0956	0(3)	E1093	0(3)	E1530	0(3)	E2217	0(3)
E0158	0(3)	E0273	0(3)	E0486	0(3)	E0700	0(3)	E0957	0(3)	E1100	0(3)	E1540	0(3)	E2218	0(3)

CPT	MUE	CPT	MUE	CPT	MUE	CPT	MUE	CPT	MUE	CPT	MUE	CPT	MUE	CPT	MUE
E2219	0(3)	E2387	0(3)	G0078	1(3)	G0276	1(3)	G0428	0(3)	G2005	1(3)	J0131	400(3)	J0583	1250(3)
E2220	0(3)	E2388	0(3)	G0079	1(3)	G0277	5(3)	G0429	1(2)	G2006	1(3)	J0132	300(3)	J0584	90(3)
E2221	0(3)	E2389	0(3)	G0080	1(3)	G0278	1(2)	G0432	1(2)	G2007	1(3)	J0133	1200(3)	J0585	600(3)
E2222	0(3)	E2390	0(3)	G0081	1(3)	G0279	1(2)	G0433	1(2)	G2008	1(3)	J0135	8(3)	J0586	300(3)
E2224	0(3)	E2391	0(3)	G0082	1(3)	G0281	1(3)	G0435	1(2)	G2009	1(3)	J0153	180(3)	J0587	300(3)
E2225	0(3)	E2392	0(3)	G0083	1(3)	G0282	0(3)	G0438	1(2)	G2010	0(3)	J0171	120(3)	J0588	600(3)
E2226	0(3)	E2394	0(3)	G0084	1(3)	G0283	1(3)	G0439	1(2)	G2011	1(2)	J0178	4(3)	J0592	12(3)
E2227	0(3)	E2395	0(3)	G0085	1(3)	G0288	1(2)	G0442	1(2)	G2012	0(3)	J0180	140(3)	J0594	320(3)
E2228	0(3)	E2396	0(3)	G0086	1(3)	G0289	1(2)	G0443	1(2)	G2013	1(3)	J0185	130(3)	J0595	12(3)
E2230	0(3)	E2397	0(3)	G0087	1(3)	G0293	1(2)	G0444	1(2)	G2014	1(3)	J0190	0(3)	J0596	840(3)
E2231	0(3)	E2402	0(3)	G0101	1(2)	G0294	1(2)	G0445	1(2)	G2015	1(3)	J0200	0(3)	J0597	250(3)
E2291	1(2)	E2500	0(3)	G0102	1(2)	G0295	0(3)	G0446	1(3)	G6001	2(3)	J0202	12(3)	J0598	100(3)
E2292	1(2)	E2502	0(3)	G0103	1(2)	G0296	1(2)	G0447	2(3)	G6002	2(3)	J0205	0(3)	J0599	900(3)
E2293	1(2)	E2504	0(3)	G0104	1(2)	G0297	1(2)	G0448	1(3)	G6003	2(3)	J0207	4(3)	J0600	3(3)
E2294	1(2)	E2506	0(3)	G0105	1(2)	G0302	1(2)	G0451	1(3)	G6004	2(3)	J0210	16(3)	J0606	150(3)
E2295	0(3)	E2508	0(3)	G0106	1(2)	G0303	1(2)	G0452	1(3)	G6005	2(3)	J0215	0(3)	J0610	15(3)
E2300	0(3)	E2510	0(3)	G0108	8(3)	G0304	1(2)	G0453	10(3)	G6006	2(3)	J0220	20(3)	J0620	1(3)
E2301	0(3)	E2511	0(3)	G0109	12(3)	G0305	1(2)	G0454	1(2)	G6007	2(3)	J0221	300(3)	J0630	8(3)
E2310	0(3)	E2512	0(3)	G0117	1(2)	G0306	4(3)	G0455	1(2)	G6008	2(3)	J0256	1600(3)	J0636	100(3)
E2311	0(3)	E2599	0(3)	G0118	1(2)	G0307	4(3)	G0458	1(3)	G6009	2(3)	J0257	1400(3)	J0637	20(3)
E2312	0(3)	E2601	0(3)	G0120	1(2)	G0328	1(2)	G0459	1(3)	G6010	2(3)	J0270	32(3)	J0638	150(3)
E2313	0(3)	E2602	0(3)	G0121	1(2)	G0329	1(3)	G0460	1(3)	G6011	2(3)	J0275	1(3)	J0640	24(3)
E2321	0(3)	E2603	0(3)	G0122	0(3)	G0333	0(3)	G0463	4(3)	G6012	2(3)	J0278	15(3)	J0641	1200(3)
E2322	0(3)	E2604	0(3)	G0123	1(3)	G0337	1(2)	G0466	1(2)	G6013	2(3)	J0280	10(3)	J0670	10(3)
E2323	0(3)	E2605	0(3)	G0124	1(3)	G0339	1(2)	G0467	1(3)	G6014	2(3)	J0282	70(3)	J0690	16(3)
E2324	0(3)	E2606	0(3)	G0127	1(2)	G0340	1(3)	G0468	1(2)	G6015	2(3)	J0285	5(3)	J0692	12(3)
E2325	0(3)	E2607	0(3)	G0128	1(3)	G0341	1(2)	G0469	1(2)	G6016	2(3)	J0287	60(3)	J0694	12(3)
E2326	0(3)	E2608	0(3)	G0129	6(3)	G0342	1(2)	G0470	1(3)	G6017	2(3)	J0288	0(3)	J0695	60(3)
E2327	0(3)	E2609	0(3)	G0130	1(2)	G0343	1(2)	G0471	2(3)	G9143	1(2)	J0289	115(3)	J0696	16(3)
E2328	0(3)	E2610	1(3)	G0141	1(3)	G0365	2(3)	G0472	1(2)	G9147	0(3)	J0290	24(3)	J0697	12(3)
E2329	0(3)	E2611	0(3)	G0143	1(3)	G0372	1(2)	G0473	1(3)	G9148	0(3)	J0295	12(3)	J0698	12(3)
E2330	0(3)	E2612	0(3)	G0144	1(3)	G0379	1(2)	G0475	1(2)	G9149	0(3)	J0300	8(3)	J0702	20(3)
E2331	0(3)	E2613	0(3)	G0145	1(3)	G0380	2(3)	G0476	1(2)	G9150	0(3)	J0330	50(3)	J0706	16(3)
E2340	0(3)	E2614	0(3)	G0147	1(3)	G0381	2(3)	G0480	1(2)	G9151	0(3)	J0348	200(3)	J0710	0(3)
E2341	0(3)	E2615	0(3)	G0148	1(3)	G0382	2(3)	G0481	1(2)	G9152	0(3)	J0350	0(3)	J0712	180(3)
E2342	0(3)	E2616	0(3)	G0166	2(3)	G0383	2(3)	G0482	1(2)	G9153	0(3)	J0360	6(3)	J0713	12(3)
E2343	0(3)	E2617	0(3)	G0168	2(3)	G0384	2(3)	G0483	1(2)	G9156	1(2)	J0364	6(3)	J0714	12(3)
E2351	0(3)	E2619	0(3)	G0175	1(3)	G0390	1(2)	G0490	1(3)	G9157	1(2)	J0365	0(3)	J0715	0(3)
E2358	0(3)	E2620	0(3)	G0176	5(3)	G0396	1(2)	G0491	1(3)	G9187	0(3)	J0380	1(3)	J0716	4(1)
E2359	0(3)	E2621	0(3)	G0177	5(3)	G0397	1(2)	G0492	1(3)	G9480	1(3)	J0390	0(3)	J0717	400(3)
E2360	0(3)	E2622	0(3)	G0179	1(2)	G0398	1(2)	G0493	1(3)	G9481	2(3)	J0395	0(3)	J0720	15(3)
E2361	0(3)	E2623	0(3)	G0180	1(2)	G0399	1(2)	G0494	1(3)	G9482	2(3)	J0400	120(3)	J0725	10(3)
E2362	0(3)	E2624	0(3)	G0181	1(2)	G0400	1(2)	G0495	1(3)	G9483	2(3)	J0401	400(3)	J0735	50(3)
E2363	0(3)	E2625	0(3)	G0182	1(2)	G0402	1(2)	G0496	1(3)	G9484	2(3)	J0456	4(3)	J0740	2(3)
E2364	0(3)	E2626	0(3)	G0186	1(2)	G0403	1(2)	G0498	1(2)	G9485	2(3)	J0461	800(3)	J0743	16(3)
E2365	0(3)	E2627	0(3)	G0219	0(3)	G0404	1(2)	G0499	1(2)	G9486	2(3)	J0470	2(3)	J0744	8(3)
E2366	0(3)	E2628	0(3)	G0235	1(3)	G0405	1(2)	G0500	1(3)	G9487	2(3)	J0475	8(3)	J0745	8(3)
E2367	0(3)	E2629	0(3)	G0237	8(3)	G0406	1(3)	G0501	1(3)	G9488	2(3)	J0476	2(3)	J0770	5(3)
E2368	0(3)	E2630	0(3)	G0238	8(3)	G0407	1(3)	G0506	1(2)	G9489	2(3)	J0480	1(3)	J0775	180(3)
E2369	0(3)	E2631	0(3)	G0239	2(3)	G0408	1(3)	G0508	1(2)	G9490	2(3)	J0485	1500(3)	J0780	10(3)
E2370	0(3)	E2632	0(3)	G0245	1(2)	G0410	6(3)	G0509	1(2)	G9678	1(2)	J0490	160(3)	J0795	100(3)
E2371	0(3)	E2633	0(3)	G0246	1(2)	G0411	6(3)	G0511	1(2)	G9685	0(3)	J0500	4(3)	J0800	3(3)
E2372	0(3)	E8000	0(3)	G0247	1(2)	G0412	1(2)	G0512	1(2)	G9978	2(3)	J0515	6(3)	J0834	3(3)
E2373	0(3)	E8001	0(3)	G0248	1(2)	G0413	1(2)	G0513	1(2)	G9979	2(3)	J0517	30(3)	J0840	18(3)
E2374	0(3)	E8002	0(3)	G0249	3(3)	G0414	1(2)	G0514	1(1)	G9980	2(3)	J0520	0(3)	J0841	24(3)
E2375	0(3)	G0008	1(2)	G0250	1(2)	G0415	1(2)	G0515	8(3)	G9981	2(3)	J0558	24(3)	J0850	9(3)
E2376	0(3)	G0009	1(2)	G0252	0(3)	G0416	1(2)	G0516	1(2)	G9982	2(3)	J0561	24(3)	J0875	300(3)
E2377	0(3)	G0010	1(3)	G0255	0(3)	G0420	2(3)	G0517	1(2)	G9983	2(3)	J0565	200(3)	J0878	1500(3)
E2378	0(3)	G0027	1(2)	G0257	1(3)	G0421	2(3)	G0518	1(2)	G9984	2(3)	J0567	300(3)	J0881	500(3)
E2381	0(3)	G0068	16(3)	G0259	2(3)	G0422	6(2)	G0659	1(2)	G9985	2(3)	J0570	4(3)	J0882	300(3)
E2382	0(3)	G0069	16(3)	G0260	2(3)	G0423	6(2)	G2000	1(3)	G9986	2(3)	J0571	0(3)	J0883	1250(3)
E2383	0(3)	G0070	16(3)	G0268	1(2)	G0424	2(2)	G2001	1(3)	G9987	2(3)	J0572	0(3)	J0884	1250(3)
E2384	0(3)	G0071	1(3)	G0269	2(3)	G0425	1(3)	G2002	1(3)	J0120	1(3)	J0573	0(3)	J0885	60(3)
E2385	0(3)	G0076	1(3)	G0270	8(3)	G0426	1(3)	G2003	1(3)	J0129	100(3)	J0574	0(3)	J0887	360(3)
E2386	0(3)	G0077	1(3)	G0271	4(3)	G0427	1(3)	G2004	1(3)	J0130	6(3)	J0575	0(3)	J0888	360(3)

CPT	MUE	CPT	MUE	CPT	MUE	CPT	MUE	CPT	MUE	CPT	MUE	CPT	MUE	CPT	MUE
J0890	0(3)	J1459	300(3)	J1885	8(3)	J2505	1(3)	J3070	3(3)	J7050	20(3)	J7326	2(2)	J7648	0(3)
J0894	100(3)	J1460	10(2)	J1890	0(3)	J2507	8(3)	J3090	200(3)	J7060	10(3)	J7327	2(2)	J7649	0(3)
J0895	12(3)	J1555	480(3)	J1930	120(3)	J2510	4(3)	J3095	150(3)	J7070	7(3)	J7328	336(3)	J7650	0(3)
J0897	120(3)	J1556	300(3)	J1931	609(3)	J2513	1(3)	J3101	50(3)	J7100	2(3)	J7329	0(3)	J7657	0(3)
J0945	4(3)	J1557	300(3)	J1940	10(3)	J2515	8(3)	J3105	4(3)	J7110	3(3)	J7330	1(3)	J7658	0(3)
J1000	1(3)	J1559	300(3)	J1942	1064(3)	J2540	75(3)	J3110	2(3)	J7120	20(3)	J7336	1120(3)	J7659	0(3)
J1020	8(3)	J1560	1(2)	J1945	0(3)	J2543	20(3)	J3121	400(3)	J7121	5(3)	J7340	1(3)	J7660	0(3)
J1030	8(3)	J1561	300(3)	J1950	12(3)	J2545	1(3)	J3145	750(3)	J7131	500(3)	J7342	10(3)	J7665	0(3)
J1040	4(3)	J1562	0(3)	J1953	300(3)	J2547	600(3)	J3230	6(3)	J7170	1800(3)	J7345	200(3)	J7667	0(3)
J1050	1000(3)	J1566	300(3)	J1955	11(3)	J2550	3(3)	J3240	1(3)	J7175	9000(1)	J7500	15(3)	J7668	0(3)
J1071	400(3)	J1568	300(3)	J1956	4(3)	J2560	16(3)	J3243	200(3)	J7177	10500(3)	J7501	8(3)	J7669	0(3)
J1094	0(3)	J1569	300(3)	J1960	0(3)	J2562	48(3)	J3245	0(3)	J7178	7700(1)	J7502	60(3)	J7670	0(3)
J1095	517(1)	J1570	4(3)	J1980	8(3)	J2590	15(3)	J3246	100(3)	J7179	9600(1)	J7503	120(3)	J7674	100(3)
J1100	120(3)	J1571	20(3)	J1990	0(3)	J2597	45(3)	J3250	4(3)	J7180	6000(1)	J7504	15(3)	J7676	0(3)
J1110	3(3)	J1572	300(3)	J2001	400(3)	J2650	0(3)	J3260	12(3)	J7181	3850(1)	J7505	1(3)	J7677	175(3)
J1120	2(3)	J1573	130(3)	J2010	10(3)	J2670	0(3)	J3262	800(3)	J7182	22000(1)	J7507	40(3)	J7680	0(3)
J1130	300(3)	J1575	650(3)	J2020	6(3)	J2675	1(3)	J3265	0(3)	J7183	9600(1)	J7508	300(3)	J7681	0(3)
J1160	3(3)	J1580	9(3)	J2060	10(3)	J2680	4(3)	J3280	0(3)	J7185	22000(1)	J7509	60(3)	J7682	0(3)
J1162	10(3)	J1595	2(3)	J2062	10(3)	J2690	4(3)	J3285	9(3)	J7186	9600(1)	J7510	60(3)	J7683	0(3)
J1165	50(3)	J1599	300(3)	J2150	8(3)	J2700	48(3)	J3300	160(3)	J7187	9600(1)	J7511	9(3)	J7684	0(3)
J1170	50(3)	J1600	0(3)	J2170	8(3)	J2704	400(3)	J3301	16(3)	J7188	22000(1)	J7512	300(3)	J7685	0(3)
J1180	0(3)	J1602	300(3)	J2175	6(3)	J2710	10(3)	J3302	0(3)	J7189	26000(1)	J7513	0(3)	J7686	0(3)
J1190	8(3)	J1610	3(3)	J2180	0(3)	J2720	10(3)	J3303	24(3)	J7190	22000(1)	J7515	90(3)	J7699	0(3)
J1200	8(3)	J1620	0(3)	J2182	300(3)	J2724	3500(3)	J3304	64(2)	J7191	0(3)	J7516	4(3)	J7799	2(3)
J1205	4(3)	J1626	30(3)	J2185	60(3)	J2725	0(3)	J3305	0(3)	J7192	22000(1)	J7517	16(3)	J7999	6(3)
J1212	1(3)	J1627	100(3)	J2186	600(3)	J2730	2(3)	J3310	0(3)	J7193	20000(1)	J7518	12(3)	J8498	1(3)
J1230	5(3)	J1628	100(3)	J2210	5(3)	J2760	2(3)	J3315	6(3)	J7194	9000(1)	J7520	40(3)	J8499	0(3)
J1240	6(3)	J1630	7(3)	J2212	240(3)	J2765	18(3)	J3316	6(3)	J7195	20000(1)	J7525	2(3)	J8501	57(3)
J1245	6(3)	J1631	9(3)	J2248	300(3)	J2770	7(3)	J3320	0(3)	J7196	0(3)	J7527	20(3)	J8510	5(3)
J1250	4(3)	J1640	672(3)	J2250	30(3)	J2778	10(3)	J3350	0(3)	J7197	6300(1)	J7599	1(3)	J8515	0(3)
J1260	2(3)	J1642	150(3)	J2260	16(3)	J2780	16(3)	J3355	0(3)	J7198	30000(1)	J7604	0(3)	J8520	50(3)
J1265	100(3)	J1644	50(3)	J2265	400(3)	J2783	60(3)	J3357	90(3)	J7200	20000(1)	J7605	0(3)	J8521	15(3)
J1267	150(3)	J1645	10(3)	J2270	15(3)	J2785	4(3)	J3358	520(3)	J7201	9000(1)	J7606	0(3)	J8530	60(3)
J1270	16(3)	J1650	30(3)	J2274	100(3)	J2786	500(3)	J3360	6(3)	J7202	11550(1)	J7607	0(3)	J8540	48(3)
J1290	60(3)	J1652	20(3)	J2278	1000(3)	J2787	1(3)	J3364	0(3)	J7203	12000(1)	J7608	0(3)	J8560	6(3)
J1300	120(3)	J1655	0(3)	J2280	8(3)	J2788	1(3)	J3365	0(3)	J7205	9750(1)	J7609	0(3)	J8562	12(3)
J1301	60(3)	J1670	2(3)	J2300	10(3)	J2790	3(3)	J3370	12(3)	J7207	7500(1)	J7610	0(3)	J8565	0(3)
J1320	0(3)	J1675	0(3)	J2310	10(3)	J2791	15(3)	J3380	300(3)	J7208	18000(1)	J7611	0(3)	J8597	4(3)
J1322	150(3)	J1700	0(3)	J2315	380(3)	J2792	450(3)	J3385	80(3)	J7209	7500(1)	J7612	0(3)	J8600	40(3)
J1324	0(3)	J1710	0(3)	J2320	4(3)	J2793	320(3)	J3396	150(3)	J7210	22000(1)	J7613	0(3)	J8610	20(3)
J1325	18(3)	J1720	10(3)	J2323	300(3)	J2794	100(3)	J3397	600(3)	J7211	22000(1)	J7614	0(3)	J8650	0(3)
J1327	99(3)	J1726	28(3)	J2325	34(3)	J2795	2400(3)	J3398	150(2)	J7296	0(3)	J7615	0(3)	J8655	1(3)
J1330	1(3)	J1729	25(3)	J2326	120(3)	J2796	150(3)	J3400	0(3)	J7297	0(3)	J7620	0(3)	J8670	180(3)
J1335	2(3)	J1730	0(3)	J2350	600(3)	J2797	333(3)	J3410	16(3)	J7298	0(3)	J7622	0(3)	J8700	120(3)
J1364	8(3)	J1740	3(3)	J2353	60(3)	J2800	3(3)	J3411	8(3)	J7300	0(3)	J7624	0(3)	J8705	22(3)
J1380	4(3)	J1741	32(3)	J2354	60(3)	J2805	3(3)	J3415	6(3)	J7301	0(3)	J7626	0(3)	J8999	2(3)
J1410	4(3)	J1742	4(3)	J2355	2(3)	J2810	20(3)	J3420	1(3)	J7303	0(3)	J7627	0(3)	J9000	20(3)
J1428	450(3)	J1743	66(3)	J2357	90(3)	J2820	10(3)	J3430	50(3)	J7304	0(3)	J7628	0(3)	J9015	1(3)
J1430	10(3)	J1744	90(3)	J2358	405(3)	J2840	160(3)	J3465	120(3)	J7306	0(3)	J7629	0(3)	J9017	30(3)
J1435	0(3)	J1745	150(3)	J2360	3(3)	J2850	48(3)	J3470	3(3)	J7307	0(3)	J7631	0(3)	J9019	60(3)
J1436	0(3)	J1746	200(3)	J2370	30(3)	J2860	170(3)	J3471	999(2)	J7308	3(3)	J7632	0(3)	J9020	0(3)
J1438	2(3)	J1750	45(3)	J2400	4(3)	J2910	0(3)	J3472	2(3)	J7309	1(3)	J7633	0(3)	J9022	168(3)
J1439	750(3)	J1756	500(3)	J2405	64(3)	J2916	20(3)	J3473	450(3)	J7310	0(3)	J7634	0(3)	J9023	140(3)
J1442	1500(3)	J1786	680(3)	J2407	120(3)	J2920	25(3)	J3475	80(3)	J7311	1(3)	J7635	0(3)	J9025	300(3)
J1443	272(3)	J1790	2(3)	J2410	2(3)	J2930	25(3)	J3480	200(3)	J7312	14(3)	J7636	0(3)	J9027	100(3)
J1444	272(3)	J1800	12(3)	J2425	125(3)	J2940	0(3)	J3485	160(3)	J7313	38(3)	J7637	0(3)	J9030	50(3)
J1447	960(3)	J1810	0(3)	J2426	819(3)	J2941	8(3)	J3486	4(3)	J7315	2(3)	J7638	0(3)	J9032	300(3)
J1450	4(3)	J1815	200(3)	J2430	3(3)	J2950	0(3)	J3489	5(3)	J7316	3(2)	J7639	0(3)	J9033	300(3)
J1451	200(3)	J1817	0(3)	J2440	4(3)	J2993	2(3)	J3520	0(3)	J7318	120(3)	J7640	0(3)	J9034	360(3)
J1452	0(3)	J1826	1(3)	J2460	0(3)	J2995	0(3)	J3530	0(3)	J7320	50(3)	J7641	0(3)	J9035	170(3)
J1453	150(3)	J1830	1(3)	J2469	10(3)	J2997	100(3)	J3535	0(3)	J7321	2(2)	J7642	0(3)	J9036	360(3)
J1454	1(3)	J1833	1116(3)	J2501	25(3)	J3000	2(3)	J3570	0(3)	J7322	48(3)	J7643	0(3)	J9039	210(3)
J1455	18(3)	J1835	0(3)	J2502	60(3)	J3010	100(3)	J7030	20(3)	J7323	2(3)	J7644	0(3)	J9040	4(3)
J1457	0(3)	J1840	3(3)	J2503	2(3)	J3030	2(3)	J7040	12(3)	J7324	2(3)	J7645	0(3)	J9041	35(3)
J1458	100(3)	J1850	14(3)	J2504	15(3)	J3060	760(3)	J7042	12(3)	J7325	96(3)	J7647	0(3)	J9042	200(3)

CPT	MUE	CPT	MUE	CPT	MUE	CPT	MUE	CPT	MUE	CPT	MUE	CPT	MUE
J9043	60(3)	J9280	12(3)	K0052	0(3)	K0842	0(3)	L0480	1(2)	L1100	2(2)	L1951	2(2)	L2395	4(2)
J9044	35(3)	J9285	200(3)	K0053	0(3)	K0843	0(3)	L0482	1(2)	L1110	2(2)	L1960	2(2)	L2397	4(3)
J9045	22(3)	J9293	8(3)	K0056	0(3)	K0848	0(3)	L0484	1(2)	L1120	3(3)	L1970	2(2)	L2405	4(2)
J9047	160(3)	J9295	800(3)	K0065	0(3)	K0849	0(3)	L0486	1(2)	L1200	1(2)	L1971	2(2)	L2415	4(2)
J9050	6(3)	J9299	480(3)	K0069	0(3)	K0850	0(3)	L0488	1(2)	L1210	2(3)	L1980	2(2)	L2425	4(2)
J9055	120(3)	J9301	100(3)	K0070	0(3)	K0851	0(3)	L0490	1(2)	L1220	1(3)	L1990	2(2)	L2430	4(2)
J9057	60(3)	J9302	200(3)	K0071	0(3)	K0852	0(3)	L0491	1(2)	L1230	1(2)	L2000	2(2)	L2492	4(2)
J9060	24(3)	J9303	90(3)	K0072	0(3)	K0853	0(3)	L0492	1(2)	L1240	1(3)	L2005	2(2)	L2500	2(2)
J9065	100(3)	J9305	120(3)	K0073	0(3)	K0854	0(3)	L0621	1(2)	L1250	2(3)	L2010	2(2)	L2510	2(2)
J9070	55(3)	J9306	840(3)	K0077	0(3)	K0855	0(3)	L0622	1(2)	L1260	1(3)	L2020	2(2)	L2520	2(2)
J9098	5(3)	J9307	80(3)	K0098	0(3)	K0856	0(3)	L0623	1(2)	L1270	3(3)	L2030	2(2)	L2525	2(2)
J9100	120(3)	J9308	280(3)	K0105	0(3)	K0857	0(3)	L0624	1(2)	L1280	2(3)	L2034	2(2)	L2526	2(2)
J9120	5(3)	J9311	160(3)	K0108	0(3)	K0858	0(3)	L0625	1(2)	L1290	2(3)	L2035	2(2)	L2530	2(2)
J9130	24(3)	J9312	150(3)	K0195	0(3)	K0859	0(3)	L0626	1(2)	L1300	1(2)	L2036	2(2)	L2540	2(2)
J9145	240(3)	J9315	40(3)	K0455	0(3)	K0860	0(3)	L0627	1(2)	L1310	1(2)	L2037	2(2)	L2550	2(2)
J9150	12(3)	J9320	4(3)	K0462	0(3)	K0861	0(3)	L0628	1(2)	L1499	1(3)	L2038	2(2)	L2570	2(2)
J9151	0(3)	J9325	400(3)	K0552	0(3)	K0862	0(3)	L0629	1(2)	L1600	1(2)	L2040	1(2)	L2580	2(2)
J9153	132(3)	J9328	400(3)	K0553	0(3)	K0863	0(3)	L0630	1(2)	L1610	1(2)	L2050	1(2)	L2600	2(2)
J9155	240(3)	J9330	50(3)	K0554	0(3)	K0864	0(3)	L0631	1(2)	L1620	1(2)	L2060	1(2)	L2610	2(2)
J9160	0(3)	J9340	4(3)	K0601	0(3)	K0868	0(3)	L0632	1(2)	L1630	1(2)	L2070	1(2)	L2620	2(2)
J9165	0(3)	J9351	120(3)	K0602	0(3)	K0869	0(3)	L0633	1(2)	L1640	1(2)	L2080	1(2)	L2622	2(2)
J9171	240(3)	J9352	40(3)	K0603	0(3)	K0870	0(3)	L0634	1(2)	L1650	1(2)	L2090	1(2)	L2624	2(2)
J9173	150(3)	J9354	600(3)	K0604	0(3)	K0871	0(3)	L0635	1(2)	L1652	2(2)	L2106	2(2)	L2627	1(3)
J9175	10(3)	J9355	105(3)	K0605	0(3)	K0877	0(3)	L0636	1(2)	L1660	1(2)	L2108	2(2)	L2628	1(3)
J9176	3000(3)	J9356	60(3)	K0606	0(3)	K0878	0(3)	L0637	1(2)	L1680	1(2)	L2112	2(2)	L2630	1(2)
J9178	150(3)	J9357	4(3)	K0607	0(3)	K0879	0(3)	L0638	1(2)	L1685	1(2)	L2114	2(2)	L2640	1(2)
J9179	50(3)	J9360	40(3)	K0608	0(3)	K0880	0(3)	L0639	1(2)	L1686	1(3)	L2116	2(2)	L2650	2(3)
J9181	100(3)	J9370	4(3)	K0609	0(3)	K0884	0(3)	L0640	1(2)	L1690	1(2)	L2126	2(2)	L2660	1(3)
J9185	2(3)	J9371	5(3)	K0669	0(3)	K0885	0(3)	L0641	1(2)	L1700	1(2)	L2128	2(2)	L2670	2(3)
J9190	20(3)	J9390	36(3)	K0672	4(3)	K0886	0(3)	L0642	1(2)	L1710	1(2)	L2132	2(2)	L2680	2(3)
J9200	20(3)	J9395	20(3)	K0730	0(3)	K0890	0(3)	L0643	1(2)	L1720	2(2)	L2134	2(2)	L2750	8(3)
J9201	20(3)	J9400	500(3)	K0733	0(3)	K0891	0(3)	L0648	1(2)	L1730	1(2)	L2136	2(2)	L2755	8(3)
J9202	3(3)	J9600	4(3)	K0738	0(3)	K0898	1(2)	L0649	1(2)	L1755	2(2)	L2180	2(2)	L2760	8(2)
J9203	180(3)	K0001	0(3)	K0740	0(3)	K0899	0(3)	L0650	1(2)	L1810	2(2)	L2182	4(2)	L2768	4(2)
J9205	215(3)	K0002	0(3)	K0743	0(3)	K0900	0(3)	L0651	1(2)	L1812	2(2)	L2184	4(2)	L2780	8(3)
J9206	42(3)	K0003	0(3)	K0800	0(3)	L0112	1(2)	L0700	1(2)	L1820	2(2)	L2186	4(2)	L2785	4(2)
J9207	90(3)	K0004	0(3)	K0801	0(3)	L0113	1(2)	L0710	1(2)	L1830	2(2)	L2188	2(2)	L2795	2(2)
J9208	15(3)	K0005	0(3)	K0802	0(3)	L0120	1(2)	L0810	1(2)	L1831	2(2)	L2190	2(2)	L2800	2(2)
J9209	55(3)	K0006	0(3)	K0806	0(3)	L0130	1(2)	L0820	1(2)	L1832	2(2)	L2192	2(2)	L2810	4(2)
J9211	6(3)	K0007	0(3)	K0807	0(3)	L0140	1(2)	L0830	1(2)	L1833	2(2)	L2200	4(2)	L2820	2(3)
J9212	0(3)	K0008	0(3)	K0808	0(3)	L0150	1(2)	L0859	1(2)	L1834	2(2)	L2210	4(2)	L2830	2(3)
J9213	12(3)	K0009	0(3)	K0812	0(3)	L0160	1(2)	L0861	1(2)	L1836	2(2)	L2220	4(2)	L2861	0(3)
J9214	100(3)	K0010	0(3)	K0813	0(3)	L0170	1(2)	L0970	1(2)	L1840	2(2)	L2230	2(2)	L2999	2(3)
J9215	0(3)	K0011	0(3)	K0814	0(3)	L0172	1(2)	L0972	1(2)	L1843	2(2)	L2232	2(2)	L3000	2(3)
J9216	0(3)	K0012	0(3)	K0815	0(3)	L0174	1(2)	L0974	1(2)	L1844	2(2)	L2240	2(2)	L3001	2(3)
J9217	6(3)	K0013	0(3)	K0816	0(3)	L0180	1(2)	L0976	1(2)	L1845	2(2)	L2250	2(2)	L3002	2(3)
J9218	1(3)	K0014	0(3)	K0820	0(3)	L0190	1(2)	L0978	2(3)	L1846	2(2)	L2260	2(2)	L3003	2(3)
J9219	0(3)	K0015	0(3)	K0821	0(3)	L0200	1(2)	L0980	1(2)	L1847	2(2)	L2265	2(2)	L3010	2(3)
J9225	1(3)	K0017	0(3)	K0822	0(3)	L0220	1(3)	L0982	1(3)	L1848	2(2)	L2270	2(3)	L3020	2(3)
J9226	1(3)	K0018	0(3)	K0823	0(3)	L0450	1(2)	L0984	3(3)	L1850	2(2)	L2275	2(3)	L3030	2(3)
J9228	1100(3)	K0019	0(3)	K0824	0(3)	L0452	1(2)	L0999	1(3)	L1851	2(2)	L2280	2(2)	L3031	2(3)
J9229	27(3)	K0020	0(3)	K0825	0(3)	L0454	1(2)	L1000	1(2)	L1852	2(2)	L2300	1(2)	L3040	2(3)
J9230	5(3)	K0037	0(3)	K0826	0(3)	L0455	1(2)	L1001	1(2)	L1860	2(2)	L2310	1(2)	L3050	2(3)
J9245	11(3)	K0038	0(3)	K0827	0(3)	L0456	1(2)	L1005	1(2)	L1900	2(2)	L2320	2(3)	L3060	2(3)
J9250	50(3)	K0039	0(3)	K0828	0(3)	L0457	1(2)	L1010	2(2)	L1902	2(2)	L2330	2(3)	L3070	2(3)
J9260	20(3)	K0040	0(3)	K0829	0(3)	L0458	1(2)	L1020	2(3)	L1904	2(2)	L2335	2(2)	L3080	2(3)
J9261	80(3)	K0041	0(3)	K0830	0(3)	L0460	1(2)	L1025	1(3)	L1906	2(2)	L2340	2(2)	L3090	2(3)
J9262	700(3)	K0042	0(3)	K0831	0(3)	L0462	1(2)	L1030	1(3)	L1907	2(2)	L2350	2(2)	L3100	2(2)
J9263	700(3)	K0043	0(3)	K0835	0(3)	L0464	1(2)	L1040	1(3)	L1910	2(2)	L2360	2(2)	L3140	1(2)
J9264	600(3)	K0044	0(3)	K0836	0(3)	L0466	1(2)	L1050	1(3)	L1920	2(2)	L2370	2(2)	L3150	1(2)
J9266	2(3)	K0045	0(3)	K0837	0(3)	L0467	1(2)	L1060	1(3)	L1930	2(2)	L2375	2(2)	L3160	2(2)
J9267	750(3)	K0046	0(3)	K0838	0(3)	L0468	1(2)	L1070	2(2)	L1932	2(2)	L2380	2(3)	L3170	2(2)
J9268	1(3)	K0047	0(3)	K0839	0(3)	L0469	1(2)	L1080	2(2)	L1940	2(2)	L2385	4(2)	L3201	1(3)
J9270	0(3)	K0050	0(3)	K0840	0(3)	L0470	1(2)	L1085	1(2)	L1945	2(2)	L2387	4(2)	L3202	1(3)
J9271	300(3)	K0051	0(3)	K0841	0(3)	L0472	1(2)	L1090	1(3)	L1950	2(2)	L2390	4(2)	L3203	1(3)

CPT	MUE	CPT	MUE	CPT	MUE	CPT	MUE	CPT	MUE	CPT	MUE	CPT	MUE	CPT	MUE
L3204	1(3)	L3640	1(2)	L3999	2(3)	L5560	2(2)	L5690	2(3)	L5970	2(2)	L6628	2(2)	L6915	2(2)
L3206	1(3)	L3649	2(3)	L4000	1(2)	L5570	2(2)	L5692	2(2)	L5971	2(2)	L6629	2(2)	L6920	2(2)
L3207	1(3)	L3650	1(2)	L4002	4(3)	L5580	2(2)	L5694	2(2)	L5972	2(2)	L6630	2(2)	L6925	2(2)
L3208	1(3)	L3660	1(2)	L4010	2(2)	L5585	2(2)	L5695	2(3)	L5973	2(3)	L6632	4(3)	L6930	2(2)
L3209	1(3)	L3670	1(3)	L4020	2(2)	L5590	2(2)	L5696	2(2)	L5974	2(2)	L6635	2(2)	L6935	2(2)
L3211	1(3)	L3671	1(3)	L4030	2(2)	L5595	2(2)	L5697	2(2)	L5975	2(2)	L6637	2(2)	L6940	2(2)
L3212	1(3)	L3674	1(3)	L4040	2(2)	L5600	2(2)	L5698	2(2)	L5976	2(2)	L6638	2(2)	L6945	2(2)
L3213	1(3)	L3675	1(2)	L4045	2(2)	L5610	2(2)	L5699	2(3)	L5978	2(2)	L6640	2(2)	L6950	2(2)
L3214	1(3)	L3677	1(2)	L4050	2(2)	L5611	2(2)	L5700	2(2)	L5979	2(2)	L6641	2(3)	L6955	2(2)
L3215	0(3)	L3678	1(2)	L4055	2(2)	L5613	2(2)	L5701	2(2)	L5980	2(2)	L6642	2(3)	L6960	2(2)
L3216	0(3)	L3702	2(2)	L4060	2(2)	L5614	2(2)	L5702	2(2)	L5981	2(2)	L6645	2(2)	L6965	2(2)
L3217	0(3)	L3710	2(2)	L4070	2(3)	L5616	2(2)	L5703	2(2)	L5982	2(2)	L6646	2(2)	L6970	2(2)
L3219	0(3)	L3720	2(2)	L4080	2(2)	L5617	2(3)	L5704	2(2)	L5984	2(2)	L6647	2(2)	L6975	2(2)
L3221	0(3)	L3730	2(2)	L4090	4(2)	L5618	4(3)	L5705	2(2)	L5985	2(2)	L6648	2(2)	L7007	2(2)
L3222	0(3)	L3740	2(2)	L4100	2(2)	L5620	4(3)	L5706	2(2)	L5986	2(2)	L6650	2(2)	L7008	2(2)
L3224	2(2)	L3760	2(2)	L4110	4(2)	L5622	4(3)	L5707	2(2)	L5987	2(2)	L6655	4(3)	L7009	2(2)
L3225	2(2)	L3761	2(2)	L4130	2(2)	L5624	4(3)	L5710	2(2)	L5988	2(2)	L6660	4(3)	L7040	2(2)
L3230	2(2)	L3762	2(2)	L4205	8(3)	L5626	4(3)	L5711	2(2)	L5990	2(2)	L6665	4(3)	L7045	2(2)
L3250	2(2)	L3763	2(2)	L4210	4(3)	L5628	2(3)	L5712	2(2)	L5999	2(3)	L6670	2(2)	L7170	2(2)
L3251	2(2)	L3764	2(2)	L4350	2(2)	L5629	2(2)	L5714	2(2)	L6000	2(2)	L6672	2(2)	L7180	2(2)
L3252	2(2)	L3765	2(2)	L4360	2(2)	L5630	2(2)	L5716	2(2)	L6010	2(2)	L6675	2(2)	L7181	2(2)
L3253	2(2)	L3766	2(2)	L4361	2(2)	L5631	2(2)	L5718	2(2)	L6020	2(2)	L6676	2(2)	L7185	2(2)
L3254	1(3)	L3806	2(2)	L4370	2(2)	L5632	2(2)	L5722	2(2)	L6026	2(2)	L6677	2(2)	L7186	2(2)
L3255	1(3)	L3807	2(2)	L4386	2(2)	L5634	2(2)	L5724	2(2)	L6050	2(2)	L6680	4(3)	L7190	2(2)
L3257	1(3)	L3808	2(2)	L4387	2(2)	L5636	2(2)	L5726	2(2)	L6055	2(2)	L6682	4(3)	L7191	2(2)
L3260	0(3)	L3809	2(2)	L4392	2(3)	L5637	2(2)	L5728	2(2)	L6100	2(2)	L6684	4(3)	L7259	2(2)
L3265	1(3)	L3891	0(3)	L4394	2(3)	L5638	2(2)	L5780	2(2)	L6110	2(2)	L6686	2(2)	L7360	1(3)
L3300	4(3)	L3900	2(2)	L4396	2(2)	L5639	2(2)	L5781	2(2)	L6120	2(2)	L6687	2(2)	L7362	1(2)
L3310	4(3)	L3901	2(2)	L4397	2(2)	L5640	2(2)	L5782	2(2)	L6130	2(2)	L6688	2(2)	L7364	1(3)
L3330	2(2)	L3904	2(2)	L4398	2(2)	L5642	2(2)	L5785	2(2)	L6200	2(2)	L6689	2(2)	L7366	1(2)
L3332	2(2)	L3905	2(2)	L4631	2(2)	L5643	2(2)	L5790	2(2)	L6205	2(2)	L6690	2(2)	L7367	2(3)
L3334	4(3)	L3906	2(2)	L5000	2(3)	L5644	2(2)	L5795	2(2)	L6250	2(2)	L6691	2(3)	L7368	1(2)
L3340	2(2)	L3908	2(2)	L5010	2(2)	L5645	2(2)	L5810	2(2)	L6300	2(2)	L6692	2(3)	L7400	2(2)
L3350	2(2)	L3912	2(3)	L5020	2(2)	L5646	2(2)	L5811	2(2)	L6310	2(2)	L6693	2(2)	L7401	2(2)
L3360	2(2)	L3913	2(2)	L5050	2(2)	L5647	2(2)	L5812	2(2)	L6320	2(2)	L6694	2(3)	L7402	2(2)
L3370	2(2)	L3915	2(2)	L5060	2(2)	L5648	2(2)	L5814	2(2)	L6350	2(2)	L6695	2(3)	L7403	2(2)
L3380	2(2)	L3916	2(3)	L5100	2(2)	L5649	2(2)	L5816	2(2)	L6360	2(2)	L6696	2(2)	L7404	2(2)
L3390	2(2)	L3917	2(2)	L5105	2(2)	L5650	2(2)	L5818	2(2)	L6370	2(2)	L6697	2(2)	L7405	2(2)
L3400	2(2)	L3918	2(2)	L5150	2(2)	L5651	2(2)	L5822	2(2)	L6380	2(2)	L6698	2(2)	L7499	2(3)
L3410	2(2)	L3919	2(2)	L5160	2(2)	L5652	2(2)	L5824	2(2)	L6382	2(2)	L6703	2(2)	L7510	4(3)
L3420	2(2)	L3921	2(2)	L5200	2(2)	L5653	2(2)	L5826	2(2)	L6384	2(2)	L6704	2(2)	L7600	0(3)
L3430	2(2)	L3923	2(2)	L5210	2(2)	L5654	2(2)	L5828	2(2)	L6386	2(2)	L6706	2(2)	L7700	2(1)
L3440	2(2)	L3924	2(2)	L5220	2(2)	L5655	2(2)	L5830	2(2)	L6388	2(2)	L6707	2(2)	L7900	0(3)
L3450	2(2)	L3925	4(3)	L5230	2(2)	L5656	2(2)	L5840	2(2)	L6400	2(2)	L6708	2(2)	L7902	0(3)
L3455	2(2)	L3927	4(3)	L5250	2(2)	L5658	2(2)	L5845	2(2)	L6450	2(2)	L6709	2(2)	L8000	6(3)
L3460	2(2)	L3929	2(2)	L5270	2(2)	L5661	2(2)	L5848	2(2)	L6500	2(2)	L6711	2(2)	L8001	4(3)
L3465	2(2)	L3930	2(2)	L5280	2(2)	L5665	2(2)	L5850	2(2)	L6550	2(2)	L6712	2(2)	L8002	4(3)
L3470	2(2)	L3931	2(2)	L5301	2(2)	L5666	2(2)	L5855	2(2)	L6570	2(2)	L6713	2(2)	L8010	4(3)
L3480	2(2)	L3933	3(3)	L5312	2(2)	L5668	2(2)	L5856	2(2)	L6580	2(2)	L6714	2(2)	L8015	4(3)
L3485	2(2)	L3935	3(3)	L5321	2(2)	L5670	2(2)	L5857	2(2)	L6582	2(2)	L6715	5(3)	L8020	4(3)
L3500	2(2)	L3956	4(3)	L5331	2(2)	L5671	2(2)	L5858	2(2)	L6584	2(2)	L6721	2(2)	L8030	2(3)
L3510	2(2)	L3960	1(3)	L5341	2(2)	L5672	2(2)	L5859	2(2)	L6586	2(2)	L6722	2(2)	L8031	2(3)
L3520	2(2)	L3961	1(3)	L5400	2(2)	L5673	4(3)	L5910	2(2)	L6588	2(2)	L6805	2(2)	L8032	2(2)
L3530	2(2)	L3962	1(3)	L5410	2(2)	L5676	2(2)	L5920	2(2)	L6590	2(2)	L6810	2(3)	L8035	2(3)
L3540	2(2)	L3967	1(3)	L5420	2(2)	L5677	2(2)	L5925	2(3)	L6600	2(2)	L6880	2(2)	L8039	2(3)
L3550	2(2)	L3971	1(3)	L5430	2(2)	L5678	2(2)	L5930	2(2)	L6605	2(2)	L6881	2(2)	L8040	1(2)
L3560	2(2)	L3973	1(3)	L5450	2(2)	L5679	4(3)	L5940	2(2)	L6610	2(2)	L6882	2(2)	L8041	1(2)
L3570	2(2)	L3975	1(3)	L5460	2(2)	L5680	2(2)	L5950	2(2)	L6611	2(3)	L6883	2(2)	L8042	2(2)
L3580	2(2)	L3976	1(3)	L5500	2(2)	L5681	2(2)	L5960	2(2)	L6615	2(2)	L6884	2(2)	L8043	1(2)
L3590	2(2)	L3977	1(3)	L5505	2(2)	L5682	2(2)	L5961	1(3)	L6616	2(2)	L6885	2(2)	L8044	1(2)
L3595	2(2)	L3978	1(3)	L5510	2(2)	L5683	2(2)	L5962	2(2)	L6620	2(2)	L6890	2(3)	L8045	2(2)
L3600	2(2)	L3980	2(2)	L5520	2(2)	L5684	2(3)	L5964	2(2)	L6621	2(2)	L6895	2(2)	L8046	1(3)
L3610	2(2)	L3981	2(2)	L5530	2(2)	L5685	4(3)	L5966	2(2)	L6623	2(2)	L6900	2(3)	L8047	1(2)
L3620	2(2)	L3982	2(2)	L5535	2(2)	L5686	2(2)	L5968	2(2)	L6624	2(2)	L6905	2(2)	L8048	1(3)
L3630	2(2)	L3984	2(2)	L5540	2(2)	L5688	2(3)	L5969	0(3)	L6625	2(2)	L6910	2(2)	L8049	6(3)

CPT	MUE	CPT	MUE	CPT	MUE	CPT	MUE	CPT	MUE	CPT	MUE	CPT	MUE	CPT	MUE
L8300	1(3)	L8684	1(3)	P9056	3(3)	Q0498	1(3)	Q5104	150(3)	V2204	2(3)	V2625	2(2)	V5213	0(3)
L8310	1(3)	L8685	0(3)	P9057	4(3)	Q0499	1(3)	Q5105	400(3)	V2205	2(3)	V2626	2(2)	V5214	0(3)
L8320	2(3)	L8686	0(3)	P9058	4(3)	Q0501	1(3)	Q5106	60(3)	V2206	2(3)	V2627	2(2)	V5215	0(3)
L8330	2(3)	L8687	0(3)	P9059	15(3)	Q0502	1(3)	Q5107	170(3)	V2207	2(3)	V2628	2(3)	V5221	0(3)
L8400	12(3)	L8688	0(3)	P9060	4(3)	Q0503	3(3)	Q5108	12(3)	V2208	2(3)	V2629	2(2)	V5230	0(3)
L8410	12(3)	L8689	1(3)	P9070	15(3)	Q0504	1(3)	Q5109	150(3)	V2209	2(3)	V2630	2(2)	V5240	0(3)
L8415	6(3)	L8690	2(2)	P9071	15(3)	Q0506	8(3)	Q5110	1500(3)	V2210	2(3)	V2631	2(2)	V5241	0(3)
L8417	12(3)	L8691	1(3)	P9073	4(3)	Q0507	1(3)	Q5111	12(3)	V2211	2(3)	V2632	2(2)	V5242	0(3)
L8420	14(3)	L8692	0(3)	P9100	12(3)	Q0508	24(3)	Q5112	120(3)	V2212	2(3)	V2700	2(3)	V5243	0(3)
L8430	12(3)	L8693	1(3)	P9603	100(3)	Q0509	2(3)	Q5113	120(3)	V2213	2(3)	V2702	0(3)	V5244	0(3)
L8435	12(3)	L8694	1(3)	P9604	2(3)	Q0510	1(2)	Q5114	120(3)	V2214	2(3)	V2710	2(3)	V5245	0(3)
L8440	4(3)	L8695	1(3)	P9612	1(3)	Q0511	1(2)	Q5115	120(3)	V2215	2(3)	V2715	4(3)	V5246	0(3)
L8460	4(3)	L8696	1(3)	P9615	1(3)	Q0512	4(3)	Q9950	5(3)	V2218	2(3)	V2718	2(3)	V5247	0(3)
L8465	4(3)	L8701	1(3)	Q0035	1(3)	Q0513	1(2)	Q9951	0(3)	V2219	2(3)	V2730	2(3)	V5248	0(3)
L8470	14(3)	L8702	1(3)	Q0081	2(3)	Q0514	1(2)	Q9953	10(3)	V2220	2(3)	V2744	2(3)	V5249	0(3)
L8480	12(3)	M0075	0(3)	Q0083	2(3)	Q0515	0(3)	Q9954	18(3)	V2221	2(3)	V2745	2(3)	V5250	0(3)
L8485	12(3)	M0076	0(3)	Q0084	2(3)	Q1004	0(3)	Q9955	0(3)	V2299	2(3)	V2750	2(3)	V5251	0(3)
L8499	1(3)	M0100	0(3)	Q0085	2(3)	Q1005	0(3)	Q9956	9(3)	V2300	2(3)	V2755	2(3)	V5252	0(3)
L8500	1(2)	M0300	0(3)	Q0091	1(3)	Q2004	1(3)	Q9957	3(3)	V2301	2(3)	V2756	0(3)	V5253	0(3)
L8501	2(3)	M0301	0(3)	Q0092	2(3)	Q2009	100(3)	Q9958	600(3)	V2302	2(3)	V2760	0(3)	V5254	0(3)
L8507	3(3)	P2028	1(2)	Q0111	2(3)	Q2017	12(3)	Q9959	0(3)	V2303	2(3)	V2761	0(2)	V5255	0(3)
L8509	1(3)	P2029	1(2)	Q0112	3(3)	Q2026	0(3)	Q9960	250(3)	V2304	2(3)	V2762	0(3)	V5256	0(3)
L8510	1(2)	P2031	0(3)	Q0113	1(3)	Q2028	0(3)	Q9961	200(3)	V2305	2(3)	V2770	2(3)	V5257	0(3)
L8511	1(3)	P2033	1(2)	Q0114	1(3)	Q2034	1(2)	Q9962	200(3)	V2306	2(3)	V2780	2(3)	V5258	0(3)
L8512	1(3)	P2038	1(2)	Q0115	1(3)	Q2035	1(2)	Q9963	240(3)	V2307	2(3)	V2781	0(2)	V5259	0(3)
L8513	1(3)	P3000	1(3)	Q0138	510(3)	Q2036	1(2)	Q9964	0(3)	V2308	2(3)	V2782	2(3)	V5260	0(3)
L8514	1(3)	P3001	1(3)	Q0139	510(3)	Q2037	1(2)	Q9966	250(3)	V2309	2(3)	V2783	2(3)	V5261	0(3)
L8515	1(3)	P7001	0(3)	Q0144	0(3)	Q2038	1(2)	Q9967	300(3)	V2310	2(3)	V2784	2(3)	V5262	0(3)
L8600	2(3)	P9010	4(3)	Q0161	66(3)	Q2039	1(2)	Q9969	3(3)	V2311	2(3)	V2785	2(2)	V5263	0(3)
L8603	4(3)	P9011	4(3)	Q0162	24(3)	Q2043	1(2)	Q9982	1(3)	V2312	2(3)	V2786	0(3)	V5264	0(3)
L8604	3(3)	P9012	12(3)	Q0163	6(3)	Q2049	0(3)	Q9983	1(3)	V2313	2(3)	V2787	0(3)	V5265	0(3)
L8605	4(3)	P9016	12(3)	Q0164	8(3)	Q2050	20(3)	Q9991	1(3)	V2314	2(3)	V2788	0(3)	V5266	0(3)
L8606	5(3)	P9017	24(3)	Q0166	2(3)	Q2052	0(3)	Q9992	1(3)	V2315	2(3)	V2790	1(3)	V5267	0(3)
L8607	20(3)	P9019	12(3)	Q0167	108(3)	Q3014	2(3)	R0070	2(3)	V2318	2(3)	V2797	0(3)	V5268	0(3)
L8609	1(3)	P9020	5(3)	Q0169	12(3)	Q3027	30(3)	R0075	2(3)	V2319	2(3)	V5008	0(3)	V5269	0(3)
L8610	2(3)	P9021	8(3)	Q0173	5(3)	Q3028	0(3)	R0076	1(3)	V2320	2(3)	V5010	0(3)	V5270	0(3)
L8612	1(3)	P9022	12(3)	Q0174	0(3)	Q3031	1(3)	V2020	1(3)	V2321	2(3)	V5011	0(3)	V5271	0(3)
L8613	2(3)	P9023	15(3)	Q0175	6(3)	Q4001	1(3)	V2025	0(3)	V2399	2(3)	V5014	0(3)	V5272	0(3)
L8614	2(3)	P9031	12(3)	Q0177	16(3)	Q4002	1(3)	V2100	2(3)	V2410	2(3)	V5020	0(3)	V5273	0(3)
L8615	2(3)	P9032	12(3)	Q0180	1(3)	Q4003	2(3)	V2101	2(3)	V2430	2(3)	V5030	0(3)	V5274	0(3)
L8616	2(3)	P9033	12(3)	Q0181	2(3)	Q4004	2(3)	V2102	2(3)	V2499	2(3)	V5040	0(3)	V5275	0(3)
L8617	2(3)	P9034	4(3)	Q0477	1(1)	Q4012	2(3)	V2103	2(3)	V2500	2(3)	V5050	0(3)	V5281	0(3)
L8618	2(3)	P9035	4(3)	Q0478	1(3)	Q4013	2(3)	V2104	2(3)	V2501	2(3)	V5060	0(3)	V5282	0(3)
L8619	2(3)	P9036	4(3)	Q0479	1(3)	Q4014	2(3)	V2105	2(3)	V2502	2(3)	V5070	0(3)	V5283	0(3)
L8621	360(3)	P9037	4(3)	Q0480	1(3)	Q4018	2(3)	V2106	2(3)	V2503	2(3)	V5080	0(3)	V5284	0(3)
L8622	2(3)	P9038	4(3)	Q0481	1(2)	Q4021	2(3)	V2107	2(3)	V2510	2(3)	V5090	0(3)	V5285	0(3)
L8625	1(3)	P9039	2(3)	Q0482	1(3)	Q4025	1(3)	V2108	2(3)	V2511	2(3)	V5095	0(3)	V5286	0(3)
L8627	2(2)	P9040	8(3)	Q0483	1(3)	Q4026	1(3)	V2109	2(3)	V2512	2(3)	V5100	0(3)	V5287	0(3)
L8628	2(2)	P9041	100(3)	Q0484	1(3)	Q4027	1(3)	V2110	2(3)	V2513	2(3)	V5110	0(3)	V5288	0(3)
L8629	2(2)	P9043	10(3)	Q0485	1(3)	Q4028	1(3)	V2111	2(3)	V2520	2(3)	V5120	0(3)	V5289	0(3)
L8631	2(3)	P9044	20(3)	Q0486	1(3)	Q4030	2(3)	V2112	2(3)	V2521	2(3)	V5130	0(3)	V5290	0(3)
L8641	4(3)	P9045	20(3)	Q0487	1(3)	Q4037	2(3)	V2113	2(3)	V2522	2(3)	V5140	0(3)	V5298	0(3)
L8642	2(3)	P9046	40(3)	Q0488	1(3)	Q4042	2(3)	V2114	2(3)	V2523	2(3)	V5150	0(3)	V5299	1(3)
L8658	3(3)	P9047	20(3)	Q0489	1(3)	Q4046	2(3)	V2115	2(3)	V2530	2(3)	V5160	0(3)	V5336	0(3)
L8659	4(3)	P9048	2(3)	Q0490	1(3)	Q4050	2(3)	V2118	2(3)	V2531	2(3)	V5171	0(3)	V5362	0(3)
L8670	3(3)	P9050	1(3)	Q0491	1(3)	Q4051	2(3)	V2121	2(3)	V2599	2(3)	V5172	0(3)	V5363	0(3)
L8679	3(3)	P9051	4(3)	Q0492	1(3)	Q4074	0(3)	V2199	2(3)	V2600	0(2)	V5181	0(3)	V5364	0(3)
L8680	0(3)	P9052	3(3)	Q0493	1(3)	Q4081	400(3)	V2200	2(3)	V2610	0(2)	V5190	0(3)		
L8681	1(3)	P9053	3(3)	Q0494	1(3)	Q4103	0(3)	V2201	2(3)	V2615	0(2)	V5200	0(3)		
L8682	2(3)	P9054	2(3)	Q0495	1(3)	Q5101	1500(3)	V2202	2(3)	V2623	2(2)	V5211	0(3)		
L8683	1(3)	P9055	2(3)	Q0497	2(3)	Q5103	150(3)	V2203	2(3)	V2624	2(2)	V5212	0(3)		

Appendix J — Inpatient-Only Procedures

Inpatient Only Procedures—This appendix identifies services with the status indicator C. Medicare will not pay an OPPS hospital or ASC when they are performed on a Medicare patient as an outpatient. Physicians should refer to this list when scheduling Medicare patients for surgical procedures. CMS updates this list quarterly. The following was updated 10/01/2019.

00176 Anesth pharyngeal surgery	01636 Anesth forequarter amput	20816 Replantation digit complete
00192 Anesth facial bone surgery	01638 Anesth shoulder replacement	20824 Replantation thumb complete
00211 Anesth cran surg hematoma	0163T Lumb artif diskectomy addl	20827 Replantation thumb complete
00214 Anesth skull drainage	0164T Remove lumb artif disc addl	20838 Replantation foot complete
00215 Anesth skull repair/fract	01652 Anesth shoulder vessel surg	20955 Fibula bone graft microvasc
00474 Anesth surgery of rib	01654 Anesth shoulder vessel surg	20956 Iliac bone graft microvasc
00524 Anesth chest drainage	01656 Anesth arm-leg vessel surg	20957 Mt bone graft microvasc
00540 Anesth chest surgery	0165T Revise lumb artif disc addl	20962 Other bone graft microvasc
00542 Anesthesia removal pleura	01756 Anesth radical humerus surg	20969 Bone/skin graft microvasc
00546 Anesth lung chest wall surg	01990 Support for organ donor	20970 Bone/skin graft iliac crest
00560 Anesth heart surg w/o pump	0202T Post vert arthrplst 1 lumbar	21045 Extensive jaw surgery
00561 Anesth heart surg <1 yr	0219T Plmt post facet implt cerv	21141 Lefort i-1 piece w/o graft
00562 Anesth hrt surg w/pmp age 1+	0220T Plmt post facet implt thor	21142 Lefort i-2 piece w/o graft
00567 Anesth CABG w/pump	0235T Trluml perip athrc visceral	21143 Lefort i-3/> piece w/o graft
00580 Anesth heart/lung transplnt	0254T Evasc rpr iliac art bifur	21145 Lefort i-1 piece w/ graft
00604 Anesth sitting procedure	0345T Transcath mtral vlve repair	21146 Lefort i-2 piece w/ graft
00632 Anesth removal of nerves	0375T Total disc arthrp ant appr	21147 Lefort i-3/> piece w/ graft
0075T Perq stent/chest vert art	0451T Insj/rplcmt aortic ventr sys	21151 Lefort ii w/bone grafts
0076T S&i stent/chest vert art	0452T Insj/rplcmt dev vasc seal	21154 Lefort iii w/o lefort i
00792 Anesth hemorr/excise liver	0455T Remvl aortic ventr cmpl sys	21155 Lefort iii w/ lefort i
00794 Anesth pancreas removal	0456T Remvl aortic dev vasc seal	21159 Lefort iii w/fhdw/o lefort i
00796 Anesth for liver transplant	0459T Relocaj rplcmt aortic ventr	21160 Lefort iii w/fhd w/ lefort i
00802 Anesth fat layer removal	0461T Repos aortic contrpulsj dev	21179 Reconstruct entire forehead
00844 Anesth pelvis surgery	0483T Tmvi percutaneous approach	21180 Reconstruct entire forehead
00846 Anesth hysterectomy	0484T Tmvi transthoracic exposure	21182 Reconstruct cranial bone
00848 Anesth pelvic organ surg	0494T Prep & cannulj cdvr don lung	21183 Reconstruct cranial bone
00864 Anesth removal of bladder	0495T Mntr cdvr don lng 1st 2 hrs	21184 Reconstruct cranial bone
00865 Anesth removal of prostate	0496T Mntr cdvr don lng ea addl hr	21188 Reconstruction of midface
00866 Anesth removal of adrenal	0543T Ta mv rpr w/artif chord tend	21194 Reconst lwr jaw w/graft
00868 Anesth kidney transplant	0544T Tcat mv annulus rcnstj	21196 Reconst lwr jaw w/fixation
00882 Anesth major vein ligation	0545T Tcat tv annulus rcnstj	21247 Reconstruct lower jaw bone
00904 Anesth perineal surgery	11004 Debride genitalia & perineum	21255 Reconstruct lower jaw bone
00908 Anesth removal of prostate	11005 Debride abdom wall	21268 Revise eye sockets
00932 Anesth amputation of penis	11006 Debride genit/per/abdom wall	21343 Open tx dprsd front sinus fx
00934 Anesth penis nodes removal	11008 Remove mesh from abd wall	21344 Open tx compl front sinus fx
00936 Anesth penis nodes removal	15756 Free myo/skin flap microvasc	21347 Opn tx nasomax fx multple
00944 Anesth vaginal hysterectomy	15757 Free skin flap microvasc	21348 Opn tx nasomax fx w/graft
0095T Rmvl artific disc addl crvcl	15758 Free fascial flap microvasc	21366 Opn tx complx malar w/grft
0098T Rev artific disc addl	16036 Escharotomy addl incision	21422 Treat mouth roof fracture
01140 Anesth amputation at pelvis	19271 Revision of chest wall	21423 Treat mouth roof fracture
01150 Anesth pelvic tumor surgery	19272 Extensive chest wall surgery	21431 Treat craniofacial fracture
01212 Anesth hip disarticulation	19305 Mast radical	21432 Treat craniofacial fracture
01214 Anesth hip arthroplasty	19306 Mast rad urban type	21433 Treat craniofacial fracture
01232 Anesth amputation of femur	19361 Breast reconstr w/lat flap	21435 Treat craniofacial fracture
01234 Anesth radical femur surg	19364 Breast reconstruction	21436 Treat craniofacial fracture
01272 Anesth femoral artery surg	19367 Breast reconstruction	21510 Drainage of bone lesion
01274 Anesth femoral embolectomy	19368 Breast reconstruction	21615 Removal of rib
01404 Anesth amputation at knee	19369 Breast reconstruction	21616 Removal of rib and nerves
01442 Anesth knee artery surg	20661 Application of head brace	21620 Partial removal of sternum
01444 Anesth knee artery repair	20664 Application of halo	21627 Sternal debridement
01486 Anesth ankle replacement	20802 Replantation arm complete	21630 Extensive sternum surgery
01502 Anesth lwr leg embolectomy	20805 Replant forearm complete	21632 Extensive sternum surgery
01634 Anesth shoulder joint amput	20808 Replantation hand complete	21705 Revision of neck muscle/rib

21740	Reconstruction of sternum
21750	Repair of sternum separation
21825	Treat sternum fracture
22010	I&d p-spine c/t/cerv-thor
22015	I&d abscess p-spine l/s/ls
22110	Remove part of neck vertebra
22112	Remove part thorax vertebra
22114	Remove part lumbar vertebra
22116	Remove extra spine segment
22206	Incis spine 3 column thorac
22207	Incis spine 3 column lumbar
22208	Incis spine 3 column adl seg
22210	Incis 1 vertebral seg cerv
22212	Incis 1 vertebral seg thorac
22214	Incis 1 vertebral seg lumbar
22216	Incis addl spine segment
22220	Incis w/discectomy cervical
22222	Incis w/discectomy thoracic
22224	Incis w/discectomy lumbar
22226	Revise extra spine segment
22318	Treat odontoid fx w/o graft
22319	Treat odontoid fx w/graft
22325	Treat spine fracture
22326	Treat neck spine fracture
22327	Treat thorax spine fracture
22328	Treat each add spine fx
22532	Lat thorax spine fusion
22533	Lat lumbar spine fusion
22534	Lat thor/lumb addl seg
22548	Neck spine fusion
22556	Thorax spine fusion
22558	Lumbar spine fusion
22586	Prescrl fuse w/ instr l5-s1
22590	Spine & skull spinal fusion
22595	Neck spinal fusion
22600	Neck spine fusion
22610	Thorax spine fusion
22630	Lumbar spine fusion
22632	Spine fusion extra segment
22633	Lumbar spine fusion combined
22634	Spine fusion extra segment
22800	Post fusion </6 vert seg
22802	Post fusion 7-12 vert seg
22804	Post fusion 13/> vert seg
22808	Ant fusion 2-3 vert seg
22810	Ant fusion 4-7 vert seg
22812	Ant fusion 8/> vert seg
22818	Kyphectomy 1-2 segments
22819	Kyphectomy 3 or more
22830	Exploration of spinal fusion
22841	Insert spine fixation device
22843	Insert spine fixation device
22844	Insert spine fixation device
22846	Insert spine fixation device
22847	Insert spine fixation device
22848	Insert pelv fixation device
22849	Reinsert spinal fixation
22850	Remove spine fixation device
22852	Remove spine fixation device
22855	Remove spine fixation device
22857	Lumbar artif diskectomy
22861	Revise cerv artific disc
22862	Revise lumbar artif disc
22864	Remove cerv artif disc
22865	Remove lumb artif disc
23200	Resect clavicle tumor
23210	Resect scapula tumor
23220	Resect prox humerus tumor
23335	Shoulder prosthesis removal
23472	Reconstruct shoulder joint
23474	Revis reconst shoulder joint
23900	Amputation of arm & girdle
23920	Amputation at shoulder joint
24900	Amputation of upper arm
24920	Amputation of upper arm
24930	Amputation follow-up surgery
24931	Amputate upper arm & implant
24940	Revision of upper arm
25900	Amputation of forearm
25905	Amputation of forearm
25915	Amputation of forearm
25920	Amputate hand at wrist
25924	Amputation follow-up surgery
25927	Amputation of hand
26551	Great toe-hand transfer
26553	Single transfer toe-hand
26554	Double transfer toe-hand
26556	Toe joint transfer
26992	Drainage of bone lesion
27005	Incision of hip tendon
27025	Incision of hip/thigh fascia
27030	Drainage of hip joint
27036	Excision of hip joint/muscle
27054	Removal of hip joint lining
27070	Part remove hip bone super
27071	Part removal hip bone deep
27075	Resect hip tumor
27076	Resect hip tum incl acetabul
27077	Resect hip tum w/innom bone
27078	Rsect hip tum incl femur
27090	Removal of hip prosthesis
27091	Removal of hip prosthesis
27120	Reconstruction of hip socket
27122	Reconstruction of hip socket
27125	Partial hip replacement
27130	Total hip arthroplasty
27132	Total hip arthroplasty
27134	Revise hip joint replacement
27137	Revise hip joint replacement
27138	Revise hip joint replacement
27140	Transplant femur ridge
27146	Incision of hip bone
27147	Revision of hip bone
27151	Incision of hip bones
27156	Revision of hip bones
27158	Revision of pelvis
27161	Incision of neck of femur
27165	Incision/fixation of femur
27170	Repair/graft femur head/neck
27175	Treat slipped epiphysis
27176	Treat slipped epiphysis
27177	Treat slipped epiphysis
27178	Treat slipped epiphysis
27181	Treat slipped epiphysis
27185	Revision of femur epiphysis
27187	Reinforce hip bones
27222	Treat hip socket fracture
27226	Treat hip wall fracture
27227	Treat hip fracture(s)
27228	Treat hip fracture(s)
27232	Treat thigh fracture
27236	Treat thigh fracture
27240	Treat thigh fracture
27244	Treat thigh fracture
27245	Treat thigh fracture
27248	Treat thigh fracture
27253	Treat hip dislocation
27254	Treat hip dislocation
27258	Treat hip dislocation
27259	Treat hip dislocation
27268	Cltx thigh fx w/mnpj
27269	Optx thigh fx
27280	Fusion of sacroiliac joint
27282	Fusion of pubic bones
27284	Fusion of hip joint
27286	Fusion of hip joint
27290	Amputation of leg at hip
27295	Amputation of leg at hip
27303	Drainage of bone lesion
27365	Resect femur/knee tumor
27445	Revision of knee joint
27448	Incision of thigh
27450	Incision of thigh
27454	Realignment of thigh bone
27455	Realignment of knee
27457	Realignment of knee
27465	Shortening of thigh bone
27466	Lengthening of thigh bone
27468	Shorten/lengthen thighs
27470	Repair of thigh
27472	Repair/graft of thigh
27486	Revise/replace knee joint
27487	Revise/replace knee joint
27488	Removal of knee prosthesis
27495	Reinforce thigh
27506	Treatment of thigh fracture
27507	Treatment of thigh fracture
27511	Treatment of thigh fracture
27513	Treatment of thigh fracture
27514	Treatment of thigh fracture
27519	Treat thigh fx growth plate
27535	Treat knee fracture
27536	Treat knee fracture
27540	Treat knee fracture
27556	Treat knee dislocation
27557	Treat knee dislocation
27558	Treat knee dislocation

27580	Fusion of knee	32200	Drain open lung lesion	32940	Revision of lung
27590	Amputate leg at thigh	32215	Treat chest lining	32997	Total lung lavage
27591	Amputate leg at thigh	32220	Release of lung	33015	Incision of heart sac
27592	Amputate leg at thigh	32225	Partial release of lung	33020	Incision of heart sac
27596	Amputation follow-up surgery	32310	Removal of chest lining	33025	Incision of heart sac
27598	Amputate lower leg at knee	32320	Free/remove chest lining	33030	Partial removal of heart sac
27645	Resect tibia tumor	32440	Remove lung pneumonectomy	33031	Partial removal of heart sac
27646	Resect fibula tumor	32442	Sleeve pneumonectomy	33050	Resect heart sac lesion
27702	Reconstruct ankle joint	32445	Removal of lung extrapleural	33120	Removal of heart lesion
27703	Reconstruction ankle joint	32480	Partial removal of lung	33130	Removal of heart lesion
27712	Realignment of lower leg	32482	Bilobectomy	33140	Heart revascularize (tmr)
27715	Revision of lower leg	32484	Segmentectomy	33141	Heart tmr w/other procedure
27724	Repair/graft of tibia	32486	Sleeve lobectomy	33202	Insert epicard eltrd open
27725	Repair of lower leg	32488	Completion pneumonectomy	33203	Insert epicard eltrd endo
27727	Repair of lower leg	32491	Lung volume reduction	33236	Remove electrode/thoracotomy
27880	Amputation of lower leg	32501	Repair bronchus add-on	33237	Remove electrode/thoracotomy
27881	Amputation of lower leg	32503	Resect apical lung tumor	33238	Remove electrode/thoracotomy
27882	Amputation of lower leg	32504	Resect apical lung tum/chest	33243	Remove eltrd/thoracotomy
27886	Amputation follow-up surgery	32505	Wedge resect of lung initial	33250	Ablate heart dysrhythm focus
27888	Amputation of foot at ankle	32506	Wedge resect of lung add-on	33251	Ablate heart dysrhythm focus
28800	Amputation of midfoot	32507	Wedge resect of lung diag	33254	Ablate atria lmtd
31225	Removal of upper jaw	32540	Removal of lung lesion	33255	Ablate atria w/o bypass ext
31230	Removal of upper jaw	32650	Thoracoscopy w/pleurodesis	33256	Ablate atria w/bypass exten
31290	Nasal/sinus endoscopy surg	32651	Thoracoscopy remove cortex	33257	Ablate atria lmtd add-on
31291	Nasal/sinus endoscopy surg	32652	Thoracoscopy rem totl cortex	33258	Ablate atria x10sv add-on
31360	Removal of larynx	32653	Thoracoscopy remov fb/fibrin	33259	Ablate atria w/bypass add-on
31365	Removal of larynx	32654	Thoracoscopy contrl bleeding	33261	Ablate heart dysrhythm focus
31367	Partial removal of larynx	32655	Thoracoscopy resect bullae	33265	Ablate atria lmtd endo
31368	Partial removal of larynx	32656	Thoracoscopy w/pleurectomy	33266	Ablate atria x10sv endo
31370	Partial removal of larynx	32658	Thoracoscopy w/sac fb remove	33300	Repair of heart wound
31375	Partial removal of larynx	32659	Thoracoscopy w/sac drainage	33305	Repair of heart wound
31380	Partial removal of larynx	32661	Thoracoscopy w/pericard exc	33310	Exploratory heart surgery
31382	Partial removal of larynx	32662	Thoracoscopy w/mediast exc	33315	Exploratory heart surgery
31390	Removal of larynx & pharynx	32663	Thoracoscopy w/lobectomy	33320	Repair major blood vessel(s)
31395	Reconstruct larynx & pharynx	32664	Thoracoscopy w/ th nrv exc	33321	Repair major vessel
31725	Clearance of airways	32665	Thoracoscop w/esoph musc exc	33322	Repair major blood vessel(s)
31760	Repair of windpipe	32666	Thoracoscopy w/wedge resect	33330	Insert major vessel graft
31766	Reconstruction of windpipe	32667	Thoracoscopy w/w resect addl	33335	Insert major vessel graft
31770	Repair/graft of bronchus	32668	Thoracoscopy w/w resect diag	33340	Perq clsr tcat l atr apndge
31775	Reconstruct bronchus	32669	Thoracoscopy remove segment	33361	Replace aortic valve perq
31780	Reconstruct windpipe	32670	Thoracoscopy bilobectomy	33362	Replace aortic valve open
31781	Reconstruct windpipe	32671	Thoracoscopy pneumonectomy	33363	Replace aortic valve open
31786	Remove windpipe lesion	32672	Thoracoscopy for lvrs	33364	Replace aortic valve open
31800	Repair of windpipe injury	32673	Thoracoscopy w/thymus resect	33365	Replace aortic valve open
31805	Repair of windpipe injury	32674	Thoracoscopy lymph node exc	33366	Trcath replace aortic valve
32035	Thoracostomy w/rib resection	32800	Repair lung hernia	33367	Replace aortic valve w/byp
32036	Thoracostomy w/flap drainage	32810	Close chest after drainage	33368	Replace aortic valve w/byp
32096	Open wedge/bx lung infiltr	32815	Close bronchial fistula	33369	Replace aortic valve w/byp
32097	Open wedge/bx lung nodule	32820	Reconstruct injured chest	33390	Valvuloplasty aortic valve
32098	Open biopsy of lung pleura	32850	Donor pneumonectomy	33391	Valvuloplasty aortic valve
32100	Exploration of chest	32851	Lung transplant single	33404	Prepare heart-aorta conduit
32110	Explore/repair chest	32852	Lung transplant with bypass	33405	Replacement of aortic valve
32120	Re-exploration of chest	32853	Lung transplant double	33406	Replacement of aortic valve
32124	Explore chest free adhesions	32854	Lung transplant with bypass	33410	Replacement of aortic valve
32140	Removal of lung lesion(s)	32855	Prepare donor lung single	33411	Replacement of aortic valve
32141	Remove/treat lung lesions	32856	Prepare donor lung double	33412	Replacement of aortic valve
32150	Removal of lung lesion(s)	32900	Removal of rib(s)	33413	Replacement of aortic valve
32151	Remove lung foreign body	32905	Revise & repair chest wall	33414	Repair of aortic valve
32160	Open chest heart massage	32906	Revise & repair chest wall	33415	Revision subvalvular tissue

33416 Revise ventricle muscle	33615 Repair modified fontan	33820 Revise major vessel
33417 Repair of aortic valve	33617 Repair single ventricle	33822 Revise major vessel
33418 Repair tcat mitral valve	33619 Repair single ventricle	33824 Revise major vessel
33420 Revision of mitral valve	33620 Apply r&l pulm art bands	33840 Remove aorta constriction
33422 Revision of mitral valve	33621 Transthor cath for stent	33845 Remove aorta constriction
33425 Repair of mitral valve	33622 Redo compl cardiac anomaly	33851 Remove aorta constriction
33426 Repair of mitral valve	33641 Repair heart septum defect	33852 Repair septal defect
33427 Repair of mitral valve	33645 Revision of heart veins	33853 Repair septal defect
33430 Replacement of mitral valve	33647 Repair heart septum defects	33860 Ascending aortic graft
33440 Rplcmt a-valve tlcj autol pv	33660 Repair of heart defects	33863 Ascending aortic graft
33460 Revision of tricuspid valve	33665 Repair of heart defects	33864 Ascending aortic graft
33463 Valvuloplasty tricusp	33670 Repair of heart chambers	33870 Transverse aortic arch graft
33464 Valvuloplasty tricusp	33675 Close mult vsd	33875 Thoracic aortic graft
33465 Replace tricuspid valve	33676 Close mult vsd w/resection	33877 Thoracoabdominal graft
33468 Revision of tricuspid valve	33677 Cl mult vsd w/rem pul band	33880 Endovasc taa repr incl subcl
33470 Revision of pulmonary valve	33681 Repair heart septum defect	33881 Endovasc taa repr w/o subcl
33471 Valvotomy pulmonary valve	33684 Repair heart septum defect	33883 Insert endovasc prosth taa
33474 Revision of pulmonary valve	33688 Repair heart septum defect	33884 Endovasc prosth taa add-on
33475 Replacement pulmonary valve	33690 Reinforce pulmonary artery	33886 Endovasc prosth delayed
33476 Revision of heart chamber	33692 Repair of heart defects	33889 Artery transpose/endovas taa
33477 Implant tcat pulm vlv perq	33694 Repair of heart defects	33891 Car-car bp grft/endovas taa
33478 Revision of heart chamber	33697 Repair of heart defects	33910 Remove lung artery emboli
33496 Repair prosth valve clot	33702 Repair of heart defects	33915 Remove lung artery emboli
33500 Repair heart vessel fistula	33710 Repair of heart defects	33916 Surgery of great vessel
33501 Repair heart vessel fistula	33720 Repair of heart defect	33917 Repair pulmonary artery
33502 Coronary artery correction	33722 Repair of heart defect	33920 Repair pulmonary atresia
33503 Coronary artery graft	33724 Repair venous anomaly	33922 Transect pulmonary artery
33504 Coronary artery graft	33726 Repair pul venous stenosis	33924 Remove pulmonary shunt
33505 Repair artery w/tunnel	33730 Repair heart-vein defect(s)	33925 Rpr pul art unifocal w/o cpb
33506 Repair artery translocation	33732 Repair heart-vein defect	33926 Repr pul art unifocal w/cpb
33507 Repair art intramural	33735 Revision of heart chamber	33927 Impltj tot rplcmt hrt sys
33510 Cabg vein single	33736 Revision of heart chamber	33928 Rmvl & rplcmt tot hrt sys
33511 Cabg vein two	33737 Revision of heart chamber	33929 Rmvl rplcmt hrt sys f/trnspl
33512 Cabg vein three	33750 Major vessel shunt	33930 Removal of donor heart/lung
33513 Cabg vein four	33755 Major vessel shunt	33933 Prepare donor heart/lung
33514 Cabg vein five	33762 Major vessel shunt	33935 Transplantation heart/lung
33516 Cabg vein six or more	33764 Major vessel shunt & graft	33940 Removal of donor heart
33517 Cabg artery-vein single	33766 Major vessel shunt	33944 Prepare donor heart
33518 Cabg artery-vein two	33767 Major vessel shunt	33945 Transplantation of heart
33519 Cabg artery-vein three	33768 Cavopulmonary shunting	33946 Ecmo/ecls initiation venous
33521 Cabg artery-vein four	33770 Repair great vessels defect	33947 Ecmo/ecls initiation artery
33522 Cabg artery-vein five	33771 Repair great vessels defect	33948 Ecmo/ecls daily mgmt-venous
33523 Cabg art-vein six or more	33774 Repair great vessels defect	33949 Ecmo/ecls daily mgmt artery
33530 Coronary artery bypass/reop	33775 Repair great vessels defect	33951 Ecmo/ecls insj prph cannula
33533 Cabg arterial single	33776 Repair great vessels defect	33952 Ecmo/ecls insj prph cannula
33534 Cabg arterial two	33777 Repair great vessels defect	33953 Ecmo/ecls insj prph cannula
33535 Cabg arterial three	33778 Repair great vessels defect	33954 Ecmo/ecls insj prph cannula
33536 Cabg arterial four or more	33779 Repair great vessels defect	33955 Ecmo/ecls insj ctr cannula
33542 Removal of heart lesion	33780 Repair great vessels defect	33956 Ecmo/ecls insj ctr cannula
33545 Repair of heart damage	33781 Repair great vessels defect	33957 Ecmo/ecls repos perph cnula
33548 Restore/remodel ventricle	33782 Nikaidoh proc	33958 Ecmo/ecls repos perph cnula
33572 Open coronary endarterectomy	33783 Nikaidoh proc w/ostia implt	33959 Ecmo/ecls repos perph cnula
33600 Closure of valve	33786 Repair arterial trunk	33962 Ecmo/ecls repos perph cnula
33602 Closure of valve	33788 Revision of pulmonary artery	33963 Ecmo/ecls repos perph cnula
33606 Anastomosis/artery-aorta	33800 Aortic suspension	33964 Ecmo/ecls repos perph cnula
33608 Repair anomaly w/conduit	33802 Repair vessel defect	33965 Ecmo/ecls rmvl perph cannula
33610 Repair by enlargement	33803 Repair vessel defect	33966 Ecmo/ecls rmvl prph cannula
33611 Repair double ventricle	33813 Repair septal defect	33967 Insert i-aort percut device
33612 Repair double ventricle	33814 Repair septal defect	33968 Remove aortic assist device

33969 Ecmo/ecls rmvl perph cannula	35001 Repair defect of artery	35518 Art byp grft axillary-axilry
33970 Aortic circulation assist	35002 Repair artery rupture neck	35521 Art byp grft axill-femoral
33971 Aortic circulation assist	35005 Repair defect of artery	35522 Art byp grft axill-brachial
33973 Insert balloon device	35013 Repair artery rupture arm	35523 Art byp grft brchl-ulnr-rdl
33974 Remove intra-aortic balloon	35021 Repair defect of artery	35525 Art byp grft brachial-brchl
33975 Implant ventricular device	35022 Repair artery rupture chest	35526 Art byp grft aor/carot/innom
33976 Implant ventricular device	35081 Repair defect of artery	35531 Art byp grft aorcel/aormesen
33977 Remove ventricular device	35082 Repair artery rupture aorta	35533 Art byp grft axill/fem/fem
33978 Remove ventricular device	35091 Repair defect of artery	35535 Art byp grft hepatorenal
33979 Insert intracorporeal device	35092 Repair artery rupture aorta	35536 Art byp grft splenorenal
33980 Remove intracorporeal device	35102 Repair defect of artery	35537 Art byp grft aortoiliac
33981 Replace vad pump ext	35103 Repair artery rupture aorta	35538 Art byp grft aortobi-iliac
33982 Replace vad intra w/o bp	35111 Repair defect of artery	35539 Art byp grft aortofemoral
33983 Replace vad intra w/bp	35112 Repair artery rupture spleen	35540 Art byp grft aortbifemoral
33984 Ecmo/ecls rmvl prph cannula	35121 Repair defect of artery	35556 Art byp grft fem-popliteal
33985 Ecmo/ecls rmvl ctr cannula	35122 Repair artery rupture belly	35558 Art byp grft fem-femoral
33986 Ecmo/ecls rmvl ctr cannula	35131 Repair defect of artery	35560 Art byp grft aortorenal
33987 Artery expos/graft artery	35132 Repair artery rupture groin	35563 Art byp grft ilioiliac
33988 Insertion of left heart vent	35141 Repair defect of artery	35565 Art byp grft iliofemoral
33989 Removal of left heart vent	35142 Repair artery rupture thigh	35566 Art byp fem-ant-post tib/prl
33990 Insert vad artery access	35151 Repair defect of artery	35570 Art byp tibial-tib/peroneal
33991 Insert vad art&vein access	35152 Repair ruptd popliteal art	35571 Art byp pop-tibl-prl-other
33992 Remove vad different session	35182 Repair blood vessel lesion	35583 Vein byp grft fem-popliteal
33993 Reposition vad diff session	35189 Repair blood vessel lesion	35585 Vein byp fem-tibial peroneal
34001 Removal of artery clot	35211 Repair blood vessel lesion	35587 Vein byp pop-tibl peroneal
34051 Removal of artery clot	35216 Repair blood vessel lesion	35600 Harvest art for cabg add-on
34151 Removal of artery clot	35221 Repair blood vessel lesion	35601 Art byp common ipsi carotid
34401 Removal of vein clot	35241 Repair blood vessel lesion	35606 Art byp carotid-subclavian
34451 Removal of vein clot	35246 Repair blood vessel lesion	35612 Art byp subclav-subclavian
34502 Reconstruct vena cava	35251 Repair blood vessel lesion	35616 Art byp subclav-axillary
34701 Evasc rpr a-ao ndgft	35271 Repair blood vessel lesion	35621 Art byp axillary-femoral
34702 Evasc rpr a-ao ndgft rpt	35276 Repair blood vessel lesion	35623 Art byp axillary-pop-tibial
34703 Evasc rpr a-unilac ndgft	35281 Repair blood vessel lesion	35626 Art byp aorsubcl/carot/innom
34704 Evasc rpr a-unilac ndgft rpt	35301 Rechanneling of artery	35631 Art byp aor-celiac-msn-renal
34705 Evac rpr a-biiliac ndgft	35302 Rechanneling of artery	35632 Art byp ilio-celiac
34706 Evasc rpr a-biiliac rpt	35303 Rechanneling of artery	35633 Art byp ilio-mesenteric
34707 Evasc rpr ilio-iliac ndgft	35304 Rechanneling of artery	35634 Art byp iliorenal
34708 Evasc rpr ilio-iliac rpt	35305 Rechanneling of artery	35636 Art byp spenorenal
34709 Plmt xtn prosth evasc rpr	35306 Rechanneling of artery	35637 Art byp aortoiliac
34710 Dlyd plmt xtn prosth 1st vsl	35311 Rechanneling of artery	35638 Art byp aortobi-iliac
34711 Dlyd plmt xtn prosth ea addl	35331 Rechanneling of artery	35642 Art byp carotid-vertebral
34712 Tcat dlvr enhncd fixj dev	35341 Rechanneling of artery	35645 Art byp subclav-vertebrl
34808 Endovas iliac a device addon	35351 Rechanneling of artery	35646 Art byp aortobifemoral
34812 Xpose for endoprosth femorl	35355 Rechanneling of artery	35647 Art byp aortofemoral
34813 Femoral endovas graft add-on	35361 Rechanneling of artery	35650 Art byp axillary-axillary
34820 Xpose for endoprosth iliac	35363 Rechanneling of artery	35654 Art byp axill-fem-femoral
34830 Open aortic tube prosth repr	35371 Rechanneling of artery	35656 Art byp femoral-popliteal
34831 Open aortoiliac prosth repr	35372 Rechanneling of artery	35661 Art byp femoral-femoral
34832 Open aortofemor prosth repr	35390 Reoperation carotid add-on	35663 Art byp ilioiliac
34833 Xpose for endoprosth iliac	35400 Angioscopy	35665 Art byp iliofemoral
34834 Xpose endoprosth brachial	35501 Art byp grft ipsilat carotid	35666 Art byp fem-ant-post tib/prl
34841 Endovasc visc aorta 1 graft	35506 Art byp grft subclav-carotid	35671 Art byp pop-tibl-prl-other
34842 Endovasc visc aorta 2 graft	35508 Art byp grft carotid-vertbrl	35681 Composite byp grft pros&vein
34843 Endovasc visc aorta 3 graft	35509 Art byp grft contral carotid	35682 Composite byp grft 2 veins
34844 Endovasc visc aorta 4 graft	35510 Art byp grft carotid-brchial	35683 Composite byp grft 3/> segmt
34845 Visc & infraren abd 1 prosth	35511 Art byp grft subclav-subclav	35691 Art trnsposj vertbrl carotid
34846 Visc & infraren abd 2 prosth	35512 Art byp grft subclav-brchial	35693 Art trnsposj subclavian
34847 Visc & infraren abd 3 prosth	35515 Art byp grft subclav-vertbrl	35694 Art trnsposj subclav carotid
34848 Visc & infraren abd 4+ prost	35516 Art byp grft subclav-axilary	35695 Art trnsposj carotid subclav

35697 Reimplant artery each	41145 Tongue removal neck surgery	43415 Repair esophagus wound
35700 Reoperation bypass graft	41150 Tongue mouth jaw surgery	43425 Repair esophagus opening
35701 Exploration carotid artery	41153 Tongue mouth neck surgery	43460 Pressure treatment esophagus
35721 Exploration femoral artery	41155 Tongue jaw & neck surgery	43496 Free jejunum flap microvasc
35741 Exploration popliteal artery	42426 Excise parotid gland/lesion	43500 Surgical opening of stomach
35800 Explore neck vessels	42845 Extensive surgery of throat	43501 Surgical repair of stomach
35820 Explore chest vessels	42894 Revision of pharyngeal walls	43502 Surgical repair of stomach
35840 Explore abdominal vessels	42953 Repair throat esophagus	43520 Incision of pyloric muscle
35870 Repair vessel graft defect	42961 Control throat bleeding	43605 Biopsy of stomach
35901 Excision graft neck	42971 Control nose/throat bleeding	43610 Excision of stomach lesion
35905 Excision graft thorax	43045 Incision of esophagus	43611 Excision of stomach lesion
35907 Excision graft abdomen	43100 Excision of esophagus lesion	43620 Removal of stomach
36660 Insertion catheter artery	43101 Excision of esophagus lesion	43621 Removal of stomach
36823 Insertion of cannula(s)	43107 Removal of esophagus	43622 Removal of stomach
37140 Revision of circulation	43108 Removal of esophagus	43631 Removal of stomach partial
37145 Revision of circulation	43112 Removal of esophagus	43632 Removal of stomach partial
37160 Revision of circulation	43113 Removal of esophagus	43633 Removal of stomach partial
37180 Revision of circulation	43116 Partial removal of esophagus	43634 Removal of stomach partial
37181 Splice spleen/kidney veins	43117 Partial removal of esophagus	43635 Removal of stomach partial
37182 Insert hepatic shunt (tips)	43118 Partial removal of esophagus	43640 Vagotomy & pylorus repair
37215 Transcath stent cca w/eps	43121 Partial removal of esophagus	43641 Vagotomy & pylorus repair
37217 Stent placemt retro carotid	43122 Partial removal of esophagus	43644 Lap gastric bypass/roux-en-y
37218 Stent placemt ante carotid	43123 Partial removal of esophagus	43645 Lap gastr bypass incl smll i
37616 Ligation of chest artery	43124 Removal of esophagus	43771 Lap revise gastr adj device
37617 Ligation of abdomen artery	43135 Removal of esophagus pouch	43775 Lap sleeve gastrectomy
37618 Ligation of extremity artery	43279 Lap myotomy heller	43800 Reconstruction of pylorus
37660 Revision of major vein	43283 Lap esoph lengthening	43810 Fusion of stomach and bowel
37788 Revascularization penis	43286 Esphg tot w/laps moblj	43820 Fusion of stomach and bowel
38100 Removal of spleen total	43287 Esphg dstl 2/3 w/laps moblj	43825 Fusion of stomach and bowel
38101 Removal of spleen partial	43288 Esphg thrsc moblj	43832 Place gastrostomy tube
38102 Removal of spleen total	43300 Repair of esophagus	43840 Repair of stomach lesion
38115 Repair of ruptured spleen	43305 Repair esophagus and fistula	43843 Gastroplasty w/o v-band
38380 Thoracic duct procedure	43310 Repair of esophagus	43845 Gastroplasty duodenal switch
38381 Thoracic duct procedure	43312 Repair esophagus and fistula	43846 Gastric bypass for obesity
38382 Thoracic duct procedure	43313 Esophagoplasty congenital	43847 Gastric bypass incl small i
38562 Removal pelvic lymph nodes	43314 Tracheo-esophagoplasty cong	43848 Revision gastroplasty
38564 Removal abdomen lymph nodes	43320 Fuse esophagus & stomach	43850 Revise stomach-bowel fusion
38724 Removal of lymph nodes neck	43325 Revise esophagus & stomach	43855 Revise stomach-bowel fusion
38746 Remove thoracic lymph nodes	43327 Esoph fundoplasty lap	43860 Revise stomach-bowel fusion
38747 Remove abdominal lymph nodes	43328 Esoph fundoplasty thor	43865 Revise stomach-bowel fusion
38765 Remove groin lymph nodes	43330 Esophagomyotomy abdominal	43880 Repair stomach-bowel fistula
38770 Remove pelvis lymph nodes	43331 Esophagomyotomy thoracic	43881 Impl/redo electrd antrum
38780 Remove abdomen lymph nodes	43332 Transab esoph hiat hern rpr	43882 Revise/remove electrd antrum
39000 Exploration of chest	43333 Transab esoph hiat hern rpr	44005 Freeing of bowel adhesion
39010 Exploration of chest	43334 Transthor diaphrag hern rpr	44010 Incision of small bowel
39200 Resect mediastinal cyst	43335 Transthor diaphrag hern rpr	44015 Insert needle cath bowel
39220 Resect mediastinal tumor	43336 Thorabd diaphr hern repair	44020 Explore small intestine
39499 Chest procedure	43337 Thorabd diaphr hern repair	44021 Decompress small bowel
39501 Repair diaphragm laceration	43338 Esoph lengthening	44025 Incision of large bowel
39503 Repair of diaphragm hernia	43340 Fuse esophagus & intestine	44050 Reduce bowel obstruction
39540 Repair of diaphragm hernia	43341 Fuse esophagus & intestine	44055 Correct malrotation of bowel
39541 Repair of diaphragm hernia	43351 Surgical opening esophagus	44110 Excise intestine lesion(s)
39545 Revision of diaphragm	43352 Surgical opening esophagus	44111 Excision of bowel lesion(s)
39560 Resect diaphragm simple	43360 Gastrointestinal repair	44120 Removal of small intestine
39561 Resect diaphragm complex	43361 Gastrointestinal repair	44121 Removal of small intestine
39599 Diaphragm surgery procedure	43400 Ligate esophagus veins	44125 Removal of small intestine
41130 Partial removal of tongue	43401 Esophagus surgery for veins	44126 Enterectomy w/o taper cong
41135 Tongue and neck surgery	43405 Ligate/staple esophagus	44127 Enterectomy w/taper cong
41140 Removal of tongue	43410 Repair esophagus wound	44128 Enterectomy cong add-on

44130	Bowel to bowel fusion	
44132	Enterectomy cadaver donor	
44133	Enterectomy live donor	
44135	Intestine transplnt cadaver	
44136	Intestine transplant live	
44137	Remove intestinal allograft	
44139	Mobilization of colon	
44140	Partial removal of colon	
44141	Partial removal of colon	
44143	Partial removal of colon	
44144	Partial removal of colon	
44145	Partial removal of colon	
44146	Partial removal of colon	
44147	Partial removal of colon	
44150	Removal of colon	
44151	Removal of colon/ileostomy	
44155	Removal of colon/ileostomy	
44156	Removal of colon/ileostomy	
44157	Colectomy w/ileoanal anast	
44158	Colectomy w/neo-rectum pouch	
44160	Removal of colon	
44187	Lap ileo/jejuno-stomy	
44188	Lap colostomy	
44202	Lap enterectomy	
44203	Lap resect s/intestine addl	
44204	Laparo partial colectomy	
44205	Lap colectomy part w/ileum	
44206	Lap part colectomy w/stoma	
44207	L colectomy/coloproctostomy	
44208	L colectomy/coloproctostomy	
44210	Laparo total proctocolectomy	
44211	Lap colectomy w/proctectomy	
44212	Laparo total proctocolectomy	
44213	Lap mobil splenic fl add-on	
44227	Lap close enterostomy	
44300	Open bowel to skin	
44310	Ileostomy/jejunostomy	
44314	Revision of ileostomy	
44316	Devise bowel pouch	
44320	Colostomy	
44322	Colostomy with biopsies	
44345	Revision of colostomy	
44346	Revision of colostomy	
44602	Suture small intestine	
44603	Suture small intestine	
44604	Suture large intestine	
44605	Repair of bowel lesion	
44615	Intestinal stricturoplasty	
44620	Repair bowel opening	
44625	Repair bowel opening	
44626	Repair bowel opening	
44640	Repair bowel-skin fistula	
44650	Repair bowel fistula	
44660	Repair bowel-bladder fistula	
44661	Repair bowel-bladder fistula	
44680	Surgical revision intestine	
44700	Suspend bowel w/prosthesis	
44715	Prepare donor intestine	
44720	Prep donor intestine/venous	
44721	Prep donor intestine/artery	
44800	Excision of bowel pouch	
44820	Excision of mesentery lesion	
44850	Repair of mesentery	
44899	Bowel surgery procedure	
44900	Drain appendix abscess open	
44960	Appendectomy	
45110	Removal of rectum	
45111	Partial removal of rectum	
45112	Removal of rectum	
45113	Partial proctectomy	
45114	Partial removal of rectum	
45116	Partial removal of rectum	
45119	Remove rectum w/reservoir	
45120	Removal of rectum	
45121	Removal of rectum and colon	
45123	Partial proctectomy	
45126	Pelvic exenteration	
45130	Excision of rectal prolapse	
45135	Excision of rectal prolapse	
45136	Excise ileoanal reservior	
45395	Lap removal of rectum	
45397	Lap remove rectum w/pouch	
45400	Laparoscopic proc	
45402	Lap proctopexy w/sig resect	
45540	Correct rectal prolapse	
45550	Repair rectum/remove sigmoid	
45562	Exploration/repair of rectum	
45563	Exploration/repair of rectum	
45800	Repair rect/bladder fistula	
45805	Repair fistula w/colostomy	
45820	Repair rectourethral fistula	
45825	Repair fistula w/colostomy	
46705	Repair of anal stricture	
46710	Repr per/vag pouch sngl proc	
46712	Repr per/vag pouch dbl proc	
46715	Rep perf anoper fistu	
46716	Rep perf anoper/vestib fistu	
46730	Construction of absent anus	
46735	Construction of absent anus	
46740	Construction of absent anus	
46742	Repair of imperforated anus	
46744	Repair of cloacal anomaly	
46746	Repair of cloacal anomaly	
46748	Repair of cloacal anomaly	
46751	Repair of anal sphincter	
47010	Open drainage liver lesion	
47015	Inject/aspirate liver cyst	
47100	Wedge biopsy of liver	
47120	Partial removal of liver	
47122	Extensive removal of liver	
47125	Partial removal of liver	
47130	Partial removal of liver	
47133	Removal of donor liver	
47135	Transplantation of liver	
47140	Partial removal donor liver	
47141	Partial removal donor liver	
47142	Partial removal donor liver	
47143	Prep donor liver whole	
47144	Prep donor liver 3-segment	
47145	Prep donor liver lobe split	
47146	Prep donor liver/venous	
47147	Prep donor liver/arterial	
47300	Surgery for liver lesion	
47350	Repair liver wound	
47360	Repair liver wound	
47361	Repair liver wound	
47362	Repair liver wound	
47380	Open ablate liver tumor rf	
47381	Open ablate liver tumor cryo	
47400	Incision of liver duct	
47420	Incision of bile duct	
47425	Incision of bile duct	
47460	Incise bile duct sphincter	
47480	Incision of gallbladder	
47550	Bile duct endoscopy add-on	
47570	Laparo cholecystoenterostomy	
47600	Removal of gallbladder	
47605	Removal of gallbladder	
47610	Removal of gallbladder	
47612	Removal of gallbladder	
47620	Removal of gallbladder	
47700	Exploration of bile ducts	
47701	Bile duct revision	
47711	Excision of bile duct tumor	
47712	Excision of bile duct tumor	
47715	Excision of bile duct cyst	
47720	Fuse gallbladder & bowel	
47721	Fuse upper gi structures	
47740	Fuse gallbladder & bowel	
47741	Fuse gallbladder & bowel	
47760	Fuse bile ducts and bowel	
47765	Fuse liver ducts & bowel	
47780	Fuse bile ducts and bowel	
47785	Fuse bile ducts and bowel	
47800	Reconstruction of bile ducts	
47801	Placement bile duct support	
47802	Fuse liver duct & intestine	
47900	Suture bile duct injury	
48000	Drainage of abdomen	
48001	Placement of drain pancreas	
48020	Removal of pancreatic stone	
48100	Biopsy of pancreas open	
48105	Resect/debride pancreas	
48120	Removal of pancreas lesion	
48140	Partial removal of pancreas	
48145	Partial removal of pancreas	
48146	Pancreatectomy	
48148	Removal of pancreatic duct	
48150	Partial removal of pancreas	
48152	Pancreatectomy	
48153	Pancreatectomy	
48154	Pancreatectomy	
48155	Removal of pancreas	
48400	Injection intraop add-on	
48500	Surgery of pancreatic cyst	
48510	Drain pancreatic pseudocyst	
48520	Fuse pancreas cyst and bowel	

48540 Fuse pancreas cyst and bowel	50328 Prep renal graft/arterial	51585 Removal of bladder & nodes
48545 Pancreatorrhaphy	50329 Prep renal graft/ureteral	51590 Remove bladder/revise tract
48547 Duodenal exclusion	50340 Removal of kidney	51595 Remove bladder/revise tract
48548 Fuse pancreas and bowel	50360 Transplantation of kidney	51596 Remove bladder/create pouch
48551 Prep donor pancreas	50365 Transplantation of kidney	51597 Removal of pelvic structures
48552 Prep donor pancreas/venous	50370 Remove transplanted kidney	51800 Revision of bladder/urethra
48554 Transpl allograft pancreas	50380 Reimplantation of kidney	51820 Revision of urinary tract
48556 Removal allograft pancreas	50400 Revision of kidney/ureter	51840 Attach bladder/urethra
49000 Exploration of abdomen	50405 Revision of kidney/ureter	51841 Attach bladder/urethra
49002 Reopening of abdomen	50500 Repair of kidney wound	51865 Repair of bladder wound
49010 Exploration behind abdomen	50520 Close kidney-skin fistula	51900 Repair bladder/vagina lesion
49020 Drainage abdom abscess open	50525 Close nephrovisceral fistula	51920 Close bladder-uterus fistula
49040 Drain open abdom abscess	50526 Close nephrovisceral fistula	51925 Hysterectomy/bladder repair
49060 Drain open retroperi abscess	50540 Revision of horseshoe kidney	51940 Correction of bladder defect
49062 Drain to peritoneal cavity	50545 Laparo radical nephrectomy	51960 Revision of bladder & bowel
49203 Exc abd tum 5 cm or less	50546 Laparoscopic nephrectomy	51980 Construct bladder opening
49204 Exc abd tum over 5 cm	50547 Laparo removal donor kidney	53415 Reconstruction of urethra
49205 Exc abd tum over 10 cm	50548 Laparo remove w/ureter	53448 Remov/replc ur sphinctr comp
49215 Excise sacral spine tumor	50600 Exploration of ureter	54125 Removal of penis
49220 Multiple surgery abdomen	50605 Insert ureteral support	54130 Remove penis & nodes
49255 Removal of omentum	50610 Removal of ureter stone	54135 Remove penis & nodes
49412 Ins device for rt guide open	50620 Removal of ureter stone	54390 Repair penis and bladder
49425 Insert abdomen-venous drain	50630 Removal of ureter stone	54430 Revision of penis
49428 Ligation of shunt	50650 Removal of ureter	54438 Replantation of penis
49605 Repair umbilical lesion	50660 Removal of ureter	55605 Incise sperm duct pouch
49606 Repair umbilical lesion	50700 Revision of ureter	55650 Remove sperm duct pouch
49610 Repair umbilical lesion	50715 Release of ureter	55801 Removal of prostate
49611 Repair umbilical lesion	50722 Release of ureter	55810 Extensive prostate surgery
49900 Repair of abdominal wall	50725 Release/revise ureter	55812 Extensive prostate surgery
49904 Omental flap extra-abdom	50728 Revise ureter	55815 Extensive prostate surgery
49905 Omental flap intra-abdom	50740 Fusion of ureter & kidney	55821 Removal of prostate
49906 Free omental flap microvasc	50750 Fusion of ureter & kidney	55831 Removal of prostate
50010 Exploration of kidney	50760 Fusion of ureters	55840 Extensive prostate surgery
50040 Drainage of kidney	50770 Splicing of ureters	55842 Extensive prostate surgery
50045 Exploration of kidney	50780 Reimplant ureter in bladder	55845 Extensive prostate surgery
50060 Removal of kidney stone	50782 Reimplant ureter in bladder	55862 Extensive prostate surgery
50065 Incision of kidney	50783 Reimplant ureter in bladder	55865 Extensive prostate surgery
50070 Incision of kidney	50785 Reimplant ureter in bladder	56630 Extensive vulva surgery
50075 Removal of kidney stone	50800 Implant ureter in bowel	56631 Extensive vulva surgery
50100 Revise kidney blood vessels	50810 Fusion of ureter & bowel	56632 Extensive vulva surgery
50120 Exploration of kidney	50815 Urine shunt to intestine	56633 Extensive vulva surgery
50125 Explore and drain kidney	50820 Construct bowel bladder	56634 Extensive vulva surgery
50130 Removal of kidney stone	50825 Construct bowel bladder	56637 Extensive vulva surgery
50135 Exploration of kidney	50830 Revise urine flow	56640 Extensive vulva surgery
50205 Renal biopsy open	50840 Replace ureter by bowel	57110 Remove vagina wall complete
50220 Remove kidney open	50845 Appendico-vesicostomy	57111 Remove vagina tissue compl
50225 Removal kidney open complex	50860 Transplant ureter to skin	57112 Vaginectomy w/nodes compl
50230 Removal kidney open radical	50900 Repair of ureter	57270 Repair of bowel pouch
50234 Removal of kidney & ureter	50920 Closure ureter/skin fistula	57280 Suspension of vagina
50236 Removal of kidney & ureter	50930 Closure ureter/bowel fistula	57296 Revise vag graft open abd
50240 Partial removal of kidney	50940 Release of ureter	57305 Repair rectum-vagina fistula
50250 Cryoablate renal mass open	51525 Removal of bladder lesion	57307 Fistula repair & colostomy
50280 Removal of kidney lesion	51530 Removal of bladder lesion	57308 Fistula repair transperine
50290 Removal of kidney lesion	51550 Partial removal of bladder	57311 Repair urethrovaginal lesion
50300 Remove cadaver donor kidney	51555 Partial removal of bladder	57531 Removal of cervix radical
50320 Remove kidney living donor	51565 Revise bladder & ureter(s)	57540 Removal of residual cervix
50323 Prep cadaver renal allograft	51570 Removal of bladder	57545 Remove cervix/repair pelvis
50325 Prep donor renal graft	51575 Removal of bladder & nodes	58140 Myomectomy abdom method
50327 Prep renal graft/venous	51580 Remove bladder/revise tract	58146 Myomectomy abdom complex

58150 Total hysterectomy	60521 Removal of thymus gland	61538 Removal of brain tissue
58152 Total hysterectomy	60522 Removal of thymus gland	61539 Removal of brain tissue
58180 Partial hysterectomy	60540 Explore adrenal gland	61540 Removal of brain tissue
58200 Extensive hysterectomy	60545 Explore adrenal gland	61541 Incision of brain tissue
58210 Extensive hysterectomy	60600 Remove carotid body lesion	61543 Removal of brain tissue
58240 Removal of pelvis contents	60605 Remove carotid body lesion	61544 Remove & treat brain lesion
58267 Vag hyst w/urinary repair	60650 Laparoscopy adrenalectomy	61545 Excision of brain tumor
58275 Hysterectomy/revise vagina	61105 Twist drill hole	61546 Removal of pituitary gland
58280 Hysterectomy/revise vagina	61107 Drill skull for implantation	61548 Removal of pituitary gland
58285 Extensive hysterectomy	61108 Drill skull for drainage	61550 Release of skull seams
58293 Vag hyst w/uro repair compl	61120 Burr hole for puncture	61552 Release of skull seams
58400 Suspension of uterus	61140 Pierce skull for biopsy	61556 Incise skull/sutures
58410 Suspension of uterus	61150 Pierce skull for drainage	61557 Incise skull/sutures
58520 Repair of ruptured uterus	61151 Pierce skull for drainage	61558 Excision of skull/sutures
58540 Revision of uterus	61154 Pierce skull & remove clot	61559 Excision of skull/sutures
58548 Lap radical hyst	61156 Pierce skull for drainage	61563 Excision of skull tumor
58575 Laps tot hyst resj mal	61210 Pierce skull implant device	61564 Excision of skull tumor
58605 Division of fallopian tube	61250 Pierce skull & explore	61566 Removal of brain tissue
58611 Ligate oviduct(s) add-on	61253 Pierce skull & explore	61567 Incision of brain tissue
58700 Removal of fallopian tube	61304 Open skull for exploration	61570 Remove foreign body brain
58720 Removal of ovary/tube(s)	61305 Open skull for exploration	61571 Incise skull for brain wound
58740 Adhesiolysis tube ovary	61312 Open skull for drainage	61575 Skull base/brainstem surgery
58750 Repair oviduct	61313 Open skull for drainage	61576 Skull base/brainstem surgery
58752 Revise ovarian tube(s)	61314 Open skull for drainage	61580 Craniofacial approach skull
58760 Fimbrioplasty	61315 Open skull for drainage	61581 Craniofacial approach skull
58822 Drain ovary abscess percut	61316 Implt cran bone flap to abdo	61582 Craniofacial approach skull
58825 Transposition ovary(s)	61320 Open skull for drainage	61583 Craniofacial approach skull
58940 Removal of ovary(s)	61321 Open skull for drainage	61584 Orbitocranial approach/skull
58943 Removal of ovary(s)	61322 Decompressive craniotomy	61585 Orbitocranial approach/skull
58950 Resect ovarian malignancy	61323 Decompressive lobectomy	61586 Resect nasopharynx skull
58951 Resect ovarian malignancy	61332 Explore/biopsy eye socket	61590 Infratemporal approach/skull
58952 Resect ovarian malignancy	61333 Explore orbit/remove lesion	61591 Infratemporal approach/skull
58953 Tah rad dissect for debulk	61340 Subtemporal decompression	61592 Orbitocranial approach/skull
58954 Tah rad debulk/lymph remove	61343 Incise skull (press relief)	61595 Transtemporal approach/skull
58956 Bso omentectomy w/tah	61345 Relieve cranial pressure	61596 Transcochlear approach/skull
58957 Resect recurrent gyn mal	61450 Incise skull for surgery	61597 Transcondylar approach/skull
58958 Resect recur gyn mal w/lym	61458 Incise skull for brain wound	61598 Transpetrosal approach/skull
58960 Exploration of abdomen	61460 Incise skull for surgery	61600 Resect/excise cranial lesion
59120 Treat ectopic pregnancy	61500 Removal of skull lesion	61601 Resect/excise cranial lesion
59121 Treat ectopic pregnancy	61501 Remove infected skull bone	61605 Resect/excise cranial lesion
59130 Treat ectopic pregnancy	61510 Removal of brain lesion	61606 Resect/excise cranial lesion
59135 Treat ectopic pregnancy	61512 Remove brain lining lesion	61607 Resect/excise cranial lesion
59136 Treat ectopic pregnancy	61514 Removal of brain abscess	61608 Resect/excise cranial lesion
59140 Treat ectopic pregnancy	61516 Removal of brain lesion	61611 Transect artery sinus
59325 Revision of cervix	61517 Implt brain chemotx add-on	61613 Remove aneurysm sinus
59350 Repair of uterus	61518 Removal of brain lesion	61615 Resect/excise lesion skull
59514 Cesarean delivery only	61519 Remove brain lining lesion	61616 Resect/excise lesion skull
59525 Remove uterus after cesarean	61520 Removal of brain lesion	61618 Repair dura
59620 Attempted vbac delivery only	61521 Removal of brain lesion	61619 Repair dura
59830 Treat uterus infection	61522 Removal of brain abscess	61624 Transcath occlusion cns
59850 Abortion	61524 Removal of brain lesion	61630 Intracranial angioplasty
59851 Abortion	61526 Removal of brain lesion	61635 Intracran angioplsty w/stent
59852 Abortion	61530 Removal of brain lesion	61645 Perq art m-thrombect &/nfs
59855 Abortion	61531 Implant brain electrodes	61650 Evasc prlng admn rx agnt 1st
59856 Abortion	61533 Implant brain electrodes	61651 Evasc prlng admn rx agnt add
59857 Abortion	61534 Removal of brain lesion	61680 Intracranial vessel surgery
60254 Extensive thyroid surgery	61535 Remove brain electrodes	61682 Intracranial vessel surgery
60270 Removal of thyroid	61536 Removal of brain lesion	61684 Intracranial vessel surgery
60505 Explore parathyroid glands	61537 Removal of brain tissue	61686 Intracranial vessel surgery

61690 Intracranial vessel surgery	63082 Remove vertebral body add-on	63307 Remov vert idrl bdy lmbr/sac
61692 Intracranial vessel surgery	63085 Remove vert body dcmprn thrc	63308 Remove vertebral body add-on
61697 Brain aneurysm repr complx	63086 Remove vertebral body add-on	63700 Repair of spinal herniation
61698 Brain aneurysm repr complx	63087 Remov vertbr dcmprn thrclmbr	63702 Repair of spinal herniation
61700 Brain aneurysm repr simple	63088 Remove vertebral body add-on	63704 Repair of spinal herniation
61702 Inner skull vessel surgery	63090 Remove vert body dcmprn lmbr	63706 Repair of spinal herniation
61703 Clamp neck artery	63091 Remove vertebral body add-on	63707 Repair spinal fluid leakage
61705 Revise circulation to head	63101 Remove vert body dcmprn thrc	63709 Repair spinal fluid leakage
61708 Revise circulation to head	63102 Remove vert body dcmprn lmbr	63710 Graft repair of spine defect
61710 Revise circulation to head	63103 Remove vertebral body add-on	63740 Install spinal shunt
61711 Fusion of skull arteries	63170 Incise spinal cord tract(s)	64755 Incision of stomach nerves
61735 Incise skull/brain surgery	63172 Drainage of spinal cyst	64760 Incision of vagus nerve
61750 Incise skull/brain biopsy	63173 Drainage of spinal cyst	64809 Remove sympathetic nerves
61751 Brain biopsy w/ct/mr guide	63180 Revise spinal cord ligaments	64818 Remove sympathetic nerves
61760 Implant brain electrodes	63182 Revise spinal cord ligaments	64866 Fusion of facial/other nerve
61850 Implant neuroelectrodes	63185 Incise spine nrv half segmnt	64868 Fusion of facial/other nerve
61860 Implant neuroelectrodes	63190 Incise spine nrv >2 segmnts	65273 Repair of eye wound
61863 Implant neuroelectrode	63191 Incise spine accessory nerve	69155 Extensive ear/neck surgery
61864 Implant neuroelectrde addl	63194 Incise spine & cord cervical	69535 Remove part of temporal bone
61867 Implant neuroelectrode	63195 Incise spine & cord thoracic	69554 Remove ear lesion
61868 Implant neuroelectrde addl	63196 Incise spine&cord 2 trx crvl	69950 Incise inner ear nerve
61870 Implant neuroelectrodes	63197 Incise spine&cord 2 trx thrc	75956 Xray endovasc thor ao repr
62005 Treat skull fracture	63198 Incise spin&cord 2 stgs crvl	75957 Xray endovasc thor ao repr
62010 Treatment of head injury	63199 Incise spin&cord 2 stgs thrc	75958 Xray place prox ext thor ao
62100 Repair brain fluid leakage	63200 Release spinal cord lumbar	75959 Xray place dist ext thor ao
62115 Reduction of skull defect	63250 Revise spinal cord vsls crvl	92941 Prq card revasc mi 1 vsl
62117 Reduction of skull defect	63251 Revise spinal cord vsls thrc	92970 Cardioassist internal
62120 Repair skull cavity lesion	63252 Revise spine cord vsl thrlmb	92971 Cardioassist external
62121 Incise skull repair	63265 Excise intraspinl lesion crv	92975 Dissolve clot heart vessel
62140 Repair of skull defect	63266 Excise intrspinl lesion thrc	92992 Revision of heart chamber
62141 Repair of skull defect	63267 Excise intrspinl lesion lmbr	92993 Revision of heart chamber
62142 Remove skull plate/flap	63268 Excise intrspinl lesion scrl	93583 Perq transcath septal reduxn
62143 Replace skull plate/flap	63270 Excise intrspinl lesion crvl	99184 Hypothermia ill neonate
62145 Repair of skull & brain	63271 Excise intrspinl lesion thrc	99190 Special pump services
62146 Repair of skull with graft	63272 Excise intrspinl lesion lmbr	99191 Special pump services
62147 Repair of skull with graft	63273 Excise intrspinl lesion scrl	99192 Special pump services
62148 Retr bone flap to fix skull	63275 Bx/exc xdrl spine lesn crvl	99356 Prolonged service inpatient
62161 Dissect brain w/scope	63276 Bx/exc xdrl spine lesn thrc	99357 Prolonged service inpatient
62162 Remove colloid cyst w/scope	63277 Bx/exc xdrl spine lesn lmbr	99462 Sbsq nb em per day hosp
62163 Zneuroendoscopy w/fb removal	63278 Bx/exc xdrl spine lesn scrl	99468 Neonate crit care initial
62164 Remove brain tumor w/scope	63280 Bx/exc idrl spine lesn crvl	99469 Neonate crit care subsq
62165 Remove pituit tumor w/scope	63281 Bx/exc idrl spine lesn thrc	99471 Ped critical care initial
62180 Establish brain cavity shunt	63282 Bx/exc idrl spine lesn lmbr	99472 Ped critical care subsq
62190 Establish brain cavity shunt	63283 Bx/exc idrl spine lesn scrl	99475 Ped crit care age 2-5 init
62192 Establish brain cavity shunt	63285 Bx/exc idrl imed lesn cervl	99476 Ped crit care age 2-5 subsq
62200 Establish brain cavity shunt	63286 Bx/exc idrl imed lesn thrc	99477 Init day hosp neonate care
62201 Brain cavity shunt w/scope	63287 Bx/exc idrl imed lesn thrlmb	99478 Ic lbw inf < 1500 gm subsq
62220 Establish brain cavity shunt	63290 Bx/exc xdrl/idrl lsn any lvl	99479 Ic lbw inf 1500-2500 g subsq
62223 Establish brain cavity shunt	63295 Repair laminectomy defect	99480 Ic inf pbw 2501-5000 g subsq
62256 Remove brain cavity shunt	63300 Remove vert xdrl body crvcl	C9606 PC H rev ac tot/subtot occl 1 ves
62258 Replace brain cavity shunt	63301 Remove vert xdrl body thrc	G0341 Percutaneous islet celltrans
63050 Cervical laminoplsty 2/> seg	63302 Remove vert xdrl body thrlmb	G0342 Laparoscopy islet cell trans
63051 C-laminoplasty w/graft/plate	63303 Remov vert xdrl bdy lmbr/sac	G0343 Laparotomy islet cell transp
63077 Spine disk surgery thorax	63304 Remove vert idrl body crvcl	G0412 Open tx iliac spine uni/bil
63078 Spine disk surgery thorax	63305 Remove vert idrl body thrc	G0414 Pelvic ring fx treat int fix
63081 Remove vert body dcmprn crvl	63306 Remov vert idrl bdy thrclmbr	G0415 Open tx post pelvic fxcture

Appendix K — Place of Service and Type of Service

Place-of-Service Codes for Professional Claims

Listed below are place of service codes and descriptions. These codes should be used on professional claims to specify the entity where service(s) were rendered. Check with individual payers (e.g., Medicare, Medicaid, other private insurance) for reimbursement policies regarding these codes. To comment on a code(s) or description(s), please send your request to posinfo@cms.gov.

01	Pharmacy	A facility or location where drugs and other medically related items and services are sold, dispensed, or otherwise provided directly to patients.
02	Telehealth	The location where health services and health related services are provided or received through telecommunication technology.
03	School	A facility whose primary purpose is education.
04	Homeless shelter	A facility or location whose primary purpose is to provide temporary housing to homeless individuals (e.g., emergency shelters, individual or family shelters).
05	Indian Health Service freestanding facility	A facility or location, owned and operated by the Indian Health Service, which provides diagnostic, therapeutic (surgical and non-surgical), and rehabilitation services to American Indians and Alaska natives who do not require hospitalization.
06	Indian Health Service provider-based facility	A facility or location, owned and operated by the Indian Health Service, which provides diagnostic, therapeutic (surgical and nonsurgical), and rehabilitation services rendered by, or under the supervision of, physicians to American Indians and Alaska natives admitted as inpatients or outpatients.
07	Tribal 638 freestanding facility	A facility or location owned and operated by a federally recognized American Indian or Alaska native tribe or tribal organization under a 638 agreement, which provides diagnostic, therapeutic (surgical and nonsurgical), and rehabilitation services to tribal members who do not require hospitalization.
08	Tribal 638 provider-based Facility	A facility or location owned and operated by a federally recognized American Indian or Alaska native tribe or tribal organization under a 638 agreement, which provides diagnostic, therapeutic (surgical and nonsurgical), and rehabilitation services to tribal members admitted as inpatients or outpatients.
09	Prison/correctional facility	A prison, jail, reformatory, work farm, detention center, or any other similar facility maintained by either federal, state or local authorities for the purpose of confinement or rehabilitation of adult or juvenile criminal offenders.
10	Unassigned	N/A
11	Office	Location, other than a hospital, skilled nursing facility (SNF), military treatment facility, community health center, State or local public health clinic, or intermediate care facility (ICF), where the health professional routinely provides health examinations, diagnosis, and treatment of illness or injury on an ambulatory basis.
12	Home	Location, other than a hospital or other facility, where the patient receives care in a private residence.
13	Assisted living facility	Congregate residential facility with self-contained living units providing assessment of each resident's needs and on-site support 24 hours a day, 7 days a week, with the capacity to deliver or arrange for services including some health care and other services.
14	Group home	A residence, with shared living areas, where clients receive supervision and other services such as social and/or behavioral services, custodial service, and minimal services (e.g., medication administration).
15	Mobile unit	A facility/unit that moves from place-to-place equipped to provide preventive, screening, diagnostic, and/or treatment services.
16	Temporary lodging	A short-term accommodation such as a hotel, campground, hostel, cruise ship or resort where the patient receives care, and which is not identified by any other POS code.
17	Walk-in retail health clinic	A walk-in health clinic, other than an office, urgent care facility, pharmacy, or independent clinic and not described by any other place of service code, that is located within a retail operation and provides preventive and primary care services on an ambulatory basis.
18	Place of employment/worksite	A location, not described by any other POS code, owned or operated by a public or private entity where the patient is employed, and where a health professional provides on-going or episodic occupational medical, therapeutic or rehabilitative services to the individual.
19	Off campus-outpatient hospital	A portion of an off-campus hospital provider based department which provides diagnostic, therapeutic (both surgical and nonsurgical), and rehabilitation services to sick or injured persons who do not require hospitalization or institutionalization.
20	Urgent care facility	Location, distinct from a hospital emergency room, an office, or a clinic, whose purpose is to diagnose and treat illness or injury for unscheduled, ambulatory patients seeking immediate medical attention.

21	Inpatient hospital	A facility, other than psychiatric, which primarily provides diagnostic, therapeutic (both surgical and nonsurgical), and rehabilitation services by, or under, the supervision of physicians to patients admitted for a variety of medical conditions.
22	On campus-outpatient hospital	A portion of a hospital's main campus which provides diagnostic, therapeutic (both surgical and nonsurgical), and rehabilitation services to sick or injured persons who do not require hospitalization or institutionalization.
23	Emergency room—hospital	A portion of a hospital where emergency diagnosis and treatment of illness or injury is provided.
24	Ambulatory surgical center	A freestanding facility, other than a physician's office, where surgical and diagnostic services are provided on an ambulatory basis.
25	Birthing center	A facility, other than a hospital's maternity facilities or a physician's office, which provides a setting for labor, delivery, and immediate post-partum care as well as immediate care of new born infants.
26	Military treatment facility	A medical facility operated by one or more of the uniformed services. Military treatment facility (MTF) also refers to certain former U.S. Public Health Service (USPHS) facilities now designated as uniformed service treatment facilities (USTF).
27-30	Unassigned	N/A
31	Skilled nursing facility	A facility which primarily provides inpatient skilled nursing care and related services to patients who require medical, nursing, or rehabilitative services but does not provide the level of care or treatment available in a hospital.
32	Nursing facility	A facility which primarily provides to residents skilled nursing care and related services for the rehabilitation of injured, disabled, or sick persons, or, on a regular basis, health-related care services above the level of custodial care to individuals other than those with intellectual disabilities.
33	Custodial care facility	A facility which provides room, board, and other personal assistance services, generally on a long-term basis, and which does not include a medical component.
34	Hospice	A facility, other than a patient's home, in which palliative and supportive care for terminally ill patients and their families is provided.
35-40	Unassigned	N/A
41	Ambulance—land	A land vehicle specifically designed, equipped and staffed for lifesaving and transporting the sick or injured.
42	Ambulance—air or water	An air or water vehicle specifically designed, equipped and staffed for lifesaving and transporting the sick or injured.
43-48	Unassigned	N/A
49	Independent clinic	A location, not part of a hospital and not described by any other place-of-service code, that is organized and operated to provide preventive, diagnostic, therapeutic, rehabilitative, or palliative services to outpatients only.
50	Federally qualified health center	A facility located in a medically underserved area that provides Medicare beneficiaries with preventive primary medical care under the general direction of a physician.
51	Inpatient psychiatric facility	A facility that provides inpatient psychiatric services for the diagnosis and treatment of mental illness on a 24-hour basis, by or under the supervision of a physician.
52	Psychiatric facility-partial hospitalization	A facility for the diagnosis and treatment of mental illness that provides a planned therapeutic program for patients who do not require full time hospitalization, but who need broader programs than are possible from outpatient visits to a hospital-based or hospital-affiliated facility.
53	Community mental health center	A facility that provides the following services: outpatient services, including specialized outpatient services for children, the elderly, individuals who are chronically ill, and residents of the CMHC's mental health services area who have been discharged from inpatient treatment at a mental health facility; 24 hour a day emergency care services; day treatment, other partial hospitalization services, or psychosocial rehabilitation services; screening for patients being considered for admission to state mental health facilities to determine the appropriateness of such admission; and consultation and education services.
54	Intermediate care facility/individuals with intellectual disabilities	A facility which primarily provides health-related care and services above the level of custodial care to individuals with Intellectual Disabilities but does not provide the level of care or treatment available in a hospital or SNF.
55	Residential substance abuse treatment facility	A facility which provides treatment for substance (alcohol and drug) abuse to live-in residents who do not require acute medical care. Services include individual and group therapy and counseling, family counseling, laboratory tests, drugs and supplies, psychological testing, and room and board.
56	Psychiatric residential treatment center	A facility or distinct part of a facility for psychiatric care which provides a total 24-hour therapeutically planned and professionally staffed group living and learning environment.
57	Non-residential substance abuse treatment facility	A location which provides treatment for substance (alcohol and drug) abuse on an ambulatory basis. Services include individual and group therapy and counseling, family counseling, laboratory tests, drugs and supplies, and psychological testing.
58-59	Unassigned	N/A

60	Mass immunization center	A location where providers administer pneumococcal pneumonia and influenza virus vaccinations and submit these services as electronic media claims, paper claims, or using the roster billing method. This generally takes place in a mass immunization setting, such as, a public health center, pharmacy, or mall but may include a physician office setting.
61	Comprehensive inpatient rehabilitation facility	A facility that provides comprehensive rehabilitation services under the supervision of a physician to inpatients with physical disabilities. Services include physical therapy, occupational therapy, speech pathology, social or psychological services, and orthotics and prosthetics services.
62	Comprehensive outpatient rehabilitation facility	A facility that provides comprehensive rehabilitation services under the supervision of a physician to outpatients with physical disabilities. Services include physical therapy, occupational therapy, and speech pathology services.
63-64	Unassigned	N/A
65	End-stage renal disease treatment facility	A facility other than a hospital, which provides dialysis treatment, maintenance, and/or training to patients or caregivers on an ambulatory or home-care basis.
66-70	Unassigned	N/A
71	Public health clinic	A facility maintained by either state or local health departments that provides ambulatory primary medical care under the general direction of a physician.
72	Rural health clinic	A certified facility which is located in a rural medically underserved area that provides ambulatory primary medical care under the general direction of a physician.
73-80	Unassigned	N/A
81	Independent laboratory	A laboratory certified to perform diagnostic and/or clinical tests independent of an institution or a physician's office.
82-98	Unassigned	N/A
99	Other place of service	Other place of service not identified above.

Type of Service

Common Working File Type of Service (TOS) Indicators

For submitting a claim to the Common Working File (CWF), use the following table to assign the proper TOS. Some procedures may have more than one applicable TOS. CWF will reject codes with incorrect TOS designations. CWF will produce alerts on codes with incorrect TOS designations.

The only exceptions to this annual update are:

- Surgical services billed for dates of service through December 31, 2007, containing the ASC facility service modifier SG must be reported as TOS F. Effective for services on or after January 1, 2008, the SG modifier is no longer applicable for Medicare services. ASC providers should discontinue applying the SG modifier on ASC facility claims. The indicator F does not appear in the TOS table because its use depends upon claims submitted with POS 24 (ASC facility) from an ASC (specialty 49). This became effective for dates of service January 1, 2008, or after.

- Surgical services billed with an assistant-at-surgery modifier (80-82, AS) must be reported with TOS 8. The 8 indicator does not appear on the TOS table because its use is dependent upon the use of the appropriate modifier. (See Pub. 100-4 *Medicare Claims Processing*

Manual, chapter 12, "Physician/Practitioner Billing," for instructions on when assistant-at-surgery is allowable.)

- TOS H appears in the list of descriptors. However, it does not appear in the table. In CWF, "H" is used only as an indicator for hospice. The contractor should not submit TOS H to CWF at this time.

- For outpatient services, when a transfusion medicine code appears on a claim that also contains a blood product, the service is paid under reasonable charge at 80 percent; coinsurance and deductible apply. When transfusion medicine codes are paid under the clinical laboratory fee schedule they are paid at 100 percent; coinsurance and deductible do not apply.

Note: For injection codes with more than one possible TOS designation, use the following guidelines when assigning the TOS:

When the choice is L or 1:

- Use TOS L when the drug is used related to ESRD; or
- Use TOS 1 when the drug is not related to ESRD and is administered in the office.

When the choice is G or 1:

- Use TOS G when the drug is an immunosuppressive drug; or
- Use TOS 1 when the drug is used for other than immunosuppression.

When the choice is P or 1:

- Use TOS P if the drug is administered through durable medical equipment (DME); or
- Use TOS 1 if the drug is administered in the office.

The place of service or diagnosis may be considered when determining the appropriate TOS. The descriptors for each of the TOS codes listed in the annual HCPCS update are:

0	Whole blood
1	Medical care
2	Surgery
3	Consultation
4	Diagnostic radiology
5	Diagnostic laboratory
6	Therapeutic radiology
7	Anesthesia
8	Assistant at surgery
9	Other medical items or services
A	Used DME
B	High risk screening mammography
C	Low risk screening mammography
D	Ambulance
E	Enteral/parenteral nutrients/supplies
F	Ambulatory surgical center (facility usage for surgical services)
G	Immunosuppressive drugs
H	Hospice
J	Diabetic shoes
K	Hearing items and services
L	ESRD supplies
M	Monthly capitation payment for dialysis
N	Kidney donor
P	Lump sum purchase of DME, prosthetics, orthotics
Q	Vision items or services
R	Rental of DME
S	Surgical dressings or other medical supplies
U	Occupational therapy
V	Pneumococcal/flu vaccine
W	Physical therapy

Appendix L — Multianalyte Assays with Algorithmic Analyses

The following tables contain the Administrative Codes for Multianalyte Assays with Algorithmic Analyses (MAAA), category I codes for Administrative Codes for Multianalyte Assays with Algorithmic Analyses (MAAA) and the most current list of Proprietary Laboratory Analysis (PLA) codes.

The following is a list of administrative codes for multianalyte assays with algorithmic analysis (MAAA) procedures that are usually exclusive to one single clinical laboratory or manufacturer. These tests use the results from several different assays, including molecular pathology assays, fluorescent in situ hybridization assays, and nonnucleic acid-based assays (e.g., proteins, polypeptides, lipids, and carbohydrates) to perform an algorithmic analysis that is reported as a numeric score or probability. Although the laboratory report may list results of individual component tests of the MAAAs, these assays are not separately reportable.

The following list includes the proprietary name and clinical laboratory/manufacturer, an alphanumeric code, and the code descriptor.

The format for the code descriptor usually includes:

- Type of disease (e.g., oncology, autoimmune, tissue rejection)
- Chemical(s) analyzed (e.g., DNA, RNA, protein, antibody)

- Number of markers (e.g., number of genes, number of proteins)
- Methodology(s) (e.g., microarray, real-time [RT]-PCR, in situ hybridization [ISH], enzyme linked immunosorbent assays [ELISA])
- Number of functional domains (when indicated)
- Type of specimen (e.g., blood, fresh tissue, formalin-fixed paraffin embedded)
- Type of algorithm result (e.g., prognostic, diagnostic)
- Report (e.g., probability index, risk score)

MAAA procedures with a Category I code are noted on the following list and can also be found in code range 81500–81599 in the pathology and laboratory chapter. If a specific MAAA test does not have a Category I code, it is denoted with a four-digit number and the letter M. Use code 81599 if an MAAA test is not included on the following list or in the Category I codes. The codes on the list are exclusive to the assays identified by proprietary name. Report code 81599 also when an analysis is performed that may possibly fall within a specific descriptor but the proprietary name is not included in the list. The list does not contain all MAAA procedures.

Proprietary Name/Clinical Laboratory/Manufacturer	Code	Descriptor
Administrative Codes for Multianalyte Assays with Algorithmic Analyses (MAAA)		
	0001M (0001M has been deleted. To report, see 81596.)	
ASH FibroSURE™, BioPredictive S.A.S	0002M	Liver disease, 10 biochemical assays (ALT, A2-macroglobulin, apolipoprotein A-1, total bilirubin, GGT, haptoglobin, AST, glucose, total cholesterol, and triglycerides) utilizing serum, prognostic algorithm reported as quantitative scores for fibrosis, steatosis, and alcoholic steatohepatitis (ASH)
NASH FibroSURE™, BioPredictive S.A.S	0003M	Liver disease, 10 biochemical assays (ALT, A2-macroglobulin, apolipoprotein A-1, total bilirubin, GGT, haptoglobin, AST, glucose, total cholesterol, and triglycerides) utilizing serum, prognostic algorithm reported as quantitative scores for fibrosis, steatosis, and nonalcoholic steatohepatitis (NASH)
ScoliScore™ Transgenomic	0004M	Scoliosis, DNA analysis of 53 single nucleotide polymorphisms (SNPs), using saliva, prognostic algorithm reported as a risk score
HeproDX™, GoPath Laboratories, LLC	0006M	Oncology (hepatic), mRNA expression levels of 161 genes, utilizing fresh hepatocellular carcinoma tumor tissue, with alpha-fetoprotein level, algorithm reported as a risk classifier
NETest (Wren Laboratories, LLC)	0007M	Oncology (gastrointestinal neuroendocrine tumors), real-time PCR expression analysis of 51 genes, utilizing whole peripheral blood, algorithm reported as a nomogram of tumor disease index
	0008M (0008M has been deleted. To report, see 81520.)	
	(0009M has been deleted)	
	(0010M has been deleted. To report, see 81539.)	
NeoLAB™ Prostate Liquid Biopsy, NeoGenomics Laboratories	▲ 0011M	Oncology, prostate cancer, mRNA expression assay of 12 genes (10 content and 2 housekeeping), RT-PCR test utilizing blood plasma and urine, algorithms to predict high-grade prostate cancer risk
Cxbladder™ Detect, Pacific Edge Diagnostics USA, Ltd.	0012M	Oncology (urothelial), mRNA, gene expression profiling by real-time quantitative PCR of five genes (*MDK, HOXA13, CDC2 [CDK1], IGFBP5,* and *CXCR2*), utilizing urine, algorithm reported as a risk score for having urothelial carcinoma
Cxbladder™ Monitor, Pacific Edge Diagnostics USA, Ltd.	0013M	Oncology (urothelial), mRNA, gene expression profiling by real-time quantitative PCR of five genes (*MDK, HOXA13, CDC2 [CDK1], IGFBP5,* and *CXCR2*), utilizing urine, algorithm reported as a risk score for having recurrent urothelial carcinoma

Proprietary Name/Clinical Laboratory/Manufacturer	Code	Descriptor
Category I Codes for Multianalyte Assays with Algorithmic Analyses (MAAA)		
Vectra® DA, Crescendo Bioscience, Inc.	81490	Autoimmune (rheumatoid arthritis), analysis of 12 biomarkers using immunoassays, utilizing serum, prognostic algorithm reported as a disease activity score (Do not report 81490 with 86140)
Corus® CAD, CardioDx, Inc.	81493	Coronary artery disease, mRNA, gene expression profiling by real-time RT-PCR of 23 genes, utilizing whole peripheral blood, algorithm reported as a risk score
AlloMap®, CareDx, Inc.	81595	Cardiology (heart transplant), mRNA, gene expression profiling by real-time quantitative PCR of 20 genes (11 content and 9 housekeeping), utilizing subfraction of peripheral blood, algorithm reported as a rejection risk score
Risk of Ovarian Malignancy Algorithm (ROMA)™, Fujirebio Diagnostics	81500	Oncology (ovarian), biochemical assays of two proteins (CA-125 and HE4), utilizing serum, with menopausal status, algorithm reported as a risk score
OVA1™, Vermillion, Inc.	81503	Oncology (ovarian), biochemical assays of five proteins (CA-125, apolipoprotein A1, beta-2 microglobulin, transferrin, and pre-albumin), utilizing serum, algorithm reported as a risk score
Tissue of Origin Test, Kit-FFPE, Cancer Genetics, Inc.	81504	Oncology (tissue of origin), microarray gene expression profiling of >2000 genes, utilizing formalin-fixed paraffin embedded tissue, algorithm reported as tissue similarity scores
PreDx Diabetes Risk Score™, Tethys Clinical Laboratory	81506	Endocrinology (type 2 diabetes), biochemical assays of seven analytes (glucose, HbA1c, insulin, hs-CRP, adiponectin, ferritin, interleukin 2-receptor alpha), utilizing serum or plasma, algorithm reporting a risk score
Harmony™ Prenatal Test, Ariosa Diagnostics	81507	Fetal aneuploidy (trisomy 21, 18, and 13) DNA sequence analysis of selected regions using maternal plasma, algorithm reported as a risk score for each trisomy
No proprietary name and clinical laboratory or manufacturer. Maternal serum screening procedures are performed by many labs and are not exclusive to a single facility.	81508	Fetal congenital abnormalities, biochemical assays of two proteins (PAPP-A, hCG [any form]), utilizing maternal serum, algorithm reported as a risk score
	81509	Fetal congenital abnormalities, biochemical assays of three proteins (PAPP-A, hCG [any form], DIA), utilizing maternal serum, algorithm reported as a risk score
	81510	Fetal congenital abnormalities, biochemical assays of three analytes (AFP, uE3, hCG (any form)), utilizing maternal serum, algorithm reported as a risk score
	81511	Fetal congenital abnormalities, biochemical assays of four analytes (AFP, uE3, hCG (any form), DIA) utilizing maternal serum, algorithm reported as a risk score (may include additional results from previous biochemical testing)
	81512	Fetal congenital abnormalities, biochemical assays of five analytes (AFP, uE3, total hCG, hyperglycosylated hCG, DIA) utilizing maternal serum, algorithm reported as a risk score
Breast Cancer Index, Biotheranostics, Inc	81518	Oncology (breast), mRNA, gene expression profiling by real-time RT-PCR of 11 genes (7 content and 4 housekeeping), utilizing formalin-fixed paraffin-embedded tissue, algorithms reported as percentage risk for metastatic recurrence and likelihood of benefit from extended endocrine therapy
EndoPredict®, Myriad Genetic Laboratories, Inc.	# ● 81522	Oncology (breast), mRNA, gene expression profiling by RT-PCR of 12 genes (8 content and 4 housekeeping), utilizing formalin-fixed paraffin-embedded tissue, algorithm reported as recurrence risk score
Oncotype DX® Genomic Health	81519	Oncology (breast), mRNA, gene expression profiling by real-time RT-PCR of 21 genes, utilizing formalin-fixed paraffin embedded tissue, algorithm reported as recurrence score
Prosigna® Breast Cancer Assay, NanoString Technologies, Inc.	81520	Oncology (breast), mRNA gene expression profiling by hybrid capture of 58 genes (50 content and 8 housekeeping), utilizing formalin-fixed paraffin-embedded tissue, algorithm reported as a recurrence risk score
MammaPrint®, Agendia, Inc.	81521	Oncology (breast), mRNA, microarray gene expression profiling of 70 content genes and 465 housekeeping genes, utilizing fresh frozen or formalin-fixed paraffin-embedded tissue, algorithm reported as index related to risk of distant metastasis
Oncotype DX® Colon Cancer Assay, Genomic Health	81525	Oncology (colon), mRNA, gene expression profiling by real-time RT-PCR of 12 genes (7 content and 5 housekeeping), utilizing formalin-fixed paraffin-embedded tissue, algorithm reported as a recurrence score
Cologuard™, Exact Sciences, Inc.	81528	Oncology (colorectal) screening, quantitative real-time target and signal amplification of 10 DNA markers (KRAS mutations, promoter methylation of NDRG4 and BMP3) and fecal hemoglobin, utilizing stool, algorithm reported as a positive or negative result (Do not report 81528 with 81275, 82274)
ChemoFX®, Helomics, Corp.	81535	Oncology (gynecologic), live tumor cell culture and chemotherapeutic response by DAPI stain and morphology, predictive algorithm reported as a drug response score; first single drug or drug combination
ChemoFX®, Helomics, Corp.	+ 81536	Oncology (gynecologic), live tumor cell culture and chemotherapeutic response by DAPI stain and morphology, predictive algorithm reported as a drug response score; each additional single drug or drug combination (List separately in addition to code for primary procedure) (Code first 81535)

Proprietary Name/Clinical Laboratory/Manufacturer	Code	Descriptor
VeriStrat, Biodesix, Inc.	81538	Oncology (lung), mass spectrometric 8-protein signature, including amyloid A, utilizing serum, prognostic and predictive algorithm reported as good versus poor overall survival
4Kscore test, OPKO Health Inc.	81539	Oncology (high-grade prostate cancer), biochemical assay of four proteins (Total PSA, Free PSA, Intact PSA, and human kallikrein-2 [hK2]), utilizing plasma or serum, prognostic algorithm reported as a probability score
CancerTYPE ID, bioTheranostics, Inc.	81540	Oncology (tumor of unknown origin), mRNA, gene expression profiling by real-time RT-PCR of 92 genes (87 content and 5 housekeeping) to classify tumor into main cancer type and subtype, utilizing formalin-fixed paraffin-embedded tissue, algorithm reported as a probability of a predicted main cancer type and subtype
Prolaris®, Myriad Genetic Laboratories, Inc.	81541	Oncology (prostate), mRNA gene expression profiling by real-time RT-PCR of 46 genes (31 content and 15 housekeeping), utilizing formalin- fixed paraffin-embedded tissue, algorithm reported as a disease-specific mortality risk score
Decipher® Prostate, Decipher® Biosciences	● 81542	Oncology (prostate), mRNA, microarray gene expression profiling of 22 content genes, utilizing formalin-fixed paraffin-embedded tissue, algorithm reported as metastasis risk score
Afirma® Gene Expression Classifier, Veracyte, Inc.	81545	Oncology (thyroid), gene expression analysis of 142 genes, utilizing fine needle aspirate, algorithm reported as a categorical result (eg, benign or suspicious)
ConfirmMDx® for Prostate Cancer, MDxHealth, Inc.	81551	Oncology (prostate), promoter methylation profiling by real-time PCR of 3 genes (GSTP1, APC, RASSF1), utilizing formalin-fixed paraffin-embedded tissue, algorithm reported as a likelihood of prostate cancer detection on repeat biopsy
DecisionDx®-UM test, Castle Biosciences, Inc.	● 81552	Oncology (uveal melanoma), mRNA, gene expression profiling by real-time RT-PCR of 15 genes (12 content and 3 housekeeping), utilizing fine needle aspirate or formalin-fixed paraffin-embedded tissue, algorithm reported as risk of metastasis
HCV FibroSURE™, FibroTest™, BioPredictive S.A.S.	81596	Infectious disease, chronic hepatitis C virus (HCV) infection, six biochemical assays (ALT, A2-macroglobulin, apolipoprotein A-1, total bilirubin, GGT, and haptoglobin) utilizing serum, prognostic algorithm reported as scores for fibrosis and necroinflammatory activity in liver
	81599	Unlisted multianalyte assay with algorithmic analysis

Proprietary Laboratory Analyses (PLA)

PreciseType® HEA Test, Immucor, Inc.	0001U	Red blood cell antigen typing, DNA, human erythrocyte antigen gene analysis of 35 antigens from 11 blood groups, utilizing whole blood, common RBC alleles reported
PolypDX™, Atlantic Diagnostic Laboratories, LLC, Metabolomic Technologies, Inc.	0002U	Oncology (colorectal), quantitative assessment of three urine metabolites (ascorbic acid, succinic acid and carnitine) by liquid chromatography with tandem mass spectrometry (LC-MS/MS) using multiple reaction monitoring acquisition, algorithm reported as likelihood of adenomatous polyps
Overa (OVA1 Next Generation), Aspira Labs, Inc, Vermillion, Inc.	0003U	Oncology (ovarian) biochemical assays of five proteins (apolipoprotein A-1, CA 125 II, follicle stimulating hormone, human epididymis protein 4, transferrin), utilizing serum, algorithm reported as a likelihood score
	(0004U has been deleted)	
ExosomeDx®, Prostate (IntelliScore), Exosome Diagnostics, Inc, Exosome Diagnostics, Inc	0005U	Oncology (prostate) gene expression profile by real-time RT-PCR of 3 genes (ERG, PCA3, and SPDEF), urine, algorithm reported as risk score
Drug-drug, Drug-substance Identification and Interaction, Aegis Sciences Corporation	0006U	Detection of interacting medications, substances, supplements and foods, 120 or more analytes, definitive chromatography with mass spectrometry, urine, description and severity of each interaction identified, per date of service
ToxProtect, Genotox Laboratories Ltd	0007U	Drug test(s), presumptive, with definitive confirmation of positive results, any number of drug classes, urine, includes specimen verification including DNA authentication in comparison to buccal DNA, per date of service.
AmHPR® H. pylori Antibiotic Resistance Panel, American Molecular Laboratories, Inc.	▲ 0008U	Helicobacter pylori detection and antibiotic resistance, DNA, 16S and 23S rRNA, gyrA, pbp1,rdxA and rpoB, next generation sequencing, formalin-fixed paraffin-embedded or fresh tissue or fecal sample, predictive, reported as positive or negative for resistance to clarithromycin, fluoroquinolones, metronidazole, amoxicillin, tetracycline, and rifabutin
DEPArray™HER2, PacificDx	0009U	Oncology (breast cancer), ERBB2 (HER2) copy number by FISH, tumor cells from formalin-fixed paraffin-embedded tissue isolated using image-based dielectrophoresis (DEP) sorting, reported as ERBB2 gene amplified or non-amplified
Bacterial Typing by Whole Genome Sequencing, Mayo Clinic	0010U	Infectious disease (bacterial), strain typing by whole genome sequencing, phylogenetic-based report of strain relatedness, per submitted isolate
Cordant CORE™, Cordant Health Solutions	0011U	Prescription drug monitoring, evaluation of drugs present by LC-MS/MS, using oral fluid, reported as a comparison to an estimated steady-state range, per date of service including all drug compounds and metabolites
MatePair Targeted Rearrangements, Congenital, Mayo Clinic	0012U	Germline disorders, gene rearrangement detection by whole genome next-generation sequencing, DNA, whole blood, report of specific gene rearrangement(s)

Proprietary Name/Clinical Laboratory/Manufacturer	Code	Descriptor
MatePair Targeted Rearrangements, Oncology, Mayo Clinic	0013U	Oncology (solid organ neoplasia), gene rearrangement detection by whole genome next-generation sequencing, DNA, fresh or frozen tissue or cells, report of specific gene rearrangement(s)
MatePair Targeted Rearrangements, Hematologic, Mayo Clinic	0014U	Hematology (hematolymphoid neoplasia), gene rearrangement detection by whole genome next-generation sequencing, DNA, whole blood or bone marrow, report of specific gene
	(0015U has been deleted)	
BCR-ABL1 major and minor breakpoint fusion transcripts, University of Iowa, Department of Pathology, Asuragen	0016U	Oncology (hematolymphoid neoplasia), RNA, BCR/ABL1 major and minor breakpoint fusion transcripts, quantitative PCR amplification, blood or bone marrow, report of fusion not detected or detected with quantitation
JAK2 Mutation, University of Iowa, Department of Pathology	0017U	Oncology (hematolymphoid neoplasia), *JAK2* mutation, DNA, PCR amplification of exons 12-14 and sequence analysis, blood or bone marrow, report of JAK2 mutation not detected or detected
ThyraMIR™, Interpace Diagnostics	0018U	Oncology (thyroid), microRNA profiling by RT-PCR of 10 microRNA sequences, utilizing fine needle aspirate, algorithm reported as a positive or negative result for moderate to high risk of malignancy
OncoTarget/OncoTreat, Columbia University Department of Pathology and Cell Biology, Darwin Health	0019U	Oncology, RNA, gene expression by whole transcriptome sequencing, formalin-fixed paraffin embedded tissue or fresh frozen tissue, predictive algorithm reported as potential targets for therapeutic agents
	(0020U has been deleted)	
Apifiny®, Armune BioScience, Inc	0021U	Oncology (prostate), detection of 8 autoantibodies (ARF 6, NKX3-1, 5'-UTR-BMI1, CEP 164, 3'-UTR-Ropporin, Desmocollin, AURKAIP-1, CSNK2A2), multiplexed immunoassay and flow cytometry serum, algorithm reported as risk score
Oncomine™ Dx Target Test, Thermo Fisher Scientific	0022U	Targeted genomic sequence analysis panel, non-small cell lung neoplasia, DNA and RNA analysis, 23 genes, interrogation for sequence variants and rearrangements, reported as presence/absence of variants and associated therapy(ies) to consider
LeukoStrat® CDx *FLT3* Mutation Assay, LabPMM LLC, an Invivoscribe Technologies, Inc Company, Invivoscribe Technologies, Inc	0023U	Oncology (acute myelogenous leukemia), DNA, genotyping of internal tandem duplication, p.D835, p.I836, using mononuclear cells, reported as detection or non-detection of FLT3 mutation and indication for or against the use of midostaurin
GlycA, Laboratory Corporation of America, Laboratory Corporation of America	0024U	Glycosylated acute phase proteins (GlycA), nuclear magnetic resonance spectroscopy, quantitative
UrSure Tenofovir Quantification Test, Synergy Medical Laboratories, UrSure Inc	0025U	Tenofovir, by liquid chromatography with tandem mass spectrometry (LC-MS/MS), urine, quantitative
Thyroseq Genomic Classifier, CBLPath, Inc, University of Pittsburgh Medical Center	0026U	Oncology (thyroid), DNA and mRNA of 112 genes, next-generation sequencing, fine needle aspirate of thyroid nodule, algorithmic analysis reported as a categorical result ("Positive, high probability of malignancy" or "Negative, low probability of malignancy")
JAK2 Exons 12 to 15 Sequencing, Mayo Clinic, Mayo Clinic	0027U	*JAK2* (Janus kinase 2) (eg, myeloproliferative disorder) gene analysis, targeted sequence analysis exons 12-15
	(0028U has been deleted)	
Focused Pharmacogenomics Panel, Mayo Clinic, Mayo Clinic	0029U	Drug metabolism (adverse drug reactions and drug response), targeted sequence analysis (ie, *CYP1A2, CYP2C19, CYP2C9, CYP2D6, CYP3A4, CYP3A5, CYP4F2, SLCO1B1, VKORC1* and rs12777823)
Warfarin Response Genotype, Mayo Clinic, Mayo Clinic	0030U	Drug metabolism (warfarin drug response), targeted sequence analysis (i.e., *CYP2C9, CYP4F2, VKORC1,* rs12777823)
Cytochrome P450 1A2 Genotype, Mayo Clinic, Mayo Clinic	0031U	*CYP1A2 (cytochrome P450 family 1, subfamily A, member 2)* (eg, drug metabolism) gene analysis, common variants (ie, *1F, *1K, *6, *7)
Catechol-O- Methyltransferase *(COMT)* Genotype, Mayo Clinic, Mayo Clinic	0032U	*COMT (catechol-O-methyltransferase)* (eg, drug metabolism) gene analysis, c.472G>A (rs4680) variant
Serotonin Receptor Genotype *(HTR2A* and *HTR2C),* Mayo Clinic, Mayo Clinic	0033U	*HTR2A (5-hydroxytryptamine receptor 2A), HTR2C (5-hydroxytryptamine receptor 2C)* (eg, citalopram metabolism) gene analysis, common variants (i.e., *HTR2A* rs7997012 [c.614-2211T>C], *HTR2C* rs3813929 [c.- 759C>T] and rs1414334 [c.551-3008C>G])
Thiopurine Methyltransferase *(TPMT)* and Nudix Hydrolase *(NUDT15)* Genotyping, Mayo Clinic, Mayo Clinic	0034U	*TPMT (thiopurine S-methyltransferase), NUDT15 (nudix hydroxylase 15)* (eg, thiopurine metabolism) gene analysis, common variants (i.e., *TPMT *2, *3A, *3B, *3C, *4, *5, *6, *8, *12; NUDT15 *3, *4, *5)*
Real-time quaking- induced conversion for prion detection (RT- QuIC), National Prion Disease Pathology Surveillance Center	0035U	Neurology (prion disease), cerebrospinal fluid, detection of prion protein by quaking- induced conformational conversion, qualitative
EXaCT-1 Whole Exome Testing, Lab of Oncology-Molecular Detection, Weill Cornell Medicine-Clinical Genomics Laboratory	0036U	Exome (ie, somatic mutations), paired formalin-fixed paraffin-embedded tumor tissue and normal specimen, sequence analyses
FoundationOne CDx™ (F1CDx), Foundation Medicine, Inc, Foundation Medicine, Inc	0037U	Targeted genomic sequence analysis, solid organ neoplasm, DNA analysis of 324 genes, interrogation for sequence variants, gene copy number amplifications, gene rearrangements, microsatellite instability and tumor mutational burden

Proprietary Name/Clinical Laboratory/Manufacturer	Code	Descriptor
Sensieva ™ Droplet 25OH Vitamin D2/D3 Microvolume LC/MS Assay, InSource Diagnostics, InSource Diagnostics	0038U	Vitamin D, 25 hydroxy D2 and D3, by LC- MS/MS, serum microsample, quantitative
Anti-dsDNA, High Salt/Avidity, University of Washington, Department of Laboratory Medicine, Bio-Rad	0039U	Deoxyribonucleic acid (DNA) antibody, double stranded, high avidity
MRDx BCR-ABL Test, MolecularMD, MolecularMD	0040U	*BCR/ABL1 (t(9;22))* (eg, chronic myelogenous leukemia) translocation analysis, major breakpoint, quantitative
Lyme ImmunoBlot IgM, IGeneX Inc, ID-FISH Technology Inc. (ASR) (Lyme ImmunoBlot IgM Strips Only)	0041U	Borrelia burgdorferi, antibody detection of 5 recombinant protein groups, by immunoblot, IgM
Lyme ImmunoBlot IgG, IGeneX Inc, ID-FISH Technology Inc (ASR) (Lyme ImmunoBlot IgG Strips Only)	0042U	Borrelia burgdorferi, antibody detection of 12 recombinant protein groups, by immunoblot, IgG
Tick-Borne Relapsing Fever (TBRF) Borrelia ImmunoBlots IgM Test, IGeneX Inc, ID-FISH Technology Inc (Provides TBRF ImmunoBlot IgM Strips)	0043U	Tick-borne relapsing fever Borrelia group, antibody detection to 4 recombinant protein groups, by immunoblot, IgM
Tick-Borne Relapsing Fever (TBRF) Borrelia ImmunoBlots IgG Test, IGeneX Inc., ID-FISH Technology Inc (Provides TBRF ImmunoBlot IgG Strips)	0044U	Tick-borne relapsing fever Borrelia group, antibody detection to 4 recombinant protein groups, by immunoblot, IgG
The Oncotype DX® Breast DCIS Score™ Test, Genomic Health, Inc, Genomic Health, Inc	0045U	Oncology (breast ductal carcinoma in situ), mRNA, gene expression profiling by real- time RT-PCR of 12 genes (7 content and 5 housekeeping), utilizing formalin-fixed paraffin-embedded tissue, algorithm reported as recurrence score
FLT3 ITD MRD by NGS, LabPMM LLC, an Invivoscribe Technologies, Inc Company	0046U	*FLT3 (fms-related tyrosine kinase 3)* (eg, acute myeloid leukemia) internal tandem duplication (ITD) variants, quantitative
Oncotype DX Genomic Prostate Score, Genomic Health, Inc, Genomic Health, Inc	0047U	Oncology (prostate), mRNA, gene expression profiling by real-time RT-PCR of 17 genes (12 content and 5 housekeeping), utilizing formalin-fixed paraffin-embedded tissue, algorithm reported as a risk score
MSK-IMPACT (Integrated Mutation Profiling of Actionable Cancer Targets), Memorial Sloan Kettering Cancer Center	0048U	Oncology (solid organ neoplasia), DNA, targeted sequencing of protein-coding exons of 468 cancer-associated genes, including interrogation for somatic mutations and microsatellite instability, matched with normal specimens, utilizing formalin-fixed paraffin-embedded tumor tissue, report of clinically significant mutation(s)
NPM1 MRD by NGS, LabPMM LLC, an Invivoscribe Technologies, Inc Company	0049U	*NPM1 (nucleophosmin)* (eg, acute myeloid leukemia) gene analysis, quantitative
MyAML NGS Panel, LabPMM LLC, an Invivoscribe Technologies, Inc Company	0050U	Targeted genomic sequence analysis panel, acute myelogenous leukemia, DNA analysis, 194 genes, interrogation for sequence variants, copy number variants or rearrangements
UCompliDx, Elite Medical Laboratory Solutions, LLC, Elite Medical Laboratory Solutions, LLC (LDT)	0051U	Prescription drug monitoring, evaluation of drugs present by LC-MS/MS, urine, 31 drug panel, reported as quantitative results, detected or not detected, per date of service
VAP Cholesterol Test, VAP Diagnostics Laboratory, Inc, VAP Diagnostics Laboratory, Inc	0052U	Lipoprotein, blood, high resolution fractionation and quantitation of lipoproteins, including all five major lipoprotein classes and subclasses of HDL, LDL, and VLDL by vertical auto profile ultracentrifugation
Prostate Cancer Risk Panel, Mayo Clinic, Laboratory Developed Test	0053U	Oncology (prostate cancer), FISH analysis of 4 genes (*ASAP1, HDAC9, CHD1 and PTEN*), needle biopsy specimen, algorithm reported as probability of higher tumor grade
AssuranceRx Micro Serum, Firstox Laboratories, LLC, Firstox Laboratories, LLC	0054U	Prescription drug monitoring, 14 or more classes of drugs and substances, definitive tandem mass spectrometry with chromatography, capillary blood, quantitative report with therapeutic and toxic ranges, including steady-state range for the prescribed dose when detected, per date of service
myTAIHEART, TAI Diagnostics, Inc, TAI Diagnostics, Inc	0055U	Cardiology (heart transplant), cell-free DNA, PCR assay of 96 DNA target sequences (94 single nucleotide polymorphism targets and two control targets), plasma
MatePair Acute Myeloid Leukemia Panel, Mayo Clinic, Laboratory Developed Test	0056U	Hematology (acute myelogenous leukemia), DNA, whole genome next-generation sequencing to detect gene rearrangement(s), blood or bone marrow, report of specific gene rearrangement(s)
	(0057U has been deleted)	
Merkel SmT Oncoprotein Antibody Titer, University of Washington, Department of Laboratory Medicine	0058U	Oncology (Merkel cell carcinoma), detection of antibodies to the Merkel cell polyoma virus oncoprotein (small T antigen), serum, quantitative
Merkel Virus VP1 Capsid Antibody, University of Washington, Department of Laboratory Medicine	0059U	Oncology (Merkel cell carcinoma), detection of antibodies to the Merkel cell polyoma virus capsid protein (VP1), serum, reported as positive or negative
Twins Zygosity PLA, Natera, Inc, Natera, Inc	0060U	Twin zygosity, genomic-targeted sequence analysis of chromosome 2, using circulating cell-free fetal DNA in maternal blood
Transcutaneous multispectral measurement of tissue oxygenation and hemoglobin using spatial frequency domain imaging (SFDI), Modulated Imaging, Inc, Modulated Imaging, Inc	0061U	Transcutaneous measurement of five biomarkers (tissue oxygenation [StO2], oxyhemoglobin [ctHbO2], deoxyhemoglobin [ctHbR], papillary and reticular dermal hemoglobin concentrations [ctHb1 and ctHb2]), using spatial frequency domain imaging (SFDI) and multi-spectral analysis

Appendix L — Multianalyte Assays with Algorithmic Analyses

Proprietary Name/Clinical Laboratory/Manufacturer	Code	Descriptor
SLE-key® Rule Out, Veracis Inc, Veracis Inc	● 0062U	Autoimmune (systemic lupus erythematosus), IgG and IgM analysis of 80 biomarkers, utilizing serum, algorithm reported with a risk score
NPDX ASD ADM Panel I, Stemina Biomarker Discovery, Inc, Stemina Biomarker Discovery, Inc d/b/a NeuroPointDX	● 0063U	Neurology (autism), 32 amines by LC-MS/MS, using plasma, algorithm reported as metabolic signature associated with autism spectrum disorder
BioPlex 2200 Syphilis Total & RPR Assay, Bio-Rad Laboratories, Bio-Rad Laboratories	● 0064U	Antibody, Treponema pallidum, total and rapid plasma reagin (RPR), immunoassay, qualitative
BioPlex 2200 RPR Assay, Bio-Rad Laboratories, Bio-Rad Laboratories	● 0065U	Syphilis test, non-treponemal antibody, immunoassay, qualitative (RPR)
PartoSure™ Test, Parsagen Diagnostics, Inc, Parsagen Diagnostics, Inc, a QIAGEN Company	● 0066U	Placental alpha-micro globulin-1 (PAMG-1), immunoassay with direct optical observation, cervico-vaginal fluid, each specimen
BBDRisk Dx™, Silbiotech, Inc, Silbiotech, Inc	● 0067U	Oncology (breast), immunohistochemistry, protein expression profiling of 4 biomarkers (matrix metalloproteinase-1 [MMP-1], carcinoembryonic antigen-related cell adhesion molecule 6 [CEACAM6], hyaluronoglucosaminidase [HYAL1], highly expressed in cancer protein [HEC1]), formalin-fixed paraffin-embedded precancerous breast tissue, algorithm reported as carcinoma risk score
MYCODART Dual Amplification Real Time PCR Panel for 6 Candida species, RealTime Laboratories, Inc, RealTime Laboratories, Inc	● 0068U	Candida species panel (C. albicans, C. glabrata, C. parapsilosis, C. kruseii, C tropicalis, and C. auris), amplified probe technique with qualitative report of the presence or absence of each species
miR-31now™, GoPath Laboratories, GoPath Laboratories	● 0069U	Oncology (colorectal), microRNA, RT-PCR expression profiling of miR-31-3p, formalin-fixed paraffin-embedded tissue, algorithm reported as an expression score
CYP2D6 Common Variants and Copy Number, Mayo Clinic, Laboratory Developed Test	● 0070U	CYP2D6 (cytochrome P450, family 2, subfamily D, polypeptide 6) (eg, drug metabolism) gene analysis, common and select rare variants (ie, *2, *3, *4, *4N, *5, *6, *7, *8, *9, *10, *11, *12, *13, *14A, *14B, *15, *17, *29, *35, *36, *41, *57, *61, *63, *68, *83, *xN)
CYP2D6 Full Gene Sequencing, Mayo Clinic, Laboratory Developed Test	+ ● 0071U	CYP2D6 (cytochrome P450, family 2, subfamily D, polypeptide 6) (eg, drug metabolism) gene analysis, full gene sequence (List separately in addition to code for primary procedure)
CYP2D6-2D7 Hybrid Gene Targeted Sequence Analysis, Mayo Clinic, Laboratory Developed Test	+ ● 0072U	CYP2D6 (cytochrome P450, family 2, subfamily D, polypeptide 6) (eg, drug metabolism) gene analysis, targeted sequence analysis (ie, CYP2D6-2D7 hybrid gene) (List separately in addition to code for primary procedure)
CYP2D7-2D6 Hybrid Gene Targeted Sequence Analysis, Mayo Clinic, Laboratory Developed Test	+ ● 0073U	CYP2D6 (cytochrome P450, family 2, subfamily D, polypeptide 6) (eg, drug metabolism) gene analysis, targeted sequence analysis (ie, CYP2D7-2D6 hybrid gene) (List separately in addition to code for primary procedure)
CYP2D7-2D6 trans-duplication/multiplication non-duplicated gene targeted sequence analysis, Mayo Clinic, Laboratory Developed Test	+ ● 0074U	CYP2D6 (cytochrome P450, family 2, subfamily D, polypeptide 6) (eg, drug metabolism) gene analysis, targeted sequence analysis (ie, non-duplicated gene when duplication/multiplication is trans) (List separately in addition to code for primary procedure)
CYP2D6 5' gene duplication/multiplication targeted sequence analysis, Mayo Clinic, Laboratory Developed Test	+ ● 0075U	CYP2D6 (cytochrome P450, family 2, subfamily D, polypeptide 6) (eg, drug metabolism) gene analysis, targeted sequence analysis (ie, 5' gene duplication/multiplication) (List separately in addition to code for primary procedure)
CYP2D6 3' gene duplication/multiplication targeted sequence analysis, Mayo Clinic, Laboratory Developed Test	+ ● 0076U	CYP2D6 (cytochrome P450, family 2, subfamily D, polypeptide 6) (eg, drug metabolism) gene analysis, targeted sequence analysis (ie, 3' gene duplication/multiplication) (List separately in addition to code for primary procedure)
M-Protein Detection and Isotyping by MALDI-TOF Mass Spectrometry, Mayo Clinic, Laboratory Developed Test	● 0077U	Immunoglobulin paraprotein (M-protein), qualitative, immunoprecipitation and mass spectrometry, blood or urine, including isotype
INFINITI® Neural Response Panel, PersonalizeDx Labs, AutoGenomics Inc	● 0078U	Pain management (opioid-use disorder) genotyping panel, 16 common variants (ie, ABCB1, COMT, DAT1, DBH, DOR, DRD1, DRD2, DRD4, GABA, GAL, HTR2A, HTTLPR, MTHFR, MUOR, OPRK1, OPRM1), buccal swab or other germline tissue sample, algorithm reported as positive or negative risk of opioid-use disorder
ToxLok™, InSource Diagnostics, InSource Diagnostics	● 0079U	Comparative DNA analysis using multiple selected single-nucleotide polymorphisms (SNPs), urine and buccal DNA, for specimen identity verification
BDX-XL2, Biodesix®, Inc, Biodesix®, Inc	● 0080U	Oncology (lung), mass spectrometric analysis of galectin-3-binding protein and scavenger receptor cysteine-rich type 1 protein M130, with five clinical risk factors (age, smoking status, nodule diameter, nodule-spiculation status and nodule location), utilizing plasma, algorithm reported as a categorical probability of malignancy
	(0081U has been deleted. To report, use 81552)	

Proprietary Name/Clinical Laboratory/Manufacturer	Code	Descriptor
NextGen Precision™ Testing, Precision Diagnostics, Precision Diagnostics LBN Precision Toxicology, LLC	● 0082U	Drug test(s), definitive, 90 or more drugs or substances, definitive chromatography with mass spectrometry, and presumptive, any number of drug classes, by instrument chemistry analyzer (utilizing immunoassay), urine, report of presence or absence of each drug, drug metabolite or substance with description and severity of significant interactions per date of service
Onco4D™, Animated Dynamics, Inc, Animated Dynamics, Inc	● 0083U	Oncology, response to chemotherapy drugs using motility contrast tomography, fresh or frozen tissue, reported as likelihood of sensitivity or resistance to drugs or drug combinations
BLOODchip®, ID CORE XT™, Grifols Diagnostic Solutions Inc	● 0084U	Red blood cell antigen typing, DNA, genotyping of 10 blood groups with phenotype prediction of 37 red blood cell antigens
	(0085U has been deleted)	
Accelerate PhenoTest™ BC kit, Accelerate Diagnostics, Inc	● 0086U	Infectious disease (bacterial and fungal), organism identification, blood culture, using rRNA FISH, 6 or more organism targets, reported as positive or negative with phenotypic minimum inhibitory concentration (MIC)-based antimicrobial susceptibility
Molecular Microscope® MMDx—Heart, Kashi Clinical Laboratories	● 0087U	Cardiology (heart transplant), mRNA gene expression profiling by microarray of 1283 genes, transplant biopsy tissue, allograft rejection and injury algorithm reported as a probability score
Molecular Microscope® MMDx—Kidney, Kashi Clinical Laboratories	● 0088U	Transplantation medicine (kidney allograft rejection), microarray gene expression profiling of 1494 genes, utilizing transplant biopsy tissue, algorithm reported as a probability score for rejection
Pigmented Lesion Assay (PLA), DermTech	● 0089U	Oncology (melanoma), gene expression profiling by RTqPCR, *PRAME* and *LINC00518*, superficial collection using adhesive patch(es)
myPath® Melanoma, Myriad Genetic Laboratories	● 0090U	Oncology (cutaneous melanoma), mRNA gene expression profiling by RT-PCR of 23 genes (14 content and 9 housekeeping), utilizing formalin-fixed paraffin-embedded tissue, algorithm reported as a categorical result (ie, benign, indeterminate, malignant)
FirstSight^{CRC}, CellMax Life	● 0091U	Oncology (colorectal) screening, cell enumeration of circulating tumor cells, utilizing whole blood, algorithm, for the presence of adenoma or cancer, reported as a positive or negative result
REVEAL Lung Nodule Characterization, MagArray, Inc	● 0092U	Oncology (lung), three protein biomarkers, immunoassay using magnetic nanosensor technology, plasma, algorithm reported as risk score for likelihood of malignancy
ComplyRX, Claro Labs	● 0093U	Prescription drug monitoring, evaluation of 65 common drugs by LC-MS/MS, urine, each drug reported detected or not detected
RCIGM Rapid Whole Genome Sequencing, Rady Children's Institute for Genomic Medicine (RCIGM)	● 0094U	Genome (eg, unexplained constitutional or heritable disorder or syndrome), rapid sequence analysis
Esophageal String Test™ (EST), Cambridge Biomedical, Inc	● 0095U	Inflammation (eosinophilic esophagitis), ELISA analysis of eotaxin-3 *(CCL26 [C-C motif chemokine ligand 26])* and major basic protein *(PRG2 [proteoglycan 2, pro eosinophil major basic protein])*, specimen obtained by swallowed nylon string, algorithm reported as predictive probability index for active eosinophilic esophagitis
HPV, High-Risk, Male Urine, Molecular Testing Labs	● 0096U	Human papillomavirus (HPV), high-risk types (ie, 16, 18, 31, 33, 35, 39, 45, 51, 52, 56, 58, 59, 66, 68), male urine
BioFire® FilmArray® Gastrointestinal (GI) Panel, BioFire® Diagnostics	● 0097U	Gastrointestinal pathogen, multiplex reverse transcription and multiplex amplified probe technique, multiple types or subtypes, 22 targets (Campylobacter [C. jejuni/C. coli/C. upsaliensis], Clostridium difficile [C. difficile] toxin A/B, Plesiomonas shigelloides, Salmonella, Vibrio [V. parahaemolyticus/V. vulnificus/V. cholerae], including specific identification of Vibrio cholerae, Yersinia enterocolitica, Enteroaggregative Escherichia coli [EAEC], Enteropathogenic Escherichia coli [EPEC], Enterotoxigenic Escherichia coli [ETEC] lt/st, Shiga-like toxin-producing Escherichia coli [STEC] stx1/stx2 [including specific identification of the E. coli O157 serogroup within STEC], Shigella/Enteroinvasive Escherichia coli [EIEC], Cryptosporidium, Cyclospora cayetanensis, Entamoeba histolytica, Giardia lamblia [also known as G. intestinalis and G. duodenalis], adenovirus F 40/41, astrovirus, norovirus GI/GII, rotavirus A, sapovirus [Genogroups I, II, IV, and V])

Proprietary Name/Clinical Laboratory/Manufacturer	Code	Descriptor
BioFire® FilmArray® Respiratory Panel (RP) EZ, BioFire® Diagnostics	● 0098U	Respiratory pathogen, multiplex reverse transcription and multiplex amplified probe technique, multiple types or subtypes, 14 targets (adenovirus, coronavirus, human metapneumovirus, influenza A, influenza A subtype H1, influenza A subtype H3, influenza A subtype H1-2009, influenza B, parainfluenza virus, human rhinovirus/enterovirus, respiratory syncytial virus, Bordetella pertussis, Chlamydophila pneumoniae, Mycoplasma pneumoniae)
BioFire® FilmArray® Respiratory Panel (RP), BioFire® Diagnostics	● 0099U	Respiratory pathogen, multiplex reverse transcription and multiplex amplified probe technique, multiple types or subtypes, 20 targets (adenovirus, coronavirus 229E, coronavirus HKU1, coronavirus, coronavirus OC43, human metapneumovirus, influenza A, influenza A subtype, influenza A subtype H3, influenza A subtype H1-2009, influenza, parainfluenza virus, parainfluenza virus 2, parainfluenza virus 3, parainfluenza virus 4, human rhinovirus/enterovirus, respiratory syncytial virus, Bordetella pertussis, Chlamydophila pneumonia, Mycoplasma pneumoniae)
BioFire® FilmArray® Respiratory Panel 2 (RP2), BioFire® Diagnostics	● 0100U	Respiratory pathogen, multiplex reverse transcription and multiplex amplified probe technique, multiple types or subtypes, 21 targets (adenovirus, coronavirus 229E, coronavirus HKU1, coronavirus NL63, coronavirus OC43, human metapneumovirus, human rhinovirus/enterovirus, influenza A, including subtypes H1, H1-2009, and H3, influenza B, parainfluenza virus 1, parainfluenza virus 2, parainfluenza virus 3, parainfluenza virus 4, respiratory syncytial virus, Bordetella parapertussis [IS1001], Bordetella pertussis [ptxP], Chlamydia pneumoniae, Mycoplasma pneumoniae)
ColoNext®, Ambry Genetics®, Ambry Genetics®	● 0101U	Hereditary colon cancer disorders (eg, Lynch syndrome, *PTEN* hamartoma syndrome, Cowden syndrome, familial adenomatosis polyposis), genomic sequence analysis panel utilizing a combination of NGS, Sanger, MLPA, and array CGH, with MRNA analytics to resolve variants of unknown significance when indicated (15 genes [sequencing and deletion/duplication], *EPCAM* and *GREM1* [deletion/duplication only])
BreastNext®, Ambry Genetics®, Ambry Genetics®	● 0102U	Hereditary breast cancer-related disorders (eg, hereditary breast cancer, hereditary ovarian cancer, hereditary endometrial cancer), genomic sequence analysis panel utilizing a combination of NGS, Sanger, MLPA, and array CGH, with MRNA analytics to resolve variants of unknown significance when indicated (17 genes [sequencing and deletion/duplication])
OvaNext®, Ambry Genetics®, Ambry Genetics®	● 0103U	Hereditary ovarian cancer (eg, hereditary ovarian cancer, hereditary endometrial cancer), genomic sequence analysis panel utilizing a combination of NGS, Sanger, MLPA, and array CGH, with MRNA analytics to resolve variants of unknown significance when indicated (24 genes [sequencing and deletion/duplication], *EPCAM* [deletion/duplication only])
	(0104U has been deleted)	
KidneyIntelX™, RenalytixAI, RenalytixAI	● 0105U	Nephrology (chronic kidney disease), multiplex electrochemiluminescent immunoassay (ECLIA) of tumor necrosis factor receptor 1A, receptor superfamily 2 (*TNFR1, TNFR2*), and kidney injury molecule-1 (KIM-1) combined with longitudinal clinical data, including *APOL1* genotype if available, and plasma (isolated fresh or frozen), algorithm reported as probability score for rapid kidney function decline (RKFD)
13C-Spirulina Gastric Emptying Breath Test (GEBT), Cairn Diagnostics d/b/a Advanced Breath Diagnostics, LLC, Cairn Diagnostics d/b/a Advanced Breath Diagnostics, LLC	● 0106U	Gastric emptying, serial collection of 7 timed breath specimens, non-radioisotope carbon-13(^{13}C) spirulina substrate, analysis of each specimen by gas isotope ratio mass spectrometry, reported as rate of $^{13}CO_2$ excretion
Singulex Clarity C.diff toxins A/B aAssay, Singulex	● 0107U	Clostridium difficile toxin(s) antigen detection by immunoassay technique, stool, qualitative, multiple-step method
TissueCypher® Barrett's Esophagus Assay, Cernostics, Cernostics	● 0108U	Gastroenterology (Barrett's esophagus), whole slide-digital imaging, including morphometric analysis, computer-assisted quantitative immunolabeling of 9 protein biomarkers (p16, AMACR, p53, CD68, COX-2, CD45RO, HIF1a, HER-2, K20) and morphology, formalin-fixed paraffin-embedded tissue, algorithm reported as risk of progression to high-grade dysplasia or cancer

© 2019 Optum360, LLC

Proprietary Name/Clinical Laboratory/Manufacturer	Code	Descriptor
MYCODART Dual Amplification Real Time PCR Panel for 4 Aspergillus species, RealTime Laboratories, Inc/MycoDART, Inc	● 0109U	Infectious disease (Aspergillus species), real-time PCR for detection of DNA from 4 species (*A. fumigatus, A. terreus, A. niger,* and *A. flavus*), blood, lavage fluid, or tissue, qualitative reporting of presence or absence of each species
Oral OncolyticAssuranceRX, Firstox Laboratories, LLC, Firstox Laboratories, LLC	● 0110U	Prescription drug monitoring, one or more oral oncology drug(s) and substances, definitive tandem mass spectrometry with chromatography, serum or plasma from capillary blood or venous blood, quantitative report with steady-state range for the prescribed drug(s) when detected
Praxis(™) Extended RAS Panel, Illumina, Illumina	● 0111U	Oncology (colon cancer), targeted *KRAS* (codons 12, 13, and 61) and *NRAS* (codons 12, 13, and 61) gene analysis utilizing formalin-fixed paraffin-embedded tissue
MicroGenDX qPCR & NGS For Infection, MicroGenDX, MicroGenDX	● 0112U	Infectious agent detection and identification, targeted sequence analysis (16S and 18S rRNA genes) with drug-resistance gene
MiPS (Mi-Prostate Score), MLabs, MLabs	● 0113U	Oncology (prostate), measurement of *PCA3* and *TMPRSS2-ERG* in urine and PSA in serum following prostatic massage, by RNA amplification and fluorescence-based detection, algorithm reported as risk score
EsoGuard™, Lucid Diagnostics, Lucid Diagnostics	● 0114U	Gastroenterology (Barrett's esophagus), *VIM* and *CCNA1* methylation analysis, esophageal cells, algorithm reported as likelihood for Barrett's esophagus
ePlex Respiratory Pathogen (RP) Panel, GenMark Diagnostics, Inc, GenMark Diagnostics, Inc	● 0115U	Respiratory infectious agent detection by nucleic acid (DNA and RNA), 18 viral types and subtypes and 2 bacterial targets, amplified probe technique, including multiplex reverse transcription for RNA targets, each analyte reported as detected or not detected
Snapshot Oral Fluid Compliance, Ethos Laboratories	● 0116U	Prescription drug monitoring, enzyme immunoassay of 35 or more drugs confirmed with LC-MS/MS, oral fluid, algorithm results reported as a patient-compliance measurement with risk of drug to drug interactions for prescribed medications
Foundation PI?, Ethos Laboratories	● 0117U	Pain management, analysis of 11 endogenous analytes (methylmalonic acid, xanthurenic acid, homocysteine, pyroglutamic acid, vanilmandelate, 5-hydroxyindoleacetic acid, hydroxymethylglutarate, ethylmalonate, 3-hydroxypropyl mercapturic acid (3-HPMA), quinolinic acid, kynurenic acid), LC-MS/MS, urine, algorithm reported as a pain-index score with likelihood of atypical biochemical function associated with pain
Viracor TRAC™ dd-cfDNA, Viracor Eurofins, Viracor Eurofins	● 0118U	Transplantation medicine, quantification of donor-derived cell-free DNA using whole genome next-generation sequencing, plasma, reported as percentage of donor-derived cell-free DNA in the total cell-free DNA
MI-HEART Ceramides, Plasma, Mayo Clinic, Laboratory Developed Test	● 0119U	Cardiology, ceramides by liquid chromatography-tandem mass spectrometry, plasma, quantitative report with risk score for major cardiovascular events
Lymph3Cx Lymphoma Molecular Subtyping Assay, Mayo Clinic, Laboratory Developed Test	● 0120U	Oncology (B-cell lymphoma classification), mRNA, gene expression profiling by fluorescent probe hybridization of 58 genes (45 content and 13 housekeeping genes), formalin-fixed paraffin-embedded tissue, algorithm reported as likelihood for primary mediastinal B-cell lymphoma (PMBCL) and diffuse large B-cell lymphoma (DLBCL) with cell of origin subtyping in the latter
Flow Adhesion of Whole Blood on VCAM-1 (FAB-V), Functional Fluidics, Functional Fluidics	● 0121U	Sickle cell disease, microfluidic flow adhesion (VCAM-1), whole blood
Flow Adhesion of Whole Blood to P-SELECTIN (WB-PSEL), Functional Fluidics, Functional Fluidics	● 0122U	Sickle cell disease, microfluidic flow adhesion (P-Selectin), whole blood
Mechanical Fragility, RBC by shear stress profiling and spectral analysis, Functional Fluidics, Functional Fluidics	● 0123U	Mechanical fragility, RBC, shear stress and spectral analysis profiling
First Trimester Screen	Fß?, Eurofins NTD, LLC, Eurofins NTD, LLC	● 0124U	Fetal congenital abnormalities, biochemical assays of 3 analytes (free beta-hCG, PAPP-A, AFP), time-resolved fluorescence immunoassay, maternal dried-blood spot, algorithm reported as risk scores for fetal trisomies 13/18 and 21

Proprietary Name/Clinical Laboratory/Manufacturer	Code	Descriptor
Maternal Fetal Screen | T1?, Eurofins NTD, LLC, Eurofins NTD, LLC	● 0125U	Fetal congenital abnormalities and perinatal complications, biochemical assays of 5 analytes (free beta-hCG, PAPP-A, AFP, placental growth factor, and inhibin-A), time-resolved fluorescence immunoassay, maternal serum, algorithm reported as risk scores for fetal trisomies 13/18, 21, and preeclampsia
Maternal Fetal Screen | T1 + Y Chromosome ?, Eurofins NTD, LLC, Eurofins NTD, LLC	● 0126U	Fetal congenital abnormalities and perinatal complications, biochemical assays of 5 analytes (free beta-hCG, PAPP-A, AFP, placental growth factor, and inhibin-A), time-resolved fluorescence immunoassay, includes qualitative assessment of Y chromosome in cell-free fetal DNA, maternal serum and plasma, predictive algorithm reported as a risk scores for fetal trisomies 13/18, 21, and preeclampsia
Preeclampsia Screen | T1?, Eurofins NTD, LLC, Eurofins NTD, LLC	● 0127U	Obstetrics (preeclampsia), biochemical assays of 3 analytes (PAPP-A, AFP, and placental growth factor), time-resolved fluorescence immunoassay, maternal serum, predictive algorithm reported as a risk score for preeclampsia
Preeclampsia Screen | T1 + Y Chromosome?, Eurofins NTD, LLC, Eurofins NTD, LLC	● 0128U	Obstetrics (preeclampsia), biochemical assays of 3 analytes (PAPP-A, AFP, and placental growth factor), time-resolved fluorescence immunoassay, includes qualitative assessment of Y chromosome in cell-free fetal DNA, maternal serum and plasma, predictive algorithm reported as a risk score for preeclampsia
BRCAplus, Ambry Genetics	● 0129U	Hereditary breast cancer-related disorders (eg, hereditary breast cancer, hereditary ovarian cancer, hereditary endometrial cancer), genomic sequence analysis and deletion/duplication analysis panel (ATM, BRCA1, BRCA2, CDH1, CHEK2, PALB2, PTEN, and TP53)
+RNAinsight™ for ColoNext®, Ambry Genetics	+● 0130U	Hereditary colon cancer disorders (eg, Lynch syndrome, PTEN hamartoma syndrome, Cowden syndrome, familial adenomatosis polyposis), targeted mRNA sequence analysis panel (APC, CDH1, CHEK2, MLH1, MSH2, MSH6, MUTYH, PMS2, PTEN, and TP53) (List separately in addition to code for primary procedure)
+RNAinsight™ for BreastNext®, Ambry Genetics	+● 0131U	Hereditary breast cancer-related disorders (eg, hereditary breast cancer, hereditary ovarian cancer, hereditary endometrial cancer), targeted mRNA sequence analysis panel (13 genes) (List separately in addition to code for primary procedure)
+RNAinsight™ for OvaNext®, Ambry Genetics	+● 0132U	Hereditary ovarian cancer-related disorders (eg, hereditary breast cancer, hereditary ovarian cancer, hereditary endometrial cancer), targeted mRNA sequence analysis panel (17 genes) (List separately in addition to code for primary procedure)
+RNAinsight™ for ProstateNext®, Ambry Genetics	+● 0133U	Hereditary prostate cancer-related disorders, targeted mRNA sequence analysis panel (11 genes) (List separately in addition to code for primary procedure)
+RNAinsight™ for CancerNext®, Ambry Genetics	+● 0134U	Hereditary pan cancer (eg, hereditary breast and ovarian cancer, hereditary endometrial cancer, hereditary colorectal cancer), targeted mRNA sequence analysis panel (18 genes) (List separately in addition to code for primary procedure)
+RNAinsight™ for GYNPlus®, Ambry Genetics	+● 0135U	Hereditary gynecological cancer (eg, hereditary breast and ovarian cancer, hereditary endometrial cancer, hereditary colorectal cancer), targeted mRNA sequence analysis panel (12 genes) (List separately in addition to code for primary procedure)
+RNAinsight™ for ATM, Ambry Genetics	+● 0136U	ATM (ataxia telangiectasia mutated) (eg, ataxia telangiectasia) mRNA sequence analysis (List separately in addition to code for primary procedure)
+RNAinsight™ for PALB2, Ambry Genetics	+● 0137U	PALB2 (partner and localizer of BRCA2) (eg, breast and pancreatic cancer) mRNA sequence analysis (List separately in addition to code for primary procedure)
+RNAinsight™ for BRCA1/2, Ambry Genetics	+● 0138U	BRCA1 (BRCA1, DNA repair associated), BRCA2 (BRCA2, DNA repair associated) (eg, hereditary breast and ovarian cancer) mRNA sequence analysis (List separately in addition to code for primary procedure)
NPDX ASD Energy Metabolism, Stemina Biomarker Discovery, Inc, Stemina Biomarker Discovery, Inc.	● 0139U	Neurology (autism spectrum disorder [ASD]), quantitative measurements of 6 central carbon metabolites (ie, α-ketoglutarate, alanine, lactate, phenylalanine, pyruvate, and succinate), LC-MS/MS, plasma, algorithmic analysis with result reported as negative or positive (with metabolic subtypes of ASD)

Proprietary Name/Clinical Laboratory/Manufacturer	Code	Descriptor
ePlex® BCID Fungal Pathogens Panel, GenMark Diagnostics, Inc, GenMark Diagnostics, Inc	● 0140U	Infectious disease (fungi), fungal pathogen identification, DNA (15 fungal targets), blood culture, amplified probe technique, each target reported as detected or not detected
ePlex® BCID Gram-Positive Panel, GenMark Diagnostics, Inc, GenMark Diagnostics, Inc	● 0141U	Infectious disease (bacteria and fungi), gram-positive organism identification and drug resistance element detection, DNA (20 gram-positive bacterial targets, 4 resistance genes, 1 pan gram-negative bacterial target, 1 pan Candida target), blood culture, amplified probe technique, each target reported as detected or not detected
ePlex® BCID Gram-Negative Panel, GenMark Diagnostics, Inc, GenMark Diagnostics, Inc	● 0142U	Infectious disease (bacteria and fungi), gram-negative bacterial identification and drug resistance element detection, DNA (21 gram-negative bacterial targets, 6 resistance genes, 1 pan gram-positive bacterial target, 1 pan Candida target), amplified probe technique, each target reported as detected or not detected
CareViewRx, Newstar Medical Laboratories, LLC, Newstar Medical Laboratories, LLC PsychViewRx Plus analysis by Newstar Medical Laboratories, LLC. To report, see (~0150U)	● 0143U	Drug assay, definitive, 120 or more drugs or metabolites, urine, quantitative liquid chromatography with tandem mass spectrometry (LC-MS/MS) using multiple reaction monitoring (MRM), with drug or metabolite description, comments including sample validation, per date of service
CareViewRx Plus, Newstar Medical Laboratories, LLC, Newstar Medical Laboratories, LLC	● 0144U	Drug assay, definitive, 160 or more drugs or metabolites, urine, quantitative liquid chromatography with tandem mass spectrometry (LC-MS/MS) using multiple reaction monitoring (MRM), with drug or metabolite description, comments including sample validation, per date of service
PainViewRx, Newstar Medical Laboratories, LLC, Newstar Medical Laboratories, LLC	● 0145U	Drug assay, definitive, 65 or more drugs or metabolites, urine, quantitative liquid chromatography with tandem mass spectrometry (LC-MS/MS) using multiple reaction monitoring (MRM), with drug or metabolite description, comments including sample validation, per date of service
PainViewRx Plus, Newstar Medical Laboratories, LLC, Newstar Medical Laboratories, LLC	● 0146U	Drug assay, definitive, 80 or more drugs or metabolites, urine, by quantitative liquid chromatography with tandem mass spectrometry (LC-MS/MS) using multiple reaction monitoring (MRM), with drug or metabolite description, comments including sample validation, per date of service
RiskViewRx, Newstar Medical Laboratories, LLC, Newstar Medical Laboratories, LLC	● 0147U	Drug assay, definitive, 85 or more drugs or metabolites, urine, quantitative liquid chromatography with tandem mass spectrometry (LC-MS/MS) using multiple reaction monitoring (MRM), with drug or metabolite description, comments including sample validation, per date of service
RiskViewRx Plus, Newstar Medical Laboratories, LLC, Newstar Medical Laboratories, LLC	● 0148U	Drug assay, definitive, 100 or more drugs or metabolites, urine, quantitative liquid chromatography with tandem mass spectrometry (LC-MS/MS) using multiple reaction monitoring (MRM), with drug or metabolite description, comments including sample validation, per date of service
PsychViewRx, Newstar Medical Laboratories, LLC, Newstar Medical Laboratories, LLC	● 0149U	Drug assay, definitive, 60 or more drugs or metabolites, urine, quantitative liquid chromatography with tandem mass spectrometry (LC-MS/MS) using multiple reaction monitoring (MRM), with drug or metabolite description, comments including sample validation, per date of service
PsychViewRx Plus, Newstar Medical Laboratories, LLC, Newstar Medical Laboratories, LLC CareViewRx analysis by Newstar Medical Laboratories, LLC. To report, see (~0143U)	● 0150U	Drug assay, definitive, 120 or more drugs or metabolites, urine, quantitative liquid chromatography with tandem mass spectrometry (LC-MS/MS) using multiple reaction monitoring (MRM), with drug or metabolite description, comments including sample validation, per date of service
BioFire® FilmArray® Pneumonia Panel, BioFire® Diagnostics, BioFire® Diagnostics	● 0151U	Infectious disease (bacterial or viral respiratory tract infection), pathogen specific nucleic acid (DNA or RNA), 33 targets, real-time semi-quantitative PCR, bronchoalveolar lavage, sputum, or endotracheal aspirate, detection of 33 organismal and antibiotic resistance genes with limited semi-quantitative results
Karius® Test, Karius Inc, Karius Inc	● 0152U	Infectious disease (bacteria, fungi, parasites, and DNA viruses), DNA, PCR and next-generation sequencing, plasma, detection of >1,000 potential microbial organisms for significant positive pathogens

Proprietary Name/Clinical Laboratory/Manufacturer	Code	Descriptor
Insight TNBCtype™, Insight Molecular Labs	● 0153U	Oncology (breast), mRNA, gene expression profiling by next-generation sequencing of 101 genes, utilizing formalin-fixed paraffin-embedded tissue, algorithm reported as a triple negative breast cancer clinical subtype(s) with information on immune cell involvement
therascreen® *FGFR* RGQ RT-PCR Kit, QIAGEN, QIAGEN GmbH	● 0154U	*FGFR3 (fibroblast growth factor receptor 3)* gene analysis (ie, p.R248C [c.742C>T], p.S249C [c.746C>G], p.G370C [c.1108G>T], p.Y373C [c.1118A>G], FGFR3-TACC3v1, and FGFR3-TACC3v3)
therascreen *PIK3CA* RGQ PCR Kit, QIAGEN, QIAGEN GmbH	● 0155U	*PIK3CA (phosphatidylinositol-4,5-bisphosphate 3-kinase, catalytic subunit alpha)* (eg, breast cancer) gene analysis (ie, p.C420R, p.E542K, p.E545A, p.E545D [g.1635G>T only], p.E545G, p.E545K, p.Q546E, p.Q546R, p.H1047L, p.H1047R, p.H1047Y)
SMASH™, New York Genome Center, Marvel Genomics™	● 0156U	Copy number (eg, intellectual disability, dysmorphology), sequence analysis
CustomNext + RNA: *APC*, Ambry Genetics®, Ambry Genetics®	+ ● 0157U	*APC (APC regulator of WNT signaling pathway)* (eg, familial adenomatosis polyposis [FAP]) mRNA sequence analysis (List separately in addition to code for primary procedure)
CustomNext + RNA: *MLH1*, Ambry Genetics®, Ambry Genetics®	+ ● 0158U	*MLH1 (mutL homolog 1)* (eg, hereditary non-polyposis colorectal cancer, Lynch syndrome) mRNA sequence analysis (List separately in addition to code for primary procedure)
CustomNext + RNA: *MSH2*, Ambry Genetics®, Ambry Genetics®	+ ● 0159U	*MSH2 (mutS homolog 2)* (eg, hereditary colon cancer, Lynch syndrome) mRNA sequence analysis (List separately in addition to code for primary procedure)
CustomNext + RNA: *MSH6*, Ambry Genetics®, Ambry Genetics®	+ ● 0160U	*MSH6 (mutS homolog 6)* (eg, hereditary colon cancer, Lynch syndrome) mRNA sequence analysis (List separately in addition to code for primary procedure)
CustomNext + RNA: *PMS2*, Ambry Genetics®, Ambry Genetics®	+ ● 0161U	*PMS2 (PMS1 homolog 2, mismatch repair system component)* (eg, hereditary non-polyposis colorectal cancer, Lynch syndrome) mRNA sequence analysis (List separately in addition to code for primary procedure)
CustomNext + RNA: Lynch *(MLH1, MSH2, MSH6, PMS2)*, Ambry Genetics®, Ambry Genetics®	+ ● 0162U	Hereditary colon cancer (Lynch syndrome), targeted mRNA sequence analysis panel *(MLH1, MSH2, MSH6, PMS2)* (List separately in addition to code for primary procedure)

Appendix M — Glossary

-centesis. Puncture, as with a needle, trocar, or aspirator; often done for withdrawing fluid from a cavity.

-ectomy. Excision, removal.

-orrhaphy. Suturing.

-ostomy. Indicates a surgically created artificial opening.

-otomy. Making an incision or opening.

-plasty. Indicates surgically formed or molded.

abdominal lymphadenectomy. Surgical removal of the abdominal lymph nodes grouping, with or without para-aortic and vena cava nodes.

ablation. Removal or destruction of a body part or tissue or its function. Ablation may be performed by surgical means, hormones, drugs, radiofrequency, heat, chemical application, or other methods.

abnormal alleles. Form of gene that includes disease-related variations.

absorbable sutures. Strands prepared from collagen or a synthetic polymer and capable of being absorbed by tissue over time. Examples include surgical gut and collagen sutures; or synthetics like polydioxanone (PDS), polyglactin 910 (Vicryl), poliglecaprone 25 (Monocryl), polyglyconate (Maxon), and polyglycolic acid (Dexon).

acetabuloplasty. Surgical repair or reconstruction of the large cup-shaped socket in the hipbone (acetabulum) with which the head of the femur articulates.

Achilles tendon. Tendon attached to the back of the heel bone (calcaneus) that flexes the foot downward.

acromioclavicular joint. Junction between the clavicle and the scapula. The acromion is the projection from the back of the scapula that forms the highest point of the shoulder and connects with the clavicle. Trauma or injury to the acromioclavicular joint is often referred to as a dislocation of the shoulder. This is not correct, however, as a dislocation of the shoulder is a disruption of the glenohumeral joint.

acromionectomy. Surgical treatment for acromioclavicular arthritis in which the distal portion of the acromion process is removed.

acromioplasty. Repair of the part of the shoulder blade that connects to the deltoid muscles and clavicle.

actigraphy. Science of monitoring activity levels, particularly during sleep. In most cases, the patient wears a wristband that records motion while sleeping. The data are recorded, analyzed, and interpreted to study sleep/wake patterns and circadian rhythms.

air conduction. Transportation of sound from the air, through the external auditory canal, to the tympanic membrane and ossicular chain. Air conduction hearing is tested by presenting an acoustic stimulus through earphones or a loudspeaker to the ear.

air puff device. Instrument that measures intraocular pressure by evaluating the force of a reflected amount of air blown against the cornea.

alleles. Form of gene usually arising from a mutation responsible for a hereditary variation.

allogeneic collection. Collection of blood or blood components from one person for the use of another. Allogeneic collection was formerly termed homologous collection.

allograft. Graft from one individual to another of the same species.

amniocentesis. Surgical puncture through the abdominal wall, with a specialized needle and under ultrasonic guidance, into the interior of the pregnant uterus and directly into the amniotic sac to collect fluid for diagnostic analysis or therapeutic reduction of fluid levels.

anastomosis. Surgically created connection between ducts, blood vessels, or bowel segments to allow flow from one to the other.

anesthesia time. Time period factored into anesthesia procedures beginning with the anesthesiologist preparing the patient for surgery and ending when the patient is turned over to the recovery department.

Angelman syndrome. Early childhood emergence of a pattern of interrupted development, stiff, jerky gait, absence or impairment of speech, excessive laughter, and seizures.

angioplasty. Reconstruction or repair of a diseased or damaged blood vessel.

annuloplasty. Surgical plication of weakened tissue of the heart, to improve its muscular function. Annuli are thick, fibrous rings and one is found surrounding each of the cardiac chambers. The atrial and ventricular muscle fibers attach to the annuli. In annuloplasty, weakened annuli may be surgically plicated, or tucked, to improve muscular functions.

anorectal anometry. Measurement of pressure generated by anal sphincter to diagnose incontinence.

anterior chamber lenses. Lenses inserted into the anterior chamber following intracapsular cataract extraction.

applanation tonometer. Instrument that measures intraocular pressure by recording the force required to flatten an area of the cornea.

appropriateness of care. Proper setting of medical care that best meets the patient's care or diagnosis, as defined by a health care plan or other legal entity.

aqueous humor. Fluid within the anterior and posterior chambers of the eye that is continually replenished as it diffuses out into the blood. When the flow of aqueous is blocked, a build-up of fluid in the eye causes increased intraocular pressure and leads to glaucoma and blindness.

arteriogram. Radiograph of arteries.

arteriovenous fistula. Connecting passage between an artery and a vein.

arteriovenous malformation. Connecting passage between an artery and a vein.

arthrotomy. Surgical incision into a joint that may include exploration, drainage, or removal of a foreign body.

ASA. 1) Acetylsalicylic acid. Synonym(s): aspirin. 2) American Society of Anesthesiologists. National organization for anesthesiology that maintains and publishes the guidelines and relative values for anesthesia coding.

aspirate. To withdraw fluid or air from a body cavity by suction.

assay. Chemical analysis of a substance to establish the presence and strength of its components. A therapeutic drug assay is used to determine if a drug is within the expected therapeutic range for a patient.

atrial septal defect. Cardiac anomaly consisting of a patent opening in the atrial septum due to a fusion failure, classified as ostium secundum type, ostium primum defect, or endocardial cushion defect.

attended surveillance. Ability of a technician at a remote surveillance center or location to respond immediately to patient transmissions regarding rhythm or device alerts as they are produced and received at the remote location. These transmissions may originate from wearable or implanted therapy or monitoring devices.

auricle. External ear, which is a single elastic cartilage covered in skin and normal adnexal features (hair follicles, sweat glands, and sebaceous glands), shaped to channel sound waves into the acoustic meatus.

autogenous transplant. Tissue, such as bone, that is harvested from the patient and used for transplantation back into the same patient.

autograft. Any tissue harvested from one anatomical site of a person and grafted to another anatomical site of the same person. Most commonly, blood vessels, skin, tendons, fascia, and bone are used as autografts.

autologous. Tissue, cells, or structure obtained from the same individual.

AVF. Arteriovenous fistula.

AVM. Arteriovenous malformation. Clusters of abnormal blood vessels that grow in the brain comprised of a blood vessel "nidus" or nest through which arteries and veins connect directly without going through the capillaries. As time passes, the nidus may enlarge resulting in the formation of a mass that may bleed. AVMs are more prone to bleeding in patients ages 10 to 55. Once older than age 55, the possibility of bleeding is reduced dramatically.

backbench preparation. Procedures performed on a donor organ following procurement to prepare the organ for transplant into the recipient. Excess fat and other tissue may be removed, the organ may be perfused, and vital arteries may be sized, repaired, or modified to fit the patient. These procedures are done on a back table in the operating room before transplantation can begin.

Bartholin's gland. Mucous-producing gland found in the vestibular bulbs on either side of the vaginal orifice and connected to the mucosal membrane at the opening by a duct.

Bartholin's gland abscess. Pocket of pus and surrounding cellulitis caused by infection of the Bartholin's gland and causing localized swelling and pain in the posterior labia majora that may extend into the lower vagina.

basic value. Relative weighted value based upon the usual anesthesia services and the relative work or cost of the specific anesthesia service assigned to each anesthesia-specific procedure code.

Berman locator. Small, sensitive tool used to detect the location of a metallic foreign body in the eye.

bifurcated. Having two branches or divisions, such as the left pulmonary veins that split off from the left atrium to carry oxygenated blood away from the heart.

Billroth's operation. Anastomosis of the stomach to the duodenum or jejunum.

bioprosthetic heart valve. Replacement cardiac valve made of biological tissue. Allograft, xenograft or engineered tissue.

biopsy. Tissue or fluid removed for diagnostic purposes through analysis of the cells in the biopsy material.

Blalock-Hanlon procedure. Atrial septectomy procedure to allow free mixing of the blood from the right and left atria.

Blalock-Taussig procedure. Anastomosis of the left subclavian artery to the left pulmonary artery or the right subclavian artery to the right pulmonary artery in order to shunt some of the blood flow from the systemic to the pulmonary circulation.

blepharochalasis. Loss of elasticity and relaxation of skin of the eyelid, thickened or indurated skin on the eyelid associated with recurrent episodes of edema, and intracellular atrophy.

blepharoplasty. Plastic surgery of the eyelids to remove excess fat and redundant skin weighting down the lid. The eyelid is pulled tight and sutured to support sagging muscles.

blepharoptosis. Droop or displacement of the upper eyelid, caused by paralysis, muscle problems, or outside mechanical forces.

blepharorrhaphy. Suture of a portion or all of the opposing eyelids to shorten the palpebral fissure or close it entirely.

bone conduction. Transportation of sound through the bones of the skull to the inner ear.

bone mass measurement. Radiologic or radioisotopic procedure or other procedure approved by the FDA for identifying bone mass, detecting bone loss, or determining bone quality. The procedure includes a physician's interpretation of the results. Qualifying individuals must be an estrogen-deficient woman at clinical risk for osteoporosis with vertebral abnormalities.

brachytherapy. Form of radiation therapy in which radioactive pellets or seeds are implanted directly into the tissue being treated to deliver their dose of radiation in a more directed fashion. Brachytherapy provides radiation to the prescribed body area while minimizing exposure to normal tissue.

breakpoint. Point at which a chromosome breaks.

Bristow procedure. Anterior capsulorrhaphy prevents chronic separation of the shoulder. In this procedure, the bone block is affixed to the anterior glenoid rim with a screw.

buccal mucosa. Tissue from the mucous membrane on the inside of the cheek.

bundle of His. Bundle of modified cardiac fibers that begins at the atrioventricular node and passes through the right atrioventricular fibrous ring to the interventricular septum, where it divides into two branches. Bundle of His recordings are taken for intracardiac electrograms.

Caldwell-Luc operation. Intraoral antrostomy approach into the maxillary sinus for the removal of tooth roots or tissue, or for packing the sinus to reduce zygomatic fractures by creating a window above the teeth in the canine fossa area.

canthorrhaphy. Suturing of the palpebral fissure, the juncture between the eyelids, at either end of the eye.

canthotomy. Horizontal incision at the canthus (junction of upper and lower eyelids) to divide the outer canthus and enlarge lid margin separation.

cardio-. Relating to the heart.

cardiopulmonary bypass. Venous blood is diverted to a heart-lung machine, which mechanically pumps and oxygenates the blood temporarily so the heart can be bypassed while an open procedure on the heart or coronary arteries is performed. During bypass, the lungs are deflated and immobile.

cardioverter-defibrillator. Device that uses both low energy cardioversion or defibrillating shocks and antitachycardia pacing to treat ventricular tachycardia or ventricular fibrillation.

care plan oversight services. Physician's ongoing review and revision of a patient's care plan involving complex or multidisciplinary care modalities.

case management services. Physician case management is a process of involving direct patient care as well as coordinating and controlling access to the patient or initiating and/or supervising other necessary health care services.

cataract extraction. Surgical removal of the cataract or cloudy lens. Anterior chamber lenses are inserted in conjunction with intracapsular cataract extraction and posterior chamber lenses are inserted in conjunction with extracapsular cataract extraction.

catheter. Flexible tube inserted into an area of the body for introducing or withdrawing fluid.

Centers for Medicare and Medicaid Services. Federal agency that oversees the administration of the public health programs such as Medicare, Medicaid, and State Children's Insurance Program.

certified nurse midwife. Registered nurse who has successfully completed a program of study and clinical experience or has been certified by a recognized organization for the care of pregnant or delivering patients.

CFR. Code of Federal Regulations.

CGMS. Continuous glucose monitoring system.

CHAMPUS. Civilian Health and Medical Program of the Uniformed Services. See Tricare.

CHAMPVA. Civilian Health and Medical Program of the Department of Veterans Affairs.

chemodenervation. Chemical destruction of nerves. A substance, for example, Botox, is used to temporarily inhibit the transfer of chemicals at the presynaptic membrane, blocking the neuromuscular junctions.

chemoembolization. Administration of chemotherapeutic agents directly to a tumor in combination with the percutaneous administration of an occlusive substance into a vessel to deprive the tumor of its blood supply. This ensures a prolonged level of therapy directed at the tumor. Chemoembolization is primarily being used for cancers of the liver and endocrine system.

chemosurgery. Application of chemical agents to destroy tissue, originally referring to the in situ chemical fixation of premalignant or malignant lesions to facilitate surgical excision.

Chiari osteotomy. Top of the femur is altered to correct a dislocated hip caused by congenital conditions or cerebral palsy. Plate and screws are often used.

chimera. Organ or anatomic structure consisting of tissues of diverse genetic constitution.

choanal atresia. Congenital, membranous, or bony closure of one or both posterior nostrils due to failure of the embryonic bucconasal membrane to rupture and open up the nasal passageway.

chondromalacia. Condition in which the articular cartilage softens, seen in various body sites but most often in the patella, and may be congenital or acquired.

chorionic villus sampling. Aspiration of a placental sample through a catheter, under ultrasonic guidance. The specialized needle is placed transvaginally through the cervix or transabdominally into the uterine cavity.

chronic pain management services. Distinct services frequently performed by anesthesiologists who have additional training in pain management procedures. Pain management services include initial and subsequent evaluation and management (E/M) services, trigger point injections, spine and spinal cord injections, and nerve blocks.

cineplastic amputation. Amputation in which muscles and tendons of the remaining portion of the extremity are arranged so that they may be utilized for motor functions. Following this type of amputation, a specially constructed prosthetic device allows the individual to execute more complex movements because the muscles and tendons are able to communicate independent movements to the device.

circadian. Relating to a cyclic, 24-hour period.

CLIA. Clinical Laboratory Improvement Amendments. Requirements set in 1988, CLIA imposes varying levels of federal regulations on clinical procedures. Few laboratories, including those in physician offices, are exempt. Adopted by Medicare and Medicaid, CLIA regulations redefine laboratory testing in regard to laboratory certification and accreditation, proficiency testing, quality assurance, personnel standards, and program administration.

clinical social worker. Individual who possesses a master's or doctor's degree in social work and, after obtaining the degree, has performed at least two years of supervised clinical social work. A clinical social worker must be licensed by the state or, in the case of states without licensure, must completed at least two years or 3,000 hours of post-master's degree supervised clinical social work practice under the supervision of a master's level social worker.

clinical staff. Someone who works for, or under, the direction of a physician or qualified health care professional and does not bill services separately. The person may be licensed or regulated to help the physician perform specific duties.

clonal. Originating from one cell.

CMS. Centers for Medicare and Medicaid Services. Federal agency that administers the public health programs.

CO₂ laser. Carbon dioxide laser that emits an invisible beam and vaporizes water-rich tissue. The vapor is suctioned from the site.

codons. Series of three adjoining bases in one polynucleotide chain of a DNA or RNA molecule that provides the codes for a specific amino acid.

cognitive. Being aware by drawing from knowledge, such as judgment, reason, perception, and memory.

colostomy. Artificial surgical opening anywhere along the length of the colon to the skin surface for the diversion of feces.

commissurotomy. Surgical division or disruption of any two parts that are joined to form a commissure in order to increase the opening. The procedure most often refers to opening the adherent leaflet bands of fibrous tissue in a stenosed mitral valve.

common variants. Nucleotide sequence differences associated with abnormal gene function. Tests are usually performed in a single series of laboratory testing (in a single, typically multiplex, assay arrangement or using more than one assay to include all variants to be examined). Variants are representative of a mutation that mainly causes a single disease, such as cystic fibrosis. Other uncommon variants could provide additional information. Tests may be performed based on society recommendations and guidelines.

community mental health center. Facility providing outpatient mental health day treatment, assessments, and education as appropriate to community members.

component code. In the National Correct Coding Initiative (NCCI), the column II code that cannot be charged to Medicare when the column I code is reported.

comprehensive code. In the National Correct Coding Initiative (NCCI), the column I code that is reported to Medicare and precludes reporting column II codes.

computerized corneal topography. Digital imaging and analysis by computer of the shape of the corneal.

conjunctiva. Mucous membrane lining of the eyelids and covering of the exposed, anterior sclera.

conjunctivodacryocystostomy. Surgical connection of the lacrimal sac directly to the conjunctival sac.

conjunctivorhinostomy. Correction of an obstruction of the lacrimal canal achieved by suturing the posterior flaps and removing any lacrimal obstruction, preserving the conjunctiva.

constitutional. Cells containing genetic code that may be passed down to future generations. May also be referred to as germline.

consultation. Advice or opinion regarding diagnosis and treatment or determination to accept transfer of care of a patient rendered by a medical professional at the request of the primary care provider.

continuous positive airway pressure device. Pressurized device used to maintain the patient's airway for spontaneous or mechanically aided breathing. Often used for patients with mild to moderate sleep apnea.

core needle biopsy. Large-bore biopsy needle inserted into a mass and a core of tissue is removed for diagnostic study.

corpectomy. Removal of the body of a bone, such as a vertebra.

costochondral. Pertaining to the ribs and the scapula.

COTD. Cardiac output thermodilution. Cardiac output measured by thermodilution method that requires heart catheterization and then injection of a thermal indicator, usually iced saline. A computer calculates the cardiac output using an equation that incorporates body temperature, injectate volume and temperature, time, and other calculated ratios over a denominator of the integral of the change in blood temperature during the cold injection, reflected by the area of the inscribed curve.

CPT. 1) Chest physical therapy. 2) Cold pressor test. 3) Current Procedural Terminology.

craniosynostosis. Congenital condition in which one or more of the cranial sutures fuse prematurely, creating a deformed or aberrant head shape.

craterization. Excision of a portion of bone creating a crater-like depression to facilitate drainage from infected areas of bone.

cricoid. Circular cartilage around the trachea.

CRNA. Certified registered nurse anesthetist. Nurse trained and specializing in the administration of anesthesia.

cryolathe. Tool used for reshaping a button of corneal tissue.

cryosurgery. Application of intense cold, usually produced using liquid nitrogen, to locally freeze diseased or unwanted tissue and induce tissue necrosis without causing harm to adjacent tissue.

CT. Computed tomography.

cutdown. Small, incised opening in the skin to expose a blood vessel, especially over a vein (venous cutdown) to allow venipuncture and permit a needle or cannula to be inserted for the withdrawal of blood or administration of fluids.

cyclophotocoagulation. Procedure done to prevent vision loss from glaucoma in which a neodymium: YAG laser is used to burn and destroy a portion of the ciliary body in order to decrease the amount of aqueous humor being produced in the eye. This procedure is only done when creating a drain for aqueous humor to reduce intraocular pressure would not be successful. Destroying portions of the ciliary body reduces the amount of fluid present in the eye.

cytogenetic studies. Procedures in CPT that are related to the branch of genetics that studies cellular (cyto) structure and function as it relates to heredity (genetics). White blood cells, specifically T-lymphocytes, are the most commonly used specimen for chromosome analysis.

cytogenomic. Chromosomic evaluation using molecular methods.

dacryocystotome. Instrument used for incising the lacrimal duct strictures.

DBS. Deep brain stimulation. Treatment for disabling neurological symptoms associated with diseases including Parkinson's. DBS requires three components: the implanted electrode, extension, and neurostimulator. Electrical impulses are sent from the neurostimulator to the implant to block tremors.

debride. To remove all foreign objects and devitalized or infected tissue from a burn or wound to prevent infection and promote healing.

definitive drug testing. Drug tests used to further analyze or confirm the presence or absence of specific drugs or classes of drugs used by the patient. These tests are able to provide more conclusive information regarding the concentration of the drug and their metabolites. May be used for medical, workplace, or legal purposes.

definitive identification. Identification of microorganisms using additional tests to specify the genus or species (e.g., slide cultures or biochemical panels).

dentoalveolar structure. Area of alveolar bone surrounding the teeth and adjacent tissue.

Department of Health and Human Services. Cabinet department that oversees the operating divisions of the federal government responsible for health and welfare. HHS oversees the Centers for Medicare and Medicaid Services, Food and Drug Administration, Public Health Service, and other such entities.

Department of Justice. Attorneys from the DOJ and the United States Attorney's Office have, under the memorandum of understanding, the same direct access to contractor data and records as the OIG and the Federal Bureau of Investigation (FBI). DOJ is responsible for prosecution of fraud and civil or criminal cases presented.

dermis. Skin layer found under the epidermis that contains a papillary upper layer and the deep reticular layer of collagen, vascular bed, and nerves.

dermis graft. Skin graft that has been separated from the epidermal tissue and the underlying subcutaneous fat, used primarily as a substitute for fascia grafts in plastic surgery.

desensitization. 1) Administration of extracts of allergens periodically to build immunity in the patient. 2) Application of medication to decrease the symptoms, usually pain, associated with a dental condition or disease.

destruction. Ablation or eradication of a structure or tissue.

diabetes outpatient self-management training services. Educational and training services furnished by a certified provider in an outpatient setting. The physician managing the individual's diabetic condition must certify that the services are needed under a comprehensive plan of care and provide the patient with the skills and knowledge necessary for therapeutic program compliance (including skills related to the self-administration of injectable drugs). The provider must meet applicable standards established by the National Diabetes Advisory or be recognized by an organization that represents individuals with diabetes as meeting standards for furnishing the services.

diagnostic procedures. Procedure performed on a patient to obtain information to assess the medical condition of the patient or to identify a disease and to determine the nature and severity of an illness or injury.

dialysis. Artificial filtering of the blood to remove contaminating waste elements and restore normal balance.

diaphragm. 1) Muscular wall separating the thorax and its structures from the abdomen. 2) Flexible disk inserted into the vagina and against the cervix as a method of birth control.

diaphysectomy. Surgical removal of a portion of the shaft of a long bone, often done to facilitate drainage from infected bone.

diathermy. Applying heat to body tissues by various methods for therapeutic treatment or surgical purposes to coagulate and seal tissue.

dilation. Artificial increase in the diameter of an opening or lumen made by medication or by instrumentation.

dissect. Cut apart or separate tissue for surgical purposes or for visual or microscopic study.

DNA. Deoxyribonucleic acid. Chemical containing the genetic information necessary to produce and propagate living organisms. Molecules are comprised of two twisting paired strands, called a double helix.

DNA marker. Specific gene sequence within a chromosome indicating the inheritance of a certain trait.

dorsal. Pertaining to the back or posterior aspect.

drugs and biologicals. Drugs and biologicals included - or approved for inclusion - in the United States Pharmacopoeia, the National Formulary, the United States Homeopathic Pharmacopoeia, in New Drugs or Accepted Dental Remedies, or approved by the pharmacy and drug therapeutics committee of the medical staff of the hospital. Also included are medically accepted and FDA approved drugs used in an anticancer chemotherapeutic regimen. The carrier determines medical acceptance based on supportive clinical evidence.

dual-lead device. Implantable cardiac device (pacemaker or implantable cardioverter-defibrillator [ICD]) in which pacing and sensing components are placed in only two chambers of the heart.

duplex scan. Noninvasive vascular diagnostic technique that uses ultrasonic scanning to identify the pattern and direction of blood flow within arteries or veins displayed in real time images. Duplex scanning combines B-mode two-dimensional pictures of the vessel structure with spectra and/or color flow Doppler mapping or imaging of the blood as it moves through the vessels.

duplication/deletion (DUP/DEL). Term used in molecular testing which examines genomic regions to determine if there are extra chromosomes (duplication) or missing chromosomes (deletions). Normal gene dosage is two copies per cell except for the sex chromosomes which have one per cell.

DuToit staple capsulorrhaphy. Reattachment of the capsule of the shoulder and glenoid labrum to the glenoid lip using staples to anchor the avulsed capsule and glenoid labrum.

Dx. Diagnosis.

DXA. Dual energy x-ray absorptiometry. Radiological technique for bone density measurement using a two-dimensional projection system in which two x-ray beams with different levels of energy are pulsed alternately and the results are given in two scores, reported as standard deviations from peak bone mass density.

dynamic mutation. Unstable or changing polynucleotides resulting in repeats related to genes that can undergo disease-producing increases or decreases in the repeats that differ within tissues or over generations.

ECMO. Extracorporeal membrane oxygenation.

ectropion. Drooping of the lower eyelid away from the eye or outward turning or eversion of the edge of the eyelid, exposing the palpebral conjunctiva and causing irritation.

Eden-Hybinette procedure. Anterior shoulder repair using an anterior bone block to augment the bony anterior glenoid lip.

EDTA. Drug used to inhibit damage to the cornea by collagenase. EDTA is especially effective in alkali burns as it neutralizes soluble alkali, including lye.

effusion. Escape of fluid from within a body cavity.

electrocardiographic rhythm derived. Analysis of data obtained from readings of the heart's electrical activation, including heart rate and rhythm, variability of heart rate, ST analysis, and T-wave alternans. Other data may also be assessed when warranted.

electrocautery. Division or cutting of tissue using high-frequency electrical current to produce heat, which destroys cells.

electrode array. Electronic device containing more than one contact whose function can be adjusted during programming services. Electrodes are specialized for a particular electrochemical reaction that acts as a medium between a body surface and another instrument.

electromyography. Test that measures muscle response to nerve stimulation determining if muscle weakness is present and if it is related to the muscles themselves or a problem with the nerves that supply the muscles.

electrooculogram (EOG). Record of electrical activity associated with eye movements.

electrophysiologic studies. Electrical stimulation and monitoring to diagnose heart conduction abnormalities that predispose patients to bradyarrhythmias and to determine a patient's chance for developing ventricular and supraventricular tachyarrhythmias.

embolization. Placement of a clotting agent, such as a coil, plastic particles, gel, foam, etc., into an area of hemorrhage to stop the bleeding or to block blood flow to a problem area, such as an aneurysm or a tumor.

emergency. Serious medical condition or symptom (including severe pain) resulting from injury, sickness, or mental illness that arises suddenly and requires immediate care and treatment, generally received within 24 hours of onset, to avoid jeopardy to the life, limb, or health of a covered person.

empyema. Accumulation of pus within the respiratory, or pleural, cavity.

EMTALA. Emergency Medical Treatment and Active Labor Act.

end-stage renal disease. Chronic, advanced kidney disease requiring renal dialysis or a kidney transplant to prevent imminent death.

endarterectomy. Removal of the thickened, endothelial lining of a diseased or damaged artery.

endomicroscopy. Diagnostic technology that allows for the examination of tissue at the cellular level during endoscopy. The technology decreases the need for biopsy with histological examination for some types of lesions.

endovascular embolization. Procedure whereby vessels are occluded by a variety of therapeutic substances for the treatment of abnormal blood vessels by inhibiting the flow of blood to a tumor, arteriovenous malformations, lymphatic malformation, and to prevent or stop hemorrhage.

entropion. Inversion of the eyelid, turning the edge in toward the eyeball and causing irritation from contact of the lashes with the surface of the eye.

enucleation. Removal of a growth or organ cleanly so as to extract it in one piece.

epidermis. Outermost, nonvascular layer of skin that contains four to five differentiated layers depending on its body location: stratum corneum, lucidum, granulosum, spinosum, and basale.

epiphysiodesis. Surgical fusion of an epiphysis performed to prematurely stop further bone growth.

escharotomy. Surgical incision into the scab or crust resulting from a severe burn in order to relieve constriction and allow blood flow to the distal unburned tissue.

established patient. 1) Patient who has received professional services in a face-to-face setting within the last three years from the same physician/qualified health care professional or another physician/qualified health care professional of the exact same specialty and subspecialty who belongs to the same group practice. 2) For OPPS hospitals, patient who has been registered as an inpatient or outpatient in a hospital's provider-based clinic or emergency department within the past three years.

evacuation. Removal or purging of waste material.

evaluation and management codes. Assessment and management of a patient's health care.

evaluation and management service components. Key components of history, examination, and medical decision making that are key to selecting the correct E/M codes. Other non-key components include counseling, coordination of care, nature of presenting problem, and time.

event recorder. Portable, ambulatory heart monitor worn by the patient that makes electrocardiographic recordings of the length and frequency of aberrant cardiac rhythm to help diagnose heart conditions and to assess pacemaker functioning or programming.

exenteration. Surgical removal of the entire contents of a body cavity, such as the pelvis or orbit.

exon. One of multiple nucleic acid sequences used to encode information for a gene polypeptide or protein. Exons are separated from other exons by non-protein-coding sequences known as introns.

extended care services. Items and services provided to an inpatient of a skilled nursing facility, including nursing care, physical or occupational therapy, speech pathology, drugs and supplies, and medical social services.

external electrical capacitor device. External electrical stimulation device designed to promote bone healing. This device may also promote neural regeneration, revascularization, epiphyseal growth, and ligament maturation.

external pulsating electromagnetic field. External stimulation device designed to promote bone healing. This device may also promote neural regeneration, revascularization, epiphyseal growth, and ligament maturation.

extracorporeal. Located or taking place outside the body.

Eyre-Brook capsulorrhaphy. Reattachment of the capsule of the shoulder and glenoid labrum to the glenoid lip.

False Claims Act. Governs civil actions for filing false claims. Liability under this act pertains to any person who knowingly presents or causes to be presented a false or fraudulent claim to the government for payment or approval.

fascia. Fibrous sheet or band of tissue that envelops organs, muscles, and groupings of muscles.

fasciectomy. Excision of fascia or strips of fascial tissue.

fasciotomy. Incision or transection of fascial tissue.

fat graft. Graft composed of fatty tissue completely freed from surrounding tissue that is used primarily to fill in depressions.

FDA. Food and Drug Administration. Federal agency responsible for protecting public health by substantiating the safety, efficacy, and security of human and veterinary drugs, biological products, medical devices, national food supply, cosmetics, and items that give off radiation.

filtered speech test. Test most commonly used to identify central auditory dysfunction in which the patient is presented monosyllabic words that are low pass filtered, allowing only the parts of each word below a certain pitch to be presented. A score is given on the number of correct responses. This may be a subset of a standard battery of tests provided during a single encounter.

fissure. Deep furrow, groove, or cleft in tissue structures.

fistulization. Creation of a communication between two structures that were not previously connected.

flexor digitorum profundus tendon. Tendon originating in the proximal forearm and extending to the index finger and wrist. A thickened FDP sheath, usually caused by age, illness, or injury, can fill the carpal canal and lead to impingement of the median nerve.

fluoroscopy. Radiology technique that allows visual examination of part of the body or a function of an organ using a device that projects an x-ray image on a fluorescent screen.

focal length. Distance between the object in focus and the lens.

focused medical review. Process of targeting and directing medical review efforts on Medicare claims where the greatest risk of inappropriate program payment exists. The goal is to reduce the number of noncovered claims or unnecessary services. CMS analyzes national data such as internal billing, utilization, and payment data and provides its findings to the FI. Local medical review policies are developed identifying aberrances, abuse, and overutilized services. Providers are responsible for knowing national Medicare coverage and billing guidelines and local medical review policies, and for determining whether the services provided to Medicare beneficiaries are covered by Medicare.

fragile X syndrome. Intellectual disabilities, enlarged testes, big jaw, high forehead, and long ears in males. In females, fragile X presents with mild intellectual disabilities and heterozygous sexual structures. In some families, males have shown no symptoms but carry the gene.

free flap. Tissue that is completely detached from the donor site and transplanted to the recipient site, receiving its blood supply from capillary ingrowth at the recipient site.

free microvascular flap. Tissue that is completely detached from the donor site following careful dissection and preservation of the blood vessels, then attached to the recipient site with the transferred blood vessels anastomosed to the vessels in the recipient bed.

fulguration. Destruction of living tissue by using sparks from a high-frequency electric current.

gas tamponade. Absorbable gas may be injected to force the retina against the choroid. Common gases include room air, short-acting sulfahexafluoride, intermediate-acting perfluoroethane, or long-acting perfluorooctane.

Gaucher disease. Genetic metabolic disorder in which fat deposits may accumulate in the spleen, liver, lungs, bone marrow, and brain.

gene. Basic unit of heredity that contains nucleic acid. Genes are arranged in different and unique sequences or strings that determine the gene's function. Human genes usually include multiple protein coding regions such as exons separated by introns which are nonprotein coding sections.

genome. Complete set of DNA of an organism. Each cell in the human body is comprised of a complete copy of the approximately three billion DNA base pairs that constitute the human genome.

habilitative services. Procedures or services provided to assist a patient in learning, keeping, and improving new skills needed to perform daily living activities. Habilitative services assist patients in acquiring a skill for the first time.

HCPCS. Healthcare Common Procedure Coding System.

HCPCS Level I. Healthcare Common Procedure Coding System Level I. Numeric coding system used by physicians, facility outpatient departments, and ambulatory surgery centers (ASC) to code ambulatory, laboratory, radiology, and other diagnostic services for Medicare billing. This coding system contains only the American Medical Association's Physicians' Current Procedural Terminology (CPT) codes. The AMA updates codes annually.

HCPCS Level II. Healthcare Common Procedure Coding System Level II. National coding system, developed by CMS, that contains alphanumeric codes for physician and nonphysician services not included in the CPT coding system. HCPCS Level II covers such things as ambulance services, durable medical equipment, and orthotic and prosthetic devices.

HCPCS modifiers. Two-character code (AA-ZZ) that identifies circumstances that alter or enhance the description of a service or supply. They are recognized by carriers nationally and are updated annually by CMS.

Hct. Hematocrit.

health care provider. Entity that administers diagnostic and therapeutic services.

hemilaminectomy. Excision of a portion of the vertebral lamina.

hemodialysis. Cleansing of wastes and contaminating elements from the blood by virtue of different diffusion rates through a semipermeable membrane, which separates blood from a filtration solution that diffuses other elements out of the blood. The blood is slowly filtered extracorporeally through special dialysis equipment and returned to the body. Synonym(s): renal dialysis.

hemodialysis. Cleansing of wastes and contaminating elements from the blood by virtue of different diffusion rates through a semipermeable membrane, which separates blood from a filtration solution that diffuses other elements out of the blood.

hemoperitoneum. Effusion of blood into the peritoneal cavity, the space between the continuous membrane lining the abdominopelvic walls and encasing the visceral organs.

heterograft. Surgical graft of tissue from one animal species to a different animal species. A common type of heterograft is porcine (pig) tissue, used for temporary wound closure.

heterotopic transplant. Tissue transplanted from a different anatomical site for usage as is natural for that tissue, for example, buccal mucosa to a conjunctival site.

HGNC. HUGO gene nomenclature committee.

HGVS. Human genome variation society.

Hickman catheter. Central venous catheter used for long-term delivery of medications, such as antibiotics, nutritional substances, or chemotherapeutic agents.

HLA. Human leukocyte antigen.

home health services. Services furnished to patients in their homes under the care of physicians. These services include part-time or intermittent skilled nursing care, physical therapy, medical social services, medical supplies, and some rehabilitation equipment. Home health supplies and services must be prescribed by a physician, and the beneficiary must be confined at home in order for Medicare to pay the benefits in full.

homograft. Graft from one individual to another of the same species.

hospice care. Items and services provided to a terminally ill individual by a hospice program under a written plan established and periodically reviewed by the individual's attending physician and by the medical director: Nursing care provided by or under the supervision of a registered professional nurse; Physical or occupational therapy or speech-language pathology services; Medical social services under the direction of a physician; Services of a home health aide who has successfully completed a training program; Medical supplies (including drugs and biologicals) and the use of medical appliances; Physicians' services; Short-term inpatient care (including both respite care and procedures necessary for pain control and acute and chronic symptom management) in an inpatient facility on an intermittent basis and not consecutively over longer than five days; Counseling (including dietary counseling) with respect to care of the terminally ill individual and adjustment to his death; Any item or service which is specified in the plan and for which payment may be made.

hospital. Institution that provides, under the supervision of physicians, diagnostic, therapeutic, and rehabilitation services for medical diagnosis, treatment, and care of patients. Hospitals receiving federal funds must maintain clinical records on all patients, provide 24-hour nursing services, and have a discharge planning process in place. The term "hospital" also includes religious nonmedical health care institutions and facilities of 50 beds or less located in rural areas.

HUGO. Human genome organization

IA. Intra-arterial.

ICD. Implantable cardioverter defibrillator.

ICD-10-CM. International Classification of Diseases, 10th Revision, Clinical Modification. Clinical modification of the alphanumeric classification of diseases used by the World Health Organization, already in use in much of the world, and used for mortality reporting in the United States. The implementation date for ICD-10-CM diagnostic coding system to replace ICD-9-CM in the United States was October 1, 2015.

ICD-10-PCS. International Classification of Diseases, 10th Revision, Procedure Coding System. Beginning October 1, 2015, inpatient hospital services and surgical procedures must be coded using ICD-10-PCS codes, replacing ICD-9-CM, Volume 3 for procedures.

ICM. Implantable cardiovascular monitor.

ileostomy. Artificial surgical opening that brings the end of the ileum out through the abdominal wall to the skin surface for the diversion of feces through a stoma.

iliopsoas tendon. Fibrous tissue that connects muscle to bone in the pelvic region, common to the iliacus and psoas major.

ILR. Implantable loop recorder.

IM. 1) Infectious mononucleosis. 2) Internal medicine. 3) Intramuscular.

immunotherapy. Therapeutic use of serum or gamma globulin.

implant. Material or device inserted or placed within the body for therapeutic, reconstructive, or diagnostic purposes.

implantable cardiovascular monitor. Implantable electronic device that stores cardiovascular physiologic data such as intracardiac pressure waveforms collected from internal sensors or data such as weight and blood pressure collected from external sensors. The information stored in these devices is used as an aid in managing patients with heart failure and other cardiac conditions that are non-rhythm related. The data may be transmitted via local telemetry or remotely to a surveillance technician or an internet-based file server.

implantable cardioverter-defibrillator. Implantable electronic cardiac device used to control rhythm abnormalities such as tachycardia, fibrillation, or bradycardia by producing high- or low-energy stimulation and pacemaker functions. It may also have the capability to provide the functions of an implantable loop recorder or implantable cardiovascular monitor.

implantable loop recorder. Implantable electronic cardiac device that constantly monitors and records electrocardiographic rhythm. It may be triggered by the patient when a symptomatic episode occurs or activated automatically by rapid or slow heart rates. This may be the sole purpose of the device or it may be a component of another cardiac device, such as a pacemaker or implantable cardioverter-defibrillator. The data can be transmitted via local telemetry or remotely to a surveillance technician or an internet-based file server.

implantable venous access device. Catheter implanted for continuous access to the venous system for long-term parenteral feeding or for the administration of fluids or medications.

IMRT. Intensity modulated radiation therapy. External beam radiation therapy delivery using computer planning to specify the target dose and to modulate the radiation intensity, usually as a treatment for a malignancy. The delivery system approaches the patient from multiple angles, minimizing damage to normal tissue.

in situ. Located in the natural position or contained within the origin site, not spread into neighboring tissue.

incontinence. Inability to control urination or defecation.

infundibulectomy. Excision of the anterosuperior portion of the right ventricle of the heart.

internal direct current stimulator. Electrostimulation device placed directly into the surgical site designed to promote bone regeneration by encouraging cellular healing response in bone and ligaments.

interrogation device evaluation. Assessment of an implantable cardiac device (pacemaker, cardioverter-defibrillator, cardiovascular monitor, or loop recorder) in which collected data about the patient's heart rate and rhythm, battery and pulse generator function, and any leads or sensors present, are retrieved and evaluated. Determinations regarding device programming and appropriate treatment settings are made based on the findings. CPT provides required components for evaluation of the various types of devices.

intramedullary implants. Nail, rod, or pin placed into the intramedullary canal at the fracture site. Intramedullary implants not only provide a method of aligning the fracture, they also act as a splint and may reduce fracture pain. Implants may be rigid or flexible. Rigid implants are preferred for prophylactic treatment of diseased bone, while flexible implants are preferred for traumatic injuries.

intraocular lens. Artificial lens implanted into the eye to replace a damaged natural lens or cataract.

intravenous. Within a vein or veins.

introducer. Instrument, such as a catheter, needle, or tube, through which another instrument or device is introduced into the body.

intron. Nonprotein section of a gene that separates exons in human genes. Contains vital sequences that allow splicing of exons to produce a functional protein from a gene. Sometimes referred to as intervening sequences (IVS).

IP. 1) Interphalangeal. 2) Intraperitoneal.

irrigation. To wash out or cleanse a body cavity, wound, or tissue with water or other fluid.

Kayser-Fleischer ring. Condition found in Wilson's disease in which deposits of copper cause a pigmented ring around the cornea's outer border in the deep epithelial layers.

keratoprosthesis. Surgical procedure in which the physician creates a new anterior chamber with a plastic optical implant to replace a severely damaged cornea that cannot be repaired.

keratotomy. Surgical incision of the cornea.

krypton laser. Laser light energy that uses ionized krypton by electric current as the active source, has a radiation beam between the visible yellow-red spectrum, and is effective in photocoagulation of retinal bleeding, macular lesions, and vessel aberrations of the choroid.

lacrimal. Tear-producing gland or ducts that provides lubrication and flushing of the eyes and nasal cavities.

lacrimal punctum. Opening of the lacrimal papilla of the eyelid through which tears flow to the canaliculi to the lacrimal sac.

lacrimotome. Knife for cutting the lacrimal sac or duct.

lacrimotomy. Incision of the lacrimal sac or duct.

laparotomy. Incision through the flank or abdomen for therapeutic or diagnostic purposes.

laryngoscopy. Examination of the hypopharynx, larynx, and tongue base with an endoscope.

larynx. Musculocartilaginous structure between the trachea and the pharynx that functions as the valve preventing food and other particles from entering the respiratory tract, as well as the voice mechanism. Also called the voicebox, the larynx is composed of three single cartilages: cricoid, epiglottis, and thyroid; and three paired cartilages: arytenoid, corniculate, and cuneiform.

laser surgery. Use of concentrated, sharply defined light beams to cut, cauterize, coagulate, seal, or vaporize tissue.

LEEP. Loop electrode excision procedure. Biopsy specimen or cone shaped wedge of cervical tissue is removed using a hot cautery wire loop with an electrical current running through it.

levonorgestrel. Drug inhibiting ovulation and preventing sperm from penetrating cervical mucus. It is delivered subcutaneously in polysiloxone capsules. The capsules can be effective for up to five years, and provide a cumulative pregnancy rate of less than 2 percent. The capsules are not biodegradable, and therefore must be removed. Removal is more difficult than insertion of levonorgestrel capsules because fibrosis develops around the capsules. Normal hormonal activity and a return to fertility begins immediately upon removal.

ligament. Band or sheet of fibrous tissue that connects the articular surfaces of bones or supports visceral organs.

ligation. Tying off a blood vessel or duct with a suture or a soft, thin wire.

lymphadenectomy. Dissection of lymph nodes free from the vessels and removal for examination by frozen section in a separate procedure to detect early-stage metastases.

lysis. Destruction, breakdown, dissolution, or decomposition of cells or substances by a specific catalyzing agent.

Magnuson-Stack procedure. Treatment for recurrent anterior dislocation of the shoulder that involves tightening and realigning the subscapularis tendon.

maintenance of wakefulness test. Attended study determining the patient's ability to stay awake.

Manchester operation. Preservation of the uterus following prolapse by amputating the vaginal portion of the cervix, shortening the cardinal ligaments, and performing a colpoperineorrhaphy posteriorly.

mapping. Multidimensional depiction of a tachycardia that identifies its site of origin and its electrical conduction pathway after tachycardia has been induced. The recording is made from multiple catheter sites within the heart, obtaining electrograms simultaneously or sequentially.

marsupialization. Creation of a pouch in surgical treatment of a cyst in which one wall is resected and the remaining cut edges are sutured to adjacent tissue creating an open pouch of the previously enclosed cyst.

mastectomy. Surgical removal of one or both breasts.

McDonald procedure. Polyester tape is placed around the cervix with a running stitch to assist in the prevention of pre-term delivery. Tape is removed at term for vaginal delivery.

MCP. Metacarpophalangeal.

medial. Middle or midline.

mediastinotomy. Incision into the mediastinum for purposes of exploration, foreign body removal, drainage, or biopsy.

medical review. Review by a Medicare administrative contractor, carrier, and/or quality improvement organization (QIO) of services and items provided by physicians, other health care practitioners, and providers of health care services under Medicare. The review determines if the items and services are reasonable and necessary and meet Medicare coverage requirements, whether the quality meets professionally recognized standards of health care, and whether the services are medically appropriate in an inpatient, outpatient, or other setting as supported by documentation.

Medicare contractor. Medicare Part A fiscal intermediary, Medicare Part B carrier, Medicare administrative contractor (MAC), or a durable medical equipment Medicare administrative contractor (DME MAC).

Medicare physician fee schedule. List of payments Medicare allows by procedure or service. Payments may vary through geographic adjustments. The MPFS is based on the resource-based relative value scale (RBRVS). A national total relative value unit (RVU) is given to each procedure (HCPCS Level I CPT, Level II national codes). Each total RVU has three components: physician work, practice expense, and malpractice insurance.

meibomian gland. Sebaceous gland located in the tarsal plates along the eyelid margins that produces the lipid components found in tears.

metabolite. Chemical compound resulting from the natural process of metabolism. In drug testing, the metabolite of the drug may endure in a higher concentration or for a longer duration than the initial "parent" drug.

methylation. Mechanism used to regulate genes and protect DNA from some types of cleavage.

microarray. Small surface onto which multiple specific nucleic acid sequences can be attached to be used for analysis. Microarray may also be known as a gene chip or DNA chip. Tests can be run on the sequences for any variants that may be present.

mitral valve. Valve with two cusps that is between the left atrium and left ventricle of the heart.

moderate sedation. Medically controlled state of depressed consciousness, with or without analgesia, while maintaining the patient's airway, protective reflexes, and ability to respond to stimulation or verbal commands.

Mohs micrographic surgery. Special technique used to treat complex or ill-defined skin cancer and requires a single physician to provide two distinct services. The first service is surgical and involves the destruction of the lesion by a combination of chemosurgery and excision. The second service is that of a pathologist and includes mapping, color coding of specimens, microscopic examination of specimens, and complete histopathologic preparation.

monitored anesthesia care. Sedation, with or without analgesia, used to achieve a medically controlled state of depressed consciousness while maintaining the patient's airway, protective reflexes, and ability to respond to stimulation or verbal commands. In dental conscious sedation, the patient is rendered free of fear, apprehension, and anxiety through the use of pharmacological agents.

monoclonal. Relating to a single clone of cells.

mosaicplasty. Multiple, small grafts composed of bone and cartilage placed to treat osteochondral defects of the knee. The grafts are cylindrical in shape and are placed in corresponding size holes made to the desired depth to fill the defect and allow for a more naturally shaped reconstruction.

multiple sleep latency test (MSLT). Attended study to determine the tendency of the patient to fall asleep.

multiple-lead device. Implantable cardiac device (pacemaker or implantable cardioverter-defibrillator [ICD]) in which pacing and sensing components are placed in at least three chambers of the heart.

Mustard procedure. Corrective measure for transposition of great vessels involves an intra-atrial baffle made of pericardial tissue or synthetic material. The baffle is secured between pulmonary veins and mitral valve and between mitral and tricuspid valves. The baffle directs systemic venous flow into the left ventricle and lungs and pulmonary venous flow into the right ventricle and aorta.

mutation. Alteration in gene function that results in changes to a gene or chromosome. Can cause deficits or disease that can be inherited, can have beneficial effects, or result in no noticeable change.

mutation scanning. Process normally used on multiple polymerase chain reaction (PCR) amplicons to determine DNA sequence variants by differences in characteristics compared to normal. Specific DNA variants can then be studied further.

myotomy. Surgical cutting of a muscle to gain access to underlying tissues or for therapeutic reasons.

myringotomy. Incision in the eardrum done to prevent spontaneous rupture precipitated by fluid pressure build-up behind the tympanic membrane and to prevent stagnant infection and erosion of the ossicles.

nasal polyp. Fleshy outgrowth projecting from the mucous membrane of the nose or nasal sinus cavity that may obstruct ventilation or affect the sense of smell.

nasal sinus. Air-filled cavities in the cranial bones lined with mucous membrane and continuous with the nasal cavity, draining fluids through the nose.

nasogastric tube. Long, hollow, cylindrical catheter made of soft rubber or plastic that is inserted through the nose down into the stomach, and is used for feeding, instilling medication, or withdrawing gastric contents.

nasolacrimal punctum. Opening of the lacrimal duct near the nose.

nasopharynx. Membranous passage above the level of the soft palate.

Nd:YAG laser. Laser light energy that uses an yttrium, aluminum, and garnet crystal doped with neodymium ions as the active source, has a radiation beam nearing the infrared spectrum, and is effective in photocoagulation, photoablation, cataract extraction, and lysis of vitreous strands.

nebulizer. Latin for mist, a device that converts liquid into a fine spray and is commonly used to deliver medicine to the upper respiratory, bronchial, and lung areas.

nerve conduction study. Diagnostic test performed to assess muscle or nerve damage. Nerves are stimulated with electric shocks along the course of the muscle. Sensors are utilized to measure and record nerve functions, including conduction and velocity.

neurectomy. Excision of all or a portion of a nerve.

neuromuscular junction. Nerve synapse at the meeting point between the terminal end of a nerve (motor neuron) and a muscle fiber.

neuropsychological testing. Evaluation of a patient's behavioral abilities wherein a physician or other health care professional administers a series of tests in thinking, reasoning, and judgment.

new patient. Patient who is receiving face-to-face care from a provider/qualified health care professional or another physician/qualified health care professional of the exact same specialty and subspecialty who belongs to the same group practice for the first time in three years. For OPPS hospitals, a patient who has not been registered as an inpatient or outpatient, including off-campus provider based clinic or emergency department, within the past three years.

Niemann-Pick syndrome. Accumulation of phospholipid in histiocytes in the bone marrow, liver, lymph nodes, and spleen, cerebral involvement, and red macular spots similar to Tay-Sachs disease. Most commonly found in Jewish infants.

Nissen fundoplasty. Surgical repair technique that involves the fundus of the stomach being wrapped around the lower end of the esophagus to treat reflux esophagitis.

nonabsorbable sutures. Strands of natural or synthetic material that resist absorption into living tissue and are removed once healing is under way. Nonabsorbable sutures are commonly used to close skin wounds and repair tendons or collagenous tissue.

obturator. Prosthesis used to close an acquired or congenital opening in the palate that aids in speech and chewing.

obturator nerve. Lumbar plexus nerve with anterior and posterior divisions that innervate the adductor muscles (e.g., adductor longus, adductor brevis) of the leg and the skin over the medial area of the thigh or a sacral plexus nerve with anterior and posterior divisions that innervate the superior gemellus muscles.

occult blood test. Chemical or microscopic test to determine the presence of blood in a specimen.

ocular implant. Implant inside muscular cone.

oophorectomy. Surgical removal of all or part of one or both ovaries, either as open procedure or laparoscopically. Menstruation and childbearing ability continues when one ovary is removed.

orthosis. Derived from a Greek word meaning "to make straight," it is an artificial appliance that supports, aligns, or corrects an anatomical deformity or improves the use of a moveable body part. Unlike a prosthesis, an orthotic device is always functional in nature.

osteo-. Having to do with bone.

osteogenesis stimulator. Device used to stimulate the growth of bone by electrical impulses or ultrasound.

osteotomy. Surgical cutting of a bone.

ostomy. Artificial (surgical) opening in the body used for drainage or for delivery of medications or nutrients.

pacemaker. Implantable cardiac device that controls the heart's rhythm and maintains regular beats by artificial electric discharges. This device consists of the pulse generator with a battery and the electrodes, or leads, which are placed in single or dual chambers of the heart, usually transvenously.

palmaris longus tendon. Tendon located in the hand that flexes the wrist joint.

paracentesis. Surgical puncture of a body cavity with a specialized needle or hollow tubing to aspirate fluid for diagnostic or therapeutic reasons.

paratenon graft. Graft composed of the fatty tissue found between a tendon and its sheath.

passive mobilization. Pressure, movement, or pulling of a limb or body part utilizing an apparatus or device.

pedicle flap. Full-thickness skin and subcutaneous tissue for grafting that remains partially attached to the donor site by a pedicle or stem in which the blood vessels supplying the flap remain intact.

Pemberton osteotomy. Osteotomy is performed to position triradiate cartilage as a hinge for rotating the acetabular roof in cases of dysplasia of the hip in children.

penetrance. Being formed by, or pertaining to, a single clone.

percutaneous intradiscal electrothermal annuloplasty. Procedure corrects tears in the vertebral annulus by applying heat to the collagen disc walls percutaneously through a catheter. The heat contracts and thickens the wall, which may contract and close any annular tears.

percutaneous skeletal fixation. Treatment that is neither open nor closed and the injury site is not directly visualized. Fixation devices (pins, screws) are placed through the skin to stabilize the dislocation using x-ray guidance.

pericardium. Thin and slippery case in which the heart lies that is lined with fluid so that the heart is free to pulse and move as it beats.

peripheral arterial tonometry (PAT). Pulsatile volume changes in a digit are measured to determine activity in the sympathetic nervous system for respiratory analysis.

peritoneal. Space between the lining of the abdominal wall, or parietal peritoneum, and the surface layer of the abdominal organs, or visceral peritoneum. It contains a thin, watery fluid that keeps the peritoneal surfaces moist.

peritoneal dialysis. Dialysis that filters waste from blood inside the body using the peritoneum, the natural lining of the abdomen, as the semipermeable membrane across which ultrafiltration is accomplished. A special catheter is inserted into the abdomen and a dialysis solution is drained into the abdomen. This solution extracts fluids and wastes, which are then discarded when the fluid is drained. Various forms of peritoneal dialysis include CAPD, CCPD, and NIDP.

peritoneal effusion. Persistent escape of fluid within the peritoneal cavity.

pessary. Device placed in the vagina to support and reposition a prolapsing or retropositioned uterus, rectum, or vagina.

phacoemulsification. Cataract extraction in which the lens is fragmented by ultrasonic vibrations and simultaneously irrigated and aspirated.

phenotype. Physical expression of a trait or characteristic as determined by an individual's genetic makeup or genotype.

photocoagulation. Application of an intense laser beam of light to disrupt tissue and condense protein material to a residual mass, used especially for treating ocular conditions.

physical status modifiers. Alphanumeric modifier used to identify the patient's health status as it affects the work related to providing the anesthesia service.

physical therapy modality. Therapeutic agent or regimen applied or used to provide appropriate treatment of the musculoskeletal system.

physician. Legally authorized practitioners including a doctor of medicine or osteopathy, a doctor of dental surgery or of dental medicine, a doctor of podiatric medicine, a doctor of optometry, and a chiropractor only with respect to treatment by means of manual manipulation of the spine (to correct a subluxation).

PICC. Peripherally inserted central catheter. PICC is inserted into one of the large veins of the arm and threaded through the vein until the tip sits in a large vein just above the heart.

PKR. Photorefractive therapy. Procedure involving the removal of the surface layer of the cornea (epithelium) by gentle scraping and use of a computer-controlled excimer laser to reshape the stroma.

pleurodesis. Injection of a sclerosing agent into the pleural space for creating adhesions between the parietal and the visceral pleura to treat a collapsed lung caused by air trapped in the pleural cavity, or severe cases of pleural effusion.

plication. Surgical technique involving folding, tucking, or pleating to reduce the size of a hollow structure or organ.

polyclonal. Containing one or more cells.

polymorphism. Genetic variation in the same species that does not harm the gene function or create disease.

polypeptide. Chain of amino acids held together by covalent bonds. Proteins are made up of amino acids.

polysomnography. Test involving monitoring of respiratory, cardiac, muscle, brain, and ocular function during sleep.

Potts-Smith-Gibson procedure. Side-to-side anastomosis of the aorta and left pulmonary artery creating a shunt that enlarges as the child grows.

Prader-Willi syndrome. Rounded face, almond-shaped eyes, strabismus, low forehead, hypogonadism, hypotonia, intellectual disabilities, and an insatiable appetite.

presumptive drug testing. Drug screening tests to identify the presence or absence of drugs in a patient's system. Tests are usually able to identify low concentrations of the drug. These tests may be used for medical, workplace, or legal purposes.

presumptive identification. Identification of microorganisms using media growth, colony morphology, gram stains, or up to three specific tests (e.g., catalase, indole, oxidase, urease).

professional component. Portion of a charge for health care services that represents the physician's (or other practitioner's) work in providing the service, including interpretation and report of the procedure. This component of the service usually is charged for and billed separately from the inpatient hospital charges.

profunda. Denotes a part of a structure that is deeper from the surface of the body than the rest of the structure.

prolonged physician services. Extended pre- or post-service care provided to a patient whose condition requires services beyond the usual.

prostate. Male gland surrounding the bladder neck and urethra that secretes a substance into the seminal fluid.

prosthetic. Device that replaces all or part of an internal body organ or body part, or that replaces part of the function of a permanently inoperable or malfunctioning internal body organ or body part.

provider of services. Institution, individual, or organization that provides health care.

proximal. Located closest to a specified reference point, usually the midline or trunk.

psychiatric hospital. Specialized institution that provides, under the supervision of physicians, services for the diagnosis and treatment of mentally ill persons.

pterygium. Benign, wedge-shaped, conjunctival thickening that advances from the inner corner of the eye toward the cornea.

pterygomaxillary fossa. Wide depression on the external surface of the maxilla above and to the side of the canine tooth socket.

pulmonary artery banding. Surgical constriction of the pulmonary artery to prevent irreversible pulmonary vascular obstructive changes and overflow into the left ventricle.

Putti-Platt procedure. Realignment of the subscapularis tendon to treat recurrent anterior dislocation, thereby partially eliminating external rotation. The anterior capsule is also tightened and reinforced.

pyloroplasty. Enlargement and reconstruction of the lower portion of the stomach opening into the duodenum performed after vagotomy to speed gastric emptying and treat duodenal ulcers.

qualified health care professional. Educated, licensed or certified, and regulated professional operating under a specified scope of practice to provide patient services that are separate and distinct from other clinical staff. Services may be billed independently or under the facility's services.

RAC. Recovery audit contractor. National program using CMS-affiliated contractors to review claims prior to payment as well as for payments on claims already processed, including overpayments and underpayments.

radiation therapy simulation. Radiation therapy simulation. Procedure by which the specific body area to be treated with radiation is defined and marked. A CT scan is performed to define the body contours and these images are used to create a plan customized treatment for the patient, targeting the area to be treated while sparing adjacent tissue. The center of the area to be treated is marked and an immobilization device (e.g., cradle, mold) is created to make sure the patient is in the same position each time for treatment. Complexity of treatment depends on the number of treatment areas and the use of tools to isolate the area of treatment.

radioactive substances. Materials used in the diagnosis and treatment of disease that emit high-speed particles and energy-containing rays.

radiology services. Services that include diagnostic and therapeutic radiology, nuclear medicine, CT scan procedures, magnetic resonance imaging services, ultrasound, and other imaging procedures.

radiotherapy afterloading. Part of the radiation therapy process in which the chemotherapy agent is actually instilled into the tumor area subsequent to surgery and placement of an expandable catheter into the void remaining after tumor excision. The specialized catheter remains in place and the patient may come in for multiple treatments with radioisotope placed to treat the margin of tissue surrounding the excision. After the radiotherapy is completed, the patient returns to have the catheter emptied and removed. This is a new therapy in breast cancer treatment.

Rashkind procedure. Transvenous balloon atrial septectomy or septostomy performed by cardiac catheterization. A balloon catheter is inserted into the heart either to create or enlarge an opening in the interatrial septal wall.

rehabilitation services. Therapy services provided primarily for assisting in a rehabilitation program of evaluation and service including cardiac rehabilitation, medical social services, occupational therapy, physical therapy, respiratory therapy, skilled nursing, speech therapy, psychiatric rehabilitation, and alcohol and substance abuse rehabilitation.

respiratory airflow (ventilation). Assessment of air movement during inhalation and exhalation as measured by nasal pressure sensors and thermistor.

respiratory analysis. Assessment of components of respiration obtained by other methods such as airflow or peripheral arterial tone.

respiratory effort. Measurement of diaphragm and/or intercostal muscle for airflow using transducers to estimate thoracic and abdominal motion.

respiratory movement. Measurement of chest and abdomen movement during respiration.

ribbons. In oncology, small plastic tubes containing radioactive sources for interstitial placement that may be cut into specific lengths tailored to the size of the area receiving ionizing radiation treatment.

Ridell sinusotomy. Frontal sinus tissue is destroyed to eliminate tumors.

RNA. Ribonucleic acid.

rural health clinic. Clinic in an area where there is a shortage of health services staffed by a nurse practitioner, physician assistant, or certified nurse midwife under physician direction that provides routine diagnostic services, including clinical laboratory services, drugs, and biologicals and that has prompt access to additional diagnostic services from facilities meeting federal requirements.

Salter osteotomy. Innominate bone of the hip is cut, removed, and repositioned to repair a congenital dislocation, subluxation, or deformity.

saucerization. Creation of a shallow, saucer-like depression in the bone to facilitate drainage of infected areas.

Schiotz tonometer. Instrument that measures intraocular pressure by recording the depth of an indentation on the cornea by a plunger of known weight.

screening mammography. Radiologic images taken of the female breast for the early detection of breast cancer.

screening pap smear. Diagnostic laboratory test consisting of a routine exfoliative cytology test (Papanicolaou test) provided to a woman for the early detection of cervical or vaginal cancer. The exam includes a clinical breast examination and a physician's interpretation of the results.

seeds. Small (1 mm or less) sources of radioactive material that are permanently placed directly into tumors.

Senning procedure. Flaps of intra-atrial septum and right atrial wall are used to create two interatrial channels to divert the systemic and pulmonary venous circulation.

sensitivity tests. Number of methods of applying selective suspected allergens to the skin or mucous.

sensorineural conduction. Transportation of sound from the cochlea to the acoustic nerve and central auditory pathway to the brain.

sentinel lymph node. First node to which lymph drainage and metastasis from a cancer can occur.

separate procedures. Services commonly carried out as a fundamental part of a total service and, as such, do not usually warrant separate identification. These services are identified in CPT with the parenthetical phrase (separate procedure) at the end of the description and are payable only when performed alone.

septectomy. 1) Surgical removal of all or part of the nasal septum. 2) Submucosal resection of the nasal septum.

Shirodkar procedure. Treatment of an incompetent cervical os by placing nonabsorbent suture material in purse-string sutures as a cerclage to support the cervix.

short tandem repeat (STR). Short sequences of a DNA pattern that are repeated. Can be used as genetic markers for human identity testing.

sialodochoplasty. Surgical repair of a salivary gland duct.

single-lead device. Implantable cardiac device (pacemaker or implantable cardioverter-defibrillator [ICD]) in which pacing and sensing components are placed in only one chamber of the heart.

single-nucleotide polymorphism (SNP). Single nucleotide (A, T, C, or G that is different in a DNA sequence. This difference occurs at a significant frequency in the population.

sinus of Valsalva. Any of three sinuses corresponding to the individual cusps of the aortic valve, located in the most proximal part of the aorta just above the cusps. These structures are contained within the pericardium and appear as distinct but subtle outpouchings or dilations of the aortic wall between each of the semilunar cusps of the valve.

sleep apnea. Intermittent cessation of breathing during sleep that may cause hypoxemia and pulmonary arterial hypertension.

sleep latency. Time period between lying down in bed and the onset of sleep.

sleep staging. Determination of the separate levels of sleep according to physiological measurements.

somatic. 1) Pertaining to the body or trunk. 2) In genetics acquired or occurring after birth.

SPECT. Single photon emission computerized tomography. SPECT images are taken after the injection of a radionuclide using a special camera containing a detector crystal, usually sodium iodide. Images are captured as the gamma radiation from the radionuclide scintillates or gives off its energy in a flash of light when coming in contact with the crystal. This type of imaging is reported for the anatomical area and purpose such as detecting liver function or myocardial perfusion after an ischemic event.

speculoscopy. Viewing the cervix utilizing a magnifier and a special wavelength of light, allowing detection of abnormalities that may not be discovered on a routine Pap smear.

speech-language pathology services. Speech, language, and related function assessment and rehabilitation service furnished by a qualified speech-language pathologist. Audiology services include hearing and balance assessment services furnished by a qualified audiologist. A qualified speech pathologist and audiologist must have a master's or doctoral degree in their respective fields and be licensed to serve in the state. Speech pathologists and audiologists practicing in states without licensure must complete 350 hours of supervised clinical work and perform at least nine months of supervised full-time service after earning their degrees.

sphincteroplasty. Surgical repair done to correct, augment, or improve the muscular function of a sphincter, such as the anus or intestines.

spirometry. Measurement of the lungs' breathing capacity.

splint. Brace or support. 1) dynamic splint: brace that permits movement of an anatomical structure such as a hand, wrist, foot, or other part of the body after surgery or injury. 2) static splint: brace that prevents movement and maintains support and position for an anatomical structure after surgery or injury.

stent. Tube to provide support in a body cavity or lumen.

stereotactic radiosurgery. Delivery of externally-generated ionizing radiation to specific targets for destruction or inactivation. Most often utilized in the treatment of brain or spinal tumors, high-resolution stereotactic imaging is used to identify the target and then deliver the treatment. Computer-assisted planning may also be employed. Simple and complex cranial lesions and spinal lesions are typically treated in a single planning and treatment session, although a maximum of five sessions may be required. No incision is made for stereotactic radiosurgery procedures.

stereotaxis. Three-dimensional method for precisely locating structures.

Stoffel rhizotomy. Nerve roots are sectioned to relieve pain or spastic paralysis.

strabismus. Misalignment of the eyes due to an imbalance in extraocular muscles.

surgical package. Normal, uncomplicated performance of specific surgical services, with the assumption that, on average, all surgical procedures of a given type are similar with respect to skill level, duration, and length of normal follow-up care.

symblepharopterygium. Adhesion in which the eyelid is adhered to the eyeball by a band that resembles a pterygium.

sympathectomy. Surgical interruption or transection of a sympathetic nervous system pathway.

tarso-. 1) Relating to the foot. 2) Relating to the margin of the eyelid.

tarsocheiloplasty. Plastic operation upon the edge of the eyelid for the treatment of trichiasis.

tarsorrhaphy. Suture of a portion or all of the opposing eyelids together for the purpose of shortening the palpebral fissure or closing it entirely.

technical component. Portion of a health care service that identifies the provision of the equipment, supplies, technical personnel, and costs attendant to the performance of the procedure other than the professional services.

tendon. Fibrous tissue that connects muscle to bone, consisting primarily of collagen and containing little vasculature.

tendon allograft. Allografts are tissues obtained from another individual of the same species. Tendon allografts are usually obtained from cadavers and frozen or freeze dried for later use in soft tissue repairs where the physician elects not to obtain an autogenous graft (a graft obtained from the individual on whom the surgery is being performed).

tendon suture material. Tendons are composed of fibrous tissue consisting primarily of collagen and containing few cells or blood vessels. This tissue heals more slowly than tissues with more vascularization. Because of this, tendons are usually repaired with nonabsorbable suture material. Examples include surgical silk, surgical cotton, linen, stainless steel, surgical nylon, polyester fiber, polybutester (Novafil), polyethylene (Dermalene), and polypropylene (Prolene, Surilene).

tendon transplant. Replacement of a tendon with another tendon.

tenon's capsule. Connective tissue that forms the capsule enclosing the posterior eyeball, extending from the conjunctival fornix and continuous with the muscular fascia of the eye.

tenonectomy. Excision of a portion of a tendon to make it shorter.

tenotomy. Cutting into a tendon.

TENS. Transcutaneous electrical nerve stimulator. TENS is applied by placing electrode pads over the area to be stimulated and connecting the electrodes to a transmitter box, which sends a current through the skin to sensory nerve fibers to help decrease pain in that nerve distribution.

tensilon. Edrophonium chloride. Agent used for evaluation and treatment of myasthenia gravis.

terminally ill. Individual whose medical prognosis for life expectancy is six months or less.

tetralogy of Fallot. Specific combination of congenital cardiac defects: obstruction of the right ventricular outflow tract with pulmonary stenosis, interventricular septal defect, malposition of the aorta, overriding the interventricular septum and receiving blood from both the venous and arterial systems, and enlargement of the right ventricle.

therapeutic services. Services performed for treatment of a specific diagnosis. These services include performance of the procedure, various incidental elements, and normal, related follow-up care.

thoracentesis. Surgical puncture of the chest cavity with a specialized needle or hollow tubing to aspirate fluid from within the pleural space for diagnostic or therapeutic reasons.

thoracic lymphadenectomy. Procedure to cut out the lymph nodes near the lungs, around the heart, and behind the trachea.

thoracostomy. Creation of an opening in the chest wall for drainage.

thyroglossal duct. Embryonic duct at the front of the neck, which becomes the pyramidal lobe of the thyroid gland with obliteration of the remaining duct, but may form a cyst or sinus in adulthood if it persists.

total disc arthroplasty with artificial disc. Removal of an intravertebral disc and its replacement with an implant. The implant is an artificial disc consisting of two metal plates with a weight-bearing surface of polyethylene between the plates. The plates are anchored to the vertebral immediately above and below the affected disc.

total shoulder replacement. Prosthetic replacement of the entire shoulder joint, including the humeral head and the glenoid fossa.

trabeculae carneae cordis. Bands of muscular tissue that line the walls of the ventricles in the heart.

trabeculectomy. Surgical incision between the anterior portion of the eye and the canal of Schlemm to drain the aqueous humor.

tracheostomy. Formation of a tracheal opening on the neck surface with tube insertion to allow for respiration in cases of obstruction or decreased patency. A tracheostomy may be planned or performed on an emergency basis for temporary or long-term use.

tracheotomy. Formation of a tracheal opening on the neck surface with tube insertion to allow for respiration in cases of obstruction or decreased patency. A tracheotomy may be planned or performed on an emergency basis for temporary or long-term use.

traction. Drawing out or holding tension on an area by applying a direct therapeutic pulling force.

transcranial magnetic stimulation. Application of electromagnetic energy to the brain through a coil placed on the scalp. The procedure stimulates cortical neurons and is intended to activate and normalize their processes.

transcription. Process by which messenger RNA is synthesized from a DNA template resulting in the transfer of genetic information from the DNA molecule to the messenger RNA.

translocation. Disconnection of all or part of a chromosome that reattaches to another position in the DNA sequence of the same or another chromosome. Often results in a reciprocal exchange of DNA sequences between two differently numbered chromosomes. May or may not result in a clinically significant loss of DNA.

trephine. 1) Specialized round saw for cutting circular holes in bone, especially the skull. 2) Instrument that removes small disc-shaped buttons of corneal tissue for transplanting.

tricuspid atresia. Congenital absence of the valve that may occur with other defects, such as atrial septal defect, pulmonary atresia, and transposition of great vessels.

turbinates. Scroll or shell-shaped elevations from the wall of the nasal cavity, the inferior turbinate being a separate bone, while the superior and middle turbinates are of the ethmoid bone.

tympanic membrane. Thin, sensitive membrane across the entrance to the middle ear that vibrates in response to sound waves, allowing the waves to be transmitted via the ossicular chain to the internal ear.

tympanoplasty. Surgical repair of the structures of the middle ear, including the eardrum and the three small bones, or ossicles.

unlisted procedure. Procedural descriptions used when the overall procedure and outcome of the procedure are not adequately described by an existing procedure code. Such codes are used as a last resort and only when there is not a more appropriate procedure code.

ureterorrhaphy. Surgical repair using sutures to close an open wound or injury of the ureter.

vagotomy. Division of the vagus nerves, interrupting impulses resulting in lower gastric acid production and hastening gastric emptying. Used in the treatment of chronic gastric, pyloric, and duodenal ulcers that can cause severe pain and difficulties in eating and sleeping.

variant. Nucleotide deviation from the normal sequence of a region. Variations are usually either substitutions or deletions. Substitution variations are the result of one nucleotide taking the place of another. A deletion occurs when one or more nucleotides are left out. In some cases, several in a reasonably close proximity on the same chromosome in a DNA strand. These variations result in amino acid changes in the protein made by the gene. However, the term variant does not itself imply a functional change. Intron variations are usually described in one of two ways: 1) the changed nucleotide is defined by a plus or a minus sign indicating the position relative to the first or last nucleotide to the intron, or 2) the second variant description is indicated relative to the last nucleotide of the preceding exon or first nucleotide of the following exon.

vascular family. Group of vessels (family) that branch from the aorta or vena cava. At each branching, the vascular order increases by one. The first order vessel is the primary branch off the aorta or vena cava. The second order vessel branches from the first order, the third order branches from the second order, and any further branching is beyond the third order. For example, for the inferior vena cava, the common iliac artery is a first order vessel. The internal and external iliac arteries are second order vessels, as they each originate from the first order common iliac artery. The external iliac artery extends directly from the common iliac artery and the internal iliac artery bifurcates from the common iliac artery. A third order vessel from the external iliac artery is the inferior epigastric artery and a third order vessel from the internal iliac artery is the obturator artery. Note orders are not always identical bilaterally (e.g., the left common carotid artery is a first order and the right common carotid is a second order. Synonym(s): vascular origins and distributions.

vasectomy. Surgical procedure involving the removal of all or part of the vas deferens, usually performed for sterilization or in conjunction with a prostatectomy.

vena cava interruption. Procedure that places a filter device, called an umbrella or sieve, within the large vein returning deoxygenated blood to the heart to prevent pulmonary embolism caused by clots.

ventricular assist device. Temporary measure used to support the heart by substituting for left and/or right heart function. The device replaces the work of the left and/or right ventricle when a patient has a damaged or weakened heart. A left ventricular assist device (VAD) helps the heart pump blood through the rest of the body. A right VAD helps the heart pump blood to the lungs to become oxygenated again. Catheters are inserted to circulate the blood through external tubing to a pump machine located outside of the body and back to the correct artery.

ventricular septal defect. Congenital cardiac anomaly resulting in a continual opening in the septum between the ventricles that, in severe cases, causes oxygenated blood to flow back into the lungs, resulting in pulmonary hypertension.

vertebral interspace. Non-bony space between two adjacent vertebral bodies that contains the cushioning intervertebral disk.

volar. Palm of the hand (palmar) or sole of the foot (plantar).

Waterston procedure. Type of aortopulmonary shunting done to increase pulmonary blood flow. The ascending aorta is anastomosed to the right pulmonary artery.

Wharton's ducts. Salivary ducts below the mandible.

wick catheter. Device used to monitor interstitial fluid pressure, and sometimes used intraoperatively during fasciotomy procedures to evaluate the effectiveness of the decompression.

wound closure. Closure or repair of a wound created surgically or due to trauma (e.g., laceration). The closure technique depends on the type, site, and depth of the defect. Consideration is also given to cosmetic and functional outcome. A single layer closure involves approximation of the edges of the wound. The second type of closure involves closing the one or more deeper layers of tissue prior to skin closure. The most complex type of closure may include techniques such as debridement or undermining, which involves manipulation of tissue around the wound to allow the skin to cover the wound. The AMA CPT® book defines these as Simple, Intermediate and Complex repair.

xenograft. Tissue that is nonhuman and harvested from one species and grafted to another. Pigskin is the most common xenograft for human skin and is applied to a wound as a temporary closure until a permanent option is performed.

z-plasty. Plastic surgery technique used primarily to release tension or elongate contracted scar tissue in which a Z-shaped incision is made with the middle line of the Z crossing the area of greatest tension. The triangular flaps are then rotated so that they cross the incision line in the opposite direction, creating a reversed Z.

ZPIC. Zone Program Integrity Contractor. CMS contractor that replaced the existing Program Safeguard Contractors (PSC). Contractors are responsible for ensuring the integrity of all Medicare-related claims under Parts A and B (hospital, skilled nursing, home health, provider, and durable medical equipment claims), Part C (Medicare Advantage health plans), Part D (prescription drug plans), and coordination of Medicare-Medicaid data matches (Medi-Medi).

Appendix N — Listing of Sensory, Motor, and Mixed Nerves

This list contains the sensory, motor, and mixed nerves assigned to each nerve conduction study to improve coding accuracy. Each nerve makes up one single unit of service.

Motor Nerves Assigned to Codes 95907-95913

I. Upper extremity, cervical plexus, and brachial plexus motor nerves
    A. Axillary motor nerve to the deltoid
    B. Long thoracic motor nerve to the serratus anterior
    C. Median nerve
        1. Median motor nerve to the abductor pollicis brevis
        2. Median motor nerve, anterior interosseous branch, to the flexor pollicis longus
        3. Median motor nerve, anterior interosseous branch, to the pronator quadratus
        4. Median motor nerve to the first lumbrical
        5. Median motor nerve to the second lumbrical
    D. Musculocutaneous motor nerve to the biceps brachii
    E. Radial nerve
        1. Radial motor nerve to the extensor carpi ulnaris
        2. Radial motor nerve to the extensor digitorum communis
        3. Radial motor nerve to the extensor indicis proprius
        4. Radial motor nerve to the brachioradialis
    F. Suprascapular nerve
        1. Suprascapular motor nerve to the supraspinatus
        2. Suprascapular motor nerve to the infraspinatus
    G. Thoracodorsal motor nerve to the latissimus dorsi
    H. Ulnar nerve
        1. Ulnar motor nerve to the abductor digiti minimi
        2. Ulnar motor nerve to the palmar interosseous
        3. Ulnar motor nerve to the first dorsal interosseous
        4. Ulnar motor nerve to the flexor carpi ulnaris
    I. Other
II. Lower extremity motor nerves
    A. Femoral motor nerve to the quadriceps
        1. Femoral motor nerve to vastus medialis
        2. Femoral motor nerve to vastus lateralis
        3. Femoral motor nerve to vastus intermedialis
        4. Femoral motor nerve to rectus femoris
    B. Ilioinguinal motor nerve
    C. Peroneal (fibular) nerve
        1. Peroneal motor nerve to the extensor digitorum brevis
        2. Peroneal motor nerve to the peroneus brevis
        3. Peroneal motor nerve to the peroneus longus
        4. Peroneal motor nerve to the tibialis anterior
    D. Plantar motor nerve
    E. Sciatic nerve
    F. Tibial nerve
        1. Tibial motor nerve, inferior calcaneal branch, to the abductor digiti minimi
        2. Tibial motor nerve, medial plantar branch, to the abductor hallucis
        3. Tibial motor nerve, lateral plantar branch, to the flexor digiti minimi brevis
    G. Other
III. Cranial nerves and trunk
    A. Cranial nerve VII (facial motor nerve)
        1. Facial nerve to the frontalis
        2. Facial nerve to the nasalis
        3. Facial nerve to the orbicularis oculi
        4. Facial nerve to the orbicularis oris
    B. Cranial nerve XI (spinal accessory motor nerve)
    C. Cranial nerve XII (hypoglossal motor nerve)
    D. Intercostal motor nerve
    E. Phrenic motor nerve to the diaphragm
    F. Recurrent laryngeal nerve
    G. Other
IV. Nerve Roots
    A. Cervical nerve root stimulation
        1. Cervical level 5 (C5)
        2. Cervical level 6 (C6)
        3. Cervical level 7 (C7)
        4. Cervical level 8 (C8)
    B. Thoracic nerve root stimulation
        1. Thoracic level 1 (T1)
        2. Thoracic level 2 (T2)
        3. Thoracic level 3 (T3)
        4. Thoracic level 4 (T4)
        5. Thoracic level 5 (T5)
        6. Thoracic level 6 (T6)
        7. Thoracic level 7 (T7)
        8. Thoracic level 8 (T8)
        9. Thoracic level 9 (T9)
        10. Thoracic level 10 (T10)
        11. Thoracic level 11 (T11)
        12. Thoracic level 12 (T12)
    C. Lumbar nerve root stimulation
        1. Lumbar level 1 (L1)
        2. Lumbar level 2 (L2)
        3. Lumbar level 3 (L3)
        4. Lumbar level 4 (L4)
        5. Lumbar level 5 (L5)
    D. Sacral nerve root stimulation
        1. Sacral level 1 (S1)
        2. Sacral level 2 (S2)
        3. Sacral level 3 (S3)
        4. Sacral level 4 (S4)

Sensory and Mixed Nerves Assigned to Codes 95907–95913

I. Upper extremity sensory and mixed nerves
   A. Lateral antebrachial cutaneous sensory nerve
   B. Medial antebrachial cutaneous sensory nerve
   C. Medial brachial cutaneous sensory nerve
   D. Median nerve
      1. Median sensory nerve to the first digit
      2. Median sensory nerve to the second digit
      3. Median sensory nerve to the third digit
      4. Median sensory nerve to the fourth digit
      5. Median palmar cutaneous sensory nerve
      6. Median palmar mixed nerve
   E. Posterior antebrachial cutaneous sensory nerve
   F. Radial sensory nerve
      1. Radial sensory nerve to the base of the thumb
      2. Radial sensory nerve to digit 1
   G. Ulnar nerve
      1. Ulnar dorsal cutaneous sensory nerve
      2. Ulnar sensory nerve to the fourth digit
      3. Ulnar sensory nerve to the fifth digit
      4. Ulnar palmar mixed nerve
   H. Intercostal sensory nerve
   I. Other

II. Lower extremity sensory and mixed nerves
   A. Lateral femoral cutaneous sensory nerve
   B. Medical calcaneal sensory nerve
   C. Medial femoral cutaneous sensory nerve
   D. Peroneal nerve
      1. Deep peroneal sensory nerve
      2. Superficial peroneal sensory nerve, medial dorsal cutaneous branch
      3. Superficial peroneal sensory nerve, intermediate dorsal cutaneous branch
   E. Posterior femoral cutaneous sensory nerve
   F. Saphenous nerve
      1. Saphenous sensory nerve (distal technique)
      2. Saphenous sensory nerve (proximal technique)
   G. Sural nerve
      1. Sural sensory nerve, lateral dorsal cutaneous branch
      2. Sural sensory nerve
   H. Tibial sensory nerve (digital nerve to toe 1)
   I. Tibial sensory nerve (medial plantar nerve)
   J. Tibial sensory nerve (lateral plantar nerve)
   K. Other

III. Head and trunk sensory nerves
   A. Dorsal nerve of the penis
   B. Greater auricular nerve
   C. Ophthalmic branch of the trigeminal nerve
   D. Pudendal sensory nerve
   E. Suprascapular sensory nerves
   F. Other

In the following table, the reasonable maximum number of studies per diagnostic category is listed that allows for a physician or other qualified health care professional to obtain a diagnosis for 90 percent of patients with that same final diagnosis. The numbers denote the suggested number of studies, although the decision is up to the provider.

Type of Study/Maximum Number of Studies

Indication	Limbs Studied by Needle EMG (95860–95864, 95867–95870, 95885–95887)	Nerve Conduction Studies (Total nerves studied, 95907-95913)	Neuromuscular Junction Testing (Repetitive Stimulation 95937)
Carpal Tunnel (Unilateral)	1	7	—
Carpal Tunnel (Bilateral)	2	10	—
Radiculopathy	2	7	—
Mononeuropathy	1	8	—
Polyneuropathy/Mononeuropathy Multiplex	3	10	—
Myopathy	2	4	2
Motor Neuronopathy (e.g., ALS)	4	6	2
Plexopathy	2	12	—
Neuromuscular Junction	2	4	3
Tarsal Tunnel Syndrome (Unilateral)	1	8	—
Tarsal Tunnel Syndrome (Bilateral)	2	11	—
Weakness, Fatigue, Cramps, or Twitching (Focal)	2	7	2
Weakness, Fatigue, Cramps, or Twitching (General)	4	8	2
Pain, Numbness, or Tingling (Unilateral)	1	9	—
Pain, Numbness, or Tingling (Bilateral)	2	12	—

Notes

Notes